Pediatric Respiratory Medicine

PEDIATRIC RESPIRATORY MEDICINE

EDITORS

LYNN M. TAUSSIG, M.D.
President and CEO
National Jewish Medical and Research Center;
Professor of Pediatrics
University of Colorado School of Medicine
Denver, Colorado

LOUIS I. LANDAU, M.D., F.R.A.C.P.
Executive Dean and Professor of Paediatrics
The Faculty of Medicine and Dentistry
University of Western Australia
Perth, WA, Australia

ASSOCIATE EDITORS

PETER N. LE SOUËF, M.D., M.R.C.P. (UK), F.R.A.C.P.
Professor of Paediatrics
University of Western Australia;
Respiratory Physician
Department of Respiratory Medicine
Princess Margaret Hospital for Children
Perth, WA, Australia

WAYNE J. MORGAN, M.D., C.M.
Professor, Pediatrics & Physiology
Associate Head for Academic Affairs
Chief, Pediatric Pulmonary Section
Department of Pediatrics
University of Arizona Health Sciences Center
Tucson, Arizona

FERNANDO D. MARTINEZ, M.D.
Swift-McNear Professor of Pediatrics
Director
Respiratory Sciences Center
University of Arizona Health Sciences Center
Tucson, Arizona

PETER D. SLY, M.D., F.R.A.C.P.
Associate Professor
University of Western Australia;
Head, Division of Clinical Sciences
TVW Telethon Institute for Child Health Research;
Respiratory Physician
Department of Respiratory Medicine
Princess Margaret Hospital for Children
Perth, WA, Australia

with 970 illustrations

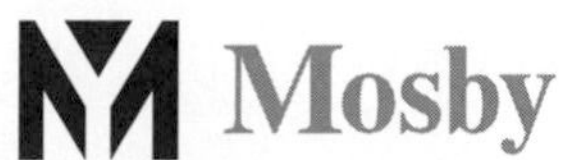

St. Louis Baltimore Boston Carlsbad Chicago Minneapolis New York Philadelphia Portland
London Milan Sydney Tokyo Toronto

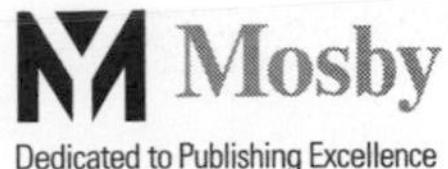

Publisher: Laura DeYoung
Managing Editor: Kathy Falk
Acquisitions Editor: Brian Morovitz
Developmental Editor: Robin Sutter
Project Manager: Carol Sullivan Weis
Project Specialist: Pat Joiner
Designer: Jen Marmarinos
Manufacturing Manager: David Graybill

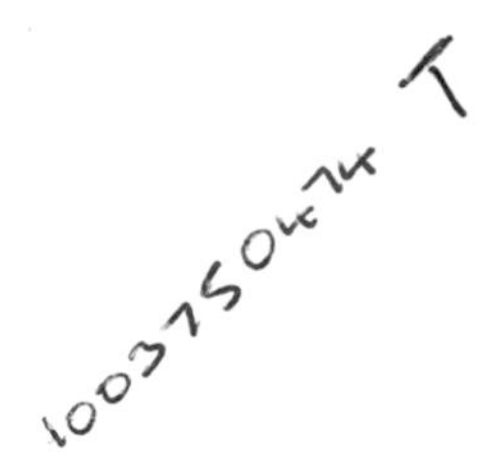

Printed in the United States of America
Composition by Top Graphics
Lithography by Top Graphics
Printing/binding by Maple-Vail Book Mfg Group

Mosby, Inc.
11830 Westline Industrial Drive
St. Louis, Missouri 63146

Library of Congress Cataloging-in-Publication Data
Pediatric respiratory medicine / editors, Lynn M. Taussig, Louis
I. Landau ; associate editors, Peter LeSouëf . . . [et al.].
p. cm.
Includes bibliographical references and index.
ISBN 0-8016-7406-9
1. Pediatric respiratory diseases. I. Taussig, Lynn M. (Lynn
Max), 1942- . II. Landau, Louis I.
[DNLM: 1. Respiratory Tract Diseases—in infancy & childhood. WS
280 P3678 1998]
RJ431.P416 1998
618.92′2—dc21
DNLM/DLC
for Library of Congress

97-46466
CIP

99 00 01 02 / 9 8 7 6 5 4 3 2

Contributors

STEVEN H. ABMAN, M.D.
Professor and Director, Pediatric Heart Lung Center
Department of Pediatrics
The Children's Hospital and University of Colorado School of Medicine
Denver, Colorado

BENOOSH AFGHANI, M.D.
Assistant Professor of Pediatrics
Pediatric Infectious Diseases
Memorial Miller Children's Hospital
Long Beach, California
University of California, Irvine
Irvine, California

MOIRA L. AITKEN, M.B., M.D., F.R.C.P.
Associate Professor of Medicine
Pulmonary and Critical Care Division
Director, Adult CF Clinic
Department of Medicine
University of Washington
Seattle, Washington

JULIAN LEWIS ALLEN, M.D.
Professor of Pediatrics and Section Chief
Pediatric Pulmonary and Cystic Fibrosis Center
Medical College of Pennsylvania and Hahnemann School of Medicine
Allegheny University of the Health Sciences
St. Christopher's Hospital for Children
Philadelphia, Pennsylvania

SANDRA D. ANDERSON, Ph.D., D.Sc.
Department of Respiratory Medicine
Royal Prince Alfred Hospital
Camperdown, New South Wales, Australia

M. INNES ASHER, M.B., Ch.B., F.R.A.C.P.
Department of Paediatrics
Faculty of Medicine and Health Science
University of Auckland
Auckland, New Zealand

EDUARDO BANCALARI, M.D.
Professor of Pediatrics
Director, Division of Neonatology
University of Miami School of Medicine
Miami, Florida

TAMAR BEN-AMI, M.D.
Chief, Section of Pediatric Radiology
Department of Radiology
University of Chicago
Chicago, Illinois

ROBERT A. BERG, M.D.
Professor of Pediatrics
Chief, Pediatric Critical Care Section
Department of Pediatrics
University of Arizona Health Sciences Center
Tucson, Arizona

MARGARITA BIDEGAIN, M.D.
Department of Pediatrics
Division of Neonatology
University of Miami School of Medicine
Miami, Florida

RICHARD D. BLAND, M.D.
Fields Professor of Pediatrics
Department of Pediatrics
University of Utah Health Sciences Center
Salt Lake City, Utah

RICHARD C. BOUCHER, M.D.
Professor of Medicine
Director
CF/Pulmonary Research and Treatment Center
University of North Carolina at Chapel Hill
Chapel Hill, North Carolina

KYLE L. BRESSLER, M.D., F.A.A.P.
Director, Pediatric Otolaryngology
University of Miami
Miami, Florida

JOHN G. BROOKS, M.D.
Professor and Chairman
Department of Pediatrics
Dartmouth Medical School;
Medical Director
Children's Hospital at Dartmouth
Lebanon, New Hampshire

MARK A. BROWN, M.D.
Assistant Professor of Clinical Pediatrics
Director, Pulmonary Training Program
Department of Pediatrics
Arizona Respiratory Sciences Center
University of Arizona Health Sciences Center
Tucson, Arizona

MICHAEL R. BYE, M.D.
Associate Professor of Clinical Pediatrics
Columbia University College of Physicians & Surgeons
Acting Director, Pediatric Pulmonary Medicine
Babies and Children's Hospital/Columbia Presbyterian Medical Center
New York, New York

KAI-HÅKON CARLSEN, M.D., Ph.D.
Professor, Medical Director
Voksentoppen Centre of Asthma and Allergy in Children
University of Oslo
Oslo, Norway

DAVID P. CARLTON, M.D.
Department of Pediatrics
University of Utah Health Sciences Center
Salth Lake City, Utah

JOHN L. CARROLL, M.D.
Associate Professor of Pediatrics
Pediatric Pulmonary Division
Department of Pediatrics
The John Hopkins Children's Center
Baltimore, Maryland

FLEMING CARSWELL, M.D.
Institute of Child Health
Bristol Royal Hospital for Sick Children
Bristol, United Kingdom

RUSSELL G. CLAYTON, Sr., D.O.
Assistant Professor
Division of Pediatric Pulmonology
Department of Pediatrics
Medical College of Pennsylvania and Hahnemann School of Medicine
St. Christopher's Hospital for Children
Philadelphia, Pennsylvania

BARRY S. CLEMENTS, M.B., Ch.B., M.R.C.P. (UK), F.R.A.C.P.
Pediatric Respiratory Physician
Princess Margaret Hospital for Children
Perth, Australia

JOHN L. COLOMBO, M.D.
Associate Professor of Pediatrics
Director
Pediatric Pulmonology and Nebraska Cystic Fibrosis Center
University of Nebraska Medical Center
Omaha, Nebraska

MOIRA L. COOPER, M.D., F.R.C.P.C.
Assistant Professor of Radiology
Dalheusie University
Department of Radiology
Izaak Walton Killam Grace Health Center
Halifax, Nova Scotia, Canada

MARY COREY, Ph.D.
Scientist
Department of Population Biology
The Hospital for Sick Children
Toronto, Ontario, Canada

ROBERT S. DAUM, M.D.
Professor of Pediatrics
Department of Pediatrics
University of Chicago
Chicago, Illinois

PAMELA B. DAVIS, M.D., Ph.D.
Professor of Pediatrics, Medicine, Microbiology & Molecular Biology, and Physiology & Biophysics
Department of Pediatrics
Case Western Reserve University School of Medicine
Cleveland, Ohio

ROBBERT de IONGH, Ph.D.
Hospital Scientist
Ciliary Studies Laboratory
Respiratory Unit (C31)
Concord Hospital
Concord, NSW, Australia;
NH&MRC Research Fellow
Department of Anatomy and Histology and Institute for Biomedical Research
The University of Sydney
Sydney, NSW, Australia

FLOYD W. DENNY, Jr., M.D.
Alumni Distinguished Professor of Pediatrics
Chairman Emeritus
University of North Carolina School of Medicine
Chapel Hill, North Carolina

ROBIN R. DETERDING, M.D.
Assistant Professor of Pediatrics
Department of Pediatrics
University of Colorado School of Medicine
Denver, Colorado

EMILY L. DOBYNS, M.D.
Assistant Professor of Pediatrics
Pediatric Critical Care
The Children's Hospital
Denver, Colorado

RICHARD L. DONNERSTEIN, M.D.
Professor of Pediatrics
Chief, Pediatric Cardiology Section
Department of Pediatrics
Steele Memorial Children's Research Center
University of Arizona Health Sciences Center
Tucson, Arizona

EDWIN C. DOUGLASS, M.D.
Professor, Department of Pediatrics
Director, Clinical Oncology
St. Christopher's Hospital for Children
Philadelphia, Pennsylvania

GREGORY P. DOWNEY, M.D., F.R.C.P. (c), M,
Associate Professor, Department of Medicine
Program Director
Division of Respirology
The University of Toronto and the Toronto Hospital
Toronto, Ontario, Canada

DWIGHT B. DuBOIS, M.D.
President
Cenetron Diagnostics, LLC
Austin, Texas

TREVOR DUKE, F.R.A.C.P.
Fellow in Intensive Care
Royal Children's Hospital
Melbourne, Victoria, Australia

DAVID EVANS, Ph.D.
Associate Professor of Clinical Public Health
Pediatric Pulmonary Division
Columbia University College of Physicians & Surgeons
New York, New York

MARK LLOYD EVERARD, M.B., Ch.B., M.R.C.P., D.M.
Consultant Paediatrician
Paediatric Respiratory Unit
Sheffield Children's Hospital
Sheffield, United Kingdom

LELAND L. FAN, M.D.
Professor of Pediatrics
Baylor College of Medicine
Houston, Texas

THOMAS WILLIAM FERKOL, Jr., M.D.
Assistant Professor of Pediatrics
Rainbow Babies and Children's Hospital
Case Western Reserve University
Cleveland, Ohio

STANLEY B. FIEL, M.D.
Professor of Medicine
Chief, Pulmonary and Critical Care Medicine
Director, Adult CF Program
Medical College of Pennsylvania and Hahnemann School of Medicine
Philadelphia, Pennsylvania

CLAUDE GAULTIER, M.D., Ph.D.
Professor of Physiology
Department of Developmental Physiology
Hospital Robert Debre
University Paria VII
Paris, France

GWENDOLYN L. GILBERT, M.D., B.S., F.R.A.C.P., F.R.C.P.A.
Clinical Professor and Director
Centre for Infectious Diseases and Microbiology Laboratory Service
Institute of Clinical Pathology and Medical Research
Westmead, New South Wales, Australia

STANLEY J. GOLDBERG, M.D.
Professor of Pediatrics
Pediatric Cardiology Section
Department of Pediatrics
Steele Memorial Children's Research Center
University of Arizona Health Sciences Center
Tucson, Arizona

CHRISTOPHER G. GREEN, M.D.
Professor and Associate Chairman
Department of Pediatrics
University of Wisconsin-Madison
Madison, Wisconsin

GEORGE GWINN, M.D.
Fellow
Allergic Disease Center
Creighton University School of Medicine
Omaha, Nebraska

THOMAS C. HAY, D.O.
Associate Professor of Radiology
Department of Radiology
The Children's Hospital
Denver, Colorado

MARK JOHN HAYDEN, M.B., Ch.B., M.R.C.P. (UK)
Clinical Research Fellow
University Department of Paediatrics
Princess Margaret Hospital
Perth, WA, Australia

ROBERT HENNING, F.A.N.Z.C.A.
Staff Specialist in Intensive Care
Royal Children's Hospital
Melbourne, Victoria, Australia

LAUREN D. HOLINGER, M.D.
Professor of Otolaryngology
Northwestern University Medical School;
Head, Pediatric Otolaryngology
Children's Memorial Hospital
Department of Pediatric Otolaryngology
Chicago, Illinois

J. ROGER HOLLISTER, M.D.
Professor and Chief
Rheumatology Section
Department of Pediatrics
University of Colorado School of Medicine
Denver, Colorado

LAURA S. INSELMAN, M.D.
Active Attending Pulmonologist and Medical Director
Respiratory Care Department and Pulmonary Function Laboratory
DuPont Hospital for Children
A.I. DuPont Institute of the Nemours Foundation
Wilmington, Delaware;
Associate Professor of Pediatrics
Jefferson Medical College of Thomas Jefferson University
Philadelphia, Pennsylvania

MICHAEL D. ISEMAN, M.D.
The Girard and Madeline Beno Chair in Mycobacterial Diseases
Chief, Clinical Mycobacteriology Service
Division of Infectious Diseases
National Jewish Medical and Research Center;
Professor of Medicine
University of Colorado School of Medicine
Denver, Colorado

ALAN K. KAMADA, Pharm.D.
Assistant Faculty Member
Clinical Pharmacology Division
Department of Pediatrics
National Jewish Medical and Research Center;
Adjoint Assistant Professor
Department of Pharmacy Practice
School of Pharmacy
University of Colorado Health Sciences Center
Denver, Colorado

ANDREW S. KEMP, M.B., B.S., F.R.A.C.P., Ph.D.
Professor
Director of Immunology
Department of Immunology
Royal Children's Hospital
Melbourne, Victoria, Australia

EDWIN L. KENDIG, Jr., M.D., Sc.D. (Hon.)
Professor Emeritus of Pediatrics
Medical College of Virginia
Health Sciences Division
Virginia Commonwealth University;
Director Emeritus
Child Chest Clinic
Medical College of Virginia Hospital;
Director Emeritus
Department of Pediatrics
St. Mary's Hospital
Richmond, Virginia

KIRK KINBERG, M.D.
Fellow
Allergic Disease Center
Creighton University School of Medicine
Omaha, Nebraska

KEVIN KIRCHNER, M.D.
Georgia Pediatric Pulmonology Associates
Atlanta, Georgia

MAX KLEIN, M.B., Ch.B., F.C.P. (S.A.)
Associate Professor
Department of Paediatrics and Child Health
University of Cape Town;
Head
Paediatric Pulmonology and Paediatric Intensive Care Services
Red Cross War Memorial Children's Hospital
Cape Town, South Africa

MICHAEL R. KNOWLES, M.D.
Professor of Medicine
Director, Adult Cystic Fibrosis Clinic
CF/Pulmonary Research and Treatment Center
University of North Carolina at Chapel Hill
Chapel Hill, North Carolina

SAILESH KOTECHA, M.A., M.R.C.P., Ph.D.
Senor Lectuer in Child Health
Department of Child Health
University of Leicester
Leicester, United Kingdom

PHILIP C. LaGESSE, M.D.
Fellow
Pediatric Pulmonary Division
Oregon Health Sciences University
Portland, Oregon

LOUIS I. LANDAU, M.D., F.R.A.C.P.
Executive Dean and Professor of Paediatrics
The Faculty of Medicine and Dentistry
University of Western Australia
Perth, WA, Australia

CELIA J. LANTERI, M.App.Sc., Ph.D.
Research Scientist
CAU, Medical School
Flinders University
Adelaide, South Australia, Australia

GARY L. LARSEN, M.D.
Senior Faculty Member
Department of Pediatrics
National Jewish Medical and Research Center;
Professor of Pediatrics
Head, Section of Pediatric Pulmonary Medicine
University of Colorado School of Medicine
Denver, Colorado

PETER N. Le SOUËF, M.D., M.R.C.P. (UK), F.R.A.C.P.
Professor of Paediatrics
University of Western Australia;
Respiratory Physician
Department of Respiratory Medicine
Princess Margaret Hospital for Children
Perth, WA, Australia

MARGARET W. LEIGH, M.D.
Professor of Pediatrics
Chief, Division of Pulmonary Medicine and Allergy
Department of Pediatrics
University of North Carolina at Chapel Hill
Chapel Hill, North Carolina

HENRY LEVISON, M.D.
Professor of Pediatrics
Hospital for Sick Children
Toronto, Canada

IAN B. MacLUSKY, M.B., F.R.C.P.
Assistant Professor and Director
Pulmonary Function and Sleep Laboratories
Division of Respiratory Medicine
Department of Paediatrics
University of Toronto, Hospital for Sick Children
Toronto, Ontario, Canada

MELVIN I. MARKS, M.D.
Executive Director
Miller Children's Hospital
Long Beach, California;
Professor and Vice Chairman
Department of Pediatrics
University of California, Irvine
Irvine, California

FERNANDO D. MARTINEZ, M.D.
Swift-McNear Professor of Pediatrics
Director
Respiratory Sciences Center
University of Arizona Health Sciences Center
Tucson, Arizona

KAREN S. McCOY, M.D.
Associate Professor
Chief, Section of Pediatric Pulmonary Medicine
The Ohio State University College of Medicine
Columbus, Ohio

ROBERT B. MELLINS, M.D.
Professor of Pediatrics
Director, Pediatric Pulmonary Division
College of Physicians & Surgeons of Columbia University
New York, New York

CRAIG M. MELLIS, M.D., M.P.H., F.R.A.C.P.
Professor of Clinical Epidemiology
Department of Respiratory Medicine
The New Children's Hospital
Westmead, New South Wales, Australia

MELANIE A. MILLER, M.D.
Instructor of Clinical Pediatrics
Department of Pediatrics
University of Chicago
LaRabida Children's Hospital & Research Center
Chicago, Illinois

WAYNE J. MORGAN, M.D., C.M.
Professor, Pediatrics & Physiology
Associate Head for Academic Affairs
Chief, Pediatric Pulmonary Section
Department of Pediatrics
University of Arizona Health Sciences Center
Tucson, Arizona

JACOPO P. MORTOLA, M.D.
Professor of Physiology
Department of Physiology
McGill University
Montreal, Quebec, Canada

ALAN RIDLEY MORTON, D.P.E., M.Sc., Ed.D.
Emeritus Professor
Department of Human Movement
University of Western Australia
Perth, Australia

ETSURO K. MOTOYAMA, M.D.
Professor of Anesthesiology, Critical Care Medicine and Pediatrics
Department of Anesthesiology
University of Pittsburgh and Children's Hospital of Pittsburgh
Pittsburgh, Pennsylvania

MICHAEL NETZEL, M.D.
Fellow
Allergic Disease Center
Creighton University School of Medicine
Omaha, Nebraska

CHRISTOPHER J.L. NEWTH, M.B., F.R.C.P.(C), F.R.A.C.P.
Professor of Pediatrics
Division of Pediatric Critical Care
Children's Hospital Los Angeles
University of Southern California School of Medicine
Los Angeles, California

BÉATRICE OBERWALDNER, P.T.
Respiratory Physiotherapist
Respiratory and Allergic Disease Division
Paediatric Department
University of Graz
Graz, Austria

HUGH M. O'BRODOVICH, M.D.
Professor and Head, Department of Pediatrics
The University of Toronto
Division of Respiratory Research
Hospital for Sick Children
Toronto, Ontario, Canada

HOWARD B. PANITCH, M.D.
Associate Professor
Department of Pediatrics
Medical College of Pennsylvania and Hahnemann School of Medicine
Alegheny University of the Health Sciences;
Attending Pulmonologist
St. Christopher's Hospital for Children
Philadelphia, Pennsylvania

CAITLIN PAPASTAMELOS, M.D.
Assistant Professor
Department of Pediatrics
Temple University School of Medicine;
Attending Pulmonologist
St. Christopher's Hospital for Children
Philadelphia, Pennsylvania

EDWARD N. PATTISHALL, M.D., M.P.H.
Director
Cardiovascular/Critical Care Research
Glaxo Wellcome, Inc.
Research Triangle Park, North Carolina;
Assistant Research Professor of Pediatrics
University of North Carolina
Chapel Hill, North Carolina

JÜRG PFENNINGER, M.D.
Director, Department of Paediatric Intensive Care
University Children's Hospital
University of Berne
Berne, Switzerland

CHRISTIAN F. POETS, M.D.
Department of Paediatric Pulmonology
Hannover Medical School
Hannover, Germany

MOBEEN H. RATHORE, M.D.
Associate Professor of Pediatrics
Chief
Division of Pediatric Infectious Disease/Immunology
University of Florida Health Science Center/Jacksonville
Director, Northeast Florida Pediatric AIDS Program
Jacksonville, Florida

C. GEORGE RAY, M.D.
IMMUNO Professor and Chairman
Department of Pediatrics
Saint Louis University School of Medicine
St. Louis, Missouri

GREGORY J. REDDING, M.D.
Professor of Pediatrics
Department of Pediatrics
University of Washington School of Medicine
Children's Hospital and Medical Center
Seattle, Washington

KYOO HWAN RHEE, M.D.
Associate Professor of Clinical Pediatrics
Pediatric Critical Care Section
Department of Pediatrics
University of Arizona Health Sciences Center
Tucson, Arizona

BERYL J. ROSENSTEIN, M.D.
Professor of Pediatrics
John Hopkins University School of Medicine
Director, Cystic Fibrosis Center
Johns Hopkins Hospital
Baltimore, Maryland

JONATHAN RUTLAND, B.Sc., M.B., B.S., F.R.A.C.P., F.C.C.P.
Consultant Thoracic Physician
Ciliary Studies Laboratory
Respiratory Unit
Concord Hospital
Concord, NSW, Australia

PAUL H. SAMMUT, M.B., B.Ch.
Associate Professor of Pediatrics
Pediatric Pulmonology & Cystic Fibrosis
Department of Pediatrics
University of Nebraska Medical Center
Omaha, Nebraska

DANIEL V. SCHIDLOW, M.D.
Professor and Senior Vice Chairman
Department of Pediatrics
Medical College of Pennsylvania and Hahnemann University School of Medicine;
Senior Vice President for Clinical Affairs
Director, Cystic Fibrosis Center
St. Christopher's Hospital for Children
Philadelphia, Pennsylvania

ZIAD M. SHEHAB, M.D.
Professor of Clinical Pediatrics
Chief, Pediatric Infectious Disease Section
Department of Pediatrics
University of Arizona Health Sciences Center
Tucson, Arizona

MICHAEL SILVERMAN, M.D., M.R.C.P., F.R.C.P.C.H.
Professor of Child Health
Department of Child Health
University of Leicester
Leicestershire, England

YAKOV SIVAN, M.D.
Director, Pediatric Intensive Care Unit
Dana Children's Hospital
Tel-Aviv Sourasky Medical Center
Tel-Aviv University, Sackler Faculty of Medicine
Tel-Aviv, Israel

THOMAS L. SLOVIS, M.D.
Chief Pediatric Imaging
Children's Hospital of Michigan;
Professor of Radiology and Pediatrics
Wayne State University School of Medicine
Department of Pediatrics Imaging
Children's Hospital of Michigan
Detroit, Michigan

PETER D. SLY, M.D., F.R.A.C.P.
Associate Professor
University of Western Australia;
Head, Division of Clinical Sciences
TVW Telethon Institute for Child Health Research;
Respiratory Physician
Department of Respiratory Medicine
Princess Margaret Hospital for Children
Perth, WA, Australia

BJARNE SMEVIK, M.D.
Consultant in Pediatric Radiology
Department of Radiology
Rikshospitalet, The National Hospital
Clinic of Pediatrics
Oslo, Norway

MICHAEL SOUTH, M.D., F.R.A.C.P.
Associate Professor
Department of Paediatrics
Melbourne University
Melbourne, Victoria, Australia

DAVID P. SOUTHHALL, M.D., F.R.C.P.
Professor of Pediatrics
Academic Department of Paediatrics
North Staffordshire Hospital Centre
University of Keele
Stoke-on-Trent, United Kingdom

RENATO T. STEIN, M.D., M.P.H.
Assistant Professor
Pediatric Pulmonary Section
Department of Pediatrics
Pontificia Universidade Catolica RS
Porto Alegre, RS, Brazil

KURT R. STENMARK, M.D.
Professor of Pediatrics
Division of Pediatric Critical Care
University of Colorado School of Medicine
Denver, Colorado

ROBERT C. STERN, M.D.
Professor of Pediatrics
Department of Pediatrics
Case Western Reserve University
Cleveland, Ohio

LAURA M. STERNI, M.D.
Assistant Professor
Department of Pediatrics
Division of Pediatric Pulmonary
Johns Hopkins University School of Medicine
Baltimore, Maryland

DENNIS C. STOKES, M.D.
Associate Professor of Pediatrics
Clinical Director
Division of Pediatric Pulmonary Medicine
Co-Director, Cystic Fibrosis Center
Department of Pediatrics
Vanderbilt University School of Medicine
Nashville, Tennessee

COLIN E. SULLIVAN, Bsc. (Med), M.B.B.S., Ph.D., F.R.A.C.P., F.A.A.
Professor of Medicine
Department of Medicine
David Read Laboratory
University of Sydney
Sydney, NSW, Australia

STANLEY J. SZEFLER, M.D.
Helen Wohlberg & Herman Lambert
Chair in Pharmacokinetics
Director of Clinical Pharmacology
National Jewish Medical and Research Center;
Professor of Pediatrics and Pharmacology
University of Colorado School of Medicine
Denver, Colorado

LYNN M. TAUSSIG, M.D.
President and CEO
National Jewish Medical and Research Center;
Professor of Pediatrics
University of Colorado School of Medicine
Denver, Colorado

ROBERT TOWNLEY, M.D.
Professor of Medicine and Microbiology
Allergic Disease Center
Creighton University School of Medicine
Omaha, Nebraska

ERIKA VON MUTIUS, M.D.
Head, Pediatric Pulmonary and Allergology
University Children's Hospital
Munich, Germany

WENDY VOTROUBEK, R.N., M.P.H.
Clinical Nurse Specialist-Pediatric Pulmonary
Department of Pediatric Pulmonary
University Medical Center
Tucson, Arizona

JEFF S. WAGENER, M.D.
Professor
Pediatric Pulmonary Section
Department of Pediatrics
University of Colorado School of Medicine
Denver, Colorado

MICHAEL A. WALL, M.D.
Professor of Pediatrics and Chief
Pediatric Pulmonary Division
Oregon Health Sciences University
Portland, Oregon

FREDERICK S. WAMBOLDT, M.D.
Director, Medical Psychiatry Clinic
Department of Medicine
National Jewish Medical and Research Center;
Associate Professor of Psychiatry
University of Colorado School of Medicine
Denver, Colorado

MARIANNE Z. WAMBOLDT, M.D.
Director, Division of Child Psychiatry
Associate Director, Department of Pediatrics
National Jewish Medical and Research Center;
Associate Chairman, Division of Child Psychiatry
Department of Psychiatry
University of Colorado School of Medicine
Denver, Colorado

JOHN O. WARNER, M.D., F.R.C.P., D.Ch.
Professor of Child Health
University of Southampton
Southampton
Hants, United Kingdom

KAREN A. WATERS, MBBS, Ph.D., F.R.A.C.P.
Clinical Senior Lecturer
David Read Laboratory
University of Sydney
Sydney, NSW, Australia

GEOFFREY A. WEINBERG, M.D.
Associate Professor of Pediatrics
Division of Infectious Diseases
University of Rochester School of Medicine & Dentistry;
Director, Pediatric HIV Program
Children's Hospital at Strong & Strong Memorial Hospital
Rochester, New York

A. CLINTON WHITE, Jr., M.D.
Associate Professor of Medicine, Family Medicine, and Microbiology & Immunology
Baylor College of Medicine
Houston, Texas

BENJAMIN S. WILFOND, M.D.
Associate Professor of Pediatrics
Co-Director, Tucson Cystic Fibrosis Center
Pediatric Pulmonary Section
Department of Pediatrics
University of Arizona Health Sciences Center
Tucson, Arizona

MARY ELLEN B. WOHL, M.D.
Professor of Pediatrics
Harvard Medical School;
Chief, Division of Respiratory Diseases
Division of Respiratory Diseases
Children's Hospital
Boston, Massachusetts

ROBERT E. WOOD, Ph.D., M.D.
Professor of Pediatrics
Director
University of North Carolina Center for Pediatric Bronchology
Department of Pediatric
University of North Carolina
Chapel Hill, North Carolina

PETER D. YORGIN, M.D.
Assistant Professor of Pediatrics
Chief, Pediatric Nephrology Section
Department of Pediatrics
Steele Memorial Children's Research Center
University of Arizona Health Sciences Center
Tucson, Arizona

MAXIMILIAN S. ZACH, M.D.
Professor of Pediatrics
Respiratory and Allergic Disease Division
Paediatric Department
University of Graz
Uni-Kinderklinik
Graz, Austria

To the Landau, Le Souëf, Martinez, Morgan, Sly, and Taussig families for their love, encouragement, patience, and understanding

Foreword

Welcome to a new textbook, *Pediatric Respiratory Medicine,* authored by authorities from around the world. We might ask what is so special about an international perspective in this age of telecommunication and frequent world congresses. A reflection on the table of contents provides an answer. Practices do differ, and insight into approaches based on varied experiences can be thought-provoking and enriching.

A FEW HISTORICAL HIGHLIGHTS

The scientific basis for insight into pulmonary diseases and their pathogenesis was initiated by the physiologist William Harvey (1678) and subsequently the chemists Priestley and Lavoisier and the microbiologists Koch and Pasteur. Later, especially after World War II, studies on aviation medicine stimulated means of measuring blood gas levels and the mechanics of respiration. Seminal advances came from the laboratories of Fenn, Otis, and Rahn in Rochester, NY; Whittenberger and Mead at the Harvard School of Public Health; Cournand and Richards, who introduced cardiac catheterization; and Lilienthal and Riley (1946), who explored some of the effects of altitude.

The crescendo of interest in respiratory physiology led to support for research centers. One of the most prominent multidisciplinary centers, at the University of California, San Francisco, greatly stimulated research and teaching in physiology, pharmacology, biochemistry, and molecular biology of cardiopulmonary disorders.

The rapid expansion of knowledge during the last half century can be attributed to the scientific renaissance made possible by public support of governmental research institutions such as the National Institutes of Health and Medical Research Councils in Great Britain, Australia, and Canada. This continuing financial support has made possible new knowledge that is summarized in this textbook.

PRINCIPLES

The first section of this book emphasizes some general principles that focus on one of the central issues for all medicine: Why did this individual become ill at this time? The answers depend on an understanding of the environment and the genetic determinants of host response. Thinking on this topic has focused on the roles of nature vs. nurture, suggesting that one or the other is a determinant of illness, when usually it is both. Arnold Rich, Professor of Pathology at Johns Hopkins, expanded the concept for infectious diseases. In his classic text, *The Pathogenesis of Tuberculosis,* he proposed the relationship as follows:

$$\text{Risk of illness} = \frac{\text{Number of infecting organisms} \times \text{Virulence}}{\text{Host defenses (native and acquired)}}$$

Much of the current information on epidemiology, genetics, and host defenses is reviewed in the first section of this text. A comprehensive discussion of specific disorders, procedures, and therapies follows, which allows the reader to use this book as an invaluable resource.

The reader will find current scholarly discussions on topics such as host defense systems and lung injury and repair. Subjects of continuing interest such as exercise physiology and responses to high altitude are exceptionally well done. Common and rare pulmonary disorders are discussed in a way that will inform the clinician and stimulate the scientist. Indeed, for the clinician-scientist this book is indispensable.

GAPS IN KNOWLEDGE

It is only fair to ask what is not found in any new textbook in 1998. The excitement of the new genetics (discovery of genes and their alleles) has spurred hope that specific interventions based on knowledge of the molecular events that lead to disease will be forthcoming.

We hope that will be in the future. It is not the case in 1998 for patients with cystic fibrosis, most immune deficiency disorders, pulmonary hypertension, and muscular dystrophies, for example.

We will not find in this book a way to prevent many viral infections. Most of us, as well as our patients, will have the same disability from upper and lower respiratory tract viruses, as has been the case for generations. The human immunodeficiency virus continues to thrive despite massive efforts to produce a vaccine.

Asthma remains a leading admitting medical diagnosis in children's hospitals in the United States. Although effective medications are available to provide symptomatic relief and environmental rearrangements can reduce the risk of exposure to allergens and irritants, we have not been successful in preventing many attacks.

Not all of the suggested interventions in purulent lung disease have been subjected to prospective, randomized clinical trials in children, although recent progress in that regard is discussed in several sections. Breathing exercises and chest physiotherapy are examples of widely used approaches that lack comparative studies with other modalities to mobilize sputum; such approaches include periodic deep breathing and enhancement of airway turbulence by simple means (i.e., "flutter") or mucolysis by inhalation of aerosols.

GLOBAL PERSPECTIVE

Upper and lower respiratory tract infections, often superimposed on malnutrition, impaired host defenses, and overcrowding plus pollution, remain the leading cause of death among the world's children who live in poverty. The important observation that the increased availability of vitamin A, especially in southeast Asia and parts of Africa and Central America, can reduce the mortality rate of measles pneumonia by half is a major public health achievement. The World Health Organization, the World Summit on Children, and UNICEF have established correction of vitamin A deficiency as a goal for the year 2000. These agencies, in cooperation with each country, are working to make ongoing immunization of children a major goal. Poliomyelitis has been eradicated in the Western hemisphere, and measles could be eliminated with universal immunization.

These last comments highlight the need for all individuals entrusted with the care of children to consider the child first but also to focus on the environment, local and global, that has such a significant role in the prevention of disease. We are challenged by the need for ever-more new knowledge and the goal of making it available for the world's children.

I cannot think of a better way for the student of pediatric pulmonology to acquire an authoritative overview of the state of the specialty than to refer to this book over and over again.

REFERENCES

Comroe JH: *Retrospectroscope: insights into medical discovery,* Ithaca, NY, 1900, Perinatology Press.

Lilienthal JL, Riley RL, Proemmel DD, Frank RE: An experimental analysis in man of the oxygen pressure gradient from alveolar air to arterial blood during rest and exercise at sea level and at altitude, *Am J Physiol* 147:199-216, 1946.

Priestley J: *Experiments and observations on different kinds of air,* vol 2, London, 1775, Johnson.

Rich AR: *The pathogenesis of tuberculosis,* ed 2, Springfield, Ill, 1951, Charles C Thomas.

Mary Ellen Avery, M.D.
Thomas Morgan Rotch Distinguished Professor of Pediatrics
Harvard Medical School
Boston, Massachusetts

Preface

From its inception, *Pediatric Respiratory Medicine* was to be an international textbook. The tremendous advances in communication, the expansion of professional societies to become more global, and the interactions among clinicians and scientists on different continents suggest that medical textbooks now need to be more international in scope, summarizing different geographic approaches to advance the understanding of health and disease.

This international approach had made it difficult to review the history of pediatric pulmonology. It would be hard to write such a history for any country, let alone for the world, and the risk of leaving out certain people or events would be great. Thus there is no separate history chapter. However, the development of pediatric pulmonology as a vibrant, distinct subspecialty probably occurred in very similar ways in countries worldwide.

A number of major influences contributed to the evolution of pediatric pulmonology as a pediatric subspecialty. These included the following:

- Growing interest by pediatricians in childhood respiratory problems, especially asthma and pneumonia
- Growth of adult pulmonology, which provided training for pediatricians and spawned an expanded interest in the research, clinical, and educational aspects of pediatric pulmonary disorders
- Discovery of cystic fibrosis and the subsequent establishment of cystic fibrosis centers
- Increasing interest by pathologists in the growth and development of the lung
- Increased interest in childhood tuberculosis in the 1950s and dramatic changes in the worldwide patterns of this disease
- Development of neonatology as a discipline and heightened interest in respiratory problems of the newborn
- Growth of academic departments of pediatrics and the desire and need for pediatric subspecialties
- Establishment of pediatric intensive care units
- Publication of textbooks and journals focusing on various respiratory illnesses of infants and children

As the discipline grew, there was progressive recognition by funding and certifying agencies. This has culminated in the establishment of certification examinations in a number of countries, enhanced funding of research programs for pediatric respiratory disorders by governmental agencies, increased focus on pediatric respiratory problems by academic societies, and proliferation of training programs.

The breadth and depth of clinical and research interests encompassed in this discipline have increased markedly over the past 3 to 4 decades. This book attempts to meet these varied interests. The chapters have been written to provide more anatomic, biochemical, pharmacologic, physiologic, cellular, and molecular information for those interested in these areas while also focusing on clinical aspects for the clinicians caring for the millions of children who suffer from respiratory disorders. Thus we trust that the book will be of benefit to "students" at all levels of training and experience. Textbooks, by the time they appear in print, are outdated. The major purpose of a textbook is to provide a relatively quick and concise overview of a topic, thereby allowing the reader to have a better foundation as he or she reads current articles that focus on more specific aspects of the subject.

Many thanks are in order. First, to our publisher, Mosby, and especially to Kathy Falk for her patience, persistence, guidance, and encouragement. Second, to all of our contributing authors for their extensive time and efforts. Finally, to the children with respiratory illnesses and their families who have helped us understand and manage these conditions and shown us courage in the face of adversity.

Lynn M. Taussig
Louis I. Landau
Peter N. Le Souëf
Fernando D. Martinez
Wayne J. Morgan
Peter D. Sly

Contents

PART TWELVE SIDS

PART THIRTEEN STRUCTURAL AND MECHANICAL ABNORMALITIES

PART FOURTEEN MISCELLANEOUS DISORDERS

PEDIATRIC RESPIRATORY MEDICINE

PART ONE

General

CHAPTER 1

Epidemiology of Respiratory Disease

Louis I. Landau

Whereas the epidemiology of individual respiratory diseases is discussed in the chapters describing those diseases, this chapter provides a perspective on a worldwide basis and discusses the changing patterns of respiratory illness over time. Epidemiology is the quantitative study of the distribution, determinants, and control of disease in populations. Research findings have an impact on the individual and society. Studies are used to identify groups at risk and to elucidate etiology rather than mechanisms. Findings may also be used to suggest effective interventions. Epidemiologic studies frequently have a temporal or geographic base within which the explanatory (independent) variables are used to explain the response (dependent) variables. Response variables over recent decades have changed dramatically. Whereas in the past, the index of the impact of disease was mortality, the index has slowly moved to hospitalization, then to morbidity, and most recently to quality-of-life issues.

Considerable differences persist in disease patterns throughout the developing and more developed countries. Infectious diseases remain a major cause of death in children in developing countries. Viral infections remain a major problem aggravating the cycle of malnutrition, ill health, infection, and continued malnutrition, and such infections have a greater effect on health in the malnourished child who has impaired immune mechanisms than on a healthy child who is not malnourished. Bacteria, particularly nontypeable *Haemophilus* species, colonize very young children in developing countries, leading to chronic suppurative infection of the upper and lower airways. Tuberculosis remains one of the major causes of morbidity and mortality in both developing and developed countries. The emergence of human immunodeficiency virus infection has once again led to an increased incidence of tuberculosis. Surprisingly, the incidence of allergies and asthma is increasing as standards of living improve. Improved standards of care have led to an increase in the median life expectancy for those with inherited disorders such as cystic fibrosis and acquired problems such as chronic neonatal lung disease; as a result, many of these conditions are becoming problems in the adult as well as the child.

The environmental factors responsible for many of the changes in the incidence of certain respiratory diseases are not clearly identified. Changes in the external environment occur with improved socioeconomic status, resulting in either increased or reduced pollution. The microenvironment changes with newer housing standards, dietary changes, and the use of numerous chemicals, such as pesticides, preservatives, and stabilizers. People's lifestyles have altered with the use of child care facilities, fad diets, changing family size, and tobacco smoking. Parental smoking is a major cause of respiratory illness in children; it has clearly been associated with abnormal lung development in fetal life, abnormal lung function after birth, and wheeze-associated respiratory illness in the early years of life, as well as asthma symptoms, bronchiolitis requiring hospitalization, and sudden infant death syndrome.

Several types of studies are undertaken to analyze the etiologic factors important in the development of disease states. These include the following:

1. Occurrence studies:
    a. Incidence: The number of new cases that develop in a population over a given period.
    b. Prevalence: The number of people with the disease in a population at any one point in time. This may fluctuate, so period prevalence is used to cover a length of time.
2. Cohort studies: The pattern in those with disease rather than the whole population. These studies are used to identify predictors and determinants of disease and provide information helpful for understanding the etiology and pathogenesis of the disease.
3. Causality studies: Hill[1] has suggested the following criteria that should be used to suggest causality:
    a. Time sequence
    b. Strength of association
    c. Dose effect
    d. Specificity
    e. Consistency
    f. Biologic plausibility
    g. Reversibility

Some of the changes in disease pattern are obvious, but others are more subtle and more difficult to document. Standardization of survey procedures, definitions, and methodology is important for identifying relationships between etiologic agents and disease states. Molecular biology is now being increasingly used in epidemiologic studies to provide a more objective basis for phenotypic expression. This new technology will certainly change the practice of epidemiology over the next decade.

SUDDEN INFANT DEATH SYNDROME

The prevalence of sudden unexpected death has generally been about 1 in 500 but varies from 1 in 50 to 1 in 2000. The reasons for these differences have not been clarified, just as the cause of death has not been identified. There have been many hypotheses relating to abnormal control of ventilation, toxins, responses to allergens, smothering, and abnormal cardiac rhythms. Epidemiologic studies have identified risk factors such as bottle-feeding, parental smoking, sleeping while in the prone position, and overheating.[2-4] These studies have not helped clinicians understand the mechanism triggering sudden infant death syndrome, but attention to these risk factors has been associated with a decreased incidence of sudden unexpected death in many communities even though the cause of the disease has not been elucidated.

CHRONIC NEONATAL LUNG DISEASE

Chronic neonatal lung disease, or bronchopulmonary dysplasia, is one of the major causes of chronic lung disease in childhood. It is associated with the improved survival of extremely low-birth-weight infants (<750 g). Chronic lung disease is associated with early ventilation and oxygen therapy of extremely immature lungs. Infants demonstrate bronchial hyperresponsiveness, and some researchers have suggested an association with asthma and atopy. This finding has not been consistent. Hagan et al[5] found that a family history of asthma was associated with an increased severity of neonatal lung disease but not an increased prevalence.

TUBERCULOSIS

The prevalence of tuberculosis remains a global emergency. It is anticipated that there will be 90 million new cases by the year 2000. This will occur in spite of dramatic advances over most of the twentieth century, when the prevalence of tuberculosis fell from 100 to 60 in 100,000 in the 1950s and then to 5 in 100,000 after the introduction of national tuberculosis programs in the 1980s and 1990s. The highest prevalence of tuberculosis currently is in Asia; in many other countries, it is seen most frequently in immigrants from Asia.

Mortality was initially an accurate guide of disease because there was a constant relationship among infection, disease, and death. Once this relationship was broken by highly effective treatment, it was necessary to use other indexes such as the tuberculin test to determine the prevalence of the disease. The standardized mortality rate fell 2% each year from 1850 to 1950, after which it fell by 11% per year. In the 1850s, the mortality rate was highest in young adults (400 in 100,000), but by the end of that century, the mortality rate was highest in older adults. With the introduction of chemotherapy, death became rare in young adults. The number of deaths from tuberculous meningitis in infants and children indicates that the disease is still a significant problem. In 1949 and 1950, more than 40% of 13 to 14 year olds in the United Kingdom were tuberculin positive,[6] whereas from 1971 to 1973, 1.14% of 13 year olds were tuberculin positive.[7] In developed countries, there has been a continued decline in infection risk; in these countries, infection with the human immunodeficiency virus is putting a new group at significant risk for tuberculosis.

The control of tuberculosis resulted from a combination of public health initiatives, including effective chemotherapy, case findings undertaken actively in high-risk groups and passively with contacts of index cases, and chemoprophylaxis for all those infected with tuberculosis but without active illness to help prevent development of the disease, which would otherwise occur in 1% to 2% of such infected individuals. These control measures have been more effectively delivered by the introduction of standardized treatment regimens, special clinics, case registration, stringent migrant screening, active follow-up of index cases, mass chest radiographic surveys, tuberculosis allowances, and an active research program. The bacille Calmette-Guérin vaccination is widely used, although considerable controversy remains regarding its effectiveness; some researchers report a 20% to 80% reduction in the disease rate, whereas others suggest negligible benefit. The benefit certainly declines as the risk of infection declines, so in developed countries the vaccination is used only in high-risk groups.[8]

RESPIRATORY INFECTIONS

Respiratory infections remain the major cause of mortality in developing countries. The relative rate of bacterial vs. viral lower respiratory illness in developing countries is difficult to determine because of the lack of sensitivity and specificity for most tests for bacterial infections. The rate of lower respiratory illness caused by bacterial vs. viral infections varies from less than 15% to more than 50%.

Studies of lung aspirates in lower respiratory illnesses in developing countries have suggested that over 60% are associated with bacterial infection, with 25% being viral.[9] Few clinical or radiologic criteria help. Guidelines from the World Health Organization suggest that coughing, indrawing, fever, and a high respiratory rate would justify the use of antibiotics; those most commonly used would be penicillin, amoxicillin, and co-trimoxazole. Even in developed countries, determining the etiology of community-acquired childhood pneumonia is difficult. Although the pneumonia is more likely to be viral, there is always concern that it could result from mycoplasma, chlamydia, or bacteria.[10] There is concern about findings regarding the etiology of lower respiratory illness in developed countries being extrapolated to developing countries.

More than one fourth of all childhood deaths in developing countries can be attributed to acute respiratory infections. Many are related to conditions preventable by immunization against diseases such as pertussis, measles, diphtheria, *Haemophilus influenzae* infection, and tuberculosis. The mortality rate can be reduced by breast-feeding, improved nutrition, and decreased indoor and outdoor pollution. However, the introduction of chemotherapy has been associated with the most rapid decline in the death rate from pneumonia.

ASTHMA AND ATOPY

The incidence of asthma and atopy is increasing in all countries that have improved standards of living, reaching prevalence rates of 30% to 40% in many developed countries. Some of this is certainly due to recognition and diagnostic transfer,[11] but there has been a real increase in the incidence of both asthma and atopy.[12] These changes have also been described in migrants moving from one lifestyle situation to another. These rapid changes are clearly due not to genetic drift but most likely to changes in the environment. As discussed elsewhere, external pollution may contribute to an allergen being more allergenic in those already sensitized, but it does not appear to be associated with the increased prevalence of atopy or allergy. Pollution is responsible for increased respiratory symptoms and bronchitis, but the rate of atopy is often lower in communities with considerable pollution. It is argued that an increased risk of atopy may be associated with the lower incidence of acute respiratory illness in early life so that T cell responses result in sensitization to allergens rather than tolerance to potentially dangerous infectious agents.[13] This concept could lead to a novel immunologic approach to the prevention of childhood asthma.[14]

ENVIRONMENTAL TOBACCO SMOKE

Passive smoking is a major cause of morbidity in early childhood. Smoking during pregnancy has been identified as a major cause of impaired lung development and lower respiratory illness from birth. It is responsible for increased hospitalizations related to lower respiratory illness in the first year of life. It is argued that at least 20% of asthma symptoms can be attributed to parental smoking.

Maternal Smoking During Pregnancy

Mothers who smoke have babies that are generally 200 g lighter than those not exposed to tobacco smoke; this effect is dose dependent and maximal later in pregnancy.[15]

Smoking during pregnancy is associated with increased rates of placenta previa, abruptio placentae, antepartum hemorrhage, and premature rupture of membranes.[16] The data on preterm births conflict despite these events that would normally predispose to preterm labor. Perinatal mortality is increased[17] when one adjusts for confounders. However, perinatal death rates in low-birth-weight babies of smokers are lower than those for babies of similar weight born to nonsmokers; this could be related to a reduced risk of respiratory distress syndrome. Anatomic studies suggest that premature babies born to smokers have more mature lungs than babies of similar gestation born to nonsmokers, possibly because of a stress-type response.

Maternal smoking during pregnancy may affect airway development and lung elastic properties in utero.[18-20] These problems manifest as increased airway resistance, decreased maximal expiratory flow, and increased lung compliance.

Asthma

According to a U.S. Environmental Protection Agency report,[21] there is evidence that passive smoking is causally associated with additional episodes and increased severity of asthma in children. The evidence is suggestive, but not conclusive, of a causal association with the incidence of new cases of asthma.

Studies of children with known asthma have shown that exposure to environmental tobacco smoke makes the condition worse.[22,23] It has been reported that reduced exposure to environmental tobacco smoke is followed by improvement in the asthma severity score.[24] Confounding may diminish the observed effect of passive smoking because parents may be less likely to smoke around their child if he or she is atopic. Asthmatic children of mothers who smoke have increased airway responsiveness to pharmacologic or physical stimulants[25] and increased characteristics of atopy such as positive responses to skin prick tests for allergens and elevated serum immunoglobulin E levels.[26]

Lower Respiratory Illness

A number of reviews have now revealed a consistent association between passive smoking and respiratory morbidity in early childhood. More recent studies[27,28] have confirmed a large number of previous studies demonstrating a significant relationship between exposure to environmental tobacco smoke and lower respiratory symptoms, lower respiratory disease, or both. Exposure to environmental tobacco smoke as measured by urinary cotinine levels is associated with admission to the hospital with lower respiratory tract infection.[29] It is sometimes difficult to differentiate antenatal exposure to cigarette smoke from postnatal exposure from maternal smoking. However, studies from China show a dose-response relationship in large numbers of infants whose fathers smoke but whose mothers do not.[30]

In many studies, day-care is associated with increased lower respiratory symptoms in infancy. However, if the mother smokes heavily, this relationship is reversed: Infants who are exposed to heavy maternal smoking because they do not attend day-care have a higher risk of lower respiratory illness than those who are not exposed to heavy maternal smoking because they do attend day-care.[31]

Lung Function

The Surgeon General's report[32] concluded, "The available data demonstrate maternal smoking reduces lung function in young children." Maternal smoking has detrimental effects on lung function in infants.[18-20] Infants who have low pulmonary function are more likely to develop lower respiratory illness during the first few years of life. Changes in lung function in later childhood are more varied. Many children have reduced expiratory flows in the mid–vital capacity range. Some have reduced 1-second forced expiratory volumes, and there are lower rates of increase in 1-second forced expiratory volumes with age in those exposed to environmental tobacco smoke, particularly if exposure is associated with other conditions such as asthma.[33-37]

Bronchial Responsiveness

Studies do not conclusively demonstrate any increase in bronchial responsiveness in normal children exposed to environmental tobacco smoke. However, increased bronchial responsiveness has been demonstrated in asthmatic children exposed to mothers who smoke.[25] Some researchers have revealed a stronger effect in girls than in boys.[38]

Sudden Infant Death

Studies of sudden infant death and environmental tobacco smoke have demonstrated a significant increase in risk for infants so exposed.[39,40] The finding is now consistent in many countries, and a dose-response relationship has been documented.

Middle Ear Disease

A consistent relationship has been documented between exposure to environmental tobacco smoke and serous otitis media.[41,42] The relationship with acute otitis media is not as strong.

ASSOCIATION BETWEEN CHILDHOOD RESPIRATORY ILLNESS AND ADULT RESPIRATORY DISEASE

Chronic lung disease in adulthood is associated with lower respiratory illness in childhood. The question arises as to whether the symptoms in early life identify the at-risk individual who continues to have problems in adult life or whether illness in early life causes lung damage that predisposes to progressive lung disease. Factors common to both include active and passive cigarette smoking, family history of respiratory disease, social conditions, and gender. Although lung damage can occur because of agents such as adenoviruses and mycoplasma or chemical irritation resulting from the aspiration of gastric contents or inhalation of toxic gases, increasing evidence indicates that significant events in fetal life lead to abnormal lung function in infancy, predisposing to early childhood respiratory illness resulting from agents such as respiratory syncytial virus and chronic airway disease in later life.[43,44]

REFERENCES

1. Hill AB: The environment and disease, *Proc Roy Soc Med* 58:295-300, 1965.

Sudden Infant Death Syndrome

2. Taylor JA, Sanderson M: A re-examination of the risk factors for sudden infant death syndrome, *J Pediatr* 126:887-891, 1995.
3. Dwyer T, Ponsonby AL: SIDS epidemiology and incidence, *Pediatr Ann* 24:350-352, 1995.
4. Ponsonby AL, Dwyer T, Kasl SV, Kasl SV, Cochrane JA: The Tasmanian SIDS case-control study: univariate and multivariate factor analysis, *Paediatr Perinat Epidemiol* 9:256-272, 1995.

Chronic Neonatal Lung Disease

5. Hagan R. Minutillo C, French N, Reese A, Landau LI, Le Souëf PN: Neonatal chronic lung disease, oxygen dependency, and a family history of asthma, *Pediatr Pulmonol* 20:277-283, 1996.

Tuberculosis

6. MRC national tuberculin survey, *Lancet* 2:775, 1952.
7. Christie PN, Sutherland I: A national tuberculin survey in Great Britain: 1971-73, *Bull Int Union Tuberc* 51:185-190, 1976.
8. Stillwell JA: Benefits and costs of the school's BCG vaccination program, *Br Med J* 1:1002-1004, 1976.

Respiratory Infections

9. Shann F: Etiology of severe pneumonia in children in developing countries, *Pediatr Infect Dis J* 5:247-251, 1986.
10. Isaacs D: Problems in determining the etiology of community acquired childhood pneumonia, *Pediatr Infect Dis J* 8:143-148, 1989.

Asthma And Atopy

11. Carman PG, Landau LI: Increased paediatric asthma admissions in Western Australia: is it a problem of diagnosis? *Med J Aust* 152:23-26, 1990.
12. Ninan TK, Russell G: Respiratory symptoms and atopy in Aberdeen school children: evidence from 2 surveys 25 years apart, *Br Med J* 304:873-875, 1992.
13. Holt P, McMennamin C, Nelson D: Primary sensitization to inhalant allergens during infancy, *Pediatr Allergy Immunol* 1:3-13, 1990.
14. Holt P: A potential vaccine strategy for asthma and allied atopic disease during early infancy, *Lancet* 344:456-458, 1994.

Environmental Tobacco Smoke

15. Butler NR, Goldstein H, Ross EM: Cigarette smoking in pregnancy: its influence on birth weight and perinatal mortality, *Br Med J* 2:127-130, 1972.
16. U.S. Department of Health and Human Services: *The health consequences of smoking for women: a report of the Surgeon General,* Washington, DC, 1983, US Government Printing Office.
17. Newnham JP: Smoking in pregnancy, *Fetal Med Rev* 3:115-132, 1991.
18. Young S, Le Souëf PN, Geelhoed GC, Stick SM, Turner KJ, Landau LI: The influence of a family history of asthma and parental smoking on airway responsiveness in early infancy, *N Engl J Med* 324:1168-1173, 1991.
19. Hanrahan JP, Tager IB, Segal MR, Tosteson TD, Castille RG, Van Vunakis H, Weiss ST, Speizer FE: The effect of maternal smoking during pregnancy on early infant lung function, *Am Rev Respir Dis* 145:1129-1135, 1992.
20. Tager IB, Hanrahan JP, Tosteson TD, Castille RG, Brown RW, Weiss ST, Speizer FE: Lung function, pre- and postnatal smoke exposure and wheezing in the first year of life, *Am Rev Respir Dis* 147:911-917, 1993.
21. U.S. Environmental Protection Agency: *Respiratory health effects of passive smoking: lung cancer and other disorders,* Washington, DC, 1992, Office of Research and Development.
22. Murray AB, Morrison BJ: Passive smoking by asthmatics: its greater effects on boys than girls and on older than younger children, *Pediatrics* 84:451-459, 1989.
23. Chilmonczyk BA, Salmun LM, Megathlin KN, Neveux LM, Palomaki GE, Knight GJ, Pulkkinen AJ, Haddow JE: Association between exposure to environmental tobacco smoke and exacerbations of asthma in children, *N Engl J Med* 32:1665-1669, 1993.
24. Murray AB, Morrison BJ: The decrease in severity of asthma in children of parents who smoke since the parents have been exposing then to less tobacco smoke, *J Allergy Clin Immunol* 91:102-110, 1993.
25. Murray AB, Morrison BJ: The effect of cigarette smoke from the mother on bronchial responsiveness and severity of symptoms in children with asthma, *J Allergy Clin Immunol* 77:575-581, 1986.
26. Weiss ST, Tager IB, Munoz A, Speizer FE: The relationship of respiratory infections in early childhood and the occurrence of increased levels of bronchial responsiveness and atopy, *Am Rev Respir Dis* 131:573-578, 1985.
27. McConnochie KM, Roghmann KJ: Breast feeding and maternal smoking as predictors of wheezing in children aged 6 to 10 years, *Pediatr Pulmonol* 2:260-268, 1986.
28. Woodward A, Douglas RMH, Miles H: Acute respiratory illness in Adelaide children: breast feeding modifies the effect of smoking, *J Epidemiol Comm Health* 44:224-230, 1990.
29. Reese AC, James IR, Landau LI, Le Souëf PN: Relationship between urinary cotinine level and diagnosis in children admitted to hospital, *Am Rev Respir Dis* 146:66-70, 1992.
30. Chen Y, Li W, Yu S: Influence of passive smoking on admissions for respiratory illness in early childhood, *Br Med J* 293:303-306, 1986.
31. Wright AL, Holberg C, Martinez FD, Taussig LM: Relationship of parental smoking to wheezing and non-wheezing lower respiratory tract illness in infancy, *J Pediatr* 118:207-214, 1991.
32. U.S. Department of Health and Human Services: *The health consequences of involuntary smoking: a report of the Surgeon General,* Washington, DC, 1986, US Government Printing Office.
33. Strachan DP, Jarvis MJ, Feyerabend C: The relationship of salivary cotinine to respiratory symptoms, spirometry, and exercise induced bronchospasm in 7 year old children, *Am Rev Respir Dis* 142:147-151, 1990.
34. Cook DG, Whincup PH, Papacosta O, Strachan DP, Jarvis MJ, Bryant A: Relation of passive smoking as assessed by salivary cotinine concentration and questionnaire to spirometric indices in children, *Thorax* 48:14-20, 1993.
35. Lebowitz MD, Holberg CJ, Knudson RJ, Burrows B: Longitudinal study of pulmonary function development in children, adolescents, and early childhood, *Am Rev Respir Dis* 136:69-75, 1987.
36. Sherrill DL, Martinez FD, Lebowitz MD, Flannery EM, Herbison GP, Stanton RW, Silva PA, Sears MR: Longitudinal effects of passive smoking on pulmonary function in New Zealand children, *Am Rev Respir Dis* 145:1136-1141, 1992.
37. Rona RJ, Chinn S: Lung function, respiratory illness, and passive smoking in British primary school children, *Thorax* 48:21-25, 1993.
38. Forastiere F, Agabiti N, Corbo GM, Pistelli R, Dell'Orco V, Ciappi G, Preucci CA: Passive smoking as a determinant of bronchial responsiveness in children, *Am J Respir Crit Care Med* 149:365-370, 1994.
39. Dwyer T, Newman NM, Ponsonby A-LB, Gibbons LE: Prospective cohort study of prone sleeping position and sudden infant death syndrome, *Lancet* 337:1244-1247, 1991.
40. Mitchell EA, Ford PRK, Stewart AW, Taylor BJ, Becroft DMO, Thompson JMD, Scriagg R, Hassal IB, Barry EMJ, Allen EM, Roberts AP: Smoking and sudden infant death syndrome, *Pediatrics* 91:893-896, 1993.
41. Etzel RA, Pattishall EN, Haley NJ, Fletcher RH, Henderson FW: Passive smoking and middle ear effusion among children in day care, *Pediatrics* 90:228-232, 1992.
42. Strachan DP: Impedance and tympanometry and the home environment and 7 year old children, *J Laryngol Otol* 104:4-8, 1990.

Association Between Childhood Respiratory Illness and Adult Respiratory Disease

43. Burrows B, Knudson RJ, Lebowitz MD: The relationship of childhood respiratory illness to adult obstructive airway disease, *Am Rev Respir Dis* 115:751-760, 1977.
44. Samet JM, Tager IB, Spiezer FE: The relationship between respiratory illness in childhood and chronic inflow obstruction in adulthood, *Am Rev Respir Dis* 127:508-523, 1983.

CHAPTER 2

Environmental Factors in Pediatric Respiratory Disease

Fernando D. Martinez

Although the phenotypic manifestation of the genetic material is the essence of biology, factors external to the genotype control its expression at all times. In its broadest sense, the "environment" is the lifetime accumulation of external effects on gene expression. This definition provides a broader view of the environment than that usually attributed to this concept. In fact, the biologic "environment" has been increasingly made synonymous with the physical surroundings: water, land, and atmosphere. This restrictive concept fails to consider the significance of the interaction between all body functions and flora and fauna (including viruses and bacteria) and the important role of the uterine milieu in determining the patterns (normal or abnormal) of fetal development.

ONTOGENIC SELECTION OF DEVELOPMENTAL PATTERNS

Strong evidence now suggests that the developmental modules assumed by the lung and the immune system during the developmental phase are not mechanically determined by only the genetic background of the individual. It has become increasingly apparent that both organs usually have the potential for alternative developmental pathways. There is little doubt that genetic factors limit these developmental choices, but for the great majority of individuals (i.e., those lying away from the extremes of the gaussian distribution of compounded polygenic influences[1]), the history of encounters with external influences determines to a large extent the final outcome. This property of phenotypic selection is probably common to all organs but should be expected to be particularly important for the immune system and for the respiratory system, which have among the widest and most active relationships with all body systems.

It is reasonable to surmise that these choices among different developmental pathways can occur only early during ontogeny, when organs and their cell components are still in a more primitive, malleable form. It is also likely that once a developmental pattern is selected, the potential for a shift back to other alternatives may be very limited. In a certain sense, "natural selection" of ontogenic pathways may behave much like the "natural selection" of species that is hypothesized to occur during evolution. If this were true, however, a mechanism would need to exist by which specific cell system selections occurring during the developmental phase would favor the individual's adaptation later in life. Although this could be a very efficient mechanism of anticipated or "preemptive" adaptation, there is very little empirical evidence that such a mechanism exists. One of the best examples of developmental responses to external stimuli during fetal life is the induced early maturation of surfactant synthesis by corticosteroid administration to the mother.[2] This "environmental" induction of a vital metabolic function seems to be useful. Increased corticosteroid production occurs naturally in association with intrauterine stress, and stressful events in the perinatal period are often associated with premature birth and sure death in the absence of a surface tension–reducing mechanism for the lung and airways. During evolution, a variety of "preemptive" adaptive responses to specific external influences may have been selected that resulted in the subsequent enhanced survival of individuals who had the potential of developing those responses.

It can be deduced from this discussion that researchers could define critical periods during which external stimuli can influence the development of the lung and the immune system in ways that would not be possible in other life periods. These stimuli may even give rise to irreversible changes in organ structure and function. An extraordinary example of this pattern of lung response to external stimuli was accidentally discovered by Kida and Thurlbeck.[3] These authors were interested in the effects of β-aminopropionitrile on lung structure and function in suckling rats. They thus designed an experiment in which an active substance dissolved in saline was injected intraperitoneally to the experimental group and in which saline was injected by the same route to control animals. When subsequently studying the elasticity and microscopic anatomy of the lungs in these two groups, the investigators noted that the control group had abnormally larger alveoli and significantly less alveoli per unit volume than untreated animals. Saline-treated animals also had higher static lung compliance than expected. When saline-treated animals and untouched animals were sacrificed early during adult life (at 8 weeks of age), Kida and Thurlbeck[3] observed that the changes in lung structure in saline-injected animals had persisted up to that age. Other researchers[4] have shown that similar changes can be elicited in the lungs of animals receiving low doses of corticosteroids, but these doses need to be administered during a very precise developmental window: from postnatal day 4 to postnatal day 13. The same doses of corticosteroids, administered at any other time, produce no significant long-term changes in lung structure or function.

Studies by Barker et al[5] have suggested that very long-term consequences of environmental influences on the lung may also occur in humans. They studied the relationship between birth weight and subsequent level of lung function. They observed that birth weight directly correlated with lung function up to 70 years later. More recently, this same group[6] reported that larger head circumference at birth was associated with higher levels of IgE later in life. There is little doubt that these two neonatal parameters (birth weight and head circumference) are determined both by genetic and environmental factors, including among the latter maternal nutrition, maternal age, and maternal exposure to noxious stimuli such as tobacco smoke. When developmental patterns of the immune and respiratory systems are altered, these external stimuli may have consequences that can still be detected decades after their initial effects.

DEVELOPMENTAL PATTERNS AND LUNG DISEASE

In this context, many chronic respiratory diseases can be considered deviations in the normal developmental design of the lung and immune systems that render the subject unable to adequately cope with the environment in which he or she is raised and lives. This chapter does not deal with the environmental factors that determine acute diseases or even exacerbations of chronic lung ailments in children. These factors are so disparate and specific to each illness that it would be impossible to discuss them in a single, introductory chapter. Instead, we are dealing with the mechanism by which external influences determine the *inception* of long-term illnesses or create the conditions for recurrent acute illnesses.

The paradigm of ontogenic natural selection that is being proposed applies to even the most extreme cases of "monogenic diseases" such as cystic fibrosis (CF). It is well known to all those involved in the care of CF patients that large phenotypic differences may exist among CF siblings who by definition have the same CF genotype. It is now clear that the CF phenotype is determined only partially (albeit substantially) by the CF genotype and that other genes and an important environmental component determine the expression of the disease, particularly in the lungs.[7] Unfortunately, few studies of the natural history of CF have addressed this issue. Nevertheless, some data suggest that maternal smoking may increase the severity of CF in school-age children.[8] It is not known whether this effect is the result of postnatal exposure to environmental tobacco smoke or maternal smoking during pregnancy.

INCEPTION OF ASTHMA AND THE ENVIRONMENT

The case can be made even more convincingly for asthma. The results of studies of twins have shown that up to half of the susceptibility to asthma is inherited. Although this suggests a strong genetic component, it also indicates that expression of the disease is modulated by the environment. Because the incidence of asthma is highest during childhood and up to three fourths of all cases develop during this period,[9] it is reasonable to assume that the described developmental paradigm applies to asthma. Recent evidence strongly suggests that this may indeed be the case (see also Chapter 61).

Emerging data suggest that the developmental pattern followed by the immune system in early life may be strongly influenced by external stimuli. Initially, T-helper (Th) cells, which play a pivotal role in determining the nature of the immune response to external stimuli, are characterized by a primitive, multipotential program of cytokine production. When stimulated, these so-called Th0 cells secrete cytokines that will later be produced exclusively by one, but not both, of the two main mature Th cell phenotypes, the so-called Th1 and Th2 subtypes. These two Th cell types are well characterized in the mouse but appear to exist more as extreme developmental poles than as two unique Th cell types in humans. Th1-like cells produce mainly interferon-γ and interleukin-2 (IL-2), whereas Th2-like cells produce (among other cytokines) IL-4, IL-5, and IL-13. Th1-like cells promote cell-mediated and immunoglobulin G–mediated (IgG-mediated) responses, and they also block the development of Th2-like responses to antigen. Conversely, Th2-like cells promote IgE-mediated responses to antigen and may block Th1-like responses as well.

Role of Exposure to Allergens in Early Life

Both genetic factors and the nature of the first encounters with antigen in early life (and even during fetal life) may profoundly affect the nature of subsequent responses to the antigen. It has been suggested, for example, that exposure to allergens, when occurring at a particular period during infancy, could drive the immune system toward a persistent Th2-like response to these same allergens. Data by Sedgwick and Holt[10] showed that in mice, development of immune tolerance is a normal phenomenon by which animals exposed to certain antigens initially develop IgE responses to those antigens but later show no IgE responses when reexposed to these same antigens. Interestingly, Holt et al[11] observed that tolerance did not develop when animals were exposed to antigens during a very precise interval during the newborn period; these animals in fact showed persistent production of specific IgE against these antigens when reexposed during adult life. Because asthma is strongly associated with high concentrations of circulating IgE against certain specific allergens during childhood, it was postulated that exposure to these allergens during critical periods in early life could block the development of immune tolerance to these allergens. This could thus predispose to persistent production of IgE against asthma-related allergens and to asthma.

This conclusion appeared to be reinforced by the finding of a relationship between sensitization to certain seasonal allergens and birth during the season of highest allergen exposure.[12] In addition, an inverse relation was reported between bedroom exposure to house dust mites during the first 2 years of life and age at the first episode of asthma in asthmatic subjects who were allergic to mites.[13] Finally, it was observed that asthmatic children who were strongly sensitized against house dust mites became symptom free when transferred for rather prolonged periods of time to a mite-free environment in the Italian Alps.[14] It was thus proposed that a causal relationship existed between exposure to house dust mite antigen during early life and the development of asthma and that prevention of exposure could be a strategy for the primary prevention of the disease.[15] Moreover, it was recently suggested that a strategy of early activation of immune tolerance by the administration of high doses of antigen could prevent sensitization to allergens,[16] with the implicit conclusion that it could also prevent the development of asthma. This proposed strategy implied the administration of antigen via the oral route, based on the assumption that this route is a much stronger inducer of tolerance, as demonstrated by the high incidence of tolerance to ingested allergenic foods such as egg or milk products.

This line of thought has had considerable influence on the design of strategies for the prevention and treatment of asthma in the last 10 years. Unfortunately, new evidence suggests that the factors determining the development of asthma are more complex than a simple cause-and-effect relationship between certain exposures and asthma inception. Data from the inland desert districts of Australia[17] and from Arizona[18] and New Mexico,[19] two arid regions of the United States, have shown that childhood asthma is not less frequent in these areas than in the coastal regions of both countries. What is particularly intriguing about these findings is that house dust mites either are found in very low numbers or are simply absent from indoor environments in these arid regions. Asthmatic children were thus very unlikely to be sensitized to house dust mites in these regions, and sensitization to other allergens such as molds or indoor pets was more prevalent. Moreover, recent preliminary reports from the islands of Cape Verde, a former Portuguese colony off the western coast of Africa, show exceedingly high home infestation with house dust mites and very low rates of wheezing associated with bronchial hyperresponsiveness.[20] In addition, recent studies have failed to show or have shown only weak associations between concentrations of house dust mites in the homes of mite-sensitive asthmatics and the severity of asthma or level of bronchial responsiveness in these subjects.[21] These data thus suggest that although exposure to allergens is very important for the development of sensitization, asthmatics seem to have the potential of becoming sensitized to many allergens in early life. Some data even suggest that asthmatic subjects have serum levels of IgE significantly higher than expected, given their parents' serum IgE levels.[22] It is thus likely that either predisposition to asthma or asthma itself (and not primarily exposure to aeroallergens) may be the main predisposing factor for allergic sensitization in chronic asthma. This may explain the tendency of asthmatics to become sensitized to multiple aeroallergens,[23] including food allergens to which they rapidly become tolerant after infancy.[24] Conversely, sensitization among nonasthmatics may be more strongly related to exposure and thus more related to the level of sensitization to different aeroallergens.

Role of Infection in Early Life

The role of infections in the inception of asthma has been one of the most intensely studied and debated issues in pediatric pulmonary medicine. Several reports starting in the early 1970s and continuing into the 1980s suggested that bronchiolitis in infancy was associated with an increased likelihood of subsequent bronchial hyperresponsiveness,[25-27] increased prevalence of wheezing,[28] and lower levels of lung function.[29] One possible explanation for these findings was that viral infections caused changes in the lungs and immune system that predisposed to the outcomes previously described. This hypothesis was attractive because it offered the possibility of a prevention strategy for asthma that was aimed at avoiding or immunizing against viral respiratory infections in early life. It soon became clear, however, that most children become infected with the most common respiratory viruses such as respiratory syncytial virus (RSV) at least once during the first 2 years of life.[30] It also became clear that certain predisposed subjects had a peculiar reaction to *infections* with RSV and other viruses and that this gave rise to specific *illnesses* such as bronchiolitis or wheezing respiratory illnesses.[31] The connection between these illnesses and the subsequent development of asthma would thus be not one of a cause-and-effect pattern but rather a pattern of response to environmental stimuli that determines both the illnesses and the subsequent development of asthma. Studies by Welliver et al[32] suggest that subjects who develop higher titers of RSV-specific IgE during acute RSV bronchiolitis are more likely to develop subsequent recurrent wheeze; such studies can be reinterpreted in this context as suggesting that a selection of clones capable of mediating a preferential Th2-like response had already occurred in these infants. It is possible that this type of immune response to viral infection may be associated with the inflammatory mediators and cells that are characteristic of asthma, although the data supporting this conjecture are not conclusive.

In the previous discussion, the assumption was made that the selection of a particular type of immune response had already occurred by the time of the first encounters with virus. It is likely, however, that this may be the case only for a minority of highly predisposed subjects. Data presently available suggest that in most children, the maturation of the Th1-like response occurs during the first year of life, and during this period, production of interferon-γ by stimulated peripheral blood Th cells is lower than that observed in adults.[33] In infants predisposed to allergies, the process of maturation of the Th1-like response may be substantially delayed.[34] It is thus tempting to speculate that in these children, a Th2-like response results from the insufficiency of the blocking action of the Th1 response.

The environmental factors that stimulate the maturation of the Th1-like response are not well understood. Recent epidemiologic data have strongly suggested an inverse relation between infections in early life and the development of allergies and asthma,[35] prompting the hypothesis that these infections may stimulate the development of a mature Th1-like response, thus protecting against IgE-mediated reactions. Although some evidence indicates that this may be the case,[36] this evidence is still very preliminary, and further studies are needed in this area.

Role of Other Environmental Factors

Unfortunately, very little is known regarding the role of other environmental factors on the inception of asthma. Some studies have suggested that younger maternal age predisposes to the development of asthma in children.[37] It is now well established that maternal age is directly related to birth weight.[38] The causes of this association are not well understood, but it has been postulated that younger mothers may compete for nutrients with their children during pregnancy.[39] There is also some evidence of a direct relationship between infant lung size and maternal age.[40] The role that maternal age plays on the development of the immune system in the fetus is unknown.

Diet in early life has been extensively investigated, but the evidence suggesting a protective role of prolonged breast-feeding on the development of asthma is not convincing. Two studies have suggested that breast-feeding may decrease the likelihood of developing wheezing in nonatopic preschool children,[41,42] but the mechanism for this protective effect is unknown. One study suggested protection by breast-feeding and food allergen avoidance on the development of asthma into the teen years,[43] but other studies have been unable to confirm this finding.[44] There is some evidence that when eaten regularly, certain foods such as fish may decrease bronchial responsiveness and the likelihood of developing asthma.[45] These data also require confirmation.

The role of indoor and outdoor contamination has been extensively studied. The only indoor factor that has been clearly linked to the development of asthma is environmental tobacco smoke,[46] but the issue is still controversial.[47] Other indoor contaminants such as nitric oxides have not been shown to be associated with an increased incidence of asthma. Paradoxically, an inverse relationship has been reported between the use of coal or wood for heating and the prevalence of bronchial hyperresponsiveness and allergies.[48] Large studies on the role of outdoor pollutants have failed to find any association with the prevalence of asthma, although a consistent association between levels of outdoor contamination with several pollutants and the prevalence of bronchitis and phlegm production has been reported.[49] Comparisons of the prevalence of asthma and allergies between highly contaminated cities in eastern Germany and less contaminated cities in western Germany, both studied immediately after the reunification of that country, have consistently shown a lower prevalence of bronchial responsiveness and allergies in the former than in the latter.[50] The factors that determine these differences are still unknown.

CONCLUSION

Many external factors regulate the expression of genotype as a specific phenotype. The paradigm that these external factors contribute to the selection of developmental pathways for the respiratory and immune system in utero and during early life offers a framework for the understanding of the complex role of the environment on the development of most childhood respiratory illnesses, especially asthma.

REFERENCES

Ontogenic Selection of Developmental Patterns

1. Weiss KM: Segregation analysis: quantitative traits in families. In Weiss KM, ed: *Genetic variation and human disease: principles and evolutionary approaches*, New York, 1993, Cambridge University Press, pp 92-116.
2. Gardner MO, Goldenberg RL: Use of antenatal corticosteroids for fetal maturation, *Curr Opin Obstet Gynecol* 8:106-109, 1996.
3. Kida K, Thurlbeck WM: Lack of recovery of lung structure and function after the administration of beta-amino-propionitrile in the postnatal period, *Am Rev Respir Dis* 122:467-475, 1980.
4. Massaro D, Teich N, Maxwell S, Massaro GD, Whitney P: Postnatal development of alveoli: regulation and evidence for a critical period in rats, *J Clin Invest* 76:1297-1305, 1985.
5. Barker DJ, Godfrey KM, Fall C, Osmond C, Winter PD, Shaheen SO: Relation of birth weight and childhood respiratory infection in adult lung function and death from chronic obstructive airways disease, *Br Med J* 303:671-675, 1991.
6. Godfrey KM, Barker DJ, Osmond C: Disproportionate fetal growth and raised IgE concentration in adult life, *Clin Exp Allergy* 24:603-605, 1994.

Developmental Patterns and Lung Disease

7. Rozmahel R, Wilschanski M, Matin A, Plyte S, Oliver M, Auerbach W, Moore A, Forstner J, Durie P, Nadeau J, Bear C, Tsui LC: Modulation of disease severity in cystic fibrosis transmembrane conductance regulator deficient mice by a secondary genetic factor, *Nat Genet* 12:280-287, 1996.
8. Smyth A, O'Hea U, Williams G, Smyth R, Heaf D: Passive smoking and impaired lung function in cystic fibrosis, *Arch Dis Child* 71:353-354, 1994.

Inception of Asthma and the Environment

9. Yunginger JW, Reed CE, O'Connell EJ, Melton J, O'Fallon WM, Silverstein MD: A community-based study of the epidemiology of asthma: incidence rates, 1964-1983, *Am Rev Respir Dis* 146:888-894, 1992.
10. Sedgwick JD, Holt PG: Down-regulation of immune responses to inhaled antigen: studies on the mechanism of induced suppression, *Immunology* 56:635-642, 1985.
11. Holt PG, Vines J, Britten D: Suppression of IgE responses by antigen inhalation: failure of tolerance mechanism(s) in newborn rats, *Immunology* 63:591-593, 1988.
12. Korsgaard J, Dahl R: Sensitivity of house dust mite and grass pollen in adults: influence of the month of birth, *Clin Allergy* 13:529-535, 1983.
13. Sporik R, Holgate ST, Platts-Mills TAE, Cogswell JJ: Exposure to house-dust mite allergen (*Der p* I) and the development of asthma in childhood, *N Engl J Med* 323:502-507, 1990.
14. Peroni DG, Boner AL, Vallone G, Antolini I, Warner JO: Effective allergen avoidance at high altitude reduces allergen-induced bronchial hyperresponsiveness, *Am J Respir Crit Care Med* 149:1442-1446, 1994.
15. Peat JK, Tovey E, Toelle BG, Haby MM, Gray EJ, Mahmic A, Woolcock AJ: House dust mite allergens: a major risk factor for childhood asthma in Australia, *Am J Respir Crit Care Med* 153:141-146, 1996.
16. Holt PG: A potential vaccine strategy for asthma and allied atopic diseases during early childhood, *Lancet* 344:1227-1228, 1994.
17. Peat JK, Toelle BG, Gray EJ, Haby MM, Belousova E, Mellis CM, Woolcock AJ: Prevalence and severity of childhood asthma and allergic sensitization in seven climatic regions of New South Wales, *Med J Aust* 163:22-26, 1995.
18. Halonen M, Stern D, Wright AL, Taussig LM, Martinez FD: *Alternaria* as a major allergen for asthma in children raised in a desert environment, *Am J Respir Crit Care Med* 155:1356-1361, 1996.
19. Sporik R, Ingram JM, Price W, Sussman JH, Honsinger RW, Platts-Mills TA: Association of asthma with serum IgE and skin test reactivity to allergens among children living at high altitude, *Am J Respir Crit Care Med* 151:1388-1392, 1996.
20. Pinto R: Personal communication.
21. Chan-Yeung M, Manfreda J, Dimich-Ward H, Lam J, Ferguson A, Warren P, Simons E, Broder I, Chapman M, Platts-Mills T, Becker A: Mite and cat allergen levels in homes and severity of asthma, *Am J Respir Crit Care Med* 152:1805-1811, 1995.
22. Burrows B, Martinez FD, Cline MG, Lebowitz MD: The relationship between parental and children's serum IgE and asthma, *Am J Respir Crit Care Med* 152:1497-1500, 1995.
23. Sears MR, Herbison GP, Holdaway MD, Hewitt CJ, Flannery EM, Silva PA: Relative risks of sensitivity to grass pollen, house dust mite and cat dander in the development of childhood asthma, *Clin Exp Allergy* 19:419-424, 1989.
24. Host A: Cow's mild protein allergy and intolerance in infancy: some clinical, epidemiological and immunological aspects, *Pediatr Allergy Immunol* 5:1-36, 1994.
25. Gurwitz D, Mindorff C, Levison H: Increased incidence of bronchial reactivity in children with a history of bronchiolitis, *J Pediatr* 98:551-555, 1981.
26. Sims DG, Downham MAPS, Gardner PS, Webb JK, Weightman D: Study of 8 year old children with a history of respiratory syncytial virus bronchiolitis in infancy, *Br Med J* 1:11-14, 1978.
27. Pullen CR, Hey EN: Wheezing, asthma, and pulmonary dysfunction 10 years after infection with respiratory syncytial virus in infancy, *Br Med J* 84:1665-1669, 1982.
28. Sherman CB, Tosteson TD, Tager IB, Speizer FE, Weiss ST: Early childhood predictors of asthma, *Am J Epidemiol* 132:83-95, 1990.
29. Voter KZ, Henry MM, Stewart PW, Henderson FW: Lower respiratory illness in early childhood and lung function and bronchial reactivity in adolescent males, *Am Rev Respir Dis* 137:302-307, 1988.
30. Glezen P, Denny FW: Epidemiology of acute lower respiratory disease in children, *N Engl J Med* 288:498-505, 1973.
31. Martinez FD, Wright AL, Taussig LM, Holberg CJ, Halonen M, Morgan WJ, Group Health Medical Associates: Asthma and wheezing in the first six years of life, *N Engl J Med* 332:133-138, 1995.
32. Welliver RC, Wong DT, Sun M, Middleton E, Vaughan RS, Ogra PL: The development or respiratory syncytial virus-specific IgE and the release of histamine in nasopharyngeal secretions after infection, *N Engl J Med* 305:841-846, 1981.
33. Martinez FD, Stern DA, Wright AL, Holberg CJ, Taussig LM, Halonen M: Association of interleukin-2 and interferon-gamma production by blood mononuclear cells in infancy with parental allergy skin tests and subsequent development of atopy, *J Allergy Clin Immunol* 96:652-660, 1995.
34. Holt PG, Clough JB, Holt BJ, Baron-Hay MJ, Rose AH, Robinson BWS, Thomas WR: Genetic "risk" for atopy is associated with delayed postnatal maturation of T-cell competence, *Clin Exp Allergy* 22:1093-1099, 1992.
35. Holt PG: Infections and the development of allergy, *Toxicol Lett* 86:205-210, 1996.
36. Martinez FD, Stern DA, Wright AL, Taussig LM, Halonen M, Group Health Medical Association: Association of non-wheezing lower respiratory tract illnesses in early life with persistently diminished serum IgE levels, *Thorax* 50:1067-1072, 1995.
37. Schwartz J, Gold D, Dockery DW, Weiss ST, Speizer FE: Predictors of asthma and persistent wheeze in a national sample of children in the United States: association with social class, perinatal events, and race, *Am Rev Respir Dis* 142:555-562, 1990.
38. Martinez FD, Wright AL, Holberg CJ, Morgan WJ, Taussig LM: Maternal age as a risk factor for wheezing lower respiratory illnesses in the first year of life, *Am J Epidemiol* 136:1258-1268, 1992.
39. Naeye RL: Teenaged and pre-teenaged pregnancies: consequences of the fetal-maternal competition of nutrients, *Pediatrics* 67:146-150, 1981.

40. Martinez FD: Maternal risk factors in asthma, *Ciba Found Symp* 6:233-243, 1997.
41. Wright AL, Holberg CJ, Taussig LM, Martinez FD: Relationship of infant feeding to recurrent wheezing at age six, *Arch Pediatr Adolesc Med* 149:758-763, 1995.
42. Burr ML, Limb ES, Maguire MJ, Amarah L, Eldridge BA, Layzell JC, Merrett TG: Infant feeding, wheezing and allergy: a prospective study, *Arch Dis Child* 68:724-729, 1993.
43. Saarinen UM, Kajosaari M: Breastfeeding as prophylaxis against atopic disease: prospective follow-up study until 17 years old, *Lancet* 346:1714, 1995.
44. Zeiger RS, Heller S: The development and prediction of atopy in high-risk children: follow-up at age seven years in a prospective randomized study of combined maternal and infant food allergen avoidance, *J Allergy Clin Immunol* 95:1179-1190, 1995.
45. Hodge L, Salome CM, Peat JK, Haby MM, Xuan W, Woolcock AJ: Consumption of oily fish and childhood asthma risk, *Med J Aust* 164:137-140, 1996.
46. Martinez FD, Cline MG, Burrows B: Increased incidence of asthma in children of smoking mothers, *Pediatrics* 89:21-26, 1992.
47. Martinez, FD: Passive smoking and respiratory disorders other then cancer. In *Respiratory health effects of passive smoking: lung cancer and other disorders*, Washington, DC, 1992, Office of Research and Development, US Environmental Protection Agency.
48. von Mutius E, Illi S, Nicolai T, Martinez FD: Relation of indoor heating with asthma, allergic sensitization, and bronchial responsiveness: survey of children in south Bavaria, *Br Med J* 312:1448-1450, 1996.
49. Dockery DW, Speizer FE, Stram DO, Ware JH, Spengler JD, Ferris BG: Effects of inhalable particles on respiratory health of children, *Am Rev Respir Dis* 139:587-594, 1989.
50. von Mutius E, Martinez FD, Fritzsch C, Nicolai T, Thiemann H-H: Differences in the prevalence of asthma and atopic sensitization between East and West Germany, *Am J Respir Crit Care Med* 149:358-364, 1994.

CHAPTER 3

Molecular Genetics and Pediatric Respiratory Medicine

Peter N. Le Souëf

Molecular genetics is a relatively new field of investigation that offers the possibility of determining the precise etiology of an inherited disease. Fully understanding the molecular basis of such a disease requires the identification of the chromosome, the gene involved, the normal deoxyribonucleic acid (DNA) sequence, the DNA variation associated with disease, the mechanism of gene expression, and the role of both the normal and the abnormal protein produced by the gene.

In pediatric respiratory disease, molecular genetics is particularly relevant because the most important respiratory diseases in children, cystic fibrosis and asthma, have genetic bases and many more respiratory diseases are likely to have heritable factors. The genetic mechanisms involved in cystic fibrosis and asthma represent the extremes in the spectrum of genetic disease. For cystic fibrosis, the pattern of inheritance is simple: A single gene is involved, mendelian laws are followed, and the phenotype is relatively easily identified in the majority of cases. For asthma, the pattern is complex, there is no clear pattern of inheritance, several genes are probably involved, interactions between genes could be expected, the environment plays a major but not fully defined role, and there is no universal definition of the condition.

The importance of molecular genetics is emphasized by the fact that the recent major advances in the knowledge of cystic fibrosis have come about because of the molecular genetic discoveries of the last few years. Previous exhaustive investigations into the biochemistry and pathology of the disease had failed to detect its true etiology. Details of the molecular basis of cystic fibrosis are presented in Chapter 67. Similar advances in understanding asthma in children may depend on the genetic basis of the disease being discovered at the molecular level. Research into these aspects of asthma is still at a very early stage.

The ability to identify genes involved in disease processes has resulted because of recent, substantial progress in DNA methodologies. This chapter describes the basic principles of genetic transmission, methodologies used to identify genes and their mutations, practical applications of the techniques for understanding respiratory disease, and examples of discoveries made to date.

GENERAL PRINCIPLES

Basic Principles

A human is the product of a mathematic formula recorded in a simple quaternary code of 3 billion units.[1,2] A pair of DNAs is the unit, and the units of DNA are contained within 46 (23 pairs) chromosomes. DNA contains the purine bases adenine (A) and guanosine (G) and the pyrimidine bases cytosine (C) and thymine (T); A always pairs with T, and C always pairs with G. DNA is grouped into genes, and there are approximately 100,000 genes in the human genome. Genes are constructed of exons, the coding regions, in which three nucleotides (a codon) code for an amino acid; introns, noncoding, intervening regions whose function is largely unknown; and several other regulating and controlling regions, including promoters, operators, enhancers, and terminators. There are 64 possible combinations of the 3 nucleotides making up a codon, and from these combinations, there are codes for 21 amino acids. There is a degree of redundancy in this process because some amino acids can be translated from up to four different codons. The genetic message in DNA is transcribed into ribonucleic acid (RNA), in which a third pyrimidine uracil (U) substitutes for T and is transmitted as messenger RNA (mRNA). Mature mRNA is transported to the cytoplasm, is decoded by transfer RNA (tRNA), and after a complex series of steps, is translated into protein in ribosomes.[1,2] RNA is relatively unstable, so to assist laboratory analysis, mRNA can be made into a corresponding strand of complementary DNA (cDNA).

Patterns of Inheritance

Simple Mendelian Inheritance

Inheritance of a disease can follow simple mendelian patterns or be complex. If a single gene is involved, inheritance can be dominant or recessive. With dominant inheritance, there is an involved parent, and half of that parent's offspring may have the same condition. With recessive inheritance, offspring exhibit a condition only when both alleles of a gene are involved. This occurs in half the offspring from an affected parent and a carrier or in a fourth of offspring from two carriers. In sex-linked recessive inheritance, a gene that can cause a characteristic or a disease occurs in the X chromosome of a male patient or both X chromosomes of a female patient. The degree to which individuals are affected by a given gene abnormality is its penetrance, and this can vary for different genes.

More recently, paternal or maternal imprinting has been described. *Imprinting* means that a gene is expressed only if it is inherited from a parent of a particular gender.[2] Imprinting is thought to occur at the time of meiosis and to involve DNA methylation, which disables future gene expression in the current but not subsequent individuals.[3] The reason for imprinting is as yet unknown.

Complex Inheritance

When a heritable disease does not have a simple inheritance pattern, there are several possible reasons, including environmental effects, interactions between a major mutation and other loci, and polygenic inheritance.

Environmental Effects. There may be an environmental effect[4] on a single locus mutation. Two individuals with an identical genotype may exhibit a different phenotype because of an interaction between the mutant allele and the environment. If an environmental exposure has a sufficiently strong effect in this circumstance, the disease may be present in one individual and not the other. For example, a child with cystic fibrosis may have no physical abnormalities in early life if respiratory infections are either vigorously treated or do not occur through lack of exposure. A child with the same mutation may have marked signs of disease if subjected to repeated respiratory infections or inadequate treatment.

Interactions. Another reason for the complexity of inheritance is interactions between a major mutation and other loci. For example, liver disease in α_1-antitrypsin deficiency is thought to depend on the alleles for liver proteases[5]; homozygous individuals accumulate an abnormal α_1-antitrypsin protein that relies on the presence of high-activity proteases for removal from the liver. Interaction between a major allele and other minor alleles is also likely with cystic fibrosis, although specific examples have not yet been elucidated at the molecular level. One plausible possibility is that the combination of cystic fibrosis genes and genes determining atopy results in more troublesome symptoms of cystic fibrosis.

Polygenic Inheritance. Complexity can also occur when inheritance is polygenic. *Polygenic inheritance* infers interaction between a number of loci, each with a small but additive effect. There may be alleles with a negative effect and others with a positive effect, the final phenotype depending on the particular combination in an individual.[6] As noted, asthma is probably a polygenic disease with strong interactions with the environment. The selection of study populations for investigations into polygenic diseases is an important issue, and the principles of such selection are discussed in the section on asthma.

FINDING GENES ASSOCIATED WITH DISEASE

Forward and Reverse Genetics

There are two basic strategies for finding genes associated with disease (Fig. 3-1). One is "forward" genetics, in which the gene is found by first identifying an abnormal protein product, determining its amino acid sequence and therefore the DNA sequence of the corresponding cDNA, locating that sequence on the genomic DNA, and from this identifying the disease gene and the its chromosome. "Reverse" genetics relies on searching the genome for the location of the gene involved and then, if necessary, determining the normal function of the gene and its product, as well as the DNA sequence variation causing disease and the function of the resulting abnormal protein product.

In pediatric respiratory disease, not many conditions allow the use of forward genetics to determine the location of involved genes. Reverse genetics was used to find the cystic fibrosis transmembrane regulator gene[7] and is being used in the search for genes associated with asthma. There are several different ways of approaching reverse genetics. One is a general or undirected search of the genome, which is used when there is no information about where the relevant gene is located. Another is the candidate gene approach, which is used to study genomic DNA or mRNA when evidence suggests that a particular gene is involved.

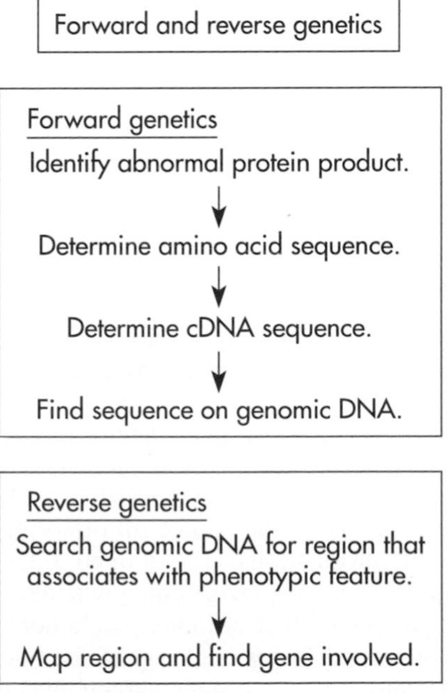

Fig. 3-1. Schematic representation of forward and reverse genetics.

This field of research is developing rapidly, and new DNA techniques are becoming available. Older, established techniques for mapping genes by physical methods such as in situ hybridization, somatic cell hybrids, and observation of the effects of chromosomal abnormalities have become less important. The advent of polymerase chain reaction (PCR) has greatly reduced the use of older molecular techniques such as Southern blot analysis of DNA fragments produced by restriction fragment length polymorphisms.

PCR has revolutionized the whole field of molecular biology, and it is now used in almost all areas.[1,2] PCR allows a length of up to about 2 kb of DNA to be amplified millions of times, and its methodology is now well known. Briefly, short DNA primers are used to demarcate the ends of the amplified segment. The primers are designed to be long enough (about 15 base pairs) to ensure that they are unique within the DNA in the initial sample. The specificity of the amplified segment is ensured because both primers should seek out unique sequences; the reaction does not work unless the primers are less than 2 or 3 kb apart on the sample of DNA. Amplification proceeds by the alternate use of high temperatures to denature the double strand and colder temperatures to allow primers to anneal to the single strand. Creation of a new double strand is then achieved by primer extension using DNA polymerase at a temperature suitable for this enzyme.[8]

Using Genetic Markers to Locate Genes Associated with Disease

Genetic Markers

Genetic markers are used in genome searches and candidate gene studies. One kind of DNA marker is a short DNA sequence that follows simple mendelian inheritance and contains one or more polymorphisms. Polymorphisms are essential because they allow pedigrees to be analyzed in families via tracking of the inheritance marker. The marker identifies alleles, DNA variations at a particular locus. Each person has two versions of the DNA at that locus. If the versions are the same, they are homozygous for that allele, and if they are different, they are heterozygous. Ideally, a marker has many alleles, each with a prevalence of around 50% in the general population. Ideally, an allele shows codominant inheritance with the disease under investigation (consistent relationship between genotype and phenotype).

Another kind of marker is a run of randomly repeated sequences, most commonly C and A ("CA repeats"). The number of repeats varies among individuals. There are enough CA repeat markers to allow a complete genome search to be undertaken.

Informativeness

For a family genetic pattern to be "informative," it must provide useful information about the inheritance pattern of a given characteristic. At the DNA level, the allele associated with the characteristic in question should be heterozygous in one of the parents. If it is heterozygous in both parents, determining the source of alleles in offspring is impossible. If the associated allele is homozygous in one parent, all offspring will inherit it, and no useful information can be derived. If the allele is homozygous in both parents, determining whether the offspring inherited it from the mother or father would not be possible.

Another important factor is clarity of the phenotype. The characteristic caused by the genetic variant must be detectable and distinguishable from characteristics with other etiologies. Cystic fibrosis is an excellent phenotype because most individuals with this condition can be identified using a simple sweat test. Asthma is an extremely difficult phenotype because it is principally a clinical diagnosis, there are no uniform definition and no diagnostic test for definitively identifying the condition, and it can lie dormant for extended periods. As discussed later, most of the molecular genetic findings concerning asthma are related to atopy.

Linkage

Linkage analysis relies on recombination, which is the spontaneous crossing-over of two chromatids, one from the mother and one from the father. This occurs at meiosis, with breakage of the DNA strands at the site of crossing and reunion of DNA between paternal and maternal ends. When two genetic loci are inherited together, they must lie close to each other and are therefore "linked." The closer the two loci, the less chance of recombination occurring between them; conversely, the greater the distance between loci, the greater the chance of them being separated by recombination. Thus if a genetic marker is commonly found to be associated with a particular disease or phenotype, the marker probably lies near the gene responsible for the disease.

Genetic distances are measured in centimorgans (cM). One centimorgan equals the distance along the chromosome corresponding to a 1% chance of recombination and averages about 1 million base pairs of DNA in the human genome. However, the number of cross-overs can vary greatly from this number, and one centimorgan can range from 100,000 to 10 million base pairs. Genes lying closer than 50 cM show direct linkage; those farther apart tend to sort independently. The extent of genetic linkage can be expressed by the recombination fraction, which is the probability that a recombination event has occurred between two genes; it is denoted by the Greek letter θ. Genes segregating independently are unlinked and have a θ of 0.5, whereas linked genes have a θ of less than 0.5. Genes located very close to one another only rarely have a recombination event between them and therefore have a θ close to zero.

Genetic linkage can be used to find genes associated with characteristics only if a family is examined because recombination events can be recognized exclusively when reproduction has occurred. The more family members examined and the more families with the same genetic association studied, the more likely that linkage can be demonstrated. In addition, linkage can be demonstrated only if the family is genetically informative (see section on informativeness). Analysis of linkage studies produces "lod scores," which are logarithms to the base of 10 of odds. The *odds* in the lod score refer to the odds that two loci are linked with a particular θ and are usually calculated for θ up to 0.5 in increments of 0.05. These calculations are complex, having originally been described by Morton in 1955,[9] and require the use of a computer-based program.[10,11] If sufficient members of an informative family or a number of informative families are studied and an appropriate polymorphic marker is used, a significant result will be obtained for a marker close to the site of the genetic variation.

Affected Sibling Pair Analysis

Sibling pair analysis can be used to detect linkage but is a much simpler approach based on the original concept of Penrose[12] and developed by Haseman and Elston.[13] It relies on the expectation that for a pair of siblings with the same phenotype, alleles are shared more often than expected if the alleles are close to the gene causing the phenotype. Sibling pair analysis is used for detecting autosomal recessive diseases. The rationale is simple: If one parent has the alleles *ab* and the other has the alleles *cd,* the children have the alleles *ac, ad, bc,* or *bd.* If one of the alleles is close to the gene associated with the phenotype, there is more than a one in four chance that affected siblings share this allele.

There are several advantages of the sibling pair method over the lod score analysis. It makes no assumptions regarding the method of inheritance and gene frequency, and because only people with clear phenotypes are chosen, it avoids the problem of incomplete penetrance. Phenocopies, however, greatly reduce the power of the analysis. Sibling pair analysis was used to map the cystic fibrosis gene to chromosome 7. A drawback of this approach is the need for large numbers of affected pairs for a genome search for genes associated with a disease. For a disease such as asthma, 100 pairs would be a small number, and 1000 pairs may be needed to detect the involved genes.

Linkage Disequilibrium

Linkage disequilibrium occurs when combinations of genetic markers are found more or less frequently than expected from their distance apart. It implies that the DNA and the markers interacting with it have been inherited together so that the distance between them is small. However, it can occur as a result of reduced recombination in that region or of a founder effect.

Linkage disequilibrium is usually used to seek an association between a disease and a particular genotypic marker. The rationale in this situation relies on the distance being short between the marker and the gene causing the disease so that recombination in successive generations is unlikely to separate the disease gene and the marker. In this situation, linkage disequilibrium is seen. When there is a large distance between the disease gene and marker, the two are likely to become separated by recombination over several generations, and no association is seen. Because of the relatively short lengths of DNA needed to ensure that the affected gene and the marker remain associated, the technique is less powerful than conventional linkage studies. Thus the use of linkage disequilibrium has limited value in detecting genes associated with disease. However, the technique can be useful in confirming the results of conventional linkage assessments. When the conventional approach detects a strong association between a gene and a marker, finding a linkage disequilibrium for that marker confirms that there is very little distance between marker and gene.

Genome Search

If there is no information about the location of a gene involved in a genetic disease, the entire human genome can be scanned using 150 to 300 DNA markers. The size of the population studied varies greatly according to the disease and the pattern of inheritance. For simple autosomal dominant inheritance with reliable penetrance, a successful genome search could be performed on a large extended family if there are sufficient affected individuals and generations. To be most economical of effort and expense, markers should be approximately 20 cM apart. Markers closer than this are not likely to produce useful information, and because more markers are needed, the search will be expensive. If expense is no object, a 10-cM search should be able to locate occasional associations missed by a 20-cM search. Markers farther apart may miss associations.

Either linkage analysis or sibling pair analysis can be used to locate regions of the genome involved in the disease process. However, when linkage has successfully identified the region containing the abnormal gene, the length of DNA of this region is still relatively long. Thus a successful linkage investigation narrows the search, but other techniques are needed to find the actual gene. This can be very difficult, and mapping of the region is needed.

Genetic Mapping

Genetic mapping is the process that establishes the location of genes. The previous section covers the first part of mapping, which is to locate the region of the genome containing the gene of interest. The next part is to locate the gene within that region, and this can mean searching a sequence of DNA of up to 2 million base pairs. One of the ways that this can be done is with multilocus linkage analysis.[10] This method uses several markers known to be from the region of interest of the genome. Because the position of the markers is usually established, one can determine the most likely position of the gene by calculating the lod score for the likelihood that the gene is located in a known position vs. a more distant position. When this lod score is plotted against position along the chromosome, the highest lod score is the place where the gene most likely is located. One of the advantages of using several markers is that whereas one or some of the markers may not be informative, others may. However, the exact position of some markers may not have been firmly established. This and the inherent lack of specificity of data generated from calculations involving recombination are reasons that the multilocus linkage method may not be particularly reliable in locating the gene unless the lod scores are especially high.

When the best estimate about the location of the abnormal gene in the chromosome has been made and the gene itself has not been identified, final localization of the gene can be difficult. With luck, useful knowledge of potential candidate genes located in the region may be obtained from several sources, including data on genes in corresponding regions in animals and data from other work mapping that region in humans. However, if there is no information about the nature of the gene, further localization is likely to involve complex and time-consuming methodologies.

The basis of the approach is to obtain a series of long lengths of overlapping so that the DNA in the region in question is all contained in at least one of the DNA strands. The set of DNA strands is called a *library* or a *contig* if all the sequences overlap and are therefore contiguous. If necessary, a library can be constructed by "walking" along the chromosome. This refers to the technique by which a subfragment of one clone is used to isolate the next set by hybridizing between overlapping genomic clones. Care is required to ensure that the extension is in the direction of interest. The technique of walking allows extension of clones into regions in which sequences and genes are unknown. Very long (around 300 kb) sequences can be replicated in yeast as "yeast artificial chromosomes," and shorter sequences can be replicated as cosmids in bacteria. So that long sections of DNA can be screened more rapidly, "jumping" can be performed. A jumping library aims to have two sequences separated by 100 to 250 kb.[14] This technique uses very low DNA concentrations and an excess of a suitable genetic marker that contains a suppressor gene and creates circular molecules of DNA.

Candidate Gene Approach

When there is reason to suspect that a particular gene is involved in the genetic process and part or all of a gene's DNA sequence is known, the gene is referred to as a *candidate gene.* A candidate gene can be studied without knowing where it is located on the genome. If DNA markers from the gene are used, linkage and sibling pair analyses can be undertaken.

Finding Mutations in Candidate Genes: Screening Methods

Single-Stranded Conformational Polymorphism

Single-stranded conformational polymorphism (SSCP) analysis was first described in 1989 and since then has become one of the most widely used screening methods for detecting mutations.[15] Mutations in several diseases have been discovered using this approach.[16-18] With SSCP analysis, primers are initially chosen so that gene segments of approximately 150 base pairs can be amplified by PCR. The resulting PCR products are then subjected to single-stranded nondenaturing gel electrophoresis.[15-17] The technique relies on abnormal DNA strands showing an altered gel migration rate compared with normal DNA (Fig. 3-2). This occurs because the tertiary structure of the single strands can be altered sufficiently with only one base change to migrate at a different rate along the gel.

The resulting single-stranded conformational polymorphisms have proved to be a sensitive method for detecting sequence changes within a PCR product.[15-18] Strands showing altered migration patterns can be sequenced[19] and the associated variation rapidly and easily identified.

Heteroduplex Analysis

Heteroduplex analysis is similar to SSCP analysis except that heteroduplexes are run on the gel. Specimens differing by as little as only one base pair from the wild-type run at different speeds and are thus detected. PCR products of 200 to 300 base pairs are used.[18] Use of this approach allows confirmation of the SSCP findings and detects most of the 10% to 20% of mutations missed by that procedure. As for SSCP, strands with abnormal migration are sequenced to determine the actual DNA variation.

Sequence analysis may indicate whether the variation is likely to be a benign polymorphism. This can be ascertained if the DNA changes indicate the likelihood of a significantly abnormal product being produced.

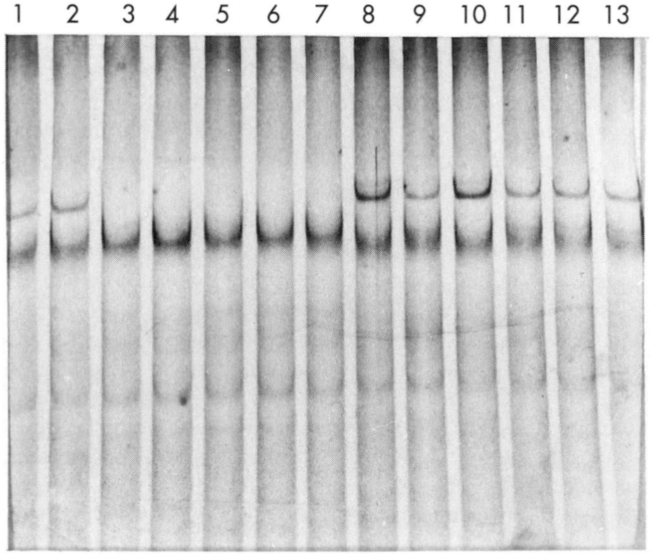

Fig. 3-2. Silver-stained polyacrylamide gel showing an altered pattern in the interleukin-4 promoter region for individuals with a C-T mutation at position –524 from the putative transcription start site. This region was amplified from the genomic DNA of different individuals using PCR and specific primers and was analyzed by SSCP. Lanes 3 through 7 show the pattern detected in normal individuals, whereas lanes 1 and 2 and 8 through 13 show the abnormal banding pattern resulting from the mutation.

Chemical Mismatch Cleavage

Chemical mismatch cleavage is another method that is available to detect mutations and can be used for larger fragments.[18] It can detect 100% of mutations in segments 1 to 2 kb long. The technique relies on the DNA strands being more susceptible to breakage ("cleavage") in places where there is a mismatch of a base pair. Osmium tetroxide reacts with mismatched T residues, and hydroxylamine reacts with mismatched C residues. These chemicals may also cause breaks in other positions, but these are much less frequent. Therefore when the DNA exposed to the chemicals is run on a gel, the strands cut at the site of the mismatch are most common and can be seen as the clearest band. The length of the DNA fragment gives the approximate location of the mutation within the original DNA segment. A similar version of this technique is the enzyme mismatch cleavage technique, which uses an enzyme to cleave the mismatch.

Sequencing

Direct sequencing of PCR products can be used to detect mutations. Sequencing is probably more expensive than the SSCP or heteroduplex techniques, but it can provide the result in one procedure. DNA segments of up to about 500 base pairs can be used for sequencing. Both radioisotope and chemiluminescent markers have been used for sequencing in either manual or fully automated sequencers.

Using Known Markers: Building Polygenic Associations

When mutations associated with disease are recognized, populations can be screened to determine the effect of the mutation on phenotype. When several mutations are known, the population can be screened for each, and their effects can be compared. If mutations coexist in the same individual, potential interactions between them can be determined.

PEDIATRIC RESPIRATORY DISEASES WITH INHERITED COMPONENTS

Cystic Fibrosis

Details of the molecular genetics of cystic fibrosis are contained in Chapter 67. As noted, cystic fibrosis is an example of a disease with a relatively simple monogenic etiology.

Asthma

Asthma as an Example of a Polygenic Disease

Studies into the genetic background of asthma at the molecular level are difficult because of the probability of a polygenic nature of inheritance and the strong effect of environment on phenotype. However, progress has been made in this area over the last few years, and there are now several genes that are directly or indirectly implicated. Before current knowledge on asthma molecular genetics is discussed, however, the problems in defining *asthma* and the selection of study populations are discussed. The approach to population selection that is presented can be considered as representative of the approach needed for polygenic diseases.

Phenotype Problems

There is no clear definition of *asthma*, and the many definitions that do exist tend to reflect the discipline of the definition's author. The most common definition is of a condition characterized by reversible airway obstruction.[20] However, some clinicians now diagnose asthma when recurrent cough is observed without clear evidence of airway narrowing.[21] Epidemiologists have considered that airway hyperresponsiveness should be part of the definition.[22,23] Cellular biologists understand asthma to be a disease of chronic airway inflammation, allergists view it as an allergic disease,[24] and immunologists consider it a disease of altered T cell function.[25] Therefore whether an individual has asthma is at times difficult to ascertain. Determining whether asthma has occurred in the past is even harder. Diagnostic criteria have changed considerably over the years, as has the awareness of asthma, so obtaining reliable pedigrees is almost impossible. For these reasons, much of the molecular genetic data on asthma to date is on immunoglobulin E–related (IgE-related) findings rather than asthma itself. Because there is a strong relationship between elevated IgE levels and both asthma and bronchial hyperresponsiveness from childhood[26] through adulthood,[27] these data are relevant and have given insight into the complexity of asthma genetics.

Selection of Study Population

To determine the genetic contribution to asthma, researchers can study normal or asthmatic populations. *Normal* in this context refers to a population representative of the general population, thereby including those with and without asthma. New "asthma genes" can be discovered by studying both normal and asthmatic populations, and interactions between environment and genetics can be investigated in each population. Each approach has its advantages and disadvantages (Table 3-1).

Normal Populations. Only normal populations can allow the population prevalence of a particular genetic variation to be determined, and this is the principle advantage of such populations. If the population is large enough and well documented, it can be used for searching the genome for the genes involved in atopy and asthma. For gathering the most informative data, studying more than one racial group and more than one environment may be an advantage if sufficient numbers are examined to allow the effects of different genes to be detected. Analyses of normal populations studied longitudinally from before birth or very early in life may provide the best opportunity for understanding the natural history of asthma, but genetic markers must be available to identify family members with particular genotypes. The main weakness of normal population studies in a polygenic disease is that involved genes may be missed; this can occur because of difficulties in defining the phenotype (i.e., asthma) but more likely occurs because too many genes produce a similar phenotype, with none being common enough to achieve the statistical significance needed for recognition. Phenocopies, which produce a similar clinical picture with a nongenetic cause, may also be common. In addition, the environmental effect, which is very strong in asthma, may swamp the effect of defects in a single gene. Finally, a genetic defect found to be important in one population or race may not exist in another.

Asthmatic Populations. The most useful families for genetic studies of asthmatic populations may be those with the clearest pedigrees, but the complexity of polygenic diseases and the advent of economical techniques for detecting mutations means that studying groups consisting of only unrelated, affected individuals also has merit. Such individuals should ideally have a clear history of asthma. Because fewer subjects are mislabeled, the population size needed for a mutation screen is minimized. Uncommon but important genetic variations are more likely to be detected because they should be more frequent in a population selected for its clarity of phenotype. Studying normal populations is still needed because the population prevalence of a given variation and the variability of penetrance of the variation should be determined. Information on families is needed for linkage studies and for confirming mendelian inheritance. Studying populations with relatively

Table 3-1 Advantages and Disadvantages of Normal and Asthmatic Populations in Studying Genes Involved in Asthma

POPULATION	ADVANTAGES	DISADVANTAGES
Normal	Studying normal populations allows the population prevalence of mutations to be determined.	Genes involved with asthma are more likely to be missed.
	Analyses of normal populations studied longitudinally from very early in life are best for understanding the natural history of asthma.	Phenocopies are more likely to cause problems.
		Environmental effects may swamp genetic effects.
		Findings may be relevant only for that population or race.
Asthmatic	Smaller populations are needed to identify involved genes.	Normal populations still need to be studied to determine the prevalence and variability of penetrance of a mutation.
	Uncommon but important mutations are more likely to be detected.	Populations with relatively clearly defined asthma are less likely to have genetic defects that tend to cause mild or moderate disease.

severe asthma may result in missing genetic defects that tend to only cause mild or moderate disease.

Specific Findings

Chromosome 6. Genes for HLA molecules are located on chromosome 6,[28] and these are involved in specific antigen recognition. This role has been recognized for many years,[29] but molecular techniques have only recently been used to detect associations.[30] Young et al[30] used such an approach to demonstrate an association between particular HLA loci and skin reactivity to environmental allergens. Overall, the importance of HLA genes in asthma genetics has yet to be determined. Current data suggest that for an antigen to be transported to a T cell, a particular HLA class II protein is needed.

Chromosome 11q. A series of papers from the Oxford Asthma Genetics Group[31-34] have established that a gene on chromosome 11q is involved with the genetics of atopy, as defined by the presence of a raised total IgE level or a positive skin or radioallergosorbent test to common aeroallergens. The gene most strongly implicated is the gene for the β-chain of the high-affinity receptor for IgE (FcεRIIβ). Initially, a genome search was undertaken in seven extended families; the search used restriction fragment length polymorphism and Southern blot analyses, and linkage was found for a DNA marker (D11S97) of chromosome 11 (11q13).[31] The findings were confirmed in a larger number of families.[32] When a series of DNA probes and an affected sibling pair analysis were used, the 11q13 gene was then found to produce an effect only if inherited from the mother.[33] Later, researchers recognized that the 11q region of the human genome corresponds to the chromosomal region in the mouse known to carry the gene for FcεRIβ. This knowledge led to studies confirming that this gene is located at 11q13[34-36] and supported the suggestion that a defect of this gene produces atopy in humans.[34,35] DNA markers from within the gene achieved the strongest linkage.[34] The receptor itself is centrally involved in the process of atopy[37] because it is found on the surface of mast cell and other immunologic cells. An association between chromosome 11q markers and raised IgE levels has been confirmed by groups in Japan, Holland, and the United States,[38,39] and an association between this region and increased airway responsiveness has been shown by an Australian group.[40] However, several other groups have failed to find linkage in similar studies.[41-45] Moffatt et al[46] have noted that care is needed in the selection of study populations with appropriate phenotypes.

An unexpected finding was that the phenotype is affected only if the abnormal 11q13 gene is derived from the mother.[33] Paternal genomic imprinting is one explanation for this observation.[3] Imprinting is used to describe the situation in which a gene from a particular parent is inactivated, perhaps at the time of meiosis.[2,3] There are several examples of either paternal or maternal imprinting for other conditions.[47] Another explanation is that the effect occurs in utero from placental influences. Several studies show a greater maternal than paternal effect for inheritance of atopy.[48]

Recently, specific mutations in the FcεRIβ gene have been reported[49,50]; the mutations appear to be associated with atopy. These findings have yet to be confirmed by another group.

Chromosome 5. Data from several groups suggest that an area on the long arm of chromosome 5 is associated with the development of atopy and in some cases, with increased airway responsiveness.[51-55] Involvement of this chromosome is expected because it has a region containing genes for several important cytokines directly involved in airway inflammation, including interleukin-4 (IL-4), IL-5, IL-9, and IL-13. Linkage between a marker on this chromosome and atopy has been found in an Amish population in the United States,[51] a Dutch population,[53] an Australian population,[54] and a population in southern England.[55] In the Dutch population, linkage was also found for increased airway responsiveness.[53] These linkage studies do not establish which gene or genes are involved, and within the region for which linkage has been reported, there are many genes with undefined sequences or function. Thus a great deal of work is still needed to completely sequence the region and determine the function of all the genes within it.

An early report suggests that a polymorphism in the promotor region of the gene for IL-4 is associated with the development of asthma.[56,57] The presence of this polymorphism has been confirmed in a preliminary study in an Australian population.[58] The effect of this polymorphism on phenotype has yet to be determined.

The gene for the β_2-adrenoreceptor is located on chromosome 5q31-32. Polymorphisms of this gene have been noted but are no more common in asthmatics than in nonasthmatics.[59] However, among the asthmatic population, those with the glycine 16 polymorphism had increased nocturnal asthma,[60] and those with the glutamic acid 27 polymorphism had increased airway responsiveness.[61]

Chromosome 14. The T cell receptor-α and T cell receptor-β gene complexes are located on chromosome 14. Linkage has recently been reported for T cell receptor-α microsatellite DNA markers and specific IgE responses.[62]

Other Genetic Diseases

Several other heritable diseases lend themselves to relatively straightforward molecular genetic analysis. These include α_1-antitrypsin[63] and cilial dysfunction. Genetic susceptibility to other respiratory diseases such as bronchiectasis, chronic bronchitis, and virus-induced wheeze in infancy may have a polygenic basis. The ability to determine a genetic basis depends on being able to clearly define phenotypes both within and among families.

PRACTICAL APPLICATIONS

As noted, molecular genetic discoveries have been responsible for major advances in understanding cystic fibrosis. This new knowledge has had practical application in the diagnosis of cystic fibrosis, both before and after birth. Whether such advances will be possible with asthma genetic studies remains to be seen.

Understanding the molecular genetics of a disease allows genotype and phenotype relationships to be ascertained in epidemiologic studies. Functional studies of mutations can be used to determine the function of the mutated gene, and this may, in some instances, provide evidence to improve the basic understanding of the disease process. Such evidence may lead to better treatment or to prevention. Gene therapy is a potential outcome, but it may be applicable only in monogenic diseases such as cystic fibrosis.

SUMMARY

Recent advances in molecular biology have allowed the genes responsible for several diseases to be identified. In respiratory medicine, cystic fibrosis has been an outstanding example, with rapid advances in understanding occurring after the identification of the gene and its mutations. Finding a gene defect that causes disease can be done either by searching the entire human genome using 150 to 300 DNA markers or by directly identifying the mutations in known genes. The former approach requires that (1) the phenotype be accurately recognized, (2) studied families have some members with and some without the disease, and (3) sufficient numbers of families be studied to allow a mathematic association to be established between genetic markers and the disease trait. This approach establishes the general location of the gene involved. The actual gene and its defect can then be found by careful mapping of the region. Discovery of the defect provides the key to understanding the nature of the disease and to planning possible strategies for prevention or treatment.

The most important respiratory disease being investigated is asthma. Many years of intensive research have failed to identify why some individuals are susceptible to asthma and others are not. Molecular genetics offers the possibility of substantial progress in this area. Studying polygenic diseases is difficult, and large populations must be analyzed. Findings so far have been interesting and relate mostly to atopy. Over the next few years, further work should reveal the most important genetic defects involved.

REFERENCES

General Principles

1. Lewin B: *Genes V,* Oxford, England, 1994, Oxford University Press.
2. Strachan T, Read AP: *Human molecular genetics,* Oxford, England, 1996, BIOS.
3. Hall JG: Genomic imprinting, *Arch Dis Child* 65:1013-1016, 1990.
4. Peat JK, Tovey E, Mellis CM, Leeder SR, Woolcock AJ: Importance of house dust mite and *Alternaria* allergens in childhood asthma: an epidemiological study in two climatic regions of Australia, *Clin Exp Allergy* 23:812-820, 1993.
5. Crystal RG, Brantly ML, Hubbard RC, Curiel DT, States DJ, Holmes MD: The alpha-1 antitrypsin gene and its mutations: clinical consequences and strategies for therapy, *Chest* 95:196-208, 1989.
6. Stuart J: Genetics and biology: a comment on the significance of the Elston-Stewart algorithm, *Hum Hered* 42:9-15, 1992.

Finding Genes Associated with Disease

7. Kerem B, Rommens JM, Buchanan JA, Markiewicz D, Cox TK, Chakravarti A, Buchwald M, Tsui LC: Identification of the cystic fibrosis gene: genetic analysis, *Science* 245:1073-1080, 1989.
8. Newton CR, Graham A: *PCR,* Oxford, England, 1994, BIOS.
9. Morton NE: Sequential tests for the detection of linkage, *Am Hum Genet* 7:277-318, 1955.
10. Ott J: *Analysis of human genetic linkage,* Baltimore, 1991, Johns Hopkins University Press.
11. Davies KE, Read AP: *Molecular basis of inherited disease,* ed 2, Oxford, England, 1992, Oxford University Press.
12. Penrose LS: The detection of autosomal linkage in data which consist of pairs of brothers and sisters of unspecified parentage, *Ann Eugen* 6:133-138, 1935.
13. Haseman JK, Elston RC: The investigation of linkage between a quantitative trait and a marker locus, *Behav Genet* 2:3-19, 1972.
14. Forrest SM, Cross GS, Speer A, Gardner-Medwin D, Davies KE: Preferential deletion of exons in Duchenne and Becker muscular dystrophy, *Nature* 329:638-640, 1987.
15. Orita M, Iwahana H, Kanazawa H, Hayashi, Sekiya T: Detection of polymorphisms of human DNA by gel electrophoresis as single-strand conformation polymorphisms, *Proc Natl Acad Sci* 86:2766-2770, 1989.
16. Ainsworth PJ, Surh LC, Coulter Mackie MB: Diagnostic single strand conformational polymorphism (SSCP): a simplified non-radioisotopic method, *Nucl Acid Res* 19:405-406, 1991.
17. Dockhorn-Dwoviczak B, Dwoviczak B, Brömmelkamp L, Bülles J, Horst J, Böcker WW: Non-isotopic detection of single strand conformational polymorphisms (PCR-SSCP): a rapid and sensitive technique in diagnosis of phenylketonuria, *Nucl Acid Res* 19:2500, 1991.
18. Cotton RGH: Current methods of mutation detection, *Mut Res* 285:125-144, 1993.
19. Brown TA: *DNA sequencing: the basics,* Oxford, England, 1994, IRL.

Pediatric Respiratory Diseases with Inherited Components

20. American Thoracic Society: Definition of asthma, *Am Rev Respir Dis* 134:704-707, 1962.
21. Phelan PD, Landau LI, Olinsky A: *Respiratory illness in children,* ed 3, Oxford, England, 1990, Blackwell.
22. Toelle BG, Peat JK, Salome CM, Mellis CM, Woolcock AJ: Toward a definition of asthma for epidemiology, *Am Rev Respir Dis* 146:633-637, 1992.
23. Holgate ST, Beasley R, Twentyman OP: The pathogenesis and significance of bronchial responsiveness in airways disease, *Clin Sci* 73:561-572, 1987.
24. Platts-Mills TAE, de Weck AL: Dust mite allergens and asthma: a worldwide problem, *J Allergy Clin Immunol* 83:416-427, 1989.
25. Marsh DG, Lockhart A, Holgate ST: *The genetics of asthma,* Oxford, England, 1993, Blackwell.
26. Sears MR, Burrows B, Flannery EM, Herbison GP, Hewitt CJ, Holdaway MD: Relation between airway responsiveness and serum IgE in children with asthma and in apparently normal children, *N Engl J Med* 325:1067-1071, 1991.
27. Burrows B, Martinez FD, Halonen M, Barbee RA, Cline MG: Association of asthma with serum IgE levels and skin-test reactivity to allergens, *N Engl J Med* 320:271-277, 1989.
28. Marsh DG, Meyers DA, Bias WB: The epidemiology and genetics of atopic allergy, *N Engl J Med* 305:1551-1559, 1981.
29. Marsh DG: Genetic and molecular analysis of human immune responsiveness to allergens. In Marsh DG, Lockhart A, Holgate ST, eds: *The genetics of asthma,* Oxford, England, 1993, Blackwell, pp 201-213.
30. Young RP, Dekker JW, Wordsworth BP, Schou C, Pile KD, Matthiesen F, Rosenberg WMC, Bell JI, Hopkin JM, Cookson WOCM: HLA-DR and HLA-DP genotypes and immunoglobulin E responses to common major allergens, *Clin Exp Allergy* 24:431-439, 1994.
31. Cookson WOCM, Sharp PA, Faux JA, Hopkin JM: Linkage between immunoglobulin E responses underlying asthma and rhinitis and chromosome 11q, *Lancet* 1:1292-1295, 1989.
32. Young RP, Sharp JA, Lynch J, Faux JA, Lathrop GM, Cookson WOCM, Hopkin JM: Confirmation of genetic linkage between atopic IgE responses and chromosome 11q13, *J Med Genet* 29:236-238, 1992.
33. Cookson WOCM, Young RP, Sandford AJ, Moffat MF, Shirakawa T, Sharp PA, Faux JA, Julier C, Le Souëf PN, Nakamura Y, Lathrop GM, Hopkin JM: Maternal inheritance of atopic IgE responsiveness on chromosome 11q, *Lancet* 340:381-384, 1992.
34. Sandford AJ, Shirakawa T, Moffat MF, Daniels SE, Ra C, Faux JA, Young RP, Nakamura Y, Lathrop GM, Cookson WOCM, Hopkin JM: Localization of atopy and beta subunit of high-affinity IgE receptor (FcεRI) on chromosome 11q, *Lancet* 341:332-334, 1993.
35. Ra C, Jouvin M-HE, Kinet J-P: Complete structure of the mouse mast cell receptor for IgE (FcepsilonR1) and surface expression of chimeric receptors (rat-mouse-human) on transfected cells, *J Biol Chem* 264:15323-15327, 1989.
36. Kuester H, Zhang L, Brini AT, MacGlashan DW, Kinet JP: The gene and cDNA for the human high affinity IgE receptor beta chain and expression of the complete human Fc epsilon R1 receptor, *J Biol Chem* 267:12782-12787, 1992.
37. Katz HR: Development-associated changes in mast cell Fc receptor expression and function. In Holgate ST, Austen KF, Lichtenstein LM, Kay AB, eds: *Asthma: physiology, immunopharmacology, and treatment,* London, 1993, Academic, pp 89-97.

38. Shirikawa T, Morimoto K, Hashimoto T, Furuyama J, Yamam M, Takai S: Linkage between atopic IgE responses and chromosome 11q in Japanese families, *Cytogenet Cell Genet* 58:197, 1991.
39. Collee JM, ten Kate LP, de Vries HG, Kliphuis JW, Bouman K, Scheffer H, Gerritsen J: Allele sharing on chromosome 11q13 in sibs with asthma and atopy, *Lancet* 342:936, 1993 (letter).
40. Van Herwerden L, Harrap SB, Wong ZYH, Abrahamson MJ, Kutin JJ, Forbes AB, Raven J, Lanigan A, Walter EH: Linkage of high-affinity IgE receptor gene with bronchial hyperreactivity even in absence of atopy, *Lancet* 346:1262-1265, 1995.
41. Lympany P, Welsh K, MacCochrane G, Kemeny DM, Lee TH: Genetic analysis using DNA polymorphism of the linkage between chromosome 11q13 and atopy and bronchial responsiveness to methacholine, *J Allergy Clin Immunol* 89:619-628, 1992.
42. Amelung PJ, Panhuysen CIM, Postma DS, Levitt RC, Koeter GH, Francomano CA, Bleecker ER, Meyers DA: Atopy and bronchial responsiveness: exclusion of linkage to markers on chromosomes on 11q and 6p, *Clin Exp Allergy* 22:1077-1084, 1992.
43. Hizawa N, Yamaguchi E, Ohe M, Itoh A, Furaya K, Ohnuma N, Kawakami Y: Lack of linkage between atopy and locus 11q13, *Clin Exp Allergy* 22:1065-1069, 1992.
44. Rich SS, Roitman-Johnson B, Greenberg B, Roberts S, Blumenthal MN: Genetic analysis of atopy in three large kindreds: no evidence of linkage to D11S97, *Clin Exp Allergy* 22:1070-1076, 1992.
45. Morton NE: Major loci for atopy? *Clin Exp Allergy* 22:1041-1043, 1992 (editorial).
46. Moffatt MF, Sharp PA, Faux JA, Young RP, Cookson WOCM, Hopkin JM: Factors confounding genetic linkage between atopy and chromosome 11q, *Clin Exp Allergy* 22:1046-1051, 1992.
47. Cooper DN, Krawczak M: *Human gene mutation*, Oxford, England, 1993, BIOS.
48. Ownby DR: Environmental factors versus genetic determinants of childhood inhalant allergies, *J Allergy Clin Immunol* 86:279-287, 1990.
49. Shirakawa T, Li A, Dubowitz M, Dekker JW, Shaw AE, Faux JA, Ra C, Cookson WOCM, Hopkin JM: Association between atopy and variants of the beta subunit of the high-affinity immunoglobulin E receptor 19, *Nat Genet* 7:125-130, 1994.
50. Hill MR, James AL, Faux JA, Ryan G, Hopkin JM, Le Souëf P, Musk AW, Cookson WOCM: Association of marked atopy and FcεR1-beta Leu181/Leu183 in general population sample, *Br Med J* 311:776-779, 1995.
51. Marsh DG, Neely JD, Breazeale DR, Ghosh B, Freidhoff LR, Ehrlich-Kautzky E, Schou C, Krishnaswamy G, Beaty TH: Linkage analysis of IL-4 and other chromosome 5q31.1 markers and total serum immunoglobulin-E concentrations, *Science* 264:1152-1156, 1994.
52. Meyers DA, Postma DS, Panhysen CIM, Xu J, Amelung PJ, Levitt RC, Bleecker ER: Evidence for a locus regulating total serum IgE levels mapping to chromosome 5, *Genomics* 23:464-470, 1994.
53. Postma DS, Bleecker ER, Amelung PJ, Holroyd KJ, Xu J, Panhuysen CIM, Meyers DA, Levitt RC: Genetic susceptibility to asthma: bronchial hyperresponsiveness coinherited with a major gene for atopy, *N Engl J Med* 333:894-900, 1995.
54. Sandford AJ, Daniels SE, James AL, Le Souëf PN, Musk AW, Cookson WOCM: Chromosome 5, markers, total serum IgE and bronchial responsiveness in a random population, *Am J Respir Crit Care Med* 151:341, 1995 (abstract).
55. Morton NE: Genetic studies on atopy and asthma in Wessex, *Clin Exp Allergy* 25(suppl 2):107-109, 1995.
56. Borish LC, Mascali JJ, Klinnert M, Leppert M, Rosenwasser LJ: Polymorphisms in the chromosome 5 gene cluster, *J Allergy Clin Immunol* 93:220, 1994 (abstract).
57. Rossenwasser LJ, Klemm DJ, Dresback JK, Inamura H, Mascali JJ, Klinnert K, Borish L: Promoter polymorphisms in the chromosome 5 gene cluster in asthma and atopy, *Clin Exp Allergy* 25(suppl 2):74-78, 1995.
58. Boyer S, Pereira E, Rye P, Goldblatt J, Sanderson C, Le Souëf P: Confirmation of the presence of a polymorphism in the interleukin-4 promoter in an asthmatic cohort, *Am J Respir Crit Care Med* 151:470, 1995 (abstract).
59. Reishaus E, Innis M, MacIntyre N, Liggett SB: Mutations in the gene encoding for the beta-2 adrenergic receptor in normal and asthmatic subjects, *Am J Respir Cell Mol Biol* 8:334-339, 1993.
60. Turki J, Pak J, Green S, Martin R, Liggett S: The Gly15 polymorphism of the beta2-adrenergic receptor predisposes to nocturnal asthma, *Am J Respir Crit Care Med* 151:342, 1995 (abstract).
61. Hall IP, Wheatley A, Wilding P, Liggett SB: Association of the Glu 27 beta2-adrenoceptor polymorphism with lower airway reactivity in asthmatic subjects, *Lancet* 345:1213-1214, 1995.
62. Moffat MF, Hill MR, Cornelius F, Schou C, Faux JA, Young RP, James AL, Ryan G, Le Souëf P, Musk AW, Hopkin JM, Cookson WOCM: Genetic linkage of the TCR-alpha/delta region to specific immunoglobulin E responses, *Lancet* 343:1597-1600, 1994.
63. Morgan K, Kalsheker N: An enhancer mutation in the α-1-antitrypsin gene associated with chronic obstructive airways disease (COAD) results in a dramatic reduction in the positive cooperative interaction between transcription factors, *Am J Respir Crit Care Med* 151:161, 1995 (abstract).

CHAPTER 4

Developmental Anatomy and Physiology of the Respiratory System

Claude Gaultier

In the first years of life, maturational changes in the respiratory system and breathing control are most marked, and respiratory disorders are particularly common and severe. Immaturity of the lung contributes substantially to the morbidity and mortality associated with prematurity. Respiratory control immaturity is involved in the pathophysiology of apnea of prematurity, apparently life-threatening events, and sudden infant death syndrome (SIDS). Immaturity of the chest wall limits the ability of infants to adapt to increased breathing loads during respiratory disorders.

Antenatal and postnatal environmental factors, such as malnutrition and chronic hypoxia, impair the development of the respiratory system and respiratory control mechanisms. Developmental abnormalities may be associated with increased vulnerability to insults such as viral infections, passive smoking, and air pollution.

Knowledge of the development of the respiratory system is currently moving from developmental anatomy and physiology to developmental cellular and molecular biology. The challenge for coming years will be to unravel the links among dysregulation in gene expression and cellular phenotypes, abnormal physiologic function, and clinical symptoms of respiratory disorders in infants and children. Improved knowledge of the underpinnings of developmental processes will improve the ability to prevent antenatal and postnatal exposure to insults and devise effective treatment strategies.

UPPER AIRWAYS

Developmental Anatomy

The configuration of the upper airways changes with growth.[1,2] In the newborn, the epiglottis is large and can cover the soft palate, forming a low epiglottic sphincter and encouraging nasal breathing ("obligatory" nasal breathing of the newborn). A horizontal position of the tongue and an elevated position of the hyoid bone and laryngeal cartilage are other specific features. Over the first 2 years of life, changes in upper airway anatomy lead to formation of a dynamic velolingual sphincter that permits buccal respiration and speech. The epiglottis, larynx, and hyoid bone move downward. The posterior portion of the tongue becomes vertical during late infancy. The facial skeleton grows vertically, and the mandible lengthens from front to back.

Developmental Physiology

Function

Newborn mammals, including human infants, have difficulty breathing through their mouths when the nasal passages are occluded. Although nasal breathing is considered obligatory in the newborn and infant, mouth-breathing can occur in the presence of nasal obstruction. Oropharyngeal structures have been examined using fluoroscopy during nasal occlusion in healthy infants.[3] Infants can breath through the mouth by detaching the soft palate from the tongue, thus opening the pharyngeal isthmus. However, the time required to establish mouth-breathing varies with age, the state of alertness, or both factors, with younger and sleeping infants responding more slowly than older and awake infants. When nasal passages are obstructed, mouth-breathing is established more slowly during rapid-eye-movement (REM) sleep than during non-REM sleep.[4,5]

Oropharyngeal dynamics in babies have been studied during life and at autopsy.[6-8] The relationship between pharyngeal pressure and oropharyngeal patency has been evaluated at autopsy in infants up to 3 months of age.[9] The closing pressure is 0.82 cm H_2O on average and is generally lower than the opening pressure. The position of the neck is a significant determinant of oropharyngeal dynamics,[10] and neck flexion is thought to play a role in the occurrence of obstructive apnea.[11] During inspiration in normal children[12] and some normal premature infants,[13] phasic activity of the genioglossus muscle is absent; when pharyngeal pressure increases, phasic genioglossus activity appears or is augmented.[13]

Nasal resistance has been measured in Caucasian and black infants during the first year of life using an adapted posterior rhinomanometric method. The percentage contribution of nasal resistance to airway resistance is significantly higher in Caucasian infants than in black infants (mean values, 49% and 31%, respectively).[14] This difference probably reflects anatomic differences in nasal structures.

Reflexes Originating in the Upper Airways

In human infants and newborn animals, reflexes originating in the upper airways can induce apnea and bradycardia.[15,16] In anaesthetized puppies, the duration of apnea elicited by water instillation into the larynx decreased as age increased.[16] Studies in unanesthetized lambs have suggested that sensitivity of the respiratory system to superior laryngeal nerve inhibition decreases with development[15]; the cause for this maturation is still unclear. In premature infants, reflex apnea has been reported to occur after instillation of water or saline into the larynx during sleep.[17-19] Prolonged apnea in preterm infants may be a pathologic extreme that extends the normal spectrum of airway protective responses to upper airway fluids.[19] The laryngeal chemoreflex has been implicated in the pathophysiology of SIDS.[20] Studies in newborn animals noted that the degree of apnea and bradycardia elicited by the laryngeal chemoreflex was increased by upper airway infection,[21] anemia,[22] and infection by the respiratory syncytial virus.[23] Such an infection is associated with central and obstructive apneas during sleep in human infants.[24] The apnea and bradycardia elicited by the laryngeal reflex in human infants increase dramatically in the presence of hypoxia because of a cardioinhibitory effect on peripheral chemoreceptors during apnea with suppression of input from pulmonary stretch receptors.[20]

During the neonatal period, stimulation of other upper airway receptors can result in apnea. Activation of upper airway mechanoreceptors by negative pressure causes apnea in puppies but not in adult dogs.[25] In human infants, trigeminal airway stimulation can elicit a response similar to that seen during the diving reflex and can include apnea and bradycardia.[26] Studies of healthy infants tested during REM sleep showed that the ventilatory response to trigeminal stimulation became increasingly blunted as the infants mature.[27]

CHEST WALL

Developmental Anatomy

Ribcage

At birth, the ribs are mainly composed of cartilage and project at right angles from the vertebral column. As a result, the ribcage is more circular than in adults[28-30] (Fig. 4-1) and lacks mechanical efficiency.[31] In adults, ribcage volume can be increased by elevating the ribs. In infants, the ribs are already elevated, which may be one reason that ribcage motion during room air breathing contributes little to tidal volume.[31] Rib orientation (see Fig. 4-1) does not change substantially until the infant acquires the ability to assume the upright posture. This changes the forces acting on the ribcage. The action of gravity on the ribs and the pull of the muscles inserted on the ribs cause the ribs to slope caudally. This leads to relative lengthening of the thoracic cavity, which loses its circular cross section to acquire the ovoid adult pattern.[29,30] The thoracic index (anteroposterior/lateral diameter) decreases significantly with age during the first 3 years of life.[30] During the same period, gradual mineralization of the ribs occurs. These changes in shape and structure are extremely important because they stiffen the ribcage.

Respiratory Muscles

In the newborn, the diaphragm seems poorly adapted to the burden of respiratory work. The angle of insertion of the diaphragm in infants is different from that in adults (i.e., almost horizontal instead of oblique). This results in decreased contraction efficiency in infants. With its open angle of insertion and small area of apposition[32] (Fig. 4-2), the flat diaphragm of the newborn seems designed to suck the chest wall inward rather than draw air into the chest cavity. In infants, the contracting diaphragm tends to pull the lower ribcage inward because of its almost horizontal insertion. For the same reason, the downward course of the contracting diaphragm is shorter, the abdominal pressure increase is smaller, and consequently, the ribcage expansion is less marked. The diaphragm tends to distort the floppy ribcage of infants, especially preterm infants (see section on thoracoabdominal motion).

With growth, there is a gradual increase in respiratory muscle bulk, as well as important changes in the composition, size, and oxidative capacity of respiratory muscle fibers. In preterm infants, the diaphragm contains less than 10% type I fibers[33] and a higher percentage of type II fibers, particularly type IIc.[34] The mean cross-sectional area of all fiber types increases after birth.[35,36] The total oxidative capacity of the diaphragm, defined as the succinyl dehydrogenase activity, is low at birth.[35,36]

Fig. 4-1. Changes in configuration and cross-sectional shape of the thorax from infancy to early childhood. (Redrawn from Openshaw P et al: *Thorax* 39:624-627, 1984.)

Developmental Physiology

Chest Wall Compliance

High chest wall compliance relative to lung compliance is an inherent characteristic of newborn mammals.[37] Few studies have investigated chest wall mechanics in infants and children.[38-40] Data on the time pattern of changes in chest wall compliance during infancy and early childhood have been recently obtained.[40] In infancy, compliance of the chest wall is nearly threefold that of the lung. By the second year of life, the increase in chest wall stiffness is such that the chest wall and lung have similar compliances, as in adults.

Thoracoabdominal Motion

Developmental changes in thoracic properties over time influence the pattern of thoracoabdominal motion during infancy and early childhood. The contribution of the ribcage to tidal breathing increases with postnatal age. Studies have found that this contribution is 34% during non-REM sleep at 1 month of age[41] and increases to adolescent levels (i.e., approximately 60%) by 1 year of age.

Chest wall muscle contraction helps stabilize the compliant infant ribcage, minimizing inward displacement of the ribs during diaphragmatic contractions. However, when the stabilizing effect of intercostal muscles is inhibited (e.g., during REM sleep), paradoxic inward motion of the ribcage occurs during inspiration (Fig. 4-3).[31,42] Full-term newborns spend more than half of their total sleep time in REM sleep, and REM sleep is even more prominent in premature infants.[43]

Asynchronous chest wall movements during REM sleep are associated with a number of mechanical derangements in healthy newborns, including a decrease in functional residual capacity (FRC),[44,45] a decrease in the transcutaneous partial pressure of oxygen,[46] and an increase in the diaphragmatic work of breathing.[47] During REM sleep, a large proportion of the force of the diaphragm is wasted in distorting the ribcage rather than effecting volume exchange. Furthermore, infants can use their abdominal muscles to optimize diaphragmatic length, and this abdominal muscle activity is inhibited during REM sleep.[48] The increase in diaphragmatic work of breathing represents a significant expenditure of calories and may con-

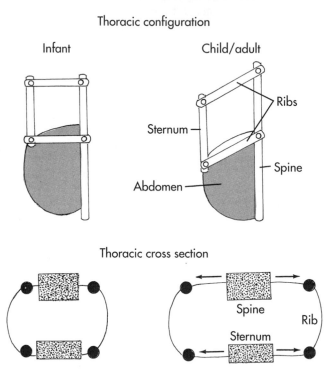

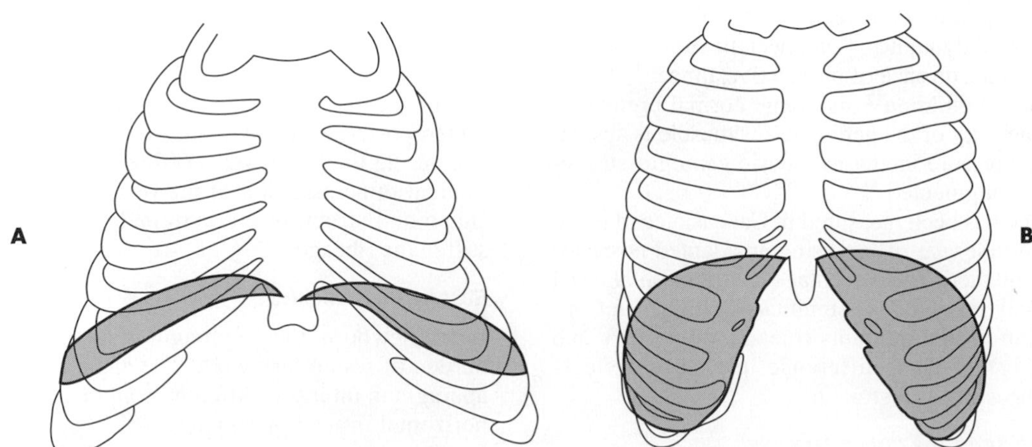

Fig. 4-2. Newborn (**A**) and adult (**B**) ribcage. The shaded areas represent the anterior projection of the diaphragm. (Redrawn from Devlieger H et al: *J Dev Physiol* 16:321-329, 1991.)

tribute to the development of diaphragmatic fatigue and ventilatory failure. Moreover, acidosis and hypoxia, both of which increase muscle fatigability, are not uncommon in sick premature infants.

With the changes in ribcage geometry and chest wall compliance that occur over time, the time spent with paradoxic ribcage motion during REM sleep decreases, nearing or reaching zero after 3 years of age.[49] In adolescents, no paradoxic movement is observed.[50]

The mechanical properties of the chest wall have clinical implications for respiratory adaptation during sleep in infants with respiratory disorders associated with increased resistive loads of breathing, such as upper airway obstruction and chronic lung diseases. In young infants suffering from such disorders, thoracoabdominal asynchronism occurs even during non-REM sleep.[51-53] As growth proceeds and the thoracic cage becomes less compliant, the increases in resistive load lead to the heightened activation of inspiratory thoracic muscles, which maintains inspiratory ribcage movement. However, inhibition of inspiratory intercostal muscles occurs during REM sleep, with the need for lower negative pressures during inspiration leading to the destabilized ribcage moving paradoxically.[54]

Pressures Generated by Respiratory Muscles and Respiratory Muscle Fatigue

Maximum pressures exerted by infants are surprisingly high compared with adult values. This is probably related to the small radius of curvature of the ribcage, diaphragm, and abdomen because according to the Laplace's law, a smaller radius results in higher pressures. Esophageal pressures of up to −70 cm H_2O have been reported during the first breath.[55] Inspiratory and expiratory pressures of about 120 cm H_2O have been recorded during crying in normal infants.[56] During late childhood and adolescence, gradual increases in maximal static inspiratory and expiratory pressures occur, with substantial differences between male and female patients at all ages.[57,58]

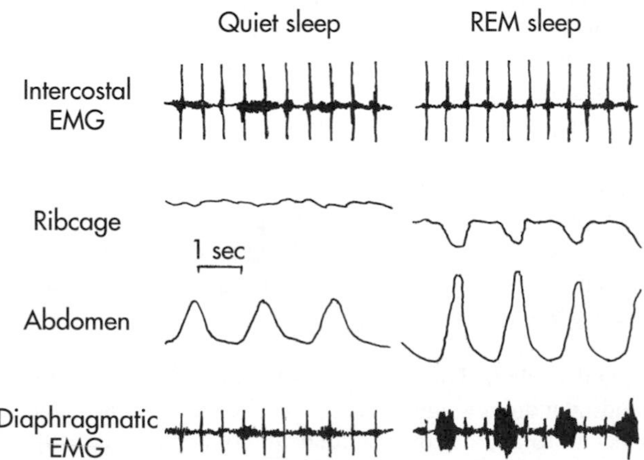

Fig. 4-3. Movement of the ribcage and abdomen measured with magnetometers and electromyograms *(EMG)* using surface electrodes on the intercostal muscles and the diaphragm of a newborn during non-REM *(left)* and during REM *(right)* sleep. During REM sleep, there is marked inward distortion of the ribcage with increased outward movement of the abdomen; the intercostal electromyogram is decreased, and the diaphragmatic electromyogram is increased. The inspiratory rate is increased. (Redrawn from Bryan AC, Gaultier CL. In Macklem PT, Roussos H, eds: *The thorax,* part B, New York, 1985, Marcel Dekker, pp 871-888.)

However, despite a relatively high maximum static inspiratory pressure, the inspiratory force reserve of respiratory muscles appears to be reduced during early infancy compared with that in adulthood because of the higher inspiratory pressures at rest.[59,60] The high pressure demand at rest in infants is due to the high minute ventilation and high metabolic rate normalized for body weight.[61] Occlusion pressure and inspiratory time measurements have been used to estimate the inspiratory pressure demand in children older than 4 years of age.[60] The ratio of mean inspiratory pressure to maximum static inspiratory pressure at FRC was 0.2 at 7 years of age (i.e., more than twice the value in adults).[59] It has been suggested that in healthy newborns the tension-time index of the diaphragm may be close to the fatigue threshold.[62]

Under any breathing conditions, two important parameters (i.e., pressure and time) determine the tension-time index, which allows the clinician to evaluate the position of the breathing pattern in relation to the critical level of muscle function or to the threshold of muscle fatigue[63-65] (Fig. 4-4). The small inspiratory force reserve places young children closer to the diaphragm fatigue threshold than older children. All conditions characterized by prolonged muscle contraction or increased pressure demand may lead to respiratory muscle fatigue. Young children with croup or epiglottitis are at especially high risk for fatigue because obstructed and prolonged inspiration is combined with a need for high pressures to produce adequate ventilation. Thus infants can develop ventilatory failure rapidly after small changes in mechanical loads. Infants are capable of using other muscles to unload (rest) the diaphragm. When the respiratory drive is increased because of

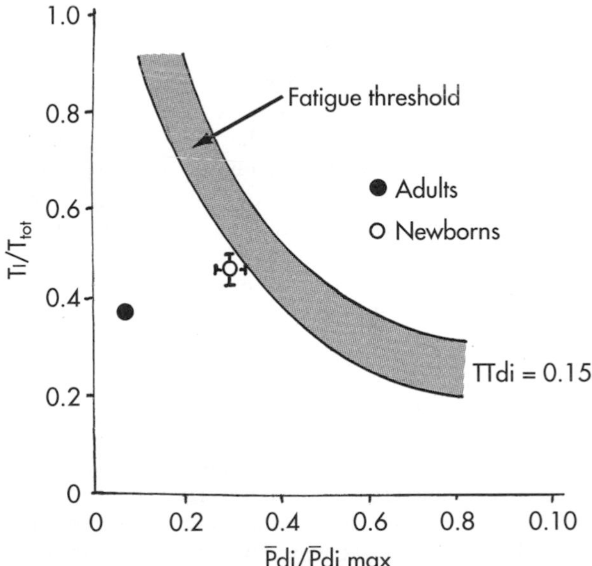

Fig. 4-4. Relationship between ratio of inspiratory time *(Ti)* over total duration of the respiratory cycle *(T_{tot})* and mean transdiaphragmatic pressure used to breathe at rest over maximal transdiaphragmatic pressure *($\bar{P}di$ max)*. The gray area defines the diaphragmatic fatigue threshold and corresponds to the so-called tension-time index of the diaphragm *(TTdi = 0.15)*. Breathing patterns below the fatiguing threshold can be obtained indefinitely. Filled circle refers to the average value for normal adults during resting breathing. Open circle is the estimated value for normal infants. Bars indicate 1 standard deviation. (Redrawn from Milic-Emili J. In Cosmi EV, Scarpelli EM, eds: *Pulmonary surfactant system,* Rome, 1983, Elsevier Science, pp 135-141.)

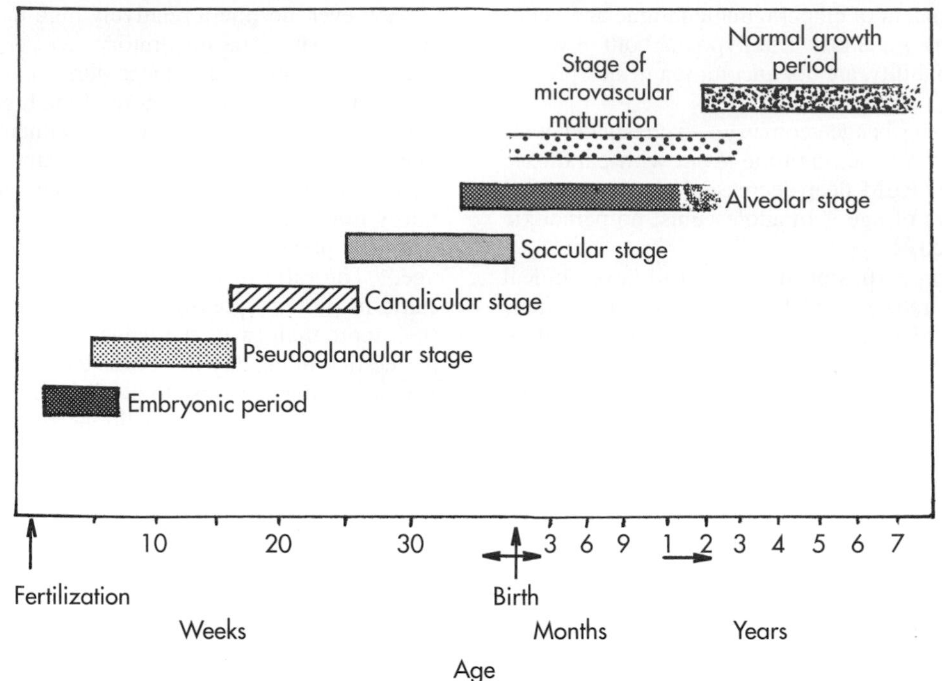

Fig. 4-5. Stages of lung development and growth with their respective timing. Open bars in the stages of alveolation and microvascular maturation indicate uncertainty as to exact timing. (Redrawn from Zeltner T, Burri P: *Respir Physiol* 67:269-282, 1987.)

carbon dioxide breathing or increased upper airway resistance, infants and young children recruit the intercostal muscles, abdominal muscles, or both sets of muscles.[48] However, this muscle recruitment aimed at preventing an increase in diaphragmatic work of breathing and diaphragmatic fatigue is suppressed during REM sleep.

The paucity of fatigue-resistant type I fibers, the high proportion of fatigue-susceptible type IIc fibers, and the low oxidative capacity of the neonatal diaphragm suggest that the muscle may be relatively prone to fatigue. This hypothesis has been contradicted by in vitro[36] and in situ findings. However, an in vivo study in rabbits found that fatigue occurred more quickly in neonatal than adult animals.[66] Thus whether fatigability of the neonatal respiratory muscles is increased compared to those of adults remains controversial.

LUNGS

Developmental Anatomy

Lung development includes growth of lung structures and maturational cell differentiation processes. Three laws govern lung development: Alveolar development occurs both before and after birth, extraacinar airway development is complete by week 16 of gestation, and arterial development follows airway development for extraacinar arteries and alveolar development for intraacinar arteries.[67] Fig. 4-5 shows the timetable of antenatal and postnatal lung development.[68]

Antenatal Lung Development

Antenatal human lung development can be subdivided into an early embryonic period, during which most organs are formed, and a fetal period that includes several stages.[68-70]

Embryonic Development of the Lung. The lung appears around day 26 as a ventral bud of the esophagus at the caudal end of the laryngotracheal sulcus. The epithelial components of the lung are thus derived from the endoderm and the enveloping connective tissue from the mesodermal germ layer. The tracheal bud rapidly divides into two branches that develop into the two main bronchi. The future airways continue to grow and branch dichotomously into the surrounding mesenchyma. By the end of the sixth week the lobar and segmental portions of the airway tree are preformed as tubes of high columnar epithelium. Simultaneously with the early stages of pulmonary organogenesis, vascular connections develop. The pulmonary arteries branch off from the sixth pair of aortic arches and descend to freshly formed lung buds, forming a vascular plexus in the surrounding mesenchyma. The pulmonary veins start to develop around the fifth week as a single evagination in the sinoatrial portion of the heart. Merging of the embryonic period into the fetal period is considered to occur on day 50. At that time, the lung resembles a small tubuloacinar gland, which is why the subsequent stage is called the *pseudoglandular stage*.

Fetal Period. The fetal period successively includes the pseudoglandular stage to week 16, the canalicular stage from weeks 24 to 26, and the saccular-alveolar stages to term.[68-70]

Pseudoglandular stage. The pseudoglandular stage is characterized by formation of the extraacinar bronchi (Fig. 4-6) and arteries. The conductive airway system is formed through continuous growth and branching. The proximal airways are lined with a high columnar epithelium (Fig. 4-7) and the distal airways with a cuboidal epithelium. The cytoplasm of airway epithelial cells is poorly differentiated and rich in glycogen. Differentiation of the airway wall occurs in a centrifugal direction, so ciliated, nonciliated, and goblet cells first appear in the proximal airways. The luminal surfaces of the columnar cells have few microvilli with or without primary rudimentary cilia.[71] Precursors for neuroendocrine cells appear during this

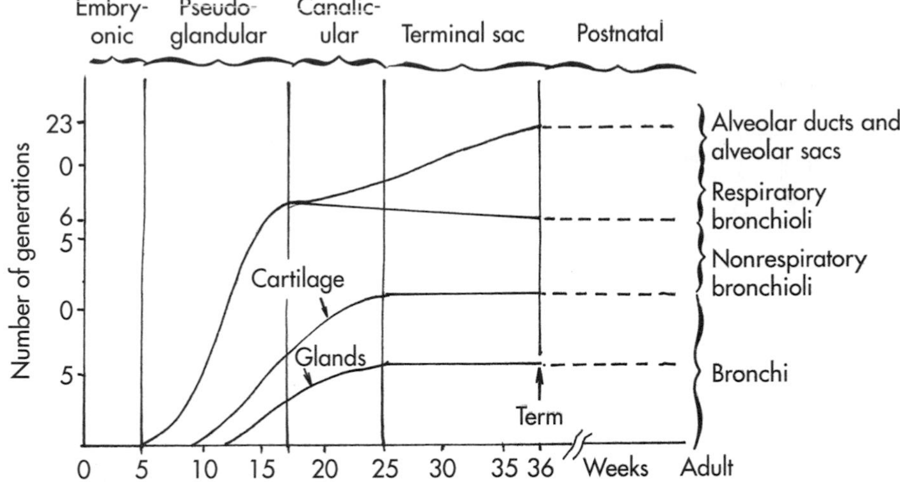

Fig. 4-6. Timetable for development of the airway tree, its generations, and typical wall structures. Generation numbers are fitted to the average airway tree of Weibel's dichotomous branching model. (Redrawn from Burri P. In Fishman P, Fisher A, eds: *Handbook of physiology,* Section 3: The respiratory system, vol 1: Circulatory and nonrespiratory functions, Bethesda, Md, 1985, Williams & Wilkins, pp 1-46.)

stage.[72] Mucus glands are also present.[73] Mesenchymal cells differentiate into chondrocytes[74] and smooth muscle cells. Capillaries are randomly distributed in the mesenchyme (Fig. 4-8). As a rule, the arteries develop and grow according to the same pattern as the airways. In contrast to the airway system, which averages 23 generations in adults, the arterial system has 28 to 30 generations. Arteries that follow the divisions of the airways are called *conventional arteries;* the smaller arteries with intermediate branchings that supply alveolar regions adjacent to airways are called *supernumerary arteries.*[75,76] By week 12, both types are present. The branching pattern of the veins matches that of the arteries.[77]

Factors Controlling Branching Morphogenesis. Epitheliomesenchymal interactions play a key role in regulating the growth and branching pattern. Transplantation experiments have shown that the mesenchyma is directly responsible for the branching pattern in the lung.[78] The branching process depends on interactions between cell-substrate adhesion molecules and underlying extracellular matrix (ECM) and intercellular adhesion molecules.[79,80] Epidermal growth factor may be an important mediator of this process.[81] The mechanisms responsible for the mesenchymal influences have not been fully elucidated but have been shown to depend on the synthesis of proteoglycans, collagen, laminin, and fibronectin.[79] Cellular attachment to the ECM is mediated by integrin receptors.[82] Branching is decreased in the presence of monoclonal antibodies against integrin receptors.[83] Integrin receptors appear to interact with fibronectin within the clefts that mark the branching points.[84] Transforming growth factor-β_1 colocalizes with fibronectin within these clefts and may regulate fibronectin deposition, thereby indirectly affecting branch formation.[85] Triamcinolone acetonide increases fetal rat airway branching in vitro.[86]

Canalicular stage. Events during the canalicular stage include acini anlage formation and epithelial cell differentiation with formation of the air-blood barrier. Production of surfactant starts toward the end of this canalicular stage. The transition from the pseudoglandular stage to the canalicular stage is marked by the appearance of rudimentary acini. *Acinus* is generally defined as the portion of gas-exchanging tissue supplied by a terminal bronchus. The acinus margins become recognizable as a result of decreased density of the mesenchyma. At the end of week 17, the newly delineated acinus is composed of the anlage of the terminal bronchiole, two to four rudimentary respiratory bronchioles, and clusters of short tubules and buds. Over the following weeks, the clusters grow by further peripheral branching and by lengthening of each tubular branch. The epithelium differentiates into two cell types: secretory cells (type 2, containing lamellar bodies) and lining cells (type 1) characterized by low junctional complexes with neighboring cells and by close contact with capillaries (see Fig. 4-7). Peripheral growth is accompanied by an increase in capillarization. Capillaries begin to develop around the airspaces, subsequently establishing close contact with the lining cells to form the prospective air-blood barrier (see Fig. 4-8).

Saccular-alveolar stages. The saccular-alveolar stage starts at weeks 24 to 26 of gestation. At this time, the fetal lung can theoretically function in air. However, because of a low level of surfactant synthesis, very premature babies are at high risk for respiratory distress syndrome. At the beginning of this stage, the airways end in clusters of thin-walled saccules. The saccules produce the last generations of airways (i.e., prospective alveolar ducts and alveolar sacs). Between weeks 28 and 36, there is a striking change in the appearance of the lung characterized by a marked decrease in interstitial tissue with thinning of saccule walls. Secondary crests divide the saccules into smaller units. The margins of the crests contain elastic fibers. The saccule walls retain their earlier double capillary network. The formation of alveoli marks the beginning of the alveolar phase. According to recent studies, alveolar develop-

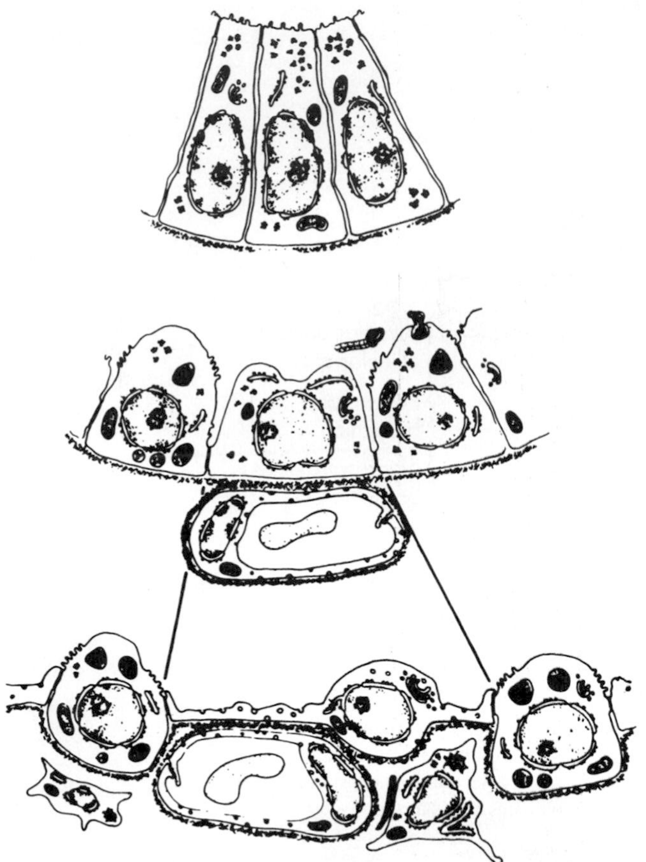

Fig. 4-7. Phases of epithelial transformation. *Top,* Pseudoglandular stage: high columnar epithelium and cells rich in glycogen. *Middle,* Canalicular stage: epithelium beginning to differentiate into two cells types, secretory (type 2, containing lamellar body) and lining cells (type 1), and characterized by the low position of the junctional complex with neighboring cells and close contact with capillaries. *Bottom,* Terminal sac stage: differentiation of type 1 and type 2 cells. (From Burri P. In Fishman P, Fisher A, eds: *Handbook of physiology,* Section 3: The respiratory system, vol 1: Circulatory and nonrespiratory functions, Bethesda, Md, 1985, Williams & Wilkins, pp 1-46.)

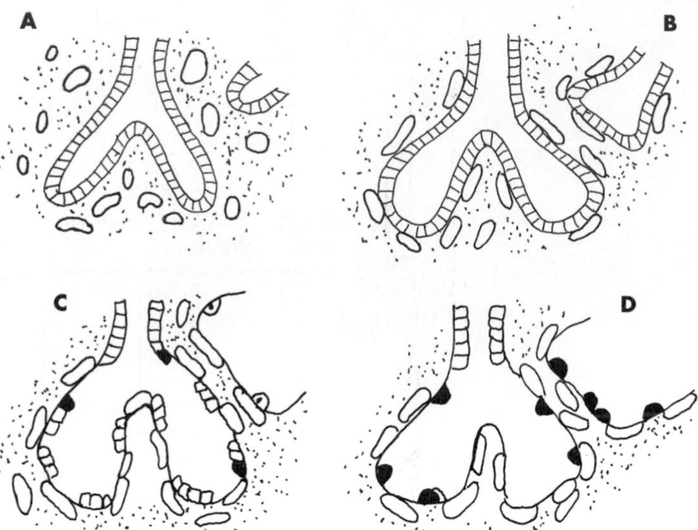

Fig. 4-8. Development of the pulmonary capillaries. **A,** Pseudoglandular stage: Capillaries are randomly distributed in mesenchyme. **B,** Beginning of the canalicular stage: Capillaries start to arrange around the epithelial tubes. **C,** Capillaries establish close contacts to the lining epithelium, which flattens to form thin air-blood barriers. **D,** Saccular stage: Epithelium is differentiated in type 1 and type 2 cells. (Redrawn from Burri P. In Fishman P, Fisher A, eds: *Handbook of physiology,* Section 3: The respiratory system, vol 1: Circulatory and nonrespiratory functions, Bethesda, Md, 1985, Williams & Wilkins, pp 1-46.)

ment starts between weeks 29 and 32.[87,88] The internal surface area of the lung increases rapidly after the onset of alveolar development, from 1 or 2 to 3 or 4 m^2 at term.[87] The number of alveoli present at birth is still controversial. Early studies[89,90] examining only one lung found numbers ranging from 17×10^6 to 24×10^6. Larger mean numbers were found more recently[87,88]: 50×10^6 and 150×10^6. Despite these discrepancies, there is no doubt that the number of alveoli is lower at birth than in adulthood (i.e., 300×10^6 to 600×10^6).[91] During the saccular and alveolar phases, intraacinar blood vessels increase in width, length, and number.

FACTORS CONTROLLING GROWTH OF THE PERIPHERAL PART OF THE LUNG. The exact mechanisms responsible for the growth and maturation of the periphery of the lung during the canalicular and saccular-alveolar stages have not been yet elucidated. They have been shown to depend on cell populations, cell-to-cell interactions, hormones, and growth factors. In rat fetal lung, epithelial cell proliferation slows during the transition between the canalicular and saccular stages.[92] This reduction in cell proliferation is accompanied by morphologic evidence of differentiation. There is increased proliferation of fibroblasts and endothelial cells. The mesenchymal tissue influences epithelial cell function. An endogenous steroid may cause fetal fibroblasts to secrete a lung maturation factor (fibroblast pneumocyte factor) that promotes lipid synthesis by type 2 cells.[93] Epithelial cell–fibroblast interactions also involve direct intercellular contact.[94] Foot processes from epithelial cells cross the basal membrane and come into close contact with fibroblasts. They are most prominent at the onset of surfactant synthesis.[95,96] The ECM contributes to the regulation of surfactant synthesis.[79] Surfactant apoprotein gene expression appears to require cell-matrix contact and cell-to-cell contact. A variety of hormones and growth factors, most notably glucocorticoids, thyroid hormone, epidermal growth factor, insulin-like growth factor,[97-99] and gastrin-releasing peptide,[100] participate in the regulation of surfactant synthesis.[101] The factors that modulate endothelial growth in the fetal lung have not been identified. Growth factors, such as transforming growth factor-β, fibroblast growth factors, and platelet-derived growth factor, may be involved.[79,102]

Postnatal Lung Development

Alveolar Development. At term, the internal surface area of the lung is to 3 to 4 m^2,[87] and the in vitro lung volume with a transpulmonary pressure of 25 cm H_2O is 150 ml.[87] Alveolar multiplication continues after birth. Early studies suggested that postnatal alveolar multiplication ends at 8 years of age.[90] However, more recent studies have shown that it is terminated by 2 years of age and may even end earlier, possibly between 1 and 2 years of age.[68,70,103] During postnatal alveolar multiplication, the capillary network of the septa is remodeled from the initial double pattern to the single pattern seen in adults.[104] This process continues after the end of alveolar multiplication, stopping between 3 and 5 years of age.[68,70] At 2 years of age, the number of alveoli varies substantially among individuals. After 2 years of age, boys have larger numbers of alveoli than girls. After the end of alveolar multiplication, the alveoli continue to increase in size until thoracic growth is completed.[103]

Factors controlling postnatal alveolar multiplication have been studied in rats. In rats, alveolar multiplication starts on day 4 and peaks between days 7 and day 12.[104,105] This period is characterized by fibroblast proliferation and accumulation of ECM components (lectin, fibronectin, elastin, collagen).[106,107] TGF-β is involved in elastin production.[108] Dexamethasone impairs postnatal alveolar multiplication by decreasing fibroblast proliferation, lectin accumulation, and acceleration of capillary remodeling.[109,110]

Airway Development. Hislop and Haworth[111] have recently described airway size and structure in the normal lungs of fetuses and infants. The mean airway lumen diameter from the main bronchi to the respiratory bronchi increases linearly with postconceptional age. Each type of airway shows a similar relative increase in diameter of 200% to 300% from birth to adulthood. The absolute amount of cartilage increases until 8 months of age. The area of the submucosal glands (expressed in relation to the lumen perimeter as millimeters squared per millimeter) increases linearly from birth to 8 months of age. The area of the hilar bronchi continues to increase until adulthood. At birth, submucosal glands are innervated by nerves containing peptides. Bronchial smooth muscle is present at birth, even at the level of respiratory bronchioles (Fig. 4-9). The bronchial smooth muscle area increases from birth to 8 months of age in all airways from the main bronchi to the respiratory bronchioles. In proximal airways only, this area increases from 8 months of age to adulthood. In premature infants, airway size is appropriate for the postconceptional age, and airways contain increased amounts of bronchial smooth muscle and goblet cells. At birth, smooth muscle is innervated by nerves containing peptides (neuropeptide-tyrosine, vasointestinal peptide, substance P, neuropeptide Y, somatostatin, and gene-related peptide).[112] Smooth muscle innervation appears to change with age because the relative number of peptide-containing nerves within the respiratory unit decreases from infancy to adulthood. No developmental changes in myosin chain isoforms have been demonstrated in human airway smooth muscle.[113]

Arterial Development. Pulmonary vascular resistance falls rapidly at birth as a result of dilation of the small muscular arteries and reduction in the amount of vascular smooth muscle in the lungs.[114] Postnatal adaptation of the pulmonary circulation is thought to be related to changes in endothelial cell function, including an increased capability for synthesis and release of endothelium-derived relaxing factor identified as nitric oxide.[115,116] Ultrastructural studies have found evidence of postnatal smooth muscle maturation with changes in contractile myofilaments[114] and the types of cytoskeletal proteins.[117] The number of arteries increases rapidly during the first 2 months of life.[118] Subsequently, arteries multiply at the same rate as alveoli, and the alveolar-arterial ratio remains fairly constant. Arterial size increases are most marked during the first 2 months of life but remain substantial during the first 4 years.

Studies of the structure of the arteries that accompany the peripheral airways have demonstrated that the respiratory bronchiolar arteries acquire a muscle coat as they increase in size during the first year of life. From birth to 6 months of age, the mean number of arteries surrounded by muscle cells is 58% among the arteries accompanying terminal bronchioli vs. only 23% among arteries accompanying alveolar ducts. These mean proportions

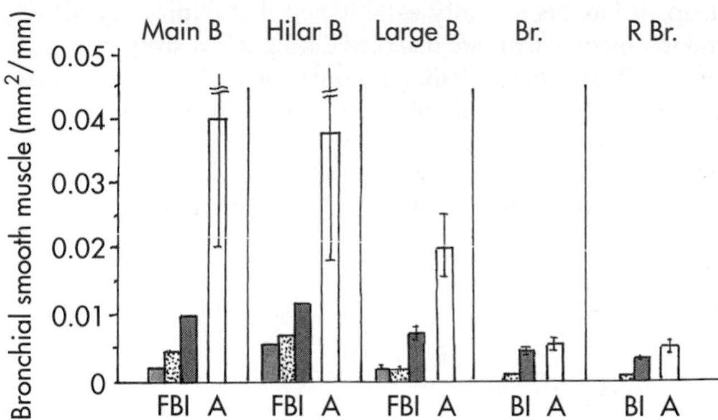

Fig. 4-9. Area of bronchial smooth muscle related to airway perimeter at four representative ages: *F,* Fetus at 22 weeks' gestation; *B,* fetus at term; *I,* infant at 8 months; *A,* adult. Bars indicate standard error of the mean. *B,* Bronchus; *Br.,* bronchioli; *R Br.,* respiratory bronchioli. (Redrawn from Hislop AA, Haworth SG: *Am Rev Respir Dis* 140:1717-1726, 1989.)

reach 92% and 40%, respectively, between 1 and 4 years of age and increase further to 96% and 71%, respectively, after 5 years.

Remodeling of the arterial wall within the acinus is accompanied by an increase in the nerve supply to the arterial wall during childhood.[119] Many respiratory unit arteries do not have accompanying nerve fibers in infants 1 to 4 months of age. The proportion of innervated vessels increases with age. In all age groups, the vasoconstricting neuropeptide tyrosine is the predominant neuropeptide associated with perivascular nerves. In infants with pulmonary hypertension, respiratory unit arteries are prematurely innervated by sympathetic-like nerve fibers. In both the normal and the pulmonary hypertensive lung, the development of sympathetic innervation seems to occur in parallel with an increase in the amount of smooth muscle in peripheral arteries.

Developmental Physiology

FRC

During breathing in the resting state, the volume of gas in the lungs at FRC represents lung oxygen stores. The FRC is determined by the static passive balance of forces between the lung and the chest wall. In infants, the outward recoil of the chest wall is very small and the inward recoil of the lung slightly less than in adults.[37] Consequently, the static passive balance of forces dictates a very low ratio of FRC over total lung capacity (TLC) in infants, which would be inadequate for gas exchange. Measured FRC and estimated TLC values in infants[120] indicate that the dynamic FRC/TLC ratio is about 40%, a value similar to that in supine adults. Thus it is very likely that in newborns and infants with little outward recoil of the chest wall, the dynamic end-expiratory volume is substantially greater than the passively determined FRC.[121]

Infants, in contrast to adults, terminate expiration at substantial flow rates[122] (Fig. 4-10). This suggests active interruption of relaxed expiration. The newborn may use two active mechanisms to slow expiration and maintain FRC. One is the postinspiratory activity of the diaphragm,[123,124] and the other is laryngeal narrowing during expiration,[125] the extreme form of which is the grunting observed in newborns with respiratory distress syndrome. Laryngeal braking of expiration has an effect like auto–positive end-expiratory pressure, which increases FRC. FRC would be expected to fall during REM sleep. It has been firmly established that expiratory airflow braking mechanisms are disabled during REM sleep in preterm infants. Postinspiratory diaphragmatic activity is reduced during REM sleep, and animal studies have demonstrated that expiratory laryngeal adduction is substantially diminished during REM sleep.[125] Furthermore, flow studies in human preterm newborns show clear evidence of expiratory braking during non-REM sleep but suggested passive airflow without expiratory braking during REM sleep.[126] The transition from dynamically maintained to passively determined end-expiratory lung volume has been estimated to occur during the second half of the first year of life.[127]

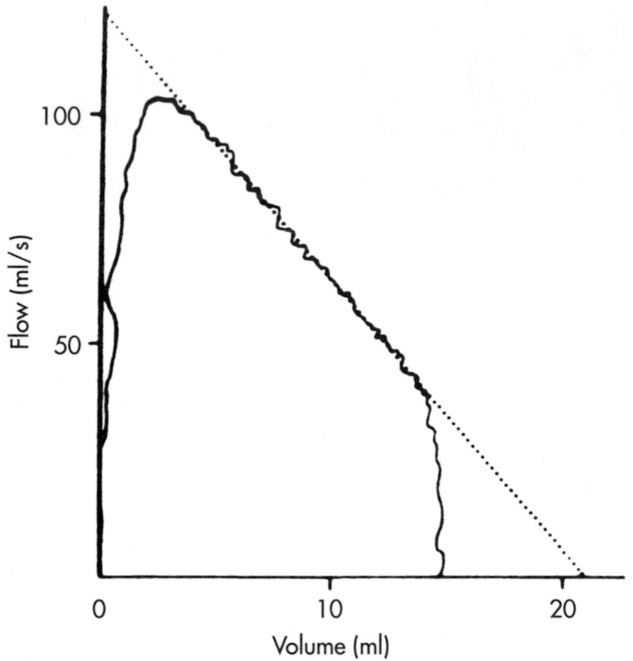

Fig. 4-10. Passive flow-volume curve in an infant, showing abrupt inspiration substantially above passive FRC. (From Le Souëf PN et al: *Am Rev Respir Dis* 129:552-556, 1984.)

Mechanical Properties of the Lung

Elastic Properties. Changes in pressure-volume relationships have been related to changes in the amount, distribution, and structure of elastin and collagen in the growing rat lung.[128] In humans, little is known about the development of the elastic properties of the lung. One study has shown that the true elastin content of the lung increases up to a plateau during the first 6 months of life.[129] Measurements of the pressure-volume relationship of the lung have been performed in excised lungs of infants and a few children[130-132] and in vivo in older children using esophageal balloons to measure transpulmonary pressure. In excised preparations, lung pressures of up to 30 cm H_2O have been used; in vivo, the TLC is taken to represent full inflation. Fig. 4-11 shows the changes in the shape of the pressure-volume curve that accompany pulmonary maturation.[133] In excised lungs, when lung volume is expressed as a fraction of the lung volume at 30 cm H_2O, there is a marked change in the overall shape of the pressure-volume curve within the age range examined. The younger lung holds a greater fraction of this volume at low pressure than the older lung. The in vivo quasistatic pressure-volume curves during deflation show that lung recoil increases with age in children older than 6 years of age.[134]

Studies in animals and in humans have shown that antenatal and postnatal environmental factors modify the elastic properties of the lungs. Protein malnutrition impairs elastin deposition in the lungs and is associated with a shift of the pressure-volume curves upward and to the left.[135] Neonates born to mothers liv-

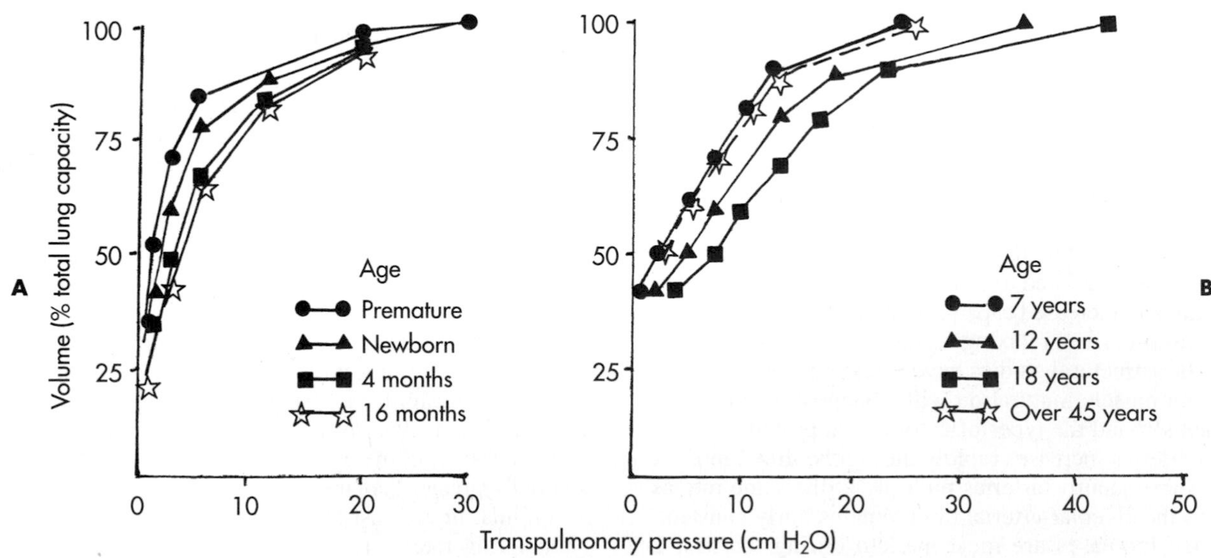

Fig. 4-11. A, Pressure-volume curves obtained from excised lungs. Curves are grouped by length. Lengths of 30 to 45, 46 to 55, 56 to 65, and 66 to 90 cm correspond to premature infants, infants 1 month of age, infants 4.4 months of age, and infants 16 months of age, respectively. **B,** Pressure-volume curves obtained from children. Heights of 115, 150, and 180 cm correspond to 6, 12, 13, and 17 years, respectively, as estimated from growth charts. (**A** data from Fagan DG: *Thorax* 31:534-543, 1976; and Fagan DG: *Thorax* 32:198-202, 1977. **B** data from Zapletal A et al: *J Appl Physiol* 40:953-959, 1986. **A** and **B** redrawn from Bryan AC, Wohl MEB. In Fishman P, Fisher A, eds: *Handbook of physiology*, Section 3: The respiratory system, vol 1: Circulatory and nonrespiratory functions, Bethesda, Md, 1985, Williams & Wilkins, pp 179-191.)

ing at high altitudes have higher total respiratory system compliance than those born to mothers living at sea level.[136]

Compliance, Resistance, and Time Constant of the Total Respiratory System. Compliance of the respiratory system increases during the first year of life. This increase has been estimated at 152%.[137] The rate of increase in lung compliance exceeds that of chest wall compliance and accounts in large part for the increase in compliance of the respiratory system during the first year of life. During the same period, total resistance of the respiratory system decreases by 42%, a noticeably less considerable modification than the change in compliance. The difference between rates of change in compliance and total resistance of the respiratory system corresponds with anatomic findings that alveolar formation is substantial during the first year of life whereas the total number of conducting airways is present at birth. In the human infant, measurements have shown that the expiratory time constant of the total respiratory system increases during the first year of life and then reaches a plateau.[138-141] This change may reflect the increase in compliance caused by rapid alveolar growth. After 1 year of age, the relative stability of this constant suggests that changes in compliance and resistance are balanced after infancy.

Flow-Resistive Properties. During postnatal life, airway growth results in increases in the radius and length of airways and in changes in the mechanical properties of airway walls. Airway compliance is greater in infants and young children than in adults. In excised preparations, the trachea of the newborn is twice as compliant as the adult trachea.[142] Radiographic studies in normal infants have shown variations of 20% to 50% in the anteroposterior diameter of the intrathoracic trachea during exertion.[143] This may be related to the decreased amount of cartilage.[111]

Measurements of airway, pulmonary, and respiratory resistance have been performed in newborns, infants, and children 5 years of age and older.[135] Airway resistance falls tenfold on average from term to adolescence. The inverse of airway resistance, airway conductance, corrected for differences in upper airway resistance and divided by the lung volume at which it was measured (specific airway conductance), decreases during the first years of life and remains constant beyond the age of 5 years (Fig. 4-12).[144,145] This profile of the specific airway conductance strongly suggests that the airways are well formed and relatively large in newborns but that during the early period of life, lung volume increases disproportionately with the size of the airways.

The total resistance of the respiratory system includes resistance of the airways, lung tissue, and chest wall. Little is known about the changes in the lung and chest wall components of total resistance. A recent study investigated growth-related changes in the viscoelastic properties of the total respiratory system by measuring pressure variations after airway occlusion in paralyzed subjects 3 weeks to 15 years of age.[146] This measure decreases during the first 2 years of life and increases after age 5. These changes have been interpreted as indicating greater influence of the lung tissue during the early period of life and greater influence of chest wall viscoelastic properties at older ages.

The distribution of resistance along the central and peripheral airways has been studied in excised lungs from infants, children, and adults.[147] The central airway conductance per gram of lung weight remained unchanged from the neonatal period to adulthood, whereas the peripheral airway conductance per gram of lung weight increased with age in subjects older than 5 years of age. These data suggest that peripheral airways may be disproportionately narrow in children younger than 5 years of age. Disproportionately low peripheral airway conductance values in infants as compared with older children should be accompanied by low maximum expiratory flows at low lung volumes. However, relatively high flows at low lung volumes have been observed in healthy, anaesthetized infants and children.[148] Furthermore, the maximum expiratory flow at FRC measured from partial expiratory flow-volume curves was higher in neonates and similar in infants compared with those reported in children and adults.[149,150] Thus physiologic data do not support the hypothesis suggested by pathologic findings that peripheral airways are disproportionately smaller in infants than in adults.

Abnormal growth of conducting airways (e.g., in lung hypoplasia) is associated with low airway resistance values during infancy.[151] Conceivably, dysregulation during the processes involved in morphogenesis (see section on the fetal period in developmental anatomy) may be responsible for the substantial interindividual variability in postnatally measured indexes of pulmonary flow-resistive properties.

Postmortem evaluations of airway size in preterm infants have shown that airway size is normally related to postconceptional age.[111] However, data obtained during childhood suggest that premature birth is associated with impaired airway growth.[152]

Gas Exchange. In the newborn, the partial pressure of oxygen in arterial blood (Pao_2) is approximately 70 mm Hg.[153] The alveolar-arterial difference in Pao_2 is about 30 mm Hg while a person breathes room air and 120 mm Hg while a person breathes oxygen.[153] The Pao_2 in arterialized blood samples rises rapidly during the first 2 years of age and then slowly up to the age of 8 years[154,155] (Fig. 4-13). Thereafter, Pao_2 values remain stable and similar to those seen in adults.[156]

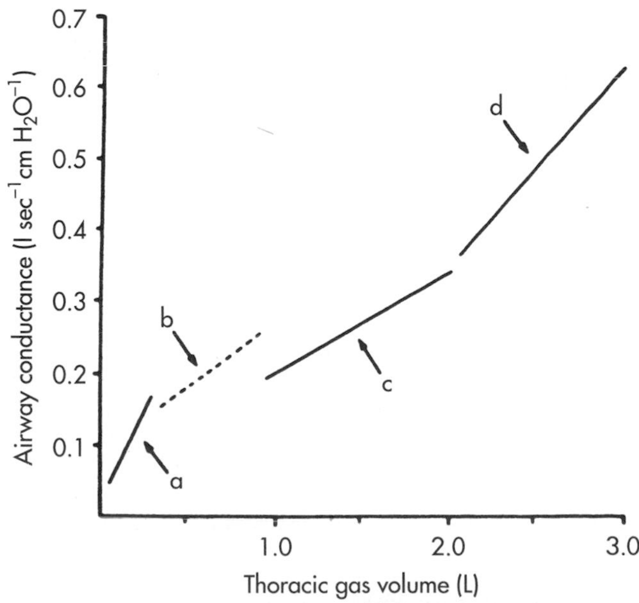

Fig. 4-12. Comparison of regression lines of airway conductance during mouth-breathing vs. thoracic gas volume from infancy to adulthood. Regression lines refer to data in infants *(a),* in children 1 to 5 years of age *(b),* and in older children *(c)* and adults *(d).* (From Bryan AC, Wohl MEB. In Fishman P, Fisher A, eds: *Handbook of physiology,* Section 3: The respiratory system, vol 1: Circulatory and nonrespiratory functions, Bethesda, Md, 1985, Williams & Wilkins, pp 179-191.)

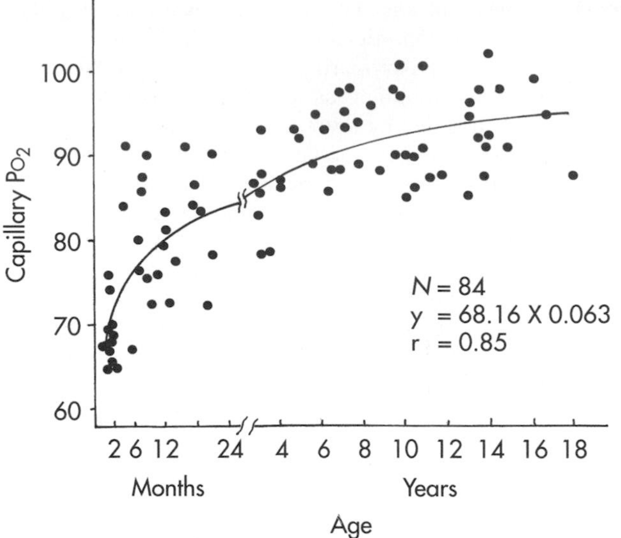

Fig. 4-13. Arterialized partial pressure of oxygen in the capillaries in 84 infants and children from 20 days to 18 years plotted against age. *X,* Age expressed in months and years. (Redrawn from Gaultier CL et al: *Bull Eur Physiol Respir* 14:287-297, 1978.)

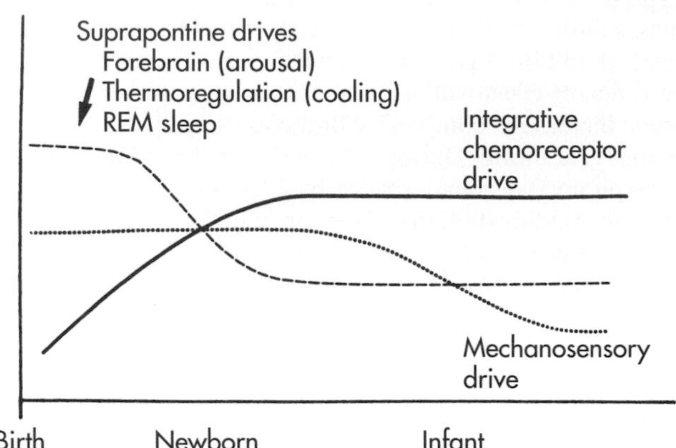

Fig. 4-14. Relative importance of different respiratory drive mechanisms after birth. (From Lagercrantz H et al. In Crystal RG, West J, eds: *The lung: scientific foundations*, New York, 1991, Raven, pp 1711-1722.)

The lung volume at which some of the intrapulmonary airways are closed (closing volume, an index of susceptibility to hypoxemia) decreases with age.[157,158] In infants and young children, the closing capacity (closing volume plus residual volume) is sometimes greater than the FRC and some areas of the lung may be closed throughout part or all of the tidal volume, resulting in impaired gas exchange.

Mechanisms that result in improvements in pulmonary gas exchange during growth have been more extensively investigated in piglets than humans. Using the multiple inert gas technique in the awake, growing piglet, researchers have shown that low PaO_2 values were due to two mechanisms: ventilation-perfusion mismatch and diffusion limitation for oxygen.[159] The impaired oxygen diffusion in piglets was related to the inadequate diffusion-perfusion equilibrium of oxygen.[160] This suggests that the capillary transit time in newborns may be too short to permit alveolar-capillary diffusion equilibrium, implying that newborns have little pulmonary vascular reserve for gas exchange. In newborns, the ratio of pulmonary diffusing capacity to FRC is close to that obtained in 11- to 13-year-old boys during submaximal exercise.[161]

The fairly low PaO_2 values in infants and young children are close to the steep part of the oxygen-hemoglobin dissociation curve. Any further decrease in PaO_2 can induce severe oxygen desaturation. During sleep, especially REM sleep, decreases in the arterial oxygen saturation (SaO_2) to less than 90% have been demonstrated in healthy full-term infants.[162] Drops to less than 90% become less common with advancing age and are not observed in healthy children older than 9 years of age.[163,164]

RESPIRATORY CONTROL

Development of the Neuronal Network Controlling Respiration

Breathing in mammals relies on a neuronal network located within three brain stem complexes (dorsal respiratory group in which nucleus of the tractus solitarius is located, ventral respiratory group, and pontine respiratory group).[165] The respiratory neuronal network receives suprapontine influences[166] from the systems involved in thermoregulation, sleep-wake and arousal patterns,[167] and circadian rhythms.

At birth, the control of breathing switches from discontinuous and metabolically less dependent fetal breathing to continuous metabolically dependent breathing. Fig. 4-14 shows the relative importance of various respiratory drive mechanisms after birth.

Although there is a substantial body of data on the control of respiration by the neuronal network in adult mammals, less is known about the structural organization of the central respiratory neurons in human newborns. The neurons of the bulbopontine respiratory complexes are probably formed during the proliferative phase between gestational weeks 10 and 20 in human fetuses. Significant differentiation of respiratory neurons and formation of the respiratory neuronal network probably also occurs during the neonatal period.[168] The dendritic spines of respiratory neurons of some brain stem nuclei (nucleus of the tractus solitarius) increase before birth, with the highest densities being observed shortly before. These dendritic spines represent areas with high synaptic densities. After birth, the density of synaptic connections decreases gradually. Interestingly, SIDS victims have higher dendritic densities in the brain stem than infants who die from other causes,[169] suggesting that brain stem immaturity is involved in the pathophysiology of SIDS.

So that the understanding of respiratory rhythm generation can be improved during the early period of life, there is a need for studies on neuronal differentiation and organization, on gene expression associated with the many different neurotransmitters that determine cell phenotypes, and on membrane proteins that affect sensitivity and responsiveness to specific stimuli.[170] Experimental studies on maturational changes in the nucleus of the tractus solitarius have shown that some neurotransmitter mechanisms (such as those involving *N*-methyl-D-aspartate receptors) are mature at birth[171] whereas other processes relevant to morphologic and bioelectrical properties are still immature.[172,173] Abnormalities in the timing of the maturation of synaptic relationships with respect to that of cellular metabolism may be involved in the pathophysiology of SIDS.

Among neurotransmitters involved in the function of the respiratory central pattern generator, some are excitatory (e.g., glutamate, aspartate), whereas others are inhibitory (e.g., γ-aminobutyric acid).[165] The central generator is controlled by neuromodulators (acetylcholine, biogenic amines, neuropeptides).[165] Inhibitory amino acids seem to be expressed at an earlier stage than excitatory amino acids.[174] There may be some dominance of inhibitory neuroactive agents terminating at the respiratory neurons before birth, possibly as a result of the low fetal Pa_{O_2} values.[174] Experiments in rabbits have shown that reorganization of synapses occurs immediately after birth. Neuropeptides increase in respiratory brain structures in the newborn rabbit compared to the fetus. This may be related to the postnatal increase in Pa_{O_2}.[175] Further peptide phenotype changes occur after birth in respiratory areas of the brain stem.[168] The plasticity of the peptide system during the early period of life may contribute to adaptation to environmental disturbances.

The fetal and perinatal environment may influence developmental processes in the brain stem. Interestingly, preliminary data have shown that chronic hypoxia during the perinatal period in rats is associated with alterations in the maturation of brain stem neuronal neurotransmitters and with a shift in the balance of excitatory and inhibitory neurotransmitters toward inhibition.[176] It has been postulated that neuronal immaturity may be the main cause of respiratory instability in the newborn. This hypothesis is consistent with the finding that brain auditory response latency is correlated with the frequency of apneas in preterm infants.[177] Brain stem auditory response latency is thought to be related to neuronal conductivity. The auditory pathways are located in the immediate vicinity of the respiratory neurons in the brain stem. Therefore maturation of the auditory pathways may parallel development of breathing pattern stability.

Pattern of Breathing, Apnea, and Periodic Breathing

Over the last decades, many studies have shown that apneas of short duration (<10 seconds) are common in early life. Apneas are more frequent in preterm than in full-term infants[178] (Fig. 4-15). Apneas in preterm infants are related to underlying oscillatory breathing patterns.[179,180] Although obstructive apneas have been reported more frequently in preterm infants, there is no consensus regarding the incidence of such events. The incidence of obstructive apneas was very low in two studies.[181,182] Higher incidences were found in other studies.[183] Upper airway obstruction may be an important risk factor for apnea in preterm infants. Continuous positive airway pressure selectively reduces obstructive apneas in preterm infants.[184] There is a general consensus that the occurrence of obstructive apneas decreases with increasing postconceptional age.[185] This may result from the improvement in extrathoracic airway stability with maturation.[186] In full-term newborns, most apneas are central.[187]

Some studies on apneas in early life have focused on variations in its occurrence across sleep states. In all such studies except one,[188] apneas were more frequent during REM sleep than during non-REM sleep in both preterm and full-term newborns[178,185,187] (see Fig. 4-15). The higher frequency of apneas during REM sleep in newborns contrasts with the fact that few apneas occur in children and adolescents, especially during stage I non-REM sleep.[189]

The observation that REM sleep is associated with greater respiratory instability than non-REM sleep during early life

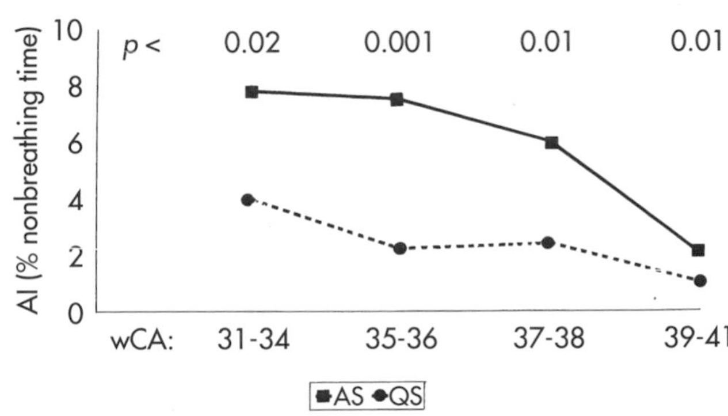

Fig. 4-15. Apnea index *(AI)* (the percentage of nonbreathing time calculated by dividing the sum of all respiratory pauses by the time spent in the given state multiplied by 100) in four groups of infants from 31 to 40 weeks' postconceptional age *(wCA)*. *p* values indicate the level of significance between sleep states. *AS,* Apnea index during active (REM) sleep; *QS,* apnea index during quiet (non-REM) sleep. (Modified from Curzi-Dascalova L, Christova-Guerguieva E: *Biol Neonate* 44:325-332,1983.)

may result either from overall immaturity of brain stem centers and the respiratory pump or from phasic inhibitory mechanisms inherent to REM sleep.[190] In preterm infants, apneic spells occur predominantly during the period of decreased spinal motoneuron excitability that occurs during REM sleep.[191] Frequent apneas during REM sleep early in life may reflect an exaggeration of normal phasic inhibitory-excitatory central mechanisms that occur during this sleep state. Irregular phasic respiratory patterns of REM sleep occur synchronously with other brain stem phasic activities, such as REMs. Tidal volume and total respiratory cycle duration decrease with increasing frequency of REMs in infants.[192] Inhibitory mechanisms during REM sleep affect the muscles involved in respiratory adaptation, such as the upper airway muscles. Upper airway muscle inhibition may increase the risk of upper airway obstruction. This may play a key role in prolonging apneic events.

Periodic breathing is frequent in preterm infants. Infants of 30 weeks' postconceptional age spend about 25% of their time in periodic breathing.[193] Periodic breathing is even more prominent at younger gestational ages. Studies of periodic breathing in full-term infants have yielded variable results. The time spent in periodic breathing was found to decrease during the first year of life.[194]

Many factors may increase the occurrence of apnea, periodic breathing, or both in neonates and infants; these include medications taken by the mother (meperidine[195]) or infant (phenothiazine[196]), metabolic disorders,[197] anemia,[22] hypoxia,[198] upper airway infections, viral infections,[23] gastroesophageal reflux,[199] hyperthermia (which increases the time spent in periodic breathing),[200] and sleep deprivation (which increases the number of obstructive events)[201] (Fig. 4-16). The influence of three of these factors (i.e., administration of meperidine to the mother, hyperthermia, and sleep deprivation) is significantly greater during REM than non-REM sleep. Therefore in infants whose homeostasis is disturbed, the risk of increased respiratory instability may be greater during REM sleep than during non-REM sleep. Any factor that increases respiratory instability is a potential risk factor for acute life-threatening events and SIDS. The sleeping position (prone or supine) was not found to affect the incidence, duration, or type of apnea in healthy infants or in infants with a history of apnea.[202]

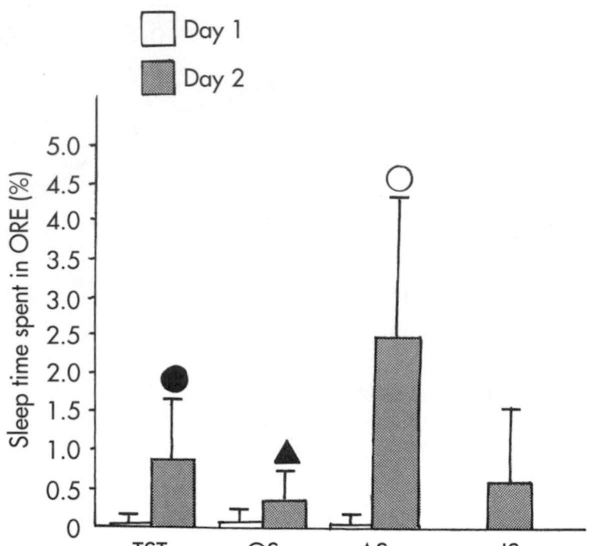

Fig. 4-16. Sleep spent in an obstructive respiratory event *(ORE)* during total sleep time *(TST)*, quiet (non-REM) sleep *(QS)*, active (REM) sleep *(AS)*, and indeterminate sleep *(IS)*. The values are expressed as percentages. Day 1 is the baseline; day 2 figures were taken after a sleep deprivation recovery nap. Bars indicate the standard deviation. Percentage of time spent in an obstructive respiratory event significantly increased after sleep deprivation during total sleep time *(full circle,* $p < 0.01$), quiet sleep *(triangle,* $p < 0.05$), and active sleep *(open circle,* $p < 0.002$). (Redrawn from Canet E et al: *J Appl Physiol* 66:1158-1163, 1989.)

Reflexes Originating from the Lung and Chest Wall

Reflexes originating from the tracheobronchial tree and within the lung parenchyma have significant effects in newborns, who differ in this respect from adults. The vagally mediated Hering-Breuer inspiratory inhibitory reflex is an important mechanism for regulating the rate and depth of respiration in newborn mammals.[203-205] The activity of this reflex can be expressed as the relative change in expiratory time after end-expiratory occlusion compared to the resting expiratory time during spontaneous breathing. This parameter has been measured during non-REM sleep in infants younger than 1 year of age. Results showed that the reflex persisted beyond the neonatal period and showed no variation in activity during the first 2 months of life.[205] Later, activity of the reflex was negatively correlated with age.[137] The reflex is less potent during REM sleep than during non-REM sleep in newborns.[206]

The functional immaturity of pulmonary irritant receptors has been reported in preterm infants younger than 35 weeks' postconceptional age.[207] Apnea occurred when the receptors were stimulated. This paradoxic response to irritants may be related to incomplete vagal myelinization.[208] Rapid lung inflation can initiate an augmented inspiratory effort, called *Head's paradoxic reflex,* which been observed during the neonatal period.

In adult animals, various reflexes that arise in the ribcage influence intercostal and phrenic motoneurons.[209] These reflexes are of potential importance in the newborn with a compliant ribcage prone to distortion during REM sleep. Ribcage distortion is associated with breathing pattern changes, including decreases in inspiratory time and tidal volume, prolongation of expiratory time, irregularity of breathing,[209-211] and even apnea.[155]

Chemoreception

Peripheral Chemoreceptors

Oxygen-sensitive chemoreceptors are activated by changes in the partial pressure of oxygen and trigger respiratory drive changes aimed at maintaining normal partial pressure levels. Studies in fetal lambs have demonstrated that peripheral chemoreceptors can be activated by further decreasing the already low fetal PaO_2.[166] The initiation of breathing at birth immediately results in a very substantial increase in PaO_2. Consequently, the chemoreceptors have to be reset at a higher PaO_2 level. The mechanisms underlying this resetting have not yet been elucidated. Recent studies in newborn rats suggest that dopamine may be involved.[212] The turnover rate of dopamine is high immediately after birth and decreases markedly a few hours later when the peripheral chemoreceptors start to reset[212] (Fig. 4-17). Resetting of peripheral chemoreceptors is essentially complete approximately 24 to 48 hours after birth in healthy human full-term newborns tested during non-REM sleep using breath-by-breath alternations in inspired oxygen[213] or single breaths of 100% oxygen.[214] Interestingly, delayed resetting of peripheral chemoreceptors has been demonstrated in kittens subjected to hypoxia during the perinatal period.[215] A similar delay has been recently reported in infants with chronic hypoxia resulting from bronchopulmonary dysplasia.[216] Because peripheral chemoreceptors play a key role in initiating the ventilatory, cardiovascular, and arousal responses to hypoxia and asphyxia, this delay may be among the factors that place infants with bronchopulmonary dysplasia at greater risk for SIDS. The ventilatory response to a single breath of 100% oxygen was not significantly different between REM and non-REM sleep in human newborns.[217]

In newborns, steady-state hypoxia produces a transient increase in ventilation followed by a decrease to or below the baseline level[218] (Fig. 4-18). The profile of this biphasic response is affected by the sleep state in preterm infants, with the initial hypoxia-induced increase in ventilation being smaller during REM than non-REM sleep.[219] The initial increase in ventilation in response to steady-state hypoxia has been ascribed to peripheral chemoreceptor stimulation, and the subsequent decrease has been ascribed to other mechanisms, including a decrease in metabolic rate, changes in lung mechanics, and the central depressant effect of hypoxia. Hypoxia may activate neurochemical mechanisms that affect breathing. Endorphins, γ-aminobutyric acid, adenosine, and dopamine have been suggested as possible neurotransmitters and modulators of hypoxia-induced depression.[220] Furthermore, chemoreception interacts with thermometabolism. The ventilatory response in kittens tested at or close to thermoneutrality increases in parallel with thermal efficiency.[221]

The carotid body response to carbon dioxide is quite different. In the newborn, the carotid body responds to rapid changes in the partial pressure of arterial carbon dioxide, even at an age when there is little sensitivity to hypoxia because resetting has not yet occurred.[222]

Central Chemoreceptors

Hypercapnia is a respiratory stimulant during late fetal life. At birth, the ventilatory response appears to be more mature than the response to hypoxia. Studies of the response of newborns to carbon dioxide have shown that the curve plotting minute ventilation against the alveolar partial pressure of carbon dioxide has a slope similar to that seen in adults, although the curve is shifted to the left because of lower resting carbon dioxide levels.[223] The tidal volume component of the ventilatory response takes on greater importance with postnatal development. The

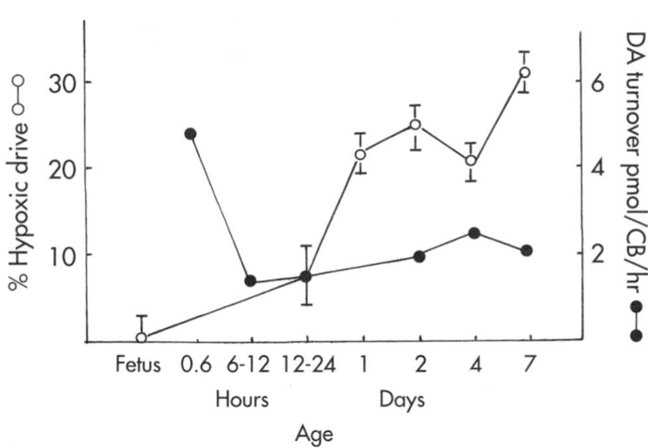

Fig. 4-17. Peripheral chemosensitivity was tested by giving oxygen to unanesthetized rat pups. Respiration was monitored using plethysmography, and the relative decrease during oxygen exposure was used as an index of peripheral chemoreceptor activity. From day 1, ventilation decreased significantly, suggesting an increase in chemoreceptor activity with increasing age. Dopamine *(DA)* turnover in the carotid bodies *(CB)* was relatively high immediately after birth and markedly decreased a few hours later. (Redrawn from Hertzberg T et al: *J Physiol* 425:211-225, 1990.)

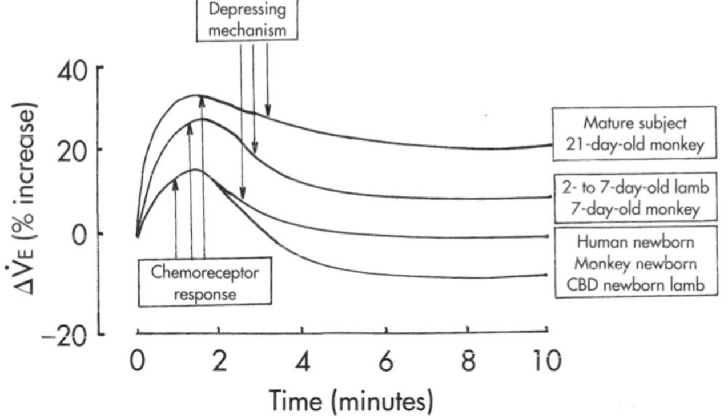

Fig. 4-18. Ventilatory response to steady-state hypoxia in the newborn. The newborn has a diphasic response to hypoxia. $\Delta\dot{V}_E$, Change in expiratory gas flow. (Redrawn from Davis GM, Bureau MA: *Clin Perinatol* 14:551-579, 1987.)

neonatal ventilatory response to carbon dioxide appears to have a number of limitations. In contrast to adults who can produce tenfold to twentyfold increases in minute ventilation in response to inhaled carbon dioxide, neonates cannot increase the minute ventilation more than 3 to 4 times the baseline level.[218,223]

Data conflict on the influence of the sleep state on the carbon dioxide–induced ventilatory response in newborns. Studies using the steady-state technique generally failed to detect any significant difference in the ventilatory response to carbon dioxide between REM and non-REM sleep.[224] In contrast, four studies using the rebreathing technique with either hyperoxic[48,225-227] or normoxic[227] gas mixtures reported a significantly decreased ventilatory response to hypercapnia during REM sleep compared with non-REM sleep in preterm and full-term newborns[225-227] (Fig. 4-19). The ventilatory response to hypercapnia varies widely among individuals and in a given individual within the same sleep state.[227] Mechanisms that contribute to the decreased ventilatory response to carbon dioxide during REM sleep include a decrease in the contribution of the ribcage to ventilation,[225] a

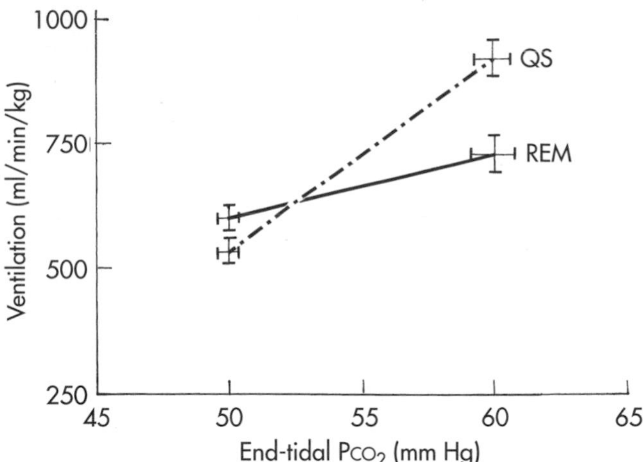

Fig. 4-19. Partial end-expiratory pressure of carbon dioxide vs. minute ventilation for REM sleep and quiet (non-REM) sleep *(QS)*. Data are means plus or minus 95% confidence intervals for position. Data are from 46 tests in five full-term babies. (Redrawn from Cohen G et al: *J Appl Physiol* 71:168-174, 1991.)

decrease in central output to the diaphragm,[48,226] and inhibition of abdominal muscle recruitment by carbon dioxide breathing during REM sleep as compared with non-REM sleep.[48]

Thermoregulation

Hypothalamic mechanisms that increase ventilation are active before birth.[228] Cooling of the skin provides a potent drive to breathing in the neonatal period. Ambient temperature is closely linked to metabolic rate, especially in the early period of life, when the basal metabolic rate is high and provides an important tonic sensory input that directly influences the stability of breathing.[229] The effects of ambient temperature changes are complex; these changes alter the metabolic rate, which is a major stimulus for breathing during the neonatal period and probably also contributes to maintain breathing in infants. Under resting conditions, the most important determinant of metabolic rate is environmental temperature. Metabolic rate is lowest when environmental temperatures are within the neutral range. In adults, thermoregulatory mechanisms are impaired during REM sleep. In contrast, in newborns, REM sleep seems to be associated with the maintenance of homeothermia in cool as well as in warm environments.[230] Metabolic responses are more active during REM sleep than during non-REM sleep.[231] A more active metabolic response during REM than non-REM sleep may increase the instability of breathing. In fact, small increases in body temperature are associated with significant increases in the time spent in periodic breathing during REM sleep but not during non-REM sleep.[200] High body temperature was associated with decreases in the threshold and latency for reflex contraction of the laryngeal adductor in newborn dogs,[232] suggesting that hyperthermia may permit reflex laryngeal closure in newborns. Interactions between developmental changes in thermoregulation and control of breathing may influence the risk of SIDS.[233]

Circadian Rhythms

Circadian rhythms are apparent for many physiologic phenomena, such as sleep-wakefulness, body temperature, release of hormones, and activity of neurotransmitters. A biologic clock in the anterior hypothalamus (i.e., the suprachiasmatic nucleus) harmonizes these rhythms. The suprachiasmatic nucleus regulates activity of the pineal gland, which produces melatonin.

Perinatal animal studies and data from human fetuses and preterm infants have shown that human circadian rhythms are present as early as 30 weeks' gestation.[234,235] In preterm infants during early life, circadian rhythmicity is present for some physiologic variables (e.g., body temperature, heart rate) but not others (e.g., respiratory rate).[236,237] The emergence of circadian variations in the respiratory rate has been studied in full-term infants.[238] The age at which the circadian pattern appears, which is characterized by a lower respiratory rate between 10 PM and 1 AM, was 1 month for REM sleep and 3 months for non-REM sleep. One study reported more frequent respiratory pauses during the early morning hours.[239]

Additional investigations are needed to gain further insight into the maturation of circadian rhythms of physiologic variables, including those related to control of breathing. Impaired maturation of the pineal gland may be involved in the pathophysiology of SIDS.[240]

Arousal Responses

Arousal from sleep is the most important protective response to danger-signaling stimuli during sleep.[167] Arousal responses to hypoxia, hypercapnia, apnea, gastroesophageal reflux, and auditory stimuli, as well as spontaneous arousals, have been studied in infants. However, whether arousal responses change with maturation remains unclear for a couple of reasons: Many studies included only infants within the peak age range of SIDS occurrence (i.e., 2 to 4 months of age), and criteria for arousal vary across studies. Different types of arousal have been considered: behavioral arousal, electroencephalographic (EEG) arousal, movement arousal,[241] and miniarousal.[185] Full-term and preterm newborns have similar rates of spontaneous arousals lasting longer than 5 seconds.[242] In full-term newborns, the rate of spontaneous behavioral arousals was similar to the rate of EEG arousals lasting longer than 2 seconds.[243]

Although apnea occurs in almost all preterm and full-term infants, little is known about the mechanisms that terminate an apneic episode. The occurrence of behavioral arousals has been studied in preterm apneic infants.[244] Less than 10% of apnea episodes ended with an arousal. Arousal was significantly more common in long vs. short, mixed vs. central, and severe vs. mild apneas. *Miniarousals,* defined as the occurrence of movements after an obstructive apnea, have been reported to prevent prolonged apnea in preterm infants.[185]

Behavioral arousal to hypercapnic stimuli has been studied in healthy infants and young children during non-REM sleep.[244-246] Hypercapnia is a potent stimulus causing arousal from non-REM sleep. All tested infants and young children had behavioral arousal from sleep when the end-tidal partial pressure of carbon dioxide was between 48 and 52 mm Hg. One study reported the occurrence of behavioral arousal at the end of a carbon dioxide rebreathing test during non-REM and REM sleep in preterm infants. Behavioral arousal occurred in only one third of tests during REM sleep vs. 93% during non-REM sleep.[48]

Compared to hypercapnia, hypoxia is less effective in causing arousal from sleep. Few studies have reported the incidence of behavioral arousal during non-REM sleep in response to hypoxic stimuli. One study in healthy infants (mean age 8.4 ± 3.2 months) found that arousal occurred consistently.[245] Only a few of the infants in the other studies exhibited arousals.[244,247,248] Thus the absence of hypoxic arousal cannot be ascribed to a deficient arousal response to hypoxia in infants. Studies in lambs have shown a delayed arousal response to severe hypoxia during REM sleep compared to non-REM sleep.[249]

Other stimuli can lead to arousal from sleep in infants. In near-term infants, the esophageal acid infusion test induced significant increases in the rate and duration of EEG arousals during REM sleep.[250] The auditory arousal threshold decreases with maturation between 44 and 52 weeks' postconceptional age.[251]

Several factors may impair arousal from sleep. Arousal was found to be less common in infants who slept in the prone rather than the supine position.[202] Drugs such as phenothiazine can depress arousal mechanisms in infants.[196] Arousal response habituation may occur with exposure to repetitive stimuli during sleep, as shown in lambs for airway obstruction.[252] Finally, sleep fragmentation or deprivation may impair arousal responses from sleep.[253]

REFERENCES

Upper Airways

1. Moss ML: The veloepiglottic sphincter and obligate nose breathing in the neonate, *J Pediatr* 67:330-331, 1965.
2. Bosma JF: Postnatal ontogeny of performances of the pharynx, larynx and mouth, *Am Rev Respir Dis* 131(suppl):510-515, 1985.
3. Rodenstein DO, Perlemuter N, Stanescu DC: Infants are not obligatory nasal breathers, *Am Rev Respir Dis* 131:343-347, 1985.
4. Swift PG, Emery JL: Clinical observations on the responses to nasal occlusion in infancy, *Arch Dis Child* 48:947-951, 1973.
5. Purcell M: Response in the newborn to raised upper airway resistance, *Arch Dis Child* 51:602-607, 1976.
6. Tonkin SL, Partridgle J, Beach D, Withey S: The pharyngeal effect of partial nasal obstruction, *Pediatrics* 63:261-271, 1979.
7. Thack BT, Stark AR: Spontaneous neck flexion and airway obstruction during apneic spells in preterm infants, *J Pediatr* 94:275-281, 1979.
8. Stark AR, Thach BT: Recovery of airway patency after obstruction in normal infants, *Am Rev Respir Dis* 123:691-693, 1981.
9. Roberts JL, Reed WT, Mathew OP, Menon AA, Thach BT: Assessment of pharyngeal airway stability in normal and micrognathic infants, *J Appl Physiol* 58:290-300, 1985.
10. Wilson SL, Thach BT, Brouillette RT, Abu-Osba YK: Upper airway patency in the human infant: influence of airway pressure and posture, *J Appl Physiol* 48:500-504, 1980.
11. Reef WR, Roberts JL, Thach BT: Factors influencing regional patency and configuration of the human infant upper airway, *J Appl Physiol* 58:635-644, 1985.
12. Jeffery B, Brouillette RT, Hunt CE: Electromyographic study of some accessory muscles of respiration in children with obstructive sleep apnea, *Am Rev Respir Dis* 129:696-702, 1984.
13. Carlo WA, Miller MJ, Martin RJ: Differential response of respiratory muscles to airway occlusion in infants, *J Appl Physiol* 59:847-852, 1985.
14. Stocks J, Godfrey S: Nasal resistance during infancy, *Respir Physiol* 34:233-246, 1978.
15. Marchal F, Corke BC, Sundell H: Reflex apnea from laryngeal chemostimulation in the sleeping premature newborn lamb, *Pediatr Res* 16:621-627, 1982.
16. Boggs DF, Bartlett D: Chemical specificity of a laryngeal apneic reflex in puppies, *J Appl Physiol* 53:455-462, 1982.
17. Davies AM, Koening JS, Thach BT: Upper airway chemoreflex responses to saline and water in preterm infants, *J Appl Physiol* 64:1412-1420, 1988.
18. Perkett EA, Vaughan RL: Evidence for laryngeal chemoreflex in some human preterm infants, *Acta Paediatr Scand* 71:969-972, 1982.
19. Pickens DL, Schefft G, Thach BT: Prolonged apnea associated with upper airway protective reflexes in apnea of prematurity, *Am Rev Respir Dis* 137:113-118, 1988.
20. Wennergren G, Hertzberg T, Milerad J, Bjure J, Lagercrantz H: Hypoxia reinforces laryngeal reflex bradycardia in infants, *Acta Paediatr Scand* 78:11-17, 1989.

21. Sessle BJ, Lucier GE: Functional aspects of the upper respiratory tract and larynx: a review, In *Sudden infant death syndrome,* New York, 1983, Academic, pp 501-529.
22. Lee JC, Dowing SE: Laryngeal reflex inhibition of breathing in piglets: influences of anemia and catecholamine depletion, *Am J Physiol* 239(1):R25-R30, 1980.
23. Lindgren C, Ling J, Graham B, Grogard J, Sundell H: Respiratory syncytial virus infection reinforces reflex apnea in young lambs, *Pediatr Res* 31:381-385, 1992.
24. Pickens DL, Schefft GL, Storch GA, Thach BT: Characterization of prolonged apneic episodes associated with respiratory syncytial virus infection, *Pediatr Pulmonol* 6:195-201, 1989.
25. Fisher JT, San'Ambrogio G: Airways and lung receptors and their reflex effects in the newborn, *Pediatr Pulmonol* 1:112-126, 1985.
26. Allen LG, Howard G, Smith JB, McCubbin JA, Weaver RL: Infant heart rate response to trigeminal airstream stimulation: determination of normal and deviant values, *Pediatr Res* 13:184-187, 1979.
27. Ramet J, Praud JP, D'Allest AM, Dehan M, Gaultier C: Cardiac and respiratory responses to trigeminal airstream stimulation during REM sleep: maturation-related changes in human infants, *Chest* 98:92-96, 1990.

Chest Wall

28. Takahashi E, Atsumi H: Age differences in thoracic form as indicated by the thoracic index, *Human Biol* 27:65-74, 1955.
29. Howatt WF, Demuth GR: Configuration of the chest wall, *Pediatrics* 25:177-184, 1965.
30. Openshaw P, Edwards S, Helms P: Changes in rib cage geometry during childhood, *Thorax* 39:624-627, 1984.
31. Bryan AC, Gautlier C: The thorax in children. In Macklem PT, Roussos H, eds: *The thorax,* New York, 1985, Marcel Dekker, pp 871-888.
32. Devlieger H, Daniel H, Marchal G, Moerman PH, Casaer P, Eggermont E: The diaphragm of the newborn infant: anatomic and ultrasonographics studies, *J Dev Physiol* 16:321-329, 1991.
33. Keens TG, Bran AC, Levison H, Lanuzzo CD: Developmental pattern of muscle fiber types in human ventilatory muscle, *J Appl Physiol* 44:909-913, 1978.
34. Maxwell LC, McCarter JM, Keuhl TJ, Robotham JL: Development of histochemical and functional properties of baboon respiratory muscles, *J Appl Physiol* 54:551-561, 1983.
35. Sieck GC, Fournier M: Developmental aspects of diaphragm muscle cells: structural and functional organization. In Haddad GG, Farber JP, eds: *Developmental neurobiology of breathing,* New York, 1991, Marcel Dekker, pp 375-428.
36. Sieck GC, Fournier M, Blanco CE: Diaphragm muscle fatigue resistance during postnatal development, *J Appl Physiol* 71:458-464, 1991.
37. Agostoni E: Volume-pressure relationships to the thorax and lung in the newborn, *J Appl Physiol* 14:909-913, 1959.
38. Gerhard T, Bancalari E: Chest wall compliance in full-term and premature infants, *Acta Paediatr Scand* 69:349-364, 1980.
39. Sharp M, Druz W, Balgot R, Bandelin V, Damon J: Total respiratory compliance in infants and children, *J Appl Physiol* 2:775-779, 1970.
40. Papastamelos C, Panitch HB, England SE, Allen JL: Developmental changes in chest wall compliance in infancy and early childhood, *J Appl Physiol* 78:179-184, 1995.
41. Hershenson MD, Colin AA, Wohl MEB, Stark AR: Change in the contribution of the rib cage to total breathing during infancy, *Am Rev Respir Dis* 141:922-925, 1990.
42. Curzi-Dascalova L: Thoraco-abdominal respiratory correlations in infants: constancy and variability in different sleep states, *Early Hum Dev* 2:25-38, 1978.
43. Curzi-Dascalova L, Peirano P, Morel-Kahn F: Development of sleep states in normal premature and full-term newborns, *Dev Psychobiol* 2:431-444, 1988.
44. Henderson-Smart DJ, Read DJC: Reduced lung volume during behavioral active sleep in the newborn, *J Appl Physiol* 46:1081-1085, 1979.
45. Walti H, Moriette G, Radvanyi-Bouvet MF, Chaussain M, Morel-Kahn F, Pajot N, Relier JP: Influence of breathing pattern on functional residual capacity in sleeping newborn infants, *J Dev Physiol* 8:167-172, 1986.
46. Martin RJ, Okken A, Rubin D: Arterial oxygen tension during active and quiet sleep, *J Pediatr* 94:271-274, 1979.
47. Guslits BG, Gaston SE, Bryan MH, England SJ, Bryan AC: Diaphragmatic work of breathing in premature human infants, *J Appl Physiol* 62:1410-1415, 1987.
48. Praud JP, Egreteau L, Benlabed M, Curzi-Dascalova L, Nedelcoux H, Gaultier C: Abdominal muscle activity during CO_2 rebreathing in sleeping neonates, *J App Physiol* 70:1344-1350, 1991.
49. Gaultier C, Praud JP, Canet E, Delaperche MF, D'Allest AM: Paradoxical inward rib cage motion during rapid eye movement sleep in infants and young children, *J Dev Physiol* 9:391-397, 1987.
50. Tabachnik E, Muller NL, Bryan AC, Levison H: Changes in ventilation and chest wall mechanics during sleep in normal adolescents, *J Appl Physiol* 51:557-564, 1981.
51. Sivan Y, Deakers TW, Newth CJL: Thoracoabdominal asynchrony in acute upper airway obstruction in small children, *Am Rev Respir Dis* 142:540-544, 1990.
52. Allen JL, Wolfson MR, McDowell K, Shaffer TH: Thoracoabdominal asynchrony in infants with airflow obstruction, *Am Rev Respir Dis* 11:33-43, 1990.
53. Allen JL, Greenspan JS, Deoras KS, Keklikian E, Wolfson MR, Shaffer TH: Interaction between chest motion and lung mechanics in normal infants and infants with bronchopulmonary dysplasia, *Pediatr Pulmonol* 11:37-43, 1991.
54. Goldman MD, Pagani M, Trang HTT, Praud JP, Sartene R, Gautlier C: Asynchronous chest wall movements during non–rapid eye movement and rapid eye movement sleep in children with bronchopulmonary dysplasia, *Am Rev Respir Dis* 147:1175-1184, 1993.
55. Karlberg P, Koch G: Respiratory studies in newborn infants, *Acta Paediatr Scand Suppl* 105:439-448, 1962.
56. Shardonofsky FR, Perez-Chada D, Carmuega E, Milic-Emili J: Airway pressures during crying in healthy infants, *Pediatr Pulmonol* 6:14-18, 1989.
57. Cook CD, Mead J, Ozalez MM: Static volume-pressures characteristics of the respiratory system during maximum effort, *J Appl Physiol* 19:1016-1022, 1964.
58. Gaultier C, Zinman R: Maximal static pressures in healthy children, *Respir Physiol* 51:45-61, 1983.
59. Gaultier C, Boule M, Tournier G, Girard F: Inspiratory force reserve of the respiratory muscles in children with chronic obstructive pulmonary disease, *Am Rev Respir Dis* 131:811-815, 1985.
60. Gaultier C, Perret L, Boule M, Buvry A, Girard F: Occlusion pressure and breathing pattern in healthy children, *Respir Physiol* 46:71-80, 1981.
61. Robertson JD, Reid DD: Standards for the basal metabolism in normal people in Britain, *Lancet* 1:940-943, 1952.
62. Milic-Emili J: Respiratory muscle fatigue and its implication in respiratory distress syndrome. In Cosmi EV, Scarpelli EM, eds: *Pulmonary surfactant system,* Rome, 1983, Elsevier Science, pp 135-141.
63. Milic-Emili J: Respiratory muscle fatigue in children. In Prakash O, ed: *Critical care of the child,* Dordrecht, Netherlands, 1984, Martinus Nijhoff, pp 87-94.
64. Bellemare F, Grassino A: Effects of pressure and timing of contraction on the human diaphragm fatigue, *J Appl Physiol* 53:1190-1193, 1982.
65. Bellemare F, Grassino A: Evaluation of human diaphragmatic fatigue, *J Appl Physiol* 53:1196-1206, 1982.
66. Le Souëf PM, England SJ, Stogryn HAF, Bryan AC: Comparison of diaphragmatic fatigue in newborn and older rabbits, *J Appl Physiol* 65:1040-1044, 1988.

Lungs

67. Reid L: The embryology of the lung. In De Reuk AVS, Porter R, Ciba Foundation, *Symposium: development of the lung,* London, 1967, Churchill Livingstone, pp 109-112.
68. Zeltner TB, Caduff JH, Gehr P, Pfenninger J, Burri PH: The postnatal development and growth of the human lung. I. Morphometry, *Respir Physiol* 67:247-267, 1987.
69. Burri PH: Development and growth of the human lung. In Fishman P, Fisher A, eds: *Handbook of physiology.* Section 3: The respiratory system, vol 1: Circulation and nonrespiratory functions, Bethesda, Md, 1985, Williams & Wilkins, pp 1-46.
70. Zeltner TB, Burri P: The postnatal development and growth of the human lung. II. Morphology, *Respir Physiol* 67:269-282, 1987.
71. Gaillard DA, Lallemand AV, Petit AF, Puchelle ES: In vivo ciliogenesis in human fetal tracheal epithelium, *Am J Anat* 1985:415-428, 1989.
72. Gutz E, Gillan JE, Bryan AC: Neuroendocrine cells in the developing human lung: morphologic and functional considerations, *Pediatr Pulmonol* 1:S21-S29, 1985.
73. Bucher U, Reid L: Development of the mucus-secreting elements in human lung, *Thorax* 16:219-225, 1961.

74. Bucher V, Reid L: Development of the intersegmental bronchial tree: the pattern of branching and development of cartilage at various stages of intra-uterine life, *Thorax* 16:207-218, 1961.
75. Hislop A, Reid L: Intra-pulmonary arterial development during fetal life: branching pattern and structure, *J Anat* 113:35-48, 1972.
76. Hislop A, Reid L: Pulmonary arterial development during childhood: branching pattern and structure, *Thorax* 28:313-319, 1973.
77. Hislop A, Reid L: Fetal and childhood development of the intrapulmonary veins in man: branching pattern and structure, *Thorax* 28:129-135, 1973.
78. Hilfer SR, Rayner RM, Brown JW: Mesenchymal control of branching in the fetal mouse lung, *Tissue Cell* 17:523-538, 1985.
79. McGowan SE: Extracellular matrix and the regulation of lung development and repair, *FASEB J* 6:2895-2904, 1992.
80. Warburton D, Lee M, Berberich MA, Bernfield M: Molecular embryology and the study of lung development, *Am J Respir Cell Mol Biol* 9:5-9, 1993.
81. Warburton D, Seth R, Shum L, Horcher PG, Hall FL, Slavkin HC: Epigenetic role of epidermal growth factor expression and signaling in embryonic mouse lung morphogenesis, *Dev Biol* 149:123-133, 1992.
82. Ruosilahti E: Integrins, *J Clin Invest* 87:1-5, 1991.
83. Roman J, Little CW, McDonald JA: Potential role of RGD-binding integrins in mammalian lung branching morphogenesis, *Development* 112:551-558, 1991.
84. Roman J, McDonald JA: Expression of fibronectin, the integrin 5, and smooth muscle actin in heart and lung development, *Am J Respir Cell Mol Biol* 6:472-480, 1992.
85. Heine UI, Munoz EF, Flanders KC, Roberts AB, Sporn MB: Colocalization of TGF-beta 1 and collagen I and III, fibronectin and glycosaminoglycans during lung branching morphogenesis, *Development* 109:29-36, 1990.
86. Massoud EAS, Harman JA, Tinder SS, Rotschild A, Thurlbeck WM: The in vitro effect of triamcinolone acetonide on branching morphogenesis in the fetal rat lung, *Pediatr Pulmonol* 14:28-36, 1992.
87. Langston C, Kida K, Reed M, Thurlbeck WM: Human lung growth in late gestation and in the neonate, *Am Rev Respir Dis* 129:607-613, 1984.
88. Hislop AA, Wigglesworth JS, Desai R: Alveolar development in the human fetus and infant, *Early Hum Dev* 13:1-11, 1986.
89. Dunnil MS: Postnatal growth of the lung, *Thorax* 17:329-333, 1962.
90. Davies G, Reid L: Growth of alveoli and pulmonary arteries in childhood, *Thorax* 25:669-691, 1970.
91. Angus GE, Thurlbeck WM: Number of alveoli in the human lung, *J Appl Physiol* 32:483-485, 1972.
92. Adamson IYR, King GM: Sex-related differences in cellular composition and surfactant synthesis of developing fetal rat lung, *Am Rev Respir Dis* 129:130-134, 1984.
93. Smith BT, Post M: Tissue interactions. In Crystal RG, West JB, eds: *The lung: scientific foundations,* New York, 1991, Raven, pp 671-676.
94. Brody JS: Cell-to-cell interactions in lung development, *Pediatr Pulmonol* 1:542-548, 1985.
95. Adamson IYR, King GM: Sex differences in development of fetal rat lung. II. Quantitative morphology of epithelial-mesenchymal interactions, *Lab Invest* 50:461-468, 1984.
96. Adamson IYR, King GM: Epithelial-interstitial cell interactions in fetal rat lung development accelerated by steroid, *Lab Invest* 55:145-152, 1986.
97. Stiles AD, D'Ercole AJ: The insulin-like growth factors and the lung, *Am J Respir Cell Mol Biol* 3:93-100, 1990.
98. Han VKM, D'Ercole AJ, Lund PK: Cellular localization of somatomedin (insulin-like growth factor) messenger RNA in the human fetus, *Science* 236:193-197, 1987.
99. Han VKM, Hill DJ, Strain AJ, Towle AC, Lauder JM, Underwood LE, D'Ercole AJ: Identification of somatomedin/insulin-like growth factor immunoreactive cells in the human fetus, *Pediatr Res* 22:245-249, 1987.
100. Sunday ME, Hua J, Dai HB, Nustrat A, Torday JS: Bombesin increases fetal lung growth and maturation in utero and in organ culture, *Am J Respir Cell Mol Biol* 3:199-205, 1990.
101. Sundell HW, Gray ME, Serenius FS, Escobedo M, Stahlman MT: Effects of epidermal growth factor on lung maturation in fetal lambs, *Am J Pathol* 100:707-726, 1980.
102. Han RN, Mawdsley C, Souza P, Tanswell K, Post M: Platelet-derived growth factors and growth-related genes in rat lung. III. Immunolocalization during fetal development, *Pediatr Res* 31:323-329, 1992.
103. Thurlbeck WM: Postnatal human lung growth, *Thorax* 37:564-571, 1982.
104. Burri PH: The postnatal growth of the rat lung. III. Morphology, *Anat Rec* 180:77-98, 1974.
105. Massaro D, Teich N, Maxwell S, Massaro GD, Whitney P: Postnatal development of alveoli: regulation and evidence for a critical periods in rats, *J Clin Invest* 76:1297-1305, 1985.
106. Clerch LB, Whitney PL, Massaro D: Rat lung lectin synthesis, degradation and activation, *Biochem J* 245:683-690, 1987.
107. Plumb DJ, Dubaybo BA, Thet LA: Changes in lung tissue fibronectin content and synthesis during postnatal lung growth, *Pediatr Pulmonol* 3:413-419, 1987.
108. McGowan SE, McNamer R: Transforming growth factor increases elastin production by neonatal rat lung fibroblasts, *Am J Respir Cell Mol Biol* 3:369-376, 1990.
109. Massaro D, Massaro GD: Dexamethasone accelerates postnatal alveolar wall thinning and alters wall composition, *Am J Physiol* 251:R218-R224, 1986.
110. Damke BM, Maenni B, Burri PH: Influence of postnatally administered glucocorticoids on rat lung growth, *Experientia* 46:A66, 1990.
111. Hislop A, Haworth SG: Airway size and structure in the normal fetal and infant lung and the effect of premature delivery and artificial ventilation, *Am Rev Respir Dis* 140(6):1717-1726, 1989.
112. Hislop AA, Wharton J, Allen KM, Polak JM, Haworth SG: Immunohistochemical localization of peptide-containing nerves in human airways: age-related changes, *Am J Respir Cell Mol Biol* 3:191-198, 1990.
113. Mohammed MA, Sparrow MP: The distribution of heavy chain isoforms of myosin in airway smooth muscle from adult and neonate humans, *Biol Chem J* 260:421-426, 1986.
114. Allen KA, Haworth SG: Human postnatal pulmonary arterial remodeling: ultrastructural studies of smooth muscle cell and connective tissue maturation, *Lab Invest* 59:702-709, 1988.
115. Abman SH, Chatfield BA, Hall SL, McMurphy IF: Role of endothelium-derived relaxing factor during transition of pulmonary circulation at birth, *Am J Physiol* 259(6 Pt 2):H1921-H1927, 1990.
116. Abman SH, Chatfield BA, Rodman DM, Hall SL, McMurphy IF: Maturational changes in endothelium-derived relaxing factor activity of ovine pulmonary arteries in vitro, *Am J Physiol* 260(4 Pt 1):L280-L285, 1991.
117. Allen KM, Haworth SG: Cytoskeletal features of immature pulmonary vascular smooth muscle cells: the influence of pulmonary hypertension on normal development, *J Pathol* 158:311-317, 1989.
118. Haworth SG, Hislop AA: Pulmonary vascular development: normal values of peripheral vascular structure, *Am J Cardiol* 52:578-583, 1983.
119. Allen KM, Wharton J, Polak JM, Haworth SG: A study of nerves containing peptides in the pulmonary vasculature of healthy infants and children and of those with pulmonary hypertension, *Br Heart J* 62:353-360, 1989.
120. Gaultier CL, Boule M, Allaire Y, Clement A, Girard F: Growth of lung volumes during the first three years of life, *Bull Eur Physiopathol Respir* 15:1103-1116, 1979.
121. Kosch PC, Stark AR: Dynamic maintenance of end-expiratory lung volume in full-term infants, *J Appl Physiol* 54:773-777, 1983.
122. Le Souëf PN, England SJ, Bryan AC: Passive respiratory mechanics in newborns and children, *Am Rev Respir Dis* 129:552-556, 1984.
123. Mortola JP, Milic-Emili J, Noworaj A, Smith B, Fox G, Weeks S: Muscle pressure and flow during expiration in infants, *Am Rev Respir Dis* 129:49-53, 1984.
124. Kosch PC, Hutchison AA, Wozniak JA, Carlo WA, Stark AR: Posterior cricoarytenoid and diaphragm activities during tidal breathing in neonates, *J Appl Physiol* 64:1968-1978, 1988.
125. Harding R, Johnson P, McClelland ME: Respiratory function of the larynx in developing sheep and the influence of sleep state, *Respir Physiol* 40:165-179, 1980.
126. Stark AR, Cohlan BA, Waggerer TB, Frantz ID, Kosch PC: Regulation of end-expiratory lung volume during sleep in premature infants, *J Appl Physiol* 62:1117-1123, 1987.
127. Colin AA, Whol MEB, Mead J, Ratjen FA, Glass G, Stark AR: Transition from dynamically maintained to relaxed end-expiratory volume in human infants, *J Appl Physiol* 67:2107-2111, 1989.
128. Nardell EA, Brody JS: Determinants of mechanical properties of rat lung during postnatal development, *J Appl Physiol* 53:140-148, 1982.

129. Keely FW, Fagan DG, Webster SI: Quantity and character of elastin in developing human lung parenchymal tissues of normal infants and infants with respiratory distress syndrome, *J Lab Clin Med* 90:981-989, 1977.
130. Fagan DG: Post-mortem studies of the semistatic volume-pressure characteristics of infant's lungs, *Thorax* 31:534-543, 1976.
131. Fagan DG: Shape changes in static V-P loops from children's lungs related to growth, *Thorax* 32:198-202, 1977.
132. Stigol LA, Vawter GF, Mead J: Studies on elastic recoil of the lung in a pediatric population, *Am Rev Respir Dis* 105:552-563, 1972.
133. Bryan AC, Whol ME: Respiratory mechanics in children. In Macklem PT, Mead J, eds: *Handbook of Physiology,* Section 3: The respiratory system, Baltimore, Md, 1986, Williams & Wilkins, pp 179-191.
134. Zapletal A, Paul T, Samanek M: Pulmonary elasticity in children and adolescents, *J Appl Physiol* 40:953-959, 1976.
135. Kalenga M, Henquin JC: Protein deprivation from the neonatal period impairs lung development in the rat, *Pediatr Res* 21:45-49, 1987.
136. Mortola JP, Rezzonico R, Fisher JT, Villena-Cabrera N, Vargas E, Gonzales R, Pena F: Compliance of the respiratory system in infants born at high altitude, *Am Rev Respir Dis* 142:43-48, 1990.
137. Marchal F, Crance JP: Measurement of ventilatory system compliance in infants and young children, *Respir Physiol* 68:311-318, 1987.
138. Marchal F, Haouzi P, Gallina C, Crance JP: Measurement of ventilatory system resistance in infants and young children, *Respir Physiol* 73:201-210, 1988.
139. Mortola JP, Fisher JT, Smith B, Fox G, Weeks S: Dynamics of breathing in infants, *J Appl Physiol* 52:1209-1215, 1982.
140. Grunstein MM, Springer C, Godfrey S, Bar-Yishay E, Vilzoni D, Incore SC, Schramm CM: Expiratory volume clamping: a new method to assess respiratory mechanics in sedated infants, *J Appl Physiol* 62:2107-2114, 1987.
141. Ratjen FA, Colin AA, Stark AR, Mead J, Wohl MEB: Changes of time constants during infancy and early childhood, *J Appl Physiol* 67:2112-2115, 1989.
142. Croteau JR, Cook CD: Volume-pressure and length-tension measurements in human tracheal and bronchial segments, *J Appl Physiol* 16:170-172, 1961.
143. Wittenborg MH, Gyepes MT, Crocker D: Tracheal dynamics in infants with respiratory distress, stridor, and collapsing trachea, *Radiology* 88:653-662, 1967.
144. Stocks J, Godfrey S: Specific airway conductance in relation to postconceptional age during infancy, *J Appl Physiol* 43:144-154, 1977.
145. Zapletal A, Samanek M, Paul T: Upstream and total airway conductance in children and adolescents, *Bull Eur Physiopathol Respir* 18:31-37, 1982.
146. Lanteri CJ, Sly PD: Changes in respiratory mechanics with age, *J Appl Physiol* 74:369-378, 1993.
147. Hogg JC, Williams J, Richardson JB, Macklem PT, Thurlbeck WM: Age as a factor in the distribution of lower-airway conductance and in the pathologic anatomy of obstructive lung disease, *N Engl J Med* 282:1283-1287, 1970.
148. Motoyama EK: Pulmonary mechanics during early postnatal years, *Pediatr Res* 11:220-223, 1977.
149. Taussig LM, Landau LI, Godfrey S, Arad I: Determinants of forced expiratory flows in newborn infants, *J Appl Physiol* 53:1220-1227, 1982.
150. Tepper RS, Morgan WJ, Cota K, Wright A, Taussig LM, GHMA Pediatricians: Physiologic growth and development of the lung during the first year of life, *Am Rev Respir Dis* 134:513-519, 1986.
151. Helms P, Stocks J: Lung function in infants with congenital pulmonary hypoplasia, *J Pediatr* 101:918-922, 1982.
152. Mansell AL, Driscoll JM, James LS: Pulmonary follow-up of moderately low birth weight infants with and without respiratory distress syndrome, *J Pediatr* 110:111-115, 1987.
153. Koch G: Alveolar ventilation, diffusion capacity and the (A-a) PO_2 difference in the newborn infant, *Respir Physiol* 4:168-192, 1968.
154. Gaultier Cl, Boule M, Allaire Y, Clement A, Buvry A, Girard F: Determination of capillary oxygen tension in infants and children, *Bull Eur Physiopathol Respir* 14:287-297, 1978.
155. Dong SH, Lik HM, Song GW, Rong ZP, Wy YP: Arterialized capillary blood gases and acid-base studies in normal individuals 29 days to 24 years of age, *Am J Dis Child* 139:1019-1022, 1985.
156. Levison HEA, Featherby EA, Weng TR: Arterial blood gases, alveolar-arterial oxygen difference, and physiologic dead space in children and young adults, *Am Rev Respir Dis* 101:972-974, 1970.
157. Mansell A, Bryan AC, Levison H: Airway closure in children, *J Appl Physiol* 33:711-714, 1972.
158. Gaultier CL, Allaire Y, Pappo A, Girard F: Etude du volume de fermeture chez l'enfant sain et atteint d'obstruction bronchique, In Hatzfeld, ed: *Distribution of pulmonary gas exchange,* Paris, 1975, Colloque INSERM 51, pp 365-372.
159. Escourrou PJL, Teisseire BP, Herigault RA, Vallez MO, Dupeyrat AJ, Gaultier Cl: Mechanism of improvement in pulmonary gas exchange during growth in awake piglets, *J Appl Physiol* 65:1055-1061, 1988.
160. Escourrou P, Qi X, Weiss M, Mazmanian GM, Gaultier CL, Herve P: Influence of pulmonary blood flow on gas exchange in piglets, *J Appl Physiol* 75:2478-2483, 1993.
161. Koch G, Eriksson BO: Effect of physical training on anatomical R-L shunt at rest and pulmonary diffusing capacity during near-maximal exercise in boys 11-13 years old, *Scand J Clin Lab Invest* 31:95-103, 1973.
162. Mok JY, McLaughlin FJ, Pintar M, Hak H, Amaro-Galvez R, Levison H: Transcutaneous monitoring of oxygenation: what is normal? *J Pediatr* 118:365-371, 1986.
163. Chipps BE, Mak H, Schuberth KC, Talamo JH, Menkes HA: Nocturnal oxygen saturation in normal and asthmatic children, *Pediatrics* 65:1157-1160, 1980.
164. Tabachnik E, Muller NL, Bryan AC, Levison H: Changes in ventilation and chest wall mechanics during sleep in normal adolescents, *J Appl Physiol* 51:557-564, 1981.

Respiratory Control

165. Bianchi AL, Denavit-Saubie M, Champagnat J: Central control of breathing in mammals: neuronal circuitry, membrane properties, and neurotransmitters, *Physiol Rev* 75:1-45, 1995.
166. Lagercrantz H, Milerad J, Walker D: Control of ventilation in the neonate. In Crystal RG, West JB, eds: *The lung: scientific foundations,* New York, 1991 Raven, pp 1711-1722.
167. Harper RM: State-dependent electrophysiological changes in central nervous system activity. In Haddad GG, Farber JP, eds: *Developmental neurobiology of breathing,* New York, 1991, Marcel Dekker, pp 521-549.
168. Lawson EE, Czyzyk-Krzeska MF, Dean JB, Millhorn DE: Developmental aspect of the neural control of breathing. In Beckerman RC, Brouillette RT, Hunt C, eds: *Developmental aspect of the neural control of breathing,* Baltimore, 1992, Williams & Wilkins, pp 1-15.
169. Quattrochi JJ, McBride PT, Yates AJ: Brainstem immaturity in sudden infant death syndrome: a quantitative rapid Golgi study of dendritic spines in 95 infants, *Brain Res* 325:39-48, 1985.
170. Millhorn DE, Szymeckel CL, Bayliss DA, Seroogy KB, Hokfelt T: Cellular, molecular, and developmental aspects of chemical synaptic transmission. In Haddad GG, Farber JP, eds: *Developmental neurobiology of breathing,* New York, 1991, Marcel Dekker, pp 11-70.
171. Schweitzer P, Pierrefiche O, Foutz AS, Denavit-Saubie M: Effects of *N*-methyl-D-aspartate (NMDA) receptor blockade on breathing pattern in newborn cat, *Dev Brain Res* 56:290-293, 1990.
172. Haddad GG: Cellular and membrane properties of brainstem neurons in early life. In Haddad GG, Farber JP, eds: *Developmental neurobiology of breathing,* New York, 1991, Marcel Dekker, pp 155-175.
173. Denavit-Saubie M, Kalia A, Pierrefiche O, Schweitzer P, Foutz AS, Champagnat J: Maturation of brain stem neurons involved in respiratory rhythmogenesis: biochemical, bioelectrical and morphological properties, *Biol Neonate* 65:171-175, 1994.
174. Lagercrantz H: Neurochemical modulation of fetal behaviour and excitation at birth. In von Euler C, Forssberg H, Lagercrantz H, eds: *Neurobiology of infant behaviour,* Stockholm, 1989, Stockholm Press, pp 19-29.
175. Lagercrantz H, Persson H, Srinivasen M, Yamamoto Y: The developmental expression of some neuropeptide genes in respiration-related areas of the rabbit brain, *J Physiol* 417:25-32, 1989.
176. Kole M, Chen J, Ramakrishna CA, Stolle JA, Neubauer JA, England SJ: Maturation of neurotransmitters in the brainstem with neonatal hypoxic exposure, *Am J Respir Crit Care Med* 149:A286, 1994.
177. Henderson-Smart DJ, Pettigrew AG, Campbell DJ: Clinical apnea and brain stem neural function in preterm infants, *N Engl J Med* 308:353-357, 1983.
178. Curzi-Dascalova L, Christova-Guerguieva E: Respiratory pauses in normal prematurely born infants: a comparison with full-term newborns, *Biol Neonate* 44:325-332, 1983.
179. Waggener TB, Stark AR, Cohlan BA, Frantz III ID: Apnea duration is related to ventilatory oscillation characteristics in newborn infants, *J Appl Physiol* 57:536-544, 1989.

180. Waggener TB, Frantz ID III, Cohlan BA, Stark AR: Mixed and obstructive apneas are related to ventilatory oscillations in premature infants, *J Appl Physiol* 66:2818-2826, 1989.
181. Thach BT, Stark AR: Spontaneous neck flexion and airway obstruction during apneic spells in preterm infants, *J Pediatr* 94:275-281, 1979.
182. Upton CJ, Milner AD, Stokes GM: Upper airway patency during apnoea of prematurity, *Arch Dis Child* 67:419-424, 1992.
183. Finer NN, Barrington KJ, Hayes BJ, Hugh A: Obstructive mixed, and central apnea in the neonate: physiologic correlates, *J Pediatr* 121:943-950, 1992.
184. Miller MJ, Carlo WA, Martin RJ: Continuous positive airway pressure selectively reduces obstructive apnea in preterm infants, *J Pediatr* 106:91-94, 1985.
185. Hoppenbrouwers T, Hodgman JE, Cabal L: Obstructive apnea associated patterns of movement, heart rate, and oxygenation in infants at low and increased risk for SIDS, *Pediatr Pulmonol* 15:1-12, 1993.
186. Duara S, Neto GS, Claure N, Gerhardt T, Bancalari E: Effect of maturation on the extrathoracic airway stability of infants, *J Appl Physiol* 73:2368-2372, 1992.
187. Guilleminault C, Ariagno R, Korobkin R, Nagel L, Baldwin R, Coons S, Owen M: Mixed and obstructive sleep apnea and near miss for sudden infant death syndrome. II. Comparison of near miss and normal control infants by age, *Pediatrics* 64:882-891, 1979.
188. Lee D, Caces R, Kwiatkowski K, Cates D, Rigatto H: A developmental study on types and frequency distribution of short apneas (3 to 15 seconds) in term and preterm infants, *Pediatr Res* 22:344-349, 1987.
189. Carskadon MA, Harvey K, Dement WC, Guilleminault C, Simmons FB, Anders TF: Respiration during sleep in children, *West J Med* 128:477-481, 1978.
190. Gaultier CL: Apnea and sleep states in newborns and infants, *Biol Neonate* 65:231-234, 1994.
191. Schulte FJ, Busse C, Eichorn N: Rapid eye movement sleep, motoneuron inhibition, and apneic spells in preterm infants, *Pediatr Res* 11:709-713, 1977.
192. Haddad GG, Lait L, Mellins RB: Determination of ventilatory pattern in REM sleep in normal infants, *J Appl Physiol* 53:52-56, 1982.
193. Parmelee AH, Stern E, Harris MA: Maturation of respiration in prematures and young infants, *Neuropediatrie* 3:294-304, 1972.
194. Kelly DH, Stellwagen LM, Kaitz E, Shannon DC: Apnea and periodic breathing in normal full-term infants during the first twelve months, *Pediatr Pulmonol* 1:215-219, 1985.
195. Hamza J, Benlabed M, Orhant E, Escourrou P, Curzi-Dascalova L, Gaultier CI: Neonatal pattern of breathing during active and quiet sleep after maternal administration of meperidine, *Pediatr Res* 32:412-416, 1992.
196. Kahn A, Hasaerts D, Blum D: Phenothiazine-induced sleep apnea in normal infants, *Pediatrics* 75:844-847, 1985.
197. Jansen AH, Chernick V: Development of respiratory control, *Physiol Rev* 63:437-483, 1983.
198. Manning DJ, Stothers JK: Sleep state, hypoxia and periodic breathing in the neonate, *Acta Paediatr Scand* 80:763-769, 1991.
199. Herbst JJ, Minton SD, Book LS: Gastroesophageal reflux causing respiratory distress and apnea in newborn infants, *J Pediatr* 95:763-768, 1979.
200. Berterottiere D, D'Allest AM, Dehan M, Gaultier C: Effects of increase in body temperature on the breathing pattern in premature infants, *J Dev Physiol* 13:303-308, 1990.
201. Canet E, Gaultier Cl, D'Allest AM, Dehan M: Effect of sleep deprivation on respiratory events during sleep in healthy infants, *J Appl Physiol* 66:1158-1163, 1989.
202. Kahn A, Grosswasser J, Sottiaux M, Rebuffat E, Franco P, Dramaix M: Prone or supine body position and sleep characteristics in infants, *Pediatrics* 91:1112-1115, 1993.
203. Farber JP: Development of pulmonary and chest wall reflexes influencing breathing. In Haddad GG, Farber JP, eds: *Developmental neurobiology of breathing,* New York, 1991, Marcel Dekker, pp 245-269.
204. Gerhardt T, Bancalari E: Maturational changes of reflexes influencing inspiratory time in newborns, *J Appl Physiol* 50:1282-1285, 1981.
205. Rabette PS, Fletcher ME, Dezateux CA, Soriano-Brucher H, Stocks J: Hering-Breuer reflex and respiratory system compliance in the first year of life: a longitudinal study, *J Appl Physiol* 76:650-656, 1994.
206. Finer NA, Abroms IF, Taeusch TW: Ventilation and sleep states in newborn infants, *J Pediatr* 89:100-108, 1976.
207. Fleming PA, Bryan AC, Bryan MH: Functional immaturity of pulmonary irritant receptors and apnea in newborn preterm, *Pediatrics* 61:515-518, 1978.
208. Sachis RN, Armstrong DL, Becker LE, Bryan AC: The vagus nerve and sudden infant death syndrome: a morphometric study, *J Pediatr* 98:278-280, 1981.
209. Shannon R: Involvement of thoracic nerve afferents in the respiratory response to chest compression, *Respir Physiol* 36:65-76, 1979.
210. Hagan RE, Bryan AC, Bryan MH, Gulston G: Neonatal chest wall afferents and regulation of respiration, *J Appl Physiol* 42:362-367, 1977.
211. Knill R, Bryan AC: An intercostal-phrenic inhibitory reflex in human newborn infants, *J Appl Physiol* 40:352-356, 1979.
212. Hertzberg T, Hellstrom S, Lagercrantz H, Pequignot JM: Resetting of arterial chemoreceptors and carotid body catecholamines in the newborn rat, *J Physiol* 425:211-225, 1990.
213. Calder NA, Williams BA, Kumar P, Hanson MA: The respiratory response of healthy term infants to breath-by-breath alternations in inspired oxygen at two postnatal ages, *Pediatr Res* 35:321-324, 1994.
214. Hertzberg T, Lagercrantz H: Postnatal sensitivity of the peripheral chemoreceptors in newborn infants, *Arch Dis Child* 62:1238-1241, 1987.
215. Hanson MA, Kumar P, Williams BA: The effect of chronic hypoxia upon the development of respiratory chemoreflexes in the newborn kitten, *J Physiol (Lond)* 411:563-574, 1989.
216. Calder NA, Williams BA, Smyth J, Boon AW, Kumar P, Hanson MA: Absence of respiratory chemoreflex responses to mild hypoxia in infants who have suffered bronchopulmonary dysplasia: implications for the risk of sudden infant death, *Pediatr Res* 35:677-681, 1994.
217. Fagenholz SA, O'Connell K, Shannon DC: Chemoreceptor function and sleep apnea, *Pediatrics* 58:31-36, 1976.
218. Davis GM, Bureau MA: Pulmonary and chest wall mechanics in the control of respiration in the newborn, *Clin Perinatol* 14:551-579, 1987.
219. Rigatto H, Kalapesi Z, Leahy FN, Durand M, McCallum M, Cates D: Ventilatory response to 100% and 15% O_2 during wakefulness and sleep in preterm infants, *Early Hum Dev* 7:1-10, 1982.
220. Moss IR, Luman JG: Neurochemicals and respiratory control during development, *J Appl Physiol* 67:1-13, 1989.
221. Bonora M, Marlot D, Gaultier H, Duron B: Effects of hypoxia on ventilation during postnatal development in conscious kitten, *J Appl Physiol* 56:1464-1471, 1984.
222. Canet E, Kianicka I, Gagne B, Bureau MA, Praud JP: Postnatal evolution of the O_2 and CO_2 peripheral chemoreflex in awake newborn lamb: a parallel evaluation, *Am J Respir Crit Care Med* 149:A287, 1994.
223. Guthrie RD, Standeart TA, Hodson WA, Woodrom DE: Sleep and maturation of eucapnic ventilation and CO_2 sensitivity in the premature primate, *J Appl Physiol* 48:347-354, 1980.
224. Gaultier CL: Breathing and sleep during growth: physiology and pathology, *Bull Eur Physiopathol Respir* 21:55-112, 1985.
225. Honma Y, Wilkes D, Bryan AC: Rib cage and abdominal contributions to ventilatory response to CO_2 infants, *J Appl Physiol* 56:1211-1216, 1984.
226. Moriette G, Van Reempts P, Moore M, Cates D, Rigatto H: The effect of rebreathing CO_2 on ventilation and diaphragmatic electromyography in newborn infants, *Respir Physiol* 62:387-397, 1985.
227. Cohen G, Xu C, Henderson-Smart D: Ventilatory response of the sleeping newborn to CO_2 during normoxic rebreathing, *J Appl Physiol* 71:168-174, 1991.
228. Walker DW: Effects of increased core temperature on fetal breathing movements and electrocortical activity in fetal sleep, *J Dev Physiol* 10:515-523, 1988.
229. Johnson P, Andews DC: The role of thermometabolism on cardiorespiratory function in postnatal life. In Gaultier C, Escourrou P, Curzi-Dascalova L, eds: *Sleep and cardiorespiratory control,* vol 227, Paris, 1991, Colloque INSERM/John Libbey, Eurotext, pp 45-53.
230. Bach V, Boufferache B, Kremp O, Maingourd Y, Libert JP: Regulation of sleep and body temperature in responses to exposure to cool and warm environment in neonates, *Pediatrics* 93:789-796, 1994.
231. Fleming JP, Levine MR, Azaz Y, Johnson P: The effect of sleep state on the metabolic response to cold stress in newborn infants, In Jones CT, ed: *Fetal and neonatal development,* Ithaca, NY, 1988, Perinatology Press, pp 643-647.
232. Haraguchi S, Fung RO, Sasaki CT: Effect of hyperthermia on the laryngeal closure reflex: implications in the sudden infant death syndrome, *Ann Otol Rhinol Laryngol* 92:24-28, 1983.
233. Fleming PJ, Levine MR, Wigfield R, Stewart AJ: Interactions between thermoregulation and the control of respiration in infants: possible relationship to sudden infant death, *Acta Paediatr Suppl* 389:57-59, 1993.

234. Rivkees SA, Reppert SM: Perinatal development of day-night rhythms in humans, *Horm Res* 37:99-104, 1992.
235. Mirmiran M, Swabb DF, Kok JH, Hofman MA, Witting W, Van Gool WA: Circadian rhythms and the suprachiasmatic nucleus, *Prog Brain Res* 93:151-163, 1992.
236. Mirmiran M, Kok JH, de Kleine MJK, Koppe JG, Overdijk J, Witting W: Circadian rhythms in preterm infants: a preliminary study, *Early Hum Dev* 23:139-146, 1990.
237. Mirmiran M, Kok JH: Circadian rhythms in early human development, *Early Hum Dev* 26:121-128, 1991.
238. Hoppenbrouwers T, Jensen D, Hodgman J, Harper R, Sterman M: Respiration during the first six months of life in normal infants. II. The emergence of a circadian pattern, *Neuropediatrie* 10:264-280, 1979.
239. Updike PA, Accurso FJ, Jones RH: Physiologic circadian rhythmicity in preterm infants, *Nurs Res* 34:160-163, 1985.
240. Weissbluth L, Weissbluth M: Sudden infant death syndrome: a genetically determined impaired maturation of the photoneuroendocrine system: a unifying hypothesis, *J Theor Biol* 167:13-25, 1994.
241. Mograss MA, Ducharme FM, Brouillette RT: Movements/arousals: description, classification, and relationship to sleep apnea in children, *Am J Respir Crit Care Med* 150:1690-1695, 1994.
242. Thoppil CK, Belan MA, Cowen CP, Matthew OP: Behavioral arousal in newborn infants and its association with termination of apnea, *J Appl Physiol* 70:2479-2484, 1991.
243. Scher MS, Richardson GA, Coble PA, Day NL, Stoffer DS: The effects of prenatal alcohol and marijuana exposure: disturbances in neonatal sleep cycling and arousal, *Pediatr Res* 24:101-105, 1988.
244. McCulloch K, Brouillette RT, Guzzetta AJ, Hunt CE: Arousal response in near-miss sudden infant death syndrome and normal infants, *J Pediatr* 101:911-917, 1982.
245. Van Der Hal AL, Rodriguez AM, Sargent CW, Platzker ACG, Keens TG: Hypoxic and hypercapnic arousal responses and prediction of subsequent apnea in apnea of infancy, *Pediatrics* 75:848-854, 1985.
246. Marcus CL, Bautista DB, Amihyia A, Davidson-Ward SL, Keens TG: Hypercapnic arousal responses in children with congenital central hypoventilation syndrome, *Pediatrics* 88:993-998, 1991.
247. Milerad J, Hertzberg T, Wennergreen G, Lagercrantz H: Respiratory and arousal response to hypoxia in apneic infants reinvestigated, *Eur J Pediatr* 148:565-470, 1989.
248. Davidson-Ward SL, Bautista DB, Keens TG: Hypoxic arousal responses in normal infants, *Pediatrics* 89:860-864, 908, 1992.
249. Fewell JE, Baker SB: Arousal from sleep during rapidly developing hypoxemia in lambs, *Pediatr Res* 22:471-477, 1987.
250. Ramet J, Egreteau L, Curzi-Dascalova L, Escourrou P, Dehan M, Gaultier C: Cardiac, respiratory, and arousal responses to an esophageal and infusion test in near-term infants during active sleep, *J Pediatr Gastroenterol Nutr* 15:135-140, 1992.
251. Kahn A, Picard E, Blum D: Auditory arousal threshold of normal and near-miss SIDS infants, *Dev Med Child Neurol* 28:299-302, 1986.
252. Fewell JE, Williams BJ, Szabo JS, Taylor BJ: Influence of repeated upper airway obstruction on the arousal and cardiopulmonary response to upper airway obstruction in lambs, *Pediatr Res* 23:191-195, 1988.
253. Phillipson EA, Bowes G, Sullivan CE, Woolf GM: The influence of sleep fragmentation on arousal and ventilatory responses to respiratory stimuli, *Sleep* 3:281-288, 1980.

CHAPTER 5

Lung Cell Biology

Kevin Kirchner, Emily L. Dobyns, and Kurt R. Stenmark

The lung consists of diverse cell types that function with one another and with the cardiovascular and hematopoietic systems to efficiently eliminate the carbon dioxide produced by cellular metabolism and to resupply the cells with oxygen. Within the adult human lung parenchyma, alveolar type I cells account for 93% to 96% of the alveolar surface area and 6% to 9% of the total cell population. Alveolar type II cells account for 4% to 7% of the alveolar surface area and 13% to 19% of the total cell population. The remainder of the cell population within the lung is about 35% to 39% endothelial cells, 34% to 40% interstitial cells (fibroblasts), and 2% to 5% macrophages.[1] Specific structural and functional duties are performed by each of these cells. Important interaction and communication among various lung cell types is ongoing and essential for normal cellular and lung function.

Airways conduct gas into and out of the alveoli and are lined with cells that optimize this process and protect the airways and distal lung parenchyma from damage. Eight different cell types line the conducting airways: ciliated cells, serous cells, basal cells, small mucous granule cells, Clara cells, neuroendocrine cells, brush cells, and mucous goblet cells.[2] Once the gas reaches the alveoli, the alveolar lining cells, interstitial cells, and endothelial cells are responsible for the maintenance of alveolar-capillary integrity and the enhancement of gas exchange. Blood vessels composed of endothelial cells, smooth muscle cells (SMCs), and adventitial fibroblasts regulate blood flow to the gas-exchange units and also actively participate in a number of other metabolic, immunologic, hemostatic, and host defense functions performed by the lung.

LUNG GROWTH AND DEVELOPMENT

Basic Concepts

The lung begins to form in humans at 21 to 24 days' gestation as a bud of the primitive foregut[3] (Fig. 5-1). This process evolves rapidly during the first, or pseudoglandular, phase of lung development, with rapid and complete formation of all the airways through the terminal bronchioles by week 16 of gestation. The lung then begins to form the primitive gas-exchanging units (acini) during the second, or canalicular, phase

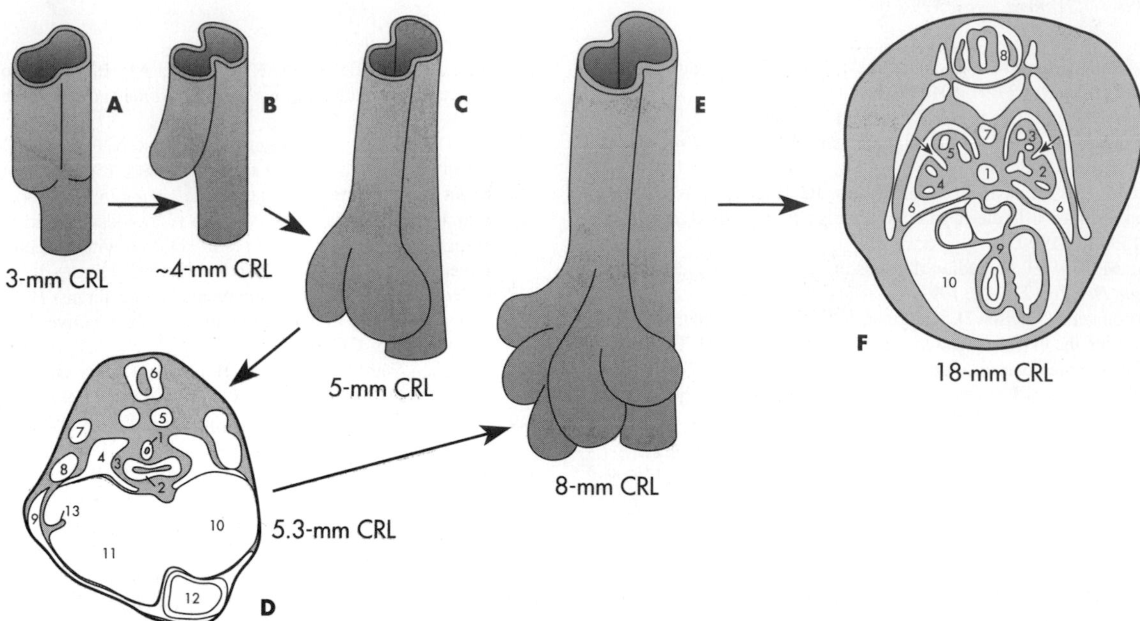

Fig. 5-1. Early development of the human lung. Budding of the lung primordium from the prospective esophagus. Crown rump length *(CRL)* of 3 to 5.3 mm corresponds to a fetal age of 24 to 48 days; an 8-mm CRL corresponds to an age of 4.5 weeks. In **A** to **C** and **E,** the epithelial tube forms as a diverticulum from the foregut by deepening of the laryngotracheal grooves. After joining each other, the grooves completely separate the trachea from the esophagus. **D** and **F,** The tubular sprouts grow into the surrounding mesenchyme. Transverse sections of the fetus **(D)** at age 28 days: *1,* Esophagus; *2,* left and right lung buds with tracheal bifurcation; *3,* lung mesenchyme; *4,* pericardioperitoneal canal; *5,* dorsal aorta; *6,* neural tube; *7,* postcardinal vein; *8,* common cardinal vein; *9,* pericardial vein; *10,* left atrium; *11,* right atrium; *12,* conus cordis; *13,* right venous valve. Transverse sections **(F)** at age 46 days: *1,* Esophagus; *2,* left upper lobe; *3* and *5,* lower lobes; *4,* middle lobe; *6,* pleural cavity; *7,* aorta; *8,* neural lobe; *9,* heart; *10,* pericardial cavity. Arrows within **F** point to oblique fissures. (**A** to **C** and **E** redrawn from Burri PH: *Ann Rev Physiol* 46:617-628,1984; **D** and **F** redrawn from Gasser RF: *Atlas of human embryos,* New York, 1975, Harper & Row, p 317.)

of development. This developmental stage is completed by about week 26 of gestation. During the final (terminal sac or alveolar) phase of lung development, the lungs prepare for gas exchange as functional type II cells capable of secreting surfactant mature and continue to increase in number and size from week 26 of gestation until term. After birth, the lung may continue to form new alveoli until sometime between 2 and 7 years of age, although most form during the first 2 years of life in humans.[4] The airways continue to increase in size but not number after week 16 of gestation.[5-7]

The mesenchyme surrounding the early lung buds contains a vascular network derived from the foregut. This mesenchyme is important not only for directing airway development but also for contributing to vascular development. Primitive vascular structures form a network with the branching airways. These vessels differentiate into arteries and later into the pulmonary arteries, which grow toward the lung bud from the sixth branchial arch. Thus the close association of airways and arteries begins early in development. As development proceeds, there is a synchronization of airway and vessel branching, implying that they respond to common mediators or that they exchange messenger molecules. Remaining separate, however, are the veins that arise within the loose mesenchyme of the lung septa.

Any disruption of the cells and processes that drive lung development can cause disturbances in lung or vascular growth, which usually present in early infancy but sometimes remain hidden until adulthood. Furthermore, many diseases or lung injuries initiate a series of cellular events that may recapitulate the events controlling cell growth in early lung development.

Mechanisms Contributing to Airway Parenchymal Growth

Mesenchymal-Epithelial Interactions

Interaction between epithelial cells and the underlying mesenchyme is essential for normal lung growth and development (Fig. 5-2). The mesenchyme signals the overlying epithelial cells to proliferate and form the airways and alveoli during development. In the mid-1960s, it was demonstrated that removing the mesenchyme from explanted fetal lung buds inhibited formation of the lung.[8] Furthermore, tracheal and bronchial mesenchyme failed to induce the formation of lung-like tissue from the esophageal portion of the foregut, and esophageal mesenchyme failed to induce branching by tracheal epithelium.[9] These studies demonstrated that both the specific primitive pulmonary epithelium and mesenchyme are programmed in concert early in development to evolve into the diverse cellular elements of the adult lung.

Integrins, syndecans, cadherins, fibronectins, and other extracellular matrix and cell surface components modulate the development of the embryonic lung in animal models.[10-18] Blocking the function of cell surface or extracellular matrix molecules inhibits branching morphogenesis in vitro. It remains

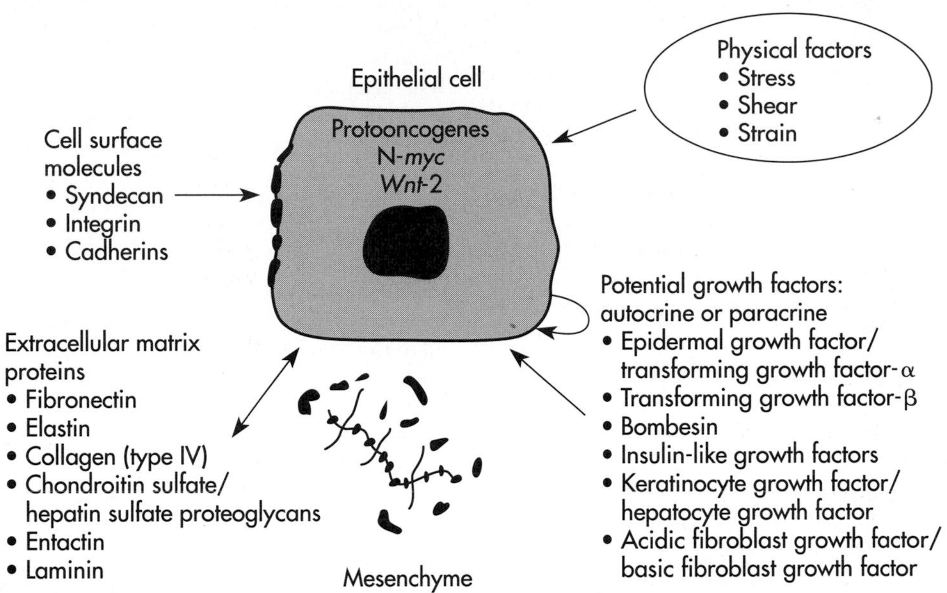

Fig. 5-2. Mesenchymal-epithelial-physicochemical factors regulating lung growth at the cellular level. Alveolar epithelial cell depicted with known nuclear transcription factors, cellular surface molecules, putative growth factors, mesenchymal matrix proteins, and physical factors that modulate differentiation and growth.

unknown, however, exactly how these components signal the epithelium to differentiate and how each extracellular matrix molecule functions in concert with the others. Inhibition of a specific component independent of the others results in histologically and biochemically similar growth inhibition in vitro. Several excellent articles have reviewed this topic.[19-23]

The primitive pulmonary epithelium originates from the endoderm when the tracheal bud evaginates during development and eventually evolves into the ciliated lining cells of the airways, airway submucous glands, airway mucous cells, Clara cells, and alveolar type I and type II cells. Although the mesenchyme is clearly essential, the exact cells and proteins involved in this complex process remain unclear. Lung bud experiments have demonstrated that surfactant apoprotein-C (SP-C), an alveolar type II cell-specific messenger ribonucleic acid (mRNA), is initially expressed in the primordial trachea, but as branching morphogenesis evolves, expression occurs only in the more distal epithelial cells.[24] Interestingly, removing a bronchial mesenchymal bud and transplanting it onto the trachea induces the tracheal epithelial cells "surrounded by" this bud to undergo branching morphogenesis and reexpress SP-C.[25]

Elastin may serve as a structural protein that is critical to alveolar formation[26,27] (Fig. 5-3). Alveoli appear to originate as outpockets through the elastin fibers that are entwined within the extracellular matrix of the interstitium ("fishnet hypothesis"). Disrupting the elastin network with the proteolytic enzyme elastase or β-amino-propionitrile, an inhibitor of elastin and collagen cross-linking, results in a lung that has distorted alveolar architecture and physiologic loss of elastic recoil.[28,29]

Growth Factors

Peptide growth factors modulate the growth and development of the pulmonary epithelium.[30,31] Studies of embryonic epithelium separated from its mesenchyme suggest that exogenous polypeptides may trigger this response. When the epithelium and mesenchyme are cultured separately on a transcellular filter that inhibits direct epithelial-mesenchymal contact, the epithelium continues to proliferate and branch, suggesting that a diffusible factor released by the mesenchyme triggers epithelial cell proliferation.[32] When embryonic epithelial tissue is cultured without mesenchyme, the proliferation and differentiation of pulmonary epithelial cells continues to occur in the presence of concentrated adult bronchoalveolar lavage fluid, acidic fibroblast growth factor (aFGF), keratinocyte growth factor (KGF), or a combination of these growth factors.[33]

Other growth factors that stimulate isolated neonatal alveolar type II cells to proliferate in vitro include transforming growth factor-α (TGF-α) and epidermal growth factor (EGF).[34] Human fetal lung epithelial cells also express the receptors, mRNA, and protein for platelet-derived growth factor (PDGR) in vitro.[35,36] In vivo, antibodies to EGF and aFGF localize to epithelial cells within infant rat lungs.[37] EGF immunoreactivity in the lungs of human fetal tissue and in acutely and chronically injured neonatal lungs has been localized to nonciliated fetal tracheal cells but not to postnatal tracheal epithelial cells.[38] Positive immunostaining for EGF was seen before and after birth in submucosal glandular cells. EGF immunoreactivity was also observed after birth in the bronchiolar epithelium of infants with chronic lung disease.

Bombesin-like peptides secreted by neuroendocrine cells within the lung may also be critical to fetal lung growth and maturation.[39,40] Neuroendocrine cells are found within the lung in clusters at airway bifurcations and as basal cells within the airway epithelium. They increase in number in more distal airways but are not found beyond the terminal bronchioles.[41] The in

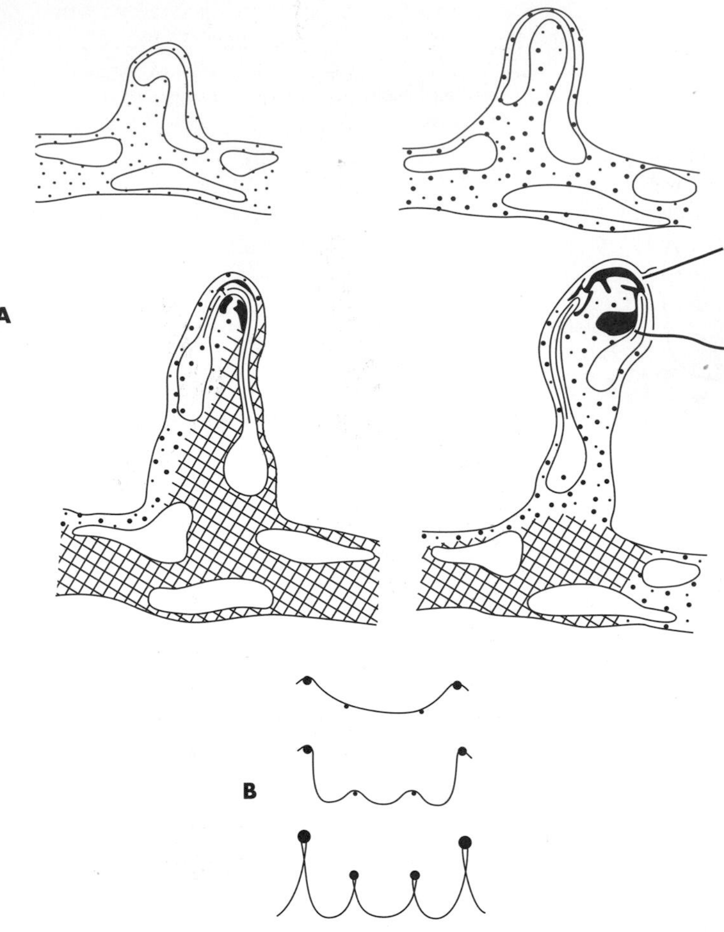

Fig. 5-3. A, Formation and capillarization on secondary septa. Patching indicates tissue; white areas indicate capillary lumina; fine dots indicate closed capillary segments; coarse dots indicate elastic tissue; black areas indicate cytoplasmic extensions of cells not yet identified. *Top left,* Lifting off of capillary loops; *top right,* stretching and narrowing of the existing capillary; *bottom left,* closing down of the capillary lumen, shutting it off from the blood circulation; *bottom right,* apparition of unidentified cells that wrap the endothelial cells. "Bridging" of capillaries by unidentified cells suggesting later recanalization. **B,** Relationship of elastic fibers to the formation of the new alveolar wall *(top);* alveolar growth results in evagination between new fibers *(middle),* producing three new alveoli from the original large, flat alveolus *(bottom).* (**A** from Burri PH: *Anat Rec* 180:77-98, 1974; **B** from Hodson WA: *Development of the lung,* Philadelphia, 1997, Marcel Dekker, p 646.)

utero administration of bombesin-like peptide activity resulted in fetal lungs that had a 70% increase in thymidine incorporation into deoxyribonucleic acid (DNA) and increased surfactant lipid biosynthesis and SP-A mRNA production.[42] Furthermore, embryonic mouse lung expresses the receptors for bombesin-like peptides during the pseudoglandular phase of development in vivo, and the exogenous administration of bombesin in vitro enhances branching morphogenesis.[43] Other evidence suggests that neuroepithelial bodies enhance airway growth.[44]

Further insights into the cellular aspects of the growth and development of the lung have come from studies in transgenic mice. A targeted mutation of the N-*myc* protooncogene, a nuclear transcription factor, in mice results in markedly underdeveloped airways and alveolar epithelium with decreased alveolar septation and terminal sac formation that is incompatible with survival.[45] Of interest, N-*myc* gene expression is often increased in human small cell carcinomas of the lung.[46,47] *Wnt*-2, a gene that encodes a protein acting as an oncogene for epithelial cells and that is important in intracellular signaling, is more active or highly expressed by mesenchymal cells during fetal lung development than in the adult lung.[48] Investigators have developed transgenic mouse models to study the cell lineage relationships of alveolar type II cells and Clara cells.[49] Interestingly, a *lac-Z* fusion gene linked to SP-C is expressed initially in the endodermal cells of the lung during the embryonic phase in mice and gradually undergoes a proximal to distal extinction of expression during in vivo development to the point where it is expressed only in alveolar type II cells after birth.[49] When a similar technique was used with a transgene flanking the Clara cell secretory protein in rats, Clara cell gene expression was observed 4 days before that seen in normal rats, suggesting that in normal rats a *cis*-acting element may be suppressing the expression of this gene in a temporal and spatial fashion, since the gene was expressed in similar locations within the lung.[50] These experiments suggest that specific epithelial cells were committed to become Clara cells before this phenomenon occurred.

Physical Mechanisms

Physical mechanisms are critical to the morphogenesis and growth of many organs.[51] Alveolar distention, ventilation, and pulmonary blood flow participate in the regulation of both antenatal and postnatal lung growth. In utero animal models and human disease correlates expand the understanding of the role of different physical mechanisms (Box 5-1). Overdistending the lung in utero by ligating the trachea or a bronchus results in a "hyperplastic" lung that contains increased DNA content per milligram of tissue and weighs more than normal lungs.[52] A corresponding human malformation that supports this observation is congenital laryngeal atresia when the lungs are overdistended with alveolar fluid and have increased alveolar surface area, lung volume, alveolar number, and elastin maturation with normal maturation of surfactant biosynthesis.[53] Similarly, polyhydramnios increases acinar complexity by a presumed mechanism of alveolar distention, although its exact effects on lung growth remain unclear.[54] Conversely, chronic drainage of the fetal lung fluid by transtracheal catheter or experimental amniotic fluid drainage results in a hypoplastic lung that has reduced volume, weight, and alveolar complexity.[55] The most critical factor that influences the severity of the hypoplasia appears to be the timing of the insult during development, although the duration of the insult clearly modulates the response.[56] Of note, oligohydramnios may have two mechanisms by which it affects alveolar growth: (1) inadequate alveolar distention secondary to loss of alveolar fluid into the amniotic sac and (2) chest wall compression secondary to insufficient levels of amniotic fluid. The human disease correlate of pulmonary hypoplasia implicating alveolar fluid insufficiency and inadequate alveolar distention is Potter's syndrome with renal agenesis and oligohydramnios.[57,58]

Another human abnormality that may be associated with significant pulmonary hypoplasia is congenital diaphragmatic hernia and massive abdominal wall defects. Infants with fatal congenital diaphragmatic hernia have fewer alveoli and smaller lung volumes than predicted when corrected for the

BOX 5-1
Physical Factors Affecting Lung Growth

Hypertrophy and hyperplasia

Laryngeal atresia
Tracheal ligation
Ventilation
Chronic maternal carbon dioxide administration

Hypoplasia

Oligohydramnios
Chronic tracheal drainage by transtracheal catheter
Potter's syndrome: ? Alveolar fluid loss or mechanical chest wall compression
Congenital diaphragmatic hernia
Massive abdominal wall defects
Phrenic nerve agenesis: decreased ventilation
Ligation of pulmonary artery and agenesis of pulmonary artery

reduction in acinar complexity.[59] Both lungs may be affected depending on the timing of the insult, with the ipsilateral lung more severely affected. Animal models of congenital diaphragmatic hernia in sheep and rats produce similar findings, and future studies will likely improve the understanding of the pathophysiology of this process at a cellular level.[60-62] Of 35 infants with fatal liver-containing abdominal wall defects and narrow thoracic cage deformities, 14 suffered marked pulmonary hypoplasia with significantly lower ratios of lung weight to body weight and chest wall circumferences, which implies that the abdominal wall contents may physically influence the growth of the chest wall and lungs.[63]

Inhibition of fetal breathing movements in sheep by spinal cord or phrenic nerve transection also results in a hypoplastic lung.[64-67] Human fetuses with congenital agenesis of the phrenic nerve have abnormal development of the diaphragm and pulmonary hypoplasia.[68] Conversely, increasing mechanical stretch in vivo by administering carbon dioxide to pregnant rat dams results in offspring that have increased alveolar surface area, thinner airspace walls, and alveolar type II cells with less cellular glycogen and increased lamellar bodies.[69]

In vitro studies also suggest that physical factors stimulate the growth of pulmonary cells. A novel dynamic study of rat fetal lung buds demonstrated that the primitive airways contract as early as the pseudoglandular phase of development and that these contractions appear to distend the more distal portions of the developing lung.[70] Cyclic mechanical stretch of human lung fibroblasts increases the cell numbers by 39% and 163% above control after 2 and 4 days in vitro.[71] Furthermore, supernatant media collected from these stretched cells induces quiescent human lung fibroblasts to proliferate independent of mechanical stretch, which suggests that physical stretch triggers the release of autocrine growth factors. Subsequent studies examining the effects of stretch on cell cultures of rat fetal epithelial and mesenchymal cells isolated during the canalicular phase of development provide evidence that fetal epithelial cells proliferate in vitro after mechanical stretch and that this response may be regulated by locally produced growth factors.[72,73] Fetal rabbit alveolar type II cells isolated at 24 days' gestation also respond to stretch by increasing both DNA and phospholipid biosynthesis, with the latter being dramatically influenced by the frequency of the stretch.[74]

After birth, physical mechanisms also modulate the growth of the lung. Children who have undergone partial lung resection for congenital lung anomalies within the first few years of life have normal lung volumes and airflows when examined several years after the surgery.[75-77] The only abnormal physiologic parameter was delayed gas emptying from the regenerated lung tissue in the hemithorax in which lung tissue was resected.[76] Using animal models of unilateral lung resection, several investigators have demonstrated that the remaining lung tissue increases rapidly in volume, DNA content, and protein content to be essentially equal to that of a sham-operated or unoperated animal.[78,79] Interestingly, some evidence suggests that airways may fail to grow to the same magnitude as the alveoli.[80,81] When a novel technique of pleural plombage was used, the growth observed after unilateral pneumonectomy appeared to be regulated by stretch of the remaining lung.[82,83]

Pulmonary blood flow is critical to the growth of the lung in utero because ligation of a pulmonary artery results in significant pulmonary hypoplasia.[84,85] Insufficient blood flow to the developing lung caused by pulmonary artery ligation may result in decreased alveolar lung fluid secretion and thus alveolar distention.[86] Pulmonary blood flow modulates lung growth after birth but is not as important as lung distention.[83]

Considerable controversy exists as to whether lung tissue is restored in adults after partial lung resection, and most believe the existing alveoli increase in size but not number beyond childhood.[78] Recently, a study reported that adult dogs who underwent right pneumonectomy (approximately a 54% reduction in lung mass) exhibited increases in the lung volume and the histologic complexity of the cellular components that were consistent with alveolar growth and not simple hyperexpansion of existing parenchyma.[87] The cellular mechanisms that transduce the physical stimuli into the phenomena of cellular growth and hypertrophy in the lung remain unknown.

Mechanisms Contributing to Lung Vascular Growth

The embryonic endothelial tubes forming the lung vasculature acquire an SMC layer as development proceeds. During this process, SMCs proliferate and exhibit developmentally regulated alterations in protein expression, including changes in extracellular matrix, cytoskeletal, contractile, and growth factor protein expression.[88] Smooth muscle is essential for the development of vascular tone, which in turn is key to circulatory regulation. Within SMCs, marked and important changes in contractile and cytoskeletal protein expression are observed during development. Major switches in isoform expression of the two major contractile proteins, actin and myosin, occur with maturation of the vascular wall. Other proteins thought to be important in the SMC contractile responses, such as calponin, aldesmin, and vinculin, also undergo major changes in isotype expression during development.[89]

Thus compared to the adult, fetal as well as newborn SMCs underexpress many of the contractile proteins thought to be important in SMC contraction.[90] The acquisition of the contractile phenotype by SMCs in the mature wall is associated with an increase in contractile capability and decreased potential for cell replication. More important, it is the unique phenotype found in fetal and neonatal SMCs that may contribute to the rapid growth responses observed in neonatal vascular wall cells in response to stress. Furthermore, in adult vascular disease states, a reversion to the fetal or neonatal phenotype is observed during the response to injury.[91]

Growth Factors

During vascular development, the bulk of smooth muscle proliferation occurs before birth. Mechanisms that control cell proliferation during development remain unclear, although this is an area of intense investigation. However, in situ hybridization and immunohistochemistry studies have demonstrated the importance of locally produced growth factors in vascular cell proliferation. Basic fibroblast growth factors (bFGFs) and aFGFs are present in vessels from embryonic to adult animals. Both of these factors are mitogenic for vascular wall cells and are potent angiogenic factors.[92] TGF-β is expressed during early lung development and colocalizes with collagen types I and III, fibronectin, and proteoglycans, suggesting a role in at least extracellular matrix protein production.[93] Other investigators have proposed a role for TGF-β in angiogenesis or new blood vessel formation. Insulin-like growth factor I (IGF-I) and IGF-II are present in fetal pulmonary arteries.[94] IGF-II is present earlier in development than IGF-I. Both stimulate the proliferation of SMCs and increase elastin and collagen synthesis.[95]

Other studies have demonstrated that at least in the very early phases of smooth muscle development, growth factors may not be necessary.[91] Embryonic rat aortic SMCs rapidly and autonomously replicate in vitro. These cells are refractory to mitogenic stimulation by known smooth muscle peptide mitogens. The precise roles for all the growth factors in vascular development and repair continue to be investigated.

Extracellular Matrix

Extracellular matrix production and accumulation is crucial for normal vascular development. During development, the extracellular matrix appears to be important in the organization of endothelial cells into tubelike precursors of capillaries (angiogenesis). A proposed mechanism is the cell-specific differentiation of endothelial cells induced by components of the extracellular matrix.[96] It has been proposed that organization of these tubelike structures results from cellular traction or contractility and matrix malleability rather than cell differentiation.[97]

Endothelial cells as well as SMCs and fibroblasts play important roles in connective tissue production. Both SMCs and endothelial cells synthesize tropoelastin, which then cross-links to form elastin. Elastin maintains the flexibility of the vessel wall. It is largely produced during the fetal and early neonatal periods, with production essentially concluded in the first decade of life. Elastogenesis is poorly understood but can be modulated by a wide variety of cytokines.[97] The elastogenic response varies dramatically with age and location. For instance, in the neonate with vascular injury, a persistence of fetal-like levels and isoforms of elastin continue to be produced in the setting of pulmonary hypertension.[98] In the adult, however, elastin production must be reactivated in response to injury; both the type of elastin produced and its location within the vessel markedly differ from that observed in fetal and neonatal vascular injury states.

In contrast to the flexibility provided by elastin, collagen provides rigidity to the vascular wall. Collagen exists in several chemical types, and changes in these types occur during lung vascular development. Collagen types III and V are most abundant in late gestation and newborn resistance–sized pulmonary arteries. With normal postnatal development, there is an increase in the high-tensile–strength type I collagen. This delay in type I collagen expression in small pulmonary blood vessels is thought to allow plasticity in the system, which is necessary in fetal and neonatal life.[99] Collagen types I, IV, and VIII are actively synthesized by endothelial cells during the angiogenic process.[97,100,101] Thus it is assumed that these collagens are necessary for the early development of blood vessels. Collagens types I and IV are necessary for endothelial cell adhesion and proliferation.[102] Although some studies suggest that collagen type V inhibits endothelial cell proliferation, changes in type IV collagen production are noted in injury states and thus are thought to be at least markers of the injured endothelial cell.[103]

In summary, much remains to be understood about the cellular aspects of lung growth and development. Most information has been obtained from animal studies. Comprehension of the mechanisms controlling normal embryonic and postnatal lung growth will probably improve the understanding of congenital lung malformations, provide insights into the reparative process after lung injury, and enhance knowledge of pulmonary cancers.

ALVEOLAR TYPE II CELL STRUCTURE AND FUNCTION

The alveolar type II cell, or type II pneumocyte, has several important functions within the lung. These functions include surfactant secretion and metabolism, repair of the pulmonary epithelium after lung injury, fluid secretion and absorption within the alveolus, and host immune functions.

Surfactant Secretion and Metabolism

Several excellent reviews have summarized the improved understanding of surfactant gene expression, apoprotein synthesis, and phospholipid synthesis and metabolism by alveolar type II cells.[104-106] The importance of surfactant in the pathogenesis of hyaline membrane disease of the newborn was first recognized in 1959.[107] Since this discovery, the understanding has advanced to the point where exogenous surfactant administration to the newborn infant with respiratory distress syndrome has become routine therapy in major medical centers throughout the world and has improved the survival rate of prematurely born infants.[108]

Research now focuses on the cellular processing of surfactant phospholipids and proteins. A recent in vitro study in the isolated perfused rat lung demonstrated that the uptake and recycling of natural surfactant are threefold higher than the uptake and recycling of exogenous bovine surfactant, which suggests that most of the exogenous surfactant may remain in the alveolar space until it is degraded and that it is not recycled like natural surfactant.[109] Important cellular stimulants of surfactant protein and phospholipid secretion include alveolar stretch and β-adrenergic agents in vivo and cyclic adenosine monophosphate (cAMP) or protein kinase C mechanisms in vitro.[110] The mechanical stretch of alveolar type II cells in vitro mediates surfactant secretion by increasing cytosolic calcium levels.[111] Alveolar type II cells that are actively dividing during a normal growth state may not be actively synthesizing and storing surfactant, which is different from the process that occurs after lung injury.[112] During development, factors that enhance surfactant phospholipid synthesis include thyroid hormone, EGF, catecholamines, cAMP, estrogens, and prolactin.[113] Factors that inhibit fetal phospholipid synthesis include testosterone and insulin.

Human disease correlates of surfactant abnormalities other than prematurity have been described. Term infants of diabetic mothers often have respiratory distress syndrome.[114] Animal models of maternal diabetes have demonstrated that fetal lungs have abnormalities in surfactant biosynthesis and decreased production of SP-A, SP-B, and SP-C.[115,116] Congenital alveolar proteinosis has recently been attributed to an SP-B deficiency.[117,118]

Several investigators have expanded the understanding of the surfactant abnormalities in acute respiratory distress syndrome, a disease process in children and adults that is somewhat similar to infant respiratory distress syndrome.[119] Recognized surfactant abnormalities include no overall change in phospholipid content but decreased amounts of phosphatidylcholine and phosphatidylglycerol and increased quantities of phosphatidylinositol, phosphatidylethanolamine, sphingomyelin, and phosphatidylserine.[120-124] When patients at risk for acute respiratory distress syndrome were examined prospectively, those who developed the syndrome had surfactant abnormalities that included reductions in phosphatidylcholine, phosphatidylglycerol, SP-A, and SP-B content.[124,125] Patients at risk who developed the syndrome had a fourfold increase in the in vitro surface tension of their endogenous pulmonary surfactant compared to normal, whereas those at risk who failed to develop the syndrome had only a twofold increase in the endogenous surface tension.[124] The technical aspects of efficient surfactant delivery to older children and adults with this syndrome remain to be determined, but preliminary investigational trials to assess the efficacy of surfactant administration had encouraging results, and additional trials are being implemented.[126-128]

Repair of the Pulmonary Epithelium after Lung Injury

An essential function of the alveolar type II cell is repair of the alveolar epithelial barrier after lung injury. Several disease processes injure the lung, but repair of the alveolus appears to be similar despite the diversity of offending agents. However, the etiologic factor likely influences the ability of the alveolar type II cell to repair the alveolus and ultimately determines whether restoration of normal lung parenchyma occurs or fibrosis develops.

Alveolar type II cells are the progenitors of alveolar type I cells, both in normal cycling of alveolar epithelium and after different types of lung injury.[110] Animal models of alveolar injury include bacterial pneumonia, nitrogen dioxide inhalation, and hyperoxic exposure.[129-132] Alveolar type I cells are more susceptible to noxious stimuli.[133] Because type I cells cover most of the alveolar surface area, loss of the alveolar-capillary barrier results in critical alterations in pulmonary gas exchange. Alveolar flooding with proteinaceous fluid ensues, and if the alveolus is not repaired, interstitial fibroblasts invade the space and fibrosis occurs.[134] Alveolar type II cells produce antioxidant defense mechanisms that include manganese superoxide dismutase, catalase, and glutathione.[135,136] An immunohistochemical study of postmortem lung tissue from infants with bronchopulmonary dyplasia demonstrated intense staining of manganese superoxide dismutase compared to that in nondiseased control tissue.[137] In spite of these mechanisms, they remain susceptible to oxidant injury.

The extracellular matrix is important in the restoration of the alveolar barrier. Elastin, a protein critical to the formation of alveolar structure and the maintenance of elastic recoil within the lungs, appears to be more vulnerable to injury in the developing lung.[138] In "infant" animal models, hyperoxia decreases the gene expression of tropoelastin, histologically decreases elastin fiber length and structure, and abnormally increases the compliance of the lungs after exposure.[139,140] Approximately two thirds of human infants with exposure to a fraction of inspired oxygen of more than 60% for more than 5 days have evidence of increased elastase in their bronchoalveolar lavage fluid and increased urinary desmosine excretion suggestive of degradation of elastin fibers.[141] In human lungs, types I, III, and IV collagen and laminin are found within the basement membrane and interstitium. In fibrotic states, increased deposition of all three collagen subtypes is observed outside the basal lamina, with primary deposition of type I collagen during the more progressive, irreversible phases of lung fibrosis.[142]

The ability of alveolar type II cells to repair the epithelial barrier is likely influenced by growth factors that trigger or inhibit the cells' ability to divide and reconstitute the alveolus. Several known growth factors stimulate alveolar type II cell growth in vitro. These include EGF, TGF-α, IGF-I, aFGF, hepatocyte growth factor, cholera toxin, and KGF.[110,143,144] Which of these factors are important in vivo is unknown. In vivo, KGF administered intratracheally to rats induces marked proliferation of alveolar type II cells in a dose-dependent fashion, and the normal rat lung constitutively expresses both KGF and recombinant KGF mRNA.[145] Whether KGF participates in normal lung growth or repair after lung injury remains unknown.

In humans with pulmonary fibrosis, histologic antibody studies have implicated several factors in the evolution of idiopathic pulmonary fibrosis. These include PDGF-α, PDGF-β, tumor necrosis factor-α (TNF-α), TGF-β, and endothelin-1.[146-151] The growth factors that stimulate or inhibit the normal reparative process in the alveolus could have important clinical implications if specific agents can be administered to enhance the ability of the lung to repair itself in the face of ongoing pulmonary injury. (See Chapter 7 for a more detailed discussion of lung injury and repair.)

Fluid Secretion and Absorption

The alveolar type II cell actively maintains fluid homeostasis within the alveolus.[110,152] During in utero growth and development, the type II cell secretes fluid into the developing alveolus, and it is theorized that this mechanism helps promote alveolar growth via physical mechanisms and possibly stimulatory growth factors within the fluid lining the primitive embryonic alveolus.[153] In vivo, the absorption of fluid from the alveolus is enhanced by β-agonists and hormones, presumably through the up-regulation of sodium-potassium adenosinetriphosphatase–sensitive sodium channels.[154-157] In vitro, human fetal lung epithelial cells form domelike cysts that have a negative luminal side, supporting the hypothesis that the alveolar fluid is secreted primarily by chloride channels actively at the basolateral membrane and passively at the apical surface.[158] At birth, the type II cell switches from a secretory cell to an absorptive cell, and studies suggest that delay of this transition results in transient tachypnea of the newborn.[159-161] After birth, the type II cell continues to absorb water through sodium channels, which may help prevent the formation of pulmonary edema.[161,162]

Host Defense Mechanisms

Alveolar type II cells exhibit characteristics suggesting that they may defend the alveolus against infection. Rat and human type II pneumocytes synthesize C3, C2, C4, C5a, and factor B in vitro; these proteins are important in inflammation, immunologic reaction, and cytotoxicity.[163] SP-A and SP-D bind *Pneumocystis carinii* and influenza virus type A, respectively, in vitro.[164,165] Incubation of rat alveolar macrophages with SP-A enhances the phagocytosis of *Staphylococcus aureus* by 70% in vitro; yet it paradoxically decreases the superoxide burst produced by alveolar macrophages in separate studies.[166,167] SP-A also increases the aggregation and opsonization of *Haemophilus influenzae* type A but not type B in vitro.[168] SP-D may also bind to alveolar macrophages to enhance the phagocytosis of microbes.[169] Alveolar type II cells also secrete three cytokines (macrophage chemoattractant protein-1, interleukin-6 [IL-6], and leukotriene B_4) and nitric oxide (NO) in vitro.[170-173] These bioactive substances may modulate the immune response in the lung. Which of these factors is most important and whether these alveolar type II cell products function in vivo remain to be determined.

AIRWAY-LINING CELLS

Growth, Development, and Maturation

At least eight different types of cells line the conducting airways and maintain the integrity of the epithelial barrier. Of these cells, Clara cells, presecretory cells, and basal cells are presumed to be responsible for the regeneration of the airway epithelial barrier.[174] Clara cells differentiate into ciliated cells in vitro.[175,176] Presecretory cells differentiate into goblet cells and ciliated cells, whereas basal cells differentiate into ciliated cells and squamous cells.[174] It is also hypothesized that presecretory cells may be precursors for basal cells or vice versa.[174] During the pseudoglandular phase of development, neuroendocrine cells are the first differentiated airway cells. They are found initially at airway branch points and may be important in branching morphogenesis.[177] Chronologically, ciliated cells, secretory cells, and basal cells differentiate afterward.[174] During in utero development, studies in rats, rabbits, and the rhesus monkey suggest that nonciliated bronchiolar epithelial cells (Clara cells) are the precursors of ciliated bronchiolar epithelial cells.[178-182] In rabbits, this transition to ciliated cells occurs over a short time immediately before and after birth.[183]

Ciliated cells first appear within the human trachea at about week 11 of gestation. Ciliogenesis progresses in a proximal to distal sequence, with the appearance of ciliated cells through the terminal bronchioles by birth in humans.[184] By week 24 of gestation the pattern and number of ciliated epithelial cells within the trachea resemble those of an adult. The percentage of ciliated cells is higher in more proximal airways, numbering about 50%, and progressively decreases in more peripheral airways.[185]

Early secretory cells begin to appear in the human trachea during weeks 12 and 13 of gestation.[186] The number increases dramatically between weeks 15 and 19 to occupy about 50% of the tracheal epithelial surface and then decreases to about 10% to 15% of the tracheal surface by 24 weeks.[184] Goblet cells, which account for about 15% of the tracheobronchial surface, are likely derived from secretory cells.[187] Goblet, serous, and basal cells begin to appear around week 16 of gestation in the human.[188] How and when the cells begin to assume secretory functions in vivo in the human remain unknown, although studies that examined tracheal mucin and lysozyme secretion from human autopsy specimens suggest that maturational changes in cellular function occur.[189]

Airway submucosal glands develop between weeks 10 and 13 of gestation as evaginations of the tracheobronchial epithelium into the surrounding airway mesenchyme.[190] Interestingly, human fetal lung fibroblasts grown in coculture with adult human tracheobronchial epithelial cells induce a similar phenomena in vitro. Epithelial cells grow into a collagen matrix and form submucosal glandlike structures in the presence of fetal lung fibroblasts but not adult lung fibroblasts.[191]

Airway Epithelial Cells: Structure and Function

Airway epithelial cells protect the conducting airways and distal lung parenchyma from injury by both physical and biochemical mechanisms and effectively maintain an interface with air that enhances gas transport to the alveolar gas-exchanging units. Each cell type within the airway has overlapping functions in some aspects and unique functions in others.

Clara cells are nonciliated, nonmucous secretory cells that are found in the trachea distally through the terminal bronchioles in humans. Clara cells in different locations within the tracheobronchial tree have slightly different secretory products. For example, distal airway cells lack the Clara cell 10-kD protein (CC10) present in proximal airway Clara cells.[192] Clara cells synthesize surfactant SP-A, SP-B, SP-D, secretory leukocyte protease inhibitor, a trypsin-like protease, uteroglobin (CC10), and β-galactosidase–binding lectin.[193] CC10 and uteroglobin may modulate the inflammatory response by inhibiting phospholipase A_2.[194,195] Secretory leukocyte protease inhibitors likely counterbalance the release of endogenous, potentially damaging proteases by neutrophils that are intermittently recruited to the airways to battle noxious factors. The surfactant apoproteins and trypsinlike proteins may be important in the defense of the lung against infectious agents. Clara cells also have abundant amounts of cytochrome P-450 and flavin-containing monooxygenases, which paradoxically seems to render these cells more susceptible to injury by noxious stimuli.[193,196] Clara cells are also important in the regeneration of the tracheal epithelium, and Clara cells and ciliated cells but not basal cells in vitro repopulate the epithelium of a denuded trachea.[197,198]

Basal epithelial cells derived from rabbit tracheal epithelium repopulate a denuded trachea with a columnar, pseudostratified epithelium that contains ciliated, basal, and goblet cells.[199,200] Basal cells are firmly attached to the basal lamina and may serve as the anchoring cells for ciliated columnar cells.[201,202]

Ciliated cells are present throughout the conducting airways and help clear the airways of infectious agents and other inert noxious factors with their rhythmic ciliary action that propels the airway surface liquid toward the oropharynx. Goblet cells likely secrete an acidic, mucin type of glycoprotein into the airway that traps pulmonary irritants within the airway surface liquid.[203] What stimulates goblet cell secretion remains unknown, but studies suggest that neutrophil elastase, cathepsin G, bacterial proteases, and irritating gases enhance secretion.[204-207] Patients with cystic fibrosis and chronic bronchitis have increased numbers of mucous cells in their airways.[203] The precise function of other epithelial cells within the airway, including brush, serous, and small mucous granule cells, remains unknown, although they likely help produce airway surface liquid.

Neuroendocrine cells within the airway occur as single epithelial cells interspersed within the epithelial layer or as clusters of cells bordered by Clara cells.[41] These clusters of cells, or neuroepithelial bodies, are often found at bronchiolar bifurcations.[208] These cells have abundant cholinesterase activity, which implies that they may be important in the regulation of airway epithelial cell secretion. They also contain important neuropeptides, including calcitonin gene–related peptide, serotonin, and bombesin.[41] These neuropeptides are likely important in the neuroregulation of both airway secretion and motor tone via the noncholinergic nonadrenergic system, and neuroepithelial bodies may be innervated by the cholinergic system.[209] The immunoreactivity of pulmonary neuroendocrine cells increases in the airways of infants with bronchopulmonary dysplasia at autopsy.[210,211] How these cells regulate antenatal and postnatal airway secretion and airway reactivity in vivo is poorly understood.

LUNG FIBROBLASTS

The major cell type in the lung interstitium is the fibroblast. Several types of fibroblasts, all derived from mesenchymal tissue, have been described within the lung.[212] These include interstitial fibroblasts, contractile interstitial cells or myofibroblasts, and pericytes. In addition to fibroblasts, the interstitium in the mature lung contains other cell types such as lymphocytes, plasma cells, and mast cells. During development, significant changes occur in the type of fibroblasts composing the interstitial compartment. In early development, a rapidly proliferating fibroblast filled with neutral lipid has been found. This has been called the *lipid interstitial cell.* This cell is frequently found adjacent to a more typical fibroblast that does not contain lipid. As the lung matures, the number of these cells gradually decreases, and in the fully mature lung, few are seen.[213] The interstitial fibroblast plays a primary role in maintaining the integrity of the alveolar compartment, through both its anatomic location and its production of collagen and other matrix components. Types I and III collagen are the major extracellular matrix secretory products of the lung fibroblast.[214] However, it is now clear that in addition to their role in the maintenance of airspace integrity, resident lung fibroblasts are very important in the generation of immune and inflammatory responses within the lung.[215] Fibroblasts actively produce a wide variety of cytokines (Box 5-2). This cytokine production enables the fibroblast to regulate not only the function of other lung fibroblasts but also the function within the lung of macrophages, lymphocytes, endothelial cells, SMCs, epithelial cells, chondrocytes, and nervous tissues. The fibroblast produces and releases other products that enable it to play an important role in regulating the lung tissue response to injury. Fibroblasts produce nitrites and nitrates, which have actions that are probably similar to those of endothelial NO. In addition, reactive oxygen species (such as superoxide), prostaglandins, and components of the alternative and classic pathways of complement (such as C1, C2, factors B and H, C4, C6, C7, C8, and C9) have also been reported. Also, as previously noted, it is clear that the fibroblast plays an important role during lung development in maturation of the alveolar epithelium. The fibroblast produces a factor that stimulates the differentiation and synthesis of pulmonary surfactant by alveolar type II cells. It is possible that at least parts of this cascade can be recapitulated in the response of the adult lung to injury.

In addition to the major types of fibroblasts described, there is much heterogeneity within the interstitial fibroblasts themselves.[216] Fibroblasts, like many other cells, consist of subpopulations with unique phenotypes and functions. Differences in morphology, expression of surface markers, antigen presentation to T cells, ability to synthesize collagen, and cytokine production in fibroblast subpopulations have been reported. It is now clear that unique subpopulations of fibroblasts demonstrate very specific responses to injury. The inflammatory responses that typically precede fibrotic induction may be controlled by one subset of resident fibroblasts. Another subset may be important for fibroblast hyperplasia and extensive extracellular matrix production, which are the hallmarks of fibrosis.[217] The development of strategies to prevent or reverse debilitating and potentially fatal lung fibrosis will require an understanding of how and why specific subsets of fibroblasts are activated in lung injury states.

BOX 5-2
Selected Cytokins Produced by Fibroblasts

IL-1α
Pro-IL-1β
IL-6
IL-8
Granulocyte-macrophage colony–stimulating factors
Granulocyte colony-stimulating factor
Macrophage colony-stimulating factor
bFGF
TGF-β
Multipotent growth factor/stem cell growth factor
PDGF
IGF-I
IGF-II
Nerve growth factor
Monocyte chemotactic protein-1/monocyte chemotactic and activating factor
β-galactoside-binding protein
Neuroleukin
Cytokine inhibitory factor
gro
Migration-stimulating factor
EGF

ENDOTHELIUM

The endothelium creates a nonthrombogenic, semipermeable barrier between the bloodstream and all extravascular tissue and fluid compartments in the lung. In addition, it influences vascular tone, hemostasis, growth, differentiation, chemotaxis, and the vascular response to injury. Thus knowledge of endothelial function is critical for understanding lung function in health and disease.

Regulation of Vascular Tone

The vasomotor tone of the blood vessel is determined by the contractile state of the SMC. The endothelial cell plays an important role in modulating SMC contractility through the synthesis, transport, and metabolism of various vasoactive substances.[218-220] Both vasodilating and vasoconstricting substances are produced by the endothelial cell. Changes in the oxygen content and chemical composition of the blood as well as alterations in pulsatile blood flow (with resultant changes in shear stress and pressure-induced distention across the vessel wall) modulate the synthesis or metabolism of vasoactive substances by the endothelial cell. Furthermore, changes in intracellular messengers such as cAMP, cyclic guanosine monophosphate (cGMP), and calcium within the endothelial cell regulate its production and the release of vasoactive mediators. Thus regulation of vascular tone is highly complex and must reflect a balance in the local production of vasodilating and constricting factors (Fig. 5-4).

Endothelial-Derived Relaxing Factor and NO

Endothelial-derived relaxing factor (EDRF), or endothelial-derived NO, is a potent vasodilator discovered in 1980 by Furchgott and Zawadzki.[221] They demonstrated that an intact endothelial lining was necessary for acetylcholine to dilate strips of arteries in an organ bath and that stimulation of en-

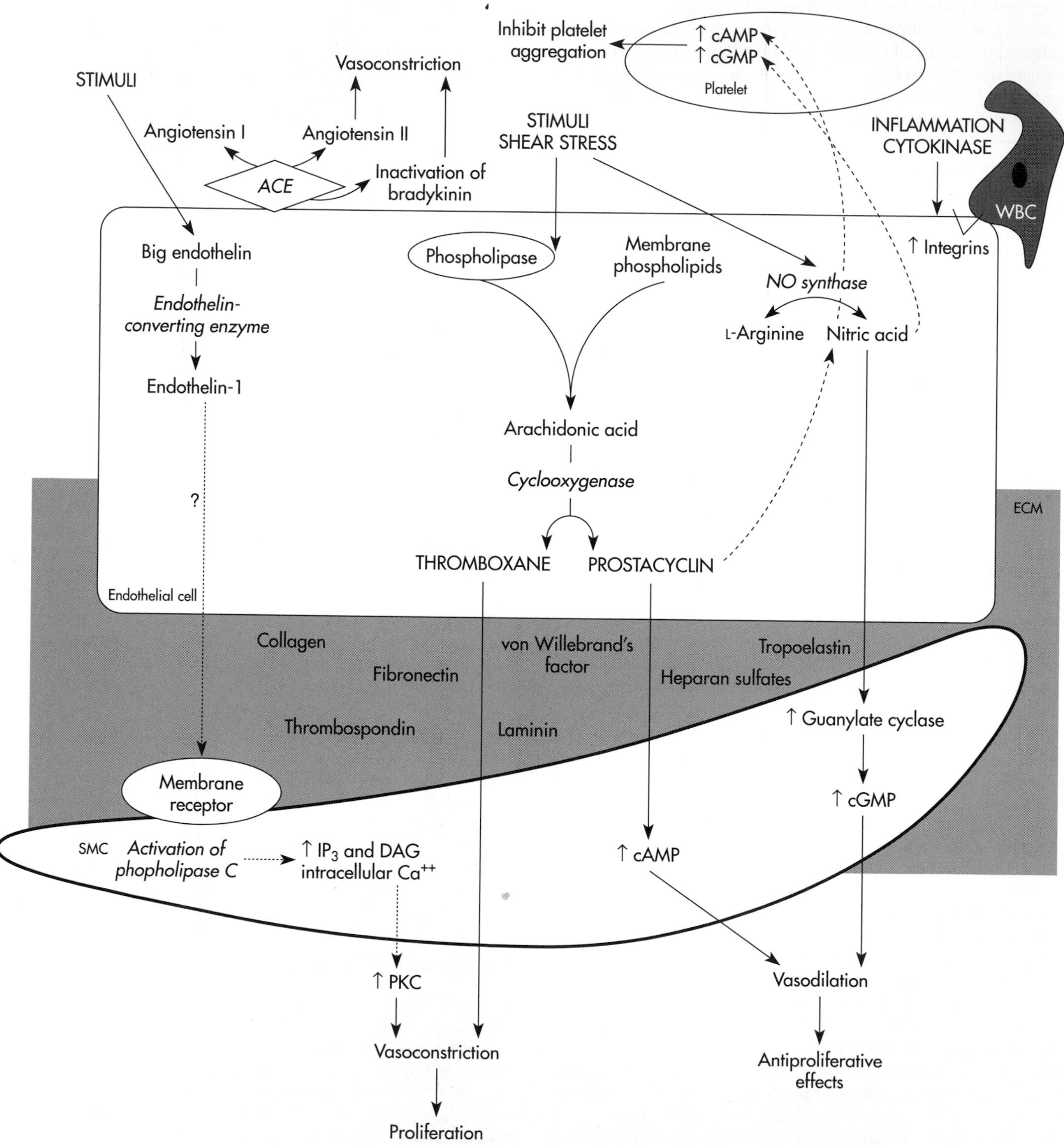

Fig. 5-4. Potential interactions between the endothelium and SMCs under normal and pathologic conditions. The endothelial cells can influence both the local vascular environment and distal vascular beds. *ACE,* Angiotensin-converting enzyme; *WBC,* white blood cell; *ECM,* extracellular matrix; *IP$_3$,* inositol triphosphate; *DAG,* diacylglycerol; *Ca^{++},* calcium; *PKC,* protein kinase C.

dothelial cell muscarinic receptors caused the release of an EDRF capable of causing the underlying smooth muscle to relax. EDRF was later identified as *endothelial-derived NO* using simultaneous chemical and bioassays demonstrating that the NO released from stimulated endothelial cells reproduced the actions of EDRF.[222,223] The actions of EDRF and endothelial-derived NO are both inhibited by hemoglobin and superoxide ions, providing further proof that they are the same compound.[224]

NO is synthesized from L-arginine through a multistep oxidation reaction catalyzed by NO synthase.[225-227] The second product of the reaction is L-citrulline. Physical forces and agonists that stimulate increases in intracellular levels of calcium (which combines with calmodulin to stimulate NO synthase) all increase the production of endothelial NO. Shear stress, acetylcholine, bradykinin, histamine, serotonin, adenosine triphosphate (ATP), adenosine diphosphate (ADP), substance P, and thrombin all stimulate endothelial NO production. NO diffuses into the underlying SMC and stimulates soluble guanylate cyclase, which increases the levels of cGMP in the SMC and triggers vasorelaxation. NO acts predominantly as a local hormone because it is rapidly inactivated by hemoglobin, a scavenger that prevents any systemic effect of NO as it escapes into the bloodstream.

It appears that the blood vessels of healthy humans are continuously dilated by NO released from endothelial cells.[228-230] NO production increases during heavy exercise and infections. Indeed, the rapid fall in blood pressure seen in endotoxin shock may result from an immediate increase in NO levels stimulated by *Escherichia coli* lipopolysaccharide.[231]

In addition to vasodilation, NO has many effects on the blood vessel. NO inhibits platelet aggregation and adhesion by increasing cGMP levels in platelets.[232] NO also inhibits SMC and fibroblast proliferation in culture.[233] This antiproliferative action may participate in limiting the smooth muscle growth that occurs with vascular injury.

Prostacyclin

Prostacyclin (prostaglandin I_2) is another potent vasodilator produced by endothelial cells.[234,235] Prostacyclin is synthesized via cyclooxygenase enzymes from the essential fatty acid, arachidonic acid, which is released from membrane phospholipids by phospholipase A_2. Prostacyclin released from the endothelial cell binds to specific receptors on SMCs (or platelets) and activates adenylate cyclase, thus increasing intracellular cAMP, which decreases intracellular levels of calcium levels and causes relaxation. The half-life of prostacyclin is short, only 6 minutes in whole blood.[236] The synthesis and secretion of prostacyclin is modulated by numerous agonists. Thrombin induces prostacyclin synthesis by modulating the intracellular accumulation of inositol triphosphate, thereby increasing intracellular calcium levels. Prostacyclin synthesis is also stimulated by histamine, bradykinin, IL-1, interferon-α, interferon-γ, activated neutrophils, and numerous other growth factors and cytokines.[219,237-240] On the other hand, aspirin, nonsteroidal antiinflammatory drugs, and cyclosporine inhibit the synthesis of prostacyclin by inhibiting the enzyme cyclooxygenase.[241,242] The release of prostacyclin is also inhibited by dexamethasone and cigarette smoke.[243]

In addition to its role as a vasodilator, prostacyclin is a potent inhibitor of platelet aggregation.[234] Prostacyclin, by inducing rises in platelet cAMP levels, is the strongest known inhibitor of platelet aggregation. It also inhibits changes in platelet shape, binding of factor VIII and fibrinogen to platelet surface receptors, platelet secretion, and the development of platelet procoagulant activity. Prostacyclin acts synergistically with EDRF to suppress platelet activation.[244] Many of the same agonists activate both prostacyclin and EDRF synthesis by increasing intracellular calcium levels.

Endothelin

In addition to the vasodilators produced by endothelial cells, several vasoconstrictors are produced.[218,219] Both the vasorelaxant and antiaggregatory activities of prostacyclin and NO are balanced by the activities of endogenously produced vasoconstrictors (Fig. 5-5). Endothelin-1 is the most potent vasoconstrictor described to date.[245,246] It is cleaved from a prepropeptide, big endothelin, by an endopeptidase, endothelin-converting enzyme. The release of endothelin-1 is stimulated by thrombin, epinephrine, and calcium ionophore. The cyclic deformation of endothelial cells in culture also results in the increased synthesis of endothelin-1. Although the exact mechanism of its actions are unknown, the current view is that endothelin-1 binds to a specific membrane receptor, causing the activation of phospholipase C, the release of inositol phosphates and diacylglycerol, and increased levels of intracellular calcium.[246] Subsequent activation of protein kinase C takes place. In addition, some of the vasoconstrictor effects of endothelin may be mediated by the release of thromboxane. More important, NO down-regulates (at least in vitro) the production of endothelin by endothelial cells.

Endothelin-1 also stimulates neutrophil adhesion to endothelial cells in culture. The neutrophil adhesion can be augmented by NO inhibitors, indicating further potential interactions between NO and endothelin-1. In addition to its potent vasoconstrictor activities, endothelin-1 is a mitogen for SMCs and fibroblasts and therefore could play a role in the vascular remodeling that accompanies some pulmonary diseases.[247,248]

Endothelin-1 can be found in low concentrations in the systemic circulation of healthy adults but at concentrations not thought to be high enough to induce hypertension. Higher concentrations are postulated to exist at the endothelial-smooth muscle junction, and therefore endothelin-1 is thought of as a local hormone. Elevated serum concentrations of endothelin-1 have been found in adults with acute respiratory distress (acute respiratory distress syndrome) and in neonates with persistent pulmonary hypertension, indicating a potential role for this vasoconstrictor in certain types of pulmonary hypertension.[249-250]

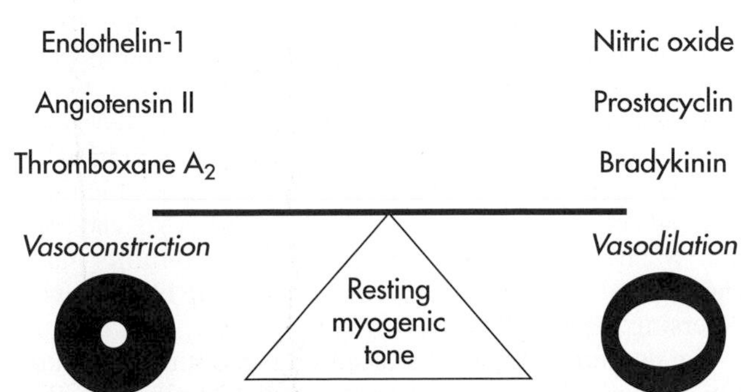

Fig. 5-5. Balance between vasodilator and vasoconstrictor production that controls the resting vascular tone. Changes in the production of products on either side of the balance may have significant effects on vascular tone.

Angiotensin and Bradykinin

Angiotensin-converting enzyme, located on the luminal surface of the endothelial cell, catalyzes the formation of angiotensin II, a potent vasoconstrictor, from its inactive precursor angiotensin I. Some 90% of this conversion occurs in the lungs. In addition to its traditional role as a vasoconstrictor, angiotensin II stimulates vascular smooth muscle hypertrophy and hyperplasia. Bradykinin, another vasoactive peptide, is also inactivated by angiotensin-converting enzyme. Bradykinin affects vascular tone directly and indirectly through the release of mediators such as NO and prostacyclin. Bradykinin also appears to have antiproliferative actions, which are probably mediated via its stimulation of NO and prostacyclin release.

Hemostatic Properties

The vascular endothelium actively participates in the regulation of the hemostatic system by secreting, synthesizing, and binding different coagulation and fibrinolytic components, lipid compounds, and glycosaminoglycans. Normally the intact vessel wall provides a thromboresistant surface. Disruption of the vessel wall exposes the extracellular matrix, which binds and activates platelets and coagulation factors, favoring a more prothrombic state. In addition, certain local stimuli may induce procoagulant factors, inhibit the production of antithrombotic factor by endothelial cells, or cause both reactions.

The endothelial cells control blood flow by modulating vascular tone through the release and metabolism of vasodilators and vasoconstrictors, as previously mentioned. Normal blood flow is important in regulating the state of activation of platelets and procoagulant factors. Low flow allows the unopposed accumulation of activated coagulation factors and platelets, which can result in the formation of a thrombus. The reestablishment of normal flow before thrombus formation appears to have dispersive effects on the procoagulant factors. The platelets can be partially inactivated by the large concentrations of locally produced EDRF and prostacyclin. 13-Hydroxyoctadecadienoic acid, which is synthesized by endothelial cells from linoleic acid, is also a potent inhibitor of platelet adhesion, aggregation, and thromboxane A_2 production.[251] Unlike prostacyclin, synthesis of 13-hydroxyoctadecadienoic acid is suppressed by thrombin and trypsin. Antithrombin III, endothelial cell surface mucopolysaccharide, activated protein C, and other circulating protease inhibitors can inactivate the activated coagulation factors circulating in the blood. In addition, endothelial cells are capable of interfering with platelet activation by inactivating norepinephrine, serotonin, and histamine.

Activated platelets release ADP, which further recruits and activates platelets, allowing the formation of a platelet clot. Ectoenzymes on the endothelial cell surface enable the endothelial cells to metabolize ADP and ATP to AMP and adenosine.[252] The conversion to adenosine both inhibits platelet function and vasodilates the vessel, increasing blood flow and dispersing the platelet clot.

The nonthrombogenic surface of the endothelium not only prevents activation and aggregation of platelets but also allows for the inactivation of thrombin and activated coagulation factors.[253] Antithrombin III is a physiologically important protein in the prevention of thrombus formation. Plasma antithrombin III inactivates thrombin by forming covalent thrombin-antithrombin complexes. Heparan sulfate, which is synthesized by and is present on the endothelial cell membranes, greatly accelerates the formation of these complexes.[254]

Inactivation of thrombin also occurs by the interaction of protein C, protein S, and thrombomodulin.[255] Protein C is synthesized in the liver, and when activated by thrombin, it activates factors Va and VIIIa. The activation of protein C occurs very slowly unless thrombomodulin, an endothelial cell surface protein, is present to bind to thrombin. Endotoxin, IL-1, TNF, and hypoxia all suppress thrombomodulin activity, likely by suppressing transcription. Protein S, which is synthesized and secreted by endothelial cells, markedly potentiates activated protein C.

Thrombin is also inactivated by binding or forming a complex with protease nexin 1, a protein secreted by endothelial cells.[256] Complex formation is accelerated by heparan sulfate on the endothelial cell surface. The thrombin-protease nexin 1 complex binds to and then is internalized by the endothelial cells. The internalized complex is then inactivated by lysosomal enzymes. The exact in vivo role of protease nexin 1 is unclear, since most thrombin is inactivated by antithrombin III.

Blood vessel injury can induce endothelial and platelet responses that enhance coagulation. For instance, thrombin can stimulate endothelial cells to express tissue factor.[257] Normally, endothelial cells express little or no tissue factor. Endotoxin, TNF, hypoxia, and leukocytes also can markedly increase tissue factor activity in endothelial cells.[258] Tissue factor reacts with calcium and factor VII to accelerate the activation of factor X. Factor Xa in turn activates factors VIII and IX. Factor IX binds to the endothelial cell surface with factor X, localizing the coagulation process and limiting the circulation of activated factors.

Injury to the endothelium can also cause denudation of the endothelial cells and thus expose the subendothelium, or basement membrane. Collagen types IV and V as well as microfibrils present in the subendothelium are all capable of causing platelet aggregation and subsequent thromboxane release. In addition, von Willebrand's factor (vWF), vitronectin, fibronectin, and thrombospondin, all proteins normally present in the subendothelium, may act as substrates for platelet attachment. vWF appears particularly important in platelet adhesion to the subendothelium. Endothelial cells are known to synthesize and secrete functionally active vWF. Platelets contain one or more surface receptors for vWF, and it is likely that platelets adhere to the subendothelium via vWF. Weibel-Palade bodies appear to be the storage sites within endothelial cells for vWF. IL-1, TNF, endotoxin, amphotoxin, thrombin, and complement C5b-9 all stimulate the short-term release of vWF.

Platelet-activating factor is a potent activator of platelets, monocytes, and polymorphonuclear leukocytes (PMNs) that is produced by endothelial cells.[259,260] It induces PMN adherence to endothelial cells and promotes chemotaxis through endothelial cell monolayers. Many cytokines, including TNF, IL-1, angiotensin II, histamine, bradykinin, and ATP, stimulate endothelial cell production of platelet-activating factor. Prostacyclin inhibits the production of platelet-activating factor.

Growth and Repair

After relatively minor injuries to the vascular endothelium, it appears that repair is achieved by the migration of adjacent endothelial cells into the wound. This is then followed by endothelial proliferation, which replaces the dead or denuded cells. More significant injuries often require or at least stimulate the migration or proliferation of medial SMCs and adventitial fibroblasts. These cell types are motile, synthesize connective tissue, and secrete collagenases and elastases and other proteases, which allows them to repair and remodel the vessel wall.[261] Endothelial cells secrete a number of growth-promoting and growth-inhibiting factors that alter SMC and fibroblast function and replication and thus play an important role in modulating vascular repair.

Endothelial cells produce a heparin-binding growth factor family of related proteins, at least five of which have been isolated and cloned. The best known members of this family are aFGF and bFGF. In addition, higher-molecular-weight forms of bFGF have been observed. Both proteins bind to cellular receptors and induce the proliferation and synthesis of DNA and the release of collagenase and plasminogen activator in endothelial cells as well as other cell types. Although the mechanism by which aFGF and bFGF are released from endothelial cells is uncertain, it is known that bFGF does bind to heparin sulfate proteoglycans in the extracellular matrix. This binding may provide a reservoir of bFGF that can be released over time by either heparinase or plasmin and may thus be important in the vascular response to injury.

Endothelial cells also produce and secrete a factor called *vascular permeability factor.* This factor promotes endothelial cell growth and blood vessel leakage and stimulates angiogenesis by binding to a receptor on the endothelial cell surface. However, unlike PDGF, aFGF, and bFGF, it does not stimulate the growth of SMCs or fibroblasts. An important physiologic stimulus of its release in vitro is tissue or local hypoxia. It is possible that under hypoxic conditions in the lung, this factor plays an important role in new blood vessel formation.

Endothelial cells secrete abluminally a PDGF-like protein that binds to specific PDGF receptors on both fibroblasts and SMCs. PDGF is mitogenic and chemotactic for SMCs, fibroblasts, and endothelial cells that express PDGF receptors (not all endothelial cells express the receptor). Various factors, including endotoxin, IL-1, IL-6, thrombin, TNF, TGF-β, and factor Xa, increase both PDGF-α and β-chain mRNA expression as well as PDGF synthesis. PDGF, in addition to its effects on smooth muscle and fibroblast growth, is vasoactive and may play a role in controlling blood vessel tone under conditions of high PDGF production.

Endothelial cells also secrete substances that may inhibit SMC proliferation. Endothelial cells secrete a heparin-like inhibitor of SMC growth that is active at low nanomolar concentrations. In addition, TGF-β is synthesized and secreted by endothelial cells and can have either growth-inhibitory or in certain situations, growth-promoting effects on underlying SMCs.

Barrier Properties

The endothelium forms a relatively impermeable membrane. The endothelial cells are linked together by semicontinuous tight junctions.[262] Gases readily diffuse through these junctions, but the blood's cellular and fluid elements are restricted. Several mechanisms of transport have been documented. Substances can also pass between the cells. Substances can be internalized from the cell surface via plasmalemma vesicles, which then associate with tubulovesicular networks within the cytoplasm of the endothelial cell. The substances are then released into the subendothelial space by the vesicles.[263,264] This transcytosis can be receptor mediated, in which case specific carrier proteins on the cell surface bind the ligand to be transported, or can be nonspecific.[265-267]

Normally blood cells do not attach or migrate through the endothelium. In response to inflammatory stimuli, all leukocytes can attach via interactions with adhesion molecule receptor-ligands, which facilitate the emigration of PMNs.[268] There are three classes of adhesion proteins: integrins, members of the immunoglobulin gene superfamily, and selectins.[269,270] Integrins, transmembrane proteins located on the surface of all leukocytes, interact with the endothelial ligand, the proteins of the immunoglobulin gene superfamily. The selectins are surface proteins expressed on both the endothelial cell and the leukocyte. These adhesion proteins can be constitutively expressed or synthesized after specific stimulation. In general, the interaction among the receptor-ligands slows movement of the PMN, allowing it to adhere to the endothelium. The PMN becomes activated by any number of cytokines and then migrates between endothelial cells.[271,272] This is an area of intense interest because of the role that PMNs play in host defense and immune surveillance.

Extracellular Matrix Production

The basement membrane on which endothelial cells lie is composed of extracellular matrix proteins secreted by the endothelial cells and SMCs, probably facilitating interactions between both cell types. The components of the extracellular matrix influence cell behavior and contribute to morphogenesis. The extracellular matrix directs cell migration, expression of gene products, and cell division and modifies cell shape and intracellular association.

Endothelial cells express receptors for fibronectin, laminin, collagen type IV, fibrinogen, and vitronectin.[273,274] These receptors allow the endothelial cells to adhere to the extracellular matrix, to proliferate, and to migrate. The expression of the receptors can be altered by growth factors, glycosaminoglycans, and inflammatory mediators present in the extracellular matrix, thereby participating in the control of vascular endothelial cell function.

Laminin is a glycoprotein to which the endothelial cells adhere using specific receptors. Laminin promotes endothelial cell adhesion, proliferation, and growth. The amount of laminin secreted by endothelial cells is increased by decreased cell density (being greatest in areas of angiogenesis) and heat stress. Laminin also influences the SMC, being involved in the maintenance of a more differentiated cell type.

Fibronectin and thrombospondin act as adhesion proteins for endothelial cells and platelets. Endothelial cells adhere, spread, and grow on fibronectin but only adhere to thrombospondin. Both proteins appear to be important in wound healing. Their synthesis increases at sites of healing and inflammation. Angiogenesis is associated with increased fibronectin mRNA signal. Both bind to heparin and heparan sulfates. Heparin decreases fibronectin synthesis.

Heparan sulfates are synthesized by the endothelial cell and are present on the cell membrane and in the extracellular matrix. They have important anticoagulant activities and act as adhesion proteins. The specific heparan sulfate present on the cell surface differs from those found in the extracellular matrix, suggesting different functions for each location. Heparin inhibits SMC proliferation and prevents collagen and elastin cross-linking. This action of heparin has been used to attenuate the remodeling process in experimental pulmonary hypertension. Dermatan sulfate is another glycosaminoglycan synthesized by endothelial cells, and it also functions in anticoagulant activities.

Elastin fragments are chemotactic for endothelial cells, indicating that the disruption of elastin fibers seen with vessel injury may act in the repair process by attracting and activating endothelial cells. Endothelial cells secrete both an elastase and an inhibitor, which together are active in vessel wall remodeling.

VASCULAR SMOOTH MUSCLE

Vascular smooth muscle was initially thought of as a very homogeneous system whose main function was maintenance of vascular tone. More recent findings have altered this thinking, so now, vascular SMCs are seen as a very heterogeneous group with diverse cellular functions.[275-277]

In addition to developmentally regulated differences in SMC phenotype, there exists both regional and local phenotype heterogeneity. Phenotypic differences and differences in the production of elastin and collagen have been demonstrated along the longitudinal axis of the aorta. More recently, phenotypically distinct SMC populations have been documented in bovine lobar and main pulmonary arteries.[277] When immunochemical techniques were used to determine SMC-specific contractile and cytoskeletal proteins, clusters of highly differentiated SMCs were found in the outer media. Adjacent to these highly differentiated SMCs were SMCs that expressed fewer cytoskeletal proteins, and in the inner media, there was a narrow band of cells negative for all SMC markers. When the same SMC markers were used, distinct SMC populations were identified in fetal, neonatal, and adult bovine main pulmonary arteries. Thus the smooth muscle layer of pulmonary vessels is composed of heterogeneous populations of SMCs, which may respond very differently to the same stimuli.

In general, the contractile or vasodilator responses of smooth muscle result from the activation of surface receptors that change membrane characteristics (i.e., depolarization or hyperpolarization). This results in the activation of second messengers, which then causes a change in ion fluxes. The culmination of this process is the functional response of the vascular SMC, which may be contraction, proliferation, secretion, or dilation.

Surface receptors on the SMC convert external stimuli into cellular responses through various signal-transduction pathways. A limited number of second messengers can stimulate many diverse responses. All transmembrane glycoprotein receptors contain an external ligand-specific region, a hydrophobic anchor traversing the membrane, and a submembranous region. Contiguity between external and internal receptor domains is necessary for the generation of transmembrane signals. Three ligand-operated receptor mechanisms have been identified. First, the ligand-operated receptor can possess an intrinsic ion channel where the transmembrane receptor complex controls the intracellular signal and the ion itself is the messenger. In the second type, the cytoplasmic region of the receptor interacts with a submembranous regulatory system (i.e., G proteins). In the third type, the receptor may express specific ligand-dependent enzymatic activity (i.e., tyrosine kinase); in this case the intrinsic catalytic activity of the receptor is the messenger. Once signal transduction is initiated, a series of signal cascades further amplify, regulate, and ultimately terminate the signal, integrating the reactions into a specific response.

The development of myogenic tone depends on the interactions between the contractile proteins myosin and actin.[278] Actin and tropomyosin are attached to the SMC membrane by membrane plaques. Myosin molecule heads are bundled together as the thick filaments. These thick filaments cycle between high- and low-affinity binding to actin in a reaction driven by ATP hydrolysis. Unlike striated muscle, in which there is a highly ordered and banded structure of these filaments, the organization of the SMC filaments (cytoskeleton) remains to be elucidated.

Changes in intracellular concentrations of free ionized calcium ions are the primary determinants of vascular smooth muscle contraction and relaxation.[279] Calcium ions from the extracellular space or from the intracellular stores enter the SMC cytoplasm and activate the enzyme myosin light chain kinase.[280] When actin is present, phosphorylation of the light chains of myosin leads to increased activity of myosin-adenosinetriphosphatase and subsequently cross-bridge formation. Myosin must be dephosphorylated by a phosphatase before relaxation can occur.

A second, calcium-independent system of SMC contraction, which is activated by specific agonists (i.e., prostaglandin F_{2a} and phorbol esters), also exists. Agonist-receptor interaction initiates G protein–mediated activation of phospholipase C. This splits phosphatidylinositol biphosphate from the cell membrane into diacylglycerol and inositol triphosphate. Inositol triphosphate is capable of releasing calcium ions from the sarcoplasmic reticulum. Diacylglycerol activates protein kinase C, which phosphorylates an undefined protein to cause contraction. The protein kinase C mechanism may be important in force maintenance in tonically reactive muscle.[280]

Many responses share the same signal-transduction system. Therefore many vasoactive substances and contractile responses can stimulate SMC proliferation. Binding of certain vasoconstrictors and growth factors to their specific receptors activates phospholipase C. This leads to the generation of inositol triphosphate and diacylglycerol, which leads to increases in intracellular calcium levels. The expression of the protooncogenes c-*fos* and c-*myc* precedes the mitogenic stimulation of quiescent cells. Expression of both protooncogenes is increased by increased levels of calcium and growth factors. In contrast, agents that stimulate the synthesis of cyclic nucleotides (cAMP, cGMP) inhibit vascular cell proliferation. The details of the forces, factors, and interactions of cell-signaling processes that operate under pathologic conditions remain to be elucidated.

REFERENCES

1. Crapo JD, Barry BE, Gehr P, Bachofen M, Weibel ER: Cell number and cell characteristics of the normal human lung, *Am Rev Respir Dis* 126:332-337, 1982.
2. Farmer SG, Hay DW: The airway epithelium. In Lenfant C, ed: *Lung biology in health and disease,* vol 55, Marcel Dekker, 1991, pp 3-39.

Lung Growth and Development

3. Thurlbeck WM: Pre- and postnatal organ development. In Chernick VS, Mellins RB, eds: *Basic mechanisms of pediatric respiratory disease: cellular and integrative,* Philadelphia, 1991, BC Decker, pp 23-35.
4. Inselman LS, Mellins RB: Medical progress: growth and development of the lung, *J Pediatr* 98:1-15, 1981.

5. Bucher U, Reid L: Development of the intrasegmental bronchial tree: the pattern of branching and development of cartilage at various stages of intrauterine life, *Thorax* 16:207-218, 1961.
6. Hislop A, Muir DCF, Jacobsen M, Simon G, Reid L: Postnatal growth and function of the preacinar airways, *Thorax* 27:265-274, 1972.
7. Horsfield K, Gordon WI, Kemp W, Phillips S: Growth of the bronchial tree in man, *Thorax* 42:383-388, 1987.
8. Spooner BS, Wessels MK: Mammalian lung development. I. Interaction in primordium formation and bronchial morphogenesis, *J Exp Zool* 175:445-454, 1970.
9. Wessells MK: Mammalian lung development. I. Interaction formation of morphogenesis of tracheal buds, *J Exp Zool* 175:455-466, 1970.
10. Arden MG, Spearman MA, Adamson IYR: Degradation of type IV collagen during the development of fetal rat lung, *Am J Respir Cell Mol Biol* 9:99-105, 1993.
11. Roman J, McDonald JA: Fibulin's organization into the extracellular matrix of fetal lung fibroblasts is dependent on fibronectin matrix assembly, *Am J Respir Cell Mol Biol* 8:538-545, 1993.
12. Roman J, McDonald JA: Potential role of RGD-binding integrins in mammalian lung morphogenesis, *Development* 112:551-558, 1991.
13. Roman J, McDonald JA: Expression of fibronectin, the α_5 integrin, and α-smooth muscle actin in heart and lung development, *Am J Respir Cell Mol Biol* 6:472-480, 1992.
14. Sannes PL, Burch KK, Khosla J, McCarthy KJ, Couchman JR: Immunohistochemical localization of chondroitin sulfate, chondroitin sulfate proteoglycan, heparan sulfate proteoglycan, entactin, and laminin in basement membranes of postnatal developing and adult rat lungs, *Am J Respir Cell Mol Biol* 8:245-251, 1993.
15. Juul SE, Kinsella MG, Wight TN, Hodson WA: Alterations in nonhuman primate *(M. nemestrina)* lung proteoglycans during normal development and acute hyaline membrane disease, *Am J Respir Cell Mol Biol* 8:299-310, 1993.
16. Brauker JH, Trautman MS, Bernfield M: Syndecan, a cell surface glycoprotein, exhibits a molecular polymorphism during lung development, *Dev Biol* 147:285-292, 1991.
17. Trautman MS, Kimelman J, Bernfield M: Developmental expression of syndecan, an integral membrane proteoglycan, correlates with cell differentiation, *Development* 111:213-220, 1991.
18. Hirai Y, Nose A, Kobayashi S, Takeichi M: Expression and role of E- and P-cadherin adhesion molecules in embryonic histogenesis. I. Lung epithelial morphogenesis, *Development* 105:263-270, 1989.
19. Liley H, Bernfield M: Mechanisms of development and repair of the lung. In Chernick VS, Mellins RB, eds: *Basic mechanisms of pediatric respiratory disease: cellular and integrative,* Philadelphia, 1991, BC Decker, pp 11-22.
20. Guzowski DE, Blau H, Bienkowski RS: Extracellular matrix in developing lung. In Scarpelli EM, ed: *Pulmonary physiology,* 1990, Philadelphia, Lea & Febiger, pp 83-105.
21. Kleinman HK, Schnaper HW: Basement membrane matrices in tissue development, *Am J Respir Cell Mol Biol* 8:238-239, 1993.
22. McGowan SE: Extracellular matrix and the regulation of lung development and repair, *FASEB J* 6:2895-2904, 1992.
23. Boushey HA, Junod A, Perruchoud AP, Wanner A, eds: Integrins and other adhesion molecules, *Am Rev Respir Dis* 148:S27-S87, 1993.
24. Shannon JM: Induction of type II cell differentiation in fetal tracheal epithelium by grafted distal lung mesenchyme, *Dev Biol* 166:600-614, 1994.
25. Shannon JM: Induction of type II cell differentiation in fetal rat tracheal epithelium by grafted pulmonary mesenchyme, *Am Rev Respir Dis* 147:A511, 1993 (abstract).
26. Loosli CG, Potter EL: Pre- and postnatal development of the respiratory portion of the human lung, *Am Rev Respir Dis* 80:5-23, 1959.
27. Amy R, Bowes D, Burri PH: Postnatal growth of the mouse lung, *J Anat* 124:131-151, 1977.
28. Kida K, Yasui S, Utsuyama M: Lung changes resulting from intraperitoneal injections of porcine pancreatic elastase in suckling rats, *Am Rev Respir Dis* 30:1111-1117, 1984.
29. Kida K, Thurlbeck WM: Lack of recovery of lung structure and function following administration of β-amino-propionitrile in the post-natal period, *Am Rev Respir Dis* 122:467-475, 1980.
30. King RJ, Jones MB, Minoo P: Regulation of lung cell proliferation by polypeptide growth factors, *Am J Physiol* 257(2 Pt 1):L23-L38 1989.
31. Uhal BD, Flowers KM, Rannels DE: Type II pneumocyte proliferation in vitro: problems and future directions, *Am J Physiol* 261(suppl):110-117, 1991.
32. Shannon JM: Transfilter induction of type II cell differentiation in fetal rat tracheal epithelium by distal pulmonary mesenchyme, *Am Rev Respir Dis* 149:A712, 1994 (abstract).
33. Deterding RR, Shannon JM: Growth factor effects on distal fetal pulmonary epithelium in vitro, *Am Rev Respir Dis* 149:A254, 1994 (abstract).
34. Ryan RM, Mineo-Kuhn MM, Kramer CM, Finkelstein JN: Growth factors alter neonatal type II alveolar epithelial cell proliferation, *Am J Physiol* 266(1 Pt 1):L17-L22, 1994.
35. Canigia I, Liu J, Han R, Buch S, Funa K, Tanswell K, Post M: Fetal lung epithelial cells express receptors for platelet-derived growth factor, *Am J Respir Cell Mol Biol* 9:54-63, 1993.
36. Buch S, Jassal D, Edelson J, Han R, Liu J, Tanswell K, Post M: Ontogeny and regulation of platelet-derived growth factor gene expression in distal fetal rat lung epithelial cells, *Am J Respir Cell Mol Biol* 11:251-261, 1994.
37. Sannes PL, Burch KK, Khosla J: Immunohistochemical localization of epidermal growth factor and acidic and basic fibroblast growth factors in postnatal developing and adult rat lungs, *Am J Respir Cell Mol Biol* 7:230-237, 1992.
38. Stahlman MT, Orth DN, Gray ME: Immunohistochemical localization of epidermal growth factor in the developing human respiratory system and in acute and chronic lung disease in the neonate, *Lab Invest* 60:539-547, 1989.
39. Cutz E, Gillan JE, Bryan AC: Neuroendocrine cells in the developing human lung: morphological and functional considerations, *Pediatr Pulmonol* 1(suppl):S21-S29, 1985.
40. Stahlman MT, Kasselberg AG, Orth DN, Gray ME: Ontogeny of neuroendocrine cells in human fetal lung. II. An immunohistochemical study, *Lab Invest* 52:52-60, 1985.
41. Scheuermann DW: Neuroendocrine cells. In Crystal RG, West JB, eds: *The lung: scientific foundations,* Philadelphia, 1991, Raven, pp 289-299.
42. King KA, Hua J, Torday JS, Drazen JM, Graham SA, Shipp MA, Sunday MA: CD-10/neutral endopeptidase 24.11 regulates fetal lung growth and maturation in utero by potentiating endogenous bombesin-like peptides, *J Clin Invest* 91(5):1969-1973, 1993.
43. Aguayo SM, Schuyler WE, Murtagh JJ Jr, Roman J: Regulation of lung branching morphogenesis by bombesin-like peptides and neutral endopeptidase, *Am J Respir Cell Mol Biol* 10:635-642, 1994.
44. Hoyt RF Jr, McNelly NA, McDowell EM, Sorokin SP: Neuroepithelial bodies stimulate proliferation of airway epithelium in fetal hamster lung, *Am J Physiol* 260(4 Pt 1):L234-L240, 1991.
45. Moens CB, Auerbach AB, Conlon RA, Joyner AL, Rossant J: A targeted mutation reveals a role for N-*myc* in branching morphogenesis in the embryonic mouse lung, *Genes Dev* 6:691-704, 1992.
46. Nau MM, Brooks BJ Jr, Carney DN, Gazdar AF, Battey JF, Sausville EA, Minna JD: Human small cell lung cancers show amplification and expression of the N-*myc* gene, *Proc Natl Acad Sci USA* 83:1092-1096, 1986.
47. Wong AJ, Ruppert JM, Eggleston J, Hamilton SR, Baylin SB, Vogelstein B: Gene amplification of c-*myc* and N-*myc* in small cell carcinoma of the lung, *Science* 233:461-464, 1986.
48. Levay-Young BK, Navre M: Growth and developmental regulation of *WNT-2 (irp)* gene in mesenchymal cells of fetal lung, *Am J Physiol* 262(6 Pt 1):L672-L83, 1992.
49. Hansbrough JR, Fine SM, Gordon JI: A transgenic mouse model for studying the lineage relationships and differentiation program of type II pneumocytes at various stages of lung development, *J Biol Chem* 268:9762-9770, 1993.
50. Hackett BP, Gitlin JD: 5′ flanking region of the Clara cell secretory protein gene specifies a unique temporal and spatial pattern of gene expression in the developing pulmonary epithelium, *Am J Respir Cell Mol Biol* 11:123-129, 1994.
51. Newman SA, Comper WD: "Generic" physical mechanisms of morphogenesis and pattern formation, *Development* 110:1-18, 1990.
52. Moessinger AC, Harding R, Adamson TM, Singh M, Kiu GT: Role of lung fluid volume in growth and maturation of the fetal sheep lung, *J Clin Invest* 86:1270-1277, 1990.
53. Wigglesworth JS, Desai R, Hislop AA: Fetal lung growth in congenital laryngeal atresia, *Pediatr Pathol* 7:515-525, 1987.
54. Cooney TP, Dimmick JE, Thurlbeck WM: Increased acinar complexity with polyhydramnios, *Pediatr Pathol* 5:183-197, 1986.
55. Collins MH, Moessinger AC, Kleinerman J, James LS, Blanc WA: Morphometry of hypoplastic fetal guinea pig lungs following amniotic fluid leak, *Pediatr Res* 20:955-960, 1986.

56. Moessinger AC, Collin MH, Blanc WA, Rey HR, James LS: Oligohydramnios-induced lung hypoplasia: the influence of timing and duration in gestation, *Pediatr Res* 20:951-954, 1986.
57. Perlman M, Williams J, Hirsch M: Neonatal pulmonary hypoplasia after prolonged leakage of amniotic fluid, *Arch Dis Child* 51:349-353, 1976.
58. Hislop A, Hey E, Reid L: The lungs in congenital bilateral renal agenesis and dysplasia, *Arch Dis Child* 54:32-38, 1979.
59. George KD, Cooney TP, Chiu BK, Thurlbeck WM: Hypoplasia and immaturity of the terminal lung unit (acinus) in congenital diaphragmatic hernia, *Am Rev Respir Dis* 136:947-950, 1987.
60. Tenbrinck R, Tibboel D, Gaillard JLJ, Kluth D, Bos AP, Lachmann B, Molenaar JC: Experimentally induced congenital diaphragmatic hernia in rats, *J Pediatr Surg* 25:426-429, 1990.
61. Pringle KC, Turner JW, Schofield JC, Soper RT: Creation and repair of diaphragmatic hernia in the fetal lamb: lung development and morphology, *J Pediatr Surg* 18:131-140, 1984.
62. DeLorimer AA, Tierney OF, Parker HR: Hypoplastic lungs in fetal lambs with surgically produced congenital diaphragmatic hernia, *Surgery* 62:12-17, 1967.
63. Argyle JC: Pulmonary hypoplasia in infants with giant abdominal wall defects, *Pediatr Pathol* 9:43-55, 1989.
64. Harding R, Hooper SB, Han VK: Abolition of fetal breathing movements by spinal cord transection leads to reductions in fetal lung liquid volume, lung growth, and IGF-II gene expression, *Pediatr Res* 34:148-153, 1993.
65. Liggins GC, Vilos GA, Campos GA, Kitterman JA, Lee CH: The effect of spinal cord transection on lung development in fetal sheep, *J Dev Physiol* 3:51-65, 1981.
66. Fewell JE, Lee CC, Kitterman JA: Effects of phrenic nerve section on the respiratory system of fetal lambs, *J Appl Physiol* 51:293-297, 1981.
67. Nagai A, Thurlbeck WM, Jansen AH, Ioffe S, Chernick V: The effect of chronic biphrenectomy on lung growth and maturation in fetal lambs, *Am Rev Respir Dis* 137:167-172, 1988.
68. Goldstein JD, Reid LM: Pulmonary hypoplasia resulting from phrenic nerve agenesis and diaphragmatic amyoplasia, *J Pediatr* 97:282-287, 1980.
69. Nagai A, Thurlbeck WM, Deboeck C, Ioffe S, Chernick V: The effect of maternal CO_2 breathing on lung development of fetuses in the rabbit, *Am Rev Respir Dis* 135:130-136, 1987.
70. McCray PB: Spontaneous contractility of human fetal airway smooth muscle, *Am J Respir Cell Mol Biol* 8:573-580, 1993.
71. Bishop JE, Mitchell JJ, Absher PM, Baldor L, Geller HA, Woodcock-Mitchell J, Hamblin MJ, Vacek P, Low RB: Cyclic mechanical deformation stimulates human lung fibroblast proliferation and autocrine growth factor activity, *Am J Respir Cell Mol Biol* 9:126-133, 1993.
72. Liu M, Skinner SJM, Xu J, Han RNN, Tanswell AK, Post M: Stimulation of fetal rat lung cell proliferation in vitro by mechanical stretch, *Am J Physiol* 263(3 Pt 1):L376-L383, 1992.
73. Liu M, Xu J, Tanswell AK, Post M: Stretch-induced growth-promoting activities stimulate fetal rat lung epithelial cell proliferation, *Exp Lung Res* 19:505-517, 1993.
74. Scott JE, Yang SY, Stanik E, Anderson JE: Influence of strain on (^{3}H)thymidine incorporation, surfactant-related phospholipid synthesis, and cAMP levels in fetal type II alveolar cells, *Am J Respir Cell Mol Biol* 8:258-265, 1993.
75. Stiles QR, Meyer BW, Lindesmith GG, Jones JC: The effects of pneumonectomy in children, *J Thorac Cardiovasc Surg* 58:394-400, 1969.
76. McBride JT, Wohl MEB, Strieder DJ, Jackson AC, Morton JR, Zwerdling RG, Griscom NT, Treves S, Williams AJ, Schuster S: Lung growth and airway function after lobectomy in infancy for congenital lobar emphysema, *J Clin Invest* 66:962-967, 1980.
77. Laros CD, Westermann CJJ: Dilatation, compensatory growth, or both after pneumonectomy during childhood and adolescence, *J Thorac Cardiovasc Surg* 93:570-576, 1987.
78. Cagel PT, Thurlbeck WM: Postpneumonectomy compensatory lung growth, *Am Rev Respir Dis* 138:1314-1326, 1988.
79. Rannels DE: The role of physical factors in compensatory growth of the lung, *Am J Physiol* 257:L179-L189, 1989.
80. McBride JT: Postpneumonectomy airway growth in the ferret, *J Appl Physiol* 58:1010-1014, 1985.
81. Kirchner KK, McBride JT: Changes in airway length after unilateral pneumonectomy in weanling ferrets, *J Appl Physiol* 68:187-192, 1990.
82. McBride JT: Lung volumes after an increase in lung distention in pneumonectomized ferrets, *J Appl Physiol* 67:1418-1421, 1989.
83. McBride JT, Kirchner KK, Russ G, Finkelstein J: Role of pulmonary blood flow in postpneumonectomy lung growth, *J Appl Physiol* 73:2448-2451, 1992.
84. Wallen LD, Perry SF, Alston JT, Maloney JE: Morphometric study of the role of the pulmonary arterial flow in fetal lung growth in sheep, *Pediatr Res* 27:122-127, 1990.
85. Wallen LD, Perry SF, Alston JT, Maloney JE: Fetal lung growth: influence of pulmonary arterial flow and surgery in sheep, *Am J Respir Crit Care Med* 149:1005-1011, 1994.
86. Wallen LD, Kulisz E, Maloney JE: Main pulmonary artery ligation reduces lung fluid production in fetal sheep, *J Dev Physiol* 16:173-179, 1991.
87. Hsia CCW, Herazo LF, Fryder-Doffey F, Weibel ER: Compensatory lung growth occurs in adult dogs after right pneumonectomy, *J Clin Invest* 94:405-412, 1994.
88. Morin FC III, Stenmark KR: State of the art: persistent pulmonary hypertension of the newborn, *Am J Respir Crit Care Med* 151:2010-2032, 1995.
89. Frid M, Shekhomin B, Koteliansky V, Glukhova M: Phenotypic changes of humans during development: late expression of heavy caldesmon and calponin, *Dev Biol* 153:185-193, 1992.
90. Frid M, Moiseeva E, Stenmark KR: Multiple phenotypically distinct smooth muscle cell populations exist in the adult and developing bovine arterial media: in vivo, *Circ Res* 75:669-681, 1994.
91. Stenmark KR, Mecham RP: Cellular and molecular mechanisms of pulmonary vascular remodeling, *Annu Rev Physiol* 59:89-144, 1997.
92. Klagsbrun M: The fibroblast growth factor family: structural and biological properties, *Prog Growth Factor Res* 1:207-235, 1989.
93. Heine U, Munoz E, Flanders K, Roberts A, Spron M: Colocalization of TGF-beta$_1$ and collagen I and III, fibronectin and glycosaminoglycans during lung branching morphogenesis, *Development* 109:29-36, 1990.
94. Han V, D'Ercole A, Lung P: Cellular localization of somatomedin (insulin-like growth factor) messenger RNA in the human fetus, *Science* 230:193-197, 1987.
95. Badesch D, Lee P, Parks W, Stenmark KR: Insulin-like growth factor I stimulates elastin synthesis by bovine pulmonary arterial smooth muscle cells, *Biochem Biophys Res Commun* 160:382-387, 1989.
96. Kubota Y, Kleinman HK, Martin GR, Lawley TJ: Role of laminin and basement membrane in the morphological differentiation of human endothelial cells into capillary-like structures, *J Cell Biol* 107:1589-1598, 1988.
97. Vernon RB, Angelio JC, Iruela-Arispe ML, Lane TF, Sage EH: Reorganization of basement membrane matrices by cellular traction promotes the formation of cellular networks in vitro, *Lab Invest* 66:536-547, 1992.
98. Stenmark KR, Mecham R, Durmowicz A, Parks W: Persistence of the fetal pattern of tropoelastin gene expression in severe neonatal pulmonary hypertension, *J Clin Invest* 93:1234-1242, 1994.
99. Durmowicz A, Parks W, Hyde D, Mecham R, Stenmark KR: Persistence, reexpression, and induction of pulmonary arterial fibronectin, tropoelastin, and type I procollagen mRNA expression in neonatal hypoxic pulmonary hypertension, *Am J Pathol* 145:1411-1420, 1994.
100. Howard PS, Myers JC, Gortien SF, Macarak EJ: Progressive modulation of endothelial phenotype during in vitro blood vessel formation, *Dev Biol* 146:325-328, 1991.
101. Iruela-Arispe ML, Diglio CA, Sage EH: Modulation of extracellular matrix proteins by endothelial cells undergoing angiogenesis in vitro, *Arterioscler Thromb* 11:805-815, 1991.
102. Underwood PA, Bennett FA: The effect of extracellular matrix molecules on the in vitro behavior of bovine endothelial cells, *Exp Cell Res* 205:311-319, 1993.
103. Ketis NV, Lawler J, Bendena WG: Extracellular matrix components affect the pattern of protein synthesis of endothelial cells responding to hyperthermia, *In Vitro Cell Dev Biol Anim* 29A:768-772, 1993.

Alveolar Type II Cell Structure and Function

104. Rooney SA: The surfactant system and lung phospholipid biochemistry, *Am Rev Respir Dis* 131:439-460, 1985.
105. Wright JR, Clements JA: Metabolism and turnover of lung surfactant, *Am Rev Respir Dis* 135:426-444, 1987.
106. Hawgood S: Pulmonary surfactant apoproteins: a review of protein and genomic structure, *Am J Physiol* 257(2 Pt 1):L13-L22, 1989.
107. Avery ME, Mead J: Surface properties in relation to atelectasis and hyaline membrane disease, *Am J Dis Child* 97:517-523, 1959.
108. Lewis JF, Jobe AH: Surfactant for the treatment of respiratory distress syndrome, *Am Rev Respir Dis* 136:1256-1275, 1987.

109. Moxley MA, Jacoby J, Longmore WJ: Uptake and reutilization of surfactant phospholipids by type II cells of isolated perfused lung, *Am J Physiol* 260(4 Pt 1):L268-βL273, 1991.
110. Mason RJ, Williams MC: Alveolar type II cells. In Crystal RG, West JB: *The lung: scientific foundations,* Philadelphia, 1991, Raven, pp 235-246.
111. Wirtz HRW, Dobbs LG: Calcium mobilization and exocytosis after one mechanical stretch of lung epithelial cells, *Science* 250:1266-1269, 1990.
112. Uhal BD, Etter MD: Type II pneumocyte hypertrophy without activation of surfactant biosynthesis after partial pneumonectomy, *Am J Physiol* 264(2 Pt 1):L153-L159, 1993.
113. Gross I: Regulation of fetal lung maturation, *Am J Physiol* 259(6 Pt 1):L337-L344, 1990.
114. Robert MF, Neff RK, Hubbell JP, Taeusch HW, Avery ME: Association between maternal diabetes and the respiratory distress syndrome in the newborn, *N Engl J Med* 294:357-360, 1976.
115. Hall-Guttentag S, Phelps DS, Warshaw JB, Floros J: Delayed hydrophobic surfactant proteins (SP-B, SP-C) expression in fetuses of streptozocin-treated rats, *Am J Respir Cell Mol Biol* 7:190-197, 1992.
116. Sugahara K, Iyama K, Sano K, Morioka T: Overexpression of pulmonary surfactant apoprotein A mRNA in alveolar type II cells and nonciliated bronchiolar (Clara) epithelial cells in streptozocin-induced diabetic rats demonstrated by in situ hybridization, *Am J Respir Cell Mol Biol* 6:307-314, 1992.
117. Nogee LM, deMello DE, Dehner LP, Colten H: Deficiency of pulmonary surfactant protein B in congenital alveolar proteinosis, *N Engl J Med* 328:406-410, 1993.
118. deMello DE, Heyman S, Phelps DS, Hamvas A, Nogee L, Cole S, Colten HR: Ultrastructure of lung in surfactant protein B deficiency, *Am J Respir Cell Mol Biol* 11:230-239, 1994.
119. Lewis JF, Jobe AH: Surfactant and the adult respiratory distress syndrome, *Am Rev Respir Dis* 147:218-233, 1993.
120. Petty TL, Reiss OK, Paul GW, Silvers GW, Elkins ND: Characteristics of pulmonary surfactant in adult respiratory distress syndrome associated with trauma and shock, *Am Rev Respir Dis* 115:531-536, 1977.
121. Petty TL, Silvers GW, Paul GW, Stanford RE: Abnormalities in elastic properties and surfactant function in adult respiratory distress syndrome, *Chest* 75:571-574, 1979.
122. Hallman M, Spragg R, Harrell JH, Moser KM, Gluck L: Evidence of lung surfactant abnormality in respiratory failure, *J Clin Invest* 70:673-683, 1982.
123. Pison U, Seeger W, Buchhorn R, Joka T, Brand M, Obertacke U, Neuhof H, Schmit-Neverburg K: Surfactant abnormalities in patients with respiratory failure after multiple trauma, *Am Rev Respir Dis* 140:1033-1039, 1989.
124. Gregory TJ, Longmore WJ, Moxley MA, Whitsett JA, Reed CR, Fowler AA, Hudson LD, Maunder RJ, Crim C, Hyers TM: Surfactant chemical composition and biophysical activity in acute respiratory distress syndrome, *J Clin Invest* 88:1976-1981, 1991.
125. Pison U, Obertacke U, Seeger W, Hawgood S: Surfactant protein A (SP-A) is decreased in acute parenchymal lung injury associated with polytrauma, *Eur J Clin Invest* 22:712-718, 1992.
126. Richman PS, Spragg RG, Robertson B, Merritt TA, Curstedt T: The adult respiratory distress syndrome: first trials with surfactant replacement, *Eur Respir J* 2:109S-111S, 1989.
127. Nosaka S, Sakai T, Yonekura M, Yoshikawa K, Surfactant for adults with respiratory failure, *Lancet* 336:947-948, 1990.
128. Weg J, Reines H, Balk R, Tharratt R, Kearney P, Killian T, Scholten D, Zaccardelli D, Horton J, Pattishall E: Safety and efficacy of an aerosolized surfactant (Exosurf) in human sepsis induced ARDS, *Chest* 100:137S(abst), 1991.
129. Pine JH, Richter WR, Esterly JR: Experimental lung injury. I. Bacterial pneumonia: ultrastructural, autoradiographic and histochemical observations, *Am J Pathol* 73:115-130, 1973.
130. Evans MJ, Cabral LJ, Stephens RJ, Freeman G: Renewal of alveolar epithelium in the rat following exposure to NO_2, *Am J Pathol* 70:175-198, 1973.
131. Kapanci Y, Weibel ER, Kaplan HP, Robinson FR: Pathogenesis and reversibility of the pulmonary lesions of oxygen toxicity in monkeys. II. Ultrastructure and morphometric studies, *Lab Invest* 20:101-118, 1969.
132. Bowden DR, Adamson IYR: Reparative changes following pulmonary cell injury: ultrastructural, cytodynamic, and surfactant studies in mice after oxygen exposure, *Arch Pathol* 92:279-283, 1971.
133. Schneeber EE: Alveolar type I cells. In Chernick VS, Mellins RB, eds: *The lung: scientific foundations,* Philadelphia,1991, Raven, pp 229-234.
134. Roman JR, McDonald JA: Cellular processes in lung repair, *Chest* 100:245-248, 1991,
135. Lewis-Molock Y, Suzuki K, Taniguchi N, Nguyen DH, Mason RJ, White CW: Lung manganese superoxide dismutase increases during cytokine-mediated protection against pulmonary oxygen toxicity in rats, *Am J Respir Cell Mol Biol* 10:133-141, 1994.
136. Sosenko IRS, Frank L: Oxidants and antioxidants. In Chernick VS, Mellins RB, eds: *Basic mechanisms of pediatric respiratory disease: cellular and integrative,* Philadelphia, 1991, BC Decker, pp 315-327.
137. Dobashi K, Asayama K, Hayashibe H, Kawaoi A, Morikawa M, Nakazawa S: Immunohistochemical study of copper-zinc and manganese superoxide dismutases in the lungs of human fetuses and newborn infants: developmental profile and alterations in hyaline membrane disease and bronchopulmonary dysplasia, *Virtuous Arch A Pathol Anat Histopathol* 423:177-184, 1993.
138. Amy R, Bowes D, Burri PH: Postnatal growth of the mouse lung, *J Anat* 124:131-151, 1977.
139. Bruce MC, Bruce EN, Janiga K, Chetty A: Hyperoxic exposure of developing rat lung decreases tropoelastin mRNA levels that rebound post-exposure, *Am J Physiol* 265(3 Pt 1):L293-L300, 1993.
140. Bruce MC, Pawlowski R, Tomachefski JF: Changes in lung elastic fiber structure and concentration associated with hyperoxic exposure in the developing rat lung, *Am Rev Respir Dis* 140:1067-1074, 1989.
141. Bruce MC, Schuyler M, Martin RJ, Starcher BC, Tomashefski JF, Wedig KE: Risk factors for the degradation of lung elastic fibers in the ventilated neonate: implications for impaired lung development in bronchopulmonary dysplasia, *Am Rev Respir Dis* 146:204-212, 1992.
142. Sheppard MN, Harrison NK: Lung injury, inflammatory mediators, and fibroblast activation in fibrosing alveolitis, *Thorax* 47:1064-1074, 1992.
143. Panos RJ, Rubin JS, Aaronsen SA, Mason RJ: Keratinocyte growth factor and hepatocyte growth factor/scatter factor are heparin-binding growth factors for alveolar type II cells in conditioned medium, *J Clin Invest* 92:969-977, 1993.
144. Mason RJ, Leslie CC, McCormick-Shannon K, Deterding RR, Nakamura T, Rubin JS, Shannon JM: Hepatocyte growth factor is a growth factor for rat alveolar type II cells, *Am J Respir Cell Mol Biol* 10:561-567, 1994.
145. Ulich TR, Yi ES, Longmuir K, Yin S, Blitz R, Morris CF, Housley RM, Pierce GF: Keratinocyte growth factor is a growth factor for type II pneumocytes in vivo, *J Clin Invest* 93:1298-1306, 1994.
146. Khalil N, O'Conner RN, Unruh HW, Warren PW, Flanders KC, Kemp A, Bereznay OH, Greenberg AH: Increased production and immunohistochemical localization of transforming growth factor-β in idiopathic pulmonary fibrosis, *Am J Respir Cell Mol Biol* 5:155-162, 1991.
147. Giaid A, Michel RP, Stewart DJ, Sheppard M, Corrin B, Hamid Q: Expression of endothelin-1 in lungs of patients with cryptogenic fibrosing alveolitis, *Lancet* 341:1550-1554, 1993.
148. Nash JRG, McLaughlin PJ, Butcher D, Corrin B: Expression of tumour necrosis factor-α in cryptogenic fibrosing alveolitis, *Histopathology* 22:343-347, 1993.
149. Piguet PF, Ribaux C, Karpuz V, Grau GE, Kapanci Y: Expression and localization of tumor necrosis factor-α and its mRNA in idiopathic pulmonary fibrosis, *Am J Pathol* 143:651-655, 1993.
150. Antoniades HN, Bravo MA, Avila RE: Platelet-derived growth factor in idiopathic pulmonary fibrosis, *J Clin Invest* 86:1055-1064, 1990.
151. Vignaud JM, Allam M, Martinet N, Pech M, Plenat F, Martinet Y: Presence of platelet-derived growth factor in normal and fibrotic lung is specifically associated with interstitial macrophages, while both interstitial macrophages and alveolar epithelial cells express c-*sis* protooncogene, *Am J Respir Cell Mol Biol* 5:531-538, 1991.
152. Welsh MJ: Epithelial Electraloy transport. In Chernick VS, Mellins RB, eds: *Basic mechanisms of pediatric respiratory disease: cellular and integrative,* Philadelphia, 1991, BC Decker, pp 162-168.
153. Bland RD, Nielson DW: Developmental changes in lung epithelial ion transport and liquid movement, *Annu Rev Physiol* 54:373-394, 1992.
154. Strang LB: Fetal lung liquid: secretion and reabsorption, *Phys Rev* 71:991-1016, 1991.
155. Chapman DL, Widdicombe JH, Bland RD: Developmental differences in rabbit lung epithelial Na^+-K^+-ATPase, *Am J Physiol* 259(6 Pt 1):L481-L487, 1990.
156. Celsi G, Wang ZM, Akusjarvi G, Aperia A: Sensitive periods for glucocorticoids' regulation of Na^+-K^+-ATPase mRNA in the developing lung and kidney, *Pediatr Res* 33:5-9, 1993.

157. O'Brodovich H, Hannam V, Rafii B: Sodium channel but neither Na^+-H^+ nor Na-glucose symport inhibitors slow neonatal lung water clearance, *Am J Respir Cell Mol Biol* 5:377-384, 1991.
158. McCray PB, Welsh MJ: Developing fetal alveolar epithelial cells secrete fluid in primary culture, *Am J Physiol* 260(4):L494-L500, 1991.
159. Gowen CW, Lawson EE, Gingras J, Boucher RC, Gatzy JT, Knowles MR: Electrical potential difference and ion transport across nasal epithelium of term neonates: correlation with mode of delivery, transient tachypnea of the newborn, and respiratory rate, *J Pediatr* 113:121-127, 1988.
160. Barker PM: Transalveolar Na^+ absorption, *Am Rev Respir Dis* 150:302-303, 1994.
161. O'Brodovich H, Hannam V, Seear M, Mullen JBM: Amiloride impairs lung water clearance in newborn guinea pigs, *J Appl Physiol* 68:1758-1762, 1990.
162. Sakuma TS, Okaniwa G, Nakada T, Nishimura T, Fujimura S, Mattay MA: Alveolar fluid clearance in the resected human lung, *Am J Respir Crit Care Med* 150:305-310, 1994.
163. Strunk RC, Eidlen DM, Mason RJ: Pulmonary alveolar type II epithelial cells synthesize and secrete proteins of the classical and alternative complement pathways, *J Clin Invest* 81:1419-1426, 1988.
164. Hartshorn KL, Crouch EC, White MR, Eggleton P, Tauber AI, Chang D, Sastry K: Evidence for a protective role of pulmonary surfactant protein D (SP-D) against influenza A viruses, *J Clin Invest* 94:311-319, 1994.
165. Zimmerman PE, Voelker DR, McCormack FX, Martin WJ: The 120 kD surface glycoprotein of *Pneumocystis carinii* is a ligand for surfactant protein A, *J Clin Invest* 86:143-149, 1992.
166. vanIwaarden F, Welmers B, Verhoef J, Haagsman HP, van Golde MGL: Pulmonary surfactant protein A enhances the host-defense mechanism of rat alveolar macrophages, *Am J Respir Cell Mol Biol* 2:91-98, 1990.
167. Katsura H, Kawada H, Konno K: Rat surfactant apoprotein A (SP-A) exhibits antioxidant effects on alveolar macrophages, *Am J Respir Cell Mol Biol* 9:520-525, 1993.
168. McNeely TB, Coonrud JD: Aggregation and opsonization of type A but not type B *Haemophilus influenzae* by surfactant protein A, *Am J Respir Cell Mol Biol* 11:114-122, 1994.
169. Kuan SH, Persson A, Parghi D, Crouch E: Lectin-mediated interactions of surfactant protein D with alveolar macrophages, *Am J Respir Cell Mol Biol* 10:430-436, 1994.
170. Crestani B, Cornillet P, Dehoux M, Rolland C, Guenounou M, Aubier M: Alveolar type II epithelial cells produce interleukin-6 in vitro and in vivo, *J Clin Invest* 94:731-740, 1994.
171. Standiford TJ, Kunkel SL, Phan SH, Rollins BJ, Strieter RM: Alveolar macrophage–derived cytokines induce monocyte chemoattractant protein-1 expression from human pulmonary type II–like epithelial cells, *J Biol Chem* 266:9912-9918, 1991.
172. Cott GR, Westcott JY, Voelkel NF: Prostaglandins and leukotriene production by alveolar type II cell in vitro, *Am J Physiol* 258(4 Pt 1):L179-L187, 1990.
173. Punjabi CJ, Laskin JD, Pendino KJ, Goller NL, Durhan SK, Laskin DL: Production of nitric oxide by rat type II pneumocytes: increased expression of inducible nitric oxide synthase following inhalation of a pulmonary irritant, *Am J Respir Cell Mol Biol* 11:165-172, 1994.

Airway-Lining Cells

174. Jetten AM: Growth and differentiation factors in tracheobronchial epithelium, *Am J Physiol* 260(6 Pt 1):L361-L373, 1991.
175. Brody AG, Hook GER, Cameron G, Jetten AM, Butterick C, Nettesheim P: The differentiation capacity of Clara cells isolated from the lungs of rabbits, *Lab Invest* 57:219-229, 1987.
176. Hook GER, Brody AR, Cameron GS, Jetten AM, Gilmore LB, Nettesheim P: Repopulation of denuded tracheas by Clara cells isolated from the lungs of rabbits, *Exp Lung Res* 12:311-330, 1987.
177. Hoyt RF, McNelly NA, Sorokin SP: Dynamics of neuroepithelial body (NEB) formation in developing hamster lung: light microscopic autoradiography after ^{3}H-thymidine labeling in vivo, *Anat Rec* 227:340-350, 1990.
178. Massaro G, Massaro D: Development of bronchiolar epithelium in rats, *Am J Physiol* 250:R783-R788, 1986.
179. Hyde DM, Plopper CG, Kass PH, Alley JL: Estimation of cell numbers and volumes of bronchiolar epithelium during rabbit lung maturation, *Am J Anat* 167:359-370, 1983.
180. Plopper CG, Alley JL, Serabjit-Singh CJ, Philpot RM: Cytodifferentiation of the nonciliated bronchiolar epithelial (Clara) cell during rabbit lung maturation: an ultrastructural and morphometric study, *Am J Anat* 167:329-357, 1983.
181. Tyler NK, Hyde DM, Hendricks AG, Plopper CG: Morphogenesis of the respiratory bronchioles during fetal lung development in the rhesus monkey, *Am J Anat* 182:215-223, 1988.
182. Tyler NK, Hyde DM, Hendricks AG, Plopper CG: Cytodifferentiation of two epithelial populations of the respiratory bronchioles during fetal lung development in the rhesus monkey, *Anat Rec* 225:297-305, 1989.
183. Plopper CG, Nishio SJ, Alley JL, Hyde DM: The role of the nonciliated bronchiolar epithelial (Clara) cell as the progenitor cell during bronchiolar epithelial differentiation in the perinatal rabbit lung, *Am J Respir Cell Mol Biol* 7:606-613, 1992.
184. Gaillard DA, Lallement AV, Petit AF, Puchelle ES: In vivo ciliogenesis in human fetal tracheal epithelium, *Am J Anat* 185:415-428, 1989.
185. Serafini SM, Michaelson ED: Length and distribution of cilia in human and canine airways, *Bull Eur Physiopathol Respir* 13:551-559, 1977.
186. deHaller R: Development of the mucus-secreting elements in the human lung. In Emery J, ed: *The anatomy of the developing lung,* London, 1969, Heinemann, pp 94-115.
187. Rhodin JA: The ciliated cell: ultrastructure and function of the human tracheal mucosa, *Am Rev Respir Dis* 93(suppl):1-15, 1966.
188. Cutz E: Cytomorphology and differentiation of airway epithelium in developing human lung. In McDowell EM, ed: *Lung carcinomas,* Edinburgh, 1987, Churchill Livingstone.
189. Boat TF, Kleinerman JI, Fanaroff AA, Stern RC: Human tracheobronchial secretions: development of mucous glycoprotein and lysozyme-secreting systems, *Pediatr Res* 11:977-980, 1977.
190. Bucher U, Reid L: Development of the mucus-secreting elements in human lung, *Thorax* 16:219-225, 1961.
191. Infeld MD, Brennan JA, Davis PB: Human fetal lung fibroblasts promote invasion of extracellular matrix by normal human tracheobronchial epithelial cells in vitro: a model of early airway gland development, *Am J Respir Cell Mol Biol* 8:69-76, 1993.
192. Singh G, Singh J, Katyal SL, Brown WE, Kramps JA, Paradis IL, Dauber JH, Macpherson TA, Squeglia N: Identification, cellular localization, isolation and characterization of human Clara cell specific 10 kD protein, *J Histochem Cytochem* 36:73-80, 1988.
193. Massaro GD, Singh G, Mason R, Plopper CG, Malkinson AM, Gail DB: Conference report: biology of the Clara cell, *Am J Physiol (Lung Cell Mol Physiol)* 199:L101-L105, 1994.
194. Singh GS, Katyal SL, Brown WE, Kennedy AL: Mouse Clara cell 10-kDa (CC10) protein: cDNA nucleotide sequence and molecular basis for the variation in progesterone binding of CC10 from different species, *Exp Lung Res* 19:67-75, 1993.
195. Singh GS, Katyal SL, Brown WE, Kennedy AL, Singh U, Wong-Chong ML: Clara cell 10 kDa protein (CC10): comparison of structure and function to uteroglobin, *Biochem Biophys Acta* 1039:348-355, 1990.
196. Devereux TR, Domin BA, Philpot RM: Xenobiotic metabolism by isolated pulmonary cell, *Pharmacol Ther* 41:243-256, 1989.
197. Brody AR, Hook GER, Cameron G, Jetten AM, Butterick C, Nettesheim P: The differentiation capacity of Clara cells isolated from the lungs of rabbits, *Lab Invest* 57:219-229, 1987.
198. Hook GER, Brody AR, Cameron GS, Jetten AM, Gilmore LB, Nettesheim P: Repopulation of denuded tracheas by Clara cells isolated from the lungs of rabbits, *Exp Lung Res* 12:311-330, 1987.
199. Inayama Y, Hook GER, Brody AR, Cameron G, Jetten AM, Gilmore LB, Gray T, Nettesheim P, *Lab Invest* 58:706-717, 1988.
200. Inayama Y, Hook GER, Brody AR, Jetten AM, Gray T, Mahler J, Nettesheim P: In vitro and in vivo growth and differentiation of clones of tracheal basal cells, *Am J Pathol* 134:539-549, 1988.
201. Evans MJ, Cox RA, Shami SG, Plopper CG: Junctional adhesion mechanism in airway basal cells, *Am J Cell Respir Biol* 3:341-347, 1990.
202. Evans MJ, Plopper CG: The role of basal cells in adhesion of columnar epithelium to airway basement membrane, *Am Rev Respir Dis* 138:481-483, 1988.
203. Leigh MW, Boat TR: Airway secretions. In Chernick VS, Mellins RB, eds: *Basic mechanisms of pediatric respiratory disease: cellular and integrative,* Philadelphia, 1991, BC Decker, pp 328-345.
204. Klinger JD, Tandler B, Liedke CM, Boat TF: Proteinases of *Pseudomonas aeruginosa* evoke mucin release by tracheal epithelium, *J Clin Invest* 74:1669-1678, 1984.

205. Kim KC, Nassiri J, Brody JS: Mechanisms of airway goblet cell mucin release: studies with cultured tracheal surface epithelial cells, *Am J Respir Cell Mol Biol* 1:137-143, 1989.
206. Boat TF, Polony I, Cheng PW: Mucin release from rabbit tracheal epithelium in response to sera from normal and cystic fibrosis subjects, *Pediatr Res* 16:792-797, 1982.
207. Kent PW: Chemical aspects of tracheal glycoproteins. In *Respiratory tract mucus,* Ciba Foundation Series 57, New York, 1978, North Holland, pp 155-170.
208. DiAugustine RP, Sonstegard KS: Neuroendocrine like (small granule) epithelial cells of the lung, *Environ Health Perspect* 55:271-295, 1984.
209. Davis PB, Kercsmar CM: Neural control of the lung. In Chernick VS, Mellins RB, eds: *Basic mechanisms of pediatric respiratory disease: cellular and integrative,* Philadelphia, 1991, BC Decker, pp 203-220.
210. Johnson DE, Wobken JD: Calcitonin gene–related peptide immunoreactivity in airway epithelial cells of the human fetus and infant, *Cell Tissue Res* 250:579-583, 1987.
211. Johnson MD, Gray ME, Stahlman MT: Calcitonin gene–related peptide in human fetal lung and in neonatal lung disease, *J Histochem Cytochem* 36:199-204, 1988.

Lung Fibroblasts

212. Phipps RP, ed: *Pulmonary fibroblast heterogeneity,* Boca Raton, Fla, 1992, CRC.
213. Brody JS, Kaplan NB: Proliferation of alveolar interstitial cells during postnatal growth: evidence of two distinct populations of pulmonary fibroblasts, *Am Rev Respir Dis* 127:763-770, 1983.
214. Breen E, Falco VM, Absher M, Cutroneo KR: Subpopulations of rat lung fibroblasts with different amounts of type I and type III collagen mRNAs, *J Biol Chem* 265:6286-6290, 1990.
215. Elias JA, Zitnik RJ, Ray P: Fibroblast immune-effector function. In Phipps RP, ed: *Pulmonary fibroblast heterogeneity,* Boca Raton, Fla, 1992, CRC, pp 295-322.
216. Silvera MR, Sempowski GD, Watta H, Penney DP, Phipps RP: Lung fibroblast heterogeneity, *J Aer Med* 6:1-21, 1993.
217. Derdak S, Penney D, Kang P, Felch M, Brown D, Phipps R: Collagen and fibronectin production by subpopulations of lung fibroblasts: evidence supporting functionally distinct fibroblast subsets in the pathogenesis of pulmonary fibrosis, *Am J Physiol* 263:L283, 1992.

Endothelium

218. Luscher TF, Ynag Z, Diederich D, Buhler FR: Endothelium-derived vasoactive substances: potential role in hypertension, atherosclerosis, and vascular occlusion, *J Cardiovasc Pharmacol* 14(6):S63-S69, 1989.
219. Vane JR, Anggard EE, Botting RM: Mechanisms of disease, *N Engl J Med* 323(1):27-36, 1990.
220. Sumpio BE, Widmann MD: Enhanced production of an endothelium-derived contracting factor by endothelial cells subjected to pulsatile stretch, *Surgery* 108:277-281, 1990.
221. Furchgott RF, Zawadzki JV: The obligatory role of endothelial cells in the relaxation of arterial smooth muscle by acetylcholine, *Nature* 288:373-376, 1980.
222. Ignarro LJ, Byrns RE, Buga GM, Wood KS: Endothelium-derived relaxing factor from pulmonary artery and vein possesses pharmacologic and chemical properties identical to those of nitric oxide radical, *Circ Res* 61:866-879, 1987.
223. Ignarro LJ, Byrns RE, Buga GM, Wood KS: Endothelium-derived relaxing factor (EDRF) released from artery and vein appears to be nitric oxide (NO) or a closely related radical species, *Fed Proc* 46:644(abst), 1987.
224. Palmer RM, Ferrige AG, Moncada S: Nitric oxide release accounts for the biological activity of endothelium-derived relaxing factor, *Nature* 327:524-526, 1987.
225. Palmer RM, Ashton DS, Moncada S: Vascular endothelial cells synthesize nitric oxide from L-arginine, *Nature* 333:664-666, 1988.
226. Mitchell JA, Hecker M, Vane JR: The generation of L-arginine in endothelial cells is linked to the release of endothelium-derived relaxing factor, *Eur J Pharmacol* 176:253-254, 1990.
227. Leaf CD, Wishnok JS, Tannenbaum SR: L-Arginine is a precursor for nitrate biosynthesis in humans, *Biochem Biophys Res Commun* 163:1032-1037, 1989.
228. Panza JA, Quyyumi AA, Brush JE Jr, Epstein SE: Abnormal endothelium-dependent vascular relaxation in patients with essential hypertension, *N Engl J Med* 323:22-27, 1990.
229. Rees DD, Palmer RM, Moncada S: Role of endothelium-derived nitric oxide in the regulation of blood pressure, *Proc Natl Acad Sci USA* 86:3375-3378, 1989.
230. Vallance P, Collier J, Moncada S: Effects of endothelium-derived nitric oxide on peripheral arteriolar tone in man, *Lancet* 2:997-1000, 1989.
231. Salvemini D, Korbut R, Anggara E, Vane J: Immediate release of a nitric oxide like factor from bovine aortic endothelial cells by *Escherichia coli* lipopolysaccharide, *Proc Natl Acad Sci USA* 87:2593-2597, 1990.
232. Radomski MW, Palmer RM, Moncada S: The anti-aggregating properties of vascular endothelium: interactions between prostacyclin and nitric oxide, *Br J Pharmacol* 92:639-646, 1987.
233. Garg UC, Hassed A: Nitric oxide generating vasodilators and 8-bromo-cyclic guanosine monophosphate inhibits mitogenesis and proliferation of cultured rat vascular smooth muscle cells, *J Clin Invest* 83:1774-1777, 1989.
234. Moncada S, Vane JR: Arachidonic acid metabolites and the interactions between platelets and blood vessel walls, *N Engl J Med* 300:1142-1147, 1979.
235. Webster BB, Marcus AJ, Jaffe EA: Synthesis of prostaglandin I_2 (prostacyclin) by cultured human and bovine endothelial cells, *Proc Natl Acad Sci USA* 74:3922-3926, 1977.
236. Orchard MA, Robinson C: Stability of prostacyclin in human plasma and whole blood: studies on the protective effect of albumin, *Thromb Haemost* 46:645-647, 1981.
237. Baenziger NL, Fogerty FJ, Mertz LF: Regulation of histamine-mediated prostacyclin synthesis in cultured human vascular endothelial cells, *Cell* 24:915-923, 1981.
238. Hong SL: Effect of bradykinin and thrombin on prostacyclin synthesis in endothelial cells from calf and pig aorta and human umbilical vein, *Thromb Res* 18:787-795, 1980.
239. Webster BB, Ley CWM, Jaffe EA: Stimulation of endothelial prostacyclin production by thrombin, trypsin and the ionophore A23187, *J Clin Invest* 62:923-930, 1978.
240. Zavoico GB, Ewenstein BM, Schafer AI, Pober JS: IL-1 and related cytokines enhance thrombin stimulated PGI_2 production in cultured endothelial cells without affecting thrombin stimulated von Willebrand factor secretion or platelet activating factor biosynthesis, *Immunology* 142:3993-3999, 1989.
241. Jaffe EA, Weksler BB: Recovery of endothelial cell prostacyclin production after inhibition by low dose aspirin, *J Clin Invest* 63:532-535, 1979.
242. Brotherton AFA, Hoak JC: Prostacyclin biosynthesis in cultured vascular endothelium is limited by deactivation of cyclooxygenase, *J Clin Invest* 72:1255-1261, 1983.
243. Reinders JH, Brinkman HJ, van Mourik JA: Cigarette smoke impairs endothelial cell prostacyclin production, *Arteriosclerosis* 6:15-23, 1986.
244. Radomski MW, Palmer RMY, Moncada S: Endogenous nitric oxide inhibits platelet adhesion to vascular endothelium, *Lancet* 2:1057-1058, 1987.
245. Hughes AD, Thum SA, Woodall N, Schachter M, Hair WM, Martin GN, Sever PS: Human vascular responses to endothelin-1: observations in vivo and in vitro, *J Cardiovasc Pharmacol* 13:S225-S228, 1989.
246. Simonson MS, Wanns Mene P, Dubyak GR, Kester M, Dunn MJ: Endothelin-1 activates the phosphoinositide cascade in cultured glomerular mesangial cell, *J Cardiovasc Pharmacol* 13(5):S80-S83, 1989.
247. Nakaki T, Nakayama M, Yamamoto S, Kato R: Endothelin-mediated stimulation of DNA synthesis in vascular smooth muscle cells, *Biochem Biophys Res Commun* 158:880-883, 1989.
248. Hahn AWA, Resink RJ, Kern F, Buhler FR: Effects of endothelin-1 on vascular smooth muscle cell phenotypic differentiation, *J Cardiovasc Pharmacol* 20(12):S33-S36, 1992.
249. Allen SW, Chatfield BA, Koppenhafer SA, Schaffer MS, Wolfe RR, Abman SH: Circulating immunoreactive endothelin-1 in children with pulmonary hypertension, *Am Rev Respir Dis* 148:519-522, 1993.
250. Rosenberg AA, Kannaugh J, Kopenhafer SL, Loomis M, Chatfield BA, Abman SH: Elevated immunoreactive endothelin-1 levels in newborn infants with persistent pulmonary hypertension, *J Pediatr* 123:109-114, 1993.
251. Yamaja-Setty BN, Berger M, Stuart MJ: 13-Hydroxyoctadeca-9,11-dienoic acid inhibits thromboxane A2 synthesis, and stimulates 12-HETE production in human platelets, *Biochem Biophys Res Commun* 148:528-533, 1987.

252. Pearson JD, Carleton JS, Gordon JL: Metabolism of adenosine nucleotides by ectoenzymes of vascular endothelial and smooth muscle cells in culture, *Biochem J* 190:421-429, 1980.
253. Rosenberg RD: Biochemistry of heparin antithrombin interactions and the physiologic role of this natural anticoagulant mechanism, *Am J Med* 87:2S-9S, 1989.
254. Preissner KT: Physiological role of vessel wall related antithrombotic mechanisms: contribution of endogenous and exogenous heparin-like components to the anticoagulant potential of the endothelium, *Haemostasis* 20:30-49, 1990.
255. Esmon CT: The roles of protein C and thrombomodulin in the regulation of blood coagulation, *J Biol Chem* 264:4743-4746, 1989.
256. Gronke RS, Bergman BL, Baker JB: Thrombin interaction with platelets: influence of platelet protease nexin, *J Biol Chem* 262:3030-3036, 1987.
257. Weiss HJ, Turitto VT, Baumgartner HR: Evidence for the presence of tissue factor activity on subendothelium, *Blood* 73:968-975, 1989.
258. Colucci M, Balconi G, Lorenzet R: Cultured human endothelial cells generate tissue factor in response to endotoxin, *J Clin Invest* 71:1893-1896, 1983.
259. Prescott SM, Zimmerman GA, McIntyre TM: Human endothelial cells in culture produce platelet-activating factor when stimulated with thrombin, *Proc Natl Acad Sci USA* 81:3534-3538, 1984.
260. McIntyre TM, Zimmerman GA, Prescott SM: Leukotrienes C4 and D4 stimulate human endothelial cells to synthesize platelet activating factor and bind neutrophils, *Proc Natl Acad Sci USA* 83:2204-2208, 1986.
261. Zhu LD, Wigle D, Hinek A, Kobayashi J, Ye C, Zuker M, Dodo H, Keeley FW, Rabinovitch M: The endogenous vascular elastase that governs development and progression of monocrotaline-induced pulmonary hypertension in rats is a novel enzyme related to the serine proteinase adipsin, *J Clin Invest* 94:1163-1171, 1994.
262. Franke WW, Goldschmidt MD, Zimbelmann R: Molecular cloning and amino acid sequence of human plakoglobin, the common junctional plaque protein, *Proc Natl Acad Sci USA* 86:4027-4031, 1989.
263. Simionescu M, Simionescu N: Endothelial transport of macromolecules: transcytosis and endocytosis: a look from cell biology, *Cell Biol Rev* 25:5-78, 1991.
264. Antohe F, Dobrila L, Heltianu C, Simionescu N, Simionescu M: Albumin-binding proteins function in the receptor-mediated binding and transcytosis of albumin across cultured endothelial cell, *Eur J Cell Biol* 60:268-275, 1993.
265. Ghinea N, Mai TV, Groyer-Picard MT, Milgram E: How protein hormones reach their target cells: receptor-mediated transcytosis of hCG through endothelial cell, *J Cell Biol* 125:87-97, 1994.
266. Horvat R, Palade GE: Thrombomodulin and thrombin localization on the vascular endothelium: their internalization and transcytosis by plasmalemmal vesicles, *Eur J Cell Biol* 61:299-313, 1993.
267. Milici AJ, Watrous NE, Stukenbrok H, Palade GE: Transcytosis of albumin in capillary endothelium, *J Cell Biol* 105:2603-2612, 1987.
268. Talbott GA, Sharar SR, Harlan JM, Winn RK: Leukocyte-endothelial interactions and organ injury: the role of adhesion molecules, *New Horizons* 2:545-554, 1994.
269. Hynes RO: Integrins: versatility, modulation and signaling in cell adhesion, *Cell* 69:11-25, 1992.
270. Smyth SS, Joneckis CC, Parise LV: Regulation of vascular integrins, *Blood* 81:2827-2843, 1993.
271. Lawrence MB, Springer TA: Leukocytes roll on a selectin at physiologic flow rates: distinction from and prerequisite for adhesion through integrins, *Cell* 65:859-873, 1991.
272. Von Andrian UH, Chambers JD, McEvoy LM: Two-step model of leukocyte-endothelial cell interaction in inflammation: distinct roles for LECAM-1 and the leukocyte β2 integrins in vivo, *Proc Natl Acad Sci USA* 88:7538-7542, 1991.
273. Tarone G, Stetanuto G, Mascarello P, Defilippi P, Altruda F, Silengo L: Expression of receptors for extracellular matrix proteins in human endothelial cells, *J Lipid Mediators* 2:S45-S53, 1990.
274. Hayashi K, Madri JA, Yurchenco PD: Endothelial cells interact with the core protein of basement membrane through beta 1 and beta 3 integrins: an adhesion modulated by glycosaminoglycan, *J Cell Biol* 119:945-959, 1992.

Vascular Smooth Muscle

275. Kocher O, Gabbiani F, Gabbiani G, Reidy M, Cokay MS, Peters H, Huttner I: Phenotypic features of smooth muscle cells during the evolution of experimental carotid artery intimal thickening, *Lab Invest* 65(4):459-470, 1991.
276. Glukhova MA, Frid MG, Koteliansky VE: Phenotypic changes of human aortic smooth muscle cells during development and in the adult vessel, *Am J Physiol* 261:78-80, 1991.
277. Frid MG, Mecham RP, Moiseeva EO, Stenmark KR: Identification of phenotypically distinct smooth muscle cell populations in mature and developing bovine pulmonary arteries, *Am Rev Respir Dis* 147(4):A492, 1993 (abstract).
278. Morgan JP, Perreault CL, Morgan KG: The cellular basis of contraction and relaxation in cardiac and vascular smooth muscle, *Am Heart J* 121:961-968, 1991.
279. van Breemen C, Saida K: Cellular mechanisms regulating [$Ca2^+$] in smooth muscle, *Annu Rev Physiol* 51:315-329, 1989.
280. Ruegg UT, Wallnofer A, Weir S, Cauvi C: Receptor-operated calcium-permeable channels in vascular smooth muscle, *J Cardiovasc Pharmacol* 14(6):S49-S58, 1989.

CHAPTER 6

Host Defense Systems of the Lung

Gary L. Larsen

From the first breath at the time of birth, the lungs must be protected from numerous insults from the environment. This defense takes many forms and has evolved to include mechanical as well as biochemical processes that work in an integrated fashion to safeguard the respiratory tract. This chapter reviews the host defense systems found in humans that protect this organ from injury. Because of this book's focus on pediatric respiratory medicine, information on the developmental aspects of the various components of lung defense is presented.

GENERAL CONCEPTS OF LUNG DEFENSE

Protection of the respiratory tract is provided by several complex but complementary processes.[1,2] The host defense systems normally prevent entry into or rapidly remove foreign material from the lungs. These systems include filtration of potential environmental pathogens from inspired air, cough to clear material from air passages, and mucociliary clearance to eliminate substances not cleared by the first two mechanisms. Both nonimmunologic and immunologic responses of the lung to potentially injurious agents commonly lead to inflammation.

FILTRATION AND DEPOSITION OF ENVIRONMENTAL PATHOGENS

The upper airway and the branching airways within the lung constitute the first line of defense against airborne particles. As ambient air containing suspended solid and liquid particles is drawn toward the gas-exchanging areas of the lung during inspiration, three major mechanisms of deposition come into play: inertial impaction, gravitational settlement, and diffusion.[3] In general, many larger particles (>10 μm) are trapped in the nose and upper airways (above the cricoid ring) as a result of inertial impaction. This mechanism of deposition is based on the principle that the inertia of a particle causes it to maintain its original direction for a distance depending on the particle's density and the square of its diameter. Thus when the stream of air changes direction or velocity, such as happens in the nasopharynx and at the divisions of larger airways within the lung, the larger and more dense particles are likely to hit the walls in these areas and be trapped. This is the primary means of deposition for the majority of larger particles within the respiratory tract. Indeed, because of this mechanism, the lung is spared the task of dealing with many large particles because they are filtered from inspired air before they penetrate the lung. Smaller particles are deposited primarily by gravitational settlement in the deeper recesses of the lung, with the speed of this process again proportional to the density of a particle and the square of its diameter. Diffusion takes place because airborne particles are displaced by the random bombardment of gas molecules, leading to collision with the airway walls. Compared to the first two processes, diffusion is responsible for a smaller percentage of total lung deposition.

Factors Influencing Particle Deposition

Regional deposition within the upper and lower respiratory tract as a function of particle size has been estimated by several investigators,[4] with one commonly cited example shown in Fig. 6-1. In this figure, deposition within the nasal, tracheobronchial, and pulmonary (area beyond the terminal bronchioles) compartments is plotted as a function of particle size. This display is based on a breathing pattern of 15 breaths/min with a tidal volume of approximately 750 ml and thus would be most appropriate for an adult or adolescent undergoing mild exercise. The alterations that might be expected in a smaller subject are discussed later.

Several factors other than particle size also influence deposition. Primary among them are flow rates during inspiration. The greater the flow rate (as seen with exertion), the greater the impaction of particles. Conversely, the probability of a particle being deposited in an airway as a consequence of gravity or diffusion increases as airflow at the mouth decreases or breath-holding occurs. Other factors that may be important include changes in the size of a particle such as occurs with either evaporation or hygroscopic growth. Electrostatic changes may also have significant effects. A change from nose to mouth breathing also alters patterns of deposition. These and other factors, including the influence of diseases of the airways on particle deposition, have been reviewed.[3]

A child's airway may be subjected to many types of insults[5] (Fig. 6-2). In this figure, the aerodynamic diameter of the par-

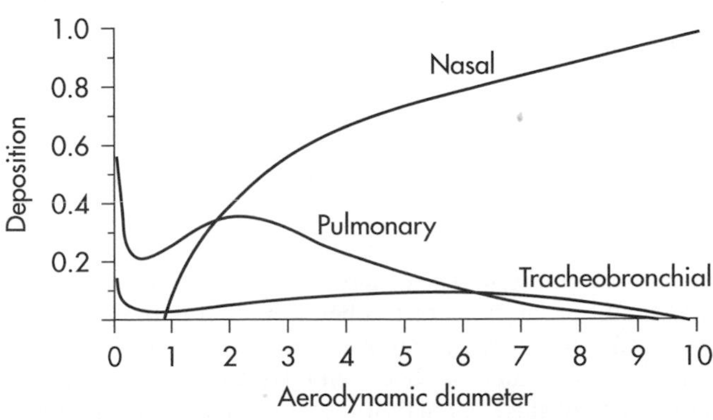

Fig. 6-1. Nasal, tracheobronchial, and pulmonary deposition fractions. See text for discussion. (From Task Group on Lung Dynamics: *Health Phys* 12:173-207, 1966.)

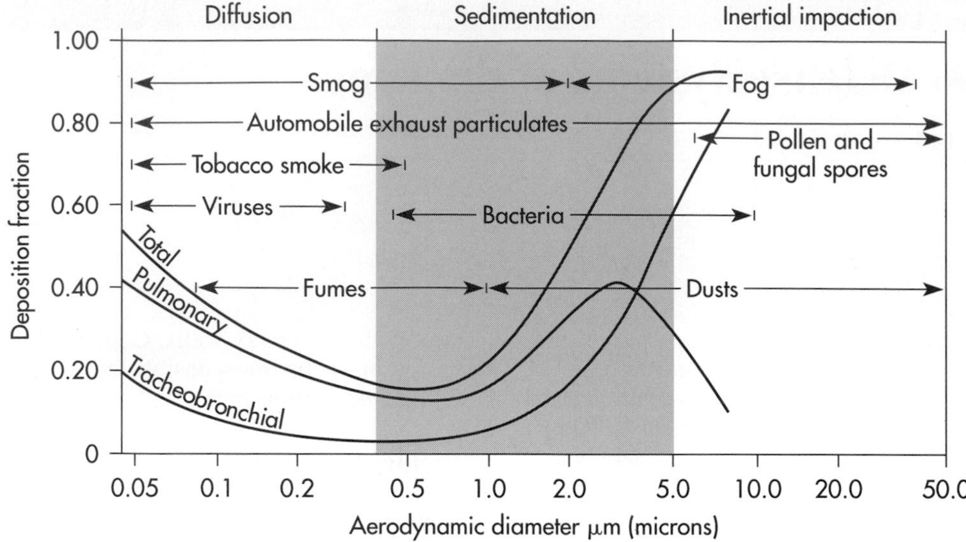

Fig. 6-2. The size-deposition relationship is shown for several stable particles of varying aerodynamic diameter for the tracheobronchial and pulmonary compartments of the lung. The total curve represents the sum from the two compartments. The deposition fractions are from the calculations of Yu et al[6] and are for mouth breathing at less than 0.25 L/s. The particle diameters over which diffusion, sedimentation, and inertial impaction are most important are displayed as is the approximate sizes of some common environmental insults. (From Dolovich MB, Newhouse MT. In Middleton E, Reed CE, Ellis EF, Adkinson NF, Yuninger JW, Busse WW, eds: *Allergy: principles and practice,* ed 4, St Louis, 1993, Mosby, pp. 712-739.)

ticles is plotted against the deposition fractions taken from the calculations of Yu et al.[6] The sizes and sites of deposition are of pathogenic importance in terms of the pulmonary symptoms produced by these insults. For example, the size of pollens leads to their deposition in the larger central airways before they reach the "pulmonary" compartment. As discussed in Chapter 61, allergic asthma in children is felt to be associated with inflammation within the central airways, with less pathology found within the gas-exchanging areas of the lung.

Changes in Particle Deposition with Growth

Studies of particle deposition have been performed primarily on adults; thus relatively little is known about particle deposition in infants and children. However, studies to date suggest that some important differences exist. For example, it has been estimated that the young child receives a potentially larger nasal dose of an aerosol than an adult because of aerosol deposition.[7] In addition, calculations based on casts of airways from infants to adults indicated that smaller (younger) subjects usually have greater tracheobronchial deposition efficiencies than larger (older) individuals.[8] For example, it has been estimated that the tracheobronchial dose per kilogram of body mass for particles with diameters of 5 μm may be 6 times higher in the resting newborn than in the resting adult if equivalent deposition efficiencies are operative above the larynx.[8] Additional predictions of tracheobronchial deposition have been made for infants, children, and adolescents.[9] Thus for most particle diameters between 0.01 and 10.0 μm and for most states of physical activity, smaller individuals probably exhibit greater tracheobronchial deposition efficiencies than larger individuals. Considering the greater ventilation capacity per kilogram of body mass for smaller subjects, this suggests that the initial deposited tracheobronchial dose for young children may be well above that for the adult.

COUGH AS A MECHANISM TO PROTECT THE AIRWAYS

Several neurally mediated reflexes help protect the airways. These reflexes, which may occur separately or together, include sneezing, coughing, and bronchoconstriction. This discussion focuses on cough because of its important role in limiting exposure to and deposition of potentially pathogenic material within the airways.

Cough must be considered an integral part of the mechanisms of airway defense against inhaled particles (e.g., dust) as well as noxious substances (e.g., cigarette smoke, ammonia fumes). Thus the cough that occurs in otherwise normal individuals within a smoke-filled environment should be considered a protective reflex that helps limit the insult to the lower respiratory tract. In addition, cough should be considered an adjunct to the normal mechanisms of mucociliary clearance (see later section), becoming especially important when usual methods of mucus clearance are impaired or overwhelmed. This section emphasizes cough as a protective defense in otherwise normal individuals. The differential diagnosis of cough is dealt with in Chapter 12, whereas specific disease states in which cough is a prominent feature are discussed in the chapters on those disorders.

Although much is known about the stimuli and disease processes that elicit cough, knowledge concerning cough receptors is incomplete and controversial. This problem is further confounded by confusion in nomenclature.[10] In addition, there is debate about which nerve fibers within the vagus nerve trunk carry the majority of sensory information.[11] Despite these problems, several general comments can be made. First, it is clear

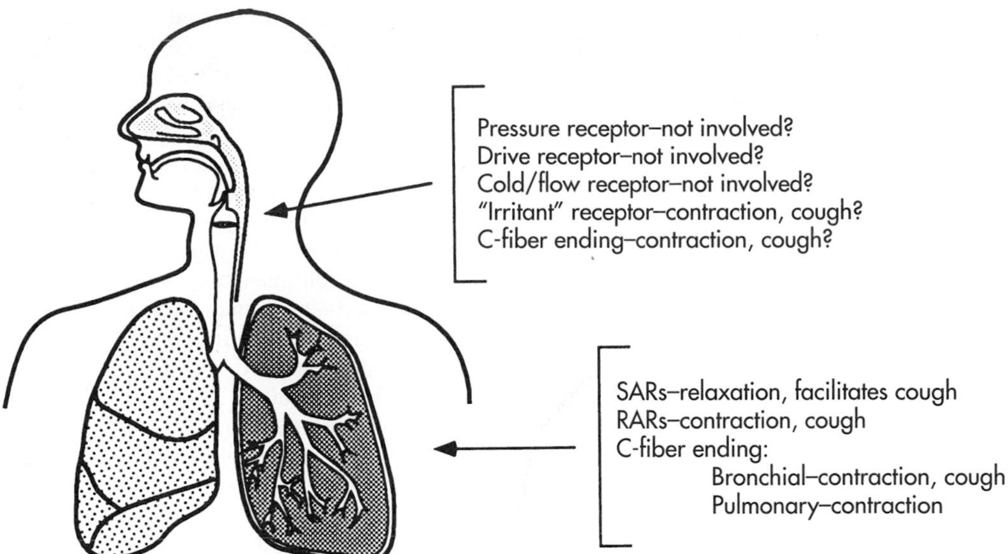

Fig. 6-3. Location and types of vagal afferent nerve endings that may be involved in initiating cough and regulating airway tone. In the larynx, "irritant" receptors have been most closely associated with cough. Within the tracheobronchial tree, rapidly adapting stretch receptors *(RARs)* may directly help mediate cough, whereas slowly adapting stretch receptors *(SARs)* are felt to facilitate cough. (From Karlson J-A, Sant'Ambrogia G, Widdicombe J: *J Appl Physiol* 65:1007-1023, 1988.)

that cough-sensitive nerves extend from the larynx to the division of the segmental bronchi. Based primarily on studies performed in animals, it appears that many nerve fibers are involved in the production of cough. Adaptations of the cough reflex seen in humans in response to different types of airway stimulation suggest that there are different receptor populations with separate afferent neuronal pathways within the airways.[12] Determining which sensory fibers are of primary importance in the human cough reflex is difficult because of a lack of both specific stimuli and specific inhibitors of different fiber types. Still, most authorities agree that more than one fiber type makes up the afferent neural fibers leading to cough and these fibers can differ from those that reflexly narrow the airways.[11,13]

Vagal afferent receptors that may be involved in cough and the regulation of airway tone have been reviewed.[11] Within the airways, the larynx and points of proximal airway branching appear to be especially important as sites where receptors initiate the cough reflex. As shown in Fig. 6-3, within the larynx, "irritant" receptors with myelinated afferents mediate cough and bronchoconstriction; less is known about laryngeal nonmyelinated afferents and their receptors. Thus when cough and bronchoconstriction have been evoked from the larynx, myelinated afferents are usually implicated, but participation of laryngeal C-fiber receptors cannot be excluded. It is helpful to divide the afferent nerve endings of the lower airways (tracheobronchial tree) into four types: slowly adapting pulmonary stretch receptors (SARs), rapidly adapting stretch or irritant receptors (RARs), pulmonary C-fiber receptors or J receptors, and bronchial C-fiber receptors.[10] Although all four types have been implicated in regulating bronchomotor tone and in mediating cough, the myelinated irritant receptors (RARs) and unmyelinated bronchial C fibers have received the most attention as initiators of cough reflexes. The SARs may not directly lead to cough but are thought to contribute in an indirect fashion through their stimulatory effect on expiratory muscles, thus functioning in a facilitating role.

In humans, much also remains to be learned about the central nervous system relay for cough reflexes.[14] However, the physiologic consequences of the efferent pathway are better understood and characterized in terms of the four phases of cough. First, inspiration may occur, leading to more efficient use of the expiratory muscles. This is followed by compression, which occurs when the rib cage and abdominal muscles contract while the glottis is closed. Compression leads to increased intrathoracic pressures, which help achieve the high airflows that occur when the glottis opens during expression, the third phase of cough. The final phase, relaxation, is characterized by expiratory muscle relaxation, leading to a fall in intrathoracic pressures.

Developmental Aspects of Cough

The development of cough has been reviewed.[15] Based on the observation that less than half of both term and premature infants cough when stimulated by direct laryngoscopy and spraying of the vocal cords with saline[16] (Fig. 6-4), there has been speculation that the peripheral receptors and central neural mechanisms mediating cough reflexes are ineffective early in life. This, combined with a musculoskeletal system that is undergoing development (e.g., compliant rib cage and airways, mechanically disadvantaged diaphragm), has led to the concern that cough is not only less common but also less effective in the neonatal period.[15] Studies in newborn animals have led to speculation that sparse RAR activity as well as lower activity of SARs in newborns contributes to the weaker response to tussigenic stimuli in the early stages of development.[17] In terms of changes with age, a cough reflex was present in 90% of infants older than 1 month[16] (see Fig. 6-4), suggesting that this potential impairment in lung defense is not long lasting in these otherwise normal subjects. This same investigation found that less than half of premature infants had cough reflexes at comparable postnatal ages.

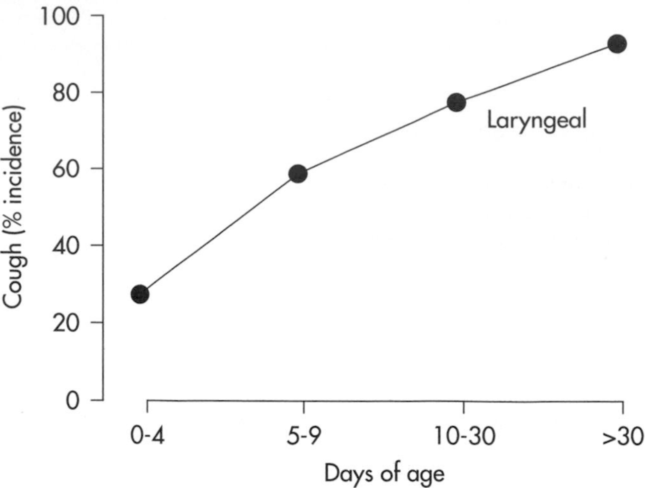

Fig. 6-4. The percent incidence of cough in full-term infants as a function of age. Stimulation of the pharynx and vocal cords was obtained by direct laryngoscopy followed by the squirting of saline onto the vocal cords. Any cough resulting from either the introduction of the scope or exposure to saline was considered a positive result. The cough reflex was present in only 27% of 63 infants within the first 4 days of life but occurred in 90% (19 of 21 infants) when the postnatal age was 2 to 11 months (greater than 30 days in the figure). (Data from Miller HC, Proud GO, Behrle FC: *Yale J Biol Med* 24:284-291, 1952. From Karlsson J-A, Sant'Ambrogia G, Widdicombe J: *J Appl Physiol* 65:1007-1023, 1988.)

MUCUS SECRETION AND CLEARANCE

A critical mechanism for removing particles from the entire system of conducting airways (nasopharynx and tracheobronchial tree) is mucociliary clearance. The contributions of the nose to lung defense have been reviewed[18] and are not addressed except to emphasize that many larger particles are removed from inspired air in the nasopharynx before they enter the lungs (see Fig. 6-1). Particles that escape this first line of defense encounter a film of mucus that covers most of the surface of the tracheobronchial epithelium. Deposition on this film leads to eventual removal from the airways as the mucus is propelled to the oropharynx, where it, along with unwanted particles, is swallowed or expectorated.

Secretory cells and their products are important for maintaining a healthy environment within the lower respiratory tract.[19] Respiratory secretions consist of a double layer on the surface of the airway epithelium. The inner layer of periciliary fluid (sol phase) is the environment in which cilia beat and is probably supplied by transepithelial ion and water transport. The outer mucous layer (gel phase) is viscous in nature. Because it is nonabsorbent to water, it may prevent dehydration of the sol phase. Respiratory mucus in the tracheobronchial tree is produced by both submucosal glands and goblet cells. The former are confined to cartilaginous airways, whereas the latter extend farther into the periphery of the conducting airways. Although goblet cells are present in the epithelia of all ciliated regions of human airways, they become progressively fewer in number in the more distal bronchioles. The submucosal glands are primarily under parasympathetic neural control, and goblet cells secrete products when directly irritated. The thickness of the mucus layer is fairly constant, at least throughout the larger airways (5 to 10 μm). It appears possible that mucus is normally secreted only in response to stimulation of the airway surface and that the small plaques generated in this fashion become the vehicles for removing trapped particles, including bacteria.[20] Mucus may appear to be a continuous sheet within the trachea because the impact of particles is greater in this larger airway and because mucus generated in all lower airways converges for clearance within the trachea. The importance of mucus in the defense of the lung was suggested by the observation that particle transport failed in the absence of mucus but was restored by the placement of autologous or heterologous mucus on the ciliated epithelium.[21]

Tracheobronchial mucus consists of a mixture of secretions from the surface epithelium and submucosal glands as well as tissue fluid transudate.[22] It is composed primarily of water (95%), glycoproteins (2% to 3%), proteoglycans (0.1% to 0.5%), and lipids (0.3% to 0.5%). The main structure of the viscoelastic hydrophilic gel is formed by glycoproteins and proteoglycans, with the former very important in giving mucus its characteristic elasticity. The lengthy glycoprotein molecules are probably intertwined, with their coils held together by weak noncovalent bonds or cross-linked into a three-dimensional network by disulfide bonds.

Ciliated cells within the tracheobronchial tree of humans have approximately 200 cilia per cell.[23] Cilia are complex structures, with their axonemes enclosed in extensions of the epithelial cell membrane[20] (Fig. 6-5). Congenital ciliary defects that cause respiratory disease and infertility as well as acquired abnormalities found in cilia are dealt with in Chapter 75.

Cilia beat in one plane with a fast, effective stroke (power stroke) followed by a recovery stroke that is 2 to 3 times slower. The normal beat frequency in several species, including humans, ranges between 12 and 22 Hz.[24] Throughout most of the beat cycle, cilia move through the periciliary fluid beneath the layer of mucus, with their tips penetrating the mucus only during the effective stroke. Cilia work not alone but as members of a metachronous wave. Although there is evidence in mammalian respiratory epithelia for nervous and hormonal control of mucus secretions, there is no convincing evidence of direct nervous or hormonal control of ciliary beat frequency. Rather, it may be that an increase in the mucus load stimulates ciliary activity.[20]

Mucociliary Clearance as a Function of Age

Cells needed for the production and clearance of mucus are present within the developing airway from a very early period of prenatal development.[25] Ciliated cells are differentiated in the proximal airways by week 13 of gestation, with differentiation proceeding centrifugally during fetal development. Ciliary activity that is coordinated begins during the saccular phase. Submucosal or bronchial glands are present in the trachea by week 10 of gestation, whereas goblet cells appear by week 13. The rate at which mucociliary clearance occurs at various postnatal ages has not been well characterized because of the difficulty of performing such studies in infants and small children. However, it is known that mucociliary clearance does decrease in older subjects. By analyzing the decrease in the bronchial radioactivity of an aerosol of resin particles labeled with technetium 99m, researchers noted that clearance was significantly lower in subjects older than 54 years of age compared with subjects 21 to 37 years of age. In addition, a significant negative correlation was obtained between the ages of the healthy subjects and their rate of mucociliary clearance.[26]

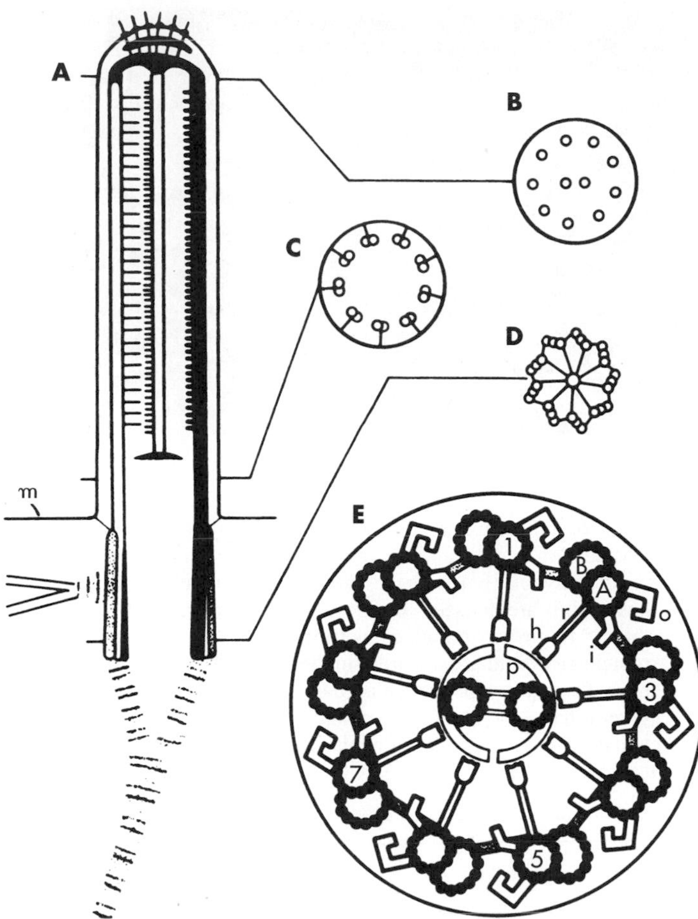

Fig. 6-5. Longitudinal (**A**) and cross-sectional (**B** to **E**) views of the structures of a cilium from the respiratory tract. **A,** Longitudinally, the ciliary shaft is surrounded by a membrane continuous with that around the cell *(m)*. The shaft terminates in a crown of claws attached to a dense cap at the tips of the longitudinal microtubules of the axoneme. The microtubules continue into the basal body, which lies in the cell's cortex and bears rootlet fibers. **B** to **D,** The structures seen in cross section depend on the level examined. A cross section from the midportion of the shaft (**E**) depicts the typical structures, including the nine doublets linked by strands of nexin *(n)*. The A subfibers of each doublet carry both outer *(o)* and inner *(i)* dynein arms that project toward the next doublet. Radial spokes *(r)* with dilated heads *(h)* can attach to projections *(p)* associated with the central microtubules. (From Sleigh MA, Blake JR, Liron N: *Am Rev Respir Dis* 137:726-741, 1988.)

PULMONARY INFLAMMATION

Nonspecific and antigen-specific (immune) mechanisms of lung defense commonly lead to an inflammatory response that is responsible for protecting this organ. Inflammation also has the potential to injure the lung,[27] but discussion of the deleterious aspects of inflammation is reserved for Chapters 25, 51, 61, and 67.

Definition and General Features of Inflammation

Inflammation is broadly defined as a nonspecific protective reaction of vascularized tissues to injury.[28] The classic clinical features of this phenomenon are related to an increase in blood flow in vessels (calor and rubor), an increase in vascular permeability and cellular infiltration (tumor), and the release of materials at the site of inflammation that leads to pain (dolor). In general, this process is self-limited and leads to the return of the tissue or organ to a normal state both structurally and functionally.

The hemodynamic changes associated with inflammation are often the first to be manifested. Vasodilation, increased blood flow, and enhanced permeability are the fundamental elements of inflammation. These alterations apparently allow the body maximal opportunity to recruit inflammatory cells and bring plasma proteins to the site of injury. This has practical importance in terms of both effectively mounting an appropriate response and limiting the process when it is no longer needed. For example, the plasma proteins may lead to resolution of the process by bringing plasma proteinase inhibitors to sites of inflammation (see later section).

The histologic picture seen in an acute inflammatory reaction within the lung is shown in Fig. 6-6. The response was produced by the instillation of C5a des Arg into the peripheral airways of normal rabbits.[29] This proinflammatory (phlogistic) fragment is generated from the fifth component of complement (C5) during complement activation through either the classic or alternative pathway and induces neutrophil chemotaxis (directed migration of neutrophils), oxygen radical generation, and neutrophil granule exocytosis.[30] The same type of inflammatory response may be seen in other vascularized tissues of the body after exposure to C5a des Arg or in the lung after exposure to other stimuli such as immune complexes and bacteria. Thus this example is meant to display the typical histologic picture of inflammation within one region of the lung (alveoli). The sequence of permeability, neutrophil accumulation, and later mononuclear phagocyte infiltration occurs before resolution of the process. Over several days, the alveoli clear, and the alveolar walls assume their normal thickness and cellularity. A similar histologic evolution in terms of progression and resolution of the process is seen in both the large and small airways.[31]

One of the fundamental features of inflammation is the redundant nature of the process. Interactions of the kinin, clotting, fibrinolytic, and complement pathways are in part responsible for this redundancy in that they each permit generation of inflammatory mediators while also allowing for amplification of the response by recruiting mediators from the other systems. In addition, a mediator or mediators with similar actions may be produced by many different cells within the lung. Therefore the inflammatory response is complex, with the possibility for generating multiple phlogistic mediators by several types of cells. This built-in redundancy both amplifies the response in a normal individual and preserves the response if one system is deficient. This latter point is best illustrated by genetic deficiencies in animals. For example, the B10.D2/nSn C5-sufficient (C5+) and B10.D2/oSn C5-deficient (C5 −) strains of congenic mice both mount inflammatory reactions to intrapulmonary challenge with *Pseudomonas aeruginosa*.[32] Although the response to this stimulus occurred earlier and was significantly greater in magnitude in the C5+ strain, there is still a sizable reaction within the lungs in the absence of C5 (Fig. 6-7).

Ontogeny of the Inflammatory Response

Knowledge about the ontogeny of inflammatory responses within the lung is limited. Most studies of ontogeny have been performed in animals, leaving researchers to speculate about

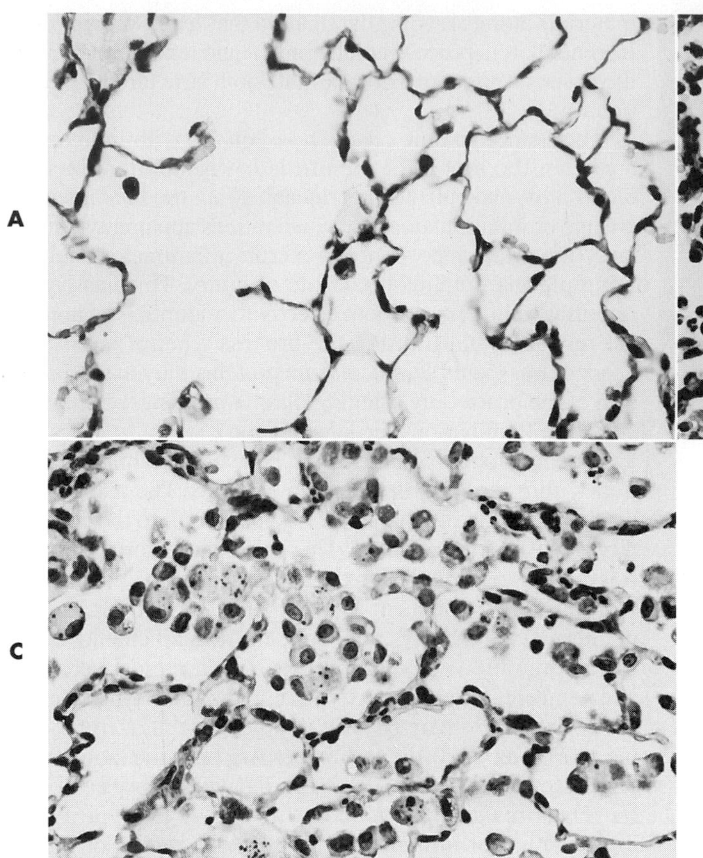

Fig. 6-6. Inflammatory response produced by instillation of C5a des Arg into the airways of rabbits. **A,** In the normal lung, resident alveolar macrophages are present in some alveoli, but neutrophils are not seen. **B,** Six hours after administration of this C5 fragment, granulocytes (primarily neutrophils) and a protein-rich fluid are apparent in the alveoli. **C,** By 24 to 48 hours the neutrophils are replaced by mononuclear cells. Over several days, the alveoli clear, and the alveolar wall returns to its normal thickness and cellularity. (From Larsen GL, Henson PM: *Ann Rev Immunol* 1:355-359, 1983.)

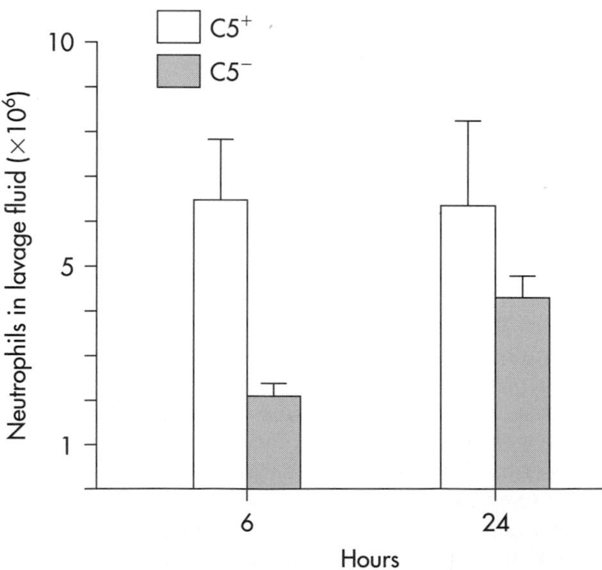

Fig. 6-7. Response of C5+ and C5 − mice to challenge with 2.5 × 10^6 *P. aeruginosa* given intratracheally. Displayed are the number of neutrophils (mean ± standard error of the mean) obtained by lavage of lungs of C5+ and C5 − mice 6 and 24 hours after bacterial challenge. In this study, the C5+ mice had an earlier and significantly greater inflammatory reaction in the lung as defined by bronchoalveolar lavage and histology. Despite the absence of C5 and an inability to produce C5 fragments, the C5 − mice still mounted an appreciable inflammatory response. (From Larsen GL, Mitchell BC, Harper TB, Henson PM: *Am Rev Respir Dis* 126:306-311, 1982.)

the relevance of the findings in humans. However, a few observations should be cited to stress that the inflammatory response has age-dependent features.

Macrophages have not been identified within the lung during the pseudoglandular and canalicular phases of fetal development.[33] In the rabbit, the influx of pulmonary macrophages into the alveoli precedes birth by several hours and occurs when phosphatidylcholine is released into the extracellular space by type II cells.[34] In terms of other inflammatory cells, some studies suggest that cellular functions (i.e., intracellular killing of organisms, oxidative metabolism, migration) of circulating human neutrophils are immature in the neonate.[35,36] In addition, newborn and perinatal animals are hyporesponsive to several vasoactive mediators as well as mediators that produce directed migration (chemotaxis) of inflammatory cells.[37] This immaturity or defect in the pulmonary inflammatory response may help explain the observation that bacterial infections of the respiratory tract are frequently encountered and can be quite severe in the young infant[36] (see Chapter 39).

Chemical Mediators of Inflammation

An *inflammatory mediator* may be defined as a chemical messenger that acts on blood vessels and cells to contribute to an inflammatory response.[28]

Vasodilation

Of the features associated with the inflammatory process, vasodilation has been the least studied. Despite this limitation, this feature is generally considered to be critically important for the full expression of an acute inflammatory reaction. In this respect, local blood flow is an important determinant of the amount of exudate produced. A number of mediators, including histamine and various eicosanoids (products of arachidonic acid metabolism), are involved in the regulation of local blood flow. For example, prostaglandins (PGs) may exert their effects in part by modulating blood flow. In addition, it is now apparent that PGs can have marked proinflammatory effects as potentiators of the effects of other mediators. PGE_2 and PGI_2 injections induce vasodilation, presumably by acting on cells of the blood vessel wall.[28] In addition, vasodilator PGs have been detected in inflammatory exudates. At physiologic concentrations, vasodilator PGs enhance the permeability effects of histamine and bradykinin.[38] A similar potentiating effect of vasodilator PGs has been noted with chemotactic factors,[39] suggesting that local vasodilation enhances the migration of neutrophils into tissue.

Other products of the cyclooxygenase pathway of arachidonic acid metabolism, such as thromboxane A_2, have vasoconstricting properties.[28] Thus the eicosanoids generated during an inflammatory process may have contrasting actions. In addition, a vasodilating PG may have effects that may be either proinflammatory or antiinflammatory. For example, PGs may inhibit leukocyte and mast cell secretion,[28] thus limiting the inflammatory response. Therefore the concentration and mix of mediators generated at a site within the lung may define the overall effect on the tissue.[40]

Altered Permeability

In many types of tissue injury, increased permeability occurs in at least two phases: an early, transient increase occurring almost immediately after an insult to the tissue and a late or second phase beginning after a variable latent period but persisting for hours or days. Evidence indicates that the early, transient permeability seen with certain types of challenges is due to the release of histamine. Mediation of the delayed phase of exudation is more complex and has been attributed to various factors, including kinins, PGs, neutrophils, and lipoxygenase products of arachidonic acid metabolism.[28]

Histamine is the mediator most often associated with an early increase in permeability after various insults to the lung. Although histamine is widely distributed, the histamine contained in mast cells within the lungs provides the primary source for acute pulmonary inflammatory reactions. Mast cells are commonly located around blood vessels and may be stimulated to release their products by several stimuli, including various drugs, allergen–immunoglobulin E (IgE) interactions, and complement fragments (C3a and C5a) produced through activation of either the alternative or the classic pathway. The concept that histamine increases vascular permeability by causing contraction of the endothelial cells of the postcapillary venule, thus creating interendothelial junctions for the passage of fluid and proteins, has been reviewed.[41]

Bradykinin can also increase vascular permeability. The generation of this mediator is complex and involves several steps and pathways.[42] First, Hageman factor (factor XII of the clotting system) is activated by contact with a negatively charged surface or by contact with a variety of biologic materials. This enzyme then activates (and is activated by) plasma kallikrein. The kinin is cleaved from kininogen by this kallikrein or kallikrein from tissues, as well as possibly by other proteases such a plasmin. Once generated, kinins are rapidly broken down in plasma and tissues by kininases and within the circulation undergo almost complete inactivation during one passage through the pulmonary circulation.[43]

Platelet-activating factor, or acetylglyceryl ether phosphorylcholine, is another mediator that can cause increases in vascular permeability as well as other proinflammatory events.[44] When inhaled into the human lung, platelet activating factor is thought to generate secondarily eicosanoids,[45] making it possible that these secondary products are responsible for some of the acute effects of this mediator. Because of its ability to aggregate rabbit platelets, this lipid was initially referred to as *platelet-activating factor.* However, it has subsequently been shown to also be a potent chemotactic factor for polymorphonuclear leukocytes. In addition, the molecule causes these cells to degranulate and stimulates an increase in oxidative metabolism. Appropriately stimulated neutrophils, eosinophils, monocytes, alveolar macrophages, and endothelial cells synthesize and release this biologically active lipid.

Several other molecules generated within the lung can increase permeability.[28] These include fibrinopeptides, fibrin degradation products, various lymphokines, and anaphylatoxins (C3a, C5a).

Cellular Infiltration

As displayed in Fig. 6-6, one of the most noticeable histologic features of an inflammatory response is accumulation of cells within the pulmonary tissue. Early in the reaction the infiltrate is predominantly neutrophils, whereas at a later time the picture is dominated by mononuclear phagocytes. The molecular mechanisms by which leukocytes migrate out of blood vessels are now being defined.[46] Central to the whole process is the concept that chemotactic factors are generated at an extravascular site and pass through the vessel wall to initiate the first step in the emigration of the cells from the vasculature: the adhesion of leukocytes to the endothelium. A number of inducible cell adhesion molecules, including endothelial-leukocyte adhesion molecule-1, have now been identified and may be critical to this process.[46]

Research in the area of inflammation has emphasized the identification of molecules that produce directed motion of inflammatory cells along a concentration gradient (chemotaxis). Some of the most potent neutrophil chemotaxins are C5 fragments.[29] These fragments are low-molecular-weight factors produced through the cleavage of C5 by a variety of endopeptidases. C5 convertases derived from the classic or alternative complement pathways cleave the 74-amino acid terminal fragment termed *C5a.* Other proteases, including plasmin, trypsin, kallikrein, and bacterial proteases, may cleave the C5 molecule at the same or a different site, generating fragments with similar biologic activities.

Within the lung, the chemotactic factors produced by alveolar macrophages after various challenges probably act with the complement system to mount a full inflammatory response. Alveolar macrophages have been recognized for some time to synthesize and secrete low-molecular-weight protein chemoattractants as well as low-molecular-weight lipids with chemoattractant activity.[47,48] One characterized mediator that is a potent chemoattractant for neutrophils in vitro and that is expressed after immune stimulation of many cell types, including macrophages, is interleukin-8 (IL-8).[49] The observation that this cytokine may also be expressed in human bronchial epithelial cells[50] again underscores the potential for redundancy of the inflammatory process.

Other specific chemoattractants for inflammatory cells include lymphokines such as IL-1 produced by monocytes and macrophages,[51] factors produced by mast cells, and lipid mediators. One potent lipid chemotactic for neutrophils is the arachidonic acid metabolite, 5,12-dihydroxyeicosatetraenoic acid, or leukotriene B_4 (LTB_4). Arachidonic acid is converted to LTB_4 and related compounds in human neutrophils, monocytes, eosinophils, and macrophages. In some leukocytes, such as the human alveolar macrophage, LTB_4 may be the major product formed from arachidonic acid.[48] In vivo, this mediator promotes the adherence of neutrophils to the blood vessel wall, leads to a polymorphonuclear leukocyte–dependent increase in vascular permeability, and is associated with accumulation of polymorphonuclear leukocytes in the skin and lung.

Within the systemic circulation, the predominant site of neutrophil margination and emigration is the postcapillary venule.[52] Although this has also been assumed to be relevant in the lung, a study within the alveoli and terminal airways of rabbits suggests that the site of neutrophil sequestration and migration may almost exclusively be within the capillary.[53] The stimulus for inflammation in this study was the activated form of C5. Before these observations can be extrapolated to other stimuli that lead to pulmonary inflammation, study of these inflammatory stimuli and their mediators must be performed. Yet the study by Downey et al[53] does raise the possibility that this pattern of leukocyte traffic may be a characteristic of the lung, reflecting the effects of hydrodynamic and geometric conditions present within the pulmonary capillaries that are unique to this vascular bed.

Oxygen Radicals

The neutrophil is armed to use both the reduced form of nicotinamide-adenine dinucleotide phosphate (NADPH) oxidase system and the granule constituents in a cooperative manner to fight invading organisms. In terms of the former, the plasma membrane of the neutrophil is the location of the enzyme NADPH oxidase that underlies this cell's ability to generate a family of reactive oxidizing chemicals, including superoxide anion, hydrogen peroxide, and the hydroxyl radical.[54] The bulk of superoxide generated by the cell dismutates to hydrogen peroxide, which is rapidly catabolized. Myeloperoxidase, an enzyme that is localized to the azurophilic granules of neutrophils and that is released in substantial amounts into the extracellular fluid when this cell is triggered, catalyzes peroxidative reactions.[55] In combination with hydrogen peroxide, myeloperoxidase can oxidize halides to their corresponding hypohalous acids. In most instances, this reaction involves chloride with the formation of hypochlorous acid (HOCl). Studies have now revealed that under a variety of conditions, human neutrophils can be triggered to generate HOCl as a major product of oxidative metabolism.[54] HOCl is a powerful oxidant that rapidly attacks biologically relevant molecules, creating a derivative group of oxidants known as *chloramines.* Although chloramines are less powerful oxidants than HOCl, they are able to chlorinate or oxidize a wide range of target molecules.[54,56] As long as hydrogen peroxide is supplied, myeloperoxidase uses plasma chloride to generate HOCl until the pool of oxidizable targets is consumed. Only then does HOCl generation come to a halt as the oxidant attacks and oxidatively autoinactivates myeloperoxidase itself.[56] Using in vitro systems, Klebanoff[55] and Test and Weiss[56] have shown that neutrophils can use the large quantities of reactive chlorinated oxidants to mediate extracellular cytotoxicity. However, it has been more difficult to implicate these oxidants in vivo. This is probably because of the fact that most in vitro systems use simple, plasma-free buffers to maximize the interactions of HOCl and the target population of cells whereas, in more physiologic surroundings, HOCl attacks both cellular targets and plasma constituents. Thus the oxidant's extracellular cytolytic potential is dissipated.

Another mechanism through which products of the respiratory burst might participate in lung defense is through the production of mediators of inflammation that potentiate an inflammatory response. A link may exist between the occurrence of aggressive oxygen species and the stimulation of eicosanoid biosynthesis.[57]

Neutrophil Granules

Neutrophils contain many storage granules, which in turn contain microbicidal substances and digestive enzymes.[35] Although three or more secretory compartments have been identified, most information concerns two types: primary and secondary granules.[58] The granules are distinguished by their protein content and the physiology of their secretory processes. Primary (azurophilic) granules are related to lysosomes and contain proteases such as elastase and cathepsins as well as several microbicidal substances, including lysozyme, myeloperoxidase, defensins,[59] and bactericidal/permeability–increasing protein. Additional cationic proteins also have microbicidal properties. In general terms, after ingestion of microorganisms into phagosomes, primary granules act as lysosomes by fusing with phagosomes to form phagolysosomes. It is felt that the contents of the primary granules are less likely than the products of secondary granules to be secreted directly into the extracellular milieu (degranulation).

The secondary (specific) granules within neutrophils are more numerous than the primary granules. The microbicidal enzyme lysozyme is found within this granule. The granules also contain lactoferrin, which may facilitate the formation of the hydroxyl radical,[60] making it a potentially important contributor to the microbicidal activity of neutrophils. Other specific granule contents include procollagenase, plasminogen activator, cytochrome *b,* histaminase, vitamin B_{12}–binding protein, and receptors for fMet-Leu-Phe, iC3b, and laminin.[58] Activation of neutrophils results in the secretion of specific granule contents into phagosomes as well as into the extracellular milieu. Thus secondary granules are thought to have more of an external secretory function in cases in which their contents modify the external environment. This modification of the environment may be important for neutrophil infiltration into tissues as well as for tissue remodeling that is part of the reparative process after an insult.

A critical part of the neutrophil's role in defense of the lung is the cell's adherence to and ingestion of particles and microorganisms by the process of phagocytosis and the subsequent killing of potentially pathogenic organisms.[58] The membrane surface components that mediate the phagocytosis of inert particles (e.g., carbon) are not well characterized. However, receptor-mediated phagocytosis can occur when microorganisms are opsonized by C3b, iC3b, or antibody. When neutrophils come in contact with such particles, there is an accumulation of actin filaments at the site of particle attachment. As the advancing pseudopod comes into contact with the particle, further receptor-opsonin interaction occurs. When the particle to be ingested is completely surrounded, the opposing pseudopods fuse to form a sealed phagosome within the cytoplasmic compartment. The contents of the phagosome fuse with primary granules to form the phagolysosome. Within the phagolysosome, defensins are major antimicrobial agents with activity against a variety of bacteria, fungi, and certain viruses.[59] The actions of these and other highly cationic proteins involves the donation of protons to form bonds with negatively charged substances at the microbial surface. Disruption of cell membrane permeability and transport mechanisms may lead to death of the cell. Other antimicrobial agents work through other mechanisms. For example, lysozyme is bactericidal because of its enzymatic cleavage of the β-1-4 bond between *N*-acetylglucosamine and *N*-acetylmuramic acid residues in bacterial cell walls. In addition to facilitating hydroxyl radical formation, lactoferrin may retard bacterial growth by binding iron so that it is not readily available to the microorganism. Elastase, a neutral protease found within primary granules, degrades proteins of gram-negative rods.[61] These and other microbicidal mechanisms of defense used by neutrophils have been reviewed.[58]

The contents of neutrophil granules also have the potential to injure the lungs and other organs.[54] Although neutrophil granules contain a large family of enzymes, their greatest potential for acting as mediators of tissue destruction probably resides in three particular enzymes: elastase and collagenase found in primary granules and gelatinase found in secondary granules. Normally, tissues are protected against injury because they are bathed in powerful plasma antiproteinases. For example, the host's primary defense against unchecked elastase-mediated damage is α_1-proteinase inhibitor, a 52-kD glycoprotein that irreversibly inhibits neutrophil elastase by forming an enzyme-inhibitor complex. Additional protection is provided by the fact the metalloproteinases (collagenase, gelatinase) are synthesized in a latent, inactive form.

NONIMMUNOLOGIC RESPONSES OF THE LUNG

Stimuli Leading to Inflammation

Stimuli that produce inflammation may do so through immunologic and nonimmunologic mechanisms. For example, the inhalation of endotoxin or noxious gases may lead to inflammation through the direct effects of the agents without participation of antigen-specific cell or humoral mechanisms directed at the stimulus. Gram-negative bacteria to which the host has been previously exposed may produce inflammation through a combination of processes. Thus endotoxin within the cell wall may serve as a stimulus for the migration of polymorphonuclear leukocytes into the site of infection.[51] When bacteria-specific antibodies are also present, an antigen-antibody complex may also initiate an inflammatory reaction. Because both processes are critical in lung defense and may provide effective deterrents only when combined, their separate components should be understood. For this reason, various aspects of nonimmune and antigen-specific defenses are considered separately. As will become apparent, some cells (e.g., macrophages, mast cells) and extracellular factors (e.g., complement) have important roles in both types of defense.

Cells of Importance in Nonimmune Responses

Some resident cells within the respiratory tract can initiate and perpetuate inflammatory reactions by virtue of their location and cellular functions. These include pulmonary macrophages, airway epithelial cells, mast cells, and polymorphonuclear leukocytes.

Pulmonary Macrophages

Macrophages are pulmonary representatives of the mononuclear phagocytic system and are present in alveoli and respiratory bronchioles (alveolar macrophages) as well as more central airways (Fig. 6-8). For simplicity, the term *pulmonary macrophage* as used in this section refers to the entire population of mononuclear phagocytes within the lung independent of the maturity of the cell and thus includes recently recruited blood monocytes as well as macrophages that have resided within the lung for several weeks. The interstitial compartment as well as the walls of conducting airways also contain macrophages.[62] These mobile cells represent a critical line of defense against injurious agents that escape clearance by the mechanisms of impaction, cough clearance, and mucociliary clearance. Many of these cells reside within the periphery of the lung, where these protective mechanisms are no longer effective because of the small size and structure of the airways.

Pulmonary macrophages have an important role in maintaining normal lung function through their ability to scavenge particulates, kill microorganisms, recruit and activate other in-

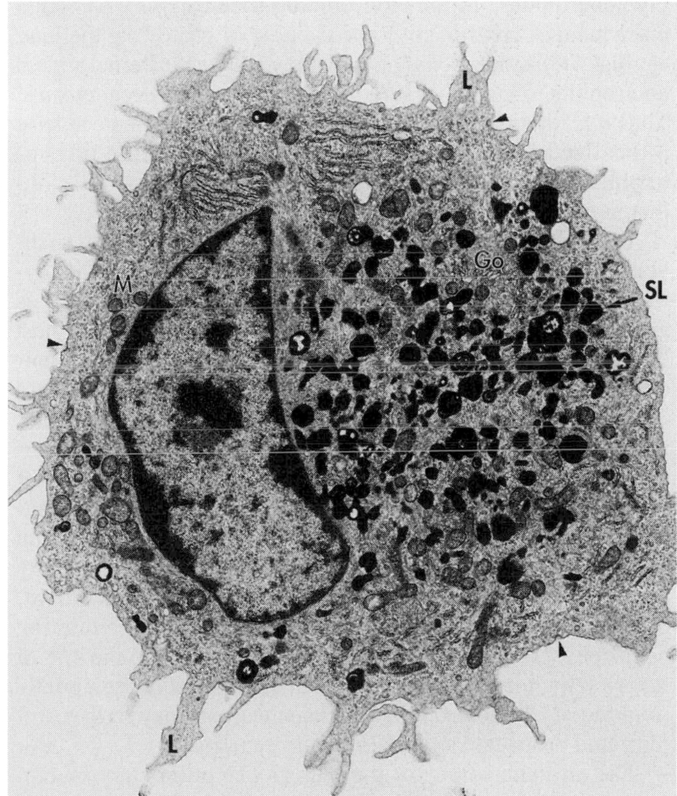

Fig. 6-8. Normal alveolar macrophage from the lung of a rabbit. The cell has a large cytoplasm-to-nuclear ratio and contains many dark cytoplasmic inclusions, the secondary lysosomes *(SL)*. Primary lysosomes are not readily apparent at this magnification. The synthetic potential of the cell is apparent from the rough endoplasmic reticulum. The secretory activity is demonstrated by the presence of Golgi apparatuses *(Go)*. Numerous mitochondria *(M)* indicate the high metabolic rate of the cell. Numerous surface folds (lamellae) are cut in cross section *(L)* and represent the active motile and phagocytic potential of this cell. At the base of the lamellae are a number of coated pits *(arrowheads)* that suggest ongoing endocytic activity. Bar = 1 um. (× 13,950.) (From Musson RA, Henson PM. In Bienenstock J, ed: *Immunology of the lung and upper respiratory tract,* New York, 1984, McGraw-Hill, pp 119-138.)

flammatory cells, and function as accessory cells in normal immune responses. A critical activity of pulmonary defense is the phagocytosis and killing of microbial organisms performed by macrophages. Pulmonary macrophages engulf particulates, including microorganisms and macromolecular debris, nonspecifically as well as through specific ligands interacting through several surface receptors, including receptors that recognize the Fc portion of most classes of Igs, CR1 and CR3 receptors, and receptors for transferrin and lactoferrin.[63] The highly ruffled plasma membrane and numerous surface folds (lamellae) indicate the active motile and phagocytic potential of this cell (see Fig. 6-8). When a particulate is phagocytized in the airway, the macrophage is usually activated to release a variety of mediators both into the phagolysosome that surrounds the ingested particle and also into the local environment of the cell. Within the cell, the respiratory oxidative burst along with lysosomal proteolytic enzymes, phagolysosomal acidification, and microbicidal cationic proteins are used to kill ingested microorganisms.[63,64] In contrast to the mechanisms of killing described for neutrophils, mature macrophages have little myeloperoxidase, so production of the hypohalide radical is not a factor in macrophage defense unless these is a source of myeloperoxidase in the environment (neutrophils). Although macrophages are thought to be capable of protecting the lung against *Staphylococcus aureus,* they may require help from neutrophils to kill *Klebsiella pneumoniae* and *P. aeruginosa.*[65] Thus it is important that macrophages be able to initiate at least a localized inflammatory response with attraction of neutrophils so that certain microorganisms can be effectively eliminated from the respiratory tract.

The secretory products of pulmonary macrophages are diverse (Box 6-1) and include oxidants, bioactive lipids, cytokines, polypeptide growth factors, and proteases as well as antiproteases.[63] These products are important not only for host defense but also for the resolution of inflammation and repair of the lung (see later section). In terms of the cell's ability to initiate and perpetuate an inflammatory response by attracting and activating other cells, experiments demonstrate that activated alveolar macrophages release factors chemotactic for neutrophils when exposed to various classes of agents, including aggregated human Ig, zymosan, and oxygen.[47,66] One such chemotactic factor is LTB_4,[48] whereas another more recently described mediator is IL-8.[49] Chemotaxins (peptide and lipid) produced by this cell are probably responsible for recruiting neutrophils as well as mononuclear phagocytes to the site of invasion by microbes, whereas chemotaxins produced directly or indirectly by neutrophils (see later section) may further amplify and propagate an inflammatory reaction.

The ultimate source of the majority of pulmonary macrophages appears to be the bone marrow.[67] Monocytes released from the bone marrow enter the lung, where they mature into tissue macrophages. The alveolar macrophage population is also replenished by local proliferation,[68] but it appears that this mechanism is not nearly as important as movement of blood monocytes from the pulmonary capillaries into the lung. In contrast to neutrophils, pulmonary macrophages normally live for longer periods in this environment (weeks to months). The factors that stimulate the influx of monocytes into the respiratory tract during the normal migration of the cell from the bone marrow as well as during inflammatory processes are not as well characterized as those that attract polymorphonuclear leukocytes from the circulation. However, these factors may include complement fragments, *N*-formylated peptides, materials from polymorphonuclear leukocytes, and lymphokines.[65]

BOX 6-1
Some Secretory Products of Pulmonary Macrophages*

Products that contribute to pulmonary defense
Toxic oxygen species
Superoxide anion
Hydrogen peroxide
Hydroxyl radical
Proteases
Elastase
Collagenase
Cathepsins
Complement components
C3
C5
Factor D
Bioactive lipids
Cyclooxygenase metabolites (PGE_2)
Lipoxygenase metabolites
Platelet-activating factor
Cytokines
IL-1
IL-8
Tumor necrosis factor

Products that resolve inflammation and repair the lung
Antioxidant
Glutathione
Antiproteases
α^1-Proteinase inhibitor
α^2-Macroglobulin
Tissue inhibitor of metalloproteinases
Polypeptide growth factors
Fibronectin
Platelet-derived growth factor
Transforming growth factor-α

*A more comprehensive list of secretory products of pulmonary macrophages may be found in Crystal.[63]

Airway Epithelial Cells

The airway epithelium has a barrier function that in itself is important in defending the lung from environmental pathogens. However, the metabolic activities of cells that line the airways may also be important in responding to potentially injurious agents. In this respect, human airway epithelial cells share with alveolar macrophages the ability to generate the products of arachidonic acid that may initiate or amplify an acute inflammatory reaction.[69] For example, one product of the 15-lipoxygenase pathway, 8,15-dihydroxyeicosatetraenoic acid, is nearly as potent as LTB_4 in its ability to produce chemotaxis of human polymorphonuclear leukocytes. As noted previously, the potent neutrophil chemoattractant IL-8 may also be expressed in human bronchial epithelial cells.[50] These metabolic properties of airway epithelial cells, coupled with the cells' strategic location within the respiratory tract, suggest that inhaled materials may stimulate the production of mediators capable of reacting to the challenge by mobilizing neutrophils to the airway. Studies using bronchial epithelial cells from species other than humans also suggest that these cells can produce chemotactic factors for other cells important in host defense and inflammatory responses, including monocytes[70] and lymphocytes.[71] In addition, fibronectin released from cultured airway epithelial cells[72] may be important in repairing the lung after an inflammatory reaction, thus preserving the lungs' structure and function (see section on resolution of inflammation). Thus epithelial cells can play a major role in lung defense and repair by modulating the inflammatory response to inhaled stimuli.

Mast Cells

Mast cells are frequently found at the interface of the internal and external environment, including the respiratory mucosal surfaces. Pulmonary mast cells are most abundant in the membranous portion of the trachea, beneath the pleura, and in the connective tissue surrounding the small airways and vessels.[73] In humans, mast cells are subdivided by neutral protease composition.[74] Mast cells with tryptase and not chymase are thought to predominate in the lung (~90%), whereas mast cells with both tryptase and chymase make up the other 10% of mast cells identified by the dispersion of mast cells from human lungs. Mast cells are a repository of several mediators with significant inflammatory potential that might limit the entry of unwanted particles into the lung. Two classes of biologically active molecules have long been recognized to be produced by these cells: preformed mediators in secretory granules and membrane-derived lipid mediators. It has been shown that cytokines are also produced by mast cells, suggesting a potential role of this cell in the growth and development of various other cell types.[75]

Although the classic mast cell secretory reaction is triggered when an allergen bridges specific IgE antibodies associated with mast cell IgE Fc receptors, it is now appreciated that in addition to allergen, several other stimuli may lead to the secretion of mediators by mast cells with tryptase and chymase. These stimuli include drugs (e.g., opiates), physical stimuli (e.g., pressure, heat, cold), neurohormones such as substance P, leukocyte-derived histamine-releasing factors, and products of complement activation such as C5a.[76] Thus mast cell activation through either nonimmunologic or immunologic mechanisms may produce mediators with many proinflammatory actions. The heterogeneity of mast cells and the potential biologic significance of these differences have been reviewed.[74,76]

Polymorphonuclear Leukocytes

Polymorphonuclear leukocytes (neutrophils, eosinophils, basophils) are normally present within the conducting airways and alveolar spaces in very small numbers and are thought to be virtually absent from the interstitial spaces of lung parenchyma.[77] However, a large number of neutrophils, estimated to be up to 3 times the circulating pool of this cell,[77] are marginated in the pulmonary vascular bed. This pool of cells as well as the circulating cells may be attracted to migrate into the lung.

As previously noted, several mechanisms may account for the recruitment of neutrophils into the respiratory tract. First, inhaled substances may directly attract neutrophils.[78] For example, chemotactic factors are present within certain microbial cell walls (formylmethionyl peptides). In addition, complement activation may result in the generation of potent neutrophil chemoattractants.[79,80] Resident alveolar macrophages may also release factors that attract neutrophils.[48] For certain inhaled stimuli, all three mechanisms may be operative and contribute to the pathologic picture.[78]

Neutrophils themselves have the potential to amplify an acute inflammatory reaction in various ways. For example, proteinases such as elastase and cathepsin G that are released from neutrophils during phagocytosis may cleave C5 to yield chemotactically active fragments. This may be especially important in patients with hereditary deficiencies of α_1-proteinase inhibitor.[81]

Once attracted into the pulmonary tissues, the actions of polymorphonuclear leukocytes include phagocytosis and the removal of particulates from the respiratory tract. The most effective phagocytosis is produced when there is opsonization of particulates with soluble material in the lung. Although the major opsonins are from the IgG class of specific antibodies (especially IgG1 and IgG3), other factors, including the complement fragment C3b, can function in this capacity. Within neutrophils, microbial killing is effected by a variety of systems, including oxygen-dependent and oxygen-independent mechanisms (cationic proteins, proteases, lysozyme).

Extracellular Factors Important in the Defense of the Lung

Although many factors with proinflammatory or antiinflammatory activity are found within the lung,[77,82] one group of proteins stand out in terms of their importance in host defense and participation in an inflammatory response: complement components.

Complement

Components of both the classic and the alternative complement pathways have been found within the lungs of nonhuman primates and humans as defined by examination of bronchoalveolar lavage fluid.[77,82,83] The third component of complement (C3) and the terminal components (C5 to C9) mediate most of the biologically important actions of this series of proteins. All are activated through both the classic and the alternative pathways.

The classic complement pathway is typically activated by antigen-antibody complexes with the involvement of IgM or the IgG1, IgG2, and IgG3 subclasses. On the other hand, the alternative complement pathway, in which the early components of the classic pathway are bypassed, can be activated by a wide variety of substances, including complex polysaccharides, lipopolysaccharide, and some immune complexes.[84] The two pathways and the complement components are displayed in Fig. 6-9, where it can be seen that activation of the alternative complement pathway yields many of the same biologically active products as activation of the classic pathway. These products include powerful chemotactic factors derived from C5 that were detailed previously. Activation of both pathways also leads to the formation of opsonins that facilitate the recognition and killing of microorganisms by phagocytic cells (iC3b). Bactericidal activity is also generated by the activation of the terminal components C5 to C9 and assembly of the membrane attack complex. The site of action of these terminal components appears to be the outer lipid membrane of gram-negative organisms.[85]

Although activation of the classic pathway is usually initiated by antigen-antibody complexes and thus may be thought of as part of the body's immunologic mechanisms of host defense (see later section), some microorganisms, including some enveloped ribonucleic viruses and certain mycoplasmas and bacteria, are also able to activate C1 (and the classic pathway) without antibody.[86] Thus both pathways may be thought of as contributing to the lung's "natural" mechanisms of defense.

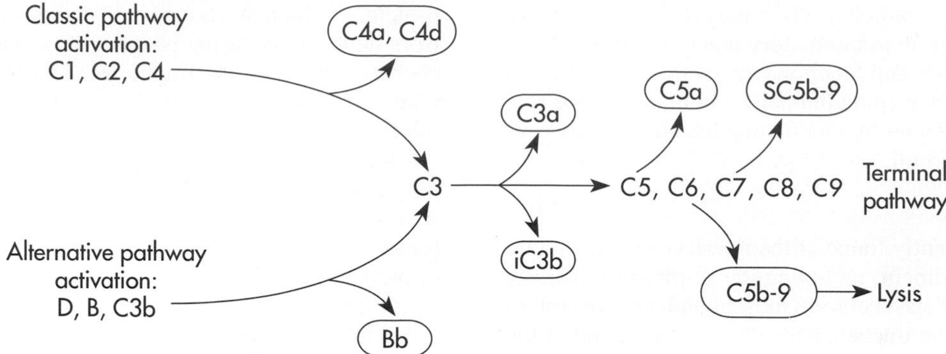

Fig. 6-9. Diagram of the major components of the complement pathways. Split products resulting from complement activation are circled. Products that are important in host defense can be produced by activation of either the classic or alternative pathway and include chemotactic factors (C5 fragments, including *C5a*), opsonins *(iC3b),* and factors with bactericidal activity (membrane attack complex, *C5b-9*). This system is an important component of the host defense response through its interactions with antibody and through mechanisms that are independent of antibody. (Courtesy Dr Patricia Giclas, National Jewish Center for Immunology and Respiratory Medicine, Denver.)

From the standpoint of ontogeny, synthesis of certain components of complement (including C3 and C5) begin in the human fetal liver during the first trimester of gestation.[87] During fetal life, the liver and other tissues continue to produce complement components. Transplacental passage of complement proteins does not occur, and the levels of immunochemically and hemolytically detectable components in normal newborn sera range between 60% and 90% of those found in adult sera. Values found in preterm infants are even lower. The concentrations of these components increase in the first few years of life until they reach normal adult levels. Overall, the activity of alternative pathway components in newborn sera is less than that of the classic pathway proteins.[88]

Other Factors

Although the complement system is a cornerstone of the noncellular host defense systems, other factors found within the pulmonary environment also contribute to the protection of the lung. The iron-binding protein transferrin is found predominately in the alveolar spaces,[89] whereas lactoferrin predominates along the airways.[90] Because iron is an essential ingredient for the survival of microorganisms, the ability of these iron-transport proteins to complex free iron in mucosal secretions and alveolar lining fluid may lead to the suppression of bacterial growth. In addition, human lactoferrin has a direct microbicidal effect on several bacteria, including *Streptococcus pneumoniae* and *E. coli.*[91] Two other components of normal bronchoalveolar lavage fluid can be thought of as nonimmune opsonins in that they have the ability to coat certain bacteria and enhance phagocytic uptake of the organism by alveolar macrophages. In this respect, fibronectin has been found to facilitate the uptake of bacteria by macrophages in vitro.[92] In addition, surfactant has been found to enhance staphylococcal phagocytosis by alveolar macrophages.[93] Other extracellular bactericidal factors of importance in pulmonary host defense (e.g., lysozymes, degradative enzymes) have been reviewed.[94]

As discussed previously, various factors within the lung can function as opsonins. For each opsonin, an opsonin-specific membrane receptor on phagocytes is responsible for binding particles coated with the opsonin. For example, iC3b is one of the most important non-Ig factors with opsonic activity, with this function mediated via two types of phagocytic receptors: CR1 and CR3. It is beyond the scope of this review to present this information in more detail. Opsonization by various factors and the membrane receptors that help mediate this host defense have been reviewed.[95]

IMMUNOLOGIC RESPONSES OF THE LUNG

Most material with antigenic potential is effectively limited from producing an immunologic response by the mechanisms of defense previously outlined. Thus for an immunologic response to occur, material must breach defense barriers and reach the responsive lymphoid tissue. When this occurs, a complex series of events transpires that subsequently provides antigen specificity to host defenses within the lung. This specificity is conferred by an elaborate system of receptors on T and B cells and through antibodies. In the context of antigen specificity, a basic function of the immune system is to differentiate "self" from "nonself" at a molecular level, thus providing additional layers of defense against foreign materials.

It is clear from several lines of investigation that the lung can function as an immune organ. Furthermore, it appears that pulmonary immune reactions are fundamentally similar to those that occur systemically.[65,96] Although the many studies in which these conclusions were drawn were performed in animal models and not humans, these conclusions appear appropriate, based on current knowledge from many sources. The lung's role as an immunologic organ has probably evolved in response to the respiratory tract's routine exposure to microbes and foreign particles that takes place with ventilation.

Overview of Normal Immunologic Responses

Generation of immune responses can be thought of in terms of three functional limbs[65]:

1. The afferent limb includes the processing and presentation of antigen to lymphatic tissue.
2. A central limb involves the interactions of immunocompetent cells that lead to the generation of effector lymphocytes.
3. The efferent limb includes the processes associated with terminal differentiation of effector lymphocytes.

The immune system ultimately exerts its effects through circulating effector cells and molecules that act at locations within the respiratory tract that may be remote from the site of the initial interaction with antigen. In this respect, the immune system consists of two major effector systems: antibody- and cell-mediated immunity. In addition to specificity of antibodies and effector lymphocytes for foreign antigens, immune responses are generally characterized by clonal expansion of antigen-reactive lymphocytes as well as memory, which leads to accelerated secondary immune responses to antigens.[96] Thus specific antibody and effector T cells may not appear for days after a nonimmune host encounters a foreign antigen that makes its way to lymphatic tissue, but specific antibody as well as sensitized T cells are more readily available in a sensitized host when the invading antigen again finds its way to the respiratory tract.

As noted, the initial phase of an immune response involves the processing, transport, and presentation of antigen to lymphocytes. This is accomplished when antigen deposited within the airways is taken up by an antigen-presenting cell, in which the antigen is processed by partial degradation. To be effective in antigen presentation, the cells must also display relevant antigenic determinants on cell surface membranes, express macromolecular gene products of the major histocompatibility complex (MHC), and secrete cytokines, including IL-1. The cells that can function in this capacity are discussed in a subsequent section.

Lymphocytes are the antigen-reactive cells of the immune system. They are distinguished primarily by certain characteristic cell surface markers called *clusters of differentiation (CD)* and by their receptors for antigen. The nomenclature of the CD markers as well as their expression as a function of T cell maturation has been reviewed in detail.[97] T cells recognize antigens by a membrane structure called the *CD3/T cell antigen receptor complex,* whereas B cells recognize antigens using surface Ig molecules. On T cells, the T cell receptor (TCR) is a disulfide-linked heterodimer composed of either α and β or γ and δ chains. Most mature T cells (more than 90% in both the blood and lungs) have an $\alpha\beta$ TCR.[98] The function of T cells expressing the $\gamma\delta$ TCR is the subject of ongoing study[99] but could include the down-regulation of immune responses to inert protein antigens presented via an intact, noninflammed epithelial surface in the respiratory tract.[100]

In a classic immune response to an exogenous antigen, the antigen-presenting cells interact with helper/inducer T cells (CD4+ cells) on which the TCR recognizes both antigen and class II MHC determinants on the cell presenting the antigen. Interaction of the two cell types, together with secretion of IL-1, leads to activation of the CD4+ cell characterized by elaboration of IL-2 and expression of IL-2 surface membrane receptors. The activated CD4+ cells undergo clonal expansion with differentiation into helper/inducer cells that can activate B cells as well as suppressor/cytotoxic T cells (CD8+ cells). In addition, activated CD4+ cells can differentiate into effectors of delayed-type hypersensitivity in that this discrete subset of cells elaborate lymphokines such as interferon-γ and migration inhibition factor, which induce the accumulation and activation of macrophages in the region of the insult.

Pulmonary Cells Important in Immunologic Responses

Antigen-Presenting Cells

Accessory or antigen-presenting cells must be able to engulf and process an antigen by partial degradation. As noted previously, they also display relevant antigenic determinants on cell surface membranes, express class II macromolecular gene products of the MHC (surface membrane HLA-DR antigens), and secrete cytokines (IL-1 and others). Within the lung, a variety of cell types, including pulmonary macrophages, dendritic cells, and B cells, might normally assume these functions. Some lung parenchymal cells (endothelial cells, alveolar epithelial cells, fibroblasts) may also function in antigen presentation under certain pathologic conditions.[101] Of these various cell types, mononuclear phagocytes[102] and dendritic cells[103] appear to be most important in terms of their antigen-presenting capabilities. Relatively speaking, compared to dendritic cells, alveolar macrophages may be less efficient antigen-presenting cells and, within the framework of their potential activities within the respiratory tract, may function more to limit than promote immunologic responses.[104] In this respect, the production of PGEs and toxic oxygen radicals by macrophages can inhibit lymphocyte proliferation.[105]

Lymphocytes

As with mononuclear phagocytes, lymphocytes are present at or near the airways extending from the nasopharynx to the alveolar spaces. Different levels of lymphatic tissue organization are identifiable in the lung and include lymph nodes (paratracheal and adjacent to major bronchi), lymphoid nodules and aggregates (throughout the submucosa of conducting airways), interstitial lymphoid tissue, and bronchoalveolar cells. The term *bronchus-associated lymphoid tissue (BALT)* has been applied to the organized tissue that is directly subjacent to the bronchial mucosa of the proximal conducting airways.[106] The nodules of lymphoid tissue that make up BALT are separated from the lumen of the airways by lymphoepithelium, a single layer of flattened epithelial cells that lack cilia and are infiltrated with lymphocytes. This structure is thought to facilitate antigen uptake. Although the contribution of BALT to local immune responses is not well defined, it may function as a repository of IgA precursor cells for the synthesis of secretory IgA.

The cellular population found within the more distal airspaces of the lung has become better defined with the use of fiberoptic bronchoscopy, with lavage as a method of sampling the cells and proteins within airways. In this respect, lymphocytes comprise approximately 7% to 10% of the cells obtained by bronchoalveolar lavage from normal humans.[77,82] Of the lymphocytes, the majority are T cells, with the overall number of T and B cells lavaged from airways closely approximating that found in peripheral blood. In addition, it appears that the relative ratio of helper to suppressor T cells in the compartment assessed by lavage is also similar to that in peripheral blood.

The extent to which immunologic responses occur in various regions of the lung depends in part on the degree of development of lymphoid tissue in different regions of the respiratory tract.[96] In this respect, immune reactions occurring at mucosal surfaces of conducting airways may be characterized by the synthesis and secretion of antibody by lymphoid cells resident in the submucosa, whereas immune responses occurring in gas-exchange units probably depend more on an influx of antigen-reactive lymphocytes that then proliferate and differentiate locally into immune effector cells.

The major effector functions of activated T cells include regulation of the various limbs of the immune response, mediation of delayed-type hypersensitivity, and production of cell-mediated cytotoxicity. These biologic function are primarily distributed between CD4+ and CD8+ cells. Different subsets of CD4+ lymphocytes are responsible for providing "help" for antibody-producing B cells, mediating delayed-type hypersensitivity reactions (via lymphokine production), inducing cytotoxic CD8+ and suppressor cells, and enhancing natural killer (NK) cell activity. Conversely, CD8+ subsets serve as suppressor cells and effect cell-mediated cytotoxicity. A more detailed description of both CD4+ and CD8+ T cell subsets is found in a review by Saltini et al.[98]

Delayed-type hypersensitivity is important in the lung's defense against viruses, fungi, mycobacteria, and other intracellular parasites.[107] As noted previously, this type of response is mediated by the subset of CD4+ cells that elaborate lymphokines, inducing the accumulation and activation of additional lymphocytes as well as mononuclear and polymorphonuclear phagocytes. Activation of macrophages in such a fashion is felt to be an important factor in the containment and elimination of intracellular parasites such as *Mycobacterium tuberculosis*. Although the initial stimulus to CD4+ activation is antigen specific, the augmented microbicidal activity of macrophages is not restricted to the immunizing organism. In this manner, the CD4+ cells that mediate delayed-type hypersensitivity bring out the important but nonspecific effector cell functions of macrophages.[105] The cellular cytotoxicity mediated by CD8+ cells is important in host defense in that it destroys virally infected host cells. Virally infected host cells display viral antigens on their surface. The CD8+ antigen-reactive cell recognizes the viral antigen as foreign and differentiates into virus-specific cytotoxic T cells.

B cells are the effectors of the humoral arm of the immune response. These cells arise from stem cells within the bone marrow and differentiate in the spleen and liver during fetal life and in the marrow during adulthood.[108] Igs synthesized by B cells serves as antigen receptors on the surface of the cell and as soluble receptors for antigens once they are secreted into the extracellular milieu. Mature B cells, characterized by the presence of Ig on surface membranes, are released into the circulation and migrate to secondary lymphatic tissue, including lymph nodes within the respiratory tract. After antigenic stimulation, B cells proliferate and differentiate into plasma cells that secrete specific antibody and into memory B cells that function in secondary anamnestic responses.

In addition to B and T cells, a third type of lymphocyte is present within the lung: the NK cell.[97,109] These lymphocytes can bind to and kill both virus-infected and tumor cells by mechanisms not yet understood. NK cells are large, granular lymphocytes that do not express on their surface the CD3 antigen or any of the known TCR chains (α, β, γ, or δ) but do express certain characteristic differentiation antigens (CD56 and CD16) and mediate cytotoxic reactions even in the absence of class I or class II MHC expression on the target cells.[110] In children, the most important role of this group of cells may be defense against viral infections. NK cells kill virus-infected host cells but not normal, uninfected cells. NK cells do not require prior exposure to antigen to respond and thus may provide an initial antiviral defense before antibodies and antigen-specific cytotoxic lymphocytes develop. Although these characteristics of NK cells suggest that they should not be included in a discussion of immunologically specific responses, it is important to note that NK cells also mediate antibody-dependent cellular cytotoxicity through a cell surface receptor located on this effector cell that binds the Fc region of Ig. Thus antibody-dependent cellular cytotoxicity provides a mechanism for NK cells to use the antigen specificity of antibodies to direct their killing activity. The cytotoxic effects of NK cells may also be increased by cytokines, including IL-2, as well as both interferon-α and interferon-γ. Because interferons are induced during viral infections, they may play a role in the antiviral immunity mediated by NK cells.

It is clear from clinical and experimental investigations that specific B and T effector cells do accumulate and function in the lung. This reaction serves to concentrate and focus cells producing antibody and specifically sensitized T cells at the site of antigen deposition. The complex network of cell-cell and cell-matrix interactions important in the margination and homing of lymphocytes to lymphoid and mucosal surfaces has recently been reviewed.[98,111]

Igs within the Respiratory Tract

All major Igs (IgG, IgA, IgM, IgE) have been identified in bronchial secretions. Their presence is felt to reflect both local synthesis as well as transudation from serum. Because of Ig's relatively low molecular weight, transudation and exudation into airway secretions may be more important for most subclasses of IgG than for the other classes of Ig (see later section). Conversely, most of the IgA, IgM, and IgE in airway secretions is probably synthesized locally. The two major Igs within the respiratory tract in terms of lung defense are IgA and IgG. In contrast to the relative amounts of Igs found within the bloodstream, the concentration of IgG relative to IgA is low in upper airway secretions but increases in the lower airways so that IgG exceeds IgA in bronchoalveolar lavage fluid.[82]

IgG

An analysis of IgG subclasses was reported on bronchoalveolar lavage fluid analysis in normal adults.[112] In this study, concentrations of IgG1 and IgG2 in lung lavage were similar to those in serum. Local IgG3 concentrations were variable in relation to values in serum, but data pertaining to IgG4 suggested preferential accumulation of this IgG subclass within the lower respiratory tract.

Well-recognized biologic activities of IgG are important in the pulmonary immune response of the respiratory tract. The formation of immune complexes either in a fluid phase or on the surface of a cell (including a bacterium and a fungus) leads to the generation of several biologically active products through the activation of complement. In addition, the IgG class of antibody (particularly IgG1 and IgG3) acts as opsonins, facilitating the recognition and killing of microorganisms by phagocytic cells. The frequency with which individuals suffering from agammaglobulinemia or hypogammaglobulinemic states develop significant pulmonary infections illustrates the important role played by this class of proteins in pulmonary defense.

IgA

Secretory IgA is the predominant Ig isotype in the respiratory tract above the larynx. As previously discussed, current evidence suggests that most of the IgA found within the upper and lower respiratory tracts is synthesized locally. Whereas approximately 90% of IgA in serum is monomeric, over 90% within the respiratory tracts is dimeric. Both the IgA1 and IgA2 subclasses are found in the respiratory tract, with the latter less susceptible to bacterial proteases.[113]

Secretory IgA consists of an IgA dimer, a joining (J) chain, and a secretory component.[65] The production of IgA at mucosal surfaces is felt to conform to the following pattern. Submucosal plasma cells synthesize the dimeric IgA with incorporation of the J chain into the molecule during this process. Secretory component is produced as a transmembrane protein by mucosal epithelial cells lining the airways. Dimeric IgA is pinocytosed into and transported across the epithelial cell to the airway lumen. During transport, dimeric IgA becomes covalently linked to the secretory component (Fig. 6-10).

The biologic activities of IgA relative to pulmonary defense have been reviewed[87] and include activation of the alternative complement pathway with the resultant generation of biologically active products as outlined in the discussion of the complement system. More important, IgA also inhibits viral binding to respiratory epithelial cells and neutralizes toxins. Regulation of antigen entry into the lymphoid tissue of the respiratory tract may also help prevent immune responses to antigens. This antibody isotype may also play a role in antibody-dependent cytotoxicity.

Ontogeny of Immunologic Responses

For the body to mount a fully developed immunologic response, several cells (e.g., macrophages, neutrophils) and mediator systems (e.g., complement pathway, products of macrophages) may be needed. The ontogeny of many of these cells and systems as they relate to lung defense have been summarized in preceding sections. It is beyond the scope of this text to review in detail the ontogeny of lymphocytes starting with fetal development. Therefore emphasis is placed primarily on the ontogenic events associated with the perinatal period and extending into childhood. Comprehensive reviews that deal with the ontogeny of immunity[114] and the developmental immunology of the lung[87] are available.

In humans, thymocytes from 9-week-old fetuses can express the γδ TCR.[115] By week 10 of fetal development, the αβ TCRs are found, followed by a progressive decrease in the number of thymocytes with γδ TCRs. T cells acquire maturational surface markers by about week 14 of gestation. Although fetal thymocytes possess several functional capabilities, detectable T cell function appears in peripheral blood lymphocytes around the time of birth. In postnatal life, lymphocytes develop in the primary lymphoid organs, namely the thymus and bone marrow. The development of diversity is felt to occur primarily in these organs, whereas clonal expansion can occur anywhere in the peripheral lymphoid tissue.[116]

The immunologic development of the human fetus has been extensively studied.[117] B cells with surface complement receptors and IgM can be detected in the fetal liver by about week 9 of gestation. By week 12, lymphocytes expressing other classes of Ig appear. During B cell ontogeny, all B cell clones arise from surface IgM-expressing progenitors. IgM synthesis can be detected as early as weeks 10 to 12, whereas IgG synthesis is demonstrated somewhat later. The synthesis of serum IgA and secretory IgA cannot be detected until week 30 of gestation.

No information is available on levels of Igs within the respiratory tract of humans as a function of development. However, Ig levels within the blood have been defined as a function of age in healthy individuals.[118] At birth, normal neonates have approximately 10% of the normal adult level of serum IgM, near-adult levels of IgG (the majority from the mother), and little or no IgA. Adult levels of IgM are achieved by 1 to 2 years of age, whereas adult concentrations of IgG are achieved by 4 to 6 years of age. Adult levels of serum IgA are not usually attained until near the time of puberty. Given that IgG is the one antibody isotype found within the lung that relies heavily on transudation from the bloodstream (see previous section), the amounts found within the lung might be expected to reflect these ontogenic differences found within the blood.

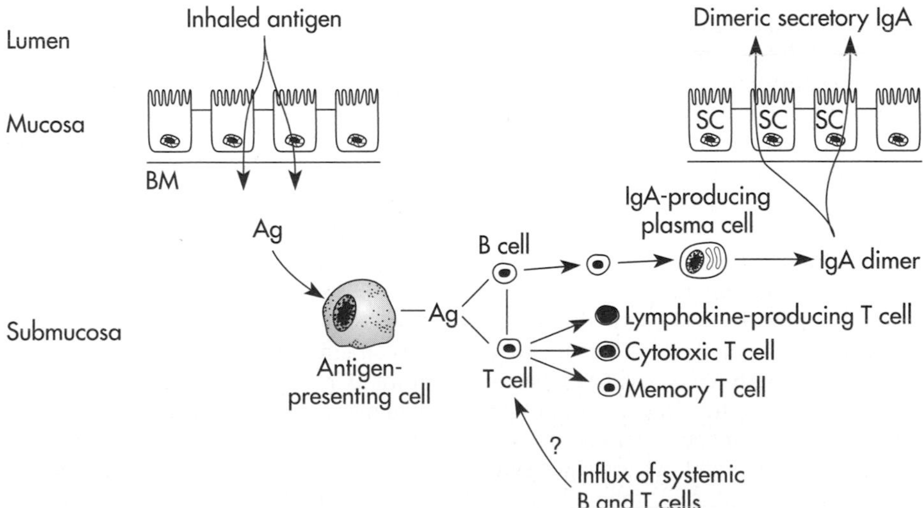

Fig. 6-10. Schematic representation of the induction, generation, and secretion of specific IgA antibody at a mucosal surface within the respiratory tract. After deposition and penetration of inhaled antigen *(Ag),* interactions occur between antigen-presenting cells and antigen-reactive lymphocytes that lead to the generation of plasma cells and effector T cells. If the plasma cell produces IgA, an IgA dimer is released from the cell and transported actively through the epithelium of serous glands via attachment to secretory component *(SC)* before release into the airway lumen. An influx of precursor lymphocytes from systemic sources may be required for a primary response, but during a secondary response, previously generated memory T and B cells may be available locally to mount an amnesic response. (From Kaltreider HB. In Murray JF, Nadel JA, eds: *Textbook of respiratory medicine,* Philadelphia, 1988, WB Saunders, pp 332-357.)

The ability to mount an antibody response in the perinatal period differs both quantitatively and qualitatively from the response in an older child or adult. The IgM response is predominant and tends to be persistent, whereas IgG and IgA antibody formation is relatively deficient.[114] This relative deficiency in IgG and IgA synthesis cannot result from a lack of precursor B cells because cells bearing these classes on their surface are present by the beginning of the second trimester. Rather, based on experimental evidence from human and nonhuman mammalian systems, the concept has arisen that there is ontogenetic dominance of suppressor T cell function early in life.[114]

RESOLUTION OF INFLAMMATION

Although a great deal of information is available on both antigen-specific and nonspecific mechanisms that initiate and perpetuate inflammation in defending the lung, much less is known about resolution of this response.[119] However, resolution of the inflammatory response is critical if injury to this organ is to be prevented. From inspection of Fig. 6-6, it is apparent that for an inflammatory response to resolve, the influx of cells must cease and injurious oxygen radicals and proteases must be inactivated. Fluids and proteins must also be removed or reabsorbed. In addition, inflammatory cells and debris must be removed and damaged cells (such as epithelial cells) replaced. As part of the reparative process, new basement membrane material may need to be laid down and epithelial cells induced to replicate.

The host has several mechanisms in place to contain an inflammatory reaction once it has been initiated. Systems known to exist for these purposes include chemotactic factor inactivator and circulating inhibitors of the neutrophil proteinases. Chemotactic factor inactivator, a major serum regulator of C5 fragment–induced neutrophil chemotaxis and neutrophil lysosomal enzyme release, may also markedly reduce the chemotactic activity caused by macrophages stimulated with phagocytic and nonphagocytic stimuli.[120] This mechanism may thus be important in limiting the neutrophilic component of an inflammatory response once it has been triggered. Also, neutrophils become "desensitized" to a chemotactic stimuli, with the resulting tachyphylaxis also contributing to termination of the influx of these cells into a tissue.[51] The major circulating inhibitors of neutrophil proteinases include α_1-proteinase inhibitor as well as α_2-macroglobulin, the tissue inhibitor of metalloproteinases, plasminogen activator inhibitor-1, α_1-antichymotrypsin, and C1 esterase inhibitor.[54] After the oxidizing environment created by the neutrophil and other inflammatory cells has dissipated, this antiproteinase screen can be reconstituted by diffusion of inhibitors from the circulation into the site of inflammation. Local synthesis of antiproteinases is also important, and cells such as monocytes and macrophages synthesize and secrete α_1-proteinase inhibitor, C1 inhibitor, plasminogen activator inhibitor, α_2-macroglobulin, and collagenase inhibitor.[121] These antiproteinases not only protect the tissue from proteolytic damage but may also prevent the persisting protease-generated formation of chemotactic factors from molecules such as C5.

Macrophages play an important role in the resolution of acute inflammation. These cells accumulate in the sites of inflammation and act as scavengers to help remove debris.[122] In helping contain the destructive potential of neutrophils, macrophages can bind and internalize the active proteases released from neutrophils.[123] Mature macrophages possess a number of receptors, including one for neutrophil elastase that may be important in this phase of the reparative process. In addition, neutrophils may be removed by macrophages in resolving inflammatory lesions. In vitro, human monocyte–derived macrophages recognize and ingest neutrophils that have undergone an aging process but not freshly isolated human neutrophils.[124] This study also suggests that a monocyte maturation process, akin to that seen during inflammation, is also necessary before macrophages recognize and remove senescent neutrophils.[124] Thus the late increase in mononuclear phagocytes that is typical of an acute inflammatory reaction may help resolve this process through ingestion of proteases and neutrophils plus removal of at least part of the tissue debris. Alveolar macrophages may also help maintain normal lung architecture through their ability to release growth factors for parenchymal cells (e.g., platelet-derived growth factor, fibronectin) and their ability to degrade the extracellular matrix.[63]

The basal lamina appears to be important for epithelial and endothelial repair. Loss of this scaffolding is one factor that may lead to permanent lung damage.[125] Knowledge is still limited in terms of signals that stimulate epithelial repair. Loss of contact with neighboring cells may stimulate mitosis and migration.[126] Type II cells may use fibronectin to link molecules of the cell and other extracellular matrix molecules.[127] Factors controlling vascular proliferation are also not well defined.[128] On the other hand, the regulation of fibroblast proliferation and collagen synthesis in lung disease has been studied in more detail.[129] Fibroblasts are influenced by contact with other fibroblasts and epithelial cells and by soluble factors produced by cells such as lymphocytes, other fibroblasts, and macrophages.[129] Macrophages appear to produce both activators and suppressors of fibroblast proliferation and collagen synthesis, with the balance of these products changing as the inflammatory process evolves.[126]

Many factors determine whether a pulmonary inflammatory response resolves after protecting the lung or persists and damages the host. A critical determinant is the nature of the insult. The physical characteristics of the agent also help determine how the inflammatory response is initiated (e.g., direct stimulation to lung parenchyma or immune or inflammatory cells, antigen presentation to immunocompetent cells, direct activation of complement). Other factors of importance include the concentration of the foreign agent as well as the length and frequency of exposure to it. In addition to inciting the inflammatory response via one of these pathways, the provoking agent certainly has an effect on the processes that control the progression and resolution of a normal inflammatory reaction. For example, inflammation may become chronic because of the persistence of the etiologic agent, such as when an intracellular parasite of low virulence survives and replicates, producing sustained inflammation. Other scenarios that lead to lung injury and influence the process of repair are discussed in Chapter 7.

CONCLUSIONS

The importance of an anatomically normal respiratory tract as well as intact humoral and cellular mechanisms for effective defense of the lung is readily apparent.[1,2,130] The pulmonary sequelae of an impaired or absent cough reflex (see Chapters 28 and 29), abnormalities of ciliary function (see Chapter 75), Ig deficiencies (see Chapters 40 and 56), and defects in oxidative metabolism in the neutrophil (see Chapter 56) all attest to the importance of these mechanisms in defending the lung against invading organisms. In general, the body is well equipped to handle challenges from the environment with a built-in redundancy in lung defense that helps ensure the integrity of the organ.

An important part of lung defense is the inflammatory reaction that can be initiated by both antigen-specific and nonspecific mechanisms. Pulmonary inflammation is generally beneficial to the host and resolves without significant sequelae because of an extensive array of checks and balances. However, it is also important to realize that when part of the checks and balances is lacking (e.g., deficiency of α_1-proteinase inhibitor), inflammation may eventually harm the host (see Chapter 78). In addition, if this programmed response goes awry (see Chapter 52), is prolonged, or is inappropriate in magnitude (see Chapter 66), lung dysfunction and irreversible injury are produced. Given the variety of environmental insults to which the lung is continuously exposed and the complexities of the processes that defend the respiratory tract, it is remarkable that lung disease is the exception. Indeed, most children never experience significant pulmonary disease because of the efficiency of these elaborate and complementary systems of defense.

REFERENCES

General Concepts of Lung Defense

1. Murray JF: Defense mechanisms. In Murray JF, ed: *The normal lung,* Philadelphia, 1986, WB Saunders, pp 313-337.
2. Reynolds HY: Pulmonary host defenses: state of the art, *Chest* 95(suppl):223S-230S, 1989.

Filtration and Deposition of Environmental Pathogens

3. Muir DCF: Particle deposition. In Crystal RG, West JB, Barnes PJ, Cherniack NS, Weibel ER, eds: *The lung: scientific foundations,* New York, 1991, Raven, pp 1839-1843.
4. Task Group on Lung Dynamics: Deposition and retention models for internal dosimetry of the human respiratory tract, *Health Phys* 12:173-207, 1966.
5. Dolovich MB, Newhouse MT: Aerosols: generation, methods of administration, and therapeutic applications in asthma. In Middleton E, Reed CE, Ellis EF, Adkinson NF, Yuninger JW, Busse WW, eds: *Allergy: principles and practice,* ed 4, St Louis, 1993, Mosby, pp 712-739.
6. Yu CP, Nicolaides P, Soong TT: Effect of random airway sizes on aerosol deposition, *Am Ind Hyg Assoc J* 40:999-1005, 1979.
7. Phalen RF, Oldham MJ, Mautz WJ: Aerosol deposition in the nose as a function of body size, *Health Phys* 57(suppl):299-305, 1989.
8. Phalen RF, Oldham MJ, Beaucage CB, Crocker TT, Mortensen JD: Postnatal enlargement of human tracheobronchial airways and implications for particle deposition, *Anat Rec* 212:368-380, 1985.
9. Phalen RF, Oldham MJ, Kleinman MT, Crocker TT: Tracheobronchial deposition predictions for infants, children and adolescents, *Ann Occup Hyg* 32(suppl):11-21, 1988.

Cough as a Mechanism to Protect the Airways

10. Korpas J, Widdicombe JG: Aspects of the cough reflex, *Respir Med* 85:3-5, 1991.
11. Karlsson J-A, Sant'Ambrogia G, Widdicombe J: Afferent neural pathways in cough and reflex bronchoconstriction, *J Appl Physiol* 65:1007-1023, 1988.
12. Morice AH, Higgins KS, Yeo WW: Adaptation of cough reflex with different types of stimulation, *Eur Respir J* 5:841-847, 1992.
13. Sheppard D, Rizk NW, Boushey HA, Bethel RA: Mechanism of cough and bronchoconstriction induced by distilled water aerosol, *Am Rev Respir Dis* 127:691-694, 1983.
14. Fuller RW: Cough. In Crystal RG, West JB, Barnes PJ, Cherniack NS, Weibel ER, eds: *The lung: scientific foundations,* New York, 1991, Raven, pp 1861-1867.
15. Leith DE: The development of cough, *Am Rev Respir Dis* 131:S39-S42, 1985.
16. Miller HC, Proud GO, Behrle FC: Variations in the gag, cough, and swallow reflexes and tone of the vocal cords as determined by direct laryngoscopy in newborn infants, *Yale J Biol Med* 24:284-291, 1952.
17. Fisher JT, Sant'Ambrogio G: Location and discharge properties of respiratory vagal afferents in the newborn dog, *Respir Physiol* 50:209-220, 1982.

Mucus Secretion and Clearance

18. Proctor DF: State of the art: the upper airways. I. Nasal physiology and defense of the lungs, *Am Rev Respir Dis* 115:97-129, 1977.
19. Jones R, Reid L: Secretory cells and their glycoproteins in health and disease, *Br Med Bull* 34:9-16, 1978.
20. Sleigh MA, Blake JR, Liron N: State of art: the propulsion of mucus by cilia, *Am Rev Respir Dis* 137:726-741, 1988.
21. Sade J, Eliezer N, Silberberg A, Nevo AC: The role of mucus in transport by cilia, *Am Rev Respir Dis* 102:48-52, 1970.
22. Clarke SW, Pavia D: Mucociliary clearance. In Crystal RG, West JB, Barnes PJ, Cherniack NS, Weibel ER, eds: *The lung: scientific foundations,* New York, 1991, Raven, pp 1845-1859.
23. Rhodin JAG: Ultrastructure and function of the human tracheal mucosa, *Am Rev Respir Dis* 93(suppl):1-15, 1966.
24. Low PMP, Luk CK, Dulfano MJ, Finch PJP: Ciliary beat frequency of human respiratory tract by different sampling techniques, *Am Rev Respir Dis* 130:497-498, 1984.
25. Mautone AJ, Cataletto MB: Mechanical defense mechanisms of the lung. In Scarpelli EM, ed: *Pulmonary physiology: fetus, newborn, child, and adolescent,* ed 2, Philadelphia, 1990, Lea & Febiger, pp 192-214.
26. Puchelle E, Zahm JM, Bertrand A: Influence of age on bronchial mucociliary transport, *Scand J Respir Dis* 60:307-313, 1979.

Pulmonary Inflammation

27. Larsen GL, Parrish DA, Henson PM: Lung defense: the paradox of inflammation, *Chest* 83S:1-5, 1983.
28. Larsen GL, Henson PM: Mediators of inflammation, *Ann Rev Immunol* 1:355-359, 1983.
29. Larsen GL, McCarthy K, Webster RO, Henson J, Henson PM: A differential effect of C5a and C5a des Arg in the induction of pulmonary inflammation, *Am J Pathol* 100:179-192, 1980.
30. Webster RO, Hong SR, Johnston RB Jr, Henson PM: Biological effects of the human complement fragments C5a and C5a des Arg on neutrophil function, *Immunopharmacology* 2:201-219, 1980.
31. Behrens BL, Clark RAF, Presley DM, Graves JP, Feldsien DC, Larsen GL: Comparison of the evolving histopathology of early and late cutaneous and asthmatic responses in rabbits after a single antigen challenge, *Lab Invest* 56:101-113, 1987.
32. Larsen GL, Mitchell BC, Harper TB, Henson PM: The pulmonary response of C5 sufficient and deficient mice to *Pseudomonas aeruginosa, Am Rev Respir Dis* 126:306-311, 1982.
33. Scarpelli EM: Lung cells from embryo to maturity. In Scarpelli EM, ed: *Pulmonary physiology: fetus, newborn, child, and adolescent,* ed 2, Philadelphia, 1990, Lea & Febiger, pp 42-82.
34. Zeligs BJ, Nerurkar LS, Bellanti JA, Zeligs JD: Maturation of the rabbit alveolar macrophage during animal development. I. Perinatal influx into alveoli and ultrastructural differentiation, *Pediatr Res* 11:197-208, 1977.
35. Falloon J, Gallin JI: Neutrophil granules in health and disease, *J Allergy Clin Immunol* 77:653-662, 1986.
36. Fick RB Jr: Cell-mediated antibacterial defenses of the distal airways, *Am Rev Respir Dis* 131(suppl):S43-S48, 1985.
37. Angle MJ, McManus LM, Pinckard RN: Age-dependent differential development of leukotactic and vasoactive responsiveness to acute inflammatory mediators, *Lab Invest* 55:616-621, 1986.
38. Williams TJ, Peck MJ: Role of prostaglandin-mediated vasodilatation in inflammation, *Nature* 270:530-532, 1977.
39. Wedmore CV, Williams TJ: Control of vascular permeability by polymorphonuclear leukocytes in inflammation, *Nature* 289:646-650, 1981.
40. Wenzel SE, Westcott JY, Smith HR, Larsen GL: Spectrum of prostanoid release after bronchoalveolar allergen challenge in atopic asthmatics and in control groups: an alteration in the ratio of bronchoconstrictive to bronchoprotective mediators, *Am Rev Respir Dis* 139:450-457, 1989.

41. Hammersen F: Endothelial contractility: does it exist? In Alltura BM, ed: *Advances in microcirculation: vascular endothelium and basement membranes,* Basel, Switzerland, 1980, Karger, pp 95-134.
42. Proud D, Kaplan AP: Kinin formation: mechanisms and role in inflammatory disorders, *Ann Rev Immunol* 6:49-83, 1988.
43. Fishman AP, Pietra GG: Handling of bioactive materials by the lung, *N Engl J Med* 291:884-890, 1974.
44. Pinckard RN, McManus LM, Hanahan DJ: Chemistry and biology of acetyl glyceryl ether phosphorylcholine (platelet activating factor). In Weissmann G, ed: *Advances in inflammation research,* New York, 1982, Raven, pp 147-180.
45. Taylor IK, Ward PS, Taylor GW, Dollery CT, Fuller RW: Inhaled PAF stimulates leukotriene and thromboxane A2 production in humans, *J Appl Physiol* 71:1396-1402, 1991.
46. Albelda SM: Endothelial and epithelial cell adhesion molecules, *Am J Respir Cell Mol Biol* 4:195-203, 1991.
47. Merrill WW, Naegel GP, Matthay RA, Reynolds HY: Alveolar macrophage-derived chemotactic factor: kinetics of in vitro production and partial characterization, *J Clin Invest* 65:268-276, 1980.
48. Martin TR, Altman LC, Albert RK, Henderson WR: Leukotriene B4 production by the human alveolar macrophage: a potential mechanism for amplifying inflammation in the lung, *Am Rev Respir Dis* 129:106-111, 1984.
49. Baggiolini M, Walz A, Kunkel SL: Neutrophil-activating peptide-1/interluekin-8: a novel cytokine that activates neutrophils, *J Clin Invest* 84:1045-1049, 1989.
50. Nakamura H, Yoshimura K, Jaffe HA, Crystal RG: Interleukin-8 gene expression in human bronchial epithelial cells, *J Biol Chem* 266:19611-19617, 1991.
51. Movat HZ: Tumor necrosis factor and interleukin-1: role in acute inflammation and microvascular injury, *J Lab Clin Med* 110:668-681, 1987.
52. Allison F Jr, Smith MR, Wood WB: Studies on the pathogenesis of acute inflammation. I. The inflammatory reaction to thermal injury as observed in the rabbit ear chamber, *J Exp Med* 102:655-667, 1955.
53. Downey GP, Worthen GS, Henson PM, Hyde DM: Neutrophil sequestration and migration in localized pulmonary inflammation: capillary localization and migration across the interalveolar septum, *Am Rev Respir Dis* 147:168-176, 1993.
54. Weiss SJ: Tissue destruction by neutrophils, *N Engl J Med* 320:365-376, 1989.
55. Klebanoff SJ: Phagocytic cells: products of oxygen metabolism. In Gallin JI, Goldstein IM, Snyderman R, eds: *Inflammation: basic principles and clinical correlates,* New York, 1988, Raven, pp 391-444.
56. Test ST, Weiss SJ: The generation and utilization of chlorinated oxidants by human neutrophils, *Adv Free Radical Biol Med* 2:91-116, 1986.
57. Lands WEM: Interactions of lipid hydroperoxides with eicosanoid biosynthesis, *J Free Radical Biol Med* 1:97-101, 1985.
58. Abramson SL, Malech HL, Gallin JI: Neutrophils. In Crystal RG, West JB, Barnes PJ, Cherniack NS, Weibel ER, eds: *The lung: scientific foundations,* New York, 1991, Raven, pp 553-563.
59. Ganz T, Selsted ME, Szklarek D, Harwig SSL, Daher K, Bainton DF, Lehrer RI: Defensins: natural peptide antibiotics of human neutrophils, *J Clin Invest* 76:1427-1435, 1985.
60. Ambruso DR, Johnston RB Jr: Lactoferrin enhances hydroxyl radical production by human neutrophils, neutrophilic particulate fractions, and an enzymatic generating system, *J Clin Invest* 67:352-360, 1981.
61. Blondin J, Janoff A: The role of lysosomal elastase in the digestion of *Escherichia coli* proteins by human polymorphonuclear leukocytes, *J Clin Invest* 58:971-979, 1976.

Nonimmunologic Responses of the Lung

62. Brain JD, Godleski JJ, Sorokin SP: Quantification, origin, and fate of pulmonary macrophages. In Brain JD, Proctor DF, Reid LM, eds: *Respiratory defense mechanisms,* New York, 1977, Marcel Dekker, pp 849-892.
63. Crystal RG: Alveolar macrophages. In Crystal RG, West JB, Barnes PJ, Cherniack NS, Weibel ER, eds: *The lung: scientific foundations,* New York, 1991, Raven, pp 527-538.
64. Hocking WG, Golde DW: The pulmonary-alveolar macrophage, *N Engl J Med* 301:580-587, 639-645, 1979.
65. Kaltreider HB: Phagocytic, antibody and cell-mediated immune mechanisms. In Murray JF, Nadel JA, eds: *Textbook of respiratory medicine,* Philadelphia, 1988, WB Saunders, pp 332-357.
66. Fox RB, Hoidal JR, Brown DM, Repine RE: Pulmonary inflammation due to oxygen toxicity: involvement of chemotactic factors and polymorphonuclear leukocytes, *Am Rev Respir Dis* 123:521-523, 1981.
67. Thomas ED, Rambergh RE, Sale GE, Sparkes RS, Golde DW: Direct evidence for bone marrow origin of the alveolar macrophage in man, *Science* 192:1016-1018, 1976.
68. Bitterman PB, Saltzman LE, Adelberg S, Ferrans VJ, Crystal RG: Alveolar macrophage replication: one mechanism for the expansion of the mononuclear phagocyte population in the chronically inflamed lung, *J Clin Invest* 74:460-469, 1984.
69. Hunter JA, Finkbeiner WE, Nadel JA, Goetzl EJ, Holtzman MJ: Predominant generation of 15-lipoxygenase metabolites of arachidonic acid by epithelial cells from human trachea, *Proc Natl Acad Sci USA* 82:4633-4637, 1985.
70. Koyama S, Rennard SI, Shoji S, Romberger D, Linder J, Ertl R, Robbins RA: Bronchial epithelial cells release chemoattractant activity for monocytes, *Am J Physiol* 257:L130-L136, 1989.
71. Robbins RA, Shoji S, Linder J, Gossman GL, Allington LA, Klassen LW, Rennard SI: Bronchial epithelial cells release chemoattractant activity for lymphocytes, *Am J Physiol* 257:L109-L115, 1989.
72. Sjoji S, Ertl RF, Linder J, Romberger DJ, Rennard SI: Bronchial epithelial cells produce chemotactic activity for bronchial epithelial cells: possible role for fibronectin in airway repair, *Am Rev Respir Dis* 141:218-225, 1990.
73. Friedman MM, Kaliner MA: Human mast cells and asthma, *Am Rev Respir Dis* 135:1157-1164, 1987.
74. Kitamura Y: Heterogeneity of mast cells and phenotypic change between subpopulations, *Ann Rev Immunol* 7:59-76, 1989.
75. Plaut M, Pierce JH, Watson CJ, Hanley-Hyde J, Nordan RP, Paul WE: Mast cell lines produce lymphokines in response to cross-linkage of FcεRI or to calcium ionophores, *Nature* 339:64-67, 1989.
76. Schwartz LB, Huff TF: Mast cells. In Crystal RG, West JB, Barnes PJ, Cherniack NS, Weibel ER, eds: *The lung: scientific foundations,* New York, 1991, Raven, pp 601-616.
77. Hunninghake GW, Gadek JE, Kawanami O, Ferrans VJ, Crystal RG: Inflammatory and immune processes in the human lung in health and disease: evaluation by bronchoalveolar lavage, *Am J Pathol* 97:149-206, 1979.
78. Von Essen SG, Robbins RA, Thompson AB, Ertl RF, Linder J, Rennard S: Mechanisms of neutrophil recruitment to the lung by grain dust exposure, *Am Rev Respir Dis* 138:921-927, 1988.
79. Fick RB Jr, Robbins RA, Squier SU, Schoderbek WE, Russ WD: Complement activation in cystic fibrosis respiratory fluids: in vivo and in vitro generation of C5a and chemotactic activity, *Pediatr Res* 20:1258-1268, 1986.
80. Robbins RA, Russ WD, Rasmussen JK, Clayton MM: Activation of the complement system in the adult respiratory distress syndrome, *Am Rev Respir Dis* 135:651-658, 1987.
81. Johnson U, Ohlsson K, Olsson I: Effects of granulocyte neutral proteases on complement components, *Scand J Immunol* 5:421-426, 1976,
82. Young KR Jr, Reynolds HY: Bronchoalveolar washings: proteins and cells from normal lungs. In Bienenstock, J, ed: *Immunology of the lung and upper respiratory tract,* New York, 1984, McGraw-Hill, pp 157-173.
83. Kolb WP, Kolb LM, Wetsel RA, Rogers WR, Shaw JO: Quantitation and stability of the fifth component of complement (C5) in bronchoalveolar lavage fluids obtained from nonhuman primates, *Am Rev Respir Dis* 123:226-231, 1981.
84. Fries LF, Winkelstein JA: The complement system. In Crystal RG, West JB, Barnes PJ, Cherniack NS, Weibel ER, eds: *The lung: scientific foundations,* New York, 1991, Raven, pp 447-468.
85. Joiner KA: Studies on the mechanism of bacterial resistance to complement-mediated killing and on the mechanism of action of bactericidal antibody, *Curr Top Microbiol Immunol* 121:99-133, 1985.
86. Winkelstein JA: Complement and natural immunity, *Clin Immunol Allergy* 3:421-439, 1983.
87. Kamani NR, Bonagura VR: Developmental immunology of the lung. In Scarpelli EM, ed: *Pulmonary physiology: fetus, newborn, child, and adolescent,* Philadelphia, 1990, Lea & Febiger, pp 140-160.
88. Johnston RB Jr, Alternburger KM, Atkinson AW, Curry RH: Complement in the newborn infant, *Pediatrics* 64(suppl):781-786, 1979.
89. Bell DY, Haseman JA, Spock A, McLennan G, Hook GER: Plasma proteins of the bronchoalveolar surface of the lungs of smokers and nonsmokers, *Am Rev Respir Dis* 124:72-79, 1981.

90. Thompson AB, Bohling T, Payvandi F, Rennard SI: Lower respiratory tract lactoferrin and lysozyme arise primarily in the airways and are elevated in association with chronic bronchitis, *J Lab Clin Med* 115:148-150, 1990.
91. Arnold RR, Brewer M, Gauthier JJ: Bactericidal activity of human lactoferrin: sensitivity of a variety of microorganisms, *Infect Immun* 28:893-898, 1980.
92. Czop JK, McGowan SE, Center DM: Opsonin-independent phagocytosis by human alveolar macrophages: augmentation by human plasma fibronectin, *Am Rev Respir Dis* 125:607-609, 1982.
93. O'Neill SJ, Lesperance E, Klass DJ: Human lung lavage surfactant enhances staphylococcal phagocytosis by alveolar macrophages, *Am Rev Respir Dis* 130:1177-1179, 1984.
94. Coonrod JD: The role of extracellular bactericidal factors in pulmonary host defense, *Semin Respir Infect* 1:118-129, 1986.
95. Ross GD: Opsonization and membrane complement receptors. In Ross GD, ed: *Immunobiology of the complement system: an introduction for research and clinical medicine,* Orlando, Fla, 1986, Academic, pp 87-114.

Immunologic Responses of the Lung

96. Kaltreider HB: Normal immune response. In Crystal RG, West JB, Barnes PJ, Cherniack NS, Weibel ER, eds: *The lung: scientific foundations,* New York, 1991, Raven, pp 499-510.
97. Lanier L: Cells of the immune response: lymphocytes and mononuclear phagocytes. In Stites DP, Terr AI, eds: *Basic and clinical immunology,* ed 7, Norwalk, Conn, 1991, Appleton & Lange, pp 61-72.
98. Saltini C, Richeldi L, Holroyd KJ, du Bois RM, Crystal RG: Lymphocytes. In Crystal RG, West JB, Barnes PJ, Cherniack NS, Weibel ER, eds: *The lung: scientific foundations,* New York, 1991, Raven, pp 459-482.
99. Augustin A, Kubo RT, Sim G-K: Resident pulmonary lymphocytes expressing the γ/δ T-cell receptor, *Nature* 340:239-241, 1989.
100. McMenamin C, Olvier J, Girn B, Holt BJ, Kees UR, Thomas WR, Holt PG: Regulation of T-cell sensitization at epithelial surfaces in the respiratory tract: suppression of IgE responses to inhaled antigens by CD3+ $TcR\alpha^-/\beta^-$ lymphocytes (putative γ/δ cells), *Immunology* 73:234-239, 1991.
101. Hance AJ: Accessory-cell–lymphocyte interactions. In Crystal RG, West JB, Barnes PJ, Cherniack NS, Weibel ER, eds: *The lung: scientific foundations,* New York, 1991, Raven, pp 483-498.
102. Brain JD: Lung macrophages: how many kinds are there? What do they do? *Am Rev Respir Dis* 137:507-509, 1988.
103. Sertl K, Takemura T, Taschachler E, Ferrans VJ, Kaliner MA, Shevach EM: Dendritic cells with antigen presenting capability reside in airway epithelium, lung parenchyma and visceral pleura, *J Exp Med* 163:436-451, 1986.
104. Kaltreider HB: Alveolar macrophages: enhancers or suppressors of pulmonary immune reactivity? *Chest* 82:261-262, 1982.
105. Nathan CF, Murray HW, Cohen ZA: The macrophage as an effector cell, *N Engl J Med* 303:622-626, 1980.
106. Bienenstock J: Bronchus-associated lymphoid tissue. In Bienenstock J, ed: *Immunology of the lung and upper respiratory tract,* New York, 1984, McGraw-Hill, pp 96-118.
107. Murray HW: Interferon-gamma, the activated macrophage, and host defense against microbial challenge, *Ann Intern Med* 108:595-608, 1988.
108. Wall R, Kuehl M: Biosynthesis and regulation of immunoglobulins, *Ann Rev Immunol* 1:393-422, 1983.
109. Robinson BWS, Pinkston P, Crystal RG: Natural killer cells are present in the normal human lung but are functionally impotent, *J Clin Invest* 74:942-950, 1984.
110. Trinchieri G: Biology of natural killer cells, *Adv Immunol* 47:187-376, 1989.
111. Woodruff JJ, Clarke LM, Chin YH: Specific cell-adhesion mechanisms determining migration pathways of recirculating lymphocytes, *Ann Rev Immunol* 5:201-222, 1987.
112. Merrill WW, Naegel GP, Olchowski JJ, Reynolds HY: Immunoglobulin G subclass proteins in serum and lavage fluid of normal subjects: quantitation and comparison with immunoglobulins A and E, *Am Rev Respir Dis* 131:584-587, 1985.
113. Mestecky J, Russell MW: IgA subclasses, *Monogr Allergy* 19:227-301, 1986.
114. Lawton AR, Cooper MD: Ontogeny of immunity. In Steihm ER, ed: *Immunologic disorders in infants and children,* ed 3, Philadelphia, 1989, WB Saunders, pp 1-14.
115. Kamani NR, Douglas SD: Structure and development of the immune system. In Stites DP, Terr AI, eds: *Basic and clinical immunology,* ed 7, Norwalk, Conn, 1991, Appleton & Lange, pp 9-33.
116. Claman HN: The biology of the immune response, *JAMA* 268:2790-2796, 1992.
117. Van Furth R, Schuit HRE, Hijmans W: The immunological development of the human fetus, *J Exp Med* 122:1173-1188, 1965.
118. Allansmith M, McClellan BH, Butterworth M, Maloney JR: The development of immunoglobulin levels in man, *J Pediatr* 72:276-290, 1968.

Resolution of Inflammation

119. Henson PM, Larsen GL, Henson JE, Newman SL, Musson RA, Leslie CC: Resolution of pulmonary inflammation, *Fed Proc* 43:2799-2806, 1984.
120. Robbins RA, Justice JM, Rasmussen JK, Russ WD, Thomas KR, Rennard SI: Role of chemotactic factor inactivator in modulating alveolar macrophage–derived neutrophil chemotactic activity, *J Lab Clin Med* 109:164-170, 1987.
121. Barbey-Morel C, Pierce JA, Campbell EJ, Perlmutter DH: Lipopolysaccharide modulates the expression of α_1 proteinase inhibitor and other serine proteinase inhibitors in human monocytes and macrophages, *J Exp Med* 166:1041-1054, 1987.
122. Musson RA, Henson PM: Phagocytic cells. In Bienenstock J, ed: *Immunology of the lung and upper respiratory tract,* New York, 1984, McGraw-Hill, pp 119-138.
123. Campbell EJ: Human leukocyte elastase, cathepsin G, and lactoferrin: family of neutrophil granule glycoproteins that bind to an alveolar macrophage receptor, *Proc Natl Acad Sci USA* 79:6941-6945, 1982.
124. Newman SL, Henson JE, Henson PM: Phagocytosis of senescent neutrophils by human monocyte–derived macrophages and rabbit inflammatory macrophages, *J Exp Med* 156:430-442, 1982.
125. Vracko R: Basal lamina scaffold: anatomy and significance for maintenance of orderly tissue structure, *Am J Pathol* 77:313-346, 1974.
126. Kuhn C III: Inflammation and repair. In Murray JF, Nadel JA, eds: *Textbook of respiratory medicine,* Philadelphia, 1988, WB Saunders, pp 289-302.
127. Torikata C, Villiger B, Kuhn C III, McDonald JA: Ultrastructural distribution of fibronectin in normal and fibrotic human lung, *Lab Invest* 52:399-408, 1985.
128. Folkman J, Klagsbrun M: Angiogenic factors, *Science* 235:442-447, 1987.
129. Clark JG, Kuhn C III, McDonald JA, Mecham RP: Lung connective tissue, *Int Rev Connect Tissue Res* 10:249-331, 1983.

Conclusions

130. Goldstein IM, Shak S: Humoral and cellular mediators of host defenses. In Murray JF, Nadel JA, eds: *Textbook of respiratory medicine,* Philadelphia, 1988, WB Saunders, pp 358-373.

CHAPTER 7

Mechanisms of Acute Lung Injury and Repair

Gregory P. Downey and Hugh M. O'Brodovich

The syndrome of acute lung injury, also known as *adult respiratory distress syndrome (ARDS),* was first alluded to by Osler[1] three quarters of a century ago and formally described by Ashbaugh et al[2] in 1967. Despite the word *adult,* this syndrome in fact has been described in patients as early as 2 weeks of age and certainly occurs in the pediatric population in a form that is indistinguishable from the adult disease.[3-5] In addition, established hyaline membrane disease in the premature infant is clinically and pathophysiologically similar to ARDS. ARDS is the result of a final common pathway initiated by a variety of local or systemic insults that lead to diffuse damage of the pulmonary parenchyma. (This chapter interchangeably uses the terms *ARDS* and *acute lung injury.*) The first clinically recognizable consequences of this injury largely ensue from an increase in the permeability of the alveolar-capillary membrane with resultant pulmonary edema.[6] Despite the accumulation of a tremendous amount of information regarding the physiologic and cellular basis of lung injury and increasingly sophisticated supportive (intensive) care, significant improvements in prognosis have lagged behind.

Although the advances in intensive care have prevented early deaths from respiratory failure, unfortunately these patients often die later from progressive multiorgan failure. This latter sequence of events, termed the *systemic inflammatory response syndrome (SIRS),* is attributable to generalized and uncontrolled activation of the inflammatory response (Fig. 7-1), leading to diffuse endothelial injury and microcirculatory dysfunction.[7] SIRS, of which lung injury is but a part, is a consequence of an abnormal host response to the inciting event, and although most commonly related to progressive infection, noninfectious disorders can result in a similar clinical syndrome.

In the last two decades, enthusiastic researchers have claimed to discover the mediator responsible for the syndrome. Unfortunately, none of these discoveries have withstood the test of time. Moreover, several therapeutic strategies targeting candidate mediators have been tested in clinical trials. Despite the enthusiasm generated in preliminary studies, it has been conclusively demonstrated that antiendotoxin,[8] anti–tumor necrosis factor-α antibodies,[9] and antagonists of interleukin-1 (IL-1)[10] are not beneficial for most patients and in fact may be detrimental. No one mediator is responsible for acute lung injury; rather, a complex interplay exists between diverse proinflammatory (e.g., lipopolysaccharide [LPS], complement products, cytokines, chemokines, reactive oxygen species, eicosanoids) and antiinflammatory (IL-10, IL-1 receptor agonist, prostaglandin I_2) mediators. It is essential that clinicians obtain a better understanding of the complexities of the acute inflammatory response in ARDS if they are to successfully intervene to prevent and ameliorate tissue injury.

CLINICAL AND PATHOLOGIC ASPECTS

The syndrome of acute lung injury is manifested by hypoxemic respiratory failure that usually arises after a latent period of 6 to 72 hours after initial exposure to one of a variety of predisposing insults.[11] During this latent period, before severe organ damage occurs, there may be a window of opportunity that has great potential for therapeutic intervention. The most common predisposing events include severe systemic infection (sepsis), shock, multiple trauma, pancreatitis, and overwhelming bacterial or viral pneumonia (Box 7-1). Despite the multiplicity of these inciting events, the resulting clinical manifestations and pathologic findings are remarkably uniform, suggesting that common pathogenic mechanisms or tissue responses exist. The initial clinical manifestations of acute lung injury include dyspnea, tachypnea, cyanosis refractory to oxygen therapy, decreased lung compliance, and radiographically evident diffuse alveolar infiltrates.[2] The most stringent criteria for ARDS include that no cardiovascular dysfunction should exist as the primary inciting cause and that the pulmonary capillary occlusion (wedge) pressure should not be elevated. As the disease state progresses, severe pulmonary hypertension often coexists.[12] Finally, in a minority of patients, refractory hypoxemia and hypercapnia supervene and become unresponsive to ventilator therapy.

It has become apparent from epidemiologic studies that a range of illness severity exists and that the prognosis varies according to the nature of the predisposing factors and the extent of lung and other organ dysfunction.[13,14] Estimates of the incidence of ARDS were originally 75 per 100,000 with an associated mortality rate of 50% to 60%. More recent data have cast some doubts on these figures and suggest that the incidence may be 1.5 to 3.5 per 100,000.[15] The apparently changing incidence rate probably reflects better initial care of the predisposing events, so fewer cases progress to lung injury severe enough to be classified as ARDS; it is likely that the initial figures represent an overestimate. With respect to the variations in mortality rate, the prognosis varies according to the predisposing cause and extent of organ dysfunction, which may differ among centers. It is hoped that the use of a standardized scoring system for lung injury[13-16] with more rigorous definitions for ARDS will help resolve these apparent discrepancies.

Because acute respiratory failure was the most clinically obvious and immediately life-threatening manifestation of ARDS, lung injury was the focal point of early investigations. However, as patients survived the initial critical period, it became evident that widespread organ dysfunction (Table 7-1), ranging from biochemical abnormalities to frank failure of multiple organs, accompanied or followed the pulmonary abnormalities.[17] This multisystem involvement (i.e., SIRS) in-

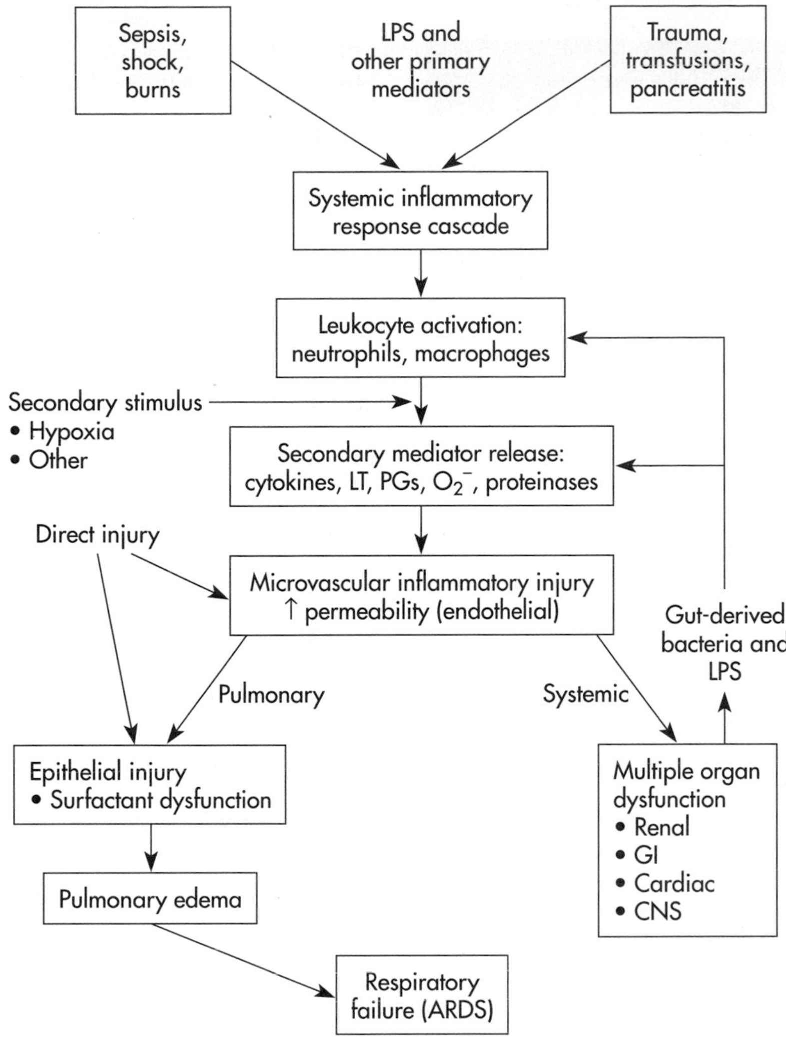

Fig. 7-1. Proposed mechanisms underlying acute lung injury (ARDS) and the SIRS. Diffuse activation of the inflammatory response cascade leads to microvascular sequestration of leukocytes and endothelial injury. In the lung, epithelial injury is a major contributing factor to pulmonary edema. *LPS,* Lipopolysaccharide; *LT,* leukotriene; *PGs,* prostaglandins; O_2^-, superoxide; *GI,* gastrointestinal; *CNS,* central nervous system.

BOX 7-1
Conditions Predisposing to Acute Lung Injury (ARDS)

Direct lung injury

Overwhelming pneumonia: bacterial, fungal, viral, mycoplasmal, *Pneumocystis*
Inhalational injuries
- Nitrogen dioxide
- Chlorine
- Sulfur dioxide
- Ammonia
- Phosgene
- Smoke

Oxygen toxicity*
Aspiration*
- Gastric contents
- Hydrocarbons
- Saltwater or fresh water

Pulmonary contusion
Radiation pneumonitis*
Embolism
- Air*
- Bone marrow (fat)

Secondary lung injury

Sepsis syndrome
- Infectious causes (bacteremia, fungemia)
- Noninfectious causes (immunologic [e.g., systemic lupus erythematosus])

Shock
Trauma
Burns
Pancreatitis
Disseminated intravascular coagulation
Effect of cardiopulmonary bypass
Diabetic ketoacidosis
Massive blood transfusion (>10 U)
Drug overdose
- Narcotics (heroin, methadone)
- Salicylates

Paraquat exposure

*These entities may have elements of direct and secondary lung injury.

Table 7-1 Multiple Organ Dysfusion Syndrome: Examples of Organ Dysfunction

SYSTEM	EVIDENCE OF DYSFUNCTION
Cardiovascular	Decreased left and right ventricular function
Renal	Oliguria, progressive azotemia
Central nervous	Confusion, agitation, seizures, coma
Hematologic	Thrombocytopenia, leukopenia, activation of the clotting and fibrinolytic cascade
Gastrointestinal	Liver: elevated aminotransferase levels, hyperbilirubinemia, loss of reticuloendothelial function
	Gastrointestinal system: hemorrhage, ileus, malabsorption

cluded dysfunction or failure of the cardiovascular system, kidneys, central nervous system, hematologic system, and gastrointestinal system. In addition to these clinically conspicuous manifestations of gastrointestinal dysfunction, the loss of the barrier function of the gut facilitates portal and eventually systemic translocation of bacterial and the release of bacterial products such as LPS.[18] Bacteremia and endotoxemia likely contribute to the overwhelming systemic activation of the inflammatory response.

At autopsy, the lungs of the patients are heavy (edematous), firm (resembling liver), congested, and diffusely atelectatic.[19] Microscopically, there is hyperemia with engorged dilated capillaries and widespread microthromboemboli; alveoli are filled with proteinaceous fluid containing red and white (neutrophils and macrophages) blood cells as well as cell fragments. There is diffuse alveolar atelectasis, and hyaline membranes (composed of fibrin strands, plasma proteins, and cell debris) are seen primarily within alveolar ducts.[20] The enormous number of neutrophils within the pulmonary capillaries, interstitium, and alveolar space is noteworthy (see later section). Evidence of injury to the endothelium and epithelium is widespread, with cellular edema, degeneration, and finally cell death leading to exposure of the underlying basement membrane of both the endothelial and epithelial surfaces. The leakage of circulating blood cells and plasma components into the interstitial and alveolar spaces indicates the loss of the alveolar-capillary membrane's barrier function. Together, these features define this as an acute inflammatory response involving the lung in a diffuse manner (hence the old term *diffuse alveolar damage*). If the patient survives this stage of the disease, a reparative phase ensues with proliferation of cuboidal epithelial cells (derived from type II pneumocytes) and increased interstitial cellular infiltrates. From 5 to 7 days after the clinical onset of ARDS, a fibrotic phase supervenes with disruption of the acinar structure and fibrosis involving the alveoli and alveolar ducts. The total lung collagen can be increased twofold to threefold,[21] illustrating the magnitude of fibrosis that occurs during this phase.

PATHOPHYSIOLOGY

Vascular and Epithelial Permeability

For this discussion, *injury* is defined physiologically as a loss of a tissue's or an organ's ability to perform its normal function. With respect to the lung, the most obvious functional consequence of injury is the inability to sustain effective gas exchange, leading to progressive hypoxemic respiratory failure and inability to remove carbon dioxide. The primary disturbance of ARDS is a type of pulmonary edema characterized by an increase in permeability of the alveolar-capillary membrane to fluid, solutes, and formed elements (cells) of the blood.[22] The accumulation of edema fluid in the interstitial and alveolar spaces contributes both directly and indirectly to decreased lung compliance and decreased functional residual capacity. Recent work has suggested that the decreased compliance is due in large part to the widespread presence of nonventilated regions of the lung,[23] which may represent as much as two thirds of the total potentially functional alveolar units; thus for the same change in airway pressure, less than the usual volume of alveolar gas is exchanged. Also, because the specific compliance of the remaining ventilated lung units is relatively normal, they are overdistended by mechanical ventilation when conventional tidal volumes and resultant high airway pressures place them at the top of their pressure-volume curve. These two factors are primarily responsible for the observed decrease in total lung compliance. There is also significant mismatching of ventilation and perfusion with inappropriate continued perfusion of areas of low or no ventilation (shunt) that results in hypoxemia. Ventilation-perfusion imbalance in areas of high ventilation and perfusion result in dead space ventilation that is increased (often markedly) in ARDS. The widespread microemboli may contribute to this elevation. In addition, the increased water content of the lung contributes both directly (by compression of vessels) and indirectly (by hypoxic pulmonary vasoconstriction) to an increased pulmonary vascular resistance.

To understand the mechanisms involved in the production of this edema, the clinician must first understand the factors regulating water and solute movement in the normal lung. Although briefly described here, a more thorough discussion of pulmonary edema is found in Chapter 57.

Normal Physiology of Transmembrane Water and Solute Movement

The movement of water and solutes out of the circulation and across the alveolar-capillary membrane is usually discussed in terms of the Starling equation.[1*] This equation describes the rate of fluid movement (J_v) across a semipermeable membrane in response to hydraulic and osmotic forces, as follows:

$$J_v = PS \cdot [(P_{mv} - P_{pmv}) - \sigma (\pi_{mv} - \pi_{pmv})]$$

Examination of the Starling equation reveals several potential mechanisms for increasing fluid flow across a membrane. The

*PS refers to the conductance of the membrane to fluid and is the product of the permeability per unit surface area (P) and the available surface area (S). P_{mv} refers to the hydrostatic pressure within the fluid-exchanging *micro*vessels (capillaries and somewhat larger vessels). P_{mv} has been only indirectly assessed. The Taylor-Gaar equation ($P_{mv} = P_{LA} + [P_{PA} - P_{LA}] \cdot 0.4$) is reasonably accurate in normal lungs but is the average pressure of all of the arteriolar, capillary, and venular regions participating in fluid exchange. These various regions may have differing values, and data also indicate that the ratio of upstream to downstream resistances varies with disease or the use of vasoactive agents. P_{pmv} refers to the *peri*micro*v*ascular pressure, which is usually negative in the normal lung and "follows" pleural pressure. σ refers to the reflection coefficient for solutes and describes the resistance to the transmembrane movement of the solute, which is therefore the ability of that solute to express its potential osmotic pressure. (If $\sigma = 1$, then the solute is always reflected, whereas if $\sigma = 0$, then it moves freely across the membrane.) π refers to the osmotic pressure generated by an "ideal" solute (i.e., $\pi = 1$) and is proportional to the solute's concentration as described by van't Hoff's law. The negative sign between the hydraulic and osmotic forces is necessary because they induce fluid movement in opposite directions.

rate of fluid movement increases in response to elevated transmembrane hydraulic pressures, altered osmotic pressures (the concentration of solutes to which the membrane is relatively impermeable), or changes in the permeability to solutes or fluid, or the amount of perfused microvascular surface area. (The term *microvascular* refers to blood vessels that participate in fluid exchange and include both alveolar and extraalveolar intrapulmonary vessels; the latter contribute approximately 30% to 50% of total lung fluid movement.)

The epithelial and endothelial membranes have markedly different reflection coefficients for solutes. The pulmonary endothelium has relatively large interendothelial spaces with effective molecular radii of approximately 40 Å. This contrasts to the interepithelial tight junctions, which have effective molecular radii of approximately 4 Å and thus make the epithelial monolayer so tight that it restricts the movement of even sodium and chloride. In normal lung endothelium, the various-sized proteins, not the ions (the endothelial reflection coefficient for sodium = 0), are the relevant solutes when considering the osmotic pressure and reflection coefficient. Just the opposite occurs for the *normal* epithelium in which ions become osmotically active solute as the reflection coefficient of sodium approaches 1. Because each 1 mOsm/L yields 19 mm Hg of osmotic pressure, the contribution of the protein (only about 1.5 mOsm/L even in plasma) is trivial compared to the electrolyte concentration of 280 mOsm/L. Once the integrity of the epithelial tight junctions is lost, changes in ionic concentrations would at best have a very transient and minimal effect on transmembrane fluid movement. Thus the maintenance of a polarized epithelial monolayer with intact tight junctions on its apical membrane is critical for normal lung function.

Altered Transmembrane Fluid Movement

A hallmark of acute lung injury syndromes is the protein-rich exudate found within the lung's interstitial and alveolar spaces. Intuitive reasoning and experimental data indicate that there must be profound increases in the epithelial and endothelial permeability to solutes. However, the classic separation of cardiogenic (high pressure) and noncardiogenic (high permeability) pulmonary edema at best is correct for only the first stages of the disease process and at worst has been an arbitrary and incorrect classification that has led to a poor understanding of the disease process. For example, it has recently been demonstrated that classic high-pressure pulmonary edema in postnatal lungs is also characterized by significant epithelial injury and that fluid can move directly from the vascular to alveolar spaces through these epithelial lesions.[24] Similarly, prematurely born infants with classic surfactant-deficiency respiratory distress syndrome (hence high-pressure pulmonary edema from markedly negative hydrostatic pressure) rapidly develop distal lung epithelial lesions with hyaline membrane formation[25] and have increased pulmonary permeability to solutes.[26] In ARDS, the high-permeability pulmonary edema is associated with leakage of protein into the alveolar space. As discussed later, these proteins and especially fibrin or fibrinogen and its degradation products rapidly cause surfactant dysfunction. The resultant increased surface tension would make perimicrovascular pressure even more negative, further promoting increases in fluid movement. Also, changes in vascular pressures or perfused surface area can greatly increase lung fluid accumulation. Not only is this obvious on a theoretic basis (see equation in previous section), but experimental data have also shown that an increase from 5 to only 10 mm Hg[27] in pulmonary arterial occlusion pressures or a doubling of pulmonary blood flow and perfused surface area[28] in the presence of increased pulmonary permeability edema markedly increases the leakage of fluid into the lungs. Therefore so that the clinician can better understand the mechanisms of edema formation during acute lung injury, better knowledge of the characteristics of membrane barrier decreases (cellular loss or intercellular integrity) and regulation of transmicrovascular hydraulic and osmotic pressures (even within the usually "normal" ranges) is required.

Cellular Mechanisms

The basic mechanisms leading to the pathologic and physiologic alterations of acute lung injury have not been clearly delineated. As the syndrome develops, an acute inflammatory response in the lung is initiated and progresses to diffuse lung injury (see Fig. 7-1). So that what goes wrong in ARDS can be illustrated, it is useful to compare a situation in which lung inflammation proceeds in a more regulated fashion, such as uncomplicated pneumococcal pneumonia.[29] Although these two entities share some similarities, several important differences become evident on closer examination. Both involve an acute inflammatory response, but in the case of pneumonia, once the inciting cause (i.e., the bacteria) has been removed, the inflammation resolves and the lung returns to its premorbid state. This implies that under most circumstances, counterregulatory mechanisms limit inflammatory damage and allow repair mechanisms to succeed (see later section). In acute lung injury syndrome, the inflammatory response is activated on a massive scale and becomes generalized (systemic) and self-propagating despite removal of the inciting cause.[30]

Direct (Toxic) Lung Injury

The term *direct (toxic) lung injury* implies the direct toxicity of a noxious substance or substances to pulmonary parenchymal tissues (primarily endothelial and epithelial cells), leading to acute lung injury syndrome without the primary requirement for activation of leukocytes. Conditions and substances known to be directly toxic to lung tissues include ingestion of hydrocarbons, radiation pneumonitis, aspiration of gastric acid, and inhalation of toxic gases (see Box 7-1). With direct injury, pulmonary endothelial or epithelial cells are damaged, leading to loss of the barrier function of the alveolar-capillary membrane, resulting in pulmonary edema. However, the fully developed acute lung injury syndrome resulting from these conditions is in many cases intensified by the secondary activation of the inflammatory cascade. An example of this overlap is pulmonary oxygen toxicity in which there may be an initial direct toxic effect on the pulmonary endothelial and epithelial cells[31] followed by secondary inflammatory damage.[32-34]

Leukocyte-Mediated Lung Injury

The most common pathway leading to acute lung injury syndrome involves the unregulated release of leukocyte-derived toxic products, including reactive oxygen species, proteolytic enzymes, products of arachidonic metabolism such as platelet-activating factor, and cationic proteins (Box 7-2). Initial attention was directed at the most abundant leukocyte, the neutrophil. It has been demonstrated in vitro and in vivo that neutrophils can be stimulated by a variety of activating agents such as LPS,[35-37] complement fragments,[38] and tumor necro-

BOX 7-2
Leukocyte-Derived Toxic Products

Oxidants (reactive oxygen species)

Superoxide anion
Hydrogen peroxide
Hydroxyl radical
Hypohalous acids (hypochlorous acid])
Chloramines
Nitric oxide
Peroxynitrite*

Proteolytic enzymes

Elastase
Gelatinase
Collagenase
Cathepsin
Lysozyme
Neuraminidase
Heparanase

Other products

Cationic proteins (defensins)

*Peroxynitrite is the reaction product of superoxide and nitric oxide.

sis factor[39] to release toxic products that injure endothelial and epithelial cells. The neutrophil has also been implicated in animal models of acute lung injury induced by the administration of endotoxin,[40] hyperoxia,[41] microembolization,[42] and mechanical ventilation.[43] In humans, much evidence (albeit indirect) implicates leukocytes in the pathogenesis of acute lung injury. Transient leukopenia, presumably from pulmonary microvascular sequestration, precedes the onset of clinically manifested lung injury,[44] and excess numbers of neutrophils are present in the pulmonary microvasculature and bronchoalveolar fluid[45] of patients with acute lung injury. Neutrophils isolated from these patients are in an activated state as assessed by the enhanced release of reactive oxygen species and lysosomal enzymes in vitro.[46] Moreover, excessive amounts of potentially injurious leukocyte products, including the proteolytic enzymes elastase[47] and collagenase,[48] have been found in lung lavage fluid. Excessive amounts of hydrogen peroxide[49] have also been found in expired air from patients with acute lung injury. Thus much evidence indicates a primary role for activated neutrophils in the pathogenesis of acute lung injury. However, it is also apparent that other inflammatory cells, including cells of the monocyte-macrophage lineage, can produce toxic products injurious to lung tissues.[50,51] Under unusual circumstances, such as in neutropenic patients,[52,53] these other types of leukocytes may be the primary sources of mediators of lung injury.

A question that must be addressed is why neutrophils, which serve a crucial physiologic function in host defense as phagocytes (a fact attested to by the propensity for infections in patients with defects in certain neutrophil functions), suddenly turn on their host. The pulmonary capillaries are the major site of the physiologic marginated pool of neutrophils, which accounts for 75% of all intravascular neutrophils.[54,55] Under physiologic circumstances, these cells exist in relative harmony with the lung; that is, their substantive armamentarium is held in check. However, in pathologic circumstances, in which there is diffuse activation of the inflammatory response, control mechanisms are overwhelmed, and these neutrophils become activated in close apposition to the alveolar-capillary membrane. The release of leukocyte-derived toxic compounds can result in immediate damage to this crucial part of the lung. Moreover, the entire cardiac output passes through the lungs, enabling the rapid delivery of additional neutrophils. When the inflammatory response is prolonged, large numbers of young neutrophils and precursor cells can be released into the circulation from the marrow to replenish those that have emigrated into the tissues, thus sustaining the inflammatory response.[56,57]

There is incomplete understanding of the pathways regulating leukocyte activation and their malfunction in inflammatory disorders. Under normal physiologic circumstances, neutrophils slowly pass through the labyrinth of the pulmonary capillary bed in a stop-and-go fashion but without prolonged stops.[58] When there is widespread activation of the inflammatory response, circulating leukocytes are exposed to chemotactic factors and other inflammatory mediators. These can be produced by several lung cells (alveolar macrophages and pulmonary endothelial and epithelial cells can release growth factors, eicosanoids, platelet-activating factor, and IL-8) and cells of the monocyte-macrophage system in other parts of the body (IL-1 and tumor necrosis factor), or the factors may be present in the circulation (complement fragments, proteins of the coagulation cascade such as fibrinopeptide B, and LPS). Circulating neutrophils exposed to these factors are retained within pulmonary capillaries (Fig. 7-2). That the capillary is the site of sequestration and emigration of neutrophils (Fig. 7-3) is unique to the lung compared to the systemic microvascular beds (where these events occur in the postcapillary venules) and may result from unique geometric and hydrodynamic constraints in the pulmonary microcirculation.[59-63]

The initial phases of neutrophil retention likely result from an increase in their mechanical rigidity secondary to alterations in the microfilament component of their cytoskeleton.[64] Because the median diameter of human pulmonary capillaries is less than that of the circulating leukocytes (5.5 vs. 8.0 μm), these rigid cells are unable to deform rapidly enough to negotiate the capillaries and are therefore retained (see Fig. 7-2). After this initial retention based on mechanical alterations, a second, more prolonged retention phase occurs secondary to increased adhesive forces between the leukocytes and endothelial cells (Fig. 7-4). In particular, adhesion* likely begins with an interaction between L-selectin on the neutrophil plasma membrane and sulfated glycoproteins on the endothelium, although the precise nature of the endothelial ligand for

*Adhesion molecules can be divided into several families, including the immunoglobulin superfamily (intercellular adhesion molecule-1 [ICAM-1], ICAM-2, and vascular cell adhesion molecule [VCAM]), the selectins (E-, L-, and P-selectins), and the integrins.[68] L-selectin is expressed by neutrophils and may mediate cell rolling and the early phase of adherence. Leukocytes express at least three types of β_2-integrins—$\alpha_L\beta_2$ (leukocyte function–associated antigen-1 [LFA-1] = CD11a/CD18), $\alpha_m\beta_2$ (Mac-1 = CD11b/CD18), and $\alpha_x\beta_2$ (gp150/95 = CD11c/Cd18)—and heterodimers composed of noncovalently associated α and β subunits, which are involved in cell-to-cell and cell-to-substratum adhesion. Macrophages and neutrophils also express β_1-integrins, such as $\alpha_4\beta_1$. Neutrophils and monocytes express a novel integrin termed the *leukocyte response integrin,* closely related to the β_3-integrin family. Counterreceptors for some of these integrins are known: ICAM-1 and ICAM-2 for $\alpha_L\beta_2$ (LFA-1); C3b, fibrinogen, and ICAM-1 for $\alpha_m\beta_2$ (Mac-1), fibrinogen for $\alpha_x\beta_2$ (gp150/95); and fibronectin and VCAM for $\alpha_4\beta_1$. These adhesion molecules are involved in many diverse cell functions that are indispensable for normal function, such as cell-to-cell and cell-to-substratum interactions, phagocytosis, and motility.[68]

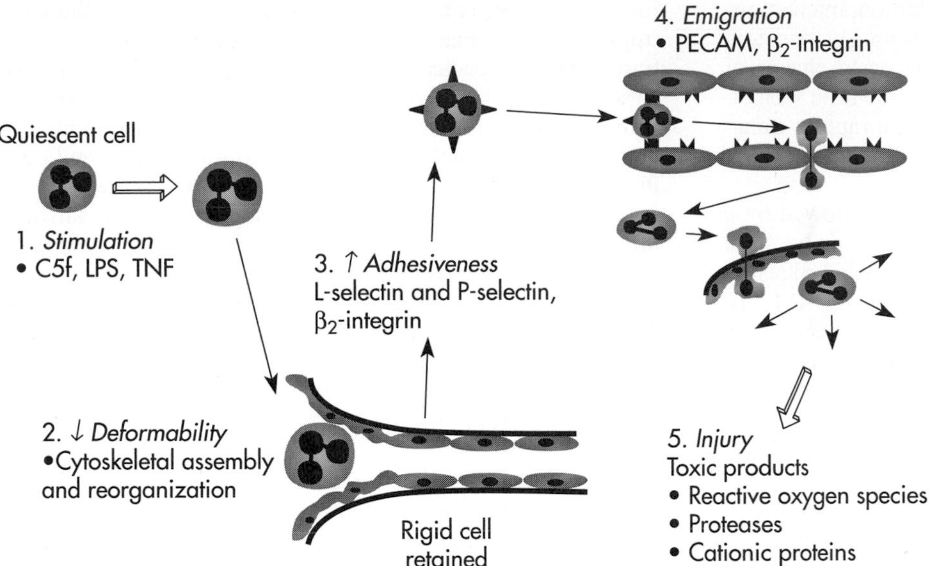

Fig. 7-2. Proposed mechanisms underlying pulmonary leukocyte sequestration and emigration in acute lung injury (ARDS). Stimulation of circulating cells leads to changes in cell deformability (increased rigidity) and increased adhesiveness, resulting in microvascular sequestration. Emigration across the endothelium, through the interstitium, across the epithelium, and into the alveolar space follows. During these processes, the release of toxic products, including reactive oxygen species, proteolytic enzymes, and cationic proteins, results in damage to the surrounding cells. *TNF,* Tumor necrosis factor; *PECAM,* platelet–endothelial cell adhesion molecule.

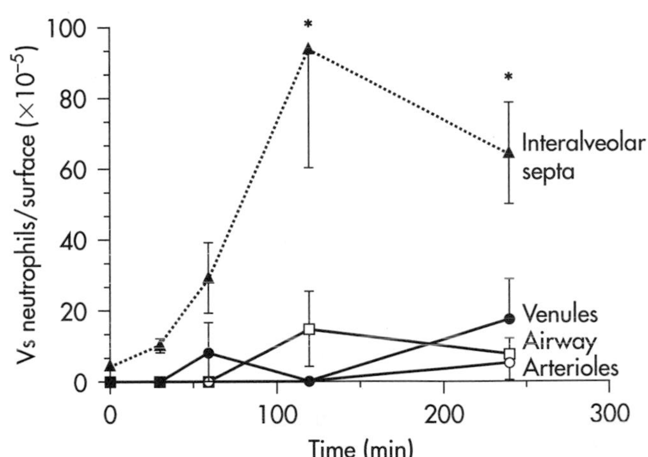

Fig. 7-3. Neutrophil sequestration and migration occurs almost exclusively in the pulmonary capillaries. Quantification of the volume of neutrophils in the four compartments is normalized to the surface area of the basal lamina of the compartment. Note that the interalveolar septum is the location of the pulmonary capillaries. Volume to surface ratio *(Vs)* of neutrophils in the interalveolar septa normalized to the surface area of the interalveolar septa is significantly increased at 60, 120, and 240 minutes and in the airways at 120 minutes. Symbols represent the mean plus or minus the standard error of the mean (in mm^3/mm^2). Asterisks indicate significant differences in $P \leq 0.05$ compared to control values. (From Downey GP et al: *Am Rev Respir Dis* 147:168-176, 1993.)

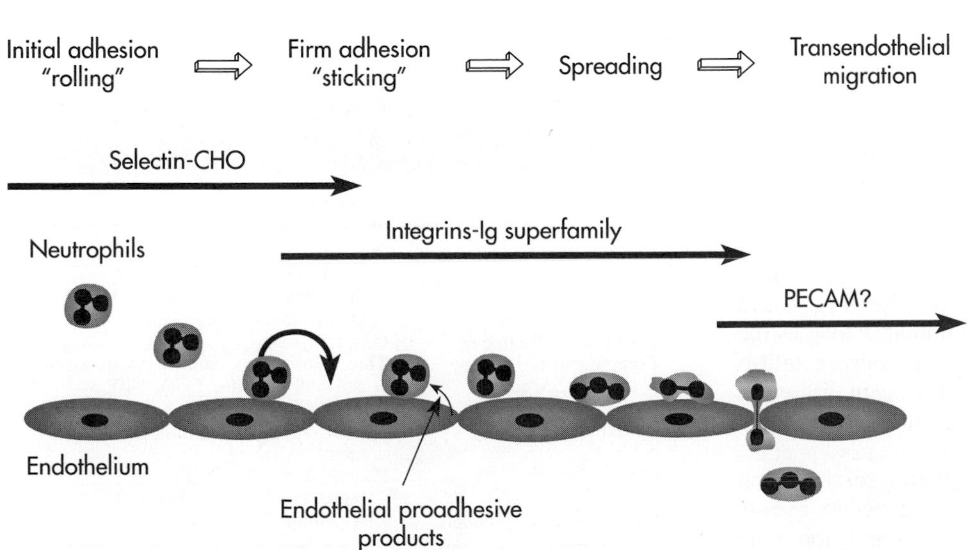

Fig. 7-4. Proposed mechanisms underlying pulmonary leukocyte adhesion and emigration in acute lung injury (ARDS). The initial low-affinity adhesive interactions are mediated by selectin-carbohydrate *(CHO)* interactions. Both L-selectin and P-selectin are involved at this stage. Slightly later, high-affinity adhesive interactions involving α_2-integrins (CD11/CD18) on the neutrophil and endothelial adhesion molecules of the immunoglobulin *(Ig)* superfamily (e.g., intercellular adhesion molecule-1) occur. Endothelial-derived lipid mediators such as platelet activating factor likely participate at this phase to promote neutrophil adhesion. Emigration across the endothelium follows and involves platelet–endothelial cell adhesion molecules *(PECAM)* in the endothelial intercellular junctions.

neutrophil L-selectin is uncertain.[65-68] In addition, interactions between endothelial P-selectin and P-selectin glycoprotein ligand on the neutrophil contribute to the early phases of adhesion.[69,70] Stores of P-selectin are contained within Weibel-Palade bodies in the endothelial cells and are rapidly transported to the plasma membrane in response to inflammatory mediators.

These initial carbohydrate interactions are followed by a higher-affinity (firm) and more prolonged interaction between leukocyte β_2-integrins (CD11/CD18) and endothelial adhesion molecule (intercellular adhesion molecule-1 [ICAM-1]). Platelet-activating factor produced by endothelial cells may act on neutrophils in close proximity, leading to potentiation of their adhesion to the endothelium.[71] As the inflammatory response progresses, there are increased synthesis and surface expression of additional endothelial adhesion molecules, including ICAM and E-selectin, that promote further adhesion of leukocytes to the pulmonary endothelium. Transmigration of neutrophils across the epithelial barrier involves the interaction of the platelet–endothelial cell adhesion molecule (localized to the intercellular junctions of endothelial cells) with cognate ligands, including the platelet–endothelial cell adhesion molecule itself, on the neutrophil plasma membrane.[72] Pulmonary microvascular sequestration, even with extravascular migration of neutrophils, is by itself insufficient to induce lung injury. Rather, additional factors such as hypoxia and exposure to activating agents or inflammatory mediators such as arachidonic acid metabolites are necessary before these sequestered and emigrating cells release sufficient amounts of toxic products to result in lung injury.[73] Once circulating cells become adherent, their behavior is altered. Specifically, if these adherent cells (either attached to the endothelium, the epithelium, or interstitial matrix proteins) are exposed to additional activating agents such as cytokines produced by alveolar macrophages, they release enormous quantities of reactive oxygen species and proteolytic enzymes,[74] thus potentiating pulmonary dysfunction.

Priming relates to the phenomenon whereby exposure of leukocytes to subthreshold levels of one agent (that do not in themselves result in activation) primes the cell so that on exposure to a secondary (activating) agent, a greatly augmented response (e.g., oxidant release) is observed.[75] In essence, the response of a primed cell to a given activating stimulus is much larger than if a naive cell was similarly exposed. For example, low concentrations of LPS do not activate neutrophils, but if these primed cells are then exposed to a second (activating) stimulus such as complement fragments, phorbol esters, or lipid mediators such as leukotriene B_4, the resultant production of superoxide is enhanced manyfold. When these in vitro observations are related to acute lung injury, the immense numbers of neutrophils sequestered within the pulmonary microvasculature combined with the altered behavior of adherent and primed leukocytes[76,77] may be one of the principal reasons for amplification and loss of control of the regulation of the early phase of the inflammatory response. Returning once more to the example of a localized pneumonia, as long as the host defense mechanisms (combined with appropriate antibiotic therapy) deal effectively with the inciting agent (bacteria), the inflammatory response does not spiral out of control, and tissue injury is minimal.

The systemic activation of the inflammatory response can be self-perpetuating, inducing a variety of secondary events that lead to further amplification and loss of regulation. One important event is a loss of the barrier function of the gastrointestinal tract that facilitates portal and eventually systemic translocation of bacterial as well as bacterial products such as LPS.[78,79] Products of these intestinally derived bacteria, such as LPS (endotoxin), gain access to the cells of the reticuloendothelial system, including hepatic (Kupffer's cells) and pulmonary macrophages, which in turn release a variety of inflammatory mediators (Table 7-2), including cytokines such as tumor necrosis factor, IL-1, and IL-8.[30] Bacterial translocation and macrophage activation are believed to play an integral role in what has been termed the *amplification phase* of the syndrome that is consequent to systemic activation of the inflammatory response.

Pulmonary Hypertension

In both the early and late phases of acute lung injury, moderate to severe pulmonary hypertension is observed and may contribute to respiratory failure. Clinically, the presence of pulmonary hypertension in patients with ARDS is associated with a poor prognosis.[12] The pathophysiologic basis of pulmonary hypertension includes functional and structural components. Pulmonary vasoconstriction is observed in the earliest stages of the acute lung injury and is likely multifactorial, with contributions from extravascular compression by edema fluid, hypoxic pulmonary vasoconstriction, the release of vasoactive compounds (including endothelin), and products of arachidonic acid metabolism such as thromboxane A_2 and leukotrienes. The source of these vasoactive metabolites is unclear, but leukocytes, platelets, endothelial cells, and other lung parenchymal cells are all possible sources.[19] Recent attention has been directed at a possible deficit in the production of vasodilator substances such as nitric oxide produced by endothelial nitric oxide synthase.[80,81] Paradoxically, although net vasoconstriction of the pulmonary vascular bed may be present, in some forms of acute lung injury the pulmonary vascular pressor response to local alveolar hypoxia is reduced or lost completely, thus aggravating the degree of hypoxemia. Morphologic studies have demonstrated that early in the genesis of acute lung injury, there is often widespread occlusion of the small pulmonary arteries and arterioles by microthromboemboli (see later section). At later stages, there is often extensive obliteration of the microvessels in conjunction with extensive remodeling of the remaining arterioles. The aggregate effects of these abnormalities combined with the changes in vasomo-

Table 7-2 Mediators Implicated in Acute Lung Injury Syndrome

CLASS OF MEDIATOR	EXAMPLES
Products of arachidonic acid metabolism	Platelet-activating factor, hydroxyeicosatetraenoic acid, thromboxanes, leukotrienes B_4 and D_4, prostaglandins E_2, and I_2
Complement fragments	C3a, C5a, $C5a_{des\ arg}$
Components of the clotting cascade	Thrombin, fibrinopeptides, plasminogen activator inhibitor, factor VIII, α_2-antiplasmin
Cytokines	IL-1, IL-2, IL-6, IL-8, tumor necrosis factor
Growth factors	Platelet-derived growth factor, transforming growth factor-β
Bacteria-derived products	LPS (endotoxin)

tor tone contribute to the ventilation-perfusion mismatching and severe pulmonary hypertension that is present in ARDS.

Coagulation and Fibrin Deposition

The coagulation and fibrinolytic cascades are activated during acute lung injury, thereby generating both thrombin and plasmin endogenously. The amount of thrombin generated in premature newborns with respiratory distress syndrome correlates with the severity of the disease.[82] As a result of the endogenous thrombin generation, intravascular fibrin deposition occurs in infants with persistent pulmonary hypertension[83] and adults with either ARDS[84] or acute respiratory failure.[85,86] The pathologic generation of thrombin and plasmin could have several effects on pulmonary circulation. These include increased pulmonary vascular resistance from the mechanical obstruction of the pulmonary vessels and the generation of vasoactive products that could both alter vascular tone and increase the permeability of the pulmonary microvascular bed to proteins.[87]

During acute lung injury, the generation of thrombin with fibrin formation is not confined to the intravascular space. Bronchoalveolar lavage samples obtained from patients with ARDS[88] document the activation of the coagulation cascade and impaired fibrinolytic capacity (Fig. 7-5). Intraalveolar fibrin deposition occurs in both neonatal[89] and adult[22] respiratory distress syndromes. This extravascular fibrin deposition occurs within the alveolar ducts and spaces, especially in areas of epithelial destruction. This fibrin formation could adversely affect gas exchange, especially if fibrin prevents the reexpansion of collapsed airspaces or the reabsorption of alveolar exudates. Furthermore, fibrinogen, fibrin monomer, and products of fibrin degradation are among the most potent inhibitors of surfactant function.[90,91]

The mechanism or mechanisms responsible for thrombin generation, fibrin deposition, and fibrin degradation are complex, and a detailed discussion is beyond the scope of this chapter. In brief, physiologic and pathophysiologic activation of the coagulation system is initiated by the exposure of blood to tissue factor (TF) (previously reflected by the extrinsic pathway). TF is expressed by several cell types, including alveolar macrophages and fibroblasts, but healthy endothelial cells do not express TF on their surfaces. However, endothelial cells in culture do express TF on their surfaces in response to a variety of stimuli, including IL-1α, tumor necrosis factor-α, thrombin, and endotoxin. The expression of TF by endothelial cells is of particular relevance because these cell surfaces have the ability to support the assembly of clotting factor components on their surface. Patients with ARDS also have increased levels and qualitative changes in the circulating von Willebrand factor antigen. These abnormalities also promote thrombosis because of the enhanced platelet–vessel wall interaction.[92]

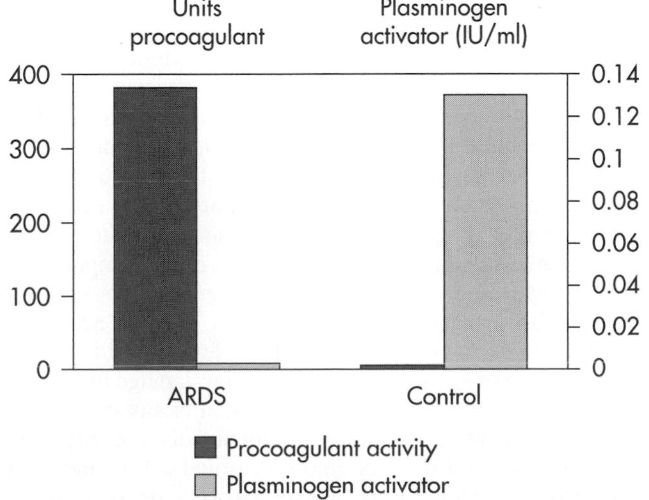

Fig. 7-5. Deposition of fibrin within the alveolar space is markedly enhanced during ARDS because of the markedly increased procoagulant and markedly decreased fibrinolytic capacity in bronchoalveolar lavage fluid. (Data from Idell S et al: *J Clin Invest* 84:695-705, 1989; and Bertozzi P et al: *N Engl J Med* 322:890-897, 1990.)

Only recently have clinicians studied the mechanisms responsible for regulating thrombin generation with resultant fibrin formation and dissolution. All the components required for fibrin formation are present in the airspaces of patients with ARDS because the alveolar edema fluid contains plasma proteins of all sizes.[93,94] Alveolar macrophages express TF activity that likely initiates a potent procoagulant effect and plays a role in postnatal lung disease.[95] However, neither are alveolar macrophages present in significant numbers in normal newborn lungs, nor do the numbers of alveolar macrophages increase after birth in infants during the course of acute respiratory distress syndrome.[96,97]

The net effect of the normal alveolar epithelial surface on the coagulation and fibrinolytic cascades is uncertain. Fetal human and animal lung epithelium in vivo and primary cultures of alveolar epithelium in vitro[98] produce glycosaminoglycans that oppose thrombin formation through the natural inhibitors of thrombin: antithrombin III and heparin cofactor II. However, there is also TF-dependent procoagulant activity in alveolar epithelial conditioned media,[98] and adult type II epithelium expresses TF on its cell surface.[99] The in vivo net effect of these opposing procoagulant and anticoagulant properties is unknown.

Abnormalities of Surfactant

Neonatal respiratory distress syndrome, characterized by a primary lack of alveolar surface active material, shares many features with acute lung injury in adults. In infants, surfactant replacement unequivocally improves the morbidity and mortality rates, whereas in adults, no such survival benefit has been apparent.[100] One reason for this lack of benefit is that most clinical trials have used synthetic surfactant material, which is inferior to natural surfactants because it lacked apoproteins.[101] However, it also appears that in ARDS, there are more complex disturbances of the alveolar surfactant system. These include a lack of functionally important phospholipid and apoprotein components and an inhibition of surfactant function by plasma proteins that have leaked into the alveolar space or by inflammatory mediators such as reactive oxygen species, proteinases, and phospholipases produced locally by inflammatory cells. An important concept,[102] advanced by Lewis et al,[100] is that the physical state of surfactant as measured by the ratio of small to large aggregates is abnormal in ARDS and that the extent of lung injury correlates with the conversion of large to small aggregates. Moreover, the mode of mechanical ventilation can influence this conversion. These authors suggest that aggregate changes contribute to the pathophysiology of ARDS and that improper mechanical ventilation may make the situation worse by accelerating this process (the "second hit theory"). The therapeutic implications are that the maintenance of alveolar surfactant in large aggregate forms (perhaps by antiproteinase administration [proteinase activity increases large aggregate conversion]), ventilation with low tidal volumes and positive end-expiratory pressures above the inflection point, or both actions may prevent progressive lung dysfunction.

Recent studies have resurrected hope in the use of surfactant in the treatment of ARDS. In animal models of acute lung injury, the administration of large quantities of natural surfactant rapidly improves gas exchange.[103,104] A recent report has documented that direct bronchoscopic administration of large quantities of surfactant to humans with ARDS results in a marked improvement in gas exchange, although this study lacked controls.[101]

Factors Limiting Inflammation and Lung Injury

Under most circumstances the inflammatory response is subject to the limitations imposed by endogenous antiinflammatory factors. Examples include the following:

1. Limitation of the microvascular sequestration of neutrophils by the endothelial production of prostaglandins I_2 and E_2 (which diminish the rigidity[105] and adhesiveness[59] of neutrophils) and the shedding of L-selectin from neutrophils (which limits the early adhesive interactions)
2. Inhibition of the production and release of toxic leukocyte-derived products, including reactive oxygen species and proteolytic enzymes by the endothelial production of prostaglandins I_2 and E_2,[106,107] and by circulating plasma proteins such as α_2-macroglobulin[108,109]
3. Interference with the action of various inflammatory mediators by naturally occurring inhibitors, such as IL-1 receptor antagonist (which prevents the binding of IL-1 with its receptor)[18,30] and IL-10 (which exerts diverse antiinflammatory effects),[110] and interference with the activation of the coagulation cascade by α_2-macroglobulin
4. Antagonism or neutralization of the toxic leukocyte-derived products (e.g., scavenging of reactive oxygen species by antioxidants, such as catalase, superoxide dismutase, and glutathione peroxidase, and neutralization of proteinases by antiproteinases, such as α_1-proteinase inhibitor)
5. Removal of effete inflammatory cells without the release of toxic enzymes by a process involving the specific recognition of apoptotic* neutrophils by macrophages[111]

Even these regulatory mechanisms can be overwhelmed or circumvented. For example, α_1-proteinase inhibitor can be inactivated by oxidation of reactive oxygen species produced by leukocytes.[112,113] Another example is the ability of adherent neutrophils to form a restricted pericellular space between their plasma membrane and the cells to which they are tightly adherent (such as endothelial or epithelial cells). In effect, this creates a microenvironment that effectively excludes inhibitory molecules and thus allows the unopposed action of proteinases and reactive oxygen species in high concentrations in close proximity to endothelial or epithelial cells.[113]

Recent observations have highlighted the physiologic importance of the antiinflammatory response.[114-116] It is believed that compounds such as IL-10 and IL-1 receptor antagonist are designed to limit inflammatory tissue injury. More important, low concentrations of these antiinflammatory cytokines in bronchoalveolar lavage fluid obtained from patients with early ARDS correlate closely with a poor prognosis.[115] (An alternative view exists, however.[116]) These findings support the notion that failure to mount a localized intrapulmonary antiinflammatory response early in the course of acute lung injury contributes to severe organ injury and a worse prognosis. This concept holds forth the potential for therapeutic augmentation of antiinflammatory responses for patients with acute lung injury and other inflammatory diseases.

In summary, despite the presence of diverse mechanisms that tend to limit inflammation, in situations in which there is massive and systemic activation of the inflammatory cascade, control mechanisms can be overwhelmed or circumvented. In these cases, tissue injury can occur.

Treatment-Related Lung Injury

Although there have been tremendous strides in the supportive care of patients with acute lung injury, it is unfortunate that some of the modalities used for treatment have their own inherent ill effects on the lung.

Hyperoxia-Induced Injury

The administration of excessive concentrations of oxygen for prolonged periods results in injury to lung cells, including the pulmonary endothelium and epithelium.[34] In animals, for example, prolonged hyperoxia produces acute lung injury and diffuse alveolar damage. Furthermore, in humans, pulmonary dysfunction after prolonged ventilation correlates better with the duration of ventilation than with the duration of the illness, suggesting that oxygen toxicity may play an important role in the progression of acute lung injury. There are many mechanisms by which hyperoxia can result in lung injury. One likely major factor is the generation of reactive oxygen species with increased mitochondrial production of these compounds related to elevated oxygen tension.[117] Also, in response to hyperoxia, alveolar macrophages release factors such as cytokines and chemotactic factors that contribute to secondary neutrophil-mediated inflammatory damage of the lung.[33,41] In normal lungs, inhalation of 100% oxygen rapidly impairs lung function: Mucociliary transport is impaired in hours, endothelial cells show morphologic damage by 1 day, and acute lung injury syndrome is fully established in a few days. Lower concentrations of oxygen (50%) cause similar damage but require longer periods of exposure. Factors that alter susceptibility to hyperoxia involve preexisting pulmonary disease, metabolic rate, corticosteroid therapy, and nutritional status, including vitamin deficiencies.[34] Finally, hyperoxia can delay healing in previously injured cells.

Ventilator-Induced Injury

Mechanical ventilation improves gas exchange in patients with ARDS. However, this supportive modality has minimal if any

---

**Apoptosis* refers to the process of programmed cell death. In contrast to necrosis, apoptosis involves well-defined nuclear alterations followed by the degradation of DNA by endonucleases. More important, the proteolytic enzymes remain within the granules and are not released into the extracellular medium when apoptotic neutrophils are ingested by cells of the reticuloendothelial system such as alveolar macrophages.

effect on the ultimate prognosis and can worsen lung damage. Although positive-pressure ventilation at normal pressures in normal mature lungs can be used for prolonged periods without inducing pulmonary damage,[118,119] the same pressures in the immature lung is associated with the development of bronchopulmonary dysplasia.[120] Patients with ARDS frequently require peak inspiratory pressures greater than 30 to 40 cm H_2O to achieve adequate oxygenation. Because this equals or exceeds the pressure required to inflate normal lungs to total lung capacity and ARDS is a very heterogenous lesion,[121] it is reasonable to believe that such ventilatory strategies might damage the more normal regions of the lung that receive a disproportionate fraction of ventilation. Indeed, according to several investigators, high inflation pressures in animal models[122] can cause pulmonary edema that is associated with an increase in the permeability of both the endothelial[123] and the epithelial[124] membranes. The damage may be a result of the increased lung volume rather than the actual increase in pressure,[125] although this remains a point of controversy. Indeed, recent reports suggest that mechanical ventilation with even low tidal volumes may induce lung injury.[126] If the lungs are allowed to deflate below the inflection point of the pressure-volume curve, the terminal airways may collapse. During the next breath, these airways may be ripped open, leading to physical damage of the epithelium.

The presence of an endotracheal tube and routine suctioning of the airways produce enough mechanical trauma to directly damage the epithelium.[127] This effect, combined with the introduction of a high-velocity stream of gas directly into the airways and the potential for hyperoxia to rapidly (within approximately 6 hours) impair mucociliary transport,[128] can result in damage to large airways and defective clearance of pulmonary secretions. This not only results in acute problems in the clearance of secretions but can also cause permanent sequelae such as airway stenosis (subglottic, bronchus intermedius) and areas of bronchiolitis obliterans.[120]

RESOLUTION AND REPAIR

Clearance of Alveolar Space Fluid

The epithelium that lines the distal regions of the lung was long considered to play only a passive role in lung fluid movement, functioning much like a piece of plastic wrap in the alveolar space, keeping the fluid that was within the interstitium from entering the airspace. This concept appears to be incorrect.[129] The fetal lung epithelium secretes fluid (chloride) by energy-dependent pathways, and the perinatal and postnatal distal lung epithelia actively absorb sodium and fluid. Indeed, it is now known that the active transport of sodium by distal lung epithelium is the predominant mode of alveolar fluid clearance at the time of birth[130,131] and in the edematous postnatal animal lung[132] and human lung.[133] The ability of the lung to concentrate airspace fluid (and actively absorb salt and water by inference) correlates with survival from pulmonary edema caused by either heart failure or ARDS[134] (Fig. 7-6).

The epithelium lining the distal (acinar) regions of the lung is largely made up of Clara cells and types I and II epithelial cells. In vitro studies have shown that the primary cultures of Clara cells[135] and mature fetal[131,136] and adult[137,138] type II alveolar epithelium transport sodium via apical sodium channels[139-144] and basolateral ouabain-sensitive sodium-potassium adenosinetriphosphatase. Although sodium transport by the alveolar epithelium shares several similarities with renal epithelial transport, including similar-sized transcripts for an epithelial sodium channel and increased sodium transport when cyclic adenosine monophosphate is increased, there are several differences. For example, sodium transport is unaffected by antidiuretic hormone.[145,146]

The ability of the distal lung epithelia to actively transport sodium and hence absorb alveolar liquid is affected by phenomena associated with acute lung injury. Nitrogen dioxide,[147] oxidants,[148,149] or activated alveolar macrophages[150] decrease lung epithelial paracellular resistance, a finding suggesting damage to the interepithelial tight junctions. A recent study[148] has also found that hydrogen peroxide is more potent in its ability to reduce alveolar epithelial monolayer resistance and ion transport when it is applied to the basal as opposed to the apical membrane. In addition to damage to reactive oxygen species, other mechanisms can affect alveolar epithelial ion transport. Coincubation of alveolar epithelium with activated alveolar macrophages decreases the amount of amiloride-sensitive sodium transport and the number of apical membrane sodium channels via a nitric oxide–dependent but antioxidant-insensitive mechanism.[51] All of these factors would be expected to decrease sodium transport. However, hyperoxia also increases lung expression of sodium-potassium adenosinetriphosphatase in whole rat lungs.[151] It is also unknown whether the new type II alveolar epithelial cells that proliferate during the recovery of ARDS have a decreased, a normal, or an increased ability to transport sodium. If repair mechanisms recapitulate ontogeny, significant differences in sodium transport are possible; the immature, in contrast to the mature, fetal

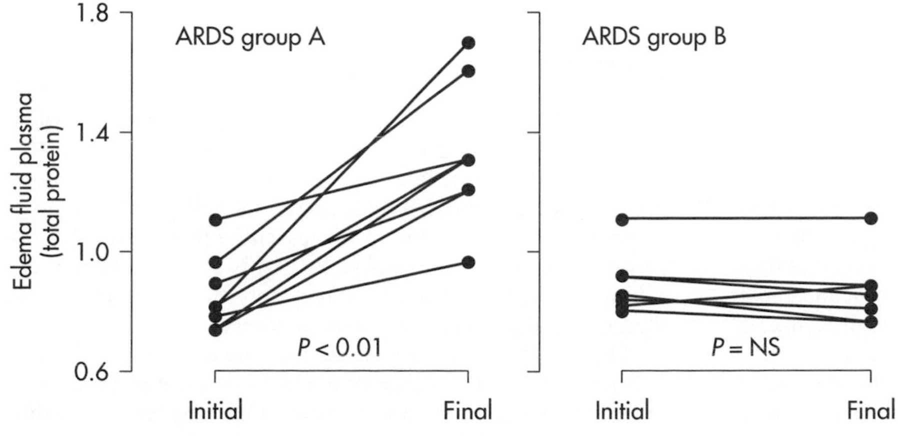

Fig. 7-6. Inability to concentrate alveolar fluid predicts mortality in ARDS. The pulmonary edema fluid and plasma protein concentration were measured in patients with ARDS at the time of intubation and approximately 6 hours later. In group A, who survived, edema fluid was concentrated in all patients, whereas in those who died (group B), edema fluid was not concentrated. Similar findings were seen in patients with high-pressure (cardiogenic) pulmonary edema. *NS,* Not significant. (From Matthay MA, Wiener-Kronish JP: *Am Rev Respir Dis* 142:1250-1257, 1990.)

lung epithelium cannot initiate sodium absorption in response to β-agonists.[152] Undoubtedly the ability of the lung to recover from alveolar pulmonary edema depends on its ability to stop certain factors from causing the injury and various stimuli from altering the sodium-transport ability of the epithelium.

Clearance of Airspace Fibrin

Cellular and inflammatory debris must be cleared from the alveolar spaces for efficient recovery from acute lung injury. Using an example of the lungs' repair processes, this section focuses on fibrin removal from the airspace. Other equally important phenomena, such as the mechanisms involved in the removal of particulates from the airspaces and airways, are discussed in detail in Chapter 6.

Thrombin is activated and fibrin is deposited within the vascular, interstitial, and alveolar spaces during acute lung injury (see previous section). As discussed in Chapter 60, complex fibrinolytic pathways are responsible for vascular recanalization in patients with pulmonary thromboembolic phenomena. Although similar mechanisms are involved in the clearance of airspace fibrin, there are also novel differences resulting from the lungs' resident cells modulating the fibrinolytic cascade.

Plasmin (derived from plasminogen within the intraalveolar plasma exudate) and elastases (derived from macrophages and neutrophils) are the predominant enzymes responsible for intraalveolar fibrinolysis. The activities of these enzymes are regulated by complex interactions of various protease/inhibitor complexes such as plasminogen activators and plasminogen activator inhibitors. The proteins that regulate intraalveolar fibrinolysis are present within the pathologic plasma exudates and are generated by some of the resident lung cells. For example, adult rat type II alveolar epithelial cells[153,154] and alveolar macrophages[155] can express urokinase-type plasminogen activator and plasminogen activator inhibitors. Plasmin itself is directly inhibited by a variety of plasma-derived antiproteases, including C1 esterase inhibitor, antithrombin III, and α_2-macroglobulin.

Adults with ARDS have defective intraalveolar fibrinolysis. The depressed fibrinolysis occurs because antiplasmins and plasminogen activator inhibitor type I are present within the alveolar space fluid.[88,156] Pulmonary fibrin accumulation during ARDS therefore results from both enhanced fibrin formation and a defective fibrin clearance. Although fibrinolytic therapy promotes recanalization of obstructed pulmonary vessels in patients with ARDS,[85] it is unknown whether enhanced intraalveolar fibrinolysis would be effective and whether it would be beneficial (perhaps decreasing lung scarring) or detrimental (perhaps enhancing the leakage of plasma into the airspaces).

Cellular Basis of Repair

The majority of mature neonatal[120] and adult[157] patients who survive acute lung injury have normal lung function. However, most adults still die from ARDS, and approximately half of the most immature infants with hyaline membrane disease develop bronchopulmonary dysplasia.[120] Thus it seems likely that there is a variation in the lung's ability to undergo efficient repair and that the incidence varies among patients and differing patient groups.

Efficient repair of the lungs' epithelia and endothelia is crucial for the restoration of normal lung function. One rapid response that can take place is a "spreading" of preexisting cells with reformation of the interepithelial tight junctions[158] and migration of endothelial cells to areas of vascular injury.[159] A second response that takes days to weeks is the regeneration of new cells. This has been extensively studied in regard to the pulmonary alveolar epithelium. In severe lung injury, the type I alveolar epithelial cells sustain widespread damage, and as repair proceeds, cuboidal cells that are morphologically similar to type II alveolar epithelial cells are seen lining the airspaces. Data from different experimental lung injury models indicate that these new cuboidal cells (presumably type II alveolar epithelium or a subpopulation thereof) subsequently differentiate into type I cells.[20,160] If the underlying elastin and collagen "scaffolding" architecture of the lung is intact, then repair of the alveolus may be successful. On the other hand, if the alveoli are fused within a protein-rich fibrin mesh and there is destruction of the underlying structure, then abnormal or incomplete repair may occur.[20] Animal experiments have demonstrated that newborn animals exposed to hyperoxia[161] or inhibitors of collagen and elastin synthesis[162] suffer from dysplastic lung growth that is not reversible (at least for the subsequent several weeks).

Pulmonary Fibrosis

In some patients with ARDS, the protein-rich edema does not rapidly disappear, and the alveolar spaces become organized by loose fibrous connective tissue that creates a pattern of intraalveolar fibrosis.[20,163,164] Indeed, the lung collagen content is abnormally high in patients dying of ARDS,[21] and as occurs in fibrosing alveolitis, the ratio of type I to type III collagen is increased in infants with bronchopulmonary dysplasia.[165] Marked proliferation of myofibroblasts and fibroblasts occurs in the areas of hyaline membrane formation.[163,164] The mechanisms and regulation of fibrosis in patients with acute lung injury are poorly understood, and the current understanding is largely based on studies of patients with fibrosing alveolitis and experimental animal models.[166]

The gross disruption of the parenchymal architecture that is apparent in the early phases of acute lung injury must be repaired for lung function to recover. The presence of fibrosis on a lung biopsy has been associated with mortality in established ARDS.[167,168] A syndrome has been described in patients with late ARDS who have persistent respiratory failure, radiographic infiltrates, and features of ongoing inflammation (fever and leukocytosis) without a source of infection. In these patients, open lung biopsy demonstrates diffuse fibroproliferation without signs of pneumonia.[169-171] Certainly the factors that facilitate resolution of the inflammatory response without fibrosis need to be delineated.

IMPLICATIONS FOR THERAPY

A detailed discussion of the therapy for acute lung injury is provided in Chapter 25. No one therapy is likely to prevent or ameliorate the multitude of disturbances observed in acute lung injury syndrome. Within limits, the acute inflammatory response is beneficial and in fact essential to survival. Therapeutic strategies must therefore be highly selective in their inhibition or interference and affect only those aspects of inflammation that contribute to tissue injury.

Any therapeutic interventions must be delivered early, between the initial appearance of the inciting result and the onset of severe physiologic abnormalities. One implication of this strategy is that patients at high risk for developing acute lung injury must be identified early, before the onset of the fully developed syndrome. Although this has been an area of intense investigation, at present, no such indicator can identify patients who will develop severe lung injury. Furthermore, given the current state of knowledge of the mechanisms of acute lung injury, it is unlikely that measuring one single marker or mediator will ever be of sufficient predictive value. Rather, it is more likely that measuring several crucial mediators, combined with an indicator of the host response to the injury, will be of most value in the stratification of risk. Examples of possible mediators that have been studied as indicators of risk include elevated complement breakdown products,[172] elevated serum antioxidant levels (e.g., superoxide dismutase, catalase, glutathione peroxidase),[173] elevated circulating endotoxin levels,[174] elevated IL-8 levels in serum[175] or bronchoalveolar lavage fluid,[176] and enhanced pulmonary microvascular retention of radiolabeled neutrophils.[45] An example of a potential indicator of host response to the injury is the level of the *N*-terminal propeptide of type III collagen, an elevation of which may predict patients at risk of progressing to severe end-stage fibrosis.[177] However, two cautionary notes must be added. First, prospective studies with appropriate disease-matched controls must be performed to validate any such indicator. Second, because the temporal progression from being at risk to the actual development of acute lung injury is not well defined, for some conditions predisposing to ARDS, a universal marker of risk may be very difficult to identify.

Prevention of Unregulated Inflammation

Besides obvious therapy directed at the primary disorder when available (e.g., appropriate antibiotic therapy for disseminated infection), possible sites for early intervention include the inhibition of neutrophil sequestration and adhesion within the pulmonary (and systemic) microvasculature. Strategies to interfere with this phase include the administration of pentoxifylline and derivatives that prevent neutrophil stiffening and pulmonary retention[178-181]; anticomplement (anti-C5a) and IL-8 antibodies, antibodies, peptides, and soluble oligosaccharides that selectively interfere with adhesion[69,182]; and antibodies to endotoxin[183] and compounds that interfere with the toxic effects of endotoxin such as deacylated LPS.[184] The most recent results of clinical trials with antiendotoxin antibodies demonstrate no benefit[8] and illustrate the point that one site of intervention may be insufficient to affect the outcome. In addition, the trend for a poorer outcome in certain subgroups receiving the antiendotoxin antibody[8] illustrates the potential risk of nonselectively interfering with cellular functions that play a critical role in normal physiologic processes.

There are several potential approaches to target events slightly later in the inflammatory cascade. These include the administration of IL-1 receptor antagonists;[19,185,186] antibodies to tumor necrosis factor,[9,187,188] soluble cytokine receptors to bind and neutralize circulating cytokines such as tumor necrosis factor or IL-1,[19] and agents that interfere with the production, release, or effects of toxic leukocyte-derived products. Examples of these types of agents include diphenylene iodonium derivatives, which inhibit the reduced form of BB nicotinamide-adenine dinucleotide phosphate, oxidase-derived reactive oxygen species[189] and inhibit the administration of exogenous antioxidants such as catalase and superoxide dismutase; *N*-acetyl cysteine;[34,190,191] proteinase inhibitors such as α_1-proteinase inhibitor[192] bactericidal permeability-inhibiting protein;[10] and low-molecular-weight elastase inhibitors[193] that may block the effect of leukocyte products after their release. Novel methods are being devised to enhance the delivery of the therapeutic agents to the respiratory system. These include the use of nebulized liposomes to allow the delivery of large proteins such as superoxide dismutase to the interior of cells[194] and to allow the use of gene therapy with transient transfection strategies,[195] with selective delivery to the respiratory tract to enhance the local production of antioxidants and antiproteinases (α_1-proteinase inhibitor).

Reversal of Specific Pathophysiologic Defects

Pulmonary hypertension is one example of a specific defect for which therapeutic interventions may be possible. In particular, continuous inhalation of nitric oxide in the range of 5 to 20 ppm has recently been reported to reduce pulmonary artery pressures and improve gas exchange for 3 to 53 days in a group of patients with ARDS and was associated with minimal toxicity.[80] Strategies to minimize or prevent ventilator-induced barotrauma such as ventilation with low tidal volumes should be included.

Facilitation of Reparative Processes

Reparative processes include the administration of exogenous surfactant[196] and agents designed to facilitate the removal of edema fluid from the alveolar space, such as agents that stimulate active sodium transport out of the alveolar space[132] (e.g., β_2-agonists) or agents that increase the intracellular level of cyclic adenosine monophosphate in alveolar epithelial cells delivered to the respiratory tract. The recent cloning of the sodium channel[197] raises the possibility of the use of targeted gene therapy with transient transfection strategies to augment active sodium transport out of the alveolar space. The prevention of extracellular collagen deposition or facilitation of its removal or remodeling would be expected to ameliorate the short- and long-term consequences of pulmonary parenchymal fibrosis.

SUMMARY

Acute lung injury syndrome (ARDS) is caused by a wide variety of initiating events. The resulting clinical picture is rather stereotypical, implying that the pathways leading to injury converge and are funneled into a final common pathway leading to lung injury. This concept holds out the possibility that selective intervention may ameliorate lung damage. In the majority of cases, acute lung injury may result from an acute inflammatory response that becomes unregulated because of the overwhelming nature of the insult and an inappropriate host response to the inciting event.

The challenge for the next decade will be to unravel at the cellular and molecular level the complexities of the inflammatory response, including reparative processes, and to target therapeutic interventions so that they will lessen the injurious consequences of inflammation while leaving the beneficial effects intact.

REFERENCES

1. Osler W: *The principles and practice of medicine,* ed 10, New York, Appleton, 1927, p 48-52.
2. Ashbaugh DG, Bigelow DB, Petty TL, Levine BE: Acute respiratory distress in adults, *Lancet* 2:319-323, 1967.
3. Holbrook PR, Taylor G, Pollack MM, Fields AI: Adult respiratory distress syndrome in children, *Pediatr Clin North Am* 27:667-685, 1980.

4. Royall JA, Levin DL: Adult respiratory distress syndrome in pediatric patients. I. Clinical aspects, pathology, and mechanisms of lung injury, *J Pediatr* 112:169-180, 1988.
5. Davis SL, Furman DP, Costarino AT: Adult respiratory syndrome in children: associated disease, course and predictors of death, *J Pediatr* 123:35-45, 1993.
6. Spragg, RG, Smith RM: Biology of acute lung injury. In Crystal RG, West JB, eds: *The lung: scientific foundations,* New York, 1991, Raven, pp 2003-2017.
7. Bone RC, Balk RA, Cerra FB, Dellinger RP, Fein AM, Knaus WA, Schein RMH, Sibbald W: ACCP/SCCM Consensus Conference: definitions for sepsis and organ failure and guidelines for the use of innovative therapies in sepsis, *Chest* 101:1644-1655, 1992.
8. Warren HS, Danner RL, Mumford RS: Anti-endotoxin monoclonal antibodies, *N Engl J Med* 326:1165-1166, 1992.
9. Fisher CJ Jr, Opal SM, Dhainaut JF, Stephens S, Zimmerman JL, Nightingale P, Harris SJ, Schein RM, Panacek EA, Vincent JL: Influence of an antitumor necrosis factor monoclonal antibody on cytokine levels in patients with sepsis, *Crit Care Med* 21:318-337, 1993.
10. Fisher CJ Jr, Slotman GJ, Opal SM, Pribble JP, Bone RC, Emmanuel G, Ng D, Bloedow DC, Catalano MA: Initial evaluation of human recombinant interleukin-1 receptor antagonist in the treatment of sepsis syndrome: a randomized, open-label, placebo-controlled multicenter trial—The IL-1RA Sepsis Syndrome Study Group, *Crit Care Med* 22:12-21, 1994.

Clinical and Pathologic Aspects

11. Fowler AA, Hamman RF, Good JT, Benson KN, Baird M, Eberle DJ, Petty TL, Heyers TM: Adult respiratory distress syndrome: risk with common predispositions, *Ann Intern Med* 99:293-298, 1983.
12. Villar J, Blazquez MA, Lubillo S, Quintana J, Manzano JL: Pulmonary hypertension in acute respiratory failure, *Crit Care Med* 17:523-526, 1989.
13. Matthay MA: The adult respiratory distress syndrome: definition and prognosis, *Clin Chest Med* 11:575-580, 1990.
14. Rocker GM, Wiseman MS, Pearson D, Shale DJ: Diagnostic criteria for adult respiratory distress syndrome: time for reappraisal, *Lancet* 1:120-123, 1989.
15. Villar J, Slutsky AS: The incidence of the adult respiratory distress syndrome, *Am Rev Respir Dis* 140:814-816, 1989.
16. Bernard GR, Artigas A, Brigham KL, Carlet J, Falke K, Hudson L, Lamy M, Legall JR, Morris A, Spragg R: The American-European Consensus Conference on ARDS: definitions, mechanisms, relevant outcomes, and clinical trial coordination, *Am J Respir Crit Care Med* 149:818-824, 1994.
17. Dorinsky PM, Gadek JE: Multiple organ failure, *Clin Chest Med* 11:581-591, 1990.
18. Giroir BP: Mediators of septic shock: new approaches for interrupting the endogenous inflammatory cascade, *Crit Care Med* 21:780-789, 1993.
19. Tomashefski JF: Pulmonary pathology of the adult respiratory distress syndrome, *Clin Chest Med* 11:593-619, 1990.
20. Bachofen M, Weibel ER: Structural alterations of lung parenchyma in the adult respiratory distress syndrome, *Clin Chest Med* 3:35-56, 1982.
21. Zapol WM, Trelstad RL, Coffey JW, Tsai I, Salvador RA: Pulmonary fibrosis in severe acute respiratory failure, *Am Rev Respir Dis* 119:547-554, 1979.

Pathophysiology

22. Katzenstein AA, Bloor CM, Leibow AA: The role of oxygen, shock, and related factors, *Am J Pathol* 85:210-222, 1976.
23. Gattinoni L, D'Andrea L, Pelosi P, Vitale G, Pesenti A, Fumagalli R: Regional effects and mechanism of positive end-expiratory pressure in early adult respiratory distress syndrome, *JAMA* 269:2122-2127, 1993.
24. Bachofen HS, Schurch S, Weibel ER: Experimental hydrostatic pulmonary edema in rabbit lungs: barrier lesions, *Am Rev Respir Dis* 147:997-1004, 1993.
25. Nilsson R, Grossmann G, Robertson B: Lung surfactant and the pathogenesis of neonatal bronchiolar lesions induced by artificial ventilation, *Pediatr Res* 12:249-255, 1978.
26. Jefferies AL, Coates G, O'Brodovich H: Pulmonary epithelial permeability in hyaline-membrane disease, *N Engl J Med* 311:1075-1080, 1984.
27. Prewitt RM, McCarthy J, Wood LDH: Treatment of acute low pressure pulmonary edema in dogs: relative effects of hydrostatic and oncotic pressure, nitroprusside, and positive end-expiratory pressure, *J Clin Invest* 67:409-441, 1981.
28. O'Brodovich H, Coates G: Effect of exercise on lung lymph flow in unanesthetized sheep with increased pulmonary vascular permeability, *Am Rev Respir Dis* 134:862-866, 1986.
29. Reynolds HY: Lung inflammation: normal host defense or a complication of some diseases, *Ann Rev Med* 38:295-323, 1987.
30. St John RC, Dorinsky PM: Immunologic therapy for ARDS, septic shock, and multiple-organ failure, *Chest* 103:932-943, 1993.
31. Crapo JD, Barry BE, Forscue HA, Shelburne J: Structural and biochemical changes in rat lungs occurring during exposures to lethal and adaptive doses of oxygen, *Am Rev Respir Dis* 122:123-143, 1980.
32. Shasby DM, Fox RB, Harada RN, Repine JE: Reduction of the oedema of acute hyperoxic lung injury by granulocyte depletion, *J Appl Physiol* 52:1237-1244, 1982.
33. Rinaldo JE, English D, Levine J, Stiller R, Henson J: Increased intrapulmonary retention of radiolabelled neutrophils in early oxygen toxicity, *Am Rev Respir Dis* 137:345-352, 1988.
34. Heffner JE, Repine JE: Pulmonary strategies of antioxidant defense, *Am Rev Respir Dis* 140:531-554, 1989.
35. Dahinden C, Galanos C, Fehr J: Granulocyte activation by endotoxin, *J Immunol* 130:857-861, 1983.
36. Smedley LA, Tonnesen MG, Sanhaus RA, Haslett C, Guthrie LA, Johnson RB, Henson PM, Worthen GS: Neutrophil mediated injury to endothelial cells: enhancement by endotoxin and essential role of neutrophil elastase, *J Clin Invest* 77:1233-1243, 1986.
37. Haslett C, Worthen GS, Giclas PAM, Morrison DC, Henson JE, Henson PM: The pulmonary vascular sequestration of neutrophils in endotoxaemia is initiated by an effect of endotoxin on the neutrophil in the rabbit, *Am Rev Respir Dis* 136:9-18, 1987.
38. Sacks T, Moldow CF, Craddock PR, Bowers TK, Jacob HS: Oxygen radical mediated endothelial cell damage by complement-stimulated leukocytes: an in vitro model of immune vascular damage, *J Clin Invest* 61:1161-1167, 1978.
39. Stevens KE, Ishizaka A, Larrick JW, Raffin TA: Tumor necrosis factor causes increased pulmonary permeability and edema: comparison to septic acute lung injury, *Am Rev Respir Dis* 137:1364-1370, 1988.
40. Brigham KL, Meyrick B: Endotoxin and lung injury, *Am Rev Respir Dis* 133:913-927, 1986.
41. Harada RN, Bowman CM, Fox RB, Repine JE: Alveolar macrophage secretions: initiators of inflammation in pulmonary oxygen toxicity? *Chest* S81:52-54, 1982.
42. Staub NC, Schultz EL, Albertine KH: Leukocytes and pulmonary microvascular injury, *Ann NY Acad Sci* 384:332-343, 1982.
43. Kawano T, Mori S, Cybulsky M, Burger R, Ballin A, Cutz E, Bryan AC: Effect of granulocyte depletion in a ventilated surfactant-depleted lung, *J Appl Physiol* 62:27-33, 1987.
44. Thommason H, Boyko WJ, Russel JA, Hogg JC: Transient leukopenia associated with adult respiratory distress syndrome, *Lancet* 1:809-812, 1984.
45. Warshawski FJ, Sibbald WJ, Driedger AA, Cheung H: Abnormal neutrophil-pulmonary interaction in the adult respiratory distress syndrome, *Am Rev Respir Dis* 133:797-804, 1986.
46. Chollet-Martin S, Jourdain B, Gibert C, Elbim C, Chastre J, Gougerot-Pocidalo MA: Interactions between neutrophils and cytokines in blood and alveolar spaces during ARDS, *Am J Respir Crit Care Med* 153:594-601, 1996.
47. Lee CT, Fein AM, Lippman M, Hotzmann H, Kimbel P, Weinbaum G: Elastolytic activity in pulmonary lavage fluid from patients with adult respiratory distress syndrome, *N Engl J Med* 304:192-196, 1981.
48. Christner P, Fein A, Goldberg S, Lippman M, Abrams W, Weinbaum G: Collagenase in the lower respiratory tract of patients with adult respiratory distress syndrome, *Am Rev Respir Dis* 131:690-695, 1985.
49. Baldwin SR, Grum CM, Boxer LA, Simon RH, Ketai LH, Devall LJ: Oxidant activity in expired breath of patients with adult respiratory distress syndrome, *Lancet* 1:11-3, 1986.
50. Jacobs RF, Tabor DR, Burks AW, Campbell CD: Elevated interleukin-1 release by human alveolar macrophages during the adult respiratory distress syndrome, *Am Rev Respir Dis* 140:1686-1692, 1989.
51. Compeau CG, Rotstein OD, Tohda H, Morunoka Y, Rafii B, Slutsby AS, O'Brodovich H: Endotoxin-stimulated alveolar macrophages impair lung epithelial Na^+ transport by an L-arg dependent mechanism, *Am J Physiol* 266:C1330-C1341, 1994.
52. Braude S, Apperley J, Krautz T, Goldman JM: Adult respiratory distress syndrome after allogenic bone-marrow transplantation: evidence for a neutrophil-independent mechanism, *Lancet* 1:1239-1242, 1985.
53. Ongibene FP, Martin SE, Parker MM, Schlesinger T, Roach P, Burch C, Shelhamer JH, Parillo JE: Adult respiratory distress syndrome in patients with severe neutropenia, *N Engl J Med* 315:547-551, 1986.

54. Hogg JC, Doerschuk CA: Leukocyte traffic in the lung, *Ann Rev Physiol* 57:97-114, 1995.
55. Doerschuk CM, Allard MF, Martin BA, MacKenzie A, Autor AP, Hogg JC: The marginated pool of the neutrophils in the lungs of rabbits, *J Appl Physiol* 63:1806-1815, 1987.
56. Van Eeden S, Miyagashima R, Haley L, Hogg JC: L-selectin expression increases on peripheral blood polymorphonuclear leukocytes during active marrow release, *Am J Respir Crit Care Med* 151:500-507, 1995.
57. Van Eeden S, Miyagashima FR, Haley L, Hogg JC: A possible role for L-selectin in the release of polymorphonuclear leukocytes from bone marrow, *Am J Physiol Heart Circ Physiol* 272:H1717-H1724, 1997.
58. Lein DC, Wagner WW, Capen RL, Haslett CL, Hanson WL, Hofmeister SE, Henson PM, Worthen GS: Physiologic neutrophil sequestration in the canine pulmonary circulation: evidence for localization in capillaries, *J Appl Physiol* 62:1236-1243, 1987.
59. Downey GP, Doherty DE, Gumbay RS, Henson J, Henson PM, Worthen GS: Enhancement of pulmonary inflammation by PGE_2: evidence for a vasodilator effect, *J Appl Physiol* 64:728-741, 1988.
60. Downey GP, Worthen GS: Neutrophil retention within model capillaries: role of cell deformability, geometry and hydrodynamic forces, *J Appl Physiol* 65:1861-1871, 1988.
61. Downey GP, Doherty DE, Schwab B, Elson EL, Henson PM, Worthen GS: Retention of leukocytes in capillaries: role of cell size and deformability, *J Appl Physiol* 69:1767-1778, 1990.
62. Erzurum SC, Downey GP, Schwab B, Elson EL, Worthen GS: Mechanisms of lipopolysaccharide-induced neutrophil retention: relative contributions of adhesive and cellular mechanical properties, *J Immunol* 149:154-162, 1992.
63. Downey GP, Worthen GS, Henson PM, Hyde DM: Neutrophil sequestration and migration in response to local instillation of C5a in the lung: capillary localization and migration across the interalveolar septum, *Am Rev Respir Dis* 147:168-176, 1993.
64. Worthen GS, Schwab B, Elson EL, Downey GP: Cellular mechanics of stimulated neutrophils: stiffening of cells induces retention in pores in vitro and lung capillaries in vivo, *Science* 245:183-186, 1989.
65. Springer TA: Adhesion receptors of the immune system, *Nature* 346:425-434, 1990.
66. Bevilacqua MP, Nelson RM: Selectins, *J Clin Invest* 91:379-387, 1993.
67. Fuhlbrigge RC, Alon R, Puri KD, Lowe JB, Springer TA: Sialylated fucosylated ligands for L-selectin expressed on leukocytes mediate tethering and rolling adhesions in physiologic flow conditions, *J Cell Biol* 135:837-848, 1996.
68. Hynes RO: Integrins: versatility, modulation, signaling in cell adhesion, *Cell* 69:11-25, 1992.
69. Mulligan MS, Paulson JC, De Frees S, Zheng Z-L, Lowe JB, Ward PA: Protective effects of oligosaccharides in P-selectin–dependent lung injury, *Science* 364:149-151, 1993.
70. Ramos CL, Kunkel EJ, Lawrence MB, Jung U, Vestweber D, Bosse R, McIntyre KW, Gillooly KM, Norton CR, Wolitzky BA, Ley K: Differential effect of E-selectin antibodies on neutrophil rolling and recruitment to inflammatory sites, *Blood* 89(8):3009-3018, 1997.
71. Lewis MS, Whatley RE, Cain P, McIntyre TM, Prescott SM, Zimmerman GA: Hydrogen peroxide stimulates the synthesis of platelet-activating factor by endothelium and induces endothelial cell–dependent neutrophil adhesion, *J Clin Invest* 82:2045-2055, 1988.
72. Xie Y, Muller WA: Molecular cloning and adhesive properties of murine platelet/endothelial cell adhesion molecule 1, *Proc Natl Acad Sci USA* 90:5569-5573, 1993.
73. Larsen GL, Webster RO, Worthen GS, Gumbay RS, Henson PM: Additive effect of intravascular complement activation and brief episodes of hypoxia in producing increased permeability in rabbit lung, *J Clin Invest* 75:902-910, 1985.
74. Nathan C, Srimal S, Farber C, Sanchez E, Kabbash L, Asch A, Gailit J, Wright SD: Cytokine-induced respiratory burst of human neutrophils: dependence on extracellular matrix proteins and CD11/CD18 integrins, *J Cell Biol* 109:1341-1349, 1989.
75. Donnelly SC, Haslett C, Dransfield I, Robertson CE, Carter DC, Ross JA, Grant IS, Tedder TF: Role of selectins in development of adult respiratory distress syndrome, *Lancet* 344:215-219, 1994.
76. Worthen GS, Haslett C, Rees AJ, Gumbay RS, Henson JC, Henson PM: Neutrophil-mediated pulmonary vascular injury: synergistic effects of trace amounts of lipopolysaccharide in C5a-induced lung injury, *Am Rev Respir Dis* 136:19-28, 1987.
77. Young SK, Worthen GS, Haslett C, Tonnesen MG, Henson PM: Interaction between chemoattractants and bacterial lipopolysaccharide in the induction and enhancement of neutrophil adhesion, *Am J Respir Cell Mol Biol* 2:523-532, 1990.
78. Cerra FB: The systemic septic response: concepts of pathogenesis, *J Trauma* 30:S169-S174, 1990.
79. Haglund U: Systemic mediators released from the gut in critical illness, *Crit Care Med* 21:515-518, 1993.
80. Rossaint R, Falke KJ, Lopez F, Slama K, Pison U, Zapol WM: Inhaled nitric oxide for the adult respiratory distress syndrome, *N Engl J Med* 328:399-405, 1993.
81. Eichacker PQ: Inhaled nitric oxide in adult respiratory distress syndrome: do we know the risks versus benefits? *Crit Care Med* 4:563-565, 1997.
82. Schmidt B, Vegh P, Weitz J, Johnston M, Caco C, Roberts R: Thrombin/antithrombin III complex formation in the neonatal respiratory distress syndrome, *Am Rev Respir Dis* 145:767-770, 1992.
83. Levin DL, Weinberg D, Perkin RM: Pulmonary microthrombi syndrome in newborn infants with unresponsive persistent pulmonary hypertension, *J Pediatr* 102:299-303, 1983.
84. Busch C, Dahlgrens B, Jakobson S, Jung B, Bodig J, Soldeen T: The use of ^{125}I–labelled fibrinogen for determination of fibrin trapping in the lungs of patients developing the microembolism syndrome, *Acta Anaesth Scand* 57(suppl):46-54, 1975.
85. Greene R, Lind S, Jantsch H, Wilson R, Lynch K, Jones R, Carvalho A, Reid L, Waltman AC, Zapol W: Pulmonary vascular obstruction in severe ARDS: angiographic alterations after IV fibrinolytic therapy, *Am J Radiol* 148:501-508, 1987.
86. Greene R, Zapol WM, Snider MT, Reid L, Snow R, O'Connell RS, Novelline RA: Early bedside detection of pulmonary vascular occlusion in acute respiratory failure, *Am Rev Respir Dis* 124:593-601, 1981.
87. Malik AB, Staub NC, eds: *Mechanisms of lung microvascular injury,* New York, 1982, New York Academy of Sciences, pp 82-97.
88. Idell S, James KK, Levin EG, Schwartz BS, Manchanda N, Maunder RJ, Maring TR, McLarty J, Fair DS: Local abnormalities in coagulation and fibrinolytic pathways predispose to alveolar fibrin deposition in the adult respiratory distress syndrome, *J Clin Invest* 84:695-705, 1989.
89. Gajl-Peczalska K: Plasma protein composition of hyaline membrane in the newborn as studied by immunofluorescence, *Arch Dis Child* 39:226-231, 1964.
90. Seeger W, Stohr G, Wolf HRD: Alteration of surfactant function due to protein leakage: special interaction with fibrin monomer, *J Appl Physiol* 58:326-338, 1985.
91. O'Brodovich H, Weitz JI, Possmayer F: Effect of fibrinogen degradation products and lung ground substance on surfactant function, *Biol Neonate* 57:325-333, 1990.
92. Carvalho ACA, Bellman SM, Saullo VJ, Quin D, Zapolr WM: Altered factor VIII in acute respiratory failure, *N Engl J Med* 307:1113-1119, 1982.
93. Holter JF, Weiland JE, Pacht ER, Gadek JE, Davis WB: Protein permeability in the adult respiratory distress syndrome: loss of size selectivity of the alveolar epithelium, *J Clin Invest* 78:1513-1522, 1986.
94. Sprung CL, Long WM, Marcial EH, Schein RMH, Parker RE, Shomer T, Brigham KL: Distribution of proteins in pulmonary edema, *Am Rev Respir Dis* 136:957-963, 1987.
95. Chapman HA, Stahl M, Allen CL, Yee R, Fair DS: Regulation of the procoagulant activity within the bronchoalveolar compartment of normal human lung, *Am Rev Respir Dis* 137:1417-1425, 1988.
96. Alenghat E, Esterly JR: Alveolar macrophages in perinatal infants, *Pediatrics* 74:221-223, 1984.
97. Jacobs RF, Wilson CB, Palmer S, Springmeyer SC, Henderson WR, Glover DM, Kessler DL, Murphy JGH, Hughes JP, Van Belle G, Chi EY, Hodson WA: Factors related to the appearance of alveolar macrophages in the developing lung, *Am Rev Respir Dis* 131:548-553, 1985.
98. O'Brodovich H, Berry L, D'Costa M, Burrows R, Andrew M: Influence of fetal pulmonary epithelium on thrombin activity, *Am J Physiol* 261:L262-L270, 1991.
99. Gross TJ, Simon RH, Sitrin RG: Tissue factor procoagulant expression by rat alveolar epithelial cells, *Am J Respir Cell Mol Biol* 6:397-403, 1992.
100. Lewis JF, Veldhuizen R, Possmayer F, Sibbald W, Whitsett J, Qanbar R, McCaig L: Altered alveolar surfactant is an early marker of acute lung injury in septic adult sheep, *Am J Respir Crit Care Med* 150:123-130, 1994.
101. Walmrath D, Gunther A, Ghofrani HA, Schermuly R, Schneider T, Grimminger F, Seeger W: Bronchoscopic surfactant administration in patients with severe adult respiratory distress syndrome and sepsis, *Am J Respir Crit Care Med* 154:57-62, 1996.

102. Seeger W, Gunther A, Walmrath HA, Grimminger F, Lasch HG: Alveolar surfactant and adult respiratory distress syndrome: pathogenetic role and therapeutic prospects, *Clin Invest* 71:177-190, 1993.
103. Eijking EP, van Daal GJ, Tenbrinck R, Luijendijk A, Sluiters JF, Hannappel E, Lachmann B: Effect of surfactant replacement on *Pneumocystis carinii* pneumonia in rats, *Intensive Care Med* 17:475-478, 1991.
104. Eijking EP, Gommers D, So KL, Vergeer M, Lachmann B: Surfactant treatment of respiratory failure induced by hydrochloric acid aspiration in rats, *Anesthesiology* 78:1145-1151, 1993.
105. Downey GP, Erzurum SC, Young SK, Schwab B, Elson EL, Worthen GS: Biophysical properties and microfilament assembly in neutrophils: modulation by cyclic AMP, *J Cell Biol* 114:1179-1190, 1991.
106. Zurier RB, Weissmann G, Hoffstein S, Kammerman S, Tai HH: Mechanisms of lysosomal enzyme release from human leukocytes. II. Effects of cAMP and cGMP, autonomic agonists, and agents which affect microtubule function, *J Clin Invest* 53:297-309, 1974.
107. Rivkin I, Rosenblatt J, Becker EL: The role of cAMP in the chemotactic responsiveness and spontaneous motility of rabbit peritoneal neutrophils, *J Immunol* 115:1126-1134, 1975.
108. Hyers TM, Kew RR, KrsekStaples J, Heuertz R, Webster RO: Regulation of neutrophil function by acute phase reactants: implications for resolution of the adult respiratory distress syndrome, *Chest* 99:7S-9S, 1991.
109. Heuertz RM, Piquette CA, Webster RO: Rabbits with elevated serum C-reactive protein exhibit diminished neutrophil infiltration and vascular permeability in C5a-induced alveolitis, *Am J Pathol* 142:319-328, 1993.
110. Trinchieri G: Cytokines acting on or secreted by macrophages during intracellular infection (IL-10, IL-12, IFN-gamma), *Curr Opin Immunol* 9:17-23, 1997.
111. Savill J, Fadok V, Henson P, Haslett C: Phagocyte recognition of cells undergoing apoptosis, *Immunol Today* 14:131-136, 1993.
112. Cambell ET, Senior RM, McDonald JA, Cox DL: Proteolysis by neutrophils: relative importance of cell-substrate contact and oxidative inactivation of proteinase inhibitors in vitro, *J Clin Invest* 70:845-852, 1982.
113. Weiss SJ: Tissue destruction by neutrophils, *N Engl J Med* 320:365-376, 1989.
114. Bone RC: Sepsis and its complications: the clinical problem, *Crit Care Med* 22:S8-S11, 1994.
115. Donnelly SC, Strieter RM, Reid PT, Kunkel SL, Burdick MD, Armstrong I, MacKenzie A, Haslett C: The association between mortality rates and decreased concentrations of interleukin-10 and interleukin-1 receptor antagonist in the lung fluids of patients with the adult respiratory distress syndrome, *Ann Intern Med* 125:191-196, 1996.
116. Parsons PE, Moss M, Vannice JL, Moore EE, Moore FA, Repine JE: Circulating IL-1ra and IL-10 are increased but do not predict the development of the acute respiratory distress syndrome in at-risk patients, *Am J Respir Crit Care Med* 155:1469-1473, 1997.
117. Turrens JF, Freeman BA, Crapo JD: Hyperoxia increases H_2O_2 release by lung mitochondria and microsomes, *Arch Biochem Biophys* 217:411-421, 1982.
118. Nash G, Bowen JA, Langlinais PC: "Respirator lung": a misnomer, *Arch Pathol* 21:234-240, 1971.
119. DeLemos R, Wolfsdorf K, Nachman R: Lung injury from oxygen in lambs: the role of artificial ventilation, *Anesthesiology* 30:609-618, 1969.
120. O'Brodovich HM, Mellins RB: Bronchopulmonary dysplasia: unresolved neonatal acute lung injury, *Am Rev Respir Dis* 132:694-709, 1985.
121. Bombino M, Gattinoni L, Pesenti A, Pistolesi M, Miniati M: The value of portable chest roentgenography in adult respiratory distress syndrome, *Chest* 100:762-769, 1991.
122. Webb HH, Tierney DF: Experimental pulmonary edema due to intermittent positive pressure ventilation with high inflation pressures, *Am Rev Respir Dis* 110:556-565, 1974.
123. Parker JC, Townsley MI, Rippe B, Taylor AE, Thigpen J: Increased microvascular permeability in dog lungs due to high peak airway pressures, *J Appl Physiol* 57(6):1809-1816, 1984.
124. O'Brodovich H, Coates G, Marrin M: Effect of inspiratory resistance and PEEP on 99mTc-DTPA clearance, *J Appl Physiol* 60(5):1461-1465, 1986.
125. Dreyfuss D, Soler P, Basset G, Saumon G: High inflation pressure pulmonary edema, *Am Rev Respir Dis* 137:1159-1164, 1988.
126. Muscadere JG, Mullen JBM, Gan K, Bryan AC, Slutsky AS: Tidal ventilation at low airway pressures can cause pulmonary barotrauma, *Am Rev Respir Dis* 145:A454, 1992.
127. Lundgren R, Horstedt P, Winblad B: Respiratory mucosal damage by flexible fiberoptic bronchoscopy in pigs, *Eur J Respir Dis* 64:24-32, 1983.
128. Boat TF: Studies of oxygen toxicity in cultured human neonatal respiratory epithelium, *J Pediatr* 95:916-919, 1979.

Resolution and Repair

129. O'Brodovich H: Epithelial ion transport in the fetal and perinatal lung, *Am J Physiol* 261:C555-C564, 1991.
130. O'Brodovich H, Hannam V, Seear M, Mullen JBM: Amiloride impairs lung water clearance in newborn guinea pigs, *J Appl Physiol* 68(4):1758-1762, 1990.
131. O'Brodovich H, Hannam V, Rafii B: Sodium channel but neither Na^+-H^+ nor Na-glucose symport inhibitors slow neonatal lung water clearance, *Am J Respir Cell Mol Biol* 5:377-384, 1991.
132. Berthiaume Y, Staub NC, Matthay MA: Beta-adrenergic agonists increase lung liquid clearance in anesthetized sheep, *J Clin Invest* 79:335-343, 1987.
133. Sakuma T, Okinawa G, Nakada T, Nishimura T, Fulimura S, Matthay MA: Alveolar fluid clearance in the resected human lung, *Am J Respir Crit Care Med* 150(2):305-310, 1994.
134. Matthay MA, Wiener-Kronish JP: Intact epithelial barrier function is critical for the resolution of alveolar edema in man, *Am Rev Respir Dis* 142:1250-1257, 1990.
135. Van Scott MR, Hester S, Boucher RC: Ion transport by rabbit nonciliated bronchiolar epithelial cells (Clara cells) in culture, *Proc Natl Acad Sci USA* 84:5496-5500,1987.
136. O'Brodovich H, Rafii B, Post M: Bioelectric properties of fetal alveolar epithelial monolayers, *Am J Physiol* 258:L201-L206, 1990.
137. Mason, RJ, Williams MC, Widdicombe JH, Sanders MJ, Misfeld DS, Berry LC Jr: Transepithelial transport by pulmonary alveolar type II cells in primary culture, *Proc Natl Acad Sci USA* 79:6033-6037, 1982.
138. Cheek JN, Kim KJ, Crandall ED: Tight monolayers of rat alveolar epithelial cells: bioelectric properties and active sodium transport, *Am J Physiol* 256:C688-C693, 1989.
139. Orser BA, Bertlik M, Fedorko L, O'Brodovich H: Non-selective cation channel in fetal alveolar type II epithelium, *Biochem Biophys Acta (Molec Cell Structure)* 1094(1):19-26, 1991.
140. Matalon S, Bauer M, Benos D, Kleyman T, Lin C, Cragoe EJ Jr, O'Brodovich H: Fetal lung epithelial cells contain two populations of amiloride-sensitive Na^+ channels, *Am J Physiol* 264:L357-L364, 1993.
141. Matalon S, Kirk KL, Bubien JK, Oh Y, Hu P, Yue G, Shoemaker R, Cragoe EJ Jr, Benos DJ: Immunocytochemical and functional characterization of Na^+ conductance in adult alveolar pneumonocytes, *Am J Physiol* 262:C1228-C1238, 1992.
142. Wang X, Kleyman T, Tohda H, Marunaka Y, O'Brodovich H: EIPA sensitive Na^+ currents in intact fetal distal lung epithelial cells, *Can J Physiol Pharmacol* 71:58-62, 1993.
143. O'Brodovich H, Ueda J, Canessa C, Rafii B, Rossier BC, Edelson J: Expression of the epithelial Na^+ channel in the developing rat lung, *Am J Physiol* 65(2 Pt 1):C491-C496, 1993.
144. Rotin DE, Bar-Sagi D, Waddell T, O'Brodovich H, Merilainen J, Lehto PV, Canessa CM, Rossier BC, Downey GP: An SH3 binding region in the epithelial Na^+ channel (αrENaC) mediates its localization at the apical membrane, *EMBO J* 13:4440-4450, 1994.
145. Cott GR, Sugahara K, Mason RJ: Stimulation of net active ion transport across alveolar type II cell monolayers, *Am J Physiol* 250:C222-C227, 1986.
146. O'Brodovich H, Rafii B, Perlon P: Arginine vasopressin and atrial natriuretic peptide do not alter ion transport by cultured fetal distal lung epithelium, *Pediatr Res* 31:318-322, 1992.
147. Cheek JM, Kim KJ, Crandall ED: NO_2 decreases paracellular resistance to ion and solute flow in alveolar epithelial monolayers, *Exp Lung Res* 16:561-575, 1990.
148. Kim KJ, Suh DJ: Asymmetric effects of H_2O_2 on alveolar epithelial barrier properties, *Am J Physiol* 264:L308-L315, 1993.
149. McBride RK, Stone KK, Marin MG: Oxidant injury alters barrier function of ferret tracheal epithelium, *Am J Physiol* 8:L165-L174, 1993.
150. Compeau CG, Tohda H, Marunaka Y, Rafii B, Rotstein O, Slutsky A, O'Brodovich H: Endotoxin-stimulated alveolar macrophages impair lung epithelial Na^+ transport by an L-arg–dependent mechanism, *Am J Physiol* 266:C1330-C1341, 1993.
151. Nici L, Dowin R, Gilmore-Hebert M, Jamieson JD, Ingbar DH: Upregulation of rat lung Na-K-ATPase during hyperoxic injury, *Am J Physiol* 261:L307-L314, 1991.
152. Brown MJ, Olver RE, Ramsden CA, Strang LB, Walters DV: Effects of adrenaline and of spontaneous labour on the secretion and absorption of lung liquid in the fetal lamb, *J Physiol (Lond)* 344:137-152, 1983.

153. Gross TJ, Simon RH, Kelly CJ, Sitrin RG: Rat alveolar epithelial cells concomitantly express plasminogen activator inhibitor-1 urokinase, *Am J Physiol* 4:L286-L295, 1991.
154. Simon RH, Gross TJ, Edwards JA, Sitrin RB: Fibrin degradation by rat pulmonary alveolar epithelial cells, *Am J Physiol* 6:L482-L488, 1992.
155. Sitrin RG, Brubaker PG, Fantone JC: Tissue fibrin deposition during acute lung injury in rabbits and its relationship to local expression of procoagulant and fibrinolytic activities, *Am Rev Respir Dis* 135:930-936, 1987.
156. Bertozzi P, Astedt B, Zenzius L, Lynch K, Lemaire F, Zapol W, Chapman HA Jr: Depressed bronchoalveolar urokinase activity in patients with adult respiratory distress syndrome, *N Engl J Med* 322:890-897, 1990.
157. Alberts WM, Priest GR, Moser KM: The outlook for survivors of ARDS, *Chest* 84:272-274, 1983.
158. Marin L, Gordon RE, Lane BP: Development of tight junctions in rat tracheal epithelium during the early hours after mechanical injury, *Am Rev Respir Dis* 119:101-106, 1979.
159. Brown LM, Ryan US, Absher M: Mathematical analysis of endothelial sibling pair cell-cell interactions using time-lapse cinematography data, *Tissue Cell* 14:651-655, 1982.
160. Adamson IYR, Bowden DH: The type 2 cell as progenitor of alveolar epithelial regeneration: a cytodynamic study in mice after exposure to oxygen, *Lab Invest* 30:35-42, 1974.
161. Shaffer SG, O'Neill D, Bradt SK: Chronic vascular pulmonary dysplasia associated with neonatal hyperoxia exposure in the rat, *Pediatr Res* 21:14-20, 1987.
162. Kida K, Thurlbeck WM: Lack of recovery of lung structure and function after the administration of β-amino-propionitrile in the postnatal period, *Am Rev Respir Dis* 122:467-475, 1980.
163. Kobashi Y, Manabe T: The fibrosing process in so-called organized diffuse alveolar damage: an immunohistochemical study of the change from hyaline membrane to membranous fibrosis, *Virchow Arch A* 422:47-52, 1993.
164. Fukuda Y, Ishizaki M, Masuda Y, Kimura G, Kawanami O, Masugi Y: The role of intraalveolar fibrosis in the process of pulmonary structural remodeling in patients with diffuse alveolar damage, *Am J Pathol* 126:171-182, 1987.
165. Shoemaker CT, Reiser KM, Goetsman BW, Last JA: Elevated ratios of type I/III collagen in the lungs of chronically ventilated neonates with respiratory distress, *Pediatr Res* 18:1176-1180, 1984.
166. Crouch E: Pathobiology of pulmonary fibrosis, *Am J Physiol* 3:L159-L184, 1990.
167. Martin C, Papazian L, Payan M-J, Saux P, Gouin F: Pulmonary fibrosis correlates with outcome in adult respiratory distress syndrome: a study in mechanically ventilated patients, *Chest* 107:196-200, 1995.
168. Suchyta MR, Clemmer TP, Elliot GC, Orme JF, Weaver LK: The adult respiratory distress syndrome: a report of survival and modifying factors, *Chest* 107:1074-1079, 1992.
169. Meduri GU, Belenchia JM, Estes RJ, Wunderink RG, El Torky M, Leeper KV: Fibroproliferative phase of ARDS: clinical findings and effects of corticosteroids, *Chest* 100:943-952, 1991.
170. Collins JF, Smith JD, Coalson JJ, Johanson WFJ: Variability in lung collagen amounts after prolonged support of acute respiratory failure, *Chest* 85:641-646, 1984.
171. Meduri GU, Chinn AJ, Leeper KV, Wunderink RG, Tolley E, Winer-Muram HT, Kare V, El Torky M: Corticosteroid rescue treatment of progressive fibroproliferation in late ARDS: patterns of response and predictors of outcome, *Chest* 105:1516-1527, 1994.

Implications for Therapy

172. Parsons PE, Giclas PC: The terminal complement complex (sC5b-9) is not specifically associated with the development of the adult respiratory distress syndrome, *Am Rev Respir Dis* 141:98-103, 1990.
173. Leff JA, Parsons PE, Day CE, Taniguchi N, Jochum M, Fritz H, Moore FA, Moore EE, McCord JM, Repine JE: Serum antioxidants as predictors of adult respiratory distress syndrome in patients with sepsis, *Lancet* 341:777-780, 1993.
174. Parsons PE, Worthen GS, Moore EE, Tate RM, Henson PM: The association of circulating endotoxin with the development of the adult respiratory distress syndrome, *Am Rev Respir Dis* 140:294-301, 1989.
175. Miller EJ, Cohen AB, Nagao S, Griffith D, Maunder RJ, Martin TR, Weiner-Kronish JP, Sticherling M, Christophers E, Matthay MA: Elevated levels of NAP-1/interleukin-8 are present in the airspaces of patients with the adult respiratory distress syndrome and are associated with increased mortality, *Am Rev Respir Dis* 146:427-432, 1992.
176. Donnelly SC, Strieter RM, Kunkel SL, Walz A, Robertson CR, Carter DC, Grant IS, Pollok AJ, Haslett C: Interleukin-8 and development of adult respiratory distress syndrome in at-risk patient groups, *Lancet* 341:643-647, 1993.
177. Clark JG, Milberg JA, Steinberg KP, Hudson LD: Type III procollagen peptide in the adult respiratory distress syndrome: association of increased peptide levels in bronchoalveolar lavage fluid with increased death, *Ann Intern Med* 122:17-23, 1995.
178. Schmalzer EA, Chien S: Filterability of subpopulations of leukocytes: effect of pentoxifylline, *Blood* 64:542-546, 1984.
179. Welsh CH, Lien D, Worthen GS, Weil JV: Pentoxifylline decreases endotoxin-induced pulmonary neutrophil sequestration and extravascular protein accumulation in the dog, *Am Rev Respir Dis* 138:1106-1114, 1988.
180. Ishizaka A, Wu Z, Stephens KE, Harada H, Hogue RS, O'Hanley PT, Raffin TA: Attenuation of acute lung injury in septic guinea pigs by pentoxifylline, *Am Rev Respir Dis* 138:376-382, 1988.
181. Seear MD, Hannam VL, Kaapa P, Usha Raj J, O'Brodovich HM: Effect of pentoxifylline on haemodynamics, alveolar fluid reabsorption and pulmonary oedema in a model of acute lung injury, *Am Rev Respir Dis* 142:1083-1087, 1990.
182. Walsh CJ, Carey PD, Cook DJ, Bechard DE, Fowler AA, Sugerman HJ: Anti-CD 18 antibody attenuates neutropenia and alveolar capillary membrane injury during gram-negative sepsis, *Surgery* 110:205-212, 1991.
183. Zeigler EJ, Fisher CJ, Sprung CL, Straube RC, Sadoff JC, Foulke GE, Wortel CH, Fink MP, Dellinger RP, Teng NNH, Allen IE, Berger HJ, Knatterund GL, LoBuglio AF, Smith CI, the HA-1A Sepsis Study Group: Treatment of gram-negative bacteremia and septic shock with HA-1A human monoclonal antibody against endotoxin: a randomized, double-blind, placebo-controlled trial, *N Engl J Med* 324:429-436, 1991.
184. Dal Nogare AR, Yarbroug WC: A comparison of the effects of intact and deacylated lipopolysaccharide on human polymorphonuclear leukocytes, *J Immunol* 144:1404-1410, 1990.
185. Ohlsson K, Bjork P, Bergenfeld M, Hageman R, Thompson RC: Interleukin-1 receptor antagonist reduces mortality from endotoxic shock, *Nature* 348:550-552, 1990.
186. Arend WP: Interleukin-1 receptor antagonist: a new member of the interleukin-1 family, *J Clin Invest* 88:1445-1451, 1991.
187. Beutler B, Milsark IW, Cerami A: Passive immunization against cachectin/tumor necrosis factor protects mice from the lethal effect of endotoxin, *Science* 229:869-871, 1985.
188. Exley AR, Cohen J, Buurman W, Owen R, Hanson G, Lumley J, Aulakh JM, Bodmer M, Riddell A, Stephens S, Perry M: Monoclonal antibody to TNF in severe septic shock, *Lancet* 335:1275-1277, 1990.
189. Cross AR, Jones OTG: The effect of the inhibitor diphenylene iodonium on the superoxide-generating system of neutrophils: specific labelling of a component polypeptide of the oxidase, *Biochem J* 237:111-116, 1986.
190. Wispe JR, Warner BB, Clark JC, Dey CR, Neuman J, Glasser SW, Crapo JD, Chang L-Y, Whitsett JA: Human Mn-superoxide dismutase in pulmonary epithelial cells of transgenic mice confers protection from oxygen injury, *J Biol Chem* 267:23937-23941, 1992.
191. Suter PM, Domenighetti G, Schaller M-D, Laverrière M-C, Ritz R, Perret C: *N*-Acetylcysteine enhances recovery from acute lung injury in man: a randomized, double-blind, placebo-controlled clinical study, *Chest* 105:190-194, 1994.
192. Redens TB, Leach WJ, Bogdanoff DA, Emerson TE: Synergistic protection from lung damage by combining antithrombin III and alpha-1 proteinase inhibitor in the *E. coli* endotoxic sheep pulmonary dysfunction model, *Circ Shock* 26:15-26, 1988.
193. Gossage JR, Kuratomi Y, Davidson JM, Lefferts PL, Snapper JR: Neutrophil elastase inhibitors SC-37698 and SC-39026, reduce endotoxin-induced lung dysfunction in awake sheep, *Am Rev Respir Dis* 147:1371-1379, 1993.
194. Tanswell AK, Olson DM, Freeman BA: Liposome-mediated augmentation of antioxidant defenses in fetal rat pneumocytes, *Am J Physiol* 258(2):L165-L172, 1990.
195. Lemarchand P, Jaffe HA, Danel C, Cid MC, Kleinman HK, Stratford-Perricaudet LD, Perricaudet M, Pavirani A, Lecocq J-P, Crystal RG: Adenovirus-mediated transfer of a recombinant human α_1-antitrypsin cDNA to human endothelial cells, *Proc Natl Acad Sci USA* 89:6482-6486, 1992.
196. Lewis JF, Jobe AH: Surfactant and the adult respiratory distress syndrome, *Am Rev Respir Dis* 147:218-233, 1993.
197. Canessa CM, Horisberger JT, Rossier BC: Epithelial sodium channel related to proteins involved in neurodegeneration, *Nature* 361:467-470, 1993.

PART TWO

Applied Physiology

CHAPTER 8

Applied Clinical Respiratory Physiology

Peter D. Sly and Mark John Hayden

BASIC PHYSIOLOGIC PRINCIPLES

Functional Anatomy of the Respiratory System

Rib Cage

The rib cage is formed by the 12 thoracic vertebrae, the 12 pairs of ribs, and the sternum and costal cartilages. Posteriorly the ribs articulate with the vertebral bodies. The head of the first, tenth, eleventh, and twelfth ribs each articulate with a single vertebra. The other ribs articulate with two vertebrae across the intervertebral disk. There is an articular surface on the tubercle of ribs 1 through 10, through which the ribs articulate with the transverse process of the vertebra to which it corresponds numerically.

Anteriorly, the first seven ribs are connected directly to the sternum via the costal cartilages and are called *true ribs.* The remaining five ribs are called *false ribs* because they are not attached directly to the sternum. The cartilages of ribs 8, 9, and 10 are joined to the cartilage of the rib above, and ribs 11 and 12 are free anteriorly. These are often called *floating ribs.*

The axis of rotation of the rib changes progressively down the thoracic cage (Fig. 8-1). The upper ribs have a pump-handle movement, with the anterior end swinging upward and outward. The lower ribs have a bucket-handle movement, with the ribs moving laterally and upward; the lowest ribs have a caliper movement, with the entire rib swinging laterally. These combinations of movements lift the rib cage as well as expand it in the anteroposterior and lateral directions. Such movement increases the transverse diameter of the rib cage, particularly at its lower end, and increases its volume. An understanding of how the ribs move is fundamental to understanding how the muscles of respiration expand the rib cage during breathing. This point is highlighted in sections discussing the individual muscle groups. The consequences of abnormalities in the rib cage are dealt with in Chapter 74.

Muscles of Respiration

Skeletal muscle is made up of fibers shaped like elongated cylinders. They vary in length from a few millimeters to more than 30 cm, and their diameter varies from 0.01 to 0.1 mm. The fibers taper at each end, where they are attached to the tendons. When examined in transmitted light, each fiber has a characteristic transverse striation of alternating dark (A) and light (I) bands (Fig. 8-2). Each fiber is covered in a fine tubular sheath known as the *sarcolemma.* The fibers are made up of a number of myofibrils, which are the active contractile components in the muscle fiber. The myofibrils have alternating dark A bands and light I bands along their length. The A and I bands for adjacent myofibrils are aligned transversely to give the muscle fiber its characteristic striations. A dark, narrow line, the Z disk, runs transversely across the middle of the I band. The segment of the fibril between two successive Z disks is termed a *sarcomere.* The sarcomere is the basic contractile unit of the muscle. Thin actin filaments are attached to the Z disk, and thick myosin filaments overlap two sets of actin filaments. Contraction of the muscle is thought to occur when cross-bridges form between the actin and myosin filaments and the actin filaments slide progressively along the myosin filaments. Muscle shortening is thought to be limited when the Z disks limit further sliding of the filaments.

When muscle excitation occurs, a propagated action potential is initiated across the muscle fibers' sarcolemmal membrane, which travels in both directions away from the centrally located myoneural junction. The action potential is an ionic current flow resulting from sequential increases in membrane sodium and potassium conductance. The action potential also spreads inward along the transverse tubular system (which is an extension of the sarcolemmal membrane). The action potential causes calcium ions to be liberated into the tubular space. During rest, muscle interaction between actin and myosin is inhibited by the troponin-tropomyosin complex, thus preventing muscle contraction. The influx of calcium ions is thought to initiate muscle contraction by combining with troponin, releasing actin and myosin from the inhibitory influence of the troponin-tropomyosin complex. The sliding filament paradigm, which has been proposed to explain skeletal muscle, explains muscle contraction in terms of the thick (myosin) and thin (actin) filaments sliding over one another, forming attachments known as *cross-bridges.* During this process, adenosine triphosphate is converted to adenosine diphosphate, with the accompanying release of energy. The cross-bridges are not static connections but actively cycle (attaching, detaching, and reattaching) during a contraction. Relaxation occurs as a result of the active transport of calcium ions into longitudinally orientated elements of the sarcoplasmic reticulum and a reversing of this process. Skeletal muscle cells typically bridge their attachment points on the skeleton. As a result, each cell is independent, the force of contraction can be increased by recruiting more cells for contraction.

The muscle fibers supplied by a single nerve fiber are known as a *motor unit.* A muscle is made up of many individual motor units, each unit consisting of many different muscle fibers. The number of muscle fibers in a motor unit varies widely among different muscles but can be as low as 2 to 10 fibers in small muscles used for delicate movements (e.g., laryngeal and extraocular muscles) and as many as 2000 fibers for large muscles such as the gastrocnemius muscle. Fibers from a single motor unit are not packed into one region of the muscle but are scattered throughout the muscle.

Muscles of Inspiration

Diaphragm. The diaphragm is the most important inspiratory muscle. It consists of three main parts: the costal diaphragm originating from the costal margin and inserting into the central tendon, the crural diaphragm originating mainly from the vertebral column and also inserting into the central tendon, and the

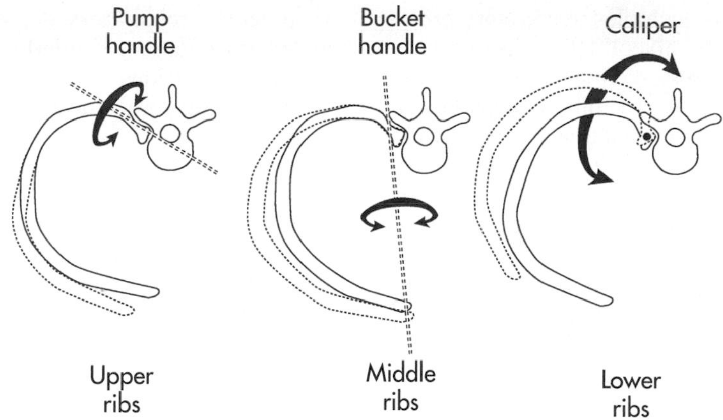

Fig. 8-1. Schematic representation of rib motion around its axis. The dotted lines represent the upper and middle ribs, and the black dot represents the lower ribs.

central tendon itself. The fibers of both muscular parts are directed axially; the costal part is apposed directly to the inner surface of the rib cage (zone of apposition).

Stimulation of the costal fibers causes a fall in pleural pressure and inflation of the lungs. Abdominal pressure rises, and the abdomen is displaced outward. The rib cage is also displaced outward. The force generated by the costal diaphragm is partly transmitted to the rib cage through the zone of apposition. This results in the rib cage being "pushed" upward and outward because of the ribs' axis of rotation. Stimulation of the crural fibers also causes a fall in pleural pressure, a rise in abdominal pressure, and outward displacement of the abdominal wall, but there is no displacement of the rib cage.

External intercostal muscles. The external intercostal muscles connect adjacent ribs and slope downward and forward. When they contract, the ribs are pulled upward and forward, resulting in an increase in both the anteroposterior and lateral diameters of the thorax.

Accessory muscles. The major accessory muscles are the scalene muscles, which elevate the first two ribs, and the sternocleidomastoid muscles, which elevate the sternum. These muscles play only a minor role in normal quiet breathing but contribute significantly at times of increased ventilatory requirements, such as during exercise or with obstructive diseases of the respiratory system (e.g., asthma). Other muscles may also help inspiration; for example, the muscles of the alae nasi flare the nostrils and reduce nasal resistance, the small muscles of the head and neck can help raise the first rib, and the pectoralis major can be used to stabilize the rib cage.

Muscles of Expiration. Quiet expiration is usually passive, but at times of increased ventilatory requirement, expiration may become an active process.

Muscles of the anterior abdominal wall. Contraction of the rectus abdominis muscle, internal and external oblique muscles, and transversus abdominis muscle causes the abdominal pressure to rise and the anterior abdominal wall to be displaced inward. This pushes the diaphragm upward and aids expiration. These muscle also contract forcefully during coughing, vomiting, and defecation.

Internal intercostal muscles. The internal intercostal muscles aid active expiration by pulling the ribs downward and inward. They also stiffen the intercostal spaces and prevent them from bulging outward.

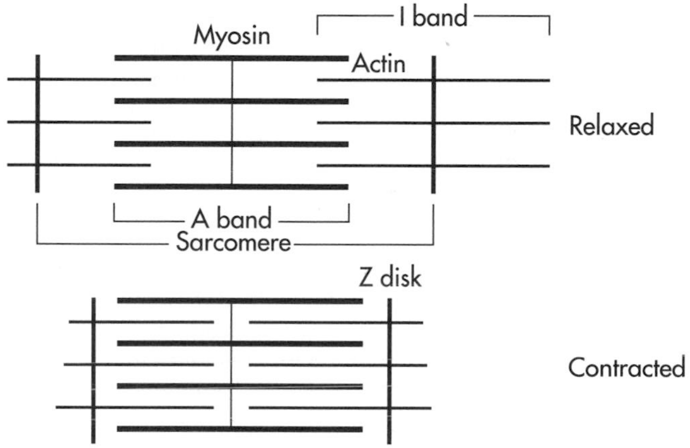

Fig. 8-2. The sarcomere in the relaxed and contracted state. Sarcomeric shortening occurs by sliding of actin over myosin filaments.

Pleura

Each lung is covered by a serous membrane arranged in the form of a closed sac called the *pleura.* A part of this serous membrane (the visceral pleura) covers the surface of the lung and lines the fissures between its lobes. The rest of the membrane (the parietal pleura) lines the inner surface of the corresponding half of the chest wall, covers a large part of the diaphragm, and is reflected over the mediastinum. Between the two layers of the pleura is a potential space called the *pleural space.* The pleural space is 10 to 15 μ wide and contains a small amount of liquid. The lymphatic system opens directly onto the parietal pleura. Active transport of pleural liquid occurs from top to bottom and from costal to mediastinal surfaces. The pleural space "couples" the chest wall to the lungs; without the intact pleural space the lungs would collapse away from the chest wall (a pneumothorax).

Lungs

Airways. The airways consist of a series of branching tubes that become narrower, shorter, and more numerous as they penetrate deeper into the lung. The trachea divides into the right and left main bronchi, which in turn divide into lobar bronchi, segmental bronchi, subsegmental bronchi, small bronchi, bronchioles, terminal bronchioles, respiratory bronchioles, alveolar ducts, and finally alveoli (Fig. 8-3). At each division, or generation, the total cross-sectional area of the tracheobronchial tree increases. The division of airways does not occur symmetrically. The tracheobronchial tree is generally divided into two parts. The airways from the trachea (generation 0) to the terminal bronchioles (generation 16) are generally known as the *conducting airways* because they have no alveoli arising from them.

The airways from the respiratory bronchioles (generations 17 through 19) and the alveolar ducts (generations 20 through 22) have increasing numbers of alveoli budding from their wall and are known collectively as the *transitional* and *respiratory zones.* The portion of lung distal to a terminal bronchus forms an anatomic unit called the *primary lobule* or *acinus.*

Gas exchange occurs only within the acini and not in the conducting airways. The total volume of the conducting airways is approximately 150 ml in adults. During expiration, 500 ml of air is forced out of the acini and through the airways. Approximately 350 ml of this air is exhaled through the nose or mouth (together with the 150 ml of air in the conducting airways), but about 150 ml remains in the conducting airways. With the next inspiration, 500 ml of air enters the alveoli, but the first 150 ml is not atmospheric air but the 150 ml left in the conducting airways at the end of the previous expiration. Thus only 350 ml of new atmospheric air enters the alveoli during one inspiration. At the end of inspiration, 150 ml of fresh air also fills the conducting airways but cannot participate in gas exchange. The volume of the conducting airways is known as the *anatomic dead space.* The ratio of dead space volume to tidal volume (V_{DS}/V_T), together with the breathing frequency, determines the alveolar ventilation. It is the alveolar ventilation that is important for gas exchange. A decrease in V_T without a corresponding increase in breathing frequency, as may occur with central respiratory depression, leads to a decrease in alveolar ventilation. Similarly, an increase in V_{DS}, such as can occur in conditions that make the conducting airways more compliant (e.g., bronchiectasis), can also lead to alveolar hypoventilation.

The cross-sectional area of the tracheobronchial tree increases with each division. This increase in area becomes very rapid in the respiratory zone (see Fig. 8-3).

During respiration, gas flows through the conducting airways by bulk flow, like water through a hose. Beyond that point, the cross-sectional area of the airways is so large that the forward velocity of the gas becomes very small. Diffusion of gas takes over as the dominant mechanism of ventilation in the respiratory zone.

Airway Smooth Muscle. In contrast to skeletal muscle cells, which are mechanically independent, smooth muscle cells must be mechanically coupled and their activation coordinated. Increases in force are produced by increases in the activation of all the coupled cells. The "tone" maintained in airway smooth muscle is an example of continuous partial activation.

There are similarities in ultrastructure, subcellular mechanisms, and contractile and regulatory proteins in striated and smooth muscle. However, there are differences in the way muscle function is regulated. For example, in smooth muscle a calcium-sensitive regulation of contraction is mediated not via a tropomyosin-troponin system but by a calmodulin-mediated, myosin-linked light-chain phosphorylation mechanism. There is still much to be defined in this field.

Smooth muscle exists in the walls of airways, where it is oriented in a spiral fashion rather than a circular fashion around the airway. The smooth muscle has been reported to make an angle of approximately 30 degrees with the cross-sectional plane.[1]

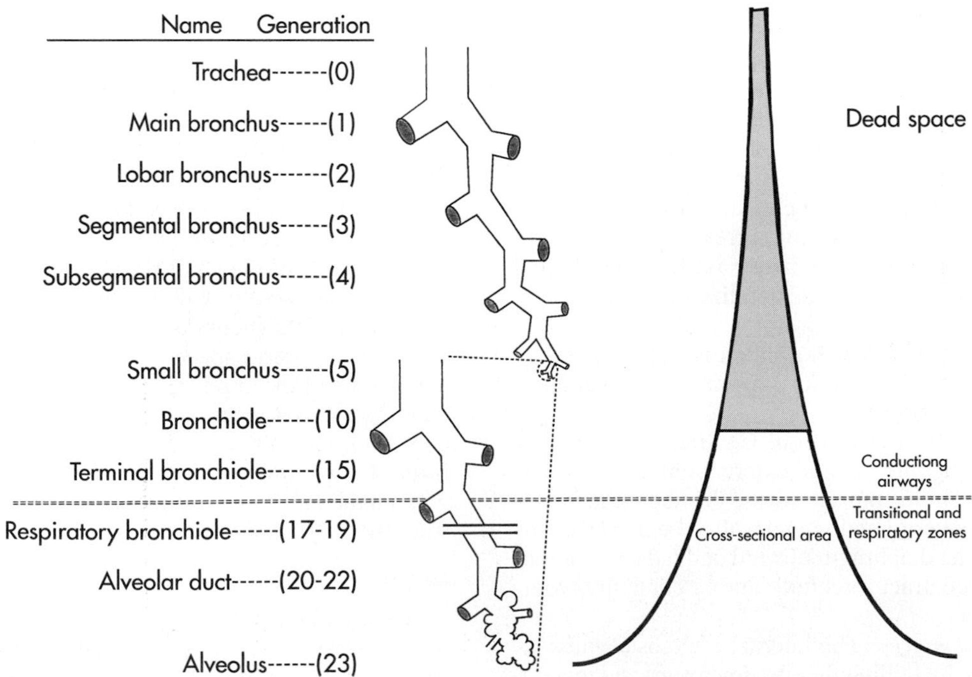

Fig. 8-3. Airway generations. Airway size decreases with increasing generations but the total cross-sectional area increases. The conducting airways (generations 0 to 16) have no gas exchange and contribute to the amount of dead space *(shaded area).*

This means that smooth muscle contraction results in both narrowing and shortening of the airways. The orientation of the smooth muscle could be very important in determining airway responsiveness to various stimuli[2] (see Part Ten).

Alveoli. The lung can be considered a collection of hundreds of millions of bubbles, each approximately 0.3 mm in diameter. The alveoli bring the air and blood into proximity to each other to facilitate gas exchange. The alveolar walls are thin and contain numerous capillaries. The alveolar-capillary membrane consists of four layers: the capillary endothelium and its basement membrane, a thin connective tissue layer, the alveolar epithelium and its basement membrane, and a surfactant lining. The alveolar epithelium consists of two types of cells: Type 1 cells, or squamous pneumocytes, are large, mature cells that do not divide, cover most of the alveolar surface, and are vulnerable to injury, and type 2 cells, or granular pneumocytes, are small, cuboidal cells packed with granules that store and synthesize surfactant. Type 2 cells differentiate into type 1 cells during growth and repair after injury.

The alveoli are inherently unstable. Because of the surface tension of the liquid lining the alveoli, relatively large forces develop that tend to collapse alveoli. The surfactant secreted by the type 2 cells profoundly lowers the surface tension of the alveolar lining fluid. This increases the compliance of the lung and reduces the work of expanding it with each breath. It also makes the alveoli more stable and less likely to collapse. Because the surface tension forces are greater within bubbles with a larger radius of curvature, there is a tendency for smaller bubbles to empty into larger ones (Fig. 8-4). This results in a reduction of alveolar surface area and a decreased ability for gas exchange. Surfactant reduces the surface tension more in smaller bubbles and prevents the collapse of smaller alveoli.

Surfactant also helps keep the alveoli dry. Surface tension forces tend to suck fluid into the alveolar spaces from the capillaries. By reducing these forces, surfactant prevents the transudation of fluid.

Infants born prematurely may suffer from a condition known as *respiratory distress syndrome*. This syndrome is thought to result from a lack of surfactant and is characterized by stiff lungs (low compliance), areas of collapsed alveoli (atelectasis), and alveoli filled with transudate. The result is a decreased capability for gas exchange (see Chapters 31 and 32).

Connective Tissues. In addition to the airways and blood vessels, the lungs consist of a network of collagen and elastin fibers within a proteoglycan matrix. These fibers form a supportive network connecting adjacent airways and alveoli. They are partly responsible for the elastic recoil of the lung, help prevent the collapse of the alveoli and airways, and promote homogeneous emptying of the lungs. The elastin fibers are thought to be largely responsible for the distensibility of the lungs at volumes in the low to middle ranges. This distensibility is reflected in the slope of the static pressure-volume curve (a reflection of the compliance of the lungs). The collagen fibers are thought to be more involved in limiting distention of the lungs, which is reflected by the plateau in the static pressure-volume curve (Fig. 8-5). The influence of the proteoglycans in the connective tissue matrix on lung distensibility is unknown.

The collapse of alveoli or airways in one area tends to pull on adjacent alveoli and airways. The adjacent structures resist this pull, which in turn tends to resist the tendency for the alveoli or airways to collapse. This relationship is known as *mechanical interdependence.*

Pulmonary Circulation

The pulmonary circulation begins at the main pulmonary artery, which receives the mixed venous blood pumped by the right ventricle. The pulmonary artery divides in a manner corresponding to the division of the tracheobronchial tree. Pulmonary arteries accompany the bronchi as far as the terminal bronchioles. Beyond that, they break up to supply the capillary bed, which lies in the walls of the alveoli, where gas exchange occurs. The oxygenated blood is collected by the small pulmonary veins that run between the lobules and eventually unite to form four large veins that drain into the left atrium. The blood supply to the lungs comes from the bronchial circulation, which is formed by systemic arteries and veins and is separate from the pulmonary circulation. The pulmonary circulation is a low-pressure system, and the arteries have thin walls containing little smooth muscle. This lessens the work of the right side of the heart as much as is feasible for efficient gas exchange to occur in the lung. If the pulmonary arteries are subjected to chronic hypoxia, the muscle in the wall hypertrophies and narrows the lumen. This increases the resistance to blood flow through the pulmonary system and results

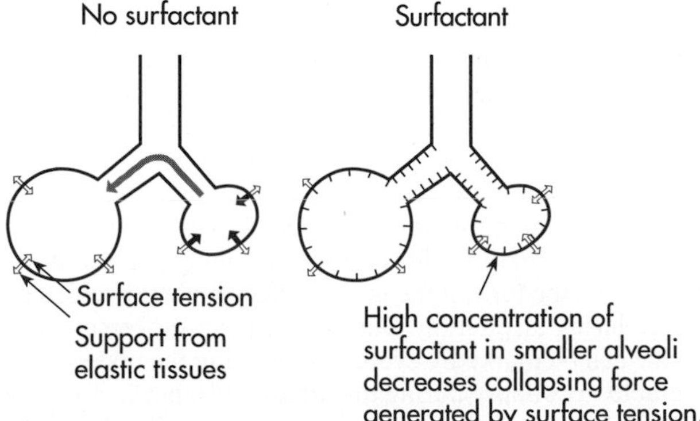

Fig. 8-4. The presence of surfactant in the alveoli decreases surface tension and prevents alveoli with a high radius of curvature (small size) from emptying into larger alveoli. (Arrow size represents the magnitude of force.)

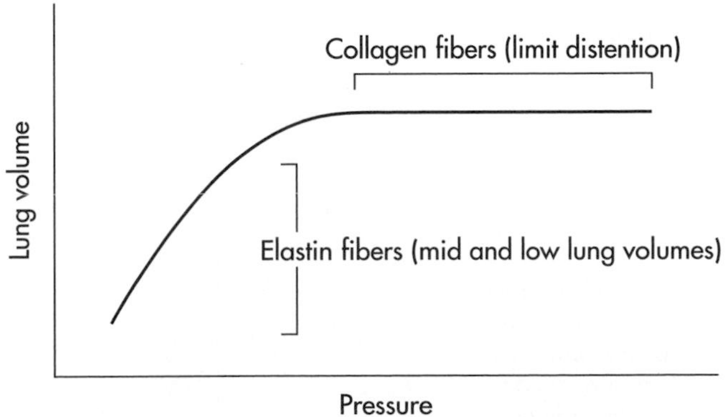

Fig. 8-5. Pressure-volume relationship of the lungs. The influence of connective tissues at different lung volumes is demonstrated.

in increased pulmonary artery pressures and an increased strain on the right side of the heart (see Part Nine).

Upper Airway

The upper airway consists of the passages for airflow between the larynx and the airway opening. Ordinarily it is composed of the nasal passages (from the nostrils to the posterior termination of the nasal septum), the nasopharynx (from the end of the nasal septum to the lower border of the soft palate), and the pharynx (from the palate to the larynx). When a person breathes through the mouth, it also includes the mouth. The nasal airway consists of two passages, each with turbinates projecting from the lateral wall into the lumen. In adults, the surface area of the functional (turbinated) portion of the nasal mucosa is around 120 cm^2, approximately double that of the trachea. The blood vessels in the nasal mucosa, especially that covering the turbinates, are arranged to provide an erectile capacity comparable to that of the male genitalia.

The following are the main anatomic features that allow the nasal passages to perform their specialized function:

1. The axis of the nasal airway is oriented at 90 degrees to that of the trachea.
2. The cross-sectional area increases from the smallest area in the respiratory tract (anterior nares) to the relatively large turbinated airway and then decreases again in the nasopharynx.
3. The anatomic arrangement of the turbinates concentrates the airflow into a relatively small stream.
4. The surface area of the turbinated airway is large.
5. The extensive vascular network gives the body the ability to vary the width of the nasal airway.

All of these features allow the nasal airway to function as an efficient air filtering and conditioning unit (Fig. 8-6).

Air Conditioning. Blood flow in the nasal mucosa is arranged in a countercurrent fashion such that air entering the nose is progressively brought to body temperature and humidity. This usually means that the air is warmed to 37° C and fully saturated with water. The transfer of heat (by turbulent convection) and water (by evaporation) to the air cools the mucosa. During expiration, some of the heat and water vapor return to the mucosa from the alveolar gas. If the nasal airway is bypassed, the mouth and pharynx can perform these air-conditioning functions almost as well as the nose. The trachea and bronchi cannot. During strenuous exercise, the nasal airway is usually bypassed, and increased minute ventilation may exceed the conditioning capacity of the mouth and pharynx. This causes drying and cooling of the lower airways and may provoke exercise-induced asthma in susceptible individuals.

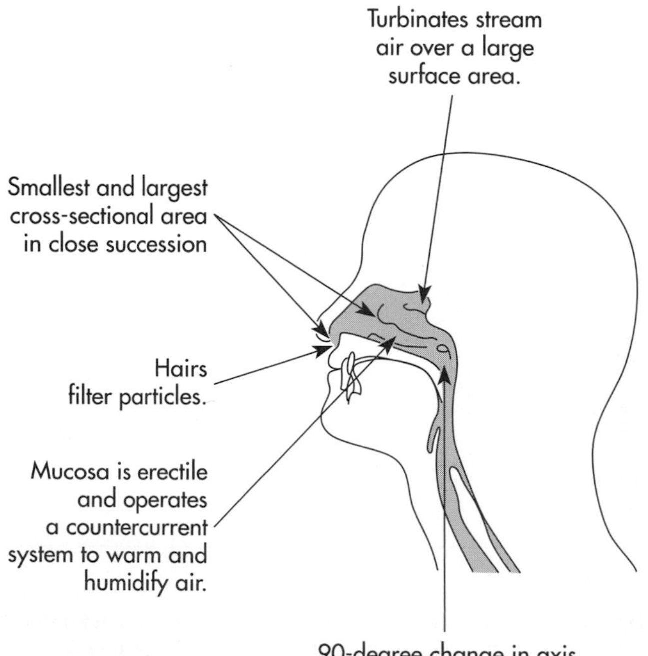

Fig. 8-6. Air filtration and conditioning factors of the upper airway.

Filtration and Cleansing. Hairs in the anterior nares block the passage of very large particles into the nose. Once inside the nose, the air is forced to pass in narrow streams close to the mucosa. The turbulent flow through the nasal airway and the changes of airstream direction force many particles to become trapped in the mucus lining the nasal mucosa. Particles with diameters greater than 10 μ are almost completely removed from the inspired air in the nose. The nasal mucosa is also capable of removing some toxic gases, especially those that are water soluble; for example, sulfur dioxide in concentrations up to 25 ppm can be removed by the nasal mucosa.

Mechanics of the Upper Airway. The nose accounts for approximately half the total respiratory resistance to airflow, but the absolute value shows marked variation among subjects. Nasal resistance varies with changes in nasal vascular congestion, posture, exercise, ambient air conditions, pharmacologic agents, and disease.

Almost all of the nasal resistance is contributed by the first 2 to 3 cm of the nasal passage (i.e., the anterior constriction [the nares and the tip of the inferior turbinate]). The turbinated passage contributes little to resistance under normal circumstances. However, if the nasal mucosa is engorged with blood, the turbinated passages can make a significant contribution to the total resistance.

The nasal vasculature is under autonomic control, reflexively responding to changing ambient air conditions. Small fluctuations occur in response to the temperature of inspired air; there is a significant increase in nasal resistance resulting from vascular engorgement when the temperature of inspired air falls below 7° C. Changes in body posture alter resistance through hydrostatic effects on the vasculature. Changing from a standing or sitting to a recumbent position increases nasal resistance. Nasal resistance is often higher through one nasal passage than the other because of differences in the degree of vascular engorgement. The high-resistance changes from one side of the nose to the other occurs in 3- to 4-hour cycles. This cycle may allow one nasal passage to recover from injury suffered in filtering and conditioning inspired air.

The most compliant region of the upper airway is the pharynx. The negative pressures generated during inspiration tend to collapse the pharynx. This region is usually protected from collapsing by the tone of the upper airway muscles, which also contract during inspiration. During rapid-eye-movement sleep, this tone can be markedly decreased, making the upper airway vulnerable to collapse during inspiration. If other factors combine to make the upper airway more prone to collapse, the syndrome of obstructive sleep apnea may be seen (see Chapter 73). Some infants are born with relatively small upper airways. This may be part of a recognized syndrome or may be a familial trait. A small upper airway has a higher resistance and may necessitate the generation of greater negative pressures to produce sufficient inspiratory flow. This results in a greater tendency for the upper airway to collapse. The same syndrome is seen in adults, especially those who are grossly obese. These people probably have deposits of fat around the upper airway that effectively "load" the upper airway and make it more likely to collapse during inspiration. Heavy alcohol use can also precipitate upper airway obstruction during inspiration, probably by decreasing the tone of the upper airway muscles that are responsible for stabilizing the upper airway.

Modeling

General Theory of Modeling

A system is any collection of physical components whose interactions with one another and with the environment are of interest. A model is something that mimics some aspect of the system; it may be a physical model or a theoretical model.

Models are constructed for many reasons. At one extreme, one may wish to have a purely empirical description of the system; that is, one may wish to have a model that behaves in a similar fashion to the system but does not have to have any structural similarity. At the other extreme, one may wish to have a detailed description of the system, with every distinct process in the system represented faithfully in the model. The construction and use of models of varying degrees of complexity are integral parts of the scientific process. Indeed, the scientific method consists of continually testing and refining models of the system being studied. The detail and completeness of the model are thus synonymous with understanding of the system. It is important to remember that no model is ever correct. Most models are initially formed, either from preconceived ideas about what the structure of the system should be or from preliminary data about how the system behaves.

In general, a model transforms an input to produce an output. This can be represented as follows:

$$Y = H \odot X \tag{1}$$

where *Y* is the output from the model, *H* is the transfer function of the model, $\odot$ is the convolution integral, and *X* is the input to the model. If one considers a pressure transducer, the pressure being measured is the input, and the electric signal coming from the transducer is the output. The process by which the transducer converts (or transforms) the pressure signal into an electric one represents the transfer function of the transducer.

Any model consists of a structure and a number of parameters. The model structure determines its qualitative behavior, and the model parameters determine its quantitative behavior.

Linear Modeling Theory

Systems may be divided into two categories: linear and nonlinear. In the real world, almost every system is nonlinear. However, many systems may be approximately linear under certain conditions. A linear model has certain useful properties that make analysis easier. The system is linear if it obeys the principle of superposition, meaning that the output from the sum of two inputs equals the sum of the outputs from the two inputs alone. Let the inputs be $x_1(t)$ and $x_2(t)$. The output is a function (*f*) of the input, as follows:

$$y_1(t) = f\{x_1(t)\} \tag{2}$$

$$y_2(t) = f\{x_2(t)\} \tag{3}$$

The linear condition requires the following for any inputs x_1 and x_2:

$$\begin{aligned} y_1(t) + y_2(t) &= f\{x_1(t)\} + f\{x_2(t)\} \\ &= f\{x_1(t) + x_2(t)\} \end{aligned} \tag{4}$$

If, in addition, the output of the system does not depend on the time when the input was applied, the system is time invariant.

Another important property of a linear system is that if the input is a sine wave, the output is also a sine wave of the same frequency, but the amplitude and phase may be altered by the system.

Even if a system is nonlinear, there may be a range of inputs over which the system can be approximated by a linear model. This is known as the *linear range* of the system.

If a system obeys these conditions, the relationship between the input and output can be investigated using techniques such as Fourier transformations.

Modeling the Respiratory System

The respiratory system consists of airways and airspaces. The most simple model of the respiratory system is a representation of a single balloon on a pipe. Thus the structure is one of a single-compartment model because it has a single degree of freedom; that is, it can move in only one dimension. Such a model can be described by a first-order linear differential equation. This model has two parameters, the elastance of the balloon and the resistance of the pipe. If the balloon in the model is inflated and allowed to empty, the relationship between the pressure applied at the opening of the model, *P(t),* and the volume in the model, *V(t),* can be written as:

$$P(t) = EV(t) + R\dot{V}(t) \tag{5}$$

where *E* is the elastance of the balloon, *R* is the resistance of the pipe, and $\dot{V}$ is the rate of change of volume (or flow at the model opening). When one measures P(t), V(t), and $\dot{V}$(t), one can calculate estimates of the elastance and resistance using regression analyses. If the model is a reasonable representation of the respiratory system, the values of resistance and elastance reflect the resistance of the airways and the elastance of the lungs.

Relaxed Expiration

During a relaxed expiration P(t) = 0, so Equation 5 changes, as follows:

$$EV(t) + R\dot{V}(t) = 0 \tag{6}$$

This can be rewritten as a first-order differential equation, as follows:

$$\delta V(t)/\delta t + E/R \cdot V(t) = 0 \tag{7}$$

$$\delta V(t)/V(t) = -E/R \cdot \delta t \tag{8}$$

This can be solved by integration to yield the following:

$$V(t) = Ae^{-t/\tau} \tag{9}$$

where *A* represents the initial volume at t = 0 and τ = R/E. This demonstrates that the volume-time profile of the single-compartment model of the respiratory system describes a single exponential, with a time constant equal to R/E during a passive "expiration."

When the volume-time profile is measured during relaxed expirations, it is not well described by a single exponential. Fitting two exponentials to the data gives a more accurate description of the data. This suggests that the passive respiratory system is not behaving as a single compartment.

In another approach, during a relaxed expiration, the pressure inside the model (PA) is greater than that measured at the airway opening (PAO) because of the pressure required to overcome the frictional resistance of moving air through the pipe (the resistive pressure). If the flow is stopped abruptly during the expiration, PAO will rapidly rise to equal PA, the value of which is determined by the elastic recoil of the model at that volume. The value of the rapid increase in PAO is equal to the resistive pressure drop across the pipe.

Measurements of PAO made during interruptions to expiratory flow in humans and animals, however, do not share this picture. In general there is a rapid initial rise in PAO, followed by a secondary, slower increase in pressure to a plateau (Fig. 8-7). A single-compartment model is inadequate for describing these data. Thus a more complex model must be developed. The next step is to increase the order of the model to a second-order model. This could be two compartments connected in series or parallel or a single compartment with viscoelastic and elastic properties. Each of these models can be made to reproduce the measured data. There is no way to identify which model best represents the system with the current input-output data. Additional input-output data are needed for this. In a series of animal experiments designed to define which two-compartment model best represented the respiratory system, PA was also measured during interruptions to airflow. According to these data, immediately after airflow interruption, PAO jumped to meet PA, and both pressures rose together to reach the plateau. The model that is most consistent with these data is the single-compartment with viscoelastic and elastic properties.[3]

Use of Modeling in the Measurement of Respiratory Mechanics

All measurements of respiratory mechanics are based on an underlying model assumption. The majority of respiratory function tests implicitly assume a lumped-parameter, linear, single-compartment model to represent the respiratory system. When one reports a value of airway resistance or lung elastance, the underlying assumption is that there is *one* value for these parameters or that the lung can be represented by the simple "balloon on a pipe" model. This assumption is rarely satisfied in real life. However, under many conditions, especially patients with normal lungs, the single-compartment model assumption is reasonably accurate and provides useful data. These issues are discussed further in Chapters 14 and 15, which deal with measurement of lung function.

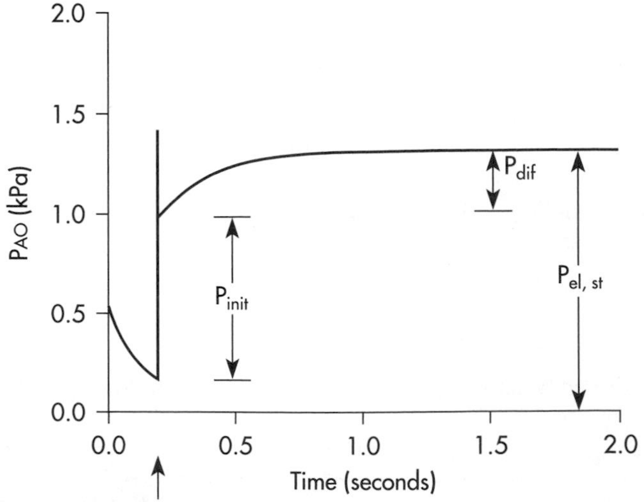

Fig. 8-7. Airway opening pressure after an expiratory flow interruption *(arrow)* demonstrating a rapid initial jump in pressure (P_{init}) and a slower secondary change. (P_{dif}) to the static elastic recoil pressure ($P_{el,st}$). (From Freezer NJ et al: *Pediatr Res* 33(3)261-266, 1993.)

Elastic Properties of the Respiratory System

The respiratory system is composed of a collection of elastic structures. When a force is applied to an elastic structure, the structure resists deformation by producing an opposing force to return the structure to its relaxed state. This opposing force is known as *elastic recoil.* In the respiratory system the pressure generated by the elastic recoil is known as the *elastic recoil pressure* (PEL). The force required to stretch an elastic structure depends on how far it is stretched, not on how rapidly it is being stretched. Similarly, the pressure required to overcome the elastic recoil of the lung depends on the lung volume above or below the elastic equilibrium volume (EEV) (i.e., the volume at which the outward recoil of the chest wall balances the inward recoil of the lungs [see later section]). The PEL divided by the lung volume gives a measure of the elastic properties of the respiratory system and is called *elastance,* as follows:

$$E = P_{EL}/V \tag{10}$$

When lung volume is plotted on the ordinate and PEL is plotted on the abscissa, the slope of the static pressure-volume curve is equivalent to the reciprocal of elastance, called *compliance.* Elastance and compliance are discussed more fully in Chapters 14 and 15.

Hysteresis

The static pressure-volume curves of the respiratory system, lungs, and chest wall are not the same during inspiration and expiration. This phenomenon is called *hysteresis* (Fig. 8-8). Hysteresis is the failure of a system to follow identical paths of response on application and withdrawal of a forcing agent. Hysteresis in the respiratory system depends on viscoelasticity, such as stress adaptation (i.e., a rate-dependent phenomenon) and on

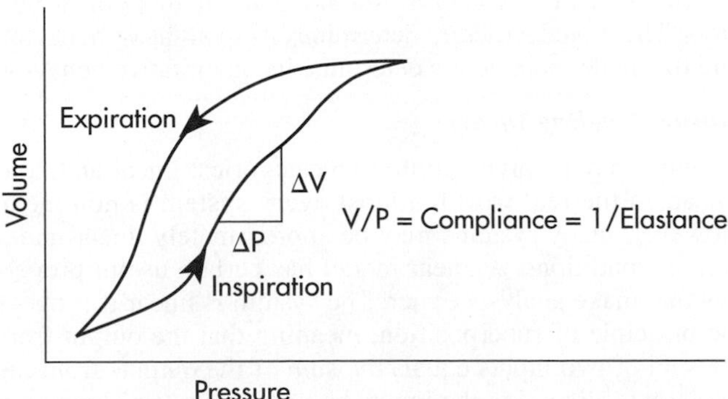

Fig. 8-8. Hysteresis in the pressure-volume curve of the lung. The area contained within the curve represents energy lost in the system. *V,* Volume; *P,* pressure; *ΔV,* change in volume; *ΔP,* change in pressure

plasticity (i.e., a rate-independent phenomenon). In the lungs, hysteresis is due mainly to surface properties and alveolar recruitment-derecruitment, whereas in the chest wall, it seems mainly related to muscles and ligaments because both skeletal muscles and elastic fibers exhibit hysteresis. Hysteresis is negligible for volume changes such as those occurring during quiet breathing. This is functionally desirable because the area of the hysteresis loop represents energy lost from the system.

Muscles of the Respiratory System

Basic Concepts of Skeletal Muscle Mechanics

Muscle Fiber Type. The three basic types of muscle fibers are distinguished by their histochemical and morphologic properties and their time course of contraction: fast-twitch, oxidative, glycolytic (FOG); fast-twitch, glycolytic (FG); and slow-twitch, oxidative (SO). The concentration of myoglobin in the FOG and SO fibers makes them red, so these fibers are also known as *fast-twitch red* and *slow-twitch red* fibers, respectively. The FG fibers have minimal myoglobin and are known as *fast-twitch white fibers* (Table 8-1).

Within a species, white fibers are frequently larger in diameter than fast red fibers, with slow red fibers intermediate in size. FG fibers are used for short-term, fast, powerful activity in which endurance and resistance to fatigue are not required. FOG fibers are used for sustained phasic activity in which resistance to fatigue is desirable. The SO fibers are sluggish but are economical contractile units most suitable for sustained tonic activity (such as the maintenance of posture, in which resistance to fatigue is of prime importance).

Most mammalian muscles contain a mixture of the three types of muscle fibers. Each motor unit of a mixed muscle is composed of a single fiber type. The contractile properties of a mixed muscle are determined by the predominant fiber type. Although three types of muscle fiber are recognized, classification of muscle based on their mechanical properties alone yields two types of muscle: fast-twitch, including both FOG and FG fibers; and slow-twitch muscle, composed of predominantly SO fibers.

The following factors are important in determining the twitch characteristics of muscles:

1. The speed of sarcomere shortening, which is proportional to the specific activity of myosin adenosine triphosphatase (ATPase) activity (which varies with myosin isotype).
2. The neural supply to the muscle: If a motor nerve that normally innervates a slow muscle is transplanted into a fast muscle and time is allowed for nerve regeneration, the muscle changes its properties from those of a fast muscle to those of a slow muscle, and vice versa.
3. The stage of muscle development: Differentiation into fast and slow fibers takes place rather late in development. In species in which the young are born mature (e.g., guinea pig), the differentiation occurs before birth, whereas in species in which the young are born immature (e.g., mouse, rat, human), the differentiation occurs after birth. The differentiation seems to involve changes in the biochemical and morphologic properties of the sarcoplasmic reticulum and transverse tubular system, which effect changes in the excitation-contraction coupling.
4. Training: Any training, particularly endurance training, can alter fiber composition and characteristics.

Thus the composition of a muscle is a dynamic property that can be altered to suit the requirements of the muscle at the time.

Muscle Mechanics. Skeletal muscle has been most successfully modeled as the following interacting components (Fig. 8-9):

1. A contractile component responsible for force generation and muscle shortening
2. A lightly damped series-elastic component representing an internal load that the muscle must overcome
3. A parallel-elastic component responsible for the passive tension produced as the muscle is stretched

During contraction, the actin and myosin filaments slide over one another, shortening the sarcomere. The force generated is a function of the degree of sarcomere shortening. As the filaments slide over one other, cross-bridges form between the fibers. These cross-bridges are independent, force-generating elements, and the force produced is a function of the number of active cross-bridges.

Length-Tension Relationship. Measurement of the force developed with activation over a range of lengths provides information about the ability of the muscle to stiffen and support loads. The "resting tension" curve is the tension produced when the muscle is passively stretched. The shape of this curve is typical of noncontractile biologic tissues and results primarily from the presence of elastin and collagen. With activation of the muscle at a given length, the tension rises to a level shown by the "total tension" curve. The difference in tension

Table 8-1 Properties of Muscle Fiber Types

PROPERTIES	FOG	FG	SO
Synonym	Fast-twitch red	Fast-twitch white	Slow-twitch red
Presence of myoglobin	Positive	Negative	Positive
Isometric-twitch contraction time	Short	Short	Long
Myosin adenosine triphosphatase activity	High	High	Low
Glycolytic enzyme system	Reasonable	Good	Poor
Mitochondrial oxidative system	Good	Poor	Good
Resistance to fatigue	Good	Poor	Very good
Movements	Sustained, phasic	Brief, rapid, powerful	Sustained, tonic

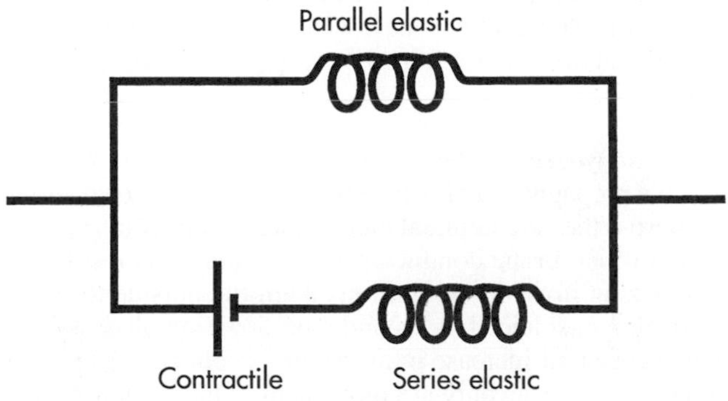

Fig. 8-9. Circuit diagram representing the mechanical properties of skeletal muscle.

between the total and resting tension curves represents the activity of the contractile element or force generator of the muscle and is known as the *active tension.* The length at which the active tension is maximal is defined as the optimal length of the muscle. The resting length of the muscle is defined as the maximal length the muscle can be stretched before passive tension develops. This length generally corresponds to the muscle's resting length in the body. When the resting muscle is stretched beyond optimal length, it exerts a passive tension that increases exponentially as a function of increasing muscle length. When the muscle is maximally stimulated at varying lengths, an isometric length-tension curve can be drawn. The *active tension* of the muscle is defined as the difference between the total tension measured and the passive tension at that length. There is an optimal muscle length, usually between 100% and 120% of the length at which isometric tension is maximal during tetanic stimulation. Comparing the tension-generating capacity of one muscle with another muscle of a different size requires expression of tension in relation to the amount of contractile material active in parallel with the muscle. This is usually done by expressing tension in terms of force per unit of a cross-sectional area of the muscle. The cross-sectional area is only roughly related to the amount of contractile material acting in parallel because it ignores variations in the density with which myofibrils are packed within individual fibers and it ignores differences in extracellular space that occupies 8% to 25% of the cross-sectional area in different muscles. When expressed this way, fast and slow muscle show no major differences in the intrinsic strength of their contractile material.

Force-Velocity Relationship. A light weight can be moved very rapidly by a muscle, whereas a heavy weight must be moved slowly. This fundamental property of muscle is known as the *force-velocity relationship.* There is an inverse curvilinear relationship between the force produced by a muscle and the velocity with which the muscle can shorten while producing that force. This can be expressed by Hill's equation, which describes a hyperbolic relationship between force and velocity, as follows:

$$(P + a)(V + b) = (P_0 + a)b \qquad (11)$$

where P is the instantaneous force of contraction, V is the velocity of shortening, P_0 is the force of contraction at zero velocity (i.e., the isometric force of contraction), and a and b are constants. The position of the force-velocity curve depends on the initial length of the muscle.

The shortening velocity of a muscle (appropriately normalized for fiber cross-sectional area and so on) reflects the average cross-bridge cycling rates, which in turn are functions of the load and the isoform of myosin expressed in that particular muscle cell.[4,5]

Electromyogram. The electromyogram is a reflection of a muscle's propagated action potential that is due to ionic current flow across the sarcolemmal membrane. An initial transient increase in membrane conductance to sodium ions results in a depolarizing flow of sodium ions from the outside to the inside of the muscle cell. A second repolarization phase follows when a transient increase in membrane conductance to potassium ions allows an outward movement of the potassium ions. Thus the action potential of a single muscle fiber is a simple biphasic waveform (i.e., a positive wave followed by a negative one). This wave is propagated along the muscle fiber with a velocity of approximately 2 to 6 m/s. The amplitude of the action potential is affected by factors such as the size of the fiber (increased with fiber diameter), the distance between the recording electrode and the discharging fiber (decreased inversely with the distance), and the conductive and capacitive properties of the intervening tissues and the electrode-tissue interface (the properties act as a low-pass filter [that is, high frequencies are progressively attenuated]). Although the action potential from each fiber is a simple biphasic wave, action potentials from nearby fibers are not synchronous and are not changing in the same direction at any particular time. Also, they are not all moving in the same direction relative to the electrode. Thus the electromyogram recorded represents a complex summation of many single-fiber action potentials.

Basic Concepts of Smooth Muscle Mechanics

Although smooth muscle does not have the same anatomic structure as skeletal muscle, biochemical and biophysical studies in the 1970s indicated that smooth muscles contract in a manner similar to skeletal muscle. However, recent physiologic studies have demonstrated that the "sliding filament" paradigm, in which the active cycling of cross-bridges is responsible for the amount of force developed (number of cross-bridges) and the force-velocity relationships (cycling rate) of muscle, cannot adequately explain the "force maintenance" properties of smooth muscle. This lead to the description of "latchbridges." *Latch* refers to a state in which force is maintained, despite a reduced cross-bridge cycling rate, by calcium-dependent cross-bridge phosphorylation.[4] Although the term *latchbridge* tends to imply that the actin and myosin filaments are locked together, this is not the case.

In a review of the regulation of smooth muscle contraction, Murphy[4] suggested that the unique properties of smooth muscle derive from a covalent regulatory mechanism whereby phosphorylation of cross-bridges is obligatory for attachment and cycling and that the fundamental myosin "motor" whose behavior is described by the sliding filament/cross-bridge hypothesis is the same in smooth and striated muscle. He presented evidence suggesting that covalent regulation in smooth muscle allows four rather than two cross-bridge states: free, attached, phosphorylated, and dephosphorylated. This hypothesis seems to explain the special properties of smooth muscle.

Length-Tension Relationships. Although skeletal muscle usually has a resting length approximating the optimal length, it has not been established whether this is also true for airway smooth muscle. Some investigators have found that airway smooth muscle is close to optimal length at the end of tidal expiration. The contractile elements of smooth muscle can develop approximately the same force as those of skeletal muscle. Skeletal muscle can shorten to approximately 65% of optimal length, whereas tracheal smooth muscle can shorten to about 10% of optimal length. The reason for this difference is not known. The ratio of myosin to actin is less in smooth muscle than in striated muscle, and well-defined sarcomeres are not present. It has been speculated that the lack of limiting Z bands allow the myosin filaments to "crawl" farther along a set of relatively long actin filaments.

Force-Velocity Relationships. Measurements of force at various velocities of contraction provide information regarding the ability of the muscle not only to support loads but also to shorten and thus do work. They also provide an index of power generation. Smooth muscle force-velocity curves are also hyperbolic and can be fitted by Hill's equation, as previously described. Force-velocity studies show that the force of contraction at zero velocity for smooth muscle is similar to the force of contraction for striated muscle but that maximum velocity values are much smaller. The maximum velocity is a convenient index of the contractility of smooth muscle as long as the shortening is limited to less than 25% of optimal length.

When a muscle is forcibly lengthened, the load may exceed the force of contraction at zero velocity. This may be the case for airway smooth muscle during inspiration. Thus a muscle that is being actively elongated may be stronger than the same muscle that is shortening. An elongating muscle also consumes less energy than the shortening muscle at equivalent velocities.

Influence of Breathing Movements on Smooth Muscle Mechanics. As diameters of airways change with inspiration and expiration, it is important to know how the smooth muscle behaves when its length is externally forced. When the muscle length is changed with amplitudes and frequencies similar to those occurring during respiration, considerable force-length hysteresis occurs. The tension in the muscle depends not only on the pattern of the imposed length cycles but also on their timing. When the muscle is repeatedly stretched, the more time between cycles, the greater the initial tension in the muscle.

Individual Respiratory Muscles

The mechanical task of the respiratory muscles differs from that of a typical limb muscle because the respiratory muscle must overcome primarily elastic and resistive impedances, whereas limb muscles contend principally with inertive impedances. Usually, respiratory muscles must repeatedly perform relatively sustained tension-generating and shortening actions, whereas limb muscles are usually required to generate short bursts of tension and shortening in executing the usual rhythmic motions of the limbs. This difference can be a determining factor for the contractile and endurance properties of the respiratory muscles. The changes in lung volume that occur during breathing indicate that different muscle are asked to begin contracting from different lengths.

Diaphragm. The diaphragm is a mixed muscle made up of approximately 21% FOG, 55% SO, and 24% FG fibers. The number of fatigue-resistant SO fibers increases in the diaphragm during infancy and has been reported to be approximately 10% in premature infants, 25% in full-term infants, and reaching the adult level (around 55%) by 2 years of age. In all species studied, including humans, the diaphragm is functionally intermediate in its rate of tension generated between fast and slow muscles. The diaphragm fibers are thought to be at optimal length at supine functional residual capacity (FRC), although maximal tension seems to occur at somewhat longer lengths.

Intercostal Muscles. The composition of the intercostal muscles is similar to that of the diaphragm. Also, the percentage of fatigue-resistant fibers is substantially reduced in premature infants and, to a lesser extent, full-term neonates, reaching adult levels by 2 years of age.

Scalenus Muscles. The scalenus muscles insert into the first rib, and contraction elevates the first rib during inspiration. These muscles have generally been regarded as accessory muscles of respiration, but they appear to contract, as indicated by the presence of action potentials, during resting breathing and should be regarded as primary respiratory muscles. There is no published data about their fiber type distribution or contractile properties.

Sternocleidomastoid Muscle. The sternocleidomastoid muscle is clearly an accessory muscle of respiration because it usually does not contract unless breaths are considerably deeper than resting tidal breaths. It appears to be made up of 65% fast-twitch and 35% slow-twitch fibers.

Abdominal Muscles. The respiratory actions of the abdominal muscles are twofold. They are primary expiratory muscles because of their direct action on the rib cage and their ability to compress the abdominal contents, forcing the diaphragm upward. They also appear to facilitate the inspiratory action of the diaphragm by contracting toward the end of expiration, pushing the diaphragm upward and optimizing its fiber length for generating tension during the subsequent inspiration. This action of the abdominal muscles occurs during the postural change from supine to upright, during voluntary hyperventilation, and during exercise.

Dynamics of Breathing

Ventilation of the lungs involves motion of the respiratory system, which is produced by the forces required to overcome the flow-resistive, inertial, and elastic properties of the lungs and chest wall. Under normal circumstances, these forces are produced by the respiratory muscles.

Flow Resistance

The force required to move a block of wood over a surface is determined by the friction between the block of wood and the surface and by the speed with which the block is moving. It is not, however, determined by the block's position. Similarly, the pressure required to produce flow between the atmosphere and alveoli and thus to overcome the frictional resistance *(fr)* of the airways is proportional to flow *($\dot{V}$)* (i.e., the rate at which volume is changing), as follows:

$$P_{mouth} - P_{alv} = P_{fr} \propto \dot{V} \quad (12)$$

The pressure required to produce a unit of flow is known as the *flow resistance (R),* as shown by the following:

$$R = P_{fr}/\dot{V} \quad (13)$$

If the respiratory system is modeled as a single compartment with a single constant elastance *(E)* and a single constant resistance *(R),* then the equation of motion describing the balance of forces acting on the system is as follows:

$$P = EV + R\dot{V} + I\dot{V} \quad (14)$$

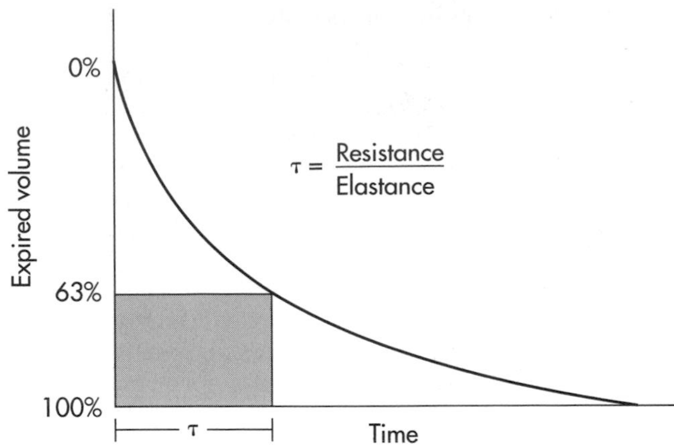

Fig. 8-10. Time constant of lung emptying.

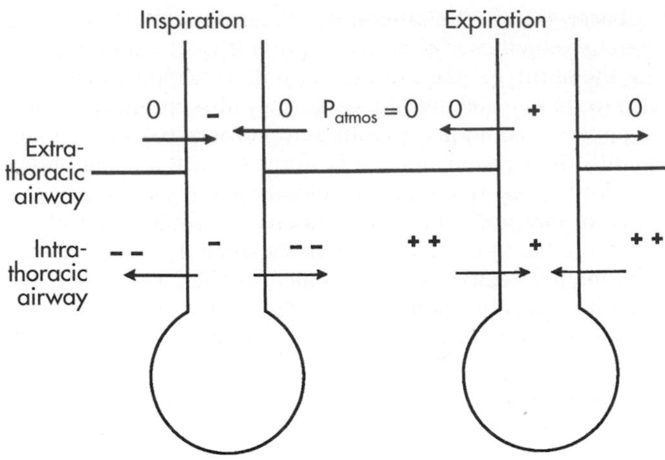

Fig. 8-11. Transmural airway pressures during inspiration and expiration, with net forces illustrating one factor leading to extrathoracic narrowing on inspiration and intrathoracic narrowing on expiration. Arrows indicate net force on airway; plus and minus signs indicate pressure relative to atmospheric pressure *(0).*

The inertance *(I)* is usually negligible and therefore ignored. During tidal respiration, approximately 90% of the pressure produced is required to overcome the elastic forces, and approximately 10% is required to overcome the flow-resistant forces.

Traditionally, it was thought that the majority of the force developed during breathing was required to move gas through the airways and that little energy was dissipated by the tissues of the respiratory system. In recent years, however, it has become increasingly apparent that the viscoelastic properties of the respiratory system contribute significantly to the behavior of that system. The energy expended moving the tissues has been called *tissue viscance* or *resistance,* although it is a nonnewtonian resistance. The anatomic structures responsible for the viscoelastic behavior of lung tissue are not known. Candidates likely to contribute to viscoelasticity include the air-liquid interface, collagen and elastin fibers, actin/myosin crossbridges, contractile (Kapanci) cells within the interstitium, and smooth muscle in the alveolar ducts. Experimental evidence is consistent with the involvement of "contractile" elements because the stress adaptation seen after an airflow interruption (a manifestation of viscoelastic behavior) increases after "constrictor" stimuli[3,6-9] and decreases after "relaxant" stimuli. Alternatively, the viscoelasticity demonstrated in many animal studies may be a reflection of the immense complexity of the lungs, with no single structure responsible.[10]

Studies in animals have demonstrated that when measured during inspiration, tissue resistance increases and airway resistance falls with increasing lung volume. Tissue resistance contributes approximately 65% of respiratory system resistance at FRC in mechanically ventilated animals and increases to as much as 95% at higher lung volumes.[11] The contribution of tissue resistance to respiratory system resistance in humans, under the same conditions, is not known, but the overall behavior of the respiratory system appears to be similar.

Driving Pressures for Respiration

Inspiration occurs when the respiratory muscles cause the alveolar pressure to be less than atmospheric pressure. Air then moves along this pressure gradient, and the lungs inflate, thus storing potential energy in the elastic structures. At the end of inspiration the respiratory muscles relax, and the elastic recoil of the respiratory system causes the alveolar pressure to be positive relative to atmospheric pressure, and expiration occurs. Under resting conditions, expiration is usually passive. At times of increased ventilatory requirements, such as during exercise, contraction of the abdominal and internal intercostal muscles can aid expiration.

Time Constant of Emptying

When the respiratory system is allowed to empty passively and the volume-time profile is measured, the time taken for volume to be reduced by 63% is known as the *time constant* (τ) of the respiratory system (Fig. 8-10). If the respiratory system is modeled as a single compartment with a single, constant elastance and a single, constant resistance, then the following occurs:

$$\tau = R/E \qquad (15)$$

Under these conditions, the volume-time profile can be represented by a single exponential decay.

In healthy adults the time constant of the passive respiratory system is approximately 0.5 second, which allows the lungs to empty to the EEV at the end of each expiration; the FRC and EEV are equal. This means that the respiratory system is relaxed at the end of expiration and that inspiration can begin as soon as inspiratory muscle activity commences. In obstructive airway diseases, such as asthma and chronic bronchitis, resistance is increased, and the expiratory time constant is longer. Therefore a longer time is required for the lungs to empty and return the respiratory system to EEV. Patients with these diseases frequently have carbon dioxide retention and an increased respiratory drive. This results in an increased respiratory rate with a decrease in the time available for expiration. Thus the respiratory system frequently does not have time to return to EEV before the next inspiration starts. This means that FRC occurs at a volume higher than EEV and that the respiratory system is not relaxed at the end of expiration but that there is a positive recoil pressure. This pressure has been called *intrinsic positive end-expiratory pressure,* or $PEEP_i$. Before inspiratory flow can begin, the inspiratory muscle must produce enough force to overcome the $PEEP_i$; thus this force is "lost" to producing inspiratory flow and represents a load that must be overcome by the inspiratory muscle. In patients with severe airway obstruction this pressure can be as high as 15 to 20 cm H_2O. The expiratory time constant is shorter in children, with values approximating 0.3 second reported in infants with normal lungs.[9] Infants with hyaline membrane disease have stiffer-than-normal lungs, with expiratory time constants reported to be as low as 0.1 second.[12]

Dynamic Change in Airway Caliber During Respiration

Airway caliber is partially dependent on the transmural pressure (Fig. 8-11). The external airway wall is subjected to interstitial pressure, which is approximately equal to pleural pressure for all intrathoracic airways. The external walls of extrathoracic airways are subjected to atmospheric pressure. The pressure inside the airway depends on the generation of the airway. During inspiration, pleural pressure is negative relative to atmospheric pressure. Alveolar pressure is approximately equal to pleural pressure, and pressure at the mouth is atmospheric. Thus there is a pressure gradient from the mouth to the alveoli. Transmural pressure for the extrathoracic airways is positive, and there is a tendency for these airways to narrow during inspiration. The transmural pressure is negative for the intrathoracic airways, causing a tendency for these airways to dilate during inspiration. The degree of change in airway caliber depends on the magnitude of the transmural pressure and the airway wall compliance. At the end of inspiration, the inspiratory muscles relax, and the elastic recoil of the respiratory system produces positive pleural and alveolar pressures (relative to atmospheric pressure). Thus there is a tendency for intrathoracic airways to narrow and extrathoracic airways to dilate during expiration.

Gas Exchange

The basic respiratory function of the respiratory system is to supply oxygen to the body and to remove excess carbon dioxide. The following are the basic steps involved in this process:

1. Ventilation, the exchange of gas between the atmosphere and the alveoli
2. Diffusion across the alveolar-capillary membranes
3. Transport of gases in the blood
4. Diffusion from the capillaries of the systemic circulation to the cells of the body
5. Use of oxygen and production of carbon dioxide within the cells (i.e., internal respiration)

Ventilation

Ventilation is the process whereby fresh, oxygen-rich gas is delivered to the alveoli and carbon dioxide is removed. As discussed earlier, the volume of gas reaching the alveoli per unit time, not the volume of gas entering and leaving the respiratory system, is the important parameter for gas exchange.

Gas Diffusion

Gas diffusion is a passive process: Gases diffuse from a site of high partial pressure to a site of low partial pressure. The flux is proportional to the area available for diffusion and to the difference in partial pressure per unit length of the diffusion pathway. Conditions that thicken the alveolar wall, the main blood-gas barrier, can interfere with diffusion. These disorders are discussed more fully in Chapter 26 and in Part Eight.

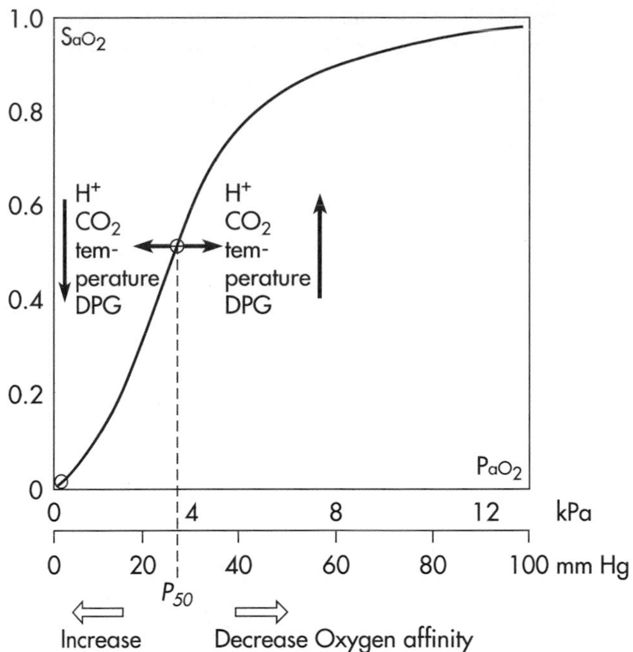

Fig. 8-12. The oxygen-hemoglobin dissociation curve, with representation of the influence of various factors on oxygen affinity. See text for details. (From Tammeling GJ et al: *Contours of breathing,* ed 2, Burlington, Ontario, Canada, 1985, Boehringer Ingelheim Pharmaceuticals.)

Gas Transport

Gas is transported in the blood via two primary methods: dissolved in plasma or combined with hemoglobin. Approximately 98% of oxygen transported in the blood is bound to hemoglobin. When oxygen combines loosely with the heme portion of hemoglobin in the lung, where the oxygen partial pressure is high, it forms oxyhemoglobin. When the oxyhemoglobin reaches the tissues, where oxygen partial pressure is low, the oxygen is released and diffuses to the cells. The binding of oxygen to hemoglobin is a nonlinear process, as demonstrated by the sigmoid oxygen-hemoglobin dissociation curve (Fig. 8-12). When hemoglobin is 100% saturated with oxygen, large changes in the partial pressure of oxygen ($Pa{O_2}$) are required before the arterial oxygen saturation ($Sa{O_2}$) falls much. However, below an $Sa{O_2}$ of about 90%, the relationship between the fall in $Pa{O_2}$ and that in $Sa{O_2}$ becomes steeper. Increases in both body temperature and arterial pH shift the oxygen-hemoglobin dissociation curve to the right, facilitating the peripheral unloading of oxygen. Normal lungs have sufficient reserve capacity to overcome the increased difficulty in loading oxygen under these circumstances. However, in the presence of a marked $\dot{V}/Q$ imbalance (see later section), rightward shifts in the oxygen-hemoglobin dissociation curve may become more significant.

Carbon dioxide is transported more readily in the blood than oxygen because carbon dioxide, being a nonpolar molecule, is highly lipid soluble. Carbon dioxide is transported in the blood in the following ways, all of which begin with the gas being dissolved in the plasma after it has diffused into the systemic capillaries from the tissues:

1. As bicarbonate ions (60% to 70%)
2. Combined with hemoglobin to form carbaminohemoglobin (15% to 30%)
3. Dissolved in plasma and red blood cells (7% to 10%)

Carbon dioxide does not bind to hemoglobin at the same site as oxygen; instead it binds directly with some of the amino groups that form the hemoglobin molecule. The carbon dioxide-hemoglobin dissociation curve is less curvilinear.

Ventilation/Perfusion Imbalance

Inhomogeneity of the ventilation/perfusion ($\dot{V}/Q$) balance in the lungs most commonly occurs in conditions that produce ventilatory inhomogeneity, such as obstructive airway diseases (e.g., asthma). $\dot{V}/Q$ mismatch results in a decrease in the transfer of oxygen to arterial blood and a decrease in carbon dioxide elimination. However, the result is a lowering of Pa_{O_2}, with a lesser increase in Pa_{CO_2}. Several factors contribute to this phenomenon. The gas tension in an individual alveolar-capillary unit depends on the ratio of ventilation to perfusion in that unit. Well-ventilated units tend to raise the oxygen tension toward that of the inspired gas (about 150 mm Hg when breathing air), whereas well-perfused units tend to lower oxygen tension toward that of the mixed venous blood (normally about 40 mm Hg). For the same reasons, the P_{CO_2} is higher in overperfused units and lower in overventilated units. The extreme case of overventilation and underperfusion results in an increase in dead space, whereas the converse results in an intrapulmonary shunt (Fig. 8-13). Mixing of the blood from units with different $\dot{V}/Q$ balances does not compensate for the different oxygen and carbon dioxide tensions because by definition, relatively more blood comes from the underventilated, overperfused units. This results in a difference between the gas tensions in the mixed pulmonary venous blood (which becomes the arterial gas tension) and the mixed alveolar gas (in reality the average tension) and is expressed as an alveolar-arterial difference. The alveolar-arterial difference is greater for oxygen than for carbon dioxide.

A lowering of the Pa_{O_2} or an increase of Pa_{CO_2} results in an increase in respiratory rate via chemoreceptor stimulation. This increase can lower the Pa_{CO_2} but cannot raise the Pa_{O_2} to the same extent. This is because of the different shapes of the blood gas content–tension curves. Because the oxygen-hemoglobin dissociation curve is almost flat at high blood oxygen contents, increasing ventilation to well-ventilated units cannot increase the blood oxygen content but does remove extra carbon dioxide from the blood passing through the well-ventilated units. This means that increasing ventilation, in the face of $\dot{V}/Q$ inhomogeneity, reduces the Pa_{CO_2} toward or below normal but does not increase the Pa_{O_2} to normal values.

Control of Breathing

The primary function of the respiratory system is gas exchange. This requires a precise regulation of blood gas concentrations, which allows for the varying requirements imposed by the different levels of demand encountered with differing levels of activity. This control system can be thought of as having two parts: a "feed-forward" component, which is related to the ventilatory requirements, and a "feedback" component, which tells the system how well it is performing. The

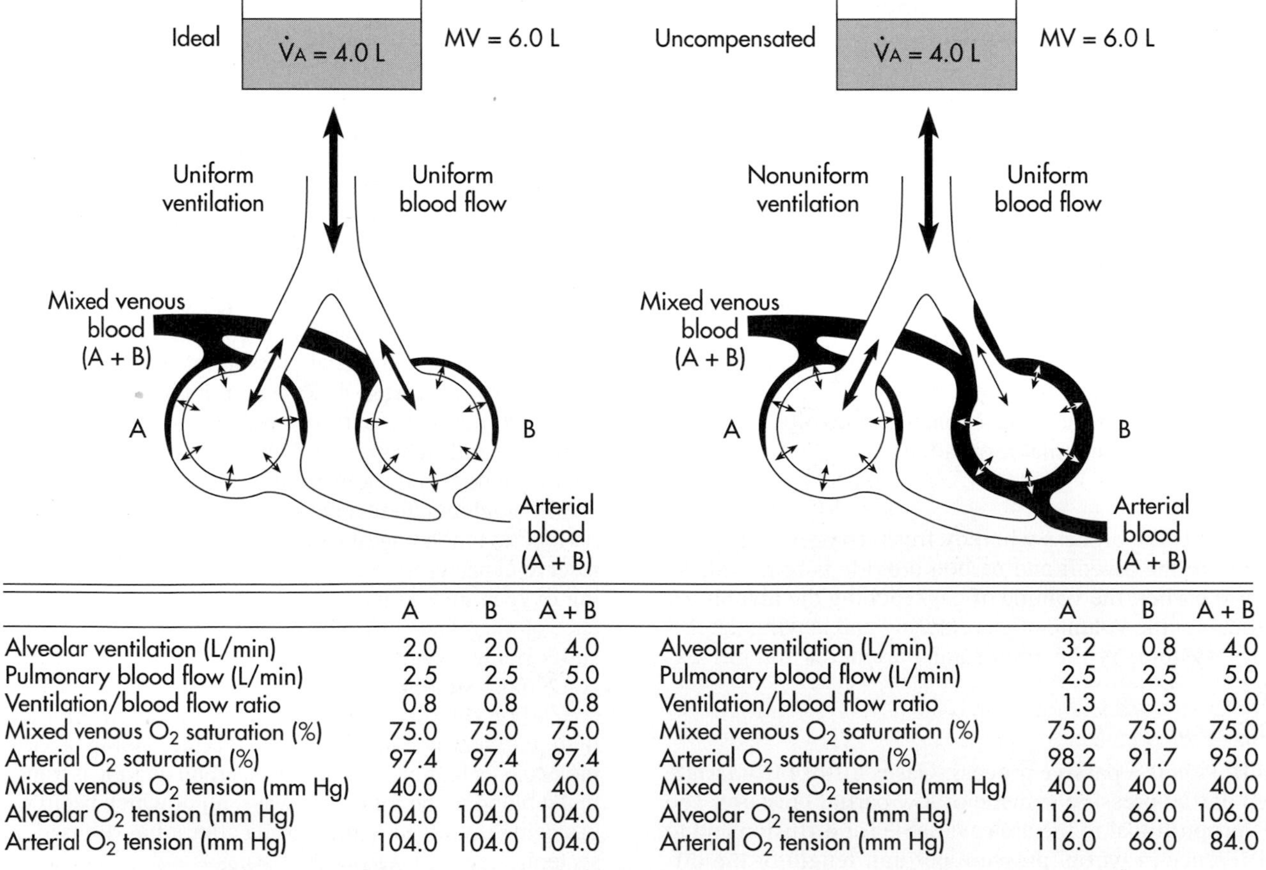

	A	B	A + B
Alveolar ventilation (L/min)	2.0	2.0	4.0
Pulmonary blood flow (L/min)	2.5	2.5	5.0
Ventilation/blood flow ratio	0.8	0.8	0.8
Mixed venous O_2 saturation (%)	75.0	75.0	75.0
Arterial O_2 saturation (%)	97.4	97.4	97.4
Mixed venous O_2 tension (mm Hg)	40.0	40.0	40.0
Alveolar O_2 tension (mm Hg)	104.0	104.0	104.0
Arterial O_2 tension (mm Hg)	104.0	104.0	104.0

	A	B	A + B
Alveolar ventilation (L/min)	3.2	0.8	4.0
Pulmonary blood flow (L/min)	2.5	2.5	5.0
Ventilation/blood flow ratio	1.3	0.3	0.0
Mixed venous O_2 saturation (%)	75.0	75.0	75.0
Arterial O_2 saturation (%)	98.2	91.7	95.0
Mixed venous O_2 tension (mm Hg)	40.0	40.0	40.0
Alveolar O_2 tension (mm Hg)	116.0	66.0	106.0
Arterial O_2 tension (mm Hg)	116.0	66.0	84.0

Fig. 8-13. *Left,* Ideal $\dot{V}Q$ matching. *Right,* Nonuniform ventilation with uniform blood flow leading to mismatch. $\dot{V}_A$, Alveolar ventilation; *MV,* respiratory minute volume. (From Comroe JH Jr et al: *The lung: clinical physiology and pulmonary function tests,* ed 2, St Louis, 1962, Mosby.)

feed-forward system includes factors such as cardiac output, carbon dioxide production, oxygen consumption, input from muscle afferents, and input from higher brain centers. The feedback system consists of the partial pressures of carbon dioxide and oxygen and the hydrogen ion concentration reaching the respiratory centers. The feed-forward system is important because it allows the respiratory centers to "anticipate" the increased ventilatory requirements (e.g., during exercise). Without this anticipation, the ability to cope with the increased ventilatory demands is substantially reduced. This concept is expanded more fully in an article by Cunningham et al.[13]

Although much of the knowledge about the interaction of changes in blood gases through control of breathing have come from studies in which the influences of carbon dioxide and oxygen have been studied separately, in the real world, these variables almost always change together. Changes in blood gas tensions are sensed by chemoreceptors located in the carotid bodies and central respiratory centers. The carotid body receptors respond to a change in either blood carbon dioxide or oxygen levels by a change in output. The impulses that reach the central respiratory control centers are identical, whether they are produced by changes in oxygen or carbon dioxide tensions. The carotid body chemoreceptors respond to a fall in Pao_2 or an increase in $Paco_2$ with an increase in output, stimulating an increased respiratory rate. Changes in $Paco_2$ also result in changes in hydrogen ion concentration, which also influences chemoreceptor output. The central chemoreceptors are influenced by the pH and carbon dioxide tensions in the cerebrospinal fluid. The output from the central chemoreceptors is thought to act independently on the respiratory control centers.

The relationship between ventilation *(V)* and alveolar carbon dioxide partial pressure (P_{ACO_2}) can be described as:

$$V = S(P_{ACO_2} - B) \quad (16)$$

where *S* is the slope of the line or sensitivity of the relationship and *B* is the intercept with the P_{ACO_2} axis (Fig. 8-14). Hypoxia increases the sensitivity without altering the intercept. At very high levels of $Paco_2$ and very low levels of Pao_2, respiratory depression occurs.

Studies investigating the control of breathing in infants have reported conflicting results, largely because of the methodological difficulties inherent in studying infants. The major difference in the control of breathing between adults and infants is in the infants' ventilatory response to hypoxia. Despite the difficulties in using appropriate methodology, it is now generally agreed that the slope of the ventilatory response to carbon dioxide, when appropriately corrected for size in infants, is the same as that in the adult.

When exposed to low oxygen mixtures, newborns respond with a brief period of hyperpnea, followed by ventilatory depression. If the neonate has been allowed to cool (or is not in a neutral thermal environment), the period of hyperpnea is not seen. The ventilatory depression in response to hypoxia persists for about a week in full-term infants and for several weeks in infants born prematurely. The mechanism for this paradoxic response remains obscure. Recent evidence favors an immaturity of the central controlling centers rather than an immaturity of the peripheral chemoreceptors. Sleep state also seems to modify the ventilatory response to hypoxia, with the paradoxic response absent during rapid-eye-movement sleep. For an in-depth discussion of control of breathing in the fetus and newborn, see Bryan et al.[14]

The state of the respiratory system is important in the translation of the signals from the respiratory center to alveolar ventilation and gas exchange. Diseases of the various components of the respiratory system are characteristically associated with increased mechanical loads. These loads may be elastic, resistive, inertial, or a combination thereof.

Diseases that increase the resistance against which the patient must breath impose resistive loads. Increased intrinsic resistive loading occurs when the peribronchial forces that act to keep the airways patent are overwhelmed, resulting in airway narrowing; when gas flow becomes turbulent, increasing energy dissipation; or when high-viscosity or high-density gases are breathed. The most common example of increased intrinsic resistive loading seen in children is asthma, although other lungs diseases, such as chronic suppurative bronchitis and emphysema, also occur. The primary ventilatory response to these disorders is usually an alteration in V_T and respiratory timing indices, although many patients with severe disease appear to tolerate a chronic increase in $Paco_2$ rather than respond appropriately, thereby conserving work of breathing. A breathing pattern with a prolonged expiratory phase is optimal for lung emptying and avoiding increases in lung volume (which would impose an increased elastic load), although a shortened inspiratory time would require higher inspiratory flows, adding to the increased resistive load.

Increased elastic loading occurs when the respiratory system is stiffer than usual; this occurs with hyaline membrane disease and interstitial lung diseases (increased lung stiffness); severe cases of obesity, ankylosing spondylitis, or kyphoscoliosis (increased chest wall stiffness); or conditions of decreased muscle performance (e.g., high quadriplegia, Guillain-

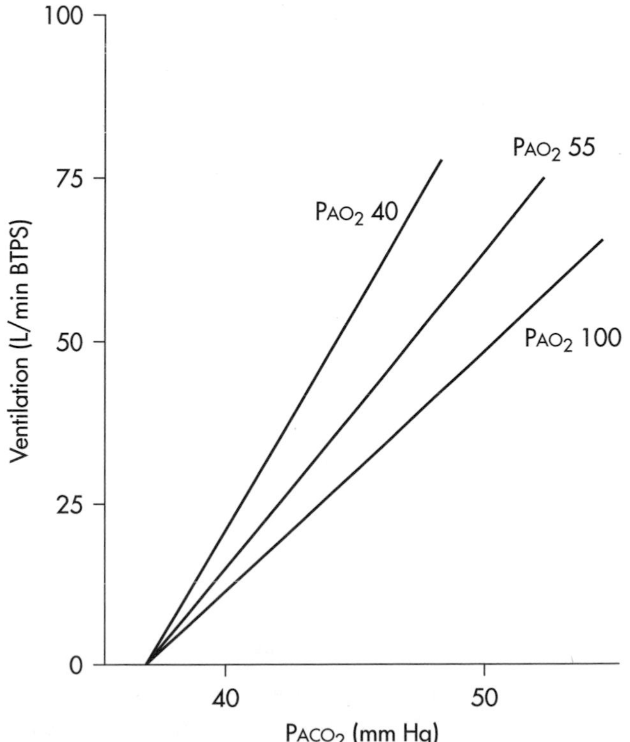

Fig. 8-14. Carbon dioxide response curves at various fixed values for P_{AO_2}. *BTPS,* Body temperature, pressure, saturated. (From Ganong WF: *Review of medical physiology,* ed 16, Norwalk, Conn, 1993, Appleton & Lange.)

Barré syndrome, botulism, muscular dystrophies). In these conditions, the ability to expand the thorax is decreased. The primary ventilatory response to these disorders is usually tachypnea; hypoxia and a relatively normal or even low Pa_{CO_2} result. Rapid, shallow breathing, which minimizes the elastic load, may be seen.

APPLIED PHYSIOLOGY

Maintenance of Lung Volume

In healthy subjects at rest, FRC occurs at the volume at which the elastic recoil of the respiratory system is zero. This volume is known as the *EEV*, or the relaxation volume.

The lungs and chest wall both contribute to the elastic properties of the respiratory system. The chest wall and the lungs are mechanically in series; thus the algebraic sum of the pressure exerted by the chest wall and lungs equals the pressure of the respiratory system. The EEV of the respiratory system occurs where the elastic recoil of the chest wall is equal and opposite to that of the lungs (Fig. 8-15). In isolation the relaxation volume of the lungs is zero; that is, there is always a tendency for the lungs to empty when there is gas in them. However, in practice, the lungs can never empty fully because small airways collapse before the lung volume becomes zero, thus trapping gas in the lungs. In healthy people the relaxation volume of the respiratory system is well above the volume at which the small airways close. Newborns have a more compliant (less stiff) chest wall. The chest wall thus has less elastic recoil to balance that of the lungs. This moves the static pressure-volume curve to the right, thus decreasing the relaxation volume of the respiratory system. Infants born prematurely also have stiff lungs. Thus at any given volume the PEL of the lungs is increased. This moves the static pressure-volume curve of the lungs, and hence that of the respiratory system, to the right, further reducing the EEV. This reduction may be marked enough so that the relaxation volume is less than the "closing volume" for small airways. This situation cannot be tolerated, and the infant remedies the situation by breathing at a higher volume than the relaxation volume. Thus FRC and relaxation volume are not necessarily interchangeable because they may not always be equivalent.

Hyperinflation

Hyperinflation refers to an increase in lung volume above that usually seen at rest. As previously discussed, the end-expiratory lung volume coincides with the EEV of the respiratory system in adults and older children with normal lungs. Hyperinflation occurs naturally in two primary settings: (1) in the presence of a significant increase in resistance and (2) in the presence of a significant decrease in elastic recoil. Both of these conditions result in an increase in the time constant of emptying of the respiratory system. If the respiratory rate required to satisfy ventilatory demands does not allow sufficient expiratory time, hyperinflation occurs. Another setting in which hyperinflation may develop is during mechanical ventilation. On theoretical grounds, an expiratory time equal to 3 times the expiratory time constant allows emptying of 95% of the end-inspiratory volume, whereas an expiratory time equal to 5 times the expiratory time constant allows emptying of 99% of the volume. In practice, if the expiratory time constant was less than 3 times the expiratory time constant, hyperinflation (manifested as the development of $PEEP_i$) develops in ventilated infants.[12]

Hyperinflation does serve a useful purpose. The increase in lung volume is associated with an increase in airway caliber secondary to mechanical interdependence. The increase in lung volume also increases the tissue viscance.[15,16] The degree to which resistance and therefore the time constant of emptying falls depends on the balance between these opposing influences. A patient with severe airflow obstruction may have so much expiratory flow limitation that these values are in fact flow limited during tidal breathing at rest. The only way that the expiratory flows can be increased at times of increased ventilatory demand, such as during exercise or febrile illnesses, is to increase lung volume, thus moving tidal breathing to a more advantageous part ot their expiratory flow-volume curve. It is not surprising therefore that hyperinflation has been found to be, at least partly, an active phenomenon.[17-19] Hyperinflation is achieved by tonic contraction of inspiratory muscles[18] and by expiratory "braking" by adduction of the vocal cords.[20]

The increase in expiratory flows made possible by hyperinflation does come at a cost. Hyperinflation puts the inspiratory muscles at a mechanical disadvantage, placing them at an in-

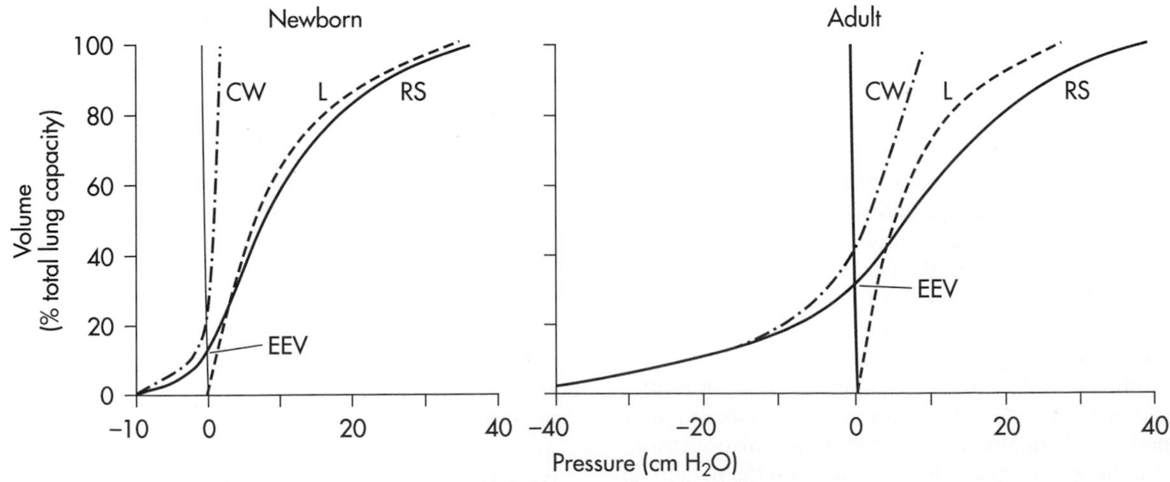

Fig. 8-15. Pressure-volume curves of the newborn and adult respiratory system *(RS)* demonstrating the effect of lung *(L)* and chest wall *(CW)* compliance on EEV. (From Agostini E: *J Appl Physiol* 14:909-913, 1959.)

efficient part of their length-tension relationships. Under these conditions, the muscle excitation must increase to produce the same external work. This results in an increase in energy consumption and a decrease in efficiency. The work of breathing also increases because although the resistive work decreases and the total resistance is less, the elastic work increases and more than offsets any gain in resistive work. In addition, actively contracting muscles run the risk of limiting their own energy supply by narrowing the feeding arteries. These factors place the inspiratory muscles at risk of developing inspiratory muscle fatigue.

Two compensatory processes have been reported that have the potential to decrease the load on the inspiratory muscles. In patients with severe chronic airflow limitation, end-expiratory lung volume has been reported to increase during exercise while the anteroposterior dimensions of the abdomen decrease because of expiratory recruitment of the abdominal muscles.[21] End-expiratory cephalad displacement of the diaphragm, secondary to contraction of abdominal muscle toward the end of expiration,[22] aids inspiration in at least two ways: It puts the muscle fibers of the diaphragm on a more favorable part of their length-tension relationship, and it stores elastic and gravitational energy in the abdominal compartment and releases it during the subsequent inspiration, performing inspiratory work and contributing to minute ventilation without increasing the activation of the diaphragm.

The expiratory braking, achieved by partial glottic adduction, "unloads" the inspiratory muscles by allowing hyperinflation to be maintained with less tonic activation of inspiratory muscles.

Forced Expiration

Expiratory Flow Limitation

Measurements during forced expiration are useful in detecting obstructive lung disease because during a forced expiration, expiratory flow is independent of the force driving the flow over most of the expired vital capacity as long as reasonable effort is made. This observation was made by plotting the pressure-flow relationships at isovolume points measured during expirations made with increasing effort (Fig. 8-16). This observation led directly to the description of the maximal expiratory flow volume curve, which emphasized that at most lung volumes, there was a limit to maximal expiratory flow. The peak flow depends largely on effort, and the flows near the residual volume may be effort dependent because some people may not be able to maintain sufficient force to maintain flow limitation at this low lung volume.

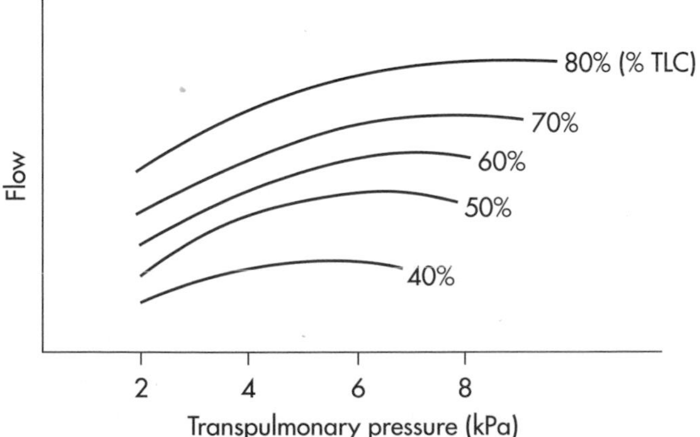

Fig. 8-16. Isovolume pressure-flow curves in a normal adult at different proportions of total lung capacity *(TLC)*. (From Tammeling GJ et al: *Contours of breathing,* ed 2, Burlington, Ontario, Canada, 1985, Boehringer Ingelheim Pharmaceuticals.)

The mechanism for expiratory flow limitation is complex. In fluid dynamic terms, a system cannot carry a greater flow than the flow for which the fluid velocity equals wave speed at some point in the system. The wave speed is the speed at which a small disturbance travels in a compliant tube filled with fluid. In the arteries, this is the speed at which the pulse propagates. In the airway the speed is higher than this, mainly because the fluid density is lower. The wave speed *(c)* in a compliant tube with an area *(A)* that depends on lateral pressure *(P)* filled with a fluid of density *(p),* is given by the following:

$$c = (A\delta P/p\delta A)^{1/2} \quad (17)$$

where $\delta P/\delta A$ is the slope of the pressure-area curve for the airway. Maximal flow is the product of the fluid velocity at wave speed and airway area, as follows:

$$\dot{V}_{max} = cA \quad (18)$$

At high lung volumes the flow-limiting site in the human airways is typically in the second and third airway generations. As lung volume decreases, flow decreases, and the flow-limiting site moves peripherally. At low lung volumes the density dependence of maximal flow is small, and the viscosity dependence is large and becomes the predominant mechanism limiting expiratory flow.

Physiology of Wheezing

Flow limitation in a compliant tube is accompanied by the "flutter" of the walls at the site of flow limitation. This flutter occurs to conserve the energy in the system because the driving pressure in excess of that required to produce $\dot{V}_{max}$ is dissipated in causing the flutter.[23,24] In the presence of airway obstruction, this flutter may become large enough to generate sound. This sound is heard as wheezing. Thus expiratory wheezing is a sign of expiratory flow limitation. However, although wheezing implies the presence of expiratory flow limitation, flow limitation can occur in the absence of detectable wheezing.[23] Gavriely et al[25] demonstrated that the transpulmonary pressures (as an indication of the effort required for breathing) required to produce wheezing were substantially greater than those required to achieve flow limitation. They concluded that this extra pressure was required to "induce flattening of the intrathoracic airways downstream from the choke point" and to induce oscillations in the airway walls.[25]

Cough

Cough is the most common natural forced expiration. Most of the forced expirations measured by clinicians are artificially produced to satisfy the clinician's desires. Cough has several practical functions. It can be stimulated by various receptors in the respiratory tract; that is, irritant receptors in the large airways stimulate cough in response to mechanical irritation (e.g., inhalation of dust, cigarette smoke, aspirated material) or respiratory infections to help clear material from the respiratory tract; irritant receptors in the larynx prevent or minimize aspiration of foreign materials into the airways; or stretch receptors in the lung parenchyma, stimulated by application of high distention pressures to the lung, limit maximal inspiration, presumably protecting the lung from overdistention and mechanical disruption. Cough can also be initiated voluntarily.

Whether cough is initiated by voluntary means or by stimulation of receptors, the first action is usually inspiration of a variable volume of air. Next, the glottis is closed simultaneously with or just after the onset of forceful expiratory muscle activity that quickly raises thoracoabdominal pressures to 100 cm H_2O or more above ambient pressure. About 0.2 second after the glottis closes, it is actively opened; subglottic pressure falls, and expiratory flow begins. Intrathoracic pressures, however, usually continue to rise; thus peak pressure usually occurs after peak flow. Expiratory flow quickly rises to "maximal" flow as central intrathoracic airways collapse. Their narrowed cross section is associated with high gas linear velocities and therefore with high shearing forces at airway walls and high kinetic energies. These conditions are probably important in suspending and clearing materials adherent to the walls. After a widely variable volume of air is expired, expiratory muscle activity diminishes abruptly, perhaps with the onset of antagonist activity of the diaphragm and other muscles; alveolar pressure falls toward ambient pressure, and flow drops toward zero, sometimes interrupted finally by glottic closure. Several coughs may follow in immediate series from high to low lung volume without intervening inspirations. This has the effect of "squeezing" secretions in the smaller airways more centrally to airways with high enough linear velocities to clear the secretions.

REFERENCES

Basic Physiologic Principles

1. Ebina M, Yaegashi H, Takahashi T, Motomiya M, Tanemura M: Distribution of smooth muscles along the bronchial tree, *Am Rev Respir Dis* 141:1322-1326, 1990.
2. Bates JHT, Martin JG: A theoretical study of the effect of airway smooth muscle orientation on bronchoconstriction, *J Appl Physiol* 69(3)995-1001, 1990.
3. Bates JH, Ludwig MS, Sly PD, Brown K, Martin JG, Fredberg JJ: Interrupter resistance elucidated by alveolar pressure measurement in open-chest normal dogs, *J Appl Physiol* 65(1):408-414, 1988.
4. Murphy RA: What is special about smooth muscle? The significance of covalent crossbridge regulation, *FASEB J* 8:311-318, 1994.
5. Schiaffino S, Reggiani C: Myosin isoforms in mammalian skeletal muscle, *J Appl Physiol* 77:493-501, 1994.
6. Sly PD, Hutchison AA: Validity of sputum eosinophilia in diagnosing co-existent asthma in children with cystic fibrosis, *Aust Paediatr J* 16(3):205-206, 1980.
7. Sly PD, Lanteri CJ: Differential responses of the airways and pulmonary tissues to inhaled histamine in young dogs, *J Appl Physiol* 68(4):1562-1567, 1990.
8. Sly PD, Lanteri CJ: Lack of vagal influence on pulmonary visco-elasticity in puppies, *Respir Physiol* 84(2):133-143, 1991.
9. Sly PD, Lanteri CJ: Site of action of hypertonic saline in the canine lung, *J Appl Physiol* 71(4):1315-1321, 1991.
10. Bates JHT, Maksym GN, Navajas D, Suki B: Lung tissue rheology and 1/f noise, *Ann Biomed Eng* 22:674-681, 1994.
11. Ludwig MS, Dreshaj I, Solway J, Munoz A, Ingram RJ: Partitioning of pulmonary resistance during constriction in the dog: effects of volume history, *J Appl Physiol* 62(2):807-815, 1987.
12. Kano S, Lanteri CJ, Pemberton PJ, Le Souëf PN, Sly PD: Fast versus slow ventilation for neonates, *Am Rev Respir Dis* 148(3):578-584, 1993.
13. Cunningham DJC, Robbins PA, Wolff CB: Integration of respiratory responses to changes in alveolar partial pressures of CO_2 and O_2 and in arterial pH. In Fishman AP, Cherniak NS, Widdicombe JB, Geiger SR, eds: *Handbook of physiology,* section 3: The respiratory system, vol 2, part 1, Control of breathing, Bethesda, Md, 1986, American Physiological Society, pp 467-528.
14. Bryan AC, Bowes G, Maloney JE: Control of breathing in the fetus and the newborn. In Fishman AP, Cherniak NS, Widdicombe JB, Geiger SR, eds: *Handbook of physiology,* section 3: The respiratory system, vol 2, part 1: Control of breathing, Bethesda, Md, 1986, American Physiological Society, pp 621-647.

Applied Physiology

15. Loring SH, Drazen JM, Smith JC, Hoppin JFG: Vagal stimulation and aerosol histamine increase hysteresis of lung recoil, *J Appl Physiol* 51(2):477-484, 1981.
16. Ludwig MS, Robatto FM, Simard S, Stamenovic D, Fredberg JJ: Lung tissue resistance during contractile stimulation: structural damping decomposition, *J Appl Physiol* 72(4):1332-1337, 1992.
17. Muller N, Bryan AC, Zamel N: Toxic inspiratory muscle activity as a cause of hyperinflation in histamine induced asthma, *J Appl Physiol* 49:863-874, 1981.
18. Martin JG, Habib M, Engel LA: Inspiratory muscle activity during induced hyperinflation, *Respir Physiol* 39(3):303-313, 1980.
19. Martin J, Powell E, Shore S, Emrich J, Engel LA: The role of respiratory muscles in the hyperinflation of bronchial asthma, *Am Rev Respir Dis* 121:441-447, 1980.
20. Collett PW, Brancatisano AP, Engel LA: Upper airway dimensions and movements in bronchial asthma, *Am Rev Respir Dis* 133:1143-1150, 1986.
21. Dodd DS, Brancatisano T, Engel LA: Chest wall mechanics during exercise in patients with severe chronic air flow obstruction, *Am Rev Respir Dis* 129:33-38, 1984.
22. Mead J, Sly P, Le Souëf P, Hibbert M, Phelan P: Rib cage mobility in pectus excavatum, *Am Rev Respir Dis* 132(6):1223-1228, 1985.
23. Gavriely N, Kelly KB, Grotberg JB, Loring SH: Forced expiratory wheezes are a manifestation of airway flow limitation, *J Appl Physiol* 62(6):2398-2403, 1987.
24. Shabtai-Musih Y, Grotberg JB, Gavriely N: Spectral content of forced expiratory wheezes during air, He, and SF_6 breathing in normal humans, *J Appl Physiol* 72(2):629-635, 1992.
25. Gavriely N, Kelly KB, Grotberg JB, Loring SH: Critical pressures required for generation of forced expiratory wheezes, *J Appl Physiol* 66(3):1136-1142, 1989.

CHAPTER 9

Exercise Physiology

Alan Ridley Morton

The trend is for children to become involved with serious sports training at progressively younger ages, with some beginning as early as 6 years of age, and teenagers are performing at world championship level in many sports, particularly swimming, tennis, and gymnastics. It is important therefore that the clinician have a good understanding of the physiologic, psychologic, and sociologic responses of children to vigorous exercise, with emphasis on the benefits and possible detrimental outcomes.

Exercise physiology is a branch of applied physiology concerned with the patient's responses to both acute and chronic exercise (training). It is concerned with these responses under various climatic, hyperbaric, and hypobaric conditions as they differ between genders and among people of different ages. In a chapter of this size, it is impossible to describe all of the physiologic changes accompanying acute and chronic exercise; therefore the major metabolic and cardiorespiratory factors are discussed only briefly.

Unfortunately, most of the research in this relatively new discipline has been performed on adults, and as a result, many of the pediatric exercise physiology questions are either unanswered or only partly answered. The reason for the lack of evidence concerning children can be explained by the reluctance of parents and ethics committees to provide consent for many of the required invasive and noninvasive procedures, such as muscle biopsies and arterial and venous blood sampling (especially when performed on a serial basis), and exposure to harsh environmental conditions and prolonged or severe exercise for what is often misconstrued as "athletic curiosity." When cross-sectional studies are performed in an effort to compare athletic children with sedentary children, it is difficult to separate training effects from genetic endowment. Nevertheless, this chapter examines the general responses to exercise and, when information is available, compares the responses of adults to those of children. This comparison will indicate any advantages that the mature child, who more closely resembles the adult, has over the immature child. This maturity difference is often evident in children of the same chronologic age who are expected to compete against one another in sports.

Humans require regular physical activity to achieve optimal growth,[1] optimal development of the heart and lungs, and optimal strength of bones, ligaments, tendons, and muscles. The child needs to play and be on the move constantly and, until a generation ago, considered *rest* a four letter word; however, this no longer appears to be true. For instance, studies in England[2,3] and Singapore[4] have indicated that the daily activity level of children today, as determined by continuous heart rate monitoring, is very low and that many children seldom undertake enough physical activity to appropriately stress the cardiopulmonary system. A sedentary lifestyle during adulthood, which is often the result of a childhood with restricted physical activity, may contribute to the development of various illnesses collectively classified as *hypokinetic diseases.* These diseases include coronary heart disease, obesity, and low back problems.[5]

It is generally accepted that the foundation for the life-long regular exercise habit should be laid down during childhood and depends on a competent school physical education program emphasizing motor skills, improvement and maintenance of fitness components, and the pleasure of participation in physical activities.[6]

It is impossible to cover the role of exercise in the prevention, management, and treatment of the various diseases in this chapter. Therefore the reader is referred to the excellent text by Bar-Or.[7]

METABOLIC RESPONSES TO ACUTE EXERCISE

Energy Systems

The muscular system, as with other systems of the body, has one source of energy for metabolism (Fig. 9-1): adenosine triphosphate (ATP), often referred to as the *universal energy currency.* ATP is a molecule that contains adenosine plus three phosphate groups in the following format:

$$\text{ADENOSINE - Pi}^{-} \sim \text{Pi}^{-} \sim \text{Pi}^{-2}$$

The last two phosphate radicals are attached by two high-energy bonds (~), each of which releases 30.7 kJ (7.3 kcal) per mole of ATP when the bond is broken to change ATP to adenosine diphosphate (ADP) or ADP to adenosine monophosphate. The provision of ATP for metabolism occurs by at least one of three metabolic systems: the phosphagen system, the lactic acid system, and the oxygen (aerobic) system.

Phosphagen System

The phosphagen system consists of the ATP store and the phosphocreatine (PC) (also called *creatine phosphate*) store (see upper section of Fig. 9-1). The ATP store in the body is small and is sufficient to allow maximal effort for about 1 to 2 seconds, but there are ways of providing more ATP to replace that being used during metabolism. Muscles cannot obtain ATP from the blood or other tissues, so they must manufacture it. To do this, they need ADP, inorganic phosphate (Pi), and energy from other chemical sources to reconstruct the ATP molecules by rephosphorylation of ADP, as follows:

$$\text{ADP + Pi (plus energy)} \rightarrow \text{ATP}$$

One method of providing more ATP is to break down another stored chemical containing a high-energy phosphate bond so that the energy released by its breakdown can be used to reconstitute ATP from ADP and Pi: PC (creatine ~ PO_3^-) de-

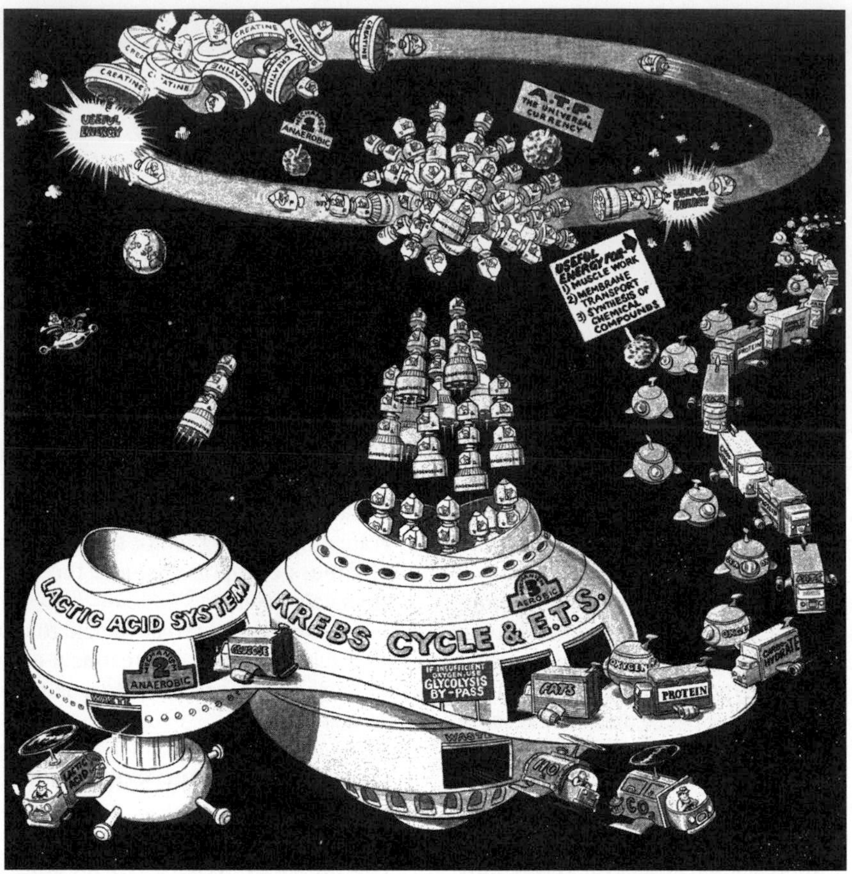

Fig. 9-1. Respresentation of the body's energy sources.

composes to creatine plus a phosphate ion plus energy. The breaking of the PC bond releases 43.3 kJ (10.3 kcal) per mole, which is considerably more than seen in the breakdown of the high-energy bonds in ATP, indicating that there is more than enough energy to reconstitute ATP. Unfortunately, the energy available from the store of PC is also very limited and is enough for only about another 5 to 8 seconds of maximal effort. That is, the ATP and PC activity, combined referred to as the *phosphagen system,* can provide energy for less than 10 seconds of maximal activity. This phosphagen system is the most rapidly available source of energy and is often termed the *immediate energy source.* It is extremely important in explosive type efforts such as throwing, hitting, jumping, and sprinting.

The system is rapidly replenished during recovery; in fact it requires about 30 seconds to replenish about 70% of the phosphagens and 3 to 5 minutes to replenish 100%. This means that during intermittent work (short periods of activity followed by rest periods), much of the phosphagen can be replenished during the recovery period and thus be used over and over again.

Lactic Acid System (Anaerobic Glycolysis)

Because the ATP-PC system can sustain intense activity for less than 10 seconds, other means of reconstituting the ATP molecule must be available. This is accomplished by the use of the other two energy systems, the lactic acid system and the oxygen system, both of which use the breakdown products of the foods ingested.

During the initial stages of exercise and during high-intensity effort, the body cannot provide sufficient oxygen to regenerate the ATP required. To allow for this, the ATP-PC and another system termed the *anaerobic glycolysis system* or *lactic acid system* provides the ATP.

The lactic acid system, also referred to as the *short-term energy source,* uses glucose or glycogen (carbohydrates), which break down to pyruvic acid; then if insufficient oxygen is available, the pyruvic acid breaks down to lactic acid. During the breakdown of glucose to lactic acid, a small amount of ATP is produced (see lower left section of Fig. 9-1). If this system is overworked, the hydrogen ions from the dissociation of lactic acid and the subsequent decrease in pH are associated with fatigue, and when the hydrogen ion concentration becomes high enough, it can decrease the contractile capacity of muscle. This system can sustain another 40 seconds of maximal work over and above that of the ATP-PC system. During glycolysis, which occurs in the cytoplasm of the cell, a complex series of enzymatic reactions occur to provide ATP. This is a slower process than in the phosphagen system. The lactic acid system results in two or three ATP molecules being made available, depending on whether glucose or glycogen is used. This system is very inefficient compared to the oxygen system, which can provide 38 molecules of ATP; however, the lactic acid system can provide these two or three ATP molecules even when the supply of oxygen to the muscle is absent.

Lactic acid can be removed during rest periods, but this is a slow process compared to the replenishment of the phosphagen stores. In fact, a large accumulation of lactate may take at least an hour to be removed.

The lactic acid system provides the majority of energy during bursts of vigorous activity that can be maintained for only 1 to 2 minutes; for example, people doing long sprints (200-, 400-, and 800-m runs) rely largely on the lactic acid system, although during these events, some energy would be provided by all three systems. Neither the ATP-PC system nor the lactic acid system require oxygen to be present, so they are classified as *anaerobic energy systems.*

Oxygen (Aerobic) System

If the level of activity is light enough to be performed for a considerable length of time, sufficient oxygen will be available to prevent pyruvic acid from breaking down to lactic acid after glycolysis. Instead, the pyruvic acid breaks down to acetylcoenzyme A, which enters the Krebs' cycle and the electron transport system and is eventually processed to form water plus carbon dioxide plus a large amount of ATP. Oxygen is required in this process, and the carbon dioxide produced is then transported to the lungs for removal from the body. Fat and protein can also be used aerobically to provide ATP (see lower section of Fig. 9-1). The aerobic system, also termed *the long-term energy source,* is the important energy system for activities lasting longer than 2 minutes (all-out efforts lasting 2 minutes receive half of their energy aerobically and half anaerobically). The higher the maximal oxygen uptake (aerobic power) by the muscles, the higher the work rate that can be sustained.

The contribution of the various energy sources during a given event or sport can be gauged by the duration of the event or effort phases in the sport. For instance, events lasting less than 6 to 10 seconds rely almost exclusively on energy provided by the ATP-PC system. In events lasting 10 to 60 seconds, most of the energy is provided via the anaerobic glycolytic pathway (lactic acid system). As the event increases to about 2 to 4 minutes, the reliance on the anaerobic pathways becomes less important, and aerobic (oxygen system) metabolism increases in importance. Events performed at a low level of intensity for prolonged periods of time, such as a marathon, use the oxygen system almost completely because the ability to provide oxygen is adequate to cover the oxygen requirements.

Summary of Energy Sources

During glycolysis, four molecules of ATP are formed from a molecule of glucose; however, two of these are expended to initiate the process by the phosphorylation of glucose, leaving a net gain of two ATP molecules. During the use of the oxygen system, there is a maximum gain of 38 molecules of ATP: 2 via glycolysis and 36 via the Krebs' cycle and electron transport system.

Although most of this discussion concerns carbohydrate use, fat and protein can also be used to provide ATP aerobically; however, only carbohydrate can be used anaerobically. Triglycerides are digested to fatty acids, which are activated in a process called *β-oxidation,* which prepares fatty acids for entrance into the Krebs' cycle by modifying them to acetylcoenzyme A. Protein is used as a substrate only in small amounts unless the available carbohydrates and fats are seriously depleted.

The use of a gram of fat as the energy substrate produces 2¼ times as much energy (37.7 kJ or 9 kcal) as 1 g of carbohydrate (16.7 kJ or 4 kcal). However, about 8% less oxygen is required to produce a given amount of energy when using carbohydrate compared to fat.

MUSCULAR SYSTEM

It appears that the number of muscle fibers is determined at birth; however, the thickness of the fibers grow about fivefold from birth and adulthood.[8] The increase in muscle girth is due almost entirely to hypertrophy or continued growth of existing muscle fibers and not by hyperplasia. In male patients, this increase is facilitated by the secretion of testosterone after sexual maturation.[9]

At birth, about 20% of the muscle fibers are type IIc (undifferentiated), whereas by the age of 6, the distribution of types I, IIa, and IIb fibers is identical to that of adults.[10] There are almost no type IIc fibers found after the child has reached 1 year of age.

Muscular strength, or the ability to exert force, is highly related to the cross-sectional area of the muscle and to lean body mass. According to Malina,[8] muscle strength increases linearly with chronologic age from early childhood to about 13 to 14 years in boys. This is followed by a period until about 20 years of age, during which there is considerable acceleration of the increase in muscular strength. The muscular strength of girls increases linearly until about 15 years, after which it tends to plateau with very little additional increase.

CARDIORESPIRATORY RESPONSES TO ACUTE EXERCISE

The cardiorespiratory system plays an important role during exercise because its response to the exercise-induced increase in metabolic rate allows the muscles to be supplied with an increased supply of oxygen, glucose, and free fatty acids to support the increase in metabolism and to remove waste products (particularly carbon dioxide and heat). This system also transports hormones, vitamins, and amino acids to their target areas so that they can help regulate the body's activities during performance at an increased metabolic rate. When the body changes from a resting state to one of maximal exercise intensity, its energy expenditure may increase more than 23 to 26 times the resting value, and the metabolic demands of the most active skeletal muscles may increase by as much as 130 to 200 times the resting value. That is, the body's rate of oxygen consumption ($\dot{V}O_2$) may increase by more than twentyfold, exhibiting a linear relationship between $\dot{V}O_2$ and the intensity of exercise or rate of work.

The increase in $\dot{V}O_2$ is accomplished by the following:

1. An increase in cardiac output ($\dot{Q}$)
2. An increase in the oxygen extraction rate by the muscles (a-$\bar{v}O_2\Delta$)
3. A redistribution of the $\dot{Q}$ so that more blood is channeled to the active tissues (skeletal and cardiac muscle) and to the skin for heat dissipation and so that reduced amounts are channeled to organs such as the gut and kidneys while maintaining the absolute flow rate to the brain (though decreased relative to the increased $\dot{Q}$)
4. An increase in ventilation
5. An increase in the lung diffusion capacity resulting from an increase in blood flow to the lungs (particularly to the upper portion) and the opening of closed alveoli
6. An increase in hematocrit because of the redistribution of fluid from the plasma to the interstitial space (hemoconcentration), thus increasing the oxygen-carrying capacity of the circulating blood

The magnitude of many of these responses changes as a result of regular, frequent, endurance-overload training sessions (chronic exercise). These changes in responses result in an increase in the maximal work capacity and a decrease in the myocardial oxygen demand for a given level of submaximal work.

Cardiovascular Response to Acute Exercise

The increase in $\dot{Q}$ during maximal work may be as much as 4 to 5 times the resting $\dot{Q}$, is linearly related to the increase in the $\dot{V}O_2$ and therefore to the work rate, and is a result of an increase in both the heart rate and the stroke volume. When the body changes from rest to a given level of submaximal exercise, the heart rate and oxygen consumption increase rapidly and reach a steady state in about 3 or 4 minutes; with cessation of exercise the heart rate decreases rapidly at first and then more gradually until the resting level is reached (Fig. 9-2, *A* and *C*). The steady-state heart rate increases linearly with an increase in $\dot{V}O_2$ from the resting level to the maximum heart rate, which can be estimated as 220 minus the age of the individual and represents a 2 ½-fold to 3-fold increase. Stroke volume increases rapidly with an increase in work rate but usually plateaus at about 40% to 60% of the maximal oxygen consumption ($\dot{V}O_{2\,max}$) and represents an approximately twofold increase. This is assuming that the exercise is performed in an upright position because the maximal stroke volume during upright exercise is very similar to the resting stroke volume in the supine position. When the body changes from resting to maximal exercise while in the supine position, there is little increase in the stroke volume. At rest a change from supine to standing results in a drop in stroke volume resulting from the effects of gravity, which tends to cause the blood to pool in the legs. This pooling decreases the central blood volume and venous return, thus reducing stroke volume.

The approximately threefold increase in a-$\bar{v}O_2\Delta$ from resting to maximal exercise is attained by increasing the number of patent capillaries, by increasing the oxygen partial pressure gradient between blood and active tissues (which results from the use of oxygen by active cells in accordance with the characteristics of the oxygen-hemoglobin dissociation curve), and by metabolically inducing an increase in blood temperature and acidity (the Bohr effect).

The blood pressure increases during exercise to ensure an adequate blood flow to critical areas such as the brain and the heart and to meet the increased requirements of the skeletal muscles. This increase occurs as a result of an increased $\dot{Q}$ value and the vasoconstriction in inactive tissues. It also occurs despite a large decrease in peripheral resistance.

The blood pressure during a given submaximal workload reaches a steady state within 3 to 4 minutes. When the steady-state blood pressure is plotted against $\dot{V}O_{2\,max}$ or the increasing workload, it follows a pattern indicating that the systolic blood pressure increases linearly, reaching a value about 1.5 to 1.6 times the resting level. Meanwhile, the diastolic pressure re-

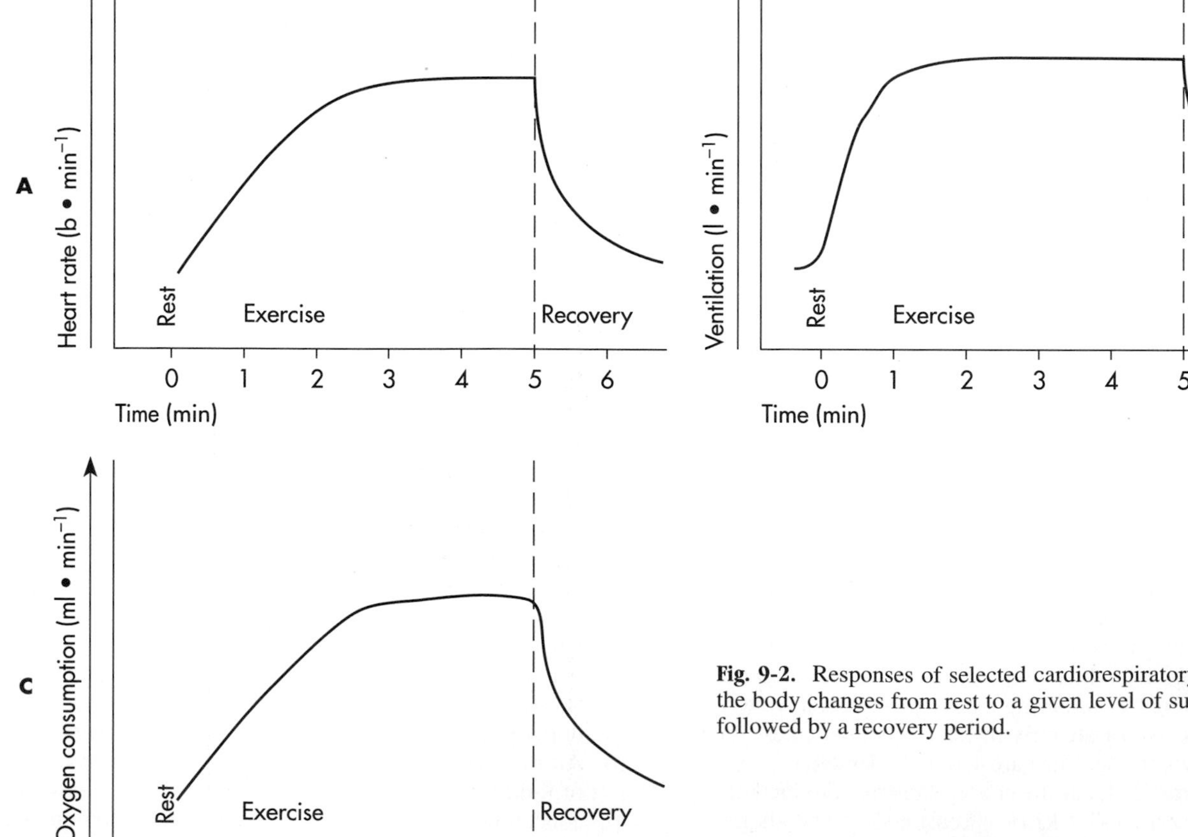

Fig. 9-2. Responses of selected cardiorespiratory parameters when the body changes from rest to a given level of submaximal exercise followed by a recovery period.

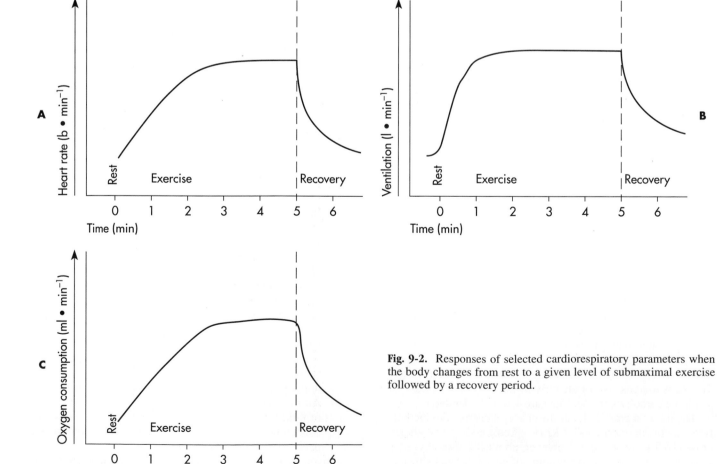

mains fairly constant or increases to about 1.1 times the resting value; under some conditions, it even decreases slightly. The mean arterial blood pressure, which is equal to the diastolic blood pressure plus one third of the pulse pressure, increases linearly to about 1.3 times the resting level.

The relatively small increases in arterial blood pressure caused by the large increase in $\dot{Q}$ is explained by the curvilinear decrease in the total peripheral resistance caused by the increasing workload. The total peripheral resistance can be reduced by about 4½-fold. This decrease in total peripheral resistance results primarily from vasodilation of the arterial vascular beds in the active muscles as a result of the metabolites released during the increased metabolism of these muscles. These metabolites override the sympathetic vasoconstrictor effects.

The myocardial oxygen consumption ($M\dot{V}O_2$), like the heart rate, increases linearly with increasing workload. The $M\dot{V}O_2$ may increase fourfold to fivefold from rest to maximal exercise because of an increase in coronary blood flow and the $a\text{-}\bar{v}O_2\Delta$ of the cardiac muscle. The myocardial $a\text{-}\bar{v}O_2\Delta$ is very high at rest and increases only slightly during exercise, whereas the coronary blood flow increases about fourfold during maximal exercise. The heart, which is only about 0.5% of the weight of the body, receives about 5% of the $\dot{Q}$.

Ventilatory Responses to Acute Exercise

The increase in the ventilatory rate from rest to a given level of submaximal exercise is very rapid at first and then becomes more gradual until a steady state is attained. Similarly, when exercise is terminated, a rapid decrease is followed by a more gradual decline until the resting ventilatory value is reached (see Fig. 9-2, *B*).

When exercise is increased from resting until maximal levels are attained, the minute ventilation increases linearly with the increase in workload up to approximately 50% to 60% of the $\dot{V}O_{2\ max}$, after which it becomes curvilinearly related, with the increase in ventilation being greater than the increase in workload. The increase in minute ventilation results from an increase in the breathing frequency, which varies from 10 to 15 breaths/min at rest to 45 to 70 breaths/min at maximal work (depending on age), and an increase in tidal volume, which may reach values as high as 50% to 60% of the vital capacity during maximal work. Both breathing frequency and tidal volume tend to increase linearly when there is an increase in workload and $\dot{V}O_2$ during light to moderate work, whereas at heavier workloads and higher $\dot{V}O_2$, the tidal volume tends to level off, and the increases in ventilation become dependent primarily on an increase in breathing frequency. The increase in ventilation increases the elastic and flow-resistive work of breathing, which increases the energy required for breathing. The energy required by the muscles of breathing is very low at rest but may increase fiftyfold during maximal exercise.[11]

The point on the ventilation-$\dot{V}O_2$ curve at which the relationship suddenly changes from linear to curvilinear is often referred to as the *respiratory compensation threshold*[12] or *ventilatory anaerobic threshold.*[13]

The ventilatory response during exercise, which increases the provision of oxygen for transport to muscle cells, also includes a threefold increase in the lung diffusion capacity. This is due primarily to an increase in the amount of blood flowing through the lung, particularly to the upper sections, as a result of more of the pulmonary capillaries becoming patent; thus the total surface area available for pulmonary gas exchange is increased. (Diffusion capacity is measured in milliliters of oxygen diffused for each millimeter of mercury of partial pressure difference between the alveolus and pulmonary blood.)

CARDIORESPIRATORY RESPONSES TO CHRONIC EXERCISE

Exercise sessions repeated every 2 or 3 days for weeks or months (endurance training) result in physiologic and morphologic adjustments that modify physical performance. Training increases the maximal work capacity, and the best measure of this capacity is the $\dot{V}O_2$. The $\dot{V}O_2$ depends on the ability of the body to take in oxygen from the environment, transport it to the active muscles, extract it from the blood, and use it for muscular work. That is, the $\dot{V}O_2$ is the maximum $\dot{Q}$ multiplied by the maximum arteriovenous oxygen difference ($a\text{-}\bar{v}O_2\Delta$).

The responses of the trained and sedentary individual differ in the parameters that modify maximal work capacity. The person in training has a higher maximal work capacity, higher $\dot{V}O_{2\ max}$, and greater maximum $\dot{Q}$; however, both the $\dot{V}O_2$ and the $\dot{Q}$ at rest and at any given level of submaximal work is essentially the same for both the trained and sedentary individual.

The increased maximum $\dot{Q}$ is a result of an increased maximum stroke volume because the maximum heart rate is changed very little and in fact may decrease as a result of endurance training. The stroke volume at rest or at any given submaximum work rate is also higher in the trained person, and because the $\dot{Q}$ is essentially the same, it is evident that the heart rate at that workload must be considerably lower.

The pattern of response for $M\dot{V}O_2$ for the trained and sedentary individual is similar to that for the heart rate responses. That is, $M\dot{V}O_2$, which is highly related to the double product (heart rate multiplied by systolic blood pressure), which in turn reflects the work of the heart, is considerably lower in the trained individual at rest and at any given level of submaximal work, whereas the maximum attainable $M\dot{V}O_2$ is very similar for the trained and sedentary individual. This indicates that the trained heart is more efficient.

The $a\text{-}\bar{v}O_2\Delta$ and oxygen use in the trained and the sedentary people is essentially the same at rest and for given levels of submaximal work; however, the maximal ability to extract and use oxygen from a given amount of blood is greater in the trained individual. This response pattern is similar to that of $\dot{Q}$ and $\dot{V}O_2$.

Systolic, diastolic, and mean blood pressures all tend to be reduced at rest or at submaximal work intensities after endurance training. The values at maximal work capacity are similar for the trained and the sedentary individual. There is a greater reduction in the peripheral resistance in trained than sedentary individuals at rest and at all levels of exercise intensity.

The changes in ventilation with increasing workload after endurance training has a pattern similar to those in the sedentary individual; however, at any submaximal workload the ventilatory rate is reduced in trained individuals. The ventilatory rate is very similar at rest, whereas the maximum ventilatory rate is greater in the trained individual. The pattern of response for pulmonary diffusion capacity is similar in the trained and the sedentary individual except that the value is greater in the trained person at rest at any given submaximal workload and at maximal work capacity.

COMPARISON OF CHILDREN AND ADULTS

An examination of sports programs for children indicates that boys and girls are for the most part, participating in games and events designed by and for adults. This is particularly true in school sports programs. The child is an "immature working machine," not a miniature adult, and because there are important differences in physiologic responses to muscular activity, children should not be expected to perform in a manner similar to adults.

Anaerobic Metabolism

Alactacid Energy Component

The concentration of the phosphagens (ATP and CP) are similar in children and adults. The rate of use of both phosphagens at workloads eliciting a given percentage of $\dot{V}O_{2\ max}$ is also similar in children and adults. Thus the alactic anaerobic processes do not differ significantly.[14-18]

Lactacid Energy Component

A child possesses lower concentrations of phosphofructokinase, the rate-limiting enzyme in glycolysis, than adults.[18] Furthermore, the child exhibits a lower maximum lactic acid level in both blood and muscle after maximal work and lower lactic acid levels at all submaximal workloads when compared to adults. This suggests that the child has a lower lactacid anaerobic capacity and is at a disadvantage in events requiring maximal use of this energy source.[15,19] Furthermore, development of this lactacid energy capacity and thus success in events dependent on this energy source are closely related to maturity level.

Aerobic Metabolism

The child's heart and lungs are smaller than the adult's when expressed in absolute terms, but the sizes are very similar if expressed relative to body size.[20] Aerobic capacity ($\dot{V}O_{2\ max}$), the usual index of endurance capacity and cardiorespiratory fitness,[21] depends on the $\dot{Q}$ and the a-$\bar{v}O_2\Delta$. The stroke volume of the heart is similar in children and adults when corrections are made for the difference in body size,[16] whereas the maximum attainable heart rate is slightly higher in children.[22,23] Because these are the components of $\dot{Q}$, it is evident that adaptation of the $\dot{Q}$ to aerobic work in the child is at least equivalent to that of the adult.

Despite the fact that maximal a-$\bar{v}O_2\Delta$ normally depends on the hemoglobin concentration in the blood and that children have a lower hemoglobin concentration than adults, the maximum a-$\bar{v}O_2\Delta$ is similar for both adults and children.[16,22,23] Eriksson[15,24] claims that this is because the child's maximum a-$\bar{v}O_2\Delta$ comes closer to the blood's oxygen-carrying capacity as a result of more active enzyme systems.[25] Children also have the ability to shunt a greater percentage of the $\dot{Q}$ through the active tissues during exercise, thus exhibiting a lower $\dot{Q}$ at any given submaximal level of oxygen uptake. This may result from a decrease in the amount of oxygen demanded by the child's smaller viscera or a decreased need for blood flow to the skin which is caused by a more ready elimination of the body's heat.[25] Systolic, mean, and even diastolic arterial blood pressures are relatively lower in children than in adults.[26,27]

In absolute terms, the pulmonary diffusion capacity is smaller in children than adults because it is dependent on the area of the alveolar membrane available for gaseous diffusion. This changes, as do lung volumes, with body size, particularly height.

The question of the equality of aerobic capabilities between adults and children, however, is one in which there is not complete agreement. For instance, Astrand[28] claims that the $\dot{V}O_{2\ max}$ in children is not as high as expected for their size and they do not have the aerobic power to handle their weight compared to adults. However, the 16- to 18-year-old boys in his study had a mean $\dot{V}O_{2\ max}$ of 3.68 L·min^{-1}, which translated into 57.6 ml·kg·$^{-1}$min^{-1}, whereas 7- to 9-year-old boys had values of 1.75 L·min^{-1} and 57 ml·kg·$^{-1}$min^{-1}. This indicates that the oxygen uptake expressed relative to body weight was the same, although the adult did have a higher aerobic power reserve. This was indicated by the adult's ability to increase the basal metabolic rate 13.5-fold, whereas the 8-year-old children demonstrated a maximum increase of only 9.4-fold.

Bar-Or[7] plotted data from a large number of studies and showed that the maximal aerobic power for boys, when expressed in liters per minute, increased continually from age 5 to 18 years, whereas for girls the values, though always slightly lower than boys, increased at about the same rate until about 14 years of age, after which it leveled off and increased no further. Because $\dot{V}O_{2max}$ is related not only to maturity but also to body size, Bar-Or[7] also compared the maximal aerobic power of individuals of different body mass and showed that it remained fairly constant for boys 5 to 18 years when expressed relative to body weight, whereas for girls the values were similar but lower up to age 10 years, after which there was a continual decline with age. Bar-Or[7] suggested that this decline may reflect an increase in body adiposity of girls during adolescence. Somewhat similar results have been reported by Andersen et al[29] and Kemper and Verschuur.[30]

The child requires a greater stride frequency than the adult when running at the same speed, and because this results in a more expensive use of energy per unit of time, the child requires a greater oxygen uptake per kilogram of body weight than the adult.[28] Providing that the child is competing only against those of similar maturity, the sporting implications are minimal.

However, the most recent view is that the aerobic capacity of children is at least equivalent to that of the adult. As Eriksson[24] claims, when participating in an aerobic activity lasting less than 1 hour, the child, like the adult, must carry and transport his or her own body weight; therefore the child is not at any real disadvantage compared to the adult.

In aerobic events requiring a work level of 70% $\dot{V}O_{2\ max}$ for longer than 1 hour, the child is at a disadvantage because of the smaller absolute and relative storage capacity for muscle glycogen.[15,16,18,31] Muscle glycogen depletion is associated with fatigue.

The mean maximum accumulated oxygen deficit, a measure of anaerobic capacity, is 58.5 and 39 ml O_2·kg^{-1}, respectively, for men and women.[32] These values are higher than those found for boys (35 ml $O_2 \cdot kg^{-1}$) and girls (40 ml $O_2 \cdot kg^{-1}$).[33] Carlson and Naughton[33] express concern over the accuracy of the values that they obtained for girls because they indicated that the reliability of the girls was poorer.

The ventilation required per liter of oxygen consumed (oxygen ventilatory equivalent) at maximal exercise decreases from 6 to 18 years. In children under 10 years of age the values for ventilatory equivalent are about 30 L/L O_2 consumed during light work and up to 40 L/L O_2 during maximal exercise. The resting adult ventilatory equivalent is 20 to 25 L/L O_2 and increases to 30 to 35 L/L O_2 during moderately heavy exercise and to 40 L/L O_2 during maximal exercise. This seems to indicate that the ventilatory system is less efficient in children, this inefficiency being more pronounced in younger children because they use smaller amounts of oxygen from given amounts of inspired air.

The respiratory frequency during maximal exercise is about 70 breaths/min in 5-year-old children. The respiratory frequency drops to 55 breaths/min and 40 to 45 breaths/min in 12 year olds and adults, respectively.[10] The young child has a shallower breathing pattern with a tidal volume/vital capacity ratio lower than that in older children and adults.

Strength

Children are at a disadvantage in events relying largely on strength because not only are children weaker than adults but they are also weaker relative to their body dimensions. According to Paterson,[34] this indicates the involvement of biologic factors that modify muscular dynamics. Astrand[28] lists three factors that affect muscle strength in aging children: (1) the increase in size of the muscles; (2) the aging process itself, which may reflect maturation of the central nervous system; and (3) the development of sexual maturity, which probably plays a dominant role for boys. For this reason, it is not very productive to include weight training for the prepubertal boy or girl because the strength gains are small until the androgenic hormones are produced in amounts sufficient to permit muscle hypertrophy.[35] It is therefore more beneficial to spend the extra time on practicing skills.[36] However, there are few detrimental effects if performed correctly, and those using weight training will certainly become stronger.[37-40] Also, learning the correct techniques of lifting is valuable in performing activities of daily living. The value of weight training in children's training programs is still not completely resolved, and many questions remain. For instance, it may be that those who commence weight training early may develop greater strength as an adult. Based on a recent review, Tanner[41] has claimed that most children and adolescents, provided that they adhere to a well-supervised, progressive strength-training program, can improve performance in other sports. This view is supported in a comprehensive review of the risks and benefits of resistance training in children by Blimkie.[42]

Thermoregulation

The human body is about 20% to 25% efficient under the best conditions; therefore most of the metabolic activity is eventually converted to heat. During vigorous exercise, a considerable heat load is imposed on the body, and bodily mechanisms, including sweating, shunting of blood through the arteriovenous anastomosis in the skin, and cutaneous vasodilation, are initiated to increase the rate of heat dissipation by evaporation, conduction, convection, and radiation.

Vigorous prolonged exercise in high temperatures and humidity can increase body core temperatures to levels high enough to cause cell and tissue destruction, which are manifested as heat illnesses such as heat cramps, heat exhaustion, and heat stroke. To prevent heat illness, people exercising in the heat should drink plenty of fluids (remembering that thirst is not an adequate guide to fluid needs); select appropriate, loose-fitting, light clothing; and cease exercise if any of the early symptoms of heat illness occur. People organizing and administering sporting events should cancel endurance events if the environmental conditions are such that the wet bulb globe temperature exceeds 28° C.[43]

The child has a larger skin surface area/body mass ratio than the adult and is therefore more susceptible to heat loss or heat gain from the environment. The child also has less mature sweat glands and thus is at a disadvantage and in possible danger when performing heavy, long-term activities in the heat and high humidity. Children are also at a disadvantage when competing in endurance swimming events in cold water. That is, children are disadvantaged when performing exercise under environmental extremes of heat or cold. Inbar et al[44] have also postulated that children are prevented from deriving the full effect of exercise-in-heat acclimatization because of some as-yet-undefined age-related factors associated with the thermoregulatory system.

Application

The differences between children and adults are important in sporting events. For example, there is a need to modify adult equipment, adult facilities, the duration of events, the number of players per team, and the rules and to use a physiologic basis for selecting the most appropriate activities for the various age groups.

For instance, when the type of activities most suitable for children are selected, evidence suggests that the child can handle short, intense (alactic) sprints or aerobic work of less than 1 hour's duration without undue stress. However, compared to adults, children perform poorly in lactacid sprint-type events lasting ½ to 1½ minutes (e.g., 200- or 400-m track events). Success in these events depends on the child's level of maturity, so children who mature late may suffer psychologically as a result of continual failure. There is no apparent reason to suggest that the child should not attempt to train this energy system.

Although the available scientific data are meager and inconclusive, the American Academy of Pediatrics has issued a position statement on children lifting weights.[45] It claims that an athlete should not attempt maximal lifts until growth is complete at about age 16 or 17; thus weight-lifting and powerlifting are contraindicated before this age. The position statement admits that a well-supervised weight training program involving submaximal resistance can enhance performance in most sports, especially after puberty. The Academy warns of the tendency for weight-lifting to result in a transient elevation of blood pressure and the suspicion that lifting very heavy weights can cause epiphysial damage in preadolescents.

The recognition of these differences between children and adults has been responsible (at last) for the realization that adult equipment and playing fields and adult game rules are not suitable for small children. As a result, some sporting associations have introduced modifications. The fields have been reduced in size, as have goal posts, balls, bats, and other playing equipment, and the duration of play and rest periods has been modified to better suit the physiologic development of the players. A study by Elliott[46] showed the need to modify the size of tennis racquets to suit the size and strength of the child. He found that children approximately 8 years of age, because they are smaller in stature and have less strength, could not handle the increases in the moment of inertia involved with the use of a larger racquet, so performance deteriorated, primarily in the strokes requiring greater total racquet movement such as the serve.

EFFECTS OF TRAINING

General Outcomes

One of the common questions related to the training of children concerns the suggestion that if training occurs during the period of rapid growth (prepuberty and puberty), there is a more marked improvement in components, such as aerobic power, than can be attained in training during adulthood. Certainly some animal studies have shown that this occurs, at least with the rat.[47]

Although some human studies[14,16,48,49] indicate that training before and during puberty produces a greater increase in the size of organs of the cardiorespiratory system than training later in life, Eriksson[16] claims that the changes in $\dot{V}O_{2\,max}$ similar. He found that in 11-year-old boys training for running, $\dot{V}O_{2\,max}$ expressed in $ml{\cdot}kg^{-1}{\cdot}min^{-1}$ improved 16%, which is similar to the increase found by Saltin et al[50] for sedentary adults. However, improvement is easier the more unfit the subject is initially, and sedentary adults are probably more unfit than sedentary children. A review by Bar-Or[51] has shown that $\dot{V}O_{2\,max}$ can be increased in children with training; however, the improvement in prepubescent children is not as great as it is in adults. This conflicts with the view of Shephard,[52] who claims that there is no immediate evidence that the training response of the prepubescent child is less than in an older person.

Another question that is frequently asked, particularly by parents, is whether hard training has any deleterious effect on the growing child. A study by Astrand et al[48] showed that in 30 Swedish girl swimmers age 12 to 16 years, who trained intensively up to 65 km/week over a number of years, the $\dot{V}O_{2\,max}$ improved to a mean value of 52 ml $O_2{\cdot}kg^{-1}{\cdot}min^{-1}$. This training also increased the size of the organs involved in the oxygen transport system, and there was no indication of any detrimental effects.

These same girls were studied for 10 years, during which time all ceased regular training and most regressed to a very sedentary lifestyle. As a result, their $\dot{V}O_{2\,max}$ decreased from a mean of 52 to 37 ml $O_2{\cdot}kg^{-1}{\cdot}min^{-1}$ (29% decrease); however, the dimensions of the lungs and heart were relatively unchanged.[49] The implication of retaining the larger heart and lungs is unknown, but others[53] have reported increased heart volumes in former top-rated endurance athletes without any accompanying medical problems. It does suggest, however, that the functional capacity of the cardiovascular system declines more markedly than its dimensions after training is ceased. This hypokinetically induced drop in $\dot{V}O_{2\,max}$ to levels lower than those of the average nonathlete creates concern regarding the long-term effects on attitude toward physical activity after participation in a demanding training program at an early age.

A representative sample of 16 of the original 30 girls then embarked, at a mean age of 23.9 years, on a 12-week retraining program to determine whether the $\dot{V}O_{2\,max}$ could be improved in this now-sedentary group of former swimmers to a greater extent than the average sedentary woman.[54] The study showed that the 12-week program increased $\dot{V}O_{2\,max}$ by 14% without an increase in heart volume and yet almost restored stroke volume to that computed for the girls during their competitive swimming period 10 years earlier. This suggests that the training effect on the pumping function of the heart may be more pronounced in former top athletes than in previously sedentary people. Although these increases in $\dot{V}O_{2\,max}$ and stroke volume are larger in other studies,[55] the studies are not quite comparable, so it is still difficult to claim that previous training in early life is of definite advantage. In fact, Pollock[56] has reviewed a large number of training studies, and his summary table indicates that a 14% gain represents an average increase in $\dot{V}O_{2\,max}$.

Because the training participation by these girls was not as good as expected and because no control group was used, Eriksson et al[57] repeated the study using the most elite girls from the 1961 study ($N = 4$). This study used a control group of women each of whom lived in the same neighborhood and was age-matched to one of the former swimmers.[57] After retraining, the former girl swimmers had a 19% increase in $\dot{V}O_{2\,max}$ when expressed in liters per minute, whereas $\dot{V}O_{2\,max}$ in the control group increased 12.5%. When $\dot{V}O_{2\,max}$ was expressed relative to body weight, the former swimmers' increase was still 19% compared to 10% for the controls. Stroke volume of the heart increased in both groups exhibiting a 33% and 26% increase for the former swimmers and the control group, respectively. This study gives some support to the hypothesis that a former athlete has a greater capability to increase aerobic power with training.

Another longitudinal study of 29 girl swimmers who started vigorous swimming at ages 8.6 and 13.7 years has been reported.[49,58] These girls were followed annually to age 16 years. At 15 years of age, 15 of the 29 were still training, thus allowing comparisons between those still in training and the 14 who had dropped out. The data showed that heart volume increased with growth in both groups; however, the girls who continued to train had larger hearts at each age. A similar pattern was evident for maximum oxygen uptake in which absolute values (in liters per minute) increased with age for both groups. However, when these values were corrected for growth, the training group again showed a slightly greater value than the nontraining group. Static lung volumes were larger than normal after only a few years of training and increased further only in relation to the increase in height.

Early training does not necessarily guarantee sporting success later in life. Nor is it a prerequisite for success. One of the conclusions drawn from the Medford Boy's Growth Study[59] was that outstanding elementary school athletes may not be outstanding in junior high and outstanding junior high school athletes may not have been outstanding in elementary school. He found that 45% of those outstanding athletes in junior high were not considered such in elementary school.

Possible Detrimental Outcomes

During training and competition, repetitive stress on a muscle, bone, or joint produces adaptations, some of which may be undesirable.[60] Extreme overuse may lead to bony and muscular hypertrophy[61] and create problems such as little leaguer's elbow, tennis arm, swimmer's shoulder, Osgood-Schlatter disease, Sever's disease, and stress fractures.[62] In the child, ligaments are stronger than the epiphyses, so injuries are more likely to involve epiphyseal problems rather than be simple sprains. This type of injury then will require a more definitive treatment, such as protection, until the epiphyses heals, but more important, epiphysial injuries are often undetected.

To prevent problems caused by overuse, many sporting associations limit the amount of time a player uses particular muscle groups; for instance, U.S. Little League baseball limits the number of innings that young players can pitch to six per week. To be successful, this system still relies on the coach placing the child's welfare above everything else, limiting the number of pitches allowed during a training session, and educating the child so that he or she restricts throwing activities when not under supervision. Similarly, restrictions have been advocated to prevent the frequent back injuries in young "fast bowlers" in cricket[63] and to prevent running injuries by limiting competitive race distances for children of various ages.[64]

Larson and McMahon[65] reported on 1338 athletic injuries in the area around Eugene, Oregon; 20% of these injuries occurred in the age groups 14 years and younger, which consisted of 60% of the participants, whereas 40% occurred in the group 15 to 18 years old, which constituted only 15% of the participants. This study indicated that the 15- to 18-year-old group is the most vulnerable to athletic injury. They found that 1.67% (23) were epiphysial injuries but claimed that although growth deformity can occur afterward, this type of injury is the exception rather than the rule. Most cases of epiphysial displacement were easily reduced with traction and gentle manual pressure, and only rarely was open reduction necessary.

Australian studies by Davidson et al[66] and Sugarman, reported by the Australian Football Schools Union,[67] also indicate the low incidence of injury in the younger children, even in collision sports such as rugby. It is only as the boys become mature and develop the muscle bulk and speed, which contribute to greater momentum and coordination, and the desire to "hit" rather than tackle that the incidence of injury becomes a real concern.

However, even if the number of injuries is less than once believed and even if, as Larson and McMahon claim, they can be successfully treated medically, prevention should be the aim. Prevention efforts will involve an adequate level of preseason conditioning and emphasis on skills to ensure correct mechanics. Tennis elbow in adults is certainly related to overuse and faulty stroke mechanics.[68] Thus all coaches should modify an activity (such as using two-handed backhand) or reduce the number of repetitions of an activity that places too much stress on young bones and joints.

Based on reports on heel cord injuries, epiphysial growth plate injuries, and other chronic joint trauma as a result of long-distance running, the American Academy of Pediatrics[69] has, in the interest of prevention, issued the following statement:

> Long distance competitive running events primarily designed for adults are not recommended for children prior to physical maturation. Under no circumstances should a full marathon be attempted by immature youths (less than Tanner Stage 5 sexual maturity rating). After pubertal development is complete, guidelines for adult distance running are appropriate.

The Australian Sports Medicine Federation[64] recommended that the maximum permitted competitive running distances for children under 12 years, 12 to 15 years, 15 to 16 years, and 16 to 17 years of age be 5 km, 10 km, a half marathon, and 30 km, respectively. Those 18 years of age and older should be permitted to run a full marathon race. The Federation also recommended that the maximum weekly training distance be no more than 3 times the recommended race distances.[64]

There is not enough evidence to prove or disprove the need to limit the amount and intensity of vigorous training; however, it appears prudent to err on the side of caution until such studies are performed. After reviewing the injury risks to children in sports, Larson and McMahon[65] drew the following conclusion:

> A more vigorous type of life will produce more wear and tear on joint surfaces than a sedentary one. However, the benefits derived by children participating in athletics, such as physical fitness, learning to meet competition and the discipline of an organized athletic program outweigh such an indefinite potential.

LEVEL OF MATURITY AND SPORTS PERFORMANCE

In sports, the different levels of performance at a given age are often the result of different levels of maturity rather than of skill. For instance, Cumming et al[70] showed that the level of performance in track-and-field events was more closely related to skeletal age than chronologic age, height, or weight. Mero et al[71] have also shown that endurance capacity and strength were greater in an athletic group than in a control group and that the athletic group demonstrated an advanced biologic maturity. Clarke[59] found that the skeletal age of children who were age 13 years chronologically varied from 8 years, 10 months to 15 years, 11 months.

Advanced maturity imparts not only an increased body size, lactacid anaerobic ability, increased ability to store glycogen, and increased strength and muscle bulk but also an increase in speed and power. Speed, which increases with age at least to the age of 18 for boys and 14 for girls, is probably due to the maturation of the nervous system.[28] Speed is related more closely to maturity level than height because at any given age, the running speed is usually not different in children of different heights, except for boys around puberty. Boys around 14 and 15 years of age have increased running speed with increased height, probably because the taller boys are more mature.

The rate of growth and development is as individual as physique, eye color, and other personal characteristics.[72] Therefore because junior sports programs should try to provide optimal participation and fair competition with a minimal risk of injury, classification on the basis of chronologic age is not satisfactory. This is especially true in events in which speed, size, and strength are important for successful performance. Probably the best criteria for matching competitors in sports should include maturity, age, height, weight, skill, and where indicated, gender. The five stages of genital development or pubic hair development as described by Tanner[73] are adequate means of scoring maturity, and certainly no one classified in stages 1 or 2 should compete against anyone classified in stages 4 or 5 regardless of chronologic age. Shaffer[72] suggests estimating maturity level simply by observing secondary sexual development, namely the axillary and pubic hair, rather than organ development. He also suggests that girls' date of menarche is often adequate for determining maturity level.

Though the early maturers may have a distinct advantage in sports at an early age, they may suffer long-term disadvantages compared to the late maturers. Late maturers who do not become "sporting dropouts" because of discouragement from continual failure often spend a great deal of time acquiring skill so that they may compete. Many of the early maturers, however, because they are bigger and stronger, spend little time developing skill. They are content to use bulk rather than finesse, and unfortunately this practice is encouraged by many so-called coaches, especially in collision sports. As a result, these early maturers often become relegated to the second team when the late maturers eventually reach a similar size and develop similar speed and strength. Because success usually promotes continued interest and effort, lack of success often leads to hatred of the specific sport and often all forms of physical activity; as a result, many early maturers terminate their sporting careers before reaching their 20s.

CONCLUSION

If the effects of regular frequent exercise are plotted on the y-axis against the amount of exercise on the x-axis, the graph would take the shape of an inverted U. That is, little or no regular exercise has detrimental effects on the child and may be associated with some of the hypokinetic diseases such as heart disease and obesity in later life. As the volume of regular exercise is increased, there are increasing benefits, including increased capacity and efficiency of the cardiorespiratory, muscular, and metabolic systems, leading to greater work capacity. If, however, the volume and intensity of regular exercise become excessive, detrimental effects, especially stress fractures, overuse injuries, and even chronic fatigue syndrome, are likely.

All children require regular exercise for normal growth and development and for the development of minimal levels of health and fitness. Although many children today have far too little exercise, there are others who begin very intensive physical training for sports at an early age. Many children in age-group sports participate in unfair competition because chronologic age alone is used as the means of classification. In collision sports, this can be dangerous for the late maturer.

The physiologic responses to acute exercise and to training are similar in children and adults, and for the most part, these responses are beneficial. The pediatrician must understand these responses and be aware of the role of exercise in the possible prevention and management of many diseases such as asthma, cystic fibrosis, diabetes mellitus, hypertension, obesity, and cerebral palsy. The pediatrician must realize that although no sport is risk free, sports-related injuries can be minimized with proper preparticipation medical screening, with supervision, and with the use of protective equipment. Activities such as weight training, weight-lifting, and long-distance running are becoming popular with children and teenagers; therefore the advice of pediatricians to parents, sport administrators, and participants concerning what is safe and what can be hazardous at various ages can be very effective in minimizing detrimental outcomes. The desirability of regular, appropriate, supervised physical training is not in question and should be recommended on the basis of improved health, fitness, and performance capabilities.

REFERENCES

1. Ekblom B: Effect of physical training on oxygen transport in man, *Acta Physiol Scand* 328:1-45, 1969.
2. Armstrong N, Balding J, Gentle P, Kirby B: Estimation of coronary risk factors in British school children: a preliminary report, *Br J Sports Med* 24(1):61-65, 1990.
3. Armstrong N, Balding J, Gentle P, Kirby B: Patterns of physical activity among 11 to 16 year old British children, *Br Med J* 301:203-205, 1990.
4. Gilbey H, Gilbey M: The physical activity of Singapore primary school children as measured by heart rate monitoring, *Pediatr Exerc Sci* 7:26-35, 1995.
5. Kraus H, Raab W: *Hypokinetic disease,* Springfield, Ill, 1961, Charles C Thomas.
6. Morton AR: Children in sport: selected considerations. In VII Commonwealth & International Conference on Sport, Physical Education, Recreation and Dance, (Conference 82). In Howell ML, Parker AW, eds: *Scientific aspects of elitism in sport,* vol 8, Brisbane, Australia, 1984, Queensland University, pp 231-240.
7. Bar-Or O: *Pediatric sports medicine for the practitioner,* New York, 1983, Springer-Verlag.

Muscular System

8. Malina RM: Growth of muscle tissue and muscle mass. In Falkner F, Tanner JM, eds: *Human growth: postnatal growth neurobiology,* New York, 1986, Plenum, pp 77-99.
9. Dubowitz V, Brooke MH: *Muscle biopsy: a modern approach to major problems in neurology,* vol 2, Philadelphia, 1973, WB Saunders.
10. Bell RD, MacDougall JD, Billeter R, Howald H: Muscle fiber types and morphometric analysis of skeletal muscle in six-year-old children, *Med Sci Sports* 12(1):28-31, 1980.

Cardiorespiratory Responses to Acute Exercise

11. Moffett DF, Moffett SB, Schauf CL: *Human physiology: foundations and frontiers,* ed 2, St Louis, 1993, Mosby.
12. Paterson DJ, Morton AR: The exercise anaerobic threshold: incorrect nomenclature, *NZ J Sports Med* 14(3):73-74, 1986.
13. Wasserman K, Whipp BJ, Koyal, SN, Beaver WL: Anaerobic threshold and respiratory gas exchange during exercise, *J Appl Physiol* 35(2):236-243, 1973.

Comparison of Children and Adults

14. Ekblom B: Effect of physical training in adolescent boys, *J Appl Physiol* 27:350-355, 1969.
15. Eriksson BO, Karlsson J, Saltin B: Muscle metabolites during exercise in pubertal boys, *Acta Paediatr Scand* 60(suppl 217):154-157, 1971.
16. Eriksson BO: Physical training, oxygen supply and muscle metabolism in 11-13 year old boys, *Acta Physiol Scand* 384(suppl):1-48, 1972.
17. Eriksson BO, Saltin B: Muscle metabolism during exercise in boys aged 11-16 years compared to adults, *Acta Paediatr Belg* 28(suppl):257-265, 1974.
18. Eriksson BO, Gollnick PD, Saltin B: Muscle metabolism and enzyme activities after training in boys 11-13 years old, *Acta Physiol Scand* 87:485-497, 1973.
19. Karlsson J: Lactate and phosphagen concentrations in working muscles in man, *Acta Physiol Scand* 358(suppl):1-72, 1971.
20. Sundberg S, Elovainio R: Cardiorespiratory function in competitive endurance runners aged 12-16 years compared with ordinary boys, *Acta Paediatr Scand* 7:987-992, 1982.
21. Zauner CW, Maksud MG, Melichna J: Physiological considerations in training young athletes, *Sports Med* 8(1):15-31, 1989.
22. Astrand PO: *Experimental studies of physical working capacity in relation to sex and age,* Copenhagen, 1952, Munksgaard.
23. Robinson S: Experimental studies of physical fitness in relation to age, *Arbeits Physiol* 10:251-323, 1938.
24. Eriksson BO: Physical activity from childhood to maturity: medical and pediatric considerations. In Landry F, Orban WAR, eds: *Physical activity and human well-being,* Miami, 1978, Symposia Specialists, pp 47-55.
25. Shephard RJ: The child in sport and physical activity: physiology comment. In Albinson JG, Andrews GM, eds: *Child in sport and physical activity,* Baltimore, 1976, University Park Press, pp 35-40.
26. Lauer RM, Burns TL, Clarke WP: Assessing children's blood pressure: considerations of age and body size—the Muscadine study, *Pediatrics* 75(6):1081-1090, 1985.
27. Bar-Or O: Importance of differences between children and adults for exercise testing and exercise prescription. In Skinner JS, ed: *Exercise testing and exercise prescription for special cases,* Malvern, Penn, 1993, Lea & Febiger, pp 57-74.
28. Astrand PO: Physiology. In Albinson JG, Andrew GM, eds: *Child in sport and physical activity,* Baltimore, 1976, University Park Press, pp 19-33.
29. Andersen KL, Seliger V, Rutenfranz J, Skrobak-Kaczynski J: Physical performance capacity of children in Norway. Part IV. The rate of growth in maximal aerobic power and the influence of improved physical education in a rural community: population parameters in a rural community, *Eur J Appl Physiol* 35:49-58, 1976.

30. Kemper HG, Verschuur R: Longitudinal study of maximal aerobic power in teenagers, *Ann Hum Biol* 14:435-444, 1987.
31. Eriksson BO, Karlsson J, Saltin B: Muscle metabolites during exercise in 13 year old boys, *Acta Paediatr Scand* 60(suppl 217):57-63, 1971.
32. Weyand PG, Cureton KJ, Conley DS, Higbie EJ: Peak oxygen deficit during one- and two-legged cycling in men and women, *Med Sci Sports Exerc* 25(5):584-591, 1993.
33. Carlson JS, Naughton GA: An examination of the anaerobic capacity of children using maximal accumulated oxygen deficit, *Pediatr Exerc Sci* 5(1):60-71, 1993.
34. Paterson DH: Physiological peculiarities of children. In Coaching Association of Canada: *Coaching science update,* Ottawa, 1979-1980, The Association.
35. Jones HE: *Motor performance and growth: a developmental study of dynamometric strength,* Berkeley, Calif, 1949, University of California Press.
36. Shaffer TE: The young athlete: new guidelines in sports medicine, *Pediatr Consult* 1(5):1-12, 1980.
37. American Academy of Pediatrics: Weight training and weight-lifting: information for the pediatrician, *Physician Sportsmed* 11(3):157-161, 1983.
38. Ramsay JA, Blimkie CJR, Smith K, Garner S, MacDougall JD, Sale DG: Strength training effects in prepubescent boys, *Med Sci Sports Exerc* 20(5):605-614, 1990.
39. Sewall L, Micheli LJ: Strength development in children, *Med Sci Sports Exerc* 16(2):158, 1984.
40. Weltman A, Janney C, Rians CB, Strand K, Berg B, Tippitt S, Wise J, Cahill BR, Katch FI: The effects of hydraulic resistance strength training in pre-pubertal males, *Med Sci Sports Exerc* 18(6):629-638, 1986.
41. Tanner SM: Weighing the risks: strength training for children and adolescents, *Physician Sportsmed* 21(6):105-116, 1993.
42. Blimkie CJR: Benefits and risks of resistance training in children. In Cahill BR, Pearl A, eds: *Intensive participation in children's sport,* Champaign, Ill, 1993, Human Kinetics, pp 133-165.
43. American College of Sports Medicine: The prevention of thermal injuries during distance running, *Med Sci Sports Exerc* 19(5):529-533, 1987.
44. Inbar O, Bar-Or O, Dotan R, Gutin B: Conditioning versus exercise in heat as methods for acclimatizing 8-10-year old boys to dry heat, *J Appl Physiol* 50(2):406-411, 1981.
45. Legwold G: Does lifting weights harm a prepubescent athlete? *Physician Sportsmed* 10(7):141-144, 1982.
46. Elliott BC: Tennis racquet selection: a factor in early skill development, *Aust J Sports Sci* 1(1):23-25, 1981.

Effects of Training

47. Montoye HJ, Nelson R, Johnson P, MacNab R: Effects of exercise in swimming endurance and organ weight in mature rats, *Res Q* 31(3):474-484, 1960.
48. Astrand PO, Engstrom L, Eriksson BO, Karlberg P, Nylander I, Slatin B, Thoren C: Girl swimmers, *Acta Paediatr Scand Suppl* 147:1-75, 1963.
49. Engstrom I, Eriksson BO, Karlberg P, Saltin B, Thoren C: Preliminary report on the development of lung volumes in young girl swimmers, *Acta Paediatr Scand* 60(suppl 217):73-76, 1971.
50. Saltin B, Hartley LH, Kilbom A, Astrand, I: Physical training in sedentary middle-aged and older men. II. Oxygen uptake, heart rate and blood lactate concentrations at submaximal and maximal exercise, *Scand J Clin Lab Invest* 24:323-334, 1969.
51. Bar-Or O: Trainability of the prepubescent child, *Physician Sportsmed* 21(6):105-116, 1989.
52. Shephard R: Effectiveness of training programmes for prepubescent children, *Sports Med* 13(3):194-213, 1992.
53. Saltin B, Grimby G: Physiological analysis of middle-aged and former athletes: comparison with still active athletes of the same age, *Circulation* 38:1104-1115, 1968.
54. Eriksson BO, Lundin A, Saltin B: Cardiopulmonary function in former girl swimmers and the effect of physical training, *Scand J Clin Lab Invest* 35:135-145, 1975.
55. Kilbom A, Astrand I: Physical training with submaximal intensities in women. II. Effects on cardiac output, *Scand J Clin Lab Invest* 28:163-175, 1971.
56. Pollock ML: The quantification of endurance training programmes. In Wilmore JH, ed: *Exercise and sport sciences reviews,* New York, 1973, Academic, pp 155-188.
57. Eriksson BO, Freychuss U, Lundin A, Thoren CAR: Effect of physical training in former female top athletes in swimming. In Berg K, Eriksson BO, eds: *Children in exercise,* ed 9, Baltimore, 1980, University Park Press, pp 116-127.
58. Eriksson BO, Thoren B: Training girls for swimming from medical and physiological points of view, with special reference to growth. In Eriksson B, Funberg B, eds: *Swimming medicine,* ed 4, Baltimore,1978, University Park Press, pp 3-15.
59. Clarke HH: *Physical and motor tests in the Medford Boy's Growth Study,* Englewood Cliffs, NJ, 1971, Prentice Hall.
60. Micheli LJ: Overuse injuries in children's sport: the growth factor, *Orthop Clin North Am* 14(2):337-360, 1983.
61. Cumming GR: Medical comment. In Albinson JG, Andrew GM, eds: *Child in sport and physical activity,* Baltimore, 1976, University Park Press, pp 67-77.
62. Stanitski CL: Combating overuse injuries: a focus on children and adolescents, *Physician Sportsmed* 21(1):87-106, 1993.
63. Foster D, Elliott B, Gray S, Herzbergh L: Guidelines for the fast bowler, *Sportscoach* 7(2):47-48, 1984.
64. Roberts DM, Morton, AR, Sinclair A: Australian Sports Medicine Federation: children in sport policy, *Sport Health* 1:19-20, 1983.
65. Larson RL, McMahon RO: The epiphyses and the childhood athlete, *JAMA* 196(7):607-612, 1966.
66. Davidson R, Kennedy J, Kennedy M, Vanderfield GK: Competitive sport in Australian schoolboys, *Aust J Sports Med* 11(4):100-102, 1979.
67. Australian Rugby Football Schools Union: *Schoolboy rugby union injuries,* Sydney, Australia, 1983, The Union.
68. Priest JD, Braden V, Gerberich SG: An analysis of players with and without pain, *Physician Sportsmed* 8:4-5, 1980.
69. American Academy of Pediatrics: Risks in long distance running in children, *Physician Sportsmed* 10(8):82-86, 1982.

Level of Maturity and Sports Performance

70. Cumming GR, Garand T, Borysyk L: Correlation of performance in track and field events with bone age, *J Pediatr* 80:970-973, 1972.
71. Mero A, Kauhanen H, Peltola E, Buoriman T, Komi P: Physiological performance capacity in different prepubescent athletic groups, *J Sports Med Physical Fitness* 30:57-66, 1990.
72. Shaffer TE: The uniqueness of the young athlete: introductory remarks, *Am J Sports Med* 8(5):370-371, 1980.
73. Tanner JM: *Growth at adolescence,* ed 2, Oxford, England, 1962, Blackwell Scientific.

CHAPTER 10

Respiration of Infants at High Altitude

Jacopo P. Mortola

High altitude is a multifactorial environmental condition that includes cold, atmospheric dryness, and increased atmospheric radiation. However, for most endotherms (mammals and birds), the factor of primary importance associated with increased altitude is the decrease in oxygen (O_2) concentration* that accompanies the drop in barometric pressure.

It is estimated that several million people live permanently in the high-altitude areas of the world[1] (i.e., above 3000 m); hence, a large number of infants are born in an environment with an O_2 concentration less than 12% and an inspired partial pressure of O_2 less than 100 mm Hg. This chapter addresses the way that high-altitude newborns cope with the low O_2 tension and, specifically, the role of the respiratory function in adapting to the environment. Before the options available to the newborn are contemplated, however, the extent to which gestation at high altitude may result in fetal hypoxemia, the consequences of high altitude on fetal development, and the newborn's adaptive mechanisms for dealing with high altitude are discussed.

Whereas the respiratory physiology of the adult highlander has been the object of many studies,[2,3] the available information on the infant highlander is little and scattered. When necessary, therefore, data derived from observations on newborn animals experimentally exposed to hypobaric or normobaric hypoxic conditions are mentioned to complement the human data.

FETAL OXYGENATION AT HIGH ALTITUDE

At sea level, the partial pressure of O_2 (Po_2) of the umbilical vein (which is the major determinant of the arterial Po_2 of the fetus [$Pao_{2\,fet}$]) is approximately 30 mm Hg (i.e., much less than the maternal value [$Pao_{2\,mat}$], about 95 mm Hg) and 5 to 10 mm Hg less than the Po_2 of the uterine venous blood. Despite major differences in the functional anatomy of the placental barrier among species, in general, the Po_2 of the umbilical vein behaves as if it was closely related to that of the uterine venous blood.[4,5] Therefore because of the shape of the oxyhemoglobin curve, almost flat above 70 mm Hg, even very high values of $Pao_{2\,mat}$ during hyperoxic breathing have minimal effects on uterine venous Po_2 and $Pao_{2\,fet}$. Conversely, during modest maternal hypoxemia, such as during jet air travel, no signs of fetal hypoxemia are apparent[6] because a drop in uterine venous Po_2 and $Pao_{2\,fet}$ is expected only when $Pao_{2\,mat}$ decreases below approximately 70 mm Hg. During chronic hypoxia, an increase in uterine oxygen delivery and placental diffusing capacity can further drop the $Pao_{2\,mat}$ threshold for fetal hypoxemia.[7]

Data on maternal and fetal oxygenation at high altitude are almost entirely derived from measurements on chronically instrumented sheep. Metcalfe et al[8] observed values of umbilical venous Po_2 in sheep fetuses at high altitude that were close to values in fetuses at sea level. Measurements performed on animals acutely exposed to 10,000 and 15,000 feet of simulated altitude indicated that $Po_{2\,fet}$ dropped by about 5 and 7 mm Hg,[9,10] respectively, slowly increasing again after several days[11]; hence, during sustained hypoxia, despite the low $Pao_{2\,mat}$, fetal oxygenation appears to be very well protected, probably by the combination of numerous compensatory factors that could include a reduction in oxygen consumption ($\dot{V}o_2$) of the nonessential fetal organs,[7] maternal hyperventilation,[12] and increases in uterine oxygen delivery, hematocrit, hemoglobin levels,[8,13] and placental mass. The last, well documented in high-altitude women,[3,14] is accompanied by morphologic and ultrastructural changes that can improve the placental diffusion capacity by shortening the diffusion distance.[15]

At high altitude, after the immediate acute drop after the onset of maternal hypoxemia, $Pao_{2\,fet}$ in the subsequent weeks gradually rises to almost, albeit not quite, the value at sea level.[11,16] There are very few data for humans. The Pao_2 from the scalp of human fetuses during delivery was almost the same at 4200 m (average, 19 mm Hg) and at sea level (21.5 mm Hg).[17]

In summary, the data available from human and, mostly, animal observations indicate that during chronic maternal hypoxemia at high altitude, $Pao_{2\,fet}$ also drops, although by only a small amount because of numerous compensatory mechanisms at the maternal, placental, and fetal level.

Hematocrit and hemoglobin concentration at birth are slightly higher in high-altitude infants,[3,18] similar to what was found in sheep studies and in newborn rats after gestation at simulated high altitude.[19] On the other hand, the reported hematocrit values of infants in Leadville, Colorado (~3100 m), are close to the upper end of the normal range.[20-22]

The concentration of fetal hemoglobin at birth was also higher in the infant highlander.[18] This erythropoietic response is one of several considerations (see later section) suggesting the presence of chronic fetal hypoxemia at high altitude despite the maternal and placental compensatory mechanisms and the minimal difference in $Pao_{2\,fet}$ from the value at sea level. At the low $Pao_{2\,fet}$, the high O_2 affinity of the fetal hemoglobin means that even minute changes in $Po_{2\,fet}$ might have sizable effects on arterial O_2 saturation.

BODY WEIGHT AT BIRTH

A reduction in infant birth weight and increased infant mortality at high altitude have been documented by numerous

*O_2 *concentration* refers to the molar concentration of O_2, milliliters of O_2 (standard temperature and pressure, dry) per milliliter of air (body temperature, pressure, saturation), which decreases with the drop in barometric pressure; fractional concentration, on the other hand, is approximately 0.21, irrespective of altitude.

studies.[14,21] Irrespective of the high-altitude population surveyed, birth weight and postnatal growth were consistently found to be lower than at low altitude.[3] In La Paz, Bolivia,* the average weight of babies born at term from women of Spanish or mixed descent was lower than that of Quechua and Aymara natives despite the opposite trend in socioeconomic status.[23] A study of white births in the United States, based on more than 12 million birth files between 1978 and 1981 and controlled for socioeconomic factors, also revealed that an infant's birth weight was inversely proportional to the altitude of the mother's residence for altitudes above 1000 m[24] (Fig. 10-1). In addition, child growth was less than it was in lowlanders,[25] a conclusion also supported by analysis of the growth pattern of well-nourished children of European ancestry living in the Bolivian Andes.[26] Because the reduced growth rate was still apparent after controlling for birth weight, it was concluded that the blunted growth of the infant highlander was the combined result of the low birth weight caused by prenatal hypoxia and the postnatal effect of altitude.[25] High-altitude mothers of infants with low birth weight also had lower hemoglobin concentrations,[21] a finding in accord with the notion of the importance of maternal oxygenation on fetal growth at high altitude.

*In La Paz, Bolivia, at an altitude of 3600 to 4050 m, the average inspired Po_2 was 93 mm Hg, and the inspiratory concentration of O_2 was 0.11 ml of O_2 (standard temperature and pressure, dry) per milliliter of air (body temperature, pressure, saturation).

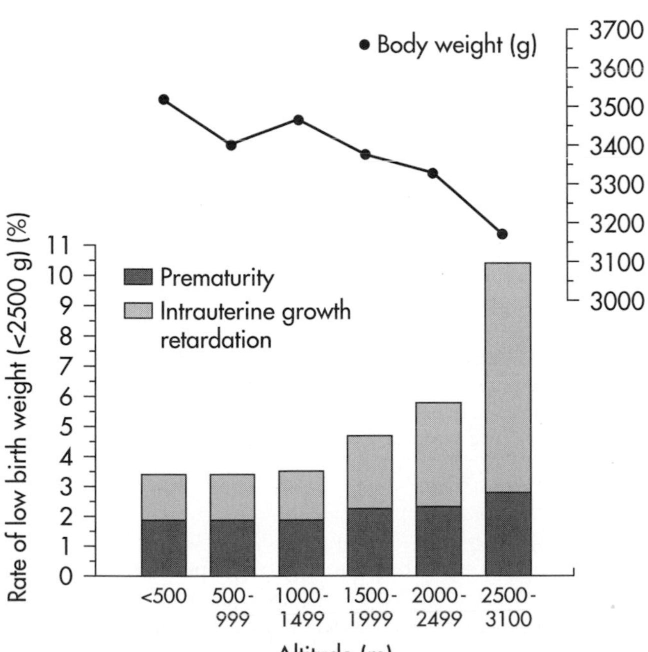

Fig. 10-1. *Top,* Mean body weight at birth for white infants in the United States as a function of the altitude of the mother's residence. *Bottom,* Rate of low birth weight (<2500 g) as a function of the altitude in infants born before 37 weeks' gestation (prematurity) or born at term (intrauterine growth retardation). Most of the increase in the rate of low birth weight with altitude is related to the group with intrauterine growth retardation. (Modified from Yip R: *J Pediatr* 11:869-876, 1987.)

The effect of maternal acclimatization before gestation on neonatal outcome has not been studied in humans. In the rat, low birth weight at high altitude was unaffected by the presence or absence of maternal acclimatization to hypoxia before gestation.[19] Indeed, ventilatory acclimatization is normally completed in a few days in the rat and in a few weeks in humans, which is probably too small a fraction of the whole gestation period to cause sizable effects on fetal development and neonatal outcome. On the other hand, during gestation at high altitude, the degree of maternal hyperventilation positively correlated with the infant's birth weight because the hyperventilation protected fetal arterial oxygenation.[12,21] This result probably reflected a fine balance between the advantages of increasing $Pao_{2\ mat}$ and the disadvantages related to the alkalosis; extreme maternal hyperventilation and alkalosis, in fact, decrease fetal oxygenation, possibly because of the Bohr effect and decreased uteroplacental perfusion.[27]

In summary, despite the well-known difficulties in determining the potential contribution of nutritional, demographic, and socioeconomic factors,[28] the evidence suggests that at high altitude in humans, as in other species, hypoxia is the primary cause of reduced birth weight and postnatal growth.

DEFENSE AGAINST HYPOXIA

Because, in mammals, O_2 transfer other than via the lungs is negligible, over a fixed period of time the total $\dot{V}o_2$ equals the difference between the quantity of O_2 inhaled (O_2 in) and the quantity of O_2 exhaled (O_2 ex), as follows:

$$\dot{V}o_2 = O_{2\ in} - O_{2\ ex} \tag{1}$$

$O_{2\ in}$ and $O_{2\ ex}$ are the product of, respectively, the inspired and expired airflow ($\dot{V}$) and the corresponding O_2 concentrations (c), as follows:

$$O_{2\ in} = \dot{V}_{1\ in} \bullet co_{2\ in} \tag{2}$$

$$O_{2\ ex} = \dot{V}_{ex} \bullet co_{2\ ex} \tag{3}$$

The difference between $\dot{V}_{in}$ and $\dot{V}_{ex}$ introduced by a respiratory quotient less than 1 is negligible; hence, both $\dot{V}_{in}$ and $\dot{V}_{ex}$ can be considered equal to minute ventilation ($\dot{V}E$). Therefore substitution of Equations 2 and 3 into Equation 1 yields the following:

$$\dot{V}o_2 = O_{2\ in} - O_{2\ ex} = \dot{V}E \bullet (co_{2\ in} - co_{2\ ex}) \tag{4}$$

It is useful to rearrange this equation, as follows:

$$\dot{V}o_2 = (\dot{V}E \bullet co_{2\ in}) \bullet [(co_{2\ in} - co_{2\ ex})/co_{2\ in}] \tag{5}$$

which states that total O_2 consumption ($\dot{V}o_2$) equals the product of ventilatory O_2 delivery ($\dot{V}E \bullet co_{2\ in}$) and the O_2 extracted from the inspired air, or O_2 extraction coefficient ($co_{2\ in} - co_{2\ ex})/co_{2\ in}$.

Equation 5 implies that the drop in $co_{2\ in}$ at high altitude can be compensated for by (1) an increase in $\dot{V}E$ (hyperpnea), (2) a drop in O_2 use (hypometabolism), (3) an increase in O_2 extraction, or (4) any combination of these factors. On acute exposure to hypoxia, the first and second responses commonly occur in both adult and newborn mammals, including humans, although hyperpnea tends to prevail among adult species and hypometabolism among newborns.[29-31]

Ventilation and Metabolism in the Infant Highlander

The values of $\dot{V}E$ measured in infants at high altitude are very close to those recorded at low altitude.[32-34] The lack of hyperpnea could have been interpreted as indicating that hypometabolism was the primary mechanism by which the infant highlander's body responded to the low levels of inspired oxygen, similar to what has been observed in the lowlander infant and many other newborn species on exposure to acute hypoxia.[29] However, this interpretation is incorrect. Comparison of both ventilatory and metabolic rates ($\dot{V}O_2$ and carbon dioxide production [$\dot{V}CO_2$]) between 1-day-old infants (Native Amerindians and mestizos) born at high altitude and infants of the same body weight born at low altitude, either from the same race or from a Caucasian population, revealed that neither parameter differed significantly; the major difference was in the O_2 extraction, which was much increased (>160%) in the highlanders[35] (Fig. 10-2). In other words, in contrast to the lowlander's response to acute hypoxia, the mechanism against the low $co_{2\,in}$ used by the infant born at high altitude was neither an increase in gas convection nor a reduction in O_2 use; rather it was a more efficient extraction of O_2 from the inspired air.

The increased O_2 extraction was observed even when breathing pure O_2,[35] which eliminates the hypoxic stimulation of the peripheral chemoreceptors. Hence, the high O_2 extraction of the neonatal highlander was interpreted as the expression of mechanisms that included not only functional but also structural adaptations to the chronic hypoxemia. This interpretation, of course, implies that fetal oxygenation during gestation was less than at sea level and that the fetus was able to recognize the hypoxemia and respond to it.

O_2 Extraction

Information on the mechanisms potentially involved in the enhanced O_2 extraction of the infant at high altitude is fragmentary and incomplete.

In 1- to 2-day-old infants at high altitude, the compliance of the respiratory system is approximately 35% higher than in infants of the same age at low altitude[34] (Fig. 10-3). Because chest wall compliance is only a minimal component of the total compliance of the respiratory system in infants,[36] the finding probably indicates an increased lung compliance. Adult highlanders have higher lung compliance than lowlanders of the same age and race,[37] whereas no increase in compliance occurs in the sojourner at high altitude.[38] Levels of lung deoxyribonucleic acid and proteins are decreased in fetuses of hypoxic rats,[19,39,40] and the process of alveolar septation is reduced in rat pups that are hypoxic during gestation[41]; fewer alveolar attachments to the bronchioles could decrease lung recoil and therefore increase lung compliance.[42] In such a case, the increased compliance at birth would be a manifestation of inhibited lung growth during the fetal period and may not necessarily be advantageous for the gas-exchange function of the neonatal lung. No measurements of pulmonary gas diffusion capacity are available in the newborn; at 4 to 6 years of age, children in La Paz, Bolivia, have higher values than children at sea level.[43]

Breathing in the infant highlander is deeper and slower than in lowlanders (Fig. 10-4), a pattern that $\dot{V}E$ being the same (see Fig. 10-2), maximizes alveolar ventilation. The deeper tidal volume is probably favored by the higher lung compliance. On the other hand, the functional basis for the tendency to a lower breathing rate and particularly a longer expiratory time is not

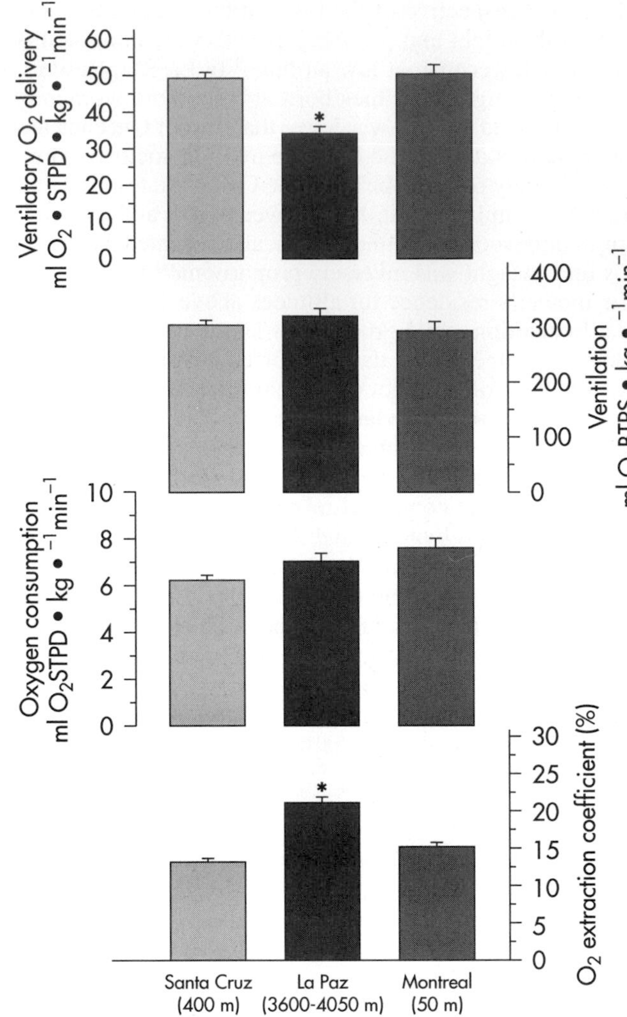

Fig. 10-2. The three parameters of Equation 5 (see text) are compared between 1-day old infants at low altitude (Santa Cruz, Bolivia, and Montreal) and high altitude (La Paz, Bolivia). Ventilatory O_2 delivery ($\dot{V}E \bullet co_{2\,in}$) is lower in the high-altitude group because of the lower $co_{2\,in}$ not compensated for by an increase in $\dot{V}E$. $\dot{V}O_2$ and $\dot{V}E$ do not significantly differ. However, at high altitude, O_2 extraction $[(co_{2\,in} - co_{2\,ex})/co_{2\,in}]$ is much higher than at low altitude. There were 30 infants in the Santa Cruz group, 30 in the La Paz group, and 25 in the Montreal group. Bars indicate 1 standard error, and asterisks indicate the significant difference between the two groups. *STPD,* Standard temperature and pressure, dry; *BTPS,* body temperature, pressure, saturation. (Data from Mortola JP et al: *Am Rev Respir Dis* 146:11-15,1992; and Mortola JP et al: *Am Rev Respir Dis* 146:1206-1209, 1992.)

clear. It cannot be attributed to a stronger pulmonary vagal inhibition. In fact, analysis of the response to brief airway occlusions indicates that the strength of the vagal Hering-Breuer expiratory-promoting reflex is reduced in high-altitude infants, presumably because of the stronger hypoxic chemical drive.[44]

In summary, in addition to the hematologic changes previously mentioned (increased hematocrit and hemoglobin levels), pulmonary factors could contribute to the enhanced O_2 extraction of the infant highlander. Because they were not observed in the lowlanders of the same ethnic group, these changes have been interpreted primarily as the effects of prenatal hypoxia rather than as genetic traits. This, of course, does

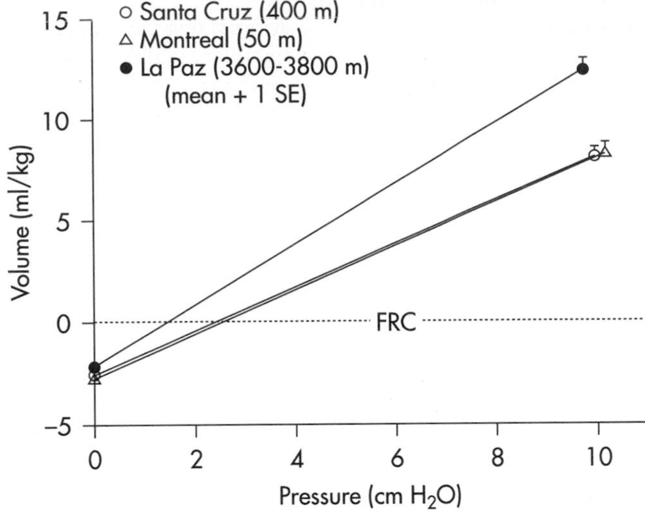

Fig. 10-3. Group average pressure-volume curve of infants studied in La Paz, Bolivia ($N = 34$); Santa Cruz, Bolivia ($N = 36$); and Montreal ($N = 33$). In the high-altitude group, compliance of the respiratory system (the slope of the pressure-volume curve) was significantly higher than in the low-altitude groups. Symbols represent group mean, and bars indicate 1 standard error *(SE)*. *FRC,* Functional residual capacity. (Modified from Mortola JP et al: *Am Rev Respir Dis* 142:43-48, 1990.)

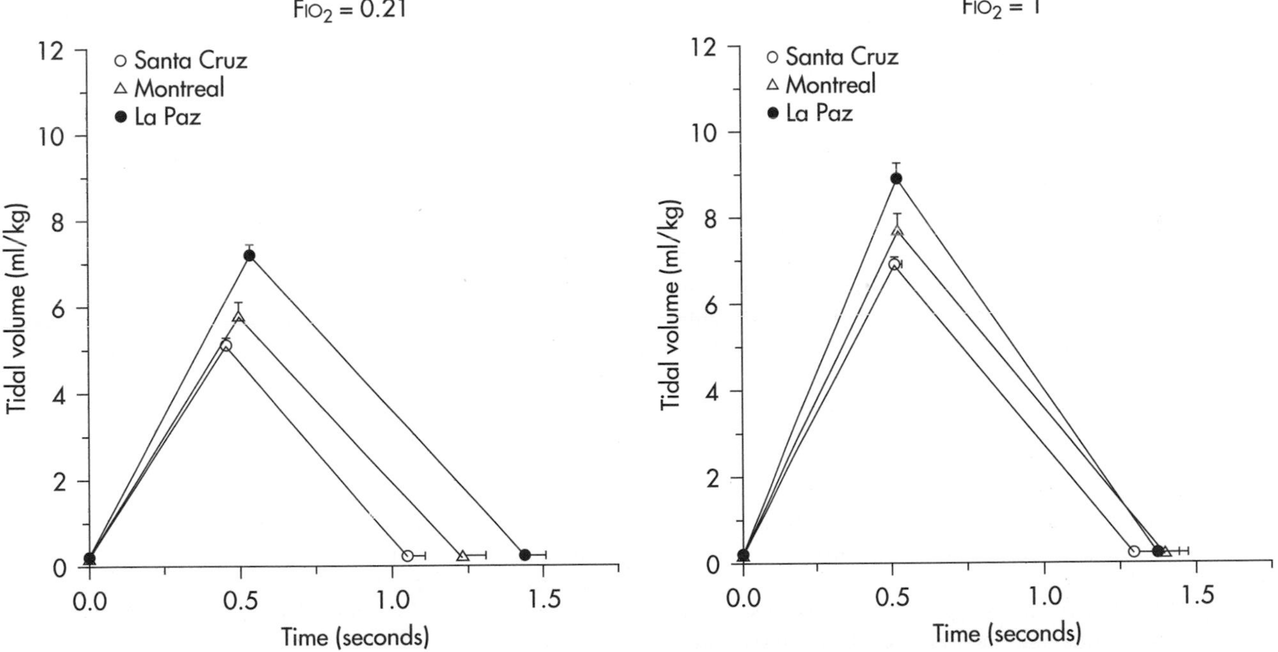

Fig. 10-4. Average spirogram during air breathing (fractional inspired O_2 [FIO_2] = 0.21) and hyperoxia ($FIO_2 = 1$) in infant highlanders (La Paz, Bolivia, $N = 30$, *filled circles*) and infant lowlanders of the same race (Santa Cruz, Bolivia, $N = 30$, *circles*) or of a Caucasian population (Montreal, $N = 25$, *triangles*). Average body weights of the three groups were comparable. With a similar minute ventilation (see Fig. 10-2), the deeper and slower pattern of the highlanders favors alveolar ventilation. Bars indicate 1 standard error. (From the data of Mortola JP et al: *Am Rev Respir Dis* 146:11-15,1992; and Mortola JP et al: *Am Rev Respir Dis* 146:1206-1209, 1992.)

not exclude the possibility that genetic factors can play a role in the respiratory adaptation of the highlander, as suggested by comparisons of some pulmonary function tests on youths highlanders of European and Andean origin.[45,46]

VENTILATORY CHEMOSENSITIVITY

At high altitude, adult natives have lower $\dot{V}E$ and PaO_2 and a higher arterial partial pressure of carbon dioxide ($PaCO_2$) than newcomers[2,47]; their $\dot{V}E$ response to hypoxia becomes apparent at lower values of inspired O_2 concentrations (FIO_2) than in lowlanders; therefore at the same FIO_2 or PaO_2, their $\dot{V}E$ is lower than in lowlanders.[3] Several indications suggest that the loss of ventilatory drive during chronic hypoxia is an acquired rather than a genetic characteristic of high-altitude populations.[2,47] It would be of interest to know to what extent the highlander's modifications of hypoxic chemosensitivity are apparent at birth as the result of the chronic fetal hypoxemia, but very few data are available, whether from human or animal studies.

The immediate effect of hyperoxia is a reduction in $\dot{V}E$[32] by a similar amount in both high- and low-altitude infants. To the extent that hyperoxia eliminates the activity of peripheral chemoafferents, the similar drop in $\dot{V}E$ would indicate a similar chemoreceptor-mediated respiratory drive in the two groups. This surprising conclusion could be explained by the fact that air breathing during the early postnatal period, even at high altitude, substantially increases PaO_2 relative to the fetal value; hence, it probably decreases chemoreceptor activity to a low value, as shown in animal studies,[48] irrespective of altitude. In older infants (2 to 6 month of age) the drop in $\dot{V}E$ with hyperoxia seemed to be more marked and sustained, but only four subjects were studied, and there were no lowlander controls.[32]

After the sudden drop in $\dot{V}E$ in hyperoxia, the infant's $\dot{V}E$ increases above the control value.[49-51] The mechanisms responsible for this response, partly contributed by a rise in $\dot{V}O_2$, are not completely understood[52]; nevertheless, the steady-state value of hyperoxic hyperpnea was identical between infants of low and high altitudes.[35]

A drop of the inspired O_2 (from an inspired pressure of 91 mm Hg to lower values) resulted in a biphasic $\dot{V}E$ response, which was similar in lowlander and highlander infants.[32] It would be of interest to compare these responses to the corresponding metabolic adjustments because the magnitude of the metabolic drop during hypoxia can influence the level of $\dot{V}E$.[53]

No study seems to have investigated the $\dot{V}E$ response to hypercapnia in high-altitude infants. Lahiri et al[32] attempted such a measurement; although both low- and high-altitude infants responded to moderate levels of carbon dioxide, their frequent awakening during the test precluded a definite quantitative comparison.

In children and adults with chronic hypoxia resulting from congenital cyanotic heart disease, there was no obvious relationship between arterial O_2 desaturation and partial pressure of carbon dioxide, the latter often maintained around the normal value.[54] This finding coincides with that from a later study documenting the poor hypoxic hyperventilation of patients with cyanotic heart disease, which could be interpreted as loss of hypoxic chemosensitivity resulting from the chronic hypoxic status.[55]

LONG-TERM EFFECTS OF NEONATAL HYPOXIA

Animal observations indicate that body growth, impaired during the prenatal and neonatal hypoxia, resumes at a higher rate on return to normoxia and that body weight eventually reaches the control value.[56,57] The phenomenon of "catch-up" growth[58] can also occur in children with growth retardation because of cyanotic heart disease when the disease is corrected.[58,59] This information can probably be extrapolated to the condition of the high-altitude infant, although specific studies have not been performed to determine whether the low birth weight of the infant highlander can be corrected on descent to low altitude.

Numerous and convincing data indicate that the blunted $\dot{V}E$ response to hypoxia of the adult highlander persists for some years after descent to sea level, although the phenomenon may not be completely irreversible.[47,60] Whether chronic hypoxia in the early phases of development would be sufficient for long-lasting effects is a question of obvious importance both from the biologic and clinical viewpoints. In humans, this could be examined in a carefully selected group of adults who were born after full-term gestation at high altitude and who migrated to low altitude during early childhood; however, the information in this respect is only anecdotal. In a study by Sørensen and Severinghaus,[61] the only two subjects who would fulfill these criteria (two high-altitude natives who moved to sea level at 2 and 7 years of age) had no response to hypoxia 16 years after they left the high-altitude area. Patients studied at least 1 year after correction of congenital tetralogy of Fallot still presented a blunted response to hypoxia[62]; a later report[55] denied the long-lasting irreversibility of the blunted $\dot{V}E$ response, but its conclusion was based on the preoperative and postoperative comparison of only three patients with congenital cardiac disease that may not have caused continuous hypoxemia before surgical correction.

Young rats exposed to hypoxia since birth exhibited a reduced $\dot{V}E$ response to hypoxia.[63] In young adult rats exposed to hypoxia only during the first week after birth, several changes in respiratory control and mechanics and pulmonary circulation were apparent[56,57,64,65]; among these, the findings of a blunted response to hypoxia and of increased lung size and lung compliance are of interest because they are considered part of the native highlander's characteristics. These changes were not seen in adult rats exposed to similar degrees of hypoxia after weaning (i.e., at a much later stage of postnatal development). Hence, these observations would corroborate the notion that the highlander's respiratory features can be acquired and are not necessarily genetic traits. In addition, they support the concept that neonatal hypoxia is both necessary and sufficient for long-term alterations in respiratory function and control.

CONCLUSIONS

At birth, the newborn at high altitude is small, but its metabolic rate and $\dot{V}E$ are comparable to those of lowlanders of the same body weight. In some respects, this fact summarizes the mechanisms against hypoxia that the highlander will use throughout life. Body growth will be slightly reduced, and the adult's body weight may be lower than it would have been at sea level. However, this is a small compromise for the advantages of protecting body functions, body temperature, and metabolic rate without the energetic cost and acid-base unbalance of strenuous hyperventilation.

The key feature of the highlander's mechanisms against hypoxia is increased O_2 extraction; this option is quite clearly manifested at birth, most likely not because of genetic characteristics but because of mechanisms triggered by the chronic fetal hypoxemia. The extent to which the pulmonary structural alterations induced by prenatal hypoxia participate in the increased O_2 extraction of the postnatal period is not clear. Unlike the hematologic and cardiovascular functions, the change in lung physiology at birth is so drastic that the structural alterations of the lung during prenatal hypoxia may not necessarily carry adaptive value after birth.

REFERENCES

1. Heath D, Williams DR: *Man at high altitude,* ed 2, Edinburgh, 1981, Churchill Livingstone.
2. Weil JV: Ventilatory control at high altitude. In Cherniack NS, Widdicombe JG, eds: *Handbook of physiology,* Section 3: The respiratory system, vol 2, part 2: Control of breathing, Bethesda, Md, 1986, American Physiological Society, pp 703-727.
3. Monge C, León-Velarde F: Physiological adaptation to high altitude: oxygen transport in mammals and birds, *Physiol Rev* 71:1135-1172, 1991.

Fetal Oxygenation at High Altitude

4. Longo LD: Respiratory gas exchange in the placenta. In Farhi LE, Tenney SM, eds: *Handbook of physiology,* Section 3: The respiratory system, vol 4: Gas exchange, Bethesda, Md, 1986, American Physiological Society, pp 351-401.
5. Wilkening RB: The placenta: O_2 transfer. In Sutton JR, Houston CS, Coates G, eds: *Hypoxia: the tolerable limits,* Indianapolis, 1988, Benchmark, pp 221-232.
6. Huch R, Baumann H, Fallenstein F, Schneider KTM, Holdener F, Huch A: Physiologic changes in pregnant women and their fetuses during jet air travel, *Am J Obstet Gynecol* 154:996-1000, 1986.
7. Edelstone DI: The fetus: responses to reduced O_2 delivery. In Sutton JR, Houston CS, Coates G, eds: *Hypoxia: the tolerable limits,* Indianapolis, 1988, Benchmark, pp 251-261.
8. Metcalfe J, Meschia G, Hellegers A, Prystowsky H, Huckabee W, Barron DH: Observations on the placental exchange of the respiratory gases in pregnant ewes at high altitude, *Q J Exp Physiol* 47:74-92, 1962.
9. Cotter JR, Blechner JN, Prystowsky H: Observations on pregnancy at altitude. I. The respiratory gases in maternal arterial and uterine venous blood, *Am J Obstet Gynecol* 99:1-8, 1967.
10. Blechner JN, Cotter JR, Hinkley CM, Prystowsky H: Observations on pregnancy at altitude. II. Transplacental pressure differences of oxygen and carbon dioxide, *Am J Obstet Gynecol* 102:794-805, 1968.
11. Makowshi EL, Battaglia FC, Meschia G, Behrman RE, Schruefer J, Seeds AE, Bruns PD: Effect of maternal exposure to high altitude upon fetal oxygenation, *Am J Obstet Gynecol* 100:852-861, 1968.
12. Moore LG, Brodeur P, Chumbe O, D'Brot J, Hofmeister S, Monge C: Maternal hypoxic ventilatory response, ventilation, and infant birth weight at 4300 m, *J Appl Physiol* 60:1401-1406, 1986.
13. Kitanaka T, Gilbert RD, Longo LD: Maternal responses to long-term hypoxemia in sheep, *Am J Physiol* 256:R1340-R1347, 1989.
14. McClung J: *Effects of high altitude on human birth: observations on mothers, placentas, and the newborn in two Peruvian populations,* Cambridge, Mass, 1969, Harvard University Press, pp 1-150.
15. Gilbert RD, Cummings LA, Juchau MR, Longo LD: Placental diffusing capacity and fetal development in exercising or hypoxic guinea pigs, *J Appl Physiol* 46:828-834, 1979.
16. Kitanaka T, Alonso JG, Gilbert RD, Siu BL, Clemons GK, Longo LD: Fetal responses to long-term hypoxemia in sheep, *Am J Physiol* 256:R1348-R1354, 1989.
17. Sobrevilla LA, Cassinelli MT, Carcelen A, Malaga JM: Human fetal and maternal oxygen tension and acid-base status during delivery at high altitude, *Am J Obstet Gynecol* 111:1111-1118, 1971.
18. Ballew C, Haas JD: Hematologic evidence of fetal hypoxia among newborn infants at high altitude in Bolivia, *Am J Obstet Gynecol* 155:166-169, 1986.
19. Gleed RD, Mortola JP: Ventilation in newborn rats after gestation at simulated high altitude, *J Appl Physiol* 70:1146-1151, 1991.
20. Howard RC, Bruns PD, Lichty JA: Studies of babies born at high altitude. III. Arterial oxygen saturation and hematocrit values at birth, *Am Med Assoc J Dis Child* 93:674-678, 1957.
21. Moore LG, Rounds SS, Jahnigen D, Grover RF, Reeves JT: Infant birth weight is related to maternal arterial oxygenation at high altitude, *J Appl Physiol* 52:695-699, 1982.
22. Niermeyer S, Shaffer EM, Thilo E, Corbin C, Moore LG: Arterial oxygenation and pulmonary arterial pressure in healthy neonates and infants at high altitude, *J Pediatr* 123:767-772, 1993.

Body Weight at Birth

23. Haas JD, Frongillo EA, Stepick CD, Beard JL, Hurtado LG: Altitude, ethnic and sex difference in birth weight and length in Bolivia, *Hum Biol* 52:459-477, 1980.
24. Yip R: Altitude and birth weight, *J Pediatr* 111:869-876, 1987.
25. Yip R, Binkin NJ, Trowbridge FL: Altitude and childhood growth, *J Pediatr* 113:486-489, 1988.
26. Greksa LP: Effect of altitude on the stature, chest depth and forced vital capacity of low-to-high altitude migrant children of European ancestry, *Hum Biol* 60:23-32, 1988.
27. Huch R: Maternal hyperventilation and the fetus, *J Perinat Med* 14:3-17, 1986.
28. Greksa LP, Spielvogel H, Caceres E: Effect of altitude on the physical growth of upper-class children of European ancestry, *Ann Hum Biol* 12:225-232, 1985.

Defense Against Hypoxia

29. Mortola JP, Rezzonico R, Lanthier C: Ventilation and oxygen consumption during acute hypoxia in newborn mammals: a comparative analysis, *Respir Physiol* 78:31-43, 1989.
30. Frappell P, Lanthier C, Beaudinette RV, Mortola JP: Metabolism and ventilation in acute hypoxia: a comparative analysis in small mammalian species, *Am J Physiol* 262:R1040-R1046, 1992.
31. Mortola JP: Hypoxic hypometabolism in mammals, *News Physiol Sci* 8:79-82, 1993.
32. Lahiri S, Brody JS, Motoyama EK, Velasquez TM: Regulation of breathing in newborns at high altitude, *J Appl Physiol* 44:673-678, 1978.
33. Cotton EK, Grunstein MM: Effects of hypoxia on respiratory control in neonates at high altitude, *J Appl Physiol* 48:587-595, 1980.
34. Mortola JP, Rezzonico R, Fisher JT, Villena-Cabrera N, Vargas E, Gonzáles R, Peña F: Compliance of the respiratory system in infants born at high altitude, *Am Rev Respir Dis* 142:43-48, 1990.
35. Mortola JP, Frappell PB, Frappell DE, Villena-Cabrera N, Villena-Cabrera M, Peña F: Ventilation and gaseous metabolism in infants born at high altitude and their responses to hyperoxia, *Am Rev Respir Dis* 146:1206-1209, 1992.
36. Mortola JP: Dynamics of breathing in newborn mammals, *Physiol Rev* 67:187-243, 1987.
37. Brody JS, Lahiri S, Simpser M, Motoyama EK, Velasquez T: Lung elasticity and airway dynamics in Peruvian natives to high altitude, *J Appl Physiol* 42:245-251, 1977.
38. Gautier H, Peslin R, Grassino A, Milic-Emili J, Hannhart B, Powell E, Miserocchi G, Bonora M, Fischer JT: Mechanical properties of the lungs during acclimatization to altitude, *J Appl Physiol* 52:1407-1415, 1982.
39. Larson JE, Thurlbeck WM: The effect of experimental maternal hypoxia on fetal lung growth, *Pediatr Res* 24:156-159, 1988.
40. Faridy EE, Sanii MR, Thliveris JA: Fetal lung growth: influence of maternal hypoxia and hyperoxia in rats, *Respir Physiol* 73:225-242, 1988.
41. Massaro GD, Olivier J, Massaro D: Short term perinatal 10% O_2 alters postnatal development of lung alveoli, *Am J Physiol* 257:L221-L225, 1989.
42. Massaro GD, Olivier J, Dzikowiki C, Massaro D: Postnatal development of lung alveoli: suppression by 13% O_2 and a critical period, *Am J Physiol* 258:L321-L327, 1990.
43. Vargas E, Beard J, Haas J, Cudkowicz L: Pulmonary diffusing capacity in young Andean high-land children, *Respiration* 43:330-335, 1982.
44. Mortola JP, Trippenbach T, Rezzonico R, Fisher JT, Diaz M, Villena-Cabrera N, Peña F: Hering-Breuer reflexes in high-altitude infants, *Clin Sci* 88:345-350, 1995.
45. Greksa LP, Spielvogel H, Caceres E, Paredes-Fernandez L: Lung function of young Aymara highlanders, *Ann Hum Biol* 14:533-542, 1987.
46. Greksa LP, Spielvogel H, Paz-Zamora M, Caceres E, Paredes-Fernández L: Effect of altitude on the lung function of high altitude residents of European ancestry, *Am J Phys Anthropol* 75:77-85, 1988.

Ventilatory Chemosensitivity

47. Severinghaus JW: Hypoxic respiratory drive and its loss during chronic hypoxia, *Clin Physiol* 2:57-79, 1972.
48. Blanco CE, Dawes GS, Hanson MA, McCooke HB: The response to hypoxia of arterial chemoreceptors in fetal sheep and new-born lambs, *J Physiol (Lond)* 351:25-37, 1984.
49. Cross KW, Warner P: The effect of inhalation of high and low oxygen concentrations on the respiration of the newborn infant, *J Physiol (Lond)* 114:283-295, 1951.
50. Davi M, Sankaran K, Rigatto H: Effect of inhaling 100% O_2 on ventilation and acid-base balance in cerebrospinal fluid of neonates, *Biol Neonate* 38:85-89, 1980.
51. Mortola JP, Frappell PB, Dotta A, Matsuoka T, Fox G, Weeks S, Mayer D: Ventilatory and metabolic responses to acute hyperoxia in newborns, *Am Rev Respir Dis* 146:11-15, 1992.
52. Daristotle L, Engwall MJ, Niu W, Bisgard GE: Ventilatory effects and interactions with change in Pa_{O_2} in awake goats, *J Appl Physiol* 71:254-260, 1991.
53. Mortola JP, Rezzonico R: Metabolic and ventilatory rates in newborn kittens during acute hypoxia, *Respir Physiol* 73:55-68, 1988.
54. Husson G, Otis AB: Adaptive value of respiratory adjustments to shunt hypoxia and to altitude hypoxia, *J Clin Invest* 36:270-278, 1957.
55. Edelman NH, Lahiri S, Braudo L, Cherniack NS, Fishman AP: The blunted ventilatory response to hypoxia in cyanotic congenital heart disease, *New Engl J Med* 282:405-411, 1970.

Long-Term Effects of Neonatal Hypoxia

56. Okubo S, Mortola JP: Long-term respiratory effects of neonatal hypoxia in the rat, *J Appl Physiol* 64:952-958, 1988.
57. Okubo S, Mortola JP: Respiratory mechanics in adult rats hypoxic in the neonatal period, *J Appl Physiol* 66:1772-1778, 1989.
58. Prader A, Tanner JM, von Harnack GA: Catch-up growth following illness or starvation, *J Pediatr* 62:646-659, 1963.
59. Gingell RL, Pieroni DR, Hornung MG: Growth problems associated with congenital heart disease in infancy. In Lebenthal E, ed: *Textbook of gastroenterology and nutrition in infancy,* vol 2, New York, 1981, Raven, pp 853-860.
60. Lahiri S: Respiratory control in Andean and Himalayan high-altitude natives. In West JB, Lahiri S, eds: *High altitude and man,* Bethesda, Md, 1984, American Physiological Society, pp 147-162.
61. Sørensen SC, Severinghaus JW: Irreversible respiratory insensitivity to acute hypoxia in man born at high altitude, *J Appl Physiol* 25:217-220, 1968.
62. Sørensen SC, Severinghaus JW: Respiratory insensitivity to acute hypoxia persisting after correction of tetralogy of Fallot, *J Appl Physiol* 25:221-223, 1968.
63. Eden GJ, Hanson MA: Effects of chronic hypoxia from birth on the ventilatory response to acute hypoxia in the newborn rat, *J Physiol (Lond)* 392:11-19,1987.
64. Okubo S, Mortola JP: Control of ventilation in adult rats hypoxic in the neonatal period, *Am J Physiol* 259:R836-R841, 1990.
65. Hakim TS, Mortola JP: Pulmonary vascular resistance in adult rats exposed to hypoxia in the neonatal period, *Can J Physiol Pharmaco* 68:419-424, 1990.

CHAPTER 11

Breathing in Unusual Environments

Michael A. Wall and Philip C. LaGesse

DIVING

A large number of medical conditions have been associated with breath-holding and scuba diving, and many texts and review articles on the subject are available.[1-4] This chapter concentrates on risk factors for injury that may be especially applicable to children with lung disease.

Gas Physics and Diving Equipment

The major risks to divers are associated with the behavior of gases in conditions of changing ambient pressure. Boyle's law states that in a closed system under conditions of constant temperature, the volume of gas is inversely proportional to the pressure applied to the system. This relationship explains one of the most potentially dangerous medical aspects of scuba diving: barotrauma associated with rapid ascent. Henry's law states that the amount of gas dissolved in a liquid at a constant temperature is proportional to the partial pressure of that gas. This law explains how blood can become supersaturated with gas, particularly nitrogen, as a scuba diver descends. On rapid ascent the nitrogen tends to come out of solution and form bubbles in blood and tissues, which may lead to the various manifestations of decompression sickness.

As a person descends from sea level, the ambient pressure increases by 1 atm for every 10 m (Fig. 11-1). In comparison, air is much less dense than water, and a person must ascend to an altitude of about 5450 m (18,000 ft) before the ambient pressure decreases to 0.5 atm. Fig. 11-1 depicts what happens to the relative volumes as a person ascends in increments of 10 m from various depths. For instance, as one goes from a depth of 30 to 20 m, the pressure decreases from 4 to 3 atm, and the volume of the system increases by a factor of 1.33. On the other hand, an ascent from 10 m to the surface leads to a doubling of volume. This is the reason that barotrauma caused by rapid expansion of gas often occurs at relatively shallow depths.

In essence, there are three ways that a human being can descend in the water (Fig. 11-2). In a submarine the hull resists compression, and the pressure inside is kept at about 1 atm. During a breath-hold dive, the respiratory system is compressed by ambient water pressure, and the volume decreases

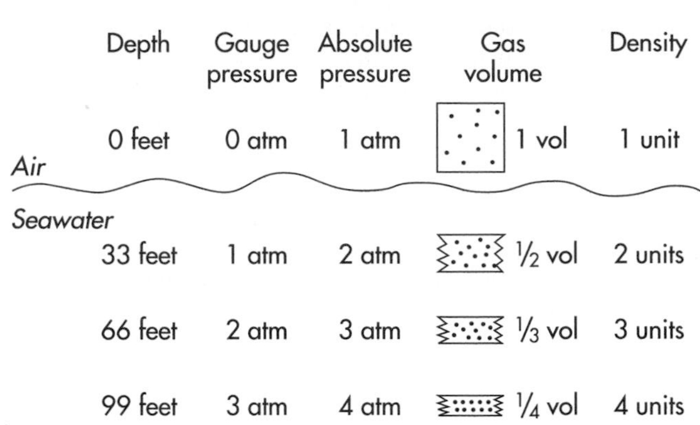

Fig. 11-1. Effect of increasing depth on relative ambient pressure and gas volume. (From Strauss RH, ed: *Diving medicine,* New York, 1976, Grune & Stratton.)

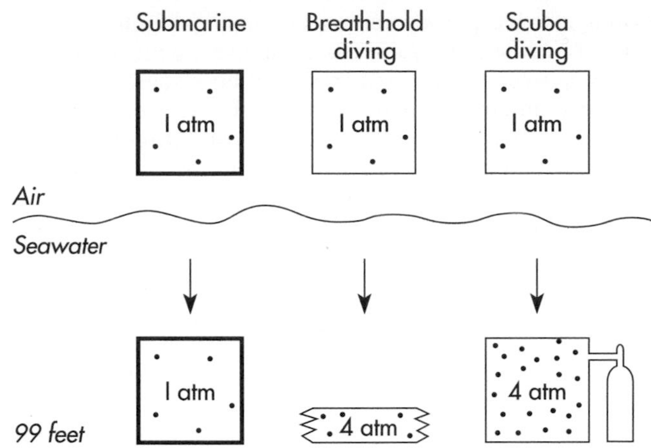

Fig. 11-2. Impact of the three methods of submersion on relative ambient pressure and gas volume. (From Strauss RH, ed: *Diving medicine,* New York, 1976, Grune & Stratton.)

according to Boyle's law. On ascent the ambient pressure decreases, and the lungs reexpand to approximately their original volume. Thus a breath-hold dive does not expose one to the risks associated with overdistention of the lungs. During scuba diving, however, one breathes compressed air at ambient pressure and maintains relatively normal lung volumes. The breathing of air at ambient pressure is made possible by the special features of scuba equipment. Typically this involves a two-stage regulator system. The first-stage regulator sits on top of the high-pressure tank and reduces the pressure from about 2000 to 5000 psi (135 to 350 atm) to 100 to 150 psi above ambient in the tubing going to the second stage. The second stage regulator is located at the mouthpiece and allows inhalation as the diver makes an inspiratory effort. At the end of inspiration, the pressure inside the lungs is equal to ambient as seen in Fig. 11-2.

Pulmonary Barotrauma

Assume that a scuba diver is breathing tidally at a lung volume of 50% of total lung capacity at a depth of 30 m with a gas pressure in the lungs of 4 atm. The diver then ascends to 10 m with the glottis and mouth tightly closed. At the new depth the pressure in the lungs is 2 atm, and the volume doubles to the total lung capacity. If the diver then ascends farther, the lung volume cannot expand to any significant degree, and transpulmonary pressure increases. At total lung capacity the transpulmonary pressure is usually 40 to 50 cm H_2O. When it reaches 80 to 100 cm H_2O, lung rupture ensues, leading to pneumothorax, pneumomediastinum, or air embolism. If a diver starts a closed-mouth rapid ascent at total lung capacity, which commonly occurs in panic situations, lung rupture occurs much sooner than if the ascent started at functional residual capacity. In fact, a rapid ascent from 2 m below the surface can cause lung rupture if one starts at total lung capacity.

For these reasons, scuba divers are instructed to ascend in one of two fashions. The usual ascent is made slowly while breathing in and out. During this ascent, the volume exhaled exceeds that inhaled on each breath, so lung rupture is avoided. If a rapid ascent is required, divers are instructed to exhale actively or keep the mouth and glottis open all the way to the surface.

Recommendations for Children with Lung Disease

Patients with obstructive lung disease may be especially prone to lung rupture during ascent from scuba diving. The reason for this is that areas of the lung communicating only poorly with the airways may not have enough time to empty before regional transpulmonary pressure rises to a level that causes rupture. This phenomenon depends on the time constant of the area in question, the relative volume in the area before ascent, and the rate of ascent. Examples of lung diseases that could predispose a diver to lung rupture include cystic fibrosis, bronchopulmonary dysplasia, and current asthma. An additional group of patients who should avoid scuba diving are those who have had a previous spontaneous pneumothorax or who have a condition that might predispose to pneumothorax (e.g., Marfan syndrome, Ehlers-Danlos syndrome). Although these patients do not have obstructive lung disease, they are thought to be at risk because lung rupture may occur at a lower transpulmonary pressure than in people without such risk factors.

Although scuba diving or snorkeling is clearly contraindicated in patients with active asthma, the recommendations are not as clear for people with mild asthma or a past history of asthma. Asymptomatic asthmatics may have abnormalities of lung function suggestive of air trapping or airway narrowing and therefore might be susceptible to pulmonary rupture. In addition, scuba diving may involve vigorous exercise while the diver breathes cool, dry air, and under these conditions, asthma may be precipitated. Various authors have made different recommendations for people with a past history of asthma who intend to dive, and the subject has been recently reviewed by Jenkins et al.[4] These conservative but realistic recommendations list the following contraindications to diving:

1. Current asthma
2. Past history of asthma with currently abnormal pulmonary function (At a minimum the subject should have normal spirometric values, including forced vital capacity, 1-second forced expiratory volume, and forced expiratory flow, mid-expiratory phase.)
3. Asthma in the past 5 years requiring medication (Other authors recommend 2 years.[2])
4. A history of exercise-induced asthma
5. Bronchial hyperresponsiveness to an inhalation challenge of hypertonic saline or cold air

As suggested, these recommendations may be quite conservative. A British survey of 104 scuba divers with asthma who had made over 12,000 dives revealed no instances of pneumothorax, air embolism, or even an asthma attack.[5] This survey was perhaps biased toward responses from asthmatics who dove without sustaining a problem, but it nonetheless indicates that the majority of asthmatics are not at high risk while diving. No legislated regulations govern diving by asthmatics.

Pulmonary Barotrauma: Signs and Symptoms

Lung rupture may cause mediastinal emphysema, pneumothorax, air embolism, or any combination thereof. The signs and symptoms of mediastinal rupture include chest pain, dyspnea, subcutaneous crepitus, dysphagia, and voice changes. Pneumothorax presents initially as sudden chest pain with dyspnea. Because air in the pleural cavity continues to expand until one reaches the surface, tension pneumothorax with decreased cardiac output is common. Air embolism is thought to result from rupture into the pulmonary veins with subsequent carriage of air bubbles into the arterial system. The bubbles lodge in small arteries virtually anywhere in the body, with the cerebral and coronary systems being the common sites. Thus air embolism may present as a sudden stroke with focal or global consequences or as a myocardial infarction.

Treatment

Mild mediastinal emphysema usually requires no treatment, although administration of oxygen may hasten its resolution. Divers thought to have a pneumothorax should be given oxygen in high concentration and transported to the nearest hospital for appropriate treatment, which may range from administration of oxygen to placement of a chest tube. Emergency, on-site relief of pressure from a tension pneumothorax may be required if cardiac output is severely impaired. Victims of suspected air embolism should be given high-concentration oxygen and transported in an emergent fashion to the nearest hyperbaric facility. In the United States, one can call the Divers Alert Network at Duke University 24 hours a day for advice and consultation ([919]684-8111).

Decompression Sickness

Decompression sickness (the bends or caisson disease) is caused by the release of nitrogen bubbles into the tissues and arterial system on ascent. During descent, nitrogen and oxygen are breathed at ambient pressure and pass into the bloodstream and tissues at progressively higher pressures. Much of the oxygen is consumed by metabolic demands, but the bulk of the nitrogen remains dissolved in a supersaturated fashion. The total amount of nitrogen dissolved in tissues increases as a function of both the depth and length of stay. Detailed tables are available to advise divers of their safe bottom time at any depth. This is the time a diver can stay at any given depth and safely ascend to the surface without making stops to decompress along the way. The signs and symptoms of decompression sickness range from pruritus and joint pain to severe neurologic dysfunction with spinal cord paralysis, stroke, cerebral edema, and death. Treatment includes the immediate administration of oxygen and transport to a hyperbaric chamber facility.

Other Medical Problems Associated with Diving

Patients with sinus disease may develop barotrauma on ascent in a fashion similar to pulmonary barotrauma. This usually presents as pain over the frontal sinuses with epistaxis and responds to conservative therapy with decongestants.[2] Recurrent otitis or serous otitis is another contraindication to breath-hold or scuba diving because barotrauma may occur during descent. The signs and symptoms range from a feeling of pressure and pain to tympanic rupture, hematotympanum, conductive hearing loss, and vertigo.[3] The etiology is an inability to equalize middle ear pressure with ambient pressure, which is usually caused by blockage or swelling of the eustachian tube. Treatment ranges from decongestants to surgery depending on the extent of injury.

ALTITUDE AND AIR TRAVEL

The major potential problem of ascent above sea level for children with lung disease is hypoxemia. Barometric pressure decreases in an exponential fashion with altitude (Fig. 11-3), although from sea level to 4000 m, the relationship is for all practical purposes linear. The most frequent questions concerning children with lung disease and altitude are about air travel in which the cabin is pressurized to an altitude of 1500 to 2400 m. The authors have also been asked to give recommendations concerning hang gliding, skiing, and the feasibility of obtaining a pilot's license.

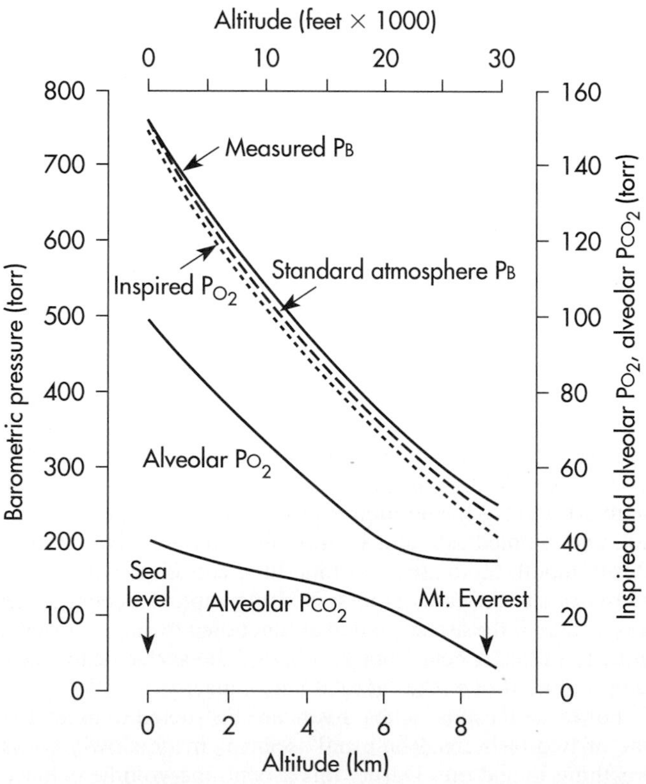

Fig. 11-3. Effect of altitude on barometric pressure (*PB*) and fraction of inspired oxygen. PO_2, Partial pressure of oxygen; PCO_2, partial pressure of carbon dioxide. (From West JB. In Crystal RG, West JB, eds: *The lung,* New York, 1991, Raven, pp 2093-2108.)

At 1500 m the alveolar oxygen partial pressure (Po_2) in a normal person will be about 74 mm Hg; at 2400 m, it will be about 60 mm Hg. Assuming a normal alveolar-arterial oxygen gradient, arterial Po_2 should be in the range of 67 to 55 mm Hg. However, normal people hyperventilate somewhat at this range of Po_2, so the real arterial Po_2 is slightly higher. For any patient with chronic lung disease a precise prediction of arterial Po_2 when going from sea level to altitude is difficult because there is considerable variation in terms of ventilatory control mechanisms and mechanical ability to hyperventilate. Nonetheless, many patients with a sea level Po_2 of 55 to 75 mm Hg will show decreases in Po_2 to the range of 38 to 50 mm Hg as they ascend to 2400 m. Regression equations have been published relating ground-level Po_2 and the 1-second forced expiratory volume to Po_2 at altitude that can serve as guidelines for clinical decision making.[6]

Several papers have been published reporting the effect of transient, altitude-related hypoxemia in adults with chronic obstructive pulmonary disease (COPD). The majority of these patients were elderly, and many had cardiovascular conditions that would not be present in children. In one study, 18% of adults with COPD who flew in commercial aircraft had transient symptoms, but none had a serious medical incident.[7] In another study the same research group showed that 12 of 18 COPD patients exposed to hypobaric pressure simulating an altitude of 2400 m had a Po_2 of less than 50 mm Hg, but none developed serious medical problems.[8] A recent review that included data from five surveys of in-flight medical emergencies showed that the incidence of any emergency is quite low (0.4 to 3.4 per 100,000 passengers) and that cardiac conditions were the most common problem.[9]

Patients already requiring preflight oxygen therapy need at least the same amount of oxygen during air travel and perhaps more. For patients who do not require preflight oxygen, the situation is not as clear. The majority of young patients whose Po_2 is greater than 55 mm Hg can tolerate the cabin altitude of air travel without supplemental oxygen with minimal discomfort. Patients whose Po_2 is less than 55 mm Hg should arrange for in-flight oxygen, but a number of such patients have ignored this advice with no adverse consequences.

In the United States, airlines are required to provide supplemental oxygen for in-flight use. However, there are no standard policies or procedures for obtaining oxygen or for the delivery system to be used. Passengers are generally not allowed to use their own delivery systems. A physician's prescription is required and must state the flow to be maintained. It should be noted that airlines are not required to provide oxygen in the terminal. Physicians and patients should contact the airline well before the departure date to ensure that oxygen will be available. The American Lung Association has published a brochure containing useful guidelines and airline-specific rules and prices.[10]

Barotrauma may be a concern for patients who have cystic lung disease or areas of the lung that communicate poorly with the airways. The latter is almost purely theoretic because it would take a very rapid ascent to overcome even a very slowly emptying time constant. If a patient had a noncommunicating cyst at sea level that was fully expanded with a regional transpulmonary pressure of 40 to 50 mm Hg, then rupture would theoretically be possible on ascent to cabin altitudes of 4000 to 8000 ft. However, recent articles concerning the medical problems encountered by patients with COPD during air travel do not mention pneumothorax,[7-9] so such events must be rare. Nonetheless, the authors routinely remind their patients with advanced cystic fibrosis or other cystic lung diseases about the symptoms of pneumothorax as they prepare for air travel.

In recent years, there has been concern from teenagers and young adults with cystic fibrosis concerning the potential altitude-associated risks of snow skiing. The summits of many resorts in the western United States are at altitudes where even sedentary patients may experience some discomfort, and with exercise, such patients may become quite dyspneic. The authors advise patients with moderate to severe obstructive lung disease that they may become rather uncomfortable skiing at altitude but note that many have chosen to ski anyway with no long-lasting consequences. The authors have also been asked by teenagers and young adults with cystic fibrosis whether they would be able to obtain a private pilot's license. In the United States, all people who wish to obtain a pilot's license must pass a physical examination administered by a Federal Aviation Administration–approved physician. In the guide for examiners, no specific statements disqualify someone with a childhood lung disease, although moderate to severe asthma and bronchiectasis are both listed as relative contraindicators.[11] Each case is considered on an individual basis by the examiners. It has become the author's policy to advise hypoxemic patients that they probably would not pass the medical examination and that their medical history and laboratory results will be forwarded on request.

Acute Altitude-Related Problems

At altitudes above approximately 2500 m, even young, well-conditioned athletes may begin to experience altitude-related problems. Above 4000 m the incidence increases to about 40% to 50%. Acute mountain sickness is a syndrome in which headache is a universal feature; other signs and symptoms include lassitude, nausea, anorexia, and palpitations. The etiology of acute mountain sickness has not been completely elucidated but appears to include factors related to hypoxia, fluid retention, and extreme physical exertion.[12] The condition is to some degree inversely related to age[13] and genetic predisposition because at the same altitude, some highly conditioned climbers develop acute mountain sickness and others do not.

Peripheral edema and chest crackles are common in people suffering from acute mountain sickness, suggesting a role for fluid retention. The headache may be related to mild cerebral edema, and the incidence of acute mountain sickness is reduced by prophylactic treatment with acetazolamide, a carbonic anhydrase inhibitor.[12] Slow acclimatization can also help reduce the incidence of the syndrome. At very high altitudes, retinal hemorrhage is common,[14] and acute mountain sickness may progress to cerebral edema and death. The only definitive treatment is rapid descent.

Acute high-altitude pulmonary edema is probably related etiologically to acute mountain sickness but can occur in the absence of headache and other typical symptoms. Unilateral pulmonary hypoplasia may be a particular risk factor in children.[15] The signs and symptoms usually start with dry cough and proceed to dyspnea; orthopnea; diffuse crackles; pink, frothy sputum; and cyanosis. The protein content of the fluid is high,[16] suggesting that capillary damage and fluid transudation are part of the pathophysiology. Slow acclimatization can help reduce the incidence of high-altitude pulmonary edema but does not eliminate it. Nifedipine may be efficacious for prevention in some climbers.[17] The only definitive treatment is rapid descent, although administration of oxygen and continuous positive airway pressure may temporarily help. If available, nitric oxide may be inhaled as an adjunct to therapy.[18]

CARBON MONOXIDE

Carbon monoxide (CO) is an odorless, colorless gas present in minute quantities in the atmosphere. CO is produced by incomplete combustion of carbon-containing compounds such as wood, hydrocarbons, and coal. Lethal concentrations of CO can be found in the blood of 50% of fire victims,[12] and all burn victims should be assumed to have CO poisoning until proved otherwise.

Disease Mechanisms

CO causes poisoning by three proposed mechanisms: (1) its high binding affinity for hemoglobin, (2) a leftward shift in the oxygen-hemoglobin dissociation curve, and (3) binding to intracellular oxygen-transport systems. CO has a binding affinity for hemoglobin 240 times that of oxygen, so the competition for binding sites is therefore heavily weighted toward CO. Thus CO poisoning causes a functional anemia so that any hemoglobin site bound by CO is virtually unavailable for oxygen binding. The presence of carboxyhemoglobin in the blood causes the binding sites that are available to bind oxygen with a higher affinity, thus causing a decrease in tissue oxygen delivery (Fig. 11-4). CO can bind to the cytochrome oxidases of the intracellular oxygen-transport system and thus cause hypoxia. Animal experiments have suggested that this mechanism of tissue damage may be relevant in CO poisoning[19-21] and in fact may explain much of the pathophysiology in this condition.

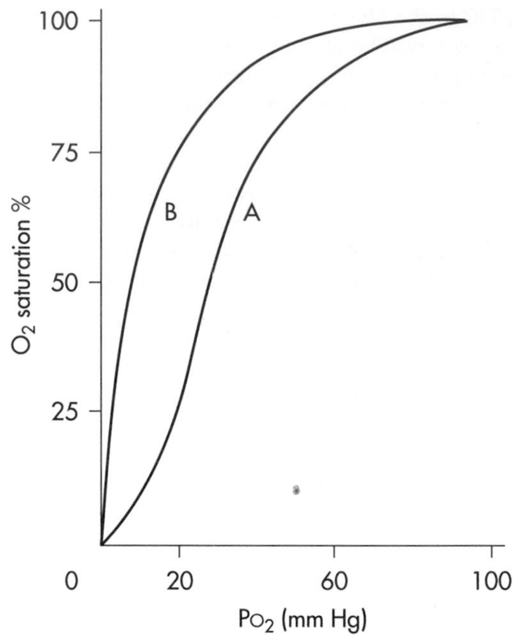

Fig. 11-4. Effect of carboxyhemoglobin on the shape of the oxygen-hemoglobin dissociation curve. *A,* No carboxyhemoglobin; *B,* 60% carboxyhemoglobin.

Clinical Manifestations

The signs and symptoms of CO poisoning vary with the concentration of carboxyhemoglobin. At levels below 10% a victim may experience dyspnea with exertion and mild headache. At levels of approximately 20%, dyspnea with exertion becomes more apparent, and headaches are described as *throbbing.* At levels of 30% to 40%, neurologic symptoms become more apparent and include severe headache, irritability, confusion, dizziness, and blurred vision. At levels of about 50%, victims may be extremely confused, dizzy, and faint. At higher levels, seizures and coma may appear, and at 60% to 80%, fatalities become common.

Assessment

As noted previously, all fire victims should be assumed to be suffering from CO poisoning until proved otherwise. Symptoms may vary considerably, and because carboxyhemoglobin is well known to be "cherry red," cyanosis is not a reliable physical finding. Spectrophotometric measurement of carboxyhemoglobin concentration is the most reliable method of diagnosis. The standard measures of oxygenation used in most emergency rooms and intensive care units are of limited use in CO poisoning. Arterial Po_2 may be normal in CO poisoning, but this finding needs to be interpreted with caution because the usual relationship between Po_2 and oxygen saturation is disrupted by a leftward shift in the oxygen-hemoglobin dissociation curve. Oxygen saturation as determined by a pulse oximeter also needs to be interpreted with caution. The standard pulse oximeter uses only the wavelengths required to measure levels of oxyhemoglobin (HbO_2) and deoxygenated hemoglobin (HbD). Oxygen saturation is then calculated as follows:

$$\%\ \text{Saturation pulse oximeter} = \frac{HbO_2}{HbO_2 + HbD} \times 100\%$$

The usual measurement of oxygen saturation by a pulse oximeter assumes that all of the hemoglobin binding sites in the blood could be bound with oxygen. As previously described, this assumption is incorrect in the setting of CO poisoning. For instance, if the carboxyhemoglobin level is 10%, only about 90% of the bindings sites in blood would theoretically be available for oxygen binding. The standard pulse oximeter will then measure the percentage of these remaining 90% of binding sites that are actually bound to oxygen. A cooximeter, on the other hand, uses more wavelengths and measures the amount of hemoglobins other than HbO_2 and HbD, such as carboxyhemoglobin and methemoglobin. Thus oxygen saturation assessed via cooximetry may be lower than that measured by pulse oximetry for the following reason:

$$\%\ \text{Saturation pulse oximeter} = \frac{HbO_2}{HbO_2 + HbD + \text{HB Other}}$$

Therapy

The only definitive therapy for CO poisoning is administration of oxygen. Oxygen significantly reduces the biologic half-life of CO (Fig. 11-5) and should be administered in high concentration via a nonrebreathing mask to all burn victims until a carboxyhemoglobin level is obtained. Hyperbaric oxygen therapy offers two theoretic advantages. As seen in Fig. 11-5, in-

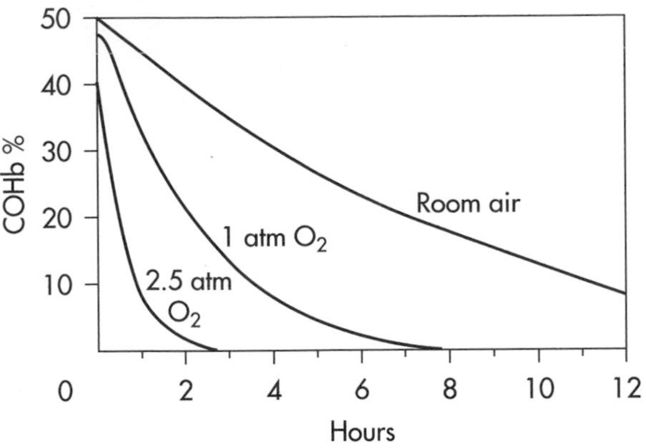

Fig. 11-5. Effect of oxygen at varying concentrations on the elimination of carboxyhemoglobin. (Modified from Winter PM, Miller JN: *JAMA* 236:1502-1504, 1976.)

creasing the pressure at which oxygen is administered further reduces the half-life of carboxyhemoglobin. In addition, hyperbaric therapy increases the amount of oxygen dissolved in the plasma to levels that can almost sustain life even in the absence of hemoglobin. Unfortunately, hyperbaric oxygen is available only in a few locales, and bedside intensive care is virtually impossible in a hyperbaric chamber, so for most patients, such therapy is impractical.

REFERENCES

Diving

1. Strauss RH, ed: *Diving medicine,* New York, 1976, Grune & Stratton.
2. Strauss RH: State of the art: diving medicine, *Am Rev Respir Dis* 119:1001-1023, 1979.
3. Melamed Y, Shupak A, Bitterman H: Medical problems associated with underwater diving, *New Engl J Med* 326:30-35, 1992.
4. Jenkins C, Anderson SD, Wong R, Veale A: Compressed air diving and respiratory disease, *Med J Aust* 158:275-279, 1993.
5. Farrell PJS, Glanvill P: Diving practices of scuba divers with asthma, *Br Med J* 300:166, 1990.

Altitude and Air Travel

6. Dillard TA, Berg BW, Rajagopal KR, Dooley JW, Mehm WH: Hypoxemia during air travel in patients with chronic obstructive pulmonary disease, *Ann Intern Med* 111:362-367, 1989.
7. Dillard TA, Beninati WA, Berg BW: Air travel in patients with chronic obstructive pulmonary disease, *Arch Intern Med* 151:1793-1795, 1991.
8. Berg BW, Dillard TA, Rajagopal KR, Mehm WJ: Oxygen supplementation during air travel in patients with chronic obstructive lung disease, *Chest* 101:638-641, 1992.
9. Gong H: Air travel and oxygen therapy in cardiopulmonary patients, *Chest* 101:1104-1113, 1992.
10. Livingstone G: *Airline travel with oxygen,* New York, 1992, American Lung Association.
11. Office of Aviation Medicine, Federal Aviation Administration: *Guide for aviation medical examiners,* Washington, DC, 1992, US Department of Transportation.
12. West WB: High altitude. In Crystal RM, West JB, eds: *The lung,* New York, 1991, Raven, pp 2093-2108.
13. Hackett PH, Rennie D, Levine HD: The incidence, importance, and prophylaxis of acute mountain sickness, *Lancet* 2:1150-1154, 1976.
14. Frayser R, Houston CS, Bryan AC, Rennie ID, Gary G: Retina hemorrhage at high altitude, *New Engl J Med* 282:1183-1184, 1970.
15. Hackett PH, Creagh CE, Grover RF, Honigman B, Houston CS, Reeves JT, Sophocles AM, Van Hardenbrock M: High altitude pulmonary edema in persons without the right pulmonary artery, *New Engl J Med* 302:1070-1073, 1980.
16. Schoene RB, Hackett PH, Henderson WR, Sage EH, Chow M, Roach RC, Mills WJ, Martin TR: High altitude pulmonary edema: characteristic of lung lavage fluid, *JAMA* 256:63-69, 1986.
17. Bartsch P, Maggiorini M, Ritter M, Noti C, Vock P, Oelz O: Prevention of high altitude pulmonary edema by nifedipine, *New Engl J Med* 325:1285-1289, 1991.
18. Scherrer U, Vollenweider L, Delabays A, Savcic M, Eichenberger U, Gian-Reto K, Firkle A, Ballmer PE, Nicod P, Bartsch P: Inhaled nitric oxide for high altitude pulmonary edema, *New Engl J Med* 334:624-629, 1996.

Carbon Monoxide

19. Spear RM, Munster AM: Burns, inhalational injury, and electrical injury. In Rogers MC, ed: *Textbook of pediatric intensive care,* Baltimore, 1987, Williams & Wilkins, pp 1323-1346.
20. Drabkin DL, Lewey RH, Bellet S, Ehrilich WH: The effect of replacement of normal body by erythrocytes saturated with carbon monoxide, *Am J Med Sci* 205:755-756, 1943.
21. Ramirez AG, Agostini JC, Goldbaum LR, Absolon KB: Lack of toxicity of transfused carboxyhemoglobin red blood cells and carbon monoxide inhalation, *Surg Forum* 25:165-168, 1974.

PART THREE

Assessment

CHAPTER 12

Clinical Assessment and Diagnostic Approach to Common Problems

Mark A. Brown and Wayne J. Morgan

For millennia the mark of the healer or physician was the ability to discern the nature of a patient's illness through careful questioning, observation, and examination. However, over the past half century or more, practitioners have for a variety of reasons come to rely more and more on technologic means of diagnosis. Although always important, the art of physical diagnosis will likely reassume greater importance in clinical practice in the future because of the growing emphasis on cost containment and the likelihood of limited access to certain technologies. This chapter focuses on clinical assessment of the respiratory system in children. There is much overlap between the respiratory examination and that of other systems, and it is assumed that the reader has mastered basic physical examination skills. Several excellent resources for the general physical examination are listed in the references.[1,2]

HISTORY

The extent and focus of the history (and physical examination) are dictated by the patient's pressing complaint. With few exceptions, there is no such thing as a "routine history and physical," both those activities being tailored to fit the particular complaint that the patient has. An extended history may not be necessary in every case. For example, it would not be necessary to inquire into the stool characteristics of a patient presenting for evaluation of snoring. Careful attention should be paid to the patient's narrative, and probing, nonleading questioning and clarification of key points follow. The exact order of elicitation is not as important as a consistent general routine covering all aspects pertinent to the patient's complaint.

Most physicians begin with the history of present illness, although in younger pediatric patients, it may be appropriate to begin with the antenatal and birth histories. Often the first step is to elicit the chief complaint with an open-ended statement or question. It is generally better not to accept a diagnosis as the reason for seeking consultation. The clinician should insist on hearing the symptoms that promoted concern in the patient's own words. Obviously, information such as the circumstances at onset, frequency, duration, and severity is important. Adapting the mnemonic device PQRST (provocation/palliation; quality; radiation; severity; timing) may be helpful in systematically characterizing a symptom. Associated symptoms such as fatigue, exercise induction or intolerance, and viral syndrome are important to note as well. The results of prior evaluations should be solicited and every effort made to obtain the actual reports or images of previous procedures, including those from pulmonary function tests. Information about previous therapies used and the response or lack thereof can provide important clues as to possible etiologies and may allow an assessment of compliance as well.

The antenatal, birth, and neonatal histories in general should be reviewed; the detail necessary depends on the individual. The duration of the pregnancy, together with any complications, including maternal medications and substance use or abuse (as well as tobacco), should be noted. The circumstances of the delivery and the neonatal course should also be reviewed.

Previous respiratory problems, including previous respiratory illnesses, hospitalizations, and pulmonary injuries (e.g., chest trauma or surgery, smoke inhalation), should be explored in detail, especially as they relate to airway instrumentation (e.g., endotracheal intubation, bronchoscopy). A history of recurrent pneumonia may suggest immunodeficiency, cystic fibrosis, anatomic abnormality, dysfunctional swallowing, or bronchiectasis. The child with a history of tracheoesophageal fistula repair is prone to tracheomalacia and gastroesophageal reflux–related disease.[3] Survivors of adult respiratory distress syndrome initially have restrictive lung disease followed later by peripheral airway obstructive disease.[4,5] Evidence of atopy, such as eczema, atopic dermatitis, hay fever or known allergies, may be important in the child with chronic cough or difficulty controlling asthma. A history of frequent infections, blood product transfusion, parental substance abuse, or poor growth may be a clue to an underlying immunodeficiency. Risk factors for human immunodeficiency virus, both iatrogenic and behavioral, should be carefully explored because this virus is the most clinically relevant immunodeficiency in many countries.

The family history may provide valuable information. It is often fruitful to probe using a variety of terms; for example, *chronic bronchitis, wheezy bronchitis,* and *asthmatic bronchitis* are all frequently used to describe asthma. There may be terms in the local vernacular, especially in areas where segments of the population use traditional healers, with whom the practitioner should become familiar. It is also important to elicit a family history of illnesses unlikely in the child, such as a parent or grandparent with recent lung cancer, because this may disclose a cause of undue anxiety about a cough or another respiratory symptom.

The social history is always important, if for no other reason than it provides a better understanding of the patient's circumstances, potentially yielding information helpful in both making a diagnosis and planning therapy (e.g., assessing the likelihood of compliance problems). Specific items to be elicited include the makeup (number, age) of the household unit and the family's living arrangements (house, trailer, apartment). School or day-care attendance or child care arrangements should be reviewed, with attention paid to the environment there as well (see later section). Hobbies may also be important, especially those involving exposure to dusts, paints, and other fumes. Even hair spray use can be clinically relevant. In a setting that preserves confidentiality, the clinician should discretely ask older children and adolescents about inhaled substances of abuse, such as tobacco, marijuana, and solvents (e.g., paint, glue, correction fluid). Of course, contact with ill individuals and travel are also pertinent.

A careful environmental history is important. The type of heating and cooling system in place should be noted. Other information such as the age of the dwelling, the presence of a basement, and recent renovations may also be useful. The number and type of animals present should be established. Many families do not consider animals kept outside, such as farm animals or birds, to be pets, so it may be better to ask about "animals" rather than "pets." It is important to inquire about exposure to potential irritants. The most common of these is smoke, either from tobacco use or use of wood for heating, cooking, or both. New composite furniture (manufactured from particle board and veneers), waterbeds, carpets, and ceiling tiles may contain volatile aldehydes that may incite asthma.

Often neglected in the pediatric patient, a review of systems can provide important information. Headache may be a sign of sinus disease or, especially if occurring in the early morning, a result of obstructive sleep apnea. Ocular symptoms such as conjunctivitis and blepharitis, as well as nasal symptoms, may indicate an atopic predisposition or in the infant a chlamydial infection. Recurrent mouth ulcers or thrush can be associated with immunodeficiency, as may chronic or recurrent ear drainage. Poor feeding, edema, shortness of breath, and exercise tolerance can be clues to the presence of congestive heart failure. Stool characteristics, abdominal bloating, and fatty food intolerance are important features of cystic fibrosis. Neurologic symptoms such as seizures or developmental delay are important in evaluating the child with apparent life-threatening events or suspected chronic or recurrent aspiration.

PHYSICAL EXAMINATION

This section focuses on the chest and respiratory system, with pertinent findings in other systems included as appropriate. For examination of other systems the reader is referred to one of the general physical examination texts listed in the references.[1,2] It is best to establish a consistent pattern for the physical examination so that part of it is not omitted. The order in which the components of the examination are presented here is arbitrary. At all times the privacy of the patient should be respected, the examination being conducted out of view (and preferably out of hearing) of other patients. In the case of adolescents the use of another staff member, the same gender as the patient, as a chaperon may be appropriate.

Upper Airway

Although not truly an airway or gas-exchanging tissue, the ear is considered part of the respiratory tract for several reasons. The middle ear and eustachian tube develop embryologically from the first pharyngeal pouch and share a contiguous mucosal surface with the respiratory tract.[6] The lining of the eustachian tube consists of ciliated pseudostratified columnar epithelium identical to the remainder of the respiratory tract.[7] Although the middle ear is lined predominantly with simple squamous or cuboidal epithelium, patches of ciliated pseudostratified columnar epithelium have been described there as well.[7] There are also cough receptors located in the external auditory canal. Thus it is important to examine the ears for foreign bodies and for signs of middle ear infection or another abnormality as a source of chronic cough.

The nasal passages are uniquely configured to perform their role as the portal for inspired air. The turbinates, and to some degree the paranasal sinuses, warm and humidify inspired air from ambient temperature and humidity to roughly body temperature and 100% relative humidity. Careful inspection of the nose can identify subtle changes indicative of local and sometimes systemic disorders. Children with inhalant allergies frequently develop a transverse nasal crease, the result of repetitive up-and-down rubbing to relieve itching and discomfort. This may be accompanied by other signs associated with allergic disease, such as dark circles under the eyes ("allergic shiners") and Dennie's sign, which is skin creases radiating from the inner canthus of the eye to approximately two thirds the length of the lower lid margin. The nasal bridge is normally straight. A deviation of the bridge may indicate a congenital abnormality or previous trauma and should prompt careful inspection of the septum for deviation and obstruction. Widening of the nasal bridge can be seen in individuals with extensive nasal polyps (Fig. 12-1). The relative patency of the passages can be assessed by asking the child to sniff (or simply listening in the younger child) while manually occluding one naris. A question of complete obstruction can be clarified by passage of a feeding tube or red rubber catheter. With congenital or acquired absence of the alar cartilage the nares may collapse with each inspiration.

The nasal passages themselves can often be visualized through the use of an otoscope and a large (4- to 5-mm) ear speculum by placing the free hand on the top of the patient's head and with the thumb gently lifting the tip of the patient's nose. Alternatively a nasal speculum can be used. The nasal mucosa, normally pink and glistening, should be inspected for edema and changes in color (inflamed or pale, boggy or gray), and the color, consistency, and odor of any secretions are noted. Obviously inflamed mucosa suggests infection, whereas pale, boggy mucosa is frequently seen in allergic rhinitis. With chronic rhinitis the mucosa may take on a grayish appearance. Foul-smelling and sometimes bloody secretions suggest a foreign body or chronic sinus disease, whereas clear secretions may occur in allergic rhinitis or early in the course of an uncomplicated upper respiratory infection. A smear of nasal secretions, stained with Hansel's stain, may be helpful, a predominance of eosinophils suggesting allergic disease and a predominance of polymorphonuclear leukocytes (especially when accompanied by a single bacterial morphology) suggesting bacterial sinus disease. No conclusions regarding the causative organism should be drawn from these results, however. The septum should be inspected for deviations, perforations, and sites of bleeding. (The nasopharynx is a common source of perceived hemoptysis.) Foreign bodies, polyps (see Fig. 12-1), and masses within the nares should be carefully sought out and inspected.

Examination of the paranasal sinuses is difficult in children younger than 10 years of age. Techniques such as transillumination and percussion not only are impeded by lack of cooperation but also may be difficult to interpret because of the relative thickness and density of the overlying soft tissues. However, it may be possible to localize the source of purulent secretions in the nose by direct inspection. Most commonly this is the middle meatus, which is located between the middle

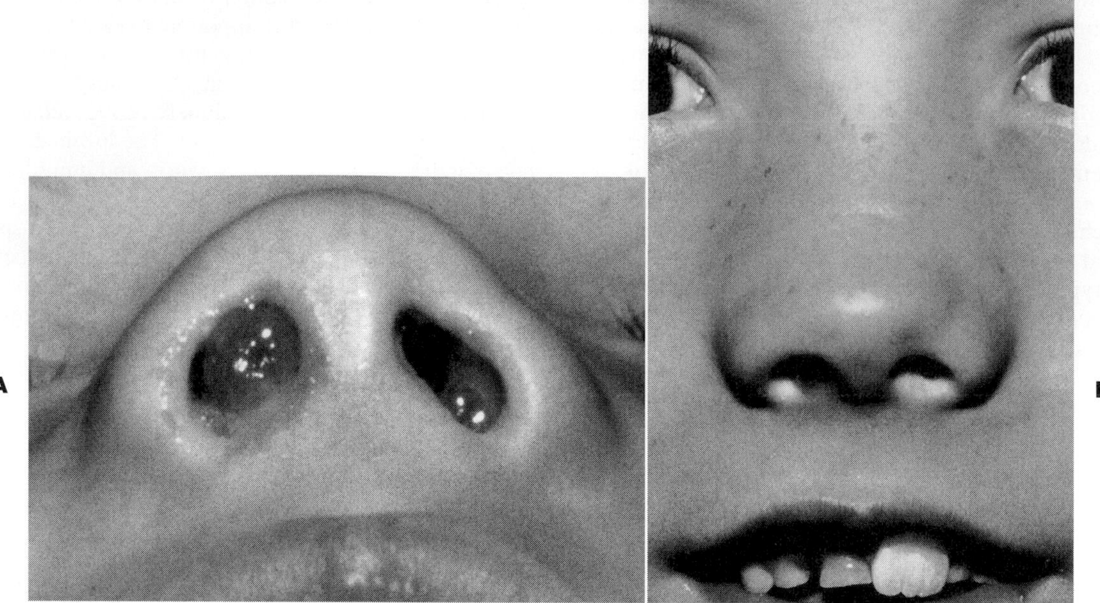

Fig. 12-1. A, Child with cystic fibrosis and a large nasal polyp. **B,** Note the widening of the nasal bridge and the polyp projecting from the right naris.

and inferior turbinates; the middle meatus drains the frontal, maxillary, and anterior ethmoid sinuses. The confluence of these three meatuses is called the *osteomeatal complex.* Obstruction from edema, a foreign body, or a polyp in this region is a frequent cause of chronic sinus disease. However, this may not be readily identified on examination; computed tomography (CT) is a more reliable means of diagnosis.

The profile of the mandible should be inspected carefully for the presence of retrognathia or micrognathia, either of which may lead to airway obstruction, especially during sleep. The state of oral hygiene, including not only of the teeth but also the oral mucosa, should be noted. The integrity of the palate should be ensured either by visualization or preferably by gentle palpation because a submucous cleft palate can easily be missed on simple inspection. The size and shape of the uvula is noted. A long uvula may cause chronic cough, whereas a bifid uvula may be a clue to an occult submucous cleft palate. The motion of the uvula and soft palate during phonation and gagging is important to note, especially in children with known neurologic abnormalities. Poor or abnormal motion may suggest palatal insufficiency or cranial nerve palsy that may be associated with dysfunctional swallowing and an increased risk of aspiration. The clinician should also note the presence and size of the tonsils as well as any other masses, especially unilateral enlargement, which can be seen in retropharyngeal or tonsillar abscess or lymphoma. Adenoidal tissue visible on the posterior pharyngeal wall ("cobblestoning") is abnormal and implies hypertrophy in association with allergic disease.

The presence or absence of foul breath should be noted. Fetid breath may indicate poor dental hygiene, a nasal foreign body, anaerobic infection, or even pneumonia.

The position of the trachea is important to note during examination of the neck. Deviation to one side may be associated with pneumothorax, neck mass, unilateral pulmonary agenesis or hypoplasia, or unilateral hyperinflation such as with foreign body or congenital cystic lung disorders. With the exception of unilateral pulmonary agenesis or hypoplasia, which causes deviation toward the involved side, the trachea is deviated away from the abnormality. The neck should be palpated for masses, thyromegaly, and adenopathy.

The character of the voice often provides important information as well. Hoarseness with or without stridor suggests an abnormality of the vocal cords such as edema, dysfunction (e.g., paresis, paralysis), or injury. A weak voice accompanied by a high-pitched inspiratory stridor but no hoarseness can result from a subglottic obstruction, whereas a muffled voice associated with a low-pitched stridor but no hoarseness suggests a supraglottic obstruction. Narrowing of the glottis itself results in hoarseness with a high-pitched stridor only on inspiration. Hoarseness or a muffled cry in a newborn is very suggestive of a congenital glottic or subglottic abnormality and should prompt further investigation, especially in infants at risk for laryngeal papillomatosis because of maternal genital papillomatosis.

Chest

Inspection

Examination of the chest, as with other areas, should begin with inspection. The general shape of the chest and the presence of any deformities are noted. The circumference of the chest, as measured at the nipple line, should be roughly equal to the head circumference in infants and is larger in older children. Barrel chest deformity, an increase in the anteroposterior dimension of the chest, is associated with obstructive lung disease. There is a good correlation between the degree of severity of this deformity and both increased lung volumes (functional residual capacity, residual volume, total lung capacity, functional residual capacity/total lung capacity, and residual volume/total lung capacity) and radiographic findings of hyperinflation in children with poorly controlled asthma.[8]

Asymmetry of the chest can be seen in children with cardiomegaly (especially with right-sided ventricular hypertrophy), pneumothorax, and scoliosis. Pectus carinatum (pigeon breast) or pectus excavatum (funnel chest) can be present to a variable degree. The latter may falsely accentuate the severity or even mimic the presence of sternal retractions. Harrison's groove or sulcus, a horizontal depression in the lower thoracic cage at the site of diaphragmatic attachment, may be seen in patients who have chronically increased work of breathing, as in pulmonary fibrosis, cystic fibrosis, or poorly controlled asthma.

Work of breathing is assessed mainly through inspection. The respiratory rate, preferably noted with the child at rest or asleep, is a fairly sensitive clinical indicator of pulmonary health (Table 12-1). However, fever and metabolic acidosis can lead to an increased respiratory rate in the absence of pulmonary disease. Nasal flaring, an attempt to reduce nasal resistance to airflow, is a manifestation of increased work of breathing, as is the use of accessory muscles of respiration such as the sternocleidomastoid muscles. Retractions or indrawing of the skin of the neck and chest are signs of increased work of breathing as well. Areas of retraction include the suprasternal notch (suprasternal retractions), the subxiphoid region (infrasternal retractions), and the costal interspaces (intercostal retractions). In infants and toddlers the sternum itself draws in during inspiration, a manifestation of the increased chest wall compliance in this age group. Because of this, other sites of retraction may be absent in this age group, whereas in the older child, suprasternal and intercostal retractions predominate.

Children with evidence of increased work of breathing are said to have dyspnea, although complaints of shortness of breath are subjective and may not be related to a true respiratory pathologic condition. Children with neuromuscular disease, quadriplegia, paralyzed hemidiaphragm, and other such conditions may complain of dyspnea associated with metabolic acidosis or fever because of their inability to effectively increase their minute ventilation, the normal response in such a setting. Dyspnea may be semiquantitated by noting the number of words a child is able to speak before having to take a breath or by asking the child to count and noting the highest number reached. Both the use of accessory muscles and dyspnea correlate closely with lung function as measured by the 1-second forced expiratory volume and oxyhemoglobin saturation in children with acute exacerbations of asthma.[9]

The respiratory pattern may also provide valuable information. It is important to remember that the respiratory pattern is set by the respiratory centers in the brain stem. Changes in the pattern can reflect responses to oxygenation state, acidosis, or alkalosis or can indicate a primary abnormality of the respiratory centers themselves. The depth of respiration should also be noted. One author has suggested that each physician establish informal "norms" for depth of respiration in children of various ages by noting the distance from the nose at which the breath can be felt on the hand.[10]

Individuals with restrictive lung disease may have shallow, rapid respirations. Hyperpnea, rapid and deep respiration, can be associated with a number of underlying problems, including hypoxia and metabolic acidosis. Alkalosis may result in slow, shallow breaths. Biot's respiration, a pattern of very irregular respirations with alternating periods of hyperpnea and apnea, can be seen in meningitis, encephalitis, and other central nervous lesions involving the respiratory centers. Cheyne-Stokes respirations are a repetitive pattern of gradually increasing and decreasing respirations over 30 seconds to 1 minute and are generally associated with coma. The relative length of the respiratory phases (the inspiratory/expiratory ratio) is significant, with the inspiratory and expiratory phases normally being approximately equal. Prolonged expiration is seen in obstructive diseases such as bronchiolitis, acute exacerbations of asthma, and cystic fibrosis. Some degree of paradoxic respiration, or abdominal ("belly") breathing, may be normal, especially in children up to 6 or 7 years of age. Prominent respirations of this type in any child, however, generally reflect a pulmonary abnormality such as pneumonia, upper airway obstruction, or obstructive lung disease.

Table 12-1 Respiratory Rates of Normal Children

	SLEEPING		AWAKE	
AGE	MEAN	RANGE	MEAN	RANGE
Waring				
6-12 mo	27	22-31	64	58-75
1-2 yr	19	17-23	35	30-40
2-4 yr	19	16-25	31	23-42
4-6 yr	18	14-23	26	19-36
6-8 yr	17	13-23	23	15-30
AGE	**BOYS**	**GIRLS**		
Iliff and Lee				
0-1 yr	31	30		
1-2 yr	26	27		
2-3 yr	25	25		
3-4 yr	24	24		
4-5 yr	23	22		
5-6 yr	22	21		
6-7 yr	21	21		
7-9 yr	20	20		
9-13 yr	19	19		
13-14 yr	19	18		
14-15 yr	18	18		
15-16 yr	17	18		
16-17 yr	17	17		
17-18 yr	16	17		

Adapted from Waring WW. In Kendig EL, Chernick V, eds: *Disorders of the respiratory tract in children*, Philadelphia, 1983, WB Saunders, pp 57-78; and Iliff A, Lee VA: *Child Develop* 23:237-245, 1952.

Palpation

Although more generally thought of in terms of the abdominal examination, palpation is important in the respiratory examination as well. It is used to confirm the visual observations of chest wall shape and excursion. Palpation is performed by placing the entire hand on the chest and feeling with the palm and fingertips. Friction rubs may be felt as high-frequency vibrations in synchrony with the respiratory pattern. Tactile fremitus, the transmission of vibrations associated with vocalization, is at times difficult to assess in children because of a lack of cooperation and a higher-pitched voice; lower-pitched vocalization is more effectively transmitted. It is best felt with the palmar aspects of the metacarpal and phalangeal joints on the costal interspaces. Decreased fremitus suggests airway obstruction, pleural fluid, or pleural thickening, whereas increased fremitus is associated with parenchymal consolidation. Occasionally a "thud" can be felt high in the chest or in the neck, a finding suggestive of a free tracheal foreign body. One can also assess chest excursion by placing the hands with the fingertips anterior and thumbs posterior and noting the degree of chest wall movement, comparing excursion of one side with the other by noting the movement of the thumbs away from the midline (the spinous processes). The point of maximal impulse, frequently shifted to the left in cardiac disease, may be shifted to the right in severe asthma, a large left-sided pleural effusion, or a tension pneumothorax. With massive left-sided atelectasis, it may be shifted to the left.

Percussion

Much like its counterpart in the musical world, percussion of the chest relies on differences in vibratory characteristics, in this case using various tissues, to produce characteristic sounds. First described by Leopold Auenbrugger in Vienna in 1761, the technique was largely ignored by the medical community until around the turn of the next century, when it was revived by Napoleon's personal physician, Corvisant. It is widely thought that Auenbrugger adapted the technique from that used by his innkeeper father to determine the level of wine in barrels, though it is not known for certain how Auenbrugger developed the idea. There are two different methods of performing percussion: direct (or immediate), in which the chest is struck directly with the finger, and indirect (or mediate), in which sound is generated by striking a finger laid on the chest. This discussion involves the indirect method only. A discussion of direct percussion can be found elsewhere.[11]

Correct technique is critical in both performing and interpreting percussion of the chest, especially in small children. Percussion is best performed with the child upright with the head in a neutral position. A single finger from one hand (the pleximeter) is placed on an interspace; care is taken to avoid contact of the other fingers and palm with the chest because contact between the chest and any other part of the nonstriking hand dampens the sound generated and leads to erroneous interpretation. The finger is then struck with a single finger from the other hand (the plexor) by holding the hand fixed and pivoting at the wrist, quickly removing the striking finger, again to avoid dampening the sound. Many examiners find it comfortable to use the long fingers of each hand for this technique. Generally the clinician strikes 2 to 3 times in each position. The force used should be consistent with each strike and should not be too strong. Excessive force may lead to an erroneous impression of hyperresonance, especially in a small child. Some have suggested the use of a reflex hammer as the plexor; this should not be done in children because it may lead to increased resonance. Sounds commonly elicited by percussion of the chest are listed in Table 12-2.

The clinician can delineate the level of the diaphragmatic leaves anteriorly and posteriorly by carefully percussing along the lower thoracic cage (Table 12-3). This can be helpful in guiding auscultation. The clinician may even be able to assess diaphragmatic excursion in older children and adults with suspected diaphragmatic dysfunction by percussing during inspiration and expiration; in adults this is normally 5 to 6 cm. The extent of the mediastinal structures can also be delineated.

Auscultation

After development of the stethoscope by Rene Laennec in 1816 and its improvement by Piorry, Williams, Cammann, and others, physicians had the ability to recognize changes in sound characteristics in the chest and to correlate these changes with specific pathophysiologic events in health and disease. (An excellent review of the history and physics of the stethoscope is available.[12]) Although the standard stethoscope does not amplify sound, by excluding extraneous environmental sounds and to some degree localizing sounds, it allows the clinician to assess gas movement within the lungs and relate changes to known associations with specific abnormalities. Thus developing expertise in interpreting auscultatory findings is very much an experiential process, and as such, there is no substitute for having listened to a large number of patients, both with and without lung disease. Audiotape programs, such as one available from the American College of Chest Physicians,[13] can be helpful in establishing a base on which to build this skill.

For most physicians the standard binaural stethoscope is adequate as long as it is in good repair. The earpieces should fit well to exclude environmental sounds. The tubing should not be cracked or kinked and ideally should be no longer than 30 cm, although many physicians accept longer lengths for ease and comfort in examining patients. The bell should be fitted with a rubber ring, and the diaphragm should be intact. Pulmonologists may find it more convenient to use a differential stethoscope, a stethoscope with two chest pieces, one connected to each earpiece, allowing simultaneous auscultation and direct comparison of sounds in different locations. However, use of the differential stethoscope requires even more practice than the standard binaural stethoscope for effective use, so it is probably not practical for the general pediatrician or family physician.

The diaphragm, which filters out low-pitched sounds, thereby isolating high-pitched sound, should be pressed tightly against the skin. In contrast, the bell should be placed lightly on the skin to preferentially isolate low-pitched sounds. If excessive pressure is applied when using the bell, the skin below the bell may be stretched taut, thereby functioning as a diaphragm and filtering out the low-pitched sounds being sought. A loud, roaring sound generally indicates inadequate contact between the chest piece and skin, especially when the bell is

Table 12-2 Sounds Elicited by Percussion of the Chest

TERM	DEFINITION
Tympany	This sound is usually heard only in the abdomen; massive pneumothorax is suggested if it is heard in the chest.
Hyperresonance	This sound is associated with emphysema or free intrapleural air.
Bellmetal resonance	Also called the *coin test,* this is a clearly transmitted metallic sound heard with a stethoscope when tapping a coin that is held flat against the chest with another coin; it indicates a pneumothorax.
Skodiac resonance	This peculiar, high-pitched sound is obtained by percussion just above the level of a pleural effusion.
Resonance	This is the normal state in the chest; it is sometimes called *vesicular resonance.*
Dullness	This sound is associated with pleural fluid or parenchymal consolidation.
Flatness	This sound can be heard by percussing over muscle; its presence in the chest suggests massive effusion.

Table 12-3 Usual Level of Diaphragm as Assesssed by Percussion

TERM	LEFT	RIGHT
Anterior	Ribs 8-10	Ribs 6 (midaxillary line)
Posterior	Ribs 8-10	Ribs 8-10

used. This can be especially problematic when examining an infant or small child unless a stethoscope with appropriate-sized chest pieces is used. Instruments with chest pieces appropriate for premature infants, infants, children, and adolescents and adults are available. The clinician should avoid listening through clothing or bed clothes and should listen (if possible) with the patient breathing slowly and deeply through the mouth in a neutral position, either upright or prone or supine.

As always, it is best to develop a consistently used pattern of examination to avoid missing areas (Fig. 12-2). The upper lobes are best heard by listening anteriorly in the infraclavicular regions, the lower lobes by listening posteriorly below the scapulae, and the right middle lobe and lingula by listening anteriorly lateral to the lower third of the sternum. All lobes can be heard in the axillae.

When auscultating, the clinician should note the amplitude of the sounds produced. It is also important to specify the timing (continuous, early, or late), pitch (high, medium, or low), and character (fine, medium, or coarse) of sounds. These sounds can be divided into breath sounds (produced by the movement of gas through the airways), voice sounds (modifications of phonation not heard distinctly in the normal state), and adventitious sounds (neither breath or voice sounds). Table 12-4 lists the most commonly heard sounds.

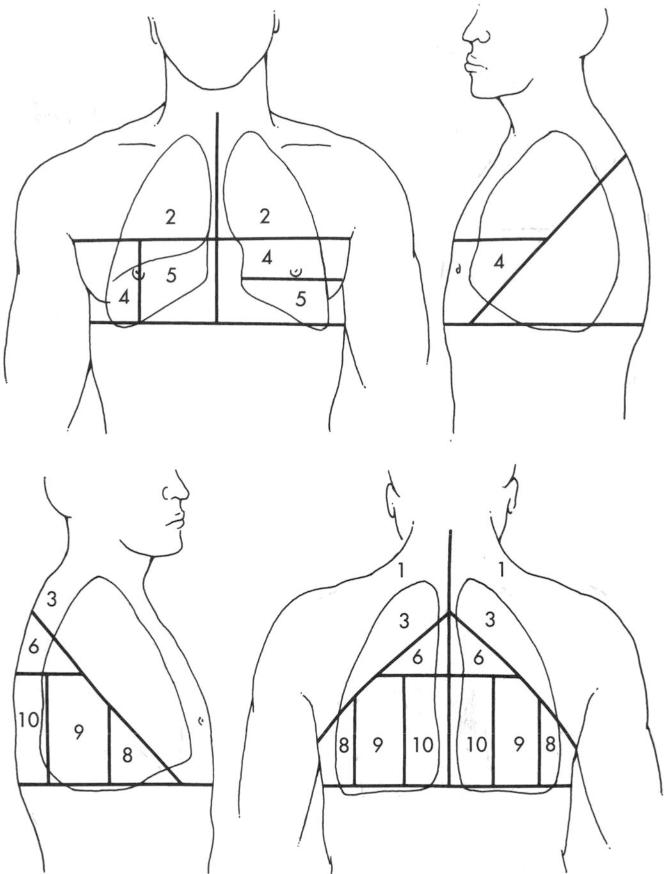

Fig. 12-2. Projections of the lobar/segmental pattern on the surface of the chest. *1,* Apical segment of the upper lobes; *2,* anterior segment of the upper lobes; *3,* posterior segment of the upper lobes; *4,* superior lingular *(left)* and lateral *(right)* segments of the middle lobe; *5,* inferior lingular *(left)* and medial *(right)* segments of the middle lobe; *6,* superior segment of the lower lobes; *8,* anterior basal segment of the lower lobes; *9,* lateral basal segment of the lower lobes; *10,* posterior basal segment of the lower lobes.

Breath Sounds. Vesicular breath sounds are the sounds heard during respiration in a healthy individual. They have a low-pitched, "whishing" quality with a relatively longer inspiratory phase and a shorter expiratory phase and are louder on inspiration. These sounds emanate from the lobar and segmental airways and are then transmitted through normal parenchyma.[14]

Bronchial breath sounds are usually louder than vesicular sounds and have short inspiratory and long expiratory phases. They are higher pitched and louder during expiration. They may be the result of consolidation or compression (i.e., airlessness) of the underlying parenchyma. A similar sound can be heard by listening directly over the trachea.

Bronchovesicular breath sounds, as the name implies, are intermediate between vesicular and bronchial sounds. The respiratory phases are roughly equal in length. This sound is felt to be indicative of a lesser degree of consolidation or compression (airlessness) than bronchial sounds. Bronchovesicular (and sometimes bronchial) breath sounds can occasionally be heard in normal individuals in the auscultatory triangle (the area in the back bound by the lower border of the trapezius, the latissimus dorsi, and the rhomboideus major muscles) and the right upper lobe.

Wheezes are continuous musical sounds, more commonly expiratory in nature, and usually associated with short inspiratory and prolonged expiratory phases. They can be of single (monophonic) or multiple (polyphonic) pitches, which are higher pitched than vesicular sounds. These can often be very difficult to distinguish from snoring and upper airway sounds such as stridor.

Stridor is a musical, monophonic, often high-pitched sound, usually thought of as inspiratory in nature; it can be expiratory as well, produced by partial obstruction of a central, typically extrathoracic airway. Its presence in both inspiration and expiration suggests severe, fixed airway obstruction.

A cardiorespiratory murmur is a localized vesicular sound that appears to be synchronized with the heartbeat, mimicking a cardiac murmur or bruit. It can be heard anywhere in the

Table 12-4 Pulmonary Auscultatory Sounds*

COMMON TERMINOLOGY	ACCP-ATS "PREFERRED" TERMINOLOGY
Breath sounds	**Breath sounds**
Vesicular sounds	Normal
Bronchial sounds	Decreased
Bronchovesicular sounds	Absent
Wheeze	
Stridor	
Cardiorespiratory murmur	
Voice sounds	
Whispered pectoriloquy	Clarity increased or decreased
Bronchophony	Intensity increased or decreased
Egophony	
Adventitious sounds	**Adventitious sounds**
Fine (subcrepitant) crackles or rales	Crackles or rales (no subclassifications)
Coarse (crepitant) crackles or rales	Wheezes or rhonchi (varying pitch, quality, intensity)
Rhonchi	Mediastinal crunch
Squawk	Pleural rub
Pleural friction rub	Pleuropericardial rub
Peristalsis	

ACCP, American College of Chest Physicians; *ATS,* American Thoracic Society.
*See text for description of terms.

chest but is frequently very dependent on body position, often disappearing with position change. It may be heard in systole, diastole, or both during quiet respiration.

Voice Sounds. The normal lung parenchyma filters vocalization so that whispered sounds are not usually heard during auscultation and normally spoken syllables are indistinct. Bronchophony is the distinct transmission of spoken syllables as the result of an underlying consolidation or compression. More severe consolidation or compression results in the transmission of whispered sounds or whispered pectoriloquy. Egophony is very similar to bronchophony but has a nasal quality as well. It may reflect an underlying effusion, consolidation or compression, or both conditions.

Adventitious Sounds. The nomenclature for adventitious sounds is perhaps the least standardized of all physical findings and therefore is prone to confusion. Synonymous terms such as *rales* and *crackles, subcrepitant* and *fine,* and *crepitant* and *course* are widely used in a variety of combinations. Because past attempts at standardization have met with variable success,[12,15] the authors have chosen to identify these sounds using several descriptors, allowing the reader to choose which to use and hopefully allowing him or her to recognize others when used by colleagues.

Fine (subcrepitant) crackles are thought to be the result of the explosive reopening of alveoli that closed during the previous exhalation or exhalations.[16] These occur exclusively during inspiration and are associated with conditions such as bronchitis, pneumonia, pulmonary infarction, and atelectasis. They can also be normal when heard in the posterior lung bases during the first few breaths on awakening. They may be imitated by rolling several strands of hair between the thumb and forefinger in front of the ear or by pulling apart Velcro. Hamman's sign, also called a *mediastinal crunch,* is the finding of crackles associated with systole and is suggestive of pneumomediastinum.

Coarse (crepitant) crackles are popping sounds likely produced by the movement of thin fluids in bronchi or bronchioles.[16] They occur early in inspiration and occasionally in expiration as well, may be audible at the mouth, and may clear or change pattern after a cough. They can sometimes be heard in the anterior lung bases during exhalation to residual volume. An example of these sounds are the crackles typically heard in patients with cystic fibrosis.

Rhonchi (sometimes more descriptively called *large airway sounds*) are gurgling or bubbling sounds usually heard during exhalation. These sounds are the result of movement of fluid within larger airways.

A squawk is a short inspiratory wheeze often heard in association with fine crackles. It is thought to result from the explosive opening and fluttering of a large airway.

In individuals with decreased or absent pleural lubricating fluid, a pleural friction rub may be heard. This loud, grating sound may come and go over a short period of time. It is usually associated with a subpleural inflammatory process.

Finally, peristalsis may sometimes be heard within the thorax, especially over the left lung base because of the proximity of the stomach and large bowel. The clinician must be alert to the possibility of acquired or congenital diaphragmatic hernia.

Other Signs and Symptoms

Occasionally, pulmonary disease is manifest by changes or signs in other organ systems. An example is digital clubbing, the broadening and thickening of the ends of the fingers and toes that occur as the result of connective tissue hypertrophy and hyperplasia[17] and increased vascularity[18] in the distal phalanges (Fig. 12-3). It may be quite subtle but can be confirmed clinically by checking for Schamroth's sign (Table 12-5). Although clubbing can be a primary finding (either idiopathic or inherited), it is usually seen in association with lung disease, heart disease, or liver or other gastrointestinal diseases as well (Box 12-1). The degree of clubbing can be quantitated by several methods as a way of following the progression of lung disease.[19,20] Clubbing may occur acutely (e.g., with a bout of severe pneumonia) but may also regress if the underlying cause is corrected. When associated with a usually painful periostosis, clubbing is one component of hypertrophic osteoarthropathy.

The pathophysiology of clubbing associated with lung disease is unclear. It may be the result of the lungs' failure to remove or inactivate a circulating fibroblast growth factor,[21] although the arachidonic acid metabolites prostaglandin F_{2a} and E have been implicated in patients with cystic fibrosis.[22] Still another theory proposes that clubbing is the result of peripheral impaction of megakaryocytes and platelets in the digits, with subsequent release of platelet-derived growth factor, which induces the histologic and anatomic changes associated with clubbing.[23]

Cyanosis, another abnormality that may be associated with lung disease, is the bluish discoloration of tissues caused by increased concentrations of reduced (unoxygenated) hemoglobin, which is purple (Box 12-2). It occurs more readily in tissues with low blood flow or higher oxygen extraction than tissues with higher flow or lower oxygen extraction. This accounts for the traditional interpretation that peripheral cyanosis (or acrocyanosis) reflects less severe hypoxemia than central cyanosis.

The use of cyanosis as a clinical indicator of hypoxemia is confounded by a number of factors. Simply identifying the cyanotic patient can be problematic because of variations in skin pigmentation, poor lighting, the presence of nail polish, or temperature extremes (especially cold). Even when cyanosis is unequivocally present or absent, inferences made regarding the oxygenation state of the patient may not be correct. Cyanosis occurs when the concentration of reduced arterial hemoglobin exceeds 3 g/dl. At this level the concentration of reduced hemoglobin in the capillary beds is generally 4 to 6 g/dl. However, the blood's oxygen-carrying capacity and therefore blood oxygen content depend primarily on total hemoglobin concentration. Thus the actual oxygen content may be normal in a cyanotic patient with polycythemia, but an anemic patient may have an abnormally low oxygen content in the absence of cyanosis. Clinical impressions of oxygenation, such as cyanosis, should therefore be verified by arterial blood gas analysis.

Pulsus paradoxus is another physical sign sometimes associated with pulmonary disease, particularly obstructive lung disease. Pulsus paradoxus is the fluctuation in arterial systolic blood pressure with the respiratory cycle, the pressure falling during inspiration and rising with exhalation. It is quantified as the difference between the systolic pressures measured during inspiration and expiration. It can be measured a number of ways, most easily by using a sphygmomanometer. It can also be qualitatively identified by observing the pressure tracing of an intraarterial catheter or the pulse tracing of a pulse oximeter. It may also be detected by palpation in patients with pulsus paradoxus greater than 20 mm Hg, signifying more severe obstructive lung disease (see later section).

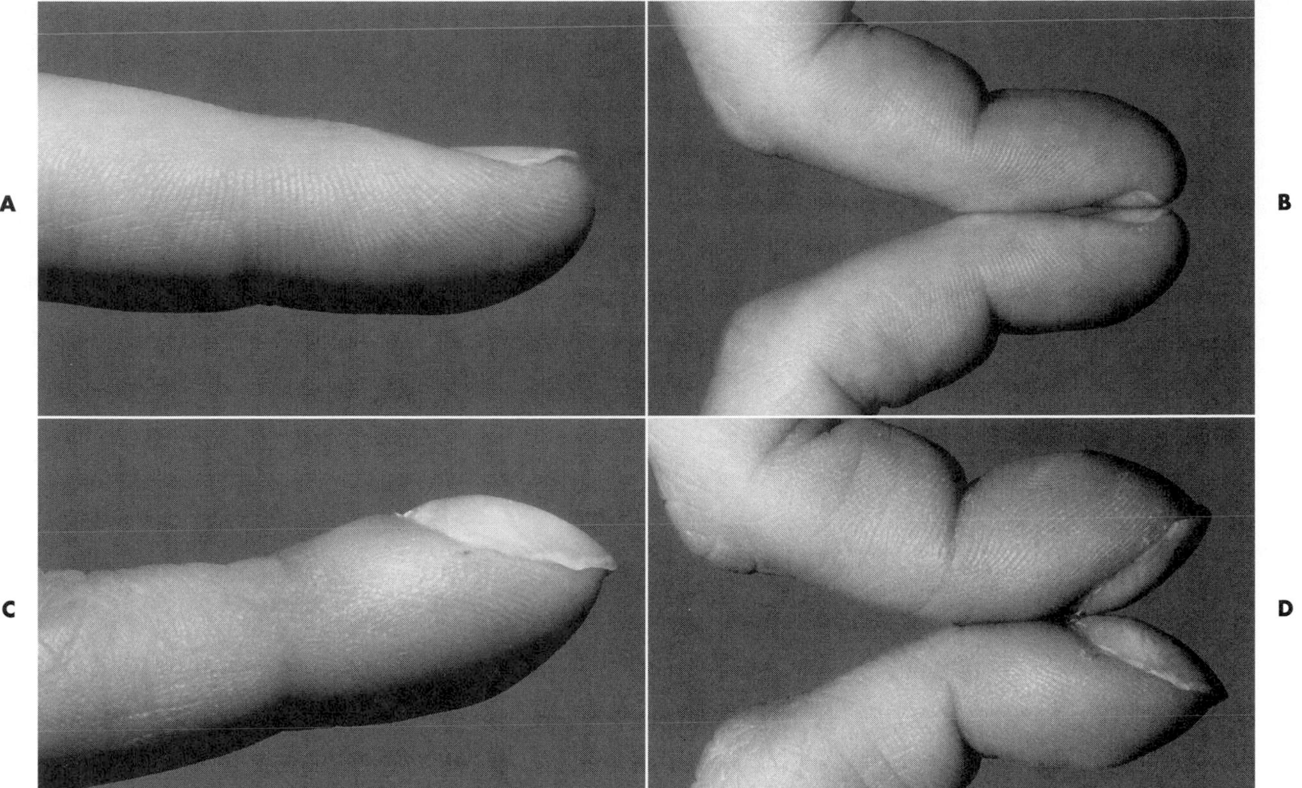

Fig. 12-3. Lateral view of the index finger and Schamroth's sign in a healthy individual (**A** and **B**) and in an individual with severe clubbing (**C** and **D**).

Table 12-5 Pulmonary "Signs"

SIGN	DEFINITION
Abrahams'	Rales and other adventitious sounds, changes in respiratory murmurs, and an increase in whispered sounds can be heard on auscultation over the acromial end of the clavicle for some time before they become audible at the apex.
Aufrecht's	Diminished breath sounds occur in the trachea just above the jugular notch in cases of tracheal stenosis.
Baccelli's	There is good conduction of a whisper in nonpurulent pleural effusions.
Bird's	There is a zone of dullness on percussion with the absence of respiratory signs in the presence of a hydatid cyst of the lung.
di'Espine's	In pulmonary tuberculosis, bronchophony over the spinous processes is heard at a lower level than in healthy people.
Ewart's	In large pericardial effusions, an area of dullness with bronchial breathing and bronchophony is found below the angle of the left scapula.
Ewing's	Dullness on percussion to the inner side of the angle of the left scapula denotes an accumulation of fluid in the pericardium behind the heart.
Fischer's	In a case of tuberculosis of the bronchial glands, if one bends the child's head as far back as possible, auscultation of the manubrium sterni sometimes reveals a continuous loud murmur caused by the pressure of the enlarged glands on the vena anonyma.
Hamman's	Crackles associated with systole is suggestive of pneumomediastinum; this sign is also called the *mediastinal crunch.*
Hoover's	A modification in the movement of the costal margins during respiration is caused by flattening of the diaphragm; this sign suggests emphysema or another intrathoracic condition causing a change in the contour of the diaphragm.
Jackson's	During quiet respiration, the movement of the paralyzed side of the chest may be greater than that of the opposite side, whereas in forced respiration, the paralyzed side moves less than the other.
Lorenz's	This sign is stiffness of the thoracic spine in early pulmonary tuberculosis.
Perez's	Rales are audible over the upper part of the chest when the arms are alternately raised and lowered; it is a common occurrence in cases of fibrous mediastinitis and aneurysm of the aortic arch.
Rotch's	Percussion dullness occurs in the fifth intercostal space on the right side in cases of pericardial effusion.
Schamroth's	In patients with clubbing, there are loss of the normal diamond-shaped aperture at the base of the nails and an increased angle at the nail tips when the dorsal surfaces of the terminal phalanges are approximated.
Skoda's	Skodaic resonance occurs.

The pathophysiology of pulsus paradoxus is likely multifactorial.[24] With wider swings in intrathoracic pressure associated with airway obstruction, there is a wider gradient between pressure within the intrathoracic and extrathoracic arterial vessels. Thus the left ventricle must generate increased force to keep the arterial pressure relatively constant. Because the ventricle does not do so in an instantaneous fashion, there is a drop in arterial pressure. The wider swing in intrathoracic pressure also results in greater right ventricular filling pressure, leading to increased right ventricular end-diastolic volume and displacement of the ventricular septum leftward. This reduces left ventricular filling, thereby reducing stroke volume and further decreasing arterial pressure during and immediately after inspiration.

BOX 12-1
Digital Clubbing

Intrapulmonary shunting and inflammation
- Bronchiectasis
- Severe pneumonia, lung abscess, or empyema
- Interstitial lung disease (autoimmune and infectious)
- Pulmonary arteriovenous malformation
- Hepatopulmonary syndrome
- Pulmonary malignancy

Cardiac and cardiovascular causes
- Cyanotic congenital heart disease
- Bacterial endocarditis

Noncardiopulmonary causes
- Inflammatory bowel disease
- Thyrotoxicosis

Familial

BOX 12-2
Cyanosis

Central cyanosis

Arterial hypoxemia
Normal levels of arterial oxygen
- Hematologic causes
  - Methemoglobin
  - Other hemoglobinopathies
- Vascular cause
  - Superior vena caval obstruction

Peripheral cyanosis

Vascular causes
- Peripheral cyanosis resulting from vasomotor instability or hypothermia
- Venous obstruction
- Shock or hypoperfusion with venous stasis

Hematologic cause
- Polycythemia

Pulsus paradoxus is useful in evaluating children with cystic fibrosis[25] and asthma, in which pulsus paradoxus of more than 15 mm Hg has been found to correlate with a 1-second forced expiratory volume of less than 60% of the predicted value.[26] It should be noted that the levels of pulsus paradoxus commonly seen with obstructive lung disease are much higher than those seen in individuals whose cardiac tamponade is the etiology of pulsus paradoxus.

EVALUATION OF THE CHILD WITH CHRONIC COUGH

Physiology

Cough is an extremely important component of pulmonary host defense. When functioning effectively, it clears bulk material from the airway. In patients with impaired mucociliary clearance either from acquired or congenital abnormalities of ciliary function or other mechanical factors, cough may be the only airway clearance mechanism available. The loss of effective cough in patients with advanced neuromuscular or neurologic disease is a critical factor in the morbidity and mortality of those disorders.

Although a seemingly simple action, cough is actually a very complex reflex involving afferent pathways in the vagus and efferent pathways in the somatic nervous system. Cough can be produced or suppressed volitionally, although it is not always completely suppressible. Although their existence has not yet been confirmed histologically (only inferred by physiology and suggested by electron micrographic studies), cough receptors are thought to be fairly widely distributed in the respiratory tract. They are found predominantly in the extrapulmonary airways (larynx, trachea, mainstem bronchi) but are also present in the external auditory canals, tympanic membranes, upper airway, pleura, pericardium, and diaphragm. Few, if any, are found in the lung parenchyma itself.

The sequence of events associated with a cough are well described. The initial phase consists of opening of the glottis and a short inspiration, which increases lung volume for the next phases. The glottis then closes, and the chest wall, abdominal, and perineal muscles contract, generating high intrathoracic and transpulmonary pressures. With the sudden opening of the glottis, there is rapid decompression of the airway with a high-velocity expulsion of gas and movement of airway contents (e.g., secretions and other solid material) proximally. In smaller airways the intrathoracic pressure generated may lead to airway closure, trapping some material distally. Thus cough primarily clears the larger, more central airways. Recognition of this phenomenon has led to alternative methods of airway clearance, such as autogenic drainage[27] and the use of positive expiratory pressure and flutter valve devices,[27,28] which are thought to be more effective at clearing the smaller, more distal airways.

Movement of material as the result of coughing occurs by three mechanisms. First, the high-velocity airflow results in a wavelike gas or liquid pumping of the mucous blanket and movement of loose mucus and other material. The increase in intrathoracic pressure causes airway compression, which squeezes some material proximally into larger airways. This is especially important peripherally, where gas velocities are insufficient to propel mucus. Finally, the vibration of the airway walls and the shearing force of the high-velocity gas flow dislodge mucus from the wall. The sounds produced by coughing are the result of the vibration of secretions and nonrigid respiratory structures.

In contrast to the beneficial airway clearing effects of cough, there are a number of potential deleterious effects as well. Extremely forceful coughing may induce bronchospasm in some individuals. With extremely forceful coughing, there may be injury to the larynx or development of an air leak such as a pneumothorax, a pneumomediastinum, or interstitial emphysema. The high intrathoracic pressures generated during coughing impede venous return to the heart, may result in transient systemic hypertension, or may induce dysrhythmias. Syncope can occur because of strenuous coughing. With very forceful coughing, rib fractures may occur. Other complications include rupture of the rectus abdominis muscles, urinary incontinence, pulmonary emboli, and kinking and knotting of venous catheters. An excellent in-depth review of cough is available.[29]

Evaluation

There are many etiologies of chronic cough in childhood (Box 12-3). Without some guidance in tailoring it to the individual, evaluation of this complaint could consume a tremendous amount of time and medical resources. The guidance needed can usually be provided by a careful history.

BOX 12-3
Persistent Cough*

- Congenital anomalies
  - Connection of the airway to the esophagus
    - Laryngeal cleft
    - Tracheoesophageal fistula
  - Laryngotracheomalacia
    - Primary laryngotracheomalacia
    - Laryngotracheomalacia secondary to vascular or other compression
  - Bronchopulmonary foregut malformation
  - Congenital mediastinal tumors
  - Congenital heart disease with pulmonary congestion
- Infection
  - Recurrent viral infection (infants and toddlers)
  - Chlamydial infection (infants)
  - Whooping cough–like syndrome
    - *Bordetella pertussis* infection
    - Chlamydial infection
    - *Mycoplasma* infection
    - Cystic fibrosis (infants and toddlers)
  - Granulomatous infection
    - Mycobacterial infection
    - Fungal infection
  - Suppurative lung disease (bronchiectasis and lung abscess)
    - Cystic fibrosis
    - Foreign body aspiration with secondary suppuration
    - Cilia dyskinesia
    - Immunodeficiency
      - Primary immunodeficiency
      - Secondary immunodeficiency (especially human immunodeficiency virus and acquired immunodeficiency syndrome)
  - Paranasal sinus infection
- Allergy and asthma
  - Asthma and cough-variant asthma
  - Allergic or vasomotor rhinitis and postnasal drip
- Aspiration (fluid material)
  - Dyskinetic swallowing with aspiration
    - General neurodevelopmental problems
    - Möbius syndrome
  - Bottle-propping and bottle in bed (infants and toddlers)
  - Gastroesophageal reflux
- Foreign body aspiration (solid material)
  - Upper airway aspiration (tonsillar, pharyngeal, laryngeal)
  - Tracheobronchial aspiration
  - Esophageal aspiration with an obstruction or aspiration resulting from dysphagia
- Physical and chemical irritation
  - Smoke from tobacco products (active and passive)
  - Wood smoke from stoves and fireplaces
  - Dry, dusty environment (hobbies and employment)
  - Volatile chemicals (hobbies and employment)
- Psychogenic or habit cough

*Longer than 3 weeks.

Onset of cough in the neonatal period is suggestive of a congenital airway malformation. In the perinatal period, abnormalities such as tracheal stenosis, laryngeal web, and tracheosophageal fistula may present with cough, whereas tracheomalacia typically results in cough later in the neonatal period. There may be an association with infectious symptoms such as TORCH (toxoplasmosis, other agents, rubella, cytomegalovirus, herpes simplex) syndrome, chlamydial infection, or pertussis; in older children, there may be an association with tuberculosis or sinusitis. The character of the cough can also provide important clues to the etiology. A continual cough, perhaps worse at night, may be found in asthma, cystic fibrosis, or other forms of bronchiectasis (especially if the cough is productive). Features suggestive of asthma (such as prolonged cough after upper respiratory tract infections, exercise, or exposure to environmental irritants) or the presence of risk factors for asthma (family history, history of prematurity) should prompt a careful evaluation for asthma or cough-variant asthma as a cause. A loud, honking cough absent during sleep is highly suggestive of a psychogenic cough, habit cough, or cough tic. History of a choking or gagging spell followed by chronic cough may promote concern over a possible aspirated foreign body, although there may be no such history, even in cases of documented foreign body aspiration. Chronic aspiration or gastroesophageal reflux as the cause of cough may be elicited by a careful neurologic and feeding history. Obviously, signs or symptoms of chronic illness, such as poor growth, recurrent fevers, and purulent sputum, should prompt a search for more severe pulmonary or systemic disease. Finally, the social history often provides information vital to elucidation of the cause. Factors such as exposure to environmental tobacco smoke, wood stoves, solvents, and dusts can explain chronic respiratory symptoms. The presence of family or school conflicts may support a suspicion of psychogenic cough.

The physical examination must be complete and carefully performed, with emphasis placed on the head and neck (transverse nasal crease, allergic shiners, boggy anasal mucosa, polyps, ear disease, foreign body in ear or nose, postnasal drip, long uvula, cobblestoning of posterior pharynx), chest (hyperinflation, wheezes, crackle, stridor), and heart (murmurs, gallops, signs of heart failure). The laboratory evaluation, which could easily be exhaustive, should be directed by findings elicited in the history and examination. Common tests include pulmonary function testing, including bronchoprovocation (pharmacologic, exercise, cold air); chest radiograph (two views, occasionally inspiratory and expiratory or lateral decubitus) and other imaging studies (CT, magnetic resonance imaging [MRI], sinus series and CT); barium esophagogram; esophageal pH monitoring; and bronchoscopy. The use of flexible vs. rigid bronchoscopy in evaluating pediatric patients has been reviewed recently[30] and bronchoscopy may be appropriate in selected patients. Unless foreign body aspiration is considered likely, flexible fiberoptic bronchoscopy is generally the procedure of choice. Laboratory studies that may be helpful include a complete blood count with differential (evaluating for leukocytosis, eosinophilia), total immunoglobulin E assay, purified protein derivative and control skin tests, sweat test, sputum culture (including culture for acid-fast bacillus and fungus), ciliary biopsy, and limited allergy skin testing (limited to locally common aeroallergens and animals and foods known to be in the child's environment). It may also be reasonable to perform an empiric trial of bronchodilators or a short course of systemic corticosteroids.

EVALUATION OF THE CHILD WITH AIRWAY OBSTRUCTION

Regardless of the etiology of the obstruction, wheezing and stridor with increased work of breathing are the cardinal manifestations of clinically significant airway obstruction. Usually the term *stridor* refers to a vibratory sound that is loudest on inspiration and is predominantly due to dynamic extrathoracic airway obstruction. In contrast, wheezing is usually produced by intrathoracic obstruction that worsens on expiration. At times, it can be difficult to distinguish between wheezing and stridor, and it should be remembered that critical airway obstruction can lead to stridor or wheeze in both phases of respiration (Box 12-4). A monophonic wheeze suggests obstruction

BOX 12-4
Airway Obstruction: Wheeze and Stridor

Inspiratory obstruction = extrathoracic

The vibratory sound produced by inspiratory obstruction is heard during inspiration, is usually monophonic, and may be high pitched as in croup or low to medium pitched as in snoring resulting from adenotonsillar hypertrophy.

- Congenital malformations
  - Nasal, nasopharyngeal, and oropharyngeal malformations
    - Retrognathia (Pierre Robin syndrome)
    - Nasal, choanal, or nasopharyngeal stenosis; tumor; mass
      - Craniopharyngioma
      - Anterior encephalocele
      - Teratoma
    - Adenotonsillar hypertrophy
    - Obesity or redundant pharyngeal tissue
    - Hypotonia (e.g., Down syndrome)
    - Oral cavity or pharyngeal tumor
    - Lingual tumor
      - Lingual thyroid tumor
      - Hemangioma
    - Neck masses
      - Bronchial cleft cyst
      - Cystic hygroma
  - Laryngeal or subglottic airway malformations
    - Laryngomalacia
    - Paralyzed vocal cords
    - Laryngeal or arytenoid cysts
    - Laryngocele
    - Subglottic stenosis
    - Subglottic hemangioma
- Infection
  - Nasal, nasopharyngeal, and oropharyngeal infection
    - Tonsillitis and peritonsillar abscess
    - Sublingual abscess (Ludwig's angina)
    - Retropharyngeal abscess
  - Laryngeal and subglottic infection
    - Epiglottitis
    - Croup (spasmodic)
    - Bacterial tracheitis (usually some expiratory wheeze)
    - Juvenile respiratory papillomatosis (early)
    - Tetanus with laryngospasm
- Foreign body or aspiration
  - Gastroesophageal reflux with edema, laryngospasm
  - Foreign body aspiration in pharynx, larynx, or subglottis
- Trauma
  - Laryngeal hematoma
  - Laryngeal burns or scalds
  - Stenosis secondary to instrumentation
  - Vocal cord paralysis after surgery
- Allergy and asthma
  - Anaphylactoid reaction to food or inhalant
  - Vocal cord dysfunction
- Metabolic problem
  - Hypocalcemia or hypomagnesemia
- Acquired tumor (rare)

Expiratory obstruction = intrathoracic

The vibratory sound produced by this obstruction is best heard on expiration and may be focal or monophonic and of low to medium pitch or may be diffuse or polyphonic and of medium to high pitch.

- Congenital malformations
  - Tracheobronchial tree malformations
    - Tracheobronchomalacia
      - Primary (focal or diffuse) tracheobronchomalacia
      - Tracheobronchomalacia secondary to compression by tumor (focal)

Expiratory obstruction = intrathoracic—cont'd

- Congenital malformations–cont'd
    - Tracheostenosis
      - VATER (vertebral defects, imperforate anus, tracheo-esophageal fistula, radial and renal dysplasia) association
      - Complete tracheal rings
  - Vascular compression (ring or sling)
    - Aberrant subclavian vein
    - Pulmonary artery sling (aberrant left pulmonary artery)
    - Right-sided thoracic aorta with left ductus arteriosus
    - Left-sided thoracic aorta with right ductus arteriosus
    - Double aortic arch
  - Dilated cardiac chamber or dilated pulmonary artery with compression
- Infection
  - Intrinsic airway narrowing
    - Bronchitis
    - Bronchiolitis
    - Laryngotracheobronchitis
    - Bacterial tracheitis
    - Bronchiectasis
    - Cystic fibrosis
    - Juvenile respiratory papillomatosis (late)
  - Extrinsic airway compression
    - Mycobacterial or fungal infection with lymph node enlargement
    - Infection of congenital foregut malformations, cysts
    - Lung abscess
- Foreign body or aspiration
  - Gastroesophageal reflux with bronchitis
  - Foreign body in airway
  - Foreign body in esophagus
- Trauma
  - Tracheobronchial burns or scalds
  - Tracheobronchial injury (blunt or penetrating)
- Allergy and asthma
  - Anaphylactoid reaction to food or inhalant
  - Asthma with inflammation or bronchospasm
- Autoimmune disease
  - Bronchiolitis obliterans after lung or bone marrow transplant
  - Idiopathic bronchiolitis obliterans
- Tumor
  - Primary airway narrowing
    - Hamartoma
    - Benign tumors (e.g., lipoma, chondroma, myoblastoma)
    - Malignant tumor
      - Bronchial adenoma
      - Bronchogenic carcinoma
      - Sarcoma
  - Extrinsic airway compression
    - Hodgkin's lymphoma
    - T cell lymphoproliferative disease with mediastinal mass
    - Sarcoma
- Pulmonary edema

Inspiratory and expiratory obstruction

When obstruction is evident in both phases of breathing, the obstruction may be variable and may simultaneously occur in both the intrathoracic and extrathoracic airways (e.g., croup with laryngotracheobronchitis). If this has not occurred, the obstruction may have become critical in nature. This is particularly the case in extrathoracic airway obstruction in which the loss of obstruction during expiration is worrisome. In contrast, in intrathoracic airway obstruction resulting from asthma and bronchitis, wheezing commonly occurs in both phases of respiration but can usually be localized to the chest as opposed to the upper airway.

of a large central airway, whereas a polyphonic wheeze reflects peripheral airway obstruction.

Although asthma is certainly the most common disorder associated with wheezing, not every child with wheezing has asthma, nor does every child with asthma wheeze. The differential diagnosis of wheezing varies significantly with the age of the child. Congenital anatomic abnormalities that produce wheezing, like those associated with cough, are generally more likely to present in early infancy rather than later. Laryngotracheomalacia is an exception, usually presenting at several weeks of age or later. Laryngomalacia and extrathoracic tracheomalacia typically present as inspiratory stridor, whereas intrathoracic tracheomalacia and bronchomalacia are associated with low-pitched expiratory wheezing. Asthma, bronchiolitis, and bronchopulmonary dysplasia all may be associated with wheezing in infancy but can generally be distinguished on historical grounds. Along with asthma, cystic fibrosis and chronic aspiration (secondary to gastroesophageal reflux or a neurologic abnormality with dysfunctional swallowing) may present as wheezing at any age. Foreign body aspiration, most commonly pulmonary but also esophageal, classically presents as a monophonic, unilateral wheeze and is unusual before 6 months of age. This diagnosis, however, should be considered regardless of history (or lack thereof). Congestive heart failure may lead to wheezing secondary to lymphatic engorgement and resultant compression of the airway within the peribronchovascular sheath. Finally, wheezing may be produced by vocal cord opposition, either volitionally (often subconsciously) or because of vocal cord dysfunction.[31]

Evaluation of the child with wheezing starts with a careful history followed by thorough examination. When present, signs and symptoms of increased work of breathing or distress may dictate swift intervention before etiologic evaluation can take place. Depending on the age of the patient and the suspected etiology, ancillary tests may be helpful. These could include imaging studies (chest radiograph, CT, MRI, esophagogram, swallowing study), pulmonary function testing with bronchoprovocation or bronchodilator response, microbiologic studies (especially for respiratory syncytial virus in infants), and an empiric trial of bronchodilators. Bronchoscopic evaluation may also be helpful.

EVALUATION OF THE CHILD WITH EXERCISE INTOLERANCE

The majority of patients with chronic lung or cardiac disease and exercise intolerance usually have a clear reason for the inability to exercise; this may include deconditioning secondary to the primary illness. Instead of deconditioning, this section addresses the apparently normal child who has a difficult time exercising and develops dyspnea with a normal workload. These patients are commonly brought to their physician because they are unable to complete physical education at school or have a difficult time on sports teams. The approach to the apparently normal child with exercise intolerance involves delineating whether the child has a cardiorespiratory problem or is simply deconditioned (Box 12-5). The history is critical in this assessment. Data regarding symptoms compatible with asthma, cystic fibrosis, or another lung condition such as preexisting bronchopulmonary dysplasia need to be obtained. Similarly, a history of congenital or acquired cardiac disease needs to be reviewed.

BOX 12-5
Exercise Intolerance

- Chronic lung disease
  - Asthma
    - Exercise-induced bronchospasm
    - Vocal cord dysfunction
    - Deconditioning resulting from exercise-induced bronchospasm
  - Other pulmonary conditions
    - Bronchopulmonary dysplasia
    - Cystic fibrosis
    - Pulmonary fibrosis
    - Other
- Congenital or acquired cardiac disease
- Deconditioning with or without obesity
- Myopathy or muscular dystrophy
- Endocrine abnormalities
  - Thyroid dysfunction
  - Cortisol insufficiency
  - Diabetes mellitus
- Other chronic illnesses

Other than deconditioning, the leading cause of exercise intolerance is a variant of asthma, exercise-induced bronchospasm (EIB).[32] Children with EIB usually complain of a tightening or pain in the chest or submental triangle after vigorous exercise. This pain may be associated with frank wheezing or cough. Usually, patients complain of difficulty breathing that does not improve on stopping the exercise but that instead worsens after they sit down to rest. The symptoms then usually subside spontaneously. On cold or dry days, the tightness and cough are worse with exercise involving free running, such as soccer, football, and hockey. Swimming and cycling seem less prone to inducing bronchospasm. Some athletes notice that they can "run through" their bronchospasm or even prevent it by doing brief sprints before competing to obtain the protective effect of exercise on further EIB. Children with EIB may also have a history of spontaneous or prolonged wheezing and cough with colds. Collateral allergic symptoms should also be sought. The physical examination may be normal, but signs of allergy and asthma should be sought. Occasionally, wheezing or hyperinflation may be found; however, in children with these signs, usually asthma has already been diagnosed. Laboratory studies such as an exercise or cold-air challenge test may be conducted both to demonstrate airway hyperreactivity and to reproduce the symptoms so that the child can confirm their nature (see Chapter 15). In contrast, a trial of a β-agonist such as albuterol before exercise may be effective in diagnosing EIB as well as assessing a treatment modality.

Cardiovascular disease leading to exercise intolerance in an apparently normal child is uncommon and is usually diagnosed based on a history of diaphoresis and dyspnea with initiation of exercise. Furthermore, dyspnea resolves with resting compared to the persistence or worsening of EIB. A history of ankle edema, palpitations, fainting, chest pain, and nocturnal symptoms such as orthopnea or paroxysmal nocturnal dyspnea should be obtained but is positive only in children with relatively severe disease. Physical examination may reveal weight loss and fatigue, a hyperactive precordium, pathologic murmurs, and evidence of hypervolemia such as hepatomegaly and peripheral edema. Electrocardiography and chest radiography are central to the laboratory assessment; however, a child with dyspnea and signs of cardiac disease should be referred to a pediatric cardiologist for clinical assessment, echocardiography, and management.

It is relatively common for the pulmonary specialist to be asked to assess a child for exercise intolerance who has neither EIB nor heart disease. These children are commonly mildly to moderately obese, have a sedentary lifestyle, and do not readily engage in sports. They are commonly assessed because of an inability to keep up with school exercise programs. Their dyspnea and fatigue usually occur during exercise such as running laps. They usually do not have chest pain or cough and do not complain of any dysphoria or tightness in the submental region. They may complain of headache, leg pain, and cramping with exercise. Lacking the symptom complexes and findings previously noted, this group may most benefit from exercise testing. The clinician can use the test to reproduce the symptoms and demonstrate that the child does not have bronchospasm. Furthermore, the child may be unable to exercise vigorously enough to successfully complete an exercise challenge test. These clinical and laboratory findings combined can be useful to reassure the family that cardiorespiratory disease is not present and that deconditioning is the main problem. An exercise program and weight-control program can then be prescribed to help the child return to an active lifestyle.

EVALUATION OF THE CHILD WITH CHEST PAIN

The child with chest pain can present a challenge for the practitioner; parental anxiety is usually high because of the concern that the child may have heart disease (Box 12-6). In fact, the majority of children with chest pain have either EIB or a musculoskeletal cause that will respond to antiinflammatory medication or nonspecific therapies.[33,34]Chest pain resulting from cardiac disease is uncommon in an apparently healthy child without other cardiac symptoms. The history should be focused after the clinician determines that the child is generally well. The pain should be characterized using the PQRST approach. The pain is described as sharp, burning, or dull and aching. It is localized, and any radiation such as from the spine through an intercostal space should be noted. Radiation to the shoulder suggests diaphragmatic irritation. Worsening of the pain with breathing or movement should be noted, as should other provocative factors. The history should include a survey of activities compatible with muscular strain such as recent trauma, contact sports, and sports such as weight training. Surprisingly, many children do not associate anterior parasternal chest pain with the fact that they just began weight training to increase their pectoral muscle bulk. Also, many children carry schoolbooks in a pack or bag slung over one shoulder, leading to shoulder girdle strain. Patients with asthma, pertussis, and cystic fibrosis may develop chest pain associated with chronic cough and repetitive trauma to the ribs and muscles of the chest wall. The history should also review recent symptoms of lung infection, allergies, asthma, and EIB. Symptoms of arthritis or joint disease should be assessed, as should any recent skin changes or weight loss. Gastroesophageal reflux with esophagitis can also present as chest pain. A history of reflux after meals or on lying down with heartburn, a bitter taste in the mouth, water brash, and sensitivity to acid, high-fat foods, or coffee can be helpful. The physical examination should be relatively complete and include an assessment of general well-being and the respiratory, cardiovascular, gastrointestinal, and musculoskeletal systems. Changes on the chest wall with swelling or any mass, particularly over the costochondral and clavicular joints, should be specifically noted. Tenderness over the site of chest pain strongly implicates a musculoskeletal process. Although acute infection such as pneumococcal pneumonia with pleurisy is usually a clear diagnosis, other infections such as histoplasmosis, coccidioidomycosis, and tuberculosis may have a slow course and present with pleuritic pain. Thus a careful chest examination for reduced air entry, crackles, or a friction rub is important. The results of chest radiography are usually normal in musculoskeletal chest pain but may be reassuring to both the parent and practitioner. Electrocardiography or stress testing is only occasionally useful in cases without additional cardiac symptoms or signs.

BOX 12-6
Chest Pain

- Musculoskeletal or soft tissue problems (most common)
  - Chronic cough (asthma, cystic fibrosis, pertussis)
  - Sports or weight training that caused muscle or joint strain
  - Blunt trauma to the ribs or joints
  - Costochondritis
  - Tietze's syndrome
  - Rheumatoid arthritis
  - Breath development, inflammation
  - Diaphragmatic pain
  - Slipping rib syndrome
- Asthma
  - Acute bronchospasm, especially with exercise
  - Pneumomediastinum
  - Pneumothorax
- Pleural inflammation
  - Viral inflammation: Bornholm disease or pleurodynia
  - Bacterial, mycobacterial, or fungal infection with pleurisy
- Gastrointestinal or abdominal problems
  - Gastroesophageal reflux
  - Gastric or duodenal ulcer
  - Diaphragmatic irritation caused by an intraabdominal process
- Cardiac problems (uncommon)
  - Aberrant coronary problems
  - Pericarditis, myocarditis, or myopathy
  - Palpitations or dysrhythmias that are confused with pain
- Pulmonary vasculature
  - Pulmonary embolus
  - Sickle cell pulmonary crisis
- Psychogenic or psychophysiologic problems

EVALUATION OF THE CHILD WITH HEMOPTYSIS

The approach to diagnosing hemoptysis in a child depends on whether there is a known preexisting disease such as cystic fibrosis.[35,36] In the previously well child with hemoptysis, the history is critical (Box 12-7). Care should be taken to ensure that the red or purple material expectorated was actually blood and not coloring from food. Afterward, the most important point is to try to determine that the bleeding truly represents respiratory bleeding from the lower respiratory tract and is not due to nasal, pharyngeal, or gastrointestinal bleeding (Table 12-6). A history of recent epistaxis, acute or recurrent tonsillitis, or throat trauma focuses attention on the upper respiratory tract. Indeed, examination of the nasopharynx by a specialist is sometimes important in ruling out a bleeding site in the upper respiratory tract. A history of gastroesophageal reflux, vomiting, liver disease, or portal hypertension focuses concern on the gastrointestinal tract as the source of the bleeding.

Although some streaking of the sputum in bacterial bronchitis or pneumonia is relatively common, true hemoptysis in

BOX 12-7
Hemoptysis

Pulmonary origin of bleeding

Infection
- Acute tracheobronchitis or severe pneumonia
- Bronchiectasis
- Erosion by an infected lymph node (mycobacteria, fungi)
- Lung abscess
- Fungal infection, including secondary mycetoma
- Parasitic infection
- Pulmonary hemorrhage in severe viral pneumonia

Foreign body aspiration

Bronchial tumor
- Primary tumor
- Secondary tumor

Autoimmune lung disease
- Idiopathic pulmonary hemosiderosis
- Goodpasture's syndrome
- Milk allergy (Heiner syndrome)
- Wegener's granulomatosis
- Other vasculitis (e.g., Churg Strauss)

Pulmonary vascular conditions
- Pulmonary embolism
- Primary pulmonary hypertension
- Obstructed pulmonary veins
- Raised left arterial pressure
  - Congestive heart failure or pulmonary edema
  - Mitral valve stenosis
  - Aortic valvular stenosis or obstruction
- Arteriovenous malformations
- Osler-Weber-Rendu disease
- Sickle cell pulmonary crisis
- Pulmonary hemorrhage in acute respiratory distress syndrome

Bronchopulmonary foregut malformations

Trauma
- Blunt trauma with pulmonary contusion or airway disruption
- Penetrating trauma

Nonpulmonary origin of bleeding

Upper airway conditions
- Epistaxis
- Sinusitis
- Adenoidal or tonsillar bleeding
- Severe pharyngitis or pharyngeal trauma
- Coagulopathy with trauma to the mouth or pharynx

Gastrointestinal conditions
- Esophagitis with gastroesophageal reflux
- Esophageal varices secondary to portal hypertension
- Gastric or duodenal ulcer
- Mallory-Weiss syndrome or esophageal erosion with severe vomiting or bulimia

Munchausen or Munchausen by proxy syndrome

Lack of bleeding

Natural and artificial coloring in food
Dyes in medicines
Nasal foreign body with dye (crayon)

the previously well child is rare. The hemoptysis should be characterized by the volume of blood (i.e., streaking vs. submassive [<240 ml] vs. massive [≥240 ml]). Whether the blood was a bright red liquid that clotted or simply old purple-brown clots should be noted. In the case of submassive and massive hemoptysis the patient may have a warm, bubbling feeling over the affected segment. The history should rigorously assess the possibility of foreign body aspiration. This may not have been a recent event because foreign bodies leading to bleeding must usually be in the respiratory tree long enough to cause chronic infection or irritation with mucosal erosion. Past respiratory illness such as remote foreign body aspiration,

Table 12-6 Differential Features of Hemoptysis and Hematemesis

HEMOPTYSIS	HEMATEMESIS
Blood is coughed up, not vomited. Retching and nausea may come from pharyngeal irritation from blood.	Blood is vomited.
A portion of the blood should be frothy.	Blood is never frothy.
Blood is usually, but not always, bright red in color.	Blood is dark red in color.
Blood is alkaline in reaction.	Blood is acid in reaction.
Hemoptysis is preceded by a gurgling noise or a sensation stimulating a cough reflex. This may be absent in massive hemoptysis.	Hematemesis is preceded by nausea and vomiting.
There is sometimes a history of past cough.	There may be history of alcoholism and/or gastric disturbances, plus clinical findings of liver disease.
There is continued blood-tinged sputum, which lasts for several days.	Blood-tinged sputum is usually absent.
Blood is mixed with pus, organisms, or macrophages; some of the macrophages may contain hemosiderin particles.	Vomited blood may contain food particles.
Anemia may or may not be present.	There are often clinical and laboratory findings of blood loss before the actual hematemesis.

From Lyons HA: *Basics of RD: ATS news,* New York, 1976, American Lung Association.

pertussis, and severe pneumonia can also be associated with hemoptysis related to bronchiectasis formation. A history of heart disease should be obtained because increased left atrial pressures or obstructed pulmonary veins can lead to bleeding. Usually, however, the cardiovascular history is negative. Physical examination is usually negative in the absence of acute lung infection or chronic lung problems such as cystic fibrosis. Focal lung changes such as reduced or lagged air entry and focal hyperinflation may suggest foreign body aspiration. Coarse crackles and reduced air entry may lead to the consideration of infection and, if accompanied by clubbing, bronchiectasis. Chest radiography is used to rule out pneumonia, gross bronchiectasis, and cavitary disease. Evidence of focal hyperaeration or atelectasis may suggest focal airway obstruction resulting from a foreign body, infected lymph node, or tumor. If the diagnosis of bronchiectasis is considered, a thin-section, high-resolution CT scan rapidly identifies the presence of these lesions. Bronchoscopy can also be used, but the site may be obscured in the presence of moderate bleeding. Bronchoscopy may be most useful after the bleeding has quieted, when lesions such as bronchial adenomas, lymph nodes eroding the mucosa, and foreign bodies can be better seen. Angiography may be used while echocardiography and cardiac catheterization may have a role in diagnosing recurrent hemoptysis with no apparent lesion. In this case the hemoptysis may result from an obstructed pulmonary vein.

EVALUATION OF THE CHILD WITH HYPOXIA

The approach to evaluating the child with evidence of tissue hypoxia requires the determination of whether the hypoxia is due to a failure of oxygen delivery or an inability of the tissues to use oxygen (Box 12-8). Failure of oxygen delivery or use may be evidenced by an alteration in global metabolism, resulting in anaerobic glycolysis with the production of a lactic acidosis, or an end-organ dysfunction (e.g., confusion secondary to cerebral hypoperfusion). A common approach has been to classify tissue hypoxia as occurring in one of four manners. The first two abnormalities lead to reduced oxygen content in the blood. The most common cause in patients with lung disease, hypoxemic hypoxia, is due to a reduced arterial partial pressure of oxygen, leading to an inadequate saturation of hemoglobin (see later section). The second is anemic hypoxia. Even with a normal arterial partial pressure of oxygen and hemoglobin saturation, anemia (reduced functional hemoglobin) leads to reduced oxygen delivery resulting from reduced oxygen capacity in the blood. This occurs in carbon monoxide poisoning, in which the hemoglobin is bound with the carbon monoxide, reducing the amount available to carry oxygen. In addition, carbon monoxide poisoning increases the affinity of hemoglobin for oxygen, further reducing oxygen delivery to the tissues. If oxygen content is adequate but signs of tissue hypoxia are present, there are two possibilities. Either the oxygen is not being delivered to the tissues, or the tissues are unable to use oxygen in aerobic metabolism. The former is called *circulatory hypoxia* and may occur globally as in shock or locally as in vascular obstruction with ischemia. The latter, histotoxic hypoxia, occurs in sepsis and cyanide poisoning of aerobic metabolism when the cells are unable to conduct aerobic glycolysis.

BOX 12-8
Tissue Hypoxia

- Hypoxemic hypoxia: low arterial partial pressure of oxygen
  - Low inspired oxygen concentration (low inspired oxygen partial pressure)
    - Low barometric pressure (high altitude)
    - Low inspired oxygen concentration (low fraction of inspired oxygen
  - Cardiorespiratory disease
    - Hypoventilation
    - Diffusion block
    - Ventilation-perfusion imbalance
    - Shunting
      - Intrapulmonary shunting
      - Extrapulmonary shunting
- Anemic hypoxia
  - Anemia
  - Carbon monoxide poisoning
- Circulatory hypoxia
  - Shock or hypoperfusion
    - Hypovolemic shock
    - Obstructive shock
    - Cardiogenic shock
    - Distributive shock
  - Local vascular obstruction
- Histotoxic hypoxia
  - Sepsis with poor oxygen use
  - Cyanide poisoning

The approach to hypoxemic hypoxia (see Box 12-8) is to divide potential causes into five categories. As in assessing tissue hypoxia, the clinician simply needs to work through the steps of the oxygenation of blood in the lung to delineate potential problems. First, a reduced inspired oxygen partial pressure leads to hypoxemia in the absence of compensatory hyperventilation. This may result from a reduced fractional concentration of oxygen secondary to oxygen consumption by combustion or of other gases in the environment. It may also occur with a reduced barometric pressure caused by increases in altitude. Hypoventilation with an increase in the level of alveolar carbon dioxide and decrease in the level of alveolar oxygen causes hypoxemia as a result of a failure to ventilate adequate oxygen into the lungs to meet the body's metabolic demands. These first two causes of hypoxemia are associated with a normal alveolar-arterial oxygen difference. Thickening of the alveolar-capillary membrane may cause the normal perfusion limitation of oxygen transfer to become diffusion limited and lead to hypoxemia. Increased cardiac output and reduced alveolar oxygen levels exacerbate this diffusion block. Areas of local hypoventilation in the lung resulting from either airway or airspace disease lead to hypoxemia secondary to a ventilation-perfusion imbalance with incomplete saturation of blood passing through these regions of the lung. Finally, blood from the systemic venous system may bypass the ventilation entirely, either because of intrapulmonary shunting with lung disease or arteriovenous fistulae or because of extrapulmonary shunting with congenital heart or great vessel malformation (cyanotic congenital heart disease). The arterial carbon dioxide level may be normal in all of these conditions except hypoventilation. This is because the healthy, well-ventilated lung can compensate for the dysfunctional lung by clearing excess carbon dioxide. Unfortunately, blood that is normally ventilated is already nearly completely saturated with oxygen, and thus healthy units cannot return arterial oxygen to normal by overcompensating for units with diffusion block, ventilation-perfusion imbalance, or shunt. Finally, shunt is commonly separated from the other causes of hypoxia because it does not respond to the administration of supplemental oxygen with a significant increase in arterial oxygen levels.

EVALUATION OF THE CHILD WITH HYPOVENTILATION

The definition of *hypoventilation* is an increase in the arterial carbon dioxide level above 45 mm Hg; it is, by definition, a respiratory acidosis. It may differ with the apparent minute ventilation, tidal volume, or respiratory rate. *Hyperpnea* and *hypopnea* refer to an apparent increase or decrease in overall breathing; however, *hyperventilation* and *hypoventilation* refer specifically to the level of arterial carbon dioxide achieved. The first step in assessing the child with hypoventilation is to try to determine whether the respiratory pump is functioning as well as expected in response to substantive lung disease or whether it is a primary or adjunctive cause of the increased arterial carbon dioxide (Box 12-9). Second, the pump may be functioning properly and delivering an adequate minute ventilation; however, there may be an increased ventilation of physiologic dead space with reduced alveolar ventilation. This may result either from a reduction in tidal volume with a fixed physiologic dead space or from an increase in physiologic dead space that is not matched by an increase in tidal volume. In either case, the dead space/tidal volume ratio increases, and alveolar ventilation is compromised, leading to carbon dioxide retention.

The differential diagnosis of airspace or airway disease that can lead to carbon dioxide retention is broad and is not addressed further here. The differential diagnosis of a failure of the respiratory pump is considered here because it may apply even in the cases in which lung disease is paramount. A useful approach is to work through the steps necessary for the maintenance of minute ventilation, starting centrally with respiratory

BOX 12-9
Hypoventilation

Reduced minute ventilation

Respiratory pump failure as a primary cause
- Central controller failures
  - Encephalopathy or brain stem dysfunction
    - Infection
    - Intoxication
    - Metabolic dysfunction or seizure
    - Tumor
    - Trauma, concussion, or hemorrhage
    - Malformation (Arnold-Chiari malformation)
  - Central hypoventilation syndrome
  - Metabolic alkalosis
- Cervical spinal cord disruption (upper motor neuron)
  - Infection
  - Tumor
  - Trauma, concussion, or hemorrhage
  - Inflammation (transverse myelitis)
  - Compression (achondroplasia, Down syndrome)
  - Multiple sclerosis
- Cervical spinal cord (lower motor neuron: cell)
  - Infection (poliomyelitis)
  - Inflammation or degeneration (transverse myelitis)
  - Vasculitis or vascular accident
  - Werdnig-Hoffman disease
- Phrenic or intercostal nerves (lower motor neuron: axon)
  - Trauma (thoracic surgery or penetrating injury)
  - Demyelinating neuropathies (Guillain-Barré syndrome)
  - Tumor
- Neuromuscular junction failure
  - Myasthenia gravis
  - Botulism
  - Aminoglycosides
  - Pseudocholinesterase deficiency
- Respiratory muscle failure
  - Muscular dystrophies
  - Extreme electrolyte abnormalities

Reduced minute ventilation—cont'd

- Respiratory muscle failure—cont'd
  - Extreme starvation or metabolic imbalance
  - Familial paralysis syndromes (e.g., hypokalemia)
- Chest wall disease or disruption
  - Flail chest
  - Restrictive chest wall disease
    - Kyphoscoliosis
    - Congenital chest wall malformation or dystrophy
    - Ankylosing spondylitis
  - Prune-belly syndrome (infancy)

Increased respiratory work with muscle fatigue
- Increased elastic work
  - Pulmonary fibrosis
  - Pulmonary edema
    - Cardiogenic edema
    - Noncardiogenic edema (adult respiratory distress sydrome)
  - Diffuse pneumonia
- Increased resistive work
  - Upper airway obstruction
  - Lower airway obstruction
- Mixed increase in elastic and resistive work

Increased minute or reduced alveolar ventilation

Increased physiologic dead space
- Increased anatomic dead space
  - Severe bronchiectasis
- Increased alveolar dead space
  - Alveolar distention or overexpansion
    - Intrathoracic airway obstructive airway disease
    - Mechanical ventilation with inadvertent positive end-expiratory pressure
  - Shock with reduced pulmonary perfusion pressures
  - Pulmonary embolus

Reduced tidal volume with normal physiologic dead space

control and ending with the respiratory muscles and chest wall (see Box 12-9). Failure may result from central controller failure or disruption of upper motor neuron function, such as in sedation or cervical cord damage. Lower motor neuron disease may occur at a cellular level, such as in poliomyelitis, or may be more peripheral resulting from damage to the phrenic nerves caused by trauma or demyelinating diseases. The neuromuscular junction may inadequately conduct the neural impulse, such as in botulism, or the muscle be unable to respond, such as in profound hypokalemia. Finally, even if the controller/feedback system is functioning and the respiratory muscles are able to respond, the chest wall itself must be able to function as a pump without reduced motion or inappropriate paradoxical motion.

REFERENCES

1. Barnes LA: *Manual of pediatric physical diagnosis,* ed 6, St Louis, 1991, Mosby.
2. DeGowin EL: *Bedside diagnostic examination: a comprehensive pocket textbook,* ed 5, New York, 1987, Macmillan.

History

3. Chetcuti P, Phelan PD, Greenwood R: Lung function abnormalities in repaired oesophageal atresia and tracheo-oesophageal fistula, *Thorax* 47:1030-1034, 1992.
4. Fanconi S, Kraemer R, Weber J, Tschaeppeler H, Pfenninger J: Long-term sequelae in children surviving adult respiratory distress syndrome, *J Pediatr* 106:218-222, 1985.
5. Tremper L, Park SM: Long-term follow-up of pediatric survivors of ARDS, *Chest* 94(suppl):74s, 1988.

Physical Examination

6. Moore KL, Peraud TVN: *The developing human,* ed 5, Philadelphia, 1977, WB Saunders, pp 193-195.
7. Michaels L: Ear. In Sternberg SS, ed: *Histology for pathologists,* New York, 1992, Raven, pp 925-949.
8. Gillam GL, McNichol KN, Williams HE: Chest deformity, residual airways obstruction and hyperinflation and growth in children with asthma, *Arch Dis Child* 45:789-799, 1970.
9. Kerem E, Canny G, Tibshirani R, Reisman J, Bentur L, Schuh S, Levison H: Clinical-physiologic correlations in acute asthma of childhood, *Pediatrics* 87:481-486, 1991.
10. Barnes LA: *Manual of pediatric physical diagnosis,* ed 6, St Louis, 1991, Mosby, p 97.
11. DeGowin EL: *Bedside diagnostic examination: a comprehensive pocket textbook,* ed 5, New York, 1987, Macmillan, pp 301-302.
12. Rappaport MB, Sprague HB: Physiologic and physical laws that govern auscultation and their clinical application, *Am Heart J* 21:257-318, 1941.
13. Kraman S: Lung sounds (audiotape), Northbrook, Ill, 1990, American College of Chest Physicians.
14. Kraman SS: Vesicular (normal) lung sounds: how are they made, where do they come from, and what do they mean? *Semin Respir Med* 6:183-191, 1985.
15. Wilkins RL, Dexter JR, Murphy RLH, DelBono EA: Lung sound nomenclature survey, *Chest* 987:886-889, 1990.
16. Murphy RLH: Discontinuous adventitious lung sounds, *Semin Respir Med* 6:210-219, 1985.
17. Bigler FC: The morphology of clubbing, *Am J Pathol* 34:237-261, 1958.
18. Lovell RRH: Observations on the structure of clubbed fingers, *Clin Sci* 9:299-321, 1950.
19. Bentley D, Moore A, Shwachman H: Finger clubbing: a quantitative survey by analysis of the shadowgraph, *Lancet* 2:164-167, 1976.

20. Waring WW, Wilkinson RW, Wiebe RA, Faul BC, Hilman BC: Quantitation of digital clubbing in children: measurement of casts of the index finger, *Am Rev Respir Dis* 104:155-174, 1971.
21. Martinez-Lavin M: Recent findings in hypertrophic osteoarthropathy, *Contemp Intern Med* 4:75-85, 1992.
22. Lemen RJ, Gates AJ, Mathe AA, Waring WW, Hyman AL, Kadowitz PD: Relationships among digital clubbing, disease severity and serum prostaglandins F2a and E concentrations in cystic fibrosis patients, *Am Rev Respir Dis* 117:639-646, 1978.
23. Dickinson CJ: The aetiology of clubbing and hypertrophic osteoarthropathy, *Eur J Clin Invest* 23:330-338, 1993.
24. McGregor M: Pulsus paradoxus, *New Engl J Med* 301:480-482, 1979.
25. Hen J, Dolan TF: Pulsus paradoxus in cystic fibrosis, *J Pediatr* 99:585-587, 1981.
26. Rebuck AS, Tomarken JL: Pulsus paradoxus in asthmatic children, *Can Med Assoc J* 112:710-711, 1975.

Evaluation of the Child with Chronic Cough

27. Pryor JA, Webber BA: Physiotherapy for cystic fibrosis: which technique? *Physiotherapy* 78:105-108, 1992.
28. Mahlmeister MJ, Fink JB, Hoffman GL, Fifer LF: Positive-expiratory-pressure mask therapy: theoretical and practical considerations and a review of the literature, *Respir Care* 36:1218-1229, 1991.
29. Banner AS: Cough: physiology, evaluation, and treatment, *Lung* 164:74-92, 1986.
30. Perez CR, Wood RD: Update on pediatric flexible bronchoscopy, *Pediatr Clin North Am* 41:385-400, 1994.

Evaluation of the Child with Airway Obstruction

31. Brugman SM, Howell JH, Rosenberg DM, Blager FB, Lack G: The spectrum of pediatric vocal cord dysfunction, *Am J Respir Crit Care Med* 149:A353, 1994.

Evaluation of the Child with Exercise Intolerance

32. Pierson WE: Exercise induced bronchospasm in children and adolescents, *Pediatr Clin North Am* 35:1031-1040, 1988.

Evaluation of the Child with Chest Pain

33. Zavaras-Angelidou KA, Weinhouse E, Nelson DB: Review of 180 episodes of chest pain in 134 children, *Pediatr Emerg Care* 8:189-193, 1992.
34. Wiens L, Sabath R, Ewing L, Gowdamarajan R, Portnoy J, Scagliotti D: Chest pain in otherwise healthy children and adolescents is frequently caused by exercise-induced asthma, *Pediatrics* 90:350-353, 1992.

Evaluation of the Child with Hemoptysis

35. Schidlow DV, Taussig LM, Knowles MR: Cystic Fibrosis Foundation consensus conference report on pulmonary complications of cystic fibrosis, *Pediatr Pulmonol* 15:187-198, 1993.
36. Pianosi P, al-Sadoon H: Hemoptysis in children, *Pediatr Rev* 17:344-348, 1996.

CHAPTER 13

Imaging of the Respiratory System

Moira L. Cooper and Thomas L. Slovis

Because new tests can be invented faster than it is decided that they are of no use, clinicians now have at their disposal a myriad of imaging methods.[1] The role of the radiologist has thus broadened from assurance of film quality, film interpretation, and reporting to the acquisition of the most correct examination by teaching physicians about new imaging techniques and their applications.

This chapter discusses the different imaging tools available and their uses in the investigation of respiratory tract problems. Specific disease entities are discussed elsewhere in this book. Rather, a basic systematic approach to the proper use of imaging is offered. In this chapter, the respiratory tract is arbitrarily divided into four anatomic regions—nasal airway, paranasal sinuses, extrapulmonary airway, and chest.

PHYSICAL PRINCIPLES OF IMAGING MODALITIES

Radiography

The x ray, the most common medium used in imaging, is a form of electromagnetic radiation. High-voltage generators produce an electron beam that, on striking a rotating anode, produces a spectrum of x rays of varying energies. The number of x rays (photons) and the shape of the energy spectrum can be manipulated with changes in output (the tube current in milliamperes [mA]), filtration, and maximum voltage across the x-ray tube (peak kilovoltage [kvP]). These x rays interact within the body in various ways depending on the thickness and density of the body part. The number of x rays that traverse the body and reach the film or another detector dictate the characteristics of the image produced.

Extrapolation from data identifying the risks of high-dose radiation (leukemia, cancer, cataract stimulation) implies that even low-dose radiation exposure from diagnostic examinations may not be innocuous. Therefore every effort must be made to limit radiation exposure, especially in the pediatric population (Table 13-1). The best way to do this is to limit the number of studies

Table 13-1 Average Radiation Dose

	DOSE (mR)
Newborn chest, two views	20
Digital newborn chest, two views	8
1-year-old chest, two views	50
Conventional chest, two views in older child	75
Digital chest, two views in older child	19
Neck, two views	100
Fluoroscopy/minute*	500-1000
CT chest standard/slice*†	1500
CT chest high-resolution/slice*†	2000
Ambient radiation/year/at sea level	100

Skin entry dose from National Council on Radiation Protection and Measurements: *Radiation protection in pediatric radiology,* NCRD Rep No 68, Bethesda, Md, 1981, The Council.
mR, Millirad (0.001 R).
*Data from Children's Hospital of Michigan, Detroit.
†Each slice is finely coned, so there should be no additive dose.

performed on a child and to tailor the imaging process to the clinical problem at hand. Other measures, such as attention to careful technique, tight coning of the primary beam, careful shielding of the gonads, and use of the newer, high-speed rare earth systems, all help decrease exposure.

Digital radiology is becoming more widely used. This technique, which needs less initial radiation because of the increased sensitivity of the cassettes, provides more constant film quality and, with its computer capabilities, postprocessing manipulation of the image. This will further reduce radiation dose by decreasing the need for repeat studies done for suboptimal penetration[2] (Fig. 13-1 and Table 13-1).

Tomography (Laminography)

This technique, achieved by moving both the x-ray tube and the film cassette, permits visualization of objects within only a defined anatomic plane (usually about 0.5 to 1 cm thick) and blurs all those above and below. The radiation dose for a complete lung study is quite high (in the rad range [i.e., >1000

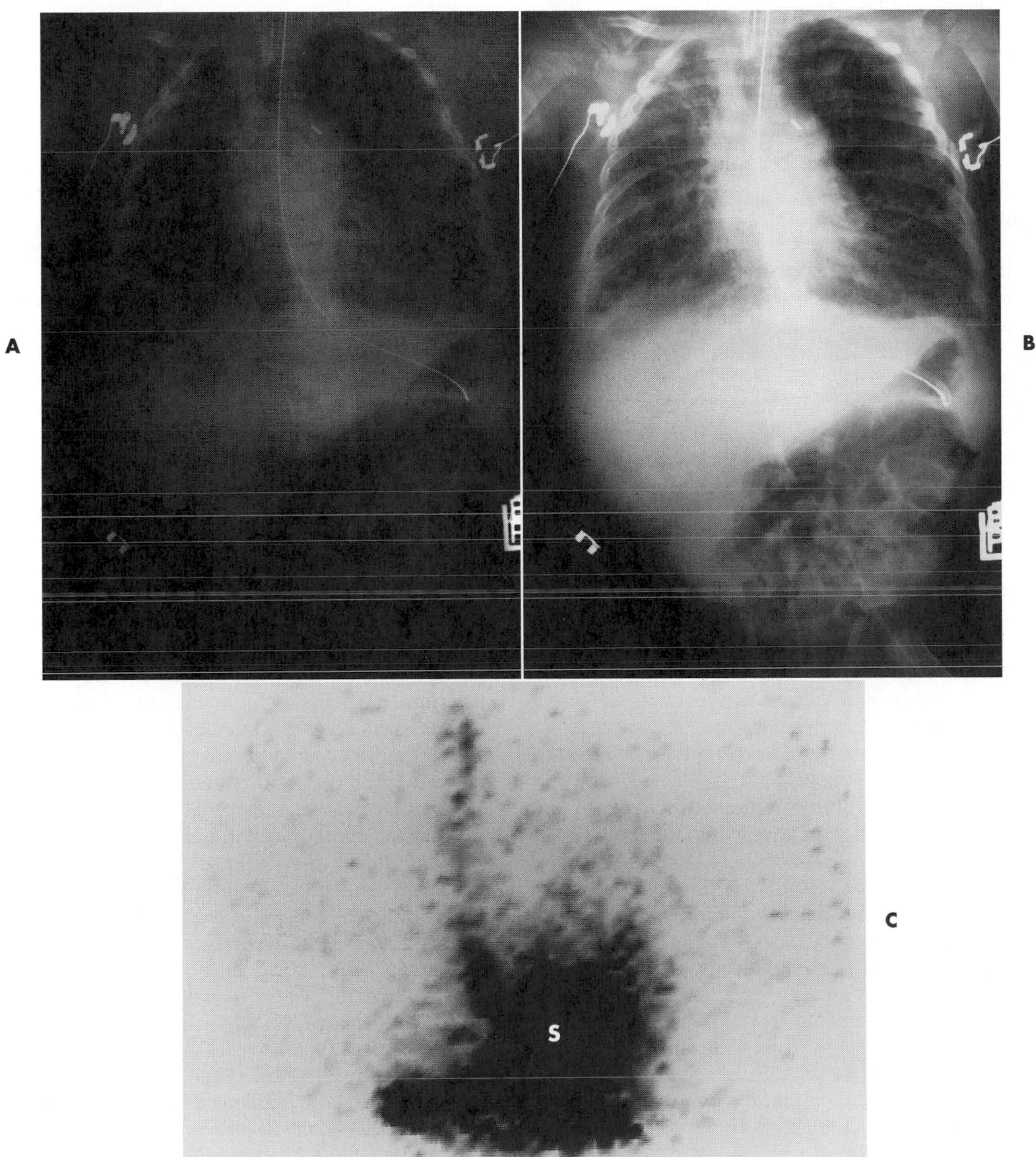

Fig. 13-1. Technologic advances. **A** and **B,** Digital radiography. Manipulation of a digitized image in a neonate with bronchopulmonary dysplasia, ductus ligation, and multiple tubes. The first film is clearly too dark **(A).** Postprocessing manipulation and reprinting of the digitized image without exposing the patient achieves an adequate exposure **(B). C,** Nuclear medicine scan. One image from a gastroesophageal reflux study reveals the stomach *(S)* with technetium-99m and reflux into the entire esophagus. This technique can show reflux into the airway.

mR]).[3] The role of tomography in imaging the pediatric respiratory tract is small and has largely been replaced by computed tomography (CT).

Fluoroscopy

Fluoroscopy uses an image intensifier to change the x rays exiting the patient into visible light that can be viewed on a television monitor. Videotapes and spot film images can be recorded for review and storage. Digitized fluoroscopy allows for postprocessing of the image without increasing the patient's exposure to radiation.

This technique permits the radiologist to dynamically view an abnormality in various projections and is quite valuable in studies designed to detect changes in airway caliber and air entry and exit from the lung. For these reasons, fluoroscopy is particularly useful in detecting a bronchial foreign body. Contrast studies of the esophagus and the bronchus as well as angiography are performed under fluoroscopic control.[4]

Nuclear Medicine

With this technique, a radioactive isotope is tagged to various pharmaceutical agents that are then given to the patient (e.g., orally, intravenously). The energy that is subsequently emitted is then guided by collimators into a scintillation camera, which produces an image. In the authors' institutions, lung perfusion scans are done with technetium-99m attached to macroaggregated albumin particles, whereas ventilation scans are performed with technetium-99m aerosol diethylenetriamine pentaacetic acid.[5] Nuclear scans are also done for gastroesophageal reflux using technetium-99m sulfa colloid mixed with infant formula or apple juice[6] (see Fig. 13-1).

The indications for pulmonary scintigraphy are largely regional perfusion and ventilation. The incidence of pulmonary embolism in children is unknown.[7] Ventilation and associated perfusion anomalies are also evident in conditions such as asthma, bronchial foreign body, cystic fibrosis, and lobar emphysema. Gallium- and indium-labeled white blood cells and technetium-99m hexamethyl propylene amine oxime–labeled white blood cells have all been used in the diagnosis of pulmonary inflammation.

In cases of malignancy, gallium-67 citrate is routinely used for the staging and follow-up of children with Hodgkin's disease and for the definition of lymphomatous involvement in the hila and mediastinum.[7] Occasionally, thallium-201 is used for this purpose. Subtle bony changes, including the presence of metastatic disease, can be picked up by a bone scan with technetium-99m methylene diphosphonate.

Ultrasound

Unlike the other imaging modalities discussed so far, ultrasound (US) uses no ionizing radiation, making its use in the pediatric population very attractive. High-energy sound waves, which are generated in the transducer, are reflected back in varying degrees and at different times by body materials and surfaces. This information is then digitized and an image generated. Because air is a very poor conductor of sound waves, the use of US in the chest is limited to the thymus and to areas of fluid or consolidation or masses that are close to the inner thoracic wall or diaphragm (Fig. 13-2).

Prenatal US has significantly enhanced the clinician's ability to diagnose congenital abnormalities of the chest, including diaphragmatic hernia, pleural effusion, and cystic adenomatoid malformation.[8] US clearly has a role in cases of a neonate or an older child whose chest radiograph is opaque and in whom the diagnosis is not clearly defined.[9] Because US is a "real-time" study, diaphragmatic motion can readily be visualized. This technique, which can be performed portably, distinguishes a mass or an effusion from a paralyzed hemidiaphragm.

Doppler US and color flow imaging use the Doppler effect, whereby sound waves change in frequency when reflected by a moving surface. This technique permits the visualization and characterization of blood vessels, blood velocity, and vascularity of a mass (see Fig. 13-2).

Computed Tomography

With CT, a receptor collects beams from a fan of x rays that have been transmitted into the patient from different directions. This information is digitized, and the thousands of pixels of data are processed to measure attenuation coefficients (density characteristics) of small areas of tissue and their positions relative to other structures in the imaged field. Various algorithms maximize spatial and contrast resolution for different purposes and body areas.

For precise evaluation of the lung anatomic structures and the secondary pulmonary lobule, high-resolution computed tomography (HRCT) is used with thin slices (1.0 to 3.0 mm) and high-contrast algorithms (bone algorithms), which have high spatial resolution[10,11] (Fig. 13-3). In a motionless object, the resolution is 0.3 to 0.5 mm.[9] In HRCT, the tube current can be lowered to minimize the extra radiation.[12] HRCT is useful for defining parenchymal disease and doing a precise study of the airway, whereas conventional CT is useful for mediastinal evaluation[13] (Fig. 13-4). Intravenous contrast enhancement is often used during imaging of the respiratory tract. This defines the great vessels in the neck and mediastinum, differentiates parenchymal from pleural processes, and characterizes the internal composition of mass lesions. Because motion is so detrimental to good images, the authors use only the low-osmolarity contrast agents, which tend to produce less burning, vomiting, and other motion-causing reactions.

Sedation is required in most younger children because it is imperative that the child remain motionless. Various sedation protocols are practiced (Box 13-1), but regardless of the protocol used, the duration of the examination, the type of pharmaceutical product, the underlying medical condition, and the necessity of the study must be weighed carefully before any child is sedated.[14-16] Helical CT and electron-beam ultrafast scanners have eliminated the need for sedation in many instances.[10,17]

Magnetic Resonance Imaging

Ionizing radiation is not used in magnetic resonance (MR) imaging; instead, images are created from information provided by the proton-density and energy-decay characteristics of different tissues. The patient is placed in a strong magnetic field, and a series of radiofrequency waves are pulsed through the body. This causes the protons, predominantly hydrogen protons, to repeatedly flip and realign. The resulting emitted radiofrequencies are then collected and digitized. Images can be created in multiple planes and weighted to demonstrate the proton density (tesla [T1]) and relaxation parameters (T2) of various tissues to different extents.[18] In most cases, an anatomic image is desired in multiple planes; therefore a T1 image is most applicable

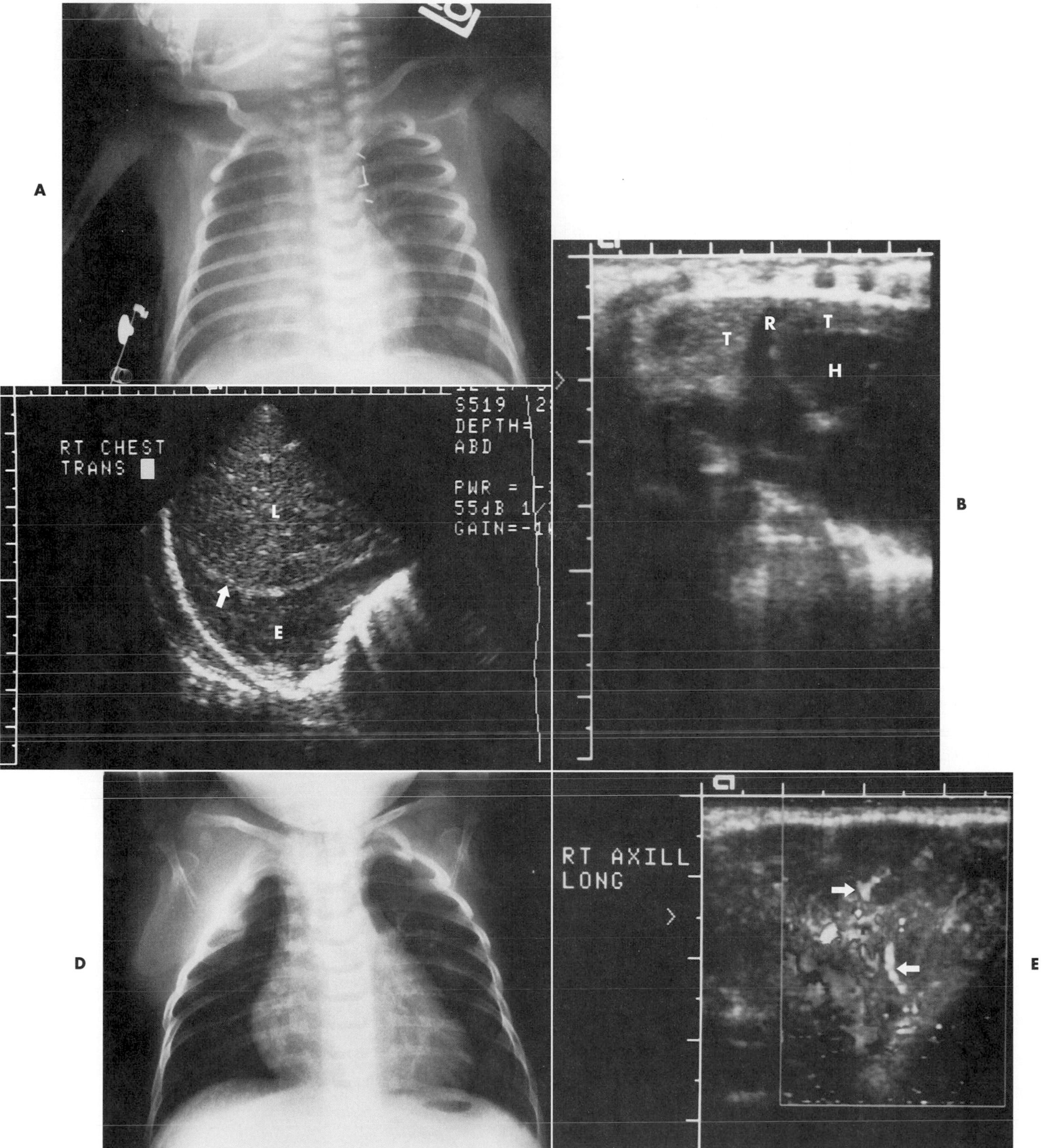

Fig. 13-2. Use of chest US. **A,** Rotated chest radiograph in a cardiac patient after surgery reveals a questionable anterior mediastinal mass. **B,** US shows the mass to be homogeneous thymus projected anteriorly and superiorly to the heart. *H,* Heart; *R,* rib artifact; *T,* thymus. **C,** Transverse US in another patient shows the diaphragm *(arrow),* liver *(L),* and a fluid complex: an empyema *(E).* **D** and **E,** Hemangioma of the chest wall. Chest film **(D)** reveals a mass of the right chest wall separating the scapula from the ribs. The ribs are deformed and osteoporotic. Color flow Doppler US **(E)** reveals the vascular nature *(arrows)* of this mass.

A

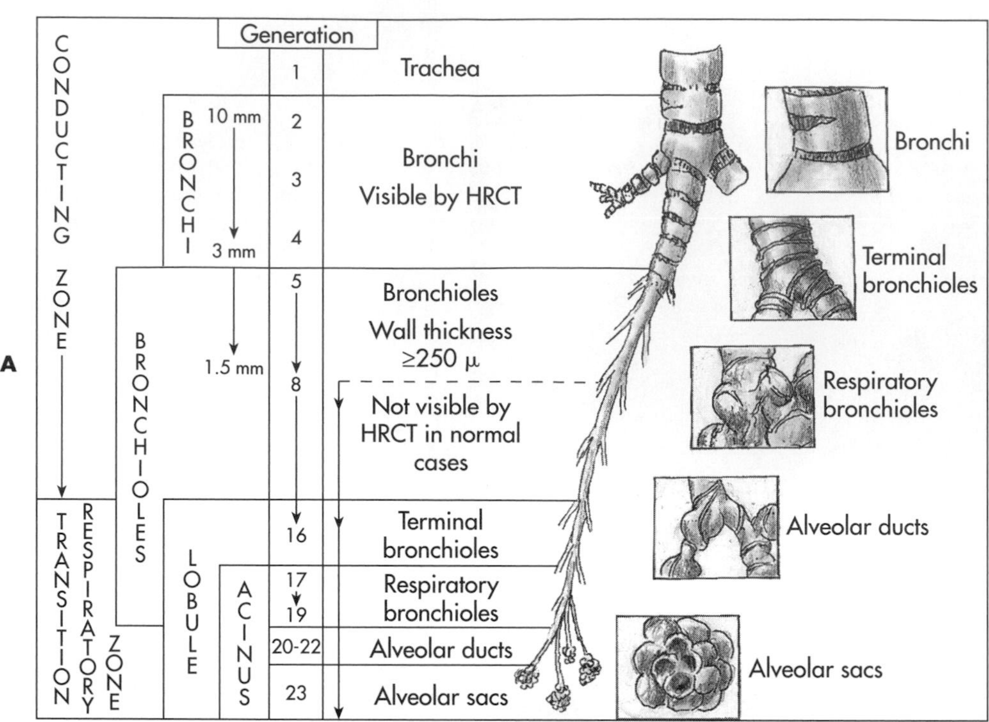
Generation
CONDUCTING ZONE
TRANSITION RESPIRATORY ZONE
BRONCHI
10 mm
3 mm
1.5 mm
BRONCHIOLES
LOBULE
ACINUS
1
2
3
4
5
8
16
17
19
20-22
23
Trachea
Bronchi
Visible by HRCT
Bronchioles
Wall thickness
≥250 μ
Not visible by
HRCT in normal
cases
Terminal bronchioles
Respiratory bronchioles
Alveolar ducts
Alveolar sacs
Bronchi
Terminal bronchioles
Respiratory bronchioles
Alveolar ducts
Alveolar sacs

B

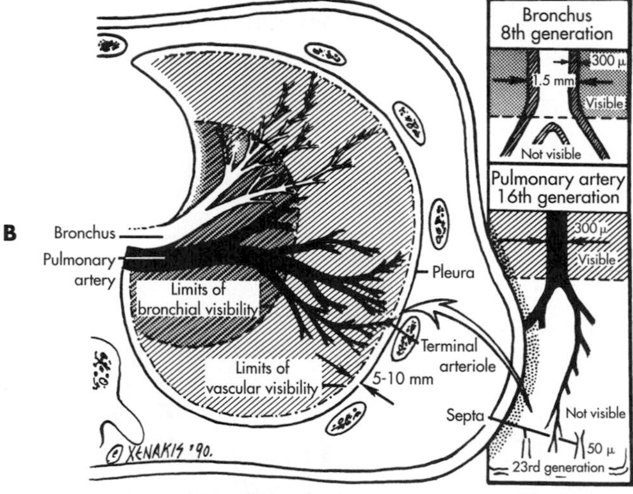
Bronchus
Pulmonary artery
Limits of bronchial visibility
Limits of vascular visibility
Pleura
Terminal arteriole
5-10 mm
Septa
© XENAKIS '90.
Bronchus 8th generation
300 μ
1.5 mm
Visible
Not visible
Pulmonary artery 16th generation
300 μ
Visible
Not visible
50 μ
23rd generation

C

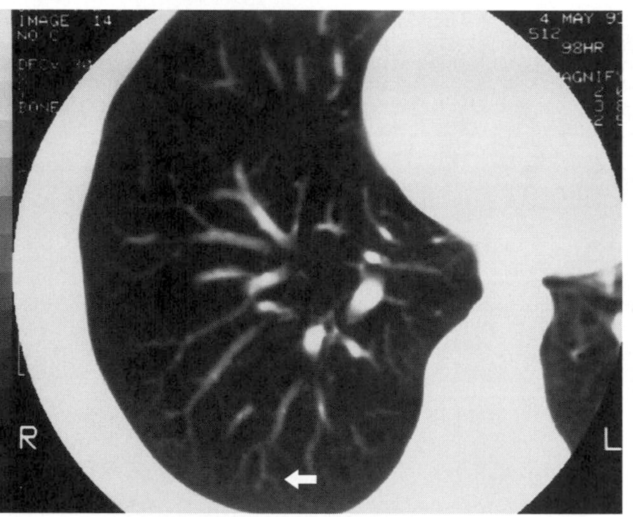
IMAGE 14
4 MAY
R
L

D

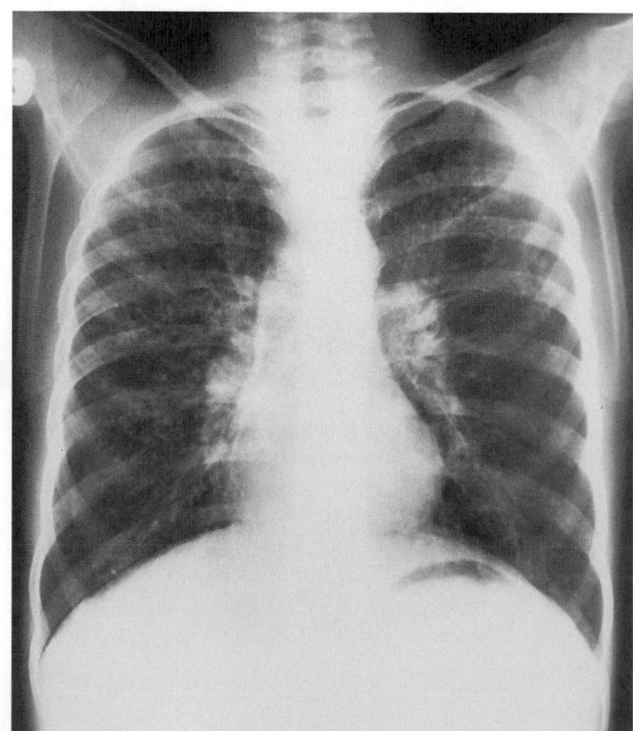

E

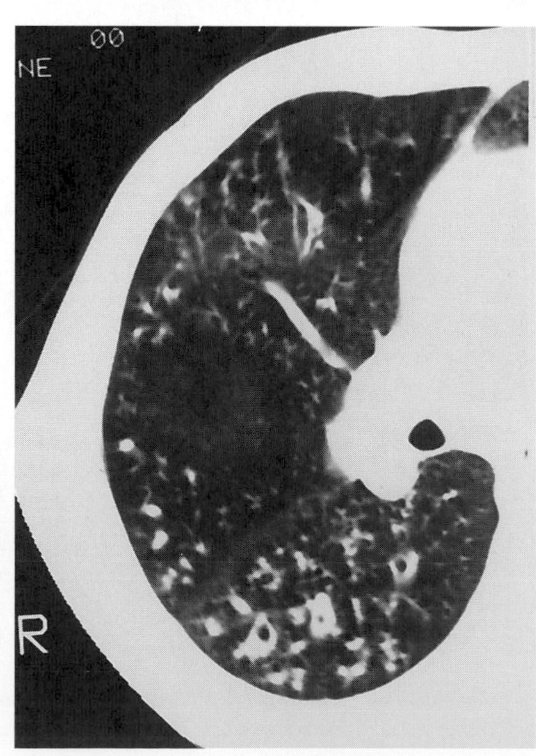
R

Fig. 13-3. Lung as demonstrated by HRCT. **A,** The normal bronchial divisions are depicted, and delineation between the divisions visible by HRCT is shown. **B,** Both vascular and bronchial anatomic structures are depicted specifying the limits of visibility on HRCT. **C,** HRCT scan showing the secondary lobule of the periphery of the lung. Each secondary lobule contains an interlobar septum *(arrow)* that is composed of connective tissue containing the pulmonary veins and lymphatic system. In the center of each septum are the lobular bronchiole and artery. The latter are visible sometimes as a "dot," whereas the normal bronchiole is not seen by HRCT. **D,** Frontal radiograph of a patient with cystic fibrosis reveals hyperexpansion, bronchial dilation, and density throughout both lung fields. **E,** HRCT scan shows diffuse bronchiectasis with large, dilated air passage in the periphery. In addition, there are thickened septa at the periphery of the lung. (**A** and **B** from Naidich DP et al, eds: *Computed tomography and magnetic resonance of the thorax,* ed 2, New York, 1991, Raven, pp 503-555.)

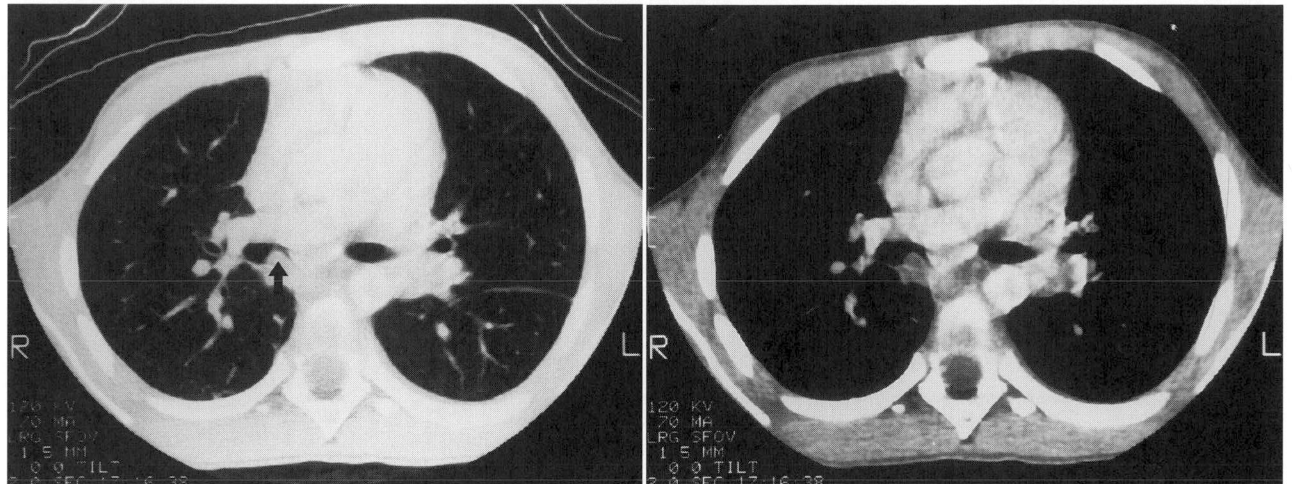

Fig. 13-4. Use of CT for mediastinal evaluation. **A,** Thin (1.5-mm) cut section (with low tube current to reduce radiation) reveals excellent resolution with increased sharpness of the vascular markings and bronchial walls. Bronchi are visible in the inner third of the lung, and vascular structures are visible nearly to the subplural surface. A mass is seen on the right mainstem bronchus *(arrow)*. **B,** Optimal setting and algorithm for the mediastinum in this contrast-enhanced examination reveal the right bronchial lesion: a bronchial adenoma.

BOX 13-1
Sedation Protocol at Children's Hospital of Michigan*

Initial doses

Chloral hydrate (orally)

50, 75, or 100 mg/kg depending on patient's weight and age and length of examination, up to the maximum of 2000 mg orally

Neonate to 2 years

Pentobarbital sodium (Nembutal) (intravenously)

3 mg/kg in patient 12 months of age and older

1 μg/kg of fentanyl if patient is not asleep 5 minutes after pentobarbital sodium

Fentanyl (intravenously)

1 μg/kg for patient of any age

Mostly for pain when used alone

Midazolam hydrochloride (Versed) (intravenously)

0.3 mg/kg once and 0.4 mg/kg once for all children 8 years and older; if patient weighs more than 50 kg, 0.2 mg/kg first and then 0.2 mg/kg or 0.3 mg/kg depending on patient's condition

Used if there is a previous adverse reaction to pentobarbital sodium (children who need 6 mg/kg or more of pentobarbital sodium and still have problems with motion during magnetic resonance imaging)

Diazepam (Valium) (orally)

0.04 mg/kg to 0.2 mg/kg (usual dose, 0.1 mg/kg; maximum dose, 10 mg) in older children undergoing magnetic resonance imaging

Supplemental doses

Chloral hydrate

If patient is not asleep 20 minutes after administration:

25 to 50 mg to equal 100 mg/kg, up to a maximum of 2000 mg

OR

μg/kg fentanyl intravenously

OR

2 μg/kg fentanyl intramuscularly

Pentobarbital sodium (Nembutal)

If patient is not asleep 5 minutes after administration:

Another 1 μg/kg of fentanyl

OR

Another intravenous dose of pentobarbital sodium that is equal to or greater than the first dose by 1 mg/kg (For example, if 3 mg/kg was given first, then 3 or 4 mg/kg should be given in the second dose.)

Guidelines for cumulative maximum dose: 10 to 12 mg/kg

Pentobarbital sodium can be given intramuscularly if the clinician is unsuccessful at initiating an intravenous administration: 6 mg/kg if the patient weighs less than 15 kg and 5 mg/kg if the patient weighs more than 15 kg

Supplemental dose in 1 hour: 2 mg/kg if the patient weighs less than 15 kg and 2.5 mg/kg if the patient weighs more than 15 kg

Fentanyl

Second dose of 1 μg/kg 5 to 10 minutes after initial dose

Then boost of 1 μg/kg every 30 to 45 minutes

Midazolam hydrochloride (Versed)

After two doses:

Another dose equal to or greater than the second by 0.1 mg/kg in 2 to 5 minutes (For example, if 0.4 mg/kg is the second dose, then 0.4 to 0.5 mg/kg should be the third dose.)

OR

1 μg/kg fentanyl intravenously after the two doses of midazolam hydrochloride

Possible boost every 30 minutes with 0.3 mg/kg of midazolam hydrochloride not to exceed a total dose of 2.1 mg/kg (inducting and supplemental)

Guidelines for cumulative induction dose: 1.5 mg/kg

Boosting

1 μg/kg fentanyl intravenously every 30 to 45 minutes with any medication regimen

0.3 mg/kg midazolam hydrochloride intravenously every 30 minutes, use with initial doses of diazepam orally and midazolam hydrochloride

*This protocol should be used only with a fully trained pediatric nurse, technologist, and physician team. The protocol is revised yearly. This version is from March 1995.

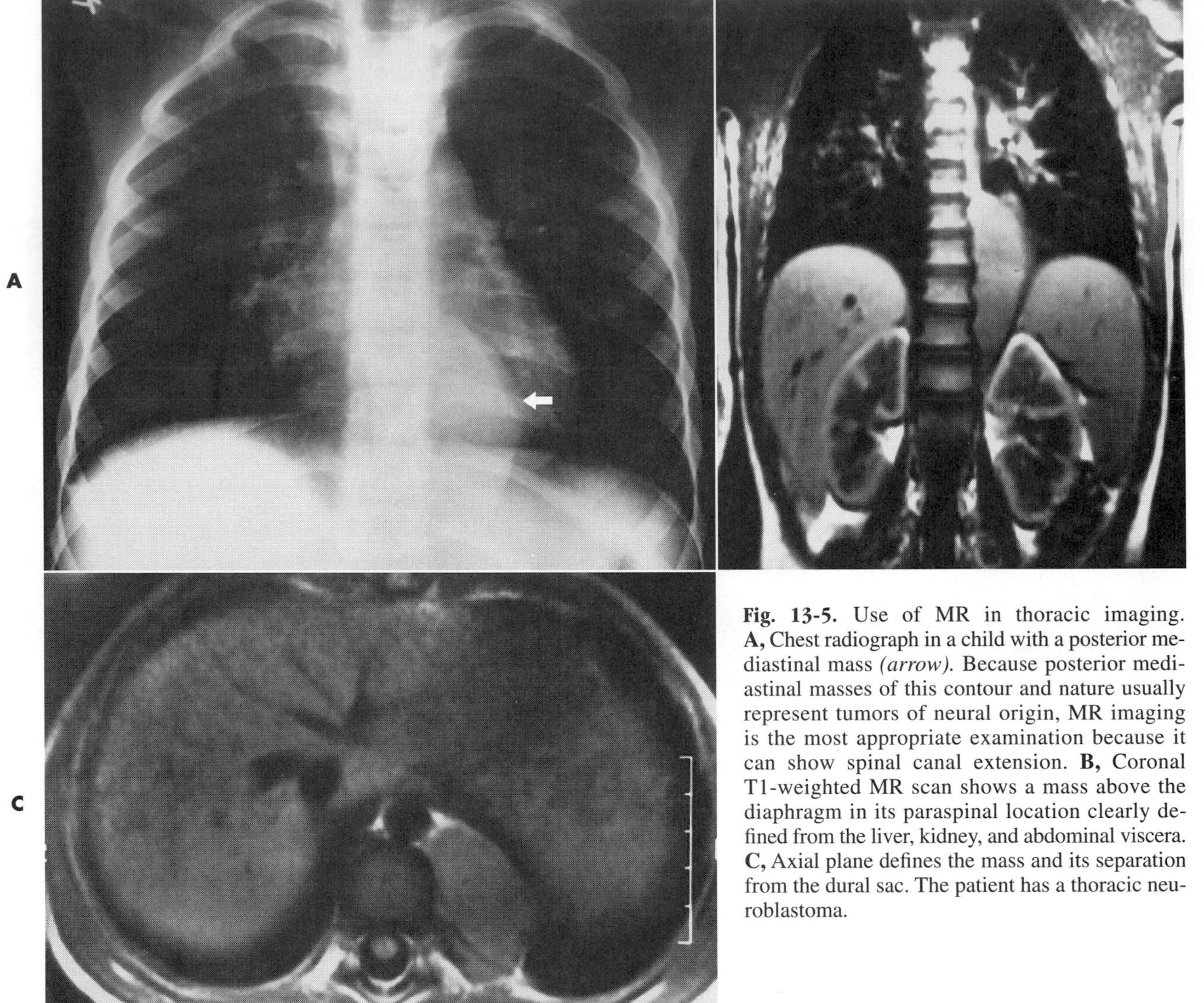

Fig. 13-5. Use of MR in thoracic imaging. **A,** Chest radiograph in a child with a posterior mediastinal mass *(arrow).* Because posterior mediastinal masses of this contour and nature usually represent tumors of neural origin, MR imaging is the most appropriate examination because it can show spinal canal extension. **B,** Coronal T1-weighted MR scan shows a mass above the diaphragm in its paraspinal location clearly defined from the liver, kidney, and abdominal viscera. **C,** Axial plane defines the mass and its separation from the dural sac. The patient has a thoracic neuroblastoma.

Table 13-2 MR vs. CT in Imaging Sinonasal Masses

PROS	CONS
CT	
Has better availability Is faster Requires less sedation Provides better bony detail Is more sensitive to calcification	Is less sensitive in differentiating between tumor and inflammation Causes beam hardening from dental devices and metallic plates Causes radiation exposure Uses iodinated contrast material with associated risk of allergic reactions
MR	
Provides more soft tissue detail Is multiplanar Can distinguish between tumor and inflammation Provides wider coverage Causes loss of bony detail Has no signal from calcium Is restricted when patient has metallic devices	Takes more time Takes more sedation and scan time Costs more Has more limited availability

(Fig. 13-5). The relative merits of CT vs. MR imaging are outlined in Table 13-2 and are discussed with reference to specific areas and problems later in this chapter. Currently, MR imaging is the cross-sectional modality of choice for the evaluation of mediastinal masses and vascular abnormalities.

Angiography and Interventional Angiography

The use of angiography, which exposes the patient to the risks of ionizing radiation, sedation, and intravascular contrast material, is decreasing in most centers. One of the new, less invasive techniques, such as MR imaging or CT, is often used instead.

In instances of vascular intervention, embolization is frequently necessary. Many conditions require the use of this technique, as follows[19] (Fig. 13-6):

> In the pediatric population, the conditions most frequently necessitating embolization include pulmonary arterial venous malformations, massive hemoptysis secondary to cystic fibrosis or bronchiectasis, uncontrolled hemorrhage from trauma or arterial venous malformation, and rarely congenital malformations such as sequestration or arterial venous shunting.

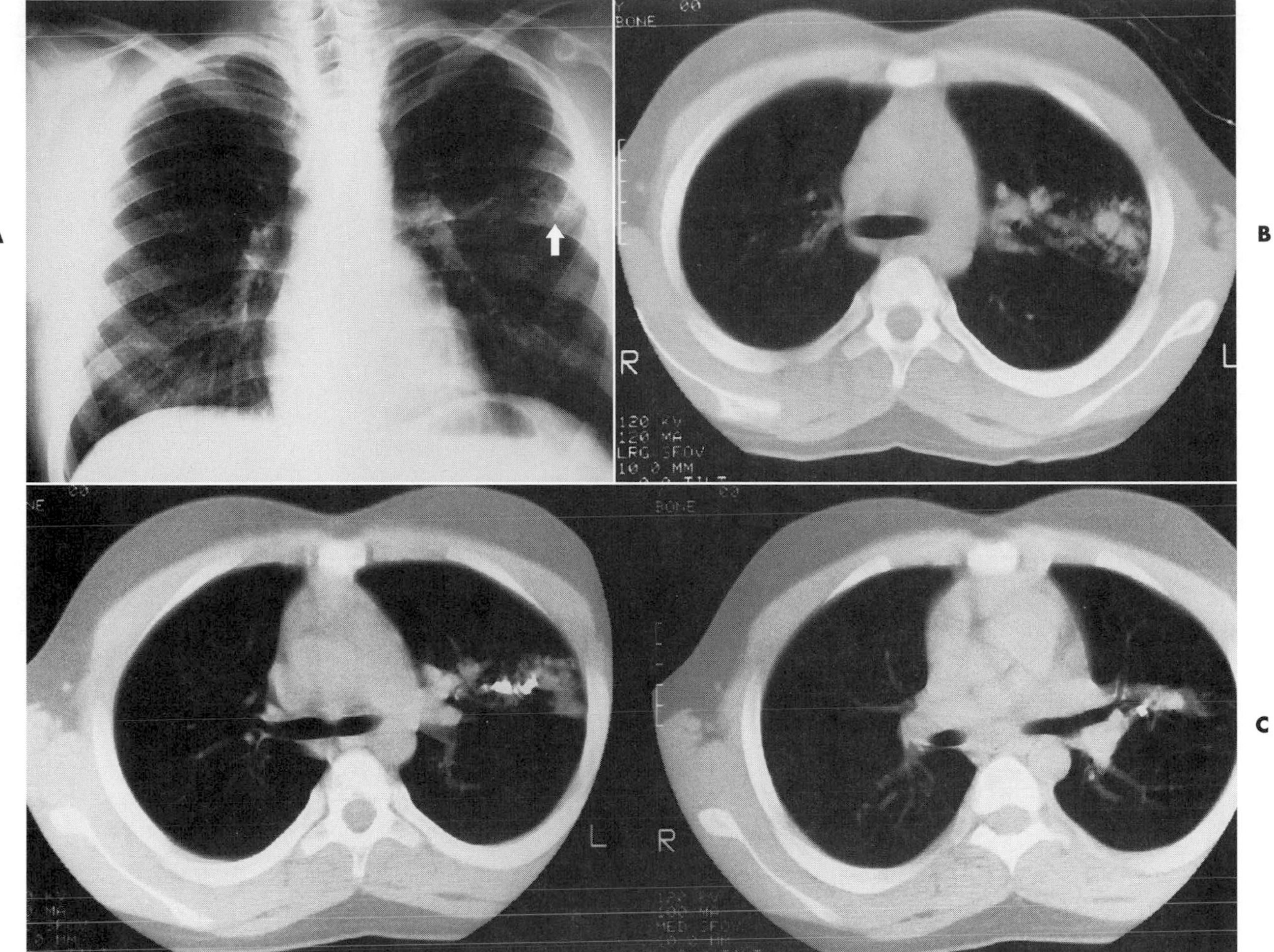

Fig. 13-6. Coordination of modalities to diagnose and treat an arterial venous malformation of the lung. **A,** Chest radiograph showing a vague serpiginous density in the left upper lobe *(arrow)*. **B,** Nonenhanced CT showing the lesion to advantage with vessels feeding from and draining toward the hilum. **C,** Postembolization CT showing coils in a few of the feeding arteries.

ANATOMIC EVALUATION OF THE RESPIRATORY TRACT

Nasal Airway

The introduction of CT, with its capability for axial, thin-sectioning imaging and its superior definition of bone, air, and soft tissue interfaces, has revolutionized imaging of the nose and nasal airway.[20] CT is the undisputed first choice for investigating the causes of nasal airway obstruction in the neonate and infant. The confirmation of choanal atresia, an important cause of neonatal respiratory distress, had been made using plain film after instillation of opaque contrast media. CT now not only provides confirmation of the clinical diagnosis but also determines the thickness of the bony plate and distinguishes between bony and membranous atresia.[21,22] With CT, other unusual sites of nasal airway obstruction, such as bony stenosis of the anterior nares or midnose hypoplasia, can be detected (Fig. 13-7). Congenital nasal masses, such as nasal encephaloceles, dermoids, and nasal gliomas, can cause rhinorrhea and nasal airway obstruction in the young infant and are also well characterized by CT[23] (Fig. 13-8).

MR imaging plays a complementary role in the investigation of nasal masses and tumors.[24-26] MR imaging, especially when enhanced with gadolinium diethylenetriamine pentaacetic acid, is superior to CT in demonstrating the extent of malignant disease. MR imaging also affords wider coverage of the head and neck in three planes. CT, however, provides better demonstration of calcium and bony detail, is less expensive, and is more widely available[25,26] (see Table 13-2). Both tests require the patient to be motionless, and in the pediatric population, this usually requires sedation. CT of the nose could be completed in less than 10 minutes, whereas an MR imaging may take up to an hour, a factor that must be considered when sedating an infant with potential airway obstruction.

Plain film radiologic examination of the nose can be used as a screening procedure for trauma.[27] Specific projections such as the anteroposterior view of the face, Waters' view, and two soft tissue laterals for the nasal spine help display the nasal bones. However, in traumatic injuries, the gross appearance of the external nose and estimation of internal form are usually of more value.[28] Visualization of more complex fractures of the sinonasal complex is provided by CT, as discussed later in the next section.[29]

In summary, although plain films can be used as a screening procedure, if imaging studies are clinically indicated to investigate nasal obstruction or trauma, CT is clearly the modality of choice. In cases of a suspected neoplasm, CT can be complemented with contrast-enhanced MR imaging.

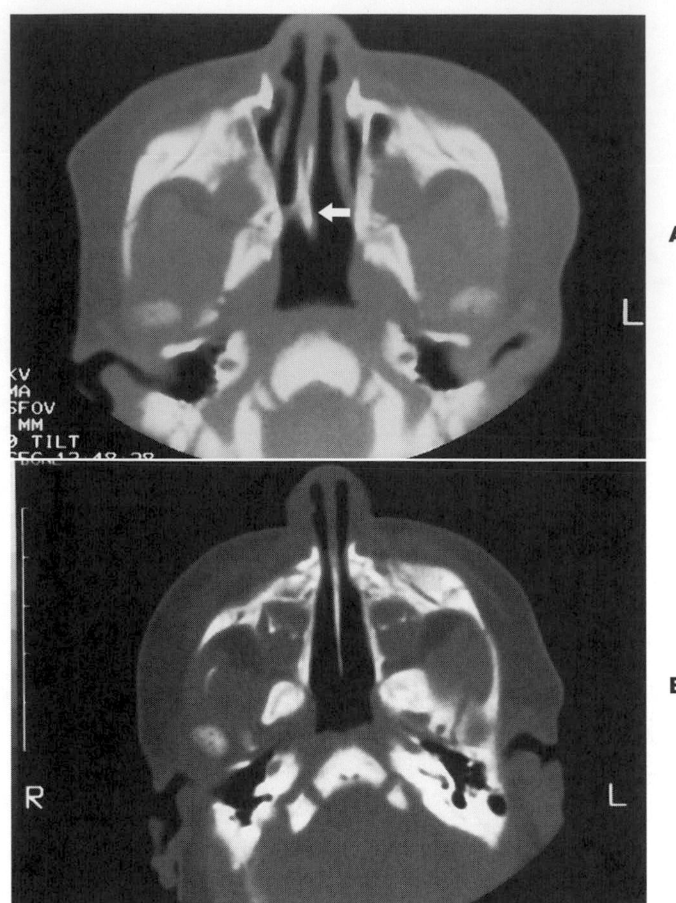

Fig. 13-7. Abnormalities of the nasal airway. **A,** CT scan through the choanal air space shows narrowing on the right. The vomer *(arrow)* is normal but deviated, and the lateral wall of the nose (palatine bone) is also normal. A thin membrane connects the two. This is a unilateral membranous choanal atresia. **B,** In another patient, the choanal air space is normal, but there is bony narrowing more anteriorly. This congenital bony stenosis is quite unusual.

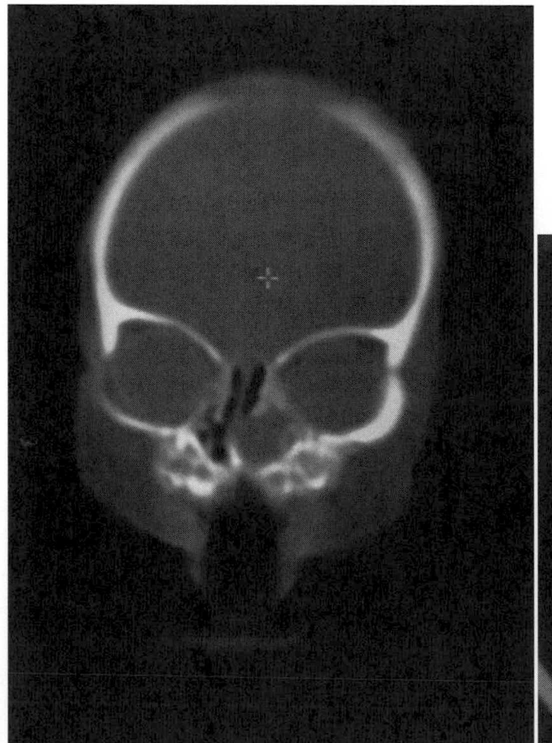

Fig. 13-8. Nasal encephalocele. Coronal **(A)** and axial **(B)** CT scans of a newborn with a large mass *(M)* extending from the brain into the nose.

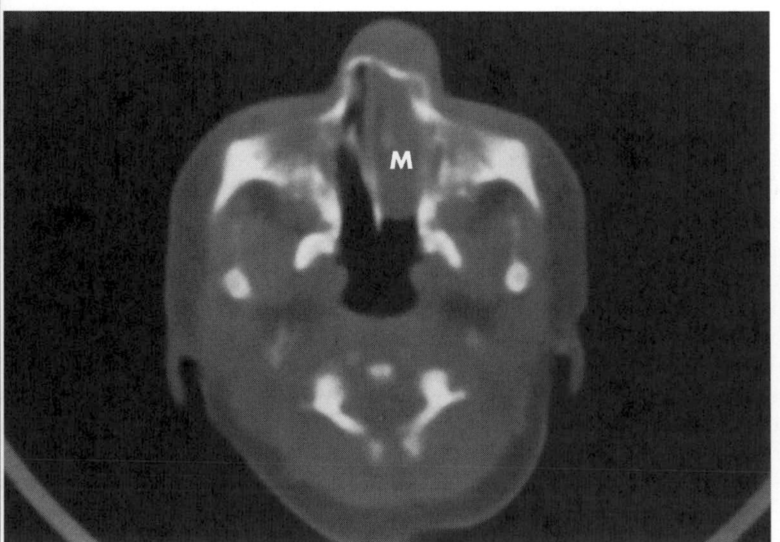

Paranasal Sinuses

The pulmonary physician should be aware of the status of the paranasal sinuses because disease in children with cystic fibrosis is common and changes in the sinuses may be associated with exacerbation of asthma. Together with occlusion of the osteomeatal complex of the maxillary sinus, abnormal mucociliary apparatus is the major pathophysiologic event in acute sinusitis. Normal motility of the cilia usually protects respiratory epithelium from bacterial invasion. In disease that affects cilia motility, sinus disease is common.

Few specific clinical signs and symptoms of sinus disease exist in the pediatric age group. In addition, there are many variations in the appearance of the developing sinuses and a high incidence of opacified sinuses in an asymptomatic population. The diagnosis and institution of therapeutic measures based solely on the findings on plain films are unfounded.[30]

The maxillary sinus is the first paranasal sinus to form, being present at birth, and the rudimentary aerated sinus is 6 to 8 cm in volume.[31] Ethmoid air cells are also present at birth. The anterior components are aerated early in the postnatal period, with pneumatization progressing in the posterior direction. Pneumatization of sphenoid sinus occurs between 7 months and 2 years of age, whereas the frontal sinuses are the last to aerate at 6 to 12 years. As was the case with the nose, CT has revolutionized the imaging of the paranasal sinuses.

Inflammatory Sinus Disease

Plain film assessment of the sinuses normally consists of the following projections: Caldwell's (occipitofrontal), Waters' (occipitomental), and lateral. Failure to obtain more than one frontal view causes the clinician to miss significant disease.[32]

These films should be done with the patient in the erect position because the only diagnostic finding of acute infection is the air-fluid level (Fig. 13-9). Although these studies may still have a role in detecting the presence of acute sinusitis, it has been repeatedly shown that they are unreliable and have produced both overestimates and underestimates of sinusitis in infants and children.[33-35] One study found discrepancies between CT and plain film findings in 74% of cases of sinusitis.[33] Minimal mucosal thickening, superimposition of soft tissues caused by slight rotation, retention cysts, and normal but small sinuses can all be mistaken for opacified sinuses on the plain film. Furthermore, the angulation required to visualize the maxillary sinuses can create double contours and mimic disease.

The plain film finding of opacification is not synonymous with infection. Children with cystic fibrosis, asthma, and thalassemia and other diseases causing extramedullary hematopoiesis all may have opacified sinuses.[36] The sinuses of these children may not be actively infected at the time of imaging.

CT of the sinuses is normally done with contiguous 3-mm coronal slices.[37] The study is performed at a low tube current so that the radiation dose, although higher than plain films, is significantly reduced. Because it yields so much more information than plain films, CT clearly is worth the added dose.[37] There still is, however, a high incidence of abnormal findings in the sinuses of asymptomatic children. Therefore like plain films, CT should not be used as the sole reason for instituting treatment.

The primary role of CT in imaging sinus disease is not simply to detect the presence or absence of inflammation but rather to define the anatomy of the sinuses and the osteomeatal unit and to distinguish among different patterns of sinonasal inflammatory disease (Fig. 13-10). This facilitates more tailored medical and surgical management.[38-42] This examination must be performed after an adequate course of medical therapy to eliminate as much mucosal inflammation as possible and allow for better definition of the underlying anatomy.

CT plays a very important role in imaging possible complications of sinus disease such as periorbital cellulitis, subperiosteal orbital abscess, epidural abscess, brain abscess, meningitis, and hematogenous spread of infection to the cavernous sinus[43,44] (see Fig. 13-10). CT can also be used during follow-up to document resolution of these complications after successful medical or surgical treatment. The use of US in the diagnosis of sinusitis has been investigated, but the reliability of

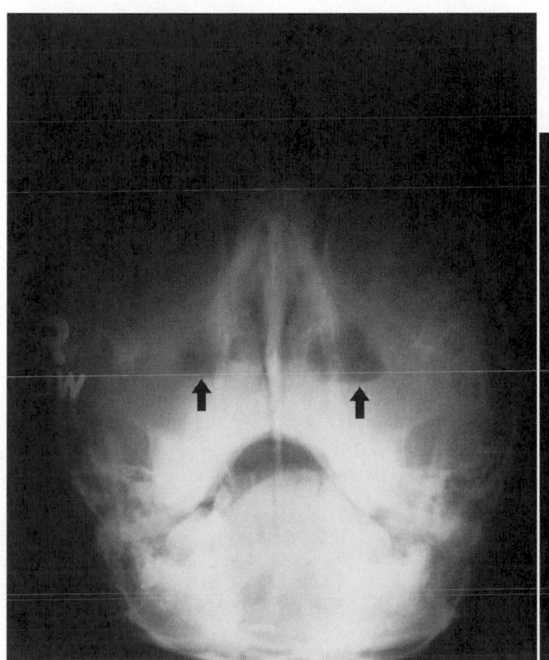

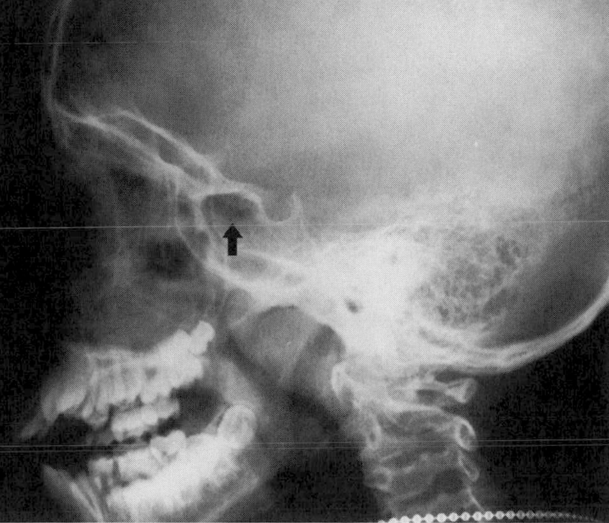

Fig. 13-9. Acute sinusitis on plain films. **A,** Waters' view of the maxillary sinuses shows bilateral air-fluid levels *(arrows)*. **B,** Lateral view in another patient shows a sphenoid air-fluid level *(arrow)*.

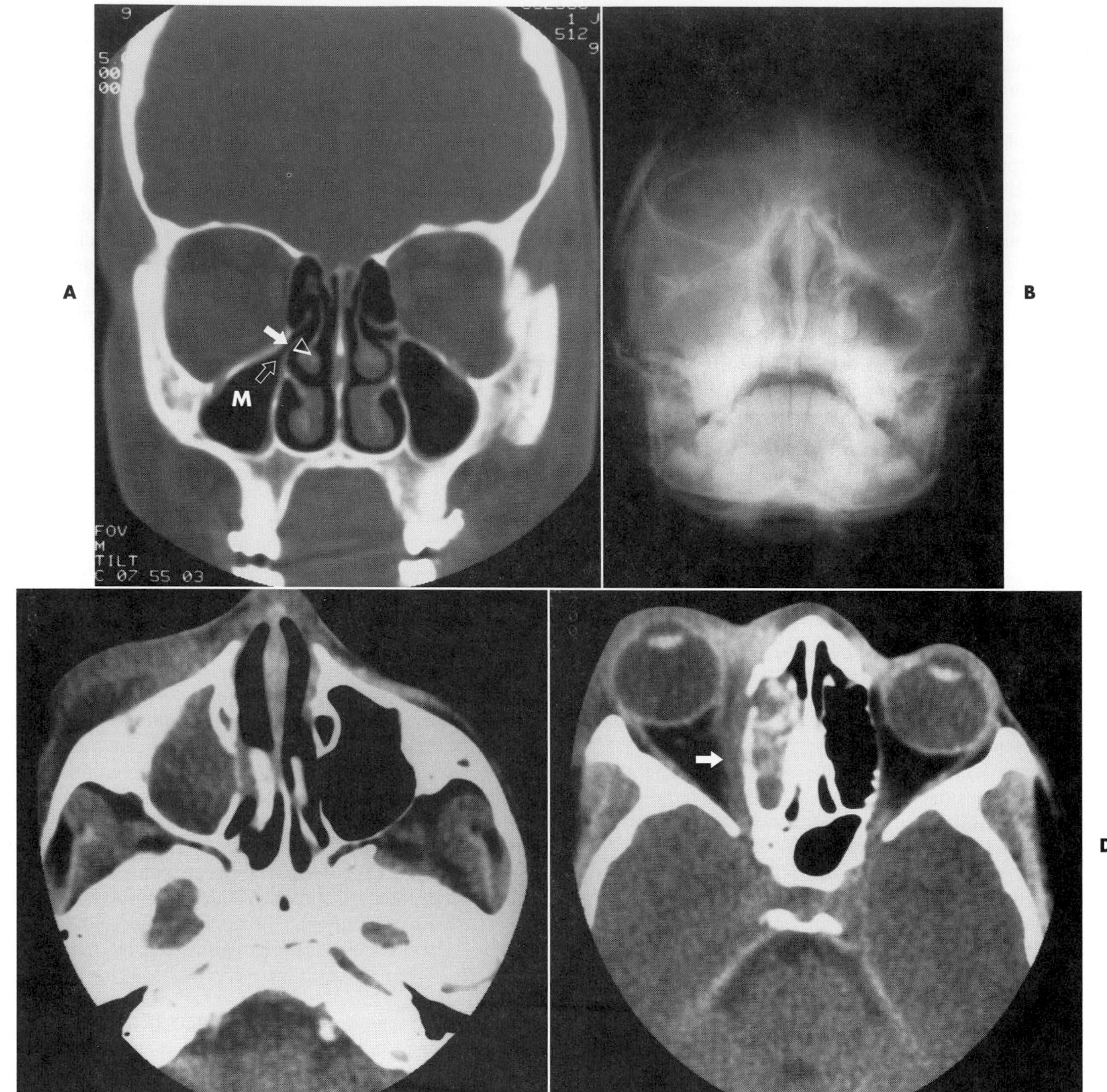

Fig. 13-10. CT evaluation of the sinuses. **A,** Normal coronal CT scan showing the air-filled maxillary sinus *(M),* ostia *(open arrow),* infundibulum *(arrow),* and middle meatus *(triangle).* The air-filled region between the infundibulum and the middle meatus is the hiatus semilunaris. The soft tissue extension between the middle meatus and the infundibulum is the uncinate process of the inferior turbinate. In this case, the structures are all normal on the right, whereas another section showed a normal left osteomeatal complex. **B,** Complication of sinus infection. Waters' view of the sinuses shows opacification of the right maxillary sinuses. Because there is no air-fluid level, it is uncertain whether this mucosal thickening is secondary to allergy or infection. **C** and **D,** Axial CT scan **(C)** shows opacification of the right maxillary sinus, and a higher section **(D)** reveals ethmoidal opacification and postseptal extension of inflammation into the right orbit. Note how the medial rectus muscle is deviated laterally *(arrow).* There is proptosis on the right. This patient had postseptal orbital cellulitis that originated from the sinuses.

this method has not been well established, and its role is not widely accepted.[45,46]

Trauma

High-resolution CT has become the accepted standard of imaging severe trauma of the nasosinus complex. The ethmoid air cells in particular are very difficult to image well without CT because the septa and laminae are poorly visualized and often obscured by associated opacification of the sinuses.

The clinical assessment, along with the initial plain films, should provide a framework that tailors the CT examination to the type and degree of trauma. A CT scan of the brain should also be obtained when the risk of associated brain injury is high. A CT scan of the temporal bones (thin, 1.5-mm coronal view with or without axial sections on bone algorithm) is recommended when the possibility of a temporal bone fracture is considered.[47] Conventional x-ray tomography (laminography), pantomography, and dental views may be occasionally useful.

Masses

Sinonasal tumors in the pediatric group are not common, and their presentation can mimic sinusitis.[26] MR imaging and CT play complementary roles in the investigation of a mass in this area. CT provides superior visualization of bony detail, such as detection of early cribriform plate erosion or calcification within a mass, whereas MR imaging, especially with adjunctive use of contrast, better defines the extent of malignant disease and distinguishes tumor from inflamed mucosa. MR imaging also permits greater evaluation of the head and neck and can detect unsuspected associated cervical disease.[48]

It is evident therefore that a combination of CT and contrast-enhanced MR imaging is best for demonstrating disease in the sinonasal complex. Table 13-2 outlines the relative merits of MR and CT in imaging sinonasal masses.

IMAGING OF THE EXTRAPULMONARY AIRWAY: PHARYNX TO THE CARINA

Imaging of the pediatric airway is usually prompted by clinical concerns of airway obstruction. The infant or child may have stridor, cough, hoarseness, an unusual cry, or a history of foreign body ingestion. High-yield imaging is performed in an infant younger than 6 months of age with stridor, persistence of stridor for more than 7 days, a history of airway manipulation, a history of foreign body aspiration or ingestion, and recurrent symptoms.

The investigation should begin with frontal and lateral plain film examination. When the initial examination needs further clarification, an anteroposterior study is performed during inspiration to prevent tracheal buckling; magnification, high-kilovoltage (high-KV), and added filtration are used to maximize visualization of the airway against the bony and soft tissue background[49,50] (Fig. 13-11). The same technique can also be used for the lateral film. It is imperative that the lateral examination be taken during inspiration and with the child's head extended. These measures prevent the creation of a pseudomass caused by bulging of the hypermobile, redundant retropharyngeal soft tissues into the pharynx[50] (Fig. 13-12). When the retropharyngeal space is truly enlarged, the etiology may be inflammatory or neoplastic or may be related to a foreign body (Box 13-2).

Visualization of an enlarged epiglottis, an enlarged aryepiglottic fold, or both structures most often means epiglottitis. (Fig. 13-13 and Box 13-2 detail the nonspecificity of this radiographic finding.[51-54]) In suspected epiglottitis, it is also critical that any chest or neck radiograph be done in an upright position. Placing the child in a supine position may cause severe distress and even apnea.

Further study of the glottic and subglottic airway should be done dynamically with airway fluoroscopy, a technique that optimizes visualization of the small pediatric airway using magnification, high-KV, small focal spot, and heavy filtration.[55] The dynamic nature of this examination permits assessment of both the structure and the function of the airway, allowing the clinician to make the diagnosis not only of structural lesions such as subglottic stenosis and hemangioma but also of laryngomalacia, tracheomalacia, and vocal cord paralysis[54,55] (Fig. 13-14). The airway, however, can react in only a few ways and the radiographic image of narrowed subglottic region also has a differential diagnosis (Box 13-3).

Glottic, subglottic, and tracheal foreign bodies may be difficult to detect because the clinical symptoms vary from wheeze or rattle to stridor. Magnification, high-KV static or fluoroscopic studies make it easier to detect foreign bodies.[56]

As an adjunct to the airway study, barium can be administered by the oral route or via a nasogastric tube in an attempt to detect a fistula. The esophagram demonstrates potential intrinsic abnormalities in the esophagus that cause respiratory problems (e.g., foreign bodies, clefts, fistulas) and also reveals the presence of a mass in the retropharyngeal or retrotracheal soft tissues[49,53] (Fig. 13-15). Fluoroscopy with the barium esophagram is also an important radiographic resource for evaluating possible vascular rings impinging on the airway[57] (Figs. 13-16 and 13-17). Full definition of a vascular abnormality is best done with MR imaging (see later section). The esophagram may also detect gastroesophageal reflux, a cause of aspiration and airway and pulmonary disease, although it does so with less sensitivity than the nuclear study. CT with the administration of intravenous contrast material to accentuate the major vessels is used primarily to evaluate masses in the neck and mediastinum. Cine or ultrafast CT, a technique using very fast exposures (0.05 to 0.1 without sedation), permits a more dynamic assessment of the airway and can successfully evaluate anomalies such as tracheomalacia and tracheal stenosis.[58-62]

MR imaging, with the benefits of multiplanar imaging and cardiac gating, provides exquisite demonstration of the thoracic vasculature and its relationship to the airway. It gives clear anatomic definition of vascular rings, pulmonary slings, and compression of the airway by enlarged vessels and cardiac chambers[63,64] (see Figs. 13-16 and 13-17). In most instances, an esophagram yields the diagnosis; in uncertain cases or those with unusual circumstances, an MR scan is an important additional study. MR imaging also complements CT in characterizing and defining mediastinal and neck masses.[57,63]

Other imaging tools can play an ancillary role in examining the airway. If a thyroid mass or an ectopic thyroid tissue is suspected, a pertechnetate thyroid scan is indicated. US is the most widely available and least expensive way of imaging superficial, small, well-defined neck masses. Color Doppler now gives added information about the vascularity of the mass and its relationship to the vessels in the neck. Tracheography, which uses a small amount of contrast material instilled in the airway, is very rarely indicated because the central airway is usually adequately seen with magnification high-KV

Text continued on p 170

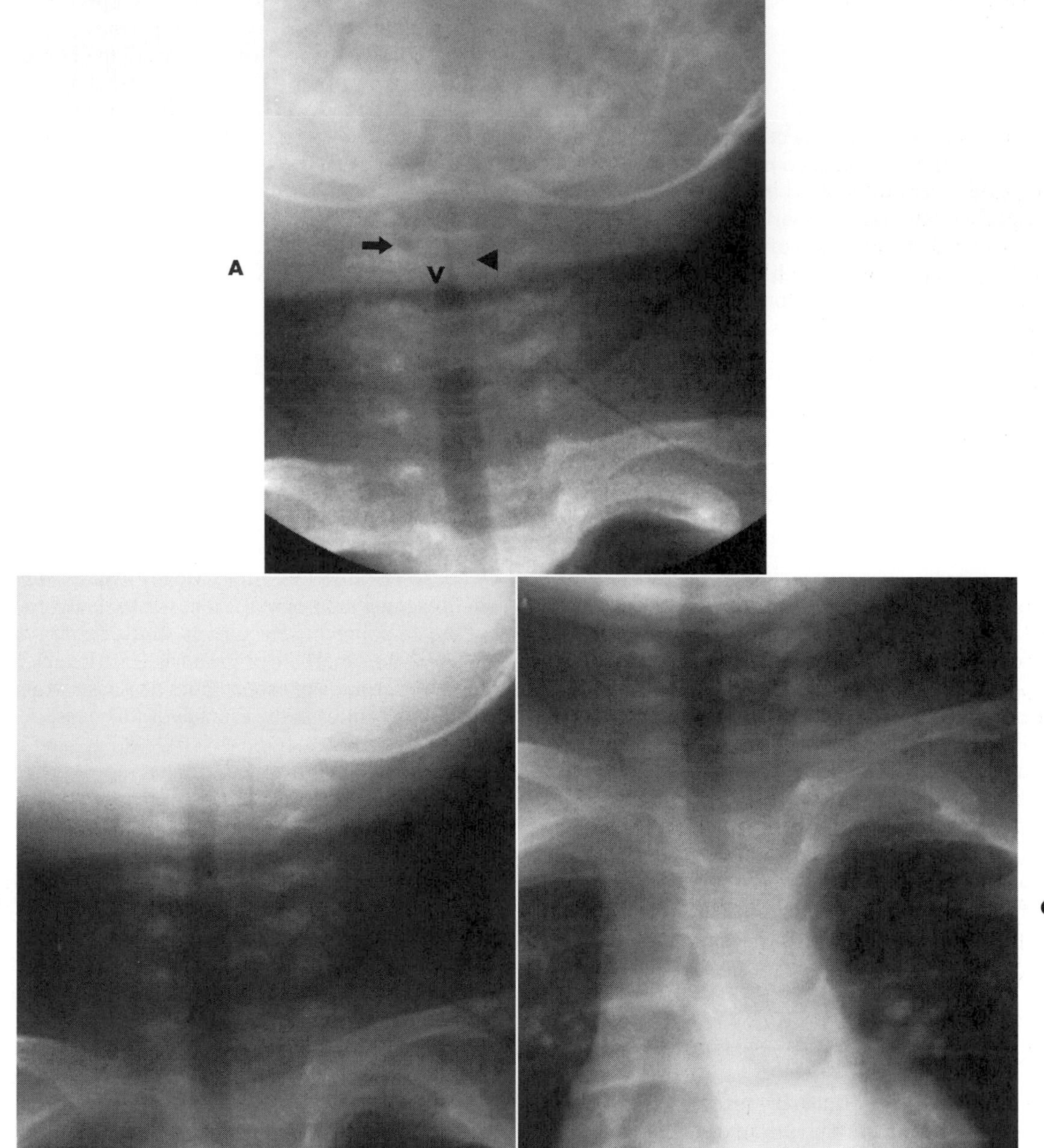

Fig. 13-11. Magnified high-KV films of the normal airway from the glottis to the carina. **A,** Frontal radiograph taken during phonation reveals the pyriform sinuses *(arrow),* the laryngeal ventricles *(arrowhead),* and the medially positioned vocal cords *(V).* Below the cords is the subglottic region that is nicely shouldered. There is symmetry. The proximal trachea is well seen, is patent, and is of uniform caliber. **B,** Frontal radiograph of the same patient with quiet breathing reveals the cords to be laterally positioned and shows a fairly uniform caliber of the airway from the vestibule to the thoracic inlet. **C,** Frontal radiograph shows the entire airway from the high cervical region to the bifurcation at the carina and right and left mainstem bronchus.

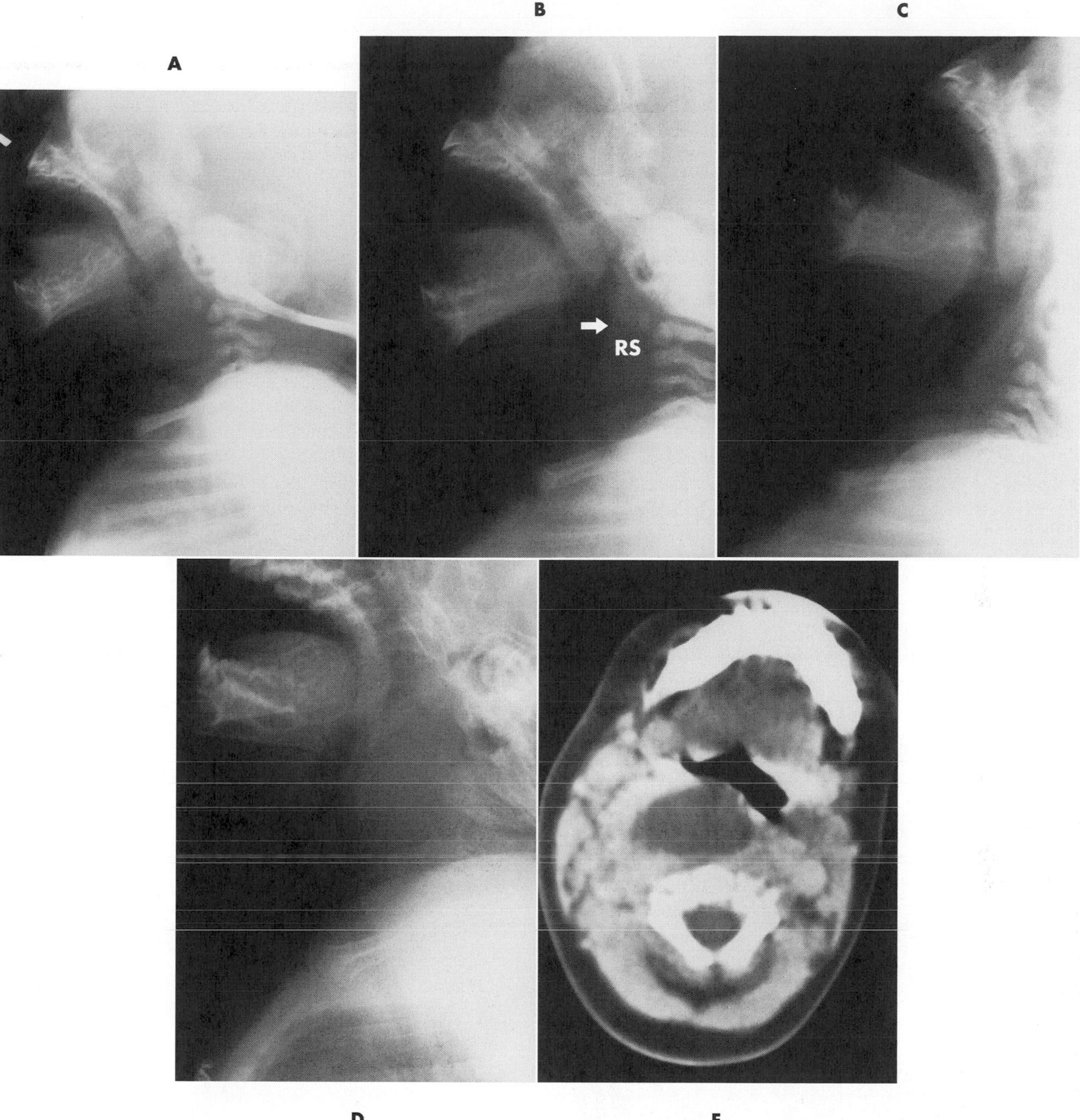

Fig. 13-12. Evaluation of the retropharyngeal space. The same infant with three different degrees of distention of the hypopharynx and extension of the neck. **A,** There is no air in the hypopharynx. **B,** There is now some air in the hypopharynx, the neck is not extended *(arrow),* and the retropharyngeal space *(RS)* is widened; the retropharyngeal space is the distance from the front of the vertebrae to the posterior air column of the hypopharynx. The size of the retropharyngeal space varies with age. In this 7-month-old child, the space can be the same size as the anteroposterior diameter of the fourth vertebral body. It is measured, however, from the back of the hypopharynx to the front of the spine, not at the level of the fourth vertebral body. **C,** With proper inspiration and extension, the retropharyngeal space clearly is within normal limits. **D** and **E,** This 6-month-old infant has stridor and fever. Despite repeated efforts of extension and inspiration, the retropharyngeal space was always bulging and enlarged. For this reason, a CT scan **(E)** was obtained. A large retropharyngeal abscess is noted anterior to the vertebral body. It is shifting the hypopharynx to the left.

BOX 13-2
Differential Diagnosis of an Enlarged Retropharyngeal Space and Epiglottis

Enlarged retropharyngeal space

Infection
Retropharyngeal abscess, phlegmon, or both infections
Cellulitis of lymphoid tissue
Tuberculosis
Tumor (most often neuroblastoma in a young child)
Foreign body aspiration

Enlarged epiglottis with or without enlarged aryepiglottic folds and increased retropharyngeal space

Angioneurotic edema
Acute infection of the epiglottis (rare)

Enlarged epiglottis with or without enlarged aryepiglottic folds

Acute infection of the epiglottis
Irritation by foreign body
Trauma
Burn
Lye ingestion
Infiltration
Kimura's disease
Sarcoid infiltration
Chronic epiglottis
Epiglottic cysts

A

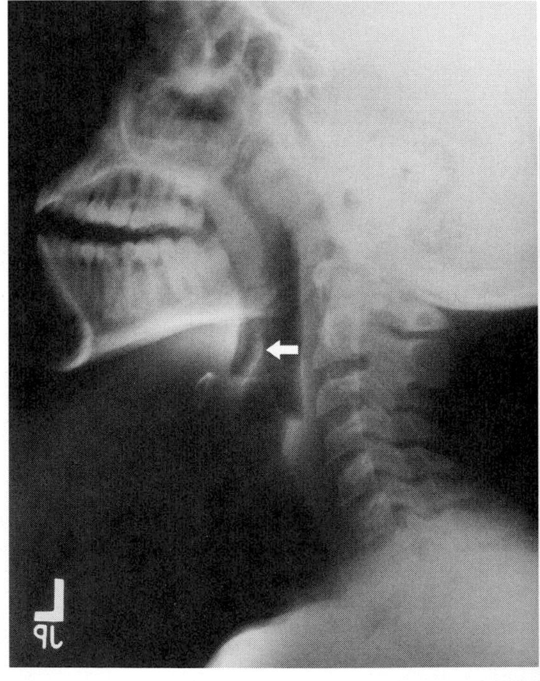

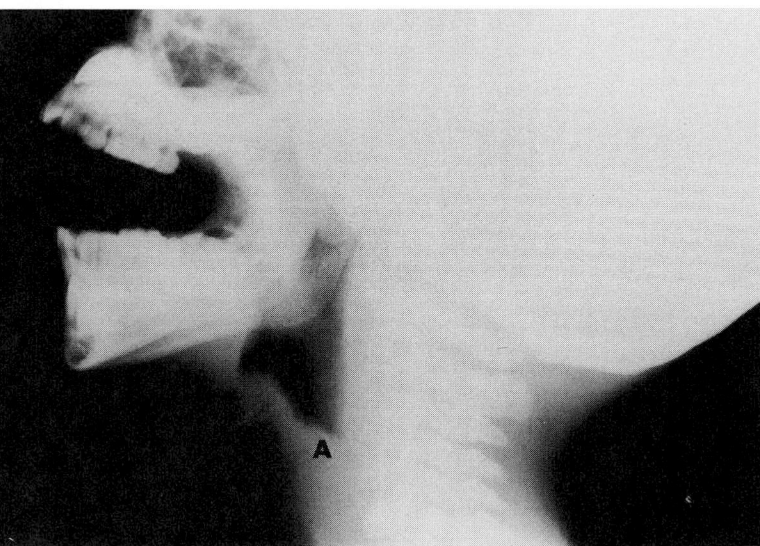

B

Fig. 13-13. Epiglottis. **A,** Normal lateral neck film in an older child reveals the thin epiglottis *(arrow)*. The aryepiglottic folds are imperceptible. Note the small retropharyngeal space. In this age group (over 3 years), the normal adult standard for the retropharyngeal space (no greater than one third of the anteroposterior diameter of the fourth vertebral body) is acceptable. **B,** Child with acute *Haemophilus influenzae* infection of the epiglottitis. At the level of the hyoid bone, there is a thick projection of soft tissue that extends back to the arytenoid cartilage *(A)*. This study shows both an enlarged epiglottis and thickened aryepiglottic folds.

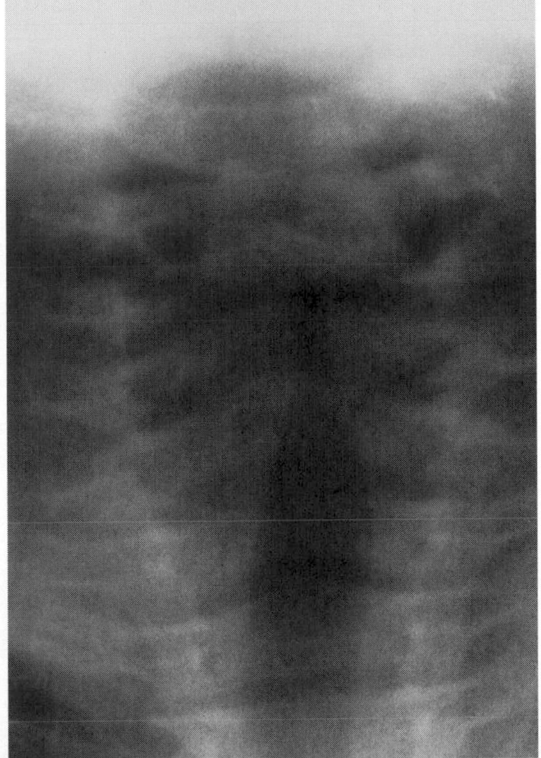

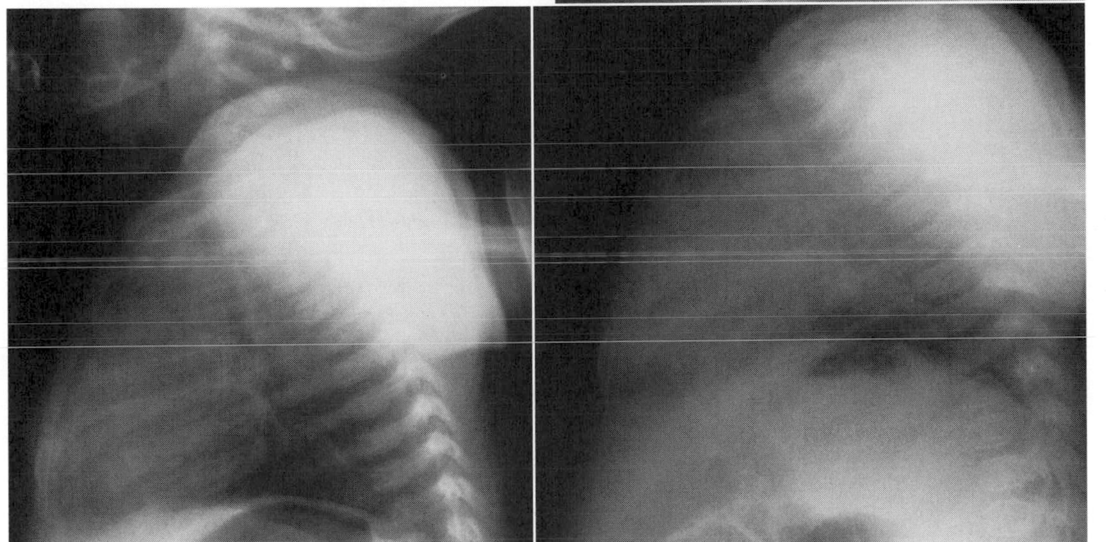

Fig. 13-14. Role of fluoroscopy for airway evaluation. **A,** A 1-year-old child with acute onset of stridor. The area below the vocal cords is constricted and almost comes to a pencil point. This is acute viral laryngeal tracheal bronchitis, or viral croup. **B** and **C,** This infant had noisy respirations. The lateral chest radiograph **(B)** was followed by another exposure **(C).** There was a great deal of dynamic change in the size of the airway but no fixed narrowing. Tracheomalacia is difficult to define because precise measurements of the airway in expiration are not readily obtainable for every age.

BOX 13-3
Differential Diagnosis of Subglottic Narrowing*

Symmetric

Laryngotracheal bronchitis (viral croup)
Tracheal stenosis
Congenital
Acquired (airway manipulation)
Subglottic hemangioma

Asymmetric

Subglottic hemangioma

*Age is crucial because subglottic hemangioma most often presents in the first 6 months of life, whereas it is uncommon to see laryngotracheal bronchitis in a patient younger than 6 months of age.

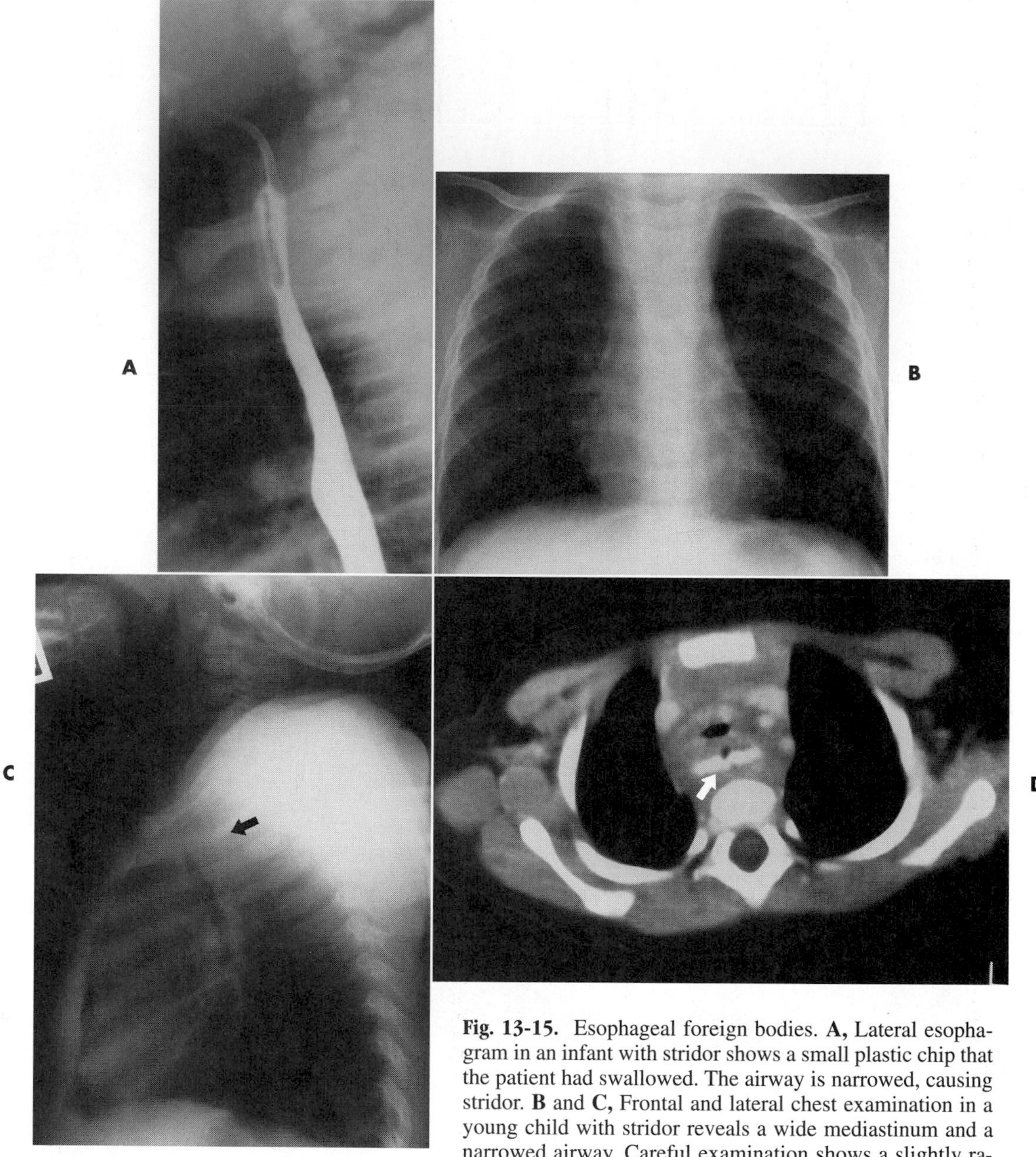

Fig. 13-15. Esophageal foreign bodies. **A,** Lateral esophagram in an infant with stridor shows a small plastic chip that the patient had swallowed. The airway is narrowed, causing stridor. **B** and **C,** Frontal and lateral chest examination in a young child with stridor reveals a wide mediastinum and a narrowed airway. Careful examination shows a slightly radiopaque density behind the airway *(arrow).* **D,** CT examination demonstrates the foreign body in the esophagus *(arrow).* The esophageal wall is thickened, and the narrowed anterior airway is secondary to mediastinal inflammation. The foreign body was a small button.

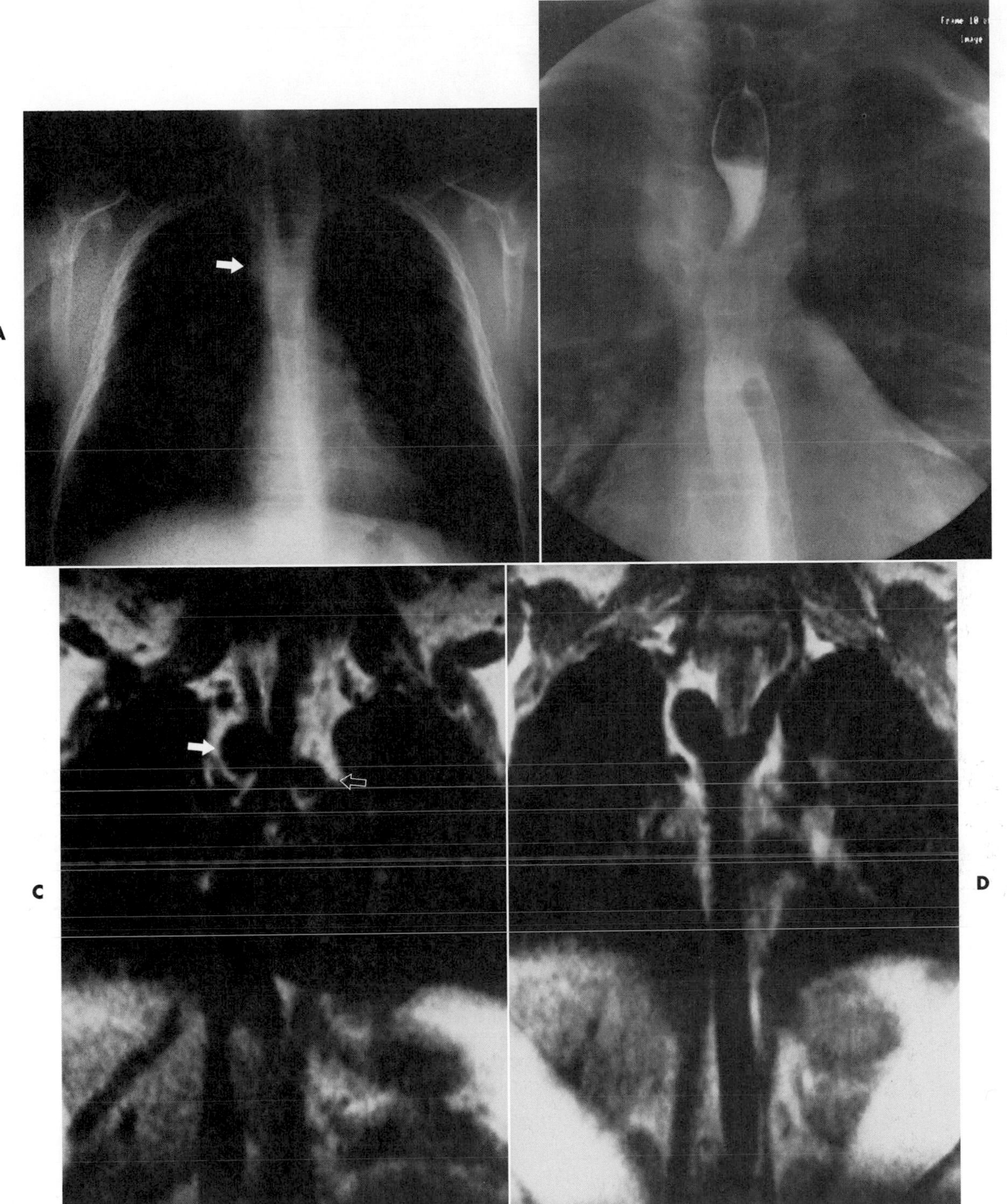

Fig. 13-16. Double aortic arch. **A,** Frontal radiograph in a 10-year-old child who had been wheezing since infancy reveals that the airway is patent but is positioned against the left pedicles. The trachea is not a midline structure, and the carina should be close to or superimposed on the right pedicles. There is also a bulge or mass on the right side *(arrow).* **B,** Frontal esophagram show a constant right-sided impression and a smaller, lower, left-sided impression. **C,** Coronal T1-weighted MR scan shows the tracheal bifurcation with the large right arch *(arrow)* and the smaller left arch *(open arrow).* Compare the right arch to the bulge in **A** and to the frontal esophagram in **B. D,** Coronal T1-weighted MR scan more posteriorly shows the joining of the right and left arches and central descent.

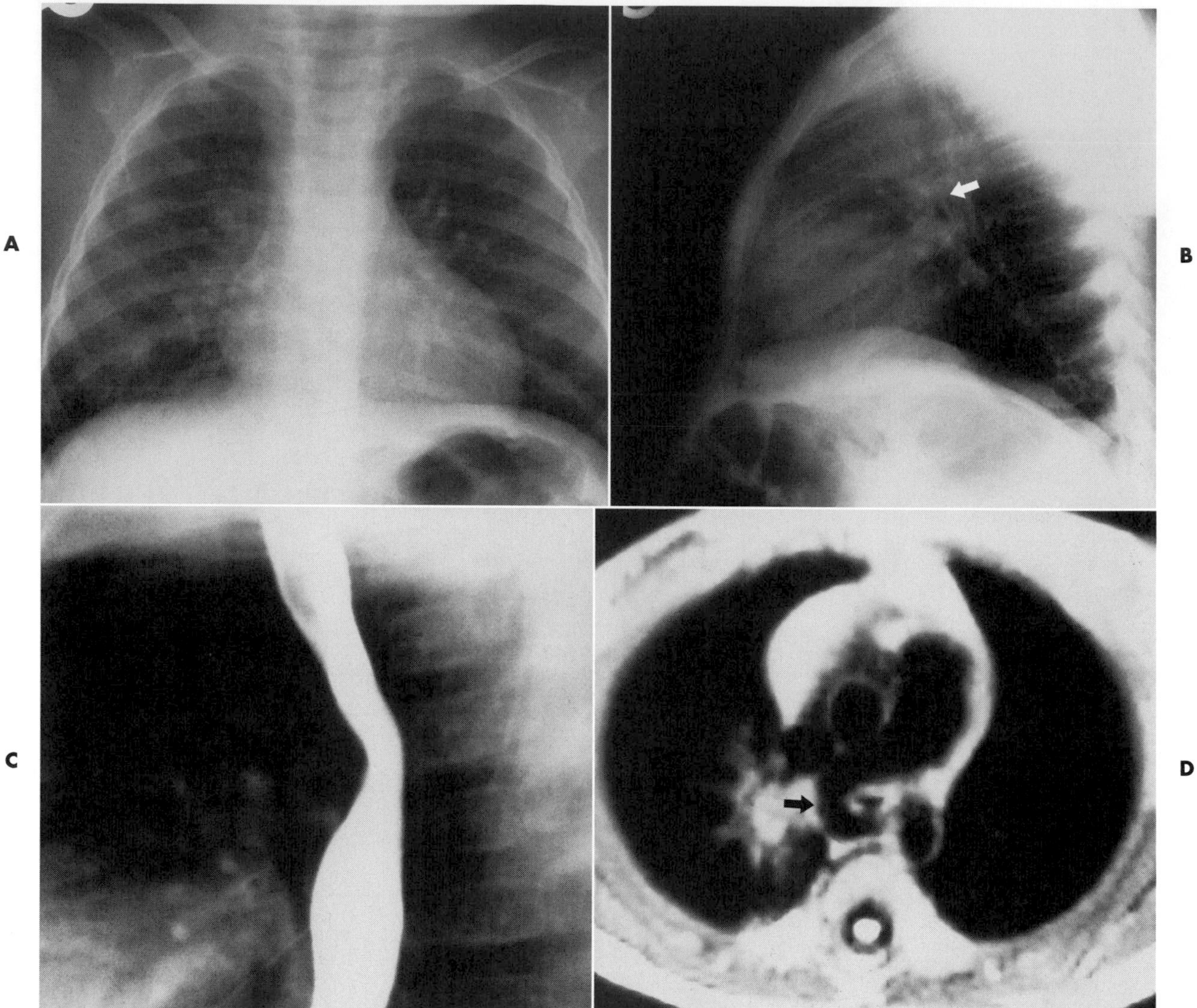

Fig. 13-17. Pulmonary sling: anomalous left pulmonary artery arising from the right pulmonary artery. **A,** Frontal chest radiograph in a child with noisy respirations reveals a properly positioned carina and no detectable abnormality. **B.** On the lateral radiograph, there appears to be anterior bowing of the trachea *(arrow)*. **C,** An esophagram confirms the bulge between the esophagus and the airway. **D,** Axial T1-weighted MR scan shows the left pulmonary artery coming off the right and encircling the trachea. The trachea is narrowed. The pulmonary sling *(arrow)* is the encircling portion of the left pulmonary artery. A frequent accompanying anomaly is stenosis of the right mainstem bronchus.

fluoroscopy. Xeroradiography has no role; the enhanced image contrast is completely overshadowed by the excessive amount of radiation exposure.

Although a variety of tools are available for imaging the pediatric airway, the mainstay is carefully constructed plain films and a fluoroscopic examination (Fig. 13-18). These imaging studies should be complementary to the judicious use of flexible fiberoptic bronchoscopy.[65]

CHEST

Plain Film

The chest x-ray film remains the foundation of any radiographic investigation of the pediatric thorax. The indications for this examination are as plentiful as the number of procedures performed in a busy pediatric radiology department. Infants and children present their own set of challenges, not only in the interpretation of the examination but also in the procurement of a technically perfect study. In interpreting the plain film, the clinician must become familiar with the normal appearance of the pediatric chest and recognize when the sometimes reluctant subject did not remain stationary in the desired position or follow breathing instructions while the examination was performed.

Before embarking on a painstaking systematic review of the radiographic findings, the clinician should first check the three *T*s: technique, traps, and tubes (Box 13-4).

Technique

Defects in technique can produce spurious findings or mask real ones.[66-70] First, the clinician should determine whether the patient is well centered. The anterior rib ends on each side should be equidistant from the ipsilateral pedicle and the spinous processes of the vertebral bodies the same distance from the right and left lateral chest walls (Fig. 13-19).

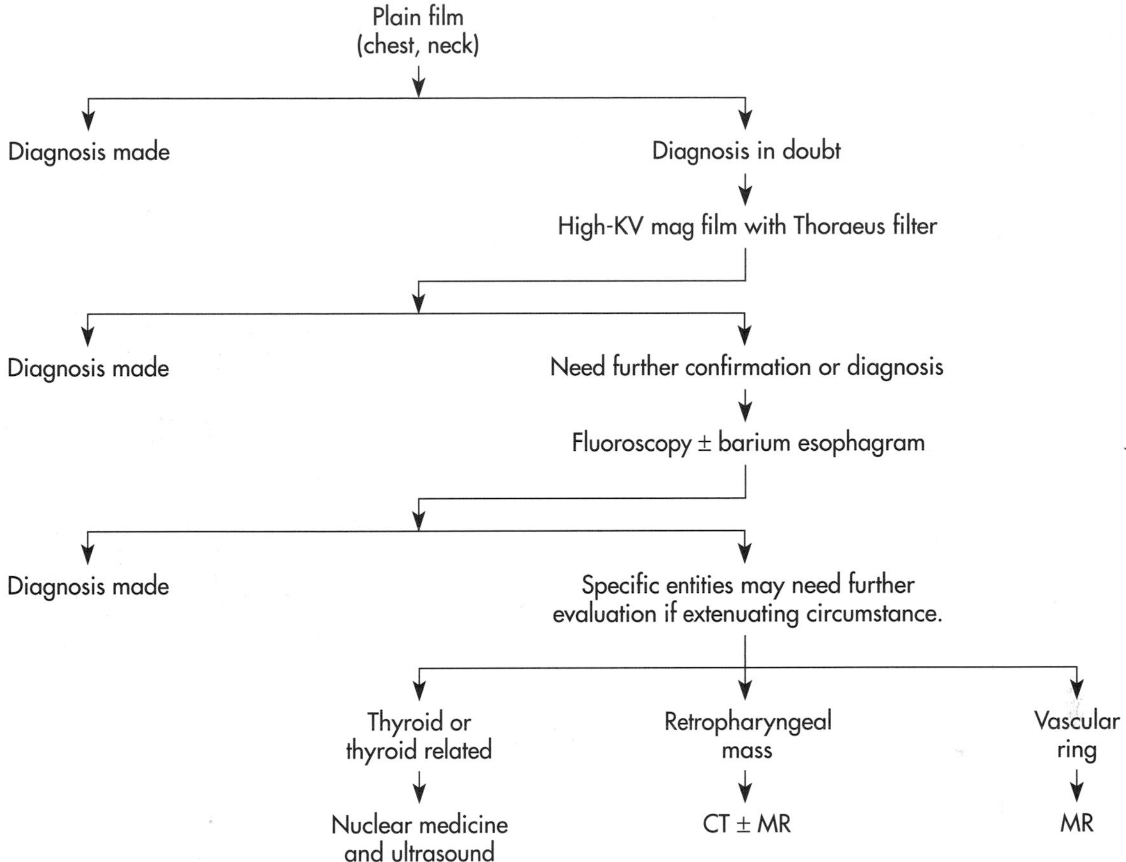

Fig. 13-18. Algorithm for imaging of the pediatric airway. *mag,* Magnification.

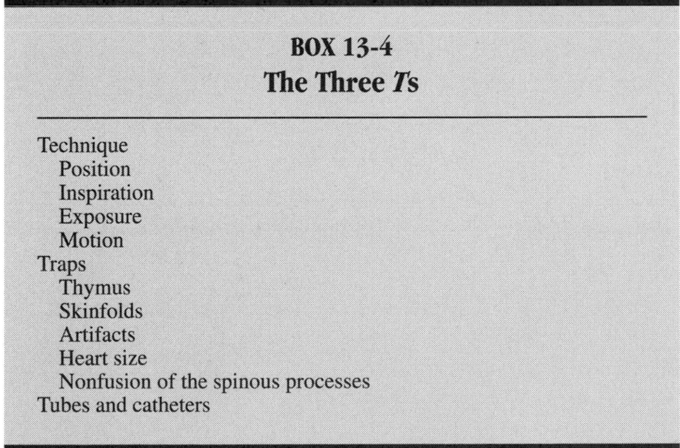

BOX 13-4
The Three *T*s

Technique
- Position
- Inspiration
- Exposure
- Motion

Traps
- Thymus
- Skinfolds
- Artifacts
- Heart size
- Nonfusion of the spinous processes

Tubes and catheters

Second, the clinician should determine whether there is adequate inspiration. Poor inspiration exaggerates heart size and gives the impression of increased alveolar and interstitial density.[67] At least five and preferably six anterior ribs should be projected above the dome of the hemidiaphragm. Buckling of the trachea, which is fixed only at the larynx and the carina, is a clue that the exposure occurred in expiration (Fig. 13-20).

Third, the radiograph should be well exposed. An optimally exposed examination must meet two criteria: The pedicles of the vertebral bodies should be seen through the heart, and the pulmonary vessels must be evident in the middle third of the lungs without bright lighting of the picture[71,72] (see Fig. 13-1).

Fourth, the clinician should determine whether there is evidence of motion. Motion causes loss of sharpness of the pulmonary vascular markings.

Traps: Normal Variants

It is very important to become familiar with the normal appearance of the pediatric chest because the chest radiograph in this age group is unique in many ways. The neonatal chest is shaped like a mound of sand: equal in anteroposterior and transverse dimensions. As growth occurs, the thorax elongates, developing an adult contour by the time the child is ready to start elementary school.

The radiologic appearance of the lungs' response to an inflammatory insult is largely dictated by several unique structural features in the lungs of infants and small children (those younger than 8 years of age). The pediatric airways collapse more easily and are both absolutely and relatively smaller than in adults.[71,73] There are less air conductance and more mucous production in the peripheral airways. Collateral ventilation is not well developed. All these features predispose to air trapping and atelectasis when the airway is inflamed[66,69,73] (Fig. 13-21).

The thymus gland is a normal structure that increases in size during childhood. Compared with the thoracic contents, its size is greatest in infancy. Its size and configuration, along with its location in the anterior and superior mediastinum, can be confusing for the unsuspecting imager (Figs. 13-22

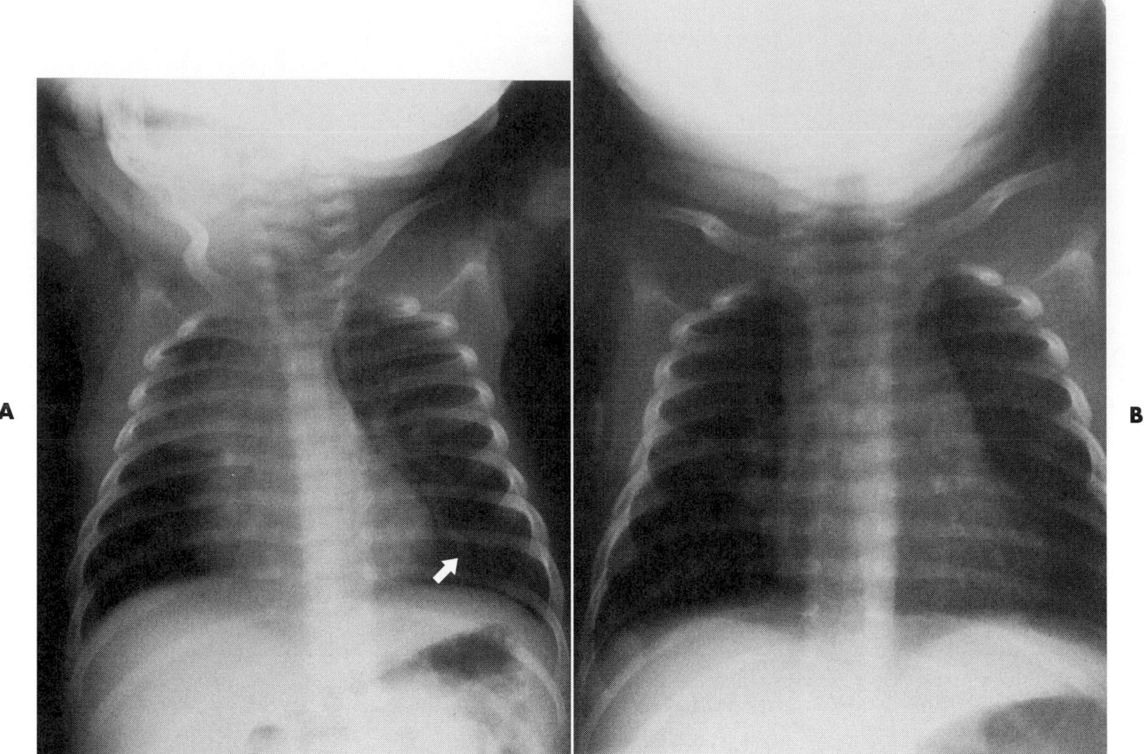

Fig. 13-19. Effects of position. **A,** A rotated chest film showing a "mass" in the right upper lobe. The anterior ribs *(arrow)* on the left are clearly closer to the ipsilateral pedicle than those on the right. There is also offset of the clavicles. **B,** A straight film shows a normal mediastinum and chest. The "mass" was the thymus.

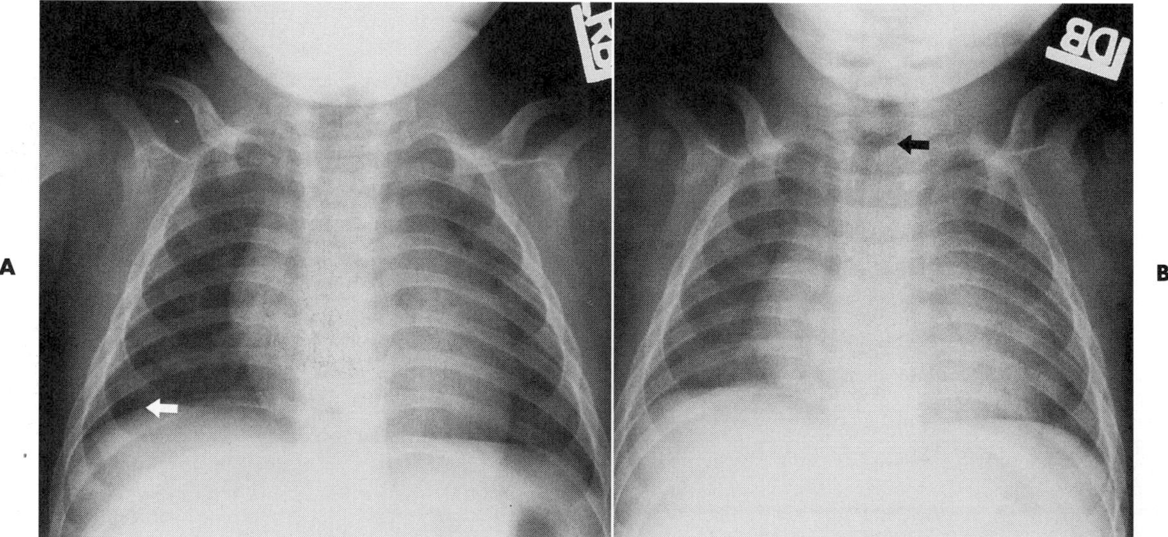

Fig. 13-20. Normal inspiratory-expiratory examination. **A,** Normal inspiratory chest film shows that the airway is patent, the carina is adjacent to the right pedicles, and there are five anterior ribs above the diaphragm. (The arrow is on the fifth rib.) **B,** An expiratory film of the same infant shows buckling of the airway *(arrow);* a horizontal, apparently larger heart; and "infiltrates in the lungs." There are only four anterior ribs above the diaphragm.

Fig. 13-21. Chlamydial pneumonia in a 5-week-old child. **A,** Frontal chest radiograph photographed to see the multiple densities throughout both lungs. The ninth anterior rib crosses the diaphragm, indicating marked hyperexpansion. Hyperexpansion can be diagnosed if it is visible on two views (i.e., nonvoluntary). **B,** Lateral view of the same patient shows the large anterior and posterior air spaces (i.e., hyperexpansion).

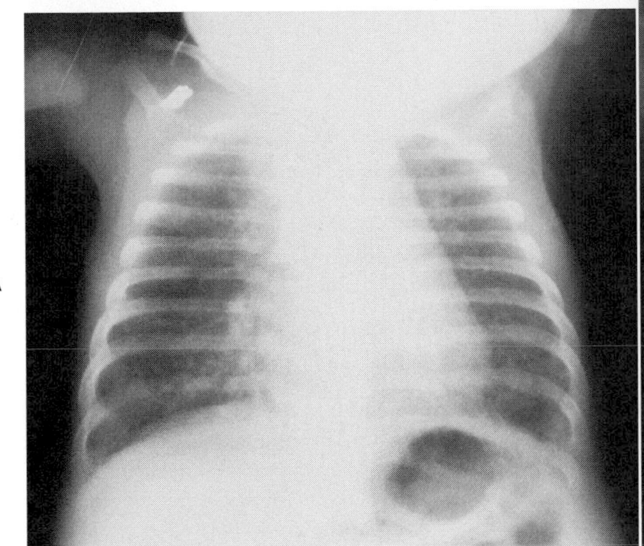

A

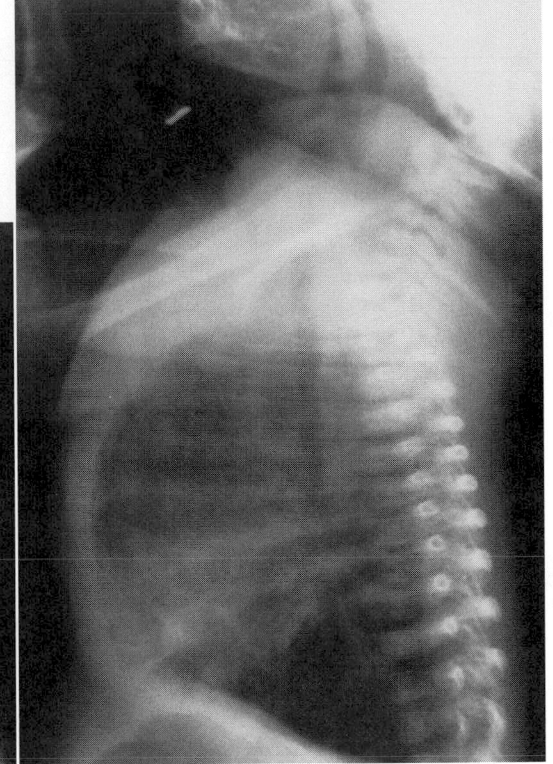

B

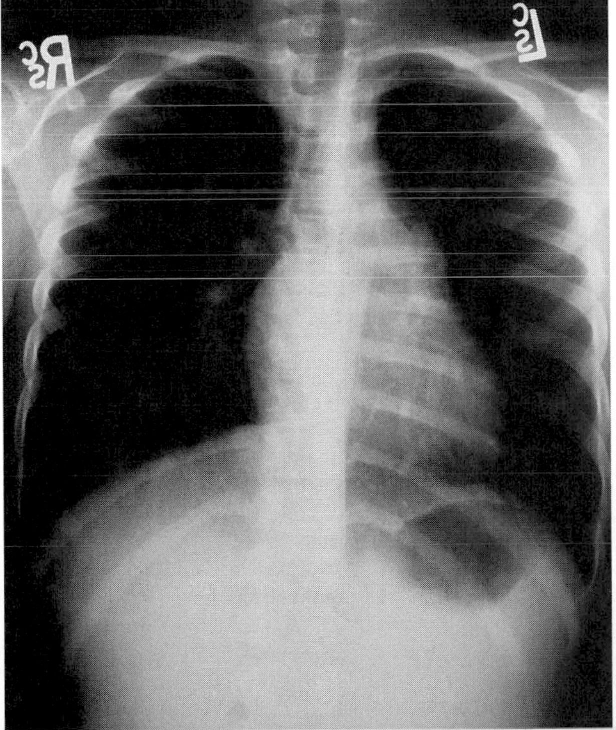

A

Fig. 13-22. Persistence of a normal thymus. **A,** This chest film of 7-year-old child was acquired for another reason, and a density was noted along the left cardiac margin above the level of the aorta. **B,** Contrast-enhanced CT scan shows the anteriorly placed density enhanced homogeneously. This is a normal residual thymus.

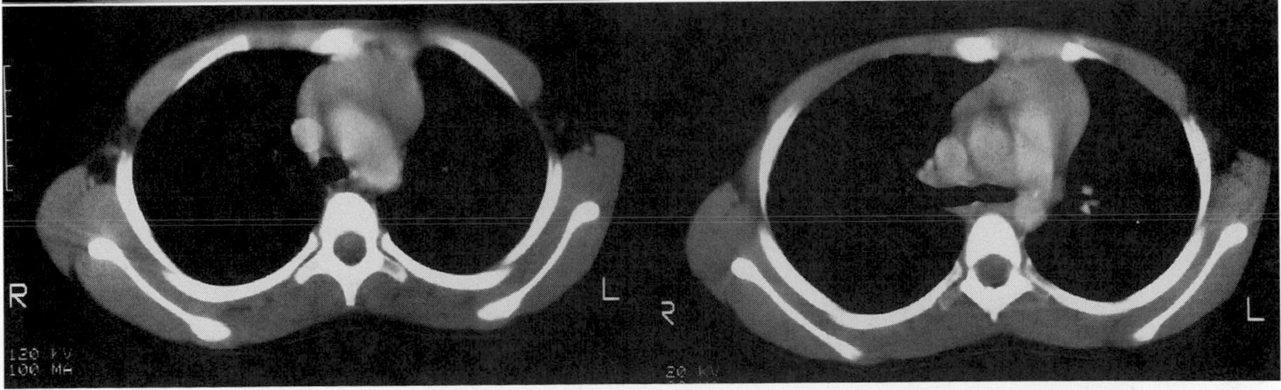

B

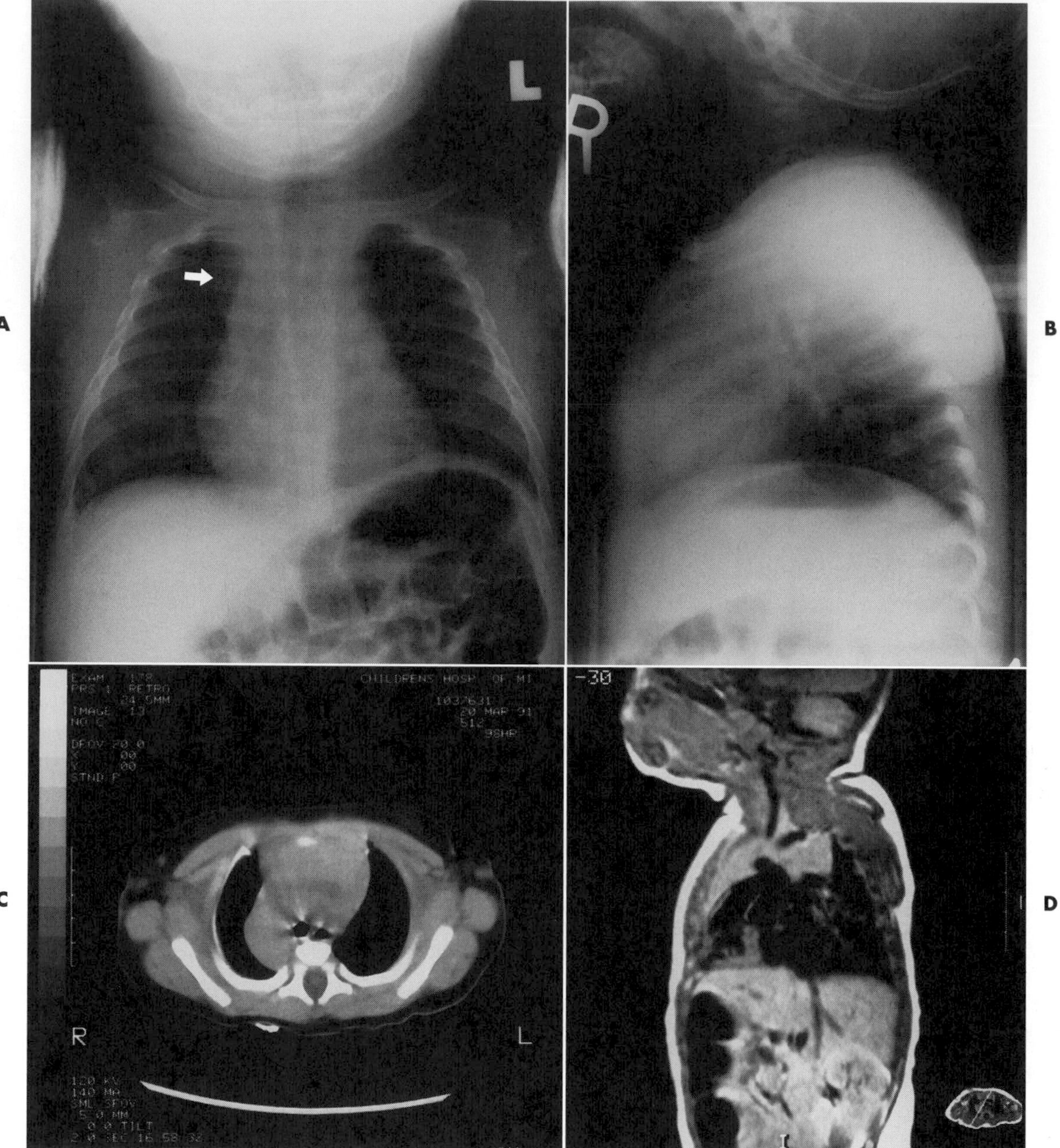

Fig. 13-23. Aberrant thymus. **A** and **B,** Right-sided mediastinal mass *(arrow)* in an infant. It is not silhouetting the heart; therefore it is not in the anterior or middle mediastinum and is posteriorly placed. On the lateral film, only the normal anteriorly placed thymus can be seen. **C,** Nonenhanced CT scan shows the anterior thymus as well as a right-sided posterior homogenous mass of the same density as the thymus. **D,** T1-weighted sagittal MR scan shows continuation of the anterior, middle, and posterior components of this aberrant thymus. (From Slovis TL et al: *Pediatr Radiol* 22:490-492, 1992.)

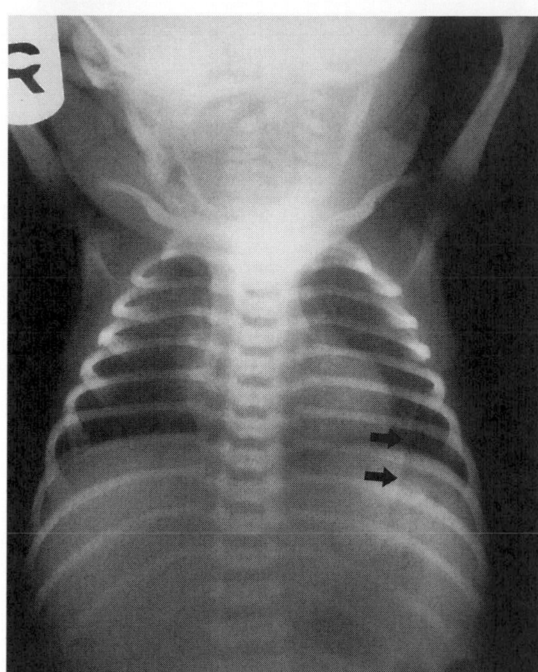

Fig. 13-24. Skinfold mimicking pneumothorax. An opacity along the left lateral thoracic cavity wall extends oblique (not in contour of a collapsed lung) *(arrows)*. There are lung markings lateral to this density, so it cannot represent a pneumothorax.

and 13-23). Several features, when meticulously sought, distinguish the normal thymus from an ominous abnormality.[74] The thymus is homogeneous and is of a density that allows visualization of the bronchovascular markings behind it. The inferior edge produces a notch on the left heart border, and there is often an insinuation of the thymus into the minor fissure on the right, which when present, appears to have the configuration of a sail.[75] If there is still doubt, an oblique projection sometimes helps because on this view, normal scalloping of the margin caused by indenting of the anterior rib ends is accentuated.

Normal skinfolds can mimic pneumothoraxes but are in fact easily distinguished by the presence of lung markings (pulmonary vessels) extending beyond the line (Figs. 13-24 and 13-25). Artifacts from immobilization devices can also be distinguished because, unlike a pneumothorax, they are very geometric and straight.

The two posterior neural arches of the spine begin to fuse posteriorly during the first year of life. The cleft between them can persist into adulthood but usually ossifies and disappears starting in the lumbar region between the ages of 3 and 5 years. The narrow vertical lucency seen on the anteroposterior projection is therefore a normal finding and should not be mistaken for a narrow trachea or a pathologic lesion (Fig. 13-26).

Vascular structures, such as the left superior intercostal vein (aortic nipple) and the ductus arteriosus, can also look like masses but do have characteristic appearances and are completely normal.[76] The heart, especially in the infant chest when viewed during suboptimal inspiration, often appears enlarged on anteroposterior examination. However, the lateral examination confirms the normal size of the cardiac silhouette.

Tubes

The clinician should always note the position of every tube, clip, suture, and monitoring device. The authors usually acquire only frontal films for follow-up in a patient whose lungs are intubated. However, if the child is experiencing unexplained airway obstruction, a lateral film is mandatory (Fig. 13-27).

Approach to Film

With an understanding of the technical problems, the anatomic variations that can be traps, and the necessity to define tubes and catheters, the clinician must develop a systematic method of interpreting the examination. This is particularly true of the subspecialist. An ABCs approach is helpful (Box 13-5). Many nonpulmonary or surgical pulmonary causes of neonatal respiratory distress are detected with this systematic approach (Box 13-6).

Abdomen

Infradiaphragmatic disease can present with respiratory tract signs and symptoms. Radiographic observations of abdominal or retroperitoneal findings may also help explain changes seen on the chest film (e.g., gallstones in a child with a large heart [Fig. 13-28]). The clinician needs to determine whether the visceral situs is correct; the visualized bowel loops are normal in size, location, and appearance; there are any unusual masses or calcifications; the diaphragm contours are regular; and there is any free air.

Bones and Soft Tissues

The clinician should look for abnormalities in the bony thorax and soft tissues. More important, unsuspected fractures are a sign of child abuse[77] (Figs. 13-29 and 13-30). Chest wall lesions may present as thoracic disease (Figs. 13-2 and 13-31).

Chest

When examining the chest, the clinician should pay special attention to the airway (patency, position, size, and shape) and the mediastinum and heart (position, size, and shape) before evaluating the lungs.

Airway

The airway is not a midline structure (see Fig. 13-16). It lies slightly to the right of midline, and the carina is seen on the frontal chest film superimposed on the right T4-5 pedicle. The position of the airway is the key to the position of the aortic arch. Especially in younger children, when the normal left arch is difficult to see, the airway must be appropriately positioned with the carina over the right pedicle. If the trachea is not in this position, a right or double arch or mass is strongly suggested (see Fig. 13-16).

The airway should be seen in its entirety from the glottis to the carina on the frontal chest film (see Figs. 13-2 and 13-15). If a portion of the airway is obliterated, the etiology should be found.

Mediastinum

It is important to look at the mediastinum as a whole rather than to look at just at the heart. Unusual contours, adenopathy, masses, and vascular abnormality need to be noted (Figs. 13-2,

Text continued on p 180

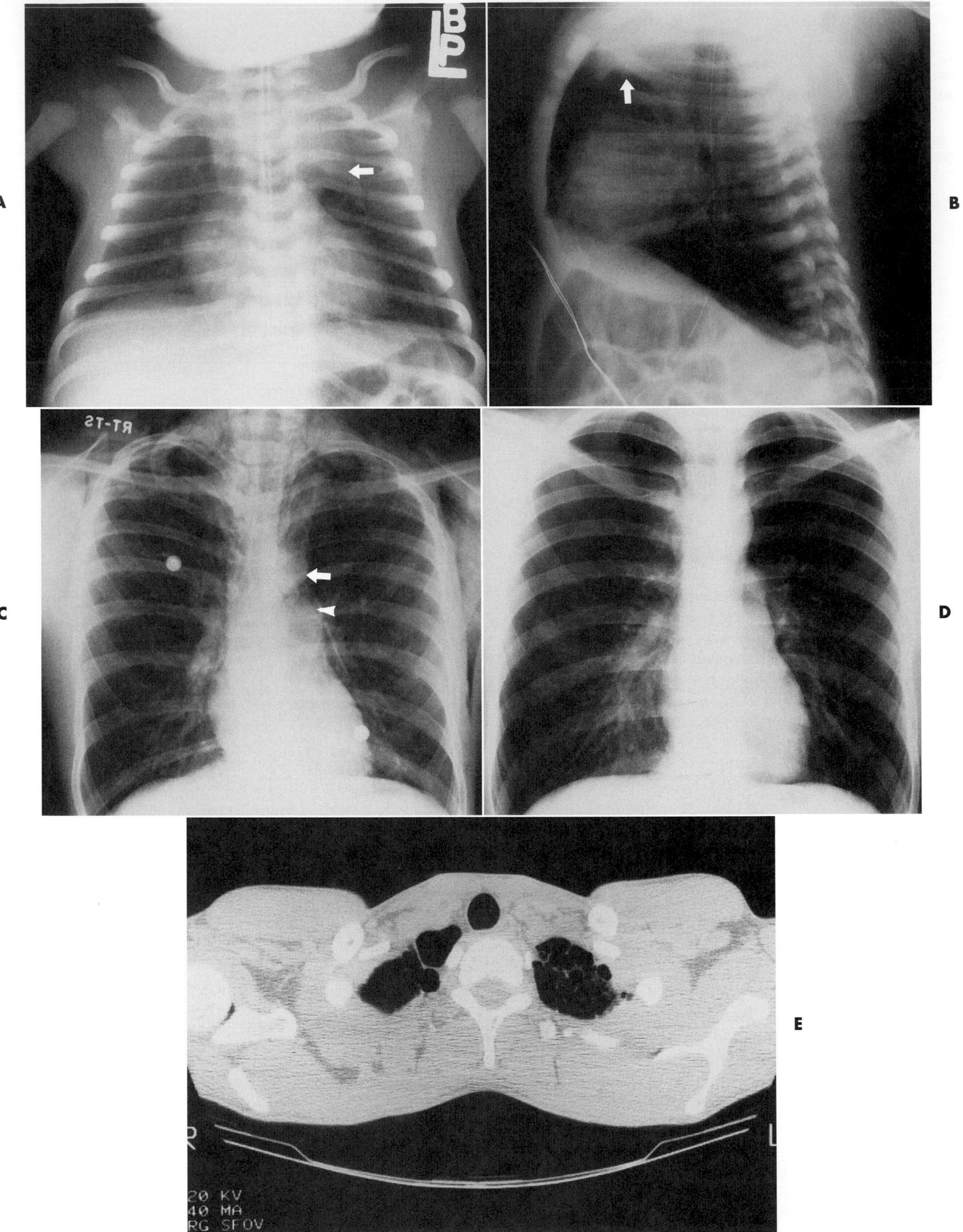

Fig. 13-25. Pneumothorax and pneumomediastinum. **A** and **B,** Frontal and lateral films of a neonate with a pneumomediastinum. The thymus *(arrows)* is elevated and surrounded by air on both views and is clearly separate from the rest of the mediastinum. Note the left skinfold; lung markings are seen lateral to the fold. **C,** Pneumomediastinum in an older child shows air in the subcutaneous tissues of the shoulders, particularly on the left, and into the neck. In addition, the mediastinum has a stranded appearance. The aortic arch *(arrow)* separates from the pulmonary artery *(arrowhead),* indicating that a pneumopericardium is also present. The pericardium attaches between the two vessels. This child had asthma. **D** and **E,** Teenager with pain in the right side of the chest. Frontal radiograph **(D)** shows no lung markings lateral to a pleural opacity extending from the diaphragm to the clavicle. There is a similar finding at the apex of the left lung, indicating bilateral pneumothoraxes. Spontaneous pneumothoraxes are frequently caused by blebs; therefore CT is indicated. The CT scan **(E)** taken after re-expansion of the lungs reveals multiple blebs at the apex of each lung.

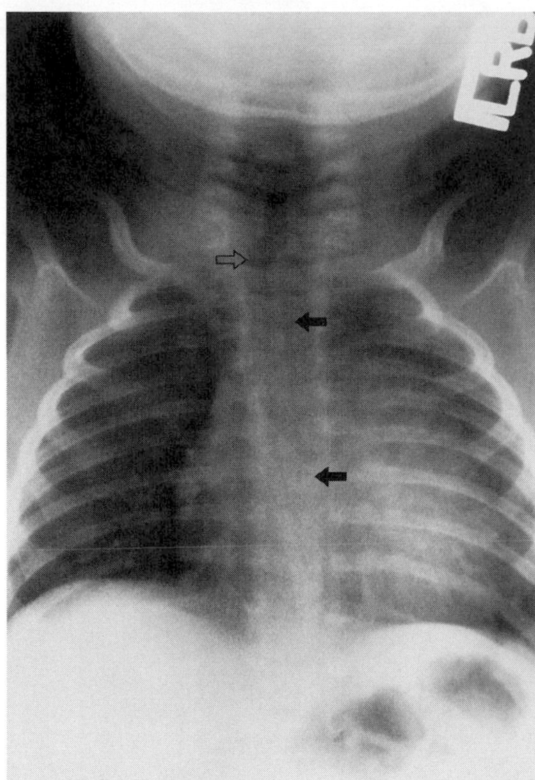

Fig. 13-26. Nonfusion of the posterior neural arches. A chest film was taken for "pneumonia" in this young infant. There is an opacity behind the left heart. Nonfusion of the spinous process *(arrows)* is a normal finding in the first years of life. Note the normal buckling of the airway to the right *(open arrow).*

Fig. 13-27. Abnormal tube position. **A,** Frontal radiograph of a neonate shows the end of the endotracheal tube *(arrow)* below the level of the clavicles in an appropriate position. The lungs have a hazy density consistent with a mild form of hyaline membrane disease. However, the child was doing poorly and a lateral film was suggested. **B,** Lateral radiograph shows that the tube *(arrow)* is not in the airway *(A)* but in the esophagus *(E).*

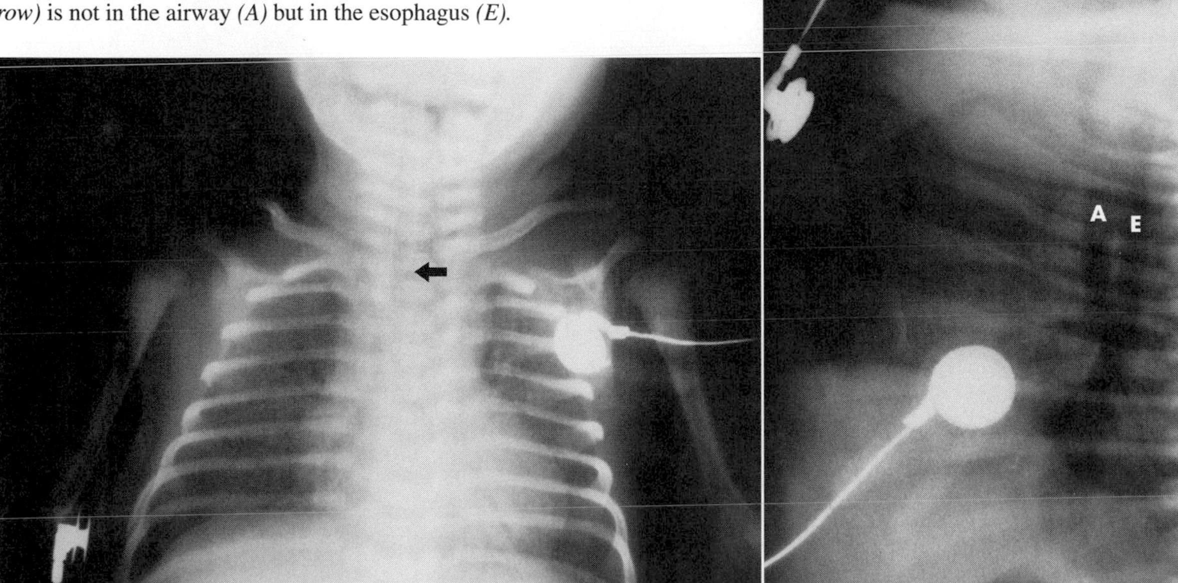

BOX 13-5
ABCs Approach to the Chest Film

A: Abdomen
  Visceral situs, masses, free air, calcifications, bowel loops, diaphragmatic contours
B: Bones (and soft tissue)
  Fractures, anomalies, masses
C: Chest
  Airway: patency, position, size, shape
  Mediastinum: position, size, shape
  Heart: position, size, shape
  Lungs: volume, vascularity, density-opacity
S: Soft tissue swelling, foreign body

From Haller JO, Slovis TL: *Pediatric radiology,* ed 2, Heidelberg, 1995, Springer-Verlag.

BOX 13-6
Nonpulmonary or Surgical Pulmonary Cases of Respiratory Distress in the Neonate

Abdominal causes

Abdominal contents in the thorax cavity (e.g., diaphragmatic hernia, intrathoracic stomach)

Bone: skeletal lesions

Rib fracture or flail chest as in osteogenesis imperfecta
Malformation such as asphyxiating thoracic dystrophy and other short rib conditions
Chest wall masses

Chest: intrathoracic

Vascular rings and slings	Bronchial obstruction
Mediastinal masses	Bronchogenic cyst
Esophageal abnormalities	Lobar emphysema
Esophageal atresia	Bronchial adenoma
H-type fistula	Atresia of bronchus
Foreign body	Adenomatoid malformation
Cardiac disease	

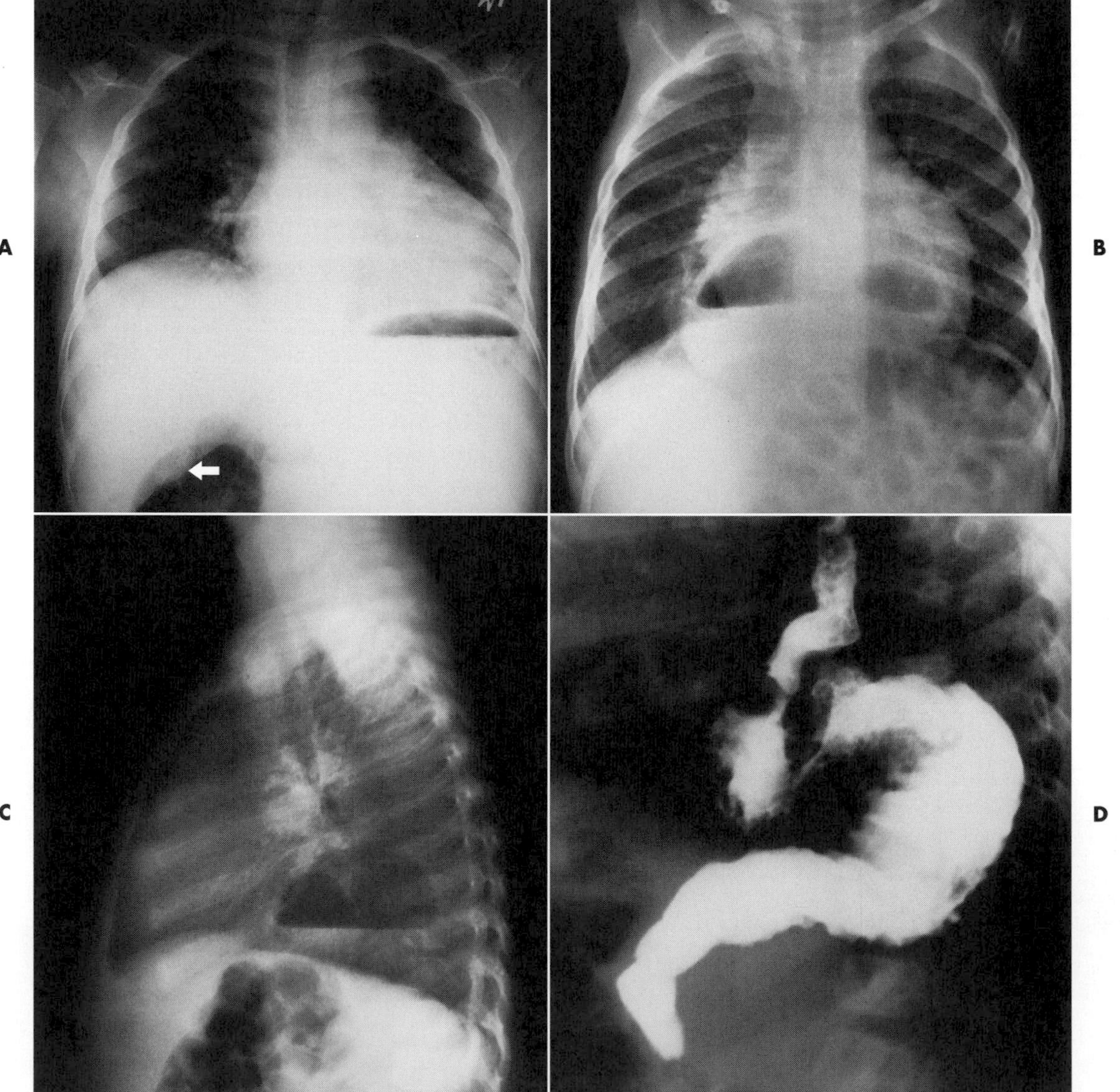

Fig. 13-28. Systematic evaluation of films. **A,** Frontal radiograph reveals cardiomegaly and opacity behind the heart, signifying pneumonia. However, close appraisal shows gallstones *(arrow)* in the right upper quadrant, defining systemic disease (sickle cell anemia). **B** and **C,** Frontal and lateral erect radiographs reveal air-fluid levels at the base of the lungs in a 1-year-old infant with tachypnea and dyspnea. Note the absence of a stomach "bubble." **D,** Lateral film of a barium swallow reveals the intrathoracic stomach. There was intermittent twisting (volvulus) of the stomach.

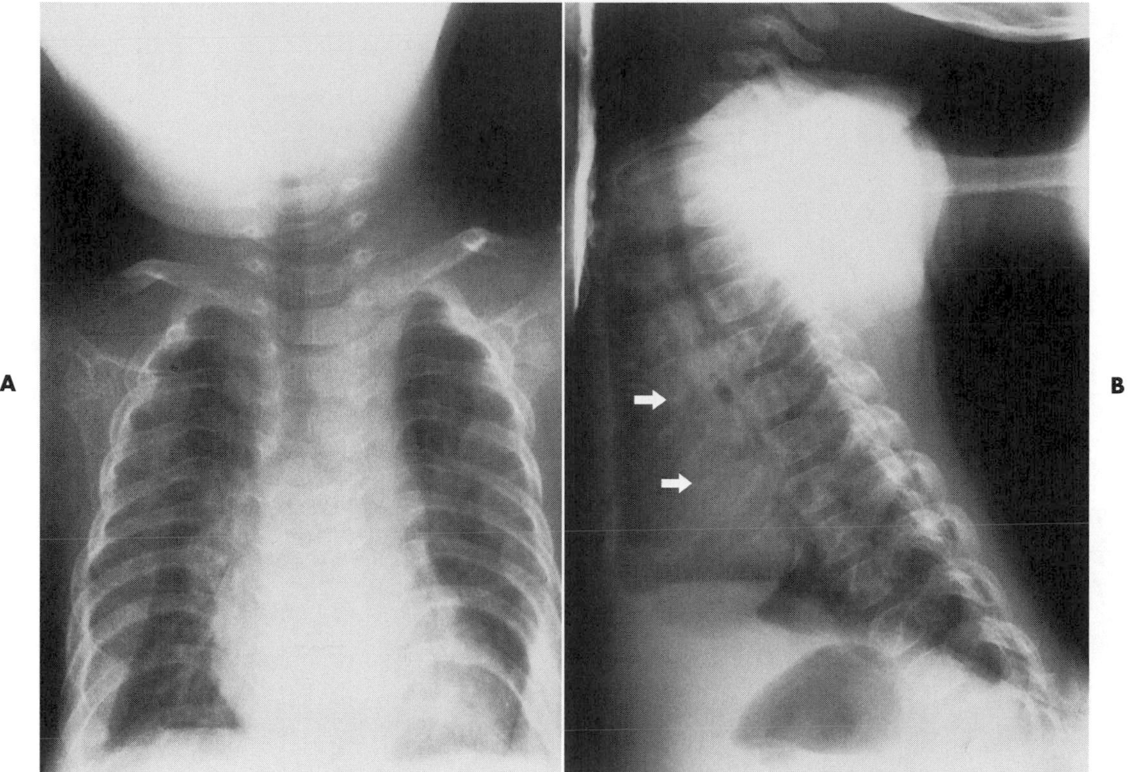

Fig. 13-29. Systematic evaluation of the chest. **A,** This young infant had mild respiratory distress. The thorax is bell shaped, and the ribs appear somewhat thickened. **B,** Lateral films show how short the ribs are. (The arrows are on the anterior ribs.) The anteroposterior diameter of the chest is very narrow. This is an example of asphyxiating thoracic dystrophy (Jeune's syndrome). The name is a misnomer because many of these children survive.

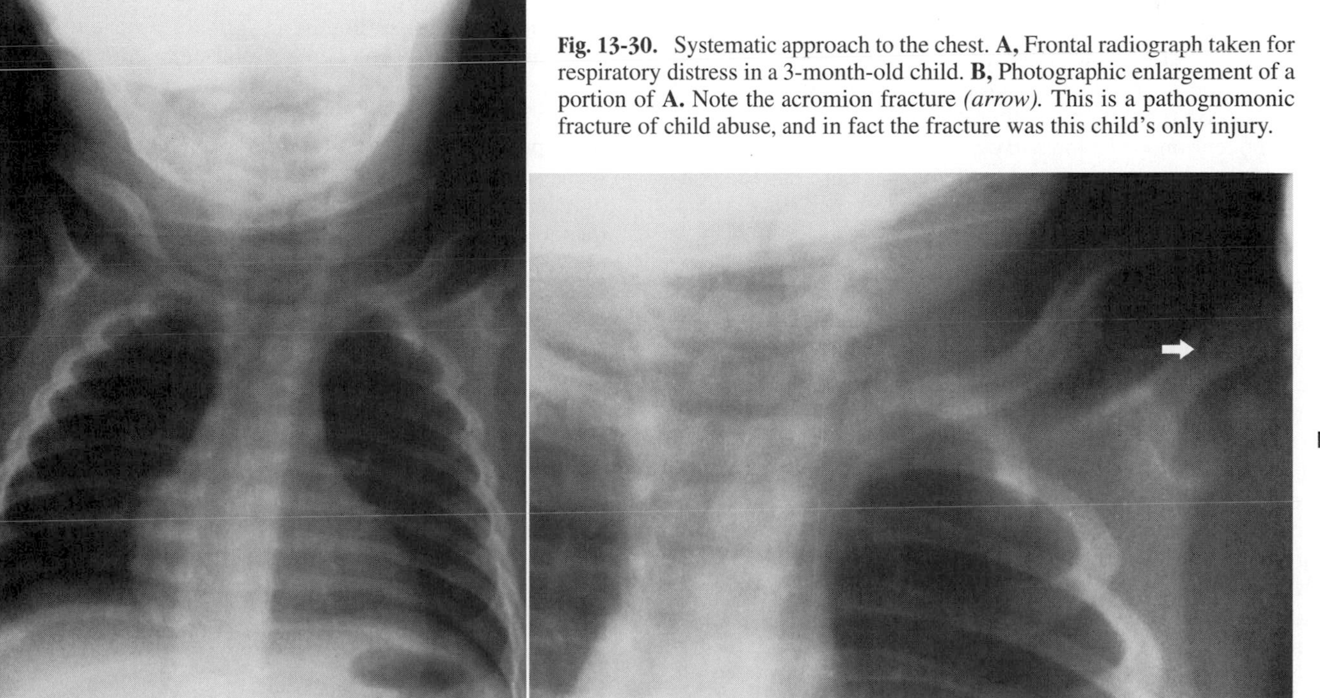

Fig. 13-30. Systematic approach to the chest. **A,** Frontal radiograph taken for respiratory distress in a 3-month-old child. **B,** Photographic enlargement of a portion of **A.** Note the acromion fracture *(arrow).* This is a pathognomonic fracture of child abuse, and in fact the fracture was this child's only injury.

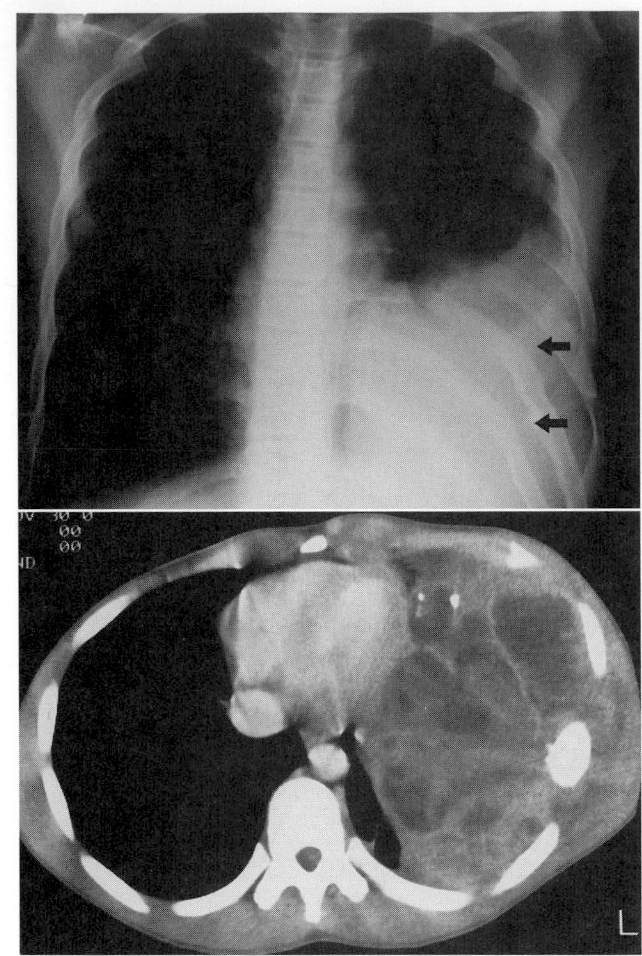

Fig. 13-31. Chest wall masses affecting the lung or presenting as respiratory problems. **A,** Chest film of a teenage boy who had difficulty breathing. There is a pleural reaction on the left and a density involving the lower half of the thoracic cavity. Careful observation shows involvement of the eighth and ninth posterior lateral left ribs *(arrows)*. **B**, Enhanced CT scan shows calcifications within the mass, involvement of the rib, and the inhomogeneous nature of this lesion. This was proved to be rhabdomyosarcoma.

13-5, 13-16, 13-22, 13-23, and 13-32). The most common mediastinal mass (see later section) is the thymus. After appreciating mediastinal contour, the clinician should use both the lateral and frontal films to determine the heart's size. In young children, the heart's size is determined better on the lateral view than on the frontal. If there is cardiac enhancement, it should occur on *both* views. By noting the site of the arch relative to the airway position, the size of the heart, and the condition of the pulmonary vascularity (see later section), the clinician can appreciate the role of cardiac disease.

Lungs

When the lungs are viewed, the most important concept is density, both within the unobscured lung and through the viscera (i.e., the heart and liver). More important, the clinician should determine whether there is a change in density (i.e., what should be black is now white). Normally the branching vessels behind the heart and the vessels at the base of the lungs through the top of the liver should be seen. The most posterior portion of the diaphragm inserts at L2, so there is a significant portion of lung that needs to be viewed below the easily visualized anterior edge of the diaphragm. (see Fig. 13-5). Alterations in density can be either increased blackness (hyperexpansion or cyst containing air) or increased opacity (soft tis-sue density where an aerated lung should be). The latter is usually caused by pulmonary consolidation, atelectasis, a mass, collections of fluid, or ectopic viscera such as an intrathoracic kidney (Fig. 13-33). When the alteration in density is such that there is opacification, a common radiographic finding is the silhouette sign. Loss of a normal mediastinal or diaphragmatic border occurs because of a contiguous opacity of similar density.

Another helpful radiographic sign when opacity is present in the lung parenchyma is the air bronchogram (Fig. 13-34). The *air bronchogram* refers to air-containing bronchi that become visible because the surrounding airspace is opacified by fluid, pneumonia, or atelectasis. Opacification of the pleural space is found in pleural effusions and in pleural inflammation (thickening). A unique type of effusion is the subpulmonic effusion in which the shape of the diaphragm appears to have been altered (Fig. 13-35). The clue to this diagnosis is that the highest point of the diaphragm is no longer in the midclavicular line but is more laterally displaced.

Increased blackness with a shift of the mediastinum or diaphragm or fissures is another form of density alteration. This is frequently found in lobar emphysema, bronchiolitis obliterans, and most commonly, a bronchial foreign body (Figs. 13-36 and 13-37). As a complication of asthma and other air-blocking diseases, pneumomediastinum and pneumothorax must be recognized (see Fig. 13-25). In each chest film, the clinician must consciously search for the lateral border of the lung against the chest wall to avoid missing a pneumothorax.

Last, the pulmonary vascularity is viewed. It diminishes in size from the central to peripheral directions but in a well exposed film is seen in the middle third of the lungs. When the vascularity becomes quite prominent, the diagnosis may be shunt vascularity, and when there is loss of distinct vascular markings, it may be interstitial edema, which is the first radiographic sign of pulmonary edema.

Text continued on p 186

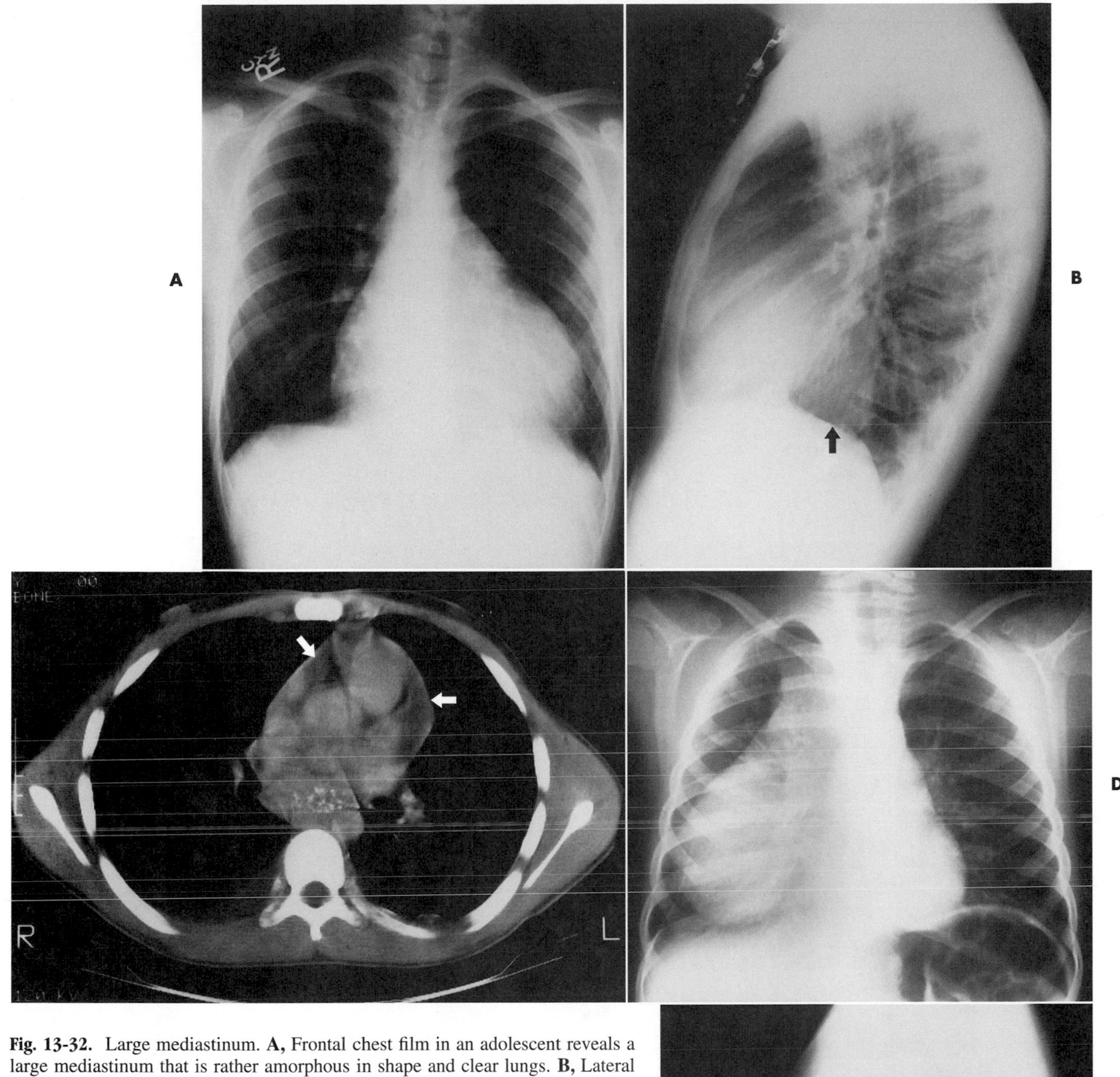

Fig. 13-32. Large mediastinum. **A,** Frontal chest film in an adolescent reveals a large mediastinum that is rather amorphous in shape and clear lungs. **B,** Lateral film adds little information except for the fact that there is a "mass" filling the posterior air space *(arrow).* **C,** Contrast-enhanced CT scan reveals the etiology of this mass and the patient's disease. There are a pericardial effusion *(arrows),* adenopathy, and calcification in the mediastinum. This patient had tuberculosis. **D** and **E,** Frontal and lateral films in a 6-year-old child with cough. There is a large mass silhouetting the right heart margin. On the lateral view **(E),** it overlies the middle mediastinum. The patient has non-Hodgkin's lymphoma.

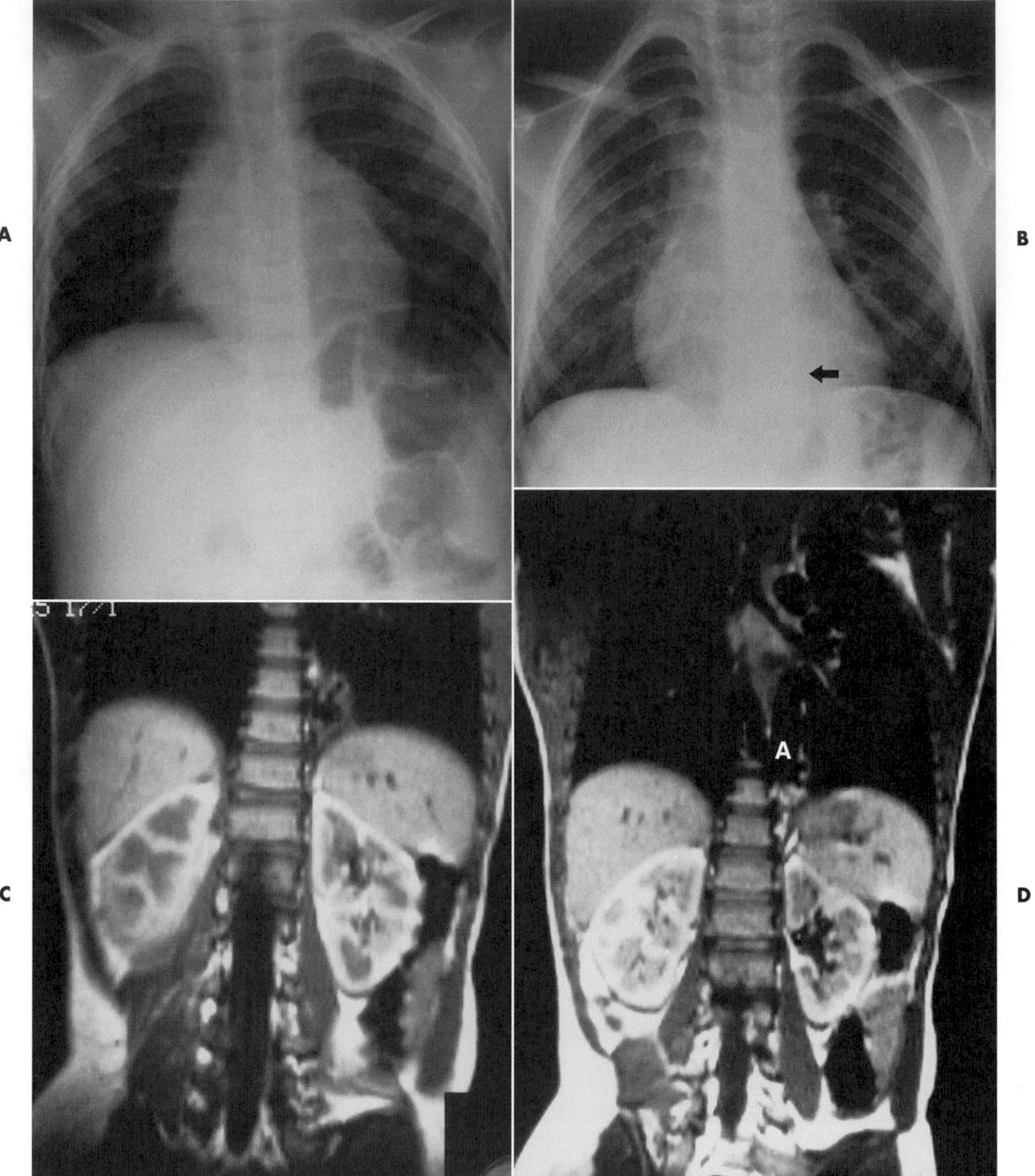

Fig. 13-33. Increased opacity within the lungs. **A,** Frontal chest film in a 4-year-old child with fever. The vessels are seen clearly behind the left side of the heart, but there is increased opacity behind the right side of the heart. This was pneumonia involving the perihilar and medial basal segments of the right lung. **B,** This 6-year-old child had a persistent density behind the left heart. On this oblique frontal film, it can be seen obliterating the diaphragm medially: the silhouette sign *(arrow)*. **C** and **D,** Because the child was not ill, an MR scan was done and revealed the mass to have multiple vessels. A somewhat anterior cut **(D)** shows the vessels coming from the aorta *(A)*. This was proved to be a sequestration.

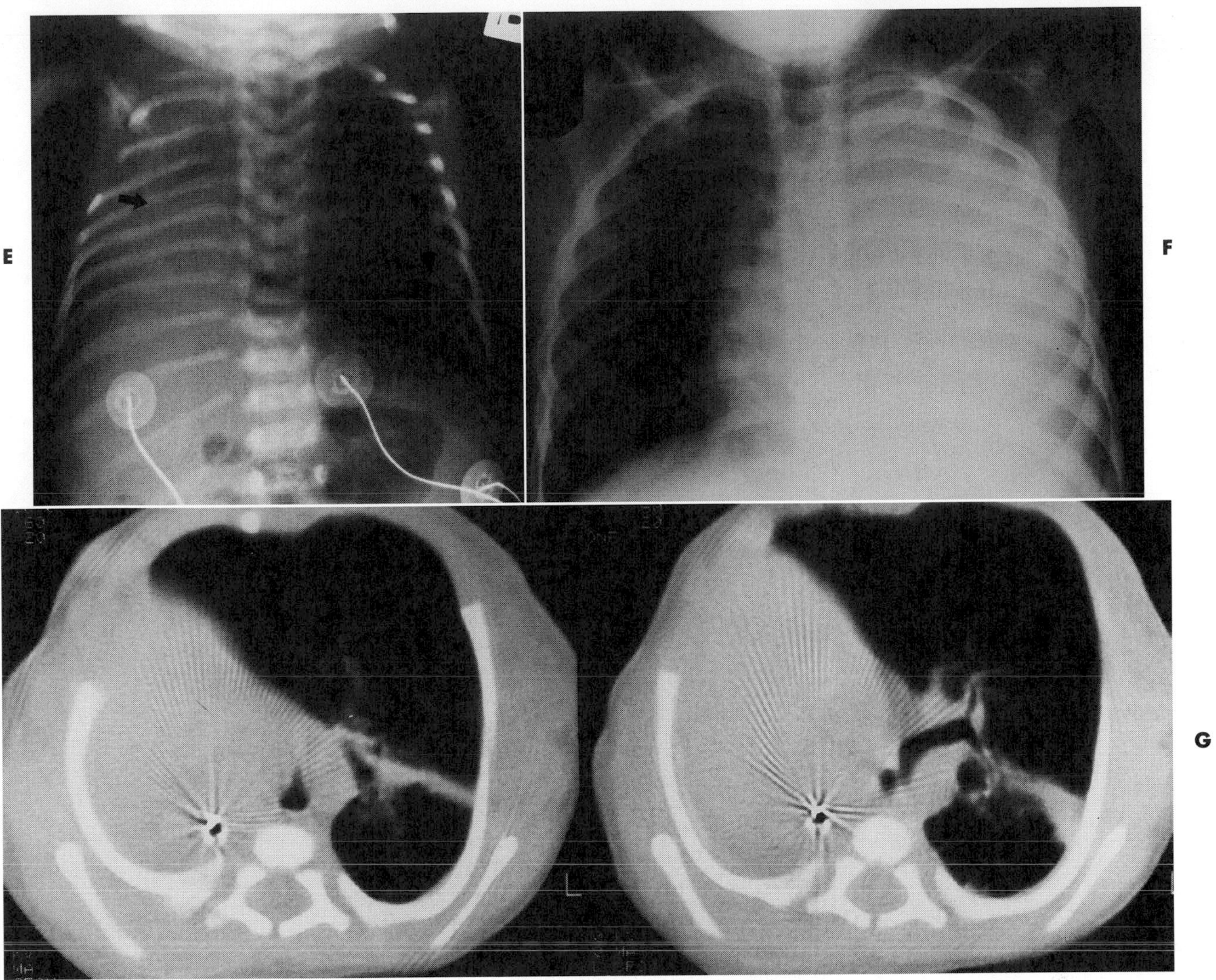

Fig. 13-33, cont'd. **E,** This newborn's chest radiograph demonstrates the silhouette sign. There is absence of the right lung, and the heart margins are obliterated. The mediastinum is shifted to the right, and there is a faint lucency in the medial portion of the right thorax *(arrow).* The change in density is crucial in understanding the lesion. The carina is not clearly demonstrated. **F,** Single frontal radiograph in a very ill 1-year-old child. The left heart border and diaphragm are obliterated (silhouette sign), but the mediastinum is not shifted (see normal right heart margin). This child had a large empyema. It could not be atelectasis because the mediastinum is not shifted into the opaque hemithorax. **G,** CT scan of the same child as in **E** shows that the nasogastric tube is displaced posteriorly and to the right. The herniation of the left lung across the midline accounts for the lucency on the plain film **(E).** There is no right mainstem bronchus, and only the left mainstem bronchus is demonstrated. The diagnosis is right pulmonary atresia.

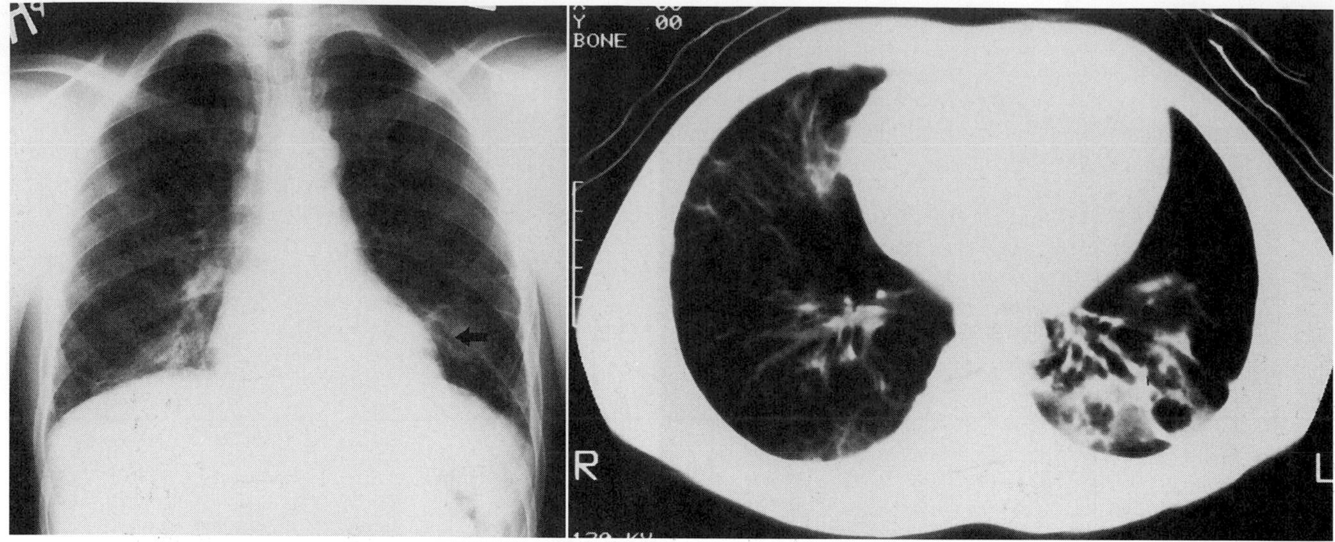

Fig. 13-34. Air bronchogram. A 12-year-old child with an immune deficiency and recurrent infections. Lymphoid interstitial pneumonitis had been histologically demonstrated. **A,** On the frontal chest film, a density is seen bilaterally, but there is an especially prominent bronchogram *(arrow)* in the left lower lobe. **B,** CT scan reveals bronchiectasis in the left lower lobe with less bronchiectasis in the right lower lobe.

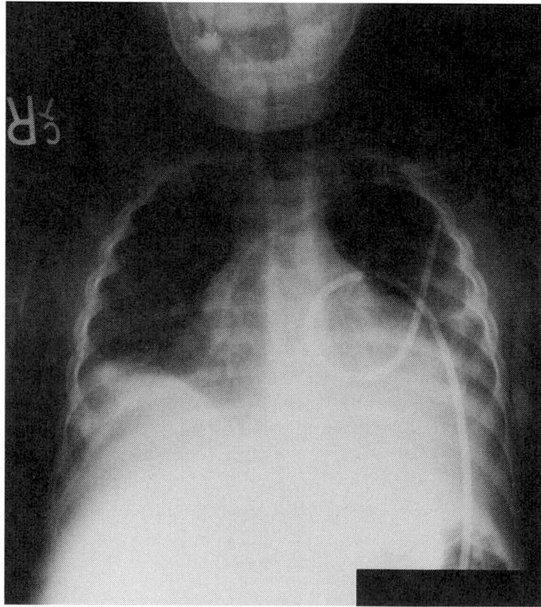

Fig. 13-35. Subpulmonic effusion. The lateral aspect of the right hemidiaphragm is higher and laterally displaced compared with the normal shape. Infiltrate in the left lower lung obscures the left hemidiaphragm.

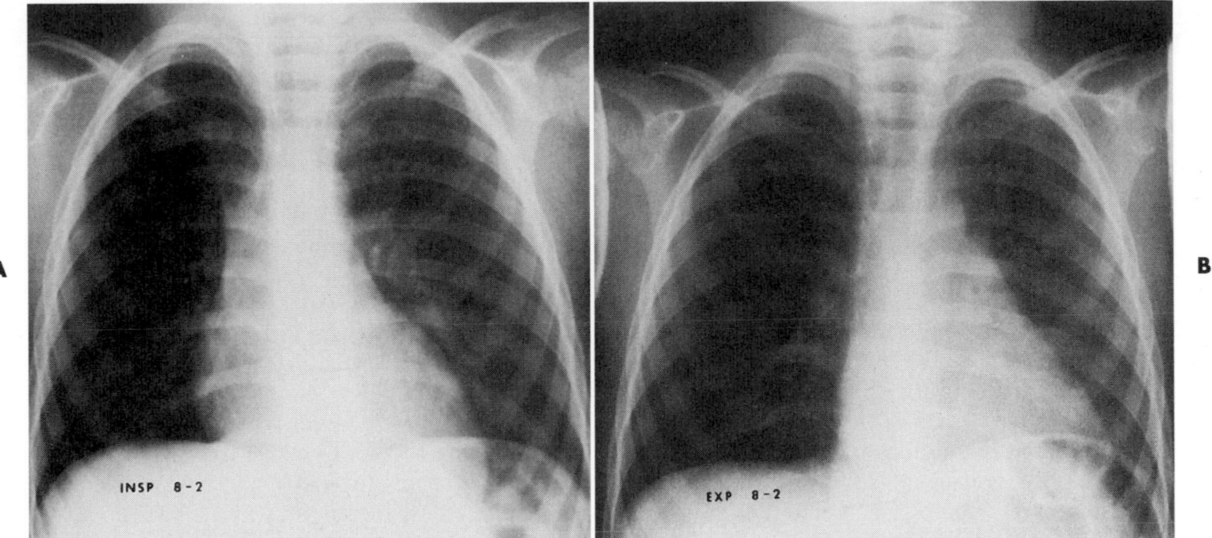

Fig. 13-36. Increased lucency in the lungs: bronchial foreign body. Inspiratory **(A)** and expiratory **(B)** films of a 2-year-old child shows that the right lung is blacker than the left and that the vessels are more difficult to see. In **A,** the mediastinum is well centered, but in **B,** the mediastinum shifts to the left. In addition, the left hemidiaphragm in **B** is higher than the right hemidiaphragm. Shifting of the mediastinum and elevation of the hemidiaphragm are signs of unequal aeration. The finding of air moving into but not leaving the right lung confirms the diagnosis. Air moves well into and out of the left lung. The foreign body in the right mainstem bronchus proved to be food.

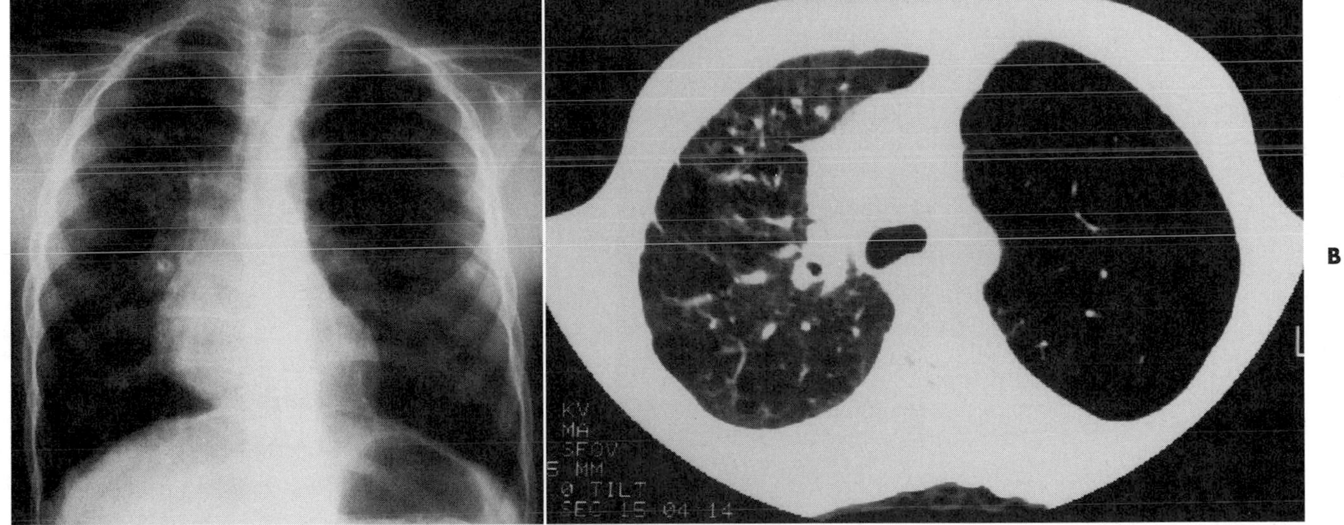

Fig. 13-37. Increased aeration. A 10-year-old girl had been born prematurely and was on a ventilator for 4 months. She developed bronchopulmonary dysplasia and persistent asthma. **A,** The plain film reveals increased blackness or lucency in the left upper lobe with a shift of the mediastinum to the right. There are also areas of opacification throughout both lungs. **B,** CT with lung windows done at the level of the carina shows the hyperexpanded left upper lobe. No bronchial obstruction was demonstrated.

IMAGING FOR COMMON PEDIATRIC RESPIRATORY PROBLEMS

In institutions where one modality or methodology is more sophisticated than another, the imaging algorithms described here should be altered. The most important requirement is an educated, experienced interpretation of whatever modality is used.

Neonate

The most important examination in the neonate is an initial two-view plain film series. The imager must rule out nonmedically treatable causes of respiratory distress; therefore the ABC approach is crucial (see Box 13-6). Subsequent chest examinations depend on the initial diagnosis, but if a medical cause of the respiratory distress is noted (e.g., hyaline membrane disease, transient tachypnea, meconium aspiration), a single view chest is usually all that is needed.[78-80]

Except when low-osmolarity contrast or barium is used for an esophagram (e.g., esophageal atresia, fistulas, vascular rings), the only other imaging tests that are indicated would be rarely a contrast bronchogram for peripheral anomalies and HRCT for the definition of congenital anomalies or extent of parenchymal disease.[81]

Child with Suspected Pulmonary Infection

In the young child (1 month to 3 years of age) with an acute fever of unknown origin, a chest film is all that is necessary (see Fig. 13-21). There is some evidence that the yield is extremely low unless there are clinical signs and symptoms of tachypnea, auscultatory findings, or more serious changes.[82-85]

In a child with chronic, recurrent, or complicated infection, the plain film again is the starting point. However, the search for an etiology also includes an esophagram for H-type fistula (Fig. 13-38), a nuclear study for gastrointestinal reflux (see Fig. 13-1), and perhaps HRCT for definition of the extent of parenchymal or bronchial disease (Figs. 13-34, 13-38, and 13-39). In systemic disorders with pulmonary infection or infiltration, HRCT reveals exceedingly useful information (extent of air trapping, cysts, parenchymal destruction, adenopathy, abscess, and calcifications)[86-88] (Box 13-7). Fig. 13-40 shows two cases in which HRCT provides for precise diagnosis and interventional drainage.

In a child with suspected complication of infection, such as empyema, abscess, or bronchiectasis, CT is the best test. Similarly, in the opaque hemithorax, CT and HRCT can differentiate among chest wall, pleural, and parenchymal disease[10,89,90] (Fig. 13-41).

Wheezing Child

Not every child who wheezes has asthma or medical pulmonary disease. The clinician and imager should be alert to hints on plain film that suggest mechanical causes for wheezing.

Any lesion around or within the airway can cause wheezing. The most frequent that the authors have observed is a lesion caused by a bronchial foreign body (Fig. 13-42), but bronchogenic cysts, bronchial adenomas, pulmonary rings and slings, and mediastinal masses have all been seen (see Figs. 13-4, 13-16, 13-17, and 13-36). It is important to look for signs of an obstructed airway in any child who has differential air trapping on chest x-ray films (Box 13-8 and Fig. 13-36).

Known asthmatics do not need a chest film with every "routine" episode. Rather, history taking, physical examination, and an appropriate, prompt therapy should be performed, and radiographs are obtained only if there are unusual findings or if the condition does not respond. Clearly, the indication for a chest film in a known asthmatic is the presence of suspected complications (e.g., pneumomediastinum, pneumothorax, complete lobar collapse) (see Fig. 13-25).

Search for Metastatic Pulmonary Disease in a Child with a Known Tumor

The most common tumors that metastasize to the lung are listed in Box 13-9. If the chest film is positive for metastatic disease, it seems logical to stop the workup at this point. When the chest film is negative, however, CT is indicated (Fig. 13-43). For detection of metastatic disease, CT with contiguous slices of intermediate thickness is probably the best.[10] In general, this can be accomplished with HRCT. The appearance on CT, however, is not specific, and granulomas may be difficult to differentiate from viable tumor.[91] In these instances, a biopsy can be performed with CT guidance.[92]

Mediastinal and Parenchymal Masses

Mediastinal masses are usually found on plain film examinations obtained for an unrelated reason. Further imaging, primarily CT and MR imaging, is then performed to determine the location, nature, and extent of the mass as well as to search for metastatic spread.[93] So that this procedure is simplified and the list of diagnostic possibilities is shortened, a compartmental approach is often used wherein the mediastinum is arbitrarily divided into anterior, middle, and posterior compartments[94] (Fig. 13-44). The mass is then placed into one compartment by determining its effect on the normal mediastinal structures and its spread (see Figs 13-5, 13-16, 13-22, 13-23, and 13-32).

The most common anterior mediastinal mass in the pediatric population is by far the normal thymus. In cases of confusion, this structure is well defined by both CT and MR.[94-97] In some cases, a normal thymus can also be characterized with US[98,99] (see Fig. 13-2).

When a mass is visualized in the anterior mediastinum, the two prime considerations are lymphoma, which is the most common, and germ cell tumors, which are distinguished by the presence of calcification and cystic changes. Lymph node masses, again primarily lymphoma and foregut duplication cysts, account for the majority of middle mediastinal masses (see Fig. 13-32). About 95% of masses in the posterior mediastinum are neurogenic in origin. Although CT is more sensitive in detecting calcification, which is common in these lesions, MR imaging is superior for detecting the extent of chest wall invasion and intraspinal extension and should be the primary test after the plain film.[74,94]

True parenchymal lung masses (i.e., excluding round pneumonia) are uncommon in infants and children.[100,101] Like mediastinal lesions, these masses also are often found incidentally. Granulomatous nodules and masses of congenital origin, such as bronchogenic cysts, sequestrations, and cystic adenomatoid malformations, are some of the more frequent lung masses in children (see Fig. 13-33).

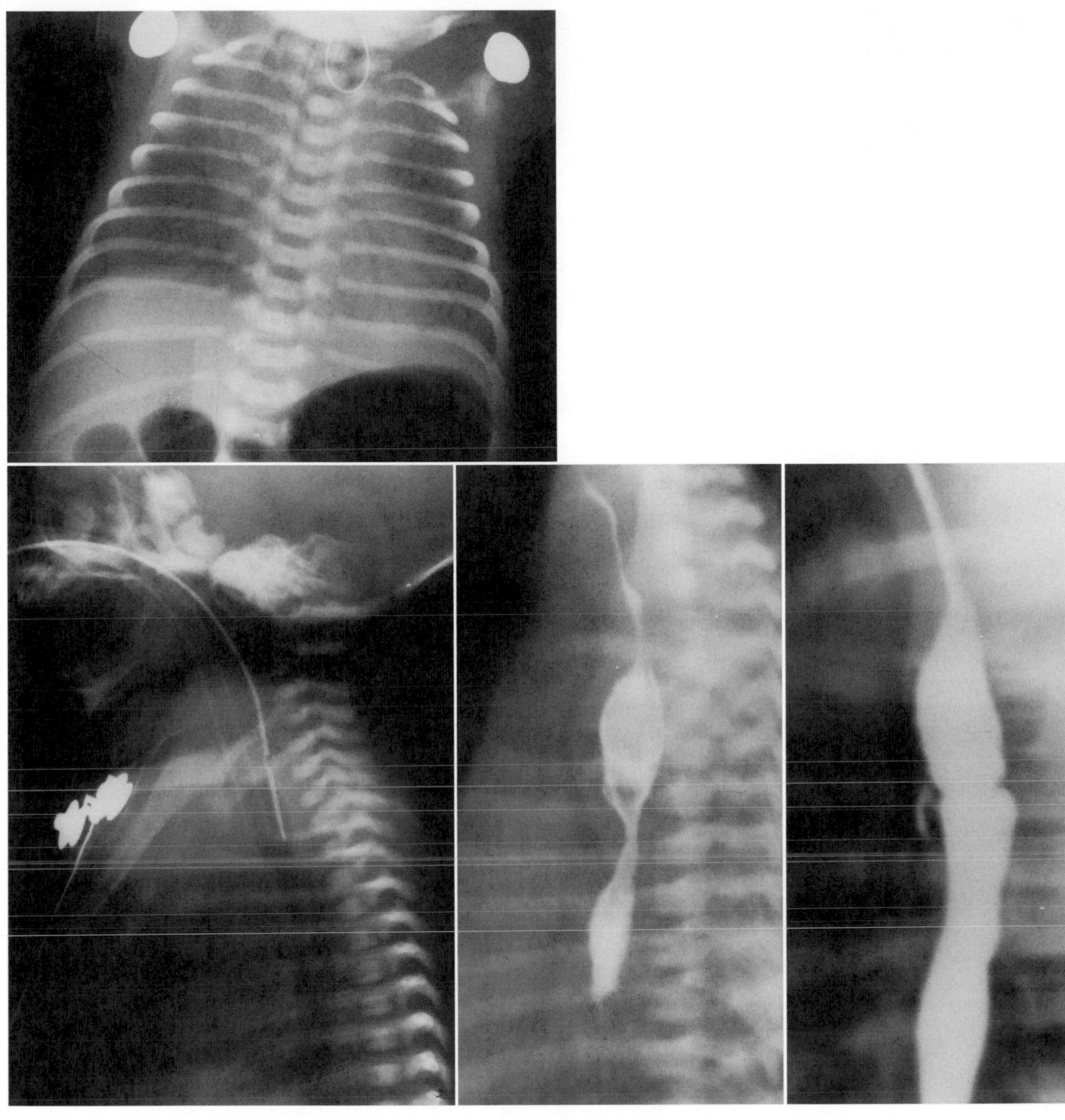

Fig. 13-38. Esophageal atresia with a recurrent fistula. **A,** Film shows the nasogastric tube coiled in the esophageal pouch of a newborn with esophageal atresia. There are air bronchograms and densities in both lungs consistent with aspiration. When the ABCs approach is used, there is clearly gas within the bowel, showing that a distal fistulous tract must be present. **B,** Lateral film demonstrating the level of the atresia by the inferior extent of the nasogastric tube. **C,** Lateral film of a postoperative esophagram shows the continual anterior bowing of the airway by a dilated proximal esophagus. Note the narrowing of the esophagus at the level of the anastomosis. Frequently, this has to be dilated. This film also helps explain why, since the pouch is dilated in utero, there is frequently abnormalities of the airway with secondary tracheomalacia. **D,** Lateral film of esophagram acquired 1 year later shows a recurrent fistula near the site of the anastomosis. The fistula fills with contrast progressing anteriorly. No contrast is seen in the airway at this time.

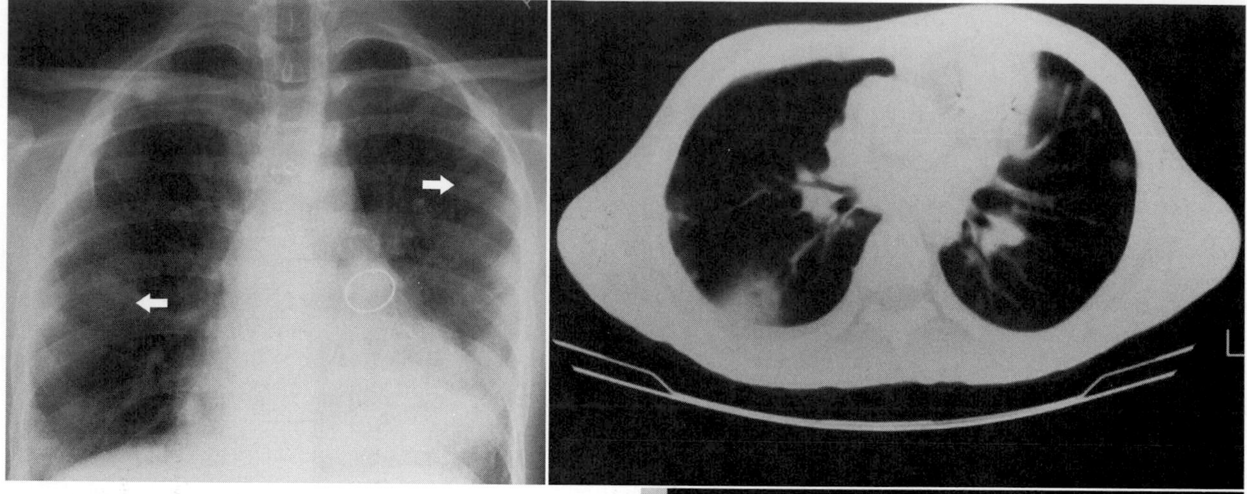

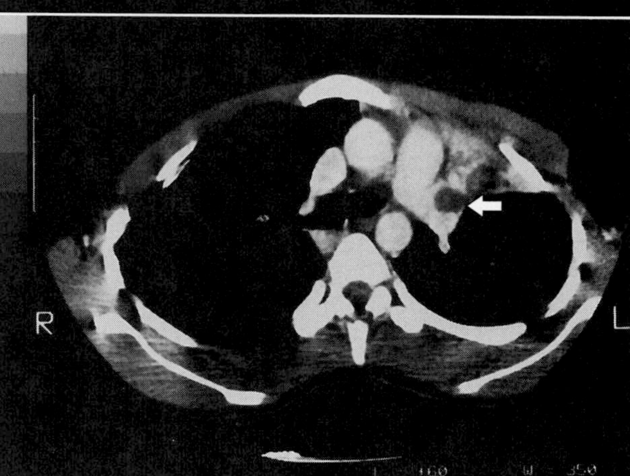

Fig. 13-39. Use of HRCT in complicated diseases. **A,** Frontal film of a teenager who has had a Rastelli operation reveals multiple nodules throughout the lungs *(arrows)*. **B,** HRCT reveals the multiple nodules primarily in the periphery of the lungs. In most instances, a vessel leads to each nodule, suggesting the diagnosis of septic pulmonary emboli. The child had dental work without prophylactic antibiotics, and his graft had become infected. **C,** Contrast-enhanced CT scan with mediastinal windows in a 14-year-old girl with ataxia telangiectasia demonstrates the reason for a persistent collapse of the left upper lobe: a bronchial adenoma *(arrow)*.

BOX 13-7
Situations in Which HRCT Provides New or Important Information*

Airspace diseases
Complicated infection
Empyema
Immune-compromised host
Tuberculosis
Pulmonary hemorrhage
Pulmonary edema
Interstitial disease
Bronchopulmonary dysplasia
Histiocytosis
Sarcoid disease
Airway
Bronchiectasis
Cystic fibrosis
Bronchiolitis obliterans
Bronchial obstruction as suggested by prolonged consolidation
Guide to biopsy or drainage
Chest film abnormality inconsistent with clinical severity of disease

*Modified from Kuhn JP: *Radiol Clin North Am* 31:533-581, 1993

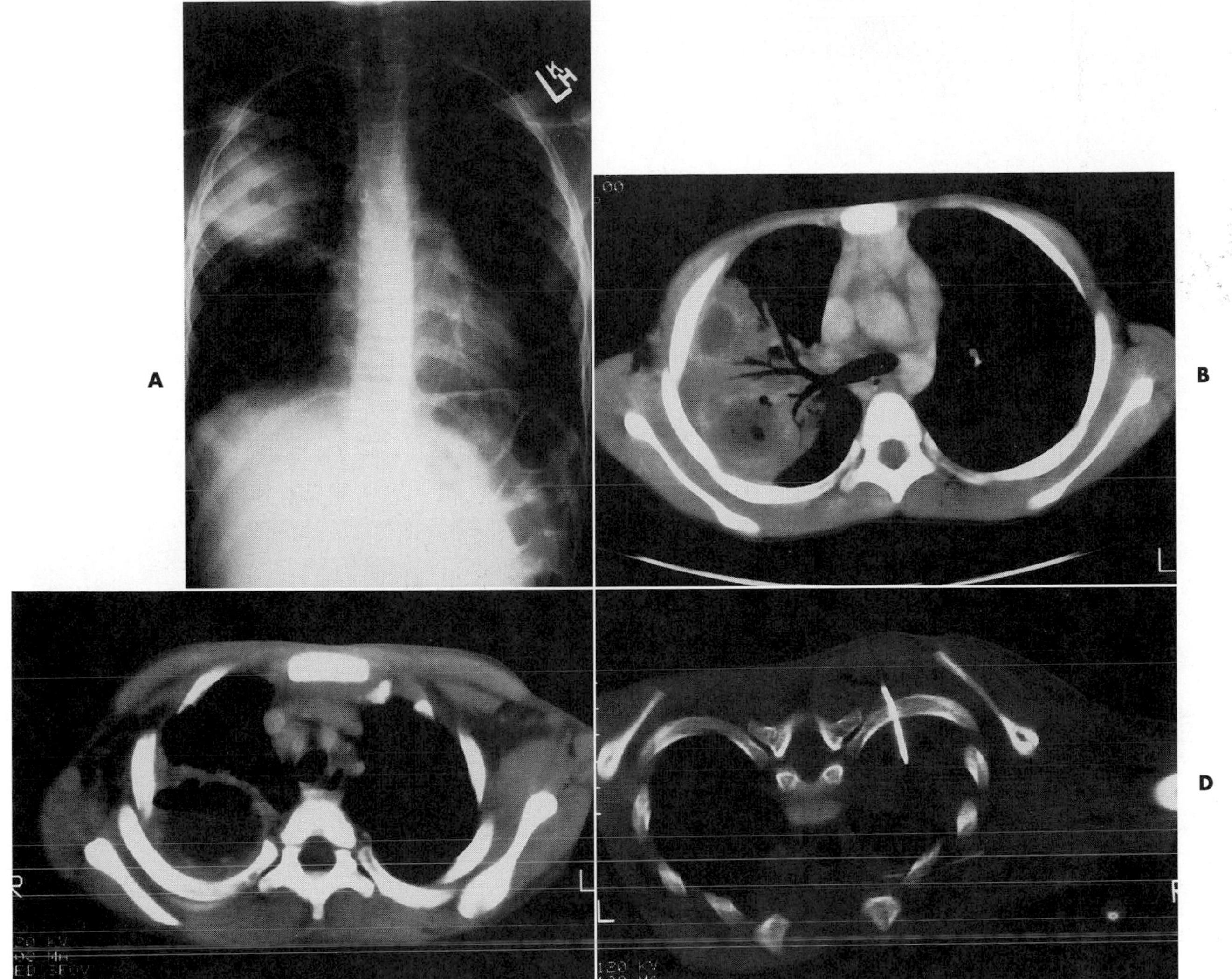

Fig. 13-40. Interventional drainage with CT guidance. **A,** Teenager with acute respiratory symptoms and a density in the right upper lobe. Because the patient was more ill than expected, CT was done. **B,** An enhanced CT study reveals air bronchograms entering the consolidation. With enhancement abscesses are also demonstrated by their low density and enhancing walls. **C** and **D,** Another child with a pulmonary lesion on the right upper lobe, this time with an air-fluid level **(C).** The air-fluid level was localized with CT, and a needle was placed within the abscess for drainage **(D).** Note that **D** is done with the patient in the prone position.

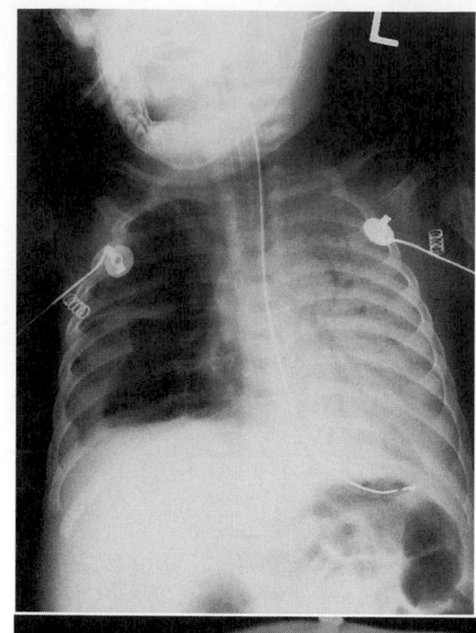

Fig. 13-41. Use of HRCT in complicated infection: pneumonococcal necrotizing pneumonia and empyema. **A,** Frontal radiograph showing diffuse air bronchograms and opacification of the left hemithorax. A pleural reaction is visible on the right. **B**, HRCT reveals multiple areas of bronchiectasis on the left. The thickened pleura on the right is seen without enhancement. **C,** Enhancement reveals the split pleural sign (i.e., separation and enhancement of the visceral and parietal pleura). The split pleural sign is diagnostic of an empyema.

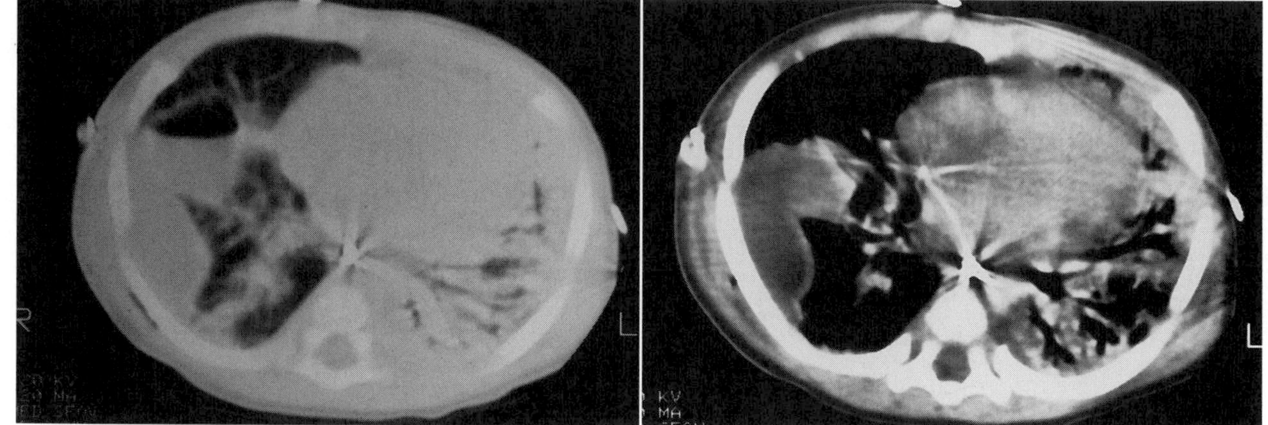

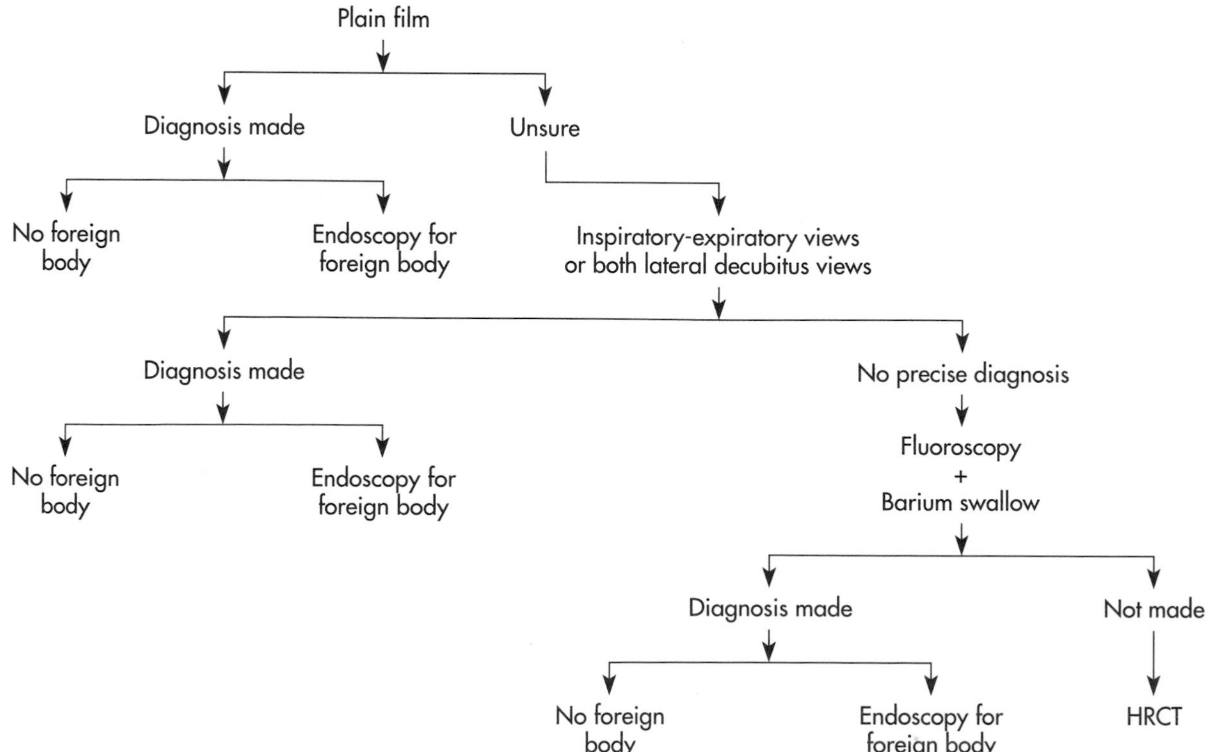

Fig. 13-42. History of possible foreign body ingestion.

BOX 13-8
Imaging Signs of an Obstructed Bronchial Airway

Differential density of the lungs
Defect in airway
Failure of air entry or exit on inspiration or expiration or on decubitus or fluoroscopic examination
Mediastinal shift on inspiration or expiration
Hilar and diaphragmatic asymmetry

BOX 13-9
Most Common Tumors that Metastasize to the Lungs

Wilms' tumor
Osteogenic sarcoma
Hepatoblastoma: hepatocellular carcinoma
Rhabdomyosarcoma
Ewing's sarcoma

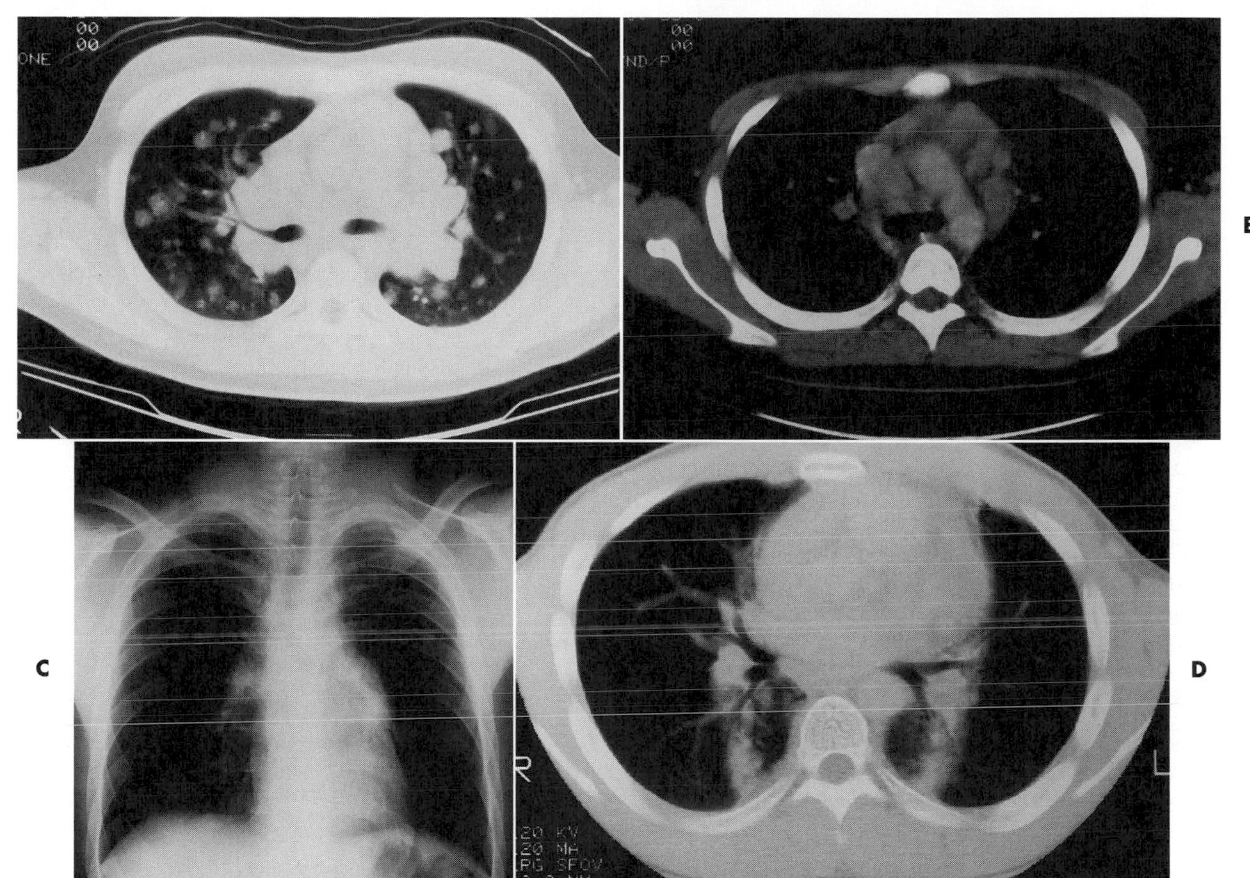

Fig. 13-43. Complication of neoplastic disease and therapy. **A** and **B,** Teenager with Hodgkin's disease. Multiple pulmonary nodules as shown by HRCT (**A**). Reconstruction to standard mediastinal windows (**B**) demonstrates mediastinal adenopathy. **C** and **D,** Frontal radiograph and CT in a 16-year-old teenager after mediastinal radiation for Hodgkin's disease. There is a density in the perihilar regions (**C**). There is radiation pneumonitis in the port of radiotherapy (**D**).

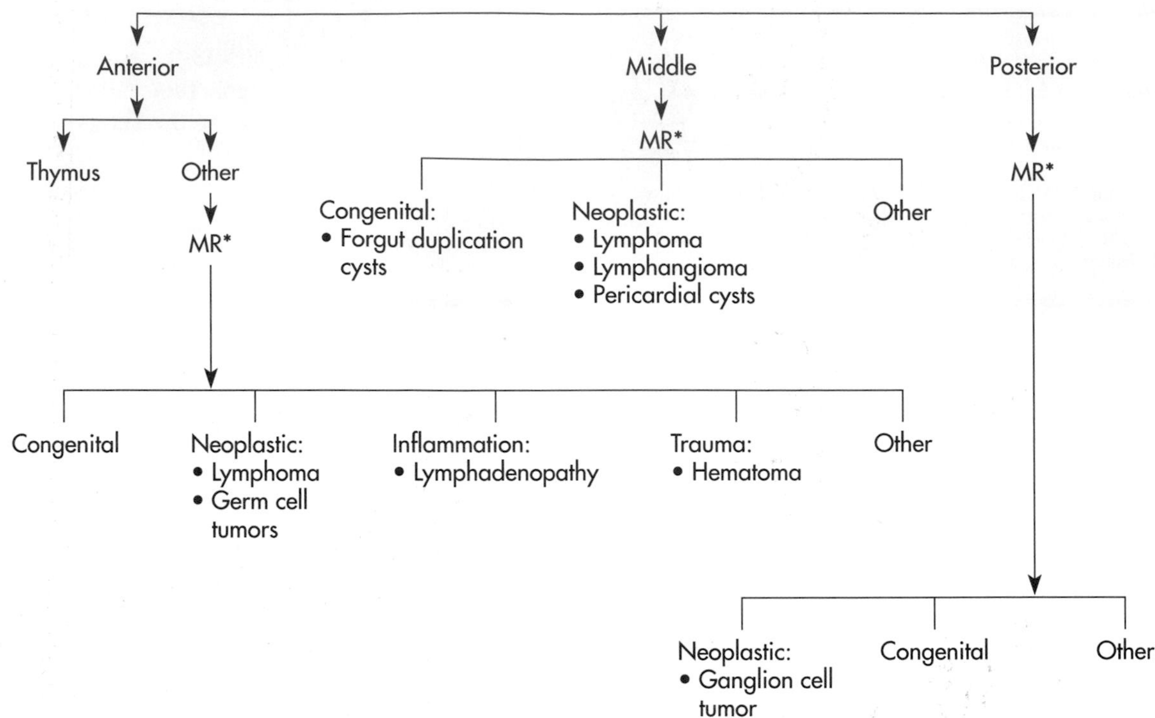

Fig. 13-44. Mediastinal masses: plain film and esophagram. Asterisks indicate that CT can be done if necessary.

REFERENCES

1. Geddes DM: The Kerley Pergamon lecture: the role of the radiologist—a chest physician's view, *Clin Radiol* 46:160-165, 1992.

Physical Principles of Imaging Modalities

2. Tarver RD, Cohen M, Broderick NJ, Conces DJ Jr: Pediatric digital chest imaging, *J Thorac Imaging* 5:31-35, 1990.
3. Bernard J, Sauvegrain J, Nahum H: Tomography of the lungs in infancy and childhood: techniques, indications and results, *Prog Pediatr Radiol* 1:59-90, 1967.
4. MacPherson RI, Hill JG, Bremann Othersen H, Tagge EP, Smith CD: Esophageal foreign bodies in children: diagnosis, treatment and complications, *AJR Am J Roentgenol* 166:919-924, 1996.
5. Papanicolaou N, Treves S: Pulmonary scintigraphy in pediatrics, *Semin Nucl Med* 10:259-285, 1980.
6. Heyman S, Kirkpatrick JA, Winter HS, Treves S: An improved radionuclide method for the diagnosis of gastroesophageal reflux and aspiration in children (milk scan), *Radiology* 131:479-482, 1979.
7. Larar GN, O'Tuama LA, Treves S: Nuclear medicine in the pediatric chest, *Radiol Clin North Am* 31:481-490, 1993.
8. May DA, Barth RA, Yeager S, Nussbaum-Blask A, Bulas DI: Perinatal and postnatal chest sonography, *Radiol Clin North Am* 31:499-516, 1993.
9. Ben-Ami TE, O'Donovan JC, Yousefzadeh DK: Sonography of the chest in children, *Radiol Clin North Am* 31:517-532, 1993.
10. Kuhn JP: High-resolution computed tomography of pediatric pulmonary parenchymal disorders, *Radiol Clin North Am* 31:533-552, 1993.
11. Lynch DA, Brasch RC, Hardy KA, Webb WR: Pediatric pulmonary disease: assessment with high-resolution ultrafast CT, *Radiology* 176:243-248, 1990.
12. Mayo JR, Jackson SA, Muller NL: High-resolution CT of the chest: radiation dose, *AJR Am J Roentgenol* 160:479-481, 1993.
13. Siegal M, Luker GD: Pediatric applications of helical (spiral) CT, *Radiol Clin North Am* 33(5):997-1022, 1995.
14. Committee on Drugs, American Academy of Pediatrics: Guidelines for monitoring and management of pediatric patients during and after sedation for diagnostic and therapeutic procedures, *Pediatrics* 89:1110-1115, 1992.
15. Frush DP, Bisset III GS: Sedation of children in radiology: time to wake up, *AJR Am J Roentgenol* 65:913-914, 1995.
16. Vade V, Sukhani R, Dolenga M, Habisohn-Schuck C: Chloral hydrate sedation of children undergoing CT & MR imaging: safety as judged by American Academy of Pediatric guidelines, *AJR Am J Roentgenol* 165:905-909, 1995.
17. Brasch RC: Ultrafast computed tomography for infants and children, *Radiol Clin North Am* 26:277-286, 1988.
18. Falaschi F, Battola L, Mascalchi M, Cioni R, Zampa V, Lencioni R, Antonelli A, Bartolozzi C: Usefulness of MR signal intensity in distinguishing benign from malignant pleural disease, *AJR Am J Roentgenol* 166:963-968, 1996.
19. Kaye RD, Grifka RG, Towbin R: Intervention in the thorax in children, *Radiol Clin North Am* 31:693-712, 1993.

Anatomic Evaluation of the Respiratory Tract

20. Asperstrand F: Radiological examination of the nasal cavity, *Radiology* 29:187-190, 1989.
21. Chinwuba C, Wallman J, Strand R: Nasal airway obstruction: CT assessment, *Radiology* 159:503-506, 1986.
22. Slovis TL, Renfro B, Watts FB, Kuhns LR, Belenky W, Spoylar J: Choanal atresia: precise CT evaluation, *Radiology* 155:345-348, 1985.
23. Barkovich AJ, Vandermarck P, Edwards MSB, Cogen PH: Congenital nasal masses: CT and MR imaging features in 16 cases, *Am J Roentgenol* 12:105-116, 1991.
24. Dillon WP, Som PM, Rosenau W: Hemangioma of the nasal vault: MR and CT features, *Radiology* 180:761-765, 1991.
25. Lloyd GAS, Lund VJ, Phelps PD, Howard DJ: Magnetic resonance imaging in the evaluation of the nose and paranasal sinus disease, *Br J Radiol* 60:957-968, 1987.
26. Brown JH, Deluca SA: Imaging of sinonasal tumors, *Am Fam Physician* 45:1653-1656, 1992.
27. Lloyd GAS: Diagnostic imaging of the nose and paranasal sinuses, *J Laryngol Otol* 103:453-460, 1989.
28. Bluestone CD, Stool SE: *Pediatric otolaryngology,* ed 2, Philadelphia, 1990, WB Saunders, pp 817-819.
29. Daly BD, Russell JL, Davidson MJ, Lamb JT: Thin section computed tomography in the evaluation of naso-ethmoidal trauma, *Clin Radiol* 41:272-275, 1990.

30. Arruda LK, Mimica IM, Sole D, Weckx LL, Schoettler J, Heiner DC, Naspitz CK: Abnormal maxillary sinus radiographs in children: do they represent bacterial infection? *Pediatrics* 85:553-558, 1990.
31. Scuderi AJ, Harnsberger HR, Boyer RS: Pneumatization of the paranasal sinuses: normal features of importance to the accurate interpretation of CT scans and MR images, *Am J Roentgenol* 160:1101-1104, 1993.
32. Samuel E: Plain radiographs and CT scans in the diagnosis of sinus disease, *Am J Roentgenol* 155:425, 1990 (letter).
33. McAlister WH, Lusk R, Muntz HR: Comparison of plain radiographs and coronal CT scans in infants and children with recurrent sinusitis, *Am J Roentgenol* 153:1259-1264, 1989.
34. Andrew WK, Swart JG: Fallibility of sinus radiographs in demonstrating ethmoid sinusitis, *S Afr Med J* 72:158, 1987 (letter).
35. Som PM, Lawson W, Biller HF, Lanzieri CF: Ethmoid sinus disease: CT evaluation in 400 cases. I. Nonsurgical patients, *Radiology* 159: 591-597, 1986.
36. Lusk RP, Lazar RH, Muntz HR: The diagnosis and treatment of recurrent and chronic sinusitis in children, *Pediatr Clin North Am* 36:1411-1421, 1989.
37. Gross GW, McGeady SJ, Kerut T, Ehrlich SM: Limited-slice CT in the evaluation of paranasal sinus disease in children, *Am J Roentgenol* 156:367-369, 1991.
38. Zinreich SJ: Paranasal sinus imaging, *Otolaryngol Head Neck Surg* 103:863-869, 1990.
39. Babbel RW, Harnsberger HR, Sonkens J, Hunt S: Recurring patterns of inflammatory sinonasal disease demonstrated on screening sinus CT, *Am J Roentgenol* 13:903-912, 1992.
40. Calhoun KH, Waggenspack GA, Simpson CB, Hokanson JA, Bailey BJ: CT evaluation of the paranasal sinuses in symptomatic and asymptomatic populations, *Otolaryngol Head Neck Surg* 104:480-483, 1991.
41. Lloyd GAS: CT of the paranasal sinuses: study of a control series in relation to endoscopic sinus surgery, *J Laryngol Otol* 104:477-481, 1990.
42. van der Veken PJV, Clement PAR, Buisseret TH, Desprechins B, Laufman L, Derde MP: CT-scan study of the incidence of sinus involvement and nasal anatomic variations in 196 children, *Rhinology* 28:177-184, 1990.
43. Gutowski WM, Mulbury PE, Hengerer AS, Kido DK: The role of C.T. scans in managing the orbital complications of ethmoiditis, *Int J Pediatr Otorhinolaryngol* 15:117-128, 1988.
44. Andrews TM, Myer CM III: The role of computed tomography in the diagnosis of subperiosteal abscess of the orbit, *Clin Pediatr* 31:37-43, 1992.
45. Reilly JS, Hotaling AJ, Chiponis D, Wald ER: Use of ultrasound in detection of sinus disease in children, *Int J Pediatr Otorhinolaryngol* 17:225-230, 1989.
46. Revonta M, Kuuliala I: The diagnosis and follow-up of pediatric sinusitis: Waters' view radiography versus ultrasonography, *Laryngoscopy* 99:321-324, 1989.
47. Kassel EE: Traumatic injuries of the paranasal sinuses, *Otolaryngol Clin North Am* 21:455-493, 1988.
48. Lund VJ, Howard DJ, Lloyd GA, Cheesman AD: Magnetic resonance imaging of paranasal sinus tumors for craniofacial resection, *Head Neck* 11:279-283, 1989.

Imaging of the Extrapulmonary Airway: Pharynx to the Carina

49. Slovis TL, Haller JO, Berdon WE, Baker DH, Joseph PM: Noninvasive visualization of the pediatric airway, *Curr Probl Diagn Radiol* 8:3-67, 1979.
50. Joseph PM, Berdon WE, Baker DH, Slovis TL, Haller JO: Upper airway obstruction in infants and small children, *Radiology* 121:143-149, 1976.
51. Watts FB Jr, Slovis TL: The enlarged epiglottis, *Pediatr Radiol* 5:133-136, 1977.
52. McHugh K, deSilva M, Kilham HA: Epiglottic enlargement secondary to laryngeal sarcoidosis, *Pediatr Radiol* 23:71, 1993.
53. Carpenter BLM, Merten DF: Radiographic manifestations of congenital anomalies affecting the airway, *Radiol Clin North Am* 29:219-240, 1991.
54. Strife JL: Upper airway and tracheal obstruction in infants and children, *Radiol Clin North Am* 26:309-322, 1988.
55. Slovis TL: Noninvasive evaluation of the pediatric airway: a recent advance, *Pediatrics* 59:872-880, 1977.
56. Svedstrom E, Puhakka H, Kero P: How accurate is chest radiography in the diagnosis of tracheobronchial foreign bodies in children? *Pediatr Radiol* 19:520-522, 1989.
57. Shackelford GD: The pediatric airway: radiology and new imaging, *Int Anesthesiol Clin* 26:3-5, 1988.
58. Ben-Ami T, Rozenman J, Yahav J, Sagy M, Barzilay Z: Computed tomography in children with esophageal and airway trauma, *J Pediatr Surg* 23:919-923, 1988.
59. Brasch RC, Gould RG, Gooding CA, Ringertz HG, Lipton MJ: Upper airway obstruction in infants and children: evaluation with ultrafast CT, *Radiology* 165:459-466, 1987.
60. Kao SC, Smith WL, Sato Y, Franken EA Jr, Kimura K, Soper RT: Ultrafast CT of laryngeal and tracheobronchial obstruction in symptomatic postoperative infants with esophageal atresia and tracheoesophageal fistula, *Am J Roentgenol* 154:345-350, 1990.
61. Griscom NT, Wohl MEB: Dimensions of the growing trachea related to age and gender, *Am J Roentgenol* 146:233-237, 1986.
62. Griscom NT: Computed tomographic determination of tracheal dimensions in children and adolescents, *Radiology* 145:361-364, 1982.
63. Auringer ST, Bisset GS III, Myer CM III: Magnetic resonance imaging of the pediatric airway compared with findings at surgery and/or endoscopy, *Pediatr Radiol* 21:329-332, 1991.
64. Donnelly LF, Bissett GS III, McDermott B: Case report: anomalous midline location of the descending aorta—a cause of compression of the carina and left mainstem bronchus in infants, *Am J Roentgenol* 164(3):705-707, 1995.
65. Berdon WE: Tracheal anomalies, vascular compression and respiratory distress: the soft and hard and long and short of it, *Pediatr Radiol* 25:S197-S198, 1995 (editorial).

Chest

66. Griscom NT: Pneumonia in children and some of its variants, *Radiology* 167:297-302, 1988.
67. Edwards DK, Higgins CB, Gilpin EA: The cardiothoracic ratio in newborn infants, *Am J Roentgenol* 136:907-913, 1981.
68. Haller JO, Slovis TL: *Pediatric radiology,* ed 2, Heidelberg, Germany, 1995, Springer-Verlag, pp 7-52.
69. Kirks DR: *Diagnostic radiology of infants and children,* ed 2, Boston, 1992, Little, Brown, pp 516-518.
70. Fletcher BD: Diagnostic radiology of the respiratory tract. In Kendig EL, Chornich V, eds: *Disorders of the respiratory tract in children,* ed 5, Philadelphia, 1990,WB Saunders, pp 102-103.
71. Burko H: Considerations in the Roentgen diagnosis of pneumonia in children, *Am J Roentgenol* 88:555-565, 1962.
72. Stone RM, Van Metter R, Senol E, Pilgrim TK: Effect of exposure variation on the clinical utility of chest radiography, *Radiology* 199:497-504, 1996.
73. Griscom NT, Wohl MEB, Kirkpatrick JA Jr: Lower respiratory infections: how infants differ from adults, *Radiol Clin North Am* 16:367-387, 1978.
74. Slovis TL, Meza M, Kuhn JP: Aberrant thymus: MR assessment, *Pediatr Radiol* 22:490-492, 1993.
75. Mulvey RB: The thymic "wave" sign, *Radiology* 81:834-838, 1963.
76. Berdon WE, Baker DH, James LS: The ductus bump: a transient physiologic mass in chest roentgenograms of newborn infants, *Am J Roentgenol* 95:91-98, 1965.
77. Kleinman PK, Marks SC, Spevak MR, Richmond JM: Fractures of the rib head in abused infants, *Radiology* 185:119-123, 1992.

Imaging for Common Pediatric Respiratory Problems

78. Wood BP, Davitt MA, Metlay LA: Lung disease in the very immature neonate: radiographic and microscopic correlation, *Pediatr Radiol* 20:33-40, 1989.
79. Yuksel B, Greenough A, Karani J, Page A: Chest radiograph scoring system for use in pre-term infants, *Br J Radiol* 64:1015-1018, 1991.
80. Arroe M: The risk of x-ray examinations of the lungs in neonates, *Acta Paediatr Scand* 80:489-493, 1991.
81. Nakano Y, Odagiri K: Use of computed radiography in respiratory distress syndrome in the neonatal nursery, *Pediatr Radiol* 19:167-168, 1989.

82. Crain EF, Bulas D, Bijur PE, Goldman HS: Is a chest radiograph necessary in the evaluation of every febrile infant less than 8 weeks of age? *Pediatrics* 88:821-824, 1991.
83. Patterson RJ, Bissett GS III, Kirks DR, Vanness A: Chest radiographs in the evaluation of the febrile infant, *Am J Roentgenol* 155:833-835, 1990.
84. Kramer MS, Roberts-Brauer R, Williams RL: Bias and 'overcall' in interpreting chest radiographs in young febrile children, *Pediatrics* 90:11-13, 1991.
85. Katz JA, Bash R, Rollins N, Cash Y, Buchanan GR: The yield of routine chest radiography in children with cancer hospitalized for fever and neutropenia, *Cancer* 68:940-943, 1991.
86. Stiglbauer R, Schurawitzki H, Eichler I, Gotz M: High resolution CT in children with cystic fibrosis, *Acta Radiol* 33:548-553, 1992.
87. Amorosa JK, Miller RW, Laraya-Cuasay L, Gaur S, Marone R, Frenkel L, Nosher JL: Bronchiectasis in children with lymphocytic interstitial pneumonia and acquired immune deficiency syndrome, *Pediatr Radiol* 22:603-607, 1992.
88. Bhalla M, Turcios N, Aponte V, Jenkins M, Leitman BS, McCauley DI, Naidich DP: Cystic fibrosis: scoring system with thin-section CT, *Radiology* 179:783-788, 1991.
89. Muller NL: Imaging of the pleura, *Radiology* 186:297-309, 1993.
90. Kuhn JP: Pediatric thorax. In Naidich DP, Zerhouni EA, Siegelman SS, eds: *Computed tomography and magnetic resonance of the thorax,* ed 2, New York, 1991, Raven, pp 503-555.
91. Keiko H, Hajume N, Touru N: CT of pulmonary metastases with pathological correlation, *Semin Ultrasound CT MRI* 16(5):379-394, 1995.
92. Kazerooni EA, Lem FT, Akra M, Martinez FJ: Risk of pneumothorax in CT-guided transthoracic needle aspiration biopsy of the lung, *Radiology* 198:371-375, 1996.
93. Mooney DP, Sargent SK, Pluta D, Mazurek P: Spiral CT: use in the evaluation of chest masses in the critically ill neonate, *Pediatr Radiol* 26:15-18, 1996.
94. Meza MP, Benson M, Slovis TL: Imaging of mediastinal masses in children, *Radiol Clin North Am* 31:583-604, 1993.
95. deGreer G, Webb WR, Gamsu G: Normal thymus: assessment with MR and CT, *Radiology* 158:313-317, 1986.
96. St Amour TE, Siegel MJ, Glazer HS, Nadel SN: CT appearance of the normal and abnormal thymus in childhood, *J Comput Assist Tomogr* 11:645-650, 1987.
97. Swischuck LE, John SD: Case report: normal thymus extending between the right brachiocephalic vein and innominate artery, *Am J Roentgenol* 166(6):1462-1464, 1996.
98. Han BK, Babcock DS, Oestreich AE: Normal thymus in infancy: sonographic characteristics, *Radiology* 170:471-474, 1989.
99. Carty H: Ultrasound of the normal thymus in the infant: a simple method of resolving a clinical dilemma, *Br J Radiol* 63:737-738, 1990.
100. Eggli KD, Newman B: Nodules, masses, and pseudomasses in the pediatric lung, *Radiol Clin North Am* 31:651-666, 1993.
101. Brown G, Shaw DG: Inflammatory pseudotumors in children: CT and ultrasound appearances with histopathological correlation, *Clin Radiol* 50:782-786, 1995.

Suggested Readings

Felman AH: *The pediatric chest: radiological, clinical and pathological observations,* Springfield, Ill, 1983, Charles C Thomas.
Fraser RG, Par JAP, Par PD, Fraser RS, Genereux GP: *Diagnosis of diseases of the chest,* ed 3, Philadelphia, 1988, WB Saunders.
Kirks DR, ed: *Practical pediatric imaging: diagnostic radiology of infants and children,* ed 2, Boston, 1991, Little, Brown.
Naidich DP, Zerhouni EA, Siegelman SS, eds: *Computed tomography and magnetic resonance of the thorax,* ed 2, New York, 1991, Raven.
Newman B, ed: *Radiol Clin North Am* 31(3): 1993.
Silverman FN, Kuhn JP, eds: *Caffey's pediatric x-ray diagnosis,* St Louis, 1992, Mosby.

CHAPTER 14

Respiratory Function Testing in Infants and Other Noncooperative Subjects

Peter D. Sly, Celia J. Lanteri, Mark John Hayden, and Wayne J. Morgan

LUNG FUNCTION TESTING IN INFANTS

Measurement of lung function in adults and older children has become a routine part of the management of respiratory diseases. Pulmonary function tests provide objective evidence regarding the nature and control of respiratory diseases and the effect of therapy and provide opportunities to study the mechanisms by which diseases alter lung function. These objective assessments have been unavailable to those managing respiratory diseases in infants until relatively recently. Many advances have been made in the last decade, and now the techniques and equipment necessary to measure lung function in infants are readily available.

This chapter is not intended to be sufficiently detailed that the reader can learn to measure lung function in infants from these pages. A more detailed guide to measuring lung function in infants has recently been published.[1] The interested reader is referred to this publication for practical details of the various tests.

Influence of Measurement Conditions on Lung Function

A major requirement for most methods of measuring lung function in infants is to have the infant sleeping. This is necessary to effect reproducible results. However, infants cannot be relied on to sleep naturally on demand or to remain asleep long enough to allow pulmonary function to be measured. Thus the majority of infant lung function tests are performed with the infant sedated, most commonly with chloral hydrate or a similar sedative. Sedating infants for pulmonary function testing is considered safe, with no reported adverse effects despite many thousands of tests having been performed throughout the world.[2] However, a fall in arterial oxygen saturation has been reported in wheezy infants sedated for pulmonary function testing,[3] so continuous monitoring of oxygen saturation is considered mandatory in such infants.

Standardization of measurement conditions must address both laboratory conditions and the infant's state with respect to factors that influence the results of respiratory function tests, such as feeding, posture, and sleep state. For a detailed description of the effects of measurement conditions, the reader is referred to a book that has been recently published by a joint working party of the American Thoracic Society and the European Respiratory Society.[1]

Measurement Techniques

The techniques used to measure pulmonary function in infants can be conveniently grouped into three groups: measures of lung volume, measures of forced expiratory flow, and measures of compliance and resistance.

Measures of Lung Volume

Knowledge of lung volume can play an important role in the respiratory care of infants and young children and can assist in the interpretation of measurements of resistance, compliance, and forced expiratory flow. Two main techniques are used for measuring lung volumes in infants: body plethysmography and gas-dilution techniques.

Body Plethysmography. In body plethysmography the infant is placed inside a rigid, closed container (a plethysmograph) and makes respiratory efforts against an occlusion at the airway opening; the respiratory efforts rarefy and compress the thoracic gas (Fig. 14-1). Calculation of the amount of gas in the thorax during occluded breathing efforts are made by applying Boyle's law. The assumptions underlying this technique are discussed more fully in Chapter 15. There are, however, a number of particular difficulties in applying these assumptions to measurements in infants. The success of the plethysmographic measurement of lung volume relies on the plethysmograph having an adequate frequency response over the range of frequencies used. In an adult plethysmograph, with a volume typically 50 to 100 times that of the adult's intrathoracic volume, the frequency response is poor below 0.2 Hz because of the thermal time constant of the box and the necessary presence of a slow leak to allow for gas expansion resulting from the heat generated by the subject. Adults and older children are asked to make occluded breathing efforts at a frequency of approximately 1 Hz. This is primarily to keep the glottic aperture open, aiding the transmission of alveolar pressure to the airway opening and minimizing the difference in airway resistance (Raw) between inspiration and expiration.[4] However, this technique ensures that the box is being operated at a frequency at which the frequency response is adequate and that gas compression within the box is essentially isothermal.

The infant plethysmograph is considerably smaller than the adult, giving it a greater surface area–to–volume ratio. Thus the mean distance over which heat diffusion must occur between any point inside the plethysmograph and its walls is greatly reduced. This in turn leads to a much reduced thermal time constant,[5] which adversely influences the frequency response of the plethysmograph in the frequency range usually encountered in infants. The thermal time constant of a 60 L plethysmograph, with metal walls, was reported to be 0.16 second.[5] Gas compression within this box was found to be polytropic (i.e., between isothermal and adiabatic) over a frequency range of 0.1 to 3 Hz. Infants, obviously, cannot be requested to breathe at a particular frequency, and the respiratory rate is likely to change during measurements, particularly those that involve giving the infant a bronchodilator or bronchial challenge agent.[5] Changes in the frequency of the occluded breath-

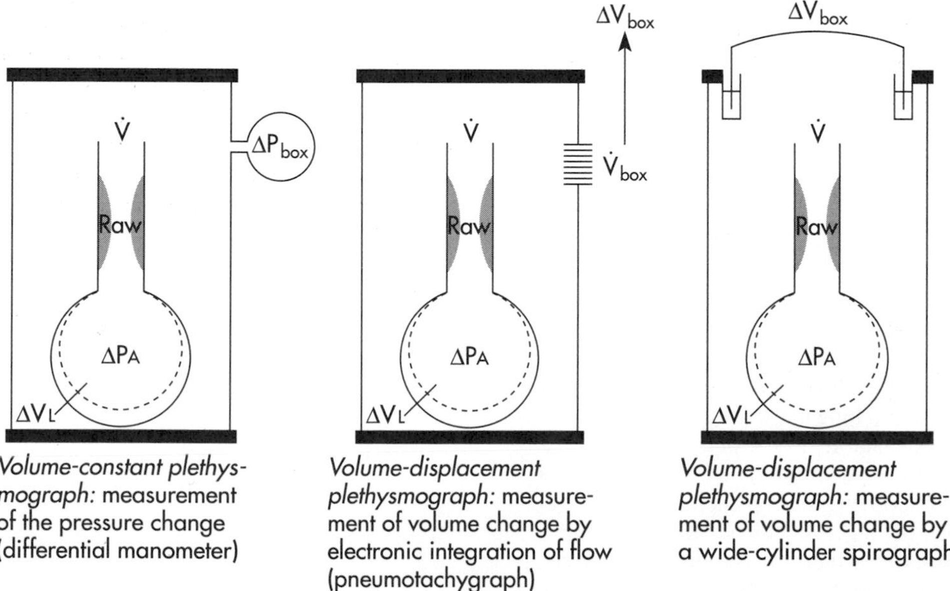

Fig. 14-1. Types of plethysmographs. Dotted lines indicate volume change by compression; solid lines indicate volume change by expansion of thoracic gas (ΔV_L). ΔV_{box}, Change in volume in plethysmograph; ΔP_{box}, change in pressure in plethysmograph; $\dot{V}$, gas flow; *Raw,* airway resistance; ΔP_A, change in alveolar pressure; ΔV_L, change in lung volume. (From Tammeling GJ, Quanjer PH: *Contours of breathing,* Burlington, Ontario, Canada, 1985, Boehringer Ingelheim Pharmaceuticals.)

ing efforts result in changes in the value of thoracic gas volume calculated simply because of the polytropic gas compression.

An alternative to the "constant-volume" plethysmograph is the "flow plethysmograph" in which a pneumotachograph measures gas flow between the plethysmograph and the exterior (see Fig. 14-1, *center*). The flow signal can be integrated to produce the volume change occurring in the box resulting from respiration (i.e., tidal volume). During occluded breathing efforts, this volume should equal the change in volume recorded in a constant-volume plethysmograph (see Chapter 15). In a flow plethysmograph the gas displacement minimizes polytropic gas compression and eliminates thermal effects. If the resistance and inertance of the pneumotach is too high, the flow signal may be damped, introducing errors into the calculations of lung function. These errors can be improved by using a screen pneumotachograph fitted flush with the plethysmograph wall without any connecting tubing or by correcting for the resistance and inertance of the pneumotachograph.[6]

In addition, transmission of the changes in alveolar pressure to the airway opening during occluded breathing efforts occurs with a time constant dependent on the Raw and upper airway compliance. Infants have higher Raw and more compliant upper airways, both of which increase the time required to transmit alveolar pressure changes to the upper airway. This problem is magnified in conditions with increased Raw, such as wheezing illnesses. Under these conditions, the airway opening pressure may markedly underestimate alveolar pressure, resulting in overestimations of thoracic gas volume and thus limiting the accuracy and usefulness of this technique in infants with airway disease.

Gas-Dilution Techniques. The most common application of the gas-dilution technique is the helium-dilution technique. This technique is based on the principle of gas equilibration between an unknown lung volume and a known volume containing helium as an indicator gas. Gas is mixed by ventilatory movements, and the lung volume is calculated from the change in helium concentration. Lung volume can also be measured using the nitrogen-washout technique. With this technique, the infant breathes from a reservoir of nitrogen-free gas, and the washout of nitrogen in the alveolar gas is measured with a rapidly responding nitrogen analyzer. These techniques are discussed in greater detail in Chapter 15.

The major problems with these techniques include the following:

1. Any leak in the circuit results in the final concentration of gas (especially helium) being artificially low, with the consequent overestimation of lung volume. For these tests the infants breathe through a face mask, increasing the possibility of leaks, which may be difficult to detect.
2. Adequate time must be allowed for the helium to be distributed throughout the lung and for the final helium concentration to become stable. In the presence of small airways and in conditions with increased Raw, the time required for equilibration may be considerable. Long equilibration times may be impractical when testing infants.
3. Gas-dilution techniques measure the lung volume readily communicating with the airway opening, which may be substantially less than the total lung volume. The response to treatments, such as bronchodilators, can be difficult to interpret because a beneficial treatment effect may be measured as a decrease in lung volume if most airways are patent or as an increase in lung volume if the bronchodilator opens previously closed airways, resulting in an increased volume of lung in communication with the airway opening.

Measures of Forced Expiratory Flow

The primary method used to measure forced expiratory flows in infants has been the rapid thoracic compression (RTC) technique. The RTC technique produces forced expiratory flows by suddenly applying a pressure to the thorax and abdomen at the end of a tidal inspiration using an inflatable thoracoabdominal jacket connected to a positive-pressure reservoir. Flow is measured at the mouth with an appropriately sized pneumotachograph attached to a mask sealed around the infant's nose and mouth.[7] Flow is integrated to obtain volume, and a flow-volume curve is constructed. Before the RTC maneuver, a reproducible end-expiratory volume (functional residual capacity [FRC]) is established from at least three tidal breaths. An RTC initiated at the end of inspiration then produces a partial expiratory flow-volume curve, with exhalation continuing to a volume below the previous FRC. RTC maneuvers are repeated at increasing jacket pressures until the pressure that produces the highest expiratory flows is determined. The maximum flow occurring at the previously established tidal FRC ($\dot{V}_{max\ FRC}$) is reported.

Use of the RTC has led to major advances in understanding the normal growth and development of the respiratory system and respiratory diseases. For example, $\dot{V}_{max\ FRC}$ shows an essentially linear increase with somatic growth and with lung volume throughout the first year of life.[8,9] Seidenberg et al[10] demonstrated that lung function abnormalities persist for up to 3 months in the absence of clinical symptoms after an episode of acute viral bronchiolitis. However, the RTC technique has not proved to be the "panacea" it initially promised to be.

The use of measurements of forced expiration rely on expiratory flow limitation being achieved. Although this may be the case with the RTC technique in infants with airway obstruction, flow limitation is unlikely to be achieved in healthy infants. Furthermore, FRC is notoriously variable in infants, even over short periods, which leads to substantial variability in the values of $\dot{V}_{max\ FRC}$ (Fig. 14-2). Many studies have consistently failed to demonstrate a bronchodilator response after therapy with inhaled β-sympathomimetics; yet many clinical studies have shown that infants can benefit from the administration of inhaled bronchodilators. One possible reason for this discrepancy is that bronchodilators alter FRC, possibly reducing hy-

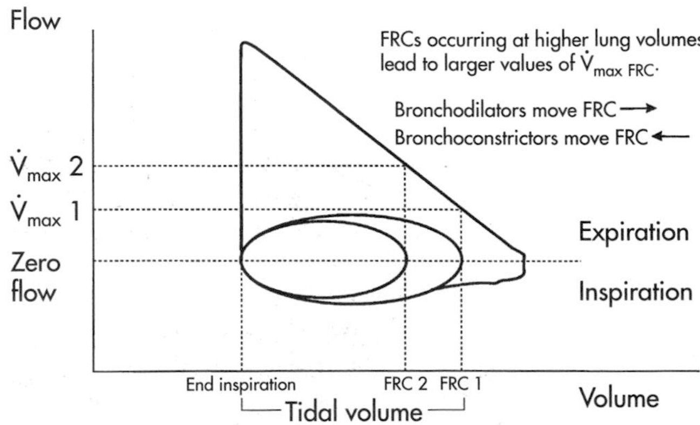

Fig. 14-2. Effect of variation of FRC on $\dot{V}_{max\ FRC}$ as calculated from a partial expiratory flow-volume curve.

perinflation. This would reduce the $\dot{V}_{max\ FRC}$, masking the expected increase after bronchodilator treatment (see Fig. 14-2).

In an attempt to overcome many of the problems with the RTC technique, Turner et al[11,12] have developed a technique whereby the lungs are inflated to a preset pressure using a pump before the RTC. They reason that the use of a standard inflation pressure reduces the variability of the measurements produced. They then measure the volume forcibly exhaled in a given time, usually 0.75 second (Fig. 14-3). This technique is analogous to the 1-second forced expiratory volume that is routinely measured in older children and adults. In addition, because the forced expiration is induced from a higher lung volume, full forced expiratory flow-volume curves appear possible (Fig. 14-4).

Early results with this technique are promising; it appears to be better able to detect abnormal lung function in infants who have wheezing or cystic fibrosis than the conventional RTC technique.[11,13] The technical details of this new technique are still being sorted out in an attempt to produce the most reliable measures of forced expiration in infants.

Measures of Resistance and Compliance

A number of techniques are available for measuring resistance and compliance in spontaneously breathing infants. The most commonly used tests are occlusion tests, which invoke the Hering-Breuer reflex, and body plethysmography. Older techniques involving the measurement of esophageal pressure as an index of pleural pressure have largely fallen out of favor for use in spontaneously breathing infants and are not discussed further. Other possibilities include the use of forced oscillation techniques.

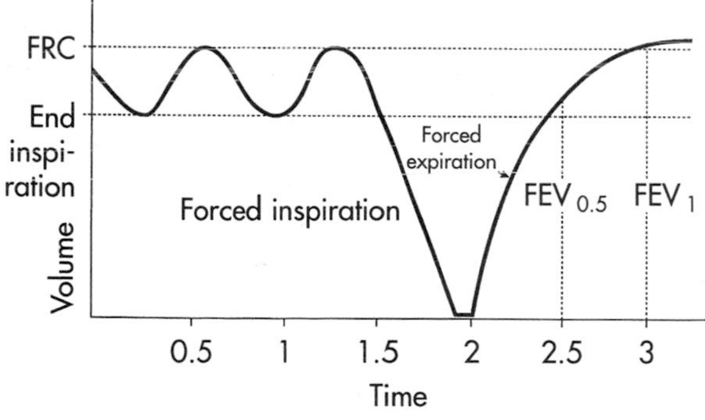

Fig. 14-3. Volume-time plot of the raised volume RTC maneuver. *$FEV_{0.5}$*, ½-second forced expiratory volume; *FEV_1*, 1-second forced expiratory volume.

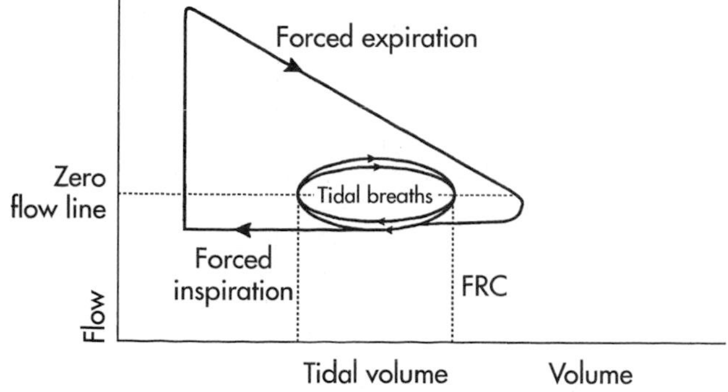

Fig. 14-4. Flow-volume plot of the raised-volume RTC maneuver.

Techniques that Invoke the Hering-Breuer Reflex. Techniques invoking the Hering-Breuer reflex rely on the assumptions that this reflex, producing complete relaxation of both inspiratory and expiratory respiratory muscles, can be elicited during airway occlusion and that airway opening pressure comes into equilibrium with alveolar pressure during the occlusion. There are two main applications of these occlusion techniques.

In the multiple-breath occlusion technique, pressure is measured at the mouth during brief airway occlusions performed on multiple breaths. Occlusions are performed at different volumes above FRC, and the individual measurements are plotted as volume vs. pressure. The slope of the line of "best fit" is the compliance of the respiratory system (Fig. 14-5).

In the single-breath occlusion technique, the airway is occluded at the end of inspiration, with the subsequent expiration occurring passively. A passive expiratory flow-volume curve is then constructed and a line fitted to the linear portion (Fig. 14-6). Compliance is calculated by dividing the total exhaled volume by the pressure at the airway opening recorded during the occlusion. The slope of the linear part of the passive flow-volume curve is equal to the reciprocal of the expiratory time constant (τrs). Resistance can be calculated by dividing the time constant by the compliance.

The problem with these techniques is ensuring relaxation of the respiratory muscles after airway occlusion and equilibration of airway opening and alveolar pressures. Generally, the presence of a plateau in airway opening pressure indicates that both of these assumptions have been satisfied. There are no firm recommendations as to how long a plateau should be maintained. However, a recent study suggests that the length of the airway occlusion can influence the values of compliance calculated from the subsequent expiration, with compliance decreasing by 0.15 ml/cm H_2O for each 0.1 second of occlusion time.[14] These data strongly argue for standardizing the length of occlusion and discarding data in which a plateau is not achieved.

Body Plethysmography. Body plethysmography is commonly used to measure Raw in adults and older children but has been modified for infants by the inclusion of a rebreathing bag containing heated, humidified, oxygen-enriched gas at body temperature, pressure, and saturation. This sophisticated technique requires a large amount of expertise and training but can produce simultaneous measurements of lung volume and Raw. However, this technique is unreliable in the presence of airway obstruction, particularly in infants because of their very compliant upper airways.

Forced Oscillation Techniques. Forced oscillation techniques are described in detail in Chapter 15. However, these techniques have been used in infants,[15,16] and impedance spectra have been measured above 4 Hz. In infants the forcing function is generally applied through a face mask and includes the impedance of the nose. When making measurements in infants, the clinician must take extreme care to prevent leaks around the face mask.

Recently, an adaptation of the forced oscillation technique has been reported for infants.[17] By applying the forcing function during a pause in breathing produced by invoking the Hering-Breuer reflex, these authors could obtain reliable impedance data from 0.5 to 20 Hz. The impedance spectra showed the same marked frequency dependence reported in

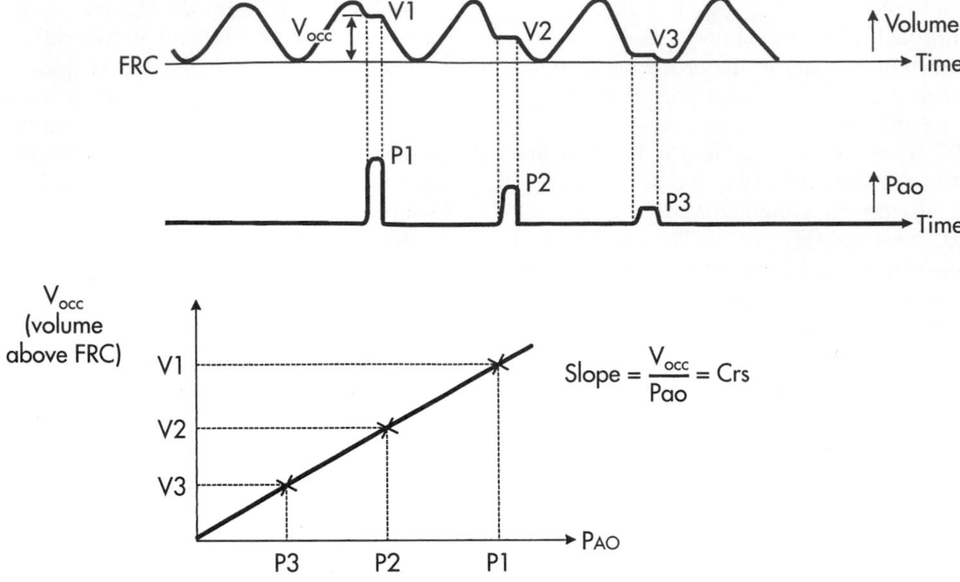

Fig. 14-5. Calculation of compliance of the respiratory system using the multiple-breath occlusion technique. V_{occ}, Volume at which occlusion is made; *V*, volume; *P*, pressure; *Pao*, pressure at the airway opening; *Crs*, compliance of the respiratory system.

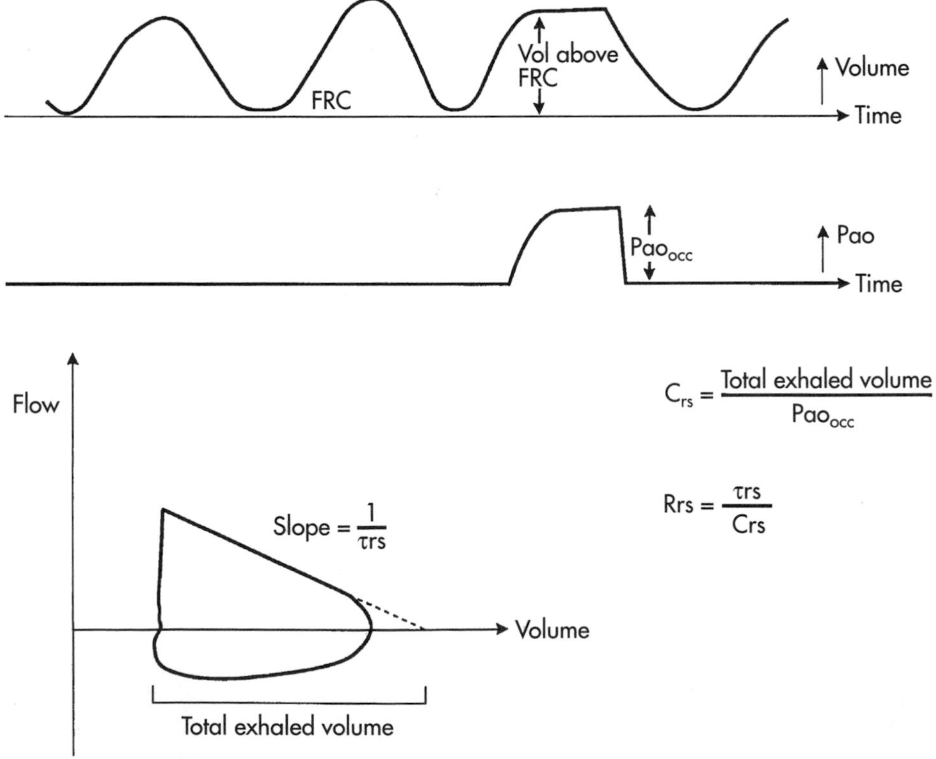

Fig. 14-6. Calculation of respiratory compliance *(Crs)* and resistance *(Rrs)* using the single-breath occlusion technique. Pao_{occ}, airway opening pressure following occlusion; *Pao*, pressure at the airway opening; τrs, expiratory time constant.

paralyzed animals[18,19] and in adults studied either during voluntary muscle relaxation[20,21] or during mechanical ventilation with paralysis.[22] Although experience with this technique is limited, it does show considerable promise and may be useful in determining the relative contributions of airway and tissue mechanical properties to the behavior of the respiratory system in infants.

Measures of Tidal Breathing Parameters

Inductance plethysmography is a noninvasive technique that is gaining popularity for measuring tidal breathing in infants. The inductance plethysmograph consists of a pair of wire bands that are usually embedded into an elastic material encircling the chest wall and abdomen. The wires are arranged in a sinusoidal fashion and are excited by an oscillator to produce an impedance proportional to the area enclosed within the band. With calibration of the impedance signal with known volume changes, it is possible to calculate changes in the cross-sectional areas of the thoracic and abdominal cavities in terms of changes in lung volume. However, the calibration is notoriously unstable and extremely sensitive to changes in body posture.

A new generation of respiratory inductance plethysmographs was introduced in the mid-1980s. These devices produce an automatic qualitative calibration during the initial period of operation. Subsequent measurements of tidal breathing excursion are related to that measured during this initial period.[23]

Martinez et al[24] recently adapted a technique previously described in adults[25] for measuring tidal breathing parameters. They measured the time to peak tidal expiratory flow (T_{ptef}) and expressed it as a percentage of total expiratory time (T_E) (Fig. 14-7). This ratio, T_{ptef}/T_E (referred to by them as *Tme/Te*), was low in infants who subsequently developed wheezing lower respiratory illnesses. Martinez et al[24] used a pneumotachograph and face mask in sedated infants to measure T_{ptef}/T_E. Stick et al[26] demonstrated that T_{ptef}/T_E could be successfully measured using an uncalibrated respiratory inductance plethysmograph during quiet sleep in infants.

The precise physiologic interpretation of T_{ptef}/T_E is unclear. In adults, T_{ptef}/T_E is correlated with airway conductance, lower values occurring with subjects with airway obstruction and low airway conductance.[25] This can be conceptualized by comparing the normally rounded shape of the expiratory limb of the flow-volume loop seen during tidal breathing (see Fig. 14-7, *left*), at which T_{ptef}/T_E approximates 0.5 with the peaked shape of the expiratory limb of a forced expiratory flow-volume curve (see Fig. 14-7, *right*), at which T_{ptef}/T_E approaches 0.15 to 0.2. For a given level of respiratory drive, as airways become more obstructed the tidal flow-volume curve becomes more like that normally seen during forced expiration, and T_{ptef}/T_E decreases. Martinez et al[24] interpreted a low premorbid value of T_{ptef}/T_E as being indicative of smaller-than-usual airways, making the infants more likely to develop wheezing illnesses with the usual respiratory tract viral infections.

However, the flow-volume curve represents an "integrated" output from the respiratory system, and factors other than airway conductance are likely to influence the expiratory flow pattern. T_{ptef}/T_E is also influenced by respiratory rate, becoming lower as respiratory rate increases and becoming lower in the prone than the lateral or supine sleeping positions.[27] Thus more research will be necessary to elucidate the physiologic meaning of T_{ptef}/T_E.

MEASUREMENT OF LUNG FUNCTION DURING MECHANICAL VENTILATION

Measurement of respiratory mechanics has the potential to provide a greater understanding of the pathogenesis of conditions leading to respiratory failure and to provide objective assessments of therapies. However, several factors must be taken into account when the measurements of respiratory mechanics are interpreted.

Influence of Measurement Conditions on Lung Function

Effects of Frequency, Flow, and Volume

Many studies have demonstrated that the respiratory system exhibits frequency-dependent behavior. The practical significance of such behavior is that the measurements of respiratory mechanics change when the ventilation frequency (i.e., the frequency "exciting" the respiratory system) changes. In general, as the exciting frequency increases, the value of resistance decreases, and the value of elastance increases[28] (Fig. 14-8).

Because a change in ventilatory requirements usually accompanies both improvements and deteriorations in clinical condition, the changes in respiratory mechanics caused by changes in ventilation frequency can mask changes resulting from a disease process. Thus the frequency-dependent behav-

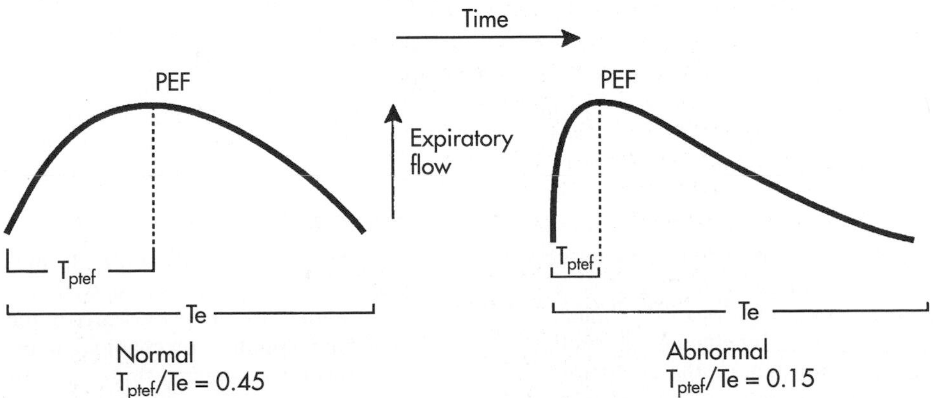

Fig. 14-7. Calculation of the ratio of time to T_{ptef}/T_E from tidal expiratory flow and time recordings. *PEF,* Peak expiratory time.

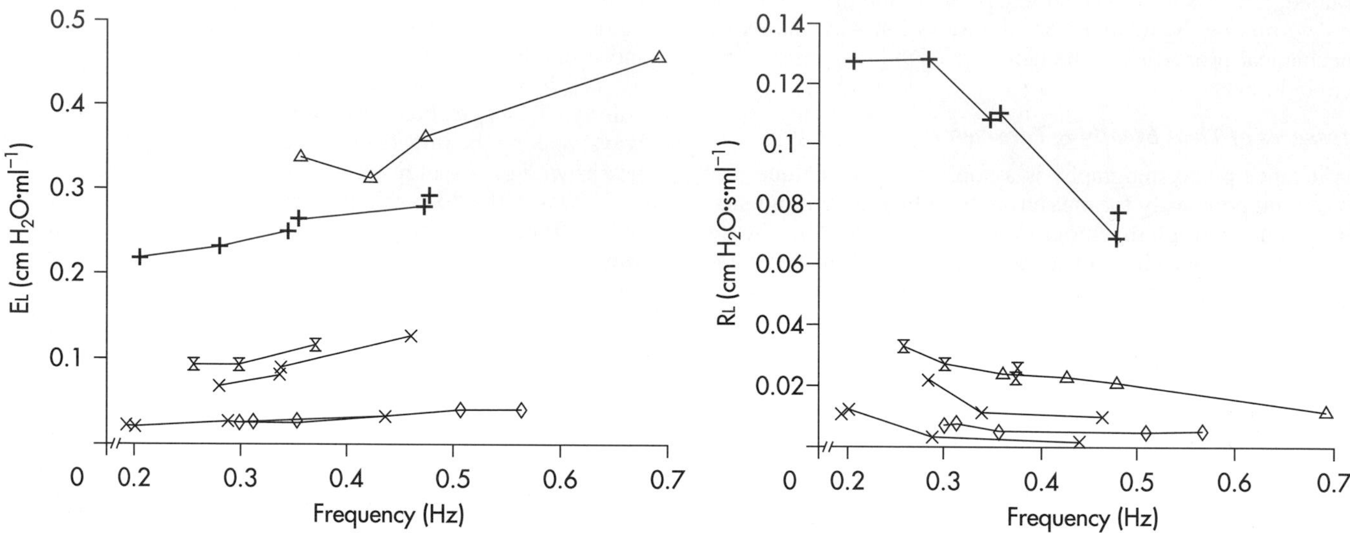

Fig. 14-8. Frequency dependence of elastance and resistance. *R*L, Resistance of the lung; *E*L, elastance of the lung. (From Nicolai TN et al: *Eur Respir* J 6:1340-1346, 1993.)

ior of the respiratory system must be considered and the measurements of respiratory function interpreted in light of the ventilator frequency.

The Raw and resistance of the endotracheal tube are flow dependent. This implies that increases in flow are accompanied by increases in the value of the resistance calculated without any fundamental change in the underlying resistive properties of the respiratory system.

The relaxed pressure-volume curve of the respiratory system has a sigmoid shape. This means that the respiratory system becomes stiffer at both high and low lung volumes. Under normal circumstances humans breathe within the "linear portion" of the pressure-volume curve, at which the compliance (or elastance) is effectively constant. If, however, ventilation begins from a low volume or extends to a high lung volume, at which point the pressure-volume curve is flatter, the compliance changes with volume.

Similarly, as the lungs are inflated, the airways are pulled open because of their attachment to the collagen matrix of the lungs. This relationship between the airways and the tissues is known as *mechanical interdependence.* This means that Raw tends to decrease as lung volume increases. In contrast, during mechanical ventilation, the resistance imposed by the tissues of the lungs and chest wall increases progressively during inspiration.[29] The effect of lung volume on total resistance depends on the relative effects of volume on Raw and tissue resistance.

The effects of frequency, flow, and volume on the measurements of respiratory mechanics must be taken into account when respiratory function is monitored in the intensive care unit. Both improvements and deteriorations in a clinical condition are likely to be accompanied by changes in ventilatory requirements. Under ideal circumstances, the ventilatory pattern remains constant so that true changes in respiratory mechanics could be monitored; however, it may not be possible or advisable to keep the ventilation pattern constant. Therefore it is important to understand the effects of frequency, flow, and volume of respiratory mechanics, no matter what measurement technique is used.

Influence of a Tracheal Tube

The presence of a tracheal tube (TT) has a number of effects on the measurement of respiratory mechanics. A TT adds a flow-dependent resistance to that of the respiratory system, the value of which depends on the internal diameter and length of the tube as well as the condition of its internal surface. A TT also bypasses the upper airway, which removes the main mechanism used by infants to maintain lung volume. Because cuffed TTs are rarely used in pediatric or neonatal intensive care units, leaks around the TT may complicate measurements of respiratory mechanics.

An important consideration is the effect of a TT on the expiratory limb of the passive flow-volume curve. Because of its flow-dependent resistance, a TT makes the expiratory limb concave to the volume axis (Fig. 14-9). In contrast, time-constant inhomogeneity causes the expiratory limb to become curvilinear in the opposite direction. In a computer model study,[30] the flow-dependent resistance of a 3.5-mm TT canceled out the curvilinear expiratory limb produced by a fourfold time-constant inhomogeneity. Thus a linear expiratory limb of a passive flow-volume curve in the presence of a TT implies some degree of time-constant inhomogeneity.

Spontaneous vs. Ventilator Breaths

For mechanically ventilated infants and children, the pressure applied to the respiratory system that is responsible for producing ventilation can be measured at the airway opening. This means that respiratory mechanics can be calculated from measurements of pressure and flow at the airway opening. During spontaneous breathing, however, the pressure applied to the respiratory system and production of ventilation is produced by the respiratory muscles and cannot be measured at the air-

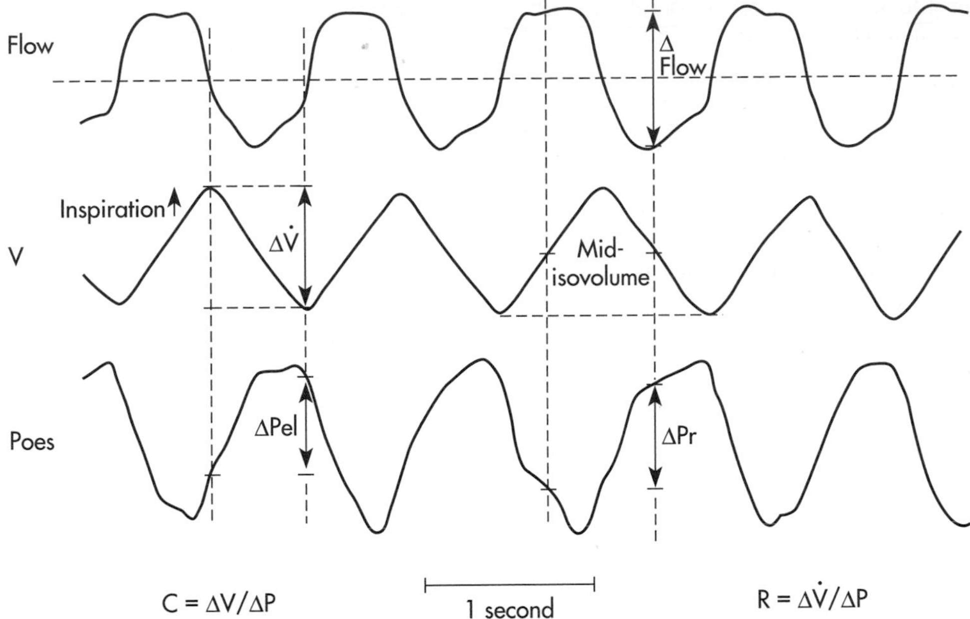

Fig. 14-9. Calculation of compliance *(C)* and resistance *(R)* with the Mead-Whittenberger technique. *V,* Volume; ΔV, change in volume; *Poes*, esophageal pressure; ΔPr, resistance pressure change; ΔP, change in pressure; $\Delta \dot{V}$, change in airflow.

way opening. Under these circumstances, it is necessary to measure transpulmonary pressure (see Chapter 15).

Influence of Leak

Leak around the TT can be a major problem for the measurement of respiratory function during mechanical ventilation. Leaks are generally pressure sensitive; that is, the leak occurs above a certain critical pressure. Because of this, the leak is more likely to occur during the inspiratory phase than during the expiratory phase. The type of ventilator used influences the effects of leak on the ventilation delivered. Volume-controlled ventilators frequently produce a constant inspiratory flow and deliver a set volume in the inspiratory time set. Leak around the TT reduces the tidal volume delivered and reduces the peak pressure but does not alter the flow profile. Time-cycled, pressure-limited ventilators produce an initially high inspiratory flow, which decreases towards zero as the peak pressure limit is approached. A leak around the TT reduces the tidal volume delivered, but the peak pressure may not be decreased. To compensate for the leak, the inspiratory flow remains positive to maintain the peak pressure. In both cases, calculating the volume by integrating the inspiratory flow passing into the TT (i.e., via a pneumotachograph) overestimates the volume delivered to the patient.

Most computerized systems for measuring lung function in mechanically ventilated subjects incorporate an automatic drift-correction procedure for the flow signal. Some drift is physiologic given that the respiratory quotient is not 1.0 (usually 0.8 in healthy lungs) (see Chapter 8). These drift-correction procedures can mask the leak and produce stable volume-time traces. However, the measurements of lung function obtained in patients with significant leaks around the TT are unreliable. Although no systematic study of the size of leak that can be tolerated has been published and some authors claim that leaks of up to 10% can be tolerated,[31] the authors' personal experience suggests that as little as 5% leak can introduce significant errors into measurements of resistance and compliance.

Measurement Techniques

A number of articles reviewing the different techniques used to measure dynamic respiratory mechanics (resistance and dynamic compliance) are available in the literature.[30,32,33] A brief description of some of the more common techniques for measuring lung function during mechanical ventilation follows. For a more detailed description and critique of these techniques, the original articles and these reviews should be consulted.

Mead-Whittenberger Technique

Traditionally the Mead-Whittenberger technique has been used to measure compliance and resistance in spontaneously breathing subjects.[34] Changes in transpulmonary pressure are related to changes in flow and volume over the tidal volume range (see Fig. 14-9). Compliance is calculated by examining points of zero flow at end inspiration and end expiration. The pressure change (ΔP) and corresponding volume change *(ΔV)* between these points can be used to determine dynamic compliance *(Cdyn):* Cdyn = $\Delta V/\Delta P$. Traditionally this is measured during expiration. Similarly, resistance *(R)* can be estimated when changes in pressure are related to changes in flow between points of equal volume in the midvolume range: R = $\Delta P/\Delta V$. Elastic forces are assumed to be equal and opposite under these conditions.

This technique assumes that resistance and compliance are constant throughout inspiration and expiration, which may be reasonable within the tidal volume range; however, this may not be true for measurements in hyperinflated or diseased subjects. This technique may be difficult to apply to ventilated subjects because the points of zero flow and midtidal volume occur at times when the pressure patterns are changing rapidly. Hand ventilation, using an anesthetic circuit, may allow a smoother pressure profile and may simplify use of this technique in mechanically ventilated subjects.

Least Squares Regression Method

The least squares regression method for measuring resistance involves relating the driving pressure of the system to the corresponding flow.[35] Driving pressure is corrected by subtracting the contribution of the elastic and viscoelastic pressure components from transpulmonary pressure. The driving pressure is then plotted against flow, and linear regression is used to determine the slope, which is the resistance of the system. This technique again assumes a linear relationship of the data.

Mortola-Saetta Method

The Mortola-Saetta method is a variation of the least squares regression technique and involves plotting P/V vs. $\dot{V}$/V. Again, the slope of this relationship is a measure of lung resistance, whereas the intercept is a measure of lung elastance.[33]

Volume-Corrected Resistance

The volume-corrected resistance technique corrects measurement of resistance from the pressure-flow relationship for changes over tidal volume range by plotting pressure/flow against volume.[36]

Forced Oscillation Technique

The forced oscillation technique involves imposing oscillatory changes in pressure (and therefore flow) at the airway opening and measuring the resulting pressure changes at the airway opening (single port) or at the body surface (double port).[37-40] This allows the calculation of respiratory impedance, which includes both the resistive and the elastic properties of the system. It is possible to examine the relationship of each of these measurements of mechanics with frequency. This technique has not yet been widely used in clinical situations; however, recent advances in computing and signal processing means that the potential of this technique may be realized in the future. For a more detailed description of the technique, the reader is referred to Chapter 15.

Interrupter Technique

The interrupter technique allows the respiratory resistance to be partitioned into components representing the conducting airways (Raw) and a peripheral phenomena, representing the tissue viscoelastic components, known as P_{dif}[30] (Fig. 14-10). When the airway is occluded during expiration, there is an initial rapid jump in pressure after occlusion (P_{init}), representing the pressure loss across the resistance of the airways. When this jump in pressure is related to flow measured immediately before occlusion, a value for the airways resistance (and any additional chest wall and TT newtonian resistance) may be obtained (Raw). A slower, secondary rise in pressure to a plateau occurs after occlusion (P_{dif}). This component represents stress recovery within the tissues and the chest wall as well as any redistribution of gas (pendelluft) occurring between different lung units. Thus this technique allows measurement of Raw, static elastance, and the viscoelastic properties of the lung from each occlusion. However, this again requires a very rapid occlusion valve and sophisticated analysis procedures to accurately extract the viscoelastic and Raw measurements.[30] Respiratory muscle activity also affects the accuracy of these measurements. This technique has been used as a research tool in children,[41-45] but it has limited clinical applications. It has been applied with some success to spontaneously breathing infants; however, the accuracy of resistance measurements may be affected by respiratory muscle activity after occlusion.

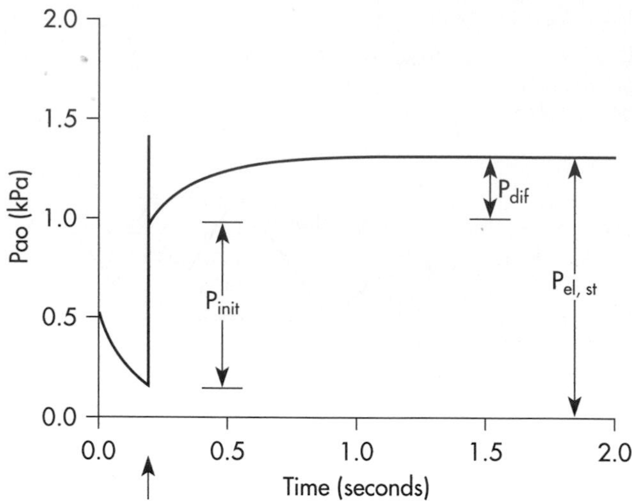

Fig. 14-10. Airway opening pressure after an expiratory flow interruption *(arrow)* demonstrating an initial rapid jump in pressure *(P_{init})* and a slower secondary change *(P_{dif})*. $P_{el, st}$, Static elastic recoil pressure. (From Freezer NJ, Nicolai T, Sly PD: *Pediatr Res* 33(3):261-266, 1993.)

Forced Deflation Technique

For the successful application of the forced deflation technique, the child needs to be intubated and deeply sedated or under general anesthesia with or without muscle relaxation. The lungs are inflated to 40 cm H_20 airway pressure (which is defined as total lung capacity) and held for 2 to 3 seconds. Inflation is performed approximately 4 times to ensure maximal recruitment of previously closed lung units and to ensure a constant volume history. After the last inflation, the lungs are opened to a negative-pressure reservoir (usually −40 cm H_2O), which produces a forced deflation of the lungs.[46,47] In healthy infants, residual volume is reached in 1 to 2 seconds, the volume exhaled being the forced vital capacity (FVC). The resultant forced expiratory flow is integrated to provide exhaled volume, and a maximum expiratory flow-volume curve is generated. Maximum expiratory flow is measured at 25% and 10% of FVC above residual volume (MEF_{25} and MEF_{10}, respectively), and the ratios of MEF_{25}/FVC and MEF_{10}/FVC are calculated. Flows measured at volumes greater than 30% of FVC above residual volume appear not to be flow limited and are therefore less reproducible. Furthermore, artifact introduced by the endotracheal tube acting as a critical orifice may occur at volumes above mid-FVC. This technique is rather invasive and would not appear to be suitable for general use in mechanically ventilated children and infants.

Multiple Linear Regression Techniques

Most techniques for measuring the mechanics of the respiratory system, including all of those previously discussed, are based on the general equation of motion for a linear single-compartment model, as follows:

$$P = EV + R\dot{V} + I\dot{V} \qquad (1)$$

That is, the driving pressure of the system *(P)* is the sum of its elastic *(EV* = elastance × volume), resistive *(R* = resistance ×

flow), and inertive (I = inertance × acceleration) components. For most practical applications the contribution of inertance in this equation is negligible and can be ignored. Thus the equation can be written as follows:

$$P = EV + R\dot{V} \tag{2}$$

When this equation is applied to the respiratory system itself, pressure measurements at end expiration, at which $\dot{V} = 0$ and $V = 0$, may not be zero, such as when positive end-expiratory pressure (PEEP) has been set by the ventilator or intrinsic positive end-expiratory pressure ($PEEP_i$) occurs because of insufficient expiratory time to allow complete expiration to FRC. In these cases a constant term *(K)* must be included in the equation to allow for calculation of this pressure during the fitting procedure. This new equation follows:

$$P = EV + R\dot{V} + K \tag{3}$$

If this equation is applied to the respiratory system during mechanical ventilation, multiple linear regression analysis may be used to determine dynamic elastance *(Ers)* (the reciprocal of compliance *[Crs]*) and dynamic resistance *(Rrs)* by relating pressure measured at the airway opening *(Pao)* to simultaneous measurements of $\dot{V}$ and V. The constant term for end-expiratory pressure ($P_{A\,EE}$) is a reflection of end-expiratory alveolar pressure.[47] Thus the equation of motion for a single-compartment model of the respiratory system follows:

$$Pao = Ers \times V + Rrs \times \dot{V} + P_{A\,EE} \tag{4}$$

$$Pao = 1/Crs \times V + Rrs \times \dot{V} + P_{A\,EE} \tag{5}$$

The mechanical properties of the respiratory system can be partitioned into components for the lungs and chest wall by measuring esophageal pressure as an index of pleural pressure. Dynamic lung elastance and lung resistance may be calculated by relating transpulmonary pressure to flow and volume. Transpulmonary pressure *(Ptp)* may be calculated by subtracting pleural pressure estimates from an esophageal catheter *(Pes)* from pressure measurements at the airway opening *(Pao)*: Ptp = Pao − Pes. In this case the constant term, *K* (as seen in equation 3), represents transpulmonary pressure at end expiration.

Values of inspiratory and expiratory mechanics can be obtained by separately analyzing the inspiratory and expiratory components of ventilated breaths. Pressure at the airway opening is pressure applied to the respiratory system regardless of whether it is during inspiration or expiration. The flow that results depends on two things: the applied pressure and the initial conditions. During a passive expiration against no equipment resistance, pressure at the airway opening is zero at all times, and the flow is quasiexponential. The fact that flow is not zero during expiration in ventilated subjects is due to the initial conditions; that is, at the start of expiration, there is gas in the lungs. During expiration against equipment resistance (e.g., pneumotach or the ventilator circuit), pressure at the airway opening is not zero and is applied to the respiratory system. Thus fitting a model to measurements of pressure at the airway opening, flow, and volume during expiration gives an estimate of expiratory mechanics.

With separate calculation of inspiratory and expiratory mechanics, the respiratory time constant (τ) for each phase may be calculated ($\tau = R \times C$ or $\tau = R/E$), and this information may be useful when the suitability of a particular ventilation pattern is examined for a particular case. If the expiratory time set on the ventilator is less than 3 times the expiratory time constant, $PEEP_i$ may develop, and hyperinflation may occur.[48]

One of the major advantages of multiple linear regression is that it produces an indication of absolute lung volume. End-expiratory pressure is a measure of end-expiratory alveolar pressure, and thus changes in lung volume can be monitored, and the development of $PEEP_i$ may be calculated by subtracting the applied pressure at the end of expiration from the end-expiratory pressure.[49] Other measurements tracking lung volume have proved difficult to use in ventilated subjects. Plethysmography is rarely practical in the intensive care unit, and gas dilution is unreliable in many disease states. Other techniques for measuring mechanics require either the standardization of lung volume by inflating to a set pressure or the assumption that the FRC can be used as a stable volume reference, which is not necessarily the case.

Although multiple linear regression is usually based on a linear single-compartment model, it determines a mean and standard deviation for each coefficient as well as visual check of the goodness of fit. These values are weighted for inspiration, expiration, and tidal volume depending on the ventilation pattern selected for analysis. More advanced fitting procedures and algorithms may also be used for sophisticated modeling of the respiratory system and tracking changes over time. Recursive multiple linear regression allows each sampled point to be calculated and updated with each additional data point instead of a single mean value. Such algorithms may have a memory function so that the influence of each point on the next may be varied.[50]

Model Assumptions

All of these techniques are based on the assumption that the respiratory system can be represented by a linear single-compartment model. Although a such a model may be a reasonable approximation of the behavior of the respiratory system at a single frequency within the tidal volume range, mechanics calculated from these techniques are ultimately only an approximation of the true system. Under extreme ventilatory conditions (high or low volumes) or diseased states the lungs' behavior is less adequately described by a single-compartment model. This topic is covered in Chapter 8.

Multiple linear regression analyses can be performed using more complicated models for the respiratory system. Under various circumstances, the model can allow for volume dependence of elastance or resistance, flow dependence of resistance, or inertance. Using a volume-dependent resistance in adults, Peslin et al[51] found a small improvement in fit, but the magnitude and direction of contribution of the volume-dependent resistance was variable. However, Rousselot et al[52] found that including such a term in their model provided a meaningful negative volume-dependent resistance in young children and an overall improvement in fit. This volume dependence should become significant only if the lung is being either overventilated, producing overdistention of some lung units, or underventilated, resulting in atelectasis. Similarly, inclusion of a volume-dependent elastance term has led to significant improvements in the model fit to data collected from premature infants and animals.[53,54] These factors must be taken into account when clinicians measure respiratory mechanics in ventilated children, particularly in the presence of abnormal lungs.

REFERENCES

Lung Function Testing in Infants

1. Stocks J, Sly PD, Tepper RS, Morgan WJ, eds: *Infant respiratory function testing,* New York, 1996, Wiley-Liss.
2. Gaultier C, Fletcher M, Beardsmore C, Motoyama E, Stocks J: Measurement conditions. In Stocks J, Sly P, Tepper R, Morgan WJ, eds: *Infant respiratory function testing,* New York, 1996, Wiley-Liss, pp 29-44.
3. Mallol J, Sly PD: Effect of chloral hydrate on arterial oxygen saturation in wheezy infants, *Pediatr Pulmonol* 5(2):96-99, 1988.
4. Peslin R: Techniques in life sciences: techniques in respiratory physiology. II. *Respir Physiol* 1-26, 1984.
5. Sly PD, Lanteri C, Bates JH: Effect of the thermodynamics of an infant plethysmograph on the measurement of thoracic gas volume, *Pediatr Pulmonol* 8(3):203-208, 1990.
6. John JD, Drefeldt B, Taskar B, Mansson C, Jonson B: Dynamic properties of body plethysmographs and effects on physiological parameters, *J Appl Physiol* 77:152-159, 1994.
7. Taussig LM, Landau LI, Godfrey S, Arad I: Determinants of forced expiratory flows in newborn infants, *J Appl Physiol* 53(5):1220-1227, 1982.
8. Hanrahan JP, Tager IB, Castille RG, Segal MR, Weiss ST, Speizer FE: Pulmonary function measures in healthy infants: variability and size correction, *Am Rev Respir Dis* 141:1127-1135, 1990.
9. Tepper S, Morgan WJ, Cota K, Wright A, Taussig LM: Physiologic growth and development of the lung during the first year of life, *Am Rev Respir Dis* 134:513-519, 1986.
10. Seidenberg J, Masters IB, Hudson I, Olinsky A, Phelan PD: Disturbance in respiratory mechanics in infants with bronchiolitis, *Thorax* 44:660-667, 1989.
11. Turner DJ, Lanteri CJ, Le Souëf PN, Sly PD: Improved detection of abnormal respiratory function using forced expiration from raised lung volume in infants with cystic fibrosis, *Eur Respir J* 7:1995-1999, 1994.
12. Turner DJ, Stick SM, Le Souëf KL, Sly PD, Le Souëf PN: A new technique to generate and assess forced expiration from raised lung volume in infants, *Am J Respir Crit Care Med* 151(5):1441-1450, 1995.
13. Turner DJ, Sly PD, Le Souëf PN: Assessment of forced expiratory volume-time parameters in detecting histamine-induced bronchoconstriction in wheezy infants, *Pediatr Pulmonol* 15(4):220-224, 1993.
14. Mallol J, Willet K, Burton P, Sly PD: Influence of duration of occlusion time on respiratory mechanics measured with the single-breath technique in infants, *Pediatr Pulmonol* 17:250-257, 1994.
15. Desager KN, Buhr W, Willemen M, van Bever HP, de Backer W, Vermeire PA, Lándsér FJ: Measurement of total respiratory impedance in infants by the forced oscillation technique, *J Appl Physiol* 41:101-106, 1991.
16. Jackson AC, Neff KM, Lutchen KR, Dorkin HL: Interpretation of respiratory system impedance (4-256 hz) in healthy infants, *Eur Respir Rev* 19:165-166, 1994.
17. Sly P, Hayden M, Petak F, Hantos Z: Measurement of low-frequency respiratory impedance in infants, *Am J Respir Crit Care Med* 154:161-166, 1996.
18. Rotger M, Peslin R, Navajas D, Farre R: Lung and respiratory impedance at low frequency during mechanical ventilation in rabbits, *J Appl Physiol* 78(6):2153-2160, 1995.
19. Hantos Z, Daroczy B, Suki B, Nagy S, Fredberg JJ: Input impedance and peripheral inhomogeneity of dog lungs, *J Appl Physiol* 72(1):168-178, 1992.
20. Barnas GM, Yoshino K, Fredberg J, Kikuchi Y, Loring SH, Mead J: Total and local impedances of the chest wall up to 10Hz, *J Appl Physiol* 68:1409-1414, 1990.
21. Barnas GM, Yoshino K, Loring SH, Mead J: Impedance and relative displacements of relaxed chest wall up to 4 Hz, *J Appl Physiol* 62:71-81, 1987.
22. Farré R, Ferrer M, Rotger M, Navajas D: Servocontrolled generator to measure respiratory impedance from 0.25 to 26 Hz in ventilated patients at different PEEP levels, *Eur Respir J* 8:1222-1227, 1995.
23. Sackner MAW, Watson H, Belsito AS, Feinerman D, Suarez M, Gonzalez G, Bizousky F, Krieger B: Calibration of respiratory inductive plethysmograph during natural breathing, *J Appl Physiol* 66:410-420, 1989.
24. Martinez FD, Morgan WJ, Holberg CJ, Taussig LM, Personnel G: Diminished lung function as a predisposing factor for wheezing respiratory illness in infants, *N Engl J Med* 319:1112-1117, 1988.
25. Morris MJ, Lane DJ: Tidal expiratory flow patterns in airflow obstruction, *Thorax* 36:135-142, 1981.
26. Stick SM, Ellis E, Le Souëf PN, Sly PD: Validation of respiratory inductance plethysmography (respitrace) for the measurement of tidal breathing parameters in newborns, *Pediatr Pulmonol* 14(3):187-191, 1992.
27. Ellis E: Unpublished observations.

Measurement of Lung Function during Mechanical Ventilation

28. Nicolai TN, Lanteri CJ, Sly PD: Frequency dependence of elastance and resistance in ventilated children with and without the chest opened, *Eur Respir J* 6:1340-1346, 1993.
29. D'Angelo E, Calderini E, Robatto FM, Bono D, Milic-Emili J: Respiratory mechanics in anesthetised paralyzed humans: effects of flow, volume, and time, *J Appl Physiol* 67:2556-2564, 1989.
30. Sly PD, Brown KA, Bates JH, Spier S, Milic EJ: Noninvasive determination of respiratory mechanics during mechanical ventilation of neonates: a review of current and future techniques, *Pediatr Pulmonol* 4(1):39-47, 1988.
31. Bhutani VK, Sivieri EM, Abbasi S, Shaffer TH: Evaluation of neonatal pulmonary mechanics and energetics: a two factor least mean square analysis, *Pediatr Pulmonol* 4(3):150-158, 1988.
32. England SJ: Current techniques for assessing pulmonary function in the newborn and infant: advantages and limitations, *Pediatr Pulmonol* 4:48-53, 1988.
33. Mortola JP, Saetta M: Measurements of respiratory mechanics in the newborn: a simple approach, *Pediatr Pulmonol* 3:123-130, 1987.
34. Mead J, Whittenberger JL: Physical properties of human lungs measured during spontaneous respiration, *J Appl Physiol* 5:779-796, 1953.
35. Mortola JP, Fisher JT, Smith B, Fox G, Weeks S: Dynamics of breathing in infants, *J Appl Physiol* 52:1209-1215, 1982.
36. Beardsmore CS, Godfrey S, Shani N, Maayan C, Baryishay E: Airway resistance measurements throughout the respiratory cycle in infants, *Respiration* 49:81-93, 1986.
37. Landser FJ, Nagels J, Demedts M, Billiet L, van de Woestijne KP: A new method to determine frequency characteristics of the respiratory system, *J Appl Physiol* 41:101-106, 1976.
38. Hantos Z, Daroczy B, Gyurkovits K: Total respiratory impedance in healthy children, *Pediatr Pulmonol* 1(2):91-98, 1985.
39. Marchal F, Haouzi P, Gallina C, Crance JP: Measurement of ventilatory resistance in infants and young children, *Respir Physiol* 73:201-210, 1988.
40. Lebecque P, Desmond K, Swartebroeckx Y, Dubois P, Lulling J, Coates A: Measurement of respiratory system resistance by forced oscillation in normal children: a comparison with spirometric values, *Pediatr Pulmonol* 10:117-122, 1991.
41. Freezer NJ, Sly PD: The pulmonary mechanics and outcome of neonates on ECMO, *Pediatr Pulmonol* 11:108-112, 1991.
42. Freezer NJ, Lanteri CJ, Sly PD: Effect of pulmonary blood flow on measurements of respiratory mechanics using the interrupter technique, *J Appl Physiol* 74(3):1083-1088, 1993.
43. Freezer NJ, Sly PD: Predictive value of measurements of respiratory mechanics in preterm infants with HMD, *Pediatr Pulmonol* 16(2):116-123, 1993.
44. Lanteri CJ, Sly PD: Changes in respiratory mechanics with age, *J Appl Physiol* 74(1):369-378, 1993.
45. Chowienczyk PJ, Lawson CP, Lane S, Johnson R, Wilson N, Silverman M, Cochrane GM: A flow interruption device for measurement of airway resistance, *Eur Respir J* 4:623-628, 1991.
46. Motoyama EK: Pulmonary mechanics during early postnatal years, *Pediatr Res* 11:220-223, 1977.
47. Motoyama EK, Fort MD, Klesh KW, Mutich RL, Guthrie RD: Early onset of airway reactivity in premature infants with bronchopulmonary dysplasia, *Am Rev Respir Dis* 136:50-57, 1987.
48. Kano S, Lanteri CJ, Pemberton PJ, Le Souëf PN, Sly PD: Fast versus slow ventilation for neonates, *Am Rev Respir Dis* 148(3):578-584, 1993.
49. Nicolai T, Lanteri C, Freezer N, Sly PD: Non-invasive determination of alveolar pressure during mechanical ventilation, *Eur Respir J* 4(10):1275-1283, 1991.
50. Lauzon AM, Bates JH: Estimation of time-varying respiratory mechanical parameters by recursive least squares, *J Appl Physiol* 71(3):1159-1165, 1991.

51. Peslin R, *da SJ,* Chabot F, Duvivier C: Respiratory mechanics studied by multiple linear regression in unsedated ventilated patients, *Eur Respir J* 5(7):871-878, 1992.
52. Rousselot JM, Peslin R, Duvivier C: Evaluation of the multiple linear regression method to monitor respiratory mechanics in ventilated neonates and young children, *Pediatr Pulmonol* 13(3):161-168, 1992.
53. Kano S, Lanteri CJ, Sly PD: Estimation of respiratory system over distension during mechanical ventilation using multiple linear regression, *Am Rev Respir Dis* 147:A127, 1993.
54. Lanteri CJ, Willet K, Kano S, Jobe AH, Ikegami M, Polk DH, Newnham JP, Kohan R, Kelly R, Sly PD: Time course of changes in lung mechanics following fetal steroid treatment, *Am J Respir Crit Care Med* 150:759-765, 1994.

CHAPTER 15

Lung Function in Cooperative Subjects

Peter D. Sly, Mark John Hayden, and Wayne J. Morgan

The measurement of pulmonary function provides an objective assessment of the state of the respiratory system and useful information for the diagnosis and management of respiratory tract illnesses in adults and children. A basic knowledge of the physiologic principles behind the tests and techniques used for making the measurements is necessary to understand the appropriate use of lung function testing and to intelligently interpret the data produced.

Many measurements of respiratory function are based on forced expiratory maneuvers. The age at which a child develops the ability to perform these maneuvers reliably has not been well studied. Le Souëf et al[1] attempted to teach children as young as 3 years old to perform standard spirometry. With intensive coaching, approximately 20% of the 3 year olds could reliably perform forced expiratory maneuvers. The percentage rose progressively with age until most children age 6 or older could perform the necessary forced expirations. Other studies have also demonstrated that most children 5 years and older are capable of performing spirometry and completing bronchoprovocation tests.[2] However, these studies have been performed in a pulmonary function laboratory by staff experienced in measuring pulmonary function in children and at a time when the child was well. A well-trained technician experienced in handling children and a laboratory setting that children do not find threatening are essential for gaining the child's confidence and producing reliable measurements of pulmonary function.[3]

This chapter deals with the basic physiologic principles of lung function testing. For applications of these tests in particular conditions, the reader is referred to the chapters dealing with those conditions.

LUNG VOLUMES

The measurement of static lung volume (i.e., the amount of gas within the lungs at any given point during inflation or deflation) can provide important information about the state of the respiratory system. Also, because the value of many parameters of lung function, including resistance, compliance, and forced expiratory flows, depends on the lung volume at which they are measured, knowledge of lung volume aids interpretation of other measures of lung function.

Subdivisions of Lung Volume

Traditionally, descriptive terms have been used to subdivide lung volumes into a number of fractions related to normal physiologic function (Fig. 15-1). By convention, each subdivision is called a *volume,* whereas any combination of two or more volumes is called a *capacity.* The more commonly used subdivisions follow:

1. *Tidal volume (VT)* is the volume of gas breathed in and out with each breath.
2. *Vital capacity (VC)* is the maximum volume that can be exhaled after a maximal inspiration (i.e., VC = VT + inspiratory reserve volume + expiratory reserve volume).
3. *Functional residual capacity (FRC)* is the amount of gas remaining in the lungs at the end of expiration (whether that expiration is during tidal breathing or during periods of increased ventilatory requirements such as exercise).
4. *Total lung capacity (TLC)* is the total amount of gas within the lungs after a maximal inspiration (TLC = FRC + inspiratory capacity).
5. *Residual volume (RV)* is the amount of gas left in the lungs after a maximal expiration (RV = TLC − VC).

The commonly used terms to subdivide lung volume are illustrated in Fig. 15-1.

With normal tidal breathing in adults and older children, the normal end-expiratory lung volume (i.e., FRC) coincides with the elastic equilibrium volume (EEV) of the respiratory sys-

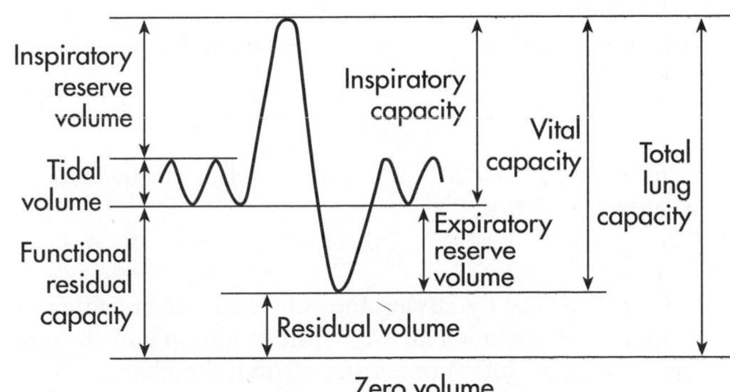

Fig. 15-1. The subdivisions of lung volume.

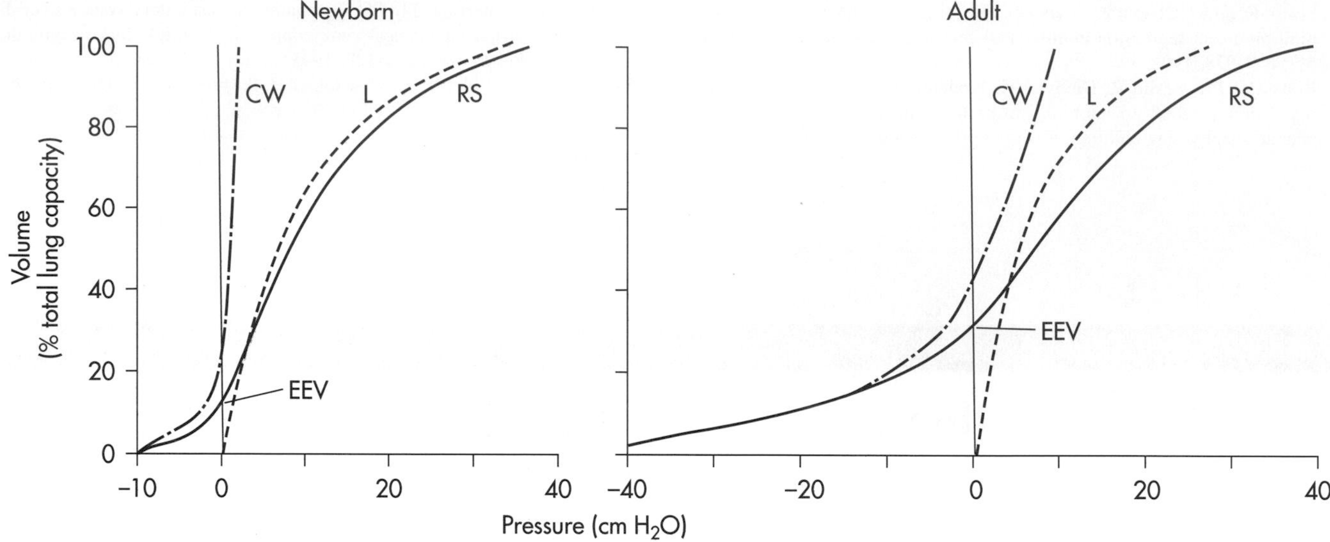

Fig. 15-2. Pressure-volume curves of the newborn and adult lung, demonstrating the effect of lung *(L)* and chest wall *(CW)* compliance on EEV. (From Agostini E: *J Appl Physiol* 14:909, 1959.)

tem. This EEV occurs where the outward elastic recoil of the chest wall is balanced by the inward elastic recoil of the lungs (Fig. 15-2). The EEV is the volume the respiratory system assumes if all muscle forces are relaxed (e.g., during passive expiration) and normally occurs at approximately 40% of VC. However, under various normal and abnormal clinical situations, FRC may be above or below EEV. At times of increased ventilatory requirements, such as during exercise or with lung disease, active expiration can push FRC below EEV. Similarly, if the recoil of the chest wall is decreased (e.g., in normal neonates) or if the lung recoil is increased, such as that seen in diseases characterized by "stiff lungs" (e.g., respiratory distress syndrome), EEV may occur at a lower lung volume, at which there is risk of closure of the small airways. Breathing from low lung volumes is inefficient because extra force is required to open the closed airways. Under these circumstances, FRC is usually actively elevated above EEV by various means, including an increased respiratory rate, thus beginning the next inspiration before EEV has been reached, and a slowed expiration caused by contracting the inspiratory muscles or adductor muscles of the glottis.

Measurement of Lung Volumes

Plethysmography

Thoracic gas volume (Vtg) at FRC is usually measured directly in a plethysmograph using techniques based on Boyle's law.[4] In other words, for a given amount of gas at a constant temperature, the product of pressure *(P)* and volume *(V)* is constant, as follows:

$$P \times V = (P + \Delta P) \times (V + \Delta V)$$

Assuming the product $\Delta P \cdot \Delta V$ is negligible, this equation can be written as follows:

$$V = -\Delta V/\Delta P \times P$$

Vtg is measured by having the subject make breathing efforts against an occluded airway while sitting in a plethysmograph. During occluded breathing efforts, the changes in intrathoracic gas volume are assumed to occur by gas compression-decompression alone. From Boyle's law, as previously expressed, the Vtg at which the occluded breathing efforts were made can be calculated, as follows:

$$Vtg = -\Delta V/\Delta P_A \times P_B$$

where ΔV is the change in gas volume during the occluded breathing efforts, which is measured with the plethysmograph; ΔP_A is the change in alveolar pressure, which is measured from changes in airway opening pressure during the occluded breathing efforts; and P_B is the barometric pressure in the room minus water vapor pressure at body temperature.

The application of Boyle's law to plethysmography is based on the following assumptions:

1. During occluded breathing efforts, there is no flow along the airways, and the changes in alveolar pressure can be represented by changes in airway opening pressure.
2. Gas compression and decompression, both within the lungs and within the plethysmograph, occur under isothermal conditions.
3. Compression of abdominal gas is negligible.

In healthy subjects seated in an adult-sized plethysmograph, these assumptions are reasonably valid. The major potential source of error comes from the compliance of the upper airways, especially the cheeks.[4] The respiratory system can be represented as two compliant compartments (i.e., the upper airways and the alveolar gas compartment) separated by a resistive element (the airways). Changes in pressure in the alveolar compartment are transmitted to the airway opening with a time constant determined by the airway resistance and the compliance of the upper airway. If either the airway resistance or the compliance of the upper airway increases, the time constant of transmission may become long enough that the changes in airway opening pressure underestimate changes in alveolar pressure, resulting in an overestimation of the true lung volume. For subjects with normal lungs, supporting the cheeks with hands is usually sufficient to ensure accurate measurements of lung volume.

The original plethysmographs were largely constant-volume, "pressure" plethysmographs. However, this type has now been largely replaced by variable-volume "flow" plethysmographs. These plethysmographs include a pneumotachograph

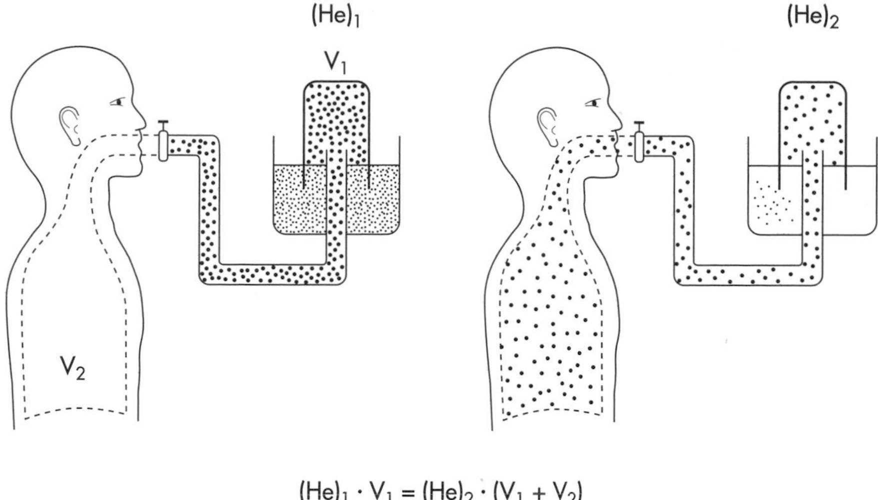

Fig. 15-3. The calculation of lung volumes using the helium-dilution technique. *He,* Helium; *V,* volume.

in the wall and measure the flow into and out of the box produced by chest wall movement during the occluded breathing efforts. This flow is then integrated to give the volume change resulting from compression of the Vtg during occluded breathing efforts. These flow plethysmographs have the advantage of an improved frequency response at low frequencies without sacrificing performance at higher frequencies. They are suitable for measuring volume variations over a wide range of amplitudes and frequencies and also allow the measurement of forced expiration within the plethysmograph.

Once Vtg has been measured, TLC and RV are calculated from Vtg and measurements of inspiratory capacity and VC. The RV may be falsely elevated if the child does not exhale fully. RV is one of the most variable of all lung function tests in children,[5] and the results must be interpreted with caution. Caution must be exercised in the measurement and interpretation of lung volumes by plethysmography in the presence of marked airway obstruction.

Gas Dilution

Alternatively, lung volumes can be measured by gas dilution. In theory, these techniques are simple, involving the measurement of the dilution of a known concentration of gas by an unknown volume (the Vtg) (Fig. 15-3). With measurement of the final gas concentration, it is possible to calculate Vtg. Although the helium-dilution method is simple to perform and is relatively inexpensive,[6] it is time consuming, has potentially limiting cooperation, and is likely to significantly underestimate the Vtg in the presence of airway obstruction.

The apparatus required for measuring lung volume by gas dilution is relatively simple; it consists of a spirometer, gas reservoir, gas analyzer, and system for supplying oxygen and removing carbon dioxide during the test. The system functions as a closed circuit, which must be free of leaks. The subject is instructed to breathe to and from the spirometer, and when a regular respiratory pattern has been established, the circuit is switched so that the subject breathes to and from the gas reservoir, which contains a known concentration of the indicator gas. By convention, the indicator gas is introduced at the end of expiration. When the gas concentration in the circuit (including the lungs) reaches a new equilibrium, the final concentration is used to calculate the new volume of the system (i.e., circuit plus lungs). Any leak in the circuit results in a falsely low final concentration and an overestimation of the end-expiratory lung volume. Gas-dilution techniques measure the part of the lung volume that is readily available for gas exchange and does not measure "trapped" gas. Therefore in subjects with significant airway obstruction, the Vtg measured by gas dilution is likely to be significantly lower than that measured by plethysmography.

RESISTANCE AND COMPLIANCE

Elastic Properties of the Respiratory System

The respiratory system is composed of a collection of elastic structures. When a force is applied to an elastic structure, the structure resists deformation by producing an opposing force to return the structure to its relaxed state. This opposing force is known as the *elastic recoil pressure.* The force required to stretch a purely elastic structure depends on how far it is stretched, not how rapidly it is being stretched. Similarly, the pressure required to overcome the elastic recoil of the lung and chest wall depends on the lung volume above or below EEV. The elastic recoil pressure *(Pel)* divided by the lung volume gives a measure of the elastic properties of the respiratory system *(elastance [E])*: E = Pel/V. The reciprocal of elastance is known as *compliance (C)* and describes how much the respiratory system is inflated for a given change in applied pressure: C = V/Pel. When lung volume is plotted on the ordinate and elastic recoil pressure is plotted on the abscissa, the slope of the pressure-volume curve is equivalent to the compliance of the respiratory system (Fig. 15-4).

Dynamics of Respiration

Ventilation of the lungs involves motion of the respiratory system, which is produced by forces required to overcome the elastic, flow-resistive, and inertial properties of the lungs and chest wall. Under normal circumstances, these forces are produced by the respiratory muscles.

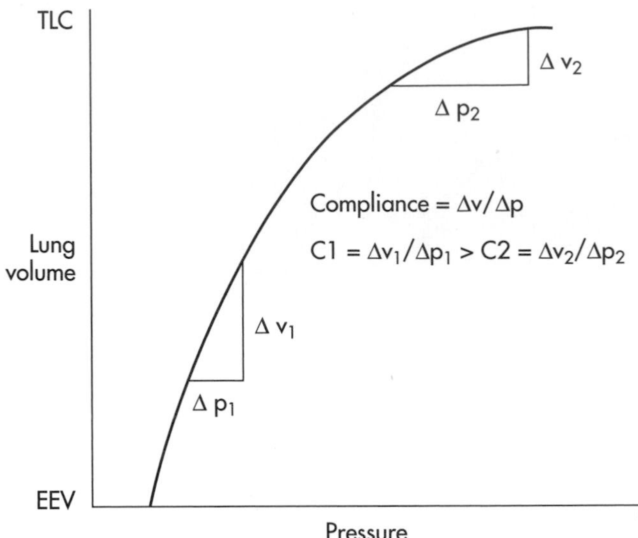

Fig. 15-4. Static pressure-volume curve of the lung allows calculation of compliance *(C),* which decreases at high lung volumes.

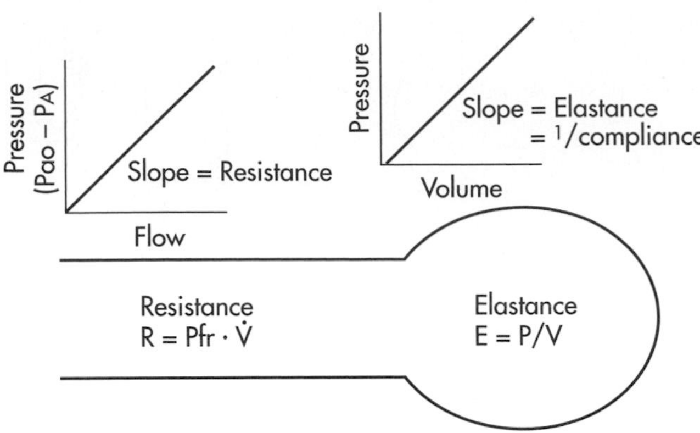

Fig. 15-5. Diagram of the single-compartment model of the lung, consisting of a resistance and compliance in series. *Pao,* Pressure at the airway opening.

The force required to move a block of wood over a surface is determined by the friction between the block of wood and the surface and by how fast the wood is moving. It is not, however, determined by the block's position. Similarly, the pressure required to produce a flow of gas between the atmosphere and the alveoli must overcome the frictional resistance of the airways. This pressure is proportional to the flow ($\dot{V}$) (i.e., the rate at which volume is changing), as follows:

$$Pao - P_A = Pfr \propto \dot{V}$$

where *Pao* is pressure at the airway opening (usually atmospheric pressure), *PA* is alveolar pressure, and *Pfr* is the pressure required to overcome frictional resistance. The pressure required to produce a unit of flow is known as the *flow resistance (R),* as follows:

$$R = Pfr/\dot{V}$$

Most commonly used tests of pulmonary function model the respiratory system as a single compartment with a single resistance and a single elastance (Fig. 15-5). The equation of motion describing the balance of forces acting on the system during ventilation follows:

$$P = EV + R\dot{V} + I\ddot{V}$$

where *P* is the applied pressure, *I* is the coefficient of inertance, *E* is elastance, $\dot{V}$ is gas flow, and $\ddot{V}$ is gas acceleration. Under most circumstances the inertance is negligible and therefore ignored. During spontaneous breathing, the applied pressure is produced by the respiratory muscles and can be measured as the transpulmonary pressure. During tidal respiration, approximately 90% of the applied pressure is required to overcome elastic forces, and approximately 10% is required to overcome flow-resistive forces.

Traditionally, the majority of the force developed during breathing has been thought to be required to move gas through the airways, with little energy dissipated by the tissues of the respiratory system. In recent years, the contribution of tissue viscoelasticity to the behavior of the respiratory system has become increasingly apparent. The energy expended moving the tissues has been called *tissue viscance* or *resistance,* although it is a non-newtonian resistance. When measured during inspiration, tissue resistance increases with increasing lung volume,[7,8] whereas airway resistance falls. Tissue resistance contributes approximately 65% of respiratory system resistance at FRC in mechanically ventilated animals and increases to as much as 95% at higher lung volumes.[8,9] The contribution of tissue resistance to respiratory system resistance in humans under the same circumstances is not known.

Measurement Techniques

Plethysmography

Airway resistance is most commonly measured in children by plethysmography. When a subject breathes within a plethysmograph, volume changes are recorded in proportion to variations in alveolar pressure and in alveolar gas volume (i.e., Vtg), provided volume changes due to other influences, such as changes in gas conditions from body temperature, pressure, and saturation within the lungs to ambient temperature and pressure (saturated) within the box, can be eliminated. Under these circumstances, the change in volume can be expressed as follows:

$$\Delta V = \Delta P_A \times Vtg/P_B$$

Alveolar pressure is the product of resistance to gas flow by flow at the airway opening *(Raw),* as follows:

$$\Delta V = (Raw + Req) \times \dot{V} \times Vtg/P_B$$

where *Req* is the resistance of the equipment connected to the airway. Calculation of airway resistance follows:

$$Raw = (\Delta V/\dot{V} \times P_B/Vtg) - Req$$

This technique has been standardized for use in adults and children and includes measuring Vtg, as previously described; opening the shutter; connecting the subject to the box or a gas-conditioning circuit through a flowmeter; and asking the patient to pant while supporting the cheeks with the hands. Panting is usually made at a frequency of 1 to 3 Hz with a V_T of 50 to 150 ml, giving a airway opening flow of 0.3 to 3.0 L/s peak to peak. Precise details are published elsewhere.[4]

Occlusion Techniques and Esophageal Manometry

Measurement of compliance in spontaneously breathing subjects requires either the subjects' relaxing the respiratory muscles against an occluded airway at various points during inspiration and expiration or the insertion of an esophageal balloon. These techniques measure compliance of the respiratory system and lung and are not commonly used in children. Thus these measurement techniques are not discussed here.

Forced Oscillation

Because the forced oscillation requires little active cooperation from the subject, it is attractive for use in children. It was introduced in the 1950s as a method for determining the impedance of the total respiratory system (Zrs) by applying sinusoidal variations in pressure to the respiratory system *(Prs)* and measuring the resulting flow.[10] In essence, Zrs is calculated from Prs/$\dot{V}$ and can be expressed as an amplitude ratio and a phase shift between the signals. This technique can also measure Zrs at different frequencies and thus represents the frequency-dependent behavior of the respiratory system (Fig. 15-6). It assumes that both the measuring system and the mechanical properties of the respiratory system are linear during the time of measurement and for the amplitude of the pressures applied.[11]

The signal applied to the respiratory system is known as a *forcing function.* Over the years a number of different forcing functions have been used to measure Zrs. The simplest consists of a single sinusoid, which measures Zrs at that (single) frequency. Measurements can be repeated at different frequencies and a picture of the frequency-dependent behavior of the respiratory system built. Alternatively, multiple sinusoids can be applied at the same time. If this approach is adopted, the clinician must carefully limit the amplitude of the resulting signal because too great an amplitude may be uncomfortable for the subject and result in nonlinear behavior of the respiratory system. Forcing functions can be optimized in a number of ways, such as ensuring that the components are not integer multiples of one another[12] or that no component is either the sum or the difference of other components.[13] Both of these optimization procedures are designed to reduce the effects of nonlinearities and to reduce harmonic distortion. For more detailed descriptions, the reader is referred to the specialized literature.

Whatever forcing function is used, some estimate of the reliability of the Zrs data is required. Reliability is generally assessed by determining the "coherence function." This is in essence the correlation between the input signal (the forcing function) and the output signal (the $\dot{V}$). Perfect correlation results in a coherence value of 1.0. By convention, Zrs is considered to be reliable if the coherence is at or above 0.95 at a particular frequency. Measurement noise reduces the reliability of Zrs, which is reflected in a decreased coherence. In this context the breathing frequency and heart rate can decrease the reliability of Zrs at those frequencies (and at their harmonics) and usually limit the lower end of the frequency spectrum that can be measured in children.[14-16]

Calculation of Zrs from data obtained using forcing functions that contain multiple frequencies is usually performed in the frequency domain. This is done using fast Fourier transformations or similar mathematic techniques. A description of the mathematics involved is beyond the scope of this chapter, but the resultant Zrs spectrum is conventionally expressed as *real* and *imaginary parts.* The real part is related to the component in phase with the pressure signal and reflects the resistive behavior of the respiratory system. The imaginary part is related to the component of flow out of phase with pressure and reflects the elastic and inertive behaviors of the respiratory system (see Fig. 15-6).

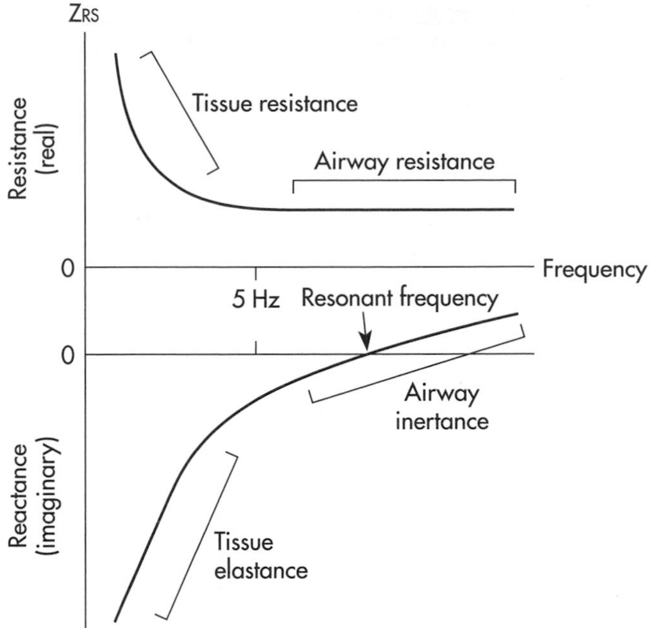

Fig. 15-6. Zrs data from the forced oscillation technique. Low-frequency data represent tissue elastance and resistance, and high-frequency data represent airway resistance and inertance. *Real* and *imaginary* are terms defining the phase relationship of the signals.

Many studies have used parameter-estimating techniques to produce values of resistance, elastance, and inertance from Zrs spectra.[16-24] These studies have demonstrated that the real part of Zrs reflects airway resistance at higher frequencies (above 5 to 10 Hz in adults and older children), whereas the low frequencies (<2 Hz) reflect the resistive properties of the lung tissues and chest wall (see Fig. 15-6). At low frequencies, the imaginary part is dominated by elastic behavior, whereas at high frequencies, inertive behavior dominates. The elastic and inertive behavior of the respiratory system are 180 degrees out of phase with each other (i.e., they have the opposite sign). The frequency at which these properties are equal and opposite and therefore cancel each other out is known as the *resonant frequency* of the respiratory system (see Fig. 15-6). This can be recognized as the frequency at which the imaginary part of Zrs crosses the zero axis. The resonant frequency has been reported to change with age and with lung disease.[14,16,25]

The use of forced oscillation in children has been limited by some of the practical problems encountered when applying this technique and by the lack of user-friendly, commercially available equipment. The following major technical problems need to be overcome:

1. Interference from the breathing frequency
2. Leak around the mouthpiece
3. Upper airway compliance

The breathing frequency causes a loss of coherence from the forcing function for up to five harmonics of the fundamental frequency. In practice, this means that no useful Zrs data are obtained at frequencies below 4 Hz in spontaneously breathing children. Adults are frequently able to hold their breath with their glottis open for long enough to measure Zrs at lower frequencies. This does not appear to be the case in most children.

Leak around the mouthpiece acts as a resistance pathway in parallel with the respiratory system. This resistance mainly affects the lower frequencies and results in overestimation of resistance and underestimation of elastance. The effect of a leak is compounded in situations in which the airway resistance is increased, such as with airway disease or during bronchoprovocation tests.

The compliance of the upper airways acts as a shunt compliance in parallel with the respiratory system. This results in shunting of the forcing function away from the respiratory system, especially at higher frequencies. This in turn results in overestimation of airway resistance and underestimation of inertance (with a shift of the resonant frequency to a higher frequency). The effect of a shunt compliance is increased in situations in which airway resistance is increased (see previous section).

MEASUREMENTS OF FORCED EXPIRATION

Measurements of forced expiration have become the major method used to detect the presence of obstructive lung disease. The use of such measurements is derived from the observation that expiratory flow is independent of the force driving flow over most of the expired VC as long as reasonable effort is made[26] (Fig. 15-7). This observation led directly to the description of the maximum expiratory flow volume (MEFV) curve, which emphasized that at most lung volumes, there was a limit to maximum expiratory flow ($\dot{V}_{max}$). The peak expiratory flow (PEF) is discussed later, and flows near RV may be effort dependent because expiratory muscle contraction may not be able to provide sufficient force to maintain flow limitation at this low lung volume.

Flow Limitation

The mechanism for expiratory flow limitation is complex. Elegant descriptions can be read in the *Handbook of Physiology* published by the American Physiological Society.[27] In fluid dynamic terms, a system cannot carry a greater flow than the flow for which fluid velocity equals wave speed at some point in the system. The wave speed is the speed at which a small disturbance travels in a compliant tube filled with fluid. In the arteries, this is the speed at which the pulse propagates. In the airway the speed is higher than this, mainly because the fluid density is lower. The wave speed *(c)* in a compliant tube with an area *(A)* that depends on a lateral pressure *(P)* filled with a fluid of density *(ρ),* is given by:

$$c = (AdP/\rho dA)^{1/2}$$

where *dP/dA* is the slope of the pressure-area curve for the airway (i.e., an expression of airway wall compliance). $\dot{V}_{max}$ is the product of the airway area and fluid velocity at wave speed, as follows:

$$\dot{V}_{max} = cA$$

At high lung volumes the flow-limiting site in the human airways is typically in the second and third airway generations. As lung volume decreases, airway caliber decreases, the flow-limiting site moves peripherally, and $\dot{V}_{max}$ decreases. At low lung volumes the density dependence of $\dot{V}_{max}$ is small, and the viscosity dependence is large and becomes the predominant mechanism limiting expiratory flow.

Flow limitation in a compliant tube is accompanied by "flutter" of the walls at the site of flow limitation.[28] This flutter conserves the energy in the system because the driving pressure in excess of that required to produce $\dot{V}_{max}$ is dissipated in causing the wall flutter. In the presence of airway obstruction, this flutter may become large enough to generate sound, which is heard as wheezing. Thus expiratory wheezing is a sign of expiratory flow limitation.

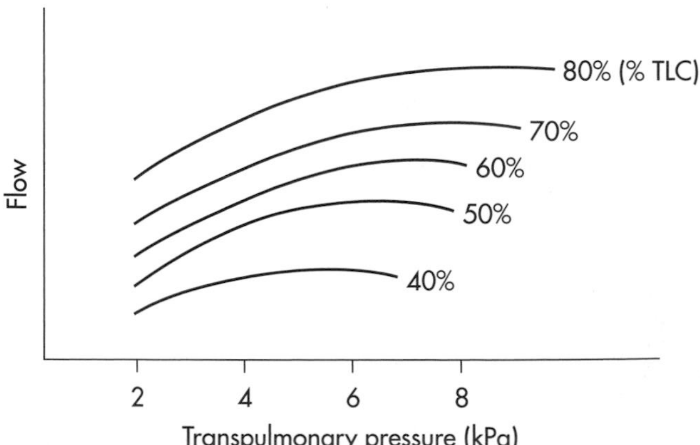

Fig. 15-7. Isovolume pressure-flow curves in a normal adult at different proportions of TLC. (From Tammeling GJ, Quanjer PH: *Contours of breathing,* Burlington, Ontario, Canada, 1985, Boehringer Ingelheim Pharmaceuticals.)

MEFV Curves

Most children can accomplish forced expiratory maneuvers by the age of 7 years. To produce reliable MEFV curves, children need to be able to give a maximal effort without hesitation for at least 3 seconds. In young children, a learning effect may be operative, so more than the standard three tests may be required to obtain consistent, representative data. The VC and the forced expiratory volume in 1 second are the most informative measures. Forced expiratory flows at lower lung volumes are more sensitive, but their variability is greater. The forced expiratory flow occurring between 25% and 75% of expired VC is frequently used as an indication of "small airway" disease. This practice is based on the assumption that the site of flow limitation is likely to exist in the small airways over this volume range. There is no direct evidence to support this assumption, especially in children. Figure 15-8 shows the relationship between the spirogram (a volume-time plot of forced expiration) and an MEFV curve.

Peak Expiratory Flow

Measurements of PEF are of value in identifying and assessing the degree of airflow limitation in epidemiologic studies and in clinical practice, where they can be helpful in monitoring the progress of disease and the effects of treatment. PEF is the maximum flow achieved during a forced expiration starting from the level of maximal lung inflation.[29]

Traditionally, PEF was not thought to be flow limited because a plateau is not seen on isovolume pressure-flow curves, presumably because of the inability of the respiratory muscles to generate sufficient force. Recently, Pedersen[30] argued that PEF is likely to match wave speed (Vws) if forced expiratory flow has a well-defined peak. He calculated wave speed from measurements of dA/dPtm and cross-sectional area *(A)*, measuring intrabronchial pressure using a pitot static probe. He proposed that using a speed index defined as the actual velocity (V/A) divided by the wave speed (Vws/A), PEF is just limited with a speed index of 1 in the central airways. Kano et al[31] demonstrated that PEF was decreased by performing forced expiration after a breath hold at TLC. They proposed that the breath hold allowed viscoelastic energy in the airway wall to be dissipated, resulting in a reduction of airway wall compliance. This would result in a reduction of dA/dPtm and a reduction in the wave speed achievable. These observations are consistent with flow limitation being achieved at PEF.

This does not, however, mean that PEF is independent of effort. The magnitude of PEF depends on how this maximum flow is reached. If expired volume from the TLC at which PEF is reached is small, PEF will be higher because at higher lung volume, the higher elastic recoil pressure and lower upstream resistance result in a greater wave speed and a higher PEF. In any interpretation of changes in PEF, the magnitude of effort and the volume at which PEF is reached are critical.

Miniature PEF meters are cheap and portable and can be used in the home. However, recent studies using explosive decompression devices and computer-controlled pumps have clearly demonstrated that the miniflow meters currently used for monitoring PEF are inaccurate, with substantial overestimation of flow in the range of 200 to 400 L/min.[32] This range is commonly encountered in pediatric practice. This error is thought to come from nonlinear characteristics of the critical orifice within the meter.[33] We have recently demonstrated a similar pattern of errors in children age 6 to 19 years when PEF measured using a miniflow meter was compared with that measured using a spirometer.[34] In theory, this error can be corrected by adjusting the scale on the flowmeter.[32]

Although PEF increases with height during childhood, at any given height, there is a wide range of normal values. This limits the usefulness of expressing a measured PEF as a percentage of predicted normal based on population studies. Thus the clinician needs to determine each child's "personal best" PEF by monitoring it for 1 to 2 weeks at a time when the child is well. This value can then be used as a basis for comparison during exacerbations of asthma.

REFERENCES

1. Le Souëf PN, La Fortune BC, Landau LI: Spirometric assessment of asthmatic children aged two to six years, *Aust NZ J Med* 16:625, 1986.
2. Sly PD, Hibbert ME: Childhood asthma following hospitalization with acute viral bronchiolitis in infancy, *Pediatr Pulmonol* 7:153-158, 1989.
3. Sly PD, Robertson CF: Pulmonary function testing in children, *Med J Aust* 150:706-707, 1989.

Lung Volumes

4. Peslin R: Body plethysmography. In Otis AB, ed: *Techniques in respiratory physiology.* Part II. Techniques in the life sciences, New York, 1984, Elsevier, pp 414/1-414/25.
5. Hutchinson AA, Erben A, Mclennan LA, Landau LI, Phelan PD: Intrasubject variability of pulmonary function testing in healthy children, *Thorax* 36:370-377, 1981.
6. Clausen JL, ed: *Pulmonary function testing in children: guidelines and controversies*, New York, 1984, Grune & Stratton.

Resistance and Compliance

7. Sly PD, Brown KA, Bates JHT, Macklem PT, Milic-Emili J, Martin JG: The effect of lung volume on interrupter resistance in cats challenged with methacholine, *J Appl Physiol* 64:360-366, 1988.
8. Ludwig MS, Dreshaj I, Solway J, Munoz A, Ingram RH: Partitioning of pulmonary resistance during constriction in the dog: effects of volume history, *J Appl Physiol* 62:807-815, 1987.
9. Sly PD, Lanteri CJ: Differential responses of the airways and pulmonary tissues to inhaled histamine in young dogs, *J Appl Physiol* 68:1562-1567, 1990.

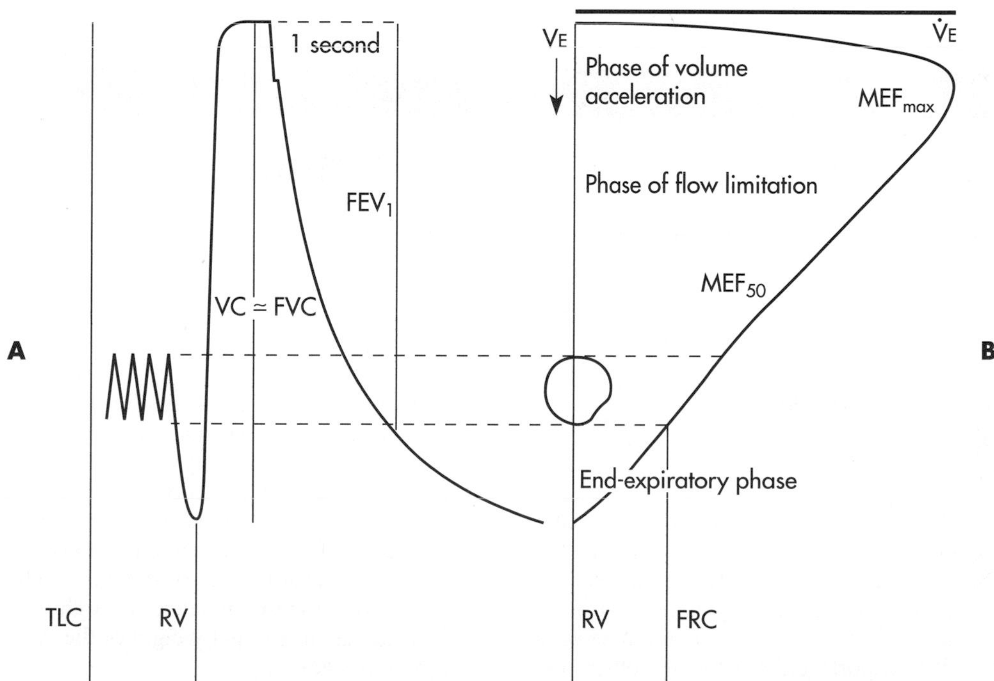

Fig. 15-8. **A,** Spirogram. **B,** MEFV curve. *FEV_1*, Forced expiratory volume in 1 second. (From Tammeling GJ, Quanjer PH: *Contours of breathing,* Burlington, Ontario, Canada, 1985, Boehringer Ingelheim Pharmaceuticals.)

10. DuBois AB, Brody AW, Lewis DH, Burgess F: Oscillation mechanics of lungs and chest in man, *Department of Pharmacology and Physiology* 8:587-594, 1955.
11. Goldman M, Knudson RJ, Mead J, Peterson N, Schwaber JR, Wohl ME: A simplified measurement of respiratory resistance by forced oscillation, *J Appl Physiol* 28(1):113-116, 1970.
12. Hantos Z, Daroczy B, Suki B, Nagy S, Fredberg JJ: Input impedance and peripheral inhomogeneity of dog lungs, *J Appl Physiol* 72(1):168-178, 1992.
13. Lutchen KR, Yang K, Kaczka DW, Suki B: Optimal ventilation waveforms for estimating low-frequency respiratory impedance, *J Appl Physiol* 75(1):478-488, 1993.
14. Clement J, Dumoulin B, Gubbelmans R, Hendriks S, van de Woestijne KP: Reference values of total respiratory resistance and reactance between 4 and 26 Hz in children and adolescents aged 4-20 years, *Bull Eur Physiopathol Respir* 23:441-448, 1987.
15. Desager KN, Buhr W, Willemen M, Van Bever HP, de Backer W, Vermeire PA, Láundsér FJ: Measurement of total respiratory impedance in infants by the forced oscillation technique, *J Appl Physiol* 41:101-106, 1991.
16. Hantos Z, Daroczy B, Gyurkovits K: Total respiratory impedance in healthy children, *Pediatr Pulmonol* 1(2):91-98, 1985.
17. Jackson AC, Neff KM, Lutchen KR, Dorkin HL: Interpretation of respiratory system impedance (4-256 hz) in healthy infants, *Eur Respir Rev* 19:165-166, 1994.
18. Farre R, Peslin R, Oostveen E, Suki B, Duvivier C, Navajas D: Human respiratory impedance from 8 to 256 Hz corrected for upper airway shunt, *J Appl Physiol* 67:1973-1981, 1989.
19. Lutchen KR, Saidel GM: Estimation of mechanical parameters in multicompartment models applied to normal and obstructed lungs during tidal breathing, *IEEE Trans Biomed Eng* 33(9):878-887, 1986.
20. Lutchen KR, Jackson AC: Reliability of parameter estimates from models applied to respiratory impedance data, *J Appl Physiol* 62(2):403-413, 1987.
21. Lutchen KR, Hantos Z, Jackson AC: Importance of low-frequency impedance data for reliably quantifying parallel inhomogeneities of respiratory mechanics [published erratum appears in *IEEE Trans Biomed Eng* 35(9):765, 1988], *IEEE Trans Biomed Eng* 35(6):472-481, 1988.
22. Lutchen KR: Optimal selection of frequencies for estimating parameters from respiratory impedance data, *IEEE Trans Biomed Eng* 35(8):607-617, 1988.
23. Lutchen KR, Jackson AC: Confidence bounds on respiratory mechanical properties estimated from transfer versus input impedance in humans versus dogs, *IEEE Trans Biomed Eng* 39(6):644-651, 1992.
24. Lutchen KR, Everett JR, Jackson AC: Impact of frequency range and input impedance on airway-tissue separation implied from transfer impedance, *J Appl Physiol* 74(3):1089-1099, 1993.
25. Solymar L, Aronsson MD, Sixt R: The forced oscillation technique in children with respiratory disease, *Pediatr Pulmonol* 1:256-261, 1985.

Measurements of Forced Expiration

26. Fry DL, Hyatt RE: Pulmonary mechanics: a unified analysis of the relationship between pressure, volume and gas flow in the lungs of normal and diseased human subjects, *Am J Med* 29:672-689, 1960.
27. Wilson TA, Rodarte JR, Butler JP: Wave-speed and viscous flow limitation. In Macklem PT, Mead J, eds: *Handbook of physiology,* Section 3: The respiratory system, Bethesda, Md, 1986, American Physiological Society, pp 55-62.
28. Gavriely N, Kelly KB, Grotberg JB, Loring SH: Forced expiratory wheezes are a manifestation of flow limitation, *J Appl Physiol* 62:2398-2403, 1987.
29. Quanjer PH, Lebowitz MD, Gregg I, eds: Peak expiratory flow: conclusions and recommendations of a working party of the European Respiratory Society, *Eur Respir J* 1993.
30. Pedersen OF: Physiological determinants of peak expiratory flow: report of the European Respiratory Society Peak Flow Working Group, *Eur Respir J* (in press).
31. Kano S, Burton DL, Lanteri CJ, Sly PD: Determination of peak expiratory flow, *Eur Respir J* 6:1347-1352, 1993.
32. Miller MR, Dickinson SA, Hitchings DJ: The accuracy of portable peak flow meters, *Thorax* 47:904-909, 1992.
33. Pedersen OF: Personal communication.
34. Sly PD, Cahill P, Willet K, Burton P: Accuracy of mini peak flow meters following changes in lung function in asthmatic children, *Br Med J* 308:572-574, 1994.

CHAPTER 16

Gas Exchange and Acid-Base Physiology

Peter D. Yorgin and Kyoo Hwan Rhee

BASIC PHYSIOLOGY OF GAS EXCHANGE AND ACID BASE

Normal Gas Exchange

In the body, gas exchange occurs by simple diffusion at the lung (pulmonary gas exchange) and at the tissue (intracellular gas exchange). Once a gas has diffused into the blood at a site of gas exchange, it is dissolved into plasma, it binds to hemoglobin (loading), or both processes occur. When a gas circulates with blood (transport) and reaches the other site of gas exchange, it is released from the blood (unloading), thus completing the process of gas exchange. Eventually, oxygen is consumed in the tissue, and carbon dioxide is eliminated through the lungs.

Oxygenation, the process by which oxygen is added to the pulmonary blood, occurs at the pulmonary alveolar level. The term *ventilation* generally refers to the removal of carbon dioxide from the alveoli. The rate of gas diffusion through the membrane is determined by several factors, including (1) the pressure difference of each gas between two sides of the membrane, (2) the solubility of the gas, (3) the surface area of the membrane, (4) the distance through which the gas must diffuse, (5) the molecular weight of the gas, and (6) the temperature of the gas.[1]

The relative rates at which different gases at the same pressure diffuse are proportional to their diffusion coefficients. Solubility and molecular weight are two important factors that determine the diffusion coefficient of a gas. If the diffusion coefficient for oxygen is 1, the relative diffusion coefficients for different gases in the body fluid are as follows: carbon dioxide, 20.3; carbon monoxide, 0.81; nitrogen, 0.53; and helium, 0.95. Therefore carbon dioxide diffuses more rapidly than oxygen across membranes. Equilibration at alveolar level, however, is roughly equal for both carbon dioxide and oxygen because the driving pressure of oxygen (partial pressure of alveolar oxygen − partial pressure of pulmonary end-capillary oxygen ≈ 100 − 40 ≈ 60 mm Hg) is much higher than that of carbon dioxide (partial pressure of pulmonary end-capillary carbon dioxide (partial pressure of alveolar carbon dioxide ≈ 45 − 40 ≈ 5 mm Hg).

In normal spontaneous respiration, oxygenation and ventilation occur simultaneously. Any change in ventilation also has an impact on oxygenation. Ventilation with fresh room air carries oxygen at about 150 mm Hg into the alveolus to oxygenate desaturated pulmonary arterial blood with a partial pressure of oxygen (Po_2) of about 40 mm Hg. The same gas delivered to the alveolus by ventilation contains effectively no carbon dioxide and allows the removal of carbon dioxide from pulmonary arterial blood with an equilibration at about 40 mm Hg. Oxygenation and ventilation, however, can be independently controlled during artificial respiration. Oxygenation improves with increased alveolar Po_2, increased pulmonary blood exposure to oxygen, or both processes. Alveolar Po_2 increases as the concentration of inspired oxygen (FIo_2) increases. Continuous positive airway pressure and positive end-expiratory pressure determine the level of positive alveolar pressure. The amount of surface area available for gas exchange increases with positive airway pressure as additional alveoli are recruited. Functionally, the recruitment of collapsed alveoli increases the cross-sectional area exposed to oxygen. Moreover, the thickness of the interstitial space, the area between the alveolar and capillary basement membranes, is also affected by alveolar pressure. Higher alveolar pressures decrease the thickness of the interstitial space, allowing more effective gas exchange. Although positive alveolar pressure improves oxygenation, it is important to note that excessive distention of the alveolus with high alveolar pressure may lead to reduced pulmonary blood flow and the development of alveolar dead space with ventilation-perfusion mismatch.

Ventilation improves with increased tidal volume, increased respiratory rate, or both. Ventilation decreases the partial pressure of carbon dioxide (Pco_2) in the alveoli, thereby maintaining a lower alveolar Pco_2 relative to the pulmonary end-capillary Pco_2. If there were no difference between alveolar Pco_2 and pulmonary end-capillary Pco_2, then diffusion of carbon dioxide from the blood into the alveoli would not occur. Because the diffusion coefficient of carbon dioxide is 20 times higher than that of oxygen, only a small gradient of Pco_2 (5 to 7 mm Hg) is required to support diffusion across the intact alveolar membrane and remove the carbon dioxide produced in intracellular metabolism.

Oxygen

Loading. Alveolar Po_2 (PAo_2) can be calculated using the following equation[2]:

$$\begin{aligned} PAO_2 &= PIO_2 - PACO_2/R + F \approx 0.21\,(760 - 47) - \frac{40}{0.8} \\ &\approx FIO_2\,(PB - P_{H_2O}) - PACO_2/R \approx 150 - 50 \\ &\approx FIO_2\,(PB - 47) - PACO_2/R \approx 100 \\ &\approx FIO_2\,(PB - 47) - \frac{40}{0.8} \end{aligned}$$

where PIo_2 is the partial pressure of oxygen in the conducting airway (150 mm Hg at sea level in room air), $PACO_2$ is the partial pressure of alveolar carbon dioxide, *R* is the respiratory exchange quotient (carbon dioxide produced/oxygen consumed ≈ 0.8), *F* is the correction factor, *PB* is the barometric pressure (760 mm Hg at sea level), and P_{H_2O} is the water vapor pressure (47 mm Hg at 37° C).

The approximate alveolar Po_2 in room air is 100 mm Hg at sea level, and the Po_2 of the venous blood entering the pulmonary end-capillary bed averages 40 mm Hg at sea level. Oxygen diffuses into the blood from alveoli with the pressure difference of approximately 60 mm Hg. The Po_2 in pulmonary end-capillary blood rises quickly to the level of alveolar Po_2. Because bronchial circulation, which accounts for 2% of the total pulmonary blood flow, bypasses pulmonary circulation (shunt flow), the Po_2 in arterial blood decreases to approximately 95 mm Hg.

Normally, about 97% of the oxygen in the blood is transported in chemical combination with hemoglobin in the red blood cells, and the remaining 3% is carried in the dissolved state in the water of plasma and cells. Thus under normal conditions, oxygen is transported to the tissues almost entirely by hemoglobin. Each hemoglobin molecule can loosely bind to four oxygen molecules. The percentage of the hemoglobin bound with oxygen increases as blood Po_2 increases. The affinity of hemoglobin for oxygen increases after the hemoglobin has previously bound with other oxygen molecules.[3] The relationship between oxygen affinity and hemoglobin is described by the oxygen-hemoglobin dissociation curve. This curve is an S-shaped curve that increases maximally between a PO_2 of 10 and 50 mm Hg. In a healthy individual, arterial blood has a Po_2 of 95 mm Hg, and the oxygen saturation is about 97%. On the other hand, a normal systemic venous Po_2 is about 40 mm Hg, and the oxygen saturation of hemoglobin is about 75%. The ability of hemoglobin to bind oxygen changes in various conditions, and the oxygen saturation may vary at the same Po_2 (Fig. 16-1, *A*). The following factors affect oxyhemoglobin affinity: the hemoglobin amino acid sequence (hemoglobinopathy, carboxyhemoglobin, methemoglobin), temperature, Pco_2, pH, and concentration of 2,3-diphosphoglycerate. For example, when blood carbon dioxide is removed by the lung and the blood pH increases, the oxygen-hemoglobin dissociation curve shifts to the left, and more oxygen binds to hemoglobin for transport (Bohr effect).[4] On the other hand, oxygen affinity to hemoglobin decreases with decreased pH and increased Pco_2 in the tissues. The oxygen-hemoglobin dissociation curve shifts to the right, and the Po_2 required to saturate 50% of functional hemoglobin increases to facilitate unloading of oxygen to the tissue (Fig. 16-1, *B*).

Transport. Once hemoglobin binds oxygen to become oxyhemoglobin, blood flow transports the oxyhemoglobin to the tissue, where oxygen is needed for efficient energy production.

The total amount of oxygen transported to the tissue is calculated as follows[5]:

$$\begin{aligned} \dot{D}o_2 &= CO \times Cao_2 \\ &= CO \times (Hgb \times Sao_2 \times 1.34) + (Pao_2 \times 0.003) \\ &\approx CO \times Hgb \times Sao_2 \end{aligned}$$

where $\dot{D}o_2$ is the total amount of oxygen delivered per minute (in liters per minute), *CO* is cardiac output (in liters per minute), Cao_2 is arterial oxygen content (in milliliters per

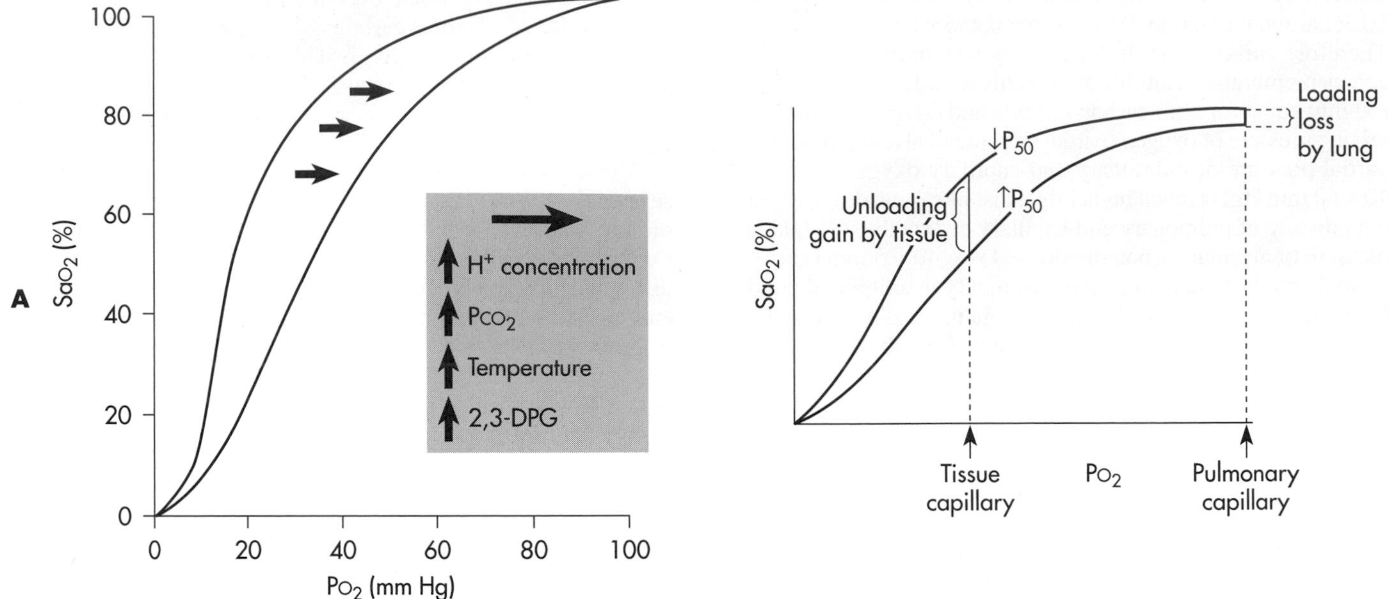

Fig. 16-1. **A,** Shift of the oxygen-hemoglobin dissociation curve to the right by an increase in the number of hydrogen ions *(H^+)*, the number of carbon dioxide molecules, the temperature, or the concentration of 2,3-diphosphoglycerate *(2,3-DPG)*. **B,** The effect on oxygen loading and unloading caused by an increase in oxygen affinity (decrease in Po_2 required to saturate 50% of functional hemoglobin [P_{50}]) and a decrease in oxygen affinity (increase in P_{50}). The loading loss and unloading loss and gain are indicated by the heights of the heavy vertical bars between the two curves. Sao_2, Arterial oxygen saturation. (From Klocke RA. In Bryan-Brown CW, Ayres SM, eds: *Oxygen transport and utilization: new horizons,* Fullerton, Calif, 1987, Society of Critical Care Medicine, p 243.)

liter), *Hgb* is hemoglobin (grams per deciliter of blood), Sao_2 is arterial oxygen saturation (percentage), and Pao_2 is the partial pressure of arterial oxygen (in millimeters of mercury). The dissolved oxygen per Po_2 per deciliter of blood is 0.003 ml/mm Hg/dl of blood.

Example: What is the amount of oxygen delivered when the cardiac output is 5.0 L/min with a hemoglobin level of 15 g/dl, an arterial oxygen saturation of 100%, and an arterial Po_2 of 100 mm Hg?

$$\begin{aligned}\dot{D}o_2 &= CO \times Cao_2\\ &= CO \times (Hgb \times Sao_2 \times 1.34) + (Pao_2 \times 0.003)\\ &= 5.0\ \text{L/min} \times \{(15\ \text{g/dl} \times 1.34) + (100\ \text{mm Hg} \times 0.003\ \text{ml/mm Hg/dl})\}\\ &= 5.0\ \text{L/min} \times \{(20.1\ \text{ml/dl}) + (0.3\ \text{ml/dl})\}\\ &= 5.0\ \text{L/min} \times \{(20.1 + 0.3)\ \text{ml/dl}\}\\ &= 5.0\ \text{L/min} \times 204\ \text{ml/L}\\ &= 1020\ \text{ml of oxygen/min}\end{aligned}$$

It is worth noting that the major factors affecting oxygen delivery include cardiac output, hemoglobin level, and oxygen saturation, whereas the effect of dissolved oxygen from arterial Po_2 is minuscule (20.1 vs. 0.3 ml/dl).

Unloading. When oxyhemoglobin reaches the low Po_2 environment in the tissue, the hemoglobin quickly unloads oxygen. The amount of oxygen unloaded depends on the Po_2 gradient between blood and tissue. When the tissue consumes more oxygen, the tissue Po_2 decreases. Thus the Po_2 gradient between the blood and tissue increases and allows the hemoglobin to unload more oxygen. If the blood Po_2 is higher than the level necessary to fully saturate hemoglobin with oxygen, however, the amount of oxygen that the hemoglobin unloads changes little (see Fig. 16-1, *B*). The Bohr effect facilitates unloading of oxygen in the tissue, where carbon dioxide and hydrogen ion levels increase, thus reducing hemoglobin's affinity for oxygen.

Carbon Dioxide

Loading. Unlike oxygen, which primarily binds with hemoglobin, carbon dioxide is carried in four different forms. First, a significant portion of carbon dioxide is transported in the dissolved state, although a small portion of the dissolved carbon dioxide is removed with a small arteriovenous difference. The amount of dissolved carbon dioxide in venous blood is 2.7 ml/dl (Pco_2 of 45 mm Hg) and 2.4 ml/dl at the level of the alveoli (Pco_2 of 40 mm Hg). Because the rate of carbon dioxide diffusion into alveoli depends on the difference between alveolar and venous blood levels of carbon dioxide, the small difference between the levels of dissolved and alveolar carbon dioxide (only 0.3 ml/dl) does not lead to clinically significant carbon dioxide removal.

Second, the dissolved carbon dioxide in the blood reacts with water to form carbonic acid. This mechanism accounts for a very small amount of carbon dioxide transport. There is a direct relationship between carbonic acid and dissolved carbon dioxide. At 37° C, each carbonic acid molecule is in equilibrium with 340 molecules of carbon dioxide. As the level of carbon dioxide increases, the level of carbonic acid also increases. Because Pco_2 and carbonic acid values are higher in venous blood than in arterial blood, venous blood is slightly more acidic (pH, 7.38) than arterial blood (pH, 7.40).

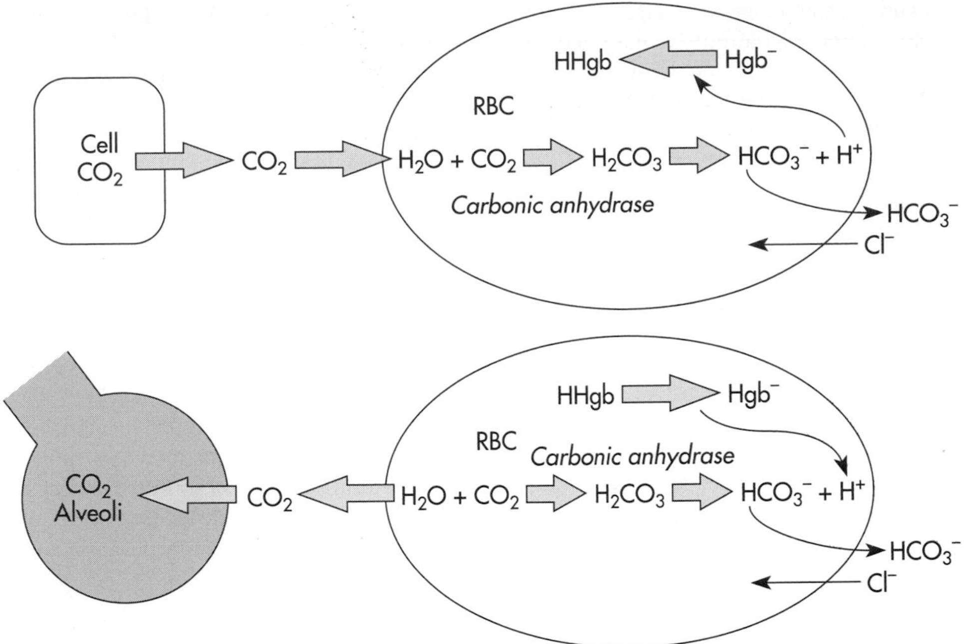

Fig. 16-2. Carbon dioxide transport is facilitated by red blood cells *(RBC)*. A major portion of the carbon dioxide produced by tissues is transported to the lungs as bicarbonate *(H_2CO_3)*. As carbon dioxide enters the red blood cell, carbonic acid *(HCO_3^-)* is formed and subsequently dissociates to form bicarbonate and a hydrogen ion *(H^+)*. As the hydrogen ion binds with hemoglobin *(Hgb)*, bicarbonate leaves the cell in exchange for chloride *(Cl^-)* (chloride shift). At the alveolar level, the red blood cell undergoes the same process in reverse. *HHgb,* Hydrogen ion bound to Hgb. (Modified from Malley WJ: *Clinical blood gases,* Philadelphia, 1990, WB Saunders, p 113.)

Third, a majority of carbon dioxide travels to the lung in the form of bicarbonate. This is a reversible reaction and accounts for about 70% of the carbon dioxide transported from the tissue to the lung. Although some of the carbon dioxide that enters the blood forms bicarbonate, the amount formed tends to be very small because of the slow reaction rate in plasma. Carbon dioxide diffuses into erythrocytes, where carbonic acid formation rapidly occurs because of carbonic anhydrase in the red blood cells (Fig. 16-2). The three carbonic anhydrase isoenzymes follow: A (also III), B (also I), and C (also II). Two isozymes, B and C, are found in red blood cells. The carbonic acid is hydrolyzed to hydrogen ions and bicarbonate. The hydrogen ion is rapidly buffered by binding to hemoglobin. Bicarbonate diffuses into the plasma via a bicarbonate chloride carrier protein while the chloride moves into the red blood cell to maintain electrochemical neutrality. Red blood cell carbonic anhydrase is so important in the transport of carbon dioxide from cells that inhibition of carbonic anhydrase would lead to profoundly elevated intracellular carbon dioxide values.

Fourth, carbon dioxide reacts directly with amine radicals of hemoglobin molecules to form the compound carbaminohemoglobin. The reaction is slow and accounts only for 20% of carbon dioxide to be removed. The loading process of carbon dioxide in the tissue is facilitated by the Haldane effect; the carbon dioxide–carrying capacity of hemoglobin increases when the oxygen molecule is unloaded at the tissue level.

Transport. Meanwhile, carbon dioxide, which is produced in the tissue, diffuses into the blood, and blood flow carries the three different forms of carbon dioxide to the lung for elimination. Blood flow is a major determining factor in gas transport when the amount of gas loaded remains constant. Besides cardiac output, blood viscosity (e.g., polycythemia) and red cell deformability (e.g., sickle cell, microcyte) affect microcirculation and play important roles in gas exchange at the tissue level.[6]

Unloading. Carbon dioxide is produced in the tissue and carried to the lung as dissolved carbon dioxide, carbonic acid, carbaminohemoglobin, and bicarbonate ions for elimination by pulmonary gas exchange. In a normal adult, normal ventilation disposes of an average of 10,000 to 15,000 mmol of carbon dioxide per day. As the dissolved carbon dioxide diffuses across the alveolar membrane, carbonic acid dissociates to form water and carbon dioxide. As the plasma carbon dioxide levels decrease, carbonic acid in the red blood cells is converted into carbon dioxide and water by carbonic anhydrase (see Fig. 16-2). Carbonic anhydrase inhibitors may increase carbon dioxide tension in the tissues and decrease carbon dioxide tension in the alveoli. A transient decrease in the rate of carbon dioxide elimination results but is rapidly overcome by compensatory mechanisms. When carbon dioxide moves out of the erythrocyte, bicarbonate moves back in exchange for chloride. The bicarbonate is necessary to replenish the bicarbonate consumed in the hydrolysis reaction. Carbaminohemoglobin unloads the carbon dioxide in the lung, where the P_{CO_2} is lower. The process of carbon dioxide loading and unloading is facilitated by the Haldane effect; the binding of oxygen with hemoglobin displaces carbon dioxide from the hemoglobin. The concept of the Haldane effect is that like the Bohr effect in oxygen carriage, the affinity of hemoglobin to carbon dioxide varies with chemical conditions such as P_{O_2}. When hemoglobin is oxygenated in the lung to release hydrogen ions, carbonic acid and ultimately carbon dioxide are produced, with the effect being a reduced affinity to carbon dioxide in the lung resulting from oxygenation (see Fig. 16-2, *bottom*). In the tissue, the hemoglobin gives up oxygen and takes up or buffers hydrogen, leading to increased affinity for carbon dioxide (see Fig. 16-2, *top*).

Abnormal Gas Exchange

When any step in the process of gas exchange between the lung and the tissue is inhibited, less oxygen reaches the tissue. The lack of oxygen causes hypoxic cellular damage. Moreover, the level of intracellular carbon dioxide increases and ultimately creates a hypercapnic acidosis. Hypoxic injury and hypercapnic acidosis can be caused by defective pulmonary gas exchange, loading, transporting, or unloading or defective tissue gas exchange. If not corrected in time, these conditions can cause irreversible tissue damage. Therefore it is important to understand the pathophysiology of the hypoxia and hypercapnia to find their causes and give specific therapy before any permanent tissue damage occurs.

Hypoxia

Pathophysiology. Cells require a continuous supply of energy to perform their functions within an organ and to maintain adequate control over membrane permeability.[7] A failure of cellular energy metabolism results in organ dysfunction and cell death as control is lost over solute and metabolite exchange across the membrane.[8]

Generation of energy occurs in both the presence and absence of oxygen, although aerobic metabolism using oxygen is the most efficient method of energy production. Approximately 20 times more energy is produced in mitochondria by oxidative phosphorylation when substrate consumption is coupled to the consumption of oxygen than when it is without oxygen.[9] Adenosine triphosphate (ATP) in mitochondria diffuses to the sites of energy use in the cytosol, where a large amount of chemical energy is released from the hydrolysis of one of ATP's high-energy phosphate bonds. The adenosinetriphosphatases (ATPases) are the enzymes that control the hydrolysis of ATP, resulting in the formation of adenosine diphosphate (ADP), inorganic phosphate *(Pi),* and a hydrogen ion *(H⁺)*, as follows:

$$ATP \rightarrow ADP + Pi + H^+$$

ADP, inorganic phosphate, and the hydrogen ion return to the mitochondria, where they serve as substrates for the formation of other ATP molecules.

An imbalance between the rate of ATP supply to the cell and the demands for energy results in intracellular accumulation of ADP, inorganic phosphate, and hydrogen ions. Changes in the concentration of these metabolites serve as feedback signals to modulate the pattern of substrate use by the cells and to promote anaerobic synthesis of ATP. The three sources of anaerobic ATP production follow: glycolysis, the creatine kinase reaction, and the adenyl kinase reaction.

Glycolysis is a universal cellular reaction to hypoxia in which glucose or glycogen is metabolized to lactate with the production of ATP. The overall reaction of glycolysis is as follows:

$$Glucose + 2\ ADP + 2\ Pi \rightarrow 2\ Lactate + 2\ ATP$$

The production of ATP by glycolysis is inefficient because only 2 mol of ATP are produced per mole of glucose consumed compared with 38 mol of ATP when glycolysis is coupled to oxidative phosphorylation.

In some organs and tissues with high metabolic demands, such as the brain, the heart, and skeletal muscle, the creatine kinase reaction is used as a ready anaerobic source of ATP in addition to that provided by glycolysis. In this reaction, phosphocreatine *(PCr)* is metabolized to creatine, transferring its high-energy phosphate bond to ATP. This reaction also helps buffer intracellular acidosis by using the hydrogen ion *(H^+)*, as follows:

$$PCr + ADP + H^+ \leftrightarrow ATP + Creatine$$

Under physiologic conditions, the creatine kinase reaction is in equilibrium. Increases in the levels of ADP and hydrogen ions during hypoxia promote the formation of ATP and creatine, whereas the opposite occurs when the supplies of ATP rise.

The third anaerobic source of energy is the adenyl kinase reaction. Two ADP molecules are converted into one ATP molecule and one adenosine monophosphate *(AMP)* molecule, as follows:

$$ADP + ADP \rightarrow ATP + AMP$$

The production of adenosine monophosphate leads to the formation of adenosine by the 5′-nucleotidase reaction. Because adenosine is a potent vasodilator, blood flow increases in the hypoxic tissue, transporting more oxygen in response to hypoxia.[10-12]

Measuring the metabolic by-products of the anaerobic reactions, such as the arterial lactate level, may be useful in monitoring the adequacy of global tissue oxygenation. These metabolic by-products, however, do not reflect the hypoxic status of individual organs because of the variable regional blood flow to each organ, changes in tissue lactate accumulation, and washout.[13] While being metabolized by various organs, lactate is released by the liver in response to circulating catecholamines. Lactate metabolism in the body is complicated, making the interpretation of a lactate value difficult.

Phosphorus-31 magnetic resonance spectroscopy can monitor ATP formation, which is indicative of the adequacy of tissue oxygenation.[14] This method has some advantages over other techniques because it measures in a noninvasive manner the level of high-energy phosphate regionally, such as in skeletal muscle, the brain, and the heart. The major drawback is that the patient needs to be in a magnetic cylinder that limits the use of other monitoring devices. Thus phosphate-31 magnetic resonance is impractical to use in a critical care setting.

Causes of Tissue Hypoxia. As mentioned earlier, each step in oxygenation, including pulmonary gas exchange, loading, transporting, and unloading and finally tissue gas exchange, may cause hypoxic cellular damage (Box 16-1).

Normally, the amount of oxygen delivered to the tissue is 3 to 4 times the amount of oxygen the tissue consumes. There is a significant reserve before the oxygen level reaches the critical point where tissue hypoxia occurs (Fig. 16-3). Therefore arterial hypoxemia, which is the state of low blood oxygen content resulting from low Po_2, does not necessarily create tissue hypoxia. As long as capillary Po_2 at the tissue level remains higher than the minimum tissue Po_2 of 20 mm Hg, there will be oxygen to diffuse from the capillary blood into the tissue for consumption (consumable oxygen).[15] Assuming that arterial Po_2, hemoglobin, tissue oxygen consumption, and oxygen diffusion rates remain constant, the blood flow through the

BOX 16-1
Causes of Hypoxia

Pulmonary gas exchange
Inadequate oxygenation of the airway
Decreased ventilation and perfusion (e.g., intrapulmonary shunt)
Disruption of alveolar-capillary diffusion (e.g., pulmonary edema, pneumonia)

Loading
Dysfunctional hemoglobin (e.g., carboxyhemoglobin, methemoglobin)
Changes in the factors shifting the oxygen-hemoglobin dissociation curve (e.g., pH, P_{CO_2}, 2,3-diphosphoglycerate level, body temperature)
Venous-to-arterial shunts ("right-to-left" cardiac shunt)

Transport
Hemoglobin and hematocrit
Red blood cell deformability
Low cardiac output: generalized or local ischemia
Tissue edema

Unloading
Changes in the factors shifting the oxygen-hemoglobin dissociation curve (e.g., pH, P_{CO_2}, 2,3-diphosphoglycerate level, body temperature)

Tissue gas exchange
Capillary "shunt" resulting from peripheral vasodilation (e.g., septic shock)
Poisoning of cellular enzymes (e.g., cyanide poisoning)
Diminished cellular metabolic capacity (e.g., beriberi)

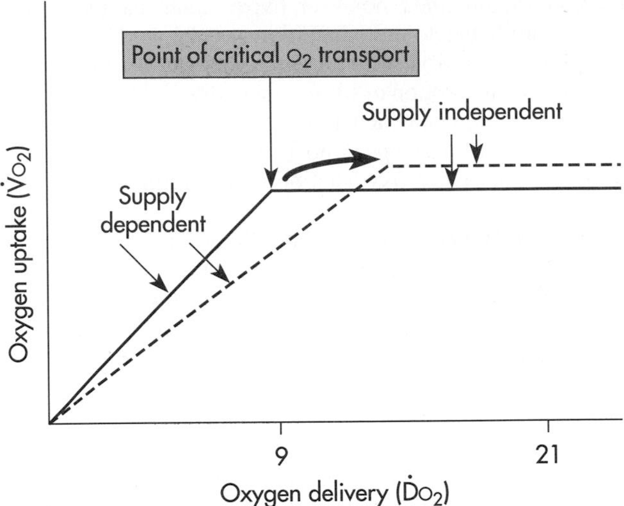

Fig. 16-3. Oxygen delivery ($\dot{D}O_2$) and uptake ($\dot{V}O_2$). In normal tissue *(solid line),* oxygen uptake becomes supply dependent until oxygen delivery reaches the point of critical oxygen transport (≈9 ml/min/kg). Beyond the critical point, however, oxygen uptake is supply independent; regardless of the delivery, oxygen uptake remains constant. Oxygen uptake in adult respiratory distress syndrome *(dashed line)* stays supply dependent until oxygen delivery increases several times higher than normal, indicating that only an increase in oxygen delivery can provide sufficient oxygen to produce normal oxygen volume values.

tissue determines capillary and venous P_{O_2} (Fick principle). Hypoxic lactic acidosis does not develop in hypoxemia when there is enough tissue perfusion to maintain capillary and venous P_{O_2} well above the minimum tissue P_{O_2} of 20 mm Hg.

In acute hypoxemia, the P_{O_2} chemoreceptors of the carotid arteries and aortic arch quickly recognize low blood P_{O_2}. The respiratory center and the heart are stimulated to increase minute ventilation and cardiac output, respectively, thereby preventing tissue hypoxia. In chronic hypoxemia with chronic lung diseases or cyanotic heart diseases, hemoglobin levels increase to maintain the amount of oxygen for transport. Mitochondria can become more efficient to produce energy with a limited oxygen supply to prevent tissue hypoxia.[16]

On the other hand, tissue ischemia, which is the state of low blood oxygen content in the tissue resulting from decreased blood flow from decreased cardiac output, vascular obstruction, or both conditions, can cause hypoxic injury even with a normal arterial P_{O_2}.[17] When cardiac output decreases, there is not enough tissue perfusion to maintain the P_{O_2} gradient for diffusion between the blood and the tissue. Thus ischemia is much worse than hypoxemia in the development of hypoxic cellular injury.[18]

Hypercapnia

Pathophysiology. Carbon dioxide is produced in the tissues as the result of aerobic metabolism and removed from the body through tissue gas exchange, loading, transport, and unloading and finally pulmonary gas exchange. The disruption of any of these processes causes carbon dioxide to accumulate in the body fluid and thus produces hypercapnia.

Because of the free diffusibility of carbon dioxide across cell membranes, a sudden increase in extracellular P_{CO_2} decreases the intracellular pH.[19] Because of the abundance of carbonic anhydrase in the cytosol, carbonic acid is formed, thus rapidly causing intracellular acidosis.[20] Most effects of hypercapnia occur at the cellular level. The reduced intracellular pH decreases oxidative metabolism and inhibits the activity of contractile elements by interfering with both excitation-contraction coupling and actin-myosin interaction.[21] Myocardial and skeletal muscle contractility decreases, although most of this impairment is reversible.[22]

In the intact animal, the depressing effect of hypercapnia is offset by the stimulating action of carbon dioxide on the central and autonomic systems. Carbon dioxide is a potent vasodilator. Hypercapnia dilates the coronary arteries and cerebral arteries and may improve blood flow through the normal myocardium and normal brain tissue. Conversely, hypercapnia reduces perfusion through the injured ischemic areas; this is the steal phenomenon.[23,24] Increased P_{CO_2} diminishes cerebral vascular tone. Cerebral blood volume increases, thereby raising intracranial pressure.[25,26] Hypercapnic acidosis constricts pulmonary arteries and renal arteries, leading to pulmonary artery hypertension and decreased renal blood flow.[27-29] Initially, the direct cardiovascular effects of hypercapnia are offset by increased sympathetic tone and catecholamine release before the hypercapnic respiratory acidosis is compensated.[30] Increased P_{CO_2}, low pH, or both shift the oxygen-hemoglobin dissociation curve to the right, which decreases oxygen affinity. When the arterial P_{O_2} is in the normal range, the rightward shift of the oxygen-hemoglobin dissociation curve is advantageous because there is easier unloading of oxygen to the tissue. However, when the arterial P_{O_2} is low, it is more difficult to load oxygen at the pulmonary alveolar-capillary level because of decreased oxygen affinity (see Fig. 16-1, *B*).

The concomitant tissue hypoxia potentiates the adverse effects of acute hypercapnic acidosis.[31] When the tissue oxygenation is maintained, however, hypercapnia and intracellular acidosis are better tolerated. With time, the acidosis resolves through the excretion of hydrogen ions from the kidneys and the increased resorption of bicarbonate ions.[32,33] Clinically, permissive hypercapnia, which allows a P_{CO_2} rise with alveolar hypoventilation, is an accepted mode of ventilation to prevent further lung injury when oxygenation is well maintained.[34-37]

Causes of Hypercapnia. Carbon dioxide is produced in the tissues as the result of aerobic metabolism and removed from the body through tissue gas exchange, loading, transport, and unloading and finally pulmonary gas exchange. According to the standard equation, arterial P_{CO_2} (Pa_{CO_2}) is proportional to carbon dioxide production ($\dot{V}_{CO_2}$) and inversely proportional to alveolar ventilation ($\dot{V}_A$):

$$Pa_{CO_2} = \frac{K\dot{V}_{CO_2}}{\dot{V}_A}$$

The constant K has the value of 0.863 mm Hg when carbon dioxide is expressed in milliliters per minute under standard conditions (dry gas at standard temperature and pressure) and alveolar ventilation is expressed in liters per minute under body conditions (saturated gas at body temperature and pressure).

The disruption of any of these processes causes the accumulation of carbon dioxide in the body fluid to produce hypercapnia (Box 16-2). In hypoxia resulting from poor perfusion through the pulmonary membrane or through the tissues, serious hypercapnia usually does not occur because carbon dioxide diffuses 20 times as rapidly as oxygen. However, in hypoxia caused by hypoventilation, carbon dioxide transfer between the alveoli and the atmosphere is affected as much as oxygen transfer. Therefore hypercapnia always accompanies hypoxia.

Diminished blood flow in circulatory deficiency removes less carbon dioxide from the tissues, resulting in tissue hypercapnia. However, the transport capacity of the blood for carbon dioxide is about 3 times that for oxygen, so tissue hypercapnia is much less severe than tissue hypoxia.

BOX 16-2

Causes of Hypercapnia

Carbon dioxide production

Increased body temperature: approximately 10% per degree of temperature
Excessive muscular activity: shivering, rigor, seizure
Physiologic stress
Sepsis
Parenteral nutrition with glucose

Decreased carbon dioxide clearance

Increased tissue carbon dioxide levels
Tissue gas exchange
Poor tissue perfusion (e.g., ischemia)
Disrupted diffusion (e.g., tissue edema)
Loading
Capillary shunt resulting from peripheral vasodilation (e.g., septic shock)
Transport
Low hemoglobin level or hematocrit
Decreased red blood cell deformability
Low cardiac output
Increased blood carbon dioxide levels
Unloading
Venous-to-arterial shunts ("right-to-left" cardiac shunt)
Pulmonary gas exchange
Decreased ventilation (e.g., respiratory depression, neuromuscular disorder, chest deformity)
Increased dead space (e.g., upper airway obstruction, lower airway obstruction: reactive airway disease)
Disruption of alveolar-capillary diffusion (e.g., pulmonary edema, pneumonia)

Acid-Base Homeostasis

It is imperative for a pulmonary physician to understand how respiratory and metabolic factors influence acid-base balance. This portion of the chapter emphasizes the concepts necessary to assess acid-base status and provides clinical examples. Comprehensive reviews of acid-base physiology can be found elsewhere.[37-40]

Buffering Systems

Slight changes in the hydrogen ion concentration of fluid-bathing cells can profoundly affect the rate of chemical reactions within the cell. Buffering of extracellular fluid is necessary because buffers can quickly limit the change in hydrogen ion concentrations; this is unlike the renal and respiratory systems, which take time to respond to changes in hydrogen ion concentration. Buffers can combine with an acid or a base and limit the change in hydrogen ion concentrations to less than the exchange that would occur without the buffer. An acid-base buffer is usually composed of two or more chemical compounds.

The major extracellular buffer is the carbon dioxide–bicarbonate system, which has two buffering molecules: carbonic acid and bicarbonate. Under appropriate conditions, the hydrogen ion (H^+) and bicarbonate (HCO_3^-) can associate to form carbonic acid (H_2CO_3). Carbonic acid in a reversible process forms water and carbon dioxide. The reaction follows:

$$H^+ + HCO_3^- \leftrightarrow H_2CO_3 \leftrightarrow H_2O + CO_2$$

If an acid is added to the carbon dioxide–bicarbonate buffering system the following reaction occurs, as follows:

$$H^+ + HCO_3^- \leftrightarrow H_2CO_3$$

If an base is added to the buffering system the following reaction occurs:

$$OH^- + H_2CO_3 \leftrightarrow H_2O + HCO_3^-$$

where OH^- is the hydroxide ion. The serum hydrogen ion concentration, which is regulated primarily by the carbon dioxide–bicarbonate buffering system, can be determined by knowing both the P_{CO_2} and the bicarbonate value. The pH is a logarithmic means of expressing hydrogen ion concentration in a solution. The pH of an acidic solution is less than 7 (hydrogen ion concentration = 10^{-7} mmol/L); a pH greater than 7 indicates that the solution is alkaline. In a healthy individual the pH of the extracellular fluid is maintained within a narrow range: 7.38 to 7.42. The determination of blood pH is helpful in the evaluation of numerous disorders, particularly pulmonary and renal disorders. The pH of blood can be directly measured using a pH probe (and the Nernst equation) or can be calculated using the Henderson-Hasselbalch equation. This equation describes the relationship between carbonic acid and bicarbonate, as follows:

$$H_2CO_3 \rightarrow H^+ + HCO_3^-$$

The equation is modified so that the concentration of hydrogen ions can be determined by knowing both the bicarbonate and carbonic acid concentrations. Because a value expressed in pH is desirable, the logarithm of both sides of the equation must be obtained, as follows:

$$-\log[H^+] = pH = pKa + \log([HCO_3^-]/[H_2CO_3])$$

where *pKa* is the pH value at which bicarbonate and carbonic acid are found in equal concentrations. *pKa* also represents the pH at which there is the greatest amount of buffering capacity available. The pKa of the carbon dioxide–bicarbonate buffering system is 6.1. At a pH of 7.40, carbonic acid concentrations are very low and cannot be easily measured. Conversely P_{CO_2} values are higher and can be easily measured. In most equations, the carbonic acid value is replaced by the solubility coefficient multiplied by P_{CO_2}. The solubility coefficient is 0.0308 for results in millimoles per liter at 37° C, as follows:

$$pH = pKa + \log([HCO_3^-]/[(0.0308)(CO_2)])$$

Because the Henderson-Hasselbalch equation can be challenging to use in clinical situations, other formulas have been developed. One such formula makes use of the fact that hydrogen ion concentrations change in a linear fashion in the pH range around 7.40 (Fig. 16-4). Accordingly, the Henderson-Hasselbalch equation can be altered to be more clinically useful, as follows:

$$H^+ \text{ concentration} \cong (K)\text{Lungs/Kidneys}$$

where *(K)* equals 24, so the following equation can be used:

$$H^+ \text{ concentration} \cong 24\ (P_{CO_2}/HCO_3^-)$$

The hydrogen ion concentration at a normal pH (7.40) is 40 mmol/L (see Fig. 16-4). A healthy individual with a P_{CO_2} of 40 mm Hg and a bicarbonate concentration of 24 mmol/L, would have a calculated hydrogen ion concentration of 40 mmol/L (normal), which equals a pH of 7.40. For any increase of 1 in the hydrogen ion concentration the pH decreases by 0.01; for any decrease of 1 in the hydrogen ion concentration, the pH increases by 0.01. For example, if the hydrogen ion concentration is 50 (an increase of 10), then the pH is 7.30 (a decrease of 0.1 pH unit).

Example: A 2-month-old boy has respiratory distress and a large infiltrate on the left lower lobe on chest radiograph. The measured pH on the blood gas is 7.16 with a measured P_{CO_2} of 63 mm Hg.

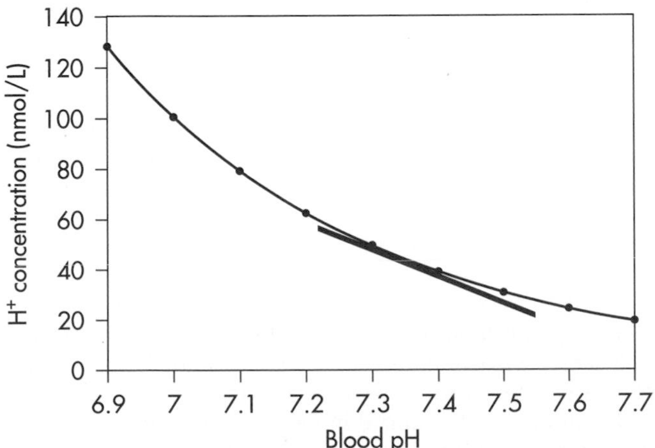

Fig. 16-4. Relative to pH, the hydrogen ion concentration (mmol/L/10^{-7}) of blood changes in a linear fashion in a limited area surrounding a pH of 7.40. The Henderson-Hasselbalch equation can be modified for easy clinical use because of this relationship.

The reported bicarbonate level (26 mmol/L) is suspected to be incorrect. What should the correct bicarbonate value be?

Solution: The equation would be arranged as follows to determine the hydrogen ion concentration:

$$H^+ \text{ concentration} = 24\ (63 \text{ mm Hg } [P_{CO_2}]/26 \text{ mmol/L } [HCO_3^-])$$

The equation would be altered in the following fashion to determine the bicarbonate concentration:

$$HCO_3^- = (K)P_{CO_2} / H^+ \text{ concentration}$$

The hydrogen ion concentration would be 64 mmol/L (equivalent to a pH of 7.16), and the correct serum bicarbonate value would be 23.6 mmol/L. In this example the initially reported bicarbonate level was incorrect.

The results of blood gas analyses are often slightly different than the results calculated using the Henderson-Hasselbalch equation because of the effect of the phosphate and protein buffering systems. The phosphate buffering system functions in much the same way as the carbon dioxide–bicarbonate buffering system. However, two compounds, $H_2PO_4^-$ and HPO_4^-, act as buffers. When a strong acid is added, the following reaction occurs:

$$HCl + Na_2HPO_4 \rightarrow NaH_2PO_4 + NaCl$$

In this reaction a strong acid (HCl) is converted into a weak acid (NaH_2PO_4) thereby causing only a minor change in pH. If a strong base is added to the buffer system the following reaction occurs:

$$NaOH + NaH_2PO_4 \rightarrow Na_2HPO_4 + H_2O$$

With this reaction a strong base (NaOH) is exchanged for a weak base (NaH_2PO_4), causing only a minor shift toward an alkaline pH. The phosphate buffering system has a pKa of 6.8, which means that there are relatively equal amounts of $H_2PO_4^-$ and HPO_4^- at a pH of 7.40. Therefore the phosphate buffering system has its best buffering capacity in the normal blood pH range. Yet the concentration of $H_2PO_4^-$ and HPO_4^- with the phosphate system is much less than that with the carbon dioxide–bicarbonate system and therefore contributes less buffering capacity. Nevertheless, phosphate contributes significantly in acid-base regulation in the kidney.

Intracellular proteins also act as potent buffers and perhaps account for as much as three fourths of all chemical buffering in the body. Some amino acids, such as histidine, form free radicals that can dissociate to form a base and hydrogen ions[41]; hydrogen ions can bind to the protein. Intracellular hydrogen ion concentrations are affected primarily by carbon dioxide, which can rapidly diffuse through the cell membrane to affect intracellular pH. Bicarbonate and hydrogen ions, which diffuse through the cell membranes more slowly, also influence intracellular pH.

Pulmonary Regulation of Acid Base

The pulmonary compensatory response to acute acidemia or alkalemia is swift. If a strong acid is added to the blood, the pH begins to drop as bicarbonate is consumed, and the P_{CO_2} begins to rise. Blood pH cannot directly influence the central respiratory center because of the blood-brain barrier. Instead, as P_{CO_2} increases, carbon dioxide levels increase in the cerebrospinal fluid (CSF) that bathes the central respiratory center (CRC). As a result, carbonic acid and hydrogen ion levels increase in the CSF. Hydrogen ions directly stimulate the CRC, causing the ventilatory rate to increase. Additional ventilatory stimuli are supplied by peripheral chemoreceptors that respond to the rising hydrogen ion concentrations. Because the lungs represent an open system by which carbon dioxide can be rapidly disposed, the blood pH is rapidly corrected toward 7.40 by decreasing the P_{CO_2} value to less than 40 mm Hg. The underlying metabolic acidosis persists until the kidneys excrete the excess acid, a process that typically takes 1 to 2 days.

If a strong base is added to the blood, the pH rapidly rises, and the carbonic acid value and P_{CO_2} decrease. Ventilatory drive decreases in response to decreased levels of hydrogen ions in the serum and CSF, causing an increase in P_{CO_2}. The compensatory response to respiratory acidosis is characterized by an increase in the P_{CO_2} until the pH is normalized at approximately 7.40. The compensatory response is limited by coincident hypoxia; as ventilation decreases the P_{O_2} does too.

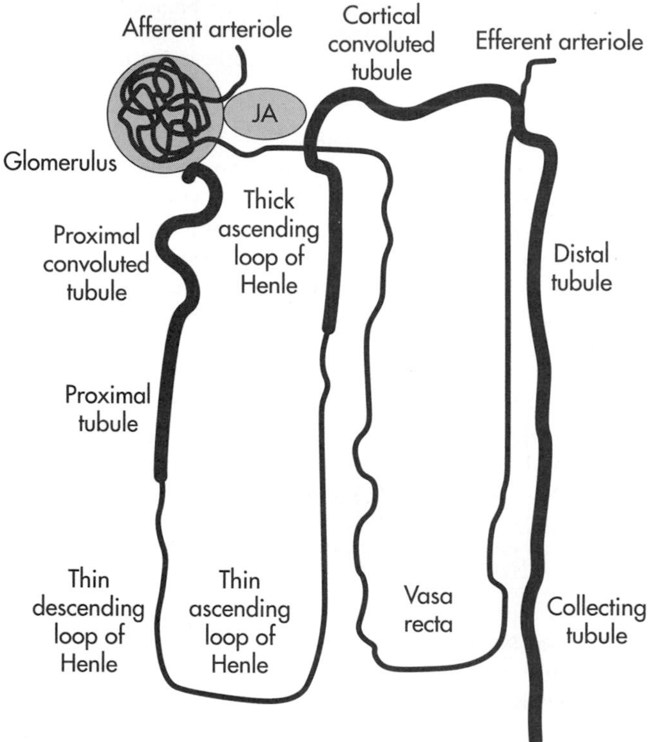

Fig. 16-5. Nephron. Blood is brought to the glomerulus by the afferent arteriole and leaves via the efferent arteriole. In some nephrons the efferent arteriole changes course, becoming the vasa recta, which courses through the interstitial area between the ascending loop of Henle and the distal/collecting tubule. *JA*, Juxtaglomerular apparatus.

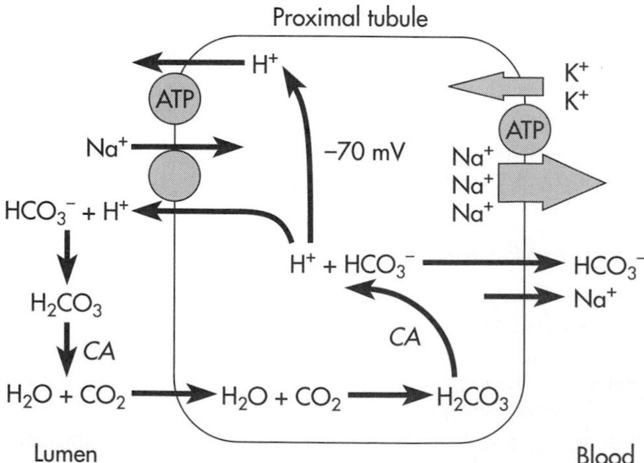

Fig. 16-6. Proximal tubule cell. Na^+, Sodium; HCO_3^-, bicarbonate; H^+, hydrogen ion; H_2CO_3, carbonic acid; *CA,* carbonic anhydrase; K^+, potassium.

Renal Regulation of Acid Base

The kidneys maintain acid-base balance via the following mechanisms: bicarbonate resorption, hydrogen ion excretion, and bicarbonate excretion. To accomplish the regulation of acid-base, the kidney must filter a large volume of blood. The kidneys receive a disproportionate amount of blood based on their weight because of their low vascular resistance.[42] In a healthy, 70-kg adult, the kidneys receive 20% to 25% of the cardiac output, which is equivalent to a renal blood flow of approximately 1 to 1.25 L/min of blood. The amount of renal blood flow relative to cardiac output is not fixed. Renal blood flow changes by a process known as *autoregulation* in response to hemodynamic alterations.

Red blood cells constitute approximately 40% of the blood volume and cannot be filtered. Accordingly, renal plasma flow is approximately 600 to 750 ml/min in an adult. A total of 100 to 120 ml/min of filtrate is derived from the plasma flow. The factors responsible for the regulation of glomerular filtration are discussed in detail elsewhere.[43] The net amount of glomerular filtrate per minute is known as the *glomerular filtration rate.*

The constituents of glomerular filtrate, including bicarbonate, are very similar to those of plasma. Yet the constitution of the filtrate is affected by the negatively charged glomerular basement membrane (GBM). The GBM is negatively charged because of the presence of heparan sulfate molecules within the GBM.[44,45] The negative charges within the GBM inhibit the movement of negatively charged ions across the membrane despite the effect of glomerular filtration pressure. As a result, the urine net charge is slightly positive as urine enters the proximal tubule. Despite the negative charges within the GBM, all small, negatively charged, nonprotein-bound molecules, including bicarbonate, are filtered. Conversely, large, negatively charged molecules, such as albumin, cannot be filtered and therefore remain in the blood.

After emerging from Bowman's capsule, the filtrate comes in contact with the convoluted proximal tubule (Fig. 16-5). The primary acid-base regulatory function of the proximal tubule is bicarbonate resorption. In an adult, approximately 3600 mmol of bicarbonate is filtered each day. The proximal tubule resorbs approximately 75% of the filtered bicarbonate. The proximal renal tubular cell cytoplasm is negatively charged because of the presence of a sodium-potassium ATPase pump in the basal membrane.[46] This pump draws out three sodium molecules in exchange for two potassium molecules (Fig. 16-6).[46,47] Because the cell is relatively rich in intracellular potassium, some of the potassium leaks back into the renal tubular capillary. The movement of sodium and potassium by the sodium-potassium ATPase pump promotes an intracellular charge of −70 mV. This large, negative intracellular charge inhibits the resorption of bicarbonate, which is negatively charged, through the cell.

Bicarbonate is reclaimed in the proximal tubule by an elegant mechanism (see Fig. 16-6). On the luminal surface, the hydrogen ion is reversibly secreted in exchange for sodium.[47,48] Sodium-independent hydrogen ion secretion also occurs via an ATP-dependent pump.[49] In the lumen, hydrogen ions combine with bicarbonate to form carbonic acid. Luminal type IV carbonic anhydrase facilitates the dehydration of carbonic acid into water and carbon dioxide.[50,51] Although bicarbonate is unable to pass into the proximal tubular cell, carbon dioxide can move into the cell, where it combines with water in the presence of intracellular carbonic anhydrase to form carbonic acid. The carbonic acid is converted into bicarbonate and hydrogen ions. The bicarbonate leaves the cell in exchange for chloride or leaves conductively with sodium across the basolateral membrane.[52] The hydrogen ion is secreted into the tubule lumen, where it once again can facilitate the resorption of bicarbonate.

Bicarbonate resorption in the proximal tubule is regulated in part by luminal bicarbonate concentration.[53] Hydrogen ion secretion is stimulated by the decrease in the hydrogen ion gradient across the luminal membrane. Hydrogen ion secretion and bicarbonate resorption are also stimulated by hypokalemia or an increase in the P_{CO_2}. An extracellular fluid overload decreases bicarbonate resorption.

The distal tubule and collecting duct resorb any remaining bicarbonate and acidify the urine. The collecting duct has two types of cells: principal and intercalated. The principal cells primarily absorb sodium in exchange for potassium. There are two types of intercalated cells: one that excretes bicarbonate and another that excretes hydrogen ions.[54] Alkalemia acts as a stimulus to increase bicarbonate secretion. Most distal renal tubular cells, however, secrete hydrogen ions. The secretion and loss of hydrogen ions indirectly increase the concentration of serum bicarbonate. Hydrogen ions in combination with chloride cannot be excreted because hydrochloric acid is a strong acid. When the urinary pH drops to below 4.5, the excretion of hydrogen ions into the tubule lumen ceases. Furthermore, the very low pH would be injurious to the renal tubule and uroepithelium. Hydrogen ions can combine with either ammonia or phosphate to buffer the urine pH.

Ammonia is produced by the conversion of glutamine to ammonia in most renal tubule cells except those in the thin segment of the loop of Henle. The secreted hydrogen ions combine with ammonia to form ammonium. The ammonium is excreted with chloride. The release of renal tubular ammonia increases with increases in hydrogen ion secretion and the formation of ammonium.

Phosphate buffering acts in a similar fashion. Approximately 20% of all filtered phosphate is not resorbed before it reaches the distal tubule. Phosphate can combine with either one or two hydrogen ions and is typically excreted with sodium. Each time that a hydrogen ion is buffered by the ammonia or phosphate buffering system, a new bicarbonate molecule is produced by the renal tubule cell and released into the blood.

Acute Buffering Processes

When there is an accumulation or loss in P_{CO_2}, the pH changes in an inverse manner within 10 minutes. Plasma bicarbonate levels alter immediately in response to the pH changes caused by either an increase or a decrease in the P_{CO_2} (Table 16-1). The immediate bicarbonate changes are modest (4 to 5 mmol) and are incomplete when compared with those caused by a chronic respiratory abnormality. The small changes in serum bicarbonate levels are due to intracellular nonbicarbonate buffers.[55,56] In addition, the production of lactic and citric acids increases slightly, thereby decreasing serum bicarbonate levels during an acute decrease in P_{CO_2}.[57,58] When there is an acute change in the pH attributed to an increase or a decrease in the bicarbonate value, the P_{CO_2} changes in response. As a result of sodium bicarbonate infusion, the P_{CO_2} changes by 2.5 mm Hg for every 0.10 change in the pH.

Chronic Buffering Processes

With any level of chronically elevated or decreased P_{CO_2}, serum bicarbonate changes cause the pH to return toward normal but not completely (Table 16-2). Several hours to days are needed

Table 16-1 Rules of Acute Respiratory Compensation

CHANGE	RULE	EXAMPLE
$\uparrow P_{CO_2}$	For every increase of 1 mm Hg, the pH decreases by 0.008 pH unit. Compensation: The HCO_3^- level increases by 0.1 mmol/L.	P_{CO_2}: 40 → 60 mm Hg pH: 7.40 → 7.24 HCO_3^-: 24 → 26 mmol/L
$\downarrow P_{CO_2}$	For every decrease of 1 mm Hg, the pH increases by 0.007 pH unit. Compensation: The HCO_3^- level decreases by 0.25 mmol/L.	P_{CO_2}: 40 → 20 mm Hg pH: 7.40 → 7.54 HCO_3^-: 24 → 19 mmol/L

HCO_3^-, Bicarbonate.

Table 16-2 Rules of Chronic Acid-Base Compensation

CHANGE	RULE	EXAMPLE
$\uparrow P_{CO_2}$	For every increase of 1 mm Hg, the pH decreases by 0.0025 pH unit. Compensation: The HCO_3^- level increases by 0.4 mmol/L.	P_{CO_2}: 40 → 60 mm Hg pH: 7.40 → 7.35 HCO_3^-: 24 → 28 mmol/L
$\downarrow P_{CO_2}$	For every decrease of 1 mm Hg, the pH increases by 0.003 pH unit. Compensation: The HCO_3^- level decreases by 0.5 mmol/L.	P_{CO_2}: 40 → 20 mm Hg pH: 7.40 → 7.46 HCO_3^-: 24 → 14 mmol/L
$\uparrow HCO_3^-$	For every increase of 1 mm Hg, the pH increases by 0.003-0.008 pH unit. Compensation: The P_{CO_2} increases by 0.2-0.9 mm Hg.	HCO_3^-: 24 → 34 mmol/L pH: 7.40 → 7.43-7.48 P_{CO_2}: 40 → 48 mm Hg
$\downarrow HCO_3^-$	For every decrease of 1 mm Hg, the pH decreases by 0.012 pH unit. Compensation: The P_{CO_2} decreases by 1.25 mm Hg.	HCO_3^-: 24 → 14 mmol/L pH: 7.40 → 7.28 P_{CO_2}: 40 → 28 mm Hg

HCO_3^-, Bicarbonate.

for the full renal response to hypocapnia to begin.[59] A decrease in PCO_2 causes a decrease in bicarbonate resorption by the renal tubule.[60-64] Hydrogen ion secretion by the proximal and distal renal tubules is also diminished.[65,66] The increase in the serum chloride level occurs because of a shift of chloride out of the red blood cells, an extracellular volume contraction, and an enhanced renal chloride resorption. When the PCO_2 rises, the kidneys compensate by secreting more hydrogen ions[67,68] and by increasing the amount of bicarbonate resorbed.[61-63,69-71]

BLOOD GAS MEASUREMENT

A blood gas determination typically consists of the following separate measurements: pH, PO_2, and PCO_2, which provide information about the respiratory, circulatory, and metabolic condition of the patient. Oxygen and carbon dioxide are the most important respiratory gases and reflect the adequacy of pulmonary gas exchange. Serum levels of bicarbonate, which are calculated based on the Siggaard-Andersen curve[72] (Fig. 16-7) and the pH, indicate the patient's acid-base status.

Even though blood gas analysis has been available for several decades,[73,74] many physicians still have difficulty interpreting the results correctly.[75] This section provides basic information regarding blood gas acquisition, determination, and physiology; yet the primary focus is on the correct interpretation of the test results.

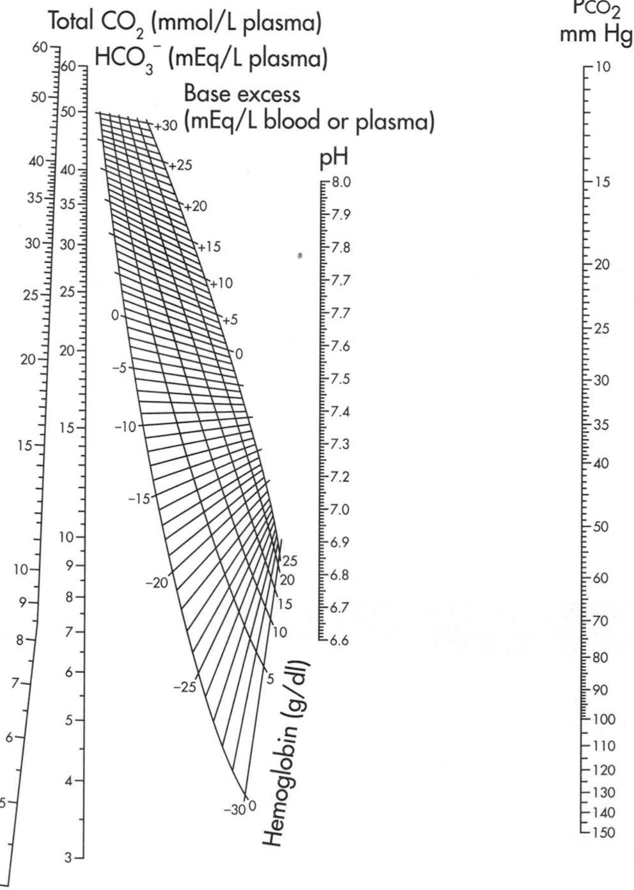

Fig. 16-7. Siggaard-Andersen alignment nomogram. *HCO_3^-*, Bicarbonate. (From Siggaard-Andersen O: *Scand J Clin Lab Invest* 15:211-217, 1963.)

Blood Gas Analysis

With a typical automated blood gas analyzer, the sample pH is determined by an electrode with an electrolytic circuit.[76] The probe is constructed of a special pH-sensitive glass that allows hydrogen ions to pass into a reference solution with a known pH (Fig. 16-8, *A*). Because of the different charge between the two solutions, an electric potential develops and is measured. At 37° C, the pH electrode registers a 61.5-mV change for each pH unit difference between a known buffer solution an a blood sample. The voltage charge can be calculated by a modification of the Nernst equation, as follows:

$$V_m = V_2 - V_1 = \frac{RT}{ZF} \ln \frac{C2}{C1}$$

where V_m is equilibrium voltage across a membrane separating two solutions containing a single ionic species, V_2 is voltage$_2$, V_1 is voltage$_1$, R is the gas constant, T is the temperature, Z is the valence of the solute, F is Faraday's constant, and C is the concentration of the solution.

The PCO_2 electrode has a internal buffer solution of sodium chloride and sodium bicarbonate that is separated from the blood by a carbon dioxide–permeable membrane (Fig. 16-8, *B*). Carbon dioxide crosses the membrane and combines with water to form carbonic acid. Hydrogen ions are produced in direct correlation with the amount of carbon dioxide crossing the membrane. The pH of the buffer is determined from the voltmeter reading and is correlated to a PCO_2 value.

Most oxygen analysis is performed by a Clark electrode, which is based on the oxidation-reduction reaction of dissolved oxygen and water (Fig. 16-8, *C*). The electrode has a positively charged silver–silver chloride terminal and a negatively charged platinum terminal. The reaction requires a constant supply of electrons, which are made available by a current flowing through a silver wire. As an electric charge is passed between the electrodes, oxygen is attracted to the platinum electrode (cathode). The oxygen reacts with the water that is consuming electrons and producing hydroxyl ions. The current that flows through the circuit is directly proportional to the amount of oxygen in the solution.

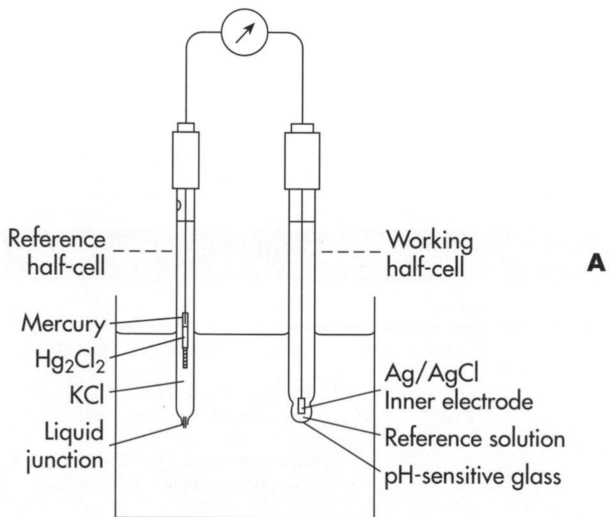

Fig. 16-8. Blood gas probes. **A,** pH probe. **B,** Carbon dioxide probe. **C,** Oxygen probe. *Hg_2Cl_2*, Mercury chloride; *KCl,* potassium chloride; *Ag/AgCl,* silver-silver chloride. (From Malley WJ: *Clinical blood gases,* Philadelphia, 1990, WB Saunders, pp 41-43.)

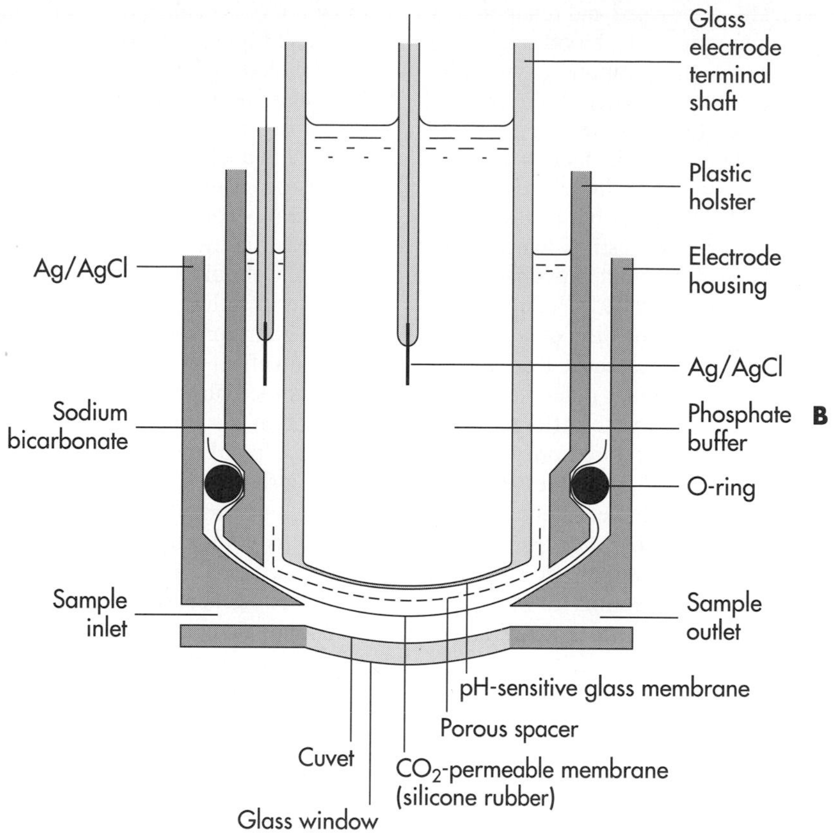

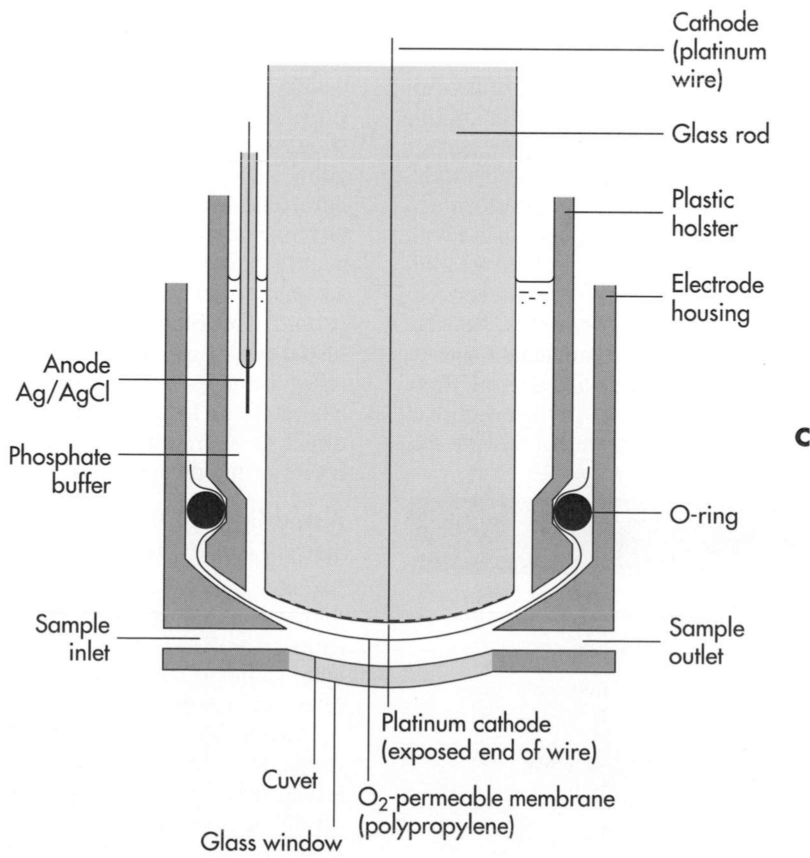

Fig. 16-8, cont'd. For legend see opposite page.

Blood gas results are typically performed and reported at a temperature of 37° C. The temperature of the blood at the time of pH determination influences ion concentrations, oxygen dissociation from hemoglobin, and gas solubility. There is a direct, positive relationship between temperature and gas pressure. If a blood specimen carried on ice to the laboratory for a blood gas analysis is not warmed to 37° C, the test results are radically altered (Table 16-3). Because most blood gas analysis machines properly warm blood before testing, temperature correction is of greatest value for patients with hyperthermia or hypothermia (less than 35° or greater than 39° C). Substantial controversies exist about the clinical application of correcting the temperature of blood specimens.[77-79] Because there are no normal blood gas values at body temperatures other than 37° C and the in vivo metabolism is adjusted with different body temperatures, interpretation of the temperature-corrected values of blood gas using the normal blood gas values at 37° C may not be valid. Therefore it is difficult to determine whether a PO_2 or PCO_2 is adequate for a patient whose core temperature is very different from 37° C. Because there are no sufficient data to support routine temperature correction for blood gas analysis, it is reasonable to use 37° C for interpretation, regardless of the patient's body temperature.

Performing Arterial Blood Gas Analysis

The radial artery is frequently chosen for arterial blood gas sampling because of the presence of the ulnar artery, which provides collateral arterial flow to the hand via the palmar arch in the event of radial artery compromise. Other sites appropriate for arterial blood gas sampling include the brachial, dorsalis pedis, and posterior tibial arteries. The ulnar artery is not frequently chosen because the median nerve is close to the ulnar artery and can be damaged when an arterial blood sample is obtained. The temporal artery is also infrequently used because of the risk of scalp necrosis resulting from emboli.[80]

Before a radial artery is selected for an arterial puncture, Allen's test or a modified Allen's test should be performed. These tests ensure that the perfusion of the patient's hand will not be compromised when a sample is obtained for arterial blood gas analysis. In Allen's test,[81] which was first described in 1929, the radial artery is occluded for 3 minutes, and the hand color is compared with that of the contralateral hand. If the color does not change, there is adequate arterial flow through the ulnar artery to perfuse the hand in the event that radial arterial flow is lost. In the second portion of the test, the ulnar artery is occluded for 3 minutes. A change in the color of the hand suggests the presence of radial artery occlusion.

The modified Allen's test[82] is performed by occluding both the ulnar and the radial arteries. The hand should be opened and closed repeatedly or massaged from the hand to the wrist to cause blanching. Pressure is released from the ulnar artery. Perfusion of the hand within 10 seconds indicates adequate collateral perfusion in the event that the radial artery is compromised. If the hand is not perfused within 10 seconds, another site should be chosen.

After concluding that perfusion of the patient's hand will not be compromised by arterial puncture, the clinician should make an effort to ensure that the blood gas sample accurately reflects the patient's respiratory and acid-base status. Hyperventilation associated with the stress of the procedure can induce profound respiratory alkalosis. If the patient is a young child, a second person should restrain and comfort the child. The use of subcutaneous lidocaine[83] or cutaneous lidocaine cream may slightly diminish the discomfort associated with the procedure.

Excessive heparin within the syringe can alter the pH of the sample by decreasing the PCO_2.[84] If a prepackaged heparin syringe is unavailable for the pediatric patient, a tuberculin syringe, a 23-gauge butterfly needle, and approximately 0.1 ml (just enough to fill the dead space) of 1000 U/ml of heparin are needed. The heparin and all of the air are expelled because both may have a deleterious effect on the reliability of the sample results.[84] For an adult, a 3-ml syringe, a 21-gauge needle, and enough 1000 U/ml heparin to fill the dead space are needed. The syringe can be modified by placing a small-gauge needle though the plunger so that the blood fills the syringe in a pulsatile manner without aspirating.[85]

The location of the artery can usually be found by palpation. In the event that the artery is not easily located by palpation, Doppler ultrasound can also be used.[86] It is often useful to mark the location of the artery using a pen. The skin should be swabbed with povidone iodine (Betadine) and allowed to dry. Sterile gloves are worn throughout the procedure. The skin should be punctured between the distal and proximal wrist creases at a 15- to 45-degree angle with the needle bevel pointed upward.[87,88] The needle should be advanced after the clinician again locates the artery using palpation. Most blood gas analyzers require a minimum volume of 0.3 to 0.5 ml of blood to perform a blood gas analysis. After the air is expelled, the sample is capped and sent to the laboratory on ice. Once the needle is removed from the artery, direct pressure should be applied for 5 minutes to reduce bleeding and prevent hematoma formation.

Table 16-3 Temperature-Correction Values for Normal Blood

°C	°F	pH	PCO_2*	PO_2*
20	68	7.65	19	27
25	77	7.58	24	37
30	86	7.50	30	51
35	95	7.43	37	70
36	97	7.41	38	75
37	99	7.40	40	80
38	100	7.39	42	85
39	102	7.37	44	91
40	104	7.36	45	97

From Shapiro BA et al. In Shapiro BA et al, eds: *Clinical application of blood gases,* ed 5, St Louis, 1994, Mosby, p 228.
*In millimeters of mercury (mm Hg).

Blood Gas Monitoring

Arterial Blood Gas Monitoring

Samples may be obtained from an artery, vein, or capillary. Samples of arterial blood can be obtained using an indwelling catheter or direct arterial puncture. When compared with the other methods, the arterial blood gas yields PO_2 results that best reflect the levels of oxygen delivered to the tissues.

An arterial cannulation is indicated for patients who require frequent sampling of arterial blood. Although the umbilical artery may be used in neonates, complications, including thrombosis, organ infarction, infection, and hemorrhage, are possible. The radial, posterior tibial, and dorsalis pedis arteries are generally suitable for cannulation. The temporal, brachial, axillary, and to a lesser degree, femoral arteries are avoided when possible because of the risk of serious complications, including cerebral embolism and thrombosis of a distal portion of a limb.[80]

Capillary Blood Gas Monitoring

Because arterial blood gas determination is painful[83] and can lead to local complications,[89] other means of assessing the P_{O_2}, P_{CO_2}, and pH were developed. Capillary blood, when properly sampled, yields results similar to those found with arterial sampling (Fig. 16-9).[83,90-93] Correlation between arterial and capillary samples vary, but generally they are best for pH, moderate for P_{CO_2}, and worst for P_{O_2}. Values for capillary blood gas (CBG) P_{O_2},[94] pH, P_{CO_2}, and carbonic acid levels may vary significantly from arterial samples[90] because of the arteriovenous mixing that occurs with capillary sampling.[95] Even though the difference between CBG and arterial blood gas results are statistically significant, the differences may not be clinically relevant when the P_{O_2} is less than 100 mm Hg.[90] Conversely, Graham and Kenny[96] concluded that because P_{O_2} levels vary dramatically during CBG sample acquisition, CBG results should not be used for P_{O_2} determination in newborns. Nevertheless CBG analyses are routinely performed in neonates and are clinically useful.

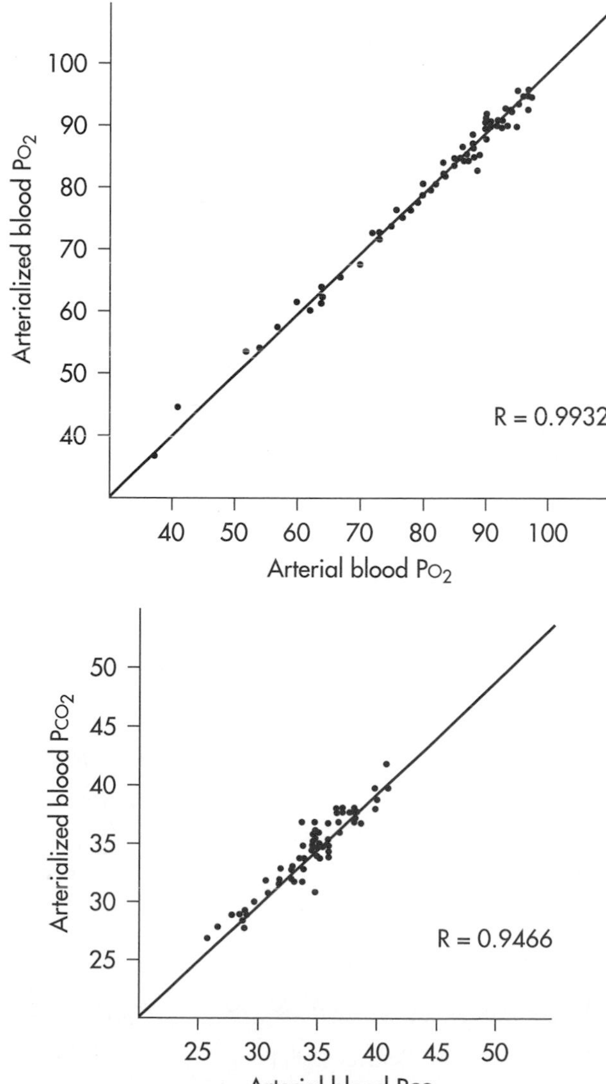

Fig. 16-9. Comparison of the capillary and arterial blood gas P_{O_2} and P_{CO_2}. *R,* Correlation coefficient. (From Canny GJ, Levison H: *Pediatr Pulmonol* 2(5):313-314, 1986.)

It is often easier to obtain a capillary blood sample than an arterial blood sample. CBG testing can be performed using blood obtained from a warmed extremity or an earlobe.[83,92] The first drop of blood is wiped away, and subsequent free-flowing drops of blood are collected into a heparinized capillary tube. Squeezing the site to encourage blood flow may distort the results. Results from earlobe samples agree very closely with those from arterial samples.[83,92] Warming was thought to be necessary to arterialize the capillary bed; however, McLain et al[97] suggested that warming of the sample site does not improve the accuracy of the results.

CBG testing is clinically useful in the management of children and adults with respiratory distress.[90,98] Finger CBG testing has been most used in the pediatric population; however, Canny and Levison[99] also demonstrated the usefulness of this technique in adolescents with chronic lung disease. CBG values have a greater potential for artifact because the blood is exposed to air during collection from a lancet wound. If the sample is collected from a slowly bleeding source, the sample begins to equilibrate with air: The P_{O_2} increases, and the P_{CO_2} decreases.

Venous Blood Gas Monitoring

Appropriately obtained samples of peripheral or central venous blood in well-perfused patients may be used to grossly reflect the arterial acid-base status.[100] When a patient's circulatory system is well perfused, the venous pH is 0.04 unit lower than the arterial pH because the venous P_{CO_2} is 5 to 7 mm Hg higher than the arterial P_{CO_2} (with relatively stable bicarbonate levels). Peripheral venous blood represents the acid-base status of local tissue, whereas central venous blood may represent the average tissue acid-base status of the whole body.[101,102] Therefore the values of venous blood gas may differ significantly from those obtained from simultaneous analysis of arterial blood gas depending on the status of tissue perfusion. The venous pH, P_{O_2}, and bicarbonate levels decrease and the P_{CO_2} increases when perfusion worsens. Application of a tourniquet may significantly distort the values of the blood gas because it decreases local perfusion.

Mixed venous blood gas samples from the pulmonary artery represent the average oxygen consumption and the acid-base status of whole body, and the values are used for hemodynamic calculation in conjunction with simultaneous arterial blood gas analysis. When blood samples are aspirated from a pulmonary artery catheter, the sample must be withdrawn slowly to prevent mixing with pulmonary end-capillary blood that contains high oxygen.

Continuous Intraarterial Blood Gas Monitoring

In 1980, Richman et al[103] reported the use of an special arterial probe and a portable gas chromatograph. However, because of the size of the instrument, it could not be used in vivo. Subsequently, smaller fiberoptic systems have been developed and successfully used to provide continuous blood gas monitoring through an indwelling intraarterial catheter.[104-107] In vivo measurement of blood gas and acid-base parameters requires the same individual components needed for conventional blood gas analysis. The major difference is that optical measurements have replaced electrochemical measurements as the transduction mechanism from blood concentrations to electrical signals. In conventional instruments the transducers are called *electrodes,* and in the new systems the transducers are called *optical sensors* or *optodes.* The optical sensors rely on a chemical interaction between the analytes (oxygen, carbon dioxide, and hydrogen ions) and indicator phase to produce an optically detectable signal. The indicator phase is chosen for its ability to affect light passing through it in a way that is proportional to the amount of analyte being measured. Light returning from the analyte chamber changes in intensity or is emitted at a different wavelength. Measuring analytes in vivo requires the transmission of light to and from a remote location, and this has been achieved using the fiberoptic system. A blood gas probe is made up of three single fiberoptic sensors and a thermocouple incorporated into a single structure.[108] These probes are usually placed through a 20-gauge angiocatheter and require a space between the wall for the sensor to allow blood sampling and measurement of an accurate intravascular blood pressure.[109] Even though numerous factors complicate the accurate acquisition of determinations from blood gas machines, preliminary data suggest that the evaluated blood gas monitoring system so far appears to be as accurate as the blood gas machines.

An obvious advantage to on-line results is the ability to immediately treat changes in the patient's condition without the delay incurred by transport, analysis, and reporting. In addition, errors resulting from poor sampling technique and incorrect transport and storage of the sample are eliminated. With in vivo systems, results are updated as often as 20 seconds, and the instruments are designed to indicate trends in changing acid-base and blood gas parameters, permitting more rapid intervention if the patient's condition starts to deteriorate. The system may also reduce blood loss. The risk of nosocomial infection, the exposure to blood, and the risks to patients should not be any different from those associated with insertion of a radial artery cannula.[110] The technology, however, is still evolving, and more work needs to be done, especially in children because of their size, before this system is accepted as one of the reliable continuous monitoring systems in patient care.

Noninvasive Techniques

Pulse Oximetry

The pulse oximeter is based on the principles of light absorption. The concentration of an unknown solute in a solvent can be determined by light absorption (Beer-Lambert law),[107] which is as follows:

$$L_{out} = L_{in} - (Dca)$$

where *L* is the intensity of light, *D* is the distance the light travels through a solution, *c* is the concentration of the solute, and *a* is the absorption coefficient of the solute.[111] All currently available pulse oximeters use two wavelengths of light, one in the red band (660 nm) and the other in the infrared band (940 nm), because the absorption characteristics of oxyhemoglobin and reduced hemoglobin are very different at these two wavelengths[112] (Fig. 16-10). A miniaturized light source is applied to an area of the body thin enough that the light can transverse a pulsating capillary bed and be sensed by a light detector located at the opposite area. The recommended site is the finger in most patients, but the palm and whole foot may be used in infants and newborns. The forehead[113] and nasal septum may be used because the anterior ethmoidal artery flow is maintained in low-flow states.[114] It is assumed that each pulsatile flow is systemic arterial flow and that there is enough hemoglobin to affect the amount of light absorption.

Each pulsation results in an increase in the distance the light has to travel, which increases the amount of light absorption. A microprocessor programmed with experimentally derived data calculates the concentration of oxyhemoglobin and reduced hemoglobin. The oxygen saturation is derived by comparing absorbencies at baseline *(BA)* and during the peak *(PA)* of a transmitted pulse at the wavelengths of 660 nm and 940 nm, respectively. The oxymetry-determined plethysmographic signal amplitudes at various saturations and the algorithm used by the microprocessor determine the oxygen saturation by the ratio of red absorbance *(R)* to infrared absorbance *(IR)*[112] (see Fig. 16-10) as follows:

$$\frac{R = PA_{660}/BA_{660}}{IR = BA_{940}/BA_{940}}$$

By using the only two wavelengths of light specifically chosen to measure oxyhemoglobin and reduced hemoglobin, the pulse oximeter determines only "functional saturation," which is the ratio of oxyhemoglobin to all functional hemoglobins capable of carrying oxygen. In contrast to the functional oxygen saturation, the "fractional saturation" measured by cooximetry on most blood gas machines gives the ratio of oxygenated hemoglobin to all other hemoglobin types, including carboxyhemoglobin and methemoglobin, which are incapable of carrying oxygen. However, these dysfunctional hemoglobins "confuse" pulse oximeters and give erroneous data. Carboxyhemoglobin absorbs very little infrared light but absorbs as much red light as oxyhemoglobin, causing patients to appear "red-cherry." To the pulse oximeter, carboxyhemoglobin looks like oxyhemoglobin at 660 nm, whereas carboxyhemoglobin is relatively transparent at 940 nm. In the presence of significant levels of carboxyhemoglobin (e.g., carbon monoxide poisoning), therefore, the pulse oximeter saturation (Spo_2) is much higher than the true saturation and may be estimated using the following equation[115,116]:

$$Spo_2 = \frac{O_2Hb + (0.9)(CO)}{\text{Total hemoglo.}} \times 100\%$$

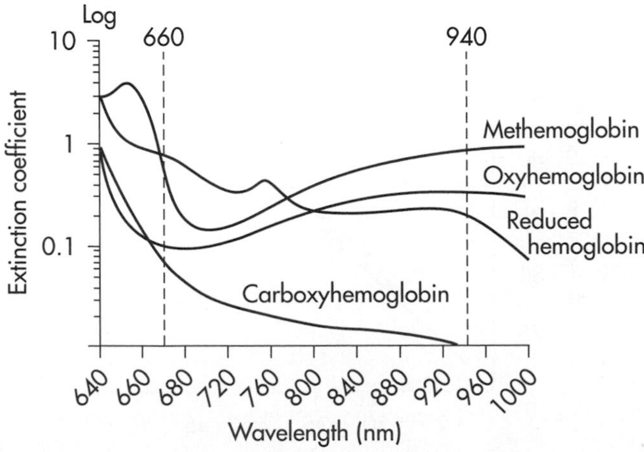

Fig. 16-10. Hemoglobin extinction curves. Transmitted light absorbance spectra of four hemoglobin species: oxyhemoglobin, reduced hemoglobin, carboxyhemoglobin, and methemoglobin. (From Pologe JA: *Int Anesthesiol Clin* 25:155-175, 1987.)

where O_2Hb is true oxyhemoglobin and *COHb* is carboxyhemoglobin.

Methemoglobin absorbs as much red light as reduced hemoglobin and more infrared light than the other hemoglobins, resulting in very dark, chocolate-colored blood with an absorbance ratio close to 1.[117,118] This ratio makes a methemoglobin Spo_2 value of 85% and gives a pulse oximeter saturation level higher than the true saturation level but to a less degree compared with carboxyhemoglobin. In suspected cases of carboxyhemoglobinemia or methemoglobinemia, an arterial sample should be sent for measurement of true saturation levels. Fetal hemoglobin differs from adult hemoglobin in the amino acid sequence of two of the four globin chains, but the difference does not affect light absorption and therefore does not affect Spo_2.[119]

Dyes and pigments affect pulse oximeter saturation.[120] Methylene blue causes a spurious fall in Spo_2 values to approximately 65% for 1 to 2 minutes. When methylene blue is used as an antidote to methemoglobin, the test results of a patient with methemoglobinemia who received methylene blue are confusing. The effect of methylene blue on laboratory oximeters is similar to its effect on pulse oximeters. Bilirubin has not been found to significantly affect Spo_2 values, although levels over 20 mg/dl affect laboratory oximeters. In very darkly pigmented individuals, the readings may be erroneously high or unobtainable (3% to 5%).[121,122] Fingernail polish worn by the patient can affect the accuracy of Spo_2 values. Blue polish absorbs red light, and black absorbs in both the red and infrared range, resulting in a decrease of 3% to 5%.[123,124]

Pulse oximeters are designed to amplify any detected pulse signal and estimate the Spo_2 values from the absorbance ratio. At the highest amplifications, an Spo_2 value can be generated from noise, including external light sources, motion artifacts, and venous pulsation. Most current models set minimum values for the signal-to-noise ratio, but case reports of nonsense Spo_2 values exist. Tricuspid regurgitation and intraaortic balloon pumps can interfere with recognition of the arterial pulse.[125,126] If the Spo_2 value has been determined erroneously from background noise or motion, the pulse rate displayed should be compared with the electrocardiogram for consistency. A low pulse wave amplitude resulting from peripheral vasoconstriction results in an inaccurate Spo_2 measurement. Shock states, vasopressors, severe edema, and peripheral vascular disease make it difficult for the sensor to distinguish true signal from background noise.[127,128] Placing the sensor on the nasal septum, warming the extremities, and using local vasodilators have been suggested as solutions.[111] In addition, electrocautery and magnetic resonance imaging scanners can cause spurious decreases in Spo_2 values or false alarms because of wide-spectrum radiofrequency emissions picked up directly by the photodetector.[129,130] A well-shielded pulse oximeter and probe protected from radiofrequency signals should be used in these environments.

The accuracy of pulse oximeters has been proved, with an overall failure rate of only 2% to 3% and 7% in the sickest patients.[131,132] However, the calibration curve does not include experimental data below an oxygen saturation of 70%. Clinical studies that test the accuracy of pulse oximetry below 70% are rare because the risk precludes gathering of data from volunteers at that level of hypoxia. The bias and precision of pulse oximetry vary widely among manufacturers at saturation values below 70%, and thus the reported values below 70% are not reliable.[133,134]

The potential dangers associated with noninvasive monitoring are relatively few. Other than rare case reports of false-positive and false-negative readings, true complications are rare. There are several reports of severe burns under probes used in magnetic resonance imaging scanners,[135,136] "suntanning" and burns in neonates,[137] burns associated with defective probes,[138] and pressure injury.[139] Most of these complications can be prevented with routine inspection of the digit to which the probe is applied.

Transcutaneous Gas Monitoring

Transcutaneous gas monitoring measures the cutaneous gas tension and oxygen and carbon dioxide tensions of heated skin. The stratum corneum, composed of lipid in a protein matrix, is normally the rate-limiting factor for gaseous diffusion and is a very efficient barrier to gas transport. When the stratum corneum is heated above 41° C, however, the physical characteristics of this layer change, creating a "diffusion window" to allow gases to diffuse readily.[140] An optimal diffusion window is predicted to occur at 44° C.[141,142] The epidermis does not affect the rate of gaseous diffusion. The dermis is a highly vascular layer with capillary vessels into the epidermis, which are dilated to increase the dermal blood flow with heating.

Cutaneous gas exchange depends both on the differences of blood and cutaneous Po_2 and Pco_2 and on blood flow to the dermal vasculature. This principle reduces the usefulness of transcutaneous gas analysis as a indicator of arterial blood gas levels but makes it a valuable monitor of peripheral perfusion. The gradients of Po_2 and Pco_2 between arterial blood and skin widen when cardiac output and peripheral perfusion decline to cause less tissue gas exchange. The transcutaneous gas index, which is the ratio of gases between the arterial blood and skin, may be useful in evaluating hemodynamic instability. The relationships between the transcutaneous Po_2 index and age or the cardiac output are shown in Table 16-4.[143] The transcutaneous Po_2 index decreases progressively with age from premature infants to elderly patients. The transcutaneous Po_2 index in adults is 0.79 during stable hemodynamic conditions but falls to less than 0.5 when the cardiac index is less than 2.2 L/min/M^2.[144] This index is relatively insensitive to probe location as long as the probe remains on the trunk. On the other hand, transcutaneous Pco_2 is always higher than arterial Pco_2, and the transcutaneous Pco_2 index increases with poor peripheral perfusion.

The transcutaneous electrode should be calibrated every 4 hours during continuous use and whenever a sensor site changes. The site of application should be moved each time to prevent possible skin burn from heated electrodes. In practical use, electrode temperature usually is limited to 44° C, and location is changed every 4 to 6 hours. Transcutaneous Po_2 on

Table 16-4 Transcutaneous Oxygen Monitoring Index

$Ptco_2$ INDEX	AGE/HEMODYNAMIC STATUS
1.14 ± 0.1	Premature infants
1.0 ± 0.1	Newborn
0.84 ± 0.1	Children
0.8 ± 0.1	Adult, cardiac index >2.2 L/min/M^2
0.7 ± 0.1	Adult, age >65 years
0.5 ± 0.1	Adult, cardiac index 1.5-2.2 L/min/M^2
0.1 ± 0.1	Adult, cardiac index <1.5 L/min/M^2

From Wahr JA, Tremper KK: *Crit Care Clin* 11:199-217, 1995.
$Ptco_2$, Transcutaneous carbon dioxide tension.

the extremities is lower than that measured on the trunk, whereas transcutaneous PCO_2 on the extremities is higher. Thus the trunk is the location of choice for transcutaneous monitoring unless clinically contraindicated. After placement of the electrode on the skin, approximately 8 to 10 minutes pass before the sensor displays a steady value. Under conditions of poor dermal perfusion, a longer time is required. If the sensor becomes dislodged, it will report the PO_2 of room air, about 150 mm Hg, and a PCO_2 of near zero. It is worth remembering that external pressure on the electrode compresses the dermal capillaries and decreases perfusion, producing false values.

Capnography and Measurement of End-Tidal Carbon Dioxide

Capnography is the technique of displaying carbon dioxide concentration changes during the respiratory cycle.[145] A capnogram, a continuous record of PCO_2 (percentage in expired gas), typically is a graphic display plotting carbon dioxide on the ordinate and time on the abscissa. A capnometer is a device that measures carbon dioxide concentrations of inspired and expired gases. The instrument used to record the PCO_2 in expired gas is called a *capnograph.*[146] Two types of devices are available to monitor carbon dioxide concentration: an infrared detector and a mass spectrometer. Infrared capnographs are used to monitor 1 individual, and a mass spectrometer is usually a centralized monitoring system serving more than 1 patient, possibly as many as 20.

Infrared capnographs use the principle that molecules containing more than one element absorb infrared radiation in a unique and characteristic manner. Because it chooses the wavelengths at which the substance of interest absorbs the most light, this principle can be used to measure the concentration of that substance in a gas mixture. Carbon dioxide strongly absorbs infrared light with a 4.28-μm wavelength (Fig. 16-11), so radiation with this wavelength is used to measure PCO_2. The infrared light of this wavelength is beamed through a calibrated carbon dioxide–filled chamber with the gas serving as a control and through a chamber with the gas to be analyzed. Infrared-sensitive photocells receive light from both chambers and calculate the concentration of carbon dioxide in the sample gas by comparing it with the known concentration of carbon dioxide in the control.[147] The amount of infrared light absorbed depends on the concentration of carbon dioxide molecules in the sample. A semiconductor, called the *detector,* is used to create an electric signal that can be processed to display the continuous carbon dioxide concentration. This infrared technique provides breath-by-breath measurement of carbon dioxide concentration with a response time of approximately 100 msec.

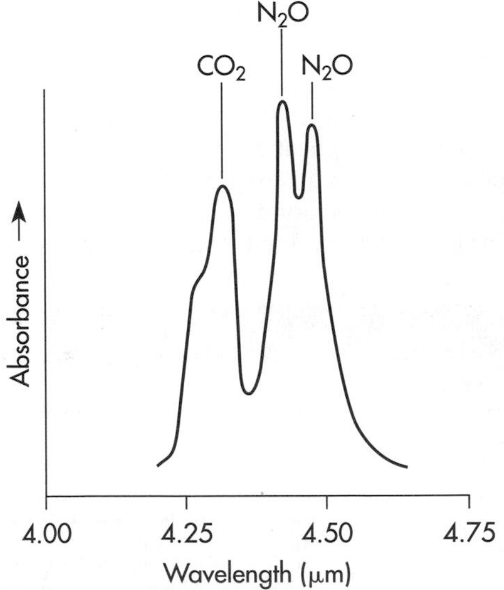

Fig. 16-11. Absorption of infrared radiation by carbon dioxide and by nitrous oxide *(N_2O)* depends on the wavelength of the radiation.

The gas to be analyzed can reach the sample chamber in one of two ways. The mainstream analyzer has a special flow-through adaptor called the *cuvette* that is mounted directly in line with the endotracheal tube and the Y-piece of ventilator (Fig. 16-12). The cuvette contains an infrared light source and photodetector, which is heated to prevent condensation. The advantages of the mainstream analyzer include a quick response time and the lack of delay and interference resulting from the long catheter used with the other technique.[148] Disadvantages include added dead space and the size and weight of the cuvette in the patient's airway, especially in infants and small children.[147] The sidestream analyzer uses suction to withdraw a continuous sample of inspired and expired gas through a capillary tube, which is connected to an adaptor, from the patient's airway to the monitor. The advantages and the disadvantages of this system are opposite to those of the mainstream system. There are some potential problems. Water vapor can interfere with the accuracy of carbon dioxide analysis. Another problem is nonlinear absorption of infrared light by carbon dioxide. The manufacturers adjust for this problem in the design of instruments. Last, background gases, such as nitrogen and nitrous oxide, can cause some absorption of the infrared light. This effect is referred to as *pressure broadening,* and most monitors compensate for this either manually or automatically.

Mass spectrometry is based on the physical principles that every gaseous substance yields unique and characteristic ions when bombarded with an electron beam and that the number of these ions produced is proportional to the concentration of the substance in the original sample.[149] Quadruple filtering and magnetic sector analysis are two methods of performing mass spectrometry. The continuously aspirated sample of a patient's respired gases travels through a tube to the mass spectrometer, usually at a site distant from the patient. An electron beam bombards the sample in an ionization chamber. Some of the gas molecules become charged ions of the original substance, and some become ion fragments of original substance. A detector plate is positioned so that ions unique to that substance strike it. Fragments hitting the detector produce an electric current proportional to the fractional concentration of the gas in the original sample. The electric current is processed by a computer that can digitize and transform the information to display it. This system can simultaneously measure the gases from as many as 20 patients. It is the only method currently available for clinical breath-by-breath measurement of all respiratory gases. The major drawback is that it must be shared by patients because of the size and expense of the system. In addition, the response time can be as long as 80 seconds (Table 16-5).

In a normal lung, carbon dioxide rapidly diffuses across the capillary-alveolar membrane when ventilation and perfusion are well matched (Fig. 16-13). End-tidal carbon dioxide pressure ($PETCO_2$), defined as the PCO_2 equivalent to airway carbon dioxide concentration at the end of an expiration, closely approximates the arterial PCO_2 in normal lungs.[150] The dispar-

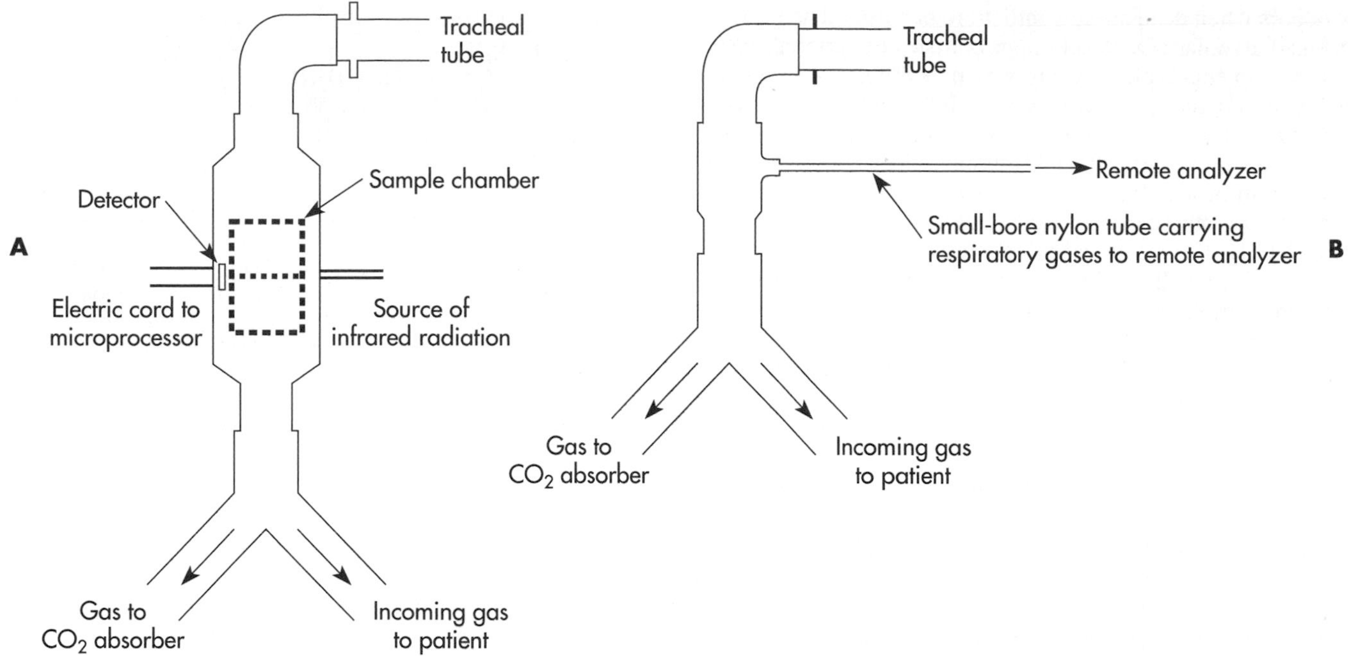

Fig. 16-12. **A,** Mainstream carbon dioxide analyzer. The sample chamber resides within the breathing circuit as close to the patient's airway as possible. Only infrared mainstream carbon dioxide analyzers are currently available. **B,** Sidestream carbon dioxide analyzer. The small-bore tube carries the sample from the airway to a distant sample chamber. All mass spectrometers and some infrared analyzers are of this variety. (From Stock MC: *Crit Care Clin* 4:511-526, 1988.)

Table 16-5 Comparison of Mass Spectrometry and Infrared Light Absorption for Breath-by-Breath Carbon Dioxide Values

ATTRIBUTE	MASS SPECTROMETRY	INFRARED LIGHT ABSORPTION
Continuous measurement	This is possible, but no other sites are analyzed because the unit is shared.	Yes, mostly dedicated units.
Delay time	The delay time is 45 seconds to 5 minutes depending on the distance from the spectrometer to the patient, the number of sites, the duration of sampling, and the assignment of priority.	The delay time is approximately 100 msec.
Gas analysis capability	All respiratory and anesthetic gases are measured.	Only molecular compounds containing more than two elements are measured.

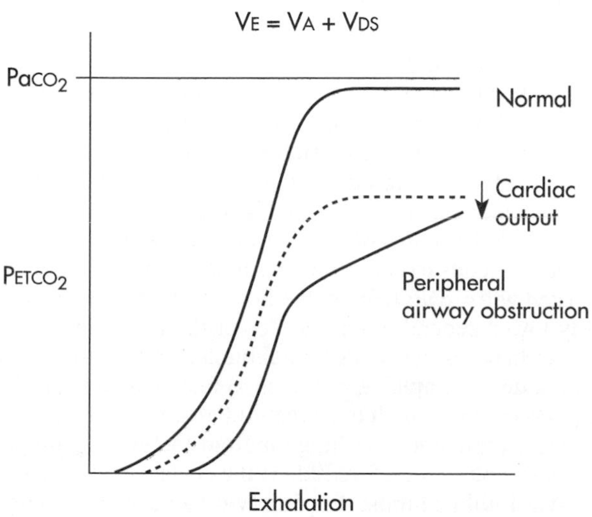

Fig. 16-13. Total ventilation (*V*E) is composed of both alveolar ventilation *(V*A*)* and dead space ventilation (*V*DS). The partial pressure of arterial carbon dioxide *($Pa{CO_2}$)* is considered the best reflection of alveolar ventilation. The end-tidal $P{CO_2}$ *($PET{CO_2}$)* is the expired $P{CO_2}$ at the end of the plateau. Increased dead space ventilation is manifested as an increased $Pa{CO_2}/PET{CO_2}$ gradient. The two most common causes of increased dead space ventilation are decreased cardiac output and lung disease. A decreased pulmonary perfusion results in more alveoli having lower $P{CO_2}$; the net result is a decreased expired $P{CO_2}$ but no change in the lung-emptying pattern. This is depicted as the dashed curve with a shape similar to normal. Lung disease involves changing emptying patterns and thus changes in the curve. (From Shapiro BA et al. In Shapiro BA et al, eds: *Clinical application of blood gases,* ed 5, St Louis, 1994, Mosby, p 259.)

ity occurs when dead space ventilation increases. The Pco_2 of perfused alveolar gas closely approximates the arterial Pco_2. However, in end-expiratory gas, which includes gas from both perfused and nonperfused alveoli, the difference between $PETCO_2$ and arterial Pco_2 becomes significant. As dead space ventilation increases, $PETCO_2$ underestimates the arterial Pco_2. Dilution with fresh, carbon dioxide–free gas, which occurs in the breathing circuit because of various reasons, lowers the $PETCO_2$. The dilutional effect may be more prominent in patients with small tidal volumes, such as infants and small children. Sampling errors may occur with leaks at the connection between the patient and the airway equipment. A falsely low $PETCO_2$ can occur with loose-fitting endotracheal tubes, which are commonly used in infants and small children. Incomplete exhalation before the next mechanical breath, which may occur with small airway obstruction, can falsely lower the $PETCO_2$. However, the waveform may give the clues of low airway obstruction. Alveolar gas may not have sufficient time to enter the patient's main airway, producing a lower $PETCO_2$ reading.

As shown in Fig. 16-14,[151] fresh, carbon dioxide–free gas fills the breathing circuit during normal inhalation, and the capnography is at zero. When exhalation starts, carbon dioxide–containing gas from the alveoli begins to enter the trachea and eventually arrives at the patient's airway. As the Pco_2 begins to rise in the airway, a sharp, smooth upstroke is produced in the capnogram, and then the slowly rising Pco_2 over time produces a nearly horizontal plateau in the graph. Near the end of the exhalation, the Pco_2 approaches the highest level on the plateau, $PETCO_2$. This is considered the best approximation of the alveolar Pco_2, estimating the arterial Pco_2. At this point, the difference between the $PETCO_2$ and arterial Pco_2 is minimal, so the $PETCO_2$ reflects the arterial Pco_2. With normal pulmonary function, the arterial Pco_2 is slightly higher than $PETCO_2$ with a difference of less than 4 mm Hg.[152] With inhalation, fresh, carbon dioxide–free gas enters the patient's airway, and the graph returns to zero until the next exhalation.

A sudden drop of the $PETCO_2$ usually comes from critical events. These include esophageal intubation,[153] airway disconnection, ventilator malfunction, and an obstructed endotracheal tube.[154] Loss of the plateau with a decreased $PETCO_2$ denotes an absence of full exhalation and may be caused by a loose-fitting endotracheal tube and a leaking or defective endotracheal tube cuff. An increase in physiologic dead space ventilation causes a progressive drop in $PETCO_2$ over time. Clinical pictures of this include low cardiac output states with severe blood loss, pulmonary embolism, and cardiopulmonary arrest. Hypothermia with decreased carbon dioxide production and hyperventilation also causes a progressive drop of the $PETCO_2$. Hyperthermia increases carbon dioxide production and $PETCO_2$ if ventilation and dead space remain constant. A rapid rise of the $PETCO_2$ may be noted in malignant hyperthermia. Acute, transient rises in the $PETCO_2$ commonly are caused by injections of bicarbonate and the release of a limb tourniquet. In addition, an acute increase in the cardiac output may increase $PETCO_2$.

A sudden rise in the baseline of the capnogram with an equal rise in the $PETCO_2$ usually suggests some contamination in the sampling device (e.g., the cuvette), and cleaning usually corrects the abnormality. A gradual rise in both the baseline and the $PETCO_2$ comes from rebreathing exhaled gas. This may be seen in partial rebreathing circuits, faulty check valves of a ventilators that allow bidirectional flow instead of unidirectional flow. Some abnormal capnographs are shown in Fig. 16-15.

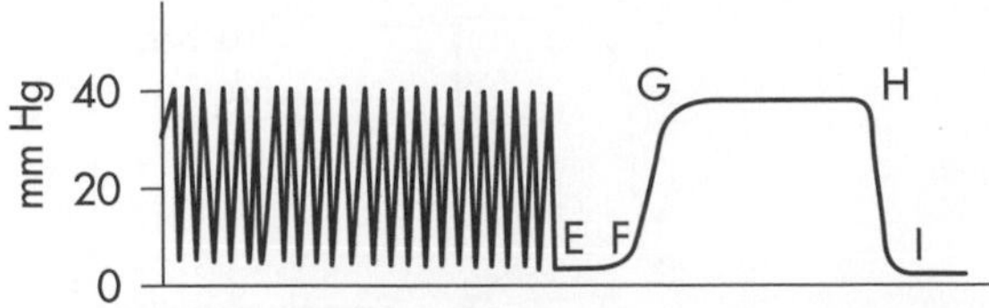

Fig. 16-14. Normal pattern of exhaled Pco_2 over time. The left portion of the trace was obtained with slow paper speed so that the $PETCO_2$ trend can be observed easily. The right side of the trace was obtained with rapid paper speed. Segment *EF* is inspiration; the Pco_2 of the inspired gas is zero. Segment *FG* is the start of exhalation, where gas is exhaled from anatomic dead space; the initial exhaled Pco_2 is very low. As increasing numbers of perfused alveoli empty, the carbon dioxide concentration rises rapidly. Segment *GH* is the alveolar plateau. The $PETCO_2$ cannot be interpreted without a clear alveolar plateau; $PETCO_2$ is read at point *H*. Segment *HI* is the beginning of inspiration. There should be no carbon dioxide in the inspired gas; thus Pco_2 falls rapidly.

The $PETCO_2$ is influenced by carbon dioxide production, alveolar ventilation, and pulmonary perfusion. Therefore the $PETCO_2$ alone does not provide adequate information of changes, so simultaneously the arterial Pco_2 should be intermittently obtained for an arterial $Pco_2/PETCO_2$ gradient to elucidate causes. Gastric gas contains negligible amounts of carbon dioxide, so the $PETCO_2$ returning from the stomach is near zero. Therefore the $PETCO_2$ can distinguish tracheal intubation from esophageal intubation because the $PETCO_2$ returning from the lung should be significantly higher than the gastric $PETCO_2$.[155] During blind nasotracheal intubation, a sudden rise of the $PETCO_2$ with a typical plateau also confirms that the endotracheal tube is in place.

Blood Gas Errors

Blood gas samples are susceptible to sampling, handling, and testing errors. The composition of the syringe with respect to the anticoagulant,[156] the pH of the anticoagulant,[157] the volume of blood to be drawn,[158] the syringe material,[84,159] and the syringe performance[160] all have been debated.

The addition of heparin to a blood sample may dilute the concentration of gases in the total sample. The major error associated with excessive heparin in the sample is a false-low Pco_2. The pH of the sample generally does not change because the effects of a decreased Pco_2 on pH are offset by the acidic pH of the heparin solution. As the sample size gets smaller, the relative contribution of the heparin becomes more significant. Syringes prepared with a crystalline heparin and an adequate size of blood sample minimize the effects of the dilution.

When a blood sample is placed in a syringe and an air bubble is included, the Po_2 of the air (approximately 158 mm Hg at sea level) tends to equilibrate with the blood.[161] When contaminated with an air bubble, the Po_2 may be falsely higher or falsely lower depending on the Po_2 of the blood sample. On the other hand, because an air bubble has practically no carbon dioxide, a sample equilibrates to falsely lower the Pco_2. The pH rises along with a decreased Pco_2. Minimizing agitation of a sample and expelling air from the syringe immediately on sampling therefore reduce the occurrence of these errors. Air bubbles must be removed within 30 seconds;

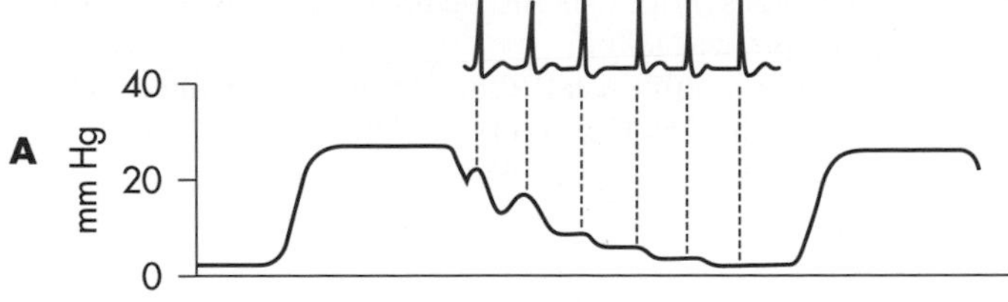

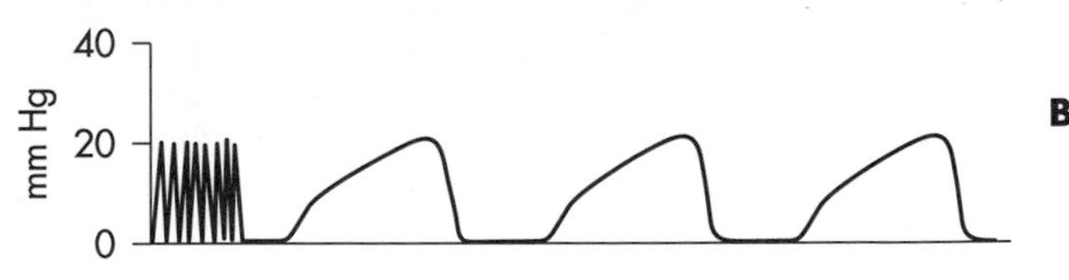

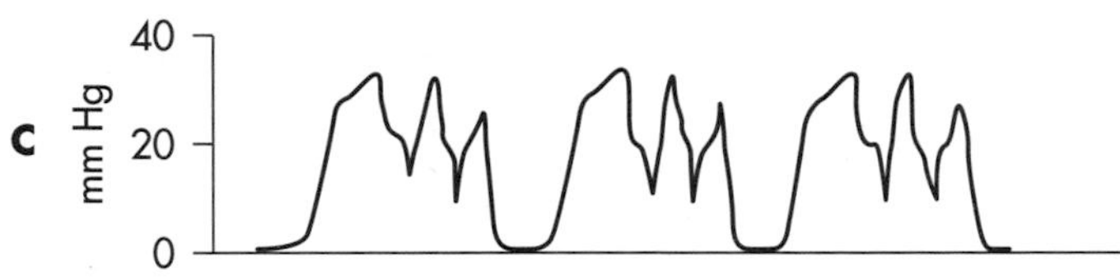

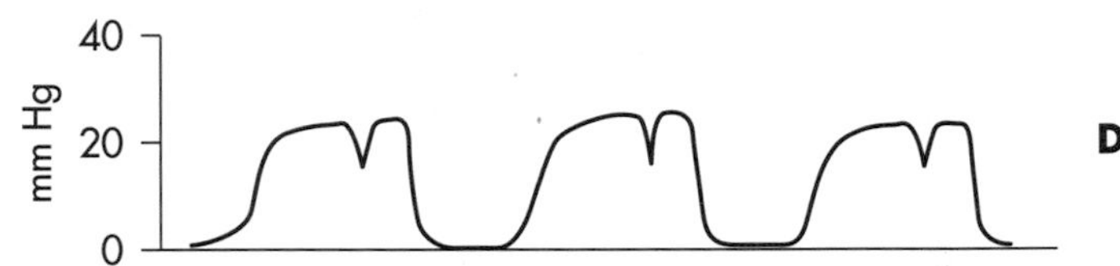

Fig. 16-15. **A,** Cardiac oscillations that result from a slow ventilatory rate (usually during mechanical ventilation). After the lungs passively empty, the pulmonary oscillation produced by the beating heart causes further gas flow from the lungs. **B,** Erratic breathing pattern. There is no alveolar plateau; thus P_{ETCO_2} cannot be obtained from this trace, although a digital display may give a spurious value. **C,** Exhaled carbon dioxide pattern consistent with obstructive lower airway disease. The increased dead space ventilation with this disease results in a slow rise of the alveolar component of the exhaled P_{CO_2} waveform. **D,** Exhaled carbon dioxide pattern characteristic of an early stage of recovery from neuromuscular blockade.

otherwise, P_{O_2} values increase and P_{CO_2} values begin to decrease.[162] Major errors can be seen in 30 minutes.

When a patient has an indwelling arterial catheter with a 1-ml dead space volume, approximately 2 ml of blood must be discarded to yield reliable results.[162] Failure to discard the blood contaminated with heparin and saline yields aberrant blood gas results.

In small infants the discard volume represents a significant amount of blood. The discard volume can be decreased by using the 3-drop method[163] or by replacing the discard volume.[164] These methods also eliminate the risk of emboli with retrograde flushing.

Blood is living tissue in which oxygen continues to be consumed and carbon dioxide continues to be produced, even after the blood is drawn into a syringe. This causes a significant effect in patients with severe leukocytosis.[165,166] If the sample is immediately placed in ice to keep it at approximately 4° C, the changes over several hours become insignificant (Table 16-6). Harsten et al[84] suggested that the results are likely to be more reliable by placing the blood gas on ice for transport to the laboratory. Conversely, Nanji and Whitlow[167] concluded that a blood gas sample is essentially unchanged if the laboratory performs the analysis within 20 minutes after the sample is drawn. Sending blood samples via a pneumatic transport device significantly alters blood gas results and therefore should be avoided.[168]

Table 16-6 In Vitro Blood Gas Changes*

	37° C	4° C
pH	0.01/10 min	0.001/10 min
P_{CO_2}	1 mm Hg/10 min	0.1 mm Hg/10 min
P_{O_2}	0.1 ml/dl/10 min	0.01 ml/dl/10 min

From Shapiro BA et al. In Shapiro BA et al, eds: *Clinical application of blood gases,* ed 5, St Louis, 1994, Mosby, p 228.
*Approximate changes with time and temperature after the sample is drawn into the syringe. A temperature of 37° C assumes that the blood remains at body temperature in the syringe. A temperature of 4° C assumes that the sample is properly iced immediately after being drawn.

Table 16-7 Predicted Effect of F_{IO_2} on Blood Oxygen Content

F_{IO_2}	PREDICTED ARTERIAL P_{O_2}
30%	150 mm Hg
40%	200 mm Hg
50%	250 mm Hg
80%	400 mm Hg
100%	500 mm Hg

From Shapiro BA et al: *Clinical application of blood gases,* ed 5, St Louis, 1994, Mosby, p 65.

INTERPRETATION OF ARTERIAL BLOOD GAS RESULTS

Oxygen

Each arterial blood gas value should first be evaluated in the context of normal values. Arterial oxygen values, which are affected by age and altitude, can also be altered by the F_{IO_2}, the condition of the alveolar air-blood barrier, and pulmonary blood flow. At sea level an arterial P_{O_2} of 97 mm Hg (range = 80 to 103 torr) is considered normal. A patient with normal lungs receiving supplemental oxygen should have an arterial P_{O_2} approximately 5 times the F_{IO_2} (Table 16-7). The arterial P_{O_2} decreases in the elderly and varies depending on whether an individual is sitting or supine.[169] The normal value for arterial P_{O_2} changes with age according to the following formulas:

$$\text{Supine arterial } P_{O_2} = 103.5 - (0.42 \times \text{Age})$$

$$\text{Sitting arterial } P_{O_2} = 104.2 - (0.27 \times \text{Age})$$

If arterial hypoxemia is present, it may be caused by hypoventilation, absolute shunting, diffusion defects, or relative shunting (Table 16-8). Hypoventilation can be rapidly diagnosed by the presence of elevated arterial PCO_2 values. Calculation of the alveolar-arterial oxygen tension gradient while the patient is breathing room air can be helpful in discriminating hypoventilation from shunting. A gradient higher than 20 mm Hg suggests shunting.

An absolute shunt is defined as blood passing form the right to the left side of the heart without being oxygenated. Absolute shunting does not respond to increases in the inspired oxygen level because the shunted blood never comes in contact with oxygen. Shunting may also occur at the level of the alveoli. Blood cannot be oxygenated when the alveolus is blocked, collapsed, or filled with fluid. There is also anatomic shunting resulting from persistent pulmonary hypertension and congenital heart defects.

When there is no right-to-left shunt, an arterial blood gas value represents pulmonary gas exchange, whereas a venous blood gas value represents tissue gas exchange. Pulmonary gas exchange relies on pulmonary function, and tissue gas exchange is affected by tissue perfusion. Therefore the interpretation of blood gas values should be different based on where the blood sample was taken.

Table 16-8 Examples of Arterial Hypoxemia

PROBLEM	EXAMPLE
Low PiO_2	Low FIO_2 and altitude
Alveolar hypoventilation (low alveolar PO_2 with increased alveolar PCO_2)	Central nervous system depression, pulmonary disease
Diffusion block	Pulmonary fibrosis
$\dot{V}/\dot{Q}$ mismatch	Pulmonary embolism
Shunt	Congenital heart disease

PiO_2, Partial pressure of oxygen in the conducting airway; $\dot{V}$, gas flow; $\dot{Q}$, blood flow.

When there is a right-to-left shunt, total cardiac output ($\dot{Q}t$) is composed of shunted blood ($\dot{Q}s$) and pulmonary end-capillary blood flow ($\dot{Q}c$) (Fig. 16-16), as follows:

$$\dot{Q}t = \dot{Q}s + \dot{Q}c$$

The total amount of oxygen ejected from the left side of the heart is equal to the amount of oxygen carried in pulmonary end-capillary blood plus the amount of oxygen carried in shunted blood, as follows:

$$\dot{Q}t \times CaO_2 = \dot{Q}c \times CcO_2 + \dot{Q}s \times C\bar{v}O_2$$

where CaO_2, CcO_2, and $C\bar{v}O_2$ are the arterial, pulmonary end-capillary, and mixed venous oxygen contents, respectively.

The shunt equation is used to solve for $\dot{Q}s/\dot{Q}t$, as follows:

$$\frac{\dot{Q}s}{\dot{Q}t} = \frac{CcO_2 - CaO_2}{CcO_2 - C\bar{v}O_2}$$

Oxygen content is measured directly or calculated according to the following formula:

$$O_2 \text{ content} = (SO_2 \times Hgb \times 1.34) + (0.003 \times PaO_2)$$

where SO_2 is the percent saturation of hemoglobin with oxygen, *Hgb* is the hemoglobin concentration, and PaO_2 is the partial pressure of arterial oxygen. The pulmonary end-capillary oxygen content cannot be measured directly unless a pulmonary CBG analysis is performed. Instead, it may be calculated by assuming that it is equivalent to the alveolar PO_2.

As shown in Fig. 16-16, the classic shunt ($\dot{Q}s/\dot{Q}t$) (i.e., anatomic shunt plus capillary shunt) is not exposed to alveolar PO_2 and therefore is not affected by FIO_2.[170] This shunt is calculated while the patient breathes 100% inspired oxygen and

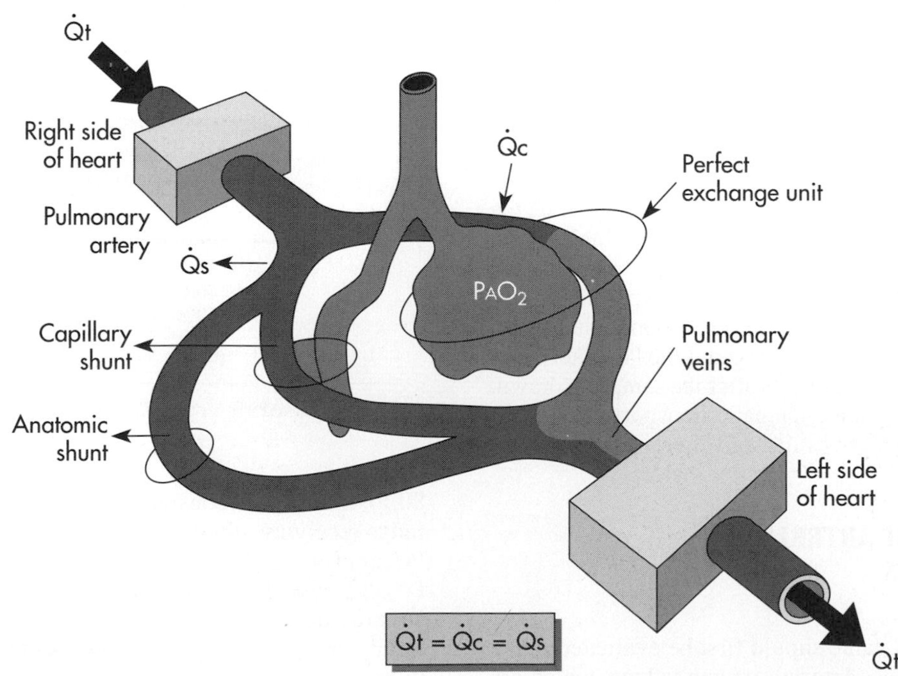

Fig. 16-16. A visual concept of physiologic shunting. PAO_2, Partial pressure of alveolar oxygen. (From Shapiro BA et al. In Shapiro BA et al, eds: *Clinical application of blood gases,* ed 5, St Louis, 1994, Mosby, p 88.)

represents only the zero gas flow/blood flow ($\dot{V}/\dot{Q}$) and not the venous admixture with low $\dot{V}/\dot{Q}$. When the patient is breathing less than 100% inspired oxygen, the calculated intrapulmonary shunt represents the venous admixture with low $\dot{V}/\dot{Q}$. This is called *physiologic shunt* ($\dot{Q}sp/\dot{Q}t$). When $\dot{Q}sp/\dot{Q}t$ is applied to patients with diseased lungs, it represents the severity of diminishment of the lung as an oxygenator. When mixed venous blood is not available, a modified version of the shunt equation can be used. The modified version of the shunt equation assumes a fixed arteriovenous oxygen difference of 5 vol %.[171]

$$\frac{\dot{Q}sp}{\dot{Q}t} = \frac{Cco_2 - Cao_2}{Cco_2 - C\bar{v}o_2 + 5.0}$$

Many studies using this principle have been published assessing the reliability of the newer oxygen tension–based indexes in reflecting $\dot{Q}sp/\dot{Q}t$[172-176] (Table 16-9). These include the alveolar-arterial Po_2 gradient ($P[A - a]o_2$), the arterial-alveolar oxygen tension ratio (Pao_2/PAo_2), the ratio of arterial oxygen tension to inspired oxygen concentration (Pao_2/Fio_2), and the respiratory index ($P[A - a]o_2/Pao_2$).[172-176] The clinical application of $P(A - a)o_2$ is limited in patients who have an arterial Po_2 much less than 150 mm Hg and in whom the Fio_2 is varied. With an arterial Po_2 less than 100 mm Hg, changes in the oxygen content increasingly become a function of changes in hemoglobin saturation rather than in dissolved oxygen. In contrast to the $P(A - a)o_2$, the Pao_2/PAo_2 is relatively unaffected by changes in the Fio_2. So that calculation of the alveolar Po_2 could be avoided, the Pao_2/Fio_2 was introduced. This index is affected by changes in arterial Pco_2 values, and values less than 2 have been reported to correlate well with $\dot{Q}sp/\dot{Q}t$ values of more than 20%. Last, $P(A - a)o_2/Pao_2$ was introduced to minimize the inherent problems of $P(A - a)o_2$, and it is a better indicator than $P(A - a)o_2$ in estimating $\dot{Q}sp/\dot{Q}t$.

Carbon Dioxide

The arterial concentration of carbon dioxide (*$Paco_2$*) is determined mainly by the degree of alveolar ventilation (*$\dot{V}A$*) in relation to the patient's carbon dioxide production (*$\dot{V}co_2$*), as follows:

$$PACO_2 \propto \frac{\dot{V}CO_2}{\dot{V}A}$$

Alveolar ventilation is lowered by increased alveolar dead space, which occurs when alveoli are ventilated but not perfused. This circumstance is reflected in a measured gradient between $PETco_2$ and mixed alveolar Pco_2. $PETco_2$ is lower than alveolar Pco_2 because of the addition of alveolar dead space gas, which does not contain carbon dioxide.[177]

Alveolar Pco_2 is difficult to measure directly, and the assumption is made that it is equal to arterial Pco_2. This assumption is valid because carbon dioxide is highly diffusible across the alveolar-capillary membrane, which quickly equilibrates alveolar Pco_2 and pulmonary end-capillary $Pcco_2$. The difference between mixed venous Pco_2 (46 mm Hg) and pulmonary end-capillary Pco_2 (40 mm Hg) is small. Consequently, even a large admixture of venous blood to the pulmonary end-capillary from a large shunt produces only a small increase in arterial Pco_2.

Under normal conditions the balance between carbon dioxide production and alveolar ventilation is set so that arterial Pco_2 is maintained at 40 mm Hg (37 to 45 mm Hg).[178] The Pco_2 is influenced by altitude, ventilation, and the condition of the alveoli. A blood gas Pco_2 of less than 37 mm Hg with a pH of more than 7.45 is consistent with hyperventilation. A patient with a blood gas Pco_2 greater than 45 mm Hg with a pH less than 7.35 probably has significant ventilatory failure. Many patients with lung disease breathe more rapidly (tachypnea) or more deeply (hyperpnea) to maintain a normal Pco_2. Small changes in Pco_2 evoke a rapid increase in ventilation to restore the Pco_2 toward normal. Stimuli such as hypoxemia, fever, anxiety, central nervous system disease, septicemia, and medications can increase ventilation,[179] whereas central nervous system depression and pulmonary disease may cause an increase in the Pco_2. The Pco_2 rises or decreases until it achieves a new equilibrium; at equilibrium, carbon dioxide production equals excretion. Because respiration is so efficient, modest changes in carbon dioxide production usually do not alter the Pco_2.

The Pco_2 levels are fastidiously maintained within a very narrow range by balancing carbon dioxide production and excretion. Carbon dioxide production increases in response to several conditions, including exercise, burns, and sepsis. Carbon dioxide production can transiently rise as a result of a sodium bicarbonate infusion. After accepting a hydrogen ion, bicarbonate can be converted into carbon dioxide and water. Therefore infusion of sodium bicarbonate can increase the Pco_2 level in an individual whose minute ventilation cannot be increased. In an individual with normal lung function, minute ventilation can be increased to compensate for the increased carbon dioxide production.

pH

Any change in the hydrogen ion concentration in blood causes a defense of the pH by compensatory mechanisms. For example, if there is a perturbation in the Pco_2, then the bicarbonate level increases or decreases to compensate for the perturbation, thereby normalizing the pH. Any change in the bicarbonate or carbon dioxide level that does not yield a significant change in the pH (because of compensatory mechanisms) is referred to as *acidosis* or *alkalosis*.

> *Example:* A neonate with respiratory distress has the following blood gas values: pH, 7.38; Pco_2, 52 mm Hg; and bicarbonate level, 29 mmol/L. In this case, the acid-base status can be described as a primary respiratory acidosis with a compensatory metabolic alkalosis.

When a primary respiratory or metabolic process overwhelms the compensatory mechanism, the blood pH changes.

Table 16-9 Comparison of Gas Exchange Index

PARAMETER	MEAN ± SD	RANGE	R VALUE
$\dot{Q}sp/\dot{Q}t$	22.3 ± 11.2	3.0-53.0	—
Estimated shunt	27.6 ± 11.3	2.7-62.3	+0.94
RI	3.1 ± 2.6	0.3-14.0	+0.74
Pao_2/PAo_2	0.3 ± 0.2	0.06-0.77	−0.72
Pao_2/Fio_2	1.8 ± 0.9	0.1-4.3	−0.71
$P(A - a)o_2$	222.8 ± 141.7	32-611	+0.62

From Cane RD et al: *Crit Care Med* 16:1243-1245, 1988.
SD, Standard deviation; *RI,* respiratory index ($P[A - a]o_2/PAo_2$); *Pao_2/PAo_2*, arterial-alveolar oxygen tension ratio; *Pao_2/Fio_2*, ratio of arterial oxygen tension to inspired oxygen concentration; *$P(A - a)o_2$*, alveolar-arterial oxygen tension.

The normal pH in the extracellular fluids is 7.40 ± 0.02 (1 standard deviation). When the pH is lower than 7.40, the patient is acidemic. When the pH is higher than 7.40, the patient is alkalemic. When there is a perturbation in the blood pH, the etiology is either respiratory or metabolic (Fig. 16-17). For example, if the patient is acidemic, there is an excess of P_{CO_2} or a decrease in the bicarbonate level.

If no compensatory process existed, recognition of the inciting problem would be quite easy. Formulas have been derived that describe the relationship between carbon dioxide and bicarbonate in acute and chronic acid-base disorders (see Tables 16-1 and 16-2). These formulas can assist in determining the primary event and the compensatory process.

In most cases the pH deviation suggests the primary process. For example, in a patient with a pH of 7.32, a bicarbonate value of 26 mmol/L, and an arterial P_{CO_2} of 52 mm Hg, acidemia exists. The elevated bicarbonate level could not have caused the acidemia, so the cause is respiratory acidosis. In this case, the renal compensatory process has not had time to correct the pH to normal.

Bicarbonate

Serum bicarbonate values are routinely calculated from known pH and carbon dioxide values using the Henderson-Hasselbalch equation. Alternatively, serum bicarbonate levels can be estimated from total carbon dioxide values. Total carbon dioxide levels can be determined by adding a strong acid to the blood. The total carbon dioxide value includes bicarbonate, carbonic acid, dissolved carbon dioxide, carbonate, and carbon dioxide bound to amino acids. Because 95% of the total carbon dioxide value is bicarbonate, the total carbon dioxide value is usually 2 mmol/L higher than the calculated bicarbonate value.

Serum bicarbonate values change in the same direction as blood carbon dioxide levels because of the hydrogen ion–accepting capacity of hemoglobin and other proteins. When carbon dioxide is bubbled through a bicarbonate solution without hemoglobin, the serum bicarbonate concentration does not change.

Example: A patient with diabetic ketoacidosis has a serum bicarbonate level of 5 mmol/L, a pH of 7.11, and a P_{CO_2} of 16.5 mm Hg. As sodium bicarbonate is infused, the carbon dioxide level rises because of a decrease in respiratory drive and the conversion of bicarbonate to water and carbon dioxide.

In children and adults, the normal serum bicarbonate value is 24 mmol/L (range 22 to 29 mmol/L). However, in newborns the values are significantly lower because of a lower bicarbonate resorption threshold in the proximal tubule and a limited ability to excrete hydrogen ions.[180] Decreased renal tubule ammonia production also contributes to the low serum bicarbonate values. Newborns typically have an alkaline urinary pH during the first week of life. The urine pH becomes acidic during the second week of life. Serum bicarbonate values are lower in preterm infants (18 to 20 mmol/L) than those born at term (20 to 22 mmol/L). The metabolic acidosis seen early in life is due in part to an expanded extracellular volume. The mild metabolic acidosis has a beneficial effect of facilitating an increase in the respiratory drive. Bicarbonate therapy is not

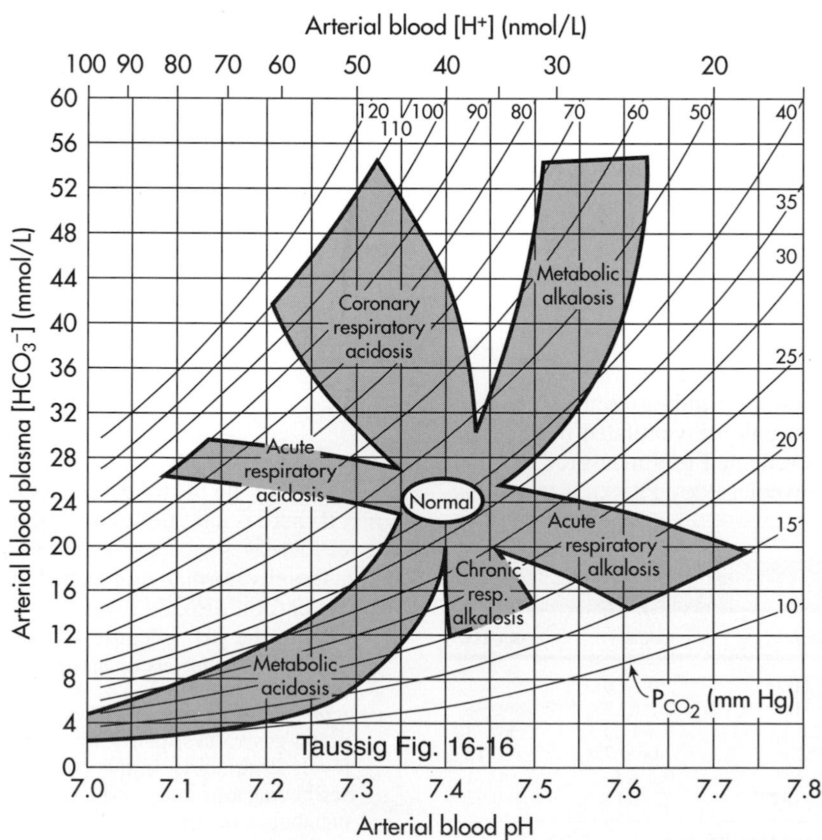

Fig. 16-17. Acid-base nomogram. The nomogram bands represent 95% confidence limits for an acid-base disorder. (From Cogan MG, Rector FC. In Brenner B, Rector FC: *The kidney,* ed 4, Philadelphia, 1991, WB Saunders, p 473.)

indicated for the treatment of physiologic metabolic acidosis because the condition resolves without treatment.

Simple Acid-Base Disorders

Acid-base problems generally fall into two broad categories: those with a single primary disorder coupled with a compensatory response (a simple acid-base disorder) and those in which two primary disorders occur together (a mixed acid-base disorder). The type of acid-base disorder can be determined by evaluating the pH, arterial P_{CO_2}, and bicarbonate level. In a simple acid-base problem, the arterial P_{CO_2} and the bicarbonate level always move in the same direction (Table 16-10). Movement of the arterial P_{CO_2} and the bicarbonate level in opposite directions indicates a mixed acid-base disorder. Assessment of the appropriateness of the compensation using Tables 16-1 and 16-2 can also be helpful in uncovering a mixed acid-base problem.

Metabolic Acidosis

The following basic mechanisms can cause serum bicarbonate levels to fall, causing metabolic acidosis[181]:

1. As an acid is added to the body fluids, bicarbonate buffers the acid, leaving less bicarbonate.
2. Bicarbonate can be lost through the gastrointestinal tract or through the kidneys.
3. Serum bicarbonate levels can be decreased by dilution with a nonbicarbonate-containing solution.

The evaluation of any metabolic acidosis should include a determination of the anion gap. The limits of electrochemical neutrality ensure that there are equal numbers of positive and negative ions. The anion gap can be determined by using the following equation:

$$Na^+ + \text{Unmeasured cations} = (Cl^- + HCO_3^-) + \text{Unmeasured anions}$$

$$\text{Anion gap} = Na^+ - (Cl^- + HCO_3^-) = \text{Unmeasured anions} - \text{Unmeasured cations}$$

Note that potassium in this formula is considered an unmeasured cation and should not be added to sodium *(Na^+)* in the calculation of the anion gap. The normal anion gap is 12 ± 4 mmol/L.[182] Under normal conditions the anion gap is constituted predominantly of negative charges on serum proteins[41] (Fig. 16-18). The anion gap is clinically useful because it can be used to determine the cause of metabolic acidosis. Patients with metabolic acidosis typically have an increased or a normal anion gap. If hydrochloric acid is added to blood, then there is a one-to-one replacement of bicarbonate for chloride, yielding a normal anion gap acidosis. The same is true for intestinal or renal loss of bicarbonate; the kidney resorbs more chloride to maintain electrochemical neutrality. If bicarbonate is replaced by an unmeasured anion and the serum chloride level remains unchanged, the anion gap increases. An increased anion gap can be caused by an increase in unmeasured anions, a decrease in unmeasured cations, or both changes (Table 16-11). A decreased anion gap is due to hypoalbumine-

Table 16-10 Simple Acid-Base Disorders

TYPE OF DISORDER	pH	Pa_{CO_2}	HCO_3^-
Metabolic acidosis	↓	↓	↓
Metabolic alkalosis	↑	↑	↑
Acute respiratory acidosis	↓	↑	↑
Chronic respiratory acidosis	↓	↑	↑
Acute respiratory alkalosis	↑	↓	↓
Chronic respiratory alkalosis	↑	↓	↓

From Schrier RW: *Renal and electrolyte disorders,* ed 3, Boston, 1986, Little, Brown, p 146.
Pa_{CO_2}, Partial pressure of arterial carbon dioxide; *HCO_3^-*, bicarbonate.

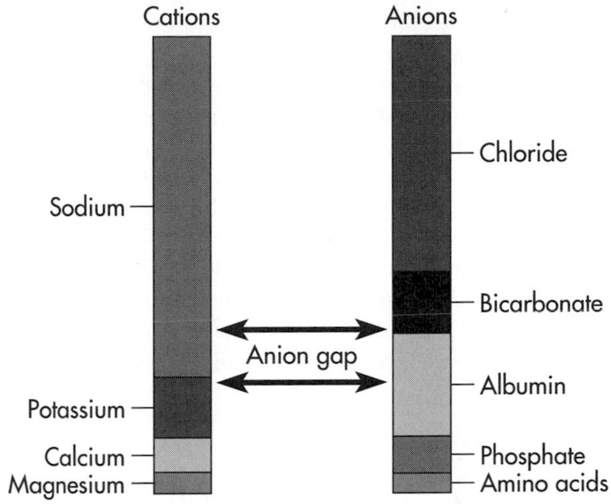

Fig. 16-18. Anion gap. Because of the demands of electrochemical neutrality, the concentration of positive and negative ions in serum must be equal. The serum sodium value is greater than that of the chloride and bicarbonate values combined. The normal ion gap, 12 ± 4 mmol/L, is composed of albumin, phosphates, and amino acids. When bicarbonate has been replaced by other anions, the anion gap is higher than normal.

Table 16-11 Causes of Anion Gap Acidosis

CAUSE	UNMEASURED ANION
Toxins and medications	
Ethanol	Lactic acid
Ethylene glycol	Oxalic acid
Isoniazid toxicity	Lactic acid
Methanol	Formic acid
Paraldehyde	Acetic acid
Salicylates	Lactic acid
Isopropyl alcohol	Oxalic acid
Lactic acidosis	Lactic acid
Uremia	Uric, oxalic, succinic, pimelic, and adipic acids
Amino acidopathies	
Maple syrup urine disease	α-Ketoisocaproic, α-keto-β methylvaleric, α-ketoisovaleric, indolacetic, acetoacetic, and β-hydroxybutyric acids
Isovaleric acidemia	Isovaleric acid
Glutaric acidemia	Glutaric, lactic, isobutyric, isovaleric, and α-methylbutyric acids
Propionyl–coenzyme A carboxylase deficiency	Propionic, methylcitric propionylglycine, acetoacetic, β-hydroxypropionate, and β-hydroxybutyric acids
Methylmalonic aciduria	Methylmalonic acid
Defects in carbohydrate metabolism	
Diabetic ketoacidosis	Acetoacetic and β-hydroxybutyric acids
Fructose-1,6-diphosphatase deficiency	Lactic and pyruvic acids
Glucose-6-phosphatase deficiency	Lactic acid
Pyruvate carboxylase deficiency	Lactic and pyruvic acids
Succinyl–coenzyme A–transferase deficiency	Acetoacetic and β-hydroxybutyric acids

mia, hypercalcemia, hyperkalemia, hypermagnesemia, or the administration of lithium.

Most of the acute change in the serum bicarbonate level is repaired by intracellular buffering processes.[183,184] Hemoglobin, phosphorous, protein, and bone[61,185] all contribute to buffering hydrogen ion. Serum chloride levels rise in response to the decrease in bicarbonate levels. In the event that metabolic acidosis persists, treatment of the underlying disorder is indicated. Sodium bicarbonate therapy is typically reserved for treatment of a hyperchloremic metabolic acidosis resulting from renal tubular acidosis, diarrhea, a ureterosigmoidostomy, or amino acid or cholestyramine infusions. Care should be taken to prevent a paradoxical decrease in cerebral pH or a decrease of the respiratory drive resulting from the increase in pH. Generally, sodium bicarbonate therapy should be used when the serum pH is less than 7.1. Because sodium bicarbonate has a sodium content of 1000 mEq/L, large doses can cause significant hypernatremia. In addition, serum potassium values fall after infusion of bicarbonate because of the movement of potassium back into cells in exchange for hydrogen ions.

Respiratory Acidosis

Any process that interferes with ventilation can cause respiratory acidosis. The causes of ventilatory failure include chronic obstructive pulmonary disease, medications, an extreme ventilation-perfusion mismatch, an extensive infiltrative process, exhaustion, neuromuscular disorders, and excessive carbon dioxide production.

Hypercapnea stimulates the secretion of hydrogen ions by the distal tubule (Fig. 16-19), which lowers the urine pH, titrates filtered buffers, and traps ammonium.[49,186] Studies with fluorescent probes demonstrate that vesicles with hydrogen ions fuse with the luminal membrane to increase hydrogen ion secretion. Bicarbonate secretion in the distal tubule is inhibited.[187] Therefore serum bicarbonate values increase. The higher bicarbonate concentration is maintained by enhanced renal bicarbonate resorption in both the proximal and distal tubules. The renal compensatory response to chronic hypercarbia usually takes 1 to 2 days. Hypercapnia also decreases proximal sodium chloride resorption and causes chloruresis.

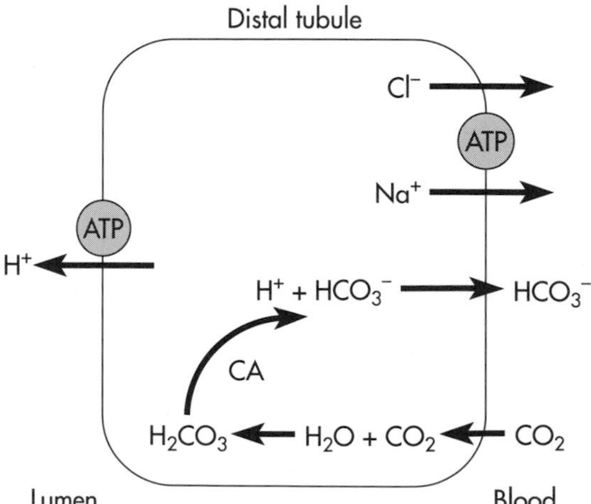

Fig. 16-19. Secretion of hydrogen ions *(H^+)* by the distal tubule allows reclamation of bicarbonate *(HCO_3^-)* when serum carbon dioxide levels are elevated. Bicarbonate cannot be resorbed into the blood until the hydrogen ion has bound to either an ammonia or phosphate molecule in the urine. *Cl^-*, Chloride; *Na^+*, sodium; *CA*, carbonic anhydrase; *H_2CO_3*, carbonic acid.

Occasionally, too much bicarbonate is generated, so the blood is alkaline as a result of nighttime hypercapnia or a renal response geared to blood P_{CO_2} rather than pH. Therefore the patient with chronic respiratory acidosis may have a modest alkalosis. In chronic respiratory acidosis the blood bicarbonate concentration increases 0.25 to 0.3 mEq/L for each elevation of 1 mm Hg in P_{CO_2} (see Table 16-2).

Metabolic Alkalosis

Metabolic alkalosis is a disorder characterized by an increase in serum bicarbonate levels, which causes an increase in the serum pH. The following mechanisms cause metabolic alkalosis: (1) intravascular volume contraction in which chloride is lost disproportionately to bicarbonate, (2) loss of hydrogen ions, and (3) net addition of bicarbonate to the extracellular space. Chloride loss (without concurrent hydrogen ion loss) most commonly occurs with gastrointestinal disease or chemical diuretic use. When hypochloremia develops, the kidney increases the resorption of bicarbonate by increasing hydrogen ion secretion by the distal tubule. The increase in bicarbonate resorption is necessary so that electrochemical neutrality is maintained while sodium is resorbed.

Metabolic alkalosis can develop when more chloride than sodium is lost from the gastrointestinal tract of patients with acute diarrhea. Chloride losses resulting from diarrhea may range from 10 to 110 mEq/L of stool. There also is a rare congenital form of chloride diarrhea in which a defect in bowel transport of chloride occurs. Chemical diuretics can cause a profound loss of chloride by the kidney. Patients with Bartter's syndrome also experience profound chloriduria. Chloride depletion causes extracellular volume contraction and increases the serum bicarbonate level.

Hydrogen ions can be lost through gastrointestinal or renal mechanisms. The secretion of hydrochloric acid in the stomach leaves a cation and bicarbonate molecule in the serum. If hydrogen ions are lost from the body, there is a net increase in serum bicarbonate values. Renal hydrogen losses can be accelerated by the presence of mineralocorticoids and diuretics.

With potassium depletion, potassium egresses from somatic cells to maintain the ratio of intracellular to extracellular potassium. As potassium egresses from the cell, hydrogen ions move in to maintain electrochemical neutrality. Sodium cannot be exchanged for potassium because all cells have a sodium-potassium pump that pumps sodium out of the cell. The movement of hydrogen ions into the cell leads to higher extracellular bicarbonate levels.

The administration of bicarbonate or substances that generate bicarbonate such as citrate, acetate, and lactate causes a rise in serum bicarbonate levels. Because the kidney can excrete bicarbonate, the alkalosis that develops in response to exogenous alkali is typically mild.

Three mechanisms act to decrease serum bicarbonate levels when metabolic alkalosis develops. There are intracellular buffering mechanisms by which the hydrogen ion, which is derived from intracellular proteins and phosphate, is released into the extracellular space. Lactic acid levels also increase and provide additional hydrogen ions for buffering.[188] The kidney can excrete bicarbonate via β-intercalated cells in the distal tubule. Compensatory respiratory acidosis is the third process by which the pH is returned toward normal; in this case the degree of compensation is somewhat limited because the arterial Po_2 also drops with hypoventilation. Nevertheless, the arterial Pco_2 can increase to approximately 55 mm Hg. With a respiratory compensation to metabolic alkalosis, the arterial Pco_2 should increase by 0.25 to 1 times the change in the concentration of bicarbonate.

Factors such as volume depletion, production of aldosterone, and potassium depletion also interfere with renal bicarbonate wasting, thus maintaining alkalosis. Volume depletion decreases the amount of glomerular filtrate delivered to the proximal tubule. Sodium and bicarbonate resorption are therefore relatively increased. In the proximal tissue aldosterone increases hydrogen ion secretion by the distal tubule. Potassium depletion increases the rate of bicarbonate resorption.[189] The intracellular hydrogen ion concentration is elevated in response to potassium depletion in all cells, including renal tubular cells; therefore hydrogen ion secretion by the renal distal tubule increases.

Occasionally, metabolic alkalosis can occur in a patient whose chronic hypercapnia resolves but whose cells cannot excrete bicarbonate rapidly enough. Conversion of large amounts lactic acid resulting from hypoperfusion can also cause metabolic alkalosis.

The effective treatment of metabolic alkalosis depends on the recognition of chloride-responsive and chloride-resistant processes. Treatment consisting of sodium or potassium chloride replacement leads to rapid resolution of the metabolic alkalosis induced by chloride depletion. Individuals with sodium chloride–resistant metabolic alkalosis either have increased mineralocorticoid activity or are potassium depleted. Hypermineralocorticoid states are typically accompanied by hypertension.

Respiratory Alkalosis

Respiratory alkalosis is caused by a process in which the pH rises in response to a decreasing Pco_2 (Box 16-3). The Pco_2 falls when ventilatory losses of carbon dioxide exceed carbon dioxide production. Generally, ventilation can be increased via central or peripheral neural stimulation, mechanical ventilation, or voluntary effort.

Buffering by hydrogen ion release from intracellular sources constitutes the first defense against respiratory alkalosis.[56] Amazingly, buffering is complete in minutes and persists for at least 2 hours.[190] In response to acute respiratory alkalosis the bicarbonate level decreases by 1 to 3 mmol/L for every decrease of 10 mm Hg in arterial Pco_2.

BOX 16-3
Causes of Respiratory Alkalosis

- Central alkalosis
  - Pain, anxiety
  - Head trauma
  - Fever
  - Pregnancy
  - Brain tumors
  - Administration of salicylates
  - Hepatic encephalopathy
- Peripheral alkalosis
  - Altitude
  - Pulmonary embolism
  - Pneumonia
  - Congestive heart failure
  - Interstitial lung disease
  - Hepatic insufficiency
  - Gram-negative sepsis
- Mechanical or voluntary hyperventilation

The kidney compensates in response to respiratory alkalosis by reducing the amount of bicarbonate generated and by excreting bicarbonate.[60] The process of renal compensation occurs within 24 to 48 hours.[59] The stimulus for the renal compensatory mechanism is not pH but rather Pco_2.[191,192] In chronic respiratory alkalosis the plasma bicarbonate level is decreased 2 to 5 mmol/L for every decrease of 10 mm Hg in Pco_2. The only means of treating respiratory alkalosis is correcting the underlying disorder responsible for causing the alkalosis.

Mixed Acid-Base Disorders

A mixed acid-base disorder is a combination of two primary acid-base disorders. Recognition of a mixed acid-base disorder often depends on a determination of whether the compensatory process was adequate and appropriate. Frequently the blood gas results fall outside of those predicted for an acid-base disorder (see Fig. 16-17). Some patients with mixed acid-base disorders may have a serious deviation of pH, whereas others may have a normal pH. When there is a significant deviation of pH, one of the two primary disorders has blocked the other's compensatory mechanism.

> *Example:* A 9-month-old boy with renal tubular acidosis is unable to take his medication because of the respiratory distress associated with respiratory syncytial virus. At admission, the results of his arterial blood gas analysis are as follows: arterial Po_2, 67 mm Hg; pH, 7.19; arterial Pco_2, 56 mm Hg; and bicarbonate level, 17 mmol/L. The diagnosis is a mixed acid-base disorder: metabolic acidosis and acute respiratory acidosis.

Occasionally the amount of compensation is excessive given the clinical situation. For example, in children with an aspirin intoxication, the arterial Pco_2 is typically lower than expected based on the acidosis caused by the aspirin alone. The excessive respiratory alkalosis is attributed to the stimulatory effect that aspirin has on ventilation.

Patients with chronic lung disease typically have high arterial Pco_2 values and an appropriate compensatory metabolic alkalosis. The addition of diuretics, which are frequently used to decrease alveolar interstitial edema, causes serum bicarbonate values to increase to levels greater than expected. The blood gas results are frequently consistent with simple metabolic alkalosis. A patient's history may be the only means by which the mixed acid-base disorder can be detected. The addition of acute respiratory acidosis makes the picture even more complicated.

> *Example:* A 15-month-old girl with bronchopulmonary dysplasia receives furosemide, 1 mg/kg/day. Her typical blood gases results are as follows: arterial Po_2, 87 mm Hg (on 0.5 L of nasal O_2); pH, 7.49; arterial Pco_2, 55 mm Hg, and bicarbonate level, 42 mmol/L. The diagnosis is a mixed acid-base disorder: chronic respiratory acidosis and compensatory metabolic alkalosis plus metabolic alkalosis resulting from a contraction alkalosis. The child then develops viral pneumonia, and the blood gas results are as follows: arterial Po_2, 67 mm Hg; pH, 7.33; arterial Pco_2, 74 mm Hg; and bicarbonate level, 39 mmol/L. If one were not familiar with the case, this would appear to be a simple acid-base problem, an acute respiratory acidosis with an incomplete compensatory metabolic alkalosis. However, with an increase of the arterial Pco_2 value by 34 mm Hg (above 40 mm Hg), one would anticipate an acute bicarbonate compensation of only 3 to 4 mmol/L. Moreover, the blood gas value falls into the predicted range for chronic respiratory acidosis.

CLINICAL CORRELATES
Differences in Acute vs. Chronic Carbon Dioxide Retention

Acute respiratory acidosis is usually caused by an abrupt decline in ventilation, which causes the Pco_2 to rise and pH to fall. A child with acute respiratory acidosis frequently is hypoxic and has tachypnea, dyspnea, and hyperpnea.

> *Example:* The arterial blood gas results obtained from a child with known severe asthma coming to the emergency room with status asthmaticus reveals a low pH, 7.25, with a high Pco_2, 85, and a slightly elevated serum bicarbonate level, 27. These results are consistent with a child who has impending respiratory failure. Most asthmatics have a mild respiratory alkalosis at the time of presentation. The elevated bicarbonate level is attributed to buffering by intracellular buffering mechanisms. The increase in the serum bicarbonate level by 1 mmol/L for every increase of 10 mm Hg in PCO_2[193] is immediate.

Renal buffering does not have a noticeable impact on the pH until 12 to 24 hours after the respiratory acidosis begins.[194] Treatment of the patient who has acute respiratory acidosis involves rapid recognition and correction of the inciting cause coupled with oxygen administration. Sodium bicarbonate should be given to preclude the serious cardiovascular affects of acidosis.

The basis for chronic respiratory acidosis is typically a decrease in alveolar ventilation. The Pco_2 is elevated; however, unlike in acute respiratory acidosis, in chronic respiratory acidosis, effective renal compensation has occurred. Therefore the serum pH is only slightly below normal. For each increase of 10 mm Hg in the Pco_2, the bicarbonate value increases by 4 mmol/L. Serum chloride values are decreased to reciprocate for the increased serum bicarbonate values. An arterial blood gas analysis obtained from a child with stable bronchopulmonary dysplasia would be remarkable for normal to slightly low pH, a markedly elevated Pco_2, and a compensatory elevated bicarbonate level. Treatment consists primarily of administration of bronchodilators, effective pulmonary cleansing, and administration of steroids (in the case of bronchopulmonary dysplasia).

Loop and thiazide diuretics are helpful in the management of chronic lung disease because excessive fluid causes pulmonary congestion. The pathophysiology of this problem can be ascribed to the excessive venous constriction caused by chronic hypercapnia. Therefore in addition to diuretic therapy, avoidance of aggressive fluid administration is advised because it can lead to pulmonary congestion and congestive heart failure.

Impact of Chronic Carbon Dioxide Retention on Buffering in CSF

CSF pH is almost entirely regulated by Pco_2 and to a lesser degree bicarbonate. Carbon dioxide easily diffuses from the blood to the CSF. Conversely, bicarbonate diffuses slowly across the blood-brain barrier and requires active transport.[195] Thus CSF pH can decrease rapidly with any acute change in Pco_2. Some investigators have attributed the stupor associated with hypercapnia to CSF acidosis,[196,197] whereas others have not found an association.[198]

Reduced Carbon Dioxide Drive

The CRC located in the medulla oblongata and pons directly controls respiration. There are three parts of the CRC. The dorsal portion of the medulla controls the rhythm of respiration. The ventrolateral area of the medulla contains cells that control the inspiration and expiration phase. The pneumotaxic center located in the pons controls the depth of inspiration.

In addition to the CRC, there are peripheral chemoreceptors that lie in close apposition to the aorta and carotid artery. The type 1 cells within the carotid body can influence the CRC through the transduction of impulses through the carotid sinus nerve.[199] Hypoxia, hypercapnia, or acidosis induces changes within the type 1 cells, thereby increasing the firing of the carotid sinus nerve.[199]

Carbon dioxide indirectly stimulates CRC activity. As the level of carbon dioxide that bathes the CRC in CSF increases, carbonic acid and hydrogen ion levels increase. Hydrogen ions have a potent direct stimulatory effect on the CRC, but because the blood-brain barrier is almost completely impermeable to hydrogen ions, only hypoxia or a change in Pco_2 stimulates the CRC. On the other hand, the peripheral chemoreceptors can respond to changes in the hydrogen ion concentration.[199]

The cause of chronic respiratory acidosis is down-regulation of the respiratory drive in the presence of long-standing respiratory disease. As respiratory acidosis develops, carbon dioxide moves across the blood-brain barrier. The excitability of the CRC is greatest over the first few hours, but the response slowly declines over 1 to 2 days. The decreased response to hypercapnia is due to the effect of the renal compensatory mechanism. As hydrogen ion concentration decreases, stimulation of peripheral chemoreceptors diminishes. Bicarbonate slowly diffuses across the blood-brain barrier, neutralizing the hydrogen ions. Ultimately, the respiratory drive is regulated by hypoxia in patients who have chronic hypercarbia. In a clinical situation in which oxygen is given to a patient with chronic hypercarbia, it is possible to extinguish the respiratory drive, causing carbon dioxide narcosis and respiratory failure. The CRC is probably better suited to a vigorous response to acute respiratory acidosis than to chronic respiratory acidosis resulting from the high energy cost of the ventilatory response.[200]

Acetazolamide Therapy for Chronic Carbon Dioxide Retention

Weaning ventilatory support for children with chronic carbon dioxide retention resulting from chronic lung disease can be difficult because of an inadequate drive to breath. The lack of a respiratory drive is due to the adaptation of the CRC to hypercarbia. Acidemia, which would also stimulate the CRC, typically has resolved because of the compensatory metabolic alkalosis. In addition, the hypoxic drive is suppressed by supplemental oxygen. Although purposeful worsening of hypoxia and hypercarbia in an effort to induce a more vigorous respiratory drive is unfeasible, induction of acidemia by acetazolamide-induced renal wasting of bicarbonate is an option.

Bicarbonate is primarily resorbed in the proximal tubule and is dependent on the presence of carbonic anhydrase, which is found in large amounts only in the convoluted proximal tubule.[201] Inhibition of carbonic anhydrase by acetazolamide yields an inability of the tubule to resorb bicarbonate. The loss of bicarbonate obligates the loss of sodium and potassium, thus causing a diuretic effect. Increased urinary bicarbonate losses cause normalization of serum bicarbonate values and acute acidemia. After the initial drop in serum bicarbonate concentration lasting 2 to 4 days, serum bicarbonate levels begin to rise. Bicarbonate can be effectively resorbed in the distal tubule by the secretion of more hydrogen ions. The secretion of additional hydrogen ions is triggered by the acidemia.

As the child becomes acidemic, the respiratory drive increases, thereby decreasing the P_{CO_2}. The expectation is that the CRC will be "reset" to cause a response to the increasing hypercarbia.

Diuretics and Contraction Alkalosis with Hypokalemia

Most chemical diuretics achieve their effect by inhibiting sodium resorption; the additional urinary sodium causes water loss. In addition, the inhibition of sodium resorption in the thick ascending limb and cortical convoluted tubule diminishes the capacity of the countercurrent exchange to create a large renal interstitial osmolarity gradient. Without a large interstitial gradient, urine cannot be concentrated.

Loop diuretics such as furosemide, bumetanide, and ethacrynic acid block the symporter within the thick ascending limb of the loop of Henle[202] (Fig. 16-20). Because of the large amount of sodium and chloride resorption attributable to the symporter, the diuresis seen with a loop diuretic is much greater than with any other class of diuretic. The symporter cotransports two molecules of chloride, one molecule of potassium, and one molecule of sodium from the tubule lumen into the cell.[203] Loop diuretics also increase the excretion of calcium and magnesium. Thiazide diuretics such as hydrochlorothiazide, metolazone, and chlorothiazide inhibit the function of the sodium-chloride pump found within the distal convoluted tubule.[204]

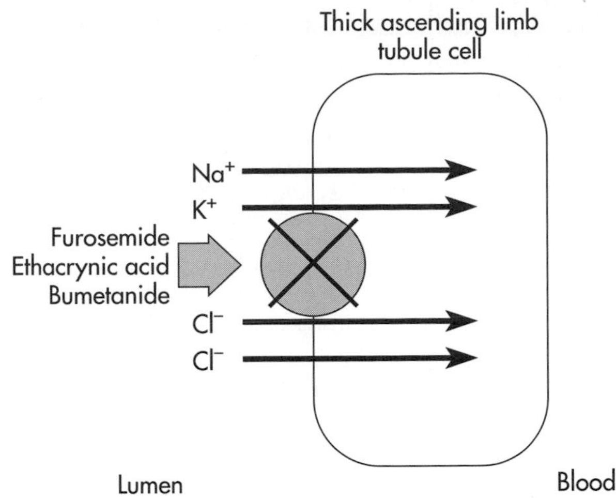

Fig. 16-20. The thick ascending limb symporter resorbs two chloride (Cl^-) molecules with one potassium (K^+) and one sodium (Na^+) molecule. Dysfunction of the symporter causes Bartter's syndrome. Loop diuretics inhibit symporter function, causing the loss of sodium, chloride, potassium, and water in the urine. Inhibition of the symporter function also decreases urinary concentration by limiting the effectiveness of the countercurrent exchange.

Bicarbonate values rise acutely with the use of loop and thiazide diuretics because of four reasons. First, the extracellular volume is depleted without increasing the total body bicarbonate content; however, because of the volume contraction, bicarbonate concentrations increase. Second, long-term use of loop and thiazide diuretics causes hypokalemic and hypochloremic metabolic alkalosis resulting from increased sodium delivery to the distal tubule, which stimulates potassium and hydrogen ion secretion independent of an aldosterone effect.[205]

Third, extravascular volume contraction causes the glomerular filtration rate to decrease. As a result, more sodium and water are resorbed in the proximal tubule. Because sodium delivery is decreased to the collecting duct, the juxtaglomerular apparatus secretes renin into the afferent arteriole. Renin cleaves angiotensinogen, thereby forming angiotensin I. Angiotensin I is converted to angiotensin II in the lungs by angiotensin-converting enzyme. Angiotensin II causes vasoconstriction and stimulates aldosterone release. Aldosterone binds to a cytoplasmic receptor found in distal renal tubular cells. The aldosterone-cytoplasmic receptor complex is translocated to the nucleus, where the gene for the sodium-potassium pump is up-regulated, transcribed, and translated. The sodium-potassium pump protein is transferred to the luminal surface, where it resorbs sodium in exchange for potassium. This exchange does not always occur on a one-to-one basis. As potassium depletion develops, hydrogen ion excretion increases so that sodium resorption can continue. Renal proton secretion decreases the hydrogen ion concentration in serum, thereby increasing pH and the serum bicarbonate level.

As plasma potassium levels begin to decrease because of diuretic-mediated potassium depletion, aldosterone levels decrease. In the distal tubule, aldosterone promotes hydrogen ion excretion in exchange for sodium. As aldosterone levels decline, the number of hydrogen ions secreted by the tubule also declines. This represents an important feedback mechanism to prevent severe hypokalemia and metabolic alkalosis.

Finally, profound hypokalemia resulting from potassium depletion causes potassium to egress from somatic cells. Because all cells have a potassium pump that keeps intracellular levels of sodium low, sodium cannot move into the cell in exchange for the potassium leaving the cell. Hydrogen ions, however, can move into the cell, thereby decreasing serum hydrogen ion concentrations. Serum bicarbonate levels rise in response.

Treatment of the hypokalemic and hypochloremic metabolic alkalosis caused by diuretics typically consists of potassium chloride or potassium-sparing diuretics. Potassium chloride therapy is advantageous in that both potassium depletion and chloride deficiency are corrected.

For example, patients who have chronic carbon dioxide retention experience a compensatory metabolic alkalosis. When diuretic therapy is added for the treatment of pulmonary disease, the serum bicarbonate value increases from its already high baseline because of contraction alkalosis and chloride and potassium depletion. The increases in the serum bicarbonate level and pH cause an increase in the P_{CO_2}. Because the patient's response to hypercapnia has already been inhibited, the P_{CO_2} rises (possibly to dangerous levels) in response to the contraction alkalosis. Only chloride replacement in the form of potassium chloride facilitates urinary bicarbonate excretion so that carbon dioxide levels can return toward baseline. Potassium-sparing diuretics do not substantially improve the contraction alkalosis-mediated hypercapnia because the chloride deficiency is not repaired.

Potassium-sparing diuretics such as spironolactone, triamterene, and amiloride increase serum potassium levels and may slightly decrease renal hydrogen ion excretion. Compliance with such therapy is generally better than with oral potassium chloride therapy.

REFERENCES

Basic Physiology of Gas Exchange and Acid Base

1. Guyton AC, Hall JE: Physical principles of gas exchange: diffusion of oxygen and carbon dioxide through the respiratory membrane. In Guyton AC, Hall JE, eds: *Textbook of medical physiology,* ed 9, Philadelphia, 1996, WB Saunders, pp 501-512.
2. O'Brodovich HM, Haddad GG: The functional basis of respiratory pathology. In Chernick V, ed: *Kendig's disorders of the respiratory tract in children,* ed 5, Philadelphia, 1990, WB Saunders, pp 3-47.
3. Comroe JH: *Physiology of respiration,* ed 2, St Louis, 1977, Mosby.
4. Siggaard-Andersen O, Garby L: The Bohr effect and the Haldane effect, *Scand J Clin Lab Invest* 31:1-8, 1973.
5. Bryan-Brown CW: Oxygen transport variables and the management of the critically ill: rationalization in pursuit of uncertainty? In Bryan-Brown CW, Ayres SM, eds: *Oxygen transport and utilization: new horizons,* Fullerton, Calif, 1987, Society of Critical Care Medicine, pp 1-11.
6. Stone HO, Thompson HK, Schmidt-Nielsen K: Influence of erythrocytes on blood viscosity, *Am J Physiol* 214:913-918, 1968.
7. Gutierrez G: Tissue oxygenation and high energy phosphate metabolism. In Shoemaker WC, Ayres SM, Grenvik A, Holbrook PR, eds: *Textbook of critical care,* ed 3, St Louis, 1995, Mosby, pp 300-305.
8. Hochachka PW, Guppy M: *Metabolic arrest and the control of biological time,* Cambridge, Mass, 1987, Harvard University Press, pp 10-35.
9. Balaban RS: Regulation of oxidative phosphorylation in the mammalian cell, *Am J Physiol* 258:C377-C389, 1990 (review).
10. Berne RM: Adenosine: an important physiological regulator, *News Physiol Sci* 1:163-167, 1986.
11. Wei HM, Kang YH, Merrill GF: Coronary vasodilation during global myocardial hypoxia: effects of adenosine deaminase, *Am J Physiol* 254:H1004-H1009, 1988.
12. Van Belle H, Goosens F, Wynants J: Formation and release of purine catabolites during hypoperfusion, anoxia, and ischemia, *Am J Physiol* 252:H886-H893, 1987.
13. Connett RJ, Gayeski TE, Honig CR: Lactate accumulation in fully aerobic working dog gracilis muscle, *Am J Physiol* 246:H120-H128, 1984.
14. Gutierrez G, Andry JM: Nuclear magnetic resonance measurements: clinical applications, *Crit Care Med* 17:73-82, 1989 (review).
15. Bryan-Brown CW, Baek SM, Makabali G, Shoemaker WC: Consumable oxygen: availability of oxygen in relation to oxyhemoglobin dissociation, *Crit Care Med* 1:17-21, 1973.
16. Longmuir IS: Tissue adaptation of hypoxia. In Bryan-Brown CW, Ayres SM, eds: *Oxygen transport and utilization: new horizons,* Fullerton, Calif, 1987, Society of Critical Care Medicine, pp 229-237.
17. Kontos HA: Regulation of the cerebral microcirculation in hypoxia and ischemia. In Bryan-Brown CW, Ayres SM, eds: *Oxygen transport and utilization: new horizons,* Fullerton, Calif, 1987, Society of Critical Care Medicine, pp 311-318.
18. Siesjö BK: Critical degrees of hypoxia and ischemia when cerebral function and metabolism are perturbed. In Bryan-Brown CW, Ayres SM, eds: *Oxygen transport and utilization: new horizons,* Fullerton, Calif, 1987, Society of Critical Care Medicine, pp 293-310.
19. Feihl F, Perret C: Permissive hypercapnia: how permissive should we be? *Am J Respir Crit Care Med* 150:1722-1737, 1994 (review).
20. Thomas RC: Experimental displacement of intracellular pH and the mechanism of its subsequent recovery, *J Physiol (Lond)* 354:3-22, 1984.
21. Orchard C, Kentish J: Effects of changes of pH on the contractile function of cardiac muscle, *Am J Physiol* 258:C967-C981, 1990.
22. Tang WC, Weil MH, Gazmuri RJ, Bisera J, Rackow EC: Reversible impairment of myocardial contractility due to hypercarbic acidosis in the isolated perfused rat heart, *Crit Care Med* 19:218-224, 1991.
23. Case RB, Greenberg H, Moskowiitz R: Alterations in coronary sinus P_{O_2} and O_2 saturation resulting from P_{CO_2} changes, *Cardiovasc Res* 9:167-177, 1975.
24. Factor SM: Pathophysiology of myocardial ischemia. In Hurst JW, eds: *The heart, arteries and veins,* ed 7, New York, 1990, McGraw-Hill, pp 940-960.
25. Lanier WL, Weglinski MR: Intracranial pressure. In Cucchiara RF, Michenfelder JD, eds: *Clinical neuroanesthesia,* New York, 1991, Churchill Livingstone, pp 77-110.
26. Hargreaves DM: Hypercapnia and raised cerebrospinal fluid pressure, *Anaesthesia* 45:1096-1097, 1990.
27. Viitanen A, Salmenperã M, Heinonen J: Right ventricular response to hypercarbia after cardiac surgery, *Anesthesiology* 73:393-400, 1990.
28. Fishman AP: The enigma of hypoxic pulmonary vasoconstriction. In Fishman AP, ed: *The pulmonary circulation: normal and abnormal,* Philadelphia, 1990, University of Pennsylvania Press, pp 109-129.
29. Bersentes TJ, Simmons DH: Effects of acute acidosis on renal hemodynamics, *Am J Physiol* 212:633-640, 1967.
30. Walley K, Lewis TH, Wood LDH: Acute respiratory acidosis decreases left ventricular contractility but increases cardiac output in dogs, *Circ Res* 67:628-635, 1990.
31. Barach AL: The adaptive function of hypercapnia. In Petty TL, ed: *Lung biology in health and disease,* New York 1978, Marcel Dekker, pp 151-162.
32. Morse JO, Kettel LJ, Diener CF, Burrows B: Effect of long-term, continuous oxygen therapy in patients with severe chronic hypercapnia, *Am Rev Respir Dis* 107:1064-1066, 1973.
33. Neff TA, Petty TL: Tolerance and survival in severe chronic hypercapnia, *Arch Intern Med* 129:591-596, 1972.
34. Hickling KG, Walsh J, Henderson S, Jackson R: Low mortality rate in adult respiratory distress syndrome using low-volume pressure-limited ventilation with permissive hypercapnia: prospective study, *Crit Care Med* 22:1568-1578, 1994.
35. Bidani A, Tzouanakis AE, Cardenas VJ Jr, Zwischenberger JB: Permissive hypercapnia in acute respiratory failure, *JAMA* 272:957-962, 1994.
36. Tuxen DV: Permissive hypercapnic ventilation, *Am J Respir Crit Care Med* 150:870-874, 1994 (review).
37. Brenner B, Rector FC: *The kidney,* ed 4, Philadelphia, WB Saunders, 1991.
38. Madias NE, Cohen JJ: Respiratory alkalosis and acidosis. In Seldin DW, Giebisch G, eds: *The kidney: physiology and pathophysiology,* ed 2, New York, 1992, Raven Press, pp 1837-2872.
39. Emmet M, Alpern RJ, Seldin DW: Metabolic acidosis. In Seldin DW, Giebisch G, eds: *The kidney: physiology and pathophysiology,* ed 2, New York, 1992, Raven Press, pp 2759-2836.
40. Schrier RW: *Renal and electrolyte disorders,* ed 3, Boston, 1986, Little, Brown, pp 141-206.
41. Guyton AC, Hall JE: Regulation of acid-base balance. In Guyton AC, Hall JE, eds: *Textbook of medical physiology,* ed 9, Philadelphia, 1996, WB Saunders, p 390.
42. Maher JF: Pathophysiology of renal hemodynamics, *Nephron* 27:215-221, 1981.
43. Guyton AC, Hall JE: In Guyton AC, Hall JE, eds: *Textbook of medical physiology,* ed 9, Philadelphia, 1996, WB Saunders, pp 315-347.
44. Kanwar YS, Farquahar MG: Presence of heparan sulfate in the glomerular basement membrane, *Proc Natl Acad Sci USA* 76:1303-1307, 1979.
45. Vernier RL, Klein DJ, Sisson SP, Mahan JD, Oegema TR, Brown DM: Heparan sulfate–rich anionic sites in the human glomerular basement membrane, *New Engl J Med* 309:1001-1009, 1983.
46. Glynn IM, Karlish SLD: The sodium pump, *Ann Rev Physiol* 37:13-15, 1975.
47. Jorgensen PL: Sodium and potassium ion pump in the kidney tubule, *Physiol Rev* 60:864-917, 1980.
48. Aronson PS: Mechanism of active H^+ secretion in the proximal tubule, *Am J Physiol* 245:F647-F659, 1983.
49. Schwartz GJ: Na^+-dependent H^+ efflux from proximal tubule: evidence for reversible Na^+-H^+ exchange, *Am J Physiol* 241:F380-F385, 1981.
50. Bank N, Aynedjian HS, Murtz BF: Evidence for a DCCD-sensitive component of proximal bicarbonate reabsorption, *Am J Physiol* 249:F636-F644, 1985.
51. Wistrand PJ: Properties of membrane-bound carbonic anhydrase, *Ann NY Acad Sci* 429:195-206, 1984.
52. Alpern RJ: Mechanism of basolateral $H^+/OH^-/HCO_3^-$ transport in the rat proximal tubule: a sodium coupled electrogenic process, *J Gen Physiol* 86:613-636, 1985.
53. Alpern RJ, Cogan MG, Rector FC Jr: Effect of luminal bicarbonate concentration on proximal acidification in the rat, *Am J Physiol* 243:F53-F59, 1982.
54. Schwartz GJ, Barasch J, Al-Awqati Q: Plasticity of epithelial polarity, *Nature* 318:368-371, 1985.
55. Elkinton JR, Singer RB, Barker ES, Clark JK: Effect in man of acute experimental respiratory alkalosis and acidosis on ionic transfers in the total body fluids, *J Clin Invest* 34:1671-1690, 1955.
56. Giebisch G, Berger L, Pitts RF: The extrarenal response to acute-acid base disturbances of respiratory origin, *J Clin Invest* 34:231-245, 1955.

57. Relman AS: Metabolic consequences of acid-base disorders, *Kidney Int* 1:347-359, 1972.
58. Sykes MK, Cooke PM: The effect of hyperventilation on excess lactate production during anesthesia, *Br J Anaesth* 37:372-379, 1965.
59. Gennari FJ, Goldstein MB, Schwartz WB: The nature of the renal adaptation to chronic hypocapnia, *J Clin Invest* 51:1722-1730, 1972.
60. Gledhill N, Beirne GJ, Dempsey JA: Renal response in short-term hypocapnia in man, *Kidney Int* 8:376-384, 1975.
61. Kurtzman NA: Relationship of extracellular volume and carbon dioxide tension in renal bicarbonate reabsorption, *Am J Physiol* 219:1299-1304, 1970.
62. Barker ES, Singer RB, Elkinton JR, Clark JK: The renal response in man to acute experimental respiratory alkalosis and acidosis, *J Clin Invest* 36:515-529, 1957.
63. Rector FC, Seldin DW, Roberts AD, Smith JS: The role of carbon dioxide tension and carbonic anhydrase activity in the renal absorption of bicarbonate, *J Clin Invest* 39:1706-1721, 1960.
64. Waring DW, Sullivan LP, Mayhew DA, Tucker JM: A study of factors affecting renal bicarbonate reabsorption, *Am J Physiol* 226:1392-1400, 1974.
65. Mello A, Malnic G: Peritubular pH and P_{CO_2} in renal tubular acidification, *Am J Physiol* 228:1766-1774, 1975.
66. Malnic G, Mello A, Giebisch G: Micropuncture study of the renal tubular hydrogen ion transport in the rat, *Am J Physiol* 222:147-158, 1972.
67. Carter NW, Seldin DW, Teng HC: Tissue and renal response to chronic respiratory acidosis, *J Clin Invest* 38:949-960, 1959.
68. Bengele HH, Graber ML, Alexander EA: Effect of respiratory acidosis on acidification by the medullary collecting duct, *Am J Physiol* 244:F89-F94, 1983.
69. Mathisen O, Monclair T, Raeder M, Kiil F: Coupling of $NaHCO_3$ and NaCl reabsorption in dog kidneys during changes in plasma P_{CO_2}, *Am J Physiol* 236:F232-F239, 1979.
70. Langberg H, Mathisen O, Holdaas H, Kiil F: Filtered bicarbonate and plasma pH as determinants of renal bicarbonate reabsorption, *Kidney Int* 20:780-788, 1981.
71. Cogan MG: Chronic hypercapnia stimulates proximal bicarbonate reabsorption by the rat, *J Clin Invest* 74:1942-1947, 1984.

Blood Gas Measurement

72. Siggaard-Andersen O: Blood acid-base alignment nomogram: scales for pH, P_{CO_2}-base excess of whole blood of different hemoglobin concentrations, plasma bicarbonate, plasma CO_2, *Scand J Clin Lab Invest* 15:211-217, 1963.
73. Severinghaus JW, Astrup PB: History of blood gas analysis. II. pH and acid-base measurements, *J Clin Monit* 1(4):259-277, 1985.
74. Severinghaus JW, Astrup PB: History of blood gas analysis. III. Carbon dioxide tension, *J Clin Monit* 2(1):60-73, 1986.
75. Hingston DM, Irwin RS, Pratter MR, Dalen JE: A computerized interpretation of arterial blood gas data: do physicians need it? *Respir Care* 27:809-815, 1982.
76. Gilbert HC, Vender JS: Arterial blood gas monitoring, *Crit Care Clin* 11(1):233-248, 1995.
77. Ream AK, Reitz BA, Silverberg G: Temperature correction of P_{CO_2} and pH in estimating acid-base status: an example of the emperor's new clothes? *Anesthesiology* 56:41-44, 1982.
78. Sessler DI: Temperature monitoring. In Miller RD, ed: *Anesthesia,* ed 4, New York, 1994, Churchill Livingstone, p 1376.
79. Reeves RB: An imidazole alphastat hypothesis of vertebrate acid base regulation: tissue carbon dioxide and body temperature of bull frogs, *Respir Physiol* 14:219-236, 1972.
80. Simmons MA, Levine RL, Lubchenco LO, Guggenheim MA: Warning: serious sequelae of temporal artery catheterization, *J Pediatr* 92:284, 1978.
81. Allen EV: Thromboangiitis obliterans: methods of diagnosis of chronic occlusive arterial lesions distal to the wrist with illustrative cases, *Am J Med Sci* 178:237-244, 1929.
82. Greenhow DE: Incorrect performance of Allen's test: ulnar flow erroneously presumed inadequate, *Anesthesiology* 37:356-357, 1974.
83. Dar K, Williams T, Altken R, Woods KI, Fletcher S: Arterial versus capillary sampling for analyzing blood gas pressures, *Br Med J* 309:24-25, 1995.
84. Harsten A, Berg B, Inerot S, Muth L: Importance of handling of samples for the results of blood gas analysis, *Acta Anaesthesiol Scand* 32:365-368, 1988.
85. McLaren RE: Blood gas techniques, *Respir Med* 87:79-80, 1993.
86. Nagabhushan A, Colella JJ, Wagner R: Use of Doppler ultrasound in performing percutaneous cannulation of the radial artery, *Crit Care Med* 4(6):327, 1976.
87. Suddaby EC, Sourbeer MO: Drawing pediatric arterial blood gases, *Crit Care Nurse* 10(7):28-31, 1990.
88. Fletcher MA, MacDonald MG, Avery GB: *Atlas of procedures in neonatology,* Philadelphia, 1983, JB Lippincott, p 63.
89. Mortensen J: Clinical sequelae from arterial needle puncture, cannulation and incision, *Circulation* 35:1118-1123, 1967.
90. Begin R, Racine T, Roy JC: Value of capillary blood gas analyses in the management of acute respiratory distress, *Am Rev Respir Dis* 112:879-881, 1975.
91. Langlands JHM, Wallace WFM: Small blood samples from ear lobe puncture: a substitute for arterial puncture, *Lancet* 2:315-317, 1965.
92. Pitkin AD, Roberts CM, Wedzicha JA: Arterialized earlobe blood gas analysis: an underused technique, *Thorax* 49(4):364-366, 1994.
93. Courtney SE, Weber KR, Breakie LA, Malin SW, Bender CV, Guo SM, Siervogel RM: Capillary blood gases in the neonates, *Am J Dis Child* 144:168-172, 1990.
94. Folger GM Jr, Kouri P, Sabbah HN: Arterialized capillary blood sampling in the neonate: a reappraisal, *Heart Lung* 9(3):521-526, 1980.
95. Wallman AA, Arora PL, Allen H, Hyde RW: Measurement of capillary oxygen tension during the breathing of 100 percent oxygen for the assessment of right-left shunts, *Am Rev Respir Dis* 98(6):1013-1020, 1968.
96. Graham G, Kenny MA: Changes in transcutaneous oxygen tension during capillary blood-gas sampling, *Clin Chem* 26(13):1860-1863, 1980.
97. McLain BI, Evans J, Dear PR: Comparison of capillary and arterial blood gas measurements in neonates, *Arch Dis Child* 63:743-747, 1988.
98. Doig WB: Value of arterialized capillary blood gas analysis in lower respiratory tract infection in childhood, *Arch Dis Child* 46:243-246, 1971.
99. Canny GJ, Levison H: The accuracy of arterialized capillary blood for the measurement of blood gas tensions in patients with lung disease, *Pediatr Pulmonol* 2(5):313-314, 1986.
100. Gambino SR, Thiede WH: Comparisons of pH in human arterial, venous and capillary blood, *Am J Clin Pathol* 32:298-300, 1959.
101. Frewen TC, Sumabat WO, Del Maestro RF: Cerebral blood flow, metabolic rate, and cross-brain oxygen consumption in brain injury, *J Pediatr* 107:510-513, 1985.
102. Gayle MO, Frewen TC, Amstrong RF, Gilbert JJ, Kronick JB, Kissoon N, Lee R, Tiffin N, Brown T: Regular venous bulb catheterization in infants and children, *Crit Care Med* 17:385-388, 1989.
103. Richman KA, Jobes DR, Schwalb AJ: Continuous in-vivo blood gas determination in man: reliability and safety of a new device, *Anesthesiology* 52(4):313-317, 1980.
104. Royston BD: Continuous monitoring of arterial blood gases. In Royston D, ed: Monitoring in anesthesiology: current standards and newer techniques, *Int Anesthesiol Clin* 31(3):1-22, 1993 (review).
105. Larson CP, Vender J, Seiver A: Multisite evaluation of a continuous intra-arterial blood gas monitoring system, *Anesthesiology* 81(3):543-552, 1994.
106. Zimmerman JL, Dellinger RP: Initial evaluation of a new intra-arterial blood gas system in humans, *Crit Care Med* 21(4):481-482, 1993.
107. Wahr JA, Tremper KK: Continuous intravascular blood gas monitoring, *J Cardiothorac Vasc Anesth* 8(3):342-353, 1994.
108. Lumsden T, Marshall WR, Divers GA, Riccitelli SD: The PB3300 intra-arterial blood gas monitoring system, *J Clin Monit* 10(1):59-66, 1994.
109. Gehrich JL, Lubbers DW, Opitz N, Hansmann DR, Miller WW, Tusa JK, Yafuso M: Optical fluorescence and its application to an intravascular blood gas monitoring system, *IEEE Trans Biomed Eng* 33:117-132, 1986.
110. Ryan DW: Limitations of invasive intravascular monitoring, *Intern Ther Clin Monit* 10:216-220, 1989.
111. Schnapp LM, Cohen NH: Pulse oximetry: uses and abuses, *Chest* 98:1244-1250, 1990 (review).
112. Pologe JA: Pulse oximetry: technical aspects of machine design, *Int Anesthesiol Clin* 25:137-153, 1987 (review).
113. Cheng EY, Hopwood MB, Kay J: Forehead pulse oximetry compared to finger pulse oximetry and arterial blood gas measurement, *J Clin Monit* 4(3):223-226, 1988.

114. Scheller J, Loeb R: Respiratory artifact during pulse oximetry in critically ill patients, *Anesthesiology* 69:602-603, 1988.
115. Barker SJ, Tremper KK: The effect of carbon monoxide inhalation on pulse oximeter signal detection, *Anesthesiology* 67:599-603, 1987.
116. Vegfors M, Lenmarken C: Carboxyhemoglobinemia and pulse oximetry, *Br J Anaesth* 66:625-626, 1991.
117. Barker SJ, Tremper KK, Hyatt J: Effects of methemoglobinemia on pulse oximetry and mixed venous oximetry, *Anesthesiology* 70:112-117, 1989.
118. Watcha MF, Connor MT, Hing AV: Pulse oximetry in methemoglobinemia, *Am J Dis Child* 143:845-847, 1989.
119. Pologe JA, Raley DM: Effects of fetal hemoglobin on pulse oximetry, *J Perinatol* 7:324-326, 1987.
120. Scheller MS, Unger RJ, Kelner MJ: Effect of intravenously administered dyes on pulse oximetry readings, *Anesthesiology* 65:550-552, 1986.
121. Emery JR: Skin pigmentation as an influence on the accuracy of pulse oximetry, *J Perinatol* 7:329-330, 1987.
122. Ries AL, Prewitt LM, Johnson JJ: Skin color and ear oximetry, *Chest* 96:287-290, 1989.
123. Cote CJ, Goldstein EA, Fuchsman WH, Hoaglin DC: The effect of nail polish on pulse oximetry, *Anesth Analg* 67:683-686, 1988.
124. Rubin AS: Nail polish color can affect pulse oximeter saturation, *Anesthesiology* 68:825, 1988 (letter).
125. Smith TC: Intra-aortic balloon pumps and the pulse oximeter, *Anaesthesia* 47:1010-1011, 1992.
126. Stewart KG, Rowbottom SJ: Inaccuracy of pulse oximetry in patients with severe tricuspid regurgitation, *Anaesthesia* 46:668-670, 1991.
127. Al Khudhairi D, Prabhu R, el Sharkawy M, Burtles R: Evaluation of a pulse oximeter during profound hypothermia: an assessment of the Biox 3700 during induction of hypothermia before cardiac surgery in pediatric patients, *Int J Clin Monit Comput* 7:217-222, 1990.
128. Clayton DG, Webb RK, Ralston AC, Duthie D, Runciman: A comparison of performance of 20 pulse oximeters under conditions of poor perfusion, *Anaesthesia* 46:3-10, 1991.
129. Block FE, Detko GJ: Minimizing interference and false alarms from electrocautery in the Nellcor N-100 pulse oximeter, *J Clin Monit* 2:203-205, 1986.
130. Waggle WA: Technique for RF isolation of a pulse oximeter in a 1.5-T MR unit, *AJNR Am J Neuroradiol* 10:208-209, 1989.
131. Moller JT, Pedersen T, Rasmussen LS, Jensen PF, Pedersen BD, Ravlo O, Rasmussen NH, Espersen K, Johannessen NW, Cooper JB: Randomized evaluation of pulse oximetry in 20,802 patients. I. Design, demography, pulse oximetry failure rate, and overall complication rate, *Anesthesiology* 78:436-444, 1993.
132. Moller JT, Johannessen NW, Espersen K, Ravlo O, Pedersen BD, Jensen PF, Rasmussen NH, Rasmussen LS, Pedersen T, Cooper JB: Randomized evaluation of pulse oximetry in 20,802 patients. II. Perioperative events and postoperative complications, *Anesthesiology* 78:445-453, 1993.
133. Severinghaus JW, Naifeh KH: Accuracy of response of six pulse oximeters to profound hypoxia, *Anesthesiology* 67:376-380, 1987.
134. Severinghaus JW, Naifeh KH, Ko SC: Errors in 14 pulse oximeters during profound hypoxia, *J Clin Monit* 5:72-81, 1989.
135. Bashein G, Syrory G: Burns associated with pulse oximetry during magnetic resonance imaging, *Anesthesiology* 75:382-383, 1991.
136. Shellock FG, Slimp GL: Severe burn of the finger caused by using a pulse oximeter during MR imaging, *Am J Roentgenol* 153:1105-1106, 1989.
137. Sobel DB: Burning of a neonate due to a pulse oximeter: arterial saturation monitoring, *Pediatrics* 89:154-155, 1992.
138. Sloan TB: Finger injury by an oxygen saturation probe, *Anesthesiology* 8:936-938, 1988.
139. Rubin MM, Ford HC, Sadoff RS: Digital injury from a pulse oximeter probe, *J Oral Macillofac Surg* 49:301-302, 1991.
140. Baumgardner JE, Graves DJ, Neufeld GR, Quinn JA: Gas flux through human skin: effects of temperature, stripping and inspired tension, *J Appl Physiol* 5:1536-1545, 1985.
141. Lucey JF: Clinical uses of transcutaneous oxygen monitoring, *Adv Pediatr* 28:27-56, 1981.
142. Lübbers DW: Theoretical basis of the transcutaneous blood gas measurements, *Crit Care Med* 9:721-733, 1981,
143. Rowe MI, Weinberg G: Transcutaneous oxygen monitoring in shock and resuscitation, *J Pediatr Surg* 14:773-778, 1979.
144. Tremper KK, Shoemaker WC: Transcutaneous oxygen monitoring of critically ill adults with and without low flow shock, *Crit Care Med* 9:706-709, 1981.
145. Hollinger CB, Hoyt JW: Capnography and respiratory monitoring. In Shoemaker WC, Ayres SM, Grenvik A, Holbrook PR, eds: *Textbook of critical care,* ed 3, St Louis, 1995, Mosby, pp 305-311.
146. Carlon GC, Ray C Jr, Miodownik S, Kopec I, Groeger JS: Capnography in mechanically ventilated patients, *Crit Care Med* 16:550-556, 1988 (review).
147. Technology Subcommittee of the Working Group on Critical Care, Ontario Ministry of Health: Noninvasive blood gas monitoring: a review for use in the adult critical unit, *Can Med Assoc J* 146:703-712, 1992.
148. Gravenstein JS, Paulus DA: Monitoring ventilation and gases. In Gravenstein JS, Paulus DA: *Clinical monitoring practice,* ed 2, Philadelphia, 1987, JB Lippincott, pp 184-196.
149. Stock MC: Noninvasive carbon dioxide monitoring, *Crit Care Clin* 4:511-526, 1988.
150. Blitt CD: Monitoring and patient safety. In Blitt CD, ed: *Monitoring in anesthesia and critical care medicine,* ed 2, New York, 1990, Churchill Livingstone, pp 48-63.
151. Swedlow DB: Capnometry and capnography: an anesthesia disaster warning system, *Semin Anesth* 5:194, 1986.
152. Snyder NV, Elliot FL, Grenvik A: Capnography. In Spencer A, ed: *Respiratory monitoring in intensive care,* New York, 1982, Churchill Livingstone, pp 100-121.
153. Linko K, Paloheimo M, Tammisto T: Capnography for detection of accidental oesophageal intubation, *Acta Anaesthesiol Scand* 27:199-202, 1983.
154. Murray IP, Modell JH: Early detection of endotracheal tube accidents by monitoring carbon dioxide concentration in respiratory gas, *Anesthesiology* 59:344-346, 1983.
155 Linko K, Paloheimo M, Tammisto T: Capnography facilitates blind nasogastric intubation, *Acta Anaesthesiol Belg* 43:117-122, 1983.
156. Crockett AJ, McIntyre E, Ruffin R, Alpers JH: Evaluation of lyophilized heparin syringes for the collection of arterial blood for acid base analysis, *Anaesth Intensive Care* 9:40-42, 1981.
157. Stein PE, Goodier DW: Effect of in vitro sodium citrate anticoagulant on results of arterial blood gas analysis, *J Clin Pathol* 39(9):1046, 1986 (letter).
158. Pretto JJ, Rochford PD: Effects of sample storage time, temperature and syringe type on blood gas tensions in samples with high oxygen partial pressures, *Thorax* 49:610-612, 1994.
159. Carter BG, Tibballs J, Hochmann M, Osborne A, Chiriano A, Murray G: A comparison of syringes to collect blood for analysis of gases, electrolytes and glucose, *Anaesth Intensive Care* 22(6):698-702, 1994.
160. Petty TL, Bailey D, Best C: A new device for arterial blood gas sampling, *JAMA* 239(19):2016-2017, 1978.
161. Biswas CK, Ramos JM, Agroyannis B, Kerr DNS: Blood gas analysis: effect of air bubbles in syringe and delay in estimation, *Br Med J* 282:923-927, 1982.
162. Preusser BA, Lash J, Stone KS, Winningham ML, Gonyon D, Nickel JT: Quantifying the minimal discard sample required for accurate arterial blood gases, *Nurs Res* 38(5)276-279, 1989.
163. Weibley RE, Riggs CD: Evaluation of an improved sampling method for blood gas analysis from indwelling arterial catheters, *Crit Care Med* 17(8):803-805, 1989.
164. Peruzzi WT, Parker MA, Lichtenthal PR, Cochran-Zull C, Toth B, Blake M: A clinical evaluation of a blood conservation device in medical intensive care unit patients, *Crit Care Med* 21(4):501-510, 1993.
165. Fox MJ, Brody JS, Weintraub LR: Leukocyte larceny: a cause of spurious hypoxemia, *Am J Med* 67:742-746, 1979.
166. Shohat M, Schonfeld T, Zaizoz R, Cohen IJ, Nitzan M: Determination of blood gases in children with extreme leukocytosis, *Crit Care Med* 16:787-788, 1988.
167. Nanji AA, Whitlow KJ: Is it necessary to transport arterial blood samples on ice for pH and gas analysis? *Can Anesth Soc J* 31(5):568-571, 1984.
168. McKane MH, Southorn PA, Santrach PJ, Burritt MF, Plevak DJ: Sending blood gas specimens through pressurized transport tube systems exaggerates the oxygen tension measurements created by the presence of air bubbles, *Anesth Analg* 81:179-182, 1995.

Interpretation of Arterial Blood Gas Results

169. Aberman A, Goldstein M, Rebuck AS: *Clinical approach to arterial blood gas interpretation and electrolytes,* Philadelphia, 1984, America College of Physicians.
170. Shapiro BA, Peruzzi WT, Kozelowski-Templin R: Assessment of the lung as an oxygenator. In Shapiro BA, Peruzzi WT, Kozelowski-Templin R, eds: *Clinical application of blood gases,* ed 5, St Louis, 1994, Mosby, pp 85-101.
171. Zetterstrom H: Assessment of the efficiency of pulmonary oxygenation: the choice of an oxygenation index, *Acta Anaesthesiol Scand* 32(7):579-584, 1988,
172. Hess D, Maxwell C: Which is the best index of oxygenation: $P_{(A-a)}O_2$, PaO_2/PAO_2 or PaO_2/FIO_2? *Respir Care* 30:961-963, 1985.
173. Maxwell C, Hess D, Shefet D: Use of the arterial/alveolar oxygen tension ratio to predict the inspired oxygen concentration needed for a desired arterial oxygen tension, *Respir Care* 29:1135-1139, 1984.
174. Covelli HD, Nessan VJ, Tuttle WK: Oxygen derived variables in acute respiratory failure, *Crit Care Med* 11:646-649, 1983.
175. Cane RD, Shapiro BA, Templin R, Walther K: The unreliability of oxygen tension based on indices in reflecting intrapulmonary shunt in critically ill, *Crit Care Med* 16:1243-1245, 1988.
176. Sganga G, Siegl JH, Coleman B, Giovannini I, Boldrini G, Pittiruti M: The physiologic meaning of the respiratory index in various types of critical illness, *Circ Shock* 17:179-193, 1985.
177. Helfaer MA, Nichols DG, Rogers MC: Developmental physiology of the respiratory system. In Rogers MC, ed: *Textbook of pediatric intensive care,* ed 2, Baltimore, 1992, Williams & Wilkins, pp 104-133.
178. Madias NE, Adrogue HJ, Horowitz GL, Cohen JJ, Schwartz WB: A redefinition of normal acid-base equilibrium in man: carbon dioxide tension as a key determinant of normal plasma bicarbonate concentration, *Kidney Int* 16(5):612-618, 1979.
179. Kaehny WD: Respiratory acid-base disorders, *Med Clin North Am* 67(4):915-928, 1983.
180. Edelmann CM Jr, Rodriguez-Soriano J, Boichis H, Gruskin AB, Acosta ML: Renal bicarbonate reabsorption and hydrogen ion excretion in normal infants, *J Clin Invest* 46:1309-1317, 1967.
181. Garella S, Chang B, Kahn SI: Dilutional acidosis: review of a concept, *Kidney Int* 8:279-283, 1975.
182. Emmett M, Nairns RG: Clinical use of the anion gap, *Medicine* 56:38-54, 1977.
183. Schwartz WB, Jensen RL, Relman AS: The disposition of acid administered to sodium depleted subjects: the renal response and the role of whole body buffers, *J Clin Invest* 33:587-597, 1954.
184. Schwartz WB, Ørning KJ, Porter R: The internal distribution of hydrogen ions with varying degrees of metabolic acidosis, *J Clin Invest* 36:373-382, 1957.
185. Burnell JM: Changes in bone sodium and carbonate in metabolic acidosis and alkalosis in the dog, *J Clin Invest* 50:327-331, 1971.
186. Jacobson HR: Medullary collecting duct acidification: effects of potassium, HCO_3 concentration, and PCO_2, *J Clin Invest* 74:2107-2114, 1984.
187. Schwartz GJ, Al-Awqati Q: Carbon dioxide causes exocytosis of vesicles containing H^+ pumps in isolated perfused proximal and collecting ducts, *J Clin Invest* 75(5):1638-1644, 1985.
188. Swan RC, Axelrod DR, Seip M, Pitts R: Distribution of sodium bicarbonate infused into nephrectomized dogs, *J Clin Invest* 34:1795-1801, 1955.
189. Roberts KE, Randall HT, Sanders HL, Hood M: Effects of potassium on renal tubular reabsorption of bicarbonate, *J Clin Invest* 34:666-672, 1955.
190. Arbus GS, Hebert LA, Levesque PR, Etsten BE, Schwartz WB: Characterization and clinical application of the "significance band" for respiratory alkalosis, *N Engl J Med* 280:117-123, 1969.
191. Cohen JJ, Madias NE, Wolf CJ, Schwartz WB: Regulation of acid base equilibrium in chronic hypocapnia: evidence that the response of the kidney is not geared to the defense of extracellular H^+, *J Clin Invest* 57:1483-1489, 1976.
192. Schwartz WB, Brackett NC, Cohen JJ: The response of extracellular hydrogen ion concentration to graded degrees of chronic hypercapnia: the physiologic limitation of the defense of pH, *J Clin Invest* 44:291-301, 1965.

Clinical Correlates

193. Brackett NC, Cohen JJ, Schwartz WB: Carbon dioxide titration curve of normal man: effect of increasing degrees of acute hypercapnia on acid base equilibration, *New Engl J Med* 272:6-12, 1965.
194. Schwartz WB, Cohen JJ: The nature of the renal response to chronic disorders of acid-base equilibrium, *Am J Med* 64(3):417-428, 1978.
195. Plum F, Siesjö BK: Recent advances in CSF physiology, *Anesthesiology* 42:708-730, 1975.
196. Bulger RJ, Schrier RW, Arend WP, Swanson AG: Spinal fluid acidosis and the diagnosis of pulmonary encephalopathy, *New Engl J Med* 274(8):433-437, 1966.
197. Posner JB, Plum F: Spinal fluid pH and neurologic symptoms in systemic acidosis, *New Engl J Med* 277(12):606-613, 1967.
198. Guisado R, Arieff AI: Neurologic manifestations of diabetic comas: correlations with biochemical alterations in the brain, *Metabolism* 24:665-679, 1975.
199. Peers C, Buckler KJ: Transduction of chemostimuli by the type 1 carotid body cell, *J Membrane Biol* 144(1):1-9, 1995.
200. Rochester DF: Respiratory muscle weakness, pattern of breathing, and carbon dioxide retention in chronic obstructive pulmonary disease, *Am Rev Respir Dis* 143(5 pt 1):901-903, 1991.
201. Maren TH, Ellison AC: A study of renal carbonic anhydrase, *Mol Pharmacol* 3:503-508, 1967.
202. Greger R, Schlatter E: Cellular mechanism of the action of loop diuretics on the thick ascending limb of Henle's loop, *Klin Wochenschr* 61:1019-1027, 1983.
203. Greger R, Schlatter E, Lang F: Evidence for electroneutral sodium chloride cotransport in the cortical thick ascending limb of Henle's loop of rabbit kidney, *Pflugers Arch* 396:308-314, 1983.
204. Burg MB: Renal handling of sodium, chloride, water, amino acids, and glucose. In Brenner BM, Rector FC, eds: *The kidney,* ed 2, Philadelphia, 1981, WB Saunders, p 328-370.
205. Bosch JP, Goldstein MN, Levitt MF, Kahn T: Effect of chronic furosemide administration on hydrogen and sodium excretion in the dog, *Am J Physiol* 232(5):F397-F404, 1977.

CHAPTER 17

Diagnostic and Therapeutic Procedures in Pediatric Pulmonary Patients

Robert E. Wood

GENERAL PRINCIPLES

Invasive procedures should be performed only when less invasive or noninvasive or less expensive procedures cannot yield the same or equivalent information. They should be performed only with the proper equipment and with sufficient numbers of trained and skilled personnel (both operator and assistants). The procedure should be performed in an appropriate setting, such as a well-equipped and staffed procedure (or operating) room or an intensive care unit, rather than at the patient's bedside.

Careful attention should be given to the timing of procedures. In general, earlier diagnosis results in earlier selection of the most effective therapy and avoids the confounding influence of empirical therapy. This should in turn result in savings of more than just money. Elective procedures should, in general, not be performed at hours that will result in significant delays in the processing of diagnostic specimens. Finally, scheduling of elective procedures to avoid meal times and to possibly coincide with normal nap times may reduce stress and strain on patients as well as parents.

Careful and appropriate monitoring of the patient's vital signs (pulse, respiratory rate, and blood pressure) and physiologic status (mental status, oxygen saturation) before, during, and after the procedure is essential. In general, one person (not the operator) should be responsible for monitoring the patient and responding to changes in status.[1]

Patients should be comfortable during and after procedures and within the limits of safety, reasonable convenience, and cost. In many, if not all, cases, this means sedation, which must be carried out with skill and with appropriate agents. If adequate provision cannot be made for safe and effective sedation and monitoring of the patient, then general anesthesia should be used.

SEDATION AND ANESTHESIA FOR PROCEDURES

Optimal sedation or anesthesia of a patient in preparation for a procedure provides for relief of anxiety and pain and also ensures that the patient remains relatively still during the procedure. Although general anesthesia can achieve all these goals, sedation can be used safely and effectively in most children for most diagnostic procedures. On the other hand, physicians should not hesitate to use general anesthesia whenever it is in the patient's best interests, whether for safety or for comfort. Examples of situations in which general anesthesia may be appropriate for procedures normally done with sedation include patients with unstable airways, patients who have been traumatized by numerous prior procedures, patients who are known to respond poorly to conventional sedation, and patients for whom a prolonged or difficult procedure is anticipated. Current anesthetic techniques have greatly reduced the risk traditionally associated with general anesthesia,[2,3] and patients should not be deprived of the benefits of general anesthesia when it is appropriate, even though it is more expensive.[4] With either general anesthesia or sedation, monitoring of the patient must not stop when the procedure is over because respiratory depression may last longer than sedation, especially when the stimulation associated with the procedure is no longer a factor.

Sedation is a state of depressed awareness between the fully conscious state and surgical anesthesia. Responsiveness to pain and other stimuli is decreased, as are reflexes. As the depth of sedation increases, respiratory drive is depressed. Careful and continuous monitoring is necessary to ensure patient safety. Current guidelines for sedation[1,5] require that vital signs, oxygenation, and the patency and adequacy of the airway be monitored continuously during sedation. *Conscious sedation* is a buzzword and refers to the level of sedation at which the patient maintains protective reflexes and response to verbal commands. Conscious sedation may be most appropriate for nonpainful procedures, such as radiographic imaging studies. In practice, many (especially younger) pediatric patients require a deeper level of sedation to safely and effectively tolerate potentially painful procedures. Therefore extra care must be taken to provide effective monitoring, and sedative agents should be chosen with regard to duration of action.

The choice of medications for pediatric sedation is an important determinant of success. Children (and their parents) are anxious about impending medical procedures. Children who must undergo repeated procedures are particularly vulnerable to psychologic trauma and should be handled with extra care.[6] Agents that partially or totally block short-term recall (e.g., benzodiazepines) can be extremely valuable. However, these agents are not in themselves usually sufficient for effective sedation for invasive procedures except perhaps at high doses. In general, both an analgesic agent and an anxiolytic agent should be used for any procedure involving pain; analgesia and sedation are not necessarily the same. Both types of agents depress the respiratory drive, and their effects may be additive.

Because children often become upset before a procedure, some form of presedation is useful if there is no contraindication such as unstable upper airway obstruction. Chloral hydrate has traditionally been used for this purpose; some concerns have been raised about this agent (potential mutagenicity in bacterial studies), but it has been approved for use in children by the American Academy of Pediatrics.[7] Other medications can be used, including oral[8] or nasal midazolam or ketamine.[9] A child who is comfortably sleepy separates more easily from a parent and can then be given additional medications to achieve the degree of sedation needed for the procedure itself. If the child is upset and crying at the time that medications are being given for sedation, larger doses will be required. Some children become excited and disinhibited when given sedative agents; this is usually only a stage through which they pass on the way to sedation, but it is more likely to be a problem if inadequate initial doses are used.

Chemical sedation is more readily controlled if the agents are given by the intravenous (IV) route because there is less uncertainty regarding absorption and the time course of the medication's effect. It may be helpful to place a lidocaine and prilocaine cream (EMLA Cream)[10] on potential IV sites before presedation to facilitate IV placement after the child has become somewhat sedate. In general, fractional dosing should be used and the patient's response assessed before additional medications are given. The response to medications such as midazolam and narcotics should be maximal within 2 to 3 minutes. Rapid infusion leads to a high concentration in the brain, with hypotension and respiratory depression or even apnea; infusion over 60 to 90 seconds is equally efficacious and safer than bolus infusion.

There are many safe and effective techniques for chemical sedation[11] (Table 17-1), and the operator should choose one or two and develop expertise with these, including a thorough knowledge of the pharmacology of the drugs, their side effects, and interactions. When there is doubt about a technique, consultation should be obtained from a pediatric anesthesiologist.

Patients (and their parents) who are under stress are more open to suggestion than they ordinarily would be; that is, they behave as though they are in a light hypnotic trance. Physicians must be aware of this phenomenon and use it for the patient's benefit. Inadvertent negative suggestions can have a dramatic impact on the patient's (or parents') behavior. One should be careful to use positive suggestion, avoiding negatives, and to prepare the patient for an experience that will be as relaxed and comfortable as possible. Children in particular are quite suggestible, and operators skilled in the techniques of hypnosis or simple distraction can often perform minor procedures with no sedation at all.[12] Because many pediatric practitioners are not necessarily skilled in these techniques, it seems most practical to combine simple relaxation and positive suggestion with chemical sedation.

Sedation diminishes protective reflexes; one of the major risks of sedation is aspiration of gastric contents. Patients should have nothing by mouth for several hours before sedation. Clear fluids may be given up to 2 hours before sedation.[13,14] Young infants may become dehydrated or hypoglycemic if they have nothing by mouth for too long, so IV fluid may be necessary before a procedure.

After completion of the procedure, the patient must be carefully monitored to ensure safe emergence from sedation. Some practitioners reverse the effect of the sedation (e.g., using naloxone, flumazenil, or both agents).[15] However, this practice may have serious shortcomings. The effect of the reversing agent may not last as long as that of the primary agent; therefore patients treated with reversing agents must be monitored even more carefully. Furthermore, extremely rapid reversal of sedation can be frightening and disorienting; it is kinder and gentler to allow the patient to awaken naturally as long as vital signs are stable. On the other hand, reversal agents should be available for use in an emergency when IV sedation is performed.

BRONCHOSCOPY

Indications

Bronchoscopy affords direct visual inspection of the upper and lower airways, and allows collection of diagnostic specimens such as washings, brushings, or biopsies. The most common indications for diagnostic bronchoscopy in pediatric patients include stridor, atelectasis, recurrent or persistent pneumonia, suspected foreign body aspiration, persistent wheezing unresponsive to medical therapy, hemoptysis, persistent cough, suspected congenital anomalies, upper airway obstruction, and suspected vocal cord paralysis. Because upper airway lesions are frequently associated with lower airway lesions,[16,17] it is

Table 17-1 Drugs Commonly Used for Pediatric Sedation

AGENT	DOSE/ROUTE	COMMENT
Diphenhydramine	1 mg/kg PO	This is a very mild sedative.
Chloral hydrate	75-100 mg/kg PO	Maximum dose is 2 g; this medication may cause gastric irritation.
Midazolam	0.75 mg/kg PO	Onset occurs in 10-20 minutes.
	0.4 mg/kg nasal	—
	0.05-0.2 mg/kg IV	Maximal effect occurs in 2-3 minutes.
Meperidine	1-4 mg/kg IV	—
Morphine sulfate	0.05-0.1 mg/kg IV	—
Fentanyl	1-3 μg/kg IV	This medication may cause rigid chest syndrome.
Ketamine*	2-10 mg/kg IM	This medication should be used with midazolam and atropine.
	1-3 mg/kg IV	—
Methohexital*	1-2 mg/kg IV	This medication provides 1-5 minutes of general anesthesia.
Pentobarbital	1-3 mg/kg IV	This medication is used primarily for imaging studies.
	2-6 mg/kg IM	—
	2-6 mg/kg PO	—
Reversal agents†		
Naloxone	Neonates: 0.01-0.1 mg/kg IV	—
	Infants < 20 kg: 0.1 mg/kg IV	—
	Children > 20 kg: 2 mg IV	—
Flumazenil	Children < 20 kg: 0.01 mg/kg IV	—
	Children > 20 kg: 0.2 mg IV	—

PO, Oral; *IM,* intramuscular.
*Agents that may require special (anesthesia) qualifications for use.
†The effect of such agents (especially reversal of respiratory depression) may not last as long as that of the primary agent; repeated doses may be required, and careful monitoring is always necessary.

usually appropriate to examine both the upper and lower airways even when the primary indication for the procedure involves the upper airway (e.g., stridor, suspected vocal cord paralysis).

Bronchoscopy can be used for therapeutic purposes as well. Extraction of foreign bodies from the airways, removal of tissue masses or other forms of airway obstructions such as mucus plugs, and therapeutic bronchopulmonary lavage are primary examples of therapeutic bronchoscopy.

Contraindications

Bronchoscopy is contraindicated when other, less invasive or less risky procedures can yield the same diagnostic information or therapeutic benefit. Relative contraindications (some of which may in themselves be indications) include massive hemoptysis, severe airway obstruction, severe hypoxemia, severe bronchospasm, and bleeding diatheses such as thrombocytopenia. All these conditions require additional care with sedation and anesthesia, instrumentation, airway management, preparation of the patient, and monitoring before, during, and after the procedure. None, however, is an absolute contraindication to bronchoscopy if the potential benefit of the procedure exceeds the potential risk. In some circumstances in which the potential benefit to the patient is marginal and the risk to medical personnel is significant (such as patients with cavitary tuberculosis), bronchoscopy may be contraindicated.

Instrumentation

Bronchoscopy may be performed with either rigid or flexible (fiberoptic) instruments. In general, depending on the training and preference of the operator and the availability of suitable instruments, either type of bronchoscope can be used for most purposes. However, there are some specific situations in which a flexible instrument has special advantages. These include examination of the lower airways in a patient who is intubated with an endotracheal or tracheostomy tube (the flexible bronchoscope can be passed through the tube without having to extubate the patient) and a patient in whom there is an unstable cervical fracture, cervical ankylosis, or mandibular hypoplasia (these conditions all make it difficult or impossible to pass a rigid bronchoscope into the trachea through the mouth). A flexible bronchoscope has a much smaller diameter than a rigid instrument and thus can be passed farther into the distal airways. Because it is flexible, it can also reach the upper lobes more easily than a rigid instrument.

There are situations in which the use of a rigid bronchoscope is necessary or more advantageous. These include the extraction of tracheal or bronchial foreign bodies and the evaluation of patients with suspected H-type tracheoesophageal fistula, laryngoesophageal cleft, and bilateral abductor paralysis of the vocal cords. Because the rigid bronchoscope is passed through the mouth, it yields a better view of the posterior aspect of the larynx and trachea than a flexible bronchoscope, which is usually passed through the nose and thus approaches the larynx from the posterior aspect, giving a better view of the anterior part of the larynx and upper trachea.

It is sometimes stated that a rigid bronchoscope affords better control of the airway than a flexible instrument because the patient's lungs can be ventilated through the rigid bronchoscope. However, there are techniques that allow continued mechanical ventilation even with a flexible bronchoscope[18,19] so that patients who have profound hypoxia or who are paralyzed can safely and effectively undergo flexible bronchoscopy. Alternatively, a flexible bronchoscope of appropriate size can be passed through or alongside an endotracheal or tracheostomy tube while positive-pressure ventilation is maintained.

Flexible Bronchoscopes

Flexible bronchoscopes are constructed of thousands of glass fibers that carry the image and illumination, and their distal tips can be angulated to direct the instrument into the desired anatomic location. Most of these instruments have a small but functional suction channel, which allows the instillation and retrieval of liquids such as saline (for diagnostic lavage or clearing secretions from the lens) and medications such as topical anesthetics or antibiotics. The most important aspect of a flexible bronchoscope is that it must be small enough to allow the patient to ventilate around it; the standard "pediatric" instrument has a diameter of 3.5 to 3.7 mm. An ultrathin instrument with a diameter of 2.2 mm (but no suction channel) is also available. The standard pediatric flexible bronchoscope can be used in patients of virtually any age, but it results in total airway obstruction in children who weigh less than 2.5 kg. The smallest "adult" flexible bronchoscope is 4.9 mm in diameter and can be used (if necessary) in children as young as about 4 years. Although the potential for airway obstruction is higher with this larger instrument, it has a larger suction channel, and the image quality is higher.

The image seen through a flexible bronchoscope is composed of several thousand points of light and color, each representing the light transmitted by a single glass fiber. Although the resolution of the flexible instrument is necessarily lower than that of a rigid bronchoscopic telescope, it is nevertheless quite adequate for diagnostic purposes. The glass fibers are fragile. Flexible bronchoscopes should be handled only by responsible, well-trained persons. A flexible bronchoscope should never be passed through a patient's mouth (even under general anesthesia and even through an endotracheal tube) without a suitable bite block in place; the cost in dollars per millisecond can be astronomical.

Rigid Bronchoscopes

Rigid bronchoscopes are essentially metal tubes; the nomenclature for their size is different from that of flexible instruments and describes the largest instrument that can be passed through the bronchoscope. A 3.5-mm flexible bronchoscope passes easily through a 3.5-mm rigid bronchoscope.

It is difficult to see well through a rigid bronchoscope unless a telescope is used. The glass rod (Hopkins) telescope[20] gives infinite resolution and good illumination. Telescopes are available with distal prisms to facilitate views of the upper lobes. The greatest advantage of a rigid bronchoscope is its relatively large inner diameter, through which one can ventilate the patient's lungs and pass a wide variety of instruments such as forceps for foreign body retrieval.

Techniques for Bronchoscopy

Bronchoscopy is usually performed with the patient supine and the bronchoscopist standing (or sitting) behind the patient's head. A flexible bronchoscope allows other positions for both the patient and bronchoscopist. For example, some bronchoscopists prefer to examine the older patient in a sitting position with the operator standing facing the patient. There are some disadvantages to this technique, including a higher probability of aspiration of oral contents during the procedure. However, if for some reason a patient is unable to assume a supine position, it is entirely correct to perform flexible bronchoscopy in any other suitable position. The entire airway should be systematically examined. Airway structure, dynamics, and contents (i.e., secretions) should be carefully noted.

Care should be taken to achieve effective topical anesthesia of the larynx before the tip of the bronchoscope is passed through the glottis. Although some bronchoscopists use transtracheal injection of lidocaine in adults, this is a dangerous practice in children and is unnecessary. For flexible bronchoscopy, simple instillation of lidocaine into one nostril (0.5 to 1 ml of 2% lidocaine) usually results in effective anesthesia of the nose and larynx. Additional lidocaine (1 ml of 2% lidocaine) is sprayed onto the larynx through the suction channel of the bronchoscope. For rigid bronchoscopy, the larynx can be directly sprayed with lidocaine after exposure with a laryngoscope. A 1% solution is used below the glottis to reduce the amount of lidocaine absorbed by the patient. The total dose should not exceed approximately 7 mg/kg.[21]

Flexible Bronchoscopy

After adequate sedation or anesthesia, the upper airway is anesthetized with topical lidocaine. The flexible bronchoscope is passed through one nostril. In some circumstances, the bronchoscope may be passed through the mouth, but this is more difficult than transnasal passage, is less informative, and risks damage to the instrument if an effective bite block is not used. Other approaches include passage through an endotracheal tube (oral or nasal), a nasopharyngeal tube, or a tracheostomy tube or stoma.

As the bronchoscope is passed into the trachea, the patient must be assessed for adequacy of ventilation and topical anesthetic effect. If necessary, supplemental oxygen can be given through the suction channel of the flexible bronchoscope, but care must be taken not to wedge the tip of the instrument into a bronchus while oxygen is being passed through the channel; this will prevent the development of a pneumothorax. The tip of the bronchoscope can be directed to systematically inspect all the airways.

Rigid Bronchoscopy

Rigid bronchoscopy is almost always performed with general anesthesia. Ventilation must be interrupted while a laryngoscope is inserted to allow the bronchoscope to reach the larynx. The tip of the bronchoscope is gently passed through the glottis and into the trachea under direct vision. When the shaft of the bronchoscope has been advanced far enough that the ventilating side holes are below the glottis, the anesthesia circuit is attached to the bronchoscope, and ventilation can be resumed. The proximal end of the bronchoscope must be covered with a lens cap to maintain pressure in the airway and prevent blowing the anesthetic gas into the operator's face. When forceps or other instruments are passed through the bronchoscope, ventilation must be interrupted unless a Venturi jet ventilation system is being used or flexible instruments are being passed through a side port.

The patient's neck must be somewhat extended and the mandible brought forward to pass a rigid bronchoscope into the trachea. The cricoid ring becomes a fulcrum about which the shaft of the bronchoscope moves, thus subjecting it to pressure and forces that can result in trauma. In contrast, a flexible bronchoscope must be small enough to allow ventilation around the instrument; it is thus harder to traumatize the subglottic space with a flexible instrument.

Bronchial Brushing

Small-diameter brushes can be passed through the suction channel of flexible bronchoscopes (or through a rigid bronchoscope) to obtain specimens containing large numbers of epithelial cells. In adults, this is often done in the evaluation of suspected malignancy (which is rare in pediatric patients). A more common use for bronchial brushing is to obtain microbiologic specimens that are (supposedly) uncontaminated by secretions from the upper airways. Microbiology specimen brushes are protected by plastic sheaths, which in turn are protected by outer sheaths and are plugged with wax.[22,23] As the catheter/brush assembly traverses the bronchoscope, the wax plug and outer catheter prevent contamination of the brush with material inside the suction channel of the bronchoscope. The assembly is passed under direct vision to near the desired location, and the inner catheter is advanced out the end of the outer catheter, dislodging the wax plug (which melts or is coughed out later). The brush is then advanced into position, and the specimen is obtained by repeatedly moving the brush against the bronchial wall; it is then withdrawn into the inner catheter. The inner catheter is withdrawn into the outer catheter, and the entire assembly is then removed from the bronchoscope. The outer catheter may then be wiped with alcohol; the inner catheter and then the brush are extended, and with sterile wire cutters, the brush is cut off into a suitable specimen container.

This technique can be used to obtain a lower airway specimen uncontaminated by secretions previously suctioned through the bronchoscope. Unfortunately, many patients aspirate oral secretions during topical anesthesia and passage of the bronchoscope, so a specimen obtained with a microbiology specimen brush is clearly not guaranteed to be uncontaminated by upper airway flora.

However, the smallest specimen brush is too large to pass through the suction channel of the pediatric flexible bronchoscope, so in most pediatric patients, the clinician must be content with direct aspirates or specimens from bronchoalveolar lavage (BAL) for microbiologic studies (see later section). If the child is large enough for a small adult bronchoscope (4.9-mm diameter; 2.0-mm suction channel), then a microbiology brush may be used. The minimum age is generally about 4 years, and even then the clinicians must exercise great caution regarding airway obstruction by the bronchoscope.

Complications of Bronchoscopy

The complications of bronchoscopy[24-30] depend on the technique and instruments used; the underlying risk factors of the patient; the skill, experience, and diligence of the bronchoscopy team; and of course, luck. The bronchoscopist should identify risk factors in advance, reduce the risk when possible, and carefully balance risk against benefit when choosing instruments and techniques.

In general, complications are classified as mechanical, physiologic, and infectious. Mechanical complications include trauma to the airway and airway obstruction and are best prevented by the careful selection and use of instruments. Rigid instruments must be large enough to allow the patient to breathe through them; during prolonged procedures, this may result in subglottic edema (uncommon with flexible instruments, which must be small enough for the patient to breathe around). If a bronchoscope is passed through an area of compressed or stenosed airway, mucosal edema or accumulation of mucus may occlude that airway after the procedure. Judicious use of systemic steroids may be indicated when the risk of edema after the procedure is high. Epistaxis or bronchial hemorrhage can result from trauma from the bronchoscope itself or from instruments passed through the bronchoscope. Perforation of the tracheobronchial mucosa may lead to air leaks (which may require the insertion of a chest tube) or hemorrhage; perforation is most common when transbronchial biopsy is performed. Hemorrhage usually is transient, and no intervention is needed except suctioning or perhaps local lavage with ice-cold saline or 1:10,000 epinephrine. Severe hemorrhage may require selective intubation of the contralateral mainstem bronchus, packing of the bronchus, or the use of a bronchial-blocking balloon catheter. Clots remaining in the airways after hemorrhage may require removal by extensive suctioning or even rigid bronchoscopy.

Physiologic complications result from alterations in gas exchange or vagal tone. Hypoxemia may develop when the airway is obstructed by the bronchoscope, when ventilation is interrupted (as during the extraction of a foreign body), or as a result of respiratory depression induced by sedation. Flooding of the airways with saline (or blood) also may lead to hypoxemia. Hypercarbia is usually the result of excessive sedation or anesthesia but may also occur in the setting of high-grade airway obstruction. Brief hypercarbia is usually of little consequence, however, and the administration of supplemental oxygen during the procedure can usually prevent or reduce the magnitude of hypoxemia.

Changes in vagal tone (usually because of insufficient topical anesthesia) can lead to bradycardia. Other cardiac dysrhythmias may occur, especially in patients with hypoxemia or preexisting cardiac problems. Laryngospasm and bronchospasm may also occur; both can be prevented or minimized by effective topical anesthesia. Similarly, ineffective topical anesthesia in the distal airways can result in severe coughing, which may then lead to mechanical trauma. On the other hand, excessive use of topical agents (usually lidocaine) can result in hypotension, seizures, and other effects. Bronchoscopy can also result in increased intracranial pressure.[31]

Infectious complications of bronchoscopy may affect either the patient or the bronchoscopy personnel; care must be taken to ensure that instruments are not contaminated from the previous patient and that proper technique is used to protect patient and personnel alike.[32-35] Although children are less likely than adults to aerosolize *Mycobacterium tuberculosis* during coughing, bronchoscopists have been infected in this way by pediatric patients; of course, other infectious agents can also be spread in this fashion. Patients may aspirate oropharyngeal secretions, thus contaminating their lower airways, and infection can be spread from one area of the lungs to another during bronchoscopy. Finally, pseudoinfections can occur when the specimens, but not the patient, are contaminated; this can result in considerable diagnostic and therapeutic confusion.[36,37]

BRONCHOALVEOLAR LAVAGE

One of the more important aspects of diagnostic bronchoscopy is the retrieval of specimens from the distal airways. Although direct aspiration of secretions from the proximal airways can be useful, a more representative and informative specimen can be obtained by washing a relatively large area of the distal airways and alveolar spaces with sterile saline. Strictly speaking, in BAL,[38,39] a sufficient volume of saline is used to ensure that the fluid subsequently aspirated contains some of the fluid lining of the alveolar surface. When relatively small volumes of saline are used, the term *bronchial lavage* is often used. In practice, especially in pediatric patients, it may be difficult to ascertain the minimum volume necessary to achieve BAL.[40] On the other hand, for the most common clinical indications in pediatric patients, it may make very little difference to the interpretation of the data whether a bronchial lavage or BAL is performed. This is especially true in the diagnosis of pulmonary infections.

Indications

BAL is performed in pediatric patients primarily to obtain a representative sample from the distal airways for microbiologic studies.[40] For example, patients with pulmonary infiltrates and presumed pulmonary infection who do not produce sputum are candidates for diagnostic BAL. On the other hand, most pediatric patients with pneumonia have a viral infection and do not require bronchoscopy or BAL; immunosuppressed patients, those who have recurrent or persistent pneumonia (including those in whom therapy has failed), or those with unusual clinical circumstances may benefit from the procedure, however. Young patients with cystic fibrosis, in whom it may be difficult to ascertain the flora of the lower respiratory tract, may also benefit.[41,42]

BAL is indicated in the investigation of interstitial pulmonary disease. Although such use in adults has been relatively disappointing in terms of the ability to make specific diagnoses of noninfectious entities, it is nevertheless reasonable to use BAL to exclude infection before the decision to perform an open lung biopsy is made.[43,44]

In addition to microbiologic studies, the content of proteins, cells, and other constituents of the airway surface fluid may be determined.[45] The cellular component may be of particular interest.[46-48]

Contraindications

There are no absolute contraindications to BAL if it is skillfully performed with suitable technique. In practice, however, bronchoscopic BAL may be difficult to safely accomplish in very small (premature) infants; if it is performed, the 3.5-mm flexible bronchoscope must be used, and because infants weighing less than 2.5 to 3 kg cannot breathe around this instrument, the procedure must be completed very rapidly and carefully. Only about half the saline used for BAL is recovered, leaving the rest in the alveolar spaces and distal airways. Although this is absorbed over several hours, significant impairment of gas exchange may result from flooding of the alveolar spaces with saline or from the airway occlusion required during the procedure.[49] Patients who are profoundly hypoxic may suffer further respiratory embarrassment as a result of BAL; the relative effect can be minimized by the use of a small instrument (which would wedge into a more distal airway, thus washing a smaller volume of lung). Patients with severe pulmonary hypertension may be at high risk for complications.[28]

Instrumentation

Successful and safe BAL requires that the saline be delivered to a discrete portion of the lungs. Therefore the delivery system, a flexible bronchoscope or a catheter, must be wedged into a bronchus. Merely instilling saline into a endotracheal tube, for example, may be unsafe or ineffective because large volumes produce respiratory distress and small volumes do not reliably reach the alveoli. In either case, the amount of saline recovered by suction is relatively small.

Techniques

BAL is most readily performed with a flexible bronchoscope,[39] which can be directed to the area of primary interest. The bronchoscope is advanced into the selected bronchus until its tip is gently wedged in place. The image of the bronchial lumen should be kept to one side (adjacent to the position of the suction port) to minimize the tendency of the bronchus to collapse around the suction port during withdrawal of fluid. Sterile saline is instilled through the suction channel; this may be done with a syringe, or if large volumes will be used, tubing from a reservoir may be connected to the suction adapter. When the desired volume has been instilled, the fluid is withdrawn using gentle suction. Some operators prefer to withdraw the fluid by hand into a syringe, whereas others withdraw the fluid by vacuum into a suction trap.

When a rigid bronchoscope is used, a catheter must be passed through the bronchoscope and wedged into position. Such catheters are small relative to a flexible bronchoscope and therefore sample a more limited region of the lung than BAL performed with a flexible bronchoscope. It may also be more difficult to direct the catheter into a specific bronchus.

Nonbronchoscopic BAL may be performed by passing a catheter through an endotracheal or tracheostomy tube.[50,51] In special circumstances, this might be done with fluoroscopic guidance, but nonbronchoscopic BAL is usually done in the setting of diffuse lung disease, when there is relatively little need to direct the catheter to a specific site. As with rigid bronchoscopes, nonbronchoscopic BAL samples a smaller site than flexible bronchoscopic BAL. Nevertheless, significant diagnostic information can often be obtained with relatively little cost and risk.

For achieving some measure of reproducibility and standardization of BAL technique in adults, the same volumes and aliquot numbers are used for each procedure. Typically, these may be three 100-ml aliquots or five 50-ml aliquots.[38] Cells migrate more slowly than soluble constituents, and the total yield of cells approaches a limit as the number of aliquots increases.[52] Various markers have been used to determine the dilution of the epithelial lining fluid (ELF); urea is used most commonly. It is assumed that urea exists in the ELF at the same concentration as in plasma; therefore the ratio of urea in BAL fluid to urea in plasma gives a measure of the dilution of ELF in the BAL fluid.[53] However, BAL does not sample a static space or volume of airway surface liquid. There is a constant exchange of fluid, electrolytes, and other soluble constituents across the airway and alveolar epithelium.[54-56] Thus the concentration of any material or cell type in the BAL fluid depends on the volume of fluid used for the lavage, the efficiency of mixing and recovery, the initial concentration in the ELF, and the rate of flux of the material or fluid into the BAL fluid during the procedure.

In pediatric subjects, there is no agreement regarding standard technique. Wedging the same size bronchoscope into an airway in children of various ages and sizes results in washing a greatly varying proportion of total lung volume. For example, in a newborn, the 3.5-mm flexible bronchoscope may wedge into a lobar bronchus, whereas in a 4-year-old child, it may wedge into a subsubsegmental bronchus. It is unclear whether using the same volume of saline in these two situations results in washing similar surface areas. Reported techniques include volumes of 0.5 to 3 ml/kg or the use of a fixed volume (usually two aliquots of 10 ml each) for each patient almost regardless of age.

In general, it is useful to perform BAL with more than one aliquot of saline. Some authorities discard the return from the first aliquot, suggesting that it represents "bronchial" rather than "alveolar" washings.[57] The composition of the first aliquot is indeed somewhat different from subsequent aliquots, but there is no practical way to obtain a pure bronchial or alveolar fraction. In pediatric practice, there is little rationale or justification for discarding the first aliquot or processing it differently because material from the proximal airways is washed distally and therefore contaminates the subsequent aliquots.

If BAL is being performed to evaluate a specific radiologic lesion, then the bronchoscope should be positioned in the appropriate bronchus. On the other hand, if there is no localized area of disease, it is advantageous to choose the lingula or right middle lobe for lavage. These bronchi are relatively long and relatively horizontal, and the tip of the bronchoscope is more likely to remain comfortably wedged in the bronchus (even with coughing) than if it is wedged into a basal segment of one of the lower lobes.

The amount of fluid returned is usually between 40% and 60% of that instilled. In patients whose bronchi collapse around the tip of the bronchoscope, there may be more difficulty achieving return of the saline. Patients under general anesthesia or on mechanical ventilation also have low returned volumes.

Complications

A significant percentage of patients who undergo BAL experience transient fever and even chills, usually beginning 4 to 6 hours after the procedure. This phenomenon is almost always self-limiting, should be anticipated, and is readily treated with antipyretics. It most likely results from absorption of toxins or inflammatory mediators from the alveolar surface and is more common in patients whose airways are inflamed.[58,59]

BAL can result in hypoxemia because residual saline in the lavaged area interferes with gas exchange until the saline has been absorbed. It may also stimulate mucus production and cough. Wedging of the bronchoscope into an airway may result in localized bleeding. If the bronchoscope is not wedged snugly, saline spills into adjacent bronchi and stimulates cough and respiratory distress.

Specimen Handling

The purpose of BAL is to obtain a specimen for analysis; the care with which the specimen is handled is as important to the success of the procedure as the techniques used to obtain the specimen. Prompt processing reduces the loss of labile substances (or organisms) or the overgrowth of microbial species.

Cells adhere to glass surfaces, and specimens collected or transported in glass containers may be depleted of their cellular content in relatively nonpredictable ways.

The analyses performed on BAL specimens should be determined by the indications for the procedure, although it makes sense to perform bacterial cultures (preferably, a quantitative culture) in almost all cases. At least a simple cytologic preparation should also be made; it is helpful to have a cytocentrifuge in the bronchoscopy laboratory and to perform a simple and quick cytologic analysis immediately because this often results in significant changes in patient management. Other cultures and diagnostic tests (e.g., antigen detection, polymerase chain reaction) can be performed according to the clinical indications. BAL can also be used for research applications,[60] and a wide variety of substances have been measured in BAL specimens from pediatric patients.

Interpretation of Findings

There are many difficulties inherent in the interpretation of findings from BAL fluid; these relate to the area of lung sampled, the (variable and usually unknown) dilution of the fluid, and the expected normal values.[38,61,62] In some cases, interpretation is simple. For example, identification of material or organisms that should not be present in normal lungs, such as the cysts of *Pneumocystis carinii,* should give a relatively unequivocal diagnosis. In the case of substances that may be found in the lungs under normal conditions, interpretation is more challenging and may depend on relative quantitation. An example is the presence of lipid in alveolar macrophages. A large amount of lipid (large intracytoplasmic droplets in a substantial percentage of cells) strongly suggests aspiration.[63] However, chronic and sometimes acute inflammation can result in the accumulation of lipid in macrophages, presumably as a result of the phagocytosis of dead neutrophils and debris. There is some suggestion that such "endogenous" lipid may be discriminated by the size of the intracytoplasmic lipid droplets and by the number of cells containing such droplets, but there is no gold standard by which such identification can be proved. If aspiration is suspected, lipid stains should be performed, but the unequivocal identification of exogenous substances (perhaps by chemical means) would be more definitive proof of aspiration.

Microbiologic diagnosis is complicated,[64] especially by the relative difficulty of ensuring that the specimen is not contaminated with oral secretions. Bacteria may contaminate the bronchoscope during passage through the nose or mouth, or they may be aspirated into the trachea as a result of topical anesthesia. Although the risk of orotracheal aspiration can be reduced by placement of the patient into a head-down position before the application of the topical anesthetic and by being careful not to suction through the instrument channel until the tip of the bronchoscope is at least at the level of the carina, the clinician can never be certain that there is no contamination (this is also true when a microbiology specimen brush is used, as discussed previously). Quantitative culture can be helpful in this regard. Clearly, there is a difference between 2000 and 2,000,000 colonies in each milliliter of BAL fluid, the latter being more consistent with pulmonary infection and the former with oral contamination. Furthermore, except in patients who have neutropenia, pulmonary infection should be accompanied by significant numbers of neutrophils in the BAL fluid. Therefore BAL specimens should be examined microscopically to ascertain the relative distribution and number of cell types. (Gram's stains are not optimal for this purpose.) The absence of inflammatory cells should make the clinician very suspicious that the bacteria in the BAL specimen are from the mouth and not the lungs. The presence of intracytoplasmic bacteria is also strong evidence of infection.[48] Care must be taken to avoid overinterpretation.[61]

The total number of cells in the BAL fluid depends on the technique used for BAL as well as the concentration of cells in the ELF. The significance of cell counts is subject to considerable uncertainty, although if the same technique is always used, the clinician may have more confidence in relative numbers. In the author's experience, the fluid from BAL performed using two 10-ml aliquots of saline in pediatric patients in whom no infection or inflammation is suspected (and in whom cultures are sterile) contains 100,000 to 300,000 cells in each milliliter, 95% of which are alveolar macrophages and 1% to 2% are neutrophils. In patients with infection, the cell numbers and the percentage of neutrophils are much higher (ranging up to 90% neutrophils). Other authors have reported similar findings.[45,47,65]

Eosinophils are rarely seen in BAL fluid from subjects free of lung disease but are seen in the BAL fluid of patients with allergic states, foreign body reactions, and parasitic diseases. Increased percentages of lymphocytes may be seen in the BAL fluid of patients with sarcoidosis and other interstitial diseases.[66,67]

INTUBATION

Indications

An artificial airway is established to bypass airway obstruction, to facilitate mechanical ventilation, or to achieve repeated access to the lower airways for suctioning. The choice of tube type depends on the indications for and the anticipated length of intubation.

Contraindications

There are no absolute contraindications to the establishment of an artificial airway. Certain factors make the procedure more difficult or risky and may mandate one or another alternative technique (including tracheostomy). Risk factors include bleeding diatheses, severe hypoxemia, cardiovascular instability, and severe airway obstruction. However, some of these are also indications for intubation. Unstable cervical fractures mandate endoscopic rather than conventional intubation because the neck must be kept immobilized. Great care must be taken if a patient requires intubation with a full stomach because the risk of aspiration is great.

Instrumentation

The essential requirements for intubation include a suitable artificial airway and a method for visualizing the larynx (i.e., a laryngoscope). In some situations, an endotracheal tube may be passed via the nose and into the trachea without exposing the larynx for direct visualization; in others, a flexible bronchoscope may be used to direct the endotracheal tube.

Intubation must be performed in an appropriate setting, with appropriate measures for monitoring the patient and for altering the approach if warranted. Rarely must a patient be intubated immediately; in most circumstances, bag and mask ventilation is sufficient until suitable preparations can be completed. Alternative methods for ventilating the patient's lung must always be available before elective intubation is attempted; these include (at least) a mask, a self-inflating resuscitation bag or an anesthesia bag with a source of compressed oxygen, and an oral airway of appropriate size.

The endotracheal tube must be the appropriate diameter for the patient's airway. Table 17-2 lists the customary tube sizes.[68] Useful approximations for the appropriate endotracheal tube size include the diameter of the fifth digit of the patient's hand or the following formula:

$$\text{Diameter in millimeters} = (\text{Age}/4) + 4$$

Tubes of this size and at least one size larger and smaller should be available before the clinician attempts intubation. In general, there should be a leak of air around the endotracheal tube no greater than 25 cm H_2O pressure to reduce the potential for trauma to the subglottic space and subglottic stenosis.[69] Depending on the indication for intubation, an endotracheal tube may have a cuff to seal the trachea around its distal end, a monitoring lumen through which gas may be sampled, both, or neither. Although cuffed tubes are rarely used in pediatric patients because the cricoid diameter is relatively small and thus there is relatively little leak around the endotracheal tube, they may be warranted if relatively high airway pressures are required to maintain ventilation. In adolescents or adults, the diameter of the endotracheal tube is relatively smaller in relation to the tracheal or cricoid diameter, and a cuff may be necessary for conventional ventilation.

Table 17-2 Suggested Endotracheal Tube Sizes*

AGE	INTERNAL DIAMETER	LENGTH	
		ORAL	NASAL
Premature	2.5-3.0 mm	8 cm	11 cm
Newborn	3.0-3.5 mm	9 cm	12 cm
6 mo	3.5 mm	10 cm	14 cm
1 yr	4.0-4.5 mm	12 cm	16 cm
2 yr	5.0-5.5 mm	14 cm	17 cm
2-4 yr	5.5-6.0 mm	15 cm	18 cm
4-7 yr	6.0-6.5 mm	16 cm	19 cm
7-10 yr	6.5-7.0 mm	17 cm	21 cm
10-12 yr	7.0-7.5 mm	20 cm	23 cm
12-16 yr	7.5-8.0 mm	21 cm	24 cm

From Chatburn RL, Lough MD: *Pediatric respiratory therapy,* ed 3, St Louis, 1985, Mosby, pp 148-191.
*NOTE: Tube size should allow an air leak at a pressure not exceeding 25 cm H_2O.

Techniques for Intubation

Preparation of the Patient

For elective intubation, the patient should have an empty stomach[14,70] and should be given appropriate medications to reduce anxiety and relieve pain. Topical anesthesia of the larynx improves patient comfort and reduces the risk of adverse reactions such as laryngospasm and severe vagal reactions. In an emergency, it is probably even more important to have effective laryngeal anesthesia to reduce the probability of gagging and emesis, which could lead to aspiration. This may be accomplished by instilling 1 to 2 ml of 2% lidocaine through the mouth or nose; effective topical anesthesia is achieved within 30 to 60 seconds. It is not necessary to apply the lidocaine directly to the glottis; the superior laryngeal nerve crosses the floor of the pyriform sinuses and is very superficial; pooling of lidocaine in the pyriform sinuses results in effective topical anesthesia. Atropine may be administered to reduce salivary secretions and to reduce the potential for vagal stimulation. Patients may have severe vagal reactions when the larynx is manipulated without effective laryngeal anesthesia, even under what appears to be a surgical level of general anesthesia.

Oral Intubation

With oral intubation the patient's neck is slightly extended, and a laryngoscope is gently inserted into the mouth. The laryngoscope should be held in the left hand and passed along the right side of the tongue. The tongue is then moved toward the left, exposing a path for visualization and passage of the endotracheal tube along the right side of the mouth. The laryngoscope blade is used to elevate the tongue; the tip of the blade is placed into the vallecula. In some circumstances, it may be necessary to elevate the epiglottis with the tip of the laryngoscope blade, but this may traumatize the epiglottis or vocal cords and is usually not necessary. The laryngoscope is lifted straight up to expose the larynx. Under direct vision, the endotracheal tube is inserted into the mouth and is guided through the glottis. It may help to stiffen the endotracheal tube with a soft-metal stylet, but the tip of the stylet should never extend beyond the end of the endotracheal tube; the use of stylets increases the risk of laryngeal trauma during intubation. Alternatively, the endotracheal tube can be stiffened by cooling it in ice for a few minutes. The tube is passed into the trachea to the desired distance, and the laryngoscope is withdrawn from the mouth.

The position of the endotracheal tube is then verified. Definitive proof that the tube is in the trachea involves demonstration of carbon dioxide in the exhaled gases. In the operating room, a capnometer is often used for this purpose; disposable indicators are also available that demonstrate a color change when exposed to carbon dioxide.[71] The more traditional and common method is to observe for chest rise and to listen for breath sounds while the patient is ventilated with an anesthesia bag; the breath sounds should be symmetric bilaterally (assuming that the patient had symmetric breath sounds before intubation). Observation of condensation of moisture in the tube during exhalation is not definitive because it can be seen with esophageal intubation as well. Success is clinically verified when the patient's condition stabilizes or improves. The tube is secured in position, and its location is definitively verified via a chest radiograph (or a flexible bronchoscope [see later section]).

In newborns, an endotracheal tube can be guided into the larynx with the index finger without using a laryngoscope. Although this method is useful in an emergency, its disadvantage is that the larynx is not visualized.

Nasal Intubation

Passage of the endotracheal tube through the nose has some advantages over oral intubation. A nasal tube leaves the mouth free so that infants can carry on nonnutritive sucking. A nasal tube is more easily secured in position and moves less than an oral tube. Because it passes behind the tongue, a nasal tube may be more comfortable than an oral tube. On the other hand, nasal intubation may be more difficult, and sometimes there may be nasal trauma. There is a small but significant incidence of sinusitis complicating nasal intubation. Some (especially inexperienced) operators may find nasal intubation more difficult; it may be useful to initially intubate orally and then to switch to a nasal tube when the patient is more stable.

Passage of a nasotracheal tube is performed in much the same fashion as oral intubation, except that the tube is first passed through one nostril to a depth such that its tip can be expected to be just above the larynx. The tube should be lubricated with a sterile, water-soluble jelly, and the nose is anesthetized with topical lidocaine before insertion of the tube. When the larynx is exposed with a laryngoscope, the tip of the tube is grasped with McGill forceps and advanced into the glottis. Alternatively, the tube can be advanced while the neck is flexed or extended to guide the tip of the tube into the glottis. An assistant advances the tube or controls the patient's head and neck. Some operators prefer to perform blind nasal intubation without laryngoscopy; in this technique the tube is inserted through the nose and advanced to a position estimated to be near the larynx. By listening to the breath sounds through the tube and observing for condensation of moisture in the tube, the clinician can estimate the location of the tip of the tube. The tube is advanced while the patient's neck is flexed or extended to, it is hoped, advance the tube into the trachea. Although this technique sounds awkward, it can be surprisingly successful when performed by experienced operators, and it may be necessary in a patient whose mouth cannot be opened. (However, see the section on endoscopic intubation for a more effective technique.)

Endoscopic Intubation

Although the standard methods for oral and nasal intubation are successful in most cases, there are clearly circumstances in which these techniques are difficult or inappropriate. These situations include patients with mandibular hypoplasia, cervical or mandibular ankylosis, masses in the mouth or neck, and severe contractures of the neck. A flexible bronchoscope provides a nearly foolproof method for accomplishing the intubation and a diagnostic evaluation of the airway.[72,73]

A flexible bronchoscope of appropriate size is passed through the endotracheal tube. The flexible bronchoscope is then passed through the nose or mouth and into the trachea. When the tip of the bronchoscope reaches the carina, the endotracheal tube is advanced over the bronchoscope until the tip of the tube is seen just above the carina. The bronchoscope is then withdrawn. Experienced operators should be able to accomplish this maneuver in 1 minute or less. Not only is the airway anatomy visualized, but the location of the tip of the endotracheal tube is also immediately verified. When the tube has been positioned and the patient's lung has been ventilated for at least 1 minute, the lower airways should be examined to ensure that there is no anatomic abnormality and that the lobar and segmental airways are patent.

Virtually any patient can undergo endoscopic intubation; intubation can be performed on a premature infant when a 2.5- or 3.0-mm endotracheal tube is used with 2.2-mm ultrathin flexible bronchoscope. The standard 3.5-mm pediatric flexible bronchoscope can be used with endotracheal tubes ranging in size from 4.5 to 6.5 mm; with larger tubes, an adult flexible bronchoscope should be used.

Although bronchoscopic intubation is simple in principle and is almost always successful, it requires a skilled and experienced operator. The procedure is difficult in patients in whom there is a mass lesion or pharyngeal collapse. Insufflation with oxygen through the suction port of the bronchoscope (or through a nasopharyngeal tube) can be very helpful; occasionally the clinician may need to use a rigid laryngoscope to lift the mandible and tongue so that the glottis can be visualized.

During bronchoscopic intubation, there is a risk of damage to the flexible bronchoscope; it is likely that more bronchoscopes are damaged in the process of intubation than with any other procedure. This is especially true of the ultrathin instruments.

Care of the Intubated Child

The endotracheal tube must be secured in place, with reasonable provision for comfort, so that it cannot easily be dislodged. Tubing attached to the endotracheal tube should be supported in a way that reduces tension on the tube. Inspired gases must be adequately humidified to prevent inspissation of secretions, and secretions should be removed from the tube by suctioning at regular intervals. Suction catheters should not routinely be passed beyond the tip of the endotracheal tube.

In a patient whose respiratory tract has been intubated for more than a few hours, additional factors must be taken into account. Phonation is impossible, and if the patient is awake and alert, some provision for effective communication may be necessary. Sedation may be appropriate for the duration of intubation because many children are frightened and uncomfortable. Chest physiotherapy should be routinely performed to help mobilize secretions to the tip of the tube. Nutritional needs must be met by routes other than the oral route.

When the patient requires intubation over a period of several days to weeks, secretions may accumulate in the tube despite regular suctioning and saline irrigation. This may require that the tube be changed. In general, however, the number of tube changes should be kept to a minimum because each change introduces the potential for trauma to the subglottic space. When prolonged intubation is contemplated, serious consideration should be given to tracheostomy.

Laryngeal Mask Airway

An alternative to endotracheal intubation that may be useful in selected circumstances is the laryngeal mask airway.[74,75] This device consists of a triangular mask (with an inflatable cuff around the perimeter) attached to a large-bore airway. The mask is inserted into the posterior pharynx; the apex of the triangle enters the proximal esophagus. The cuff is inflated to seal the mask around the larynx and the base of the tongue. The laryngeal mask airway may be used for short-term anesthesia or for endoscopic procedures performed under general anesthesia when the supraglottic airway does not need to be examined.

TRACHEOSTOMY

A tracheostomy is an artificial airway inserted surgically into the cervical trachea. The terms *tracheostomy* and *tracheotomy* (the latter referring to the surgical placement of the tracheostomy tube) are used interchangeably in practice. Tracheostomy tubes may be maintained indefinitely and are generally comfortable (once the postoperative period is over). They may be removed and replaced with relative ease and allow the patient to swallow and to phonate.

Indications

The primary indication for tracheostomy is the maintenance of a long-term artificial airway. Although endotracheal tubes may be maintained in infants and young children for weeks to several months, placement of a tracheostomy tube reduces the risk of laryngeal damage. In patients with large pharyngeal tumors or severe subglottic obstructions, tracheostomy may be the only method of establishing a safe and secure airway. Finally, in some patients with chronic laryngeal incompetence, a tracheostomy may be performed to facilitate pulmonary cleansing.

Contraindications

There are few absolute contraindications to the placement of a tracheostomy except perhaps the presence of tumor or infection in the surgical field. Coagulation defects and unusual anatomic conditions (including significant tracheal obstruction by the innominate artery) make tracheostomy more difficult and may warrant delay until the underlying condition is corrected.

Instrumentation

Tracheostomy tubes may be constructed of metal or plastic; the plastic tubes are more common today. Metal tubes and large plastic tubes used in adults typically have a removable inner cannula, which must be removed and cleaned several times each day. Because of the small diameter of the tubes used in infants and young children, most nonmetallic pediatric tracheostomy tubes do not have inner cannulas. The tube size (diameter and length) must be matched to the airway dimensions of the patient. There is a bewildering array of tube types on the market, and virtually all can be customized for the particular needs of the patient.

Technique

Tracheotomy is a surgical procedure; details of technique may be found in standard surgical texts. In brief, an incision is made over the cervical trachea, avoiding the thyroid isthmus and associated vessels. The incision is extended by blunt dissection to the anterior tracheal wall. The trachea is usually entered between the second and third (or third and fourth) tracheal rings; in children, one ring often must be divided. A suitable tube is inserted through the tracheal incision and secured in place.[76,77]

It may be difficult to reinsert the tracheostomy tube if it becomes dislodged before healing of the incision and establishment of a mature track, especially if the ends of the cartilage ring that was cut in the operation resume their normal position. Therefore it is customary to place retraction sutures around the ends of the cut cartilage ring; these are left in place until the tube is successfully changed (usually after 5 to 7 days) and it is verified that the track is stable. In an emergency recannulation, these retraction sutures can be used to pull the ends of the cartilage ring laterally, thus dilating the track so that the tube can be reinserted.

Alternative techniques exist for placing a tracheostomy tube, although they are not readily applicable in infants and young children. In brief, these involve transtracheal needle puncture followed by passage of a guidewire and a dilator; the tracheostomy tube is placed in much the same fashion as an over-the-wire vascular catheter.[78,79]

In an emergency, cricothyroidotomy[80] may be used to place an artificial airway into the trachea below the larynx. A horizontal incision is made directly over the cricothyroid membrane (identified by feel just at the inferior margin of the thyroid cartilage). After dilation with a suitable instrument, a tube is passed into the trachea. Because cricothyroidotomy risks laryngeal damage, the patient should undergo formal surgical revision and placement of a conventional tracheostomy as soon as it is feasible if there is a continuing need for the tracheostomy tube.

Complications

Immediate complications of tracheotomy include hemorrhage, air leak (pneumothorax, pneumomediastinum, or subcutaneous emphysema), and possibly damage to the recurrent laryngeal nerves. Displacement of the tube before the track has healed may have disastrous consequences if the patient does not have a functional airway.

Long-term complications include the development of granulation tissue, which may completely obstruct the suprastomal trachea; bleeding from the track, which is usually minimal but may be massive from the creation of a tracheoinnominate fistulas; respiratory distress resulting from obstruction or dislodgment of the tube; and trauma to the lower airways from suction catheter trauma. Infection is a constant risk because the normal defenses of the upper airway are bypassed.

Care of the Child with a Tracheostomy

A tracheostomy tube interferes with the normal humidification of inspired air. The inspired air should be humidified to reduce the risk of inspissation of secretions in the airways or the tracheostomy tube; a mist collar should be used in infants most of the time. After some months, many patients can tolerate nonhumidified air more easily, but some provision should still be made for adding humidification at least part of the time. "Artificial noses" are small devices that attach to the tracheostomy tube, condense some moisture during exhalation, and evaporate it on inspiration; these may be quite useful,[81] and they also filter the inspired air.

Patients with tracheostomies require assistance clearing secretions from the airways and in keeping the tube patent. Dry mucus has the consistency of dry rubber cement and can occlude a tracheostomy tube with lethal consequences. Therefore suctioning of the tube on a regular basis is essential. Suction catheters can traumatize the airway; this leads to increased mucus production, mucus stasis, and sometimes bronchial stenosis.[82] Suctioning should be performed only deeply enough to clear the tracheostomy tube; chest physiotherapy and cough should clear the bronchi of secretions.

Tracheostomy tubes should be changed at regular intervals (typically once a week). Caregivers must learn the techniques involved.[83] Metal tracheostomy tubes have very thin walls, and an obturator must be used during insertion to prevent the tube from cutting the tissue. However, obturators should not be used with plastic tubes because they are not necessary to prevent tissue damage and they obstruct the airway during insertion. If difficulty is encountered during attempted insertion of the tube (sterile, water-soluble lubricant should always be used), a suction catheter passed through the tube can be used as a guidewire in the same fashion as a guidewire with a vascular catheter. It is a good practice to have a spare tube one size smaller than the usual tube because in an emergency, it may be necessary to use a smaller tube to reestablish an airway.

The tracheostomy tube must be secured to the patient's neck with an appropriate strap. Various materials are used, ranging from adjustable Velcro straps to simple twill tape. The strap must be tight enough to prevent accidental decannulation but not so tight that it is uncomfortable. Materials must always be kept close at hand to cut or remove the strap and replace the tracheostomy tube quickly in case of emergency. An emergency kit should contain a clean tube of the appropriate size with straps already in place and ready to be secured, another tube one size smaller, a suction catheter, lubricating jelly, and scissors.

Because of the risk of catastrophic airway obstruction if the tracheostomy tube becomes dislodged or obstructed, infants and young children with tracheostomies must be monitored carefully. Unfortunately, there is no entirely satisfactory way to do this. Cardiorespiratory monitors may respond to airway occlusion only after the child has become sufficiently hypoxic to become apneic, whereas pulse oximeters have a very high rate of false alarms. Nevertheless, caregivers must be well trained to detect and respond quickly and appropriately to emergencies by suctioning, giving positive-pressure breathing, changing the tracheostomy tube on an emergency basis, and providing the basic elements of resuscitation. The preparation of a child and family for home care with a tracheostomy is complex and demanding.[84]

Tracheostomy tubes should be sized to fit the needs of the patient. In very young infants, the internal diameter of the tube should be large enough to minimize airway resistance, with relatively little concern for the child's ability to vocalize around the tube. Most full-term newborns do well with a tube with an internal diameter of 3 to 3.5 mm. The end of the tube must not touch the carina, but the tube must be long enough that it lies parallel to the tracheal axis. A short tube often pushes into the posterior membranous portion of the trachea, producing partial expiratory obstruction; this also places the child at risk of developing granulation tissue at the tip of the tube. The tube size must be increased to keep pace with the child's growth. It also becomes more important to allow for some air movement around the outside of the tube to facilitate phonation.

At some point, it may become feasible to provide the patient with a one-way ("speaking") valve on the tracheostomy tube. This allows the child to breathe in through the tube but forces expired air through the glottis, thus facilitating both phonation and improved clearance of secretions.[85] There must be sufficient airway around the tube for effective airflow; expiratory pressures greater than 10 cm H_2O are not well tolerated. On the other hand, some children with severe tracheomalacia or bronchomalacia benefit greatly from the enhanced expiratory resistance provided by the speaking valve.

Most patients with tracheostomies develop some granulation tissue at the superior margin of the stoma[86]; this may progress to complete obstruction of the suprastomal trachea with potentially lethal consequences. It is prudent to examine the airway with a bronchoscope at regular intervals[17,87] to assess for this complication as well as to evaluate the patient's readiness for possible decannulation.[88] Although there is controversy about how aggressively to remove small to medium suprastomal granulations, it is clear that near-total obstruction places the child at risk of serious complications.

Specific criteria for decannulation include the ability to breathe adequately without support and an anatomic and functionally patent airway.[87] Endoscopic examination of the airway before decannulation is virtually mandatory, and the airway should be examined with the tracheostomy tube removed. Some authors prefer to place a series of increasingly smaller tracheostomy tubes in preparation for decannulation, culminating in a small, plugged tube. In this author's experience, however, endoscopic evaluation followed if necessary by degranulation and immediate decannulation is almost always successful. If the airway is obstructed by granulation tissue or the collapse of the anterior tracheal wall,[89] then smaller tracheostomy tubes will not solve the problem. If the airway structure and dynamics appear adequate, the child should be observed in the hospital for 48 hours; the stoma usually closes very rapidly (often within hours), and a true emergency may arise if the child needs recannulation. In a small percentage of children, a persistent tracheocutaneous fistula requires surgical closure at a later date. Some children require laryngeal or tracheal reconstruction before successful decannulation.

THORACENTESIS

Indications

The accumulation of fluid in the pleural space often poses diagnostic problems that may be directly addressed by analysis of the fluid. Pleural effusions that are very small or that on clinical grounds are clearly the result of simple mechanical processes may not require thoracentesis. Examples of the latter include patients with congestive heart failure or severe hypoproteinemia. On the other hand, if infectious or malignant disease is suspected, then analysis of the fluid is warranted.[90]

Contraindications

If the diagnostic importance is sufficiently high, there are no absolute contraindications to thoracentesis. However, certain situations (i.e., thrombocytopenia) make the procedure more risky. Because children need sedation for thoracentesis, hypoxic patients are at greater risk from respiratory depression during the procedure. Careful attention to the patient's physiologic condition, continuous monitoring, and correction of risk factors amenable to correction (e.g., platelet transfusion) reduce the risk. It may not always be possible to determine the location of the diaphragm from simple radiographs, so there is some risk of puncturing the liver or spleen if the needle is placed too low.

Instrumentation

In brief, thoracentesis involves inserting a needle through the intercostal space and into the pleural space. If the goal is merely to obtain a specimen for diagnostic purposes, especially if the fluid is not loculated, then a simple needle of suitable length and diameter can be used. If the goal is to withdraw a substantial volume of pleural fluid, then use of a plastic catheter (passed over a small needle or through a larger needle) is more suitable. If an IV catheter (catheter over the needle) is used, it must be long enough to reach the pleural space and should be large enough that even highly viscous fluid can be withdrawn through it. Generally, a 16- or 18-gauge catheter should be used.

Radiographic evaluation before attempted thoracentesis is needed to determine the relative volume of fluid and its mobility or lack thereof. If the entire hemithorax is opacified, it may sometimes be difficult to ascertain the amount of fluid present and the position of the diaphragm; a computed tomographic or ultrasound scan can be very helpful in identifying the hemithorax. Small or loculated fluid collections are best located with ultrasound; the most appropriate site can be marked before skin preparation so that the needle can be inserted directly into the fluid.

Technique

The patient should be prepared with appropriate sedation and monitored carefully. Because fluid moves with gravity, it is usually most effective to perform the procedure with the patient sitting erect (usually leaning slightly forward and supported on pillows or an overbed table). Alternatively, in a supine patient the needle can be placed in the posterior axillary line with the patient very near the edge of the procedure table. The level of fluid is determined by percussion. The most common site for the insertion of the needle is the seventh intercostal space in the midaxillary or posterior axillary line; this may be modified according to the clinical situation (with ultrasound guidance if necessary).

After appropriate skin cleansing and disinfection and sterile draping, a small-gauge needle is used to infiltrate lidocaine into the track intended for the larger needle. The needle, which is attached to a syringe containing 1 to 2 ml of lidocaine, is inserted perpendicularly to the skin and advanced to the rib and then up and over the top of the rib, thus avoiding the neurovascular bundle, which follows the inferior margin of the rib. The needle should be held with the fingers against the skin so that if the patient moves, the operator's hand and the needle move in the same direction at the same time. The needle is carefully advanced with the other hand, which may be used to alternately gently withdraw and inject lidocaine. As soon as pleural fluid appears in the syringe, the depth of the needle is marked, and the needle is withdrawn. Then the larger needle/catheter is inserted in the same track, and gentle suction is applied as the needle reaches the marked depth. When fluid is obtained, the needle/catheter is advanced slightly into the pleural space, and the needle is withdrawn, leaving the catheter in the pleural space. A three-way stopcock is then attached to facilitate repeated aspiration with a syringe or drainage into a reservoir. When the desired amount of fluid has been withdrawn, the catheter is removed, and the site is dressed with a simple dressing; pressure dressings are seldom necessary. If fluid is not obtained with the probing needle, it may be because the fluid is loculated and the needle has been placed in the wrong position (the clinician should consider ultrasound guidance or try one interspace higher) or because what appears to be pleural fluid may in fact be pleural thickening.

An alternative technique is to use a large-bore needle (after the probing needle has been used to provide local anesthesia and locate the pleural fluid) through which a plastic catheter is passed. Once the needle enters the pleural space, the catheter is advanced and the needle withdrawn. Yet another technique is to use a catheter advanced over a guidewire that has in turn been passed into the pleural space over a needle[90,91] (see the section on the placement of chest tubes).

Complications

The complications of thoracentesis include bleeding, pneumothorax, and infection. Although the absolute risk of bleeding is small, it may be prudent to ensure that clotting mechanisms are normal before thoracentesis. Pneumothorax may occur if the needle is advanced too far, especially if the patient moves or coughs. An upright chest radiograph should be obtained after the procedure to evaluate for air leak. In patients with massive accumulations of pleural fluid, removal of large volumes can lead to unilateral pulmonary edema or hypotension. (As the pulmonary vascular bed in the previously collapsed or compressed lung fills with blood, the blood pressure may fall.) These complications seem to be more likely when the fluid has been present for a long time; there are no specific guidelines as to how much fluid may be safely withdrawn in a given patient.[92,93] Clearly, if the volume of fluid in the pleural space is sufficient to cause respiratory distress, then at least enough should be removed to relieve the distress. Purulent fluid should be drained as completely as possible; if the fluid is highly purulent it will also be highly viscous, and it may be necessary to insert a large-bore chest tube to achieve adequate drainage.

Specimen Handling

Specimens of pleural fluid should be sent for total and differential cell count, appropriate cultures, and determination of total protein content. Because pleural fluid often contains considerable amounts of fibrin, it is useful to collect some of the fluid into a tube containing an anticoagulant and to use this tube for cell counts and other determinations. Other analyses may be performed, including (but not limited to) amylase, glucose, and pH, depending on the clinical setting.

Interpretation of Findings

See Chapter 63.

TUBE THORACOSTOMY

Indications

A chest tube[90,91] is placed to remove air or fluid from the pleural space. In contrast to simple thoracentesis, which may also be used to treat pleural effusion or pneumothorax, a chest tube is left in place to enable drainage over a period of time. The size and type of tube are determined by the quantity and nature of the material to be drained; small tubes are suitable for the treatment of a pneumothorax, whereas much larger tubes may be required to drain an empyema. In rare circumstances, a chest tube may be placed prophylactically in anticipation of life-threatening pneumothorax or pleural fluid accumulation.

Contraindications

If the accumulation of pleural fluid or air is immediately life threatening, there are no contraindications to chest tube placement. Factors that make the procedure more risky include uncorrected thrombocytopenia, clotting factor deficiencies, extensive infections or tumors involving the chest wall, and severe scoliosis or other anatomic deformities.

Instrumentation

The essential instruments for chest tube placement include a suitable tube, the equipment with which the chest wall is penetrated, and a closed drainage system to which the tube is connected. Chest tubes, depending on their intended purpose, range in size from a 20-gauge IV catheter to 30-French (9.5 mm diameter) or larger. The tip of the tube is smooth to prevent trauma to the lung, and the proximal end must be capable of attaching to a drainage system. For a simple pneumothorax, a through-the-needle plastic catheter may be suitable, although such relatively thin-walled catheters may kink. Another disadvantage of such simple tubes is that there is only one hole (at the end); if the single hole becomes occluded, the tube becomes nonfunctional. In most cases, it will be more appropriate to use a tube designed to be passed over a guidewire because such tubes not only are stronger but also have more than one hole through which air or fluid may drain. When fluid is to be drained, a larger-diameter tube is more appropriate, depending on the viscosity of the fluid.

Drainage systems consist of tubing and a reservoir along with some mechanism to maintain a negative intrathoracic pressure. The most common (and simplest) system includes a chamber into which fluid drains; this chamber is connected to another reservoir containing sterile water, and the tubing from the first chamber extends some distance below the surface of the water in the second chamber. This arrangement allows fluid and air to escape, but prevents flow of air back into the pleural space. The second chamber can be attached to a vacuum line to maintain a continuous negative pressure; this may be important in the management of pleural air leaks.

For emergency treatment of a pneumothorax when a closed, water-sealed drainage system is unavailable or inappropriate, a simple one-way valve may be attached to the chest tube.[94] When intrathoracic pressure increases, air escapes through the valve, but it cannot reenter the chest. Such systems can be lifesaving but should in most situations be converted to appropriate water-seal drainage as soon as feasible.

Technique

There are two general techniques for chest tube insertion: percutaneous placement and surgical placement.

Percutaneous Insertion

Catheters may be inserted either through a large-bore needle or over a guidewire; in either case, the technique is very similar to that for simple thoracentesis. After suitable skin preparation and local anesthesia, the needle is inserted through the intercostal space along the superior margin of the rib. When the pleural space is reached, the catheter (or guidewire) is advanced and the needle withdrawn. The needle may be directed initially to guide the catheter or wire into the desired location (generally posteriorly for drainage of fluid and anteriorly for drainage of air).

The technique for placement of an over-the-wire catheter is analogous to that for a similar vascular catheter. After insertion of the guidewire through the probing needle, the needle is removed. A sharp scalpel (#11 blade) is used to make a small incision at the point of insertion, and the track is dilated by passing a dilator over the wire. Because the dilator is quite stiff, it should not be passed deeply into the thorax, but its tip must penetrate the parietal pleura. The dilator is removed, and the selected catheter is then threaded over the guidewire and advanced into the chest. The catheter should be grasped very close to the chest wall as it is advanced to prevent kinking of the guidewire. When the tube has been advanced to the desired depth, the guidewire is removed, and the tube is connected to a closed sterile drainage system.

Surgical Insertion

The chosen site is prepared as for thoracentesis. After instillation of local anesthetic, a skin incision just long enough to accommodate the chest tube is made approximately 2 cm below the intended insertion site. The skin is pulled upward so that the incision overlies the puncture site. A surgical clamp is used to penetrate the intercostal space just above the rib and to dilate the wound so that the tube can be passed. The tip of the tube is grasped with the clamp, inserted through the track, and advanced into position after the clamp is removed. Alternatively, a chest tube with an internal trocar may be used instead of the surgical clamp. The trocar has a sharp point and may be used to penetrate the intercostal space as well as to facilitate the passage of the tube itself. Great care must be taken, however, when a trocar is used in this fashion so that penetration of the lung is avoided. The tube or trocar must be held with the gloved hand very close to the chest wall so that it cannot advance farther than intended once the pleura is penetrated. The tube is advanced over the trocar, which is then removed.

When the tube is in place, the tension on the skin overlying the insertion site is released, creating a subcutaneous track for the tube. This reduces the risk of air leakage around the insertion site and allows the tube to exit the chest on an oblique angle rather than perpendicularly. A purse-string suture should be placed around the tube, and the tube should be anchored to the chest wall with another suture or suitable taping. The tube should be secured so that accidental traction on the tube neither pulls the tube from the patient's chest nor moves the tube within the chest (which is painful).

Removal of Chest Tubes

A chest tube placed to drain a pleural effusion is usually left in place until the daily volume of drainage is minimal, whereas that placed for treatment of a pneumothorax is left until there has been no air leak for at least 24 hours. If the tube does not drain the pleural space adequately, it may require repositioning or replacement.

It is prudent to clamp a chest tube for some period of time before its removal. If fluid or air then reaccumulates within the pleural space, it is necessary to unclamp only the tube. When the tube is to be removed, any sutures attached to the tube are removed, the entrance site is covered with sterile gauze impregnated with petroleum jelly, and the tube is withdrawn. Before the tube is pulled, it should be rotated to break up adhesions between the tube and the lung. Gentle pressure is maintained over the insertion site during and after withdrawal. The tube should be withdrawn promptly to prevent entrance of air into the pleural space through the proximal side holes in the tube once they exit the chest. The purse-string suture, if used, is pulled tight and tied, and a pressure dressing is applied. A chest film with the patient sitting erect is obtained after removal of the tube to ensure that there is no residual pneumothorax.

Complications

The complications of chest tube insertion are essentially the same as those of thoracentesis and include bleeding, damage to the neurovascular bundle, perforation or laceration of the lung, and infection. If the drainage system to which the tube is connected is mishandled, ascending infection may contaminate the pleural cavity. Likewise, disconnection of the tube from its underwater seal may result in a large pneumothorax.

PERCUTANEOUS NEEDLE ASPIRATION OF THE LUNG

Before the advent of flexible bronchoscopy and BAL, the only way to obtain a specimen from the distal airways involved rigid bronchoscopy, open lung biopsy, or percutaneous needle aspiration.[95-97] Although needle aspirations are seldom performed today, this is the only way except open biopsy to guarantee that there is no chance of contamination of the specimen by upper respiratory tract flora.

Indications

Percutaneous needle aspiration may be indicated when it is necessary to obtain a specimen from the distal airways and alternative methods, such as flexible bronchoscopy, are not available or for some reason are contraindicated. Patients with pulmonary consolidation or lesions located close to the pleura are the most appropriate candidates. Very small volumes of specimen are obtained and may be examined by microscope or a variety of microbiologic techniques. Percutaneous needle aspiration of lung lesions may be desirable in the investigation of possible malignancy or granulomatous disease.

Contraindications

Patients with noncorrectable bleeding disorders should not undergo percutaneous needle aspiration. Other factors that increase risk include pulmonary hypertension and positive-pressure ventilation. Percutaneous needle aspiration should not be performed through a pleural effusion.

Technique

The technique for percutaneous needle aspiration is very similar to that for thoracentesis. However, the object is for the needle to traverse the visceral pleura in the area of the parenchymal lesion. Sedation and local anesthesia are used as for thoracentesis. A needle of suitable size and length is attached to a syringe containing 1 to 2 ml of sterile, nonbacteriostatic saline. The needle is advanced to a position just short of the pleura. Cooperative patients are requested to hold the breath (most children will not do so, of course), and then the needle is rapidly advanced across the pleura. As quickly as possible, the contents of the syringe are injected, and then the plunger of the syringe is withdrawn to aspirate as much material as possible into the syringe (usually this amounts to only a few drops). The needle and syringe are then rapidly withdrawn. This entire process should take only 2 to 3 seconds; a longer time increases the risk of laceration of the pleura and pneumothorax.

Transtracheal aspiration[98] is a related procedure that has been performed for similar indications. This procedure, which is rarely performed since the advent of flexible bronchoscopy, involves passage of a catheter through a needle that has been inserted through the cricothyroid membrane, and then secretions are aspirated from the airway. Fatal complications have been reported,[99] and the procedure does not guarantee that the specimen is not contaminated with oral secretions. Transtracheal aspiration should not be performed in infants and young children.

In the investigation of deeper parenchymal lesions for suspected malignancy, especially in older patients, a very thin, flexible needle can be used to reduce the risk of laceration of the lung. Fluoroscopy (preferably biplane fluoroscopy) or computerized tomography should be used to guide the needle into the lesion. If warranted, a cutting needle may be used to obtain a small specimen of lung parenchyma for histologic examination. This procedure increases the risk of bleeding and air leak.

Complications

Pneumothorax is an obvious risk of percutaneous needle aspiration. Usually, the air leak is small and requires no therapy, but insertion of a chest tube is sometimes required. The risk of bleeding is somewhat higher than that for thoracentesis.

PLEURAL BIOPSY

Indications

Biopsy of the parietal pleura is indicated in the evaluation of pleural disease not diagnosed by thoracentesis or other methods. Most commonly, malignancy or mycobacterial disease is suspected. Pleural fluid is usually present when a pleural biopsy is considered.

Contraindications

Patients with uncorrectable bleeding disorders should not undergo pleural biopsy.

Instrumentation

A pleural biopsy needle (Cope or Abrams) consists of an outer cannula that is perforated near its tip, a cutting trocar, and a stylet. The Abrams needle is generally preferred.[90]

Technique

The patient is prepared as for thoracentesis. Because the biopsy needle is relatively large, a small skin incision is made with a scalpel (#11 blade). The needle with the cutting trocar and stylet in place is then passed through the parietal pleura. The stylet is withdrawn; a syringe can be attached to withdraw pleural fluid and confirm the position of the needle tip. The cutting trocar is rotated (Abrams) or withdrawn (Cope) to the open position, and the needle is withdrawn so that the opening in the outer cannula engages pleural tissue. The cutting trocar is then rotated (or advanced) to the closed position so that the biopsy specimen is held within the core of the trocar (it may be recovered by aspiration into the syringe or by removal of the cannula). Several specimens can be obtained in the same site by rotating the outer cannula and repeating the biopsy process. The operator should consider the orientation of the cutting port and avoid taking a biopsy toward the inferior aspect of the rib above the puncture site (to avoid cutting the neurovascular bundle).[100]

Complications

Pneumothorax and bleeding are the two most common complications. Care must be taken to avoid the neurovascular bundle by inserting the biopsy needle through the inferior part of the intercostal space and to avoid taking a biopsy in the superior aspect of the site.

THORACOSCOPY

There have been rapid advances in endoscopic instrumentation and technique in recent years. Many thoracic procedures that previously required open surgical approaches can now be performed with endoscopic visualization and manipulation. Continued miniaturization of instruments will ensure that pediatric patients are not deprived of the benefits of such minimally invasive diagnoses and surgery.[101]

One potential limitation of thoracoscopy is that the patient must be able to tolerate one-lung anesthesia. The lung must be at least partially deflated to visualize the pleural surfaces. In pediatric patients, this may present technical problems in airway management. Patients with respiratory failure or insufficiency may be poor candidates for thoracoscopy. However, they are also poor candidates for thoracotomy, and in some cases, thoracoscopy can be informative even if the lung cannot be deflated.

Indications

Diagnostic thoracoscopy[102] is indicated in the evaluation of complicated pleural effusions (especially if malignancy is suspected), persistent pneumothorax, subpleural lung nodules, and mediastinal or pleural nodes or masses. In addition, thoracoscopic techniques may be indicated for lung biopsy or for the achievement of pleurodesis.[103,104]

Contraindications

As previously noted, the inability of the patient to tolerate one-lung anesthesia may make thoracoscopy inappropriate. Obliteration of the pleural space may make it impossible. As with other invasive procedures, uncorrected bleeding disorders increase the risk of hemorrhage.

Instrumentation

Thoracoscopy involves direct visualization of the intrathoracic contents through a rigid telescope inserted through the intercostal space. The telescopes are similar to those used for rigid bronchoscopy. A variety of ancillary instruments are available to manipulate the lung and intrathoracic contents. The telescopes and other instruments are passed through trocars, which allow an instrument to be removed and reinserted as necessary.

Technique

Thoracoscopy is a surgical procedure requiring general anesthesia. In general, more than one trocar (often three) is inserted into the thoracic cavity; one is used for a telescope, and others are used to manipulate the lung. Placement of the trocars depends on the area of interest. The lung is at least partially deflated, grasped with forceps, and pulled or pushed aside to achieve adequate visualization. The presence of pleural adhesions may complicate the inspection.

In addition to visual inspection, specimens of lung, pleura, or lymph nodes may be obtained with a variety of biopsy instruments. Hemostasis can be achieved by electrocautery, staples, sutures, or laser. Because the entire pleural surface can be visualized, thoracoscopy may be more versatile than limited thoracotomy when a lung biopsy is required.

LUNG BIOPSY

When other diagnostic methods have failed, histologic examination of lung tissue may be required. There are two techniques for obtaining such a specimen: transbronchial biopsy and open lung biopsy. Because of technical limitations, transbronchial biopsy is not frequently used in pediatric patients, although it plays a critical role in the management of patients after lung transplant. Transbronchial biopsy specimens are very small, and histologic diagnosis is not as easily made as with an open biopsy.

Indications

Lung biopsy may be indicated in the evaluation of interstitial or other diffuse infiltrative diseases, nodular disease, and sometimes, suspected infection. Lung biopsy is indicated in the evaluation of suspected malignancy and suspected rejection after lung transplantation.[105,106] In general, bronchoscopy with BAL should be performed before open lung biopsy. In most cases, the pertinent diagnostic information from bronchoscopy and BAL is available within 24 hours, and the more invasive procedure (if it is necessary) is not delayed long. If the information is urgently required (as in a lung transplant) or if only a transbronchial biopsy is desired, then biopsy and BAL are performed at the same time.

Contraindications

If lung biopsy is the only way to achieve the necessary diagnosis, then there are no absolute contraindications to biopsy, but the technique may be dictated by the clinical circumstances. The risk of pneumothorax after transbronchial biopsy is much higher, for example, in patients on positive-pressure ventilation.

Instrumentation

Transbronchial biopsy is performed with flexible forceps passed through a bronchoscope.[107] These devices induce a substantial amount of crush artifact in the specimen obtained. The smallest available forceps are approximately 1 mm in diameter and can be used with the standard (3.5-mm) flexible bronchoscope. Unfortunately, the small size of the specimens obtained with this instrument severely limit the practical applications of the technique. The largest forceps available are approximately 2.5 mm in diameter and require the use of a flexible bronchoscope 6 mm in diameter.

Technique

Lung biopsy may be performed surgically or by thoracoscopy. An advantage of these techniques is that the lung surface can be examined and the specimen is much larger than that obtained by transbronchial biopsy. Automatic stapling devices are used to detach the specimen and seal the cut edges of the lung.

Transbronchial biopsy should be performed with fluoroscopic guidance, both to ensure that the selected area of the lung is being sampled and to reduce the risk of pleural perforation. The flexible bronchoscope is advanced to the desired bronchus, and the forceps are passed through the suction channel. The closed forceps are advanced to the desired depth, retracted slightly, opened, and then advanced to meet gentle resistance before closing. A slight tug should be felt and may be viewed on the fluoroscope if tissue is obtained. The specimen is placed immediately into either fixative or saline; if the specimen floats, it is more likely to contain alveolar tissue. Multiple specimens are usually obtained to ensure that an adequate amount of tissue is available for analysis.

Complications

Lung biopsy always carries the risk of hemorrhage, air leak, or both, and the overall risks are higher in patients with respiratory failure or multiorgan failure. The incidence of pneumothorax after transbronchial biopsy is relatively small and depends somewhat on the technique used and the nature of the lung disease (the risk is higher in patients with poor compliance). Deaths from massive hemorrhage have occurred after transbronchial biopsy. Infectious complications of transbronchial biopsy are those associated with bronchoscopy, and the incidence of complications may be increased if atelectasis results from bronchial obstruction caused by blood clots due to bleeding from the biopsy sites. Good pulmonary cleansing to clear the airways of clots after transbronchial biopsy reduces the incidence of complications.

NASAL MUCOSAL BIOPSY AND BRUSHING

The nasal mucosa consists of ciliated epithelium nearly identical to that of the trachea and bronchi. Therefore the nose is an important site for diagnostic evaluation of generalized mucosal abnormalities.

Indications

Patients suspected of having primary ciliary dyskinesia may undergo nasal mucosal biopsy for functional and ultrastructural evaluation of ciliary function.

Contraindications

There are essentially no contraindications to nasal biopsy. However, a biopsy taken during the course of a viral infection may reveal abnormalities that would not be present otherwise and that are not relevant to the patient's underlying condition.[108,109]

Instrumentation

Ciliated cells can be obtained with a small brush about 1 to 2 mm in diameter or with a small curette. The latter is more likely to yield intact pieces of epithelium.

Technique

Under normal circumstances, the anterior third of the nasal epithelium is squamous, whereas the more posterior two thirds is ciliated. The biopsy should be obtained from an area of ciliated epithelium; the most appropriate area is at least halfway along the inferior turbinate, preferably under this structure. The specimen is placed into tissue culture medium for examination by light microscopy for ciliary beat frequency and pattern or by electron microscopy. Functional analysis should take place as soon as possible because ciliary activity may decrease rapidly in traumatized cells; in general, ciliary activity is less likely to be demonstrable in individual cells than along the border of a patch of epithelial surface where the cells are more intact. Patients with primary ciliary dyskinesia have cilia that beat very slowly and incoordinately or not at all; the cilia may appear rigid. Specimens that appear to be abnormal should be processed for electron microscopy. A diagnosis of ciliary dysfunction should not be made in the absence of ultrastructural confirmation and may be complicated by environmental or infectious influences.

SPUTUM EXAMINATION

The examination of sputum is an important aspect of pulmonary diagnosis, at least in patients who produce sputum.[110] Invasive procedures to obtain specimens from the lower respiratory tract should usually be deferred until sputum has been evaluated. Unfortunately, sputum specimens may be difficult to obtain from children.

Indications

Sputum should be examined whenever productive cough is part of the complex of symptoms. A productive cough implies the presence of an abnormal quantity of respiratory secretions (or inadequate clearance). Induced sputum specimens may be useful in the diagnosis of diffuse lung diseases and certain infectious diseases such as tuberculosis. Sputum may be examined microscopically as well as by microbiologic methods.

Technique

There are two problems associated with sputum examination: obtaining a specimen and ensuring that the specimen comes from the lower respiratory tract. Even though they may have copious tracheal secretions and a cough that sounds productive, young children are usually unable to expectorate the specimen. A common practice therefore is to obtain a swab from the posterior pharynx while attempting to induce a cough. Although this may be successful (the swab will obviously have a sample of mucus, which may be green or yellow), it is not always certain that such a specimen comes from the lungs and not from the nasopharynx. There is a relatively poor correlation, at least in young children, between the results of such "gag sputum" specimens and specimens obtained by bronchoscopy and BAL. Microscopic examination of the specimen for the presence of alveolar macrophages can help determine whether the specimen is indeed from the lower respiratory tract.

In older patients who do not have a productive cough, it may still be possible to induce sputum by the inhalation of an aerosol (especially an ultrasonic aerosol) of saline (hypertonic or isotonic).[111] This procedure may place medical personnel at some risk, and they should be protected by appropriate procedures from the aerosol generated by the patient's cough.

To reduce the probability of contamination of the sputum specimen with oral secretions, the specimen should ideally be collected after the mouth is rinsed with water and not within an hour or so of a meal. The patient should be instructed to provide sputum rather than saliva, although it may be possible to separate material that appears to be sputum from saliva after expectoration. It is standard in many microbiology laboratories to remove saliva by washing the sputum specimen with sterile saline before processing it.

Sputum may be examined microscopically as a wet mount by placing it under a coverslip on a microscope slide, or it may be smeared and stained with a variety of stains, depending on the purpose of the examination. Although Gram's stain is usually used in the microbiology laboratory, this is not an effective stain for study of cell types. Wright's or Giemsa stains are useful for evaluating inflammatory cells and eosinophils and identifying alveolar macrophages (the absence of which suggests that the specimen may not have come from the lower respiratory tract). The presence of numerous neutrophils does not in itself prove that the specimen came from the lungs, but the presence of large numbers of squamous epithelial cells does suggest heavy contamination with oral secretions.

REFERENCES

1. American Academy of Pediatrics Committee on Drugs: Guidelines for monitoring and management of pediatric patients during and after sedation for diagnostic and therapeutic procedures, *Pediatrics* 89:1110-1115, 1992.

Sedation and Anesthesia for Procedures

2. Desmonts JM: Have anesthesia-related mortality and morbidity decreased in the last 30 years? Evaluation based on a review of epidemiologic studies, *Bull Acad Natl Med* 178:1537-1547, 1994.
3. Berthoud MC, Reilly CS: Adverse effects of general anaesthetics, *Drug Saf* 7:434-459, 1992 (review).
4. Squires RH, Morriss F, Schluterman S, Drews B, Galyen L, Brown KO: Efficacy, safety, and cost of IV sedation versus general anesthesia in children undergoing endoscopic procedures, *Gastrointest Endosc* 41:99-104, 1995.
5. Council on Scientific Affairs, American Medical Association: The use of pulse oximetry during conscious sedation, *JAMA* 270:1463-1468, 1993 (review).
6. Zuckerberg AL: Perioperative approach to children, *Pediatr Clin North Am* 41:15-29, 1994 (review).
7. American Academy of Pediatrics Committee on Drugs and Committee on Environmental Health: Use of chloral hydrate for sedation in children, *Pediatrics* 92:471-473, 1993.
8. Feld LH, Negus JB, White PF: Oral midazolam preanesthetic medication in pediatric outpatients, *Anesthesiology* 73:831-834, 1990.
9. Abrams R, Morrison JE, Villasenor A, Hencmann D, Da Fonseca M, Mueller W: Safety and effectiveness of intranasal administration of sedative medications (ketamine, midazolam, or sufentanil) for urgent brief pediatric dental procedures, *Anesth Prog* 40:63-66, 1993.
10. Gajraj NM, Pennant JH, Watcha MF: Eutectic mixture of local anesthetics (EMLA) cream, *Anesth Analg* 78:574-583, 1994 (review).
11. Cote CJ: Sedation for the pediatric patient: a review, *Pediatr Clin North Am* 41:31-58, 1994 (review).
12. Olness K: Hypnosis in pediatric practice, *Curr Prob Pediatr* 12:1-47, 1981.
13. Sandhar BK, Goresky GV, Maltby JR, Shaffer EA: Effect of oral liquids and ranitidine on gastric fluid volume and pH in children undergoing outpatient surgery, *Anesthesiology* 71:327-330, 1989.
14. Schreiner MS, Triebwasser A, Keon TP: Ingestion of liquids compared with preoperative fasting in pediatric outpatients, *Anesthesiology* 72:593-597, 1990.
15. Baktai G, Szekely E, Marialigeti T, Kovacs L: Use of midazolam ("Dormicum") and flumazenil ("Anexate") in paediatric bronchology, *Curr Med Res Opin* 12:552-559, 1992.

Bronchoscopy

16. Gonzalez C, Reilly JS, Bluestone CD: Synchronous airway lesions in infancy, *Ann Otol Rhinol Laryngol* 96:77-80, 1987.
17. Wood RE: Spelunking in the pediatric airways: explorations with the flexible fiberoptic bronchoscope, *Pediatr Clin North Am* 31:785-799, 1984.
18. McKenzie B, Wood RE, Bailey A: Airway management for unilateral lung lavage in children, *Anesthesiology* 70:550-553, 1989.
19. Bailey AG, Valley RD, Azizkhan RG, Wood RE: Anaesthetic management of infants requiring endobronchial argon laser surgery, *Can J Anaesth* 39:590-593, 1992.
20. Gans SL, Berci G: Advances in endoscopy of infants and children, *J Pediatr Surg* 6:199-223, 1971.
21. Amitai Y, Zylber Katz E, Avital A, Zangen D, Noviski N: Serum lidocaine concentrations in children during bronchoscopy with topical anesthesia, *Chest* 98:1370-1373, 1990.
22. Wimberley N, Faling LJ, Bartlett JG: A fiberoptic bronchoscopy technique to obtain uncontaminated lower airway secretions for bacterial culture, *Am Rev Respir Dis* 119:337-343, 1979.
23. Chastre J, Fagon JY, Bornet-Lecso M, Calvat S, Dombret MC, al Khani R, Basset F, Gibert C: Evaluation of bronchoscopic techniques for the diagnosis of nosocomial pneumonia, *Am J Respir Crit Care Med* 152:231-240, 1995.
24. Credle WF, Smiddy JF, Elliot RL: Complications of fiberoptic bronchoscopy, *Am Rev Respir Dis* 109:67-72, 1974.
25. Lockhart CH, Elliot JL: Potential hazards of pediatric rigid bronchoscopy, *J Pediatr Surg* 19:239-242, 1984.
26. Hoeve LJ, Rombout J, Meursing AE: Complications of rigid laryngobronchoscopy in children, *Int J Pediatr Otorhinolaryngol* 26:47-56, 1993.
27. Schnapf BM: Oxygen desaturation during fiberoptic bronchoscopy in pediatric patients, *Chest* 99:591-594, 1991.
28. Wagener JS: Fatality following fiberoptic bronchoscopy in a two-year-old child, *Pediatr Pulmonol* 3:197-199, 1987.
29. Weiss SM, Hert RC, Gianola FJ, Clark JG, Crawford SW: Complications of fiberoptic bronchoscopy in thrombocytopenic patients, *Chest* 104:1025-1028, 1993.
30. Lindahl H, Rintala R, Malinen L, Leijala M, Sairanen H: Bronchoscopy during the first month of life, *J Pediatr Surg* 27:548-550, 1992.
31. Peerless JR, Snow N, Likavec MJ, Pinchak AC, Malangoni MA: The effect of fiberoptic bronchoscopy on cerebral hemodynamics in patients with severe head injury, *Chest* 108:962-965, 1995.
32. Nelson KE, Larson PA, Schraufnagel DE, Jackson J: Transmission of tuberculosis by flexible fiberbronchoscopes, *Am Rev Respir Dis* 127:97-100, 1983.
33. Hanson PJ, Collins JV: AIDS and the lung. I. AIDS, aprons, and elbow grease: preventing the nosocomial spread of human immunodeficiency virus and associated organisms, *Thorax* 44:778-783, 1989.
34. Prakash UB: Does the bronchoscope propagate infection? *Chest* 104:552-559, 1993.
35. Gillis S, Dann EJ, Berkman N, Koganox Y, Kramer MR: Fatal *Haemophilus influenzae* septicemia following bronchoscopy in a splenectomized patient, *Chest* 104:1607-1609, 1993.
36. Siegman-Igra Y, Inbar G, Campus A: An "outbreak" of pulmonary pseudoinfection by *Serratia marcescens, J Hosp Infect* 6:218-220, 1985.
37. Gubler JG, Salfinger M, von Graevenitz A: Pseudoepidemic of nontuberculous mycobacteria due to a contaminated bronchoscope cleaning machine: report of an outbreak and review of the literature, *Chest* 101:1245-1249, 1992.

Bronchoalveolar Lavage

38. Baughman RP, ed: *Bronchoalveolar lavage,* St Louis, 1992, Mosby.
39. Reynolds HY: State of the art: bronchoalveolar lavage, *Am Rev Respir Dis* 135:250-263, 1987.
40. Wood RE: Bronchoalveolar lavage in infants and children. In Baughman RP, ed: *Bronchoalveolar lavage,* St Louis, 1992, Mosby, pp 26-38.
41. Wood RE: Treatment of CF lung disease in the first two years, *Pediatr Pulmonol* 4(suppl):68-70, 1989.
42. Balough K, McCubbin M, Weinberger M, Smits W, Ahrens R, Fick R: The relationship between infection and inflammation in the early stages of lung disease from cystic fibrosis, *Pediatr Pulmonol* 20:63-70, 1995.
43. deBlic J, Blanche S, Danel C, Le-Bourgeois M, Caniglia M, Scheinmann P: Bronchoalveolar lavage in HIV infected patients with interstitial pneumonitis, *Arch Dis Child* 64:1246-1250, 1989.
44. Fan LL: Evaluation and therapy of chronic interstitial pneumonitis in children, *Curr Opin Pediatr* 6:248-254, 1994 (review).
45. Midulla F, Villani A, Merolla R, Bjermer L, Sandstrom T, Ronchetti R: Bronchoalveolar lavage studies in children without parenchymal lung disease: cellular constituents and protein levels, *Pediatr Pulmonol* 20:112-118, 1995.
46. Ratjen F, Bredendiek M, Zheng L, Brendel M, Costabel U: Lymphocyte subsets in bronchoalveolar lavage fluid of children without bronchopulmonary disease, *Am J Respir Crit Care Med* 152:174-178, 1995,
47. Riedler J, Grigg J, Stone C, Tauro G, Robertson CF: Bronchoalveolar lavage cellularity in healthy children, *Am J Respir Crit Care Med* 152:163-168, 1995.
48. Sole-Violan J, Rodriguez de Castro F, Rey A, Martin-Gonzalez JC, Cabrera-Navarro P: Usefulness of microscopic examination of intracellular organisms in lavage fluid in ventilator-associated pneumonia, *Chest* 106:889-894, 1994.
49. Burns DM, Shure D, Francoz R, Kalafer M, Harrell J, Witztum K, Moser KM: The physiologic consequences of saline lobar lavage in healthy human adults, *Am Rev Respir Dis* 127:695-701, 1983.

50. Acourt CH, Carrard CS, Crook D, Bowler I, Conlon C, Peto T, Anderson E: Microbiological lung surveillance in mechanically ventilated patients, using nondirected bronchial lavage and quantitative culture, *Q J Med* 86:635-648, 1993.
51. Koumbourlis AC, Kurland G: Nonbronchoscopic bronchoalveolar lavage in intubated, mechanically ventilated infants: technique, efficacy, and applications, *Pediatr Pulmonol* 15:257-263, 1993.
52. Brain JD, Frank R: Alveolar macrophage adhesion: wash electrolyte composition and free cell yield, *J Appl Physiol* 34:75-80, 1973.
53. Rennard SI, Basset G, Lecossier D, ODonnell KM, Pinkston P, Martin PG, Crystal RG: Estimation of volume of epithelial lining fluid recovered by lavage using urea as marker of dilution, *J Appl Physiol* 60:532-538, 1986.
54. Kelly CA, Fenwick JD, Corris PA, Fleetwood A, Hendrick DJ, Walters EH: Fluid dynamics during bronchoalveolar lavage, *Am Rev Respir Dis* 138:81-84, 1988.
55. Cheng PW, Boat TF, Shaikh S, Wang OL, Hu PC, Costa DL: Differential effects of ozone on lung epithelial lining fluid volume and protein content, *Exp Lung Res* 21:351-365, 1995.
56. Von Wichert P, Joseph K, Muller B, Franck WM: Bronchoalveolar lavage: quantitation of intraalveolar fluid? *Am Rev Respir Dis* 147:148-152, 1993.
57. Rennard SI, Ghafouri M, Thompson AB, Linder J, Vaughan W, Jones K, Ertl RF, Christensen K, Prince A, Stahl MG, Robbins RA: Fractional processing of sequential bronchoalveolar lavage to separate bronchial and alveolar samples, *Am Rev Respir Dis* 141:208-217, 1990.
58. Pugin J, Suter PM: Diagnostic bronchoalveolar lavage in patients with pneumonia produces sepsis-like systemic effects, *Intensive Care Med* 18:6-10, 1992.
59. Pereira W, Kovnat DM, Khan MA, Iacovino JR, Spivack ML, Snider GL: Fever and pneumonia after flexible fiberoptic bronchoscopy, *Am Rev Respir Dis* 112:59-64, 1975.
60. Workshop summary and guidelines: investigative use of bronchoscopy, lavage, and bronchial biopsies in asthma and other airway diseases, *J Allergy Clin Immunol* 88:808-814, 1991.
61. Stanley MW, Mrak RE, Bardales RH: Detached single cilia: another potential pseudomicrobe seen in bronchoalveolar lavage specimens, *Diagn Cytopathol* 13:225-228, 1995.
62. Cantral DE, Tape TG, Reed EC, Spurzem JR, Rennard SI, Thompson AB: Quantitative culture of bronchoalveolar lavage fluid for the diagnosis of bacterial pneumonia, *Am J Med* 95:601-607, 1993.
63. Colombo JL, Hallberg TK: Recurrent aspiration in children: lipid-laden alveolar macrophage quantitation, *Pediatr Pulmonol* 3:86-89, 1987.
64. Bonten MJ, Gaillard CA, Wouters EF, van Tiel FH, Stobberingh EE, van der Geest S: Problems in diagnosing nosocomial pneumonia in mechanically ventilated patients: a review, *Crit Care Med* 22:1683-1691, 1994.
65. Ratjen F, Bredendiek M, Brendel M, Meltzer J, Costabel U: Differential cytology of bronchoalveolar lavage fluid in normal children, *Eur Respir J* 7:1865-1870, 1994.
66. Chadelat K, Baculard A, Grimfeld A, Tournier G, Boule M, Boccon Gibod L, Clement A: Pulmonary sarcoidosis in children: serial evaluation of bronchoalveolar lavage cells during corticosteroid treatment, *Pediatr Pulmonol* 16:41-47, 1993.
67. Daniele RP, Elias JA, Epstein PE, Rossman MD: Bronchoalveolar lavage: role in the pathogenesis, diagnosis, and management of interstitial lung disease, *Ann Intern Med* 102:93-108, 1985.

Intubation

68. Chatburn RL, Lough MD: Mechanical ventilation. In Lough MD, Dershuk CF, Stern RC, eds: *Pediatric respiratory therapy,* ed 3, St Louis, 1985, Mosby, pp 148-191.
69. Sherman JM, Nelson H: Decreased incidence of subglottic stenosis using an "appropriate-sized" endotracheal tube in neonates, *Pediatr Pulmonol* 6:183-185, 1989.
70. Cote CJ: NPO after midnight for children: a reappraisal, *Anesthesiology* 72:589-592, 1990.
71. Bhende MS, Thompson AE: Evaluation of an end-tidal CO_2 detector during pediatric cardiopulmonary resuscitation, *Pediatrics* 95:395-399, 1995.
72. Wood RE: Pitfalls in the use of the flexible bronchoscope in pediatric patients, *Chest* 97:199-203, 1990.
73. Rucker RW, Silva WJ, Worcester CC: Fiberoptic bronchoscopic nasotracheal intubation in children, *Chest* 76:56-58, 1979.
74. Brimacombe J: The advantages of the LMA over the tracheal tube or facemask: a meta-analysis, *Can J Anaesth* 42:1017-1023, 1995.
75. Pinosky M: Laryngeal mask airway: uses in anesthesiology, *South Med J* 89:551-555, 1996 (review).

Tracheostomy

76. Kenigsberg K: Tracheostomy in infants, *Semin Thorac Cardiovasc Surg* 6:196-199, 1994 (review).
77. Hotaling AJ, Robbins WK, Madgy DN, Belenck WM: Pediatric tracheotomy: a review of technique, *Am J Otolaryngol* 13:115-119, 1992.
78. Chendrasekhar A, Ponnapalli S, Duncan A: Percutaneous dilatational tracheostomy: an alternative approach to surgical tracheostomy, *South Med J* 88:1062-1064, 1995.
79. Toursarkissian B, Fowler CL, Zweng TN, Kearney PA: Percutaneous dilational tracheostomy in children and teenagers, *J Pediatr Surg* 29:1421-1424, 1994.
80. Bainton CR: Cricothyrotomy, *Int Anesthesiol Clin* 32:95-108, 1994.
81. Hay R, Miller WC: Efficacy of a new hygroscopic condenser humidifier, *Crit Care Med* 10:49-51, 1982.
82. Azizkhan RG, Lacey SR, Wood RE: Acquired symptomatic bronchial stenosis in infants: successful management using an argon laser, *J Pediatr Surg* 25:19-24, 1990.
83. Hazinski MF: Pediatric home tracheostomy care: a parent's guide, *Pediatr Nurs* 12:41-48, 1986.
84. Hotaling AJ, Zablocki H, Madgy DN: Pediatric tracheotomy discharge teaching: a comprehensive checklist format, *Int J Pediatr Otorhinolaryngol* 33:113-126, 1995.
85. Dettelbach MA, Gross RD, Mahlmann J, Eibling DE: Effect of the Passy-Muir valve on aspiration in patients with tracheostomy, *Head Neck* 17:297-302, 1995.
86. Prescott CAJ: Peristomal complications of pediatric tracheostomy, *Int J Pediatr Otorhinolaryngol* 23:141-149, 1992.
87. Benjamin B, Curley JWA: Infant tracheotomy: endoscopy and decannulation, *Int J Pediatr Otorhinolaryngol* 20:113-121, 1990.
88. Willis R, Myer C, Miller R, Cotton RT: Tracheotomy decannulation in the pediatric patient, *Laryngoscope* 97:764-765, 1987.
89. Azizkhan RG, Lacey SR, Wood RE: Anterior cricoid suspension and tracheal stomal closure for children with cricoid collapse and peristomal tracheomalacia following tracheostomy, *J Pediatr Surg* 28:169-171, 1993.

Thoracentesis

90. Light RW: *Pleural diseases,* ed 2, Philadelphia, 1990, Lea & Febiger.
91. Iberti TJ, Stern PM: Chest tube thoracostomy, *Crit Care Clin* 8:879-895, 1992.
92. Light RW, Jenkinson SG, Minh VD, George RB: Observations on pleural fluid pressures as fluid is withdrawn during thoracentesis, *Am Rev Respir Dis* 121:799-804, 1980.
93. Mahfood S, Hix WR, Aaron BL, Blaes P, Watson DC: Reexpansion pulmonary edema, *Ann Thorac Surg* 45:340-345, 1988 (review).

Tube Thoracostomy

94. Heimlich HJ: Heimlich valve for chest drainage, *Med Instrum* 17:29-31, 1983.

Percutaneous Needle Aspiration of the Lung

95. Hughes JR, Sinha DP, Cooper MR, Shah KV, Bose SK: Lung tap in childhood: bacteria, viruses, and mycoplasmas in acute lower respiratory tract infections, *Pediatrics* 44:477-485, 1969
96. Sanders C: Transthoracic needle aspiration, *Clin Chest Med* 13:11-16, 1992 (review).
97. Chaudhary S, Hughes WT, Feldman S, Sanyal SK, Coburn T, Ossi M, Cox F: Percutaneous transthoracic needle aspiration of the lung: diagnosing *Pneumocystis carinii* pneumonitis, *Am J Dis Child* 131:902-907, 1977.
98. Baran D, Cordier N: Usefulness of transtracheal puncture in the bacteriological diagnosis of lung infections in children, *Helv Paediatr Acta* 28:391-399, 1973.
99. Schillaci RF, Iacovoni VE, Conte RS: Transtracheal aspiration complicated by fatal endotracheal hemorrhage, *N Engl J Med* 295:488-490, 1976.

Pleural Biopsy

100. Tomlinson JR, Sahn SA: Invasive procedures in the diagnosis of pleural disease, *Semin Respir Med* 9:30-36, 1987 (review).

Thoracoscopy

101. Bullard KM, Adzick S: Pediatric thoracoscopy: a new vista, *Pediatr Pulmonol* 22(2):129-135, 1996 (review).
102. Mathur PN: Medical thoracoscopy, *J Bronchol* 1:144-151, 1994.
103. Yim AP, Low JM, Ng SK, Ho JK, Liu KK: Video-assisted thoracoscopic surgery in the paediatric population, *J Paediatr Child Health* 31:192-196, 1995.
104. Harris RJ, Kavuru MS, Rice TW, Kirby TJ: The diagnostic and therapeutic utility of thoracoscopy: a review, *Chest* 108:828-841, 1995 (review).

Lung Biopsy

105. Scott JP, Higenbottam TW, Smyth RL, Whitehead B, Helms P, Fradet G, de Leval MR, Wallwork J: Transbronchial biopsies in children after heart-lung transplantation, *Pediatrics* 86:698-702, 1990.
106. Kurland G, Noyes BE, Jaffe R, Atlas AB, Armitage J, Orenstein DM: Bronchoalveolar lavage and transbronchial biopsy in children following heart-lung and lung transplantation, *Chest* 104:1043-1048, 1993.
107. Shure D: Transbronchial biopsy and needle aspiration, *Chest* 95:1130-1138, 1989.

Nasal Mucosal Biopsy and Brushing

108. Boat TF, Carson JL: Ciliary dysmorphology and dysfunction: primary or acquired? *N Engl J Med* 323:1700-1702, 1990.
109. Carson JL, Collier AM, Hu SS: Acquired ciliary defects in nasal epithelium of children with acute viral upper respiratory infections, *N Engl J Med* 312:463-468, 1985.

Sputum Examination

110. Mehta AC, Marty JJ, Lee FY: Sputum cytology, *Clin Chest Med* 14:69-85, 1993.
111. Ognibene FP, Gill VJ, Pizzo PA, Kovacs JA, Godwin C, Suffredini AF, Shelhamer JH, Parrillo JE, Masur H: Induced sputum to diagnose *Pneumocystis carinii* pneumonia in immunosuppressed pediatric patients, *J Pediatr* 115:430-433, 1989.

PART FOUR

Therapeutic Principles

CHAPTER 18

Pharmacology of the Lung and Drug Therapy

Alan K. Kamada and Stanley J. Szefler

Lung pharmacology is a diverse topic. Not only are a number of pharmacologic properties involved in the administration of drugs to the lung, but the lung itself is a complex site for drug delivery and metabolism. Simple factors such as the timing of doses can have a profound effect on the pharmacologic response to selected medications. In pediatric practice, age- and size-related patient variables must also be considered.

This chapter reviews basic principles of pharmacology that pertain to the lung and therapeutic dosing strategies in pediatric patients. Asthma, which has received increased attention in recent years, serves as the focus. After the chapter is an appendix of commonly used medications used in pediatric pulmonary medicine. Pharmacologic treatments of specific disease entities are covered in the relevant chapters.

THE LUNG AS A SITE FOR DRUG DELIVERY

The lung is a complex site for the administration of medications. Delivery depends on a number of factors, including the desired tissue site of action. The lung can be divided into four basic anatomic components—airways, vasculature, innervation, and interstitium—each of which has its own subcomponents. Successful delivery to these sites depends on a number of different variables that are directly affected by the relevant anatomic structures. The choice of target site is important in achieving the goal of therapy (e.g., eradicating infection, attaining bronchodilation, reducing inflammation).

Airways

The airways, simply thought of as a series of narrowing and branching tubes, consist of cartilaginous bronchi, membranous bronchioles, and terminal gas-exchanging ducts or alveoli.[1] These can be subdivided into their various cross-sectional components, which include the epithelium, lamina propria, smooth muscle, and submucosal connective tissue. The β-adrenergic receptors of smooth muscle are theoretically the target site for the β-adrenergic agonist bronchodilators. Inflammatory cells or other cells such as epithelial lining cells or infectious organisms may also be the actual target cells for drug delivery. For example, lymphocytes, currently thought to play an important role in the pathogenesis and severity of asthma, are the target cells of glucocorticoid therapy. Finally, the bifurcations resulting from the branching of the airways and the reductions in airway caliber with each branching provide unique challenges to drug delivery by the inhaled route of administration.

Vasculature

The blood supply of the lungs and airways, the bronchial arteries, originates from either the aorta or the intercostal arteries. The functional pulmonary circulation is a complex network of arteries, arterioles, capillaries, venules, and veins. Blood flows from the pulmonary artery to the arteries of the lung and then to the capillaries, where gas exchange occurs in the alveoli. From there, the oxygenated blood returns via the venules, veins, and pulmonary vein and then to the circulation of the body. In general, the vasculature follows adjacent to the branching airways; however, at the periphery of the lung the veins branch away to pass between the lobules, whereas the arteries and bronchi continue down the centers of the lobules.[2] Because of the vast numbers of alveoli present, the majority of the total blood volume and surface area are present in the capillaries in the walls of the alveoli.[1] This has implications not only for drug therapy with regards to therapeutic effects but also for drug-induced toxicities because the entire blood volume circulates through the lungs and comes into contact with this vast surface area (see Chapter 30).

Innervation

Innervation of the lung has been well described with regards to the adrenergic and cholinergic pathways. Although abnormalities of these pathways have been described in asthma, such as enhanced α-adrenoreceptor function, impaired β-receptor function, and enhanced cholinergic responses, all of which ultimately result in bronchoconstriction, there is increasing evidence that neural mechanisms may contribute to the airway inflammation associated with the disease.[3,4] In addition to the classic cholinergic and adrenergic pathways, a nonadrenergic, noncholinergic pathway has been implicated as being important in regulating the tone and secretions of the airways and vasculature.[3,4] Increased attention has been focused on this "neurogenic inflammation" and neuropeptides and their regulation, such as the bronchodilator peptides that include vasoactive intestinal peptide, peptide histidine isoleucine, and peptide histidine methionine; the potent bronchoconstrictors such as substance P, neurokinin A, and calcitonin gene–related peptide; and the peptidases angiotensin-converting enzyme and neural endopeptidase.[5] As information regarding neuropeptides and their roles in the pathogenesis of relevant diseases is obtained, newer treatment modalities targeting these mechanisms may be instituted.

Interstitium

Pulmonary interstitium, which surrounds the blood vessels, consists of loose connective tissue (primarily collagen and elastic fibers[6]) and is generally sparse under normal conditions. Although comprising a small volume, changes in vascular permeability may result in a dramatic expansion of the perivascular interstitium, which is a major storage compartment for excess extravascular fluid in the initial stages of pulmonary edema.[7] Thus although it is not normally a target site for drug therapy, the interstitium can clearly be important in the pathogenesis of lung disorders.

ROUTES OF DRUG DELIVERY

Before any medication can be effective, it must be delivered to its site of action in the target tissues. A number of methods can be used to effectively deliver medication. These can be broadly divided into the topical and systemic routes of administration. Topical administration includes the inhalation of aerosols delivered by the commonly used metered dose inhalers, dry powder inhalers, and nebulized solutions. Systemic delivery consists of vascular distribution after oral and parenteral administration. Each of these routes has advantages and disadvantages. The inhaled route of administration is discussed in greater detail in Chapter 19.

Inhaled Administration

The inhaled route of administration is generally preferred over systemic routes because medications are delivered directly to the site of action, bypassing the need for absorption as with orally administered medications. Smaller doses are required, and a more rapid onset of action can be obtained.[8] Any potential systemic adverse effects can also be minimized or avoided, provided that the drug has a low degree of systemic activity and absorption. Thus the inhaled route of administration appears to be advantageous over systemic delivery (Table 18-1).

The inhaled route for drug delivery is affected by a variety of physiologic and physicochemical factors. Not only must the inhaled medication be contained within particles small enough to be aerosolized, but the particles within the aerosol must also be of proper diameter to be inhaled, avoid impaction with the pharynx, and travel down through the bifurcations of the bronchi to the smaller airways, which is the target site for most inhaled medications.[9,10] Because infants and young children have smaller lungs and airways, the delivery of medications via inhalation can be considered more difficult in this population than in adults. Diseased airways, which have reduced conductance and airflow, may cause further difficulties in achieving adequate drug delivery.

Deposition of particles in the airways occurs via basic physical mechanisms. Large particles (those >5 μm in diameter) impact on the pharynx and wall of the larger airways because of the inertia of the inhaled particle (inertial impaction), and small particles (those <5 μm in diameter) deposit in the small airways as a result of gravitational sedimentation.[9,10] Other factors, such as brownian movement and electrostatic forces, play lesser roles in the deposition of particles in the respiratory tract. Even smaller particles (those generally <1 μm in diameter) are often too small to be deposited and retained in the airways and are exhaled. Thus the "respirable range" of aerosol particles consists of those larger than 1 μm and smaller than 5 μm in diameter.

Drugs for inhalation must first be solubilized in a delivery vehicle, which, it is hoped, does not have adverse effects of its own.[11] Some highly desirable medications for inhaled administration are not water soluble and thus require unique and innovative delivery vehicles. Liposomes have been proposed as delivery vehicles for targeting various water-insoluble medications, such as glucocorticoids and cyclosporin, to the lung.[12,13]

The delivery device itself must produce aerosols containing particles of an appropriate size, between 1 and 5 μm in diameter, as previously mentioned. Several studies have demonstrated that the different brands of metered dose inhalers and nebulizers can produce varying aerosol characteristics, rates of output, output, and residual volumes[14-17] and that some single lots of nebulizers may even demonstrate widely variable characterstics.[18,19] This can have profound implications when the optimal delivery device is selected for critical medications, such as pentamidine.[20,21]

Each type of inhaled drug–delivery device has advantages and disadvantages (Table 18-2). With drug delivery from metered dose inhalers, the potential for local or systemic adverse effects can be minimized with proper technique and spacer devices. The benefits of spacer devices include less need for coordinating inhalation and actuation for proper use (as with breath-actuated devices), the time needed for the propellant to evaporate, retention of the larger nonrespirable particles, and reduction of particle velocity.[22] If a drug has a poor topical-to-systemic potency ratio, however, an increase of systemic adverse effects can be observed because of better pulmonary deposition.

Metered dose inhalers, the established standard of aerosolized drug administration, will eventually be phased out because of the increasing concern over the effect of chlorofluorocarbons on the Earth's ozone layer.[23] Although the chlorofluorocarbon propellants used in metered dose inhalers

Table 18-1 Topical and Systemic Routes of Drug Delivery

ROUTE	ADVANTAGES	DISADVANTAGES
Topical: inhaled	Drug is delivered directly to site of action. Drug bypasses absorption. Route provides reduced incidence of adverse effects.	Coordination is often required for optimal use and delivery. Route may be inconvenient. Administration may be inconsistent.
Systemic: oral	Drug is easy to administer. Route is convenient. Drug can be inexpensive.	There are potential problems with absorption. There is potential for first-pass metabolism. Drug interactions can occur. There is increased incidence of adverse effects. There is limited exposure at site of action.
Intravenous	Drug has 100% bioavailability. Route provides rapid onset of action.	Route is inconvenient. Administration is costly. Aseptic technique is required. There is potential for drug interactions. There is increased incidence of adverse effects. There is limited exposure at site of action.

represent a minute fraction of the total worldwide production and use, new methods for drug delivery will be needed as fluorocarbons become less accessible and potentially less cost-effective.

Several such examples are the dry powder inhalers, which include the Spinhaler (Fisons, Rochester, NY) and newer devices such as the Turbuhaler (AB Draco, Södertälje, Sweden), Diskhaler (Glaxo Wellcome, Research Triangle Park, NC), and Rotahaler (Glaxo Wellcome, Research Triangle Park, NC). All are similar in that they are breath-actuated devices that deliver a dry, micronized powder of medication to the lungs; they also may be easier to use because they theoretically have less airflow resistance compared with the Spinhaler.[24] Some suggest, however, that high flow rates may be required to optimally actuate these devices,[8,22] a potential problem for young children and infants as well as patients whose lungs are acutely obstructed. A benefit of newer dry powder inhalers may be better lung deposition[25] with similar or even improved total bioavailability compared with metered dose inhalers[25,26]; however, some have suggested that these devices can provoke coughing and that increased bioavailability may alter the risk for systemic adverse effects. The Turbuhaler and Diskhaler are among the devices that contain multiple doses.

Finally, the drug must be delivered to the site of action in concentrations sufficient to produce therapeutic effects. For example, although the delivery of antibiotics topically to the lung in patients with cystic fibrosis may appear to be advantageous, thick mucus secretions can minimize effective delivery to the target tissue, making systemic therapy more beneficial. As mentioned previously, delivery of medications to the lung of pediatric patients can be considered more difficult because of the smaller airways. Other topical delivery systems, such as the sublingual and transdermal routes, are available; however, these do not yet have applications in pediatric pulmonary practice.

Oral Administration

The oral route of drug administration requires absorption from the gastrointestinal tract as an initial step. Although this route may often be more convenient than the inhaled route, especially for younger children, a number of factors can adversely influence its use.

First, a drug given orally must be bioavailable from the gastrointestinal tract. Epinephrine, for example, is not administered orally because of rapid metabolism in the gastrointestinal mucosa and liver, making the drug ineffective. If a drug can be administered orally, other drugs or food can affect the gastric emptying time or the drug absorption itself. For example, the bioavailability of theophylline can be affected by the specific sustained-release formulation, administration with meals, and patient variables such as gastric motility and absorption from the gastrointestinal tract.[27] Although sustained-release formulations are designed to affect the rate but not the extent of absorption, differences have been observed.[27] Patient factors that can affect gastrointestinal motility and absorption (e.g., dumping syndromes or ostomies, which greatly shorten gastrointestinal transit time) can also adversely affect the bioavailability of medications. Even postural changes can affect the absorption of theophylline. One study in normal subjects demonstrated significantly lower serum theophylline concentrations when subjects remained in the supine compared with the standing position, for 12 hours after a 400-mg oral dose of aminophylline.[28]

The second factor that influences oral administration is the incidence of adverse effects. The stimulatory effects of β-adrenergic agonists are greater after systemic compared with inhaled administration. For both terbutaline and oral albuterol, studies have shown significantly more adverse effects and increased heart rate and tremor but similar efficacy when intravenous administration is compared with inhaled administration.[29,30] Thus an increased number of adverse effects does not necessarily indicate increased efficacy. A medication given orally must therefore be active with a low degree of adverse effects.

Parenteral Administration

Parenteral routes of administration include the subcutaneous, intramuscular, and intravenous routes. For these routes to be viable, a medication must be water soluble or in suspension. The intravenous route of administration bypasses the absorption step, resulting in 100% bioavailability. Another advantage is the rapid onset of action. These routes of drug administration may not always be viable because of inconvenience and cost. Also, the drug's adverse effects are not reduced compared with the effects after oral administration. Other disadvantages with parenteral routes are patient discomfort, the need for sterile conditions, and potential risks to health care practitioners from

Table 18-2 Inhaled Drug–Delivery Devices

DELIVERY DEVICE	ADVANTAGES	DISADVANTAGES
Metered dose inhaler	Standard of therapy	Need for coordination Phase-out of fluorocarbon propellants
Metered dose inhaler with spacer device	Reduced topical effects Reduced systemic drug absorption Increased pulmonary drug deposition	Cost of spacer Need to clean spacer
Dry powder inhaler	Actuation by breath Possible increased pulmonary drug deposition compared with metered dose inhaler	Possible provocation of cough Possible requirement for high flow rates Some single-dose units only
Nebulizer	Ease of use Efficient delivery	Inconvenience for some patients Need for water-soluble drug Need to clean nebulizer High cost (air compressors and ultrasonic) Possible inconsistent drug delivery (jet) Possibility of chemical breakdown of drug (ultrasonic) Potential mechanical difficulties (ultrasonic)

blood-borne pathogens. In some cases, however, these routes of administration may be the only way to achieve therapeutic concentrations at the target tissues, such as with some anti-infective agents and in emergency situations with asthmatic patients.

DRUG DISTRIBUTION

The distribution of systemically administered medications is important in that the drugs must be available to the target tissues. A mathematics parameter known as the *volume of distribution (Vd)* relates a drug's plasma concentration *(C)* to the concentration in the tissues and is defined by the following equation:

$$Vd = \frac{Dose}{C}$$

However, this does not necessarily provide insight into the drug's concentration at the relevant target tissue sites. A drug's volume of distribution, known from population values, allows calculation of the loading dose *(LD)* required to give a specified peak plasma drug concentration (C_p), as follows:

$$LD = Vd \cdot C_p$$

With oral dosing, the bioavailability of the particular drug and dosage form must also be considered. For some medications, such as theophylline, a "therapeutic range," which balances the desired therapeutic effects with the unwanted toxic effects, has been developed.[31,32] In the case of theophylline, the traditionally regarded therapeutic range (10 to 20 μg/ml) has been reassessed, and new guidelines recommend lower concentrations (5 to 15 μg/ml).[33,34]

The volume of distribution is related to the drug's lipophilicity, plasma protein binding, and route of elimination. A highly lipophilic medication, which tends to distribute and bind more widely to body tissues, generally has a larger volume of distribution and is metabolized in the liver.[35] Drugs that are highly protein bound or have large molecules and thus remain primarily in the plasma tend to have smaller volumes of distribution and are excreted unchanged by the kidney.[35] Factors affecting these parameters, such as competitive protein binding by other medications or metabolic changes that can affect protein binding (pH, serum albumin concentration, disease states that affect affinity of binding to albumin), can influence the drug's volume of distribution and can result in changes in therapeutic effect or toxicity.

For example, the physiologic effect of drugs that are highly protein bound can be significantly altered by small changes in protein binding and increases of the free or active drug concentration. An example of such a drug, although not particularly relevant to pediatric pulmonary practice, is phenytoin. Phenytoin is approximately 90% protein bound.[36] With just 10% of the total drug concentration present as free drug, a clinically significant effect on its therapeutic effects and toxicities can result from small changes of 1% to 2% in protein binding. This becomes more important and can result in a more dramatic effect because phenytoin demonstrates saturable elimination pathways.

For drugs that distribute to highly perfused tissues (as opposed to adipose tissue), dosing is often based on ideal body weight. Examples of such drugs are aminoglycoside antibiotics and, on occasion, theophylline. Finally, differences among drugs themselves can manifest as differences in distribution to specific tissues. It has been demonstrated in an animal model that methylprednisolone achieves higher concentrations in the lung and persists for a longer period of time than prednisolone.[37,38] This may result in a therapeutic benefit of methylprednisolone over prednisolone during treatment of inflammatory conditions of the lung.

ELIMINATION

Drugs are eliminated from the body via two general pathways. They are either metabolized in the liver or excreted in the urine. As alluded to previously, the route of elimination is affected to some degree by the lipophilicity and size of the drug molecule. Drug metabolism can occur in body tissues besides the liver; however, this is usually to such a small extent that the effect on the total body clearance is minimal. A notable exception are glucocorticoids, which are thought to be metabolized in all body tissues.[39] In most instances, the total body clearance of a drug is the sum of both the hepatic and renal clearances. If a steady-state serum drug concentration (C_{ss}) is desired, the clearance *(Cl)* must be known so that the maintenance dose *(MD)* can be calculated, as follows:

$$MD = Cl \cdot C_{ss} \cdot t$$

where *t* is the dosing interval. Clearance can also be calculated directly with detailed pharmacokinetics studies. After the serum concentration vs. time curve is plotted after a dose of a given drug, the clearance is calculated as follows:

$$Cl = \frac{Dose}{AUC}$$

where *AUC* is the area under the serum concentration vs. the time curve. The AUC is most commonly calculated using the trapezoidal rule, which involves dividing the serum concentration vs. the time curve into a series of trapezoids and calculating their areas (Fig. 18-1). The AUC is the sum of the areas of these trapezoids, and approximated by the following equation[40]:

$$AUC = \tfrac{1}{2}(C_1 + C_2)(t_2 - t_1) + \tfrac{1}{2}(C_2 + C_3)(t_3 - t_2) + \tfrac{1}{2}(C_3 + C_4)(t_4 - t_3) + \tfrac{1}{2}(C_{n-1} + C_n)(t_n - t_{n-1})$$

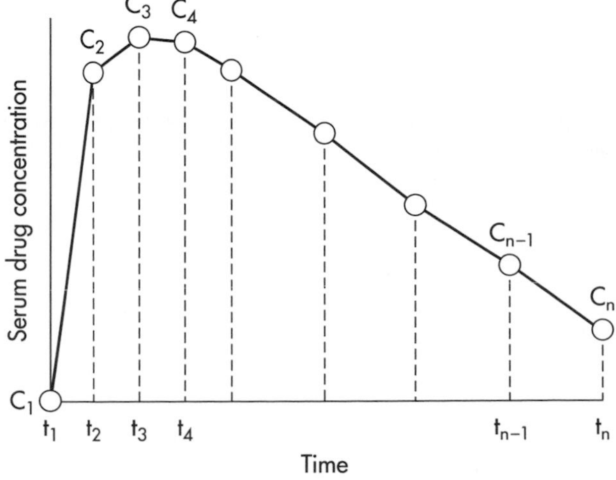

Fig. 18-1. Division of a serum drug concentration vs. time curve into a series of trapezoids for calculation of its AUC using the trapezoidal rule.

Hepatic Clearance

Hepatic elimination of medications often occurs via the cytochrome P-450 pathway, as with theophylline. This pathway is important because it is susceptible to a number of drug interactions and is influenced by a number of disease states, resulting in both acceleration and reduction in drug metabolism (Table 18-3). For example, theophylline, a drug with a low therapeutic index, requires close monitoring and appropriate dosage adjustment to maintain therapeutic concentrations and prevent toxic concentrations. Of special consideration are the anticonvulsant agents phenytoin, phenobarbital, and carbamazepine, which enhance the metabolism of theophylline and glucocorticoids,[41-43] and the macrolide antibiotics, which cause reduced theoph-ylline and methylprednisolone clearance.[42,44-47]

Clearance and inactivation of drugs occur via other metabolic pathways. The β-adrenergic agonist albuterol, for example, undergoes conjugation in humans and glucuronidation in other species.[48] Drug clearance via these metabolic pathways is influenced by hepatic blood flow and the intrinsic capacity of liver enzymes to metabolize drugs.[49] Disease states that affect these factors can result in changes in drug metabolism. The most common disease state affecting the hepatic elimination of drugs is liver disease, which invariably results in reduced drug elimination. For example, theophylline elimination can be significantly altered by liver cirrhosis, acute hepatitis, cholestasis, and cor pulmonale.[27,50] Glucocorticoids, however, are extensively metabolized throughout the body.[39] Thus liver disease has a minor impact on total body elimination, and dosage adjustments are not necessary. Other disease states can affect a drug's metabolism. Prednisolone elimination is enhanced in children with cystic fibrosis compared with children without the disease.[51] Elimination of other drugs metabolized via hepatic glucuronosyltransferase and biliary secretion are thought to be enhanced in cystic fibrosis as well, with oxidative metabolism unaffected.[52]

Renal Clearance

Renal drug clearance is a function of three mechanisms: glomerular filtration, tubular secretion, and tubular reabsorption. These mechanisms are influenced by plasma drug concentration and protein binding, urine flow and pH, and the general degree of kidney function and thus can affect the renal elimination of drugs.[49] For some drugs such as aminoglycoside antibiotics, estimates of creatinine clearance based on serum creatinine concentrations allow for a relatively accurate estimation of drug clearance and required dosing regimens.

First- and Zero-Order Elimination

Most drugs are metabolized by first-order elimination; that is, the rate of metabolism is proportional to the amount of drug in the body. A constant fraction of the drug in the body is metabolized per unit time. This constant is known as the *elimination rate constant* (k_e). The amount of drug removed *(R)* depends on the amount of drug present in the body *(A)* and is defined by the following equation:

$$R = k_e \cdot A$$

The elimination rate constant can be calculated from a drug's clearance *(Cl)* and volume of distribution *(Vd),* as follows:

$$k_e = \frac{Cl}{Vd}$$

For some drugs, elimination pathways may become saturated. Thus metabolism occurs at a fixed rate (k_m) or demonstrates

Table 18-3 Drugs and Disease States that Alter Theophylline Clearance

FACTOR	INCREASES CLEARANCE BY APPROXIMATELY
Carbamazepine	60%
Phenobarbital	25%
Phenytoin	75%
Rifampin	80%
Smoking	50%
Diet (low carbohydrate, high protein diet, or high degree of char-broiled meat)	Of clinical significance only if the changes in diet are extreme and for a prolonged period of time
Hyperthyroidism	≈20%
FACTOR	**DECREASES CLEARANCE BY APPROXIMATELY**
Allopurinol (high doses)	20%
Cimetidine	50%
Ciprofloxacin	30%
Clarithromycin	17%
Erythromycin	25%
Interferon-α (recombinant)	50%
Methotrexate	20%
Mexiletine	20%
Oral contraceptives	30%
Propranolol	20%
Thiabendazole	65%
Troleandomycin	50% (25% with low dose therapy)
Bronchopulmonary dysplasia	Variable effect, but may be profound
Diet (high carbohydrate, low protein diet, or high degree of dietary xanthines)	Of clinical significance only if the changes in diet are extreme and for a prolonged period of time
Heart failure	Variable effect, but may be profound
Hepatic failure	Variable effect, but may be profound
Hypothyroidism	40%
Sustained fever (>105° F for >24 hr)	Up to 50%

From Hendeles L et al: *J Pediatr* 120:177-183, 1992.

zero-order elimination. With zero-order elimination, the amount of drug removed depends not on the amount of drug in the body but on the amount of time involved and can be described as follows:

$$R = k_m \cdot \text{Time}$$

Most drugs demonstrate first-order elimination, with zero-order elimination observed in some patients as the dose is increased. A small fraction of the population may demonstrate zero-order theophylline metabolism even with therapeutic doses, and a number of cases of this phenomenon have been reported.[53] In such cases, changes in dosage do not correspond to proportional changes in serum concentration as they would if the drug demonstrated first-order elimination. Rather, small dosage increases can result in large increases in serum concentrations and possibly toxicity. Patients who demonstrate zero-order theophylline metabolism at concentrations within or close to the therapeutic range must be identified and then followed by close monitoring and careful dosage titration to maintain safe concentrations and prevent toxicities.

RECEPTOR PHARMACOLOGY

Receptors are biologic units, specific protein recognition sites, that bind or interact with molecules and determine the cellular response to such molecules at target tissues. These molecules commonly include drugs but also consist of endogenous hormones, neurotransmitters, mediators, and peptides. Receptor types include cell surface receptors and intracellular receptors. An example of each receptor site particularly relevant to respiratory diseases is the β-adrenergic receptor (cell surface receptor) and glucocorticoid receptor (intracellular receptor).

Surface Receptors

Cell surface receptors, structurally consisting of polypeptide chains folded and crossing back through cell surface membranes several times, are known as *G protein–coupled receptors* because they interact with a guanine nucleotide regulatory protein.[54] Among these are the β-adrenergic receptors, adenosine receptor subtypes, and muscarinic receptor subtypes. The β-adrenergic receptor family consists of β_1- and β_2-subtypes as well as the recently identified β_3-subtype.[55]

Stimulation of β-adrenergic receptors results in a variety of effects. These include β_1 or chronotropic effects, and β_2 or smooth muscle relaxation effects. This stimulation of β_2-adrenergic receptors of the respiratory smooth muscle makes β-adrenergic agonist agents useful in the treatment of asthma. The mechanisms by which β-adrenergic agonists result in bronchodilation are well understood. Stimulation of the receptors activates adenylate cyclase and increases the level of intracellular cyclic adenosine monophosphate. This is followed by activation of protein kinase A, inhibition of myosin phosphorylation, and lowering of intracellular calcium concentrations, which ultimately results in relaxation of airway smooth muscle.

Selectivity of an adrenergic agonist agent between β_1- and β_2-adrenergic effects results in a lesser incidence of the undesirable β_1 or chronotropic effects. Although it was once popular belief that β_1-adrenergic receptors existed only in heart tissue and β_2-adrenergic receptors were found only in lung tissue, radioligand-binding studies have demonstrated that each receptor subtype exists in both cardiac and lung tissue in almost equal proportions.[56] Stimulation of β_3-receptors, which are found in adipose tissue, is thought to result in the metabolic responses of adipocytes, muscle, and the gastrointestinal tract.[57]

A number of factors regulate β-adrenergic receptors. Desensitization resulting from chronic catecholamine stimulation has been described as resulting from "uncoupling" of the receptor and G protein,[58] a process reversed by glucocorticoids.[59] Down-regulation, or reduced receptor binding, resulting from chronic exposure to agonist agents has also been observed.[58] A number of mechanisms of this poorly understood process have been proposed, including agonist-promoted receptor degradation, a loss of ligand-binding capacity by activated receptors, and an agonist-induced decline in receptor synthesis.[58,60]

Although receptor down-regulation may play a role in tachyphylaxis to β-adrenergic agonists and perhaps the widely publicized potential for detrimental effects after regular use of these agents in treating asthma,[61,62] the clinical importance of such effects remains to be elucidated. Other factors, such as the inflammatory mediators phospholipase A_2, platelet-activating factor, leukotrienes B_4 and C_4, 15-lipoxygenase products, oxygen metabolites, and cytokines, may also affect β-adrenergic receptor expression and function and ultimately control of severe asthma.[63]

Conversely, the up-regulation of β-adrenergic receptors by glucocorticoids and thyroid hormones has been described.[58] Functionally, glucocorticoids, which are necessary for normal β-adrenergic receptor function, reduce the threshold for receptor stimulation[64] and potentiate the bronchodilatory effects of agonist agents.[65-68] A twofold to threefold increase in the number of lung β-adrenergic receptors has been observed after the administration of glucocorticoids.[69-71] This is thought to result from increases in the rate of transcription- and receptor-specific messenger ribonucleic acid in cells.[72,73] Glucocorticoids can also increase the responsiveness of desensitized cells to β-adrenergic agonists.[59,74,75]

Intracellular Receptors

The glucocorticoid receptor is an example of an intracellular receptor (Fig. 18-2). This receptor is in both the cytoplasm and the nucleus of the cell. Through mechanisms not clearly understood, glucocorticoids enter the cell, where they interact with the glucocorticoid receptor and begin the chain of events that results in their biologic effects. Once in the cell, binding of the glucocorticoid molecule to the receptor is preceded by a number of processes.

The first step involved in the binding of free glucocorticoid within the cell to the glucocorticoid receptor appears to be phosphorylation of the soluble receptor.[76-78] After this is the binding of two 90-kD proteins,[79] which are from the family of heat shock proteins elicited by stressors,[80,81] to the receptor, with binding of one hsp56 protein to the two hsp90 proteins.[82,83] Once it is bound to these proteins, the receptor complex can bind to the glucocorticoid. It is thought that the receptor, when bound to hsp90, is stabilized in a high-affinity state for glucocorticoids.[84] Activation or transformation, the next step, is thought to result from a conformational change in the receptor that may result from dissociation of the receptor-hormone from the heat shock proteins. Dimerization of two receptor-hormone complexes may also occur before nuclear translocation.[85]

Once translocated into the nucleus, the glucocorticoid receptor–hormone complex can now bind to deoxyribonucleic

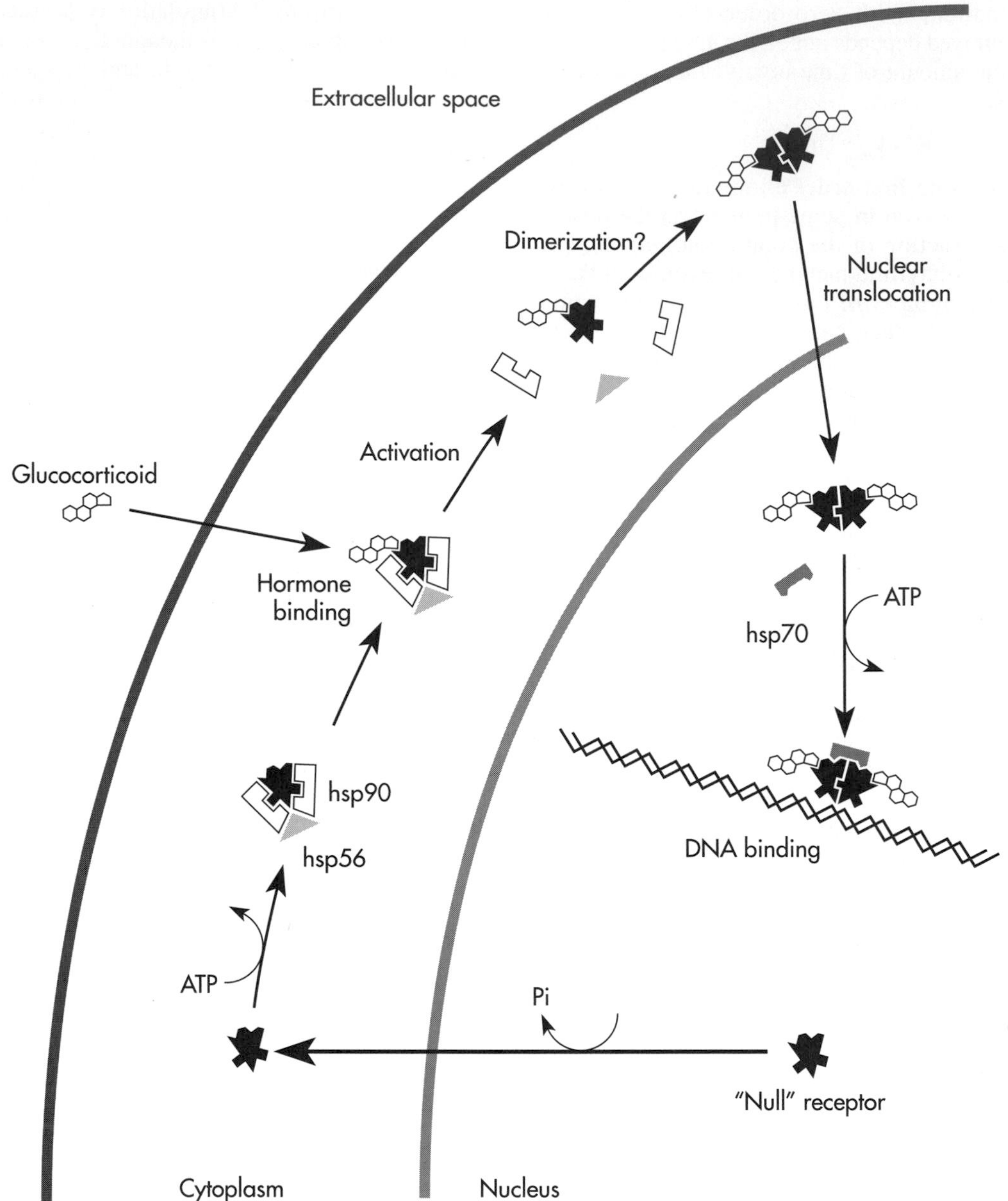

Fig. 18-2. Glucocorticoid receptor and its functional components within the cell. See text for details. *ATP,* Adenosine triphosphate; *DNA,* deoxyribonucleic acid; *Pi,* inorganic phosphate.

acid (DNA) and exert its biologic effects. Several endogenous and exogenous factors, including interferon-γ, lipopolysaccharide, thioredoxin, phosphoglyceride, epidermal growth factor receptor, transfer ribonucleic acid, protein kinase C, and other proteins, are thought to regulate the glucocorticoid receptor.[86-88] Interleukin-2 and interleukin-4 are thought to play a role in the reduced glucocorticoid receptor–binding affinity observed in the peripheral blood mononuclear cells of asthmatic patients who fail to respond to glucocorticoid treatment.[89,90]

PHARMACODYNAMICS

Pharmacodynamics relates to the chemical and biochemical effects of a drug as they pertain to its mechanism of action. A drug's pharmacodynamics can be measured with regards to its onset of action, peak effect, duration of effects, and offset of action. For example, a number of factors alter the pharmacodynamics of glucocorticoids. Changes in the basic glucocorticoid structure, which result in differences in absorption, distribution, receptor affinity, and elimination, can affect the magnitude and duration of the drug's effects.[91] Thus a drug's pharmacokinetics influences its pharmacodynamics, although this relationship is not always well understood. One might assume that changes in a drug's concentration or the dose administered would result in proportional changes in its clinical effect.

In a study investigating glucocorticoid response as tyrosine aminotransferase activity in an animal model, a tenfold increase in dose resulted in only a 50% increase in peak effect and a doubling of the duration of effect.[91] Further study using a similar model demonstrated that frequent smaller doses were more effective than larger single doses in prolonging the duration of effect.[92] Other studies have demonstrated a similar disproportion between changes in dosage and response. A study using lymphocytopenic effect as a measure of glucocorticoid response showed a 33% increase in peak effect and a 20% increase in duration of effect after a sixfold increase in prednisolone dose.[93] In a model of methylprednisolone pharmacodynamics measured by whole blood histamine suppression, similar durations of effect were observed with a single 40-mg dose and a 20-mg dose followed by a 5-mg dose 8 hours later.[94] Therefore it is not entirely surprising that low doses of glucocorticoids can achieve similar therapeutic effects compared with higher doses.[95,96] This may be one factor that explains the greater beneficial effect of inhaled glucocorticoid therapy compared to oral therapy.

Although numerous cellular and biochemical effects of glucocorticoids have been demonstrated, it is still unclear as to which are important in the mechanism of action. Thus there are no good markers of the effects of glucocorticoids at their site of action. Clinicians treating asthmatic patients are left with functional markers, such as bronchial hyperresponsiveness and pulmonary function, and changes in airway cellularity as measures of the effects of glucocorticoid therapy. Peripheral (blood, sputum) markers of lung inflammation that bypass the need for invasive procedures such as bronchoalveolar lavage and bronchial biopsy would be useful in determining the response to glucocorticoid treatment. Two substances, soluble interleukin-2 receptor and eosinophil cationic protein, are being studied as potential peripheral markers of inflammatory processes and allergic disease.[97-101]

DRUG ACTION

Several strategies can be used to combat disease. Asthma, for example, has two distinct mechanisms, bronchoconstrition and increased bronchial hyperresponsiveness, that are thought to result from inflammation within the lungs and airways (Fig. 18-3).

Bronchodilation

Asthma was once thought to result primarily from bronchoconstriction.[102] In recent years, however, new information regarding the pathogenesis of the disease has led to an emphasis on the inflammatory component of treatment.[33,34] Nevertheless, relief of symptomatic bronchoconstriction continues to play an important role in the treatment of asthma.

There are, in theory, two ways that bronchodilation can be achieved. Direct bronchodilation is one mechanism, and the other is reversal or blocking bronchoconstriction. The bronchodilator medications commonly used in the treatment of asthma include β-adrenergic agonist agents, such as albuterol, and theophylline. β-Adrenergic agonists act by stimulating β-adrenergic receptors and, through the chain of events previously discussed, result in relaxation of the bronchial smooth muscles and inhibition of mediator release from inflammatory cells.

Theophylline was once thought to act by the inhibition of cyclic nucleotide phosphodiesterases, which results in increases in the levels of cyclic adenosine monophosphate or cyclic guanosine monophosphate and ultimately smooth muscle relaxation.[103] The exact mechanism or mechanisms for the therapeutic effects of theophylline remain in question; however, a number of effects, including enhancement of β-adrenergic effects or independent effects, adenosine receptor antagonism, prostaglandin antagonism, stimulation of catecholamine release, inhibition of mast cell mediator release, and improvement of diaphragmatic contractility, have been proposed. Nevertheless, the result is essentially the same as for the β-adrenergic agonist agents (e.g., bronchodilation).

A major difference between the two medications, however, is the time course of their effects. β-Adrenergic agonists act rapidly; however, these effects tend to be short-lived, gener ally lasting 4 to 6 hours. Thus these agents are effective only against the immediate asthmatic response after single-allergen bronchial challenge or a trigger exposure. Conversely, theophylline is thought to be effective against the late asthmatic response[104] and may increase the amount of allergen required to elicit an immediate response.[104,105] These results have been disputed, however.[106] Neither medication is thought to provide benefit against the bronchial hyperreactivity or inflammation associated with the disease, although a role for theophylline has been suggested.[107,108] Another factor differentiating β-adrenergic agonists and theophylline is the increased risk for toxicity and the numerous drug interactions with theophylline.

Bronchoprotection

Bronchoprotection can be considered a protective effect against asthmatic responses after exposure to known triggers such as allergens or nonspecific stimuli such as histamine, methacholine, and exercise. In this respect, β-adrenergic agonists do provide partial benefit, if only for the immediate response. Newer long-acting β-adrenergic agonists, such as salmeterol and formoterol, block both the immediate and late asthmatic responses; thus they can be considered advantageous over presently available agents.[109-111] Salmeterol has also been suggested to have antiinflammatory effects of its own based on observations in an animal model and a study in humans.[112,113] The benefits of theophylline with regards to bronchoprotective effects, as discussed in the previous section, remain in question. Pretreatment with cromolyn sodium and presumably nedocromil sodium provides benefit on the immediate and late asthmatic responses after exposure to allergens and other bronchospastic agents.[114-121]

Anticholinergic agents such as ipratropium bromide provide some protection against the nocturnal asthma symptoms thought to result from changes in the cholinergic tone during sleep.[122,123] However, these agents provide little or no benefit against asthmatic responses to allergen and no benefit on bronchial hyperresponsiveness.[122] In fact, a "rebound" hyperresponsiveness has been observed after discontinuation.[124] Glucocorticoids as well as hydrocortisone and its synthetic derivatives are beneficial in the treatment of asthma because they protect against the late asthmatic response after allergen exposure and decrease bronchial hyperresponsiveness.[125,126] When new medications are evaluated for their use in treating asthma, one of the first items studied is their potential bronchoprotective effects when administered before challenge in animal or human models.

Resolution of Inflammation

Resolution of the inflammatory process within the lungs and airways is the ultimate goal of antiasthma therapy because this can be considered a "cure" for the disease. This process of healing may be prolonged, however, requiring symptomatic relief in the meantime. The current measures of inflammation are crude and do not adequately reveal the degree of inflammation within the lung. Bronchial hyperresponsiveness or hy-

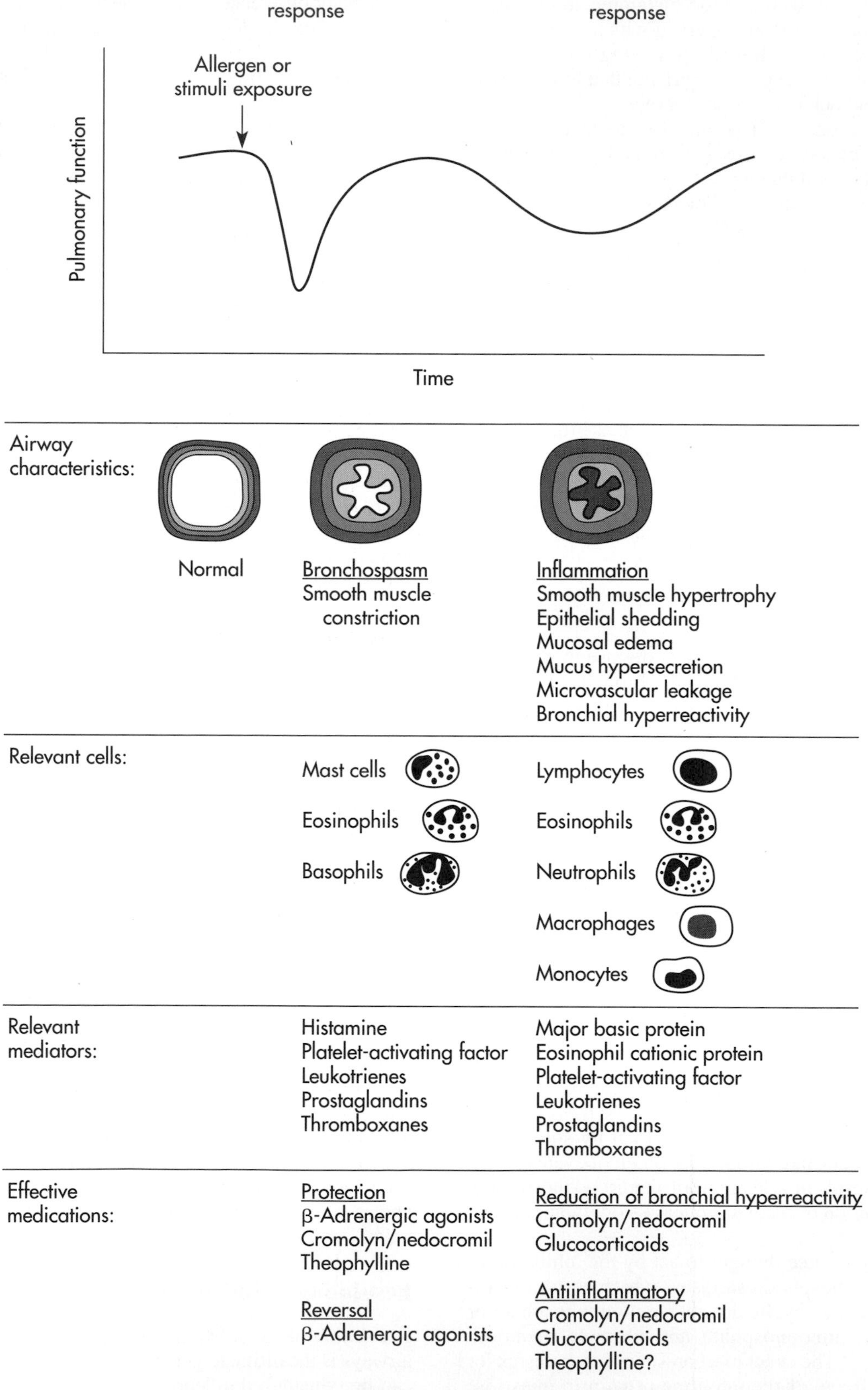

Fig. 18-3. Characteristics of asthmatic airways (pathophysiologic, relevant cells, and relevant mediators) in the immediate and late asthmatic responses to allergens and triggers and their effective treatment with medications.

perreactivity is often used as a measure of disease activity. The degree of reactivity, commonly measured as the provocative dose or concentration of a substance (often methacholine or histamine) that is required to elicit a 20% drop in the 1-second forced expiratory volume (PD_{20} or PC_{20}), has been correlated to the severity of asthma and medication requirements.[127-129] This measurement, however, sheds light only on the ongoing functional abnormality in the lung and airways and can be affected by environmental conditions such as viral respiratory infections and exposure to relevant allergens.[130-132] Furthermore, bronchial hyperresponsiveness may be slowly resolving or irreversible even after active inflammation is controlled.

The close association of airway inflammation and bronchial hyperresponsiveness has led to an emphasis on antiinflammatory medication in the treatment of asthma.[33,34,125] These include cromolyn sodium, nedocromil, and the most potent agents, glucocorticoids. Indeed these agents are beneficial in preventing and reversing the development of bronchial hyperresponsiveness.[133] As mentioned in the previous section, there is no direct measure of their antiinflammatory effects in the lung with the exception of invasive procedures such as bronchial lavage and biopsy. Assessment of the response to treatment is often based on changes in bronchial hyperresponsiveness and pulmonary function, which may not directly reflect the inflammatory process within the lung. These parameters are commonly examined to determine the potential long-term beneficial effects of new asthma medications. As mentioned in a previous section, peripheral markers of lung inflammation would be useful in determining responses to the various antiasthma medications.

Glucocorticoids, particularly when inhaled, reduce the number of inflammatory cells observed in the airways of asthmatic patients[134-137] and have become the gold standard for antiinflammatory agents. In fact, the antiinflammatory effects of glucocorticoids (i.e., changes in airway inflammatory cells) are associated with increased symptom control and reduced bronchial hyperresponsiveness.[134-137] Another potential benefit is the inhibition of plasma exudation, presumably resulting from reduced microvascular leakage and respiratory membrane permeability.[138,139] This may explain the relatively rapid reversal in control after discontinuation of inhaled glucocorticoid therapy.

CHRONOPHARMACOLOGY

For disease processes that exhibit biologic rhythms, a relatively new discipline known as *chronopharmacology* has emerged. In this discipline the timing of therapeutic modalities is used to optimize their effect on disease control. Asthma is an example of such a disease, since many patients demonstrate nocturnal worsening of pulmonary function. Etiologies for this nocturnal worsening and therapies designed to prevent the deterioration of pulmonary function during the evening hours have been investigated.

In patients with nocturnal asthma exacerbations, the following occur:

1. The number of peripheral blood eosinophils is higher than in asthmatics without nocturnal symptoms.[140]
2. Eosinophil counts are higher during the night than during the day.[141]
3. A lower concentration of methacholine is required to elicit a 20% drop in the forced expiratory volume in 1 second at 4 AM compared with 4 PM.[142]
4. The leukocytes demonstrate a reduced β-adrenergic receptor density and responsiveness at 4 AM vs. 4 PM.[143]
5. The total number of leukocytes, neutrophils, and eosinophils in bronchoalveolar lavage fluid is elevated at 4 AM vs. at 4 PM, corresponding to the observed reduction in the 1-second forced expiratory volume.[144]

Thus therapies designed to prevent these changes may be useful in treating nocturnal asthma. Early studies have demonstrated that the timing of glucocorticoid doses is important in the overall daytime control of asthma.[145,146] Alternative modalities include single daily doses of theophylline given in the evening to protect against the nocturnal decline in pulmonary function[147,148] and doses of glucocorticoids given at the unconventional time of 3 PM, which provides greater protection from nighttime worsening than when given at 8 PM or the more conventional 8 AM dosing.[145,149]

AGE-RELATED CHANGES

A number of variables, which may change with growth and development, can affect the absorption, distribution, and elimination of drugs. The airways are developed by week 16 of gestation, and growth in terms of the multiplication of alveoli occurs during the first few years after birth.[150] The changes in pulmonary arteries, primarily a reduction in the thickness of the vessel walls, occur rapidly during the first 3 days of age.[150] Thus with the exception of growth (in terms of size), no major changes in lung development would affect drug disposition.

Absorption

Absorption of drug from the gastrointestinal tract is influenced by a number of factors, including gastric acidity, gastrointestinal motility, mucosal membrane permeability, bacterial flora, enzyme activity, biliary function, and diet.[151] These factors change with aging and in turn affect the rate and extent of drug absorption.[152] As acid secretory capacity matures during the first few days of life, gastric acidity changes from a pH of 8 to 6 during the neonatal period, nears adult values for the first month of life, and then increases until adult values are attained at age 3 to 7 years of age.[151,153] Therefore drugs that are weak acids should be more slowly absorbed in children than in adults because of the decreased gastric acidity. Conversely, better gastric absorption of weak bases should be observed in pediatric patients. Data consistent with these theories include increased bioavailability of penicillin and ampicillin in children compared with adults and delayed absorption and reduced bioavailability of phenobarbital, phenytoin, and acetaminophen.[153] Phenobarbital absorption has also been correlated to age.[154]

Although much is known regarding gastric acidity in neonates and young children, limited information is available regarding other factors that may affect drug absorption. Gastric emptying time is prolonged in the neonate and infant and approaches adult values at 6 to 8 months of age.[153] Similarly, intestinal transit time can be prolonged because peristalsis is irregular,[155] a potential problem for sustained-release products such as theophylline and oral albuterol. These factors can influence drug absorption, as can the episodes of diarrhea common in this age group. Biliary function, which develops during the first month of life,[156] and the development of intestinal bacterial flora may also influence the absorption of drugs.

Distribution

A drug's volume of distribution relates to its plasma concentration, which is affected by body composition. Thus age-related changes in body composition can affect the distribution of drugs. Neonates have a higher proportion of body mass in the form of water compared with older children and adults. The proportion of total body water decreases from 75% to 85% in the neonatal period to 55% in adulthood.[153] The result of such differences is manifested as higher loading dose requirements for drugs that distribute to total body water in infants and young children. Unlike total body water, body fat increases with age.[151] This results in smaller volumes of distribution for lipophilic drugs in young children.

Protein binding, as discussed in a previous section, also influences the distribution of drugs. Neonatal serum concentrations of albumin, the major binding protein, is approximately 80% of adult values and increases to normal within the first year of life.[151] Because only free drug is considered active, a lower serum albumin concentration and a lower proportion of bound drug can result in greater pharmacologic and possibly toxic effects with drug concentrations that appear to be therapeutic. The binding affinity of albumin for some drugs, including theophylline, appears to be decreased in the neonate as well.[157]

Elimination

In general, neonates are thought to demonstrate a reduced enzyme capacity for metabolizing drugs, which increases with age.[151,153] Insufficiencies of elimination pathways are often compensated for by metabolism via alternative pathways, as seen in neonatal methylation of theophylline to caffeine.[158] The differences in renal drug clearance between children and adults may not result from intrinsic enzyme capacities or quantity but can be attributed to changes in body composition (i.e., proportion of liver tissue).

Like hepatic enzyme activity, renal function (renal blood flow, glomerular filtration, and tubular function), when normalized for body surface area, is reduced in infants and children compared with adults. After birth, increased cardiac output and reductions in intrarenal vascular resistance result in increased kidney perfusion and increased renal function. However, this increase in renal function during the first week of life is not observed in premature newborns. Glomerular filtration, which is developed to a greater degree than tubular function at birth, gradually increases to adult values by 3 years of age. Premature infants have lower filtration rates than full-term infants, and their filtration capacity develops more slowly. Differences in renal drug clearance between children and adults are thought to correspond to maturation of renal function.[153] These points highlight the need for individualization of doses based on desired drug concentrations and therapeutic and toxic effects for drugs cleared primarily by the kidney.

NEW DRUGS ON THE HORIZON

A number of new pulmonary drugs are being investigated and may soon be available in the United States. Some are available in other countries.

Long-Acting β-Adrenergic Agonists

Two inhaled β-adrenergic agonist agents with a prolonged duration of action compared with presently available agents are salmeterol and formoterol. These agents share properties of the shorter-acting agents in that they are rapid acting, although with a slightly slower onset of action,[159] and provide protection from immediate responses after allergen challenge. Formoterol and salmeterol also have a long duration of action, which allows protection from late asthmatic responses after allergen exposure and more convenient twice-daily dosing.[109-112,160] These properties can be attributed to the lipophilic nature of these drugs, resulting in a longer half-life and increased affinity for the receptor.

Inhaled Glucocorticoids

Budesonide, probably the most well studied of the inhaled glucocorticoids, is available in Europe and Canada and is now available in the United States. Its advantage over other agents may be an improved topical to systemic potency ratio,[161,162] which may reduce the risk for systemic adverse effects with inhaled administration. A factor increasing the complexity of its evaluation, however, is its delivery device, which may provide twice the amount of drug to the lung than with conventional metered dose inhalers.[25] Advantages that would be desirable in a new inhaled glucocorticoid include high tissue affinity (lipophilic), low oral bioavailability, and of course, a high intrinsic glucocorticoid potency.[163] Fluticasone propionate shares these properties and may demonstrate even greater potency. Other glucocorticoids being developed include butixocort propionate, and mometasone.[163-165]

Nedocromil Sodium

Nedocromil sodium is thought to share similar properties to cromolyn sodium; however, it is a distinctly different chemical entity. Like cromolyn, it is effective as a prophylactic agent given before allergen exposure, preventing immediate and late asthmatic responses; it may have antiinflammatory effects as well.[116-120,166]

Leukotriene Modifiers

Leukotrienes are potent mediators involved in the inflammatory process (vascular permeability, mucus secretion, attraction and activation of cells) as well as bronchoconstriction.[167,168] Leukotriene receptor antagonist (zafirlukast, montelukast, pranlukast) and 5-lipoxygenase inhibitors (zileuton) have been developed to attenuate the effects of leukotrienes. These agents inhibit late responses to inhaled allergen and postallergen-induced bronchial responsiveness, attenuation of bronchoconstriction after exercise, and aspirin ingestion in aspirin-sensitive individuals. Although improvement of pulmonary function and symptoms have been demonstrated in patients with mild to moderate asthma during treatment with leukotriene modifiers, further study is required to determine their role in asthma therapy.[169]

Loop Diuretics

Interest in the use of loop diuretics for the treatment of asthma has increased in recent years. A number of investigations demonstrating beneficial effects in preventing challenge-induced bronchoconstriction have been published since the first study, which demonstrated that inhaled furosemide is effective in protecting against exercise-induced bronchoconstriction.[170] Protective effects have subsequently been demonstrated against early and late asthmatic responses induced by various antigens.[171,172] Unfortunately, furosemide, the most potent loop diuretic examined, has not demonstrated efficacy on improving nonspecific bronchial hyperresponsiveness in asthmatics.[173,174] Preliminary studies suggest that these drugs are well tolerated and may provide significant steroid-sparing effect; however, the results of long-term trials are awaited.[175]

New Phosphodiesterase Inhibitors

Theophylline has been a mainstay in the treatment of asthma for many years; however, renewed concern over its toxicities has led to a decline of its use in recent years.[41] This is reflected in the various asthma-treatment guidelines, which recommend theophylline as a second-, third-, or even fourth-line agent.[33,34] One of theophylline's mechanisms, as previously mentioned, is thought to occur via inhibition of phosphodiesterases, which may result in reduced inflammatory cell activity and reduced airway smooth muscle tone. Interest in developing an "improved" theophylline has led to research into more specific and potent enzyme inhibitors. Although it is early in the development process, some agents have already demonstrated limited efficacy and hold promise for the future.[176,177]

Steroid-Sparing Agents

A number of potential antiinflammatory agents have been investigated in recent years for their steroid-sparing effect in severe steroid-dependent asthma and are reviewed elsewhere.[133,178] These "alternative" asthma therapies include methotrexate, troleandomycin, intravenous γ-globulin, gold salts, interferon-γ, colchicine, hydroxychloroquine, and dapsone. Although efficacy has been demonstrated in some cases, further study in double-blind, placebo-controlled fashion is needed. It appears that each of these medications contributes to efficacy in approximately 33% to 50% of the study populations. Perhaps selective consideration for therapy would increase the efficacy of the individual agents.

INNOVATIVE STRATEGIES FOR THE FUTURE

As mechanisms for diseases become better understood, newer therapies designed to alter specific defects will be developed. These include new bronchodilators and glucocorticoids for inhalation, immunomodulators, inhibitors of mediator synthesis, new classes of medications, and gene therapy. Drug delivery will also be affected, and clinicians can expect to see liposome-drug formulations for the inhalation of water-insoluble medications and new devices for inhalation therapy, such as breath-actuated dry powder inhalers.

Immunomodulators

The immunologic mechanisms for diseases have received increased attention in recent years. In asthma, for instance, eosinophil and T cell activation and the expression of cytokines are thought to play important roles in the pathophysiology of the disease.[179] Several studies have demonstrated correlations between the number of T cells in bronchoalveolar lavage fluid and biopsy specimens and activation markers to the severity of asthma and the subjects' atopic status.[180-184] T cells and eosinophils have even been implicated as contributing to the pathogenesis of cystic fibrosis.[185] New therapies directed at various immunologic pathways are being investigated, and even old medications are being reevaluated for their potential role as immunomodulators.

Theophylline, for instance, may exert some of its beneficial effects in asthma as a result of changes in T cell populations. One study demonstrated increases in the numbers of CD4 and CD8 lymphocytes in the peripheral blood of mild asthmatics after theophylline treatment at low serum concentrations.[186] Another study demonstrated that withdrawal of theophylline in asthmatics resulted in decreases in the number of CD8DR and CD4/CD25 T cell populations, possibly indicating that theophylline induces a switch of the T-helper (Th) cells from the Th2 to Th1 subset and reverts back to Th2 when the drug is discontinued.[187] This Th2 subpopulation is thought to be the predominant T cell found in the bronchoalveolar lavage fluid of atopic asthmatics,[188] appears to be selectively activated in atopic asthmatics,[189] and may be involved in the etiology of abnormalities of the glucocorticoid receptor in peripheral blood mononuclear cells from "steroid-resistant" asthmatics.[89,90]

Cyclosporin and a more potent immunosuppressant agent FK506 have been proposed[190-192] and studied for their use in asthma as a result of their selective inhibition of T cell activation.[193-199] These agents have also been investigated for antiinflammatory activity resulting from their action on adhesion molecules.[200,201] Clearly, as the pathophysiologies of diseases become better understood, so will the mechanisms of the medications used to treat them.

Adhesion Molecules

The research on and understanding of adhesion molecules has vastly increased in recent years, leading to speculation regarding their involvement in allergic inflammatory disorders. Adhesion molecules are glycoproteins expressed on the surface of cells. These proteins have multiple functions that include promoting adhesion of cells to one another, activating cells, and promoting cell migration and infiltration.[202] Adhesion molecules promote the migration of leukocytes from the vascular to the extravascular compartments, promote antigen-specific T cell recognition, are involved in stimulating T cell activation, stimulate the effector mechanisms of the activated T cells, stimulate the proliferation of cells, and regulate cell growth.[202-204]

Adhesion molecules are divided into the following groups or families based on their structure: the immunoglobulin supergene family, the integrins, and the selectins.[203] The expression and activation of various adhesion molecules are induced by a number of inflammatory mediators, many of which have been implicated in the pathogenesis of asthma.[202] Increased expression of intercellular adhesion molecule-1 was detected in the bronchial biopsy specimens from symptomatic asthmatics,[205] and up-regulation of adhesion molecules was observed in T cells from the blood and bronchoalveolar lavage fluid after allergen challenge of sensitized individuals.[206] Also, antiinflammatory medications used in the treatment of asthma affect the expression of various adhesion molecules, providing further evidence for their role in the disease.

For example, cromolyn sodium inhibits the induction of E-selectin, a member of the selectin family of adhesion molecules, by substance P,[207] and glucocorticoids inhibit expression of intercellular adhesion molecule-1, a member of the immunoglobulin supergene family of adhesion molecules, by interleukin-1–induced cells.[208] Medications thought to be beneficial in refractory asthma (i.e., cyclosporin, methotrexate, gold) have also demonstrated effects on the expression of adhesion molecules.[209-211] Thus adhesion molecules may play an important role in the pathogenesis of inflammatory diseases, and therapies directed at blocking the molecules and inhibiting their expression may be useful in the treatment of such diseases.

Gene Therapy

With the identification and characterization of genetic mutations as the bases for diseases such as with cystic fibrosis, there has been increased research and speculation into gene therapy as a therapeutic modality.[212,213] The gene for cystic fibrosis is autosomal recessive. When mutated, a 1480 amino acid protein responsible for chloride transport across membranes, known as the *cystic fibrosis transmembrane conductance regulator (CFTR),* is dysfunctional, resulting in the various pulmonary and gastrointestinal manifestations of the disease. This mutation most commonly results from a deletion of three base pairs, which ultimately leads to the absence of an amino acid, phenylalanine, at position 508.[214]

Gene therapy involves the use of a vector, usually a virus, to introduce and express the appropriate gene sequence into the host. This technique has been successfully pursued and is being investigated for the treatment of adenosine deaminase deficiency.[215] Simply put, it involves incorporating the gene of choice into the viral DNA, which after infecting the host, can result in expression of the appropriate proteins by host cells. Thus the recent identification and cloning of the normal human CFTR gene sequence was an important step in transforming gene therapy for cystic fibrosis into a reality.

These procedures are not without risk, however. Dividing cells are required for incorporation into the host DNA; thus the use of retroviruses, which have a high rate of transfer, have been suggested. Integration into host DNA is mutagenic and can be carcinogenic through oncogenes and interference with tumor-suppressor genes.[213] Adenovirus has also been suggested because it naturally infects lung epithelia[213] and because foreign genes can readily be inserted.[216] It already has been used to introduce human CFTR into the lung epithelium of rats.[217] Although this would appear to be an advantage, the adenovirus does not integrate into the genome of the lung epithelial stem cell, and it is lost with the turnover of epithelial cells or degradation and necessitates repeated reinfection.[213] Other disadvantages include a possible replication of competent virus as a result of recombination with wild-type virus and potential inflammatory reactions induced by the virus protein.[213] Nevertheless, gene therapy remains a promising adjunct.

Membrane-Derived Lipid Mediators

Leukotrienes, prostaglandins, and thromboxanes are lipoxygenase and cyclooxygenase metabolites of arachidonic acid and are derived from the phospholipid membranes of inflammatory cells. Prostaglandins undergo further breakdown to prostaglandin D_2 and prostaglandin F_{2a}, two potent bronchoconstrictors and potentiators of airway hyperresponsiveness.[218-220] Another cyclooxygenase product is thromboxane A_2, which is produced by the many inflammatory cells in the lung and based on animal models, may be involved in bronchoconstriction and the development of inflammation and airway hyperresponsiveness.[221,222]

Sulfidopeptide leukotrienes (leukotrienes C_4, D_4, and E_4) constitute slow-reacting substance of anaphylaxis and are products of the lipoxygenase-breakdown pathway of arachidonic acid. These leukotrienes are liberated during the inflammatory processes and have a potent effect on bronchoconstriction and presumably airway inflammation and hyperresponsiveness.[167,168] Platelet-activating factor is liberated early in the cell membrane by phospholipase and is a mediator of bronchoconstriction, airway hyperreactivity, edema, and cellular changes associated with generalized inflammatory responses.[223] Clearly, these products can be important in the biochemical and physiologic changes of asthma. Lipoxygenase inhibitors, synthetase inhibitors, and specific receptor antagonists for these products have been developed, and continued study will determine their role in the treatment of disease.

Drug Delivery

A number of mechanisms designed to optimize drug delivery have been developed or are being investigated. These include the use of prodrugs, alternative delivery devices, and liposomes as vehicles for delivery of the medications to their relevant sites of action.

Prodrugs

Prodrugs are molecules that are chemically related to a medication; however, they are not usually active. The purpose of such entities is often to bypass presystemic first-pass metabolism after oral administration, which would normally inactivate the parent active medication. After oral administration, the molecule is then biotransformed to its active form. Although the purpose is not that of a traditional prodrug, prednisone is an example of such a chemical entity. Prednisone itself has no activity; however, it rapidly undergoes interconversion via reduction of the 11-keto group to the form prednisolone, which is active.[224,225]

A newer example of this is the bronchodilator bambuterol (Fig. 18-4). Bambuterol, now available in Europe, is a biscarbamate ester prodrug of terbutaline that has a high affinity for lung tissue and displays presystemic metabolic stability.[226] Although in itself inactive, bambuterol is slowly converted via hydrolysis to terbutaline, its active form.[226-228] Thus bambuterol can be considered a sustained-release formulation of terbutaline, which allows for more convenient once-daily dosing.[229-231]

Delivery Devices

The delivery of medications by the inhaled route is complex and is affected by numerous factors. Obviously, coordination is required by patients to properly actuate a metered dose inhaler. Spacer devices bypass the need for precise coordination between actuation and inhalation. To further minimize the need for coordination, breath-actuated metered dose inhalers have been developed. This includes the Autohaler device (3M Pharmaceuticals, St. Paul), which is essentially a metered dose inhaler with a cocking lever and baffle that expels the aerosol when inhalation pressure opens the baffle and triggers the device. This can result in improved drug delivery in patients with poor inhaler technique.[232] With the expected phase-out of pressurized metered dose inhalers because of the anticipated chlorofluorocarbon ban, these devices may become obsolete, al-

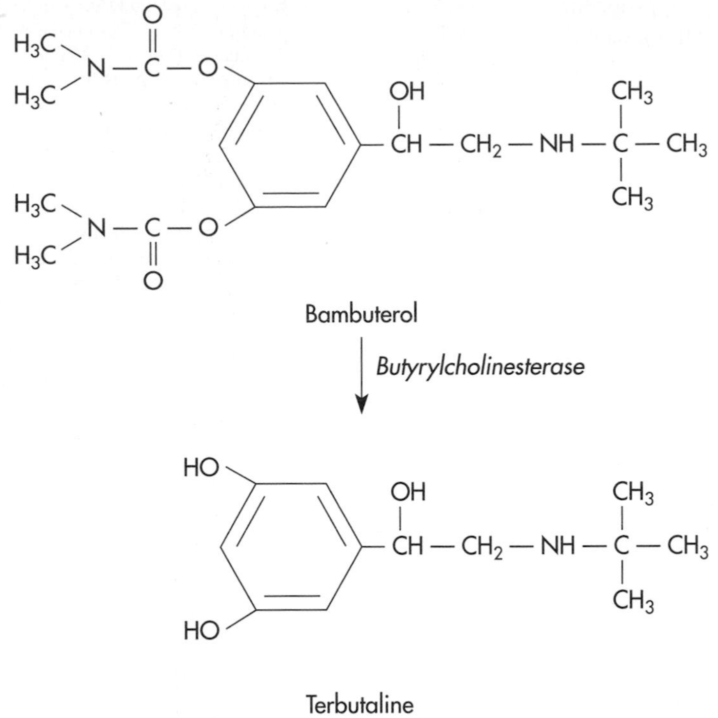

Bambuterol

Butyrylcholinesterase

Terbutaline

Fig. 18-4. Chemical structures of the prodrug bambuterol and its active form terbutaline after metabolism via butyrylcholinesterase.

though alternative propellants are being developed. The need for coordination and the need for chlorofluorocarbon propellants are overcome by the use of dry powder inhalers. These devices were discussed in a previous section and are described in greater detail in Chapter 19.

Ultrasonic nebulizers have been available for many years. These devices vary from the more common "jet" nebulizers in that the aerosol is produced by a piezoelectric crystal vibrating at a high frequency and creating a "fog" from the solution.[233] Ultrasonic nebulizers may be advantageous in that a much denser aerosol with considerably smaller particles (higher aerosol output) is produced[234]; however, whether these small aerosol particles contain a significant amount of medication has not been well studied and remains unclear. Other disadvantages and concerns would be that the heat and vibration produced may cause a chemical breakdown of the medication to be nebulized, that mechanical problems may occur with such devices, and that the cost of such devices is high. Ultrasonically nebulized distilled water, through mechanisms still unknown, provokes bronchoconstriction and is often used as a model to evaluate the protective effects of medications.

Liposome-Delivery Vehicles

Drugs that may be beneficial to treat respiratory diseases often do not have intrinsic physicochemical properties that allow for their delivery via optimal routes such as inhalation. For example, lipophilic medications such as cyclosporin and glucocorticoids are not easily solubilized without the addition of detergents and other agents and thus are not easily administered by nebulizer. Often, alternative formulations, such as those designed for intravenous or perhaps intranasal use, are used for inhaled administration. Although these products are solutions or suspensions and are easily given via nebulizer, they are not without some risk with no guarantee for therapeutic effects.[11] To overcome these disadvantages, researchers must investigate the incorporation of such water-insoluble medications into liposomes.

Liposomes are lipid vesicles containing an aqueous volume. Medications investigated thus far for incorporation into liposome-drug complexes include cyclosporin, glucocorticoids, amphotericin B, and antiviral agents.[13,235-237] Liposomes have also been suggested as a possible alternative delivery system for gene therapy in cystic fibrosis.[213] Aerosolized liposomes, given chronically, have been demonstrated to be without risk in an animal model.[12] Further investigation is required to determine the effect of liposomes on humans when administered over a long period, on the stability of medications, and on the delivery of such medications to the desired target site of action.

Aerosolized Antibiotics

A recent review succinctly summarized the use of inhaled antibiotics in the treatment of cystic fibrosis and the concerns associated with this therapy.[238] Indications for such treatment were maintenance or prevention of declines of the patient's status, adjunct therapy to intravenous antibiotics, treatment of acute episodes, and prevention and treatment of *Pseudomonas* colonization. Potential side effects with aerosolized antibiotic treatment include bacterial resistance resulting from low concentrations of the inhaled antibacterial agent, selection of difficult organisms, local irritation, and allergies. None of these appears to be a significant factor.

Inhaled tobramycin, recently shown to be an effective treatment,[239] has the advantages of being relatively inexpensive, having increased intrinsic activity against *Pseudomonas aeruginosa,* having fewer problems with resistance, and being less nephrotoxic compared with gentamicin.[238] Other important factors (aside from antibiotic selection) include the drug formulation, the selection of the appropriate nebulizer and compressor, and the patient's breathing technique.[239] To overcome the variability of these factors, researchers are investigating new delivery systems such as micronized antibiotic powder for inhalation.[240]

REFERENCES

The Lung as a Site for Drug Delivery

1. Staub NC, Albertine KH: The structure of the lungs relative to their principal function. In Murray JF, Nadel JA, eds: *Textbook of respiratory medicine,* Philadelphia, 1988, WB Saunders, pp 12-36.
2. West JB: Structure and function: how the architecture of the lung subserves its function. In West JB, ed: *Respiratory physiology,* ed 3, Baltimore, 1985, Williams & Wilkins, pp 1-10.
3. Barnes PJ: Airway inflammation and autonomic control, *Eur J Respir Dis* 69(suppl 47):80-87, 1986 (review).
4. Casale TB: Neuromechanisms of asthma, *Ann Allergy* 59:391-399, 1987 (review).
5. Casale TB: Neuropeptides and the lung, *J Allergy Clin Immunol* 88:1-14, 1991 (review).
6. Comper WD, Laurent TC: Physiological function of connective tissue polysaccharides, *Physiol Rev* 58:255-315, 1978 (review).
7. Staub NC: Pulmonary edema, *Physiol Rev* 54:678-811, 1974 (review).

Routes of Drug Delivery

8. Newman SP, Clarke SW: Aerosols in therapy. In Morén F, Newhouse MT, Dolovich MB, eds: *Aerosols in medicine: principles, diagnosis and therapy,* Amsterdam, 1985, Elsevier Science, pp 289-312.
9. Brain JD, Valberg PA: Deposition of aerosol in the respiratory tract, *Am Rev Respir Dis* 120:1325-1373, 1979 (review).
10. Summers QA: Inhaled drugs and the lung, *Clin Exp Allergy* 21:259-268, 1991 (review).
11. Kamada AK, Szefler SJ: Inhaled therapy in infants: why not nebulize glucocorticoids? *Pediatr Pulmonol* 13:198-199, 1992 (editorial).
12. Myers MA, Thomas DA, Straub L, Soucy DW, Niven RW, Kaltenbach M, Hood CI, Schrier H, Gonzalez-Rothi RJ: Pulmonary effects of chronic exposure to liposome aerosols in mice, *Exp Lung Res* 19:1-19, 1993.
13. Waldrep JC, Scherer PW, Knight V: Experimental lung therapy using drug-liposome aerosols, *Am Rev Respir Dis* 147:A289, 1993 (abstract).
14. Bouchikhi A, Becquemin MH, Bignon J, Roy M, Teillac A: Particle size study of nine metered dose inhalers, and their deposition probabilities in the airways, *Eur Respir J* 1:547-552, 1988.
15. Mercer TT, Goddard RF, Flores RL: Output characteristics of several commercial nebulizers, *Ann Allergy* 23:314-326, 1965.
16. Kradjan W, Lakshminarayan S: Efficiency of air compressor–driven nebulizers, *Chest* 85:512-516, 1985.
17. Hess D, Horney D, Snyder T: Medication-delivery performance of eight small-volume, hand-held nebulizers: effects of diluent volume, gas flow rate, and nebulizer model, *Respir Care* 34:717-723, 1989.
18. Alvine GF, Rodgers P, Fitzsimmons KM, Ahrens RC: Disposable jet nebulizers: how reliable are they? *Chest* 101:316-319, 1992.
19. Hollie MC, Malone RA, Skufca RM, Nelson HS: Extreme variability in aerosol output of the deVilbiss 646 jet nebulizer, *Chest* 100:1339-1344, 1991.
20. Thomas SHL, O'Dougherty MJ, Page CJ, Nunan TO, Bateman NT: Which apparatus for inhaled pentamidine? A comparison of pulmonary deposition via eight nebulizers, *Eur Respir J* 4:616-622, 1991.
21. Mason JW, Miller WC: What nebulizer should be used to aerosolize pentamidine for *Pneumocystis carinii* pneumonia? *Respir Care* 34:218-220, 1989.
22. Byron PR: Inhalation devices. In D'Arcy PF, McElnan JC, eds: *The pharmacy and pharmacotherapy of asthma,* Chichester, England, 1989, Ellis Horwood, pp 135-159.
23. Epsein SW: Is the MDI doomed to extinction? *Chest* 103:1313, 1993 (editorial).
24. Morén F: Aerosol dosage forms and formulations. In Morén F, Newhouse MT, Dolovich MB, eds: *Aerosols in medicine: principles, diagnosis and therapy,* Amsterdam, 1985, Elsevier Science, pp 262-287.
25. Thorsson L, Edsbäcker S, Conradson T-B: Lung deposition of budesonide from Turbuhaler® is twice that from a pressurized metered-dose inhaler P-MDI, *Eur Respir J* 7:1839-1844, 1994.
26. Hindle M, Newton DAG, Chrystyn H: Relative bioavailability of salbutamol to the lung after inhalation by metered dose inhaler and dry powder inhaler, *Thorax* 48:433-434, 1993 (abstract).
27. Glynn-Barnhart A, Hill M, Szefler SJ: Sustained release theophylline preparations: practical recommendations for prescribing and therapeutic drug monitoring, *Drugs* 35:711-726, 1988.
28. Warren JB, Cuss F, Barnes PJ: Posture and theophylline kinetics, *Br J Clin Pharmacol* 19:707-709, 1985.
29. Thiringer G, Svedmyr N: Comparison of infused and inhaled terbutaline in patients with asthma, *Scand J Respir Dis* 57:17-24, 1976.
30. Francis PWJ, Krastius IRB, Levison H: Oral and inhaled salbutamol on prevention of exercise-induced bronchospasm, *Pediatrics* 66:103-108, 1980.

Drug Distribution

31. Mitenko PA, Ogilvie RI: Rational intravenous doses of theophylline, *N Engl J Med* 289:600-603, 1973.
32. Levy G, Koysooko R: Pharmacokinetic analysis of the effect of theophylline on pulmonary function in asthmatic children, *J Pediatr* 86:789-793, 1975.
33. National Asthma Education Program, Expert Panel Report: *Guidelines for the diagnosis and management of asthma,* Pub No 91-3042, Bethesda, Md, 1991, United States Department of Health and Human Services, Public Health Service, National Institutes of Health, National Heart, Lung, and Blood Institute.
34. International Asthma Project: *International consensus report of the diagnosis and management of asthma,* Pub No 92-3091, Bethesda, Md, 1992, United States Department of Health and Human Services, Public Health Service, National Institutes of Health, National Heart, Lung, and Blood Institute.
35. Nierenberg DW, Melmon KL: Introduction to clinical pharmacology. In Melmon KL, Morrelli HF, Hoffman BB, Nierenberg DW, eds: *Melmon and Morrelli's clinical pharmacology: basic principles in therapeutics,* ed 3, New York, 1992, McGraw-Hill, pp 1-51.
36. Tozer TN, Winter ME: Phenytoin. In Evans WE, Schentag JJ, Jusko WJ, eds: *Applied pharmacokinetics: principles of therapeutic drug monitoring,* ed 3, Vancouver, Wash, 1992, Applied Therapeutics, pp 25-1–25-44.
37. Vichyanond P, Irvin CG, Larsen GL, Szefler SJ, Hill MR: Penetration of corticosteroids in the lung: evidence for a difference between methylprednisolone and prednisolone, *J Allergy Clin Immunol* 84:867-873, 1989.
38. Greos LS, Vichyanond P, Bloedow DC, Irvin CG, Larsen GL, Szefler SJ, Hill MR: Methylprednisolone achieves higher concentrations in the lung than prednisolone: a pharmacokinetic analysis, *Am Rev Respir Dis* 144:586-592, 1991.

Elimination

39. Martin LE, Harrison C, Tanner RJN: Metabolism of beclomethasone dipropionate by animal and man, *Postgrad Med J* 51(suppl 4):11-20, 1975.
40. Gibaldi M, Perrier D, eds: *Pharmacokinetics,* ed 2, New York, 1982, Marcel Dekker, pp 445-449.
41. Hendeles L, Weinberger M, Szefler S, Ellis E: Safety and efficacy of theophylline in children with asthma, *J Pediatr* 120:177-183, 1992 (review).
42. Szefler SJ, Ellis EF, Brenner M, Rose JQ, Spector SL, Yurchak AM, Andrews F, Jusko WJ: Steroid-specific and anticonvulsant interaction aspects of troleandomycin-steroid therapy, *J Allergy Clin Immunol* 69:455-460, 1982.
43. Bartoszek M, Brenner AM, Szefler SJ: Prednisolone and methylprednisolone kinetics in children receiving anticonvulsant therapy, *Clin Pharmacol Ther* 42:424-432, 1987.
44. Kamada AK, Hill MR, Brenner AM, Szefler SJ: Effect of low-dose troleandomycin on theophylline clearance: implications for therapeutic drug monitoring, *Pharmacotherapy* 12:98-102, 1992.
45. Weinberger M, Hudgel D, Spector S, Chidsey C: Inhibition of theophylline clearance by troleandomycin, *J Allergy Clin Immunol* 59:228-231, 1977.
46. Ball BD, Hill MR, Brenner M, Sanks R, Szefler: Effect of low-dose troleandomycin on glucocorticoid pharmacokinetics and airway hyperresponsiveness in severely asthmatic children, *Ann Allergy* 65:37-47, 1990.

47. LaForce CF, Szefler SJ, Miller MF, Ebling W, Brenner M: Inhibition of methylprednisolone elimination in the presence of erythromycin therapy, *J Allergy Clin Immunol* 72:34-39, 1983.
48. Martin LE, Hobson JC, Page JA, Harrison C: Metabolic studies of salbutamol ^{3}H: a new bronchodilator in rat, rabbit, dog and man, *Eur J Pharmacol* 14:183-199, 1971.
49. Staubus AE: Biopharmaceutics and pharmacokinetics: general principles. In Knoeben JE, Anderson PO, eds: *Clinical drug data,* ed 6, Hamilton, Ill, 1988, Drug Intelligence, pp 13-27.
50. Hendeles L, Weinberger M: Theophylline. In Middleton E Jr, Reed CE, Ellis EF, Adkinson NF Jr, Yuninger JW, Busse WW, eds: *Allergy: principles and practice,* ed 4, St Louis, 1993, Mosby, pp 816-855.
51. Dove AM, Szefler SJ, Hill MR, Jusko WJ, Larsen GL, Accurso FJ: Altered prednisolone pharmacokinetics in patients with cystic fibrosis, *J Pediatr* 120:789-794, 1992.
52. Kearns GL, Mallory GB Jr, Crom WR, Evans WE: Enhanced hepatic drug clearance in patients with cystic fibrosis, *J Pediatr* 117:972-979, 1990.
53. Butts JD, Secrest B, Berger R: Nonlinear theophylline pharmacokinetics: a preventable cause of iatrogenic theophylline toxic reactions, *Arch Intern Med* 151:2073-2077, 1991.

Receptor Pharmacology

54. Barnes PJ: Molecular biology of receptors, *Q J Med* 83:339-353, 1992 (review).
55. Emorine LJ, Marullo S, Briend-Sutren M-M, Patey G, Tate K, Delavier-Klutchko C, Strosberg AD: Molecular characterization of the human β_3-adrenergic receptor, *Science* 245:1118-1121, 1989.
56. Hedberg A, Kempf F, Josephson M, Molinoff PB: Coexistence of $beta_1$ and $beta_2$ adrenergic receptors in the human heart: effects of treatment with receptor antagonists or calcium entry blockers, *J Pharmacol Exp Ther* 234:561-568, 1985.
57. Fraser CM, Nelson HS, Middleton E Jr: Adrenergic agents. In Middleton E Jr, Reed CE, Ellis EF, Adkinson NF Jr, Yuninger JW, Busse WW, eds: *Allergy: principles and practice,* ed 4, St Louis, 1993, Mosby, pp 778-815.
58. Wang H-Y, Hadcock JR, Malbon CC: β-Adrenergic receptor regulation: new insights on biochemical and molecular mechanisms, *Receptor* 1:13-32, 1990 (review).
59. Samuelson WM, Davies AO: Hydrocortisone-induced reversal of β-adrenergic receptor uncoupling, *Am Rev Respir Dis* 130:1023-1026, 1984.
60. Hadcock JR, Malbon CC: Down-regulation of beta-adrenergic receptors: agonists induced reduction in receptor mRNA levels, *Proc Natl Acad Sci USA* 85:5021-5025, 1988.
61. Sears MR, Taylor DR, Print CG, Lake DC, Li Q, Flannery EM, Yates DM, Lucas MK, Herbison GP: Regular inhaled beta-agonist treatment in bronchial asthma, *Lancet* 336:1391-1396, 1990.
62. Spitzer WO, Suissa S, Ernst P, Horwitz RI, Habbick B, Cockroft D, Boivin J-F, McNutt M, Buist AS, Rebuck AS: The use of β-agonists and the risk of death and near death from asthma, *N Engl J Med* 326:501-506, 1992.
63. Barnes PJ: Beta-adrenoreceptors and asthma, *Clin Exp Allergy* 23:165-167, 1993 (editorial).
64. Heltianu C, Simionescu M, Simionescu N: Histamine receptors of the microvascular endothelium revealed *in situ* with a histamine-ferritin conjugate: characteristic high-affinity binding sites in venules, *J Cell Physiol* 93:357-364, 1982.
65. Townley RG, Daley D, Selenke W: The effects of corticosteroids on the β-adrenergic receptors in bronchial smooth muscle, *J Allergy* 45:118-125, 1970.
66. Geddes BA, Jones TR, Dvorsky RJ, Lefcoe NM: Interaction of glucocorticoids and bronchodilators on isolated guinea pig tracheal and human bronchial smooth muscle, *Am Rev Respir Dis* 110:420-427, 1974.
67. Dvorsky-Gebauer RJ: Potentiation of bronchodilators by glucocorticoids, *Lancet* 2:306-307, 1976.
68. Davies C, Conolly ME: Tachyphylaxis to β-adrenoreceptor agonists in human bronchial smooth muscles: studies *in vitro, Br J Clin Pharmacol* 40:417-423, 1980.
69. Lee TP, Reed CE: Effects of steroids on the regulation of the levels of cyclic AMP in human lymphocytes, *Biochem Biophys Res Commun* 78:998-1004, 1977.
70. Mano K, Akbarzadeh A, Townley RG: Effect of hydrocortisone on β-adrenergic receptors in lung membranes, *Life Sci* 25:1925-1930, 1979.
71. Fraser CM, Venter JC: The synthesis of β-adrenergic receptors in cultured human lung cells: induction by glucocorticoids, *Biochem Biophys Res Commun* 94:390-397, 1980.
72. Collins S, Caron MG, Lefkowitz RJ: β-Adrenergic receptors in smooth muscle cells are transcriptionally regulated by glucocorticoids, *J Biol Chem* 263:9067-9070, 1988.
73. Hadcock JR, Malbon CC: Regulation of β-adrenergic receptors by "permissive" hormones: glucocorticoids increase steady-state levels of receptor mRNA, *Proc Natl Acad Sci USA* 85:8415-8519, 1988.
74. Hui KK, Connolly ME, Tashkin DP: Reversal of human lymphocyte β-adrenoreceptor desensitization by glucocorticoids, *Clin Pharmacol Ther* 32:566-571, 1982.
75. Ellul-Micallef R, Fenech FF: Effect of intravenous prednisolone in asthmatics with diminished adrenergic responsiveness, *Lancet* 2:1269-1271, 1975.
76. Sando JJ, LaForest AC, Pratt WB: ATP-dependent activation of L-cell glucocorticoid receptors to the steroid binding form, *J Biol Chem* 254:4772-4778, 1979.
77. Sando JJ, Hammond ND, Stratford CA, Pratt WB: Activation of thymocyte glucocorticoid receptors to the steroid binding form, *J Biol Chem* 254:4779-4789, 1979.
78. Nielsen CJ, Sando JJ, Pratt WB: Evidence that dephosphorylation inactivates glucocorticoid receptors, *Proc Natl Acad Sci USA* 74:1398-1402, 1977.
79. Denis M, Wikström A-C, Gustaffson JA: The molybdate-stabilized nonactivated glucocorticoid receptor contains a dimer of Mr 90,000 non–hormone-binding protein, *J Biol Chem* 262:11803-11806, 1987.
80. Sanchez ER, Faber LE, Henzel WJ, Pratt WB: The 56-59-kilodalton protein identified in untransformed steroid receptor complexes is a unique protein that exists in cytosol in complex with both the 70- and 90-kilodalton heat shock proteins, *Biochemistry* 29:5145-5152, 1990.
81. Renoir JM, Radanyi C, Faber LE, Baulieu EE: The non–DNA-binding heterooligomeric form of mammalian steroid hormone receptors contains a hsp90-bound 59-kilodalton protein, *J Biol Chem* 265:10740-10745, 1990.
82. Joab I, Radanyi C, Renoir M, Buchou T, Catelli M-G, Binart N, Mester J, Baulieu E-E: Common, non–hormone binding component in nontransformed chick oviduct receptors of four steroid hormones, *Nature* 308:850-853, 1984.
83. Sanchez E, Toft DO, Schleisinger MJ, Pratt DB: Evidence that the 90-kDa phosphoprotein associated with the untransformed L-cell glucocorticoid receptor is a murine heat shock protein, *J Biol Chem* 260:12398-12401, 1985.
84. Nemoto T, Ohara-Nemoto Y, Denis M, Gustafsson J-Å: The transformed glucocorticoid receptor has a lower steroid-binding affinity than the nontransformed receptor, *Biochemistry* 29:1880-1886, 1990.
85. Muller M, Renkawitz R: The glucocorticoid receptor, *Biochem Biophys Acta* 1088:171-182, 1991 (review).
86. Salkowski CA, Vogel SN: IFN-γ increases glucocorticoid receptor expression in murine macrophages, *J Immunol* 148:2770-2777, 1992.
87. Salkowski CA, Vogel SN: Lipopolysaccharide increases glucocorticoid receptor expression in murine macrophages: a possible mechanism for glucocorticoid-mediated suppression of endotoxicity, *J Immunol* 149: 4041-4047, 1992.
88. Bodine PV, Litwack G: The glucocorticoid receptor and its endogenous regulators, *Receptor* 1:83-119, 1990.
89. Sher ER, Leung DYM, Surs W, Kam JC, Zeig G, Kamada AK, Harbeck R, Szefler SJ: Steroid resistant asthma: cellular mechanisms contributing to inadequate response to glucocorticoid therapy, *J Clin Invest* 93:33-39,1994.
90. Kam JC, Szefler SJ, Surs W, Sher ER, Leung DYM: Combination IL-2 and IL-4 reduces the glucocorticoid receptor binding affinity and T cell response to glucocorticoids, *J Immunol* 151:3460-3466,1993.

Pharmacodynamics

91. Boudinot FD, D'Ambrosio A, Jusko WJ: Receptor-mediated pharmacodynamics of prednisolone in the rat, *J Pharmacokinet Biopharm* 14:469-493, 1986.
92. Nichols AI, Boudinot FD, Jusko WJ: Second generation model for prednisolone pharmacodynamics in the rat, *J Pharmacokinet Biopharm* 17:209-227, 1989.

93. Oosterhuis B, Ten Berge IJM, Schellenkens PTA, Van Boxtel CJ: Concentration-dependent effects of prednisolone on lymphocyte subsets and mixed lymphocyte cultures in humans, *J Pharmacol Exp Ther* 243:716-722, 1987.
94. Reiss WG, Slaughter RL, Ludwig EA, Middleton E, Jusko WJ: Steroid dose sparing: pharmacodynamic responses to single vs. divided doses of methylprednisolone in man, *J Allergy Clin Immunol* 85:1058-1066, 1990.
95. Hummel S, Lehtonen L, Adolph J, Gronke K, Kandt D, Losbach H, Mohorn M, Possner S, Rabe U, Seelig U, Slapke J, Wenz W, Winterstein K-H, Glende M, Meiske W, Hirsjärvi-Lahti T: Comparison of oral-steroid sparing by high-dose and low-dose inhaled steroid in maintenance treatment of severe asthma, *Lancet* 340:1483-1487, 1992.
96. Bowler SD, Mitchell CA, Armstrong JG: Corticosteroids in acute severe asthma: effectiveness of low doses, *Thorax* 47:584-587, 1992.
97. Lai CKW, Chan CHS, Leung JCK, Lai K-N: Serum concentrations of soluble interleukin 2 receptors in asthma: correlation with disease activity, *Chest* 103:782-786, 1993.
98. Lasalle P, Sergant M, Delneste Y, Gosset P, Wallaert B, Zandecki M, Capron A, Joseph M, Tonnel AB: Levels of soluble IL-2 receptor in plasma from asthmatics: correlations with blood eosinophilia, lung function, and corticosteroid therapy, *Clin Exp Immunol* 87:266-271, 1992.
99. Fahy JV, Lui J, Wong H, Boushey HA: Cellular and biochemical analysis of induced sputum from asthmatic and from healthy subjects, *Am Rev Respir Dis* 147:1126-1131, 1993.
100. Virchow J-C Jr, Hage U, Kortsik C, Matthys H, Kroegel C: Sputum ECP levels distiguish between broncial asthma and COPD, *J Allergy Clin Immunol* 91:179, 1993 (abstract).
101. Tomassini M, Magrini L, De Petrillo G, Adriani E, Bonini S: Serum levels of eosinophil cationic protein and allergen exposure, *J Allergy Clin Immunol* 91:180, 1993 (abstract).

Drug Action

102. American Thoracic Society Committee on Diagnostic Standards for Nontuberculous Respiratory Diseases: Definitions and classification of chronic bronchitis, asthma and pulmonary emphysema, *Am Rev Respir Dis* 85:762-768, 1962.
103. Rall TW: Drugs used in the treatment of asthma: the methylxanthines, cromolyn sodium, and other agents. In Goodman AG, Rall TW, Nies AS, Taylor P: *Goodman and Gilman's the pharmacologic basis of therapeutics,* ed 8, New York, 1990, Pergamon, pp 618-637.
104. Pauwels R, Van Renterghem D, Van Der Straeten M, Johannesson N, Persson CGA: The effect of theophylline and enprofylline on allergen-induced bronchoconstriction, *J Allergy Clin Immunol* 76:583-590, 1985.
105. Martin GL, Atkins PC, Dunsky EH, Zweiman B: Effects of theophylline, terbutaline, and prednisone on antigen-induced bronchospasm and mediator release, *J Allergy Clin Immunol* 66:204-212, 1980.
106. Cockroft DW, Murdock KY, Gore BP, O'Byrne PM, Manning P: Theophylline does not inhibit allergen-induced increase in airway hyperresponsiveness to methacholine, *J Allergy Clin Immunol* 83:913-920, 1989.
107. Magnussen H, Reuss G, Jörres R: Theophylline has a dose-related effect on the airway response to inhaled histamine and methacholine in asthmatics, *Am Rev Respir Dis* 136:1163-1167, 1987.
108. McWilliams BC, Menendez R, Kelley HW, Howick J: Effects of theophylline on inhaled methacholine and histamine in asthmatic children, *Am Rev Respir Dis* 130:193-197, 1984.
109. Simons FER, Soni NR, Watson WTA, Becker AB: Bronchodilator and bronchoprotective effects of salmeterol in young patients with asthma, *J Allergy Clin Immunol* 90:840-846, 1992.
110. Ullman A, Svedmyr N: Salmeterol, a new long acting inhaled β-2-adrenoreceptor agonist: a comparison with salbutamol, *Thorax* 43:674-678, 1988.
111. Midgren B, Melander B, Perrson G: Formoterol, a new, long-acting β_2 agonist, inhaled twice daily, in stable asthmatic subjects, *Chest* 101: 1019-1022, 1992.
112. Johnson M: The pharmacology of salmeterol, *Lung* 168(suppl):115-119, 1990.
113. Lötvall J, Lunde H, Ullman A, Törnqvist H, Svedmyr N: Twelve months, treatment with inhaled salmeterol in asthmatic patients: effects on β_2-receptor function and inflammatory cells, *Allergy* 47:477-483, 1992.
114. Cockcroft DW, Murdock KY: Comparative effects of inhaled salbutamol, sodium cromoglycate and beclomethasone dipropionate on allergen-induced early asthmatic responses, late asthmatic responses, and increased bronchial hyperresponsiveness, *J Allergy Clin Immunol* 79:734-740, 1987.
115. Booij-Noord H, Orie NGM, De Vries K: Immediate and late bronchial obstructive reactions to inhalation of house dust and protective effects of disodium cromoglycate and prednisolone, *J Allergy Clin Immunol* 48:344-354, 1971.
116. Crimi N, Palermo F, Oliveri R, Cacopardo B, Vandieri C, Mistretta A: Adenosine-induced bronchoconstriction: comparison between nedocromil sodium and sodium cromoglycate, *Eur J Respir Dis 69*(suppl 147):258-262, 1986.
117. del Bono L, Dente FL, Patalano F, del Bono N: Protective effect of nedocromil sodium and sodium cromoglycate on bronchospasm induced by cold air, *Eur J Respir Dis 69*(suppl 147):268-270, 1986.
118. Bauer CP: The protective effect of nedocromil sodium in exercise-induced asthma, *Eur J Respir Dis 69*(suppl 147):252-254, 1986.
119. Crimi E, Brusasco V, Brancantisano M, Losurdo E, Crimi P: Adenosine-induced bronchoconstriction: premedication with chlorpheniramine and nedocromil sodium, *Eur J Respir Dis 69*(suppl 147):255-257, 1986.
120. Dahl R, Pederson B: Influence of nedocromil sodium on the dual airway response after allergen challenge: a double-blind, placebo-controlled study, *Eur J Respir Dis 69*(suppl 147):263-265, 1986.
121. Rebelić: M: Nedocromil sodium and exercise induced asthma in adolescents, *Eur J Respir Dis 69*(suppl 147):266-267, 1986.
122. Gross NJ: Ipratropium bromide, *N Engl J Med* 319:486-494, 1988 (review).
123. Postma DS, Keyzer JJ, Koeter GH, Sluiter HJ, De Vries K: Influence of parasympathetic and sympathetic nervous systems on nocturnal asthma, *Clin Sci* 69:281-288, 1985.
124. Newcomb R, Tashkin DP, Hui KK, Conolly ME, Lee E, Dauphinee B: Rebound hyperresponsiveness to muscarinic stimulation after chronic therapy with an inhaled muscarinic antagonist, *Am Rev Respir Dis* 132:12-15, 1985.
125. Barnes PJ: A new approach to the treatment of asthma, *N Engl J Med* 321:1517-1527, 1989 (review).
126. Sertl K, Clark T, Kaliner M: Corticosteroids: their biologic mechanisms and application to the treatment of asthma, *Am Rev Respir Dis* 141(suppl):S1-S96, 1990.
127. Juniper EF, Frith PA, Hargreave FE: Airway responsiveness to histamine and methacholine: relationship to minimum treatment to control symptoms of asthma, *Thorax* 36:575-579, 1981.
128. Murray AB, Ferguson AC, Morrison B: Airway responsiveness to histamine as a test for overall severity of asthma, *J Allergy Clin Immunol* 68:119-124, 1981.
129. Hargreave FE, Ryan G, Thomson NC, O'Byrne PM, Latimer K, Juniper EF, Dolovich J: Bronchial responsiveness to histamine or methacholine in asthma: measurement and clinical significance, *J Allergy Clin Immunol* 68:347-355, 1981 (review).
130. Busse WW: Respiratory infections: their role in airway responsiveness and the pathogenesis of asthma, *J Allergy Clin Immunol* 85:671-683, 1990 (review).
131. Platts-Mills TAE, Tovey ER, Mitchell EB, Moszoro H, Nock P, Wilkins SR: Reduction of bronchial hyperreactivity during prolonged allergen avoidance, *Lancet* 2:675-678, 1982.
132. Boulet L-P, Cartier A, Thomson NC, Roberts RS, Dolovich J, Hargreave FE: Asthma and increases in nonallergic bronchial responsiveness from seasonal pollen exposure, *J Allergy Clin Immunol* 71:399-406, 1983.
133. Szefler SJ: Anti-inflammatory drugs in the treatment of allergic disease, *Med Clin North Am* 76:953-975, 1992 (review).
134. Djukanović: R, Wilson JW, Britten KM, Wilson SJ, Walls AF, Roche WR, Howarth PH, Holgate ST: Effect of an inhaled corticosteroid on airway inflammation and symptoms of asthma, *Am Rev Respir Dis* 145:669-674, 1992.
135. Laitinen LA, Laitinen A, Haahtela T: A comparative study of the effects of an inhaled corticosteroid, budesonide, and a β_2-agonist, terbutaline, on airway inflammation in newly diagnosed asthma: a randomized double-blind, parallel-group controlled trial, *J Allergy Clin Immunol* 90:32-42, 1992.

136. Burks C, Power CK, Norris A, Condez A, Schmekel B, Poulter LW: Lung function and immunopathological changes after inhaled corticosteroid therapy in asthma, *Eur Respir J* 5:73-79, 1992.
137. Duddridge M, Ward C, Hendrick DJ, Walters EH: Changes in bronchoalveolar lavage inflammatory cells in asthmatic patients treated with high dose inhaled beclomethasone dipropionate, *Eur Respir J* 6:489-497, 1993.
138. Van De Graaf EA, Out TA, Roos CM, Jansen HM: Respiratory membrane permeability and bronchial hyperreactivity in patients with stable asthma: effects of therapy with inhaled steroids, *Am Rev Respir Dis* 143:362-368, 1991.
139. Boschetto P, Rogers DF, Fabbri LM, Barnes PJ: Corticosteroid inhibition of airway microvascular leakage, *Am Rev Respir Dis* 143:605-609, 1991.

Chronopharmacology

140. Calhoun WJ, Bates ME, Schrader L, Sedgwick JB, Busse WW: Characteristics of peripheral blood eosinophils in patients with nocturnal asthma, *Am Rev Respir Dis* 145:577-581, 1992.
141. Dahl R: Diurnal variation in the number of circulatory eosinophil leukocytes in normal controls and asthmatics, *Acta Allergol* 32:301-303, 1977.
142. Martin RJ, Cicutto LC, Ballard RD: Factors related to the nocturnal worsening of asthma, *Am Rev Respir Dis* 141:33-38, 1990.
143. Szefler SJ, Ando R, Cicutto LC, Surs W, Hill MR, Martin RJ: Plasma histamine, epinephrine, cortisol, and leukocyte β-adrenergic receptors in nocturnal asthma, *Clin Pharmacol Ther* 49:59-68, 1991.
144. Martin RJ, Cicutto LC, Smith HR, Ballard RD, Szefler SJ: Airways inflammation in nocturnal asthma, *Am Rev Respir Dis* 143:351-357, 1991.
145. Reinberg A, Halberg F, Falliers CF: Circadian timing of methylprednisolone effects in asthma boys, *Chronobiologica* 1:333-347, 1974.
146. Reinberg A, Gervais P, Choussade M, Fraboulet G, Duburgue B: Circadian changes in the effectiveness of corticosteroids in eight patients with allergic asthma, *J Allergy Clin Immunol* 71:425-433, 1983.
147. Martin RJ, Cicutto LC, Ballard RD, Goldenheim PD, Cherniak RM: Circadian variations in theophylline concentrations and the treatment of nocturnal asthma, *Am Rev Respir Dis* 139:475-478, 1989.
148. D'Alonzo GE, Smolensky MH, Feldman S, Gianotti LA, Emerson MB, Staudinger H, Steinijans VW: Twenty-four hour lung function in adult patients with asthma: chronoptimized theophylline therapy once-daily dosing in the evening vs. conventional twice-daily dosing, *Am Rev Respir Dis* 142:84-90, 1990.
149. Beam WR, Weiner DE, Martin RJ: Timing of prednisone and alterations of airways inflammation in nocturnal asthma, *Am Rev Respir Dis* 146:1524-1530, 1992.

Age-Related Changes

150. Thurlbeck WM: Growth, aging, and adaptation. In Murray JF, Nadel JA, eds: *Textbook of respiratory medicine,* Philadelphia, 1988, WB Saunders, pp 37-46.
151. Boreus LO: *Principles of pediatric clinical pharmacology,* New York, 1982, Churchill Livingstone.
152. Besunder JB, Reed M, Blumer JL: Principles of drug biodisposition in the neonate: a critical evaluation of the pharmacokinetic-pharmacodynamic interface, *Clin Pharmacokinet* 14:189-216, 1983.
153. Milsap RL, Hill MR, Szefler SJ: Special pharmacokinetic considerations in children. In Evans WE, Schentag JJ, Jusko WJ, eds: *Applied pharmacokinetics: principles of therapeutic drug monitoring,* ed 3, Vancouver, Wash, 1992, Applied Therapeutics, pp 10-1-10-32.
154. Heimann G: Enteral absorption and bioavailability in children in relation to age, *Eur J Clin Pharmacol* 18:43-50, 1980.
155. Signer E, Fridirich R: Gastric emptying in newborns and young infants, *Acta Pediatr Scand* 64:525-530, 1975.
156. Murphy GM, Signer E: Progress report: bile acid metabolism in infants and children, *Gut* 15:151-163, 1974.
157. Morselli PL: Clinical pharmacokinetics in neonates, *Clin Pharmacokinet* 1:81-91, 1976.
158. Tserng KY, King KC, Takieddine FN: Theophylline metabolism in premature infants, *Clin Pharmacol Ther* 29:594-600, 1981.

New Drugs on the Horizon

159. Beach JR, Young CL, Stenton SC, Avery AJ, Walters EH, Hendrick DJ: A comparison of the speeds of action of salmeterol and salbutamol in reversing methacholine-induced bronchoconstriction, *Pulmonol Pharmacol* 5:133-135, 1992.
160. Pearlman DS, Chervinsky P, LaForce C, Seltzer JM, Southern DL, Kemp JP, Dockhorn RJ, Grossman J, Liddle RF, Yancey SW, Cocchetto DM, Alexander WJ, Van As A: A comparison of salmeterol with albuterol in the treatment of mild-to-moderate asthma, *N Engl J Med* 327:1420-1425, 1992.
161. Brattsand R, Thalen R, Roempke K, Gruvstad E: Development of new glucocorticosteroids with a very high ratio between topical and systemic activities, *Eur J Respir Dis* 63(suppl 122):62-73, 1982.
162. Johansson S-Å, Andersson K-E, Brattsand R, Gruvstad E, Hedner P: Topical and systemic glucocorticoid potencies of budesonide and beclomethasone dipropionate in man, *Eur J Clin Pharmacol* 22:523-529, 1982.
163. Brattsand R, Axelsson BI: New inhaled glucocorticosteroids. In Barnes PJ, ed: *New drugs for asthma,* ed 2, London, 1992, IBC Technical Services, pp 193-208.
164. Barnes PJ: New drugs for asthma, *Eur Respir J* 5:1126-1136, 1992 (review).
165. Richards IM, Shields SK, Griffin RL, Fidler SF, Dunn CJ: Novel steroid-based inhibitors of lung inflammation, *Clin Exp Allergy* 22:432-439, 1992 (review).
166. Thomson NC: Nedocromil sodium: an overview, *Respir Med* 83:269-276, 1989 (review).
167. Dahlen SE, Hansson G, Hedqvist P, Bjorck T, Gramstrom E, Dahlen B: Allergen challenge of lung tissue from asthmatics elicits bronchial contraction that correlates with the release of leukotrienes C4, D4 and E4, *Proc Natl Acad Sci USA* 80:1712-1716, 1983.
168. Drazen JM, Austen KF: Leukotrienes and airway responses, *Am Rev Respir Dis* 136:985-988, 1987.
169. Expert Panel Report 2, National Asthma Education and Prevention Program: *Guidelines for the diagnosis and management of asthma,* Pub No 97-4051, Bethesda, Md, 1997, US Department of Health and Human Services, National Institutes of Health, National Heart, Lung, and Blood Institute.
170. Bianco S, Vaghi A, Robuschi M, Pasargiklian M: Prevention of exercise-induced bronchoconstriction by inhaled frusemide, *Lancet* 2:252-255, 1988.
171. Bianco S, Pieroni MG, Refini RM, Rottoli L, Sestini P: Protective effect of inhaled furosemide on allergen-induced early and late asthmatic reactions, *N Engl J Med* 321:1069-1073, 1990.
172. Verdiani P, Di Stefania C, Baronti A, Bianco S: Protective effect of inhaled furosemide on the early response to antigen and subsequent change in airway reactivity in atopic patients, *Thorax* 45:377-381, 1990.
173. Grubbe RE, Hopp R, Dave NK, Brennan B, Bewtra A, Townley R: Effect of inhaled furosemide on the bronchial response to methacholine and cold air hyperventilation challenges, *J Allergy Clin Immunol* 85:881-884, 1990.
174. Nichol GM, Alton EW, Nix A, Geddes DM, Chung KF, Barnes PJ: Effect of inhaled furosemide on metabisulfite- and methacholine-induced bronchoconstriction and nasal potential difference in asthmatic subjects, *Am Rev Respir Dis* 142:576-580, 1990.
175. Bianco S, Pieroni MG, Refini RM, Robuschi M, Vaghi A, Sestini P: Inhaled loop diuretics as potential new anti-asthma drugs, *Eur Respir J* 6:130-134, 1993 (review).
176. Giembycz MA, Dent G: Prospects for selective cyclic nucleotide phosphodiesterase inhibitors in the treatment of bronchial asthma, *Clin Exp Allergy* 22:337-344, 1992 (review).
177. Torphy TJ, Undem BJ: Phosphodiesterase inhibitors: new opportunities for the treatment of asthma, *Thorax* 46:512-523, 1991 (review).
178. Szefler SJ: Alternative therapy in severe asthma: rationale and guidelines for applications (review), Update No 11. In Middleton E Jr, Reed CE, Ellis EF, Adkinson NF Jr, Yuninger JW, eds: *Allergy principles and practice,* ed 3, St Louis, 1991, Mosby, pp 1-14.

Innovative Strategies for the Future

179. Corrigan CJ, Kay AB: T cell and eosinophils in the pathogenesis of asthma, *Immunol Today* 13:501-507, 1992 (review).

180. Kelly CA, Stenton SC, Ward C, Bird G, Hendrick DJ, Walters EH: Lymphocyte subsets in bronchoalveolar lavage fluid obtained from stable asthmatics, and their correlations with bronchial responsiveness, *Clin Exp Allergy* 19:169-175, 1988.
181. Corrigan CJ, Kay AB: CD4 T-lymphocyte activation in acute severe asthma: relationship to disease severity and atopic status, *Am Rev Respir Dis* 141:970-977, 1990.
182. Bradley BL, Azzawi M, Jacobson M, Assooufi B, Collins JV, Irani A-MA, Schwartz LB, Durham SR, Jeffery PK, Kay AB: Eosinophils, T-lymphocytes, mast cells, neutrophils, and macrophages in bronchial biopsy specimens from atopic subjects with asthma: comparison with biopsy specimens from atopic subjects without asthma and normal control subjects and relationship to bronchial hyperresponsiveness, *J Allergy Clin Immunol* 88:661-674, 1991.
183. Walker C, Kaegi MK, Braun P, Blaser K: Activated T cells and eosinophilia in bronchoalveolar lavages from subjects with asthma correlated with disease severity, *J Allergy Clin Immunol* 88:935-942, 1991.
184. Robinson DS, Bentley AM, Hartnell A, Kay AB, Durham SR: Activated memory T helper cells in bronchoalveolar lavage fluid from patients with atopic asthma: relation to asthma symptoms, lung function, and bronchial responsiveness, *Thorax* 48:26-32, 1993.
185. Azzawi M, Johnston PW, Majumdar S, Kay AB, Jeffery PK: T lymphocytes and activated eosinophils in airway mucosa in fatal asthma and cystic fibrosis, *Am Rev Respir Dis* 145:1477-1482, 1992.
186. Ward AJM, McKenniff M, Evans JM, Page CP, Costello JF: Theophylline: an immunomodulatory role in asthma? *Am Rev Respir Dis* 147:518-523, 1993.
187. Kidney J, Dominguez M, Taylor PM, Rose M, Chung KF, Barnes PJ: Immunomodulation by theophylline in asthma: demonstration by withdrawal of therapy, *Am J Respir Crit Care Med* 151:1907-1914, 1995.
188. Robinson DS, Hamid Q, Ying S, Tsicopoulos A, Barkans J, Bentley AM, Corrigan C, Durham SR, Kay AB: Predominant T_{H2}-like bronchoalveolar T-lymphocyte population in atopic asthma, *N Engl J Med* 326:298-304, 1992.
189. Bellini A, Vittori E, Marini M, Ackerman V, Mattoli S: Intraepithelial dendritic cells and selective activation of Th2-like lymphocytes in patients with atopic asthma, *Chest* 103:997-1005, 1993.
190. Morley J: Cyclosporin A in asthma therapy: a pharmacological rationale, *J Autoimmunol* 5(suppl A):265-269, 1992.
191. Cyclosporin in chronic severe asthma, *Lancet* 339:338-339, 1992 (editorial).
192. Calderón E, Lockey RF, Bukantz SC, Coffey RG, Ledford DK: Is there a role for cyclosporine in asthma? *J Allergy Clin Immunol* 89:629-636, 1992.
193. Lapa e Silva JR, Baker D, Scheper RJ, Vargaftig BB, Pretolani M: Effects of FK-506 and nedocromil sodium on the bronchial inflammatory infiltrate of actively sensitized guinea pigs, *Am Rev Respir Dis* 147:A65, 1993 (abstract).
194. Nizankowska E, Soja J, Pinis G, Bochenek G, Sladek K, Domagala B, Pajak A, Szczeklik A: Treatment of steroid-dependent asthma with cyclosporin, *Am Rev Respir Dis* 147:A294, 1993 (abstract).
195. Elwood W, Lötvall JO, Barnes PJ, Chung KF: Effect of dexamethasone and cyclosporin A on allergen-induced airway hyperresponsiveness and inflammatory cell responses in sensitized Brown-Norway rats, *Am Rev Respir Dis* 145:1289-1294, 1992.
196. Yukawa T, Arima M, Terashi Y, Sagara H, Makino S: The effect of inhaled cyclosporine A on allergen-induced late asthmatic response and increase of airway hyperresponsiveness in guinea pig experimental models of asthma, *Am Rev Respir Dis* 145:A420, 1992 (abstract).
197. Finnerty N, Sullivan TJ: Effect of cyclosporine on corticosteroid dependent asthma, *Allergy Clin Immunol* 87:297, 1991 (abstract).
198. Alexander AG, Barnes NC, Kay AB: Trial of cyclosporin in corticosteroid-dependent chronic severe asthma, *Lancet* 339:324-328, 1992.
199. Szczeklik A, Nizankowska E, Dworski R, Domagala B, Pinis G: Cyclosporin for steroid-dependent asthma, *Allergy* 46:312-315, 1991.
200. Zaragoza RH, Medina LM, Hill MR: Cyclosporin-A effects on the regulation of neutrophils adhesion molecules, *J Allergy Clin Immunol* 91:215, 1993 (abstract).
201. Zaragoza RH, Medina LM, Young SK, Hill MR: Potential anti-inflammatory effects of cyclosporin A, *J Allergy Clin Immunol* 89:287, 1992 (abstract).
202. Calderón E, Lockey RF: A possible role for adhesion molecules in asthma, *J Allergy Clin Immunol* 90:852-865, 1992 (review).
203. Springer TA: Adhesion receptors of the immune system, *Nature* 346:425-434, 1990 (review).
204. Adhesion molecules in the diagnosis and treatment of inflammatory disease, *Lancet* 336:1351-1352, 1990.
205. Ando N, Fukuda T, Nakajima H, Makino S: Expression of intercellular adhesion molecule-1 (ICAM-1) is upregulated in the bronchial mucosa of symptomatic asthmatics, *J Allergy Clin Immunol* 89:214, 1992 (abstract).
206. Pacheco K, Dresback J, Rosenwasser L: Upregulation of adhesion molecules by allergen challenged T cells from blood and BAL, *J Allergy Clin Immunol* 91:185, 1993 (abstract).
207. Thompson HL, Burbelo PD, Segui-Real B, Yamada Y, Metcalfe DD: Laminin promotes mast cell attachment, *J Immunol* 146:2323-2327, 1989.
208. Rothlein R, Czajkowski M, O'Neill MM, Marlin SD, Mainolfi E, Merluzzi VJ: Induction of intercellular adhesion molecule 1 on primary and continuous cell lines by pro-inflammatory cytokines, *J Immunol* 141:1665-1669, 1988.
209. Petzelbauer P, Stingl G, Wolff K, Volc-Platzer B: Cyclosporin A suppresses ICAM-1 expression by papillary endothelium in healing psoriatic plaques, *J Invest Dermatol* 96:362-369, 1991.
210. Cronstein BN, Eberle MA, Gruber H, Levin RI: A novel antiinflammatory action of methotrexate (MTX): MTX increases adenosine release from connective tissue cells and thereby inhibits neutrophil (PMN) function, *FASEB* J 5:A510, 1991 (abstract).
211. Corkill MM, Krikham BW, Haskard DO, Barbatis C, Gibson T, Panayi GS: Gold treatment of rheumatoid arthritis decreases synovial expression of the endothelial leukocyte adhesion receptor ELAM-1, *J Rheumatol* 18:1453-1460, 1991.
212. Tizzano EF, Buchwald M: Cystic fibrosis: beyond the gene to therapy, *J Pediatr* 120:337-349, 1992 (review).
213. Coutelle C, Caplen N, Hart S, Huxley C, Williamson R: Gene therapy for cystic fibrosis, *Arch Dis Child* 68:437-443, 1993 (review).
214. Koch C, Høiby N: Pathogenesis of cystic fibrosis, *Lancet* 341:1065-1069, 1993 (review).
215. Culver KW, Anderson WF, Blaese RM: Lymphocyte gene therapy, *Human Gene Ther* 2:107-109, 1991.
216. Collins FS: Cystic fibrosis: molecular biology and therapeutic implications, *Science* 286:774-779, 1992.
217. Rosenfeld MA, Yoshimura K, Trapnell BC, Yoneyama K, Rosenthal ER, Dalemans W, Fukayama M, Bargon J, Stier LE, Stratford-Perricaudet L, Perricaudet M, Guggio WB, Pavirani A, Lecocq J-P, Crystal RG: In vivo transfer of the human cystic fibrosis transmembrane conductance regulator gene to the airway epithelium, *Cell* 68:143-155, 1992.
218. Hardy CC, Robinson C, Tattersfield AE, Holgate ST: The bronchoconstrictor effect of inhaled prostaglandin D_2 in normal and asthmatic men, *N Engl J Med* 311:209-213, 1984.
219. Fish JE, Jameson LS, Albright A, Norman PS: Modulation of the bronchomotor effects of chemical mediators by prostaglandin F_{2a} in asthmatic subjects, *Am Rev Respir Dis* 130:571-574, 1984.
220. Fuller RW, Dixon CMS, Dollery CT, Barnes PJ: Prostaglandin D_2 potentiates airway responsiveness to histamine and methacholine, *Am Rev Respir Dis* 133:252-254, 1986.
221. Kleeberger SR, Kolbe J, Adkinson NF Jr, Peters SP, Spannhake EW: Thromboxane contributes to the immediate antigenic response of canine peripheral airways, *J Appl Physiol* 63:1589-1595, 1987.
222. Chung KF, Aizawa H, Becker AB, Frick O, Gold WM, Nadel JA: Inhibition of antigen-induced airway hyperresponsiveness by a thromboxane synthetase inhibitor (OKY 046) in allergic dogs, *Am Rev Respir Dis* 134:258-261, 1986.
223. Barnes PJ, Chung KF, Page CP: Platelet activating factor as a mediator of allergic disease, *J Allergy Clin Immunol* 81:919-934, 1988 (review).
224. Jenkins JS, Sampson PA: Conversion of cortisone to cortisol and prednisone to prednisolone, *Br Med J* 2:205-207, 1967.
225. Rose JQ, Yurchak AM, Jusko WJ: Dose dependent pharmacokinetics of prednisone and prednisolone in man, *J Pharmacokinet Biopharm* 9:389-417, 1981.
226. Ryerfeldt A, Nilsson E, Tunek A, Svensson LA: Bambuterol: uptake and metabolism in guinea pig isolated lung, *Pharm Res* 5:151-155, 1988.

227. Tunek A, Svennson LA: Bambuterol, a carbamate ester of terbutaline, as inhibitor of cholinesterases in human blood, *Drug Metabol Dispos* 16:759-764, 1988.
228. Tunek A, Levin E, Svennson LA: Hydrolysis of 3H-bambuterol, a carbamate prodrug of terbutaline, in blood from humans and laboratory animal in vitro, *Biochem Pharmacol* 37:3867-3876, 1988.
229. Holstein-Rathlou NH, Laursen LC, Madsen F, Svendsen UG, Gnosspelius Y, Weeke B: Bambuterol: dose response study of a new terbutaline prodrug in asthma, *Eur J Clin Pharmacol* 30:7-11, 1986.
230. Sitar DS, Warren CP, Aoki FY: Pharmacokinetics and pharmacodynamics of bambuterol, a long-acting bronchodilator pro-drug of terbutaline, in young and elderly patients with asthma, *Clin Pharmacol Ther* 52:297-306, 1992.
231. Sitar DS, Aoki FY, Warren CP, Knight A, Grossman RF, Alexander M, Soliman S: A placebo-controlled dose-finding study with bambuterol in elderly patients with asthma, *Chest* 103:771-776, 1993.
232. Newman SP, Weisz AWB, Talaee N, Clarke SW: Improvement of drug delivery with a breath actuated pressurized aerosol for patients with poor inhaler technique, *Thorax* 46:712-716, 1991.
233. Mercer TT: Production of therapeutic aerosol: principles and techniques, *Chest* 80(suppl):813-818, 1981 (review).
234. Lourenço RV, Cotromanes E: Clinical Aerosols. I. Characterization of aerosols and their diagnostic uses, *Arch Intern Med* 142:2163-2172, 1982 (review).
235. Gilbert BE, Wyde PR, Wilson SZ: Aerosolized liposomal amphotericin B for treatment of pulmonary and systemic Cryptococcus neoformans infections in mice, *Antimicrob Agents Chemother* 36:1466-1471, 1992.
236. Gilbert BE, Six HR, Wilson SZ, Wyde PR, Knight V: Small particle aerosols of enviroxime-containing liposomes, *Antivir Res* 9:355-365, 1988.
237. Vadiei K, Lopez-Bernstein G, Perez-Soler R, Luke DR: In vitro evaluation of liposomal cyclosporin, *Int J Pharmaceut* 57:133-138, 1989.
238. Littlewood JM, Smye SW, Cunliffe H: Aerosol antibiotic treatment in cystic fibrosis, *Arch Dis Child* 68:788-792, 1993.
239. Ramsey BW, Dorkin HL, Eisenberg JD, Gibson RL, Harwood IR, Kravitz RM, Schidlow DV, Wilmott RW, Astley SJ, McBrunie MA, Wentz K, Smith AL: Efficacy of aerosolized tobramycin in patients with cystic fibrosis, *N Engl J Med* 328:1740-1746, 1993.
240. Goldman JM, Boyston SM, O'Connor S, Meigh RE: Inhaled micronised gentamicin powder: a new delivery system, *Thorax* 45:939-940, 1990.

APPENDIXES

The following appendixes list inhaled medications that are commonly used to treat pediatric respiratory disorders.

Appendix 18-1 Recommended Doses for β-Adrenergic Agonists*

FORMULATION	DOSAGE	COMMENTS
For acute exacerbations		
Albuterol		
Metered dose inhaler (90 μg/actuation)	2 actuations inhaled every 5 min for a total of 12 actuations	Response should be monitored via peak flows or spirometry; if improved, dosage is decreased to 4 actuations every hr; if not improved, patient should switch to nebulizer.
Nebulizer solution, 0.5% (5 mg/ml)	0.10-0.15 mg/kg/dose up to 5 mg inhaled every 20 min for 1-2 hr; minimum dose: 1.25 mg	If improved, dosage should be decreased to 1 treatment every 1-2 hr; if not improved, continuous inhalation should be used.
	0.5 mg/kg/hr by continuous nebulization, maximum dosage: 15 mg/hr	—
Metaproterenol		
Metered dose inhaler (650 μg/actuation)	2 actuations inhaled	Frequent high-dose administration has not been evaluated; not interchangeable with albuterol or terbutaline.
Nebulizer solution, 5% (50 mg/ml)	0.1-0.3 ml (5-15 mg) inhaled via nebulizer	Dose should not exceed 15 mg.
Terbutaline		
Metered dose inhaler (200 μg/actuation)	2 actuations inhaled every 5 min for a total of 12 actuations	—
Injectable solution, 0.1% (1 mg/ml) in 0.9% sodium chloride	0.01 mg/kg up to 0.3 mg injected subcutaneously every 2-6 hr as needed	Inhaled bronchodilator is preferred.
	10 μg/kg intravenously over 10 min as loading dose, then 0.4 μg/min increased as needed by 0.2 μg/min	Inhaled bronchodilator is preferred; final maintenance dosage should be 3-6 μg/kg/min.
Epinephrine		
Injectable solution 1:1000 (1 mg/ml)	0.01 mg/kg up to 0.3 mg injected subcutaneously every 20 min for a total of 3 doses	Inhaled bronchodilator is preferred.
For chronic therapy		
Albuterol		
Metered dose inhaler (90 μg/actuation)	2 actuations inhaled every 4-6 hr	—
Dry powdered inhaler (200 μg/capsule)	Contents of one capsule inhaled every 4-6 hr	—
Nebulizer solution, 0.5% (5 mg/ml)	0.10-0.15 mg/kg up to 5 mg in 2 ml 0.9% sodium chloride inhaled via	—

From National Asthma Education Program, Expert Panel Report: *Guidelines for the diagnosis and management of asthma,* Pub No 91-3042, Bethesda, Md, 1991, United States Department of Health and Human Services, Public Health Service, National Institutes of Health, National Heart, Lung and Blood Institute; and *Drug facts and comparisons,* 1993, St Louis, 1993, Facts & Comparisons.

*Doses should be adjusted if used in children outside the indicated age ranges.

Appendix 18-1 Recommended Doses for β-Adrenergic Agonists*—cont'd

FORMULATION	DOSAGE	COMMENTS
For chronic therapy—cont'd		
Albuterol—cont'd		
Oral syrup	0.1-0.2 mg/kg orally every 8 hr, maximum: 12 mg/day (2-6 yr)	—
	2 mg orally every 6-8 hr, maximum: 24 mg/day (6-14 yr)	—
	2-4 mg orally every 6-8 hr, maximum: 32 mg/day (≥12 yr)	—
Oral tablet, plain	2 mg orally every 6-8 hr, maximum: 24 mg/day (6-12 yr)	—
Oral tablet, extended release	4-8 mg orally every 12 hr, maximum: 32 mg/day (≥12 yr)	—
Bitolterol		
Metered dose inhaler (370 μg/actuation)	2 actuations inhaled every 8 hr, maximum: 2 treatments in 4 hr or 3 treatments in 6 hr (>12 yr)	—
Nebulizer solution 0.2% (2 mg/ml)	0.50-0.75 ml (1.0-1.5 mg) inhaled via nebulizer every 4-6 hr, maximum: 8 mg/day (>12 yr)	—
Pirbuterol		
Metered dose inhaler (650 μg/actuation)	2 actuations inhaled every 4-6 hr, maximum: 12 actuations/day (≥12yr)	—
Metaproterenol		
Metered dose inhaler (650 μg/actuation)	2-3 actuations inhaled every 6-8 hr (>12 yr)	—
Nebulizer solution, 5% (50 mg/ml)	0.2-0.3 ml (10-15 mg) in 2.5 ml 0.9% sodium chloride inhaled via nebulizer every 6-8 hr (>12 yr)	—
Oral syrup	1.3-2.6 mg/kg/day orally divided over 6-8 hr (>6 yr)	—
	10 mg orally every 6-8 hr (6-9 yr)	—
	20 mg orally every 6-8 hr (>9 yr)	—
Salmeterol		
Metered dose inhaler (25 μg/actuation)	2 actuations inhaled every 12 hr (≥12 yr)	—
Terbutaline		
Metered dose inhaler (200 μg/actuation)	2 actuations inhaled every 4-6 hr (≥12 yr)	—
Oral tablet	2.5 mg orally every 8 hr, maximum: 7.5 mg/day (12-15 yr)	
	2.5-5.0 mg orally every 6 hr, maximum: 15 mg/day (>15 yr)	—

Appendix 18-2 Estimated Comparative Daily Doses for Inhaled Corticosteroids in Children

DRUG	LOW DOSE	MEDIUM DOSE	HIGH DOSE
Beclomethasone dipropionate (42, 84 μg/actuation)	84-336 μg	336-672 μg	>672
Budesonide (Turbuhaler) (200 μg/actuation)	100-200 μg	200-400 μg	>400 μg
Flunisolide (250 μg/actuation)	500-750 μg	1000-1250 μg	>1250 μg
Fluticasone propionate (44, 100, 220 μg/actuation)	88-176 μg	176-440 μg	>440 μg
Triamcinolone acetonide (200 μg/actuation)	400-800 μg	800-1200 μg	>1200

From Expert Panel Report 2, National Asthma Education and Prevention Program: *Guidelines for the diagnosis and management of asthma,* Pub No 97-4051, Bethesda, Md, 1997, US Department of Health and Human Services, National Institutes of Health, National Heart, Lung, and Blood Institute.

Appendix 18-3 Recommended Doses*

DRUG	FORMULATION	DOSAGE
Inhaled medications		
Ipratropium bromide	Metered dose inhaler (18 μg/actuation)	2 actuations inhaled 4 times daily, maximum: 12 actuations/day (>12 yr)
Cromolyn sodium	Metered dose inhaler (800 μg/actuation)	2 actuations inhaled 4 times daily (≥5 yr)
	Nebulizer solution (20 mg/2 ml ampule)	20 mg inhaled via nebulizer 4 times daily (>12 yr)
Nedocromil sodium	Metered dose inhaler (1.75 mg/actuation)	2 actuations inhaled 4 times daily (>12 yr)
Leukotriene modifiers		
Zafirlukast	Oral tablet	20 mg orally 2 times daily (≥12 yr)
Zileuton	Oral tablet	600 mg orally 4 times daily (≥12 yr)

From *Drug facts and comparisons: 1993,* St Louis, 1993, Facts & Comparisons.
*Doses should be adjusted if used in children outside the indicated age ranges.

Appendix 18-4 Algorithm for Dosing Theophylline

Initial dosage
Adults and children >1 yr:
12-14 mg/kg/day up to 300 mg/day

↓

After 3 days, *if tolerated,* increase dose to:

Incremental dose increase
Adults and children ≥45 kg: 400 mg/day
Children <45 kg: 16 mg/kg/day up to 400 mg/day

↓

After 3 days, *if tolerated,* increase dose to:

Final dose before measurement of serum theophylline concentration (STC)
Adults and children ≥45 kg: 600 mg/day
Children <45 kg: 20 mg/kg/day up to 600 mg/day

↓

Check expected peak STC when no doses have been missed, added, or taken at unequal dosing intervals for at least 3 days.

Dosage adjustment based on STC

Peak STC	*Recommendations*
<7.5 μg/ml	Increase dose by ~25% and recheck STC for further dosage adjustments.
7.5-9.9 μg/ml	If tolerated, increase dose by ~25%.
10.0-14.9 μg/ml	If tolerated, maintain dose and recheck STC at 6- to 12-month intervals.
15.0-19.9 μg/ml	Consider decreasing dose by ~10% to maintain greater margin of safety.
20.0-24.9 μg/ml	Decrease dose ~10%-25% and recheck STC after 3 days.
25.0-30.0 μg/ml	Skip the next dose, decrease subsequent doses by ~25%, and recheck STC after 3 days.
>30.0 μg/ml	Skip the next 2 doses, decrease subsequent doses by ~50%, and recheck STC. Administer activated charcoal until STC <20.0 μg/ml.

From Hendeles L et al: *J Pediatr* 120:177-183, 1992 (review).

CHAPTER 19

Aerosol Therapy and Delivery Systems

Mark Lloyd Everard and Peter N. Le Souëf

PRINCIPLES OF AEROSOL MEDICATION DELIVERY

Inhalation of aerosolized medications for therapeutic purposes has been used for many centuries[1] and is currently the mainstay of therapy for patients with a variety of respiratory conditions. Inhalation of smoke from the burning of plants such as thorn apple *(Datura stramonium)* has been used since ancient times. In recent centuries, "asthma cigarettes" were popularized in which anticholinergic constituents of plant products such as stramonium leaves and deadly nightshade *(Atropa belladonna)* were aerosolized during smoking.[1] Devices specifically designed to aerosolize therapeutic products were developed in the second half of the nineteenth century (Fig. 19-1), and with increasingly effective medications and delivery systems, this form of therapy has become the route of choice for many respiratory conditions.

Until recently, aerosolized medications have been used predominantly to treat diseases of the respiratory tract such as asthma and chronic bronchitis. More recently, conditions such as *Pneumocystis carinii* pneumonia and the endobronchial sepsis characteristic of cystic fibrosis have also been treated using this route. The principle benefit of using aerosolized rather than systemic therapy in these situations is that medication is delivered directly to its site of action. This permits the following:

1. More rapid onset of action
2. Increased therapeutic index with less potential for systemic side effects because the aerosolized dose is lower than the systemic doses required for a comparable effect
3. Barriers to effective therapy, such as poor gastrointestinal availability and first-pass metabolism by the liver, to be bypassed

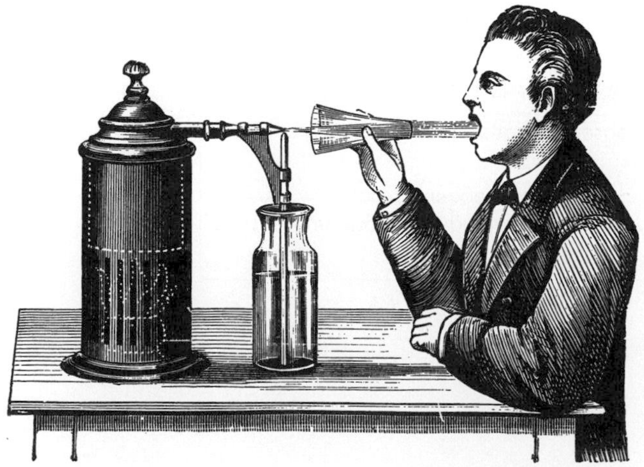

Fig. 19-1. Steam-driven aerosol delivery system (atomizer) from the early part of the twentieth century.

Recently, there has been considerable interest in other benefits that might be derived from using aerosols to administer medications. For pulmonary disease, a prolonged duration of action is possible by modifying the structure of the medications or delivering them in liposomes or other forms of encapsulation that release medication over a period of time.[2,3] Such strategies potentially simplify therapy and may permit more sustained levels within the airways.

The list of agents delivered as aerosols to or via the lungs is continually expanding, recent inclusions being products such as vaccines, interferons, chemotherapeutic agents, and recombinant deoxyribonucleic acid products such as deoxyribonuclease.[4,5] It is also now appreciated that the lung provides an enormous absorptive area and that a wide variety of medications acting systemically might be administered via this route. Medications such as adrenaline administered as a fluid bolus are already administered via this route, but a variety of additional medications, particularly peptides such as insulin, might also be administered via the respiratory tract.[5,6]

Importance of Understanding the Principles of Aerosol Medication Delivery

The dose delivered to the lungs of patients often has little to do with prescribed dose.[7] Aerosol delivery systems are generally inefficient because of highly variable medication delivery to the lower respiratory tract. This variability results from both patient factors and factors relating to the delivery system. The dose delivered from a nominated dose might vary thirtyfold or more depending on the delivery system used and factors related to the patient's use of that system. Such variability would generally not be tolerated for other routes of delivery such as oral or intravenous administration, but it is only recently that clinicians have started to consider the dose reaching the lungs rather than the prescribed dose. This situation has arisen largely because the most widely used medications, the β_2-sympathomimetics, have a very high therapeutic index when inhaled and are generally used in supramaximum doses. As a result, these medications produce therapeutic responses despite wide variations in the efficiency of the delivery system and suboptimal inhalation techniques. For other medications, such as inhaled steroids and sodium cromoglycate, both the devices and the technique used are likely to contribute to the therapeutic response; hence the delivered rather than the prescribed dose becomes very important.

With increasingly potent and expensive medications, appropriate, efficient, and reproducible delivery systems should be developed to maximize efficacy and minimize the cost and the potential for harm. Meanwhile, to optimize therapy using current delivery systems, clinicians must understand the principles that influence the delivery of medications to the lower respiratory tract and appreciate the advantages and limitations of the delivery systems.

Deposition of Aerosols in the Respiratory Tract

When an aerosol is inhaled, particles may be exhaled or deposited anywhere within the respiratory tract from the nose or mouth to the alveoli. The quantity of medication deposited and the distribution of deposition are influenced by the following:

1. The physical properties of the aerosol
2. The mechanisms of deposition
3. The pattern of inhalation and, to a lesser extent, exhalation
4. Anatomic considerations and intersubject and intrasubject variation
5. The disease process affecting the structure of the respiratory tract

Aerosols

An aerosol is a suspension of solid or liquid particles in a gaseous phase. Medication may be suspended as "dry" solid particles or contained within a liquid droplet, either in solution or in suspension.[8] Most aerosols produced by jet or ultrasonic nebulizers contain medication in solution, whereas droplets produced by most metered dose inhalers (MDIs) contain medication particles suspended in liquid composed predominantly of chlorofluorocarbons (CFCs). Once generated, the characteristics of aerosols can change rapidly.[9,10] This is particularly true for the aerosol generated by MDIs. At the actuator, the droplets are large and have a high velocity. Within a few seconds, evaporation of propellant and deceleration resulting from air resistance result in smaller, slow-moving particles composed essentially of medication particles surrounded by propellant in a gaseous form.[4,11,12] For wet aerosols from nebulizers, similar changes can also occur quite rapidly. The concentration of medication in the droplets exiting the nebulizer is essentially that of the solution from which it is formed, but drying of droplets or hygroscopic growth can occur rapidly, resulting in particles shrinking or increasing in size.[13,14] Substantial changes in the size of droplets can occur before inhalation when, for example, lengths of tubing are placed between the device and patient. Significant changes resulting from hygroscopic growth may also take place after inhalation as the droplets are warmed and subject to almost 100% relative humidity within the respiratory tract.[2,4,9,10,15]

The diameter of particles that can exist in the form of an aerosol covers more than five orders of magnitude from 0.005 to 100 μm,[8] but for therapeutic purposes, particles between 1 and 5 μm are generally deemed to be in the respirable range (i.e., they penetrate into the lower respiratory tract and have a high probability of deposition),[4] although some droplets of 10 μm or more deposit within the lungs. Indeed, maximal deposition in the larger conducting airways is likely to occur in the range of 5 to 8 μm.[2,9,16,17] This window is defined by the ability of the respiratory tract to effectively exclude larger particles from the lower respiratory tract and the low probability of deposition of particles in the range 0.1 to 1 μm.[4,10,15,18] Although the likelihood of deposition, particularly in alveolar regions, increases again below 0.1 μm, such aerosols are difficult to generate, and such particles are individually able to carry very little medication.

Examples of substances within this range are cigarette smoke, which has particles generally in the range 0.01 to 0.6 μm; neutrophils, which have a diameter of approximately 7 μm; and pollens, which have a range of 10 to 100 μm.[15] The challenge for those developing aerosol-delivery systems is to efficiently produce particles within the respirable range. As discussed later, aspects such as targeting specific regions of the lung (e.g., the alveoli or tracheobronchi) and reproducing doses are becoming increasingly important.

Description of an Aerosol

To simplify the description of an aerosolized particle that may be irregular in shape, the clinician can use a single value known as the *aerodynamic diameter.* This value is the diameter of a fictitious sphere of unit density that has the same settling (gravitational) velocity[8,9,19] (Fig. 19-2). More important, particles of the same aerodynamic diameter not only have the same settling velocity but also behave identically in any situation in which they are traveling as a particle in an aerosol. The use of this parameter avoids complex descriptions of particles that might otherwise include details such as shape, dimension, and density. The distribution of aerodynamic diameters within an aerosol can be determined in a variety of ways.

For a monodispersed aerosol, all particles have the same size, shape, and density and hence can be described by a single aerodynamic diameter. However, therapeutic aerosols usually contain particles covering a wide range of aerodynamic diameters, and they are generally described in terms of their mass median aerodynamic diameter (MMAD) and the geometric standard deviation (GSD).[4,8-10,19]

The MMAD is the aerodynamic diameter such that half the droplet mass is contained in smaller droplets and half in larger. The GSD gives an indication of the spread of particle sizes and is defined by the ratio of the diameter of the particle on the 84.2th percentile (the particle larger than 84.2% of all the particles) to the median diameter (Fig. 19-3). For a monodisperse aerosol, in which all the particles are of the same shape and size, the GSD is 1, although for practical purposes aerosols with GSDs less than 1.22 are regarded to behave as monodisperse aerosols.[8-10,19] This distinction is important because most work in the biomedical field has used monodisperse aerosols, and as such, patterns of deposition for a given MMAD are likely to be significantly different from that of a polydisperse therapeutic aerosol of the same MMAD.[2,9,10,17]

The relationship between particle numbers and mass distribution is shown in Fig. 19-3. Because the mass of a spherical droplet is related to the cube of its radius, a 10-μm droplet contains 1000 times the mass of a 1-μm droplet. Consequently,

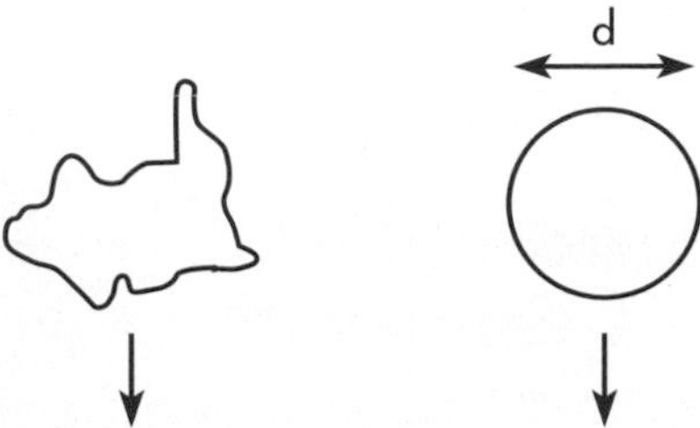

Fig. 19-2. Aerodynamic diameter *(d)* of any particle is the diameter of a fictitious sphere of unit density that has the same settling (gravitational) velocity.

for polydispersed aerosols, there are numerically many more droplets smaller than the MMAD than there are greater than this value; indeed for a polydispersed aerosol, as little as 10% of droplets by number might be greater in size than the MMAD. Particles within many therapeutic aerosols approximate to a log normal distribution; that is, when the number of droplets of a given size are plotted against size, the plot appears skewed, but the size distribution becomes normally distributed if plotted against the logarithm of size. However, many MDIs and dry powder inhalers (DPIs) do not produce particles with a log normal distribution but have a bimodal or even multimodal polydispersed distribution and hence do not have a linear relationship between size and cumulative percentage.

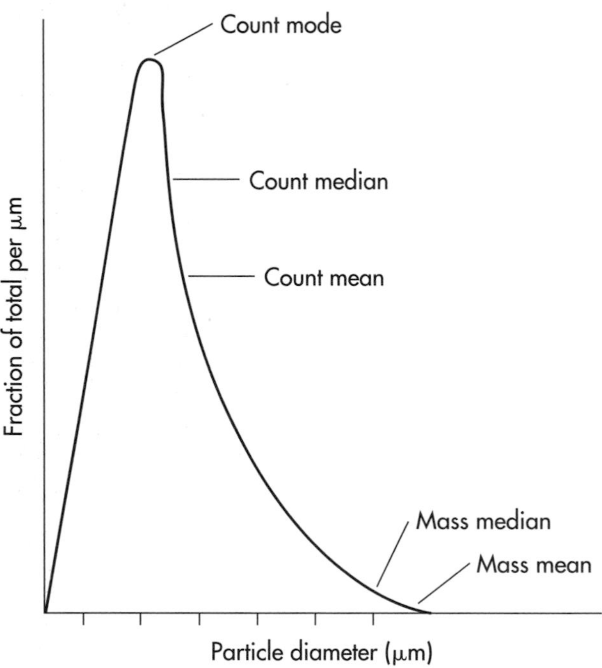

Fig. 19-3. Relationship between particle numbers and mass distribution for a polydisperse aerosol.

Measurement of Particle Size

Information relating to the size distribution of the particles of an aerosol generated by therapeutic delivery systems is frequently quoted by manufacturers and in scientific publications. It is important that the limitations and appropriateness of the method used to derive this data be considered when such material is read. A number of recent reviews would be valuable for centers wishing to be involved in this area.[20,21]

There are many methods of measuring the size of particles contained in an aerosol,[15,21] but the two most widely used methods in the assessment of therapeutic aerosols are light scattering systems (principally laser diffraction) (Fig. 19-4, *A*) and inertial impaction systems (Fig. 19-4, *B*).[20,21]

Laser diffraction involves passing an aerosol through a laser beam. The beam of light is scattered by the particles in the aerosol, and refraction occurs as light passes through nonopaque particles. The scattered light is collected by a series of detectors, and the resultant signals are converted into information relating to the volume distribution of particles within the aerosol, from which information related to the mass distribution is derived.[20,22] Inertial impaction devices take the form of liquid impingers or cascade impactors. Air is drawn through the devices at a constant flow. This may be between 5 and 60 L/min depending on the device. The airflow passes through a series of stages before it passes through an absolute filter. The velocity of the airflow increases between each successive stage as the connecting jets narrow. Particles from an aerosol introduced into this airflow impact on plates contained in each stage. The stage at which a particle impacts is determined by its aerodynamic diameter; large particles impact on upper stages, whereas smaller particles pass through to lower stages before being deposited by impaction or being collected by the absolute filter. The particle size distribution is then derived from assaying the quantity of medication on each stage and knowing the cutoff for aerodynamic diameters of each stage.[15,21]

The principal advantage of the impaction approach is that it provides information on the distribution of medication. This is important for aerosols derived from medication suspensions such as nebulized steroid preparations and most MDI preparations. The medication in such aerosols may not be evenly dis-

A

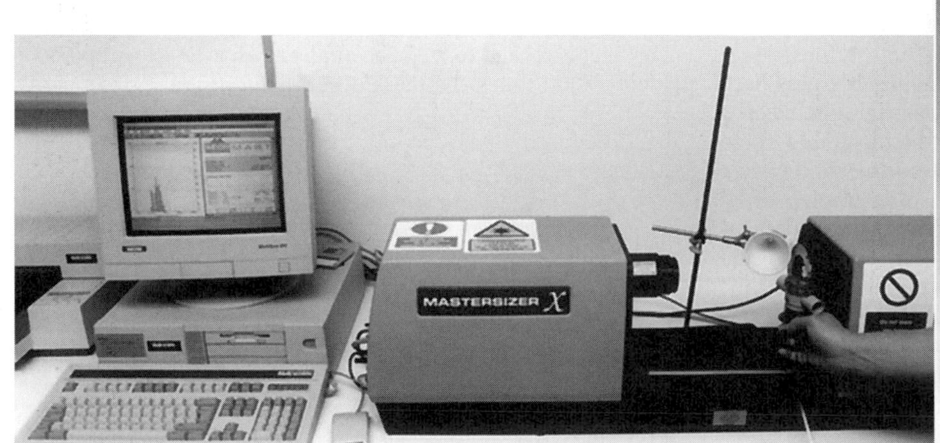

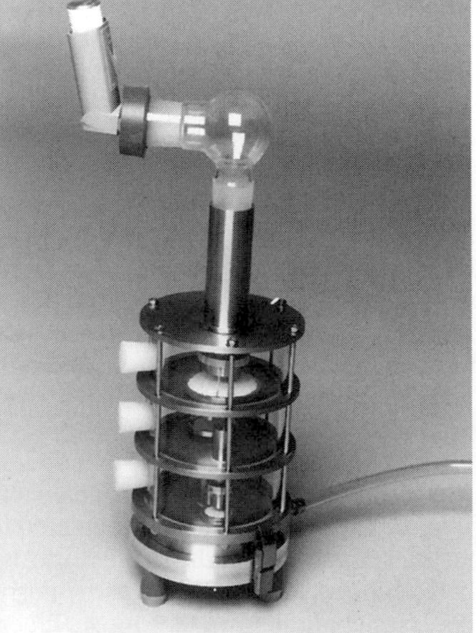

B

Fig. 19-4. Malvern laser particle sizer (Malvern Instruments UK) **(A)** and Astra multistage liquid impinger (Copley, Nottingham, UK) **(B).**

tributed amongst droplets, with some droplets having no medication and others, particularly larger ones, carrying the bulk of the aerosolized medication.

Such techniques are relatively cheap but are very time consuming compared with laser light scattering. There are also problems with assessing volatile aerosols because drying occurs as a result of the constant airflow through the device. For example, when jet nebulizers are assessed, they produce a significantly lower MMAD than that generated by the nebulizer.[20,21] For MDIs, which generate an evolving aerosol, the size of the inlet throat can greatly alter the resultant distribution. A large throat permits greater evaporation of propellant with less loss through impaction and hence results in a lower MMAD. These and other changes resulting from differences in operating flows mean that significantly different MMADs can be produced by using different impactors.[21] Other potential problems such as particles bouncing off stages and being reentrained into the airflow also need to be considered when using these devices.

Laser systems are expensive but are very convenient, producing results rapidly; their advantage is that they can measure particle sizes as the aerosol leaves the device without secondary artifacts resulting from drying. For nonvolatile aerosols generated by jet nebulizers, agreement has been produced when comparing laser diffraction and impaction methods.[20] For MDIs, measurements can be made using a laser system, but there are problems caused by the propellant cloud altering the light transmission. More important, the aerosol evolves rapidly; hence results are determined by the distance from the laser and are therefore difficult to interpret.

For wet aerosols generated by jet or ultrasonic nebulizers from solutions, laser diffraction is the method of choice. Despite the problems related to selection of throats and evolution of aerosol through the device, inertial impaction techniques are the standard method of assessing MDIs.[21] Attempts are being made to standardize methods and to correlate in vitro results with behavior in subjects, but much work is still required.

For DPIs, inertial impaction methods are generally used, but these have lacked flexibility because they generally operate at a single flow, whereas the particle size distribution of DPIs varies considerably with the inspiratory flow. Recent work has attempted to address this problem by the calibration of certain impingers at different flows. Laser particle sizing has been used occasionally for DPIs[23] but there are problems (e.g., when the disaggregated and residual agglomerated powder have different densities). Again, prediction of lung deposition cannot yet be made with great accuracy using particle size measurements. The respirable dose obtained from in vitro studies generally significantly overestimates the dose delivered to the lungs of patients.

Mechanisms of Deposition

An appreciation of the mechanism by which particles deposit is essential if other aspects of aerosol therapy are to be understood. Unlike the gastrointestinal tract, the respiratory tract is designed to exclude particles through methods such as filtration in the upper airway, mucociliary clearance, and cough. As previously noted, therapeutic aerosols are generally in the range 1 to 10 μm, and in this range the two major mechanisms of deposition are inertial impaction and gravitational sedimentation.[4,10,15,19,24] Other potentially relevant factors include diffusion, interception, and electrostatic attraction.

Inertial Impaction

A particle traveling through a gas has its own momentum; the greater the mass or velocity, the greater its momentum (Fig. 19-5, *A*). With any change in the direction of airflow, such as in the pharynx or at a bifurcation within the lower respiratory

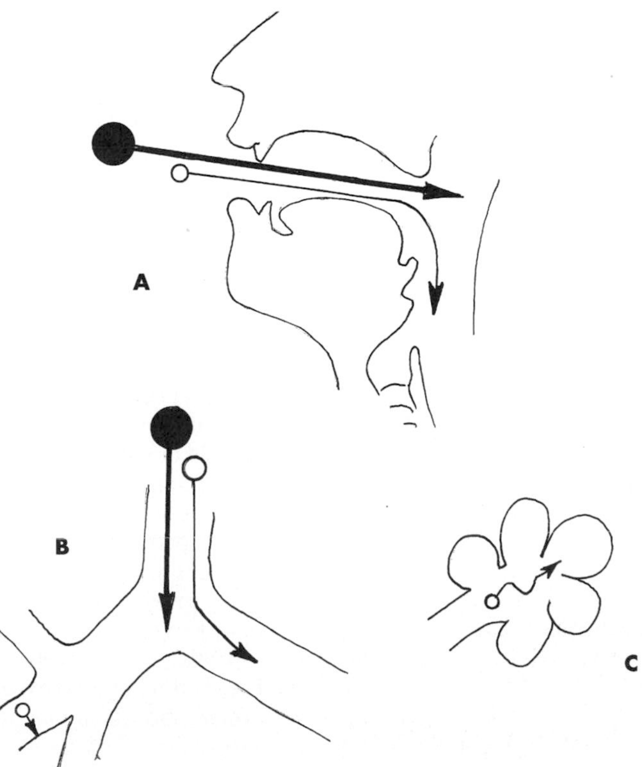

Fig. 19-5. Mechanisms of deposition within the respiratory tract. **A,** Impaction. **B,** Sedimentation. **C,** Diffusion.

tract, particles tend to continue in their original direction. Whether the particle impacts or follows the direction of airflow depends on the relative influences of its momentum and the drag of the gas flow. Even when the patient is mouth-breathing, the momentum of particles larger than 10 μm ensures that most deposit in the pharynx, whereas particles smaller than 3 μm have such low inertia with quiet breathing that the majority do not deposit because of impaction. Impaction is the predominant mechanism operating in the larger central airways, but as the overall cross-sectional area of successive generations increases, the velocity of airflow decreases, and the likelihood of deposition resulting from impaction also decreases peripherally.

Sedimentation

For smaller particles reaching the distal airways, sedimentation resulting from the effect of gravity is believed to be the major process resulting in deposition (Fig. 19-5, *B*). Because settling of such particles is relatively slow (e.g., 125 mm/s for a 2-μm particle vs. 2900 mm/s for a 10-μm particle[15]), the quantity deposited increases with time, and this is the basis of the 10-second breath-holding recommendation frequently given when using MDIs. The rate of settling declines with time because of previous losses; hence significantly fewer particles deposit in the tenth second compared with the first. Although impaction is the predominant mechanism of deposition in the central airways, sedimentation probably contributes a significant proportion, especially with a period of breath-holding.[24]

Diffusion

For particles of 0.1 to 0.5 μm, the rate of settling is so slow (e.g., 2.1 mm/s for a 0.2-μm particle[15]) that even with prolonged breath-holding, deposition resulting from sedimentation is very low (Fig. 19-5, *C*). Below the particle size of 1 μm, displacement of particles resulting from diffusion increases, and this becomes the dominant mechanism. Diffusion occurs as a result of the random collision of gas molecules with particles. For a 0.2-μm particle, displacement resulting from motion is 37 mm/s, increasing to 570 mm/s for a 0.01-μm particle.[15] Consequently, the probability of an inhaled particle depositing in the respiratory tract reaches a minimum at around 0.5 μm and then increases again.

Interception

When a particle has a similar diameter to the airway through which it is passing, it may deposit because of interception. This is generally not important for spherical droplets, but for elongated objects, such as inorganic fibers, it can become important and has potential therapeutic applications.[2,10]

Electrostatic Charge

Many therapeutic aerosols carry an electric charge and can induce an opposite change on the airway wall, potentially leading to enhanced deposition. The role of this factor, if any, and indeed any possible use of it for therapeutic purposes have not been investigated in depth.[2,4,15,25] Most aerosols do not carry a large charge per particle. Hence electrostatic charge is unlikely to play a major role in deposition for most therapeutic aerosols.

Conclusions

Aerosol deposition is not an even "blanket" but occurs in "hot spots."[2,9,10] Impaction can be predicted at bifurcations, and this results in much greater deposition at these sites than along the lumen of the large airways. In peripheral airways, gravity causes uneven distribution resulting from sedimentation.[9] Another example of uneven deposition is reduced delivery of medication to the upper lobes compared with the lower lobes when the patient is erect. This appears to result partly from reduced ventilation in the upper lobes relative to the lower lobes.[26,27] Medication delivery to the upper lobes appears to be improved when aerosol is inhaled in the supine position, which has been attributed to improved ventilation in this position.[26] However, reduced ventilation of the upper lobes alone is not sufficient to fully explain the relatively lower medication delivery, and other factors, such as differences in anatomy, are also important in medication delivery.[7,27] The significance of uneven deposition is unclear, but the potential problems have been illustrated by breakthrough *P. carinii* infection in the upper lobes of some patients receiving nebulized pentamidine prophylaxis. This has been attributed to the relatively lower doses received by the upper lobes,[26] although recent work has suggested that other factors such as relative medication resistance may be important.[28]

Targeting of medications to specific regions of the respiratory tract has been frequently been discussed, but this subject has become important only recently. Until recently the only active step toward targeting was the use of spacing devices with MDIs to reduce upper airways deposition. More recently, targeting deposition to regions within the lower respiratory tract has become topical.[2,9] For highly soluble medications, including most bronchodilators, it is possible that targeting is unimportant and that redistribution of medication from the central to the peripheral airways occurs through the pulmonary and bronchial circulations.[9,29] For medications with poor absorption (e.g., antibiotics) or those with specific peripheral effects but unpleasant side effects if deposited centrally (e.g., pentamidine), understanding factors that might permit targeting becomes important if maximal benefit is to be derived from this route of administration.

Predicting Patterns of Deposition

One might predict that large particles, rapid inspiratory flows, and shallow breaths would enhance deposition in more central airways and that small particles, low inspiratory flows, larger volumes, and breath-holding would minimize upper airway deposition and maximize deposition in the small airways and alveoli. A considerable amount of theoretic and practical work concerning the pattern of deposition of particles in adults supports these suggestions. A large number of mathematic models have been described and used to predict the pattern of deposition of particles in the airways of adults. These have been refined and developed on the basis of experimental work using monodispersed nonvolatile aerosols, largely by researchers in the field of industrial hygiene,[4,15,18,24,30] and are believed to provide reasonably accurate predictions of deposition patterns for particles of a given MMAD. Fig. 19-6 illustrates the probability of a particle of a particular size depositing in a given compartment of the respiratory tract. The exact pattern for aerosol of any given MMAD depends on factors such as age, respiratory pattern, and airway obstruction.

Mathematic models exist for children and infants,[31-36] but there is little in vivo experimental work; hence the limitations of these models are unknown. On the other hand, therapeutic aerosols are almost always polydispersed, and one cannot use the calculated MMAD and described models to accurately predict the pattern of deposition.[9,10] The total lung deposition obtained when a particular device is used has been assessed in a

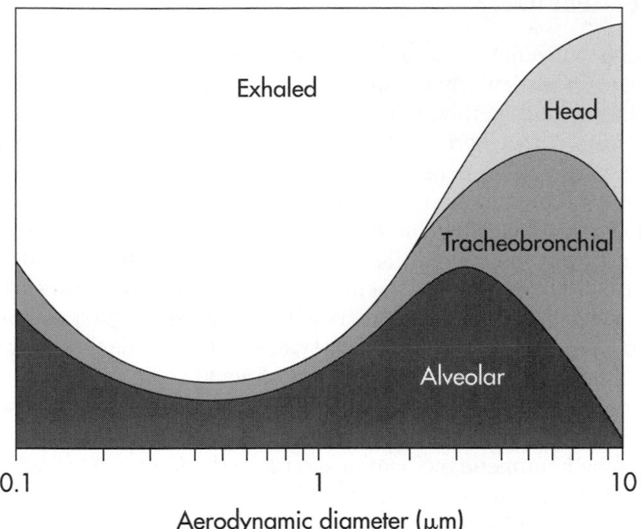

Fig. 19-6. Schematic pattern of deposition for particles of different aerodynamic diameters. The actual pattern depends on factors such as age, inspiratory flow, breath-holding, and the presence of respiratory disease.

number of indirect ways, including the measurement of medication in blood and urine,[37-40] but these studies do not provide information on the pattern of deposition within the lung. Assessment of deposition for therapeutic aerosols has generally involved the use of indirect radiolabeling techniques in which the radiolabel is assumed to travel with the medications. Ethical and technical aspects of such studies have recently been reviewed.[41,42] A major problem with this approach is the lack of standardization of the methods used to quantify lung deposition, which makes comparison of results obtained in different centers very difficult. Furthermore, the current approach appears to be to perform deposition studies with each new device. It would be highly desirable if the probable deposition pattern of a device could be predicted from the aerosol characteristics assessed in vitro. An attempt to do this with the polydispersed aerosols generated by jet nebulizers suggests that a reasonable approximation can be made regarding the relative proportions depositing in the upper and lower airways and the peripheral to central deposition within the lungs based on the MMAD as measured by a laser particle sizer.[43] However, total deposition cannot be directly inferred from these results. It is not yet possible to do the same for MDIs and DPIs, and predictions of lung deposition based on the MMAD or respirable dose as measured by inertial impaction measurements generally significantly overestimate the lung dose.

Breathing Pattern and Anatomic Considerations

Inspiratory Flow

One can predict that rapid inhalation will impart particles with greater inertia and enhance deposition in the upper airways and large central airways. For this reason, slow inhalations are recommended for most delivery systems, including jet nebulizers and MDIs, although the importance of low inspiratory flow when using MDIs has been questioned and may be much less important than good coordination.[40,44] For current DPIs, the energy imparted by the patient's effort is used to overcome the strong forces of attraction that exist among particles around 2 μm in size.[9] The greater the effort, the greater the disaggregation and hence the greater the number of respirable particles. Consequently, these devices are at their most efficient in delivering medication to the lower respiratory tract when inspiratory flows are maximum, the increased velocity of particles being more than offset by the increase in respirable particles.[37,45,46]

Inspiratory Volumes

Deep inspiratory breaths are likely to enhance peripheral deposition.[4,9] Bulk transport of gas can carry particles to approximately the bronchioles with a deep inspiration. Convective mixing aided by cardiac impulses is involved in carrying particles deeper into the peripheries.[10] For DPIs, large-volume breaths are generally used to generate high inspiratory flows. For MDIs, large inspiratory breaths are recommended, although the balance of evidence suggests that starting from functional residual capacity is as effective as inhaling from residual volume. An example of failure to achieve effective delivery resulting from insufficient inspiratory volume occurs in patients using MDIs who stop inhaling when the cold propellants hit the pharynx.[11] There is little work addressing the subject of inspiratory patterns on medication delivery from jet nebulizers. Evidence suggests that tidal breathing delivers quantities similar to those delivered by slow, deep breaths with breath-holding.[47,48] This is probably because the total dose inhaled is reduced when a constant driving gas flow is used because of the periods spent breath-holding. Also, much of a deep breath simply contains entrained air without additional medication.[49,50] Utilization of such patterns when using interrupters, which deliver medication only during inspiration, and possibly when using auxiliary holding chambers probably enhances medication delivery. However, this approach remains to be tested and would increase the inconvenience for the patient.

Breath-Holding

As previously noted, breath-holding enhances deposition resulting from sedimentation, and this increase particularly enhances deposition in the peripheries of the lung. For practical purposes, however, the only delivery system that benefits from breath-holding appears to be the MDIs. Breath-holding with jet nebulizers increases wastage unless dosimetric nebulizers are used. The suggestion has been made that the high inspiratory flows used with DPIs result in deposition of the majority of the particles through impaction and hence a breath-holding pause is not necessary,[9,16,46] but others, using a pharmacokinetic method, suggested that a breath-holding pause is valuable.[51]

Nose vs. Mouth

The nose performs a number of functions, including humidification of inspired air and filtration of particulate matter.[15] Deposition in the nose results predominantly from impaction through turbulence created at the internal ostium. Hence nasal filtration is greater for larger particles and is very low for particles smaller than 2 μm, and filtration is increased as the inspiratory flow increases. Deposition studies using jet nebulizers in adults have shown that the nose does filter considerably more medication than the mouth, resulting in significantly lower delivery of medication to the lungs.[52] This is probably the case for children but may not be the case for infants.

Intersubject and Intrasubject Variation

Radiolabel deposition studies have shown that for all devices the dose of medication delivered to the lungs of subjects varies considerably. The relative contribution of differences in inhalation techniques and variations in anatomy is debatable. The contribution of anatomic variation and changes in flow appears to be reduced when smaller particles (less than 3 μm) are inhaled because losses resulting from impaction are small.[2] Deposition of medication from currently available devices can vary considerably even when used by the same subject, and such intrasubject variation should be considered if deposition studies are planned.[53]

Obstructive Airway Disease

With obstructive airway disease, the pattern of aerosol deposition becomes more central as the disease progresses, with increasingly prominent hot spots.[4,9,12,54] Because of turbulence in the irregular and narrowed airways, particles deposit because of inertial impaction. Particles that do penetrate into the peripheries of lungs with airway disease are more likely to be deposited than they would in normal airways, but far fewer particles penetrate into these regions; hence the quantity of medication deposited peripherally is reduced.[10] This increasingly central pattern of deposition is a sensitive index of airway obstruction, and these changes can be observed well before spirometric changes are evident. The effect of turbulence is lower for finer particles, so the use of finer aerosols to enhance peripheral delivery in those with obstructive disease is theoretically possible.

Clearance from the Lungs

Particles, solutions, and suspensions can be cleared from the respiratory tract through mucociliary clearance or transport through bronchial or alveolar epithelium into the bronchial and pulmonary circulations. The route and speed of clearance depend on the site of deposition and the nature of the substance deposited.* Such issues are likely to become increasingly important as the range of medications administered via the lungs increases.

MEDICATION-DELIVERY SYSTEMS

Inadequate or incomplete instruction of patients or their parents frequently results in suboptimal therapy. This situation has arisen partly as a result of conflicting opinions regarding the optimal use of particular devices. The principles underlying each group of delivery systems are relatively straightforward, and understanding these systems and the mechanisms by which inhaled particles deposit within the airways prevents much of the confusion that exists in this area. Table 19-1 summarizes the advantages and disadvantages of the different systems that are used.

*References 2, 5, 9, 12, 55, and 56.

Table 19-1 Role of Inhaler Systems

SYSTEM	ADVANTAGES	DISADVANTAGES
Nebulizer	Tidal breathing Use by patient of any age Large doses Wide range of medications	Expensive and inconvenient equipment Time-consuming method Preservatives, pH, osmolality
MDI	Convenience Use with chambers by patients of all ages Limited dose	Technique problems Lack of pure medication Replacement of CFCs
DPI	Convenience	Effort-dependent efficiency

Jet Nebulizers

Jet nebulizers have long been one of the mainstays of aerosol therapy, particularly in asthma (Fig. 19-7). In the past, jet nebulizers were inefficient in terms of medication delivery. Furthermore, the reproducibility of both the dose delivered and the particle size generated was poor, even among nebulizers from the same batch.[22,50,57] Recommendations for use have generally been aimed at maximum output of medication from inefficient systems rather than convenience of the patient.[50] Because of the improvements in other delivery systems, such as the use of holding chambers with face masks,[50,51] there may no longer be a place for these devices in the routine therapy of asthma and even in the treatment of acute asthma.[58] Patients are likely to continue to use nebulizers in acute asthma because current medication formulations allow high doses of β_2-sympathomimetic medications to be easily delivered by nebulizer. Higher doses of these medications per actuation of an MDI or a DPI would potentially reverse this situation.

For other conditions, jet nebulizers are being used to deliver an increasing range of medications that cannot be delivered in other forms, such as inhaled antibiotics. Often this is because large doses are needed and these cannot be accommodated by MDIs, but it is also because the development costs of formulations for MDI delivery are high. Although powder systems could be used for many of these medications,[23,59] development costs are also likely to be a problem. Pharmaceutical companies do not perceive a commercial benefit from developing such systems because sales are likely to be low. This situation might change if clinicians deemed such therapies to be of sufficient value that they could convince companies of the benefits to patients. If optimal therapeutic benefit is to be derived from administering these medications via jet nebulizers, an understanding of the principles involved is important. Certain manufacturers are also improving designs to increase efficiency and reproducibility so that many of the shortcomings of these devices are being addressed.

Generating Droplets in the Respirable Range

Jet nebulizers have been used in various forms for many decades, and all designs are based on the Bernoulli principle.[14,19] A jet of air is forced through a narrow orifice, creating a vacuum as it expands beyond the orifice. Fluid is drawn up into the region of low pressure via the Venturi effect. The fluid becomes entrained into the airflow, creating long filaments of liquid that then break into droplets as a result of the effects of surface tension.[14] The majority of these primary droplets are too large to penetrate beyond the upper airway, and if they were to leave the nebulizer, they would represent wasted medication. To prevent this wastage, modern small-volume therapeutic nebulizers use a baffle placed between the jet orifice and the patient.[14,19] Smaller droplets cam follow the airstream around the baffle as the majority of droplets impact on the baffle and fall back into the nebulizer bowl to be renebulized. For some nebulizers, estimates suggest that over 99% of primary droplets impact on the baffle and can be renebulized.

The design of the baffle is one of the determinants of nebulizer performance. The more effective the baffle within the nebulizer, the smaller the MMAD of the aerosol. However, because this reduction in MMAD is achieved by retaining all but the finest droplets and hence reducing the mass output,[14] nebulization times increase considerably as the MMAD falls.

Most nebulizers represent a compromise between keeping nebulization times as short as possible and producing an aerosol with a reasonable MMAD. In certain situations such as targeting medication to the lung peripheries, MMADs at the lower end of the respirable range are desired. These can be achieved by more effective internal baffles and acceptance of longer nebulization periods. Alternative approaches include using an external baffle or drying the aerosol.[31,60] An external baffle may take many forms, but one of its simplest forms consists of a one-way valve between the nebulizer and the mouthpiece. Such baffles do not increase nebulization times because the droplets removed are not available to be renebulized, but they do reduce the dose delivered to the patients because much of the nebulized medication collects in the baffle. Drying chambers use relatively dry air to reduce the size of droplets before they reach patients by causing the solvent to evaporate.

Operating Conditions

Apart from the basic design, aerosol characteristics can be greatly influenced by operating conditions. In particular, the MMAD of an aerosol generated by a nebulizer is greatly influenced by the driving gas flow. The higher the flow, the greater the velocity of primary droplets and the greater the momentum of particles of a given aerodynamic diameter. Consequently, the MMAD of droplets able to pass around the baffle falls. If the rate of primary droplet generation remained constant, the nebulizer output would fall. However, the increased energy input provided by the higher flow also results in a greater rate of generation of smaller primary droplets, which more than compensates for the loss of larger droplets impacting on the baffle. The net result is a greater rate of medication delivery contained in an aerosol with a lower MMAD. However, the aerosol concentration (mass of medication per liter of aerosol) usually increases only slightly as the flow increases and may indeed fall at the highest flows because the increased output is contained in a larger volume of aerosol.[50]

For most nebulizers, a flow of at least 6 L/min through the nebulizer is required to minimize medication delivery times and produce desirable MMADs. For a given nebulizer, the flow generated depends on the pressure applied. Hence when portable compressors are assessed, the important parameter is the flow generated through a given nebulizer, not the flow generated with no resistance in place.[4,61]

The "dead volume" of most nebulizers is in the region of 1 ml.[4] Consequently, if an initial fill volume of 2 ml is used, more than 50% of the medication placed in the nebulizer remains in the nebulizer. Because of the increase in solution concentration with time, the residual 1 ml contains significantly more than half the initial mass of medication. The amount of medication delivered can be increased by diluting the 2 ml, for example, to 4 ml with saline.[4,11] In this case the residual 1 ml contains over one fourth of the original medication mass, but diluting the solution significantly also increases the nebulization time. Diluting solutions in this way is probably not necessary for medications such as bronchodilators and is undesirable for other medications in terms of convenience and patient compliance. Better-designed nebulizers with much smaller dead volumes are desirable so that smaller fill volumes can be used.[50]

Solution Viscosity and Suspensions

Theoretic considerations predict that the MMAD of the primary droplets increases with increasing viscosity and surface tension.[14] However, experimental evidence suggests that for most medication suspensions, viscosity and surface tension do not have a systematic effect on the MMAD of the aerosol leaving the nebulizer.[53,62] Viscosity does, however, significantly influence the rate of medication delivery.[47,63] For more viscous suspensions such as antibiotics, nebulization periods may be excessive with standard compressors; hence compressors that can generate flows through the nebulizer of at least 8 L/min are generally recommended.

For suspensions such as inhaled steroids, the medication contained within the droplets need not be distributed at equal concentrations in each droplet, as is the case for solutions. Indeed, the medication tends to be distributed predominantly in larger droplets. A higher proportion of medication is contained within the respirable range at higher flows, and again more powerful compressors are generally advocated.

Changes in Output with Time

Airflow through the nebulizer not only imparts energy to generate droplets but also causes fluid to evaporate from the enormous surface area of the droplets being generated.[4] Consequently, the concentration of the solution increases with time, and this is significant within a few minutes.[64] Nebulization is

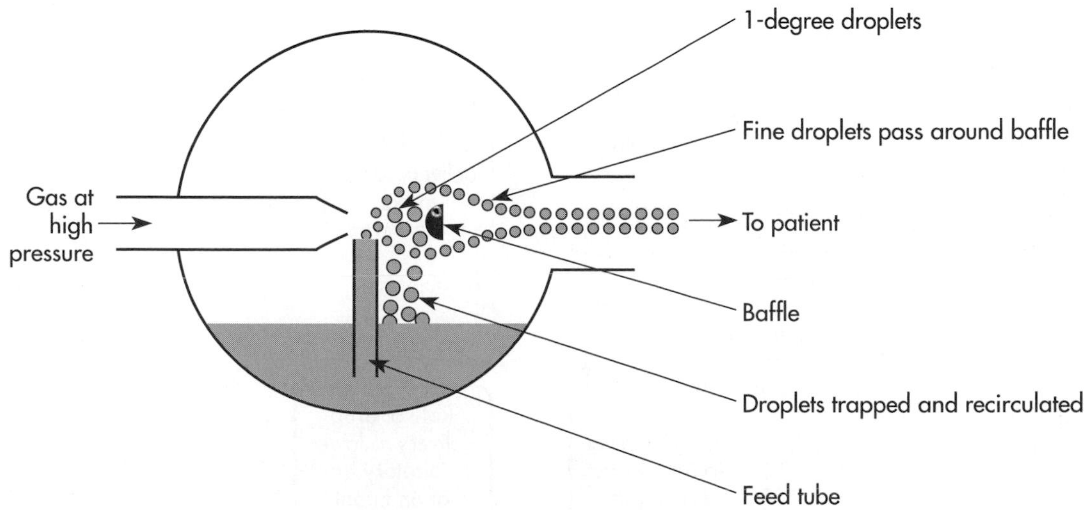

Fig. 19-7. Aerosol generation by a jet nebulizer.

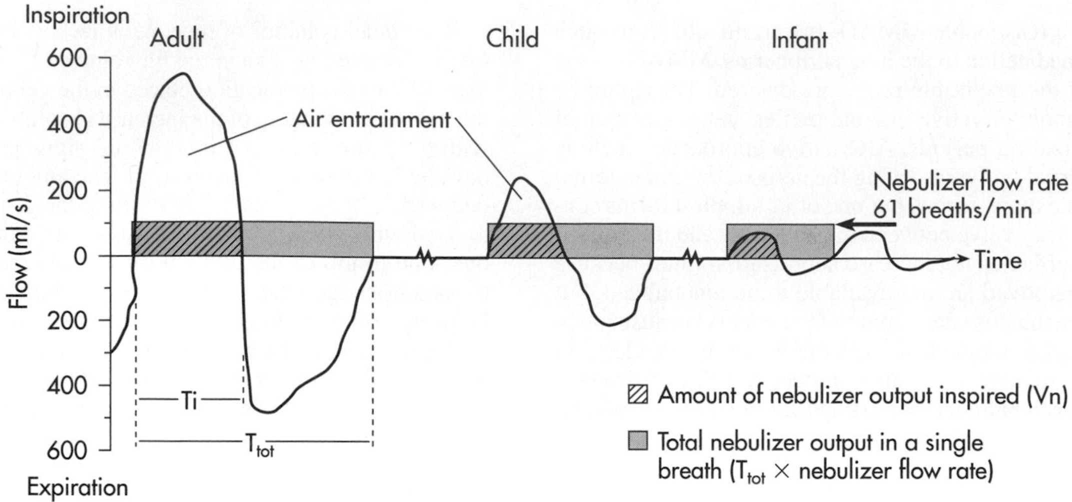

Fig. 19-8. Effect of air entrainment on medication delivery. Aerosol concentration is greatest at low tidal volumes and is reduced by entraining air at higher tidal volumes. *Ti,* Inspiratory time; *Ttot* , time for one breath. (From Collis GG et al: *Lancet* 336:341-343, 1990.)

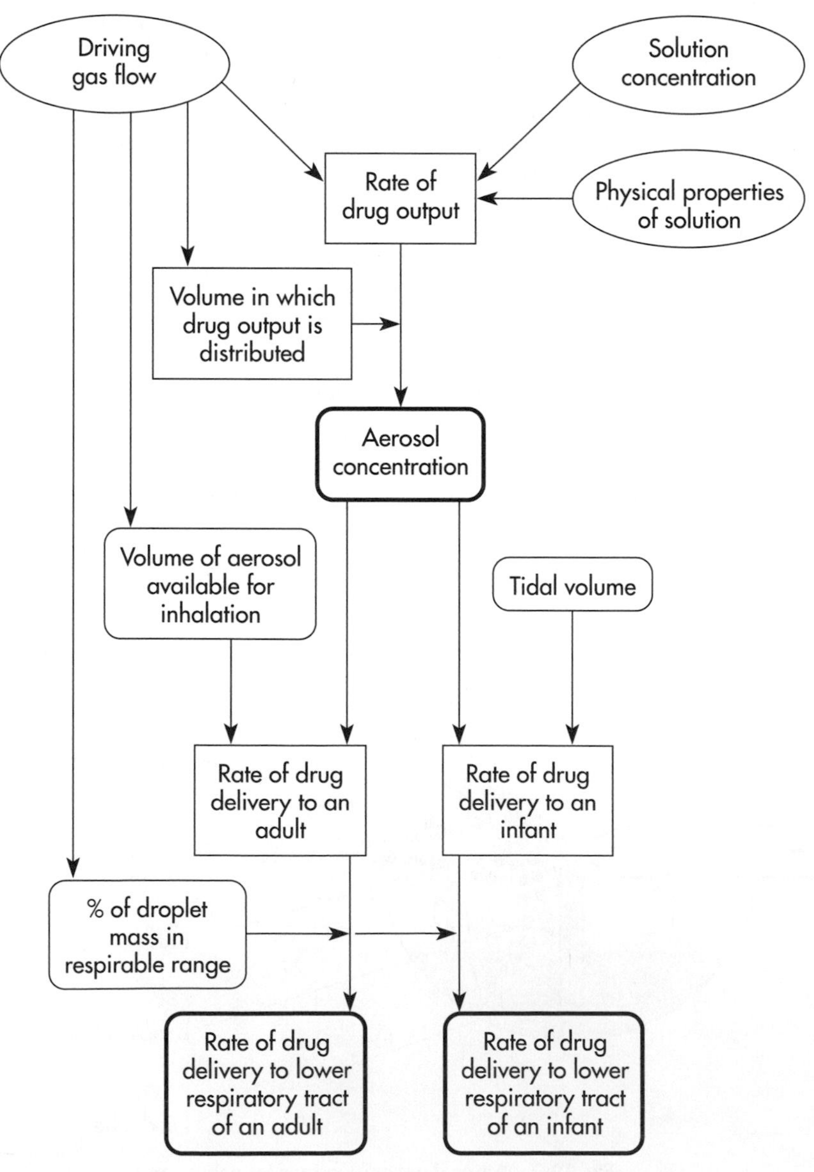

Fig. 19-9. Factors influencing the rate of medication delivery from jet nebulizers. (From Everard ML et al: *Thorax* 50:517-519, 1995.)

also accompanied by a significant fall in the temperature of the fluid being nebulized.[4,13,14] This fall in temperature is also accompanied by a fall in MMAD.[13]

Air Entrainment

For an infant inhaling from a close-fitting nebulizer mask, the driving gas flow exceeds the peak inspiratory flow so that the entire breath is composed of aerosol derived from the nebulizer (Fig. 19-8). The inhaled dose per breath is the product of the tidal volume and aerosol concentration. Because the inspiratory flow of an adult exceeds the flow of gas through the nebulizer, much of the inhaled air contains not aerosol but entrained air and therefore does not increase medication delivery. Therefore the dose inhaled by an adult in a given period of continuous nebulization is very similar to that inhaled by a young child who also entrains air with inspiratory flows exceeding nebulizer flows. Consequently, the greatest dose per kilogram from a given nebulizer bowl dose is inhaled by infants and young children.[49,50] As previously noted, the lung dose is the product of the inhaled dose and the percentage of that dose depositing in the lungs. More work is required to determine the pattern of deposition of therapeutic aerosols in infancy and childhood, but a recent study in children has found that the lung dose corrected for total lung capacity was inversely related to height.[65] Factors determining the rate of medication delivery have recently been discussed and are illustrated in Fig. 19-9.[50]

Paradoxical Bronchoconstriction

Bronchoconstriction can be induced by preservatives, nonosmolar solutions, and acidic solutions.[66] Because of the large doses used and the rapid onset of action, this is rarely a problem with β_2-agonists but is occasionally a problem with other medications. Single-dose packaging has been introduced for many medications. These solutions are generally preservative free and usually, but not always, isotonic. However, many are still significantly acidic.

Recommendations for Nebulizer Use

Tidal breathing is generally used for continuous-flow jet nebulizers because no other pattern of breathing has been shown to be superior.[47,48] A mouthpiece is desirable because nasal breathing from a face mask significantly reduces the dose delivered to the lungs.[52] Some patients (adults as well as children) still breathe through the nose even when using a mouthpiece, and for them a noseclip or face mask may be necessary.

High driving gas flows (6 to 8 L/min) are recommended for conventional nebulizers to produce aerosols with low MMADs and to maximize the dose contained in droplets smaller than 5 to 7 μm. A fill volume of 3 to 4 ml is frequently recommended to maximize output. Tapping the nebulizer bowl after the output becomes intermittent increases the medication output.[64] Unfortunately, maximizing output by tapping or diluting solutions increases the nebulization time.[64]

Alternative strategies are desirable if nebulized therapy is to be made more convenient. Nebulizers with smaller dead volumes that obviate the need to dilute solutions and the use of more concentrated solutions would both lead to shorter treatment times. The benefit of this approach was demonstrated in a study in which it was shown that inhaling five breaths generated from a concentrated solution of a bronchodilator produced the same clinical effect as inhaling for 5 minutes from a diluted solution[67]; the increased rate of medication delivery using more concentrated solutions has been demonstrated in radiolabeled deposition studies.[68] Marketing of more concentrated solutions is unlikely to happen for existing medications because of the need to obtain approval from regulating authorities, but this should be considered for future products.

Wastage of medication during expiration is another source of inefficiency, and for conventional jet nebulizers, this can be countered with manually operated interrupters that stop nebulization during exhalation[11] or that use storage chambers.[69,70] These are obviously desirable for expensive medications such as antibiotics.

Recent Advances in Jet Nebulizers

The delivery and particle size output from jet nebulizers have been extremely variable even within the same batch of the same make. Recently, manufacturers have started to address this problem by using improved plastics and molding techniques.

Newer Venturi-type nebulizers are now coming on the market; these nebulizers "entrain" air through the nebulizing chamber during inhalation[71,72] and result in increased output during inspiration and reduced losses during expiration.

In an attempt to improve the predictability of lung doses, authorities now recommended that certain medications such as deoxyribonuclease and pentamidine be delivered with certain nebulizers. Regulatory bodies are likely to pay increasing attention to delivery systems, which will lead to improvements in terms of the reproducibility of medication delivery to the lower respiratory tract. It will, however, be some time until delivery systems will predictably deliver a given dose to a particular region of the lung.

Ultrasonic Nebulizers

Ultrasonic nebulizers are becoming increasingly popular because they are quiet and have a high output. The best portable devices appear to be at least as effective as jet nebulizers; the slightly larger particle size is offset by the increased output.[4,73,74] Medication output is minimal except during inhalation, minimizing this source of wastage, although dead volumes can be significant. Fluid is aerosolized resulting from energy supplied by a piezoelectric crystal that vibrates when a current is passed through it. The median diameter of aerosols generated by these devices is determined by the frequency of vibration[4,14] and can be affected by the viscosity. As the technology improves and reliability problems are overcome, pocket-sized devices will become available. They are not suitable for suspensions such as steroids[72] because relatively little medication is delivered despite a high output of solution or for viscous medications such as antibiotics because little medication leaves the nebulizer. Unlike jet nebulizers, which result in cooling, ultrasonic nebulizers cause an increase in fluid temperature, and this is a potential problem with some medications such as proteins that may be denatured. As with jet nebulizers, particle size and rate of output can vary among devices of the same design.[11]

Metered Dose Inhalers

MDIs have been in use for nearly 40 years and remain very popular because of their convenience. Each canister contains micronized medication (i.e., particles of medication that have been reduced [usually in a cyclone mill] to approximately 2 to 3 μm). These medication particles are usually suspended, rather than dissolved, in propellants, some of which are still CFCs. CFCs are rapidly being replaced with hydrofluoroalkanes (HFAs). The canisters also contain a surfactant to reduce aggregation within the chamber and to lubricate the valve stem.[4] A metering valve holds usually 25 to 100 μL of the propellant/medication suspension depending on the medication formulation and dose. The volume of the valve is also an important variable. Low-volume valves are generally better than higher-volume valves because the variability of medication dose is substantially lower with the lowest-volume valves. During actuation, the metering chamber is closed to the canister and open to the atmosphere. The rapid reduction in pressure within the chamber leads to explosive boiling of the propellants, or "flashing," and this propels the contents of the canister out through the actuator. The droplets leaving the actuator contain one or more medication particles covered in propellant and surfactant. They travel at up to 30 m/s and are larger than 30 μm.[4,12] The particles rapidly decelerate because of resistance of the air, and the propellant evaporates.

To be used efficiently, devices must first be shaken vigorously because they are designed so that medication and propellant separate out very rapidly within the MDI.[75,76] Most recommendations advise patients to exhale, coordinate actuation with the onset of inhalation, inhale slowly (over at least 2 seconds) and breath-hold for up to 10 seconds.[9,29,77] Two studies suggested that rapid inhalation does not significantly reduce the dose delivered to the lungs, although the pattern was more central.[40,44] A third study suggested that inhaling at only 10 L/min was optimal.[39] There appears to be no advantage in exhaling to residual volume rather than functional residual capacity before inhaling.[9,19,39,77]

Problems with MDIs

The biggest problem with MDIs is the difficulty that patients find in coordinating actuation of the MDI and inhalation,[4,11] although many other errors in technique are described.[11] Further problems include limited range of medication delivery, limited dose per actuation, potential toxicity problems, and an impending ban on CFCs. MDIs account for approximately 0.5% of the world's CFC production,[78] but their use for therapeutic purposes has already been banned in some countries and likely to be universal by the year 2000. Intense efforts are being made to find suitable replacements, and HFAs appear most promising. CFCs have potential toxic effects, particularly on the cardiovascular system, but available evidence suggests that, as MDIs are currently used, these effects are not significant. The propellants and surfactants can cause cough and bronchoconstriction in a significant proportion of asthmatics.[79] The way in which MDIs are handled can significantly affect the dose delivered,[76] adding to the variability in delivered dose.

Holding Chambers and Spacers

The use of add-on devices in the form of spacers or holding chambers (enclosed chambers with valves) can solve problems with coordination, can greatly reduce deposition of medication in the throat (important for steroids), and for some chambers, can increase the dose delivered to the lungs compared with an optimally used MDI.[4,11,51,80] The medication output from these chambers depends on several factors, including valve size and design,[4,11,51] and in vitro data comparing performance are available.[43,51] For young children, five tidal breaths can achieve therapeutic effects similar to those produced by large-volume breaths with breath-holding,[81] but once again, therapeutic effects need not reflect the delivered doses if supramaximum doses are used. Clinical effects with inhaled steroids have been reported in preterm infants using holding chambers with facemasks.

Dry Powder Inhalers

As with MDIs, DPIs use micronized particles (i.e., medication that has been ground into 2- to 3-μm particles). Unfortunately, particles of this size have very strong forces of attraction, which cause them to aggregate.[14,19,37] Devices currently use the patient's inspiratory effort to disaggregate the particles. This effort is augmented by using lactose carriers and grids (Rotahaler, Dischaler), using rotating turbines (Spinhaler), or spheronizing the powder and using spiral channels (Turbuhaler).[4,11] The maximum flow that can be generated varies with each device and is determined by the resistance within the particular device. Although some patients may comment that they are most comfortable using devices with a lower resistance, the efficiency of a device depends on other factors. Currently, the most efficient device appears to be the Turbuhaler, which has a relatively high resistance; consequently, peak inspiratory flows are generally lower than when other devices are used.[11] For all devices, the efficiency of disaggregation depends on the energy put into the system by the patient; hence maximal inspiratory effort should be used. There is evidence that even at the highest flows used, the increased amount of medication available in small particles offsets any increased losses resulting from impaction.[9,37,45,46] Patients should first exhale, taking care not to exhale through the device because this can blow powder out and introduce moisture into the device, which may reduce its efficiency. The patient should then inhale as fast as possible, taking care not to tip the powder out before inhaling. The importance of breath-holding is unclear. The very high inspiratory flows and large inspiratory volumes may cause virtually all the aerosol to be deposited through impaction, and there may be no need for breath-holding.[9,16,46] However, other researchers, using a pharmacokinetic method, have found a breath-holding pause to be valuable.[37] As with other types of devices, problems with reproducibility of dose are a feature of DPIs.

SPECIAL CONSIDERATIONS

Infants

Bronchodilator responsiveness in infancy has been difficult to demonstrate, and possible explanations have included (1) lack of bronchial smooth muscle; (2) lack of mature β-adrenoreceptors; (3) failure to deliver adequate medication; and (4) in infancy, failure of most conditions causing airway obstruction to respond to bronchodilators. The last of these possibilities is perhaps the most likely explanation. The first two are unlikely because bronchoconstriction can be induced by histamine and other stimuli and this bronchoconstriction can be effectively prevented by inhaled β_2-sympathomimetics. Recently, studies have indicated that the dose inhaled by an infant, although not necessarily deposited in the lungs, is much greater than that inhaled by an adult if it is corrected for body weight because the total inspiratory breath of an infant contains aerosol, whereas an adult inhales considerable quantities of entrained air that effectively dilutes the aerosol.[49,50,51]

However, a number of technical and anatomic factors might reduce medication delivery to the lungs. Failure to use a close-fitting face mask can result in a considerable reduction in the inhaled dose.[51] Quietly breathing infants are likely to breathe through their noses, which may reduce aerosol delivery to the lower respiratory tract compared with mouth-breathing, although this may not be the case for infants. The suggestion that infants inhale more medication when screaming, leading to enhanced delivery to the lungs, is incorrect.[82] Whether nose-rather than mouth-breathing is more effective at filtering aerosols in infancy is unknown. Modeling studies suggest that upper airway deposition is relatively greater in infancy than in adults, but tracheobronchial deposition may still be greater than in adults when corrected for weight.[9,32,35,36] Confirmation via research is awaited. Within the lungs, deposition of aerosols in infants is likely to be more central than that observed in adults even in healthy lungs,[9,31,36] and this tendency may be enhanced in the presence of airway obstruction. Hence much must still be determined concerning optimal medication delivery from nebulizers in infancy.

Because of problems associated with the use of jet nebulizers in infancy, which include being poorly tolerated by infants because of the noise and relatively long treatment times, alternative forms of delivery systems have been sought. Currently, the most useful systems appear to be MDIs used with holding chambers and facemasks.[51] Treatment periods are much shorter, although they still cause distress in a significant number of toddlers and infants. Again, when quiet, the infants breathe through the nose, and if infants are screaming and upset, medication delivery is likely to be negligible. Such systems have been used for all age groups, including preterm infants.

Ventilator Circuits

Traditionally, jet nebulizers were used to deliver medication to patients through ventilator circuits, but there are many problems with this form of therapy. The most important is the inefficiency of such systems. Recently, newer and more effective approaches have been adopted. The most common is the use of MDIs with suitable adaptors. The most efficient of these appears to be chambers of approximately 150 ml, which appear to be suitable for all patients from preterm baby to adult.[83-85] Medication delivery via endotracheal tubes is also possible using ultrasonic nebulizers.[85,86] Doses approaching 100% of the nominal dose can be delivered into the lower respiratory tract by actuating the medication through a catheter passed through the endotracheal tube.[87] However, there is considerable concern that delivering high concentrations of surfactants, such as oleic acid, directly onto the respiratory mucosa can cause severe epithelial damage.

Future Developments

The observation that the dose placed in a nebulizer has little to do with the lung dose[7] applies to all current delivery systems. Wide variations have been noted among subjects using the same device and among devices of the same type. Each MDI formulation is different, and differences in medication delivery could be expected with different formulations. With increasingly potent medications, regulatory authorities will pay increasing attention to the delivery systems, with performance in vivo as well as in vitro being assessed. Commercial and regulatory pressures to produce efficient devices with more reproducible delivery of medication to the lungs should lead to the development of new generations of novel delivery systems. With time, aerosol therapy should become a increasingly valuable route by which a wide variety of medications can be accurately and reproducibly administered.

REFERENCES

Principles of Aerosol Medication Delivery

1. Sakula A: A history of asthma, *J R Coll Physicians Lond* 22:35-44, 1988.
2. Gonda I: Targeting by deposition. In Hickey AJ, ed: *Pharmaceutical inhalation aerosol technology*, New York, 1992, Marcel Dekker, pp 61-82.
3. Taylor KMG, Newton JM: Liposomes for controlled delivery of drugs to the lung, *Thorax* 47:257-259, 1992.
4. Dolovich M: Physical principles underlying aerosol therapy, *J Aerosol Med* 2:171-186, 1989.
5. Wood RE, Knowles MR: Recent advances in aerosol therapy, *J Aerosol Med* 7:1-11, 1994.
6. Byron PR, Patton JS: Drug delivery via the respiratory tract, *J Aerosol Med* 7:49-75, 1994.
7. Smaldone GC, Fuhrer J, Steigbigel RT, McPeck M: Factors determining pulmonary deposition of aerosolized pentamidine in patients with human immunodeficiency virus infection, *Am Rev Respir Dis* 143:727-737, 1991.
8. Heyder J: Definition of an aerosol, *J Aerosol Med* 4:217-221, 1991.
9. Brain JD, Blanchard JD: Mechanisms of particle deposition and clearance. In Moren F, Dolovich MB, Newhouse MT, Newman SP, eds: *Aerosols in medicine: principles, diagnosis and therapy*, ed 2, Amsterdam, Netherlands, 1993, Elsevier, pp R117-R125.
10. Gonda I: Aerosols for delivery of therapeutic and diagnostic agents to the respiratory tract, *Crit Rev Ther Drug Carrier Syst* 6:273-313, 1990.
11. Selroos O: Bronchial asthma, chronic bronchitis and pulmonary parenchymal diseases. In Moren F, Dolovich MB, Newhouse MT, Newman SP, eds: *Aerosols in medicine: principles, diagnosis and therapy*, ed 2, Amsterdam, Netherlands, 1993, Elsevier, pp 261-289.
12. Summers QA: Inhaled drugs and the lung, *Clin Exp Allergy* 21:259-265, 1991.
13. Phipps PR, Gonda I: Droplets produced by medical nebulizers: some factors affecting their size and solute concentrations, *Chest* 97:1327-1332, 1990.
14. Swift DL: Aerosol and humidity therapy: generation and respiratory deposition of therapeutic aerosols, *Am Rev Respir Dis* 122(suppl):71-77, 1980.
15. Brain JB, Valberg PA: State of the art: deposition of aerosol in respiratory tract, *Am Rev Respir Dis* 120:1325-1371, 1979.
16. Clay MM, Clarke SW: Effect of nebuliser aerosol size on lung deposition in patients with mild asthma, *Thorax* 42:190-194, 1987.
17. Martonen TB, Katz I: Deposition patterns of polydispersed aerosols within the human lungs, *J Aerosol Med* 6:251-274, 1993.
18. Heyder J, Armbruster L, Gebhart J, Grein E, Stahlhofen W: Total deposition of aerosol particles in the human respiratory tract for nose and mouth breathing, *J Aerosol Sci* 6:311-328, 1975.
19. Lourenco RV, Cotromanes E: Clinical aerosols. I. Characterisation of aerosols and their diagnostic uses, *Arch Intern Med* 142:2163-2172, 1982.
20. Clark AR: The use of laser diffraction for evaluation of the aerosol clouds generated by medical nebulizers, *Int J Pharmacol* 115:69-78, 1995.
21. Dolovich M: Measurement of particle size characteristics of metered dose inhaler (MDI) aerosols, *J Aerosol Med* 4:251-263, 1991.
22. Newman SP, Pellow PGD, Clark SW: Droplet size distributions of nebulised aerosols for inhalation therapy, *Clin Phys Physiol Meas* 7:139-146, 1986.
23. Everard ML, Devadason SG, Le Souëf PN: An alternative aerosol delivery system for amiloride, *Thorax* 50:746-749, 1995.
24. Chan TL, Lippmann M: Experimental measurements and empirical modelling of the regional deposition of inhaled particles in humans, *Am Ind Hyg Assoc J* 41:399-409, 1980.
25. Hashish AH, Bailey AG, Williams TJ: Selective deposition of pulsed charged aerosols in the human lung, *J Aerosol Med* 7:167-171, 1994.
26. Baskin M, Abd A, Ilowite J: Regional deposition of aerosolised pentamidine: effects of body position and breathing pattern, *Ann Intern Med* 113:677-683, 1990.
27. O'Riordan TG, Smaldone GC: Aerosols as indices of regional ventilation, *J Aerosol Med* 7:111-117, 1994.

28. O'Riordan TG, Smaldone GC: Regional deposition and regional ventilation during inhalation of pentamidine, *Chest* 105:396-401, 1994.
29. Ryrfeldt A: The bronchial circulation: a significant local distribution system in the lung in inhalation therapy? *J Aerosol Med* 3:165-168, 1990.
30. Stahlhofen W, Gebhart J, Heyder J: Experimental determination of regional deposition of aerosol particles in the human respiratory tract, *Am Ind Hyg Assoc J* 41:385-398, 1980.
31. Knight V, Yu CP, Gilbert BE, Divine GW: Estimating the dosage of ribavirin aerosol according to age and other variables, *J Infect Dis* 158:443-448, 1988.
32. Phalen RF, Oldham MJ, Kleinman MT, Crocker TT: Tracheobronchial deposition predictions for infants, children and adolescents, *Ann Occup Hyg* 32:11-21, 1988.
33. Swift DL: Age-related scaling for aerosol and vapour deposition in the upper airways of humans, *Health Phys* 57(suppl 1):293-297, 1989.
34. Thomas RG: Regional human lung dose after inhalation of radioactive particles at ages one month to adulthood, *Ann Occup Hyg* 32(suppl 1):1025-1033, 1988.
35. Xu GB, Yu CP: Effects of age on deposition of inhaled aerosols in human lung, *Aerosol Sci Technol* 5:349-357, 1986.
36. Yu CP, Xu GB: Predicted deposition of diesel particles in young humans, *J Aerosol Sci* 18:419-429, 1987.
37. Auty RM, Brown K, Neale MG, Snashall PD: Respiratory tract deposition of sodium cromoglycate is highly dependent upon technique of inhalation using the Spinhaler, *Br J Dis Chest* 81:371-380, 1987.
38. Borgstrom L, Newman SP, Weisz A, Moren F: Pulmonary deposition of inhaled terbutaline: comparison of scanning gamma camera and urinary excretion methods, *J Pharm Sci* 81:753-755, 1992.
39. Hindle M, Newton DAG, Chrystyn H: Investigations of an optimal inhaler technique with the use of urinary salbutamol excretion as a measure of relative bioavailability to the lung, *Thorax* 48:607-610, 1993.
40. Newman SP, Steed KP, Hooper G, Kallen A, Borgstrom L: Lung deposition of pressurised terbutaline sulphate aerosols compared by two techniques, *J Aerosol Med* 7:111-117, 1994.
41. Everard ML: Studies using radio-labelled aerosols in children, *Thorax* 49:1259-1266, 1994.
42. Thomas SHL, Batechelor S, O'Doherty MJ: Therapeutic aerosols in children, *Br Med J* 307:245-247, 1993.
43. Clark AR: In-vitro assessment of spacer and reservoir devices. In Dalby RN, Evans RM, eds: *Respiratory drug delivery II,* Lexington, Ky, 1992, University of Kentucky Press, pp 470-482.
44. Newman SP, Clark AR, Talee N, Clarke SW: Pressurised aerosol deposition in the human lung with and without an "open" spacer, *Thorax* 44:706-710, 1989.
45. Borgstrom L, Bondesson E, Moren F, Newman SP: Lung deposition of budesonide inhaled via Turbuhaler: a comparison with terbutaline sulphate, *Eur Respir J* 7:69-73, 1994.
46. Pedersen S: How to use a Rotahaler, *Arch Dis Child* 61:11-14, 1986.
47. Newman SP, Woodman G, Clarke SW: Deposition of carbenicillin aerosols in cystic fibrosis: effects of nebuliser system and breathing pattern, *Thorax* 43:318-322, 1988.
48. Zainudin BM, Tolfree SEJ, Short M, Spiro SG: Influence of breathing pattern on lung deposition and bronchodilator response to nebulised salbutamol in patients with stable asthma, *Thorax* 43:987-991, 1988.
49. Collis GG, Cole CH, Le Souëf PN: Dilution of nebulised aerosols by air entrainment in children, *Lancet* 336:341-343, 1990.
50. Everard ML, Clark AR, Milner AD: Drug delivery from jet nebulisers, *Arch Dis Child* 67:586-591, 1992.
51. Everard ML, Clark AR, Milner AD: Drug delivery from holding chambers with attached facemask, *Arch Dis Child* 67:580-585, 1992.
52. Everard ML, Hardy JG, Milner AD: Comparison of nebulised aerosol deposition in the lungs of health adults after oral and nasal inhalation, *Thorax* 48:1045-1046, 1993.
53. Thomas SHL, O'Doherty MJ, Page CJ, Nunan TO: Variability in the measurement of nebulized aerosol deposition in man, *Clin Sci* 81:767-775, 1991.
54. Anderson PJ, Dolovich MB: Aerosols as diagnostic tools, *J Aerosol Med* 7:77-88, 1994.
55. Bennett WD, Ilowite JS: Dual pathway clearance of 99m Tc-DTPA from the bronchial mucosa, *Am Rev Respir Dis* 139:1132-1138, 1989.
56. Hof VIM, Patrick G: Particle retention and clearance, *J Aerosol Med* 7:39-47, 1994.

Medication-Delivery Systems

57. Alvine GF, Rogers P, Fitzsimmons KM, Aherns RC: Disposable nebulisers: how reliable are they? *Chest* 101:316-319, 1992.
58. Newhouse MT: Emergency department management of life-threatening asthma: are nebulizers obsolete? *Chest* 103:661-663, 1993 (editorial).
59. Goldman JM, Bayston SM, O'Connor S, Meigh RE: Inhaled micronised gentamicin powder: a new delivery system, *Thorax* 45:939-940, 1990.
60. Everard ML, Milner AD: A drying chamber for use with small volume jet nebulisers, *Respir Med* 89:567-569, 1995.
61. Newman SP, Pellow PGD, Clark SW: The flow-pressure characteristics of compressors used for inhalation therapy, *Eur J Respir Dis* 71:122-126, 1987.
62. Newman SP, Pellow PGD, Clark SW: Drop sizes from medical atomisers (nebulisers) for drug solutions with different viscosities and surface tensions, *Atomisat Spray Technol* 3:1-11, 1987.
63. Newman SP, Pellow PGD, Clay MM, Clark SW: Evaluation of jet nebulisers for use with gentamicin, *Thorax* 40:671-676, 1985.
64. Everard ML, Evans M, Milner AD: Is tapping jet nebulisers worthwhile? *Arch Dis Child* 70:538-539, 1994.
65. O'Doherty MJ, Thomas SHL, Gibb D, Page CJ, Harrington C, Duggan C, Nunan TO, Bateman NT: Lung deposition of aerosol nebulised pentamidine in children, *Thorax* 48:220-226,1993.
66. Beasley R, Rafferty A, Holgate ST: Adverse reactions to the non-drug constituents of nebuliser solution, *Br J Clin Pharmacol* 25:283-287, 1988.
67. Durrani FK, Richards W, Church JA, Roberts MJ, Keen TG: Evaluation of a new, shorter method of administration of adrenergic aerosols in the treatment of asthma, *Ann Allergy* 61:147-150, 1988.
68. O'Doherty MJ, Thomas SHL, Page CJ, Bradbeer C, Nunan TO, Bateman NT: Pulmonary deposition of nebulised pentamidine isethionate: effect of nebuliser type, dose and volume fill, *Thorax* 45:460-464, 1990.
69. Thomas SHL, Langford JA, George RDG, Geddes DM: Improving the efficiency of drug administration with jet nebulisers, *Lancet* 1:126, 1988 (letter).
70. Marshall LM, Francis PW, Khafagi FA: Aerosol deposition in cystic fibrosis using an aerosol conservation device and a conventional jet nebulizer, *J Paediatr Child Health* 30:65-67, 1994.
71. Mercer TT, Goddard RF, Flores RL: Effect of auxiliary air flow on the output characteristics of compressed-air nebulisers, *Ann Allergy* 27: 211-217, 1969.
72. Nikander K: Drug delivery systems, *J Aerosol Med* 7:S19-S24, 1994.
73. Thomas SHL, O'Doherty MJ, Graham A, Blower PJ, Geddes DM, Nunan TO: Pulmonary deposition of nebulised amiloride in cystic fibrosis: comparison of two nebulisers, *Thorax* 46:717-721, 1991.
74. Thomas SHL, O'Doherty MJ, Page CJ, Nunan TO, Bateman NT: Which apparatus for inhaled pentamidine? A comparison of pulmonary deposition via eight nebulisers, *Eur Respir J* 4:616-622, 1991.
75. Edman P: Pharmaceutical formulations: suspensions and solutions, *J Aerosol Med* 7:S3-S6, 1994.
76. Everard ML, Devadason SG, Le Souëf PN: Factors affecting total and "respirable" dose delivered by a salbutamol metered dose inhaler, *Thorax* 50:517-519, 1995.
77. Newhouse MT, Dolovich MD: Current concepts: control of asthma by aerosols, *New Engl J Med* 315:870-874, 1986.
78. Hauck HR: Do medical CFCs threaten the environment? *J Aerosol Med* 4:169-180, 1991.
79. Engel T: Patient-related side effects of CFC propellants, *J Aerosol Med* 4:163-167, 1991.
80. Konig P: Spacer devices used with metered-dose inhalers: breakthrough or gimmick? *Chest* 88:276-284, 1985.
81. Pool JB, Greenough A, Gleeson JGA, Price JF: Inhaled bronchodilator treatment via the nebuhaler in young asthmatic patients, *Arch Dis Child* 63:288-291, 1988.

Special Considerations

82. Murakami G, Igarashi T, Adachi Y, Matsuno M, Adachi Y, Sawai M, Yoshizumi A, Okada T: Measurement of bronchial hyperreactivity in infants and preschool children using a new method, *Ann Allergy* 64:383-387, 1990.
83. Everard ML, Stammers J, Hardy JG, Milner AD: New aerosol delivery system for neonatal ventilator circuits, *Arch Dis Child* 67:826-830, 1992.

84. Fuller HD, Dolovich MB, Posmituck G, Wong Pack W, Newhouse MT: Pressurised aerosol versus jet aerosol to mechanically ventilated patients, *Am Rev Respir Dis* 141:440-444, 1990.
85. Grigg J, Arnon S, Jones T, Clark A, Silverman M: Delivery of therapeutic aerosols to intubated babies, *Arch Dis Child* 67:25-30, 1992.
86. Thomas SHL, O'Doherty MJ, Page CJ, Treacher DF, Nunan TO: Delivery of ultrasonic nebulized aerosols to a lung model during mechanical ventilation, *Am Rev Respir Dis* 148:872-877, 1993.
87. Taylor RH, Lerman J, Chambers C, Dolovich M: Dosing efficiency and particle-size characteristics of pressurised metered dose inhaler aerosols in narrow catheters, *Chest* 103:920-944, 1993.

CHAPTER 20

Chest Physiotherapy

Maximilian S. Zach and Béatrice Oberwaldner

The term *chest physiotherapy (CPT)* stands for a spectrum of physical and mechanical interventions aimed at interacting therapeutically with acute and chronic respiratory disorders. Experience shows that CPT in children differs in many aspects from that in adults.[1] Consequently, pediatric CPT is a specialized branch of the entire CPT spectrum that is tailored to the specific needs of newborns, infants, and children. In practice, a major part of pediatric CPT is dedicated to airway clearance, but many chest physiotherapists have also acquired competence in a variety of other caregiving strategies.

CPT FOR AIRWAY CLEARANCE

CPT for airway clearance is a spectrum of mechanical techniques for the noninvasive clearance of excessive secretions or aspirated material from the airways. Because it physically addresses the respiratory tract, CPT can be seen as a therapeutic application of respiratory physiology.

CPT is used to prevent or treat the mechanical, infectious, and biochemical sequelae of accumulated intrabronchial material.[2] Such obstructive material (in most cases, secretions) increases the resistance to airflow and the work of breathing and can cause hyperinflation and atelectasis, maldistribution of ventilation, and ventilation-perfusion mismatch. Accumulation of secretions and the resulting complications facilitate infection. Microorganisms and host-mediated inflammatory responses release proteolytic enzymes that damage the airway epithelium and wall, further impairing mucociliary and cough clearance.[3] Thus intrabronchial accumulation of secretions can initiate a vicious circle of infection, impaired clearance, and progressive airway damage. In such conditions, CPT may not only have antiobstructive effects but also prevent or delay tissue damage. A theoretic third therapeutic benefit from CPT should be improved access to the bronchial mucosal surface; after effective removal of secretions, a larger portion of inhaled medications should penetrate to the airway epithelium.

The most important features of each CPT technique are its effectiveness and safety. Techniques for long-term treatment should be easy to teach to patients and caregivers; they should not fatigue the patient but rather should be time efficient and comfortable.[4] Practical applicability and cost-effectiveness demand that techniques be based on patient participation rather than on expensive equipment. One possible exception to this rule could be the very ill and exhausted patient; in this case, each technique that offers some benefit is acceptable, even if it involves expensive machinery, regular expert assistance, or both.

CPT Techniques

Conventional CPT

The term *conventional CPT* is used for a spectrum of traditional techniques that were described in the early 1960s and, at least in part, stem from practices developed as early as 1934.[5] Basically, conventional CPT is a therapeutic regimen intended to be applied by a physiotherapist or trained caregiver. However, some techniques can be self-administered by the patient.

Techniques. The techniques can be differentiated into those for mobilizing secretions and those for transporting secretions. They are combined for tailoring individually targeted treatment sessions.

Postural drainage. Postural drainage is based on the concept of gravity-assisted mobilization and transport of secretions. The patient is positioned to drain each segment of the lungs or a group of segments. These traditional positions, established by practical experience and guided by the anatomy of the bronchial tree, are summarized and illustrated in relevant textbooks.[5,6] For older children and adults, positioning for postural drainage is assisted by using frames, tilt tables, or pillows; postural drainage for an infant is administered by positioning the child over the knees of the therapist (Fig. 20-1). In the actively cooperating patient, postural drainage can be complemented by thoracic expansion exercises and by breathing control. In infants and toddlers, chest percussion, vibration, and compression can be applied during postural drainage.

Thoracic expansion exercises. Intended to aid in the mobilization of secretions, thoracic expansion exercises are deep inspirations with a 3-second hold at total lung capacity followed by a relaxed expiration. There should be a pause for breathing control after four deep breaths to avoid hypocapnia. To expand particular areas of the patient's rib cage, the physiotherapist using proprioceptive stimuli teaches locally emphasized in-

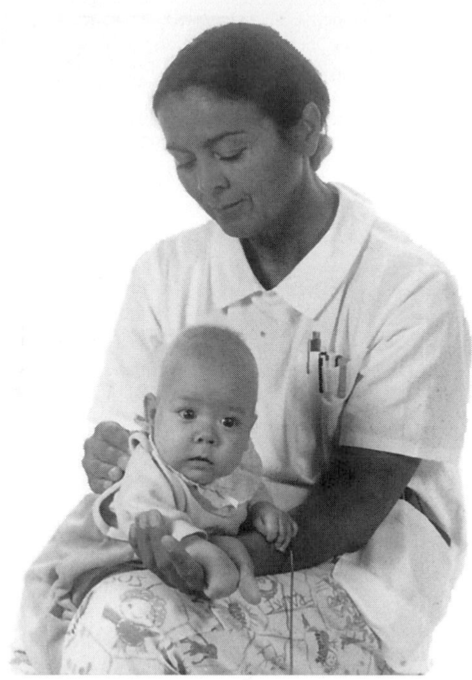

Fig. 20-1. Postural drainage position for the posterior upper lobe segments of an infant.

spirations. Consequently, one can distinguish unilateral lower, bilateral lower, posterior lower, and apical thoracic expansion. Experienced therapists can effect thoracic expansion in preterm and newborn infants by positioning with manual inspiratory assistance. Laughing and crying are effective for thoracic expansion in infants and children.

Manual hyperinflation. In mechanically ventilated lungs, an increase in volume is achieved by manual hyperinflation. The size of the bag, flow rate of gas, level and control of inspiratory pressure, and use of positive end-expiratory pressure are all important technical details that determine the efficacy and safety of this technique.[1]

Breathing control. Breathing control is needed to help the patient recover between other, more energy-consuming CPT maneuvers and reduce breathlessness; it is tidal breathing with the patient using the lower chest while relaxing the upper chest and shoulders. The patient exhales as quietly as possible by sinking the lower ribs down and then breathes in gently. The terms *diaphragmatic breathing* and *abdominal breathing* are often used for describing this technique.

Chest percussion. Intended to mobilize secretions, clapping is manual percussion with cupped hands by means of a quick flexion and extension of the wrist. In infants, the therapist's cupped hand is replaced by the fingertips or a small, cushioned face mask. Although chest percussion is essentially a physiotherapist-administered technique, patients can be taught to do self-clapping. In addition, mechanical percussors have been developed to allow for percussion administered by the patient or by a caregiver who is less experienced or is physically handicapped.

Chest vibration. Chest vibration also aims to mobilize secretions. With the hands on the patient's thorax, the therapist produces vibrations of the chest wall during expiration. This technique can be combined with chest compression.

Chest compression. As a support for the patient's own expiration, chest compression is intended to mobilize and transport secretions. In older patients, the chest is compressed by the therapist's arms that are wrapped around it or by manual pressure on the sternum, the lateral lower parts of the rib cage, or both. In infants, the chest is compressed by one or both hands; after the expiratory squeeze, the subsequent inspiration can be supported by thoracic expansion.

Assisted coughing. With impaired mucociliary clearance, coughing remains the patient's own compensatory mechanism for transporting secretions. Usually, a patient coughs spontaneously as soon as secretions have been mobilized. An attending physiotherapist can manually support the patient's chest during coughing.

Frequently, the pressure waves produced by chest percussion, vibration, or both techniques also activate the cough reflex. Experienced therapists can induce coughing by applying gentle digital pressure to the trachea in the suprasternal notch. Coughing should continue until airways have been cleared from all mobilized sputum. Care must be taken to avoid mobilization without complete expectoration because this leads to erroneous shifting of secretions from one part of the lower respiratory tract to the other.

Suction. In patients with artificial airways, the transport of secretions is mechanically hampered by the endotracheal tube or the tracheostomy cannula. In addition, the underlying disease, concomitant medication, or both can reduce the activity of the cough reflex. In these cases, suction must substitute for coughing. The catheter is introduced into the artificial airway and advanced no more than 1 cm beyond without suction. Then suction is applied while the catheter is slowly rotated and withdrawn. Correct performance of the suction procedure is essential for minimizing negative side effects. Details to be considered are preoxygenation, instillation of saline before the suction procedure, diameter of the suction catheter in relation to the size of the trachea, length and gradation of the catheter, position and number of the side holes, magnitude of the negative pressure applied, duration of the suction procedure, and manual or mechanical hyperinflation after suctioning.[1,7] Suction procedure policies regarding most of these technical details differ among centers.[8] In some patients whose lungs have not been intubated and who cough ineffectively or not all, the larynx and upper trachea can be cleared by deep pharyngeal suctioning.

Physiologic Background. The efficacy of postural drainage for clearing the lower respiratory tract and improving lung functions has been documented in several studies.[9-15] It has remained unclear whether this improved drainage results from gravity or depends on a posture-effected redistribution of ventilation.[16,17] Such posture-induced redistribution of ventilation is age dependent and differs between children and adults.[18] With few exceptions,[19] the therapeutic value of postural drainage has been established by studies of adults; thus it remains unclear whether and to what extent these findings are also valid for children. In some pediatric patients, a head-down tilt may cause gastroesophageal reflux; whether this is of clinical relevance remains to be determined.[20]

The rationale for using thoracic expansion exercises is based on the concept that high lung volumes enhance air entry behind partially obstructing mucous plugs. With a deep inspiration, airways are distended enough for inspired air to pass on toward the periphery; furthermore, airflow through collateral channels is enhanced.[17] Breathing exercises were shown to increase the partial pressure of arterial oxygen in postoperative patients.[21]

Breathing control is a strategy for economizing the energy cost of breathing (i.e., for achieving the necessary gas exchange with minimal effort).[5]

The scientific and physiologic bases of chest percussion have remained undefined. Some researchers have shown a deterioration of lung function and arterial oxygen tension with clapping,[22,23] but others, by incorporating clapping into more complex CPT regimens, did not observe such negative effects.[24,25] Pressure waves produced by clapping, vibrations, and compression may induce bronchospasm in patients with hyperreactive airways.[12,26] Although the relevant literature has thus far focused on whether chest percussion has negative side effects, it has remained unclear whether and how percussion achieves a therapeutic effect. Conclusive studies to document the efficacy of clapping per se are lacking. Whether clapping produces transthoracic pressure waves that shake secretions from the airway walls or mobilizes secretions by stimulating the cough reflex remains to be shown. Experienced pediatric chest physiotherapists claim that chest percussion has its maximal efficacy in infants and loses its therapeutic value progressively with increasing age. This observation complies with a concept of transthoracic pressure waves that decrease in efficacy with increasing size and stiffness of the chest. There is no evidence that CPT performed with mechanical percussors is more effective than manual clapping.[27-29] Consequently, patients and parents may choose between these two percussion techniques based on their personal perception of comfort, benefit, convenience, and practicability.[29]

Isolated mechanical chest vibration as a technique for mobilizing excess bronchial secretions was investigated in a radioaerosol study, but results remained inconclusive.[30] Another investigation of patients with atelectasis documented a vibration-effected increase in the partial pressure of arterial oxygen.[31] It appears that many of the existing questions related to chest percussion may also apply to chest vibration.

Chest compression also lacks a specific scientific background; as a technique for supporting the patient's expiration, however, it finds some physiologic basis in the mechanisms of a forced expiratory maneuver.

The efficacy of coughing for transporting secretions is also based on the mechanisms of forced expiration; these mechanisms are discussed in more detail in the next section. In some patients, coughing may be as effective as more complex CPT techniques for clearing secretions from airways.[32-34] Such findings, however, might not apply to patients with instability of the airway wall (i.e., bronchiectatic airway wall damage).[35] In such a situation, the high positive transthoracic pressures, which are developed during a cough, can result in complete airway collapse, thereby interrupting the expiratory airstream through the bronchus.[36] Because this occurs frequently, the forced expiration technique (FET) and other related CPT methods might be more effective than coughing; this speculation is based on the finding that the transpulmonary pressures developed with coughing exceed those occurring in a forced expiratory maneuver.[37]

Suction interrupts mechanical ventilation and thereby effected gas exchange, can facilitate bacterial contamination of the lower respiratory tract, and can cause atelectasis, suction trauma, and other complications.[38] Deep suctioning damages the airway by effecting suction biopsy of the mucosa.[39] If it occurs repeatedly, such suction trauma can result in airway obstruction by granulation tissue and scarring, a complication most frequently found at the entry into the segmental bronchi of the right lower lobe. Consequently, suction depth is a critical detail of the procedure. In addition, suctioning should be performed only when necessary; any suction routine with fixed time intervals should be avoided. Manual or mechanical hyperinflation after suctioning is recommended to prevent suction-induced atelectasis; bagging increases the compliance of the respiratory system.[40]

Practical Aspects. For clinical application, these techniques can be combined into different individually tailored CPT sessions. Therapist-administered techniques such as postural drainage, chest percussion, vibration, and compression, with assisted coughing or suction, are routinely applied in infants and small children and remain the only available CPT approach in this age group. Older patients can cooperate with breathing control and thoracic expansion exercises, or they can be trained in one of the self-administered techniques discussed later. Parents of children with chronic conditions are trained by an experienced therapist to competently administer conventional CPT at home.

Properly performed conventional CPT is neither painful nor unpleasant for children; thus after a short adaptation period, it is usually well tolerated. A treatment session can be time consuming, especially with generalized lung disease in which postural drainage must be performed for all lung segments.

FET and Active Cycle of Breathing Techniques

The FET was first described in England in the late 1970s.[41,42] As a self-administered technique for clearing the airways, it was first and most extensively studied in patients with cystic fibrosis (CF), but it can also be applied to other chronic disorders with abundant intrabronchial secretions. The active cycle of breathing techniques incorporates the FET into a sequence of thoracic expansion exercises and breathing control.[43]

Technique. In the FET, the forced expiratory maneuver used for mobilizing and transporting secretions has the form of a "huff." For producing a huff, the patient, using chest wall and abdominal muscles, exhales forcefully but not violently through the open mouth. Care must be taken to keep the glottis open. For loosening secretions in the periphery, a huff should cover the range from middle to low lung volume; subsequently, lung volume of huffing can be adjusted to the momentary location of the transported secretions. As soon as secretions reach the upper airways, they can be raised by a huff from high lung volume. The expiratory flow rate used varies individually with the airflow obstruction and compressibility of airways; huffs must be long enough to effectively move secretions. The FET is performed while the patient is in gravity-assisted positions or sitting.

The active cycle of breathing techniques adheres to the following sequential protocol: breathing control, thoracic expansion exercises, breathing control, thoracic expansion exercises, breathing control, FET (one or two huffs), and breathing control. This sequence can be repeated until all secretions are removed; individual modifications can adapt the protocol to each disease situation.

Physiologic Background. Like coughing, the FET uses expiratory airflow for mobilizing and transporting secretions, thus applying the physiology of a forced expiration.[44,45] The technique attempts to mobilize secretions from the periphery by having the patient huff in a low lung volume. The efficacy of the technique depends on the upstream movement of the equal pressure points in the airways. With an ongoing forced expiration, the dynamic compression of airways creates a wave of choke points that run upstream toward the periphery. A mucous plug, once reached and caught by such a choke point, is propelled downstream by the ongoing expiratory airflow (Fig. 20-2). In addition, the expiratory airflow velocity increases locally with this dynamic compression of the airway; accumulated intrabronchial secretions are mobilized by markedly increased shearing forces and intensified gas-liquid interactions. Recent radioaerosol studies indicate that coughing and the FET lose effectiveness progressively from the central airways to the periphery of the lung.[34] The influence of the viscoelasticity of secretions on their clearance by cough and FET remains a matter of debate; although some in vitro studies found that clearance decreases with increasing spinnability and adhesivity, other in vivo radioaerosol investigations failed to demonstrate such correlations.[34,46]

The FET is a well-investigated technique. It produces more sputum than conventional CPT in a shorter period of time.[41] Two studies comparing the efficacy of the FET and positive expiratory pressure (PEP) mask therapy have arrived at somewhat contradictory results.[14,47] Airway clearance by the FET can result in a statistically significant improvement of lung function.[15] A fall in oxygen saturation, occasionally observed with conventional CPT, can be prevented with the use of the entire active cycle of breathing techniques.[48]

Practical Aspects. The FET is an effective, self-administered CPT technique that remains independent of any mechanical adjunct. Children as young as of 3 to 4 years of age can be taught to huff; blowing games can assist training in this age group.

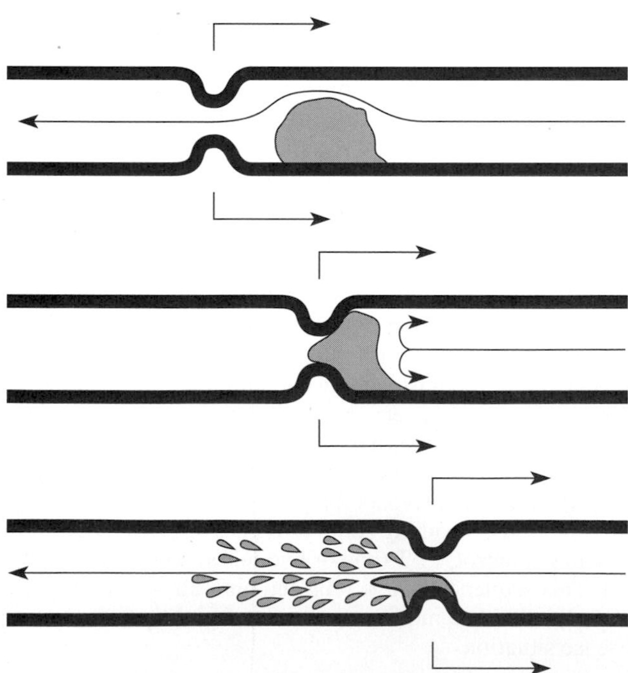

Fig. 20-2. Mobilization of mucus by a forced expiration. *Top,* The choke point moves upstream and approaches the mucous plug. *Middle,* The mucous plug is caught in the choke point. *Bottom,* The expiratory airstream ejects the mucus through the choke point.

Autogenic Drainage

Autogenic drainage (AD) is a self-administered CPT technique developed in Belgium and first described in the early 1980s.[49] The accumulated clinical experience with this technique stems mainly from its application in the treatment of CF.

Technique. AD is a special breathing technique that commences at low lung volumes (i.e., in the expiratory reserve volume) and then with mobilization of secretions is first elevated to the level of tidal breathing. With the accumulation of secretions in more central airways, the AD breathing level is further elevated into the inspiratory reserve volume, and finally, secretions are raised by a huff. The single inspiration and expiration of AD breathing exceeds the tidal volume dimension. Each inspiration is followed by a short pause; each expiration, performed with an open mouth and glottis, is mildly forced but simultaneously tries to avoid compression-induced interruption of airflow. Massively forced expiratory maneuvers and coughing are avoided. AD is usually performed with the patient in a sitting position.

Physiologic Background. AD can be seen as a modification of the FET, so comparable physiologic principles apply. The technique aims to individually determine an "ideal" expiratory flow rate that is still high enough for mobilizing and transporting secretions but still low enough for avoiding positive transthoracic pressures of such magnitude that destabilized bronchi are occluded. Clearly, such a compromise is determined by the most collapsible airway segments in the system. By commencing at low volumes and by approaching high lung volumes in a stepwise manner, the technique tries to follow the movement of mobilized secretions.

There is a discrepancy between the widespread clinical application of this technique in Europe and the paucity of controlled investigations of its value. One prospective study in CF patients indicates that the technique is clearly more effective than spontaneous coughing.[50] Another investigation found AD to be as effective as the active cycle of breathing techniques at clearing mucus in patients with CF.[51] Other relevant articles are descriptive.[52] So far, the relative value of AD compared to most other self-administered techniques remains to be defined.

Practical Aspects. Because the patient must develop significant proprioceptive abilities for feeling the movement of secretions and the occlusion of bronchi, it takes considerable time to properly learn this technique. Furthermore, a daily AD routine also tends to require more time than CPT by some other techniques. On the other hand, AD is less energy consuming and is less prone to induce bronchospasm than more aggressive forms of CPT.[50]

PEP Mask Therapy

PEP mask therapy uses the same concept as pursed-lips breathing; as a CPT technique, it was developed in Denmark in the late 1970s[47] and has found widespread acceptance. Basically, it is a self-administered CPT technique for the treatment of CF, but it may also be of some value in other conditions that produce abundant endobronchial secretions.

Technique. The PEP mask is a cushioned anesthesiology mask connected to a one-way breathing valve. An endotracheal tube adaptor for neonates is plugged into the outlet of the valve and serves as an expiratory resistor. A set of such resistors with different internal diameters allows for individual variation of the stenosis. Other types of resistors are also offered by some manufacturers.

Therapy is performed with the patient seated with the elbows resting on a table and the mask pressed tightly but comfortably over the mouth and nose (Fig. 20-3). Using diaphragmatic breathing, the patient inspires a volume larger than the tidal volume and then exhales actively but not forcefully to functional residual capacity. The resistor is chosen individually for achieving a PEP from 10 to 20 cm H_2O and an inspiratory-to-expiratory ratio of 1:3 to 1:4. A manometer connected to the outlet part of the valve allows monitoring of expiratory pressures and serves as a visual feedback to the patient. From 10 to 20 such breathing cycles are performed with the mask in place; then the mask is removed, and secretions are raised by a huff. Ideally, this sequence of PEP breaths, followed by huffing, is repeated until the airways are cleared from all mobilized secretions.

In an attempt to facilitate aerosol distribution to the peripheral airways, PEP breathing can be combined with aerosol inhalation.[53] In such a case, a mouthpiece can substitute for the mask.

Physiologic Background. It is believed that exhaling against resistance can create enough backpressure to maintain the patency of unstable airways. This theory is supported by recent work that demonstrated a marked attenuation of dynamic airway compression by PEP.[54] Thus PEP mask therapy can be used to treat patients with obstructive lung disease complicated by instability of the airway wall (i.e., bronchiectasis). PEP mask therapy is thought to increase collateral airflow to areas where the airways are obstructed by secretions, thereby facilitating subsequent expiratory mobilization of mucus.

PEP mask therapy is a well-studied technique. In some comparative investigations, it was found to be superior to other CPT techniques in terms of sputum production and other clinical measures.[47,55,56] A recent radioaerosol study showed PEP mask therapy in combination with FET to be more effective in terms of mucus clearance than FET alone.[57] Other authors either failed to find significant differences when comparing PEP mask therapy with other forms of CPT or found PEP mask therapy to be somewhat less effective.[14,58-62] PEP mask therapy has been reported to cause various changes of lung functions, such as an increased partial pressure of oxygen and tidal volume and a decreased residual volume and work of breathing.[47,55,63,64] From the sum of these published data, one can conclude that PEP mask therapy is effective for clearing airways of excess secretions in chronic lung disorders, especially CF. However, its relative value, when compared to other properly performed CPT techniques, needs to be more clearly defined.

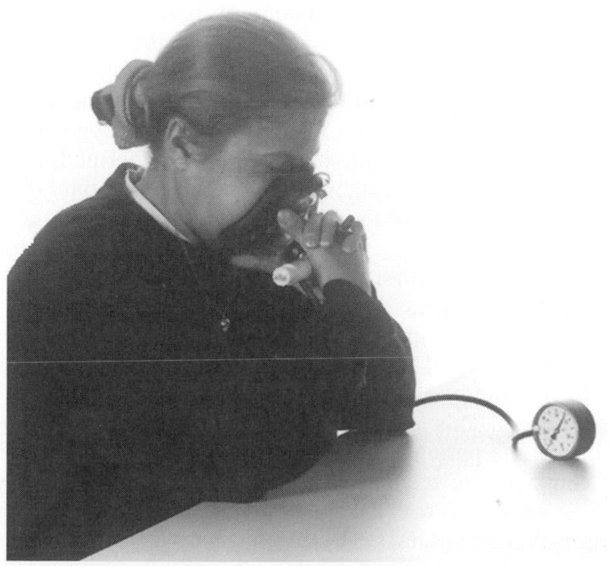

Fig. 20-3. PEP mask therapy.

Practical Aspects. PEP mask therapy is an attractive technique for patients with chronic lung disease who depend on a self-administered method for clearing their airways that is not time consuming. PEP mask therapy sessions typically take only half of the time required for a conventional CPT session but raise equivalent quantities of sputum.[65] In addition, the patient does not depend on cumbersome equipment such as percussors or tilt tables for effective self-treatment. PEP mask therapy can be taught to children beginning at approximately 4 years of age.

High-Pressure PEP Mask Therapy

High-pressure PEP mask therapy, developed in Austria in the early 1980s, incorporates forced expiratory maneuvers into PEP mask technique.[66] Like the Danish technique, it can be used by patients with CF and other chronic respiratory conditions that produce excessive bronchial secretions.

Technique. The instrument used for this technique is the same as that described in the previous section, but it is equipped with another manometer for monitoring higher pressures. Again, therapy is performed with the patient seated with the elbows resting on a table and the shoulders moved close to the neck to cover and support the lung apexes. PEP breathing for 8 to 10 cycles is done as described in the previous section; then the patient inhales to total lung capacity and subsequently performs a forced expiratory maneuver against the stenosis. Effected mobilization of secretions usually results in coughing at low lung volume. After expectorating sputum, the patient repeats the same sequence of breathing maneuvers until no more sputum is produced. Care must be taken not to terminate these forceful expirations before residual volume is reached; the sustained expiratory pressures achieved usually range between 40 and 100 cm H_2O.

The dimension of the expiratory resistor is determined individually by a spirometer-assisted method.[66] For this purpose, the outlet of the PEP mask is connected to a spirometer, and the patient performs forced expiratory vital capacity maneuvers through a series of resistors with different internal diameters (Fig. 20-4).

Physiologic Background. The effects of high-pressure PEP mask therapy are speculatively explained by increased collateral airflow to underventilated lung regions; air expired from there mobilizes obstructing secretions. In addition, a forced expiration against a marked resistive load tends to squeeze pendelluft from hyperinflated into obstructed and atelectatic lung units. Mobilization of mucous plugs might be supported by backpressure-effected dilation of airways. As in the FET,

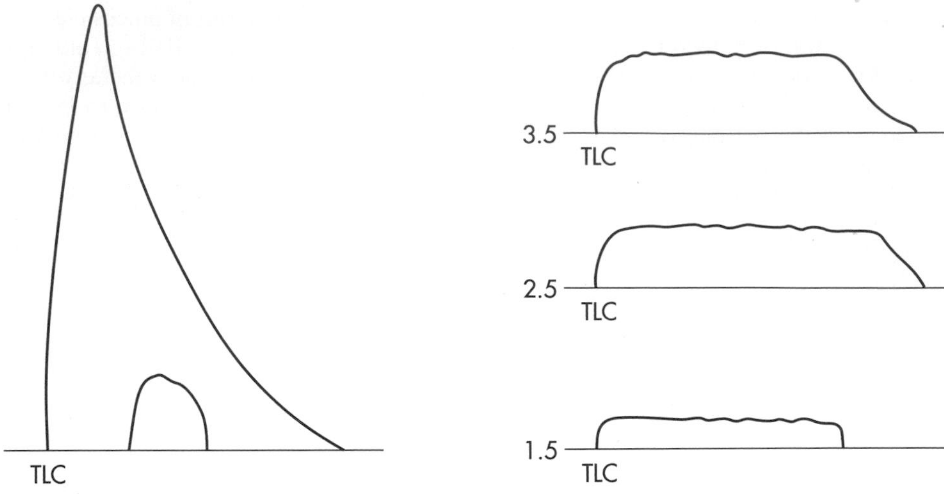

Fig. 20-4. Finding the optimal expiratory resistor for high-pressure PEP mask therapy. Patient with CF, age 15 years. *Left,* Maximum expiratory flow-volume curve of a patient with CF. *Right, top,* With a 3.5-mm internal diameter resistor, there is a stenosis-effected plateau formation, but the terminal portion of the tracing is still curvilinear (inhomogeneous emptying of different lung units). *Right, middle,* With a 2.5-mm internal diameter resistor, there is a plateau at a lower flow rate, and the terminal portion of tracing has straightened. *Right, bottom,* With a 1.5-mm internal diameter resistor, the patient terminates expiration before the residual volume is reached. The 2.5-mm resistor is chosen for further treatment. *TLC,* Total lung capacity.

upstream movement of the equal pressure points with the ongoing forced expiration and a progressive incorporation of the peripheral airways into the compressed downstream segment appear to be prerequisites for efficacy. Consequently, incomplete maneuvers, either caused by the choice of an inappropriate resistor or by an incorrectly performed technique, result in impaired airway clearance.[66]

High-pressure PEP mask therapy is a relatively well-investigated technique, but studies published so far have been limited to CF patients. In a long-term investigation, the technique decreased airway obstruction and hyperinflation.[66] In hospitalized patients, high-pressure PEP mask therapy resulted in a stepwise improvement of lung function, and these changes correlated to the weight of produced sputum.[67] When compared to AD, the technique produced more sputum in a shorter period of time.[50] So far, no investigation has compared PEP mask to high-pressure PEP mask therapy.

Practical Aspects. To avoid prolonged use of suboptimal resistors, patients using this technique need regular reevaluation by specialized therapists who are supported by a well-equipped center. Backpressure-induced airway distention imposes some stress on airway walls; consequently, high-pressure PEP mask therapy occasionally induces bronchospasm in patients with airway hyperreactivity.[50,68] Such patients should either use another CPT technique or adopt a routine of bronchodilator premedication. As evident from substantial clinical experience, the technique carries no increased risk of pneumothorax.[68] Because it takes considerable expiratory muscle strength and endurance to repeatedly exhale forcefully against a marked resistive load, high-pressure PEP mask therapy is an energy-consuming technique that does not meet the needs of an exhausted patient.

From the viewpoint of the patient, the technique is attractive because it involves highly effective but brief treatment sessions. The technique can be used properly and safely by most patients older than 5 years.

Other Techniques

This section briefly summarizes other CPT techniques that are too new to have found widespread acceptance or, like physical exercise, that clear airways as a side effect.

Oral High-Frequency Oscillation Therapy. Oral high-frequency oscillation has developed from high-frequency oscillatory ventilation. An eccentric cam piston or the diaphragm of a loudspeaker produces sine wave oscillations that are superimposed on normal tidal breathing. Oscillation of airway walls is thought to mobilize secretions. In contrast to high-frequency oscillations of the chest wall, however, oral high-frequency oscillation therapy does not enhance tracheal mucus clearance in relevant animal studies.[69] In one study of healthy subjects, oral high-frequency oscillation increased mucociliary clearance.[70] In patients with CF, this technique was as effective as conventional CPT in enhancing sputum expectoration.[71] Another study has shown this technique to be no more effective than other CPT methods.[72] It follows that the efficacy of this technique has remained ill-defined. No guidelines have yet been established on how to fine-tune the technique to the patient or the disease state.

High-Frequency Chest Compression Therapy. High-frequency chest compression therapy has been recently developed, introduced, and investigated.[73] It is applied by a device that consists of a vinyl-coated polyester inflatable vest, which covers the entire torso of the patient, and a variable air-pulse delivery system. This apparatus applies high-frequency compressions to the patient's chest to mobilize secretions. The "best" compression frequencies for an individual are thought to be those associated with the highest expiratory flow rates and the largest expired volumes. These frequencies are determined by measuring the airflow and volume at the mouth during tidal breathing while the patient receives high-frequency chest compression therapy at frequencies between 5 and 22 Hz.

One long-term study found this new technique to be superior to conventional CPT in terms of the lung function of CF patients.[73] Other investigators found both techniques equally effective in improving lung functions and sputum expectoration in hospitalized patients with CF.[74] In patients whose lungs were mechanically ventilated, this technique was as effective and safe as conventional CPT.[75] The relative value of high-frequency chest compression, when compared to other self-administered CPT techniques, remains to be evaluated. One obvious practical drawback is that this technique depends on expensive and cumbersome equipment.

Flutter Therapy. Flutter therapy tries to combine PEP breathing and oral high-frequency oscillation. Self-administered flutter treatment is performed by breathing through a pipelike instrument; in the pipe's outlet, a steel ball oscillates in the expiratory airstream and thus serves as a variable resistive load. The therapeutic value of this new instrument and technique is thus far unclear, and there is a discrepancy between widespread clinical use and paucity of controlled studies. Results of a comparative study indicate that the active cycle of breathing techniques raises more sputum than flutter therapy in patients with CF.[76,77] Another study in CF patients found the flutter technique to be more effective than conventional CPT in raising sputum.[78] There might be an optimal oscillation frequency for each individual, and patients might benefit from fine-tuning the technique to their disease situations; so far, however, there are no objective guidelines for determining an individual optimal frequency.

Physical Exercise. Strenuous physical exercise and sports can facilitate expectoration of sputum in patients with CF.[79] Several mechanisms may contribute to this effect: Exercise-induced hyperventilation accelerates mucociliary clearance[80,81] and increases gas-liquid pumping in airways filled with secretions; subtle, submersion-induced chest compression occurs with swimming, and other sports occasionally cause chest shaking and vibration.

In some children with CF, regular physical exercise may effectively substitute for CPT.[82] In adults with CF, however, CPT produces more sputum than exercise.[83] From these seemingly discrepant study results, one can conclude that sports may probably substitute for CPT in some patients with mild lung disease. However, these patients still need to be trained in a CPT technique to clear their airways when they are unable to exercise. For more severely diseased patients, CPT and physical exercise should be considered complementary rather than competing treatment strategies.

Indications and Contraindications

General Aspects

Indications. In general, CPT for airway clearance should be considered in all disease situations that have expected or already established complications from accumulated intrabronchial secretions or aspirated material. CPT is then prescribed to substitute for the patient's failing mucociliary and cough clearances. Efficient intervention by CPT should be preceded by a clear analysis of the prevailing mechanisms of the patient's disease. Because several pathophysiologic variations can occur within the frame of one diagnostic entity, it seems prudent to base the use of pediatric CPT on an analysis of disease mechanisms rather than on general diagnostic classifications.

CPT is targeted to the intrathoracic airways and thus can interact only with bronchial pathology. It is effective mainly for the clearance of the central airways and loses its efficacy progressively toward the periphery. With the possible exception of some breathing exercises and positioning, CPT has no place in the treatment of alveolar, interstitial, vascular, and pleural disease.

CPT is also indicated on diagnostic grounds when secretions from the lower respiratory tract are a more relevant substrate for bacteriologic investigation than a throat swab. Effective clearance of airways by CPT is a prerequisite for the application of therapeutic aerosols that address the bronchial mucosa.

Contraindications. The decision against applying CPT, like the decision for applying CPT, should be based on a detailed understanding of the disease. When contemplating contraindications, the clinician should remember that CPT involves a variety of mechanical interventions with different and specific risks and benefits. For example, some disease situations might preclude the use of chest percussion, vibration, and compression but not thoracic expansion exercises.

Some components of CPT are contraindicated when they threaten to cause significant hemorrhage (in bleeding disorders, some cases of vascular surgery, massive intrabronchial bleeding) or cardiac dysrhythmias (in various forms and stages of cardiac disease or surgery). Occasionally, conditions of the chest wall (trauma, infections, neoplasms, rickets, and other disorders with increased risk of rib fracture) reduce or even forbid effective mechanical access to the patient's thorax.

The critically ill child with raised intracranial pressure presents a special CPT problem inasmuch as CPT might be needed to prevent deterioration in respiratory functions but might also cause further acute rises in intracranial pressure. In this case, special CPT management with more frequent but shorter treatment periods is advisable.[84] The head-down position is contraindicated, and endotracheal suction should be reduced to a minimum.[1]

Some forms of CPT might cause bronchospasm in patients with airway hyperreactivity.[12,26] Such cases can be managed by bronchodilator premedication or by tailoring of an individual CPT regimen to avoid more aggressive mechanical irritations of the intrathoracic airways.

Specific Disorders

Acute Conditions. With few exceptions, CPT should always be considered for the treatment of atelectasis or local hyperinflation despite whether the condition occurred as a complication of bronchiolitis, bronchial asthma, aspiration, pneumonitis, bronchial stenosis, or intubation and mechanical ventilation.[24,85,86]

Children with uncomplicated acute bronchiolitis or acute severe asthma do not benefit from CPT.[87,88] Similarly, there is no reason to prescribe CPT for children with croup or epiglottitis.[1] CPT is, at best, useless in acute pneumonia with lobar or segmental consolidation,[89,90] a finding that is not surprising when the predominantly alveolar localization of the inflammatory process is considered. Foreign body aspiration is routinely treated by bronchoscopy; however, CPT performed over several days after the removal of the foreign body often produces an uncomplicated recovery.[1]

Because an endotracheal tube interrupts the mucociliary escalator and hampers cough clearance, CPT should be considered for any child whose lungs are ventilated mechanically for more than a few hours. In mechanically ventilated lungs, intrabronchial accumulation of secretions is further enhanced by mucus inspissation, which is caused by fluid restriction and the use of diuretics, by the suppression of cough resulting from sedatives and neuromuscular blockage, and by poor humidification of inspired gas. Thus CPT is important in neonatology, pediatric intensive care, and pediatric surgery. For cases of lobar atelectasis or unilateral lung collapse in newborns, infants, and children whose lungs are mechanically ventilated, most centers have developed some routine of nonendoscopic bronchial lavage; such procedures usually consist of saline instillation, bagging, expiratory vibration, and chest compression followed by endotracheal suctioning.[91]

In neonatology, CPT might be prescribed for premature infants with hyaline membrane disease whose lungs are ventilated and for neonates with meconium aspiration syndrome, aspiration of food, and any other disorder requiring mechanical ventilation. Because CPT has potentially serious side effects in this patient group,[92,93] it should always be applied on an as-needed and not on a routine basis. Properly performed CPT removes secretions, improves oxygenation, and prevents postextubation atelectasis in newborns with respiratory disease.[86,94,95] A prerequisite for applying CPT effectively and safely in premature infants and newborns is a profound knowledge of the special respiratory anatomy and physiology in this age group; specifically, the therapist should modify the approach to match an extremely compliant thorax, a special mechanical situation of the diaphragm, the closing airways, an age-specific interrelation of body position and distribution of ventilation, and an actively elevated functional residual capacity. Respiratory care of the newborn is described in more detail in relevant textbooks and manuals.[1,96,97]

In the pediatric intensive care unit, CPT is often needed after the repair of congenital cardiac defects, after pulmonary surgery, and for patients with congenital diaphragmatic hernia, gastroschisis, exomphalos, and tracheoesophageal fistula.[1] In addition, patients with intubated and ventilated lungs and with severe neurologic disorders or various critical medical conditions benefit from CPT. The preoperative and postoperative CPT management of children undergoing cardiac and transplantation surgery requires specialized knowledge and experience.[1] Treatment frequency should be determined and adjusted on the basis of careful and repeated reassessment of the individual. Any chest physiotherapist working in a pediatric intensive care unit must be profoundly familiar with the special environment, its staff, machinery, and techniques. CPT strategies for intensive care are described and discussed in a special textbook.[98]

Chronic Diseases. CPT has a traditional position in the treatment of CF.[3] A recent meta-analysis of relevant studies confirmed that CPT effects significantly greater sputum clearance in CF patients than no treatment.[99] Other forms of chronic suppurative lung disease, such as localized bronchiectasis, primary ciliary dyskinesia, and some cases of agammaglobulinemia, also benefit from daily CPT. In addition, neurologically handicapped children, who chronically aspirate secretions and food, often need regular CPT. Occasionally, CPT should be prescribed for a child with bronchopulmonary dysplasia or any other chronic respiratory problem characterized by excess intrabronchial secretions. In contrast, the asthma syndrome constitutes no routine indication for CPT.

OTHER FACETS OF CPT

In addition to airway clearance, the CPT team of a pediatric respiratory center may be involved in other caregiving programs as well as diagnostic and therapeutic procedures. Such involvement differs substantially among hospitals and centers and regions and countries, the most relevant modifying factor being the availability of other specialized health care professionals such as respiratory therapists, specialized technicians, nurses, and medical doctors. Thus the subsequent list, which is based on local experience, intends to stimulate a possible wider perspective on the job description of pediatric chest physiotherapists. In the United States, the respiratory therapist is responsible for many of the same areas as the chest physiotherapist in Europe.

Breathing Exercises

Breathing exercises encompass a wide spectrum of therapeutically applied breathing patterns and body positions. One end of this spectrum is characterized by the breathing maneuvers for airway clearance, maneuvers needed for properly inhaling an aerosol, and maneuvers for adapting a patient's breathing pattern to various physical activities. On the spectrum's other end are ill-defined and occasionally obscure breathing maneuvers that have managed to survive in some institutions and physiotherapy schools in spite of lacking any physiologic basis or scientific proof of efficacy.

Muscle Training and Exercise Programs

Training programs, especially when targeted on chest and shoulder girdle, can increase respiratory muscle endurance.[100] In addition, body-building exercises may increase upper body muscle mass. By disguising disease-related chest deformities, this effect might improve a patient's body image. Chronic obstructive lung disease affects posture and thoracoabdominal musculature; targeted exercise programs may counteract this development and help the patient maintain good posture and mobility. Under the guidance of an experienced chest physiotherapist, any patient may find an easier and safer access to such programs.

Exercise programs, either organized in the form of repeated sports lessons or as a training camp, can improve the respiratory status of pediatric patients with chronic lung disease.[79,82] In addition, the chest physiotherapists conducting these programs gain valuable insight into patients' respiratory status, exercise tolerance, compliance with medication, and psychosocial problems and habits.

Aerosol Therapy

A pediatric respiratory center must provide a wide spectrum of techniques for aerosol delivery, ranging from nebulizers to dry powder or metered dose inhalers to spacers. The efficacy and safety of aerosol therapy depend on the meticulous standards for the maintenance of equipment, hygiene, dosing, and training patients and parents to perform inhalation techniques. Within a medical center, many health care professionals administer aerosol therapy, but quality control and adoption of new techniques are the responsibilities of the center's chest physiotherapists. Other responsibilities include updating other health care professionals on new techniques and equipment and organizing individual or group training sessions for patients and parents.

Lung Function Testing

Pediatric chest physiotherapists should be trained in recording and interpreting several simple and straightforward lung function tests such as spirometry, flow-volume curves, peak expiratory flow, transcutaneously measured blood gas tension, and pulse oximetry. This enables them to closely monitor the patient's therapy, thereby introducing an additional factor of control and safety. Because of their special expertise in training children to perform complex breathing maneuvers, they frequently succeed in obtaining valid lung function recordings in very young children.

Assistance with Other Diagnostic and Therapeutic Procedures

With the widespread introduction of flexible fiberoptic bronchoscopy, the pediatric airway has become more easily accessible for the pediatric pulmonologist. Incorporation of the chest physiotherapist into the endoscopy team provides the opportunity to further improve personal knowledge about this organ system. With time, the chest physiotherapist develops into a valuable assistant for the endoscopist. Occasionally, bronchoscopic lavage is performed for the removal of impacted intrabronchial secretions.[101] In such cases, simultaneously performed CPT might increase the sputum yield of the procedure. Besides endoscopy, the chest physiotherapist can offer assistance with exercise testing and in the sleep laboratory.

Long-Term Oxygen Therapy

Long-term oxygen therapy can be applied via a concentrator or, for supporting the patient's mobility, via a portable system (small tank or liquid oxygen container). Minitracheostomies may facilitate oxygen delivery to the patient. The caregiving system required for prescribing long-term oxygen therapy may be set up, maintained, and updated by the center's CPT team.

Tracheostomy Care

A small group of children with complex congenital or acquired lesions of the upper respiratory tract or progressive neuromuscular disease require tracheostomy for securing the patency of the upper airway or for applying long-term mechanical ventilation. Pediatric tracheostomy care is a comprehensive treatment encompassing many important details such as selection of the ideal cannula, the changing and proper fixation of cannulas, suction, humidification, the use of filters and valves, and the training of parents and other caregivers. Chest physiotherapists can be responsible for such a program; in fact, some modern concepts for pediatric tracheostomy care have been developed by chest physiotherapists.[102]

Home Mechanical Ventilation

Home mechanical ventilation has been widely accepted as a caregiving strategy for children with chronic respiratory insufficiency related to etiologies such as bronchopulmonary dysplasia, spinal muscular atrophy, phrenic nerve paralysis, diaphragmatic hernia, thoracic and abdominal wall deformities, high-level myelodysplasia and spinal cord injury, childhood myopathies, and central hypoventilation syndrome.[103-105] Home mechanical ventilation can be applied via a tracheostomy or through the nose or the mouth. Specifically pediatric guidelines for home mechanical ventilation have recently been developed.[106] As with tracheostomy care, the success and safety of a home mechanical ventilation program depend on the availability of a comprehensive and highly specialized treatment plan and on the meticulous training of parents. Again, such programs can be organized and carried out by a center's CPT service.

Psychologic Support

Many pediatric chest physiotherapists find themselves as patient- and parent-elected troubleshooters for psychosocial problems. By frequently talking to patients and by touching them, they gain the confidence of patients and parents and become profoundly familiar with their personal problems, which is especially important when working with children who suffer from chronic respiratory disease. With this type of knowledge, the chest physiotherapist often provides a vital, albeit unofficial, link among patients, parents, and staff.

SCIENTIFIC BASIS OF CPT

Relevant Problems and Misconceptions

Efficacy

Over 2 decades ago, a conference on the scientific basis of CPT was opened by the statement that CPT lacks an established scientific basis and evidence of lasting clinical benefit.[107] Since then, various aspects of CPT have been subject to prospective and controlled clinical studies. However, many techniques and methodologic details have thus far remained empirical. That the proponents of specific techniques tend to champion their methods at symposia and meetings has not helped clarify the situation; thus controversy still reigns in the field.[4] It follows that the scientific basis of CPT is still fragile and incomplete.

Evaluating the efficacy of CPT is a difficult task because numerous confounding variables cannot be eliminated from such studies. Each CPT technique consists of several methodologic components; different therapists and centers often tend to emphasize different parts of the technique and neglect others. When comparing the performance of CPT among centers, one finds major technical differences, a situation that illustrates an urgent need for standardization. Consequently, comparative studies of different techniques frequently find that a technique is most effective where it was developed or is most intensively practiced. Because of the pathophysiologic heterogeneity of diagnostic entities and the methodologic heterogeneity of CPT techniques, the "best" CPT technique appears to be a misconception, and the ongoing search for such a technique is ineffectual. It may be more appropriate to evaluate which CPT regimens are more effective for individuals rather than evaluating whether any one technique is the most effective for all patients and disease situations.[108] However, research aimed at improving the efficacy of CPT by better matching the specific pathophysiologic and methodologic details does not exist yet.

Physiologic Basis

Another handicap for establishing a more substantial scientific basis of CPT is the incomplete understanding of each technique's physiologic basis. Most techniques have been developed by trial and error at the bedside; traditionally, therapists have focused on whether, not how, a specific technique works. Any future concept of tailoring specific CPT techniques to individual patients and disease situations requires a clearer understanding of the mechanisms responsible for each technique's efficacy.

CPT Studies

Short-Term Studies

Short-term studies evaluate the effects of one or a few treatment sessions. Their potential clinical relevance is based on the speculation that a specific, documented short-term effect of CPT might alter the disease course. So far, clinicians have been unable to determine which diagnostic technique can most accurately assess the CPT-effected removal of secretions.

Sputum Weight. One of the simplest and most straightforward strategies is to quantify expectorated sputum by its weight. Contamination by saliva might introduce some error, but such an error progressively loses significance with increasing sputum volumes. Clearly, one cannot investigate a technique for emptying a ketchup bottle when the bottle contains hardly any ketchup in the first place.[109] For adolescents and adults, a daily sputum volume in excess of 30 ml must be obtained for documenting the efficacy of CPT.[109,110]

Lung Function Measurements. Assessment of lung function and blood gases is another traditional approach to the evaluation of short-term CPT effects. Numerous studies have documented beneficial lung function changes after the application of different CPT techniques, but many attempts to correlate the dimension of lung function changes to the weight of raised sputum have remained unsuccessful.[9,12,33] One recent study of CF patients, however, finally established such a cause-and-effect relationship.[67] This traditional difficulty in documenting a lung function–sputum weight correlation is most likely explained by airway-related noise. CPT-effected shifting of secretions from one lung unit to the other without complete expectoration, therapy-induced bronchospasm in patients with airway hyperreactivity, and occasionally applied concomitant medications are all confounding variables that tend to disguise the potentially beneficial effects of sputum expectoration on lung function. Blood gas measurements might be particularly sensitive to this type of noise.

Radioaerosol Studies. Radioaerosol studies are considered a promising strategy for assessing the effects of CPT.[111] Treatment-effected movements of the inhaled tracer are observed directly with a gamma camera. One handicap of this diagnostic approach, which particularly applies to children, is the radiation. Another caveat relates to the maldistribution of ventilation that invariably develops with any intrabronchial accumulation of secretions: Inhaled tracer particles tend to deposit least in the most obstructed lung units, which on the other hand, should benefit most from CPT.

Other Diagnostic Techniques. Occasionally, the effects of CPT can be directly observed when CPT is applied in the course of an endoscopic investigation. With few exceptions, conventional chest radiographs are too insensitive for direct visualization of accumulated intrabronchial secretions. However, they remain the routine diagnostic approach for assessing the effects of CPT on segmental or lobar atelectasis.

Long-Term Studies

The long-term effects of repeatedly applied CPT on chronic respiratory disease can be evaluated only by long-term studies. Such studies are extremely difficult to perform because the long-term course of chronic respiratory disease is usually variable and characterized by exacerbations, remissions, and the effects of other concomitant treatment strategies. Another limitation is introduced by patients, who often do not comply with CPT recommendations.[112] For obvious ethical reasons, it is frequently impossible to set up an equally diseased control group without CPT. In spite of all these limitations, a few studies, performed mainly with CF patients, have tried to establish a scientific basis for the long-term prescription of CPT in chronic pediatric lung disease.[66,73,113,114]

Conclusions

In summary, the relevant literature provides some first fragments for a scientific basis of pediatric CPT but also illustrates the urgent need for additional controlled investigations. Thus clinical and scientific audits should be an integral part of CPT practice.[115]

ORGANIZATIONAL ASPECTS

Professional Situation

At present, CPT-related organizational concepts, required level of specialization, interaction with other health care professionals, legal and administrative basis for practice, and employment conditions all differ widely among countries, medical schools, and hospitals. For example, some overlap exists, but there are also some important differences between the professional concepts of *CPT* and *respiratory therapy,* the former being of predominantly European and the latter of North American origin. One end of the professional spectrum is characterized by a profoundly structured and highly trained CPT team in the organizational framework of a pediatric respiratory center; on the other end, a specialized CPT service is completely absent. In the latter case, some CPT techniques are applied by other health care professionals or, occasionally, by physiotherapists from other pediatric subspecialties. Whether such CPT, which might lack quality and therapeutic intensity, should be prescribed at all or whether it threatens to produce more complications than benefits remains a matter of discussion. In some countries, employment of chest physiotherapists is characterized by hospital-based services; in other countries, many physiotherapists, including those who specialize in CPT, work in private practice, a situation that may impede the intensive interaction between other caregivers and the physiotherapist. The prerequisites for establishing an effective pediatric CPT service are the specialized theoretic and practical training courses that are offered by physiotherapy schools and training hospitals and that include a major pediatric component.

Improving the Efficacy of CPT

When pediatric CPT is based within the framework of a pediatric respiratory center, intensive interaction between the chest physiotherapists and all other health care professionals is mandatory for improving the efficacy of treatment. A "respiratory progress chart" for each patient can assist the health care team in monitoring the disease and patient responses to CPT.[116]

Such written documentation also intensifies the flux of information between medical physicians and physiotherapists. In addition, all members of the CPT team should take part in patient- and problem-related staff conferences for maximal integration into all relevant caregiving programs. Various delivery systems aimed at correcting CPT misallocations are developed and evaluated.[117]

Other health care professionals, including medical physicians, often have no clear knowledge of CPT and its potential indications, contraindications, and risks. Thus the buildup of an effective CPT service includes ongoing education of professionals and administrators. Another important factor for improving the efficacy of a center's CPT team is an intensive exchange of thoughts and visits with other pediatric CPT groups.

REFERENCES

1. Parker A: Paediatrics. In Webber BA, Pryor JA, editors: *Physiotherapy for respiratory and cardiac problems,* Edinburgh, 1993, Churchill Livingstone, pp 281-318.

CPT for Airway Clearance

2. Zach MS, Oberwaldner B: Chest physiotherapy: the mechanical approach to antiinfective therapy in cystic fibrosis, *Infection* 15:381-384, 1987 (review).
3. Zach MS: Lung disease in cystic fibrosis: an updated concept, *Pediatr Pulmonol* 8:188-202, 1990 (review).
4. Hardy KA: A review of airway clearance: new techniques, indications, and recommendations, *Respir Care* 39:440-452, 1994 (review).
5. Webber BA: *The Brompton hospital guide to chest physiotherapy,* ed 5, Oxford, England, 1988, Blackwell.
6. Waring WW: Diagnostic and therapeutic procedures. In Chernick V, Kendig EL, editors: *Kendig's disorders of the respiratory tract in children,* Philadelphia, 1990, WB Saunders, pp 77-96.
7. Young CS: Recommended guidelines for suction, *Physiotherapy* 70:106-108, 1984.
8. Young CS: Airway suctioning: a study of paediatric physiotherapy practice, *Physiotherapy* 74:13-15, 1988.
9. Cochrane GM, Webber BA, Clarke WS: Effect of sputum on pulmonary function, *Br Med J* 2:1181-1183, 1977.
10. Wong JW, Keens TG, Wannamaker EM, Crozier DN, Levison H, Aspin N: Effect of gravity on tracheal mucus transport rates in normal subjects and in patients with cystic fibrosis, *Pediatrics* 60:146-152, 1977.
11. Bateman JRM, Newman SP, Daunt KM, Pavia D: Regional lung clearance of excessive bronchial secretions during chest physiotherapy in patients with stable chronic airways obstruction, *Lancet* 1:294-297, 1979.
12. Feldman J, Traver GA, Taussig LM: Maximal expiratory flows after postural drainage, *Am Rev Respir Dis* 119:239-245, 1979.
13. Sutton PP, Parker RA, Webber BA, Newman SP, Garland N, Lopez-Vidriero MT, Pavia D, Clarke SW: Assessment of the forced expiration technique, postural drainage and directed coughing in chest physiotherapy, *Eur J Respir Dis* 64:62-68, 1983.
14. Hofmeyr JL, Webber BA, Hodson ME: Evaluation of positive expiratory pressure as an adjunct to chest physiotherapy in the treatment of cystic fibrosis, *Thorax* 41:951-954, 1986.
15. Webber BA, Hofmeyr JL, Morgan MDL, Hodson ME: Effects of postural drainage: incorporating the forced expiration technique, on pulmonary function in cystic fibrosis, *Br J Dis Chest* 80:353-359, 1986.
16. Mellins RS: Pulmonary physiotherapy in the pediatric age group, *Am Rev Respir Dis* 110:137-142, 1974 (review).
17. Menkes H, Britt J: Rationale for physical therapy, *Am Rev Respir Dis* 122(suppl 2):127-131, 1980 (review).
18. Davies H, Helms P, Gordon J: Effect of posture on regional ventilation in children, *Pediatr Pulmonol* 12:227-232, 1992.
19. Hardy KA, Wolfson MR, Schidlow DV, Schaffer TH: Mechanics and energetics of breathing in newly diagnosed infants with cystic fibrosis: effect of combined bronchodilator and chest physical therapy, *Pediatr Pulmonol* 6:103-108, 1989.
20. Button BM, Heine RG, Catto-Smith AG, Olinsky A: Acute effects of postural drainage on gastro-oesophageal reflux in infants with cystic fibrosis, *Pediatr Res* 36(1 pt 2):9A, 1994.
21. Hedstrand U, Liw M, Rooth G, Ögren CH: Effect of respiratory physiotherapy on arterial oxygen tension, *Acta Anaesth Scand* 22:349-352, 1978.
22. Connors AF, Hammon WE, Matin RJ, Rogers RM: Chest physical therapy: the immediate effect on oxygenation in acutely ill patients, *Chest* 78:559-564, 1980.
23. Wollmer P, Ursing K, Midgren B, Eriksson L: Inefficiency of chest percussion in the physical therapy of chronic bronchitis, *Eur J Respir Dis* 66:233-239, 1985.
24. Mackenzie CF, Shin B, McAslan TC: Chest physiotherapy: the effect on arterial oxygenation, *Anesth Analg* 57:28-30, 1978.
25. May DB, Munt PW: Physiologic effects of chest percussion and postural drainage in patients with stable chronic bronchitis, *Chest* 75:29-32, 1979.
26. Rochester DF, Goldberg SK: Techniques of respiratory physical therapy, *Am Rev Respir Dis* 122:133-146, 1980 (review).
27. Maxwell M, Redmond A: Comparative trial of manual and mechanical percussion technique with gravity-assisted bronchial drainage in patients with cystic fibrosis, *Arch Dis Child* 54:542-544, 1979.
28. Pryor JA, Parker RA, Webber BA: A comparison of mechanical and manual percussion as adjunct to postural drainage in the treatment of cystic fibrosis in adolescents and adults, *Physiotherapy* 67:140-141, 1981.
29. Bauer ML, McDougal J, Schoumacher RA: Comparison of manual and mechanical chest percussion in hospitalized patients with cystic fibrosis, *J Pediatr* 124:250-254, 1994.
30. Pavia D, Thomson ML: A preliminary study of the effect of a vibrating pad on bronchial clearance, *Am Rev Respir Dis* 113:92-96, 1976.
31. Holody B, Goldberg HS: The effect of mechanical vibration physiotherapy on arterial oxygenation in acutely ill patients with atelectasis or pneumonia, *Am Rev Respir Dis* 124:372-375, 1981.
32. Rossman CM, Waldes R, Sampson D, Newhouse MT: Effect of chest physiotherapy on the removal of mucus in patients with cystic fibrosis, *Am Rev Respir Dis* 126:131-135, 1982.
33. DeBoeck C, Zinman R: Cough versus chest physiotherapy: a comparison of the acute effects on pulmonary function in patients with cystic fibrosis, *Am Rev Respir Dis* 129:182-184, 1984.
34. Hasani A, Pavia D, Agnew JE, Clarke SW: Regional lung clearance during cough and forced expiration technique (FET): effects of flow and viscoelasticity, *Thorax* 49:557-561, 1994.
35. Zach MS, Oberwaldner B, Forche G, Polgar G: Bronchodilators increase airway instability in cystic fibrosis, *Am Rev Respir Dis* 131:537-543, 1985.
36. Smaldone GC, Itoh H, Swift DL, Wagner HN: Effect of flow-limiting segments and cough on particle deposition and mucociliary clearance in the lung, *Am Rev Respir Dis* 120:747-758, 1979.
37. Langlands J: The dynamics of cough in health and in chronic bronchitis, *Thorax* 22:88-96, 1967.
38. Young CS: A review of the adverse effects of airway suction, *Physiotherapy* 70:104-106, 1984.
39. Bailey C, Kattwinkel J, Teja K, Buckley T: Shallow versus deep endotracheal suctioning in young rabbits: pathologic effects on the tracheobronchial wall, *Pediatrics* 82:746-751, 1988.
40. Jones AYM, Hutchinson RC, Oh TE: Effects of bagging and percussion on total static compliance of the respiratory system, *Physiotherapy* 78:661-666, 1992.
41. Pryor JA, Webber BA, Hodson ME, Batten JC: Evaluation of the forced expiration technique as an adjunct to postural drainage in treatment of cystic fibrosis, *Br Med J* 2:417-418, 1979.
42. Pryor JA, Webber BA: An evaluation of the forced expiration technique as an adjunct to postural drainage, *Physiotherapy* 65:304-307, 1979.
43. Webber BA, Pryor JA: Physiotherapy skills: techniques and adjuncts. In Webber BA, Pryor JA, editors: *Physiotherapy for respiratory and cardiac problems,* Edinburgh, 1993, Churchill Livingstone, pp 113-171.
44. Mead J, Turner JM, Macklem PT, Little JB: Significance of the relationship between lung recoil and maximum expiratory flow, *J Appl Physiol* 22:95-108, 1967.
45. Macklem PT, Mead J: The physiological basis of common pulmonary function tests, *Arch Environ Health* 14:5-9, 1967 (review).

46. King M, Zahm JM, Pierrot D, Vaquez-Girod S, Puchelle E: The role of mucus gel viscosity, spinnability, and adhesive properties in clearance by simulated cough, *Biorheology* 26:737-745, 1989.
47. Falk M, Kelstrup M, Andersen JB, Kinoshita T, Falk P, Stovring S, Gothgen J: Improving the ketchup bottle method with positive expiratory pressure, PEP, in cystic fibrosis, *Eur J Respir Dis* 65:423-432, 1984.
48. Pryor JA, Webber BA, Hodson ME: Effect of chest physiotherapy on oxygen saturation in patients with cystic fibrosis, *Thorax* 45:77-78, 1990.
49. Chevallier J: Autogenic drainage. In Lawson D, editor: *Cystic fibrosis: horizons,* New York, 1984, John Wiley & Sons, p 235.
50. Pfleger A, Theissl B, Oberwaldner B, Zach MS: Self-administered chest physiotherapy in cystic fibrosis: a comparative study of high-pressure PEP and autogenic drainage, *Lung* 170:323-330, 1992.
51. Miller S, Hall DO, Clayton CB, Nelson R: Chest physiotherapy in cystic fibrosis: a comparative study of autogenic drainage and the active cycle of breathing techniques with postural drainage, *Thorax* 50:165-169, 1995.
52. Schöni MM: Autogenic drainage: a modern approach to physiotherapy in cystic fibrosis, *J Roy Soc Med* 82(suppl 16):32-37, 1989 (review).
53. Andersen JB, Klausen NO: A new mode of administration of nebulized bronchodilator in severe bronchospasm, *Eur J Respir Dis* 63(suppl 119):97-100, 1982.
54. Al-Nahhas A, Hoffmeyer B, Takis C, Obeid E, Pichurko B: Dynamic airway compression limiting forced vital capacity is attenuated by positive airway pressure in severe cystic fibrosis, *Am J Respir Crit Care Med* 149(4 pt 2):A675, 1994.
55. Tonnesen P, Stovring S: Positive expiratory pressure (PEP) as lung physiotherapy in cystic fibrosis: a pilot study, *Eur J Respir Dis* 65:419-422, 1984.
56. Christensen EF, Nedergaard T, Dahl R: Long-term treatment of chronic bronchitis with positive expiratory pressure mask and chest physiotherapy, *Chest* 97:645-650, 1990.
57. Falk M, Mortensen J, Kelstrup M, Lanng S, Larsen L, Ulrik CS: Short-term effects of positive expiratory pressure and the forced expiration technique on mucus clearance and lung function in CF, *Pediatr Pulmonol* (suppl 9):268, 1993.
58. Tyrrell JC, Hiller EJ, Martin J: Face mask physiotherapy in cystic fibrosis, *Arch Dis Child* 61:598-611, 1986.
59. VanAsperen PP, Jackson L, Hennessy P, Brown J: Comparison of a positive expiratory pressure (PEP) mask with postural drainage in patients with cystic fibrosis, *Aust Paediatr J* 23:283-284, 1987.
60. Kaminska TM, Pearson SB: A comparison of postural drainage and positive expiratory pressure in the domiciliary management of patients with chronic bronchial sepsis, *Physiotherapy* 74:251-254, 1988.
61. Steen HJ, Redmond AO, O'Neill D, Beattie F: Evaluation of the PEP mask in cystic fibrosis, *Acta Paediatr Scand* 80:51-56, 1991.
62. VanderSchans CP, VanderMark TW, DeVries G, Piers DA, Beekhuis H, Dankert-Roelse JE, Postma DS, Koeter GH: Effect of positive expiratory pressure breathing in patients with cystic fibrosis, *Thorax* 46:252-256, 1991.
63. Groth S, Stafanger G, Dirksen H, Andersen JB, Falk M, Kelstrup M: Positive expiratory pressure (PEP mask) physiotherapy improves ventilation and reduces volume of trapped gas in cystic fibrosis, *Bull Eur Physiopathol Respir* 21:339-343, 1985.
64. VanderSchans CP, deJong W, deVries G, Postma DS, Koeter GH, VanderMark TW: Effect of positive expiratory pressure on breathing pattern in healthy subjects, *Eur Respir J* 6:60-66, 1993.
65. Mahlmeister MJ, Fink JB, Hoffman GL, Fifer LF: Positive-expiratory-pressure mask therapy: theoretical and practical considerations and a review of the literature, *Respir Care* 36:1218-1229, 1991 (review).
66. Oberwaldner B, Evans JC, Zach MS: Forced expirations against a variable resistance: a new chest physiotherapy method in cystic fibrosis, *Pediatr Pulmonol* 2:358-367, 1986.
67. Oberwaldner B, Theissl B, Rucker A, Zach MS: Chest physiotherapy in hospitalized patients with cystic fibrosis: a study of lung function effects and sputum production, *Eur Respir J* 4:152-158, 1991.
68. Zach MS, Oberwaldner B: Effect of positive expiratory pressure breathing in patients with cystic fibrosis, *Thorax* 47:66-67, 1992.
69. King M, Phillips DM, Zidulka A, Chang HK: Tracheal mucus clearance in high-frequency oscillation, *Am Rev Respir Dis* 130:703-706, 1984.
70. George RJD, Johnson MA, Pavia D, Agnew JE, Clarke SW, Geddes DM: Increase in mucociliary clearance in normal man induced by oral high frequency oscillation, *Thorax* 40:433-437, 1985.
71. Natale JE, Pfeifle J, Homnick DN: Comparison of intrapulmonary percussive ventilation and chest physiotherapy: a pilot study in patients with cystic fibrosis, *Chest* 105:1789-1793, 1994.
72. Pryor JA, Wiggins J, Webber BA, Geddes DM: Oral high frequency oscillation (OHFO) as an aid to physiotherapy in chronic bronchitis with airflow limitation, *Thorax* 44:350P, 1989.
73. Warwick WJ, Hansen LG: The long-term effect of high-frequency chest compression therapy on pulmonary complications of cystic fibrosis, *Pediatr Pulmonol* 11:265-271, 1991.
74. Arens R, Gozal D, Omlin KJ, Vega J, Boyd KP, Woo MS, Keens TG: Comparative efficacy of high frequency chest compression and conventional chest physiotherapy in hospitalized patients with cystic fibrosis, *Pediatr Pulmonol* (suppl 9):267, 1993.
75. Whitman J, VanBeusekom R, Olson S, Worm M, Indihar F: Preliminary evaluation of high-frequency chest compression for secretion clearance in mechanically ventilated patients, *Respir Care* 38:1081-1087, 1993.
76. Pryor JA, Webber BA: Physiotherapy for cystic fibrosis: which technique? *Physiotherapy* 78:105-108, 1992 (review).
77. Pryor JA, Webber BA, Hodson ME, Warner JO: The flutter VRP1 as an adjunct to chest physiotherapy in cystic fibrosis, *Respir Med* 88:677-681, 1994.
78. Konstan MW, Stern RC, Doershuk CF: Efficacy of the flutter device for airway mucus clearance in patients with cystic fibrosis, *J Pediatr* 124:689-693, 1994.
79. Zach MS, Purrer B, Oberwaldner B: Effect of swimming on forced expiration and sputum clearance in cystic fibrosis, *Lancet* 2:1201-1203, 1981.
80. Wolff RK, Dolovich MB, Obminski G, Newhouse MT: Effects of exercise and eucapnic hyperventilation on bronchial clearance in man, *J Appl Physiol Respir Environ Physiol* 43:46-50, 1977.
81. Oldenburg FA, Dolovich MB, Montgomery JM, Newhouse MT: Effects of postural drainage, exercise and cough on mucus clearance in chronic bronchitis, *Am Rev Respir Dis* 120:739-745, 1979.
82. Zach M, Oberwaldner B, Häusler F: Cystic fibrosis: physical exercise versus chest physiotherapy, *Arch Dis Child* 57:587-589, 1982.
83. Salh W, Bilton D, Dodd M, Webb AK: Effect of exercise and physiotherapy in aiding sputum expectoration in adults with cystic fibrosis, *Thorax* 44:1006-1008, 1989.
84. Prasad A, Tasker R: Guidelines for the physiotherapy management of critically ill children with acutely raised intracranial pressure, *Physiotherapy* 76:248-250, 1990.
85. Marini JJ, Pierson DJ, Hudson LD: Acute lobar atelectasis: a prospective comparison of fiberoptic bronchoscopy and respiratory therapy, *Am Rev Respir Dis* 119:971-978, 1979.
86. Finer NN, Moriartey RR, Boyd J, Phillips HJ, Stewart AR, Ulan O: Postextubation atelectasis: a retrospective review and a prospective controlled study, *J Pediatr* 94:110-113, 1979.
87. Webb MSC, Martin JA, Cartlidge PHT, Ng YK, Wright NA: Chest physiotherapy in acute bronchiolitis, *Arch Dis Child* 60:1078-1081, 1985.
88. Asher MJ, Douglas C, Airy M, Andrews D, Trenholme A: Effects of chest physical therapy on lung function in children recovering from acute severe asthma, *Pediatr Pulmonol* 9:146-151, 1990.
89. Graham WGB, Bradley DA: Efficacy of chest physiotherapy and intermittent positive-pressure breathing in the resolution of pneumonia, *N Engl J Med* 299:624-627, 1978.
90. Britton S, Bejstedt M, Vedin L: Chest physiotherapy in primary pneumonia, *Br Med J* 290:1703-1704, 1985.
91. Galvis AG, Reyes G, Nelson WB: Bedside management of lung collapse in children on mechanical ventilation: saline lavage-simulated cough technique proves simple, effective, *Pediatr Pulmonol* 17:326-330, 1994.
92. Purchit DM, Caldwell C, Levkoff AH: Multiple rib fractures due to physiotherapy in a neonate with hyaline membrane disease, *Am J Dis Child* 129:1103-1104, 1975.
93. Fox WW, Schwartz JG, Shaffer TH: Pulmonary physiotherapy in neonates: physiologic changes and respiratory management, *J Pediatr* 92:977-981, 1978.
94. Etches PC, Scott B: Chest physiotherapy in the newborn: effect on secretions removed, *Pediatrics* 62:713-715, 1978.

95. Finer NN, Boyd J: Chest physiotherapy in the neonate: a controlled study, *Pediatrics* 61:282-285, 1978.
96. Koff PB, Eitzman D, Neu J: *Neonatal and pediatric respiratory care,* ed 2, St Louis, 1993, Mosby.
97. Aloan CA: *Respiratory care of the newborn,* ed 1, Philadelphia, 1987, JB Lippincott.
98. Mackenzie CF, Imle PC, Ciesla N: *Chest physiotherapy in the intensive care unit,* ed 2, Baltimore, 1989, Williams & Wilkins.
99. Thomas J, Cook DJ, Brooks D: Chest physical therapy management of patients with cystic fibrosis: a meta-analysis, *Am J Respir Crit Care Med* 151:846-850, 1995.

Other Facets of CPT

100. Keens TG, Krastins JRB, Wannamaker EM, Levison H, Crozier DN, Bryan AC: Ventilatory muscle endurance training in normal subjects and patients with cystic fibrosis, *Am Rev Respir Dis* 116:853-860, 1977.
101. Rothman BF, Walker LH, Stone RT, Seguin FW: Bronchoscopic limited lavage for cystic fibrosis patients, *Ann Otol Rhinol Laryngol* 91:641-642, 1982.
102. Oberwaldner B, Zobel G, Zach M: Pädiatrische Tracheostomapflege (paediatric tracheostomy care), *Monatsschr Kinderheilkd* 140:206-215, 1992.
103. Estournet-Mathiaud B, Barois A: Home treatment of severe bronchopulmonary dysplasias: oxygen therapy and assisted ventilation, *Eur Respir Rev* 2:304-307, 1992.
104. Goldberg AJ: Myopathies in patients under two years of age, *Eur Respir Rev* 2:308-311, 1992.
105. Barois A, Estournet-Mathiaud B: Ventilatory support at home in children with spinal muscular atrophies (SMA), *Eur Respir Rev* 2:319-322, 1992.
106. Kacmarek RM: Home mechanical ventilatory assistance for infants, *Respir Care* 39:550-560, 1994 (review).

Scientific Basis of CPT

107. Petty TL: Physical therapy, *Am Rev Respir Dis* 110:129-131, 1974.
108. Williams MT: Chest physiotherapy and cystic fibrosis: why is the most effective form of treatment still unclear? *Chest* 106:1872-1882, 1994 (review).
109. Murray JF: The ketchup-bottle method, *N Engl J Med* 300:1155-1157, 1979.
110. Selsby DS: Chest physiotherapy may be harmful in some patients, *Br Med J* 298:541-542, 1989.
111. Pavia D: The role of chest physiotherapy in mucus hypersecretion, *Lung* (suppl):614-621, 1990 (review).
112. Passero MA, Remor B, Salomon J: Patient-reported compliance with cystic fibrosis therapy, *Clin Pediatr* 20:264-268, 1981.
113. Desmond KJ, Schwenk WF, Thomas E, Beaudry PH, Coates AL: Immediate and long-term effects of chest physiotherapy in patients with cystic fibrosis, *J Pediatr* 103:538-542, 1983.
114. Reisman JJ, Rivington-Law B, Corey M, Marcotte J, Wannamaker E, Harcourt D, Levison H: Role of conventional physiotherapy in cystic fibrosis, *J Pediatr* 113:632-636, 1988.
115. Webber BA: Evaluation and inflation in respiratory care, *Physiotherapy* 77:801-804, 1991 (review).

Organizational Aspects

116. Thomson KM, Dyson AJ, Schonell M: Respiratory progress chart, *Physiotherapy* 66:88-89, 1980.
117. Steller JK, Haney D, Burkhart J, Fergus L, Giles D, Hoisington E, Kester L, Komara J, McCarthy K, McCann B, Meredith R, Orens D, the Section of Respiratory Therapy: Physician-ordered respiratory care vs. physician-ordered use of a respiratory therapy consult service: early experience at the Cleveland Clinic Foundation, *Respir Care* 38:1143-1154, 1993.

CHAPTER 21

Assisted Ventilatory Support and Oxygen Treatment

Yakov Sivan, Jürg Pfenninger, and Christopher J.L. Newth

The concept of respiratory support encompasses a wide variety of means and methods by which the function of respiration and gas exchange is assisted. This can range from enrichment of the inspiratory fraction of inspired oxygen (FIO_2) by only oxygen supply to full ventilatory support, which also replaces the act of breathing and gas delivery to the alveoli. However, there are fundamental differences in the mechanics and the physiologic processes between spontaneous unaided breathing and the replacement of this process by mechanical devices. The most crucial difference is the fact that the normal mechanism is based on negative-pressure ventilation (NPV), whereas the most common practice of ventilatory support involves the application of positive airway pressure to the airways and lungs during inspiration. This not only affects the operation and function of respiration but also has major effects on other systems, especially the cardiovascular system. Even the use of oxygen supplementation alone may have deleterious effects.

The practical goal of assisted ventilatory support is the use of mechanical means to continuously supply the hemoglobin and cells with adequate amounts of oxygen and to wash out carbon dioxide with minimal complications and adverse effects until the patient can take over and manage these tasks again unaided. Under normal physiologic conditions the rate of oxygen transport to the microcirculation, defined as the product of the cardiac output and the arterial oxygen content, is more than sufficient to sustain aerobic metabolism. However, during respiratory failure, aerobic metabolism becomes limited by the oxygen supply as the rate of oxygen transport falls. This results in a linear relationship between the rate of oxygen transport and oxygen consumption and has been labeled *pathologic supply dependency.*[1-3] Hence the major aim of assisted respiratory support is to provide enough oxygen to maintain adequate oxygen transport so that the oxygen consumption stays above the anaerobic threshold.

OXYGEN ADMINISTRATION AND THERAPY

Oxygen is the most common and most important therapeutic agent in the management of hypoxemia and tissue hypoxia. Oxygen added to the inspired gas is especially helpful in the treatment of hypoxemia caused by ventilation-perfusion ($\dot{V}/\dot{Q}$) mismatching with low $\dot{V}/\dot{Q}$ ratios. Oxygen may also improve arterial oxygenation caused by an alveolar-pulmonary capillary diffusion defect, although this mechanism is uncommon as the major or sole underlying pathophysiology in infants and children. When the pathophysiologic mechanism is pure intrapulmonary right-to-left shunting of blood, oxygen therapy is of very limited benefit, if at all. Although the living organism uses oxygen all the time, when oxygen is administered at enriched concentrations, it may cause severe complications and thus should be viewed as any other drug. Therefore oxygen should be used only when clinically indicated and in the amount required, which should be closely monitored.

Oxygen-Delivery Systems

A variety of methods are available for the delivery of oxygen to infants and children (Table 21-1). Low-flow systems provide oxygen at flow rates that are below the maxim inspiratory flow of the patient—less than 10 L/min. The inspired gas is diluted with room air, and the FIO_2 that enters the airways is affected by the relationships among oxygen flow, patient's inspiratory flow, and pattern of breathing. High-flow systems deliver oxygen at flow rates above the patient's requirement so that the patient's breathing pattern and flow do not affect the FIO_2.

Head boxes (hoods) are commonly used for infants and small children. This system disturbs the small child the least because it does not have direct contact with the face, although moisture "raining out" on the walls may obscure the patient's head from easy observation. The hood size should be adjusted to the patient's size. This is an open system, and with high oxygen flow, the FIO_2 may be 0.8 or even higher. A high flow is required to wash out carbon dioxide. An oxygen blender is used to titrate the FIO_2 inside the hood; the FIO_2 should be measured by an oxygen monitor. Children who are too big for hoods but who do not tolerate face masks can be put into an oxygen tent. The FIO_2 in a tent is unpredictable and usually does not exceed 0.35. Many children do not tolerate tents, which separate them from their parents and the environment. Oxygen tents also leave the patient damp from the "rainout." For the same reason, the child is often obscured from caregivers by heavy condensation on the tent walls.

Nasal cannulas are used in infants and children. The flow rate is limited to about 6 L/min because higher flows dry the nasal mucosa, irritate the patient, and are thus poorly tolerated. The FIO_2 at the nasopharynx varies greatly according to the magnitude of room-air entrainment, which depends on the relationship between cannula flow rate and the minute ventilation. However, this FIO_2 is not measurable for clinical use. A high FIO_2 may result when the system flow exceeds the patient's inspiratory flow and minute ventilation, so the flow rate needs to be adjusted according to the patient's partial pressure of arterial oxygen (PaO_2) or saturation with arterial blood oxygen (SaO_2) measured noninvasively.

Table 21-1 Inspired FIO_2 for Commonly Used Oxygen-Delivery Systems (in Infants and Children)

SYSTEM OXYGEN	FLOW RATE	FIO_2
Head box	20.0-40.0 L/min	0.21-0.80
Oxygen tent	—	0.21-0.35
Nasal cannula	0.25-6.0 L/min	0.21-0.50
Simple face mask	1.0-6.0 L/min	0.21-0.50
Nonrebreathing mask	4.0-10.0 L/min	0.50-1.00
Venturi mask	4.0-12.0 L/min	0.24-0.40

Similarly, simple face masks that cover the nose and mouth deliver an FIO_2 between 0.28 and 0.5 depending on the same relationship. A flow of 5 to 6 L/min is required to wash out carbon dioxide. This flow rate is usually less than the patient's inspiratory flow, so room air is entrained. Under these circumstances, the FIO_2 must also vary with the pattern of breathing. Therefore accurate measurement of the delivered FIO_2 is not practical.

Nonrebreathing masks have one-way valves that separate inhaled and exhaled gas so that inspired gas originates only from the delivery system. The latter contains a reservoir bag that supplies the patient's entire tidal volume (V_T). Thus, high FIO_2 levels, close to 1.0, can be reached.

Venturi masks entrain air at a constant magnitude for a preset oxygen flow rate using Bernoulli's principle. These are high-flow devices in which the FIO_2 depends on the ratio of oxygen to entrained air, provided that the patient's inspiratory flow rate does not exceed the total flow. These type of masks enable higher total flow rates to be delivered at a fixed FIO_2 for a set oxygen flow rate.

The FIO_2 needed to alleviate hypoxemia is usually determined empirically by trial and error. Several simplified formulas for clinical use are commonly used as measures of the efficiency of gas exchange and define the relationship among alveolar (PAO_2), inspired (FIO_2), and arterial (PaO_2) oxygen tensions. PAO_2 can be estimated from the modified alveolar gas equation:

$$PAO_2 = FIO_2 \times (PB - PH_2O) - PaCO_2/R$$

where PB is barometric pressure, P_{H_2O} is water vapor pressure (usually 47 mm Hg), and R is respiratory exchange ratio (assumed to be 0.8), which is the ratio of carbon dioxide production to oxygen consumption.

The simplified formulas used for clinical practice include the calculation of the difference of the partial pressures of alveolar and arterial oxygen, the PaO_2/PAO_2 ratio, and the PaO_2/FIO_2 ratio. If these relationships are relatively constant at different FIO_2 levels, calculating them for one FIO_2 theoretically enables the clinician to predict the PaO_2 from any other FIO_2 and thus titrate the FIO_2 without repeatedly sampling arterial blood gas. Unfortunately, these shortcuts have proved to be only partially reliable for clinical use. A major limitation is that these relationships change unpredictably with changes in FIO_2, so they do not allow satisfactory prediction of changes in PaO_2 with changes in FIO_2 and thus do not obviate the need for arterial blood gas sampling.[4,5] This limitation is more evident with the difference of the partial pressures of alveolar and arterial oxygen than with the PaO_2/PAO_2 and PaO_2/FIO_2 ratios. The last two remain more stable with changes in the FIO_2. A PaO_2/PAO_2 ratio below 0.75 is compatible with pulmonary gas exchange dysfunction.[5] In general, oxygen therapy should be started when the PaO_2 is below 60 mm Hg on room air or at even higher PaO_2 levels when respiratory distress exists.

HYPERBARIC OXYGEN THERAPY

Hyperbaric oxygen (HBO) is the inhalation of 100% oxygen at pressures greater than atmospheric. The therapeutic potential of HBO has been promoted for more than a century, but only in the last 20 years has it become a standard of respiratory care in selected situations.[6,7] As a result, in 1990, there were more than 200 clinical HBO units in the United States compared with 37 in 1976. The indications for HBO therapy are summarized in Box 21-1.

Physiologic Aspects

Two laws of physics are particularly pertinent with HBO: Boyle's law and Henry's law. Boyle's law states that the product of pressure and volume is a constant. Thus the volume of a closed gas space is inversely proportional to the absolute pressure around the space. Henry's law states that the amount of gas dissolved in a liquid is proportional to the absolute pressure applied to the liquid. During HBO, the body behaves like a liquid, dissolving considerable amounts of oxygen.

HBO treatment causes physiologic effects. When the gas pressure is increased to 3 to 5 atm, the partial pressure of oxygen (PO_2) is increased 3 to 5 times. At these pressures, while a person is breathing 21% oxygen, the partial pressure of inspired oxygen increases to 500 mm Hg and is as high as 2280 to 3800 mm Hg at an FIO_2 of 1.0. This significantly expands the mass action of oxygen, which may be important in certain chemical reactions (e.g., when competing with the high affinity of carbon monoxide [CO] for hemoglobin). During HBO, the amount of oxygen dissolved in plasma becomes larger, and the oxygen content and delivery increase. With 3 atm and an FIO_2 of 1.0, the PO_2 is $3 \times 760 = 2280$ mm Hg (ignoring water vapor pressure); the amount of oxygen dissolved in the plasma is thus 2100×0.003 vol%/mm Hg = 6.3 vol% (about 10.0 vol% at 5 atm). Other physiologic effects of HBO include vasoconstriction with reduction of edema and compartment pressures[8-11]; enhancement of host defense mechanisms, particularly in immunocompromised patients[6,7]; enhanced killing of anaerobic microorganisms[12]; bubble reduction in arterial gas embolism (AGE) and decompression sickness (DCS) (Boyle's law); and enhanced neovascularization and collagen production, especially in postradiation ischemic tissues.[13]

Technical Aspects

HBO therapy can be supplied with either a monoplace (one patient) chamber or a multiplace (multiperson) chamber. Multiplace chambers are advantageous because they permit ready access to the patient via the secondary chamber without depressurizing the treatment chamber, but they require more staffing personnel. In the monoplace chamber, the patient lies supine, and communication is achieved via an intercom. Critically ill patients who need close monitoring and assisted ventilation are easier to treat in a multiplace chamber. Chamber pressures typically range from 3 to 5 atm, and treatment duration usually is 90 to 120 minutes. Treatment of AGE and DCS may require up to 6 hours.[6]

Ventilators may exhibit altered performance (especially decreased VT and minute ventilation) when used in a hyperbaric environment and may require modifications.[6,7,14] Careful control of assisted ventilation is very important.

BOX 21-1
Indications for HBO Therapy

Emergency conditions

Air or gas embolism
Decompression sickness
Carbon monoxide or cyanide poisoning
Gas gangrene
Necrotizing soft tissue infections
Acute traumatic ischemia or crush injury
Ischemic grafts and flaps

Chronic conditions

Enhancement of healing in selected problem wounds
Refractory osteomyelitis
Radiation necrosis

Data from Weaver LK: *Respir Care* 37:720-738, 1992; Tibbles PM: *N Engl J Med* 334:1642-1648, 1996; and the Committee Report of the Undersea and Hyperbaric Medical Society, Bethesda, Md, 1989, The Committee.

Uses

Arterial Gas Embolism (AGE)

AGE may complicate medical procedures and diving.[15-18] In diving, AGE occurs as pressure decreases during ascent and gas expands. When this expansion exceeds the rate of gas elimination through the airways, the alveoli may disrupt, and gas enters the pulmonary circulation to be carried to the systemic circulation, from which it may reach the brain and coronary arteries.[6,7,18] AGE presents as acute neurologic changes, including loss of consciousness, hemiplegia, abnormal mentation, and seizures. This situation is an emergency, and prompt treatment with HBO is important. The effectiveness of HBO in AGE is based on numerous reports but not on prospective randomized studies.[14,18-20]

Decompression Sickness (DCS)

Most cases of DCS occur in divers breathing compressed gas at increased ambient pressure when they return to lower pressure too rapidly.[7,20] When a diver is exposed to increased ambient pressure, the amount of nitrogen dissolved in tissues increases. The reduction in pressure that occurs when the diver ascends causes nitrogen to move from tissues to the blood and to be eliminated by the lungs. If this occurs too rapidly, bubbles may form in the bones, cartilage, nerves, and blood, obstructing the microcirculation.[6,20] Patients have bone and joint pains, paresthesias, signs of pulmonary congestion, and neurologic changes resulting from brain edema. HBO reduces the size of the air bubbles, which alleviates microvascular obstruction, and the 100% oxygen replaces nitrogen in bubbles and tissues. This results in reduction of brain edema and clinical improvement.

CO Poisoning

CO binds to hemoglobin, forming carboxyhemoglobin, and also to cytochromes. Controversy still exists about whether HBO compared with 100% normobaric oxygen is the treatment of choice in CO poisoning. The rationale behind the use of HBO is that it amplifies the ability of oxygen to compete with CO on hemoglobin sites, thereby significantly reducing the carboxyhemoglobin half-life. It also increases oxygen delivery because dissolved oxygen becomes substantial. HBO facilitates the reversal of CO-cytochrome binding, thereby improving cellular oxygenation. The most common indication for HBO therapy in CO poisoning is unconsciousness and central nervous system depression.[6]

Side Effects and Complications

The most common complication of HBO therapy is barotrauma, which occurs in cavities that do not communicate and therefore do not equilibrate with the environment. This most commonly happens in the middle ear when the eustachian tube fails to open, and the patient has pain and even tympanic membrane rupture. The risk is higher in patients whose lungs are intubated, and preventive myringotomy has been suggested.[6,7] The same problem with reverse-pressure gradients occurs during the withdrawal of HBO therapy when the cavity pressure is higher then the environmental pressure. If this occurs distal to an obstructed airway, severe lung barotrauma can ensue. Oxygen toxicity causes the central nervous system complications of seizures and coma. This occurs especially when the patient is exposed to 100% HBO for longer than 2 to 3 hours, as in some treatment protocols of DCS and AGE.[21] Having the patient breathe 21% oxygen air for short periods (air breaks) diminishes the risk and extends the time the patient can be treated.

Other complications may arise from inadequate monitoring of critically ill patients and of equipment, especially ventilators, in chambers where the access of the attendant is impaired.

MANUAL VENTILATION

Hand ventilation with a bag and mask is a standard technique for emergency ventilatory support and resuscitation. Two major types of devices exist: anesthesia bags and self-inflatable bags. The anesthesia bags are powered with oxygen and deliver an F_{IO_2} of 1.0. They have the safety factor of being inoperable without their oxygen source. The self-inflatable bags deliver an F_{IO_2} from 0.5 to 0.9[22] but have the disadvantage or danger of inflating even when the oxygen supply is unknowingly disconnected, such that the F_{IO_2} is 0.21. The performance of hospital resuscitation personnel is unsatisfactory with the anesthesia bag, suggesting that this equipment should be avoided except in operating rooms[23] and by skilled operators in intensive care units. Mask-bag ventilation of infants and children can be performed successfully by the self-inflatable bag. In most cases, hyperventilation occurs because of a tendency to use excessive pressure and rate. A pressure-relief (pop-off) valve is thus essential to limit peak inspiratory pressure (PIP) to prevent barotrauma and gastric distention. However, in patients with noncompliant or highly resistant respiratory systems, the pressure required to inflate the lungs may exceed the pop-off relief pressure. In this situation the bag must have a means to lock and exclude the valve so that high inflating pressures can be used—this is the routine during the initial phase of resuscitation because pressures required for adequate ventilation during cardiopulmonary resuscitation usually exceed the pop-off limits.[24,25] The pop-off valve must also provide an audible signal that gas is being vented,[26] and its relief pressure should be set to 40 ± 10 cm H_2O for children and should not exceed 45 cm H_2O for newborns. Currently available devices vent gas at pressures varying from 38 to 106 cm H_2O.[22] By use of a tail reservoir, the F_{IO_2} can be increased to attain the minimum of 0.85 specified by the International Organization for Standards and the American Heart Association for a bag-valve resuscitator.[26]

The capability of attaching a positive end-expiratory pressure (PEEP) device to maintain end-expiratory pressure is important in patients receiving high PEEP during mechanical ventilation. Acute deterioration may occur when these patients are switched from the ventilator with high PEEP to bag–endotracheal tube (ETT) ventilation without PEEP for transport purposes or even for short periods, such as for ETT suctioning.

A prototype volume-controlled resuscitator has been tested in 25 infants.[27] Although this technique may cause less hyperventilation compared with the self-inflating bag, its usefulness still needs to be proved. The laryngeal mask is a new type of oral airway that forms a seal around the larynx and obviates the need for intubation. Its use in difficult tracheal intubations in children has been reported,[28,29] and it may well be a useful tool for caregivers lacking intubation skills.

ARTIFICIAL AIRWAY

Oropharyngeal Airways

The use of an oropharyngeal airway is indicated for the unconscious infant or child if procedures to open the airway (e.g., head tilt–chin lift) fail to provide a clear, unobstructed airway.[24] In conscious patients, the oropharyngeal airway may induce vomiting. Proper selection of size is important to achieve good separation of the tongue from the back of the pharynx. A full range of sizes are available from the premature infant to the adult, but the choice of size (unlike ETT) is by trial and error.

Laryngeal Mask Airways

Laryngeal mask airways have proved to be a major advance in the management of the airway. The primary roles for this method of airway management are related to control of the difficult airway that is not easily visualized and control of the airway in a patient with or without respiratory failure who requires flexible fiberoptic bronchoscopy. This technique allows visualization of the vocal cords and the immediate subglottic structures, which are usually obscured by an ETT.

Nasopharyngeal Airways

The placement of nasopharyngeal airways through the larger nasal passage, with the tip just above the epiglottis, can bypass significant upper airway obstruction secondary to hypertrophied tonsils and adenoids, retrognathia, or floppy hypopharyngeal tissues without the need for tracheal intubation. In chronic situations, the continuous flow of air and oxygen at up to 10 L/min can be added for further relief.[30]

Endotracheal Tubes

Ventilation via an ETT is the most effective and safest ventilatory method.[24] Indications for endotracheal intubation include (1) provision of positive-pressure ventilation (PPV) for the management of respiratory failure, (2) relief of upper airway obstruction (e.g., croup, epiglottitis), and (3) provision of airway protection when central nervous system control of ventilation is inadequate.

It is crucial to select the proper size of the ETT before intubation (Table 21-2). The following equation is useful for patients who are 1 year of age and older:

$$\text{ETT size (inner diameter in millimeters)} = \frac{\text{Age in years} + 16}{4}$$

An alternative method of tube size selection is based on a multicenter study that demonstrated that the child's length can predict correct ETT size more accurately than the child's age.[24,31,32] When the appropriate-size tubes are used, they cause very little damage to the tracheal mucosa. In children with up-

Table 21-2 Size of ETTs and Suction Catheters

AGE	INTERNAL DIAMETER	LENGTH TO MAXILLARY GUMLINE*	SUCTION CATHETER
Preterm	2.5-3.0 mm	7-8 cm	6 Fr
Newborn	3.0-3.5 mm	9 cm	6 Fr
1-6 months	3.5 mm	10 cm	8 Fr
6-18 months	4.0 mm	11 cm	8 Fr
1½-2 years	4.5 mm	12 cm	8 Fr
3-4 years	5.0 mm	14 cm	10 Fr
5-6 years	5.5 mm	16 cm	10 Fr
7-9 years	6.0 mm	18 cm	10 Fr
10-12 years	6.5 mm	20 cm	10 Fr
13-15 years	7.0-7.5 mm	21-22 cm	10 Fr
Adult female	7.5-8.0 mm	22-24 cm	12 Fr
Adult male	8.5-9.0 mm	22-24 cm	14 Fr

*A total of 1 to 2 cm should be added for the length from the tip to the nares for nasal ETT.

per airway obstruction the tube size should be 0.5 to 1.0 mm smaller than specified here. Also, children with certain diseases such as Down syndrome and achondroplasia are more likely to develop subglottic edema after intubation, so smaller tubes should be considered.

Problems that may occur during endotracheal intubation are hypoxemia, vomiting and aspiration, bradycardia, esophageal intubation, and endobronchial intubation. In a controlled situation a pulse oximeter and a cardiorespiratory monitor should be used, the stomach should be emptied, and atropine, 0.02 mg/kg (minimum 0.1 mg), may be administered. It is very important to make sure that all the necessary equipment is at hand before beginning the procedure. This equipment includes an oxygen source; an appropriate-size tube and tubes that are 0.5 mm smaller and 0.5 mm larger; a stylet; McGill's forceps; a suction system, including a Yankauer tip and a suction catheter of appropriate size to fit into the ETT; a resuscitation bag with face mask; an appropriate-size laryngoscope; airway; fixation tape; medications to facilitate intubation; a resuscitation cart if available; and an end-tidal capnometer, which provides immediate feedback to all of a successfully placed ETT by its signal. Muscle relaxants should be administered only by personnel who are experienced with pediatric intubation when control of the airways with bag and mask ventilation is possible and when the patient does not have upper airway obstruction.

A useful mnemonic for preparation for intubation is STATICS, as follows:

S Scope (laryngoscope)
T Tube (ETT)
A Airway
T Tape (for fixation)
I Introducer (stylet)
C Connector (adaptor)
S Suction (Yankauer)

Once the ETT is placed and PPV provided, chest movements should be observed for symmetry and breath sounds auscultated over both lungs. In contrast to oral tubes, nasal ETTs allow better fixation, are more comfortable, and may be associated with lower rates of accidental extubation and of sliding down into the mainstem bronchi. However, nasotracheal intubation is more difficult in pediatric patients, so if there is urgency, the airway should be quickly controlled by orotracheal intubation with or without the use of a stylet. The tube can later be changed to a nasal one at leisure. On the other hand, this carries the risks of an additional intubation and laryngeal damage. Contraindications for the nasal route include thrombocytopenia and coagulation disorders (risk of significant nasal bleeding) and head trauma with suspected basal skull fracture (risk of penetration of ETT into the skull, risk of sinusitis with meningitis).

Maintaining the Artificial Airway

Great care should be given to the small ETT that connects the child or small infant to the ventilator or bag. Because the small child has a short trachea, there is little room for error in ETT placement. Even a small up or down movement of the ETT may result in accidental extubation or one-lung intubation, both having the potential for serious consequences. The narrow pediatric trachea requires a small-diameter ETT, which is prone to plugging and obstruction. So that these complications can be avoided, infants and children whose lungs are intubated must be cared for only by experienced personnel and must never be left unattended. Clinical observations needing to be checked routinely and indicating that the ETT is patent and is in the right position include equal breath sounds, symmetry of chest expansion, and lack of coughing (tip of ETT "tickling" the carina). The depth of the ETT insertion should be determined before the intubation according to the age of the patient (see Table 21-2). However, the predicted lengths are not always reliable for the individual, and the rate of tube malpositioning based on clinical assessment alone may be as high as 15%.[33,34] Hence endotracheal intubation should be followed by a specific technique for verifying ETT position. The most common technique is chest radiography. The tip of the ETT should be below the clavicle and above the carina, optimally lying midtrachea. Alternative methods for noninvasive assessment of ETT position have been investigated. A recent development is an ETT in which a magnet is imbedded at a specified distance from the tip of the ETT. A hand-held device is placed at the suprasternal notch and then activated. If the ETT is in the correct position, the light on the device turns green. In a study that evaluated the usefulness of this technique in newborns, ETT position was assessed by the magnet technique in 36 patients after intubation compared with 45 whose ETT position was not checked by the magnet. In both groups, chest radiography was then taken. Repositioning of the ETT after intubation was needed in 6 of 36 patients (17%) compared with 20 of 45 controls (44%).[35] This study emphasized the usefulness of the technique but also its weakness, which is that it does not eliminate the need for radiography. In addition, although simple, this method cannot differentiate tracheal from esophageal intubation.[36,37] Another technique used to assess the ETT position is direct visualization of the tip of the ETT in relation to the carina using a small-diameter flexible fiberoptic bronchoscope. Although this technique has the advantage of easy assessment of repositioning during the visualization, it is less common because it requires experience and skill. The radiographic method is by far the most commonly used, although it carries the potential risks of radiographic radiation sequelae and is more expensive and time consuming. After the ETT position has been confirmed, the length of the ETT from the mouth or nares together with the ETT size should be displayed at the bedside.

ETTs are cuffed or noncuffed. In infants, the cricoid is the narrowest portion of the airway. It is circular, and a fair seal can be accomplished without a cuff using the round ETT. In older children and adults, the glottis is the narrowest portion, and because it is ovoid, an uncuffed tube does not create a seal. A small air leak around the ETT during PPV is desirable because it minimizes subglottic damage.[38] When the low-pressure cuff is inflated, it reduces or prevents ventilator-supplied air leak around the ETT and may also decrease the risk of aspiration. The inflated cuff generates pressure on the tracheal wall. Ischemia of the mucosa is proportional to the cuff pressure over 20 to 25 cm H_2O, which is the perfusion pressure of the tracheal mucosa and submucosa.[39] A common clinical practice is to estimate the cuff pressure by palpating the cuff reservoir. This, however, has been found unreliable compared with the objective measurement of cuff pressure using a manometer.[40] Another common practice is to inflate the cuff until no air leak is present and add 0.5 to 1.0 ml. One study showed that bronchial aspiration could still occur by inflating the cuff only to prevent air leaks.[41] In most pediatric intensive care units, noncuffed tubes are routinely used in infants and children younger than 8 years old (ETT inner diameter size, 3.0 to 6.0 mm) to minimize laryngeal injury, whereas cuffed tubes are used in older children. Air leakage, however, can cause significant difficulties during assisted ventilation of children with acute restrictive lung disease or increased airway resistance because major air loss occurs during positive-pressure inspiration. In such cases, reintubation with a cuffed ETT is indicated. Even in small children, the use of cuffed ETT is not associated with higher rates of postextubation subglottic narrowing when careful ETT care and size selection are used.[42] Thus, the cuff should be deflated and reinflated on a regular basis each day. The occluding volume and pressure may vary from day to day according to the amount of edema and possible expansion (or deflation) of air inside the cuff.

HUMIDIFICATION

1. The absolute humidity of a gas is the total amount of moisture in the gas.
2. Relative humidity is the ratio of the absolute humidity to the maximum amount of water that the gas could contain at the same temperature (stated as a percentage).

Physiologic Considerations

Under normal circumstances, the nose and upper airways heat and moisturize inspired gas with a continuous temperature and humidity gradient extending from the tip of the nose to at least as far as the carina[43] (Fig. 21-1). The warmer a gas, the higher its potential for containing water in the gaseous state. The highly vascular nasal cavity provides gas to the lungs containing 44 mg/L at 37° C (warmed from room temperature). Most of the heat loss from the respiratory tract occurs as a result of vaporization of water. Heat lost in this way may cause a drop in body temperature, particularly in vulnerable populations, such as infants and young children.[44] Breathing dry, nonhumidified gas causes serious complications of the airways: destruction of cilia and mucous glands, resulting in impaired function of the mucociliary elevator, which leads to sputum retention and atelectasis.[45,46] Nonhumidified gas also damages the basement membrane and cells of the airway and causes desquamation of cells, hyperemia, mucosal ulceration, and bronchoconstriction in susceptible individuals. A gas that is not fully saturated in the airways also absorbs water from the environment, including secretions, thus drying them up. On the other hand, excessive artificial humidification of inspired gases may add heat and water to the body, cause pulmonary changes in infants and children,[47,48] and impair mucociliary elevator function.[49]

Because medical gas is dry, it has to be humidified before reaching the patient. The amount of humidification required in patients with bypassed upper airways is not always clear because most studies have been reported from animal models, whereas those reported from humans suffer from methodologic drawbacks.[49] The American National Standards Institute[50] requires that "patients with bypassed upper airway receive a minimum of 30 mg/L of moisture necessary to prevent inspissation of secretions and mucosal damage," whereas the British Standards Institute[51] recommends a minimum of 33 mg/L for adults. Based on the assumption that it is desirable to mimic the conditions obtained during natural nasal breathing, it is recommended that the output of any therapeutic gas-delivery system be matched to the normal inspiratory conditions occurring at its point of entry into the respiratory system.[52] If the levels of heat and humidity are less than those normally encountered at the entry point, a potentially harmful humidity deficit may occur. If the levels are above normal, fluid overload and patient discomfort may result. When an ETT is used, the normal warming and humidification mechanisms of the upper airway

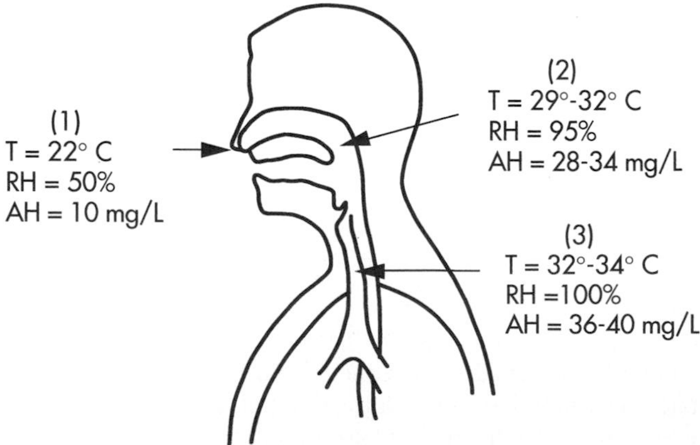

Fig. 21-1. Normal temperature *(T)*, relative humidity *(RH)*, and absolute humidity *(AH)* of inspired gas at various locations in the respiratory system. These locations correspond to points of entry of therapeutic gases delivered through *(1)* masks, nasal cannulas, tents, and head boxes; *(2)* nasal catheters and airways; and *(3)* ETTs and tracheostomy tubes. The normal inspired gas conditions shown are suggested heat and humidity levels for gas delivered by these devices. (Modified from Chatburn RL, Primiano FP Jr: *Respir Care* 32:249-253, 1987.)

are bypassed. Gas delivered through an ETT therefore should be warmed to 32° to 34° C at approximately 100% relative humidity, whereas gas delivered at the nose should be warmed to at least room temperature and humidified to at least 50% relative humidity. The gas delivered to patients whose lungs are intubated is ideally at 37° C with 100% relative humidity. However, because there is a gradual decrease in temperature in the gas-delivery circuit from the humidifier to the patient, the gas leaving the humidifier loses heat and moisture, and condensation occurs in the circuit. This is not usually a problem in patients using masks or hoods but becomes a major difficulty in patients whose lungs are ventilated because condensed water poses a risk of accidental tracheal lavage and also provides a vector for nosocomial infections. So that these complications can be avoided, water traps should be used in the circuit.

Some insensible water loss normally occurs through pulmonary ventilation. Therefore it is not necessarily desirable to completely prevent water loss from the airways during mechanical ventilation with humidification.[43,53]

Modern humidifiers use servomechanisms to control gas temperature where the temperature probe is placed at the airway opening. This helps keep the gas temperature more stable but does not solve the problem of water condensation inside the tubing. So that the latter can be avoided, long, thin heating wires have been developed that are placed inside the delivery circuit. These decrease heat loss and cooling (and thus condensation) during the flow of gas from the humidifier to the patient.

Types of Humidifiers

Cold-Water Humidifiers

Humidifiers are devices that provide gas with water vapor (i.e., water in the gaseous state). In the most simple and least effective ones, gas flows over the surface of water at room temperature and takes up only a scant amount of water. When the gas is directed through the water, bubbling takes place, thereby increasing the interface between water and gas, and the efficacy of humidification[43,53] is much improved (Fig. 21-2). The gas leaving the humidifier can achieve a relative humidity of nearly 100%. However, the gas is unheated, and its absolute humidity is low. When this gas reaches the airways beyond the tip of an ETT, it warms up, resulting in a decreased and an unsatisfactory level of relative humidity. Therefore this type of humidifier is not suitable for patients with bypassed upper airways and is used only in spontaneously breathing children whose lungs are not intubated and who need supplemental oxygen (oxygen masks, head boxes, nasal cannula).

Hot-Water Humidifiers

Hot-water humidifiers are similar to the cold-water humidifiers but also contain a heating source. These humidifiers deliver gas fully saturated with water vapor at a set temperature above the room temperature and are thus appropriate for use with ventilators and bypassed airways.[53] Heated humidifiers should meet the requirements of the American National Standards Institute of an output humidity level of at least 30 mg H_2O/L.[43,50,53] Although gas leaves the ventilator-humidifier system fully saturated with an absolute humidity of more than 30 mg/L of water, it cools a little along the circuit tubes of the breathing circuit, resulting in condensation and a decrease of absolute humidity. When the gas reaches the tip of the ETT, it warms up, and the relative humidity decreases (see Fig. 21-2). The gas then may absorb water from the airways, drying some secretions. So that overheating and burns to the airway can be prevented,[54] the heated humidifier is servocontrolled to keep the gas temperature constant and has an alarm mechanism that alerts caregivers when the temperature becomes too high or the water level becomes too low. Guidelines for clinical use include the following: The humidifier temperature should not exceed 37° C, the temperature should be monitored as near to the patient's airway as possible, and the alarm settings should be set no higher than 37° C and no lower than 30° C.[43,53,55] Hot-water humidifiers also are commonly used in small infants whose lungs are not intubated when they are receiving oxygen therapy by a head box. The heated gas prevents cooling and hypothermia.

The hot-air humidifiers containing heating wires inside the tubing deliver saturated gas with a much higher absolute humidity. The usefulness and safety of this development has been questioned, especially when the gas warms in the tubing to above the humidifier's temperature. In this case the absolute humidity remains high and constant; yet the relative humidity in the airways may be reduced, resulting in drying of secretions and plugging in the airways and the ETT.[56]

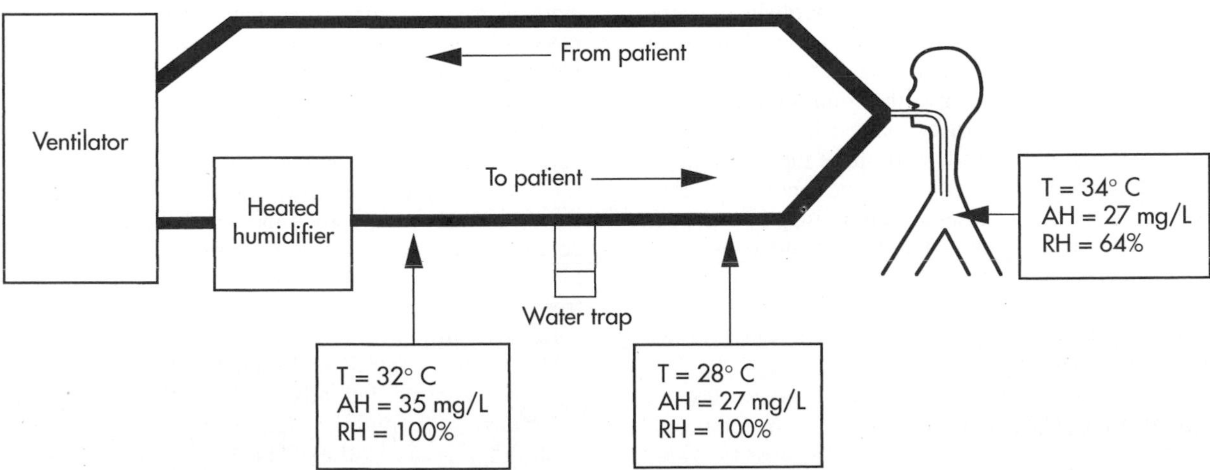

Fig. 21-2. Changes in gas temperature *(T)*, absolute humidity *(AH)*, and relative humidity *(RH)* during the passage of gas from the ventilator-humidifier system to the airways.

Nebulizers

Unlike humidifiers, which produce water vapor (water in the gaseous state), nebulizers produce water droplets within gas (aerosol). There are several types of nebulizers, and they differ by the methods by which the water droplets are generated and by the size of the droplets. They may cause excessive humidification and thus are not used in bypassed airways. They are used to deliver medication to the airways and in jet ventilation.[57] This topic is covered in depth in Chapter 19.

Heat and Moisture Exchangers

Heat and moisture exchange (HME) devices operate as "artificial noses" and are able to humidify inspired gas to a level close to that of normal nose breathing without active humidification and heating. They can be used when a high minute volume of ventilation is not required, suggesting that this type of gas conditioning may be especially useful for pediatric patients.[49,58-60] They are small and easy to use and operate by conserving heat and moisture during expiration and returning them to the inspired gas similar to the way that the normal upper airway does.[49] Some HME devices have filtering properties that offer protection from microorganisms.[61,62] Heat and moisture exchangers are less effective than active heating and humidification but are significantly better than no humidification.[48,63] Another disadvantage is that they add dead space, so only heat and moisture exchangers with small dead spaces designed specifically for pediatric patients should be used in this age group. In two prospective studies of adults whose lungs were mechanically ventilated in an intensive care unit (albeit using high minute volumes of ventilation), ETT and tracheostomy tube occlusions (including one death) were more common in the HME group compared with the heated humidifier (control) group.[61,64] Thick, tenacious secretions also occurred mainly in the HME group, and hypothermia was more frequent.[65] No information exists to support HME safety in pediatric patients whose lungs are ventilated. Moreover, the advantages of simplicity and less nursing work can be offset by a significantly increased work of breathing (WOB) with the HME devices. Therefore the American Academy for Respiratory Care has recently stated that the use of HME is contraindicated for patients with thick, copious, or bloody secretions and in patients with body temperatures less than 32° C or with large VT values.[55] Hence heat and moisture exchangers are useful for transport and may be considered for some long-term ventilator-dependent children. Nevertheless, recent unpublished experience from many pediatric intensive care units has shown that heat and moisture exchangers can be safely used in children whose lungs are ventilated as long as the contraindications are considered, the heat and moisture exchanger is replaced daily, and patients are closely observed. With these measures, nursing and respiratory therapy care of the humidification systems, as well as the risk for nosocomial infection, may be reduced. At present, the experience with heat and moisture exchangers in infants and small children (younger than 4 years of age) is too limited to recommend their use, particularly because the dead space of these devices is sufficiently large to cause further respiratory compromise.

MECHANICAL VENTILATION

The first mode of mechanical ventilatory support was intended to imitate natural breathing by exerting negative pressure on the chest in an effort to expand the lungs and generate negative intrapulmonary pressure "sucking" gas into the lungs. NPV was superseded by a more effective mode, PPV, which is the active insufflation of the lungs by the forceful delivery of gas. Although known and practiced for more than a century, this technique was not widely used until the late 1950s. PPV has become the standard and most common mode of assisted ventilation and has undergone continual improvements with the incorporation of microprocessors, electronic sensors, and feedback mechanisms into the machines. However, because of significant adverse effects related directly to the application of positive pressure to the airways and lungs, neophyte operators often look at the ventilator pressure settings without reference to the patient's chest and abdominal movement. This may result in significant hyperventilation or hypoventilation. In addition, attempts to prevent barotrauma have resulted in new techniques, including high-frequency oscillation (HFO), high- frequency jet ventilation (HFJV), liquid ventilation (LV), intratracheal ventilation, and extracorporeal ventilatory support.

Positive-Pressure Ventilation

The ventilator is connected to a source of breathing gas and delivers breaths to the patient via a circuit connected to an ETT. Breathing circuits being used by most ventilators have both inhalation and exhalation lines. During inhalation, the exhalation valve must remain closed to prevent loss of gases intended for the patient. The valve opens to permit the exhaled breath to exit through the exhalation port until the airway pressure has been reduced to the desired level. The ventilator provides control of the patient's variables and can be adjusted to the patient's need with safety limits imposed on certain adjustments.

The relationship of the parameters and variables in the respiratory system is based on the equation of gas motion,[66] as follows:

$$\text{Muscle pressure} + \text{Ventilator pressure} = \text{Volume/Compliance} + \text{Resistance} \times \text{Flow}$$

The combined muscle and ventilator pressures cause volume and flow to be delivered to the patient in amounts dependent on the compliance and resistance. The latter are assumed to be constants and are thus parameters. Pressure, volume, and flow change with time and hence are variables. If the patient's ventilatory muscles are not in use, the muscle pressure is zero, and the ventilator generates all the pressure required. On the other hand, during a spontaneous breath, ventilator pressure is zero. In between, an infinite number of combinations are possible, and these are related to the various partial ventilatory-support modes.[66]

There are several basic modes of PPV, which differ by the variable used to start and end the inspiration and expiration (i.e., volume, pressure, flow, time). The variable that controls the ventilator in a specified mode (controller) is the independent variable, and the others become dependent. Usually, three of these are set and the fourth results from the other three and from the patient's compliance and resistance. The controlling variables follow:

1. Pressure controllers: When the PIP and the PEEP are set, the volume depends on the patient's respiratory mechanics (compliance and resistance).
2. Volume controllers: The VT of each breath is set and does not change when system mechanics change. The pressure in the system is the dependent and changing variable.

3. Time controllers: Inspiratory and expiratory times are controlled, whereas both pressure and volume waveforms are affected by changes in lung mechanics.

The current group of positive-pressure ventilators fit into one of these categories.

Pressure-Cycled Ventilators

The inspiratory phase terminates at the instant that a preset end-inspiratory pressure is attained (not to be confused with pressure-limited mode of ventilation). Examples are Bennett PR-1 and PR-2 ventilators. These are the most simple machines but are now rarely used in pediatric intensive care units.

Volume-Cycled Ventilators

With volume-cycled ventilators (Table 21-3), the inspiratory phase terminates when the preset VT has been delivered. Examples are Bennett MA-I and MA-II, Puritan-Bennett 7200, and Bear 1 and 5 ventilators. A disadvantage of these ventilators in pediatric patients is the compression volume, which is the volume of gas lost in the ventilator circuit from tube expansion and gas compression. This loss is in direct relationship to the PIP and thus changes when lung compliance deteriorates. Because even relatively small-volume losses become very significant in small children, new pediatric circuits have been developed with small-diameter, short-inspiratory line, rigid tubing. These circuits minimize the compressible volume to no greater than 1 ml/cm H_2O (compared with 4 ml/cm H_2O in regular adult tubing). Even with these measures, the volume loss may be significant. For example, a set VT of 70 ml is required for a 5-kg infant when the PIP is 20 cm H_2O. The patient receives 50 ml (10 ml/kg), and 20 ml is lost in ventilating the circuit. When compliance deteriorates and the PIP increases to 40 cm H_2O to deliver the same 70 ml/breath, the lost VT increases to about 40 ml, and the patient receives only 30 ml/breath, an additional 40% loss. In addition, valves may open slowly in synchronized intermittent mandatory ventilation (SIMV) modes in older ventilators, causing a lack of synchrony between patient effort and ventilator response. These factors make this type of ventilator less suitable to infants and small children.

Time-Cycled Ventilators

With time-cycled ventilators (see Table 21-3), the inspiratory time (TI) and flow rate are set and inspiration is terminated by TI. VT is the product of these two variables (VT = TI × Flow). Examples are the InfantStar, Baby Bird, Healthdyne ventilators, Sechrist ventilators, BP 200, and Bear Cub ventilators. In these types of ventilators the PIP is preset to allow the time-cycled, pressure-limited mode of ventilation. Because the maximum available flow in these ventilators is usually less than 30 to 40 L/min, they do not provide adequate flow rates for children weighing over 20 to 25 kg. Another disadvantage is that when compliance decreases, it may not be appreciated that VT has also decreased.

Table 21-3 Commonly Used Modes of Ventilation in Children

MODE	SIMV	TCPLV
Type of ventilator	Volume cycled	Time cycled
VT	Set	Variable
Peak pressure	Variable	Set
Rate	Set or variable	Set or variable
TI	Variable	Set (I:E variable) Variable (I:E set)
I:E ratio	Variable	Set (TI variable) Variable (TI set)
Flow wave	Set but variable	Set

SIMV, Synchronized intermittent mandatory ventilation; *TCPLV,* time-cycled, pressure-limited ventilation; *TI,* inspiratory time; *I:E,* inspiratory-expiratory ratio.

Combined Ventilators

Some newly developed ventilators can be used as either volume- or time-cycled, pressure-limited ventilators. Examples are Siemens Servo 900C and Servo 300, Dräger Evita 4, Hamilton Amadeus and Veolar, Puritan Bennett 7200, Newport Breeze and Wave, and V.I.P. Bird.

Modes of Mechanical Ventilation

Controlled Mechanical Ventilation

Controlled mechanical ventilation (CMV) is a mode of ventilator operation in which all breaths are delivered by the ventilator at a preset frequency and flow rate (Fig. 21-3). This includes both preset volume (volume-controlled ventilation) and preset pressure (pressure-controlled ventilation). Because the volume-controlled mode was the first to be used in positive-pressure ventilators,[67] the term *CMV* refers to this type. It may also signify "controlled mandatory ventilation," whereas pressure-controlled ventilation is sometimes called *pressure-controlled ventilation* (see Table 21-3). Neither CMV nor PCV allows spontaneous breaths, so they are used only in patients who cannot breathe on their own (e.g., those under neuromuscular blockage).

Assist/Control Ventilation

Assist/control ventilation (ACV) is a mode in which mandatory breaths are delivered at a set frequency, volume (or pressure), and flow (Fig. 21-4). Between the machine-initiated breaths, the patient can trigger the ventilator and receive a breath at the preset volume (or pressure) with the same limits and cycle variables as the machine-triggered breaths.[68-70] If the patient does not trigger the ventilator, the machine delivers a breath at the predetermined frequency (see Fig. 21-4). The sensitivity of patient triggering is determined by the clinician. A high sensitivity (shallow inspiratory effort) may cause unintentional triggering of mandatory breaths, and a low sensitiv-

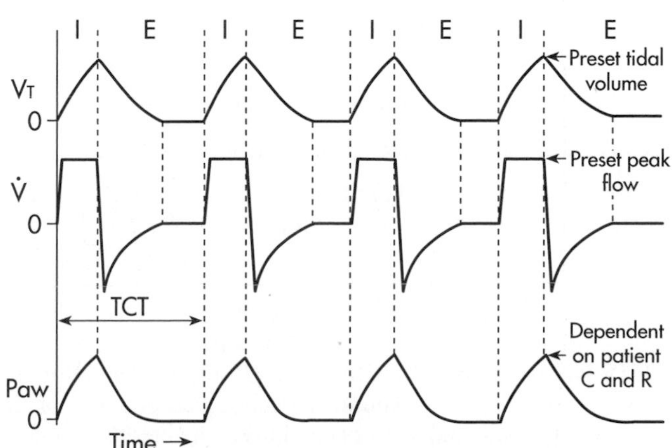

Fig. 21-3. Flow, pressure, and volume during CMV. All breaths are ventilator breaths and are evenly spaced. *I,* Inspiration; *E,* expiration; *VT,* tidal volume; *V̇,* gas flow; *Paw,* airway pressure; *TCT,* total cycle time; *C,* compliance; *R,* resistance.

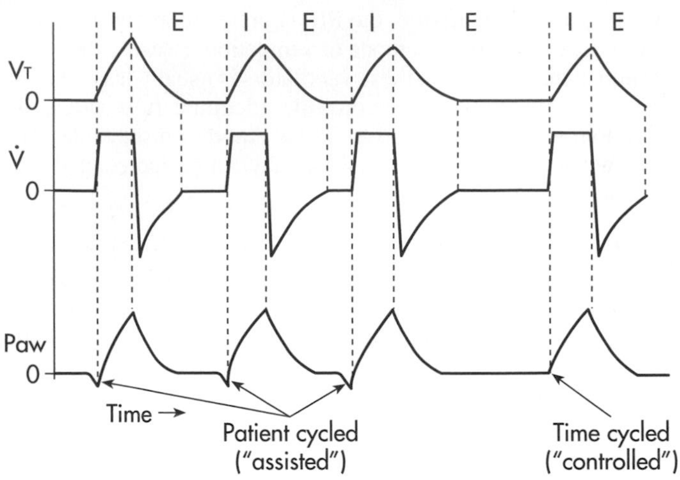

Fig. 21-4. Flow, pressure, and volume during ACV. Ventilator breaths may be patient triggered or ventilator controlled. When the patient fails to trigger the ventilator and the preset cycle time has elapsed, the ventilator delivers a mandatory breath. *I,* Inspiration; *E,* exhalation; *VT,* tidal volume; *V̇,* gas flow; *Paw,* airway pressure.

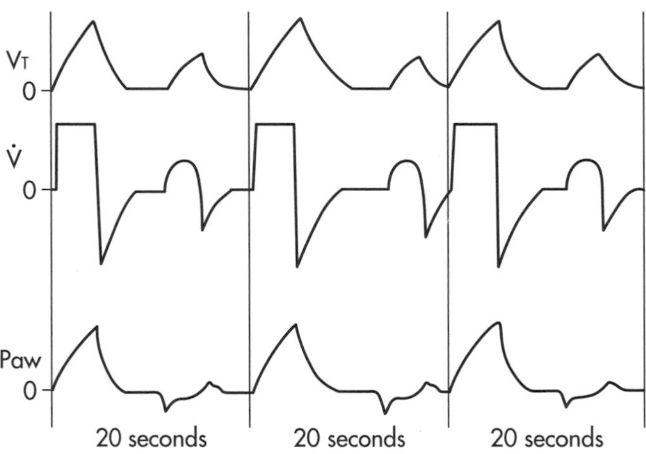

Fig. 21-5. Flow, pressure, and volume during IMV. *VT,* Tidal volume; *V̇,* gas flow; *Paw,* airway pressure.

ity may increase the WOB needed to open a demand valve to increase the gas flow for patient inspiration.[71]

(Synchronized) Intermittent Mandatory Ventilation

Intermittent mandatory ventilation (IMV) is a mode of ventilation in which mandatory machine breaths are delivered at a set frequency and volume. Between machine breaths, the patient can breathe spontaneously from either a continuous flow of gas or a demand system[68-72] (Fig. 21-5). Because spontaneous breaths may not synchronize with machine breaths, SIMV was developed. In SIMV (Fig. 21-6), the ventilator creates a timing window around the scheduled delivery of the mandatory breath and attempts to deliver the breath in concert with the patient's inspiratory effort[68-70,73,74] (see Fig. 21-6, *A*). If no inspiratory effort occurs during this time, the ventilator delivers the mandatory breath at the scheduled time (see Fig. 21-6, *B*). Some ventilators can use this principle on pressure mode, which is sometimes called *pressure-SIMV.*

Time-Cycled, Pressure-Limited Ventilation

In time-cycled, pressure-limited ventilation, the rate and TI (or inspiratory-expiratory [I:E] ratio) are preset. A preset PIP limit is determined such that excessive pressure is not produced and the risk of barotrauma is reduced. The peak pressure generated in the system may (Fig. 21-7, *A*) or may not (Fig. 21-7, *B*) reach the limit pressure. Its disadvantage is that when compliance decreases, VT falls. To increase ventilation, the clinician should increase the pressure limit. Augmenting the PEEP decreases the delivered VT because it depends on the level of PIP above PEEP; therefore the PIP must also be increased if the VT is to be held constant.

Pressure-Controlled, Inverse-Ratio Ventilation

Pressure-controlled, inverse-ratio ventilation (PC-IRV) is a particular version of PCV in which all breaths are pressure limited and time cycled and the inspiration is longer than expiration.[68-70,75] The I:E ratio is increased to 4:1. IRV was first applied to newborns in 1971 when Reynolds[76] described improvements in infants with hyaline membrane disease (HMD) whose lungs were ventilated with prolonged TI. This was later confirmed by others,[77-79] then in adults with adult respiratory distress syndrome (ARDS),[75,80,81] and only later in pediatric patients.[82]

IRV is most effective in conditions resulting in unstable or collapsed alveoli secondary to surfactant deficiency, classically in ARDS. The prolonged TI stabilizes alveoli, recruits already collapsed alveoli, and allows for more even distribution of gas, resulting in improved gas exchange.[75,83] The use of IRV allows for decreases in both PEEP and PIP levels (Fig. 21-8). The VT with PC-IRV is generated at a constant pressure throughout the TI. The inspiratory flow decelerates once the set PIP is reached (Fig. 21-9). The PIP, frequency, and TI (or I:E ratio) are the ventilator-set parameters, and the VT is the dependent variable.[75,84] It has been suggested that the decelerating flow waveform accompanying a true square-wave pressure pattern improves oxygenation in oleic acid–injured canine lungs[85] and in human lungs and contributes to the success of IRV.[6,11,75,82]

However, increasing TI and inverting the I:E ratio significantly increases the mean airway pressure (MAP) and may cause an increase in the PEEP above the set level (inadvertent PEEP, "auto-PEEP").[86-88] Inadvertent PEEP is a relatively common but seldom-appreciated ocurrence,[86,87,89,90] and neither the presence nor the magnitude of inadvertent PEEP is apparent during usual ventilator monitoring. Cole et al[91] compared the pulmonary and hemodynamic effects of IRV with conventional ventilation using PEEP. PEEP levels of 9 to 19 cm H_2O were needed to achieve results equal to those of IRV with lower set PEEP levels, and this equaled the amount of the inadvertent PEEP. Hence IRV achieved no superiority over ventilation with a conventional I:E ratio (1:1 or less) with high PEEP. There were no differences in adverse effects. The beneficial effects on pulmonary gas exchange attributed to IRV could result entirely from the presence of additional occult PEEP.[86,87] Moreover, the explanation that IRV improves gas exchange by recruiting collapsed alveoli and preventing further collapse also holds for the use of high PEEP.[92,93] Thus IRV should be compared with more conventional modes of ventilation with the same MAP. If both techniques are equivalent in a specific patient with regards to MAP, gas exchange, and adverse effects, the use of PEEP may be theoretically advantageous because it normalizes physiologic parameters (functional residual capacity [FRC]) and improves respiratory system compliance. If

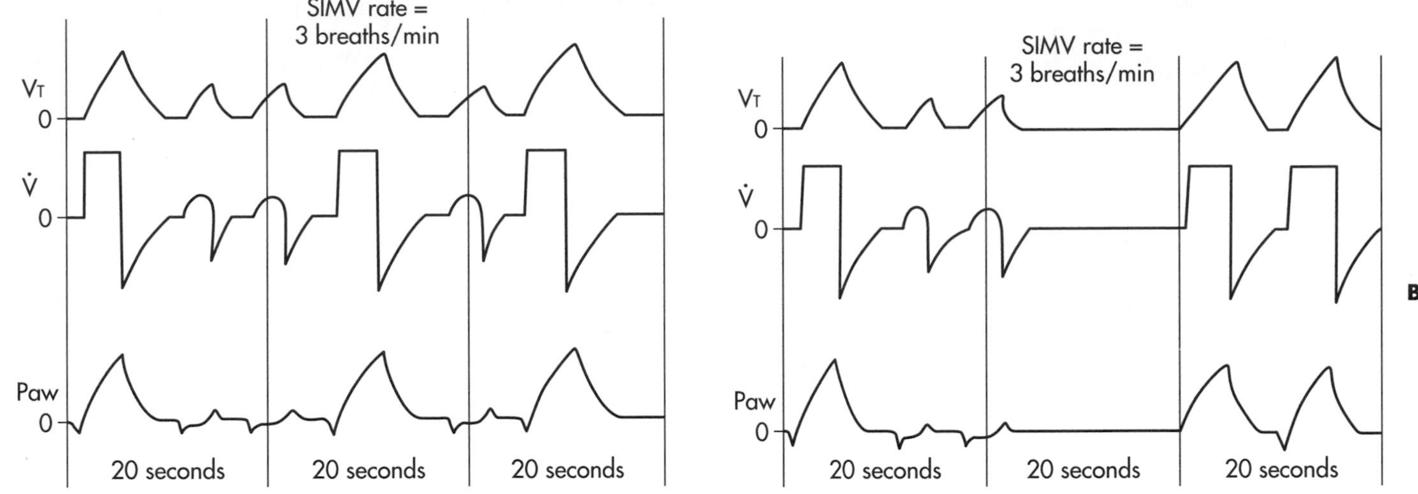

Fig. 21-6. Flow, pressure, and volume during SIMV. *VT,* Tidal volume; $\dot{V}$, gas flow; *Paw,* airway pressure. **A,** There are three ventilator breaths in a minute. The ventilator delivers the mandatory breath after the patient has remained apneic for a scheduled time (60 seconds per set rate). The patient then resumes breathing and triggers a synchronized breath. **B,** There are still three ventilator breaths in a minute. Ventilator breaths are synchronized with the patient's breaths. The elapsed time between ventilator breaths may vary.

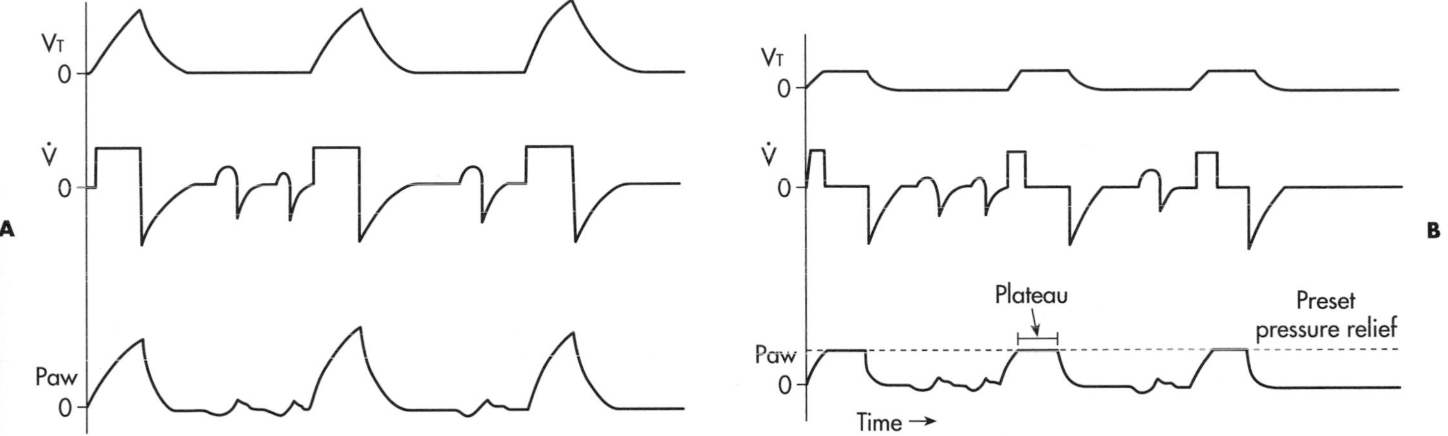

Fig. 21-7. Time-cycled, pressure-limited ventilation. *VT,* Tidal volume; $\dot{V}$, gas flow; *Paw,* airway pressure. **A,** Pressure limit is not reached. **B,** Pressure limit is reached.

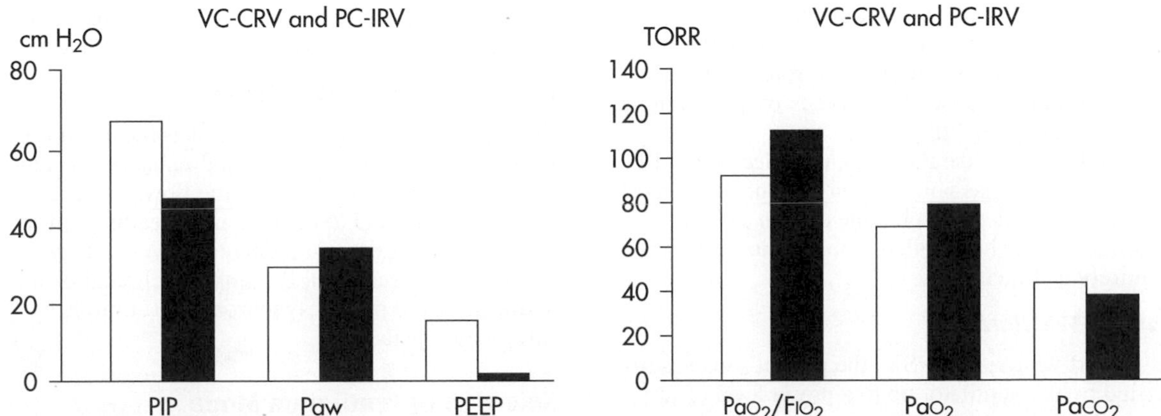

Fig. 21-8. Flow, pressure, and volume during CPAP. *VC-CRV,* Volume-controlled, conventional-ratio ventilation. *TORR,* mm Hg.

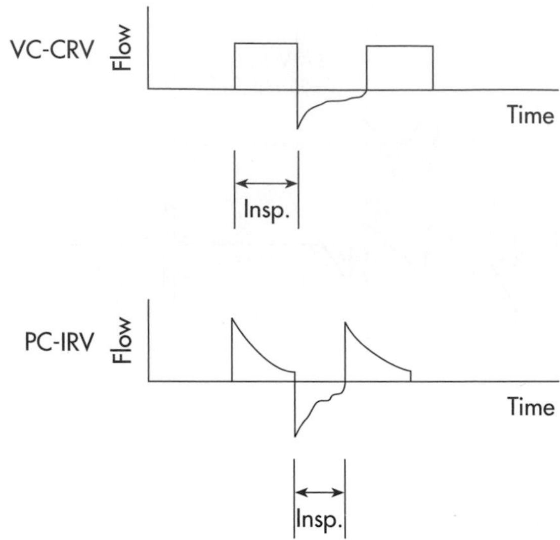

Fig. 21-9. The different basic inspiratory flow waveforms available with mechanical ventilation. At a preset peak flow the TI varies so that the area under the curve and therefore the delivered VT are the same. *VC-CRV,* Volume-controlled, conventional-ratio ventilation.

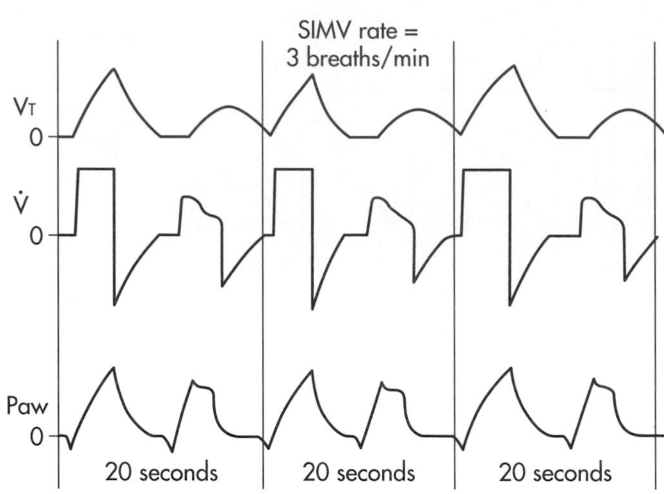

Fig. 21-10. Comparison of airway pressure and blood gas levels between PC-IRV and volume-controlled, conventional-ratio ventilation. *VT,* Tidal volume; *V̇,* gas flow; *Paw,* airway pressure. (Modified from Tharratt RS et al: *Chest* 94:755-762, 1988.)

PEEP is required, it is better to use it knowingly and in quantified amounts than unknowingly as auto-PEEP. Whether a lengthened TI and especially an inverse I:E ratio are beneficial when total MAP is held constant is still controversial.[86,87,91,94,95]

A further problem with PC-IRV is that it can result in a significant decrease in cardiac output.[86] Hence the improvement of Pa_{O_2} is counterbalanced by the decline of oxygen transport, and no net improvement in tissue oxygen delivery and gas flow is achieved.[86] Thus patients on PC-IRV are more likely to need invasive monitoring and inotropic support.

Studies that have shown the beneficial effects of PC-IRV traditionally used volume ventilation for comparison. However, when PCV with decelerating flow and a conventional I:E ratio was compared with IRV, no benefit was found for the latter.[86]

On the other hand, proponents of PC-IRV suggest that it recruits closed alveolar units in a more homogeneous manner than volume-controlled ventilation with conventional ratios and PEEP. It allows decreases in PEEP and especially PIP when these variables are at high levels that compromise the respiratory and other systems.[75,79] When PC-IRV is used, the MAP can be increased to improve oxygenation and lower the PIP. Overinflation from a high PIP is a major factor responsible for pulmonary parenchymal damage, especially barotrauma,[96] and may result in significant shear forces at the alveoli.[97] PC-IRV may reduce these shear forces by producing a more even inflation at lower PIP levels.

Besides physiologic considerations, a clear effect of PC-IRV on outcome and mortality has not yet been shown. Hence most investigators suggest using this technique only in patients after more conventional modes have failed. The decision as to when to use it is entirely a clinical one.

Pressure-Support Ventilation

In pressure-support ventilation (PSV) the patient's inspiratory effort is assisted by the ventilator up to a preset level of inspiratory pressure. This allows the patient to determine his or her own rate, TI, and VT.[68-70,73,74] PSV may be used alone or with SIMV (Fig. 21-10). Most pediatric patients have uncuffed ETT, so there may be a leak around these tubes. The leak usually varies with the child's position. In PSV the ventilator pressure is maintained until the inspiratory flow rate decreases. If the leak around the ETT exceeds this flow rate, pressure support is maintained throughout the respiratory cycle, resulting in sudden high pressure during exhalation.[98] Experience in children has shown that this hazard can be prevented by setting the pressure support limit time to 0.1 seconds beyond the set TI.[99]

Mandatory Minute Ventilation

In mandatory minute ventilation the patient can breathe spontaneously. Yet the ventilator ensures that a minimum level of minute ventilation, set by the clinician, is always achieved.[68-70,100]

Continuous Positive Airway Pressure

During continuous positive airway pressure (CPAP), ventilation occurs spontaneously without ventilator breaths, and positive pressure is maintained throughout the respiratory cycle such that exhalation is against an expiratory valve (Fig. 21-11). CPAP requires a continuous flow of gas that is 2 to 3 times the minute ventilation to prevent the rebreathing of exhaled gas. The flow can be delivered by an ETT or a face mask and also by nasal prongs, which are used mainly in preterm newborns and young infants.

Proportional-Assist Ventilation

Proportional-assist ventilation assists the patient in proportion to his or her breathing effort and enhances patient-ventilator synchrony. In this new mode, the flow, volume, and pressure all are proportional to the patient's breathing effort. However, the lungs of patients with decreased ventilatory drive may be further underventilated. Preliminary clinical data from adults show improved patient synchrony and comfort.[101,102] Pediatric information is lacking.

Selection of Ventilation Mode

The lungs of patients with severe respiratory failure are usually ventilated in a fully controlled mode, in which the ventilator per-

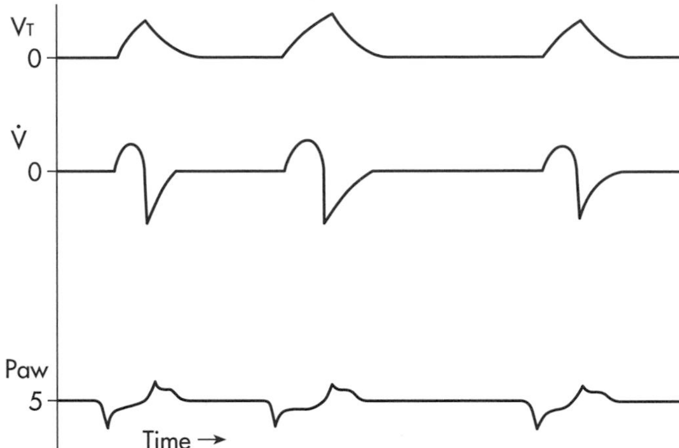

Fig. 21-11. Flow patterns in IMV (volume-controlled, conventional-ratio ventilation) and PC-IRV. $\dot{V}$, Gas flow; *Paw,* airway pressure.

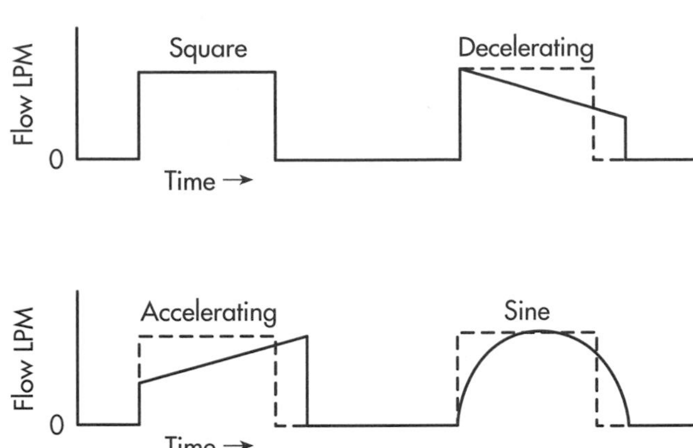

Fig. 21-12. PSV with SIMV. Both mechanical breaths and pressure-supported breaths coexist. *LPM,* Liter per minute.

forms all the WOB and controls the rate, depth, and pattern of gas delivery. Patients who need less aggressive respiratory assistance may receive only partial ventilatory support, in which both the ventilator and the patient share the WOB. CMV and PCV are used only for full support. In ACV the majority of work is done by the ventilator, and the patient's work is minimal and applied only to create the negative inspiratory pressure required to trigger the ventilator. SIMV and PSV allow a broader range of available ventilatory support that can be easily modified. Hence these modes are widely used in nonparalyzed patients and during weaning from mechanical ventilation. PSV has received considerable attention in recent years. Breathing through an ETT and a ventilator circuit (added to address the need to open a demand valve during inspiration) increases the WOB of spontaneous breaths, especially in children because of the small ETT. PSV can compensate for this additional WOB during weaning from mechanical ventilation.[103] Compared with ACV and SIMV, PSV allows for the delivery of equivalent amounts of VT but at lower PIPs.[104] This is due to the negative pressure component of the spontaneous breaths. Although the overall pressure over time may be similar to that of SIMV, the combination of ventilator and patient driving forces for each breath lowers the PIP. If the clinician adjusts the PSV level and adds this mode to SIMV, it is possible to titrate the amount of work performed by the spontaneously breathing patient to a greater extent than is possible by any other available mode.[105-107] Two basic approaches to PSV are being used: low-level PSV, which uses 2 to 10 cm H_2O of pressure to overcome the resistance imposed by the ETT, and high-level PSV, in which the pressure may range above 40 cm H_2O to provide an alternative form of substantial ventilatory support that may be more comfortable to the patient.[108] A recent study of six children who underwent cardiac surgery showed that the application of 5 to 10 cm H_2O of pressure support resulted in increased VT, decreased breathing rate, and decreased WOB.[109] Nevertheless, a difference in outcome using the various approaches has not been demonstrated, although only a few studies of PSV in children exist. The most common modes used in pediatric patients are SIMV (in patients who do not breathe spontaneously, SIMV is equivalent to CMV); PCV; time-cycled, pressure-limited ventilation; and PSV.

Flow Waveform

Several gas-delivery waveforms are available on mechanical ventilation. The basic and most commonly used are square, sine, and decelerating (Fig. 21-12). The distribution of the gas flow varies with different flow patterns. However, at present, justification for the use of various waveforms under specific clinical settings is lacking. Attempts to establish physiologic effects of various waveforms have failed to define substantial differences, and no good evidence shows the clear superiority of one waveform over another.[110-112] Nevertheless, peak inspiratory flow must meet the patient's peak inspiratory demands.[71]

Patient Ventilator Monitoring and Alarms

Cardiorespiratory monitoring of patients whose lungs are ventilated is a standard of care. The major goals of monitoring are to (1) continuously measure the ventilatory indexes that enhance the understanding of the underlying pathophysiology, aid in diagnosis, and guide management; (2) provide alarms that alert clinicians to significant changes in the patient's condition; (3) provide alarms that alert clinicians to significant changes in the ventilator limits or settings; and (4) provide trends that assist in the assessment of the therapeutic response and prognosis.[4,113]

Ventilator Monitoring

The incorporation of microprocessors into ventilators and monitoring devices extends the alarm capabilities almost infinitely. The variables necessary for clinical decision making are pressure, flow, volume, rate, and FIO_2 monitored in the ventilator circuitry[114] (Box 21-2). However, although guidelines exist for initiating and terminating mechanical ventilation, the therapeutic approach and specific aspects of ventilatory management must be individualized according to the underlying pathophysiology and the therapeutic goals.

Alarms should warn of malfunctions of the ventilator system or physiologic or pathologic changes in the patient that affect the assisted ventilation[114] (Box 21-3). Setting the alarms' limits is done at the same time as setting the ventilator's parameters. Most ventilators have battery backup in case of elec-

BOX 21-2
Variables to be Monitored on Mechanical Ventilators

Pressure
PIP
MAP
PEEP

Volume
Exhaled VT (machine breath)
Exhaled VT (spontaneous breath)
Minute volume of ventilation

Flow
Machine flow
Spontaneous flow (optional)

Timing
I:E ratio
Rate (set)
Rate (spontaneous) (optional)

Gas concentration
FIO_2

Temperature
Inhaled gas temperature

BOX 21-3
Events that Should Trigger Ventilator Alarms

Immediately life-threatening events if left unattended for even a short time
Power failure
Absence of gas delivery
Loss of gas source pressure
High pressure (PIP, PEEP)
Low PIP (pressure-limited ventilation)
Low VT (volume ventilation)
Loss of PEEP
Timing failure

Potentially life-threatening events if left unattended for a longer time
Humidifier high or low temperature
Humidifier that is out of water
High rate (autocycling)
Low rate
Excessive rate
Incompatible set parameters (e.g., I:E ratio)

tric power failure. A high-pressure alarm may indicate ETT obstruction. An alarm indicating low pressure or one indicating low exhaled volume may signify a leak in the patient's circuit or a disconnection. A low-PEEP alarm may indicate disconnection of the patient's circuit. An alarm should sound when the set control-variable parameters are incompatible (e.g., when the time set for inspiration is too short to allow the set VT to be delivered at the set flow rate).

Most ventilators have a button to silence the sound. However, the period of silence should be limited to 60 or 120 seconds, and there should be a visual guide to the cause of the alarm (e.g., excessive peak pressure, inability to maintain PEEP). These safety features alert the clinician that the cause for the alarm still exists.

Patient Respiratory System Monitoring

Respiratory monitoring is one of the most important components of care of patients with respiratory failure. This by itself may be an indication for admission to a pediatric intensive care unit because continuous monitoring has the potential to alert the clinician to sudden deleterious changes and thus allow for timely intervention. All patients with moderate to severe respiratory failure should be monitored for gas exchange and preferably for respiratory mechanics. Monitoring of pediatric patients requires an individual approach based on physical examination, noninvasive techniques, and selective careful application of invasive measures.

Physical Examination

Respiratory rate is an easy variable to monitor in infants and children whose lungs are not ventilated. This variable is reliable mainly during sleep and may vary significantly in awake situations. Breathing rate changes significantly with age, so normal values for age should be referenced. Breathing pattern, chest retractions, and breathing asynchrony all may characterize respiratory status. Clinical scoring systems based on skin color, breathing pattern, breath sounds, the presence or absence of pulsus paradoxus, and cerebral function have been developed for common acute respiratory failure situations in infants and children (Table 21-4), including acute asthma attacks and acute upper airway obstruction.[115-118]

Invasive Monitoring

Invasive respiratory monitoring of patients in respiratory failure is based on arterial blood gas analysis. This analysis remains the gold standard, even now that good noninvasive methods have emerged. Obtaining an arterial blood gas sample either is a painful procedure or requires an indwelling arterial catheter, which may have complications. Another major disadvantage is that arterial blood gas analysis provides only intermittent data and may miss sudden changes. Efforts have been made to develop intravascular electrodes for continuous PaO_2 and partial pressure of arterial carbon dioxide ($PaCO_2$) monitoring. However, at present, these are still of an experimental and preliminary nature.[4,119,120] An additional problem is that arterial blood gas values are affected by the patient's crying or altered ventilation just before arterial blood gas sampling. In the sedated child whose lungs are ventilated and who has an indwelling arterial line, this usually does not occur. In some more severe situations, saturation with venous (pulmonary artery) oxygen is also used. However, this is less commonly performed in children and requires pulmonary artery catheterization.

Noninvasive Monitoring

Chest Radiography. Although clinicians do not unanimously agree, it appears appropriate to do routine daily chest radiographs in children whose lungs are intubated and mechanically ventilated. Of 538 routine daily chest radiographs in one series of 74 adults in the intensive care unit,[33] major findings, defined as those requiring immediate diagnostic or therapeutic intervention, were detected in 13 patients (17.6%). However, the fraction of new major findings determined solely by the chest films as a percentage of total films was small (18 of 538, or 3.4%). ETT malposition was the most common major finding, followed by central venous line malpositioning, pneumothorax, and pleural effusion. The clinical value of routine chest radiographs in a pediatric intensive care unit has also been demonstrated.[121] It is reasonable to assume that tube malpositioning is encountered more frequently in infants and small children than in adults because there is less room for error in the adult age group.

Oxygenation. The introduction of easy-to-use and relatively accurate noninvasive monitors has reduced the frequency of arterial gas sampling in children. In addition to the electrocardiogram (ECG) and respiration, most infants and children whose lungs are ventilated are monitored for $Sa{O_2}$ by pulse oximetry ($Sp{O_2}$). One concern about pulse oximetry in pediatric intensive care unit patients is the decreased accuracy at low saturation levels, resulting in significant overestimation or underestimation of the true $Sa{O_2}$ when oxygen saturation falls below 75% to 80%.[122-125] Pulse oximetry is quite accurate at $Sa{O_2}$ levels above 85%, with 95% confidence limits of approximately ±4%.[4] However, because of the shape of the oxygen-hemoglobin dissociation curve with its characteristic flat section at $Pa{O_2}$ levels above 60 mm Hg, largely discrepant oxygen tensions may be related to a single level of pulse oximetry reading (Fig. 21-13). This may be even more pronounced when the curve is shifted to the right or left because of changes in pH, temperature, and levels of 2,3-diphosphoglycerate or because of the presence of fetal hemoglobin in small infants. When 14 pulse oximeters were evaluated and their $Sp{O_2}$ values were compared with $Sa{O_2}$ values measured simultaneously with drawn blood samples, it was found that both the error in accuracy (mean $Sp{O_2} - Sa{O_2}$) and the error in precision (standard deviation of the differences) remained below 3% for an $Sa{O_2}$ greater than 83% but were increased to 8% and 5%, respectively, for deeper hypoxia.[126] Inaccuracies may also occur in the presence of jaundice, elevated levels of carboxyhemoglobin, and skin pigmentation[127,128] and during the loss of a reliable waveform in low perfusion states. The latter problem may be partially overcome with the new combined pulse oximeters, which also simultaneously monitor the pulse rate from chest electrodes. This pulse oximeter disregards measurements when peripheral and central pulse rates do not agree. The pulse oximeter does not alert the clinician to hyperoxygenation, a situation that may be dangerous in preterm infants. Thus infants of this age group should be monitored by the transcutaneous $P{O_2}$ technique, which has been found reliable for newborns whose skin is very thin.[122]

Ventilation. Two techniques are available for noninvasive carbon dioxide monitoring: the transcutaneous electrode and capnography. Devices measuring the transcutaneous $P{CO_2}$ have been available for use for more than a decade. Data from neonatal and pediatric intensive care units reveal that transcutaneous $P{CO_2}$ values are higher than $Pa{CO_2}$ values.[129,130] In a study of 134 children receiving mechanical ventilation, skin perfusion at the site of the transcutaneous electrode was found to significantly influence the accuracy of transcutaneous $P{CO_2}$ measurements.[131] In infants and children with normal skin perfusion (capillary refill time <3 seconds), the mean difference between transcutaneous $P{CO_2}$ and $Pa{CO_2}$ was only 0.2 mm Hg (standard deviation of 5.4) compared with 4.1 (standard deviation of 9.9) in patients with decreased skin perfusion. Hence this technique may not be applicable to patients with low skin perfusion.

End-tidal carbon dioxide pressure (P_{ETCO_2}), measured as the plateau value of an exhaled carbon dioxide display, closely approximates the $Pa{CO_2}$ and may be used to measure $Pa{CO_2}$ noninvasively and continuously (Fig. 21-14, *A*). Although end-tidal carbon dioxide monitoring by capnography is routinely

Table 21-4 Clinical Score for Acute Asthma in Infants and Children

	0	1	2
Cyanosis	None	In room air	In $F{IO_2}$ = 0.4
Inspiratory breath sounds	Normal	Unequal	Decreased
Accessory muscle use	None	Moderate	Maximal
Expiratory wheezing	None	Moderate	Marked
Cerebral status	Normal	Depressed/agitated	Coma

A score of 5 or more than 5 indicates impending respiratory failure. A score of 7 or more than 7 indicates respiratory failure.

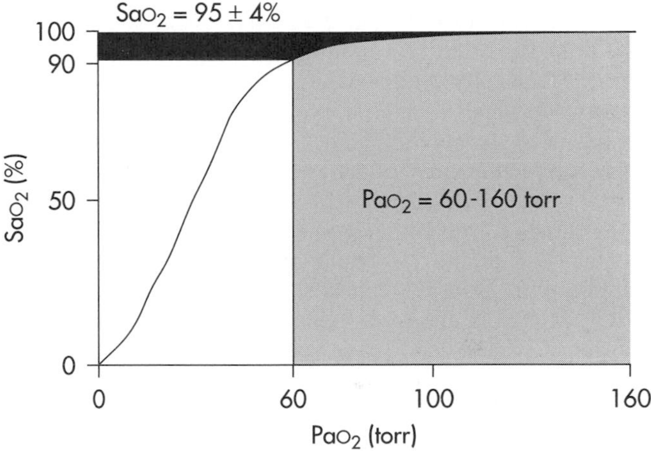

Fig. 21-13. The oxygen-hemoglobin dissociation curve. Because oximeters have 95% confidence limits for an $Sa{O_2}$ of ±4%, an oximeter reading of 95% could represent a $Pa{O_2}$ of 60 mm Hg ($Sa{O_2}$, 91%) or 160 mm Hg ($Sa{O_2}$, 99%). (Modified from Tobin MJ: *Am Rev Respir Dis* 138:1625-1642, 1988.)

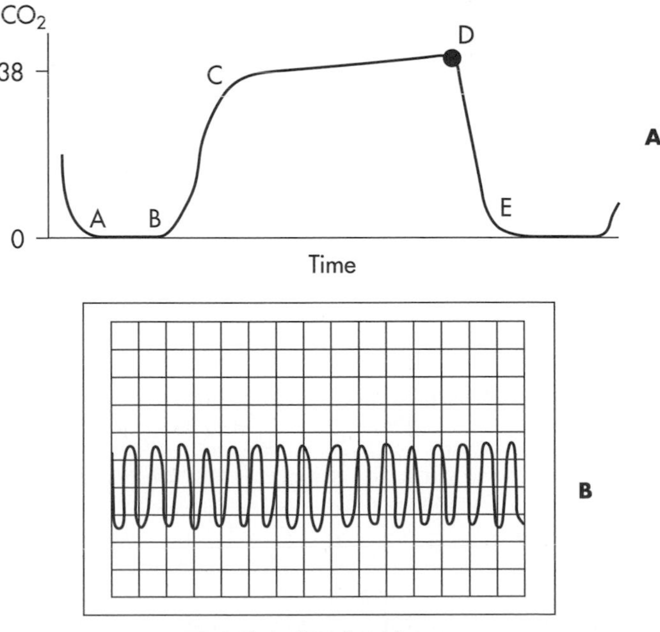

Fig. 21-14. Carbon dioxide waveform recorded from a capnometer. **A,** *A-B,* Inspiratory phase. Carbon dioxide level is nearly zero. *B-C,* Expiration starting with dead space exhalation. *C-D,* Alveolar gas resulting in the plateau phase. *D,* End-tidal carbon dioxide value. *D-E,* Inspiration resumes with rapid decrease of carbon dioxide level to zero *(E)*. **B,** No plateau is seen in a child breathing at a high rate. Inspiration restarts before the pure alveolar phase is reached.

used for healthy infants and children in sleep laboratories, its use to assess Pa_{CO_2} is limited to following trends in children requiring assisted ventilation by cardiorespiratory diseases that affect gas exchange and $\dot{V}/\dot{Q}$ matching.[132] This could explain why capnography has not been widely used in pediatric intensive care units. Several investigators have suggested that P_{ETCO_2} is not applicable to children with severe $\dot{V}/\dot{Q}$ mismatching and that correction factors should be used.[133,134] The gap between the Pa_{CO_2} and the P_{ETCO_2} is caused partly by uneven ventilation and nonhomogeneous pulmonary capillary blood distribution. An error in recording may also result from the lack of an alveolar plateau (which is necessary for end-tidal recording). This is more likely to occur in small children who breath spontaneously at relatively high rates and small V_T (Fig. 21-14, *B*). In a study of 134 infants and children whose lungs were mechanically ventilated and in whom only end-tidal carbon dioxide values were used, it was possible to define the limitations of the technique.[131] The P_{ETCO_2} was found to be a reliable and accurate method for Pa_{CO_2} assessment as long as the Pa_{O_2}/Pa_{O_2} ratio was greater than 0.3 (Fig. 21-15). In children whose lungs were ventilated and who had a Pa_{O_2}/P_{AO_2} ratio less than 0.3, the P_{ETCO_2} could still be used but only for detecting trends in $PaCO_2$ changes. When a sudden drop in the P_{ETCO_2} occurs and the Pa_{CO_2} is unchanged, the clinician should suspect increased dead space ventilation. This is typical for pulmonary vascular disease or pulmonary embolism. In this situation, some alveoli are not perfused, so their P_{ACO_2} stays low, resulting in low end-tidal carbon dioxide levels. During cardiac arrest, circulation ceases, and the P_{ETCO_2} gradually falls (while Pa_{CO_2} rises), reappearing only when pulmonary circulation is restored by effective resuscitation. Hence P_{ETCO_2} monitoring can be used to assess the extent to which resuscitative measures maintain pulmonary perfusion. The presence of an end-tidal carbon dioxide waveform ensures that the ETT is in the airway during mechanical ventilation or after intubation. A decline of the P_{ETCO_2} of 10 mm Hg or more without any changes in ventilation or hemodynamic status in a child whose head was badly injured usually signifies a marked compromise or cessation of cerebral blood flow. The major advantages of the noninvasive carbon dioxide monitoring techniques are that they do not require blood sampling (except for verifying accuracy) and they provide continuous readings so that a change in ventilatory status is quickly appreciated.

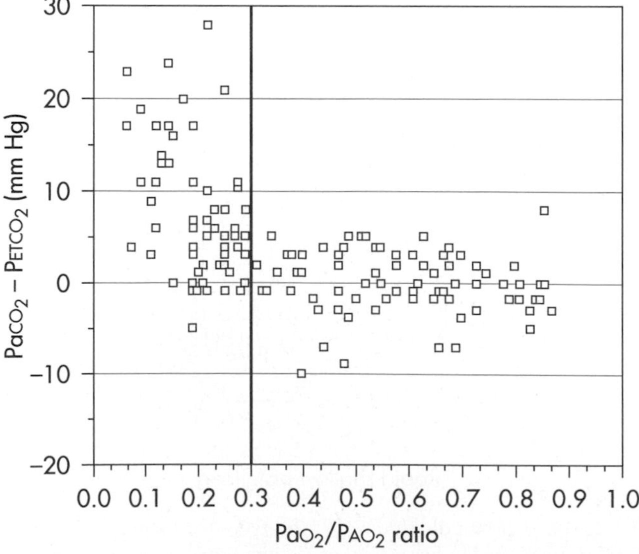

Fig. 21-15. Relationship of Pa_{CO_2} − P_{ETCO_2} difference to the Pa_{O_2}/P_{AO_2} ratio in children whose lungs are ventilated. The P_{ETCO_2} is significantly different from the Pa_{CO_2} when the Pa_{O_2}/P_{AO_2} ratio falls below 0.3. (Modified from Sivan Y et al: *Pediatr Pulmonol* 12:153-157, 1992.)

Pulmonary Mechanics and Lung Volumes. The sophisticated assessment of pulmonary function is a demanding task in infants and children whose lungs are mechanically ventilated and whose condition is unstable. Monitoring of respiratory compliance and resistance, as well as lung volumes, can assist the clinician to (1) optimize ventilator settings, (2) indicate the course of the disease, (3) assess the effectiveness of treatment modalities and medications, and (4) obtain a better understanding of the physiology of the disease. Obtaining pulmonary function measurements in children whose lungs are ventilated was once considered experimental and therefore was performed in only a few laboratories. With the incorporation of microprocessors and electronic sensors and the availability of automated systems, this area has developed to the stage of clinical bedside practice.[135,136] The discussion that follows is limited only to the basic concepts and the potential applications of this relatively new area.

The total respiratory resistance and compliance of the lungs and chest wall can be measured using an esophageal balloon and a pneumotachograph placed at the proximal end of the ETT. This allows for pressure-volume curves that can be displayed and for calculations of respiratory resistance and respiratory compliance. This technique has several limitations that are not different from those encountered in patients whose lungs are not ventilated.[135] The average pleural pressure necessary for calculations is not always possible to obtain, and the technique is highly dependent on accurate placement of the esophageal catheter. Therefore the "occlusion" technique has become more commonly used, especially in infants and children whose lungs are ventilated. If the clinician measures alveolar pressure at a known lung volume at which no flow occurs, static respiratory compliance can be determined. Alveolar pressure can be obtained by measuring pressure at the proximal end of the ETT during relaxation of the respiratory muscles against an occluded ETT (zero gas flow). The concept uses the Hering-Breuer reflex in infants but is easily performed also in older patients whose lungs are ventilated by occluding the expiratory port long enough to allow the airway pressure to reach a constant value and equilibrate alveolar with the proximal ETT pressure. This technique may be applicable especially to infants and children whose lungs are ventilated for acute respiratory failure because they are usually heavily sedated or under neuromuscular blockade, so the respiratory muscles are not activated and end-inspiratory relaxation is easily achieved. Measuring the slope and intercepts of the passive expiratory flow-volume curve obtained after the release of an expiratory occlusion allows respiratory compliance, respiratory resistance, and the time constant to be obtained from a single occlusion procedure (Slope = Time constant = Respiratory resistance × Respiratory compliance). The technique is highly reproducible and requires only transient disruptions of mechanical ventilation.[135]

Forced expiration can be performed by either the rapid thoracic compression ("squeeze") technique[138,139] or the deflation technique.[140,141] These yield forced flow-volume curves and may also be used to measure the maximum flow rate at FRC and flow limitation.[142-144] The principles, methodology, and limitations of the techniques are discussed elsewhere.[136] Nevertheless, it should be noted that the deflation method was developed specifically for infants and children whose lungs are intubated and that it may be advantageous in this population.

The FRC is an important parameter in the respiratory management of infants and children whose lungs are ventilated. Its determination is essential for the rational monitoring of mechanical ventilation in infants and children.[145] However, its use has been limited because the existing methods for FRC measurements are cumbersome. The techniques that use body plethysmography and measure thoracic gas volume cannot be applied to the sick child whose lungs are ventilated, whereas the helium-rebreathing methods add compliance and sometimes resistance to the ventilatory-respiratory system and may interfere with the ventilatory pressures delivered to the patient. FRC determination by the open-circuit nitrogen-washout technique has proved to be very accurate and easily reproducible in infants and children whose lungs are ventilated.[146] However, the technique is limited to patients whose lungs are ventilated at an FIO_2 no greater than 0.7 and who do not have a leak around the ETT.

CLINICAL CONSIDERATIONS IN VENTILATOR MANAGEMENT

The broad indications for initiating mechanical ventilation are summarized in Box 21-4. Acute respiratory failure is the most common cause for assisted ventilatory support. It may present as arterial hypoxemia, hypercapnia, or both conditions. The decision to initiate mechanical ventilation not only depends on the presence of one of these but is greatly influenced by the cause of the respiratory insufficiency, the disease process, and the goals for the patient. Hence in acute respiratory failure caused by a severe asthmatic attack, mechanical ventilation starts at worse arterial blood gas values than for a rapidly progressing neuromuscular disease, such as Guillain-Barré syndrome. For acute asthma, mechanical ventilation is more complicated, and a reasonable delay in initiating it may cause an improvement after the aggressive administration of medications and possibly sodium bicarbonate to correct the acidosis. However, there is no benefit in waiting once acute respiratory failure has occurred in progressive Guillain-Barré syndrome. Common causes for initiation of mechanical ventilation not directly related to respiratory insufficiency are the "shock state," in which assisted ventilation reduces the rate of lactic acid production and WOB, and intracranial pressure elevation. Therefore the commonly used laboratory criteria for initiation of mechanical ventilation (a $PaCO_2$ >50 to 55 mm Hg or a PaO_2 <50 mm Hg with an FIO_2 >0.6) apply mainly to acute alveolar-interstitial pulmonary disorders but not to many other clinical situations.

BOX 21-4
General Indications for Initiating Mechanical Ventilation

Established or imminent respiratory failure resulting from the following:
- Intrinsic pulmonary disease
- Hypoventilation and apnea caused by central nervous system malfunction

Defective ventilatory pump (muscle weakness, chest trauma)
Supranormal hyperventilation (pulmonary hypertension, increased intracranial pressure)
Prophylactic indications (after surgery)
Postresuscitation for circulatory arrest
Reduction of WOB

Mode of Mechanical Ventilation

Even the most sophisticated ventilator cannot adjust the flow, pressure, and distribution of gas as well as the normally functioning respiratory system during spontaneous breathing. An abundant amount of research has focused on comparisons of pulmonary gas exchange during different modes of PPV and on the question of which of the ventilatory modes is superior in different clinical situations. There is no clear-cut choice as to the best method of ventilatory support for most children with respiratory failure. Studies in adults have shown that there is very little difference in patients undergoing SIMV or PSV with respect to distribution of ventilation and perfusion.[147] The lungs of infants and small children are usually ventilated in a pressure-limited mode, although both pressure and volume modes can be used for all ages. The recognition that high positive pressure is a major risk factor for pulmonary damage has increased the preference for pressure modes even in older children with severe respiratory failure who require extensive ventilatory support, even at the cost of increased carbon dioxide and lower-than-optimal oxygenation (permissive hypercapnia or hypoxemia). These occur when lung compliance is significantly decreased, resulting in a decreased V_T for controlled pressure variables. CPAP mode is used mainly during weaning from mechanical ventilation except in preterm infants with HMD and apnea of prematurity.

Ventilator Adjustment

Several parameters should be considered when the ventilator settings are adjusted. Patient age and weight, the specific disease, and the underlying pathophysiology are important. These influence variables such as the flow rate, V_T, and minute volume of ventilation. The main ventilator manipulations to improve oxygenation are V_T, flow, and PEEP for volume-limited ventilation and PIP, T_I, and PEEP for pressure-limited ventilation. Augmenting any of these variables and using inspiratory pause (inspiratory pressure plateau, inspiratory hold) increase the MAP and may improve gas exchange in severe respiratory failure with severe $\dot{V}/\dot{Q}$ mismatching. However, the question of which variable manipulation is most advantageous for improving oxygenation is rarely clear. The answer is highly dependent on the underlying pathophysiology and the specific disease. Theoretically, augmenting the MAP by increasing variables that correct physiologic abnormalities, such as the FRC in cases of ARDS, may be advantageous. However, this is not always true. For example, when lung disease is not homogeneous and relatively unaffected areas coexist with severely damaged lung regions, increasing the PEEP and PIP may have unwitting effects on the relatively good lung units with overdistention and decreased compliance. In such situations, augmenting variables that increase T_I may be advantageous. All these measures also have potential consequences by increasing the likelihood for pulmonary barotrauma and adverse cardiovascular effects.

V_T and PIP

As a general guideline in patients with mild to moderate respiratory failure, starting with PIP of 20 to 24 cm H_2O in pressure mode is reasonable. In volume mode, a V_T of 10 to 15 ml/kg (compared with normal VT of 5 to 7 ml/kg) is usually started, which takes into consideration the compliance of the circuit and compressibility of the gas. Ventilators that measure the exhaled VT may be more informative because some of the preset VT may be wasted in the circuit and leak around the ETT so that the delivered VT is always smaller than the set VT. However, measurements of VT from devices with flow sensors on the ETTs are likely to be more accurate than volumes measured within the ventilator because they are not altered by compressive losses. In more severe situations when the respiratory compliance is significantly decreased, the PIP should be increased. The specific disease and the clinician's approach dictate the policy of ventilator adjustment. This is apparent in children whose lungs are mechanically ventilated for status asthmaticus or ARDS. The traditional approach has favored normalization of arterial blood gas levels using a high VT (10 to 15 ml/kg) regardless of peak pressure. To lower the complication rates associated with high pressures, controlled hypoventilation (permissive hypercapnia) has been suggested in cases in which deliberate hypoventilation with correction of hypoxemia and pH (with sodium bicarbonate) is applied.[148,149] On the other hand, hyperventilation and hypocapnia are pursued in cases of elevated intracranial pressure and postoperative pulmonary hypertension.

Rate

The initial ventilator rate should be at least equal to the physiologic normal breathing rate for age and then adjusted according to the specific goal based on the arterial carbon dioxide tension. This normal breathing rate is sufficient for a child with a close-to-normal cardiorespiratory status (e.g., children whose lungs are ventilated because of neuromuscular diseases). However, normal rates may not be sufficient for children with cardiorespiratory failure with metabolic or respiratory acidosis.

PEEP

The effectiveness of PEEP is due to increasing the FRC in restrictive lung diseases. This represents the recruitment of otherwise closed terminal airspaces and the prevention of alveolar collapse. The PEEP thereby decreases $\dot{V}/\dot{Q}$ mismatching and intrapulmonary shunting and increases the MAP. These effects result in improved oxygenation,[93,150] allowing for lower FIO_2 levels. The physiologic PEEP is considered to be 2 to 4 cm H_2O; thus this level of PEEP should be used in mild to moderate cases when the upper airways are bypassed. The use of higher or lower levels depends on the specific disease process or on the measurement of FRC. Data from ventilated children with acute restrictive lung disease show that the clinically chosen PEEP often fails to normalize FRC, whereas in some cases overinflation may ensue.[151] Overinflation may increase dead space, affect venous return to the right atrium, and enhance barotrauma. PEEP also affects the compliance of the respiratory system.[152,153] A wide variety of techniques have been suggested for PEEP optimization, but because of technical limitations and disagreements on the definition of the "best PEEP," none has become a practical tool.[153-156] Adjusting the PEEP to the level that results in maximal oxygen transport requires invasive procedures and pulmonary artery cannulation. Therefore much effort has been focused on noninvasive methods. The noninvasive PEEP optimization techniques are based on maximizing pulmonary compliance. This has been associated with maximal oxygen transport. Normalizing FRC while maintaining saturation above 90% has also been suggested as the best noninvasive method for titrating PEEP.[157] These approaches have been criticized because cardiac output and hence oxygen delivery, which accompanies high levels of PEEP, are reduced and also because repeated measurement of FRC is not yet an easy bedside procedure. A simple clinical guideline for PEEP titration in acute respiratory failure secondary to acute restrictive lung disease is to adjust the PEEP to the level at which the FIO_2 can be lowered to nontoxic levels without compromising cardiovascular performance and circulation.

Time Variables and Patient-Ventilator Synchronization

In pressure modes of mechanical ventilation, either the TI or the I:E ratio is set by the clinician. The other variable is dependent and is automatically determined according to the set time variable and the respiratory rate. The time required for the alveoli to fill and for the pressure to equilibrate within the respiratory system depends on the resistance to gas flow and the respiratory compliance. The product of resistance and compliance is defined as the time constant of the respiratory system and is a measure of the time required for the alveoli to reach 63% of the final volume. Three to five time constants are needed for the alveoli to fill between 95% and 99%; hence a shorter TI does not allow the entire VT to be delivered to the alveoli. The normal time constant may vary with age, from as low as 0.1 seconds in infants to 0.5 seconds in adults. Therefore a TI of 0.5 or longer is usually acceptable for ventilating the lungs of infants and children. During airway and pulmonary diseases, the resistance, compliance, and thus time constant change significantly. Moreover, the time constant may vary among different parts of the lungs. A reasonable approach comparable with physiologic breathing is to set the TI to around 0.7 seconds. This allows an I:E ratio of at least 1:2 for frequencies not exceeding 30 breaths/min and an I:E ratio of not less than 1:1 for rates of no more than 45 breaths/min. When the ventilator rate exceeds these numbers and an inverted I:E ratio mode of ventilation is not required, the TI needs to be shortened. For example, at a rate of 60 breaths/min, a TI of 0.5 seconds or less is required to provide an I:E ratio of 1:1. This may require an increase of flow (and pressure) to deliver a sufficient VT.

In volume modes of ventilation the time variables depend totally on the set variables (VT, frequency, flow) and on the resistance and compliance of the respiratory system. In cases in which the TI available by the set rate is insufficient for delivery of the set VT, the flow and the pressure limit should be adjusted, or the clinician should compensate and decrease VT, frequency, or both factors.

The expiratory time constant is usually longer than the TI constant because of the higher resistance during exhalation. This becomes even more clinically significant during airway diseases such as acute bronchiolitis, asthma, and bronchopulmonary dysplasia. When the expiratory time is less than three to five expiratory time constants, the alveoli may not empty, and overinflation and air trapping occurs with increased PEEP (inadvertent PEEP, auto-PEEP). This can be dealt with by prolonging the expiratory time, by decreasing ventilator rate, or by performing both actions.

Another variable that can be adjusted is the inspiratory plateau time (inspiratory pause, inspiratory hold). In certain ventilators, it is possible to hold inspiration and delay the initiation of exhalation after the VT has been delivered. In its extreme, this mode generates an inverse I:E ratio. An inspiratory plateau is useful in diseases in which the time constant of the alveoli is prolonged. These alveoli require a longer TI for filling, and the inspiratory hold allows for redistribution of gas to these slow-filling alveoli. However, coexisting alveoli with a normal time constant are endangered by prolonged periods of positive pressure, and their mean pressure increases significantly and unnecessarily, which may result in barotrauma and adverse cardiovascular effects.

Much effort has been devoted to trials to optimally synchronize a patient's respiratory efforts and ventilator breaths. Synchronous ventilation is believed to improve VT and minute volume. On the other hand, during nonsynchronized ventilation, assisted ventilation may be inefficient, and adverse consequences, including an increase in WOB, restlessness, agitation, and barotrauma, may occur. When the goal is to gain full control of patient ventilation, sedation and muscle paralysis are used. However, in many situations and especially during weaning, harmonized ventilatory synchrony is crucial. The modes of mechanical ventilation used to improve synchronization are SIMV, pressure-SIMV, ACV, and PSV. The lungs of infants and small children are usually ventilated in the time-cycled, pressure-limited mode, and these patients can breathe between ventilator breaths. These patients and especially newborns have a tendency to change their respiratory pattern during breathing. A method to trigger the ventilator via the infant's own respiratory efforts using an external capsule attached to the baby's abdominal wall allows for better synchronization.[158,159] Triggering of the ventilator by changes in transthoracic impedance has similar potential. Unfortunately, these techniques, like triggering of airway pressure, are relatively slow compared with the fast respiratory rates of infants and children. In this respect, flow triggering initiated from a flow-sensing device on the ETT appears more sensitive and hence faster.[160] Four flow-triggered infant ventilators were recently rigorously evaluated using an infant lung model,[161] with significant differences noted for delay time, trigger pressure, and trigger work at each PEEP level. Patient-triggered ventilation from flow sensing decreases the WOB in newborns.[162] Flow-triggered ventilators do have the drawback in pediatric practice of autocycling resulting from flow compensation to maintain PEEP levels in the presence of an airway leak.[163] In such cases, lowering the sensitivity setting of the ventilator, lowering the PEEP level, or using both actions may decrease autocycling or necessitate reintubation with a larger or cuffed[42] ETT.

FIO_2

When mechanical ventilation is started for respiratory failure, the FIO_2 should be 1.0. Only after the PaO_2 is obtained and the noninvasive SpO_2 is monitored should the FIO_2 be titrated down to the lowest suitable level.

Immediately after the patient has been connected to the ventilator, clinical assessment of ventilatory support should be performed by the evaluation of chest excursions, air entry, breathing sounds, and the color of the skin. After a short time of stabilization, arterial blood gases should be measured, preferably with SpO_2 and end-tidal carbon dioxide values noted at the same time. The ventilator variables are then readjusted, and the noninvasive oxygen and carbon dioxide monitors can be used. It is important to recognize that very low $PaCO_2$ levels (<20 or 25 mm Hg) decrease blood flow to the brain and should be avoided unless a clear indication exists.

WEANING FROM MECHANICAL VENTILATION

Weaning of ventilatory support depends not only on the patient's respiratory status but also on the recovery of other systems, such as the brain (level of consciousness) and heart (hemodynamic stability). In general, discontinuation of mechanical ventilation can be considered when the following conditions have been met: (1) The patient is stable, (2) the underlying disease and its complications have improved, (3) ventilator support is minimal compared with the patient's spontaneous breathing, and (4) the FIO_2 is low (≤0.4).

During weaning, the ventilator share of the total ventilation is gradually decreased, whereas the patient's share is increased. Some ventilators have continuous flow of gas in the circuit, so the patient can easily inhale between ventilator breaths. Other ventilators have intermittent-flow circuits, and the patient needs to apply an effort to generate a negative pressure below the PEEP pressure to open a demand valve and allow flow for a spontaneous inspiration between the ventilator mandatory breaths. The additional work imposed by the need to open a demand valve is generally small and clinically insignificant. Nevertheless, in some small infants and in patients who are in borderline condition for weaning, this may be clinically important.[164,165] Switching such patients to continuous-flow ventilators may facilitate weaning. Some modern types of ventilators have the ability for both continuous and demand flow patterns (e.g., the time-cycled, pressure-limited InfantStar, the Newport series ventilators). The gradual decrease in the ventilator's mandatory breaths is usually undertaken during SIMV or time-cycled, pressure-limited modes of ventilation until no ventilator breaths are used (i.e., CPAP). As previously discussed, pressure-support mode may also be incorporated into either of these modes when the amount of the ventilator support is gradually decreased.[106,107] Ventilatory muscle fatigue during respiratory overload may be a contributing factor in the inability to wean patients from prolonged mechanical ventilatory support.[108,166] In these cases, weaning (which is reloading of WOB back to the patient) may not be ideal with volume-cycled ventilation. During weaning on SIMV, the patient takes unassisted breaths between volume-assisted or volume-controlled breaths. The load on the patient is increased by decreasing the ventilator-mandatory breaths. However, the pressure-volume characteristics of this spontaneous breathing are often abnormally high because of the increased airway resistance and the reduced lung compliance.[108] During PSV, the muscle reloading process occurs with every breath, resulting in a more normal pressure-volume relationship. This may provide a more physiologic reloading pattern to recovering ventilatory muscles after prolonged mechanical ventilation and thus may be useful in patients who are undergoing long-term weaning and who are difficult to make comfortable.[108] Results of a recent study in children[109] agree with studies performed in adults. Nevertheless, there is not enough data from controlled studies in children to prefer this method to the more traditional method of gradual-rate decrease on SIMV. It is also not clear whether PSV results in a decreased need for sedation, a faster weaning process, or improved outcome.

CPAP is a useful test of the patient's ability to support his or her own ventilation. CPAP is not an indispensable step during weaning, and the lungs of pediatric patients recovering from acute respiratory failure (e.g., postoperative recovery, drug overdose) can usually be extubated, bypassing the CPAP step. Such an alternative to CPAP is to connect the patient to a T-piece system without a PEEP device for a short time before

BOX 21-5
Weaning from Mechanical Ventilation

Stable condition
- Underlying cause for respiratory failure has reversed.
- Fever (if present) has declined.
- Pain, electrolyte, and acid-base abnormalities have been corrected.

Physiologic assessment

PAO_2 to PaO_2 difference at $FIO_2 = 1.0$	<300 to 350 mm Hg
PaO_2 (at FIO_2 <0.4)	>60 mm Hg
$PaCO_2$	<50 mm Hg
$\frac{\dot{V}_{DS}}{V_T}$	<0.6
Vital capacity*	>10 to 15 ml/kg
Maximum negative inspiratory pressure*	<−20 to −30 cm H_2O

Trial-and-error method
- Respiratory rate, effort, SpO_2, and PCO_2 (transcutaneous PCO_2 is optional) should be continuously monitored and verified by arterial blood gas analysis.
- FIO_2 should decrease.
- PEEP should decrease.
- Ventilator rate (IMV) should decrease.

CPAP mode or connection of the patient to a T-piece with an FIO_2 <0.4
- Blood gas factors should be monitored at 15 to 30 minutes and before extubation.

Extubation and delivery of humidified oxygen via mask or head box

$\dot{V}_{DS}$, Dead space ventilation.
*Applicable to older, cooperative children.

extubation. However, it is more common to put the patient on CPAP for a short time before extubation. CPAP also is used commonly in the weaning of children with chronic respiratory failure or when malacia of the airways is a major factor. During recovery from either acute or chronic airflow obstruction or with rapid, spontaneous respirations, intrinsic PEEP (or auto-PEEP) may present a problem with a marked increase in the WOB.[163] It has been calculated that applied PEEP should be at 80% of auto-PEEP to decrease the WOB while the infant or child adapts to the load or the load decreases (as in recovering asthma).

Several physiologic variables can predict when an older child or adult is ready for CPAP or T-piece system ventilation and extubation. However, infants and young children cannot cooperate, and trial-and-error methods must be used (Box 21-5).

When the clinician elects to use a CPAP trial, the patient breathes spontaneously; the FIO_2 is less than 0.4, and the CPAP level is less than 5 cm H_2O. If the patient is stable during this phase, extubation may be attempted. Clinicians do not always agree on how long the trial should last because CPAP may increase the WOB (and the risk of weaning failure) by the need to breath through an ETT and circuit, which has a higher resistance than the patient's nonintubated airway; or by the need to open a demand valve during each inspiration in ventilators that do not use continuous flow (e.g., Siemens Servo 900C).

Most clinicians take the attitude (gained from experience) that if patients cannot tolerate the small additional WOB imposed by CPAP for several hours, they will be unlikely to sustain unaided ventilation when their lungs are extubated. After extubation, humidified oxygen should be supplied by either a head box or face mask.

USE OF MEDICATIONS TO FACILITATE MECHANICAL VENTILATION

ETTs and PPV may cause considerable physical and emotional discomfort and even pain initially. Thus sedation of children whose lungs are mechanically ventilated is the rule, although some small infants do without it. Sedation with or without muscle paralysis facilitates mechanical ventilation and thus improves oxygenation and may even decrease gas flow by minimizing the patient's activity.[167] It also enables diaphragmatic rest, which allows restoration of diaphragmatic high-energy compounds. The most commonly used medications for sedation are narcotics and benzodiazepines. Morphine, 0.1 mg/kg, or fentanyl, 1 to 2 μg/kg, may be used in repeated doses and may be increased if initial doses are ineffective. Diazepam and the shorter-acting midazolam can be given in doses of 0.1 to 0.2 mg/kg. The actions of the narcotics and benzodiazepines can be reversed by naloxone and flumazenil, respectively. A more efficient technique may be to administer these medications in continuous intravenous infusions after a loading dose. This prevents fluctuations in both medication serum concentrations and the patient's tranquility. However, excessive or inadequate levels may result. Regular starting infusion rates are 10 to 50 μg/kg/hr for morphine, diazepam, and midazolam. If sedation is not adequate with these rates, another loading dose can be given and the infusion rate increased. Either narcotics or benzodiazepines, and especially their combination, may cause cardiovascular depression. During the weaning process, sedation should be decreased to a minimum or discontinued.

Nondepolarizing neuromuscular blocking agents are frequently used in infants and children whose lungs are ventilated. Indications for their use include (1) adjunct heavy sedation to protect the child from injury related to agitation and combativeness, (2) inefficient ventilation because of patient-ventilator asynchrony, (3) head trauma with subsequent elevated intracranial pressure, and (4) very low lung compliance in which full control of ventilation is required. For many years the medication of choice in most adult and pediatric intensive care units was pancuronium bromide given as needed by intermittent intravenous injections.[168] In recent years, the administration of pancuronium or one of the new shorter-acting drugs, vecuronium or atracurium, has been extended to continuous intravenous infusion for patients with severe respiratory failure whose lungs are mechanically ventilated.[169-172] This mode of administration, although simpler and less time consuming for nurses, is complicated by the need to monitor the depth of neuromuscular blockade. During continuous intravenous infusion, overdose may easily develop and should be avoided by periodically allowing the partial return of muscle function, by frequently using a peripheral nerve stimulator, or by doing both.[173] Several reports[174-176] have raised the issue of prolonged neuromuscular weakness and even paralysis after a few days of neuromuscular relaxants administration in adults and children. Neurologic examination, electrophysiologic studies, and muscle biopsies have documented a diverse assortment of abnormal findings.[173] Two patterns of neuromuscular dysfunction secondary to the use of muscle relaxants have been reported. One is persistent neuromuscular junction blockade secondary to accumulation of the medication or one of its metabolites most commonly observed in patients with renal failure.[170,173] The second pattern in poorly understood and is attributed to generalized myopathy with histopathologic findings of atrophy, necrosis, and regeneration of muscle fibers. This pattern has been associated with prolonged use of neuromuscular blocking agents, especially with the concomitant use of corticosteroids.[172,177-180] Recovery from this type of neuromuscular dysfunction may take weeks or months. It is therefore recommended that corticosteroids not be administered for uncertain or unproved indications during prolonged neuromuscular blockade.[173] This association may present a major problem for children mechanically ventilated for acute asthma in which muscle paralysis is very commonly used to achieve ventilator-patient synchronization and improve ventilation. However, although the neuromuscular complication does occur in children, it may be that the incidence is lower than in asthmatic adults.

Neuromuscular blocking agents have neither analgesic nor sedative effects. The paralyzed patient can feel and hear everything but cannot react—an experience that is even more frustrating and stressful. Therefore all patients under neuromuscular blockade should receive adequate amounts of sedation and analgesic treatment.

PHYSIOTHERAPY AND ENDOTRACHEAL SUCTIONING DURING MECHANICAL VENTILATION

An ETT and the use of PPV impairs mucociliary clearance and hampers effective cough. In the patient whose lungs are ventilated, this may lead to plugging of tenacious secretions in the airways and atelectasis. Chest physiotherapy (CPT) and endotracheal suctioning enhance migration of secretions from the periphery of the lungs to the major airways from where they are suctioned. Although this may seem theoretically obvious, much controversy exists regarding CPT and positioning in patients whose lungs are ventilated. One study of children who underwent cardiac surgery showed that when tracheal suctioning was preceded by CPT, the rate of atelectasis was much greater than it was for suctioning alone.[181] A thorough discussion of CPT and its rationale, efficacy, and techniques is given in Chapter 20. Some implications of CPT and tracheal suctioning in the infant and child whose lungs are intubated and ventilated are discussed here.

First, unlike CPT in the patient whose lungs are not ventilated, CPT should always be followed by suctioning. The frequency of tracheal suctioning depends on the rate and amount of sputum produced and on the patient's underlying disease and its severity. Most pediatric intensive care units have routines for scheduled suctioning. However, more frequent suctioning may be needed when signs of accumulated secretions in the airway occur. These signs are decreased chest movements, increased PIP in volume modes of ventilation, decreased air movement, and increasing dyspnea. Suctioning involves disconnection from the ventilator circuit, and therefore it should last for as short a time as possible. The condition of some patients with severe respiratory failure may deteriorate even during short suctioning. The effect of endotracheal suctioning on arterial blood gas values was examined in 25 children whose lungs were mechanically ventilated and who had an FIO_2 less than 0.6.[182] Saturation and PaO_2 fell significantly after suctioning. This drop was easily prevented by preoxygenation with 100% oxygen for 1 minute and intermittent hyperventilation between suction passes. These observations have important implications, especially in children with respiratory failure who have already low or borderline presuction PaO_2 values. In patients on high PEEP (>6 cm H_2O), presuction and postsuction ventilation should be performed manually with a PEEP valve attached to the hand bag ventilation system.

Complications of CPT and tracheal suctioning in infants and children whose lungs are ventilated include hypoxemia, atelectasis, damage to the mucosa of major airways caused by excessive negative suction pressure, pneumothorax from the high inflation pressure applied during presuction bagging, bradydysrhythmias secondary to vagal reflex, and increased intracranial pressure secondary to coughing.

COMPLICATIONS OF ASSISTED VENTILATORY SUPPORT

Although PPV and oxygen therapy are often lifesaving, they are sources for serious complications and adverse effects. Complications directly related to mechanical ventilation occur in at least one fourth of patients. In a recent prospective survey of 500 patients in the pediatric intensive care unit,[183] the duration of intubation and mechanical ventilation had the strongest association with complications and became significant when both exceeded 72 hours (Tables 21-5 and 21-6). These complications develop secondary to PPV, the artificial airway, the use of high FIO_2 levels, the effects on defense mechanisms against infections, and the effect of isolation and dependence on machine and medical personnel. The complications can be divided into those that result from breathing gas with high FIO_2, those that result from the ETT and that are limited to the upper airways and the subglottic area, adverse effects to the lower airways and the lung parenchyma, and complications provoked on other systems, especially the cardiovascular system.

Complications of High FIO_2 Levels (Oxygen Toxicity)

Oxygen is a drug and has the potential to harm the patient. The harmful effects are due to two basic mechanisms: cytotoxic effects that occur mainly in the lungs and are generically termed *pulmonary oxygen toxicity* and effects that are secondary to the physical and physiologic properties of high FIO_2.

Table 21-5 Complications of ETTs

COMPLICATION	CAUSE
Dislodgment and accidental extubation	Poor ETT securing
ETT obstruction	Tenacious secretions, inadequate suctioning
Palatal grooves and clefts	Pressure of tube on palate
Decubitus nasal erosion and stricture	Pressure of tube on nares
Dental complications	Pressure of tube on gums
Subglottic stenosis	Pressure of tube and irritation of subglottic area
Respiratory system infections	Presence of foreign body, ineffective cough, mucociliary transport
Sinusitis	Obstruction of sinus drainage
Tracheal strictures and granulomas	Mucosal damage from ETT

Table 21-6 Rate of Complications Directly Related to Mechanical Ventilation in 500 Infants and Children

COMPLICATION	NUMBER	PERCENTAGE
Atelectasis	39	7.8
Air leak (pneumothorax, pneumomediastinum)	34	6.8
Tissue damage	17	3.4
Accidental extubation	16	3.2
Endobronchial intubation	12	2.4
Postintubation stridor	12	2.4
Lung infection	10	2.0
Blockage of ETT	4	0.8
Ventilator malfunction	2	0.4

From Rivera R, Tibballs J: *Crit Care Med* 20:193-199, 1992.

The pathophysiology of pulmonary oxygen toxicity is discussed elsewhere. The toxic manifestations are related to the PO_2 in the gas being breathed. Because PO_2 is directly related to the FIO_2 and to the atmospheric pressure, breathing a gas with an FIO_2 of 0.5 in a hyperbaric chamber at 2 atm has the same harmful effect as breathing it with an FIO_2 of 1.0 at 1 atm. Pulmonary oxygen toxicity is related to the duration of exposure and to the level of FIO_2. FIO_2 levels below 50% to 60% are considered safe. When a patient breathes 100% oxygen, symptoms may appear even after 12 to 24 hours. The first symptoms are due to an alteration in the tracheal clearance of secretions and manifest as nonproductive cough, dyspnea, and chest pain. After 36 to 48 hours, gas exchange deteriorates with an increase in the alveolar-arterial oxygen difference and decrease in lung compliance. Over the next phase (50 to 60 hours), epithelial permeability increases, and the surfactant is inactivated, resulting in noncardiogenic pulmonary edema and ARDS. The time required for these complications to develop is much longer when FIO_2 is reduced.

Another complication of high FIO_2 is absorption atelectasis from denitrogenation of alveoli in patients with lower airway obstruction. Administration of 100% oxygen washes out nitrogen that may be keeping the alveoli open, converting poorly ventilated lung units (regions with low $\dot{V}/\dot{Q}$ ratios) into unventilated areas (shunt).[184,185] Retrolental fibroplasia is a complication of high FIO_2 and elevated PaO_2 in premature infants.

Upper Airway and ETT Complications

An ETT is a foreign body inside the upper airway and trachea. A wide range of complications may result even with meticulous nursing care (see Table 21-5). An ETT that is too large for the airway, a cuff that has been overinflated, excessive movement of the head and neck, and repeated intubations increase the friction of the ETT against tissues and may interfere with mucosal perfusion. This can result in subglottic ischemia, leading to subglottic edema and even scarring and stenosis with postextubation upper airway obstruction.[186-188] Measures used to minimize these complications include proper selection of tube size, nasal (as opposed to oral) intubation, use of an ETT fixation technique (which prevents movements of the tube), and monitoring of the ETT cuff pressure. A gas leak around the ETT at inflation pressures of 25 to 40 cm H_2O indicates that the pressure of the ETT against the subglottic area is not too high. Nevertheless, this does not guarantee protection from the development of subglottic damage.

Unplanned or Accidental Extubations

The frequency of an unplanned or accidental extubation is a measure of the excellence of patient care in any intensive care unit, irrespective of the age of patients or their illness. It is also one of the most serious events that can occur in patients whose lungs are mechanically ventilated. It may lead to severe hypoxemia and the need for emergency reintubation in patients whose condition is unstable, some of whom may have not been fasted. The rate of accidental extubation in pediatric and neonatal intensive care units ranges between 1% and 13% of patients whose lungs are mechanically ventilated, with a little over 1 such event per 100 ventilated days[180,189-191] in a pediatric intensive care unit. Newborns appear to have a lower incidence, at 0.4 unplanned extubations per 100.[186] With a strong, multidisciplinary approach to care, unplanned extubation rates of 0.2 to 0.6 per 100 can be achieved and sustained. In about 50% of cases of accidental extubation in a pediatric intensive care unit, reintubation is not needed, which implies that some patients' lungs are ventilated longer than necessary. Risk factors for unplanned extubation include inadequate sedation, the performance of a procedure, inadequate arm restraints, and inadequate tube fixation.[180,186] The last is probably the most crucial. Different techniques of tube fixation are used in different pediatric intensive care units. ETT fixation with a cloth tape, which is replaced daily, around the head minimizes ETT movement and accidental extubation but has the disadvantage of pasting the cloth tape to patient's hair (Fig. 21-16). Oral (as opposed to nasal) tubes are also believed to be more prone for accidental extubation. Unplanned extubation is even more serious in children whose lungs are intubated but not ventilated because usually intubation in these children is performed for acute upper airway obstruction (e.g., epiglottitis). Such an event may result in complete upper airway obstruction and require a difficult reintubation, which may damage the upper airway even further. Because these lungs are not mechanically ventilated, these patients are also neither under neuromuscular blockade nor too heavily sedated. Great care should be given to restrain the arms so that these patients cannot reach the ETT.

ETTs can cause decubitus ulcers of the lips, mouth, and nares, particularly if the tube is taped tightly against the angle of the mouth or the nares. Ulcers can cause permanent deformation and provide a locus for infection. So that tissue damage is minimized, the tube should be affixed to the face in such a manner that it does not impinge on the edge of the nostril. The tube should be angulated from the nostril and parallel to the long axis of the nasal cavity.[180] A complication that occurs mainly in patients with nasotracheal tubes is obstruction of the orifice of the paranasal sinuses. This is a source of acute sinusitis occurring primarily in the maxillary sinuses of patients

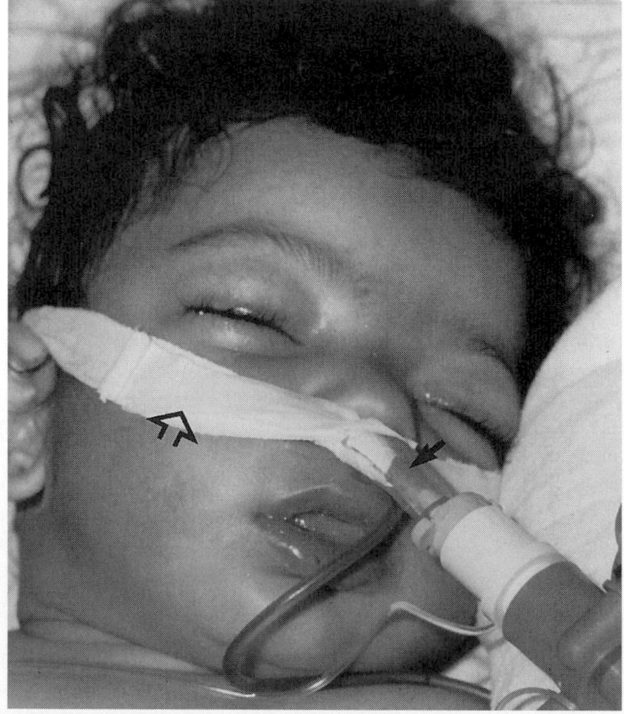

Fig. 21-16. ETT fixation with a cloth tape *(open arrow)* around the head to minimize ETT movement and accidental extubation. A brace around the external part of the ETT *(solid arrow)* prevents kinking.

whose lungs are intubated for more than 5 days. Most of the cases resolve spontaneously after removal of the ETT.[192,193]

Blockage of the ETT resulting from secretions or kinking occurs in 1.0% to 22.6% of children whose lungs are ventilated. Fatal results have been reported.[180,185,194] Adequate humidification, frequent suctioning, CPT, and the use of a brace to prevent tube kinking minimize this complication.

Adverse Effects to the Lower Respiratory System

The application of positive pressure to the lungs is a nonphysiologic process that modifies physiologic mechanisms, leading to adverse effects known as *barotrauma* and *volutrauma* (see Table 21-6). These are manifested as leakage of air from airspaces, leakage of fluid and protein out of the vascular bed, or both types of leaks. Pulmonary air leak, the most obvious clinical consequence of lung injury induced by PPV,[195] is manifested as the presence of pulmonary interstitial emphysema, subcutaneous emphysema, pneumomediastinum, pneumothorax, pneumopericardium, and pneumoperitoneum. The occurrence of pneumothorax or bronchopleural fistula significantly affects lung function, and these complications are associated with an increased mortality rate. High PIP, PEEP, and MAP and prolonged TI are also major causative factors. Some controversy exists as to which of these variables is most critical. The effects of these variables are highly dependent on the inspiratory and expiratory time constants of the alveolar units. High PIP levels distend primarily alveoli with shorter time constants because they reach equilibrium rapidly, thereby subjecting them to barotrauma more than the alveoli with slow filling time constants. A high PEEP increases the end-expiratory alveolar pressure and volume of all alveoli. However, those with prolonged expiratory time constants (airway obstruction diseases) may not have enough time to deflate before inspiration restarts, which results in overinflation with high end-expiratory pressures (auto-PEEP). A high VT with alveolar overdistention, even with relatively low pressures, has also been implicated as a major determinant.[196]

Although PEEP is used clinically to minimize the decreased oxygenation associated with pulmonary edema, excessive PIP and PEEP not only increase filtration pressures across pulmonary vessels and enhance edema formation but may also decrease pulmonary blood flow.[197] Animal studies have shown that microvascular permeability increases secondary to a high PIP (>40 cm H_2O) and VT. This occurs as a result of damage to both the epithelial and the endothelial barriers. Marked increases in microvascular pressure, pulmonary lymph flow, and protein leakage are observed when a high PIP (60 cm H_2O) was used compared with a low PIP.[192,197,198] Thus both mechanisms contribute to increased extravascular lung water and edema formation, which decreases lung compliance.

Vascular Changes

Adult and pediatric studies have shown histologic findings of pulmonary hypertension after prolonged mechanical ventilation.[199]

Nosocomial Infections

Infants and children whose lungs are ventilated in the pediatric intensive care unit are at higher risk for nosocomial respiratory infections than other hospitalized patients.[200] The incidence of nosocomial lung infection has dramatically increased with the use of prolonged mechanical ventilation. When the duration of intubation was relatively short (1 to 6 days), 2.3% in a series of 500 children[180] and 2.7% in a series of 2093 children[201] developed nosocomial pneumonia. However, in series of newborns, infants, and children whose lungs were ventilated for a mean of 8 to 15 days, the rate was 17%.[188,202] This rate becomes even higher when assisted ventilation lasts 14 days or longer. Physiologic disruption to mucociliary function and difficulties with artificial clearing of secretions and debris from the airway are causative factors. Routine analysis of tracheal aspirates is important for early detection of respiratory infection. The accuracy of direct tracheal suction for cultures has been questioned, and peripheral bronchial aspirates may be needed to differentiate nosocomial pneumonia from ETT colonization.[199] Despite careful hygienic measures, colonization of the oropharynx and the digestive tract is always present. Both sites are potential sources for pneumonia during mechanical ventilation; the only question that remains is which organism predominates. It has recently been suggested that oropharyngeal decontamination with instillation of a paste containing a combination of antibiotics reduces lower respiratory tract infections in adults whose lungs were mechanically ventilated.[203,204] However, it is as yet premature to commit to such a routine in all infants and children whose lungs are ventilated until further prospective trials in pediatric patients are completed.

Cardiovascular Adverse Effects

Positive airway pressures directly affect cardiac output and the vascular pressures and resistances in the pulmonary circulation.[192,205] During PPV, the intrathoracic pressure increases during the inspiratory phase, which leads to compression of the vena cava; hence venous return is reduced. This preload reduction may further lead to decreased cardiac output at low blood volumes. When PEEP is applied, the intrathoracic pressure and transmural pressure on alveolar vessels and great veins remain high throughout the respiratory cycle, resulting in increased pulmonary vascular resistance and pulmonary hypertension, which lead to a chain of hemodynamic consequences: increased right ventricular afterload and diastolic pressure, leftward displacement of the interventricular septum, and reduced stroke volume, resulting in decreased cardiac output.[192]

Adverse Effects to Other Systems

The combination of decreased venous return and decreased MAP caused by mechanical ventilation with high PIP and PEEP increases cerebral blood volume and decreases cerebral perfusion pressure in patients susceptible to intracranial hypertension. This is most commonly encountered in patients with severe head trauma, some of whom suffer also from acute lung injury and are subjected to high PPV.[206]

Consequently, the decreased cardiac output affects the perfusion of other organs. Decreased renal blood flow combined with the increase in the secretion of antidiuretic hormone in patients whose lungs are mechanically ventilated is responsible for decreased urine output and creatinine clearance.[207,208] Similar effects and decreased hepatic perfusion pressure have been suggested in adults whose lungs are mechanically ventilated when a very high PEEP was applied.[209]

Summary

In summary, all components of PPV have adverse effects, which are imposed mainly on the respiratory and cardiovascular systems. Minimizing ventilator-induced lung injury requires that the lowest possible PIP and VT be maintained, which has led to the concept of permissive hypercapnia (see later section). Nevertheless, the price of this guideline is the use of high FIO_2 in severe respiratory failure. Because it is usually agreed that an FIO_2 below 0.6 is safe, this principle is easy to apply within this range of FIO_2. The considerations in severe situations when high pressures are weighed against high oxygen levels are more complicated and depend on many other factors, such as the specific lung disease, the control of carbon dioxide and acidosis, the duration of mechanical ventilation, the hemodynamic state, and the involvement of other systems.

VENTILATION ISSUES SPECIFIC TO NEONATAL LUNG DISEASES

Hyaline Membrane Disease

HMD is characterized by pulmonary surfactant deficiency and transudation of plasma proteins into the alveolar spaces.[210] The result is a reduction of compliance with normal resistance (i.e., a respiratory system with a short time constant) and a tendency to develop atelectasis at early stages of the disease. If there is no rapid resolution of HMD with early weaning from the respirator, later stages of the disease may show elements of bronchopulmonary dysplasia (i.e., increased airway resistance). The main goals of respiratory therapy in HMD are therefore restoration of FRC by the application of PEEP (in the form of CPAP or in conjunction with mechanical ventilation), securing of adequate alveolar ventilation, and substitution of pulmonary surfactant.

Because the severity of HMD can vary considerably, the therapeutic approach should include administration of oxygen, CPAP, conventional mechanical ventilation with or without surfactant administration, and high-frequency ventilation (HFV). Indications for conventional mechanical ventilation are usually severe impairment of gas exchange (FIO_2 >0.6 to 0.8 to maintain an SpO_2 >85% to 90%), severe global respiratory failure ($PaCO_2$ >60 mm Hg, pH <7.2), and apnea. The details of how conventional mechanical ventilation should be performed are still controversial and include the route of intubation (orotracheal vs. nasotracheal), level of PEEP or FIO_2, respiratory rates and inspiratory and expiratory times, VT or maximum inspiratory pressures, target blood gases, and use of neuromuscular blocking agents and sedative medications.[211] Basically, the lung should be kept open by the application of PEEP throughout the respiratory cycle to prevent shearing forces in the terminal bronchioles, and ventilation should be as gentle as possible with minimally acceptable gas exchange. This may be a $PaCO_2$ in the range of 60 mm Hg, pH of 7.2, and SpO_2 of 87% to 92% with evidence of good cardiac output and normal hemoglobin concentration. Today's trends in ventilation are a small VT (5 to 7.5 ml/kg), rapid respiratory rates (inspiratory or expiratory times in the range of 0.3 seconds), and patient-triggered ventilation, which is possible with newly developed transthoracic impedance or inspiratory flow–sensing devices.[212] Weaning from mechanical ventilation is usually performed via (synchronized) IMV to CPAP by ETT and possibly administered by nasal prongs at the end. Administration of methylxanthines before stopping respiratory support may be helpful, particularly in tiny infants.

The introduction of surfactant in the treatment of HMD has significantly reduced the mortality rate, duration of mechanical ventilation, and incidence of pulmonary air leak syndromes.[213] However, exogenous surfactant is not indicated in all cases of HMD. The high cost of surfactant justifies a treatment only in moderately to severely ill infants on mechanical ventilation with FIO_2 values greater than 0.55 to 0.6. With regard to mechanical ventilation, changes in pulmonary mechanics must be anticipated after administration of surfactant, and rapid adaptation of respiratory settings is mandatory to prevent iatrogenic lung injury secondary to markedly improved compliance.

Complications of mechanical ventilation in HMD include acute life-threatening pulmonary air leak syndromes or barotrauma (e.g., pneumothorax, pneumomediastinum, pneumopericardium, pulmonary interstitial emphysema) and the more chronic type of pulmonary injury typified by bronchopulmonary dysplasia. Another type of acute lung injury volutrauma has gained recent clinical interest. Volutrauma is thought to result from overstretching of lung units with subsequent disruption of the alveolar-capillary membranes and permeability pulmonary edema. Ventilation with low VT is therefore recommended.[214]

Meconium Aspiration Syndrome

In meconium aspiration syndrome (MAS), a mixture of parenchymal pulmonary disease and obstruction of the small airways is present, which may result in a very nonhomogeneous lung.[215,216] In patients in whom airway obstruction predominates, time constants are long, which must be considered to prevent pulmonary overexpansion during mechanical ventilation. Another important and often coexisting problem of MAS is persistent pulmonary hypertension of the newborn, which may result in poor systemic oxygenation resulting from right-to-left shunting through the fetal channels.[217] A major strategy for lowering pulmonary vascular resistance is to achieve alkalosis (pH, 7.45 to 7.5) by respiratory means (increased alveolar ventilation), metabolic means (administration of sodium bicarbonate), or both. Unfortunately, both measures have side effects. Particularly, increasing minute ventilation may lead to volutrauma if large VT values are used or to pulmonary overexpansion if the respiratory rate on the ventilator is increased inappropriately, no longer permitting total expiration and causing inadvertent PEEP. In addition to conventional mechanical ventilation, other forms of treatment have been developed, including "pulmonary" vasodilation, systemic vasoconstriction (noradrenaline), HFV, and ultimately, extracorporeal membrane oxygenation (ECMO). With regard to pulmonary vasodilators (e.g., tolazoline, nitroglycerin, prostacyclin), it must be stressed that these medications also reduce systemic vascular resistance. This might in turn reduce myocardial perfusion and thus myocardial performance and possibly leave the ratio of systemic vascular resistance to pulmonary vascular resistance unaltered. An exception might be inhaled nitric oxide because it is rapidly metabolized and has therefore no systemic effect.[218,219] Another alternative might be represented by intravenous magnesium sulfate (or chloride), which also is well tolerated hemodynamically.[220] The conditions at which a switch from conventional mechanical ventilation to HFV or even ECMO should be considered are generally inadequate oxygenation with an FIO_2 greater than 0.95 and an MAP greater than 20 to 25 cm H_2O. This is expressed as an oxygenation index of greater than 40 (Oxygenation index = MAP [in cm H_2O] × FIO_2 [in %] ÷ PaO_2 [in mm Hg]).[221]

Complications of mechanical ventilation in MAS are essentially the same as those in HMD with the exception that pneumothorax seems to be a frequent event during primary resuscitation in the delivery room and that pulmonary interstitial emphysema is not as frequent as in HMD. Bronchopulmonary dysplasia may occur after MAS but takes a less severe course probably because the lungs are damaged at a more mature state than in HMD.

SPECIAL TYPES OF ASSISTED VENTILATION

Positive-Pressure Mask Ventilation by the Bilevel PPV System

Positive-pressure mask ventilation is a technique of noninvasive PPV. A major stimulus for the development of this method of respiratory support was the need to operate easy-to-use home ventilators. Nasal mask ventilation was therefore initially used for the treatment of adults with sleep apnea, chronic obstructive pulmonary disease, and neuromuscular diseases with chronic alveolar hypoventilation.

Method of Operation

The bilevel PPV system provides noninvasive positive-pressure ventilatory assistance to spontaneously breathing patients. This is a flow-cycled, pressure-limited device coupled with a nasal or a face mask. The mode of operation is comparable with the combination of pressure-support mode with PEEP. The system delivers different positive airway pressures during inspiration and exhalation (termed *inspiratory positive airway pressure [IPAP]* and *expiratory positive airway pressure [EPAP]*, respectively). The inspiratory pressure is the support pressure, and the expiratory positive pressure is analogous to the PEEP (when both inspiratory and expiratory pressures are equal, the mode of ventilation is CPAP).

The system is flow cycled; that is, it responds to the patient's inspiratory effort through the use of a flow transducer.[222] At the initiation of respiration, a change in the level of circuit flow exceeding 40 ml/s for more than 30 msec causes the machine to impose a preset IPAP. As the inspiratory flow decreases toward the end of inspiration, the pressure supported breath is terminated in synchrony with the patient's breathing pattern. The pressure in the circuit then drops to a preset EPAP for the exhalation period. The device cycles between the set IPAP and EPAP levels in response to patient triggering. Hence the patient controls his or her own respiratory frequency and inspiratory flow, whereas the device augments the patient's VT.[219] A backup rate may be set to ensure a minimum breathing rate in case of apnea. The proportion of each IPAP-EPAP cycle spent at IPAP can be controlled, ranging from 10% to 90%.

Some of the ordinary intensive care ventilators can also be used for mask ventilation. However, machines developed specifically for this purpose (e.g., BiPAP, Respironics; DP90, Taema; PB335, Puritan-Bennett and Companion 320 I/E, Puritan-Bennett) are easier to use, have only one arm of ventilation circuit (inspiratory), and are much cheaper. Humidification is not always required and may be added for the specific patient by a humidifier. Most commonly, nasal masks are used for positive-pressure mask ventilation; full face masks are also available. Both types are available in a variety of sizes. Supplemental oxygen can be entrained through a porthole in the mask or at the proximal end of the circuit.

The bilevel PPV may be advantageous compared with CPAP by providing pressure support during inspiration, thereby having the potential to decrease WOB. Studies in adults have shown that improvement in respiratory indexes during bilevel PPV were related to the reduction in inspiratory muscle energy expenditure. This suggests that bilevel PPV can reduce the energy costs of breathing in respiratory failure comparable to that observed during assisted ventilation via an ETT.[219,223]

Clinical Applications

Adult studies have shown promising results with positive-pressure mask ventilation by the bilevel PPV method in a variety of clinical situations (Box 21-6), including selected cases of acute respiratory failure[224]; weaning from assisted ventilation after acute exacerbations of chronic conditions, such as chronic obstructive pulmonary disease[225]; respiratory failure from neuromuscular diseases[222]; and home ventilation for obstructive sleep apnea. Reports of bilevel PPV in children followed reports in adults and showed its usefulness in similar clinical conditions.[219,220,226]

In acute situations, bilevel PPV minimizes the need for intubation and reintubation in pediatric patients with mild to moderate respiratory insufficiency.[223] Children whose condition deteriorates after extubation and who are considered for reinstitution of assisted ventilation because of weakness or clinically significant atelectasis are good candidates and may benefit from this noninvasive technique.[223] Another group are patients who have recovered from acute respiratory failure to a point where only minimal support is required but needed for longer periods (days or weeks). The lungs of these patients may be extubated and put on bilevel PPV. Children who are in the chronic recovery phase of ARDS may be in this category. Similarly, older children with muscular dystrophy or neuromuscular disorders may benefit from respiratory support after scoliosis or other orthopedic surgery by this technique.

In a study of 15 children with chronic respiratory failure (11 with neuromuscular diseases and 4 with cystic fibrosis),[220] bilevel PPV improved general well-being and respiratory status. In 87% of these children, significant improvement was observed in vital signs, arterial carbon dioxide levels, and serum bicarbonate levels. Bilevel PPV has also been used successfully in patients with cystic fibrosis awaiting lung transplantation.

BOX 21-6

Potential Indications for Positive-Pressure Mask Ventilation

Acute respiratory failure

Mild to moderate cases
Facilitation weaning from mechanical ventilation
Respiratory distress or failure after extubation
Significant or symptomatic atelectasis after extubation

Subacute respiratory failure*

Self-limiting neuromuscular disorders (e.g., Guillain-Barré syndrome)
Period after acute respiratory failure (e.g., chronic ARDS)

Chronic respiratory failure

"Bridging" of patients to lung transplantation
Home ventilation
Obstructive sleep apnea syndrome

*Subacute respiratory failure indicates a condition that usually starts with acute respiratory failure and improves to a state at which minimal mechanical support is needed for a prolonged period (weeks or months).

Children with obstructive sleep apnea syndrome and nocturnal hypoventilation may be excellent candidates for home use of bilevel PPV.[220,227] In these cases, bilevel PPV can be used intermittently (i.e., only during sleep periods). Nocturnal ventilatory assistance is believed to improve oxygenation and ventilation at this time and also respiratory muscle performance during daytime (unassisted) breathing.

Nasal masks are preferred to full face masks because these are smaller and allow the patient to speak. Full face masks are used when patients breathe mainly through their mouths and when mouth leaks become significant.

Before the initiation of positive-pressure mask ventilation, the patient should be evaluated for cooperation and for the adequacy of cough and gag reflexes to prevent aspiration. This is most important when the full face mask is used, especially because vomiting into the mask may obstruct the airways and cause aspiration.

Complications and Limitations

Complications are minimal.[220,223] Intolerance of the nasal mask is an important cause for failure of positive-pressure mask ventilation, especially in infants and small children. Other causes of failure include confused and combative patients, failure to relieve hypoxemia (the disease is too severe), and the presence of excessive tracheobronchial secretions.

The most common side effect with mask ventilation is the development of pressure skin irritations from the mask, which may progress to pressure sores and excoriations. The mask size and application should therefore be carefully adjusted. This problem may be ameliorated by applying a patch of wound care dressing over the bridge of the nose before instituting the mask.[220,221]

High-Frequency Ventilation

HFV is a strategy of respiratory support in which rates greater than 4 times the normal respiratory rate (i.e., > 200 cycles/min) and a VT in the range of the anatomic dead space are used.[228] Two types of HFV can be distinguished, as follows:

1. Systems with active expiration, such as high frequency oscillation (HFO), in which air is sucked out of the lungs during expiration
2. Systems with passive expiration, such as high frequency jet ventilation (HFJV), in which expiration is due entirely to the elastic recoil of the lungs

In general, HFO performs at higher rates (10 to 15 Hz) than HFJV (3 to 7 Hz), and for this reason, the VT can be kept smaller during HFO, which may represent an advantage of this method (i.e., less volutrauma). In other words, a higher MAP can theoretically be achieved without excessive PIP and alveolar overdistention. Another advantage of HFO is that the same ETT can be used as during conventional mechanical ventilation. This is not the case with HFJV, in which specially manufactured tubes must be used with a channel for the injection of gas. Alternatively, injector cannulas might be used, which are introduced into the free lumen of the ETT. However, this cannula might lead to expiratory airway obstruction with the danger of severe pulmonary overinflation. Mechanisms of gas exchange during HFV include convection, Taylor dispersion, asymmetric velocity profiles, interregional (including cardiogenic) mixing, and molecular diffusion.[229] One of the major effects observed during HFV is the excellent washout of carbon dioxide, which is particularly welcome in infants with pulmonary hypertension, and often rapid and dramatic improvement in oxygenation.

With the introduction of HFV, new complications of respiratory therapy in the form of necrotizing tracheobronchitis have been observed.[230] However, necrotizing tracheobronchitis is probably due to poor humidification, the poor circulatory status of the infant or child, a high MAP, and a shearing injury to the jet. With the development of effective humidification systems, this complication has virtually disappeared. One major indication for HFV is failure to achieve adequate gas exchange with conventional mechanical ventilation at a "reasonable price" (i.e., barotrauma and volutrauma, cardiovascular compromise). This includes mainly newborns with severe MAS, HMD, and ARDS resulting from streptococcal group B septicemia with oxygenation indexes in the range of 40 and more.[231-234] These disease entities initially require a high MAP (generally in the range of 20 to 25 cm H_2O) to keep the lung open and minimize potential lung injury.[235] The second major indication, particularly for HFO, is pulmonary interstitial emphysema of premature infants on mechanical ventilation, a complication with a very high mortality rate.[236,237] In these cases a low MAP strategy is indicated. However, if this option is chosen, the infant should not receive neuromuscular blocking agents or heavy sedation, thus allowing spontaneous respiratory activity. Otherwise, the so-called choke point with inadequately low MAP may cause problems in oxygenation.[238]

Experience with HFO in children with ARDS is still limited but promising.[239,240] Conventional ventilation for severe ARDS in children has produced disappointing results, with mortality rates of 42% to 75% reported in various series. A combination of a ventilation index ($Pa{CO_2}$ × PIP × Frequency/1000) greater than 40 and an oxygenation index (MAP × $F{IO_2}$ × 100/$Pa{O_2}$) greater than 40 has been associated with a 77% chance of mortality in patients older than 1 month of age with severe ARDS.[241] In a controlled, prospective, randomized study, Arnold et al[239,240] showed that high-frequency oscillatory ventilation benefited children with severe ARDS, although the mortality rate was not altered. When the outcome was ranked as survival without severe chronic lung disease or survival with severe chronic lung disease, HFO patients had significantly better outcomes than patients on conventional ventilation. In addition, HFO was found to achieve improved oxygenation without hemodynamic compromise.

Permissive Hypercapnia and Other Ventilatory Strategies for Reducing Iatrogenic Lung Injury

Iatrogenic lung injury can be subdivided into barotrauma and volutrauma. Whereas barotrauma is manifested by extraalveolar air (e.g., pneumothorax, pulmonary interstitial emphysema), volutrauma is a form of injury resembling ARDS, with disruption of the alveolar-capillary membrane and hyaline membrane formation (permeability pulmonary edema). In experimental animals, ARDS can be produced by mechanical ventilation alone with large VT.[211] ARDS under these circumstances is thought to result from cyclic overstretching of lung structures. Another contributing factor to lung damage during PPV is the cyclic closing and reopening of alveoli with resultant shear injury, related to allowing areas of the lung to collapse at the end of exhalation. Another possibility would be an extremely high local pH (>7.8) leading to necrosis of bronchiolar and alveolar epithelium.[242] In addition to optimal humidification and tracheobronchial toileting, new strategies to prevent iatrogenic lung injury in already severely compromised lungs have been suggested. These new "protective strategies" assume that outcome might improve if lung injury secondary to overdistention at end inhalation and to shear forces at the beginning of inhalation is minimized and include the following:

1. Maintenance of open lung units throughout the respiratory cycle but particularly during expiration by adequate PEEP (i.e., PEEP level above the inflection point on the pressure-volume curve of the respiratory system) to reduce shearing forces during repeated opening of the small airways
2. Ventilation with a low VT in the range of 5 to 7.5 ml/kg (to prevent volutrauma)
3. Driving pressures of less than 20 cm of water above PEEP (to prevent barotrauma)

In sick lungs, FRC and VT have to be related to open and recruitable parts of the lung and not to the whole lung, like they are under normal conditions of health. Particularly with ARDS (but probably also with other pulmonary diseases) the lung has diseased areas that are always closed to either ventilation or perfusion and therefore are excluded from gas exchange.[243] A strategy to prevent overdistention of the lung is real-time monitoring of pressure-volume loops, which should not show any flattening (i.e., decreased compliance) at the end of inspiration.[244] However, preventing this means restricting VT and preventing intrinsic PEEP by too-rapid respiratory rates, which in turn reduces minute ventilation; eventually there is insufficient washout of carbon dioxide.

This has led to the concept of permissive hypercapnia, in which $Pa{CO_2}$ levels of 60 to 100 mm Hg and pH levels of 7.2 or greater are accepted.[164,245] In adults, this concept seems to have improved outcome from ARDS[148,246]; experience in children is still limited[247] but promising in that hypercarbia itself does not appear to be harmful.[248] However, it must be stressed that permissive hypercapnia can be used only in patients without acute intracranial or pulmonary hypertension because of the deleterious effects of acute respiratory acidosis in these conditions.

In a prospectively randomized study of 53 adults with ARDS the effect of such a "protective ventilation strategy" on mortality was compared to conventional mechanical ventilation.[400] The latter consisted of maintaining the lowest possible PEEP, V_T of 12 ml per kg and normalization of arterial CO_2 (35-38 mm Hg). The "productive strategy" was associated with improved survival at 28 days, a higher rate of weaning from mechanical ventilation and a lower rate of barotrauma. However, in another recent randomized study of 120 adults with ARDS, a protective strategy did not reduce mortality.[401] The morbidity was even increased implicating that such strategies are not warranted for routine use in patients who do not require significantly high inspiratory pressures.

ECMO and Carbon Dioxide Removal

ECMO is a technology for the management of life-threatening cardiopulmonary failure, supporting gas exchange by circulating blood through an externalized artificial lung. Although the technology borrows significantly from cardiopulmonary bypass, ECMO is only partial bypass; hence the efficiency of gas exchange is limited. Moreover, the procedure is expensive and labor intensive and is associated with life-threatening complications.

Use in Newborns

Most causes of severe reversible cardiorespiratory failure associated with a high predicted mortality rate (meconium aspiration/perinatal asphyxia, pneumonia, ARDS, pulmonary hypoplasia as seen in congenial diaphragmatic hernia, perioperative period of some types of congenial heart disease) are complicated by severe pulmonary hypertension of the newborn ("persistent fetal circulation"). A variety of innovative respiratory support techniques have recently emerged as useful therapies for many newborns in this situation. Nevertheless, a number of such conditions respond poorly to these therapies, so these infants remain at risk for high predicted mortality. Therefore the major indications for ECMO in newborns are as follows:

1. Severe reversible failure that is unresponsive or poorly responsive to HFO, inhaled nitric oxide, or both
2. Deterioration in circulatory function despite aggressive circulatory resuscitation with volume and inotropic agents

Selection criteria for ECMO are continually evolving, but a number of generally accepted exclusion criteria follow:

1. Birth weight below 2 kg
2. Gestational age below 33 weeks
3. More than 10 to 14 days of maximal ventilation
4. Intraventricular hemorrhage
5. Irreversible abnormality in any organ system

Systemic heparinization of the patient is required. Most patients managed with ECMO undergo the treatment via the venoarterial route (which provides both cardiac and pulmonary support), necessitating ligation of both the carotid artery and the internal jugular vein. Increasing experience with venovenous bypass through a double-lumen catheter has demonstrated the efficiency of this latter technique for pulmonary support alone. Although immediate changes in cerebral blood flow have been documented,[249] there is not yet any observed intermediate ill effect of ligation of one carotid artery.[250] More widespread use of venovenous bypass should significantly reduce the concern about potential for long-term vascular complications in surviving patients.

Most patients treated with ECMO are critically ill and often moribund, but their condition quickly stabilizes during ECMO treatment. Because ECMO treatment is seen as the only chance of survival, well-controlled clinical trials to confirm the use of this mode of treatment are limited.[251]

The performance of newborn ECMO requires a large commitment from the hospital and staff. Because of the cost of staff training and patient treatment, the complexity of the treatment, and the potential life-threatening hazards, centers performing neonatal ECMO are generally established on a regional basis to provide an adequate patient population for the center and to ensure the continued proficiency of the staff.

Pediatric and Adult Use

Indications are still unclear for ECMO or extracorporeal carbon dioxide removal in pediatric and adult patients with potentially reversible cardiopulmonary diagnoses. The problem is complicated by the heterogeneity of diseases in these older patients. There is a longer duration of ECMO for the pediatric patient vs. the newborn, which probably reflects this difference in disease pathophysiology.[252] The largest single diagnostic category has been reported as viral pneumonia,[253] but this was presumptive and not proved by culture. Morris et al[254] undertook a randomized study in adults with acute respiratory failure. $ECCO_2$ (a form of venovenous ECMO) was compared with a computer-driven, standard-therapy protocol for assisted ventilation. There was no difference in survival rates between the groups. At present, these techniques should be considered experimental in these age groups and should be used with clinical research projects to evaluate indications and outcomes.

Home Mechanical Ventilation

Children and infants who cannot be weaned from mechanical ventilation and who are otherwise stable are candidates for chronic ventilatory support at home. They can be divided into three dependency groups: (1) the least dependent—children with nocturnal hypoventilation who are ambulant and ventilator independent during the day, (2) intermediate—children with chronic lung disease who are completely ventilator dependent but less physically handicapped, and (3) the most dependent—children with high cervical cord disease or with neuromuscular diseases.

Exact numbers of the incidence of home ventilation are not available, although it seems that the rate is rapidly increasing. As many as 395 ventilator-dependent children from Pennsylvania and Illinois were reported in 1983.[255] The rate depends on the environment and availability of supportive services. In the United Kingdom, the incidence of chronic ventilator-dependent children (either at home or at institutions) was found to be surprisingly low—a total of 35 cases from 1983 to 1987.[256] However, this report was based on voluntary reporting and is likely to be an underestimate. Advances in technology, medical knowledge, and the development of medical equipment specifically designed for home care needs, as well as psychologic and cost considerations, are responsible for the growing preference for this therapy. As much as $80,000 per child per year may be saved by home ventilation compared with chronic treatment in acute care hospitals.[257] Chronic home ventilation differs from intensive care unit ventilation, both in the basic needs of the patient and in the lack of caregivers with the necessary skills to provide the frequent attention to the details of home mechanical ventilation.

When considering home ventilation for a child, the clinician should evaluate the patient's stability, parental cooperation, and the availability of medical care. The underlying disease and its course are important when a ventilator-dependent child has the potential for weaning at home. The basic principles, the organization of home therapy, and family education and training are discussed in Chapter 24.

In 1991 the American Thoracic Society listed the criteria that must be fulfilled by children who are candidates for home ventilation[258] (Box 21-7). The etiologies of chronic respiratory failure in pediatric patients who are treated at home are mainly those that are secondary to bronchopulmonary dysplasia, congenital anomalies, and tracheobronchomalacia for infants, whereas in children older than 1 year of age, the main groups are chronic congenital and acquired neuromuscular diseases followed by spinal cord injuries and airway and pulmonary diseases[259] (Box 21-8).

In home settings, assisted ventilation is generally provided to patients with stable cardiopulmonary systems. The decision as to which ventilator and mode of ventilation to provide depends on the underlying disease and on available patient care resources. The mode of ventilation is usually IMV, which allows the patient to breathe spontaneously between the ventilator-mandatory breaths. Another option is the ACV volume mode,[260] which is more suitable to patients who can initiate a breath but cannot create the critical negative pressure required to inhale an acceptable VT. NPV may be suitable for children who do not require 24-hour assisted ventilation and who do not need tracheostomies. However, careful selection should be exercised because this mode may induce upper airway obstruction and recurrent aspiration. Pressure-cycled pneumatic ventilators have also been used. They are more easily portable and are not subject to electric power failure. However, they are less reliable over the long term and are not widely used. Volume-cycled ventilators are preferred; their advantages are that they require no compressor and oxygen can be easily added. They are also easier to adjust, but they are subject to power failure.[261] A self-inflating resuscitation bag should always be available in case of power failure or another emergency. During home ventilation, PEEP and high FIO_2 are usually not used. Most home-ventilated infants and children do not require supplemental oxygen. Nevertheless, the home ventilator should have the capability of adding oxygen in a controlled and reasonably precise manner. Many ventilator-dependent children need supplemental oxygen during exacerbations of pulmonary status, which are usually caused by respiratory infections.

Home ventilation does have risks. Although the home-ventilated child is less susceptible for nosocomial respiratory infections than the ventilator-dependent child in the hospital, infection is still a major problem because of the chronic nature of the disease and the presence of a tracheostomy tube. There is greater risk of accidental death because there are fewer people to act as observers and electronic surveillance is minimal. The main causes for death in home-ventilated infants and children are ventilator disconnection, accidental decannulation, obstructed tracheostomy cannula, hemorrhage caused by erosion of the cannula into a blood vessel, bouts of pulmonary hypertension, sepsis, and pneumonia.[256] Other causes are associated with progression of the primary disease. In one series of 54 home-ventilated children (33 PPV and 21 NPV),[262] there were 17 deaths over a 20-year period, including 3 from ventilator disconnection.

BOX 21-7
Criteria for Consideration of Home Mechanical Ventilation in Children

Cardiopulmonary stability
Positive trend in weight gain and growth curve
Stamina periods of play while lungs are ventilated
Freedom from frequent respiratory infections

Modified from American Thoracic Society statement: Home mechanical ventilation of pediatric patients, *ARRD* 141:258-259, 1991.

BOX 21-8
Most Common Etiologies of Chronic Respiratory Failure in Home-Ventilated Infants and Children

Neurologic disorders (peripheral)
- Neuromuscular genetic: myopathies, muscular dystrophies, anterior horn cell disease
- Neuromuscular acquired: Guillain-Barré syndrome, infant botulism
- Traumatic cord injuries
- Myelomeningocele
- Diaphragmatic (phrenic nerve) paralysis: congenital, postoperative

Neurologic disorders (central): central hypoventilation syndrome, encephalopathies
Respiratory disorders: bronchopulmonary dysplasia, laryngomalacia, tracheobronchomalacia, restrictive lung disease
Congenital anomalies

The death rate for home ventilation can be decreased by providing electronic monitoring at home. It is recommended that infants and small children who cannot breathe effectively for at least 4 to 6 hours independent of mechanical ventilation be monitored by apnea/bradycardia home monitors during sleep.[259]

NONCONVENTIONAL AND EXPERIMENTAL MODES

Synchronized Independent Lung Ventilation

Synchronized independent lung ventilation (SILV) should be considered in patients with severe single lung disease or even with bilateral disease when one lung is significantly more affected than the other.

In these circumstances, conventional PPV can be much less effective and even hazardous because the gas is preferentially directed toward the less-affected lung, thereby overexpanding it and providing little benefit to gas exchange in the affected lung. An increase of VT in one lung may cause greater $\dot{V}/\dot{Q}$ mismatching and further lead to barotrauma in the less-affected lung.[263]

The development of double-lumen ETTs suitable for pediatric patients has permitted the application of independent lung ventilation in infants and children.[260,264] SILV requires two ventilators that can be used together in an electronic "master-slave" connection and synchronized for each breath. The synchronization is important for preventing ventilation disorders, lung herniation to the contralateral side, and mediastinal shift that can compromise venous return to the right atrium.[260,265]

SILV allows the physician to selectively provide appropriate pressures, PEEP, volume, and flow to each lung. It also allows easy isolation of infected secretions from the affected lung without the need to perform selective intubations or bronchoscopy.

In a large series of 55 patients, including 18 newborns and 23 infants,[260] the clinical criteria for starting SILV were unilateral lung disease, severe hypoxemia requiring an FIO_2 greater than 0.8, and a PEEP greater than 10 cm H_2O to obtain a PaO_2 of 50 to 80 mm Hg. Application of SILV resulted in rapid improvement in PaO_2 (Fig. 21-17). When the effect of PEEP was studied in 8 newborns, further improvement was noted when PEEP was independently set to each lung. No changes in the vocal cords, larynx, trachea, or bronchi were noted in up to 120 hours of SILV with double-lumen tubes. Nevertheless, the most critical aspect of this technique is the availability of appropriate-sized double-lumen ETTs with an outer diameter appropriate for age but with an inner diameter that neither promotes mucous impaction nor significantly increases resistance to gas flow.

Negative-Pressure Ventilation

NPV is the type of ventilation in which the surface of the thorax is exposed to subatmospheric pressure during inspiration.[266] This subatmospheric pressure expands the ribcage, thereby creating a pressure gradient for gas to move from the mouth and nose to the alveoli.

NPV originated more than a century ago. Woillez in 1876 developed a manually driven negative-pressure respirator.[264] This was later replaced by the "iron lung," which was the mainstay of pediatric mechanical ventilation during the epidemics of poliomyelitis of the 1930s and 1940s.[267,268] During the 1960s and the early 1970s, NPV was adapted for newborns with idiopathic respiratory distress syndrome of the newborn (HMD); an Isolette respirator, in which the infant's body was enclosed in an air-tight, negative-pressure chamber while the head was enclosed in a separate chamber to which humidified gas was added at atmospheric pressure, was used.[269,270]

Negative-pressure respirators have two basic components: (1) a chamber in which the subatmospheric pressure is generated during inspiration and (2) the pump that generates this pressure. Some chambers cover only a part of the thorax and abdomen, whereas others cover the entire body with the exception of the head. Three modes of ventilation can be used, as follows:

1. Cyclic negative pressure. A set negative pressure is generated to assist inspiration, but expiration is totally passive. During exhalation, the chamber pressure is converted back to atmospheric. This is the most commonly used mode.
2. Negative/positive pressure. This mode is same as cyclic NPV with the addition of a positive chamber pressure during exhalation.
3. Continuous negative pressure. Subatmospheric chamber pressure is applied during both inspiration and expiration. The magnitude (amplitude) of the negative pressure varies during the breathing phases so that a negative (subatmospheric) end-expiratory pressure is maintained. The negative end-expiratory pressure thus increases the expiratory lung volume like PEEP does.

NPV has some physiologic effects that differ from PPV. There is much discrepancy in reports regarding the effects of NPV on cardiac output. Theoretically, NPV increases both venous return to the heart and left ventricular afterload, thereby having combined effects on cardiac output. Nevertheless, compared with PPV, NPV has only minor effects on the cardiovascular system.[264] In an animal model of acute lung injury, when PPV and NPV achieved the same therapeutic results, NPV was associated with smaller drops in cardiac output.[271] It may be that the high-frequency, negative-pressure ventilator (i.e., Hayek Oscillator) has even less effect on the cardiovas-

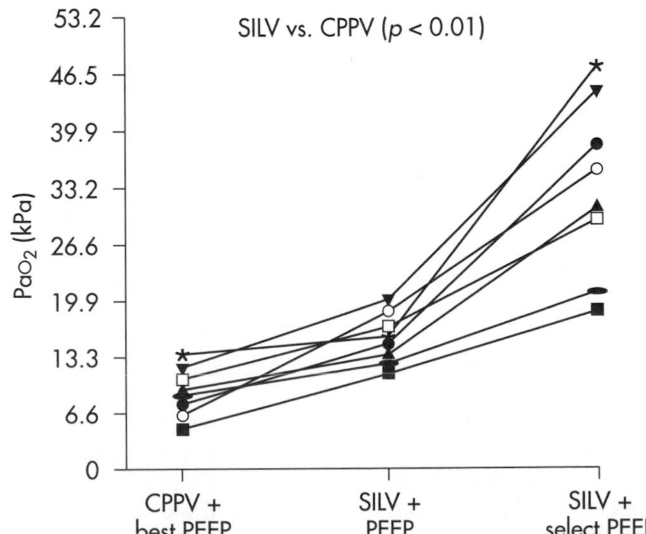

Fig. 21-17. Improvement in PaO_2 in eight newborns and preterm infants using SILV. PaO_2 was further improved when PEEP was selectively applied to each lung. *CPPV,* Continuous positive-pressure ventilation. (Modified from Marraro G: *Crit Care Clin* 8:131-145, 1992.)

cular system and could be a good mode of ventilation after Fontan's procedure, for example.

Whereas PPV bypasses the upper airways, NPV tends to adduct the vocal cords and narrow the laryngeal airway.[272] When the patient assists inspiration even slightly, the latter upper airway obstruction is usually abolished, probably because of activation of the upper airway muscles. Thus NPV may require patient cooperation or bypassing of the upper airways. The latter significantly limits the use of this technique because once the patient needs an ETT or a tracheostomy, it is easier to use PPV rather than NPV.

Although NPV was reported to be useful in neonates with respiratory distress syndrome, at present the ventilatory treatment of choice in both neonates and older children is PPV. It remains to be shown in prospectively designed studies that NPV can substitute for conventional PPV in newborns and children with acute respiratory failure. Guidelines for the institution of NPV and the limitations of the technique need to be clearly defined. Barotrauma still occurs with NPV: 10% in one neonatal series.[267] The technique also requires a proper seal around the infant's neck, which may result in decubitus wounds. A major disadvantage of NPV is that it impedes easy access to the patient and thus appropriate therapies for the respiratory and other systems.

Extrapolation from adult studies and some experience from the pediatric age group suggests that NPV may be considered for infants and children who need chronic ventilatory assistance for neuromuscular and chest wall diseases.[264] This may also apply to children whose lungs are chronically ventilated at home especially when the need is for intermittent support (e.g., central hypoventilation). The common denominator for success in these situations is that the chronic respiratory failure is secondary to "pump failure" (peripheral or central) and does not result from intrinsic lung or airway disease.

Liquid Ventilation

The use of liquid instead of gas to carry oxygen to the lungs for gas exchange has been under laboratory investigation in animal models for almost 3 decades. The first trials used oxygenated silicone oil[273] and hyperbarically oxygenated saline[274] as media. In the early 1970s, Shaffer and Moskowitz[275] developed techniques to use normobaric perfluorocarbon for LV and normal gas exchange. Researchers from that laboratory later reported that LV was effective in preterm and newborn animals.[276-278] The first human trial of perfluorocarbon LV was reported from the same laboratory by Greenspan et al[279] in 1990. They were able to use the technique to ventilate the lungs of three preterm infants for short periods, showing some improvement in pulmonary function and gas exchange.

Theory

After equilibration to 1 atm with pure oxygen, perfluorocarbon can carry 45 to 55 ml of oxygen per 100 ml of solvent, which is equivalent to an FIO_2 of 0.45 to 0.55. The oxygen-enriched perfluorocarbon is inhaled and exhaled in tidal fashion and makes direct contact with the alveolar surface. Perfluorocarbon has a low surface tension,[280] and because of the air-fluid interface, surface tension is eliminated, with a resultant increase in lung compliance. Hence LV may be a promising technique for lung diseases in which the main pathologic condition results from lack of or abnormal levels of surfactant (e.g., respiratory distress syndrome of the neonate and ARDS, respectively).

The liquid is minimally absorbed by the pulmonary capillaries and is excreted by the lungs. Studies in animals have shown that perfluorocarbon does not induce adverse effects on the lung parenchyma despite prolonged retention of this material in the tissues.[281-283] Furthermore, intravenous administration of perfluorochemicals (for blood substitution) has caused few adverse sequelae in humans.[284,285] Adverse effects on cardiac output during LV are similar to those that occur with conventional gas ventilation[286,287] and also respond to vascular volume expansion.[288]

Technique

The technique is simple and constitutes pouring of oxygenated perfluorocarbon into the trachea and then draining it. In their first human trial of three newborn infants, Greenspan et al[279] placed the oxygenated perfluorocarbon in an inspiratory reservoir that was suspended 20 to 40 cm above the infant (Fig. 21-18). The system was attached to the ETT via a Y-piece that was also connected to a calibrated expiratory reservoir suspended 20 cm below the infant. A total of 15 ml/kg of perfluorocarbon was delivered to the lungs and removed by gravity with each breath at a frequency of 3 to 5 breaths/min. The height of the inspiratory reservoir was altered to maintain a filling time of 5 seconds, and each V_T was held within the lungs for approximately 10 seconds. Using short periods of LV, arterial blood gas analysis showed improvement in two of three infants and deterioration in one (Fig. 21-19). Respiratory system compliance measured from pressure-volume loops improved in all three infants, whereas resistance improved in two of the three and deteriorated in one. In a recent study,[289] the lungs of six rabbits with acute respiratory failure induced by saline lavage were ventilated with perfluorocarbon and were compared with the lungs of rabbits with the same pathologic

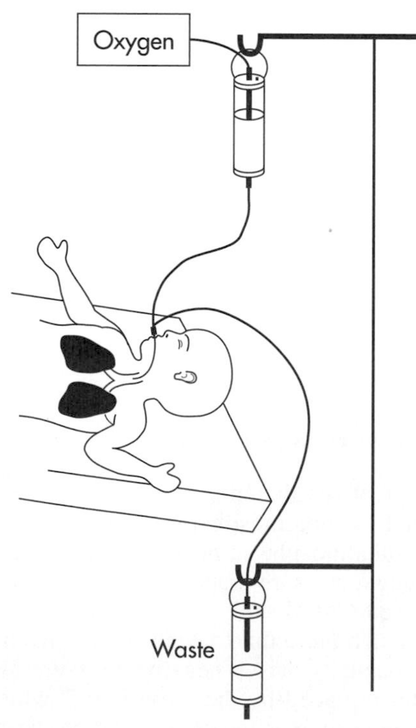

Fig. 21-18. LV system. (Modified from Greenspan JS et al: *J Pediatr* 117:106-111, 1990.)

condition whose lungs were ventilated with either saline or conventional PPV with the same VT rate and PEEP levels. After 3 hours of ventilation with 100% oxygen, the $Pa{O_2}$ was significantly higher in the perfluorocarbon group.

A simpler and more appealing approach is that of partial LV or perfluorocarbon-assisted gas exchange. The lungs are inflated with 30 ml/kg of perfluorocarbon, and at the end of exhalation, conventional mechanical ventilation is resumed. Hirschl et al[290] have reported on their preliminary experience using partial LV in 19 adults, children, and newborns with severe respiratory failure on extracorporeal life support. These treatments were associated with a decrease in the alveolar-arterial oxygen gradient and an increase in statistic lung compliance, with 11 (58%) survivors. Other studies have recently confirmed this observation in newborns[291] and children with acute respiratory failure,[292,293] showing improved values even when pediatric patients on ECMO were included. New controlled, multicenter clinical trials are currently under progress. In spite of these encouraging preliminary results, LV is not yet a clinical tool, and more clinical trials are awaited to see whether this new technique can find its niche among other new modes of ventilatory support.

Intratracheal Pulmonary Ventilation

Intratracheal pulmonary ventilation (ITPV) is a technique for respiratory support described by Muller et al[294] and Kolobow et al.[295] The technique is still in development,[296,297] but its advantages are that it allows a great reduction of dead space ventilation and that the physician can also use higher respiratory rates, thereby achieving good oxygenation and carbon dioxide washout without exposing the lungs to the damage of high PPV. No ventilators on the market are specifically designed for ITPV, although the technique can be used with some existing ventilators. A thorough discussion of this experimental technique is beyond the scope of this chapter.

In the simplest form of ITV, a small catheter is introduced through the ETT so that the tip rests at or near the carina. ITV can be used with CPAP or IMV. In ITPV, all fresh gas is continuously introduced at the level of the carina through the intratracheal catheter, and dead space is thus reduced. The ETT is for exhalation only, and this is controlled by a valve. The valve sets the frequency and the I:E ratio. When the expiration valve is closed, all the gas enters the lungs; when it is open, the gas from the lung plus the continuous flow from the IPTV catheter are exhaled through the ETT. A high gas flow increases the intratracheal pressure. Therefore tracheal pressure should be monitored, and ventilator pressures should be reduced accordingly. For continuous monitoring of the pressure at the carina, a double-lumen ETT or a second catheter needs to be inserted. This is the biggest limitation of the technique. Continuous monitoring of exhaled carbon dioxide allows calculation of the carbon dioxide washout through the following equation:

$$\dot{V}CO_2 = \dot{V}E \times FECO_2$$
$$\dot{V}CO_2 = \text{Carbon dioxide production}$$

where $\dot{V}E$ is the minute volume of ventilation and $FECO_2$ is the exhaled carbon dioxide concentration. This further allows for the calculation of the dead space ($\dot{V}DS$), as follows:

$$\dot{V}DS = VT - \left(\frac{\dot{V}CO_2 \times 760}{PaCO_2 \times f}\right)$$

where f is the respiratory frequency. From this equation the gas flow required in the intratracheal catheter can be estimated: At an I:E ratio of 1:1, half of the catheter-introduced gas flows during inspiration, and half flows during expiration. The gas flow should be set at the following: $4 \times \dot{V}DS \times$ Frequency. When the I:E ratio equals 1:2, the flow rate is set at the following: $6 \times \dot{V}DS \times$ Frequency.

The apparatus is combined with a positive-pressure ventilator, which is used for ventilation monitoring and not for assisted respiration. The minute volume of ventilation is read from the ventilator, but because the readout includes total gas flow (inspiratory and expiratory), true pulmonary ventilation is dependent on I:E ratio and can be calculated by the following equation:

$$\dot{V}E_{pulm} = \dot{V}E_{pulm} + \dot{V}E_{bias} \times \frac{I}{(I+E)}$$

where $\dot{V}E_{pulm}$ is the minute volume of pulmonary ventilation, $\dot{V}E_{bias}$ is the minute volume of bias flow ventilation, I is inspiration, and E is expiration. All pressures, including PIP, MAP, and PEEP, are read directly. The last is adjusted by gas flow.

The initiation of ITPV starts with IMV, then the catheter flow rate is increased gradually while the ventilator contribution is decreased until all gas flow originates in the intratracheal catheter. Switching back from ITPV to IMV is done in a similar manner. The periods in which both IMV and ITPV operate together are termed *hybrid ventilation.* Because it is difficult to estimate the pulmonary volume of ventilation with ITPV, continuous monitoring of transcutaneous or end-tidal carbon dioxide is mandatory.

ITPV is useful in an animal model of low lung volume similar to pulmonary hypoplasia and in an animal model of diffuse lung injury. Kolobow et al[295] were able to reduce the VT in normal sheep up to 1 ml/kg of body weight with a PIP of only 2 to 3 cm H_2O above the PEEP. The frequency was at least 120 breaths/min. In sheep that underwent resection of lung lobes with reduction of the lung volume to as low as 12%, ITPV was successful with low FIO_2 and PIP levels. When the animals' lungs were ventilated by the conventional modes, they did not survive.[289] Ravenscraft et al[298] have had some success using tracheal gas insufflation as a supplement to volume-limited ventilation in critically ill patients. The technique of ITPV is still in the experimental stage, and its applicability in various diseases states has yet to be demonstrated.

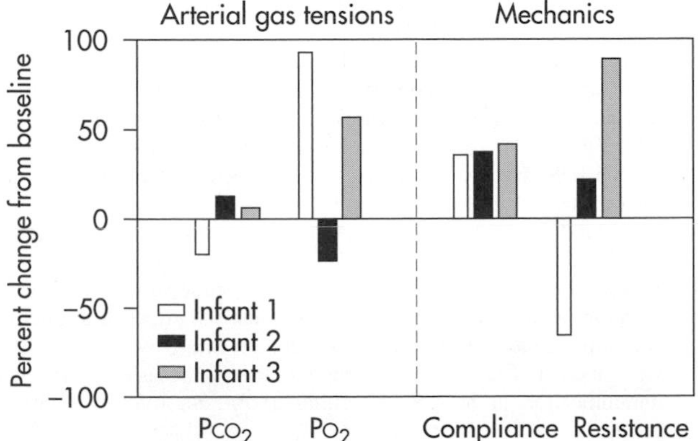

Fig. 21-19. Percent change from baseline in arterial PO_2, PCO_2, and respiratory compliance and resistance in three infants during LV. (Modified from Greenspan JS et al: *J Pediatr* 117:106-111, 1990.)

REFERENCES

1. Powers SR, Manual R, Neclerio M, English M, Marr C, Leather R, Ueda H, Williams G, Custead W, Dutton R: Physiological consequences of positive end-expiratory pressure (PEEP) ventilation, *Ann Surg* 178:265-272, 1973.
2. Danek SJ, Lynch JP, Weg JG, Dantzker DR: The dependence of uptake on oxygen delivery in the adult respiratory distress syndrome, *Am Rev Respir Dis* 122:387-395, 1980.
3. Dantzker DR, Foresman B, Gutierrez G: Oxygen supply and utilization relationships: a reevaluation, *Am Rev Respir Dis* 143:675-679, 1991.

Oxygen Administration and Therapy

4. Tobin MJ: Respiratory monitoring in the intensive care unit, *Am Rev Respir Dis* 138:1625-1642, 1988.
5. Hess D, Maxwell G: Which is the best index of oxygenation: $P(A - a)O_2$, PaO_2/PAO_2, or PaO_2/FIO_2? *Respir Care* 30:961-964, 1985.

Hyperbaric Oxygen Therapy

6. Weaver LK: Hyperbaric treatment of respiratory emergencies, *Respir Care* 37:720-738, 1992.
7. Tibbles PM, Edelsberg JS: Hyperbaric-oxygen therapy, *N Engl J Med* 334:1642-1648, 1996.
8. Bird AD, Telfer ABM: Effect of hyperbaric oxygen on limb circulation, *Lancet* 1:355-356, 1965.
9. Nylander G, Nordstrom H, Eriksson E: Effects of hyperbaric oxygen on edema formation after a scald burn, *Burns* 10:193-196, 1984.
10. Nylander G, Lewis D, Nordstrom H, Larsson J: Reduction of postischemic edema with hyperbaric oxygen, *Plast Reconstr Surg* 76:596-603, 1985.
11. Strauss MB, Hargens AR, Gershuni DH, Greenberg DA, Crenshaw AG, Hart GB, Akeson WH: Reduction of skeletal muscle necrosis using intermittent hyperbaric oxygen in a model compartment syndrome, *J Bone Joint Surg* 65:656-662, 1983.
12. Hill GB, Osterhout S: Experimental effects of hyperbaric oxygen on selected clostridial species. I. In vitro studies, *J Infect Dis* 125:17-25, 1972.
13. Hunt TK, Pai MP: The effect of varying ambient tensions on wound metabolism and collagen synthesis, *Surg Gynecol Obstet* 135:561-567, 1972.
14. Blanch PB, Desautels DA, Gallagher TJ: Deviations in function of mechanical ventilators during hyperbaric compression, *Respir Care* 36:803-814, 1991.
15. Marini JJ, Culver BH: Systemic gas embolism complicating mechanical ventilation in the adult respiratory distress syndrome, *Ann Intern Med* 110:699-703, 1990.
16. Murphy BP, Harfold FJ, Cramer FS: Cerebral air embolism resulting from invasive medical procedures: treatment with hyperbaric oxygen, *Ann Surg* 201:242-245, 1985.
17. Kindwall EP: Massive surgical embolism treated with brief recompression to six atmospheres followed by hyperbaric oxygen, *Aerospace Med* 44:663-666, 1973.
18. Bond GF: Arterial gas embolism. In Avis JC, Hunt TK, eds: *Hyperbaric therapy,* Bethesda, Md, 1977, Underseas Medical Society, pp 141-152.
19. Armon C, Deschamps C, Adkinson C, Fealey RD, Orszulak TA: Hyperbaric treatment of cerebral air embolism sustained during an open-heart surgical procedure, *Mayo Clin Proc* 66:565-571, 1991.
20. Davis C, Elliott DH: Treatment of decompression disorders. In Bennet PB, Elliott DH, eds: *The physiology and medicine of diving,* ed 3, London, 1982, Bailliere, Tindall & Cox, pp 473-487.
21. Myers RA, Schnitzer BM: Hyperbaric use: update 1984, *Postgrad Med* 76:83-86, 1984.

Manual Ventilation

22. Finer NN, Barrington KJ, Al-Fadley F, Peters KL: Limitations of self-inflating resuscitators, *Pediatrics* 77:417-420, 1986.
23. Kanter RK: Evaluation of mask-ventilation in resuscitation of infants, *Am J Dis Child* 141:761-763, 1987.
24. Emergency Cardiac Care Committee and Subcommittees, American Heart Association: Guidelines for cardiopulmonary resuscitation and emergency cardiac care. VI. Pediatric advanced life support, *JAMA* 268:2262-2275, 1992.
25. Hirschman AM, Kravath RE: Venting vs. ventilating: a danger of manual resuscitation bags, *Chest* 82:369-370, 1982.
26. Standards and guidelines for cardiopulmonary resuscitation (CPR) and emergency cardiac care (ECC), *JAMA* 255:2841-2973, 1986.
27. Kissoon N, Frewen T, Tiffin N: Prototype volume-controlled resuscitator for neonates and infants, *Crit Care Med* 18:1430-1434, 1990.
28. Ravalia A, Goddard JM: The laryngeal mask and difficult tracheal intubation, *Anaesthesia* 45:168, 1990.
29. Ebata T, Nishiki S, Masuda A, Amaha K: Anaesthesia for Treacher Collins syndrome using a laryngeal mask airway, *Can J Anaesth* 38:1043-1045, 1991.

Artificial Airway

30. Klein M, Reynolds LG: Relief of sleep-related oropharyngeal airway obstruction by continuous insufflation of the pharynx, *Lancet* 1:935-939, 1986.
31. Luten RC, Wears RL, Broselow J, Zaritsky A, Barnett TM, Lee T, Bailey A, Vally R, Brown R, Rosenthal B: Length-based endotracheal tube and emergency equipment selection in pediatrics, *Ann Emerg Med* 21:900-904, 1992.
32. Lubitz DS, Seidel JS, Chameides L, Luten RG, Zaritsky AL, Campbell FW: A rapid method for estimating weight and resuscitation drug dosages from length in the pediatric age group, *Ann Emerg Med* 17:576-581, 1988.
33. Hall JB, White SR, Karrison T: Efficacy of daily routine chest radiographs in intubated, mechanically ventilated patients, *Crit Care Med* 19:689-693, 1991.
34. Brunel SW, Coleman DL, Schwartz DE, Peper E, Cohen NH: Assessment of routine chest roentgenogram and the physical examination to confirm endotracheal tube position, *Chest* 96:1043-1045, 1989.
35. Costello S, Lui K, Perelman M, Frank J: Non-invasive determination of endotracheal tube position in neonates, *Pediatr Res* 23(suppl):230A, 1988.
36. Crone RK, Anday EK, Bohn DJ, Epstein MF, Fletcher AB, Fox WW, Frantz ID, Raphaely RC, Thompson AE, McCormic W: Nonradiographic, transcutaneous determination of tracheal tube position: results of multicenter preclinical evaluation, *Pediatr Res* 21:199A, 1987.
37. Enler AJ: Verifying endotracheal tube placement with the Trachmate intubation system, *Pediatr Nurs* 15:390-392, 1988.
38. Whited RE: A prospective study of laryngotracheal sequelae in long term intubation, *Laryngoscope* 94:367-377, 1984.
39. Joh S, Matsuura H, Kotani Y, Sugiyama K, Hirota Y, Kiyomitsu Y, Kubota Y: Changes in tracheal blood flow during endotracheal intubation, *Acta Anaesthesiol Scand* 31:300-304, 1987.
40. Fernandez R, Blanch L, Mancebo J, Bonsoms N, Artigas A: Endotracheal tube cuff pressure assessment: pitfalls of finger estimation and need for objective measurement, *Crit Care Med* 18:1423-1426, 1990.
41. Badenhorst C: Changes in tracheal cuff pressure during respiratory support, *Crit Care Med* 15:300-302, 1987.
42. Deakers TW, Reynolds G, Stretton M, Newth CJL: Cuffed endotracheal tubes in pediatric intensive care, *J Pediatr* 125:57-62, 1994.

Humidification

43. Chatburn RL, Primiano FP Jr: A rational basis for humidity therapy, *Respir Care* 32:249-253, 1987.
44. Fonkalsrud EW, Calmes S, Barcliff LT, Barrett CT: Reduction of operative heat loss and pulmonary secretions in neonates by use of heated and humidified anaesthetic gases, *J Thorac Cardiovasc Surg* 80:718-723, 1980.
45. Burton JDK: Effects of dry anaesthetic gases on the respiratory mucus membrane, *Lancet* 1:235-238, 1962.
46. Forbes AR: Temperature, humidity and mucus flow in the intubated trachea, *Br J Anaesth* 46:29-34, 1974.
47. Bissonnette B, Sessler DI, LaFlamme P: Intraoperative temperature monitoring sites in infants and children and the effect of inspired gas warming on esophageal temperature, *Anesth Analg* 69:192-196, 1989.
48. Bissonnette B, Sessler DI, LaFlamme P: Passive and active inspired gas humidification in infants and children, *Anesthesiology* 71:350-354, 1989.
49. Shelly MP: Inspired gas conditioning, *Respir Care* 37:1070-1080, 1992.
50. American National Standards Institute: *Specifications for humidifiers and nebulizers for medical use,* Publ No ANSI Z79:9, New York, 1979, The Institute.

51. British Standards Institution: *Specifications for humidifiers for use with breathing machines,* BS 4494, London, 1970, The Institution.
52. Chatburn RL: Physiologic and methodological issues regarding humidity therapy, *J Pediatr* 114:416-420, 1989.
53. Berry FA Jr, Hughes-Davies DI, DiFazio CA: A system for minimizing respiratory heat loss in infants during operation, *Anesth Analg* 52:170-175, 1973.
54. Klein EF Jr, Graces SA: "Hot pot" tracheitis, *Chest* 65:225-226, 1974.
55. Branson RD, Campbell RS, Chatburn RL, Covington J: AARC clinical practice guideline: humidification during mechanical ventilation, *Respir Care* 37:887-890, 1992.
56. Miyao H, Hirokawa T, Miyasaka K, Kawazoe T: Relative humidity, not absolute humidity, is of great importance when using a humidifier with a heating wire, *Crit Care Med* 20:674-679, 1992.
57. Carlon GC, Barker RL, Benua RS: Airway humidification with high-frequency jet ventilation, *Crit Care Med* 13:114-117, 1985.
58. Shelly M, Bethune W, Latimer RD: A comparison of five heat and moisture exchangers, *Anaesthesia* 41:527-532, 1986.
59. Weeks DB, Ramsey FM: Laboratory investigation of six artificial noses for use during endotracheal anesthesia, *Anesth Analg* 62:758-763, 1983.
60. Ogino M, Kopotic R, Mannino FL: Moisture-conserving efficacy of condenser humidifiers, *Anaesthesia* 40:990-995, 1985.
61. Misset B, Escudier B, Rivara D, Leclercq B, Nitenberg G: Heat and moisture exchanger vs. heated humidifier during long-term mechanical ventilation: a prospective randomized study, *Chest* 100:160-163, 1991.
62. Mebius C: Heat and moisture exchangers with bacterial filters: a laboratory evaluation, *Acta Anaesthesiol Scand* 36:572-576, 1992.
63. Bissonnette B, Sessler DI: Passive inspired gas humidification increases thermal steady-state temperatures in anesthetized infants, *Anesth Analg* 69:783-787, 1989.
64. Martin C, Perrin G, Gevaudan MJ, Saux P, Gouin F: Heat and moisture exchangers and vaporizing humidifiers in the intensive care unit, *Chest* 97:144-149, 1990.
65. Shelly MP, Lloyd GM, Park GR: A review of the mechanisms and methods of humidification of inspired gas, *Intensive Care Med* 14:1-9, 1988.

Mechanical Ventilation

66. Chatburn RL: Classification of mechanical ventilators, *Respir Care* 37:1009-1025, 1992.
67. Engstrom CG: The clinical application of prolonged controlled ventilation, *Acta Anaesthesiol Scand Suppl* 13:1-52, 1963.
68. Sassoon CSH: Positive pressure ventilation: alternate modes, *Chest* 100:1421-1429, 1991.
69. Sassoon CSH, Mahuette CK, Light RW: Ventilator modes old and new, *Crit Care Clin* 6:605-634, 1990.
70. Hotchkiss RS, Wilson RS: Mechanical ventilatory support, *Surg Clin North Am* 63:417-438, 1983.
71. Marini JJ, Rodriguez RM, Lamb V: The inspiratory work-load of patient-initiated mechanical ventilation, *Am Rev Respir Dis* 134:902-909, 1986.
72. Weisman IM, Rinaldo JE, Rogers RM, Sanders MH: Intermittent mandatory ventilation, *Am Rev Respir Dis* 127:641-647, 1983.
73. Branson RD, Chatburn RL: Technical description and classification of modes of ventilator operation, *Respir Care* 37:1026-1044, 1992.
74. Heenan TJ, Downs JB, Douglas ME, Ruiz BC, Jumper L: Intermittent mandatory ventilation: is synchronization important? *Chest* 77:598-602, 1980.
75. Lain DC, DiBenedetto, Morris SL, Van Nguyen A, Saulters R, Causey D: Pressure control inverse ratio ventilation as a method to reduce peak inspiratory pressure and provide adequate ventilation and oxygenation, *Chest* 95:1081-1088, 1989.
76. Reynolds EO: Effect of alteration in mechanical ventilation settings on pulmonary gas exchange in hyaline membrane disease, *Arch Dis Child* 46:152-159, 1971.
77. Boros SJ: Variations in inspiratory:expiratory ratio and airway pressure wave form during mechanical ventilation: the significance of mean airway pressure, *J Pediatr* 94:114-117, 1979.
78. Spahr RC, Klein AM, Brown DR, MacDonald HM, Holzman IR: Hyaline membrane disease: a controlled study of inspiratory to expiratory ratio in its management by ventilator, *Am J Dis Child* 134:373-376, 1980.
79. Gurevitch MJ, Van Dyke J, Young ES, Jackson K: Improved oxygenation and lower peak airway pressure in severe adult respiratory distress syndrome: treatment with inverse ratio of ventilation, *Chest* 89:211-213, 1986.
80. Manginello F, Grassi A, Schechner S, Krauss A, Auld P: Evaluation of methods of assisted ventilation in hyaline membrane disease, *Arch Dis Child* 53:878-881, 1978.
81. Tharratt RS, Allen RP, Albertson TE: Pressure controlled inverse ratio ventilation in severe adult respiratory failure, *Chest* 94:755-762, 1988.
82. Greaves TH, Cramolini GM, Walker DH, Airola VM II, Parks S, Hodge D, Birek A: Inverse ratio ventilation in a 6-year-old with severe post-traumatic adult respiratory distress syndrome, *Crit Care Med* 17:588-589, 1989.
83. Boysen PG, McGough E: Pressure-controlled and pressure support ventilation: flow patterns, inspiratory time, and gas distribution, *Respir Care* 33:126-143, 1988.
84. *Servo Ventilator 900 C operating manual,* ed 4 (English edition), Solna, Sweden, 1985, Siemens-Elena AB Ventilator Division S-171.
85. Modell HI, Cheney FW: Effects of inspiratory flow pattern on gas exchange in normal and abnormal lungs, *J Appl Physiol* 42:1103-1107, 1979.
86. Duncan SR, Rizk NW, Raffin TA: Inverse ratio ventilation: PEEP in disguise? *Chest* 92:390-392, 1987.
87. Pepe PE, Marini JJ: Occult positive end-expiratory pressure in mechanically ventilated patients with airflow obstruction, *Am Rev Respir Dis* 126:166-170, 1982.
88. Chan K, Abraham E: Effects of inverse ratio ventilation on cardiorespiratory parameters in severe respiratory failure, *Chest* 102:1556-1561, 1992.
89. Brown DG, Pierson DJ: Auto-PEEP is common in mechanically ventilated patients: a study of incidence, severity, and detection, *Respir Care* 31:1069-1074, 1986.
90. Rossi A, Gottfried SB, Zocchi L, Higgs BD, Lennox S, Calverley PM, Begin P, Grassino A, Milic-Emili J: Measurement of static compliance of the total respiratory system in patients with acute respiratory failure during mechanical ventilation, *Am Rev Respir Dis* 131:672-677, 1985.
91. Cole AG, Weller SF, Sykes MK: Inverse ratio ventilation compared with PEEP in adult respiratory failure, *Intensive Care Med* 10:337-339, 1984.
92. Suter PM, Schlobohm RM: Determination of functional residual capacity during mechanical ventilation, *Anesthesiology* 41:605-607, 1974.
93. Katz JA, Ozanne GM, Zinn SE, Fairley HB: Time course and mechanisms of lung-volume increase with PEEP in acute respiratory failure, *Anesthesiology* 54:9-16, 1981.
94. Kacmarek RM, Hess D: Pressure-controlled, inverse-ratio ventilation: panacea or auto-PEEP? *Respir Care* 35:945-948, 1990.
95. Abraham E, Yoshihara G: Cardiorespiratory effects of pressure controlled inverse ratio ventilation in severe respiratory failure, *Chest* 96:1356-1359, 1989.
96. Haake R, Schlichtig R, Ulstad DR, Henschen RR: Barotrauma, *Chest* 91:608-613, 1987.
97. Hughes JMB, Hoppin FG, Mead J: Effect of lung inflation on bronchial length and diameter in excised lungs, *J Appl Physiol* 32:25-35, 1972.
98. Black JW, Grover BS: A hazard of pressure support ventilation, *Chest* 93:333-335, 1988.
99. Becker E: Mechanical ventilation in children, *Chest* 97:254, 1990.
100. Hewlett AM, Platt AS, Terry G: Mandatory minute volume, *Anesthesia* 32:163-169, 1977.
101. Younes M: Proportional-assist ventilation: a new approach to ventilatory support, *Am Rev Respir Dis* 145:114-120, 1992.
102. Younes M, Puddy A, Roberts D, Light RB, Quesada A, Taylor K, Oppenheimer L, Cramp H: Proportional-assist ventilation: results of an initial clinical trial, *Am Rev Respir Dis* 145:121-129, 1992.
103. Brochard L, Rua F, Lorino H, Lemaire F, Harf A: Inspiratory pressure support compensates for additional work of breathing caused by the endotracheal tube, *Anesthesiology* 75:739-745, 1991.
104. Tokioka H, Saito S, Takahashi T, Kinjo M, Saeki S, Kosaka F, Hirakawa M: Effectiveness of pressure support ventilation for mechanical ventilatory support in patients with status asthmaticus, *Acta Anaesthesiol Scand* 36:5-9, 1992.
105. Brochard L, Harf A, Lorino H, Lemaire F: Inspiratory pressure support prevents diaphragmatic fatigue during weaning from mechanical ventilation, *Am Rev Respir Dis* 139:513-521, 1989.
106. MacIntyre NR: Respiratory function during pressure support ventilation, *Chest* 89:677-683, 1986.
107. MacIntyre N: Pressure support ventilation: effects on ventilatory reflexes and ventilatory muscle workloads, *Respir Care* 32:447-453, 1987.

108. MacIntyre NR: Pressure support: coming of age, *Semin Respir Med* 14:293-298, 1993.
109. Tokioka H, Kinjo M, Hirakawa M: The effectiveness of pressure support ventilation for mechanical ventilatory support in children, *Anesthesiology* 78:880-884, 1993.
110. Kacmarek RM: Essential gas delivery features of mechanical ventilators, *Respir Care* 37:1045-1055, 1992.
111. Baker AB, Babington PCB, Colliss BR, Cowie RW: Effects of varying inspiratory flow waveforms and time in intermittent positive pressure ventilation, *Br J Anaesth* 49:1221-1233, 1977.
112. Abraham E, Yoshihara G: Cardiorespiratory effects of pressure controlled ventilation in severe respiratory failure, *Chest* 98:1445-1449, 1990.
113. Weil MH: Patient evaluation, "vital signs," and initial care. In Shoemaker WC, Thompson WL, eds: *Critical care, state of the art,* Fullerton, Calif, 1980, Society of Critical Care Medicine, pp (A)1-31.
114. American Association for Respiratory Care: Consensus statement on the essentials mechanical ventilators: 1992, *Respir Care* 37:1000-1008, 1992.
115. Heiser MS, Downs JJ: Acute respiratory failure in infants and children due to lower respiratory tract obstructive disorders. In Shoemaker WC, Thompson WL, Holbrook PR, eds: *Textbook of critical care,* Philadelphia, 1988, WB Saunders, pp 535-549.
116. Kilham H, Gillis J, Benjamin B: Severe upper airway obstruction, *Pediatr Clin North Am* 34:1-14, 1987.
117. Sivan Y, Deakers TW, Newth CJL: Thoraco-abdominal asynchrony in acute upper airway obstruction in small children, *Am Rev Respir Dis* 142:540-544, 1990.
118. Klein M: Croup, epiglottitis and the febrile dysphagia syndrome, *S Afr J Cont Med Educ* 4:45-51, 1986.
119. Barker SJ, Tremper KK, Hyatt J, Zaccari J, Heitzmann HA, Holman BM, Pike K, Ring LS, Teope M, Thaure TB: Continuous fiberoptic arterial oxygen tension measurements in dogs, *J Clin Monit* 3:48-52, 1987.
120. Deakers TW, Steward DJ, Newth CJL: Evaluation of a continuous intra-arterial blood gas monitor in critically ill children, *Am J Respir Crit Care Med* 149(4):A1075, 1994.
121. Hauser GJ, Pollack MM, Sivit CJ, Taylor GA, Bulas DI, Guion CJ: Routine chest radiographs in pediatric intensive care: a prospective study, *Pediatrics* 83:465-470, 1989.
122. Fanconi S, Doherty P, Edmonds JF, Barker GA, Bohn DJ: Pulse oximetry in pediatric intensive care: comparison with measured saturations and transcutaneous tension, *J Pediatr* 107:362-366, 1985.
123. Sendak MJ, Harris AP, Donham RT: Accuracy of pulse oximetry during arterial desaturation in dogs, *Anesthesiology* 68:111-114, 1988.
124. Severinghaus JW, Naifeh KH: Accuracy of response of six pulse oximeters to profound hypoxemia, *Anesthesiology* 67:551-558, 1987.
125. Sidi A, Rush W, Gravenstein N, Ruiz B, Paulus DA, Davis RF: Pulse oximetry fails to accurately detect low levels of arterial hemoglobin oxygen saturation in dogs, *J Clin Monit* 3:257-262, 1987.
126. Hannhart B, Haberer JP, Saunier C, Laxenaire MC: Accuracy and precision of fourteen pulse oximeters, *Eur Respir J* 4:115-119, 1991.
127. Jubran A, Tobin MJ: Reliability of pulse oximetry in titrating supplemental therapy in ventilator-dependent patients, *Chest* 97:1420-1425, 1990.
128. Lawson D, Norley I, Korbon G, Loeb R, Ellis J: Blood flow limits and pulse oximeter signal detection, *Anesthesiology* 67:599-603, 1987.
129. Monaco F, Nickerson BG, McQuitty JC: Continuous transcutaneous and carbon dioxide monitoring in pediatric ICU, *Crit Care Med* 11:765-766, 1982.
130. Bhat R, Diaz-Blanco J, Chaudhry U, Vidyasagar D: Recent instrumentation, *Pediatr Clin North Am* 33:503-522, 1986.
131. Sivan Y, Eldadah M, Cheah TE, Newth CJL: Estimation of arterial carbon dioxide by end-tidal and transcutaneous Pco_2 measurements in ventilated children, *Pediatr Pulmonol* 12:153-157, 1992.
132. Luft WC, Loeppy JA, Mostyn DM: Mean alveolar gases and alveolar-arterial gradients in pulmonary patients, *J Appl Physiol* 46:534-540, 1979.
133. Epstein MF, Cohen AR, Feldman HA, Raemer DB: Estimation of $Paco_2$ by two noninvasive methods in the critically ill newborn infant, *J Pediatr* 106:282-286, 1985.
134. Watkins AMC, Weidling AM: Monitoring end-tidal CO_2 in neonatal intensive care, *Arch Dis Child* 62:837-839, 1987.
135. England SJ: Current techniques for assessing pulmonary function in the newborn and infant: advantages and limitations, *Pediatr Pulmonol* 4:48-53, 1988.
136. Hammer J, Newth CJL: Infant lung function testing in the intensive care unit, *Intensive Care Med* 21:744-752, 1995.
137. Reference deleted in pages.
138. Taussig LM, Landau LI, Godfrey S, Arad I: Determinants of forced expiratory flows in newborn infants, *J Appl Physiol* 53:1220-1227, 1982.
139. Morgan WJ, Geller DE, Tepper RS, Taussig LM: Partial expiratory flow-volume curves in infants and young children: state of the art, *Pediatr Pulmonol* 5:232-243, 1988.
140. Hammer J, Numa A, Newth CJL: Albuterol responsiveness in infants with respiratory failure caused by respiratory syncytial virus infection, *J Pediatr* 127:485-490, 1995
141. Hammer J, Newth CJL: Effort and volume dependence of forced-deflation flow-volume relationships in intubated infants, *J Appl Physiol* 80:345-350, 1996
142. Taussig LM: Maximal expiratory flows at functional residual capacity: a test of lung function for young children, *Am Rev Respir Dis* 116:1031-1038, 1977.
143. Newth CJL, Amsler B, Anderson GP, Morley J: The effect of varying inflation and deflation pressures on the maximal expiratory deflation flow-volume relationship in anesthetized rhesus monkeys, *Am Rev Respir Dis* 144:807-813, 1991.
144. Hammer J, Sivan Y, Deakers TW, Newth CJL: Flow limitation in anesthetized rhesus monkeys: a comparison of rapid thoracoabdominal compression and forced deflation techniques, *Pediatr Res* 39:539-546, 1996.
145. Shannon DC: Rational monitoring of respiratory function during mechanical ventilation, *Intensive Care Med* 15:S13-S16, 1989.
146. Sivan Y, Deakers TW, Newth CJL: An automated bedside method for measuring functional residual capacity by nitrogen washout in mechanically ventilated children, *Pediatr Res* 28:446-450, 1990.

Clinical Considerations in Ventilator Management

147. Valentine DD, Hammond MD, Downs JB, Sears NJ, Sims WR: Distribution of ventilation and perfusion with different modes of mechanical ventilation, *Am Rev Respir Dis* 143:1262-1266, 1991.
148. Dworkin G, Kattan M: Mechanical ventilation for status asthmaticus in children, *J Pediatr* 114:545-549, 1989.
149. Hickling KG, Henderson S, Lackson R: Low mortality associated with permissive hypercapnia in severe adult respiratory distress syndrome, *Intensive Care Med* 16:372-377, 1990.
150. Shapiro BA: Airway pressure therapy for acute restrictive pulmonary pathology. In Shoemaker WC, Thomson WL, eds: *Critical care: state of the art,* vol 2, Fullerton, Calif, 1981, Society of Critical Care Medicine, pp (B)1-31.
151. Sivan Y, Deakers TW, Newth CJL: Functional residual capacity in ventilated infants and children, *Pediatr Res* 28:451-454, 1990.
152. Sivan Y, Deakers TW, Newth CJL: Effect of positive end-expiratory pressure on pulmonary compliance in children with acute respiratory failure, *Pediatr Pulmonol* 11:103-107, 1991.
153. Richardson P, Carlsrom JR: Effect of end-expiratory lung volume on lung mechanics in normal and edematous lungs, *Respiration* 47:90-97, 1985.
154. Suter MP, Fairley HB, Isenberg MD: Optimum end-expiratory airway pressure in patients with acute pulmonary failure, *N Engl J Med* 292:284-289, 1975.
155. Suter PM, Fairley HB, Isenberg MD: Effect of tidal volume and positive end-expiratory pressure on compliance during mechanical ventilation, *Chest* 73:158-162, 1978.
156. Falke KJ: Do changes in lung compliance allow the determination of optimal PEEP? *Anaesthetist* 29:165-168, 1980.
157. East TD, Veen JCC, Pace NL, McJames S: Functional residual capacity as a noninvasive indicator of optimal positive end-expiratory pressure, *J Clin Monit* 4:91-98, 1988.
158. Mehta A, Callan K, Wright BM, Stacey TE: Patient triggered ventilation in the newborn, *Lancet* 2:17-19, 1986.
159. Greenough A, Pool J: Neonatal patient triggered ventilation, *Arch Dis Child* 63:394-397, 1988.
160. Sassoon CSH: Mechanical ventilator design and function: the trigger variable, *Respir Care* 37:1056-1069, 1992.
161. Nishimura M, Hess D, Kacmarek RM: The response of flow-triggered infant ventilators, *Am J Respir Crit Care Med* 152:1901-1909, 1995.
162. Jarreau P-H, Moriette G, Mussat P, Mariette C, Mohanna A, Harf A, Lorino H: Patient-triggered ventilation decreases the work of breathing in neonates, *Am J Respir Crit Care Med* 153:1176-1181, 1996.

163. Bernstein G, Knodel E, Heldt GP: Airway leak size in neonates and autocycling of three flow-triggered ventilators, *Crit Care Med* 23:1739-1744, 1995.

Weaning from Mechanical Ventilation

164. Gibney RT, Wilson R, Pontoppodian H: Comparison of work of breathing on high gas flow and demand valve continuous positive airway pressure systems, *Chest* 82:692-695, 1982.
165. Henry WC, West GA, Wilson RS: A comparison of the oxygen cost of breathing between a continuous-flow CPAP system and a demand-flow CPAP system, *Respir Care* 28:1273-1281, 1983.
166. Marini JJ: The physiologic determinants of ventilator dependence, *Respir Care* 31:271-281, 1986.

Use of Medications to Facilitate Mechanical Ventilation

167. Palmisano BW, Fisher DM, Willis M, Gregory GA, Ebert PA: The effect of paralysis on oxygen consumption in normoxic children after cardiac surgery, *Anesthesiology* 61:518-522, 1984.
168. Roizien MF, Feeley TW: Pancuronium bromide, *Ann Intern Med* 88:64-68, 1978.
169. Hansen-Flaschen J, Cowen J, Raps C: Neuromuscular blockade in the intensive care unit: more than we bargained for, *Am Rev Respir Dis* 147:234-236, 1993.
170. Hansen-Flaschen JH, Brazinsky S, Basile C, Lanken PN: Use of sedating drugs and neuromuscular blocking agents in patients requiring mechanical ventilation for respiratory failure: a national survey, *JAMA* 266:2870-2875, 1991.
171. Klessig HT, Geiger HJ, Murray MJ, Coursin DB: A national survey on the practice patterns of anesthesiologist intensivists in the use of muscle relaxants, *Crit Care Med* 20:1341-1345, 1992.
172. Eldadah MH, Newth CJL: Vecuronium by continuous infusion for neuromuscular blockade in infants and children, *Crit Care Med* 17:989-992, 1989.
173. Tuxen DV: Permissive hypercapnic ventilation, *Am J Respir Crit Care Med* 150:870-874, 1994.
174. Sergado V, Caldwell JE, Matthay MA, Sharma ML, Gruenke LD, Miller RD: Persistent paralysis in critically ill patients after long-term administration of vecuronium, *N Engl J Med* 327:524-528, 1992.
175. Rossiter A, Souney PF, McGowen S, Carvajal P: Pancuronium-induced prolonged neuromuscular blockade, *Crit Care Med* 19:1583-1587, 1991.
176. Gooch JL, Suchyta MR, Balbierz JM, Petajan JH, Clemmer TP: Prolonged paralysis after treatment with neuromuscular blocking agents, *Crit Care Med* 19:1125-1131, 1991.
177. Griffin D, Fairman N, Coursin D, Rawsthorne L, Grossman JE: Acute myopathy during treatment of status asthmaticus with corticosteroids and steroidal muscle relaxants, *Chest* 102:510-514, 1992.
178. Danon MJ, Carpenter S: Myopathy with thick filament loss following prolonged paralysis with vecuronium during steroid treatment, *Muscle Nerve* 14:1131-1139, 1991.
179. Hirano M, Ott BL, Raps EC, Minetti C, Lennihan L, Libbey NP, Bonilla E, Mays AP: Acute quadriplegic myopathy: a complication of treatment with steroids, nondepolarizing blocking agents, or both, *Neurology* 42:2082-2087, 1992.
180. Torres CF, Maniscalo WM: Muscle weakness and atrophy following prolonged paralysis with pancuronium bromide in neonates, *Ann Neurol* 18:403A, 1985.

Physiotherapy and Endotracheal Suctioning during Mechanical Ventilation

181. Reines HD, Sade RM, Bradford BF, Marshall J: Chest physiotherapy fails to prevent postoperative atelectasis in children after cardiac surgery, *Ann Surg* 195:451-455, 1982.
182. Kerem E, Yatsiv I, Goitein KJ: Effect of endotracheal suctioning on arterial blood gases in children, *Intensive Care Med* 16:95-99, 1990.

Complications of Assisted Ventilatory Support

183. Rivera R, Tibballs J: Complications of endotracheal intubation and mechanical ventilation in infants and children, *Crit Care Med* 20:193-199, 1992.
184. Suter PM, Fairley HB, Schlobohm RM: Shunt, lung volume, and perfusion during short periods of ventilation with oxygen, *Anesthesiology* 43:617-627, 1975.
185. Wagner PD, Laravuso RB, Uhl RR, West JB: Continuous distributions of ventilation-perfusion ratios in normal subjects breathing air and 100% O_2, *J Clin Invest* 54:54-68, 1974.
186. Joshi VV, Mandavia SG, Stern L, Wiglesworth FW: Acute lesions induced by endotracheal intubation, *Am J Dis Child* 124:646-649, 1972.
187. Otherson HB: Intubation injuries of the trachea in children, *Ann Surg* 189:601-606, 1979.
188. Abbott TR: Complications of prolonged nasotracheal intubation in children, *Br J Anaesthesiol* 40:347-352, 1968.
189. Little LA, Koenig JC Jr, Newth CJL: Factors affecting accidental extubations in neonatal and pediatric intensive care patients, *Crit Care Med* 18:163-165, 1990.
190. Scott PH, Eigen H, Moye LA, Geotgitis J, Laughlin JJ: Predictability and consequences of spontaneous extubation in a pediatric ICU, *Crit Care Med* 13:228-232, 1985.
191. Orlowski JP, Ellis NG, Amin NP, Crumrine RS: Complications of airway intrusion in 100 consecutive cases in a pediatric ICU, *Crit Care Med* 8:324-331, 1980.
192. Salord F, Gaussorgues P, Marti-Flich J, Sirodot M, Allimant C, Lyonnet D, Robert D: Nosocomial maxillary sinusitis during mechanical ventilation: a prospective comparison of orotracheal versus the nasotracheal route for intubation, *Intensive Care Med* 16:390-393, 1990.
193. Pedersen J, Schurizek BA, Melsen NC, Juhl B: The effect of nasotracheal intubation on the paranasal sinuses: a prospective study of 434 intensive care patients, *Acta Anaesthesiol Scand* 35:11-13, 1991.
194. Striker TW, Stool S, Downes JJ: Prolonged nasotracheal intubation in infants and children, *Arch Otolaryngol* 85:210-213, 1967.
195. Parker JC, Hernandez LA, Peevy KJ: Mechanisms of ventilator-induced lung injury, *Crit Care Med* 21:131-143, 1993.
196. Pierson DJ: Complications associated with mechanical ventilation, *Crit Care Clin* 6:711-724, 1990.
197. Parker JC, Hernandez LA, Longenecker GL, Peevy K, Johnson W: Lung edema due to high peak airway pressures in dogs: role of increased microvascular filtration pressure and permeability, *Am Rev Respir Dis* 142:321-328, 1990.
198. Dreyfuss D, Basset G, Soler P, Saumon G: Intermittent positive pressure hyperventilation with high inflation pressures produce pulmonary microvascular injury in rats, *Am Rev Respir Dis* 132:880-884, 1985.
199. Takamura T: Histopathological study of the adverse effects of prolonged respiratory therapy of the neonate lung, *Acta Pathol Jpn* 31:199-210, 1981.
200. Donowitz LG: High risk of nosocomial infection in the pediatric critical care patient, *Crit Care Med* 14:26-28, 1986.
201. Milliken J, Tait GA, Ford-Jones EL, Mindorff CM, Gold R, Mullins G: Nosocomial infections in a pediatric intensive care unit, *Crit Care Med* 16:233-237, 1988.
202. Barzilay Z, Mandel M, Keren G, Davidson S: Nosocomial bacterial pneumonia in ventilated children: clinical significance of culture-positive peripheral bronchial aspirates, *J Pediatr* 112:421-424, 1988.
203. Pugin J, Auckenthaler R, Lew DP, Suter PM: Oropharyngeal decontamination decreases incidence of ventilator-associated pneumonia: a randomized placebo-controlled double-blind clinical trial, *JAMA* 265:2704-2710, 1991.
204. Rodriquez-Roldan JM, Altuna-Cuesta A, Lopez A, Carrilo A, Garcia J, Leon J, Martinez-Pellus AJ: Prevention of nosocomial lung infection in ventilated patients: use of antimicrobial pharyngeal nonabsorbable paste, *Crit Care Med* 18:1239-1242, 1990.
205. Biondi JW, Schulman DS, Matthay RA: Effects of mechanical ventilation on right and left ventricular function, *Clin Chest Med* 9:55-71, 1988.
206. Shapiro HM, Marshall LF: Intracranial pressure responses to PEEP in head-injured patients, *J Trauma* 18:254-256, 1978.
207. Marquez JM, Douglas ME, Downs JB, Wu WH: Renal function and cardiovascular responses during positive airway pressure, *Anesthesiology* 50:393-398, 1979.
208. Baratz RA, Philbin DM, Patterson RW: Plasma antidiuretic hormone and urinary output during continuous positive-pressure breathing in dogs, *Anesthesiology* 34:510-513, 1971.
209. Bonnet F, Richard C, Glaser P, Lafay M, Guesde R: Changes in hepatic flow induced by continuous positive pressure ventilation in critically ill patients, *Crit Care Med* 10:703-705, 1982.

Ventilation Issues Specific to Neonatal Lung Diseases

210. Farrel PM, Avery ME: Hyaline membrane disease, *Am Rev Respir Dis* 111:657-688, 1975.
211. Carlo WA, Martin RJ: Principles of neonatal assisted ventilation, *Pediatr Clin North Am* 33:221-237, 1986.
212. Hird MF, Greenough A: Patient triggered ventilation using a flow triggered system, *Arch Dis Child* 66:1140-1142, 1991.
213. Yee WFH, Scarpelli EM: Surfactant replacement therapy, *Pediatr Pulmonol* 11:65-80, 1991.
214. Dreyfuss D, Soler P, Basset G, Saumon G: High inflation pressure pulmonary edema, *Am Rev Respir Dis* 137:1159-1164, 1988.
215. Wisell TE, Tuggle JM, Turner BS: Meconium aspiration syndrome: have we made a difference? *Pediatrics* 85:715-721, 1990.
216. Davey AM, Becker JD, Davis JM: Meconium aspiration syndrome: physiological and inflammatory changes in a newborn piglet model, *Pediatr Pulmonol* 16:101-108, 1993.
217. Spitzer AL, Davis J, Clark WT, Bernbaum J, Fox WW: Pulmonary hypertension and persistent fetal circulation in the newborn, *Pediatr Clin North Am* 15:389-413, 1988.
218. Roberts JD, Polaner DM, Lang P, Zapol WM: Inhaled nitric oxide in persistent pulmonary hypertension of the newborn, *Lancet* 340:818-819, 1992.
219. Kinsella JP, Neish SR, Shaffer E, Abman SH: Low-dose inhalational nitric oxide in persistent pulmonary hypertension of the newborn, *Lance*t 340:819-820, 1992.
220. Abu-Osba YK, Galal O, Manasra K, Rejjal A: Treatment of severe persistent pulmonary hypertension of the newborn with magnesium sulfate, *Arch Dis Child* 67:31-35, 1992.
221. Oritz RM, Cilley RE, Bartlett RH: Extracorporeal membrane oxygenation in pediatric respiratory failure, *Pediatr Clin North Am* 34:39-46, 1987.

Special Types of Assisted Ventilation

222. Akingbola OA, Servant GM, Custer JR, Palmisano JM: Noninvasive bi-level positive pressure ventilation: management of two pediatric patients, *Respir Care* 38:1092-1098, 1993.
223. Brochard L, Pleskwa F, Lemaire E: Improved efficacy of spontaneous breathing with inspiratory pressure support, *Am Rev Respir Dis* 136:411-415, 1987.
224. Pennock BE, Kaplan PD, Carlin BW, Sabangan JS, Magovern JA: Pressure support ventilation with a simplified ventilatory support system administered with a nasal mask in patients with respiratory failure, *Chest* 100:1371-1376, 1991.
225. Waldhorn RE: Nocturnal nasal intermittent positive pressure ventilation with bi-level positive airway pressure (BiPAP) in respiratory failure, *Chest* 101:516-521, 1992.
226. Fortenberry JD, Del Toro J, Jefferson LS, Evey L, Haase D: Management of pediatric acute hypoxemic respiratory insufficiency with bi-level positive pressure (BiPAP) nasal mask ventilation, *Chest* 108:1059-1064, 1995.
227. Padman R, Lawless S, Von Nessen S: Use of BiPAP by nasal mask in the treatment of respiratory insufficiency in pediatric patients, *Pediatr Pulmonol* 17:119-123, 1994.
228. Froese AB, Bryan AD: High frequency ventilation, *Am Rev Respir Dis* 135:1363-1974, 1987.
229. Wetzel RC, Gioia FR: High frequency ventilation, *Pediatr Clin North Am* 34:15-38, 1987.
230. Mammel MD, Boros S: Airway damage and mechanical ventilation: a review and commentary, *Pediatr Pulmonol* 3:443-447, 1987.
231. Baumgart S, Hirschl RB, Butler SZ, Coburn CE, Apitzer AR: Diagnosis-related criteria in the consideration of extracorporeal membrane oxygenation in neonates previously treated with high-frequency jet ventilation, *Pediatrics* 89:491-494, 1992.
232. Carter JM, Gerstmann DR, Clark RH, Snyder G, Cornish JD, Null Jr DM, deLemos RA : High-frequency oscillatory ventilation and extracorporeal membrane oxygenation for the treatment of acute neonatal respiratory failure, *Pediatrics* 85:159-164, 1990.
233. Varnholt V, Lasch P, Suske G, Kachel W, Brands W: High frequency oscillatory ventilation and extracorporeal membrane oxygenation in severe persistent pulmonary hypertension of the newborn, *Eur J Pediatr* 151:769-774, 1992.
234. Pfenninger J, Tschaeppeler H, Wagner BP, Weber J, Zimmerman A: The paradox of adult respiratory distress syndrome in neonates, *Pediatr Pulmonol* 10:18-24, 1991.
235. McCulloch PR, Forkert PG, Froese AB: Lung volume maintenance prevents lung injury during high frequency oscillatory ventilation in surfactant-deficient rabbits, *Am Rev Respir Dis* 137:1185-1192, 1988.
236. Clark RH, Gerstmann Dr, Null DM, Yoder BA, Cornish JD, Glasier CM, Ackerman NB, Bell RE, Delemos RA: Pulmonary interstitial emphysema treated by high-frequency oscillatory ventilation, *Crit Care Med* 14:926-930, 1986.
237. Keszler M, Donn SM, Bucciarelli RL, Alverson DC, Hart M, Lunyong V, Modanlou HD, Noguchi A, Pearlman SA, Puri A: Multicenter controlled trial comparing high-frequency jet ventilation and conventional mechanical ventilation in newborn infants with pulmonary interstitial emphysema, *J Pediatr* 119:85-93, 1991.
238. Bryan AC, Slutsky AS: Lung volume during high frequency oscillation, *Am Rev Respir Dis* 133:928-930, 1986.
239. Arnold JH, Truog RD, Thompson JE, Fackler JC: High-frequency oscillatory ventilation in pediatric respiratory failure, *Crit Care Med* 21:272-279, 1993.
240. Arnold JH, Hanson JH, Toro-Figuero LO, Gutiérrez J, Berens RJ, Anglin DL: Prospective, randomized comparison of high-frequency oscillatory ventilation and conventional mechanical ventilation in pediatric respiratory failure, *Crit Care Med* 22:1530-1539, 1994.
241. Rivera RA, Butt W, Shann F: Predictors of mortality in children with respiratory failure: possible indications for ECMO, *Anaesth Intensive Care* 18:385-389, 1990.
242. Kolobow T, Gattinoni L, Fumagalli R, Arosio P, Pesenti A, Solca M, Chen V: Carbon dioxide and the membrane artificial lung: their roles in the prevention and treatment of respiratory failure, *Trans Am Soc Artif Intern Organs* 28:20-23, 1982.
243. Gattinoni L, Pesenti A, Bombino M, Baglioni S, Rivolta M, Rossi G, Fumagalli R, Marcolin R, Mascheroni D: Relationships between lung computed tomographic density, gas exchange, and PEEP in acute respiratory failure, *Anesthesiology* 69:824-832, 1988.
244. Fisher JB, Mammel MC, Coleman JM, Bing DR, Boros SJ: Identifying lung over-distension during mechanical ventilation by using volume-pressure loops, *Pediatr Pulmonol* 5:10-14, 1988.
245. Pesenti A: Target blood gases during ARDS ventilatory management, *Intensive Care Med* 16:349-351, 1990.
246. Hickling KG: Ventilatory management of ARDS: can it affect outcome? *Intensive Care Med* 16:219-226, 1990.
247. Reynolds EM, Ryan DP, Doody DP: Permissive hypercapnia and pressure-controlled ventilation as treatment of severe adult respiratory distress syndrome in a pediatric burn patient, *Crit Care Med* 21:944-947, 1993.
248. Goldstein B, Shannon DC, Todres ID: Supercarbia in children: clinical course and outcome, *Crit Care Med* 18:166-168, 1990.
249. Schumacher RE, Barks JDE, Johnston MV, Donn SM, Scher MS, Roloff DW, Bartlett RH: Right sided brain lesions in infants following extracorporeal membrane oxygenation, *Pediatrics* 82:155-161, 1988.
250. Hofkosh D, Thompson AE, Nozza RJ, Kemp SS, Bowen A, Feldman HM: Ten years of extracorporeal membrane oxygenation: neurodevelopmental outcome, *Pediatrics* 87:549-555, 1991.
251. O'Rourke PP, Crone RK, Vacanti JP, Ware JH, Lillegei CW, Parad RB, Epstein MF: Extracorporeal membrane oxygenation and conventional medical therapy in neonates with persistent pulmonary hypertension of the newborn: a prospective randomized study, *Pediatrics* 84:957-963, 1989.
252. Green TP, Moler FW, Goodman DM: Probability of survival after prolonged extracorporeal membrane oxygenation in pediatric patients with acute respiratory failure, *Crit Care Med* 23:1132-1139, 1995.
253. O'Rourke PP: Pediatric ECMO: is there a problem? In Tibboel D, van den Voort E, eds: *Update Intensive Care Emerg Med* 25:312-321, 1996.
254. Morris A, Wallace C, Menlove R, Clemmer TP, Orme Jr. JF, Weaver LK, Dean NC, Thomas F, East TD, Pace NL: Randomized clinical trial of pressure-controlled inverse ratio ventilation and extracorporeal CO_2 removal for adult respiratory distress syndrome, *Am J Respir Crit Care Med* 149:295-305, 1994.
255. Children with handicaps and their families: case example—the ventilator dependent child, *Report on the Surgeon General's workshop,* DDHS Pub No PHS-83-50194, Washington, DC, 1983, US Department of Health and Human Services.
256. Robinson RO: Ventilator dependency in the United Kingdom, *Arch Dis Child* 65:1235-1236, 1990.
257. Fields AI, Rosenblatt A, Pollack MM, Kaufman J: Home care cost-effectiveness for respiratory technology-dependent children, *Am J Dis Child* 145:729-733, 1991.

258. American Thoracic Society: Home mechanical ventilation of pediatric patients, *Am Rev Respir Dis* 141:258-259, 1991.
259. Schreiner MS, Donar ME, Kettrick RG: Pediatric home mechanical ventilation, *Pediatr Clin North Am* 34:47-60, 1987.
260. O'Donohue WJ, Giovannoni RM, Goldberg AI, Keens TG, Make BJ, Plummer AL, Prentice WS: Long term mechanical ventilation: guideline for management in the home and at alternate community sites: report of the Ad Hoc Committee, Respiratory Care section, American College of Chest Physicians, *Chest* 90(suppl):1S-37S, 1986.
261. Banaszak EF, Travers H, Frazie M, Vinz T: Home ventilator care, *Respir Care* 26:1262-1268, 1981.
262. Frates RC, Splaingard ML, Smith EO, Harrison GM: Outcome of home mechanical ventilation in children, *J Pediatr* 106:850-856, 1985.

Nonconventional and Experimental Modes

263. Marraro G: Simultaneous independent lung ventilation in pediatric patients, *Crit Care Clin* 8:131-145, 1992.
264. Marraro G, Marinari M, Rataggi M: The clinical application of synchronized independent lung ventilation (S.I.L.V.) in pulmonary disease with unilateral prevalence in pediatrics, *Int J Clin Monit Comput* 4:123-129, 1987.
265. East TD, Pace NL, Westenskov DR: Synchronous versus asynchronous differential lung ventilation with PEEP after unilateral acid aspiration in the dog, *Crit Care Med* 11:441-444, 1983.
266. Levine S, Levy S, Henson D: Negative-pressure ventilation, *Crit Care Clin* 6:505-530, 1990.
267. Brahdy MB, Lenarsky M: Treatment of respiratory failure in acute epidemic poliomyelitis, *Am J Dis Child* 46:705-729, 1933.
268. Brahdy MB, Lenarsky M: Respiratory failure in acute epidemic poliomyelitis, *J Pediatr* 8:420-433, 1936.
269. Stern L, Ramos AD, Outerbridge EW, Beaudry PH: Negative pressure artificial respiration: use in treatment of respiratory distress syndrome of the newborn, *Can Med Assoc J* 102:595-601, 1970.
270. Linsao LS, Levison H, Swyer PR: Negative pressure artificial respiration: use in treatment of respiratory distress syndrome of the newborn, *Can Med Assoc J* 102:602-606, 1970.
271. Skaburskis M, Helal R, Zidula A: Hemodynamic effects of external continuous negative pressure ventilation compared with those of continuous positive pressure ventilation in dogs with acute lung injury, *Am Rev Respir Dis* 136:886-891, 1987.
272. Scharf SM, Feldman NT, Goldman MD, Haut HZ, Bruce E, Ingram R: Vocal cord closure: a cause of upper airway obstruction during controlled ventilation, *Am Rev Respir Dis* 117:391-397, 1978.
273. Clark LC Jr, Gollan F: Survival of mammals breathing organic liquids equilibrated with at atmospheric pressure, *Science* 152:1755-1756, 1966.
274. Kylstra JA, Paganelli CV, Lanphier EH: Pulmonary gas exchange in dogs ventilated with hyperbarically oxygenated liquid, *J Appl Physiol* 21:177-184, 1966.
275. Shaffer TH, Moskowitz GD: Demand-controlled liquid ventilation of the lungs, *J Appl Physiol* 36:208-213, 1974.
276. Shaffer TH, Lowe CA, Bhutani VK, Douglas PR: Liquid ventilation: effects on pulmonary function in distressed meconium-stained lambs, *Pediatr Res* 18:49-53, 1984.
277. Shaffer TH, Rubenstein D, Moskowitz GD, Delivoria-Papadopulos M: Gaseous exchange and acid-base balance in premature lambs during liquid ventilation since birth, *Pediatr Res* 10:227-231, 1976.
278. Foust R III, Tran NN, Cox C, Miller TF Jr, Greenspan JS, Wolfson MR, Shaffer TH: Liquid assisted ventilation: an alternative ventilatory strategy for acute meconium aspiration injury, *Pediatr Pulmonol* 21:316-322, 1996.
279. Greenspan JS, Wolfson MR, Rubenstein SD, Shaffer TH: Liquid ventilation of human preterm neonates, *J Pediatr* 117:106-111, 1990.
280. Sargent JW, Seffl RJ: Properties of perfluorinated liquid, *Fed Proc (Fed Am Soc Exp Biol)* 29:1699-1703, 1970.
281. Forman DL, Bhutani VK, Hilfer SR, Shaffer TH: A fine structure study of the liquid-ventilated newborn rabbit, *Fed Proc* 43:647, 1984.
282. Modell JG, Tham MK, Modell JH, Calderwood HW, Ruiz BC: Distribution and retention of perfluorocarbon in mice and dogs after injection or liquid ventilation, *Toxicol Appl Pharmacol* 26:86-92, 1973.
283. Calderwood HW, Ruiz BC, Tham MK, Modell JH, Saga SA, Hood CI: Residual levels and biochemical changes after ventilation with perfluorinated liquid, *J Appl Physiol* 39:603-607, 1975.
284. Mitsuno T, Ohyanagi H, Naito R: Clinical studies of a perfluorochemical whole blood substitute (Fluoso-DA): summary of 186 cases, *Ann Surg* 195:60-69, 1982.
285. Ohyanagi H, Toshima K, Sekita M, et al: Clinical studies of a perfluorochemical whole blood substitute: safety of Fluoso-DA (20%) in normal human volunteers, *Clin Ther* 2:306-312, 1979.
286. Lowe CA, Tuma RF, Sivieri EM, Shaffer TH: Liquid ventilation: cardiovascular adjustment with secondary hypercalcemia and acidosis, *J Appl Physiol* 47:1051-1056, 1979.
287. Lowe CA, Shaffer TH: Pulmonary vascular resistance with the perfluorocarbon-filled lung, *J Appl Physiol* 60:154-159, 1986.
288. Fuhrman BP: Perfluorocarbon liquid ventilation: the first human trial, *J Pediatr* 117:73-74, 1990 (editorial).
289. Tutuncu AS, Faithfull NS, Lachmann B: Comparison of ventilatory support with intratracheal perfluorocarbon administration and conventional mechanical ventilation in animals with acute respiratory failure, *Am Rev Respir Dis* 148:785-792, 1993.
290. Hirschl RB, Pranikoff T, Gauger P, Schreiner RJ, Dechert R, Bartlett RH: Liquid ventilation in adults, children and full-term neonates, *Lancet* 346:1201-1202, 1995.
291. Leach CL, Greenspan JS, Rubenstein SD, Shaffer TH, Wolfson MR, Jackson JC, DeLemos R, Fuhrman BP: Partial liquid ventilation with perflubron in premature infants with severe respiratory distress syndrome: the LiquiVent Study Group, *N Engl J Med* 12(335):761-767, 1996.
292. Gauger PG, Pranikoff T, Schreiner RJ, Moler FW, Hirschl RB: Initial experience with partial liquid ventilation in pediatric patients with the acute respiratory distress syndrome, *Crit Care Med* 24:16-22, 1996.
293. Hirschl RB, Pranikoff T, Gauger P, Schreiner RJ, Dechert R, Bartlett RH: Liquid ventilation in adults, children, and full-term neonates, *Lancet* 4(346):1201-1202, 1995.
294. Muller E, Kolobow T, Mandava S, Jones M, Vitale G, Aprigliano M, Yamada K: Intratracheal pulmonary ventilation (ITPV). A new technique to ventilate lungs as small as 12% of normal, *Pediatr Res* 29:326A, 1991.
295. Kolobow T, Muller E, Mandava S, Jones M, Vitale G, Aprigliano K, Yamada K: Intratracheal pulmonary ventilation (ITPV): a new technique, *Pediatr Res* 29:31A, 1991.
296. Nahum A, Burke WC, Ravenscraft SA, Marcy TW, Adams AB, Crooke PS, Marini JJ: Lung mechanics and gas exchange during pressure control ventilation in dogs: augmentation of CO_2 elimination by intratracheal catheter, *Am Rev Respir Dis* 146:965-973, 1992.
297. Nahum A, Ravenscraft SA, Nakos G, Burke WC, Adams AB, Marcy TW, Marini JJ: Tracheal gas insufflation during pressure control ventilation: effects of catheter position, diameter and flow rate, *Am Rev Respir Dis* 146:1411-1418, 1992.
298. Ravenscraft SA, Burke WC, Nahum A, Marcy TW, Adams AB, Nakos G, Marini JJ: Intratracheal gas insufflation augments alveolar ventilation in patients, *Am Rev Respir Dis* 145:529A, 1992.

CHAPTER 22

Pediatric Cardiopulmonary Resuscitation

Robert A. Berg

The prophet Elisha revived a child who "was dead" by putting "his mouth upon his mouth, his eyes upon his eyes and his hands upon his hands: and stretched himself upon the child; and the flesh of the child waxed warm . . . and the child opened his eyes."

2 Kings, 4:34-35

This verse from the Bible may be the first case report of successful cardiopulmonary resuscitation (CPR), describing a child who was resuscitated from apparent death. Because cardiac arrests are more common in adults than children, most of the clinical series and almost all of the clinical studies regarding various aspects of CPR involve adults. Animal experiments of cardiac arrest and various aspects of CPR usually use ventricular fibrillation models. On the other hand, most cardiac arrests in children are secondary to hemodynamic collapse or respiratory arrest rather than primary ventricular fibrillation.[1-20] Therefore guidelines for CPR in children have largely been extrapolated from data obtained in adults or in animal models of questionable relevance.

CPR in children differs from that in adults. Children are anatomically and physiologically unlike adults. In particular, the chest wall configuration and compliance are not the same. Perhaps more important, the etiology and pathogenesis of cardiac arrests in children are different.[1-20]

EPIDEMIOLOGY

Most adults suffer cardiac arrest secondary to cardiac ischemia from atherosclerotic heart disease. In contrast, the etiologies of pediatric cardiac arrests are diverse. Cardiac arrests in children usually occur secondary to profound hypoxia or acidosis resulting from a respiratory problem or circulatory shock. Prolonged hypoxia, prolonged acidosis, or both conditions impair cardiac function and ultimately lead to cardiac arrest. Therefore the myocardium and the rest of the body generally suffer significant hypoxic-ischemic insults before cardiac arrest.

Ventricular fibrillation is noted only in approximately 10% (range from none to 23%) of children in cardiac arrest.[3,13,14,16,18,21-24] Asystole, severe bradycardia, and electromechanical dissociation (or "pulseless electrical activity") are most frequently observed. These clinical data are consistent with electrophysiologic findings in an animal model of asphyxial cardiac arrest.[25]

PHYSIOLOGY OF CPR

Cardiorespiratory physiology during CPR differs dramatically from that during normal spontaneous cardiac function. Cardiac output can be attained by either a thoracic pump mechanism or a cardiac compression mechanism.[1,26,27] A classic example of the thoracic pump mechanism is "cough CPR." Patients in ventricular fibrillation can maintain an adequate cardiac output for some time simply by coughing in a sustained rhythmic manner.[28] High intrathoracic pressure tends to propel arterial blood out of the thorax (e.g., to the brain and abdomen). Venous blood may also flow retrograde into the abdominal inferior vena cava, but valves in the jugular system and upper and lower extremities tend to limit retrograde venous flow. In addition, thin-walled veins tend to collapse and create resistance to retrograde venous flow, whereas thick-walled arteries tend to maintain patency and encourage anterograde flow.

The classic example of the cardiac compression model is open-chest cardiac massage. The heart is compressed, and blood is ejected into the arterial system. Even with open-chest cardiac massage, however, retrograde venous flow occurs because of simultaneous ventricular and atrial compression, the former leading to atrioventricular valve closure and the latter to atrial emptying to an area of less resistance.[29,30]

In certain circumstances (e.g., animals with large anteroposterior chest diameters, patients with severe thoracic air trapping, patients with insufficient force of chest compressions), the thoracic pump mechanism may predominate as the main mechanism of cardiac output during CPR.[1,26-28,31] Such circumstances limit the ability to compress the heart. Echocardiographic data suggest that cardiac compression generally occurs during CPR in adults.[32,33] In children, compliant chest walls and narrow anteroposterior chest diameters favor direct cardiac compression. Perhaps these anatomic factors explain the higher cardiac outputs and higher coronary and cerebral blood flows generally observed in animal models using smaller and more immature animals.[34,35]

PEDIATRIC BASIC LIFE SUPPORT

Diagnosis of Cardiac Arrest

Apnea and pulselessness in an unresponsive child suggest cardiac arrest and should lead to the initiation of CPR. In the prehospital setting the first observer is usually a parent or another caretaker. Panic is common. Observations of respiratory effort, pulse, and responsiveness are often neglected.[36,37] Because cardiac arrests are rare in children, even medical personnel are rarely calm or experienced. Hypotensive and even normotensive children may be inappropriately categorized as "pulseless," suggesting "cardiac arrest."[38,39] In severe hypothermia, high-dose vasopressor therapy, or severe circulatory shock, peripheral pulses may be especially difficult to palpate despite adequate central arterial pressures.

Accurate diagnosis clearly leads to more appropriate therapy. A child with ventricular fibrillation needs prompt defibrillation.[1] On the other hand, an apparently apneic, pulseless, unresponsive child may need only rescue breathing. The latter scenario is common in a delivery room.

Airway Management

During CPR, rescue breathing is most efficient via an endotracheal tube.[1] Nevertheless, mouth-to-mouth and mouth-to-nose ventilation and hand-bag-valve ventilation can provide adequate respiratory support. Too often experienced hospital personnel waste invaluable time seeking the optimal mask size while they should be providing mouth-to-mouth ventilation. Although adequate ventilation can generally be provided by either the mouth-to-mouth or bag-valve-mask technique, active chest compressions may limit the effectiveness of these methods.

Because airway management is discussed in more detail in Chapter 16, only a few issues are discussed here. The larynx of a child is smaller, more cephalad, and more anterior than that of an adult. Because of the small oropharynx and the differences in laryngeal position, endotracheal intubation of a child in cardiac arrest can be difficult even for inexperienced clinicians. In particular, hyperextension of the neck as performed in adults is often counterproductive. Availability of, and knowledge regarding, the appropriate endotracheal tube and suction catheter size are additional important issues. The appropriate endotracheal tube width approximates the width of the child's fourth finger, or pinkie, or the width of the external naris. The internal diameter of the endotracheal tube can also be estimated by the following formula[1,40]:

$$4 + \frac{\text{Age (Years)}}{4}$$

This equation is more useful for children 2 years and older. An appropriate lip-to-tip distance is generally 3 times the internal diameter of the endotracheal tube.

Recent investigations have established that resuscitators can rapidly estimate the child's length and weight using a standard resuscitation tape (Figs. 22-1 and 22-2). The resuscitator then can select appropriate sizes of resuscitation equipment, including the endotracheal tube and suction catheters, as well as appropriate medication doses.[40-42] Alternatively, a "code card" or "code sheet" can provide typical equipment sizes and medication doses for weight, age, or both factors

Even after successful endotracheal intubation with an appropriate endotracheal tube, tube malpositioning can create great problems. The trachea of a newborn is only approximately 5 cm long; yet the tip of the endotracheal tube moves 1 to 3 cm with simple flexion and extension of the baby's neck.[43,44] If the endotracheal tube is not well secured at the lip or nostril, the potential for movement is obviously even greater. It is not surprising that the highly stressed intubationist frequently places the tip of the endotracheal tube far into the right mainstem bronchus. It is also common to inadvertently extubate the lungs because the child's head is allowed to hyperextend (e.g., when the child is lifted onto a gurney).

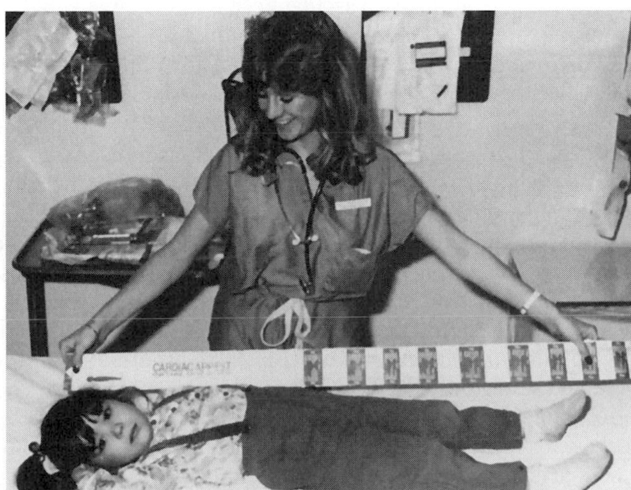

Fig. 22-1. The tape is placed next to the child to ascertain which sector corresponds to her length. (From Lutitz PS et al: *Ann Emerg Med* 17[6]:576-581, 1988.)

Breathing

The most recent recommendations of the American Heart Association (AHA) regarding assisted ventilation during basic life support focus on slowing the inspiratory time to 1 to 1½ s/breath.[1] Concerns were raised regarding the high inspiratory pressures that occur with short inspiratory times during mouth-to-mouth or bag-valve-mask ventilation. These pressures can result in gaseous overdistention of the stomach with the potential for compromise of ventilatory efforts as well as regurgitation and aspiration.

Circulation: Chest Compressions

Successful resuscitation from cardiac arrest depends on adequate myocardial and cerebral perfusion during CPR.[45-48] Effective chest compressions are a major determinant of myo-

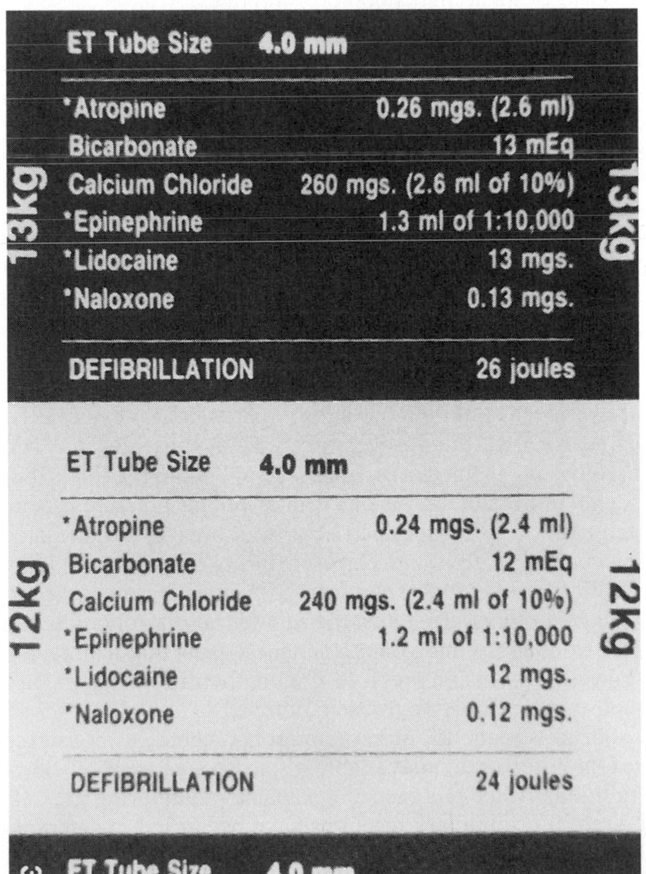

Fig. 22-2. Sector of tape indicating average weight, endotracheal tube size, and doses for a child of this length. (From Lutitz PS et al: *Ann Emerg Med* 17[6]:576-581, 1988.)

cardial and cerebral perfusion during CPR.[26,27,49] Typically, in the hospital the most experienced resuscitators focus on endotracheal intubation or "running the code." External chest compressions are frequently provided by one of the less experienced health care providers. Chest compressions may be discontinued during endotracheal intubation, intravenous access, and evaluation of the electrocardiogram. In addition, experimental data from animal models of CPR as well as clinical data in adults and children suggest that basic CPR is often performed poorly and at slow rates.[49-51] Attention to the details of chest compression deserves a higher priority in the resuscitation of children in cardiac arrest.

Effective chest compressions depend on adequate compression force, duty cycle, and rate of compression.[1] The AHA recommends compressing the chest of an infant a third to half the total depth of the chest (approximately ½ to 1 inch). According to the AHA recommendations, this may be performed either with two or three fingers on the lower sternum or with two hands encircling the thorax and thumbs on the sternum. Animal data, as well as anecdotal reports and an autopsy study, suggest that the latter is a more effective technique.[52-55] The author, who has clinical experience with infant cardiac arrest victims and central arterial pressure monitoring, agrees with these data. When chest compressions are performed on infants with this technique, firm support must be placed behind the infant's back.

The portion of the circulatory cycle in the chest-compression phase determines the duty cycle. The recommended duty cycle is 50%. Chest compression rates of at least 100 per minute are recommended for infants and children.[1] Duty cycles of 50% are easier to attain at higher compression rates. Also, because cardiac output equals stroke volume multiplied by heart rate, maintaining a compression rate of at least 100 per minute somewhat compensates for the limited "stroke volume" during CPR.

In children approximately 1 to 8 years of age, chest compressions should be provided by the heel of the hand along the lower sternum with the long axis of the heel parallel to that of the sternum. The fingers should be held up off the ribs while the heel of the hand remains in contact with the sternum. In children, as with infants, the chest should be compressed approximately a third to half the total depth of the chest. The child must be lying on a firm surface for the chest compressions to be effective.[1]

The effectiveness of chest compressions can be monitored in several ways. If direct monitoring of arterial pressure is being performed, the aortic relaxation, or diastolic, pressure should be maintained at more than 20 to 30 mm Hg.[47,48,56] If direct monitoring of arterial and central venous pressure is being performed, the coronary perfusion pressure can be calculated. The coronary arteries are perfused during the relaxation phase of CPR (diastole).[57] The coronary perfusion pressure is the aortic diastolic pressure minus the right atrial diastolic pressure. Data from adults and young animals suggest that maintaining a coronary perfusion pressure of more than 15 to 25 mm Hg is important for effective resuscitation.[48,56]

For most patients, direct arterial and central venous pressure monitoring is unavailable at the time of cardiac arrest. Traditionally, the presence of a palpable pulse during CPR and the return of pupillary reactions have been used to determine the effectiveness of CPR. Data from animal studies and children demonstrate that pulsations may result from retrograde flow in the venous system as well as antegrade flow in the arterial system.[29,30,58] Nevertheless, the strength of peripheral pulsations may indicate the force and therefore the effectiveness of chest compressions. Presumably the return of pupillary activity suggests the reestablishment of effective cerebral blood flow.

Data from animal models and adult cardiac arrest victims suggest that measurements of end-tidal carbon dioxide (CO_2) are useful predictors of coronary perfusion pressure, cardiac output, and effective resuscitation.[59-68] During the low-flow state of CPR, the major determinant of end-tidal CO_2 level is pulmonary blood flow. Pulmonary blood flow, in turn, reflects the cardiac output produced by chest compressions. When the end-tidal CO_2 concentration is less than 10 mm Hg, CPR is inadequate, and the victim almost never survives.[64,65,68] End-tidal CO_2 monitoring can also verify appropriate endotracheal tube placement.[69]

Capnometry during CPR after asphyxial cardiac arrest is somewhat different from that after ventricular fibrillation. Experimental data suggest that the end-tidal CO_2 value may be very high during the first few breaths after an asphyxial cardiac arrest. During asphyxia, alveolar CO_2 may rise, thereby resulting in high end-tidal CO_2 levels for several breaths.[70] After the first few breaths, capnometry reflects pulmonary blood flow and cardiac output and is a useful monitor of the effectiveness of CPR. The administration of sodium bicarbonate during cardiac arrest may increase the end-tidal CO_2 concentration without reflecting any increase in pulmonary blood flow because of increases in the level of pulmonary venous CO_2.[1]

CIRCULATION: CARDIOPULMONARY BYPASS

Dalton et al[71] provided emergency extracorporeal membrane oxygenation (ECMO) to 17 children who suffered cardiac arrest in the pediatric intensive care unit. Of the 17, 11 required CPR for more than 15 minutes and cannulation for ECMO during active CPR lasting 42 to 110 minutes. A total of 6 of these 11 survived to hospital discharge. Rapid emergency provision of ECMO in a well-equipped ECMO-center intensive care unit appears to be an effective adjunct to CPR.

VASCULAR ACCESS

Establishing vascular access during pediatric cardiac arrest is difficult, yet necessary, for the administration of medications and fluids.[1] Theoretically, vascular access into a large vein that drains into the superior vena cava is optimal for the delivery of medications during CPR. The lack of valves in the inferior vena cava results in to-and-fro blood flow during external chest compressions. Valves in the superior vena caval system tend to minimize this problem. Therefore medications infused into the inferior vena caval system can take longer to reach the heart and systemic circulation. In some models, medication administration via the central venous route results in a more rapid onset of action and higher peak concentrations than administration via the peripheral route.[72-75] Any potential minor benefits of central venous or superior vena caval drainage on medication administration are probably less important than the rapid and safe administration of intravascular medication.[1] Inferior venal caval access via the saphenous vein, tibial bone marrow, or femoral vein may be easier and safer than venous access near the head or neck while ventilation and chest compressions are being provided. Medication administered via the peripheral or femoral vein during CPR should probably be followed by a fluid flush to more rapidly move the medications into the central circulation.[76]

Physicians and prehospital personnel can usually attain intraosseous access for pediatric arrest victims in less than 1 minute.[77,78] If reliable vascular access cannot be achieved within 90 seconds, intraosseous vascular access should be established.[1] The technique for intraosseous access is relatively easy and safe. The bone marrow cavity is effectively a noncollapsible vein, even in the presence of shock or cardiac arrest. Although almost any needle can be used, a bone marrow needle with a stylette is recommended to prevent needle obstruction from a core of bony cortex. The proximal tibia, distal femur, and anterior superior iliac spine are all acceptable sites that are easily accessible during resuscitation. The needle should be twisted into, rather than shoved through, the bone marrow. Evidence of successful entry into the bone marrow includes the lack of resistance (or "give") after the needle passes through the cortex, the needle's ability to remain upright without support, aspiration of bone marrow into a syringe, and free flow of the infusion without significant subcutaneous infiltration.[77-79]

Almost any medication that can be administered into a vein can be safely infused into the bone marrow. All medications recommended for pediatric advanced life support can be safely and effectively administered via the intraosseous route. The onset of action of medications and plasma concentrations are similar after intraosseous and peripheral venous administration during CPR.[1,77-79]

Even this relatively safe procedure can result in rare complications. Osteomyelitis, fractures, extravasation of toxic medications (e.g., epinephrine, calcium, sodium bicarbonate), and compartment syndrome with resultant amputation have been described.[1] Microvascular pulmonary fat and bone marrow emboli have been demonstrated but do not appear to be clinically significant.[80]

ENDOTRACHEAL MEDICATION ADMINISTRATION

Endotracheal intubation may be easier to obtain than vascular access during pediatric CPR. Lidocaine, atropine, naloxone, and epinephrine (mnemonic: LANE) are common resuscitation medications that have been successfully administered via the endotracheal tube.[1] On the other hand, sodium bicarbonate and calcium are poorly absorbed and may be very irritating to the airways and lung parenchyma, so they should not be administered via the endotracheal route. Absorption of medications into the circulation after endotracheal administration depends on dispersion over the respiratory mucosa, pulmonary blood flow, and matching of ventilation to perfusion.[81-83] Droplets of medication that remain on the endotracheal tube obviously do not help the patient's condition. Poor cardiac output with inadequate chest compressions results in inadequate pulmonary blood flow and therefore poor delivery of the medication to the heart and systemic circulation. Pulmonary edema, pneumonitis, and airway disease also affect the pharmacokinetics of endotracheally administered medications.[78] The vasoconstrictive effects of epinephrine may limit local pulmonary blood flow and thereby diminish medication uptake and delivery.[84-86]

Case reports and the author's clinical experiences have indicated that endotracheal administration of epinephrine can be effective and lifesaving.[87,88] However, in animal studies, plasma epinephrine concentrations and physiologic effects varied widely after endotracheal administration.[81,85,89,90] An endotracheal epinephrine dose approximately 10 times higher than that reached during intravenous administration is generally needed to obtain peak plasma concentrations. This higher dose is not without danger. After resuscitation, a prolonged depot effect occurs and may result in profound hypertension and tachycardia. After an asphyxial episode, the extra myocardial oxygen demand resulting from tachycardia and the increased afterload may not be well tolerated. On the other hand, the usual intravenous dose of epinephrine is generally ineffective via the endotracheal tube in asystolic adults.[84]

Based on these data, the AHA recommends that any route of vascular medication administration, including intraosseous or peripheral access, is preferable to endotracheal administration.[1] If, however, epinephrine is to be administered via the endotracheal tube during the resuscitation of children, the suggested initial dosage is 10 times the usual intravenous dose. On the other hand, for infants the recommended endotracheal epinephrine dose is the same as the intravenous dose, 0.1 ml/kg of 1:10,000 solution, because the depot effect can result in prolonged severe hypertension, severe hypertension can lead to intracranial hemorrhage in neonates, most neonatal resuscitations are successful with the present recommendations, and there are no data regarding the safety or efficacy of high-dose epinephrine via endotracheal tubes in neonates.

MEDICATIONS

Medications commonly used for CPR in children are epinephrine, atropine, calcium chloride 10%, sodium bicarbonate, and lidocaine. The doses and indications for these medications are listed in Table 22-1.

Table 22-1 Common CPR Medications

MEDICATION	IV DOSE	INDICATIONS
Epinephrine	0.1 ml/kg of 1:10,000 (0.01 mg/kg) Second dose or dose via ETT: 0.1 mg/kg of 1:1,000 (0.1 mg/kg)	Cardiac arrest: asystole, pulseless arrest; symptomatic bradycardia
Atropine	0.2 ml/kg = 0.02 ml/kg (minimum: 0.1 mg; maximum: 1.0 mg)	Symptomatic bradycardia unresponsive to effective oxygenation, ventilation, and treatment with epinephrine
Calcium chloride 10%	0.2 ml/kg = 20 ml/kg	Hypocalcemia, hyperkalemia, hypermagnesemia, calcium channel blocker toxicity
Sodium bicarbonate	1 mEq/kg = 1 ml/kg of 8.4% solution = 0.5 ml/kg of 4.2% solution	Hypercalcemia, tricyclic antidepressant toxicity, severe metabolic acidosis unresponsive to oxygenation and hyperventilation
Lidocaine	1 ml/kg	Symptomatic VT or ventricular ectopy, VF/pulseless VT unresponsive to defibrillation and epinephrine

ETT, Endotracheal tube; *VT,* ventricular tachycardia; *VF,* ventricular fibrillation.

Epinephrine

Epinephrine is an endogenous catecholamine with potent α- and β-adrenergic stimulating properties. The efficacy of epinephrine administration during CPR is directly related to its α-adrenergic effects.[91,92] Arterial vasoconstriction leads to higher aortic diastolic pressure, thereby increasing the coronary perfusion pressure. Higher coronary perfusion pressure results in higher myocardial blood flow and myocardial oxygen delivery. During CPR, epinephrine is a potent peripheral vasoconstrictor but has minimal cerebral vasoconstrictive effects. Therefore during CPR, epinephrine administration results in higher cerebral perfusion pressure, cerebral blood flow, and cerebral oxygen delivery.[93-97] The epinephrine dose recommended for cardiac arrest is 0.1 ml/kg of 1:10,000 solution by the intravenous or intraosseous route (0.01 mg/kg). As previously noted, the recommended dose of epinephrine by the endotracheal route is 0.1 ml/kg of 1:1000 solution (0.1 mg/kg) in children. The effect of catecholamines may be depressed by acidosis and hypoxemia; therefore optimizing ventilation, oxygenation, and circulation is important.[98,99]

Although the efficacy of epinephrine during CPR for cardiac arrest is due to its α-adrenergic properties, some pediatric patients who are pulseless may not be in true cardiac arrest. In these patients, a pulse pressure may not be palpable in the periphery, and the patient may have bradycardia. In such cases, the medication's β-adrenergic–stimulating properties (inotropic and chronotropic effects) may be important.

The optimum dose of epinephrine for cardiac arrest in children or adults is not well established. Studies in animals and people suggest that much higher doses can improve coronary and cerebral blood flow and perfusion pressures.[93,94,96,97,100] Unfortunately, randomized controlled trials in animals and humans have been less promising with regard to improving survival and neurologic outcome with higher doses of epinephrine.[101-105] Studies in animals suggest that high doses sometimes cause a lethal toxic hyperadrenergic state immediately after the return of spontaneous circulation.[106] High epinephrine doses can also cause increased postresuscitation myocardial dysfunction[107] and histopathologic evidence of myocardial necrosis.[108] Wide interpatient variability in catecholamine pharmacokinetics and pharmacodynamics is well established for critically ill and normal children.[109-111] Similar intersubject variability exists in those resuscitated during cardiac arrest.[112-115] A lifesaving dose for one patient may be life threatening to another.

The AHA recommendations for second and subsequent doses of epinephrine have been somewhat inconsistent. For adults the AHA recommends the following[1]:

1. The second and subsequent doses should be either the same as the first dose (1 mg), or escalating doses of 1, 3, and 5 mg should be provided every 3 to 5 minutes.
2. An intermediate epinephrine dose of 2 to 5 mg should be provided every 3 to 5 minutes, or a high dose (0.1 mg/kg) should be provided every 3 to 5 minutes.

The AHA classifies these recommendations as class IIb, indicating that they are "acceptable, possibly helpful." In contradistinction, the epinephrine dosage recommendations for second and subsequent epinephrine doses in children, whether intravenous, intraosseous, or endotracheal, are 0.1 mg/kg (0.1 ml/kg of 1:1000 solution). Finally, neonatal recommendations are the most conservative: 0.01 mg/kg (0.1 ml/kg of 1:10,000 solution) for all doses.

Clearly the therapeutic endpoint regarding epinephrine dosage during CPR for cardiac arrest is adequate myocardial oxygen delivery. If a patient is in the pediatric intensive care unit and arterial and central venous pressures are monitored continuously, the epinephrine dosage should be titrated to an adequate coronary perfusion pressure (aortic diastolic pressure minus central venous diastolic pressure). If the coronary perfusion pressure is less than 15 to 25 mm Hg and CPR is unsuccessful, more effective chest compressions or a higher epinephrine dose may be indicated. Once the coronary perfusion pressure is maintained at a level higher than 25 mm Hg, higher doses of epinephrine are probably unnecessary and may be harmful.

Epinephrine infiltration into subcutaneous tissue may result in severe local ischemia and ulceration. Therefore epinephrine should be infused through a secure intravenous line, preferably into the central circulation. Epinephrine is inactivated in alkaline solutions and thus should not be mixed with sodium bicarbonate. The adverse effects of epinephrine include tachycardia, severe hypertension, ventricular ectopy, and excessive vasoconstriction compromising organ blood flow.

Atropine

Atropine is a parasympatholytic agent that accelerates sinus and atrial pacemakers and increases atrioventricular conduction. Severe bradycardia or ventricular asystole commonly results from hypoxia, ischemia, or both conditions. The efficacy of atropine therapy in the treatment of these rhythms is unclear. The AHA recommends providing adequate oxygenation and ventilation first and then administering epinephrine for severe bradycardia or ventricular asystole secondary to hypoxic-ischemic events. Atropine is recommended for the uncommon event of symptomatic bradycardia with atrioventricular block. In addition, atropine is recommended to prevent vagally mediated bradycardia during attempts at endotracheal intubation.

The recommended dose of atropine is 0.02 mg/kg with a minimum dose of 0.1 mg and a maximum dose of 0.5 mg in a child and a maximum dose of 1.0 mg in an adolescent. The dose may be repeated in 5 minutes to a maximum of 1.0 mg in children and 2.0 mg in adolescents.[1]

Calcium

Calcium has an essential intermediary role in myocardial and vascular smooth muscle excitation-contraction coupling. Increases in calcium tend to enhance the systolic function and impair the diastolic function of the myocardium. Also, increases in calcium raise systolic vascular resistance via contraction of vascular smooth muscle. However, increases in intracellular calcium levels have been implicated as an active mediator of cell death. Calcium administration has not been shown to improve outcome from cardiac arrest.[116-118] Therefore the AHA does not recommend routine administration of calcium in the resuscitation of asystolic patients.[1] Calcium is recommended for the treatment of documented hypocalcemia and should be considered for the treatment of hyperkalemia, hypermagnesemia, and overdose from calcium channel blockers.

The AHA recommends a dose of 5 to 7 mg/kg of elemental calcium despite limited information regarding optimum dosage.[1] Calcium chloride (10%) provides slightly greater bioavailability of calcium than calcium gluconate. A total of

0.2 ml/kg of 10% calcium chloride (i.e., 20 mg/kg) by slow infusion is recommended and may be repeated in 10 minutes if required.

Sodium Bicarbonate

Metabolic acidosis often accompanies cardiac arrest. Catecholamines are less effective during metabolic acidosis.[98,99] However, most studies have failed to demonstrate that administration of sodium bicarbonate improves the outcome of cardiac arrest. The highest treatment priorities for the infant or child in cardiac arrest include provision of oxygenation, ventilation, and restoration of effective systemic perfusion. After the effectiveness of these factors is ensured and epinephrine has been provided, sodium bicarbonate may be considered for the patient in prolonged cardiac arrest.

Sodium bicarbonate may have several adverse effects. Hypernatremia and hyperosmolarity may result from excessive administration. The acute hyperosmolarity may decrease systemic vascular resistance and thereby decrease coronary perfusion pressure. In premature babies, acute administration of hyperosmolar solutions may result in intracranial hemorrhage. Administration of sodium bicarbonate without adequate ventilation may transiently elevate CO_2 tension and worsen preexisting respiratory acidosis.

An important practical matter during cardiac arrest is physicochemical medication incompatibility. Frequently the patient has only one venous access site. Administration of bicarbonate can inactivate catecholamines, and more important, calcium precipitates when mixed with bicarbonate. Therefore intravenous tubing must be carefully irrigated before and after infusions of sodium bicarbonate. Excessive administration of sodium bicarbonate may result in metabolic alkalosis, producing a leftward shift of the oxyhemoglobin dissociation curve with impaired oxygen delivery. Excessive administration of sodium bicarbonate may also result in an acute intracellular shift of potassium, a decreased plasma ionized calcium concentration, a decreased ventricular fibrillation threshold, and impaired cardiac function. The AHA suggests that sodium bicarbonate be considered when shock is associated with documented metabolic acidosis.[1] However, the AHA notes that this is a class IIb recommendation (i.e., it is "acceptable and possibly helpful"). If sodium bicarbonate is used, the initial dose recommendation is 1 mEq/kg (1 ml/kg of 8.4% solution) via the intravenous or intraosseous route. A dilute solution (0.5 mEq/ml) may be used in neonates.[1]

Lidocaine

Lidocaine is the antidysrhythmic medication of choice for the treatment of ventricular ectopy, ventricular tachycardia, and ventricular fibrillation. Lidocaine suppresses ventricular ectopy and raises the threshold for ventricular fibrillation.[1] The recommended dose is 1.0 mg/kg intravenously. During cardiac arrest, only bolus infusions should be used. When prolonged therapy with lidocaine is necessary to suppress ventricular ectopy, a continuous intravenous infusion of 20 to 50 μg/kg/min is recommended.[1]

The toxic-to-therapeutic ratio of lidocaine is narrow. Myocardial and circulatory depression are important toxic effects. Central nervous system toxicity may also occur, producing slurred speech, altered consciousness, muscle twitching, and seizures. Lidocaine clearance is reduced in the presence of shock, congestive heart failure, and cardiac arrest; therefore lidocaine infusion rates should not be greater than 20 μg/kg/min in such circumstances.

Oxygen

High-concentration oxygen, preferably 100%, should be administered as soon as possible to all patients in cardiac arrest. This increases arterial oxygen tension and hemoglobin saturation if ventilation is supported and improves tissue oxygenation when circulation also is maintained.

Dopamine

Dopamine hydrochloride is a chemical precursor of norepinephrine with α-agonist and β-agonist activity. In addition, specific dopaminergic receptors dilate renal and mesenteric blood vessels at low doses. Dopamine has direct agonist effects on both types of receptors and acts indirectly by increasing the norepinephrine concentration in synaptic clefts.[1,119]

Dopamine appears to be less effective than epinephrine at improving hemodynamics during CPR. However, dopamine may be effective in preventing cardiac arrest in patients with shock or in treating postresuscitation myocardial dysfunction. There is a wide interpatient variability in dopamine pharmacokinetics and pharmacodynamics. Generally, infusions of dopamine initially stimulate dopaminergic receptors to dilate the renal and mesenteric blood vessels, whereas higher doses have predominantly β-adrenergic effects with increased heart rate and myocardial contractility. The highest dopamine infusion rates cause prominent α-agonist activity, resulting in peripheral vasoconstriction and increased blood pressure. Doses as low as 0.5 μg/kg/min produce increases in cardiac output in many pediatric patients. The appropriate dopamine infusion rate must be titered to the desired effect. Generally, doses between 2 and 20 μg/kg/min result in improved cardiac output.[1,119,120]

The adverse effects of dopamine are similar to those of epinephrine: tachycardia, hypertension, ventricular ectopy, excessive systemic vasoconstriction, and excessive pulmonary vasoconstriction. Dopamine should not be mixed with sodium bicarbonate because the dopamine may be slowly inactivated.

Dobutamine

Dobutamine hydrochloride is a synthetic catecholamine with predominantly β-agonist activity. Because dobutamine has minimal α-agonist effects, it is of no use during CPR for cardiac arrest. However, its potent inotropic activity may be helpful in preventing cardiac arrest in children with myocardial dysfunction.[109-111] Dobutamine is also a useful agent in the treatment of postresuscitation myocardial dysfunction.[121,122]

There is wide interpatient variability with regard to dobutamine's pharmacokinetics and pharmacodynamics. The recommended dose range according to the AHA is 2 to 20 μg/kg/min, although doses as low as 0.5 μg/kg/min frequently improve myocardial function.[1,109]

Intravenous Fluids

In animal models of cardiac arrest, fluid resuscitation is not beneficial during CPR if the animal was volume replete before the cardiac arrest. However, intravascular volume depletion is not rare among children in cardiac arrest. In particular, children with severe dehydration, septic shock, and trauma frequently have intravascular volume depletion. These patients may be pulseless because of inadequate cardiac preload. Fluid resuscitation alone or fluid resuscitation with catecholamine infusions may save the child's life in such circumstances. Volume resuscitation may be provided with either crystalloid solutions (normal saline or Ringer's lactate) or colloid solutions (5% albumin). The administration of 20 ml/kg intravenous volume boluses of crystalloid solution are recommended for children with trauma and circulatory collapse. After 40 ml/kg of crystalloid solutions are infused, a 10 ml/kg red blood cell transfusion is recommended.[1]

Volume resuscitation should not be provided with hypotonic solutions or solutions containing dextrose. Hypotonic solutions rapidly disperse through the extravascular and intracellular spaces and therefore result in less effective intravascular volume repletion. In addition, hypotonic solutions may result in hyponatremia with resultant cerebral edema. Resuscitation with a dextrose-containing solution may lead to hyperglycemia and counterproductive osmotic diuresis. Hyperglycemia has been implicated as a mediator of worse neurologic outcome after cardiac arrest.[1]

APPROACH TO THE APNEIC, PULSELESS, AND UNRESPONSIVE CHILD

The initial diagnostic approach to an unresponsive child is to evaluate the airway, breathing, and circulation (ABC). If the child is apneic and pulseless, basic life support should be provided immediately. As soon as possible, the cardiac rhythm should be confirmed in more than one lead.

If the patient has asystole, CPR should be continued. As soon as possible an endotracheal tube should be placed and the patient's lungs hyperventilated with 100% oxygen. Intravenous or intraosseous access should be promptly provided. A total of 0.1 ml/kg of 1:10,000 epinephrine should be infused via the intravenous or intraosseous route. When no vascular access is available, 0.1 ml/kg of 1:1000 epinephrine may be instilled via the endotracheal tube. If the patient has not been successfully resuscitated within 3 minutes, rescuers should first ensure that chest compressions are adequate and then may provide up to 0.1 ml/kg of 1:1000 epinephrine (0.1 mg/kg) every 3 to 5 minutes.

If there is electrical activity on the electrocardiogram (i.e., pulseless electrical activity, previously known as *electromechanical dissociation*), the rescuers should attempt to identify and treat potential causes while continuing to provide effective CPR. In particular, hypoxemia, severe acidosis, severe hypovolemia, tension pneumothorax, cardiac tamponade, and profound hypothermia should be considered possible causes.

If the patient has ventricular fibrillation or pulseless ventricular tachycardia, defibrillation must be provided as soon as possible. The recommended dose for initial defibrillation is 2 joules/kg. If this is not effective, the patient should immediately receive 4 joules/kg twice in succession, if necessary. If the patient does not respond to electroshock therapy, rescuers should continue effective CPR, secure an endotracheal tube airway, hyperventilate with 100% oxygen, and attempt to obtain vascular access. As soon as possible after attempts to defibrillate, epinephrine should be provided at 0.1 ml/kg of 1:10,000 solution (0.01 mg/kg) by the intravenous or intraosseous route. Alternatively, 0.1 ml/kg of 1:1,000 solution (0.1 mg/kg) may be provided via the endotracheal tube. Approximately 30 to 60 seconds after epinephrine infusion, electroshock therapy with 4 joules/kg may be provided. If this is unsuccessful, 1.0 mg/kg of lidocaine may be infused by the intravenous or intraosseous route, followed 30 to 60 seconds later by another attempt at defibrillation with 4 joules/kg. Epinephrine doses should be repeated every 3 to 5 minutes, and the AHA recommends that the second and subsequent doses be provided at 0.1 ml/kg of 1:1000 solution (0.1 mg/kg).

SYMPTOMATIC BRADYCARDIA

Bradycardia may result in poor cardiac output despite normal blood pressure. In initially assessing a child with severe bradycardia, the rescuer should establish that airway function, ventilation, and oxygenation (ABC) are adequate. If the child has severe cardiorespiratory compromise (poor perfusion, hypotension, and respiratory difficulties), chest compressions are recommended when the heart rate is less than 80 beats/min in an infant or less than 60 beats/min in a child. Intravenous or intraosseous access should be obtained, and 0.01 mg/kg of epinephrine should be infused (0.1 ml/kg of 1:10,000 solution). Epinephrine doses should be repeated every 3 to 5 minutes during CPR. If the severe cardiorespiratory compromise does not respond to these measures, treatment with atropine 0.02 mg/kg (minimum dose of 0.1 mg and maximum dose of 0.5 mg for a child, 1.0 mg for an adolescent) may be considered.

POSTRESUSCITATION MYOCARDIAL DYSFUNCTION

Postresuscitation myocardial dysfunction is well described in children after hypoxic-ischemic events and cardiac arrest.[121,122] These patients benefit from treatment with inotropic support. Recent studies in animals demonstrate myocardial dysfunction at 2 and 5 hours after cardiac arrest, which improves within 24 hours.[123] Dobutamine infusion can ameliorate the myocardial dysfunction.[121-123] Persistent circulatory dysfunction after cardiac arrest may also result from insufficient intravascular volume and loss of peripheral vascular tone, which can be treated with fluid resuscitation and vasoactive agents, respectively. Prevention of secondary insults is a hallmark of critical care management.

OUTCOME

The outcome of pediatric cardiac arrests in hospitals is discouraging. Although more than 50% of patients who are apneic and pulseless undergo successful initial resuscitation, only 9% to 33% survive to discharge.[2-4,6-8,10] Outcomes from cardiac arrests in the prehospital settings are even more dismal.

Research in animal models clearly demonstrates that successful resuscitation from cardiac arrest depends on the duration of the cardiac arrest before CPR is provided, establishment of adequate myocardial blood flow with CPR, and early defibrillation in the case of ventricular fibrillation.[34,53,83,85,112] Similarly, clinical research indicates that the success of CPR improves when the cardiac arrest is witnessed, bystander CPR is provided, adequate coronary perfusion pressures are obtained, the initial rhythm is ventricular fibrillation, and early defibrillation is provided in the case of ventricular fibrillation.[47,124-127] Although most of these clinical data are from studies in adults, the limited information available regarding children in cardiac arrest is consistent with these findings.[4,14,18,20]

PREVENTION OF CARDIAC ARREST

Many of the causes of cardiac arrest in children, such as motor vehicle accidents, submersions, bicycle accidents, firearm accidents, and falls from buildings, are preventable. These events are eminently preventable with safer cars, passive restraints, safer pool area designs, safely fenced pool areas, bicycle helmets, and limitations on the availability of firearms. In addition, many children in cardiac arrests initially have hemodynamic shock, respiratory failure, or septic shock. Improved prehospital care, earlier treatment, and more effective treatment may prevent cardiac arrest.

REFERENCES

1. Emergency Cardiac Care Committee and Subcommittees, American Heart Association: Guidelines for cardiopulmonary resuscitation and emergency cardiac care, *JAMA* 268:2171-2298, 1992.
2. Ehrlich R, Emmett SM, Rodriguez-Torres R: Pediatric cardiac resuscitation team: a six year study, *J Pediatr* 84:152-155, 1974.
3. DeBard ML: Cardiopulmonary resuscitation: analysis of six years' experience and review of the literature, *Ann Emerg Med* 10:408-416, 1981.
4. Friesen RM, Duncan P, Tweed WA, Bristow G: Appraisal of pediatric cardiopulmonary resuscitation, *Can Med Assoc J* 126:1055-1058, 1982.
5. Lewis JK, Minter MG, Eshelman SJ, Witte MK: Outcome of pediatric resuscitation, *Ann Emerg Med* 12:297-299, 1983.
6. Gillis J, Dickson D, Rieder M, Steward D, Edwards J: Results of inpatient pediatric resuscitation, *Crit Care Med* 14:469-471, 1986.
7. Wark H, Overton JH: A paediatric "cardiac arrest" survey, *Br J Anaesth* 56:1271-1274, 1984.
8. Ludwig S, Kettrick RG, Parker M: Pediatric cardiopulmonary resuscitation, *Clin Pediatr* 23:71-85, 1984.
9. Nichols DG, Kettrick RG, Dwedlow DB, Lee S, Passman R, Ludwig S: Factors influencing outcome of cardiopulmonary resuscitation in children, *Pediatr Emerg Care* 2:1-5, 1986.
10. Zaritsky A, Nadkarni V, Geston P, Fuenl K: CPR in children, *Ann Emerg Med* 16:1107-1111, 1987.
11. von Seggern K, Egar M, Fuhrman BP: Cardiopulmonary resuscitation in a pediatric ICU, *Crit Care Med* 14:275-277, 1986.
12. Bos AP, Polman A, Vander Voort E, Tibboel D: Cardiopulmonary resuscitation in paediatric intensive care patients, *Intensive Care Med* 18:109-111, 1992.
13. Eisenberg M, Bergner L, Hallstrom A: Epidemiology of cardiac arrest and resuscitation in children, *Ann Emerg Med* 12:672-674, 1983.
14. Torphy DE, Minter MG, Thompson BM: Cardiorespiratory arrest and resuscitation in children, *Am J Dis Child* 138:1099-1102, 1984.
15. Rosenberg NM: Pediatric cardiopulmonary arrest in the emergency department, *Am J Emerg Med* 2:497-499, 1984.
16. Losek JD, Hennes H, Glaeser PW, Hendley G, Nelson DB: Prehospital care of the pulseless, nonbreathing pediatric patient, *Am J Emerg Med* 5:370-374, 1987.
17. Tsai A, Kallsen G: Epidemiology of pediatric prehospital care, *Ann Emerg Med* 16:284-292, 1987.
18. Fiser DH, Wrape V: Outcome of cardiopulmonary resuscitation in children, *Pediatr Emerg Care* 3:235-237, 1987.
19. Thompson JE, Bonner B, Lower GM: Pediatric cardiopulmonary arrests in rural populations, *Pediatrics* 86:302-306, 1990.
20. O'Rourke PP: Outcome of children who are apneic and pulseless in the emergency room, *Crit Care Med* 14:466-468, 1986.

Epidemiology

21. Hickey RW, Cohen DM, Strausbaugh S, Dietrich AM: Pediatric patients requiring CPR in the prehospital setting, *Ann Emerg Med* 25(4):495-501, 1995.
22. Appleton GO, Cummins RO, Larson MP, Graves JR: CPR and the single rescuer: at what age should you "call first" rather than "call fast"? *Ann Emerg Med* 25(4):492-494, 1995.
23. Mogayzel C, Quan L, Graves JR, Tiedeman D, Fahrenbruch C, Herndon P: Out-of-hospital ventricular fibrillation in children and adolescents: causes and outcomes, *Ann Emerg Med* 25(4):484-491, 1995.
24. Hazinski MF: Is pediatric resuscitation unique? Relative merits of early CPR and ventilation versus early defibrillation for young victims of prehospital cardiac arrest, *Ann Emerg Med* 25(4):540-543, 1995.
25. Berg RA, Kern KB, Otto CW, Samson RA, Sanders AB, Ewy GA: Ventricular fibrillation in a swine model of acute pediatric asphyxial cardiac arrest, *Resuscitation* 33:147-153, 1996.

Physiology of CPR

26. Maier GW, Tyson GS Jr, Olsen CO, Keienstein KH, Davis JW, Conn EH, Sabiston DC Jr, Rankin JS: The physiology of external cardiac massage: high impulse cardiopulmonary resuscitation, *Circulation* 70:86-101, 1984.
27. Feneley MP, Maier GW, Kern KB: Influence of compression rate on initial success of resuscitation and 24-hour survival after prolonged manual cardiopulmonary resuscitation in dogs, *Circulation* 77:240-250, 1988.
28. Criley JM, Blaufuss AH, Kissel GL: Cough-induced cardiac compression: self-administered form of cardiopulmonary resuscitation, *JAMA* 236:1246-1250, 1976.
29. Weale FE, Rothwell-Jackson RL: The efficiency of cardiac massage, *Lancet* 1:990-992, 1962.
30. Connick M, Berg RA: Femoral venous pulsations during open-chest cardiac massage, *Ann Emerg Med* 24:1176-1179, 1994.
31. Deshmukh HG, Weil MH, Gudipati CV, Trevino RP, Bisera J, Rackow EC: Mechanism of blood flow generated by precordial compression during CPR. I. Studies on closed chest precordial compression, *Chest* 95:1092-1099, 1989.
32. Higano ST, Oh JK, Ewy GA, Seward JB: The mechanism of blood flow during closed chest cardiac massage in humans: transesophageal echocardiographic observations, *Mayo Clin Proc* 65:1432-1440, 1990.
33. Kuhn C, Juchems R, Frese W: Evidence for the "cardiac pump theory" in cardiopulmonary resuscitation in man by transesophageal echocardiography, *Resuscitation* 22:275-282, 1991.
34. Dean JM, Koehler RC, Schleien CL, Atchison D, Gervais H, Berkowitz I, Traystman R: Improved blood flow during prolonged cardiopulmonary resuscitation with 30% duty cycle in infant pigs, *Circulation* 84:896-904, 1991.
35. Schleien CL, Dean JM, Koehler RC, Michael JR, Chantarojansiri T, Traystman R, Rogers M: Effect of epinephrine on cerebral and myocardial perfusion in an infant animal preparation of cardiopulmonary resuscitation, *Circulation* 73:809-817, 1986.

Pediatric Basic Life Support

36. Cavallaro DL, Melker RJ: Comparison of two techniques for detecting cardiac activity in infants, *Crit Care Med* 11:189-190, 1983.
37. Lee CJ, Bullock LJ: Determining the pulse for infant CPR: time for a change? *Mil Med* 156:190-199, 1991.
38. Kisting M, Goetting MG: The misdiagnosis of pediatric cardiac arrest: pseudo-electromechanical dissociation in children, *Acad Emerg Med* 1:A87, 1994 (abstract).
39. Paradis NA, Martin GB, Goetting MG, Rivers EP, Feingold M, Nowak RM: Aortic pressure during human cardiac arrest: identification of human pseudo-electromechanical dissociation, *Chest* 101:123-128, 1992.
40. King BR, Baker MD, Braitman LE, Seidl-Friedman J, Schreiner MS: Endotracheal tube selection in children: a comparison of four methods, *Ann Emerg Med* 22:530-534, 1993.
41. Luten RC, Wears RL, Broselow J, Zaritsky A, Barnett TM, Lee T, Bailey A, Vally R, Brown R, Rosenthal B: Length based endotracheal tube selection in pediatrics, *Ann Emerg Med* 21:900-904, 1992.
42. Lubitz PS, Seidel JS, Chamedes L, Luten RC, Zaritsky AL, Campbell FW: A rapid method for estimating weight and resuscitation medication dosages from length in the pediatric age group, *Ann Emerg Med* 17:576-581, 1988.
43. Todres ID, de Bros F, Kramer SS, Moylan FMB, Shannon DC: Endotracheal tube displacement in the newborn infant, *J Pediatr* 57:126-127, 1976.
44. Donn SM, Kuhn LR: Mechanism of endotracheal tube movement with change of head position in the neonate, *Pediatr Radiol* 9:939-940, 1980.

45. Michael JR, Guerci AD, Koehler RC, Shi AY, Tsitlik J, Chandra N, Niedermeyer E, Rogers MC, Traystman RJ, Weisfeldt ML: Mechanisms by which epinephrine augments cerebral and myocardial perfusion during cardiopulmonary resuscitation in dogs, *Circulation* 69:822-835, 1984.
46. Halpern HR, Helperin HR, Tsitlik JE, Guerci AD, Mellits ED, Levin HR, Shi AY, Chandra N, Weisfeldt: Determinants of blood flow to vital organs during cardiopulmonary resuscitation in dogs, *Circulation* 73:539-550, 1986.
47. Sanders AB, Ewy GA, Taft T: Prognostic and therapeutic importance of the aortic diastolic pressure in resuscitation from cardiac arrest, *Crit Care Med* 12:871-873, 1984.
48. Paradis NA, Martin GB, Rivers EP: Coronary perfusion pressure and the return of spontaneous circulation in human cardiopulmonary resuscitation, *JAMA* 263:1106-1113, 1990.
49. Kern KB, Sanders AB, Raife J, Milander MM, Otto CW, Ewy GA: A study of chest compression rates during cardiopulmonary resuscitation in humans: the importance of rate-directed chest compressions, *Arch Intern Med* 152:145-149, 1992.
50. Berg RA, Sanders AB, Milander M, Tellez D, Liu P, Beyda D: Efficacy of audio-prompted rate guidance in improving resuscitator performance of cardiopulmonary resuscitation on children, *Acad Emerg Med* 1:35-40, 1994.
51. Milander MM, Hiscok PS, Sanders AB, Kern KB, Berg RA, Ewy GA: Effects of audible tone-guided chest compressions on hemodynamics of cardiopulmonary resuscitation, *Circulation* 86:1-235, 1992.
52. Menegazzi JJ, Auble TE, Nicklas KA, Hosack GM, Rack L, Goode JS: Two-thumb versus two-finger chest compression during CPR in a swine infant model of cardiac arrest, *Ann Emerg Med* 22:240-243, 1993.
53. Todres ID, Rogers MC: Methods of external cardiac massage in the newborn infant, *J Pediatr* 86:781-782, 1975.
54. David R: Closed chest cardiac massage in the newborn infant, *Pediatrics* 81:552-554, 1988.
55. Thaler MM, Stobie GHC: An improved technique of external cardiac compression in infants and young children, *N Engl J Med* 269:606-610, 1963.
56. Niemann JT, Criley JM, Rosenborough JP, Niskanen RA, Alferness C: Predictive indices of successful cardiac resuscitation after prolonged arrest and experimental cardiopulmonary resuscitation, *Ann Emerg Med* 14(6):521-528, 1985.
57. Kern KB: Retrograde coronary blood flow during cardiopulmonary resuscitation: an intracoronary Doppler evaluation, *Am Heart J* 128:490-499, 1994.
58. Niemann JT, Rosborough JP, Hausknecht M, Garner D, Criley JM: Pressure-synchronized cineangiography during experimental cardiopulmonary resuscitation, *Circulation* 64:985-991, 1981.
59. Sanders AB, Atlas M, Ewy GA, Kern KB, Bragg S: Expired CO_2 as an index of coronary perfusion pressure, *Am J Emerg Med* 3:147-149, 1985.
60. Weil MH, Bisera J, Trevino RP, Rackow EC: Cardiac output and end-tidal carbon dioxide, *Crit Care Med* 13:907-909, 1985.
61. Garnett AR, Ornato JP, Gonzalez ER, Johnson EB: End-tidal carbon dioxide monitoring during cardiopulmonary resuscitation, *JAMA* 257:512-515, 1987.
62. Gudipati CV, Weil MH, Bisera J, Deshmukh HG, Rackow EC: Expired carbon dioxide: a noninvasive monitor of cardiopulmonary resuscitation, 77:234-239, 1988.
63. Kern KB, Sanders AB, Voorhees WD, Babbs CF, Tackee WA, Ewy GA: Changes in expired end-tidal carbon dioxide during cardiopulmonary resuscitation in dogs: a prognostic guide for resuscitation efforts, *J Am Coll Cardiol* 13:1184-1189, 1989.
64. Sanders AB, Ewy GA, Braggs S, Atlas M, Kern KB: Expired Pco_2 as a prognostic indicator of successful resuscitation from cardiac arrest, *Ann Emerg Med* 14:948-952, 1985.
65. Sanders AB, Bern KB, Otto CW, Milander MM, Ewy GA: End-tidal carbon dioxide monitoring during cardiopulmonary resuscitation, *JAMA* 262:1347-1351, 1989.
66. Falk JL, Rackow EC, Weil MH: End-tidal carbon dioxide concentration during cardiopulmonary resuscitation, *N Engl J Med* 318:607-611, 1988.
67. Ornato JP, Garnett AR, Glausser FL: Relationship between cardiac output and the end-tidal carbon dioxide tension, *Ann Emerg Med* 19:1104-1105, 1990.
68. Callaham M, Barton C: Prediction of outcome of cardiopulmonary resuscitation from end-tidal carbon dioxide concentration, *Crit Care Med* 18:358-362, 1990.
69. Bhende MS, Thompson AE: Evaluation of an end-tidal CO_2 detector during pediatric cardiopulmonary resuscitation, *Pediatrics* 95:395-399, 1995.
70. Berg RA, Henry C, Otto CW, Sanders AB, Kernk B, Hilwig RW, Ewy GA: Initial end-tidal CO_2 is markedly elevated during cardiopulmonary resuscitation after asphyxial cardiac arrest, *Ped Emerg Care* 12(4):245-248, 1996.

Circulation: Cardiopulmonary Bypass

71. Dalton HG, Siewers RD, Fuhrman BP, Nido PD, Thompson AE, Shaver MG, Dowhy M: Extracorporeal membrane oxygenation for cardiac rescue in children with severe myocardial dysfunction, *Crit Care Med* 21:1020-1028, 1993.

Vascular Access

72. Emerman CL, Pinchak AC, Hancock D, Hagen JF: Effect of injection site on circulation times during cardiac arrest, *Crit Care Med* 16:1138-1141, 1988.
73. Kuhn GJ, White BC, Swetnam RE, Mumey JF, Rydesky MF, Tintinalli JE, Krome RL, Hoehner P: Peripheral versus central circulation time during CPR: a pilot study, *Ann Emerg Med* 10:417-419, 1981.
74. Barsan WG, Levy RC, Weir H: Lidocaine levels during CPR: differences after peripheral venous, central venous, and intra-cardiac injections, *Ann Emerg Med* 10:73-78, 1981.
75. Hedges JR, Barsan WB, Doan LA, Joyce SM, Lukes SJ, Dalsey WC, Nishiyama H: Central versus peripheral intravenous routes in cardiopulmonary resuscitation, *Am J Emerg Med* 2(5):385-390, 1981.
76. Emerman CL, Pinchak AC, Hancock D, Hagen JF: The effect of bolus injection on circulation times during cardiac arrest, *Am J Emerg Med* 8:190-193, 1990.
77. Fiser DH: Intraosseous infusion, *N Engl J Med* 322:1579-1581, 1990.
78. Spivey WH: Intraosseous infusions, *J Pediatr* 111:639-643, 1987.
79. Berg RA: Emergency infusion of catecholamines into bone marrow, *Am J Dis Child* 138:810-811, 1984.
80. Orlowski JP, Julius CJ, Petras RE, Porembka DT, Gallagher JM: The safety of intraosseous infusions: risks of fat and bone marrow emboli to the lungs, *Ann Emerg Med* 18:1062-1067, 1989.

Endotracheal Medication Administration

81. Hahnel JH, Lindner KH, Ahnefeld FKW: Endobronchial administration of emergency drugs, *Resuscitation* 7:261-272, 1989.
82. Elam JO: The intrapulmonary route for CPR drugs. In Safar P, ed: *Advances in cardiopulmonary resuscitation,* New York, 1977, Springer-Verlag, p 132-140.
83. Mace SE: Effect of technique of administration on plasma lidocaine levels, *Ann Emerg Med* 15:552-556, 1986.
84. Quinton DN, O'Byrne G, Aitkenhead AR: Comparison of endotracheal and peripheral intravenous adrenaline cardiac arrest: is the endotracheal route reliable? *Lancet* 1:828-829, 1987.
85. Orlowski JP, Gallagher JM, Porembka DT: Endotracheal epinephrine is unreliable, *Resuscitation* 19:102-113, 1990.
86. Tang W, Weil MH, Gazmuri RJ, Sun S, Duggal C, Bisera J: Pulmonary ventilation/perfusion defects induced by epinephrine during cardiopulmonary resuscitation, *Circulation* 84:2101-2107, 1991.
87. Greenberg MI, Roberts JR, Baskin SI: Use of endotracheally administered epinephrine in a pediatric patients, *Am J Dis Child* 135:767-768, 1991.
88. Lindemann R: Resuscitation of the newborn: endotracheal administration of epinephrine, *Acta Paediatr Scand* 73:210-212, 1984.
89. Ralston SH, Tacker WA, Showen L, Carter A, Babbs CF: Endotracheal versus intravenous epinephrine during electromechanical dissociation with CPR in dogs, *Ann Emerg Med* 14:1044-1048, 1985.
90. Hornchen U, Schuttler J, Stoeckel H, Eichelkraut W, Hahn N: Endobronchial instillation of epinephrine during cardiopulmonary resuscitation, *Crit Care Med* 15:1037-1039, 1987.

Medications

91. Redding JS, Pearson JW: Evaluation of drugs for cardiac resuscitation, *Anesthesiology* 24:203-207, 1963.
92. Otto CW, Yakaitis RW, Blitt CD: Mechanism of action of epinephrine in resuscitation from asphyxial arrest, *Crit Care Med* 9:321-324, 1993.

93. Brown CG, Werman HA, Davis EA, Hobson J, Hamlin RL: The effect of graded doses of epinephrine on regional myocardial blood flow during cardiopulmonary resuscitation in swine, *Circulation* 75:491-497, 1987.
94. Kosnik JW, Jackson RE, Keats S, Tworek RM, Freeman SB: Dose-related response of centrally administered epinephrine on the change in aortic diastolic pressure during closed-chest massage in dogs, *Ann Emerg Med* 14:204-208, 1985.
95. Ralston SHJ, Voorhees WD, Babbs CF: Intrapulmonary epinephrine during prolonged cardiopulmonary resuscitation: improved regional blood flow and resuscitation in dogs, *Ann Emerg Med* 13:79-86, 1984.
96. Chase PB, Kern KB, Sanders AB, Otto CW, Ewy GA: Effects of graded doses of epinephrine on both noninvasive and invasive measures of myocardial perfusion and blood flow during cardiopulmonary resuscitation, *Crit Care Med* 21:413-419, 1993.
97. Berkowitz ID, Gervais H, Schleien CL, Koehler RC, Dean JM, Traystman RJ: Epinephrine dosage effects on cerebral and myocardial blood flow in an infant swine model of cardiopulmonary resuscitation, *Anesthesiology* 75:L1041-L1050, 1991.
98. Stokke DB, Anderson PK, Brinklov MN, Nedergaard OA, Hole P, Rasmussen N: Acid-base interactions with noradrenaline-induced contractile response of the rabbit isolated aorta, *Anesthesiology* 60:400-404, 1984.
99. Cingolani HF, Faulkner SL, Mattiazzi AR, Bender HW, Graham TP: Depression of human myocardial contractility with "respiratory" and "metabolic" acidosis, *Surgery* 77:427-432, 1975.
100. Gonzales ER, Ornato JP, Garnett AR, Levine R, Young DS, Tacht EM: Dose-dependent vasopressor response to epinephrine during CPR in human beings, *Ann Emerg Med* 18:920-926, 1989.
101. Stiell IG, Hebert PC, Weitzman BN, Wells GA, Raman S, Stark RI, Higginson LA, Ahuja J, Dickinson GE: High-dose epinephrine in adult cardiac arrest, *N Engl J Med* 327:1045-1050, 1992.
102. Brown CG, Martin DR, Pepe PE, Steuven H, Cummins RO, Gonzalez E, Jastremski M: A comparison of standard-dose and high-dose epinephrine in cardiac arrest outside the hospital, *N Engl J Med* 327:1051-1055, 1992.
103. Callaham ML, Madsen CD, Barton CW, Saunders CE, Pointer J: A randomized clinical trial of high-dose epinephrine and norepinephrine vs. standard-dose epinephrine in prehospital cardiac arrest, *JAMA* 268:2667-2772, 1992.
104. Lindner KH, Ahnefeld KFW, Prengal AW: Comparison of standard and high-dose adrenaline in the resuscitation of asystole and electromechanical dissociation, *Anaesthesiol Scand* 35:253-256, 1991.
105. Lipman J, Wilson W, Kobilski S, Scribante J, Lee C, Kraus P, Cooper J, Barr J, Moyes D: High-dose adrenaline in adult in-hospital asystolic cardiopulmonary resuscitation: a double-blind randomised trial, *Anaesth Intens Care* 21:192-196, 1993.
106. Berg RA, Otto CW, Kern KB, Sanders AB, Hilwig RW, Hansen KK, Ewy GA: High dose epinephrine results in greater early mortality after resuscitation from prolonged cardiac arrest in pigs: a prospective, randomized study, *Crit Care Med* 22:282-290, 1994.
107. Tang W, Weil MH, Sun S, Noc M, Yang L, Gazmuri RJ: Epinephrine increases the severity of postresuscitation myocardial dysfunction, *Circulation* 92(10):3089-3093, 1995 (abstract now published as an article).
108. Neumar R, Bircher N, Kadovsky A, Sim K, Xaio F, Katz L, Ebmeyer U, Safar P: Myocardial necrosis after high-dose epinephrine during CPR, *Ann Emerg Med* 22:892, 1993 (abstract).
109. Berg RA, Donnerstein RL, Padbury JF: Dobutamine infusions in stable critically ill children: pharmacokinetics and hemodynamic effects, *Crit Care Med* 21:678-686, 1993.
110. Gutgesell HP, Paouet M, Duff DF, McNamara DG: Evaluation of left ventricular size and function by echocardiography: results in normal children, *Circulation* 56:457-462, 1977.
111. Perkin RM, Levin DL, Webb R, Aquino A, Reedy J: Dobutamine: a hemodynamic evaluation in children with shock, *J Pediatr* 200(6):977-983, 1982.
112. Kern KB, Elchisak MA, Sanders AB, Badylak SF, Tacker WA, Ewy GA: Plasma catecholamines and resuscitation from prolonged cardiac arrest, *Crit Care Med* 17:786-791, 1989.
113. Lindner KH, Strohmenger HU, Prengel AW, Ensinger H, Goertz A, Weichel T: Hemodynamic and metabolic effects of epinephrine during cardiopulmonary resuscitation in a pig model, *Crit Care Med* 20:1020-1026, 1992.
114. Huyghens LP, Calle PA, Moerman EJ, Bogaert MG, Buylaert WA: Plasma concentrations of epinephrine during CPR in the dog, *Ann Emerg Med* 20:239-242, 1991.
115. Wortsman J, Paradis NA, Martin GB, Rivers EP, Goetting MG, Nowaki RI, Cryer PE: Functional responses to extremely high plasma epinephrine concentrations in cardiac arrest, *Crit Care Med* 21:692-697, 1993.
116. Stueven H, Thompson B, Aprahamian C, Tonfeldt DJ, Kastenson E: The effectiveness of calcium chloride in refractory electromechanical dissociation, *Ann Emerg Med* 14:626-629, 1985.
117. Stueven H, Thompson B, Aprahamian C, Tonfeldt DJ, Kastenson E: Lack of effectiveness of calcium chloride in refractory asystole, *Ann Emerg Med* 14:630-632, 1985.
118. Harrison E, Amey B: The use of calcium in cardiac resuscitation, *Am J Emerg Med* 3:267-273, 1983.
119. Seri I: Cardiovascular, renal, and endocrine actions of dopamine in neonates and children, *J Pediatr* 126:333-344, 1995.
120. Padbury JF, Agata Y, Raylen BG, Ludlow JK, Polk DH, Goldblatte E, Pescetti J: Dopamine pharmacokinetics in critically ill newborn infant, *J Pediatr* 220:293-298, 1986.
121. Lucking SE, Pollack MM, Fields SI: Shock following generalized hypoxic-ischemic injury in previously healthy infants and children, *J Pediatr* 108:359-364, 1986.
122. Hildebrand CA, Hartmann AG, Arcinue EL, Gomez RJ, Bing RJ: Cardiac performance in pediatric near-drowning, *Crit Care Med* 16:331-335, 1988.

Postresuscitation Myocardial Dysfunction

123. Kern KB, Hilwig RW, Berg RA, Rhee KR, Sanders AB, Otto CW, Ewy GA: Postresuscitation left ventricular systolic and diastolic dysfunction: treatment with dobutamine, *Circulation* 95:2610-2613, 1997.

Outcome

124. Kerber RE: Statement on early defibrillation from the Emergency Cardiac Care Committee, American Heart Association, *Circulation* 83:2233, 1991.
125. Weaver WD, Cobb LA, Hallstrom AP, Rahrenbeuch C, Copass MK, Ray R: Factors influencing survival after out-of-hospital cardiac arrest, *J Am Coll Cardiol* 7:752-756, 1986.
126. Cummins RO, Eisenberg MS, Hallstrom AP, Litwin PE: Survival of out-of-hospital cardiac arrest with early initiation of cardiopulmonary resuscitation, *Am J Emerg Med* 3:114-118, 1985.
127. Ritter G, Wolfe RA, Goldstein S, Landis JR, Vasu CM, Acheson A, Leighton R, Medendrop SVB: The effect of bystander CPR on survival of out-of-hospital cardiac arrest victims, *Am Heart J* 110:932-937, 1985.

CHAPTER 23

Lung Transplantation

John O. Warner

Physicians of all men are most happy; what good success soever they have, the world proclaimeth, and what faults they commit, the earth covereth.

Francis Quarles, 1592-1644, Nicocles IV

The recognition received by physicians in previous centuries is now directed at surgeons and particularly transplant surgeons. The experience of witnessing a child in terminal respiratory failure miraculously given new life after a lung transplant can only inspire even the most hardened observer. The general public finds the media coverage of such dramas intensely compelling. However, the inevitable disasters that occur in transplant programs tend to receive less, if any, publicity. In such circumstances, it is difficult to present a balanced perspective of the pros and cons of lung transplantation. However, even those most committed to transplantation have begun to accept that there are two sides to the problem. Indeed one recent article published on the topic was entitled "Pediatric Lung Transplantation: The Agony and the Ecstasy."[1]

HISTORY

The first attempt at a single lung transplant in humans was made as far back as 1963. The recipient was far from suitable, having unresectable lung cancer, and died from sepsis and the breakdown of the bronchial anastomosis 18 days after surgery.[2] Over the subsequent 20 years, many attempts were made, but there were no long-term survivors. Over 50% of the recipients died from breakdown of the bronchial anastomosis.[3] Thus attention has focused on combined heart and lung transplantation, which was first successfully performed in patients with pulmonary vascular disease in 1981.[4] This was rapidly followed by its use in end-stage respiratory disease, particularly cystic fibrosis.[5,6] Much of the success of this procedure must be attributed to the introduction of cyclosporine (Cyclosporin A) into clinical practice, which dramatically ameliorated the problems of rejection.[7]

By 1992, over 500 successful heart and lung transplants had been performed throughout the world.[8] Initially, perioperative mortality was high, and later, obliterative bronchiolitis leading to severe recurrences of respiratory problems and eventual death occurred in a high percentage of longer-term survivors.[9] However, in recent years, survival has improved, with the actuarial survival rates ranging from 60% to 78% after 1 year and 60% to 73% after 2 years.[8] The figures for children with similar conditions are similar to those for adults. By far, the largest number of pediatric transplants have been for cystic fibrosis, in which actuarial survival was recently reported as 67% at 1 year, 61% at 2 years, and 54% at 3 years.[10] This compares with the survival rates of 69% after 1 year, 52% after 2 years, and 49% after 3 years for adults with cystic fibrosis after heart and lung transplant.[11]

With the exponential growth of heart transplant centers, particularly in the United States, further development of heart and lung transplantation became seriously inhibited because of a shortage of donor organs. This led to the reevaluation of isolated lung transplantation.[12] In heart and lung transplantation the tracheal anastomosis is supported by the coronary artery to bronchial collaterals, but this inevitably means that a block of three organs was required for one patient. One solution to this problem was to adopt the "domino procedure,"[13] which involves the use of the recipient's heart in a second recipient. There were several advantages to this procedure in that the donor domino heart had a conditioned right ventricle ideal for recipients who already had raised pulmonary vascular resistance. Furthermore, the heart had been thoroughly studied before removal to ensure that it was healthy and that the ischemia time was short because both operations were performed simultaneously in the same unit. Furthermore, tissue typing could also be done prospectively.

The other possibility investigated was that of returning to isolated lung transplantation. During the late 1970s in Toronto, experimental work on bronchial anastomotic breakdown culminated in the eventual report in 1986 of a successful single lung transplant for pulmonary fibrosis.[14] This was rapidly followed by similar procedures for chronic obstructive pulmonary disease[15] and primary pulmonary hypertension.[16] However, many recipients, particularly those with chronic pulmonary sepsis, were unsuitable for single lung transplants, which has led since 1990 to the increasing use of bilateral lung transplants.[17] Relatively little data are published on lung transplantation in children, although there is a suggestion that mortality and morbidity may be higher in the younger age group than in adults.[18] Thus most published information in children relates to combined heart and lung transplantation.

There is now a published series of isolated lung transplantation in children involving 79 patients who underwent 88 transplant procedures at St. Louis Children's Hospital, Missouri, which gives actuarial survivals after 12, 24, and 48 months of 69%, 67%, and 60%, respectively. More importantly, survival improved appreciably during the course of the program. Thus, the 12-month survival for the first 18 months was 42% compared with 78% after the first 18 months. There was no difference in survival between children younger than 3 and older children and adults. Younger children had a lower frequency of acute rejection and none developed obliterative bronchiolitis. As in all previous studies, the major late complication was obliterative bronchiolitis and occurred in 27% of the patients, playing a role in 64% of the late deaths. The reasons for transplants were, in order of frequency: cystic fibrosis, pulmonary vascular disease, and interstitial lung disease. There were 9 who had retransplants, most commonly for obliterative bronchiolitis.[19]

PATIENT SELECTION

Obviously the key selection criterion is the patient's limited life expectancy with a severely impaired quality of life. In general, a life expectancy of less than 2 years has been considered realistic.[20] However, perhaps this figure should be higher because there is a lengthy waiting period for suitable donor organs.[21] The relationship between longevity and lung function is more difficult to establish. In cystic fibrosis a 1-second forced expiratory volume of less than 30% of predicted normal indicates the need to consider transplantation. However, female patients, particularly those beyond adolescence, have a worse prognosis and might require referral at an earlier stage of lung function deterioration.[22] Additional criteria that have been applied in cystic fibrosis include a Shwachman score of less than 40, a 12-minute walk of less than 800 m, and an oxygen saturation of less than 90%.[10] More recently, a prognostic index including FEV_1% predicted, FVC% predicted, short stature, high white cell count, and chronic liver disease as evidenced by hepatomegaly have been incorporated into a combined prognostic index that has given a better prediction of short-term outcome. However, this has yet to be validated outside the center that developed it.[23]

The list of contraindications to transplantation has decreased progressively over the years. Initially, it was felt that previous thoracic surgery, including pleurodesis and even pleurectomy, were absolute contraindications, but this is no longer the case, although there are higher risks of complications in such circumstances.[8] Pleural adhesions can be assessed by computed tomographic scanning before transplant to aid the surgeon.[24] The use of systemic steroids before surgery has been associated with poor healing of airway anastomoses, so they should be reduced to as low a dose as possible. However, there is increasing evidence that this practice is not essential. It may be necessary to maintain the administration of steroids in patients with fibrosing alveolitis so that their health does not deteriorate before transplant.[8] Diabetes mellitus is also no longer a contraindication to transplantation. Indeed, in cystic fibrosis the survival figures are every bit as good in patients with as without associated diabetes.[11] However, established cirrhosis of the liver, which occurs in 5% of patients with cystic fibrosis, is a contraindication unless lung transplantation is combined with liver transplantation. This practice has been successful in a very small number of cases.[25] Some units consider that lung colonization with *Pseudomonas cepacia* is a contraindication to transplant because of a high mortality rate resulting from recolonization of the transplanted lungs.[26] However, others consider that such colonization is a relative risk factor and that it should not necessarily be a prime criterion for rejection from a program.[27]

Perhaps the prime contraindication to surgery is severe psychosocial disorder in the child, the family, or both. Such disorders inevitably lead to poor compliance with therapy and omission of immunosuppression after the transplant. Invasive pulmonary *Aspergillosis* infection, mycobacterial infections, and renal failure are additional major contraindications[10] (Box 23-1).

There has been inevitable concern that patients with systemic disease will have a recurrence of the disease in the transplanted organs. This concern has been allayed in cystic fibrosis; the airway mucosal bioelectric potential difference is normal in the transplanted airway and abnormal only above the airway anastomosis.[28] Likewise, there is not necessarily any contraindication to transplant in patients with pulmonary fibrosis related to systemic disorders such as systemic lupus erythematosus. However, associated renal involvement may preclude transplantation.[8]

BOX 23-1
Indications and Contraindications for Transplantation

Indications
Single lung
Pulmonary fibrosis
Obliterative bronchiolitis
Emphysema
Double lung or heart and lung
Cystic fibrosis
Bronchiectasis
Pulmonary vascular disease

Relative contraindications
Psychosocial problems
Liver cirrhosis
Renal disease
Dependence on ventilator

Individuals with very poor nutrition require some rehabilitation before surgery, although this is often extremely difficult, if not impossible. Nevertheless, in cystic fibrosis the use of nocturnal gastrostomy drip feeding can achieve improved nutrition.[3,11]

As transplant centers proliferate and the number of patients considered suitable for transplant increases, attrition rates on waiting lists become ever greater. Indeed the mean waiting time at the Hospital for Sick Children, Great Ormond Street in London, has increased from 3.3 months in 1990 to over 10 months in 1993.[1] This has led to the concept of a "window of opportunity" during which transplants should be considered when the patient is sick enough to require such surgery but healthy enough to have a reasonable chance of success.[29]

TECHNICAL ASPECTS

The donor and recipient are matched by ABO blood group compatibility, body size, and usually cytomegalovirus serologic status.[10,11] However, HLA incompatibility can be circumvented with immunosuppressive drugs. The donor lungs must be in good condition and demonstrate good gas exchange with a reasonably good chest radiograph and bacteriologically clear aspirate from the airways. The maximum ischemia time acceptable after retrieval of organs is 4 to 5 hours.[3,8,10] A variety of techniques have been proposed for ex vivo preservation of organs procured from some distance away from the donor. One recommendation has been cooling of the donor using cardiopulmonary bypass before harvest of the organs, which has lengthened the acceptable ischemia time from 4 to 5 hours.[8]

SURGICAL CONSIDERATIONS

The choice among heart and lung, single lung, and bilateral lung transplant depends partly on the underlying disease and the experience and preference of the surgeon. In general, single lung transplant is suitable only for interstitial lung diseases and perhaps pulmonary hypertension. The choice between double lung and heart and lung transplant in patients with chronic pulmonary sepsis, such as that in cystic fibrosis, may be dictated by age (see Box 23-1). Bronchial anastomoses for bilateral transplants involve a greater risk of ischemic complications, particularly in small children. Thus heart and lung transplant may be preferred in the younger child.[10]

POSTOPERATIVE MANAGEMENT

This chapter does not elaborate on the surgical aspects of postoperative care or indeed on operative techniques. Clearly the preeminent therapy is immunosuppression. At present, cyclosporine remains the mainstay of suppression of allograft rejection.[7] This drug is lipophilic and therefore is poorly absorbed in patients with cystic fibrosis.[30] With the marked variations in bioavailability, blood level monitoring is essential. Nephrotoxicity is the main side effect of concern, and inadequate dosing inevitably leads to rejection. Other complications of therapy include hypertension, hyperkalemia, hepatotoxicity, gingival hyperplasia, hirsutism, and convulsions.[8] The aim is to achieve a blood medication level of 500 ng/ml in the first month after surgery. Thereafter, doses are reduced to maintain a level between 250 and 350 ng/ml.

There is a continuing need for new immunosuppressive regimens to try to improve long-term survival from lung transplantation. Several new agents are being developed. In addition to Cyclosporin A, extra immunosuppression is achieved by Azathioprine and perioperatively with the administration of Methylprednisolone, antithymocyte globulin, antilymphocyte globulin and monoclonal antibodies to a range of receptors on T cells. Notably there are now phase III studies in renal transplantation of a monoclonal agent directed against the alpha chain of the IL-2 receptor. Resistant rejection episodes have been treated with additional Methotrexate and by the use of inhaled Cyclosporin. Newer immunosuppressive agents include Tacrolimus (FK 506), Mycophenolate mofetil, Sirolimus (Rapamycin), and a Rapamycin derivative SDZ-RAD. All of the immunosuppressive agents function by interacting with intracellular binding proteins termed *immunophilins*. The complexes block the calcium-dependent signal transduction pathways initiated by activation of T-cell receptors. This leads to inactivation of the T cells that initiate the rejection process.[31]

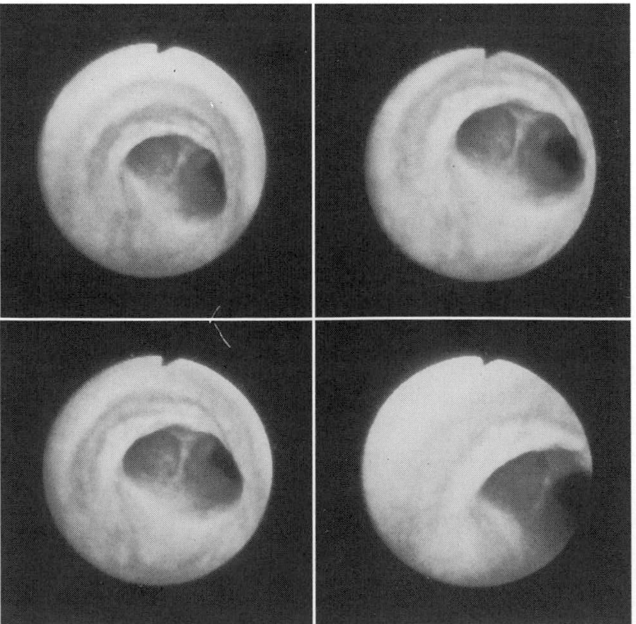

Fig. 23-1. Fiberoptic bronchoscopy. Views of the tracheal anastomosis in a 14-year-old girl who had cystic fibrosis and who had a heart and lung transplantation for end-stage lung disease.

Monitoring for rejection is based predominantly on the regular measurements of lung function as well as the use of bronchoscopy, bronchoalveolar lavage, and transbronchial biopsy as soon as any changes in lung function occur[32] (Figure 23-1). Bronchoscopy, bronchoalveolar lavage, and transbronchial biopsy are required to distinguish infection from rejection. No reliable immunologic tests indicate when rejection is occurring and distinguish it from infection. However, this appears to be an area that is open for further research.[33]

COMPLICATIONS

Mortality in the early posttransplant period is associated mostly with acute pulmonary rejection and infection with the additional complications related to surgery. After the first 3 months, morbidity and mortality are due principally to obliterative bronchiolitis. Another complication is tracheal stenosis at the anastomotic site, which is sometimes associated with generalized bronchomalacia that may proceed to obliterative bronchiolitis.[34] The side effects of cyclosporine sometimes create difficulties, and diabetes mellitus may be highlighted by the use of steroids. With longer use, there is concern about the increased incidence of lymphoma and other malignancies related to Epstein-Barr virus.[35]

Acute Rejection

Acute pulmonary rejection is common after transplant, with rates over 50% being reported.[8] It is associated with the development of increasing breathlessness, cough, and low-grade pyrexia, with either crackles or wheezes being heard over the lung fields. Lung function is diminished, and chest radiographs show abnormalities in three fourths of cases. However, none of these features, which range from interstitial shadowing to consolidation and pleural effusion, is specific for rejection.[36,37] Because none of these features is distinguishable from infection, bronchoalveolar lavage and bronchial biopsy are used to confirm the diagnosis. However, although bronchoalveolar lavage aids in the detection of microbial organisms and thus infection, such detection does not necessarily exclude rejection: No cells from lavage fluid are associated with rejection. However, transbronchial biopsy has been well defined and has proved extremely useful for indicating rejection in both adults and children. In the latter population, transbronchial biopsy is 88% sensitive for acute rejection and 60% sensitive for chronic rejection. Specificities for these problems have been 91% and 100%, respectively.[32] The characteristic feature is a dense perivascular cuffing by mononuclear cells.[38]

Treatment of acute rejection involves intensified immunosuppression, which is accomplished by increasing the dosage of cyclosporine and giving high doses of prednisolone. Antithymocyte globulin and T-cell receptor antibodies are sometimes administered.[8]

Infectious Complications

In an immunosuppressed individual, there is inevitably a high risk of infection. Indeed bacterial pneumonia is very common in the postoperative period. However, virtually any organism can be involved, and the range is identical to that in any other immunosuppressed individual. Thus once suspicion of infection arises, a very broad spectrum of antibacterial, protozoal, fungal, and viral medications must be used. If examination of sputum cultures does not identify the causative agent, the results from bronchoalveolar lavage and transbronchial biopsy become essential for guiding therapy.[8,32]

Cytomegalovirus is one of the most common causes of infection in the 1- to 2-month postoperative period. Matching of cytomegalovirus status in the donor and recipient reduces this problem. Treatment with ganciclovir with or without cytomegalovirus hyperimmune globulin has resulted in some therapeutic success.[39]

Obliterative Bronchiolitis

Obliterative bronchiolitis is the most feared long-term complication of lung transplantation. In the early days of transplant programs, it was the cause of high morbidity and mortality in long-term survivors. The exact pathogenesis is still unknown, but efficient treatment of rejection episodes has appreciably reduced its frequency.[8,40] It is assumed to result from a chronic rejection phenomenon; a chronic inflammatory process focuses around bronchioles, progressively obliterating the lumen and producing severe obstructive disease (Figure 23-2). The problem can arise between 3 months and 2 years after surgery and sometimes progresses very rapidly. It is characterized by progressive shortness of breath and cough with wheezing. A typical feature on examination is fine end-inspiratory crackles over the lung fields. Lung function studies reveal a severe obstructive ventilatory defect, with the flow-volume curve being particularly useful in showing dramatically decreased flows at low lung volume with little or no response to bronchodilators.[8] Treatment involves increased immunosuppression. However, for up to half the patients, the disease is progressive; only retransplantation gives any chance of survival.

PSYCHOSOCIAL ISSUES

For patients with chronic respiratory disorders, it is either lung transplantation or death within 2 years. Lung transplantation is often viewed as a consequence of therapeutic failure. Thus by the time that a child and family are referred to a transplant unit, their anxiety is enormous. The selection procedure, which is protracted, can only heighten the anxiety. For some, this procedure ends in rejection from the program. For those who are accepted into the program, there are the agonizing wait and a continuing inexorable decline in lung function. The attrition on waiting lists is as high at 50%, with ever-increasing waiting times for suitable organs to become available.[1]

There is an overwhelming desire to prolong life at all costs in the hope that organs will become available. This has often led to suboptimal management of patients entering a terminal phase of illness. It becomes imperative to decide when to provide relief from pain and distress even though this may reduce the patient's survival time and chance of a transplant.[41]

Once the transplant has occurred, patients must overcome many obstacles before the outcome is considered successful. For some, transplantation represents an unbelievable improvement in the quality of life and the possibility to experience an almost normal existence. However, the patient must nevertheless undergo continual intensive follow-up and therapy. For patients with cystic fibrosis, treatment for the pancreatic insufficiency must continue, and other complications of the disease may still occur. Researchers need to carefully review quality of life not only in the success stories but also in the many others who enter programs and then die at various stages during the procedure[41] (Figure 23-3).

Some work has been done in relation to liver transplantation. The relatives of patients who had died either after being turned down for a transplant or during or after transplant an-

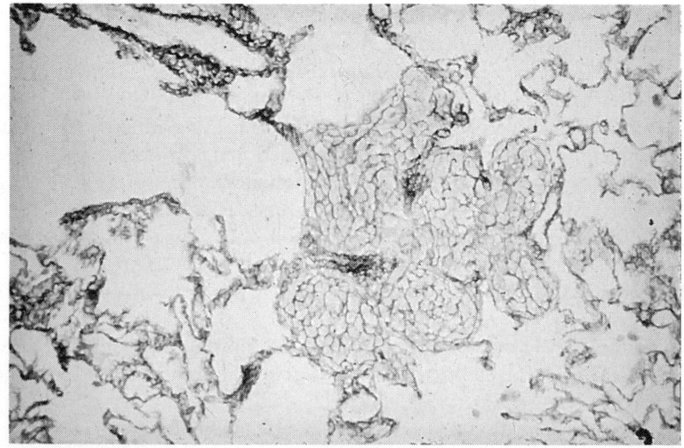

Fig. 23-2. Histology of end-stage obliterative bronchiolitis with collapsed alveoli around a scarred bronchiole and areas of overinflation.

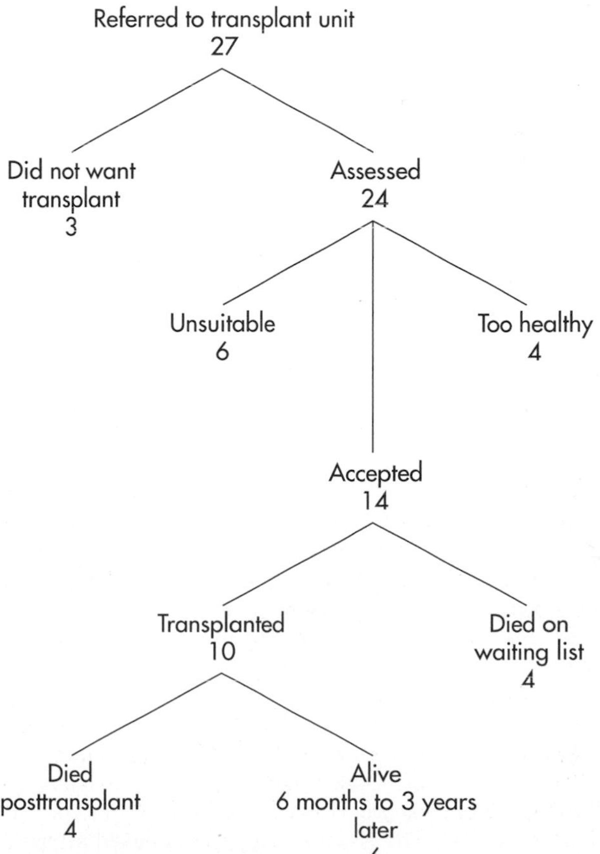

Fig. 23-3. Outcome of 27 pediatric referrals for transplant assessment to the author's unit. (Redrawn from Warner JO: *Arch Dis Child* 66:1013-1017, 1991.)

swered a detailed questionnaire. Over one third of respondents believed that the patient would have been better off if he or she had not entered the transplant program. Over half of the relatives found the death more difficult to accept because the patient had been involved in the program. Nevertheless, many felt that at least everything possible had been done to save the patient's life.[42]

It is also important to consider the psychosocial issues in relation to the relatives of the organ donor. There is again relatively little in the literature on this topic. In a study of 11 families, 5 of whom had given permission for a relative to become an organ donor and 6 of whom had not, most relatives were unaware of the wishes of the deceased in relation to organ donation. Some of the relatives who refused regretted their decision later. However, remorse was also encountered in the group who had given permission, although positive feelings were rather more common in that group than in the group who rejected donation. The authors of this study felt that there was still a need to review the system of organ acquisition and in particular to clarify the laws in relation to preassigned consent for organ donation. Despite the majority of the population feeling very positive about organ donation, very few actually expressed their wishes to the family regarding what should happen to their organs in event of death.[43]

A legitimate question is whether the suffering experienced by many who failed to benefit from transplantation can be offset by the dramatic success achieved for a few. Open debate of this issue is still required. From the author's experience, a 60% success rate for transplantation conceals the fact that only 22% of those referred to the program actually benefit from it[41] (Figure 23-3).

RESEARCH SPIN-OFFS FROM TRANSPLANTATION

After lung transplantation, denervation persists below the level of the airway anastomosis. This denervation has been associated with bronchial hyperresponsiveness to methacholine.[44] However, inhalation of capsaicin more consistently causes bronchodilation rather than bronchoconstriction, which is the tendency in asthmatic subjects. No relationship exists between methacholine and capsaicin responses either in asthmatics or transplant patients, and in the transplant subjects the responsiveness was unrelated to the degree of inflammation found in the airways on transbronchial biopsy. These observations support the current view that bronchial hyperresponsiveness is a phenomenon independent of asthma. Furthermore, local axon reflexes within the airways are more important than parasympathetic or sympathetic innervation.[45] Also, diurnal variation in lung function after transplantation is identical to that in normal subjects; therefore the variation does not depend on intact neural connections.[46]

Perhaps the most fascinating information has come from the effects of transplantation on asthma. Two nonasthmatic recipients of asthmatic lungs developed asthma after transplantation. However, two asthmatic recipients of normal lungs did not develop asthma within 3 years after transplantation. According to Corris and Dark,[47] these observations indicate that asthma is a local disease. However, alternative interpretations of the data exist. The immunosuppression used after transplantation inevitably suppresses any systemic manifestations that might promote the development of asthma in an asthmatic receiving normal lungs. However, in situations in which inflamed asthmatic airways are transplanted into a normal host who is then immunosuppressed, the systemic mechanisms that prevent the development of asthma allow the local airway inflammation to get out of control. Thus the interpretation could be the exact opposite of that suggested by the original publication. It would be interesting to review similar data from individuals who have received a single or a double lung rather than a heart and lung transplant. There is no doubt that insights into the mechanisms of lung disease in other systemic disorders will occur.

THE FUTURE

The goal in the management of any patient with a chronic respiratory disorder is to prevent a decline in lung function and therefore avoid heart and lung transplantation. However, for the foreseeable future the demand for transplant will outweigh the provision of donor organs. This has led to consideration of live related donors. One group has pioneered lobar transplant from living related donors into children with end-stage pulmonary disease.[48] Whether the ethics of this procedure will ever be resolved is dubious.[49] This has led to the idea of investigating nonhuman donors (xenotransplantation). Uncontrollable humoral rejection usually accompanies cross-species transplantation, and the very few attempts from baboon to man have failed.[1] The development of transgenic mice expressing a human cell surface molecule that prevents the activation of human complement gives some optimism for the possibility that such animals might be bred to generate suitable transplant organs. There is little doubt that more about this approach will be heard over the next decade.[50]

REFERENCES

1. Whitehead BF, DeLeval MR: Pediatric lung transplantation: the agony and the ecstasy, *Thorax* 49:437-439, 1994.

History

2. Hardy JD, Webb WBWR, Dalton ML, Walker GR: Lung homotransplantation in man: report of the initial case, *JAMA* 186:1065, 1963.
3. Kirby TJ, Mehta A: Lung transplantation: state of the art, *Appl Cardio-Pulmon Pathophysiol* 4:263-271, 1992.
4. Reitz BA, Wallwork JL, Hunt SA, Pennock JL, Billingham ME, Oyer BE, Stinson EB, Shumway NE: Heart and lung transplantation: successful therapy for patients with pulmonary vascular disease, *N Engl J Med* 306:557-564, 1982.
5. Penketh A, Higenbottam T, Hakim N, Wallwork JL: Heart/lung transplantation in patients with end stage lung disease, *Br Med J* 296:311-314, 1987.
6. Scott J, Higenbottam T, Hutter RJ, Hodson M, Stewart S, Penketh A: Heart/lung transplantation for cystic fibrosis, *Lancet* 2:192-194, 1988.
7. Borell JF, Kiss ZL: The discovery and development of cyclosporin (Sandimmune), *Transplant Proc* 23:1867-1874, 1991.
8. Heritier F, Madden B, Hodson M, Yacoub M: Lung allograft transplantation: indications, pre-operative assessment and post-operative management, *Eur Respir J* 5:1262-1278, 1992 (review).
9. Burke CM, Theodore J, Baldwin JC, Tazelaar HD, Morris AJ, McGregor C, Shumway NE, Robin ED, Jamieson SW: Twenty-eight cases of human heart/lung transplantation, *Lancet* 1:517-519, 1986.
10. Whitehead BF: Heart/lung transplantation in patients with cystic fibrosis, *Paediatr Respir Med* 216-219, 1994.
11. Madden B, Hodson M, Tsang P, Radley-Smith R, Khaghani A, Yacoub MY: Intermediate term results of heart/lung transplantation for cystic fibrosis, *Lancet* 339:1583-1587, 1992.
12. Lung transplantation, *Lancet* 339:1021-1022, 1992 (editorial).
13. Yacoub MY, Banner NR, Khaghani A, Fitzgerald M, Madden B, Tsang V, Radley-Smith R, Hodson M: Heart/lung transplantation for cystic fibrosis and subsequent domino heart transplantation, *J Heart Lung Transplant* 9:459-467, 1990.

14. The Toronto Lung Transplant Group: Lung transplantation for pulmonary fibrosis, *N Engl J Med* 314:1140-1145, 1986.
15. Trulock EP, Egan TM, Kouchoukos N, Kaiser LR, Pasque MK, Ettinger N, Cooper JD: Single lung tranpslantation for severe chronic obstructive pulmonary disease, *Chest* 96:738-742, 1989.
16. Trulock EP, Cooper JD, Kaiser LR, Pasque MK, Ettinger NA, Washington University Lung Transplantation Group: Unilateral lung transplantation for pulmonary hypertension, *Am Rev Respir Dis* 143A:467, 1991 (abstract).
17. Pasque MK, Cooper JD, Kaiser LR, Haydock DA, Triantafillou A, Trulock EP: Improved technique for bilateral lung transplantation, *Ann Thorac Surg* 49:785-791, 1991.
18. Metras D, Kreitmann B, Shennib H, Noirdevc M: Lung transplantation in children, *J Heart Lung Transplant* 11:S282-S285, 1992.
19. Sweet SC, Spray TL, Huddleston CB, Mendeloff E, Canter CE, Balzer DT, Bridges ND, Cohen AH, Mallory GB: Pediatric lung transplantation at St. Louis Children's Hospital, 1990-95, *Am J Respir Crit Care Med* 155:1027-1035, 1997.

Patient Selection

20. Whitehead B, Helms P, Goodwin M, Martin I, Scott JP, Smyth RL, Higenbottam TW, Wallwork J, Elliott M, DeLeval M: Heart/lung transplantation for cystic fibrosis. II. Outcome, *Arch Dis Child* 66:1022-1026, 1991.
21. Warner JO: Heart/lung transplantation for cystic fibrosis: commentary, *Arch Dis Child* 66:1026, 1991.
22. Kerem E, Reisman J, Corey M, Kammy GJ, Levison H: Prediction of mortality in patients with cystic fibrosis, *N Engl J Med* 326:1187-1191, 1992.
23. Hayllar KM, Williams SGJ, Wise AE, Pouria S, Lombard M, Hodson ME, Westaby D: A prognostic model for the prediction of survival in cyctic fibrosis, *Thorax* 52:313-317, 1997.
24. Morrison DL, Maurer JR, Grossman RF: Pre-operative assessment for lung transplantation, *Clin Chest Med* 11:207-215, 1990.
25. Wallwork J, Williams R, Calne RM: Transplantation of the liver, heart and lungs for primary biliary cirrhosis and primary pulmonary hypertension, *Lancet* 2:182-185, 1987.
26. Snell GI, deHowos A, Krajden M, Winton T, Maurer JR: *Pseudomonas cepacia* in lung transplant recipients with cystic fibrosis, *Chest* 103:466-471, 1993.
27. Egan JJ, McNeil K, Bookless B, Gould K, Corris P, Higenbottam T, Webb AK, Woodcock AA: Post-transplantation survival of cystic fibrosis patients infected with *Pseudomonas cepacia, Lancet* 344:552-553, 1994.
28. Wood A, Higenbottam T, Jackson M, Scott J, Stewart S, Wallwork J: Airway mucosal bio-electric potential difference in cystic fibrosis after lung transplantation, *Am Rev Respir Dis* 140:1645-1649, 1989.
29. Marshall SE, Kramer ER, Lewiston NG, Starnes VA, Theodore J: Selection and evaluation of recipients for heart/lung transplantation, *Chest* 98:1488-1494, 1990.

Postoperative Management

30. Cooney GF, Fiel SB, Shaw LM, Cavarocchi NC: Cyclosporin bioavailability in heart/lung transplant candidates with cystic fibrosis, *Transplantation* 49:821-823, 1990.
31. Briffa N, Morris RE: New immuno-suppressive regimens in lung transplantation, *Eur Respir J* 10:2630-2367, 1997.
32. Whitehead B, Scott JP, Helms P, Malone M, Macrae D, Higenbottam TW, Smyth RL, Wallwork J, Elliott M, De-Leval M: Technique and use of trans-bronchial biopsy in children and adolescents, *Pediatr Pulmonol* 12:240-246, 1992.
33. Report of ATS Workshop on Lung Transplantation, *Am Rev Respir Dis* 147:772-776, 1993.

Complications

34. Novick RJ, Ahmad D, Menkis AH: The importance of acquired diffuse broncho-malacia in heart/lung transplant recipients with obliterative bronchiolitis, *J Thorac Cardiovasc Surg* 101:643-648, 1991.
35. Ho M, Jaffe R, Miller G, Breinig MK, Dummer JS, Makowka L, Atchison RW, Karrer F, Nalesnik MA, Starzl TE: The frequency of Epstein-Barr virus infection and associated lympho-proliferative syndrome after transplantation and its manifestations in children, *Transplantation* 45:719-727, 1988.
36. Millet B, Higenbottam TW, Flower CDR, Stewart S, Wallwork J: The radiographic appearances of infection and acute rejection of the lung after heart/lung transplantation, *Am Rev Respir Dis* 140:62-67, 1989.
37. Herman SJ: Radiologic assessment after lung transplantation, *Clin Chest Med* 11:333-346, 1990.
38. Higenbottam TW, Stewart S, Penketh A, Wallwork J: Trans-bronchial lung biopsy for the diagnosis of rejection in heart/lung transplant recipients, *Transplant* 46:532-539, 1988.
39. Hutter JA, Scot J, Wreghitt T, Higenbottam T, Wallwork J: The importance of cytomegalovirus in heart/lung transplant recipients, *Chest* 95:627-631, 1989.
40. Theodore J, Starnes VA, Lewiston NJ: Obliterative bronchiolitis, *Clin Chest Med* 11:309-321, 1990.

Psychosocial Issues

41. Warner JO: Heart/lung transplantation: all the facts, *Arch Dis Child* 66:1013-1017, 1991.
42. Heyink J, Tymstra T: Liver transplantation: the shadow side, *Fam Pract* 7:233-237, 1990.
43. Tymstra T, Heyink J, Preium J, Slooff MJH: Experience of bereaved relatives who granted or refused permission for organ donation, *Fam Pract* 9:141-144, 1992.

Research Spin-Offs from Transplantation

44. Hathaway TJ, Higenbottam TW, Morrison JFJ, Clelland CA, Wallwork J: Effects of inhaled capsaicin in heart/lung transplant patients and asthmatic subjects, *Am Rev Respir Dis* 148:1233-1237, 1993.
45. Barnes PJ: Asthma is an axon reflex, *Lancet* 1:242-245, 1986.
46. Morrison FJ, Higenbottam TW, Hathaway TJ, Clelland CA, Scott JP, Wallwork J: Diurnal variation in FEV_1 after heart/lung transplantation, *Eur Respir J* 5:834-840, 1992.
47. Corris PA, Dark JH: Aetiology of asthma: lessons from lung transplantation, *Lancet* 341:1369-1371, 1993.

The Future

48. Starnes VA, Barr ML, Cohen RG: Lobar transplantation: indications, techniques and outcome, *J Thorac Cardiovasc Surg* 108:403-411, 1994.
49. Shaw LE, Miller JD, Slutsky AS, Maurer JR, Puskas JD, Patterson GA, Singer PA: Ethics of lung transplantation with live donors, *Lancet* 338:678-681, 1991.
50. White D, Wallwork J: Xeno-grafting: probability, possibility or pipe dream, *Lancet* 342:879-880, 1993.

CHAPTER 24

Issues In Home Care

Wendy Votroubek

Home care is an attempt to normalize the life of a chronically or seriously ill child in a family and community by providing the necessary medical care with the least disruption of the child's life. The success of the home care experience depends on thorough discharge planning and understanding of the home care plan.

The provision of home care for the chronically ill child is not a new phenomenon. Parents and caregivers have been caring for their ill children at home for years. Home care of the patient with pulmonary disease has taken on new dimensions in recent years because of the many advances in health care that have significantly increased the quantity of life and in many instances the quality as well.[1] In the early 1980s, parents and the health care industry advocated for these children who were once cared for in the hospital, allowing them to receive cost-effective care at home, assisting in the normalization of life.[2-4]

Home care is not appropriate for every child.[5] The clinician must understand what needs to be considered before discharge and the aspects of care with which family and caregivers need to be familiar to safely care for the child at home.

CRITERIA AND PLANNING FOR HOME CARE

The success of home care depends on the patient, family, additional caregivers, and equipment providers. The patient must be medically stable before discharge: The child should not require frequent medical or equipment changes within a 24-hour period, all coexistent medical disease should be well controlled, and the patient should not require emergency treatment.

The involvement of a multidisciplinary team is required. Team members include the primary care physician, pediatric pulmonologist, pediatric pulmonary nurse specialist, social worker, respiratory therapist, representative of the durable medical equipment company, member of the certified or licensed home care agency, and (skilled) family members.[6,7] Other team members that might be involved are the physical therapist, occupational therapist, speech therapist, dietitian, psychologist, and other physician subspecialists when indicated. Support systems (e.g., support groups, relatives, friends) are encouraged because of the stress associated with home care for technologically dependent children.

The family must be willing and able to care for the child at home and motivated to learn care issues. The family members will likely assume additional roles as part-time nurse, therapist, and care manager. The professionals and family must develop workable and realistic goals for home care and the aspects of care to be taught before discharge. Families need to be given a clear and accurate description of care needs, including the physical, social, and psychologic aspects. They should also be made aware of the possible stresses and appropriate support system to facilitate transition and adaptation.[8-11] It should also be made clear to the family that the health care team is available for support, and they should know who to call with questions or concerns.[12,13]

Social worker involvement is critical so that funding sources can be identified. Ongoing involvement is necessary, especially since sources may change after discharge from the hospital. All agreements and arrangements for care need to be made while the child is still hospitalized. These arrangements include durable medical equipment, supplies, home nursing, nurses, and therapists. Durable medical equipment companies must be willing to work with the family and funding source, guarantee continuous availability, maintain and replace equipment, and be available for equipment service on a 24-hour basis. Both the nurses and the therapist should have pediatric expertise, be familiar with the various home equipment, and assist the family with coordinating care for the child.[14]

Thorough teaching for all caregivers, including home care nurses, is necessary before discharge. Family members should be required to demonstrate all aspects of care. It is recommended that flowsheets documenting education and demonstration of skills of care be developed.[15-17] If the child is technologically dependent, use of a transitional care unit for education, observation, and assessment of skills may be needed. It is also helpful for parents to have an out-of-hospital overnight pass or for them to room in or stay overnight in the hospital before discharge to provide care for their child.[18]

Other issues that must be addressed before discharge include the appropriateness of the patient's residence and identification of local care providers.[19] The home must be safe, accessible, and conducive to all aspects of care. If electricity is required for equipment, there must be adequate power to maintain equipment and household appliances. If the child is ventilator dependent, an electrician may be required to evaluate the structure for accommodation of electric equipment.[20,21]

Local care providers need to be acquainted with the child before discharge. A primary care physician must be identified and must be familiar with the child's status, equipment needs, providers, and plans for alternative methods of care in case of emergency or failure of the home care plan. The local providers also need to be aware of an alternative care plan in case of emergency or failure of the existing plan.

OXYGEN THERAPY

Home supplemental oxygen therapy is used for a variety of pulmonary disorders, including pulmonary hypertension, cystic fibrosis, bronchopulmonary dysplasia, and ventilator dependency. The type of oxygen system used in the home is based on the dosage, the system's mobility, safety, cost, the patient's preference, the duration of therapy, reimbursement constraints, and supplies available from the durable medical equipment provider.[22,23] Patients requiring oxygen concentrations greater than 40% require special considerations and may not be suitable candidates for home oxygen therapy.

The three oxygen sources typically used in the home are gas, liquid, and concentrators. Gas oxygen is provided in various-sized cylinders made from aluminum or steel. Application is often limited to patients who have limited mobility or need a small amount of oxygen for less than 15 hours/day. "E" cylinders are used for portability in conjunction with a large tank or oxygen concentrator. These cylinders are heavy (more than 15 lb empty), are awkward to transport, and must be secured in a wheeled cart or frame attached to the back of a wheelchair. They are unsuitable for the ambulatory oxygen-dependent person or a parent who must manage other young children in addition to an oxygen-dependent baby (Tables 24-1 to 24-3).

Oxygen tanks are an ideal backup system for an oxygen concentrator because they can be used in case of a power outage. A bank of oxygen cylinders can be used for positive-pressure ventilators with a high gas requirement. They are useful in outlying areas where oxygen delivery is often infrequent and unreliable or in communities where liquid systems are unavailable or electric power is unreliable. Caregivers must take care not to damage to a tank or regulator because damage can cause sudden venting, which can propel the tank like a missile because of exceedingly high pressures.[24] In addition, an open flame or cigarette smoking is not allowed near oxygen in the home because of the danger of fire.

Oxygen concentrators are electrically powered devices that extract oxygen from room air and deliver it to the patient in concentrations between 93% and 95%. Concentrators generally provide only low-flow oxygen (up to 2 to 3 L/min.). They cannot be used with Venturi masks or medication nebulizers. Concentrators are rather large and bulky and are inappropriate for portable use. If a concentrator is used, cylinder oxygen should be available for portability and in case of equipment malfunction or power failure.

Liquid oxygen is a low-pressure oxygen system that can be used with any low-flow oxygen-delivery device. It is expensive but the most cost effective and convenient method for patients with low or moderate continuous flow needs.[25] A typical stationary reservoir is capable of holding 40 lb of oxygen and allows up to 4 days of continuous flow at 2 L/min. Because of the portability of the system through the use of a relatively lightweight reservoir (9 to 13 lb), it is the system of choice for ambulatory patients; it offers no advantages for the homebound patient (see Tables 24-1 to 24-3).

Systems that release short pulses of oxygen at the beginning of the inspiratory cycle are also available. They can be built into the oxygen reservoir or portable unit or contained separately on a special belt pack.[26] Oxygen use with demand systems may be as low as one seventh that required with nasal prongs.[27] Substantial oxygen savings with demand systems have also been demonstrated for patients with restrictive lung disease. Despite the cost savings, some patients are bothered by the clicking noise that accompanies activation.

Oxygen-delivery methods include the tracheostomy mask, nasal cannulas, masks, and transtracheal catheters. Tracheostomy masks provide a humidified source of either room air or oxygen for a child with a tracheostomy. Potential problems exist if the mask becomes dislodged at night; occasionally parents may have to put mittens (without a thumb) on the child to prevent removal.

Nasal cannulas are advantageous for oxygen-dependent patients of all ages because of minimal restrictions to visual or auditory stimulation and movement, an important consideration for infants and young children. A nasal cannula can be held in place with a headband, Velcro straps, tape, or clear surgical adhesive dressing (e.g., OpSite, Tegaderm). Special neonatal and pediatric cannulas are available for young children; makeshift cannulas can also be made by cutting off the nasal prongs, making a slit between the two holes, and positioning the slit below the nares. Flowmeters with small calibrations are needed for young children because their flow rates are usually so much lower. The Timeter (Allied Health Care Products, St. Louis) (0.1 to 1 L/min, 0.125 to 3 L/min; 25 to 200 cc min) or the Veriflow (Veriflow, Richmond, Calif.) (0.125 to 3.5 L/min; 0.03125 to 0.5 L/min) are available for the regulation of very low flow rates.[24] Nasal cannulas are appropriate for low-flow use only; they are not recommended for higher flows because of irritation and difficulty maintaining oxygenation.

Table 24-1 Oxygen Flow Time: Small "E" Cylinder*

PRESSURE GAUGE READING	FLOW 1	2	3	4	5
2200 psi	10	5	3.5	2.5	2
1600 psi	7.5	3.75	2.5	1.5	1.25
1100 psi	5	2.5	1.75	1.25	1
500 psi	2.5	1.25	0.75	0.5	0.25

*The average oxygen usage time is based on a continuous flow rate in liters per minute. The figures are approximate and should be used only as a general guide. Individual usage times may vary.

Table 24-2 Oxygen Flow Time: Large Cylinder*

PRESSURE	FLOW 0.125	0.25	0.5	0.75	1	2	3	4
GAUGE READING	DAYS				HOURS			
2200 psi	37	18	10	6.0	4.5	55	36	26
2000 psi	33	16	8	5.5	4.0	50	32	24
1800 psi	30	15	8	5.0	3.5	45	28	22
1600 psi	27	13	7	4.0	3.0	40	25	18
1400 psi	23	12	6	3.5	2.5	34	22	16
1000 psi	17	8	4	2.5	1.5	24	16	12
800 psi	13	7	3	2.0	1.25	18	12	9
600 psi	10	5	2	1.5	1.0	13	9	7

*The average oxygen usage time is based on a continuous flow rate in liters per minute. The figures are approximate and should be used only as a general guide. Individual usage times may vary.

Table 24-3 Oxygen Flow Time: Liquid Oxygen Systems*†

	HOURS		DAYS	
FLOW	SPRINT	STROLLER	LIBERATOR 20	LIBERATOR 30
0.25	20	54	36	50
0.5	11	27	18	25
0.75	7	18	12	18
1	6	10	11.5	17.5
15	4	8	7.5	11.5
2	3	6	5.5	9
2.5	2	5	4.5	7
3	1	4	3.5	6
4	—	3	2.5	4.5
5	—	2.5	2	3.5
6	—	2	1.5	3

*The average oxygen usage time is based on a continuous flow rate in liters per minute. The figures are approximate and should be used only as a general guide. Individual usage times may vary.
†Sprint, Stroller, and Liberator systems are products of Cryogenics Associates, New Prague, Minn.

Oxygen masks are occasionally used in the home but are not typically used in the infant and pediatric patient. Masks may cause claustrophobia, interfere with eating and talking, and require high flow rates to achieve an acceptable level of oxygenation.

Hoods or tents are rarely used in the home. Although tents permit greater freedom of movement for the child, they can be frightening. They also usually require higher flow rates, which are a fire hazard.

Transtracheal oxygen therapy provides oxygen via a transtracheal catheter using the trachea as its own reservoir. Less oxygen is lost to ambient air; thus oxygenation can be achieved with a flow rate a quarter to half that required with a standard nasal cannula, offering distinct advantages for the oxygen-dependent patient.[28,29] The catheters are inserted on the anterior chest and tunneled up to the trachea. Complications include obstruction of the catheter from mucus balls, increased loss of catheter tract after catheter displacement, bronchospasm, and hoarseness.[24,30] Patients with cystic fibrosis are usually considered poor candidates for transtracheal oxygen because of copious sputum production.

CYSTIC FIBROSIS

The management of patients with cystic fibrosis includes many aspects of home care, from home intravenous antibiotic therapy to chest physiotherapy (CPT). Health care providers have been using home intravenous therapy for years to prevent long-term hospital stays in patients with cystic fibrosis. There is no doubt that home intravenous antibiotic therapy is cost effective.[31,32] Patients also enjoy the many benefits of home treatment, including increased independence, continued school attendance or employment, and minimal disruption of the family routine. Although many studies document no significant difference in pulmonary function and weight,[33-35] there are questions regarding the overall efficacy of home care, especially in patients with more severe disease.[36] It is unclear whether the rest, prepared meals, or frequent professional CPT make the difference for the hospitalized patient, but there is concern that for certain patients, home care is only minimally effective.[37,38] Thus patients with cystic fibrosis who receive home care need to be carefully chosen with consideration of both their medical and social needs.[39]

When home intravenous antibiotic therapy is used, venous access remains an important factor in predicting compliance and overall success. Some patients may be able to use peripheral catheters for smaller veins. Others, because of problems maintaining venous access, may require midline catheters,[40,41] peripherally inserted central catheters,[42] implantable venous access devices,[43,44] or central venous catheters.

The other significant component of cystic fibrosis home therapy is airway clearance technique. In most patients, some form of airway clearance is prescribed and performed on a daily basis. Many patients have used the traditional methods of percussion and postural drainage as part of their daily routine and hospital care since early childhood. For patients who have problems with compliance, however, alternative techniques are available.[45] The different methods include CPT or percussion and postural drainage, percussion devices (including vibrators), percussion vests, the forced expiratory technique (FET), positive end-expiratory pressure valves, autogenic drainage, and the active cycle of breathing technique (ACBT).

Traditional CPT, which consists of postural drainage with percussion, vibration, or both techniques, has long been advocated as the mainstay of airway clearance in patients with cystic fibrosis. CPT quickly improves the maximum expiratory flow rate,[46] forced vital capacity, and forced expiratory volume.[47-49] CPT may be effective in enhancing sputum clearance from the central airways, but it appears to have little obvious effect on the more peripheral airways. Other investigators have shown no consistent improvement in lung function after CPT[50] (see Chapter 20).

Compliance with traditional CPT can be limited because of the time involved, the discomfort, and the need for a second person.[51] Methods exist to assist patients in independence: Both lightweight vibrators and hand-held percussors are available. Vibrators can be adapted for vibration over all lung fields and can be as effective as therapist-administered chest percussion and vibration.[52,53]

Percussion vests consist of an air-pulse generator and an inflatable vest that oscillates against the chest wall, producing high-frequency chest wall oscillation. Studies have shown that there are increases in PFTs[54] and that the device is as effective as CPT in improving PFTs, weight gain, and sputum expectoration.[55] The treatment usually consists of a 30-minute session at different frequencies during the aerosol treatment; postural drainage does not appear to be necessary during the high-frequency chest wall oscillation therapy. The high-frequency vest does seem to promote self-care but is costly, especially for patients with limited funding sources. It may, however be an adequate and cost-effective alternative in the hospital.[56]

The FET uses one or two forced exhalations, or "huffs," from middle to low lung volumes followed by relaxed diaphragmatic breathing. During the FET, the patient maintains an open glottis, preventing the problem of dynamic compression of the airways, which may inhibit mucociliary clearance. FET is helpful in clearing the central airways only down to the seventh generation,[57] but it does clear that part of the bronchial tree when used with postural drainage.[58]

In FET the patient takes a medium-sized inhalation and then breathes out forcefully through an open mouth, without closure of the glottis, until the chest wall and abdominal muscles contract. The process is repeated 2 or 3 times with huffs from middle to low lung volumes.[59,60] It is thought that more secretions are mobilized at this range. Relaxation and diaphragmatic breathing follow, so worsening bronchospasm, which may occur during the forced exhalation maneuvers, can be avoided. The FET does not require any caregivers for assistance after the patient has been instructed. It is hoped that because of this independence, compliance is better than with conventional CPT.

Another independent method of airway clearance is the ACBT. It consists of three breathing techniques: breathing control, thoracic expansion exercises, and the FET[45] (see previous paragraphs). Breathing control involves gentle breathing using the lower chest. Breathing control, also known as *diaphragmatic breathing,* involves breathing at a normal tidal volume and rate. Thoracic expansion exercises are deep breathing exercises emphasizing inspiration with a relaxed expiration. Because lung volume is increased, more air flows through the small airways and collateral ventilation channels and helps loosen secretions.[61] The FET is one or two huffs combined with breathing control. A cycle is repeated until effective huffing in three consecutive cycles has remained dry sounding and nonproductive.

Lung function improves when the ACBT is used[62]; there seems to be no increase in airflow obstruction in patients with cystic fibrosis.[63] ACBT can be taught to children at about 8 or 9 years of age. Huffing can be introduced using blowing games.

Autogenic drainage is a self-performed method of CPT that provides independence for the patient. It relies on controlled breathing to achieve the greatest possible airflow throughout the bronchi to enhance mucus clearance. The three phases used are unstick, collect, and evacuate.[64] The unstick phase involves a slow, deep inspiration through the nose, a 2- to 3- second breath-hold, and a passive or relaxed expiration while the glottis, throat, and mouth are kept open. The expiratory force remains balanced to prevent airway compression and obstruction. The second phase of collecting mucus is achieved by deepening inspiration and expiration. The longer the exhalation, the greater the distance the secretions are transported. In the last phase, the flow starts from about the middle of the inspiratory reserve capacity, and after small bursts of coughing, the mucus is expectorated. A treatment session usually takes 30 to 45 minutes; some patients may spend nearly 2 hours a day performing this technique. It usually takes 10 to 20 hours to teach the principles, with additional sessions to check patient understanding. The age at which this technique can be mastered is somewhere between 4 and 8 years.

Autogenic drainage improves pulmonary function to a greater degree than traditional CPT, possibly because of improved mucus clearance.[65] Autogenic drainage also seems to increase airflow, but this is seen only in patients with pressure-dependent airway collapse.[66] However, no evidence correlates the increase in flow to an increase in the clearance of bronchial secretions.[63]

Positive expiratory pressure (PEP) is a technique used to open and recruit obstructed lung tissue, allowing air to move behind secretions and assist in their mobilization. PEP is based on the premise of collateral ventilation with the application of expiratory pressure.[67] This increase in collateral ventilation enables ventilation to occur in peripheral airways that are obstructed during tidal volume breathing, thus increasing the likelihood of a productive cough.[68,69]

When using PEP, patients should not forcibly exhale and empty their lungs. Lung volumes should be kept up, and the functional residual capacity should rise a little while breathing against the resistance. Both forced exhalation (huff) and breathing controls are combined with PEP to help the patient mobilize, transport, and expectorate the loosened secretions.[70] Low-pressure PEP can be obtained either through a mouth valve or mask at pressures from 10 to 20 cm H_2O. Low-pressure PEP can also be combined with high-pressure PEP, oscillating PEP, autogenic drainage, or the huff technique to obtain an expiratory flow in airways of different sizes.[71]

When used with the FET, PEP appears to be as effective as postural drainage with FET for clearing secretions.[72,73] When used with a mask, the PEP technique is superior to conventional physiotherapy in maintaining pulmonary function[74]; however, there is only a slight change in total lung capacity, vital capacity, tidal volume, and residual volume when PEP is used.[67]

The flutter VRPI (Varioraw, Geneva) is a relatively new device for intermittent expiratory positive pressure.[45,75] The device combines the effects of PEP, oral high-frequency oscillation, and active breathing exercises. The size of a tobacco pipe, it relies on a ball bearing resting on a conical canal that is displaced during expiration, the result of equilibrium among expiratory pressure, gravity on the steel ball bearing, and angle of the valve itself. Patients take a deep breath and then breathe out normally through the valve using the abdominal muscles and relaxing the upper chest and shoulders. Patients then repeat the process up to 20 minutes, varying the angle either upward or downward to vary the frequency of oscillation to that most effective for the individual.

Studies are rather limited because the flutter is a relatively new method of airway clearance. Lyons et al[76] found less sputum volume produced with "flutter only" treatments compared with flutter and CPT treatments. Konstan et al,[77] however, found that the amount of sputum expectorated with the flutter was over 3 times that expectorated with either voluntary cough or postural drainage. The use of flutter as an adjunct to the ACBT is also being studied. Preliminary data indicate an increase in the 1-second forced expiratory volume and forced expiratory flow after 50% of vital capacity has been expelled but no change in either the forced vital capacity or forced expiratory flow after 75% of vital capacity has been expelled.[63]

TRACHEOSTOMY

Children receive tracheostomies for a variety of conditions, including laryngeal lesions (subglottic stenosis), extralaryngeal lesions (cystic hygroma), and neurologic lesions (bilateral vocal cord palsy), and for long-term mechanical ventilation. The underlying goal of a tracheostomy is to maintain an open airway. Obstruction of the tracheostomy tube therefore has the potential for being a life-threatening emergency. Because of this risk, it is imperative that parents and other caregivers in the home be taught proper management of a child with a tracheostomy. Fatalities can occur when untrained caregivers fail to provide appropriate care during an emergency.

Aspects of tracheostomy care that parents and caregivers must learn before discharge include tube changes, stoma site care, safety concerns, cardiopulmonary resuscitation, use of the Ambu bag (if part of the medical equipment), suctioning, humidification, and speech production.[78,79] Tracheostomy changes are performed regularly to maintain airway patency, reduce the incidence of infection, and prevent the formation of large tissue granulomas around the stoma. The frequency varies from 3 times a week to once a month according to the institution and the patient's needs.[80,81] Regular and frequent changes give the family the ability and confidence to intervene if the tube comes out accidentally. Parents should also be able to describe the sequence to follow if the tracheostomy tube is difficult to insert. This is a rare but life-threatening occurrence. The steps include repositioning the child's head, using a tracheostomy tube one size smaller or a suction catheter, and notifying emergency services.

Other emergency issues and safety concerns include symptoms of infection, bleeding, symptoms of respiratory distress, tube occlusion, and accidental decannulation. Infections cause changes in the odor and color of mucus. Physicians need to be notified if these persist more than 24 hours. Blood-tinged mucus may indicate either too-frequent suctioning or trauma after a tube change. Parents should notify the physician if bright red blood is suctioned from the tube. Bleeding, difficulty inserting a tracheostomy tube, or a reduction in vocalization may indicate granuloma formation at the stoma and may indicate the need for visualization of the airway pursuant to removal of potential scar tissue or granuloma.

Symptoms of respiratory distress include increased respiratory rate, increased work of breathing, a change in color (pale, dusky, blue), or all of these. Parents should call emergency services or go to the nearest emergency room if they notice these symptoms.

Life-threatening occlusion is apparent when the child displays symptoms of respiratory distress and a suction catheter cannot be passed to the end of the tube despite several attempts and saline instillation fails. This situation requires an immediate tube change. Accidental decannulation also requires immediate tube placement. Because many infants and children with upper airway problems have little airway reserve, if replacement of the dislodged tube is impossible, a smaller tube should be inserted.[82]

The tracheostomy is suctioned as needed to remove secretions; the frequency varies considerably depending on the character and amount of secretions. Too-frequent suctioning causes increased sputum production. Hyperventilation with 100% oxygen before and after suctioning may be required to prevent hypoxia.[82] The suction catheter should be inserted only to the end of the tracheostomy tube. Inserting the catheter past the end of the tube can cause increased secretions and, most important, injury to airway tissue. Families may also use a bulb syringe to suction the tip of the tracheostomy tube. This is helpful when secretions are coughed up but cannot be cleared from the tube. Bulb syringes must be cleaned thoroughly with warm soapy water every 24 hours.

Daily home care issues for the child with a tracheostomy include feeding, bathing, playing, baby-sitters, safety tips, humidification, emergency awareness, and care (including cardiopulmonary resuscitation).[83] Depending on the age and size of the child, an apnea monitor is required. Caregivers should have a travel kit (Box 24-1) when the child is away from home, even for short trips.[84] Portable suction devices such as bulb syringes or DeLee mucus suction traps as well as battery-operated suction machines should be included in this kit.

Communication is also an important concern for the child with a tracheostomy. If the child is ventilator dependent, air leaks around the tracheostomy tube permit the patient to speak during inhalation. Speech occurs when enough of the ventilator-delivered tidal volume escapes around the tube and passes through the vocal cords.[81] If a cuffed tracheostomy tube is used and the patient is able to spontaneously breathe for a short time and protect their airway, the tube cuff can be deflated, or a fenestrated tracheostomy tube inserted. The placement of a Passy-Muir Speaking Valve either in the circuit or on the trachea allows the patient to speak during exhalation (Passy-Muir, Irvine, Calif.)[85] (Fig. 24-1). Another option is the Olympic Trach-Talk (Olympic Medical, Seattle).[86]

Some form of humidification of inspired air is necessary for a patient with a tracheostomy tube because the nose and mouth

BOX 24-1
Travel Kit for a Child with a Tracheostomy

Shoulder bag
Suction machine (battery operated)
DeLee mucus suction trap
Suction catheters
Tracheostomy tube and tube that is one size smaller (with ties in place)
Tracheostomy ties
Normal saline (individual vials)
Hydrogen peroxide
Water
Pipe cleaners
Gloves, hand cleaner (alcohol wipes), or tissues
Money for a pay phone (or calling card) and card with name of doctor

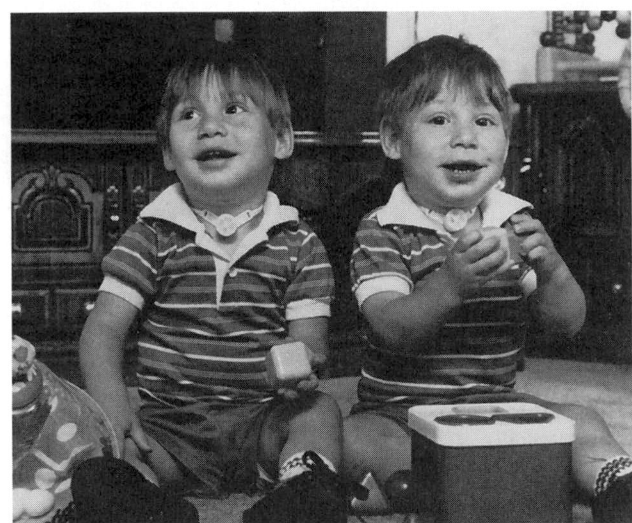

Fig. 24-1. Passy-Muir speaking valve.

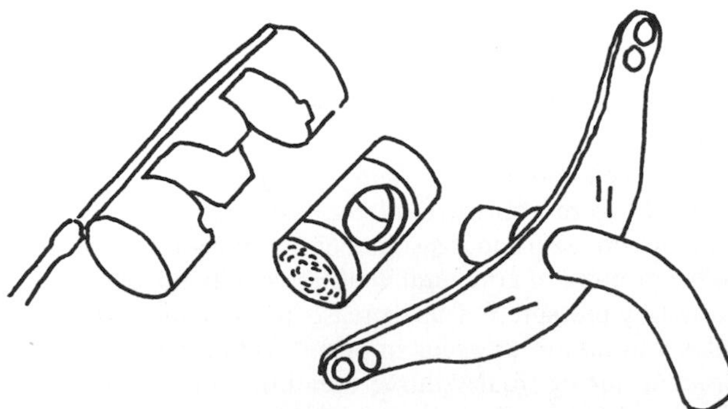

Fig. 24-2. Artificial nose. *Center,* Thermal humidifying unit, or "artificial nose." *Left,* Optional oxygen attachment. *Right,* Tracheostomy tube to which artificial nose attaches. (From Turner J et al, eds: *Handbook of adult and pediatric respiratory home care,* St Louis, 1994, Mosby, p 289.)

are bypassed. If the patient is ventilator dependent, the humidifier part of the ventilator circuit warms and moisturizes inspired air. If the patient's lungs are not being ventilated, other systems are needed. Tracheostomy collars are available but are difficult to use if the patient is not homebound. Vaporizers or room humidifiers may be acceptable but must be cleaned daily. The instillation of saline drops provides humidification when the patient is not at home. Another alternative is the artificial nose or in-line condensers: corrugated filter–like devices that fits snugly either over the end of the tracheostomy tube or between the exhalation valve and the patient. During exhalation, moisture from exhaled air condenses on the filter surface. During inhalation, air passes back through the moisture-laden filter and is warmed and humidified, replicating the natural function of the upper airway.[81] Artificial noses are especially helpful for children with smaller tracheostomy tubes or those in whom secretions build up on the inside of the tracheostomy tube (Fig. 24-2).[87]

There is an ongoing controversy regarding clean (nongloved, washed hands), clean and gloved, and sterile and gloved suctioning technique. With clean suctioning the disposable catheters are frequently reused. As long as the infant is not extremely young and is not prone to frequent infections, the caregiver may prefer to use the simplest and least expensive method. If the child develops a respiratory infection, however, clean and gloved or sterile and gloved techniques should be instituted.[88] Still another method is "cath-n-sleeve" catheters. These catheters have a sleeve extending to about 1 inch beyond the catheter tip so that caregivers can use their bare hands while still maintaining sterile technique.

Another controversial issue is the reuse of suction catheters. The major concern is fear of infection from the introduction of new or additional numbers of bacteria, potentially leading to pneumonia. Some caregivers rinse the catheter after suctioning, using one to three catheters a day.[89] Others sterilize or soak the catheters in bactericidal solution at the end of the day and then reuse them. No matter which standard is practiced, proper handwashing is necessary to prevent contamination from a person to a person or an inanimate object to a person.

MECHANICAL VENTILATION

The goals for long-term ventilatory support at home are to optimize the child's quality of life, ensure the medical safety of the child, use respiratory equipment safely and properly, and prevent or minimize complications.[90,91] Discharge planning for mechanically ventilated children, especially those on positive-pressure ventilation, is a complex process taking 2 to 4 weeks in the best of circumstances.[92,93]

Children's lungs can be ventilated at home using a variety of assisted ventilation units. These include the negative-pressure ventilation (NPV) systems, diaphragmatic pacing, positive-pressure ventilation with a nasal mask or tracheostomy, and continuous positive airway pressure (CPAP) with a nasal mask. The type of ventilation unit used depends on the diagnosis, pathologic condition, and size of the child.

Negative-Pressure Ventilation

NPV incorporates a vacuum source or bellows attached to a shell or tank that decreases the pressure surrounding the patient's chest and abdomen. This pressure change causes the diaphragm to descend and the thorax to increase in diameter, allowing air movement into the lungs, as in normal respiration.[94] The advantages of NPV devices are that they do not require an artificial airway in most patients and are easy to operate.[95] Disadvantages include esophageal reflux and the possibility of upper airway obstruction and obstructive sleep apnea from lack of synchronous upper airway tone. Candidates for NPV must have a compliant chest wall to ensure ventilation and must be medically stable to tolerate periods off the device. NPV is frequently used for nighttime support only to stabilize respiratory reserve.[96]

The chest-shell (cuirass) ventilator uses a dome-shaped shell that fits over the patient's anterior chest and abdomen. Negative pressure is generated within the chest shell, expanding the chest. Cuirass ventilators can provide effective ventilation in older children and adolescents, often without a tracheostomy. Infants and young children, however, may require a tracheostomy because of airway collapse during sleep.[97-99] Because the major benefit of NPV is that a tracheostomy may not be needed, little advantage exists for infant and young children. In addition, the smallest commercial shell produced fits children approximately 4 years of age. Therefore use of this technique is not possible for young children.

Home care issues with the chest shell include skin care, comfort, and portability. Comfort is a concern because of the necessity for a supine sleep position. Irritation and skin sores can develop at points of sealing, especially in patients with gross deformities. The use of powder or cornstarch and a T-shirt under the shell may prevent irritation.

The "raincoat" or wrap is another NPV device. It is essentially a poncho covering a shell-like grid placed on the patient's chest, encompassing either the entire body or only the upper body. Certain patients need a back brace to help prevent a rocking motion of the grid. The disadvantages are that the patient has to be supine or reclining, thus making it uncomfortable and potentially difficult for pediatric patients.

The iron lung is a self-contained NPV device. This "body tank" is an airtight cylinder that surrounds the entire body from the neck to the feet with an electrically powered bellows system to produce NPV pressure.[100] The full body chamber is not appropriate for most children or adolescents because patients can feel claustrophobic inside the tank. Nursing care is also difficult because of patient inaccessibility. Battery capabilities are not available, and the weight makes them a rather permanent device.[101]

Pneumobelts and rocking beds rely on the mechanical movement of the diaphragm to aid in ventilation. The pnuemobelt, a corsetlike belt attached to a positive-pressure generator, allows the patient more freedom of movement but requires the patient to be in an upright position.[102] It is used mainly as a daytime ventilatory aid during meals or wheelchair use.[103] Rocking beds rely on motion to alternately apply and remove pressure on the diaphragm and assist ventilation. They are simple to operate and maintain and do not require any invasive technology. The present use is rather limited. Disadvantages include size, the patient's inability to tolerate the rocking motion and confinement, and disturbed sleep.

Diaphragmatic Pacing

Diaphragmatic pacing, or bilateral pacing to the thoracic phrenic nerves, is another method of supporting ventilation in pediatric patients. Used as an alternative or supplement to mechanical ventilation, pacing is appropriate in children with quadriplegia or inadequate central respiratory drive (congenital and late-onset central hypoventilation syndrome and central hypoventilation secondary to Chiari type II malformation).[104,105]

Bilateral pacing to the thoracic phrenic nerves offers many advantages over traditional mechanical ventilation. For children requiring ventilatory support during the day, pacing promotes maximal independence and the ability to perform age-appropriate activities. It is common for these patients to engage in various sports and hobbies. Exercise does need to be in performed moderation, though, because the pacer rate does not increase despite increased metabolic needs.[106] Children who are quadriplegic also enjoy this method because it allows normalcy in the wheelchair without the need for a portable ventilator. Bilateral pacing in pediatric patients is typically used with the minimum daytime use of 12 to 15 hours a day with additional ventilatory support by mechanical ventilation.[107] However, pacing can provide overnight ventilation for patients needing only nighttime support, eliminating the need for mechanical ventilation.

Home care issues for children receiving diaphragmatic pacing include care of the pacer itself and the tracheostomy. A tracheostomy may be necessary to allow nighttime mechanical ventilation.[108,109] In such a case, a backup ventilator is required for patient support. Parents are instructed to examine the child's diaphragmatic excursion daily and follow a sequence of events in case of problems. These include replacing the battery and antenna and changing to the backup transmitter if problems occur.[107] Families need to be aware of any potential problems with both the implanted or electric components and need to understand the importance of daily monitoring. It is important that physicians with considerable experience and substantial expertise work with the family.

Another pacing concern is the cost and limited availability of centers performing diaphragmatic pacing.[109] Included in the cost are external components (transmitter and antennas), internal components (electrodes, receivers, and anodes), and a month-long intensive care hospitalization. Indirect costs to the family include batteries, transportation to the appropriate center, and lodging. When compared, however, to long-term home mechanical ventilation, the cost becomes negligible.

Positive-Pressure Ventilation

The most commonly used approach for home mechanical ventilation is the positive-pressure ventilator (see Chapter 21).[22,92,110] In this category, two types of ventilation are commonly used: volume-limited ventilation and time-cycled, pressure-limited ventilation. In the volume-limited mode the ventilator delivers a preset volume of air during the inspiratory cycle.[18] In contrast in the pressure-limited mode the ventilator delivers flow until a preset pressure is reached.[87] An example of a classic pressure-limited ventilator used for supportive ventilation in the home is the bilevel positive airway pressure (BiPAP) system, which has a limited maximum pressure of 20 to 22 cm H_2O. Two mechanical ventilators commonly used in the home are the LP10 (Aequitron Medical, Minneapolis) and PLV100 (Lifecare, Phoenix), which can be used in either the volume- or pressure-limited mode. These types of ventilators are relatively easy to operate and cost less than many other systems. They weigh less than 40 lb and can be battery operated, an important feature in allowing greater mobility in respiratory support in case of power failure.[92,111]

As previously noted, the available ventilation modes include assist-control, intermittent mandatory ventilation, synchronized intermittent mandatory ventilation, and pressure-limited modes. Ventilation using a volume-limited mode may be inadequate for patients who develop air leaks around the tracheostomy during the expiratory phase.[108] This can lead to substantial loss of ventilation and hypoxia or hypercapnia. In contrast, pressure-limited ventilators may not have this problem; however, many of the ventilators in the pressure-limited mode have a relatively short inspiratory phase. One way around this is to use the ventilator in the volume-limited mode with a pressure "pop-off."[20,22,112] This allows the tidal breath to be determined by the volume ventilator, but a pressure plateau can be achieved using a pop-off valve.[108] Alarms used in the home indicate disconnections, low and high system pressures, and mechanical failure. When BiPAP or other ventilators are used in the pressure-limited mode, it is important to note that the alarm system must be sensitive enough to detect disconnection.[113]

One disadvantage of positive-pressure ventilation in the home can be the requirement of an artificial airway or tracheostomy. Because the underlying goal of the tracheostomy is to provide an open airway, obstruction of the tracheostomy is a life-threatening emergency. Before discharge, caregivers need to become experts in the management of the tracheostomy (see section on tracheostomies). Another issue in home positive-pressure ventilation is the fact that many home ventilators have valves that are difficult to open to initiate the breath even at the highest sensitivity settings. This can make synchronization difficult for small infants or children who are weak because of a neuromuscular disorder. In many cases, provision of a bypass flow system using a compressor, intermittent mandatory ventilation bag, and H-valve may improve the patient's work of breathing during spontaneous respiration.[18,112]

Backup ventilator support must be available in the home. Patients who require 24-hour ventilation, those who tolerate only very short periods without ventilator support, and those who live a significant distance from medical support need a second fully operational ventilator in the home.[20,22] Supplemental oxygen is also required if the patient's fraction of inspired oxygen is greater than 0.21. Parents and caregivers should be trained in ventilator maintenance, troubleshooting, and emergency care before discharge. Daily routines for equipment maintenance include ventilator checks, cleaning and changing of the ventilator circuits, and cleaning of the suction machine and resuscitation bag.

Noninvasive Positive-Pressure Ventilation

Noninvasive positive-pressure ventilation (NIPPV) is another method for providing positive-pressure ventilation without a tracheostomy.[114-117] For patients who suffer from neuromuscular weakness or restrictive chest wall disease, this technique may provide better acceptance and comfort than the invasive technique.[118-120] A tracheostomy may be necessary if the patient is unable to protect the airway or handle secretions. The type of ventilators used are either volume or pressure support, depending on the prognosis and the predicted level of dependency on mechanical ventilation.

The three types of interfaces used for NIPPV include the nasal mask, the mouthpiece, and the face mask. Nasal masks may be appropriate for nighttime use but may require custom masks for the pediatric patient.[101,121] Irritation of the skin, nasal bridge, and mucous membranes may also occur. A mouthpiece with a lip seal or a custom orthodontic interface may be preferable for daytime use because it is not obtrusive and allows the patient to talk and eat but still provides the convenience of assisted ventilation.[122] However, it may pose a compliance issue for pediatric patients. Face masks offer better control of leakage but are poorly tolerated, especially during long-term ventilation at home. Face masks can also be expensive because they are custom made and in pediatric patients may require frequent adjustments. No single mask or device matches the needs of all patients; its usually best to try each type to determine which is the easiest to use for a particular patient.

Care issues for patients with NIPPV include skin care, especially with a poorly fitting nasal or face mask; gastrointestinal inflation, especially for patients on volume ventilation; and upper airway dryness. Patients also need to be assessed on a regular basis for worsening disease and increased dependency on mechanical ventilation, necessitating either combined methods of NIPPV or tracheostomy ventilation.[123]

Continuous Positive Airway Pressure

CPAP is the application of positive pressure to the airways to prevent upper airway collapse. Used primarily for obstructive sleep apnea, CPAP is administered via a mask similar to that used for NIPPV but without inspiratory pressure; instead, a continuous positive pressure is generated.[124,125] BiPAP (see Chapter 21) is similar to CPAP with higher pressures applied during inspiration than during expiration, a backup respiratory rate, and a set inspiratory and expiratory ratio.[112] It is indicated for patients who require high levels of CPAP, have extended periods of apnea, or need additional respiratory support.

CPAP and BiPAP can be administered in the home via a tracheostomy or a mask or nasal pillows held in place with head straps.[18] Masks and pillows are available in pediatric sizes, as are custom-made masks derived from commercially available equipment. As in NIPPV, no one type of mask or device is best for patients. It is recommended that clinicians try each type to find the best fit for a patient.

Technical problems include mouth leaks, which can be remedied by the use of chin straps, and nasal obstruction or stuffiness (especially during viral rhinitis), which can be treated with humidification, nasal decongestant spray, or both therapies. Mouth air leaks can be treated with the use of chin straps. Some patients also complain of claustrophobic sensations, which can be prevented by the use of the nasal pillows. Hand restraints may be needed with young children who resist mask administration or pull the mask off during sleep. Before discharge, the patient and family members need to be well versed in both the technical and safety aspects of care.

REFERENCES

1. Perrin JM: Chronically ill children in America, *Caring* 4:16, 1985.
2. Cabin B: Cost effectiveness of pediatric home care, *Caring* 48-51, 1985.
3. Weston BE, Keefe JA: Pediatric home care and public policy, *Caring* 12:60-64, 1993.
4. Whitesal E, Carlin P, Cimo D: *Getting it started and keeping it going: a workbook and video,* New Orleans, 1987, Children's Hospital.
5. DeWitt PR, Jansen MT, Davidson Ward SL, Lew CD, Bowman CM, Platzker ACG, Keens TG: Obstacles to discharge of ventilator dependent children from the hospital to home, *Am Rev Respir Dis* 139:196A, 1989 (Abstract).

Criteria and Planning for Home Care

6. Bedore B, Leighton L: Comprehensive home management, *Caring* 8:50-55, 1989.
7. McCoy PA: Discharge planning. In McCoy P, Votroubek W, eds: *Pediatric home care: a comprehensive approach,* Gaithersburg, Md, 1989, Aspen.
8. Aday LA, Wegener DH: Home care for ventilator-assisted children: implications for the children, their families, and health policy, *CHC* 17:112-120, 1988.
9. Quint RD, Chesterman E, Crain LS, Winkleby M, Boyce WT: Home care for ventilator-dependent children, *Am J Dis Child* 144:1238-1241, 1990.
10. Scharer K, Dixon DM: Managing chronic illness: parents with a ventilator-dependent child, *J Pediatr Nurs* 4:236-247, 1989.
11. Wegener DH, Aday LA: Home care for ventilator-assisted children: predicting family stress, *Pediatr Nurs* 15:371-376, 1989.
12. Kirkhart KA, Steele NF, Pomeroy M, Auguzza R, French W, Gates AJ: Louisiana's ventilator assisted care program: case management services to link tertiary with community-based care, *CHC* 17:106-111, 1988.
13. Lobosco AF, Eron NB, Bobo T, Kril L, Chalanick K: Local coalitions for coordinating services to children dependent on technology and their families, *CHC* 20:75-86, 1991.
14. Anguzza RA: Case management: more than cost containment, *Continuing Care* 26-28, 1988.
15. Anas N: Discharge planning and home management for the ventilator-assisted infant, *J Home Health Care Pract* 2(2):53-59, 1990.
16. Hazlett DE: A study of pediatric home ventilator management: medical, psychosocial, and financial aspects, *J Pediatr Nurs* 4(4)284-294, 1989.
17. McCoy PA: Health history, interviewing, nursing process, care plan, and documentation. In McCoy PA, Votroubek W, eds: *Pediatric home care: a comprehensive approach,* Gaithersburg, Md, 1990, Aspen.
18. Baroni DM: Home sweet home, *J Respir Care Pract* 3:87-90, 1996.
19. Anguzza RA: Pediatric home ventilation, *J Respir Care Pract* 3:81-84, 1996.
20. Davidson-Ward SL, Keens TG: Ventilatory management at home. In Ballard RA, ed: *Pediatric care of the ICN graduate,* Philadelphia, 1988, WB Saunders, pp 166-176.
21. Goldberg AI, Faure EAM, Vaughn CJ, Snarski R, Seleny FL: Home care for life-supported persons: an approach to program development, *J Pediatr* 104:785-795, 1984.

Oxygen Therapy

22. O'Donohue WJ Jr, Givannoni RM, Goldberg AI, Keens TG, Make BJ, Plummer AC, Prentice WS: Long-term mechanical ventilation: guidelines for management in the home and at alternate community sites, *Chest* 90(suppl):1-37, 1986.
23. Peterson P: *Good if not great travel with oxygen,* Philadelphia, 1996, Raven.
24. McDonald G: Home oxygen therapy. In Turner J, McDonald G, Larter N, eds: *Handbook of adult and pediatric respiratory home care,* St Louis, 1994, Mosby.
25. McPherson SP: *Respiratory home care equipment,* Dubuque, Iowa, 1988, Daedalus Enterprises, Kendall/Hunt.
26. O'Donohue J: The future of home oxygen therapy, *Respir Care* 33:1125, 1988.
27. Herrick TW, Yeager H: Home oxygen therapy, *Am Fam Physician* 39:157, 1989.
28. Hill D: Transtracheal oxygen: setting up a home care program, *Caring* 44-47, 1995.
29. Papcke-Benson K: Transtracheal oxygen therapy, *IACFA* 11-13, 1992.
30. Christopher KL, Spofford BT, Petrun MD, McCarty DC, Goodman JR, Petty TL: A program for transtracheal oxygen delivery, *Ann Intern Med* 107(6):802-808, 1987.

Cystic Fibrosis

31. Kane RE, Jennison K, Wood C, Black PG, Herbst JJ: Cost savings and economic considerations using home intravenous antibiotic therapy for cystic fibrosis patients, *Pediatr Pulmonol* 4:84-89, 1988.
32. Rucker R, Harrison G: Outpatient IV medications in the management of CF, *Pediatrics* 54:358-360, 1974.
33. Gilbert J, Robinson T, Littlewood JM: Home intravenous antibiotic treatment in cystic fibrosis, *Arch Dis Child* 63:512-517, 1988.

34. Martinez MA, Votroubek W, Hoefle K, Lemen KJ: Efficacy of respiratory home care versus inpatient care for cystic fibrosis patients, *Am Rev Respir Dis* 135:A194, 1987.
35. Davis SH: Outpatient management of pulmonary exacerbations in children with cystic fibrosis, *Semin Pediatr Infect Dis* 1:393-403, 1990.
36. Donati MA, Guenette G, Auerbach H: Prospective controlled study of home and hospital therapy of cystic fibrosis pulmonary disease, *J Pediatr* 11:28-33, 1987.
37. Bosworth DG, Nielson DW: Home treatment of *Pseudomonas* pneumonia in cystic fibrosis is not as effective as in-hospital treatment, *Am Rev Respir Dis* 147:A580, 1993.
38. Bosworth DG, Nielson DW: Effectiveness of home versus hospital care in the routine treatment of cystic fibrosis, *Pediatr Pulmonol* 24:42-47, 1998.
39. Hammond LJ, Caldwell S, Campbell PW: Cystic fibrosis, intravenous antibiotics, and home therapy, *J Pediatr Health Care* 5:24-30, 1991.
40. Hadaway LC: A midline alternative to central and peripheral venous access, *Caring* 45-46, 1990.
41. Harwood IR, Greene LM, Kozakowski-Koch JA, Rasor JS: New peripherally inserted midline catheter: a better alternative for intravenous antibiotic therapy in patients with cystic fibrosis, *Pediatr Pulmonol* 12:233-239, 1992.
42. Pharmacia Deltec: *Patients' choices for venous access,* St Paul, Minnesota, 1990, Pharmacia Deltec.
43. McKee J: Future dimensions in vascular access: peripheral implantable ports, *J Intravenous Nurs* 14(6):387-393, 1991.
44. Winters V, Peters B, Coila S, Jones L: A trial with a new peripheral implanted vascular access device, *Oncol Nurs Forum* 17(6):891-896, 1990.
45. Hardy KA: A review of airway clearance: new techniques, indications, and recommendations, *Respir Care* 39(5)440-452, 1994.
46. Feldman U, Traver GA, Taussig LM: Maximal expiratory flows after postural drainage, *Am Rev Respir Dis* 119:139-245, 1979.
47. Maxwell M, Redmond A: Comparative trial of manual and mechanical percussion technique with gravity-assisted bronchial drainage in patients with cystic fibrosis, *Arch Dis Child* 54(7):542-544, 1979.
48. Baran D, Van Bogaert E: *Chest physical therapy in cystic fibrosis and chronic obstructive pulmonary diseases,* Ghent, Belgium, 1977, Eur.
49. Tecklin JS, Holsclaw DS: Evaluation of bronchial drainage in patients with cystic fibrosis, *Phys Ther* 55:1081-1084, 1975.
50. Zapletal A, Stefanova J, Horak J, Vavrova V, Samanek M: Chest physiotherapy and airway obstruction in patients with cystic fibrosis: a NPV report, *Eur J Respir Dis* 64:426, 1983.
51. Possero MA, Remor B, Salomon J: Patient-reported compliance with cystic fibrosis therapy, *Clin Pediatr (Phila)* 20(4):264-268, 1981.
52. Hartsell M: Chest physiotherapy and mechanical vibration, *J Pediatr Nurs* 2:135-137, 1987.
53. Maxwell M, Redmond A: Comparative trial of manual and mechanical percussion technique with gravity-assisted bronchial drainage in patients with cystic fibrosis, *Arch Dis Child* 54:542-544, 1979.
54. Warwick WJ, Hansen IG: The long-term effect of high-frequency chest compression on pulmonary function on patients with cystic fibrosis, *Pediatr Pulmonol* 11:265-271, 1991.
55. Ahrens R, Gozal D, Omlin KJ, Vega J, Boyd KP, Keens TG, Woo MS: Comparative efficacy of high frequency chest compression and conventional chest physiotherapy in hospitalized patients with cystic fibrosis, *Pediatr Pulmonol* 9(suppl):239, 1993.
56. Ahrens R, Gozal D, Omlin KJ, Vega J, Boyd KP, Keens TG, Woo MS: Comparison of high frequency chest compression and conventional chest physiotherapy in hospitalized patients with cystic fibrosis, *Am J Respir Crit Care Med* 150:1154-1157, 1994.
57. Sutton PP: Chest physiotherapy: time for reappraisal, *Br J Dis Chest* 82:127-137, 1988.
58. Reisman JJ, Rivington-Law B, Corey M, Marcotte J, Wannamaker E, Harcourt D, Levison H: Role of conventional physiotherapy in cystic fibrosis, *J Pediatr* 113(4):632-636, 1988.
59. Pryor JA, Webber BA, Hodson ME, Batten JC: Evaluation of the forced expiration technique as an adjunct to postural drainage in treatment of cystic fibrosis, *Br Med J* 2(6187):417-418, 1979.
60. Pryor J: The forced expiratory technique. In Pryor J, ed: *Respiratory care,* London, 1991, Churchill Livingstone, pp 79-100.
61. Webber BA: The active cycle of breathing techniques, Royal Brompton and National Heart Hospital, London, *CF News,* 1990.
62. Webber BA, Hofmeyr JL, Morgan MDL, Hodson ME, Batten JC: *Effects of postural drainage incorporating the forced expiration technique, on pulmonary function in cystic fibrosis: proceedings of the 13th Annual Meeting of the European Working Group for Cystic Fibrosis,* Jerusalem, 1985, p 24.
63. Pryor JA, Webber BA: Physiotherapy for cystic fibrosis: which technique? *Physiotherapy* 78(2):105-108, 1992.
64. Chevaillier J: Autogenic drainage. In Lawson D, ed: *Cystic fibrosis:* horizons, Chichester, Mass, 1984, John Wiley, pp 235.
65. Giles DR, Wagener JS, Accurso FJ, Butler-Simon N: Short-term effects of postural drainage with clapping vs autogenic drainage on oxygen saturation and sputum recovery in patients with cystic fibrosis, *Chest* 108:952-954, 1995.
66. Schoni MH: Autogenic drainage: a modern approach to physiotherapy in cystic fibrosis, *J R Soc Med* 82(16):32-37, 1989.
67. Groth S, Stafanger G, Dirksen H, Andersen JB, Falk M, Kelstrup M: Positive expiratory pressure (PEP-mask) physiotherapy improves ventilation and reduces volume of trapped gas in cystic fibrosis, *Bull Eur Physiopathol Respir* 21:339-343, 1985.
68. Anderson JB, Quis I, Kenni T: Recruiting collapsed lung through channels with positive end expiratory pressure, *Scand J Respir Dis* 60:260-266, 1979.
69. Hofmeyr JL, Webber BA, Hodson ME: Evaluation of positive expiratory pressure as an adjunct to chest physiotherapy in the treatment of cystic fibrosis, *Thorax* 41:951-954, 1986.
70. Mahlmeister MJ, Fink JB, Hoffman GL, Fifer LF: Positive-expiratory-pressure mask therapy: theoretical and practical considerations and a review of the literature, *Respir Care* 36(11):1218-1229, 1991.
71. Lannefors L: Different ways of using positive expiratory pressure to loosen and mobilize pulmonary secretions, *Cystic Fibrosis Informer* 9(1), 1993.
72. Mortensen J, Falk M, Groth S, Jensen C: The effects of postural drainage and positive expiratory pressure physiotherapy on tracheobronchial clearance in cystic fibrosis, *Chest* 100:1350, 1991.
73. Falk M, Kelstrup M, Anderson JB, Kinoshita T, Falk P, St Vring S, G'thgen I: Improving the ketchup bottle method with positive expiratory pressure, PEP, *Eur J Respir Dis* 65:423-432, 1984.
74. McIlwaine PM, Wong LTK, Peacock D, et al: Long-term comparative trial of conventional postural drainage and percussion vs. positive expiratory pressure physiotherapy in the treatment of cystic fibrosis, *J Pediatr* 131:570-574, 1997.
75. Lindemann H: Zum Stellenwert der Physiotherapie mit dem VRP 1-Desitin ("Flutter") [The value of physical therapy with VRP1 ("Flutter")], *Pneumologie* 46(12):626-630, 1992.
76. Lyons E, Chatham K, Campbell IA, Prescott RJ: Evaluation of the Flutter Vrp1 device in young adults with cystic fibrosis, *Thorax* 47:237P, 1992.
77. Konstan MWK, Stern RC, Doershuk CF: Efficacy of the flutter in airway mucus clearance in cystic fibrosis patients, *J Pediatr* 124:689-693, 1994.

Tracheostomy

78. Carabott J, Kipling D, Manger G, King-Pankratz H: Teaching families tracheotomy care, *Can Nurse* 87:21-22, 1991.
79. Sherman LP, Rosen CD: Development of a preschool program for tracheostomy dependent children, *Pediatr Nurs* 16(4):357-361, 1990.
80. Hazinski MF: Pediatric home tracheostomy care: a parent's guide, *Pediatr Nurs* 12(1):41-48, 69, 1986.
81. Mizumori N, Nelson E, Prentice W, Withey L: Mechanical ventilation in the home. In Turner J, McDonal G, Larter N, eds: *Handbook of adult and pediatric respiratory home care,* St Louis, 1994, Mosby.
82. Whaley LF, Wong D: The child with disturbance of oxygen and carbon dioxide exchange. In Whaley LF, Wong D, eds: *Nursing care of infants and children,* St Louis, 1991, Mosby.
83. University of Colorado Health Sciences Center: *Home tracheostomy care for infants and young children,* 1989, Learner Managed Designs.
84. Peirson GS: Home care protocols for pediatric tracheostomy patients, *Caring* 6:38-42, 1993.
85. Passy V: Passy-Muir tracheostomy speaking valve, *Otolaryngol Head Neck Surg* 95:247-248, 1986.
86. Fornataro-Clerici L: Aerodynamic characteristics of tracheostomy speaking valves, *J Speech Hear Res* 36:529-532, 1993.

87. Mallory GB, Stillwell PC: The ventilator-dependent child: issues in diagnosis and management, *Arch Phys Med Rehabil* 72:43-55, 1991.
88. Kaufman J, Hardy-Ribakow D: What parents need to know about trach care, *RN* 51:99-104, 1988.
89. Kuhn S, ed: *Tracheostomy home care for children,* ed 3, Los Angeles, 1990, Department of Nursing, Children's Hospital of Los Angeles.

Mechanical Ventilation

90. Frates RC, Splaingard ML, Smith EO, Harrison GM: Outcome of home mechanical ventilation in children, *J Pediatr* 106:850-856, 1985.
91. Schreiner MS, Donar ME, Kettrick RG: Pediatric home mechanical ventilation, *Pediatr Clin North Am* 34(1)47-60, 1987.
92. Kacmarek RM, Spearman CB: Equipment used for ventilatory support in the home, *Respir Care* 31:311-328, 1986.
93. Steele NF, Harrison B: Technology-assisted children: assessing discharge preparation, *J Pediatr Nurs* 1(3):150-158, 1986.
94. Thomson A: The role of negative pressure ventilation, *Arch Dis Child* 77:454-458, 1997.
95. Splaingard ML, Frates RC, Jefferson LS, Rosen CL, Harrison GM: Home NPV pressure ventilation: report of 20 years of experience in patients with neuromuscular disease, *Arch Phys Med Rehabil* 66:239-242, 1985.
96. Hoeppner VH, Cockcroft DW, Dosman JA, Cotton DJ: Nighttime ventilation improves respiratory failure in kyphoscoliosis, *Am Rev Respir Dis* 129:240-243, 1984.
97. Bach JR, Alba AS: Management of chronic alveolar hypoventilation by nasal ventilation, *Chest* 97:52-57, 1990.
98. Ellis ER, Bye TP, Bruderer JW, Sullivan CE: Treatment of respiratory failure during sleep in patients with neuromuscular disease, *Am Rev Respir Dis* 135:148-152, 1987.
99. Sheerson J: Home ventilation, *Br J Hosp Med* 46:393-395, 1991.
100. Becker EA, Shea TA: Airway and ventilation accessories. In Johnson DL, Giovannoni RM, Driscoll SA, eds: *Ventilator assisted patient care,* Gaithersburg, Md, 1986, Aspen.
101. Bach JR, Alba AS, Saporito LR: Intermittent positive pressure ventilation via the mouth as an alternative to tracheostomy for 257 ventilator users, *Chest* 103:174-182, 1993.
102. Miller HJ, Thomas E, Wilmot CB: Pneumobelt use among high quadriplegic population, *Arch Phys Med Rehabil* 69:369-372, 1988.
103. Hill NS: Use of NPV pressure ventilation, rocking beds, and pneumobelts, *Respir Care* 39:532-549, 1994.
104. Brouillette RT, Ilbawi MN, Klemka-Walden L, Hunt CE: Stimulus parameters for phrenic nerve pacing in infants and children, *Pediatr Pulmonol* 4:33-38, 1988.
105. Weese-Mayer DE, Morrow AS, Brouillette RT, Ilbawi MN, Hunt CE: Diaphragm pacing in infants and children, *Am Rev Respir Dis* 139:974-979, 1989.
106. Weese-Mayer DE, Hunt CE, Brouillette RT, Silvestri JM: Diaphragm pacing in infants and children, *J Pediatr* 120(1):1-8, 1992.
107. Brouillette RT, Ilbawi MN, Hunt CE: Phrenic nerve pacing in infants and children: a review of experience and report on the usefulness of phrenic nerve stimulation studies, *J Pediatr* 102(1):32-39, 1983.
108. Keens TG, Jansen MT, DeWitt PK, Ward SL: Home care for children with chronic respiratory failure, *Semin Respir Med* 11(3):269-281, 1990.
109. Moxham J, Shneerson JM: Diaphragmatic pacing, *Am Rev Respir Dis* 148:533-536, 1993.
110. Goldberg AI: The regional approach to home care for life supported persons, *Chest* 86:345-346, 1984.
111. Lynch M: Home care of the ventilator-dependent child, *CHC* 19(3):169-173, 1990.
112. Kacmarek RM: Home mechanical ventilatory assistance for infants, *Respir Care* 39(5):550-565, 1994.
113. Shneerson J: Home ventilation, *Br J Hosp Med* 46:393-395, 1991.
114. Bach JB, O'Brien J, Krotenberg R, Alba AS: Management of end stage respiratory failure in Duchenne muscular dystrophy, *Muscle Nerv* 10:177-182, 1987.
115. Ellis ER, Bye PTP, Bruderer JW, Sullivan CE: Treatment of respiratory failure during sleep in patients with neuromuscular disease: positive pressure ventilation through a nose mask, *Am Rev Respir Dis* 135:148-152, 1987.
116. Leger P, Jennequin J, Gerard M, Robert D: Home positive pressure ventilation via nasal mask for patients with neuromuscular weakness or restrictive lung or chest-wall disease, *Respir Care* 34:73-79, 1989.
117. Kinnear WJM: Nasal intermittent positive pressure ventilator. In Kinnear WJM, ed: *Assisted ventilation at home,* Oxford, England, 1994, Oxford University Press.
118. Branthwaite MA: Non-invasive and domiciliary ventilation: positive pressure techniques, *Thorax* 46:208-212, 1991.
119. Meyer TJ, Hill NS: Noninvasive positive pressure ventilation to treat respiratory failure, *Ann Intern Med* 120:760-770, 1994.
120. Pierson DJ: Controversies in home respiratory care: conference summary, *Respir Care* 39(4):294-308, 1993.
121. Leger P, Jennequin J, Gerard M, Robert D: Home positive pressure ventilation via nasal mask for patients with neuromuscular weakness or restrictive lung or chest-wall disease, *Respir Care* 34:73-77, 1989.
122. Leger P: Noninvasive positive-pressure ventilation at home, *Respir Care* 39:501-510, 1994.
123. Leger P, Jennequin J, Gerard M, Lassonnery S, Robert D: Home positive pressure ventilation via nasal mask for patients with neuromusculoskeletal disorders, *Eur Respir J* 2(7):640-645, 1989.
124. Guilleminault C, Nino-Murcia G, Heldt G, Baldwin R, Hutchinson D: Alternative treatment to tracheostomy in obstructive sleep apnea syndrome: nasal continuous positive airway pressure in young children, *Pediatrics* 78(5):797-802, 1986.
125. Kandall K: Respiratory therapy devices. In Turner J, McDonald G, Larter N, eds: *Handbook of adult and pediatric respiratory home care,* St Louis, 1994, Mosby.

PART FIVE

Respiratory Insults and Intensive Care

CHAPTER 25

Lung Trauma: Toxin Inhalation and ARDS

Robert Henning and Trevor Duke

BURN INHALATION INJURY

Burns are the third most common cause of accidental death in childhood in the industrialized world after road accidents and drowning.[1] Approximately 40,000 children per year are admitted to the hospital in the United States because of burns, and 1300 die.[2] Fortunately, these numbers are decreasing.[3] Although the incidence of inhalation injury is lower in burned children than in adults (3% vs. 10%), children with inhalation injury are more likely to die or have a longer hospital stay than those without it,[1] even though those with inhalation injury tend to have a larger percentage of burned body surface area than those without it. Inhalation injury increases the mortality rate by up to 20%, and pneumonia increases it by up to 40%. When both are present, the mortality rate increases by up to 60% at all ages.[4] Respiratory failure is by far the most common cause of death in the first hour after burn injury.[5]

Respiratory system function may be impaired after smoke inhalation damage to any level of the system, from the supraglottic structures to the large and small airways, alveoli, pulmonary circulation, chest wall, respiratory muscles, and respiratory center with its neural connections. Mucosal swelling in the mouth, pharynx, and larynx may completely obstruct ventilation, whereas cast formation and mucosal edema in the small and medium-sized airways may impair gas exchange. Alveolar edema and intrapulmonary blood flow redistribution also impair oxygen transfer. Alveolar ventilation is reduced by chest wall edema from skin burns and respiratory center depression caused by carbon monoxide or cyanide toxicity. The exact pattern of damage to an individual with a respiratory injury varies widely and depends on environment factors such as the heat and chemical composition of the smoke and the presence of particles and steam and on victim factors such as age, conscious state, and previous illness.

Thermal Injury

Damage to the trachea, bronchi, and lung parenchyma resulting from heat is uncommon in clinical practice. Only 1 of 697 patients reviewed by Pruitt et al[6] had thermal injury of the trachea, and in that patient, damage was limited to the immediate subglottic area.

Inhalation of hot, dry gas (350° to 500° C) in experimental animals results in direct mucosal injury to the mouth, nose, pharynx, and larynx, but thermal injury to the trachea is mild and limited to the upper trachea. This is because the low specific heat of the inhaled gas and the large heat-exchanging surfaces of the upper airway result in cooling of the gas before it reaches the midtrachea. Flame burns (e.g., from explosion) may result in severe mucosal injury to the upper trachea, but mild burns to the lower trachea do not injure lung parenchyma. Inhalation of steam, which has a high specific heat, severely burns the whole trachea and may cause severe lung parenchymal injury.[7,8] Similarly, air saturated with water vapor at a lower temperature (e.g., 70° to 95° C) causes more severe and extensive airway injury than dry air at the same temperature.[9]

The inhalation of hot gas causes erythema, edema, hemorrhage, and ulceration of the mucosa.[7] The edema increases over 48 to 72 hours after the patient receives the burns, during which time severe and progressive upper airway obstruction may occur because of edema of the buccal or oropharyngeal mucosa, larynx, and epiglottis and of the tracheal mucosa, especially in the subglottic area. Less swelling occurs in the tongue than surrounding tissues, and the swelling occurs later, although the tongue may become fixed because of swelling of its soft tissue attachments.

Complete airway obstruction may occur within hours because of massive mucosal edema of the laryngopharynx, laryngeal surface of the epiglottis, and mucosa over the arytenoid and aryepiglottic fold.[7] Direct visualization of the larynx may become impossible because of mucosal edema and fixation of the tongue and mandible.

Scald injuries to the upper airway occur occasionally in toddlers who may attempt to drink hot coffee or may have a container of hot water spilled on their face.[10] In some cases, such injury causes only mild mucosal edema with moderate stridor that resolves over 3 to 4 days without treatment or with the administration of nebulized epinephrine. In severe cases, there may be severe obstructive supraglottic edema and eschar formation, which require tracheal intubation or tracheostomy.[10]

The mucosal injury caused by heat may be exacerbated by chemical damage resulting from water-soluble products, such as ammonia (NH_3), acetic acid, formic acid, and chlorine. These products are released by the burning and pyrolysis of organic materials.[11] (Pyrolysis is heat-induced, nonoxidative decomposition of plastics and other organic materials.)

Chemical Injury

Smoke consists of particles suspended in a mixture of gases. The particles vary in size from less than 5 μm to more than 5 mm in diameter and consist of carbon and partly burned organic material often coated with toxic products of pyrolysis, such as acrolein, NH_3, and hydrogen chloride (HCl) as well as ketones and organic acids.

Although the smaller particles may be carried to the small airways, most smoke particles are large and are deposited in the nasopharynx, larynx, or trachea, where they can cause damage because of their large heat content or the toxins on their surface. Deposition of smoke particles causes mucosal damage, with suppression of ciliary activity (especially by aldehydes), mucosal ulceration, submucosal edema, and increased mucous production.

Construction of buildings, cars, and furniture as well as combustible household items involves natural products such as wood, cotton, and silk as well as a wide range of synthetic materials. Some of the toxin products of partial combustion of these materials are discussed in Table 25-1.

The exact composition of gases in smoke depends on the combustible materials, the amount of oxygen present at the site, and the temperature of the fire. The local concentration of oxygen and the temperature vary with time during a fire and with the distance from the seat of the fire. Thus in an experimental reconstruction of the Stardust Nightclub fire in Dublin in 1981, in which 48 people died, temperatures near the origin of the fire rose to 1100° C within 2 minutes, and oxygen concentrations fluctuated in the range of 2% to 15% over 6 minutes. In general, the conversion of complex molecules to simpler molecules increases with temperature.

Toxic chemicals in smoke affect mainly the respiratory control center, large and small airways, alveoli, and pulmonary vessels. Surfactant production, alveolar macrophage activity, and airway ciliary activity are especially vulnerable.

The main groups of toxic materials in smoke are irritant gases with high water solubility such as HCl, acrolein, and NH_3; irritants with low water solubility such as phosgene and the oxides of nitrogen; asphyxiants such as hydrogen cyanide and carbon monoxide; and systemic toxins such as antimony, cadmium, chlorobenzene, and propionitrile.[12,13] HCl gas and acrolein cause intense upper airway irritation and coughing, which stimulate increased ventilation, resulting in increased exposure of the lower airway and lung parenchyma to other toxins as well as to the narcotic gases carbon monoxide, carbon dioxide, and hydrogen cyanide. Alveolar ventilation increases on first exposure to smoke and then decreases to low levels because of depression of the central nervous system, including the respiratory center.[12]

The water-soluble irritants also cause reflex laryngospasm, which may reduce the exposure of the lower airway to toxins, sometimes at the expense of severe or fatal hypoxia.[13] Aldehydes such as acrolein and acetaldehyde are found in high concentrations in wood smoke. They denature proteins and thus injure the alveolar endothelium, increasing its permeability and causing pulmonary edema. They also decrease ciliary and macrophage activity,[14] resulting in impaired defense against bacterial infection. Acrolein also causes reversible wheezing.[13]

The extremes of pH due to dissolution of HCl or NH_3 in mucosal water cause necrosis of cells and severe airway edema. This may be rapidly fatal if it involves the larynx and causes wheezing or pulmonary edema if it spreads more distally. In survivors of more prolonged exposure, tracheitis, bronchitis, and bronchiectasis may be found.[13]

Table 25-1 Source of Toxic Products in Smoke

SMOKE COMPONENT	SOURCE
Carbon monoxide	Wood, cotton, paper, silk, wool, polyvinyl chloride, polyurethane, acrylics, petroleum products
Cyanide	Wool, nylon, melamine, polyurethane
Acrolein	Wood, paper, cotton, acrylics, petroleum products
NH_3	Wool, nylon, melamine
Acetic acid	Petroleum products, wood, paper, cotton
HCl	Polyvinyl chloride
Oxides of nitrogen	Wallpaper, nitrocellulose products
Phosgene	Polyvinyl chloride
Formaldehyde	Wallpaper, melamine, wood, paper, cotton

The less soluble irritants such as nitrogen dioxide and phosgene cause lower airway and alveolar injury. Nitrogen dioxide dissolves slowly in mucosal water to form nitrous acid and nitric acid, whereas phosgene forms HCl. The inhalation of nitrogen dioxide or phosgene damages cell membranes, causing epithelial cell death (especially in the terminal bronchioles and alveoli), mucosal ulceration, and profuse pulmonary edema.[11] After an asymptomatic period of 3 to 30 hours, cough and dyspnea appear, followed 4 to 6 weeks later by fever, increased dyspnea, and productive cough. Lung biopsy at that stage may show bronchiolitis obliterans.

The systemic absorption of lipophilic compounds such as long-chain and cyclic hydrocarbons may be accelerated by surfactant, increasing their systemic toxicity and damage to pulmonary capillary endothelium.[12]

Disease Mechanisms

Mucosal Cell Injury

Heat and toxic chemicals, whether in gaseous form or adsorbed onto carbon particles, damage the luminal membrane of mucosal cells by denaturing membrane proteins, leading to cell rupture. Injury to the mucosal cells and basement membrane disrupts the barrier to bacterial entry, permitting more widespread disruption of the respiratory tract as well as bacterial migration into the circulation.

Impaired Ciliary Activity

Any factor that injures mucosal cells also reduces the transport of mucus with its entrapped particles, bacteria, and debris toward the larynx. In addition, smoke constituents such as aldehydes impair ciliary activity without causing cellular injury.

Mucosal Blood Flow and Edema

Irritant gases in smoke, especially the water-soluble irritants, increase mucus production; the volume of secretion is further increased by a rise in bronchial mucosal blood flow[15] up to twelvefold. This increase is thought to be mediated by calcitonin–gene-related peptide and substance P.[15]

Direct injury to the mucosal capillary endothelial cell membranes by heat or chemical toxins in smoke destroys the membrane sodium-potassium adenosinetriphosphatase with consequent influx of sodium ions and water. The endothelial cells become more spherical, obstructing the lumen and opening intercellular spaces. This increases capillary permeability and mucosal edema.[16]

Extravascular Lung Water

Although some studies in humans and animals have failed to demonstrate an increase in extravascular lung water (EVLW) measured by the double-indicator dilution technique[17] after smoke inhalation, other studies have shown that lung lymph flow increases after smoke inahlation[18] and that edema may be detectable at autopsy. This edema was undetectable during life by the double-indicator dilution method.[19]

Together, increased mucus production, reduced ciliary transport, mucosal edema, and the accumulation of cellular debris and soot particles lead to partial or complete obstruction of the large and small airways. They also lead to atelectasis.

Mast cell activation and the consequent release of mediators such as leukotrienes C_4, D_4, and E_4 also contribute to airway obstruction by causing airway smooth muscle contraction and by increasing mucus production and mucosal capillary permeability.[20]

Platelet Activating Factor

Platelet activating factor (PAF) is a phospholipid synthesized in many cell types, including lung endothelial cells, alveolar macrophages, and type II pneumocytes as well as granulocytes, monocytes, mast cells, and platelets in response to stimuli such as tumor necrosis factor, leukotrienes, thrombin, bradykinin, and adenosine triphosphate.[21] PAF appears to have a major role in the pathogenesis of smoke inhalation injury. PAF antagonists prevent the pulmonary lipid peroxidation, atelectasis, and intrapulmonary neutrophil accumulation caused by smoke inhalation.[22]

Neutrophil polymorphonuclear leukocytes are activated rapidly after major skin burns and inhalation injury[23] and aggregate in pulmonary capillaries, releasing proteolytic and other enzymes as well as free oxygen radical products of the oxidative burst. These damage the alveolar capillary endothelium as well as type I and type II pneumocytes.

The concentration of thromboxane A_2 increases rapidly after inhalation injury, associated with a decrease in platelet count and an increase in EVLW. Thromboxane A_2–induced platelet sequestration in the lung may contribute to lung injury by forming platelet thrombi in small vessels and releasing mediators such as PAF.[22,24,25]

Gas Exchange

Inhalation injury causes a progressive reduction in the partial pressure of arterial oxygen (PaO_2) and an increase in the alveolar-arterial difference in the partial pressure of oxygen ($PAO_2 - PaO_2$) starting 30 minutes after the insult.[26] Although alveoli are filled with fluid and debris, true shunt contributes much less to the $PAO_2 - PaO_2$ than ventilation-perfusion ($\dot{V}/\dot{Q}$) inequality.

In the first 24 hours after the injury, the blood flow through a low $\dot{V}/\dot{Q}$ compartment (<0.1) increases as the perfusion of well-ventilated alveoli decreases and a small true shunt appears because of the occlusion of the small airways by edema, mucus, and debris. At that time, administration of 100% oxygen doubles the true shunt and abolishes the low $\dot{V}/\dot{Q}$ compartment, probably because of absorption atelectasis.[24]

The ratio of volume of dead space to tidal volume increases in the first 4 hours after injury and then decreases to normal. Thus the early $\dot{V}/\dot{Q}$ inequality appears to be the result of a redistribution of intrapulmonary blood flow, whereas after 4 hours, the progressive increase in $\dot{V}/\dot{Q}$ inequality is caused by airway obstruction.

Surfactant

Inhalation of smoke and other toxins causes the proliferation of type II pneumocytes.[8] Although some animal studies have failed to demonstrate a reduction in the phosphatidylcholine content of bronchoalveolar lavage (BAL) fluid after smoke inhalation,[27] the consensus now is that smoke injury and thermal (steam) injury of the lungs reduces surfactant activity, trebles the minimal surface tension, and abolishes the normal hysteresis of the surface tension-surface area curve[28-30] (Fig. 25-1).

Because most patients with burn inhalation injury have also suffered skin burns, the effect of those burns on surfactant production may also reduce lung compliance. The sera of animals with burns over 30% of the body surface area inhibits surfactant production by cultured type II pneumocytes in vitro.[31]

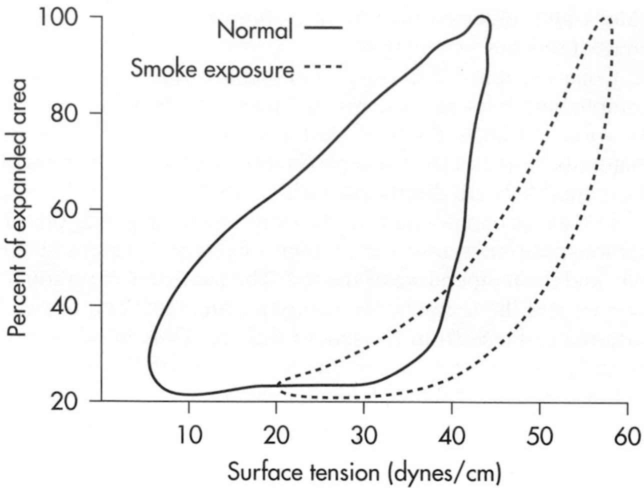

Fig. 25-1. Effect of smoke exposure on the surface tension of lung extracts. (From Niemann GF et al: *Ann Surg* 191:171-181, 1980.)

Pulmonary Effects of a Skin Burn

Cutaneous burns impair gas exchange, reduce lung compliance, and produce diffuse pulmonary infiltrates on chest radiograph in the absence of inhalation injury. Within 10 minutes of a 40% skin burn in anesthetized rats, there is intense vasoconstriction of the pulmonary arterioles and venules, with intravascular clumping of erythrocytes, partially or completely destroying capillaries as well as opening pulmonary arteriovenous anastomoses.[32] Complement activated by the burn wound causes neutrophil sequestration in pulmonary capillaries. The neutrophils release proteases, peroxidase, and other enzymes from liposomes as well as free oxygen radicals from their oxidative burst, resulting in damage to the pulmonary capillary endothelium.[33] Pulmonary lymph flow increases because of increased capillary permeability and the effects of increased capillary hydrostatic pressure, which may be caused by the constriction of pulmonary venules that follows the burn.[33]

Pathology

Airway Injury. Soot may be visible below the vocal cords in about 30% of patients with inhalation injury.[34] The degree of mucosal injury depends on the severity of smoke exposure. In the first 48 hours after mild smoke exposure, there may be only mild erythema and edema of the supraglottic and subglottic mucous membranes, but in children who die in the fire, there may be coagulative necrosis of the tracheal mucosa and superficial submucosa.[35] In general, if there is significant injury to the subglottic airway, very severe edema of the supraglottic structures develops with massive swelling of the epiglottis, aryepiglottic folds, and ventricular folds such that the airway is severely obstructed and visualization of the larynx becomes extremely difficult.[34] In moderate to severe smoke injury the tracheal mucosa may show patchy necrosis and separation, with preservation of mucosal cells only in folds and crypts.[35,36] An inflammatory cell response with edema and neutrophil influx begins within 2 hours of injury.[36] Pseudomembranes consisting of fibrin, sloughed mucosal cells, mucus, and cellular debris form in the trachea and bronchi. Bacterial colonization of the injured mucosa is detectable by 72 hours.[36] Healing occurs by proliferation of the mucous gland cells or by metaplasia of preserved epithelial cells.[37] Complete healing of the airway may take 4 weeks in moderately severe smoke injury, and in addition to the original mucosal injury, there may be residual circumferential scarring at the level of an endotracheal tube tip caused by recurrent trauma and secondary infection.

Lung Parenchyma. In the first 48 hours, intercellular junctions in the capillary endothelium widen, and edema fluid accumulates in the interalveolar septa. Marginated polymorphonuclear lymphocytes are seen in the capillaries, and hemorrhage and edema fill the alveoli.[37] Over the next 24 hours, necrosis of type I pneumocytes occurs, leaving a bare alveolar basement membrane. The alveoli are lined by pseudomembranes consisting of fibrin and cellular debris with some alveolar macrophages. Over the next 7 days, the remaining type II pneumocytes proliferate and cover the basement membrane, especially in subpleural alveoli and alveoli close to bronchi and pulmonary vessel branches.[37] Provided that the lung reticulin fiber framework remains intact, restoration of the normal architecture is still possible, but frequently the proliferation of fibroblasts and the consolidation of immature collagen into mature collagen result in fibrous tissue formation with distortion or obliteration of alveoli. Narrowing of the lumens of the small bronchi and bronchioles by inflammatory cells and fibrous tissue results in bronchiolitis obliterans in some cases.[37,38]

Asphyxia

Oxygen concentrations are low when there is fire in a closed space (2% close to the fire and 12% 14 m away in the Stardust Nightclub fire). Although hypoxia stimulates respiration, it also causes cerebral injury and subsequent cerebral edema; 6% to 8% oxygen causes collapse, unconsciousness, and death if untreated.[12] The asphyxiant effects of hypoxia are synergistic with those of carbon monoxide and cyanide.

Carbon Monoxide

Carbon monoxide is produced by partial combustion and pyrolysis of a variety of organic materials (see Table 25-1). Its avidity for hemoglobin is 200 to 280 times that of oxygen. Carbon monoxide reduces the amount of hemoglobin available for oxygen carriage, thereby reducing the content of oxygen in blood, and shifts the dissociation curve of the remainder to the left, reducing hemoglobin's ability to release oxygen to the tissues. Pulse oximetry does not reflect the reduction of oxygen carriage caused by carbon monoxide. Thus a pulse oximeter may read 96% saturation even when the carboxyhemoglobin concentration is as high as 44% (reducing oxygen content by 44%).

The effect of carbon monoxide poisoning may be acute or delayed. The acute effects are equivalent to those of an acute global hypoxemic insult. The organs most severely affected are the brain, heart, kidneys, and splanchnic system. The myocardial depression caused by carbon monoxide poisoning reduces the cardiac output and blood pressure and adds an ischemic insult to the effects of reduced blood oxygen content.[39] The onset of the delayed effects of carbon monoxide poisoning may occur 1 to 240 days after exposure. A wide range of effects has been reported, from apathy and gait disturbance to dementia, choreoathetosis, seizures, and coma.[40] The pathogenesis of this delayed injury is uncertain; possible explanations include evolution of the original acute hypoxic-ischemic insult to the brain, binding of carbon monoxide to brain cytochromes, and lipid peroxidation in cerebral neurons triggered by carbon monoxide. None of these explanations fit all of the observed facts, and each has its proponents.[39]

Cyanide

Cyanide is produced by the pyrolysis of organic materials, including silk, nylon, plastics, and polyurethane. A cyanide concentration of 110 to 135 parts per million (ppm) causes death after 30 to 60 minutes, whereas 180 ppm causes death in 10 minutes.[12] Cyanide binds competitively to cytochrome α-α_3, blocking mitochondrial oxidative phosphorylation and oxygen use. Lactic acid production increases, and cells in many organs are injured by the failure of adenosine triphosphate production; those most rapidly injured are located in organs with high metabolic rates such as the brain and heart. Brain injury causes respiratory center depression and alveolar hypoventilation, whereas myocardial injury causes failure in systemic oxygen transport. Cyanide toxicity increases alveolar ventilation, increasing the intake of hydrogen cyanide, carbon monoxide, and other smoke toxins.

Clinical Manifestations

Of patients with skin burns, an inhalation injury is more likely to be present in those with facial burns, conjunctivitis, or rhinorrhea and those trapped in a closed space (e.g., in a burning automobile). An inhalation injury is more likely to be present in a child with a larger area than a smaller area of burned body surface, but this is a weak association.[24] Stridor, wheezing, dyspnea, cough, and hoarse voice are rarely present on arrival at the hospital, and children rarely expectorate soot-laden sputum.

In a child with facial burns, a history of being found in a closed space, or burns over a large area of the body's surface, the major diagnostic issues at the time of presentation follow:

1. Is carbon monoxide or cyanide poisoning present?
2. Is upper airway obstruction present now or likely to occur in the next few hours?[41]

The presence of carbon monoxide poisoning may be suspected from the history of entrapment in a closed area, a history of unconsciousness from which the child may have recovered, hypotension or pulmonary edema, or the presence of cyanosis, hallucination, confusion, headache, or convulsion. Cherry-red coloration of mucous membranes is far less common than cyanosis in patients with carbon monoxide poisoning.[42]

When cyanide intoxication is present, the child may be stuporous or comatose and have hypotension, tachycardia, flushed skin, and slow, gasping respiration. Venous blood may be bright red because of poor oxygen use.[8]

One sign of supraglottic injury and impending airway obstruction is low-pitched stridor that may be inspiratory, expiratory, or both. Swallowing may be impaired, and the child may drool; saliva pooling in the pharynx may exacerbate the stridor. The child may prefer sitting to lying. Swelling around the glottis may produce a hoarse or muffled voice. There may be tracheal tug as well as sternal and intercostal retraction when obstruction is marked.

Cyanosis may be difficult to assess in the presence of skin burns, especially facial and oropharyngeal burns. Pulse oximetry may not reliably estimate arterial saturation when the skin perfusion is poor as a result of hypovolemia or the extremity is very edematous. In these circumstances, the clinician must rely on other signs of adequate gas exchange or measure blood gases directly in an arterial blood sample.

Dyspnea and cough may be present at the fire scene but may disappear when the child is removed from the smoky atmosphere, only to return after several hours as lower airway and parenchymal tissue inflammation increases. The child may have shallow tachypnea resulting from lung parenchymal disease or hyperpnea resulting from metabolic acidosis if shock or cyanide or carbon monoxide poisoning are present.[41]

Wheezing resulting from edema, mucus production, and separation of sloughed mucosa in the intrathoracic large and small airways may appear after a few hours and is exacerbated by cast formation. Gas trapping with chest hyperinflation and pulsus paradoxus may increase in severity over the next 96 hours.

Chest auscultation is often difficult in the presence of extensive skin burns, but areas of reduced air entry and focal or diffuse wheezes and crackles may be detectable. In small infants, there may be few signs other than hyperinflation, wheezing, tachypnea, poor air entry, and sometimes apnea.

A sudden increase in respiratory distress, especially with signs of large airway obstruction such as stridor, cyanosis, or widely transmitted wheeze that may be unilateral, may represent a life-threatening airway obstruction resulting from the movement of a cast or separation of the piece of sloughed mucosa requiring urgent bronchoscopy. It may also be a sign of pneumothorax resulting from the rupture of alveoli in a hyperinflated area of lung. Signs of mediastinal shift such as displacement of the trachea or apex beat may not be detectable in the presence of significant burn edema. The clinician needs to perform urgent chest radiographic studies or, in the extremely urgent situation, needle thoracentesis of the hemithorax in which air entry is less audible. If no pneumothorax is detected, urgent bronchoscopy is indicated. Examination of the pharynx may reveal extensive swelling and mucosal sloughing but is not a reliable way of estimating the likely severity of upper airway obstruction.[41]

Investigation of Inhalation Injury

If smoke inhalation is suspected when a child is brought to the hospital, blood is immediately taken to measure the levels of carboxyhemoglobin and plasma cyanide. Although cyanide concentration may be useful for planning therapy, there is little relationship between patient outcome and carboxyhemoglobin level at presentation because carbon monoxide causes mortality by acting at sites other than hemoglobin and because the carboxyhemoglobin concentration on arrival at the hospital depends on the time elapsed since exposure and the concentration of oxygen inhaled in the meantime.[42] Thus a high carboxyhemoglobin concentration may indicate the need for further treatment such as normobaric or hyperbaric oxygen (HBO), but the history of the fire conditions and repeated assessments of higher mental functions are better guides to therapy when the carboxyhemoglobin concentration is low.[41] In many hospitals, it is difficult to obtain the results of a cyanide assay in time for the administration of an antidote to be useful, so the decision to administer the sodium nitrite and sodium thiosulfate often depends on the history of smoke exposure and the presence of physical signs of cyanide toxicity and metabolic acidosis. Smoke from burning buildings, furniture, and automobile interiors generally contains cyanide as well as carbon monoxide, and intoxication with these two poisons often occurs together,[43] so if the carboxyhemoglobin concentration is high on admission, administration of nitrites and sodium thiosulfate is justified.[41,43,44]

Assessment of Upper Airway Obstruction

The following pieces of information are needed for management of this condition:

1. Is functionally important airway obstruction present now?
2. Is upper airway obstruction increasing such that intervention will probably be needed to protect the airway?

To obtain the answer to the first question, a competent observer makes frequent serial observations to assess for the clinical signs of upper airway obstruction and acquires information on gas exchange from pulse oximetry and blood gas analysis.

Several factors may contribute to hypercapnia in a child with inhalation injury; these factors include hypoventilation resulting from upper airway or severe lower airway obstruction or from depression of the respiratory drive caused by hypoxic cerebral injury, cyanide or carbon monoxide poisoning, opiate drugs, or head trauma sustained during the fire. Splinting of the chest by edema, circumferential eschar formation, or pain also causes hypoventilation.

In most patients with inhalation injury, the partial pressure of carbon dioxide in the arterial blood ($Pa{CO_2}$) is normal or low.[41] A normal or high $Pa{CO_2}$ implies impending respiratory failure by one of the previously mentioned mechanisms, often combined with $\dot{V}/\dot{Q}$ inequality. Hypoxemia may result from pure hypoventilation or may result from $\dot{V}/\dot{Q}$ inequality or intrapulmonary shunt (see previous section), both of which may be caused by the destruction of small airways or an injury to the lung parenchyma.

For answering the second question, the most useful investigation is fiberoptic laryngoscopy and bronchoscopy. Direct visualization of the upper airway gives definitive information about the presence and extent of mucosal injury, airway narrowing, and the presence of obstructive casts and slough. Although the severity of injury and the amount and duration of airway protection needed are not predictable when laryngoscopy and bronchoscopy are performed at admission,[45] the degree of swelling and the optimal timing of tracheal intubation can be judged by sequential bronchoscopies in the first 72 hours. Laryngoscopy at the time of extubation may be used to assess airway patency and the likelihood of successful extubation.[41]

Fiberoptic laryngoscopy using a 3.5- to 4-mm laryngoscope under local anesthesia may be used repeatedly in small children in the emergency department and in the burn unit after light sedation. In intubated patients, fiberoptic bronchoscopy may be useful for tracheobronchial toilet and lavage (both for therapeutic purposes and for the identification of pathogens when bronchopneumonia occurs) and for the surveillance of casts in the large airway. Rigid bronchoscopy is needed to remove slough, casts, or rarely, accumulations of soot[41] in cases of sudden severe large airway obstruction.

After tracheal extubation, patients with inhalation injury are more likely to have ulceration and swelling at the level of the true vocal cords, interarytenoid area, anterior commissure, cricoid cartilage, and endotracheal tube tip than patients intubated for a similar time for other reasons.[46] Although in some burn units, bronchoscopy is routinely performed in all patients after extubation for inhalation injury, others use it to assess the progress of anatomic obstruction when clinical signs of significant obstruction are present.[47]

Spirometry

Spirometry and meaningful flow-volume curves are generally impossible to measure in children younger than 6 years of age, especially in the presence of facial burns, pain, distress, and a depressed conscious state. In older children and adults with inhalation injury, the first change in lung mechanics detected by spirometry is usually a reduction in the 1-second forced expiratory volume (FEV_1) and a reduction in the ratio of FEV_1 to vital capacity (FEV_1/VC), which is detectable in the first 6 hours after injury.[41,48] This is due to mucosal injury to the large and small intrathoracic airways. When these changes occur or the patient's condition becomes symptomatic, bronchoscopic evaluation of the anatomic lesion is indicated.

Over the next 72 hours, a progressive restrictive ventilation defect appears, with reduction in forced vital capacity and stabilization of the FEV_1/VC ratio. The magnitude of this restrictive defect is related to the percentage of the body surface burned, the degree of fluid retention, and the reduction in oncotic pressure[48] and represents the progressive development of adult respiratory distress syndrome (ARDS).

Flow-Volume Loops

When flow-volume loops can be obtained, they may occasionally be a useful adjunct to clinical and blood gas and bronchoscopic data in assessing the severity and rate of progression of airway obstruction. In particular, in extrathoracic airway obstruction, maximal inspiratory flows are limited, and when glottic and supraglottic obstruction is severe, a sawtooth expiratory pattern may be seen[46] (Fig. 25-2). In the presence of severe intrathoracic obstruction, dynamic limitation of expiratory flow is seen with upward concavity of the expiratory flow curve.

Patients with severe respiratory distress at presentation need clinical assessment of the airway, and if necessary, steps should be taken to protect the airway (e.g., with an endotracheal tube) and maintain alveolar ventilation (e.g., by positive-pressure ventilation). When these are secured, the tests that are urgently needed are a chest radiographic study and an arterial blood gas analysis, and if airway obstruction is present after

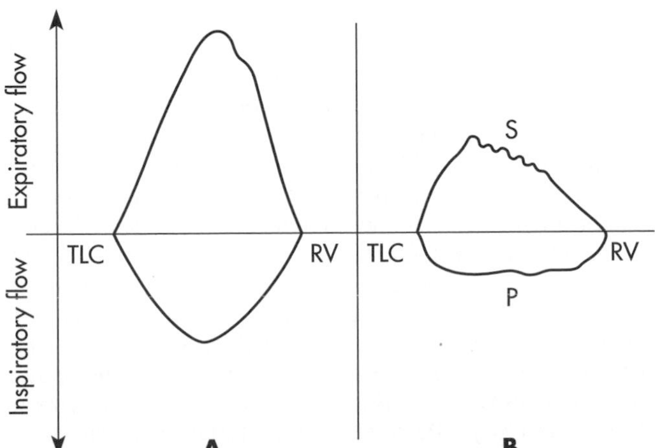

Fig. 25-2. Flow-volume loops. **A,** Normal loop. **B,** Loop in a patient with upper airway burns, showing a sawtooth expiratory flow pattern *(S)* and an inspiratory plateau *(P)* characteristic of variable extrathoracic obstruction. *TLC,* Total lung capacity; *RV,* residual volume.

tracheal intubation, fiberoptic bronchoscopy may be used to assess and remove slough and debris. Blood carboxyhemoglobin and cyanide concentrations should be measured. Measurements of lung mechanics may be useful for monitoring the progress of the lower airways and alveolar disease after these measures have been taken.

When respiratory distress is less severe or absent in a child at risk of inhalation injury, the most useful guides to management are repeated physical examination, chest radiographic studies, blood gas analyses, and fiberoptic laryngoscopy. Lung mechanics measurements may be used to assess more subtle airway and parenchymal injury in older children.

Radiologic Investigations

Information that may affect the management or prognosis can be obtained from the plain chest radiograph, computed tomographic or magnetic resonance scans of the chest and trachea, and bronchoscopy. Although the diagnosis of inhalation injury is based on the history and physical examination, chest radiographic findings of lung overdistention with a flattened diaphragm offer confirmatory evidence (Fig. 25-3). If gas exchange deteriorates and dyspnea and the respiratory rate increase, a plain chest radiograph may reveal a pneumothorax, a collapsed lung or lobe, pulmonary edema, an endotracheal tube displaced downward into a bronchus,[49] consolidation consistent with the onset of secondary bacterial bronchopneumonia, or signs of a pleural effusion.

The plain chest radiograph is an insensitive index of the amount of EVLW present,[50] but knowledge of the amount of EVLW is not needed for patient management. The clinician needs to know the magnitude of gas exchange and lung elastance abnormalities and the fact that they are not caused by some remediable cause such as pneumonia, pneumothorax, or pleural effusion. If necessary, a high left atrial pressure causing pulmonary edema can be ruled out by inserting a balloon-tipped pulmonary artery catheter and measuring the pulmonary capillary wedge pressure. Computed tomographic scan or air or dye-contrast bronchography may be used to define the site and length of tracheobronchial stenosis during the recovery phase after inhalation injury.

Management of Inhalation Injury

The priorities in the acute management of any patient with an inhalation injury are the maintenance of an adequate airway, breathing, and circulation; establishment of venous access; and exclusion of carbon monoxide and cyanide poisoning. All patients should be given high-flow (>10 L/min) oxygen by mask, and the stomach should be decompressed with a nasogastric tube because acute gastric dilation with its attendant risks of regurgitation-aspiration and impairment of venous return and diaphragmatic movement is very common in children with skin burns and inhalation injury.

Airway

Assessment of upper airway injury has already been discussed. Tracheal intubation should be performed if significant airway obstruction appears early after the injury because the swelling and obstruction are likely to increase over the next 2 to 3 days. In general, it is safer to intubate early than later, when it is more difficult to visualize the larynx, identify landmarks, and enter the trachea. Inhalational anesthesia is used for tracheal intubation, as for any patient with upper airway obstruction.

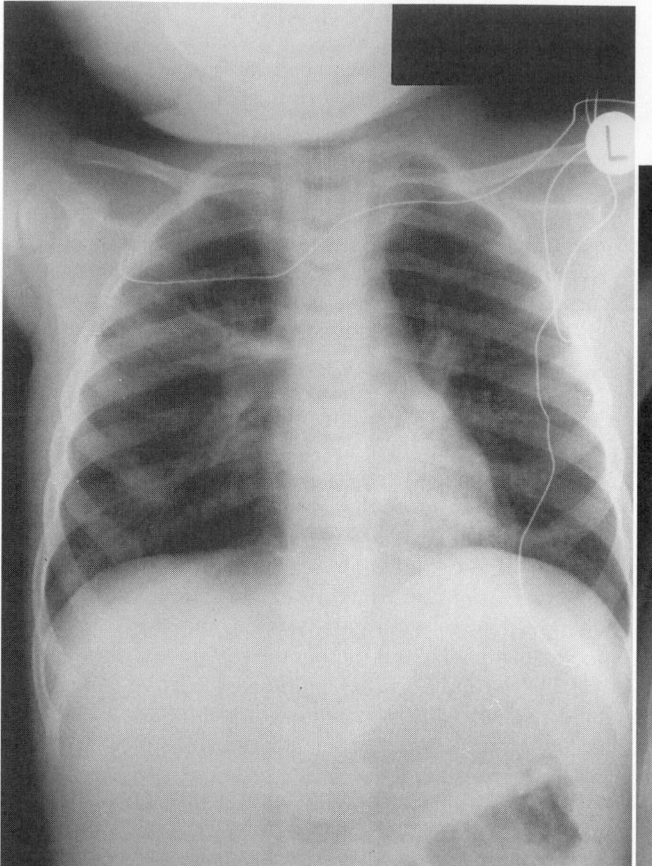

Fig. 25-3. Chest radiographs of a 3-year-old child with burn inhalation. **A,** Radiograph taken 6 hours after the injury shows areas of atelectasis. **B,** In a radiograph taken 5 days after injury, there are widespread alveolar infiltrates with patchy atelectasis and areas of overinflation.

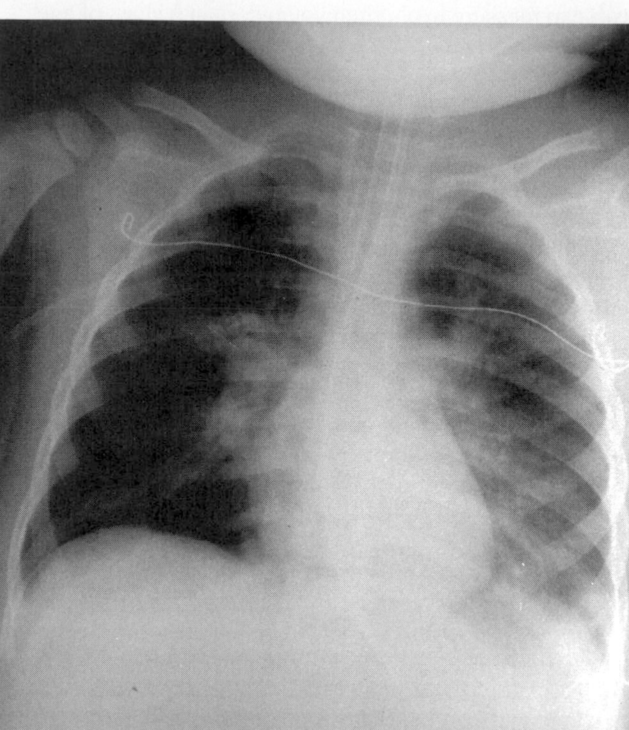

Endotracheal tube fixation and patency are critically important in these patients because reinsertion of a dislodged or blocked endotracheal tube may become impossible when edema is at its maximum and emergency tracheostomy may be extremely difficult and dangerous in the presence of neck burns. Nasotracheal tubes are more readily secured than orotracheal tubes, provided that there is no contraindication such as basal skull fracture or severe coagulopathy. Adequate humidification, frequent tracheal suction, and close nursing observation are essential to the successful management of a child with inhalation injury of the airway.

A child who is suspected of suffering from inhalation injury but in whom airway obstruction is minimal should be observed very closely in a well-lit ward and with the diagnostic measures already discussed. There is no evidence of a therapeutic benefit from mist tents or steroids in these circumstances.[51] Although nebulized adrenalin may reduce the severity of the large and small airway obstruction caused by edema, its use may not benefit the patient if it merely postpones tracheal intubation to a time when it becomes difficult or dangerous.

If tracheal intubation is impossible or the laryngeal inlet cannot be seen, the safest options are (1) passage of an orotracheal tube over a fiberoptic laryngoscope and (2) needle or surgical cricothyroidotomy in a child older than 12 years and needle cricothyroidotomy in a child younger than12 years.[51]

Gas Exchange. Hypoxemia and the $P_{AO_2} - Pa_{O_2}$ increase over the first 72 hours after inhalation injury. In the first 12 hours after the injury, the basis of treatment is high-flow oxygen by mask. In patients whose Pa_{O_2} continues to deteriorate despite the administration of oxygen by mask, tracheal intubation and continuous positive airway pressure (CPAP) or intermittent positive-pressure ventilation (IPPV) with positive end-expiratory pressure (PEEP) are used.[52] After 12 hours, any possible beneficial effect of a high fraction of inspired oxygen (F_{IO_2}) on carbon monoxide elimination is outweighed by the risk of pulmonary oxygen toxicity, so every attempt should be made to keep the F_{IO_2} below 0.5. This may involve permitting a Pa_{O_2} of 45 to 50 mm Hg and using high levels of PEEP or high-frequency ventilation. Apart from a few details, the management of impaired gas exchange resulting from lung parenchymal injury in smoke inhalation is the same as that for ARDS (see section on ARDS). In severe inhalation injury the institution of IPPV and PEEP before the appearance of hypoxemia results in better short-term survival than the commencement of IPPV/PEEP later, when hypoxemia appears.[53] There is some evidence that in inhalation injury, high-frequency ventilation may provide better gas exchange than conventional ventilation, with lower airway pressures, less barotrauma, and a lower F_{IO_2}.[54-56] The progression of ARDS is not the only cause of hypoxemia in inhalation injuries. Atelectasis and sputum retention resulting in large airway obstruction by casts increases the $P_{AO_2} - Pa_{O_2}$ gradient and may be improved by bronchoscopic removal of the casts and airway toilet. A pneumothorax caused by airway obstruction and air trapping may exacerbate the hypoxemia. Escharotomy abolishes the hypoventilation and the restrictive lung defect resulting from circumferential chest burns.[51]

Wheezing. Most wheezing after inhalation injury is due to mucosal edema, increased mucus production, and cast formation in the large and small intrathoracic airways; smooth muscle contraction is less often a significant factor. In children with reactive airways, irritant components of smoke such as NH_3, chlorine, and acrolein may provoke wheezing by stimulating type C sensory nerves within the respiratory tract mucosa. These sensory nerve fibers then release neuropeptides such as substance P and neurokinins A and B, which increase mucus production and vascular permeability, cause bronchoconstriction, and may activate mast cells.[57] Thus although the use of bronchodilator drugs such as β_2-sympathomimetics may not affect the $P_{AO_2} - Pa_{O_2}$ or lung mechanics when most wheezing is due to narrowing of large airways or the presence of airway casts or mucus plugs (and indeed may increase the $P_{AO_2} - Pa_{O_2}$ by impairing hypoxic pulmonary vasoconstriction), a therapeutic trial of nebulized albuterol may be worthwhile. The use of corticosteroids for wheezing is justifiable only in patients who are known asthmatics or in patients dependent on exogenous steroids.[51] Their use in others who wheeze merely exposes such patients to the risks of sepsis and gastric hemorrhage without demonstrable benefit. When a wheeze is widely transmitted, bronchoscopy may be needed to exclude large airway obstruction by casts or mucous plugs.

Sepsis. The use of prophylactic antibiotics has not been shown to affect mortality or morbidity in a controlled trial in adults with inhalation injury[58] and is not recommended in major burn units.[8,51] In children who die after burn injury, secondary bronchopneumonia becomes an increasingly important cause of death as the time between injury and death increases, causing 6% of deaths in the first week and 42% after the third week.[59] Routine bacteriologic surveillance (e.g., serial blood and tracheal aspirate cultures) may demonstrate only the bacterial colonization of the trachea and recurrent transient bacteremias, which are normal in inhalation injury and skin burns, respectively.[60] Therefore culture specimens should be taken only when there is clinical suspicion of pneumonia (e.g., new fever, rising white blood cell count with an increasing number of immature neutrophils, deteriorating gas exchange, appearance of new alveolar opacities on chest radiograph).

In this case, cultures of blood and possibly bronchoscopic or blind BAL[61] tracheal aspirate should be taken. The decision to start antibiotics is based on the likelihood that this new group of signs is due to pneumonia. The antibiotics chosen should be those to which the organisms that most commonly cause pneumonia in these children (*Staphylococcus aureus* and gram-negative bacilli, including *Pseudomonas*) are sensitive.[58,60]

Steroids. Although there is conflicting evidence from animal models about the efficacy of steroids given after smoke exposure on survival and other indexes of inhalation injury,[62-64] controlled trials in humans have failed to demonstrate any benefit.[58,65] Indeed, in one trial the mortality rate of the steroid treated group was 4 times and the incidence of serious infection 3 times those of the control group.[65] The prophylactic use of steroids in inhalation injury is not recommended.[8]

Exogenous Surfactant. Although surfactant activity in lung lavage fluid decreases after inhalation injury and decreased activity is associated with atelectasis, reduced lung compliance, and high-permeability pulmonary edema,[66] a controlled trial of the administration of artificial surfactant did not reduce surface tension or pulmonary edema in an animal model of inhalation injury.[67]

Carbon Monoxide and Cyanide Poisoning

Carbon monoxide poisoning should be suspected in any patient who has suffered smoke exposure in a closed space such as within a building or an automobile or who was unconscious at the fire scene. Such a child should be given high-flow oxygen by mask. The lungs of a child who has been unconscious should be intubated to permit the administration of 100% normobaric oxygen. If the carboxyhemoglobin concentration measured on admission to the hospital is greater than 30%, the clinician should consider the use of HBO therapy. A decision for or against HBO is based on a balance between the likely gains vs. the risks.

There have been no completed prospective, randomized, controlled trials of HBO vs. normobaric oxygen therapy in humans with carbon monoxide toxicity, although one trial still in progress appears to show that HBO reduces the incidence of delayed neuropsychiatric sequelae after carbon monoxide poisoning.[68] There are numerous anecdotal reports and nonrandomized trials, but a great deal of controversy exists about these results.[40] HBO therapy may be considered if it can be achieved with minimal risk to the child (i.e. the airway, breathing, and circulation are stable and can be kept stable in the hyperbaric chamber). Otherwise, normobaric 100% oxygen should be continued for 12 hours or until the blood carboxyhemoglobin concentration is less than 30%.[51]

Any patient with heavy smoke exposure and metabolic acidosis should be treated with cyanide antidotes, especially if the victim was exposed to smoke in a closed space, if there was loss of consciousness, or if on arrival at the hospital the conscious state was depressed or carboxyhemoglobin concentration was high. The recommended antidotes (available as the Lilly Cyanide Antidote Kit in the United States) consist of intravenous sodium nitrite, 6 mg/kg to a maximum of 300 mg, and sodium thiosulfate, 250 mg/kg to a maximum of 12.5 g over 20 minutes and repeated within 30 to 60 minutes if necessary. Methemoglobin concentrations should be monitored during treatment and should remain less than 10%. Amyl nitrite pearls are available for inhalation if venous access is delayed.[69,70]

Long-Term Respiratory Complications of Inhalation Injury

A large airway complication is tracheal stenosis that may involve short or long segments of the trachea and major bronchi. These lesions are most often seen at and below the tip of an endotracheal or tracheostomy tube and at the level of a tube cuff; they are more common after tracheostomy than after nasotracheal intubation.[71] Compression of the mucosal blood supply and trauma from tube movement and the recurrent impact of suction catheters on injured mucosa, plus the effects of secondary bacterial infection eroding down to and through cartilage, may explain this residual scarring. Repeated balloon dilation or resection and reanastomosis may be feasible in lesions involving a short segment of the trachea that cause disabling symptoms despite conservative treatment, but lesions involving long segments are a more difficult problem in that no surgical treatment is uniformly effective despite case reports of the success of various forms of tracheoplasty using costal cartilage, pericardium, or other tissue.[72] Such lesions can be prevented with the use of the following actions: Cuffed tracheal and tracheostomy tubes should be avoided where possible, tracheal tubes should be well fixed to prevent movement within the trachea, the tube should be of the smallest diameter through which the child can breathe without excessive respiratory effort, and suction catheters should not be passed routinely beyond the tip of the tracheal tube.

Bronchiectasis is occasionally seen, possibly because of the direct effect of irritant gases plus secondary infection.[6] Bronchiolitis obliterans organizing pneumonia has also been found and may result from the effects of toxic constituents of smoke such as the oxides of nitrogen.[38]

A prospective study of 14 children recovering from inhalation injury found normal lung mechanics in 36%, airway obstruction in 36%, a restrictive defect in 21%, and combined restrictive and obstructive defects in 7% of the patients 2.6 ± 1.9 years after injury.[73]

BLAST INJURY TO THE LUNGS AND HEART

In an explosion, large amounts of gas are produced very rapidly. A shock wave of very high pressure spreads radially away from the point of the explosion. The height of the pressure wave decreases with the cube of the distance from the explosion. The movement of the pressure wave also creates a wind pressure in the direction of its movement on objects in its path, which summates with the wave pressure on surfaces facing the explosion. Thus 15 feet from a 125-lb charge of high explosive the peak pressure may be 13 atm, whereas at 50 feet, it is only 0.7 atm of excess pressure.[74]

The effects of explosions on the body follow:

1. Primary resulting from the impact of the shock wave on the lungs, bowel, and ears
2. Secondary resulting from the impact of missiles accelerated by the expanding pressure wave
3. Tertiary resulting from acceleration of the body or body parts by the blast wind

The primary effect is due to high-velocity distortion of the chest wall by the blast pressure wave. This effect produces low-velocity shear waves that tear the places where the lung parenchyma is attached to the large vessels and bronchi. It also produces high-frequency compression waves reflected at the interface of air and blood or tissue, causing large forces at the capillary level (with tearing of capillaries, arterioles, and venules)[75] and creating fistulas between the alveoli and pulmonary veins. This results in systemic air emboli to vital organs, including the brain and heart.[76]

Low-velocity shear waves cause subpleural hemorrhages along the ribs and in the costopleural angles.[74] Laceration of the lung surface may also occur along the ribs. Subpleural petechial hemorrhages may become confluent and extensive. In the injured area, alveolar septa are disrupted; alveoli and bronchioles are filled with blood.[74,77] Partial obstruction of bronchi with a clot may result in air trapping or atelectasis, especially at the lung bases.[78]

Over the 24 hours after injury, alveolar, bronchial, and interstitial hemorrhages become more extensive, and fibrinous alveolar exudate and interstitial edema appear in nearly all areas of the lung.[77] Hypoxemia may increase because of true shunt (from continued perfusion of blood-filled alveoli) as well as $\dot{V}/\dot{Q}$ inequality,[75] which may result from partial filling of the alveoli and partial obstruction of the bronchi and bronchioles. Secondary bacterial pneumonia may complicate recovery after 3 to 4 days.[79]

Signs of blast injury include dyspnea, tachypnea, hemoptysis, chest pain, and cyanosis increasing in severity over 2 to 3 days after the explosion. There may be cough, which may become productive over 2 to 3 days. Partial bronchial obstruction with air trapping may cause expiratory wheezing and a hyperinflated chest.[78] On auscultation, there may be locally reduced air entry resulting from alveolar hemorrhage or hemothorax; diffuse crackles and wheezes may be heard. There may also be unilateral hyperresonance and displacement of the trachea and apex beat resulting from a pneumothorax. A fever may appear 1 or 2 days after the explosion. The signs of systemic gas emboli depend on the locations of the emboli. Emboli to the brain may cause a depressed conscious state, seizures, and focal neurologic deficits. Coronary emboli cause chest pain of myocardial ischemia, hypotension, and tachycardia and a third heart sound. Gas bubbles may be seen in the retinal vessels at funduscopy.

The plain chest radiograph is normal in many cases. Alveolar hemorrhage or edema may cause patchy or diffuse alveolar infiltrates that appear 2 to 4 hours after the injury, increase in severity over 1 to 2 days, and usually disappear over the next week.[76] Areas of atelectasis and overinflation may also be seen at the lung bases.[78] Pneumothorax, pneumomediastinum, and pneumatoceles may appear; the latter may take more than a week to resolve.[76]

Management

All blast victims should receive supplemental oxygen by mask, and their airway, breathing, circulation, and associated injuries should be assessed. The respiratory rate and pattern and hemoglobin saturation (by pulse oximetry) should be monitored; the blood pressure, electrocardiogram, and patient's conscious state should also be evaluated. Tracheal intubation may be needed if the airway or spontaneous breathing is inadequate. Mechanical ventilation carries the risk of increasing the size of pneumothoraxes and producing systemic gas emboli and is better avoided or minimized as far as is tolerable. In particular, a high peak airway pressure and high PEEP should be avoided if possible, even at the expense of permitting the Pa_{CO_2} to rise (and the pH to fall as low as 7.1) and the Pa_{O_2} to fall as low as 50 mm Hg. The FI_{O_2} should be kept below 50% if possible.

Because of the risks of mechanical ventilation, aggressive fluid replacement therapy, which may exacerbate pulmonary edema, should be modified, and general anesthesia, which increases mortality in blast victims, should be avoided (possibly in favor of local or regional anesthesia) in the first 48 hours after the injury. Although conservative management of airway hemorrhage is preferable because of the risks of exacerbating bleeding, barotrauma, and gas emboli, bronchoscopy may be needed to clear clots obstructing the large airways.

In patients with systemic gas emboli, the FI_{O_2} should be increased to 100% (if necessary by tracheal intubation). The administration of HBO, considered the treatment of choice for this complication, is effective in ameliorating the effects of cerebral air embolus even 11 hours after embolization.[76] At hyperbaric pressures, the obstructive gas bubbles are compressed, and administration of 100% oxygen encourages nitrogen removal from bubbles, whereas a high capillary P_{O_2} increases the diffusion of oxygen from perfused capillaries to cells supplied by nonperfused capillaries.[80] Mannitol may also be effective for treating gas emboli.[76] Early use of extracorporeal membrane oxygenation (ECMO) in patients requiring IPPV for blast injury of the lung may minimize the risk of air embolus and barotrauma, although heparin administration for ECMO may pose a severe risk of hemorrhage from torn lung blood vessels.

Outcome

Blast injury of the lung is present in 47% of victims who die at the scene of terrorist bombings. The most common lung-related cause of immediate death is massive coronary or systemic air embolism. Late death, mainly resulting from ARDS, occurs in 3.7% of initial survivors of blast lung.[81]

BLUNT INJURY OF THE LUNG

Epidemiology

Among children in U.S. cities, 40% to 66% of chest injuries are blunt injuries,[82,83] whereas in other countries such as Northern Ireland and South Africa, 85% to 91% are blunt injuries.[84,85] Most blunt chest trauma is due to motor vehicle accidents, but a few cases are caused by falls. The overall mortality rate for children with chest injuries is about 14%, decreasing from 23% in children younger than 5 years to 8.3% in children 10 to 15 years.[84] Most of these children have associated injuries, and chest injury is the sole cause of death in only 3%.[84] Two thirds of children with chest injury are boys, and the median age is 6 years.[83,85]

Disease Mechanisms

During most automobile collisions, the velocity of chest wall distortion is low (<33 mph) and produces large-amplitude, low-velocity shear waves in tissue with gross distortion of the lungs. These cause laceration and contusion of the area of the lung underlying the ribs and laceration of the main and lobar bronchi and vessels, the main sites of tissue movement.

During high-velocity collisions, in addition to shear waves, high-amplitude stress waves travel through the lung at the speed of sound and are reflected at tissue interfaces such as the airways and alveolar walls, doubling the wave pressure locally in areas away from the chest wall. Stress waves injure perihilar and peribronchial regions and the medial lung border.[86]

In many cases, pulmonary laceration is the major injury, with tearing of small blood vessels and flooding of the nearby airways and alveoli with blood.[87] Stress waves cause disruption of the alveoli, airways, and pulmonary vessels distant from the site of impact but no laceration. The presence of blood in the alveoli impairs surfactant production, resulting in reduced fluid clearance and atelectasis, which may be exacerbated by splinting resulting from pain, hemothorax, or pneumothorax. Free blood also completely or partially obstructs the small airways and may spill over into the bronchial tree from the contused area to nearby uninjured areas. Mucus production is increased, and ciliary clearance is impaired by free blood.[88]

Bleeding may continue for 24 hours or more after injury, so lung consolidation and atelectasis become more dense and widespread. Associated injuries include bleeding or major air leaks into the pleural cavity (hemothorax, pneumothorax, or bronchopleural fistula). Tears in the airway occur anywhere from the glottis to the major bronchi, causing pneumothorax or subcutaneous or mediastinal emphysema as well as airway obstruction and collapse of a lobe or lung.

Although the pain of rib fractures may limit voluntary inspiration, the presence of a flail chest does not usually in itself contribute to the impaired gas exchange found in lung trauma, contrary to early belief. In fact, despite paradoxical movement of the flail segment of ribs, ventilation on that side may be greater than on the noninvolved side.[89]

Atelectasis and the flooding of airways and alveoli with blood and proteinaceous fluid reduce the regional lung volume, the regional alveolar ventilation, and the $\dot{V}/\dot{Q}$ ratio in the contused areas of lung.[90] The functional residual capacity is reduced and remains so for some months after injury.[91] There is not enough small airway destruction in most patients to cause wheezing or hyperinflation of the affected side, and the FEV_1/VC ratio remains in the normal range.[91] Static lung compliance is reduced, and work of breathing increased.[88-90]

Much of the $P_{AO_2} - Pa_{O_2}$ in a child with a contused lung is caused by true shunt resulting from continued perfusion of the flooded, unventilated alveoli. Variability in the intensity of hypoxic pulmonary vasoconstriction among individuals means that children with the same proportion of total lung volume contused have widely varying shunt fractions and $P_{AO_2} - Pa_{O_2}$ values. Those with the smallest increase in pulmonary vascular resistance after blunt chest injury have the greatest increase in shunt fraction and vice versa.[92]

In almost all patients with symptomatic pulmonary contusions, capillary permeability is increased to some extent.[93] In low-velocity shear wave injury, the leaky vessels are localized to the area of impact or laceration (e.g., adjacent to ribs), whereas in higher-velocity stress wave injuries, capillaries over a wide area of lung leak fluid and protein into the interstitium and alveoli. If large quantities of resuscitation fluid are given to replace lost blood in a child with multiple trauma, the resulting increase in lung water will be greater and more widespread in lungs that have suffered a high-velocity blow than a lower-velocity blow.

Complications

Complications may occur at or shortly after impact. They include flail chest; airway injuries; and lung laceration, pneumothorax or hemothorax (already discussed), and lung hematomata, which do not delay functional recovery, although radiologic recovery may take weeks to months.[87] Pneumatoceles, often containing some fluid, develop hours after injury and resolve over several weeks. They may be entirely asymptomatic or may be associated with dyspnea, disordered gas exchange, and locally reduced breath sounds.[94,95] Pulmonary fibrosis visible on computed tomographic scan may develop over weeks to months, occasionally causing reduced ipsilateral lung volumes and (in adults) long-term respiratory disability.[96,97] Nosocomial pneumonia may occur, especially in children with pulmonary hematoma, atelectasis, or preexisting upper respiratory infections; in those who require tracheal intubation for several days; and in those with severe shock. Posttraumatic empyema is uncommon in childhood.[85] Prophylactic antibiotics are not indicated in children with lung contusions.[88,98]

Signs of Pulmonary Contusion

Any child with a history of severe blunt injury such as a fall or a high-velocity motor vehicle accident (including a pedestrian or cyclist injury) should be suspected of suffering from pulmonary contusion and must be investigated accordingly. There may be skin contusions on the chest wall. Although early cyanosis often implies the presence of a pneumothorax or hemothorax, tachypnea may develop early, even in the absence of air or blood in the pleural cavity. Hemoptysis is uncommon but indicates bronchial hemorrhage.

Rib fractures and flail chest are often absent in children despite severe injuries to the lungs or heart because the very flexible ribs of the child can deform greatly without breaking. Ipsilateral chest wall movement is often reduced on arrival at the hospital, and reduced air entry, inspiratory crackles, and sometimes focal wheezes may develop in the next few hours.

Investigation

The straight anteroposterior chest radiograph (Fig. 25-4) performed urgently as part of the initial assessment of any trauma patient may reveal little evidence of lung contusion, although rib fractures, hemothorax, or pneumothorax may be evident. Later, chest radiographs may show discrete spherical densities or an expanding confluent density in the contused area of lung. When there is doubt about the nature of a lung opacity seen on plain radiograph, a computed tomographic scan of the lungs demonstrates the nature and extent of any injury, including lung lacerations, much earlier than the plain radiograph, although any clinically significant contusion will be visible on plain radiograph. To exclude foreign body aspiration (including large food particles) as a cause of segmental or lobar atelectasis in a child with multiple trauma who has vomited, bronchoscopy may be needed. Maintenance of gas exchange during bronchoscopy may be difficult in severe lung contusion, and extreme care must be taken to keep the neck in a neutral position during bronchoscopy in any child who has a significant head injury or who has suffered a high-velocity deceleration injury unless spinal cord injury can be excluded with confidence.

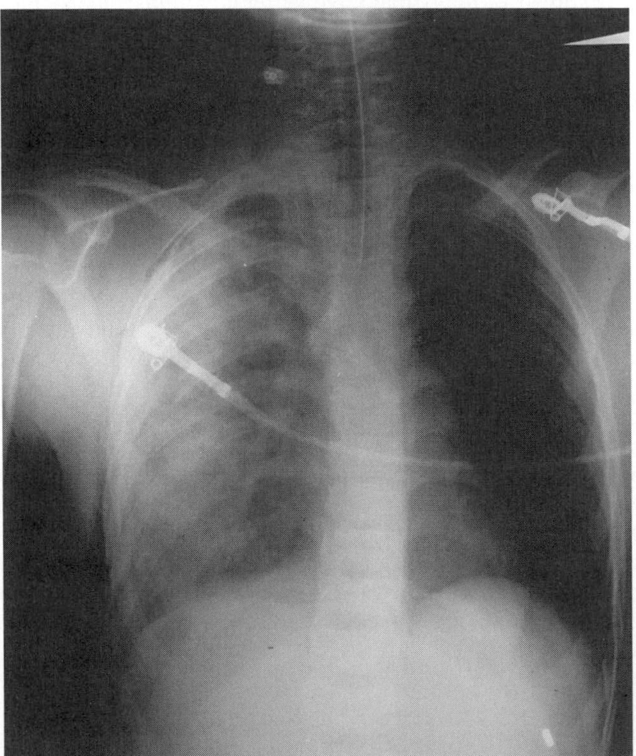

Fig. 25-4. Chest radiograph showing extensive contusion of the right lung as well as rib fractures and subcutaneous emphysema in a 12-year-old pedestrian struck by an automobile.

Blood gas analysis should be performed very early in all children with significant blunt injuries and may give the first indication (after the history and examination) of the presence of lung contusion.[98] The child's vital signs on oximetry should be monitored. Also, the clinician should perform regular physical examinations and blood gas analyses, total and differential white cell counts, and bacterial cultures of the tracheal aspirate.

Management

Oxygen

Any victim of significant blunt trauma should receive high-flow oxygen by mask, at least until cardiorespiratory stability is secured, because most of these patients have some degree of $P_{AO_2} - Pa_{O_2}$.

Respiratory Support

An awake child with an isolated lung contusion who can maintain a patent airway and can cough well because of adequate analgesia is likely to be managed successfully without tracheal intubation or mechanical ventilation.[88] Gas exchange may be supported in such a child by CPAP via a nasopharyngeal tube in infants or nasal mask in older children and adolescents.

A child who has impaired consciousness because of head injury or who has other injuries, a compromised airway, shock, or a reduced ability to breathe deeply, cough, or cooperate with physiotherapy because adequate analgesia cannot be delivered is likely to develop secondary respiratory failure, atelectasis, and nosocomial pneumonia. This child's lungs should be intubated prophylactically and gently mechanically ventilated, at least during the first 24 hours after injury. The mortality rate of patients who require intubation and ventilation is higher (27%) than that of those managed without intubation (0.4%) because of associated head injury and shock.[99] Barotrauma is a major risk from application of high pressures or large tidal volumes (>10 ml/kg) to ruptured airways or overinflated lung segments. For this reason, ventilator airway pressures and tidal volume should be minimized by allowing the Pa_{CO_2} to rise (permissive hypercapnia[100]) until the blood pH approaches 7.2 and the Pa_{O_2} approaches 50 mm Hg, with an F_{IO_2} of 0.5, if the child's associated injuries (such as head injury) or shock state permits.

Ventilation of the normal lung with or without application of CPAP to the contused lung has been used to control air leaks and ongoing major bronchial hemorrhage with flooding of the normal lung and to minimize overinflation of normal areas of the lung.[101,102] High-frequency jet ventilation may be required to maintain gas exchange in the presence of multiple air leaks.

Fluid Management

Overhydration exacerbates pulmonary edema in the contused lung, but inadequate blood volume replacement markedly increases mortality and morbidity in traumatic and hemorrhagic shock by prolonging tissue ischemia, especially in the liver and bowel mucosa, thereby causing translocation of endotoxin and gut bacteria into the bloodstream as well as activation of inflammatory mediators.[103] In isolated lung injuries, careful replacement of blood volume by aliquots of colloid or crystalloid using conventional endpoints of blood pressure, skin perfusion, urine output, and metabolic acidosis is sufficient. However, in massive lung contusion, monitoring of cardiac output and left atrial pressure using a Swan-Ganz catheter may be needed for adequate precision in fluid replacement.[88]

Other Measures

Steroids may increase mortality and impair bacterial clearance from the contused lung and thus are not indicated.[88,89,98,104] Tube thoracostomy is indicated for pneumothoraxes that are large or increasing in size. Close clinical and radiologic monitoring without thoracentesis is appropriate for small, stable pneumothoraxes. Adequate pain relief using local anesthetic nerve blocks and intravenous opiates is essential to ensure adequate chest expansion and coughing. Early vigorous chest physiotherapy is also important to prevent the complications of atelectasis and nosocomial pneumonia.

LIPOID PNEUMONIA AND HYDROCARBON PNEUMONITIS

Exogenous lipoid pneumonia occurs in children in the following circumstances:

1. In toddlers and preschool age children, exploratory ingestion of liquid hydrocarbons, including kerosene, turpentine, gasoline, dry cleaning fluids, furniture polish, and lighter fluid
2. In teenagers and older children, abuse of solvents, including inhalation of aromatic hydrocarbons such as xylene and toluene as well as gasoline and petroleum spirit-based paint
3. In the patient with mental retardation and debility or a history of forced ingestion of the oil,[105] silent aspiration into the lungs of liquid paraffin administered orally for constipation (This is the so-called adult type of lipoid pneumonia.)

Accidental Ingestion in the Preschool Child

From 1985 through 1989, 129,024 children younger than 6 years in the United States ingested hydrocarbons; of those, 5 died and 168 suffered major effects. This represents 3.3% of all poison exposures in this age group and 4% of all deaths resulting from poisoning.[106] Hydrocarbon ingestion occurs when the child, often a boy between 12 months and 5 years of age, drinks the liquid from a bottle (frequently a soft drink bottle) stored within reach.

Lung injury resulting from kerosene ingestion is becoming less common as a cause of death. A study in Brisbane, Australia, found no child deaths resulting from kerosene in 15 years, although it had been the leading cause of child poisoning deaths in that community in 1950. The change is due to reduced household use and storage of kerosene in the last 30 years and to legislation that enforces a blue coloring of kerosene to indicate its toxicity.[107] In the United States, however, ingestion remains a significant cause of morbidity, as does ingestion of lighter fluid and mineral seal oil (a major constituent of furniture polish).[106]

Substance Abuse

The intentional inhalation of volatile organic chemicals for recreational use[108] is mainly a phenomenon of the preteen and early teenage years. When it persists to late teenage and adult life, it is often an indicator of a psychosocial problem. Among a group of U.S. high school seniors in 1988, 17% had inhaled solvents at some time, 3% in the past month, and 0.2% did so daily. These figures probably underestimate the true incidence of the practice, which is more prevalent in those who drop out of school before their senior year.[109]

Although pulmonary injury is not a prominent cause of death among solvent abusers, pulmonary edema has been found at postmortem in gasoline sniffers. Liquid gasoline causes mucosal injury when ingested,[110] but it seems more likely that cardiogenic pulmonary edema is the cause of these postmortem findings.[108] The edema results from ventricular fibrillation caused by sensitization of the myocardium to endogenous catecholamines from aromatic hydrocarbons in the gasoline.

Inhalation of solvents by bagging (spraying into a plastic bag and inhaling) is more likely than inhalation by huffing (spraying onto a cloth held to the mouth) to lead to asphyxial injury. Such injury may include myocardial depression with consequent pulmonary edema and hypoxic brain injury, including seizures (with subsequent vomiting and aspiration of gastric contents).

The toxicity of solvent abuse mainly involves the kidneys (gasoline, toluene, carbon tetrachloride); central nervous system, including neuropsychiatric disorders (benzene, toluene, xylene); bone marrow (benzene); heart (fluorinated hydrocarbons, gasoline, toluene); and peripheral nerves (toluene, *n*-hexane). In lung injury caused by paint sniffing, nonhydrocarbon components of the paint, such as aluminum and silica, may cause more pulmonary damage than the hydrocarbon components.[111]

Expiratory wheezing has been found in adolescents examined within hours of inhaling toluene. A group of 37 chronic glue sniffers had significantly higher residual volumes than a group of controls of similar age, although the FEV_1 and the FEV_1/VC ratio were not different from those of the controls. In lung specimens obtained at autopsy from three chronic glue sniffers who died of traumatic injuries, there were changes suggesting panacinar emphysema, mononuclear infiltration and thickening of some alveolar septa but thinning and rupture of others, smooth muscle hypertrophy in the terminal bronchioles, widespread mucus plugging, and papillomatous hypertrophy of bronchiolar submucosal tissue.[112]

Adult-Type Lipoid Pneumonia

Adult-type lipoid pneumonia is commonly seen in debilitated, chronically ill adults who have taken oil-containing medications such as mineral oil for constipation or oily nosedrops.[113] In children who are debilitated or who suffer from neuromuscular disease, viscous oils, including mineral oil and cod liver oil, may be aspirated silently. Forced oral administration of any oily preparation can lead to aspiration of the oil, sometimes causing the child's death.[105] Silent aspiration of oil-based lip gloss and oily nosedrops has also been reported in children.[113,114]

Physical Properties of Hydrocarbons

Petroleum distillates and turpentine, which account for the majority of respiratory injuries from hydrocarbons, consist of mixtures of aromatic and C_5 to C_6 aliphatic hydrocarbons. The risk of lung injury after ingestion of these products depends on their viscosity and surface tension, whereas lightly volatile components evaporate at body temperature, displacing oxygen from alveoli and causing transient hypoxemia.[115]

Low surface tension and low viscosity reduce the effectiveness of the laryngeal and epiglottic reflexes at preventing entry of the ingested or regurgitated hydrocarbon into the trachea and encourages spreading from the proximal airways to the terminal bronchioles and alveoli. In addition, they reduce the effectiveness of surfactant in vitro and in vivo,[116] predisposing to atelectasis and pulmonary edema.

Aliphatic hydrocarbons shorter than C_6 cause more pulmonary endothelial damage than longer-chain molecules, and in animal experiments, the mortality rate decreases rapidly as the viscosity of the hydrocarbon increases.[115] Thus low-viscosity compounds such as gasoline, turpentine, mineral seal oil (in furniture polish), petroleum ether, lighter fluid, and toluene are far more toxic than more viscous hydrocarbons such as fuel oil, lubricating oil, mineral oil, and petroleum jelly.

Signs and Symptoms

Respiratory symptoms occur in 25% to 40% of the preschoolers ingesting low-viscosity hydrocarbons (kerosene, mineral seal oil). Choking, coughing, and gagging are followed by increasing tachypnea with alar flaring and an expiratory grunt within minutes of ingestion. Fever and intercostal retraction may appear within 30 minutes or may be delayed for 1 to 2 days.[117,118] The fever may be high (41° C), and in cases of significant lung injury, there is usually tachycardia.[118] Auscultatory signs may be absent, even in patients with cyanosis and severe respiratory distress,[117] or there may be crackles, wheezes, and reduced breath sounds in the lung bases, sometimes associated with dullness to percussion.[119] The odor of kerosene or another hydrocarbon may be detectable on the breath or clothing.

Because many hydrocarbons are central nervous system depressants and gastric mucosal irritants, children seen more than 30 minutes after ingestion may be drowsy or semiconscious. Vomiting with inhalation of gastric contents may contribute to further lung injury. The presence of gross pulmonary edema, especially if associated with cardiomegaly and hepatomegaly, implies massive hydrocarbon aspiration and the combination of direct lung toxicity with myocardial depression.[119]

Respiratory signs may disappear within 24 to 48 hours in mild cases, but when complications such as ARDS, secondary bacterial infection, or pneumatoceles ensue, the child may remain symptomatic for 10 days or more.[118,120] In particular, the fever may persist for up to 3 weeks.[118]

Disease Mechanisms

Because children who die after hydrocarbon ingestion do so after some hours, the available evidence on early pathologic effects comes from animal experiments. The effects of tracheal instillation of 0.3 ml/kg of kerosene in rats are shown in Table 25-2. The earliest histologic effects appear to be on the pulmonary vessels; an inflammatory exudate and signs of bronchial injury appear later.[121]

In the rabbit, intense alveolar hemorrhage and edema are seen within 15 minutes of kerosene instillation into the trachea. These changes appear in a patchy fashion over both lungs. Later, neutrophils are found in the alveolar fluid.[122] The prominence of hemorrhage and edema implies that the endothelium of pulmonary capillaries is a major site of injury by these solvents.[123]

Autopsy examination of the lungs of children who die soon after hydrocarbon aspiration also show vascular congestion, alveolar hemorrhage, and edema with later changes of vascular thromboses, interstitial and alveolar inflammatory exudate, and atelectasis and necrosis of the bronchial, bronchiolar, and alveolar walls.[117] In massive ingestion, these changes may extend very rapidly over the whole lung within hours of the event, leaving very little air-containing lung.[122] Later, the alveoli become lined with thick hyaline membranes and contain profuse fibrinous clot with erythrocytes, cellular debris, and macrophages containing small oil droplets. The lining of bronchioles is shed into the lumen.

Areas of hyperinflation and emphysematous bullae visible at autopsy can also be seen on chest radiograph.[118] These may be caused by air trapping because of the ball-valve effect of bronchial mucosal edema and sloughed bronchial mucosa. Large pneumatoceles, mainly involving the lower lobes, have been reported to occur uncommonly in children after kerosene ingestion. These pneumatoceles appear after 6 to 13 days in children age 1 to 5 years who have persistent respiratory symptoms for up to 10 days. They remain visible on radiographs for 1 to 8 months despite the absence of respiratory symptoms. They appear in consolidated areas of the lung, may be single or multiple, and may contain fluid. Pneumothorax, pneumomediastinum, pneumopericardium, subcutaneous emphysema, and pleural effusions have also been reported in children after hydrocarbon ingestion.[124]

Aspiration of more viscous aliphatic hydrocarbons such as mineral oil causes less acute toxicity, with no evidence of endothelial injury. At first, lipid-filled macrophages occupy the alveoli and interalveolar septa as well as the lymphatic vessels and regional lymph nodes. Later, the macrophages disappear, and foreign body granulomas form with fibrosis and giant cells; extracellular oil droplets may be found.[113]

The intensity of lung tissue reaction to animal and vegetable oils is proportional to the amount of free fatty acid present. Generally, this is greater in animal fats (e.g., cod liver oil) than in vegetable oils. Free fatty acids produce a severe injury with tissue necrosis, hemorrhage, vascular thrombosis, neutrophil infiltration, and later, fibrosis, which may obliterate alveoli and cause thickening of the walls of the small muscular arteries.[113,125] Paraffin granulomas may be found in debilitated patients who aspirate mineral oil or oily nosedrops. These form a mass lesion with indistinct borders, often in the posterior axillary segment of the upper lobe, and disappear slowly when oil ingestion ceases.[125,126]

Bacterial clearance from animal lungs is impaired by hydrocarbon ingestion, and secondary infection with aerobic and

Table 25-2 Pathologic Changes after Tracheal Instillation of Kerosene

TIME	CHANGE
1 hour	Engorgement of large and medium-sized vessels
4 hours	Engorgement of alveolar capillaries
24 hours	Peribronchial inflammation
	Focal areas of alveolar inflammatory exudate and consolidation
72 hours	Early resolution of alveolar exudate
7 days	Resolution of consolidation
	Persistence of some peribronchial inflammation
14 days	Persistence of vascular engorgement
	Resolution of most alveolar and peribronchial inflammation

anaerobic bacteria may follow hydrocarbon inhalation. However, animal studies and clinical experience in children have not found a major role for bacterial infection in this condition.[117] The routine use of prophylactic antibiotics is not recommended in lipoid pneumonia.[117,119,127] In debilitated patients, active infection with atypical mycobacteria occasionally complicates lipid aspiration. In experimental animals, lipids appear to enhance the pathogenicity of myocobacteria.[125,128]

The most important effects of hydrocarbon aspiration follow:

1. Alveolar and interstitial hemorrhage as well as leak of proteinaceous fluid from pulmonary capillaries. These two factors reduce the available alveolar surface area, completely filling some alveoli. The effect of this produces a large intrapulmonary shunt (up to 80% virtual shunt), possibly with a smaller component of $\dot{V}/\dot{Q}$ inequality,[19] and increases the respiratory system elastance and work of breathing.
2. Inhibition of surfactant by hydrocarbon, which increases the alveoli edema and results in atelectasis and a further increase in elastance. In addition, this loss of surfactant activity may contribute to small airway closure.[116]
3. Injury to the mucosa of bronchioles and small bronchi, which results in partial obstruction of these airways, possibly contributing to small airway closure in expiration and resultant gas trapping.[121] Small doses of kerosene injected into the trachea of dogs cause a small, insignificant leftward movement of the pressure-volume curve, whereas larger doses (0.3 ml/kg) move the curve downward to the right. It seems likely that the overall effect depends on the balance between gas trapping as a result of bronchial injury and alveolar filling with blood and proteinaceous fluid. Areas of gas trapping and areas of alveolar flooding are seen with small and large kerosene doses, but alveolar flooding becomes more prominent with larger doses. When gas trapping predominates, the lungs are overinflated, and the pressure-volume curve shifts to the left. When alveolar flooding predominates, the lungs become noncompliant, and the pressure-volume curve shifts down and to the right.[121] In 17 asymptomatic children examined 8 to 14 years after hydrocarbon ingestion, 82% had residual abnormalities in at least one pulmonary function test. The main abnormality was an increased resistance in the small airways, which was indicated by a high volume of isoflow and inhomogeneity of ventilation shown by an increased slope of phase III of the single-breath nitrogen test.[129] There was also evidence of residual air trapping. These abnormalities were not found in another study of 3 children followed up 8 to 10 years after ingestion.[130]
4. Pulmonary vascular endothelial injury and perivascular inflammation, which cause vascular thromboses and eventually endarteritis obliterans.[125] By reducing the total cross-sectional area of pulmonary vessels, this increases pulmonary vascular resistance, raising pulmonary artery pressure to 50% of systemic arterial pressure during the acute illness.[123]
5. In the first hour after inhalation of a volatile solvent, possible displacement of oxygen from the alveoli by the solvent vapor, causing hypoxemia. In the past it was suggested that hematogenous spread of hydrocarbon from the bowel caused the lung injury. This theory has been disproved by a series of animal experiments involving esophageal ligation and gastric instillation of solvent. It appears that aspiration is the main, if not the only, route of delivery of hydrocarbon to the lung when the usual amounts of hydrocarbon (<30 ml) are ingested. Aspiration occurs at the moment of ingestion rather than later, after vomiting.[131]

Radiologic Changes

Radiologic changes are a more sensitive indicator of lung injury than symptoms. Radiologic abnormalities are seen in 75% of infants who ingest hydrocarbons, but only 25% to 50% of these become symptomatic.[132,133] Although radiologic changes may appear within 30 minutes of ingestion,[117] chest radiographs taken in the first 2 hours may be deceptively clear or may show only mild hyperinflation of part or all of the lungs.[118] Most patients with hydrocarbon lung injury have radiologic signs within 12 hours[117] (Fig. 25-5). Fine, punctate, perihilar densities extend and coalesce, becoming coarse areas of consolidation involving mostly the lower lobes.[117,118,122] Regions of air trapping may be present in the periphery of the lung, and pneumothorax, pneumomediastinum, or pleural effusion may be seen. In most children, the chest radiograph changes disappear within a few days after the respiratory symptoms have resolved. In some cases, radiologic signs may persist for months, especially when pneumatoceles or paraffin granulomas are present. Even these eventually disappear completely.[124,126]

Investigations

In some cases in which there is doubt about the cause of pneumonia from the history, physical examination, and chest radiograph, the presence of fat-laden macrophages in sputum,

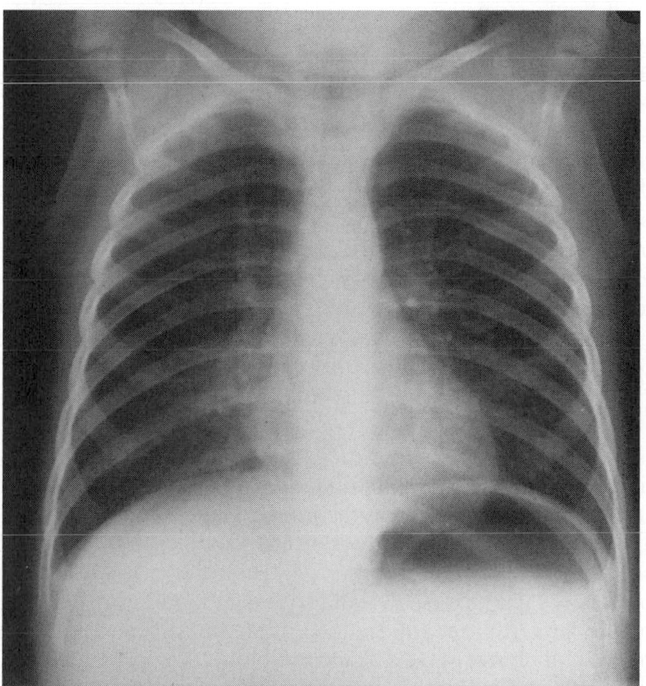

Fig. 25-5. Chest radiograph of a 2-year-old child 4 hours after ingestion of kerosene and one episode of vomiting. Fine reticulonodular opacities are most marked in the lower lobes and right middle lobe. Some alveolar opacities are also evident.

tracheal aspirate, BAL fluid, or an open biopsy specimen from the lung may indicate hydrocarbon inhalation as the cause. This is more likely to be necessary in an older, debilitated child with a swallowing disorder.

Management

Management consists of monitoring for signs of respiratory distress and injury to the heart, brain, liver, and kidneys with supportive treatment as required.

Decontamination

Induction of vomiting, nasogastric lavage, and mineral or olive oil gavage are contraindicated in any child who has ingested an oil or a hydrocarbon because these procedures are associated with an increased incidence of lipoid pneumonia.[131,134] Even the presence of a cuffed endotracheal tube does not guarantee protection of the lungs from vomited hydrocarbon. Although large quantities of activated charcoal may bind kerosene and turpentine,[115] its use is so frequently associated with vomiting that it is not justified in children with hydrocarbon ingestion.

Respiratory Management

Frequent reevaluation of clinical signs, especially in the first 72 hours, and monitoring of respiratory rate, heart rate, and hemoglobin saturation indicate the progress of respiratory failure. Monitoring of arterial blood gases by intraarterial catheter may be needed in severe cases. The chest radiograph excludes pneumothorax and pneumopericardium in the event of sudden clinical deterioration. Decisions about changes in respiratory care are based on clinical needs rather than on radiographic changes.

Oxygen should be given by mask to any child with respiratory distress, cyanosis, or a low hemoglobin saturation. If the saturation remains below 80% despite the administration of high-flow oxygen by mask and is deteriorating or if the child's respiratory rate is rising rapidly without radiologic evidence of pneumothorax, then tracheal intubation and CPAP or mechanical ventilation may be needed. High levels of CPAP, peak airway pressure, and PEEP have a serious risk of pneumothorax, pneumopericardium, or air leak from overinflated areas of the lungs.[123,135] Minimization of this risk requires that airway pressures and tidal volume be no greater than those needed to maintain an arterial pH above 7.1[136] and a PaO_2 above 50 mm Hg. The FIO_2 should be kept below 0.5 if possible. If mechanical ventilation fails to control the respiratory failure, ECMO may be used. Survivors have been reported after the use of ECMO in children with hydrocarbon aspiration.[135]

Other Measures

Steroids have no place in the treatment of hydrocarbon inhalation; human and animal studies have shown no benefit from their use,[115,127,137] and the impaired mononuclear cell response in the lung caused by steroids may increase the risk of secondary bacterial pneumonia.[127] The routine use of antibiotics is not justified.[117,127] Rather, clinical monitoring, bacteriologic surveillance, and frequent total and differential white blood cell counts should guide antibiotic therapy. Culture of fluid obtained by bronchoscopic or nonbronchoscopic BAL via an endotracheal tube may give a more accurate guide to the infecting organism when there is evidence of developing bacterial pneumonia. In a child who has aspirated a highly volatile oil such as mineral seal oil, naphthalene, or xylene, electrocardiographic monitoring may be justified because of the risk of myocardial irritability. Catecholamines, bronchodilators, and inotropic agents should be avoided whenever possible because they can provoke ventricular ectopic beats and ventricular fibrillation in these circumstances. Wheezing in these children is due to structural damage to the bronchial and bronchiolar walls, and there is no evidence to support the use of bronchodilators. Renal, liver, and myocardial function should be assessed by clinical observation, biochemical testing, and cardiac ultrasound examination in the first 2 hours after ingestion and after 24 hours in severe cases.

Prognosis

In the United States from 1985 through 1989, there were 5 deaths among 129,000 cases of hydrocarbon ingestion,[106] a mortality rate of about 0.01% of children with respiratory symptoms resulting from hydrocarbon ingestion.[106,117] The majority of children deteriorated over the first 24 hours and then improved and became asymptomatic over 3 to 4 days. In more severely affected children, symptoms may persist for 10 days or more, but in other children, the condition may progress to intractable respiratory failure over 2 to 3 days.[135] Some infants have been reported to die after 1 to 2 months of progressive respiratory failure with extensive lung consolidation and recurrent pneumothoraxes.[105]

LUNG INJURY IN NEAR-DROWNING

Epidemiology

Drowning is one of the leading causes of accidental death in childhood. In the United States, it is estimated that 1000 children younger than 5 years of age drown each year.[138] In the United Kingdom the annual incidence is 0.7 per 100,000 children, of whom 68% are younger than 5 years of age.[139] In Australia, drowning is the second most common cause of accidental death in children.[140] Drowning occurs most commonly in children under the age of 5 years and between the ages of 15 and 24 years. Boys drown 4 times more frequently than girls.[141] Data are incomplete, and estimates vary markedly, but near-drownings are believed to be 3 to 5 times—some say up to 500 times[142]—as common as drownings. Among young children, freshwater accidents are more common than saltwater accidents.

Children younger than 5 years of age are most likely to drown in backyard swimming pools, farm ponds, and drains. Buckets and rubbish bins are another risk for toddlers whose undeveloped coordination and high center of gravity allow them to fall inside head-down and prevent them from righting themselves.[143] Bathtubs are also a major source of immersion injury for toddlers, sometimes associated with child abuse.[144,145] In one series, a previous child abuse report had been filed for 25% of children injured in bathtubs.[146] Hot tubs and spas are also hazards. The common etiologic factors in most childhood immersion accidents are the presence of one of these hazards and a momentary lapse in adult supervision.[143,147,148] Teenagers are more likely to drown in saltwater. Etiologic factors include diving into shallow water, with associated spinal cord injury; voluntary hyperventilation; bravado; and alcohol use.

Medical conditions, particularly epilepsy[149] and some cardiac dysrhythmias,[150] remain risk factors for drowning throughout childhood and call for increased supervision by caregivers.

Disease Mechanisms

Drowning is a multisystem hypoxic-ischemic insult. The degree of hypoxic-ischemic brain injury determines the outcome in near-drowning. The lung injury induced by immersion can involve hypoxia to the lung parenchyma as well as aspiration of water, debris, gastric contents, or bacteria. Alveolar disruption with loss of surfactant and atelectasis, as well as pulmonary edema, airway obstruction with foreign particles, an inflammatory reaction with the development of ARDS, and secondary infection, may occur

Drowning occurs without aspiration of water in only about 10% of victims; in this group, hypoxia results primarily from laryngospasm and apnea.[151] In the majority who do aspirate fluid, it has been estimated that most survivors aspirate 22 ml/kg or less.[152] Vomiting occurs in half of children during cardiopulmonary resuscitation, whereas aspiration of gastric contents is present in up to 70% of acutely drowned patients at autopsy.[153] Aspiration of particulate matter can obstruct small or large bronchi. Particulate matter can include sand,[154] mud, undigested food, and other debris. Active inhalation rather than passive flow of fluid is believed to be the main determinant of the volume aspirated.

The composition of the aspirated water influences the pathophysiologic changes in the lungs. Even small-volume aspiration produces hypoxemia, which is the common result of both freshwater and saltwater immersion. In freshwater aspiration, pulmonary surfactant is washed out and diluted,[155] leading to atelectasis. Loss of surface-active material and disruption of alveolar cells[156] can cause the pulmonary capillaries to leak, leading to pulmonary edema. Perfusion of these collapsed and fluid-filled alveoli results in intrapulmonary shunting and hypoxemia.

Evidence from experiments suggests that in saltwater aspiration, pulmonary surfactant is less affected, although it may sometimes be inactivated. The hypertonicity of aspirated fluid causes an osmotic shift of protein-rich fluid from the capillaries into the alveoli. This results in pulmonary edema, $\dot{V}/\dot{Q}$ mismatching, and hypoxemia. Victims of saltwater drownings have a higher incidence of pulmonary edema than victims of freshwater drownings[157]; otherwise, the clinical differences between the two types of immersion accidents are minimal.[158] In an animal study, Orlowski et al[159] found no difference in the cardiovascular effects resulting from the tracheal instillation of hypotonic, isotonic, or hypertonic solutions at 20 ml/kg. In all groups, there was an immediate fall in cardiac output and an increase in pulmonary capillary wedge pressure, central venous pressure, and pulmonary vascular resistance. Similar results occurred in animals exposed to a period of anoxia. The authors concluded that the cardiovascular changes of near-drowning are a direct result of anoxia and are not dependent on the tonicity of the fluid.

The electrolyte abnormalities proposed on the basis of animal experiments include hypernatremia in saltwater immersion, hyponatremia, hyperkalemia, and hemolysis in hypotonic immersions. These are rarely seen in victims reaching the hospital.[160] This is probably because the amount of fluid aspirated is usually small. The redistribution of fluid in saltwater near-drowning, in particular, can lead to a relative depletion of the intravascular volume. Large-volume freshwater aspiration may lead to an increase in blood volume because of absorption of fluid into the circulation. Fluid overload can occur in all types of drowning because of the absorption of large volumes of swallowed water from the gastrointestinal tract, pulmonary absorption of aspirated fluid, increased levels of circulating antidiuretic hormone because of brain and lung injury, and iatrogenic causes.

Pulmonary edema and atelectasis may reduce lung compliance in near-drowning victims. Partial obstruction of smaller bronchi and respiratory bronchioles by inhaled particles,[161] airway mucosal edema, smooth muscle contraction, and increased mucus production caused by gastric acid and other inhaled irritants may increase airway resistance.

Hypoxic-ischemic injury to the lung parenchyma contributes to the inactivation of pulmonary surfactant, increased pulmonary vascular resistance and pulmonary hypertension, and the development of ARDS. ARDS develops within 1 to 48 hours in about 40% of near-drowning victims[161] because of a combination of the direct lung injury, the global hypoxic insult, sepsis, and the host inflammatory response (see section on ARDS).

Infection is believed to play a part in the pulmonary injury of only a minority of near-drownings.[160] There have been some reports, however, of specific organisms being involved; such reports warrant consideration. Three children were reported to have developed fever, neutropenia, and cardiovascular collapse in the second 12 hours after hospital admission; in these children, *Streptococcus pneumoniae* was isolated from blood cultures and cultures of endotracheal tube aspirate taken both at the time of and 18 hours after admission.[162] The origin of the pneumococci is probably the upper respiratory tract. Invasion may occur because of the diminished local defenses related to lung injury and the compromised general immunity related to the global hypoxic-ischemic insult. The authors suggested that in cases of near-drowning, an antibiotic to which *Pneumococcus* is sensitive should be chosen. A case report of two children who drowned in hot tubs warned of the risk of *Pseudomonas aeruginosa*,[163] which colonizes warm water. In a retrospective study of 40 near-drowning cases, Bohn et al[164] found a relationship among hypothermia (including therapeutically induced hypothermia), neutropenia, and sepsis. The organisms isolated from blood cultures included *P. aeruginosa, S. aureus,* and *Escherichia coli.* The development of sepsis may result from the aspiration of the normal flora of the mouth and upper respiratory tract, aspiration of organisms from the medium in which immersion occurred, colonization of endotracheal tubes and invasive monitoring lines, or the translocation of bacteria and toxins through the gastrointestinal tract mucosa compromised by hypoxia.

Assessment of the Near-Drowning Victim

Initial management of the child who has drowned involves basic and advanced life support. The taking of a detailed history can be delayed until the airway is clear of vomitus and is secured, ventilation and oxygenation are adequate, independent circulation is established, and a nasogastric tube is passed. From the child's family and the rescuers, the clinician should elicit information about possible associated injuries, predisposing medical or social conditions, the duration of immersion, the temperature of the water, the cardiac rhythm and rate during resuscitation, cardiotonic medication administered, the nature and adequacy of initial resuscitation, episodes of vomiting, and the child's neurologic response. The examination should establish the need for ventilatory assistance, whether it is because of inadequate oxygenation or alveolar hypoventilation, an inability to protect the airway because of central nervous system depression, or a hemodynamic instability. Wheezing or asymmetry of air entry may suggest bronchial obstruction with foreign particles. A neurologic examination should assess and document the child's conscious state (the motor response to verbal or painful stimuli), pupillary size, and reaction to light and the presence of the cough and gag reflexes in the unconscious patient. Any child who has been retrieved unconscious from a river, swimming pool, or shallows of a beach, especially an older child and especially if there is a history of a dive or fall, should be assumed to have cervical spine trauma until it is proved otherwise. Cervical spine radiographs should be taken and the neck immobilized with a rigid collar or by tape and sandbags.

The initial assessment of pulmonary injury should include pulse oximetry and arterial blood gas analysis with calculation of the $PAO_2 - PaO_2$ gradient. A chest radiograph may show areas of atelectasis or gas trapping resulting from foreign body aspiration, pulmonary edema, and after ventilation, signs of barotrauma (Fig. 25-6). If the history suggests the possibility of large particle aspiration or if the clinical or radiologic findings suggest airway obstruction, fiberoptic bronchoscopy can be performed through the endotracheal tube. Rigid bronchoscopy may be required for airway obstruction by large particles. The patient should receive 100% oxygen and sedation during bronchoscopy, and topical anesthesia of the airway should be provided to prevent coughing and associated rises in intracranial pressure.

The extent of cardiovascular monitoring depends on the severity of the aspiration injury. After a severe global hypoxic-ischemic injury, depressed myocardial function leads to cardiogenic pulmonary edema and a reduced cardiac output. Generalized capillary leaking of proteinaceous fluid exacerbates the pulmonary edema and causes peripheral edema involving the chest wall, which reduces respiratory system compliance. An arterial cannula should be inserted for continuous blood pressure monitoring and frequent assessment of arterial blood gases in all patients with impaired gas exchange. Central venous pressure does not reflect left-sided cardiac filling pressures in patients with lung disease, increased pulmonary vascular resistance, or right-sided heart failure.[165] In the presence of hypoxic-ischemic myocardial injury, plasma expansion therapy and inotropic support can be titrated to the optimum pulmonary capillary wedge pressure and cardiac output by using a balloon-tipped pulmonary artery catheter, although in the presence of capillary leak, pulmonary edema occurs at "normal" wedge pressures. The difficulty of inserting a pulmonary artery catheter and the additional risk of infection, thrombosis, vessel perforation, and dysrhythmia must be weighed against the value of the information provided. Metabolic acidosis with high lactate levels reflects both the global hypoxic insult before resuscitation as well as ongoing poor tissue perfusion, so serial measurements of acid base and plasma lactate may be more useful than single measurements to monitor the child's response to therapy.[166] Gastric tonometry and measurement of gastric intramural pH may provide a minimally invasive measure of tissue oxygenation,[167] but their usefulness is unproved in children.

The total and differential white cell counts can indicate the development of infection in children involved in near-drownings,[164] although the white cell count may be raised for 3 to 4 days because of severe hypoxia alone, and transient hypoxic bone marrow depression succeeded by a leukocytosis with many immature neutrophils often follows prolonged cardiac arrest. Bacteriologic surveillance should include blood cultures and BAL fluid analysis if there are clinical or laboratory signs of sepsis. Monitoring of plasma electrolytes helps guide fluid administration.

Management

Primary management requires attention to airway patency, breathing, and circulation (see also section on ARDS). If the patient is hypoxemic, oxygen should be given. If apnea or hypoventilation is present, assisted ventilation is required. The best treatment for aspiration-induced hypoxia is the application of CPAP.[168,169] CPAP can be administered in a spontaneously breathing patient by face mask or endotracheal tube or as PEEP associated with pressure support or intermittent mandatory modes of ventilation. The application of PEEP is

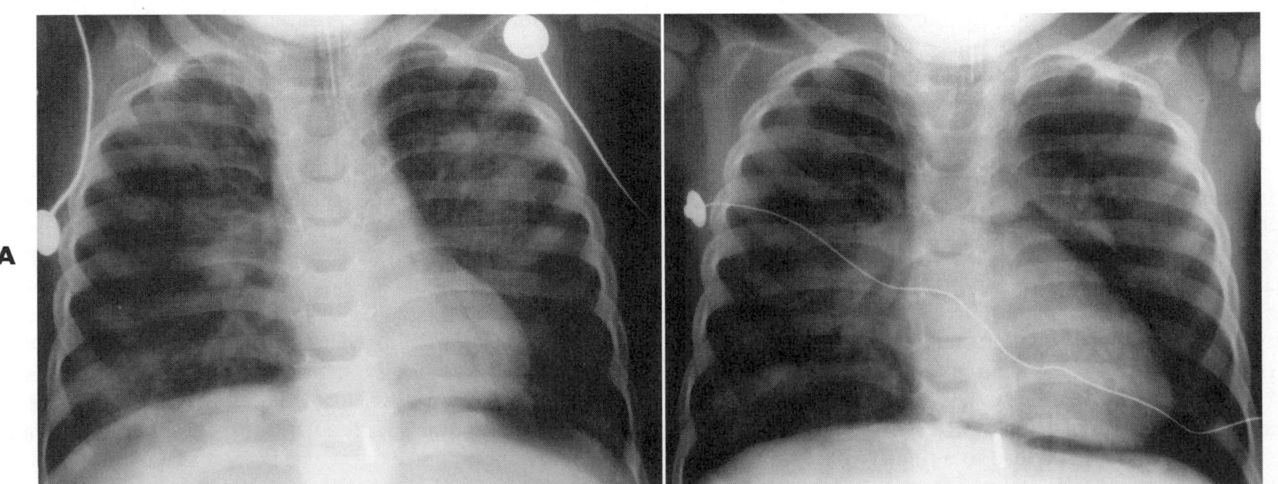

Fig. 25-6. Chest radiographs of a 2-year-old child after near-drowning in fresh water. **A,** At 2 hours after immersion, the radiograph shows widespread alveolar infiltrates, especially in the upper lobes and right middle lobe. **B,** Some 36 hours later, the radiograph shows more widespread alveolar opacity with pneumomediastinum, pneumopericardium, and right-sided pneumothorax.

indicated for borderline oxygenation and for the maintenance of safe levels of arterial oxygenation (Pa_{O_2} > 45 to 50 mm Hg), but the inspired oxygen concentration is reduced to nontoxic levels (<60%). High levels of PEEP can exacerbate intracranial hypertension by retarding cerebral venous drainage and may impair the systemic venous return and cardiac output. Newer modes of respiratory support, such as high-frequency oscillation ventilation (HFOV), have not been subjected to controlled trials in drowning but may help reduce barotrauma. If there is severe barotrauma or the child's lungs cannot be adequately ventilated and there is no evidence for irreparable severe brain dysfunction, ECMO support is indicated.

Corticosteroids have no beneficial effect on ARDS[170] and may be harmful. Based on the reports of pneumococcal sepsis in children involved in near-drownings, prophylactic penicillin may be indicated.[162] Development of penicillin resistance in pneumococci is extremely uncommon during a short course of penicillin prophylaxis, and benzyl penicillin is effective against most strains of community-acquired pneumococcus. Although there is evidence of a higher risk of *Pseudomonas* infections in hot tub drownings than in other forms of near-drowning, the prophylactic use of third-generation cephalosporins is associated with a significant risk of infection with antibiotic-resistant gram-negative organisms. If there is evidence of infection, analysis of BAL fluid may help identify the pulmonary pathogens.[171] The role of surfactant-replacement therapy in the management of pulmonary injury of near-drowning remains unproved.

Outcome

There are several good population-based reviews on the outcome of immersion accidents in children,[139,172] including one on neurologic sequelae,[173] and some large case series examining the prognostic factors.[174,175] The primary determinant of the ultimate prognosis of a child victim of near-drowning remains the degree of hypoxic-ischemic brain injury. A critical evaluation has shown that techniques of brain resuscitation aimed at aggressive treatment of intracranial hypertension, barbiturate coma, and induced hypothermia have not improved outcome.[163] The prognosis for recovery of respiratory function is generally good in survivors, although abnormalities of airflow obstruction or mild restrictive lung disease have been described. There have been isolated case reports of pulmonary interstitial fibrosis after near-drowning in fresh water.[176] Massive lung fibrosis has been reported,[177] and in one case, transient miliary pneumonitis developed 6 weeks after near-drowning in muddy water. Lung biopsy in this case showed granulomata containing algae and pollen grains.[178]

CHEMICAL AND PARTICULATE LUNG INJURY

Major lung injury resulting from the inhalation of noxious gases, chemicals, and particulates is less common in children than in adults. In adults, chemical pneumonitis is most commonly associated with industrial accidents. The most common causative agents are hydrogen sulfide, phosgene,[179] sulfur dioxide,[180] nitrogen oxides,[181] cadmium, nickel, and other metal fumes.[182] The epidemiology of inhalation in children predominantly reflects the availability of noxious substances within the home. Pulmonary injury in children has been reported after the inhalation of chlorine, talcum powder, detergent powders, and mercury and the aspiration of activated charcoal. Children with asthma are particularly susceptible to respiratory irritants; chlorine, NH_3, nitrogen dioxide, and sulfur dioxide have been reported as precipitants of airway obstruction.

Chlorine

Chlorine is an irritant gas that can damage the tracheobronchial tree and lung parenchyma. Its use in households as a component of cleaning agents and swimming pool disinfectant[183,184] means that it is frequently encountered by children. Pulmonary toxicity from chlorine inhalation has been reported in children of all ages.[185-187] There have been reports of voluntary chlorine inhalation in adolescents.[185,188,189]

Disease Mechanisms

Chlorine gas is more dense than air and dissipates slowly, leading to prolonged exposure. Chlorine is estimated to be 20 times more toxic as an oxidizing agent and irritant than HCl. It is irritating to the eyes and skin and causes bronchoconstriction, airway inflammation, and alveolar injury. Inhalation of 40 to 60 ppm can produce pneumonitis and pulmonary edema. Cellular toxicity results from the reaction of molecular chlorine with water, forming reactive oxygen species. This leads to the oxidation of functional molecular side chains in cells. The reaction of chlorine with tissue water also forms HCl and hydrochlorous acid. The net equation follows:

$$2\,Cl_2 + 2\,H_2O \longleftrightarrow 4\,HCl + O_2$$

The HCl produced causes tissue irritation and cell necrosis. Because the formation of toxic products requires water, damage is most severe in tissues with a high water content, such as the mucosa of the conjunctival sac and the respiratory tract. Pathologic examination of the lungs of patients who have died after chlorine gas exposure shows denudation of alveolar and bronchial epithelium, alveolar edema, hyaline membrane formation, and pulmonary intravascular thrombi.[190]

Clinical Presentation

Symptoms begin within minutes of exposure to more than 5 ppm. They include irritation of the eye, nose, and upper respiratory tract. Wheezing develops early. Paroxysmal cough, dyspnea, lacrimation, chest discomfort, mucus production, palpitations, dizziness, headache, and nausea are the major symptoms at presentation.[187,191] Wheeze and tachypnea are early signs. Stridor resulting from laryngeal edema may be present. Cough with frothy sputum, cyanosis, and crackles on auscultation suggest severe lung injury and pulmonary edema and usually develop within the first 24 hours after exposure.[183] The onset of pulmonary edema may be rapid. Respiratory alkalosis is most common in mild exposure, but persistent hyperchloremic metabolic acidosis may occur.[183,187,192] The presence of hypercarbia or hypoxemia with an increased P_{AO_2}–P_{aO_2} indicates severe respiratory involvement. A depressed conscious state, most probably resulting from hypoxemia, has been reported in severely affected children.[183] Spirometry in the acute stages shows an obstructive pattern with a fall in the FEV_1 and the FEV_1/VC ratio.[191,193] Reduction of the functional residual capacity indicates pulmonary edema.[194,195] Lung compliance is reduced, and there is intrapulmonary right-to-left shunting. The chest radiograph may be normal at presentation or may show evidence of airflow obstruction with hyperinflation or pulmonary edema with interstitial markings and perihilar alveolar opacities. Ventricular dysrhythmias,[185] and poor tissue perfusion requiring the infusion of plasma expanders[183] have been reported.

Management

Supplemental oxygen is the only treatment required in most cases. Nebulized albuterol and intravenous aminophylline have been given for bronchospasm, although caution must be exercised with the latter because of the risk of dysrhythmias.[185] Corticosteroids may be effective in reducing airflow obstruction.[196] In one retrospective, uncontrolled case series, nebulized sodium bicarbonate was used to treat 86 patients after acute chlorine gas inhalation,[197] and none developed pulmonary edema or required ventilatory support.

If hypoxemia resulting from pulmonary edema persists despite oxygen therapy, CPAP (delivered by mask, nasopharyngeal catheter, or endotracheal tube) or IPPV with PEEP may be needed. PEEP may not be advantageous if the predominant pulmonary abnormality is airflow obstruction and air trapping resulting from bronchospasm, rather than pulmonary edema, although a trial of CPAP or IPPV with PEEP is justified if gas exchange is deteriorating despite conservative therapy. Patients with airflow obstruction may generate their own "auto-PEEP," and this may be an indication for positive-pressure support. Tracheal intubation and assisted ventilation are required when hypoxemic or hypercapnic respiratory failure, a depressed conscious state, or severe upper airway obstruction occurs. Fluid intake should be limited because iatrogenic overhydration exacerbates the alveolar and airway edema. Serial blood gases and continuous cutaneous oximetry should be used in all children with respiratory signs. Observation for 24 hours is indicated for all children who have had significant exposure. Prophylactic antibiotics have not been shown to be beneficial.

Pulmonary Sequelae

Several studies have documented persistent obstructive pulmonary abnormalities in adults after acute chlorine exposure.[191,193] Some 2 weeks after minimally symptomatic exposure, 18 adults had diminished FEV_1 and a maximum midexpiratory flow rate. Those with the greatest reduction from predicted values were those with the most severe symptoms after exposure and those with a past medical history of smoking or asthma.[191] Airway reactivity may persist for many years after exposure.[193,198] The problem with these and other studies is the lack of a control group or detailed knowledge of preexposure lung function in exposed individuals. It is not known whether preexisting bronchial hyperreactivity accounts for the apparently high prevalence of persistent airflow obstruction after chlorine exposure. Schwartz et al[193] found that residual volume was reduced years after exposure and suggested that acute airway inflammation may result in longer-term peribronchial fibrosis. This may stiffen the bronchioles and cause them to be more resistant to closure during exhalation, permitting continued exhalation at low lung volumes and a reduced residual volume.

Givan et al[187] reported impaired lung function in an infant after acute chlorine exposure. This child had recurrent episodes of wheezing and cough with airflow obstruction that was responsive to bronchodilators and that resolved over a 2-year period. Children who have significant exposure to chlorine require follow-up for the assessment of pulmonary function and treatment if symptomatic airflow obstruction develops.

Ammonia

Liquid NH3 is a component of household cleaning products, but exposure to NH_3 gas with inhalational injury is rare in childhood. NH_3 is highly water soluble and in aqueous solution forms a potent alkali, ammonium hydroxide. Exposure to high concentrations of NH_3 causes liquefactive necrosis of the mucous membranes and submucosal tissues of the upper respiratory tract. This results in laryngeal edema and inflammation, mucous hypersecretion, mucosal sloughing, tracheitis, and bronchoconstriction. Pulmonary edema may result from massive exposure or may develop after the relief of upper airway obstruction.

Severe lacrimation, pharyngeal irritation, cough, and stridor may develop within minutes of exposure. Upper airway obstruction may be severe and require endotracheal intubation. Treatment is supportive and is similar to that for chlorine inhalation. Bronchodilators are indicated for airflow obstruction. Corticosteroids have not been shown to be of definite benefit but probably should be given for symptomatic upper airway obstruction. Nebulized adrenaline may reduce laryngeal edema and maintain a patent airway without tracheal intubation. Although most patients recover, long-term pulmonary function abnormalities and bronchiectasis have been found in adults after acute NH_3 gas inhalation.[199,200]

Alkaline Laundry Detergents

By a mechanism similar to that of NH_3, sodium carbonate–containing laundry detergents have caused upper respiratory tract obstruction.[201] Children drool and experience stridor 1 to 5 hours after ingestion of the powder. Most vomit after ingestion. One child reported to have inhaled detergent developed symptoms immediately. At endoscopy, there was edema of the pharynx, epiglottis, and larynx. Tracheal intubation may be required for airway management.[201] Caustic burns may be associated with corneal injury.

Talcum Powder

Talc inhalation is a common problem that affects primarily infants up to the age of 2 years. Exposure occurs most commonly at times of diaper changes. Some reports have suggested that the similar appearance of baby powder containers to nursing bottles is a etiologic factor.[202] Aspiration of talc has caused severe respiratory distress and death in young children.[203,204] The mortality rate may be up to 20% in cases severe enough to require assisted ventilation.[204]

Disease Mechanisms

Talc is a powder of hydrous magnesium silicate ($Mg_3Si_4O_{10}H_2O$). It consists of a layer of magnesium hydroxide between two silica sheets that slide past each other, giving the slippery feel. The mean particle size is less than 5 μm. Inhaled talc causes airway obstruction, drying of the respiratory mucosa, impairment of the ciliary clearing mechanism, and inflammation.[205] Inflammatory infiltrates in biopsy and autopsy specimens consist of mononuclear and giant cells filled with crystalline doubly refractile bodies.[206] Hyaline membrane formation, obliteration of small bronchi and alveoli, and fibrotic changes are also seen.

Children usually develop cough and respiratory distress immediately after inhalation. Sometimes, the onset of symptoms is delayed for several hours.[207] Cardiorespiratory arrest has been reported after massive aspiration.[204] Many children have minimal or transient symptoms. Wheezes, crackles, and tachypnea are common. A chest radiograph may show hyperinflation with patchy infiltrates. Hypoxemic respiratory failure should be treated like other causes of severe respiratory distress syndrome: with supplemental oxygen, PEEP, fluid restriction, and assisted ventilation (see section on ARDS). Sedation and paralysis may be required. Barotrauma has been reported in talc inhalation.[205] Corticosteroids have been used to modify the inflammatory response. BAL has been used therapeutically to clear debris obstructing large airways, but whether the benefit of this procedure outweighs the risks is unknown.

Complete resolution of pulmonary lesions with normal lung function at follow-up has been reported in survivors even after massive aspiration, although a combined restrictive-obstructive pulmonary function defect may occur.

Activated Charcoal

The use of activated charcoal has become widespread in the treatment of toxic ingestions and overdoses. Activated charcoal with its huge surface area is able to absorb a wide range of chemicals and decrease their absorption from the gastrointestinal tract. It can also increase the clearance from the systemic circulation of several substances that have an enterohepatic circulation.[208] However, activated charcoal is not a benign substance, and there has been substantial morbidity and several reports of deaths resulting from aspiration pneumonia associated with its use. Some clinical aspects of drug intoxication make the nasogastric administration of charcoal particularly hazardous. The patient may have a depressed conscious state or have seizures with poor airway protection or may be combative and uncooperative, resulting in malpositioning or dislodgment of the nasogastric tube. The ingested poison may cause vomiting by a central effect or from gastric irritation, gastric stasis, or intestinal ileus. Gastrointestinal obstruction may be caused by a solid charcoal bolus.[209] Multiple doses of charcoal in patients with impaired bowel motility[210] or even a single dose after the administration of ipecac[211] is likely to be especially dangerous.

Disease Mechanisms

When aspirated, the thick charcoal suspension may cause obstruction of the large[211] and small airways.[212] Gas trapping and barotrauma are common features. Pneumonitis with all the features of ARDS may develop. This may be exacerbated by the aspiration of gastric contents. Autopsy findings have shown lung parenchymal scarring with bronchiectasis, bronchiolectasis, and bronchiolitis obliterans. Large amounts of residual charcoal are found in the airways and alveoli associated with an inflammatory reaction that includes giant cells,[212] alveolar macrophages, and histiocytes. Regional lymph nodes also show charcoal deposition within histiocytes. Diffuse pulmonary thromboembolism has also been reported.

Clinical Features and Management

Charcoal aspiration produces severe respiratory failure. Tachypnea, dyspnea, wheezing, and cyanosis may increase in severity in the 48 hours after aspiration. Wheezes and crackles are audible widely over the chest, and areas of reduced air entry may be found in the presence of obstruction of the large airways. Radiologic findings of lung infiltrates (Fig. 25-7) may underestimate the extent of lung affected. ARDS may develop despite relatively normal early chest radiographs.[213] Bronchoscopy and tracheobronchial toilet may be useful.[211,212] Copious charcoal-laden secretions may be aspirated from the trachea for many days after the inhalation episode. β-Sympathomimetic agonists have been used to treat wheeze after aspiration, but the reversibility of airflow obstruction is probably minimal. After charcoal aspiration, bacterial colonization of endotracheal tube secretions may be associated with systemic evidence of sepsis.[210,212,213] Management should include bacteriologic surveillance of blood and tracheal aspirate and appropriate antibiotic treatment if infection is likely.

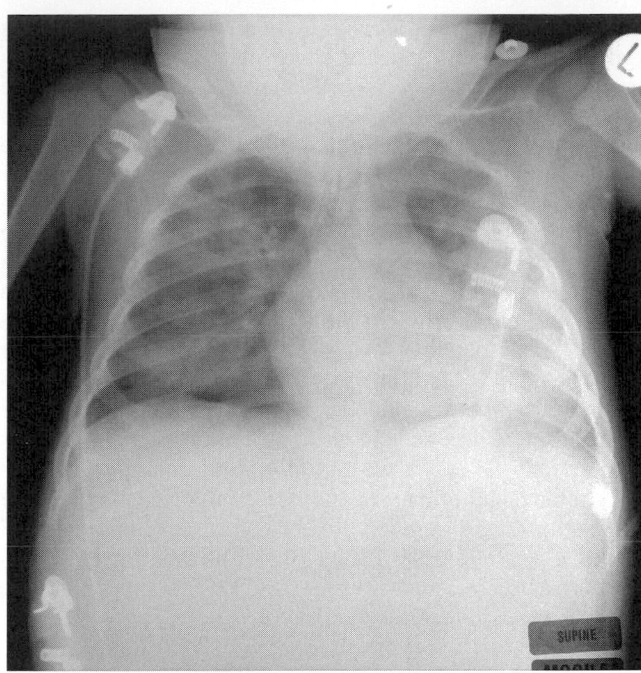

Fig. 25-7. Chest radiograph of a 2-year-old child 1 hour after vomiting and aspiration of activated charcoal. Note the very widespread alveolar opacities.

Activated charcoal should be use cautiously in childhood ingestions. In most cases of suspected poisoning in children, the lung disease that may be induced by aspiration carries a far higher risk of mortality and morbidity than the ingested poison.

Mercury

Mercury vapor inhalation is a very rare condition in childhood but causes severe acute respiratory distress and is commonly fatal.[214] The heating of mercury has been used to separate gold from gold ore and form a gold-mercury amalgam. Children have developed progressive pulmonary failure within hours of exposure; this failure is clinically and pathologically similar to other causes of ARDS. There is one report of HFOV being successfully used to maintain gas exchange in an infant with this condition.[215]

ACUTE RESPIRATORY DISTRESS SYNDROME

ARDS is a clinical syndrome with multiple etiologies. The hallmark is an acute change in lung function characterized by pulmonary edema resulting from increased alveolar-capillary permeability. This results in severe hypoxemia, decreased lung compliance, and the appearance of bilateral pulmonary infiltrates on chest radiograph. Inflammation plays a part in the pathogenesis, and fibrosis occurs in the lung parenchyma during resolution. Alveolar injury is diffuse but not uniform throughout the lung.

ARDS may occur after direct or indirect lung injury. Septicemia, near-drowning, hypovolemic shock, and closed-space burn injury were the most common antecedent illnesses in children reported by Pfenninger et al.[216] ARDS is also seen in immunocompromised children after treatment for malignancy[217]; in association with respiratory infections, including mycoplasma,[218] respiratory syncytial virus,[219] and herpesvirus[220] infections; and after major head injury,[221] multiple trauma, asphyxia,[222] and chemical aspiration. Studies of adults indicate that patients with multiple predisposing conditions (e.g., trauma, multiple transfusions, disseminated intravascular coagulation) are at a much greater risk of developing ARDS than those with a single risk factor.[223] The lung injury associated with cardiopulmonary bypass and ECMO support has the pathophysiologic features of ARDS.

Disease Mechanisms

The pathology of ARDS has been extensively reviewed by Bachofen and Weibel.[224] In the initial stage, there is damage to and edema of the interalveolar septa. There is extensive destruction of type I alveolar epithelial cells. Although on electron microscopy, the endothelial cell basement membrane appears relatively intact, this barrier becomes permeable to plasma proteins, and interstitial edema results. Proteinaceous fluid first collects within the peribronchial and perivascular connective tissue, then within the alveolar septa, and later in the alveoli. Edema fluid contains erythrocytes, leukocytes, fibroblasts, macrophages, cell debris, albumin, globulins, and amorphous material comprising strands of fibrin. Hyaline membranes form along the inner surface of the alveoli. As the alveoli and interstitium fill with exudate, the gas-exchanging and mechanical properties of the lung deteriorate. There are reduced lung volumes and poor compliance with $\dot{V}/\dot{Q}$ mismatching, intrapulmonary shunting, and increased dead space.[225,226]

Microthrombosis of pulmonary vessels occurs as a result of intravascular coagulation, pulmonary vascular congestion, and the sequestration of neutrophils and platelets that plug the pulmonary capillaries. This further exacerbates endothelial damage, high pulmonary vascular resistance, and $\dot{V}/\dot{Q}$ mismatching.

In the first days of ARDS the capillary endothelial and alveolar epithelial barrier are reduced in thickness by cellular necrosis. By the end of the first week, there is regeneration of the endothelium, and the destroyed type I pneumocytes that line the alveoli are replaced by the marked proliferation of thicker, cuboidal, type II pneumocytes. This phase of ARDS may result in complete resolution of the process or may progress to interstitial fibrosis. Fibrosis commences after the first week and particularly involves the alveolar walls. Pulmonary fibrosis rapidly and progressively obliterates the alveoli, alveolar ducts, and pulmonary interstitial space, which also is expanded by edema fluid and inflammatory cells. The apposition between the alveolar epithelium and capillary endothelium is then separated by bulky type II pneumocytes and fibroblasts in the alveolar septum and interstitium. In advanced cases of ARDS, when thickening of the alveolar wall is extensive, gas exchange is too impaired to support life. Intraalveolar hemorrhage may be focally present in some cases but is generally not severe. Although alveolar damage is widespread in ARDS, the lung is not uniformly affected. Computed tomography of patients with ARDS shows the distribution of lung collapse to be mainly in the dependent regions.[227]

Although the predisposing causes of ARDS are known and the histopathologic changes well characterized, there is still uncertainty as to the exact role and timing of the mediators involved. Neutrophils probably have a central role in the genesis of endothelial injury.[228] They are sequestered early into the lung, drawn to the lung by chemotactic components of the complement cascade (C5a), prostaglandins, tumor necrosis factor, leukotrienes, and PAF. Neutrophils release interleukin-1 and toxic oxygen radicals that cause cell destruction. Oxygen-derived free radicals, such as hydrogen peroxide and the hydroxyl radical, are bactericidal agents, which may produce host membrane damage by causing lipid peroxidation or by making target proteins more susceptible to proteolytic cleavage. Oxygen radicals also inhibit the action of α_1-antitrypsin, allowing unopposed activity of elastase and other proteolytic enzymes, which are capable of degrading elastin, collagen, proteoglycans, fibronectin, and structural components of basement membranes and the intercellular matrix. Neutrophils stimulate the production of arachidonic acid metabolites—prostaglandin, thromboxanes, and leukotrienes—some of which cause increased capillary permeability, vasoconstriction, and platelet aggregation and are chemotactic for neutrophils.

Large numbers of platelets are present in pulmonary capillaries in ARDS. They aggregate, causing increased microvascular hydrostatic pressure, and release arachidonic acid metabolites. The number of alveolar macrophages increases greatly. These cells produce cytokines such as tumor necrosis factor and the interleukins, which cause tissue damage.

The role of PAF in acute lung injury has been reviewed by Anderson et al.[229] PAF is produced by endothelial cells, type II pneumocytes, marginating neutrophils, and alveolar macrophages. PAF causes microvascular leakage and margination of leukocytes and contributes to the development of intravascular coagulation in lung capillaries.

Role of Pulmonary Hypertension

Zapol and Snider[226] found pulmonary artery hypertension and elevated pulmonary vascular resistance in 30 patients with ARDS associated with increased right ventricular stroke work. In adults[226] and children[225] with ARDS, pulmonary artery pressure and vascular resistance gradually fall after several days in survivors but increase progressively in those who die. Severe pulmonary hypertension can result in right ventricular failure and a low cardiac index. Right ventricular dilation leads to a leftward septal shift, impairing left ventricular diastolic filling. Coronary blood flow to the right ventricle decreases, producing myocardial ischemia and further compromising right ventricular function.

Inhaled nitric oxide administered by inhalation to children with ARDS causes a significant fall in pulmonary artery pressure and intrapulmonary shunting and an increase in the cardiac index, up to a dose of 20 ppm.[230] Intrapulmonary shunting decreases because inhaled nitric oxide preferentially dilates the pulmonary vessels that supply ventilated alveoli, increasing their blood flow at the expense of less well ventilated parts of the lung. Above 20 ppm, there was no further increase in oxygenation or beneficial effect on pulmonary hemodynamics. No controlled trial of nitric oxide in ARDS has yet been reported, but this therapy is widely used to improve gas exchange and right ventricular performance.

Role of Secondary Infection and Multiple Organ Failure

ARDS may be associated with organ failure of other systems as a result of the same insult (e.g., brain failure and ARDS after the hypoxic-ischemic injury of near-drowning). Renal failure, gastrointestinal hemorrhage, disseminated intravascular coagulation, impaired liver function, bone marrow suppression, and altered cerebral function are commonly associated with severe ARDS,[231] especially during the late stages. In the initial description of the sepsis syndrome by Bone et al,[232] 25% of 191 patients developed ARDS. Pfenninger et al[216] described 20 children with ARDS, of whom 60% had coagulation failure, 40% had renal failure, 40% had brain dysfunction, and 30% had hepatic or gastrointestinal failure. Nonsurvivors had more organ systems failing than those who survived.

Infection may occur in children with ARDS as part of the presenting illness, or it may be nosocomially acquired from indwelling catheters or endotracheal tubes or endogenously acquired secondary to gut ischemia or the use of broad-spectrum antibiotics. Bacteremia was present in 45% of Bone's patients but did not influence the patient's outcome.[232] In Pfenninger's study,[216] 15% of the children with multiple organ dysfunction developed culture-proven septicemia and died. Although culture-proven bacterial infection is common in patients with multiple organ system failure, it is not a prerequisite. The lung is the most common source of sepsis at autopsy in adults with clinical sepsis but negative blood cultures.

The roles of gastrointestinal tract mucosal ischemia and loss of barrier function in the development of multiple organ failure are yet to be fully elucidated, but there is evidence that gut ischemia is associated with the translocation of bacteria, endotoxin, and other bacterial toxins and the activation of neutrophils, which may affect distant organs, including the lungs. Gut mucosal ischemia may occur in ARDS secondary to hypoxemia or inadequate cardiac output with redistribution of blood flow away from the gut and toward other vital organs such as the brain and heart.

Clinical Manifestations

After the event or illness that precipitates ARDS, there may be clinical signs of respiratory distress, or the signs may develop later, commonly in the first 48 hours. Tachypnea is the first sign, at which stage the chest radiograph is often normal. Chest retractions, expiratory grunt, alar flaring, and cyanosis may also be present. Initially, there is respiratory alkalosis. Later, there is severe hypoxemia with a large $PAO_2 - PaO_2$ difference and a rising $PaCO_2$. The lungs become noncompliant with diffuse bilateral infiltrates on the chest radiograph (Fig. 25-8). The final phase involves widespread bilateral consolidation with hypoxemia in 100% oxygen and severe hypercarbia as well as respiratory and often metabolic acidosis. Multiple organ failure often ensues. Not all patients progress at the same rate or to the same extent. The condition may partially or completely resolve at any stage.

Management

The prevention of ARDS should be one aim of the treatment of all critically ill children. The principles of management are to treat the underlying cause if possible, ensure adequate tissue oxygenation, and prevent complications.

Investigating for Treatable Causes

Many factors cause a child's ARDS. For some children, there is no specific treatment. Treatable causes such as infection

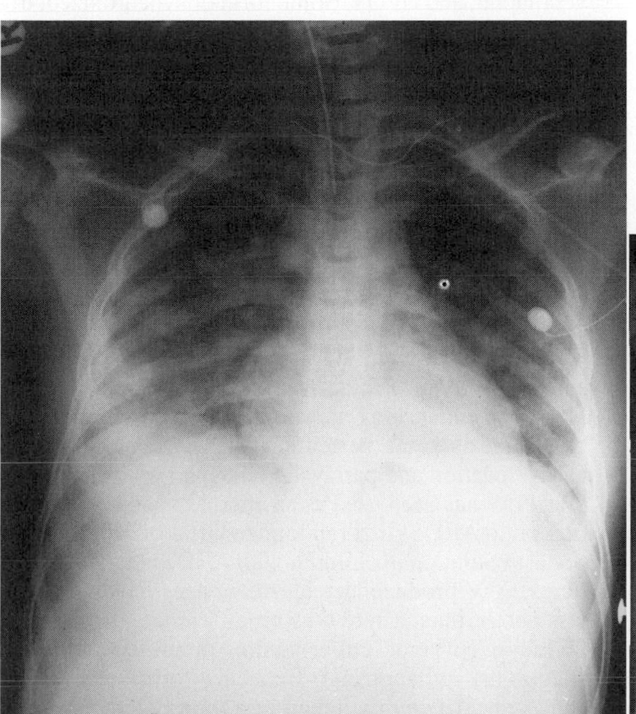

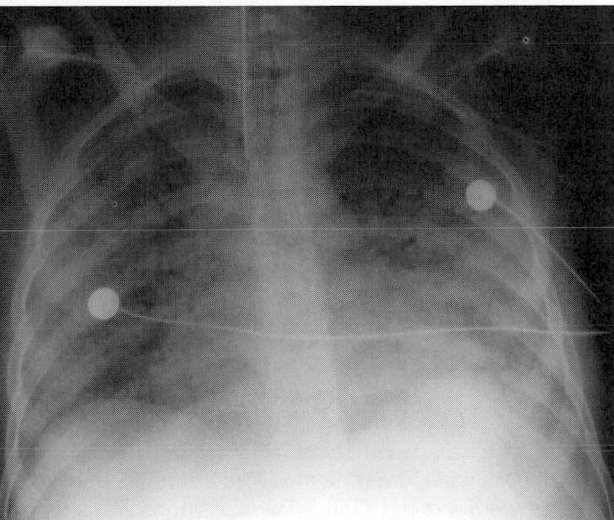

Fig. 25-8. Chest radiographs of a 12-year-old girl with ARDS associated with acute hepatic failure. **A,** Radiograph 2 days after onset. There are widespread alveolar opacities, mostly in the lower zones. **B,** Radiograph 4 days after onset. There is widespread consolidation with air bronchograms and alveolar and interstitial opacities.

should be identified and treated. The search for primary or secondary lung infection may require culture of tracheal aspirates, BAL fluid, or lung biopsy specimens. Lung biopsy may be clinically useful in adults with ARDS who are on ventilators, but lung biopsy has not been compared with less invasive methods in prospective trials.[233] BAL can be performed safely in such patients.[234] The most common finding in BAL fluid in patients with ARDS is increased numbers of polymorphonuclear leukocytes, making up nearly 80% of the total cell population (normal, <5%). The one type of ARDS that may respond to corticosteroid therapy is characterized by an increased number of eosinophils in BAL fluid or by peripheral eosinophilia.[235] Prophylactic antibiotics are not beneficial in ARDS, but potential bacterial pathogens found in BAL fluid should be treated. Lung fluid should also be cultured for viruses. Herpes simplex virus was identified in the tracheal aspirates of 30% of 46 adults with ARDS, in whom it was associated with the need for more prolonged respiratory support and an increased mortality rate than was the case in patients in whom the BAL fluid did not grow the virus.[220] Herpes simplex virus has also been found in the lungs of patients with burn injury.[236] The role of reactivation of this virus in ARDS is unclear, and prophylactic antiviral agents are not indicated, but acyclovir may be useful if the virus is present. BAL fluid may also have other opportunistic pathogens, such as *Pneumocystis carinii,* which may present with acute respiratory failure in children with known or unsuspected impaired immunity.

Ensuring Adequate Tissue Oxygenation

The therapy for ARDS is based on support for the cardiorespiratory system to maintain adequate PaO_2, $PaCO_2$, and tissue perfusion. This involves attention to ventilation strategy as well as cardiac output and tissue oxygenation. Ventilatory support maintains arterial oxygenation at a safe level while preventing pulmonary oxygen toxicity and additional lung trauma resulting from excessive ventilatory volumes or pressures. PEEP was first used successfully to treat pulmonary edema in 1938[237] and has since improved the outcome in ARDS.[238] Despite this initial success in a controlled trial of adults at risk of ARDS, the early application of PEEP at 8 cm H_2O did not reduce the incidence of the syndrome.[239] PEEP is applied to increase lung volume, keep alveoli open, and recruit collapsed alveoli and small airways. It improves arterial oxygenation in ARDS. The theoretically optimum level of PEEP would be one that allows a reduction in FIO_2 to a safe level (less than 0.5), does not impair venous return to the heart or reduce cardiac output, does not impair cerebral venous drainage or increase intracranial pressure, and optimizes arterial oxygenation.

PEEP may reduce cardiac output in children[240] and adults[241] with ARDS. The mechanism is likely to be both a decrease in systemic venous return and an increase in right ventricular pressure load. The latter causes a leftward shift of the interventricular septum with a reduction in filling[241] and an impaired systolic ejection function of the left ventricle. By increasing alveolar volume, PEEP increases the resistance to flow through the alveolar capillaries and therefore increases right ventricular afterload. PEEP of at least 15 cm H_2O reduces the cardiac index in adults.[241] In children without cardiorespiratory disease, Clough et al,[240] using Doppler measurements of cardiac output, found a fall in cardiac output of 3.7% at 5 cm H_2O of PEEP, 6.7% at 10 cm H_2O, and 15.9% at 15 cm H_2O. There was a wide variation in subjects studied, but there was a trend toward a greater fall in cardiac output for a given level of PEEP with increasing age. Ideally, the level of PEEP chosen would be based on the measurement of cardiac output and calculated oxygen delivery. PEEP levels should be gradually increased to achieve acceptable arterial saturation with nontoxic FIO_2 levels (<0.5), and the effect of PEEP on hemodynamics should be monitored clinically, if measurement of cardiac output, mixed venous PO_2, or oxygen consumption are unavailable.[242] Titration of PEEP against clinical measures is inexact. Hypotension often does not become apparent until cardiac output substantially falls.[243]

PEEP improves compliance by opening collapsed alveoli. If PEEP levels are too high, however, overdistention of already opened alveoli may lead to a reduction in compliance. According to Sivan et al,[244] in children with acute respiratory failure, the level of PEEP that normalized the functional residual capacity was within 4 cm H_2O of the PEEP at which static respiratory compliance was maximal; in most cases, this was the same value. Their data also showed that the best compliance was not achieved when the PEEP level was chosen by clinical judgment alone. In addition to an assessment of optimal tissue oxygen delivery, an assessment of maximal static compliance may be helpful in choosing the level of PEEP.

PEEP may increase cerebral venous pressures and intracranial pressure by increasing the intrathoracic pressure and impairing cerebral venous drainage. This is particularly important in children with brain injury. In an animal model,[245] when a lesion causing raised intracranial pressure is associated with diffuse lung injury, the rise in intracranial pressure and reduction in cerebral perfusion pressure with increasing levels of PEEP are not as great as when the lungs are normal. However, the high levels of PEEP that reduce cardiac output and require blood volume expansion may lead to reduced cerebral perfusion pressure with resultant cerebral ischemia as well as volume overload, which may cause cerebral edema.

Other strategies of ventilation include a control-assist mode of ventilation, IPPV with or without paralysis, intermittent mandatory ventilation, permissive hypercapnia, inverse ratio ventilation, and HFOV. Some form of synchronized, triggered, pressure-limited ventilation has been advocated[242] (e.g., pressure support, synchronized intermittent mandatory ventilation). The potential benefits of these modes of ventilation are limitation of acute rises in intrapulmonary pressures that occur with unsynchronized patient breaths, improved patient comfort, and avoidance of adverse effects of muscle relaxant medications, such as prolonged muscular weakness after the medications have been ceased. Many children with severe ARDS are unable to achieve adequate oxygenation at safe levels of FIO_2 and peak pressures without muscle relaxation, in which case pressure-limited IPPV is required.

Inverse-ratio ventilation increases the mean airway pressure by prolonging the inspiratory time.[246] This type of ventilation can enhance oxygenation after conventional ventilation has failed in some patients with ARDS[247] but may require heavy sedation and paralysis.[242]

HFOV has been used as an alternative to conventional ventilation in ARDS. In a randomized trial of HFOV vs. conventional ventilation in children with ARDS, Arnold et al[248] found that HFOV produced greater increases in oxygenation with less barotrauma. There was no difference in other outcomes, including survival. Other studies in adults with ARDS also suggest that although high-frequency forms of ventilation may achieve preset ventilation criteria for oxygenation and gas exchange at lower inspired oxygen concentrations and lower peak pressures, there is no beneficial effect on survival.[249] HFOV may be more likely to improve outcome if instituted as an early rather than a late rescue therapy.[250,251] The use of high-frequency ventilation in pediatric respiratory disease has been recently reviewed by Clark.[252]

Ventilation in the prone position in infants and children with ARDS has resulted in improved oxygenation at lower levels of inspired oxygen.[253] This strategy is based on the findings of Gattinoni et al[227] that atelectasis occurred mainly in dependent parts of the lung. Regular turning from the supine to the prone position may reduce dependent atelectasis and intrapulmonary shunt. In older children who need mechanical ventilation, the lateral decubitus position can be used; this position has been advocated for patients with hypoxemia unresponsive to other medical interventions.[242]

Large tidal volumes, high peak airway pressures, and inspired oxygen concentrations above 0.6 have been implicated as causes of lung injury. Because of the smaller lung volume available for gas exchange in ARDS, the use of tidal volumes as small as 6 ml/kg is likely to be associated with fewer pulmonary and hemodynamic complications.[254] These small, relatively normal areas of lung are overinflated and are exposed to high positive inspiratory pressures unless low volume and pressure-limited ventilation are used. Low tidal volumes have been combined with relatively low ventilatory rates to produce controlled hypoventilation with permissive hypercapnia. Permissive hypercapnia (accepting a $Paco_2$ up to 80 mm Hg and arterial pH above 7.15) is aimed at avoiding barotrauma and volutrauma. It is now an established and widely recommended stategy,[242] although there are no controlled trials to show that it improves outcome.

Outcome

The mortality rate from ARDS is about 50%,[255] and the morbidity in survivors is substantial. In three of the largest pediatric series reported, there were 19 deaths in 42 patients (45%).[216,217,222] A total of 9 of the deaths were due to severe brain injury. There were 4 deaths in which culture-proven septicemia was a major factor. Of the 23 survivors, 16 were normal, but 5 had moderate or severe neurologic deficits, including hemiparesis, seizures, and developmental delay; 1 had significant impairment of respiratory function resulting from interstitial pneumonitis; and 1 had ongoing morbidity from preexisting dermatomyositis.

At long-term follow-up of respiratory function in nine children who survived ARDS,[256] three had recurrent respiratory symptoms consisting of moderate exertional dyspnea and cough, two had radiographic evidence of pulmonary fibrosis, and all had abnormal pulmonary function tests. The abnormalities consisted of ventilation inequalities in eight patients. The ventilation inequalities shown by multiple-breath nitrogen washout curves and obstructive airway disease were found in two patients. One child had residual restrictive lung disease. There was a mild degree of hypoxemia in seven of the children.

REFERENCES

Burn Inhalation Injury

1. Ryan CA, Shankowsky HA, Tredget EE: Profile of the paediatric burn patient in a Canadian burn centre, *Burns* 18:267-272, 1992.
2. Rossignol AM, Locke JA, Burke JF: Paediatric burn injuries in New England, USA, *Burns* 16:41-48, 1990.
3. Forjuoh SN, Smith GS: Case-fatality rates by body part affected and trends in hospitalized burns in Maryland, 1981-90, *Burns* 19:387-391, 1993.
4. Shirani KZ, Pruitt BA, Mason AD: The influence of inhalation injury and pneumonia on burn mortality, *Ann Surg* 205:87-92, 1987.
5. Robinson MD, Seward PN: Thermal injury in children, *Pediatr Emerg Care* 3:266-270, 1987 (review).
6. Pruitt BA, Flemma RJ, DiVicenti FC, Foley FD, Mason AD: Pulmonary complications in burn patients: a comparative study of 697 patients, *J Thorac Cardiovasc Surg* 59:7-20, 1970.
7. Moritz AR, Henriques FC, McLean R: The effects of inhaled heat on the air passages and lungs: an experimental investigation, *Am J Pathol* 21:311-331, 1945.
8. Loke J, Matthay RA, Walker-Smith GJ: The toxic environment and its medical implications with special emphasis on smoke inhalation. In Loke J, ed: *Pathophysiology and treatment of inhalation injuries.* In Lenfant C, ed: *Lung biology in health and disease,* vol 34, New York, 1988, Marcel Dekker, pp 453-504 (review).
9. Stone HH, Rhame DW, Corbitt JD, Given KS, Martin JD: Respiratory burns: a correlation of clinical and laboratory results, *Ann Surg*165:157-168, 1967.
10. Hudson DA, Jones L, Rode H: Respiratory distress secondary to scalds in children, *Burns* 20:434-437, 1994.
11. Wald PH, Balmes JR: Respiratory effects of short-term, high-intensity toxic inhalations: smoke, gases, and fumes, *J Intensive Care Med* 2:260-278, 1987 (review).
12. Davis JWL: Toxic chemicals versus lung tissue: an aspect of inhalation injury revisited, *J Burn Care Rehabil* 7:213-222, 1986 (review).
13. Crapo RO: Causes of respiratory injury. In Haponik EF, Munster AM, eds: *Respiratory injury: smoke inhalation and burns,* New York, 1990, McGraw-Hill, pp 47-60 (review).
14. Charnock EL, Meehan JJ: Postburn respiratory injuries in children, *Pediatr Clin North Am* 27:661-676, 1980 (review).
15. Herndon DN, Traber DL: Pulmonary circulation and burns and trauma, *J Trauma* 30:S41-S44, 1990.
16. Demling RH: Burn edema. I. Pathogenesis, *J Burn Care Rehabil* 3:138-148, 1982.
17. Tranbaugh RF, Elings VB, Christensen JM, Lewis FR: Effect of inhalation injury on lung water accumulation, *J Trauma* 23:597-604, 1983.
18. Herndon DN, Traber DL, Niehaus GD, Linares HA, Traber LD: The pathophysiology of smoke inhalation injury in a sheep model, *J Trauma* 24:1044-1051, 1984.
19. Prien T, Traer LD, Herndon DN, Stothert JC, Lubbesmeyer HJ, Traber DL: Pulmonary edema with smoke inhalation undetected by indicator dilution technique, *J Appl Physiol* 63:907-911, 1987.
20. Hill ML, Szeffer SJ, Larsen GL: Asthma pathogenesis and the implications for therapy in children, *Pediatr Clin North Am* 39:1205-1224, 1992.
21. Koltai M, Hosford D, Braquet PG: Platelet-activating factor in septic shock, *New Horiz* 1:87-95, 1993.
22. Ikeuchi H, Sakano T, Sanchez J, Mason AD, Pruitt BA: The effects of platelet-activating factor (PAF) and a PAF antagonist (CV-3988) on smoke inhalation injury in an ovine model, *J Trauma* 32:344-350, 1992.
23. Videnes H, Bjerknes R: Activation of polymorphonuclear neutrophilic granulocytes following burn injury: alteration of FC-receptor complement receptor expression and of opsono-phagocytosis, *J Trauma* 36:161-167, 1994.
24. Pruitt BA, Cioffi WG, Shimazu T, Ikeuchi H, Mason AD: Evaluation and management of patients with inhalation injury, *J Trauma* 30:S63-S68, 1990.
25. Huang Y-S, Li AON, Yang ZC: Effect of smoke inhalation injury on thromboxane levels on platelet counts, *Burns* 14:440-446, 1988.
26. Sharar SR, Heimbach DM, Howard M, Hildebrandt J, Winn RK: Cardiopulmonary responses after spontaneous inhalation of Douglas fir smoke in goats, *J Trauma* 28:164-170, 1988.
27. Prien T, Strohmaier W, Gasser H, Richardson JA, Traber DL, Schlag G: Normal phosphatidylcholine composition of lung surfactant 24 hours after inhalation injury, *J Burn Care Rehabil* 10:38-44, 1989.
28. Clark WR, Webb WR, Wax S, Nieman G: Inhalation injuries: the pathophysiology of acute smoke inhalation, *Surg Forum* 28:177-179, 1977.
29. Liu Z-Y, Li N, Chu P-F, Yang C-C, Shui J-T: Pulmonary surfactant activity after severe steam inhalation in rabbits, *Burns* 12:330-336, 1986.

30. Traber DL, Herndon DN: Pathophysiology of smoke inhalation. In Haponik EF, Munster AM, eds: *Respiratory injury: smoke inhalation and burns,* New York, 1990, McGraw-Hill, pp 61-71.
31. Li JJ, Bramlet SG, Carter EA, Burke JF: The rat organotypic culture: an in-vitro model for studying surfactant metabolism abnormalities, *J Trauma* 31:174-181, 1991.
32. Hayashi M, Bond TP, Guest MM, Linares H, Wells CH, Larson DL: Pulmonary microcirculation following full-thickness burns, *Burns* 5:227-235, 1979.
33. Shirani KZ, Moylan JA, Pruitt BA: Diagnosis and treatment of inhalation injury in burn patients. In Loke J, ed: *Pathophysiology and treatment of inhalation injuries.* In Lenfant C, ed: *Lung biology in health and disease*, New York, 1988, Marcel Dekker, pp 239-280.
34. Hunt JL, Agee RN, Pruitt BA: Fiberoptic bronchoscopy in acute inhalation injury, *J Trauma* 15:641-648, 1975.
35. Judkins KC, Brander WL: Respiratory injury in children: the histology of healing, *Burns* 12:357-359, 1986.
36. Hubbard GB, Langlinais PC, Shimazu T, Okerberg CV, Mason AD: The morphology of smoke inhalation injury in sheep, *J Trauma* 31:1477-1486, 1991.
37. Linares HA, Herndon DN, Traber DL: Sequence of morphologic events in experimental smoke inhalation, *J Burn Care Rehabil* 10:27-37, 1989.
38. Epler GR, Colby TV, McLoud TC, Carrington CB, Gaensler EA: Bronchiolitis obliterans organizing pneumonia, *New Engl J Med* 312:152-158, 1985.
39. Seger D, Welch L: Carbon monoxide controversies: neuropsychologic testing, mechanism of toxicity, and hyperbaric oxygen, *Ann Emerg Med* 24:242-248, 1994 (review).
40. Tibbles PM, Perrotta PL: Treatment of carbon monoxide poisoning: a critical review of human outcome studies comparing normobaric oxygen with hyperbaric oxygen, *Ann Emerg Med* 24:269-276, 1994 (review).
41. Haponik EF: Clinical and functional assessment. In Haponik EF, Munster AM, eds: *Respiratory injury: smoke inhalation and burns,* New York, 1990, McGraw-Hill, pp 137-178.
42. Gorman DF, Runciman WB: Carbon monoxide poisoning, *Anaesth Intensive Care* 19:506-511, 1991 (review).
43. Clark CJ, Campbell D, Reid WH: Blood carboxyhaemoglobin and cyanide levels in fire survivors, *Lancet* 1:1332-1335, 1981.
44. Silverman SH, Purdue GF, Hunt JL, Bost RO: Cyanide toxicity in burned patients, *J Trauma* 28:171-174, 1988.
45. Bingham HG, Gallagher TJ, Powell MD: Early bronchoscopy as a predictor of ventilatory support for burned patients, *J Trauma* 27:1286-1288, 1987.
46. Haponik EF, Meyers DA, Munster AM, Smith PL, Britt EJ, Wise RA, Bleecker ER: Acute upper airway injury in burn patients: serial changes of flow-volume curves and nasopharyngoscopy, *Am Rev Respir Dis* 135:360-366, 1987.
47. Schneider W, Berger A, Mailänder P, Tempka A: Diagnostic and therapeutic possibilities for fibreoptic bronchoscopy in inhalation injury, *Burns* 14:53-57, 1988.
48. Whitener DR, Whitener LM, Robertson KJ, Baxter CR, Pierce AK: Pulmonary function measurements in patients with thermal injury and smoke inhalation, *Am Rev Respir Dis* 122:731-739, 1980.
49. Teixidor HS, Rubin E, Novick GS, Alonso DR: Smoke inhalation: radiologic manifestations, *Radiology* 149:383-387, 1983.
50. Peitzman AB, Shires GT, Teixidor HS, Curreri PW, Shires GT: Smoke inhalation injury: evaluation of radiographic manifestations and pulmonary dysfunction, *J Trauma* 29:1232-1238, 1989.
51. Sharar SR, Heimbach DM, Hudson LD: Management of inhalation injury in patients with and without burns. In Haponik EF, Munster AM, eds: *Respiratory injury: smoke inhalation and burns,* New York, 1990, McGraw-Hill, pp 195-214 (review).
52. Davies LK, Pulton TJ, Modell JH: Continuous positive airway pressure is beneficial in treatment of smoke inhalation, *Crit Care Med* 11:726-729, 1983.
53. Cox CS, Zwischenberger JB, Traber DL, Minifee PK, Navaratnam N, Haque AK, Herndon DN: Immediate positive pressure ventilation with positive end-expiratory pressure (PEEP) improves survival in ovine smoke inhalation injury, *J Trauma* 33:821-827, 1992.
54. Cioffi WG, Graves TA, McManus WF, Pruitt BA: High-frequency percussive ventilation in patients with inhalation injury, *J Trauma* 29:350-354, 1989.
55. Rodeberg DA, Maschinot NE, Housinger TA, Warden GD: Decreased pulmonary barotrauma with the use of volumetric diffusive respiration in pediatric patients with burns, *J Burn Care Rehabil* 13:506-511, 1992.
56. Nieman GF, Cigada M, Paskanik AM, Del Pozzo J, Clark WR, Camporesi EM, Hakim TS: Comparison of high-frequency jet to conventional mechanical ventilation in the treatment of severe smoke inhalation injury, *Burns* 20:157-162, 1994.
57. Cross CE, Halliwell B: Biological consequences of general environmental contaminants. In Crystal RG, West JB, eds: *The lung: scientific foundations,* New York, 1991, Raven, pp 1961-1973.
58. Levine BA, Petroff PA, Slade CL, Pruitt BA: Prospective trials of dexamethasone and aerosolized gentamicin in the treatment of inhalation injury in the burned patient, *J Trauma* 18:188-192, 1978.
59. Linares HA: Autopsy findings in burned children. In Carvajal HF, Parks DH, eds, *Burns in children: pediatric burn management*, St Louis, 1988, Mosby, pp 287-302.
60. Carvajal HF: Septicemia and septic shock. In Carvajal HF, Parks DH, eds: *Burns in children: pediatric burn management,* St Louis, 1988, Mosby, pp 228-251.
61. Koumbourlis AC, Kurland G: Non-bronchoscopic bronchoalveolar lavage in mechanically ventilated infants: technique, efficacy, and applications, *Pediatr Pulmonol* 15:257-262, 1993.
62. Dressler DP, Skornik WA, Kupersmith S: Corticosteroid treatment of experimental smoke inhalation, *Ann Surg* 183:46-52, 1976.
63. Beeley JM, Crow J, Jones JG, Minty B, Lynch RD, Pryce DP: Mortality and lung histopathology after inhalation lung injury, *Am Rev Respir Dis* 133:191-196, 1986.
64. Nieman GF, Clark WR, Hakim T: Methylprednisolone does not protect the lung from inhalation injury, *Burns* 17:384-390, 1991.
65. Moylan JA: Diagnostic techniques and steroids, *J Trauma* 19(suppl): 917, 1979.
66. Nieman GF, Clark WR, Wax SD, Webb WR: The effect of smoke inhalation on pulmonary surfactant, *Ann Surg* 191:171-181, 1980.
67. Feldbaum DM, Wormuth D, Nieman GF, Paskanik M, Clark WR, Hakim TS: Exosurf treatment following wood smoke inhalation, *Burns* 19:396-400, 1993.
68. Thom SR, Traber RL, Mendiguren I, Clark JM, Hardy KR, Fisher AB: Delayed neurological sequelae following carbon monoxide poisoning, *Ann Emerg Med* 23:612-613, 1994 (abstract).
69. Ellenhorn MJ, Barceloux DG: *Medical toxicology: diagnosis and treatment of human poisoning,* New York, 1988, Elsevier, pp 829-835.
70. Kirk MA, Gerace R, Kulig KW: Cyanide and methemoglobin kinetics in smoke inhalation victims treated with the cyanide antidote kit, *Ann Emerg Med* 22:1413-1418, 1993.
71. Lund T, Goodwin CW, McManus WF, Shirani KZ, Stallings RJ, Mason AD, Pruitt BA: Upper airway sequelae in burn patients requiring endotracheal intubation or tracheostomy, *Ann Surg* 201:374-382, 1985.
72. Majeski JA, Schreiber JT, Cotton R, MacMillan BG: Tracheoplasty for tracheal stenosis in the pediatric burned patient, *J Trauma* 20:81-86, 1980.
73. Desai MH, Mlcak RP, Robinson E, McCauley RL, Carp SS, Robson MC, Herndon DN: Does inhalation injury limit exercise endurance in children convalescing from thermal injury? *J Burn Care Rehabil* 14:12-16, 1993.

Blast Injury to the Lungs and Heart

74. Zuckerman S: Experimental study of blast injuries to the lungs, *Lancet* 1940, pp 219-226.
75. Maynard RL, Cooper GJ, Scott R: Mechanisms of injury in bomb blasts and explosions. In Westaby S, ed: *Trauma: pathogenesis and treatment,* Oxford, England, 1989, Heinemann, pp 30-41.
76. Stapczynski JS: Blast injuries, *Ann Emerg Med* 11:687-694, 1982.
77. Brown RFR, Cooper GJ, Maynard RL: The ultrastructure of rat lung following acute primary blast injury, *Int J Exp Pathol* 74:151-162, 1993.
78. Dean DM, Thomas AR, Allison RS: Effects of high-explosive blast on the lungs, *Lancet* 1940, pp 224-226.
79. Wang CY, Yap BH, Delikan AE: Melioidosis pneumonia and blast injury, *Chest* 103:1897-1899, 1993.
80. Pierce EC: Specific therapy for arterial air embolism, *Ann Thorac Surg* 29:300-303, 1980.
81. Frykberg ER, Tepas JJ: Terrorist bombings: lessons learned from Belfast to Beirut, *Ann Surg* 208:569-576, 1988.

Blunt Injury of the Lung

82. Meller JL, Little AG, Shermeta DW: Thoracic trauma in children, *J Trauma* 34:329-331, 1993.
83. Rielly JP, Brandt ML, Mattox KL, Pokorny WJ: Thoracic trauma in children, *J Trauma* 34:329-331, 1993.
84. Smyth BT: Chest trauma in children, *J Pediatr Surg* 14:41-47, 1979.
85. Roux P, Fisher RM: Chest injuries in children: an analysis of 100 cases of blunt chest trauma from motor vehicle accidents, *J Pediatr Surg* 27:551-555, 1992.
86. Cooper GJ, Taylor DEM: Biophysics of impact injury to the chest and abdomen, *J Roy Army Med Corps* 135:58-67, 1989.
87. Wagner RB, Crawford WO, Schimpf PR: Classification of parenchymal injuries of the lung, *Radiology* 167:77-82, 1988.
88. Demling RH, Pomfret EA: Blunt chest trauma, *New Horiz* 1:402-421, 1993.
89. Shackford SR: Blunt chest trauma: the intensivist's perspective, *J Intensive Care Med* 1:125-136, 1986.
90. Oppenheimer L, Craven KD, Forkert L, Wood LDH: Pathophysiology of pulmonary contusion in dogs, *J Appl Physiol* 47:718-728, 1979.
91. Kishikawa M, Yoshioka T, Shimazu T, Sugimoto H, Yoshioka T, Sugimoto T: Pulmonary contusion causes long-term respiratory dysfunction with decreased functional residual capacity, *J Trauma* 31:1203-1208, 1991.
92. Wagner RB, Slivko B, Jamieson PM, Dills MS, Edwards FH: Effect of lung contusion on pulmonary hemodynamics, *Ann Thorac Surg* 52:51-57, 1991.
93. Putensen C, Waibel U, Koller W, Putensen-Himmer, Hörmann C: Assessment of changes in lung microvascular permeability in posttraumatic acute lung failure after direct and indirect injuries to lungs, *Anesth Analg* 74:790-792, 1992.
94. Fagan CJ, Swischuk LE: Traumatic lung and paramediastinal pneumatoceles, *Radiology* 120:11-18, 1976.
95. Galea MH, Williams N, Mayell MJ: Traumatic pneumatocele, *J Pediatr Surg* 27:1523-1524, 1992.
96. Kishikawa M, Minami T, Shimazu T, Sugimoyo H, Yoshioka T, Katsurada K, Sugimoto T: Laterality of air volume in the lungs long after blunt chest trauma, *J Trauma* 34:908-912, 1993.
97. Livingstone DH, Richardson JD: Pulmonary disability after severe blunt chest trauma, *J Trauma* 30:562-566, 1990.
98. Jackinczyk K: Blunt chest trauma, *Emerg Med Clin North Am* 11:81-96, 1993.
99. Richardson JD, Adams L, Flint LM: Selective management of flail chest and pulmonary contusion, *Ann Surg* 196:481-486, 1982.
100. Nightingale P: Pressure controlled ventilation: a true advance? *Clin Intensive Care* 5:114-122, 1994.
101. Inoue H, Suzuki I, Iwasaki M, Ogawa J-I, Koide S, Shohtsu A: Selective exclusion of the injured lung, *J Trauma* 34:496-498, 1993.
102. Frame SB, Marshall WJ, Clifford TG: Synchronized independent lung ventilation in the management of pediatric unilateral pulmonary contusion: case report, *J Trauma* 29:395-397, 1989.
103. Turnage RH, Guice KS, Oldham KT: Pulmonary microvascular injury following intestinal reperfusion, *New Horiz* 2:463-475, 1994.
104. Richardson JD, Woods D, Johanson WG, Trinkle JK: Lung bacterial clearance following pulmonary contusion, *Surgery* 86:730-735, 1979.

Lipoid Pneumonia and Hydrocarbon Pneumonitis

105. de Oliveira GA, Del Caro SR, Bender Lamego CM, Mercon de Vargas PR, Vervloet VEC: Radiographic plain film and CT findings in lipoid pneumonia in infants following aspiration of mineral oil used in the treatment of partial small bowel obstruction by *Ascaris lumbricoides*, *Pediatr Radiol* 15:157-160, 1985.
106. Litovitz T, Manoguerra A: Comparison of pediatric poisoning hazards: an analysis of 3.8 million exposure incidents, *Pediatrics* 89:999-1006, 1992.
107. Pearn J, Nixon J, Ansford A, Corcoran A: Accidental poisoning in childhood: five year urban population study with 15 year analysis of fatality, *Br Med J* 288:44-46, 1984.
108. Vale JA, Meredith TJ: Solvent abuse. In Haddad LM, Winchester JF, eds: *Clinical management of poisoning and drug overdose*, Philadelphia, 1983, WB Saunders, pp 801-804.
109. Schonberg SK: Substance use and abuse. In McAnarney ER, Kreipe RE, Orr DP, Comerci GD, eds: *Textbook of adolescent medicine*, Philadelphia, 1992, WB Saunders, pp 1063-1077.
110. Janssen S, Van der Gest S, Meijer S, Uges DRA: Impairment of organ function after oral ingestion of refined petrol, *Intensive Care Med* 14:238-240, 1988.
111. Engstrand DA, England DM, Huntington RW: Pathology of paint-sniffer's lung, *Am J Forensic Med Pathol* 7:232-236, 1986.
112. Schikler KN, Lane EE, Seitz K, Collins WM: Solvent abuse associated pulmonary abnormalities, *Adv Alcohol Subst Abuse* 3:75-81, 1984.
113. Bartlett JG: Lipoid pneumonia, In Baum GL, Wolinsky E, eds: *Textbook of pulmonary diseases*, ed 4, Boston, 1989, Little, Brown, pp 557-563.
114. Becton DL, Lowe JE, Falletta JM: Lipoid pneumonia in an adolescent girl secondary to use of lip gloss, *J Pediatr* 105:421-423, 1984.
115. Ellenhorn MJ, Barceloux DG: *Medical toxicology: diagnosis and treatment of human poisoning*, New York, 1988, Elsevier, pp 940-947.
116. Giammona ST: Effects of furniture polish on pulmonary surfactant, *Am J Dis Child* 113:658-663, 1967.
117. Eade NR, Taussig LM, Marks MI: Hydrocarbon pneumonitis, *Pediatrics* 54:351-357, 1974.
118. Griffin JW, Daeschner CW, Collins VP, Eaton WL: Hydrocarbon pneumonitis following furniture polish ingestion, *J Pediatr* 45:13-26, 1954.
119. Arena JM: Hydrocarbon poisoning: current management, *Pediatr Ann* 16:879-883, 1987.
120. Stones DK, van Niekerk CH, Cilliers C: Pneumatoceles as a complication of paraffin pneumonia, *S Afr Med J* 72:535-537, 1987.
121. Scharf SM, Prinsloo I: Pulmonary mechanics in dogs given different doses of kerosene intratracheally, *Am Rev Respir Dis* 126:695-700, 1982.
122. Lesser LI, Weens HS, McKey JD: Pulmonary manifestations following ingestion of kerosene, *J Pediatr* 23:352-364, 1943.
123. Zucker AR, Berger S, Wood LDH: Management of kerosene-induced pulmonary injury, *Crit Care Med* 14:303-304, 1986.
124. Bergeson PS, Hales SW, Lustgarten MD, Lipow HW: Pneumatoceles following hydrocarbon ingestion, *Am J Dis Child* 129:49-54, 1975.
125. Spencer H: Radiation injuries to the lung and lipid pneumonia. In Spencer H, ed: *Pathology of the lung*, ed 4, Oxford, England, 1984, Pergamon, pp 517-525.
126. Scott PP: Hydrocarbon ingestion: an unusual cause of multiple pulmonary pseudotumors, *South Med J* 82:1032-1033, 1989.
127. Brown J, Burke B, Dajani AS: Experimental kerosene pneumonia: evaluation of some therapeutic regimens, *J Pediatr* 84:396-401, 1974.
128. Cox EG, Heil SA, Kleiman MB: Lipoid pneumonia and *Mycobacterium smegmatis*, *Pediatr Infect Dis* J 13:414-415, 1994.
129. Gurwitz D, Kattan M, Levison H, Culham JAG: Pulmonary function abnormalities in asymptomatic children after hydrocarbon pneumonitis, *Pediatrics* 62:789-794, 1978.
130. Taussig LM, Castro O, Landau LI, Beaudry PH: Pulmonary function 8 to 10 years after hydrocarbon pneumonitis, *Clin Pediatr* 16:57-59, 1977.
131. Gerarde HW: Toxicological studies on hydrocarbons. V. Kerosene, *Toxicol Appl Pharmacol* 1:462-474, 1959.
132. Cachia EA, Fenech FF: Kerosene poisoning in children, *Arch Dis Child* 39:502-504, 1964.
133. Daeschner CW, Blattner RJ, Collins VP: Hydrocarbon pneumonitis, *Pediatr Clin North Am* 4:243-253, 1957.
134. Erwin ME: Petroleum distillates and turpentine. In Haddad LM, Winchester JF, eds: *Clinical management of poisoning and drug overdose*, Philadelphia, 1983, WB Saunders, pp 771-779.
135. Scalzo AJ, Weber TR, Jaeger RW, Connors RH, Thompson MW: Extracorporeal membrane oxygenation for hydrocarbon aspiration, *Am J Dis Child* 144:867-871, 1990.
136. Feihl F, Perret C: Permissive hypercapnia: how permissive should we be? *Am J Respir Crit Care Med* 150:1722-1737, 1994.
137. Wolfsdorf J, Kundig H: Dexamethasone in the management of kerosene pneumonia, *Pediatr Res* 7:432, 1973 (abstract).

Lung Injury in Near-Drowning

138. Waller AE, Baker SP, Szocka A: Childhood injury deaths: national analysis and geographic variations, *Am J Pub Health* 79:310-315, 1989.
139. Kemp A, Sibert JR: Drowning and near drowning in children in the United Kingdom: lessons for prevention, *Br Med J* 304:1143-1146, 1992.

140. The Consultative Council on Obstetric and Paediatric Mortality and Morbidity: *Annual report for 1993,* Melbourne, 1993, Victorian Government.
141. Fiser DH: Near-drowning, *Pediatr Rev* 14:148-151, 1993.
142. Orlowski JP: Drowning, near-drowning and ice-water drowning, *JAMA* 260:390-391, 1988 (editorial).
143. Jumbelic MI, Chambliss M: Accidental drowning in 5-gallon buckets, *JAMA* 263:1952-1953, 1990.
144. Griest KJ, Zumwall RE: Child abuse by drowning, *Pediatrics* 83:41-46, 1989.
145. Pearn J, Nixon J: Bathtub immersion accidents involving children, *Med J Aust* 1:211-213, 1977.
146. Lavelle JM, Shaw KN, Seidl T, Ludwig S: Ten year review of pediatric bathtub near-drownings: evaluation for child abuse and neglect, *Ann Emerg Med* 25:344-348, 1995.
147. Pearn J, Nixon J: Swimming pool immersion accidents: an analysis from the Brisbane drowning study, *Med J Aust* 1:432-437, 1977.
148. Quan L, Gore EJ, Wentz K: Ten-year study of pediatric drownings and near-drownings in King County, Washington: lessons in injury prevention, *Pediatrics* 83:1035-1040, 1989.
149. Pearn J: Epilepsy and drowning in childhood, *Br Med J* 1:1510-1511, 1977.
150. Harris EM, Knapp JF, Sharma V: The Romano-Ward syndrome: a case presenting as near drowning with a clinical review, *Pediatr Emerg Care* 8:272-275, 1992.
151. Modell JH: Drowning, *New Engl J Med* 328:253-256, 1993.
152. Modell JH, Davis JH: Electrolyte changes in human drowning victims, *Anesthesiology* 30:414-420, 1969.
153. Fuller RH: The 1962 Wellcome prize essay: drowning and postimmersion syndrome—a clinicopathologic study, *Milit Med* 128:22-36, 1963.
154. Bonilla-Santiago J, Fill WL: Sand aspiration in drowning and near drowning, *Radiology* 128:301-302, 1978.
155. Giammona ST, Modell JH: Drowning by total immersion: effects on pulmonary surfactant of distilled water, isotonic saline, and sea water, *Am J Dis Child* 114:612-616, 1967.
156. Giammona ST: Drowning: pathophysiology and management, *Curr Prob Pediatr* 1:1-33, 1971.
157. Modell JH, Moya F, Newby EJ: The effects of fluid volume in seawater drowning, *Ann Intern Med* 67:68-80, 1967.
158. Christensen DW, Dean JM, Seltzer NA: Near drowning. In Rogers MA, ed: *Textbook of pediatric intensive care,* ed 2, Baltimore, 1992, Williams & Wilkins.
159. Orlowski JP, Abulleil MM, Phillips JM: The hemodynamic and cardiovascular effects of near-drowning in hypotonic, isotonic and hypertonic solutions, *Ann Emerg Med* 18:1044-1049, 1989.
160. Modell JH, Graves SA, Ketover A: Clinical course of 91 consecutive near-drowning victims, *Chest* 70:231-238, 1976.
161. Fuller RH: The clinical pathology of human near-drowning, *Proc Roy Soc Med* 56:33-38, 1963.
162. Vernon DD, Banner W, Cantwell GP, Holzman BH, Bolte RG, Dean JM: *Streptococcus pneumoniae* bacteremia associated with near-drowning, *Crit Care Med* 18:1175-1176, 1990.
163. Tron VA, Baldwin VJ, Pirie GE: Hot tub drownings, *Pediatrics* 75:789-790, 1985.
164. Bohn DJ, Bigger WD, Smith CR, Conn AW, Barker GA: Influence of hypothermia, barbiturate therapy, and intracranial pressure monitoring on morbidity and mortality of near drowning, *Crit Care Med* 14:529-534, 1986.
165. Swan HJC: The role of hemodynamic monitoring in the management of the critically ill, *Crit Care Med* 3:83-89, 1975.
166. Vincent J-L, Dufaye P, Berre J, Leeman M, Degaute J-P, Kahn RJ: Serial lactate determinations during circulatory shock, *Crit Care Med* 11:449-451, 1983.
167. Grum CM: Tissue oxygenation in low flow states and during hypoxemia, *Crit Care Med* 21:S44-S49, 1993.
168. Linder KH, Dick W, Lotz P: The delayed use of positive end-expiratory pressure (PEEP) during respiratory resuscitation following near drowning with fresh or salt water, *Resuscitation* 10:197-211, 1983.
169. Modell JH, Calderwood HW, Ruiz BC, Downs JB, Chapman RJ: Effects of ventilatory patterns on arterial oxygenation after near-drowning in sea water, *Anesthesiology* 40:376-384, 1974.
170. Bernard GR, Luce JM, Sprung CL: High-dose corticosteroids in patients with the adult respiratory distress syndrome, *New Engl J Med* 317:1565-1570, 1987.
171. Cook DJ, Brun-Buisson C, Guyatt GH, Sibbald WJ: Evaluation of new diagnostic technologies: bronchoalveolar lavage and the diagnosis of ventilator-associated pneumonia, *Crit Care Med* 22:1314-1322, 1994.
172. Pearn J, Nixon J, Wilkey I: Fresh-water drowning and near-drowning accidents involving children: a five-year population study, *Med J Aust* 2:942-946, 1976.
173. Pearn J, Bart RD, Yamaoka R: Neurologic sequelae after childhood near-drowning: a total population study from Hawaii, *Pediatrics* 64:187-191, 1979.
174. Frates RC: Analysis of predictive factors in the assessment of warm-water near-drowning in children, *Am J Dis Child* 135:1006-1008, 1981.
175. Fandel I, Bancali E: Near-drowning in children: clinical aspects, *Pediatrics* 58:573-579, 1976.
176. Glauser FL, Smith WR: Pulmonary interstitial fibrosis following near-drowning and exposure to short-term high oxygen concentrations, *Chest* 68:373-375, 1975.
177. Noguchi M, Kimula Y, Ogata T: Muddy lung, *Am J Clin Pathol* 83:240-244, 1985.
178. Mangge H, Plecko B, Grubbauer HM, Popper H, Smolle-Juttner F, Zack M: Late-onset miliary pneumonitis after near drowning, *Pediatr Pulmonol* 15:122-124, 1993.

Chemical and Particulate Lung Injury

179. Snyder RW, Mishel HS, Christensen GC: Pulmonary toxicity following exposure to methylene chloride and its combustion product, phosgene, *Chest* 102:1921, 1992 (letter).
180. Riechelmann H, Maurer J, Kienast K, Hafner B, Mann WJ: Respiratory epithelium exposed to sulphur dioxide: functional and ultrastructural alterations, *Laryngoscope* 105:295-299, 1995.
181. Tse RL, Bockman AA: Nitrogen dioxide toxicity: report of four cases in firemen, *JAMA* 212:1341-1344, 1970.
182. White CS, Templeton PA: Chemical pneumonitis, *Radiol Clin North Am* 30:1231-1243, 1992.
183. Heidemann SM, Goetting MG: Treatment of acute hypoxemic respiratory failure caused by chlorine exposure, *Pediatr Emerg Care* 7:87-88, 1991.
184. Wood BR, Colombo JL, Benson BE: Chlorine inhalation toxicity from vapors generated by swimming pool chlorinator tablets, *Pediatrics* 79:427-430, 1987.
185. Edwards IR, Temple WA, Dobbinson TL: Acute chlorine poisoning from a high school experiment, *NZ Med J* 96:720-721, 1983.
186. Flete J, Calvo C, Juniga J: Intoxication of 76 children by chlorine gas, *Hum Toxicol* 5:99-100, 1986.
187. Givan DC, Eigen H, Tepper RS: Longitudinal evaluation of pulmonary function in an infant following chlorine gas exposure, *Pediatr Pulmonol* 6:191-194, 1989.
188. Dewhurst F: Voluntary chlorine inhalation, *Br Med J* 282:565-566, 1981.
189. Rafferty P: Voluntary chlorine inhalation: a new form of self-abuse? *Br Med J* 281:1178-1179, 1980.
190. Adelson L, Kaufman J: Fatal chlorine poisoning: report of two cases with clinicopathologic correlation, *Am J Clin Pathol* 56:430-442, 1971.
191. Hasan FM, Gehshan A, Fuleihan FJD: Resolution of pulmonary dysfunction following acute chlorine exposure, *Arch Environ Health* 38:76-79, 1983.
192. Szerlip HM, Singer I: Hyperchloremic metabolic acidosis after chlorine inhalation, *Am J Med* 77:581-582, 1984.
193. Schwartz DA, Smith DD, Lakshminarayan S: The pulmonary sequelae associated with accidental inhalation of chlorine gas, *Chest* 97:820-825, 1990.
194. Kaufman J, Burkons D: Clinical roentgenologic, and physiologic effects of acute chlorine exposure, *Arch Environ Health* 23:29-34, 1971.
195. Charan NB, Lakshminarayan S, Myers GC: Effects of accidental chlorine exposure on pulmonary function, *West J Med* 143:333-336, 1985.

196. Chester EH, Kaimal J, Payne CB: Pulmonary injury following exposure to chlorine gas: possible beneficial effects of steroid treatment, *Chest* 72:247-250, 1977.
197. Bosse GM: Nebulized sodium bicarbonate in the treatment of chlorine gas inhalation, *J Toxicol* 32:233-241, 1994.
198. Moore BB, Sherman M: Chronic reactive airway disease following acute chlorine gas exposure in an asymptomatic atopic patient, *Chest* 100:855-856, 1991.
199. Kass I, Zamel N, Dobry CA: Bronchiectasis following ammonia burns of the respiratory tract, *Chest* 62:282-285, 1972.
200. Leduc D, Gris P, Lheureux P: Acute and long-term respiratory damage following inhalation of ammonia, *Thorax* 47:755-757, 1992.
201. Einhorn A, Horton L, Altieri M, Ochsenschlager D, Klein B: Serious respiratory consequences of detergent ingestions in children, *Pediatrics* 84:472-474, 1989.
202. Mofenson HC, Greensher J, DiTomasso A, Okun S: Baby powder: a hazard, *Pediatrics* 68:265-266, 1981.
203. Motomatsu K, Adachi H, Uno T: Two infant deaths after inhaling baby powder, *Chest* 75:448-450, 1979.
204. Brouillette F, Weber ML: Massive aspiration of talcum powder by an infant, *Can Med Assoc J* 119:354-355, 1978.
205. Reyes de la Rocha S, Brown MA: Normal pulmonary function after baby powder inhalation causing adult respiratory distress syndrome, *Pediatr Emerg Care* 5:43-48, 1989.
206. Cruthirds TP, Cole FH, Paul RN: Pulmonary talcosis as a result of massive aspiration of baby powder, *South Med J* 70:626-628, 1977.
207. Pairaudeau PW, Wilson RG, Hall MA, Milne M: Inhalation of baby powder: an unappreciated hazard, *Br Med J* 302:1200-1201, 1991.
208. Levy G: Gastrointestinal clearance of drugs with activated charcoal, *New Engl J Med* 307:676-678, 1982.
209. Atkinson SW, Young Y, Trotter GA: Treatment with activated charcoal complicated by gastrointestinal obstruction requiring surgery, *Br Med J* 305:563, 1992.
210. Givens T, Holloway M, Wason S: Pulmonary aspiration of activated charcoal: a complication of its misuse in overdose management, *Pediatr Emerg Care* 8:137-140, 1992.
211. Pollack MM, Dunbar BS, Holbrook PR, Fields AI: Aspiration of activated charcoal and gastric contents, *Ann Emerg Med* 10:528-529, 1981.
212. Elliott CG, Colby TV, Kelly TM, Hicks HG: Charcoal lung: bronchiolitis obliterans after aspiration of activated charcoal, *Chest* 96:672-674, 1989.
213. Harris CR, Filandrinos D: Accidental administration of activated charcoal into the lung: aspiration by proxy, *Ann Emerg Med* 22:1470-1473, 1993.
214. Moutinho ME, Tompkins AL, Rowland TW, Banson BB, Jackson AH: Acute mercury vapor poisoning: fatality in an infant, *Am J Dis Child* 135:42-44, 1981.
215. Moromisato DY, Anas NG, Goodman G: Mercury inhalation poisoning and acute lung injury in a child: use of high-frequency oscillatory ventilation, *Chest* 105:613-615, 1994.

Adult Respiratory Distress Syndrome

216. Pfenninger J, Gerber A, Tschappeler H, Zimmermann A: Adult respiratory distress syndrome in children, *J Pediatr* 101:352-357, 1982.
217. Nussbaum E: Adult-type respiratory distress syndrome in children: experience with seven cases, *Clin Pediatr* 22:401-406, 1983.
218. Dixon C: Mycoplasmal pneumonia and ARDS: a complication to be recognized, *J Natl Med Assoc* 73:549-552, 1981.
219. Bachmann DC, Pfenninger J: Respiratory syncytial virus triggered adult respiratory distress syndrome in infants: a report of two cases, *Intensive Care Med* 20:61-63, 1994.
220. Tuxen DV, Cade JF, Mcdonald MI, Buchanan MRC, Clark RJ, Pain MCF: Herpes simplex virus from the lower respiratory tract in adult respiratory distress syndrome, *Am Rev Respir Dis* 126:416-419, 1982.
221. Milley JR, Nugent SK, Rogers MC: Neurogenic pulmonary edema in childhood, *J Pediatr* 94:706-709, 1979.
222. Lyrene RK, Truog WE: Adult respiratory distress syndrome in a pediatric intensive care unit: predisposing conditions, clinical course, and outcome, *Pediatrics* 67:790-795, 1981.
223. Pepe PE, Potkin RT, Reus DH, Hudson LD, Carrico CJ: Clinical predictors of the adult respiratory distress syndrome, *Am J Surg* 144:124-130, 1982.
224. Bachofen M, Weibel ER: Structural alterations of lung parenchyma in the adult respiratory distress syndrome, *Clin Chest Med* 3:35-36, 1982.
225. Katz R, Pollack M, Spady D: Cardiopulmonary abnormalities in severe acute respiratory failure, *J Pediatr* 104:357-364, 1984.
226. Zapol WM, Snider MT: Pulmonary hypertension in severe acute respiratory failure, *New Engl J Med* 296:476-480, 1977.
227. Gattinoni L, Pesenti A, Bombino M, Baglioni S, Rivolta M, Rossi F: Relationships between lung computed tomographic density, gas exchange, and PEEP in acute respiratory failure, *Anesthesiology* 69:824-832, 1988.
228. Rinaldo JE, Rogers RM: Adult respiratory-distress syndrome: changing concepts of lung injury and repair, *New Engl J Med* 306:900-909, 1982.
229. Anderson BO, Bensard DD, Harken AH: The role of platelet activating factor and its antagonists in shock, sepsis and multiple organ failure, *Surg Gynecol Obstet* 172:415-424, 1991.
230. Abman SH, Griebel JL, Parker DK, Schmidt JM, Swanton D, Kinsella JP: Acute effects of inhaled nitric oxide in children with severe hypoxemic respiratory failure, *J Pediatr* 124:881-888, 1994.
231. Bell RC, Coalson JJ, Smith JD, Johanson WG: Multiple organ system failure and infection in adult respiratory distress syndrome, *Ann Intern Med* 99:293-298, 1983.
232. Bone RC, Fisher CJ, Clemmer TP, Slotman GJ, Metz CA, Balk RA: Sepsis syndrome: a valid clinical entity, *Crit Care Med* 17:389-393, 1989.
233. Canver CC, Mentzer RM Jr: The role of open lung biopsy in early and late survival of ventilator-dependent patients with diffuse idiopathic lung disease, *J Cardiovasc Surg* 35:151-155, 1994.
234. Steinberg KP, Mitchell DR: Maunder RJ, Milberg JA, Whitcomb ME, Hudson LD: Safety of bronchoalveolar lavage in patients with adult respiratory distress syndrome, *Am Rev Respir Dis* 148:556-561, 1993.
235. Allen JN, Pacht ER, Gadek JE, Davis WB: Acute eosinophilic pneumonia as a reversible cause of non-infectious respiratory failure, *New Engl J Med* 321:569-574, 1989.
236. Nash G, Foley FD: Herpetic infections of the middle and lower respiratory tract, *Am J Clin Pathol* 54:857-863, 1970.
237. Barach AL, Martin J, Eckman M: Positive pressure respiration and its application to the treatment of acute pulmonary edema, *Ann Intern Med* 12:754-795, 1938.
238. Shapiro BA, Cane RD, Harrison RA: Positive end-expiratory pressure therapy in adults with special reference to acute lung injury: a review of the literature and suggested clinical correlation, *Crit Care Med* 12:127-141, 1984.
239. Pepe PE, Hudson LD, Carrico CJ: Early application of positive end-expiratory pressure in patients at risk of adult respiratory distress syndrome, *New Engl J Med* 311:281-286, 1984.
240. Clough JB, Duncan AW, Sly PD: The effect of sustained positive airway pressure on derived cardiac output in children, *Anaesth Intensive Care* 22:30-34, 1994.
241. Jardin F, Farcot J, Boisante L, Curien N, Margairaz A, Bourdarias JP: Influence of positive end-expiratory pressure on left ventricular performance, *New Engl J Med* 304:387-392, 1981.
242. Kollef MH, Schuster DP: The acute respiratory distress syndrome, *New Engl J Med* 332:27-37, 1995.
243. Pollack MM, Fields AI, Holbrook PR: Cardiopulmonary parameters during high PEEP in children, *Crit Care Med* 8:372-376, 1980.
244. Sivan Y, Deakers TW, Newth CJ: Effect of positive end-expiratory pressure on respiratory compliance in children with acute respiratory failure, *Pediatr Pulmonol* 11:103-107, 1991.
245. Aidinis SJ, Lafferty J, Shapiro HM: Intracranial pressure responses to PEEP, *Anesthesiology* 45:275-286, 1976.
246. Marcy TW, Marini JJ: Inverse ratio ventilation in ARDS: rationale and implementation, *Chest* 100:494-504, 1991.
247. Gurevitch MJ, van Dyke J, Young ES, Jackson K: Improved oxygenation and lower peak airway pressure in severe adult respiratory distress syndrome: treatment with inverse ratio ventilation, *Chest* 89:211-213, 1986.

248. Arnold JH, Hanson JH, Toro-Figuero LO, Gutierrez J, Berens RJ, Anglin DL: Prospective, randomized comparison of high-frequency oscillatory ventilation and convectional mechanical ventilation in pediatric respiratory failure, *Crit Care Med* 22:1530-1539, 1994.
249. Clark RH: High-frequency ventilation in acute pediatric respiratory failure, *Chest* 105:652-653, 1994.
250. Smith DW, Frankel LR, Derish MT, Moody RR, Black LE III, Chipps BE, Mathers LH: High-frequency jet ventilation in children with the adult respiratory distress syndrome complicated by pulmonary barotrauma, *Pediatr Pulmonol* 15:279-286, 1993.
251. Rosenberg RB, Broner CW, Peters KJ, Anglin DL: High-frequency ventilation for acute pediatric respiratory failure, *Chest* 104:1216-1221, 1993.
252. Clark RH: High-frequency ventilation, *J Pediatr* 124:661-670, 1994.
253. Murdoch IA, Storman MO: Improved arterial oxygenation in children with the adult respiratory distress syndrome: the prone position, *Acta Paediatr* 83:1043-1046, 1994.
254. Leatherman JW, Lari RL, Iber C, Ney AL: Tidal volume reduction in ARDS: effect on cardiac output and arterial oxygenation, *Chest* 99:1227-1231, 1991.
255. Nunn JF: Adult respiratory distress syndrome. In Nunn JF, ed: *Nunn's applied respiratory physiology,* ed 4, Oxford, England, 1993, Butterworth-Heinemann, pp 505-517.
256. Fanconi S, Kraemer R, Weber J, Tschaeppeler H, Pfenninger J: Long-term sequelae in children surviving adult respiratory distress syndrome, *J Pediatr* 106:218-222, 1985.

CHAPTER 26

Respiratory Failure

Robert Henning and Michael South

This chapter covers the pathophysiologic mechanisms that lead to respiratory failure, including abnormalities of gas transport, respiratory muscle fatigue, extravascular lung water, and interactions between the circulatory and respiratory systems. The pathophysiology of individual lung diseases is covered in the relevant chapters.

Definition

Respiratory failure is defined as the impaired ability of the respiratory system to maintain adequate oxygen and carbon dioxide homeostasis.[1] In respiratory failure, the respiratory system may be unable to transfer the volumes of oxygen and carbon dioxide required by the body's metabolism or may be able to do so only at the expense of abnormal concentrations of oxygen and carbon dioxide in arterial blood.

The criteria for the diagnosis of respiratory failure are arbitrarily chosen. Commonly used criteria are a partial pressure of arterial carbon dioxide ($Paco_2$) of 50 mm Hg or a partial pressure of arterial oxygen (Pao_2) of less than 60 mm Hg in a subject breathing air at sea level. The absolute level of Pao_2 below which progressive respiratory failure ensues may be above or below 60 mm Hg, depending on the inspired oxygen concentration (Fio_2), barometric pressure, the age of the patient, and the patient's prior blood gas status.[2] Although specific criteria for the diagnosis of respiratory failure have been proposed in newborns and older children suffering from specific conditions such as Guillain-Barré syndrome and parenchymal lung disease,[3] these criteria are useful only as guides for further interventions. The label of *respiratory failure* does not in itself assist in the identification of appropriate treatment or the prognosis.

The exact point at which further treatment such as mechanical ventilation is indicated depends on the rate of deterioration, the child's response to deteriorating respiratory system function (e.g., apnea, increased respiratory effort), the child's age, and any associated illness. For example, mechanical ventilation would be started for a lesser degree of blood gas abnormality in a preterm baby, a child with septic shock, or a child with an intracranial hemorrhage than in a fit teenager with asthma.

As Boxes 26-1 through 26-3 show, respiratory failure may be caused by disorders at any point in the respiratory system. This includes the respiratory center in the brain stem and its sensory inputs via the spinal cord, motor nerve roots, nerve trunks, and respiratory muscles; the thoracic cage and pleura; the large and small airways; the gas-exchanging surfaces; and the lung interstitium and pulmonary vessels.

Examples of a lesion at a single site in the respiratory system are acute obstruction of the trachea by a foreign body and acute neuromuscular blockade by muscle relaxants. More commonly, abnormalities at different levels of the respiratory system combine to produce respiratory failure. For example, atelectasis with acute asthma or Guillain-Barré syndrome reduces the gas-exchanging surface, narrows the small airways, and produces motor nerve root disorder. Respiratory muscle fatigue frequently exacerbates respiratory failure in disorders of the chest wall and respiratory tree, especially if the latter are of long duration. In such cases, therapeutic efforts to alleviate the respiratory failure may be aimed at either or both aspects of failure in the respiratory system. For example, respiratory failure resulting from muscle fatigue in cystic fibrosis may be managed by oxygen therapy, antibiotics, and postural drainage, with or without nocturnal ventilation via a nasal mask for the muscle fatigue.

Lesions at a second site are often responsible for acute exacerbations of chronic respiratory failure. For example, acute viral bronchitis may cause daytime hypoxemia in a child with

BOX 26-1
Central Nervous System Causes of Respiratory Failure

- Medications
  - Narcotics
  - Sedatives
  - General anesthetic agents
  - Diuretics that cause metabolic alkalosis (e.g., furosemide)
  - Sodium bicarbonate
  - Prostaglandin E_1
  - Poisoning
- Metabolic conditions
  - Hypoxia
  - Extreme hypercapnia
  - Severe alkalosis
  - Hyperglycemia
  - Hypoglycemia
  - Hyponatremia
  - Hypocalcemia
  - Hyperammonemia, including Reye's syndrome and urea cycle disorders, and some organic acidemias, including maple syrup urine disease
  - Medium-chain acyl-coenzyme A dehydrogenase deficiency
  - Leigh disease
  - Cerebral edema of any cause
- Infections
  - Meningitis
  - Encephalitis
  - Brain abscess
  - Bulbar poliomyelitis
- Postinfectious demyelinating disorders of the brain stem
- Brain stem malformations
  - Syringobulbia
  - Arnold-Chiari malformation
  - Encephalocele
  - Joubert's syndrome
  - Dandy-Walker syndrome
- Bony abnormalities affecting the brain stem
  - Achondroplasia
  - Osteogenesis imperfecta
- Bulbar hemorrhage
- Brain stem trauma and raised intracranial pressure of any cause
- Seizures
- Central alveolar hypoventilation

BOX 26-2
Neuromuscular Disorders Causing Respiratory Failure

- Medications
  - Muscle relaxants
  - Anticholinesterases
  - Aminoglycosides
  - Dantrolene
  - Glucocorticoids
  - Heavy metal poisoning
- Metabolic conditions
  - Severe hypophosphatemia
  - Hypokalemia or hyperkalemia
  - Hypermagnesemia
  - Uremia
  - Carnitine deficiency
  - Acid maltase deficiency
  - Acute intermittent porphyria
- Infections
  - Poliomyelitis
  - Tetanus
  - Botulism
  - Diphtheria
- Trauma
  - Spinal cord trauma
  - Phrenic nerve trauma
  - Diaphragm trauma
- Other
  - Myasthenia gravis
  - Muscular dystrophy
  - Hoffman-Werdnig syndrome
  - Kugelberg-Welander syndrome
  - Guillain-Barré syndrome
  - Prolonged starvation
  - Multiple sclerosis
  - Polyneuropathy of critical illness
  - Dermatomyositis or polymyositis
  - Envenomations (tick, tetrodotoxin, snake)

BOX 26-3
Pulmonary Causes of Respiratory Failure

Disorders of bellows function

- Chest wall
  - Kyphoscoliosis
  - Asphyxiating thoracic dystrophy
  - Collodion skin
  - Circumferential chest burns
  - Chest wall edema
- Pleura
  - Hemothorax
  - Pleural effusion
  - Pneumothorax: open or closed
  - Bronchopleural fistula
- Lung
  - Pulmonary hypoplasia

Airway disorders

- Upper airway obstruction
  - Nose
  - Pharynx
  - Larynx
  - Trachea
  - Bronchi

Airway disorders—cont'd

- Small airway obstruction
  - Asthma
  - Viral bronchiolitis
  - Bronchiolitis obliterans
  - Inhalation injury to small airways

Lung parenchymal disorders

- Pneumonia
- Pulmonary edema
- Pulmonary fibrosis
- Pulmonary alveolar proteinosis

Pulmonary vascular disorders

- Primary pulmonary hypertension
- Pulmonary arteriovenous malformations
- Pulmonary embolism

congenital alveolar hypoventilation syndrome, and atelectasis or bronchopneumonia may precipitate severe respiratory failure in a teenager with severe kyphoscoliosis.

Classification of Respiratory Failure

There are two types of respiratory failure[2]:

1. Nonventilatory (type 1) respiratory failure, in which hypoxemia is present while the Pa_{CO_2} is low or normal
2. Ventilatory (type II) respiratory failure, in which both hypoxemia and hypercapnia are present

In both types, hypoxemia is present to some extent; both can occur during the course of a single illness, and both can result from ventilation-perfusion ($\dot{V}/\dot{Q}$) inequality. The causes of hypoxemia in a person breathing air at sea level are hypoventilation, right-to-left shunt, $\dot{V}/\dot{Q}$ inequality, and diffusion block. These causes are discussed more fully later. The amount of hypoxemia attributable to each of these mechanisms varies from one disease to another. The contribution of each cause varies among patients with one disease and during the course of an illness in one patient.

HYPOVENTILATION

Hypoventilation (reduced alveolar ventilation) causes hypoxemia by increasing the partial pressure of carbon dioxide in alveolar gas (P_{ACO_2}) (type II respiratory failure) because Pa_{CO_2} is inversely proportional to the alveolar ventilation and directly proportional to the body's rate of producing carbon dioxide.

As P_{ACO_2} increases, it displaces oxygen from the alveolar gas so that the partial pressure of oxygen in alveolar gas (P_{AO_2}) (and therefore Pa_{O_2}) decreases, as is shown from the alveolar gas equation, which follows:

$$P_{AO_2} = P_{IO_2} - P_{ACO_2}/R + [P_{ACO_2} \times F_{IO_2} \times (1 - R)/R]$$

where P_{IO_2} is the partial pressure of oxygen in inspired gas, and *R* is the respiratory quotient (approximately 0.8 in children on a normal diet). Thus a patient who is hypercapnic is always hypoxemic unless he or she is receiving supplemental oxygen. Pure hypoventilation may result from neuromuscular, central nervous system, or chest wall disease. If these conditions persist, especially if they lead to reduced tidal volume (V_T) and reduced sighing, small airway closure and atelectasis are likely to ensue, with consequent $\dot{V}/\dot{Q}$ inequality, shunt, or both. Thus hypoventilation alone is a relatively uncommon cause of carbon dioxide retention, except in acute conditions.[4]

In type I respiratory failure, disordered gas exchange is due to $\dot{V}/\dot{Q}$ inequality, shunt, or impaired diffusion. Hypoventilation alone can produce a type II pattern of respiratory failure (e.g., opiate-induced hypoventilation), but most commonly this pattern is caused by $\dot{V}/\dot{Q}$ inequality with an inadequate compensatory increase in alveolar ventilation. The inadequate response to hypercapnia may result from insensitivity of the chemoreceptors or of the respiratory center to changes in the Pa_{CO_2} (e.g., in central alveolar hypoventilation syndrome) or from failure of communication between the brain stem and respiratory muscles (as in neurologic disease); it may also occur because disorders of the airways, lung parenchyma, chest wall, and respiratory muscles prevent these structures from responding to increased neutral output from the respiratory center. Hypoxemia and extreme hypercapnia may themselves depress central respiratory drive.

Respiratory drive and the resulting neuromuscular response may be adequate when the dynamic compliance of the respiratory system is high but may become inadequate when compliance decreases. This is especially important in a young infant, whose compliant rib cage and horizontal rib position reduce the mechanical efficiency of the respiratory muscles in expanding the thoracic volume. Respiratory muscle fatigue and distortion of the chest wall may also impair the ability of the respiratory system to increase the minute ventilation and restore Pa_{CO_2} in the presence of $\dot{V}/\dot{Q}$ inequality, shunt, or diffusion defects.[5]

The newborn's ventilatory response to carbon dioxide is similar to the older child's and adult's, but unlike the response in older children and adults, the carbon dioxide response in the newborn is depressed by hypoxemia.[6,7] The newborn with recurrent apnea is less able than older infants to sustain inspiratory effort in the face of increased inspiratory loads.[8] These properties of the immature respiratory system may contribute to carbon dioxide retention in the presence of lung disease.

As hyperinflation increases in obstructive conditions such as asthma and bronchiolitis, the precontraction length of the diaphragmatic muscle fibers decreases, so the force of contraction decreases, resulting in a reduced V_T and raised Pa_{CO_2}.[9] At any level of alveolar ventilation, depending on the mechanical characteristics of the respiratory system, there are combinations of respiratory rate and V_T at which respiratory work is minimized but at which gas exchange is not optimal.[9] When alveolar ventilation and work of breathing are low, the combination of rate and V_T selected may optimize gas exchange, but at higher levels of V_T and work of breathing, mechanical loading is adjusted to reduce respiratory work at the expense of gas exchange.[10] For example, when the respiratory system elastance decreases in pneumonia, the work of breathing is minimized when the respiratory pattern is a shallow tachypnea. In this pattern, however, the dead space to tidal volume ratio (V_D/V_T) is high. When elastance is severely increased, the increase in the dead space to tidal volume ratio resulting from extreme tachypnea may result in reduced alveolar ventilation and therefore raised P_{ACO_2} and reduced P_{AO_2}.

Acute vs. Chronic Respiratory Failure

Acute respiratory failure is an immediately life-threatening condition that develops over minutes to hours (e.g., a tension pneumothorax resulting from a fractured rib). Chronic respiratory failure is a potentially life-threatening condition that develops over months to years (e.g., the gradually deteriorating gas exchange in a child with kyphoscoliosis resulting from muscular dystrophy).

RESPIRATORY MUSCLE FAILURE

The integrity of the pumping action of the respiratory muscles is as essential to life as the actions of the cardiac muscle; yet more is known about the actions of the heart under normal and pathologic conditions than about the actions of the respiratory muscles. Only in the last 20 years have detailed investigations into respiratory muscle function been conducted. The muscles of the respiratory pump have a large reserve, and they can sustain high levels of contraction and hence ventilatory work over prolonged periods. At rest, only 10% to 15% of diaphragmatic muscle motor units are active.[11] However, the muscles may become weak and fail under a number of conditions.

Weakness of the respiratory muscles may contribute to alveolar hypoventilation and respiratory failure in the following circumstances:

1. Respiratory muscle weakness secondary to fatigue from increased work of breathing is a common contributing factor to alveolar hypoventilation in many thoracic or pulmonary disorders. For example, in a child with severe acute asthma, the progression to respiratory failure occurs when the diaphragm becomes fatigued and cannot maintain the increased work of breathing caused by increased airway resistance.
2. Respiratory muscle weakness may be the primary and sole cause of alveolar hypoventilation. An example is a patient with severe infantile botulism.
3. A mixture of these two circumstances may occur. For example, a patient with Duchenne muscular dystrophy may be able to sustain the work of normal breathing but may not be able to do so when the work of breathing is increased by pulmonary disease, such as pneumonia. Alveolar hypoventilation occurs with less severe pulmonary consolidation than it would in a previously normal patient.

Normal Respiratory Muscle Function

The primary muscle of inspiration is the diaphragm, which is innervated from cervical spinal roots 3 to 5. Diaphragmatic contraction leads to inspiration by two main mechanisms: a simple, pistonlike caudal displacement of the dome of the diaphragm and elevation of the lower ribs into which the diaphragm inserts as the muscle sheet contracts across the relatively incompressible abdominal contents. The upper ribs are raised by mechanical coupling, and because of the oblique attachments of the ribs, the transverse diameter of the chest increases as the ribs rise. In infants, the compliant chest wall limits the latter effect.[12]

Other inspiratory muscles include the sternocleidomastoid, scalene, internal intercostal, and external intercostal muscles. These muscles are usually inactive during quiet respiration but become recruited as increased effort is required by exercise or pulmonary disease. These accessory inspiratory muscles make the ribs more horizontal and raise the rib cage. In infants, these muscles have a limited ability to support inspiration because the ribs are almost horizontal at rest.[13-15] The rib cage develops a more adult configuration by about 2 years of age, but before this age, the intercostal muscles play an important role in preventing deformation of the compliant chest wall during inspiration.[16,17]

The abdominal muscles (external and internal oblique, rectus abdominis, and transversus abdominis) and the interosseous internal intercostal muscles were traditionally considered expiratory in their action. They can certainly cause expiration and are used in forced expiratory activities such as coughing. However, the main action of these muscles is probably to increase the efficiency of inspiration. Two mechanisms enable them to do this. Contraction pulls the rib cage down and inward; if this occurs beyond the point at which the elastic recoil of the chest wall exceeds the collapsing force of the lungs (i.e., below functional residual capacity [FRC]), kinetic energy is stored in the rib cage, which assists the next inspiration.[18] Abdominal muscle contraction also pushes the diaphragm upward to a point where the muscle fibers reach their optimal resting length for maximal contraction during the next inspiration (see later section).

During quiet respiration, usually only the diaphragm is active, but as the need for alveolar ventilation increases (e.g., in exercise) or the work required to maintain ventilation increases (e.g., in obstructive airway disease), first the accessory inspiratory muscles and then the so-called expiratory muscles are recruited into use.

The stimulus for muscle contraction begins in the central nervous system and is transmitted as an axonal action potential to the neuromuscular junction. The release of acetylcholine from the small neuronal end plate at its synapse with the muscle cell membrane greatly amplifies the signal and, by opening cationic channels, causes muscle cell depolarization. The change in membrane polarity reaches the tubular sarcoplasmic reticulum, and calcium ions are released. Free calcium ions combine with troponin, a protein that prevents actin and myosin filaments from reacting. Calcium causes troponin to change its physical configuration, and the actin and myosin filaments can then slide over one other, shortening the muscle and generating force. Relaxation occurs when calcium is pumped back into the sarcoplasmic reticulum. Both the sliding reaction of actin and myosin filaments and the return of calcium to the sarcoplasmic reticulum are active steps requiring hydrolysis of adenosine triphosphate (ATP).

In addition to producing ventilation of the alveoli, the respiratory muscles have a number of other functions, including stabilization of the compliant chest wall in infants; expulsive efforts such as coughing, sneezing, vomiting, and defecation; and stabilization of the chest and abdomen in motor activities involving the trunk.

Developmental Biology of Respiratory Muscles and Susceptibility to Fatigue

As noted previously, differences in chest wall configuration and compliance between young infants and older children can place normal infants at a disadvantage when trying to meet the increased ventilatory requirements imposed by pulmonary disease or increased metabolic demands. Differences in the microstructure and properties of the respiratory neuromuscular system of infants may also be important.

In older children and adults, each muscle fiber in the diaphragm is innervated by only one motoneuron, and each motoneuron innervates 200 to 300 muscle fibers. Each fiber of the neonatal diaphragm receives innervation from several motoneurons, and this persists for the first few weeks of life.[19] The significance of this polyneural innervation is unknown, but it may have a role in reducing the susceptibility to diaphragmatic fatigue.

In newborn rats, the quantity of acetylcholine released by the diaphragmatic neuronal end plates in response to an action potential is less than that released in adult rats.[20] At high frequencies of stimulation, the neonatal diaphragmatic neuromuscular junction may be prone to transmission failure.

Skeletal muscle fibers, including those of the diaphragm, may be classified into two basic groups, type I or II, according to histochemical and electrophysiologic characteristics. Type I fibers do not stain in the myofibrillar adenosinetriphosphatase reaction, have a high capacity for oxidative phosphorylation, develop their maximal force generation slowly ("slow-twitch"), and are resistant to fatigue.[21] Type II fibers rapidly develop their maximal force generation ("fast-twitch"), but this group may be subdivided according to other properties. Type IIa fibers have intermediate oxidative phosphorylation and are fatigue resistant. Type IIb fibers have poor oxidative phosphorylation and fatigue easily. Type IIc fibers are found only in fetal and neonatal diaphragmatic muscle; they are highly oxidative and resistant to fatigue. Type IIh fibers are also found only in fetal and neonatal muscle and probably represent a transition phase from type IIa to IIb fibers[22,23] (Fig. 26-1).

There are certainly differences in the fiber composition between adults and newborns, but the extent and importance of these differences, particularly with regard to the fatigability of the diaphragm, has been the subject of some controversy. Initial investigations[21] suggested that young infants have lower proportions of type I fibers and that overall the neonatal diaphragm has a reduced ability for oxidative phosphorylation and hence an increased tendency to fatigue. More recently, it has been demonstrated[22-24] that some of these observations may have resulted from postmortem changes. In fresh specimens of neonatal diaphragm, there are fewer type I fibers, but these are replaced by the highly oxidative and fatigue-resistant type IIc fibers.

In vitro and in vivo studies of diaphragmatic action in humans and animals also have conflicting results. There is some evidence that the infantile diaphragm can generate forces as great as those in adults,[25] but other evidence suggests that the maximal force generated increases with postnatal age.[22] In vitro, fetal diaphragm muscle strips suffer fatigue less than strips from adults.

The best tests of force generation in the diaphragm rely on voluntary, or stimulated, maximal respiratory efforts, neither of which are practicable in young children with pulmonary disease. Indirect evidence that diaphragmatic fatigue occurs comes from studies of the electromyographic power spectrum in premature infants.[26]

Many researchers now believe that diaphragmatic fatigue is a more common feature of thoracopulmonary disease in infants than in adults but that this is probably a result more of the mechanical disadvantages caused by chest wall configuration and compliance than of an increased tendency to fatigue in the diaphragm muscle itself.

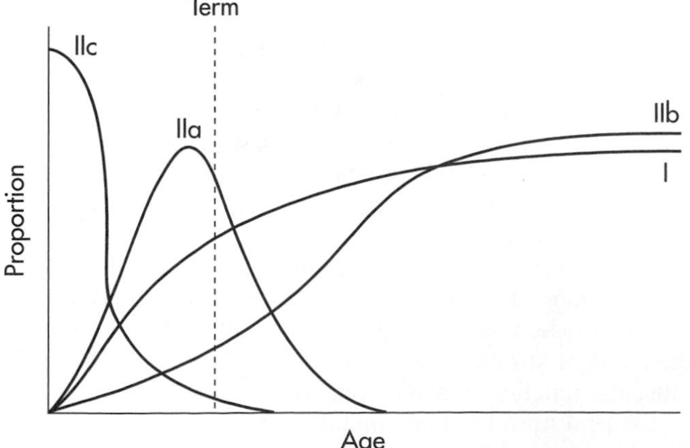

Fig. 26-1. Changes with age in the proportion of the skeletal muscle fibers in the baboon diaphragm. Figures are unavailable for the human diaphragm but are thought to be similar.

The biochemical events leading to muscle fatigue are complex. Fatigue may occur in a number of ways, including depletion of acetylcholine at the neuromuscular junction, depletion of ATP or of substrates used to generate ATP within muscle (glycogen, glucose, free fatty acids), reduced rate of calcium release from the sarcoplasmic reticulum, and reduced supply of substrate to the muscles because blood flow does not match demands. When subjected to greatly increased workloads, the diaphragm may require a blood flow rate that is 10 to 20 times greater than resting rates to meet its metabolic demands.[27,28]

Some evidence indicates that once the diaphragm begins to fatigue, there is a reduction in central nervous system respiratory drive to this muscle. This limits fatigue but may contribute to respiratory failure if other respiratory muscles cannot help maintain the ventilatory requirements.

Causes of Respiratory Muscle Fatigue

A number of factors other than age may influence respiratory muscle function and increase the tendency to fatigue. These follow:

1. Diseases of the central and peripheral nervous system, the neuromuscular junction, and skeletal muscle (see Boxes 26-1 and 26-2) affect diaphragmatic muscle function and in some cases cause alveolar hypoventilation.
2. Compression caused by lung hyperexpansion may impair blood flow to the diaphragm (e.g., in severe asthma). Low cardiac output, such as that occurring in several severe pulmonary conditions (see later section on cardiorespiratory interactions) may also limit the required increase in diaphragmatic blood flow.[29]
3. The force of diaphragmatic contraction is proportional to the mass of the muscle. Low diaphragmatic muscle mass may occur in states of malnutrition,[30] and provision of sufficient nutrition to achieve positive nitrogen balance can be difficult in ill infants, particularly preterm babies.[31] Reduced body muscle mass is a feature of some chronic respiratory disorders. The mass of the diaphragm and the maximal force of contraction are reduced in some adults with chronic obstructive airway disease. Respiratory muscle function in chronic pediatric respiratory disorders, such as cystic fibrosis, has not been studied.
4. Hypoxemia and hypercapnia lead to reduced muscle contractility and increase the tendency to fatigue.[32,33] If these abnormalities exist as a result of pulmonary disease, a vicious cycle of deterioration ensues.
5. Metabolic derangements, including hypophosphatemia,[34] hypocalcemia,[35] and hypomagnesemia,[36] can all lead to reduced diaphragmatic contractility.
6. Viral infection may reduce skeletal muscle force generation, and one study showed significant reductions in respiratory muscle strength during acute viral upper respiratory tract infections in normal adults.[37] The impact of viral infection on respiratory muscle function in patients with chronic pulmonary disease or in children has not been studied.
7. Bacterial infections, including pneumococcal sepsis,[38] and gram-negative infection with endotoxic shock[39] significantly reduce diaphragmatic contractile force in ani-

mals. There is little experimental evidence for this in humans.

Summary

There is still much to be learned about respiratory muscle function in infants and children. An infant's diaphragm is almost certainly more prone to fatigue than an adult's, but this probably results mostly from mechanical factors, with microstructural differences playing a lesser role.

A wide range of thoracopulmonary and other disorders may impair respiratory muscle function, leading to respiratory failure. Improved knowledge of how and why the respiratory muscles fail may lead to new modes of therapy.

DISORDERS OF GAS TRANSPORT

Gas exchange between tissue cells and the atmosphere may become inadequate because of a failure in oxygen and carbon dioxide exchange between inspired gas and mixed venous blood or because of abnormalities in oxygen and carbon dioxide carriage in blood and the exchange of oxygen and carbon dioxide between blood and tissue cells. Inadequacy of alveolar ventilation manifests itself as increased $Pa{CO_2}$, whereas disorders of oxygenation increase the difference in the partial pressure of oxygen between alveolar gas and arterial blood ($PA{O_2} - Pa{O_2}$). This difference may be considered equivalent to an admixture of venous blood to the oxygenated blood emerging from the pulmonary capillaries. Venous admixture includes the effects of anatomic shunt, diffusion defects, and perfusion of lung units with low $\dot{V}/\dot{Q}$.[40]

Causes of Venous Admixture

Anatomic right-to-left shunt (Fig. 26-2) is the volume of venous blood entering the aorta. This includes desaturated blood from the bronchial and thebesian veins as well as abnormal extrapulmonary shunts (intracardiac shunts and shunts via the ductus arteriosus) and intrapulmonary shunts.

The bronchial and thebesian veins drain into the pulmonary circulation distal to the gas-exchanging vessels in the alveoli (physiologic shunt), reducing the $Pa{O_2}$ below the partial pressure of end-capillary oxygen ($Pc'{O_2}$). The bronchial veins (which contain deoxygenated blood) drain into the pulmonary veins (which contain oxygenated blood), and the thebesian veins drain into the cavity of the left ventricle. In normal adults, this obligatory shunt represents less than 1% of the cardiac output and reduces the $Pa{O_2}$ by approximately 5 mm Hg.[41]

Extrapulmonary Shunt

In children with congenital heart disease, venous blood may enter the arterial circulation at the level of the atria via a patent foramen ovale or an atrial septal defect; this may also occur across a ventricular septal defect or a patent ductus arteriosus when the pulmonary artery pressure is high or if there is common mixing of venous and arterial blood (e.g., in a univentricular heart or a truncus arteriosus).

In the absence of structural cardiac abnormalities, venous blood may enter the arterial circulation via the foramen ovale or ductus arteriosus, provided that these structures are not permanently closed, when the pulmonary vascular resistance is high (e.g., in meconium aspiration syndrome[42] or hyaline membrane disease [HMD] in the newborn). The foramen ovale

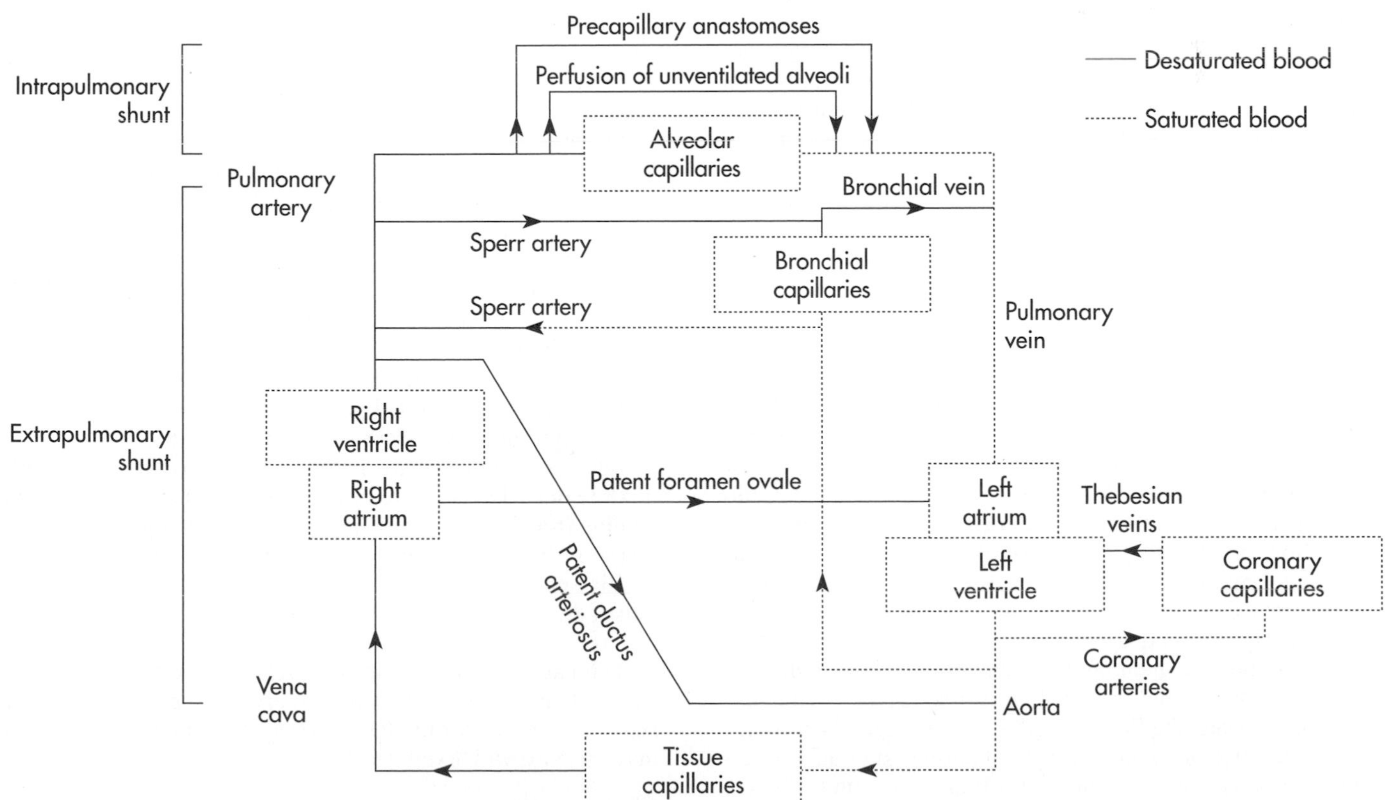

Fig. 26-2. Diagram of the circulation showing the intrapulmonary and extrapulmonary right-to-left shunts.

is closed functionally by 2 hours of age in the normal human but retains the ability to open in 30% of children and adults when right atrial pressure exceeds left atrial pressure.[43] Extrapulmonary right-to-left shunts of 27% to 73% (mean, 52%) have been measured by cardiac catheterization in meconium aspiration syndrome,[44] and a $P_{AO_2} - Pa_{O_2}$ difference of more than 610 mm Hg has been reported resulting from these shunts.[45]

In most cases of HMD, shunting via the ductus arteriosus plays a minor role in the production of arterial hypoxemia, representing only 4% of cardiac output and less than 10% of total venous admixture,[46] although in some cases of persistent pulmonary hypertension of the newborn associated with HMD, shunting via the ductus arteriosus is responsible for significant right-to-left shunting in the presence of severe hypoxemia, hypercapnia, or acidosis. The improvement in Pa_{O_2} with increasing F_{IO_2} in these circumstances is attributable to a reduction in pulmonary vascular resistance, which is caused by the increased F_{IO_2} with consequent reduction in the shunt.[47]

Intrapulmonary Shunt

An intrapulmonary shunt may take the form of discrete extraalveolar arteriovenous connections or may involve blood that transverses completely unventilated alveoli. Except in the case of pulmonary arteriovenous malformations, the most common malformations of the pulmonary circulation, the existence of true anatomic shunt vessels passing from the pulmonary artery to the pulmonary vein remains controversial. Some 36% to 47% occur as part of Osler-Weber-Rendu disease, whereas others appear as isolated congenital abnormalities. Shunts as large as 79% of the cardiac output have been reported in children with pulmonary arteriovenous malformations, and the Pa_{O_2} is less than normal in 80% of cases.[48] Von Hayek[49] in 1960 reported the existence of "sperr" arteries that form a network linking the bronchial arteries to the pulmonary artery and the pulmonary artery to the bronchial veins (and thence to the pulmonary veins, bypassing the alveoli). These muscular bypass channels may regulate the flow of desaturated blood into the systemic circulation (see Fig. 26-2).

Although some investigators have described muscular arterial connections between the bronchial and pulmonary arteries that appear in infancy and disappear by adulthood[50] and the presence of vessels that transmit 60- to 200-μ glass microspheres has been shown in postmortem specimens,[51-53] a careful histologic study by Hislop and Reid[54] did not find any precapillary arteriovenous connections in the lungs of 18 normal children. However, a study using intravenously infused krypton-81m in infants and children with recurrent apnea appeared to show blood traversing the lung without perfusing gas-exchanging surfaces during apneic episodes.[55] This may imply that functional pulmonary arteriovenous connections exist, although the histologic evidence is inconclusive. It has been suggested that functional arteriovenous shunts, opening acutely, may explain the rapid onset of arterial desaturation occurring early in apneic spells.[56]

Intrapulmonary shunting in infants is due mainly to the perfusion of airspaces not involved in gas exchange.[57] In the normal term neonate, the $P_{AO_2} - Pa_{O_2}$ is greater than it is in adults, mainly because of intrapulmonary shunting, although in normal term babies, unventilated alveoli are not found after the first few hours of life.[58] In preterm infants in whom there is no clinical or radiologic evidence of lung disease, the $P_{AO_2} - Pa_{O_2}$ is 400 mm Hg at 26 weeks after conceptional age and 250 mm Hg at 32 weeks.[59] Perfusion of immature terminal airspaces where there are few alveoli may contribute to this venous admixture.[59,60]

The collapse of small airways in infants as a result of incomplete smooth muscle and cartilage development in the bronchial wall[61] and low airway conductance is thought to predispose to the closure of some small airways in expiration.[62,63] The pressures needed to open a closed airway are greater than those that caused it to close: The reduction in airway pressure distal to a point of closure and the stability of a fluid meniscus formed at the site of an airway closure tend to keep the airway closed.[64] Airway closure prevents the ventilation of alveoli supplied by that airway: The blood perfusing those alveoli amounts to a right-to-left shunt.

Routes of collateral ventilation among groups of alveoli (which might assist in the reexpansion of collapsed alveoli) are poorly developed in infancy. Kohn's pores appear gradually with increasing postnatal age, and Lambert's channels between terminal bronchioles and adjacent alveoli appear after the age of 7 years.[65]

Gas trapping resulting from small airway closure appears to be common in small infants (especially in preterm infants,[66,67] in whom it is associated with a large $P_{AO_2} - Pa_{O_2}$ that decreases with increasing age as the thoracic trapped gas volume decreases).[67] Intrapulmonary shunt resulting from perfusion of the unventilated trapped gas compartment contributes to the $P_{AO_2} - Pa_{O_2}$ in these infants. In full-term infants, the $P_{AO_2} - Pa_{O_2}$ approaches zero by 2 weeks of age as thoracic gas volume (and gas trapping) decreases, whereas in preterm infants, the $P_{AO_2} - Pa_{O_2}$ remains elevated despite a decreasing thoracic gas volume at several months of age, presumably because atelectasis contributes both to the declining thoracic gas volume and to the $P_{AO_2} - Pa_{O_2}$.[67]

In neonates with meconium aspiration syndrome, right-to-left shunting is the main cause of arterial hypoxemia.[42] Total shunts of 27% to 73% of cardiac output have been measured in these infants.[44] Although some of the venous admixture occurs at the level of the ductus arteriosus and foramen ovale in the presence of pulmonary hypertension, much venous admixture is attributable to intrapulmonary shunt, with perfusion of collapsed lung segments or of lung units containing trapped gas whose composition approaches that of mixed venous blood.[41]

Intrapulmonary shunt accounts for much of the $P_{AO_2} - Pa_{O_2}$ in atelectasis, pneumonia, and adult respiratory distress syndrome (ARDS) in children and adults, mainly because of continued perfusion of unventilated alveoli. In pneumococcal pneumonia, this continued perfusion is due to impairment of hypoxic pulmonary vasoconstriction, possibly by bacterial products or by immune mediators.[68,69] Most of the venous admixture in ARDS is due to pure shunt, only a small proportion coming from low $\dot{V}/\dot{Q}$ lung units. The commonly observed increase in Pa_{O_2} and reduction in $P_{AO_2} - Pa_{O_2}$ with the use of positive end-expiratory pressure in ARDS are due to a reduction of the shunt caused by decreased perfusion of unventilated alveoli.[70]

The cause of venous admixture in cystic fibrosis varies from patient to patient. In some patients, intrapulmonary shunt accounts for most of the $P_{AO_2} - Pa_{O_2}$, and the degree of shunt may increase with exercise.[71]

$\dot{V}/\dot{Q}$ Inequality

$\dot{V}/\dot{Q}$ inequality is the most important cause of arterial hypoxemia in practice. The concentration of oxygen in the alveoli of a lung unit and in the pulmonary venous blood draining that unit depends on the partial pressure of oxygen in the inspired gas and desaturated pulmonary artery blood perfusing that unit as well as on the ratio of $\dot{V}/\dot{Q}$. The same applies to carbon dioxide.[41]

The P_{AO_2} is determined by the pressure of inspired oxygen, the P_{ACO_2}, and the respiratory quotient, whereas P_{ACO_2} is determined largely by alveolar ventilation and the body's rate of producing carbon dioxide (see earlier section). When the blood flow to a lung unit decreases (and therefore the $\dot{V}/\dot{Q}$ ratio increases), the P_{AO_2} and the Pc'_{O_2} of oxygen of that unit approach the partial pressure of oxygen (P_{O_2}) of inspired gas (150 mm Hg when breathing room air). When the ventilation of a lung unit decreases (and the $\dot{V}/\dot{Q}$ ratio decreases), the P_{AO_2} and Pc'_{O_2} of that unit approach the P_{O_2} of mixed venous blood. When all the units in a lung have a $\dot{V}/\dot{Q}$ ratio of 1, the Pa_{O_2} is approximately 100 mm Hg, and the $P_{AO_2} - Pa_{O_2}$ is 10 to 20 mm Hg in adults breathing room air at sea level[72] in the absence of shunt or diffusion defect.

When some units have a $\dot{V}/\dot{Q}$ ratio less than 1, the blood emerging from those units has a P_{O_2} approaching 40 mm Hg and a partial pressure of carbon dioxide (P_{CO_2}) approaching 45 mm Hg. Because of the shape of the oxygen-hemoglobin dissociation curve, increasing the Pc'_{O_2} of high $\dot{V}/\dot{Q}$ units cannot significantly increase the concentration of oxygen in end-capillary blood (Cc'_{O_2}) and therefore cannot compensate for the low Cc'_{O_2} of blood emerging from low $\dot{V}/\dot{Q}$ units, particularly because low $\dot{V}/\dot{Q}$ units contribute more blood flow than high $\dot{V}/\dot{Q}$ units.

In a spontaneously breathing subject, increased alveolar ventilation stimulated by chemoreceptors prevents the Pa_{CO_2} from rising. (Indeed the Pa_{CO_2} may be lower than normal because of a ventilatory response to arterial hypoxemia.) Because the carbon dioxide response curve is approximately linear in the working range—in fact it is hyperbolic (see Fig. 26-12)—increasing alveolar ventilation to the high $\dot{V}/\dot{Q}$ units can remove enough carbon dioxide to compensate for the high Pa_{CO_2} in the low $\dot{V}/\dot{Q}$ units (see section on the effect of $\dot{V}/\dot{Q}$ inequality on carbon dioxide). However, if alveolar ventilation does not increase in response to a raised Pa_{CO_2} (e.g., because of a central nervous system or neuromuscular disorder or because of mechanical ventilation in a child), increased $\dot{V}/\dot{Q}$ inequality also increases Pa_{CO_2}.

Effect of $\dot{V}/\dot{Q}$ Inequality on Carbon Dioxide Transfer. Although carbon dioxide transfer is less affected by $\dot{V}/\dot{Q}$ inequality than oxygen transfer, $\dot{V}/\dot{Q}$ inequality is the most common cause of hypercapnia in lung disease.[4] The main reasons follow:

1. Both oxygen and carbon dioxide are gases of intermediate solubility; their transfer is less efficient in the presence of $\dot{V}/\dot{Q}$ inequality than the transfer of very soluble or very insoluble gases (Fig. 26-3).
2. Although in the presence of $\dot{V}/\dot{Q}$ inequality, increasing the ventilation of high $\dot{V}/\dot{Q}$ units can lower the P_{CO_2} and thereby the Pa_{CO_2} in these units, the carbon dioxide dissociation curve is hyperbolic rather than linear in the normal operating range so that high $\dot{V}/\dot{Q}$ units may be unable to wash out enough carbon dioxide to compensate for the failure of low $\dot{V}/\dot{Q}$ units to eliminate carbon dioxide.[4]

Furthermore, the altered Pa_{O_2} and pH and the increased work of breathing associated with lung disease contribute to respiratory muscle fatigue and limit the maximal alveolar ventilation of which the patient is capable.

A lung with $\dot{V}/\dot{Q}$ inequality cannot transfer as much oxygen and carbon dioxide as a lung with a $\dot{V}/\dot{Q}$ ratio of 1, all else being equal. If the same amounts of oxygen and carbon dioxide are being transferred, the Pa_{O_2} will be lower and Pa_{CO_2} will be higher than in a lung with homogenous $\dot{V}/\dot{Q}$ ratios, all else being equal.[41]

In a computer model of a lung in which some compartments were ventilated in series (e.g., via pendelluft or Kohn's pores or in which some alveoli arise from more proximal bronchioles), West[73] found that carbon dioxide transfer is reduced more than oxygen transfer. This was because a "parasitic" alveolus that receives all of its inspired gas from a second alveolus is effectively rebreathing gas with a P_{O_2} of approximately 110 mm Hg and a P_{CO_2} similar to that of mixed venous blood. Although oxygen transfer from this parasitic alveolus is almost normal, carbon dioxide transfer is low. Carbon dioxide removal may be less efficient in a lung in which series ventilation of alveoli is prominent (e.g., centrilobular emphysema) than in a lung with other forms of $\dot{V}/\dot{Q}$ mismatch.

If all of the observed $P_{AO_2} - Pa_{O_2}$ is due to $\dot{V}/\dot{Q}$ inequality and none is due to shunt, breathing 100% oxygen should correct the hypoxemia. This is because if the low $\dot{V}/\dot{Q}$ units are ventilated even a little, their nitrogen content is washed out over several minutes so that their alveoli contain only oxygen, carbon dioxide, and water vapor, as follows:

$$P_{AO_2} = P_B - P_{H_2O} - P_{ACO_2}$$

where P_B is barometric pressure and P_{H_2O} is the saturated vapor pressure of water at 37° C (47 mm Hg). This method may be used to determine how much of the observed $P_{AO_2} - Pa_{O_2}$ is due to $\dot{V}/\dot{Q}$ inequality and how much is due to shunt.[74] Inaccuracy may be introduced into this method, converting some low $\dot{V}/\dot{Q}$ units with partly obstructed airways to true shunt because of absorption atelectasis. This has been predicted in theory and observed in adults using the multiple inert gas technique of $\dot{V}/\dot{Q}$ quantitation[75] and in newborn lambs,[76] but it is not seen in adults with bacterial pneumonia.[69]

In a patient with a given degree of $\dot{V}/\dot{Q}$ inequality, the Pa_{O_2} is reduced further by a low partial pressure of venous oxygen

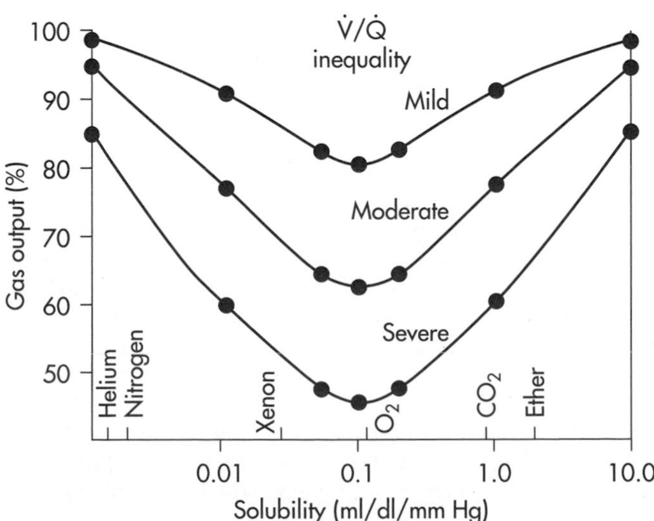

Fig. 26-3. Effect of $\dot{V}/\dot{Q}$ inequality on the transfer of gases of different solubilities in the lung. $\dot{V}/\dot{Q}$ inequality has a greater effect on the transfer of gases of intermediate solubility, such as oxygen, than on the transfer of more soluble gases, such as carbon dioxide, or less soluble gases. (From West JB: *N Engl J Med* 284:1232-1236, 1971.)

($P\bar{v}O_2$). $P\bar{v}O_2$ particularly influences lung units with a low $\dot{V}/\dot{Q}$ ratio or shunt. Measures aimed at raising the $P\bar{v}O_2$ (e.g., by raising cardiac output or reducing whole-body oxygen consumption [$\dot{D}O_2$]) may raise PaO_2 in conditions in which shunt and low $\dot{V}/\dot{Q}$ ratio are prominent (e.g., pneumonia, ARDS).[69,70] Cardiac output may be increased (at the expense of increased myocardial oxygen demand) by the use of plasma volume expansion, vasodilator medications (which improve left ventricular performance by reducing afterload), or inotropic medications such as dopamine.

None of these methods is ideal, however. Plasma volume expansion may increase the water content of the lung, thereby increasing respiratory system elastance and impairing gas diffusion. Vasodilator medications dilate systemic and pulmonary vessels indiscriminately and may increase perfusion and oxygen delivery ($\dot{D}O_2$) to nonessential tissues such as muscle at the expense of essential tissues such as the brain and heart. Some vasodilator medications such as glyceryl trinitrate and sodium nitroprusside may impair hypoxic pulmonary vasoconstriction (HPV), increasing $P_AO_2 - PaO_2$ in the presence of lung disease.[77] Catecholamines such as dopamine, which are used for their inotropic effect, also increase the body's rate of producing oxygen and carbon dioxide, mainly by their effect on fat catabolism.[78] Dopamine and dobutamine both reduce PaO_2 by about 10 mm Hg in patients with severe lung disease by increasing the perfusion of unventilated lung units (shunt) and of low $\dot{V}/\dot{Q}$ lung units.[79]

The use of any of these measures intended to improve oxygenation by raising mixed venous PO_2 depends on whether the potential gains are greater than the potential disadvantages. Trial and error—titrating dose against effect with close observation of blood gases, mixed venous PO_2, and indicators of organ function (conscious state, urine output, and plasma lactate concentration)—is the method generally used.

Causes of $\dot{V}/\dot{Q}$ Inequality. The phasic nature of alveolar ventilation and pulmonary blood flow and the difference in frequency of these two flows mean that instantaneous ventilation and perfusion of the lung are frequently unequal,[80] although the $\dot{V}/\dot{Q}$ ratio averaged over a period of minutes may be equal to 1. In fact, at low inspiratory flow rates, the ratio of ventilation per alveolus at the lung apex compared to ventilation at the base is about 0.6, but this ratio approaches 1 (i.e., ventilation becomes more evenly distributed) as inspiratory flow rate increases.[81] The effect of this is an even greater maldistribution of the $\dot{V}/\dot{Q}$ ratio throughout the lungs at high inspiratory flow rates.

The effect of short-term fluctuations in the $\dot{V}/\dot{Q}$ ratio on gas exchange is buffered by the FRC.[72] For example, after a stepwise reduction in the $\dot{V}/\dot{Q}$ ratio of a lung unit, the PO_2 and PCO_2 in the alveolar gas and end-capillary blood in that lung unit exponentially approach values closer to those in mixed venous blood. The larger the alveolar gas volume in relation to the alveolar ventilation and blood flow, the slower the exponential change. When a series of stepwise changes in the $\dot{V}/\dot{Q}$ ratio in alternating directions occur, the larger the alveolar gas volume (or FRC), the smaller the amplitude of the fluctuations in PO_2 and PCO_2 in alveolar gas and end-capillary blood.

Regional $\dot{V}/\dot{Q}$ Inequality. In the adult lung, blood flow decreases rapidly from the base to the apex, whereas alveolar ventilation decreases less rapidly (Fig. 26-4). Thus the $\dot{V}/\dot{Q}$ ratio is much higher at the lung apex than at the base, and much of the pulmonary blood flow passes through lung units whose $\dot{V}/\dot{Q}$ ratio is less than 1 and whose end-capillary PO_2 is correspondingly low.[41] This means that in the normal upright adult, gas exchange is less efficient than it would be if the $\dot{V}/\dot{Q}$ ratio were 1 in all lung units. Similarly, in the adult lying supine, both ventilation and blood flow increase from ventral to dorsal, whereas in the adult subject lying on one side, both ventilation and blood flow are greater in the dependent lung.

Children differ in the following respects:

1. Because a child's pulmonary artery pressure is similar to an adult's but the child's lung is smaller, more of the child's lung is perfused continuously throughout the cardiac cycle because the pressure in the pulmonary capillaries remains higher than the intraalveolar pressure surrounding the capillaries, even close to the apex of the lung. Because of the child's smaller lung dimensions, the head of hydrostatic pressure that is distending vessels in the lung base is less than that in the adult, so the difference in the vascular radius between the lung base and apex and therefore the difference in pulmonary vascular resistance between the lung base and apex are less and pulmonary blood flow is more evenly distributed over the lung.[58] This effect is often seen in children with high pulmonary artery pressures resulting from left-to-right cardiac shunt or from pulmonary venous hypertension. In these children, blood flow to the lung apex is increased, and flow to the lung bases is reduced.[82]
2. In children younger than 18 years of age, ventilation is distributed preferentially to the upper areas of lung and away from dependent areas.[83]

In young children, the closing volume is higher than the FRC.[84] Airways in dependent areas of the lung are the first to close during expiration and the last to reopen during inspiration, so in infants, inspired gas preferentially ventilates nondependent areas of lung. In humans of all ages, as preinspiratory lung volume decreases below the closing volume, ventilation inhomogeneity increases. Regional variability in static mechanical properties within the lung (especially in elastic recoil) may explain some of the reduced ventilation of the lung bases in children.[85]

The net effect of these two differences is that there is less $\dot{V}/\dot{Q}$ inequality in the lungs of the normal child and adolescent than in the adult. Also, in an adult with unilateral lung disease,

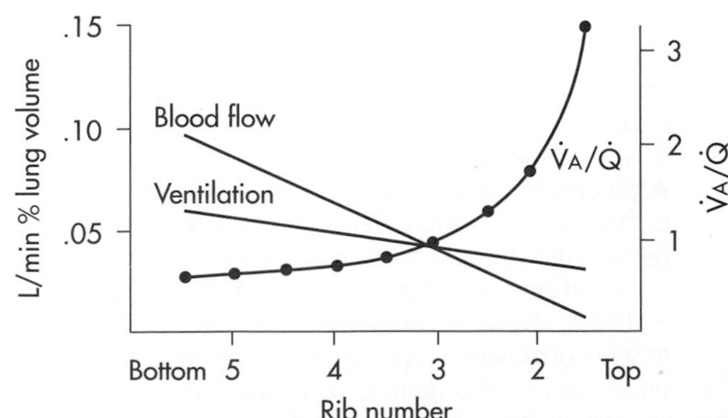

Fig. 26-4. Distribution of ventilation, blood flow, and $\dot{V}/\dot{Q}$ ratio from the base to the apex of the upright lung. *$\dot{V}A/\dot{Q}$*, Alveolar ventilation/perfusion ratio. (From West JB: *Ventilation, blood flow and gas exchange*, ed 3, Oxford, England, 1977, Blackwell, p 30.)

the P_{AO_2} (Pa_{O_2} is greater with the diseased lung in a dependent position, but in a child up to the age of 18 years, the P_{AO_2}–Pa_{O_2} is greater with the diseased lung uppermost.[86,87]

In an adult with unilateral drug disease, gas exchange (especially oxygenation) is consistently better when the patient lies with the normal lung dependent than when the patient lies supine or with the diseased lung dependent. This strategy results in a greater improvement in oxygenation than in carbon dioxide elimination.[88] In contrast, children with unilateral lung disease are managed with the diseased lung dependent, in which position the Pa_{O_2} is usually higher than when the diseased lung is uppermost. Conventional treatment of unilateral pulmonary interstitial emphysema includes managing the child in the decubitus position with the abnormal lung down.[89]

In some newborns, gas trapping in the first few days of life is associated with a raised $P_{AO_2} - Pa_{O_2}$.[43,67] This gas trapping may occur in narrow compliant airways in which occlusive bubbles readily form, and the relative lack of collateral ventilation channels in the newborn lung may contribute to the resulting regional hypoventilation[90] and to $\dot{V}/\dot{Q}$ inequality.

Role of HPV in $\dot{V}/\dot{Q}$ Inequality. Constriction of pulmonary vessels in response to alveolar hypoxia decreases the arterial hypoxemia that occurs with regional alveolar hypoventilation and thereby reduces the $P_{AO_2} - Pa_{O_2}$ in situations of $\dot{V}/\dot{Q}$ inequality and shunt. The smaller the hypoxic segment of lung, the more powerful the HPV and the greater the diversion of blood flow from the hypoxic segment.[91] Thus HPV plays a greater role in the reduction of venous admixture when the hypoxic segments are small and scattered than when a lobe is hypoxic (Fig. 26-5).

According to micropuncture studies, the vessels that constrict in response to hypoxia are the small pulmonary arteries and veins,[92] with the precapillary pulmonary arteries being the most important site of HPV.[93] The principal stimulus to HPV is low

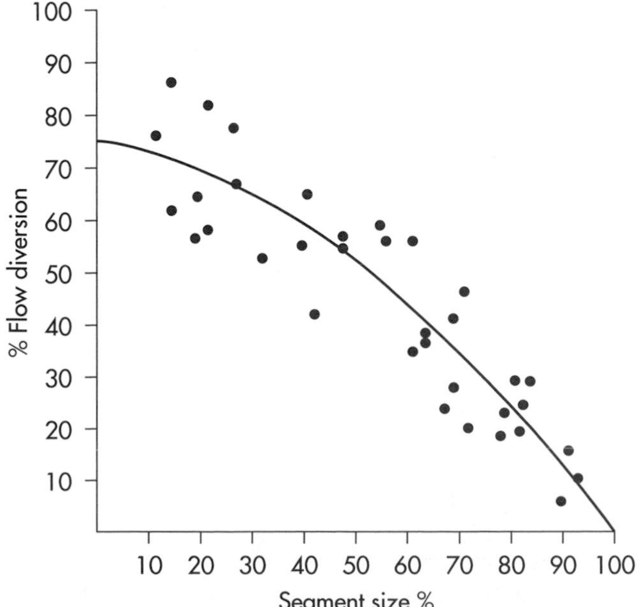

Fig. 26-5. Effectiveness of HPV as the size of the hypoxic segment of lung increases. (From Marshall BE et al: *J Appl Physiol* 51:1543-1551, 1981.)

P_{AO_2}.[58] A major reduction in the mixed venous P_{O_2} can reduce the effectiveness of HPV by reducing the Pa_{O_2} in well-ventilated areas of lung more than in less well-ventilated regions and diverting blood flow to hypoxic areas of the lung, thereby reducing the Pa_{O_2}.[94] Measures that increase the $P\bar{v}_{O_2}$ by increasing cardiac output or by reducing the $\dot{V}_{O_2}$ (e.g., by cooling or the use of muscle relaxants) may therefore be expected to increase the Pa_{O_2} in patients with shunt or $\dot{V}/\dot{Q}$ inequality.[94]

Although the adequate stimulus to HPV (low P_{AO_2}) is known, the nature of the sensor and the mode of stimulus transmission to the vascular smooth muscle cells have not been identified for certain. It appears that some form of chemical messenger is involved: A pulmonary artery to which some lung tissue is adherent contracts in response to hypoxia, and a pulmonary artery from which all lung has been stripped will not contract.[95] Possible chemical messengers include leukotrienes C_4 and D_4 (inhibitors of which suppress HPV),[96] the calcium slow channel (facilitation of calcium entry into cells augments HPV),[97] and oxygen radicals.[93]

Inhibition of endothelial nitric oxide (NO) production by hypoxia is likely to be a major contributor to HPV. NO is an important endothelium-derived relaxing factor that is produced in the pulmonary vascular endothelium and diffuses into the subjacent smooth muscle cells. There it activates guanylate cyclase, which increases the intracellular level of cyclic guanosine monophosphate and results in relaxation of vascular smooth muscle.[98,99] The relaxation of pulmonary vascular smooth muscle induced by NO is impaired by chronic hypoxia but may be restored by the administration of L-arginine, a NO precursor.[100] NO production is reduced by hypoxia in both the adult and the fetal pulmonary arteries.[101,102] However, because the primary stimulus to HPV is in the alveolar gas phase, it is not clear how the stimulus is transmitted to the vascular endothelium to inhibit NO production.

In adults with ARDS, inhaled NO acts as a selective pulmonary vasodilator, reducing pulmonary artery pressure without reducing systemic blood pressure. It also dilates the pulmonary arteries supplying the well-ventilated lung units more than the pulmonary arteries in less well-ventilated units, thereby improving $\dot{V}/\dot{Q}$ matching and increasing Pa_{O_2}.[103]

Lung units with low $\dot{V}/\dot{Q}$ ratios have high P_{ACO_2} values as well as low P_{AO_2} values. An increased P_{CO_2} acts as a pulmonary vasoconstrictor in these lung units, augmenting the effect of the low P_{AO_2}, although the raised P_{CO_2} and its accompanying low pH are each a weaker vasoconstrictor stimulus than hypoxia. The P_{CO_2} in the pulmonary artery, not the alveoli, is the main carbon dioxide vasoconstrictor stimulus.[104]

HPV in the newborn is more vigorous than in the adult and is triggered at a higher P_{AO_2} threshold;[105] despite this, the $P_{AO_2} - Pa_{O_2}$ in the newborn remains higher than in the adult for some days after birth.[59]

$\dot{V}/\dot{Q}$ Inequality in Lung Disease

Neonates. In HMD, early studies using urinary-alveolar nitrogen gradients were unable to demonstrate significant $\dot{V}/\dot{Q}$ mismatch,[106] so all of the observed $P_{AO_2} - Pa_{O_2}$ was attributed to right-to-left shunt, both intrapulmonary shunt and that at the level of the foramen ovale and ductus arteriosus. More recent data show the existence of appreciable $\dot{V}/\dot{Q}$ inequality as well as a shunt component in HMD; up to 40% of the cardiac output passes through high $\dot{V}/\dot{Q}$ lung units, and about 3% passes through low $\dot{V}/\dot{Q}$ units.[107,108] It has been suggested that the commonly observed reduction in P_{AO_2}, which follows a decrease in F_{IO_2} in infants with HMD, means that $\dot{V}/\dot{Q}$ inequality is a major cause of hypoxemia in this condition.[109] However, because extrapulmonary shunting occurs in both HMD and meconium aspiration syndrome and because the amount of shunting is greater at high pulmonary artery pressures, the reduction of F_{IO_2} may increase venous admixture by lowering the P_{AO_2} and thereby increasing HPV, total pulmonary vascular resistance, and the amount of the extrapulmonary shunt. Continuous positive airway pressure increases the total perfusion of lung units with high $\dot{V}/\dot{Q}$ in HMD by recruiting the alveoli of low $\dot{V}/\dot{Q}$ units into the high $\dot{V}/\dot{Q}$ compartment,[107] although it does not appear to recruit completely unventilated alveoli, whose perfusion continues to represent intrapulmonary shunt.[108]

$\dot{V}/\dot{Q}$ inequality contributes significantly to venous admixture in meconium aspiration syndrome,[57] although extrapulmonary shunting at the level of the ductus arteriosus and foramen ovale as well as intrapulmonary shunt cause most of the venous admixture in this condition. In atelectasis and pneumonia in the newborn, there is evidence from animal experiments that inflammatory mediators suppress the local HPV response and thereby exacerbate the arterial desaturation caused by $\dot{V}/\dot{Q}$ inequality to a greater extent than in adults.[90]

Children

ASTHMA. $\dot{V}/\dot{Q}$ inequality is the major source of hypoxemia in asthma, with very little contribution from shunt.[110-112] As the severity of the asthma attack increases, the proportion of the cardiac output that traverses low $\dot{V}/\dot{Q}$ units increases from 10% to 28%.[111,112] In some asymptomatic asthmatic adults, up to 50% of lung units lie behind closed airways. These units have a small $\dot{V}/\dot{Q}$ ratio (i.e., nonshunt) because of collateral ventilation.[110] Although this issue has not been addressed in children, it is possible that shunt may be more prominent in infants, whose collateral ventilation pathways are less well developed.[90]

Adults with moderately severe asthma have a bimodal distribution of $\dot{V}/\dot{Q}$ ratio in the lungs even when their condition is asymptomatic (Fig. 26-6): one peak at $\dot{V}/\dot{Q} = 1$ and another of low $\dot{V}/\dot{Q}$ ratio (approximately 0.1).[110] During an acute asthma attack, it appears that there is no relationship between the 1-second forced expiratory volume (absolute or percent predicted) and measures of $\dot{V}/\dot{Q}$ inequality,[112] possibly because spirometric findings are determined by the resistances of large airways, whereas gas exchange may be more influenced by edema, mucus production, and muscular contraction in small airways.[113] There is also little relationship between the clinical severity of asthma and the degree of $\dot{V}/\dot{Q}$ mismatch, so a patient with the most severe clinical evidence of asthma may have the same $\dot{V}/\dot{Q}$ inequality as a patient with the least clinically severe attack.[113]

Inhaled albuterol abolishes $\dot{V}/\dot{Q}$ inequality in asthmatic children after histamine challenge.[114] $\dot{V}/\dot{Q}$ inequality is unaffected by nebulized albuterol[112] but is exacerbated by intravenous albuterol, intravenous terbutaline,[115] and nebulized isoproterenol[110,112] in adult asthmatics. The difference in effect on $\dot{V}/\dot{Q}$ distribution between the inhaled and the intravenous route is thought to result from the fact that pulmonary vasodilator medications given intravenously dilate the vessels supplying all lung units, including underventilated units, impairing HPV, whereas inhaled pulmonary vasodilator medications act preferentially on well-ventilated lung units to which they have greater access. Thus inhaled NO reduces the $\dot{V}/\dot{Q}$ inequality and $P_{AO_2} - Pa_{O_2}$ in ARDS,[103] and inhaled halothane causes less $\dot{V}/\dot{Q}$ inequality than intravenous sodium nitroprusside for the same total reduction in pulmonary vascular resistance[116] in dogs with pulmonary atelectasis. Infusion of glyceryl trinitrate

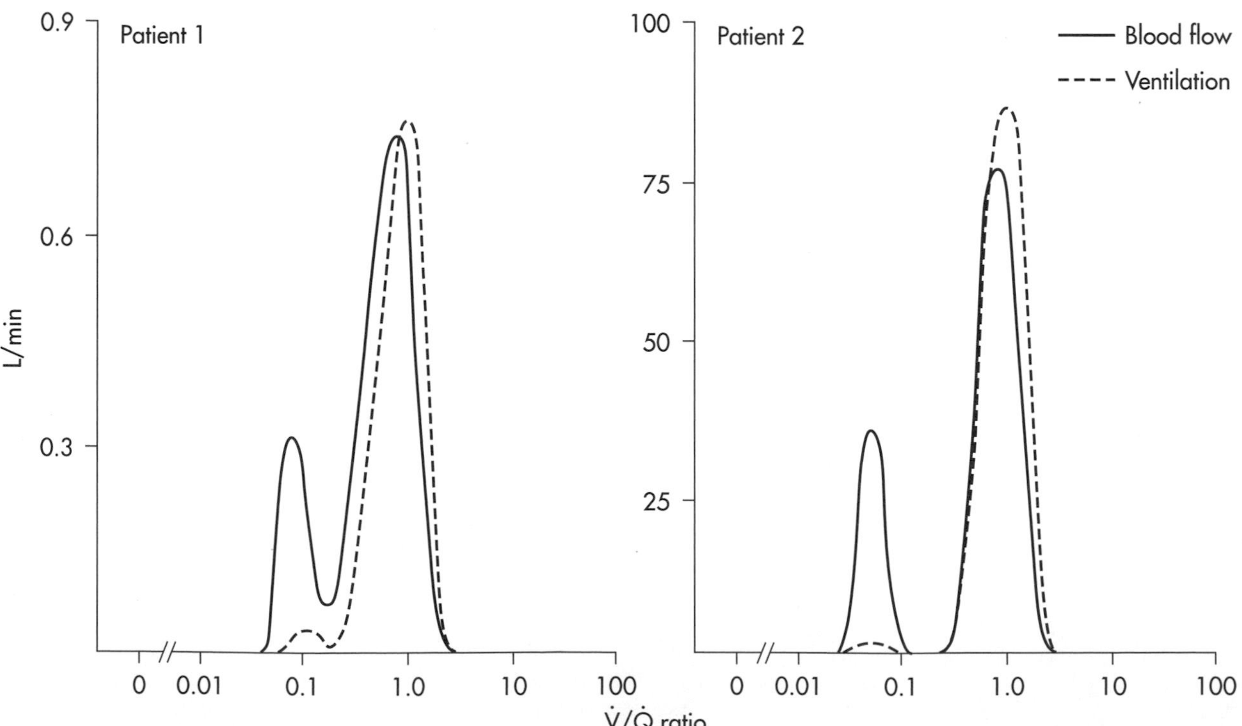

Fig. 26-6. Distribution of ventilation and blood flow between lung units of different $\dot{V}/\dot{Q}$ ratios in two patients with asthma. Note that there is some perfusion of lung units with low $\dot{V}/\dot{Q}$ ratios ($\dot{V}/\dot{Q}$ = 0.1) but that there was no perfusion of lung units with $\dot{V}/\dot{Q}$ = 0 (shunt). (From Wagner PD: *Am Rev Respir Dis* 118:511-524, 1978.)

or prostaglandin E_1 increases the $\dot{V}/\dot{Q}$ inequality and $PAO_2 - PaO_2$ in patients with ARDS.[77] Inhalation of 100% oxygen in asthma increases the $PAO_2 - PaO_2$, either by causing absorption atelectasis in low $\dot{V}/\dot{Q}$ units or by reducing HPV.[111]

Cystic fibrosis. Although intrapulmonary shunt is the main source of $PAO_2 - PaO_2$ in some patients with cystic fibrosis, $\dot{V}/\dot{Q}$ inequality makes a major contribution to hypoxemia in others. The effect of exercise also varies from patient to patient. In some, exercise reduces $\dot{V}/\dot{Q}$ inequality, whereas in others, $\dot{V}/\dot{Q}$ inequality is increased or converted to shunt. Despite an apparent increase in venous admixture with exercise in cystic fibrosis, the PaO_2 is not necessarily reduced.[71] Vasodilator medications reduce the PaO_2 by impairing HPV in cystic fibrosis.[117]

Pneumonia. The role of $\dot{V}/\dot{Q}$ inequality in producing venous admixture varies from patient to patient. In about half of patients with pneumonia, $\dot{V}/\dot{Q}$ inequality makes the major contribution, and shunt is less important.[69] HPV is relatively ineffective at reducing the perfusion of underventilated alveoli in pneumonia.[68,69]

ARDS. Although the majority of patients with ARDS show evidence of some $\dot{V}/\dot{Q}$ inequality,[118] most of the venous admixture found in this condition is due to shunt, and only a small proportion comes from $\dot{V}/\dot{Q}$ mismatch[70] (Fig. 26-7). The shunt fraction appears to be directly related to the amount of pulmonary edema present.

The use of positive end-expiratory pressure ventilation does not reduce the amount of extravascular lung water in ARDS[113] but improves PaO_2 by reducing the blood flow to unventilated alveoli. However, it also increases alveolar dead space by increasing the ventilation of unperfused alveoli.[70]

During the resolution of ARDS, shunts gradually decrease via conversion to normal $\dot{V}/\dot{Q}$ units without passing through a phase of low $\dot{V}/\dot{Q}$ ratio.[113] As the cardiac output increases in ARDS, the shunt fraction also increases, possibly because the raised $P\bar{v}O_2$ resulting from increased cardiac output suppresses HPV in unventilated areas of the lungs. In fact, the effects of raised $P\bar{v}O_2$ on shunt fraction and on end-capillary PO_2 tend to cancel each other out, so PaO_2 does not change as cardiac output increases.[113]

Diffusion Block

In practice it is difficult to separate the contribution of diffusion block to hypoxemia from that of $\dot{V}/\dot{Q}$ inequality because the two almost always occur together. The rates of diffusion of oxygen and carbon dioxide between blood and alveolar gas follows Fick's law:

$$\dot{Q} = k(P_1 - P_2) \times A/T$$

where $\dot{Q}$ is the rate of diffusion of the gas in milliliters per minute, k is a constant, $P_1 - P_2$ is the partial pressure difference of the gas between the alveolus and blood, A is the total area of the alveolar membrane, and T is the thickness of the alveolar membrane. Thus any reduction in the partial pressure gradient for a gas (e.g., resulting from high $PACO_2$ or low $P\bar{v}CO_2$ in the case of carbon dioxide), thickened alveolar-capillary membrane (e.g., resulting from pulmonary edema), or reduced surface area (e.g., resulting from atelectasis) reduces the rate at which that gas is transferred. Carbon dioxide diffuses through the alveolar membrane 20 times faster than oxygen.

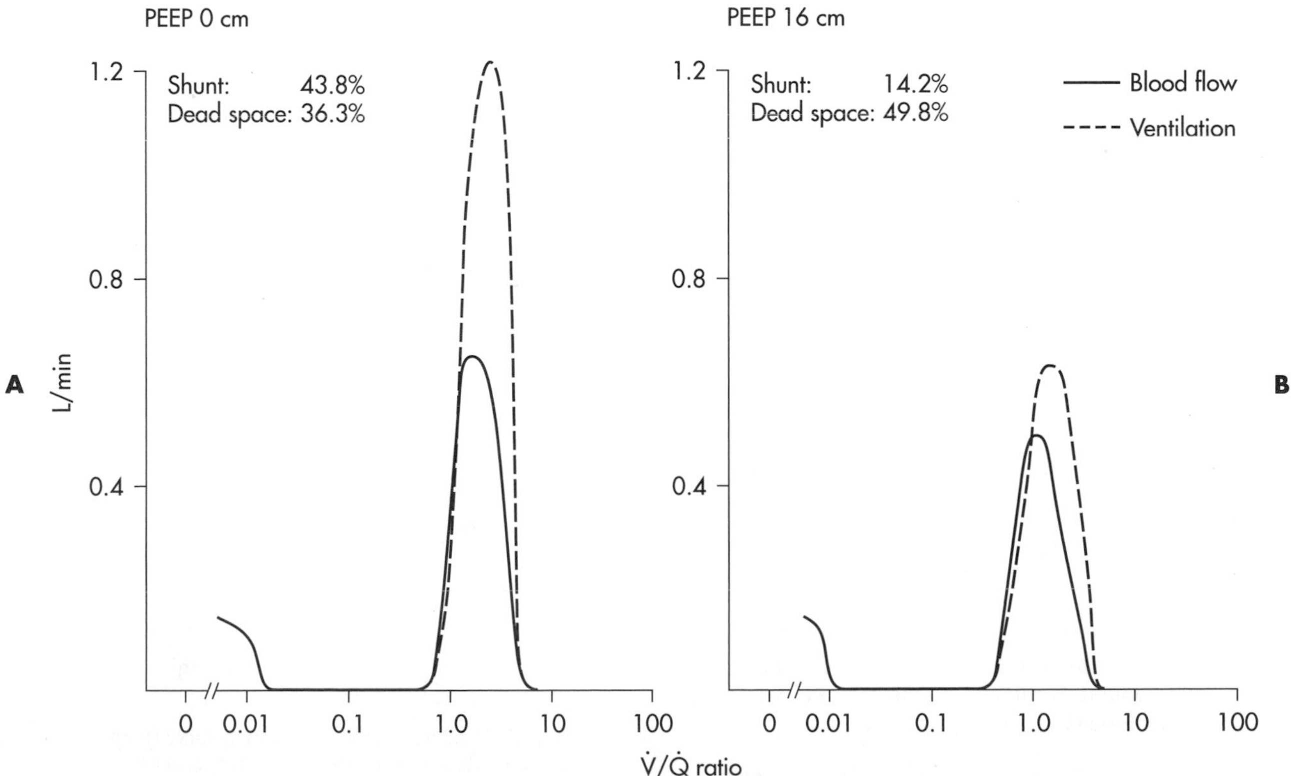

Fig. 26-7. Distribution of ventilation and blood flow between lung units of different $\dot{V}/\dot{Q}$ ratios in ARDS, showing the large contribution of shunt **(A)**. Positive end-expiratory pressure *(PEEP)* improves oxygenation in ARDS by reducing the perfusion of shunt blood flow at the expense of an increase in dead space ventilation **(B)**. (From Dantzker DR: *Am Rev Respir Dis* 120:1039-1052, 1979.)

The passage of oxygen from the alveolus into the blood and thence into red cells to attach to hemoglobin takes a finite minimum time. Each red cell remains in the pulmonary capillary an average of 0.75 second.[41] Normally the hemoglobin is loaded with oxygen by the time it is a third of the way through the pulmonary capillary. However, the time taken for hemoglobin loading is greater when the alveolar membrane is thickened or its area reduced, when the partial pressure gradient is reduced by a low PAO_2 (e.g., at high altitude), and when the circulation transit time is reduced (e.g., in a hyperdynamic circulation).

The diffusion characteristics of the normal lung as measured by the diffusing capacity for carbon monoxide ($\dot{D}LCO$) remain almost constant throughout life.[43] In HMD (in which the alveolar membrane is thickened and the total alveolar area reduced by atelectasis), some studies have shown a reduction in the $\dot{D}LCO$ lasting more than 72 hours after birth despite an increase of the FRC to normal in that time.[119] However, other studies have demonstrated no difference in the $\dot{D}LCO$ between babies with HMD and normal newborns.[72]

A significant reduction in the $\dot{D}LCO$ standardized for total lung capacity has been demonstrated in a variety of childhood illnesses in which the lungs are affected. These include interstitial pulmonary fibrosis,[120] Henoch-Schönlein purpura,[121] the active phase of childhood connective tissue disorders (including juvenile rheumatoid arthritis, systemic lupus erythematosus, and dermatomyositis),[122] interstitial pneumonitis after bone marrow transplantation,[123] amiodarone-induced pneumonitis,[124] and the acute phase of histoplasmosis.[125]

Because $\dot{D}LCO$ and $\dot{V}/\dot{Q}$ inequality have not been studied simultaneously in these conditions, the contribution to hypoxemia of a reduced diffusion capacity independent of $\dot{V}/\dot{Q}$ inequality is not certain. In adolescents and young adults with cystic fibrosis, the presence of a reduced diffusion capacity is associated with marked airflow obstruction and severe arterial desaturation on exercise,[126] although $\dot{V}/\dot{Q}$ inequality makes a much greater contribution than impaired diffusion to hypoxemia in cystic fibrosis.[71]

Oxygen Transport

Oxygen is carried in blood in the dissolved form or as an attachment to hemoglobin for the dissolved form,

$$\text{Dissolved } O_2 = (0.03 \times PO_2) \text{ ml of } O_2/L \text{ of blood}$$

When the PaO_2 is 100 mm Hg, 3 ml of dissolved oxygen is carried per liter of blood for the attached form,

$$O_2 \text{ carried by Hb} = \text{Hb} \times 1.34 \times \% \text{ saturation}/100$$

where *Hb* is the hemoglobin concentration in grams per liter. When the hemoglobin concentration is 150 g/L and the saturation is 100%, hemoglobin carries approximately 200 ml of oxygen per liter of blood.

The oxygen content of arterial blood (CaO_2) is determined by the total cardiac output (Q_T), the physiologic shunt (Q_{PS}), and the oxygen content of mixed venous blood ($C\bar{v}O_2$), plus the end-capillary blood ($Cc'O_2$):

$$CaO_2 = [Q_{PS} \times C\bar{v}O_2 + (Q_T - Q_{PS}) \times Cc'O_2] \times 1/Q_T$$

This assumes that the end-capillary blood comes from lung units with a $\dot{V}/\dot{Q}$ ratio of 1. The physiologic shunt is the total venous admixture needed to produce the observed $PAO_2 - PaO_2$. Part of this shunt is true shunt, and part is "virtual shunt" resulting from perfusion of low $\dot{V}/\dot{Q}$ lung units.

After the mixing of end-capillary and shunt blood, the resulting PaO_2 is determined by the total CaO_2 and the shape of the oxygen-hemoglobin dissociation curve. By Fick's law of diffusion, it is the PO_2 gradient from systemic capillaries to mitochondria rather than the oxygen content of blood that drives the diffusion of oxygen from capillaries to tissues.

Hemoglobin

The production of hemoglobin F ($\alpha_2\gamma_2$), the major hemoglobin of fetal life, declines after 35 weeks' gestation. At term, hemoglobin F accounts for 50% to 60% of the total hemoglobin production, and by 12 weeks after term, it accounts for 5% of hemoglobin production. Adult hemoglobin (hemoglobin A [$\alpha_2\beta_2$]) accounts for 5% to 10% of hemoglobin production at 20 weeks' gestation and 35% to 50% at birth.[127]

Each molecule of hemoglobin can carry four molecules of oxygen, and each gram of hemoglobin carries 1.34 ml of oxygen when fully saturated. The saturation of hemoglobin as the PO_2 varies is described by the oxygen-hemoglobin dissociation curve (Fig. 26-8), whose position is defined by the PO_2 at which the hemoglobin is 50% saturated (P_{50}). The normal P_{50} of hemoglobin A at 37° C and pH of 7.4 is 27 mm Hg. If the curve is shifted to the left (low P_{50}), the percentage of hemoglobin saturation at a given PO_2 is increased. If the alveolar PO_2 is normal, a low P_{50} does not affect oxygen loading in the lungs because the PAO_2 is on the plateau part of the curve, both at a normal (see Fig. 26-8, point *A*) and a low P_{50} (see Fig. 26-8, point *B*). However, in the tissues, the hemoglobin saturation is higher at a prevailing capillary PO_2 when the curve is shifted to the left (see Fig. 26-8, point F) than when

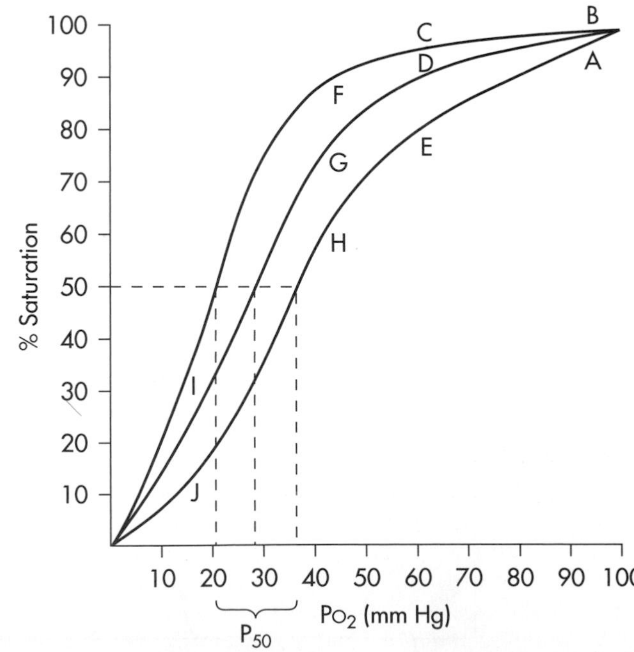

Fig. 26-8. Normal hemoglobin saturation curve (points *G, D,* and *B*), showing the effect of the leftward shift (points *I, F, C,* and *B*) and rightward shift (points *J, H, E,* and *A*) of the curve on the percentage of saturation at different PO_2 values. The dotted lines show the PO_2 values at which hemoglobin is 50% saturated *(P_{50})* of the three curves. See text for details.

the P_{50} is normal (see Fig. 26-8, point *G*). This means that less oxygen is released by the hemoglobin to supply the tissues.

The dissociation curve is shifted to the left by alkalemia, hypothermia, and the presence of hemoglobin F, whose P_{50} is 19 mm Hg. Acidemia, a high Pco_2, hyperthermia, and 2,3-diphosphoglycerate (2,3-DPG) shift the curve to the right. When the dissociation curve is shifted to the right, oxygen is unloaded more readily in the tissues (see Fig. 26-8, points *A* to *H*), but in the presence of a low PAO_2, oxygen loading in the alveolar capillaries is less effective (see Fig. 26-8, points *H* to *E*) than with a normal curve (see Fig. 26-8, points *G* to *B*). In mild hypoxemia, tissue extraction of oxygen is greater when the curve is shifted to the right. (The vertical height between points E [arterial] and H [venous] is greater than that between points D and G.) In severe hypoxemia, however, extraction is greater when the curve is shifted to the left. (The vertical height between points F [arterial] and I [venous] is greater than that between points H and J.)[128]

As previously mentioned, 2,3-DPG bound to hemoglobin shifts the dissociation curve to the right. The major stimulus to the production of 2,3-DPG from the glycolytic pathway in red cells via the Rapoport-Luebering shunt is the hydrogen ion concentration in red cells. At a low Po_2, the hydrogen ion concentration in red cells falls because the buffering capacity of deoxyhemoglobin is greater than that of oxyhemoglobin. In chronic hypoxia of more than 24 hours' duration, this reduction causes an increase in 2,3-DPG production, with a consequent rightward shift of the dissociation curve and enhanced tissue extraction of oxygen.[128] Similarly, hyperventilation (e.g., during a moderately severe asthma attack) reduces the hydrogen ion concentration in red cells and increases 2,3-DPG production.[129]

When the Pco_2 increases, the oxygen-hemoglobin dissociation curve shifts to the right, reducing the percentage of saturation at any given Po_2 and promoting the unloading of oxygen. This effect (the Bohr effect) is mediated mostly by a pH change. In a lung with appreciable $\dot{V}/\dot{Q}$ inequality, the $PAO_2 - Pao_2$ gradient is larger with a curve shifted to the left and smaller with a curve shifted to the right.[130]

Hemoglobin Concentration

Erythropoiesis is regulated by erythropoietin, a cytokine produced in the kidney in response to tissue hypoxia resulting from anemia, hypoxemia, or reduced oxygen carriage (e.g., by carbon monoxide poisoning)[131] but probably not by low cardiac output.[128] As the hematocrit increases, $\dot{D}o_2$ to the tissues increases up to a maximum (Fig. 26-9) and then decreases because blood viscosity and therefore vascular resistance also increase with hematocrit. The amount by which tissue blood flow is reduced by these changes differs among organs.

Transport of Oxygen in Tissues

As arterial blood passes through tissue arterioles and capillaries, oxygen diffuses from the vessels toward the mitochondria (and some extramitochondrial sites), where it is consumed. The Po_2 in normally functioning mitochondria and the minimum mitochondrial Po_2 needed for tissue survival are not known, although a Po_2 of 1 mm Hg or less has been found in working skeletal muscle, isolated perfused working organs, and isolated mitochondria during maximal performance.[132] The rate of oxygen diffusion from capillaries to mitochondria follows Fick's law:

$$\dot{V}o_2 = \dot{D}o_2 \times (Pco_2 - PMo_2)$$

where Pco_2 and PMo_2 are the partial pressures of oxygen in the capillary and mitochondria, respectively,[132] and $\dot{D}o_2$ is the diffusing capacity of the tissue for oxygen. The diffusion capacity is related to the capillary density around the mitochondrion and inversely related to the amount of tissue edema.

The oxygenation of a tissue depends mainly on the oxygen carriage in blood, blood flow through that tissue, and capillary surface area available for oxygen transfer.[133] Red cell flow through a capillary network is under neural, hormonal, and local metabolic control. When the Cao_2 decreases, the oxygen supply to the mitochondria can be maintained by recruiting more capillaries, increasing red cell flow through the capillaries that are already open, or extracting more oxygen from the blood and reducing the oxygen content of blood leaving the capillary network.

The integrated circulatory response of the body to hypoxemia is the net result of neurohumoral and metabolic influences on the cardiovascular system. In all systemic capillary beds, hypoxemia causes vasodilation via the effects of metabolites on vascular smooth muscle, especially in the brain, heart, and working skeletal muscle, which are critically dependent on oxygen for survival and which extract a large proportion of the oxygen presented to them. The peripheral chemoreceptors mediate an increase in the heart rate and cardiac output and vasoconstriction in nonvital organs (e.g., splanchnic bed, resting muscle), which maintains the blood pressure despite vasodilation in the brain and heart and thereby diverts available oxygen toward the vital organs. Perfusion of the brain with hypoxic blood tends to increase the heart rate, stroke volume, and cardiac output.[134] Therefore in hypoxemia, the blood pressure (and organ perfusion pressure) is maintained, and $\dot{D}o_2$ to vital organs is preserved at the expense of nonvital organs.

The response of infants to hypoxemia is qualitatively similar to that of adults, although newborns appear better able to tolerate a lower $\dot{V}o_2$ than older infants, with less metabolic acidosis and oxygen debt, possibly because of a greater ability to restrict the amount of oxygen used for growth.[135] In chronically hypoxemic infants, $\dot{D}o_2$ is augmented by increasing the hematocrit and the tissue capillary density, and growth is re-

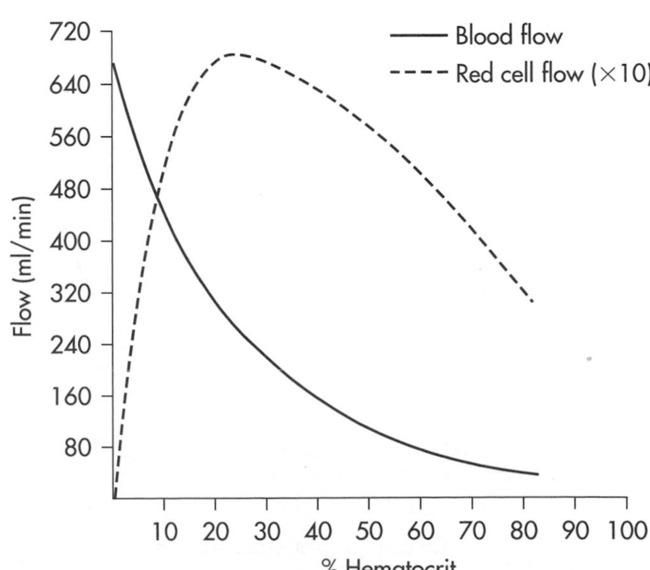

Fig. 26-9. Effect of hematocrit on blood flow and $\dot{D}o_2$ (red cell flow). (Adapted from Crowell JW, Smith EE: *J Appl Physiol* 22:501-504, 1967.)

stricted to make oxygen available for the increased cardiorespiratory work required in hypoxemia.[136]

Whole-body $\dot{D}O_2$ is defined as follows:

$$\dot{D}O_2 = \text{Cardiac output} \times CaO_2$$

whereas whole-body $\dot{V}O_2$ may be calculated from the Fick principle, as follows:

$$\dot{V}O_2 = \text{Cardiac output} \times (CaO_2 - CvO_2)$$

In the normal human, as $\dot{D}O_2$ decreases, $\dot{V}O_2$ remains constant until a critical level of $\dot{D}O_2$ is reached, after which any further reduction in $\dot{D}O_2$ causes a reduction in $\dot{V}O_2$. The critical level of $\dot{D}O_2$ is independent of whether $\dot{D}O_2$ is reduced by hypoxemia, anemia, or low cardiac output.[128] In a resting adult, the critical $\dot{D}O_2$ is 6 to 8 ml/kg/min. In a resting newborn, it has been estimated to be 12 to 15 ml/kg/min, and in older children, it lies between these two ranges.[128]

As intercapillary distance increases, the critical level of $\dot{D}O_2$ also increases, especially in hypoxic hypoxia[137] (Fig. 26-10). Intercapillary distance varies from tissue to tissue (e.g., being greater in adipose tissue than in the heart). It is also increased by tissue edema and vasoconstriction and is reduced by capillary recruitment (e.g., by increased blood pressure or blood volume expansion or local vasodilation). This means that tissues are more vulnerable to hypoxemia when their capillary density is low (e.g., in the presence of hypotension, hypovolemia, vasoconstriction, or edema).

In the splanchnic circulation, the critical $\dot{D}O_2$ is higher than that of the whole animal, so splanchnic $\dot{V}O_2$ becomes supply dependent at a higher level of $\dot{D}O_2$ than in the rest of the body.[138] This is particularly important as the splanchnic circulation undergoes vasoconstriction (and therefore reduction in $\dot{D}O_2$) early in the body's response to hypoxia. Thus hepatic and bowel dysfunction (such as gastric bleeding, paralytic ileus, altered liver enzyme levels, and transmucosal leakage of colonic organisms and endotoxin) are found in severe acute hypoxemia.[139]

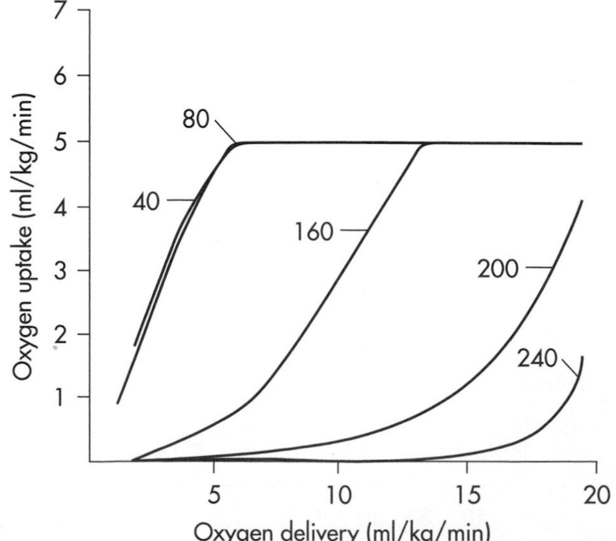

Fig. 26-10. Effect of intercapillary distance on the relationship between $\dot{V}O_2$ and $\dot{D}O_2$. Tissue $\dot{V}O_2$ is markedly reduced at any level of $\dot{D}O_2$ when the intercapillary distance is greater than 80 μm. (From Schumacker PT, Samsel RW: *J Appl Physiol* 67:1234-1244, 1989.)

The normal biphasic relationship may not occur in conditions such as ARDS, sepsis, pulmonary hypertension, and a variety of other respiratory illnesses in critically ill adults, including pneumonia, cardiogenic pulmonary edema, and chronic obstructive pulmonary disease. In these conditions, the $\dot{V}O_2$ is linearly related to $\dot{D}O_2$ over a wide range of $\dot{D}O_2$, often without a $\dot{V}O_2$ plateau being found.[140,141] It has yet to be proved that this so-called supply dependency is a real phenomenon rather than an artifact caused by mathematic coupling in the calculation of $\dot{D}O_2$ and $\dot{V}O_2$ or by spontaneous or iatrogenic catechol-induced variation in metabolic rate.[142]

Metabolic Consequences of Tissue Hypoxia. When the supply of oxygen is adequate for the needs of the tissues, the reduced form of nicotinamide adenine dinucleotide (NADH) that is produced by glycolysis and the tricarboxylic acid cycle is oxidized by electron transport enzymes within the mitochondria (Fig. 26-11). Oxidation of 1 mol of glucose consumes 6 mol of oxygen and produces 6 mol of carbon dioxide and 36 mol of ATP. When the supply of oxygen to the mitochondrion ceases (i.e., below a capillary PO_2 of 20 mm Hg[143]), NADH is not oxidized by the electron transport chain. The surplus NADH reduces pyruvic acid to lactic acid, which then dissociates, as follows:

$$\text{Lactate} - H^+ = H^+ + \text{Lactate}$$

where H^+ is the hydrogen ion. A total of 2 mol of ATP are produced by anaerobic glycolysis per mole of glucose oxidized. Hydrogen ions from the dissociation of lactic acid are partly buffered within the cell and partly in the extracellular compartment, but intracellular and extracellular pH both fall to some extent, and lactate diffuses into the extracellular fluid.

The immediate threat to life from severe hypoxemia comes from its effects on the brain and heart. Minimum levels of ATP and phosphocreatine in the brain are reached within 2 minutes of the onset of severe hypoxemia.[144] The major effects of ATP depletion follow:

1. Hydrolysis of ATP to adenosine monophosphate (AMP) via adenosine diphosphate. AMP is converted to hypoxanthine, which on restoration of oxygen supply, can form the highly toxic superoxide radical. Loss of the nucleotide pool results in prolonged ATP depletion after oxygenation is restored.
2. Loss of potassium from cells, with the influx of sodium, calcium, chloride, and water and consequent cell swelling and loss of extracellular fluid volume.
3. Accumulation of calcium in the mitochondria and cytosol caused by failure of ATP-dependent pumps, which results in membrane lipolysis with consequent cell membrane damage; membrane protein phosphorylation resulting in the dysfunction of membrane receptors and ion channels and the formation of toxic free radicals of oxygen; breakdown of the cytoskeleton; and disaggregation of axonal microtubuli.[144]

Carbon Dioxide Transport

Carbon dioxide is produced by catabolism in the mitochondria and in the cytosol of tissue cells. Adults produce about 3 ml/kg/min, children produce 4.8 ml/kg/min,[145] term newborns produce 5 ml/kg/min, and preterm newborns produce 9 ml/kg/min.[146] Carbon dioxide production is increased by any factor that increases metabolic rate (e.g., exercise, food digestion and absorption, fever, sepsis, trauma [including major surgery and burns]). Catabolism of fat produces about 25% less carbon dioxide per kilojoule (36 ml/kJ) than catabolism of carbohydrate (47 ml/kJ)[147] and is therefore the preferred energy source in patients in whom carbon dioxide elimination is critically limited. About 20 times as much carbon dioxide is produced per mole of ATP during anaerobic catabolism of carbohydrate than by aerobic metabolism. Carbon dioxide is quite fat soluble and therefore crosses cell and capillary membranes rapidly and diffuses from mitochondria and cytosol to blood in tissue capillaries according to Fick's law, as follows:

$$\dot{Q}CO_2 = k \times A/D \times (PmCO_2 - PcCO_2)$$

where $\dot{Q}CO_2$ is the volume of carbon dioxide diffusing from mitochondria to capillaries per minute, *k* is a constant, *A* is the

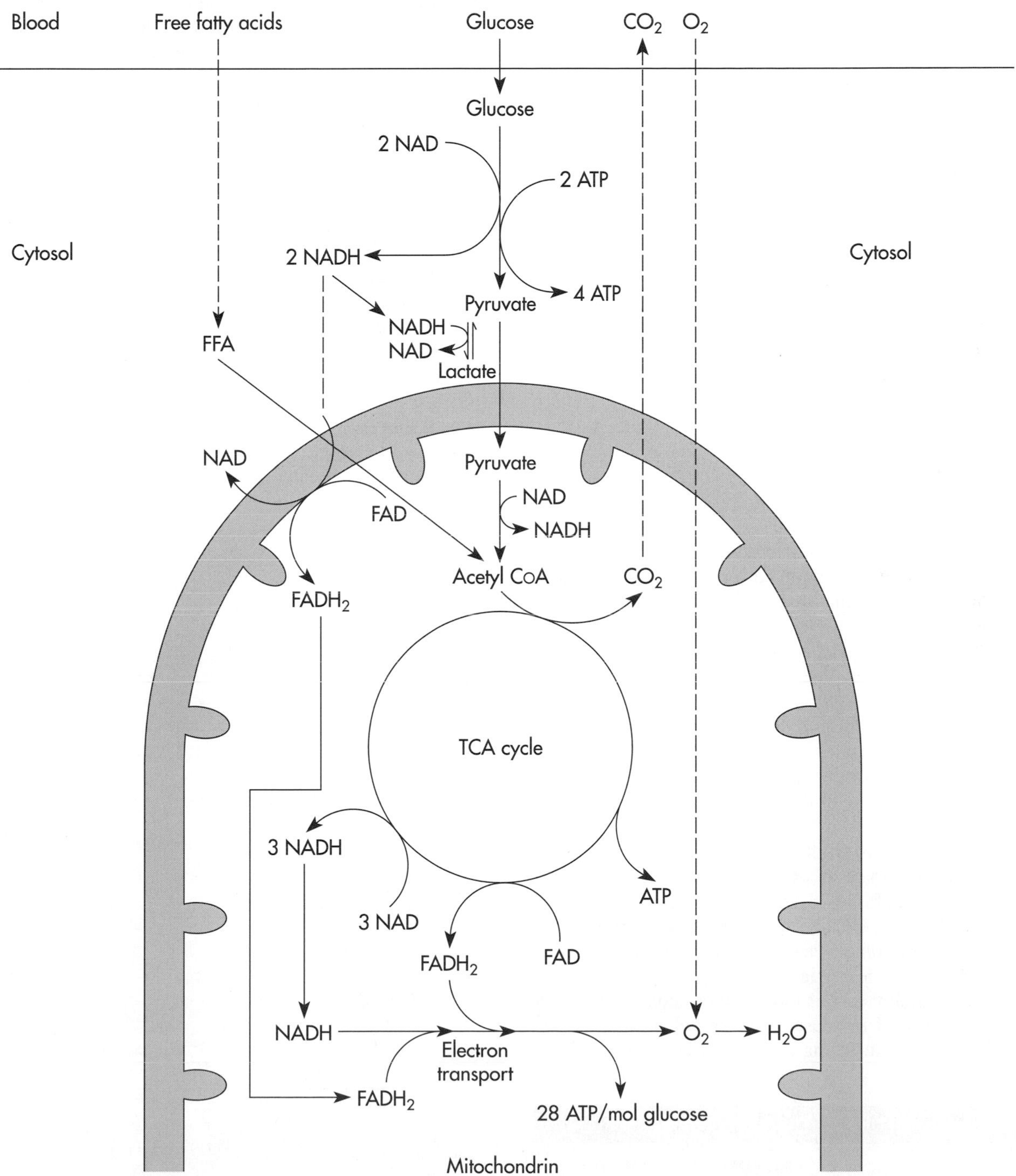

Fig. 26-11. Catabolism of glucose and free fatty acids *(FFA)* to produce energy in the form of ATP, showing the glycolytic pathway in the cytosol and the tricarboxylic acid *(TCA)* cycle in the mitochondrion and the sites of oxygen use and carbon dioxide production. In aerobic conditions, 36 mol of ATP are produced per mole of glucose, and when oxygen supply to the mitochondrion fails, a net 2 mol of ATP are produced per mole of glucose. *NAD,* Nicotinamide adenine dinucleotide; *CoA,* coenzyme A; *$FADH_2$,* reduced form of flavin adenine dinucleotide; *FAD,* flavin adenine dinucleotide.

mean area across which diffusion takes place, D is the mean diffusion distance from the mitochondria to the capillary blood, $Pm\text{CO}_2$ is the $P\text{CO}_2$ in the mitochondrion, and $Pc\text{CO}_2$ is the partial pressure of oxygen in capillary blood. Thus if $P\text{CO}_2$ in capillary blood increases (either because $Pa\text{CO}_2$ increases or because tissue blood flow is very sluggish as a result of low cardiac output or vasoconstriction), then mitochondrial $P\text{CO}_2$ must increase, the volume of carbon dioxide diffusing from mitochondria to capillaries per minute must decrease, or both effects occur. The determinants of $Pa\text{CO}_2$ are the alveolar ventilation and the body's carbon dioxide production per unit time, which in turn depends on the body's metabolic rate and respiratory quotient.

Carbon Dioxide Carriage in Blood

The volume of carbon dioxide carried in arterial blood (480 ml/L)[148] is much greater than the amount of oxygen carried (211 ml/L).[149] Carbon dioxide is carried in three different forms. Carbon dioxide is carried as dissolved carbon dioxide, as follows:

$$\text{Dissolved } CO_2 = (0.72 \times P\text{CO}_2) \text{ ml } CO_2\text{/L of blood}$$

Carbon dioxide is about 20 times as water soluble as oxygen.[148] As carbamino compounds, carbon dioxide combines reversibly with —NH_2 residues on hemoglobin and plasma proteins to form carbamino compounds, as follows:

$$CO_2 \underset{(1)}{\longleftrightarrow} \text{R—NH—COOH} \underset{(2)}{\longleftrightarrow} \text{R—NH—COO}^- + H^+$$

The hydrogen ion (H^+) from reaction 2 is buffered mainly by hemoglobin and plasma proteins.[149]

As bicarbonate, when carbon dioxide diffuses into red cells in the tissues, the red cell enzyme carbonic anhydrase catalyses the formation of carbonic acid (H_2CO_3), as follows:

$$CO_2 + H_2O \underset{(3)}{\longleftrightarrow} H_2CO_3 \underset{(4)}{\longleftrightarrow} H^+ + HCO_3^-$$

Hydrogen ions from reaction 4 are buffered mainly by hemoglobin, and bicarbonate (HCO_3^-) diffuses out of cells in exchange for chloride. Water enters the red cells, which therefore expand in the tissue capillaries and shrink again as carbon dioxide leaves the cell in the lungs. Most carbon dioxide in arterial blood (and most of the arteriovenous carbon dioxide difference) is transported as plasma bicarbonate, which is formed in the red cell (Table 26-1). Because the amount of carbonic anhydrase in red cells greatly exceeds the requirements, more than 90% inhibition of the enzyme activity makes no difference to carbon dioxide carriage.[148]

Reduced hemoglobin carries more carbon dioxide than oxyhemoglobin because of increased carbaminohemoglobin formation and increased buffering capacity (the Haldane effect)

Table 26-1 Carbon Dioxide Transport to the Lungs

	CARRIED IN ARTERIAL BLOOD	EXCRETED BY LUNGS
Dissolved carbon dioxide	5%	10%
Carbaminohemoglobin	5%	30%
Bicarbonate	90%	60%

From West JB: In West JB, ed: *Physiological basis of medical practice,* ed 12, Baltimore, 1991, Williams & Wilkins, pp 538-545.

(Fig. 26-12). This effect is responsible for 35% to 40% of carbon dioxide carriage in the fetus and adult.[150]

In the lungs, all of these processes are reversed, and carbon dioxide diffuses from red cells and plasma across the alveolar membrane into the alveoli. As previously mentioned, the process of diffusion is not instantaneous but takes a finite time. Similarly, the reactions involved in carbon dioxide transport take a finite time: Bicarbonate-chloride exchange takes 400 to 500 msec to achieve 90% completion, and the Haldane effect takes 250 to 300 msec to 90% completion.[148] Because each red cell spends 0.4 to 1.2 seconds in the pulmonary capillary, these finite times mean that carbon dioxide transfer is incomplete when the red cell leaves the lung capillary. This contributes less than 1 mm Hg to $P\text{ACO}_2 - P\text{ACO}_2$ in normal lungs at rest and about 6 mm Hg in normal lungs on maximal exercise,[151] and it may produce significant respiratory acidosis when regional pulmonary vasoconstriction in lung disease diverts the cardiac output through relatively few capillaries and red cell transit times are shortened.[148]

Effects of Raised $Pa\text{CO}_2$

Effects on the Central Nervous System. Carbon dioxide depresses neuronal excitability in a way similar to that of gases such as helium and nitrous oxide. Neuronal intracellular pH depression caused by carbon dioxide (see later section) also depresses neuronal activity. In particular, reduced excitation of the reticular activating system causes unconsciousness, and depression of the respiratory center causes hypoventilation and apnea. In dogs, no narcotic effect is evident below a $Pa\text{CO}_2$ of 95 mm Hg, but a $Pa\text{CO}_2$ greater than 245 mm Hg causes anesthesia.[152]

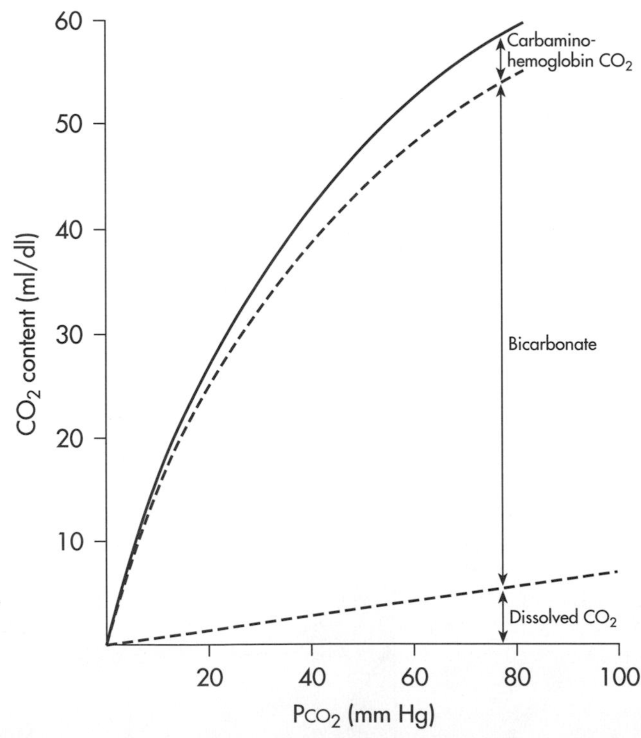

Fig. 26-12. Carbon dioxide dissociation curve for whole blood *(continuous line).* Oxyhemoglobin *(upper dotted line)* carries less carbon dioxide as carbamino compounds than reduced hemoglobin (Haldane effect). The dissociation curve is virtually a straight line over the normal physiologic range of $P\text{CO}_2$. (Adapted from Swenson ER, Hlastala MP. In Chernick V, Mellins RB, eds: *Basic mechanisms of pediatric respiratory disease: cellular and integrative,* Philadelphia, 1991, BC Decker, p 148.)

Carbon dioxide diffuses rapidly across the blood-brain barrier, whereas the bicarbonate concentration in cerebrospinal fluid takes 12 to 24 hours to equilibrate with plasma.[153] Over the range of 20 to 100 mm Hg, an increasing $Pa{CO_2}$ causes cerebral vasodilation as a result of an altered pH of the brain extracellular fluid. This results in increased cerebral blood flow, intracranial blood volume, and intracranial pressure. After several days of hypercapnia, pumping of bicarbonate into the cerebrospinal fluid by the choroid plexus epithelial cells returns the pH of cerebrospinal fluid to normal. Cerebral blood flow approaches normal,[154] and the cerebral vasodilator response to further increases in $Pa{CO_2}$ is blunted.[155]

Effects on the Cardiovascular System. Acute hypercapnia[156] reduces myocardial contractility by acutely reducing intracellular pH in the myocardial cell. Myocardial contractility (rate and magnitude of pressure development and maximal extent of shortening) reaches a minimum after 2 minutes of hypercapnia and returns to about 66% of control values after 14 minutes of hypercapnia.[157] Superimposed on this negative inotropic effect are systemic vasodilation resulting from a direct depressant effect of carbon dioxide on vascular smooth muscle as well as the intense sympathetic discharge provoked by hypercapnia and its resulting tachydysrhythmias, including supraventricular tachycardia and ventricular extrasystoles.[156]

Hypercapnia increases blood flow to the brain and heart, and hypocapnia reduces blood flow to both vital organs. Hypercapnia also increases skin, splanchnic, and liver blood flow[158] and reduces flow to skeletal muscle.[40] When extreme hypercapnia persists for several hours, myocardial depression reduces cardiac output, causing decreased blood flow to all organs.[40]

Respiratory Effects of Hypercapnia. Hypercapnia affects respiration in several ways, as follows:

1. Increased $PA{CO_2}$ displaces oxygen, reducing the $PA{O_2}$ and thereby the $Pa{O_2}$.
2. The Bohr effect occurs (see previous section).
3. Hypercapnia causes pH-dependent pulmonary vasoconstriction.
4. Skeletal muscle performance (including the performance of the diaphragm and other respiratory muscles) is depressed by hypercapnia. This effect appears to be mediated by a low intracellular pH in the myocytes.[159]

Salt and Water Retention. Salt and water retention are often seen in chronic hypercapnia, possibly as a result of high right atrial pressure in cor pulmonale. The resulting reduced glomerular filtration rate and raised renal vein pressure and aldosterone levels tend to reduce sodium and water excretion despite the countervailing influence of atrial natiuretic peptide.[156]

Acid-Base Effects of Hypercapnia. Carbonic acid (H_2CO_3) dissociates to form hydrogen ion and bicarbonate (HCO_3^-) according to the Henderson-Hasselbalch equation, as follows:

$$pH = pKa + \log (HCO_3^-/H_2CO_3)$$

which may be modified as follows:

$$pH = pKa + \log(HCO_3^-/0.03 \times P{CO_2})$$

where *pKa* is the negative logarithm of the dissociation coefficient of H_2CO_3.

A buffer is most effective at a pH equal to its pKa. Carbonic acid and bicarbonate are an effective buffer pair in body fluids despite their pKa (6.1) differing markedly from 7.4, because the concentration of carbon dioxide can be controlled by the respiratory system and the concentration of bicarbonate can be controlled by the kidneys. Because changing the concentration ratio of any buffer pair automatically changes the ratios of all other buffer pairs, variation in the carbonic acid–bicarbonate ratio is the means by which the body controls its own pH.

Carbon dioxide, being fat soluble, crosses cell membranes more rapidly than bicarbonate, which is hydrophilic. On entering cells, carbon dioxide is hydrated to form carbonic acid, which dissociates, forming hydrogen ions and lowering intracellular pH. Any variation of body pH (especially intracellular pH) on either side of a narrow optimum range reduces enzyme-substrate binding, enzyme activity, and the regulatory activity of proteins, including hormone receptors, membrane proteins, and structural proteins. In many cases, the effect of pH is mediated by changes in the dissociation of imidazole side chains of histidine, with resulting effects on protein subunit association, protein folding, and the proteins' active site.[160]

Infusion of bicarbonate has been recommended in the past to correct metabolic acidosis in hypercapnic asthmatic patients.[161,162] However, sodium bicarbonate infusion increases blood $P{CO_2}$ and reduces intracellular pH in the brain, liver, and skeletal muscle, both in humans with metabolic acidosis and in animals.[163] When sodium bicarbonate is added to closed systems from which carbon dioxide cannot be removed (such as the human with severe hypercapnic respiratory failure), extracellular and intracellular carbon dioxide concentrations increase, and intracellular pH falls, with the ill effects previously described. Therefore bicarbonate infusion is not recommended in respiratory failure.

In children as in adults, pH is inversely proportional and the bicarbonate concentration is directly proportional to the $P{CO_2}$ over the range of 15 to 90 mm Hg.[148,164] The pH decreases by 0.01 pH unit for each increase of 1 mm Hg in the $P{CO_2}$, whereas the bicarbonate level increases by 0.2 mM/L for each increase of 1 mm Hg in the $P{CO_2}$.[148]

In response to an increase in the $Pa{CO_2}$, the cells of the proximal renal tubule increase their reabsorption of bicarbonate by increasing sodium-bicarbonate cotransport across the basal membrane and increasing hydrogen ion–sodium antiport activity across the luminal membrane.[165] In the presence of hypocapnia, bicarbonate reabsorption by the proximal tubule is suppressed, and acid secretion (i.e., of ammonium and nonvolatile acid) is reduced. The net effect is a minor loss of bicarbonate in the urine and significantly reduced urine acidification.[148] These renal responses are minimal until at least 1 hour after a stepwise change in $Pa{CO_2}$ and are not complete for 4 to 6 days,[153] and full compensation depends on the adequacy of renal function.

The ability of the newborn to compensate for hypercapnia is limited by a lower renal bicarbonate threshold in the first year of life (21.5 to 22.5 mM/L) than in adulthood (24 to 28 mM/L), although the maximum rate of absorption in the newborn and the adult are similar.[166] In addition, the human neonate is less able to secrete titratable acid and ammonium than the adult, which further limits the infant's ability to compensate for respiratory acidosis up to the age of 2 years.[166] In the normal term neonate, urine cannot be acidified below a pH of 6.0.[167]

Supercarbia. Despite the limited ability of human infants and children to compensate for respiratory acidosis, long-term follow-up of children who have suffered episodes of "supercarbia" ($Paco_2$ > 150 mm Hg) has not demonstrated any adverse neurodevelopmental effects attributable to the episode of extreme hypercapnia.[168,169]

LUNG WATER AND PULMONARY EDEMA

Pulmonary edema is the accumulation of abnormal amounts of fluid in the extravascular spaces of the lung and is common in many conditions. The primary site of pathology may be pulmonary (e.g., aspiration pneumonitis) or elsewhere (e.g., cardiomyopathy). Although many diverse conditions can lead to pulmonary edema, they all do this via at least one of a small number of mechanisms. The presence of excess fluid in the airspaces decreases lung compliance, increases airway resistance, and impedes gas exchange; hence respiratory failure is a common endpoint.

Water Turnover in the Normal Lung

The normal lung is approximately 80% water by weight. Approximately 25% of this water is within the pulmonary circulation, and the remaining (extravascular) water is within the interstitial spaces and pulmonary lymphatics.[170] Less than 0.5 µm of tissue separates water that is under hydrostatic pressure in the capillary circulation from the alveolar airspaces; therefore maintenance of the barrier that prevents water from flooding the airspaces is critical to the preservation of alveolar gas exchange.

Water distribution at the level of the alveolar-capillary gas exchange unit can be considered as being in four compartments: vascular, interstitial, alveolar, and lymphatic. There is a continual flux of water from the vascular compartment, via the interstitial compartment, to the lymphatic compartment. This compartmental model allows consideration of normal and pathologic mechanisms but is an oversimplification of the real situation. In the normal lung, alveolar arterioles and venules contribute significantly to the water flux from the circulation to the pulmonary lymphatic system, and some of the water that passes from the vascular compartment to the interstitium is reabsorbed into the circulation at other locations.

The vascular compartment is separated from the interstitial space by the capillary endothelium, which is thought to be relatively permeable to water and small molecules but not to circulating proteins. The alveolar compartment is separated from the interstitial space by its epithelium, which is much less permeable to fluids and solutes. The alveolar-capillary interstitial space is continuous with that of the perivascular and peribronchial regions and thus with the lymphatic system that drains these spaces.

Pulmonary arterial pressure produces a positive hydrostatic pressure within the vascular compartment, whereas the forces of elastic recoil probably produce a subatmospheric pressure within the lung interstitium. This hydrostatic pressure difference tends to move fluid out of the capillary circulation into the interstitial space. However, because the endothelial membrane is impermeable to macromolecules, an osmotic gradient tends to keep water within the vascular compartment. The hydrostatic force varies considerably from the highest to the lowest point in the lungs, but on average, it exceeds the osmotic force. Hence there is a small, continuous flux of fluid from the vascular compartment to the interstitial space. Because the alveolar epithelial membrane is relatively impermeable, this fluid tracks to the perivascular and peribronchial interstitium, where it flows into the pulmonary lymphatic system.

The capillary endothelial and alveolar epithelial membranes are composed of single layers of cells. At the point where the two layers touch, the basement membranes are fused, and there is no true interstitial space. Where the two layers are not in direct contact, there is an interstitial space consisting of a matrix of proteins and proteoglycans.[171,172] The passage of water and solutes between the compartments is determined by the membrane structures, and the flow through the interstitium is affected by the properties of the matrix. Substances may cross membranes either between the cells or through them. The endothelial and epithelial membranes vary in both their transcellular and pericellular permeability.

The endothelial membrane is formed from a homogeneous cell type with relatively permeable cell-to-cell junctions (gap junctions, tight junctions, and zonula adherens), and most flux occurs between the cells. Transcellular fluid and solute flux can occur,[173] but the degree to which it contributes to the permeability of the endothelial membrane is controversial.

The alveolar epithelial membrane is made up from two different cell types (types I and II), and they vary in their mechanisms of transcellular fluid transport. The epithelial membrane is characterized by tight apposition at the cell-to-cell junctions. The membrane has well-developed mechanisms for the active transcellular transport of ions and hence water. In fetal life the active transport of chloride into the alveolar space leads to the secretion of fluid into the alveoli. This is the source of the "lung fluid" that passes up the airway and into the amniotic cavity.[174] In postnatal life, the active transport of sodium out of the airspace results in reabsorption of water that may have leaked into the alveolus.[175] This mechanism becomes more active during healing after alveolar injury. Type II alveolar cells may be more active in the reabsorption of sodium and water than the type I cells, and this fits with the observation that type II cells are not prominent until toward the end of fetal maturation but are very prominent in the healing lung.

Pulmonary edema occurs when the rate of fluid flux out of the vascular compartment exceeds the rate at which it can be cleared from the lung. A number of safety mechanisms help prevent the accumulation of excessive amounts of extravascular water. First, if an increased amount of fluid but not protein passes from the vascular to the interstitial compartment, then the osmotic gradient between the compartments increases and encourages fluid to remain within the circulation. This mechanism cannot occur if there is a pathologic increase in endothelial protein permeability. Second, the perivascular interstitium has limited capacitance, and fluid accumulation quickly increases the interstitial hydrostatic pressure and thus reduces the flux of water. Third, the pulmonary lymphatic system has a tremendous reserve capacity and can clear interstitial fluid formation at a rate at least 10 times the basal level.[170,176] Fourth, accumulation of interstitial fluid leads to hyperpnea (possibly by the stimulation of juxtacapillary J receptors), and increased breathing movements augment pulmonary lymphatic flow.

Formation of Pulmonary Edema

Pulmonary edema occurs when the rate of fluid flux from the vascular to the interstitial compartment exceeds the rate at which it can be cleared by reabsorption or by the lymphatic system. It is thought that a phase of interstitial edema appears first and that later, fluid leaks through the epithelial membrane to form alveolar edema.

The route by which interstitial fluid leaks into the alveolus is still uncertain. It may be that fluid breaches the cell-to-cell junctions of the alveolar epithelial membrane,[177] or it may be that fluid tracks to the peribronchiolar interstitium and then through the more permeable epithelium of the terminal bronchioles and back into the alveoli.[176,178,179] In lung injury from noxious substances that have been inhaled (e.g., toxic gas) or aspirated (e.g., gastric acid), direct leak through the damaged alveolar epithelium is most likely.

Etiology of Pulmonary Edema

The various causes of pulmonary edema (Box 26-4) may be classified by primary abnormality into two types: increased hydrostatic pressure (Box 26-5) or increased permeability. Although convenient, this classification ignores the fact that in many conditions, both types of edema coexist. For example, the edema associated with increased pulmonary microvascular hydrostatic pressure in left-sided heart failure is often exacerbated by an increase in capillary endothelial permeability brought about by stretching of the porous cell-to-cell junctions. In inflammatory lung diseases such as ARDS and pneumonia, in which the permeability of the capillary endothelium to proteins increases, the osmotic gradient that resists fluid flux into the interstitium is reduced. The resulting increase in extravascular lung water is greatly exacerbated by increases in capillary hydrostatic pressure (e.g., resulting from left ventricular dysfunction or the administration of plasma expanders). If colloid plasma expanders are infused as the capillary permeability is increased, the colloid molecules (human serum albumin, gelatin, dextran, and starch) enter the interstitial space; when the endothelium again becomes impermeable to protein and colloids, the osmotic gradient between the plasma and lung interstitium remains low, and the duration of pulmonary edema is prolonged.[180]

More details on the mechanisms of pulmonary edema formation, clinical features, and management are given in the chapters dealing specifically with the relevant conditions, but some miscellaneous conditions are covered here.

BOX 26-4
Causes of Pulmonary Edema Classified by Mechanism

Increased hydrostatic pressure gradient

Increased capillary pressure (see Box 26-5)
Decreased interstitial pressure
  Upper or lower airway obstruction
  Lung reexpansion

Increased permeability

Pneumonia (bacterial or viral)
ARDS
Generalized sepsis
Aspiration
Near-drowning
Inhalation of smoke or toxic gases
Thermal inhalation injury
Oxygen toxicity
Hypersensitivity reactions

Decreased oncotic pressure gradient

Decreased intravascular oncotic pressure
  Hypoalbuminemia
  Water overload
Increased interstitial oncotic pressure secondary to increased permeability

Decreased lymphatic drainage

Congenital pulmonary lymphangiectasis
Decreased drainage after lung transplantation

Uncertain or mixed pathogenesis

Neurogenic pulmonary edema
Narcotic abuse

Increased Permeability of the Alveolar-Capillary Membrane

Increased permeability of the alveolar-capillary membrane may occur as a direct result of the primary disease mechanism (e.g., inhaled toxins, bacterial toxins) or the effects of circulating mediators (e.g., cytokines, eicosanoids, complement). Neutrophil adhesion to the pulmonary capillary endothelium, which is mediated by selectin or integrin complexes or by platelet-activating factor on the endothelial cell membrane, leads to the release of proteases or oxygen-derived free radicals. Depletion of endothelial cell ATP production caused by oxidant damage impairs the membrane sodium-potassium pump, leading to osmotically induced cell swelling. Disassembly of the cytoskeleton as a result of paucity of ATP contributes to the endothelial cells' becoming globular in shape, opening up intercellular tight junctions, and increasing microvascular permeability.[181]

Decreased Oncotic Pressure Gradient

Hypoproteinemia, either as a primary condition (e.g., in liver disease or malnutrition) or as a result of water overload, does not usually lead to pulmonary edema. However, it may exacerbate the edema associated with other conditions. For example,

BOX 26-5
Causes of Increased Capillary Pressure Classified by Primary Site

Increased systemic arterial pressure

Aortic coarctation
Renal hypertension

Increased left atrial pressure

Mitral valve disease
Cor triatriatum

Increased pulmonary venous pressure

Obstructed anomalous pulmonary venous drainage
Pulmonary venoocclusive disease
Mediastinal tumor or fibrosis

Increased left ventricular end-diastolic pressure

Aortic valve disease
Left ventricular outflow obstruction
Cardiomyopathy (including anthracycline toxicity)
Myocarditis
Myocardial ischemia
Pericarditis or effusion
Dysrhythmias

excessive infusion of crystalloid solutions greatly increases extravascular lung water in a patient with raised capillary hydrostatic pressure caused by left ventricular failure.

Decreased Interstitial Pressure

A small number of children with acute obstruction, particularly of the upper airway (e.g., laryngotracheobronchitis, epiglottitis, laryngospasm) develop pulmonary edema.[182] This can occur after even very brief periods of obstruction[183] and is often manifested only after the obstruction has been relieved by endotracheal intubation. A simplistic view of the etiology suggests that decreased interstitial hydrostatic pressure tends to draw water across the capillary endothelium into the interstitial space. The reason that fluid enters the alveolar airspace is less clear, as is the reason that often the edema appears only after removal of the obstruction. Other factors that may be important include an increase in capillary endothelial permeability caused by hypoxia and a shift of blood from the systemic to the pulmonary circulation as a result of circulating catecholamines.

Neurogenic Pulmonary Edema

Brain injury from a variety of causes (e.g., trauma, hypoxia-ischemia, meningitis) is sometimes complicated by the development of pulmonary edema. The mechanisms have not been well studied in humans, but a number of experimental animal models of brain injury have given some insight into the causes.

The pathogenesis of neurogenic pulmonary edema is thought to result mainly from increased capillary hydrostatic pressure, but the relatively high protein content of the edema fluid suggests that the increased permeability of the alveolar-capillary membrane may also be important. The main feature of neurogenic pulmonary edema is the activation of both the neural and humoral components of the sympathetic nervous system.[184,185] Generalized vasoconstriction leads to a shift of circulating volume to the pulmonary circulation. Systemic vasoconstriction increases left ventricular afterload, and relative left ventricular failure tends to increase pulmonary capillary pressure. The increased permeability, previously documented, may result from stretching of the porous cell-to-cell junctions or from endothelial damage caused by some circulating mediators (not yet proved). The hemodynamic disturbances described can be transient; yet the features of pulmonary edema can persist for much longer. This suggests that the circulatory changes may be the initial event and that damage to the capillary endothelium with protein leakage causes the condition to persist.

Disturbances in Lung Function Caused by Pulmonary Edema

The development of pulmonary edema profoundly affects the mechanical and gas-exchanging properties of the lungs. Lung compliance is reduced by several mechanisms. The presence of large amounts of interstitial edema reduces the distensibility of the lungs and promotes the collapse of the alveoli and small airways. Flooding of the alveoli with fluid physically disrupts the surfactant layer at the air-fluid interface, and the presence of protein and cellular debris impairs the activity of surfactant.[186,187] These effects lead to greatly increased surface tension in the fluid lining of small airspaces and tend to collapse these spaces (atelectasis). Airway resistance is increased by the physical presence of fluid in the small airways and by the compression of the small airways by fluid that has accumulated in the peribronchial interstitium. The combined effects of reduced lung compliance and increased airway resistance greatly increase the work of respiration, which may lead to respiratory muscle fatigue and respiratory failure.

The gas-exchanging properties of the lung are impaired by the presence of pulmonary edema. Interstitial edema probably causes only a small reduction in gas exchange because the fused basement membranes of the alveolar-capillary membrane prevent accumulation of fluid at this point. Alveolar edema significantly impairs oxygenation. Lung units may be unventilated because they are flooded with fluid or because the airways supplying them are obstructed. Blood flow to unventilated lung units may be reduced by hypoxic vasoconstriction, but significant $\dot{V}/\dot{Q}$ mismatch usually remains with consequent hypoxemia.

Hyperventilation with hypocapnia is a common feature in the early course of pulmonary edema. Arterial hypoxemia and anxiety probably provoke increased ventilation. Stimulation by edema of the J receptors in the airways also leads to rapid, shallow respirations.

Pulmonary arterial hypertension is a frequent feature of pulmonary edema. It may lead to right-sided heart failure if sufficiently severe. Pulmonary hypertension is probably a result of hypoxic vasoconstriction in poorly ventilated lung units and direct vascular compression from edema in the perivascular interstitium.

Summary

Pulmonary edema is a feature of many conditions of diverse etiology. The effects on lung mechanics and gas exchange make it one of the common causes of respiratory failure.

CARDIORESPIRATORY INTERACTIONS

Interactions among the functions of the circulatory and respiratory systems are very complex.[188] The functions of the respiratory system have a modest effect on cardiac function under normal conditions, and this effect may vary qualitatively or quantitatively if there is respiratory or cardiac disease.

Physiologic Cardiorespiratory Interactions

Diagrams of the circulatory and respiratory system often show the right and left sides of the heart as two separate pumps connected in series via the circulation of the lungs. This is obviously a gross oversimplification. The facts that the two sides of the heart share a common muscular septum, share common circular muscle fibers, and are enclosed together in the pericardial cavity (Fig. 26-13) mean that they do not act independently. Similarly the fact that the two sides of the heart and the pulmonary circulation are contained, along with the rest of the lung tissues, within the closed thoracic cavity means that changes in lung volume and intrathoracic pressure influence circulatory function.

The output from either cardiac ventricle is determined by its venous filling (preload), the force of muscular contraction (contractility), and the pressure gradient against which it has to eject (afterload). The afterload is determined by the transmural pressure gradient, which is the difference in pressure between

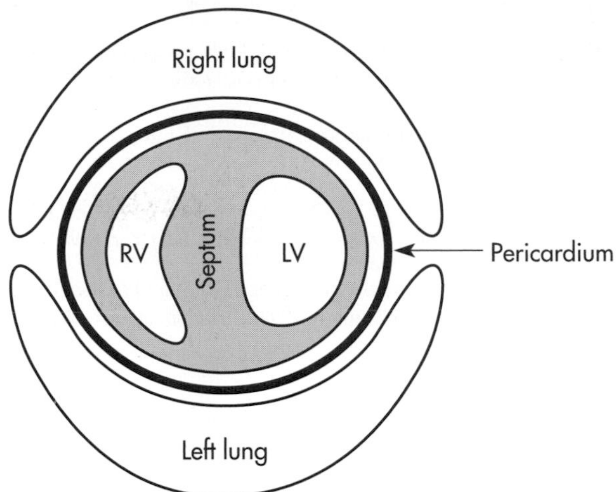

Fig. 26-13. Diagrammatic cross section of the cardiac ventricles and lungs, which interact during respiration and the cardiac cycle. The right ventricle *(RV)* and left ventricle *(LV)* share a common septum, and the right is wrapped around the left. The muscle fibers of the free walls of the two ventricles are in continuity. The pericardial sac surrounds the two ventricles and in turn is surrounded by the lungs, pleura, and chest wall. See text for details of this interaction. (From Robotham JL. In Montenegro HD, ed: *Chronic obstructive pulmonary disease*, New York, 1984, Churchill Livingstone, pp 183-217.)

the ventricular cavity and the surrounding intrathoracic pressure. The output of either ventricle may also be influenced by the pressure or volume of the other ventricle. The anatomic reasons for this ventricular interdependence have already been outlined.

Changes in intrathoracic pressure have differing effects on the preload and afterload of the two ventricles. The capacitance vessels (veins), which supply the right ventricle, lie outside the thoracic cavity, whereas the arterial circulation that the ventricle supplies is within this cavity. The reverse is true for the left ventricle.

Effects of Spontaneous Respiration in a Healthy Subject

Table 26-2 outlines how inspiration and a fall in intrathoracic pressure affect circulatory function in a healthy subject. Several of the effects cancel each other out, but the overall results are a transient increase in right ventricular output and a decrease in output from the left ventricle. The cyclic respiratory effects are easily seen in the pressure waveform trace from a peripheral systemic arterial catheter in a spontaneously breathing subject. Systolic arterial pressure varies up to 10 mm Hg between inspiration and expiration.

Because the ventricles are connected in series, such differences in output cannot be sustained. In a prolonged inspiration, the output from the left ventricle falls initially (because of the mechanisms previously outlined), and then within 3 or 4 cardiac cycles, it rises again as the increased output from the right ventricle reaches the left. The effects of expiration and a rise in intrathoracic pressure are essentially the reverse of those seen in inspiration.

Apart from breath-holding (apnea), neither respiratory phase is prolonged. The cyclic changes in ventricular output with respiration merge from one breath into the next, and the observed changes in cardiac output depend to some degree on the relative cardiac and respiratory rates.

Table 26-2 Effects of a Normal Inspiration

EFFECT	MECHANISM (BECAUSE OF A FALL IN INTRATHORACIC PRESSURE
Increase in right ventricular preload	Increase in the pressure gradient from the systemic veins to the right atrium
Increase in right ventricular afterload	Increase in the transmural pressure gradient of the right ventricle
Decrease in right ventricular afterload	Distention of the pulmonary vascular bed and reduction in its resistance to flow
Decrease in left ventricular preload	Distention of the pulmonary vasculature and a fall in the pressure gradient from the pulmonary veins to the left atrium
Increase in left ventricular preload	Fall in left atrial pressure and increase in the pressure gradient from the pulmonary venous return to the left atrium
Decrease in left ventricular filling	Increased right ventricular filling with ventricular interdependence from septal shift
Increase in left ventricular afterload	Increased transmural pressure gradient of the left ventricle

NOTE: The second and third effects tend to cancel each other out, as do the fourth and fifth.

Cardiovascular Effects of Pathologic Pulmonary Conditions

Many respiratory conditions are complicated by pulmonary arterial hypertension. The way that pulmonary hypertension reduces left ventricular filling and increases right ventricular afterload can profoundly affect cardiac function, and this subject is discussed in detail in Chapter 59.

Respiratory conditions that lead to reduced lung compliance (e.g., pneumonia, HMD, pulmonary fibrosis) or increased airway resistance (e.g., asthma, bronchiolitis, emphysema) lead, for any given level of respiratory effort, to greater swings in intrathoracic pressure than would occur in a child with normal lungs. These swings are manifested as indrawing of the soft tissues and even the ribs in the relatively compliant chest wall of a child with these conditions. These large swings persist while normal or increased respiratory effort is maintained but diminish as respiratory muscle fatigue ensues.

The effects of obstructed expiration on the cardiovascular system are similar to those of Valsalva's maneuver. Venous return and flow in the pulmonary system are severely reduced by the high intrathoracic pressure early in expiration, but there is a small initial increase in cardiac output and blood pressure as a result of expulsion of blood from the lungs and compression of the left ventricle and thoracic aorta. The reduced venous return then reduces the cardiac output and blood pressure, provoking a baroreceptor response to tachycardia and vasoconstriction that causes a rebound hypertension when the forced expiration is released and venous return increases.

Obstructed inspiration causes cardiovascular effects similar to those of a Müller maneuver (forced inspiration against a closed glottis). Low intrathoracic pressure increases systemic venous return and expands the pulmonary blood volume, but venous return to the left ventricle, the systemic cardiac output, and the blood pressure decrease early in inspiration but approach normal later in inspiration.

Conditions causing hyperinflation of the lungs and high airway resistance (e.g., asthma) can lead to substantial changes in cardiac performance. Increased negative pressure during inspiration and positive pressure during active expiration lead to big swings in intrathoracic pressure and exaggeration of the normal cyclic changes in right and left ventricular preload and afterload.[189] The variation in left ventricular stroke volume leads to a palpable swing in systolic systemic arterial pressure with respiration.[190] This pulsus paradoxus is an exaggeration of the normal pattern. In severe airway obstruction, pulmonary vascular resistance is increased by elevated lung volume, hypoxic vasoconstriction, and acidosis.

Respiratory Effects of Cardiovascular Disorders

Increased left atrial pressure resulting from reduced left ventricular contractility or compliance, pulmonary venous obstruction, mitral valve disease, pericardial disease, or hypervolemia causes pulmonary edema and affects lung mechanics and gas exchange (see earlier section). As the cardiac output decreases, increased tissue oxygen extraction reduces the mixed venous Po_2. The consequent reduction in pulmonary end-capillary Po_2 (and therefore Pao_2) is greater for lung units with normal $\dot{V}/\dot{Q}$ ratios than in those with high or low $\dot{V}/\dot{Q}$ ratios.[191] Although the mixed venous Pco_2 also increases when the cardiac output is low, the rapid diffusion of carbon dioxide across the alveolar membrane means that the $Paco_2$ is not normally increased by a reduction in cardiac output.[192]

Reduction in cardiac output also decreases the pulmonary pressure, increasing the proportion of lung units that are unperfused (PA > Pa: zone 1), especially in the uppermost parts of the lung and increasing the alveolar dead space. In practice, this is only important in the upright position. As previously described, a decrease in respiratory muscle blood flow as a result of low cardiac output contributes to respiratory muscle fatigue when the work of breathing is increased.

Effects of High Cardiac Output

In severe exercise, the cardiac output is very high, and pulmonary transit time is reduced. Diffusion limitation reduces the pulmonary end-capillary Po_2 and increases the $PAo_2 - Pao_2$. During short bursts of severe exercise in trained athletes, the Pao_2 falls below 75 mm Hg.[193] The high cardiac output found in septic shock is associated with reduced oxygen extraction and a high mixed venous Po_2, so the effect on Pao_2 of diffusion limitation as a result of high cardiac output is not as pronounced in these patients. In the presence of lung disease, inotropic drugs that increase the cardiac output tend to increase the $PAo_2 - Pao_2$ and reduce the Pao_2 by increasing the perfusion of unventilated alveoli and of low $\dot{V}/\dot{Q}$ lung units.[194]

REFERENCES

1. Sykes MK, McNicol MW, Campbell EJM: *Respiratory failure,* ed 2, Oxford, 1976, Blackwell, pp ix-xii.
2. Martin L: Respiratory failure, *Med Clin North Am* 61:1369-1396, 1977 (review).
3. Downes JJ, Fulgencio T, Raphaely RC: Acute respiratory failure in infants and children, *Pediatr Clin North Am* 19:423-445, 1972 (review).

Hypoventilation

4. West JB: Causes of carbon dioxide retention in lung disease, *N Engl J Med* 284:1232-1236, 1971 (review).
5. Hershenson MB: The respiratory muscles and chest wall. In Beckerman RC, Brouillette RT, Hunt CE, eds: *Respiratory control disorders in infants and children,* Baltimore, 1992, Williams & Wilkins, pp 28-46.
6. Kurth CD, Hutchison AA, Caton DC, Davenport PW: Maturational and anesthetic effects on apneic thresholds in lambs, *J Appl Physiol* 67:643-647, 1989.
7. Rigatto H, de la Torre Verduzco R, Cates DB: Effects of O_2 on the ventilatory response to CO_2 in preterm infants, *J Appl Physiol* 39:896-899, 1975.
8. Gerhardt T, Bancalari E: Apnea of prematurity. I. Lung function and regulation of breathing, *Pediatrics* 74:58-62, 1984 (review).
9. Cherniack NS, Altose MD: Respiratory responses to ventilatory loading. In Hornbein TF, ed: *Regulation of breathing,* vol 2. In Lenfant C, executive ed: *Lung biology in health and disease,* New York, 1981, Marcel Dekker, pp 905-964 (review).
10. Yamashiro SM, Daubenspeck JA, Lauritsen TN, Grodins FS: Total work rate of breathing optimization in CO_2 inhalation and exercise, *J Appl Physiol* 38:702-709, 1975.

Respiratory Muscle Failure

11. Sieck GC, Fournier M: Diaphragm motor unit recruitment during ventilatory and nonventilatory behaviors, *J Appl Physiol* 66:2539-2545, 1989.
12. Gerhardt T, Bancalari E: Chest wall compliance in full-term and premature infants, *Acta Paediatr Scand* 69:359-364, 1980.
13. Openshaw P, Edwards S, Helms P: Changes in rib cage geometry during childhood, *Thorax* 39:624-627, 1984.
14. Hershenson MB, Stark AR, Mead J: Action of the inspiratory muscles of the rib cage during breathing in infants, *Am Rev Respir Dis* 139:1207-1212, 1989.
15. Hershenson MB, Colin AA, Wohl ME, Stark AR: Changes in the contribution of the rib cage to tidal breathing during infancy, *Am Rev Respir Dis* 141:922-925, 1990.
16. Davi M, Sankaran K, Maccallum M, Cates D, Rigatto H: Effect of sleep state on chest distortion and on the ventilatory response to CO, *Pediatr Res* 13:982-986, 1979.
17. Pascucci RC, Hershenson MB, Sethna NF, Loring SH, Stark AR: Chest wall motion of infants during spinal anesthesia, *J Appl Physiol* 68:2087-2091, 1990.
18. Grimby G, Goldman M, Mead J: Respiratory muscle action inferred from rib cage and abdominal V-P partitioning, *J Appl Physiol* 41:739-751, 1976.
19. Gordon H, Van Essen DC: Specific innervation of muscle fiber types in a developmentally polyinnervated muscle, *Dev Biol* 111:42-50, 1985.
20. Kelly SS: The effect of age on neuromuscular transmission, *J Physiol (Lond)* 274:51-62, 1978.
21. Keens TG, Bryan AC, Levison H, Ianuzzo CD: Developmental pattern of muscle fiber types in human ventilatory muscles, *J Appl Physiol* 44:909-913, 1978.
22. Maxwell LC, McCarter RJ, Kuehl TJ, Robotham JL: Development of histochemical and functional properties of baboon respiratory muscles, *J Appl Physiol* 54:551-561, 1983.
23. Maxwell LC, Kuehl TJ, McCarter RJ, Robotham JL: Regional distribution of fiber types in developing baboon diaphragm muscles, *Anat Rec* 224:66-78, 1989.
24. Maxwell LC, Kuehl TJ, Robotham JL, McCarter RJ: Temporal changes after death in primate diaphragm muscle oxidative enzyme activity, *Am Rev Respir Dis* 130:1147-1151, 1984.
25. Akabas SR, Bazzy AR, DiMauro S, Haddad GG: Metabolic and functional adaptation of the diaphragm to training and resistive loads, *J Appl Physiol* 66:529-535, 1989.
26. Bellemare F, Bigland-Ritchie B: Central components of diaphragmatic fatigue assessed by phrenic nerve stimulation, *J Appl Physiol* 62:1307-1316, 1987.
27. Robertson CH Jr, Foster GH, Johnson RL Jr: The relationship of respiratory failure to the oxygen consumption of lactate production by an distribution of blood flow among respiratory muscles during increasing inspiratory resistance, *J Clin Invest* 59:31-42, 1977.
28. Rochester DF, Bettini G: Diaphragmatic blood flow and energy expenditure in the dog: effect of inspiratory air flow resistance and hypercapnia, *J Clin Invest* 57:661-672, 1976.
29. Aubier M, Trippenbach T, Roussos C: Respiratory muscle fatigue during cardiogenic shock, *J Appl Physiol* 51:499-508, 1981.
30. Arora NS, Rochester DF: Respiratory muscle strength and maximal voluntary ventilation in undernourished patients, *Am Rev Respir Dis* 126:5-8, 1982.

31. Wilson DC, McClure G, Dodge JA: The influence of nutrition on neonatal respiratory muscle function, *Intensive Care Med* 18:105-108, 1992.
32. Watchko JF, Standaert TA, Woodrum DE: Diaphragmatic function during hypercapnia: neonatal and developmental aspects, *J Appl Physiol* 62:768-775, 1987.
33. Watchko JF, LaFramboise WA, Standaert TA, Woodrum DE: Diaphragmatic function during hypoxemia: neonatal and developmental aspects, *J Appl Physiol* 60:1599-1604, 1986.
34. Aubier M, Murciano D, Lecocguic Y, Viires N, Jacquens Y, Squara P, Pariente R: Effect of hypophosphatemia on diaphragmatic contractility in patients with acute respiratory failure, *N Engl J Med* 313:420-424, 1985.
35. Aubier M, Viires N, Piquet J, Murciano D, Blanchet F, Marty C, Gherardi R, Pariente R: Effects of hypocalcemia on diaphragmatic strength generation, *J Appl Physiol* 58:2054-2061, 1985.
36. Dhingra S, Solven F, Wilson A, McCarthy DS: Hypomagnesemia and respiratory muscle power, *Am Rev Respir Dis* 129:497-498, 1984.
37. Mier-Jedrzejowicz A, Brophy C, Green M: Respiratory weakness during upper respiratory tract infections, *Am Rev Respir Dis* 138:5-7, 1988.
38. Boczkowski J, Dureuil B, Branger C, Pavlovic D, Murciano D, Pariente R, Aubier M: Effects of sepsis on diaphragm function in rats, *Am Rev Respir Dis* 138:260-265, 1988.
39. Hussain SNA, Simkus G, Roussos C: Respiratory muscle fatigue: a cause of ventilatory failure in septic shock, *J Appl Physiol* 58:2033-2040, 1985.

Disorders of Gas Transport

40. Nunn JF: *Applied respiratory physiology,* ed 4, Oxford, England, 1993, Butterworth-Heinemann, p 178.
41. West JB: Pulmonary gas exchange. In West JB, ed: *Best and Taylor's physiological basis of medical practice*, ed 12, Baltimore, 1991, Williams & Wilkins, pp 546-559.
42. Katz VL, Bowes WA: Meconium aspiration syndrome: reflections on a murky subject, *Am J Obstet Gynecol* 166:171-183, 1992 (review).
43. Polgar G, Weng TR: The functional development of the respiratory system from the period of gestation to adulthood, *Am Rev Respir Dis* 120:625-695, 1979.
44. Fox WW, Gewitz MH, Dinwiddie R, Drummond WH, Peckham GJ: Pulmonary hypertension in the perinatal aspiration syndromes, *Pediatrics* 59:205-211, 1977.
45. Spitzer AR, Davis J, Clarke WT, Bernbaum J, Fox WW: Pulmonary hypertension and persistent fetal circulation in the newborn, *Clin Perinatol* 15:389-413, 1988 (review).
46. Murdock AI, Kidd BSL, Llewellyn MA, Reid MM, Swyer PR: Intrapulmonary venous admixture in the respiratory distress syndrome, *Biol Neonate* 15:1-7, 1970.
47. Cotton RB: Pathophysiology of hyaline membrane disease (excluding surfactant). In Polin RA, Fox WM, eds: *Fetal and neonatal physiology,* Philadelphia, 1992, WB Saunders, pp 885-894.
48. Burke CM, Safai C, Nelson DP, Raffin TA: Pulmonary arteriovenous malformations: a critical update, *Am Rev Respir Dis* 134:334-339, 1986 (review).
49. Von Hayek H: *The human lung,* New York, 1960, Hafner, pp 282-287 (translated by VE Krahl).
50. Robertson B: Postnatal formation and obliteration of arterial anastomoses in the human lung, *Pediatrics* 43:971-979, 1969.
51. Jaykka S: Precapillary bypass and sudden infant death, *Lancet* 2:1315, 1971 (letter).
52. Wilkinson MJ, Fagan DG: Postmortem demonstration of intrapulmonary arteriovenous shunting, *Arch Dis Child* 65:435-437, 1990.
53. Tobin CE: Arteriovenous shunts in the peripheral pulmonary circulation in the human lung, *Thorax* 21:197-204, 1966.
54. Hislop A, Reid L: Pulmonary arterial development during childhood: branching pattern and structure, *Thorax* 28:129-135, 1973.
55. Southall DP, Samuels MP, Talbert DG: Recurrent cyanotic episodes with severe arterial hypoxaemia and intrapulmonary shunting: a mechanism for sudden death, *Arch Dis Child* 65:953-961, 1990.
56. Poets CF, Samuels MP, Southall DP: Potential role of intrapulmonary shunting in the genesis of hypoxemic episodes in infants and young children, *Pediatrics* 90:385-391, 1992 (review).
57. Krauss AN, Soodalter JA, Auld PAM: Adjustment of ventilation and perfusion in the full-term normal and distressed neonate as determined by urinary alveolar nitrogen gradients, *Pediatrics* 47:865-869, 1971.
58. Hoffman JIE, Heymann MA: Normal pulmonary circulation. In Scarpelli EM, ed: *Pulmonary physiology: fetus, newborn, child and adolescent,* ed 2, Philadelphia, 1989, Lea & Febiger, pp 233-256.
59. Woodrum DE, Oliver TK, Hodson WA: The effect of prematurity and hyaline membrane disease oxygen exchange in the lung, *Pediatrics* 50:380-386, 1972.
60. Hansen TN, Corbet AJS, Kenny JD, Courtney JD, Rudolph AJ: Effects of oxygen and constant positive pressure breathing on $aADCO_2$ in hyaline membrane disease, *Pediatr Res* 13:1167-1171, 1979.
61. Sinclair-Smith CC, Emery JL, Gadsdon D, Dinsdale F, Baddeley J: Cartilage in children's lungs: a quantitative assessment using the right middle lobe, *Thorax* 31:40-43, 1976.
62. Burnard ED, Grattan-Smith P, Picton-Warlow CG, Grauaug A: Pulmonary insufficiency in prematurity, *Aust Paediatr J* 1:12-38, 1965.
63. Bhutani VK, Rubenstein SD, Shaffer TH: Pressure-volume relationships of tracheae in fetal newborn and adult rabbits, *Respir Physiol* 43:221-231, 1981.
64. Martinez FD: Sudden infant death syndrome and small airway occlusion: facts and a hypothesis, *Pediatrics* 87:190-198, 1991 (review).
65. Thurlbeck WM: Postnatal growth and development of the lung, *Am Rev Respir Dis* 111:803-844, 1975 (review).
66. Krauss AN, Auld PAM: Pulmonary gas trapping in premature infants, *Pediatr Res* 5:10-16, 1971.
67. Thibeault DW, Poblete E, Auld PAM: Alveolar-arterial O_2 and CO_2 differences and their relation to lung volume in the newborn, *Pediatrics* 41:574-587, 1968.
68. Light RB, Mink SN, Wood LDH: Pathophysiology of gas exchange and pulmonary perfusion in pneumococcal lobar pneumonia in dogs, *J Appl Physiol* 50:524-530, 1981.
69. Lampron N, Lemaire F, Teisseire B, Harf A, Palot M, Matamis D, Lorino AM: Mechanical ventilation with 100% oxygen does not increase intrapulmonary shunt in patients with severe bacterial pneumonia, *Am Rev Respir Dis* 131:409-413, 1985.
70. Dantzker DR, Brook CJ, Dehart P, Lynch JP, Weg JG: $\dot{V}/\dot{Q}$ distributions in the adult respiratory distress syndrome, *Am Rev Respir Dis* 120:1039-1052, 1979.
71. Dantzker DR, Patten GA, Bower JS; Gas exchange at rest and during exercise in adults with cystic fibrosis, *Am Rev Respir Dis* 125:400-405, 1982.
72. Truog WE: Pulmonary gas exchange. In Chernick V, Mellins RB, eds: *Basic mechanisms of pediatric respiratory disease: cellular and integrative,* Philadelphia, 1991, BC Decker, pp 114-128.
73. West JB: Gas exchange when one lung region inspires from another, *J Appl Physiol* 30:479-487, 1971.
74. Berggren S: The oxygen deficit of arterial blood, *Acta Physiol Scand (Suppl)* 11:1-92, 1942 (review).
75. Dantzker DR, Wagner PD, West JB: Instability of lung units with low $\dot{V}/\dot{Q}$ ratios during O_2 breathing, *J Appl Physiol* 38:886-895, 1975.
76. Parks CR, Alden ER, Woodrum DE, Standaert TA, Hodson WA: Gas exchange in the immature lung. II. Method of estimation and maturity, *J Appl Physiol* 36:108-112, 1974.
77. Radermacher P, Santak B, Becker H, Falke KJ: Prostaglandin E_1 and nitroglycerin reduce pulmonary capillary pressure but worsen $\dot{V}/\dot{Q}$ distributions in patients with adult respiratory distress syndrome, *Anesthesiology* 70:601-606, 1989.
78. Chiolero P, Flatt JP, Revelly JP, Jequier E: Effects of catecholamines on oxygen consumption and oxygen delivery in critically ill patients, *Chest* 100:1676-1684, 1991 (review).
79. Rennotte MT, Reynaert M, Clerbaux T, Willems E, Roeseleer J, Veriter C, Rodenstein D, Frans A: Effects of two inotropic drugs, dopamine and dobutamine, on pulmonary gas exchange in artificially ventilated patients, *Intensive Care Med* 15:160-165, 1989.
80. Lenfant C: Time-dependent variations of pulmonary gas exchange in normal man at rest, *J Appl Physiol* 22:675-684, 1967.
81. Milic-Emili J: Topographical inequality of ventilation. In Crystal RG, West JB, eds: *The lung: scientific foundations,* vol 1, New York, 1991, Raven, pp 1043-1051 (review).
82. Friedman WF, Sahn DJ, Hirschklau MJ: A review: newer, non-invasive cardiac diagnostic methods, *Pediatr Res* 11:190-197, 1977.
83. Davies H, Helms P, Gordon I: Effect of posture on regional ventilation in children, *Pediatr Pulmonol* 12:227-232, 1992.
84. Mansell A, Bryan C, Levison H: Airway closure in children, *J Appl Physiol* 33:711-714, 1972.

85. Crawford ABH, Paiva M, Engel LA: Uneven ventilation. In Crystal RG, West JB, Barnes PJ, Cherniack NS, Weibel ER, eds: *The lung: scientific foundations,* New York, 1991, Raven, pp 1031-1041.
86. Davies H, Kitchman R, Gordon I, Helms P: Regional ventilation in infancy: reversal of adult pattern, *New Engl J Med* 313:1626-1628, 1985.
87. McCann EM, Goldman SL, Brady JP: Pulmonary function in the sick newborn infant, *Pediatr Res* 21:313-325, 1987.
88. Remolina C, Khan AU, Santiago TV, Edelman NH: Positional hypoxaemia in unilateral lung disease, *New Engl J Med* 304:523-525, 1981.
89. Cohen RS, Smith DW, Stevenson DK, Moskowitz PS, Graham CB: Lateral decubitus position as therapy for persistent focal pulmonary interstitial emphysema in neonates: a preliminary report, *J Pediatr* 104:441-443, 1984.
90. Truog WE: Pulmonary gas exchange in the developing lung. In Polin RA, Fox WW, eds: *Fetal and neonatal physiology,* Philadelphia, 1992, WB Saunders, pp 842-852.
91. Marshall BE, Marshall C, Benumoff J, Saidman LJ: Hypoxic pulmonary vasoconstriction in dogs: effects of lung segment size and oxygen tension, *J Appl Physiol* 51:1543-1551, 1981.
92. Raj JU, Chen P: Role of eicosanoids in hypoxic vasoconstriction in isolated lamb lungs, *Am J Physiol* 253:H626-H633, 1987.
93. Voelkel NF: Mechanisms of hypoxic pulmonary vasoconstriction, *Am Rev Respir Dis* 133:1186-1195, 1986.
94. Benumof JL, Pirlo AF, Johanson I, Trousdale FR: Interaction of PvO_2 with PAO_2 on hypoxic pulmonary vasoconstriction, *J Appl Physiol* 51:871-874, 1981.
95. Lloyd TC: Hypoxic pulmonary vasoconstriction: role of perivascular tissue, *J Appl Physiol* 25:560-565, 1968.
96. Morganroth ML, Reeves JT, Murphy RC, Voelkel NF: Leukotriene synthesis and receptor blockers block hypoxic pulmonary vasoconstriction, *J Appl Physiol* 56:1340-1346, 1984.
97. McMurtry IF: BAY K 8644 potentiates and A23187 inhibits hypoxic vasoconstriction in rat lungs, *Am J Physiol* 249:H741-H746, 1985.
98. Palmer RMJ, Ferrige AG, Moncada S: Nitric oxide release accounts for the biological activity of endothelium-derived relaxing factor, *Nature* 327:524-526, 1987.
99. Roberts JD, Chen T-Y, Kawai N, Wain J, Dupuy P, Shimouchi A, Bloch K, Polaner D, Zapol WM: Inhaled nitric oxide reverses pulmonary vasoconstriction in the hypoxic and acidotic newborn lamb, *Circ Res* 72:246-254, 1993.
100. Eddahibi S, Carville C, Raffestin B, Adnot S: In vivo administration of L-arginine restores endothelium dependent relaxant activity in the pulmonary circulation of chronically hypoxic rats, *Am Rev Respir Dis* 145:A208, 1992.
101. Johns RA, Linden JM, Peach MJ: Endothelium-dependent relaxation and cyclic GMP accumulation in rabbit pulmonary artery are selectively impaired by moderate hypoxia, *Circ Res* 65:1508-1515, 1989.
102. Shaul PW, Farrar MA, Zellers TM: Oxygen modulates endothelium-derived relaxing factor production in fetal pulmonary arteries, *Am J Physiol* 262:H355-H364, 1992.
103. Rossaint R, Falke KJ, Lopez F, Slama K, Pison U, Zapol WM: Inhaled nitric oxide for the adult respiratory distress syndrome, *New Engl J Med* 328:399-405, 1993.
104. Dawson CA: Role of pulmonary vasomotion in physiology of the lung, *Physiol Rev* 64(2):544-616, 1984 (review).
105. Custer JR, Hales CA: Influence of alveolar oxygen on pulmonary vasoconstriction in newborn lambs versus sheep, *Am Rev Respir Dis* 132:326-331, 1985.
106. Corbet AJS, Ross JA, Beaudry PH, Stern L: $\dot{V}/\dot{Q}$ relationships as assessed by $aADN_2$ in hyaline membrane disease, *J Appl Physiol* 36:74-81, 1974.
107. Landers S, Hansen TN, Corbet AJS, Stevener MJ, Rudolph AJ: Optimal constant positive airway pressure assessed by arterial alveolar difference for CO_2 in hyaline membrane disease, *Pediatr Res* 20:884-889, 1986.
108. Hand IL, Shepard EK, Krauss AN, Auld PAM: $\dot{V}/\dot{Q}$ abnormalities in the preterm infant with hyaline membrane disease: a two-compartment model of the neonatal lung, *Pediatr Pulmonol* 9:206-213, 1990.
109. Hansen T, Corbet A: Disorders of the transition. In Taeusch HW, Ballard RA, Avery ME, eds: *Schaffer and Avery's diseases of the newborn,* ed 6, Philadelphia, 1991, WB Saunders, pp 948-514.
110. Wagner PD, Dantzker DR, Iacovoni VE, Tomlin WC, West JB: $\dot{V}/\dot{Q}$ inequality in asymptomatic asthma, *Am Rev Respir Dis* 118:511-524, 1978.
111. Rodriguez-Roisin R, Ballester E, Roca J, Torres A, Wagner PD: Mechanisms of hypoxemia in patients with status asthmaticus requiring mechanical ventilation, *Am Rev Respir Dis* 139:732-739, 1989.
112. Ballester E, Reyes A, Roca J, Guitart R, Wagner PD, Rodriguez-Roisin R: $\dot{V}/\dot{Q}$ mismatching in acute severe asthma: effects of salbutamol and 100% oxygen, *Thorax* 44:258-267, 1989.
113. Wagner PD, Rodriguez-Roisin R: Clinical advances in pulmonary gas exchange, *Am Rev Respir Dis* 143:883-888, 1991 (review).
114. Hedenstierna G, Freyschuss U: Assessment of $\dot{V}/\dot{Q}$ distribution of multiple insert gas elimination techniques: its application in the child, *Eur Respir J* 2(suppl 4):181S-184S, 1989.
115. Ringstead CV, Eliasen K, Andersen JB, Heslet L, Quist J: $\dot{V}/\dot{Q}$ distributions and central hemodynamics in chronic obstructive pulmonary disease: effects of terbutaline administration, *Chest* 96:976-983, 1989.
116. Johnson D, Hurst T, Mayers I: Insufflated halothane increases venous admixture less than nitroprusside in canine atelectasis, *Anesthesiology* 77:301-308, 1992.
117. Davidson A, Bossuyt A, Dab I: Acute effects of oxygen, nifedipine and diltiazem in patients with cystic fibrosis and mild pulmonary hypertension, *Pediatr Pulmonol* 6:53-59, 1989.
118. Markello R, Winter P, Olszowka A: Assessment of $\dot{V}/\dot{Q}$ inequalities by arterial-alveolar nitrogen differences in intensive care patients, *Anesthesiology* 37:4-15, 1972.
119. Bose C, Wood B, Bose G, Donlon D, Friedman M: Pulmonary function following positive pressure ventilation initiated immediately after birth in infants with respiratory distress syndrome, *Pediatr Pulmonol* 9:244-250, 1990.
120. Zapletal A, Houstek J, Samanek M, Copova M, Paul T: Lung function in children and adolescents with idiopathic interstitial pulmonary fibrosis, *Pediatr Pulmonol* 1:154-166, 1985.
121. Chaussain M, de Boissieu D, Kalifa G, Epelbaum S, Niaudet P, Badoual J, Gendrel D: Impairment of lung diffusion capacity in Schönlein-Henoch purpura, *J Pediatr* 121:12-16, 1992,
122. Cerveri I, Bruschi C, Ravelli A, Zoia MC, Fanfulla F, Zonta L, Pellegrini G, Martini A: Pulmonary function in childhood connective tissue diseases, *Eur Respir J* 5:733-738, 1992.
123. Springmeyer SC, Silvestri RC, Flournoy N, Kosanke CW, Peterson DL, Huseby JS, Hudson LD, Storb R, Thomas ED: Pulmonary function of marrow transplant patients. I. Effects of marrow infusion, acute graft-versus-host disease and interstitial pneumonitis, *Exp Hematol* 12:805-810, 1984.
124. Adams GD, Kehoe R, Lesch M, Glassroth J: Amiodarone-induced pneumonitis: assessment of risk factors and possible risk reduction, *Chest* 93:254-263, 1988.
125. Kritski AL, Lemle A, de Souza GRM, de Souza RV, Nogueira SA, Pereira NG, Bethlem NM: Pulmonary function changes in the acute stages of histoplasmosis, with follow-up, *Chest* 97:1244-1245, 1990.
126. Lebecque P, Lapierre J-G, Lamarre A, Coates AL: Diffusion capacity and oxygen desaturation effects on exercise in patients with cystic fibrosis, *Chest* 91:693-697, 1987.
127. Glader BE, Naiman JL: Erythrocyte disorders in infancy. In Taeusch HW, Ballard RA, Avery ME, eds: *Schaffer and Avery's diseases of the newborn,* ed 6, Philadelphia, 1991, WB Saunders, pp 79-828.
128. Lister G, Fahey JT: Oxygen transport. In Chernick V, Mellins RB, eds: *Basic mechanisms of pediatric respiratory disease: cellular and integrative,* Philadelphia, 1991, BC Decker, pp 129-144.
129. Ranney HM, Rapaport SI: The red blood cell. In West JB, ed: *Best and Taylor's physiological basis of medical practice,* ed 12, Baltimore, 1991, Williams & Wilkins, pp 369-382.
130. Turek Z, Kreuzer F: Effect of shifts of the O_2 dissociation curve upon alveolar-arterial O_2 gradients in computer models of the lung with $\dot{V}/\dot{Q}$ mismatching, *Respir Physiol* 45:133-139, 1981.
131. Taetle R, Rapaport SI: Hemopoiesis. In West JB, ed: *Best and Taylor's physiological basis of medical practice,* ed 12, Baltimore, 1991, Williams & Wilkins, pp 339-348.
132. Dantzker DR: Physiological and biochemical indicators of impaired tissue oxygenation. In Reinhart K, Eyrich K, eds: *Clinical aspects of O_2 transport and tissue oxygenation,* Berlin, 1989, Springer-Verlag, pp 182-194.
133. Gaehtgens P: Microcirculatory control of tissue oxygenation. In Reinhart K, Eyrich K, eds: *Clinical aspects of O_2 transport and tissue oxygenation,* Berlin, 1989, Springer-Verlag, pp 44-52.

134. Bredle DL: Circulatory compensation as a response to hypoxia. In Reinhart K, Eyrich K, eds: *Clinical aspects of O_2 transport and tissue oxygenation,* Berlin, 1989, Springer-Verlag, pp 53-63.
135. Sidi D, Kuipers JRG, Teitel D, Heymann MA, Rudolph AM: Developmental changes in oxygenation and circulatory responses to hypoxemia in lambs, *Am J Physiol* 245:H674-H682, 1983.
136. Teitel D, Sidi D, Bernstein D, Heymann MA, Rudolph AM: Chronic hypoxemia in the newborn lamb: cardiovascular, hematopoietic and growth adaptations, *Pediatr Res* 19:1004-1010, 1985.
137. Schumacker PT, Samsel RW: Analysis of oxygen delivery and uptake relationships in the Krogh tissue model, *J Appl Physiol* 67:1234-1244, 1989.
138. Nelson DP, King CE, Dodd SL, Schumacker PT, Cain SM: Systemic and intestinal limits of O_2 extraction in the dog, *J Appl Physiol* 63:387-394, 1987.
139. Leach RM, Treacher DF: Oxygen transport: the relation between oxygen delivery and consumption, *Thorax* 47:971-978, 1992 (review).
140. Danek SJ, Lynch JP, Weg JG, Dantzker DR: The dependence of oxygen uptake on oxygen delivery in the adult respiratory distress syndrome, *Am Rev Respir Dis* 122:387-395, 1980.
141. Dorinsky PM, Costello JL, Gadek JE: Relationships of oxygen uptake and oxygen delivery in respiratory failure not due to the adult respiratory distress syndrome, *Chest* 93:1013-1019 1988.
142. Vilar J, Slutsky AS, Hew E, Aberman A: Oxygen transport and oxygen consumption in critically ill patients, *Chest* 98:687-692, 1990.
143. Bryan-Brown CW, Baek S, Makabali G, Shoemaker WC: Consumable oxygen: availability of oxygen in relation to oxyhemoglobin dissociation, *Crit Care Med* 1:17-21, 1973.
144. Lundgren J, Siesjo BK: Mechanisms of hypoxia-ischemia. In Holbrook PR, ed: *Textbook of pediatric critical care,* Philadelphia, 1993, WB Saunders, pp 1-1.
145. Lindahl SGE: Oxygen consumption and carbon dioxide elimination in infants and children during anaesthesia and surgery, *Br J Anaesth* 62:70-76, 1989.
146. Dechert R, Wesley J, Schafer L, LaMond S, Beck T, Coran A, Bartlett RH: Comparison of oxygen consumption, carbon dioxide production, and resting energy expenditure in premature and full-term infants, *J Pediatr Surg* 20:792-798, 1985.
147. McLean JA, Tobin G: *Animal and human calorimetry,* Cambridge, 1987, Cambridge University Press, p 24-49.
148. Swenson ER, Hlastala MP: Carbon dioxide transport and acid-base balance: tissue and cellular. In Chernick V, Mellins RB, eds: *Basic mechanisms of pediatric respiratory disease: cellular and integrative,* Philadelphia, 1991, BC Decker, pp 145-161.
149. West JB: Gas transport to the periphery. In West JB, ed: *Physiological basis of medical practice,* ed 12, Baltimore, 1991, Williams & Wilkins, pp 538-544.
150. Bauer C, Schroder E: Carbamino compounds of haemoglobin in human adult and foetal blood, *J Physiol* 227:457-471, 1972.
151. Johnson RL, Ramanathan M: Buffer equilibria in the lungs. In Seldin DW, Giebisch G, eds: *The kidney: physiology and pathophysiology,* New York, 1985, Raven, pp 149-171.
152. Eisele JH, Eger EI, Muallem M: Narcotic properties of carbon dioxide in the dog, *Anesthesiology* 28:856-865, 1967.
153. Cohen JJ, Madias NE: Respiratory alkalosis and acidosis. In Seldin GW, Giebisch G, eds: *The kidney: physiology and pathophysiology,* New York, 1985, Raven, pp 1641-1661.
154. Patterson JL, Heyman H, Whatley DT: Cerebral circulation and metabolism in chronic pulmonary emphysema, *Am J Med* 12:382-387, 1952.
155. Levasseur JE, Wei EP, Kontos HA, Patterson JL: Responses of pial arterioles after prolonged hypercapnia and hypoxia in the awake rabbit, *J Appl Physiol* 46:89-95, 1979.
156. Madias NE, Adrogue HJ: Respiratory acidosis and alkalosis. In Adrogue HJ, ed: *Contemporary management in critical care: acid-base and electrolyte disorders,* New York, 1991 Churchill Livingstone, pp 37-53.
157. Cingolani HE, Koretsune Y, Marban E: Recovery of contractility and pH during respiratory acidosis in ferret hearts: role of $Na^+ - H^+$ exchange, *Am J Physiol* 259(3 pt 2):H843-H848, 1990.
158. Hughes RL, Mathie RT, Campbell D, Fitch W: Effect of hypercarbia on hepatic blood flow and oxygen consumption in the greyhound, *Br J Anaesth* 51:289-296, 1979.
159. Weinberger SE, Schwartzstein RM, Weiss JW: Hypercapnia, *New Engl J Med* 321:1223-1231, 1989.
160. Somero GN: Protons, osmolytes and fitness of internal milieu for protein function, *Am J Physiol* 251:R197-R213, 1986 (review).
161. Menitove SM, Goldring RM: Combined ventilator and bicarbonate strategy in the management of status asthmaticus, *Am J Med* 74:898-901, 1983.
162. Lakshminaryan S, Sahn SA, Petty TL: Bicarbonate therapy in severe acute respiratory acidosis, *Scand J Respir Dis* 54:128-131, 1973.
163. Arieff AI: Indications for use of bicarbonate in patients with metabolic acidosis, *Br J Anaesth* 67:165-177, 1991 (review).
164. Engel K, Dell RB, Rahill WJ, Denning CR, Winters RW: Quantitative displacement of acid-base equilibrium in chronic respiratory acidosis, *J Appl Physiol* 24:288-295, 1968.
165. Ruiz OS, Arruda JAL, Talor Z: Na-HCO3 cotransport and Na-H antiporter in chronic respiratory acidosis and alkalosis, *Am J Physiol* 256:F414-F420, 1989.
166. Schwartz GJ: Acid-base homeostasis. In Edelman CM, ed: *Pediatric kidney disease,* ed 2, Boston, 1992, Little, Brown, pp 201-230.
167. Anand SK: Maturation of renal function. In Taeusch HW, Ballard RA, Avery ME, eds: *Schaffer and Avery's diseases of the newborn,* ed 6, Philadelphia, 1991, WB Saunders, pp 841-847.
168. Goldstein B, Shannon DC, Torres ID: Supercarbia in children: clinical course and outcome, *Crit Care Med* 18:166-168, 1990.
169. Horbein TF: Respiratory obstruction with oxygenation apnea, *Anesthesiology* 24:880-883, 1963.

Lung Water and Pulmonary Edema

170. Staub NC: Pulmonary edema, *Physiol Rev* 54:678-811, 1974.
171. Taylor AE, Parker JC: Pulmonary interstitial spaces and lymphatics. In Fishman AP, Fisher AB, eds: *Handbook of physiology,* Section 3: The respiratory system, Bethesda, Md, 1985, American Physiological Society, pp 167-230.
172. Bert JL, Pearce RH: The interstitium of microvascular exchange. In Renkin EM, Michael CC, eds: *Handbook of physiology,* Section 2: The cardiovascular system, Bethesda, Md, 1984, American Physiological Society, pp 521-547.
173. Palade GE: The microvascular endothelium revisited. In Simionescu M, ed: *Endothelial cell biology in health and disease,* New York, 1988, Plenum, pp 3-22.
174. Olver RE, Strang LB: Ion fluxes across the pulmonary epithelium and the secretion of lung liquid in the fetal lamb, *J Physiol* 241:327-357, 1974.
175. Basset G, Crone C, Saumon G: Fluid absorption by rat lung in situ: pathways for sodium entry in the luminal membrane of alveolar epithelium, *J Physiol* 384:325-345, 1987.
176. Staub NC: The pathogenesis of pulmonary edema, *Prog Cardiovasc Dis* 25:53-80, 1980.
177. Staub NC, Nagano H, Pearce ML: Pulmonary edema in dogs, especially the sequence of fluid accumulation in lungs, *J Appl Physiol,* 22:227-240, 1967.
178. Staub NC: Pathways for fluid and solute fluxes in pulmonary edema. In Fishman AP, Renkin EM, eds: *Pulmonary edema,* Bethesda Md, 1979, American Physiological Society, pp 113-124.
179. Gee MH, Staub NC: Role of bulk fluid flow in protein permeability of the dog lung alveolar membrane, *J Appl Physiol* 42:144-149, 1977.
180. Rosen B, Rosen AL, Sehgal HL, Sehgal LR, Gould SA, Moss GS: Hemorrhage and resuscitation. In Rippe JM, Irwin RS, Alpert JS, Fink MP, eds: *Intensive care medicine,* ed 2, Boston, 1991, Little, Brown, pp 1435-1443.
181. Turnage RH, Guice KS, Oldham KT: Pulmonary microvascular injury following intestinal reperfusion, *New Horiz* 2:463-475, 1994.
182. Travis KW, Todres ID, Shannon DC: Pulmonary edema associated with croup and epiglottitis, *Paediatrics* 59:695-698, 1977.
183. Meyer KD, Chaudhry MR: Flash pulmonary edema secondary to upper airway obstruction, *Am Heart J* 122(2):576-577, 1991.
184. Mackay EM: Experimental pulmonary edema, *Proc Soc Exp Biol* 74:695-740, 1950.
185. Chen HI, Sun SC, Chai CY: Pulmonary edema and hemorrhage resulting from cerebral compression, *Am J Physiol* 224:223-229, 1973.
186. Nitta K, Kobayashi T: Impairment of surfactant activity and ventilation by proteins in lung edema fluid, *Respir Physiol* 95(1):43-51, 1994.

187. Kobayashi T, Nitta K, Ganzuka M, Inui S, Grossmann G, Robertson B: Inactivation of exogenous surfactant by pulmonary edema fluid, *Pediatr Res* 29(4 pt 1):353-356, 1991.

Cardiorespiratory Interactions

188. Robotham JL: Cardiorespiratory interactions. In Rogers MC, eds: *Textbook of pediatric intensive care,* vol 1, Williams & Wilkins, 1987, pp 299-326.
189. Permutt S: Physiologic changes in the acute asthma attack. In Austin KF, Lichtenstein LM, eds: *Asthma physiology, immunopharmacology, and treatment,* New York, 1973, Academic, pp 15-48.
190. Buda AJ, Pinsky MR, Ingels NB, Daughters GT, Stinson EB, Alderman EL: Effect of intrathoracic pressure on left ventricular performance, *N Engl J Med* 301:453-459, 1979.
191. West JB, Wagner PD: $\dot{V}/\dot{Q}$ relationships. In Crystal RG, West JB, Barnes PJ, Cherniak NS, Weibel ER, eds: *The lung: scientific foundations,* New York, 1991, Raven, pp 1289-1305.
192. Mecher CE, Rackow EC, Astiz ME, Weil MH: Venous hypercarbia associated with severe sepsis and systemic hypoperfusion, *Crit Care Med* 18:585-589, 1990.
193. Dempsey JA, Hanson PG, Henderson KS: Exercise-induced arterial hypoxaemia in healthy human subjects at sea level, *J Physiol* 355:161-175, 1984.
194. Rennotte MT, Reynaert M, Clerbaux T, Willems E, Roeseleer J, Veriter C, Rodenstein D, Frans A: Effects of two inotropic drugs: dopamine and dobutamine on pulmonary gas exchange in artificially ventilated patients, *Intensive Care Med* 15:160-165, 1989.

CHAPTER 27

Foreign Body Aspiration

Kyle L. Bressler, Christopher G. Green, and Lauren D. Holinger

The propensity of small children to place objects into their mouths is well known. Many of these objects are aspirated. The collection of recovered foreign bodies at the Children's Memorial Hospital, Chicago, while under the direction of Dr. Paul H. Holinger, numbered over 5000. This included a diverse group of objects ranging from organic matter to metallic trinkets.

Foreign body aspiration attracts a great deal of attention, some of it for the novelty of the aspirated items. However, the danger of a foreign body should never be minimized; the National Safety Council[1] reports that each year in the United States there are approximately 2900 deaths from suffocation after ingestion of foreign bodies. The majority of these fatalities occur soon after the aspiration, with the patient never having been seen by a physician other than a coroner. Two thirds of all deaths related to foreign body ingestion occur in the home.

In addition to the danger of the aspiration episode itself, foreign body removal, despite technologic advances, remains a technically challenging procedure because of the size of the airways in which the foreign bodies are lodged. Most patients with this problem are younger than 4 years of age.[2,3]

DISEASE MECHANISMS

A child's fascination with placing objects in the mouth begins soon after grasping becomes effective. Aspiration does not become a significant problem until later, however, when children are able to walk and run, occasionally with objects in their mouths. Other contributing factors include improper preparation of food (pieces being too large, bones not being removed), an immature swallowing mechanism, hasty eating and drinking, playing while eating, talking with food in the oral cavity, small objects within grasping distance, and improper supervision of small children playing near infants. Older children commonly force objects in their younger siblings' mouths. Only careful supervision can lessen the chance of aspiration.

Organic material is the most frequent foreign body found in the airway. Nuts and beans are commonly removed, with peanuts the most common single item.[2,4] Nuts should not be given to children younger than age 5 to 6 years because this group does not have fully developed oral motor control or the molar teeth to chew them. Children who have diminished perception and sensation are at increased risk of aspiration.

Changes in toys and their component materials have altered the type of foreign bodies. Metal jacks have been supplanted by the small plastic parts of larger toys such as Lite-Brite pegs and Lego blocks. These parts are often radiolucent, making diagnosis difficult, although some manufacturers have altered the composition of their products so that they are more radiopaque. An overlooked source of foreign body aspiration is surgically placed objects. Silastic airway stents and items used to plug bronchoscope holes have been misplaced in the airway. These cases, although unusual, point out the need for intense concentration and attention to detail during procedures in or near the airway.

Unfortunately, many victims of foreign body aspiration never survive the first few minutes. Most often, these involve aspirated food objects. "Round" foods, such as hot dogs, nuts, and grapes, are most likely to cause asphyxiation.[5] Other factors that can contribute to a food object's ability to occlude an airway include a smooth or slippery surface, compressibility, and failure to break apart easily. Dried beans and peas can cause delayed airway obstruction because they swell with the absorption of moisture. More warning labels and education are needed to alert caregivers to the potential risks of feeding these foods to children.

CLINICAL MANIFESTATIONS

Children who aspirate foreign objects have a variety of presenting signs and symptoms. Often, a diagnosis of exclusion is made, and patients may see several physicians before the foreign body is identified.

The greatest factor in delayed diagnosis is the lack of a clear history. Because most aspirations occur in small children, communication after the event is problematic. For example, although the episode may have been witnessed by an older child, that child may be afraid of repercussions because he or she may have given the patient a forbidden object. It is common for an older sibling to admit to witnessing an aspiration days or weeks after the event.

Usually, three distinct clinical phases occur after a foreign body is aspirated. The first is the period immediately after the aspiration. There may be coughing, gagging, choking, stridor, and wheezing. A cyanotic episode may also occur. Many caregivers seek medical attention for the patient during this phase.

After this initial phase is a quiescent period. This asymptomatic period can last from minutes to months depending on the location of the foreign body, the degree of airway obstruction, and the inflammatory reaction to the material aspirated. During this phase, the foreign body can easily change location, with a subsequent change in signs and symptoms.

The third phase is a renewed symptomatic period. In this period, children are brought to the health care facility after an unwitnessed aspiration event. During this phase, airway inflammation or infection results in symptoms such as cough, sputum production, fever, wheezing, and rarely, hemoptysis. Unfortunately, many of the signs and symptoms can be confused with other clinical entities (Box 27-1). Clinical manifestations vary based on the location where the object comes to rest in the airway.

Laryngeal Foreign Body

Laryngeal foreign bodies that cause complete obstruction result in sudden death unless they are dislodged within minutes. Partially obstructive objects may cause hoarseness, aphonia, croupy cough, odynophagia, hemoptysis, wheezing, and dyspnea. These symptoms can be secondary to the foreign body itself or may result from a residual laryngeal reaction from a foreign body that has migrated to the trachea. An esophageal foreign body may cause similar symptoms. Two mechanisms are responsible: The first is periesophageal reaction resulting in inflammation with anterior displacement of the posterior laryngeal tissue, and the second is secretion overflow with resultant laryngeal symptoms.

BOX 27-1
Differential Diagnosis of Aspirated Foreign Body

Reactive airway disease	Empyema
Pneumonia	Croup
Tracheobronchial tumor	Bronchitis
Tracheomalacia	Psychogenic cough
Bronchomalacia	

Tracheal Foreign Body

Unique signs of tracheal foreign bodies include the audible slap, the palpable thud, and the asthmatoid wheeze. The audible slap is best heard at the open mouth during a cough. The asthmatoid wheeze is best heard with the ear at the patient's mouth. This sign is especially significant if there is a history of initial choking and gagging. Esclamado and Richardson[6] showed that the incidence of complications in the laryngotracheal foreign body group is at least 4 to 5 times greater than that reported for all aspirated foreign bodies.

Bronchial Foreign Body

The most common symptoms of bronchial foreign bodies are coughing and wheezing. Hemoptysis and dyspnea may also be present. At first, obstructive foreign bodies cause emphysema; later, atelectasis, pneumonia, pulmonary edema, and eventually, empyema may occur. Organic materials are more likely to cause an intense inflammatory reaction with large amounts of granulation tissue and pus (Fig. 27-1). Any of the late manifestations of bronchial foreign body aspiration may be obscured by prior treatment with antibiotics or steroids.

The physical signs of bronchial foreign bodies vary. Careful auscultation of the chest is essential. Auscultation must be carried out in a systematic fashion. The examiner should pay close attention to the symmetry of breath sounds because decreased breath sounds over a lobe or segment may be the only finding in certain cases. All lung fields should be assessed for the presence or absence of adventitial breath sounds, particularly wheezing. Asymmetric wheezing is a strong indicator of unilateral bronchial obstruction. Symmetric wheezing may be noted in cases of foreign bodies. Therefore symmetric wheezing should not be assumed to result from asthma. The two-headed stethoscope is especially helpful because it allows simultaneous examination of both sides of the chest.[7]

Depending on the size, shape, and location of the foreign body, breath sounds may vary. Most foreign bodies end up in the right bronchus because it is wider and originates at a less acute angle from the trachea.[2] Secretions may shift from one location to another, affecting what the examiner hears. The foreign body itself may shift position and cause a variation in the aeration distal to the object. Jackson and Jackson[8] divided such obstruction into four types (Fig. 27-2). The most common type of obstruction is the check-valve (see Fig. 27-2, *B* and *C*). In this situation, breath sounds are diminished over the affected area. There may be localized wheezing noted on inspiration. If no air escapes on expiration, no wheezing occurs. In some patients, forced expiration leads to expiratory wheezing.

The stop-valve obstruction is the next most common (see Fig. 27-2, *D*). In such cases, breath sounds are diminished over the affected area. The bypass valve phenomenon is less common (see Fig. 27-2, *A*). If airflow is not impeded, no change in breath sounds and no adventitial sounds occur. If there is some diminution of airflow past the foreign body, localized wheezing and diminished breath sounds are noted over the affected area.

In Jackson and Jackson's representation,[8] the foreign body remains in one bronchus. Foreign bodies in the lower trachea, however, may shift from one bronchus to the other and give rise to a variety of signs and symptoms. Multiple foreign bodies in a single patient may also exist, further confusing the issue.

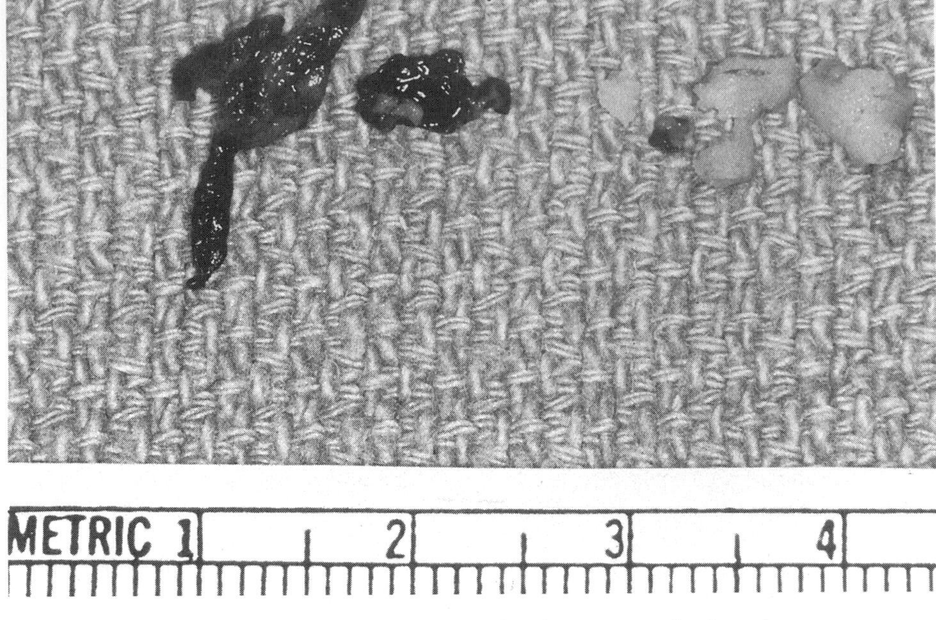

Fig. 27-1. Peanut fragments with granulation tissue removed at bronchoscopy.

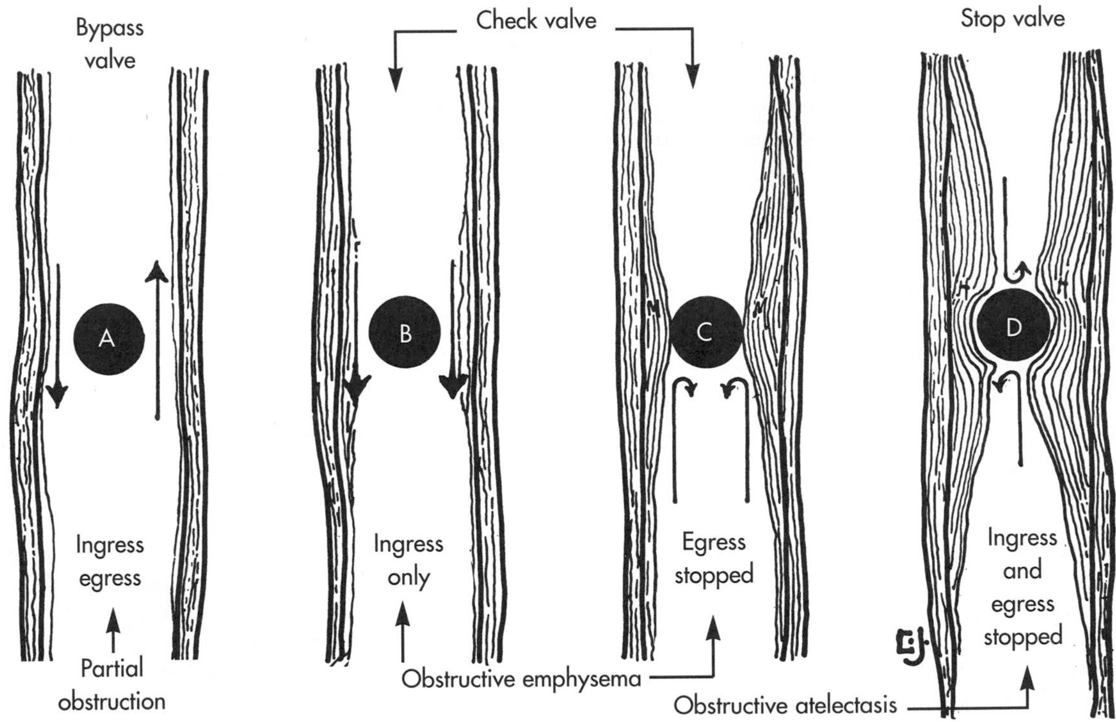

Fig. 27-2. Schematic illustrations of the three types of bronchial obstruction clinically encountered. *Type 1,* Bypass valve obstruction. **A,** The foreign body permits the passage of air in and out on inspiration and expiration so that no collapse or emphysema occurs in the tributary lung. *Type 2,* Check-valve obstruction. **B** and **C** represent the same foreign body in different phases of the respiratory cycle. **B,** The swollen mucosa has retreated because of enlargement of the bronchial lumen on inspiration. At the beginning of expiration, the bronchial wall contracts sufficiently to bring the swollen mucosa into contact with the foreign body. **C,** This valvelike closure traps the air in the subjacent lung or portion of lung, which becomes emphysematous from repetition of the valvular action at each respiratory cycle. This is obstructive emphysema. *Type 3,* Stop-valve obstruction. **D,** A foreign body is embedded in swollen mucosa, completely obstructing a bronchus at all stages of respiration. Absorption of the air results in collapse of the subjacent lung. This condition is obstructive atelectasis. If a main bronchus is obstructed, massive collapse of the corresponding lung occurs. *Type 4,* A fourth type was omitted from the schema for clarity. In check-valve obstruction, the reverse of type 2, air is forced out on expiration, especially the forced expiration of cough, but ingress is checked by the ball-valve action of the foreign body. This hastens atelectasis, and this type quickly merges into type 3. (From Jackson C, Jackson CL: *Bronchoesophagology,* Philadelphia, 1950, WB Saunders, p 17.)

RADIOGRAPHIC ASSESSMENT

Radiographic studies provide valuable information to the endoscopist. Not only can they document the presence of a foreign body, but also they act as an aid in extraction. Studies that are incomplete or of poor quality may lead to errors or a delay in diagnosis. Although many foreign bodies are radiolucent, special techniques may help establish a diagnosis.

Appropriate studies and careful techniques are critically important in accurately locating an aspirated foreign body. Two studies that form the basis of assessment are the lateral soft tissue neck radiograph and the chest series.

If a laryngeal or tracheal foreign body is suspected, a lateral neck radiograph may provide useful information. Esclamado and Richardson[6] showed that with a laryngeal or tracheal foreign body, the neck radiograph is more likely to be abnormal than the chest series. With high-quality neck radiographs, the caliber of the airway can be clearly seen. When the arms and shoulders are held down and backward, a single lateral radiograph can profile the air column in both the larynx and trachea. However, extreme care must be taken because the patient is at risk for life-threatening airway obstruction.

In cases of suspected foreign body aspiration, a standard chest series should include anteroposterior and lateral end-inspiratory views as well as an end-expiratory radiograph. Radiographs should be carefully examined for local atelectasis, local hyperinflation, and visible foreign bodies. Expiratory radiographs delineate postobstructive hyperinflation because of air trapping behind the foreign object and subsequent failure of the trapped air to empty on exhalation (Fig. 27-3). This can cause mediastinal shift to the uninvolved side. Unfortunately, expiratory radiographs are often unsuccessful in small children.[9] In these cases, decubitus radiographs or fluoroscopy may provide additional information. Most airway foreign bodies are radiolucent, and some cases present with a bypass valve phenomenon. Therefore a normal chest series does not rule out the presence of a foreign body in the airway. In the face of a suggestive history, bronchoscopy is performed.[10]

Bronchography is occasionally used as a diagnostic tool. In this technique, contrast media is instilled directly into the airway to demonstrate the relationship of a foreign object to the bronchial tree. Bronchography can help localize a radiolucent plastic foreign body that is beyond the range of endoscopic visualization.

For radiopaque objects lodged far in the lung periphery, simultaneous biplane fluoroscopy is used to visualize the object during extraction. The equipment is located in the cardiac catheterization laboratory. This important technique may serve as a "last chance" to remove a foreign body endoscopically; thoracotomy is the only alternative if endoscopic efforts fail.

Although computed tomography and magnetic resonance imaging have revolutionized medicine in the last decade, they have little value in the diagnosis and management of foreign body aspiration. Magnetic resonance imaging has been used to diagnose a previously unidentified bronchial foreign body.[11] However, because of the young age of the patients, the time and expense involved, and the risk of sedation (or general anesthesia) in a patient with pulmonary compromise, the use of these modalities in foreign body aspiration remains limited.

MANAGEMENT

Acute Aspiration: Complete Obstruction

In a witnessed foreign body aspiration with acute airway obstruction, the Heimlich maneuver is the procedure of choice. Currently, this maneuver is recommended for children older than 1 year of age. For infants younger than 1 year, chest thrusts and back blows are indicated.[12] Unlike adults, younger children may not be able to respond to the question traditionally asked of suspected aspiration victims: "Can you speak?" Blind finger sweeping in the oropharynx is contraindicated in infants because the foreign body may become lodged in the larynx, converting a partial obstruction into a complete one. This maneuver may also force the foreign body into the esophagus, where it may compress the trachea against the upper sternum.

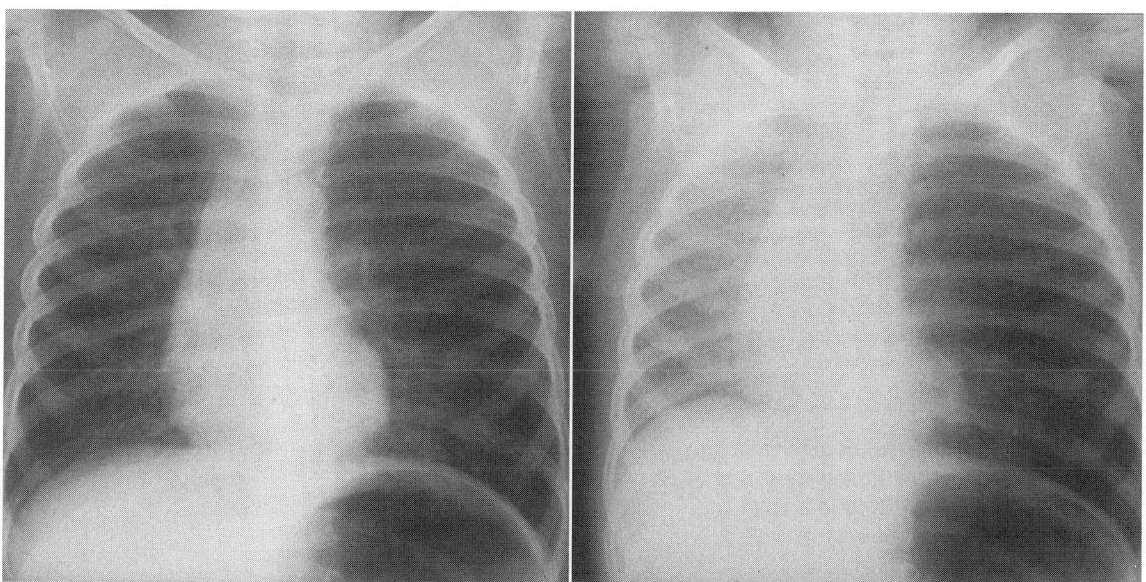

Fig. 27-3. Anteroposterior inspiratory *(left)* and expiratory *(right)* chest radiographs. Air trapping in the left lung is caused by a peanut in the left mainstem bronchus.

Questionable Foreign Body Aspiration: Flexible vs. Rigid Bronchoscopy

Because the diagnosis of foreign body aspiration is not always obvious, bronchoscopy may initially serve as a diagnostic procedure. In this setting, either flexible or open-tube (rigid) endoscopy is indicated. Selection of a particular technique depends on physician expertise and experience in a particular geographic area.

If a foreign body in a child is confirmed by physical examination or radiographic studies or if the endoscopist has a high index of suspicion that a foreign body is present, open-tube bronchoscopy is the preferred technique for removal. The same holds true if a foreign body is noted on flexible endoscopic examination.[13] The flexible bronchoscope is not the instrument of choice for bronchial foreign body removal for several reasons: limited suction, lack of ventilatory capability, limited instrumentation, and lack of airway control. A unique indication for flexible bronchoscopy is a nonradiopaque peripheral foreign body that cannot be seen with a rigid bronchoscope. In this situation, inserting a flexible instrument through an open-tube bronchoscope may greatly assist in making a diagnosis.

Rigid Bronchoscopy

Removal of an aspirated foreign body through a rigid bronchoscope is the treatment of choice. Other methods are to be discouraged. In general, a suspected airway foreign body should be removed as soon as possible. Haste should not preclude having the necessary equipment and experienced operating room personnel available. If the proper conditions are not available, consideration should be given to transferring the patient to another facility.

Airway foreign body removal can be a technically demanding exercise. Removal is facilitated by careful preparation. This includes checking equipment for malfunction before the procedure as well as having backup equipment available. If possible, a duplicate of the aspirated foreign body is obtained. This facilitates forceps selection by allowing practice attempts to grasp the duplicate.

Two methods of extraction through a rigid bronchoscope are available. The first is forceps removal through a distal lighted bronchoscope. This technique offers a large variety of forceps and superior tactile feedback. The second method is foreign body extraction with an optical forceps system. This system with fiberoptic lighting and telescopic viewing offers an improved "look" at the aspirated object and serves as an excellent teaching tool. Neither method is superior; the endoscopist should have experience with both.

Regardless of the technique used, difficulties may be encountered in rigid bronchoscopic foreign body extraction. Objects may fragment or strip off the forceps in the larynx. A large laryngeal forceps should always be available to deal with this possibility. Occasionally, forceps may be unable to grab a particular foreign body. In these cases a balloon catheter placed distally or a stone basket used to encircle the object may be helpful.[14,15]

In all cases, no more than 1½ hours should be spent attempting to remove an aspirated foreign object. Occasionally, edema or bleeding may obscure the endoscopist's view and necessitate stopping a procedure prematurely. In this situation, antibiotics and corticosteroids are administered and the patient brought back to the operating room in 3 to 4 days for another attempt at removal. Rarely, an object may be aspirated that is too large to be removed endoscopically. In this situation, a combined endoscopic and external cervical approach is used.[16] Although this requires a tracheal incision to remove the foreign body, no long-term sequelae should be expected. An endoscopist and two assistants are required to perform this technique successfully.

Most patients who undergo removal of airway foreign bodies have an uneventful postoperative course. For patients who have a long-standing foreign body extracted, productive postoperative coughing may occur as secretions trapped behind the object are released. Hemoptysis from disrupted granulation tissue may also be seen. Antibiotics are not administered after surgery unless the patient was being treated with them beforehand. Also, postoperative chest radiographs are not routinely ordered. This is obviated by a "second-look" bronchoscopy, in which the bronchi are examined immediately after the initial removal to check for remnant material or an additional foreign object.

Alternative Therapies

In the past, methods other than endoscopy have been advocated for the treatment of aspirated foreign bodies. Burrington and Cotton[17] introduced a technique of bronchodilator inhalation followed by postural drainage and percussion. This technique was continued up to 4 days before bronchoscopy. A subsequent report, however, found that this technique had only a 25% success rate compared with an 89% success rate with bronchoscopy.[18] In addition, the authors reported an episode of cardiopulmonary arrest secondary to foreign body migration. Because of the great risk of complications and low success rate, bronchodilation and postural drainage are not recommended.

Another therapy not advisable is expectant management of aspirated foreign bodies. The chance of a complication increases while waiting for an object to be coughed up: The object may migrate, or the inflammatory response becomes more intense. Even in objects thought to be dissolvable, bronchoscopy should be performed. Hard candy, which theoretically should melt away, may cause an intense inflammatory reaction. The hazard of leaving a potential irritant in the airway outweighs the risks of rigid bronchoscopy performed by experienced personnel.

OUTCOME

Airway foreign bodies can be removed with a low rate of complications. Potential complications after removal are listed in Box 27-2. Delay in diagnosis has a marked effect on the rate of complications, probably greater than any other factor.[19] This is significant because at least 25% of patients with the presenting symptom of an aspirated foreign body have complications at least 1 week after the aspiration occurred.[2,3] This delay

BOX 27-2

Complications after Airway Foreign Body Removal

Acute airway obstruction	Laryngeal lacerations
Pneumomediastinum	Bronchial stenosis
Pneumothorax	Tracheoesophageal fistula
Massive hemoptysis	Distal bronchiectasis
Laryngeal edema	

is not always attributable to caregiver negligence because many patients have been seen previously by a physician. Unfortunately, a low index of suspicion for an airway foreign body can lead to tragedy, as exemplified by two reported cases of death after undiagnosed foreign body aspiration.[20]

REFERENCES

1. National Safety Council: *Accident facts,* Itasca, Ill, 1992, The Council, p 32.
2. Holinger PH: Foreign bodies in the air and food passages, *Trans Am Acad Ophthalmol* 66:193-219, 1962.
3. Kim IG, Brummitt WM, Humphrey A, Siomra SW, Wallace WB: Foreign body in the airway: a review of 202 cases, *Laryngoscope* 83:347-354, 1973.

Disease Mechanisms

4. Mantel K, Burteandt I: Tracheobronchial foreign body aspiration in childhood: a report on 224 cases, *Eur J Pediatr* 145:211-216, 1986.
5. Harris CS, Baker SP, Smith GA, Harris RM: Childhood asphyxiation by food: a national analysis and overview, *JAMA* 251(17):2231-2235, 1984.

Clinical Manifestations

6. Esclamado RM, Richardson MA: Laryngotracheal foreign bodies in children: a comparison with bronchial foreign bodies, *Am J Dis Child* 141:259-262, 1987.
7. Parsons DS, Kearns D: The two-headed stethoscope: its use for ruling out airway foreign bodies, *Int J Pediatr Otorhinolaryngol* 22:181-185, 1991.
8. Jackson C, Jackson CL: *Diseases of the air and food passages of foreign body origin,* Philadelphia, 1936, WB Saunders, p 135.

Radiographic Assessment

9. Griffiths DM, Freeman NV: Expiratory chest x-ray examination in the diagnosis of inhaled foreign bodies, *Br Med J* 288:1074-1075, 1984.
10. Suedstrom E, Puhakka H, Kero P: How accurate is chest radiography in the diagnosis of tracheobronchial foreign bodies in children? *Pediatr Radiol* 19:520-522, 1989.
11. O'Uchi T, Tokumaru A, Mikami I, Yamasoba T, Kikuchi S: Value of MR imaging in detecting a peanut causing bronchial obstruction, *Am J Radiol* 159:481-482, 1992.

Management

12. Chameides L, ed: *Textbook of pediatric advanced life support,* Dallas, 1988, American Heart Association, pp 16-19.
13. Wood RE, Gauderer MWL: Flexible fiberoptic bronchoscopy in the management of tracheobronchial foreign bodies in children: the value of a combined approach with open tube bronchoscopy, *J Pediatr Surg* 19:693-698, 1984.
14. Kosloske AM: The Fogarty balloon technique for the removal of foreign bodies from tracheobronchial tree, *Surg Gynecol Obstet* 155:72-73, 1982.
15. Moss R, Kanchanapoon V: Stone basket extraction of a bronchial foreign body, *Arch Surg* 121:975, 1985 (letter).
16. Swensson EE, Rah KH, Kim MC, Brooks JW, Salzberg AM: Extraction of large tracheal foreign bodies through a tracheostoma under bronchoscopic control, *Ann Thorac Surg* 39(3):251-253, 1985.
17. Burrington JD, Cotton EK: Removal of foreign bodies from the tracheobronchial tree, *J Pediatr Surg* 7:119-122, 1972.
18. Law DK, Kosloske AM: Management of tracheobronchial foreign bodies in children: a reevaluation of postural drainage and bronchoscopy, *Pediatrics* 58:362-367, 1976.

Outcome

19. Liancai M, Ping H, Dequiang S: The causes and complications of late diagnosis of foreign body aspiration in children: report of 210 cases, *Arch Otolaryngol Head Neck Surg* 117:876-879, 1991.
20. Humphries CT, Wagener JS, Morgan WJ: Fatal prolonged foreign body aspiration following an asymptomatic interval, *Am J Emerg Med* 6:611-613, 1988.

CHAPTER 28

Aspiration Syndromes

John L. Colombo and Paul H. Sammut

Although Hippocrates noted the hazards of aspiration in 400 BC, it was not until Mendelson's classic description[1] in 1946 that clinicians appeared to recognize the widespread nature of aspiration lung injury. Much has been learned in the past 50 years about the effects of aspiration of foreign materials into the respiratory tract. However, the diagnosis and treatment, particularly of chronic aspiration, remain a challenge in pediatric and adult medicine.

The term *aspiration pneumonia* is often used as a generic description of several clinical syndromes. The clinical findings depend on host factors as well as the quantity and type of material aspirated (Table 28-1). Any individual may suffer from one or more of these processes. Aspiration is a common event, sometimes causing acute symptoms but probably more frequently occurring silently, even in normal individuals.[2] At the other end of the spectrum is massive aspiration that causes acute respiratory failure. This typically occurs with gastric contents. This chapter first addresses massive aspiration and infectious complications of aspiration. Foreign bodies, near-drowning, and hydrocarbon aspiration are discussed in Chapters 25 and 27.

Because it is often impossible to definitively prove that aspiration is the cause of existing lung disease, a large element of clinical judgment is required. A first step in clinical diagnosis is to recognize both the clinical manifestations of aspiration (see Table 28-1) and conditions that predispose to aspiration (Box 28-1).

ACUTE, LARGE-VOLUME ASPIRATION

Disease Mechanisms

Aspiration of gastric contents can have a broad range of pathologic and physiologic consequences, depending especially on the pH and volume of the aspirate and the amount of particulate material (see Table 28-1). Most information on patho-

Table 28-1 Syndromes of Aspiration Injury

SYNDROME/CLINICAL FINDINGS	SUBSTANCES	MAJOR PATHOPHYSIOLOGIC EVENTS
Large airway obstruction	Large solids (meat, peanut)	Atelectasis
Atelectasis	Large-bolus liquids or large particles (gastric contents)	Hypoxemia
Asphyxia ("cafe coronary")		Hypercapnia
Atelectasis or hyperinflation		Bronchitis, bronchiectasis, pneumonia
Pneumothorax		Death
Wheeze, cough		
Apnea or laryngospasm		
Acute chemical injury	Gastric contents (pH < 2.5, small particles)	Pulmonary edema
Diffuse infiltrates	Toxic exogenous liquids (hydrocarbons)	Shock
Adult respiratory distress syndrome	Toxic gases	Hypoxemia
Apnea or laryngospasm		Hemorrhagic pneumonia
Tracheobronchitis		Alveolar consolidation with polymorphonuclear neutrophil leukocytes, fibrin
		Mucosal sloughing
Infectious injury (acute or chronic)	Nasal or oral secretions	Necrotizing pneumonia
Pneumonia/bronchopneumonia	Gastric contents (hospitalized patients)	Alveolar consolidation with polymorphonuclear neutrophil leukocytes, exudate
Abscess	Exogenous contaminated materials	Bacteria (anaerobic or mixed anaerobic and aerobic), gram-negative bacilli in hospital-acquired abscess
Empyema or effusion		
Ventilator-associated pneumonia		
Recurrent chemical injury	Oral, nasal, or gastric contents	
Bronchitis or bronchiolitis		Granulomatous inflammation
Bronchopneumonia or pneumonia		Fibrosis
Atelectasis		Interstitial inflammation
Wheezing, cough		Lipoid pneumonia
Apnea or laryngospasm		Meat or vegetable fibers
Gastroesophageal reflux		Bronchiolitis obliterans

BOX 28-1
Conditions Predisposing to Aspiration Lung Injury

Anatomic and mechanical

Nasoenteric tube
Tracheostomy
Endotracheal tube
Micrognathia
Macroglossia
Cleft palate
Laryngeal cleft
Tracheoesophageal fistula
Vascular ring
Gastroesophageal reflux
Achalasia (cricopharyngeal)
Collagen vascular disease (scleroderma, dermatomyositis)
Tumors, masses (foreign body, abscess)

Neuromuscular

Depressed consciousness (e.g., general anesthesia, drug intoxication, head trauma, seizure, central nervous system infection)

Neuromuscular—cont'd

Immaturity of swallowing (prematurity)
Cerebral palsy
Hydrocephalus
Increased intracranial pressure
Vocal cord paralysis
Dysautonomia
Muscular dystrophy
Myasthenia gravis
Guillain-Barré syndrome
Werdnig-Hoffmann disease

Miscellaneous

Poor oral hygiene or gingivitis
Trauma to pharynx

physiologic consequences is derived from animal studies. Aspiration of large particles can produce acute airway obstruction and severe hypoventilation. Smaller particle or liquid aspirates induce hypoxemia via a variety of mechanisms, including reflex airway closure, hemorrhagic pneumonitis, destruction and dilution of surfactant with secondary atelectasis, and pulmonary edema from extravasation of intravascular fluids and protein. Mendelson's classic study[1] described the "asthma-like reaction" of obstetric patients who had aspirated large amounts of gastric contents. In subsequent animal studies he and others showed that large-volume acid aspiration (≥ 1 ml/kg, pH < 2.5) caused severe hypoxemia secondary to these pathophysiologic changes. With acid aspiration, these events are typically more severe and last longer than neutral liquids. Localized areas of atelectasis occur within a few minutes after acid aspiration.[3] Other early histologic findings include epithelial degeneration of the bronchi, pulmonary edema, and hemorrhage with necrosis of type I alveolar cells followed by acute infiltration of neutrophils and fibrin in alveolar spaces. Over the next 24 to 36 hours a marked increase of neutrophil infiltration results in alveolar consolidation, and mucosal sloughing may be seen in the airways. This correlates with the clinical findings of fever and increased infiltrates on chest radiographs. Hyaline membranes may be seen after 48 hours. Reparative processes, including the regeneration of bronchial epithelium, proliferation of fibroblasts, and decreased acute inflammation, begin by 72 hours. Lungs from animals obtained 2 to 3 weeks after acid aspiration show parenchymal scarring with macrophages, lymphocytes, and hemosiderin, often with bronchiolitis obliterans.[4]

Physiologic changes typically occur significantly later, and the inflammatory response is more prolonged after aspiration of small particles than after liquids. Intravascular fluid shifts into the lungs within minutes with liquid aspiration and usually after 3 to 4 hours with small particles. With smaller-volume aspiration of either acid or gastric juices, acute interstitial pneumonia develops, followed by chronic airway inflammation, interstitial thickening, granuloma formation, and fibrosis.[5] The critical volume for severe pneumonitis is estimated at 0.8 ml/kg.[6]

Infection does not usually play a primary role in aspiration of gastric contents. However, such aspiration may impair pulmonary defenses, predisposing to secondary bacterial pneumonia.

Clinical Manifestations and Management

The diagnosis of massive aspiration pneumonia usually involves a witnessed inhalation of vomit or tracheal suctioning of gastric contents. In the absence of such events, the diagnosis depends on noting compatible clinical and radiographic findings in a patient at risk for aspiration. Early bronchoscopy has been reported to be a useful diagnostic adjunct for finding gastric contents grossly or microscopically in the tracheobronchial tree or for finding localized erythema.[7] The management of patients with massive aspiration includes supportive measures of oxygen, mechanical ventilation with positive end-expiratory pressure, and prevention of further aspiration. Bronchoscopy and lavage are useful when significant particulate aspiration is suspected, rigid bronchoscopy being necessary for larger particles. There is no value in lavage for liquid aspiration or in attempts to neutralize aspirated acid.[4] Intravascular volume should be maintained; there is no apparent advantage of colloid over crystalloid.[8]

Numerous animal and human studies show treatment with corticosteroids to be beneficial,[9] ineffective, or harmful.[4] Although corticosteroids may be beneficial when given very close to the time of massive aspiration,[9] it is generally recommended that they not be used.[10]

Outcomes

Mortality

Mortality rates as high as 40% to 80% have been reported with massive aspiration.[11] However, more recent reports involving children and adults had a mortality rate of 5% and no deaths with involvement of three or fewer lobes.[12] Prevention should be the goal, but with conservative support and careful observation for complications, a good outcome is likely when massive aspiration does occur.

Infectious Complications

Aspiration of stomach contents into the lungs is associated with subsequent pleuropulmonary infections in as many as 50% of patients.[13] The risk is increased with the conditions listed in Box 28-2. The originating site of bacterial pathogens is usually the oropharynx, but colonizing organisms from the stomach have been increasingly implicated. However, the bacteriology of aspiration pneumonia is more often determined by the presence or absence of preexisting disease. Detection of superimposed infection can be difficult, and its treatment depends on the clinical setting.

Table 28-2 Colonizing Organisms of the Pharynx

AGE	PREDOMINATING ORGANISMS
Birth-1 day	*Streptococcus salivarius*
1 day-1 year	*Staphylococcus* species
	Neisseria species
	Veillonella species
	Actinomyces species
	Nocardia species
	Fusobacterium species
	Bacteroides species
	Corynebacterium
	Candida species
	Coliforms
1-12 years	Anaerobes
(deciduous dentition)	*Streptococcus mutans*
	Streptococcus sanguis
13-16 years	*Bacteroides melaninogenicus* and spirochetes, which reach adult levels

BOX 28-2
Conditions Predisposing to Infectious Complications of Aspiration

- Gingivitis
- Decayed teeth
- Gastric outlet or intestinal obstruction
- Enteral tube feeding
- Prolonged hospitalization
- Endotracheal intubation
- Use of antacids/H_2 blockers

Early clinical features of aspiration include fever, coughing and wheezing, leukocytosis, and infiltrates seen radiologically. The subsequent development of infection should be suspected if deterioration occurs with some or all of these findings, particularly after initial improvement. Supporting evidence should be sought with cultures, radiographs, and serial white blood cell counts.

The presence of artificial airways and nasogastric or orogastric tubes increases the risk of aspiration pneumonia because of their effects on swallowing. Oropharyngeal flora, which vary depending on the age of the patient (Table 28-2) or prior antibiotic use, are usually responsible for the infections.

As with adults, in children older than 1 year of age, anaerobic organisms predominate over aerobic organisms by a ratio of between 3:1 and 10:1. However, *Bacteroides melaninogenicus* and the spirochetes are present in fewer numbers in the oropharyngeal flora in children younger than 13 to 16 years of age.[14] Transtracheal aspirate cultures from children with aspiration pneumonia implicate anaerobes almost as frequently as in adults.[15] The predominant anaerobes are *B. melaninogenicus,* fusobacteria, and *Bacteroides fragilis.* The predominant aerobic bacteria are alphahemolytic streptococci, *Escherichia coli, Klebsiella pneumoniae,* and *Staphylococcus aureus.*

When aspiration occurs in an institutionalized patient or in a patient previously receiving broad-spectrum antibiotic therapy, nosocomial and facultative organisms predominate. These include *E. coli, Proteus* species, and *Pseudomonas aeruginosa.*[16]

Anaerobic organisms have been isolated from nearly all cases of pulmonary abscesses in both children and adults.[17] Hospitalized patients or those who have received prior antibiotics are more likely to develop an abscess of the lung as a nosocomial disease. In these cases, *E. coli, Klebsiella* species, and *Pseudomonas* species, as well as yeast and fungi, are more commonly responsible, with less contribution from anaerobes.

Management

Prevention is the most effective form of therapy. Gum and dental diseases should be appropriately treated. Decisions involving the placement of gastric or airway tubes must include consideration of the risk of aspiration pneumonia. Maintenance of low gastric volumes may reduce the risk of gastroesophageal reflux (GER) and aspiration. Increasing the stomach pH increases bacterial colonization rates and hence the risk of pneumonia. Controversy exists, however, in the preferential use of sucralfate over antacids to lower this risk.

No controlled studies evaluate the empiric use of available antibiotics in gastric aspiration, and good outcomes have been recorded without their use.[12] In general, antibiotics should be withheld unless there are strong risk factors for bacterial infection or until signs of superimposed infection have emerged. The choice of antimicrobial therapy in these cases should be guided by the clinical situation. In the previously healthy individual, in whom anaerobic bacteria are most likely to predominate, initial therapy with penicillin, ampicillin, or clindamycin is recommended. Other agents used with success include metronidazole and cefoxitin. In the treatment of pneumonia in children with underlying chronic disease, institutionalized patients, and those having received prior broad-spectrum antibiotic therapy, a second- or third-generation cephalosporin should be considered. In immunocompromised patients, a combination of an aminoglycoside and a synthetic penicillin or cephalosporin such as ceftazidime might be initiated until culture results are available to guide more specific therapy. Chest percussive therapy in the presence of lung abscesses may assist drainage, and early drainage of empyema also is recommended.

RECURRENT, SMALL-VOLUME ASPIRATION AND GER

In addition to quantity and quality of aspirated material, the variables of host and frequency probably play a larger role with recurrent, small-volume aspiration (also termed *microaspiration* or *silent aspiration*). It appears that small-volume aspiration into the lungs is a relatively common event, with normal adults aspirating oropharyngeal secretions during sleep.[2] A high incidence of aspiration has also been shown among patients with tracheostomies[18] and endotracheal tubes.[19] Nasogastric tubes have been associated with increased aspiration based on pneumonia occurrence and autopsies[20] but not in a small series of children using a radioisotope marker.[21] Although a relationship among recurrent aspiration, GER, and respiratory disease has been noted for several years, the specific interactions of these events remain uncertain.

Disease Mechanisms

Often it is difficult to establish a relationship between small-volume aspiration and pulmonary disease. This may result from the low sensitivity of tests detecting such intermittent aspiration and the low specificity of tests documenting aspiration as the cause of existing disease. It is generally easier to detect GER, and this may be the reason that lung disease is more commonly associated with it. This is further complicated by the fact that patients with swallowing abnormalities frequently also have GER. Therefore clinical studies often do not differentiate among GER, dysfunctional swallowing, and small-volume aspiration. However, it is important to remember that GER and aspiration may occur independently of each other.

BOX 28-3
Mechanisms for the Association of GER and Respiratory Disease

GER causing respiratory disease

Aspiration
- Direct effect: tracheitis, bronchitis, pneumonia, atelectasis
- Reflex from irritation of the trachea or upper airway, laryngospasm, bronchospasm
- Indirect effect: Inflammation or another alteration predisposing to airway hyperreactivity
- Esophageal: airway reflex without aspiration

Respiratory disease causing GER

- Diaphragm flattening and changes in abdominopleural pressure gradient
- Effects of medication (e.g., theophylline) causing decreased lower esophageal sphincter pressure

Depending on the criteria used for diagnosis, 25% to 80% of children with chronic respiratory disease have abnormal GER.[22] Possible mechanisms involved in this relationship are listed in Box 28-3. Historically, the relationship of GER to lung disease was presumed to be caused by aspiration, but elucidation of the gastroesophageal airway reflexes brought this mechanism to the forefront. With further studies of small-volume aspiration, there appears to be more acceptance of the importance of both major mechanisms.[23] In addition, airway inflammation from aspiration may predispose to or accentuate airway hyperreactivity.

Reflex bronchoconstriction from esophageal acidification has been demonstrated in both animals[24] and humans.[25] However, 10 ml of acid infused into the cat esophagus produced less than one third of the increase in total lung resistance evoked by 0.05 ml of acid instilled in the trachea. Both reactions appear to be vagally mediated.[24] In a study of nine asthmatic children, four patients with positive Bernstein's tests[25] (epigastric pain after esophageal acid infusion but not with saline) developed wheezing when 30 ml of 0.1 N hydrogen chloride was infused into the distal esophagus during sleep, but five patients with negative Bernstein's tests studied similarly showed no respiratory effect. Esophageal acidification can also increase nonspecific airway hyperreactivity without necessarily causing a change in baseline pulmonary mechanics.[26] However, human esophageal acid perfusion studies do not preclude the occurrence of associated acid aspiration.

Other GER-associated respiratory disorders are listed in Box 28-4. Obstructive, or mixed, apnea appears to be more common than central apnea.[27] Reflex central apnea is produced

BOX 28-4
Disorders Associated with GER

Asthma	Bronchiolitis obliterans
Chronic cough or wheeze	Apnea, bradycardia
Pneumonia, bronchitis	Acute, life-threatening events
Atelectasis	Stridor
Bronchiectasis	Hoarseness
Pulmonary fibrosis	Laryngomalacia

in premature animals with tracheal instillation of milk and hypotonic fluids but not with saline or tracheal fluid.[28] In most clinical studies, although significant GER was detected, overt vomiting was uncommon.

Improvement after antireflux therapy is often relied on to establish the relationship between GER and respiratory disease.[29,30] Such studies offer strong support for the importance of aspiration and GER in pulmonary disease. However, most are retrospective and uncontrolled.

Two prospective, controlled studies in adults with pulmonary disease showed significant pulmonary improvement with either medical or surgical treatment of GER.[31,32] Medical treatment with H_2-receptor antagonists produced significant respiratory improvement compared with placebo but less than seen in a surgically treated group. There were significantly fewer pulmonary symptoms and a decreased need for pulmonary medications, especially corticosteroids,[32] in the treated groups but no change in the results of pulmonary function tests.

It is also possible that respiratory diseases and their treatment can provoke GER. More negative intrathoracic pressure and increased abdominal pressure induced by coughing may increase the likelihood of reflux. Hyperinflation and diaphragmatic flattening with secondary stretching of the crura can also predispose to reflux. However, no increased reflux was found during provoked bronchospasm in adults with both asthma and GER.[33] Theophylline decreases lower esophageal sphincter pressure.[34] Positional changes associated with postural drainage and chest physiotherapy may increase the likelihood of GER.

Assessment and Diagnosis

Evaluation begins with a detailed history and physical examination. The patient or caregivers should be asked about the timing of symptoms in relation to feedings and position changes, spitting or vomiting, irritability in an infant, epigastric discomfort in an older child, and nocturnal symptoms of coughing or wheezing. It is important to remember that coughing or gagging may be minimal or absent in a child with a depressed cough reflex. Observation of the child during feeding is essential when the diagnosis of aspiration is being considered. Particular attention should be given to nasopharyngeal reflux, difficulty with sucking or swallowing, and associated coughing and choking. The palate, tongue, and oropharynx should be inspected for gross abnormalities and stimulated to assess the gag reflex. Drooling or the excessive accumulation of secretions in the mouth suggests dysphagia or esophageal motility disorder. Auscultation may reveal transient wheezes or crackles after feeding, particularly in the dependent lung segments.

A plain chest radiograph is the initial study for a child suspected of having recurrent aspiration. A patient with "classic" radiographic findings is shown in Fig. 28-1. Although segmental or lobar infiltrates localizing to dependent areas may be common, there is a wide variety in radiographic findings. In 22 children with known recurrent aspiration, chest radiographs showed localized infiltrates involving no more than two lobes in 41%, diffuse infiltrates in 27%, and bronchial wall thickening or hyperinflation in only 18%.[35] The chest radiograph was normal in 14% of these patients. A computed tomographic scan may be helpful in diagnosing lipoid pneumonia (Fig. 28-2).

Numerous other tests are available for detecting GER or aspiration (Table 28-3). A properly performed barium esophagram may demonstrate reflux into the nasopharynx or direct aspiration to the trachea. It may be difficult to differentiate aspiration through the vocal cords during swallowing from that through a laryngoesophageal cleft. The esophagram is most useful in detecting anatomic problems, including vascular rings, strictures, hiatal hernias, and tracheoesophageal fistulae without atresia (H type). The last may be difficult to demonstrate. The esophagram also yields qualitative information on esophageal motility and, when extended, on gastric emptying. The short observation time renders the esophagram relatively insensitive for detecting aspiration and GER. Because physiologic reflux episodes may occur, it can also be nonspecific.[36] However, if repetitive free GER is noted, it is probably unnecessary to do further tests for GER.

A modified barium swallow, using videofluoroscopy imaging, is the standard study for evaluating the swallowing mechanism. Because it uses different textures and quantities of liquid barium or foods laced with barium, it is a sensitive and detailed test for evaluating aspiration and defining food textures and techniques that can be used to reduce aspiration.[37]

The gastroesophageal scintiscan (Fig. 28-3), or milk scan, is more physiologic and sensitive than the barium esophagram in detecting GER. Some investigators have found that it can detect aspiration in as many as 25% of children with chronic respiratory symptoms,[38] whereas others have found it relatively insensitive.[39] These differences may relate to variability in techniques and populations studied. The scintiscan is particularly useful for measuring gastric emptying time. Its main disadvantages are the inability to detect anatomic abnormalities, possible insensitivity for aspiration, and cost.[40]

Another proposed use of radioisotopes in diagnosing aspiration is the "salivagram," which uses a small volume of concentrated marker placed on the tongue[41] or a continuous oral infusion of labeled fluid.[42] More studies of these and other methods are necessary to determine their usefulness for detecting significant aspiration.

Esophageal pH monitoring after an acidic meal was described by Tuttle and Grossman in 1958.[43] Although this test has a sensitivity as high as 92%, it is nonspecific, detecting episodes in up to 31% of patients not having pathologic GER.[36] Monitoring of esophageal pH for 18 to 24 hours is often considered to be the gold standard for detecting significant GER. When performed with high and low esophageal pH probes, it can detect upper and lower esophageal reflux, the duration and frequency of reflux episodes, and nocturnal reflux. It may also detect a temporal relationship with respiratory abnormalities when combined with polygraph studies. Disadvantages include cost (it often requires hospitalization), inability to detect nonacid (e.g., postprandial) reflux, and pos-

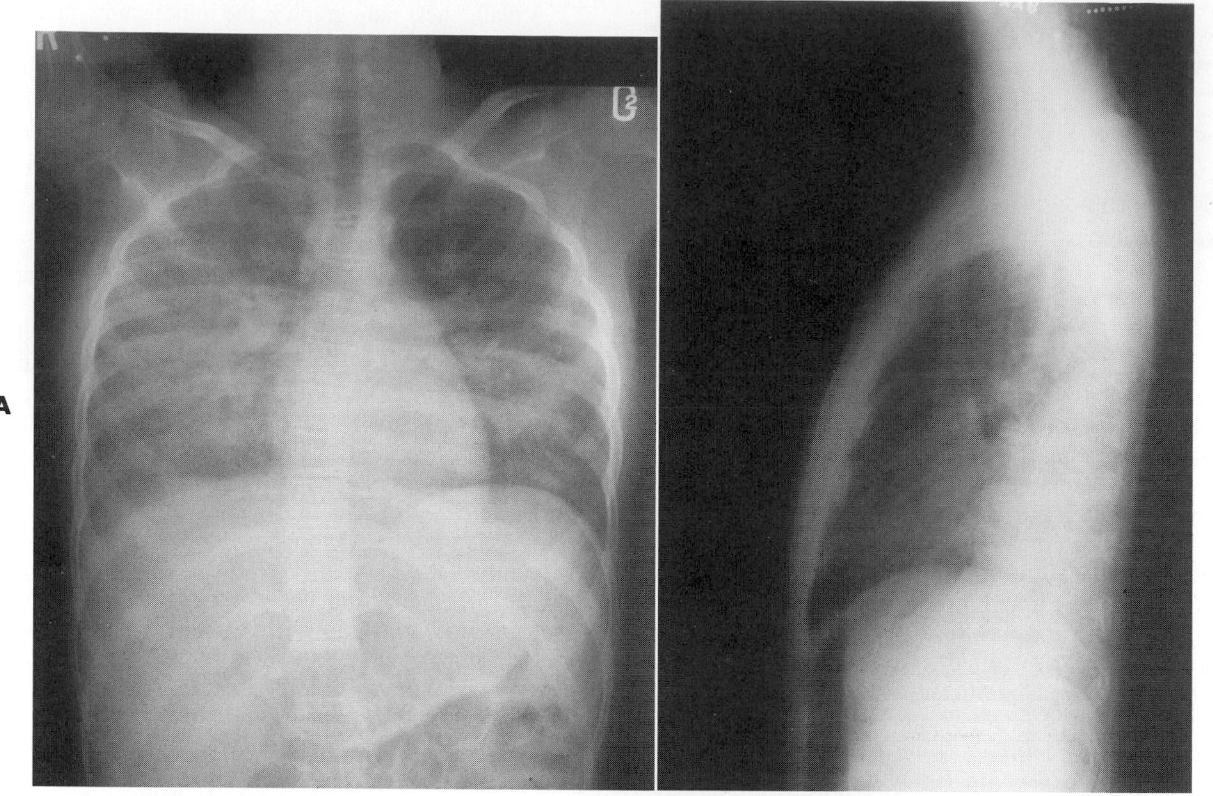

Fig. 28-1. Posteroanterior (**A**) and lateral (**B**) chest radiographs of a 15-year-old patient with mental retardation and recurrent aspiration. The "classic" findings of dependent area consolidations in the lower lobes and posterior segment right upper lobe are demonstrated.

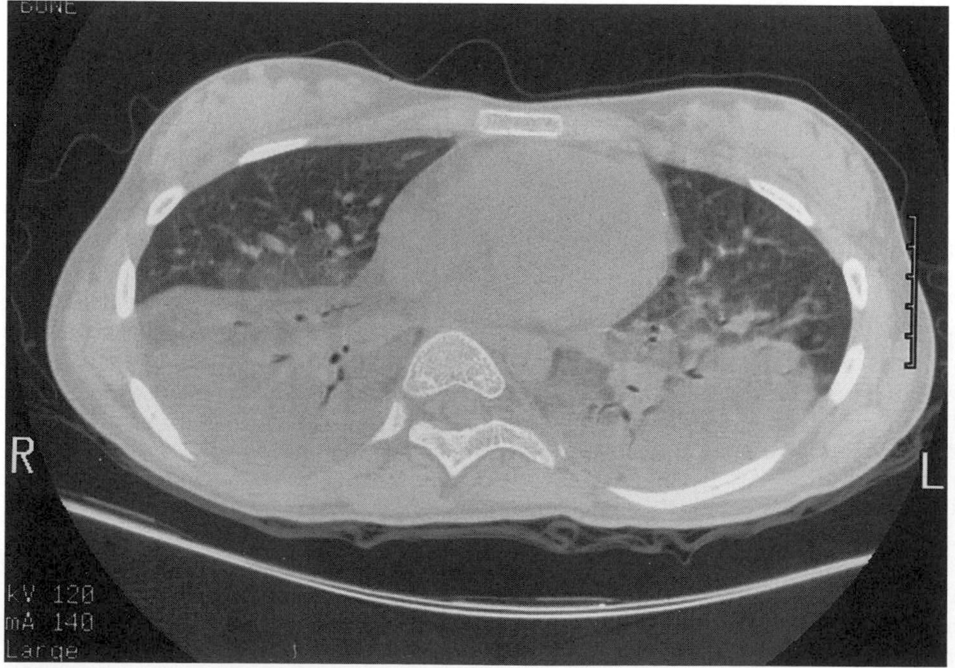

Fig 28-2. Computed tomographic scan through the midthorax of the same patient as in Fig. 28-1. The density of consolidation measured −35 to −40 Hounsfield units, which is consistent with lipoid pneumonia.

sible effects of the catheter resting in the nasopharynx and esophagus. For better detection of postprandial reflux, alternating normal and acid feedings during the monitoring has been suggested.[44]

Esophageal acid perfusion provocation was a reliable diagnostic test in associating GER with stridor in a report of five patients.[45] However, it is difficult to determine whether the stridor is indirectly provoked from esophageal pain. An acid drink followed by histamine challenge may detect children at risk for GER-triggered asthma.[46]

Esophagoscopy alone is very insensitive for detecting GER; however, when combined with biopsy, it is quite sensitive (97%), with a reported specificity of 87%.[36] It does not detect aspiration.

Table 28-3 Diagnostic Tests for GER and Aspiration*

TEST	RELATIVE SPECIFICITY
GER	
Esophageal biopsy	Moderate
Short-term esophageal pH	Low
Gastroesophageal scintiscan	Moderate
Prolonged esophageal pH	High
Barium esophagram	Low
Esophagoscopy without biopsy	High
Esophageal motility	Low
Aspiration	
Modified barium swallow	High
Salivagram	High
Bronchial washings for:	
Lipid-laden macrophage (qualitative)†	Low
Lipid-laden macrophage (quantitative)†	High
Sugars, food particles†	High
Gastroesophageal scintiscan	High
Dye studies†	High
Barium esophagram	Moderate

*Ranked from most to least sensitive.
†These tests can also indicate GER in patients with strictly intragastric feedings.

Tracheobronchial aspirates can be examined for numerous entities to evaluate for aspiration. For patients with artificial airways, the most common test uses placement of an oral dye and visual examination of tracheal secretions for the presence of staining.[18,47] The detection of aspiration in children whose lungs are endotracheally intubated ranges from 16% when 2 to 4 drops of dye were instilled to approximately 80% when larger aliquots were instilled. Quantitation of lactose in tracheal aspirates has been studied to detect aspiration in lactose-fed, ventilator-dependent infants.[48]

The finding of lipid in alveolar macrophages has long been associated with lipid aspiration pneumonia.[49] Simply sighting lipid-laden macrophages is probably a very nonspecific finding. However, semiquantification of these macrophages appears to significantly increase the specificity of this test for children.[50] Lipid-laden macrophages are observed within 6 hours after milk instillation into the rabbit airway. They disappear rapidly, 1 to 2 days after a single milk instillation and somewhat more slowly after repeated instillations.[51] It should be remembered that these cells may be observed with endogenous lipoid pneumonia, particularly with bronchial obstruction and with intravenous lipid infusion therapy.[52]

Bronchial washings can also be examined for food fibers,[53] antibovine antibodies, and bovine casein.[54] There has been limited experience with these tests, so further study is required to determine their usefulness in clinical situations.

The diagnosis of recurrent, small-volume, aspiration-induced lung injury remains a challenge. Often the best that the clinician can achieve is to demonstrate that aspiration occurs and that existing lung disease is probably caused by aspiration, often by exclusion of other processes.

Management

Chronic aspiration often occurs as part of an underlying medical condition. Therapy should be directed toward the under-

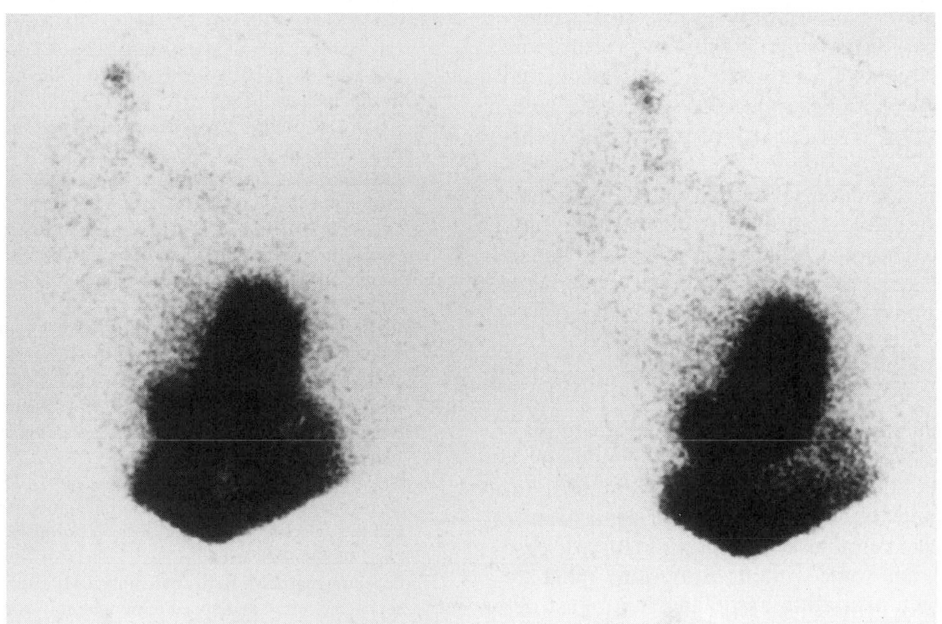

Fig. 28-3. Gastroesophageal scintiscan (milk scan) using technetium-99 mixed in milk feeding. This shows radioactive technetium in the stomach, tracheobronchial tree, and right upper lung field. With this study it is not possible to tell whether the aspiration occurred with swallowing or after GER.

lying problem. The degree of intervention should be guided by the frequency and severity of respiratory problems.

Aspiration can occur secondary to pharyngeal, laryngeal, or esophageal motor discoordination; reflux of stomach contents; or a combination thereof. In the presence of mild swallowing dysfunction, a simple alteration of feeding techniques, such as using only thickened foods, may significantly decrease the risk of aspiration. Good oral hygiene and antibiotic treatment of upper respiratory tract infections can decrease the risk of complications in aspiration. In patients with profound neurologic impairments or in those with anatomic problems, more extensive therapy may be necessary. Surgical correction of craniofacial abnormalities may improve swallowing, and procedures to compensate for laryngeal nerve paralysis have been described, although with varying success rates.[54] Because artificial airways can exacerbate aspiration, the benefits should clearly outweigh the risks when a tracheostomy is considered. In the most severe cases unresponsive to the previously mentioned maneuvers, laryngeal diversion or ablation can be considered.[55] The treatment of aspiration associated with GER is directed toward the management of the latter problem. In infants, various positions may decrease or increase the likelihood of GER,[56] but in light of the association of the prone position with possible suffocation,[57] the risk-to-benefit factors must be considered. The effectiveness of thickened feedings in the presence of GER is controversial. Continuous tube feedings avoid high intragastric pressures, reducing the likelihood of GER. Medications to reduce GER have included prokinetic drugs, such as bethanechol and metoclopramide. However, these have not found widespread acceptance because of significant side effects and questionable efficacy. Cisapride may have a role, but it is yet unclear. Better control and fewer side effects have been achieved with H_2-blocking agents, and these drugs would appear to be a reasonable first-line medical therapy.

Failed medical therapy may warrant surgical intervention. Nissen's and Thal's fundus wrap procedures have been used most frequently in children, with variable success rates. Pneumonia recurs in up to 40%[58] and appears to be highest in children with profound neurologic disability. A lower risk of pneumonia recurrence is reported in children with fewer neurologic abnormalities.[59] Placement of a gastrostomy was associated with more postoperative complications than when it was combined with fundoplication.[60] A high risk of pneumonia recurrence also persists after jejunostomy.[61]

In summary, chronic aspiration has myriad causes, and a thorough evaluation for the etiology of this disorder is necessary. Once the etiology is determined, management needs to be tailored to the individual, generally using a conservative approach, with surgical intervention used only after medical failure.

CONCLUSION

In spite of many recent advances in detecting and treating aspiration, many questions remain unanswered. Do children aspirate more than adults, and how might aspiration during childhood affect future lung function? How much aspiration is normal, and what are the variables contributing to lung disease in some children with and some without aspiration? What are the differences between aspiration associated with gastroesophageal reflux and that associated with dysfunctional swallowing? Better understanding of these issues should enable clinicians to further improve management of children with this problem.

REFERENCES

1. Mendelson CL: The aspiration of stomach contents into the lungs during obstetric anesthesia, *Am J Obstet Gynecol* 52:191-205, 1946.
2. Huxley EJ, Viroslav J, Gray WR, Pierce AK: Pharyngeal aspiration in normal adults and patients with depressed consciousness, *Am J Med* 64:564-568, 1978.

Acute, Large-Volume Aspiration

3. Hamelberg W, Bosomworth PP: Aspiration pneumonitis: experimental studies and clinical observations, *Anesth Analg* 43(6):669-677, 1964.
4. Wynne JW, Modell JH: Respiratory aspiration of stomach contents, *Ann Intern Med* 87:466-474, 1977.
5. Moran TJ: Milk-aspiration pneumonia in human and animal subjects, *Arch Pathol* 55:286-301, 1953.
6. Raidoo DM, Rocke DA, Brock-Utne JG, Marszalek A, Engelbrecht HE: Critical volume for pulmonary acid aspiration: reappraisal in a primate model, *Br J Anaesth* 65:248-250, 1990.
7. Campinos L, Duval G, Couturier M, Brage D, Pham J, Gaudy JH: The value of early fiberoptic bronchoscopy after aspiration of gastric contents, *Br J Anaesth* 55:1103-1105, 1983.
8. Peitzman AB, Shires T, Illner H, Shires GT: Pulmonary acid injury, effects of positive end-expiratory pressure and crystalloid vs. colloid fluid resuscitation, *Arch Surg* 117:662-668, 1982.
9. Sukumaran M, Granada MJ, Berger HW, Lee M, Reilly TA: Evaluation of corticosteroid treatment in aspiration of gastric contents: a controlled clinical trial, *Mt Sinai J Med* 47(4):335-340, 1980.
10. Wynne JW, DeMarco FJ, Hood I: Physiological effects of corticosteroids in foodstuff aspiration, *Arch Surg* 116:46-49, 1981.
11. Morgan JG: Pathophysiology of gastric aspiration, *Int Anesthesiol Clin* 15:1-11, 1977.
12. Hickling KG, Howard R: A retrospective survey of treatment and mortality in aspiration pneumonia, *Intensive Care Med* 14:617-622, 1988.
13. Bynum LJ, Pierce AK: Pulmonary aspiration of gastric contents, *Am Rev Respir Dis* 114:1128-1136, 1976.
14. Busch DE: Anaerobes in infections of the head and neck and ear, nose, and throat, *Rev Infect Dis* 6:S115-S122, 1984.
15. Brook I, Finegold SM: Bacteriology of aspiration pneumonia in children, *Pediatrics* 65:1115-1120, 1980.
16. Brook I: Microbiology of empyema in children and adolescents, *Pediatrics* 85(5):722-726, 1990.
17. Brook I, Finegold SM: Bacteriology and therapy of lung abscess in children, *Pediatrics* 94:10-12, 1979.

Recurrent, Small-Volume Aspiration and GER

18. Cameron JL, Reynolds J, Zuidema GD: Aspiration in patients with tracheostomies, *Surg Gynecol Obstet* 136:68-70, 1973.
19. Goodwin SR, Graves SA, Haberkern CM: Aspiration in intubated premature infants, *Pediatrics* 75:85-88, 1985.
20. Alessi DM, Berci G: Aspiration and nasogastric intubation, *Otolaryngol Head Neck Surg,* 94(4):486-489, 1986.
21. Bar-Maor JA, Lam M: Does nasogastric tube cause pulmonary aspiration in children? *Pediatrics* 87(1):113-114, 1991.
22. Orenstein SR, Orenstein DM: Gastroesophageal reflux and respiratory disease in children, *J Pediatr* 112(6):847-858, 1988.
23. Sontag SJ: Gut feelings about asthma: the burp and the wheeze, *Chest* 99(6):1321-1324, 1991.
24. Boyle JT, Tuchman DN, Altschuler SM, Nixon TE, Pack AI, Cohen S: Mechanisms for the association of gastroesophageal reflux and bronchospasm, *Am Rev Respir Dis* 131(suppl):S16-S20, 1985.
25. Davis RS, Larsen GL, Grunstein MM: Respiratory response to intraesophageal acid infusion in asthmatic children during sleep, *J Allergy Clin Immunol* 72(4):393-398, 1983.
26. Herve P, Denjean A, Jian R, Simonneau G, Duroux P: Intraesophageal perfusion of acid increases the bronchomotor response to methacholine and to isocapnic hyperventilation in asthmatic subjects, *Am Rev Respir Dis* 134:986-989, 1986.
27. de Ajuriaguerra M, Radvanyi-Bouvet MF, Huon C, Moriette G: Gastroesophageal reflux and apnea in prematurely born infants during wakefulness and sleep, *Am J Dis Child,* 145:1132-1136, 1991.
28. Downing SE, Lee JC: Laryngeal chemosensitivity: a possible mechanism for sudden infant death, *Pediatrics* 55(5):640-649, 1975.
29. Martinez DA: Sequelae of antireflex surgery and profoundly disabled children, *J Pediatr Surg* 27(2):261-273, 1992.

30. Malfroot A, Vandenplas Y, Verlinden M, Piepsz A, Dab I: Gastroesophageal reflux and unexplained chronic respiratory disease in infants and children, *Pediatr Pulmonol* 3:208-213, 1987.
31. Ekstrom T, Lindgren BR, Tibbling L: Effects of ranitidine treatment on patients with asthma and a history of gastro-oesophageal reflux: a double blind crossover study, *Thorax* 44:19-23, 1989.
32. Larrain A, Carrasco E, Galleguillos F, Sepulveda R, Pope CE: Medical and surgical treatment of nonallergic asthma associated with gastroesophageal reflux, *Chest* 99(6):1330-1335, 1991.
33. Ekstrom T, Tibbling L: Can mild bronchospasm reduce gastroesophageal reflux? *Am Rev Respir Dis* 139:52-55, 1989.
34. Berquist WE, Rachelefsky GS, Rowshan N, Siegel S, Kate R, Welch M: Quantitative gastroesophageal reflux and pulmonary function in asthmatic children and normal adults receiving placebo, theophylline, and metaproterenol sulfate therapy, *J Allergy Clin Immunol* 73(2):253-258, 1984.
35. Colombo JL: Pulmonary aspiration. In Hilman BC, ed: *Pediatric respiratory disease,* Philadelphia, 1993, WB Saunders, pp 432-434.
36. Meyers, WF, Roberts CC, Johnson DG, Herbst JJ: Value of tests for evaluation of gastroesophageal reflux in children, *J Pediatr Surg* 20(5):515-520, 1985.
37. Donner MW: Radiologic evaluation of swallowing, *Am Rev Respir Dis* 131(suppl):S20-S23, 1985.
38. McVeagh P, Howman-Giles R, Kemp A: Pulmonary aspiration studied by radionuclide milk scanning and barium swallow roentgenography, *Am J Dis Child* 141:917-921, 1987.
39. Fawcett HD, Hayden CK, Adams JC, Swischuk LE: How useful is gastroesophageal reflux scintigraphy in suspected childhood aspiration? *Pediatr Radiol* 18(4):311-313, 1988.
40. Colon AR, DiPalma JS: The brass standard, *Am J Dis Child* 146:895-896, 1992.
41. Heyman, S, Respondek M: Detection of pulmonary aspiration in children by radionuclide "salivagram," *J Nucl Med* 30:697-699, 1989.
42. Silver KH, Van Nostrand D: Scintigraphic detection of salivary aspiration: description of a new diagnostic technique and case reports, *Dysphagia* 7:45-49, 1992.
43. Tuttle SG, Grossman MI: Detection of gastroesophageal reflux by simultaneous measurement of intraluminal pressure and pH, *Proc Soc Exp Biol* 98:225-227, 1958.
44. Orenstein SR: Controversies in pediatric gastroesophageal reflux, *J Pediatr Gastroenterol Nutr* 14:338-348, 1992.
45. Orenstein SR, Kocoshis SA, Orenstein DM, Proujansky R: Stridor and gastroesophageal reflux: diagnostic use of intraluminal esophageal acid perfusion (Bernstein test), *Pediatr Pulmonol* 3:420-424, 1987.
46. Wilson NM, Charette L, Thomson AH, Silverman M: Gastro-oesophageal reflux and childhood asthma: the acid test, *Thorax* 40:592-597, 1985.
47. Goitein KJ, Rein AJJT, Gornstein A: Incidence of aspiration in endotracheally intubated infants and children, *Crit Care Med* 12(1):19-21, 1984.
48. Moran JR, Block SM, Lyerly AD, Brooks LE, Dillard RG: Lipid-laden alveolar macrophage and lactose assay as markers of aspiration in neonates with lung disease, *J Pediatr* 112(4):643-645, 1988.
49. Moran TJ: Experimental food aspiration pneumonia, *Arch Pathol* 52:350-354, 1951.
50. Colombo JL, Hallberg TK: Recurrent aspiration in children: lipid-laden alveolar macrophage quantitation, *Pediatr Pulmonol* 3:86-89, 1987.
51. Colombo JL, Hallberg TK, Sammut PH: Time course of lipid-laden pulmonary macrophages with acute and recurrent milk aspiration in rabbits, *Pediatr Pulmonol* 12:95-98, 1992.
52. Recalde A, Nickerson B, Vegas M, Scott CB, Landing BH, Warburton D: Lipid-laden macrophages in tracheal aspirates of newborn infants receiving intravenous lipid infusions: a cytologic study, *Pediatr Pathol* 2:25-34, 1984.
53. Ristagno RL, Kornstein MJ, Hansen-Flaschen JH: Diagnosis of occult meat aspiration by fiberoptic bronchoscopy, *Am J Med* 80(1):154-156, 1986.
54. Muller W, Rieger C, von der Hardt H: Increased concentrations of milk antibodies in recurrent pulmonary aspiration in infants and young children, *Acta Paediatr Scand* 74:660-663, 1985.
55. Sato I: Detection of α S1-casein in vomit from bottle-fed babies by enzyme-linked immunosorbent assay, *Int J Legal Med* 105:127-131, 1992.
56. Blister A, Krespi YP, Oppenheimer RW: Surgical management of aspiration, *Otolaryngol Clin North Am* 21(4):743-750, 1988.
57. Orenstein S, Whitington P, Orenstein D: The infant seat as treatment for gastroesophageal reflux, *N Engl J Med* 309:760-763, 1983.
58. Engelberts A, de Jonje G: Choice of sleeping position for infants: possible association with cot death, *Arch Dis Child* 65:462-467, 1990.
59. Smith CD, Othersen HB, Gogan NJ, Walker JD: Nissen fundoplication in children with profound neurological disability: high risks and unmet goals, *Ann Surg* 215(6):654-658, 1992.
60. Fung KP, Seagram G, Pasieka J, Trevmen C, Maclida H, Scott B: Investigational and outcome of 121 infants and children requiring Nissen fundoplication for the management of gastroesophageal reflux, *Clin Invest Med* 13(5):237-246, 1990.
61. Weltz CR, Morris JB, Mullen JL: Surgical jejunostomy in aspiration risk patients, *Ann Surg* 215(2):140-145, 1992.

CHAPTER 29

Respiratory Effect of Anesthesia and Sedation

Etsuro K. Motoyama

Over the last decade the role of the pediatric pulmonologist as an expert in fiberoptic bronchoscopy in infants and children has been established. Consequently, the opportunity for pediatric pulmonologists to use intravenous sedatives and hypnotic medications, as well as local anesthetics, has increased considerably. In addition, the evaluation and management of pediatric patients in intensive care settings, either as an intensivist or a consultant, require a knowledge of pharmacology, especially the effects on respiration, of sedatives, narcotics, muscle relaxants, and anesthetics. Furthermore, recent interest in and development of new and innovative pulmonary function testing in young infants necessitate that the pediatric pulmonologist have better knowledge of and skills in the sedation, monitoring, and handling of infants with medication-induced cardiopulmonary compromise.

This chapter reviews the effects on respiration of medications that pediatric pulmonologists commonly encounter and provides a general guide for management and patient safety. In general, specific data on the respiratory effects of sedatives and anesthesia-related medications in human infants and children are limited, and these effects must often be inferred from data in animals and adult humans. A detailed description and discussion of the pharmacology, pharmacokinetics, and pharmacodynamics of related medications are beyond the scope of this chapter, and readers are referred to standard textbooks in pharmacology and anesthesiology.[1-4]

INHALED ANESTHETICS

Pharmacology and Clinical Use

The pediatric pulmonologist rarely administers inhaled or volatile anesthetics. However, he or she may deal with infants and children under general anesthesia for various procedures (e.g., fiberoptic bronchoscopy, bronchoalveolar lavage, transbronchial biopsy). Volatile anesthetics are commonly used for inhalation induction because infants and children fear needlesticks. All inhaled anesthetics except nitrous oxide are potent myocardial depressants, and their administration requires extreme caution, even by experienced pediatric anesthesiologists.

Halothane

Since the 1960s, halothane has been the preferred agent for inducing anesthesia in infants and children. Because of its relatively mild odor, halothane is relatively well accepted by young patients. It is not a desirable agent, however, because it causes myocardial depression, bradycardia, decreased cardiac output, hypotension, and dysrhythmias. A significant fraction of inhaled halothane (15% to 20%) is metabolized in the liver, where sensitization and hepatic damage may occur.[2] The minimum alveolar concentration (MAC) is the amount of inhaled anesthetic required to prevent half of subjects from responding to a painful stimulus by gross purposeful movement.[5] For halothane, the MAC is about 1% at 6 to 12 months of age, but as with other inhaled anesthetics, this decreases with age. The MAC of halothane in young adults is about 0.75%.[6]

Isoflurane

Since its introduction in the early 1980s, isoflurane has been widely accepted because of its metabolic stability, and it causes less irritation of the myocardium than halothane.[2] However, isoflurane is not suitable as an inhalational induction agent in children because of its pungent odor and irritant effect on the airways, resulting in oxygen desaturation.[7] Halothane thus remained the agent of choice for inhalational induction until recently, when sevoflurane replaced it in most industrialized countries (see later discussion). In clinical practice, halothane or sevoflurane is often switched to isoflurane after induction for the maintenance of anesthesia. The MAC of isoflurane is about 1.9% at 1 year of age and 1.6% in older children.[8]

Recently, two new halogenated ethers, desflurane and sevoflurane, have been introduced for clinical use. They have a rapid onset of anesthesia and emergence because of the considerably lower blood solubility.

Desflurane

Desflurane is structurally similar to isoflurane and possesses similar characteristics in terms of metabolic stability, relative lack of myocardial irritability, and pungent odor. With its extremely low blood/gas partition coefficient (0.42), anesthetic induction and emergence are extremely rapid.[9] Desflurane, however, is unsuitable for inhalation induction in children because it causes a very high incidence of breath-holding, coughing, excessive secretions, and severe laryngospasm with oxygen desaturation.[10,11] The boiling point of desflurane (23.5° C) is much lower than that of other volatile anesthetics, and a special vaporizer is required. In addition, it has low anesthetic potency (MAC, 8% to 9%) and thus is relatively more expensive. Despite these limitations, desflurane is almost ideal for the maintenance of and emergence from anesthesia.[12] Because recovery is so rapid, the patient tends to become confused and excited, especially if a proper postanesthetic analgesia is not provided.

Sevoflurane

Sevoflurane, recently released for clinical use in North America and Europe, also has a low blood/gas partition coefficient (0.59). Unlike desflurane, it has a pleasant, nonirritating odor. Induction time is somewhat shorter than with halothane, airway irritation is minimal, and recovery is rapid.[13] The MAC in children is 2.5%. Sevoflurane appears to be less irritating to the myocardium and produces less depression at equipotent concentrations.[14] Compared to isoflurane and desflurane, the biotransformation of sevoflurane (2.9%) is relatively high and produces free inorganic fluoride. The fluoride level, however, rarely increases to nephrotoxic levels and drops off rapidly during the recovery period to subnephrotoxic levels.[13]

Nitrous Oxide

Nitrous oxide is a gaseous anesthetic with a pleasant odor. It potentiates other anesthetics, reduces the requirement of potent inhaled anesthetics, and helps increase the rate of uptake.[6] It is frequently used with potent inhaled anesthetics or with intravenous agents such as narcotics and sedatives. Nitrous oxide has a low potency, and in situations in which maximal oxygenation is essential, such as during bronchoscopy, its use in effective concentrations (50% or more) is not practical. Although nontoxic during short exposure, prolonged exposure to nitrous oxide can lead to hazards such as miscarriage, bone marrow suppression, and teratogenicity.[6]

Effect on Control of Breathing

Most sedatives, narcotics, and anesthetics depress ventilation. They variably affect minute ventilation ($\dot{V}_E$) and its components: the tidal volume (V_T), respiratory frequency (*f*), mean inspiratory flow rate (V_T/T_I), and inspiratory duty cycle (T_I/T_{TOT}), in which T_I is the inspiratory time, and T_{TOT} is the total respiratory cycle duration. $\dot{V}_E$ can be expressed in the following manner:

$$\dot{V}_E = V_T \times f$$

OR

$$\dot{V}_E = V_T/T_I \times T_I/T_{TOT}$$

All inhaled anesthetics are potent respiratory depressants in a dose-dependent manner. This subject has been reviewed extensively,[15,16] but information on human infants and children remains limited.

Response to Carbon Dioxide Levels

At resting ventilation, all inhaled anesthetics in clinical use produce variable degrees of ventilatory depression and an increase in the arterial or end-tidal partial pressure of carbon dioxide (P_{CO_2}). The carbon dioxide response curve (ventilatory response to inhaled carbon dioxide) shifts progressively to the right with decreasing slopes as the concentration of anesthetics is increased[17] (Fig. 29-1). The

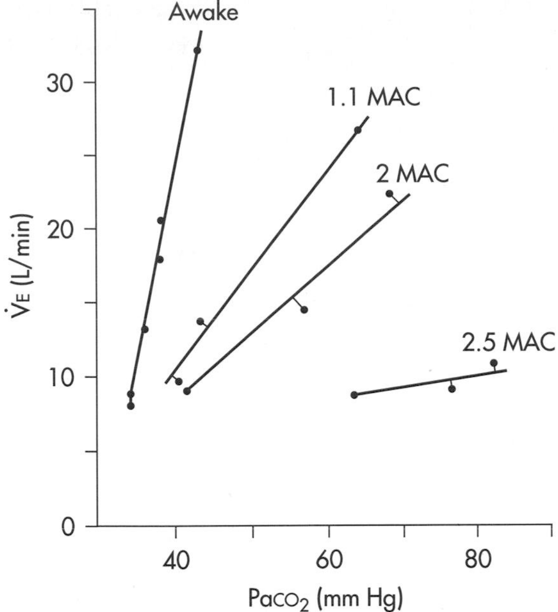

Fig. 29-1. Carbon dioxide response curve for halothane. Family of steady-state carbon dioxide response curves in one subject who was awake and under three levels of halothane anesthesia. Note the progressive decrease in ventilatory response to arterial P_{CO_2} *(Pa_{CO_2})* with increasing anesthetic depth *(MAC).* (Data from Munson ES et al: *Anesthesiology* 27:716-728, 1966.)

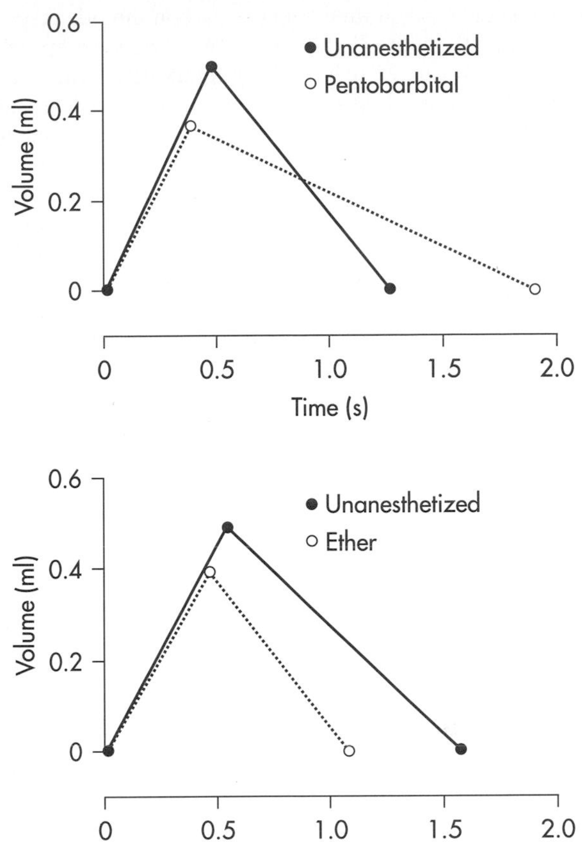

Fig. 29-2. Schematic summary of changes in the average respiratory cycle in a group of newborn rabbits before and after pentobarbital sodium anesthesia *(top)* and before and during ether anesthesia *(bottom).* Measurements were obtained during spontaneous room air breathing. Zero on the time axis indicates the onset of inspiration. The VT/TI is represented by the slope of the ascending limb of the spirogram. (From Milic-Emili J: *Int Anesthesiol Clin* 15:39-58, 1977.)

decrease in V̇E is, in general, associated primarily with the reduction of VT.[16]

Studies in adult volunteers using the occlusion technique[18] and the timing component analysis[19] indicate that the reduction in VT with anesthetics is due mostly to a reduction in the neural drive of ventilation (VT/TI, airway occlusion pressure at 0.1 second).[20,21] TI tends to decrease with anesthesia, but the T_I/T_{TOT} is relatively unaffected. In newborn rabbits, light diethyl ether anesthesia does not decrease the VT/TI, and it decreases expiratory time (TE) relative to TI, resulting in an increase in the T_I/T_{TOT}, respiratory frequency, and V̇E. Light pentobarbital anesthesia does not affect the VT/TI in newborn rabbits, but in contrast to ether, the TI decreases, and the TE increases. Consequently, the V̇E decreases because of a reduced T_I/T_{TOT} (Fig. 29-2). With deeper anesthesia using both ether and pentobarbital, the VT/TI eventually decreases in a dose-dependent fashion.[22,23] It is not clear whether such changes in the T_I/T_{TOT} are species specific or are related to age. In newborn lambs, halothane (0.85 MAC) decreases the VT and V̇E and increases the P_{CO_2}.[24]

In several studies in children 2 to 5 years of age, ventilation was reasonably well maintained at very light levels of general anesthesia (i.e., 0.5% halothane).[25-27] In higher surgical levels of anesthesia (1.0% to 1.5%, 1.0 to 1.5 MAC), however, ventilation was depressed in a dose-dependent fashion, and hypercapnia resulted. A reduced V̇E was associated with a reduced VT and increased respiratory frequency. The neural respiratory drive was depressed, as evidenced by a reduced VT/TI, whereas the T_I/T_{TOT} tended to increase without changes in the TI,[26,27] or it decreased slightly.[25] In infants younger than 12 months of age, ventilatory depression was more pronounced, and no increase in the T_I/T_{TOT} was seen, partly because of high chest wall compliance and pronounced thoracic deformity compared with older children.[27]

Ventilatory Response to Hypoxemia

In dogs, ventilatory response to hypoxemia is diminished or abolished in a dose-dependent fashion by inhaled anesthetics.[28,29] Knill and Gelb[30] demonstrated that under light halothane anesthesia in adult volunteers, hypoxic ventilatory response was disproportionately depressed by halothane compared with hypercapnia. At 1.1 MAC of halothane, hypoxic ventilatory response was completely abolished, whereas the response to hypercapnia was about 40% of the control in the awake state.

Even at a subanesthetic or trace level (0.1 MAC), halothane attenuated the hypoxic ventilatory response markedly (to 30% of control), whereas the hypercapnic response was essentially unaffected.[30] Subsequent studies from the same laboratory[31,32] showed a similar effect with 0.1 MAC of other potent volatile anesthetics, such as isoflurane and enflurane. The site of halothane's action appears to be at the peripheral chemoreceptors as seen by the rapid response in humans[32] and the direct measurement of neuronal chemoreceptor output in cats.[33] The effect of subanesthetic levels of halothane on hypercapnic ventilatory response is minimal because carbon dioxide response is predominantly controlled by the central chemoreceptors.

Recently, Temp et al[34,35] challenged these finding by demonstrating that 0.1 MAC of isoflurane had no demonstrable ventilatory effect on hypoxia. On the other hand, Dahan et al[36] confirmed the previous findings by Knill and Gelb.[30] The reason for the conflicting findings is unclear but is probably related to the contribution of the awake vs. sleep state in which these investigations were conducted.[37] The effect of a trace amount (0.05 to 0.1 MAC) of anesthetics on ventilation in infants and children is unknown, although a very high incidence of hypoxemia (>40%) in otherwise healthy infants and children without apparent hypocapnia in the postanesthetic period may suggest a blunted hypoxic ventilatory drive caused by a trace amount of anesthetics.[38]

Response to Loading

When an extrinsic load is imposed on an awake individual, ventilation is maintained by increased inspiratory effort.[18] This response is greatly diminished or abolished by the effect of anesthetics,[39,40] narcotics,[41] and barbiturates.[42] In patients with chronic obstructive airway disease, hypercapnia may develop, even though normocarbia may be maintained when they are awake.[43]

In children under light halothane anesthesia (0.5%) the addition of the resistive load initially decreases the VT. However, the VT returns to baseline within 5 minutes.[26]

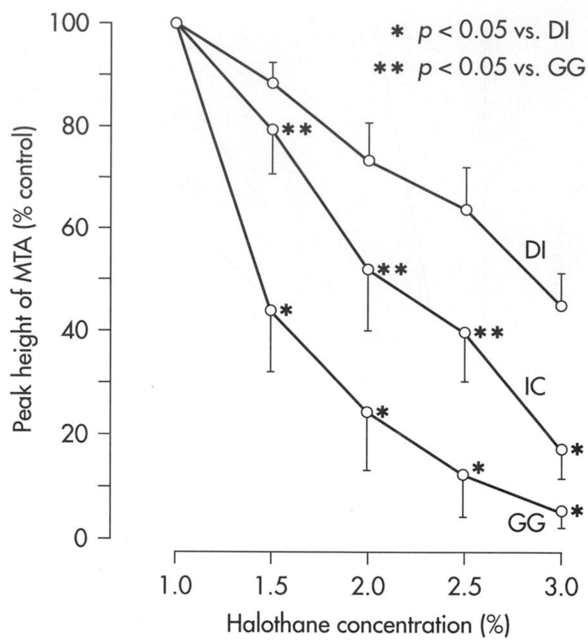

Fig. 29-3. Decrease in the phasic inspiratory muscle activity expressed as peak height of moving time average *(MTA)* in percent changes from control (1% halothane) during halothane anesthesia in adult cats. Values are mean ± standard error of the mean. *DI,* Diaphragm; *GG,* genioglossus muscle; *IC,* external intercostal muscles. (From Ochiai R et al: *Anesthesiology* 70:812-816, 1989.)

Differential Sensitivity of Inspiratory Muscles

The three groups of inspiratory muscles responsible for normal tidal inspiration are the diaphragm, external intercostal muscles, and upper airway muscles. The pharyngeal muscles (e.g., genioglossus and geniohyoid muscles) have basal tone, keep the tongue in the anterior position, and maintain the patency of the pharyngeal airway. In addition, these muscles contract with the diaphragm and widen the caliber of the pharynx during inspiration. The laryngeal dilators, especially the posterior cricoarytenoid muscles, also contract synchronously with the diaphragm and widen the glottic aperture.

All inspiratory muscle activities are depressed by the effect of inhaled anesthetics, but the sensitivity of the three muscle groups to the depressant effect of anesthetics differs considerably. Intercostal activity is more easily depressed by inhaled anesthetics such as diethyl ether[44] and halothane.[45] Using electromyography in adults, Drummond[46] demonstrated the presence of both tonic and phasic inspiratory activities in the scalene, sternocleidomastoid, and external intercostal muscles. Anesthetic induction with thiopental sodium completely abolished the tonic activities of these muscles. Drummond[46] postulated that the loss of tonic activity might contribute to reduced functional residual capacity (FRC) during general anesthesia.

Recent studies indicate that the genioglossus muscle is easily depressed during natural sleep by ethanol ingestion and by general anesthetics.[47-49] Ochiai et al[50] studied the differential sensitivity of the three inspiratory muscle groups in intact cats. They demonstrated that the genioglossus muscle was the most sensitive and the diaphragm was the least sensitive, or most resistant, muscle to the depressant effect of inhaled anesthetics. The sensitivity of the intercostal muscles to anesthetics was intermediate between the diaphragm and the genioglossus (Fig. 29-3).

The clinical impression has been that infants and young children are more susceptible to upper airway obstruction under general anesthesia, indicating that their upper airway muscles may be more sensitive to the depressant effect of anesthetics than adults'. In a more recent study, Ochiai et al[51] demonstrated a similar differential sensitivity of the three inspiratory muscle groups to halothane. Furthermore, they found that in 2-month-old kittens, the genioglossus muscle was significantly more sensitive to anesthetic depression than this muscle in adult cats, whereas the sensitivity of the diaphragm and intercostal muscles did not significantly differ from that of adults. Morphologic and physiologic studies indicate immaturity of the hypoglossal-genioglossus system in kittens compared to the phrenic-diaphragm or spinal-intercostal system.[52,53] Studies of respiratory control in response to acute hypoxia suggest that in terms of the development of its respiratory-control mechanism, a 2-month-old kitten is equivalent to a human 2- to 4-day-old infant.[53] Recent clinical studies with inductive plethysmography in children and adults undergoing general anesthesia indicate that the differential sensitivity of inspiratory muscles to anesthetics in humans is similar to that in cats.[54-56]

Effects on Respiratory Mechanics

Pressure-Volume Relationships

General anesthesia with or without muscle relaxants results in a significant reduction in the compliance of the lungs and thorax in adult humans soon after anesthetic induction in the supine position,[57,58] whereas the FRC was unchanged during anesthesia in the sitting position.[59] The physiologic mechanism of this phenomenon had puzzled anesthesiologists and physiologists for many years. Eventually, de Troyer and Bastenier-Geens[60] demonstrated in healthy adult volunteers that partial muscle paralysis with pancuronium depressed the outward recoil of the thorax immediately but not the inward recoil of the lungs. This change altered the balance between the outward recoil of the thorax and inward recoil of the lungs; consequently, the FRC diminished. The subsequent reduction in lung compliance resulted from a reduced FRC and airway closure. These authors postulated that in the awake state, thoracic inspiratory muscles have an intrinsic tone that maintains the outward recoil and rigidity of the thorax. In the cat, respiratory muscles, especially the external (inspiratory) intercostal muscles, are abundantly supplied with muscle spindles,[61] and some of the respiratory muscle spindles have a tonic rather than a rhythmic activity.[62] Intercostal muscles are more sensitive than the diaphragm to the depressant effect of anesthetics[50] and muscle relaxants.[60] General anesthesia or muscle relaxation would therefore abolish inspiratory muscle tone, reducing outward thoracic recoil, FRC, and eventually lung compliance.

In infants, the continuous muscle tone of the thorax is particularly important in maintaining FRC because the thorax is extremely compliant and lacks the intrinsic rigidity needed to oppose the elastic recoil of the lungs. In infants and young children under general endotracheal anesthesia with halothane, Fletcher et al[63] demonstrated that compliance of the respiratory system decreased about 35%, a value similar to that reported in adults under similar conditions.[57,64] This reduction occurred both during spontaneous breathing and during manual ventilation with a low VT after muscle relaxants were administered. Positive end-expiratory pressure was carefully avoided. When the VT was doubled, however, compliance returned to the preanesthetic control levels. These findings agree with previous findings in adults[60,65] and support the hypothesis that anesthesia reduces the thoracic (external intercostal muscle) tone and outward recoil of the thorax with consequent reduction in the FRC. The finding that a larger VT increases compliance also indicates that the FRC or relaxation volume decreases to the lower, flatter portion of the pressure-volume curve.

FRC

In awake individuals, the FRC decreases from about 50% of the total lung capacity in the upright posture to about 40% in the recumbent position. With most general anesthetics, the FRC decreases further immediately after the induction of anesthesia but remains at the lower level thereafter.[64,66] In healthy young adults, the FRC during anesthesia is reduced 9% to 25% from that in the awake state.[57,67-72] In older individuals, the average reduction in the FRC is higher (30%), at least partly because of the lower elastic recoil pressure of the lungs and increased closing capacity.[73]

Because of the more compliant thorax in infants and children, general anesthesia and muscle relaxation are expected to produce significant reductions in the FRC. In newborn lambs that are anesthetized with light halothane anesthesia (0.75%) and are spontaneously breathing, the VT and $\dot{V}$E decrease significantly with a 32% reduction in the FRC.[24] In children between 6 and 18 years of age, Dobbinson et al[74] found a marked and significant reduction in the FRC (a 35% reduction from awake controls) as measured with helium dilution during methoxyflurane anesthesia with D-tubocurarine. The average decrease in FRC among those younger than 12 years of age was 46%. Studies by Fletcher et al[63] on compliance in infants and young children (see previous section) also suggest a significant reduction in the FRC. Henderson-Smart and Read[75] have shown a 30% reduction in the thoracic gas volume in infants in whom the sleeping pattern changed from non–rapid eye movement to rapid eye movement. Motoyama et al[76] reported moderate decreases in the FRC (46%) in children as measured with helium dilution and a marked reduction (71%) in infants under halothane anesthesia and muscle paralysis approaching the relaxation volume in the newborn that was reported by Agostoni.[77] On the other hand, Thorsteinsson et al[78] found that the FRC in infants and children under halothane anesthesia and paralysis, as measured with a sulfur hexafluoride multiple-breath washout technique, was not significantly different from normal values obtained in sleeping infants and children by a number of authors.[79-81] The reason that the FRC is not reduced is somewhat puzzling but may be explained in part by the fact that in this study, the subjects were ventilated with 5 cm H_2O of positive end-expiratory pressure until immediately before the sulfur hexafluoride washout to control the volume history.

Effects on Pulmonary Gas Exchange

General anesthesia is associated with an increase in alveolar dead space and the alveolar-arterial difference in the partial pressure of oxygen.[82-84] A reduction of FRC associated with general anesthesia appears to be a major cause of altered distribution of ventilation.[85] All inhaled anesthetics depress hypoxic pulmonary vasoconstriction in vitro,[86,87] which may also contribute to an increase in venous admixture during general anesthesia. The effect of inhaled anesthetics on hypoxic pulmonary vasoconstriction, however, has been inconclusive in vivo.[88] Intravenous anesthetics and sedatives (opioids, barbiturates, and benzodiazepines) do not have detectable effects on hypoxic pulmonary vasoconstriction either in vitro or in vivo.[87,89-93]

Effects on Mucociliary Function

The cilia in the respiratory tract play an important role in the removal of mucus, foreign particles, and cell debris and are an important defense mechanism of the respiratory system. These cilia move in a synchronous and whiplike fashion at a rate of 600 to 1300 times per minute and propel the mucus and particles on the mucous blanket toward the airway opening at the rate of 1.5 to 2.0 cm/min.[94]

Ciliary function is affected by the thickness of the mucous layer and other factors that can occur with dehydration or infection. In vitro, viral infection reduces ciliary motion as much as 50%, and repeated infection in vitro can destroy ciliated epithelial cells completely.[95] Breathing of warm air with 50% humidity maintains normal ciliary motion, whereas inhalation of dry air for only 3 hours causes complete cessation of mucus movement. Ciliary activity can be restored by breathing warmed, humidified air.[96,97] Breathing of 100% oxygen and controlled positive-pressure ventilation also affect ciliary function.[98-100] Inflation of an endotracheal tube cuff also suppresses tracheal mucus velocity.[101]

Inhaled anesthetics can diminish the rate of mucus clearance, either by reducing the ciliary motion directly or by altering the quality, quantity, or both factors of the mucus produced. Forbes and Horrigan[102] studied the clearance of radioactive droplets from the dog trachea and found a dose-related depression of ciliary activity with halothane and enflurane anesthesia but not with diethyl ether. Using tantalum powder in the airways, the same group of investigators[100] found delayed mucus clearance during and even 6 hours after discontinuation of anesthesia with halothane or ether and mechanical ventilation. In a separate study, the same authors[103] found that thiopental depresses the mucociliary clearance to a similar extent as volatile anesthetics. These findings suggest that anesthesia adversely affects mucociliary clearance, especially in patients with abnormal pulmonary function. The effect of anesthetics on mucociliary function in infants and children has not been reported.

INTRAVENOUS AGENTS

Various sedative-hypnotic agents can be used for sedation, premedication, or the induction of general anesthesia. Usually, these agents are used intravenously, but the transmucosal (oral, nasal, and rectal) and intramuscular routes are also used.

Propofol

Pharmacology and Clinical Use

Propofol is an alkylphenol introduced into clinical practice as a general anesthetic and a sedative. Because propofol is insoluble in aqueous solution, it is formulated as a 1% solution in 10% soybean oil, 2.25% glycerol, and 1.2% egg phosphatide. After a single intravenous injection, the blood concentration of propofol decreases rapidly because of redistribution and elimination; the initial distribution half-life is 2 to 8 minutes.[104,105]

Propofol is primarily a hypnotic and has no analgesic effect. Pain may occur on injection but can be minimized by injecting the medication into a large vein, administering the medication slowly, or pretreating the site with lidocaine before injection.[106] The bolus dose for induction of anesthesia in adults is usually 1 to 2.5 mg/kg followed by continuous infusion of 80 to 150 μg/kg/min combined with nitrous oxide or opiates.[105] The induction dose in children is higher than in adults because of the larger central compartment and higher clearance rate[107] and ranges from 2.5 to 4.0 mg/kg.[108,109] The continuous infusion rate varies but is usually between 100 and 200 μg/kg/min.

The cardiovascular effects include a reduced blood pressure, cardiac output, systemic vascular resistance, and heart rate.[105,110,111] Myoclonus may be seen in children with propofol induction. Recovery is quicker than that with thiopental.[112] Administration is associated with fewer episodes of postoperative emesis than with inhaled anesthetics, making propofol suitable for outpatient surgical procedures.[113,114]

Propofol has also been used as a sedative for fiberoptic bronchoscopy and other diagnostic procedures. Propofol sedation with topical anesthesia (4% lidocaine), however, was frequently associated with moderate hemoglobin desaturation (< 90%) in adults.[115-117] The dose required for sedation is much less than that for general anesthesia.[115]

Respiratory Effects

Propofol is a potent respiratory depressant. Anesthetic induction with propofol (2.5 mg/kg) causes respiratory depression and a high incidence of apnea (>30 seconds' duration), both in adults[118] and in children.[108,118,119] The incidence of prolonged apnea was more frequent than with other intravenous induction agents, such as thiopental, and was further increased if a patient had been given opiates before propofol infusion.[118,120]

In patients premedicated with narcotics and studied with respiratory inductance plethysmography, a single intravenous dose of propofol (2.5 mg/kg) was associated with a reduction in $\dot{V}_E$, V_T, and V_T/T_I, but T_I/T_{TOT} and respiratory frequency did not significantly change.[121] The degree of ventilatory depression was similar to that with thiopental (4 mg/kg). A small but significant reduction in FRC occurred with propofol but not with thiopental.[121]

Continuous infusion of a moderate dose of propofol (100 (μg/kg/min) is associated with an apparent reduction in the neural respiratory drive, with a 40% reduction in the V_T. Respiratory frequency is somewhat increased. A higher dose of infusion (200 μg/kg/min) results in a further reduction in V_T but no change in respiratory rate.[122] The ventilatory response to carbon dioxide is also decreased significantly in adults. At an infusion rate of 100 μg/kg/min the slope of carbon dioxide response curve indicates a 59% reduction. The degree of ventilatory depression is similar to that of 1 MAC halothane or that after a brief infusion of 3 mg/kg/min of thiopental.[105] Doubling of the infusion rate (200 μg/kg/min) is not associated with a further decrease in the slope of the carbon dioxide response curve. The blood level of propofol, however, has not been measured.[122] In another study, infusion of a relatively low level (50 μg/kg/min) of propofol was associated with a moderate rise in the arterial P_{CO_2} (39 to 52 mm Hg). A higher rate of infusion (120 μg/kg/min) did not increase the arterial P_{CO_2} any further, indicating an alinear ventilatory dose response to carbon dioxide.[119] Ventilatory response to hypoxia was also depressed.[118]

The ventilatory effects of propofol infusion for conscious sedation is controversial. Blouin et al[123] studied hypoxic response before and during propofol infusion for conscious sedation in healthy male volunteers using an isocapnic rebreathing method. At a pulse-oximetric saturation (Sp_{O_2}) of 90%, the $\dot{V}_E$ and V_T decreased to about 50% of control. Furthermore, the slope of the hypoxic ventilatory response curve decreased from 0.88 L min^{-1}% $Sp_{O_2}^{-1}$ to 0.17 L min^{-1}% $Sp_{O_2}^{-1}$. On the other hand, Rosa et al[124] found no changes in $\dot{V}_E$, V_T, frequency, or timing components during minor surgery with local anesthesia and propofol sedation.

Benzodiazepines

Pharmacology and Clinical Use

Benzodiazepines have hypnotic, sedative, amnestic, anxiolytic, anticonvulsant, and centrally produced muscle relaxant properties. Hypnosis and unconsciousness may be induced by using large doses. Unlike other hypnotic and sedative medications, benzodiazepines are not general neuronal depressants. Benzodiazepines exert their effects by occupying the benzodiazepine receptors that modulate the γ-aminobutyric acid receptor, the major inhibitory neurotransmitter in the central nervous system. Benzodiazepines are metabolized in the liver via a hepatic microsomal oxidation or glucuronide conjugation.[105]

The onset and duration of action of a benzodiazepine depend on its lipid solubility. Midazolam and diazepam have a higher lipid solubility and a more rapid onset of action after a single bolus injection (30 to 60 seconds) than lorazepam (60 to 120 seconds).[105]

At sedative doses, benzodiazepines affect respiration only minimally. As the dose is increased, however, sedation progresses to hypnosis and then stupor. In general, benzodiazepines increase the seizure threshold to local anesthetics. The cardiovascular effects of benzodiazepines, including a slight decrease in systemic blood pressure secondary to a decrease in systemic vascular resistance, are mild.[3]

Respiratory Effects

As with most intravenous anesthetics and sedatives, benzodiazepines produce ventilatory depression in a dose-dependent fashion. The ventilatory depression after midazolam (0.15 mg/kg) is almost identical to that of diazepam (0.3 mg/kg).[125] The onset of ventilatory depression after a single intravenous injection of midazolam (0.1 to 0.2 mg/kg) is rapid (about 3 minutes) and lasts for 1 to 2 hours.[126] Blouin et al[127] reported a 40% reduction in the $\dot{V}_E$ and a significant reduction in the hypoxic ventilatory response.

In a large series of clinical trials for anesthetic induction with midazolam, about 20% of adults became apneic. The incidence is similar to that of thiopental.[128] After the administration of midazolam (0.1 mg/kg intravenously), Montravers et al[129] observed frequent central apnea followed by a fivefold increase in supraglottic airway resistance, which was often associated with obstructive apnea. The supraglottic resistance remained significantly elevated for 20 minutes.

Reports on the respiratory effects of benzodiazepines in infants and children are limited. Midazolam seems innocuous as a preoperative sedative for healthy infants and children because it usually does not produce sleep or deep sedation. A fall in Spo_2, however, has been reported during midazolam sedation for outpatient echocardiography in infants.[130] Yaster et al[131] reported a case of respiratory arrest in a 14-month-old toddler after intravenous midazolam (0.11 mg/kg) and fentanyl (0.2 μg/kg) for sedation, probably because of the medications' multiplicative effects on respiratory depression. The effect of transmucosal midazolam in infants younger than 5 months of age has not been reported.

Midazolam

Midazolam is a water-soluble, short-acting benzodiazepine. It is metabolized in the liver; <1% is excreted in the urine unchanged. Midazolam is the most commonly used benzodiazepine for perioperative sedation and has been administered by the transmucosal (oral, nasal, and rectal), intravenous, and intramuscular routes. Because of the decreased bioavailability of this medication, the transmucosal doses must be much higher than the intravenous or intramuscular doses. Intravenous doses of 0.1 mg/kg, oral doses of 0.5 to 0.75 mg/kg,[132-134] nasal and sublingual doses of 0.2 to 0.3 mg/kg,[135-137] and rectal doses of 0.3 mg/kg[138,139] are satisfactory for sedating children. Nasal transmucosal administration has the advantage of rapid absorption and prompt onset of the sedative-hypnotic effect (7 to 10 minutes).[135] The peak plasma concentration is achieved in about 10 minutes.[130,140] The stinging sensation and bitter taste of midazolam with nasal medication are major problems. The bitter taste is somewhat masked by mixing it with fruit-scented syrup and administering the combination orally. Orally administered midazolam takes 20 to 30 minutes to be effective. Recovery of normal activity occurs in 30 to 45 minutes.[130]

Midazolam has been used successfully for conscious sedation in patients undergoing fiberoptic bronchoscopy.[141] Acceptability to both the operators and patients is high and is comparable to that with propofol,[115] although the recovery is slower than with propofol.[116,117] For sedation in children undergoing gastrointestinal endoscopy, midazolam (0.1 to 0.15 mg/kg intravenously) is just as effective as diazepam (0.2 to 0.4 mg/kg).[142]

By 1990, more than 80 accidental deaths had been attributed to use of midazolam sedation outside the operating room in the United States alone. Some 78% of these deaths were respiratory in nature, and in 57% of these cases, opioids had been administered simultaneously. Most deaths occurred in patients breathing spontaneously with or without supplemental oxygen but with inadequate monitoring and preparation for resuscitation.[143]

Flumazenil

Flumazenil is a benzodiazepine receptor ligand and a competitive antagonist to the benzodiazepines. It is the first benzodiazepine antagonist available for clinical use. Flumazenil (3 μg/kg) reverses the ventilatory depression and depression of the hypoxic ventilatory drive produced by midazolam (0.1 to 0.2 mg/kg).[125,144] The plasma half-life is about 60 minutes, much shorter than all the benzodiazepines used clinically. There is the potential danger of resedation if a sufficient concentration of agonist remains after the antagonist has cleared.[145]

Barbiturates

Pharmacology and Clinical Use

In the past, barbiturates were used extensively as hypnotic and sedative agents, especially for preoperative sedation. More recently, however, barbiturates have been replaced largely by medications such as benzodiazepines and short-acting synthetic opioids. Because of respiratory depression and other side effects, barbiturates are used only for a few specialized purposes, including anesthetic induction (thiopental, thiamylal, methohexital) and anticonvulsive therapy (phenobarbital).

Respiratory Effects

Barbiturates depress ventilatory response to carbon dioxide and $\dot{V}_E$.[146] In one study of adults, the induction dose of thiopental (4 mg/kg) was associated with a decrease in the $\dot{V}_E$, V_T, and V_T/T_I, but respiratory frequency and T_I/T_{TOT} were not significantly affected.

In light pentobarbital anesthesia in newborn rabbits, $\dot{V}_E$ decreases solely because of a decrease in respiratory T_I/T_{TOT} resulting from both a decrease in T_I and an increase in T_E (see Fig. 29-2). With increasing doses of pentobarbital, the neural drive (V_T/T_I) eventually decreases.[23] Hypoxic ventilatory response is also depressed, even with the small dose of pentobarbital (2 mg/kg) used for preoperative medication.[146]

Upper airway and tracheal reflexes remain intact under barbiturate anesthesia and sedation unless very large doses are used.[147] Therefore irritation of the upper airways caused by instrumentation or the insertion of oral airways, laryngeal mask airways, or endotracheal tubes may provoke laryngospasm or bronchospasm.[148]

Thiopental

Thiopental sodium, a short-acting thiobarbiturate, has been the most popular agent for the intravenous induction of anesthesia. It is useful for diagnostic and operative neurologic procedures because it decreases intracranial pressure.[6] Awakening is quiet with a relatively low incidence of nausea. Adults require 4 mg/kg of thiopental for induction of anesthesia, and an inverse relationship exists between the induction dose and age; young infants require 7 mg/kg for anesthetic induction.[149]

Methohexital

Methohexital sodium, a methylated oxybarbital, is an ultra-short-acting barbiturate that is 2 to 3 times more potent than thiobarbiturates such as thiopental.[6] Hiccups occur frequently after intravenous injection.[120] Although the primary route of administration is intravenous (1 to 2 mg/kg), it has also been administered rectally (20 to 30 mg/kg) in infants and young children in whom intravenous access was not obtained before the induction of general anesthesia. The deep sedation or sleep induced by rectal methohexital usually lasts 20 or 30 minutes, although drowsiness may continue for several more hours. As with other barbiturates, methohexital has no analgesic properties. Its use in the presence of pain or strong noxious stimulation may result in excitement.

Chloral Derivatives

Pharmacology and Clinical Use

In pediatric practice, chloral hydrate has been used most commonly to induce conscious or deep sedation for various nonsurgical procedures, including infant pulmonary function testing. In vivo, chloral hydrate is rapidly metabolized by aldehyde reductase, alcohol dehydrogenase, and aldehyde dehydrogenase to form trichloroethanol, the pharmacologically active metabolite. Both chloral hydrate and trichloroethanol are sufficiently lipid soluble that they can enter cells throughout the body. Trichloroethanol is conjugated mainly with glucuronic acid in the liver and mostly excreted in the urine. If the process of conjugation is limited, trichloroethanol is further oxidized to form pharmacologically inactive trichlo-roacetic acid, which is excreted in urine.[150,151] In Europe, triclofos sodium, the phosphate ester of trichloroethanol (to which triclofos is rapidly hydrolyzed), is also used for sedation. A total of 1 g of triclofos is pharmacologically equivalent to 660 mg of chloral hydrate.[152] Triclofos results in less gastric irritation and has a less unpleasant taste than chloral hydrate; therefore it is more acceptable for oral administration in infants.[152,153]

In adults the plasma half-life of trichloroethanol ranges between 4 and 8 hours.[153] A recent study showed that after a single oral dose of chloral hydrate (50 mg/kg), the plasma half-life of trichloroethanol in children in the intensive care setting was similar to that in adults. In contrast, the plasma half-life of preterm and full-term infants was 3 to 4 times greater, with considerable interindividual variations, especially among preterm infants.[154,155]

The single, hypnotic dose of chloral hydrate commonly used in infants is 30 to 50 mg/kg. For pulmonary function testing a dose of up to 100 mg/kg is often used.[155] Overdose and adverse effects have been reported both in adults and in children.[156]

Respiratory Effects

The effects of chloral derivatives on respiration and gas exchange have been studied in neonates, infants, and young children after single-dose administration. The dose range was 50 to 100 mg/kg for chloral hydrate and 75 to 100 mg/kg for triclofos.

Neonates. Lees et al[157] compared 13 unsedated neonates (7 healthy, 6 apnea prone) during natural sleep and 31 apnea-prone neonates sedated with chloral hydrate. The end-tidal P_{CO_2} was similar in all groups. Ventilatory response to added carbon dioxide was the same in each group. Blunting of the carbon dioxide response, however, was reported in 2 of 12 full-term neonates younger than 5 days of age who had normal carbon dioxide responses during natural sleep. The baseline $\dot{V}_E$ after sedation was increased in these neonates. With added carbon dioxide, they developed tachypnea and oxygen desaturation.[158] This discrepancy in ventilatory response may be related to unpredictable variations in pharmacokinetics as well as changes in respiratory mechanics, including upper airway obstruction with sedation.[154,155,159]

Infants and Children. In healthy infants (6 to 54 weeks of age) during sedated sleep with chloral hydrate, indexes of breathing were essentially unchanged except for the V_T, which was only slightly decreased compared with that during natural sleep.[160] In another study,[161] a small but significant increase in respiratory frequency occurred, but no change in the V_T was seen.

In 10 infants and young children (4 to 19 months of age), the respiratory effects of triclofos-induced sleep were compared with those of natural sleep.[161] There were very small but statistically significant changes in respiratory frequency, heart rate, and oxygen saturation, but the changes were not considered clinically important. The Hering-Breuer inflation reflex, as evidenced by a change in the T_E after end-inspiratory airway occlusion, was not affected after triclofos administration in 66 healthy infants 4 to 8 weeks of age.[162] Thoracic gas volume, respiratory system compliance, conductance, and time constant under chloral hydrate sedation were unchanged in 10 healthy infants 6 to 54 weeks of age compared to the values in 10 infants of comparable age and birth weight during natural sleep.[160] In a double-blind, repeated-measure, dose-response study involving 26 healthy but uncooperative young children (21 to 42 months of age) during dental procedures, Wilson[163] noted a significant increase in end-tidal P_{CO_2} (approximately 5 mm Hg) with 70 mg/kg of chloral hydrate compared with placebo or a lower dose (25 and 50 mg/kg). This result may be related more to the difference between the excitement (with hypocapnia and possible sampling error) and sedation than to the degree of ventilatory depression. The method of end-tidal gas sampling was not reported.

In 10 infants 7 to 26 weeks of age recovering from viral bronchiolitis (3 with a mild decrease in the arterial oxygen saturation while awake in room air), a fall in the arterial oxygen saturation developed in all but 1 after sedation with chloral hydrate (70 to 100 mg/kg). These findings indicate no margin of safety in those with abnormal lung function.[164]

In laboratory animals, hypnotic doses of chloral hydrate depress the genioglossus muscle and may contribute to upper airway obstruction,[159] effects also seen with inhaled anesthetics.[50,51] Young children with a history of obstructive sleep apnea are at high risk of developing significant if not life-threatening upper airway obstruction after a regular dose of chloral hydrate.[159,165] It is extremely important therefore to perform a thorough history and physical examination in infants and young children before sedation.

Ketamine

Pharmacology and Clinical Use

Ketamine is a phencyclidine derivative that produces dissociation of the cortex from the limbic system. Ketamine produces dose-related anesthesia and analgesia. After the injection of ketamine, patients stare, exhibit nystagmus, and lapse into a dissociative and cataleptic state with eyes wide open. There may be coordinated but purposeless motions of the head, arms, legs, and trunk. Salivation and lacrimation are often increased, requiring anticholinergic medications, such as atropine and glycopyrrolate.

Ketamine is metabolized by the hepatic microsomal enzymes responsible for most medication detoxification. In newborn rats the onset of ketamine anesthesia is rapid and the duration prolonged; with maturation, the onset is prolonged and the duration shortens.[166] Similar age-related changes have been observed in children.[3,6]

Ketamine is particularly suited for sedation in children who are excited or upset before the induction of general anesthesia or in children undergoing relatively noninvasive procedures requiring immobilization, such as radiologic procedures, cardiac catheterization, dressing changes, and dental procedures.[105] Infants and children seem to have fewer adverse responses on emerging from anesthesia (i.e., hallucination and nightmare) than adults.[167] Ketamine may be administered intravenously (2 mg/kg), intramuscularly (2 mg/kg), or rectally (6 to 10 mg/kg).[168]

Respiratory Effects

Ketamine has a minimal respiratory depressant effect on adults except for a transient ventilatory depression lasting less than 3 minutes. In children, rectal ketamine (9 mg/kg) preceded by nasal midazolam (0.2 mg/kg) for diagnostic or short surgical procedures does not change ventilation or oxygen saturation.[139] A transient depressant effect, however, has been reported in children after bolus injection. In nine children between the ages of 6 and 10, ketamine 2 mg/kg intravenously followed by an infusion of 40 (μg/kg/min) failed to alter the resting $\dot{V}_E$, V_T, respiratory rate, or end-tidal P_{CO_2}. However, the slope of the carbon dioxide response curve decreased significantly. Both $\dot{V}_E$ and respiratory rate at a hypercapnic state (end-tidal P_{CO_2}, 60 mmHg) decreased.[169] In a retrospective study of cardiac catheterization in children with meperidine-promethazine premedication, 5 of 157 patients, all of whom were infants and young children (1 to 38 months of age), developed what appeared to be central apnea with oxygen desaturation after ketamine administration.[170]

There is some evidence that newborn animals are more sensitive to ketamine than adults. Eng et al[171] examined the respiratory depression produced by maternally administered ketamine in the newborn monkey. Two of three newborn monkeys whose mother received 2 mg/kg of ketamine failed to sustain ventilation.[15]

Opioids

Pharmacology and Clinical Use

Opioids, or narcotics, are frequently used for analgesia, sedation, and anesthesia in infants and children. Clinically, neonates are more sensitive to the effect of narcotics than children and adults. At the same plasma concentration, the brain concentration of morphine in neonates may be 2 to 4 times more than that in adults, probably because neonates have a more permeable blood-brain barrier and increased perfusion.[3,6,172] The elimination half-life in neonates is significantly increased compared with that in older infants and children.[3,173]

Respiratory Effects

All narcotics depress ventilation dose dependently. Narcotic overdosage is associated with a marked reduction in $\dot{V}_E$, with the characteristic slow respiratory frequency and normal or increased V_T.[15] In adults, morphine (0.1 to 0.2 mg/kg) decreases $\dot{V}_E$ 11% to 13% because of a reduction in the V_T, respiratory frequency, or both factors.[174,175] Morphine displaces the ventilatory response curve of carbon dioxide to the right and decreases its slope, primarily because of its direct depressant action on the brain stem respiratory centers.[176] Apneic threshold and resting end-tidal P_{CO_2} are increased.[15] Morphine (and presumably other opioids) depresses hypoxic ventilatory drive and also blunts the increased neural drive against increased inspiratory loads.[177]

In the classic study by Way et al,[178] a small dose of morphine (0.05 mg/kg), which is innocuous in adults, produced respiratory depression in neonates younger than 4 days of age. This difference in sensitivity to morphine was not found with meperidine, a highly lipid-soluble opioid.[178] The difference appears to result from the immature blood-brain barrier and increased permeability for relatively lipid-insoluble morphine into the brain tissue. The finding that the ratio of brain to plasma concentrations of morphine decreased with age in rats supports this hypothesis.[179] In addition, endogenous opioid activity may be increased in neonates and may contribute to the depressant effect of exogenous opioids because naloxone, a narcotic antagonist, shortens apneic spells and stimulates the hypoxic ventilatory response in neonates but not in older infants.[180]

A recent study suggests that sensitivity to fentanyl is not increased in infants older than 3 months of age.[181] During the recovery phase of nitrous oxide–fentanyl anesthesia, when nitrous oxide was discontinued and the patients were allowed to breathe spontaneously, the elevation of transcutaneous P_{CO_2} was correlated with increasing plasma fentanyl concentrations but did not differ among infants, children, and adults. Indeed, the incidence of apnea was higher in adults than in infants at the same plasma levels of fentanyl.[181]

The ventilatory depressant effects of opioids are increased or prolonged with the presence of other central nervous system depressants, such as inhaled anesthetics, barbiturates, and benzodiazepines.[143,180,182] Bailey et al[143] studied the effect of small doses of fentanyl (2 μg/kg) and midazolam (0.05 mg/kg) in adult volunteers. Midazolam alone produced no significant respiratory effect. Fentanyl alone produced hypoxemia (Sp_{O_2} <90%) in about half of subjects and significantly depressed the ventilatory response to carbon dioxide but did not produce apnea. The combination of fentanyl and midazolam, on the other hand, significantly increased the incidence of hypoxemia (11 of 12 subjects) and apnea (6 of 12) but did not depress the ventilatory response to carbon dioxide any further than fentanyl alone.

A high dose of some opioids, particularly fentanyl and sufentanil, increase chest wall rigidity and may severely compromise ventilation.[183,184] A more recent study in 13 infants younger than 6 months of age who were intubated and mechanically ventilated without sedation or muscle relaxants did not find any decrease in respiratory system compliance after a bolus injection of fentanyl (4 μg/kg).[185] Probably the apparent chest wall rigidity and the difficulty in ventilation in the previous reports resulted in part from upper airway obstruction.

Morphine

Morphine has been used frequently in infants and children for the relief of pain and for sedation. In a therapeutic dose (0.1 mg/kg), it causes analgesia in patients in pain without loss of consciousness. Morphine, like all other narcotics, depresses respiration with minimal circulatory effects, provided that the patient is not hypovolemic. Morphine is metabolized in the liver and largely excreted in the urine. Neonates younger than 1 week of age, compared with older infants, demonstrated longer elimination half-lives (6.8 vs. 3.9 hours) and slower clearance (6.3 vs. 23.8 ml/kg/min).[173] The combination of lower clearance and longer elimination half-life may explain a prolonged duration of action in young neonates.

Meperidine

Meperidine is a synthetic opioid also used extensively in the pediatric population. Its analgesic potency is about a hundredth that of morphine. Unlike morphine, which has a low lipid solubility, meperidine penetrates the blood-brain barrier readily because of its high lipid solubility. Meperidine is also metabolized in the liver. In newborn animals, the plasma half-life of meperidine is about twice as long as it is in adult rats. Neonates excrete 25% to 40% of a dose of meperidine in about 48 hours.[6,186]

Fentanyl

Fentanyl is a potent synthetic opioid used extensively in infants and children for analgesia, sedation, and anesthesia. Fentanyl is highly lipid soluble and rapidly crosses the blood-brain barrier. It is 50 to 100 times more potent than morphine and has minimal hemodynamic effects in clinical dosage. Preterm infants have a significantly prolonged elimination half-life (17.7 ± 0.3 hours) compared to that in children (4 to 7 hours), and respiratory depression lasts longer than in full-term neonates.[187] Full-term neonates also have a longer elimination half-life and less clearance than infants over 3 months of age and children.[188] The sedative dose is 1 to 3 μg/kg, which can be repeated as clinically indicated.

Sufentanil

Sufentanil is also a highly lipophilic compound that is distributed rapidly and completely to all body tissues. Sufentanil is 5 to 10 times more potent than fentanyl. Like fentanyl, sufentanil does not produce a significant hemodynamic effect.

Alfentanil

Alfentanil is a fentanyl analog with a lower lipid solubility, smaller volume of distribution, and much shorter duration of action. Alfentanil is about one fifth to one third as potent as fentanyl. It is a strong respiratory depressant, but information concerning its effect on the control of breathing has been limited.

LOCAL ANESTHETICS

Local anesthetics are administered to infants and children for regional anesthesia and pain relief. They are also given intravenously and topically for rigid and fiberoptic laryngoscopy and bronchoscopy. Local anesthetics can be subdivided into two classes of compounds: ester type (procaine, chloroprocaine, tetracaine) and amide type (lidocaine, mepivacaine, bupivacaine). Ester forms of local anesthetics are hydrolyzed in plasma primarily by plasma cholinesterase, whereas amide forms of medications are metabolized primarily in the liver.[6]

In the neonate, the ability to hydrolyze local anesthetics is decreased compared with the ability in adults because plasma cholinesterase levels are decreased.[189] Although the neonate can metabolize lidocaine,[190] the capability for conjugation reaction is not well developed in the neonatal liver and does not reach adult levels until about 3 months of age.[6,191-193] Another clinically important factor affecting the pharmacokinetics of local anesthetics is the level of plasma protein and protein binding. Because plasma protein binding is important in determining the unbound, free fraction of local anesthetics, lower plasma protein concentrations in the neonate result in more anesthetic remaining in the active form, with a greater risk of medication toxicity.[194] The rate of plasma decay of lidocaine and mepivacaine are similar in adults and neonates. However, the plasma levels needed to produce cardiorespiratory depression in neonates are about half those in adults.[6] Because the rate of absorption of local anesthetics through the upper airway epithelia is extremely rapid, the pulmonologist must exercise extreme caution in not overdosing topical anesthetics during bronchoscopy. Recommended upper limits of local anesthetic medications are shown in Table 29-1.

Table 29-1 Doses of Local Anesthetic Agents in Children

AGENT	PLAIN SOLUTION	SOLUTION WITH EPINEPHRINE
Chloroprocaine	15 mg/kg	15 mg/kg
Procaine	10-15 mg/kg	10-15 mg/kg
Lidocaine	5 mg/kg	10 mg/kg
Mepivacaine	5 mg/kg	7 mg/kg
Etidocaine	3 mg/kg	3-4 mg/kg
Bupivacaine	3 mg/kg	3 mg/kg
Tetracaine	2 mg/kg	2 mg/kg
Prilocaine	5-7 mg/kg*	7-9 mg/kg

From Rice LJ, Hannallah RS: In Motoyama EK, ed: *Smith's anesthesia for infants and children,* ed 5, St Louis, 1990, Mosby, p 396.
*Total not to exceed 600 mg.

MONITORING AND PATIENT SAFETY

As outlined in the guidelines recently published by the American Academy of Pediatrics,[195] the safety of infants and children under sedation is of the utmost importance. Presedation assessment should include a physical examination and observation of vital signs; in addition, other unusual physical findings should be noted. The patient should be monitored with qualified personnel dedicated to monitoring during the procedure.

Infants and children under conscious or unconscious sedation must be monitored continuously with a pulse oximeter until they are fully awake. Electrocardiography and other means of automated monitoring of vital signs may be used as supplements but not as substitutes for pulse oximetry. If not continuously recorded, vital signs should be measured at baseline and at frequent intervals thereafter and should be recorded on the patient's medical record or a flowsheet designed for this purpose.

Avoidance of the unnecessary and potentially dangerous transfer of deeply sedated infants and children requires that sedation be administered at the location where the procedure is to be performed. Infants and children should not be released home after sedation until they are fully arousable and capable of swallowing or drinking. In addition, parents should be advised that the child may be drowsy and unsteady for several hours after sedation and therefore should not be left unattended until the child has fully recovered normal control of body movement.[155]

CONCLUSION

The responses of infants and children, especially neonates, to anesthetics and various sedatives differ from those of adults for multiple reasons. Differences include the maturity of the control mechanism of breathing, the patency of upper airways under sedation or anesthesia, respiratory mechanics (both the thorax and lungs), and the early development of hepatic enzyme systems and body compartments that significantly affect the pharmacokinetics and pharmacodynamics of sedatives, opiates, and anesthetics. Also, the respiratory system effects of many medications that are frequently used in infants and children are not well understood because of the technical and ethical difficulties involved with studying this young population. The recent increased interest in infant respiratory mechanics and respiratory physiology among pediatric pulmonologists and neonatologists, together with the advanced technology and instrumentation for clinical and scientific determinations as highlighted by the recent position paper,[196] raises the hope that more information on the respiratory effects of sedatives and anesthetics will be elucidated soon.

REFERENCES

1. Miller RD, ed: *Anesthesia,* ed 4, New York, 1994, Churchill Livingstone.
2. Motoyama EK: Maintenance of anesthesia in infants and children. In Motoyama EK, ed: *Smith's anesthesia for infants and children,* ed 5, St Louis, 1990, Mosby, pp 291-312.
3. Gregory G: Pharmacology. In Gregory G, ed: *Pediatric anesthesia,* ed 3, New York, 1994, Churchill Livingstone, pp 13-45.
4. Gilman AG, Rall TW, Nies AS, Taylor P: *Goodman and Gilman's the pharmacological basis of therapeutics,* ed 8, New York, 1990, Pergamon.

Inhaled Anesthetics

5. Stanski DR: Monitoring depth of anesthesia. In Miller RD, ed: *Anesthesia,* ed 4, New York, 1994, Churchill Livingstone, pp 1127-1159.
6. Cook DR, Davis PJ: Pharmacology of pediatric anesthesia. In Motoyama EK, ed: *Smith's anesthesia for infants and children,* ed 5, St Louis, 1990, Mosby, pp 157-197.
7. Sampio MM, Crean PM, Keilty SR, Black GW: Changes in oxygen saturation during isoflurane anesthesia in children, *Br J Anaesth* 62:199-201, 1989.
8. LeDez KM, Lerman J: The minimum alveolar concentration (MAC) of isoflurane in preterm neonates, *Anesthesiology* 67:301-307, 1987.
9. Rampil IJ, Lockhart SH, Zwass MS, Peterson N, Yasuda N, Eger EI II, Weiskoph RB, Damask MC: Clinical characteristics of desflurane in surgical patients: minimum alveolar concentration, *Anesthesiology* 74:429-433, 1991.
10. Taylor RH, Lerman J: Induction and recovery characteristics of desflurane in children, *Can J Anaesth* 39:6-13, 1992.
11. Zwass MC, Fisher DM, Welborn LG, Cote CJ, Davis PJ, Dinner M, Hannallah RS, Liu LMP, Sarner J, McGill WA, Alifimoff JK, Embree PB, Cook DR: Induction and maintenance characteristics of anesthesia with desflurane and nitrous oxide in infants and children, *Anesthesiology* 76:373-378, 1992.
12. Davis PJ, Cohen IT, McGowan FX, Latta K: Recovery characteristics of desflurane versus halothane for maintenance of anesthesia in pediatric ambulatory patients, *Anesthesiology* 80:298-302, 1994.
13. Sarner JB, Levine M, Davis PJ, Lerman J, Cook DR, Motoyama EK: Clinical characteristics of sevoflurane in children: a comparison with halothane, *Anesthesiology* 82:38-46, 1995.
14. Lerman J, Burrows FA, Oyston JP, Gallergher TM, Miyasaka K, Volgiesi G: The minimum alveolar concentration (MAC) and cardiovascular effects of halothane, isoflurane and sevoflurane in newborn swine, *Anesthesiology* 73:712-721, 1990.
15. Hickey RF, Severinghaus JW: Regulation of breathing: drug effect. In Hornbein TF, ed: *Lung biology in health and disease: regulation of breathing,* New York, 1981, Marcel Dekker, pp 2251-2312.
16. Pavlin EG, Hornbein TF: Anesthesia and the control of ventilation. In Geiger SR, ed: *Handbook of physiology,* ed 2, Section 3. The respiratory system, vol 2, Bethesda, Md, 1986, American Physiological Society, pp 793-813.
17. Munson ES, Larson CP, Babad AA, Regan MJ, Buechel DR, Eger EI: The effects of halothane, fluroxene, and cyclopropane on ventilation: a comparative study in man, *Anesthesiology* 27:716-728, 1966.
18. Whitelaw WA, Derenne J-P, Milic-Emili J: Occlusion pressure as a measure of respiratory center output in conscious man, *Respir Physiol* 23:181-199, 1975.
19. Milic-Emili J, Grunstein MM: Drive and timing components of ventilation, *Chest* 70:131-132, 1976.
20. Derenne JP, Couture J, Iscoe S, Whitelaw WA, Milic-Emili J: Occlusion pressures in men rebreathing CO_2 under methoxyflurane anesthesia, *J Appl Physiol* 40:805-814, 1976.
21. Wahba WM: Analysis of ventilatory depression by enflurane during clinical anesthesia, *Anesth Analg* 59:103-109, 1980.
22. Thach BT, Wyszogrodski I, Milic-Emili J: Effect of ether on control of rate and depth of breathing in newborn rabbits, *J Appl Physiol* 40:281-286, 1976.
23. Goldberg MS, Milic-Emili J: Effect of pentobarbital sodium on respiratory control in newborn rabbits, *J Appl Physiol* 42:845-851, 1977.
24. Robinson SL, Richardson CA, Willis MM, Gregory GA: Halothane anesthesia reduces pulmonary function in the newborn lamb, *Anesthesiology* 62:578-581, 1985.
25. Murat I, Delleur MM, Maggee K, Saint-Maurice C: Changes in ventilatory patterns during halothane anaesthesia in children, *Br J Anaesth* 57:569-572, 1985.
26. Lindahl SGE, Yates AP, Hatch DJ: Respiratory depression in children at different end tidal halothane concentrations, *Anaesthesia* 42:1267-1275, 1987.
27. Benameur M, Goldman MD, Ecoffey C, Gaultier C: Ventilation and thoracoabdominal asynchrony during halothane anesthesia in infants, *J Appl Physiol* 74:1591-1596, 1993.
28. Weiskopf RB, Raymond LW, Severinghaus JW: Effects of halothane on canine respiratory response to hypoxia with and without hypercarbia, *Anesthesiology* 41:350-360, 1974.
29. Hirshman CA, McCullough RE, Cohen PJ, Weil JV: Depression of hypoxic ventilatory response by halothane, enflurane and isoflurane in dogs, *Br J Anaesth* 49:957-963, 1977.
30. Knill RL, Gelb AW: Ventilatory response to hypoxia and hypercapnia during halothane sedation and anesthesia in man, *Anesthesiology* 49:244-251, 1978.
31. Knill RL, Manninen PH, Clement JL: Ventilation and chemoreflexes during enflurane sedation and anaesthesia in man, *Can Anaesth Soc J* 26:353-360, 1979.
32. Knill RL, Clement JL: Variable effects of anaesthetics on the ventilatory response to hypoxaemia in man, *Can Anaesth Soc J* 29:93-99, 1982.
33. Davies RO, Edwards MW, Lahiri S: Halothane depresses the response of carotid body chemoreceptors to hypoxia and hypercapnia in the cat, *Anesthesiology* 57:153-159, 1982.
34. Temp JA, Henson LC, Ward DS: Does a subanesthetic concentration of isoflurane blunt the ventilatory response to hypoxia? *Anesthesiology* 77:1116-1124, 1992.
35. Temp JA, Henson LC, Ward DS: Effect of subanesthetic minimum alveolar concentration of isoflurane on two tests of the hypoxic ventilatory response, *Anesthesiology* 80:739-750, 1994.
36. Dahan A, van den Elsen MJLJ, Berkenbosch A, DeGoede J, Olievier ICW, van Kleef JW, Bovill JG: Effects of subanesthetic halothane on the ventilatory responses to hypercapnia and acute hypoxia in healthy volunteers, *Anesthesiology* 80:727-738, 1994.
37. Robotham JL: Do low dose anesthetic agents alter ventilatory control? *Anesthesiology* 80:723-726, 1994.
38. Motoyama EK, Glazener C: Hypoxemia after general anesthesia in children, *Anesth Analg* 65:267-272, 1986.
39. Nunn JF, Ezi-Ashi TI: The respiratory effects of resistance to breathe in anesthetized man, *Anesthesiology* 22:174-178, 1966.
40. Isaza GD, Posner JD, Altose MD, Kelsen SG, Cherniak NS: Airway occlusion pressure in awake and anesthetized goats, *Respir Physiol* 27:87-98, 1976.
41. Kryger MH, Jacob O, Dosman J, Macklem PT, Anthonisen NR: Effect of meperidine on occlusion pressure response to hypercapnia and hypoxia with and without external inspiratory resistance, *Am Rev Respir Dis* 114:333-340, 1976.
42. Savoy J, Arnup ME, Anthonisen NR: Response to external inspiratory resistive loading and bronchospasm in anesthetized dogs, *J Appl Physiol* 53:355-360, 1982.
43. Pietak S, Weenig CS, Hickey RF, Fairley HB: Anesthetic effects on ventilation in patients with chronic obstructive pulmonary disease, *Anesthesiology* 42:160-166, 1975.
44. Guedel AE, ed: *Inhalation anesthesia,* ed 2, New York, 1951, Macmillan.

45. Tusiewicz K, Brayan AC, Froese AB: Contribution of changing rib cage-diaphragm interaction to the ventilatory depression of halothane anesthesia, *Anesthesiology* 47:327-337, 1977.
46. Drummond GB: Reduction of tonic ribcage activity by anesthesia with thiopental, *Anesthesiology* 67:695-700, 1987.
47. Remmers JE, deGroot WJ, Sauerland EK, Anch AM: Pathogenesis of upper airway occlusion during sleep, *J Appl Physiol* 44:931-938, 1978.
48. Bonora M, Shields GI, Knuth SL, Bartlett D Jr, St John WM: Selective depression by ethanol of upper airway respiratory motor activity in cats, *Am Rev Respir Dis* 130:156-161, 1984.
49. Nishino T, Kochi T, Yonezawa T, Honda Y: Response of recurrent laryngeal, hypoglossal, and phrenic nerves to increasing depth of anesthesia with halothane or enflurane in vagotomized cats, *Anesthesiology* 63:404-409, 1985.
50. Ochiai R, Guthrie R, Motoyama EK: Effects of varying concentrations of halothane on the activity of the genioglossus, intercostals and diaphragm in cats: an electromyographic study, *Anesthesiology* 70:812-816, 1989.
51. Ochiai R, Guthrie R, Motoyama EK: Differential sensitivity of halothane anesthesia on the genioglossus, intercostals, and diaphragm in kittens, *Anesth Analg* 74:338-344, 1992.
52. Brozanski BS, Guthrie RD, Volk EA, Cameron WE: Postnatal growth of genioglossal motoneurons, *Pediatr Pulmonol* 7:133-139, 1989.
53. Watchko JF, Klesh KW, O'Day TL, Weiss MG, Guthrie RD: Genioglossal recruitment during acute hypoxia and hypercapnia in kittens, *Pediatr Pulmonol* 7:235-243, 1989.
54. Motoyama EK, Cohen IT: Continuous positive airway pressure (CPAP) improves airway patency and ventilation during inhalation induction in children, *Anesthesiology* 77:A1198, 1992.
55. Ochiai R, Ueda E, Motoyama EK, Takeda J, Fukushima K: Inspiratory muscle incoordination during halothane anesthesia in man, *Anesthesiology* 81:A1418, 1994.
56. Ochiai R, Ueda E, Motoyama EK, Takeda J, Fukushima K: Inspiratory muscle incoordination during sevoflurane anesthesia in man, *Anesth Analg* 78:S325, 1994.
57. Westbrook PR, Stubbs SE, Sessler AD, Rehder K, Hyatt RE: Effects of anesthesia and muscle paralysis on respiratory mechanics in normal man, *J Appl Physiol* 34:81-86, 1973.
58. Rehder K, Mallow JE, Fibuch EE, Krebill DR, Sessler AD: Effects of isoflurane anesthesia and muscle paralysis on respiratory mechanics in normal man, *Anesthesiology* 44:477-485, 1974.
59. Rehder K, Sittipong R, Sessler AD: The effects of thiopental-meperidine anesthesia with succinylcholine paralysis on respiratory mechanics in normal man, *Anesthesiology* 41:477-485, 1974.
60. de Troyer A, Bastenier-Geens J: Effects of neuromuscular blockade on respiratory mechanics in conscious man, *J Appl Physiol* 47:1162-1168, 1979.
61. Critchlow V, von Euler C: Intercostal muscle spindle activity in the intercostal muscle, *J Physiol (Lond)* 168:820-847, 1963.
62. Corda MC, von Euler C, Lennerstrand G: Reflex and cerebellar influences on I and on " rhythmic" and "tonic" K activity in the intercostal muscle, *J Physiol (Lond)* 184:898-923, 1966.
63. Fletcher M, Ewert M, Stack C, Hatch DJ, Stocks J: Influence of tidal volume on respiratory compliance in anesthetized infants and young children, *J Appl Physiol* 68:1127-1133, 1990.
64. Rehder K, Marsh HM: Respiratory mechanics during anesthesia and mechanical ventilation. In Macklem PT, Mead J, eds: *Handbook of physiology,* Section 3: The respiratory system, vol 3, part 1. Mechanics of breathing, Bethesda, Md, 1986, American Physiological Society, pp 737-752.
65. Hedenstierna G, McCarthy GS: Airway closure and closing pressure during mechanical ventilation, *Acta Anaesth Scand* 24:299-304, 1980.
66. Rehder K: Anesthesia and the mechanics of respiration. In Covino BG, Fozzard HA, Rehder K, Strichartz G, eds: *Effects of anesthesia,* Bethesda, Md, 1985, American Physiological Society, pp 91-106.
67. Laws AK: Effects of induction of anesthesia and muscle paralysis on functional residual capacity of the lungs, *Can Anaesth Soc J* 15:325-331, 1968.
68. Don HF, Wahba M, Cuadrado L, Kelkar K: The effects of anesthesia and 100 percent oxygen on the functional residual capacity of the lungs, *Anesthesiology* 32:521-529, 1970.
69. Rehder K, Hatch DJ, Sessler AD, March HM, Fowler WS: Effects of general anesthesia, muscle paralysis, and mechanical ventilation on pulmonary nitrogen clearance, *Anesthesiology* 35:591-601, 1971.
70. Hewlett AM, Hulands GH, Nunn JF, Milledge JS: Functional residual capacity during anaesthesia. III. Artificial ventilation, *Br J Anaesth* 46:495-503, 1974.
71. Rehder K, Sessler AD, Rodarte JR: Regional intrapulmonary gas distribution in awake and anesthetized-paralyzed man, *J Appl Physiol* 42:391-402, 1977.
72. Juno P, March HM, Knopp TJ, Rehder K: Closing capacity in awake and anesthetized-paralyzed man, *J Appl Physiol* 44:238-244, 1978.
73. Bergman NA: Distribution of inspired gas during anesthesia and artificial ventilation, *J Appl Physiol* 18:1085-1089, 1963.
74. Dobbinson TL, Nisbet HIA, Pelton DA, Levison H, Volgyesi G: Functional residual capacity (FRC) and compliance in anaesthetized paralyzed children, *Can Anaesth Soc J* 20:322-333, 1973.
75. Henderson-Smart DJ, Read DJC: Reduced lung volume during behavior active sleep in the newborn, *J Appl Physiol* 46:1081-1085, 1979.
76. Motoyama EK, Brinkmeyer SD, Mutich RL, Walczak SA: Reduced FRC in anesthetized infants and children: effect of low PEEP, *Anesthesiology* 57:A418-419, 1982.
77. Agostoni E: Volume-pressure relationship of the thorax and lung in the newborn, *J Appl Physiol* 14:909-913, 1959.
78. Thorsteinsson A, Jonmarker C, Larsson A, Vilstrup C, Verner O: Functional residual capacity in anesthetized children: normal values and values in children with cardiac anomalies, *Anesthesiology* 73:786-881, 1990.
79. Gaultier C, Boule M, Allaire Y, Clement A, Girard F: Growth of lung volumes during the first three years of life, *Bull Eur Physiopathol Respir* 15:1103-1116, 1979.
80. Bar-Yishay E, Shulman DL, Beardsmore CS, Godfrey S: Functional residual capacity in healthy preschool children lying supine, *Am Rev Respir Dis* 135:954-956, 1987.
81. Gerhardt T, Reifenberg L, Hehre D, Feller R, Bancalari E: Functional residual capacity in normal neonates and children up to 5 years of age determined by a N_2 washout method, *Pediatr Res* 20:668-671, 1986.
82. Nunn JF, Hill DH: Respiratory dead space and arterial to end-tidal CO_2 tension difference in anaesthetized man, *J Appl Physiol* 15:383-389, 1960.
83. Nunn JF: Factors influencing the arterial oxygen tension during halothane anaesthesia with spontaneous respiration, *Br J Anaesth* 38:327-341, 1964.
84. Nunn JF, Bergman NA, Coleman AJ: Factors influencing the arterial oxygen tension during anaesthesia with artificial ventilation, *Br J Anaesth* 37:898-914, 1964.
85. Nunn JF: Anesthesia and pulmonary gas exchange. In Covino BJ, Fossard HA, Rehder K, Strichartz G, eds: *Effects of anesthesia,* Bethesda, Md, 1985, American Physiological Society, pp 137-147.
86. Sykes MK, Loh L, Seed RF, Kafer ER, Chakrabarti MK: The effect of inhalational anaesthetics on hypoxic pulmonary vasoconstriction and pulmonary vascular resistance in the perfused lungs of the dog and cat, *Br J Anaesth* 44:776-788, 1972.
87. Bjertnase L: Hypoxia-induced vasoconstriction in isolated perfused lungs exposed to injectable or inhalation anaesthetics, *Acta Anaesth Scand* 21:133-147, 1977.
88. Marshall BE, Marshall C: Anesthesia and pulmonary circulation. In Covino BJ, Fozzard HA, Rehder K, Strichartz G, eds: *Effects of anesthesia,* Bethesda, Md, 1985, American Physiological Society, pp 121-136.
89. Susmano A, Passovoy M, Carlton RA: Comparison of the effects of two anaesthetic agents on the production of hypoxic pulmonary hypertension in dogs, *Am Heart J* 84:203-207, 1972.
90. Benumof JL, Wahrenbrock EA: Local effects of anaesthetics on regional hypoxic pulmonary vasoconstriction, *Anesthesiology* 43:525-532, 1975.
91. Bjertanase L, Hauge A, Kriz M: Hypoxia-induced pulmonary vasoconstriction: effects of fentanyl following different route of administration, *Acta Anaesth Scand* 24:53-57, 1980.
92. Bjertanase L, Mundal R, Hauge A, Nicolaysen A: Vascular resistance in atelectatic lungs: effects of inhalation anaesthetics, *Acta Anaesth Scand* 24:109-118, 1980.
93. Gibbs JM, Johnson H: Lack of effect of morphine and buprenorphine on hypoxic pulmonary vasoconstriction in the isolated perfused cat lung and perfused lobe of the dog lung, *Br J Anaesth* 50:1197-1201, 1978.
94. Lichtiger M, Landa JF, Hirsch JA: Velocity of tracheal mucus in anesthetized women undergoing gynecological surgery, *Anesthesiology* 41:753-756, 1976.
95. Kilburn KH, Salzano JV, eds: Symposium on structure, function and measurement of respiratory cilia, *Am Rev Respir Dis* 93(suppl):1-184, 1966.

96. Forbes AR: Temperature, humidity and mucous flow in the intubated trachea, *Br J Anaesth* 46:29-34, 1974.
97. Hirsch JA, Tokayer JL, Robinson MJ, Sackner MA: Effects of dry air and subsequent humidification on tracheal mucous velocity in dogs, *J Appl Physiol* 39:242-246, 1975.
98. Wolfe WG, Ebert PA, Sabiston DC: Effects of high oxygen tension on mucociliary function, *Surgery* 72:246-252, 1972.
99. Sackner MA, Landa J, Hirsch J, Zapata A: Pulmonary effects of oxygen breathing, *Ann Intern Med* 82:40-43, 1975.
100. Forbes AR, Gamsu G: Lung mucociliary clearance after anesthesia and spontaneous and controlled ventilation, *Am Rev Respir Dis* 120:857-862, 1979.
101. Sackner MA, Hirsch J, Epstein S: Effects of cuffed endotracheal tube on tracheal mucus velocity, *Chest* 68:774-777, 1975.
102. Forbes AR, Horrigan RW: Mucociliary flow in the trachea during anesthesia with enflurane, ether, nitrous oxide, and morphine, *Anesthesiology* 46:319-321, 1977.
103. Forbes AR, Gamsu G: Depression of lung mucociliary clearance by thiopental and halothane, *Anesth Analg* 58:387-389, 1979.

Intravenous Agents

104. Kay NH, Sear JW, Upington J, Cockshott ID, Douglas EJ: Disposition of propofol in patients undergoing surgery: a comparison in men and women, *Br J Anaesth* 58:1075-1079, 1986.
105. Reves G, Glass PSA, Lubarsky DA: Nonbarbiturate intravenous anesthetics. In Miller RD, ed: *Anesthesia,* ed 4, New York, 1994, Churchill Livingstone, pp 247-289.
106. Morton NS: Abolition of injection pain due to propofol in children, *Anaesthesia* 45:70, 1990 (letter).
107. Marsh B, White M, Morton N, Kenny GNC: Pharmacokinetic model driven infusion of propofol in children, *Br J Anaesth* 67:41-48, 1991.
108. Hannallah RS, Baker SB, Casey W: Propofol: effective dose and induction characteristics in unpremedicated children, *Anesthesiology* 74:217-219, 1991.
109. Westrin P: The induction dose of propofol in infants 1 to 6 months of age and in children 10 to 16 years of age, *Anesthesiology* 74:455-558, 1991.
110. Coates DP, Monk CR, Prys-Roberts C, Turtle M: Hemodynamic effects of infusion of the emulsion formulation of propofol during nitrous oxide anesthesia in humans, *Anesth Analg* 66:64-70, 1987.
111. Short SM, Aun CS: Hemodynamic effects of propofol in children, *Anesthesia* 46:783-785, 1991.
112. Mirakhur RK: Induction characteristics of propofol in children: comparison with thiopentone, *Anaesthesia* 43:593-598, 1988.
113. Martin TM, Nicholson SC, Bargas MS: Propofol anesthesia reduces emesis and airway obstruction in pediatric outpatients, *Anesth Analg* 76:144-148, 1993.
114. Weir PM, Munro HM, Reynolds PI, Lewis IH, Wilton NCT: Propofol infusion and the incidence of emesis in pediatric outpatient strabismus surgery, *Anesth Analg* 76:760-764, 1993.
115. Randell T: Sedation for bronchofiberscopy: comparison between propofol infusion and intravenous boluses of fentanyl and diazepam, *Acta Anaesth Scand* 36:221-225, 1992.
116. Crawford M, Pollock J, Anderson K, Glavin RJ, Macintire D, Vernon D: Comparison of midazolam with propofol for sedation in outpatient bronchoscopy, *Br J Anaesth* 70:419-422, 1993.
117. Clarkson K, Power CK, O'Connell F, Pathmakanthan S, Burke CM: A comparative evaluation of propofol and midazolam as sedative agents in fiberoptic bronchoscopy, *Chest* 104:1029-1031, 1993.
118. Taylor MB, Ground RM, Mulrooney PD, Morgan M: Ventilatory effect of propofol during induction of anaesthesia, *Anaesthesia* 41:816-820, 1986.
119. Sanderson JH, Blades JF: Multicentre study of propofol in day case surgery, *Anaesthesia* 43(suppl):70-73, 1988.
120. Gold M, Abram EC, Herrington C: A controlled investigation of propofol, thiopental and methohexitone, *Can J Anaesth* 34:478-483, 1987.
121. Grounds RM, Maxwell DL, Taylor MB, Aber V, Royston D: Acute ventilatory changes during I.V. induction of anaesthesia with thiopentone or propofol in man, *Br J Anaesth* 59:1098-1102, 1987.
122. Goodman NW, Black AMS, Carter JA: Some ventilatory effects of propofol as sole anesthetic agent, *Br J Anaesth* 59:1497-1503, 1987.
123. Blouin RT, Seifert HA, Babenco HD, Conard PF, Gross JB: Propofol depresses the hypoxic ventilatory response during conscious sedation and isohypercapnia, *Anesthesiology* 79:1177-1182, 1993.
124. Rosa G, Conti G, Orsi P, D'Alessandro F, La Rosa L, Di Giugno G, Gasparetto A: Effects of low dose propofol administration on central respiratory drive, gas exchanges and respiratory pattern, *Acta Anaesth Scand* 36:128-131, 1992.
125. Foster A, Gardaz JP, Suter PM, Gumperle M: Respiratory depression by midazolam and diazepam, *Anesthesiology* 53:494-497, 1980.
126. Gross JB, Zebrowski ME, Carel WD, Gardner S, Smith TC: Time course of ventilatory depression after thiopental and midazolam in normal subjects and in patients with chronic obstructive pulmonary disease, *Anesthesiology* 58:540-544, 1983.
127. Blouin RT, Conard PF, Perreault BS, Gross JB: Flumazenil reverses midazolam-induced depression of hypoxic ventilatory drive, *Anesthesiology* 77:A1216, 1992.
128. Reves JG, Fragen RJ, Vinik R, Greenblatt DJ: Midazolam: pharmacology and uses, *Anesthesiology* 62:310-324, 1985.
129. Montravers P, Dureuil B, Desmonts JM: Effects of i.v. midazolam on upper airway resistance, *Br J Anaesth* 68:27-31, 1992.
130. Latson LA, Cheatham JP, Gumbiner CH, Kugler JD, Danford DA, Hofshire JP, Honts J: Midazolam nose drops for outpatient echocardiography sedation in infants, *Am Heart J* 121:209-210, 1991.
131. Yaster M, Nichols DG, Deshpande JK, Wetzel RC: Midazolam-fentanyl intravenous sedation in children: case report of respiratory arrest, *Pediatrics* 86:463-467, 1990.
132. Feld LH, Negus JB, White PF: Oral midazolam preanesthetic medication in pediatric outpatients, *Anesthesiology* 73:831-834, 1990.
133. van der Walt JH, Jacob R, Murrell D, Bentley M: The perioperative effects of oral premedication in children, *Anaesth Intensive Care* 18:5-10, 1990.
134. McMillan CO, Spahr-Schopfer IA, Sikich N, Hartley E, Lerman J: Premedication of children with oral midazolam, *Can J Anaesth* 39:545-550, 1989.
135. Wilton NCT, Leigh J, Rosen DR, Pandit AU: Preanesthetic sedation of preschool children using intranasal midazolam, *Anesthesiology* 69:972-975, 1988.
136. Karl HW, Keifer AT, Rosenberger JL, Larach MG, Ruffle JM: Comparison of the safety and efficacy of intranasal midazolam or sufentanil for preinduction of anesthesia in pediatric patients, *Anesthesiology* 78:885-891, 1993.
137. Karl HW, Rosenberger JL, Larach MG, Ruffle JM: Transmucosal administration of midazolam for premedication of pediatric patients: comparison of the nasal and sublingual routes, *Anesthesiology* 78:885-891, 1993.
138. Saint-Maurice C, Meistelman C, Rey E, Esteve C, de Lauture D, Olive G: The pharmacokinetics of rectal midazolam for premedication in children, *Anesthesiology* 65:536-538, 1986.
139. Saint-Maurice C, Landais A, Delleur MM, Esteve C, MacGee K, Murat I: The use of midazolam in diagnostic and short surgical procedures in children, *Acta Anaesth Scand* 92(suppl):39-41, 1990.
140. Walbergh EJ, Willis RJ, Eckhert J: Plasma concentrations of midazolam in children following intranasal administration, *Anesthesiology* 74:233-235, 1991.
141. Kurland J, Noyes BE, Jaffe R, Atlas AB, Armitage J, Orenstein DM: Bronchoalveolar lavage and transbronchial biopsy in children following heart-lung and lung transplantation, *Chest* 104:1043-1048, 1993.
142. Tolia V, Fleming SL, Kauffman RE: Randomized, double-blind trial of midazolam and diazepam for endoscopic sedation in children, *Dev Pharmacol Ther* 14:141-147, 1990.
143. Bailey PL, Pace NL, Ashburn MA, Moll JWB, East KA, Stanley TH: Frequent hypoxemia and apnea after sedation with midazolam and fentanyl, *Anesthesiology* 73:826-830, 1990.
144. Gross JB, Weller RS, Conard P: Flumazenil antagonism of midazolam-induced ventilatory depression, *Anesthesiology* 75:179-185, 1991.
145. Lauven P, Schwilden H, Stoeckel H, Greenblatt DJ: The effects of a benzodiazepine antagonist RO 15-1788 in the presence of stable concentrations of midazolam, *Anesthesiology* 63:61-64, 1985.
146. Hirshman CA, McCullough RE, Cohen PJ, Weil JV: Effect of pentobarbital on hypoxic ventilatory drive in man: a preliminary study, *Br J Anaesth* 47:963-968, 1975.
147. Harrison GA: The influence of different anesthetic agents on the response to respiratory tract irritation, *Br J Anaesth* 34:804-811, 1962.
148. Brown GW, Patel N, Ellis FR: Comparison of propofol and thiopentone for laryngeal mask insertion, *Anaesthesia* 46:771-772, 1991.

149. Jonmarker C, Westrin P, Larsson S, Werner O: Thiopental requirements for induction of anesthesia in children, *Anesthesiology* 67:104-107, 1987.
150. Gorecki DKJ, Hindmarsh KW, Hall CA, Mayers DJ, Sankaran K: Determination of chloral hydrate metabolism in adult and neonate biological fluids after single-dose administration, *J Chromatogr* 528:333-341, 1990.
151. Reimche LD, Sankaran K, Hindmarsh KW, Kasian GF, Gorecki DKJ, Tan L: Chloral hydrate sedation in neonates and infants: clinical and pharmacologic considerations, *Dev Pharmacol Ther* 12:57-64, 1989.
152. Sellers EM, Long-Sellers M, Koch-Weser J: Comparative metabolism of chloral hydrate and triclofos, *J Clin Pharmacol* 18:456-461, 1978.
153. Breimer DD: Clinical pharmacokinetics of hypnosis, *Clin Pharmacokinet* 2:93-109, 1977.
154. Mayers JD, Hindmarsh KW, Sankaran K, Gorecki DKJ, Kasian GF: Chloral hydrate disposition following single-dose administration to critically ill neonates and children, *Dev Pharmacol Ther* 16:71-77, 1991.
155. Gaultier C, Fletcher ME, Beardsmore C, England S, Motoyama E: Respiratory function measurements in infants: measurement conditions, *Eur Respir J* 8:1057-1066, 1995.
156. Graham SR, Day RD, Lee D, Fulde GW: Overdose with chloral hydrate: a pharmacological and therapeutic review, *Med J Aust* 149:686-688, 1988.
157. Lees MH, Olsen GD, McGilliard KL, Newcomb JD, Sunderland CO: Chloral hydrate and the carbon dioxide chemoreceptor response: a study of puppies and infants, *Pediatrics* 70:447-450, 1982.
158. Sallent A, Cross KM, Wozniak JA, Brown CD, Kosch PC: Effect of chloral hydrate on minute ventilation and CO_2 responsiveness in normal newborns, *Pediatr Res* 31:A364, 1992.
159. Hershenson M, Brouillette RT, Olsen E, Hunt CE: The effect of chloral hydrate on genioglossus and diaphragmatic activity, *Pediatr Res* 18:516-519, 1984.
160. Turner DJ, Morgan SEG, Landau LI, Le Souëf PN: Methodological aspects of flow-volume studies in infants, *Pediatr Pulmonol* 8:289-293, 1990.
161. Jackson EA, Rabbette PS, Desateux C, Hatch DJ, Stocks J: The effect of triclofos sedation on respiratory rate, oxygen saturation, and heart rate in infants and young children, *Pediatr Pulmonol* 10:40-45, 1991.
162. Rabbette PS, Desateux CA, Fletcher ME, Costeloe KL, Stocks J: Influence of sedation on the Hering-Breuer inflation reflex in healthy infants, *Pediatr Pulmonol* 11:217-222, 1991.
163. Wilson S: Chloral hydrate and its effects on multiple physiological parameters in young children: a dose-response study, *Pediatr Dent* 14:171-177, 1992.
164. Mallol J, Sly PD: Effect of chloral hydrate on arterial oxygen saturation in wheezy infants, *Pediatr Pulmonol* 5:96-99, 1988.
165. Biban P, Baraldi E, Pettenazzo A, Filippone M, Zacchello F: Adverse effect of chloral hydrate in two young children with obstructive sleep apnea, *Pediatrics* 92:461-463, 1993.
166. Waterman AE, Livingston A: Effects of age and sex on ketamine anaesthesia in the rat, *Br J Anaesth* 50:885-889, 1978.
167. Sussman DR: A comparative evaluation of ketamine anesthesia in children and adults, *Anesthesiology* 40:459-464, 1974.
168. Idvall J, Holasek J, Stenberg P: Rectal ketamine for induction of anaesthesia in children, *Anaesthesia* 38:60-64, 1983.
169. Hamza J, Eccofey C, Gross JB: Ventilatory response to CO_2 following intravenous ketamine in children, *Anesthesiology* 70:422-425, 1989.
170. Greene CA, Gillette PG, Fyfe DA: Frequency of respiratory compromise after ketamine sedation for cardiac catheterization in patients <21 years of age, *Am J Cardiol* 68:1116-1117, 1991.
171. Eng M, Bonica JJ, Akamatsu TJ, Berges PU, Ueland K: Respiratory depression in newborn monkeys at caesarian section following ketamine administration, *Br J Anaesth* 47:963-967, 1985.
172. Koren G, Butt W, Chinyanga H, Soldin S, Tan YK, Pape K: Postoperative morphine infusion in newborn infants: assessment of disposition characteristics and safety, *J Pediatr* 107:963-967, 1985.
173. Lynn AM, Slattery JT: Morphine pharmacokinetics in early infancy, *Anesthesiology* 66:136-139, 1987.
174. Seed JC, Wallenstein SL, Houde RW, Bellville JW: A comparison of the analgesic and respiratory effects of dihydrocodeine and morphine in man, *Arch Int Pharmacodyn Ther* 116:293-339, 1958.
175. Smith TC, Stechen GW, Zeigler L, Wollman OH: Effects of premedicant drugs on respiration and gas exchange in man, *Anesthesiology* 28:883-890, 1967.
176. Tabatabai M, Kitahata LM, Collins JG: Disruption of the rhythmic activity of the medullary respiratory neurons and phrenic nerve by fentanyl and reversal by nalbuphine, *Anesthesiology* 70:489-495, 1989.
177. Weil JV, McCullough RE, Kline JS, Sodal IE: Diminished ventilatory response to hypoxia and hypercapnia after morphine in normal man, *N Engl J Med* 292:1103-1106, 1975.
178. Way WL, Costley EC, Way EL: Respiratory sensitivity of the newborn infant to meperidine and morphine, *Clin Pharmacol Ther* 6:454-461, 1965.
179. Kupferberg HJ, Way EL: Pharmacological basis for the increased sensitivity of the newborn rat to morphine, *J Pharmacol Exp Ther* 141:105-112, 1963.
180. Baily PL, Stanley TH: Intravenous opioid anesthetics. In Miller RD, ed: *Anesthesia,* ed 4, New York, 1994, Churchill Livingstone, pp 291-387.
181. Hertzka RE, Gauntlett IS, Fisher DM: Fentanyl-induced ventilatory depression: effects of age, *Anesthesiology* 70:213-218, 1989.
182. Bailey PL, Andriano KP, Pace NL, Westenskow DR, Stanley TH: Small doses of fentanyl potentiate and prolong diazepam induced respiratory depression, *Anesth Analg* 63:A183, 1984.
183. Scamman FL: Fentanyl-O_2-N_2O rigidity and pulmonary compliance, *Anesth Analg* 62:332-334, 1983.
184. Arandia HY, Patil VU: Glottic closure following large doses of fentanyl, *Anesthesiology* 66:574-575, 1987.
185. Irazuzta J, Pascucci R, Perlman N, Wessel D: Effects of fentanyl administration on respiratory system compliance in infants, *Crit Care Med* 21:1001-1004, 1993.
186. Mirkin BL: Perinatal pharmacology: placental transfer, fetal localization, and neonatal disposition of drugs, *Anesthesiology* 43:156-170, 1975.
187. Collins C, Koren G, Crean P, Klein J, Roy WL, MacLeod SM: Fentanyl pharmacokinetics and hemodynamic effects in preterm infants during ligation of patent ductus arteriosus, *Anesth Analg* 64:1078-1080, 1985.
188. Koehntop DE, Rodman JH, Brundage DM, Hegland MG, Buckley JJ: Pharmacokinetics of fentanyl in neonates, *Anesth Analg* 65:227-232, 1986.

Local Anesthetics

189. Ecobichon DJ, Stephens DS: Perinatal development of human blood esterases, *Clin Pharmacol Ther* 14:44-47, 1973.
190. Blankenbaker WL, DiFazio CA, Berry FA Jr: Lidocaine and its metabolites in the newborn, *Anesthesiology* 42:325-330, 1975.
191. Levy G: Pharmacokinetics of fetal and neonatal exposure to drugs, *Obstet Gynecol* 58:S6-S16, 1981.
192. Besunder JB, Reed MD, Blumer JL: Principles of drug biodisposition in the neonate: a critical evaluation of the pharmacokinetic-pharmacodynamic interface. I. *Clin Pharmacokinet* 14:189-216, 1988.
193. Besunder JB, Reed MD, Blumer JL: Principles of drug biodisposition in the neonate: a critical evaluation of the pharmacokinetic-pharmacodynamic interface. II. *Clin Pharmacokinet* 14:261-286, 1988.
194. Alifimoff JK, Cote CJ: Pediatric regional anesthesia. In Cote CJ, Ryan JF, Todres ID, Goudsouzian NG, eds: *A practice of anesthesia for infants and children,* ed 2, Philadelphia, 1993, WB Saunders, pp 429-449.

Monitoring and Patient Safety

195. Committee on Drugs, American Academy of Pediatrics: Guidelines for monitoring and management of pediatric patients during and after sedation for diagnostic therapeutic procedures, *Pediatrics* 89:1110-1115.

Conclusion

196. Joint Committee of the ATS Assembly on Pediatrics and the ERS Paediatric Assembly: Respiratory mechanics in infants: physiologic evaluation in health and disease, *Am Rev Respir Dis* 147:476-496, 1993.

CHAPTER 30

Drug-Induced Pulmonary Disease

Russell G. Clayton, Sr., and Daniel V. Schidlow

Almost 100 pharmacologic agents can cause or aggravate pulmonary disease. With few exceptions, most reports of drug-induced pulmonary disease concern adults. The incidence of such disease in the pediatric population is very difficult to estimate.

The signs and symptoms of drug-induced lung disease and the appearance of chest radiographs often mimic those of the pulmonary complications of the underlying disease. Furthermore, the onset of lung disease occurs long after the medication has been administered or even discontinued. Thus it is difficult to establish cause-and-effect relationships.

Conditions associated with drug-induced pulmonary disease include pneumonitis, pulmonary fibrosis, obliterative bronchiolitis, noncardiogenic pulmonary edema, pulmonary hemorrhage, and airway hyperreactivity. The clinical presentation is variable and ranges from a slow, gradual onset to a rapidly progressive illness. Outcomes range from complete resolution to severe disability and death.

INTERSTITIAL PNEUMONITIS AND FIBROSIS

Many pharmacologic agents can cause interstitial lung disease (Table 30-1). Most of these drugs are cytotoxic antibiotics and antimetabolites used in treating oncologic and rheumatologic disease. It is difficult to definitely ascribe the presence of fibrosis to a specific agent because many medications and radiotherapeutic agents are frequently used concomitantly in oncology patients. Fibrosis can also occur as a complication of rheumatologic disease.

In general, the underlying mechanisms leading to pneumonitis and fibrosis are similar regardless of the causative agent. Oxidant injury occurs from increased free radical generation or inhibition of glutathione and other cellular defenses against oxidant injury. Cellular damage prompts inflammatory processes that lead to fibrosis. Some medications directly stimulate the mechanisms of inflammation.

Pneumonitis and fibrosis caused by pharmacologic agents share clinical, radiographic, and histologic features. The most frequent presenting complaints are dyspnea, particularly with exertion; nonproductive cough; and chest pain. The onset may be acute but is more commonly gradual. Tachypnea, crackles, digital clubbing, fever and nonspecific rash can develop any time in the course of the disease.[1]

The typical radiographic appearance consists of bilateral reticular infiltrates. Randomly distributed alveolar infiltrates can also occur; specific patterns of distribution may implicate specific agents.[2] Pulmonary nodules can also develop. Computed tomography (CT), particularly high-resolution CT, is more sensitive in discovering early, more subtle changes. Irregular linear opacities with or without nodules and ground-glass opacity are visualized, even if the plain radiograph is normal.[3] Gallium-67 scintigraphy allows the earliest detection of this disease process by delineating areas of alveolar inflammation with increased radionuclide uptake.[4] Restrictive disease with low lung volumes and decreased carbon monoxide diffusing capacity (DLCO) is evident in pulmonary function tests.[1]

Arterial hypoxemia and respiratory alkalosis are common. Examination of bronchoalveolar lavage (BAL) fluid typically contains a predominance of lymphocytes, but the fluid may be acellular. A preponderance of polymorphonuclear leukocytes can be present early in the course of the disease.[5] Cytotoxic changes, such as cytomegaly, nuclear hyperchromasia, bizarre cell shape, prominent nucleoli, multinucleation, and cytoplasmic eosinophilia, are often found during examination of BAL fluid.[6] Interstitial mononuclear infiltration, fibrosis, and atypia are among the most prominent features on histologic examination.[7]

Bleomycin causes the highest incidence of associated pneumonitis. This agent is considered the prototype of a toxic medication capable of inducing pulmonary disease.[8] Bleomycin analogs, as well as other cytotoxic medications (see Table 30-1), have similar clinical and pathologic features. Bleomycin is an antibiotic used in the treatment of testicular tumors and lymphoma. It is found in higher concentrations in lung tissue because of a relative lack of hydrolases that inactivate it within the lung and make this organ particularly susceptible to toxicity. Tissue damage is probably due to oxidant injury that overwhelms the protective effects of the antioxidant glutathione.[9] This toxicity increases when supplemental oxygen is used, especially in high concentrations,[8] and when a cumulative dose of 100 units is exceeded. A logarithmic increase in lung disease is noted at cumulative doses exceeding 450 units. Toxicity is enhanced if the patient receives radiotherapy or if bleomycin is given as a bolus infusion or in combination with other cytotoxic agents.[8] Clinical and radiographic findings are consistent with those of pneumonitis. Intrapulmonary nodules, in addition to the aforementioned findings, can be seen on plain radiographs and on CT.[10,11] An abnormal DLCO often precedes clinical disease.[12] However, this finding varies in patients who have received bleomycin, and it does not have a prognostic significance. Histologic changes initially include endothelial damage and alveolar type I cell necrosis, followed by metaplastic type II cells, lymphocytic infiltration, fibroblast proliferation, and eventually, fibrosis.[13] Discontinuation of bleomycin attenuates or reverses the disease process. Clinical and functional improvement has been noted in some cases after treatment with glucocorticoids, but response varies.[14] Except in mild cases, the prognosis is poor.

Toxicity resulting from sterile carmustine (BCNU), a nitrosourea used in the treatment of gliomas, is also similar to bleomycin in its clinical presentation. Lung disease is induced by the inhibition of glutathione reductase in the alveolar

Table 30-1 Medications Associated with Pneumonitis and Fibrosis

MEDICATION	ESTIMATED FREQUENCY	SUSPECTED MECHANISM	RISK FACTORS
Bleomycin	Sporadic	Oxidant injury; concentrates in lung resulting from sparse hydrolases	Radiation therapy, high fraction of inspired oxygen, administration as a bolus or with other cytotoxic agents, dose exceeding 450 units
Mitomycin	Sporadic	Same as bleomycin	Frequent doses, concurrent or consecutive administration of vinblastine or vindesine
Cyclophosphamide	Sporadic	Same as bleomycin	Administration of multiple medications
Busulfan	Sporadic	Same as bleomycin	Duration of treatment
Melphalan	Sporadic	Same as bleomycin	?
Chlorambucil	Sporadic	Same as bleomycin	?
Sterile carmustine (BCNU)	Frequent	Inhibition of glutathione reductase	Dose exceeding 900-1500 mg/m^2, concurrent administration of cyclophosphamide
Methotrexate	Sporadic	?	Frequent doses, administration of multiple medications, withdrawal of corticosteroids
Amiodarone	Frequent	Damage from accumulated phospholipid, oxidant injury, iodide damage, organelle dysfunction	High doses
Nitrofurantoin	Rare	Oxidant injury	Long-term use
Gold	Rare	?	?
Penicillamine	Rare	?	?

macrophages.[15] The incidence of lung disease from this medication reaches a 20% incidence at doses of 900 to 1200 mg/m^2 and up to a 50% incidence at doses above 1500 mg/m^2. Fibrosis occurs at lower doses if high-dose cyclophosphamide is concurrently administered.[8] The onset of disease after the initiation of therapy ranges from as early as 9 days to as late as 12 years. Clinical, radiographic, and pulmonary function findings are typical of drug-induced pneumonitis. Treatment with corticosteroids does not prevent disease. The prognosis for affected individuals is poor. Ambroxol, a drug that decreases the migration of neutrophils, lymphocytes, and macrophages, may lower toxicity when given with sterile carmustine.[8]

Methotrexate is a folic acid antagonist used to treat malignant and rheumatologic processes. Pneumonitis and fibrosis are more likely to develop if doses exceed 20 mg/week, but lung disease has occurred in patients receiving doses as low as 7.5 to 15 mg/week.[16] The underlying cause of lung disease is unknown, but it probably involves the direct stimulation of inflammatory processes. Clinical and radiographic manifestations of pulmonary disease, as well as the findings of pulmonary function tests, are consistent with those of pneumonitis. Histologic examination reveals unusual pathologic features such as eosinophilic infiltration and granuloma formation.[10] Cessation of the medication often leads to reversal of the disease process, and corticosteroid therapy aids in the resolution.[17] The prognosis is favorable.

Therapy with amiodarone, an antianginal and antidysrhythmic agent, has a reported incidence of associated pulmonary disease of up to 60%, and the mortality rate is up to 33%.[18] Toxicity is dose dependent and related to the duration of maintenance therapy. Amiodarone inhibits phospholipase A,[19] with a subsequent increase in phospholipid content[20] that may cause cellular damage in the lung.[21] However, cells containing phospholipids have been found in specimens from patients who do not have lung disease, and phospholipid accumulation may simply reflect a coincident effect of drug exposure.[22] Other proposed mechanisms for lung injury include oxidant injury, cellular or organelle dysfunction as a result of the amphiphilic nature of amiodarone, or damage from iodides on the amiodarone molecule.[23] The clinical presentation is typical for drug-induced pneumonitis. Plain radiographs and CT display a distinct and prominent interstitial pattern, perhaps as a result of the presence of iodide in the lamellar bodies. Gallium-67 radionuclide scanning is strongly positive in affected patients and is often the most sensitive and specific diagnostic test.[24] In patients with amiodarone-induced lung disease, a low DLCO is the first sign of abnormal pulmonary function, often preceding clinical symptoms.[25] Characteristic lamellar cytoplasmic inclusion bodies, representing intracellular phospholipids, are seen on histologic examination, and examination of BAL fluid reveals macrophages that have a typical "foamy" appearance.[18] Lung disease often resolves after the drug is discontinued. If the onset of lung disease is insidious, resolution of disease is often slower or incomplete.[18] Administration of corticosteroids may hasten resolution in some patients.

Nitrofurantoin is an antibiotic used to treat urinary tract infections. Pulmonary toxicity can occur in patients who receive the drug for over 6 months.[26] The mechanism for lung damage is probably oxidant injury[27]; patients receiving supplemental oxygen often have more severe damage. Partial or complete resolution of clinical disease often occurs after the medication has been discontinued, although pulmonary function abnormalities may persist indefinitely. Glucocorticoids are indicated in cases of progressive disease despite the cessation of administration.[26]

HYPERSENSITIVITY PNEUMONITIS

Gold salts, methotrexate, nitrofurantoin, and imipramine are among a group of medications that have been implicated in causing hypersensitivity pneumonitis (Box 30-1). The underlying mechanism for drug-induced hypersensitivity pneumonitis is thought to be an antigenic stimulation of lymphocytes.[28] Whether the drug itself acts as the antigen or whether it stimulates antigen formation is unknown.

The prevalent signs and symptoms are progressive dyspnea, especially during exertion, and nonproductive cough accompanied by fever, myalgia, and dermatitis. Symptoms may occur suddenly after an initial dose but more commonly de-

BOX 30-1
Medications Associated with Hypersensitivity Pneumonitis

Occasional causes	Rare causes—cont'd
Gold salts	Nitrofurantoin
Methotrexate	Nonsteroidal antiinflammatory medications (e.g., aspirin, ibuprofen)
Amiodarone	Penicillamine
Rare causes	Phenytoin
Nitrofurantoin	Procarbazine
Imipramine	Pyrimethamine
Azathioprine	Chloroquine
Bleomycin	Dapsone
Carbamazepine	Sulfadoxine
Chlorambucil	Sulfasalazine
Cyclophosphamide	Vinblastine
Dantrolene	Vindesine
Mitomycin	

velop slowly during chronic administration.[28] Tachypnea and crackles are usually present.

Chest radiographs show infiltration of varying degrees. Arterial hypoxemia and hypocarbia are usually present. Leukocytosis, eosinophilia, and elevated levels of immunoglobulin E have also been reported.[28] A predominance of lymphocytes is found in BAL fluid.[29] In both peripheral blood and BAL specimens, the majority of lymphocytes are T-suppressor cells, resulting in an inverse helper/suppressor ratio.[28] Histologic examination reveals a characteristic confluence of eosinophils in alveoli. Interstitial tissues and airways also contain eosinophils, but there is no evidence of vascular changes.[7] A histologic variant consisting of interstitial eosinophilia with no alveolar eosinophils occasionally occurs in association with nitrofurantoin[30] and gold[31] therapy. Fibrosis and other cellular features of chronic interstitial pneumonia are present.

Discontinuation of the causative medication and supportive therapy usually result in improvement. Corticosteroids have been used in severe cases with good results.[26] Occasionally, residual restrictive disease persists and in some cases, progresses despite cessation of the drug and steroid therapy.[28] Symptoms tend to recur if the drug is reintroduced.

PULMONARY EDEMA

A small group of medications (Box 30-2) have been associated with the development of noncardiogenic pulmonary edema. In these cases, dyspnea occurs acutely and often progresses to respiratory failure. Tachypnea and crackles are found on physical examination. The third heart sound is absent, and the end-diastolic pulmonary capillary wedge pressure is normal, suggesting a noncardiogenic cause. The findings on chest radiographs are consistent with those of pulmonary edema. Hypoxemia can be severe.

Salicylates have been reported to cause pulmonary edema, usually when drug ingestion exceeds 30 mg/kg.[32] Hydrochlorothiazide has also been implicated as causing pulmonary edema, especially in women.[33] The underlying mechanism is unknown.

Tocolytic agents such as terbutaline and ritodrine have been associated with the development of pulmonary edema in pregnant women.[34] Two mechanisms have been proposed. A reversal of vasodilation can occur after the drug is withdrawn,

BOX 30-2
Medications Associated with Noncardiogenic Pulmonary Edema

Salicylates	Naloxone
Hydrochlorothiazides	Mitomycin
Haloperidol	Cyclophosphamide
Lidocaine	Methotrexate
Tocolytics	Deferoxamine (Desferrioxamine)
Terbutaline	Heroin
Ritodrine	Methadone
Tricyclic antidepressants	Cocaine

causing a sudden increase in pulmonary blood flow. Alternatively, the activation of complement can cause alveolar capillary leak.[16] Associated risk factors for pulmonary edema during pregnancy include twin gestation, fluid overload, anemia, and use of corticosteroids.

Tricyclic antidepressants can cause alveolar capillary leak as a result of a direct toxic effect that causes degeneration of the alveolar epithelium and capillary endothelium.[35] The incidence of pulmonary edema increases at medication levels that exceed 2000 ng/ml.

Deferoxamine (Desferrioxamine), an iron-chelating agent, can cause pulmonary edema when given in a continuous infusion for over 48 hours.[36] Alveolar capillary injury is thought to occur because of the accumulation of free radicals produced by the continued interaction of deferoxamine and iron.[37]

PULMONARY HEMORRHAGE

The use of exogenous surfactants, anticoagulants, and penicillamine has been associated with pulmonary hemorrhage. Anticoagulant drugs in normal doses very rarely cause of pulmonary hemorrhage. Streptokinase administration has been implicated as a cause of pulmonary hemorrhage in a man with unresolved pneumonia who received thrombolytic therapy for myocardial infarction.[38] The concomitant use of heparin and streptokinase or other anticoagulants may increase the risk of anticoagulant-induced pulmonary hemorrhage.

The role of exogenous surfactant as a cause of pulmonary hemorrhage is controversial. Some studies have found evidence of an increased incidence of pulmonary hemorrhage in infants treated with surfactant,[39,40] whereas a separate trial comparing treated and untreated infants failed to show any difference in the incidence of this phenomenon.[41] Pulmonary hemorrhage does not appear to be related to a bleeding diathesis in infants treated with surfactant[42] but may result from a rapid decrease in pulmonary vascular resistance.

Penicillamine has been associated with a syndrome similar to Goodpasture's that is characterized by acute dyspnea, cough, hemoptysis, and hematuria.[43] Severe hypoxemia and renal failure usually occur. The chest radiograph shows diffuse alveolar opacities consistent with hemorrhage. The histologic appearance of the lung is similar to that in Goodpasture's syndrome, but immunofluorescence studies do not show complement or immunoglobulin deposition in the basement membrane. Serum antibodies to glomerular basement membrane have been described in only one case.[43] Treatment with steroids appears to hasten improvement.

AIRWAY HYPERREACTIVITY

Several medications have the potential to induce or exacerbate airway hyperreactivity in susceptible individuals (Box 30-3). Symptoms of airway hyperreactivity, such as dyspnea and chest pain, occur acutely after the administration of the medication or gradually worsen with chronic use. Affected individuals usually have a previous history of reactive airway disease. Tachypnea and wheezing are present during acute episodes. Chest radiographs are normal or may show hyperinflation. Provocation tests using the medication in question can be performed when the diagnosis is in doubt.[1]

Aspirin is a classic example of a bronchospasm-inducing agent; 78% of adults with asthma and nasal polyps experience airway hyperreactivity after aspirin administration.[44] Other nonsteroidal antiinflammatory drugs such as ibuprofen and naproxen elicit a similar response in aspirin-sensitive individuals.[45] Nonacetylated salicylates, however, do not induce bronchospasm in these patients.[46]

The mechanism responsible for producing airway hyperreactivity most likely involves the modulation of arachidonic acid metabolism. Metabolites to the lipoxygenase pathway produce leukotrienes or limit the production of prostaglandins normally synthesized from the cyclooxygenase pathway.[47] Treatment includes the usual asthma therapy and the avoidance of acetylated salicylates and nonsteroidal antiinflammatory drugs.

Nonselective β-receptor antagonists such as propranolol induce or exacerbate airway hyperreactivity, presumably by inhibiting airway smooth muscle β-receptors. This effect is especially dramatic in people with asthma.[48] In addition, β-blockade may down-regulate cholinergic pathways, resulting in a greater bronchodilation response to cholinergic antagonists in affected individuals.[49]

Dipyridamole administered during thallium imaging studies induces bronchospasm by increasing the cellular concentration of adenosine.[50] Pretreatment with theophylline is protective. Inhalation of pentamidine[51] and beclomethasone[52] has also been associated with bronchospasm. Albuterol inhalation before administration of pentamidine via aerosol may be protective,[53] although one study failed to show any benefit.[54]

OTHER MANIFESTATIONS

Bronchiolitis obliterans has been reported with penicillamine[7,43] and gold[55] therapy. Penicillamine-induced bronchiolitis obliterans is found in patients treated for connective tissue disorders but not in those treated for Wilson's disease. Presenting symptoms are cough and dyspnea without fever. The lungs appear normal or hyperinflated or exhibit reticular opacities on chest radiograph. Histologic examination reveals polypoid masses of granulation tissue filling and obstructing small bronchi and bronchioles. An acquired autoimmune reaction may be responsible for these changes. Another possibility is that penicillamine may impair the healing of tissue damaged by the underlying connective tissue disease by causing abnormal collagen cross-linking.[7]

Pleural effusions have been noted in association with drug-induced lupus erythematosus.[5] The effusions are often bilateral and characteristically have an exudate. The effusions usually resolve after withdrawal of the medication.

Cough without underlying lung abnormalities occurs in 15% of patients receiving angiotensin-converting enzyme inhibitors.[55] The underlying mechanism is unknown.

BOX 30-3
Medications Associated with Airway Hyperreactivity

Cyclophosphamide	β-Blockers
Nitrofurantoin	Dipyridamole
Aspirin	Carbamazepine
Ibuprofen	Cocaine and cocaine alkaloid
Naproxen	Pentamidine (inhaled)
Sulfasalazine	Beclomethasone (inhaled)

ILLICIT DRUG USE

Cocaine and cocaine alkaloid (crack) have been associated with severe bronchospasm, atelectasis, pneumothorax, pneumomediastinum, pulmonary edema, and pulmonary hemorrhage.[56-58] Heroin overdose can lead to pulmonary edema; the mechanism is not clear.[59] Intravenous drug use is associated with particulate embolism and pulmonary talcosis.[56] The effects of second-hand inhalation of cocaine alkaloid on children is unknown.

REFERENCES

Interstitial Pneumonitis and Fibrosis

1. Gregory SA, Grippi MA: The clinical diagnosis of drug-induced pulmonary disorders, *J Thorac Imaging* 6:8-18, 1991.
2. Cooper JA, White DA, Matthay RA: Drug-induced pulmonary disease. I. Cytotoxic drugs, *Am Rev Respir Dis* 133:321-340, 1986.
3. Carson CW, Cannon GW, Egger MJ, Ward JR, Clegg DO: Pulmonary disease during the treatment of rheumatoid arthritis with low dose pulse methotrexate, *Semin Arthritis Rheum* 16:186-195, 1987.
4. Aronchick JM, Gefter WB: Drug-induced pulmonary disease: an update, *J Thorac Imaging* 6:19-29, 1991.
5. Rosenow EC, Myers JL, Swenson SJ, Pisani RJ: Drug-induced pulmonary disease: an update, *Chest* 102:239-250, 1992.
6. Crystal RG, Reynolds HY, Kalica AR: Bronchoalveolar lavage: report of an international conference, *Chest* 90:122-131, 1986.
7. Smith GJ: The histopathology of pulmonary reactions to drugs, *Clin Chest Med* 11:95-117, 1990.
8. Kreisman H, Wolkove N: Pulmonary toxicity of antineoplastic therapy, *Semin Oncol* 19:508-520, 1992.
9. Ohnuma T, Holland JF, Masuda H: Microbiologic assay of bleomycin: inactivation, tissue distribution, and clearance, *Cancer* 33:1230-1238, 1974.
10. Cohen MB, Austin JH, Smith-Vaniz A, Lutzky J, Grimes MM: Nodular bleomycin toxicity, *Am J Clin Pathol* 92:101-104, 1989.
11. Santrach PJ, Askin FB, Wells RJ, Azizkhan RG, Merten DF: Nodular form of bleomycin-related pulmonary injury in patients with osteogenic sarcoma, *Cancer* 64:806-811, 1989.
12. Snyder LS, Hertz MI: Cytotoxic drug-induced lung injury, *Semin Respir Infect* 3:217-228, 1988.
13. Ginsberg SJ, Comis RL: The pulmonary toxicity of antineoplastic agents, *Semin Oncol* 9:34-51, 1982.
14. White DA, Stover DE: Severe bleomycin-induced pneumonitis: clinical features and response to corticosteroids, *Chest* 86:723-728, 1984.
15. Arrick BA, Nathan CF: Glutathione metabolism as a determinant of therapeutic efficacy: a review, *Cancer Res* 44:4224-4232, 1984.
16. Cannon GW: Antirheumatic drug reactions in the lung, *Bailliere Clin Rheum* 7:147-171, 1993.
17. Furst DE, Kremer JM: Methotrexate in rheumatoid arthritis, *Arthritis Rheum* 31:305-314, 1988.
18. Martin WJ II, Rosenow EC III: Amiodarone pulmonary toxicity: recognition and pathogenesis. I. *Chest* 93:1067-1075, 1988.
19. Martin WJ II, Rosenow EC III: Amiodarone pulmonary toxicity: recognition and pathogenesis. II. *Chest* 93:1242-1248, 1988.
20. Heath MF, Costa-Jussa FR, Jacobs JM, Jacobson W: The induction of pulmonary phospholipidosis and the inhibition of lysosomal phospholipidoses by amiodarone, *Br J Exp Pathol* 66:391-397, 1985.

21. Weltzein HV: Cytolytic and membrane-perturbing properties of lysophosphatidylcholine, *Biochem Biophys Acta* 559:259-287, 1979.
22. Martin WJ, Standing JE: Amiodarone pulmonary toxicity: quantitative evidence for a cellular phospholipidosis, *J Pharm Exp Ther* 22:423-434, 1989.
23. Adams PC, Gibson GJ, Morley AR, Wright AJ, Corris PA, Reid DS, Cambell RW: Amiodarone pulmonary toxicity: clinical and subclinical features, *Q J Med* 59:449-471, 1986.
24. Magro SA, Lawrence EC, Wheeler SH, Krafchek J, Lin HT, Wyndham CR: Amiodarone pulmonary toxicity: prospective evaluation of serial pulmonary function tests, *J Am Coll Cardiol* 12:781-788, 1988.
25. Zhu YY, Botvinick E, Dae M, Golden J, Hattner R, Scheinman M: Gallium lung scintigraphy in amiodarone pulmonary toxicity, *Chest* 93:1126-1131, 1988.
26. Witten CM: Pulmonary toxicity of nitrofurantoin, *Arch Phys Med Rehabil* 70:55-57, 1989.
27. Martin WJ, Powis GW, Kachel DL: Nitrofurantoin-stimulated oxidant production in pulmonary endothelial cells, *J Lab Clin Med* 105:23-29, 1985.

Hypersensitivity Pneumonitis

28. Evans RB, Ettensohn DB, Fawaz-Estrup F, Lally EV, Kaplan SR: Gold lung: recent developments in pathogenesis, diagnosis, and therapy, *Semin Arthritis Rheum* 16:196-205, 1987.
29. Costabel U, Schmitz-Schaumann MM, Matthys H: Bronchoalveolar T-cell subsets in gold lung: evidence for a hypersensitivity reaction, *Chest* 87:135, 1985 (letter).
30. Rosenow EC, De Remee RA, Dines DE: Chronic nitrofurantoin pulmonary reaction, *N Engl J Med* 279:1258-1264, 1968.
31. Winterbauer RH, Wilske KR, Wheelis RF: Diffuse pulmonary injury associated with gold treatment, *N Engl J Med* 294:919-923, 1976.

Pulmonary Edema

32. Heffner JE, Sahn SA: Salicylate-induced pulmonary edema, *Ann Intern Med* 95:405-409, 1981.
33. Kavaru MS, Ahmad M, Amirthalinggam KN: Hydrochlorothiazide-induced acute pulmonary edema, *Cleve Clin J Med* 57:181-184, 1990.
34. Pisani RJ, Rosenow EC: Pulmonary edema associated with tocolytic therapy, *Ann Intern Med* 110:714-718, 1989.
35. Roy TM, Ossorio MA, Cipolla LM, Fields CL, Snider HL, Anderson WH: Pulmonary complications after tricyclic antidepressant overdose, *Chest* 96:852-856, 1989.
36. Tenenbein M, Kowalski S, Sienko A, Bowden DH, Adamson IY: Pulmonary toxic effects of continuous desferrioxamine administration in acute iron poisoning, *Lancet* 339:699-701, 1992.
37. Adamson IY, Sienko A, Tenenbein M: Pulmonary toxicity of deferoxamine in iron-poisoned mice, *Toxicol Appl Pharmacol* 120:13-19, 1993.

Pulmonary Hemorrhage

38. Disler LJ, Rosendorff A: Pulmonary hemorrhage following intravenous streptokinase for acute myocardial infarction, *Int J Cardiol* 29:387-390, 1990.
39. Long W, Corbet A, Cotton R, Houle L, Schiff D: A controlled trial of synthetic surfactant in infants weighing 1250 g or more with respiratory distress syndrome, *N Engl J Med* 325:1696-1703, 1991.
40. Pappin A, Shenker N, Hack M, Redline RW: Extensive intraalveolar pulmonary hemorrhage in infants dying after surfactant therapy, *J Pediatr* 124:621-626, 1994.
41. Smyth J, Allen A, Sankavan K: Effects of two rescue doses of Exosurf Neonatal in 221 500-749 gram infants, *Pediatr Res* 29:330A, 1991.
42. Long W, Corbet A, Allen A, McMillan D, Boros S, Vaughan R, Gerdes J, Houle L, Edwards K, Schiff D: Retrospective search for bleeding diathesis among premature newborn infants with pulmonary hemorrhage after synthetic surfactant treatment, *J Pediatr* 120:S45-S48, 1992.
43. Zitnik RJ, Cooper J: Pulmonary disease due to antirheumatic agents, *Clin Chest Med* 11:139-150, 1990.

Airway Hyperreactivity

44. Slepian IK, Mathews KP, McLean JA: Aspirin-sensitive asthma, *Chest* 87:386-391, 1985.
45. Mathison DA, Stevenson DD, Simon RA: Precipitating factors in asthma, *Chest* 87:50S-54S, 1985.
46. Stevenson DD, Hougham AJ, Schrank PF, Goldlust MB, Wilson RR: Salsalate cross-sensitivity in aspirin-sensitive patients with asthma, *J Allergy Clin Immunol* 86:749-758, 1990.
47. Slepian IK, Mathews KP, McLean JA: Aspirin-sensitive asthma, *Chest* 87:386-391, 1985.
48. Maclagan J, Ney UM: Investigation of the mechanism of propanolol-induced bronchoconstriction, *Br J Pharmacol* 66:409-418, 1979.
49. Gross NJ, Skorodin MS: State of the art: anticholinergic, antimuscarinic bronchodilators, *Am Rev Respir Dis* 129:856-870, 1984.
50. Lette J, Cerino M, Laverdiere M, Tremblay J, Prenovault J: Severe bronchospasm followed by respiratory arrest during thallium-dipyridamole imaging, *Chest* 95:1345-1347, 1989.
51. Toronto Aerosolized Pentamidine Study (TAPS) Group: Acute pulmonary effects of aerosolized pentamidine, *Chest* 98:907-910, 1990.
52. Shim CS, Williams MH: Cough and wheezing from beclomethasone dipropionate aerosol are absent after triamcinolone acetonide, *Ann Intern Med* 106:700-703, 1987.
53. Quieffin J, Hunter J, Schecter MT, Lawson L, Ruedy J, Pare P: Aerosol pentamidine-induced bronchoconstriction, *Chest* 100:624-627, 1991.
54. Katzman M, Meade W, Lglar K, Rachlis A, Berger P, Chan CK: High incidence of bronchospasm with regular administration of aerosolized pentamidine, *Chest* 101:79-81, 1992.

Other Manifestations

55. Fort JG, Scovern H, Abruzzo JL: Intravenous cyclophosphamide and methylprednisolone for the treatment of bronchiolitis obliterans and interstitial fibrosis associated with cryotherapy, *J Rheumatol* 15:850-854, 1988.

Illicit Drug Use

56. McCarroll KA, Roszler MH: Lung disorders due to drug abuse, *J Thorac Imaging* 6:30-35, 1991.
57. Khalsa ME, Tashkin DP, Perrochet B: Smoked cocaine: patterns of use and pulmonary consequences, *J Psychoactive Drugs* 24:265-272, 1992.
58. Ettinger NA, Albin RJ: A review of the respiratory effects of smoking cocaine, *Am J Med* 87:664-668, 1989.
59. Stern WZ, Subbaro K: Pulmonary complications of drug addiction, *Semin Roentgenol* 18:213-220, 1983.

PART SIX

Respiratory Disorders of Neonates and Infants

CHAPTER 31

Respiratory Disorders of the Newborn

Eduardo Bancalari and Margarita Bidegain

HYALINE MEMBRANE DISEASE

Hyaline membrane disease (HMD), also known as *respiratory distress syndrome,* is the most common cause of respiratory failure in the premature infant. In spite of major advances in the understanding of its pathophysiology and treatment, HMD has been a major cause of morbidity and mortality in premature infants born before week 32 of gestation. The introduction of exogenous surfactant as a mode of prevention or treatment has changed the clinical course of this disease and has considerably decreased the morbidity and mortality rates. Although many disorders can manifest with "respiratory distress" in the neonate, the term *respiratory distress syndrome* is used to characterize the respiratory disease that occurs in the premature infant as a result of an insufficient amount or insufficient activity of surfactant in the alveolar surface.

Incidence

The incidence of HMD increases as gestational age decreases. In the premature infant under 29 weeks' gestation, the reported incidence is higher than 50%.[1] Above 34 weeks' gestation, only 5% of the infants are affected. Besides gestational age, other factors may influence the incidence of HMD. In boys, androgens cause a delay in lung maturation with decreased surfactant production by type II pneumocytes.[2] This can explain the higher incidence of HMD in male compared with female premature infants. Black preterm infants develop HMD less frequently than white infants of similar gestational age, and the condition is less severe.[1] Maternal diabetes is another risk factor for the development of HMD in offspring. This is probably related to a decrease in the level of surfactant proteins, which results in surfactant dysfunction.[3] Perinatal asphyxia and birth by cesarean section are also factors that increase the incidence of HMD.[4,5] On the other hand, prolonged rupture of membranes[6] and other causes of chronic fetal stress such as maternal hypertension, maternal drug abuse, and chronic congenital infections tend to decrease the incidence of HMD.[7] Antenatal administration of steroids[8,9] or thyrotropin-releasing hormone[10] to the mother also decreases the incidence of HMD.

Pathogenesis

The most important pathologic and functional alteration in the lungs of infants with HMD is a decrease in lung volume caused by diffuse alveolar collapse.[11] Classically, HMD has been attributed to the lack of surfactant in an immature lung.[12] Lung development starts at 3 to 4 weeks' gestation with the formation of the trachea from the esophagus. At 24 weeks, the terminal airspaces start to develop, with approximation of the respiratory epithelium and capillaries and differentiation of type I and II pneumocytes. From this time, gas exchange is possible in the developing lung, but the distance between capillaries and airspaces is still 2 or 3 times larger than in the adult. After 30 weeks, subdivision of terminal bronchioles continues to occur, with alveolar formation starting at 32 to 34 weeks. All these morphologic changes are accompanied by the development of numerous biochemical functions that play a major role in lung function.

Surfactant

Surfactant appears in the fetal lung at 23 to 24 weeks, when osmophilic inclusions can be first detected in the type II pneumocytes. However, adequate amounts of surfactant are not secreted until 30 to 32 weeks' gestation, when the incidence of HMD markedly decreases.

As originally described by Avery and Mead in 1959,[12] surfactant reduces surface tension in the alveolar spaces, facilitating lung expansion and preventing alveolar collapse during expiration. It may also aid in the prevention of pulmonary edema and participate in lung defense against infections.[13,14] Surfactant is composed mainly of phospholipids but also contains proteins and carbohydrates. Phosphatidylcholine is the most abundant phospholipid in surfactant, representing 80% of the total mass of lipid components, and it is essential for surfactant's surface tension–lowering properties. The other phospholipids in surfactant are phosphatidylglycerol, phosphatidylinositol, phosphatidylserine, phosphatidylethanolamine, and sphingomyelin, but their exact role in surfactant function is still unclear. Surfactant proteins A, B, and C constitute 10% of pulmonary surfactant. They contribute to the proper function of surfactant by facilitating the formation of phospholipid films at the air-fluid interface of the alveolus and participating in the recycling of surfactant, among other roles.[15]

After undergoing synthesis in the type II pneumocyte, pulmonary surfactant is physically arranged in the form of macromolecular aggregates. In the type II cell, surfactant is in the form of lamellar bodies, but after its secretion into the alveolar space, it acquires the form of tubular myelin, with strong surface-active properties[15,16] (Fig. 31-1).

In the very immature infant, in addition to surfactant deficiency, an excessively compliant chest wall and weakness of the respiratory muscles can contribute to alveolar collapse. This collapse leads to a decrease in the ventilation-perfusion relationship, thus producing a pulmonary shunt with progressive arterial hypoxemia that can lead to metabolic acidosis. Both hypoxemia and acidosis can produce vasoconstriction of the pulmonary vessels with a decrease in pulmonary blood flow. Type II pneumocytes may be affected by this decrease, further reducing their capacity to produce surfactant. Pulmonary vascular hypertension may produce right-to-left shunt-

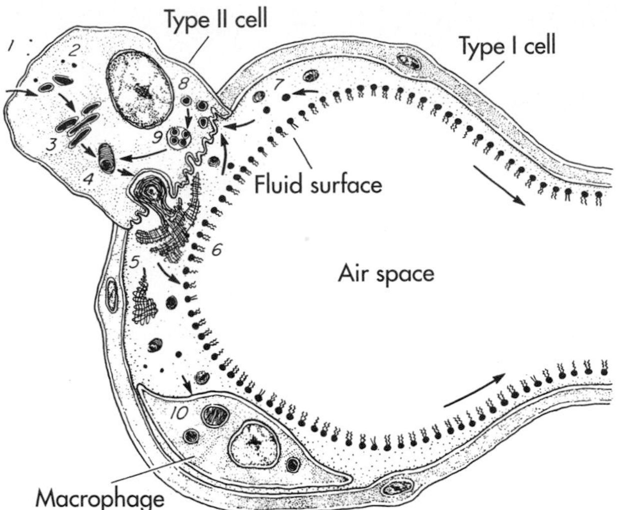

Fig. 31-1. Surfactant system. Surfactant is synthesized from precursors *(1)* in the endoplasmic reticulum *(2)* and via the Golgi apparatus *(3)*, acquiring the form of lamellar bodies *(4)*. In the alveoli, where it is present as tubular myelin *(5)*, surfactant is then recycled as small vesicles *(7)* into the type II cell by using endosomes *(8)* and multivesicular bodies *(9)*. Some surfactant is also taken up by alveolar macrophages *(10)*. (From Hawgood S, Clements JA: *J Clin Invest* 86:1-6, 1990.)

ing through both the foramen ovale and the ductus arteriosus, worsening the hypoxemia.

The pulmonary blood flow, which is initially decreased, may subsequently increase because of a reduction in pulmonary vascular resistance and persistence of an open ductus arteriosus. This excessive pulmonary blood flow, in addition to an increased vascular permeability, may result in accumulation of fluid and proteins in the interstitial and alveolar spaces. Surfactant can be inactivated by proteins in the alveolar space.[17]

The presence of both intrapulmonary and extrapulmonary shunting explains the characteristic hypoxemia in infants with HMD. Atelectasis (with impaired ventilation in some areas) and an increase in dead space caused by poor perfusion of other portions of the lung can elevate the partial pressure of arterial carbon dioxide ($Paco_2$) in the more severe cases. The premature infant with HMD responds to the loss in lung volume and increase in $Paco_2$ by increasing the respiratory rate. Hypoxemia, if severe, leads to progressive acidosis, which might contribute to further pulmonary vasoconstriction with damage to type II cells, and in this way perpetuates a vicious circle. If present, perinatal asphyxia and arterial hypotension worsen the metabolic acidosis (Fig. 31-2).

Alterations in Pulmonary Function

A reduction in functional residual capacity (FRC) and a marked decrease in lung compliance are characteristics of HMD.[18] Some alveoli are collapsed because of surfactant deficiency, whereas others are occupied by fluid, therefore explaining the decrease in FRC. In response to this, the premature infant with HMD frequently develops a grunting respiration that retards expiration and protects against further loss in FRC. Lung compliance is markedly reduced to values that are frequently below 0.5 ml/cm H_2O/kg of body weight,[19] less than half the normal value.

Pathology

At autopsy, classic macroscopic findings consist of lungs that appear solid and congested with diffuse atelectasis. Microscopically, hyaline membranes line most of the remaining airspaces (Fig. 31-3). These hyaline membranes consist of an exudate of plasma proteins leaked through damaged capillaries.

Clinical Presentation

The clinical signs of HMD usually appear in the first minutes or hours of life in the affected premature infant (Table 31-1). The signs are characterized by a progressive increase in the respiratory rate as well as subcostal and sternal retractions, grunting, cyanosis, and a bilateral decrease in breath sounds. The chest radiograph shows increased density of both lung fields with fine granularity, air bronchograms, and elevation of the diaphragm. Often, a marked radiographic improvement can be observed after treatment with exogenous surfactant (Fig. 31-4). The oxygen requirement of these infants varies depending on the severity of the disease course. Characteristically, arterial blood gas analysis reveals hypoxemia and hypercarbia and occasionally a mild metabolic acidosis.

Other causes of respiratory distress in the newborn should be considered in the differential diagnosis. These include pneumonia, congenital heart disease and other congenital anomalies, anemia, polycythemia, and hypothermia.

Without intervention with exogenous surfactant, the severity of the condition increases during the first 2 or 3 days of life, although individual variations exist. After this initial period, if there are no complications, the respiratory status begins to improve, and in infants older than 32 to 33 weeks' gestation, lung function usually normalizes by 1 week of life. In smaller infants, especially those whose gestational age is below 26 to 28 weeks, most of whom require mechanical ventilation, the clinical course is generally prolonged and is frequently complicated by barotrauma, patent ductus arteriosus (PDA), nosocomial infections, and intraventricular hemorrhage. The use of exogenous surfactant has dramatically changed the natural course of the disease by rapidly decreasing the oxygen requirements and reducing the incidence of gas leaks (see section on surfactant replacement therapy).

Prevention

Because HMD occurs primarily in the premature infant, prevention of prematurity is the most effective way to avoid this disease, but this is not possible in many cases. Major advances have taken place in the last years in the prevention of HMD by accurate antenatal prediction of lung maturation and in the use of hormones to accelerate fetal lung maturation.

Antenatal Prediction of Lung Maturation

In 1973, Gluck and Kulovich[7] described the relationship of lecithin and sphingomyelin in the amniotic fluid as indicators of fetal lung maturity. This is possible because fetal lung fluid is an important component of the amniotic fluid. The incidence of HMD is only 0.5% when the lecithin-sphingomyelin ratio is 2 or more, but it is close to 100% when the ratio is lower than 1.

A rapid test (shake test) to determine whether surfactant is present in amniotic fluid was described by Clements et al[20] in 1972. It is based on the ability of pulmonary surfactant to generate stable foam in the presence of ethanol. This test has a

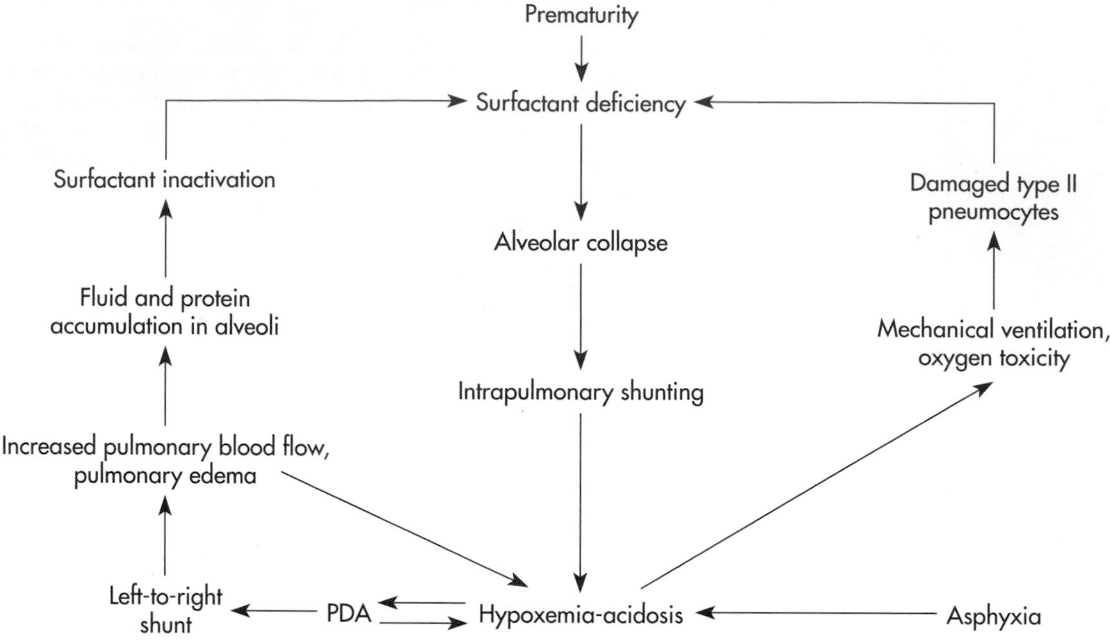

Fig. 31-2. Pathophysiology of HMD. *PDA,* Patent ductus arteriosus.

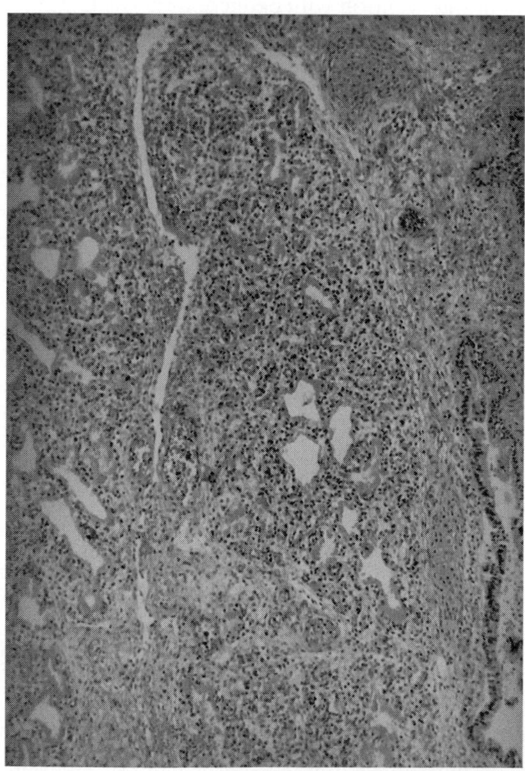

Fig. 31-3. Microscopic findings at autopsy in an infant with HMD, showing diffuse alveolar collapse with hyaline membranes lining the few remaining dilated airspaces.

high predictive value for HMD when applied to uncontaminated amniotic fluid.

Phosphatidylglycerol usually appears in the amniotic fluid at about 36 weeks' gestation. Its presence is also an indicator of lung maturity.[21]

Induction of Fetal Lung Maturation

Many hormones positively or negatively influence lung maturation. Agents that can accelerate lung maturation are corticosteroids, thyroid hormones, epidermal growth factor, and cyclic adenosine monophosphate. These substances may act by stimulating the synthesis of surfactant.[22] Of all these, steroids were evaluated the most frequently in clinical trials. Several studies performed in animals and humans have shown that the antenatal administration of steroids decreases the incidence and severity of HMD.[8,9,23] Steroids act by binding to specific receptors in the lung cells and thus stimulating the production of phosphatidylcholine by type II cells. This process takes time, and for this reason, steroids are less effective if administered less than 24 hours before delivery. They are also less effective beyond 34 weeks' gestation, and their effect appears to diminish after 7 to 10 days of administration. Although initial data suggest that the combined antenatal use of steroids with thyrotropin-releasing hormone could further reduce the incidence or severity of HMD,[10] recent publications did not confirm the beneficial effect of this antenatal hormone.[24,25]

Management

In addition to the administration of exogenous surfactant, the general management of infants with HMD includes careful stabilization, proper monitoring of cardiopulmonary function, adequate respiratory support, and thermal, metabolic, and nutritional support.

Resuscitation in the Delivery Room

Because perinatal asphyxia can further compromise the production of pulmonary surfactant, a skilled neonatal resuscitation team must be present at the delivery of all preterm infants. Hypothermia should be avoided by keeping the infants in a neutral thermal environment in which oxygen consumption is reduced to a minimum. All these infants should be admitted to

Table 31-1 Neonatal Respiratory Distress: Differential Diagnosis

	PREDISPOSING FACTORS	GESTATIONAL AGE	DISTRESS SEVERITY	INITIATION OF SYMPTOMS	HYPOXEMIA	HYPERCAPNIA	RESPONSE TO O_2	RESPONSE TO IPPV	BREATH SOUNDS	SIGNS OF INFECTION	CHEST RADIOGRAPH	COURSE*
HMD	Prematurity	Preterm	+++ to ++++	First hours	++ to ++++	+ to +++	++	Improved	Decreased crackles	Negative	Hazy, granular air bronchogram	2-5 days
TTN	Cesarean section, maternal overhydration	Full term Near term	++	First hours	+	— +	+++	Not indicated	Crackles	Negative	Hazy, vascular markings Cardiomegaly	↑1-3 days
Pneumonia	Maternal infection	Preterm Full term	++ to ++++	First day or later	++ to ++++	+ to ++	++	Variable, possible improvement	Decreased crackles	Positive	Patchy or granular Pleural effusion	3-7 days
MAS	Fetal distress	Full term Postterm	++ to +++	From birth	+ to ++++	+ to +++	++	Variable, possible improvement	Crackles, bronchial sounds	Negative	Patchy Hyperinflation	3-7 days
PPHN	Asphyxia: MAS Sepsis Hypoplastic lungs	Full term	++ to +++	First day	++++	— +	+ to ++++	Improved with hyperventilation Worsening with excessive pressure	Variable	Negative or positive	Variable (depends on underlying condition)	1-5 days
Pulmonary gas leak	Positive-pressure ventilation	Preterm Full term	+ to ++++	Variable	+ to ++++	+ to ++++	++	Variable	Decreased, asymmetric	Negative	Lung collapse Mediastinal shift	Until drained
CHD ↑PBF	Unknown	Full term Preterm	+ to +++	Variable: 2-3 days	+	+ to ++	++	Variable, possible improvement	Normal or crackles	Negative	Hazy, vascular markings Cardiomegaly	↑Until corrected
↓PBF	Unknown	Full term Preterm	— +	First day	++ to ++++	—	— +	None Worsening with excessive pressure	Normal	Negative	Dark, vascular markings	↓Until corrected 31-31

*Uncomplicated course.
O_2, Oxygen; *IPPV*, intermittent positive-pressure ventilation; *TTN*, transient tachypnea of the newborn; *MAS*, meconium aspiration syndrome; *PPHN*, persistent pulmonary hypertension of the newborn; *CHD*, congestive heart disease; *PBF*, pulmonary blood flow.

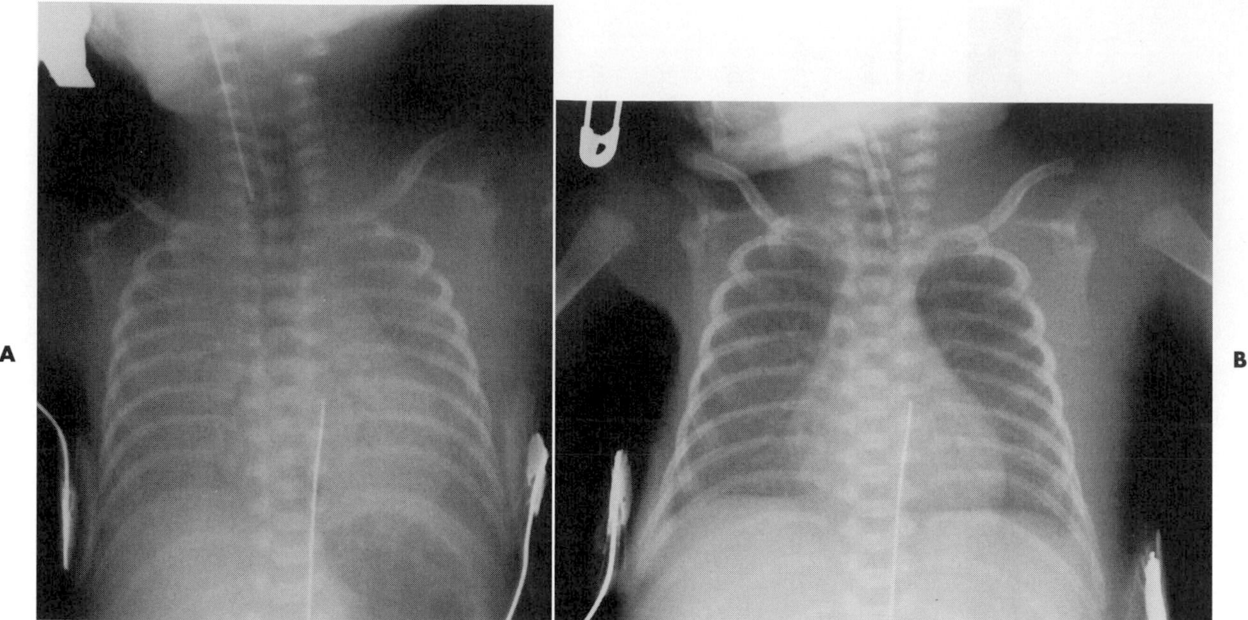

Fig. 31-4. Chest radiographs of an infant with HMD. **A,** Shortly after birth, a diffuse ground-glass appearance resulting from atelectasis with air bronchograms can be observed. **B,** Radiographic improvement with better aeration is evident after treatment with exogenous surfactant.

a neonatal intensive care setting, where continuous monitoring of heart rate, respiratory rate, blood pressure, arterial blood gases, and metabolic parameters is possible.

Oxygenation

Transcutaneous oxygen electrodes and pulse oxymetry have become important coadjuvants for the monitoring of arterial oxygenation. Although neither is a substitute for arterial blood gas analysis, they provide continuous information and are not invasive.[26] They allow early detection of complications such as pneumothorax, and they also reflect how the infant responds to different procedures such as endotracheal intubation, suction, and surfactant administration. The partial pressure of arterial oxygen (Pao_2) should be kept as much as possible between 50 and 80 mm Hg and the oxygen saturation between 90% and 94%; prolonged hyperoxia should be avoided because it is a risk factor for the development of retinopathy of prematurity.[27]

Mechanical Ventilatory Support

Larger infants, particularly those weighing more than 1500 g, with mild to moderate hypoxemia and minimal hypercarbia usually respond well to the administration of oxygen and do not require ventilatory assistance. Infants with HMD in need of mechanical ventilation have persistent hypoxemia (Pao_2 <50 mm Hg), are not responsive to the administration of supplemental oxygen, and usually have respiratory acidosis. In these infants, especially those with no or minimal hypercarbia, the use of continuous positive airway pressure (CPAP) is an effective form of treatment.[28] CPAP increases the FRC and stabilizes the airspaces, preventing their collapse during expiration. CPAP appears to be specially effective in larger infants (≥1200 g) and reduces oxygen requirements and the need for mechanical ventilation.[29,30] Although the idea of using prophylactic CPAP in premature infants at risk for HMD has been suggested, two clinical trials have failed to demonstrate a clear beneficial effect.[31,32]

In infants in whom CPAP does not work, particularly very small premature infants or those with hypoventilation and hypercarbia, intermittent positive-pressure ventilation is required after endotracheal intubation. Pressure-limited, time-cycled ventilators are preferentially used in neonates when mechanical ventilation is required. The respiratory failure and hypoxemia in infants with HMD are due mainly to an intrapulmonary shunt caused by perfusion of poorly ventilated airspaces (see Fig. 31-2). Therefore alveolar recruitment is required to obtain adequate oxygenation, and this can be achieved by increasing the mean airway pressure, which is a function of the inspiratory time, peak inspiratory pressure, and positive end-expiratory pressure. The use of a long inspiratory time (over 0.5 second) should be avoided because it can lead to alveolar rupture and gas leaks. Especially in infants with high oxygen requirements, the use of short inspiratory times and high rates appears to reduce both the incidence of pulmonary gas leak and the mortality rate.[33-36] In most infants, an inspiratory time of 0.25 to 0.50 second is sufficient to achieve adequate gas exchange. The use of positive end-expiratory pressure is an effective way of maintaining the FRC, and pressures of 4 to 6 cm H_2O are usually required during the acute phase of HMD. When hypercarbia is present, an increase in the peak inspiratory pressure or a decrease in the positive end-expiratory pressure improves the tidal volume and minute ventilation. In addition, the respiratory rate can be increased, but excessive rates must be avoided to prevent gas trapping, especially in infants with increased airway resistance.

Weaning from intermittent positive-pressure ventilation can be a long and difficult process, particularly in infants with very low birth weights. Methylxanthines such as theophylline and caffeine act as respiratory stimulants and can facilitate weaning.[37] Immediately after extubation, particularly in the very small preterm infant, the use of nasal CPAP can also improve the success rate of weaning.[38]

High-frequency ventilation is another therapeutic alternative that has been evaluated in neonates with severe HMD. Three randomized clinical trials have failed to demonstrate clear beneficial effects with the use of this therapy in infants with uncomplicated HMD when compared with conventional ventilation.[39-41] More recent publications reported a decreased incidence of chronic lung disease in neonates with HMD who received high-frequency oscillatory or jet ventilation compared with infants treated with conventional ventilation.[42-44] Therefore the use of high-frequency ventilation in neonates with HMD is still a matter of controversy, with the exception of infants who develop pulmonary interstitial emphysema (PIE), who are more likely to benefit from its use.[45]

So that pulmonary barotrauma can be reduced by eliminating asynchrony between the infant's own respiratory efforts and the mechanical breaths, patient-triggered ventilation has been used in patients with HMD. Although in theory this mode of ventilation could reduce the incidence of barotrauma and chronic lung disease and facilitate weaning, it has shown only a modest advantage over conventional ventilation in the very small premature infant.[46-49]

More information about mechanical ventilation can be found in Chapter 21.

Acid-Base Balance

Metabolic acidosis should be prevented because it interferes with the production of surfactant, increases pulmonary vascular resistance, and may have deleterious effects on the cardiovascular system. However, rapid infusions of sodium bicarbonate should be avoided because this medication may increase the incidence of intraventricular hemorrhage.[50] Severe metabolic acidosis in the course of HMD is most commonly a manifestation of perinatal asphyxia, sepsis, intraventricular hemorrhage, or circulatory failure. It is therefore essential to promptly investigate and correct the cause. If the metabolic acidosis is severe, a continuous infusion of sodium bicarbonate or acetate may be used.

Blood Pressure and Fluid Management

Pulmonary edema plays a role in the pathophysiology of HMD, and these infants tend to have a low urine output during the first 48 hours, followed by a diuretic phase with weight loss. Fluid overload should be avoided, and fluid intake is usually started at 60 to 80 ml/kg/day and then increased gradually over the next few days, although great individual variations exist. Higher fluid intake may be necessary especially in the infant with a very low birth weight and high insensible water losses. Fluid intake must be adjusted according to changes in weight, urine output, and serum electrolyte levels. The use of phototherapy, low ambient humidity, and radiant warmers increases fluid requirements. Excessive administration of fluids during the first days may contribute to the development of PDA[51] and bronchopulmonary dysplasia.[52] Because spontaneous diuresis has been described before improvement in respiratory status, the use of diuretics during the course of HMD has been evaluated. In a prospective, blinded trial, no beneficial effects in pulmonary function were observed with the prophylactic administration of furosemide; furthermore, the use of diuretics produced undesirable volume depletion in some infants.[53] Thus the use of diuretics in HMD is not a standard form of treatment, and if used, they must be evaluated on an individual basis, taking into consideration the hemodynamic status of the infant.

Careful monitoring of arterial blood pressure is essential in these patients. Arterial hypotension, if present, facilitates right-to-left shunting through an open ductus arteriosus, thus contributing to the hypoxemia. Perinatal asphyxia, sepsis, and hypovolemia are the most common conditions that can produce hypotension and if suspected, should be treated accordingly. It is important to avoid the excessive use of fluids in an attempt to correct hypotension and to consider the use of pressors, such as dopamine and dobutamine.

Nutrition

Adequate nutritional support is essential for these infants and can be achieved during the first days of life by the use of parenteral nutrition. Oral feedings can be started as soon as the infant is clinically stable and the respiratory distress resolved.

Antibiotics

Neonatal pneumonia, particularly that caused by group B streptococci, should always be considered in the differential diagnosis of HMD, particularly in larger infants with respiratory failure. The following perinatal conditions are associated with an increased incidence of infection in the premature infant: prolonged rupture of membranes, maternal fever during labor, fetal tachycardia, leukocytosis or leukopenia, hypotension, and acidosis. Before findings from blood cultures become available, especially when some of these risk factors are present, the use of ampicillin and an aminoglycoside is recommended.

Surfactant Replacement Therapy

After extensive animal experimentation[54] and multiple prospective, controlled clinical trials that demonstrated the efficacy of exogenous surfactant in the treatment of HMD[55-57] and its approval by the Food and Drug Administration in 1990, the use of surfactant has become a conventional form of therapy for these infants.

Two surfactant preparations have been predominantly used in the United States: a synthetic form composed of dipalmitoyl phosphatidylcholine, hexadecanol, and tyloxapol (Exosurf Neonatal) and a semisynthetic product (Survanta, which is a modified bovine surfactant extract). Several other surfactant preparations, including natural, synthetic, and semisynthetic forms, are used worldwide. In most cases, surfactant is administered in a liquid form through the endotracheal tube. Studies comparing natural vs. synthetic surfactants have shown faster improvement in arterial oxygenation and less air leak complications in infants treated with natural surfactants.[58-60]

A few clinical trials have addressed the question of whether the prophylactic administration of surfactant to all premature infants under a certain gestational age offers substantial advantages over rescue treatment, an approach in which surfactant is administered only to infants with confirmed HMD. Although no beneficial effects were found with the use of prophylactic surfactant in these trials, more recent clinical trials suggest that infants who received surfactant as prophylaxis required less oxygen and mechanical ventilation and also had a better survival rate than infants who received rescue therapy.[61-64] Theoretically, the administration of surfactant before the signs of HMD are established might allow more satisfactory distribution throughout the lung. On the other hand, rescue treatment avoids the exposure to surfactant in many infants who would never develop HMD and reduces the cost.

After its administration, exogenous surfactant rapidly improves arterial oxygenation and the alveolar-arterial oxygen difference, reducing the requirements of ventilatory support

(Fig. 31-5). The changes in lung mechanics that occur in response to surfactant administration are less consistent. In infants whose lungs are mechanically ventilated, studies have failed to show early changes in lung compliance that could explain the rapid improvement in oxygenation, and the studies documented a significant increase in lung compliance only 24 hours after surfactant administration.[65,66] However, spontaneously breathing infants demonstrated a significant increase in compliance within 1 hour after surfactant instillation. The authors speculated that changes in compliance were not observed during mechanical breaths because the lungs are overdistended and operating in the flat portion of the pressure-volume curve.[67] Measurements of lung volume after surfactant administration suggest that the rapid improvement in oxygenation is due to an increase in FRC.[68-70]

Clinical trials have shown that the use of exogenous surfactant significantly reduces the incidence of pulmonary gas leaks and decreases neonatal mortality rates.[57,71] In addition, infants who receive surfactant have an increase likelihood of survival without bronchopulmonary dysplasia compared with patients treated with placebo.[57,72] Surfactant replacement therapy has, however, failed to produce a later decrease in the incidence of PDA, intracranial hemorrhage, and necrotizing enterocolitis.

A clinical trial in 1991 raised the concern about pulmonary hemorrhage as a possible side effect of exogenous surfactant, although the difference between the control and treatment groups was not statistically significant.[73] Later, a multicenter trial of exogenous surfactant in infants weighing 500 to 699 g found the incidence of pulmonary hemorrhage to be significantly higher in the treatment group.[74] Pulmonary hemorrhage in these infants could be caused by increased left-to-right ductal shunting after pulmonary vascular resistance decreases after surfactant administration.

Future research on exogenous surfactant will have to evaluate the efficacy and indications of different surfactant preparations. Dosing and long-term safety must also be investigated.

Complications

PDA

The incidence of PDA in the premature infant with HMD may be as high as 90%.[75] With the survival of smaller infants and the use of exogenous surfactant, early PDA as a complication of HMD has become an increasing problem in the management of the very-low-birth-weight infant during the first days of life.[75] Factors that may determine the failure of the ductus arteriosus to close in the premature infant are hypoxemia caused by respiratory failure, increased production of prostaglandins,[76] and increased sensitivity of the ductus to the dilating effects of prostaglandin E_2.[77] Sepsis has also been associated with an increased risk of PDA, which is also mediated by elevated circulatory levels of prostaglandins.[78]

A PDA is associated with a left-to-right shunt and increased pulmonary blood flow and pulmonary artery pressure.[79,80] This increase in pulmonary blood flow produces a decrease in lung compliance that improves after PDA ligation.[81] The increased pulmonary blood flow may lead to left ventricular failure and pulmonary edema and adversely affect lung fluid balance.[82] Leakage of plasma proteins into the alveolar space may inhibit surfactant function.[17] This deterioration of pulmonary function increases oxygen requirements and mechanical ventilation. The physical examination generally reveals crackles and an active precordium, bounding pulses with a wide pulse pressure, poor peripheral perfusion, and in most but not all cases, a systolic heart murmur best heard below the left clavicle.

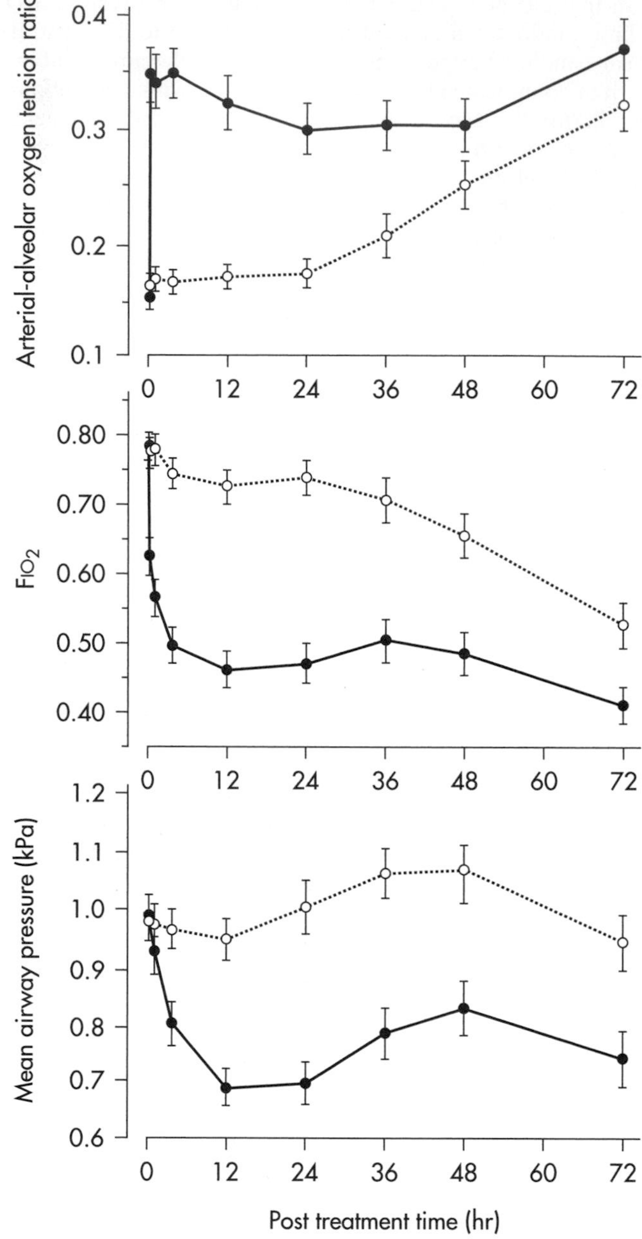

Fig. 31-5. Mean values for the arterial-alveolar oxygen tension ratio, fraction of inspired oxygen (FIO_2), and mean airway pressure before and after treatment with exogenous surfactant *(closed circles)* or air placebo *(open circles)* in infants with HMD. (From Horbar JD et al: *N Engl J Med* 320:959-965, 1989.)

Radiographically, evidence of pulmonary edema is observed, often in association with cardiomegaly (Fig. 31-6). As soon as it is clinically suspected, the presence of a PDA should be confirmed by Doppler echocardiography, and proper treatment should be promptly initiated. This consists of fluid restriction, adequate respiratory support, and treatment with indomethacin if possible. If closure of the PDA can not be achieved with medical treatment, surgical ligation should be considered. Any symptomatic PDA should be closed as soon

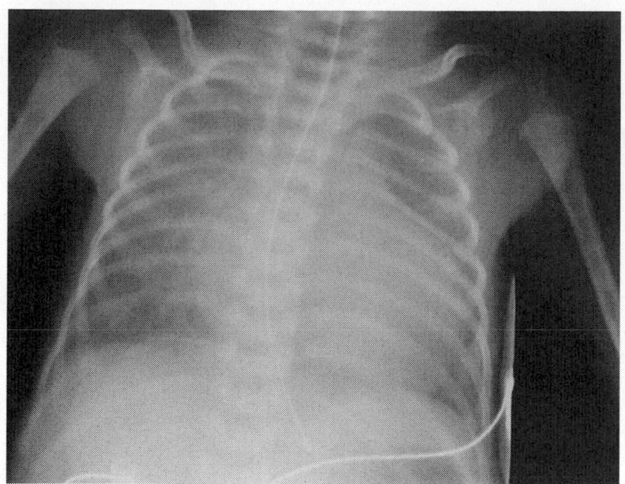

Fig. 31-6. Chest radiograph showing cardiomegaly and pulmonary edema in an infant with PDA.

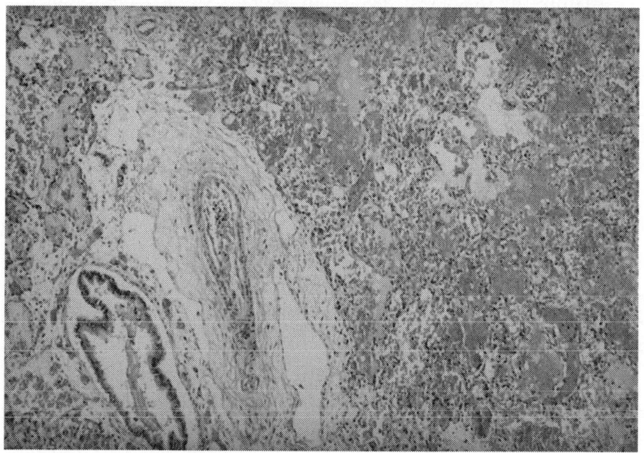

Fig. 31-7. Microscopic findings in an infant with pulmonary hemorrhage. Abundant red blood cells are seen in the pulmonary interstitium and inside the airspaces.

as possible because the presence of a ductus is associated with a higher incidence of chronic lung disease.[83]

Hemorrhagic Pulmonary Edema

Most cases of pulmonary hemorrhage in the newborn are secondary to severe pulmonary edema as a complication of HMD and PDA. The incidence of pulmonary hemorrhage in premature infants with HMD is approximately 1%, although at autopsy it is much higher, around 55%.[84] The hemorrhagic fluid in the airspaces most likely represents a capillary filtrate coming from the interstitial space, as demonstrated by Cole et al.[85] Histologically, pulmonary hemorrhage can present as either interstitial or alveolar hemorrhage. The interstitial form is characterized by hemorrhage in the pleural, interlobular septal, peribronchial, perivascular, and alveolar wall areas. When the hemorrhage is alveolar, red cells fill the airspaces and extend into the bronchioles and bronchi[86] (Fig. 31-7).

The associated predisposing factors are often perinatal asphyxia, hypothermia, hypoglycemia, congestive heart failure, coagulopathy, pneumonia, and excessive fluid administration.[85] Pulmonary hemorrhage has also been related to the use of exogenous surfactant,[73] although at autopsy the incidence of pulmonary hemorrhage was not different in infants treated with surfactant or air placebo.[84] In infants receiving surfactant replacement therapy, increased left-to-right shunt through the ductus arteriosus[75] can lead to hemorrhagic pulmonary edema.

Pulmonary hemorrhage complicating HMD is usually observed in the first 5 to 7 days of life. When massive, pulmonary hemorrhage can be a catastrophic event. There is a sudden deterioration of the respiratory status that is generally associated with bradycardia, metabolic acidosis, and shock. Hemorrhagic fluid is seen coming from the nose and the mouth or through the endotracheal tube. The chest radiograph commonly shows a diffuse opacification of both lung fields.

The immediate management of pulmonary hemorrhage consists mainly of providing adequate ventilatory support. Increasing the airway pressures, particularly the positive end-expiratory pressure, can prevent further bleeding. Transfusions of red blood cells and fresh frozen plasma may be necessary to replace volume losses, but fluid restriction is indicated when the hemorrhage is due to left ventricular failure. If the cause of pulmonary edema and hemorrhage is a PDA, it should be treated promptly, as should any other underlying cause.

TRANSIENT TACHYPNEA OF THE NEWBORN

Also known as *wet lung syndrome* or *respiratory distress syndrome type II,* transient tachypnea of the newborn (TTN) was first described by Avery et al in 1966.[87] This original description was based on a group of predominantly full-term newborns, who presented with tachypnea soon after birth and had similar radiographic findings with a benign clinical course. This transient respiratory symptomatology was attributed to a delayed resorption of alveolar fluid, which reduced lung compliance and caused a mild impairment in gas exchange.

Incidence

TTN affects 1% to 2% of all newborns,[88] especially full-term infants. Several perinatal risk factors, including elective cesarean section,[89] excessive administration of fluids to the mother during labor,[90] male gender, and macrosomia, have been linked to the development of TTN.[88] In addition, meta-analysis of several clinical trials show that delayed clamping of the umbilical cord also increases the incidence.[91]

Pathogenesis

The removal of fetal lung liquid at birth is an essential step in the newborn's adaptation to extrauterine life. The clearance of such liquid has been attributed at least in part to the mechanical compression of the chest at birth.[92] Besides this "squeezing" of fluid from the lungs into the trachea and mouth, other mechanisms seem to play a more important role in the removal of lung liquid.

A antenatal reduction in fetal lung liquid has been demonstrated in fetal lambs[93] and appears to result from a shift of fluid from the lung lumen into the interstitium.[94] The process of labor appears to be important in this antenatal redistribution and absorption of lung liquid,[95] and this could explain, at least in part, the higher incidence of TTN observed after elective cesarean section.

The cause of reduced secretion of fetal lung liquid during labor is still poorly understood. Although it has been proposed that the reduction could result from an elevated plasma concentration of epinephrine during labor,[96] blockade of β-adrenergic receptors in fetal rabbits[97] does not prevent this resorption of lung liquid.

With the influx of air into the lungs at birth, there are displacement of fluid and a decrease in the hydrostatic pressure in the pulmonary circulation, which facilitate the resorption of fluid into the pulmonary vasculature. In fetal lambs, about 10% of the lung fluid leaves the alveolar space through the lymphatic system.[94] Therefore any condition that increases hydrostatic pressure in the pulmonary vasculature can interfere with the appropriate resorption of fluid into the pulmonary circulation. This can explain the higher incidence of TTN observed after excessive administration of fluids to the mother and after delayed clamping of the umbilical cord. Mild left ventricular dysfunction has also been described in infants with TTN.[98]

Evaluation of lung function in newborns demonstrated that thoracic gas volume measurements were higher after vaginal delivery than after cesarean section.[99] This reduction in the gaseous component of the total lung volume probably results from an excessive amount of liquid in the lung after operative delivery.

The perfusion of alveoli that are fluid filled or decreased in size by interstitial water can lead to a mild to moderate degree of hypoxemia, which is frequently observed in infants with TTN. This hypoxemia is sometimes accompanied by a transient hypercarbia that is probably related to an increase in pulmonary resistance.[99]

Clinical Presentation

In infants who are only a few hours old (see Table 31-1), TTN usually presents with respiratory symptomatology characterized mainly by tachypnea. The respiratory rate commonly fluctuates between 80 and 120 breaths/min. Retractions, nasal flaring, grunting, and cyanosis can also be present. Classically, TTN affects full-term infants, particularly those who are large for gestational age, although it can affect larger premature infants. Most of these infants have a perinatal history with risk factors for the development of TTN, such as elective cesarean section or excessive administration of fluids to the mother. In addition to respiratory distress, these newborns may have a barrel chest and coarse breath sounds.

The results of arterial blood gas analysis may be normal, although they frequently show a mild to moderate degree of hypoxemia, but these patients usually require less than 40% oxygen to maintain adequate arterial oxygenation. Occasionally, hypoxemia is accompanied by mild hypercarbia, but both conditions tend to be transient and disappear within the first 24 to 48 hours.

The chest radiograph is characteristic. There are prominent, usually ill-defined central markings branching out from the hila. These markings suggest vascular engorgement.[87] The interlobar fissures may appear prominent, and small pleural effusions can be seen. The cardiac silhouette is usually enlarged (Fig. 31-8). All these findings are transient and usually disappear in 48 to 72 hours.

Probably the most challenging step in establishing the diagnosis is ruling out other pathologic conditions with similar clinical presentations. Because TTN occurs predominantly in full-term newborns, it is very important to rule out pneumonia, especially that caused by group B streptococci. In infants with pneumonia, the perinatal history may be consistent with that of infection, such as maternal fever or prolonged rupture of membranes. Such infants also frequently have other clinical signs of infection, such as arterial hypotension, temperature instability, leukocytosis, and leukopenia. Other important differential diagnoses to be considered are meconium aspiration syndrome (MAS), HMD (particularly in the large premature infant), congenital heart disease and other congenital anomalies, and pulmonary gas leaks.

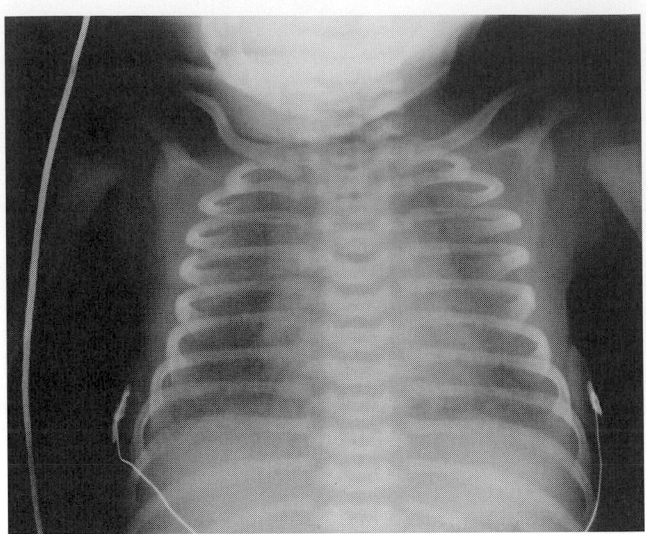

Fig. 31-8. Radiographic findings in an infant with TTN. Increased bilateral markings with prominent interlobar fissures and small pleural effusions are observed. The heart appears slightly enlarged.

The clinical course of infants with TTN is benign. The tachypnea and the radiographic abnormalities usually resolve in 24 to 72 hours.

Management

Because of the benign course of TTN, treatment consists mostly of proper stabilization, adequate monitoring, and careful evaluation to rule out other, more serious conditions. Oxygen should be provided as necessary to maintain normal oxygenation, and generally, mechanical ventilation is not required. Fluid restriction is usually indicated until the symptoms resolve; oral feedings can be started as soon as the infant is able to tolerate them. Diuretics have not been shown to affect the clinical course of the disease.[100] The use of antibiotics is indicated in cases in which the diagnosis of neonatal pneumonia is suspected and until the cultures and the clinical evaluation of the infant permit the clinician to rule out this diagnosis.

NEONATAL PNEUMONIA

Because of its grave prognosis, neonatal pneumonia should always be considered in the differential diagnosis in newborns with respiratory distress. During early onset neonatal sepsis, the lung is one of the most frequent organs involved. Pneumonia in the newborn period can be acquired during intrauterine life, at the time of delivery, or after birth. Although the most common etiology is bacterial infection, it can be caused by different microorganisms, including viruses and fungi.

Incidence

The incidence of congenital and neonatal pneumonia found at autopsy in live-born infants varies from 20% to 32%[101,102] and is similar in term and premature infants. In infants who survive, the incidence is difficult to establish because of the frequent inability to make a definitive diagnosis. The radiographic incidence of pneumonia was 4% among term infants born to mothers with documented amnionitis.[103] In a prospective study of 19,596 newborns, the incidence of early onset pneumonia was 1.79 per 1000 live births.[104] A higher incidence has been described in black infants[101] and in infants born to low-income families.[105]

Etiology and Pathogenesis

The agents and mechanisms of pulmonary infection differ depending on the type of neonatal pneumonia.

Transplacentally Acquired Pneumonia

Transplacentally acquired pneumonia includes the neonatal pneumonia seen in the context of a systemic infection in the mother, such as those caused by rubella virus, cytomegalovirus, *Treponema pallidum,* and occasionally *Listeria monocytogenes.* Many of these infants are stillborn or die in the first days of life.

A hematogenous spread to the fetus from a mother with sepsis or bacteremia is the mechanism of infection in transplacentally acquired pneumonia. A classic example would be pneumonia alba, which is occasionally seen as one of the manifestations of congenital syphilis.

Pneumonia Acquired from Colonization of the Amniotic Fluid or Birth Canal

Classically, the responsible microorganism infects the infant via an ascending route from the vaginal canal, usually producing chorioamnionitis, especially after a prolonged rupture of membranes during labor. The infection may also be acquired without evidence of chorioamnionitis during the passage through the birth canal.

In this type of infection, group B streptococci are responsible for the majority of cases of neonatal pneumonia and sepsis in the United States and Europe.[104,106,107] The rate of maternal vaginal colonization with this bacteria at the time of delivery is approximately 20%, and early onset group B streptococcal disease affects 1.8 per 1000 live newborns.[108] Mothers of affected infants usually have complications such as preterm delivery, prolonged labor, prolonged rupture of membranes, and intrapartum fever. In early onset disease, the infants have symptoms at or shortly after delivery, which suggests that most of these infections begin in utero.[108]

Other microorganisms included in this group are *Escherichia coli, Klebsiella* species, *Haemophilus influenzae, Enterobacter* species, *L. monocytogenes, Chlamydia trachomatis, Ureaplasma urealyticum, Candida* species, and herpes simplex virus. When neonatal pneumonia is associated with chorioamnionitis in the mother, aspiration of infected amniotic fluid is probably the main mechanism of infection. This is suggested by the presence of amniotic debris and maternal leukocytes in the histologic examination of the lungs.[109] However, chorioamnionitis per se is not always associated with pneumonia, and other factors, such as fetal asphyxia, seem to play an important role. Evidence of fetal asphyxia is frequently present at autopsy in infants with intrauterine pneumonia.[110] If present, asphyxia can trigger gasping respiratory movements in the fetus that can cause the aspiration of contaminated amniotic fluid.

Any obstetric factors that predispose to chorioamnionitis can also favor the development of neonatal infection. In the case of group B streptococci, the rate of symptomatic early onset disease with pneumonia is considerably increased if there is premature onset of labor,[111] prolonged rupture of membranes, prolonged labor, or maternal postpartum bacteremia.[112]

When the infant acquires the infection during passage through the vaginal canal, the aspiration of infected materials is the route of infection. In these infants the histologic presentation is similar to that in older children and adults (i.e., bronchopneumonia with evidence of bronchitis and bronchiolitis, pleuritis, alveolar hemorrhage, and occasionally pulmonary necrosis with the presence of bacteria).[110] In group B streptococcal pneumonia, hyaline membranes, similar to those observed in HMD, can be found in sections of the lungs.[113]

The cytopathic effects of herpes simplex virus can be observed in the lungs of infants with pneumonia caused by herpes infection.

Pneumonia Acquired after Birth

In infants who remain hospitalized after birth, particularly if the lungs require mechanical ventilation, infection may be transmitted from contaminated personnel or equipment. *Staphylococcus aureus;* coagulase-negative staphylococci; *Pseudomonas, Proteus, Serratia, Enterobacter,* and *Candida* organisms; and respiratory syncytial virus are among the most frequent pathogens that cause nosocomial pneumonia in these high-risk infants. If the patient has been discharged home, viral pneumonias such as those produced by respiratory syncytial virus or adenovirus may occur during the first month of life. *C. trachomatis,* although acquired at birth, usually manifests later, producing afebrile pneumonia during the first 3 months of life.[114]

In nosocomial pneumonia, several mechanisms of infection can be implicated, including contact with contaminated personnel, inhalation of infected aerosols in the nursery, use of contaminated respiratory equipment, and hematogenous dissemination from bacteremia or a distant source. The histologic presentation varies depending on the etiologic agent. *S. aureus* and *Klebsiella pneumoniae* may produce extensive tissue damage with microabscesses, empyema, and pneumatoceles.[115] *E. coli,* a necrotizing agent, may also produce pneumatoceles.[116] In pneumonia caused by *Candida* species, yeasts and pseudohyphae can be observed on postmortem examination of lung tissue (Fig. 31-9).

Clinical Presentation

Transplacentally acquired pneumonia is usually symptomatic shortly after birth (see Table 31-1). There may be a history of antenatal complications such as intrauterine growth retardation or fetal distress during labor. Respiration is likely to be depressed at birth, so these infants require resuscitation and frequently, mechanical ventilation. Besides the classic signs of respiratory distress with retractions, grunting, tachypnea, and cyanosis, such infants commonly have other signs of congenital infection, such as low birth weight, hepatosplenomegaly, petechiae, and neurologic abnormalities. Total immunoglobulin M blood levels are usually elevated, and serologic tests for

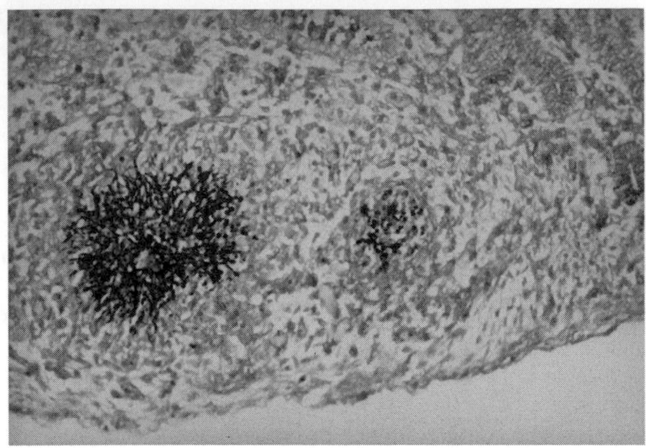

Fig. 31-9. Neonatal pneumonia caused by *Candida* organisms. Picture shows periodic acid–Schiff staining of a fungal abscess with budding yeasts and pseudohyphae.

specific etiologic agents should be performed when congenital infection is suspected.

When pneumonia has been acquired from contaminated amniotic fluid or in the birth canal, the infant may not be affected in the first hours after birth, so a high index of suspicion should be maintained in every newborn with risk factors for neonatal infection. Neonatal pneumonia can present with overt or subtle clinical signs. Classic signs are those related to the respiratory system, such as respiratory distress, cyanosis, and crackles found during the physical examination. Perhaps more important are the subtle signs, the most common being apnea, lethargy, hypotension, tachycardia or bradycardia, poor peripheral perfusion, and temperature instability. These clinical manifestations usually appear during the first 24 hours of life but sometimes are present at birth. In premature infants who have respiratory distress and a chest radiograph suggestive of HMD, the possibility of pneumonia is sometimes impossible to exclude. For this reason, appropriate cultures should be performed and antibiotic therapy started in any patient who is suspected of having HMD and who has perinatal risk factors and clinical or laboratory signs suggestive of infection.

The chest radiograph in infants with pneumonia most commonly shows bilateral diffuse densities or may have a granular appearance, like that of HMD, especially in the case of group B streptococcal pneumonia (Fig. 31-10). Radiographic changes may be present at birth or rapidly progress in severity during the first hours of life, sometimes to a complete opacification of both lungs.

The white blood cell count can reveal leukopenia or leukocytosis, frequently with a leftward shift in the differential count. A positive urine latex agglutination assay for group B streptococci can point the clinician to the diagnosis, but there is a high incidence of false-positive and false-negative results. Blood should always be drawn for culture, and when the results are positive, they confirm the diagnosis, but negative results do not rule out the possibility of pneumonia. In one review of early onset neonatal pneumonia, the findings from blood cultures showed the presence of organisms in only 46% of 35 cases cases.[104]

The presence of white blood cells and bacteria in Gram's stain of early tracheal aspirates suggests pneumonia, and the bacteria grown in these aspirates correlates well with the those

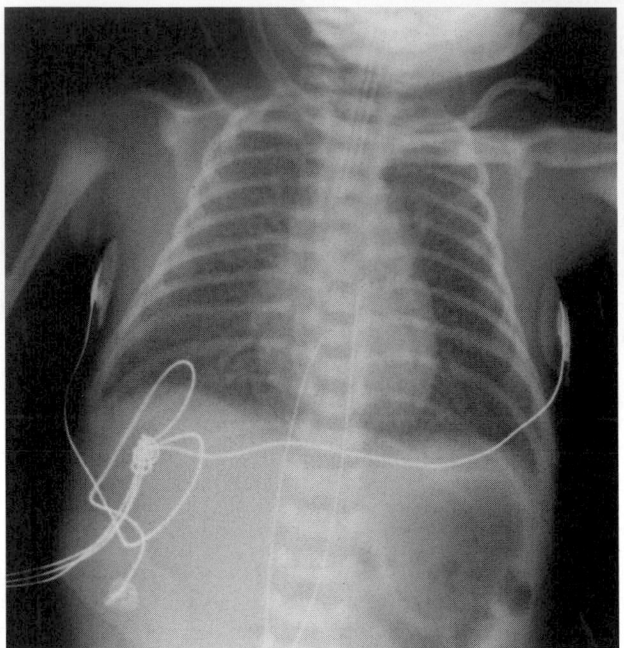

Fig. 31-10. Chest radiograph of an infant with group B streptococcal pneumonia. Note the bilateral diffuse densities, which are similar to those observed in infants with HMD.

found in simultaneously performed blood cultures.[117,118] However, in the case of nosocomial pneumonia, findings from tracheal aspirates may not be helpful in making the diagnosis. In neonates whose lungs are chronically ventilated, positive findings from tracheal aspirates occurred with equal frequency among infants suspected of having pneumonia and in the control group.[119] If a pleural effusion is present, bacteriologic studies of pleural fluid can also be diagnostic.

Regarding nosocomial infections, any infant should be suspected of having pneumonia; this is particularly true of an infant with a low birth weight whose lungs require mechanical ventilation and whose respiratory status has deteriorated. Increased requirements of oxygen and ventilatory support, any signs of systemic infection, a change in the characteristics of the tracheal secretions, the colonization of tracheal secretions with an unusual microorganism, and a worsening of the chest radiograph are the most common signs of nosocomial pneumonia. A high index of suspicion should be maintained in these infants because some of the most frequent nosocomial infections, such as those caused by *Candida* organisms or coagulase-negative staphylococci, usually have a subacute presentation with vague symptoms.[120,121] If nosocomial pneumonia is suspected, a complete blood count and appropriate cultures from blood, trachea, urine, and if possible, cerebrospinal fluid should be obtained before treatment is initiated.

Management

The goal of treatment should be to achieve adequate antibiotic coverage while providing good supportive care. Proper stabilization of the infant, adequate oxygenation and ventilation, hemodynamic status, temperature control, and fluid management are essential for the recovery of the patient; they also help prevent complications such as pulmonary hypertension, gas leaks, and chronic lung disease.

The choice of antibiotics frequently has to be made before cultures are available and is based mainly on the age of the infant and the presence of risk factors for a certain etiologic agent. During the first 5 to 7 days of life, the use of ampicillin and an aminoglycoside provides adequate coverage for group B streptococci, *L. monocytogenes,* and the most frequent, gram-negative bacteria. Later, if nosocomial pneumonia is suspected and the etiology is unknown, coverage for *Staphylococcus* organisms is necessary, as is the use of aminoglycosides or broad-spectrum cephalosporins for gram-negative bacteria. If *Candida* pneumonia is strongly suspected, the use of amphotericin is indicated. Herpes simplex pneumonia should be considered, especially in the infant who becomes ill 5 to 7 days after birth and has risk factors or other manifestations of herpetic infection. Acyclovir is the treatment of choice for this infection. After the initial phase, the antibiotics can be changed according to the results of the cultures or the clinical course of the disease. Antibiotics are usually continued for 10 to 14 days. The use of granulocyte transfusions or intravenous immunoglobulin for the treatment of neonatal infections is still controversial.

Complications

Pulmonary hypertension can complicate the course of neonatal pneumonia.[122] In group B streptococcal infection, exposure of type III antigen to blood components within the vascular space can promote the adherence of neutrophils to the endothelial cells.[123] These neutrophils can liberate inflammatory mediators, vasoactive substances such as thromboxane and leukotrienes, that constrict the pulmonary blood vessels.[124-126]

Septic shock is another frequent complication and is often the cause of death in these infants. Also, PIE and other types of gas leaks can develop at any time of the clinical course, particularly when mechanical ventilation is required. Pulmonary hemorrhage secondary to vascular damage and pulmonary hypertension can also complicate the evolution of neonatal pneumonia.[85]

Neonatal pneumonia caused by *U. urealyticum* has been related to the development of chronic lung disease in the premature infant.[127,128]

Outcome

The overall mortality rate for early onset neonatal pneumonia has been estimated to be around 29% but is much lower in late-onset pneumonia.[104] Infants who die of early onset pneumonia are more likely to be premature and have a rapid clinical deterioration and a radiographic picture resembling severe HMD.[104] In infants who survive, the severe lung injury related to the inflammatory process plus the damage produced by prolonged mechanical ventilation and oxygen toxicity places them at high risk for developing chronic lung disease.

MECONIUM ASPIRATION SYNDROME

MAS is one of the most common causes of respiratory failure in infants born at term or after term. Meconium is present in the amniotic fluid in approximately 10% of all deliveries, but in less than half of such infants, meconium is present below the vocal cords when the airway is visualized immediately after birth.[129-131] The presence of meconium in the amniotic fluid is extremely uncommon in preterm deliveries.[132] Only 10% to 30% of all infants with meconium in the trachea develop respiratory failure, but the risk and the severity are considerably increased when the meconium is thick or particulate.[129,133,134] Some infants born through meconium-stained fluid develop respiratory illness even when no meconium is visualized below the vocal cords at birth.

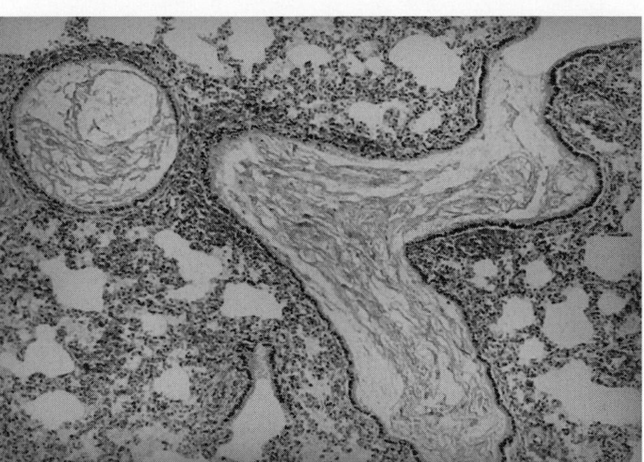

Fig. 31-11. Meconium filling the lumen of the distal airways of an infant who died from MAS.

Pathogenesis

The passage of meconium into the amniotic fluid is frequently associated with some degree of fetal distress, but it may also occur in normal or breech deliveries without evidence of asphyxia.[131,134-136] In cases of asphyxia the elimination of meconium into the amniotic fluid seems to result from increased intestinal motility produced by the hypoxic stress. The hypoxia and acidosis can also induce deep fetal respiratory efforts that increase the likelihood of aspiration of meconium-contaminated fluid into the lower airways.

Because a relatively small amount of fluid is moved by the fetus during normal respiratory activity, it is uncommon for large amounts of meconium to be aspirated into the distal airways before birth, although meconium is occasionally found in the lungs of stillborn infants.[137,138] In contrast, a large intrathoracic negative pressure is generated at the time of birth, and any material present in the nasopharynx or trachea can be aspirated into the distal airways (Fig. 31-11). For this reason, it has been proposed that aspiration of massive amounts of meconium can be prevented by effective nasopharyngeal suctioning performed immediately after birth and preferably before the infant takes the first breath of air.

Clinical Presentation

Infants who aspirate meconium are born mostly at or after term (see Table 31-1) and frequently have a history of fetal distress, low Apgar scores, and meconium-stained amniotic fluid.[132,133] Their skin, nails, and umbilical cords are also meconium stained. They have signs of respiratory distress shortly after birth, with tachypnea, intercostal retractions, and cyanosis if not given supplemental oxygen. The chest appears overdistended and is frequently barrel shaped with a protruding sternum. The breath sounds are usually obscured by coarse bronchial sounds, and expiration can be prolonged, thereby indicating small airway obstruction. The chest radiograph shows patchy areas of increased density in both lungs, sometimes confluent and alternating with hyperlucent areas (Fig. 31-12). The diaphragm is occasionally depressed, and pneumomediastinum and pneumothorax are frequent radiographic findings.[139,140]

Analysis of arterial blood during the first hour of life may reveal some degree of metabolic acidosis that reflects perinatal asphyxia. The arterial oxygen tension is always lower than normal unless the infant is given supplemental oxygen. The severity of the hypoxemia depends on the degree of the pulmonary damage, and the hypoxemia is aggravated by pulmonary hypertension, which may result in right-to-left shunting through the foramen ovale and ductus arteriosus. The $Pa{CO_2}$ is commonly elevated and in the more severe situations may require the use of mechanical ventilation to correct the alveolar hypoventilation and respiratory acidosis.[141]

Infants with severe MAS have frequent complications, many of which may be life threatening. Pneumomediastinum, pneumothorax, or both conditions occur in 10% to 15% of infants with MAS who require mechanical ventilation.[134] The high incidence of gas leak probably results from small airway obstruction that leads to gas trapping and uneven distribution of inspired gas. The risk is increased by the high transpulmonary pressure generated by the infant or required on the mechanical ventilator to achieve adequate ventilation. Parenchymal inflammation and damage caused by the meconium may also increase the potential for alveolar rupture. Persistent pulmonary hypertension of the newborn (PPHN) with right-to-left shunting is also a frequent complication in infants with MAS and is discussed later.

Another complication of severe MAS is secondary bacterial infection. No data are available in infants, but in experimental animals, meconium enhances bacterial growth in the lung.[142] Because of similarities in the clinical and radiographic manifestations of aspiration of meconium and bacterial pneumonia, it is not always easy to diagnose a superimposed bacterial infection during the acute phase of MAS, so the clinician must have a high index of suspicion. Also, infants who become infected in utero have a higher incidence of perinatal asphyxia and meconium aspiration.[131] Infants with severe MAS who require prolonged mechanical ventilation can also develop subglottic stenosis secondary to the presence of the endotracheal tube.[143]

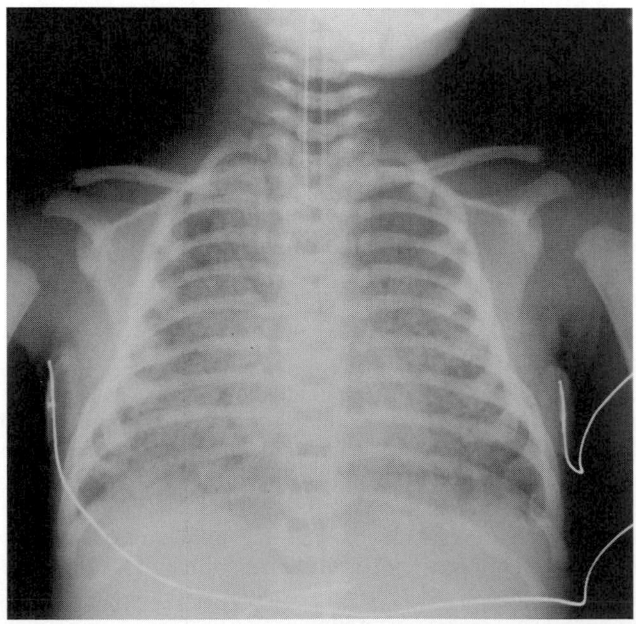

Fig. 31-12. Chest radiograph of an infant with MAS. Patchy areas of increased density are observed in both lungs.

The clinical course of MAS depends on the severity of the pulmonary involvement and on the occurrence of complications, such as PPHN, infection, and pneumothorax, that can delay recovery. Although mild cases may require only oxygen supplementation for a few hours or days, infants with severe respiratory failure require mechanical ventilation for several days or even weeks and have a high mortality rate. In a series of infants with MAS, approximately 30% required mechanical ventilation; the overall mortality rate was 4.2%.[134]

Soon after birth it is difficult to predict the clinical course of an infant's condition. In general, infants who have large amounts of thick meconium in the trachea and grossly abnormal chest radiographs have a more severe subsequent disease course, but this is not always the case.[144]

Pulmonary Function

Few studies describing the changes in pulmonary function associated with aspiration of meconium have been reported. When thick particulate meconium is aspirated into the small airways, the airways become partially obstructed, resulting in gas trapping and overinflation distal to the obstruction. The obstruction can also result in a decreased ventilation-perfusion ratio that is manifested by hypoxemia. The increased airway resistance and reduced lung compliance produce increased work of breathing that in turn causes the alveolar hypoventilation and carbon dioxide retention observed in the more severe cases of meconium aspiration. When the small airways are completely obstructed, the alveolar gas distal to the obstruction is reabsorbed, and the alveoli collapse, thus increasing the intrapulmonary shunting and arterial hypoxemia. This is favored when the infant requires high oxygen concentrations. The presence of meconium in the airways can also trigger an inflammatory reaction in the bronchial and alveolar epithelium, resulting in a diffuse chemical pneumonitis. This can reduce the diffusing capacity and may contribute to the hypoxemia seen in these patients.[145]

Neonates with severe MAS have a marked reduction in dynamic lung compliance.[146] This can be secondary to the changes in lung elasticity caused by the inflammatory reaction produced by the meconium, to inactivation of alveolar surfactant, and to the significant increase in airway resistance found in most of these infants.[147,148] Minute ventilation is usually increased as a consequence of an increased respiratory rate, but because the tidal volume is reduced, there is an increase in dead space ventilation, and alveolar ventilation is decreased, leading to carbon dioxide retention.[143,149]

Management

The infant with MAS frequently has some degree of fetal asphyxia. For this reason, the respiratory course is complicated by dysfunction of multiple organ systems, especially the central nervous, cardiovascular, and renal systems.

In infants with evidence of respiratory failure, an arterial blood gas analysis and a chest radiograph should be obtained as soon as possible. The inspired oxygen concentration must be adjusted to maintain the $Pa{O_2}$ above 70 mm Hg or the oxygen saturation above 95%. Some degree of metabolic acidosis is frequently observed as a result of perinatal asphyxia. If persistent, this must be corrected to decrease the risk of pulmonary hypertension. In infants who remain hypoxemic despite the use of high inspired oxygen concentrations or in infants in whom the $Pa{CO_2}$ rapidly increases above 50 to 60 mm Hg, it is necessary to use intermittent positive-pressure ventilation. Because of the reduced lung compliance and increased airway resistance, these infants often require high peak inspiratory pressures. This, plus the meconium-induced lung damage, makes pneumothorax a relatively frequent complication. Because most of these infants are hyperactive and restless, it is often necessary to use sedation or even neuromuscular blockade, at least during the first 24 to 48 hours of mechanical ventilation, until the infant is stable and the peak airway pressure in the ventilator can be reduced.[150]

In infants with severe respiratory failure who do not respond to conventional mechanical ventilation, the use of high-frequency ventilation using jet ventilators or oscillators can improve gas exchange and arterial blood gas levels.[151] This is usually indicated when the patient develops pulmonary hypertension with extrapulmonary right-to-left shunting and severe hypoxemia. Because meconium aspiration can inactivate alveolar surfactant, the administration of exogenous surfactant has been successfully used in some of these infants.[152,153]

As mentioned before, the risk of bacterial infection is increased in infants with MAS, but the clinical diagnosis of a superimposed infection is difficult. When bacterial pneumonia is suspected because of fever, an abnormal white blood cell count, or a deterioration in respiratory function and the appearance on radiograph, blood and tracheal cultures should be obtained and antibiotic therapy initiated. There is no clear evidence to justify the use of prophylactic antibiotics in meconium aspiration, but some clinicians elect to administer antibiotics until the acute respiratory failure subsides.

The severity of the respiratory failure should not cause the physician to overlook other complications that frequently occur as a consequence of perinatal asphyxia. As mentioned before, central nervous system, cardiovascular, renal, and metabolic function should be monitored closely, and any alteration must be promptly corrected.

Prevention

The prevention of MAS must start before birth by taking all the necessary precautions to reduce the risk of fetal distress. In the presence of meconium-stained amniotic fluid, intrapartum saline amnioinfusion reduces the risk of meconium aspiration by the fetus and also the incidence of fetal acidemia at birth.[154,155] This beneficial effect may result from dilution of the meconium by the amnioinfusion and from correction of a possible cord compression secondary to oligohydramnios.

When meconium appears in the amniotic fluid or upper airway at the time of birth, the first concern should be to reduce the risk of aspiration into the more distal airspaces and thereby prevent the subsequent pulmonary involvement. Based on experience published in the literature suggesting that early suctioning of the airway could reduce the risk of MAS,[156,157] the recommended approach has been to suction the nasopharynx with a large catheter or a suction bulb, if possible before the chest emerges from the birth canal. This is followed by visualization of the vocal cords by direct laryngoscopy and endotracheal suctioning if thick meconium is present below the vocal cords. The aspiration must be repeated until all meconium is removed from the larger airways. The suction of the airway can be accomplished using a number of mechanical devices.[158] Mouth suction should be avoided to prevent aspiration of contaminated material by the operator.

Recently, there has been controversy regarding the approach to the meconium-stained infant. Some clinicians suggest that infants whose breathing is not depressed at birth and who have thin meconium should not be exposed to the possible risks of endotracheal suctioning because the incidence of MAS is extremely low.[159-161] In fact, some have even proposed that early nasopharyngeal suctioning before the infant emerges from the birth canal may not be of benefit.[162] Because it is a relatively simple, risk-free procedure, most clinicians still recommend early suctioning of the nasopharynx to reduce the risk of aspiration into the lower airways when there is any evidence of meconium in the amniotic fluid.

Although most infants with MAS survive without sequelae, long-term follow-up studies have demonstrated an increased prevalence of hyperreactive airway disease similar to that in premature infants with chronic lung disease.[163,164]

PERSISTENT PULMONARY HYPERTENSION OF THE NEWBORN

PPHN was originally described by Siassi et al[165] in a group of infants without significant lung disease. Today, most cases occur in infants with pulmonary pathologic conditions such as MAS, with sepsis and pneumonia, and with lung hypoplasia such as that which occurs in congenital diaphragmatic hernia.

Pathogenesis

In the normal neonate, pulmonary vascular resistance decreases rapidly after birth in response to an increase in lung volume, blood pH, oxygen tension, and concentration of vascular dilating prostaglandins.[166,167] This reduction produces a fall in the pulmonary artery and right ventricular pressures that results in the cessation of right-to-left shunting through the foramen ovale and the ductus arteriosus. This normal process can be altered in response to hypoxia, acidosis, infection, or pulmonary hypoplasia and a decreased vascular cross-sectional area. In these conditions, the pulmonary artery pressure remains elevated to values that may surpass systemic blood pressure, maintaining the right-to-left shunting through the foramen ovale and ductus arteriosus.[168] This results in severe arterial hypoxemia that is relatively unresponsive to increased concentrations of inspired oxygen. The elevated pressure in the right ventricle frequently produces tricuspid regurgitation that increases the likelihood of shunting at the atrial level. This may be aggravated by the papillary muscle necrosis in the tricuspid valve that occurs in some infants who suffer severe perinatal asphyxia.[169]

Postmortem examination of the pulmonary circulation in a group of infants who died of PPHN demonstrated an increase in vascular smooth muscle and extension into the peripheral vascular bed; thus these infants may have suffered an antenatal insult that altered the pulmonary vasculature, which prevented normal adaptation after birth.[170] Other factors that may predispose an infant to PPHN are antenatal exposure to prostaglandin inhibitory drugs[171,172] and polycythemia.[173] Increased concentrations in serum or tracheobronchial secretions of a number of prostanoids and inflammatory mediators such as leukotrienes, thromboxane, and platelet-activating factor have been described in infants with PPHN. All these substances are potent vasoconstrictors and are therefore likely to play an important role in the pathogenesis of this syndrome.[174-176]

The magnitude of the right-to-left shunt in infants with PPHN is determined by the pressure gradient between the two circulations. Therefore systemic hypotension secondary to sepsis or asphyxia increases the severity of the shunting and the hypoxemia.[177]

Clinical Presentation and Diagnosis

Most infants with PPHN are born at term and have evidence of perinatal asphyxia and meconium aspiration or neonatal infection (see Table 31-1). This syndrome occurs only occasionally in preterm infants or in neonates with no lung disease. In some cases the infant is hypoxemic from birth, but more often there is a period of adequate oxygenation that may last for minutes or a few hours. During the first few hours after birth, there are a progressive deterioration in arterial oxygen tension and frequently an increase in carbon dioxide tension. The progressive hypoxemia becomes unresponsive to further increases in inspired oxygen concentration and frequently is disproportionate to the degree of pulmonary involvement. In most cases, large fluctuations in the Pao_2 also occur spontaneously or in response to physical stimulation and activity of the infant. In infants with ductal right-to-left shunting a difference between preductal and postductal oxygenation confirms the presence of a shunt at that level. The echocardiographic demonstration of high pulmonary artery pressure, tricuspid regurgitation, and shunting through the foramen ovale and ductus arteriosus confirms the diagnosis of PPHN.[178]

Prevention and Management

The management of PPHN poses one of the most difficult challenges in neonatal intensive care. Prevention and correction of predisposing factors such as perinatal asphyxia, sepsis, and polycythemia should be the first steps. Correction of hypoxemia and acidosis, both potent pulmonary vasoconstrictors, should also be pursued aggressively. The arterial oxygen tension must be maintained over 100 mm Hg to prevent hypoxemia during spontaneous fluctuations in oxygenation. A small degree of metabolic and respiratory alkalemia can result in a marked reduction in shunting and an improvement in oxygenation.[179,180] Hyperventilation is accomplished by inducing large tidal volumes and high respiratory rates on the ventilator, possibly resulting in gas trapping and excessive alveolar pressure. This may in turn impede venous return and pulmonary blood flow and worsen the hemodynamic condition of the patient.[181] In the more severe cases of PPHN, the use of high-frequency ventilation can markedly improve carbon dioxide elimination and oxygenation but can also induce gas trapping and an excessively increasing alveolar pressure.[182-185] Prolonged hyperventilation and hypocapnia have also been associated with poor neurodevelopmental outcome, which is most likely related to the decrease in cerebral blood flow induced by the hypocapnia.[186,187]

Cardiovascular support also plays an important role in the management of infants with PPHN. Medications such as dopamine, isoproterenol, and dobutamine are frequently used to increase arterial blood pressure and improve cardiac output.[179,188] Calcium infusion can improve myocardial function, particularly when hyperventilation decreases the levels of plasma ionized calcium.[189] Sedation and muscle relaxation are also used in infants whose spontaneous activity interferes with mechanical ventilation, resulting in deterioration of gas exchange.[150] A number of vasodilators have been used in PPHN, but none has been shown to alter the final outcome.[190] The major limitation with medications such as α-adrenergic blockers, calcium channel blockers, and prostacyclin is their lack of specificity; therefore they induce systemic hypotension. Prostaglandin D_2, a selective pulmonary vasodilator in fetal animals, was used in a group of infants with PPHN, but the results were also disappointing.[191] Recently, encouraging results have been reported using inhaled nitric oxide, a potent vasodilator that is rapidly inactivated in the blood and therefore has minimal or no systemic effect.[192-194] Because nitric oxide is a gas that is delivered into the airways, it reaches the better ventilated portions of the lung, preventing the ventilation-perfusion mismatch that can occur when vasodilators are administered systemically. The administration of inhaled nitric oxide to infants with PPHN results in a rapid improvement in oxygenation in more than half of patients and reduces the need for extracorporeal membrane oxygenation.[195-197]

Infants who do not respond to management can be treated with extracorporeal membrane oxygenation.[198,199] The survival rate with this mode of therapy in most centers is better than 90%, but because of the possible complications and long-term sequelae, this procedure is still used only as a last resort.[185,200,201]

The final outcome of neonates with PPHN depends on the underlying condition, the severity of the disease course, and the effectiveness of management. Although most infants survive, many require ventilatory support for long periods, and a few have central nervous system sequelae related to episodes of severe hypoxia and the hypocapnia induced by hyperventilation.[187,202] Some infants develop chronic lung disease as a result of pulmonary damage produced by infection or the aspiration of meconium or as a result of the aggressive mechanical ventilation required to maintain adequate gas exchange.

PULMONARY GAS LEAKS

A major complication in infants with respiratory failure, especially those who need assisted ventilation (see Table 31-1), is lung rupture and gas leak. Rupture of the terminal airways leads to the accumulation of extraalveolar gas, PIE, pneumomediastinum, pneumothorax, subcutaneous emphysema, or gas embolization of the lymphatic system and pulmonary and systemic circulations.

Pulmonary Interstitial Emphysema

PIE results from relative hyperinflation and commonly represents the first step in the progression to extraalveolar gas accumulation. It is important because of the significant pathophysiologic alterations it causes and the fact that it can progress to more severe forms of extraalveolar gas leak (Fig. 31-13).

Pathogenesis

PIE is caused by a dissection of gas from ruptured overdistended terminal airways or alveoli into the pulmonary interstitium. The amount of interstitial gas is variable. PIE can occur spontaneously in infants with parenchymal lung disease but more frequently occurs as a complication of mechanical ventilation.

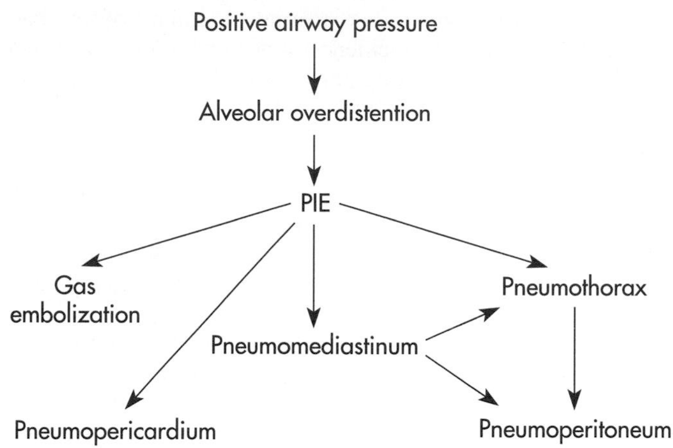

Fig. 31-13. Progression of pulmonary gas leak. (From Bancalari E, Goldman SL. In Milunsky A et al, eds: *Advances in perinatal medicine,* New York, 1989, Plenum, p 151.)

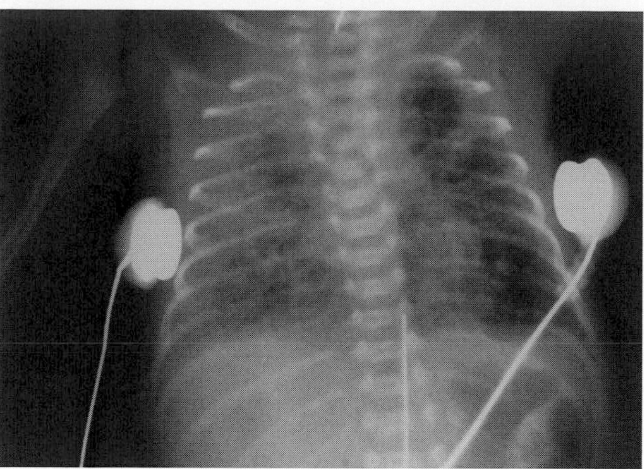

Fig. 31-14. PIE. Fine, bubbly appearance of the lungs in an infant with severe HMD. (From Bancalari E, Goldman SL. In Milunsky A et al, eds: *Advances in perinatal medicine,* New York, 1989, Plenum, p 154.)

To understand the pathophysiology of PIE, the clinician must consider that the alveoli of the newborn are less apt to compensate for excessive pressure and volume than those of the older individual. In the adult, interalveolar pores (pores of Kohn) can act as "pop-off" valves that allow higher intraalveolar pressures to equilibrate with adjacent alveoli in instances when the intraalveolar pressure is not uniform. However, these communicating pores are decreased in number and size in the newborn. Because during mechanical ventilation the pressure is not transmitted to all alveoli uniformly, the newborn has a larger propensity for developing alveolar rupture. This is further exaggerated by the presence of meconium, blood, or other particulate matter that can exacerbate the uneven aeration. It has been postulated that alveolar rupture and PIE develop when there is a large pressure gradient between the alveolus and the adjacent vascular bed.[203] However, because of experimental work using rabbits, it appears that the absolute amount of intrapulmonary pressure generated is directly responsible for the development of PIE. It appears that not only pressure but also mechanical stress resulting from overdistention of alveoli are essential in the development of alveolar rupture.[204] Once alveoli have ruptured, gas enters the adjacent interstitial tissue, where it can dissect along the perivascular (particularly pulmonary venous) sheaths to the hilum of the lung. When the volume of gas in the interstitium is large enough, the resulting perivascular pressure can produce vascular collapse, thus obstructing the pulmonary circulation.

Incidence

The incidence of PIE in infants with very low birth weights was reported to be 32%.[205] A significant reduction in the incidence of PIE, as low as 7%, has been reported with the use of exogenous surfactant in infants with HMD.[57,72] In patients requiring conventional mechanical ventilation, the use of high rates and short inspiratory times appears to reduce the incidence of gas leak, including PIE.[36]

Diagnosis

Initially, the development of PIE is rarely associated with demonstrable changes in cardiorespiratory function, but when the PIE is severe and diffuse, deterioration of the respiratory status occurs with hypoxemia and hypercarbia. The chest radiograph confirms the diagnosis: The lungs have a fine, bubbly appearance, sometimes with larger lucent areas (Fig. 31-14).

Management

Management consists primarily of preventing progression to other forms of gas leak by using the lowest effective airway pressures and short inspiratory times in the ventilator. Randomized clinical trials comparing conventional mechanical ventilation with high-frequency ventilation have failed to show a reduction in the incidence of PIE with the use of high-frequency ventilation.[39-41] However, more recent studies suggest that the use of high-frequency ventilation can be effective in the treatment of PIE[45] and could also reduce the incidence of PIE in infants with severe HMD.[206]

For unilateral PIE, selective intubation of the mainstem bronchus in the unaffected side[207] or positioning of the infant with the involved side down[208] may be beneficial. In the case of severe PIE, especially when it has progressed to the formation of large cysts, surgical resection of the affected lobe should be considered.[209]

Pneumomediastinum

Pneumomediastinum, a collection of gas within the pleural boundaries of the mediastinum, can occur spontaneously or as a complication of mechanical ventilation.

Pathogenesis

Gas is thought to enter the mediastinum after moving along the vascular sheaths toward the hilum of the lung and from there, rupturing through the pleura into the mediastinal area. Another cause of pneumomediastinum is traumatic perforation of the pharynx or esophagus.[210] The incidence in well newborns is about 2%[211] but is significantly higher in infants with pulmonary pathologic conditions.[212]

Diagnosis

Pneumomediastinum is symptomatic only if the collection of gas is under sufficient pressure to compress adjacent structures such as the heart or blood vessels, producing cardiorespiratory decompensation. The diagnosis is made radiographically by a radiolucency around the heart, which makes the heart borders appear more distinct.

Management

There is no specific treatment for pneumomediastinum.

Pneumothorax

Pneumothorax is the accumulation of gas in the pleural space between the parietal and visceral pleura. When the pressure of this gas is greater than the atmospheric pressure, the pneumothorax is considered to be "under tension." Although pneumothorax can occur spontaneously, it is one of the most common manifestations of pulmonary barotrauma in neonates requiring mechanical ventilation.

Pathogenesis

Pneumothorax in the neonate is thought to be produced in most cases by movement of gas caused by the mediastinum rupturing through the mediastinal pleura into the pleural space. A large pneumothorax can produce significant deleterious effects on cardiac output and can increase pulmonary vascular resistance. As the pneumothorax increases in size, compensatory mechanisms can no longer prevent decreases in cardiac output and systemic blood pressure. The decrease in cardiac output can be explained by the increased intrathoracic pressure that decreases venous return to the heart and also can act as a cardiac tamponade. In addition, lung collapse increases pulmonary vascular resistance[213] and contributes to the decrease in cardiac output. Several of these factors also affect ventilation and oxygenation and account for the respiratory changes associated with pneumothorax. Increasing amounts of pleural gas result in a decrease in tidal volume that can initially be compensated for by an increase in respiratory rate but if severe leads to decreased minute ventilation and hypercarbia. As lung volume is decreased and some areas are collapsed, there is an increased ventilation-perfusion mismatch, resulting in an intrapulmonary shunt and hypoxemia.

Intracranial pressure usually increases as a result of an increase in arterial blood pressure, obstruction of venous return, and increased cerebral blood flow. In the premature infant, these factors can increase the risk of intraventricular hemorrhage.[214]

Incidence

The incidence of spontaneous, asymptomatic pneumothorax in the newborn has been reported to be 1%.[211] Pneumothoraces are more frequent in infants with specific lung pathologic conditions that require mechanical ventilation. Before the introduction of surfactant, the incidence of pneumothorax in patients with HMD treated with CPAP alone was close to 20%.[215] In infants with HMD who required mechanical ventilation but did not receive surfactant, the incidence of pneumothorax was 18% when a rate of 60 breaths/min and a short inspiratory time were used, but the incidence was significantly higher (33%) in infants treated with a slow respiratory rate and longer inspiratory time.[35] The use of high-frequency ventilation in infants with HMD has not affected the incidence of pneumothorax.[40,42]

The introduction of exogenous surfactant in the management of infants with HMD has produced a dramatic reduction in the incidence of pneumothorax to a rate as low as 3% to 10% in the treated infants.[56,57,74] Early administration of surfactant seems to be important in reducing the incidence of pneumothorax. When prophylactic administration of surfactant was compared with rescue treatment in infants of less than 30 weeks' gestation, the incidence of pneumothorax was 7% in the prophylaxis group compared with 18% in the infants treated several hours after birth.[62,216]

Diagnosis

Clinically, the signs of pneumothorax in the neonate are variable. Although most spontaneously occurring pneumothoraces are asymptomatic, significant clinical deterioration indicates the diagnosis when pneumothorax is associated with lung disease or mechanical ventilation.

Spontaneously breathing infants who develop large pneumothoraces demonstrate the classic signs of respiratory failure, including cyanosis, grunting, intercostal and substernal retractions, tachypnea, and nasal flaring. These signs are sometimes difficult to evaluate in infants whose lungs are ventilated and in whom the only obvious sign of pneumothorax may be abrupt deterioration of the arterial blood gas levels. On physical examination, a pneumothorax is suggested by asymmetric chest expansion, downward displacement of the liver, and decreased heart and breath sounds on the side of the pneumothorax. The latter sign is particularly unreliable in the small premature infant whose breath sounds are easily heard uniformly all over the chest. A pneumothorax is frequently followed by an increase in respiratory rate, heart rate, and arterial blood pressure.[217]

A tension pneumothorax may be associated with shift in the heart sounds to the contralateral side. Frequently there are significant changes in the vital signs in an infant in whom a tension pneumothorax develops.

The chest radiograph is the best method of confirming the diagnosis. If the radiograph is taken with the infant in a supine position with an anteroposterior view, the pneumothorax can be seen as a crescent-shaped lucency along the lateral aspect of the thorax (Fig. 31-15) without lung markings extending into the lucent area. Care must be taken not to confuse a skinfold or blanket with this type of appearance. These "artifacts" can fre-

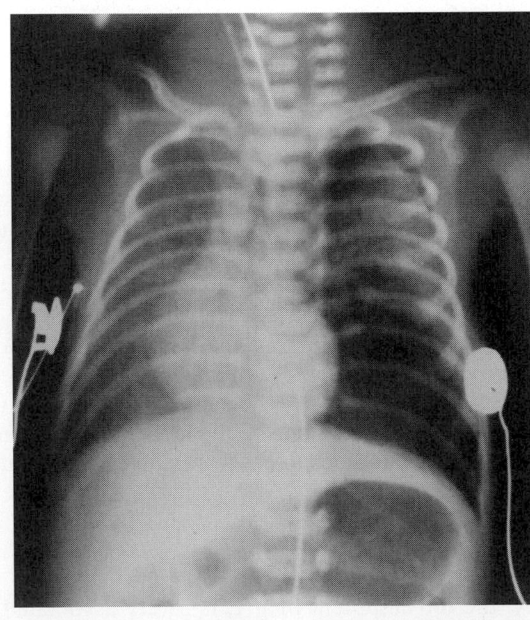

Fig. 31-15. Pneumothorax. Small crescent-shaped lucency is seen on the left at the level of the apex. (From Bancalari E, Goldman SL. In Milunsky A et al, eds: *Advances in perinatal medicine,* New York, 1989, Plenum, p 156.)

quently be recognized because they extend below the diaphragm. If the lungs do not collapse because of poor compliance or if the accumulation of extrapulmonary gas is anterior, the crescent-shaped lucency may not be present, and the only suggestion of a pneumothorax is a generalized decreased density on the side of the extrapulmonary gas. A medial pneumothorax appears as a lucency just to the right or left of the heart borders. In these cases, the presence of a pneumothorax can be ascertained by obtaining a "cross-table" lateral film. This method should be reserved for the infant who is too unstable to rotate to the decubitus position because the anterior lucency may be difficult to distinguish from a pneumomediastinum.

The presence of a tension pneumothorax is recognized because the mediastinum is shifted to the opposite side, the intercostal spaces are widened, and the diaphragm is flattened on the ipsilateral side (Fig. 31-16). If bilateral tension pneumothoraces occur simultaneously, there may be no shift of the mediastinum, but the bilaterally increased pressure compresses the heart, resulting in a smaller cardiac silhouette. Even with a tension pneumothorax, a noncompliant lung in an infant with HMD may not completely collapse. Transillumination of the chest with a fiberoptic light source is a very useful adjunct for diagnosing pneumothorax,[218] particularly in small premature infants in whom physical examination is unreliable. The thin chest wall of such infants allows for a demonstration of the "halo" of light that indicates extrapulmonary gas. Transillumination of the chest in larger infants with thicker chest walls occasionally gives false-negative results. Thus a radiographic examination should not be omitted because of a negative transillumination. However, with significant clinical deterioration, treatment should not be delayed for radiographic confirmation if a diagnosis of pneumothorax is suspected and supported by transillumination.

Management

When the diagnosis of pneumothorax is suspected, the plan for treatment is based on the following considerations: the size of the pneumothorax, the extent of the infant's respiratory deterioration, and the use of positive-pressure ventilation. A pneumothorax diagnosed in an infant with no symptoms does not require specific therapy, but the infant should be observed closely for possible signs of respiratory decompensation.

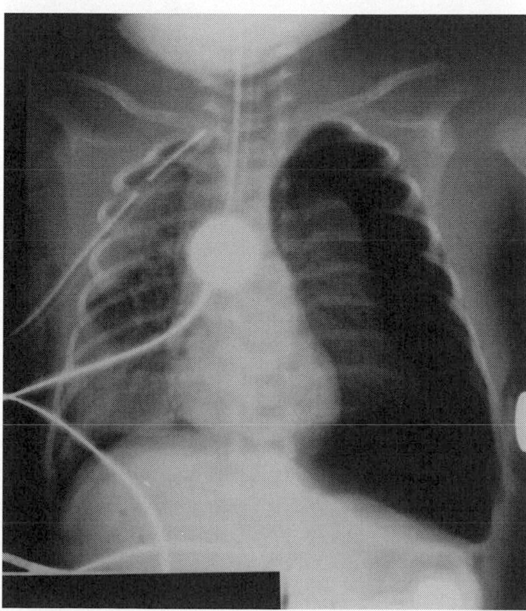

Fig. 31-16. Left tension pneumothorax. Tension is indicated by the contralateral shift of the mediastinum, small heart size, and depressed left diaphragm. (From Bancalari E, Goldman SL. In Milunsky A et al, eds: *Advances in perinatal medicine,* New York, 1989, Plenum, p 162.)

If the pneumothorax is associated with cardiorespiratory symptoms, immediate treatment is indicated. Evacuation can be accomplished by needle aspiration or by thoracostomy with chest tube insertion. The administration of 100% oxygen can accelerate the reabsorption of gas. This is based on the fact that breathing 100% oxygen will "wash out" nitrogen from the body, including the tissues surrounding the pneumothorax. This causes a gradient, facilitating faster absorption of the nitrogen from the gas collection into the bloodstream. Because of the risk of retinopathy of prematurity, this method should not be used in preterm infants. Needle aspiration is indicated only as a temporizing measure in an infant who has a tension pneumothorax or who requires positive-pressure ventilation. In these cases, the immediate placement of a chest tube is indicated. The thoracostomy tube should then be attached to an underwater seal so that air will not be drawn into the pleural space. If the volume of the pneumothorax is relatively small, the negative pressure maintained by the underwater seal is sufficient to evacuate the extrapulmonary gas. However, if there is a large volume of gas or if there is a continuous gas leak, negative pressure (15 to 20 cm H_2O) should be applied to the system to ensure complete evacuation. When there is no further drainage, the negative pressure can be discontinued, and if no reaccumulation occurs, the chest tube can be clamped and removed in 24 hours. In infants with severe pulmonary disease requiring high positive airway pressures, it may be advisable to delay the removal of the chest tube until the infant is weaned from mechanical ventilation.

Outcome

Pneumothorax is a potentially fatal complication, but if diagnosed and treated promptly, it may have only minimal consequences. The keys to preventing a poor outcome are a high index of suspicion in infants at risk and the proper equipment and personnel for effectively diagnosing and treating the disorder.

Pneumopericardium

Although the pericardial sac is not in direct communication with the pleural space, extrapulmonary gas can collect in the pericardium. This form of gas leak is not common.

Pathogenesis

The mechanism of gas entry seems to be directly from the pulmonary interstitial air, traveling along the great vessels into the pericardial sac.[219] The physiologic effects of a pneumopericardium are essentially those of cardiac tamponade. Increased pressure around the heart interferes with diastolic filling, resulting in increased central venous pressure and decreased cardiac output. This produces arterial hypotension with a narrow pulse pressure.

Diagnosis

The clinical signs of pneumopericardium in the neonate are variable, and most are nonspecific. A small pneumopericardium may develop without any significant change in the infant's cardiorespiratory status, being noticed only incidentally on the chest radiograph. When gas is accumulated under tension, an increase in respiratory distress and hypoxemia is observed, and heart sounds become distant with a decrease in arterial and pulse pressure. An increase in the central venous pressure may also be noticed. Pneumopericardium is rarely isolated because it is most commonly associated with other forms of gas leak.

The diagnosis of pneumopericardium must be suspected in any infant in whom there is an acute clinical deterioration of mechanical ventilation. A decrease in both pulse pressure and mean arterial blood pressure should alert the clinician to this diagnosis. The chest radiograph confirms the diagnosis by showing a gas lucency surrounding the heart on the anteroposterior and lateral films (Fig. 31-17).

Management

When a pneumopericardium is symptomatic, immediate drainage is imperative. Decompression can be accomplished by needle aspiration, but continuous drainage via placement of a pericardial catheter is necessary in most cases to prevent reaccumulation of gas. Without treatment, the mortality rate approaches 70%, and even with pericardiocentesis, the mortality rate remains high (20% to 60%).[220]

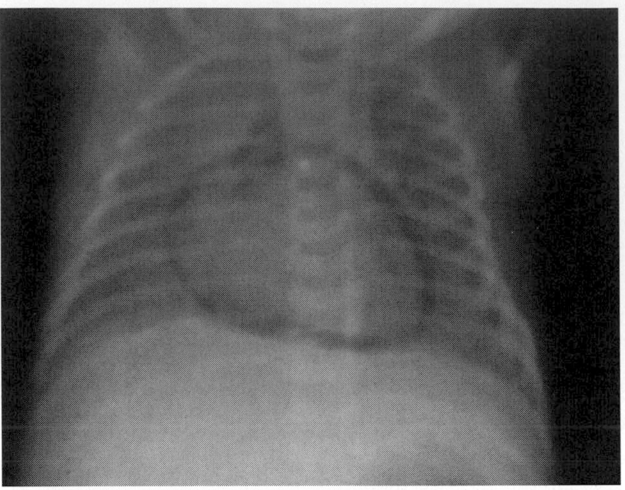

Fig. 31-17. Pneumopericardium. The heart is clearly outlined by a collection of gas in the pericardium. (From Bancalari E, Goldman SL. In Milunsky A et al, eds: *Advances in perinatal medicine,* New York, 1989, Plenum, p 163.)

Pneumoperitoneum

Free gas in the peritoneal cavity, previously considered evidence of bowel perforation, is now recognized as a possible complication of ventilator therapy and not necessarily the result of a perforated viscera. In infants whose lungs are ventilated for HMD, the reported incidence was 1.7% before the introduction of surfactant.[221]

Pathogenesis

Although the diaphragm separates the thorax from the peritoneal cavity, there are potential areas through which gas can cross from one cavity to the other. Free gas in the mediastinum or pleural space can dissect caudally along the perivascular and periesophageal tissue sheaths into the retroperitoneal space and thence into the peritoneum.

Diagnosis

The signs of pneumoperitoneum secondary to pulmonary gas leak are nonspecific. Commonly, there is abdominal distention, which may be severe enough to compromise ventilation by elevating the diaphragm. The clinical setting in which pneumoperitoneum occurs is characteristic: The infant is receiving high ventilatory pressures and usually has evidence of intrathoracic gas leak before the discovery of intraperitoneal free gas. The development of pneumoperitoneum is not usually associated with clinical deterioration unless the volume of gas is massive enough to compromise ventilation. The diagnosis is confirmed radiographically (Fig. 31-18). Unfortunately, no specific radiographic signs accurately define the presence or absence of visceral perforation.

Management

Pneumoperitoneum secondary to pulmonary gas leak usually requires no specific treatment. Rather, attention should be directed at preventing or decompressing the intrathoracic gas collection that leads to the pneumoperitoneum. Once gas is present in the peritoneum, no treatment is necessary unless a perforated viscera is suspected or unless there is significant tension that can be relieved by needle aspiration.

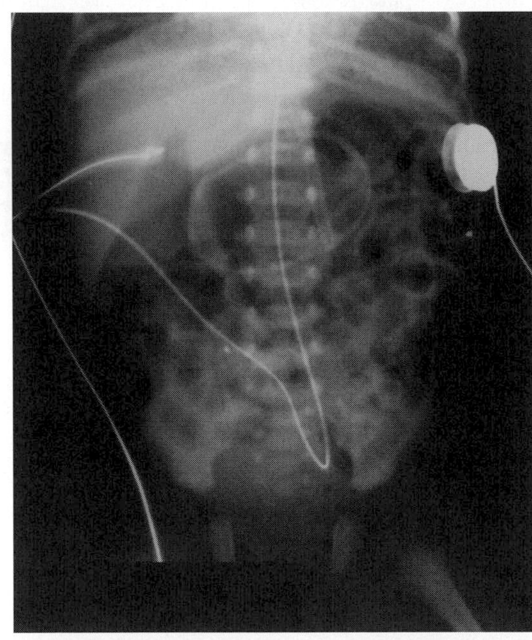

Fig. 31-18. Pneumoperitoneum. The wall of the stomach is distinct, indicating the presence of an abnormal collection of gas within the peritoneal cavity surrounding the stomach. (From Bancalari E, Goldman SL. In Milunsky A et al, eds: *Advances in perinatal medicine,* New York, 1989, Plenum, p 164.)

Gas Embolization

Intravascular gas embolism is the rarest but most catastrophic consequence of acute pulmonary barotrauma. Gregory and Tooley[222] were the first to report a case of gas embolism in a newborn who had HMD and who was receiving positive-pressure ventilation.

Pathogenesis

Gas embolism is thought to result from functional alveolar-capillary fistulas. In spontaneously breathing infants, the pres-

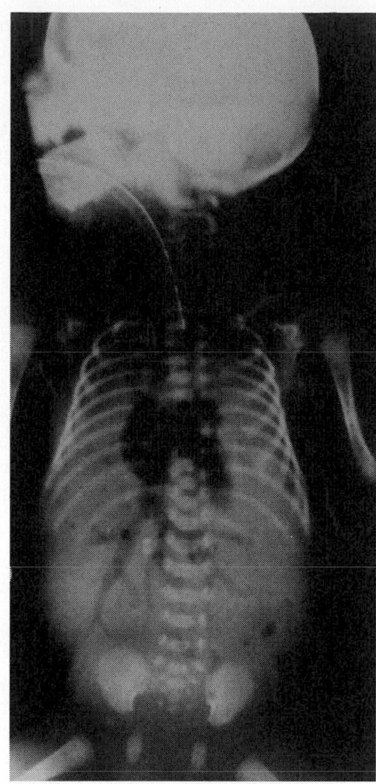

Fig. 31-19. Gas embolization. Postmortem radiograph of a premature infant who died suddenly while requiring high ventilatory pressures. Gas can be seen within the heart and in some intraabdominal veins. (From Bancalari E, Goldman SL. In Milunsky A et al, eds: *Advances in perinatal medicine,* New York, 1989, Plenum, p 129.)

sure in the pulmonary capillary bed is grater than that in the alveolus. However, with the application of positive airway pressure, this gradient is reversed, favoring the movement of gas from the alveolus into the vascular space. Once in the vascular space, the gas can travel to all parts of the body, including the cerebral and cardiac circulations, leading to rapid death from vascular obstruction.

Diagnosis

Most of the cases reported are of premature infants receiving relatively high airway pressures. Characteristically, these infants have radiographic evidence of other forms of gas leak before the development of gas embolism. Clinically, they have acute cardiovascular deterioration with development of pallor or cyanosis, bradycardia, and hypotension. Often, the diagnosis is made when gas bubbles are withdrawn from an artery or a venous catheter during the clinical deterioration. The diagnosis is confirmed radiographically with demonstration of gas shadows within the heart chambers and vascular tree (Fig. 31-19).

Massive gas embolism is invariably fatal. Thus treatment must be viewed as preventive: The lowest possible ventilatory pressures should be used to prevent alveolar rupture and gas leak.

WILSON-MIKITY SYNDROME

Wilson-Mikity syndrome was first described in 1960 and is characterized by late-onset progressive respiratory distress that occurs in small preterm infants. In contrast to chronic lung disease, it presents in infants without severe initial respiratory distress syndrome.[223,224] The respiratory symptoms usually begin between 1 and 4 weeks of age and last several weeks or months, after which most infants recover gradually. Radiographically, the lungs have a cystlike appearance with diffuse streaks of increased density resembling the changes observed in infants with chronic lung disease. On histologic examination the lungs show areas of hyperinflation alternating with areas of collapse and septal thickening, but in contrast with infants with chronic lung disease, these infants do not show significant changes in the airway epithelium. The etiology and pathogenesis of Wilson-Mikity syndrome are not known, but congenital infections have been mentioned as possible causes. This condition is seldom diagnosed today in spite of the fact that the surviving rate of very small infants has increased.

REFERENCES

Hyaline Membrane Disease

1. Hulsey TC, Alexander GR, Robillard PY, Annibale DJ, Keenan A: Hyaline membrane disease: the role of ethnicity and maternal risk characteristics, *Am J Obstet Gynecol* 168:572-576, 1993.
2. Torday J: Cellular timing of fetal lung development, *Semin Perinatol* 16(2):130-139, 1992.
3. Hall Guttentag S, Phelps DS, Floros J: Surfactant protein regulation and diabetic pregnancy, *Semin Perinatol* 16(2):122-129, 1992.
4. Goldberg JD, Cohen WR, Friedman EA: Cesarean section indication and the risk of respiratory distress syndrome, *Obstet Gynecol* 57:30-32, 1981.
5. Hjalmarson O, Krantz ME, Jacobsson B, Sorensen SE: The importance of neonatal asphyxia and caesarean section as risk factors for neonatal respiratory disorders in an unselected population, *Acta Pediatr Scand* 71:403-408, 1982.
6. Chiswick ML: Prolonged rupture of membranes, preeclamptic toxemia and respiratory distress syndrome, *Arch Dis Child* 51:674-679, 1976.
7. Gluck L, Kulovich MV: Lecithin-sphingomyelin ratios in amniotic fluid in normal and abnormal pregnancy, *Am J Obstet Gynecol* 115:539-546, 1973.
8. Crowley P, Chalmers I, Keirse MJNC: The effects of corticosteroid administration before preterm delivery: an overview of the evidence from controlled trials, *Br J Obstet Gynecol* 97:11-25, 1990.
9. Collaborative Group on Antenatal Steroid Therapy: Effect of antenatal dexamethasone administration on the prevention of respiratory distress syndrome, *Am J Obstet Gynecol* 141:276-286, 1981.
10. Ballard RA, Ballard PL, Creasy RK, Padbury J, Polk DH, Bracken M, Moya FR, Gross I: Respiratory disease in very low birth weight infants after prenatal thyrotropin-releasing hormone and glucocorticoid, *Lancet* 339:510-515, 1992.
11. Gribetz I, Frank NR, Avery ME: Static volume pressure relations of excised lungs of infants with hyaline membrane disease, newborns and stillborn infants, *J Clin Invest* 38:2168-2175, 1959.
12. Avery ME, Mead J: Surface properties in relation to atelectasis and hyaline membrane disease, *Am J Dis Child* 97:517-523, 1959.
13. Wright JR, Clements JA: Metabolism and turnover of lung surfactant, *Am Rev Respir Dis* 135:426-444, 1987 (review).
14. Van Iwaarden F, Welmers B, Verloef J, Haagsman HP, Van Golde LMG: Pulmonary surfactant protein A enhances the host-defense mechanisms of rat alveolar macrophages, *Am J Respir Cell Mol Biol* 2:91-98, 1990.
15. Hawgood S, Clements JA: Pulmonary surfactant and its apoproteins, *J Clin Invest* 86:1-6, 1990 (review).
16. King RJ, Clements JA: Surface active materials from dog lung. II. Composition and physiological correlations, *Am J Physiol* 223:715-726, 1972.
17. Ikegami M, Jobe A, Berry D: A protein that inhibits surfactant in respiratory distress syndrome, *Biol Neonate* 50:121-129, 1986.
18. McCann EM, Goldman SL, Brady JP: Pulmonary function in the sick newborn infant, *Pediatr Res* 21:313-325, 1987.
19. Dreizzen E, Migdal M, Praud JP, Magny JF, Dehan M, Chambille B, Gaultier C: Passive compliance of total respiratory system in preterm newborn infants with respiratory distress syndrome, *J Pediatr* 112:778-781, 1988.

20. Clements JA, Platzker ACG, Tierney DF, Hobel CG, Greasy RK, Margolis AJ, Thibeault DW, Tooley WH, Oh W: Assessment of the risk of the respiratory distress syndrome by a rapid test for surfactant in amniotic fluid, *N Engl J Med* 286:1077-1081, 1972.
21. Hallman M, Kulovich MV, Kirkpatrick E, Sugarman RG, Gluck L: Phosphatidylinositol and phosphatidylglycerol in amniotic fluid: indices of lung maturity, *Am J Obstet Gynecol* 125:613-617, 1976.
22. Kresch HC, Gross I: The biochemistry of fetal lung surfactant, *Clin Perinatol* 14:481-507, 1987.
23. Liggins GC, Howie RN: A controlled trial of antepartum glucocorticoid treatment for prevention of the respiratory distress syndrome in premature infants, *Pediatrics* 50:515-525, 1972.
24. ACTOBAT Study Group: Australian collaborative trial of antenatal thyrotropin-releasing hormone (ACTOBAT) for prevention of neonatal respiratory disease, *Lancet* 345:877-882, 1995.
25. Crowther CA, Hiller JE, Haslam RR, Robinson JS, the ACTOBAT Study Group: Australian collaborative trial of antenatal thyrotropin-releasing hormone: adverse effects at 12-month follow-up, *Pediatrics* 99:311-317, 1997.
26. Hay WW Jr, Thilo E, Brockway Curlander J: Pulse oximetry in neonatal medicine, *Clin Perinatol* 18(3):441-472, 1991.
27. Flynn JT, Bancalari E, Sim E, Goldberg RN, Feuer W, Cassady J, Schiffman J, Feldman H, Bachynski B, Buckley E, Roberts J, Gillings D: A cohort study of transcutaneous oxygen tension and the incidence and severity of retinopathy of prematurity, *N Engl J Med* 326:1050-1054, 1992.
28. Gregory GA, Kitterman JA, Phibbs RH, Tooley WH, Hamilton WK: Treatment of idiopathic respiratory distress syndrome with continuous positive airway pressure, *N Engl J Med* 284:1333-1340, 1971.
29. Rhodes PG, Hall RT: Continuous positive airway pressure delivered by face mask in infants with the idiopathic respiratory syndrome: a controlled study, *Pediatrics* 52:1-5, 1973.
30. Fanaroff AA, Cha CC, Sosa R, Crumrine RS, Klaus MH: Controlled trial of continuous negative external pressure in the treatment of severe respiratory distress syndrome, *J Pediatr* 83:921-928, 1973.
31. Drew JH: Immediate intubation at birth of the very low birthweight infant, *Am J Dis Child* 136:207-210, 1982.
32. Han VKM, Beverley DW, Clarson C, Sumabat WO, Shaheed WA, Brabyn DG, Chance GW: Randomized controlled trial of very early continuous distending pressure in the management of preterm infants, *Early Hum Dev* 15:21-32, 1987.
33. Spahr RC, Klein AM, Brown DR, MacDonald HM, Holzman IR: Hyaline membrane disease: a controlled study of inspiratory to expiratory ratio and its management by ventilator, *Am J Dis Child* 134:373-376, 1980.
34. Heicher DA, Kasting DS, Harrod JR: Prospective clinical comparison of two methods for mechanical ventilation of neonates: rapid rate and short inspiratory time versus slow rate and long inspiratory time, *J Pediatr* 98:957-961, 1981.
35. Oxford Region Controlled Trial of Artificial Ventilation (OCTAVE) Study Group: Multi-centre randomized controlled trial of high versus low frequency positive pressure ventilation, *Arch Dis Child* 66:770-775, 1991.
36. Pohlandt F, Saule H, Schroder H, Leonhardt A, Hornchen H, Wolff C, Bernsau U, Oppermann HC, Obladen M, Feilen KD, the Study Group: Decreased incidence of extra-alveolar air leakage or death prior to air leakage in high versus low rate positive pressure ventilation: results of a randomised seven-centre trial in preterm infants, *Eur J Pediatr* 151:904-909, 1992.
37. Durand DJ, Goodman A, Ray P, Ballard RA, Clyman RI: Theophylline treatment in the extubation of infants weighing less than 1250 grams: a controlled trial, *Pediatrics* 80:684-688, 1987.
38. Higgins RD, Richter SE, Davis JM: Nasal continuous positive airway pressure facilitates extubation of very low birth weight neonates, *Pediatrics* 88:999-1003, 1991.
39. Carlo WA, Chatburn RL, Martin RJ: Randomized trial of high-frequency jet ventilation versus conventional ventilation in respiratory distress syndrome, *J Pediatr* 110:275-282, 1987.
40. The Hifi Study Group: High frequency oscillatory ventilation compared with mechanical ventilation in the treatment of respiratory failure in preterm infants, *N Engl J Med* 320:88-93, 1989.
41. Carlo WA, Siner B, Chatburn RL, Robertson S, Martin RJ: Early randomized intervention with high frequency jet ventilation in respiratory distress syndrome, *J Pediatr* 117:765-770, 1990.
42. Clark RH, Gerstmann DR, Null DM, deLemos RA: Prospective randomized comparison of high-frequency oscillatory and conventional ventilation in respiratory distress syndrome, *Pediatrics* 89:5-12, 1992.
43. Keszler M, Modanlou HD, Brundo S, Clark FI, Cohen RS, Ryan RM, Kaneta MK, Davis JM: Multicenter controlled clinical trial of high-frequency jet ventilation in preterm infants with uncomplicated respiratory distress syndrome, *Pediatrics* 100:593-599, 1997.
44. Bhuta T, Henderson-Smart DJ: Elective high-frequency oscillatory ventilation versus conventional ventilation in preterm infants with pulmonary dysfunction: systematic review and meta-analyses, *Pediatrics* 100(5):1-7, URL: http://www.pediatrics.org, 1997.
45. Kesszler M, Donn SM, Bucciarelli RL, Alverson DC, Hart M, Lunyong V, Modanlou HD, Noguchi A, Pearlman SA, Puri A, Smith D, Stavis R, Watkins MN, Harris TR: Multicenter controlled trial comparing high-frequency jet ventilation and conventional mechanical ventilation in newborn infants with pulmonary interstitial emphysema, *J Pediatr* 119:85-93, 1991.
46. Greenough A, Milner AD: Respiratory support using patient triggered ventilation in the neonatal period, *Arch Dis Child* 67:69-71, 1992 (review).
47. Hummler H, Gernhardt T, Gonzalez A, Claure N, Everett R, Bancalari E: Influence of different methods of synchronized mechanical ventilation on ventilation, gas exchange, patient effort, and blood pressure fluctuations in premature neonates, *Pediatr Pulmonol* 22:305-313, 1996.
48. Cleary JP, Bernstein G, Mannino FL, Heldt GP: Improved oxygenation during synchronized intermittent mandatory ventilation in neonates with respiratory distress syndrome: a randomized, crossover study, *J Pediatr* 126:407-411, 1995.
49. Bernstein G, Mannino FL, Heldt GP, Callahan JD, Bull DH, Sola A, Ariagno RA, Hoffman GL, Frantz ID III, Troche BI, Roberts JL, Dela Cruz TV, Costa E: Randomized multicenter trial comparing synchronized and conventional intermittent mandatory ventilation in neonates, *J Pediatr* 128:453-463, 1996.
50. Goldberg RN, Chung D, Goldman SL, Bancalari E: The association of rapid volume expansion and intraventricular hemorrhage in the preterm infant, *J Pediatr* 96:1060-1063, 1980.
51. Bell EF, Warburton D, Stonestreet BS, Oh W: Effect of fluid administration on the development of symptomatic patent ductus arteriosus and congestive heart failure in premature infants, *N Engl J Med* 302:598-604, 1980.
52. Van Marter LJ, Leviton A, Alred EN, Pagano M, Kuban K: Hydration during the first days of life and the risk of bronchopulmonary dysplasia in low birth weight infants, *J Pediatr* 116:942-949, 1990.
53. Green TP, Johnson DE, Bass JL, Landrum BG, Ferrara B, Thompson T: Prophylactic furosemide in severe respiratory distress syndrome: blinded prospective study, *J Pediatr* 112:605-612, 1988.
54. Enhorning G, Robertson B: Lung expansion in the premature rabbit fetus after tracheal deposition of surfactant, *Pediatrics* 50:58-66, 1972.
55. Horbar JD, Soll RF, Sutherland JM, Kotagal U, Philip AGS, Kessler DL, Little GA, Edwards WH, Vidyasagar D, Raju TNK, Jobe AH, Ikegami M, Mullett MD, Myerberg DZ, McAuliffe TL, Lucey JF: A multicenter randomized, placebo-controlled trial of surfactant therapy for respiratory distress syndrome, *N Engl J Med* 320:959-965, 1989.
56. Soll RF, Hoekstra RE, Fangman JJ, Corbet AJ, Adams JM, James S, Schulze K, Oh W, Roberts JD, Dorst JP, Kramer SS, Gold J, Zola EM, Horbar JD, McAuliffe TL, Lucey JF, The Ross Collaborative Surfactant Prevention Study Group: Multicenter trial of single-dose modified bovine surfactant extract (Survanta) for prevention of respiratory distress syndrome, *Pediatrics* 85:1092-1102, 1990.
57. Long W, Thompson T, Sundell H, Schumacher R, Volberg F, Guthrie R, The American Exosurf Neonatal Study Group I: Effects of two rescue doses of a synthetic surfactant on mortality rate and survival without bronchopulmonary dysplasia in 700 to 1350 gram infants with respiratory distress syndrome, *J Pediatr* 118:595-605, 1991.
58. Horbar JD, Wright LL, Soll RF, Wright EC, Fanaroff AA, Korones SB, Shankaran S, Oh W, Fletcher BD, Bauer CR, Tyson JE, Lemons JA, Donovan EF, Stoll BJ, Stevenson DD, Papile LA, Philips J III: A multicenter randomized trial comparing two surfactants for the treatment of neonatal respiratory distress syndrome, *J Pediatr* 123:757-766, 1993.

59. Hudak ML, Farrel EE, Rosenberg AA, Jung AL, Auten RL, Durand DJ, Horgan MJ, Buckwald S, Belcastro MR, Donohue PK, Carrison V, Maniscalco WW, Balsn MJ, Torres BA, Miller RR, Jansen RD, Graeber JE, Laskay KM, Matteson EJ, Egan EA, Rody AS, Martin DJ, Riddlesberger MM, Montgomery P: A multicenter randomized, masked comparison trial of natural versus synthetic surfactant for the treatment of respiratory distress syndrome, *J Pediatr* 128:396-406, 1996.
60. Vermont-Oxford Neonatal Network: A multicenter, randomized trial comparing synthetic surfactant with modified bovine surfactant extract in the treatment of neonatal respiratory distress syndrome, *Pediatrics* 97:1-6, 1996.
61. Dunn MS, Shenan AT, Zayack D, Possmayer F: Bovine surfactant replacement therapy in neonates of less than 30 weeks' gestation: a randomized controlled trial of prophylaxis versus treatment, *Pediatrics* 87:377-386, 1991.
62. Kendig JW, Notter RH, Cox C, Reubens LJ, Davis JM, Maniscalco WM, Sinkin RA, Bartoletti A, Dweck HS, Horgan MJ, Risemberg H, Phelps DL, Shapiro DL: A comparison of surfactant as immediate prophylaxis and as a rescue therapy in newborns of less than 30 weeks' gestation, *N Engl J Med* 324:865-871, 1991.
63. Kattwinkel J, Bloom BT, Delmore P, Davis CL, Farrell E, Friss H, Jung AL, King K, Mueller D: Prophylactic administration of calf lung surfactant extract is more effective than early treatment of respiratory distress syndrome in neonates of 29 through 32 weeks' gestation, *Pediatrics* 92:90-98, 1993.
64. Morley CJ: Systematic review of prophylactic vs rescue, *Arch Dis Child* 77:F70-F74, 1997.
65. Bhutani VK, Abbasi S, Long WA, Gerdes JS: Pulmonary mechanics and energetics in preterm infants who had respiratory distress syndrome treated with synthetic surfactant, *J Pediatr* 120:S18-S24, 1992.
66. Couser RJ, Ferrara B, Ebert J, Hoekstra RE, Fangman JJ: Effects of exogenous surfactant therapy on dynamic lung compliance during mechanical breathing in preterm infants with hyaline membrane disease, *J Pediatr* 116:119-124, 1990.
67. Davis JM, Veness-Meehan K, Notter RH, Bhutani VK, Kemdig JW, Shapiro DL: Changes in pulmonary mechanics after the administration of surfactant to infants with respiratory distress syndrome, *N Engl J Med* 319:476-479, 1988.
68. Svenningsen NW: Pulmonary functional residual capacity and lung mechanics in surfactant-treated infants, *Semin Perinatol* 16:181-185, 1992.
69. Edberg KE, Ekstrom-Jodal B, Hallman M, Hjalmarsson O, Sandberg K, Silberberg AC: Immediate effects on lung function of instilled human surfactant in mechanically ventilated newborn infants with IRDS, *Acta Pediatr Scand* 79:750-755, 1990.
70. Cotton RB, Olsson T, Law AB, Parker RA, Linstrom DP, Silberberg AR, Sundell HW, Sandberg K: The physiologic effects of surfactant treatment on has exchange in newborn premature infants with hyaline membrane disease, *Pediatr Res* 34:495-501, 1993.
71. Corbet A, Bucciarelli R, Goldman S, Mammel M, Wold D, Long W, The American Exosurf Study Group I: Decreased mortality rate among small premature infants treated at birth with a single dose of synthetic surfactant: a multicenter controlled trial, *J Pediatr* 118:277-284, 1991.
72. Bose C, Corbet A, Bose G, Garcia-Prats J, Lombardy L, Wold D, Donion D, Long W: Improved outcome at 28 days of age for very low birth weight infants treated with a single dose of a synthetic surfactant, *J Pediatr* 117:947-953, 1990.
73. Long W, Corbet A, Cotton R, Courtney S, McGuiness G, Walter D, Watts J, Smyth J, Bard H, Chernick V, The American Exosurf Neonatal Study Group I, The Canadian Exosurf Neonatal Study Group: A controlled trial of synthetic surfactant in infants weighing 1250 g or more with respiratory distress syndrome, *N Engl J Med* 325:1696-1703, 1991.
74. Stevenson D, Walther F, Long W, Sell M, Pauly T, Gong A, Easa D, Pramanik A, LeBlanc M, Anday A, Dhanireddy R, Burchfield D, Corbet A, The American Exosurf Neonatal Study Group I: Controlled trial of a single dose of synthetic surfactant at birth in premature infants weighing 500 to 699 grams, *J Pediatr* 120:S3-S12, 1992.
75. Clyman RI, Jobe A, Heymann M, Ikegami M, Roman C, Payne B, Mauray F: Increased shunt through the patent ductus arteriosus after surfactant replacement therapy, *J Pediatr* 100:101-107, 1982.
76. Seyberth HW, Muller H, Wille L, Pluckthun DW, Ulmer HE: Recovery of prostaglandin production associated with reopening of the ductus arteriosus after indomethacin treatment in preterm infants with respiratory distress syndrome, *Pediatr Pharmacol* 2:127-141, 1982.
77. Clyman RI: Ontogeny of the ductus arteriosus response to prostaglandins and inhibitors of their synthesis, *Semin Perinatol* 4:115-124, 1980.
78. Gonzalez A, Sosenko IRS, Chandar J, Hummler H, Claure N, Bancalari E: Influence of infection on patent ductus arteriosus and chronic lung disease in premature infant weighing 1000 grams or less, *J Pediatr* 128:470-478, 1996.
79. Perez Fontan JJ, Clyman RI, Mauray F, Heymannn MA, Roman C: Respiratory effects of a patent ductus arteriosus in premature newborn lambs, *J Appl Physiol* 63:2315-2324, 1987.
80. Clyman RI, Mauray F, Heymann MA, Roman C: Cardiovascular effects of patent ductus arteriosus in preterm lambs with respiratory distress, *J Pediatr* 111:579-587, 1987.
81. Gerhardt T, Bancalari E: Lung compliance in newborns with patent ductus arteriosus before and after surgical ligation, *Biol Neonate* 38:96-105, 1980.
82. Stevenson JG: Fluid administration in the association of patent ductus arteriosus complicating respiratory distress syndrome, *J Pediatr* 90:257-261, 1977.
83. Rojas MA, Gonzalez A, Bancalari E, Claure N, Poole C, Silva-Neto G: Changing trends in the epidemiology and pathogenesis of neonatal chronic lung disease, *J Pediatr* 126:605-610, 1995.
84. Van Hauten J, Long W, Mullett M, Finer N, Derleth D, McMurray B, Peliowski A, Walker D, Wold D, Sankaran K, Corbet A, The American Exosurf Neonatal Study Group I, the Canadian Exosurf Neonatal Study Group: Pulmonary hemorrhage in premature infants after treatment with synthetic surfactant: an autopsy evaluation, *J Pediatr* 120:S40-S44, 1992.
85. Cole V, Normand ICS, Reynolds EOR, Rivers RPA: Pathogenesis of hemorrhagic pulmonary edema and massive pulmonary hemorrhage in the newborn, *Pediatrics* 51:175-187, 1973.
86. Esterly JR, Oppenheimer EH: Massive pulmonary hemorrhage in the newborn, *J Pediatr* 69:3-11, 1966.

Transient Tachypnea of the Newborn

87. Avery ME, Gatewood OB, Brumley G: Transient tachypnea of newborn, *Am J Dis Child* 111:380-385, 1966.
88. Rawlings JS, Smith FR: Transient tachypnea of the newborn, *Am J Dis Child* 138:869-871, 1984.
89. Patel DM, Donovan EF, Keenan WJ: Transient respiratory difficulty following cesarean delivery, *Biol Neonate* 43:146-151, 1983.
90. Singhi C, Chookang E: Maternal fluid overload during labour: transplacental hyponatremia and risk of transient neonatal tachypnoea in term infants, *Arch Dis Child* 59:1155-1158, 1984.
91. Halliday HL: Other acute lung disorders. In Sinclair JC, Bracken MB, eds: *Effective care of the newborn infant,* New York, 1992, Oxford University Press, p 369.
92. Karlberg P, Adams FH, Geubele F, Wallgren G: Alteration of the infant's thorax during vaginal delivery, *Acta Obstet Gynecol* 41:223-229, 1962.
93. Kitterman JA, Ballard PL, Clements JA, Mescher EJ, Tooley WH: Tracheal fluid in fetal lambs: spontaneous decrease prior to birth, *J Appl Physiol* 47:985-989, 1979.
94. Bland RD, Hansen TH, Haberken CM, Bressack MA, Hazinski TA, Usha Raj J, Goldberg RB: Lung fluid balance in lambs before and after birth, *J Appl Physiol* 53:992-1004, 1982.
95. Bland RD, Bressack MA, McMillan DD: Labor decreases the lung water content of newborn rabbits, *Am J Obstet Gynecol* 135:364-367, 1979.
96. Brown MJ, Olver RE, Ramsden CA, Strang LB, Walters DV: Effects of adrenaline and of spontaneous labour on the secretion and absorption of lung liquid in the fetal lamb, *J Physiol* 344:137-152, 1983.
97. McDonald JV, Gonzales LW, Ballard PL, Pitha J, Roberts JM: Lung beta-adrenoreceptor blockade affects perinatal surfactant release but not lung water, *J Appl Physiol* 60:1727-1733, 1986.
98. Halliday HL, McLure G, McReid M: Transient tachypnoea of the newborn: two distinct clinical entities, *Arch Dis Child* 56:322-325, 1981.
99. Milner AD, Saunders RA, Hopkin IE: Effects of delivery by caesarean section on lung mechanics and lung volume in the human neonate, *Arch Dis Child* 53:545-548, 1978.

100. Wiswell MT, Rawlings JS, Smith FR, Goo ED: Effect of furosemide on the clinical course of transient tachypnea of the newborn, *Pediatrics* 75:908-910, 1985.

Neonatal Pneumonia

101. Fujikura T, Froehlich LA: Intrauterine pneumonia in relation to birth weight and race, *Am J Obstet Gynecol* 97:81-84, 1967.
102. Anderson GS, Green CA, Neligan GA, Newell DJ, Russell JK: Congenital bacterial pneumonia, *Lancet* 2:585-587, 1962.
103. Yoder PR, Gibbs RS, Blanco JD, Castaneda YS, St Clair PJ: A prospective, controlled study of maternal and perinatal outcome after intra-amniotic infection at term, *Am J Obstet Gynecol* 145:695-701, 1983.
104. Webber S, Wilkinson AR, Lindsell D, Hope PL, Dobson SRM, Isaacs D: Neonatal pneumonia, *Arch Dis Child* 65:207-211, 1990.
105. Naeye RL, Dellinger WS, Blanc WA: Fetal and maternal features of antenatal bacterial infections, *J Pediatr* 79:733-739, 1977.
106. Vesikari T, Janas M, Gronroos P, Tuppurainen N, Renlund M, Kero P, Koivisto M, Kunnas M, Heinonen K, Nyman R, Pettay O, Osterlund K: Neonatal septicaemia, *Arch Dis Child* 60:542-546, 1985.
107. Christensen KK, Christensen P, Hagerstrand I, Linden V, Nordbring F, Svenningsen N: The clinical significance of group B streptococci, *J Perinat Med* 10:133-145, 1982.
108. Dillon HC, Khare S, Gray BM: Group B streptococcal carriage and disease: a 6-year prospective study, *J Pediatr* 110:31-36, 1987.
109. Davies PA: Pathogen or commensal? *Arch Dis Child* 55:169-170, 1980.
110. Bernstein J, Wang J: The pathology of neonatal pneumonia, *Am J Dis Child* 101:350-363, 1961.
111. Pass MA, Gray BM, Khare S, Dillon HC: Prospective studies of group B streptococcal infections in infants, *J Pediatr* 95:437-443, 1979.
112. Becroft DM, Farmer K, Mason GH, Morris MC, Stewart JH: Perinatal infections by group B beta-haemolytic streptococci, *Br J Obstet Gynecol* 83:960-966, 1976.
113. Katzenstein A, Davis C, Braude A: Pulmonary changes in neonatal sepsis due to group B beta-hemolytic streptococcus: relation to hyaline membrane disease, *J Infect Dis* 133:430-435, 1976.
114. Rettig PJ: Infections due to *Chlamydia trachomatis, Pediatr Infant Dis J* 5:449-457, 1986 (review).
115. Papageorgiou A, Bauer CR, Fletcher BD, Stern L: *Klebsiella* pneumonia with pneumatocele formation in a newborn infant, *Can Med Assoc J* 109:1217-1219, 1973.
116. Kunh JP, Lee SB: Pneumatoceles associated with *Escherichia coli* pneumonias in the newborn, *Pediatrics* 51:1008-1011, 1973.
117. Sherman MP, Chance KH, Goetzman BW: Gram stains of tracheal secretions predict neonatal bacteremia, *Am J Dis Child* 138:848-850, 1984.
118. Sherman MP, Goetzman BW, Ahlfors CE, Wennberg RP: Tracheal aspiration and its clinical correlates in the diagnosis of congenital pneumonia, *Pediatrics* 65:258-263, 1980.
119. Thureen PJ, Moreland S, Rodden DJ, Merenstein GB, Levin M, Rosenberg AA: Failure of tracheal aspirate cultures to define the cause of respiratory deterioration in neonates, *Pediatr Infect Dis J* 12:560-564, 1993.
120. Munson DP, Thompson TR, Johnson DE, Rhame FS, VanDrumen N, Ferrieri P: Coagulase-negative staphylococcal septicemia: experience in a newborn intensive care unit, *J Pediatr* 101:602-605, 1982.
121. Baley JE, Kliegman RM, Fanaroff AA: Disseminated fungal infections in very low-birth-weight infants: clinical manifestations and epidemiology, *Pediatrics* 73:144-152, 1984.
122. Shankaran S, Farooki ZQ, Desai R: Beta-hemolytic streptococcal infection appearing as persistent fetal circulation, *Am J Dis Child* 136:725-727, 1982.
123. Mc Fall TL, Zimmerman GA, Augustine NH, Hill HR: Effect of group B streptococcal type-specific antigen on polymorphonuclear leukocyte function and polymorphonuclear leukocyte–endothelial cell interaction, *Pediatr Res* 21:517-523, 1987.
124. Runkle B, Goldberg RN, Streitfeld MM, Clark MR, Buron E, Setzer ES, Bancalari E: Cardiovascular changes in group B streptococci sepsis in the piglet: response to indomethacin and relationship to prostacyclin and thromboxane A2, *Pediatr Res* 18:874-878, 1984.
125. Goldberg RN, Suguihara C, Streitfeld MM, Bancalari A, Clark MR, Bancalari E: Effects of a leukotriene antagonist on the early hemodynamic manifestations of group B streptococcal sepsis in piglets, *Pediatr Res* 20:1004-1008, 1986.
126. Hammerman C, Komar K, Abu-Khudair H: Hypoxic vs septic pulmonary hypertension, *Am J Dis Child* 142:319-325, 1988.
127. Cassell GH, Waites KB, Crouse DR, Rudd PT, Canupp KC, Stagno, S, Cutter GR: Association of *Ureaplasma urealyticum* infection of the lower respiratory tract with chronic lung disease and death in very-low-birth-weight infants, *Lancet* 2:240-245, 1988.
128. Holtzman RB, Hageman JR, Yogev R: Role of *Ureaplasma urealyticum* in bronchopulmonary dysplasia, *J Pediatr* 114:1061-1063, 1989.

Meconium Aspiration Syndrome

129. Gregory GA, Gooding CA, Phibbs RH, Tooley WH: Meconium aspiration in infants: a prospective study, *J Pediatr* 85:848-852, 1974.
130. Gregory GA: Aspiration syndromes in infants, *Int Anesthesiol Clin* 15:97-105, 1977.
131. Wiswell TE, Henley MA: Intratracheal suctioning, systemic infection, and the meconium aspiration syndrome, *Pediatrics* 89:203-206, 1992.
132. Matthews TG, Warshaw JB: Relevance of the gestational age distribution of meconium passage in utero, *Pediatrics* 64:30-31, 1979.
133. Rossi EM, Philipson EH, Williams TG, Kalhan SC: Meconium aspiration syndrome: intrapartum and neonatal attributes, *Am J Obstet Gynecol* 161:1106-1110, 1989.
134. Wiswell TE, Tuggle JM, Turner BS: Meconium aspiration syndrome: have we made a difference? *Pediatrics* 85:715-721, 1990.
135. Miller FC, Sacks DA, Yeh SY, Paul RH, Schifrin BS, Martin CB Jr, Hon EH: Significance of meconium during labor, *Am J Obstet Gynecol* 122:573-580, 1975.
136. Fujikura T, Klionsky B: The significance of meconium staining, *Am J Obstet Gynecol* 121:45-50, 1975.
137. Block MF, Kallenberger DA, Kern JD, Nepveux RD: In utero meconium aspiration by the baboon fetus, *Obstet Gynecol* 57:37-40, 1981.
138. Brown BL, Gleicher N: Intrauterine meconium aspiration, *Obstet Gynecol* 57:26-29, 1981.
139. Gooding CA, Gregory GA: Roentgenographic analysis of meconium aspiration of the newborn, *Radiology* 100:131-135, 1971.
140. Yeh TF, Harris V, Srinivasan G, Lilien L, Pyati S, Pildes RS: Roentgenographic findings in infants with meconium aspiration syndrome, *JAMA* 242:60-63, 1979.
141. Vidyasagar D, Yeh TF, Harris V, Pildes RS: Assisted ventilation in infants with meconium aspiration syndrome, *Pediatrics* 56:208-213, 1975.
142. Bryan CS: Enhancement of bacterial infection by meconium, *Johns Hopkins Med J* 121:9-13, 1967.
143. Bancalari E, Berlin JA: Meconium aspiration and other asphyxial disorders, *Clin Perinatol* 5:317-334, 1978.
144. Yeh TF, Harris V, Srinivasan G, Lilien L, Pyati S, Pildes RS: Roentgenographic findings in infants with meconium aspiration syndrome, *JAMA* 242:60-62, 1979.
145. Holtzman RB, Banzhaf WC, Silver RK, Hageman JR: Perinatal management of meconium staining of the amniotic fluid, *Clin Perinatol* 16:825-838, 1989.
146. Yeh TF, Lilien LD, Barathi A, Pildes RS: Lung volume, dynamic lung compliance, and blood gases during the first 3 days of postnatal life in infants with meconium aspiration syndrome, *Crit Care Med* 10:588-592, 1982.
147. Tran N, Lowe C, Sivieri EM, Shaffer TH: Sequential effects of acute meconium obstruction on pulmonary function, *Pediatr Res* 14:34-38, 1980.
148. Clark DA, Nieman GF, Thompson JE, Paskanik AM, Rokhar JE, Brendenberg CE: Surfactant displacement by meconium free fatty acids: an alternative explanation for atelectasis in meconium aspiration syndrome, *J Pediatr* 110:765-770, 1987.
149. Tyler DC, Murphy J, Cheney FW: Mechanical and chemical damage to lung tissue caused by meconium aspiration, *Pediatrics* 62:454-459, 1978.
150. Runkle B, Bancalari E: Acute cardiopulmonary effects of pancuronium bromide in mechanically ventilated newborn infants, *J Pediatr* 104:614-617, 1984.
151. Davis JM, Richter SE, Kendig JW, Notter RH: High-frequency jet ventilation and surfactant treatment of newborns with severe respiratory failure, *Pediatr Pulmonol* 13:108-112, 1992.
152. Paranka MS, Walsh WF, Stancombe BB: Surfactant lavage in a piglet model of meconium aspiration syndrome, *Pediatr Res* 31:625-628, 1992.

153. Auten RL, Notter RH, Kendig JW, Davis JM, Shapiro DL: Surfactant treatment of full-term newborns with respiratory failure, *Pediatrics* 87:101-107, 1991.
154. Sadovsky Y, Amon E, Bade ME, Petrie RH: Prophylactic amnioinfusion during labor complicated by meconium: a preliminary report, *Am J Obstet Gynecol* 161:613-617, 1989.
155. Wenstrom KD, Parsons MT: The prevention of meconium aspiration in labor using amnioinfusion, *Obstet Gynecol* 73:647-651, 1989.
156. Carson BS, Losey RW, Bowes WA, Simmons MA: Combined obstetric and pediatric approach to prevent meconium aspiration syndrome, *Am J Obstet Gynecol* 126:712-715, 1976.
157. Ting P, Brady JP: Tracheal suction in meconium aspiration, *Am J Obstet Gynecol* 122:767-771, 1975.
158. Bent RC, Wiswell TE, Chang A: Removing meconium from infant tracheae: what works best? *Am J Dis Child* 146:1085-1089, 1992.
159. Linden N, Aranda JV, Tsur M, Matoth I, Yatsiv I, Mandelberg H, Rottem M, Feigenbaum D, Ezra Y, Tamir I: Need for endotracheal intubation and suction in meconium-stained neonates, *J Pediatr* 112:613-615, 1988.
160. Cunningham AS, Lawson EE, Martin RJ, Phildes RS: Tracheal suction and meconium: a proposed standard of care, *J Pediatr* 116:153-154, 1990.
161. Cunningham AS: When to suction the meconium-stained newborn? *Contemp Pediatr* 1:91-109, 1993.
162. Falciglia HS, Henderschott C, Potter P, Helmchen R: Does DeLee suction at the perineum prevent meconium aspiration syndrome, *Am J Obstet Gynecol* 167:1243-1249, 1992.
163. MacFarlane PI, Heaf DP: Pulmonary function in children after neonatal meconium aspiration syndrome, *Arch Dis Child* 63:368-372, 1988.
164. Swaminathan S, Quinn J, Stabile MW, Bader D, Platzker ACG, Keens TG: Long-term pulmonary sequelae of meconium aspiration syndrome, *J Pediatr* 114:356-361, 1989.

Persistent Pulmonary Hypertension of the Newborn

165. Siassi B, Goldberg SJ, Emmanouilides GC, Higashino SM, Lewis E: Persistent pulmonary vascular obstruction in newborn infants, *J Pediatr* 78:610-615, 1971.
166. Rudolph AM: Fetal and neonatal pulmonary circulation, *Am Rev Respir Dis* 115:11-18, 1977.
167. Rudolph AM: High pulmonary vascular resistance after birth. I. Pathophysiologic considerations and etiologic classification, *Clin Pediatr* 19:585-590, 1980.
168. Drummond WH, Peckham GJ, Fox WW: The clinical profile of the newborn with persistent pulmonary hypertension, *Clin Pediatr* 16:335-341, 1977.
169. Setzer E, Ermocilla R, Tonkin I, John E, Sansa M, Cassady G: Papillary muscle necrosis in a neonatal autopsy population: incidence and associated clinical manifestations, *J Pediatr* 96:289-294, 1980.
170. Haworth SG, Reid L: Persistent fetal circulation: newly recognized structural features, *J Pediatr* 88:614-620, 1976.
171. Manchester D, Margolis HS, Sheldon RE: Possible association between maternal indomethacin therapy and primary pulmonary hypertension of the newborn, *Am J Obstet Gynecol* 126:467-469, 1976.
172. Wilkinson AR, Aynsley-Green A, Mitchell MD: Persistent pulmonary hypertension and abnormal prostaglandin E levels in preterm infants after maternal treatment with naproxen, *Arch Dis Child* 54:942-945, 1979.
173. Fouron JC, Hebert F: The circulatory effects of hematocrit variations in normovolemic newborn lambs, *J Pediatr* 82:995-1003, 1973.
174. Stenmark KR, James SL, Voelkel NF, Toews WH, Reeves JT, Murphy RC: Leukotriene C4 and D4 in neonates with hypoxemia and pulmonary hypertension, *N Engl J Med* 309:77-80, 1983.
175. Hammerman C, Lass N, Strates E, Komar K, Bui K-C: Prostanoids in neonates with persistent pulmonary hypertension, *J Pediatr* 110:470-472, 1987.
176. Caplan MS, Hsueh W, Sun X-M, Gidding SS, Hageman JR: Circulating plasma platelet activating factor in persistent pulmonary hypertension of the newborn, *Am Rev Respir Dis* 142:1258-1262, 1990.
177. Belik J, Baron K, Light RB: The effect of an increase in systemic arterial pressure in the newborn with right ventricular hypertension, *Pediatr Res* 28:603-608, 1990.
178. Zellers T, Gutgesell HP: Noninvasive estimation of pulmonary artery pressure, *J Pediatr* 114:735-741, 1989.
179. Drummond WH, Gregory GA, Heymann MA, Phibbs RA: The independent effects of hyperventilation, tolazoline, and dopamine on infants with persistent pulmonary hypertension, *J Pediatr* 98:603-611, 1981.
180. Schreiber MD, Heymann MA, Soifer SJ: Increased arterial pH, not decreased $Paco_2$, attenuates hypoxia-induced pulmonary vasoconstriction in newborn lambs, *Pediatr Res* 20:113-117, 1986.
181. Wung JT, James S, Kilchevsky E, James E: Management of infants with severe respiratory failure and persistence of the fetal circulation, without hyperventilation, *Pediatrics* 76:488-494, 1985.
182. Bancalari A, Gerhardt T, Bancalari E, Suguihara C, Hehre D, Reifenberg L, Goldberg RN: Gas trapping with high frequency ventilation: jet versus oscillatory ventilation, *J Pediatr* 110:617-622, 1987.
183. Kohelet D, Perlman M, Kirpalani H, Hanna G, Koren G: High-frequency oscillation in the rescue of infants with persistent pulmonary hypertension, *Crit Care Med* 16:510-516, 1988.
184. Carlo WA, Beoglos A, Chatburn RL, Walsh MC, Martin RJ: High-frequency jet ventilation in neonatal pulmonary hypertension, *Am J Dis Child* 143:233-238, 1989.
185. Carter MJM, Gerstmann DR, Clark MRH, Snyder MG, Cornish JD, Null DM, DeLemos RA: High-frequency oscillatory ventilation and extracorporeal membrane oxygenation for the treatment of acute neonatal respiratory failure, *Pediatrics* 85:159-164, 1990.
186. Ferrara B, Johnson DE, Chang PN, Thompson TR: Efficacy and neurologic outcome of profound hypocapneic alkalosis for the treatment of persistent pulmonary hypertension in infancy, *J Pediatr* 105:457-461, 1984.
187. Bifano EM, Pfannenstiel A: Duration of hyperventilation and outcome in infants with persistent pulmonary hypertension, *Pediatrics* 81:657-661, 1988.
188. Hegyi T, Hiatt IM: Tolazoline and dopamine therapy in neonatal hypoxia and pulmonary vasospasm, *Acta Paediatr Scand* 69:101-103, 1980.
189. Bifano E, Kavey R-E, Pergolizzi J, Slagle T, Bergstrom W: The cardiopulmonary effects of calcium infusion in infants with persistent pulmonary hypertension of the newborn, *Pediatr Res* 25:262-265, 1989.
190. Stevenson DK, Kasting DS, Darnall RA, Ariagno RL, Johnson JD, Malachowski N, Beets CL, Sunshine P: Refractory hypoxemia associated with neonatal pulmonary disease: the use and limitations of tolazoline, *J Pediatr* 95:595-599, 1979.
191. Soifer SJ, Clyman RI, Heymann MA: Effects of prostaglandin D2 on pulmonary arterial pressure and oxygenation in newborn infants with persistent pulmonary hypertension, *J Pediatr* 112:774-777, 1988.
192. Roberts JD, Polaner DM, Lang P, Zapol WM: Inhaled nitric oxide in persistent pulmonary hypertension of the newborn, *Lancet* 340:818-819, 1992.
193. Zayek M, Cleveland D, Morin FC III: Treatment of persistent pulmonary hypertension in the newborn lamb by inhaled nitric oxide, *J Pediatr* 122:743-750, 1993.
194. Kinsella JP, Neish SR, Ivy DD, Shaffer E, Abman SH: Clinical responses to prolonged treatment of persistent pulmonary hypertension of the newborn with low doses of inhaled nitric oxide, *J Pediatr* 123:103-108, 1993.
195. The Neonatal Inhaled Nitric Oxide Study Group: Inhaled nitric oxide in full-term and nearly full-term infants with hypoxic respiratory failure, *N Engl J Med* 336:597-604, 1997.
196. Roberts JD, Fineman JR, Morin FC III, Shaul PW, Rimar S, Schrieber MD, Polin RA, Zwass MS, Zayek MM, Gross I, Heyman A, Zapol WM (for the Inhaled Nitric Oxide Study Group): Inhaled nitric oxide and persistent pulmonary hypertension of the newborn, *N Engl J Med* 336:605-610, 1997.
197. Kinsella JP, Truog WE, Walsh WF, Goldberg RN, Bancalari E, Mayock DE, Redding GJ, deLemos RA, Sardesai S, McCurnin DC, Moreland SG, Cutter GR, Abman SH: Randomized, multicenter trial of inhaled nitric oxide and high-frequency oscillatory ventilation in severe, persistent pulmonary hypertension of the newborn, *J Pediatr* 131:55-62, 1997.
198. Bartlett RH, Gazzaniga AB, Toomasian J, Corwin AG, Roloff D, Rucker R: Extracorporeal membrane oxygenation (ECMO) in neonatal respiratory failure, *Ann Surg* 204:236-245, 1986.
199. O'Rourke PP, Crone RK, Vacanti JP, Ware JH, Lillehei CW, Parad RB, Epstein MF: Extracorporeal membrane oxygenation and conventional medical therapy in neonates with persistent pulmonary hypertension of the newborn: a prospective randomized study, *Pediatrics* 84:957-963, 1989.
200. Lott IT, McPherson D, Towne B, Johnson D, Starr A: Long-term neurophysiologic outcome after neonatal extracorporeal membrane oxygenation, *J Pediatr* 116:343-349, 1990.

201. Mendoza JC, Shearer LL, Cook LN: Lateralization of brain lesions following extracorporeal membrane oxygenation, *Pediatrics* 88:1004-1009, 1991.

202. Marron MJ, Crisafi MA, Driscoll JM Jr, Wung JT, Driscoll YT, Fay TH, James LS: Hearing and neurodevelopmental outcome in survivors of persistent pulmonary hypertension of the newborn, *Pediatrics* 90:392-396, 1992.

Pulmonary Gas Leaks

203. Macklin, MT, Macklin CC: Malignant interstitial emphysema of the lungs and mediastinum as an important occult complication in many respiratory diseases and other conditions: an interpretation of the clinical literature in light of laboratory experiment, *Medicine* 23:281-358, 1944.

204. Caldwell EJ, Powell RD Jr, Mullooly JP: Interstitial emphysema: a study of physiologic factors involved in experimental induction of the lesion, *Am Rev Respir Dis* 102:516-525, 1970.

205. Hart SM, McNair M, Gamsu HR, Price JF: Pulmonary interstitial emphysema in very low birth weight infants, *Arch Dis Child* 58:612-615, 1983.

206. HiFO Study Group: Randomized study of high-frequency oscillatory ventilation in infants with severe respiratory distress syndrome, *J Pediatr* 122:609-619, 1993.

207. Brooks JG, Bustamante SA, Koops BL, Hilton S, Cooper D, Wesenberg RL, Simmons MA: Selective bronchial intubation for the treatment of localized pulmonary interstitial emphysema in newborn infants, *J Pediatr* 91:648-652, 1977.

208. Swingle HM, Eggert LD, Bucciarelli RL: New approach to management of unilateral tension pulmonary interstitial emphysema in premature infants, *Pediatrics* 74:354-357, 1984.

209. Bauer CR, Brennan MJ, Doyle C, Poole CA: Surgical resection for pulmonary interstitial emphysema in the newborn infant, *J Pediatr* 93:656-661, 1978.

210. Touloukian RJ, Beardsley GP, Ablow RC, Effman EL: Traumatic perforation of the pharynx in the newborn, *Pediatrics* 59:1019-1022, 1977.

211. Steele RW, Metz JR, Bass JW, Dubois JJ: Pneumothorax and pneumomediastinum in the newborn, *Radiology* 98:629-632, 1971.

212. Ogata ES, Gregory GA, Kitterman JA, Phibbs RH, Tooley WH: Pneumothorax in the respiratory distress syndrome: incidence and effect on vital signs, blood gases and pH, *Pediatrics* 58:177-183, 1976.

213. Simmons DH, Linde LM, Miller JH, O'Reilly RJ: Relation between lung volume and pulmonary vascular resistance, *Circ Res* 9:465-471, 1961.

214. Dykes FD, Lazzarra A, Ahmann P, Blumenstein B, Scheartz J, Brann AW: Intraventricular hemorrhage: a prospective evaluation of etiopathogeneses, *Pediatrics* 66:42-49, 1980.

215. Hall RT, Rhodes PG: Pneumothorax and pneumomediastinum in infants with idiopathic respiratory distress syndrome receiving continuous positive airway pressure, *Pediatrics* 55:493-496, 1975.

216. The OSIRIS Collaborative Group: Early versus delayed neonatal administration of a synthetic surfactant: the judgement of OSIRIS, *Lancet* 340:1363-1369, 1992.

217. Goldberg RN: Sustained arterial blood pressure elevation associated with pneumothoraces: early detection via continuous monitoring, *Pediatrics* 68:775-777, 1981.

218. Kuhns LR, Bednareck FJ, Wyman ML, Roloff DW, Borer RC: Diagnosis of pneumothorax or pneumomediastinum in the neonate by transillumination, *Pediatrics* 56:355-360, 1975.

219. Varano LA, Maisels MJ: Pneumopericardium in the newborn: diagnosis and pathogenesis, *Pediatrics* 53:941-944, 1974.

220. Brans YW, Pitts M, Cassady G: Neonatal pneumopericardium, *Am J Dis Child* 130:393-396, 1976.

221. Madansky DL, Lawson EE, Chernick V, Taeusch HW: Pneumothorax and other forms of air leak in newborns, *Am Rev Respir Dis* 120:729-737, 1979.

222. Gregory GA, Tooley WA: Gas embolism in hyaline membrane disease, *N Engl J Med* 282:1141-1142, 1970.

Wilson-Mikity Syndrome

223. Wilson MG, Mikity VG: A new form of respiratory disease in premature infants, *Am J Dis Child* 99:489-499, 1960.

224. Hodgman JE, Mikity VG, Tatter D, Cleland RS: Chronic respiratory distress in the premature infant: Wilson-Mikity syndrome, *Pediatrics* 44:179-195, 1969.

CHAPTER 32

Chronic Respiratory Complications of Prematurity

Sailesh Kotecha and Michael Silverman

CHRONIC LUNG DISEASE: BACKGROUND

Terminology

The term *chronic lung disease (CLD),* used to describe the aftermath of prematurity and its treatment on the respiratory system, is deliberately vague. It implies a wide spectrum of disorders affecting the upper and lower respiratory tract, the result of the complex interaction of antenatal and postnatal factors. Although the use of the term *disease* may seem to indicate the possibility of a clear all-or-none definition, *CLD* encompasses a range of clinical, physiologic, pathologic, and developmental problems that extend from marginally significant at one extreme to fatal at the other. The vagueness of the term serves to hide the ignorance of many aspects of the pulmonary outcomes of prematurity.

Unlike the well-defined condition bronchopulmonary dysplasia (BPD),[1] CLD can be defined a number of ways to suit particular purposes. It is worth exploring the history of the ideas of the respiratory consequences of prematurity to draw attention to the themes that permeate this chapter.[2]

CLD has risen in importance since the advent of effective care for preterm babies. Until the 1960s and the introduction of mechanical ventilation, the survival of infants of very low birth weight (VLBW) was rare. (A VLBW infant weighs less than 1500 g at birth.) No chronic disease was therefore possible. When Northway et al[1] described the chronic clinical and radiologic features of CLD in the preterm survivors of mechanical ventilation and high inspired oxygen therapy, defining the term *BPD,* they created a series of controversies that continue today. The most vehement arguments ranged over the importance of barotrauma and oxygen toxicity as causes of lung injury in the neonate. The ignorance of the mechanisms and consequences of CLD has moved to a more sophisticated level because the multiple, interacting causes exert effects that vary in both their pathophysiologic basis and clinical features throughout infancy, childhood, and adolescence.

To some extent, the definitions of *CLD* reflect the applications of the term (Table 32-1). It has become clear that *BPD* (chronic oxygen dependency with certain characteristic radiologic features at 28 days of age) has become a less useful term because of the survival of infants at ever-lower gestational ages. Most infants who weigh less than 1000 g at birth are still oxygen dependent after 4 weeks. Thus the continually varying level of risk of an adverse long-term outcome for VLBW infants is still defined according to a single criterion: the need for oxygen therapy.[3] The suggestion of Shennan et al[3]—36 weeks of gestational age represents the best compromise—seems realistic. This cutoff point may vary with local need, secular trends, and changes in the epidemiology of CLD.

Risk prediction is vitally important both for clinical decision making and maximization of statistical power in clinical trials of preventive interventions, such as surfactant therapy. The estimates of the risk of CLD, as implied by Fig. 32-1, become more accurate as the infant ages (i.e., becomes closer to actually having CLD). Thus long-term risk prediction is likely to be least accurate in the immediate postnatal period. Improved risk prediction is a prerequisite for effective trials of preventive interventions.[4-7] Predictions based only on early lung function measurement are likely to be little better than those made only on birth weight.[8]

Diagnostic Overlap

CLD includes not only BPD but also several purely neonatal disorders such as Wilson-Mikity syndrome (Table 32-2). Clinically and radiologically, this disorder is very similar to classic BPD (Northway type IV), except for a lack of mechanical ventilation in its early postnatal course. Some pathologists deny any specific histologic features. Within the restricted category of BPD, at least two types are recognized: type 1 with "gray" lungs on chest radiographs and type 2 with classic radiologic changes.[9] There are other clinical distinguishing features (see Table 32-2). The role of developmental lung disorders such as pulmonary hypoplasia and of common clinical problems such as gastroesophageal reflux (GER) with aspiration is clearly complex. Such problems often contribute to CLD, but unless they are unless strikingly obvious, they do not usually warrant

Table 32-1 Definition of CLD

APPLICATION	DEFINITION
Recognition of clinical abnormality	
Individuals	Definition based on the presence or quantification of clinical features such as hospital readmission or abnormal lung function in infancy
Groups	Statistical definition based on the quantification of excess morbidity
Risk prediction for clinical intervention	Criteria dependent on the risk of possible interventions (For example, the need for a fraction of inspired oxygen at 40% at 4 weeks would justify low-risk intervention; the prediction of intermittent positive-pressure ventilation at term might justify a very risky procedure.)
Audit	
Clinical efficacy	All-or-none definitions such as BPD, which may be useful
Financial cost of care	Statistical definition based on excess respiratory morbidity (e.g., excess "bed days" as a result of all respiratory causes in premature infants)
Long-term health care planning	Definitions according to risk of need for long-term management, such as need for dormiciliary oxygen therapy
Death certification	Histopathologic criteria

Table 32-2 Clinical Disorders that Are Within the Spectrum of CLD or that Contribute to Morbidity

DISORDERS	COMMENT
Neonatal disorders	
Developmental abnormalities	Pulmonary hypoplasia, intrauterine infection
BPD	
Type I	Small "gray" lungs on chest radiograph
Type II	Classic Northway type IV
Wilson-Mikity syndrome	Similarity to type II BPD, without preceding RDS
Chronic pulmonary insufficiency of prematurity	Similarity to type I BPD, without preceding RDSG
Recurrent pulmonary aspiration	Gastroesophageal reflux, which often accompanies CLD
Disorders of later infancy in which morbidity rate may be greater in preterm infants	
Wheezing disorders	Excess lower respiratory tract morbidity, which is seen in infants born prematurely and can be considered epidemiologically as a form of CLD
Defects of host defense	Very rare incidence, apart from cystic fibrosis
Develomental anomalies	Excess incidence of congenital heart disease in infants with CLD

RDS, Respiratory distress syndrome.

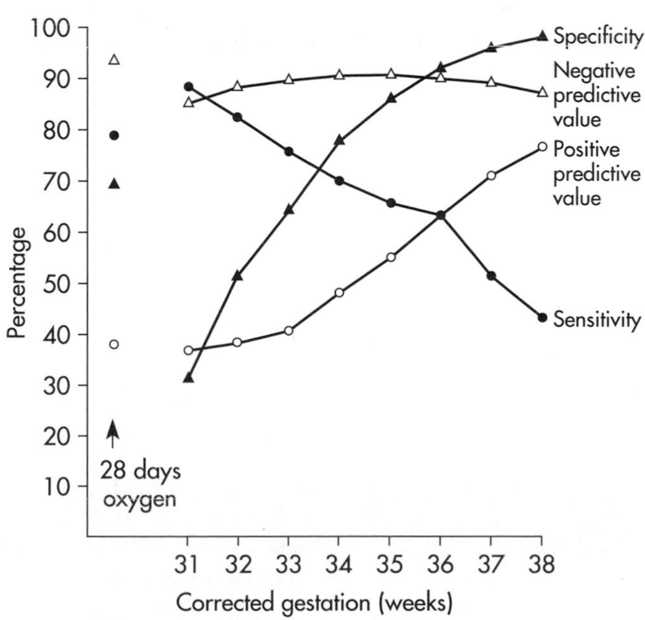

Fig. 32-1. Prediction of pulmonary morbidity in infancy based on the need for oxygen therapy at corrected gestational ages. Morbidity was defined as oxygen therapy at term, respiratory tract surgery, wheezing, at least two hospitalizations for acute lower respiratory tract illness, and clinical or radiologic changes. (From Shennan AT et al: *Pediatrics* 82:527-532, 1988.)

an independent diagnostic label. Recognizing their contribution may be important in understanding the etiology of CLD, its management, and its prognosis.

Diagnostic overlap is even more of a problem in later infancy, when infants of preterm birth tend to have greater morbidity in a range of clinical situations (see Table 32-2). For instance, because at least 30% to 60% of preschool children suffer from recurrent lower respiratory illness, mostly with wheezing,[10-12] the symptom is common in children born prematurely. Preterm infants are in fact at increased risk,[13-16] but it would be fruitless to try to define a level of morbidity that distinguishes "ordinary" wheezing lower respiratory illness from CLD. In clinical practice and increasingly in clinical epidemiology, a problem-orientated approach is more useful than one based on categoric, diagnostic labels. The same argument applies to the other disorders in Table 32-2.

This chapter uses the term *CLD* to encompass both a range of well-characterized syndromes and an overall increase in respiratory tract morbidity in infancy and later life.

Epidemiology

The prevalence of CLD varies widely. Crude figures, even when adjusted for birth weight, are difficult to interpret and hence are of only limited value except as starting points for further exploration. Terminologic inexactitude and diagnostic overlap produce so much "noise" that signals relating to important risk factors are difficult to discern. In the well-known eight-center, comparative study of VLBW infants in the United States,[17] strict diagnostic criteria were applied. Even so, major differences in the prevalence of CLD were observed that were not explained by different mortality rates within the institutions or by differences in birth weight, race, or gender. The authors speculated that the differences in 28-day oxygen requirements, which varied between 21% and 42%, might be accounted for by early postnatal management practices. At the center with the lowest incidence, nasal continuous positive airway pressure was instituted early for all symptomatic infants, and mechanical ventilation (without muscle paralysis) was commenced only when the partial pressure of carbon dioxide (Pco_2) had risen to 60 mm Hg. Local variations in management may therefore have influenced the long-term outcome.

In another large, multicenter study in the United States, the incidence of CLD varied from 3% to 33% of all preterm infants and up to 50% of those who had respiratory distress syndrome (RDS).[18] By taking a complete, clearly defined VLBW population, Kraybill et al[19] eliminated selection and diagnostic bias but came to the conclusion that although most of the variation between centers was due to differences in birth weight, about one third was due to other factors, differences in treatment being the prime suspect. Their overall incidence of classic BPD in VLBW infants was 22%. A number of the general factors that could affect the incidence of CLD are listed in Box 32-1.

Against this uncertainty, secular trends in birth weight–adjusted prevalence have clearly occurred. Within single institutions, increased survival of VLBW infants has been associated with a rise in CLD in the whole population (but not necessarily as a proportion of survivors), whereas for larger infants, the figures have fallen markedly[20] (Table 32- 3). Interestingly, despite or perhaps because of longer survival times, the prevalence of CLD has not fallen in the very smallest babies, those who weight less than 750 g at birth.[21] Although much of the change in prevalence may be accounted for by the factors listed in Box 32-1, specific changes in perinatal care have brought overall survival benefits to preterm babies, increasing the risk in some cases of severe CLD.[22] The reduction in RDS by obstetric and early neonatal interventions has played a major part (see Chapter 31).

Early perinatal interventions have been exhaustively reviewed.[23-25] Corticosteroids have been used to accelerate lung maturation for many years, but their effect on the incidence of CLD is inconsistent and at most marginal,[23] although survival is significantly enhanced. Although long-term adverse effects have not been demonstrated in humans,[23] a number of animal studies have shown persistent,[26] transient,[27] or no effects[28] from fetal corticosteroid exposure. There are little data on human lung growth.[29]

BOX 32-1
Factors Determining the Prevalence and Variations in Diagnostic Criteria in an Institution

- Population base of community
  - Social factors
  - Environmental factors
  - Age and health structure of community
  - Ethnic mix of population
- Referral patterns of neonatal unit
  - Obstetric population (high or low risk)
  - Obstetric practices
  - Postnatal referrals from units with less expertise
- Morbidity of patients
  - Early morbidity
  - Maturity of population
  - Complication rate
  - Early mortality rate
- Quality of care
  - Quality and quantity of medical and nursing staff
  - Quality of equipment
  - Use of protocols based on scientific data

Table 32-3 Percentage of Infants with Stage IV BPD and RDS Treated with Positive-Pressure Ventilation and Oxygen for More Than 24 Hours

	1962-1965 BIRTH WEIGHT (G)				1989 BIRTH WEIGHT (G)			
	<1000	1000-1500	>1500	TOTAL	<1000	1000-1500	>1500	TOTAL
BPD/RDS								
Survivors	0/0 (0)	1/2 (50)	3/11 (27)	4/13 (31)	22/30 (73)	8/34 (24)	3/47 (6)	33/111 (30)
Nonsurvivors	0/3 (0)	2/5 (40)	3/11 (27)	5/19 (26)	3/5 (60)	0/2	1/1 (100)	4/8 (50)
TOTAL	0/3 (0)	3/7 (43)	6/22 (27)	9/32 (28)	25/35 (71)	8/36 (22)	4/48 (8)	37/119 (31)

From Northway WH et al: *Arch Dis Child* 65:1076-1081, 1990.

The combination of thyroid-releasing hormone with antenatal corticosteroids seems unlikely to reduce the incidence of severe RDS and BPD any more effectively than steroids alone.[30] Compared with control infants (VLBW infants whose mothers had been treated with thyroid-releasing hormone in addition to corticosteroids), the relative risk for classic BPD in the active group was reduced to 0.4 (18 of 55 vs. 44 of 48).

The use of surfactant has had a marginal, if any, overall effect on the prevalence of CLD,[24,25] in part because increases in the overall survival rate create a larger population at risk of long-term complications.[20,24,25,31] Only the prophylactic use of natural surfactant has been associated with a significant fall of 11% (confidence interval [CI], 3.1% to 18.6%) in the absolute incidence of BPD.[24] Sequential studies in a single center, although less satisfactory in design than randomized controlled trials, also support a reduction in CLD after prophylactic natural surfactant.[31] A fall in oxygen requirement was reported in infants weighing less than 1000 g at birth after the introduction of prophylactic natural surfactant: from 75% to 50% at 28 days, 55% to 35% at 36 weeks, and 49% to 26% at discharge. However, an analysis of a large multicenter study of prophylactic surfactant showed that in the very smallest babies (<700 g), the reduced incidence of acute lung disease uncovered a high risk of CLD without antecedent acute disease and the need for mechanical ventilation, suggesting a different etiology for CLD in the smallest babies. Perhaps this late-onset type of CLD, which falls into the category of Wilson-Mikity syndrome, will become more common as surfactant therapy becomes routine. Its pathogenesis and management may differ from that of "classic" BPD. The very long-term consequences of surfactant therapy have yet to be determined. One study suggests that lung function in infancy may be less disturbed in treated than in control infants,[32] but another study found no difference in clinical outcome.[33] Both studies were biased by the lower survival rate in the placebo-treated infants.

One of the main advantages of population studies is the identification of risk factors, which can then be subjected to detailed investigation, often by randomized, controlled trial. The potential for bias in identifying risk factors from small, poorly controlled samples is largely a consequence of the "network" of interrelated risks in neonatal medicine (Fig. 32-2). The possibilities of bias are numerous and explain some of the conflicting results that have been reported from outcome studies. Many early studies identified mechanical ventilation and oxygen therapy as major risk factors for BPD on the basis of comparative outcome studies of infants whose lungs were mechanically ventilated compared with controls whose lungs were not ventilated. Such studies were confounded by the interaction of factors illustrated in Fig. 32-2 and biased by the selection of unrepresentative samples of the population. The analysis of Kraybill et al[4] illustrates some pitfalls. A crude analysis of the risk factors for oxygen dependency at 28 days of age in babies weighing less than 1000 g at birth indicated significant risks associated with low gestational age, male gender, high rate of ventilation at 96 hours of age, and low arterial P_{CO_2} at 96 hours of age. However, logistic regression analysis left male gender and low arterial P_{CO_2} as the only independent factors (the latter being a weak association).

The age at which the risk of an adverse outcome is determined may be important, not only because lung pathology, symptoms, and lung function may become less obvious with time,[14,34,35] but also because it is possible that the risk factors for acute lung damage (classic BPD) may differ from those of CLD later in childhood. The CLD could, for instance, be determined to a greater extent by disturbed long-term growth related to prematurity itself,[36,37] whereas acute lung damage might result from mechanical ventilation.[38]

Secular trends in prevalence almost certainly affect the assessment of risk because classic BPD is more common and may have a different spectrum of risk factors in VLBW infants, who are increasingly represented in the most recent studies. This can lead to bias if there is a parallel change in some important aspect of management, such as the earlier introduction of lipid-based intravenous feeding regimens.[22] Even the definition of risk factors may be important. One cannot for instance assume that low birth weight (LBW) and prematurity are equivalent, since Rona et al[39] showed in a cross-sectional study that at school age, decreased lung function was the predominant outcome for children of LBW for age, whereas prematurity led to an increase in symptoms, confirming the longitudinal data of Chan et al.[40] Finally, neonatal death from respiratory causes may itself introduce major selection bias into the analysis of the risk of CLD by removing from the equation the possible major risk factors for the severest form of CLD.

The analysis of risk should be based on studies of complete populations, using simple clinical variables to avoid bias[41] and appropriate types of statistical analysis to eliminate confusion.[4] It may then be possible to start to predict risk[4-8] for early intervention or to identify specific factors with a view to identifying remediable causes of BPD.[4,22,40,41]

The public health burden of CLD has yet to be calculated. Studies revealing that certain percentages of preterm babies

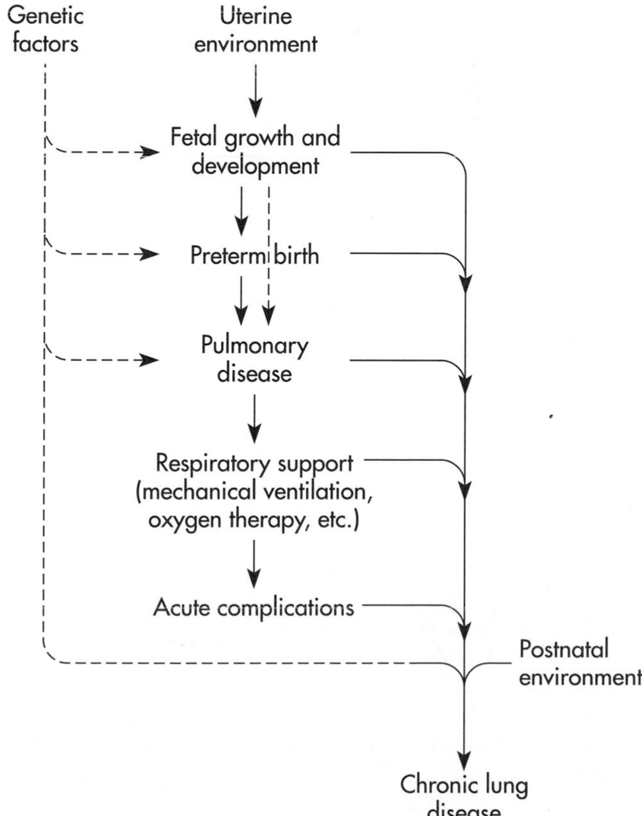

Fig. 32-2. There is a great deal of interaction among risk factors in CLD.

cough, wheeze, or require readmission to the hospital are of little intrinsic interest unless they provide information that can be used in planning or calculating the cost of health care provision. Domiciliary oxygen therapy clearly has such implications.[42,43] The effect of therapeutic or preventive regimens using surfactant and corticosteroids on the overall cost of neonatal care has been assessed.[44] The budgetary and ethical results of this study are at variance: It is cheapest to give no antenatal steroids or postnatal surfactant because of the high early mortality rate but clinically and ethically better to use both because the chance for healthy long-term survival is then far greater.

Models

The epidemiologic model used for this chapter is represented in Fig. 32-2. Its applications have already been discussed.

As a framework for understanding the interactions of growth and repair that underpin the disorder and are described by techniques in pathology, the evolution of CLD is considered in four overlapping stages representing early inflammation, its resolution, repair and modeling, and finally lung growth and development (Fig. 32-3). The earliest stages relate to acute neonatal lung disease and its management (see Chapter 31). The evidence to support this general scheme (see section on pathology) is based on a combination of histopathologic data collected in infants who die, supported by cytologic findings from bronchoalveolar lavage in infants whose lungs are ventilated and by developmental physiology later in life. Animal models have provided support for this analysis.[45]

The value of this model lies not only in its contribution to understanding the pathogenesis of CLD but also in its management. Because the disorder has such a huge clinical spectrum—from fatal cardiorespiratory failure in the neonate to the mildest symptoms and dysfunction in the school child who had a premature birth—and because it covers such a wide age range, therapeutic schemes must be tailored to the various clinicopathologic stages. It is convenient to separate the management of the acute stage in the neonatal unit from the management of CLD in the infant at home. By the end of the first year, when repair and remodeling may be largely completed and growth tracks along the channel thereby determined,[46] management issues again alter, focusing on symptom management and health maintenance rather than potentially preventive measures and health enhancement.

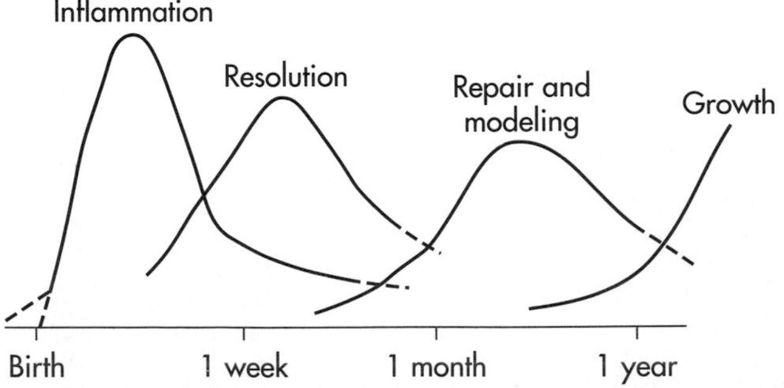

Fig. 32-3. Speculative model of the clinicopathologic phases of CLD.

PATHOLOGY

The pathologic changes associated with CLD are almost entirely based on the study of infants at autopsy. It is difficult to be certain that the lesions seen at autopsy are relevant in the living child with CLD. In these studies, diffuse alveolar damage with reversible bronchiolar necrosis is seen in the early stages; interstitial fibrosis predominates later in the disease.

Macroscopic Appearance

During acute RDS, the lung is firm with a smooth surface that, during the second week, becomes more irregular if CLD is evolving; the lung weighs approximately 25% to 75% more than expected.[47] By the third and fourth weeks the lung surface has a cobblestone appearance as a result of variable underlying alveolar distention and collapse. As the reparative process progresses during the ensuing weeks and months as a result of atelectasis, emphysema, fibrosis, and growth, deep fissuring into the lung depths may occur (Fig. 32-4, *A*). The fissuring may resemble the major normal fissures of the lung. During the second year of life, a smooth surface contour returns, with only the deepest fissures remaining.

Microscopic Changes

Histologically, CLD is characterized by an early exudative inflammatory phase followed by a subacute fibroproliferative phase of resolution and finally a chronic fibroproliferative phase[47] (Table 32-4 and Fig. 32-4, *B* to *D*) characterized by growth and remodeling. Microscopically, during the inflammatory phase, the most frequent finding is extensive residual hyaline membranes[48] with superimposed bronchiolar necrosis and obliterative, reparative bronchiolitis. Cystic dilation of bronchioles and alveolar ducts may be a prominent feature. Narrowing of the lumina of the bronchioles and alveolar ducts may occur as a result of peribronchiolar and intrinsic edema, hyaline membranes, inflammatory debris, and fibroplasia. During the subacute, fibroproliferative stage of resolution, which occurs from the second to fourth weeks of life, there is progressive replacement of the hyaline membrane with interstitial and perialveolar fibrosis. The septal walls are thickened, and myofibroblast proliferation is seen by electron microscopy.[48] Type II pneumocyte hyperplasia lines the restructured alveolar walls. During the ensuing month, remodeling occurs. Hyaline membranes are no longer seen, but interstitial fibrosis of varying severity is evident. Emphysematous areas are interspersed with areas of collapsed alveoli.

Recently, Van Lierde[49] has identified two pathologic patterns from the study of infants with CLD at autopsy. In the interstitial type there is marked interstitial fibrosis without significant airway abnormalities. Infants with this type have little or no emphysematous change. In the second group, the bronchiolar type, marked airway lesions and emphysema are noted. Although no differences were seen between these groups in birth weight, gestational age, or initial chest radiograph, the bronchiolar group had worse initial pulmonary function and required more supplemental oxygen and ventilatory support than the interstitial group. These two groups probably reflect the two pathologic extremes because most infants had a mixed picture of interstitial and bronchiolar changes.

Table 32-4 Evolution of CLD

STAGE	PATHOLOGIC STAGE	PATHOLOGIC FEATURES
Inflammation/resolution	Exudative, early reparative	Hyaline membranes: bronchial necrosis, bronchiolitis obliterans, bronchiolectasis Early septal fibrosis
Resolution/repair	Subacute, fibroproliferative	Bronchiolitis obliterans, bronchiolectasis Residual hyaline membranes (rare) Type II cell hyperplasia and regeneration Perialveolar duct fibrosis Increasing interstitial fibrosis, smooth muscle proliferation Overexpanded and collapsed acini
Growth/rmodeling	Chronic, fibroproliferative	Interstitial fibrosis, smooth muscle proliferation Honeycombed lung Vascular wall thickening Lack of bronchiolitis obliterans and bronchiolectasis

Adapted from Wigglesworth JS, Singer DB, eds: *Textbook of fetal and perinatal pathology,* Oxford, England, 1991, Blackwell.

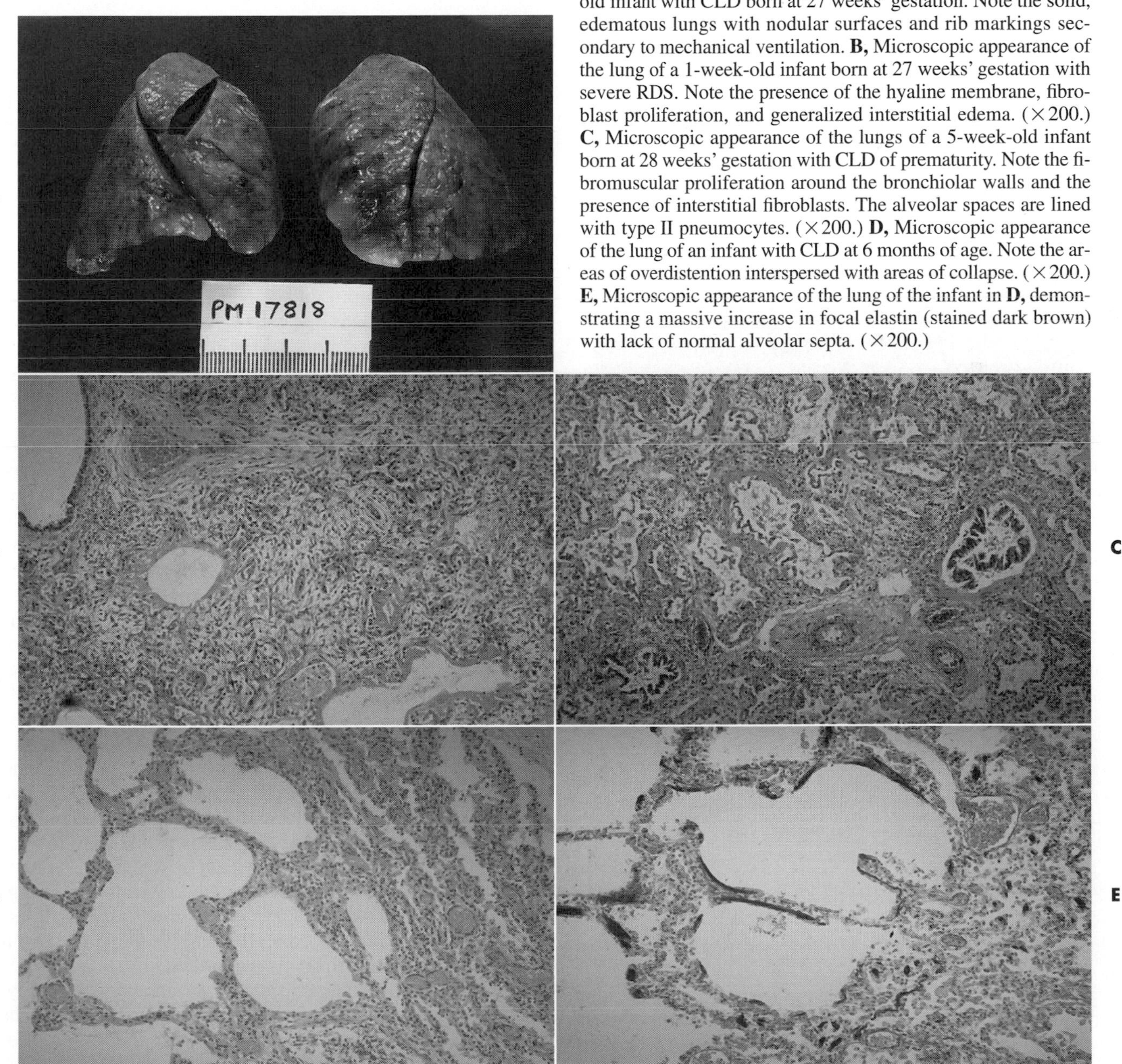

Fig. 32-4. A, Macroscopic appearance of the lungs of a 5-week-old infant with CLD born at 27 weeks' gestation. Note the solid, edematous lungs with nodular surfaces and rib markings secondary to mechanical ventilation. **B,** Microscopic appearance of the lung of a 1-week-old infant born at 27 weeks' gestation with severe RDS. Note the presence of the hyaline membrane, fibroblast proliferation, and generalized interstitial edema. (×200.) **C,** Microscopic appearance of the lungs of a 5-week-old infant born at 28 weeks' gestation with CLD of prematurity. Note the fibromuscular proliferation around the bronchiolar walls and the presence of interstitial fibroblasts. The alveolar spaces are lined with type II pneumocytes. (×200.) **D,** Microscopic appearance of the lung of an infant with CLD at 6 months of age. Note the areas of overdistention interspersed with areas of collapse. (×200.) **E,** Microscopic appearance of the lung of the infant in **D,** demonstrating a massive increase in focal elastin (stained dark brown) with lack of normal alveolar septa. (×200.)

The cell population of the airways of preterm infants whose lungs were ventilated has been defined using bronchoalveolar lavage.[50-53] Early in the development of RDS, few cells are seen in the bronchoalveolar lavage fluid of preterm newborn delivered by elective cesarean section. By day three, the cell numbers increase, the predominant cell being the neutrophil. As recovery from RDS occurs, neutrophil numbers decline, but if CLD evolves, neutrophil numbers appear to persist (see Fig. 32-7, *A*).[50-55] The cellular mechanisms are discussed in more detail later.

In infants who recover from CLD, Hislop and Haworth[56] and Hislop et al[57] found that none of the 17 infants they studied at autopsy had classic fibrotic changes but that all had reduced alveolar numbers and increased smooth muscle hypertrophy in the small airways; this suggests that normal alveolation had been disrupted. In infants who died early from RDS, the pulmonary arteries resembled those from the fetal state, whereas the pulmonary arteries of infants with CLD had a more mature structure, although muscle extended farther than normal into the smaller vessels. Marked pulmonary artery muscular hypertrophy similar to that seen in fetal life was seen in infants who died from cor pulmonale. A reduction in the density of small pulmonary arteries, compatible with alveolar hypoplasia, has recently been reported.[58]

Epithelial dysplasia is common after the repair of lung injury. It may be patchy or complete. There may be almost total replacement by squamous metaplasia in the extreme and marked basement membrane thickening[59] (Fig. 32-5).

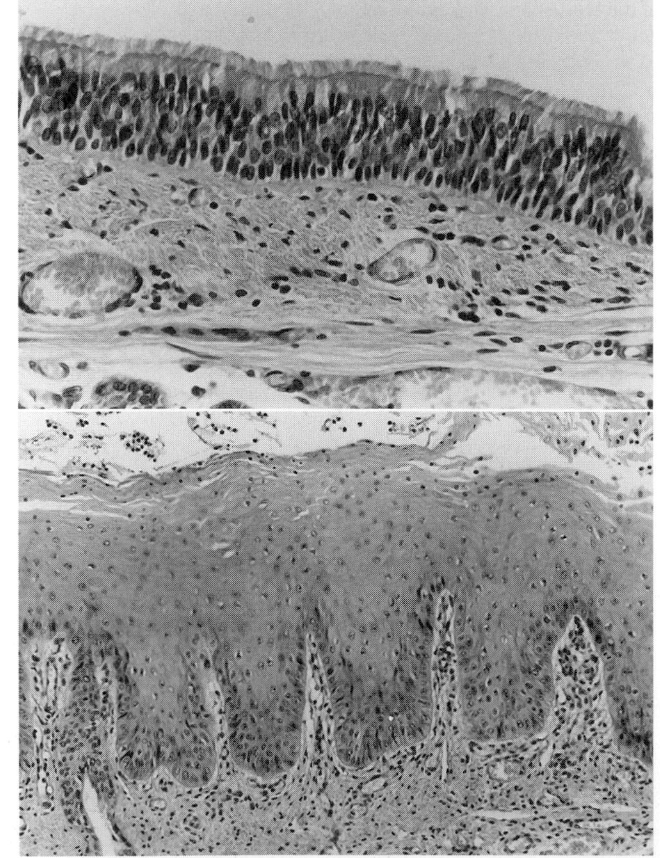

Fig. 32-5. **A,** Photomicrograph showing grade 0, normal, ciliated tracheal epithelium. (Hematoxylin-eosin, ×240.) **B,** Photomicrograph showing grade 4, mature, keratinizing, stratified squamous epithelium that is markedly thickened. It was taken from an infant with severe CLD. (Hematoxylin-eosin, ×100.)

RISK FACTORS AND PATHOGENESIS

Although the etiology of CLD is unknown, since the earliest description of BPD by Northway,[1] many of the risk factors have been identified. Multivariate analysis has demonstrated that CLD is more common in the extremely premature infant when compared with mature infants, and other independent risk factors include male gender, nonblack race, surfactant deficiency, oxygen toxicity, barotrauma resulting from mechanical ventilation (including air leaks), sepsis, patent ductus arteriosus (PDA), and fluid overload. The significance of many of these risk factors is unknown, but animal models have been used to identify the importance of some. In particular, several groups have focused their attention on the relative importance of oxygen toxicity and barotrauma to the pathogenesis of CLD. As discussed earlier, these factors might be important causes of acute lung damage, but with healing by remodeling and growth, the long-term risk of CLD depends on the degree of prematurity and the degree of disruption of the normal pattern of alveolation in late fetal life and infancy.

Oxygen Toxicity

Oxygen is toxic to mammalian lungs. Many groups have developed animal models based on mice, rats, rabbits, and premature baboons to demonstrate that lung injury comparable with that seen in human CLD can be achieved by hyperoxic exposure.[60-65] Pappas et al[61] exposed newborn mice to 80% oxygen at atmospheric pressure and noted significant pulmonary injury with an increase in the pulmonary interstitial compartment and later an increase in parenchymal and peribronchiolar pulmonary fibrosis. Merritt[66] demonstrated that in bronchoalveolar lavage of newborn guinea pigs exposed to hyperoxia, the alveolar macrophages had enhanced chemotactic activity and that after an initial depression, neutrophils also had increased chemotactic activity. Furthermore, the bronchoalveolar lavage fluid had increased elastases and growth factor activity when compared with that in control animals. Similar observations were made in preterm guinea pigs by Kelly et al.[67] In this species, 95% oxygen is rapidly fatal in preterm animals (40% survival at 4 days) compared with term animals (80% survival). In the preterm baboon, possibly the best model for human CLD, 100% oxygen causes an illness similar to systemic inflammatory response syndrome within 96 hours and does not always lead to BPD.[63] When term and preterm rabbits were exposed to hyperoxia, the term rabbits responded with an increase in the concentrations of antioxidant enzymes, including superoxide dismutase, catalase, glutathione peroxidase, and glucose-6-phosphate dehydrogenase. The preterm animal was unable to mount a similar response to hyperoxia and as a result developed more marked lung injury.[68] There are late effects of neonatal oxygen exposure on alveolation and lung mechanics in the rat.[69] These include a reduction in the number of alveoli in adults with enlargement of alveolar dimensions and a concomitant reduction in elastic lung recoil that persists to old age (Fig. 32-6). Similar changes are seen in human CLD (see Fig. 32-4). Another study suggests that airway wall thickening after remodeling leads to increased bronchial responsiveness in rats.[65] Neonatal rats are born without alveoli, so they act as a good model of the human preterm infant.

The mechanism whereby inadequate antioxidant activity results in pulmonary injury is poorly understood. It is postulated that under hyperoxic conditions, the production rate of oxygen free radicals, which include superoxides, singlet oxygen, and hydroxyl radicals, is markedly increased such that the normal antioxidant system is unable to cope with the increased load, particularly in preterm infants, who may be less able to respond by increasing the production of antioxidant enzymes. Toxic effects in the lung that are presumed to be mediated by free radicals include cytotoxic effects on the endothelial and epithelial cells of the lung parenchyma and on the alveolar macrophages; inhibition of surfactant synthesis; inhibition of the pulmonary vascular response to hypoxia; inhibition of normal lung repair by fibroblasts, resulting in altered collagen and elastin deposition; and inhibition of normal lung development, resulting in decreased alveolation.

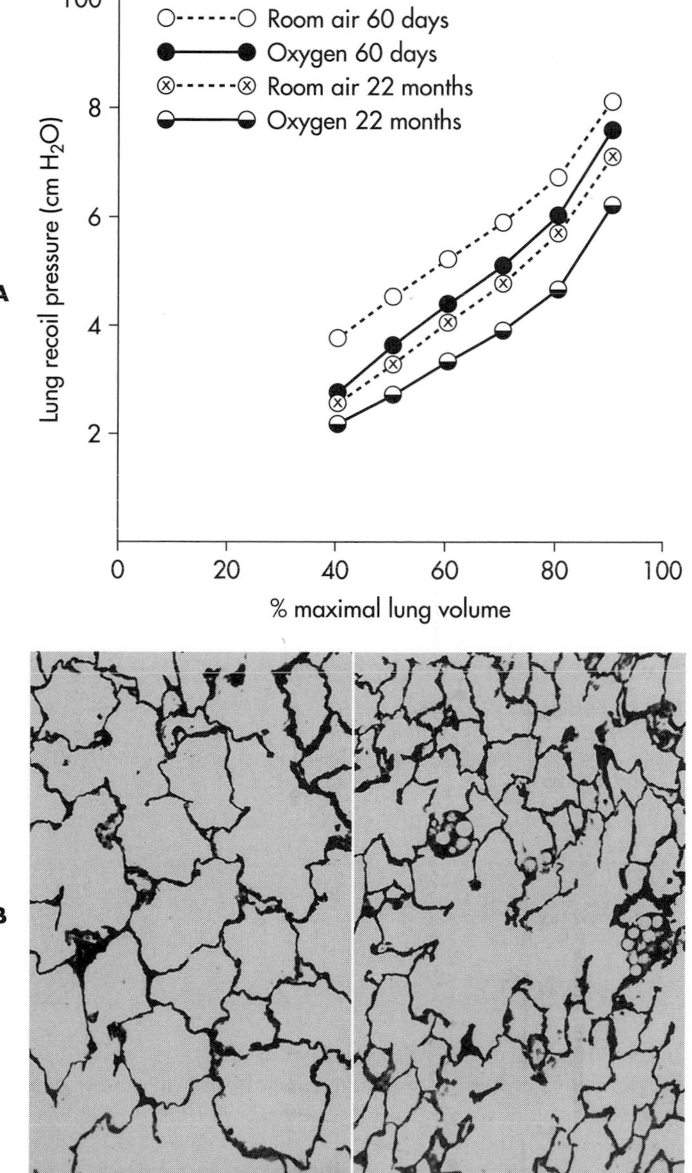

Fig. 32-6. A, Lung elastic recoil pressures with saline expansion at 40%, 50%, 60%, 70%, 80%, and 90% of maximum lung volume. Rats reared in room air, in comparison to those exposed to hyperoxia over the first 8 days of life, have a significantly greater elastic recoil pressure as adults (60 days) and during aging (22 months) ($p > 0.01$). **B,** Light micrographs of lung parenchyma of 22-month-old rats receiving room air *(right)* or suffering from hyperoxia *(left)* during the first 8 days of life. Both panels were taken at the same magnification. (From Thibeault DW et al: Pediatr Pulmonol 9:96-108, 1990.)

One approach to preventing hyperoxic pulmonary injury may be to increase the antioxidant system by the exogenous delivery of antioxidant enzymes. Walther et al[70] investigated the role of exogenous bovine superoxide dismutase given to one of twin premature lambs, with the other twin acting as a control. All lambs were exposed to hyperoxia but were normocapnic. The influx of neutrophils and macrophages into the lung was reduced, as was cellular injury, in the treated group when compared with the control group. In a double-blind, controlled trial, Rosenfeld et al[71] treated 45 premature human infants with bovine superoxide dismutase and detected reduced oxygen dependency in the treated group. A basic unanswered question is how exogenous antioxidant enzymes are effective because in vivo they mainly function intracellularly. For enhancement of intracellular delivery of antioxidant enzymes, a nontoxic preparation of superoxide dismutase has been covalently bound to heparin-like molecules and given parenterally. Selective binding to the surface of endothelial cells, including those of the pulmonary vasculature, occurs via the cells' surface heparin receptors. Another approach to augmenting the pulmonary cells' antioxidant system is to deliver superoxide dismutase encapsulated in liposomes.[72] The therapeutic benefits derived from such approaches remain to be seen.

Furthermore, antioxidant defense is provided by specific nutrients such as vitamins A, E, and C; β-carotene; sulphur-containing amino acids; and cofactors copper, zinc, selenium, and iron.[73] Supplementation with these factors may further augment the antioxidant system. Vitamin A may be particularly important to the regeneration of damaged epithelial cells. One study has shown a beneficial effect if premature infants receive supplements of vitamin A.[74] Vitamin E supplementation has not reduced the incidence of CLD, but it probably acts in synergism with other antioxidant systems. Depressed levels of the important antioxidant glutathione have been noted on the first day after birth in the bronchoalveolar lavage fluid of infants who later developed CLD.[75] The nonenzymatic antioxidants, including ceruloplasmin and uric acid, clearly have an important role in the defense against lung injury mediated by oxygen-free radicals, but further work is required with large clinical trials to evaluate the relevance of supplementation of high-risk infants with antioxidants against the development of CLD. There are potential dangers to the administration of large doses of single antioxidants. If this is done, free radicals may be simply passed down the chain to the next deficient step in the chain or even accumulate in increased amounts.

Barotrauma

In their pathologic description of CLD, Taghizadeh and Reynolds[76] found a significant association between the most severe pathologic changes of CLD and peak inspiratory pressures of more than 35 cm H_2O during mechanical ventilation. Using newborn piglets, Davis et al[77] investigated the relative contribution made to the pathogenesis of CLD by barotrauma and oxygen toxicity. Of the four groups investigated, the groups exposed to 100% oxygen with or without hyperventilation developed the most significant lung injury. Animal lungs normally ventilated in air developed no injury, and the group hyperventilated in air developed intermediate lung injury. The conclusions are that hyperoxia causes the most significant inflammatory and histologic changes but the barotrauma alone may also result in a lesser degree of lung injury. However, the importance of barotrauma to the development of CLD is provided by several studies. Premature lambs whose lungs were supported by mechanical ventilation developed more severe lung injury than lambs allowed to mature while supported by their placentae.[78] Similarly, using preterm lambs, Penn et al[79] have demonstrated the susceptibility of tracheal segments to mechanical ventilation. Because bronchomalacia is one of the long-term adverse outcomes of CLD, this form of barotrauma could be very important. It is likely that the smaller airways are similarly affected by mechanical ventilation.

The mechanism of barotrauma-induced lung injury is not known. This is further hindered by the lack of an adequate animal model of barotrauma. In premature baboons, the use of mechanical ventilation and the development of RDS has been associated with the release of platelet activating factor–like activity in the bronchoalveolar lavage fluid.[80] Mediators may therefore play a part in the development of pulmonary injury. Pulmonary edema may occur as a result of direct overdistention of the airways, resulting in a change in the permeability of endothelial and epithelial cells.[81-83] Hyperventilation leads to excessive surfactant consumption and could tip the balance where production is marginal.[84,85] Attempts to reduce barotrauma in human preterm infants by using high-frequency oscillatory ventilation have resulted in a reduced incidence of CLD compared to when conventional intermittent positive-pressure ventilation is used.[86]

The evidence therefore suggests that barotrauma significantly contributes to the development of CLD. Although the exact mechanisms of lung injury resulting from barotrauma are unknown, attempts to reduce barotrauma in human preterm infants may result in a reduced incidence of CLD.[86] High-frequency oscillatory ventilation has been shown experimentally to reduce the risk of BPD in preterm baboons,[87] although in another study, oxygen toxicity rather than mode of ventilation seemed to be the major cause of BPD.[88]

Infection

The role of infection in the pathogenesis of CLD is unclear. A multivariate analysis by Cooke[22] demonstrated that bacterial sepsis was more frequent in infants who developed CLD. Particular attention has focused on the organism *Ureaplasma urealyticum.* In animal models, infection of mice with isolates of *U. urealyticum* from newborn humans resulted in self-limiting infection.[89] However, when mice are infected with *U. urealyticum* and exposed to hyperoxia, the pulmonary lesions are more severe and the mortality rate is increased compared with infected mice exposed to air.[90] This organism is isolated more frequently in VLBW infants and is not associated with either mode of delivery or prolonged rupture of placental membranes.[91] Whether *U. urealyticum* is isolated from surface swabs, nasopharyngeal aspirates, gastric aspirates, or endotracheal aspirates, the incidence of CLD in those with positive isolates is increased when compared with the incidence in culture-negative infants. Infection may contribute to the early development of inflammation in the lung or to inactivation of surfactant within the lung.

PDA and Fluid Overload

An association has been noted by many workers between PDA and CLD.[92-94] However, a controlled, randomized study of prophylactic ligation of PDA did not demonstrate a significant improvement in oxygen dependency.[95]

A multicenter, multivariate, risk-adjusted, case-control study reported an association between an increased fluid intake within 96 hours of birth and oxygen dependency at 30 days of age.[96] Similarly, in their prospective study, van Marter et al[93] compared the medical practices of three different centers managing preterm infants with birth weights less than 1751 g. They reported that the center with the highest incidence of CLD administered higher-than-expected rates of colloids during the first 4 days of life. It has been proposed that increased fluid intake, either by direct means or by an increase in the incidence of PDA, may worsen any coexistent pulmonary edema, thus reducing pulmonary compliance. The subsequent increase in ventilatory requirements, including oxygen toxicity and barotrauma, may further exacerbate the ongoing acute lung injury. However, when Lorenz et al[97] randomized 88 infants weighing 750 to 1200 g to receive either low or high fluid intake, no difference was noted in the relative incidence of CLD between the two groups. Similarly, Kraybill et al[4] did not find an association between the development of CLD and weight loss, furosemide, or pancuronium therapy in 147 surviving infants weighing 751 to 1000 g.

Other Risk Factors

The incidence of CLD is related to the gestational age of premature infants, with the incidence increasing as gestation decreases. However, because not all premature infants develop RDS or CLD and near-term infants may develop CLD, it appears that the immaturity of the lungs predisposes the infant to the development of CLD. It is therefore not surprising to note an association between LBW and CLD because these are the infants most likely to have immature lungs. For reasons that are unclear, male infants are more prone to both RDS and CLD. Similarly, the incidence of CLD is decreased in nonwhite races. Both gender and race are independent factors for the development of CLD. An increased incidence of CLD has been reported in infants from families with atopy.[98-100] This association was not confirmed by Chan et al.[101]

POSSIBLE CELLULAR MECHANISMS IN THE PATHOGENESIS OF CLD

Although many of the risk factors contributing to the pathogenesis of CLD have been identified, no entirely suitable animal model of CLD encompasses all of them. However, animal models based on fibrosis resulting from hyperoxia or from drugs such as bleomycin, together with data from investigations of adults with pulmonary fibrosis, have provided an insight into the pathogenesis of fibrosis in the human lung.[45,102]

Cellular Responses

Interstitial fibrosis, atelectasis, emphysema, and alveolar type II cell hyperplasia are characteristic results of CLD. Prolonged exposure to hyperoxia results in initial swelling with subsequent necrosis and sloughing of ciliated cells of the bronchi and bronchioles.[103] In the alveoli, oxidant injury destroys up to 50% of the capillary bed endothelium, and type II cell hyperplasia occurs as a result of necrosis of type I alveolar cells, which is also due to oxidant injury. Type II cells line the alveolar wall and transform to functioning, gas-exchanging type I cells.[104,105] The alveolar epithelium remains largely intact during the injurious and resolution phases.[103,104]

In premature monkeys, Jackson et al[106] have shown that during the development of RDS, there is an initial increase in the number of neutrophils but not in the number of alveolar macrophages when compared with the numbers in healthy controls and fetuses of similar gestational ages. During recovery, the concentrations of macrophages increased tenfold with no additional increase in neutrophil numbers. In bronchoalveolar lavage fluid of human infants whose lungs were ventilated, few cells are seen on the first day of life, but the number increases by 72 to 96 hours.[50,55] The predominant cell at this stage is the neutrophil. With resolution of RDS the neutrophil numbers decrease but persist if the infant develops CLD (Fig. 32-7). Ogden et al[50] have demonstrated that the number of alveolar macrophages is significantly increased in infants with RDS at 96 hours compared with the number in infants who later develop CLD but is decreased in CLD at 4 and 5 weeks of age (see Fig. 32-7). Surfactant treatment of preterm infants results in an earlier increase in the number of alveolar macrophages. This postnatal increase may result from the arrival of endogenous or exogenous phospholipid in the epithelial lining fluid of the neonatal lung.[107]

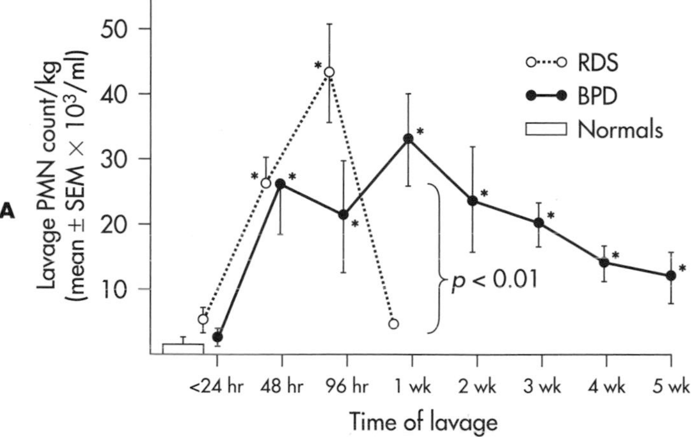

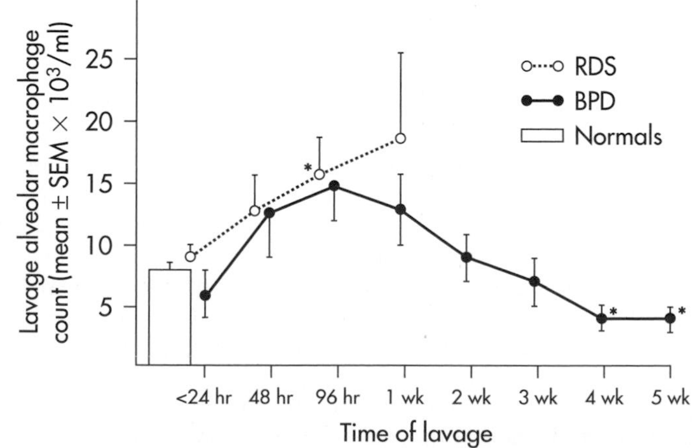

Fig. 32-7. Newborn lung lavage. **A,** Absolute neutrophil *(PMN)* count divided by body weight in kilograms (mean ± standard error of the mean *[SEM]* × 10^3/ml) at each lavage. **B,** Absolute alveolar macrophage count (mean ± standard error of the mean × 10^{-5}) at each lavage. Asterisks indicate significant difference from normal control subjects ($p < 0.05$) by analysis of variance and Duncan's multiple range test. (From Ogden BE et al: *Am Rev Respir Dis* 130:817-821, 1984.)

Elastases

Cellular and biochemical mediators are likely to be important in the pathogenesis of CLD. The release of elastases by neutrophils results in proteolytic lung damage, particularly if there is an imbalance between the levels of proteolytic enzymes and inhibitors of these enzymes, including α_2-antiproteinase and tissue inhibitor of metalloproteinases. The ratio of neutrophil elastase and α_1-antiproteinases is similar at birth in the bronchoalveolar lavage fluid of normal controls, infants who recover from RDS, and infants who subsequently develop CLD. The ratio remains static in infants who recover from RDS but increases markedly in infants who develop CLD.[50,108,109] Furthermore, α_1-antiproteinases are inactivated by free radicals released by neutrophils exposed to hyperoxia. Elastase activity and the ratio of elastase and α_1-antiproteinase are significantly decreased after dexamethasone treatment for 72 hours in infants whose lungs are ventilated and who have CLD.[108-110] However, no decrease is noted in the concentration of α_1-antiproteinase inhibitor or fibronectin, an extracellular glycoprotein that has multiple functions, including fibroblast chemotaxis.

Cytokines

The most likely candidates for control of growth and development of the lungs are cytokines. Cytokines are extracellular signaling molecules that modify the behavior of adjacent cells (paracrine) or the cells of origin (autocrine). Any disturbance of the normal growth and development of the lung leads to a cascade of cell-to-cell interactions mediated by cytokines within the lung.

Proinflammatory Cytokines

Inflammation appears to play an important role in the evolution of CLD. In experimental models, inflammation appears to be mediated by the proinflammatory cytokines tumor necrosis factor-α, interleukin-1 (IL-1), and IL-6.

Experimentally induced pulmonary fibrosis in animal models is contributing to the understanding of the pathogenesis of lung fibrosis in humans. In rats treated intratracheally with bleomycin, there is an early and transient secretion of IL-1 by alveolar macrophages, followed by a more sustained release of IL-6 by macrophages.[111,112] After pretreatment of rats with a combination of recombinant tumor necrosis factor-α and IL-1, exposure to 100% oxygen results in markedly reduced lung injury and a markedly reduced mortality rate, whereas cytokine alone provides no protection.[113] The combination probably provides protection by inducing antioxidant enzymes.[114] In human preterm infants, preliminary results from various groups indicate that the numbers of proinflammatory cytokines are increased in infants who develop CLD compared with the numbers in infants who recover from RDS.[110,115]

IL-8. IL-8, a neutrophil chemotactic agent, induces neutrophil degranulation and elicits a weak respiratory burst, resulting in the release of oxygen free radicals. It is released by a wide variety of cells, including monocytes, macrophages, neutrophils, epithelial cells, and fibroblasts. Hyperoxia increases the expression of IL-8 in monocytes exposed to 100% oxygen.[116] In fibrosing alveolitis, in which the neutrophil is the predominant cell in the bronchoalveolar lavage fluid, the concentration of IL-8 increases when compared with the concentration in controls. Similarly, in adult RDS (systemic inflammatory response syndrome), which has many similarities with neonatal RDS, the most prevalent cell in the bronchoalveolar fluid is the neutrophil.[117] The levels of IL-8 in the bronchoalveolar lavage fluid of patients with systemic inflammatory response syndrome are increased. Preliminary results from infants with CLD indicate that the concentrations of IL-8 are increased in infants with CLD compared with those in infants who recover from RDS.[115,118]

Growth Factors. Progressive inflammation and fibrosis are central to the pathogenesis of CLD. Alveolar macrophages are thought to mediate the fibrotic response in the pathogenesis of lung fibrosis, at least in idiopathic pulmonary fibrosis in adults, via the release of an array of cytokines, including the profibrotic cytokines transforming growth factor-β (TGF-β) and platelet-derived growth factor-B (PDGF-B). There is only limited information about the relevance of these cytokines to the pathogenesis of CLD.

TGF-β acts on fibroblasts to increase the transcription of fibronectin and procollagen, with a resultant increase in the levels of the associated proteins. TGF-β also inhibits the synthesis of proteases and increases the synthesis of antiproteases,[119] thus decreasing the degradation of the existing extracellular matrix. In animal models, TGF-β promotes wound repair and fibrosis,[120] although this is not due to enhanced fibroblast proliferation. Exposing two different strains of mice to bleomycin, Hoyt and Lazo[121] demonstrated that the strain of mice that developed more severe fibrosis had increased transcription of TGF-β, fibronectin, and procollagen (I and III). Similarly, Khalil et al[122,123] showed a peak in total lung levels of TGF-β on day 7, followed by a peak in the levels of collagen at day 10 in rats treated with bleomycin. Ultimately, intense TGF-β staining by immunocytochemistry was marked in areas of fibroconnective tissue deposition. Hyperplastic type II cells were intensely stained, as were alveolar macrophages when present. From the distribution of TGF-β, these researchers concluded that TGF-β may be predominately secreted by epithelial cells.[122,123]

PDGF-B is a potent chemoattractant and mitogen for fibroblasts. Although, collagen synthesis and deposition appear to be under the influence of TGF-β,[119] the contraction of the deposited collagen matrix is promoted by PDGF-B.[120]

During hyperoxic exposure of rats to 85% oxygen, the basal level of PDGF-B messenger ribonucleic acid increases 2.5-fold above control levels by day 3. This increase precedes the deoxyribonucleic acid synthesis seen on day 7, thus implying a causal role for PDGF-B in the cellular proliferative response in hyperoxia.[124] In recent studies, total PDGF-B levels were increased in the bronchoalveolar lavage fluid of preterm human infants who develop CLD when compared with the levels in preterm infants who recover from RDS.[125,126] Furthermore, the PDGF-B content in bronchoalveolar lavage fluid decreased significantly in the CLD group after 7 days of treatment with dexamethasone.

Other Cytokines. Increasing numbers of cytokines are being recognized as contributing toward the pathogenesis of pulmonary fibrosis.[127] Only a few that may have an important role in the evolution of CLD are mentioned here. Fibroblast growth factors are a family of cytokines with a high affinity for heparin; they induce the production of a collagenase, which is vital to the migration of capillary endothelial cells into the preexisting extracellular matrix and are among the most potent inducers of neovascularization. Insulin-like growth factors (somatomedins) are a family of small peptides that act as progression factors and thus complement PDGF-B in promoting the replication of fibroblasts, with the subsequent deposition of collagen. Macrophage inflammatory protein-1 is a heparin-binding cytokine released by macrophages in response to bacterial endotoxin; it is mildly chemotactic for neutrophils but stimulates them to produce an oxidative burst, with a resultant release of free oxygen radicals.

Fibronectin

Fibronectin is not strictly a cytokine, but with collagen, elastin, laminins, and proteoglycans, it is a constituent of the extracellular matrix.[128] Secreted in the soluble plasma form by hepatocytes and in the cellular form by macrophages, fibroblasts, and epithelial cells, fibronectin appears to be important in maintaining the cell-to-cell and cell-to-substratum attachments of the epithelial and endothelial cells in the lung. Both forms have similar functions. During lung injury, fibronectin functions as potent fibroblast chemoattractant and as an attachment and a competence growth factor for fibroblasts. Fibronectin transcription is increased in animal models of pulmonary fibrosis induced by bleomycin and in adults with idiopathic pulmonary fibrosis. In infants with CLD, the concentration of fibronectin in bronchoalveolar lavage fluid is increased when compared with controls who develop RDS and subsequently recover.[108,129,130] Therefore it has been proposed that basement membrane denuded during lung injury exposes fibronectin, which acts as a potent chemoattractant for fibroblasts and macrophages. There has been no documented inhibitor of fibronectin synthesis. There is certainly marked thickening of the basement membrane during remodeling after acute neonatal lung injury.[59] The topic has been little investigated.

Possible Model

In the premature lung, respiratory failure resulting from asphyxia, infection, inflammation, surfactant deficiency, and physiologic immaturity leads to the need for mechanical ventilation and oxygen therapy. Injury occurs as a result of oxygen toxicity and barotrauma, with possible contributions from infection, air leaks, and fluid overload.

Acute inflammation results in the release of proinflammatory cytokines and the neutrophil chemoattractant IL-8. Neutrophils are clearly important mediators of acute inflammation. The migration of neutrophils from the bloodstream to the lung occurs as a result of a series of complex interactions between the adhesion molecules on the surfaces of both the endothelial cells and neutrophils (Fig. 32-8). Endothelial cells activated by tumor necrosis factor-α and IL-1 express specific surface adhesion molecules that interact with constitutively expressed neutrophil surface adhesion molecules, leading to margination or "rolling" on the vessel wall. Local generation of neutrophil-activating cytokines, including IL-8, after expression of appropriate adhesion molecules on the surfaces of both neutrophils and endothelial cells leads to the migration of neutrophils to the lung.[131]

The activated neutrophils release proteolytic enzymes, including elastases, that result in proteolytic lung injury. An imbalance between the proteolytic enzymes and antiproteinases, including α_1-antiproteinases, further potentiates this proteolytic lung damage. Supplemental oxygen results in the release of oxygen free radicals, which has widespread effects, includ-

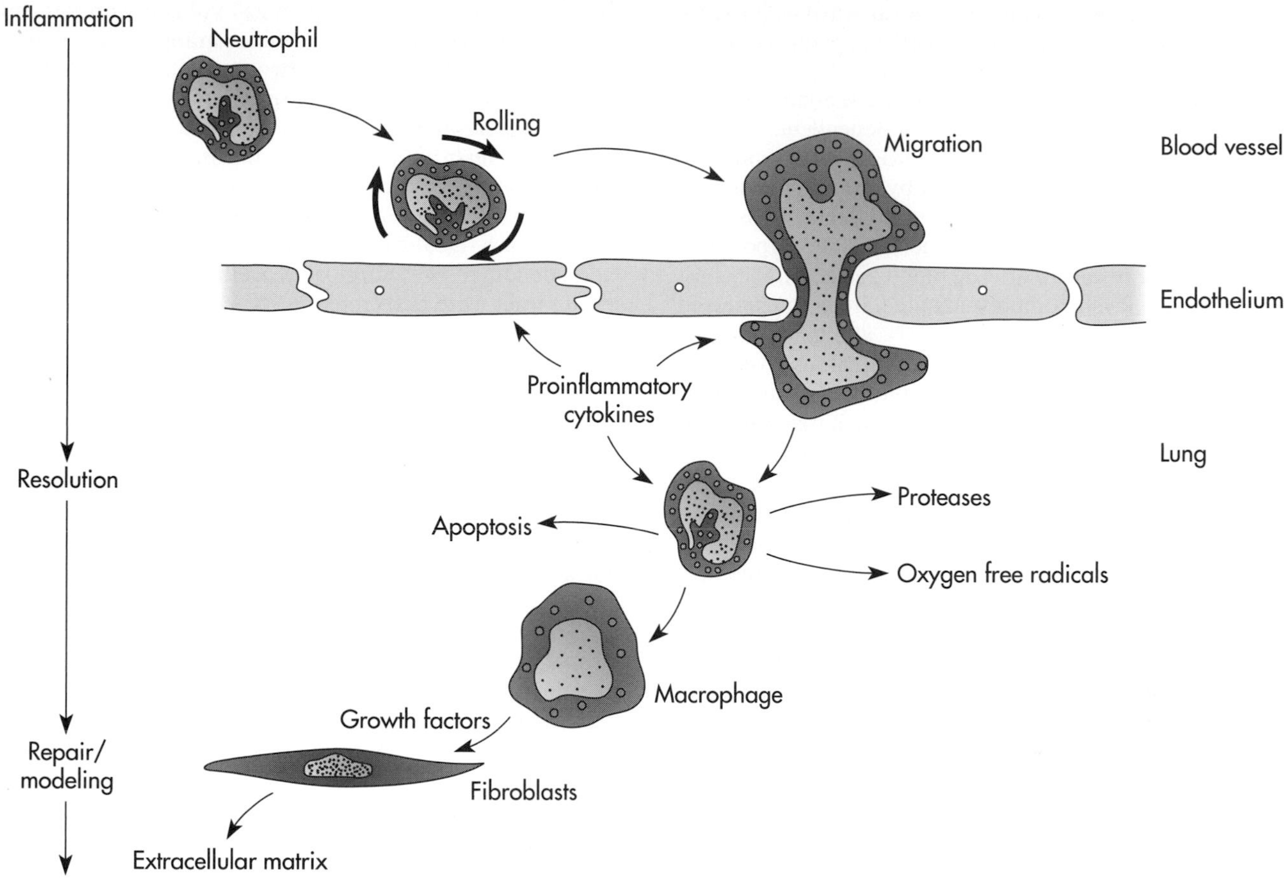

Fig. 32-8. Speculative model for the pathogenesis of CLD at the cellular level.

ing cytotoxicity of endothelial and epithelial cells, inhibition of surfactant, and inhibition of normal lung repair by fibroblasts. This destruction is further potentiated by a lack of adequate enzymatic and nonenzymatic antioxidant activity. Oxygen free radicals contribute further to the destruction of pulmonary tissues by inactivating antiproteinases and increasing the imbalance between proteolytic and antiproteolytic enzymes. Inadequate host defenses to free radicals also result in acute lung injury (Chapter 63). Additional airway damage probably occurs as a result of direct barotrauma of mechanical ventilation.

With time, resolution commences with the recruitment of macrophages to the injured lung tissues, possibly because of the chemoattractant properties of fibronectin, which is exposed by denuded basement membrane. Alveolar macrophages release an array of cytokines, including the profibrotic TGF-β and PDGF-B. Under the influence of PDGF-B, fibroblasts are recruited to the site of injury and undergo proliferation. TGF-β increases the transcription of both fibronectin and procollagen, thus resulting in the deposition of interstitial fibrotic tissue. TGF-β restores the ratio of proteolytic enzymes and antiproteinases by preventing the synthesis of proteolytic enzymes but promoting the synthesis of antiproteolytic enzymes. Other cytokines such as fibroblast and insulin-like growth factors contribute to the remodeling process by promoting neovascularization and acting as progression factors for fibroblasts.

Summary

In summary, inflammation, resolution, and healing with remodeling are essential features in the pathogenesis of CLD (see Fig. 32-3). Much research has focused on the development of pulmonary fibrosis in animal models and interstitial pulmonary fibrosis in human adults. Limited knowledge is available in human preterm infants, although many groups are now focusing on the pathogenesis of CLD in preterm infants at the cellular and molecular levels. Most of the previously discussed issues have been extrapolated from various animal models and research devoted to adults with pulmonary fibrosis. The exact significance of the mechanisms remains to be seen.

CLINICAL FEATURES OF CLD OF PREMATURITY

Neonatal Unit

In infants in whom classic BPD evolves, Northway[1] recognized four stages of clinical, radiologic, and pathologic change. Stage I is typified by the clinical, radiologic, and pathologic features of RDS (see Chapter 31). During stage II, which occurs during days 4 to 10 of age, either the infant's respiratory status improves, or the condition progresses to stage III. In infants who recover from RDS, a reduction in inspired oxygen levels, peak inspiratory pressures, and minute volume is possible. After weaning from mechanical ventilation and a variable period of supplemental oxygen (most frequently administered via a head box or if prolonged by nasal cannulae), the infant is weaned to room air. In infants whose condition does not improve, the lungs become less compliant, and ventilatory requirements may increase. Pulmonary interstitial emphysema and other air leaks, including pneumothorax and pneumomediastinum, may develop. The chest radiograph shows increasing opacification with or without air leaks. In infants who die during this stage, thick exudation into the airways with patchy bronchiolar and alveolar epithelial cell necrosis is seen at autopsy.

During stage III, occurring between the second and third weeks of age, the infant remains oxygen dependent. The respiratory status may slowly improve or progress to respiratory failure, particularly if it is complicated by chronic pulmonary interstitial emphysema, infection, or hemodynamically significant PDA. Compensated respiratory acidosis and hypoxemia are noted from the results of arterial blood gas tests. The chest radiograph shows cystic emphysematous areas interspersed with areas of reticular strands, atelectasis, and consolidation. Histologically, at autopsy, areas of emphysematous alveoli are seen adjacent to areas of atelectatic alveoli. Healing commences, and the necrotic bronchial and bronchiolar epithelial cells are replaced by mucosal metaplasia and hyperplasia.

In stage IV, occurring after 4 weeks of age, the infant is in stable or progressive respiratory failure. An infant whose respiratory status is stable is weaned from mechanical ventilation and supplemental oxygen over the ensuing weeks and months; many of these infants require long-term domiciliary supplemental oxygen. However, in an infant whose condition continues to deteriorate, ventilatory needs increase, requiring increased amounts of inspired oxygen, peak inspiratory pressure, and minute volume. The condition may be complicated by right-sided heart failure and pulmonary hypertension. The prognosis is poor. The chest radiograph usually demonstrates persistent CLD with hyperinflated and cystic lungs, particularly in the lower lobes, and in the most severe cases, striking areas of atelectasis and scarring. The pathologic features have been described.

In many infants who remain oxygen dependent the radiograph does not have the classic appearance of stage IV disease. More frequently the chest radiograph shows homogeneous or patchy, ill-defined pulmonary opacities lacking any coarse reticulation ("small gray lungs"). This radiographic appearance has been classified as type I CLD with type II disease, showing similar radiographic changes to Northway's stage IV bronchopulmonary disease[9] (Fig. 32-9). This simpler classification is useful at 1 month of age because type I disease has a better prognosis than type II disease, which more frequently follows pulmonary interstitial emphysema. Many other radiographic features, including segmental atelectasis resulting from mucus plugging and upper lobe shadowing secondary to repeated aspiration, are commonly seen (see Fig. 32-9).

Infant and Preschool Child

A useful and practical definition of CLD is a simple one of oxygen dependency at 36 weeks' corrected gestation.[3] Therefore the typical infant diagnosed as suffering from CLD is usually a preterm infant who has needed supportive mechanical ventilation, including supplemental oxygen, during the neonatal period for RDS. Clinically, features of obstructive airway disease are evident. An abnormally increased respiratory rate with retractions and a variable degree of hypoxemia (in air) are noted. The arterial P_{CO_2} may be raised. At discharge, these infants may require domiciliary oxygen. The infant may eat poorly, and weight gain is usually inadequate. Vomiting and GER are common. The chest radiograph may show changes compatible with CLD, including cystic, consolidated, fibrotic, and atelectatic areas (see Fig. 32-9). Pulmonary function tests demonstrate an increased airway resistance, low dynamic compliance, and a variable thoracic gas volume with gas-mixing inefficiency (see later section). Echocardiography may demonstrate right ventricular hypertrophy with evidence of pulmonary hypertension and tricuspid regurgitation.

The differential diagnosis of obstructive airway disease in infancy is dealt with in Chapter 63. In addition to intrathoracic disorders, it includes a number of upper airway disorders such as laryngomalacia and tracheomalacia, subglottic stenosis, laryngeal webs, vascular rings, and enlarged tonsils and adenoids.[132,133] Surgical procedures on the upper respiratory tract were performed in 30% of VLBW infants in one study.[133]

Exacerbations of respiratory symptoms are common in infants born prematurely, especially those with CLD. Potentially the most serious exacerbating factor is viral infection. In a series of 40 infants who were born prematurely and who needed mechanical ventilation for respiratory insufficiency, 70% had one or more episodes of pneumonia or bronchitis during the first 2 years of life.[134] A direct relationship was noted between the presence of CLD and respiratory infections. In a 4-month prospective study of children younger than 2 years of age with CLD, 27 of 30 children had one or more respiratory illnesses.[135] Respiratory syncytial virus was isolated from 59% of the children, and 70% of these required hospitalization. Adenovirus is particularly troublesome because it may result in bronchiolitis obliterans, which may make CLD irreparable. Whooping cough (pertussis) has been more commonly reported in infants born prematurely in surveys in the United Kingdom,[40] possibly because of a past reluctance to administer vaccine to this vulnerable group. A full immunization program is vital for preterm infants.

Other causes of exacerbations include aspiration events, heart failure, and "wheezy" episodes. Apneic events or sleep-disordered breathing with hypoxemic spells frequently complicate the situation.

Sudden infant death has been reported more frequently in infants with BPD. One small study suggested an odds ratio of 8 (11% mortality) in comparison with healthy infants weighing less than 1000 g at birth.[136] In the authors' experience of 100 very severe cases of CLD in which the infants were dependent on domiciliary oxygen therapy, one infant died suddenly and unexpectedly. In a multicenter trial of corticosteroids for CLD, there was a 3.4% mortality (7 of 209) from sudden unexpected death in infancy.[137]

Adolescent and Adult

A large number of infants with CLD who survive to childhood, adolescence, and adulthood have some degree of pulmonary dysfunction. Most studies of these populations are biased by extreme selectivity, inadequate control data, and small numbers. Yu et al[138] studied 16 survivors of CLD at a mean age of 8.4 years (range, 7.2 to 9.6 years) and reported an 81% prevalence of wheezing. Respiratory symptoms are most troublesome in the preschool years and seem to decline thereafter.[139] One study of a population-based cohort of 120 LBW children and 100 full-term controls studied at the age of 7 found troublesome cough with colds to be the only persistent symptom[40]; wheeze was no longer a problem. Exercise tolerance has been studied in small numbers of children. "Normal" preterm children have no limitation,[140] but 10-year-old survivors of BPD are commonly reported to develop exercise-induced asthma, hypoxemia, and hypercapnia.[141]

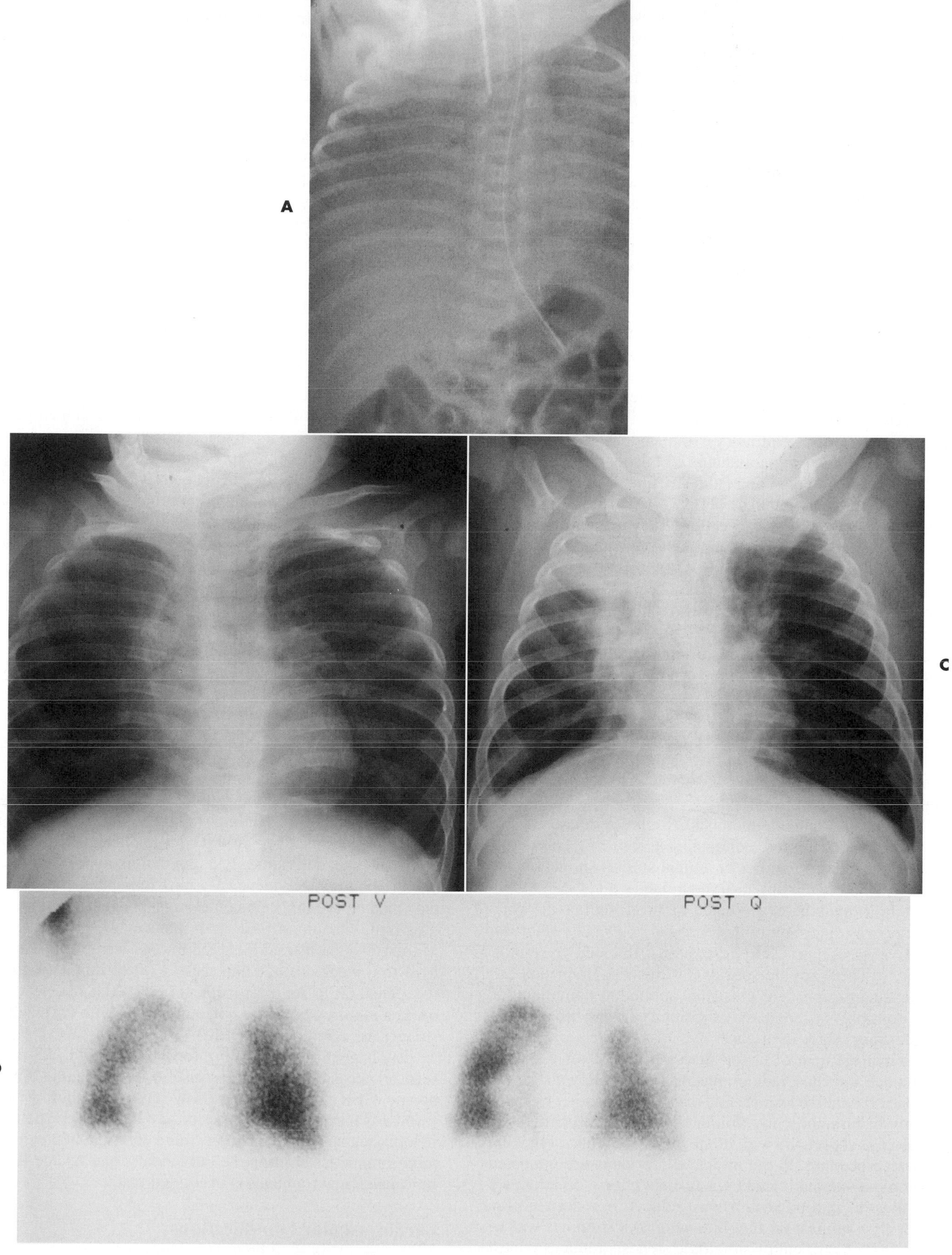

Fig. 32-9. Chest radiographs in CLD of prematurity. **A,** Type I CLD (small gray lungs) in an infant born at 27 weeks' gestation who is 4 weeks of age. **B,** Type II CLD with classic changes in a VLBW infant at 2 weeks of age. **C,** Segmental atelectasis *(right upper lobe)* resulting from mucus plugging in an infant born at 27 weeks' gestation who is 4 months of age. **D,** Patchy, matched defects of ventilation *(V)* by krypton-81m inhalation and perfusion *(Q)* by technetium-99m infusion in a child with severe CLD. *POST,* Posterior view.

Most adult survivors of CLD have a degree of pulmonary dysfunction, including hyperinflation, airway obstruction, and airway hyperresponsiveness.[2] However, LBW infants who never had any neonatal respiratory abnormalities have a degree of respiratory dysfunction when they reach middle childhood.[34-37,132] Lung function tends to improve with age, however.[34] The long-term outcome is unknown, but recent evidence linking fetal and infantile somatic and pulmonary development with CLD in adulthood suggests that chronic airway disease with accelerated aging processes may be in store for infants with CLD.[142]

ACQUIRED UPPER RESPIRATORY TRACT COMPLICATIONS

Disorders of the intrathoracic airways are important and common in infants with CLD. They include subglottic stenosis, laryngeal granulomas, laryngomalacia and tracheomalacia, vocal cord paralysis, and laryngeal perforation resulting from direct endotracheal tube trauma. In one series of 196 bronchoscopies in 132 neonates with respiratory complications, the most common findings were laryngomalacia or tracheomalacia (24%), tracheal obstruction resulting from stricture or granulation tissue (17%), obstructive mucus plugs (17%), tracheobronchitis (8%), and laryngeal perforation (2%).[143] Vocal cord paralysis secondary to thoracic surgery should be considered.

The true incidence of subglottic stenosis is unknown and probably varies according to local practice. In one study, it was reported in 5 from 845 newborns who required artificial ventilation.[144] In the authors' experience over a 15-year period, surgical procedures that were performed to relieve severe obstruction and that used shouldered orotracheal tubes have been performed on only 6 of 1200 VLBW babies whose lungs were mechanically ventilated. Arguments rage concerning the cause of upper airway damage. Direct laryngeal and tracheal trauma is likely to lead to shedding of the respiratory epithelium with subsequent reepithelialization and squamous metaplasia, scarring, and contraction.[47,59]

Large airway damage includes stricture, granuloma, cyst formation, and excessive collapsibility resulting from bronchomalacia.[145-147] A number of animal studies show how airway collapsibility (compliance) decreases with age.[148] Airway collapsibility may be exacerbated by bronchodilators, which reduce airway smooth muscle tone, and conversely stabilized by active smooth muscle contraction induced by methacholine.[138] There are big species differences. Tracheomegaly may result from positive pressures applied to compliant airways, possibly exacerbated by the trend of using bronchodilators at earlier stages of disease.

The management of upper airway pathology may require lateral neck and chest radiographs, barium swallow to exclude extrinsic obstructive lesions, and direct visualization by laryngoscopy or bronchoscopy to identify specific abnormalities. Tracheobronchography with dilute, nonionic contrast medium is a safe procedure. In the infant whose lungs are intubated, weaning may be facilitated by a 24-hour course of corticosteroids. Postextubation stridor was reduced in a double-blind trial, with a suggestion that late subglottic stenosis was reduced.[149] Management of subglottic stenosis remains controversial, but the experience in Liverpool, England, suggests that conservative treatment with tracheostomy achieved success in 73% of patients; corrective surgery and laser treatment are reserved for the more difficult cases.[150] Tracheobronchial stenosis is less amenable to effective treatment.[151]

EXTRAPULMONARY COMPLICATIONS

Growth and Nutrition Problems

Several controlled and uncontrolled studies have demonstrated suboptimal growth in survivors with CLD. Although weight and length are appropriate for gestational age at birth, they are commonly at or below the third percentile at 40 weeks' corrected gestation. As the pulmonary status improves, accelerated growth is seen in infants who recover from CLD. Infants with CLD may fail to grow satisfactorily because of increased work of breathing, hypoxemia, GER, poor feeding with inadequate nutritional intake, heart failure, neurodevelopmental handicap, and socioeconomic factors (including inadequate parenting skills and emotional deprivation).

Hypoxemia appears to be particularly detrimental to growth in infants with CLD. Groothuis et al[152] noted that when oxygen was abruptly and inadvisably discontinued by the parents of 7 infants, weight gain dramatically decreased to a mean of 1.4 g/day compared with 16.0 g/day in 15 infants who continued to receive supplemental oxygen. Growth restarted when oxygen recommenced, but infants failed to catch up with their peers. It would be unethical to try to repeat this "natural" experiment in a controlled manner, but the conclusion—adequate oxygenation is a prerequisite for adequate growth—seems clear. Factors other than hypoxemia are important because under other circumstances (e.g., cyanotic congenital heart disease), growth may be satisfactory with lower values of oxygen saturation than occur in CLD.

Infants with CLD have increased energy expenditure, particularly resulting from increased work of breathing secondary to abnormal lung mechanics. Improved growth may be obtained by increasing the caloric intake of these infants and, if necessary, by increasing the caloric density of their food. Vomiting, heart failure, and feeding difficulties may contribute to undernutrition and growth failure.

Gastroesophageal Reflux

GER is common in infants with CLD. It may manifest by obvious vomiting, poor feeding, failure to thrive, or irritability, but in some cases, even mild possetting is absent. Pulmonary effects include deteriorating lung function, hypoxic spells, and overt radiographic evidence of aspiration. Other complications may include anemia, hematemesis, esophageal stricture, laryngospasm, chronic stridor, and apnea.[153-155] Hrabovsky and Mullett[153] demonstrated that symptoms were usually evident by 4 to 6 weeks of age and that 14 of 22 infants with CLD (64%) had GER. An improvement in growth and a decrease in oxygen requirement were noted in infants with CLD who had surgery for symptomatic GER.[156,157]

Esophageal pH monitoring for 24 hours and radionuclide scan on occasion are the most useful investigations for diagnosing GER.[158] Barium swallow and meal should be performed if mechanical obstruction is suspected. Hypertrophic pyloric stenosis is, for example, more common in preterm than term infants. Examining the bronchoalveolar lavage fluid for lipid-laden macrophages is of limited value.

Cardiovascular Complications

Heart failure is common in infants with CLD and is often overlooked. Contributory factors include pulmonary hypertension, right and left ventricular hypertrophy, right-to-left shunting through the foramen ovale (particularly as the right atrial pressure rises as a consequence of pulmonary hypertension), and systemic hypertension. Persistent PDA often complicates the early course of CLD and contributes to respiratory failure. A high index of suspicion is required in these patients because there are many similarities between exacerbations of pulmonary dysfunction resulting from infection and those resulting from cardiac failure and because one condition may lead to the other. Poor feeding, tachypnea, increased oxygen requirements, and inappropriate weight gain may be present. Hepatomegaly is a late sign and is difficult to elicit in infants with obstructive airway disease. Treatment with additional supplemental oxygen, fluid restriction, and diuretics may be necessary.

The possibility that unsuspected congenital heart disease may predispose to CLD should always be considered.[159] Of the authors' 75 patients with severe CLD dependent on domiciliary oxygen therapy, 2 had structural heart disease requiring surgical procedures within the first year of life. In both cases, clinical status improved markedly in the postoperative period. Another factor in the development of pulmonary hypertension in CLD is the presence of systemic pulmonary shunt vessels, which have been described by two groups.[160,161] Histologically these have been demonstrated as dilated bronchial arteries.[162] The relevance of these vessels is unclear, as is the appropriate means of management.

Pulmonary hypertension is the most important cardiovascular complication of CLD. It can lead to cor pulmonale, which was in the past a major cause of death in CLD. There are two components: variable, oxygen sensitive (hypoxic) vasoconstriction and a relatively fixed component. Recent observations suggest that even in the presence of high concentrations of inspired oxygen, a further variable element can be uncovered by the use of inhaled nitric oxide. The underlying structural basis for pulmonary hypertension has been described by Hislop et al[57] and Hislop and Haworth.[163]

The developmental history of hypoxic vasoconstriction has not been studied in human infants, but there is an increase with age in newborn rabbits.[164] There are great interindividual differences also[165] (Fig. 32-10), and experimentally, a number of physiologic factors such as cardiac output, acid-base balance, and mixed venous oxygen tension may affect it over the short-term period.[166]

Noninvasive diagnostic methods of investigation include echocardiography with continuous-wave Doppler flow measurements and (rarely) radionuclide angiography. Cardiac catheterization is risky and should be performed only if required for the diagnosis of structural disease or a life-threatening complication.

In the past, M-mode echocardiography was extensively used to investigate the natural history and management of pulmonary hypertension in CLD.[167,168] Halliday et al[167] established the importance of an oxygen-sensitive element to pulmonary hypertension, with a clear implication that adequate oxygenation was an important aspect of management. Abman et al[165] used cardiac catheterization to study oxygen-dependent infants with CLD and made the very important observation that there were great individual differences in the response to oxygen (see Fig. 32-10). Even mild degrees of hypoxemia were associated with unacceptable pulmonary artery pressure in some individuals. A very poor prognosis (50% mortality rate) was found in 10 infants with pulmonary hypertension who were unresponsive to oxygen therapy.[160]

Cardiac catheterization has been used in a number of studies.[165,169-171] These studies have indicated significant disparities between the measurements made during catheterization and M-mode and Doppler ultrasound techniques.

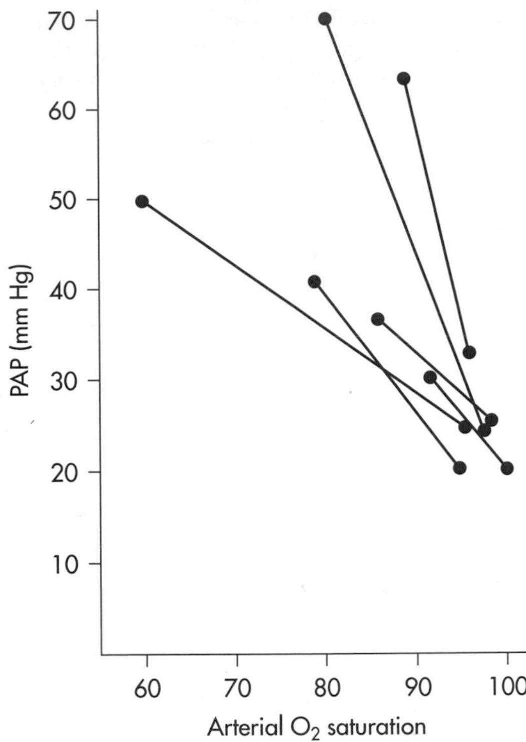

Fig. 32-10. Relationship of mean pulmonary artery pressure *(PAP)* to systemic arterial oxygen saturation in infants with BPD, measured during cardiac catheterization. There are great individual differences in both the degree of oxygen-sensitive (reversible) pulmonary hypertension and the fixed component that remains when hypoxia is abolished. (From Abman SH et al: *Pediatrics* 75:80-84, 1985.)

Recent advances in echocardiography suggest that indirect methods of assessing pulmonary artery pressure using Doppler time intervals (e.g., the ratio of pulmonary artery acceleration time and right ventricular ejection time)[172] or the more direct method for determining right ventricular pressure in the presence of tricuspid regurgitation[173-175] may be more reliable and practical for monitoring children and their responses to oxygen therapy in clinical practice.

Neurodevelopmental Problems

Because infants with CLD come from the smallest, sickest population of preterm infants, it is not surprising that neurodevelopmental problems are relatively common. Although direct comparability among studies is impossible, most studies appear to suggest that half the survivors are free of any handicap at follow-up but that half are either moderately or severely handicapped, cerebral palsy being the most frequent condition reported. Furthermore, 4% of survivors in studies reviewed by Bregman and Farrell[176] were blind as a result of severe retinopathy of prematurity. This is likely to be an underestimate because many studies exclude from follow-up any infants with significant retinopathy of prematurity. Similarly, not all studies reported the presence of sensorineural hearing loss, but the prevalence appears to be approximately 4% in survivors of CLD.[176]

Of particular importance in CLD are feeding problems and control of breathing. Many infants with CLD exhibit dysphagia. This rarely has an obvious mechanical or even neurologic cause but seems to be an acquired behavioral problem, probably on the basis of swallowing difficulties during weaning from tube to bottle food. Hypoxia during feeding may complicate matters.[177,178] Later in infancy, fear of lumpy foods may complicate feeding.

Sleep-disordered breathing is generally secondary to mechanical disturbances and is enhanced by upper airway floppiness or obstruction. However, hypoxic arousal mechanisms may not work as well in preterm infants,[179] which in a condition known to be associated with a greater likelihood of hypoxemia[178,180] is clearly a potentially life-threatening complication.

CLINICAL PULMONARY PHYSIOLOGY

Background

Lung Development and Disease

Disturbances in lung mechanics and gas exchange in CLD must be measured against the changing pattern imposed by growth and development (see Chapter 4). Abnormalities of lung function may be the result of CLD or its complications, may be causally related (see Fig. 32-2), or may be independently associated with CLD (see Table 32-2). Disturbed physiology changes with time[34]; follow-up studies have reached early adulthood,[2] but it is likely that abnormalities persist for the patient's lifetime, possibly accelerating the aging process itself.[150]

Physiologic Measurement

Functional assessment has several purposes (Table 32-5) and requires methods appropriate to the age group concerned (Table 32-6). The most important and widely used physiologic measurements relate to gas exchange and especially oxygenation because appropriate oxygen therapy appears to be the key to the successful long-term outcome of established CLD.

Gas Exchange

Pathophysiology

By definition, hypoxemia is a feature of BPD and therefore of the early stages of CLD. The degree of severity varies with the stage of disease, so in the severest cases of BPD in the neonatal unit, artificial ventilation with 100% oxygen is required. The factors leading to hypoxemia follow:

1. Mechanical disturbance leading to alveolar underventilation, as indicated by raised values for the arterial P_{CO_2}, and in the chronic state, a compensatory increase in the bicarbonate concentration (positive base excess)
2. Ventilation-perfusion mismatching, which can be measured by calculating the degree of right-to-left shunting, assuming that there is no extrapulmonary shunt
3. Extrapulmonary shunt through the foramen ovale in the presence of pulmonary hypertension in the first few months of life
4. Abnormalities of control of breathing, leading to episodic breathing, apnea or hypopnea, or chronic underventilation

In practice, these processes interact to produce the characteristic instability of arterial oxygenation from which children with CLD seem to suffer (Fig. 32-11).

There are several important consequences of hypoxemia (Table 32-7). The most important is pulmonary vasoconstriction; although a structural basis for increased pulmonary vascular resistance is undoubtedly present in many children with CLD,[163] a reactive, oxygen-sensitive element is almost always detectable too.[160,165,167,174] The mechanism of the reversible element of pulmonary vascular resistance is unclear. Even in the presence of 100% oxygen during mechanical ventilation, a reversible element can still be demonstrated by a response to inhaled nitric oxide (Fig. 32-12). The large individual differences

Table 32-5 Assessment of Pulmonary Function

PURPOSE	EXAMPLE OF MEASUREMENT
Assessment of severity of disease	Blood gas estimation, oxygen saturation by oximetry
Nature of pathophysiology	Lung mechanics
Response to therapy	Bronchodilator response; pulmonary vascular response to oxygen
Detection of complications	Sleep monitoring; echocardiography
Research	
Risk factors	Lung mechanics related to neonatal factors
Therapeutic trials	Airway function after corticosteroid therapy
Mechanics	Bronchial responsiveness

Table 32-6 Lung Function at Different Ages*

	APPROPRIATE TYPE OF INVESTIGATION		
PURPOSE	INFANT	PRESCHOOL CHILD	SCHOOL CHILD
Lung mechanics			
Airway function	Squeeze method with or without pump, *forced deflation maneuver, plethysmography*	Oscillation method	Forced expiratory maneuvers, *plethysmography*
Lung compliance	Occlusion technique, *esophageal balloon*	Weighted spirometer method	Quasistatic methods, *esophageal balloon*
Lung volume and gas mixing	Helium dilution, nitrogen washout, *plethysmography*	Helium dilution, nitrogen washout	Plethysmography, *helium dilution*
Gas exchange	Arterial blood gas test, oximetry	Oximetry	Oximetry, exercise physiology
Bronchial responsiveness	Bronchodilators only using squeeze method	Bronchodilator or constrictor using transcutaneous oxygen tension to measure response	Bronchodilator or constrictor challenge with forced expiration
Breathing during sleep	Polysomnography with oximetry *(with or without esophageal pH monitoring)*	Oximetry with movement detector, *infrared video camera*	Standard methods

*Methods in italics are technically complex or invasive.

in the degree of pulmonary vascular oxygen responsiveness among individuals[165] (see Fig. 32-10) imply either the need to measure the effect in each infant or to maintain a level of oxygenation above which hypoxic vasoconstriction is abolished in all infants with CLD. There is presumably a critical level of pulmonary hypertension at which right atrial pressure exceeds left atrial pressure, leading in young infants to shunting across the foramen ovale. The long-term benefits of a reduction in pulmonary vascular resistance include better right ventricular function[181] and probably (although as yet unproved) increased long-term survival.

Acute hypoxic airway narrowing has been demonstrated in two physiologic studies.[182,183] Because the large airways are normally exposed to ambient concentrations of oxygen, the effect must occur in peripheral airways, where gas mixing in CLD may be poor, leading to localized hypoxia, or the effect must be the result of hypoxemia. The contribution of hypoxic airway narrowing to clinical disease is unknown but clearly represents a potential vicious cycle when added to any underlying disorder of lung mechanics in CLD (see Fig. 32-11).

Adverse event
• Sleep
• Feeding
• Aspiration
• Interrupted O_2 supply

Hypoxia

↑ Pulmonary vascular resistance

↑ Airway obstruction

↓ Central drive

Fig. 32-11. Interacting cycles of hypoxia. The cycles may be broken by termination of the adverse event or by arousal of the infant.

Control of breathing may be disturbed in some infants with CLD. Sleep-disordered breathing with more frequent and prolonged pauses than normal is found in general in babies who had been born prematurely.[184-186] The hypoxic arousal response was abnormal in 8 of 12 infants in one study of CLD.[179] The significance of the finding is unclear, but these results could provide an explanation for sudden unexpected death in CLD.[136] Recent studies showed that spontaneous desaturations during sleep are more likely if the usual level of oxygenation is low, a complex way of demonstrating that the oxygen-hemoglobin dissociation curve is not linear.[180,187] Whether growth failure in hypoxic infants with CLD is related to sleep disruption is unclear.[152]

The pattern of hypoxemia during sleep, feeding, and wakefulness changes with age during infancy. Early in infancy, oxygen-dependent babies with CLD become more hypoxic during feeding,[177,178] but from about 6 months of age, their lungs generally oxygenate better. Postural effects on oxygenation are also more marked in young infants, with falls in the partial pressure of arterial oxygen of 7.5 to 15 mm Hg in the supine position in infants recovering from RDS.[188,189] Acute viral infections may be associated with transiently worse hypoxemia, especially if lower respiratory tract symptoms develop. A decline in the arterial oxygen saturation occurs 1 to 2 days before the onset even of upper respiratory tract symptoms in oxygen-dependent infants. The mechanism is unknown but provides a useful warning. Other major complications such as

Table 32-7 Consequences of Hypoxia in CLD

TARGET	ACUTE EFFECTS	LONG-TERM EFFECTS
Airways	Increased airway resistance	Smooth muscle hypertrophy
Pulmonary vasculature	Increased pulmonary vascular resistance with or without shunt via the foramen ovale	Cor pulmonale
Central nervous system	Arousal or apnea with sleep disturbance	Sudden unexpected death, growth failure

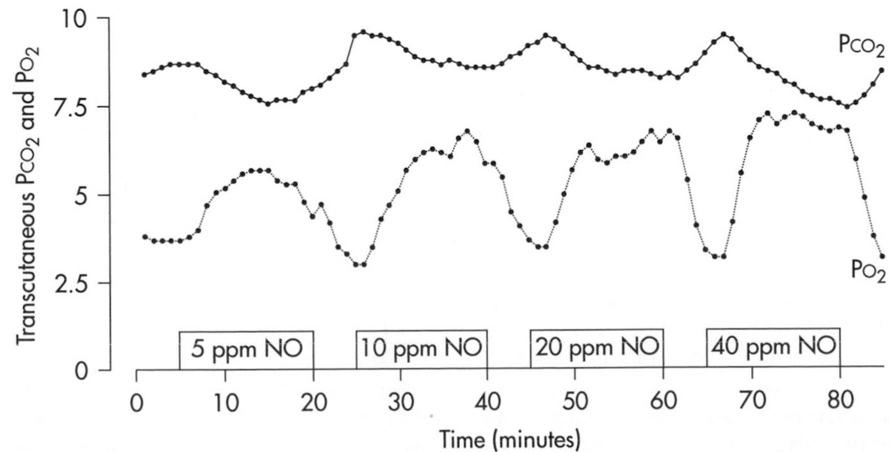

Fig. 32-12. Effect of nitric oxide *(NO)* on the partial pressures of transcutaneous oxygen *(P_{O_2})* and carbon dioxide *(P_{CO_2})* on an 12-week-old infant whose lungs are mechanically ventilated and who is receiving 100% oxygen for severe CLD of prematurity. An increasingly brisk and quantitatively greater change in the partial pressure of oxygen was induced by increasing concentrations of nitric oxide. The partial pressure tended to decline, with a longer time constant during administration of nitric oxide. (From Mupanemunda R: Unpublished observation.)

pulmonary aspiration and heart failure may be detected by worsening respiratory symptoms with increased hypoxemia. Whether chronic mild hypoxemia may persist to school age or is exacerbated by exercise remains to be confirmed.[141]

Clinical Measurement

Full arterial blood gas measurement is indicated only during the early phase of severe CLD with respiratory failure or during an acute exacerbation. Radial artery puncture through anesthetized skin should be performed by an expert, ideally while the infant sleeps. The disturbance caused by the infant often renders all but the value of the base excess useless. Because the latter is measurable from a capillary sample, in the absence of an indwelling arterial cannula, arterial sampling is an unrewarding exercise that should be performed only if the information obtained is likely to affect clinical decision making.

The advent of oximetry has rendered most other techniques obsolete. Certainly, transcutaneous monitors are useful only for detecting trends.[190] The effects of age and sleep state need to be taken into account.[191] Recording oximeters provide the information relevant to the management of oxygen therapy. However, operators should be familiar with their mode of operation (beat-to-beat or averaging) and the detection of motion artifact. For domiciliary use, oximetry is preferable to the more complex and less relevant transcutaneous monitors.[43,192]

Lung Mechanics and Lung Volumes

Neonatal Intensive Care

For technical reasons, there have been few measurements of lung volumes during neonatal intensive care. Although difficult, measurements of lung mechanics have been made, most commonly as part of trials of medication therapy or techniques of mechanical ventilation. Both static compliance (using the occlusion technique) and dynamic lung compliance (using an esophageal balloon) are low at this stage. The precise interpretation of these data is unclear because compliance is volume dependent and dynamic compliance is frequency dependent; both measurements are therefore influenced by the technique of mechanical ventilation itself. Some of the problems inherent in intensive care measurements have recently been reviewed.[193,194]

Resistance cannot reliably be measured by the single-breath technique under intensive care conditions because of the alinear characteristics of the respiratory system and endotracheal tube.[195] Very high pulmonary resistance values have been demonstrated by the esophageal balloon technique, even allowing for the endotracheal tube. The main value of such observations has been in relation to clinical trials of diuretics, bronchodilators, or corticosteroids (see later section). By briefly applying a powerful negative pressure of about 100 cm H_2O to the endotracheal tube, Motoyama et al[196] devised a system for producing maximal expiratory flow-volume curves in infants whose lungs are ventilated and used the technique to demonstrate bronchodilator responsiveness.

The site of airway obstruction cannot be determined from this type of study. Anatomically, there are abnormalities of both the large central airways and the small peripheral airways with major dynamic changes in resistance that are demonstrable (see later section).

From a practical viewpoint, few simple techniques can reliably provide information about lung mechanics during intensive care.[194] Responses to therapeutic interventions and changes in disease state can be determined more precisely using ventilatory or gas-exchange measurements[197] or their combination in such indexes as the ventilatory efficiency index.[198] A sequential trial of intermittent positive-pressure ventilation guided by a pulmonary mechanics monitor failed to demonstrate a reduction in CLD.[199]

Infants

A wide range of physiologic measurements have been made on freely breathing infants with CLD, but again there are many technical limitations,[194] especially in infants who require continuous oxygen therapy. The short-term variability of lung function tests is great in infants with BPD.[200] Sedation for lung function testing often worsens hypoxemia. Interpretation of data is affected by the normalization procedures used to compare infants with CLD to healthy infants or to compare one age group or disease state with another. If, for instance, body weight is used to correct lung volume or compliance measurements, differences in body mass index (weight/length) affect the results. Most simple normalization procedures implicitly assume a linear relationship (without any intercept) between lung function and body size; this is rarely the case. However, subject comparisons over short periods of time are not affected by these constraints, so short-term clinical trials are possible.

Lung volumes measured by helium dilution or nitrogen washout underestimate the functional residual capacity (FRC) in the presence of poor gas mixing. Values of FRC are invariably reported as low in the first 6 months of life in infants with CLD compared with those in healthy infants or controls whose lungs are ventilated,[35] exceeding the normal value by 12 months. The authors have found helium equilibration times to be as long as 12 minutes in severe CLD; measurements taken over shorter times tend to underestimate the FRC. Plethysmographic lung volumes, which detect all of the gas within the chest, are higher than normal,[201,202] again recovering to normal by 12 months. One direct comparison of the two methods[203] illustrates this discrepancy, showing that preterm infants whose condition was symptomatic (although not specifically with CLD) had a greater difference and therefore by implication more "gas trapping" than full-term infants or infants whose condition was asymptomatic. "True" lung volume cannot therefore be determined. Nevertheless, changes in "lung volume" over short periods have been used to measure response to treatment, although the physiologic interpretation of the change may be very speculative.

During the later part of infancy, FRC normalizes or may even exceed normal values,[200-204] suggesting true hyperinflation. The increase in FRC may result from worsening obstructive airway disease or a loss of elastic recoil as a consequence of alveolar underdevelopment and hence overenlargement and remodeling of the lungs with removal of excess collagen and elastin.

Lung mechanics has been extensively measured in groups of infants with and without CLD. Respiratory system compliance is always low,[200] returning toward normal by 1 to 3 years of age.[200,205] The weighted spirometer technique is worth considering in infants.[206] Resistance values are mostly high, an indication of the severity but not the site of airway obstruction.[203] Changes in resistance (or its reciprocal, conductance) with age can be judged only in relation to changes in lung volume with growth and disease. Specific airway conductance is low in infancy (about 60% of that predicted) and increases only a little in CLD over the first 3 years of life to about 70% of that predicted.[200,204,207] In healthy VLBW infants, plethysmographic airway resistance is lowest at about 6 months of age, improving thereafter.[202,208] The authors have shown that airway function seems to "track" from 12 months to 9 years in preterm infants.[46]

Flow-volume curves occurring during tidal breathing and generated by the squeeze technique in infants with CLD are clearly abnormal, exhibiting severe flow limitation, even at rest. Measured values of maximum flow at FRC of around 50% of the reference value with little improvement over the first year have been reported by Tepper et al.[209]

The concept of a single value for compliance or resistance hides the fascinating process of dynamic airway function. Changes in cross-sectional area and hence resistance and changes in wall elastance and hence maximum sustainable flow[210] may be brought about because of structural abnormalities in the airways, such as bronchomalacia[145] or airway wall thickening with glandular or smooth muscle hypertrophy,[47] because of developmental changes[148] or because of the administration of bronchodilator or bronchoconstrictor agents. With the use of computed tomographic scans, dynamic tracheal narrowing during tidal breathing is far greater in infants with CLD (63%) than in control infants (9%).[146] These observations have been confirmed using different techniques.[147]

The work of breathing in CLD is markedly increased as a result of mechanical factors combined with an increase in overall metabolic rate.[211] This is not a simple relationship between pulmonary mechanics and total metabolic rate.[212,213]

School-Age and Older Children

Many studies of preterm babies have been taken through to school age, although the numbers with classic BPD in these groups is small.[36,37,40,101,132] The general conclusions are that preterm babies at school age have reductions in the 1-second forced expiratory volume and forced vital capacity, which are largely matched, suggesting mainly restriction rather than obstruction as the basic mechanical problem. There is an increase in the total lung capacity and the ratio of residual volume and total lung capacity (to 0.4 to 0.45 compared with a predicted value of 0.22), a reduction to about half in specific airway conductance. These studies suggest that children with BPD are little different from the other preterm cohort members whose lungs have or have not been ventilated and that prematurity is the main determinant of functional impairment at school age (Fig. 32-13). To interpret earlier studies in which selected groups of children with BPD differed from healthy control children as implying that there are long-term effects from BPD is to be swayed by selection bias.

One longitudinal physiologic study that demonstrated tracking in airway function from the age of 8 to 12 months through 9 years[46] is explained by the model illustrated in Fig. 32-14. The resolution and remodeling of acute lung injury are largely complete by 1 year, and further changes in lung function represent subsequent growth. At school age, the physiologic findings of restrictive disease with a large residual volume are compatible with a reduced alveolar component, perhaps resulting from the disturbed alveolation associated with prematurity. This hypothesis awaits confirmation because no methods for measuring alveolar number or surface area in the living child are available.

Northway et al[214] have provided data on lung function in late adolescence that indicate persistent, largely reversible airway obstruction affecting the large and small airways and persistent overinflation resulting from small airway disease. The latter could represent narrowed peripheral airways or a loss of elastic recoil. Airways responsiveness to methacholine or a β_2-agonist were found in 52% of the group, and fixed obstruction was found in 24%. This contrasts with the findings in preterm and term controls, in whom 31% and 17% of the airways, respectively, were reactive to methacholine but there was no fixed obstruction.

The presence and interpretation of airway responsiveness in children who were born prematurely is controversial. In a small study, Bertrand et al[99] found increased methacholine responsiveness in children born prematurely and their mothers, suggesting that premature labor was itself due to excessive familial smooth muscle responsiveness, a finding confirmed by Riedel et al.[100] These findings were not confirmed in a population study of LBW infants and their mothers,[101] although a marginal increase in bronchial responsiveness was reported in the LBW group to a much lesser degree than might be ex-

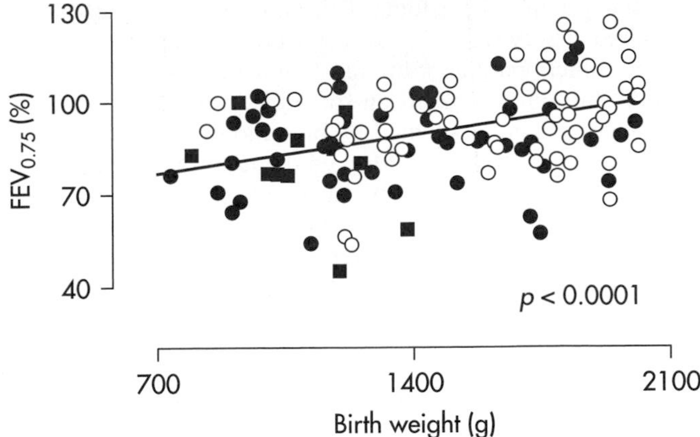

Fig. 32-13. Association between height-corrected predicted $FEV_{0.75}$ (percentage of reference value) at 7 years plotted according to birth weight. Except perhaps at the very lowest weights, the predominant effect on $FEV_{0.75}$ (forced expiratory volume 0.75) was birth weight and not neonatal respiratory therapy. Open circles indicate lack of neonatal respiratory therapy ($N = 68$); closed circles indicate neonatal respiratory therapy (oxygen and mechanical ventilation combined) ($N = 52$); closed squares indicate oxygen dependency at 30 days of life ($N = 10$). (From Chan KN et al: *Arch Dis Child* 64:1284-1293, 1989.)

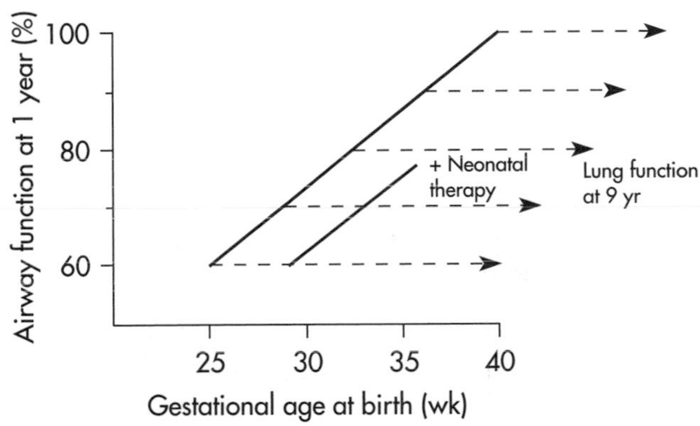

Fig. 32-14. Tracking of infant lung function. Airway function at 1 year of age depends on gestational age (or birth weight) and to a lesser extent neonatal therapy *(heavy lines)*. Thereafter, airway function seems to "track."

pected in groups with asthma. This may simply be a reflection of altered airway caliber or airway wall thickness.

For clinical purposes, the most valuable measurements in school children are based on forced expiration; these measurements are supplemented by bronchodilator challenge to assess acute reversibility. Marked deviation from normal is an indicator for more detailed assessment with plethysmography, which is supplemented as indicated by specialist imaging (computed tomography or ventilation-perfusion scans). Exercise testing may reveal additional abnormalities such as exercise-induced asthma or exercise-induced hypoxemia and hypercapnia.[141]

MANAGEMENT

General Aspects of Management

Background

CLD is rare in infants weighing more than 1500 g at birth. Because pulmonary disability occurs in the smallest, sickest infants, it is almost always accompanied by other disorders; sensory and neurodevelopmental handicaps, growth impairment and nutritional difficulty, congenital anomalies, and cardiovascular problems are among the most prominent. Only the aspects that have a bearing on pulmonary disease are considered in this chapter, but it is a prerequisite of good care that management should be carried out by a team and not by a disparate group of independent experts. Discharge from the hospital requires careful joint planning by hospital and community health professionals, even for infants who do not require domiciliary oxygen therapy, aerosol therapy, or tube (gavage) feeding. Avoidance of cigarette smoke, minimal contact with other preschool children,[215] attention to immunization programs, and ready access to the hospital in an emergency are all important. There is no evidence that apnea monitoring is of any value, although some parents demand a monitor for their own peace of mind. Where a monitor is provided for high-risk infants (e.g., those who have had apneic attacks, have GER, or are oxygen dependent), cardiopulmonary resuscitation should be taught and simple suction equipment provided. Domiciliary oxygen therapy and monitoring are discussed later.

Hospital visits should be kept to a minimum. This means that the pulmonologist, follow-up team, nutritionist, speech therapist, home-care nurse, and possibly the pediatric cardiologist or echocardiographer should all be available for consultation at a joint clinic.

The rational management of CLD presupposes an understanding of the mechanisms of the disease and its resolution. This information is rarely available. Management also requires data from clinical trials of sufficient power to provide valid results. Much of clinical practice is still based on consensus or local custom, but where possible, the conclusions of scientifically valid data are preferred to anecdotal studies to back up management schemes.

Two thorough reviews of therapy of CLD have recently been published.[24,216]

Growth and Nutrition Problems

The frequent occurrence of poor growth in CLD has been discussed (see section on clinical features). Contributory factors may include behavioral feeding problems, swallowing disorders, GER, chronic hypoxemia, and heart failure. Excessive use of diuretics to control respiratory or heart failure may impair growth, presumably as a result of a critical reduction in the extracellular fluid volume or total body sodium levels, even in the absence of hyponatremia. There are no nutritional deficiencies that are specific to infants with CLD. Corticosteroid therapy has a temporary growth-suppressing effect.

After remediable causes have been identified and treated, caloric supplementation can be achieved by increasing feed density. This appears, in the authors' experience, to have little benefit. Carbohydrate supplements alone may exacerbate respiratory failure by increasing the metabolic rate; lipid-carbohydrate combinations should be used. A speech therapist skilled in infant feeding problems may be able to retrain the child who has a behavioral or neurologic feeding disorder. It is the authors' impression that very small stature in infants with severe, chronically oxygen-dependent BPD is a manifestation of a fundamental disorder of somatic growth, of which failure of resolution of neonatal lung "injury" leading to CLD may be a component.

GER

The relationship between GER and respiratory symptoms in infants is not easy to disentangle. GER is certainly common in preterm infants in general and in infants with CLD in particular[153] (see section on clinical features). Obvious xanthine-resistant apnea, massive aspiration, recurrent vomiting, or failure to thrive may draw attention to it. A causal relationship between GER and hypoxic spells in CLD has never been demonstrated, although both are common in CLD. It is the authors' experience that GER is a sequel to, rather than a cause of, obstructive apneic spells.

Some clinicians prefer to institute simple medical management (e.g., posture, food thickening with carob extract and agar-based demulcents), pursuing further investigations if this fails. Failure of simple medical therapy should be followed by the addition of parakinetic drugs such as cisapride (0.2 mg/kg 3 to 4 times/day before feeding), although a recent controlled trial did not show it to be better than simple food thickening.[217] Diarrhea is a common side effect. H_2-blockers should be used if there is evidence of esophagitis. Fundoplication should be considered if symptomatic reflux continues despite such therapy. Several observational studies have shown improvement in such patients.[153,156,157]

Cardiovascular Complications

Clinical features that suggest impending heart failure, usually secondary to severe pulmonary hypertension, include excessive or sudden weight gain and increased breathlessness or hypoxemia (or an increase in oxygen requirement) and on physical examination, edema and hepatomegaly. Chest radiographs may show cardiac enlargement.

Oxygen therapy is the mainstay of management. In the absence of an echocardiographic assessment to demonstrate the presence and reversibility of pulmonary hypertension and to determine the appropriate target level of arterial oxygen saturation in individuals, clinicians should aim for a target level of 94% to 96%.[160,165] Many subjects can be safely managed, at least for short periods, below this range, provided that they are not highly sensitive to hypoxic vasoconstriction. Diuretic therapy should be instituted or increased if the features of heart failure occur. For short-term therapy, furosemide is useful; long-term use may lead to nephrocalcinosis.[218] A combination of a thiazide with a potassium-sparing diuretic (spironolactone or amiloride) is more appropriate for long-term treatment. It is often difficult to establish the correct dosage. Excessive sodium excretion may cause alarming hyponatremia within the first week of treatment, whereas subsequent growth failure relieved only by sodium supplementation is often a problem. The separate effects of diuretic therapy on pulmonary function are considered later.

Pulmonary vasodilators have very unpredictable effects in babies with severe oxygen-unresponsive pulmonary hypertension.[169] These infants should be individually evaluated by a pediatric cardiologist either during cardiac catheterization or by using reliable echocardiographic measurements. Both nifedipine[219] and hydralazine[160] may have effects additional to oxygen, the latter having adverse effects in infants with abnormal systemic pulmonary shunt vessels.[161,162] Both agents affect systemic vascular resistance too. Experimentally disodium cromoglycate (cromolyn sodium) is effective via the intravenous or aerosol route in lambs,[220,221] although this is controversial[222]; personal observations in babies suggest that it does not have a useful role. Nitric oxide may have a role in the persistently hypoxic neonate with CLD in the neonatal unit (see Fig. 32-12). However, there is no evidence for enhanced long-term survival.

Systemic hypertension has been recorded in oxygen-dependent infants with CLD; it is occasionally severe enough to lead to left ventricular hypertrophy. In one study, 13 of 30 infants had a systolic pressure higher than 113 mm Hg,[223] and 6 received antihypertensive therapy for a mean of 3.7 months. The hypertension resolved. Electrocardiography may not be sensitive enough to detect left ventricular hypertrophy. Echocardiography should be performed in hypertensive children with CLD. The cause of systemic hypertension is unknown, but segmental renal disease, renal vascular complications of prematurity, long-term inotropic support (or even theophylline therapy), and possibly hyperoxia might be contributory factors. Left ventricular hypertrophy is a common finding at autopsy.[47,224]

Unsuspected congenital heart disease was found in association with CLD by two groups.[159,171] This sort of observation implies that severe CLD should be seen as a marker of other, causally important anomalies or defects.

Respiratory Management

For almost all modes of respiratory therapy, there are no definite indications, no objective methods of evaluating the response in individuals (except in the very short term), and no randomized clinical trials of adequate power. Moreover, when any of these defects has been remedied, the information applies only to a specific stage of CLD (e.g. ventilated BPD or wheezy infants), and the results cannot be generalized throughout this evolving disorder.

Bronchodilators

One of the striking pathologic features of CLD is airway smooth muscle hypertrophy.[56] It would therefore seem reasonable to expect bronchodilator agents (β_2 agonists, anticholinergic agents, and methylxanthines) to be effective. Little is known, however, of the ontogeny of β receptors or muscarinic-receptor subtypes in preterm babies or even healthy infants, so no one can predict the long-term outcome of stimulating these receptors during a period of rapid pulmonary development. The β-agonist controversy should promote caution. Neuroendocrine cell hypoplasia suggests a role for nonadrenergic, noncholinergic mechanisms in CLD.[225,226]

Moreover, there is reason to suppose that airway smooth muscle tone may be important in stabilizing the compliant airway of the neonate to minimize dynamic changes during breathing (see previous section). The removal of this tone could render airways more collapsible, with adverse effects on expiratory flow during spontaneous breathing, or more distensible, with the potential for enhanced tracheomegaly during positive-pressure ventilation (see later section). Bronchodilation might also remove the potential focal protective function of narrowed airways.[227] There is no logical basis for their use, except that these drugs are often effective in relieving airway obstruction in other situations.

In addition to these unknowns, the appropriate dose and means of administration of bronchodilators have not been determined (see Chapter 18). For ventilator-dependent infants, the most effective method for delivering aerosol is probably by metered dose inhaler (MDI) and small volume spacer (such as the Aerochamber).[228-230] Jet and ultrasonic nebulizers are extremely inefficient.[231-233] For older infants whose lungs are extubated, all methods of delivery are certainly inefficient.[234] The choice of device has recently been reviewed.[235] The nose acts as an all too effective filter.[236] In wheezy infants, in general, nebulized bronchodilators often have transient adverse effects on oxygenation and airway function.[237-241] The effect is not seen when an MDI is used.[242] Changes in air entrainment during infancy mean that drugs administered by jet nebulizer are available in relatively high doses to young infants.[243]

There is only one satisfactory study of methylxanthines, which found that in 4-month-old oxygen-dependent infants, 4 days of oral theophylline therapy gave significant benefits in lung mechanics and work of breathing.[244] The open, placebo-controlled study of a single oral dose of caffeine[245] showed significant short-term mechanical benefits during mechanical ventilation. One other brief open study of theophylline gave a marginal result.[246]

Whether given by nebulizer or by the oral or subcutaneous route, in every study, β agonists have produced short-term improvements in lung mechanics as measured by a variety of techniques. Three studies of single doses of nebulized salbutamol given to ventilator-dependent infants younger than 1 month of age have shown clear benefits in terms of respiratory system compliance and resistance.[247-249] In infants who have CLD and whose lungs are mechanically ventilated, reversible airway disease was demonstrated by changes in maximum forced expiration after nebulized metaproterenol[196] and by measurements of classic lung mechanics.[250] The only full-scale clinical trial of bronchodilators in preterm infants concerns symptomatic (i.e., wheezy) infants who were born prematurely, not infants specifically with CLD.[251] This was an open, sequential study of β_2 agonists administered by MDI. Symptomatic and physiologic improvements were demonstrated.

The results for the nebulized anticholinergic agents atropine and ipratropium bromide are similarly positive but of limited significance. There is evidence that ventilator-dependent babies with CLD respond to single doses of nebulized ipratropium bromide,[250] but again, long-term randomized trials in CLD are awaited. One double-blind, randomized trial in older preterm infants whose conditions were symptomatic was effective,[252] although the same authors caution its use in infants whose condition is asymptomatic.[253] There is weak evidence for synergy between β agonists and anticholinergic agents.[254]

In practice, salbutamol (albuterol) or ipratropium bromide given by MDI and small volume spacer may be used for ventilator-dependent infants, older infants with CLD who have severe airway obstruction, and wheezy infants with CLD. There is little to support the use of bronchodilators in acute viral episodes in infancy in general and even less in acute viral exacerbations of CLD.

There are no dosage regimens, but the authors have noted that salbutamol (albuterol), 200 to 400 μg every 4 to 6 hours, and ipratropium bromide, 80 to 160 μg every 6 hours, do not seem to cause undue tachycardia or any detectable side effects. The efficacy of treatment can be judged only by general clinical features or the ventilatory efficiency index during mechanical ventilation.[197] Short-term measurements of lung function may lend support but are generally too variable over days or weeks to guide long-term therapy in individual cases.

Antiinflammatory Agents

Data on sodium cromoglycate (cromolyn sodium) are sparse and consist of one open study on ventilator-dependent infants that suggested cytologic improvement,[255] a pilot study that showed no benefit,[256] and one properly conducted, double-blind, randomized, controlled trial in older preterm infants symptomatic at follow-up.[257] In the last study, there was a significant reduction in symptoms after 3 weeks of treatment by MDI and spacer.

The pharmacologic effects of corticosteroids on the lungs can be considered at the molecular or cellular level, at the functional or physiologic level, and at the level of clinical disease. There are data on all these outcomes of corticosteroid therapy in preterm infants. The common theme of most studies is the antiinflammatory action of corticosteroids. There are, however, several other potentially relevant actions, some studied only in animal models, including enhancement of β_2-receptor density, increased transduction of the genes for several antioxidant enzymes, altered gene expression for a variety of cytokines and growth factors, enhanced surfactant production, and suppression of inducible nitric oxide synthase. The data on corticosteroids are extensive, but for bronchodilators, the risk-benefit ratio has not been fully determined. The information has recently been reviewed.[258]

Clinical trials of systemic corticosteroids in established CLD (BPD) have been thoroughly reviewed by Ehrenkranz and Mercurio.[24] Nine randomized, controlled trials of parenteral or oral dexamethasone have been reported for infants age 2 to 6 weeks.[259-267] All except two[260,265] were devoted exclusively to babies whose lungs were intubated. In the United Kingdom, a collaborative trial, by far the largest (285 babies), covered a wide clinical spectrum of disease. The main outcomes in most trials were speed of extubation and duration of oxygen therapy. Extubation was clearly facilitated in all but one study,[263] but the overall duration of oxygen therapy and hospitalization were in general unaffected.

Administration and dosage regimens are poorly worked out. Dexamethasone is the most popular corticosteroid in neonatal practice, and parenteral (usually intravenous) administration is the usual route. There has been no attempt to perform dose-ranging studies, and although the variation in starting dosage among studies is small, 0.5 to 1 mg/kg of body weight per day in divided doses, the duration of therapy varies widely from 3 to 42 days. A comparison of different regimens was carried out in only one study.[261] Despite known differences among corticosteroids in the degree of penetration into the lungs after parenteral administration, no study of this important aspect of therapy has been reported in young infants.

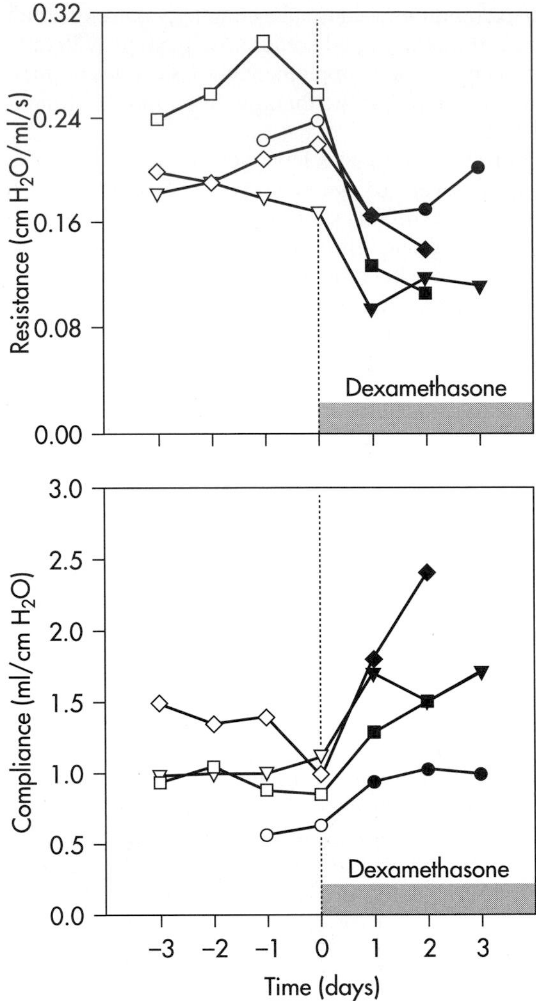

Fig. 32-15. Dexamethasone and ventilator-dependent CLD at 3 weeks. Changes in lung mechanics occur within 24 hours. (From Brundage KL et al: *Pediatr Pulmonol* 12:162-169, 1992.)

Pulmonary mechanics have been reported in a number of small, mainly sequential observations.[259,267-270] Individually, these studies have major flaws, but their consistency is remarkable. Within 12 to 72 hours, falls in respiratory resistance of about 30% and increases in compliance of 60% to 70% are typically seen (Fig. 32-15).

Attempts to understand the mechanism of corticosteroid action in CLD have lead to a bewildering number of measurements of cytokines and other cell products in bronchoalveolar lavage fluid or tracheal aspirate. This is definitely a growth area. Sadly, the majority of observations were not designed to answer any useful hypotheses. Again, there are methodological defects in many studies: inadequate control data, sequential observations, lack of attention to the expression of bronchoalveolar lavage fluid concentrations (by reference to a reliable denominator), and very variable and small patient groups. The most comprehensive and carefully conducted study showed parallel changes in tracheal fluid neutrophil cell counts, cell products, lung mechanics, and clinical status within 3 days of starting dexamethasone therapy in a randomized, controlled trial.[267]

The use of topical corticosteroids in established CLD (BPD) is reported in three observational studies of topical corticosteroid therapy for infants whose lungs have been mechanically ventilated, who have CLD, and whose lungs are intubated[270-272] and can do no more than encourage those who wish to establish properly designed clinical trials. The potential range of devices, medications, and doses is huge, although there are now sufficient data from human and model lung experiments to devise regimens for clinical trials.[228-230]

Corticosteroids are often used in older infants and children, but very little data are available to support the authors' clinical observations that infants with symptomatic, oxygen-dependent CLD benefit from topical corticosteroid therapy. In a formal clinical trial, infants who were born prematurely whose condition was symptomatic benefited from a reduction in wheeze and cough during topical corticosteroid therapy (beclomethasone, 100 μg twice a day for 6 weeks by MDI, spacer, and face mask).[273] However, symptomatic 7-year-old schoolchildren of LBW with increased bronchial responsiveness did not benefit from a similar regimen, suggesting that at that age and airway inflammation did not contribute to their disease.[274]

Adverse effects of corticosteroids are obviously a major concern. Brief and probably insignificant systolic hypertension, hyperglycemia, and neutrophilia are reported in many of the dexamethasone trials. Of more concern is the evidence of adrenal suppression of up to 1 month's duration even after 1 week of therapy.[275,276]

Gastrointestinal perforation has been reported.[277,278] Whether this rare complication can be safely prevented by the routine use of H_2-blocking agents during dexamethasone therapy remains to be investigated.

One of the most worrisome potential effects of corticosteroids on the growing lung is suppression of alveolar development. There are certainly effects on somatic growth and lung morphology from brief exposures of neonatal rats to modest doses of dexamethasone.[279,280] Measurements of lung function in infants and children exposed to antenatal dexamethasone do not suggest any persistent adverse effects.[281,282] However, the studies are small, are open to bias, and depend on an assumption that lung function is equivalent to lung growth. Transient growth suppression is demonstrable by knemometry, with apparent catch-up after cessation of steroid treatment.[283]

Diuretics

In addition to their cardiovascular indications (see previous section), diuretics are frequently used to treat the pulmonary problems of CLD. The role of diuretics has been extensively reviewed.[24,284] Their efficacy is based on experimental reductions in pulmonary vascular resistance and in extravascular lung water in experimental animals by furosemide treatment. In CLD, there is evidence of a disturbance in water balance[285-286] and peribronchial edema.[287] The mechanism of clinical improvement in response to diuretics is unclear. Local actions on the distribution of lung water and on the pulmonary vasculature may be as important as renal effects on total body water levels. For instance, furosemide has a number of such actions.[284] Potential actions on the airway epithelium are especially interesting because they open the possibility that aerosol therapy may be effective, thus avoiding troublesome renal actions.[288]

There is striking uniformity of the results of clinical trials with furosemide (1 mg/kg once or twice a day intravenously or 2 mg/kg twice a day orally) despite the variety of trial designs and methods of measuring outcome. All results demonstrate an increase in pulmonary or respiratory system compliance, and some also demonstrate falls in resistance and oxygen requirement over intervals of between 1 hour and 8 days of therapy.[288-290] The rapid onset suggests a local effect,[288,291] a conclusion supported by the presence of changes in lung mechanics in the absence of measurable diuresis.[290]

Three of four studies on the combination of thiazide and spironolactone (chlorothiazide, 20 mg/kg, or hydrochlorothiazide, 1.5 to 2 mg/kg every 12 hours, with spironolactone, 1.5 mg/kg every 12 hours by mouth) showed significant improvements in compliance with variable improvements in resistance and oxygen requirement, albeit to a less marked extent than the changes found after furosemide.[292-294] One study using a lower dose[295] found no significant effect, despite diuresis. There are no dose-ranging studies. In the authors' clinical experience (with chlorothiazide, 10 to 25 mg/kg twice a day, and amiloride, 0.2 to 0.5 mg/kg twice a day), some adjustments of dose are often necessary.

The conclusion from these small studies (8 of 9 studies had 21 or fewer subjects) is that diuretics are effective over periods of up to 8 weeks. Long-term side effects may be troublesome. Furosemide enhances calcium excretion and often leads to nephrocalcinosis and osteopenia. Electrolyte imbalance is common, and serum electrolyte measurements must be performed twice a week. Alternate-day therapy should be considered. The combination of thiazide and spironolactone leads to lower calcium levels and potassium loss but may cause troublesome hyponatremia soon after the onset of therapy.

A trial of diuretic therapy for 1 to 2 weeks is indicated for the following:

1. Chronic ventilator-dependent cases
2. Infants on very low-flow oxygen therapy (100 ml/min or less) who are to be discharged home shortly
3. Sudden deterioration or sudden weight gain

There is no standard weaning process. The authors simply allow infants to "outgrow" their therapy and withdraw when the dose has fallen below the accepted therapeutic range.

Miscellaneous Therapies

Antiinfective agents are commonly used to treat episodes of "sepsis" in the neonatal intensive care unit. Most infective pulmonary exacerbations later in childhood have a viral etiology, respiratory syncytial virus being an especially virulent agent.[144] The use of ribavirin in such infants, although recommended in North America, is rarely used in the United Kingdom. Its use is reviewed in Chapter 38. In the authors' experience of 80 1-year-old infants with CLD who had received low-flow domiciliary oxygen therapy, 27 were readmitted to the hospital with acute exacerbations over their first year; 16 of these were due to respiratory syncytial virus. There were 8 other admissions for medical or surgical conditions. Ribavirin was not used; all infants recovered without complication, and none needed mechanical ventilation. Antibiotics are indicated only for specific reasons: high index of suspicion of bacterial disease, host defense defect, and cystic fibrosis–like pattern of illness with frequent severe exacerbations. There are no clinical trials to back up these assertions.

Respiratory Failure

The management of CLD consists largely of attempting to identify remediable causes of respiratory failure or (in milder cases) respiratory dysfunction and trying to tackle them. Respiratory failure itself, defined as the failure of the respiratory system to adequately exchange oxygen and carbon dioxide for whatever reason, often needs to be tackled directly by mechanical ventilation and oxygen therapy. The classification and causes of respiratory failure in general are discussed in Chapters 19 and 21.

Upper airway obstruction is often overlooked as a cause of weaning failure in infants whose lungs have been intubated for a prolonged period. If laryngeal or subglottic edema is suspected, a short course of corticosteroids may be effective.[296] In modern neonatal practice, clinically significant structural (as opposed to transient) upper airway damage is rare. Of the 75 most severe cases of CLD in the authors' practice in 6 years—those who were discharged home on low-flow oxygen therapy—none had a long-term structural or mechanical upper airway disorder, although several have had transient upper airway obstructive symptoms during viral respiratory tract infections.

Mechanical Ventilation

Mechanical ventilation has a role in the etiology of acute lung injury (see previous section), but its role in CLD is speculative. The safest technique has not been established despite large clinical trials. There are even less data to guide the neonatologist in the ventilatory management of established CLD.[297] No clinical trials of techniques of mechanical ventilation have been reported. Devices would be welcome that could allow the clinician to avoid intubation. A resurgence of interest in continuous or intermittent negative extrathoracic pressure holds promise.[298]

Oxygen Therapy

Appropriate oxygenation is essential. Too little oxygen is clearly harmful, but excess has adverse effects too. These include toxic effects on the airway epithelium, including inhibition of ciliary action; possibly systemic hypertension; and the physical, emotional, and economic costs on the child, family, and society for unduly prolonged treatment.

The optimum level of oxygen saturation is likely to be higher than 90% and, in the absence of full cardiovascular monitoring to justify a lower level, should be 94% to 96% (see previous section). It is unknown whether brief hypoxic spells during feeding or interruption of the oxygen supply or during apneic pauses has a cumulative long-term effect on cardiovascular function, neurodevelopmental progress, or growth regulation. It seems prudent to supply sufficient oxygen to prevent even brief changes in saturation below 90% because this provides a safety margin at the upper end of the oxygen-hemoglobin dissociation curve for those "natural" variations in breathing resulting from feeding, posture, the sleep state, crying, and upper respiratory infection that may depress the partial pressure of arterial oxygen and therefore the arterial oxygen saturation.[177-180] There are no data from controlled trials, only some observational support, to justify these figures.[187]

There are several techniques for administering oxygen to infants with CLD (Table 32-8). Each has its advocates. Once progress from a head box is possible, the authors prefer a nasopharyngeal end-hole cannula (size 5 French) used according to the technique of Shann et al,[299] rather than a short cannula.[300] The authors have used all of these techniques for specific circumstances, and a flexible approach seems advisable. A gravitational system described by Zinman et al[301] is sometimes valuable.

Domiciliary therapy[43,192,302-304] is most conveniently and cheaply provided by an oxygen concentrator with a low-flow meter (range about 100 to 1000 ml/min or 25 to 200 ml/min), but backup cylinders and portable devices are also needed for emergencies and for mobility. A liquid oxygen-based system is under trial and may prove more flexible. The supervision of a dedicated home care nursing team in collaboration with other community health professionals is advantageous.

Monitoring is vital (Table 32-9). The limitations of transcutaneous devices have been discussed. They may be useful in the hospital but are too inaccurate, slow responding, and technically demanding for domiciliary use. Oximeters in averaging mode have allowed safe and stable domiciliary therapy and have arguably been responsible for the enormous recent improvement in long-term prognosis. The frequency of monitoring may vary depending on the stability of the patient's condition (see Table 32-9).

Table 32-8 Devices for Delivering Oxygen Therapy to Infants Whose Tracheas Are Not Intubated

DEVICE	COMMENT
Head box	Technique is traditional but very restrictive. Concentrations up to 95% oxygen are possible. Oxygen supply is variable, thus resulting in the need for an alternative supply during many procedures, feeding, and cuddling.
Short nasal prongs	Prongs become easily displaced. Technique is ineffective during mouth-breathing or upper respiratory tract illness. Technique causes little nasal irritation. Technique allows procedures without a break in oxygenation.
Nasopharyngeal cannula (end hole)	Technique is effective for infants needing <60% to 70% fraction of inspired oxygen. There is a continuous supply of oxygen during nose- or mouth-breathing and during feeding, procedures, and cuddles. Technique is more effective than the use of short prongs. Cannula irritates some infants, causing nasal mucus production and blockage.
Gravitational concentration in semienclosed crib	Technique may be worth considering during weaning if oxygen is required only for sleep or during upper respiratory tract illness if nasal devices are ineffective.

Table 32-9 Oxygen Monitoring

SETTING	MONITORING ACTION
Neonatal intensive care unit	Continuous oximetry with intermittent arterial or arterialized capillary blood gas analysis measured daily or on alternate days and as indicated by a change in state
Low-dependency unit	Daily oximetry to include a complete 3- to 4-hour cycle of feeding, wakefulness, and sleep
Home	Twice-weekly oximetry (or less frequent if the child's condition is stable in the long term) to provide a printed record of complete 4- to 6-hour cycle of feeding, wakefulness, and sleep; repeated with reduced oxygen supply if the arterial oxygen saturation is persistently >95% Daily or continuous monitoring for brief periods during upper respiratory tract illness

Implicit in oxygen monitoring is the need for regular echocardiographic assessment of the pulmonary circulation because one of the primary aims of oxygen therapy is to reduce pulmonary vascular resistance to normal levels. The authors recommend an echocardiographic evaluation before discharge from the hospital and at 3-month intervals thereafter until oxygen therapy ceases. Measurements are made on each occasion of right ventricular systolic times (ratio of right ventricular acceleration time and ejection time) and, where possible (50% of cases), right ventricular systolic pressure from the tricuspid regurgitant jet both in and out of oxygen therapy during sedated sleep. The information is particularly useful during weaning from oxygen therapy.

The indications for referral to the hospital for reassessment or readmission follow:

1. Sudden or gradual decline in arterial oxygen saturation requiring a marked increased in oxygen flow
2. Frequent catheter blockage resulting from nasal obstruction
3. Hypoxic spells or an acute life-threatening event

Monitoring should continue for 2 to 3 months after withdrawal of oxygen because secondary deterioration may occur and is often precipitated by a viral respiratory tract infection. It is probable that oxygen saturation never reaches truly "normal" values (98% to 100%) in children who have had prolonged severe CLD in infancy.

Management Protocols

With individual institutions, management protocols evolve by consensus and experience backed up by scientific data. As such, change is inevitable. Protocols should be seen as advisory and not prescriptive. Examples of a consensus approach to the management of ventilator-dependent respiratory failure and symptomatic infantile CLD are given in Figs. 32-16 and 32-17.

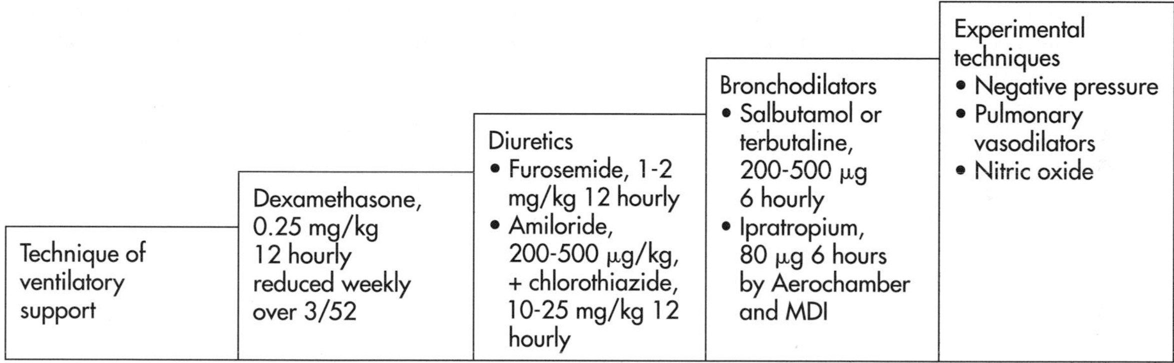

Monitor:
- Blood gases
- Blood pressure if using dexamethasone
- Chest radiograph and treat focal problem
- Blood film and count and treat infections early
- Growth
- Pulmonary vascular resistance and pressure by echocardiogram and Doppler

Fig. 32-16. Suggested stepwise approach to persistent ventilator-dependent respiratory failure in the neonatal intensive care unit.

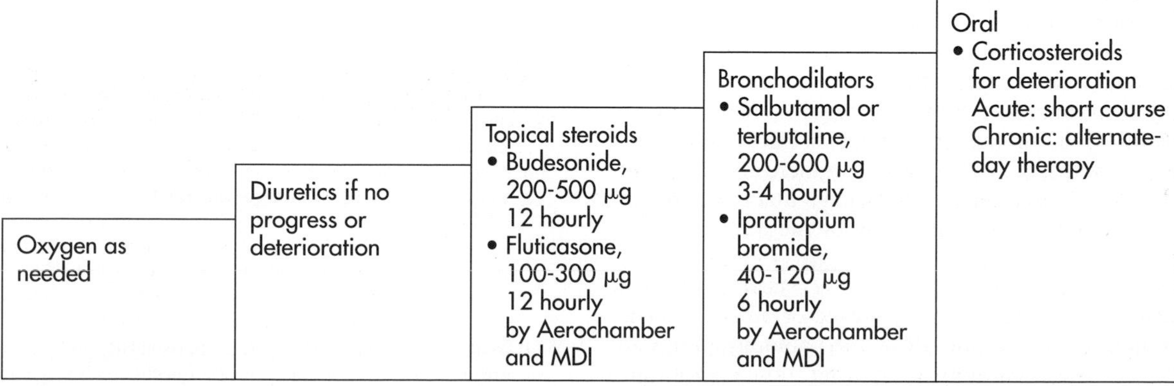

- This plan assumes that all other treatable conditions have been dealt with.
- Acute episodes after 6/12 can be managed as for "infantile asthma."

Fig. 32-17. Suggested stepwise management plan for oxygen-dependent infants whose conditions are symptomatic.

Domiciliary management demands the sort of guided self-management approach that has become the norm in the management of asthma (see Chapter 64). Thus parents can be provided with information, training (in oxygen administration, cardiopulmonary respiration, and the use of inhaler devices), and written instructions that allow them to vary their child's therapy according to clear guidelines and within agreed limits.

FUTURE DIRECTIONS

Prevention

The short-term outcome of preterm birth has already been improved considerably by interventions such as antenatal corticosteroid and thyroid-releasing hormone therapy and the early use of surfactant for babies at risk of RDS (see Chapter 31). Given the fact that the long-term outcome at school age appears to be more closely related to prematurity itself than to acute lung injury, the prospects for preventive intervention, assuming that prematurity cannot be prevented, are more speculative.

Therapeutic interventions deserving more careful evaluation include agents that enhance surfactant production, such as inositol therapy, an effective treatment that has not become widely accepted, and the more effective use of antioxidants to minimize damage by free radicals.[24] The role of *U. urealyticum* has never been formally tested by a controlled trial of appropriate antibiotic therapy. Early antiinflammatory therapy has so far meant one early trial of dexamethasone, with good effect on classic BPD.[305] With a better understanding of the mechanisms of neutrophil influx, their roles, and the factors hastening the resolution of inflammation, specific targeting with antiadhesion molecules or antibodies to cytokines may be possible.

Techniques of respiratory support that reduce barotrauma may be beneficial, and attention to "peripheral" issues such as fresh-gas temperature and humidity are important.[306] It is unlikely that improvements in technique will have more than a marginal effect, although positive-pressure ventilation by endotracheal tube is the mainstay of therapy.[307]

Mechanisms

If early inflammatory processes are central to short-term lung damage, then unraveling them will be important. The mechanisms involved in the development and resolution of inflammation hold the key because inflammation enhances surfactant inactivation and free radical damage and adds to the mechanical changes that require further damaging levels of mechanical support and oxygen therapy.

Many medications used to treat symptomatic conditions have unknown effects on the growing lungs. This is an important area of future research. It appears that there are long-term adverse effects of prematurity itself; agents that can enhance alveolation and speed the remodeling of the lungs in CLD would be an asset.

The putative stages of CLD (see Fig. 32-3) can be verified only by histologic means. Biopsy material or other evidence collected noninvasively would allow the pathophysiology to be determined more accurately, permitting more appropriate therapy than the present blunderbuss methods allow.

Clinical Care

Most aspects of care are open to scientific inquiry. These include the techniques of ventilatory support for established CLD; targeting of medication to the lungs; appropriate use of corticosteroids, bronchodilators, and diuretics at each stage of CLD; role of GER in individual cases; and validity of echocardiographic and Doppler determination of pulmonary artery pressure in relation to oxygen therapy. Many of these require multicenter trials of the type that have recently become common in neonatal practice. It is unlikely that single centers can do more than develop new ideas and techniques and collect the information from pilot studies, which can be used to justify large, expensive trials.

Long-Term Outcome

It is a concern to many that prematurity itself and CLD in particular lead to "second-class" lungs in later childhood and adult life.[308] Unless long-term, population-based cohort studies are planned, the true outcome may not be known. Moreover, the risk factors for lung disease in adults who had been born prematurely may be different from the risk factors for pulmonary symptoms, dysfunction, or even death in childhood. If these factors remain unidentified, clinicians will miss the opportunity to examine them and intervene.

In these days of health economics for all, the long-term public health and economic implications of CLD should be evaluated lifelong so that informed decisions can be made in the future.

REFERENCES

Chronic Lung Disease: Background

1. Northway WH, Rosan RC, Porter DY: Pulmonary disease following respiratory therapy of hyaline membrane disease: bronchopulmonary dysplasia, *N Engl J Med* 276:357-368, 1967.
2. Northway WH: Introduction to bronchopulmonary dysplasia, *Clin Perinatol* 19:489-495, 1992.
3. Shennan AT, Dunn MS, Ohlsson A, Lennox K, Hoskins EM: Abnormal pulmonary outcomes in premature infants: prediction from oxygen requirement in the neonatal period, *Pediatrics* 82(5):527-532, 1988.
4. Kraybill EN, Runyan DK, Bose CL, Khan JH: Risk factors for chronic lung disease in infants with birthweights of 751-1000 grams, *J Pediatr* 115:115-120, 1989.
5. Sinkin RA, Cox C, Phelps DC: Predicting risk for bronchopulmonary dysplasia: selection criteria for clinical trials, *Pediatrics* 86:728-736, 1990.
6. The International Neonatal Network: The CRIB (clinical risk index for babies) score: a tool for assessing initial neonatal risk and comparing the performance of neonatal intensive care units, *Lancet* 342:193-198, 1993.
7. Hansen TWR, Wallach M, Dey AN, Boivin P, Vohr B, Oh W: Prognostic value of clinical and radiological status on day 28 of life for subsequent course in very low birthweight (<1500g) babies with bronchopulmonary dysplasia, *Pediatr Pulmonol* 15:327-331, 1993.
8. Freezer N, Sly PD: Predictive value of measurement of respiratory mechanics in preterm infants with HMD, *Pediatr Pulmonol* 16:116-123, 1993.
9. Hyde I, English RE, Williams JD: The changing pattern of chronic lung disease of prematurity, *Arch Dis Child* 64:448-451, 1989.
10. Strachan DP: The prevalence and natural history of wheezing in early childhood, *J Roy Coll Gen Pract* 35:182-184, 1985.
11. Wright AL, Taussig LM, Ray CG, Harrison HR, Holberg CJ, The Group Health Medical Associates: The Tucson children's respiratory study. II. Lower respiratory tract illness in the first year of life, *Am J Epidemiol* 129:1232-1246, 1989.
12. Tager IB, Hanrahan JP, Tosteson TD, Castile RG, Brown RW, Weiss ST, Speizer FE: Lung function, pre- and post-natal smoke exposure, and wheezing in the first year of life, *Am Rev Respir Dis* 147:811-817, 1993.
13. Bowman E, Yu VYH: Continuing morbidity in extremely low birthweight infants, *Early Hum Dev* 18:165-174, 1989.

14. Yuksel B, Greenough A: Persistence of respiratory symptoms into the second year of life: predictive factors in infants born preterm, *Acta Paediatr* 81:832-835, 1992.
15. Frischer T, Kuehr J, Meinert R, Karmans W, Barth R, Hermann-Kunz E, Urbanek R: Relationship between low birthweight and respiratory symptoms in a cohort of primary school children, *Acta Paediatr* 81:1040-1041, 1992.
16. Von Mutius E, Nicolai T, Martinez FD: Prematurity as a risk factor for asthma in preadolescent children, *J Pediatr* 123:223-229, 1993.
17. Avery ME, Tooley WH, Keller JB, Hurd SS, Bryan MH, Cotton RB: Is chronic lung disease in low birthweight infants preventable? A survey of eight centres, *Pediatrics* 79:26-30, 1987.
18. Farrell PM, Palta M: Bronchopulmonary dysplasia. In Farrell PM, Taussig LM, eds: *Bronchopulmonary dysplasia and related chronic respiratory disorders: a report of 19th Ross Conference on Paediatric Research,* Columbus, Ohio, 1986, Ross Laboratories, pp 1-7.
19. Kraybill EN, Bose C, Diercole J: Chronic lung disease in infants with very low birth weight, *Am J Dis Child* 141:784-788, 1987.
20. Northway WH: Bronchopulmonary dysplasia: then and now, *Arch Dis Child* 65:1076-1081, 1990.
21. Hack M, Fanaroff AA: Outcomes of extremely low birth weight infants between 1982 and 1988, *N Engl J Med* 321:1642-1647, 1989.
22. Cooke RWI: Factors associated with chronic lung disease in preterm infants, *Arch Dis Child* 60:776-779, 1991.
23. Crowley P: Promoting pulmonary maturity. In Enkin M, Chalmers I, eds: *Effective care in pregnancy and childbirth,* Oxford, England, 1991, Oxford University Press, pp 746-764.
24. Ehrenkranz RA, Mercurio MR: Bronchopulmonary dysplasia. In Sinclair JC, Bracken MB, eds: *Effective care of the newborn infant,* Oxford, England, 1992, Oxford University Press, pp 399-424.
25. Ng PC: The effectiveness and side effects of dexamethasone in preterm infants with bronchopulmonary dysplasia, *Arch Dis Child* 68:330-336, 1993.
26. Beck JC, Mitzner W, Johnson JW, Hutchins GM, Foidart JM, London WT, Palmer AE, Scott R: Betamethasone and the rhesus fetus: effect on lung morphometry and connective tissue, *Pediatr Res* 15:235-240, 1981.
27. Mitzner W, Johnson JW, Beck J, London W, Sly D: Influence of betamethasone on the development of mechanical properties in the fetal rhesus monkey lung, *Am Rev Respir Dis* 125:233-238, 1982.
28. Adamson IYR, King GM: Postnatal development of rat lung following retarded fetal lung growth, *Pediatr Pulmonol* 4:230-236, 1988.
29. Wong YC, Beardsmore CS, Silverman M: Antenatal dexamethasone and subsequent lung growth, *Arch Dis Child* 57:536-538, 1982.
30. Ballard RA, Ballard PL, Creasy RK, Padbury J, Polk DH, Bracken M, Moya FR, Gross I: Respiratory disease in very low birthweight infants after prenatal thyrotropin-releasing hormone and glucocorticoid, *Lancet* 339:510-515, 1992.
31. Hudak BB, Egan EA: Impact of lung surfactant therapy on chronic lung disease in premature infants, *Clin Perinatol* 19:591-601, 1992.
32. Abbassi S, Bhutani VK, Gerdes JS: Long term pulmonary consequences of respiratory distress syndrome in preterm infants treated with exogenous surfactant, *J Pediatr* 122:446-452, 1993.
33. Couser RJ, Ferrara TB, Wheeler W, McNamara J, Fade B, Johnson K, Hoekstra RE: Pulmonary follow-up 2.5 years after a randomised, controlled, multiple dose bovine surfactant study of preterm newborn babies, *Pediatr Pulmonol* 15:163-167, 1993.
34. Blaney M, Keren E, Whyte H, O'Brodovich H: Bronchopulmonary dysplasia: improvement in lung function between 7 and 10 years of age, *J Pediatr* 118:201-206, 1991.
35. Gerhardt T, Hehre D, Feller R, Reifenberg L, Bancalari E: Serial determination of pulmonary function in infants with chronic lung disease, *J Pediatr* 110:448-456, 1987.
36. Mansell AL, Driscoll JM, James LS: Pulmonary follow-up of moderately low birthweight infants with and without respiratory distress syndrome, *J Pediatr* 110:111-115, 1987.
37. Chan KN, Noble-Jamieson CM, Elliman A, Bryan EM, Silverman M: Lung function in children of low birthweight, *Arch Dis Child* 64:1284-1293, 1989.
38. Yuksel B, Greenough A: Neonatal respiratory support and lung function abnormalities at follow up, *Respir Med* 86:97-100, 1992.
39. Rona RJ, Gulliford MC, Chinn S: Effects of prematurity and intrauterine growth on respiratory health and lung function in childhood, *Br Med J* 306:817-820, 1993.
40. Chan KN, Elliman A, Bryan EM, Silverman M: Respiratory symptoms in children of low birthweight, *Arch Dis Child* 64:1294-1304, 1989.
41. Kirplani H, Schmidt B, Gaston S, Santos R, Wilkie R: Birthweight, early passive respiratory system mechanics, and ventilator requirements as predictors of outcome in premature infants with respiratory failure, *Pediatr Pulmonol* 10:195-198, 1991.
42. Thilo EH, Comito J, McCullis D: Home oxygen therapy in the newborn: cost and parental acceptance, *Am J Dis Child* 141:766-768, 1987.
43. Silverman M: Domiciliary oxygen therapy for children, *J Roy Coll Phys* 26:125-127, 1992.
44. Egberts J: Estimated costs of different treatments of respiratory distress syndrome in a large cohort of preterm infants of less than 30 weeks of gestation, *Biol Neonate* 61(suppl):59-65, 1992.
45. de Lemos RA, Coalson JJ: The contribution of experimental models to our understanding of the pathogenesis and treatment of bronchopulmonary dysplasia, *Clin Perinatol* 19:521-539, 1992.
46. Chan KN, Wong YC, Silverman M: Relationship between infant lung mechanics and childhood lung function in children of very low birthweight, *Pediatr Pulmonol* 8:74-81, 1990.

Pathology

47. Stocker JT: The respiratory tract. In Stocker JT, Dehner LP, eds: *Pediatric pathology,* Philadelphia, 1992, JB Lippincott, pp 533-541.
48. Anderson WR, Engel RR: Cardiopulmonary sequelae of reparative stages of bronchopulmonary dysplasia, *Arch Pathol Lab Med* 107:603-608, 1983.
49. Van Lierde S, Cornelis A, Devlieger H, Moerman P, Lauweryns J, Eggermont E: Different patterns of pulmonary sequelae after hyaline membrane disease: heterogeneity of bronchopulmonary dysplasia? A clinicopathological study, *Biol Neonate* 60:152-162, 1991.
50. Ogden BE, Murphy SA, Saunders GC, Pathak D, Johnson JD: Neonatal lung neutrophils and elastase/proteinase inhibitor imbalances, *Am Rev Respir Dis* 130:817-821, 1984.
51. Merritt TA, Stuard D, Puccia J, Wood B, Edward DK, Finkelstein J, Shapiro DL: Newborn tracheal aspirate cytology: classification during respiratory distress syndrome and bronchopulmonary dysplasia, *J Pediatr* 98:949-956, 1981.
52. Merritt TA, Puccia J, Stuard D: Cytologic evaluation of pulmonary effluent in neonates with respiratory distress syndrome and bronchopulmonary dysplasia, *Acta Cytologica* 25:632-639, 1981.
53. Grigg J, Arnon S, Silverman M: Fractional processing of sequential bronchoalveolar lavage fluid from intubated babies, *Eur Respir J* 5:727-732, 1992.
54. Clement A, Chadelat F, Sardet A, Grimfeld A, Tournier G: Alveolar macrophage status in bronchopulmonary dysplasia, *Pediatr Res* 23:470-473, 1988.
55. Arnon S, Grigg J, Silverman M: Pulmonary inflammatory cells in ventilated preterm infants: effect of surfactant treatment, *Arch Dis Child* 69:44-48, 1993.
56. Hislop AA, Haworth SG: Airway size and structure in the normal fetal and infant lung and the effect of premature delivery and artificial ventilation, *Am Rev Respir Dis* 140:1717-1726, 1989.
57. Hislop AA, Wigglesworth JS, Desai R, Aber V: The effects of preterm delivery and mechanical ventilation on human lung growth, *Early Hum Dev* 15:147-164, 1987.
58. Gorenflo M, Vogel M, Obladen M: Pulmonary vascular changes in bronchopulmonary dysplasia: a clinicopathologic correlation in short- and long-term survivors, *Pediatr Pathol* 11:851-866, 1991.
59. Gau GS, Ryder TA, Mobberley MA: Iatrogenic epithelial change caused by endotracheal intubation of neonates, *Early Hum Dev* 15:221-229, 1987.

Risk Factors and Pathogenesis

60. Bonikos DS, Bensch KG, Northway WH Jr: Oxygen toxicity in the newborn: the effect of chronic continuous 100 percent oxygen on the lungs of newborn mice, *Am J Pathol* 85:623-635, 1976.
61. Pappas CT, Obara H, Bensch KG, Northway WH Jr: Effect of prolonged exposure to 80% oxygen on the lung of the newborn mouse, *Lab Invest* 48:735-748, 1983.
62. Randell SH, Mercer RR, Young SL: Neonatal hyperoxia alters the pulmonary alveolar and capillary structure of 40 day old rats, *Am J Pathol* 136:1259-1266, 1990.

63. de Lemos RA, Coalson JJ, Gerstmann DR, Kuehl TJ, Null DM Jr: Oxygen toxicity in the premature baboon with hyaline membrane disease, *Am Rev Respir Dis* 136:677-682, 1987.
64. Lorenzo AV: The preterm rabbit: a model for the study of acute and chronic effects of premature birth, *Pediatr Res* 19:201-205, 1985.
65. Hershenson MB, Garland A, Kelleher MD, Zimmerman A, Hernandez C, Solway J: Hyperoxia-induced airway remodelling in immature rats, *Am Rev Respir Dis* 146:1294-1300, 1992.
66. Merritt TA: Oxygen exposure in the newborn guinea pig lung lavage cell populations: chemotactic and elastase response—a possible relationship to neonatal bronchopulmonary dysplasia, *Pediatr Res* 16:798-805, 1982.
67. Kelly FJ, Town GI, Phillips GJ, Holgate ST, Roche WR, Postle AD: The preterm guinea pig: a model for the study of neonatal lung disease, *Clin Sci* 81:439-446, 1991.
68. Frank L, Sosenko IRS: Failure of premature rabbits to increase antioxidant enzymes during hyperoxic exposure: increased susceptibility to pulmonary oxygen toxicity compared to term rabbits, *Pediatr Res* 29:292-296, 1991.
69. Thibeault DW, Mabry S, Rezaiekhaligh M: Neonatal pulmonary oxygen toxicity in the rat and lung changes, *Pediatr Pulmonol* 9:96-108, 1990.
70. Walther FJ, Wade AB, Warburton D: Ontogeny of antioxidant enzymes in the fetal lamb lung, *Exp Lung Res* 17:39-45, 1991.
71. Rosenfeld W, Evans H, Concepciou L, Jhavevi R, Schaeffer H, Friedman A: Prevention of bronchopulmonary dysplasia by administration of bovine superoxide dismutase in preterm infants with respiratory distress syndrome, *J Pediatr* 105:781-785, 1984.
72. Tanswell AK, Freeman BA: Liposome-entrapped antioxidant enzymes prevent lethal O_2 toxicity in the newborn rat, *J Appl Physiol* 63:347-352, 1987.
73. Frank L: Antioxidants, nutrition and bronchopulmonary dysplasia, *Clin Perinatol* 19:541-562, 1992.
74. Shenai JP, Kennedy KA, Chytil F, Stahlman MT: Clinical trial of vitamin A supplementation in infants susceptible to bronchopulmonary dysplasia, *J Pediatr* 111:269-277, 1987.
75. Grigg J, Barber A, Silverman M: Bronchoalveolar lavage fluid glutathione in intubated premature infants, *Arch Dis Child* 69:49-51, 1993.
76. Taghizadeh A, Reynolds EO: Pathogenesis of bronchopulmonary dysplasia following hyaline membrane disease, *Am J Pathol* 82:241-264, 1976.
77. Davis JM, Dickerson B, Metlay L, Penney DP: Differential effects of oxygen and barotrauma on lung injury in the neonatal piglet, *Pediatr Pulmonol* 10:157-163, 1991.
78. Solca M, Kolobow T, Huang H, Pesenti A, Buckhold D, Pierce JE: Management of the antenatal preterm fetal lung in the prevention of respiratory distress syndrome in lambs, *Biol Neonate* 44:93-101, 1983.
79. Penn RB, Wolfson MR, Shaffer TM: Effect of ventilation on mechanical properties and pressure-flow relationships of immature airways, *Pediatr Res* 23:519-524, 1988.
80. Meredith KS, de Lemos RA, Coalson JJ, King RJ, Gerstmann DR, Kumar R, Kuehl TJ, Winter DC, Taylor A, Clark RH: Role of lung injury in the pathogenesis of hyaline membrane disease in premature baboons, *J Appl Physiol* 66:2150-2158, 1989.
81. Dreyfuss D, Soler P, Basset G, Saumon G: High inflation pressure pulmonary edema: respective effects of high airway pressure, high tidal volume and positive end expiratory pressure, *Am Rev Respir Dis* 137:1159-1164, 1988.
82. Webb HH, Tierney DF: Experimental pulmonary edema due to intermittent positive pressure ventilation with high inflation pressures: protection by positive end expiratory pressure, *Am Rev Respir Med* 110:556-565, 1974.
83. Coalson JJ, Kuehl TJ, Prihoda TJ, de Lemos RA: Diffuse alveolar damage in the evolution of bronchopulmonary dysplasia in the baboon, *Pediatr Res* 24:357-366, 1988.
84. Oyarzun M, Clements JA, Baritussio A: Ventilation enhances pulmonary alveolar clearance of radioactive dipalmitoyl phosphatidyl choline in liposomes, *Am Rev Respir Dis* 121:709-721, 1980.
85. Wyszogrodoski I, Kyei-Aboagye K, Taeusch HW Jr, Avery ME: Surfactant inactivation by hyperventilation: conservation by end-expiratory pressure, *J Appl Physiol* 38:461-466, 1975.
86. Clark RH, Gerstmann DR, Null DM, de Lemos RA: Prospective randomized comparison of high-frequency oscillatory and conventional ventilation in respiratory distress syndrome, *Pediatrics* 89:5-12, 1992.
87. Coalson JJ, Winter VT, Gerstmann DR, Idell S, King RJ, Delemos RA: Pathophysiologic, morphometric, and biochemical studies of the premature baboon with bronchopulmonary dysplasia, *Am Rev Respir Dis* 145:872-881, 1992.
88. Gerstmann DR, Delemos RA, Coalson JJ, Clark RH, Wiswell TE, Winter DC, Kuehl TT, Meredith FS, Null DM: Influence of ventilatory technique on pulmonary baroinjury in baboons with hyaline membrane disease, *Pediatr Pulmonol* 5:82-91, 1988.
89. Rudd PT, Cassell GH, Waites KB, Davis JK, Duffy LB: *Ureaplasma urealyticum* pneumonia: experimental production and demonstration of age-related susceptibility, *Infect Immunol* 57:918-925, 1989.
90. Crouse DT, Cassell GH, Waites KB, Foster JM, Cassady G: Hyperoxia potentiates *Ureaplasma urealyticum* pneumonia in newborn mice, *Infect Immunol* 58:3487-3493, 1990.
91. Cassel GH, Waites KB, Crouse DT, Rudd PT, Canupp KC, Stagno S, Cutter GR: Association of *Ureaplasma urealyticum* infection of the lower respiratory tract with chronic lung disease and death in very-low-birth-weight infants, *Lancet* 2:240-245, 1988.
92. Brown ER: Increased risk of bronchopulmonary dysplasia and patent ductus arteriosus, *J Pediatr* 95:865-866, 1979.
93. Van Marter LJ, Pagano M Allred EN, Leviton A, Kuban KC: Rate of bronchopulmonary dysplasia as a function of neonatal intensive care practices, *J Pediatr* 120:938-946, 1992.
94. Van de Bor M, Verloove Vanhorick SP, Brand R, Ruys JH: Patent ductus arteriosus in a cohort of 1338 preterm infants: a collaborative study, *Paediatr Perinatol Epidemiol* 2:328-336, 1988.
95. Cassady G, Crouse D, Kirklin J, Strange MJ, Joiner CH, Godoy G, Odrezin GT, Cutter GR, Kirklin JK, Pacifico AD: A randomised controlled trial of very early prophylactic ligation of the ductus arteriosus in babies who weigh 1000 g or less, *N Engl J Med* 320:1511-1516, 1989.
96. Palti M, Gabbert D, Weinstein MR, Peters ME: Multivariate assessment of traditional risk factors for chronic lung disease in very low birth weight neonate, *J Pediatr* 119:285-292, 1991.
97. Lorenz JM, Klienman LI, Kotagal UR, Reller MD: Water balance in very low birth weight infants: relationship to water and sodium intake and effect on outcome, *J Pediatr* 101:423-432, 1982.
98. Nickerson BF, Taussig LM: Family history of asthma in infants with bronchopulmonary dysplasia, *Pediatrics* 65:1140-1144, 1980.
99. Bertrand J-M, Riley SP, Popkin J, Coates AL: The long-term pulmonary sequelae of prematurity: the role of familial airway hyperreactivity and the respiratory distress syndrome, *N Engl J Med* 312:742-745, 1985.
100. Riedel F, Achenbach U, Rieger CHL: Prematurity and maternal bronchial hyperresponsiveness, *J Perinat Med* 17:151-155, 1989.
101. Chan KN, Noble-Jamieson CM, Elliman A, Bryan EM, Aber V, Silverman M: Airway responsiveness in low birthweight children and their mothers, *Arch Dis Child* 63:905-910, 1988.

Possible Cellular Mechanisms in the Pathogenesis of CLD

102. Finkelstein JN, Horowitz S, Sinkin RA, Ryan RM: Cellular and molecular responses to lung injury in relation to induction of tissue repair and fibrosis, *Clin Perinatol* 19:603-620, 1992.
103. Evans MJ: Oxidant gases, *Environs Health Perspex* 55:85-95, 1984.
104. Theta LA, Para SC, Shelburne JD: Sequential changes in lung morphology during the repair of acute oxygen-induced lung injury in adult rats, *Exp Lung Res* 11:209-228, 1988.
105. Tryka AF, Witschi H, Gosslee DG, McArthur AH, Clapp NK: Patterns of cell proliferation during recovery from oxygen injury, *Am Rev Respir Dis* 133:1055-1059, 1986.
106. Jackson JC, MacKenzie AP, Chi EY, Standaert TA, Truog WE, Hodson WA: Mechanisms for reduced total lung capacity at birth and during hyaline membrane disease in premature newborn monkeys, *Am Rev Respir Dis* 142:413-419, 1990.
107. Jacobs RF, Wilson CB, Palmer S: Factors related to the appearance of alveolar macrophages in the developing lung, *Am Rev Respir Dis* 131:548-553, 1985.
108. Gerdes JS, Harris MC, Polin RA: Effects of dexamethasone and indomethacin on elastase, alpha 1-proteinase inhibitor, and fibronectin in bronchoalveolar lavage fluid from neonates, *J Pediatr* 113:727-731, 1988.

109. Merritt TA, Cochrane CG, Holcomb K, Bohl B, Hallman M, Strayer D, Edward DK, Gluck L: Elastance and alpha 1-proteinase inhibitor activity in tracheal aspirates during respiratory distress syndrome: role of inflammation in the pathogenesis of bronchopulmonary dysplasia, *J Clin Invest* 72:656-666, 1983.
110. Yoder MC, Chua R, Tepper R: Effect of dexamethasone on pulmonary inflammation and pulmonary function of ventilator-dependent infants with bronchopulmonary dysplasia, *Am Rev Respir Dis* 143:1044-1048, 1991.
111. Kovacs EJ, Kelly J: Secretion of macrophage-derived growth factor during acute lung injury by bleomycin, *J Leukocyte Biol* 137:1-14, 1985.
112. Jordana M, Richards C, Irving LB, Gauldie J: Spontaneous *in vitro* release of alveolar macrophage cytokines after the intratracheal instillation of bleomycin in rats, *Am Rev Respir Dis* 137:1135-1140, 1988.
113. Frank L, Yam J, Roberts RJ: The role of endotoxin in protection of adult rats from high oxygen lung toxicity, *J Clin Invest* 61:269-275, 1978.
114. Frank L, Summerville J, Massaro D: Protection from oxygen toxicity with endotoxin: role of antioxidant enzymes of the lung, *J Clin Invest* 65:1104-1110, 1980.
115. Groneck P, Gotze-Speer B, Oppermann M, Eiffert H, Speer CP: Association of pulmonary inflammation and increased microvascular permeability during the development of bronchopulmonary dysplasia: a sequential analysis of inflammatory mediators in respiratory fluids of high risk preterm neonates, *Pediatrics* 93:712-718, 1994.
116. Metinko AP, Kunkel SL, Standiford TS, Strieter RM, Anoxia-hyperoxia induces monocyte-derived interleukin-8, *J Clin Invest* 90:791-798, 1992.
117. Donelly SC, Strieter RM, Kunkel SL, Walz A, Robertson CR, Carter DC, Grant IS, Pollok AJ, Haslett C: Interleukin-8 and development of adult respiratory distress syndrome in at-risk patient groups, *Lancet* 341:643-647, 1993.
118. Kotecha S, Chan B, Azam N, Silverman M, Shaw RJ: Increase in interleukin-8 and soluble intercellular adhesion molecule-1 in bronchoalveolar lavage fluid from premature infants who develop chronic lung disease, *Arch Dis Child* Fetal Neonatal Ed:F90-F96, 1995.
119. Sporn MB, Roberts AB, Wakefield LM, de Crombrugghe B: Recent advances in the chemistry and biology of transforming growth factor beta, *J Cell Biol* 105:1039-1045, 1987.
120. Shaw RJ: The role of lung macrophages at the interface between chronic inflammation and fibrosis, *Respir Med* 85:267-273, 1991.
121. Hoyt DG, Lazo JS: Alterations in pulmonary mRNA encoding procollagens, fibronectin and transforming growth factor beta precede bleomycin-induced pulmonary fibrosis in mice, *J Pharmacol Exp Ther* 246:765-771, 1988.
122. Khalil N, O'Connor RN, Unruh HW, Warren PW, Flandres KC, Kemp A, Bereznay OH, Greenberg AH: Increased production and immunohistochemical localization of transforming growth factor-beta in idiopathic pulmonary fibrosis, *Am J Respir Cell Mol Biol* 5:155-162, 1991.
123. Khalil N, Bereznay O, Sporn M, Greenberg AH: Macrophage production of transforming growth factor beta and fibroblast collagen synthesis in chronic pulmonary inflammation, *J Exp Med* 170:727-737, 1989.
124. Fabisiak JP, Evans JN, Kelly J: Increased expression of PDGF(B) (*c*-sin) mRNA in rat lung precedes DNA synthesis and tissue repair during chronic hyperoxia, *Am J Respir Cell Mol Biol* 1:181-189, 1989.
125. Watts CL, Fanaroff AA: Platelet derived growth factor (PDGF) is increased in lung secretions during the first week of life in infants who develop bronchopulmonary dysplasia, *Pediatr Res* 33:349A, 1993.
126. Watts CL, Fanaroff AA: Platelet derived growth factor response to dexamethasone in infants with bronchopulmonary dysplasia, *Pediatr Res* 33:349A, 1993.
127. Kelley J: Cytokines of the lung, *Am Rev Respir Dis* 141:765-788, 1990.
128. Watts CL, Fanaroff AA: Fibronectin: a role in respiratory distress syndrome and bronchopulmonary dysplasia, *Sem Perinatol* 16:162-169, 1992.
129. Gerdes JS, Yoder MC, Douglas SD, Paul M, Harris MC, Polin RA: Tracheal lavage and plasma fibronectin relationship to respiratory distress syndrome and development of bronchopulmonary dysplasia, *J Pediatr* 108:601-606, 1986.
130. Watts CL, Bruce MC: Effect of dexamethasone therapy on fibronectin and albumin levels in lung sections of infants with bronchopulmonary dysplasia, *J Pediatr* 121:597-607, 1992.
131. Streiter RM, Lukacs NW, Standiford TJ, Kunkel SL: Cytokines and lung inflammation: mechanisms of neutrophil recruitment to the lung, *Thorax* 48(7):764-769, 1993.

Clinical Features of CLD of Prematurity

132. Hakulinen AL, Heinonen K, Lansimies E, Kiekara O: Pulmonary function and respiratory morbidity in school-age children born prematurely and ventilated for neonatal respiratory insufficiency, *Pediatr Pulmonol* 8:226-232, 1990.
133. Fan LL, Flynn JW, Pathak DR: Risk factors predicting laryngeal injury in intubated neonates, *Crit Care Med* 11:431-433, 1983.
134. Mortensson W, Lindroth M, Jonsson S, Sernningsen U: Chest radiography and pulmonary mechanics in ventilator treated low birth weight treated infants, *Acta Radiologica [Diagn] (Stockh)* 24:71-79, 1983.
135. Groothuis JR, Gutierrez KM, Lauer BA: Respiratory syncytial virus infection in children with bronchopulmonary dysplasia, *Pediatrics* 82:199-203, 1988.
136. Werthammer J, Brown ER, Neff RK, Taeusch HW: Sudden infant death syndrome in infants with bronchopulmonary dysplasia, *Pediatrics* 69:301-304, 1982.
137. Jones R, Wincott E, Elbourne D, Grant A: Controlled trial of dexamethasone in neonatal chronic lung disease: a 3-year follow-up, *Pediatrics* 96(5 Pt 1):897-906, 1995.
138. Yu EY, Orgill AA, Lim SB, Bajuk B, Astbury J: Growth and development of very low birthweight infants recovering from bronchopulmonary dysplasia, *Arch Dis Child* 58:791-794, 1983.
139. Lindroth M, Mortensson W: Long-term follow-up of ventilator treated low birthweight infants. I. Chest x-ray, pulmonary mechanics, clinical lung disease and growth, *Acta Pediatr Scand* 75:819-826, 1986.
140. Driscoll DJ, Kleinberg F, Heise CT, Staats BA: Cardiorespiratory function in asymptomatic survivors of neonatal respiratory distress syndrome, *Mayo Clin Proc* 62:695-700, 1987.
141. Bader D, Ramos AD, Lew CD, Platzker ACG, Stabile MW, Keens TG: Childhood sequelae of infant lung disease: exercise and pulmonary function abnormalities after bronchopulmonary dysplasia, *J Pediatr* 110:693-699, 1987.
142. Barker DJP: Fetal and neonatal origins of adult disease, *Br Med J* 150-164, 1992.

Acquired Upper Respiratory Tract Complications

143. Lindahl H, Rintala R, Malinen L, Leijala M, Sairanen H: Bronchoscopy during the first month of life, *J Pediatr Surg* 27:548-550, 1992.
144. Marcovich M, Pollauf F, Burian K: Subglottic stenosis in newborns after mechanical ventilation, *Prog Pediatr Surg* 21:8-19, 1987.
145. Bhutani VK: Tracheobronchial abnormalities complicating bronchopulmonary dysplasia, *J Pediatr* 112:843-844, 1988.
146. McCubbin M, Frey EE, Wagener JS, Tribby R: Large airway collapse in bronchopulmonary dysplasia, *J Pediatr* 114:304-307, 1989.
147. McCoy KS, Bagwell CE, Wagner M, Sallent J, O'Keefe M, Kosch PC: Spirometric and endoscopic evaluation of airway collapse in infants with bronchopulmonary dysplasia, *Pediatr Pulmonol* 14:23-27, 1992.
148. Panitch HP, Deoras KS, Wolfson MR, Shaffer TH: Maturational changes in airway smooth muscle structure function relationships, *Pediatr Res* 31:151-156, 1992.
149. Couser RJ, Ferrara TB, Falde B, Johnson K, Schilling CG, Hoekstra RE: Effectiveness of dexamethasone in preventing extubation failure in preterm infants at increased risk for airway edema, *J Pediatr* 121:591-596, 1992.
150. Bowdler DA, Rogers JH: Subglottic stenosis in children: a conservative approach, *Clin Otolaryngol* 12:383-388, 1987.
151. Albert D: Management of suspected tracheobronchial stenosis in ventilated neonates, *Arch Dis Child* 72:F1-F2, 1995.

Extrapulmonary Complications

152. Groothuis JR, Rosenberg AA: Home oxygen promotes weight gain in infants with bronchopulmonary dysplasia, *Am J Dis Child* 141:992-995, 1987.
153. Hrabovsky E, Mullett MD: Gastro-oesophageal reflux in a premature infant, *J Pediatr Surg* 21:583-587, 1986.
154. Orenstein SR, Orenstein BM: Gastro-oesophageal reflux and respiratory disease in children, *J Pediatr* 112:847-858, 1988.

155. Nielson TW, Heldt GP, Tooley WA: Stridor and gastro-oesophageal reflux in infants, *Pediatrics* 85:1034-1039, 1990.
156. Giuffre RM, Rubin S, Mitchell I: Anti-reflux surgery in infants with bronchopulmonary dysplasia, *Am J Dis Child* 141:648-651, 1987.
157. Jolley SR, Halpern CT, Sterling CE, Feldman BH: The relationship of respiratory complications from gastroesophageal reflux to prematurity in infants, *J Pediatr Surg* 25:755-757, 1990.
158. Malfroot A, Vandenplas Y, Verlinden M, Piepsz A, Dab I: Gastroesophageal reflux and unexplained chronic respiratory disease in infants and children, *Pediatr Pulmonol* 3:208-221, 1987.
159. Abman SH, Accurso FJ, Bowman CM: Unsuspected cardiopulmonary abnormalities complicating bronchopulmonary dysplasia, *Arch Dis Child* 59:966-970, 1984.
160. Goodman G, Perkin RM, Awas NG, Sperling DR: Pulmonary hypertension in infants with bronchopulmonary dysplasia, *J Pediatr* 112:67-72, 1988.
161. Ascher DP, Rosen P, Null DM, de Lemos RA, Wheller JJ: Systemic to pulmonary collaterals mimicking patent ductus arteriosus in neonates with prolonged ventilatory courses, *J Pediatr* 107:282-284, 1985.
162. Tomashevsky JF, Oppermann HC, Vawter GF: Bronchopulmonary dysplasia: a morphometric study with emphasis on the pulmonary vasculature, *Pediatr Pathol* 24:69-87, 1984.
163. Hislop AA, Haworth SG: Pulmonary vascular damage and the development of cor pulmonale following hyaline membrane disease, *Pediatr Pulmonol* 9:152-161, 1990.
164. Ficke CD, Hansen TN: Hypoxic vasoconstriction increases with postnatal age in lungs from newborn rabbits, *Circ Res* 60:297-303, 1987.
165. Abman SH, Wolfe RR, Accurso FJ, Koops BL, Bowman CM, Wiggins JW Jr: Pulmonary vascular response to oxygen in infants with severe bronchopulmonary dysplasia, *Pediatrics* 75:80-84, 1985.
166. Domino KB, Chen L, Alexander CM, Williams JJ, Marshall C, Marshall BE: Time course and responses of sustained hypoxic pulmonary vasoconstriction in the dog, *Anaesthia* 60:562-566, 1984.
167. Halliday H, Dumpit FS, Brady JC: Effects of inspired oxygen on echocardiographic assessment of pulmonary vascular resistance and myocardial contractility in bronchopulmonary dysplasia, *Pediatrics* 65:536-540, 1980.
168. Fouron JC, Le Guennec JC, Villemant D, Perreault G, Davignon A: Value of echocardiography in assessing the outcome of bronchopulmonary dysplasia of the newborn, *Pediatrics* 65:529-535, 1980.
169. Bush A, Busst CM, Knight WB, Hislop AA, Haworth SG, Shinebourne EA: Changes in pulmonary circulation in severe bronchopulmonary dysplasia, *Arch Dis Child* 65:739-745, 1990.
170. Newth CJL, Gow RM, Rowe RD: The assessment of pulmonary arterial pressures in bronchopulmonary dysplasia by cardiac catheterisation and M-mode echocardiography, *Pediatr Pulmonol* 1:58-63, 1985.
171. Berman W, Yabek SM, Dillon T, Burstein R, Corlew S: Evaluation of infants with bronchopulmonary dysplasia using cardiac catheterisation, *Pediatrics* 70:708-712, 1982.
172. Evans NJ, Archer LNJ: Doppler assessment of pulmonary artery pressure during recovery from hyaline membrane disease, *Arch Dis Child* 66:802-804, 1991.
173. Skinner JR, Boys RJ, Hunter S, Hey EN: Non-invasive assessment of pulmonary artery pressure in healthy neonates, *Arch Dis Child* 66:386-390, 1991.
174. Benatar A, Clarke J, Silverman M: Echocardiographic studies in chronic lung disease of prematurity, *Arch Dis Child* 72:F14-F19, 1995.
175. Gill AB, Weindling AM: Pulmonary artery pressure changes in the very low birth weight infant developing chronic lung disease, *Arch Dis Child* 68:303-307, 1993.
176. Bregman J, Farrell EE: Neurodevelopmental outcome in infants with bronchopulmonary dysplasia, *Clin Perinatol* 19:673-694, 1992.
177. Singer L, Martin RJ, Hawkins SW, Benson-Szekely LJ, Yamashita TS, Carlo WA: Oxygen desaturation complicates feeding in infants with bronchopulmonary dysplasia after discharge, *Pediatrics* 90:380-384, 1992.
178. Garg M, Kurzner SI, Bautista DB, Keens TG: Clinically unsuspected hypoxia during sleep and feeding in infants with bronchopulmonary dysplasia, *Pediatrics* 81:635-642, 1988.
179. Garg M, Kurzner SI, Bautista D, Keens TG: Hypoxic arousal responses in infants with bronchopulmonary dysplasia, *Pediatrics* 82: 59-63, 1988.
180. Zinman R, Blanchard PW, Vachon F: Oxygen saturation during sleep in patients with bronchopulmonary dysplasia, *Biol Neonate* 61:69-75, 1992.

Clinical Pulmonary Physiology

181. Alpert BE, Gainey MA, Schidlow DV, Capitanio MA: Effect of oxygen on right ventricular performance evaluated by radionuclide angiography in two young patients with chronic lung disease, *Pediatr Pulmonol* 3:149-152, 1987.
182. Tay-Uyboco JS, Kwiatowski K, Cates DB, Kavanagh L, Rigatto H: Hypoxic airway constriction in infants of very low birth weight recovering from moderate to severe bronchopulmonary dysplasia, *J Pediatr* 115:456-459, 1989.
183. Teague WG, Pian MS, Heldt GP, Tooley WH: An acute reduction in the fraction of inspired oxygen increases airway constriction in infants with chronic lung disease, *Am Rev Respir Dis* 137:861-865, 1988.
184. Dransfield DA, Spitzer AR, Fox WW: Episodic airway obstruction in premature infants, *Am J Dis Child* 137:441-443, 1983.
185. Miller MJ, Carlo WA, DiFiore JM, Martin RJ: Airway obstruction during periodic breathing in premature infants, *J Appl Physiol* 64:2469-2500, 1988.
186. Poets CF, Southall DP: Patterns of oxygenation during periodic breathing in preterm infants, *Early Hum Dev* 26:1-12, 1991.
187. McEvoy C, Durand M, Hewlett V: Episodes of spontaneous desaturations in infants with chronic lung disease at two different levels of oxygenation, *Pediatr Pulmonol* 15:140-144, 1993.
188. Martin RJ, Herrell N, Rubin D, Fanaroff A: Effect of supine and prone positions on arterial oxygen tension in the preterm infant, *Pediatrics* 63:528-531, 1979.
189. Wagaman MJ, Shutack JG, Moomjian AS, Schwartz JG, Shaffer TH, Fox WW: Improved oxygenation and lung compliance with prone positioning of neonates, *J Pediatr* 74:787-791, 1979.
190. Rome ES, Stork EK, Carlo WA, Martin RJ: Limitations of transcutaneous Po_2 and Pco_2 monitoring in infants with bronchopulmonary dysplasia, *Pediatrics* 74:217-220, 1984.
191. Hoppenbrouwers T, Hodgman JE, Arakawa K, Durand M, Cabal LA: Transcutaneous oxygen and carbon dioxide during the first half year of life in premature and normal term infants, *Pediatr Res* 31:73-79, 1992.
192. MacFadyen U: Home oxygen treatment, *Paediatr Respir Med* 1(3):10-14, 1993.
193. England SJ: Current techniques for assessing pulmonary function in the newborn and infant: advantages and limitations, *Pediatr Pulmonol* 4:48-53, 1988.
194. ATS/ERS statement: Respiratory mechanics in infants: physiologic evaluation in health and disease, *Eur Respir J* 6:269-310, 1993 and *Am Rev Respir Dis* 147:474-496, 1993.
195. Prendiville A, Thomson A, Silverman M: Effect of tracheobronchial suction on respiratory resistance in intubated preterm babies, *Arch Dis Child* 61:1178-1183, 1986.
196. Motoyama EK, Fort MD, Klesh KW, Mutich RL, Guthrie RD: Early onset of airway reactivity in premature infants with bronchopulmonary dysplasia, *Am Rev Respir Dis* 136:50-57, 1987.
197. Lee H, Arnon S, Silverman M: Bronchodilator aerosol administration by metered dose inhaler and spacer in subacute neonatal respiratory distress syndrome, *Arch Dis Child* 70:218-222, 1994.
198. Kwong MS, Egan EA, Notter RH, Shapiro DL: Double blind trial of calf lung surfactant extract for the prevention of hyaline membrane disease in extremely premature infants, *Pediatrics* 76:585-592, 1985.
199. Rosen WC, Mammel MC, Fisher JB, Coleman JB, Bing DR, Holloman KK, Boros SJ: The effects of bedside pulmonary mechanics testing during infant mechanical ventilation: a retrospective analysis, *Pediatr Pulmonol* 16:147-152, 1993.
200. Nickerson BG, Durand DJ, Kao L: Short-term variability of pulmonary function tests in infants with bronchopulmonary dysplasia, *Pediatr Pulmonol* 6:36-41, 1989.
201. Moriette G, Gaudebout C, Clement A, Boule M, Bion B, Relier JP, Gaultier C: Pulmonary function at 1 year of age in survivors of neonatal respiratory distress, *Pediatr Pulmonol* 3:242-250, 1987.
202. Wong YC, Beardsmore CS, Silverman M: Pulmonary sequelae of neonatal respiratory distress in very low birthweight infants: a clinical and physiological study, *Arch Dis Child* 57:418-424, 1982.

203. Yuksel B, Greenough A: Relationship of symptoms to lung function abnormalities in preterm infants at follow up, *Pediatr Pulmonol* 11:202-206, 1991.
204. Arad I, Bar Yishay E, Eyal F, Gross S, Godfrey S: Lung function in infancy and childhood following neonatal intensive care, *Pediatr Pulmonol* 3:29-33, 1987.
205. Morray JP, Fox WW, Kettrick RG, Downes JJ: Improvement in lung mechanics as a function of age in the infant with severe bronchopulmonary dysplasia, *Pediatr Res* 16:290-294, 1982.
206. Tepper RS, Pagtakhan RD, Taussig LM: Noninvasive determination of total respiratory system compliance in infants by the weighted-spirometer method, *Am Rev Respir Dis* 130:461-466, 1984.
207. Gerhardt T, Reifenberg L, Goldberg RN, Bancalari E: Pulmonary function in preterm infants whose lungs were ventilated conventionally or by high-frequency oscillation, *J Pediatr* 115:121-126, 1989.
208. Yuksel B, Greenough A: Lung function in 6-20 month old infants born very preterm but without respiratory troubles, *Pediatr Pulmonol* 14:214-221, 1992.
209. Tepper RS, Morgan WJ, Cota K, Taussig LM: Expiratory flow limitation in infants with bronchopulmonary dysplasia, *J Pediatr* 109:1040-1046, 1986.
210. Wohl MEB: Lung mechanics in the developing human infant. In Chernick V, Mellins RB: *Basic mechanisms of pediatric respiratory disease: cellular and integrative,* ed 5, Philadelphia, 1989, BC Decker, pp 89-99.
211. Wolfson MR, Bhutani VK, Shaffer TH, Bowen FW: Mechanics and energetics of breathing helium in infants with bronchopulmonary dysplasia, *J Pediatr* 104:752-757, 1984.
212. Kurtzner SI, Garg M, Bautista DB, Sargent CW, Bowman CM, Keens TG: Growth failure in bronchopulmonary dysplasia: elevated metabolic rates and pulmonary mechanics, *J Pediatr* 112:73-80, 1988.
213. Kao LC, Durand DJ, Nickerson BG: Improving pulmonary function does not decrease oxygen consumption in infants with bronchopulmonary dysplasia, *J Pediatr* 112:616-621, 1988.
214. Northway WH, Moss RB, Carlisle KB, Parker BR, Popp RL, Pitlick PT, Eichler I, Lamm RL, Brown BW: Late pulmonary sequelae of bronchopulmonary dysplasia, *N Engl J Med* 323:1793-1799, 1990.

Management

215. Isaacs D: Cold comfort for the catarrhal child, *Arch Dis Child* 65:1295-1296, 1990.
216. Rush MG, Hazinski TA: Current therapy of bronchopulmonary dysplasia, *Clin Perinatol* 19:563-590, 1992.
217. Greally P, Hampton FJ, MacFadyen UM, Simpson H: Gaviscon and carob compared with cisapride in gastro-oesophageal reflux, *Arch Dis Child* 67:618-621, 1992.
218. Hufnagle KG, Khan SN, Penn D, Cacciarelli A, Williams P: Renal calcifications: a complication of long-term furosemide therapy in preterm infants, *Pediatrics* 70:360-363, 1982.
219. Brownlee JR, Beegman RH, Rosenthal A: Acute hemodynamic effects of nifedipine in infants with bronchopulmonary dysplasia and pulmonary hypertension, *Pediatr Res* 24:186-190, 1988.
220. Taylor BJ, Fewell JE, Kearns GL: Pulmonary vascular response to aerosolised cromolyn sodium and repeated episodes of isocapnic alveolar hypoxia in lambs, *Pediatr Res* 23:513-518, 1988.
221. Taylor BJ, Fewell JE, Kearns GL, Hill DE: Cromolyn sodium decreases the pulmonary vascular response to alveolar hypoxia in lambs, *Pediatr Res* 20:834-837, 1986.
222. Frantz EG, Schreiber MD, Soifer SJ: Cromolyn sodium does not prevent hypoxic-induced pulmonary hypertension in newborn and young lambs, *J Dev Physiol* 10:555-565, 1988.
223. Abman SA, Warady BA, Lum GM, Koops BL: Systemic hypertension in infants with bronchopulmonary dysplasia, *J Pediatr* 104:929-931, 1984.
224. Melnick G, Pickoff AS, Ferrer PL, Peyser J, Bancalari E, Gelband H: Normal pulmonary vascular resistance and left ventricular hypertrophy in young infants with bronchopulmonary dysplasia: an echocardiographic and pathologic study, *Pediatrics* 66:589-596, 1980.
225. Johnson DE, Lock JE, Elde RP, Thompson TR: Pulmonary neuroendocrine cells in hyaline membrane disease and bronchopulmonary dysplasia, *Pediatr Res* 16:446-454, 1982.
226. Gillan JE, Cutz E: Abnormal pulmonary bombesin immunoreactive cells in Wilson-Mikity syndrome (pulmonary dysmaturity) and bronchopulmonary dysplasia, *Pediatr Pathol* 13:165-180, 1993.
227. Stocker JT: Pathologic features of long-standing "healed" bronchopulmonary dysplasia: a study of 28 3-40 month old infants, *Human Pathol* 17:943-961, 1986.
228. Grigg J, Arnon S, Jones T, Clark A, Silverman M: Delivery of therapeutic aerosols to intubated babies, *Arch Dis Child* 67:25-30, 1992.
229. Arnon S, Grigg J, Nikander K, Silverman M: Delivery of micronised budesonide suspension by metered dose inhaler and jet nebulizer into a neonatal ventilator circuit, *Pediatr Pulmonol* 13:172-175, 1992.
230. Rozycki HJ, Byron PR, Dailey K, Gutcher GR: Evaluation of a system for the delivery of inhaled beclomethasone dipropionate to intubated neonates, *Dev Pharmacol Ther* 16:65-70, 1991.
231. Cameron D, Clay M, Silverman M: Evaluation of nebulizers for use in neonatal ventilator circuits, *Crit Care Med* 18:866-870, 1990.
232. Cameron D, Arnot R, Clay M, Silverman M: Aerosol delivery in neonatal ventilator circuits: a rabbit lung model, *Pediatr Pulmonol* 10:208-213, 1991.
233. Flavin M, MacDonald M, Dolovich M, Coates G, O'Brodovich H: Aerosol delivery to the rabbit lung with an infant ventilator, *Pediatr Pulmonol* 2:35-39, 1986.
234. Salmon B, Wilson NM, Silverman M: How much aerosol reaches the lungs of wheezy infants and toddlers? *Arch Dis Child* 64:401-403, 1990.
235. Barry P, O'Callaghan C: Inhaler devices for preschool children, *Paediatr Respir Med* 1:20-23, 1993.
236. Everard ML, Hardy JG, Milner AD: Comparison of nebulised aerosol deposition in the lungs of healthy adults following oral and nasal inhalation, *Thorax* 48:1045-1046, 1993.
237. O'Callaghan C, Milner AD, Swarbrick A: Paradoxical deterioration in lung function after nebulised salbutamol in wheezy infants, *Lancet* 2:1424-1425, 1986.
238. Prendiville A, Green S, Silverman M: Paradoxical response to salbutamol in wheezy infants, *Thorax* 42:85-91, 1987.
239. Seidenberg J, Mir Y, Von Der Hardt H: Hypoxaemia after nebulised salbutamol in wheezy infants: the importance of aerosol acidity, *Arch Dis Child* 66:672-675, 1991.
240. Ho L, Collis G, Landau LI, Le Souëf PN: Effect of salbutamol on oxygen saturation in bronchiolitis, *Arch Dis Child* 66:1061-1064, 1991.
241. Connett G, Lenney W: Prolonged hypoxaemia after nebulised salbutamol, *Thorax* 48:574-575, 1993.
242. Yuksel B, Greenough A: Comparison of the effects on lung function of different methods of bronchodilator administration, *Respir Med* 88:229-233, 1994.
243. Collis GG, Cole CH, Le Souëf PN: Dilution of nebulised aerosols by air entrainment in children, *Lancet* 336:341-343, 1990.
244. Kao LC, Durand DJ, Phillips BL, Nickerson BG: Oral theophylline and diuretics improve pulmonary mechanics in infants with bronchopulmonary dysplasia, *J Pediatr* 111:439-444, 1987.
245. Davis JM, Bhutani VK, Stefano JL, Fox WW, Spitzer AR: Changes in pulmonary mechanics following caffeine administration in infants with bronchopulmonary dysplasia, *Pediatr Pulmonol* 6:49-52, 1989.
246. Rooklin AR, Moomjian AS, Shutack JG, Schwartz JG, Fox WW: Theophylline therapy in bronchopulmonary dysplasia, *J Pediatr* 95:882-884, 1979.
247. Rotschild A, Solimano A, Puterman M, Smyth J, Sharma A, Albertheim S: Increased compliance in response to salbutamol in premature infants with developing bronchopulmonary dysplasia, *J Pediatr* 115:984-991, 1989.
248. Stefano JL, Bhutani VK, Fox WW: A randomised, placebo-controlled study to evaluate the effects of oral albuterol on pulmonary mechanics in ventilator-dependent infants at risk of developing BPD, *Pediatr Pulmonol* 10:183-191, 1991.
249. Denjean A, Guimaraes H, Migdal M, Miramand JL, Deland M, Gaultier C: Dose-related bronchodilator response to aerosolized salbutamol (albuterol) in ventilator dependent premature infants, *J Pediatr* 120:974-999, 1992.
250. Wilkie RA, Bryan MH: Effect of bronchodilators on airway resistance in ventilator-dependent neonates with chronic lung disease, *J Pediatr* 111:278-282, 1987.

251. Yuksel B, Greenough A, Maconochie I: Effective bronchodilator treatment by a simple spacer device for wheezy premature infants, *Arch Dis Child* 65:782-785, 1990.
252. Yuksel B, Greenough A: Ipratropium bromide for symptomatic preterm infants, *Eur J Pediatr* 150:854-857, 1991.
253. Yuksel B, Greenough A, Green S: Paradoxical response to nebulized ipratropium bromide in preterm infants asymptomatic at follow up, *Respir Med* 85:189-194, 1991.
254. Brundage KL, Mohsini KG, Froese AB, Fisher JT: Bronchodilator response to ipratropium bromide in infants with bronchopulmonary dysplasia, *Am Rev Respir Dis* 142:1137-1142, 1990.
255. Stenmark KR, Eyzaguirre M, Remigio L et al: Recovery of platelet activating factor and leukotrienes from infants with severe bronchopulmonary dysplasia: clinical improvement with cromolyn treatment, *Am Rev Respir Dis* 131:236A, 1985.
256. Watterberg KL, Murphy S, Neonatal Cromolyn Study Group: Failure of cromolyn sodium to reduce the incidence of bronchopulmonary dysplasia: a pilot study, *Pediatrics* 91:803-806, 1993.
257. Yuksel B, Greenough A: Inhaled sodium cromoglycate for preterm children with respiratory symptoms at follow up, *Respir Med* 86:131-134, 1992.
258. Silverman M: Chronic lung disease of prematurity: are we too cautious with steroids? *Eur J Paediatr* 153:S30-S35, 1994.
259. Avery GB, Fletcher AB, Kaplan M, Brudno DS: Controlled trial of dexmethasone in respirator-dependent infants with bronchopulmonary dysplasia, *Pediatrics* 75:106-111, 1985.
260. Collaborative Dexamethasone Trial Group: Dexamethasone therapy in neonatal chronic lung disease: an international placebo-controlled trial, *Pediatrics* 88:421-427, 1991.
261. Cummings JJ, D'Eugenio DB, Gross SJ: Controlled trial of dexamethasone in preterm infants at high risk for bronchopulmonary dysplasia, *N Engl J Med* 320:1505-1510, 1989.
262. Harkavy KL, Scanlon JW, Chowdhry PR, Grylack LJ: Dexamethasone for chronic lung disease in ventilator and oxygen dependent infants: a controlled trial, *J Pediatr* 115:979-983, 1989.
263. Kazzi NJ, Brans YW, Poland RL: Dexamethasone effects on the hospital course of infants with bronchopulmonary dysplasia who are dependent on artificial ventilation, *Pediatrics* 86:722-727, 1990.
264. Mammel MC, Green TP, Johnson DE, Thompson TR: Controlled trial of dexamethasone therapy in infants with bronchopulmonary dysplasia, *Lancet* 1:1356-1358, 1983.
265. Noble-Jamieson CM, Regev R, Silverman M: Dexamethasone in neonatal chronic lung disease: pulmonary effect and intracranial complications, *Eur J Pediatr* 148:365-367, 1989.
266. Ohlsson A, Calvert SA, Hosking M, Shennan AT: Randomised controlled trial of dexamethasone treatment in very-low-birthweight infants with ventilator dependent chronic lung disease, *Acta Paediatr* 81:751-756, 1992.
267. Yoder MC, Chua R, Tepper R: Effect of dexamethasone on pulmonary inflammation and pulmonary function of ventilator-dependent infants with bronchopulmonary dysplasia, *Am Rev Respir Dis* 143:1044-1048, 1991.
268. Brundage KL, Mohsini KG, Froese AB, Walker CR, Fisher JT: Dexamethasone therapy for bronchopulmonary dysplasia improved respiratory mechanics without adrenal suppression, *Pediatr Pulmonol* 12:162-169, 1992.
269. Gladstone IM, Ehrenkrantz RA, Jacobs HC: Pulmonary function tests and fluid balance in neonates with chronic lung disease during dexamethasone treatment, *Pediatrics* 84:1072-1076, 1989.
270. Pappagallo M, Blondheim D, Bhutani V, Abbasi S: Effect of inhaled dexamethasone in ventilator dependent preterm infants, *Pediatr Res* 27:219A, 1990.
271. Dunn MS, Magnani L, Belaiche M: Inhaled corticosteroids in severe bronchopulmonary dysplasia, *Pediatr Res* 25:213A, 1989.
272. La Force WR, Brudno DS: Controlled trial of beclomethasone dipropionate by nebulisation in oxygen-dependent and ventilator-dependent infants, *J Pediatr* 122:285-288, 1993.
273. Yuksel B, Greenough A: Randomised trial of inhaled steroids in preterm infants with respiratory symptoms at follow up, *Thorax* 47:910-913, 1992.
274. Chan KN, Silverman M: Increased airway responsiveness in children of low birthweight at school age: effect of topical corticosteroids, *Arch Dis Child* 69:120-124, 1993.
275. Arnold JG, Leslie GI, Williams G, Rack P, Silink M: Adrenocortical responsiveness in neonates weaned from the ventilator with dexamethasone, *Aust Pediatr J* 23:227-229, 1987.
276. Kari MA, Heinonen K, Ikonen RS, Koivisto M, Raivio KO: Dexamethasone treatment in preterm infants at risk for bronchopulmonary dysplasia, *Arch Dis Child* 68:566-569, 1993.
277. Ng PC: The effectiveness and side-effects of dexamethasone in preterm infants with bronchopulmonary dysplasia, *Arch Dis Child* 68:330-336, 1993.
278. O'Neill EA, Chwals WJ, O'Shea MD, Turner CS: Dexamethasone treatment during ventilator dependency: possible life-threatening gastrointestinal complications, *Arch Dis Child* 67:10-11, 1992.
279. De Souza SW, Adlard BPF: Growth of suckling rats after treatment with dexamethasone or cortisol, *Arch Dis Child* 48:519-522, 1973.
280. Massaro D, Teich N, Maxwell S, Massaro GD, Whitney P: Postnatal development of alveoli: regulation and evidence for a critical period in rats, *J Clin Invest* 76:1297-1305, 1985.
281. Wiebicke W, Poynter A, Chernick V: Normal lung growth following antenatal dexamethasone treatment for respiratory distress syndrome, *Pediatr Pulmonol* 5:27-30, 1988.
282. Wong YC, Beardsmore CS, Silverman M: Antenatal dexamethasone and subsequent lung growth, *Arch Dis Child* 57:536-538, 1982.
283. Gibson AT, Pearse RG, Wales JKH: Growth retardation after dexamethasone administration: assessment by knemometry, *Arch Dis Child* 69:505-509, 1993.
284. Rush MG, Hazinski TA: Current therapy of bronchopulmonary dysplasia, *Clin Perinatol* 19:563-590, 1992.
285. Hazinski TA, Blalock WA, Engelhardt B: Control of water balance in infants with bronchopulmonary dysplasia: role of endogenous vasopressin, *Pediatr Res* 23:86-88, 1988.
286. Rao M, Eid N, Herrod L, Parekh A, Steiner P: Anti-diuretic hormone response in children with bronchopulmonary dysplasia during episodes of acute respiratory distress, *Am J Dis Child* 140:825-828, 1986.
287. Bland RD: Edema formation in the newborn lung, *Clin Perinatol* 9:593-611, 1982.
288. Engelhardt B, Elliott S, Hazinski TA: Short- and long-term effects of furosemide on lung function in infants with bronchopulmonary dysplasia, *J Pediatr* 109:1034-1039, 1986.
289. Barnes PJ: Diuretics and asthma, *Thorax* 48:195-196, 1993.
290. McCann EM, Lewis K, Deming DD, Donovan MJ, Brady JP: Controlled trial of furosemide therapy in infants with chronic lung disease, *J Pediatr* 106:957-962, 1985.
291. Rush MG, Engelhardt B, Parker RA, Hazinski TA: Double-blind, placbo-controlled trial of alternate-day furosemide therapy in infants with chronic bronchopulmonary dysplasia, *J Pediatr* 117:112-118, 1990.
292. Kao LC, Warburton D, Sargent CW, Platzker AC, Keens TG: Furosemide acutely decreases airways resistance in chronic bronchopulmonary dysplasia, *J Pediatr* 103:624-629, 1983.
293. Kao LC, Warburton D, Cheng MH, Cedeno C, Platzker A, Keens TG: Effect of oral diuretics on pulmonary mechanics in infants with chronic bronchopulmonary dysplasia, *Pediatrics* 74:37-44, 1984.
294. Albersheim SG, Solimano AJ, Sharma AK, Smyth JA, Rotschild A, Wood BJ, Sheps SB: Randomized, double-blind, controlled trial of long-term diuretic therapy for bronchopulmonary dysplasia, *J Pediatr* 115:615-620, 1989.
295. Engelhardt B, Blalock WA, Don Levy S, Rush M, Hazinski TA: Effect of spironolactone-hydrochlorothiazide on lung function in infants with chronic bronchopulmonary dysplasia, *J Pediatr* 114:619-624, 1989.
296. Ferrara TB, Georgieff MK, Ebert J, Fisher JB: Routine use of dexamethasone for prevention of postextubation respiratory distress, *J Perinatol* 9:287-290, 1989.
297. Truog WE, Jackson JC: Alternative modes of ventilation in the prevention and treatment of bronchopulmonary dysplasia, *Clin Perinatol* 19:621-647, 1992.
298. Samuels MP, Southall DP: Negative extrathoracic pressure in treatment of respiratory failure in infants and young children, *Br Med J* 299:1253-1257, 1989.
299. Shann F, Gatchalian S, Hutchinson R: Nasopharyngeal oxygen in children, *Lancet* 2:1238-1240, 1988.
300. Vian NE, Prudent LM, Stevens DP, Weeter MM, Maisels J: Regulation of oxygen concentration delivered to infants via nasal cannulas, *Am J Dis Child* 143:1458-1460, 1989.

301. Zinman R, Franco I, Pizzuti-Daechsel R: Home oxygen delivery systems for infants, *Pediatr Pulmonol* 1:325-327, 1985.
302. Campbell AN: Low flow oxygen therapy in infants, *Arch Dis Child* 58:795-798, 1983.
303. Sauve RS, McMillan DD, Mitchell I, Creighton D, Hindle NW, Young L: Home oxygen therapy: outcome of infants discharged from NICU on continuous treatment, *Clin Pediatr* 28:113-118, 1989.
304. Hudak BB, Allen MC, Hudak ML, Loughlin GM: Home oxygen therapy for chronic lung disease in extremely low-birth-weight infants, *Am J Dis Child* 143:357-360, 1989.

Future Directions

305. Yeh TF, Torre JA, Rastogi A, Anyebuno MA, Pildes RS: Early postnatal dexamethasone therapy in premature infants with severe respiratory distress syndrome: a double blind, controlled study, *J Pediatr* 117:273-282, 1990.
306. Tarnow-Mordi WO, Sutton P, Wilkinson AR: Inadequate humidification of respiratory gases during mechanical ventilation of the newborn, *Arch Dis Child* 61:698-700, 1986.
307. Bancalari E, Sinclair JC: Mechanical ventilation. In Sinclair JC, Bracken MB, eds: *Effective care of the newborn infant,* Oxford, England, 1992, Oxford University Press, pp 200-220.
308. Wohl M-E: Bronchopulmonary dysplasia in adulthood, *N Engl J Med* 323:1834-1836, 1990.

Suggested Readings

Hanson MA, Spencer JAD, Rodeck CH, Walters D, eds: *Fetus and neonate,* vol 2, Breathing, Cambridge, England, 1994, Cambridge University Press.

Holtzman RB, Frank L: Bronchopulmonary dysplasia, *Clin Perinatol* 19(3): 489-694, 1992.

CHAPTER 33

Apnea of Prematurity and Apparent Life-Threatening Events

John G. Brooks

Apnea is the most common disorder of control of breathing in newborns and infants. Although respiratory pauses are normal at any age, they must be considered pathologic or at least potentially dangerous if they are prolonged (duration >20 seconds) or associated with bradycardia or hypoxemia.[1,2] Apnea is a clinical sign, not a diagnosis. The isolated or repetitive occurrence of apnea may be idiopathic or may indicate the presence of some other pathologic process. Apnea during the first year of life can be appropriately divided into neonatal apnea, which occurs primarily in prematurely born infants and is predominantly apnea of prematurity, and the more heterogeneous category of apparent life-threatening events (ALTEs), which usually occur after the immediate neonatal period and after the initial neonatal hospitalization.

A large part of the particular susceptibility of young infants to apnea is related to the development of control of breathing that occurs over the first few months of life.[3,4] Most full-term infants respond to mild to moderate hypercapnia with appropriate and effective increases in ventilation in a pattern very similar to that in adults.[5] In contrast, the hypoxic ventilatory response in the first few days (weeks in prematurely born infants) is unique and much less effective.[6] Mild hypoxemia (fraction of inspired oxygen, 0.15) in newborns usually results in 1 to 2 minutes of increased minute ventilation, followed by a decrease in ventilation to less than baseline. Some, but probably not all, of the decrease is proportional to an associated decrease in metabolic rate. Other inhibitory reflexes are uniquely present or potent in newborns. In infants younger than 37 weeks' postconceptional age, stimulation of the vagally innervated airway irritant receptors inhibits respiration rather than causing rapid, shallow breathing, like it does in the more mature individual.[7] The laryngeal chemoreceptor reflex, which inhibits respiration in response to stimulation by various nonisotonic fluids in the larynx, has a markedly greater potency and clinical importance in the newborn than in the adult.[8] The weaker respiratory drive in preterm infants is likely due in part to central nervous system immaturity with decreased neural arborization and myelination.

APNEA OF PREMATURITY

Recurrent apnea and periodic breathing in prematurely born infants are clinically important manifestations of immaturity of respiratory control. Because the prevalence of apnea of prematurity is clearly inversely related to gestational age at birth,[9] with the increasing survival of very immature infants, apnea of prematurity is a very common diagnosis in the neonatal intensive care unit and one that can be associated with significant morbidity.

Definition

Although there is no universally agreed-on definition of *apnea of prematurity,* most clinicians would characterize it as respiratory pauses of 20 seconds or longer or pauses of a shorter duration if accompanied by bradycardia or hypoxemia; the bradycardia and hypoxemia are not associated with any identifiable underlying cause and occur in prematurely born infants who are also demonstrating periodic breathing and are usually less than 37 weeks' postconceptional age. In contrast to apnea of prematurity, *periodic breathing* is defined as respiratory pauses of 3 to 10 seconds separated by periods of regular breathing of no longer than 20 seconds; this occurs in a repeating pattern of at least three cycles. There may be a continuum of expression of a similar mechanism of respiratory periodicity ranging from repeating oscillations of tidal volume magnitude to periodic breathing to apnea of prematurity.[10,11] Apnea of prematurity is a diagnosis of exclusion and can be established only after all other possible causes of apnea have been ruled out.

Incidence and Natural History

The prevalence of apnea of prematurity varies inversely with gestational age at birth[9,12-14] and is summarized in Table 33-1. The data in this table suggest that the prevalence is higher in the 1990s because of the increasing survival of very small premature infants. Precise determination of the prevalence is impossible because many of the smallest infants are intubated and mechanically ventilated from the time of birth until they reach a postconceptional age at which the condition is less common.

The prevalence of periodic breathing and polysomnographically documented apnea in premature infants is much higher than the prevalence of apnea of prematurity and appears to approach 100%.[14,15] Hard copy recordings of cardiorespiratory patterns of premature infants document more episodes of apnea and bradycardia than are likely to be documented on the nursing care records,[15-17] but there is no evidence that use of the more sensitive detection modality has any positive impact on outcome. There are very little good data about the age of onset and age of disappearance of apnea of prematurity because interventions such as mechanical ventilation and administration of methylxanthines may eliminate or postpone its appearance. According to Henderson-Smart,[9] in the 1% of infants who developed apnea of prematurity, defined as three or more episodes of apnea lasting 20 seconds or longer identified by impedance monitoring, it began within the first 2 days of life in 77% of 249 live inborn, nonselected infants and within the first 7 days of life in more than 98% of this affected group. The age of onset was not related to the presence or absence of birth asphyxia. For this study, the infants were monitored 10 days after their last clinically significant apneic episode, which occurred before 37 weeks' postconceptional age in 92% of infants and before 40 weeks' postconceptional age in 98% of infants.

Table 33-1 Prevalence of Apnea of Prematurity

INVESTIGATOR	POPULATION	PREVALENCE	DETECTION
Henderson-Smart[9]	All births (N = 25,154)	1%	Observation
Henderson-Smart and Cohen[13]	GA: 30-31	54%	—
	GA: 32-33	14%	
	GA: 34-35	7%	
Jones and Lukeman[12]	GA: 32 (N = 362)	28%	Nurses' observation
Barrington and Finer[14]	GA: >34 (N = 20) (no acute medical problems)	65%	Clinical observation

GA, Gestational age (in weeks).

Pathophysiology

Apneic episodes can be classified as central (diaphragmatic), obstructive, or mixed.[18] Particularly in the most premature infants, airway obstruction, usually at the level of the pharynx, is an important component of apnea of prematurity.[19-22] In mixed apnea, the obstructive component may precede or follow the central component. During central apnea, no inspiratory efforts are observed. The central and obstructive components may reflect decreased respiratory center output to the diaphragm and upper airway musculature, respectively. The effects of apnea of prematurity on respiratory gas exchange and cardiovascular function can be significant. Hypoxemia and hypercarbia develop progressively during each apneic episode.[23-25] The accompanying bradycardia can be secondary to hypoxemia or may be a reflex response directly associated with the apnea.[26-28] Perlman and Volpe[29] have documented decreased cerebral blood flow during moderate and severe apneic episodes (heart rate <120 and <80 beats/min, respectively). The clinical significance of these changes has not been proved.

A variety of theories to explain the etiology have been proposed and include central nervous system immaturity, upper airway vulnerability to obstruction, exaggerated upper airway protective reflex,[30] and immature respiratory drive.[31] There is evidence that each of these mechanisms exists in premature infants to a greater degree than in term infants. In prematurely born infants an inverse relationship between apnea frequency and brain stem maturation, as assessed by brain stem auditory-evoked response conduction times, has been reported and supports the concept of some aspect of brain immaturity as a major contributor to apnea of prematurity.[32] More immature infants have less robust ventilatory responses to inspired carbon dioxide[5] and may have paradoxical inhibitory responses to the stimulation of pulmonary irritant receptors.[7] Data conflict as to whether respiratory chemosensitivity is less in premature infants with apnea of prematurity than in equally premature infants who do not experience recurrent apnea.[33,34] The hypoxic ventilatory response in premature infants is much less robust than in older infants and usually involves a significant component of hypoxic ventilatory depression.[6] The upper airway of the premature infant lacks some of the structural and functional support that serves to more effectively maintain airway patency in older infants.[35] In addition, some upper airway reflexes, such as the laryngeal chemoreceptor reflex, are more likely to result in apnea and bradycardia in premature than in older infants.[8,30] Waggener et al[10] have demonstrated that the respiratory pauses seen in premature infants represent exaggerated underlying oscillatory breathing patterns. This applies to both mixed and obstructive apneas.[11] The underlying oscillation can be diminished by breathing enriched oxygen concentrations up to 40%, which results in a decrease in the breath-to-breath variability of instantaneous minute ventilation.[36] Gerhardt and Bancalari[33] compared 18 preterm infants with apnea to 18 equally premature infants who were free of apnea and found that the apneic group had a lesser ventilatory response to carbon dioxide; however, there was no difference between the two groups with regard to pulmonary mechanics or oxygenation.

Differential Diagnosis

Numerous causes of recurrent neonatal apnea must be ruled out before the diagnosis of apnea of prematurity, the most common, can be established.[37,38] The major causes of neonatal apnea are summarized in Box 33-1. In addition to apnea of prematurity, conditions most likely to cause apnea in the first 24 hours include infection, seizures, respiratory distress syndrome, metabolic derangements, thermal stress, severe perinatal asphyxia, and depressant medications administered to the

BOX 33-1
Neonatal Apnea: Differential Diagnosis

Infectious causes
Sepsis
Meningitis
Pneumonia

Neurologic causes
Seizure disorders
Intracranial hemorrhage
Kernicterus

Respiratory causes
Respiratory distress syndrome
Respiratory muscle weakness
Hypoxemia
Pneumonia

Cardiac causes
Hypoxemia
Patent ductus arteriosus
Pulmonary congestion

Metabolic causes
Hypoglycemia
Hypocalcemia
Hyponatremia

Metabolic causes—cont'd
Hypernatremia
Dehydration

Miscellaneous causes
Gastroesophageal reflux
Hypotension
Hypothermia
Hyperthermia
Congenital anomalies
Anemia
Perinatal asphyxia

Iatrogenic causes
Overhydration or underhydration
Inappropriate heating or cooling
Medication-induced respiratory depression or respiratory muscle weakness
Maternal medications (e.g., depressants, β-blockers)

Developmental cause
Apnea of prematurity

mother or infant in the immediate perinatal period. The relationship between anemia and apnea of prematurity has not been fully clarified. Several reports document a decreased number of respiratory pauses in anemic premature infants experiencing periodic breathing after they received transfusions of packed red blood cells, increasing the hematocrit.[39-41] However, no published reports document a decrease in clinically significant apneic episodes after transfusion in a baby with apnea of prematurity. Thus although it is likely that correction of significant anemia decreases the risk of apnea of prematurity, this has not yet been fully established. Likewise, gastroesophageal reflux has been proposed as a cause of neonatal apnea, but a temporal association has been difficult to prove with simultaneous monitoring of esophageal pH and respiratory pattern.[42] One subgroup of premature infants developed apnea, bradycardia, or both conditions (sometimes with significant cyanosis) only during or immediately after feedings.[30] Gastroesophageal reflux and stimulation of the laryngeal chemoreceptors probably contribute to these events, although feeding-associated hypoxemia may also be a contributing factor.[43-45] Premature infants who experience recurrent bradycardia without setting off apnea alarms may be experiencing recurrent upper airway obstruction and should be considered for this possibility.

The diagnosis of apnea of prematurity is made by considering and excluding all other causes of neonatal apnea. In infants whose postconceptional age is greater than 36 to 37 weeks, the index of suspicion for other causes of the apnea and the extent of the efforts to rule out other causes must be significantly heightened. On very rare occasions, a clinical picture of recurrent apnea and periodicity of breathing in an apparently otherwise healthy infant may be seen in infants of 40 weeks' postconceptional age or even 1 to 2 weeks beyond term. This is extremely unusual, but it probably represents a delayed form of apnea of prematurity.

Management

Because of the high prevalence of apnea of prematurity, all infants younger than 35 weeks' gestational age should have electronic cardiorespiratory monitoring for at least the first week of life. The appropriate evaluation of a premature infant who develops recurrent apnea depends on the severity of the apnea, the postconceptional and postnatal ages at onset, and the associated clinical findings. The evaluation should be based on ruling out the known causes of neonatal apnea, which are summarized in Box 33-1. The more severe the episode and particularly the more mature the infant, the more extensive the appropriate evaluation.

The appropriate management for secondary apnea is to treat the underlying cause. When significant obstructive apnea is suspected, careful attention should be paid to proper positioning of the head, and these infants should usually be nursed in the prone position unless they have artificial airways. Any patient with recurrent apnea must be carefully monitored, and if the spells are severe and represent central apnea, the infant's breathing must be supported with mechanical ventilation as long as there is a recurrence or a high risk of recurrence of the severe apnea, even if an underlying cause is identified.

The treatment for apnea of prematurity is largely nonspecific and consists of techniques of mechanically or pharmacologically stimulating the infant's breathing. Because hypoxemia, hypothermia, and hyperthermia are all associated with apnea, it is essential that they be ruled out initially and that normoxia and normothermia be maintained.

The simplest intervention, which is appropriate for mild apneic episodes occurring only occasionally, is tactile stimulation. This should be gentle and can be done intermittently (by hand) or continually or can be done by placing the infant on an irregularly oscillating water bed. The next level of intervention may consist of nasal continuous positive airway pressure (CPAP), which is especially effective when there is a significant obstructive component to the recurrent apnea. A total of 2 to 5 cm H_2O is effective in reducing the frequency of obstructive and mixed apnea.[46,47] CPAP may have no effect on pure central apnea. Nasal CPAP is likely to interfere with the infant's ability to feed. Severe apneic episodes may require bag- and mask-assisted ventilation or oxygen or both.

Methylxanthines are the mainstay of the pharmacologic management of apnea of prematurity.[48-55] After an initial loading dose (5 mg/kg of theophylline or 10 to 20 mg/kg of caffeine), maintenance doses should be initiated (2 mg/kg of theophylline every 8 hours or 10 mg/kg of caffeine once a day). Blood levels should be measured about 48 hours after the loading dose and approximately weekly thereafter. A very premature infant has a significantly longer serum half-life for methylxanthines, so lower doses may be appropriate. There is no true "therapeutic range" for the methylxanthines for their stimulative effect on the respiratory system, but blood levels over 10 to 15 mg/L should be avoided because of increased difficulty with side effects. A great deal of variability exists among infants with regard to susceptibility to toxicity. The primary undesirable effects of methylxanthine therapy are increased oxygen consumption, hyperglycemia, tachycardia, gastrointestinal distress, jitteriness, and at very high levels, seizures. Diuresis is another effect but may be desirable in some patients. For a given serum concentration, caffeine may have fewer side effects than theophylline. This difference may be explained by the fact that in premature infants, there is some conversion of theophylline to caffeine. For this reason, particularly when higher doses are required in premature infants, caffeine is preferable to theophylline as a therapy for apnea of prematurity. Despite some concern based on studies in developing animals, no human data indicate adverse long-term effects of methylxanthine therapy in premature neonates. Transfusions of packed red blood cells may be considered in significantly anemic infants with apnea of prematurity.[39-41] Some infants with severe apnea of prematurity, particularly those who are very premature, require mechanical ventilation.

After 7 to 10 days without significant apnea, methylxanthine therapy should be discontinued. Infants who have had 7 to 10 days free of any significant episodes with documented insignificant methylxanthine levels can be discharged if they meet all other discharge criteria. Infants who meet the other discharge criteria but continue to have mild apnea of prematurity and/or who are still receiving methylxanthine therapy, can appropriately be discharged with home cardiorespiratory monitors.[56,57] Once the infant has been apnea free for about 2 weeks, the methylxanthines can be stopped. When infants have been free of apnea for 2 weeks off methylxanthines, home monitoring can be discontinued. The family and caretakers must understand that the monitor is being used as an alternative to prolonged hospitalization and that it is not being used to prevent sudden infant death syndrome (SIDS). Although prematurity is a risk factor for SIDS, apnea of prematurity per se is not. Infants who have had apnea of prematurity are at increased risk of redeveloping apnea when they become infected with respiratory syncytial virus.[57]

APPARENT LIFE-THREATENING EVENTS

Infants who experience ALTEs have received much attention because of the possibility that they are at increased risk of subsequent morbidity and mortality.[58] Although this adverse prognosis is real for a very small subgroup of those who experience ALTEs,[59] the majority of infants may be at no increased risk compared with the general population.

The ALTE terminology refers to infants who experience episodes that are frightening to the observer and usually consist of some combination of cyanosis or pallor, increased or decreased muscle tone, and apnea that is usually central and occasionally obstructive.[57] The observers often think that the infant is dead or nearly dead. Some of these episodes are associated with choking or gagging. Previous terminology for the same sort of episode includes *aborted crib death* and *near-miss SIDS,* both of which are inappropriate because they imply a misleadingly close association between this type of incident and SIDS.

The term *apparent life-threatening event* refers to a chief complaint, the reason that the infant is brought to medical attention. After appropriate evaluation, a diagnosis such as ALTE resulting from seizures, ALTE resulting from gastroesophageal reflux, or idiopathic ALTE (sometimes referred to as *apnea of infancy*) should be assigned. Approximately 50% of infants who have ALTEs are assigned to the idiopathic category.[60-63]

There are many different causes and expressions of ALTEs, so this chief complaint includes a very heterogeneous group of clinical conditions and characteristics. In addition, this episode is usually witnessed only by a frightened, nonmedical observer, so the accuracy of the description may be limited. Despite these limitations, every infant with a history of ALTEs must be carefully considered and appropriately evaluated. Several published studies document the wide disparity between parental reports of ALTEs and simultaneous cardiorespiratory records that do not indicate a life-threatening situation.[64-67] Similar discrepancies between nurse-reported apnea and hard-copy cardiorespiratory tracings have been documented.[68]

The reported prevalence of infants who have experienced ALTEs varies from 0.05% to 6.0% of the general population.[63,69-73] The higher prevalence includes all ALTEs,[73] whereas the lowest prevalence comes from population-based studies and includes only severe ALTEs.[71] A positive history of ALTEs is reported in 4% to 27% of infants who die of SIDS.[70,73,74]

Physiologic Studies

Many studies of cardiorespiratory function in infants with ALTEs have been carried out, but the results are generally conflicting and therefore inconclusive. The varied results are most likely a consequence of differences in study populations and methodology. The probably inappropriate justification for most of these investigations is the hope that studying infants with ALTEs would elucidate physiologic abnormalities that would explain the mechanisms of SIDS. This justification is, however, fallacious because most infants with ALTEs do not die of SIDS, so there is no assurance that abnormalities in the group with ALTEs have any relevance to SIDS. The most consistent respiratory abnormalities among the reported studies of infants who have been referred to infant apnea centers because of severe idiopathic ALTEs include increased numbers of respiratory pauses compared with age-matched controls[75-78] and documentation that some infants with ALTEs have blunted ventilatory and arousal responses to hypoxia.[79] The baseline oxygenation[80] and ventilatory response to hypercapnia[81-84] in these infants with severe idiopathic ALTEs do not appear to be depressed. A variety of cardiac rhythm disturbances have been reported in single studies, but none has been confirmed.[60,85-88] Two of the three published studies that have considered brain stem auditory-evoked responses in infants with ALTEs have reported normal peak and interpeak latencies.[88-90] This brief summary of the physiology of infants with ALTEs includes only studies that were controlled and that looked only at populations with idiopathic severe ALTEs.

Studies of the demographics and epidemiology of ALTEs reveal that up to 26% of infants in this population are born prematurely[60-62,91,92] (a slightly lower percentage of premature infants are reported from populations limited to severe idiopathic ALTEs[69,70,93-95]), the median age at presentation is about 2 months, and there is a slight male predominance. The combined prevalence of SIDS among other family members of infants with ALTE is about 11%.[93-95]

The distribution of diagnoses of ALTEs based on combined data from seven published studies of 865 infants with ALTEs follows[60-63,91,92,96]:

Neurologic problems (especially seizures)	12%
Gastroesophageal reflux	28%
Infection	6%
Cardiac problems	1%
Metabolic problems	2%
Upper airway obstruction	2%
Idiopathic causes	47%

An expanded differential diagnosis of ALTEs is summarized in Box 33-2. Most pulmonary or systemic infections can present with apnea in young infants. As many as 15% to 20%

BOX 33-2
ALTEs: Differential Diagnosis

Normal causes

Mild periodic breathing during sleep
Occasional 5- to 15-second episode of central apnea during sleep
Occasional or rare mild choking with overaggressive sucking during feedings

Acute conditions

Infection
- Sepsis or meningitis
- Respiratory syncytial virus
- Pertussis
- Other respiratory infections

Medication-induced conditions
Postanesthetic conditions

Chronic conditions

Gastroesophageal reflux and/or pharyngeal incoordination stimulating sensitive laryngeal chemoreceptors

Chronic conditions—cont'd

Seizure
Other neurologic disorders
- Central nervous system tumor
- Subdural hemorrhage
- Arnold-Chiari–associated apnea

Cardiac dysrhythmia
Abnormalities of respiratory drive
- Immature respiratory center
  - Apnea of prematurity
- Respiratory center dysfunction
  - Central hypoventilation syndrome (Ondine's curse)
  - Obstructive sleep apnea

Vocal cord paralysis
Tracheomalacia
Vascular ring
Child abuse
Munchausen's syndrome by proxy
Idiopathic causes

of infants hospitalized with respiratory syncytial virus experience apnea, usually in the early days of the infection.[97-102] The mechanism by which gastroesophageal reflux results in apnea involves stimulation of the chemoreceptors in the larynx, which are sensitive to nonphysiologic pH and chloride concentrations.[8,30,103] The response of young infants to stimulation of these receptors is apnea, bradycardia, and central pooling of blood resulting in pallor. This response may also include marked, abrupt limpness. These reflex responses are more potent in the youngest infants. The more mature response of older infants and children includes swallowing to clear the stimulating substance from the receptors. If an electroencephalogram and the history suggest a seizure, it cannot be established whether the seizure caused the apnea or the severe apnea caused the seizure, but treatment is appropriate nonetheless. The apnea may rarely be the only manifestation of a seizure (i.e., apneic seizure).[104-106] The differential diagnoses in Box 33-2 are the bases for the evaluation of patients with ALTEs.

Follow-Up

On rare occasions the presenting episode is sufficiently severe to result in devastating long-term impairment.[107,108] In addition, controlled follow-up studies of infants with ALTEs at 1 to 3 years of age have demonstrated a small increased prevalence of abnormal neurodevelopmental function,[109] gross motor impairment,[110] and lower mental and psychomotor scores by the Bailey scales[111] compared to control children. The combined subsequent deaths of 776 infants with ALTEs in eight different series was 1.0%.[58] At least 6 of the 10 deaths were attributed to SIDS. Of 295 infants diagnosed with apnea of infancy (severe episode during sleep with no identifiable cause) the mortality rate was 3.0%.[58] A total of 6 of the 9 deaths were attributed to SIDS. Although SIDS is the predominant cause of death among infants with ALTEs, only about 5% of SIDS victims have been noted to experience ALTEs before their deaths. Because of the heterogeneity of the population with ALTEs, subgroup-specific mortalities have important clinical use. Data conflict about the mortality rate of infants who experience ALTEs in the first 4 to 7 days of life: up to 50% mortality.[71,112,113] There are no adequate published data to determine whether ALTEs occurring with the infant awake have a different prognosis than those occurring during sleep,[62,114] although there is a suggestion that severe episodes during sleep have a more ominous prognosis. Infants who experience repeated severe episodes during sleep may have a subsequent mortality rate of 28%.[59] In most cases the second severe episode occurred within 3 weeks of the first severe episode. Those who experience one severe episode during sleep have an 8% to 10% mortality rate.[115] Infants who have seizure disorders and recurrent severe idiopathic ALTEs (i.e., those requiring cardiopulmonary resuscitation or vigorous stimulation) may have a subsequent mortality rate of 57.0% (four of seven infants).[59]

Clinical Management

Each infant who has a history of an ALTE must be taken very seriously, even if he or she seems perfectly normal when seen. First, the clinician must consider whether any immediate intervention is necessary to ensure adequate cardiorespiratory function. Second, the clinician must try to determine, based on a careful history, whether the ALTE represents an abnormal event or is an overreaction to a normal event (much less common). If the ALTE is not an overreaction to a normal occurrence, then an effort should be made to identify a specific cause and then treat it, if possible. Except in occasional cases when the infant has been fine for at least 5 to 7 days since the event, hospitalization is indicated for observation, evaluation, parent counseling, and intervention and observation of the event in case the ALTE recurs and requires medical intervention. Finally, the clinician must decide whether specific intervention (e.g., anticonvulsants) or nonspecific intervention (e.g., home monitoring) is appropriate. The general purposes of the initial evaluation are (1) to try to observe the events if they recur; (2) to look for direct or indirect laboratory or physical signs of recurrence, hypoventilation, or recurrent hypoxemia; and (3) to use the careful taking of a history, physical examination, and other diagnostic tools to identify a specific cause of the ALTE. Issues to pursue in the initial history of the presenting episode include the infant's state of consciousness before, during, and after the event; duration of the episode; associated changes of color; muscle tone; movements; and respiratory efforts during the episode. The specific components of the intervention and the speed and pattern of the infant's response to stimulation must be carefully documented. The clinician must clarify the relationship of the ALTE to feeding and ask about the presence of any other associated sounds (e.g., choking, stridor) or associated symptoms (e.g., mild upper respiratory infection). It is very important to obtain the history about the event from the individual who was directly involved. If this was a baby-sitter, for example, it is important to talk to him or her. Points of importance in the past history include evidence of previous life-threatening episodes, abnormal breathing patterns, feeding problems, seizures, perinatal insults, other medical problems, medications, and a family history of apnea, infant deaths, seizures, and other cardiopulmonary problems. A complete physical examination should be performed with great care, with particular attention to the neurologic portion, the upper and lower airways, and the cardiac system. The infant should be carefully observed during sleep and during feeding for any respiratory difficulty or irregularity.

The minimal evaluation of infants hospitalized for evaluation consists of a careful history and physical examination, a complete blood count with differential (to look particularly for severe anemia or lymphocytosis suggestive of pertussis), a serum bicarbonate assay obtained as soon as possible after the event, and continuous cardiorespiratory monitoring. If there are monitor alarms, it is of greatest importance to assess the infant before intervention to determine whether the alarm is real or false. Additional workup is appropriate if the event was at least moderately severe or if other specific diagnoses are strongly suggested by the history or physical examination. The most common additional laboratory tests include electroencephalogram, electrocardiogram, chest radiograph, and serum electrolyte analysis. Additional evaluation of the heart, upper airway, adequacy of ventilation, oxygenation, and gastroesophageal function may be appropriate. Polysomnography consists of continuous measurement over a period of at least several hours of some combination of pulse oximetry, capnography, electroencephalogram, airflow at the nose and mouth, and esophageal pH. Polysomnography may be necessary to diagnose sleep hypoventilation, obstructive apnea, or apneic seizures but is unnecessary for most patients. Long-term recording of cardiorespiratory function (pneumogram) is not indicated because it is not a screening test for SIDS and a "normal" result is not helpful in the decision about whether to use a home monitor. "Event recording" (i.e., obtaining a permanent record of the cardiorespiratory function just before, during, and just after each alarm) may be helpful in some patients who are having recurrent alarms when it is not clear whether they are true or false alarms.[116] Event recordings can be done in the home or in the hospital but should be used only on select patients. An often used and cost-effective approach to hospitalization of infants with ALTEs involves prompt evaluation with the laboratory assessments previously mentioned and unless there is strong evidence for some specific cause of the ALTE, discharging the patient with a home monitor after 1 to 2 days of hospitalization, assuming that there is no ongoing apnea or bradycardia.[57] This approach involves rather liberal use of home monitors, but it is cost-effective because hospitalization can be brief. If these patients have recurrent alarms at home, additional evaluation is often indicated. If they have no further bothersome alarms at home, they can be spared additional evaluation, and the monitor can be stopped after 2 to 3 months without significant alarms. Some argue that all home monitoring should be performed with "smart monitors," those with a storage capability, to provide an ongoing record of whether the monitor is being used regularly. Such an approach adds significantly to the cost of home monitoring in many cases.

The 1986 recommendations of the National Institutes of Health's Consensus Conference on Infantile Apnea and Home Monitoring[57] for the use of home monitors have become the current national standard of care. All infants were placed in one of three categories with regard to the appropriateness of home monitoring. Infants with ALTEs for whom monitoring or alternative therapy was definitely indicated were those who had experienced severe ALTEs perceived to require mouth-to-mouth resuscitation or vigorous stimulation. A second group consisting of normal infants and asymptomatic premature infants was considered inappropriate for home monitors. The largest group are those who fit in neither of the first two categories (e.g., those with moderate ALTEs, a sibling of an infant with SIDS); for these infants the decision about home monitoring should be made on an individual basis with careful attention to the wishes of the family after fully informing them about the risks, benefits, liabilities, and limitations of home monitoring. The parents and other caretakers of any infant for whom a home monitor is prescribed must be fully trained in basic infant cardiopulmonary resuscitation, the use and trouble shooting of the home monitor, the reasons for monitoring, the planned duration of the monitoring, and alarms to report immediately and to report electively to the health care team. There must be 24-hour medical and technical backup for these families, and they must have a telephone. They must be fully instructed in the importance of careful observation and documentation of the condition of the infant at the time of each alarm before they intervene. Any specific underlying disease process that might contribute to the ALTE should be appropriately treated. Infants for whom a specific cause is identified (e.g., seizure, obstructive apnea, gastroesophageal reflux) may still be at increased risk of sudden, unexpected death.[58]

Primary care practitioners should be sensitive to the occurrence and management of ALTEs and should acknowledge and provide the extra degree of support often required by families who feel that their infants almost died. Practitioners should stay current with the understanding of the mechanisms of ALTEs and the relationship between ALTE and SIDS, should be aware of the significant limitations and liabilities of the use of home monitors, and should ensure that appropriate teaching and ongoing support are available to affected families.

REFERENCES

1. Kelly DH, Stellwagen LM, Kaitz E, Shannon DC: Apnea and periodic breathing in normal full-term infants during the first twelve months, *Pediatr Pulmonol* 1:215-219, 1985.
2. Weese-Mayer DE, Morrow AS, Conway LP, Brouillette RT, Silvestri JM: Assessing clinical significance of apnea exceeding fifteen seconds with event recording, *Pediatrics* 117:568-574, 1990.
3. Jansen AH, Chernick V: Fetal breathing and development of control of breathing: a brief review, *J Appl Physiol* 70:1431-1446, 1991.
4. Lagercrantz H: Neuromodulators and respiratory control in the infant, *Clin Perinatol* 14:683-695, 1987.
5. Rigatto H, Brady JP, de la Torre Verduzco R: Chemoreceptor reflexes in preterm infants. II. The effect of gestational and postnatal age on the ventilatory response to inhaled carbon dioxide, *Pediatrics* 55:614-620, 1975.
6. Rigatto H, Kalapesi Z, Leahy FN, Durand H, MacCollum M, Cates D: Ventilatory response to 100% and 15% O_2 during wakefulness and sleep in preterm infants, *Early Hum Dev* 7:1-10, 1982.
7. Fleming PF, Bryan AC, Bryan MH: Functional immaturity of pulmonary irritant receptors and apnea in newborn preterm infants, *Pediatrics* 61:515-518, 1978.
8. Donnelly DF, Haddad GG: Respiratory changes induced by prolonged laryngeal stimulation in awake piglets, *J Appl Physiol* 61:1018-1024, 1986.

Apnea of Prematurity

9. Henderson-Smart DJ: The effect of gestational age on the incidence and duration of recurrent apnoea in newborn babies, *Aust Paediatr J* 17:273-276, 1981.
10. Waggener TB, Stark AR, Cohlan BA, Frantz ID III: Apnea duration is related to ventilatory oscillation characteristics in newborn infants, *J Appl Physiol* 57:536-544, 1984.
11. Waggener TB, Frantz ID III, Cohlan BA, Stark AR: Mixed and obstructive apneas are related to ventilatory oscillations in premature infants, *J Appl Physiol* 66:2818-2826, 1989.
12. Jones RAK, Lukeman D: Apnoea of immaturity, *Arch Dis Child* 57:766-768, 1982.

13. Henderson-Smart DJ, Cohen G: Apnoea in the newborn infant, *Aust Paediatr J* 22(suppl):63-66, 1986.
14. Barrington K, Finer N: The natural history of the appearance of apnea of prematurity, *Pediatr Res* 29(4):372-375, 1991.
15. Glotzbach SF, Baldwin RB, Lederer NE, Tansey PA, Ariagno RL: Periodic breathing in preterm infants: incidence and characteristics, *Pediatrics* 84(5):785-792, 1989.
16. Southall DP, Levitt GA, Richards JM, Jones RAK, Kong C, Farndon PA, Alexander JR, Wilson AJ: Undetected episodes of apnea and bradycardia in preterm infants, *Pediatrics* 72:542-552, 1983.
17. Hageman JR, Holmes D, Suchy S, Hunt CE: Respiratory pattern at hospital discharge in asymptomatic preterm infants, *Pediatr Pulmonol* 4:78-83, 1983.
18. Dransfield DA, Spitzer AR, Fox WW: Episodic airway obstruction in premature infants, *Am J Dis Child* 137:441-443, 1983.
19. Thach BT, Stark AR: Spontaneous neck flexion and airway obstruction during apneic spells in preterm infants, *Pediatrics* 94(2):275-281, 1979.
20. Milner AD, Boon AW, Saunders RA, Hopkin IE: Upper airways obstruction and apnoea in preterm babies, *Arch Dis Child* 55:22-25, 1980.
21. Mathew OP, Roberts JL, Thach BT: Pharyngeal airway obstruction in preterm infants during mixed and obstructive apnea, *Pediatrics* 100(6):964-968, 1982.
22. Ruggins NR, Milner AD: Site of upper airway obstruction in preterm infants with problematical apnoea, *Arch Dis Child* 66:787-792, 1991.
23. Marshall TA, Kattwinkel J: Functional residual capacity and oxygen tension in apnea of prematurity, *Pediatrics* 98(3):479-482, 1981.
24. Hiatt IM, Hegyi T, Indyk L, Dangman BC, James LS: Continuous monitoring of Po_2 during apnea of prematurity, *Pediatrics* 98(2):288-291, 1981.
25. Abu-osba YK, Brouillette RT, Wilson SL, Thach BT: Breathing pattern and transcutaneous oxygen tension during motor activity in preterm infants, *Am Rev Respir Dis* 125:382-387, 1982.
26. Storrs CN: Cardiovascular effects of apnoea in preterm infants, *Arch Dis Child* 52:534-540, 1977.
27. Fenichel GM, Olson BJ, Fitzpatrick JE: Heart rate changes in convulsive and nonconvulsive neonatal apnea, *Ann Neurol* 7(6):577-582, 1980.
28. Henderson-Smart DJ, Butcher-Puech MC, Edwards DA: Incidence and mechanism of bradycardia during apnoea in preterm infants, *Arch Dis Child* 61:227-232, 1986.
29. Perlman JM, Volpe JJ: Episodes of apnea and bradycardia in the preterm newborn: impact on cerebral circulation, *Pediatrics* 76(3):333-338, 1985.
30. Pickens DL, Schefft G, Thach BT: Prolonged apnea associated with upper airway protective reflexes in apnea of prematurity, *Am Rev Respir Dis* 137:113-118, 1988.
31. Miller MJ, Martin RJ: Apnea of prematurity, *Clin Perinatol* 19(4):789-807, 1992.
32. Henderson-Smart DJ, Pettigrew AG, Campbell DJ: Clinical apnea and brain-stem neural function in preterm infants, *N Engl J Med* 308(7):353-357, 1983.
33. Gerhardt T, Bancalari E: Apnea of prematurity. I. Lung function and regulation of breathing, *Pediatrics* 74(1):58-66, 1984.
34. Upton CJ, Milner AD, Stokes GM: Response to tube breathing in preterm infants with apnea, *Pediatr Pulmonol* 12:23-28, 1992.
35. Tonkin S: Sudden infant death syndrome: hypotheses of causation, *Pediatrics* 55:650-661, 1975.
36. Weintraub Z, Alvaro R, Kwiatkowski K, Cates D, Rigatto H: Effects of inhaled oxygen (up to 40%) on periodic breathing and apnea in preterm infants, *J Appl Physiol* 72:116-119, 1992.
37. Marchal F, Bairam A, Vert P: Neonatal apnea and apneic syndromes, *Clin Perinatol* 14(3):509-529, 1987.
38. Brouillette RT, Weese-Mayer DE, Hunt CE: Breathing control disorders in infants and children, *Hosp Pract* 25:82-96, 1990.
39. DeMaio JG., Harris MC, Deuber C, Spitzer AR: Effect of blood transfusion on apnea frequency in growing premature infants, *Pediatrics* 114(6):1039-1041, 1989.
40. Sasidharan P, Heimler R: Transfusion-induced changes in the breathing pattern of healthy preterm anemic infants, *Pediatr Pulmonol* 12:170-173, 1992.
41. Joshi A, Gerhardt T, Shandloff P, Bancalari E: Blood transfusion effect on the respiratory pattern of preterm infants, *Pediatrics* 80(1):79-84, 1987.
42. de Ajuriaguerra M, Radvanyi-Bouvet MF, Huon C, Moriette G: Gastroesophageal reflux and apnea in prematurely born infants during wakefulness and sleep, *Am J Dis Child* 145:1132-1136, 1991.
43. Yu VYH: Cardiorespiratory response to feeding in newborn infants, *Arch Dis Child* 51:305-309, 1976.
44. Patel BD, Dinwiddie R, Kumar SP, Vox WW: The effects of feeding on arterial blood gases and lung mechanics in newborn infants recovering from respiratory disease, *Pediatrics* 90(3):435-438, 1977.
45. Herrell N, Martin RJ, Fanaroff A: Arterial oxygen tension during nasogastric feeding in the preterm infant, *Pediatrics* 96:914-916, 1980.
46. Miller, MJ, Waldemar AC, Martin RJ: Continuous positive airway pressure selectively reduces obstructive apnea in preterm infants, *Pediatrics* 106:91-94, 1985.
47. Ryan CA, Finer NN, Peters KL: Nasal intermittent positive-pressure ventilation offers no advantages over nasal continuous positive airway pressure in apnea of prematurity, *Am J Dis Child* 143:1196-1198, 1989.
48. Muttitt SC, Tierney AJ, Finer NN: The dose response of theophylline in the treatment of apnea of prematurity, *Pediatrics* 112(1):115-121, 1988.
49. Carrier O, Pons G, Rey E, Richard M, Moran C, Badoual J, Olive G: Maturation of caffeine metabolic pathways in infancy, *Clin Pharmacol Ther* 44(2):145-150, 1988.
50. Mehta PN, Panitch HB, Wolfson MR, Shaffer TH: Dissociation between the effects of theophylline and caffeine on premature airway smooth muscle, *Pediatr Res* 25(5):446-448, 1991.
51. Le Guennec J, Billon B, Pare C: Maturational changes of caffeine concentrations and disposition in infancy during maintenance therapy for apnea of prematurity: influence of gestational age, hepatic disease, and breast-feeding, *Pediatrics* 76(5):834-840, 1985.
52. Sims ME, Yau G, Rambhatla S, Cabal L, Wu PYK: Limitations of theophylline in the treatment of apnea of prematurity, *Am J Dis Child* 139:567-570, 1985.
53. DeCarolis MP, Romagnoli C, Muzil U, Tortorolo G, Chiarotti M, DeGiovanni N, Carnevale A: Pharmacokinetic aspects of caffeine in premature infants, *Dev Pharmacol Ther* 16:117-122, 1991.
54. Roberts JL, Mathew OP, Thach BT: The efficacy of theophylline in premature infants with mixed and obstructive apnea and apnea associated with pulmonary and neurologic disease, *J Pediatr* 100:968-970, 1982.
55. Uauy R, Shapiro DL, Smith B, Warshaw J: Treatment of severe apnea in premature with orally administered theophylline, *Pediatrics* 55:595-598, 1975.
56. Meadow W, Mendex D, Lantos J, Hipps R, Ostrowski M: What is the legal "standard of medical care" when there is no standard medical care? A survey of the use of home apnea monitoring by neonatology fellowship training programs in the United States, *Pediatrics* 89(6):1083-1087, 1992.
57. National Institutes of Health: Concensus Development Conference on Infantile Apnea and Home Monitoring, *Pediatrics* 79:292-299, 1987.

Apparent Life-Threatening Events

58. Brooks JG: Apparent life-threatening events and apnea of infancy, *Clin Perinatol* 19:809-838, 1992.
59. Oren J, Kelly D, Shannon D: Identification of a high-risk group for sudden infant death syndrome among infants who were resuscitated for sleep apnea, *Pediatrics* 77:495-499, 1986.
60. Kahn A, Blum D: Home monitoring of infants considered at risk for the sudden infant death syndrome, *Eur J Pediatr* 139:94-100, 1982.
61. Jeffery H, Rahilly R, Read D: Multiple causes of asphyxia in infants at high risk for sudden infant death, *Arch Dis Child* 58:92-100, 1983.
62. Rowland T, Donnelly J, Landis J, Lemoine M, Sigelman D, Tanella C: Infant home apnea monitoring, *Clin Pediatr* 26:383-387, 1987.
63. Sankaran K, McKenna A, O'Donnell M, Ninan A, Kasian G, Skwarchuk J, Bingham W: Apparent life-threatening prolonged infant apnea in Saskatchewan, *West J Med* 150:292-295, 1989.
64. Jeffery H, Cunningham R, Cubis A, Read D: New methods to separate artifacts from normal and defective breathing patterns in sleep-states, if infants are monitored at home, *Aust NZ J Med* 11:406-411, 1981.
65. Krongrad E, O'Neill L: Near miss sudden infant death syndrome episodes? A clinical and electrocardiographic correlation, *Pediatrics* 77:811-815, 1986.
66. Nathanson I, O'Donnell J, Commins M: Cardiorespiratory patterns during alarms in infants using apnea/bradycardia monitors, *Am J Dis Child* 143:476-480, 1989.
67. Steinschneider A, Santos V: Parental reports of apnea and bradycardia: temporal characteristics and accuracy, *Pediatrics* 88:1100-1105, 1991.

68. Graff M, Soriano C, Rovell K, Hiatt M, Hegyi T: Undetected apnea and bradycardia in infants, *Pediatr Pulmonol* 11:195-197, 1991.
69. Wennergren G, Milerad J, Lagerkranatz H, Karlberg P, Svenningsen N, Sedin G, Andersson D, Grogaard J, Bjure J: The epidemiology of SIDS and attacks of lifelessness in Sweden, *Acta Paediatr Scand* 76:898-906, 1987.
70. Damus K, Pakter J, Krongrad E, Standfast S, Hoffman H: Postnatal medical and epidemiological risk factors for the sudden infant death syndrome. In Harper R, Hoffman H, eds: *Sudden infant death syndrome: risk factors and basic mechanisms,* New York, 1984, PMA, pp 187-201.
71. Polberger S, Svenningsen N: Early neonatal sudden infant death and near death of full-term infants in maternity wards, *Acta Paediatr Scand* 74:861-866, 1985.
72. Davis N, Bakke K: Evaluation of a home apnea monitoring program, *Perinatol Neonatol* 7:15-18, 1983.
73. Mandell F: Cot death among children of nurses: observations of breathing patterns, *Arch Dis Child* 56:312-314, 1981.
74. Norvenius S: Sudden infant death syndrome in Sweden in 1973-1977 and 1979, *ACTA Paedriatr Scand Suppl* 333:1-138, 1987.
75. Guilleminault C, Ariagno R, Korobkin R, Nagel L, Baldwin R, Coons S, Owen M: Mixed and obstructive sleep apnea and near-miss for sudden infant death syndrome. II. Comparison of near miss and normal control infants by age, *Pediatrics* 64:882-891, 1979.
76. Kelly D, Shannon D: Periodic breathing in infants with near-miss sudden infant death syndrome, *Pediatrics* 63:355-360, 1979.
77. Kahn A, Blum D, Waterschoot P, Engelman E, Smets P: Effects of obstructive sleep apneas on transcutaneous oxygen pressure in control infants, siblings of sudden infant death syndrome victims, and near miss infants: comparison with the effects of central sleep apneas, *Pediatrics* 70:852-857, 1982.
78. Bazz A, Haddad G, Chang S, Mellins R: Respiratory pauses during sleep in near-miss sudden infant death syndrome, *Am Rev Respir Dis* 128:973-976, 1983.
79. Van der Hal A, Rodriguez A, Sargent C, Platzker A, Keens T: Hypoxic and hypercapnic arousal responses and prediction of subsequent apnea in apnea of infancy, *Pediatrics* 75:848-854, 1985.
80. Kahn A, Blum D, Engelman E, Waterschoot P: Effects of central apneas on transcutaneous Po_2 in control subjects, siblings of victims of sudden infant death syndrome and near miss infants, *Pediatrics* 69:413-418, 1982.
81. Fagenholz S, O'Connell K, Shannon D: Chemoreceptor function and sleep state in apnea, *Pediatrics* 58:31-36, 1976.
82. Haddad G, Leistner H, Lai T, Mellins R: Ventilation and ventilatory pattern during sleep in aborted sudden infant death syndrome, *Pediatr Res* 15:879-883, 1981.
83. Coleman J, Mammel M, Reardon C: Hypercarbic ventilatory responses of infants at risk for SIDS, *Pediatr Pulmonol* 3:226-230, 1987.
84. Parks Y, Paton J, Beardsmore C, Macfadyen U, Thompson J, Goodenough P, Simpson H: Respiratory control in infants at increased risk for sudden infant death syndrome, *Arch Dis Child* 64:791-797, 1989.
85. Kelly D, Shannon D, Liberthson R: The role of the QT interval in the sudden infant death syndrome, *Circulation* 55:633-635, 1977.
86. Haddad G, Epstein M, Epstein R, Mazza N, Mellins R, Krongrad E: The QT interval in aborted sudden infant death syndrome infants, *Pediatr Res* 13:136-138, 1979.
87. Leistner H, Haddad G, Epstein R, Lai T, Epstein M, Mellins R: Heart rate and heart rate variability during sleep in aborted sudden infant death syndrome, *J Pediatr* 97:51-55, 1980.
88. Orlowski J, Nodar R, Lonsdale D: Abnormal brainstem auditory evoked potentials in infants with threatened sudden infant death syndrome, *Cleve Clin Q* 46:77-81, 1979.
89. Gupta P, Guillerminault C, Dorfman L: Brainstem auditory evoked potentials in near-miss sudden infant death syndrome, *J Pediatr* 98:791-794, 1981.
90. Kileny P, Finer N, Sussman P, Schopflocher D: Auditory brainstem responses in sudden infant death syndrome: comparison of siblings, "near-miss" and normal infants, *J Pediatr* 101:225-227, 1982.
91. Davis J, Metrakos K, Andra J: Short reports: apnoea and seizures, *Arch Dis Child* 61:791-806, 1986.
92. Simpson H, MacFadyen U, Paton J: "Near-miss" or "near-myth" for sudden infant death syndrome? Clinical observations of 57 infants, *Aust Paediatr J* 22(suppl):47-51, 1986.
93. Guilleminault C, Boeddiker M, Schwab D: Detection of risk factors for "near miss SIDS" events in full-term infants, *Neuropediatrics* 13:29-35, 1982.
94. Rosen C, Forst J, Harrison G: Infant apnea: polygraphic studies and follow-up monitoring, *Pediatrics* 71:731-736, 1983.
95. Dunne K, Matthews T: Near-miss SIDS: clinical findings and management, *Pediatrics* 79:889-893, 1987.
96. Rahilly P: Review of "near-miss" sudden infant death syndrome and results of simplified pneumographic studies, *Aust Paediatr J* 22(suppl):53-54, 1986.
97. Abreu ES, Brezinova V, Simpson H: Sleep apnoea in acute bronchiolitis, *Arch Dis Child* 57:467-472, 1982.
98. Anas N, Boettrich C, Hall C, Brooks J: Clinical and laboratory observations, *J Pediatr* 100:65-68, 1982.
99. Bruhn F, Mokrohisky S, McIntosh K: Apnea associated with respiratory syncytial virus infections in young infants, *J Pediatr* 90:382-386, 1977.
100. Colditz P, Henry R, DeSilva L: Apnoea and bronchiolitis due to respiratory syncytial virus, *Aust Paediatr J* 18:53-54, 1982.
101. Pickens D, Schefft G, Storch G, Thach B: Characterization of prolonged apneic episodes associated with respiratory syncytial virus infection, *Pediatr Pulmonol* 6:195-201, 1989.
102. Church, NR, Anas HG, Hall CB, Brooks JG: Respiratory syncytial virus related apnea in infants: demographics and outcome, *Am Dis Child* 138:247-250, 1984.
103. Boggs DF, Bartlett D: Chemical specificity of a laryngeal apneic reflex in puppies, *J Appl Physiol* 53:455-462, 1982.
104. Navelet Y, Wood C, Robieux C, Tardieu M: Seizures presenting as apnoea, *Arch Dis Child* 64:357-359, 1989.
105. Wantanabe K, Hara K, Milyazaki S, Hakamada S, Kuroyanagi M: Apneic seizures in the newborn, *Am Dis Child* 136:980-984, 1982.
106. Nelson D, Wilmington D, Ray C: Respiratory arrest from seizure discharges in limbic system, *Arch Neurol* 19:199-207, 1968.
107. Constantinou J, Gillia J, Ouvrier R, Rahilly P: Hypoxic-ischemic encephalopathy after near-miss sudden infant death syndrome, *Arch Dis Child* 64:703-708, 1989.
108. Beal S: Apparent life-threatening events with serious sequelae in infants and young children, *J Paediatr Child Health* 28:151-155, 1992.
109. Korobkin R, Guilleminault C: Neurologic abnormalities in near miss for sudden infant death syndrome infants, *Pediatrics* 64:369-374, 1979.
110. Deykin E, Bauman M, Kelly D: Apnea of infancy and subsequent neurologic, cognitive and behavioral status, *Pediatrics* 73:638-645, 1984.
111. Black L, Steinschneider A, Shehe P: Neonatal respiratory instability and infant development, *Child Dev* 50:561-564, 1979.
112. Burchfield D, Rawlings J: Sudden deaths and apparent life-threatening events in hospitalized neonates presumed to be healthy, *Arch Dis Child* 145:1319-1322, 1991.
113. Duffty P, Bryan H: Home apnea monitoring in "near-miss" sudden infant death syndrome (SIDS) and in siblings of SIDS victims, *Pediatrics* 70:69-74, 1982.
114. Kelly D, Shannon D, O'Connell K: Care of infants with near-miss sudden infant death syndrome, *Pediatrics* 61:511-514, 1978.
115. Kelly DH, Shannon DC: Sudden infant death syndrome and near sudden infant death syndrome: a review of the literature, 1964-1982, *Pediatr Clin North Am* 29(5):1241-1261, 1982.
116. Weese-Mayer DE, Brouillette RT, Morrow AS, Conway LP, Klemka-Walden LM, Hunt CE: Assessing validity of infant monitor alarms with event recording, *J Pediatr* 115:702-708, 1989.

PART SEVEN

Disorders with Known or Suspected Infectious Causes

CHAPTER 34

Infections of the Upper Respiratory Tract

M. Innes Asher

THE COMMON COLD

The common cold is an acute, highly infectious viral disease characterized by nasal stuffiness, sneezing, coryza, throat irritation, and little or no fever; it occurs many times each year in each person. Despite related medical names, the term *the common cold* best describes this illness. The term *coryza* applies to the symptom of nasal inflammation and discharge. Because of the symptoms occurring in the throat, the term *rhinitis* is too specific. *Nasopharyngitis* applies to nasal symptoms with definite pharyngitis (see later section), which is not specifically part of the common cold.

Disease Mechanisms

The common cold may be caused by 1 of over 100 different viral types; the major ones are listed in Box 34-1. The main clinical difference among colds induced by different viruses is in the duration of the incubation period.[1] Other types of organisms that occasionally cause the common cold syndrome include *Mycoplasma pneumoniae, Coccidiodes immitis, Histoplasma capsulatum, Bordetella pertussis, Chlamydia psittaci,* and *Coxiella burnetii.*

The pathophysiology of the common cold is understood from studies done in adults because few have been done on children. The common cold arises usually from inhalation or self-inoculation of viruses onto the nasal mucosa or occasionally onto the conjunctival surface. The cells of the local respiratory epithelium become infected, with the infection spreading locally, resulting in an increase in the amount of nasal secretions. There is usually submucosal edema followed by shedding of the ciliated epithelial cells. Nasal mucociliary transport is markedly reduced. There may be an increase in the number of neutrophils in the epithelium and lamina propria. The nasal discharge has a high protein content and often becomes mucopurulent because of desquamated epithelial cells and polymorphonuclear leukocytes. Interferon is produced locally to help control the infection.

During the common cold, the greatest concentration of virus is in the nasal secretions, with little found in secretions from coughing, talking, or saliva. Therefore the greatest amount of virus comes from sneezing, nose blowing, and secretions from the nose transmitted on contaminated hands. Children may have a greater concentration of virus and tend to shed virus for longer periods than adults. Viral shedding is maximal 2 to 7 days after inoculation, although some shedding may continue for another 2 weeks. The epithelium regenerates after the fifth day.

Serum antibody and secretory antibody develop from the infection and appear to be protective against reinfections. Clinically abortive colds may be reinfection colds with early antibody recall.

The reduced nasal mucociliary transport remains slightly impaired for about a month. Children who have four to six colds in a winter may have constantly impaired mucociliary transport.

Clinical Manifestations

Most children have several colds each year. Although older children have an illness similar to that of adults, in infants, these symptoms and signs may be more varied. The minimal symptoms that define the diagnosis are nasal discharge, nasal obstruction, and throat irritation. At the onset of symptoms, there is a feeling of chilliness on exposure to cold, dryness and irritation in the nose, and a scratchy throat. This progresses rapidly to nasal stuffiness or obstruction, sneezing, watery nasal discharge, throat irritation, watering eyes or eye irritation, coughing, occasional muscular aches, general malaise, anorexia, and sometimes, low-grade fever.[1] After 1 to 3 days, the nasal secretions may become thicker and purulent. Persistent nasal discharge may lead to excoriation around the nose. If nasal obstruction occurs, it leads to mouth-breathing, aggravating the irritation of the throat. The usual duration of the illness is about 7 days, but lingering nasal discharge may persist for 2 weeks or more.

In infants the onset is more likely to be associated with a fever of 38° to 39° C (100.4° to 102.2° F). The baby may be irritable and restless, and the nasal obstruction may significantly interfere with both feeding and sleeping. Vomiting and diarrhea may also occur.

The uncomplicated common cold has a uniformly excellent outcome with complete recovery. However, complications are common and include acute otitis media, otitis media with effusion, tonsillitis, sinusitis, and lower respiratory tract infection.

Investigations. The clinical features and exposure history are specific, and no investigations are required. However, if viral studies are done, nasopharyngeal culture usually recovers the

BOX 34-1
Viral Causes of the Common Cold

Most common cause
Rhinoviruses

Common causes
Parainfluenza viruses
Respiratory syncytial virus
Coronaviruses

Occasional causes
Adenoviruses
Echoviruses
Coxsackieviruses
Influenza viruses
Reoviruses
Herpesviruses

virus, except coronaviruses and some rhinoviruses, which require special techniques. The early symptoms of many illnesses such as pertussis, epiglottitis, measles, and diphtheria are similar to those of the common cold, but in a short time, the other features of the specific illness appear. Allergic rhinitis may need to be distinguished from the common cold in the child with "recurrent colds." Assessment of the family history, possible allergic triggers, nasal eosinophilia, and the serum immunoglobulin E (IgE) help confirm or exclude this diagnosis.

Objective evidence of pharyngitis indicates that the patient does not have the common cold. Persistence of nasal symptoms or signs suggests a subacute or chronic illness such as adenoiditis or sinusitis.

Management

The common cold in children usually resolves quickly, and no specific therapy is indicated in the majority of cases. Most well-designed studies have failed to show benefits over placebo for common cold preparations used in naturally acquired infection.[2] However, many parents seek treatment, and there is a vast array of treatments available, especially over the counter (OTC). When the child feels miserable and has a fever and irritated throat, an analgesic or antipyretic may be used if the child is over the age of 6 months; these include acetaminophen (Paracetamol), 10 mg/kg/dose four to six hourly (maximum, 60 mg/kg/day) in infants up to 6 months, 15 mg/kg/dose (maximum, 90 mg/kg/day) in children older than 6 months, and 6 g maximum dose in older children.

In infants, nasal obstruction may be relieved by isotonic saline nosedrops, which can moisten irritated nasal mucosa, loosen nasal secretions, and induce sneezing. Gentle aspiration of the nasal secretion using a blunt syringe or suction can provide temporary relief for an infant. Use of concentrated capsules of eucalyptus for inhalation to clear the nose is contraindicated in young children; these can be highly dangerous if applied incorrectly to the face.[3]

Frequent intake of fluid helps relieve the irritated throat. Environmental tobacco smoke aggravates all the symptoms and should be avoided. No studies have directly evaluated the effects of humidifiers on the symptoms of the common cold, but they possibly provide some relief from nasal stuffiness. There is no place for the administration of antibiotics in the uncomplicated common cold.

The effectiveness of OTC cold medications for children with colds has never been established,[4] despite their extensive use. (There are over 800 OTC preparations available in the United States.) By the time a parent seeks treatment the cold is likely to improve in the next few days despite any medication. In the few randomized, controlled trials of antihistamine-decongestant combinations in children with the common cold, no difference was found between active drug and placebo groups; most children in all groups improved regardless of whether they received the medication or placebo.[5] These medications confer no protection against the development of otitis media.[6]

Decongestants are commonly used locally or orally in an attempt to reduce nasal obstruction by sympathomimetic vasoconstriction. Their potential side effects are a concern, especially in young children. Excessive use of sprays and drops with vasoconstrictive medications can lead to rebound obstruction, which prolongs the illness. The associated drying effect could lead to a further decrease in mucociliary clearance. These medications, if used at all, should be given only at bedtime and discontinued after 3 days.

Antihistamines do not alter the natural history of the common cold. The side effects may aggravate the symptoms: increased dry mouth, nasal stuffiness, and possibly agitation. Because of the sedative effects of most antihistamines, a child may go to sleep more readily.

Interferon has been tried experimentally but cannot be recommended for use in children. Intranasally administered interferon-α_2 is variably effective in preventing rhinovirus colds in clinically controlled trials in adults, but adverse effects are common.[7] Interferon-α_2 is not effective in naturally occurring colds secondary to coronavirus.

Intranasal nedocromil sodium has had beneficial effects in rhinovirus infections in healthy volunteers, but any benefit in naturally occurring colds has yet to be demonstrated. Zinc gluconate lozenges are ineffective.[8]

Efforts to control the spread of the common cold are usually impractical; reducing the spread of nasal secretions would be the goal. Preliminary studies using virucidal nasal paper tissues suggested a reduction in spread of rhinovirus colds in the family setting, but this result has not been compared with those from other practical measures.[8a] For children with undue susceptibility to complications, contact with crowds or infected people should be avoided.

PHARYNGITIS AND TONSILLITIS

Pharyngitis is an inflammatory illness of the mucous membrane and underlying structures of the throat; it is invariably associated with the symptom of sore throat. It includes tonsillitis, tonsillopharyngitis, and nasopharyngitis. The inflammation frequently also involves the nasopharynx, uvula, and soft palate. Pharyngitis with nasal symptoms (sometimes called *nasopharyngitis)* is usually caused by a virus, whereas pharyngitis without nasal symptoms can be caused by a wide variety of infectious agents. It is important to recognize and treat streptococcal tonsillopharyngitis, which can proceed to rheumatic fever.

Disease Mechanisms

When an infectious agent is inoculated into the pharyngeal or tonsillar tissue, localized inflammation occurs. This may occur de novo or as a complication of the common cold when the etiologic agent is more likely to be viral. A list of etiologic agents is presented in Boxes 34-2 and 34-3. The inflammation causes erythema of the pharynx, the tonsils, or both structures. Exudate typically occurs with only some organisms, including adenovirus, herpes simplex virus, *Streptococcus pyogenes, Corynebacterium diphtheriae, Arcanobacterium haemo-lyticum,* Epstein-Barr virus, and *Candida* species. Ulceration is usually seen only with herpes simplex virus and enterovirus.

The pharyngeal involvement may be overshadowed by other symptoms, such as cough and coryza when the infecting organism is the parainfluenza virus and fever, exanthem, and meningitis when the infecting organisms is an enterovirus.

The tonsillopharyngeal involvement with marked exudate caused by Epstein-Barr virus looks similar to that caused by group A streptococci. It appears that bacterial adhesion is the cause of this tonsillitis.[9]

Primary and recurrent herpes simplex virus infection occasionally has associated pharyngitis.[10] In almost all instances, there are herpes lesions in the anterior mouth and externally around the mouth.

BOX 34-2
Viral Agents in Pharyngitis and Tonsillitis

Common causes

Adenovirus types 1 to 7, 7a, 9, 14 to 16
Influenza virus types A and B
Parainfluenza virus types 1 to 4
Enteroviruses: coxsackievirus types A and B, echovirus type A
Epstein-Barr virus

Uncommon causes

Respiratory syncytial virus
Rhinoviruses
Rotaviruses
Herpes simplex virus
Measles virus
Reovirus
Cytomegalovirus
Rubella virus
Poliovirus

BOX 34-3
Other Agents in Pharyngitis and Tonsillitis

Common bacteria

Streptococcus pyogenes

Uncommon bacteria

Corynebacterium diphtheriae
Haemophilus influenzae
Neisseria meningitidis
β-Hemolytic streptococci B, C, and G
Bacteroides species
Peptostreptococcus species
Fusobacterium species
Bacteroides melaninogenicus
Corynebacterium ulcerans
Corynebacterium diphtheriae
Corynebacterium pyogenes
Actinomyces species
Francisella tularensis
Legionella pneumophila
Neisseria gonorrhoeae
Leptospira species
Treponema pallidum
Borrelia species
Streptobacillus moniliformis
Yersinia enterocolitica
Streptococcus pneumoniae
Salmonella typhi

Other organisms

Coxiella burnetii
Mycoplasma pneumoniae
Mycoplasma hominis
Chlamydia pneumoniae strain TWAR
Candida species
Toxoplasma gondii

Clinical Manifestations

Children of any age and either gender can develop pharyngitis and tonsillitis. The onset is usually sudden with fever, sore throat, and anorexia. There may be headache, nausea, vomiting, lassitude, and sometimes abdominal pains. With viral infection, there are often other signs of respiratory tract infection, with more or less systemic involvement. The cervical lymph nodes are enlarged and tender. There is moderate to severe pharyngeal erythema, and there may be follicles, ulcers, petechiae, and generalized exudate. Petechial lesions on the soft palate may occur with *S. pyogenes,* Epstein-Barr virus, measles virus, and rubella virus.

Pharyngitis is self-limited, lasting 4 to 10 days, and it has an excellent prognosis. However, in 0.3% to 3.0% of untreated *S. pyogenes* throat infections, the serious complication of rheumatic fever results. Retropharyngeal abscess or parapharyngeal abscess may complicate bacterial tonsillitis or pharyngitis; rarely, septicemia or toxic shock syndrome may occur.

In all cases of acute pharyngitis, streptococcal disease must be considered. Various clinical factors (exposure, season, incubation period, age of patient, and associated clinical findings) may distinguish among causative organisms in large epidemiologic studies, but in the individual child the clinical distinction of streptococcal pharyngitis from viral pharyngitis is unreliable. If there is an obvious nasal infection, ulceration, or conjunctivitis, the etiology is most likely viral. In a child under the age of 4 years, pharyngitis with no exudate is almost always viral. In a child older than 4 years of age, pharyngitis with exudate or fever is most likely caused by *S. pyogenes,* but other bacteria may mimic this condition.[11,12]

Investigations. A throat swab is necessary to define the presence or absence of *S. pyogenes.* An adequate swab of the inflamed tonsillar area is required. There are now rapid methods for detecting group A streptococcal antigen. Individual kits vary in their sensitivity, ranging from 31% to 93%, but have generally high specificity. The results may be obtained in about 10 minutes, making this test available for the office. Generally, if this test is negative, a throat swab should be cultured on two-plate anaerobic trimethoprim-sulfamethoxazole blood agar to give the best yield of *S. pyogenes.* Therapy is withheld pending the results of the throat culture. If the rapid test is not available, a throat culture should be taken.

Management

Symptomatic relief may be obtained from drinking warm fluids or in the older child, saltwater gargles. An analgesic is appropriate when discomfort is troublesome: acetaminophen (Paracetamol), 10 mg/kg/dose four to six hourly (up to 6 months), 15 mg/kg/dose four hourly (older than 6 months), and 6 g maximum in an older child. Simple lemon-based throat lozenges may be soothing, but ones that contain potentially toxic substances should be avoided. Decongestants and antihistamines have no place in the treatment of pharyngitis and tonsillitis. Several studies have shown that penicillin provides relief of symptoms, but other studies have not.[13]

Antibiotics are used to treat *S. pyogenes;* the aim is to prevent the development of rheumatic fever. The goal of antibiotic therapy is adequate treatment of *S. pyogenes* and elimination of nasopharyngeal carriage. Various effective regimens are used, but penicillin remains the treatment of choice[14,15] because of efficacy and low cost. Penicillin can be effective in preventing rheumatic fever even when therapy is started up to 9 days after the onset of the acute illness. Although the conventional oral dosage regimen is penicillin V, 250 mg 3 to 4 times a day,[16] a twice-daily dose of 250 mg, if reliably given, is as effective.[17] In children over 12 years of age, a higher dose of 500 mg twice a day is recommended.[17] Intramuscular benzathine penicillin is very effective and should be considered for children who are particularly unlikely to complete a course of oral treatment: benzathine penicillin intramuscularly, 0.6 megaunits for a child weighing less than 30 kg, 0.9 megaunits for a child weighing 30 to 45 kg, 1.2 megaunits for a child weighing over 45 kg. Erythromycin would be used if penicillin allergy is a concern because it is as effective as penicillin: erythromycin estolate or erythromycin ethylsuccinate, 40 mg/kg/day in three or four doses. All drugs should be used for 10 days to achieve effective eradication of *S. pyogenes.* The efficacy of penicillin in eliminating *S. pyogenes* from the tonsils and pharynx has not diminished after 40 years of use.[15] However, the failure rate in practice may be at least as high as 18% in certain communities. Ampicillin and amoxicillin are associated with a 95% risk of skin rash in infectious mononucleosis[16]; therefore they are not recommended in the treatment of pharyngitis.

In recent years, cephalosporins have been studied in some communities, where they have been found to be at least as effective as penicillin.[18] Bacteriologic and clinical failure rates are even lower than with penicillin or with erythromycin, and the cause of this is debated.[18] The following cephalosporins may be equally effective with penicillin when used for 10 days: cephalexin, cephadrine, cefadroxil, cefaclor, cefuroxime axetil, cefixime, cefprozil, loracarbef, ceftibuten, cefpodoxime proxetil, and cefetamet pivoxil. The cheapest agent should be used. Cefadroxil is effective in a dose of 30 mg/kg (maximum, 1000 mg once a day).[17] Potential disadvantages of cephalosporins are that they cover a broader spectrum of bacteria than is necessary, they have potential side effects, and the cost is high. The place of cephalosporins in the management of bacterial sore throats will become clearer in the next decade as more studies are undertaken.

The course of oral antibiotic must be 10 days; courses of shorter duration are associated with lack of effective treatment. A child must complete a full 24 hours of therapy before returning to school or day-care; otherwise he or she remains infectious to other children.[19]

BOX 34-4
Isolates in Deep Neck Abscesses

Streptococcus pyogenes
Staphylococcus aureus
γ-Hemolytic streptococci
α-Hemolytic streptococci
Streptococcus viridans
Enterococcus faecalis
Haemophilus influenzae
Haemophilus parainfluenzae
Haemophilus species
Escherichia coli
Klebsiella pneumoniae
Moraxella catarrhalis
Eikenella corrodens
Bacillus subtilis
Oral anaerobes
Peptostreptococcus species
Peptostreptococcus anaerobius
Peptostreptococcus asaccharolyticus
Staphylococcus saccharolyticus
Microaerophilic streptococci
Veillonella parvula
Eubacterium lentum
Propionibacterium acnes
Clostridium species
Fusobacterium species
Fusobacterium necrophorum
Fusobacterium nucleatum
Bacteroides species
Bacteroides capillosus
Bacteroides distasonis
Bacteroides asaccharolyticus
Bacteroides fragilis
Bacteroides intermedius
Bacteroides melaninogenicus
Bacteroides oralis
Bacteroides ruminicola
Arachnia propionica
Bifidobacterium species
Lactobacillus species

RETROPHARYNGEAL, PARAPHARYNGEAL, AND PERITONSILLAR ABSCESS

Deep abscesses in the neck may cause serious problems because of local pressure or destruction. They are classified by location into peritonsillar abscess (also known as *quinsy*), retropharyngeal abscess, and parapharyngeal abscess.

The three types of abscess have a similar microbiology (Box 34-4). The most common aerobic isolates are *S. pyogenes* and *Staphylococcus aureus.* Anaerobic isolates are very common in the appropriate cultures, which is not surprising because anaerobic bacteria are the predominant organisms in the oropharynx. Polymicrobial infections are frequent.[20,21]

Peritonsillar Abscess

Peritonsillar abscess is limited medially by the fibrous wall of the tonsil capsule and laterally by the superior constrictor muscle. Pus may be found in a single pocket or in several pockets. The cause of its presence is often not clear, but pus may follow severe tonsillitis with extension through the fibrous capsule. It occurs usually in adolescents and is rare in young children.

Clinical features include sore throat (occasionally with unilateral pain), malaise, low-grade fever, chills, dysphagia, and reduced oral intake. Trismus can result from irritation and reflex spasm of the internal pterygoid muscle. A muffled voice can result from edema, impairing movement of the palate. There may be signs of toxicity, drooling, and sometimes dehydration. The soft palate and uvula are displaced away from the affected side by swelling. The tonsil is displaced medially, and there is ipsilateral tender cervical adenopathy. Untreated peritonsillar abscess may spontaneously rupture into the mouth or extend into the pterygomaxillary space with potentially fatal complications.

Investigations

Identification of the organism from aspirated pus is highly desirable. The peripheral white cell count is elevated, with a predominance of neutrophils.

Management

A combination of antibiotic therapy and drainage of the abscess is required. Penicillin is usually used to treat *S. pyogenes* and oral anaerobes. Clindamycin may be considered. Definitive management must include drainage of the abscess. Results appear to be as good with single-needle aspiration as with acute incision and drainage or acute tonsillectomy.[22,23]

Parapharyngeal Abscess

Parapharyngeal abscess is also known as *pterygomaxillary space abscess.* The clinical manifestations are determined by the structures involved around the abscess cavity. A posterior compartment abscess may result in medial displacement of the lateral pharyngeal wall and parotid space swelling, and extension can result in serious local nerve and life-threatening vascular complications. An anterior compartment abscess can cause trismus from irritation of the internal pterygoid muscle. The source of the abscess is often unclear, but it seems likely to result from extension of infection from nearby tissues.

Clinical features include tender cervical swelling, induration and erythema of the side of the neck, sore throat, dysphagia, trismus, hoarseness, malaise, chills, and possibly, a low-grade fever. In addition to evidence of toxicity, there may be respiratory distress, medial displacement of the lateral pharyngeal wall and inferior tonsil pole, and drooling. Sometimes the presentation is a high cervical mass palpable in the neck that progresses to fluctuance. Other signs arise if there is further extension or complications. Initially a parapharyngeal abscess may be difficult to differentiate from a peritonsillar abscess, but the latter is usually less toxic and has obvious palatal fluctuance.

Investigations

The peripheral white cell count is elevated, with a predominance of neutrophils. Radiographs may be helpful. A submental vertex skull radiograph typically shows pharyngeal fullness on the side of the abscess. An anteroposterior view of the upper airway shows ipsilateral edema and obliteration of the pyriform sinus.

Management

The definitive treatment is incision and drainage and intravenous antibiotic therapy. The incision should be external, with sufficient exposure for ligation of the common carotid artery in case it is eroded. Internal incision runs a high risk of respiratory obstruction.

Retropharyngeal Abscess

A retropharyngeal abscess can form in the potential space between the middle and deep layers of cervical fascia. The infection may result from suppurative adenitis of the lymph nodes in the retropharyngeal space, local trauma, or foreign body aspiration, resulting in edema, cellulitis, or an obstructing mass.

Clinical manifestations include dysphagia, drooling, airway stridor, dyspnea, tachypnea, stiff neck, and ipsilateral cervical adenopathy. There is midline or unilateral swelling of the posterior pharynx.

Investigations

The peripheral white blood cell count is increased, with a predominance of neutrophils. The lateral neck radiograph may show posterior pharyngeal edema and a convex mass containing air. The cervical vertebrae may be retroflexed secondary to extensions of the abscess. Computed tomographic scans distinguish deep neck abscesses from cellulitis of the neck and can define any extension into adjacent areas.

Management

Intravenous antibiotics and incision and drainage are the necessary treatments. When the abscess is small, a peroral incision with the patient positioned to minimize aspiration may be satisfactory; a large abscess may need external incision.

OTITIS MEDIA

Otitis media is a very common condition in childhood. In the United States alone, acute otitis media is responsible for more than 11 million physician encounters per year in children under the age of 5 years. The widespread use of antibiotics for this condition has drastically reduced the previously fairly common suppurative complications of otitis media, but now otitis media with effusion has become more common. There are three categories of otitis media: acute otitis media, otitis media with effusion (secretory otitis media), and chronic suppurative otitis media, including perforation.

Disease Mechanisms

Otitis media may occur de novo; more commonly, it occurs as a complication of the common cold. It is particularly common in the preschool child. The eustachian tubes in a young child are shorter, wider, straighter, and more horizontal and patulous than in the older child, allowing more ready access of organisms to the middle ear. Acute otitis media occurs when viral infection causes respiratory epithelium injury in the nasopharynx, which is colonized with pathogenic bacteria, leading to hyperemia and edema of the eustachian tubes with consequent obstruction. Bacteria may arise in the middle ear by positive or negative forces through the eustachian tube or occasionally through the bloodstream or by direct spread through a damaged tympanic membrane. The inflammation of the tympanic membrane and infected inflammatory exudate in the middle ear are caused primarily by bacteria with polymorphonuclear leukocytes and edema.

Acute otitis media may occur in the context of infection with recognized respiratory viruses such as respiratory syncytial virus, influenza viruses, adenoviruses, parainfluenza viruses, enteroviruses (coxsackievirus, echovirus), rhinoviruses,[24] and even herpes simplex virus type 1 and cytomegalovirus.[25] Viral infection in isolation is a rare cause of otitis media (5%), but up to 20% of cases are combined viral and bacterial infections.[24] The remainder are caused by bacteria alone. Bacterial causes of acute otitis media are listed in Box 34-5. Bacteria are isolated from middle ear fluid by tympanocentesis in about two thirds of cases of acute otitis media and otitis media with effusion. The most common isolate is *Streptococcus pneumoniae,* accounting for up to half of cases, and nontypeable *Haemophilus influenzae* and *Moraxella catarrhalis* account for up to a quarter each. *S. pyogenes* is isolated very uncommonly (about 2%). Two or more organisms are found in about 7% of cases. A different organism may be found in each ear in about 20% of children with bilateral otitis media. *M. pneumoniae* and *Chlamydia trachomatis* are rare causes of otitis media. In neonates, there may be a higher incidence of *S. aureus* and gram-negative bacilli[26] than in older children, especially in babies in neonatal intensive care units who have had prolonged nasotracheal intubation.

If there is vascular compromise of the drum, a perforation results, and it usually heals after the infection subsides. In 20% of cases the acute otitis media progresses to otitis media with persistent effusion. Some 50% of such patients recover after 3 months, but about in 5% the condition persists after 12 months.

Chronic suppurative otitis media is diagnosed in ongoing chronic infection associated with chronic perforation. Organisms isolated in chronic suppurative otitis media are listed in Box 34-6.

BOX 34-5
Bacterial Causes of Acute Otitis Media

Common causes

Streptococcus pneumoniae serotypes 1, 3, 4, 6, 7, 9, 14, 15, 18, 19, and 23
Nontypeable *Haemophilus influenzae* and *Haemophilus influenzae* type b
Moraxella catarrhalis
Streptococcus pyogenes

Rare causes

Enteric bacteria
Staphylococcus aureus
Staphylococcus epidermidis
Pseudomonas aeruginosa

BOX 34-6
Isolates in Chronic Suppurative Otitis Media

Pseudomonas aeruginosa
Staphylococcus aureus
Enteric gram-negative bacilli
Mixed aerobic and anaerobic bacteria
Mycobacterium tuberculosis

Clinical Manifestations

Acute Otitis Media. Otitis media is particularly common in the preschool child and more common in boys than girls. Exclusive breast-feeding for at least 4 months appears to protect against otitis media in the first 12 months of life.[27] A higher rate of all forms of otitis media is found in the New Zealand Maori,[28] Australian Aborigines, Alaskan Eskimos, and North American Indians.

Acute otitis media typically presents with generalized symptoms of malaise, earache, and often, fever. An older child complains of muffled hearing, a sense of fullness, and discomfort of the ear. In a younger child, there are more likely to be systemic signs such as high fever, nausea, vomiting, loss of appetite, malaise, generalized muscle pain, nasal congestion, flushed face, and occasionally, diarrhea and restlessness. The pain may be severe and accentuated by swallowing. Occasionally there may be throbbing tinnitus. The fever, pain, and tinnitus may worsen, but there is immediate relief of pain and systemic symptoms if the drum ruptures and the pus drains. Purulent drainage stops in 1 to 2 days with the residual dry perforation, which heals in 3 weeks to 6 months. Ear pulling in the absence of other symptoms is not related to ear infection.[29]

The diagnosis of otitis media is made by appropriate otoscopic examination. A strong light source and adequate magnification are necessary. If possible, debris in the canal is removed. The mobility of the drum should be tested, ideally by occluding the external canal completely with a large ear speculum and using pneumatic otoscopy.

Typical signs of acute otitis media are retraction, diminished light reflex, and poor mobility of the drum. The light reflex may completely disappear, and the drum starts to become opaque. There is injection of vessels around the margin of the tympanic membrane and adjoining external auditory canal skin. The tympanic membrane moves but with pain. The drum then becomes red, and the pars tensa becomes thick and convex and bulges, with loss of landmarks. In young children, there may be swelling of the posterosuperior aspect of the adjacent external auditory canal skin. As the condition progresses, the drum becomes convex, tense, and whitish, and it bulges, with no mobility and hyperemic vessels on the periphery. There may be yellowish necrotic areas. Hearing impairment becomes worse, and there may be tenderness over the mastoids. The drum may rupture in the pars tensa, causing a gush of purulent material, blood, or serosanguinous fluid. The perforation is generally small and does not enlarge.

If purulent conjunctivitis is present, it is most likely due to nontypeable *H. influenzae,* and this influences antibiotic choice. *M. pneumoniae* is a more likely cause if pneumonia is present. Although viral infection may be associated with otitis media, there is no clinical way of distinguishing between viral and bacterial otitis media. *C. trachomatis* is an infrequent cause of otitis media.

There is a 20% incidence of intracranial or intratemporal complications with acute otitis media; although most cases spontaneously resolve, antibiotic therapy is indicated to prevent serious bacterial complications. With the use of antibiotics, infection is usually arrested before the drum ruptures.

Otitis Media with Effusion. After acute otitis media, up to 20% of cases progress to otitis media with effusion. A large number are transient, with episodes varying in duration and severity. Sometimes, there is recurrence of otitis media with effusion when acute otitis media does not recur. With otitis media with effusion, there is fluctuating hearing loss, which may have an adverse effect on speech, language, and cognitive development, although there seems to be catch-up to normal by age 7 years. The diagnosis is made by persistence of middle ear effusion without signs of inflammation and may be related to infection, tubal obstruction, allergic or immunologic disorders, enlarged adenoids, or rarely, nasopharyngeal tumors. Bacteria are recovered from about 30% of patients who have otitis media with effusion after myringotomy or tympanostomy tube insertion, and there is a similar spectrum to acute otitis media. It is unclear whether the bacteria contribute to the production or persistence of fluid or whether they are simply colonizers.

Chronic Suppurative Otitis Media. The presentation is with otorrhea and deafness. Some 5% of cases of acute otitis media result in perforation, and 20% of these persist.

Other Complications. Extension of the inflammation and infection beyond the mucoperiosteal lining of the middle ear may result in mastoiditis or meningitis (especially with *H. influenzae*). The symptoms and signs of acute mastoiditis may be subtle, especially if they are partially treated by antibiotics or if the tympanic membrane is ruptured. The recurrence of pain and the presence of copious purulent discharge associated with low-grade fever suggest mastoiditis. Usually, there is tenderness over the mastoid process, and there may be edema of the mastoid periosteum, sometimes with postauricular pitting. In the external auditory canal, there is a sagging bulge in the posterior superior wall.

Differential Diagnosis. The acute symptoms of otitis media need to be distinguished from those of acute systemic illness, particularly in a patient with otitis media with effusion. The specific diagnosis can usually be made by noting the general symptoms and performing an adequate and complete inspection of the tympanic membrane. There can be difficulties when the external canal or debris within it does not allow adequate visualization. The diagnosis of neonatal otitis media is difficult. The tympanic membrane often appears thickened and opaque during the first few weeks of life and lies in an extremely oblique position, making it difficult to distinguish it from the canal wall. This may result in overdiagnosis of otitis media in the neonate. The ear canal is particularly compliant, with positive pressure simulating the movement of the tympanic membrane. This may make it difficult to diagnose acute otitis media.

Hyperemia of the tympanic membrane can occur with crying, trauma to the external auditory canal, or mild upper respiratory tract infections. These situations can be distinguished from acute otitis media because other abnormal features of the drum would be lacking in them. Myringitis bullosa can be confused with otitis media. Otalgia may be caused by referred pain from infections in the adenoids, tonsils, teeth, nasopharynx, hypopharynx, or larynx through the tenth cranial nerve. Tumors of the palate, nasopharynx, or base of the skull eventually occlude one or both eustachian tubes.

Investigations. There is a poor correlation between qualitative and semiquantitative cultures of the nose and throat and those of the middle ear. Tympanocentesis is the only reliable way of detecting middle ear pathogens, but it is seldom done in practice; it tends to be a research tool.

Tympanometry gives an objective, reproducible measure of middle ear function. It is particularly useful in situations in which otoscopy is difficult or unreliable, but in the infant under 6 months of age, it can be unreliable because of collapsing ear canals. The findings of otitis media with effusion are of a type B (flat) tympanogram or C2 (peak at less than -200 mm H_2O).

When acute otitis media has classic symptoms and signs, making the diagnosis is not difficult. However, uncommonly acute otitis media may have no symptoms or less impressive signs of inflammation. Sometimes, the tympanic membrane is difficult to visualize. In this situation the clinical distinction from asymptomatic otitis media and otitis media with effusion is difficult. The critical factors are whether there is otoscopic evidence of middle ear effusion and whether there are signs of acute inflammation. If otoscopic examination cannot be satisfactorily completed, tympanography is indicated.

Management

Patients with otitis media are treated as outpatients if there is no systemic infection, unless there is major vomiting requiring hospitalization. Children should be allowed to rest until the fever has resolved for 24 hours. Pain relief with acetaminophen (Paracetamol) is indicated.

Redness of the drum with no other signs of inflammation in the presence of a common cold may indicate viral otitis media. Alternatively, it may be the first sign of bacterial otitis media. Complications of bacterial otitis media are so serious that every child with acute inflammation should be seriously considered for antibiotics. The only indication for withholding antibiotics is a situation in which there is redness and no other sign of inflammation and the child can be reliably monitored daily by otoscopy or the parent bringing the child between visits if the condition deteriorates. A patient with otitis media should be reexamined at regular intervals until the condition completely resolves.

The choice of antibiotics for acute otitis media is determined by the known likely pathogens and local sensitivity patterns. Other factors influencing choice of therapy include the age of the patient, likelihood of compliance with the dosing frequencies, hypersensitivity to antibiotics, the cost of the antibiotics, and the patient's previous experience with the medication.[30]

Amoxicillin, 40 mg/kg/day in three doses, is the usual first choice of treatment. If the patient is allergic to penicillin, trimethoprim-sulfamethoxazole is the usual alternative (8 mg of trimethoprim and 40 mg of sulfamethoxazole per kilogram per day in two doses). If the child has had no symptomatic response within 3 days, a change of an antibiotic is indicated. Alternatives are amoxicillin-clavulanate potassium, 40 mg/kg/day in three doses; cefixime, 8 mg/kg/day in one or two doses[31]; and erythromycin-sulfisoxazole, 50 mg/kg/day in four doses. Cefaclor (40 mg/kg/day in two or three doses) is less efficacious. If the child is vomiting, a single intramuscular dose of ceftriaxone, 50 mg/kg/day, is equally effective with 10 days of oral amoxicillin.[32] All these antibiotic regimens seem to have comparable efficacy in resolving the clinical features of acute otitis media, but their ability to eradicate bacteria varies markedly. The increasing prevalence of penicillin-resistant pneumococci is a concern. Paradoxically, there can be a good clinical response to amoxicillin despite the presence of middle ear pathogens that produce β-lactamase, and this antibiotic is the first choice.

When antibiotics are given early, the length of the symptomatic period may be reduced. However, the clinical outcome may not be specific for predicting bacteriologic outcome. Bacteriologic failure occurs most often in children under 18 months of age.[33] Incomplete eradication could be one reason that otitis media with effusion may develop. The duration of oral antibiotic therapy should be 10 days, but shorter courses are under study. Recurrent attacks of acute otitis media may be prevented by the use of antibiotic prophylaxis.

In acute otitis media in the neonate, special vigilance is required. If there is accompanying systemic infection, hospital admission with parenteral therapy covering *S. aureus* and gram-negative bacilli is indicated.

There is no consistent evidence from randomized, controlled trials that nasal decongestants, mucolytic agents, or antihistamines help prevent or treat any form of otitis media.[34] Vasoconstrictor nosedrops in experimental studies appear to increase the patency of the eustachian tubes; with clinical use, the number of treatment failures appears to be unaltered. If nosedrops are used, it should be for 3 days only in children over the age of 6 months.

Myringotomy is indicated when there is severe, persistent pain and failure to respond to initial antibiotic therapy or when there is a complication of otitis media with an intact drum or persistent conductive hearing loss. In clinical practice, myringotomy is seldom performed despite these indications.

The management of otitis media with effusion must be one of the most controversial topics in pediatrics. Because 50% of cases resolve naturally in 3 months, one could argue for no treatment at all apart from regular otoscopic checks. Otitis media with effusion is commonly treated with low-dose antibiotics for 2 to 4 weeks. This may have some effect on bacterial triggers of the effusion and may prevent occurrences of acute otitis media.

The practice of inserting of tympanostomy tubes is highly controversial.[35] Insertion must not be taken lightly because there are complications, including purulent discharge, granulation tissue, chronic perforation, retraction pockets, atrophic scars, and tympanosclerosis. There is concern about the widespread use of this treatment, which has become the most common operation performed in childhood in industrialized countries. In the United States, in children under the age of 15 years, 5 per 1000 children per year of these operations are done. There is general agreement that if otitis media with effusion has been present for 1 year with decreased hearing, myringotomy with insertion of tympanostomy tubes is indicated. This can result in improvement in hearing (average, 12 decibels) in the short term, but there is no evidence that there is a beneficial effect on development or behavior. At the time of insertion of tympanostomy tubes, the clinician should do a preoperative assessment, including a history of hearing difficulty or speech or learning problems, documentation of significant hearing impairment, and pneumatic otoscopy and tympanometry.

A debate on whether steroids provide added benefit in otitis media with effusion has reopened. Some studies show that prednisone plus antibiotics for 1 to 2 weeks may provide short-term improvement.[36,37] However, the effusion may recur. The long-term benefits of this treatment are unclear. Because the natural history of otitis media with effusion is to fluctuate and often resolve spontaneously, lengthy use of high-dose steroids cannot be recommended as a safe, effective therapy.

Eustachian tube inflation by mechanical means, using nasal balloons (Otovent), appears to be associated with short-term improvement in otoscopic findings in 3- to 10-year-old children compared with findings in controls.[38] Its place in the treatment of otitis media with effusion has yet to be established.

Ototopical antibiotics are indicated when there is long-standing otorrhea and no underlying tissue abnormality. These drops should be avoided in acute otitis media because they may aggravate complications.

The management of otitis media with effusion must be subject to further randomized, controlled trials with standardized clinical criteria so that the roles of antibiotics, steroids, and tympanostomy tubes can be clarified.[35]

ADENOIDECTOMY AND TONSILLECTOMY

Elective surgical removal of the adenoids and tonsils was once widely performed, usually with the hope of reducing the frequency of recurrent sore throats. The scientific basis of this practice is not well established. Children from age 3 to 8 years normally have up to nine respiratory tract infections a year. Prospective objective monitoring of symptoms has demonstrated lower rates than a review of symptoms reported from prior history.[39] The rate for tonsillectomy and adenoidectomy has been falling over the last 2 decades.

The most important indication for adenotonsillectomy is obstructive sleep apnea, which can be serious and even life threatening. Removal of both tonsils and adenoids is usually of marked clinical benefit.[40] Tonsillar or adenoidal size is not always a reliable indicator of the potential benefit of tonsillar removal.

When there is recurrent sore throat, the indication for tonsillectomy is far from clear. There may be some benefit to children who have frequent, well-documented episodes of sore throat: more than five episodes over 2 years.[39] Whereas adenotonsillectomy has been used to treat peritonsillar abscess, there is no clear advantage to drainage alone.[22]

Adenoidectomy is often recommended in conjunction with other treatments for recurrent and chronic otitis media. One randomized, controlled trial has demonstrated that adenoidectomy and bilateral myringotomy (without tympanostomy tubes) are beneficial in children 4 to 8 years old who were severely affected by chronic otitis media with effusion.[41]

SINUSITIS

Sinusitis is a bacterial infection of the paranasal sinuses that uncommonly complicates the common cold. The advent of antibiotics has dramatically altered the occurrence and complication of sinusitis; before antibiotics, surgical treatment of sinusitis was required and was frequently lifesaving.

Disease Mechanisms

Infection can occur in any of the paranasal sinuses as they develop. The ethmoid and maxillary sinuses are present at birth, and the sphenoidal and frontal sinuses are not significantly developed until 5 to 6 years. Although the full development of the frontal sinuses may take 20 years, sinus disease in postpubertal adolescents is similar to that in adults. The four paired paranasal sinuses communicate with the anterior nose, with which they form a system of narrow channels.

The mucosa of the sinuses, like that of the nose, is a continuous ciliated columnar epithelium with goblet cells and is covered in part by a mucous blanket. A continual flow of mucus from the frontal, maxillary, and anterior ethmoid sinuses is propelled toward the ostia and then posteriorly to the nasopharynx. The mucus contains IgA, IgG, IgM, and lysozyme, and the paranasal sinuses are usually sterile. Damage to mucociliary function allows for the inoculation of large numbers of pathogens into the sinuses, which causes infection. Once started, sinus infection is aggravated by further inflammation of the ostium of the sinuses, resulting in progressive obstruction.

In children, sinusitis almost always occurs as a complication of the common cold. The viral infection inflames the mucosa and causes damage to nasal ciliated epithelial cells, encouraging infection with bacteria colonizing the upper respiratory tract. Other irritants, such as swimming underwater and drying of the mucosa during winter in cold climates, can set the stage for sinus infection. Host factors predisposing to sinusitis include respiratory allergies, dental infections or extractions, defects of ciliary function, cystic fibrosis, immunodeficiency, and anatomic problems.

The organisms causing sinusitis are listed in Box 34-7. The most common causes are *S. pneumoniae, H. influenzae,* and *M. catarrhalis.* These organisms, along with *S. aureus* and *S. pyogenes,* account for over 90% of cases of sinusitis in children. In adolescents, penicillin-sensitive anaerobes become more common. There may be a vast array of enteric gram-negative and other bacilli recovered, mostly from those who have had antibiotic therapy before culture.[42]

Clinical Manifestations

Acute sinusitis is heralded by failure of common cold symptoms to resolve after 10 days.[43,44] Sometimes, the sinusitis can be more acute and have severe initial symptoms: fever greater than 39° C and purulent nasal discharge. Acute sinusitis in-

BOX 34-7
Causes of Sinusitis

Aerobic bacteria

Haemophilus influenzae
Streptococcus pneumoniae
Moraxella catarrhalis
Staphylococcus aureus
Streptococcus pyogenes
α-Hemolytic and nonhemolytic streptococci
Staphylococcus epidermidis
Alcaligenes species
Escherichia coli
Klebsiella pneumoniae
Pseudomonas aeruginosa
Serratia species
Diphtheroids
Enterococci
Neisseria species
Haemophilus species
Proteus species
Acinetobacter species
Citrobacter species
Eikenella corrodens

Anaerobic bacteria

Peptococcus species
Peptostreptococcus species
Bacteroides species
Veillonella species
Fusobacterium species
Bifidobacterium species
Propionibacterium species

Other organisms

L-forms
Mixed: aerobes and anaerobes
Mixed: *Haemophilus influenzae* with other organisms
Mycoplasma pneumoniae
Other (rhinovirus, adenovirus, *Aspergillus* species, other fungi)

Fungi

Aspergillus species
Zygomycetes
Drechslera spicifera
Bipolaris species
Curvularia lunata

volves symptoms persisting from 10 to 30 days, and after this time, it is categorized as *subacute* or *chronic.* Sinusitis is more common in boys. In preschool children the disease involves only the maxillary and ethmoid sinuses. Older children have more specific complaints than younger children.

The main symptom is rhinorrhea (80%), which is frequently purulent but can be serous or watery. In a minority of patients, there are fever, cough (especially at night), pain, headache, sore throat, periorbital swelling, vomiting, and occasionally, malodorous breath. Sinus tenderness is uncommon in children. Posterior pharyngeal pus is not usually seen in acute sinusitis and is very uncommon in chronic sinusitis. Periorbital swelling is usually a sign of acute ethmoid sinusitis. Acute sinusitis is more frequently unilateral, and chronic sinusitis is usually bilateral. In chronic sinusitis the symptoms may be minimal: vague unwellness with some persistent signs of upper respiratory tract infection.

The outlook of sinusitis in otherwise healthy children receiving adequate treatment is excellent. Untreated sinusitis can progress to orbital infection, meningitis, osteomyelitis, cavernous sinus thrombosis, and abscesses of the epidura, subdura, or brain.[45]

The relationship between sinus disease and lower respiratory tract infections or asthma is controversial. The extent to which sinus disease may aggravate or even cause lower respiratory tract symptoms or disease is unclear; the possible mechanisms are also unclear.[46,47] Nevertheless, treating sinus disease may improve lower respiratory tract symptoms.

The differential diagnosis includes foreign bodies in the nose, cysts in the maxillary antra, nasal structural defects, palatal defects, dental infections, and infection of the adenoids.

Investigations. In acute sinusitis, clinicians seldom undertake investigations. Nasal culture reveals the organism in the majority of cases, but it should be obtained with careful technique. A vasoconstrictor such as phenylephrine hydrochloride 0.25% should be applied to the anterior nose, and bilateral cultures should be obtained under direct vision using a wire cotton swab touching material as it comes from the sinus ostium. In children who have neurologic complications or in whom treatment fails, antral puncture for aerobic and anaerobic culture can be lifesaving.

Some cases of sinusitis have an elevated erythrocyte sedimentation rate. In acute sinusitis, the number of band neutrophils may be increased.

Imaging of the sinuses may be useful to provide support for a clinical diagnosis. Lateral plain radiographic views and occipitomental projections should be done in young children, and in older children, Caldwell's and basal projections should be done as well. Sinus radiographs should not be obtained until symptoms have been present for at least 10 days. When the child is younger than 6 months of age, opacification of the ethmoid air cells is normal. When the child is under the age of 1 year, opacification or thickening of the mucosa of the maxillary sinuses may also be normal. Therefore these views are not recommended until after these ages. With sinusitis, opacification is seen, and the maxillary sinuses and air-fluid level are also visualized.

Ultrasonography has been used as an alternative, but it is not of value unless there is one normal air-filled maxillary sinus for comparison. Computed tomographic scan is helpful when the findings of the plain films are equivocal or negative, when the child has chronic or recurrent disease, or when complications are suspected.[48,49]

Management

Analgesics such as acetaminophen may be useful for controlling headache, pain, or fever. The primary treatment is antibiotics, which should be started before the results of investigations are known. Amoxicillin, 40 mg/kg/day in four doses, is adequate for *S. pneumoniae* and the majority of *H. influenzae* and *M. catarrhalis.* In communities with high β-lactamase-producing *H. influenzae* and *M. catarrhalis,* the following antibiotics should be considered: amoxicillin-clavulanate potassium (40 mg/kg/day in three doses), trimethoprim-sulfamethoxazole (8 mg of trimethoprim and 40 mg of sulfamethoxazole per kilogram per day in two or three doses), and cefaclor (40 mg/kg/day in three doses). These drugs should be considered as first line if the sinusitis is recurrent, fails to improve, or is a more complicated infection with high fever or periorbital swelling. A brisk response to treatment is expected in 3 to 4 days, in which case a 10-day course of treatment is satisfactory. If the response is slower, up to 1 month of treatment may be necessary to eradicate the infection.

If there are bacterial complications of sinusitis, the child should be hospitalized and given parenteral antibiotics. Initially, intravenous cefuroxime (100 mg/kg/day in three divided doses) is recommended; however, if *S. aureus* is a major concern, oxacillin or nafcillin should be added. Therapy should be adjusted on the basis of response to treatment and the results from culture.

Vasoconstrictive drugs are often used locally or systemically in an attempt to relieve obstruction at the sinus ostia to help establish drainage, but there is no evidence supporting their effectiveness. Moreover, the drying effect of systemically active drugs on the mucous blanket might be deleterious. Topical medications can cause rebound vasodilation. These medications should be used only when there is considerable pain and then for no more than 3 days.

Surgical drainage is rarely necessary in children. It is indicated only if there is lack of response to maximal medical therapy and continuing symptoms or if there are neurologic complications.

VIRAL CROUP

Acute upper airway obstruction in children is most commonly caused by viral infection and is labeled *viral croup.* There have been various terms for this condition. The more specific diagnostic name, *acute laryngotracheitis,* defines the site of inflammation, which always involves the larynx and trachea; if it is believed to extend to the bronchi, the name *laryngotracheobronchitis* is used. Spasmodic croup and recurrent croup are often regarded as separate diagnoses but may be part of the spectrum of the same condition.

Croup is uncommon in the first 6 months of life, and under this age preexisting abnormalities of the upper airway such as subglottic stenosis or hemangioma should be considered. These lesions may also be the cause of prolonged stridor because viral croup rarely lasts more than 10 to 14 days.

Disease Mechanisms

The symptoms and signs result from inflammation in the larynx, trachea, and sometimes the bronchi. They are almost always caused by viral infection. The causative viruses are listed in Box 34-8.

The parainfluenza viruses cause most cases of croup, with type 1 being most common, type 3 less common, and type 2 infrequent. Respiratory syncytial virus and several of the adenoviruses infrequently cause croup, as does influenza virus type A, which induces a particularly severe form. Rhinoviruses, enteroviruses, herpes simplex virus, and reovirus have been associated with mild cases of croup. Morbilli (measles) virus may cause upper airway obstruction resulting from laryngotracheitis, sometimes severe enough to require intubation, and there may be complicating bacterial tracheitis. Rarely the vesicular eruption of varicella may involve the larynx. Mild "viral" croup may also be caused by *M. pneumoniae* infection. One case of *Cryptosporidium* laryngotracheitis has been described in an infant in Papua New Guinea.

Diphtheria must be considered if the child has not been immunized against *C. diphtheriae.* This organism may cause a membranous obstructive laryngitis.

BOX 34-8
Viral Causes of Acute Laryngotracheitis

Common causes	Uncommon causes
Parainfluenza virus types 1 to 3	Adenoviruses
Influenza virus types A and B	Rhinoviruses
Respiratory syncytial virus	Enteroviruses
	Herpes simplex virus
	Reovirus
	Morbilli (measles) virus

After inhalation of the virus, the cells of the local respiratory epithelium become infected. There is marked edema of the lamina propria, submucosa, and adventitia accompanied by cellular infiltration with histiocytes, lymphocytes, plasma cells, and polymorphonuclear leukocytes.

There is redness and swelling of the involved airway, most marked in the lateral walls of the trachea just below the vocal cords. The subglottic trachea is surrounded by the fixed cricoid cartilage, forcing the inflammatory swelling to encroach on the internal airway lumen, narrowing it or reducing it to a slit. The infant's glottis and subglottic region are normally narrow, and a small decrease in diameter results in a large increase in airway resistance and a decrease in airflow. As the airway diameter enlarges with growth, the impact of the subglottic airway swelling is reduced.

Obstruction to airflow through the upper airway results in stridor and difficulty breathing and progresses to hypoxia when the obstruction is severe. Hypoxia with mild obstruction indicates lower airway involvement and ventilation-perfusion mismatch resulting from lower airway obstruction or lung parenchymal infection or even fluid.[50] Hypercapnia occurs as a late change as hypoventilation progresses with obstruction.

Clinical Manifestations

Viral croup is a very common condition, affecting about 15% of children. It is most common between 6 months and 5 years of age, with a peak prevalence in the second year of life; the youngest reported patient is 3 months of age.[50a] The full picture of viral croup is rare over the age of 10 years. Boys are affected more often than girls. There is a seasonal occurrence; a peak in autumn is associated with parainfluenza virus.

Typically the illness starts with rhinorrhea, sore throat, and mild fever for a few days. Then the child develops a characteristic barking cough, hoarseness, and inspiratory stridor with or without low-grade fever.

An increasing severity of obstruction is evident with increasing heart and respiratory rate, flaring of alar nasi, and indrawing, especially suprasternal, intercostal, and sternal in the younger child or infant. Increasing chest wall retractions occur as the pleural pressure becomes increasingly negative and correlates with the severity of the upper airway obstruction.[51] Ribcage and abdominal asynchrony occurs as the condition deteriorates.[52]

As progressive hypoxia develops, the child is anxious or restless or may have depressed consciousness or cyanosis. One study has shown the respiratory rate to be the best indicator of hypoxemia.[50] The clinician should use these signs, which have formed the basis of a number of croup severity scores, to regularly reassess the child for evidence of increased airway obstruction.

On auscultation, breath sounds are normal with no added sounds except transmission of the stridor. Occasionally, there may be wheezing, indicating severe narrowing, bronchitis, or possibly coexistent asthma.

Becoming upset or worried may decrease the child's ability to manage the airway obstruction. Therefore physical examination should be limited to the respiratory tract and reasonable exclusion of other diagnostic possibilities. Investigations are intrusive and should be avoided when possible.

Most children have mild illness, requiring no specific management. Symptoms may last 7 to 14 days. By the time medical attention is sought the airway obstruction often does not progress but usually lasts 4 more days. However, in a minority of children the airway obstruction progresses to become severe. Among children hospitalized for viral croup, less than 1% require intubation. Rarely, idiopathic pulmonary edema occurs in severe obstruction,[53] presumably on a similar basis as that seen in some cases of epiglottitis (see next section).

The term *spasmodic croup* has been used to define a sudden onset of symptoms at night in a child who has been well. The symptoms are identical to viral croup but without fever, last for hours rather than days, and are seldom life threatening. The child may be well during the day and have attacks on 3 to 4 successive evenings. During the first attack, it is difficult to make an accurate diagnostic distinction from viral croup. The direct laryngoscopic appearance shows pale, watery edema of subglottic tissues. There is an association with the same viruses that cause viral croup, although it has been suggested that spasmodic croup represents allergic reaction to viral antigen rather than direct infection.[55] There is no proof of this hypothesis.

About half the cases of croup progress to recurrent croup (at least 2 episodes), usually typical spasmodic croup. In a few individuals, more than 50 episodes have been described. More of these children are boys; more have asthma, hay fever, eczema, and positive allergy prick tests; and more come from families with a history of atopy or croup than children with nonrecurrent croup.[54] Pulmonary function studies have demonstrated lower expiratory flow rates, and increased airway responsiveness to histamine has been documented on inspiratory and expiratory flow-volume loops. Reduced serum IgA levels have been found in some individuals, but the significance of this finding is unclear.[55]

The differential diagnosis includes any condition that causes obstruction in the region of the larynx. The most important are epiglottitis and laryngeal foreign body aspiration, both of which require emergency treatment. Acute angioedema usually presents with other evidence of swelling of the face and neck. Other conditions to be considered are retropharyngeal and peritonsillar abscess, bacterial tracheitis, subglottic stenosis, infectious mononucleosis, laryngeal diphtheria, and paraquat poisoning.

Investigations. Investigations are seldom necessary in straightforward viral croup. When there is severe obstruction, neck radiographs or blood tests cause anxiety in the child, which may precipitate critically poor gas exchange. Pulse oximetry may support the clinical suspicion of hypoxia but should not be used as the only means of clinical assessment.

If a lateral neck radiograph is deemed necessary to exclude epiglottitis or foreign body inhalation in a child whose airway is severely obstructed, it should be done in the presence of medical staff able to resuscitate a child with upper airway obstruction. However, epiglottitis is usually diagnosed clinically and confirmed under direct vision in the intensive care unit.

When radiography has been done, specific abnormalities are seen in 40% to 50% of cases (see Chapter 13). Posteroanterior neck radiographs may show a very narrowed subglottic region. In lateral neck radiographs, there may be widening of the hypopharynx and haziness in the subglottic region. Radiographic changes do not reliably reflect the severity of airway obstruction.

Management

Most children with viral croup have only mild airway obstruction that spontaneously settles; therefore no specific treatment is indicated. Usually, these children can be treated at home. A commonly used home treatment is to sit the child in the bathroom with a parent with a hot shower running in the belief that the warm mist will help the breathing. Provided that the child is reassured rather than frightened by this treatment, there is no harm, and the child may feel more comfortable, but benefits have not been demonstrated in controlled trials.[56] Cold or hot moisture should be avoided because it is distressing.

In the child with obvious indrawing, anxiety, or other evidence of moderate or severe airway obstruction, it is vital to use a careful nonintrusive approach. A parent should stay with the child, and all interactions with the child should appear calm and reassuring. Mist treatment in the hospital is no longer recommended, and it may increase the child's anxiety.

Mild hypoxia with an oxygen saturation lower than 93% is common and closely correlated to the respiratory rate. Correction of mild hypoxia is usually unnecessary. When there are clinical signs of hypoxia such as restlessness, marked tachycardia, and cyanosis, oxygen therapy is indicated. At the same time, treatment to relieve the obstruction is needed. Admission to the pediatric intensive care unit is indicated for children with signs of hypoxia or progressive severity of obstruction.

Corticosteroids. Corticosteroids have been introduced to relieve the obstruction. The theoretic mechanism of action of the steroids is suppression of local inflammatory reaction, shrinkage of lymphoid swelling, and reduction in capillary permeability. The place of steroids in the management of viral croup has been debated for 30 years but still has not been clarified completely. Although there are a large number of studies of steroids in croup, many are inadequately designed.

Among the well-designed studies (randomized, double blind, placebo controlled with appropriate definition of cases and monitoring), a variety of inclusion and exclusion criteria, clinical scores, and steroid regimens were used. A recent meta-analysis of the better studies[57] supports the use of steroids in children hospitalized with croup. Their use is associated with a significantly increased number of cases showing clinical improvement at 12 and 24 hours after treatment and a significantly reduced incidence of endotracheal intubation. These findings have been confirmed by two subsequent studies. A further study has shown that successful extubation can be achieved earlier without the need for reintubation in children to whom steroids were administered.[58]

When the viral croup is severe enough for the child to be admitted to an intensive care unit, the child should receive steroids. Children with mild disease not admitted to the hospital do not need steroids. Indications for the use of corticosteroids in children whose condition lies between these extremes are still subject to debate. Although studies have shown improvement in hospitalized children who have moderate or severe croup and who are not admitted to the intensive care unit, the majority of these children get better by themselves. It is unknown whether the improvement with steroids is really clinically significant. Pediatricians must still use clinical judgment to decide. A full cost benefit and safety analysis of steroid management has not been undertaken. Additional large, prospective, double-blind, randomized, controlled trials are required. These should have clear diagnostic criteria, uniform entry criteria, a validated index of severity, an adequate standardized steroid dosage, and clinically relevant outcome measures.

There has been considerable variation in the regimens of corticosteroids administered to children hospitalized with viral croup. A higher initial dose of steroid is associated with a larger number of patients whose condition improves at 12 hours. The dose depends on the preparation used. High-dose dexamethasone has now been widely used, with a single dose of 0.6 mg/kg administered intramuscularly being definitively effective.[59,60] Doses less than this may be equally effective[61]; a recent study showed that oral dexamethasone in a dose of 0.15 mg/kg is as effective as 0.3 or 0.6 mg/kg in relieving symptoms and results in a similar duration of hospitalization in children with croup.[61a] The oral route of administration may be equally effective, but further study is required to confirm this. A few studies demonstrate benefit from prednisone in a lower cortisol equivalent dose than dexamethasone,[62] suggesting that the subglottic antiinflammatory activity of prednisone is stronger than that of dexamethasone, but this requires further study. Methylprednisolone administered intramuscularly and intravenously has also been used with benefit.[62a]

In some studies, repeated doses of steroid varying between 6 and 24 hours after the initial dose have been given. The efficacy of more than one dose compared with a single dose has not been studied, but it appears that a single dose is sufficient in the majority of cases. The maximal effect of steroids is reached 6 hours after administration, and dexamethasone has a biologic half-life of 36 to 54 hours. It is logical to give only one dose of dexamethasone because croup usually improves naturally 1 to 2 days after presentation to medical care, so the need for further intervention will have passed. If prednisone is used, its shorter biologic half-life (12 to 18 hours) suggests the likelihood that a second dose may be necessary.

There is no evidence of any ill effects of one dose of corticosteroids used in viral croup. However, there may be complications with steroids used inadvertently for diagnoses mimicking viral croup, such as epiglottitis, so the clinician must be certain of the diagnosis before administering them. A low incidence of pneumonia has been reported in steroid-treated croup, but it does not appear to be any greater than the natural incidence of pneumonia complicating viral croup.

There have been two recent placebo-controlled studies of nebulized budesonide in viral croup[63,64] and one further study with a comparison oral dexamethasone.[64a] In young children who have croup with a range of severities, prompt and important clinical improvement has been demonstrated with nebulized budesonide. The rapid effect suggests a more rapid onset of action resulting from direct access to affected tissues, possibly causing α-adrenergic vasoconstriction. The decision to use oral or injected corticosteroid or nebulized budesonide should take into account the cost of each preparation, the ease of administration and the probable frequency of steroid use.[65]

Epinephrine. Epinephrine (adrenaline) was first introduced for viral croup in 1971. It is thought to stimulate α-adrenergic receptors in subglottic mucosa, producing vasoconstriction, resulting in less hyperemia and edema of the larynx and subglottic region. This results in increased airway diameter within 30 minutes. However, the effect is short lived, lasting about 2 hours because of dispersion of the epinephrine.

The first use of this treatment was with racemic epinephrine hydrochloride (Vaponefrin, equivalent to 2.25% epinephrine base), a mixture of equal parts of the inactive D-isomer and the active L-isomer. In some early studies,[66] this treatment was given with intermittent positive-pressure breathing, but a similar effect is seen without it.[67] Racemic epinephrine is not readily available in some countries, and it has been replaced by the use of L-epinephrine solution, which is cheaper.[68]

Epinephrine does not alter the natural history of the airway obstruction. Therefore when the effects wear off, rebound may occur: The obstruction may be either as bad as before or worse if the overall condition is deteriorating. It is dangerous to discharge a child with croup who has been given nebulized epinephrine before ensuring that there is no rebound; the child should be observed for 6 hours after the dose. This medication is used to provide immediate symptomatic relief in patients with moderate and severe croup and in those admitted to the intensive care unit in an attempt to avert the need for intubation.

Epinephrine is given via a nebulizer with a face mask and is driven with oxygen. The usual dose in infants weighing 10 kg is 5 mg, which may be given as 5 ml of 1:1000 solution of L-epinephrine or as 0.5 ml of 2.25% solution (22.5 mg/ml) of racemic epinephrine solution, which contains 5 mg of L-isomer. The latter is diluted with isotonic saline to a 3- to 5-ml volume. In young infants, graded doses based on body weight are appropriate: 0.5 ml/kg of 1:1000 L-epinephrine to a maximum of 5 ml of 2.25% solution or 0.05 ml/kg to a maximum of 0.5 ml of racemic epinephrine. Doses may be repeated every 2 hours or even more often. Adverse reactions have not been reported.

Other Treatments. Intravenous fluids are not usually required in viral croup, but if a child is unable to drink, intravenous maintenance fluids may be indicated. Admission to the intensive care unit is indicated when there is restlessness, anxiety, marked tachycardia, or cyanosis or when the child is tiring. In this situation, epinephrine and corticosteroids should be administered.

Despite vigorous treatment with epinephrine and steroids, a child occasionally progresses to critical airway obstruction necessitating endotracheal intubation. This should be performed by a pediatric anesthetist or intensive care pediatrician experienced in endotracheal intubation using inhalational anesthesia. Intubation should be maintained until an air leak develops, indicating a reduction of airway edema, or until a maximum of 5 days pass, at which time a trial of extubation is attempted. Rarely tracheostomy may be the only method of providing an alternative airway.

EPIGLOTTITIS

Epiglottitis is a very serious infection of the epiglottis and supraglottic structures that results in acute airway obstruction and high risk of death if untreated. It is rare but must be considered in a child with dyspnea and stridor. Although epiglottitis occurs mainly in children, it can occur at any age.

Disease Mechanisms

Acute epiglottitis is almost always caused by *H. influenzae* type B (Hib), which can be cultured from direct epiglottic swabs or blood cultures. Other causative organisms listed in Box 34-9 are usually bacteria[69,70] but occasionally viruses[71-73] or *Candida* organisms.[74]

Direct invasion by Hib causes cellulitis with marked edema of the epiglottis, aryepiglottic folds, ventricular bands, and arytenoids. There is a large potential space for the accumulation of inflammatory cells and edema fluid where the stratified squamous epithelium is loosely adherent to the anterior surface and the superior third of the posterior portion of the epiglottis. There is diffuse infiltration with polymorphonuclear leukocytes, hemorrhage, edema, and fibrin deposition, and microabscesses may form. As edema increases, the epiglottis curls posteriorly and inferiorly, causing airway obstruction. Inspiration tends to draw the inflamed supraglottic ring into the laryngeal inlet. Infection of the supraglottic larynx may extend but does not usually reach the subglottis or the laryngeal lymphatic system.

Clinical Manifestations

Epiglottitis is rare; it most commonly occurred in children under the age of 5 years in whom the annual incidence varied from region to region, up to 22.7 per 100,000 per year. With the introduction of Hib vaccination, it has virtually disappeared. The risk of epiglottitis may vary among populations, with Alaskan Eskimos and Navaho Indians having higher risk than other American populations, whereas Aborigines in Australia have a lower risk than the non-Aboriginal population.[75] There is no clear seasonal incidence. There is a slight male predominance. The mean age is about 40 months, with about 75% of cases occurring between 1 and 5 years.

Up to half of the children have preceding upper respiratory tract symptoms. The onset of epiglottitis is typically abrupt, with early toxicity. The duration of symptoms before presentation to the hospital is usually less than 24 hours. The child has symptoms caused by supraglottic swelling and airway obstruction.

There are a very sore throat, difficulty swallowing because of pain, respiratory distress, drooling, a choking sensation, irritability, restlessness, and anxiety. The temperature is high, usually between 38.8° and 40° C (101.8° to 104° F). Sighing respirations, mild stridor, retractions, and mild tachypnea occur. Less common symptoms and signs are cough, which may be harsh, and occasionally, barking, delirium, lethargy, hoarseness or aphonia, vomiting, chills, anorexia, cervical adenopathy, wheezing, and hypotonia.

The child naturally assumes a posture that maximizes the diameter of the obstructed airway: sitting and leaning forward with hyperextension of the neck and protrusion of the chin. A few may have shock with cyanosis, prostration, and loss of consciousness.

Children with epiglottitis are at risk for total airway obstruction. The enlarged, inflamed supraglottic ring can progress to respiratory obstruction with unexpected suddenness. The exact mechanism is not clear, and the early view that the swollen epiglottis collapses into the laryngeal inlet may be incorrect. Epiglottitis progresses to death in about 7% of children who do not have secured airways. With accurate early recognition and elective intubation, the mortality rate should approach zero. Most deaths occur in transit to hospital or in the first few hours after arrival.

BOX 34-9
Causes of Epiglottitis

Common cause

Haemophilus influenzae type B

Rare causes

Staphylococcus aureus
Haemophilus influenzae type A and nontypeable *Haemophilus influenzae*
Haemophilus parainfluenzae
Streptococcus pneumoniae
Streptococcus pyogenes group A
Streptococcus groups B and C
Streptococcus viridans
Bacillus species
Mycobacterium tuberculosis
Varicella-zoster virus
Herpes simplex virus type 1
Parainfluenza virus type 3
Influenza virus type B

Causes in an immunodeficient host

Pseudomonas aeruginosa
Candida tropicalis
Candida albicans
Candida species
Herpes simplex virus type 2 (neonate)

Complications are uncommon.[76] Evidence of pneumonia or atelectasis is sometimes seen on the chest radiograph. Other findings may include exudative tonsillitis, cervical lymphadenitis, and otitis media. Meningitis, septic arthritis, and pericarditis occurring with epiglottitis are rare; routine lumbar puncture is unnecessary.

The diagnosis is often clear from the specific clinical signs. However, it is sometimes difficult to differentiate epiglottitis from severe viral croup of a more rapid onset. Distinguishing features include the absence of spontaneous cough and the presence of drooling and agitation.[77] Toxicity, high fever, and sore throat may also occur with bacterial tracheitis, uvulitis, and retropharyngeal or parapharyngeal abscess. Nasopharyngeal diphtheria is now rare but may mimic acute epiglottitis and is associated with serosanguinous discharge. Noninfectious causes mimicking epiglottitis include angioedema, a pharyngeal burn, and a foreign body that is in the valleculae or larynx or that penetrates the posterior pharyngeal tissues.

Chronic epiglottic enlargement may be seen with neck radiotherapy for cancer, granulomatous lymphangitis, or lymphangiectasis and in infection with the human immunodeficiency virus.[78] The chronicity of symptoms makes these conditions easily distinguishable from acute epiglottitis. Similarly, congenital anomalies of the airway and laryngeal papillomatosis are usually quite distinct.

Investigations. Investigations should be left until the airway is secured (see later section). The diagnosis is confirmed under direct visualization. Detection of the responsible organism is important for guiding antibiotic management. Direct culture of supraglottic tissues reveals the causative organism in the majority of patients. The blood culture is positive for Hib in about 70% of cases. Blood leukocyte counts, mainly polymorphonuclear leukocytes, are increased. The numbers of immature neutrophils are increased in most cases. The level of

C-reactive protein is usually raised. Capsular antigen such as Hib has been detected using counterimmunoelectrophoresis or latex particle agglutination assay, but it adds little to the workup.

Lateral radiographic views of the soft tissues of the neck may be needed if a laryngeal foreign body is suspected, but the patient's airway must be carefully monitored throughout the procedure. The best view of the anatomic structures of the upper airway is obtained with the patient upright. The hypopharynx is dilated, and the normal cervical lordosis may be replaced by a straight or kyphotic contour. The valleculae are narrowed and may be obliterated. A thickened mass of tissue extends from the valleculae to the arytenoid muscles (see Chapter 13).

Management

Because of the high risk of complete airway obstruction, great care should be taken in treating epiglottitis. Once a doctor suspects this diagnosis, the child should be constantly attended by an individual skilled in resuscitation using the appropriate equipment for airway stabilization and ventilatory support. Delays of 2 to 3 hours have proved fatal. Every effort should be made to reduce the time needed to secure a patient's airway and initiate antibiotic therapy. During this waiting interval, unnecessary stress for the child should be prevented, the throat should not be examined, and radiographic confirmation is usually omitted. Extensive clinical assessment, transport delay, and blood tests should be eliminated.

The airways should be secured as early as possible after diagnosis. A large body of literature attests to the safety and efficacy of elective nasotracheal intubation, which is the treatment of choice. A short period of airway maintenance is usually all that is required. A nasotracheal tube that is 0.5 mm smaller than that predicted by the patient's age is recommended. Expert nursing care is essential to prevent inadvertent extubation, particularly in the first 12 to 18 hours. The criteria for extubation include being afebrile and swallowing comfortably. Repeat examination of the epiglottis and supraglottic structures by direct laryngoscopy or fiberoptic bronchoscopy is not normally necessary. Complications occurring after extubation may be laryngeal edema and subglottic granulations. Long-term complications of nasotracheal intubation are rare. Tracheostomy is lifesaving but has been replaced by safer nasotracheal intubation.

In about 10% of children with epiglottitis in whom there is severe airway obstruction, idiopathic pulmonary edema may occur before or after insertion of endotracheal tubes.[53] The hypothetical mechanism is an increased pulmonary blood flow secondary to airway obstruction, causing markedly negative intrapleural pressure with increased venous return to the right side of the heart and decreased left ventricular output. These changes increase the pulmonary microvascular pressure and produce pulmonary hyperemia and edema. Endotoxemia may play a role in altering vascular permeability, but it is not a necessary prerequisite. Continuous positive airway pressure in intubated patients may decrease the occurrence of pulmonary edema.

Until the results of sensitivity tests are known, the child should be treated with an intravenous antibiotic to cover the majority of possible isolates. Increasing numbers of *H. influenzae* produce β-lactamase (up to one third in some communities); therefore initial treatment is usually a second-generation cephalosporin such as cefuroxime (if meningitis not present) or a third-generation cephalosporin such as cefotaxime or ceftriaxone. If the isolate is proved to be susceptible, ampicillin, a cheaper agent, may be substituted. If group A *S. pyogenes* is isolated from the airway, penicillin is the drug of choice. When *S. aureus* is isolated, a semisynthetic penicillinase-resistant penicillin or glycopeptide such as vancomycin should be used depending on sensitivity patterns. Erythromycin should be used for *C. diphtheriae.*

No controlled studies address the duration of antibiotic treatment, but a course of 7 days of intravenous administration (until the child is afebrile for 48 hours) followed by oral therapy is commonly used. Ceftriaxone in a single daily dose of 100 mg/kg for 5 days is effective.[79]

Although there have been some recommendations to use corticosteroids, no controlled data support their use; in fact, they may be hazardous because of the side effects. Therapy with inhaled epinephrine has no benefit: it helps only in viral croup.

Secondary disease can occur in household contacts of epiglottitis. Epiglottitis has also occurred in household contacts of meningitis resulting from Hib. Rifampin (Rifampicin) prophylaxis eradicates nasopharyngeal carriage and is recommended as follows: a dosage of 20 mg/kg/day (600 mg maximum per dose) for 4 days for all members of a patient contact group when the index case has invasive Hib and there is at least one contact who is 4 years of age or younger. For patients younger than 2 years of age, prophylaxis is required for the child and all household contacts.[80]

Prevention of invasive Hib infection is now universally recommended using one of the approved polysaccharide conjugate vaccine regimens for children up to 5 years of age. These vaccines are highly effective in lowering the incidence of invasive epiglottitis resulting from Hib.[81,82]

BACTERIAL TRACHEITIS

Bacterial tracheitis usually presents as severe upper airway obstruction, most often in a child who has had viral croup for several days. Alternative names are *membranous laryngotracheobronchitis, pseudomembranous croup,* and *membranous croup.*[83]

Disease Mechanisms

Direct bacterial infection of the tracheal mucosa is caused by the organisms listed in Box 34-10. *S. aureus* is the most common bacteria reported.[84] Influenza virus, parainfluenza virus, and enterovirus have been isolated in children with bacterial tracheitis, suggesting that bacterial invasion may occur in an airway already inflamed by viral infection. Bacterial tracheitis is a recognized complication of measles, with a recent outbreak reported.[84a]

The bacterial infection causes a diffuse inflammatory process of the larynx, trachea, and bronchi with mucopurulent exudate and semiadherent "membranes" within the trachea. These membranes contain numerous neutrophils and cellular debris and cause major obstruction.

Clinical Manifestations

Bacterial tracheitis most commonly occurs in children in the age group vulnerable to viral croup. The initial clinical features are similar to those of viral croup, but there is a high fever (usually greater than 38.5° C), the child appears toxic, and there is severe airway obstruction. About half of cases

BOX 34-10
Causes of Bacterial Tracheitis

Common causes

Staphylococcus aureus
Haemophilus influenzae type b and nontypeable *Haemophilus influenzae*
Streptococcus pneumoniae
Klebsiella pneumoniae

Rare causes

Streptococcus pyogenes group A
Pseudomonas species
Moraxella catarrhalis

have clinical or radiographic evidence of pneumonia. A rare complication is toxic shock syndrome.

The differential diagnosis includes severe laryngotracheobronchitis (viral croup), laryngeal or tracheal foreign body aspiration, or epiglottitis. Bacterial tracheitis has a longer duration, a more typical barking cough than epiglottitis, and no drooling. Diphtheria was once a serious consideration as the most common cause of "membranous croup" that produces severe airway obstruction because of adherent membranes that separate from the airway wall with difficulty, causing bleeding.

Investigations. Bacterial cultures of tracheal secretions reveal the organism. The results from blood cultures are usually negative. White cell counts may be high or normal.

Endoscopy reveals thick mucopus and sloughed epithelium. The epithelium forms a sheetlike pseudomembrane that separates easily from the airway wall without hemorrhage and sometimes extends from the trachea to the major bronchi.

A lateral neck radiograph shows subglottic narrowing and often reveals findings of radiopaque material in the airway lumen (pseudomembrane).[85] This may be confused with foreign body.

Management

In a child suspected of having bacterial tracheitis, management should occur in a pediatric intensive care unit. Intubation is usually needed to relieve the airway obstruction, which takes days to resolve. Intermittent positive-pressure breathing is sometimes needed. Repeated suctioning is usually required because of the thick secretions and their tendency to form crusts, with intubation lasting 3 to 11 days. Sometimes, repeat endoscopic removal of the pseudomembrane is required. Occasionally, tracheostomy is needed if endotracheal tube management of secretions proves too difficult.

Nebulized epinephrine or corticosteroids do not relieve the acute airway obstruction. Intravenous antibiotics are vital, and should be directed initially against the four common pathogens until the results of tracheal cultures are known. The usual choice is oxacillin (150 mg/kg/day with four equal doses given every 6 hours) and a third-generation cephalosporin such as cefotaxime (150 mg/kg/day with four equal doses given every 6 hours) until the results of cultures and sensitivities are known. Alternatively, cefuroxime may be used. The duration of therapy should be at least 1 week.

With effective early management children should make a complete recovery from this severe illness.

RECURRENT RESPIRATORY PAPILLOMATOSIS

Juvenile recurrent respiratory papillomatosis (also known as *laryngeal papillomatosis*), a condition with benign, wartlike tumors in the respiratory tract, is usually associated with upper airway obstruction. It occurs at all ages, with about half of all cases appearing in the pediatric age group. It is characterized by the growth of papillomatous lesions, particularly in the larynx, that have a high rate of recurrence after excision.

Disease Mechanisms

It is now recognized that human papillomavirus (HPV) causes most cases of recurrent respiratory papillomatosis. The evidence for HPV etiology has been demonstrated by electron microscopy, immunocytochemistry, isolation of HPV sequences by Southern blot analysis, and in situ complementary deoxyribonucleic acid hybridization using as probes the radiolabeled deoxyribonucleic acids of HPV. Only types 6 and 11 of HPV have been identified by the latter technique.[86] The clinical presentation and course of the disease have not been definitively linked to a particular HPV type.

The replicating virus may cause overgrowth of squamous epithelial cells. The papillomata are multiple projections, each with a connective tissue stalk covered by well-differentiated stratified squamous epithelium. The viral antigen is localized in the nuclei of cells in the very superficial layers. The tumors are benign but present obstructive problems because of their localization in the vocal cords or other sites. At presentation, papillomata are usually present on one or both vocal cords with the anterior commissure, supraglottis, or subglottis also commonly affected.

There is debate about the mechanism of infection with HPV. The same types of HPV that cause perineal condylomata in women also cause juvenile recurrent respiratory papillomatosis. For a long time, it has been assumed that a child acquires the infection during the birth process from the mother with perineal condylomata. A minority of cases fit this mode of acquisition. However, there are many children in whom there is no evidence of maternal HPV infection. In these children the source of infection remains obscure. Host susceptibility has been investigated in a limited number of patients, and one child has been found to have IgG_2 subclass deficiency.[87]

Clinical Manifestations

Recurrent respiratory papillomatosis can occur at any age, with the youngest reported patient being 1 month of age.[88] In the pediatric age group, about half of patients have symptoms within the first year of life, although clinical recognition of the disease is often delayed. Patients usually come to medical attention late, with some degree of airway obstruction, including stridor, together with hoarseness or a weak cry. Life-threatening upper airway obstruction may occur. Although the lesions are usually localized within the larynx, spread to other areas (pharynx, esophagus, trachea, and lung parenchyma) may occur and indicates a more pessimistic outlook.[88] When the lung parenchyma is involved, death is the most common outcome; papillomata may destroy lung tissues as they grow, commonly with multiple nodular and cystic lesions. Pneumothorax can occur after the development of cystic pneumatoceles, presumably from the ball-valve effect of a nodular lesion.[89]

The most usual course of the disease is for the papilloma to continue to grow locally despite surgical removal and without significant spread. Over time the majority of cases in children undergo spontaneous remission (analogous to skin warts). It was traditionally believed that the onset of puberty is associated with remission, although this view has been challenged.

Malignant change to squamous cell carcinoma has been reported, although the majority occurs in adults. The now-abandoned treatment of these lesions with radiotherapy has been implicated in ensuing malignancies in the pediatric age group.

The condition is diagnosed by inspection of the larynx, either by indirect means such as fiberoptic laryngoscopy in an office or by more formal laryngoscopy and bronchoscopy when tissue biopsies can be taken. The virus signal can be identified in the tissue biopsy, but its intensity does not generally correlate with the clinical behavior of the disease.

Multiple endoscopies are usually required for further investigation and management, and flexible bronchoscopy is the method of choice for surveillance. Although ultrasound examination of the airway correlates with laryngoscopic findings, it is seldom used in clinical practice.

Management

Recurrent respiratory papillomatosis is frustrating to treat because lesions are often recurrent and sometimes aggressive. The focus of management is to ensure a safe airway without causing irreversible long-term scarring, especially affecting the voice. Total removal of the disease is impossible in most cases because undeclared viral infection occurs in apparently normal adjacent areas and the degree of destruction necessary to clear the field would in most cases require too great a degree of tissue damage.

In particularly aggressive phases of the disease, total removal may require laryngoscopies with excision as often as twice a week. The frequency of the surgery is dictated entirely by how rapidly the papilloma regrows and is individualized for each patient. All patients can expect multiple endoscopies and surgical removal (the record being 341).

The most widely used surgical method for removing recurrent respiratory papilloma is use of the carbon dioxide laser, which acts as a very precise "knife," vaporizing the papilloma, minimizing damage to the underlying larynx. However, it does not prevent regrowth any better than the older surgical methods, such as direct removal or suction diathermy. In the hands of experienced endoscopists, there is a low to moderate incidence of laryngeal scarring.[90] Photodynamic therapy has been used, pretreating the patient with a hematoporphyrin derivative and then subjecting the lesion to an argon dye laser beam at a 630-nm wavelength.[91] If possible, tracheotomy should be avoided because of seeding of the disease to the tracheotomy site.

Historically, clinicians have used numerous other therapeutic modalities, including cryotherapy, painting of the lesions with podophyllin and antimetabolites, vaccines, and immunotherapy. Overall, the results have been poor.

Interferon-α with surgery has been used in recurrent respiratory papillomatosis and has had somewhat disappointing results. Most studies have shown a dramatic decrease in the frequency of regrowth immediately after beginning such treatment. Unfortunately the initial benefit has not been sustained, and in most cases, regrowth gradually occurs. In one large multicenter, randomized study,[92] interferon was neither of curative nor of substantial value as an adjunctive agent after 1 year of treatment. In only a few patients has the disease been eradicated. In a more recent study of 66 patients,[93] there was a 33% sustained complex remission rate, leading the authors to suggest a 6-month trial of interferon-α in children requiring surgery at 2- to 3-month intervals. Although this agent is moderately well tolerated, the almost universal side effects of mild influenza-like symptoms are unpleasant, and the frequent parenteral mode of delivery is disliked, particularly in the younger age group. Other side effects commonly seen are anorexia, palmar erythema, and a mild rise in the levels of transaminase. There is one report of medication-induced systemic lupus erythematosus after interferon treatment of juvenile recurrent respiratory papillomatosis for 7 years.[94] Interferon therapy may be used in particularly aggressive disease. In less severe cases, its use is questionable; it should not be continued beyond 12 months unless the disease responds.

Acyclovir has been tried in a small number of cases, although its mechanism of action remains obscure.[95,96] It may decrease the extent of respiratory papillomatosis in patients with recalcitrant disease, but its beneficial effect appears to be insufficient to counteract rebound disease when interferon is abruptly stopped. The place for acyclovir in long-term management has yet to be established.

REFERENCES

The Common Cold

1. Tyrrel DA, Cohen S, Schlarb JE: Signs and symptoms in common colds, *Epidemiol Infect* 111:143-156, 1993.
2. Sperber SJ, Hayden FG: Chemotherapy of rhinovirus colds, *Antimicrob Agents Chemother* 32:409-419, 1988 (review).
3. Blake KD: Dangers of common cold treatment in children, *Lancet* 341:640, 1993 (letter).
4. Smith MBH, Feldman W: Over-the-counter cold medications: a critical review of clinical trials between 1950 and 1991, *JAMA* 269:2258-2263, 1993 (review).
5. Hutton N, Wilson MH, Mellits ED, Baumgardner R, Wilson LS, Bonnucceli C, Holtzman NA, DeAngelis C: Effectiveness of an antihistamine-decongestant combination for young children with the common cold: a randomized, controlled clinical trial, *J Pediatr* 118:125-130, 1991.
6. Bluestone CD, Connell JT, Doyle WJ, Hayden FG, Naclerio RM: Symposium: questioning the efficacy and safety of antihistamines in the treatment of upper respiratory tract infection, *Pediatr Infect Dis J* 7:215-242, 1988.
7. Hayden FG, Kaiser DL, Albrecht JK: Intranasal recombinant alfa-2b interferon treatment of naturally occurring common colds, *Antimicrob Agents Chemother* 32:224-230, 1988.
8. Farr BM, Conner EM, Betts RF, Oleske J, Minnefor A, Gwaltney JM: Two randomized controlled trials of zinc gluconate lozenge therapy of experimentally induced rhinovirus colds, *Antimicrob Agents Chemother* 31:1183-1187, 1987.

8a. Farr BM, Hendley JO, Kaiser DL, Gwaltney JM: Two randomized controlled trials of virucidal nasal tissues in the prevention of natural upper respiratory infections, *Am J Epidemiol* 128:1162-1172, 1988.

Pharyngitis and Tonsillitis

9. Stenfors LE, Raisanen S: The membranous tonsillitis during infectious mononucleosis is nevertheless of bacterial origin, *Int J Pediatr Otorhinolaryngol* 26:149-155, 1993.
10. McMillan JA, Weiner LB, Higgins AM, Lamparella VJ: Pharyngitis associated with herpes simplex virus in college students, *Pediatr Infect Dis J* 12:280-284, 1993.
11. Gerber MA, Randolph MF, Martin NJ, Rizkallah MF, Cleary PP, Kaplan EL, Ayoub EM: Community-wide outbreak of group G streptococcal pharyngitis, *Pediatrics* 87:598-603, 1991.
12. Karpathios T, Drakonaki S, Zervoudaki A, Coupari G, Fretzayas A, Kremastinos J, Thomaidis T: *Arcanobacterium haemolyticum* in children with presumed streptococcal pharyngotonsillitis or scarlet fever, *J Pediatr* 121:735-737, 1992.
13. Middleton DB, D'Amico F, Merenstein JH: Standardized symptomatic treatment versus penicillin as initial therapy for streptococcal pharyngitis, *J Pediatr* 113:1089-1094, 1988.
14. Marcovitch H: Sore throats, *Arch Dis Child* 65:249-250, 1990.

15. Markowitz M, Gerber MA, Kaplan EL: Treatment of streptococcal pharyngotonsillitis: reports of penicillin's demise are premature, *J Pediatr* 123:679-685, 1993 (review).
16. Committee on Infectious Diseases, American Academy of Pediatrics: *Report of the Committee on Infectious Diseases,* ed 22, Elk Grove Village, Ill, 1991, American Academy of Pediatrics.
17. Bass JW: Antibiotic management of group A streptococcal pharyngotonsillitis, *Pediatr Infect Dis J* 10:S43-S49, 1991 (review).
18. Pichichero ME: Cephalosporins are superior to penicillin for treatment of streptococcal tonsillopharyngitis: is the difference worth it? *Pediatr Infect Dis J* 12:268-274, 1993 (review).
19. Snellman LW, Stang HJ, Stang JM, Johnson DR, Kaplan EL: Duration of positive throat cultures for group A streptococci after initiation of antibiotic therapy, *Pediatrics* 91:1166-1170, 1993.

Retropharyngeal, Parapharyngeal, and Peritonsillar Abscess

20. Brook I: Microbiology of retropharyngeal abscesses in children, *Am J Dis Child* 141:202-204, 1987.
21. Jokipii AMM, Jokipii L, Sipila P, Jokinen K: Semiquantitative culture results and pathogenic significance of obligate anaerobes in peritonsillar abscesses, *J Clin Microbiol* 26:957-961, 1988.
22. Ophir D, Bawnik J, Poria Y, Porat M, Marshak G: Peritonsillar abscess: a prospective evaluation of outpatient management by needle aspiration, *Arch Otolaryngol Head Neck Surg* 114:661-663, 1988.
23. Stringer SP, Schaefer SD, Close LG: A randomized trial for outpatient management of peritonsillar abscess, *Arch Otolaryngol Head Neck Surg* 114:296-298, 1988.

Otitis Media

24. Sung BS, Chonmaitree T, Broemeling LD, Owen MJ, Patel JA, Hedgpeth DC, Howie VM: Association of rhinovirus infection with poor bacteriological outcome of bacterial-viral otitis media, *Clin Infect Dis* 17:38-42, 1993.
25. Chonmaitree T, Owen MJ, Patel JA, Hedgpeth D, Horlick D, Howie VM: Presence of cytomegalovirus and herpes simplex virus in middle ear fluids from children with acute otitis media, *Clin Infect Dis* 15:650-653, 1992.
26. Burton DM, Seid AB, Kearns DB, Pransky SM: Neonatal otitis media: an update, *Arch Otolaryngol Head Neck Surg* 119:672-675, 1993.
27. Duncan B, Ey J, Holberg CJ, Wright AL, Martinez FD, Taussig LM: Exclusive breast-feeding for at least 4 months protects against otitis media, *Pediatrics* 91:867-872, 1993.
28. Giles M, Asher I: Prevalence and natural history of otitis media with perforation in Maori school children, *J Laryngol Otol* 105:257-260, 1991.
29. Baker RB: Is ear pulling associated with ear infection? *Pediatrics* 90:1006-1007, 1992.
30. Giebink GS, Canafax DM, Kempthorne J: Antimicrobial treatment of acute otitis media, *J Pediatr* 119:495-500, 1991 (review).
31. Bluestone CD: Review of cefixime in the treatment of otitis media in infants and children, *Pediatr Infect Dis J* 12:75-82, 1993.
32. Green SM, Rothrock SG: Single dose intramuscular ceftriaxone for acute otitis media in children, *Pediatrics* 91:23-30, 1993.
33. Carlin SA, Marchant CD, Shurin PA, Johnson CE, Super DM, Rehmus JM: Host factors and early therapeutic response in acute otitis media, *J Pediatr* 118:178-183, 1991.
34. Cantekin EI, Mandel EM, Bluestone CD, Rockette HE, Paradise JL, Stool SE, Fria TJ, Rogers KD: Lack of efficacy of a decongestant-antihistamine combination for otitis media with effusion ("secretory" otitis media) in children, *N Engl J Med* 308:297-301, 1983.
35. Glue ear, *Lancet,* 340:1324-1325, 1992 (editorial).
36. Daly K, Giebink SG, Batalden PB, Anderson RS, Le CT, Lindgren B: Resolution of otitis media with effusion with the use of stepped treatment regimen of trimethoprim-sulfamethoxazole and prednisone, *Pediatr Infect Dis J* 10:500-506, 1991.
37. Rosenfeld RM: New concepts for steroid use in otitis media with effusion, *Clin Pediatr* 31:615-621, 1992.
38. Blanshard JD, Maw AR, Bawden R: Conservative treatment of otitis media with effusion by autoinflation of the middle ear, *Clin Otolaryngol* 18:188-192, 1993.

Adenoidectomy and Tonsillectomy

39. Paradise JL, Bluestone CD, Bachman RZ, Colborn DK, Bernard BS, Taylor FH, Rogers KD, Schwarzbach RH, Stool SE, Friday GA, Smith IH, Saez CA: Efficacy of tonsillectomy for recurrent throat infection in severely affected children: results of parallel randomized and nonrandomized clinical trials, *N Engl J Med* 310:674-683, 1984.
40. Brouilette RT, Fernbach SK, Hunt CE: Obstructive sleep apnea in infants and children, *J Pediatr* 100:31-40, 1982.
41. Gates GA, Avery CA, Prihoda TJ, Cooper JC: Effectiveness of adenoidectomy and tympanostomy tubes in the treatment of chronic otitis media with effusion, *N Engl J Med* 317:1444-1451, 1987.

Sinusitis

42. Tinkleman DG, Silk HJ: Clinical and bacteriologic features of chronic sinusitis in children, *Am J Dis Child* 143:938-941, 1989.
43. Wald ER, Guerra N, Byers C: Upper respiratory tract infections in young children: duration of and frequency of complications, *Pediatrics* 87:129-133, 1991.
44. Wald ER: Sinusitis in children, *N Engl J Med* 326:319-323, 1992 (review).
45. Rosenfeld EA, Rowley AH: Intracranial complications of sinusitis, other than meningitis, in children: 12 year review, *Clin Infect Dis* 18:750-754, 1994.
46. Irvin CG: Sinusitis and asthma: an animal model, *J Allergy Clin Immunol* 90:521-523, 1992.
47. Bardin PG, van Heerden BB, Joubert JR: Absence of pulmonary aspiration of sinus contents in patients with asthma and sinusitis, *J Allergy Clin Immunol* 86(1):82-88, 1990.
48. Barnes PD, Wilkinson RH: Radiographic diagnosis of sinusitis in children, *Pediatr Infect Dis J* 10:628-629, 1991.
49. Lusk RP, ed: *Pediatric sinusitis,* New York, 1992, Raven, p 17.

Viral Croup

50. Newth CJL, Levison H, Bryan AC: The respiratory status of children with croup, *J Pediatr* 81:1068-1073, 1972.
50a. Davison FW: Acute laryngeal obstruction in children, *JAMA* 171:1301-1305, 1959.
51. Wagener JS, Landau LI, Olinsky A, Phelan PD: Management of children hospitalized for laryngotracheobronchitis, *Pediatr Pulmonol* 2:159-162, 1986.
52. Sivan Y, Deakers TW, Newth CJL: Thoracoabdominal asynchrony in acute upper airway obstruction in small children, *Am Rev Respir Dis* 142:540-544, 1990.
53. Kanter RK, Watchko JF: Pulmonary edema associated with upper airway obstruction, *Am J Dis Child* 138:356-358, 1984.
54. Cohen B, Dunt D: Recurrent and non-recurrent croup: an epidemiological study, *Aust Paediatr J* 24:339-342, 1988.
55. Zach MS: Airway reactivity in recurrent croup, *Eur J Respir Dis* 64(suppl 128):81-87, 1983.
56. Henry R: Moist air in the treatment of laryngotracheitis, *Arch Dis Child* 58:577, 1983.
57. Kairys SW, Olmstead EM, O'Connor GT: Steroid treatment of laryngotracheitis: a meta-analysis of the evidence from randomized trials, *Pediatrics* 83:683-693, 1989.
58. Tibballs J, Shann FA, Landau LI: Placebo-controlled trial of prednisolone in children intubated for croup, *Lancet* 340:745-748, 1992.
59. Kuusela A-L, Vesikari T: A randomized double-blind, placebo-controlled trial of dexamethasone and racemic epinephrine in the treatment of croup, *Acta Paediatr Scand* 77:99-104, 1988.
60. Super DM, Cartelli NA, Brooks LJ, Lembo RM, Kumar ML: A prospective randomized double-blind study to evaluate the effect of dexamethasone in acute laryngotracheitis, *J Pediatr* 115:323-329, 1989.
61. Skolnik NS: Treatment of croup, *Am J Dis Child* 143:1045-1049, 1989 (review).
61a. Geelhold GC, Macdonald WBG: Oral dexamethasone in the treatment of croup: 0.15 mg/kg versus 0.3 mg/kg versus 0.6 mg/kg, *Pediatr Pulmonol* 20:362-368, 1995.
62. Meuleman J, Katz P: The immunological effects, kinetics, and use of glucocorticosteroids, *Med Clin North Am* 69:805-817, 1985.
62a. Eden A, Larkin VP: Corticosteroid treatment of croup, *Pediatrics* 33:768-769, 1964.
63. Husby S, Agertoft L, Mortensen S, Pedersen S: Treatment of croup with nebulised steroid (budesonide): a double blind, placebo controlled study, *Arch Dis Child* 68:352-355, 1993.
64. Klassen TP, Feldman ME, Watters LK, Sutcliffe T, Rowe PC: Nebulized budesonide for children with mild-to-moderate croup, *N Engl J Med* 331:285-289, 1994.
64a. Geelhold GC, Macdonald WBG: Oral and inhaled steroids in croup: a randomized, placebo-controlled trial, *Pediatr Pulmonol* 20:355-361, 1995.
65. Landau LI, Geelhoed CG: Aerosolized steroids for croup, *N Engl J Med* 331:322-323, 1994.

66. Taussig LM, Castro O, Beaudry PH, Fox WW, Bureau M: Treatment of laryngotracheobronchitis (croup): use of intermittent positive-pressure breathing and racemic epinephrine, *Am J Dis Child* 129:790-793, 1975.
67. Fogel JM, Berg J, Gerber MA, Sherter CB: Racemic epinephrine in the treatment of croup: nebulization alone versus nebulization with intermittent positive pressure breathing, *J Pediatr* 101:1028-1031, 1982.
68. Waisman Y, Klein BL, Boenning DA, Young GM, Chamberlain JM, O'Donnell R, Ochenschlager DW: Prospective randomized double-blind study comparing L-epinephrine and racemic epinephrine aerosols in the treatment of laryngotracheitis (croup), *Pediatrics* 89:302-305, 1992.

Epiglottitis

69. Lacroix J, Ahronheim G, Arcand P, Gauthier M, Rousseau E, Girouard G, Lamarre A: Group A streptococcal supraglottitis, *J Pediatr* 109:20-24, 1986.
70. Rosenfeld RM, Fletcher MA, Marban SL: Acute epiglottitis in a newborn infant, *Pediatr Infect Dis J* 11:594-595, 1992.
71. Grattan-Smith T, Forer M, Kilham H, Gillis J: Viral supraglottitis, *J Pediatr* 110:434-435, 1987.
72. Nadel S, Offit PA, Hodinka RL, Gesser RM, Bell LM: Upper airway obstruction in association with perinatally acquired herpes simplex virus infection, *J Pediatr* 120:127-129, 1992.
73. Narasimhan N, van Stralen DW, Perkin RM: Acute supraglottitis caused by *Varicella, Pediatr Infect Dis J* 12:619-620, 1993.
74. Balsam D, Sorrano D, Barax CH: *Candida* epiglottitis presenting as stridor in a child with HIV infection, *Pediatr Radiol* 22:235-236, 1992.
75. Hanna JN, Wild BE, Sly PD: The epidemiology of acute epiglottitis in children in Western Australia, *J Pediatr Child Health* 28:459-464, 1992.
76. Molteni RA: Epiglottitis: incidence of extraepiglottic infection—report of 72 cases and review of the literature, *Pediatrics* 58:526-531, 1976.
77. Mauro RD, Poole SR, Lockhart CH: Differentiation of epiglottitis from laryngotracheitis in the child with stridor, *Am J Dis Child* 142:679-682, 1988.
78. Diamant EP, Dische RM, Barzilai A, Hodes DS, Peters VB: Chronic epiglottitis in a child with acquired immunodeficiency syndrome, *Pediatr Infect Dis J* 11:770-771, 1992.
79. Knight GJ, Harris MA, Parbari M, O'Callaghan MJ, Masters IB: Single daily dose ceftriaxone therapy in epiglottitis, *J Paediatr Child Health* 28:220-222, 1992.
80. Gilbert GL, MacInnes SJ, Guise IA: Rifampicin prophylaxis for throat carriage of *Haemophilus influenzae* type b in patients with invasive disease and their contacts, *Br Med J* 302:1432-1435, 1991.
81. Wenger JD, Pierce R, Deaver KA, Plikaytis BD, Facklam RR, Broome CV, *Haemophilus influenzae* Vaccine Efficacy Study Group: Efficacy of *Haemophilus influenzae* type b polysaccharide-diphtheria toxoid conjugate vaccine in US children aged 18-59 months, *Lancet* 338:395-398, 1991.
82. Broadhurst LE, Erickson RL, Kelley PW: Decreases in invasive *Haemophilus influenzae* diseases in US army children, 1984 through 1991, *JAMA* 269:227-231, 1993.

Bacterial Tracheitis

83. Nelson WE: Bacterial croup, *J Pediatr* 105:52-55, 1984.
84. Henry RL, Mellis CM, Benjamin B: Pseudomembranous croup, *Arch Dis Child* 58:180-183, 1983.
84a. Manning SC, Ridenour B, Brown OE, Squires J: An epidemic of upper airway obstruction, *Otolaryngol Head Neck Surg* 105:415-418, 1991.
85. Han BK, Dunbar JS, Striker TW: Membranous laryngotracheobronchitis (membranous croup), *Am J Roentgenol* 133:53-58, 1979.

Recurrent Respiratory Papillomatosis

86. Levi JE, Delcelo R, Alberti VN, Torloni H, Villa LL: Human papillomavirus DNA in respiratory papillomatosis detected by in situ hybridisation and the polymerase chain reaction, *Am J Pathol* 135:1179-1184, 1989.
87. Perrick D, Wray BB, Leffell MS, Harmon JD, Porubsky ES: Evaluation of immunocompetency in juvenile laryngeal papillomatosis, *Ann Allergy* 65:69-72, 1990.
88. Quiney RE, Hall D, Croft CB: Laryngeal papillomatosis: analysis of 113 patients, *Clin Otolaryngol* 14:217-225, 1989.
89. Anderson KC, Roy TM, Fields CL, Collins LC: Juvenile laryngeal papillomatosis: a new complication, *South Med J* 86:447-449, 1993.
90. Saleh EM: Complications of treatment of recurrent laryngeal papillomatosis with the carbon dioxide laser in children, *J Laryngol Otol* 106:715-718, 1992.
91. Abramson AL, Shikowitz MJ, Mullooly VM, Steinberg BM, Amella CA, Rothstein HR: Clinical effects of photodynamic therapy on recurrent laryngeal papillomas, *Arch Otolaryngol Head Neck Surg* 118:25-29, 1992.
92. Healy GB, Gelber RD, Trowbridge AL, Grundfast KM, Ruben RJ, Price KN: Treatment of recurrent respiratory papillomatosis with human leukocyte interferon, *N Engl J Med* 319:401-407, 1988.
93. Leventhal MD, Kashima HK, Mounts P, Thurmond L, Chapman S, Buckley S, Wold D, Papilloma Study Group: Long-term response of recurrent respiratory papillomatosis to treatment with lymphoblastoid interferon alfa-N1, *N Engl J Med* 325:613-617, 1991.
94. Tolaymat A, Leventhal B, Sakarcan A, Kashima H, Monteiro C: Systemic lupus erythematosus in a child receiving long-term interferon therapy, *J Pediatr* 120:429-432, 1992.
95. Aguado DL, Pinero BP, Betancor L, Mendez A, Banales EC: Acyclovir in the treatment of laryngeal papillomatosis, *Int J Pediatr Otorhinolaryngol* 21:269-274, 1991.
96. Endres DR, Bauman NM, Burke D, Smith RJ: Acyclovir in the treatment of recurrent respiratory papillomatosis: a pilot study, *Ann Otol Rhinol Laryngol* 103:301-304, 1994.

CHAPTER 35

Acute, Chronic, and Wheezy Bronchitis

Erika von Mutius and Wayne J. Morgan

Bronchitis is a clinical respiratory problem that is common in childhood. It occurs as an acute illness generally secondary to a viral upper respiratory tract infection as well as a chronic component of underlying asthma, cystic fibrosis, foreign body aspiration, immunodeficiency, immotile cilia syndrome, and other conditions. Low-grade airway inflammation occurs secondary to inhalable noxious agents such as passive smoke or various environmental pollutants. In children, unlike in adults, chronic bronchitis per se is not considered a final diagnosis.

Because of its frequent occurrence, it would seem that bronchitis should be easily characterized and defined. However, the primary and at times exclusive manifestation of the disease is cough, a symptom of little diagnostic specificity. No noninvasive laboratory tests are available to specifically diagnose bronchitis in young children. The self-limited course of acute bronchitis as well as the missing definition of *chronic bronchitis* have limited pathologic investigation and characterization of the disease in childhood. In adults, *chronic bronchitis* is defined as a condition of chronic or recurrent productive cough that is present on most days for 3 months a year for 2 years.[1] Whether this definition can be applied to childhood bronchitis remains unclear. Thus no generally agreed-on definition of *acute, chronic, recurrent,* or *wheezy bronchitis* in childhood exists.[2] Furthermore, the clinical presentation of children with asthma, wheezy bronchitis, and recurrent and chronic bronchitis overlaps considerably. A diagnosis of bronchitis should therefore cautiously be considered.[3] It has the potential to divert the pediatrician from detecting a more specific respiratory condition.

Several studies have demonstrated the importance of childhood respiratory problems in the development of chronic pulmonary disease in adulthood.[4-7] Despite these limitations, it seems important to understand bronchitis in its various forms. This chapter attempts to provide this perspective by focusing on acute bronchitis, the symptom complex of chronic bronchitis, and the relationship among asthma, wheezy bronchitis, and chronic bronchitis.

ACUTE BRONCHITIS

Acute Viral Bronchitis

Viruses produce most attacks of acute bronchitis.[8] Rhinovirus, respiratory syncytial virus, influenza virus, parainfluenza virus, adenovirus, rubeola virus, and the paramyxoviruses all have been identified as etiologic agents.[9,10] Although the clinical pattern of viral bronchitis is similar regardless of the causative organism, certain clinical features help determine the etiology. Acute bronchitis almost universally occurs with measles, the respiratory symptoms being associated with significant conjunctivitis and high fever and preceding the appearance of the pathognomonic Koplik's spots and exanthem. Respiratory syncytial virus in infants is likely to induce moderate to severe bronchiolitis. Influenza virus is frequently associated with moderately high fever and myalgias. Attacks of acute bronchitis can occur at any time during the year but are most common in the winter, when the respiratory virus season peaks.[11] A knowledge of which pathogens are currently endemic is helpful but not conclusive etiologic evidence.

Because acute bronchitis is usually a mild and self-limited condition, the pathology is ill-defined because of the lack of tissue to study. Mucous gland activity increases, and desquamation of the ciliated epithelium occurs. Infiltration of polymorphonuclear leukocytes into the airway walls and lumen contributes to a purulent appearance of the secretions. Because this leukocytic migration is a nonspecific response to airway damage, purulent sputum does not necessarily imply bacterial superinfection.[12]

Acute bronchitis usually follows symptoms of upper respiratory tract infection such as serous rhinitis and pharyngitis. The cough usually appears 3 to 4 days after the rhinitis. The cough is initially harsh and dry but frequently evolves into a loose cough with significant sputum production. Because young children do not expectorate but generally swallow the mucus, vomiting associated with cough paroxysms can occur. Chest pain secondary to a progressive severity and production of sputum with cough may be a prominent complaint in older children.

Auscultation of the chest is usually unremarkable in the early stages. As the cough progresses, variable rhonchi, harsh breath sounds, wheezes, or a combination thereof may be heard. Crackles are infrequent. Chest radiographs are normal or may have increased bronchial markings. Generally, the symptoms resolve within 10 to 14 days. If the clinical signs persist beyond 2 to 3 weeks, a chronic condition should be suspected. Occasionally, a secondary bacterial infection occurs.

Therapy for acute viral bronchitis is largely supportive. In fact, most patients recover uneventfully without any treatment. Adequate rest, proper humidification of ambient air, adequate fluid intake, and treatment of fever with acetaminophen, if necessary, are sufficient in other patients. The use of cough suppressants should be discouraged and cough encouraged because of the productive nature of the cough. Antibiotics should be reserved for conditions in which a bacterial infection is highly suspected or preferably has been proved.

Acute Bacterial Bronchitis

Mycoplasma pneumoniae has occasionally been identified as an organism producing acute bronchitis in school-age children and adolescents.[10,13] There are no characteristic clinical findings. Positive cold hemagglutination titers associated with a concomitant rise in specific *Mycoplasma* titers confirm the diagnosis. Treatment with erythromycin or tetracycline in children over 9 years of age can be effective.

In unimmunized children, infections with *Bordetella pertussis* and *Corynebacterium diphtheriae* are associated with a characteristic tracheobronchitis. During the catarrhal stage of pertussis, symptoms of upper respiratory tract infection, such as rhinitis, conjunctivitis, low-grade fever, and cough, predominate. As the paroxysmal stage develops, episodes of coughing increase in number and severity. Characteristically, repetitive series of forceful coughs during a single expiration are followed by a sudden massive inspiratory effort, which produces the whoop. This cough eventually dislodges thick, tenacious mucus. Posttussive emesis associated with the paroxysms is a characteristic symptom even in the child without whoop. The pathologic findings of pertussis bronchitis include infiltration of the mucosa with lymphocytes and polymorphonuclear leukocytes. Furthermore, necrosis of the midzonal and basilar layers of the mucosa has been observed. Leukocytosis with an absolute lymphocytosis occurs characteristically at the end of the catarrhal stage and the beginning of the paroxysmal stage. Culture and fluorescent antibody tests of secretions can confirm the diagnosis. Treatment of pertussis is largely supportive. Erythromycin may eliminate pertussis organisms from the nasopharynx within 3 to 4 days, thereby decreasing spread of the disease. Given within 14 days of the onset of illness, erythromycin may abort pertussis. However, once paroxysms of cough develop, this medication has little effect on the course of the illness.[14]

Progressive cough and lung disease starting at a few weeks of age in conjunction with conjunctivitis or blepharitis is highly suggestive of chlamydial infection. Diagnosis can be made by culture, fluorescent antibody, or serology studies, and therapy with erythromycin is usually effective. Infection with *Ureaplasma* organisms may closely mimic chlamydial disease.[15] Although difficult to diagnose, these infections may respond to a therapeutic trial with erythromycin.

CHRONIC, RECURRENT, AND WHEEZY BRONCHITIS

The persistence of signs and symptoms of acute bronchitis or frequent recurrences should initiate an attempt to identify an underlying illness. Clinicians do not generally agree on a definition of chronic or recurrent bronchitis in childhood. Factors that must be defined are where the isolated, recurrent episodes end and the chronic state begins and how many episodes are "too many." For the purpose of this discussion, *chronic bronchitis* is defined as the symptom complex of chronic (greater than 1 month) or recurrent (at least four) episodes of productive cough per year that may be associated with wheezing or crackles on auscultation.

The chronicity and recurrence of the condition suggests either that an endogenous susceptibility or increased response to acute airway injury exists or that continuing exposure to noxious environmental agents produces the symptoms. Host factors include a variety of underlying illnesses, whereas exogenous factors affect susceptible and normal airways as well. An airway that suffers an insult responds in a limited number of ways.[3] Inflammation, edema, increased sputum production, and disordered mucus clearance occur in varying degrees and produce cough. Depending on the severity of the airway damage and the resulting increase in airflow resistance, wheezing may also be present. In subjects with bronchial hyperresponsiveness, acute airway injury may furthermore trigger bronchial obstruction, also leading to cough and wheeze. Thus cough and wheezing are nonspecific symptoms that reflect airway damage and narrowing without regard to mechanism and etiology.

This overlap of syndromes has created considerable confusion in clinical as well as in epidemiologic studies of chronic bronchitis in childhood and has limited assessment of its prevalence. When restricting the definition of *chronic bronchitis* to a productive cough that received medical therapy and lasted more than 2 weeks, Peat et al[16] found an overall prevalence of 14% to 24% in Australian children. Other definitions of *chronic* or *recurrent bronchitis* have led to widely different estimates of its prevalence (Table 35-1). The overlap of syndromes and the lack of tissue studied have furthermore hampered pathologic investigation of chronic bronchitis in childhood.

Clinical Assessment and Differential Diagnosis

The diagnosis of chronic bronchitis should occur in two phases (Box 35-1). The first is consideration and identification of several well-defined respiratory disorders according to a staged management protocol (Box 35-2). The second but simultaneous phase is elimination or modification of exogenous factors that produce or maintain the child's illness. Diagnostic tests selected on the bases of the child's history, the incidence of the suspected disease, the morbidity to the patient, and the costs are performed. At the same time, the parents are encouraged to avoid exposing the child to irritants such as cigarette smoke or recurrent viral respiratory tract infections in daycare centers.

Phase I: Differential Diagnosis

Asthma

Asthma is the most likely diagnosis in a child with recurrent or chronic bronchitis. Burrows and Lebowitz[17] showed in an epidemiologic survey in the United States that 74% of children with a diagnosis of chronic bronchitis were wheezing. Moreover, skin test reactivity was associated with symptoms of bronchitis. When subjects in whom asthma was first diagnosed between the ages of 10 and 20 were prospectively investigated, a prior diagnosis of chronic bronchitis was found to be an independent risk factor for asthma, more reflecting the natural history of the disease than estimating the risk for developing it.[18] Boule et al[19] found decreased dynamic compliance with evidence of air trapping and increased airway reactivity in 29 children with recurrent bronchitis. Conversely, chronic cough in children without any clinical evidence of asthma or another respiratory disease has been associated with exercise-induced airway hyperreactivity.[20] Both the cough and airway hyperreactivity were relieved by oral theophylline therapy. This overlap of the clinical presentations of asthma and chronic bronchitis has made the distinction between these conditions very difficult.

Wheeze in relation to viral infections has been labeled *wheezy bronchitis* only in an attempt to differentiate it from asthma because of additional precipitating factors and different age distributions of the disease.[21] Recent evidence suggests that it may be appropriate to use the term *asthma* to describe most, if not all, wheezing illness in childhood. There are several reasons for this approach. In an Australian study, both children with wheezy bronchitis (wheeze with viral infections only) and children with asthma differed from a control population in several atopic markers.[22] Furthermore, no difference in the genetic backgrounds of either condition could be found.[23] Finally, the clear demonstration that asthma was both underdiagnosed and undertreated[24,25] was in part held to be attributable to the use of terms such as *wheezy* or *asthmatoid bronchitis*. The authors therefore discouraged a label other than *asthma*. The prognosis and pathophysiologic features of each condition may differ, however. The outcome of childhood wheeze after 25 years was significantly worse for adults with a diagnosis of childhood asthma compared with those with a diagnosis of wheezy bronchitis (i.e., wheezing with viral infections only).[26] Lower levels of lung function in the first months of life precede and predict the development of wheezing respiratory illnesses during the first 3 years of life.[27-29] Thus in a certain number of infants, wheezing respiratory illnesses may rely on anatomic abnormalities such as initial

Table 35-1 Prevalence of Childhood Bronchitis

REFERENCE	STUDY	PREVALENCE	ASTHMA : BRONCHITIS RATIO
Burrows et al[5]	1977: Arizona children (chronic)	46.4%	1:1.6
Peat et al[16]	1980: Sydney children (acute and chronic)	20%	1:3
Dockery et al[69]	1980/1981: children living in six U.S. cities (acute and chronic)	3.6% to 10.0%	1:0.7 to 1:2.4
von Mutius et al[76]	1989/1990: East German children (recurrent)	30.9%	1:4.2
von Mutius et al[74]	1989/1990: West German children (recurrent)	15.9%	1:1.7

BOX 35-1
Differential Diagnosis of Chronic and Recurrent Bronchitis

Phase I: specific etiologies

Asthma
Preexisting lung disease
- Respiratory distress syndrome and bronchopulmonary dysplasia
- Postinfectious bronchiectasis

Cystic fibrosis
Foreign body aspiration
- Intrathoracic or extrathoracic airway
- Esophagus

Aspiration syndromes
- Abnormal enteropulmonary communications (e.g., laryngeal cleft)
- Dysfunction of swallowing
- Gastroesophageal reflux

Airway compression
- Weakened wall (e.g., tracheomalacia)
- Extrinsic compression (e.g., vascular ring)

Congenital heart disease
Immunodeficiency
Primary cilia abnormalities

Phase II: nonspecific airway irritation

Exposure to recurrent respiratory tract infections in day-care centers
Cigarette smoke
- Passive smoke exposure
- Active smoking

Air pollution
- Outdoor secondary to particulate matter, automobile exhaust, and other pollutants
- Indoor secondary to wood burning, irritants, and chemicals

BOX 35-2
Diagnostic Evaluation

Initial assessment

History
- Assessment of the presence of cough, wheezing, and lower respiratory tract infections
- Identification of specific symptoms of possibly underlying respiratory conditions

Physical examination
- Assessment of general well-being, height, weight, chest circumference, and signs of chronic airway disease
- Notice of worrisome signs such as clubbing

Laboratory
- No tests in acute bronchitis
- Complete blood count and differential, immunoglobulin E level, sweat chloride test, and chest radiograph
- Skin prick tests to assess atopy and specific allergens
- Skin tests for tuberculosis and fungal infection
- Baseline pulmonary function testing and response to bronchodilators or bronchial challenge
- Chlamydial culture, serology, or both tests in infants younger than 6 months of age

Therapy
- Bronchodilators
- Chest physiotherapy and management of gastroesophageal reflux
- Trial of erythromycin in infants and school-age children

Follow-up

Interim history
- Response to therapeutic trial
- Repeat of questions about specific symptoms of possible underlying respiratory conditions

Interim physical examination
- Improvement of findings after therapeutic trial
- Unexpected changes in pulmonary status

Laboratory
- Barium swallow, high-kilovolt airway films
- Measurement of levels of immunoglobulin G and its subclasses
- Assessment of cilia

Therapy
- If patient is doing well, continuation of bronchodilators and physiotherapy for 1 month and then consideration of trial off medication
- If patient is not doing well, consideration of parental compliance by starting theophylline and measuring the medication level
- If patient is not doing well, consideration of a trial of antibiotics

lower airway diameters and lengths or alterations of the lung parenchyma and may disappear with lung maturation. Wheezing illnesses continuing beyond infancy and the development of asthma may be determined by a child's susceptibility to become atopic.[30] For clinical practice, infants with recurrent wheezing illnesses and atopic stigmata such as eczema, elevated immunoglobulin E (IgE) levels, or a family history of atopy may be more likely to develop asthma in later years, whereas nonatopic wheezing infants who have been exposed to environmental noxious agents such as maternal smoking may have a better prognosis. However, a diagnosis of wheezy bronchitis should not prevent the pediatrician from initiating a therapeutic trial of bronchodilators.

A history of wheezing in children with recurrent or chronic bronchitis that responds to bronchodilator therapy or occurs with exercise, cold air, laughter, or exposure to allergens should be considered evidence of asthma. Nocturnal cough apart from colds or cough with exercise is suggestive of airway hyperreactivity. A family history of asthma or allergy may further add to the diagnosis of asthma. Evidence of allergy such as positive skin prick tests, elevated serum IgE levels, blood eosinophilia, or more than 20% eosinophils in sputum examined with Hansell's stain can support the diagnosis of asthma. However, airway hyperreactivity can exist without concomitant allergy. Thus the absence of atopy should not obviate a therapeutic trial of bronchodilators.

Pulmonary function tests can be performed in children as young as 5 years of age. The measurement of a peak flow rate, if not complete spirometry, allows the baseline assessment of airway obstruction. Increased peak flow variability or a significant bronchodilator response adds to the diagnosis. Furthermore, airway reactivity to different physical stimuli such as exercise or cold air or to pharmacologic agents such as methacholine or histamine can be determined. The availability of relatively inexpensive peak flowmeters and spirometers should make the measurement of pulmonary function an integral part of the assessment of every child with chronic airway disease.

A trial of bronchodilator therapy is useful in both the diagnosis and management of children with asthma. However, long-term therapy should be aimed at reducing airway inflammation by administering medications such as cromolyn, nedocromil, and inhaled steroids.

Preexisting Pulmonary Disease

Congenital abnormalities and airway injury acquired early in life can predispose children to subsequent pulmonary disease. Considering and identifying such early pulmonary insults may be crucial in understanding the clinical course of some chronic airway diseases. Infants who survive neonatal respiratory distress syndrome are at higher risk for developing respiratory illnesses in the first year of life and beyond.[31-34] The risk is highest for children who require mechanical ventilation and subsequently develop bronchopulmonary dysplasia but is also increased in children who have a history of respiratory distress syndrome but no bronchopulmonary dysplasia. In a significant number of these children, airway hyperreactivity, exercise-associated desaturation, cough, and wheezing can be demonstrated.[32,33,35,36]

Early lung injury by chlamydial, viral, or *B. pertussis* infection is associated with long-term pulmonary sequelae[37,38] and may leave a child vulnerable to repeated lower respiratory tract infections. This increased susceptibility may be attributable to the induction of airway hyperreactivity, preexisting small airways, or a fixed small airway obstruction. In some cases, pneumonia caused by the adenovirus, respiratory syncytial virus, measles virus, or *B. pertussis* may lead to the development of bronchiectasis. This condition should be suspected in a child who has a history of sustained productive cough exacerbated by a postural change or who has digital clubbing.

Cystic Fibrosis

Cough is the most constant symptom of pulmonary involvement in cystic fibrosis. At first, the cough may be dry and hacking, but eventually, it becomes loose and productive. Sometimes the disease remains asymptomatic for long periods, or the infant seems to have prolonged acute respiratory infections. Accompanying symptoms of gastrointestinal malabsorption, such as bulky, greasy stools and failure to gain weight despite a large food intake, should alert the pediatrician to the diagnosis of cystic fibrosis. Thus serial documentation of weight and height measurements should be part of every follow-up of children with chronic respiratory conditions. Furthermore, a diagnosis of cystic fibrosis should be considered in children with increased anteroposterior diameters of the chest, generalized hyperresonance, digital clubbing, and bronchiectasis. Cystic fibrosis is the diagnosis most tragic to miss in children with chronic or recurrent bronchitis because early initiation of therapy may alter the course of the illness and early diagnosis can alert the parents to the risk of having other children with the same disease. Thus a sweat chloride determination should be obtained in every child with chronic or recurrent bronchitis.

The sweat test should be performed using the quantitative pilocarpine iontophoresis to collect sweat and to analyze its chloride content. Because this method requires care and accuracy, it should be performed by a center that does these tests frequently.[39] The amount of sweat collected should be measured and reported. For reliable results, at least 75 mg—preferably 100 mg—of sweat should be analyzed. Because of low sweat rates, accurate testing may be difficult in the first weeks of life. More than 60 mEq/L of chloride in sweat is diagnostic of cystic fibrosis.

Foreign Body Aspiration

Foreign bodies aspirated into and retained in the tracheobronchial tree should always be considered in the differential diagnosis of chronic bronchitis.[40] A careful history and a high index of suspicion are important for the identification of this condition. Sudden violent cough, wheezing, and gagging may occur, but after the aspiration of small foreign bodies, the onset may be insidious or overlooked, and a persistent cough and wheezing may be the only presenting signs. Occasionally, persistent or recurrent pneumonia that does not completely clear with adequate antibiotic therapy may lead to the diagnosis. Unsuspected foreign bodies have been identified as the cause of chronic respiratory illness in a significant number of children. They may produce chronic airway inflammation, distal atelectasis, bronchiectasis, and severe lung damage and may thus distract from an accurate diagnosis. Physical examination, especially differential auscultation with a binaural stethoscope, can be helpful.[3] Decreased breath sounds are found over the affected side; delayed air entry into the involved lobe, regional prolongation of exhalation, and a louder wheezing can be heard. Inspiratory-expiratory and decubitus chest radiographs confirm the physical findings and may show unilateral obstructive emphysema or atelectasis. Bronchoscopy should always be performed if the possibility of a foreign body aspiration exists.

Aspiration Syndromes

A history of cough with feeding is suggestive of conditions associated with recurrent aspiration of feedings or gastric contents after reflux. "Bottle propping" (i.e., propping the bottle up in the crib so that the infant can drink while falling asleep) can cause chronic cough in infants and toddlers. Furthermore, chronic irritation of the airway subsequent to feeding can occur in conditions such as an H-type tracheoesophageal fistula, a laryngeal cleft, and dysfunctional swallowing mechanisms such as familial dysautonomia, submucous cleft palate, cerebral palsy, and muscular dystrophy.[41] If very small amounts of material are aspirated or aspiration occurs primarily during sleep, chronic cough, wheezing, and rattling breathing may be the only presenting signs. The extent of pulmonary injury after aspiration is in part determined by the pH, the amount, and the particulate content (milk or other foods) of the aspirate.[42] Wolfe et al[43] has proposed that chronic aspiration produces airway erythema with disruption of the normal tracheal clearance. Increased mucus production and a subsequent "wet" cough could then mimic the clinical appearance of chronic bronchitis.

Nocturnal cough may indicate the presence of gastroesophageal reflux. The pathophysiologic changes in chronic pulmonary disease subsequent to reflux may be attributable to microaspirations of refluxed material into the lungs or to reflex bronchoconstriction when acid is present in the lower esophagus. Chronic respiratory illness may also be seen in patients who have undergone repair of esophageal atresia. The prevalence of annual bouts of bronchitis was 74% in children under 15 years of age in an Australian center.[44] Multiple factors, including recurrent inhalation of gastric or esophageal contents, structural instability of the major airways, and abnormal airway epithelium, may contribute to these problems.

Swallowing as well as esophageal anatomy and function can be assessed with a barium swallow and esophagram. The documentation of gastroesophageal reflux may require prolonged pH monitoring.

Airway Compression

Chronic airway compression can lead to a chronic, dry, irritative cough. Extrathoracic lesions such as laryngomalacia and subglottic hemangioma lead to collapse during inspiration, with a resulting characteristic inspiratory stridor. These conditions are rarely mistaken for chronic bronchitis. Tracheomalacia and intrathoracic airway compression, however, result in collapse on expiration with wheezing. Functional or structural abnormalities of the tracheal cartilages have been reported in primary tracheomalacia, whereas vascular rings or slings as well as perihilar adenopathy and mediastinal tumors account for intrathoracic airway compression. Irrespective of the underlying condition, the wheezing is most obvious with forced exhalation during cough and laughing. In addition, lower respiratory tract infections worsen both the cough and the wheezing because of increased airway resistance upstream to the obstruction, resulting in a more dynamic collapse.

Physical examination may demonstrate a wheeze and prolonged expiration. Differential auscultation with a binaural stethoscope can be helpful in further localizing the abnormality, and the findings on auscultation are similar to those of a foreign body aspiration. High-energy airway radiographs with filtration can demonstrate airway narrowing. Airway compression by an abnormal vessel may be seen on an esophagram, and echocardiography may confirm the diagnosis of an aberrant vessel such as a double aortic arch. Chest computed tomographic scanning, particularly spiral computed tomography, can be useful in delineating vascular and other compressions of the central airways. The ease with which flexible fiberoptic bronchoscopy can now be conducted by skilled and experienced bronchoscopists makes this a most useful study in assessing children with suspected extrinsic airway compression.[45] Before surgical correction, magnetic resonance imaging can be used to definitely outline the vascular anatomic structures without requiring intravascular contrast medium or x-ray exposure.[46]

Congenital Heart Disease

Wheezing and chronic airway obstruction can be major manifestations of pulmonary edema. Narrowing of both large and small airways may underlie this condition. Although peribronchiolar cuffs of fluid would be expected to lead to increases in airway closure and resistance, morphometric studies provide no support for the notion that interstitial lung edema compresses airways.[47] They suggest that alveolar or airway luminal edema may be responsible for the increase in resistance with edema. Small airways contribute a relatively greater proportion of the total airway resistance in infants. This becomes important in the assessment of young children with known "mild" heart disease such as ventricular septal defect or patent ductus arteriosus and left-to-right-shunts. A trial of diuretics and more aggressive management of the pulmonary congestion may relieve symptoms. However, Hordof et al[48] found no improvement until repair of the lesion was carried out despite vigorous cardiotonic therapy. In addition, some children with interstitial edema as a result of left-sided heart failure with a variety of underlying diseases, such as cor triatriatum, mitral stenosis, and congenital hypoplastic left heart syndrome, have also had recurrent wheezy attacks. The differentiation between primary and secondary lung disease in this situation requires an effective communication among the cardiologist, pulmonologist, and child's pediatrician.

Infections

An additional factor important for the recurrence or maintenance of airway inflammation is the frequency of lower respiratory tract infections. The average number of infections in the infant and preschool child varies but can be as high as 8 to 10 per year. Children with frequent infections of the upper and lower respiratory tract are prone to subsequent respiratory viral infections, predominantly of the lower respiratory tract.[49] Whether this increased susceptibility is attributable to minor abnormalities in immune response mechanisms, small airway size, or altered airway reactivity remains to be elucidated. Repeated and prolonged episodes of lower respiratory tract infections should always alert the pediatrician to consider an underlying cause, most frequently airway hyperreactivity.

Other infectious agents may cause chronic bronchitis. Infections with *Chlamydia* or *Ureaplasma* organisms can lead to progressive cough and lung disease in infants. *B. pertussis* can cause airway damage and an unremitting chronic cough in infants and preschool children. *M. pneumoniae* should be considered a possible causative agent in school-age children. Furthermore, mycobacterial or fungal infection must be ruled out as a cause of chronic cough and wheezing. Delayed hypersensitivity skin testing and fungal serologies can aid in the diagnosis. The chest radiographs may reveal enlarged hilar nodes or parenchymal infiltrates.

Immunodeficiency

Recurrent respiratory disease represents the main clinical expression in children with humoral immunodeficiency syndromes such as common variable hypogammaglobulinemia, common variable immunodeficiency, or X-linked infantile (Bruton's) agammaglobulinemia.[50] Bronchitis is not the only manifestation of these conditions, but there are associated recurrent episodes of pneumonia, sinusitis, and otitis media. Therefore a thorough evaluation of the child's history and a careful physical examination provide important clues for the diagnosis.

In addition, minor abnormalities in humoral defense mechanisms such as isolated and combined IgG subclass deficiencies, in particular IgG_2 subclass deficiency, have been described in children with recurrent bronchitis.[51-53] Antibodies against polysaccharide antigens, the main determinants of encapsulated bacteria, are found mainly in the IgG_2 subclass. It has been reported that children with recurrent bronchitis and recurrent infections show a decreased humoral immune response to *Haemophilus influenzae* type b and to pneumococcal type 3 polysaccharide antigen.[54,55] The significance of selective IgA deficiency remains unknown.

Primary Abnormalities of Cilia

Chronic airway disease may be produced by cilia defects. Cilia and their supporting structures contain several proteins. A great variety of genetic abnormalities can therefore lead to some form of ciliary dyskinesis. Abnormal mucociliary clearance results in chronic bronchitis and eventually in bronchiectasis as a late complication. In addition, the absence of ciliary clearance from the middle ears, eustachian tubes, and sinus cavities results in an increased incidence and greater severity of chronic otitis media and sinusitis.[56] A positive family history and situs inversus (Kartagener's syndrome) may add to the diagnosis. Electron microscopy of cilia obtained from nasal or bronchial biopsy can detect structural abnormalities of the cilia. Functional abnormalities can be observed by examining the beating of cilia with a phase-contrast microscope in fresh specimens of mucosa.[57]

Phase II: Exogenous Factors Contributing to the Development of Chronic or Recurrent Bronchitis

Having ruled out the diagnoses previously discussed, it is important to identify other factors that may produce chronic or recurrent bronchitis. Moreover, these factors not only contribute to the development of bronchitis but may also maintain symptoms of bronchitis in other, better-defined conditions such as asthma. Exogenous factors such as increased exposure to infectious diseases in day-care centers, passive smoke, or air pollution may need other endogenous predisposing factors to produce bronchitis in certain affected children. Most of these factors are theoretically amenable to therapy by avoiding the exposure.

Child Care Setting

The frequency of infection in a particular child relates to his or her susceptibility regarding the degree of exposure to viral infections. The risk of developing lower respiratory tract infections has been reported to increase up to twofold or more for children between 4 months and 3 years of age who are in child care situations involving the presence of three or more unrelated children.[58] In the same study, the presence of siblings was also associated with risks of lower respiratory tract infections of a magnitude similar to the risks of exposure to unrelated children but only in the first 6 months of life. Another case-control study has furthermore shown a similar risk for the development of lower respiratory tract infections requiring hospitalization in children younger than 2 years of age whose care situations involved the presence of more than six children.[59] These findings underline the importance of including epidemiologic aspects in the evaluation of a child with chronic or recurrent bronchitis. Also, they suggest that children with a known susceptibility to chronic airway disease such chronic or recurrent bronchitis, asthma, bronchopulmonary dysplasia, or cystic fibrosis should avoid exposure to repeated respiratory infections in large day-care settings.

Cigarette Smoke

Cigarette smoking has been identified as the major cause of obstructive lung disease among adults in the United States. In children and in young adults who have recently taken up smoking, increases in the prevalence of respiratory symptoms such as cough, phlegm production, and shortness of breath have been reported.[60,61] Among young teenagers, functional impairment attributable to smoking may be found after as little as 1 year of smoking 10 or more cigarettes a week.[62]

Passive smoke exposure may produce effects similar to those elicited by active smoking. However, several differences both between active and passive forms of exposure and among the individuals exposed need to be considered.

Approximately half of the smoke produced by a cigarette is sidestream smoke. Compared with the concentration of mainstream smoke inhaled, the concentration of smoke components inhaled by a passively exposed subject is small. However, the mean diameter of particles from sidestream smoke is smaller than that of mainstream smoke. Furthermore, the level of respirable particulate substance in an "average" indoor smoking environment is greater than the levels of total particulates considered safe in outdoor pollution monitoring.[63]

The individual susceptibility may be an important determinant of the possible adverse effects of passive smoke exposure on respiratory morbidity. Among adults a self-selection process occurs, whereby those more susceptible to the irritant effects of tobacco smoke either never start or quit smoking. Passively exposed infants and children may include a disproportionate number of subjects prone to developing chronic airway disease subsequent to exposure.

Several studies have noted that children exposed to environmental tobacco smoke are at considerably higher risk of having acute lower respiratory tract illnesses and chronic respiratory symptoms, such as cough, phlegm, and wheezing, than unexposed children.[64-68] The majority of studies found that the effect was stronger among children whose mothers smoked than among those whose fathers smoked.[65-68] In addition, several studies also reported a dose-response relationship between degree of exposure (number of cigarettes smoked) and the risk of acute and chronic respiratory illness.[68] These findings support the existence of a causal explanation for the association. There is also convincing evidence that the risk inversely correlates with age; infants no older than 3 months of age are reported to be 3.3 times more likely to have lower respiratory illnesses if their mothers smoke 20 or more cigarettes per day than infants of nonsmoking mothers.[68] A relative risk of 1.5 to 2.0 has been reported in older infants and young children. This decrease in risk may be attributed to a decrease in illness frequency, maturation of the respiratory tract and immune system, or decreased contact between mother and child with age.

Smoking caregivers in a child care setting can add to the risk of developing lower respiratory tract infections regardless of maternal smoking status. In a recent study, an increased risk for wheezing lower respiratory tract infections of up to threefold or more has been demonstrated in young children who were in a child care setting with a smoking caregiver after controlling for maternal smoking and other risk factors.[58] These findings illustrate the potential interaction of environmental factors in eliciting airway irritation and acute and chronic respiratory disease.

In the adolescent, active smoking becomes a significant problem. Determinants of the initiation of smoking seem to be related to parental smoking, peer and sibling smoking, and personality. Every child and young adult with symptoms of chronic and recurrent bronchitis should be asked about personal smoking habits in a confidential setting; the clinician should realize that the history is of questionable validity if parents or siblings are present. The impact of passive smoke exposure on the development of the presenting symptoms can thus be assessed. In addition, preventing initiation of smoking in children at risk for chronic lung disease may be possible. The clinician should vigorously discourage any smoking in the child's environment.

Air Pollution

Air pollution with high levels of sulfur dioxide and particulate matter has long been associated with respiratory morbidity in children and adults.[69-72] A study of school children in England found increased rates of respiratory illness among children living in areas with high pollution with sulfur dioxide and particulate matters. A follow-up study of these children 4 years later, after the introduction of a clean-air program, demonstrated major reductions in air concentrations of particulate matters and a decline in respiratory morbidity among the school children.[70] The American Six Cities Study reported a positive correlation of the prevalence of bronchitis and chronic cough with exposure to particulate matter in relatively small concentrations.[69] A twofold increased prevalence of recurrent bronchitis was furthermore demonstrated in an area with high air pollution from sulfur dioxide and particulate matter in East Germany when compared with a less polluted region in West Germany.[73,74] Increased prevalences of respiratory symptoms have also been reported in children exposed to heavy car traffic.[75] The reasons for such an increase are unknown. Recent findings of an association among high concentrations of sulfur dioxide, particulate matter, and nitrogen dioxide with upper respiratory tract infections suggest that air pollutants may not only produce irritative symptoms but also enhance susceptibility to common infections and subsequent lower respiratory tract infections.[76]

In addition to outdoor pollutants, the indoor environment should be assessed for every child with symptoms of chronic and recurrent bronchitis. In particular, wood-burning stoves have been associated with acute respiratory illnesses.[77] Chronic airway irritation by noxious agents may furthermore be found with formaldehyde emissions from chipboards[78] and with activities such as house remodeling, artistic endeavors, and hobbies.

Therapeutic Approaches in Chronic and Recurrent Bronchitis

In the absence of a specific diagnosis, several therapeutic options are helpful in the management of a child with chronic or recurrent bronchitis. Exogenous factors that may be irritating the airways and contributing to the development of chronic and recurrent bronchitis can be identified and subsequently avoided. In preschool children with chronic airway disease, exposure to recurrent infections should be minimized; hence the parents should, whenever possible, avoid child care at large day-care settings. Every caregiver, in particular the mother, should be discouraged from smoking because merely smoking in another room may not adequately protect the child. The indoor environment can furthermore be screened for potential irritating agents such as wood-burning stoves or irritant glazes emitted from chipboards or chemicals used in housekeeping or hobbies.

Because many cases of chronic and recurrent bronchitis, regardless of the presence or absence of wheeze, may represent reactive airway disease, bronchodilator therapy should be considered. This can be used as a diagnostic trial and instituted either with a β-adrenergic agonist such as albuterol or with theophylline. β-Adrenergic agents have less toxicity and a more rapid onset of action, whereas compliance with a proposed treatment can be estimated by determinations of theophylline concentrations. Both kinds of bronchodilators improve mucociliary clearance. Cromolyn sodium can be an effective treatment for the preschooler with chronic cough after exercise or chronic nocturnal cough.

When a child has a productive cough, coarse crackles on auscultation, roentgenographic changes consistent with increased mucus production, then postural drainage may be helpful.[3] This can be easily taught to the parents by having them use a sealed infant anesthetic mask as a percussor. This gives very effective percussion without the need for long practice in effecting hand-cupping techniques. Bronchodilation before chest physiotherapy may be useful in increasing mucus clearance and reducing reactive bronchospasm.

In the child who continues to cough despite bronchodilator treatment and chest physiotherapy, the institution of antibiotic treatment may be considered in an effort to decrease the pathogenic bacterial or mycoplasmal colonization of the airways that can perpetuate the clinical findings of chronic and recurrent bronchitis. The selection of a specific antibiotic should be based on the child's age and the suspected pathogens. A prolonged course may be needed. In infants and school-age children, erythromycin can be effective in treating chlamydial and mycoplasmal infections. In preschoolers, the broad coverage of agents such as amoxicillin against *H. influenzae,* pneumococci, and streptococci may be useful. However, initiation of antibiotic therapy should not distract the pediatrician from detecting a more specific respiratory condition.

In infancy, the feeding history should be reviewed, and overfeeding and bottle-propping discouraged. Simple measures to treat potential gastroesophageal reflux such as upright positioning several hours after feeding may be of use, though their efficacy has not been proved.

Because of possible sequelae extending into adulthood, children with chronic or recurrent respiratory illnesses need referral to specialized centers so that underlying respiratory illnesses can be identified and so that the children can participate in close follow-up care. Long-term care by physicians familiar with the child allows more extensive investigation for more specific entities. For example, whereas the clinician might obtain a sweat chloride test early, biopsy to rule out ciliary abnormality would usually not be performed unless the disease has an unusually severe or unremitting course. Furthermore, close follow-up is essential in all children needing regular or repeated treatment.

SUMMARY

Bronchitis is a common, though poorly defined, symptom complex consisting of cough, increased mucus production, and wheezing. It occurs as an acute and chronic illness, but its validity as a single disease entity when occurring chronically is questionable. Most attacks of acute bronchitis are produced by viruses and have a benign, self-limited course. When evaluating a child with chronic or recurrent bronchitis, the clinician should first focus on identifying specific disease entities while assessing exogenous factors that may contribute to a nonspecific presentation. Such illnesses include preexisting lung disease, atopy, and aspiration syndromes; exposure to recurrent infections and indoor or outdoor pollutants such as passive smoke and particulate matter is an exogenous contributing factor. It will always be crucial to recognize and keep in mind the close relationship between asthma and chronic, recurrent, or wheezy bronchitis in childhood.

REFERENCES

1. American Thoracic Society: Definitions and classification of chronic bronchitis, asthma, and pulmonary emphysema, *Am Rev Respir Dis* 85:762-768, 1962.
2. Taussig LM, Smith SM, Blumenfeld R: Chronic bronchitis in childhood: what is it? *Pediatrics* 67:1-5, 1981.
3. Morgan WJ, Taussig LM: The chronic bronchitis complex in children, *Pediatr Clin North Am* 31:851-864, 1984.
4. Barker DJP, Osmond C: Childhood respiratory infection and adult chronic bronchitis in England and Wales, *Br Med J* 293:1271-1275, 1986.
5. Burrows B, Knudson RJ, Lebowitz MD: The relationship of childhood respiratory illness to adult obstructive airway disease, *Am Rev Respir Dis* 115:751-759, 1977.
6. Phelan D: Does adult chronic obstructive lung disease really begin in childhood? *Br J Dis Chest* 78:1-9, 1984.
7. Strachan DP, Anderson HR, Bland JM, Peckham C: Asthma as a link between chest illness in childhood and chronic cough and phlegm in young adults, *Br Med J* 296:890-893, 1988.

Acute Bronchitis

8. Glezen WP, Denny FW: Epidemiology of acute lower respiratory disease in children, *N Engl J Med* 288:498-505, 1973.
9. Denny FW, Clyde WA: Acute lower respiratory tract infections in nonhospitalized children, *J Pediatr* 108:635-646, 1986.
10. Gooch WM III: Bronchitis and pneumonia in ambulatory patients, *Pediatr Infect Dis* J 6:137-140, 1987.

11. Ayres JG: Seasonal pattern of acute bronchitis in general practice in the United Kingdom, 1976-83, *Thorax* 41:106-110, 1986.
12. Loughlin GM: Bronchitis. In Chernick V, Kendig EL, eds: *Disorders of the respiratory tract in children,* Philadelphia, 1983, WB Saunders, pp 349-359.
13. Denny FW, Clyde WA, Glezen WP: *Mycoplasma pneumoniae* disease: clinical spectrum, pathophysiology, epidemiology and control, *J Infect Dis* 123:74-92, 1971.
14. Bass JW: Erythromycin for treatment and prevention of pertussis, *Pediatr Infect Dis* J 5:154-157, 1986.
15. Stagno S, Brasfield DM, Brown MD, Cassell GH, Pifer LL, Whitley RJ, Tiller RE: Infant pneumonitis associated with cytomegalovirus, *Chlamydia, Pneumocystis* and *Ureaplasma:* a prospective study, *Pediatrics* 68:322-329, 1981.

Chronic, Recurrent, and Wheezy Bronchitis

16. Peat JK, Woolcock AJ, Leeder SR, Blackburn CR: Asthma and bronchitis in Sydney school children, *Am J Epidemiol* 11:721-727, 1980.
17. Burrows B, Lebowitz MD: Characteristics of chronic bronchitis in a warm, dry region, *Am Rev Respir Dis* 112:365-370, 1975.
18. Dodge R, Burrows B, Lebowitz MD, Cline MG: Antecedent features of children in whom asthma develops during the second decade of life, *J Allergy Clin Immunol* 92:744-749, 1993.
19. Boule M, Gaultier C, Tournier B, Allaire Y, Girard F: Lung function in children with recurrent bronchitis, *Respiration* 38:127-134, 1979.
20. Cloutier MM, Loughlin GM: Chronic cough in children: a manifestation of airway hyperreactivity, *Pediatrics* 67:6-12, 1981.
21. Wilson NM: Wheezy bronchitis revisited, *Arch Dis Child* 64:1194-1199, 1989.
22. Williams H, McNichol KN: Prevalence, natural history and relationship of wheezy bronchitis and asthma in children: an epidemiological study, *Br Med J* 4:321-325, 1969.
23. Sibbald B, Horn ME, Gregg I: A family study of the genetic basis of asthma and wheezy bronchitis, *Arch Dis Child* 55:354-357, 1980.
24. Anderson HR, Cooper JS, Bailey PA, Palmer JC: Influence of morbidity, illness label, and social, family and health service factors on drug treatment of childhood asthma, *Lancet* 2:1030-1032, 1981.
25. Speight ANP, Lee DA, Hey EN: Underdiagnosis and undertreatment of asthma in childhood, *Br Med J* 286:1256-1258, 1983.
26. Godden DJ, Ross S, Abdalla M, McMurray D, Douglas A, Oldman D, Friend JAR, Legge JS, Douglas JG: Outcome of wheeze in childhood: symptoms and pulmonary function 25 years later, *Am J Respir Crit Care Med* 149:106-112, 1994.
27. Martinez FD, Morgan WJ, Wright AL, Holberg CJ, Taussig LM, GMHA Personnel: Diminished lung function as a predisposing factor for wheezing respiratory illness in infants, *N Engl J Med* 319:1112-1117, 1988.
28. Martinez FD, Morgan WJ, Wright AL, Holberg C, Taussig LM, GMHA Personnel: Initial airway function is a risk factor for recurrent wheezing respiratory illnesses during the first three years of life, *Am Rev Respir Dis* 143:312-316, 1991.
29. Tager IB, Hanrahan JP, Tosteson TD, Castile RG, Brown RW, Weiss ST, Speizer FE: Lung function, pre- and post-natal smoke exposure, and wheezing in the first year of life, *Am Rev Respir Dis* 147:811-817, 1993.
30. Sears MR, Burrows B, Flannery EM, Herbison GP, Hewitt CJ, Holdaway MD: Relation between airway responsiveness and serum IgE in children with asthma and in apparently normal children, *N Engl J Med* 325:1067-1071, 1991.
31. Bryan MH, Hardie MJ, Reilly BJ, Sawyer RR: Pulmonary function studies during the first year of life in infants recovering from respiratory distress syndrome, *Pediatrics* 52:169-178, 1973.
32. Galdes-Sebaldt M, Sheller JR, Grogaard J, Stahlman M: Prematurity is associated with abnormal airway function in childhood, *Pediatr Pulmonol* 7:259-264, 1989.
33. von Mutius E, Nicolai T, Martinez FD: Prematurity as a risk factor for asthma in preadolescent children, *J Pediatr* 123:223-229, 1993.
34. Wong YC, Beardsmore CS, Silverman M: Pulmonary sequelae in neonatal respiratory distress in very low birth weight infants: a clinical and a physiological study, *Arch Dis Child* 57:418-424, 1982.
35. Bader D, Ramos AD, Lew CD, Platzker ACG, Stabile MW, Keens TG: Childhood sequelae of infant lung disease: exercise and pulmonary function abnormalities after bronchopulmonary dysplasia, *J Pediatr* 110:693-699, 1987.
36. Gibson RL, Jackson JC, Twiggs GA, Redding GJ, Truog WE: Bronchopulmonary dysplasia: survival after prolonged mechanical ventilation, *Am J Dis Child* 142:721-725, 1988.
37. Sly PD, Soto-Quiros ME, Landau LI, Hudson I, Newton-John H: Factors predisposing to abnormal pulmonary function after adenovirus type 7 pneumonia, *Arch Dis Child* 59:935-939, 1984.
38. Warner JO, Marshall WC: Crippling lung disease after measles and adenovirus infection, *Br J Dis Chest* 70:89-94, 1976.
39. Littlewood JR: The sweat test, *Arch Dis Child* 61:1041-1043, 1986.
40. Cotton, E, Yasuda K: Foreign body aspiration, *Pediatr Clin North Am* 31:937-941, 1984.
41. Fisher SE, Painter M, Milmoe G: Swallowing disorders in infancy, *Pediatr Clin North Am* 28:845-853, 1981.
42. Hamelberg W, Bosomworth P: Aspiration pneumonitis: experimental studies and clinical observations, *Anesth Analg* 43:669-676, 1964.
43. Wolfe JE, Bone RC, Ruth WE: Diagnosis of gastric aspiration by fiberoptic bronchoscopy, *Chest* 70:458-459, 1976.
44. Chetcuti P, Phelan PD: Respiratory morbidity after repair of oesophageal atresia and tracheo-oesophageal fistula, *Arch Dis Child* 68:167-170, 1993.
45. Wood RE, Postma D: Endoscopy of the airway in infants and children, *J Pediatr* 112:1-6, 1988.
46. Vogl T, Wilimzig C, Hofmann U, Hofmann D, Dresel S, Lissner J: MRI in tracheal stenosis by innominate artery in children, *Pediatr Radiol* 21:89-93, 1991.
47. Michel RP, Zocchi L, Rossi A, Cardinal GA, Ploy-Song-Sang Y, Poulsen RS, Milic-Emili J, Staub NC: Does interstitial lung edema compress airways and arteries? A morphometric study, *J Appl Physiol* 62:108-115, 1987.
48. Hordof AJ, Mellins RB, Gersony WM, Steeg CN: Reversibility of chronic obstructive lung disease in infants following repair of ventricular septal defect, *J Pediatr* 92:187-191, 1977.
49. Isaacs D, Clarke JR, Tyrrell DAJ, Valman HB: Selective infection of lower respiratory tract by respiratory viruses in children with recurrent respiratory tract infections, *Br Med J* 284:1746-1749, 1982.
50. Watts WJ, Bachhuber Watts M, Dai W, Cassidy JT, Grum CM, Weg JG: Respiratory dysfunction in patients with common variable hypogammaglobulinemia, *Am Rev Respir Dis* 134:699-703, 1986.
51. De Baets F, Kint J, Pauwels R, Leroy J: IgG subclass deficiency in children with recurrent bronchitis, *Eur J Pediatr* 151:274-278, 1992.
52. Shackelford PG, Polmar SH, Mayus JL, Johnson WL, Corry JM, Nahm MH: Spectrum of IgG2 subclass deficiency in children with recurrent infections: prospective study, *J Pediatr* 108:647-653, 1986.
53. Smith TF, Morris EC, Bain RP: IgG subclasses in nonallergic children with chronic chest symptoms, *J Pediatr* 105:896-900, 1984.
54. Ambrosino DM, Umetsu DT, Siber GR, Howie G, Goularte TA, Michaels R, Martin P, Schur PH, Noyes J, Schiffman G, Geha RS: Selective defect in the antibody response to *Haemophilus influenzae* type b in children with recurrent infections and normal serum IgG subclass levels, *J Allergy Clin Immunol* 81:1175-1179, 1988.
55. De Baets F, Pauwels R, Schramme I, Leroy J: IgG subclass specific antibody response in recurrent bronchitis, *Arch Dis Child* 66:1378-1382, 1991.
56. Turner JAP, Corkey CWB, Lee YJC, Levison H, Sturgess J: Clinical expressions of immotile cilia syndromes, *Pediatrics* 67:805-810, 1981.
57. Rutland J, Cole PJ: Noninvasive sampling of nasal cilia for measurement of beat frequency and study of ultra-structure, *Lancet* 2:564-565, 1980.
58. Holberg CJ, Wright AL, Martinez FD, Morgan WJ, Taussig LM: Child day care, smoking by caregivers, and lower respiratory tract illness in the first 3 years of life, *Pediatrics* 91:885-892, 1993.
59. Anderson LJ, Parker RA, Strikas RA, Farrar JA, Gangarosa EJ, Keyserling HL, Sikes RK: Day-care center attendance and hospitalization for lower respiratory tract illness, *Pediatrics* 82:300-308, 1988.
60. Bewley BR, Halil T, Snaith AH: Smoking by primary schoolchildren: prevalence of and associated respiratory symptoms, *Br J Prev Soc Med* 27:150-153, 1973.
61. Seely JE, Zuskin E, Bouhuys A: Cigarette smoking: objective evidence for lung damage in teen-agers, *Science* 172:741-743, 1971.
62. Woolcock JA, Peat JK, Leeder SR, Blackburn CRB: The development of lung function in Sydney children: effects of respiratory illness and smoking—a ten year study, *Eur J Respir Dis Suppl* 65:1-137, 1984.
63. Repace JL, Lowrey AH: Indoor air pollution, tobacco smoke and public health, *Science* 208:464-472, 1980.

64. Martinez FD, Cline M, Burrows B: Increased incidence of asthma in children of smoking mothers, *Pediatrics* 89:21-26, 1992.
65. McConnochie KM, Roghmann KJ: Breast feeding and maternal smoking as predictors of wheezing in children age 6 to 10 years, *Pediatr Pulmonol* 2:260-268, 1986.
66. Ogston SA, Florey C, Walker CM: Association of infant alimentary and respiratory illness with parental smoking and other environmental factors, *J Epidemiol Community Health* 41:21-25, 1987.
67. Woodward A, Douglas RM, Graham NMH, Miles H: Acute respiratory illness in Adelaide children: breast feeding modifies the effect of passive smoking, *J Epidemiol Community Health* 44:224-230, 1990.
68. Wright AL, Holberg C, Martinez FD, Taussig LM: Relationship of parental smoking to wheezing and nonwheezing lower respiratory tract illness in infancy, *J Pediatr* 118:207-214, 1991.
69. Dockery DW, Speizer FE, Stram DO, Ware JH, Spengler JD, Ferris BG Jr: Effects of inhalable particles on respiratory health of children, *Am Rev Respir Dis* 139:587-594, 1989.
70. Lunn JE, Knowelden J, Roe JW: Patterns of respiratory illness in Sheffield junior schoolchildren: a follow-up study, *Br J Prev Soc Med* 24:223-228, 1970.
71. Pope CA, Dockery DW: Acute health effects of PM10 pollution on symptomatic and asymptomatic children, *Am Rev Respir Dis* 145:1123-1128, 1992.
72. Ware JH, Ferris BG Jr, Dockery DW, Spengler JD, Stram DO, Speizer FE: Effects of ambient sulfur oxides and suspended particles on respiratory health of pre-adolescent children, *Am Rev Respir Dis* 133:834-842, 1986.
73. von Mutius E, Fritzsch C, Weiland SK, Roell G, Magnussen H: Prevalence of asthma and allergic disorders among children in united Germany: a descriptive comparison, *Br Med J* 305:1395-1399, 1992.
74. von Mutius E, Martinez FD, Fritzsch C, Nicolai T, Roell G, Thiemann HH: Prevalence of asthma and atopy in two areas of West and East Germany, *Am J Respir Crit Care Med* 149:358-364, 1994.
75. Wjst M, Reitmeir P, Dold S, Wulff A, Nicolai T, von Loeffelholz-Colberg E, von Mutius E: Road traffic and adverse effects on respiratory health in children, *Br Med J* 307:596-600, 1993.
76. von Mutius E, Sherrill DL, Fritzsch C, Martinez FD, Lebowitz MD: Air pollution and upper respiratory symptoms in children in East Germany, *Eur Respir J* 8(5):723-728 1995.
77. Honicky RE, Osborne JS, Akpom CA: Symptoms of respiratory illness in young children and the use of wood-burning stoves for indoor heating, *Pediatrics* 75:587-593, 1985.
78. Krzyzanowski M, Quackenboss JJ, Lebowitz MD: Chronic respiratory effects of indoor formaldehyde exposure, *Environ Res* 52:117-125, 1990.

CHAPTER 36

Acute Lower Respiratory Tract Infections: General Considerations

Floyd W. Denny, Jr.

Acute respiratory infections (ARIs) are the most common infection of the human host.[1] The majority of these are of the upper respiratory tract, but infections of the lower respiratory tract (acute lower respiratory infections [ALRIs]) are sufficiently frequent to pose almost daily problems for the clinician caring for children.

Large numbers of different microorganisms are capable of infecting the lower respiratory tract, producing several respiratory syndromes and illnesses that are on a wide spectrum of severity. Most of these illnesses are mild, and patients suffering from them are appropriately cared for in an ambulatory setting, but a small number are ill enough to require hospitalization, and some die.

CLASSIFICATION

A useful classification of ALRIs in children, shown in Fig. 36-1, is predicated on categorizing the respiratory tract *below* the epiglottitis as part of the lower tract. A description of the criteria that can be used in delineating the four clinical syndromes is shown in Table 36-1. Specific agents have been associated with certain syndromes, but infections may not be limited to a single anatomic region, and several syndromes can occur in the same child at the same time or during the course of a single illness. Despite these shortcomings, the use of the clinical syndromes as diagnostic tools is helpful. Lower respiratory infections (LRIs) can also have a variety of complications, are a

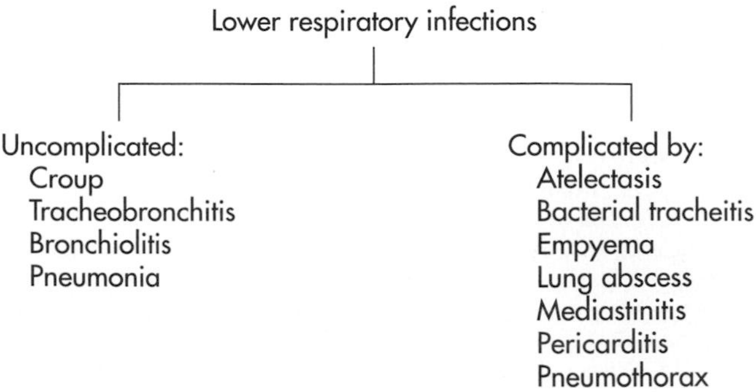

Fig. 36-1. Classification of ALRIs.

Table 36-1 Clinical Syndromes in Childhood LRIs

SYNDROME	SYMPTOMS AND SIGNS
Croup	Hoarseness, cough, inspiratory stridor with laryngeal obstruction
Tracheobronchitis	Cough, lack of laryngeal obstruction or audible wheezing but inspiratory or expiratory wheezes possibly heard on auscultation
Bronchiolitis	Expiratory wheezing, fine inspiratory crackles with or without tachypnea, air trapping, substernal retractions
Pneumonia	Crackles and/or evidence of pulmonary consolidation on physical examination or radiograph

major problem in children with diminished host defenses, and occasionally accompany generalized infections such as rubeola and varicella. Such infections are infrequent problems for the clinician and are not considered further in this chapter. Further discussion of these unusual infections and some specific common respiratory syndromes and agents can be found in chapters dedicated to them.

EPIDEMIOLOGY

Etiology

Box 36-1 lists the viruses that commonly infect the lower respiratory tracts of children. Those listed as having a defined role have attained this classification from numerous studies over many years. Isolation of these agents from the upper respiratory tract in association with specific illness syndromes has been consistent. The fact that all of the agents, with the exception of the adenoviruses, are isolated infrequently from well children has strengthened this association. Finally, repeated studies have shown that infected and ill children develop specific circulating antibodies, further associating temporally specific agents with episodes of illness. Of the viruses listed in Box 36-1 the respiratory syncytial virus (RSV) is clearly the most important, although the parainfluenza viruses and the influenza viruses are also major causes of disease. Coronaviruses and rhinoviruses, classified as having an undefined role, are associated primarily with infections of the upper respiratory tract, but the rhinoviruses have been isolated infrequently from patients with severe LRI.[2] The measles virus and occasionally the rubella virus are capable of causing severe LRIs but are found infrequently in developed countries.

Box 36-2 lists the bacteria that commonly infect the lower respiratory tracts of children. *Mycoplasma pneumoniae* has been recognized for many years as a common cause of tracheobronchitis and pneumonia, mostly in school-age children.[3] *Chlamydia pneumoniae* has been recognized more recently as a cause of infections that appear to be similar to those produced by *M. pneumoniae,* but more studies need to be done to more precisely establish the role of *C. pneumoniae* in ALRIs in children.[4] *Haemophilus influenzae* and *Streptococcus pneumoniae* are listed as having incompletely defined roles as causes of ALRIs. Historically, these bacteria were major causes of severe ALRIs in children. Several factors contribute to the lack of understanding of their overall role in respiratory infections. With the exception of epiglottitis (caused by *H. influenzae* type b) and lobar pneumonia in the older child (caused by *S. pneumoniae*), neither bacterium is associated with specific disease syndromes, as is the case with several viruses, *M. pneumoniae,* and *C. pneumoniae.* The problem is compounded by the carriage of *H. influenzae* and *S. pneumoniae* in the upper respiratory tracts in a high percentage (up to 20% and 50%, respectively) of normal children in the United States at certain ages and during certain seasons.[5-9] These bacteria are not the cause of uncomplicated upper respiratory tract infections. The failure of anticapsular polysaccharide antibodies to develop in young children has also hampered etiologic studies.

Studies showing antibody responses to various components of *S. pneumoniae* have been reported in recent years, but so far, none has clarified the role of this bacterium as a cause of community-acquired pneumonia.[10-13] At present, in the absence of epiglottitis or lobar pneumonia in the older child, the only way to implicate *H. influenzae* and *S. pneumoniae* as causes of ALRIs in children is to isolate them from the blood or pleural space or directly from the lung by percutaneous aspiration. Because of these difficulties, it is not yet possible to assign a precise role for those bacteria as causes of ALRI in children. Although it seems probable that they are less important than other agents, the previously mentioned studies are showing that these organisms may play a more important role than previously suspected. It is clear that they are extremely important in infections in children in developing countries (see later section).

Several bacteria, listed as uncommon causes in the United States, have been extremely important historically as causes of severe ALRIs. Fortunately, they are infrequently seen in the 1990s. Group A streptococci have reappeared recently as a cause of severe LRIs but are still a rather unusual cause of these infections.[14]

Box 36-3 lists the microorganisms that are uncommon causes of ALRIs or are found usually under special circumstances. The human immunodeficiency virus is the most notable example of this in the 1990s. The other viruses listed usually cause infections in newborns or in children with depressed host defenses. *Chlamydia trachomatis* and the group B streptococci are causes of ALRIs, occasionally very severe disease, in the very young child. *Legionella pneumophila,* a common cause of pneumonia in adults, is found infrequently in children. *Staphylococcus aureus,* at one time a common cause of

BOX 36-1
Viruses that Cause ALRIs in Children

Common causes
Defined role
Adenoviruses
Enteroviruses
Influenza viruses types A and B
Parainfluenza viruses types 1 to 3
Respiratory syncytial virus
Undefined role
Coronaviruses
Rhinoviruses

Uncommon causes in the United States
Measles virus
Rubella virus

BOX 36-2
Bacteria that Cause ALRIs in Children

Common causes
Defined role
Chlamydia pneumoniae
Mycoplasma pneumoniae
Incompletely defined role
Haemophilus influenzae
Streptococcus pneumoniae

Uncommon causes in the United States
Bordetella pertussis
Corynebacterium diphtheriae
Hemolytic streptococci, groups A, C, and G
Mycobacterium tuberculosis

BOX 36-3
Agents Causing ALRIs in Children in Uncommon or Special Circumstances

Viruses
Cytomegalovirus
Epstein-Barr virus
Herpes simplex virus
Human immunodeficiency virus
Varicella-zoster virus

Fungi
Blastomyces dermatitidis
Candida species
Coccidioides immitis
Cryptococcus neoformans
Histoplasma capsulatum
Malassezia furfur
Zygomycetes

Bacteria
Actinomyces species
Anaerobes
Atypical mycobacteria
Chlamydia trachomatis
Enterobacteriaceae
Group B streptococci
Legionella pneumophila
Listeria monocytogenes
Nocardia species
Rickettsiae
Staphylococcus aureus

Protozoa
Cryptosporidium
Pneumocystis carinii
Strongyloides stercoralis
Toxoplasma gondii

pneumonia in children, especially in newborns, is now an infrequent cause of ALRIs. Several of the fungi and protozoa cause frequent coinfections or superinfections in patients with acquired immunodeficiency syndrome or other patients with depressed host defenses. Infections with these agents occur very infrequently in normal children.

Role of Respiratory Viruses and *M. pneumoniae* as Causes of ALRIs in Nonhospitalized Children

As mentioned earlier, several respiratory viruses and *M. pneumoniae* are widely recognized as causes of ALRIs in children. Some diagnostic tools are available for rapidly detecting infecting agents in patients with ALRIs, but they are not readily available to many clinicians and are expensive. Certain agents are associated with certain syndromes and occur in children of a specific age and in certain seasons. Thus if the age of the child, the clinical syndrome, and the season of the year are known, a reasonable estimate of the causative agent can be frequently made. Fig. 36-2 graphically demonstrates the relationships of these elements to the causative agent. Observations made during a study of ALRIs in nonhospitalized children in Chapel Hill, North Carolina, demonstrated the quantitative relationships of these elements and are used as examples and illustrations in the following sections.[15] The examples given are representative of studies done in other parts of the United States.

Age and Gender Incidence

The age- and gender-specific attack rates for total ALRIs and the four clinical syndromes are shown in Fig. 36-3. The incidence of all ALRIs during the first 2 years of life was 20 to 25 cases per 100 children per year. It declined steadily with age, so in the 9- to 15-year age group, it was about 5 cases per 100 children per year. Data strictly comparable with these are not available, but the studies by Foy et al[16] in a prepaid medical care group in Seattle are close enough to allow comparison. They reported the combined incidence of pneumonia, bronchiolitis, and croup in children younger than 5 years of age as follows (per 100 per year):

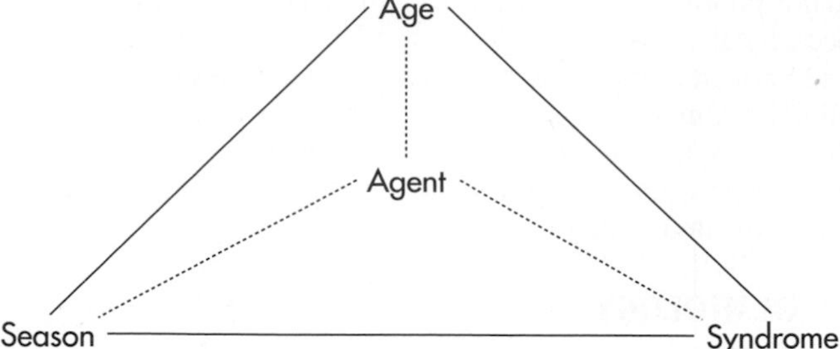

Fig. 36-2. The relationship of the agent causing ALRI to the clinical syndrome, the season of the year, and the age of the patient.

Number	Child's age
4.3	0 to 5 months
6.6	6 to 11 months
5.6	1 year
4.4	2 to 3 years
2.7	4 to 5 years

Procedural differences account for at least part of the differences between the two sets of data. These incidences are to be compared with those reported by Berman et al[17] for total ALRIs (7.0 per 100 per year) in children younger than 15 years of age in Cali, Colombia. Berman et al[17] speculated that this figure underestimated the incidence of ALRIs in the community. In the top frame of Fig. 36-3, the predominance of ALRIs in boys younger than 9 years of age is made clear; the risk was similar in both genders after that age. The overall relative risk for boys vs. girls was 1.25:1. The lower ALRI rate in the first 6 months of life compared with that for the second 6 months should be noted. In the four lower frames of Fig. 36-3, with the exception of bronchiolitis, the age-specific rates for the clinical syndromes were different from those of total ALRIs and were also different from one another.

Croup. The rate for croup was low during the first 6 months of life; there were no cases during the first month, and the rate for the second month was only 1.5 per 100 per year. Thereafter, the rate reached its peak of about 5 per 100 per year during the second year of life. The rate declined after that, and croup was unusual after children started school. Although age-specific incidence rates for croup in the Seattle Study were 3 to 5 times lower than these, the relative incidence of croup in various age groups in both studies was similar, with the peak occurrence in the 1- to 2-year-old group. Croup occurs more frequently in boys than girls. Between the ages of 6 and 12 months, boys were at the greatest risk, 1.73 times more than girls.

Tracheobronchitis. Tracheobronchitis also occurred more frequently in the first 2 years of life (5 to 7 per 100 per year) but also tended to occur frequently in 9- to 15-year-old children (2.6 per 100 per year). The relative risk for boys was only slightly higher than for girls (1.18:1). Childhood tracheobronchitis has not been well defined, so comparable incidence figures are not available.

Bronchiolitis. The age-specific attack rates for bronchiolitis differ sharply from those of the other syndromes but not

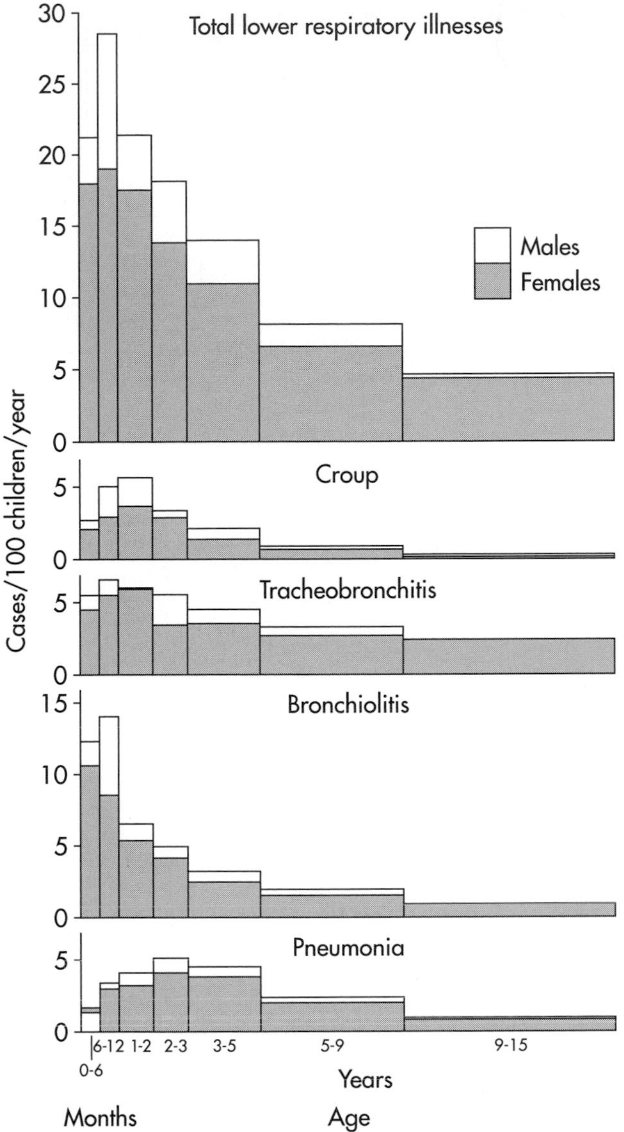

Fig. 36-3. Age- and gender-specific rates for total LRI and respiratory syndromes, 1964 to 1975. The rate for boys is represented by the entire column; that for girls is represented by the gray portion. The overall rate not shown. (From Denny FW, Clyde WA Jr: *Pediatr Res* 17:1026-1029, 1983.)

from ALRIs generally. Wheeze-associated respiratory infection regardless of age reached a peak rate in the second 6 months of life (11.6 per 100 per year); these rates decreased sharply in the second year (6.1 per 100 per year), but the condition continued as a significant problem through the early school years and reached 0.9 per 100 per year in 9- to 15-year-old children. Boys were 1.35 times more likely to develop bronchiolitis than girls. Comparable incidence data are not readily available. In one of the few outpatient studies, an attack rate for bronchiolitis in children younger than 6 years of age was 2 per 100 per year.[16] The incidence of bronchiolitis more strictly defined as wheeze, hyperinflation, and fine inspiratory crackles heard on auscultation was highest in the first 6 months of life; this rate was 2½ times that observed in the second half of the first year. Bronchiolitis was diagnosed infrequently after 2 years of age, probably because of differing criteria for this diagnosis used by clinicians, a controversial point.

Pneumonia. The age-specific attack rates for pneumonia had yet another pattern. The peak of 4.7 per 100 per year was not reached until the third year of life, but the rate in the 3- to 5-year-old group was almost as high (4.2 per 100 per year), and in 5- to 9-year-old children, it was 2.2 per 100 per year. Boys had pneumonia 1.17 times more frequently than girls. The Seattle data are those most comparable to these studies; Foy et al[16] reported rates of 3.0 to 4.2 per 100 per year in preschool children. These figures correspond well with the attack rate of 3.6 per 100 per year in the Chapel Hill studies. There were differences, however, in certain rates within the group up to 6 years of age. The peak rate in Seattle occurred in the second half of the first year, whereas the peak rate in Chapel Hill came later. This disparity is probably explained by procedural differences in the two studies, such as greater use of radiographs as diagnostic tools in Seattle.

Association of Respiratory Agents and Syndromes

The association between respiratory syndromes and certain infecting agents is well established. Fig. 36-4 shows the occurrence of the four respiratory syndromes in children with ALRI resulting from specific agents. Fig. 36-5 shows the occurrence of specific agents in children with different syndromes. The influenza viruses were not prominent causes of pneumonia, as reported by Glezen.[18] Influenza type A virus was not isolated frequently, probably because of the relatively insensitive isolation system used. These two figures show the association between agents and syndromes across all age groups. When corrected for age, these associations become more dramatic.

Of all the agents studied, parainfluenza virus type 3 was most closely associated with all syndromes. Croup was caused predominantly by the parainfluenza viruses, especially type 1. The cause of bronchiolitis was most frequently RSV. Tracheobronchitis was associated with RSV, *M. pneumoniae,* and the influenza viruses. RSV and *M. pneumoniae* were common causes of pneumonia.

Age Distribution of Children with LRIs

In addition to being associated with specific clinical syndromes the respiratory infecting agents also cause infection in children at rather specific ages, as shown in Fig. 36-6. At times, these incidences differed to a marked degree. In all instances, with the exception of the adenoviruses, rates during the first 3 months of life were lower than in later months. The patterns of the curves for RSV and parainfluenza virus type 3 were similar, except that RSV rates were higher in the first few years. In comparison, infection with the parainfluenza virus type 1 occurred in slightly older children, and adenovirus infections occurred almost exclusively in the first 5 years of life. Infection with the influenza viruses occurred commonly in all age groups; influenza viruses types A and B, along with strains that were not typed, were grouped. The rates for *M. pneumoniae* infections show an entirely different age distribution. No isolates were made in children younger than 3 months of age, and the peak rates occurred in school-age children.

A comparable study of children from middle-income families in Seattle[16] reflected a lower percentage of RSV isolates from infants younger than 2 years of age, as did the study in

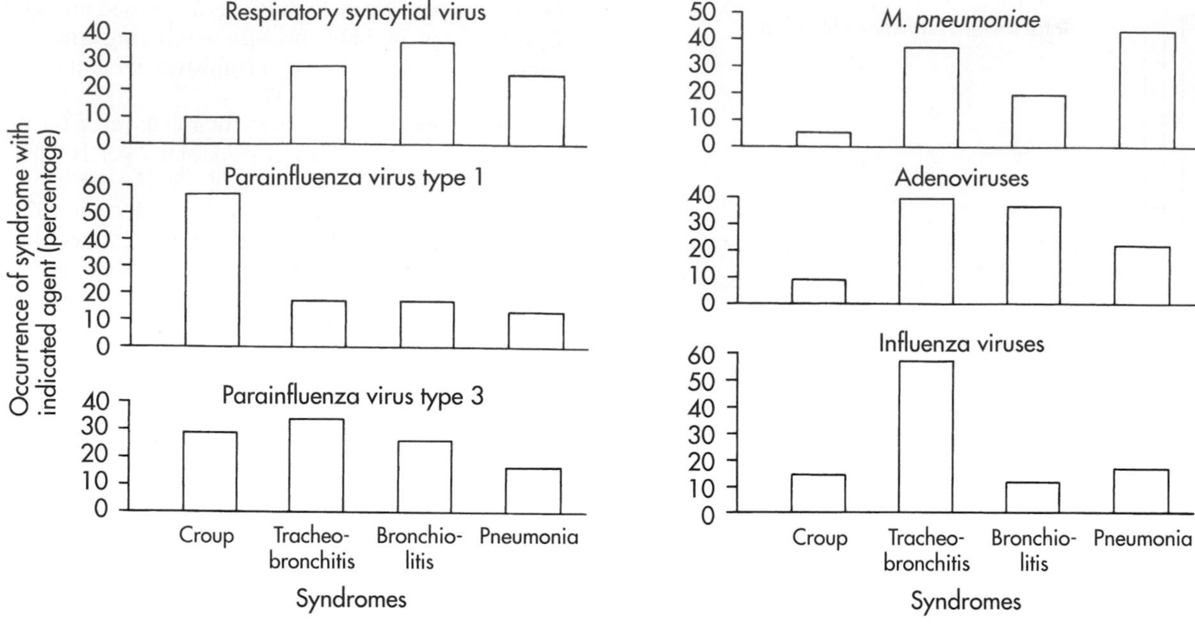

Fig. 36-4. Occurrence of four respiratory syndromes in children with lower respiratory illness related to certain agents. Note that RSV was most likely to cause bronchiolitis; when recovered, it had an almost 40% chance of association with bronchiolitis. Each agent demonstrates different patterns. (From Denny FW, Clyde WA Jr: *Pediatr Res* 17:1026-1029, 1983.)

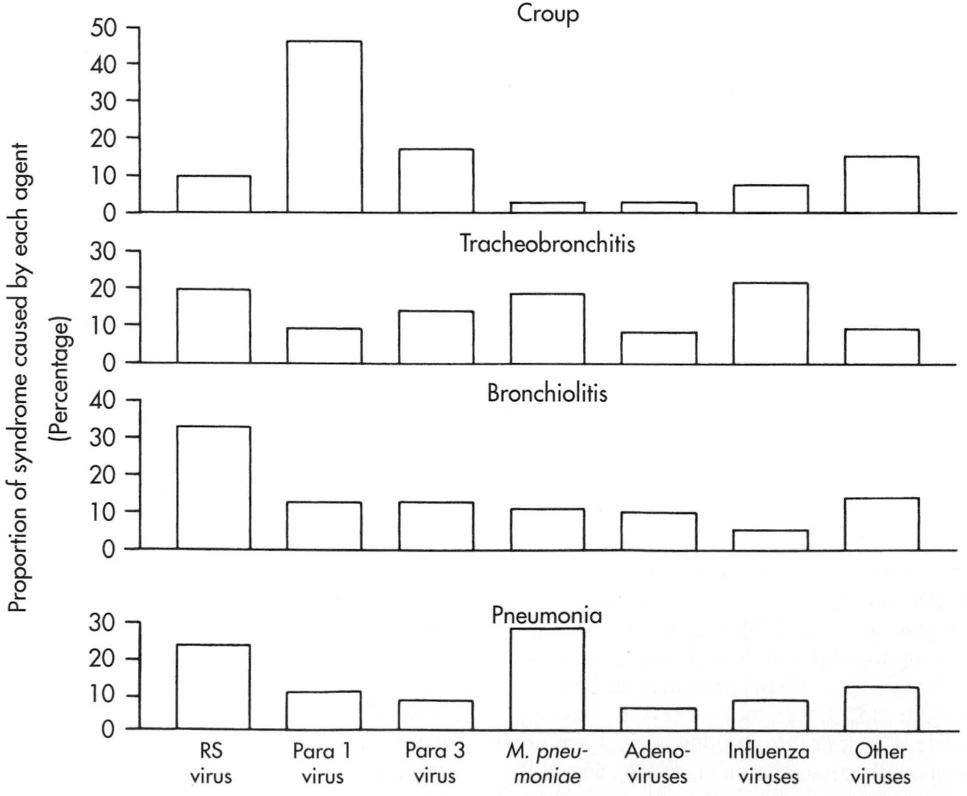

Fig. 36-5. Associations between principal agents and four respiratory syndromes. Note that almost half the cases of croup are caused by parainfluenza virus type 1 *(Para 1 virus)* but that all of the agents share fairly equally in tracheobronchitis. *RS virus,* RSV; *Para 3 virus,* parainfluenza virus type 3. (From Denny FW, Clyde WA Jr: *J Pediatr* 108:635-646, 1986.)

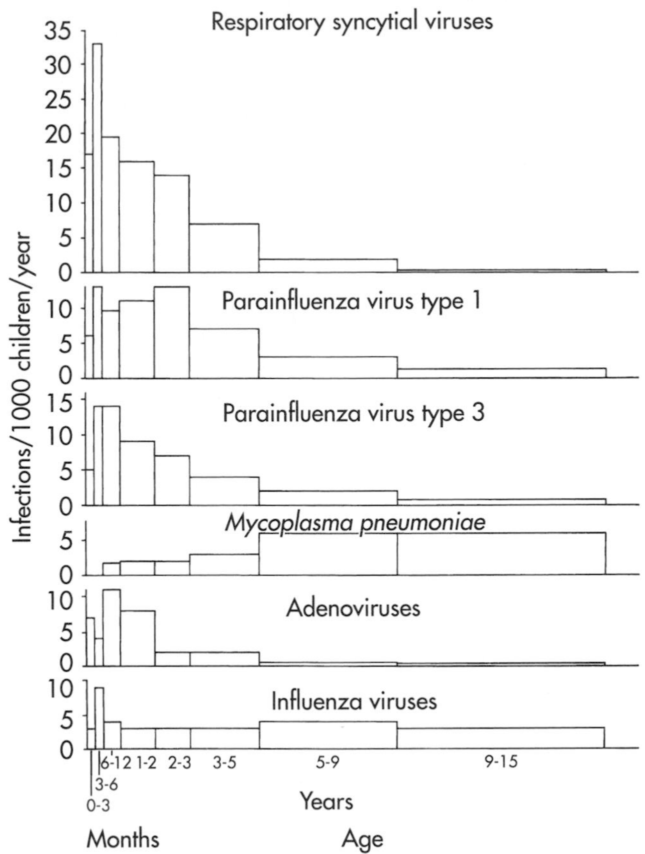

Fig. 36-6. Age-specific rates of children with LRIs caused by certain agents. (From Denny FW, Clyde WA Jr: *Pediatr Res* 17:1026-1029, 1983.)

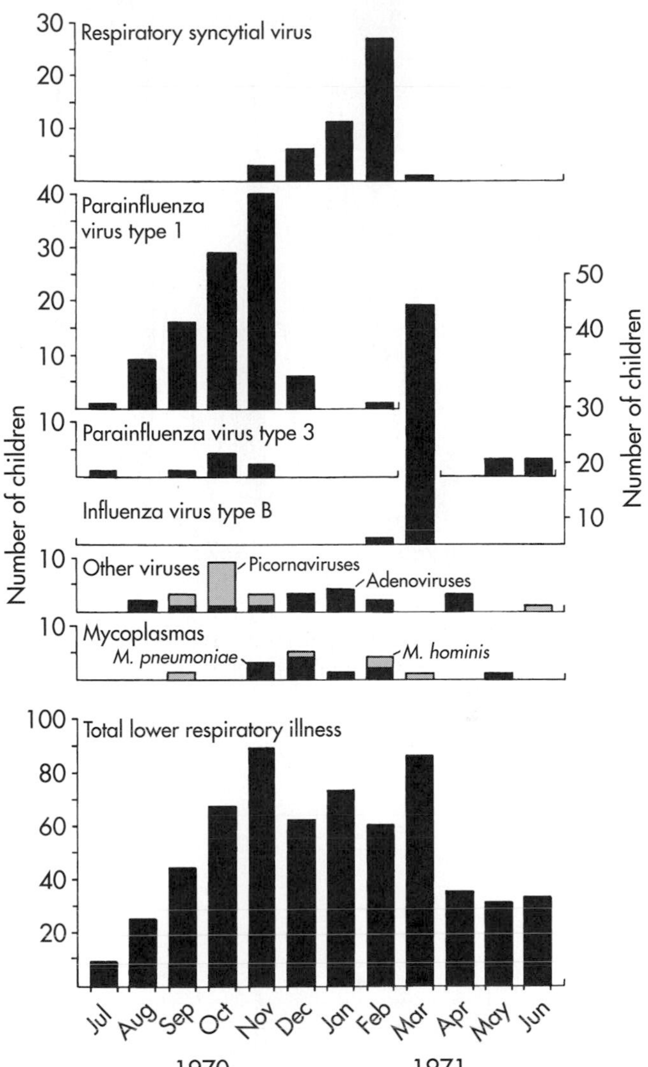

Fig. 36-7. Number of agents isolated by month from children with LRI seen in office practice in 1970 and 1971. Note the propensity of some agents to cause rather discreet outbreaks at times when other agents were present in only small numbers. (From Denny FW, Clyde WA Jr: *J Pediatr* 108:635-646, 1986.)

Tecumseh, Michigan[19]; however, the latter study included upper respiratory tract illnesses. In contrast, reports of hospitalized children have shown a different age distribution of RSV disease. In the author's hospital, 50% of children hospitalized with ALRIs caused by RSV were in the first 3 months of life.[20] In the office setting, less than 5% of children with RSV infections were in this age group, a pattern similar to that observed by Chanock and Parrott[21] in Washington, D.C. This information emphasizes the importance of determining the source of patient data (denominators) in interpreting the impact of specific infections or illnesses.

Seasonal Occurrence of Syndromes and Agents

The respiratory agents and consequently their associated syndromes frequently have characteristic seasonal patterns. A striking example of this (Fig. 36-7) shows the monthly occurrence of various agents in relationship to the occurrence of total ALRIs. Parainfluenza virus type 1 caused a large outbreak, primarily of croup, in the autumn. This was followed by a winter epidemic of RSV disease and a spring outbreak caused by influenza virus type B. All of this occurred against a low-level background of infections caused by other agents. The tendency of viral agents not to cause simultaneous epidemics in a community has been observed also by Glezen[22] in Houston.

Space does not permit a detailed presentation of the seasonal occurrence of all of the respiratory agents and syndromes. An example in Fig. 36-8, however, shows the seasonal incidence of bronchiolitis and the isolation of RSV. The close association between the yearly winter-spring outbreaks of RSV infections with the peak occurrence of bronchiolitis is clearly demonstrated. The small numbers of isolations of RSV during several respiratory seasons probably represent the use of insensitive tissue culture systems at these times. However, there are smaller outbreaks of bronchiolitis that cannot be correlated with the isolation of this agent but were related to other agents, including parainfluenza virus types 1 and 3 and *M. pneumoniae* (e.g., summer and autumn 1972). Fig. 36-9 shows a similar close association of croup and the parainfluenza viruses. A total of 9 of the 15 outbreaks of croup were associated with parainfluenza virus infections; 4 were associated with infections with the influenza viruses, RSV, or *M. pneumoniae.* The agents responsible for two of the outbreaks are unknown. Croup occurs most often in the fall, when parainfluenza virus infections commonly occur. Pneumonia and tracheobronchitis also occur in seasonal patterns that are peculiar to each syndrome and the causative agent.

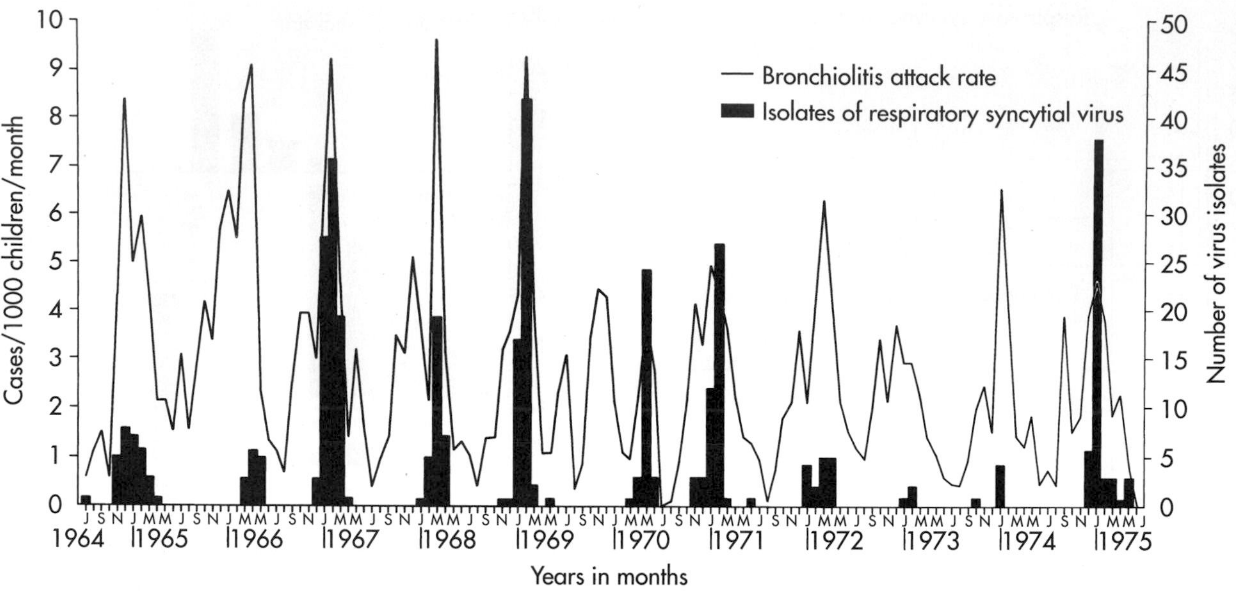

Fig. 36-8. Epidemics of bronchiolitis in children of all ages correlated with RSV isolation. Virus isolates are from all patients with LRI. (From Henderson FW et al: *J Pediatr* 95:183-190, 1979.)

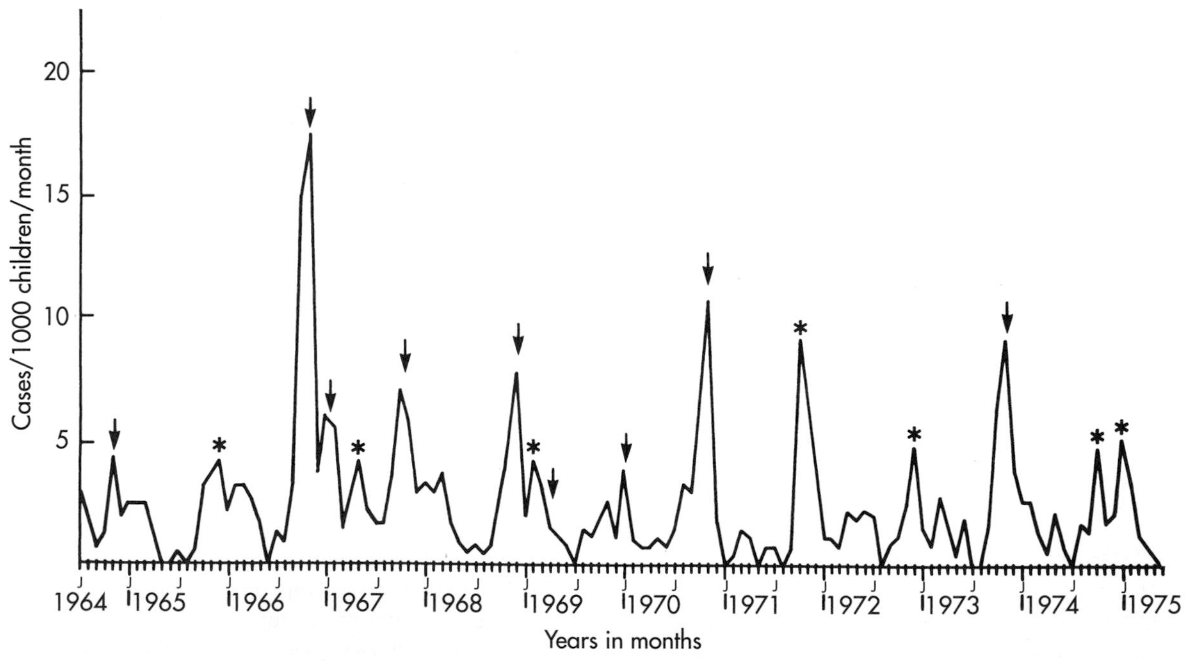

Fig. 36-9. Epidemics of croup in children from birth to 5 years of age. Arrows indicate months in which parainfluenza viruses were prevalent. Asterisks mark peaks when other agents were prevalent or when no agent was isolated in sufficient numbers to implicate it. Of 15 sharp outbreaks of croup, 9 could be attributed to parainfluenza viruses and 4 to influenza viruses, RSV, or *M. pneumoniae*. Only 2 outbreaks could not be associated with these agents. In April 1969, there were 14 isolates of parainfluenza virus type 3, with no increase in the incidence of croup, possibly reflecting a weak association. (From Denny FW et al: *Pediatrics* 71:871-876, 1983.)

Combined Roles of Agents, Age, and Season on Incidence Rates

The separate effects of the infecting agent, age, and gender of the host, relationship of agents and syndromes, and season on the expression of ALRIs in children has been shown. Figs. 36-10 through 36-12 demonstrate the interaction of these various factors; data from all 11 years of the study are presented by month. The impact of yearly variations in the seasonal occurrence of agents is blunted by presenting the data in this manner. The scales on the vertical axes of the three figures are the same to allow comparison of the rates of illness and agent isolation among age groups.

Total ALRIs and the syndromes are more common in younger children, and the rates of all decline with age. The association of the winter-spring occurrence of RSV with bronchiolitis in younger children is clearly shown, as is the association of croup and parainfluenza virus type 1 in early autumn. Parainfluenza virus type 3 and the adenoviruses are the most ubiquitous of the agents, occurring in most months of the year. The adenoviruses, however, were isolated rarely in school-age children, whereas parainfluenza virus type 3 continued to cause some illness in this group. The autumn-winter occurrence of *M. pneumoniae* in school-age children is also shown, as is the impact in all age groups of the winter-spring occurrence of the influenza viruses.

Risk Factors

Age. Young age is probably the greatest risk in the incidence and severity of ALRIs in children. All studies in developed and developing countries show that the incidence is related inversely to age. Children younger than 5 years of age are at greatest risk.[23,24] Some studies, such as those in North Carolina, have shown that the incidence of ALRIs is reduced in children in the first few months of life. The cause of this is unknown, but the presence of passive antibodies from the mother and less exposure to infected contacts probably play a role.

Crowding. Respiratory infections, for the most part, are spread by direct contact or large droplets from the respiratory tract and are thus more likely to occur during conditions that foster close contact. This has been demonstrated for all forms of crowding: number of siblings, room occupancy, population density, and probably day-care attendance.[5] Most crowding would be expected primarily to increase the incidence but might play a role in increasing the severity in situations in which crowding is so intense that the infecting dose of microorganisms is large. It is speculated that this might play a role in the increase in severity of ARIs in developing countries.[25]

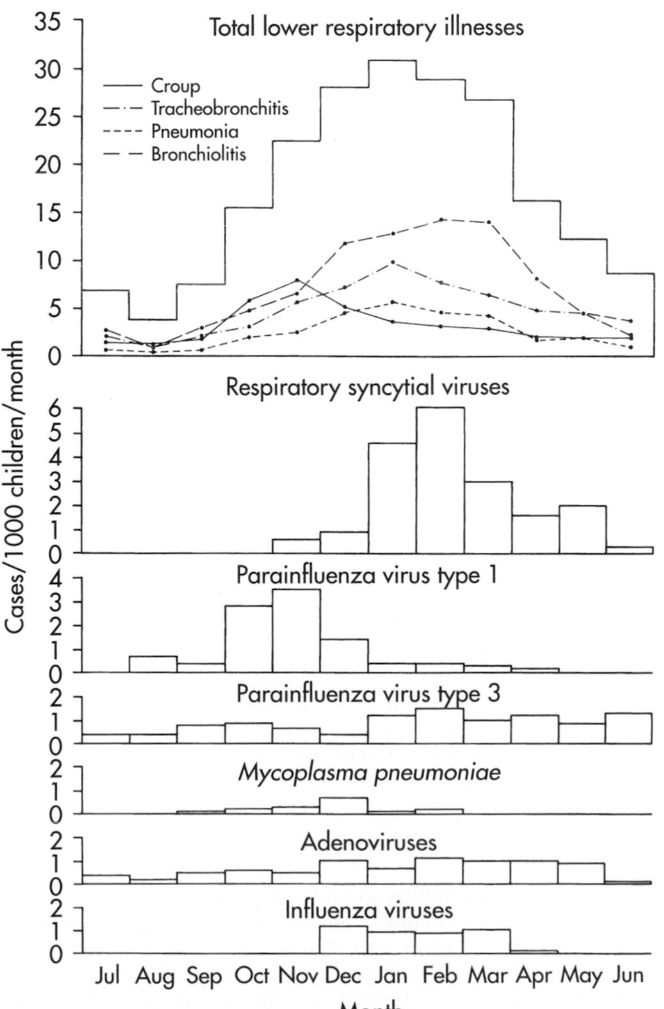

Fig. 36-10. Monthly rates of total LRIs, four syndromes, and infections caused by certain agents in children from birth to 2 years of age. (From Denny FW, Clyde WA Jr: *Pediatr Res* 17:1026-1029, 1983.)

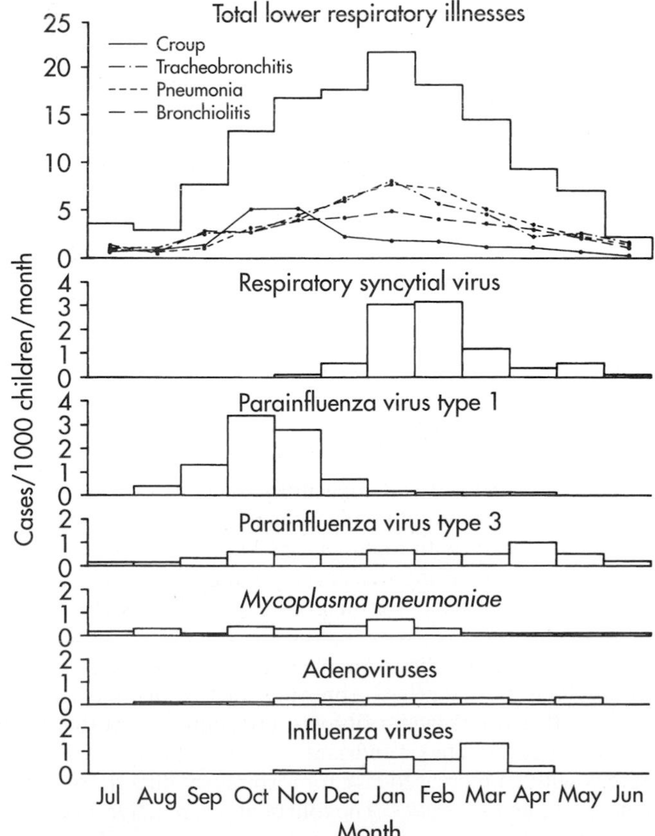

Fig. 36-11. Monthly rates of total LRIs, four syndromes, and infections caused by certain agents in children from 2 to 5 years of age. (From Denny FW, Clyde WA Jr: *J Pediatr* 108:635-646, 1986.)

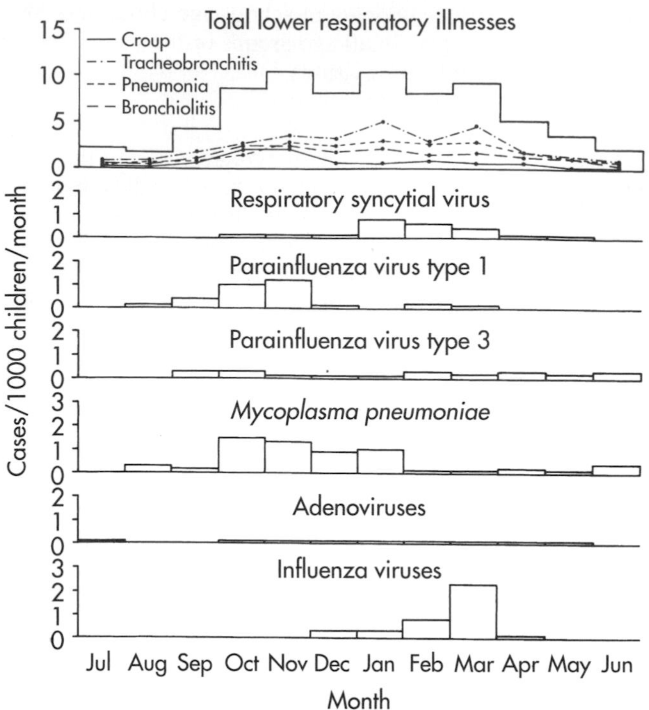

Fig. 36-12. Monthly rates of total LRIs, four syndromes, and infections caused by certain agents in children from 5 to 9 years of age. (From Denny FW, Clyde WA Jr: *J Pediatr* 108:635-646, 1986.)

Gender. The role of gender as a risk factor has received little attention. Data suggest only slight and probably insignificant differences in incidences between boys and girls for upper respiratory tract infections.[26] There are clear-cut gender differences for ALRIs, with a preponderance of disease occurring in boys, suggesting that the risk is to increased severity.[15] The reason for these differences is not known. They may have pathogenetic significance and may be related to airway size, airway function, and immune status, but this is of little help to the pediatrician in managing children with ARIs.

Inhaled Pollutants. Inhaled pollutants have received much attention in the past few years.[25] Although studies vary somewhat in the degree of risk caused by passive tobacco smoke, both for increased incidence and for increased severity, there is increasingly strong evidence that passive smoking is an important risk factor.[27,28] The impact of passive smoking appears to be greatest in the child younger than 1 year of age and is related most closely with maternal smoking. There is also evidence that wood-burning stoves and possibly the use of gas for cooking are responsible for increasing the risk of ARIs.[29,30]

Anatomic Abnormalities, Metabolic and Genetic Diseases, and Immunologic Deficiencies. Abnormalities such as tracheoesophageal fistulas, cystic fibrosis, congenital heart disease, and immunodeficiency syndromes are associated to varying degrees with an increased risk for respiratory infections, both in incidence and severity.[31] The role of atopy, reactive airways, or both factors in increasing the risk for respiratory infection is controversial. There seems to be a relationship between respiratory infections and asthma, but the "chicken and egg" relationship is unclear. The same is true for the relationship between atopy and bronchiolitis or possibly croup.[32-34] These relationships are considered further in their own sections.

Nutrition, Including Breast-Feeding. It seems probable that malnutrition is important in increasing the risk for ARIs, especially in developing countries.[25] Because malnutrition is often associated with other risk factors such as crowding and inhaled pollutants, it has not been possible to clearly define its role. The reports of the role of vitamin A deficiency in increasing the risk for ARIs is of interest but needs further study to assess its importance.[10] Breast-feeding appears to be important in developing counties in reducing the risk for ARIs, but the data relating to a protective effect in developed countries are contradictory.[35] Results of studies show only small or no reductions in the incidence of all respiratory infections but do suggest that the severity of infections might be decreased in young breast-fed infants. It is clear that the effect of nutrition on the risk for ARIs, including breast-feeding and other forms of feeding, needs increased attention.

Social and Economic Factors. It is difficult, if not impossible, to separate the various social and economic factors that may have an impact on the occurrence of ARIs, but low social class is linked clearly with increased risk.[23,24] Crowding, malnutrition, and inhaled pollutants, all found in low socioeconomic classes, especially in developing countries, are contributing factors. The role of stress is receiving increasing attention and could be a contributing factor, particularly when the stress is associated with being poor.[36]

Issues in Pathogenicity and Pathophysiology

The issues of pathogenicity and pathophysiology peculiar to specific diseases and associated with specific organisms are addressed in other chapters. However, several issues in the pathogenesis and pathophysiology of ALRIs are important to the overall understanding of these infections.

Definition of *Bronchiolitis*. The issues that have been raised about the definition of *bronchiolitis* are well demonstrated by quoting from two published sources as follows:

In 1976, McIntosh[37] wrote:

> Clinicians who care for small children all know what [bronchiolitis] means: an acute illness characterized by profuse rhinorrhea, cough, dyspnea, and wheeze. . . . . On x-ray examination, there is hyperexpansion, occasionally atelectasis, and often a slight bilateral perihilar infiltrate. The term bronchiolitis is usually reserved for this syndrome when it occurs in children under 12 mo. Over this age it is often called wheezy bronchitis, asthmatoid bronchitis, or sometimes just asthma. The disease at various ages of childhood nevertheless forms a continuum, and there is no precise age where one can point to a change from bronchiolitis to something else.

In 1992, Welliver and Cherry[33] addressed the issue as follows:

> In the past, bronchiolitis and infectious asthma were sometimes considered distinct entities. However, further study seems to indicate that they are quite similar in terms of clinical presentation, pathologic findings, mechanisms of pathogenesis, and long-term prognosis, whereas differences between the two in terms of etiologic agents precipitating illness episodes or in terms of response to therapy are more a function of patient age than of any underlying disease process.

Role of Atopy, Reactive Airways, or Both Factors. The role of atopy and reactive airways has been an important issue in bronchiolitis. Although it is clear that certain agents, especially RSV, can cause wheezing associated infection in children in the absence of atopy or reactive airways, it seems equally clear that such infections are more severe or tend to recur more frequently in children who are atopic or have reactive airways. This issue is addressed very well by Welliver and Cherry[33] as follows:

> A unifying concept of the pathogenesis of bronchiolitis incorporating the above findings can be formulated. Bronchiolitis occurs as a result of infection of individuals in early life who have hyperreactive airways. Mild forms of illness occur in those individuals who are not immunologically hypersensitive to viral antigen. In contrast, both severe forms of bronchiolitis and recurrent episodes of wheezing occur, according to currently available data, in those individuals who, in addition to having increased airway reactivity, also manifest IgE-mediated hypersensitivity to one or more viral antigens. Increased airway reactivity is an inheritable trait, frequently acquired in association with a tendency to atopy. The concept of increased airway reactivity as the fundamental defect in bronchiolitis therefore may explain the frequency of repeated wheezing episodes, the long-term abnormalities of pulmonary function, and the possible association of bronchiolitis with atopy.

Others consider that bronchiolitis and asthma are distinct entities in children with wheeze-associated respiratory infections, and this is further discussed in Chapters 38 and 61. Some would argue that bronchiolitis occurs in infants younger than 6 to 12 months of age who have preexisting risk factors or who have been exposed to viruses, particularly RSV. One of the risk factors is asthma.

The same issues have been raised in some cases of croup. Some children have recurrent bouts of croup, and most of these are diagnosed as spasmodic croup, although in recent years little effort has been made to separate these cases from those of infectious croup. In the past the diagnosis of spasmodic croup was reserved for young children, usually boys, who had recurrent bouts described as follows: The episodes always occur at night, there are low fever and only mild upper respiratory symptoms, the onset is sudden, and the infection responds well to the administration of moist air. Similar but usually milder bouts may occur for several nights. There is some evidence that recurrent or spasmodic croup is due to hyperactive airways, probably on an atopic basis.[32]

Bacterial Superinfections

Bacterial superinfection has also been a contentious issue in the pathogenesis and management of children with ALRIs. There has been widespread belief that bacterial superinfections are common complications of viral pneumonia. Although some such complications do occur, they are not common and are usually restricted to a few rather predictable circumstances. It has been recognized that patients with influenza virus infections do have bacterial superinfections, usually with *S. pneumoniae, S. aureus, H. influenzae,* and in the past, group A streptococci.[38] These superinfections are uncommon, but when they occur, they can be devastating. It has not been demonstrated that pneumonia resulting from the other respiratory viruses is frequently complicated by bacterial infections. Studies with RSV infections have shown that such occurrences are unusual.[39] Because bacteria can cause primary pulmonary infections that are difficult to separate from viral infections, the clinical caregiver is faced with a dilemma in some instances; this usually results in the administration of appropriate antibiotics.

A similar issue presents occasionally with children with croup. In the days before antibiotics, there were frequent descriptions of a syndrome termed *laryngotracheobronchitis* caused by the same bacteria. The isolation of viruses was not possible, so the relationship to the respiratory viruses is unknown. This syndrome disappeared in the 1940s, only to reappear in 1979 as the renamed *bacterial tracheitis.*[40] It is postulated, but not proved, that the syndrome is initiated by a viral infection. This complication is not common, but because of its severity, it should be kept in mind by clinicians caring for children.

Tracheobronchitis as a Clinical Entity

Tracheobronchitis as a clinical syndrome has not been widely recognized by physicians. The studies in North Carolina called attention to a large group of children who had cough and who may have had inspiratory and/or expiratory noises on auscultation but who did not have laryngeal obstruction, did not have audible wheeze or crackles.[41] Such patients fit into a separate epidemiologic picture because their condition is caused by several respiratory viruses, especially RSV (in young children); *M. pneumoniae* (in older children); and the influenza viruses (in children of all ages). The recognition of this syndrome is important because the infection of most of these patients can be managed without antibiotics.

Age Occurrence of Infection from Influenza Viruses and M. pneumoniae

Most respiratory agents produce ALRIs in preschoolers, and the rate of infection is related inversely to the age of the child. There are notable exceptions: the influenza viruses, *M. pneumoniae,* and possibly *C. pneumoniae.* The influenza viruses cause infections in patients of all ages, apparently because the virus has the ability and tendency to change the nature of its antigenic structure.[38] Thus immunity to the influenza viruses does not play a large role in protecting the older host, as is the case with most other respiratory viruses. *M. pneumoniae* has a very different age distribution, causing most illness in school-age children, with only rare or occasional clinical infections in preschoolers.[3] Young children are infected frequently but develop only circulating antibodies. Repeated infections stimulate the development of cellular immunity, which apparently promotes the clinical expression of disease.[42] Infections resulting from *Chlamydia* species apparently have the same age distribution as *Mycoplasma* infections, but the reason for this has not been demonstrated.[4]

Implications

Many ill children seen by the primary care physician have acute respiratory ailments. Many of these involve only the upper respiratory tract, and throat swabs processed for the rapid detection of group A streptococcal carbohydrate ("rapid strep test") or cultured on sheep blood agar for the isolation and identification of group A streptococci are the most important guides for antibiotic therapy. Making this decision when the illness involves the lower respiratory tract is more complex. Because of the lack of quick, easy, and inexpensive methods for identifying etiologic agents in these patients, the clinician has only clinical and epidemiologic tools to aid in the decision of whether to use antibiotics. If the clinical syndrome, the age and gender of the patient, and season of the year are considered, a good estimation of cause can be made; this should lead to more precise and effective use of antibiotics.[15,43]

Croup. Most cases of croup[44] are caused by viruses, especially the parainfluenza viruses. *M. pneumoniae* is an infrequent cause; other bacteria such as *Corynebacterium diphtheriae* are rarely involved. Because parainfluenza virus type 1, the most common cause of croup, is isolated predominantly in the autumn, this is the croup season. Croup occurs rarely in the first few months of life and reaches its peak occurrence in the second year; it occurs predominantly in boys. Most cases of croup are mild and require only supportive treatment, but occasionally a child has findings, although consistent with laryngeal obstruction, that require different management. The child with epiglottitis probably is infected with *H. influenzae* type b, and the infection should be treated accordingly. Very rarely a patient with laryngeal obstruction suggesting croup or epiglottitis may have bacterial laryngotracheobronchitis caused by *S. aureus, S. pneumoniae, H. influenzae,* or group A streptococci. Thus with few exceptions, the clinician can diagnose croup with clinical and epidemiologic tools and be reasonably confident that the decision to withhold antibiotics is correct.

Tracheobronchitis. Physicians have long recognized that a productive cough can be present without other findings of lower respiratory tract involvement, but tracheobronchitis[41] as a separate disease entity has been described only recently. The agents involved are viruses and *M. pneumoniae*. All of these agents can cause tracheobronchitis, but RSV, *M. pneumoniae,* and the influenza viruses are most commonly isolated. These agents have definite age and seasonal patterns, thus dictating the age of patients with tracheobronchitis and the seasons when these infections occur. RSV infection occurs in young children in winter and spring, the influenza viruses in all age groups in the winter and spring, and *M. pneumoniae* in school-age children in the autumn. Although erythromycin and the tetracyclines are effective in *M. pneumoniae* infections, supportive treatment is all that is required in most children with tracheobronchitis.

Bronchiolitis. Bronchiolitis[45] and other wheezing LRIs are the most common ALRI syndromes in small children. They are caused frequently by RSV, although all other respiratory agents can cause wheezing. Bronchiolitis occurs in the winter and spring during RSV epidemics in young infants. ALRIs with wheezing in school-age children in the autumn are frequently related to *M. pneumoniae*. This syndrome is not caused by other bacteria. The management of bronchiolitis is supportive in most cases; data to support the use of bronchodilators are lacking. Ribavirin is effective against RSV in vitro and has been reported to ameliorate illnesses caused by this agent.[39] It is not recommended for general use.

Pneumonia. Bacteria other than *M. pneumoniae* are unusual causes of croup, tracheobronchitis, and bronchiolitis. In children with one of these syndromes, when all other clinical and epidemiologic data are compatible with an uncomplicated infection, the clinician is justified in withholding antibiotics. The role of bacteria other than *M. pneumoniae* in pneumonia[46] is much less clear, presenting the clinician with a somewhat different challenge. There are several circumstances that may suggest methods of management. To begin, RSV and the influenza viruses are the most common causes of pneumonia in young children. The older child with lobar pneumonia probably is infected with *S. pneumoniae.* The presence of significant amounts of pleural fluid suggests an etiologic agent other than *M. pneumoniae* or a virus. *M. pneumoniae* infections occur in school-age children and are usually characterized by the gradual onset of symptoms, notably cough. Pulmonary infiltrates are usually of interstitial or bronchopneumonia character, involving one of the lower lobes. The demonstration of high (greater than1:128) or rising titers of cold hemagglutinins suggests the diagnosis. The simultaneous presence of several children with similar findings in a community usually indicates an epidemic of *M. pneumoniae* disease and simplifies management in similar patients for the duration of the epidemic. In the absence of clinical and epidemiologic data suggesting viral or *M. pneumoniae* pneumonia, the severity of illness is probably the best guide to management; the child who is severely ill should receive antimicrobial treatment until recovery or until studies indicate that such treatment is unnecessary. The child with mild pneumonia, when a respiratory virus is commonly causing disease in other children in the community, can be safely observed without antibiotic therapy.

Conclusions. In determining the general applicability of these guidelines, the physician should keep in mind that most of the observations discussed were made in a small city in North Carolina. Certain correlations, however, have been constant regardless of where studies were performed. RSV, parainfluenza viruses types 1 and 3, *M. pneumoniae,* the adenoviruses, and the influenza viruses have consistently been the most common infecting agents. The age-related rate of agents, the age-related syndromes, and the association of certain agents and particular syndromes have also been consistent, as has the predominance of ALRIs in boys. The epidemiologic aspect most variable and most likely to differ among geographic locations is the seasonal occurrence of infections with specific agents. In general, the trends presented are similar to those reported by other investigators in the United States, but may differ in other parts of the world. In the tropics, for example, ALRIs tend to be more frequent during the rainy season. The presence of regional laboratories capable of identifying the agents causing current respiratory tract infections in various geographic areas would be of immense help to the practicing pediatrician. The Centers for Disease Control and Prevention have performed this task for many years for the United States and reports the isolation of influenza viruses in *Morbidity and Mortality Weekly Report;* occasionally, RSV isolations have also been reported. Several laboratories around the country report the isolation of respiratory disease agents in local communities.

It seems likely that *S. pneumoniae* and *H. influenzae* are not major causes of ALRIs in developed countries. This may not be true in developing countries, and clinicians caring for children in these areas should be aware of the role that these two bacteria may play in the excessive morbidity and mortality among children with ALRIs, especially in pneumonia.

The type of data presented is important for reasons other than the management of acute illness. The quantitative roles of the various agents are well demonstrated. RSV is clearly the most important cause of ALRIs in children and should receive the most attention from investigators. Of the other agents discussed, the influenza and parainfluenza viruses and *M. pneumoniae* are the most important. The age-specific occurrence of agents suggests the populations in which preventive measures could help. For example, RSV and parainfluenza virus type 3 infections occur very early in life, and if preventive measures are to be effective, they must be applied before or shortly after birth. In contrast, illnesses caused by *M. pneumoniae* are not common in preschool children, so methods to prevent these could be delayed. It is readily apparent that RSV and parainfluenza virus type 3 cause frequent and at times severe disease when circulating antibodies are present. This suggests that preventive measures designed to provoke such antibody, unless in very high titers, might not be successful.

A review of this kind would not be complete without mention of the possible role of acute ALRIs on the subsequent health of children's lungs.[31] Infections, along with reactive airways (with or without atopy) and inhaled pollutants (mostly cigarette smoke), are important risk factors in the development of chronic lung disease. Bronchiolar involvement in early life, and possibly involvement of other anatomic sites, based on a predisposition to respiratory illness of both genetic and intrauterine origin, is probably associated with decrements of pulmonary function in later childhood.

ALRIs in Hospitalized Children

The overwhelming majority of children with ALRIs can be satisfactorily cared for outside of the hospital. Although the criteria for hospitalization vary greatly among societies, communities, and individual health care personnel, general guidelines can be made in the following categories for those who are not usually cared for at home:

1. Patients at the end of the severity spectrum of community-acquired ALRIs
2. ALRIs acquired nosocomially
3. ALRIs that are caused by unusual microorganisms or that occur in children with altered host defenses

This section does not present in detail the cases of ALRI in which the patients are hospitalized; these patients are discussed in other sections addressing the specific infections. Instead, a general overall view showing where this group of patients fits into the big picture of ALRIs is presented.

Severe Community-Acquired Infections

Few children with croup, tracheobronchitis, bronchiolitis, or pneumonia are ill enough to require hospitalization. Occasionally, a child with severe infectious croup develops sufficient laryngeal obstruction to require hospital treatment or the insertion of an airway. The child with bacterial tracheitis, which occurs rarely, always requires immediate specific treatment and attention to a proper airway. Children with uncomplicated tracheobronchitis rarely require hospital care. The hospitalization of children with bronchiolitis is an interesting phenomenon. Although RSV infections are less frequent in the first few months of life than in later months, most children hospitalized with RSV bronchiolitis are younger than 3 months of age. The precise reason for this is unknown, but the small size of the infant airway probably is a major factor. Small children with cardiac and pulmonary abnormalities are also at increased risk for severe bronchiolitis and usually require hospitalization. Infants of parents who smoke are more likely to be admitted to the hospital with bronchiolitis. Patients with pneumonia pose the greatest problem. The inability to determine the precise etiology by clinical and epidemiologic means and the realization that some of these patients have a treatable infection usually lead the clinician to be more cautious. This probably results in a greater number of hospitalizations in patients with pneumonia than in children with other syndromes. Regardless of the reason for hospitalization, the microbial etiology of the ALRIs in these patients is usually the same as in those cared for at home, and the recommendations for management remain the same. The availability of rapid diagnostic techniques for several of the respiratory agents has simplified the diagnosis and hence the management. The prime example are methods for rapidly identifying the RSV in infants with severe bronchiolitis or pneumonia, suggesting candidates who may be considered for treatment with ribavirin.

Children with altered host defenses can and do have infections with the same organisms that infect normal children. These infections are not unusually severe most of the time, but there is an increasing number of reports of severe and even fatal infections in such patients.[2,39,47] Such children should, of course, be cared for in the hospital.

Nosocomial Infections

Under certain circumstances, nosocomial infections can be a large problem. Because the agents that commonly cause ALRI also cause upper respiratory infections, which are more frequent, nosocomial spread is not frequently demonstrated by multiple cases of ALRIs. As a general rule the respiratory viruses cause more nosocomial infections than bacteria. Among the respiratory viruses, RSV is clearly the most contagious in the hospital; there are reports of infections in up to 45% of hospital contacts.[39] Nosocomial spread by the parainfluenza and influenza viruses has also been reported.[47,48] Adenoviruses and enteroviruses apparently cause fewer problems.

The nosocomial spread of common respiratory bacteria does not appear to be as much of a problem, partly because of the effectiveness of antibiotics in eradicating the infective organism. The long incubation period of *M. pneumoniae* infections probably precludes the recognition of spread of this organism in the hospital, although it has caused multiple infections in closed populations, such as school children and military populations.[3] The difficulty in diagnosing ALRIs resulting from *S. pneumoniae* or *H. influenzae* precludes any study of the spread of these organisms in the hospital, but the familial spread of *S. pneumoniae* has been described.[49]

The nosocomial spread of the agents causing ALRIs is a particular problem among patients with altered host defenses, including patients with cystic fibrosis.[50] Some aspects of such patients with ALRI are addressed in the next section or in special chapters devoted to the special entities.

ALRIs in Uncommon or Special Circumstances

Box 36-3 lists the microbial agents that cause ALRI in children in uncommon or special circumstances. Infections with these agents occur infrequently in normal children but can be very important when they do occur. Pneumonia is the usual syndrome seen under these circumstances. Although infections with some of these special agents have characteristic clinical findings, most are notable because they are severe or simply do not "fit the picture" of uncomplicated community-acquired infections. Infections with these special organisms are a particular problem in children with altered host defenses. The common use of adrenal corticosteroids and other medications that alter host defenses, especially in organ transplantation, are the most likely underlying reasons that host defenses are depressed.

ALRIs in Developing Countries

More children under 5 years of age in developing countries die from ALRIs than from any other single disease entity.[23,25,51-53] Every 7 seconds a child in the third world dies of an ARI, usually pneumonia. Of the 14 million children under 5 years of age who die each year in the third world, 4.24 million, 30%, die from respiratory tract infections: 840,000 from measles, 400,000 from pertussis, and 3 million from pneumonia. Because respiratory infections are the greatest problem in small children, this discussion pertains only to children under 5 years of age. Interpretation of available literature on this subject is compromised by the great diversity of the data sources and the inability to evaluate accurately how many of the differences are due to methodologic problems related to patient selection, study design, or laboratory methods. In spite of this difficulty, it is clear that ALRIs are a far greater problem in developing countries than in developed ones.

Incidence and Severity

The incidence of total respiratory tract infections in young children is very similar throughout the world where data have been collected. In studies sponsored by the Board on Science and Technology for International Development (BOSTID) of the National Research Council in 10 developing countries, the incidence of total respiratory infections varied between 6.6 and 8.7 per child per year with one outlier of 14.3.[24] Pio et al[51] reported incidence rates in developing countries of 4.2 to 7.9 per child per year. These figures are not greatly different from those reported from Michigan, Washington, and Ohio, which varied from 4.5 to 7.0 per child per year.[1,16,19] In contrast to the overall incidence of respiratory infections, the incidence of severe ALRIs is far greater in third-world children. The BOSTID studies recorded rates of all LRIs, mostly pneumonia, of up to 29.6 per 100 children per year. Pio et al[51] reported incidence rates for pneumonia in three developing countries of 5.3 to 25.6 per 100 children per year. These are to be compared with rates of pneumonia of 3.6 in North Carolina and 3.0 in Washington.[15,16] Case fatality rates for children with ALRIs in developing countries are remarkably high. Pio et al[51] reported rates of 2.7% to 12.3% in hospitalized children. The BOSTID studies reported by Selwyn[24] showed rates of 3.2% to 15.8%.

The figures for deaths are even more impressive. A study reported by the Institute of Medicine estimated the mortality rates from ARIs in some developing nations to be as high as 1500 per 100,000 children under 1 year of age and up to 500 per 100,000 for children 1 to 4 years of age.[54] Although these figures are only estimates, they are reinforced by data reported by Pio et al,[51] which showed that deaths in infants resulting from pneumonia and influenza were 173.6 and 251.0 in Egypt and Guatemala, respectively, compared with 0.7 and 1.1 per 100,000 live births in France and the Netherlands, a rate 150 to 300 times greater in the developing countries.

The number of visits to outpatient clinics or admissions to hospital with respiratory infections is another marker of severity. Table 36-2 shows that in certain developing countries, 30.1% to 60.7% of clinic visits and 31.5% to 35.8% of hospital admissions were due to ARIs.[51] The proportion of a child's time ill with respiratory infections is still another way to demonstrate morbidity. In her summary of the BOSTID studies, Selwyn[24] reported that children in seven developing countries were ill with ARIs 21.7% to 40.1% of the time. The same studies showed that children were ill from LRIs from 0.3% to 14.4% of the time.

Etiology

The same viruses and bacteria that cause LRIs in developed countries cause them in many developing countries. The principal viruses are RSV, parainfluenza viruses, influenza viruses, and adenoviruses. The bacteria are *S. pneumoniae, H. influenzae,* and *S. aureus.* As in developed nations, in developing countries, most respiratory infections are due to viruses, involve only the upper respiratory tract, and are mild and self-limiting, but many LRIs do occur and are generally more severe; many are life threatening.

Viral Agents. The isolation of respiratory viruses from hospitalized and nonhospitalized children has been reported from many developing countries. Variations in isolation techniques, choice of patients, and interpretations of data make estimates of the quantitative roles of each virus very difficult, but the same viruses are isolated wherever studies have been done.[24,25] Berman[25] has summarized the proportion of respiratory infections produced by the viruses as follows: RSV, 15% to 20%; parainfluenza viruses, 7% to 10%; influenza viruses types A and B, 5%; and adenoviruses, 2% to 4%. Recent studies have not shown as large a relative role for the influenza viruses in developing countries as has been estimated in the United States. This is probably because of the difficulty of isolating these viruses. In spite of the paucity of data to estimate roles of respiratory viruses in illnesses in developing countries, there is strong evidence that they have a major role.

Bacterial Agents. Establishing the role of bacteria as causes of LRIs in children in developing countries has been as difficult to determine as establishing their role in developed countries. Carriage of *S. pneumoniae* and *H. influenzae* in a large number of normal children, the lack of association of these agents with characteristic syndromes in most cases, and the failures of young children to develop antibodies to capsular

Table 36-2 Third-World Children with Respiratory Infections Admitted to Outpatient Clinics or Hospitals

COUNTRY	ADMISSIONS
Admitted to outpatient clinics	
Brazil	41.8%
Nigeria	30.1%
Thailand	60.7%
Iraq	39.3%
Admitted to hospital	
Bangladesh	35.8%
Burma	31.5%
Pakistan	33.6%
Zambia	34.0%

Adapted from Pio A et al. In Douglas RM, Kerby-Eaton E, eds: *Acute respiratory infections in childhood: proceedings of an international workshop,* Sydney, August 1984, University of Adelaide, pp 3-17.

polysaccharide have hampered studies. This problem is more complex in developing countries, where carriage of these bacteria can be very high. In Papua New Guinea, studies have shown that carriage was established at a very early age and reached 100% before 3 months of age. Carriage was established somewhat earlier for *S. pneumonia* than for *H. influenzae*.[51] Thus the children had the opportunity to become infected with the bacteria even if it is not understood why a particular child becomes infected. At this time the isolation of these agents from the blood or from percutaneous aspirates from the pleural space or lung is the only reliable way of establishing bacteria as causative agents. Berman[25] has summarized available literature showing the results of lung aspirates on children with pneumonia (Table 36-3). *S. pneumonia* and *H. influenzae* were frequent isolates. *S. aureus* was rather inconsistently reported, placing some doubt as to its role. The interpretation of these data, showing bacterial isolates in 62% of instances, is difficult because of the bias in patient selection. Furthermore, isolation of bacteria from the lung does not demonstrate the nature of their role in the pathogenesis of disease. The failure to isolate bacteria in 38% of patients suggests that agents other than those isolated played an important role as well. In summarizing the role of isolation of bacteria from the blood in children with ALRIs in developing countries, Berman[25] reported that blood cultures were relatively infrequently positive in contrast to lung aspirates.

Studies on further classification of *S. pneumoniae* and *H. influenzae* have produced interesting results.[25] The *H. influenzae* isolates have been classified as type b, typeable but not type b, and nontypeable; the relative distribution varies with individual studies. Data are limited from studies of serotyping *S. pneumoniae* isolates, but prominent among serotypes reported have been types 6, 14, 19, 5, 1, 16, and 31, with the types varying greatly with country of origin. Information on serotypes of both *S. pneumoniae* and *H. influenzae* is important because these data are needed to guide the development of new rapid immunologic diagnostic tests and effective vaccines.

Viral vs. Bacterial Infections. It is interesting to speculate on the relative importance of viral infections and bacterial infections causing ALRIs in developing countries. In a study of candidates for vaccine development, the Institute of Medicine[54] estimated the relative frequency and severity of infections caused by four agents in the developing world's children: parainfluenza viruses, RSV, *H. influenzae,* and *S. pneumoniae* (Table 36-4). The estimated case-fatality rate for bacterial pneumonia caused by *S. pneumoniae* and *H. influenzae* is more than 50 times higher than that for infection caused by respiratory viruses, but the estimated number of deaths resulting from bacterial pneumonia is only 2 to 4 times higher than that resulting from viral infections. Table 36-5 shows the estimated contribution of the four agents to the annual deaths of third-world children. Thus it is clear that viral and bacterial infections contribute greatly to the excessive mortality rate of third-world children.

Limited information is available on the interaction of viruses and bacteria in the production of severe illnesses. As mentioned earlier, the influenza virus is the only respiratory virus for which there is widely accepted evidence that it predisposes the host to superimposed bacterial infections. Data available from studies with RSV suggest that bacterial superinfections are unusual. In spite of this, there is widespread belief in developing countries that bacterial pneumonia after (and caused by) viral infections is common and is the cause of many severe infections. Studies in Papua New Guinea have shown that documented viral infections occurred concurrently in two thirds of bacterial infections diagnosed by isolation of a bacterial pathogen from lung or blood.[25] In Pakistan, 26% of children infected with RSV also had bacteremia infection with *H. influenzae* or *S. pneumoniae*.[25] Some 54% of the cases of bacteremia caused by *H. influenzae* infection and 47% of the cases of bacteremia caused by *S. pneumoniae* infections were associated with viral infection.

Unfortunately these studies do not clarify the relationship between viral and bacterial LRIs. Possibilities for this relationship are as follows:

1. Viral and bacterial infections are common and can occur simultaneously but are not related.
2. Viral infections result in a reduction of host defenses, which predisposes to superimposed bacterial infections and more severe disease.
3. Bacterial infections predispose the host to viral infections.
4. Simultaneous viral and bacterial infections, regardless of their relationship, have an additive effect and produce more severe disease.

The answers to these questions await future studies.

Table 36-3 Isolation of Bacterial Pathogens*

BACTERIUM ISOLATED	POSITIVE
S. pneumoniae	27%
H. influenzae	27%
S. aureus	17%
TOTAL	62%

Adapted from Berman S: *Rev Infect Dis* 13(suppl 6):S454-S462, 1991 (review).
*From 1096 lung aspirates from hospitalized children with ALRIs.

Table 36-4 Relative Case Frequencies of Cases of Respiratory Infections

CATEGORY	PARAINFLUENZA VIRUSES	RSV	*H. INFLUENZAE*	*S. PNEUMONIAE*
Mild	500	300	—	—
Moderate	100	100	—	—
Severe	10	10	7	7
Death	1	1	1	1

Adapted from Institute of Medicine: *New vaccine development: establishing priorities,* vol 2, *Diseases of importance in developing countries,* Washington, DC, 1986, National Academy Press, pp 46-62.

Table 36-5 Annual Deaths from ARIs*

PATHOGEN	DEATHS
Parainfluenza viruses	5.5%
RSV	7.0%
H. influenzae	11.5%
S. pneumoniae	22.5%

Adapted from Institute of Medicine: *New vaccine development: establishing priorities,* vol 2, *Diseases of importance in developing countries,* Washington, DC, 1986, National Academy Press, pp 46-62.
*Does not include influenza viruses.

Risk Factors

Risk factors that might increase the incidence and severity of ALRIs in nonhospitalized children in developed countries include age; crowding; male gender; inhaled pollutants; anatomic abnormalities; metabolic disease and immunologic deficiencies; malnutrition, including lack of breast-feeding; and certain social and economic factors. These same risk factors are present in developing countries, at times in very exaggerated incidences.[24,25] Crowding, inhaled pollutants, malnutrition, and extreme poverty are all found in abundance in developing countries and can play a role in the incidence and severity of ALRIs. Malnutrition, so common in developing countries, probably plays a major role in reducing the host defenses of children. The precise role of malnutrition is unknown, but there is increasing evidence that vitamin A deficiency may be an important factor. Low birth weight, found in 20% to 40% of births in some developing countries, is also associated with severe infections. Much work needs to be done to more precisely clarify the role of risk factors in ARIs, especially in third-world children.

What Is Known

Near the end of the studies sponsored by BOSTID, the state of knowledge of respiratory infections in the third world was explored.[55,56] Box 36-4 summarizes knowledge about the etiologic agents, clinical disease, and epidemiology of these infections. It seems clear that pneumonia is the most important clinical syndrome, but knowledge of its precise etiology and pathogenesis is limited. It does appear, however, that good case management is appropriate and lifesaving in some instances. Because malnutrition and poverty can affect so many things, it is clear that there is little agreement regarding the main risk factors in severe ALRIs in the developing world.[57]

Research Needs

Knowledge about ALRIs in developing countries is fragmentary at best. Thus clinicians need to know more about them. Box 36-5 outlines some of the research needs for ALRIs in developing countries.[57] If the burden of ALRIs in developing nations is to be reduced, it is clear that more and better epidemiologic studies about the natural history of these infections are needed. Physiologic risks such as prematurity, chronic neonatal lung disease, and congenital abnormalities all need to be investigated. Vaccines against nontypeable *H. influenzae* and *S. pneumoniae* should be investigated. The possibility of using maternal immunity in preventing disease early in life should be explored. Measles and pertussis are still problems. Touching all of these, however, are the technically difficult and expensive methods for accurately and quickly identifying etiologic agents. More work is needed in this regard. Under operational research, more about how to deliver oxygen to sick children, the use of bronchodilators, and fluid maintenance should be studied. The treatment of young children needs to be improved. More about the knowledge, attitudes, and practices of mothers and other health care givers in a widely diverse group of cultural circumstances needs to be elucidated.

Possibly the most important thing that needs to be known about ARI in developing countries concerns the pathogenesis of these infections. Until the pathogenesis is understood (see Box 36-5), adequate prevention and treatment of these conditions will be impossible. Rather recent studies have described pathologic lesions in the lungs of malnourished children that are characteristic of those resulting from vitamin A deficiency.[58] There is widespread belief, and practice, that bacterial invasions follow other respiratory viral infections, but the data that will support this contention are not available. As already emphasized, the role of the carriage of *H. influenzae* and *S. pneumoniae* remains speculative and should be studied. Finally, the role of unidentified risk factors in the pathogenesis

BOX 36-4
Respiratory Infections in Third-World Children

Etiologic agents

Similarities occur all over world.
Viruses include RSV, parainfluenza viruses types 1 and 3, adenoviruses, and influenza viruses types A and B.
Bacteria include *S. pneumoniae, H. influenzae* types b and non-b, and nontypeable *H. influenzae.*

Clinical disease

Pneumonia is a big problem.
Events leading to severe disease complex are largely unknown.
Good case management is beneficial.

Epidemiology

The incidence of total respiratory infections is remarkably constant all over the world.
Only severity and mortality are increased.
Risk factors include age, malnutrition, and poverty.

BOX 36-5
Future Research of Respiratory Infections in Third-World Children

Prevention and epidemiology

- Risk factor reduction
  - Malnutrition
  - Crowding
  - Physiologic risks
  - Inhaled pollutants
- Infections in infants
- Vaccines
  - *S. pneumoniae* and *H. influenzae*
  - Maternal immunity
  - Measles and pertussis vaccines
  - Diagnostic capability

Case management

- Operational research
  - Oxygen-delivery systems
  - Use of bronchodilators
  - Fluid maintenance
- Treatment of infants
- Early detection and treatment
- Antibiotics
  - Appropriate medications, doses, and schedules
  - Compliance
  - Adverse reactions
  - Bacterial resistance
- Assessment of knowledge, attitudes, and practices of mothers

Pathogenesis

- Autopsies or equivalent examinations
- Methods for assessing diagnosis
- Role of anatomic factors and functions
- Viruses vs. bacteria
- Role of carriage of *S. pneumoniae* and *H. influenzae*
- Role of risk factors

needs to be sought. In the author's opinion, the role of malnutrition as a depressor of the immune system and in vitamin A deficiency is the most promising avenue to be explored.

SUMMARY AND CONCLUSIONS

The problem of ARIs is an immense one, especially in third-world children, and the ability to cope with ARIs is not as great as could be desired. In the past few years, more has been learned about this problem, but not nearly enough is being done. In 1984, Chretien et al[59] said the following:

> No matter who is responsible, the situation represents seriously misplaced priorities. The lack of recognition of the problem, the lack of funds, and the lack of programs have led to an international tragedy of almost unprecedented magnitude.
>
> Properly organized research programs into the etiologic agents involved in ARI, together with data collection on other contributing factors, including demographic, geographic, climatic, and social factors, are needed so that effective programs of prevention and treatment can be mounted.
>
> Although attention is beginning to be focused on these areas, it must be expanded. The health professions are certainly capable of providing the expertise and resources to meet the challenge. What is needed is motivation. If, through neglect on the part of the medical profession, policy makers, governments, and health agencies, this problem is not tackled soon, the international tragedy may become an international scandal.

The author agrees with this statement but is very fearful that the situation remains much the same today as it was in 1984.

REFERENCES

1. Dingle JH, Badger GF, Jordan WS Jr: *Illness in the home: a study of 25,000 illnesses in a group of Cleveland families,* Cleveland, 1964, Press of Western Reserve University, pp 33-96.

Epidemiology

2. McMillan JA, Werner LB, Higgins AM, MacKnight K: Rhinovirus infection associated with serious illness among pediatric patients, *Pediatr Infect Dis J* 12:321-325, 1993.
3. Denny FW, Clyde WA Jr, Glezen WP: *Mycoplasma pneumoniae* disease: clinical spectrum, pathophysiology, epidemiology and control, *J Infect Dis* 123:74-92, 1971.
4. Grayston JT: *Chlamydia pneumoniae:* strain TWAR, *Chest* 95:664-669, 1989 (review).
5. Denny FW, Collier AM, Henderson FW: Acute respiratory infections in day care, *Rev Infect Dis* 8:527-532, 1986.
6. Gray BM, Converse GM III, Dillon HG Jr: Epidemiological studies of *Streptococcus pneumoniae* in infants: the effects of season and age on pneumococcal acquisition and carriage in the first 24 months of life, *Am J Epidemiol* 116:692-703, 1982.
7. Gray BM, Converse GM III, Dillon HG Jr: Epidemiological studies of *Streptococcus pneumoniae* in infants: acquisition, carriage and infection during the first 24 months of life, *J Infect Dis* 142:923-933, 1980.
8. Henderson FW, Collier AM, Sanyal MA, Watkins JM, Fairclough DL, Clyde WA Jr, Denny FW: A longitudinal study of respiratory viruses and bacteria in the etiology of acute otitis media with effusion, *N Engl J Med* 306:1377-1383, 1983.
9. Loda FA, Colllier AM, Glezen WP, Strangert K, Clyde WA Jr, Denny, FW: Occurrence of *Diplococcus pneumoniae* in the upper respiratory tract of children, *J Pediatr* 87:1087-1093, 1975.
10. McIntosh K, Halonen P, Ruuskanen O: Report of a workshop on respiratory viral infection: epidemiology, diagnosis, treatment, and prevention, *Clin Infect Dis* 16:151-164, 1993.
11. Jalonen E, Paton JC, Koskela M, Kerttula Y, Leinonen M: Measurement of antibody responses to pneumolysin: a promising method for the presumptive aetiological diagnosis of pneumococcal pneumonia, *J Infect Dis* 19:127-134, 1989.
12. Kalin M, Lindberg AA: Antibody response against the type specific capsular polysaccharide in pneumonococcal pneumonia measured by enzyme linked immunosorbent assay, *Scand J Infect Dis* 17:25-32, 1985.
13. Forgie IM, O'Neill KP, Lloyd-Evans N, Leinonen M, Campbell H, Whittle HC, Greenwood BM: Etiology of acute lower respiratory tract infections in Gambian children. II. Acute lower respiratory tract infections in children ages one to nine years presenting at the hospital, *Pediatr Infect Dis J* 10:42-47, 1991.
14. Bisno AL: Group A streptococcal infections and rheumatic fever, *N Engl J Med* 325:783-793, 1991 (review).
15. Denny FW, Clyde WA Jr: Acute lower respiratory tract infections in non-hospitalized children, *J Pediatr* 108:635-646, 1986.
16. Foy HM, Cooney MK, Maletzky AJ, Grayston JT: Incidence and etiology of pneumonia, croup and bronchiolitis in preschool children belonging to a prepaid medical care group over a four-year period, *Am J Epidemiol* 97:80-92, 1973.
17. Berman S, Duenas A, Bedoya A, Constain V, Leon S, Borrero I, Murphy J: Acute lower respiratory tract illnesses in Cali, Colombia: a two-year ambulatory study, *Pediatrics* 71:210-218, 1983.
18. Glezen WP: Serious morbidity and mortality associated with influenza epidemics, *Epidemiol Res* 4:25-44, 1982.
19. Monto AS, Cavallaro JJ: The Tecumseh study of respiratory illness. II. Patterns of occurrence of infection with respiratory pathogens, 1965-1969, *Am J Epidemiol* 94:280-289, 1971.
20. Loda FA, Clyde WA Jr, Glezen WP, Senior RJ, Sheaffer CI, Denny FW Jr: Studies on the role of viruses, bacteria and *M. pneumoniae* as causes of lower respiratory tract infections in children, *J Pediatr* 72:161-176, 1968.
21. Chanock RM, Parrott RH: Acute respiratory diseases in infancy and childhood: present understanding and prospects for prevention, *Pediatrics* 36:21-39, 1965.
22. Glezen WP: Viral pneumonia as a cause and result of hospitalization, *J Infect Dis* 147:765-770, 1983.
23. Graham NMH: The epidemiology of acute respiratory infections in children and adults: a global perspective, *Epidemiol Rev* 12:149-178, 1990 (review).
24. Selwyn BJ on behalf of the Coordinated Data Group of BOSTID Researchers: The epidemiology of acute respiratory tract infections in young children: comparison of findings from several developing countries, *Rev Infect Dis* 12(suppl 8):S870-S888, 1990.
25. Berman S: Epidemiology of acute respiratory infections in children in developing countries, *Rev Infect Dis* 13(suppl 6):S454-S462, 1991 (review).
26. Monto AS, Ullman BM: Acute respiratory illness in an American community, *JAMA* 227:164-169, 1974.
27. Health effects of environmental tobacco smoke exposure. In *The health consequences of involuntary smoking: a report of the Surgeon General,* Rockville, Md, 1986, US Department of Health and Human Services, Public Health Service, pp 17-118,
28. Committee on Passive Smoking, Board of Environmental Studies and Toxicology, National Research Council: *Effects of exposure to environmental tobacco smoke on lung function and respiratory symptoms in environmental tobacco smoke: measuring exposures and assessing health effects,* Washington, DC, 1986, National Academy Press, pp 202-209.
29. Honicky RE, Osborne JS III, Akpom CA: Symptoms of respiratory illness in young children and the use of wood-burning stoves for indoor heating, *Pediatrics* 75:587-593, 1985.
30. Melia RJW, Florey CV, Altman DG, Swan AV: Association between gas cooking and respiratory disease in children, *Br Med J* 2:149-152, 1977.
31. Strope GL, Stempel DA: Risk factors associated with the development of chronic lung disease in children, *Pediatr Clin North Am* 31:757-771, 1984.
32. Zach MS, Schnall RP, Landau LI: Upper and lower airway hyperactivity in recurrent croup, *Am Rev Respir Dis* 121:979-983, 1980.
33. Welliver RC, Cherry JD: Bronchiolitis and infectious asthma. In Feigin RD, Cherry JD, eds: *Textbook of pediatric infectious diseases,* ed 3, Philadelphia, 1992, WB Saunders, pp 245-254.
34. Welliver RC, Wong DT, Middleton E Jr, Sun M, McCarthy N, Ogra PL: Role of parainfluenza virus–specific IgE in pathogenesis of croup and wheezing subsequent to infection, *J Pediatr* 101:889-896, 1982.
35. Frank AL, Taber LH, Glezen WP, Kasel GL, Wells CR, Paredes A: Breast-feeding and respiratory virus infection, *Pediatrics* 70:239-245, 1982.
36. Graham NMH, Douglas RM, Ryan P: Stress and acute respiratory infection, *Am J Epidemiol* 124:389-401, 1986.

37. McIntosh, K: Bronchiolitis and asthma: possible common pathogenetic pathways, *J Allergy Clin Immunol* 57:595-604, 1976.
38. Leigh MW, Carson JL, Denny FW Jr: Pathogenesis of respiratory infections due to influenza virus: implications for developing countries, *Rev Infect Dis* 13(suppl 6):S501-S508, 1991 (review).
39. Hall CB: Respiratory syncytial virus. In Feigin RD, Cherry JD, eds: *Textbook of pediatric infectious diseases,* ed 3, Philadelphia, 1992, WB Saunders, pp 1633-1656.
40. Jones R, Santos JI, Overall JC: Bacterial tracheitis, *JAMA* 242:721-726, 1979.
41. Chapman RS, Henderson FW, Clyde WA Jr, Collier AM, Denny FW: The epidemiology of tracheobronchitis in pediatric practice, *Am J Epidemiol* 114:786-797, 1981.
42. Fernald GW, Collier AM, Clyde WA Jr: Respiratory infections due to *Mycoplasma pneumoniae* in infants and children, *Pediatrics* 55:327-335, 1975.
43. Denny FW: Acute respiratory infections in children: etiology and epidemiology, *Pediatr Rev* 9:135-146, 1987 (review).
44. Denny FW, Murphy TF, Clyde WA Jr, Collier AM, Henderson FW: Croup: an 11-year study in pediatric practice, *Pediatrics* 71:871-876, 1983.
45. Henderson FW, Clyde WA Jr, Collier AM, Denny FW: The etiologic and epidemiologic spectrum of bronchiolitis in pediatric practice, *J Pediatr* 95:183-190, 1979.
46. Murphy TF, Henderson FW, Clyde WA Jr, Collier AM, Denny FW: Pneumonia: an eleven year study in a pediatric practice, *Am J Epidemiol* 113:12-21, 1981.
47. Hall CB: Parainfluenza viruses. In Feigin RD, Cherry JD, eds: *Textbook of pediatric infectious diseases,* ed 3, Philadelphia, 1972, WB Saunders, pp 1613-1626.
48. Glezen WP, Cherry JD: Influenza viruses. In Feigin RD, Cherry JD, eds: *Textbook of pediatric infectious diseases,* ed 3, Philadelphia, 1992, WB Saunders, pp 1688-1704.
49. Dowling JN, Sheeke PR, Feldman HA: Pharyngeal pneumococcal acquisitions in "normal" families: a longitudinal study, *J Infect Dis* 124:9-17, 1971.
50. Feigin RD, Matson DO: The compromised host. In Feigin RD, Cherry JD, eds: *Textbook of pediatric infectious diseases,* ed 3, Philadelphia, 1992, WB Saunders, pp 960-989.
51. Pio A, Leowski J, Ten Dam HG: The magnitude of the problem of acute respiratory infections. In Douglas RM, Kerby-Eaton E, eds: *Acute respiratory infections in childhood: proceedings of an international workshop,* Sydney, Australia, August 1984, University of Adelaide, pp 3-17.
52. Denny FW, Loda FA: Acute respiratory infections are the leading cause of death in children in developing countries, *Am J Trop Med Hyg* 35:1-2, 1986.
53. Grant JP: *The state of the world's children, 1993,* published for UNICEF, Oxford, England, 1993, Oxford University Press, p 1-89.
54. Institute of Medicine: *New vaccine development: establishing priorities,* vol 2, *Diseases of importance in developing countries,* Washington, DC, 1986, National Academy Press, p 46-62.
55. Bale JR: Etiology and epidemiology of acute respiratory tract infections in children in developing countries: creation of a research program to determine the etiology and epidemiology of acute respiratory tract infection among children in developing countries, *J Infect Dis* 12(suppl 8):S861-S866, 1990.
56. McIntosh K: Etiology and epidemiology of acute respiratory tract infection in children in developing countries: overview of the symposium, *J Infect Dis* 12(suppl 8):S867-S869, 1990.
57. Denny FW Jr, Bale JR: The BOSTID Research Program: future research needs. In Gadomski A, ed: *Acute lower respiratory infection and child survival in developing countries: understanding the current status and directions for the 1990s—proceedings of a workshop held August 2-3, 1989, in Washington, DC,* Baltimore, Md, 1989, Johns Hopkins University School of Hygiene and Public Health, p 73-79.
58. Anderson VM, Turner T: Histopathology of childhood pneumonia in developing countries, *Rev Infect Dis* 13(suppl 6):S470-S476, 1991.

Summary and Conclusions

59. Chretien J, Holland W, Macklem P, Murray J, Woolcock A: Acute respiratory infections in children: a global public-health problem, *New Engl J Med* 310:982-984, 1984.

CHAPTER 37

Viral Infections of the Lower Respiratory Tract

Dwight B. Dubois and C. George Ray

Worldwide it is estimated that 3 to 5 million children die annually as a result of acute respiratory disease. Viral infections are the greatest contributors to this mortality rate, either directly or indirectly. A common clinical dilemma occurs in reliably discerning treatable causes, such as bacteria, from viral agents that may not be susceptible to specific therapies. Often, the choice is made to treat nearly all young patients who have an acute lower respiratory illness (LRI) with an antibiotic in case a bacterial agent is involved. Such therapy is useless in viral disease and has not been shown to alter the risk of bacterial superinfection; furthermore, such a practice can result in the selection of more resistant organisms if secondary infection does occur.

Capabilities have emerged that, if properly used with thoughtful clinical assessment, can provide a timely, specific diagnosis of many viral LRIs. In addition, specific antiviral therapy is available for some viral infections and may reduce both the morbidity and the mortality rates.

The term *lower respiratory illness* is defined here as the presence of crackles, rhonchi, or wheezes on physical examination or as infiltrates on a chest radiograph. Childhood asthma may be initially difficult to discriminate from LRI in some patients; indeed, both conditions can be present simultaneously.

Although 60% or more of LRIs are primarily viral[1] (Table 37-1), the concern often remains as to whether bacterial infection is present, either as a primary problem or a complication of viral infection. Of the bacteria, *Streptococcus pneumoniae* is by far the most common, followed by *Haemophilus influenzae* and *Staphylococcus aureus.* Clinical features that suggest these causes include an abrupt onset or a change in symptoms over a few to several hours, toxicity, and radiographic findings of parenchymal consolidation, pleural effusions, or both. White blood cell counts are of variable help, but extreme leukocytosis (>20,000 cells/mm^3) or increased polymorphonuclear band counts (>2000 cells/mm^3) suggest possible bacterial involvement. However, such findings are not abso-

Table 37-1 Major Causes of Acute Lower Respiratory Tract Illnesses

SYNDROME	VIRUSES	NONVIRAL AGENTS	ESTIMATED PERCENTAGE CAUSED BY VIRUSES
Epiglottitis	Rare	*Haemophilus influenzae, Streptococcus pyogenes, Streptococcus pneumoniae, Neisseria meningitidis, Corynebacterium diphtheriae*	5-10
Laryngitis and croup	Parainfluenza viruses, influenza viruses, adenoviruses, respiratory syncytical virus, rhinoviruses, coronaviruses, echoviruses	Rare	90
Laryngotracheitis and laryngotracheobronchitis	Same as for laryngitis and croup	*Haemophilus influenzae, Staphylococcus aureus*	90
Bronchitis	Parainfluenza viruses, influenza viruses, respiratory syncytial virus, adenoviruses	*Bordetella pertussis, Bordetella parapertussis, Haemophilus influenzae, Mycoplasma pneumoniae, Chlamydia pneumoniae*	80
Bronchiolitis	Respiratory syncytial virus, parainfluenza viruses, influenza viruses, adenoviruses	*Chlamydia trachomatis, Chlamydia pneumoniae, Mycoplasma pneumoniae*	90
Pneumonia	Same as for bronchiolitis	*Mycoplasma pneumoniae, Chlamydia trachomatis, Chlamydia pneumoniae, Streptococcus pneumoniae, Haemophilus influenzae, Staphylococcus aureus, Legionella* species, *Neisseria meningitidis,* mixed aerobic and anaerobic flora*	70-80

*Aspiration-related and lung abscess.

lute; severe viral infections can produce leukocytosis and variable shifts to the left. Conversely, overwhelming bacterial pneumonia can present with ominous leukopenia. The magnitude of fever is thought by some to be helpful in determining the possible presence of a bacterial infection; however, viral LRI can also provoke high fevers, which may persist for several days or more.

Other nonviral agents include *Chlamydia trachomatis, Chlamydia pneumoniae, Mycoplasma pneumoniae, Mycobacterium tuberculosis,* deep mycoses, and *Pneumocystis carinii. C. trachomatis* pneumonia is common among infants between 2 weeks and 6 months of age, accounting for an estimated 10% to 15% of LRIs in this group. Characteristically, the onset of respiratory symptoms is insidious over several days, the infant is usually afebrile, and air trapping with interstitial infiltrates is often apparent on chest radiographs. Symptomatic *M. pneumoniae* infections are uncommon in children younger than 5 years of age; however, they frequently cause pneumonia among children in the 5- to 19-year age group.[2] *C. pneumoniae* infections appear to follow clinical and age-specific patterns similar to those of *M. pneumonia* infections, but more data are needed before such a comparison can be confirmed.[3] Tuberculosis and deep mycoses should be considered when the symptoms and radiographic abnormalities insidiously progress over days to weeks. Finally, *P. carinii* infections are suggested in patients who have progressive hypoxemia (often without significant hypercarbia), alveolar infiltrates, and significant risk factors such as congenital or acquired immunodeficiency, malignancy, and severe protein malnutrition.

Despite these differential diagnostic possibilities, viral infections remain the most common causes of pediatric LRIs, especially among children younger than 5 years of age.[4] Of these, respiratory syncytial virus (RSV); parainfluenza virus types 1, 2, and 3; influenza virus types A and B; and adenoviruses comprise the majority.[5] Rhinoviruses, human coronaviruses (HCVs), influenza virus type C, and parainfluenza virus type 4 are known to have roles in upper respiratory disease, but relatively little is known about their contribution to LRI. Other viruses, such as Epstein-Barr virus (EBV), cytomegalovirus (CMV), and human herpesvirus-6 (HHV-6), have been associated occasionally with LRI, either as primary pathogens or as possible cofactors with other agents. All three increase in overall importance in the setting of immunocompromise; this is especially true for CMV.[6] Measles virus has a long history as a significant cause of LRI. Although eradication of this virus seems possible, it remains a significant problem in underdeveloped nations.

RESPIRATORY SYNCYTIAL VIRUS

Of all the causes of childhood LRI, RSV is the most common. It is responsible for at least 60% of severe LRIs among children younger than 5 years of age. Outbreaks occur annually, usually commencing in the northern hemisphere any time between October and April, and last for at least 12 weeks. Infants younger than 2 years of age are most frequently and severely affected; an estimated 5 of every 1000 infants born are hospitalized for RSV disease during the first year of life. Of these, 8% may require intubation and ventilation. The mortality rate in hospitalized patients is between 0.5% and 1.5% but rises to 3.5% or greater among infants with underlying cardiac or chronic pulmonary disease.[7] The mortality rate in infants with congenital heart disease and pulmonary hypertension has been reported to be 73%.[8] Children receiving cancer chemotherapy have a 15% mortality rate, which rises to 40% in those with immunodeficiency syndromes.[9] In Houston, the risk of acquiring RSV infection in the first year of life has been calculated to be 68.8 per 100 children, and about half of all children had experienced at least two RSV infections during the first 2 years of life.[10] Other studies have confirmed the ready transmission of RSV in hospitals and high rates of secondary transmission in households, including by adults.[11] These studies have also demonstrated that naturally acquired immunity to reinfection is imperfect; in fact, reinfection may occur in the same infant in the first or second year with resultant severe illness. However, when a third infection occurs early in life, its severity is usually reduced.[12] The reasons for this susceptibility to reinfection are not yet clear. One possibility is that antigenic variants may play some role in evading immune surveillance. Based on antigenic and nucleic acid analysis, two major groups, designated *A* and *B*, and several subgroups, including variants within the subgroups, have been described.[13] In general, it appears that group A infections are associated with more severe disease.[14]

Clinical Features

In infants, the first symptoms are usually manifested by nasal stuffiness and coryza. Over 1 to 3 days, the infection progresses downward in the respiratory tract, with cough being a predominant manifestation. At most, the illnesses expressed may be predominantly croup, tracheobronchitis, bronchiolitis, pneumonia, or some combination thereof. Fig. 37-1 depicts the usual progression of illness severity, with a plateau at the peak of illness, which lasts an average of 10 days; then gradual improvement occurs. The duration of illness can be prolonged; 3 to 7 weeks can pass before hypoxemia resolves. Fever may be absent or present, sometimes above 38° C for several days. At the height of symptoms, retractions, air trapping, expiratory and often inspiratory wheezes, and rhonchi are common. Crackles may also be detected. Chest radiographs often show hyperinflation and perihilar interstitial infiltrates. Atelectasis or lobar collapse, usually involving the right upper lobe, is seen in 26% or more of hospitalized infants.[15] The prominent laboratory findings are hypoxemia and hypercarbia. White blood cell counts vary, and may be elevated with a "shift to the left" if severe hypoxemia is present.

Complications include progressive pulmonary failure, cor pulmonale, and a risk of bacterial superinfection. If the infant's clinical status suddenly deteriorates at any time during the acute or convalescent stages, bacterial superinfection must be seriously considered. Apneic episodes are also seen in approximately 18% of infants, especially among those who are very young and prematurely born.[16] In this group, the apnea can occur with few or no other respiratory symptoms; however, the nonspecific findings of listlessness, irritability, and poor feeding may be observed. Some of these infants die suddenly and unexpectedly. Some of the reasons for severe illness with well-established viral LRIs such as RSV are illustrated in Fig. 37-2. Although not specific for RSV infection, the common findings of terminal airway obstruction and interstitial inflammation can be drastic.

Another unusual complication of acute RSV infections is cardiac dysrhythmias, especially supraventricular tachycardia. In infants with structurally normal hearts, these dysrhythmias appear to be self-limited.[17] Myocarditis, central nervous system dysfunction, and macular or maculopapular exanthems have also been reported; however, these are rare.

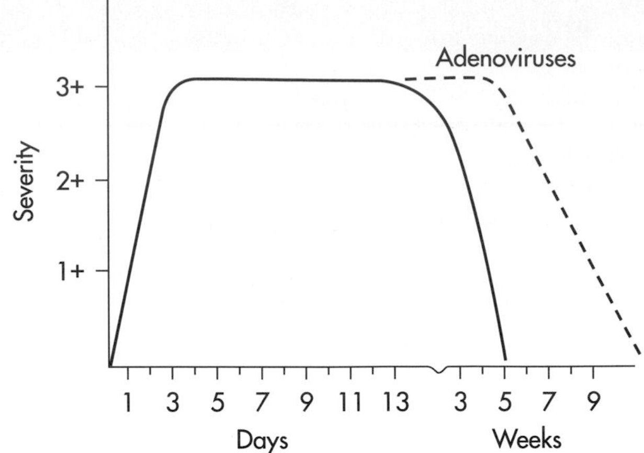

Fig. 37-1. Natural history of lower respiratory tract illnesses caused by RSV and parainfluenza viruses, as measured by severity and duration in normal patients. The prodrome with upper respiratory symptoms usually progresses to lower tract involvement over 1 to 3 days. Maximal severity persists as a "plateau" phase for 7 to 21 days (average, 10 days), followed by progressive recovery in the succeeding few weeks. The hatched line illustrates the similar but more protracted course often seen with severe adenovirus infections.

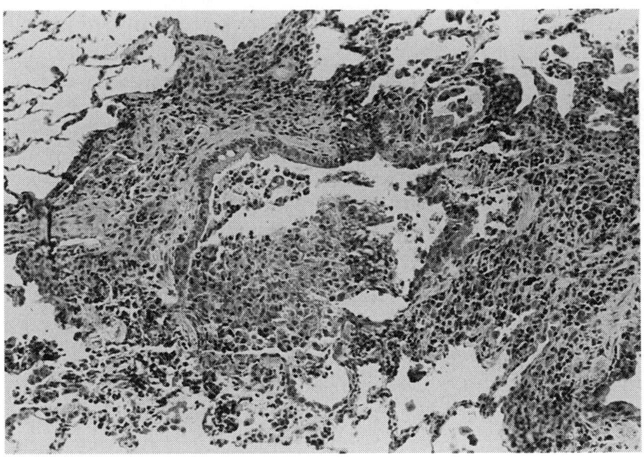

Fig. 37-2. Photomicrograph demonstrating bronchiolar inflammation, exudation, and dramatic interstitial mononuclear cell infiltrates in a case of RSV infection. (×100.) (From Ray CG. In Sherris JC, ed: *Medical microbiology: an introduction to infectious diseases,* ed 2, New York, 1990, Elsevier.)

Diagnosis

Serologic testing is available, but because of its relative insensitivity and the delay in diagnosis involved, it is not the procedure of choice. RSV can be shed from the upper respiratory tract for up to 6 days before the appearance of respiratory distress, and shedding continues for an average of 6 to 7 days (range, 1 to 20 days) thereafter.[18] In immunocompromised patients, the virus may be shed for 45 days or longer. Cultures of the nasopharynx can readily establish the diagnosis; however, detection by this method usually requires 5 to 9 days of incubation. Immunofluorescent detection of RSV antigen in exfoliated nasopharyngeal cells or enzyme-linked immunoassays of nasopharyngeal secretions have now become the diagnostic tests of choice. These methods are rapid, are relatively inexpensive, and have sensitivities and specificities of 90% or greater compared with cell culture. Cultures are used primarily for patients with negative rapid tests or unusual instances in which multiple viral agents are suspected.

Management

When eating and drinking become difficult for the patient, adequate fluids usually need to be provided via an intravenous route. Humidified oxygen is also given when hypoxemia is present, usually beginning at a concentration of 30% to 40%. In severe cases, the oxygen concentration is increased as guided by blood gas determinations. If there is clinical evidence of progressive respiratory failure, endotracheal intubation with mechanical ventilatory assistance is required.

Bronchodilators, such as albuterol, may also be tried but must be administered cautiously and discontinued if no clear-cut benefit can be demonstrated. Corticosteroids have no demonstrated role in treatment. Also, there is no scientific support for the routine use of antibiotics in these situations[19]; antibiotics are reserved for use only when a proven or presumed bacterial superinfection is present.

Ribavirin, a synthetic nucleoside, has been somewhat effective in several studies of severe RSV pneumonia and bronchiolitis,[20] but debate continues regarding its actual benefits and indications for use.[21,22] It is administered continuously for 18 to 20 hr/day for 3 to 8 days (sometimes longer) as a small-particle (<4-μ) aerosol, usually while a patient is using a mask or placed in an oxygen hood. Shorter, more intense treatments of 2 hours 3 times/day have also been suggested.[23] Although adverse effects are rarely associated with such therapy, there are significant disadvantages. The drug can cause crystalline deposits in ventilator tubing and valves, resulting in sudden, dangerous rises in expiratory pressure. The risks can be minimized by close monitoring with attention to flow through the aerosol generator, frequent tubing change and cleaning of the expiratory valve, and avoidance of one-way valves and filters.[24] Another disadvantage of ribavirin aerosol treatment is expense. The present estimated cost for the medication and its administration in the hospital is over $1100 per day. In view of the uncertainties that have been raised, the American Academy of Pediatrics Committee on Infectious Diseases now states that the use of ribavirin aerosol may be considered for patients at high risk for RSV disease as follows[25]:

1. Infants with cyanotic or complicated congenital heart disease, including pulmonary hypertension or bronchopulmonary dysplasia, cystic fibrosis, or another chronic lung disease (Previously healthy premature infants [younger than 37 weeks' gestational age] and those younger than 6 weeks of age are also at greater risk for severe RSV disease but less so than patients with underlying disease.)
2. Children with immunodeficiency, including those with acquired immunodeficiency syndrome or severe combined immunodeficiency; recent transplant recipients; and patients undergoing cancer chemotherapy
3. Infants who are severely ill with or without mechanical ventilation (usually as guided by the partial pressure of arterial oxygen, increasing values for the partial pressure of arterial carbon dioxide, and response to other therapies)
4. Hospitalized patients who may be at increased risk of progression to a complicated course because they are younger than 6 weeks of age or have an underlying condition, such as multiple congenital anomalies or certain neurologic or metabolic diseases (e.g., cerebral palsy, myasthenia gravis)

There has been a recent resurgence of interest in prophylaxis and the treatment of RSV infection by passive immunotherapy. Intravenous preparations of human immunoglobulin with high antibody titers to RSV have been tested in a cotton rat model; the results are encouraging.[26] Studies are now ongoing in high-risk human populations, but it is too soon to draw conclusions.[27] A further advance in this area will likely be in extending the current development of monoclonal antibodies derived from chimeric mouse-human hybridomas, possibly even for topical use in the respiratory tract.[28] No safe, effective means of active immunization is currently available; however, several subunit vaccines are being developed.

PARAINFLUENZA VIRUSES

The parainfluenza viruses represent the second most common cause of LRI in children younger than 5 years of age.[4] Parainfluenza virus type 3 is the most common cause of LRI among this group. Such infections can be seen at any time during the year but are most common in the spring and summer.[5] Localized outbreaks of upper respiratory illness, bronchitis, and croup caused by parainfluenza virus types 1 or 2 frequently occur in the autumn and early winter. Parainfluenza virus type 4 is rarely detected and has been associated primarily with upper respiratory symptoms.

The clinical course of parainfluenza virus infection is similar to that described for RSV as depicted in Fig. 37-1. Diagnostic approaches primarily include culture and direct antigen detection by immunofluorescence or enzyme-linked immunoassays. The specificity of rapid immunofluorescence is high (>90%), but sensitivity ranges from 60% to 80%.

The basic principles of management for parainfluenza LRIs are the same as those described for RSV. Types 1 and 3 are also susceptible in vitro to ribavirin, but no controlled clinical trials yet support its use in these infections.

INFLUENZA VIRUSES

The epidemiology of influenza virus types A and B is generally well known: rapidly evolving outbreaks that usually occur during the cooler months of the year. Both types can cause serious, lethal LRI in infants and children.[29] The clinical course contrasts with that of RSV and parainfluenza viruses in that fever, malaise, and often myalgia usually develop and rapidly become more severe over 12 to 24 hours. Nasal congestion, cough, and subsequent respiratory distress often do not appear until a day or two after the onset of systemic symptoms. Although the overall duration of the acute illness (3 to 7 days) is somewhat shorter than with RSV or parainfluenza viruses, the convalescent phase often lasts several weeks, and rapid deterioration as a result of bacterial superinfection can occur at any time in the course. Rarely, patients may develop a rapidly progressive, overwhelming viral pneumonia resulting in death within 2 to 3 days after the initial onset.

Diagnosis and basic management are similar to those described for RSV and parainfluenza viruses. Oral amantadine hydrochloride is somewhat effective in treating influenza A but is useless in influenza B. If begun within 24 to 48 hours of onset and continued for 5 to 7 days, it may reduce the duration of fever and systemic symptoms and result in a more rapid improvement of peripheral airways function.[30] It also has use as a prophylactic in high-risk children during influenza A outbreaks. A related drug, rimantadine, is also effective and appears to produce fewer adverse effects than amantadine.[31] The rapid development of viral resistance to both amantadine and rimantadine has been observed, particularly when either medication is used in households for the simultaneous treatment of symptomatic infection and contact prophylaxis.[32]

Like the parainfluenza viruses, influenza virus types A and B are susceptible to ribavirin in vitro. Volunteer studies have also suggested that ribavirin is clinically effective in both types of infection; however, it is neither licensed nor routinely recommended for such use.

Influenza virus type C has been reported to cause outbreaks of febrile respiratory illnesses, especially among pediatric clinic patients and children younger than 3 years of age. A survey by Dykes et al[33] in Los Angeles detected a 64% prevalence of antibodies to this virus among children 5 years of age and younger. However, longitudinal studies have not supported a significant role for influenza virus type C in LRI, at least among those from birth to 3 years of age.[5]

The combination vaccines for influenza virus types A and B are evaluated annually and reformulated as necessary to antigenically match the strains expected to circulate widely. Their protective efficacy varies from year to year, ranging between 50% and 95% in immunologically normal individuals older than 6 months of age. Efficacy in the first 6 months of life is not known, and the influenza vaccine is not recommended for this group; otherwise, annual immunization commencing in the autumn is appropriate in persons of all ages, except those who have experienced anaphylactic reactions to chickens or eggs. Two doses administered 1 month apart are recommended for children receiving the vaccine for the first time.

Children who especially should be immunized annually against influenza include those with chronic pulmonary, cardiac, hematologic, immunologic, and metabolic conditions and youngsters receiving long-term salicylate therapy. In addition, household contacts of these high-risk children and other caregivers (e.g., nurses, physicians, therapists) should be targeted. If an annual immunization is missed and a significant exposure is subsequently suspected (e.g., during a documented outbreak), immunization followed immediately by chemoprophylaxis with amantadine or rimantadine for 2 weeks after the vaccine schedule of one or two doses has been completed can provide "bridging" protection until there is a vaccine response.

ADENOVIRUSES

Adenoviruses are very common causes of fevers, upper respiratory illnesses, and conjunctivitis in young children. Fortunately, they produce LRI only occasionally and sporadically. Adenoviral pneumonia, most commonly caused by types 3, 5, and 7, initially progresses much like the pneumonia described for RSV and parainfluenza viruses (see Fig. 37-1), but the illnesses can be extremely severe and can last for several weeks. Risk factors for severe, potentially lethal disease include immunocompromise, congenital heart disease, and protein-calorie malnutrition. During the acute phase, chest radiographs often reveal extensive consolidation, particularly in perihilar areas. These findings, along with a frequent occurrence of high fevers, leukocytosis, and multisystem involvement, can make it difficult to discern such infections from bacterial conditions. Other systemic manifestations that sometimes develop include hepatic dysfunction, encephalopathy, coagulopathies, measles-like exanthems, and diarrhea.[34]

The diagnosis is confirmed by the detection of the virus in tissues such as lung aspirate or biopsy specimens. Because asymptomatic shedding from the throat or gastrointestinal tract is common in young children, isolation of the virus from the throat must be regarded as diagnostically supportive but not confirmatory, and isolation from stools or rectal swabs needs to be interpreted even more cautiously. Serologic studies of paired acute and convalescent sera obtained at least 2 weeks apart may further aid in confirming the diagnosis. Rapid detection has been used, including immunofluorescence and immunoenzyme assays. Such methods are generally quite specific, but sensitivity ranges between 30% and 60%.

Supportive management is all that can be offered at present. These patients must be followed closely because they are at high risk for bacterial superinfection for many weeks. They can also sustain permanent pulmonary sequelae, including pulmonary fibrosis, bronchiolitis obliterans, recurrent wheezing, and bronchiectasis.[35-37] Young age and a previous measles-like illness, as well as nutritional or immunologic deficiencies, have been reported to be risk factors.[36] The persistence of adenoviral antigens and the sustained expression of adenovirus genes in the airway epithelium have been proposed as causes.[37,38]

HUMAN CORONAVIRUSES

The role of HCV strains in LRIs is not well understood. The two strains detected most commonly are OC43 and 229E. It appears that HCV OC43 infections produce cough in addition to nasal symptoms in adults.[39] In children, sore throat, cough, coryza, and fever have been observed, and pulmonary crackles were noted in 5% of patients.[39] HCV infections have also been associated with acute attacks of wheezing in children with asthma.[40] Perhaps the most provocative of pediatric studies is that reported from England by Isaacs et al.[41] They used an enzyme-linked immunosorbent assay to detect HCV antigens in 30% of 108 acute respiratory episodes experienced by 30 children younger than 6 years of age who had a history of at least 10 recurrent respiratory illnesses in the preceding year. In addition, 29% of 51 acute respiratory episodes experienced by the siblings of these patients were also associated with HCV. Interestingly, 30% of the HCV infections detected in the former group were associated with LRI symptoms, including wheezy bronchitis, whereas none of the siblings with HCV had LRI findings. Most infections were due to HCV 229E, and peaks occurred in the late autumn, early winter, and early summer. Family studies in Seattle have shown that increased levels of antibodies to HCV strains OC43 and 229E occur more frequently during the winter[42]; children were apparently infected 3 times more often than adults, and serologic evidence suggesting reinfection was frequently observed over 3 years. Recently, prospective serologic studies among children in the first 3 years of life in Tucson, Arizona, failed to demonstrate a significant primary role for HCV in LRI.[5]

RHINOVIRUSES

The rhinovirus group is composed of at least 100 unique serotypes that are widely known as the agents responsible for many of the upper respiratory ("common cold") symptoms in adults and older children. Rhinoviruses have been isolated from infants and children hospitalized with LRIs but not at rates that differ significantly from children without respiratory illnesses.[43] The usual incubation period is 2 to 3 days, and the acute symptoms usually last 3 to 7 days. In one retrospective study, the clinical features of 44 rhinovirus culture–positive children with respiratory symptoms, who were either hospitalized or seen in an emergency department, included bronchiolitis or pneumonia; sometimes, both conditions were found (32 patients). The majority of patients were younger than 12 months of age. Although infrequent, LRIs in children infected with rhinoviruses were indistinguishable from those caused by RSV.[44] Rhinoviruses may also have a role in triggering episodes of acute asthma.[45]

The diagnosis of rhinovirus infections depends on culture of the agent in tissue culture because no rapid diagnostic test is yet available. Technical difficulties of identifying rhinoviruses in diagnostic specimens may contribute to an underestimation of their role as causes of LRI. The treatment of rhinovirus infections consists of supportive care; no antiviral medications are recommended at this time.

HERPESVIRUSES

Although uncommon as pulmonary pathogens in healthy children, all members of the herpesvirus family (herpes simplex virus [HSV] types I and II, varicella-zoster virus [VZV], CMV, EBV, and HHV-6) can cause LRI in immunocompromised patients, generally hematogenously spread as part of a systemic infection. CMV is primarily of concern in the recipients of allogeneic bone marrow transplants. However, normal children with lower respiratory tract symptoms can also have positive cultures for CMV. Serologic studies do not generally support a primary role for CMV in LRI among healthy children[5]; however, pneumonia associated with acute, primary, systemic CMV infection in otherwise normal infants has been reported.[46]

CMV pneumonitis in the recipients of bone marrow most frequently results from reactivation of latent virus and less often by transmission via blood products to seronegative patients. Graft-versus-host disease is a significant risk factor for the development of CMV pneumonitis; thus autologous and syngeneic recipients of bone marrow transplant are rarely affected. CMV pneumonitis commonly presents as a primary pulmonary process characterized by fever, tachypnea, and progressive pulmonary distress. Diffuse, bilateral pulmonary infiltrates are generally seen on chest radiographs. The diagnosis can be made by culture of the virus from bronchoalveolar lavage fluid or from lung tissue. The advent of prophylaxis with ganciclovir in high-risk patients has greatly reduced the incidence of CMV during the first 3 months after bone marrow transplantation.[47] Ganciclovir is less effective in treating CMV pneumonitis in patients after disease is clinically apparent.

Herpes simplex pneumonitis is most commonly seen as part of perinatally acquired disseminated infections but can also be transmitted during resuscitative efforts. Immunocompromise of any type is also a risk factor for HSV pneumonitis at all ages.

Varicella pneumonitis is a life-threatening complication of primary VZV infection in neonates, immunocompromised patients, and rarely, healthy children. VZV is spread by aerosolized respiratory secretions, and the initial round of viral replication occurs in the lungs. A primary wave of viremia then occurs and is followed by further viral replication in lymphatic tissue. Characteristic cutaneous lesions erupt after a secondary viremia. Varicella pneumonitis generally develops 2 to 5 days after the outbreak of a rash.[48] The clinical and radiographic manifestations vary. Asymptomatic miliary lung lesions (especially in adult varicella) may later become apparent as calcified foci. In others patients, a mild interstitial pneumonia is present, which may be overshadowed by a severe bacterial pneumonia caused by organisms such as group A streptococci or *S. aureus.* These are often accompanied by effusions and empyemas and can be extremely difficult to treat. Varicella alone can cause a progressive, lethal pneumonia in immunocompromised patients.

The transmission of VZV to neonates occurs when primary maternal chickenpox occurs within 3 weeks of parturition. Transplacental transfer of maternal antibody specific for VZV is minimal if the onset of illness occurs fewer than 5 days before birth. If maternal varicella develops within 5 days before to 2 days after delivery, systemic disease and pneumonitis can develop in the neonate, with an estimated case fatality rate of 5%.[49]

The diagnosis of varicella in normal hosts is generally made by clinical observation. Culture or immunofluorescence staining of vesicular lesions is important in immunocompromised hosts to rule out disseminated herpes simplex infections. Serologic antibody tests are useful for assessing immune status. γ-Globulin preparations containing high titers of anti-VZV activity are effective in preventing varicella if given soon after exposure. Neonates and immunocompromised children are candidates for this treatment.[49] Acyclovir is the drug of choice in treating high-risk patients and reduces the severity of illness if administered within 2 days of the outbreak of a rash. It is expected that the newly licensed, live VZV vaccine will eventually result in a significant reduction of these frequently complicated issues.

Like the other herpesviruses, EBV produces life-long infections and causes a variety of clinical syndromes, including infectious mononucleosis, central nervous system illnesses, malignant lymphoproliferative diseases, and nasopharyngeal carcinoma. Pneumonitis can occur as part of primary EBV infection but is uncommon, although perhaps underdiagnosed. In a group of 113 normal children with documented EBV-induced mononucleosis, 6 children, all younger than 4 years of age, developed pneumonia during the illness.[50] Pneumonia was self-limited in all cases. The diagnosis of primary EBV infection is made on clinical grounds in conjunction with serologic tests for heterophil antibody or IgM anti-VCA antibody.

HHV-6, the usual causative agent of roseola infantum, has been suggested as a possible cause of some cases of interstitial pneumonitis in recipients of bone marrow transplants.[51] This virus is one of the most ubiquitous of human viruses: More than 90% of the population becomes infected by 2 years of age. Detection of HHV-6 by culture is not routinely available, but the diagnosis of primary infection can be made by evidence of serologic conversion. Reactivation is difficult to document because a majority of healthy individuals have evidence of continuous viral replication in the salivary glands and blood. HHV-6 is not thought to cause pneumonia in normal persons, and no specific therapy is available.

MEASLES VIRUS

Otitis media and pharyngitis are normal components of the early phase of measles infection. Bronchitis is common, and occasionally, severe laryngitis may occur. Pneumonia caused by the measles virus probably occurs in at least 50% of children. In most cases, it is a mild bronchopneumonia and is recognized only by nonspecific lower respiratory signs and hyperinflation on chest radiograph. In other cases the inflammation is more extensive, leading to diffuse infiltrates or even segmental or lobar consolidation on chest radiographs.

Children with measles are prone to secondary bacterial infection with organisms such as pneumococcus, *H. influenzae, S. aureus,* and *Streptococcus pyogenes.* This is particularly important in developing countries, where infection secondary to measles is a major cause of death in young children. Measles may also have a deleterious effect on the course of tuberculosis in malnourished infants.

The immunodeficient child is prone to develop a progressive and fatal infection that evolves around 3 weeks after exposure. The clinical manifestations start with a fever, and there may be an atypical rash. Nonspecific respiratory symptoms and signs evolve over 2 to 3 days. The chest radiograph generally show coarse nodular infiltrates, and air leaks are common.

The diagnosis is usually made on culture from nasopharyngeal secretions or bronchoalveolar lavage fluid. Occasionally, a lung biopsy may be necessary. The histopathologic picture is most often that of giant cell pneumonia with inflammatory cell exudate and thickening of the alveolar walls with inflammatory cells. The alveolar lining cells are transformed and contain intranuclear and intracytoplasmic inclusions.[52]

Measles pneumonia can be prevented in the immunodeficient host by active community immunization. Those exposed should have immunoglobulin as soon as possible after exposure.

Modified measles does occur in the partially immune host and presents with fever and an itchy maculopapular rash, particularly over the wrists and ankles. Respiratory involvement is relatively common in this type of measles presenting with dyspnea and widespread crackles heard on auscultation. The chest radiograph shows hilar adenopathy with nodular infiltrates and frequently, a pleural effusion.[53]

HANTAVIRUS

In 1993, an outbreak of acute febrile illness progressing within 3 to 5 days to respiratory failure and shock was noted in the southwestern United States. The hallmark of this syndrome, the hantavirus pulmonary syndrome, is unexplained severe noncardiogenic pulmonary edema occurring in previously healthy persons.

Subsequent studies have implicated at least three different hantaviruses, which are primarily maintained as zoonotic agents in rodent reservoirs.[54] As of February 1996, 128 cases of hantavirus pulmonary syndrome had been reported from 24 states in the United States, with a mortality rate of 50% to 75%. Hantavirus pulmonary syndrome has also been documented in Canada, Brazil, Argentina, and Paraguay. Only 8 of the episodes have been reported in people 16 years of age or younger, and no patient was younger than 11 years of age.[55] The diagnosis can be made by serologic tests, polymerase chain reaction study of frozen tissues, immunochemistry, or paraffin-embedded tissues. No specific therapy has proved efficacious; however, intravenous ribavirin has been suggested based on in vitro data and experience with other hantaviruses.

SIMULTANEOUS INVOLVEMENT BY MULTIPLE PATHOGENS

Other viruses, *C. trachomatis,* or *M. pneumoniae* can also be detected in a significant number of young children with infections caused by RSV. In the Tucson Childrens' Respiratory Study,[56] 10.9% of previously healthy patients with RSV infection were coinfected with another potential pathogen as documented by culture or antigen detection, and the proportion became even greater when serologic results were also extensively used for diagnosis. The clinical diagnosis and outcomes were no different among patients with RSV alone compared with those already coinfected with additional agents. Routine searches for coinfecting agents when a primary pathogen such as RSV is identified are not recommended for otherwise healthy infants and children. Such extensions of a diagnostic workup are best reserved for patients who are known to have significant underlying illnesses or patients whose clinical course is not congruent with that expected for the pathogen detected.

PROSPECTS FOR PREVENTION AND TREATMENT

Current knowledge concerning the major causes of viral LRIs and their epidemiology and diagnosis has matured remarkably. Exciting advances are now being made in the critical areas of immunopathogenesis, molecular virology, and antiviral therapy. Future discoveries will surely provide even more rational approaches to prevention and treatment, including specifically designed peptide vaccines that can more appropriately recruit specific T-cell populations as allies in long-lasting protection. Other emerging strategies include enhancement of host defenses by cytokine manipulation and novel applications of older concepts, such as specific antibodies for prophylaxis and treatment. There is considerable cause for optimism, in contrast to the state of affairs described by Andrewes more than 3 decades ago, when he suggested that clinicians should perhaps accept these infections as "one of the stimulating risks of being mortal."[57]

REFERENCES

1. Wright AL, Taussig LM, Ray CG, Harrison HR, Holberg CJ, The Group Health Medical Associates: The Tucson Children's Respiratory Study. II. Lower respiratory tract illness in the first year of life, *Am J Epidemiol* 129:1232-1246, 1989.
2. Denny FW, Clyde WA: Acute lower respiratory tract infection in non-hospitalized children, *J Pediatr* 108:635-646, 1986.
3. Grayston JT: Infections caused by *C. pneumoniae* strain TWAR, *Clin Infect Dis* 15:757-763, 1992.
4. Berman S, McIntosh D: Selective primary health care: strategies for control of disease in the developing world. XXI. Acute respiratory infections, *Rev Infect Dis* 7:674-691, 1985.
5. Ray CG, Holberg CJ, Minnich LL, Shehab ZM, Wright AL, Taussig LM, The Group Health Medical Associates: Acute lower respiratory illnesses during the first three years of life: potential roles for various etiologic agents, *Pediatr Infect Dis J* 12:10-14, 1993.
6. Pollard RB: Cytomegalovirus infections in renal, heart, heart-lung and liver transplantation, *Pediatr Infect Dis J* 7:S97-S102, 1988.

Respiratory Syncytial Virus

7. Groothuis JR, Gutierrez KM, Lauer BA: Respiratory syncytial virus infection in children with bronchopulmonary dysplasia, *Pediatrics* 82:199-203, 1988.
8. Macdonald NE, Hall CB, Suffin SC, Alexson C, Harris PJ, Manning JA: Respiratory syncytial viral infection in infants with congenital heart disease, *N Engl J Med* 307:397-400, 1982.
9. Hall CB, Powell KR, MacDonald NE, Gala CL, Menegus ME, Suffin SC, Cohen HJ: Respiratory syncytial viral infection in children with compromised immune function, *N Engl J Med* 315:77-81, 1986.
10. Glezen WP, Parades A, Allison JE, Taber LH, Frank AL: Risk of respiratory syncytial virus infection for infants from low income families in relationship to age, sex, ethnic group and maternal antibody level, *J Pediatr* 98:708-715, 1981.
11. Hall CB, Douglas RG: Modes of transmission of respiratory syncytial virus, *J Pediatr* 99:100-103, 1981.
12. Glezen WP, Taber LH, Frank AL, Kasel JA: Risk of primary infection and re-infection with respiratory syncytial virus, *Am J Dis Child* 140:543-546, 1986.
13. Storch GA, Hall CB, Anderson LJ, Park CS, Dohner DE: Antigenic and nucleic acid analysis of nosocomial isolates of respiratory syncytial virus, *J Infect Dis* 167:562-566, 1993.
14. McConnochie KM, Hall CB, Walsh EE, Roghmann KJ: Variation in severity of respiratory syncytial virus with subtype, *J Pediatr* 117:52-62, 1990.
15. Simpson W, Hacking PM, Court DSM, Gardner PS: The radiological findings in respiratory syncytial virus infection in children. II. The correlation of radiological categories with clinical and virological findings, *Pediatr Radiol* 2:155-160, 1974.
16. Bruhn FW, Mokrohisky ST, McIntosh K: Apnea associated with respiratory syncytial virus infection in young infants, *J Pediatr* 90:382-386, 1977.

17. Donnerstein RL, Berg RA, Shehab Z, Ovadia M: Complex atrial tachycardias and respiratory syncytial virus infections in infants, *J Pediatr* 125:23-28, 1994.
18. Hall CB, Douglas RG, Geiman JM: Respiratory syncytial infection in infants: quantitation and duration of shedding, *J Pediatr* 89:11-15, 1976.
19. Hall CB, Powell KR, Schnabel KC, Gala CL, Pincus PH: Risk of secondary bacterial infection in infants hospitalized with respiratory syncytial viral infection, *J Pediatr* 113:266-271, 1988.
20. La Via WV, Marks MI, Stutman HR: Respiratory syncytial virus puzzle: clinical features, pathophysiology, treatment, and prevention, *J Pediatr* 121:L503-L510, 1992.
21. Moler FW, Steinhart CM, Ohmit SE, Stidham GL: Effectiveness of ribavirin in otherwise well infants with respiratory syncytial virus–associated respiratory failure, *J Pediatr* 128:422-428, 1996.
22. Randolph AG, Wang EEL: Ribavirin for respiratory syncytial virus lower respiratory tract infection: a systematic overview, *Arch Pediatr Adolesc Med* 150:942-947, 1996.
23. Englund JA, Piedra PA, Ahn Y-M, Gilbert BE, Hiatt P: High-dose, short duration ribavirin aerosol therapy compared with standard ribavirin therapy in children with suspected infection, *J Pediatr* 125:635-641, 1994.
24. Smith DW, Frankel LR, Mathers LH, Tang ATS, Ariagno RL, Prober CG: A controlled trial of aerosolized ribavirin in infants receiving mechanical ventilation for severe respiratory syncytial virus infection, *N Engl J Med* 325:24-29, 1991.
25. Committee on Infectious Diseases, American Academy of Pediatrics: Reassessment of the indications for ribavirin therapy in respiratory syncytial virus infections, *Pediatrics* 97:137-140, 1996.
26. Prince GA, Horswood RL, Chanock RM: Quantitative aspects of passive immunity to respiratory syncytial virus in infant cotton rats, *J Virol* 55:517-520, 1985.
27. Groothuis JR, Simoes EAF, Levin MJ, Hall CB, Long CE, Rodriquez WJ, Arrobio J, Meissner HC, Fulton DR, Welliver RC, Tristram DA, Siber GR, Prince GA, Van Raden M, Hemming VG, Respiratory Syncytial Virus Immune Globulin Study Group: Prophylactic administration of respiratory syncytial virus immune globulin to high-risk infants and young children, *N Engl J Med* 329:1524-1576, 1993.
28. Groothuis JR: The role of RSV neutralizing antibodies in the treatment and prevention of respiratory syncytial virus infection in high-risk children, *Antiviral Res* 23:1-10, 1994 (review).

Influenza Viruses

29. Troendle JF, Demmler GJ, Glezen WP, Finegold M, Romano MJ: Fatal influenza B virus pneumonia in pediatric patients, *Pediatr Infect Dis J* 11:117-121, 1992.
30. Van Voris LP, Betts RF, Hayden FG, Christmas WA, Douglas RG: Successful treatment of naturally occurring influenza A/USSR/77 HIN1, *JAMA* 245:1128-1131, 1981.
31. Tominack RL, Hayden FG: Rimantadine hydrochloride and amantadine hydrochloride use in influenza A virus infection, *Infect Dis Clin North Am* 1:459-478, 1987.
32. Hayden FG, Belshe RB, Clover RD, Hay AJ, Oakes MG, Soo W: Emergence and apparent transmission of rimantadine-resistant influenza A virus in families, *N Engl J Med* 321:1696-1702, 1989.
33. Dykes AC, Cherry JD, Nolan CE: A clinical, epidemiologic serologic, and virologic study of influenza C virus infection, *Arch Intern Med* 140:1295-1298, 1980.

Adenoviruses

34. Murtagh P, Cerqueiro C, Halac A, Avila M, Kajon A: Adenovirus type 7 respiratory infections: a report of 29 cases of acute lower respiratory disease, *Acta Paediatr* 82:557-561, 1993.
35. Simil S, Linna O, Lanning P, Heikkinen E, Ala-Houhala M: Chronic lung damage caused by adenovirus type 7: a ten-year follow-up study, *Chest* 80:127-131, 1981.
36. Sly PD, Soto-Quiros ME, Landau LI, Hudson I, Newton-John H: Factors predisposing to abnormal pulmonary function after adenovirus type & pneumonia, *Arch Dis Child* 59:935-939, 1984.
37. Macek V, Sorli J, Kopriva S, Marin J: Persistent adenoviral infection and chronic airway obstruction in children, *Am J Respir Crit Care Med* 150:7-10, 1994.
38. Matsuse T, Hayachi S, Kuwano K, Keunecke H, Jeffries WA, Hogg JC: Latent adenoviral infection in the pathogenesis of chronic airways obstruction, *Am Rev Respir Dis* 146:177-184, 1992.

Human Coronaviruses

39. Hendley JO, Fishburne HB, Gwaltney JM: Coronavirus infections in working adults: eight-year study with 229E and OC43, *Am Rev Respir Dis* 105:805-811, 1972.
40. McIntosh K, Ellis EF, Hoffman LS, Lybass TG, Eller JJ, Fulginiti VA: The association of viral and bacterial respiratory infections with exacerbations of wheezing in young asthmatic children, *J Pediatr* 82:578-590, 1973.
41. Isaacs D, Flowers D, Clarke JR, Valman HB, MacNaughton MR: Epidemiology of coronavirus respiratory infections, *Arch Dis Child* 58:500-503, 1983.
42. Schmidt OW, Allan ID, Cooney MK, Foy HM, Fox JP: Rises in titers of antibody to human coronaviruses OC43 and 229E in Seattle families during 1975-1979, *Am J Epidemiol* 123:862-868, 1986.

Rhinoviruses

43. Portnoy B, Eckert HL, Salvatore MA: Rhinovirus infection in children with acute lower respiratory disease: evidence against etiological importance, *Pediatrics* 35:899-905, 1965.
44. McMillan JA, Weiner LB, Higgins AM, MacKnight K: Rhinovirus infection associated with serious illness among pediatric patients, *Pediatr Infect Dis J* 12:321-325, 1993.
45. Mertsola J, Ziegler T, Ruuskanen O, Vanto T, Koivikko A, Halonen P: Recurrent wheezy bronchitis and viral respiratory infections, *Arch Dis Child* 66:124-129, 1991.

Herpesviruses

46. Stagno S, Brasfield DM, Brown MB, Cassell GH, Pifer LL, Whitley RJ, Tiller RE: Infant pneumonitis associated with cytomegalovirus, *Chlamydia, Pneumocystis,* and *Ureaplasma:* a prospective study, *Pediatrics* 68:322-329, 1981.
47. Goodrich JM, Bowden RA, Fisher L, Keller C, Schoch G, Meyers JD: Ganciclovir prophylaxis to prevent cytomegalovirus disease after allogeneic marrow transplant, *Ann Intern Med* 118:173-178, 1993.
48. Feldman S, Lott L: Varicella in children with cancer: impact of antiviral therapy and prophylaxis, *Pediatrics* 80:465-472, 1987.
49. Miller E, Cradock-Watson JE, Ridehalgh MKS: Outcome in newborn babies given anti–varicella-zoster immunoglobulin after perinatal maternal infection with varicella-zoster virus, *Lancet* 2:371-374, 1986.
50. Andiman WA, McCarthy P. Markowitz RI, Cormier D, Horstmann DM: Clinical, virologic, and serologic evidence of Epstein-Barr virus infection in association with childhood pneumonia, *J Pediatr* 99:880-886, 1981.
51. Cone RW, Hackman RC, Huang MLW, Bowden RA, Meyers JD, Metcalf M, Zeh J, Ashley R, Corey L: Human herpesvirus 6 in lung tissue from patients with pneumonitis after bone marrow transplantation, *N Engl J Med* 329:156-161, 1993.

Measles Virus

52. Lewis MJ, Cameron AH, Shah KJ, Purdham DR, Mann JR: Giant cell pneumonia caused by measles and methotrexate in childhood leukaemia in remission, *Br Med J* 1:330-331, 1978.
53. Laptook A, Wind E, Nussbaum M, Shenker IR: Pulmonary lesions in atypical measles, *Pediatrics* 62:42-46, 1978.

Hantavirus

54. Butler JC, Peters CJ: Hantaviruses and hantavirus pulmonary syndrome, *Clin Infect Dis* 19:387-395, 1994.
55. Khan AS, Ksiazek TG, Peters CJ: Hantavirus pulmonary syndrome, *Lancet* 347:739-741, 1996.

Simultaneous Involvement by Multiple Pathogens

56. Ray CG, Minnich LL, Holberg CJ, Shehab ZM, Wright AL, Barton LL, Taussig LM, The Group Health Medical Associates: Respiratory syncytial virus–associated lower respiratory illnesses: possible influence of other agents, *Pediatr Infect Dis J* 12:15-19, 1993.

Prospects for Prevention and Treatment

57. Andrewes CH: The complex epidemiology of respiratory virus infections, *Science* 146:1274-1277, 1964.

CHAPTER 38

Acute Bronchiolitis and Pneumonia in Infancy Resulting from the Respiratory Syncytial Virus

Mark Lloyd Everard

The respiratory syncytial virus (RSV) is probably unique in its ability to cause annual epidemics of respiratory disease.[1-4] Although the virus can reinfect individuals throughout life,[5-8] its greatest impact is on young infants, and it is responsible for the majority of cases of acute viral bronchiolitis and pneumonia in this age group.

During any particular epidemic, a large proportion of the population develops an RSV respiratory tract infection,[7] but in infancy the risk of infection is significantly greater, with more than 50% of infants being infected.[1,9-11] Almost all infants are infected by the virus by the end of their second winter,[1,10] and half experience two infections during their first two winters.[10] For most infants, symptoms are relatively mild—only upper respiratory tract symptoms—but up to 10% develop acute bronchiolitis, the frequency varying with the definition used. In most cases the bronchiolitis is mild enough to be managed in the community, but between 0.5% and 1.5% of all infants are admitted to the hospital with RSV bronchiolitis during the winter epidemic after their birth.[1,9,12] Those age 1 to 4 months are at particular risk of severe infection[1,9,12-14] and hospitalization.

RSV infections in infancy are of considerable importance for a number of reasons. Although the mortality rate in hospitalized, previously healthy infants is very low,[15,16] the acute morbidity rate is significant. Despite improved outcome with improved supportive care, RSV still poses a particular threat to those with certain at-risk conditions, which include immunodeficiencies, chronic lung disease of prematurity, and congenital heart disease associated with pulmonary hypertension.[15-18] The annual influx of infants with RSV infections places great strains on pediatric services every winter. It has been estimated that around 90,000 such infants are admitted to the hospital each year in the United States alone, and in 1985, it was estimated that the associated annual cost was in excess of $300 million.[19] Prospective studies have found a significant increase in the reported prevalence of respiratory symptoms in children who have been admitted to the hospital with a clinical diagnosis of bronchiolitis.[20,21] Although these symptoms are usually not severe enough to cause admission to the hospital and are restricted to early childhood,[22] it is clear that the RSV is associated with a considerable amount of chronic as well as acute respiratory morbidity. Unfortunately, there is no immediate prospect of preventing these annual epidemics.

CLINICAL SYNDROMES

RSV infections are common and can affect any part of the respiratory tract. In the upper respiratory tract, RSV usually induces coryzal symptoms and is a common cause of otitis media. It undoubtedly causes exacerbations of asthma in adults and older children and is responsible for a number of cases of croup in young children.

In infants the most common lower respiratory tract manifestation is acute bronchiolitis, although RSV is also the most common cause of pneumonia in this age group. In children younger than 2 years of age, it is also the major cause of virus-induced wheeze. It can be difficult to clearly differentiate these three entities, particularly in the older infant and young child. Such distinctions may be arbitrary, but it is increasingly recognized that there are a number of distinct entities associated with wheeze and airways obstruction in infancy.[23] It is likely that many of the controversies surrounding the etiology, pathology, and treatment will persist if these separate entities are not clearly differentiated. Differences in categorizing RSV infection and lower respiratory tract symptoms makes it very difficult to compare results from different studies using a label such as *bronchiolitis* to describe very different patient populations. The similarities in clinical manifestations exhibited by infants who develop any one of these clinical entities may simply result from the airway's limited repertoire of responses. Inflammation within the airways can induce airways obstruction resulting from the secretion of mucus, exudation into the airways, mucosal edema, and varying degrees of bronchospasm irrespective of the underlying immunologic process.

To avoid controversy, some studies[16,24] chose to group all young children infected with RSV who develop lower respiratory symptoms irrespective of symptoms such as wheeze. Although such studies are very valuable in providing a comprehensive picture of RSV infection in this age group, they tend to obscure important subgroups of patients. It is well known that the virus can induce severe life-threatening apneas in young infants with or without other evidence of lower respiratory tract involvement.[15,25-27] Apneas are more common in infants born prematurely and in younger infants.[15,25,26] It is also increasingly recognized that the virus can present with the clinical picture of acute septicemia.[27-29]

Acute Bronchiolitis

Despite the frequency and importance of acute bronchiolitis, a number of controversies still surround its diagnosis and optimal management, most of which stem from differences in defining the condition. In the United Kingdom, Australia, and parts of Europe, the term *acute bronchiolitis* is limited to infants with the following clinical pattern.[30-32] Upper respiratory tract symptoms with coryza and cough precede the relatively abrupt onset of lower respiratory symptoms by 2 to 3 days. Fever is common but frequently subsides early in the course of the illness and may be absent when the child is taken to the hospital. The onset of lower respiratory symptoms is manifested by dyspnea with an irritating cough. Difficulty feeding and agitation resulting from hypoxia are common. Wheeze may be present. Tachypnea, hyperinflation of the chest with downward displacement of the liver, and subcostal recession are typically present. Auscultation reveals widespread bilateral *crepitations,* which may be accompanied by wheezes on auscultation.

If a chest radiograph is obtained, it usually provides evidence of hyperinflation, which may be particularly evident on the lateral film, and in 10% or more of cases the films have opacities indicating atelectasis or infiltrates. The diagnosis is essentially a clinical diagnosis. Hence infants whose condition fits the clinical picture but who have areas suggestive of consolidation on the chest radiograph are still labeled as having acute bronchiolitis rather than pneumonia. Most infants admitted to the hospital with this clinical picture are younger than 6 months of age. Although older infants may also develop the same clinical picture, illness severe enough to result in hospital admission is less common. In much of North America and parts of Europe, the term *bronchiolitis* is generally applied to all conditions involving expiratory wheeze and evidence of a respiratory viral infection such as rhinorrhea and cough.[33] Some would limit the diagnosis to infants younger than 1 year of age, but many would include children up to 2 years of age or even older. This definition includes many infants excluded by the definition previously discussed and excludes others who would be included.

These differences in definition account for some of the differences in management observed around the world. Most infants admitted to the hospital with acute bronchiolitis, as previously defined, are younger than 6 months of age, and there is little or no improvement when bronchodilators are administered. If a wider definition is used, many, if not most, of those included are older infants and toddlers, who may respond more often to therapies such as bronchodilators.

RSV Pneumonia

The definition of *pneumonia* in this age group is also the cause of some controversy. Typically the infant has cough, tachypnea, and fever. Hyperinflation is not a feature, and there is little to be heard on auscultation, although some crepitations may be heard. The chest radiograph provides evidence of consolidation but without evidence of hyperinflation. In North America, the presence of changes on the chest radiograph frequently leads to a label of *pneumonia,* even with the clinical picture of acute bronchiolitis as previously defined; in the United Kingdom and Australia, the label is determined by the specific clinical picture as previously noted. Infants with RSV pneumonia tend to be older than 6 months of age.[27]

EPIDEMIOLOGY

The RSV is a ribonucleic acid virus belonging to the pneumovirus family. It is closely related to the paramyxoviruses but differs in a number of important respects.[34] It is most closely related to the bovine RSV, which causes an illness similar to bronchiolitis in young calves. The virus was first isolated from a chimpanzee in 1956 and was originally called the *chimpanzee coryza virus.* Before long, it became clear that this virus was responsible for outbreaks of respiratory disease in infants; it was renamed because of if its predilection for the respiratory system and its tendency to produce syncytia when inoculated into human cell lines.

The virus has shown evidence of antigenic heterogeneity for many years as assessed by neutralization kinetics using animal sera, but all strains appeared closely related, and it was felt that they behaved epidemiologically as a single serotype.[35] More recently, two major subgroups of RSV were identified: A and B; these are subdivided into six and three subgroups respectively.[36,37] During an epidemic, both groups A and B tend to cocirculate, as do their subgroups,[38,39] and this heterogeneity may contribute to the annual outbreaks.

Only the F, or fusion, glycoprotein and G, or attachment, glycoproteins appear to play a role in the induction of neutralizing antibodies.[34] Strain variation is most marked in the G glycoprotein.[34,39] The F protein is less variable, with significant cross-reactivity to this antigen across subgroups.[34] It has been suggested that more subtle heterogeneity will become evident with time as more complex tools of molecular biology are applied to the virus, but at present it appears that heterogeneity is only one aspect contributing to the frequent reinfections that occur throughout life. For example, 73% of adults experimentally reinfected with the same strain of virus on a number of occasions over a 2-year period had two or more infections[40]; half were reinfected within 2 months.

RSV causes respiratory disease in all parts of the world. Without fail, it produces yearly outbreaks of disease.[1-4] In temperate climates, the outbreaks commence in late autumn and early winter, rising rapidly to a peak and then falling away by late spring. Isolation of the virus in the summer is uncommon, although not rare. In tropical and subtropical climates, epidemics tend to occur during the rainy season. It is still unclear why the epidemics follow such a regular pattern, and the trigger for each epidemic remains to be defined. The onset of the epidemic each year may be altered by other epidemics caused by agents such as influenza virus type A. The virus infects individuals of all ages.[5-8] Infection usually results in symptomatic illness, since the RSV is rarely isolated from individuals who have no respiratory symptoms.[1] RSV infections of the lower respiratory tract do occur in adults and may be severe. Recent epidemiologic and clinical studies have implicated the virus in upsurges of respiratory morbidity and mortality in the elderly population.[41] However, as previously noted, the most visible evidence of the annual epidemics is the surge in infants with lower respiratory tract disease.

The incubation period before the onset of symptoms appears to be 3 to 8 days. The spread of infection appears to occur via large droplets or fomites. These droplets are transmitted to the hands and fingers, and self-inoculation then occurs with transmission of virus into the eyes or nose,[42] which acts as a portal to the respiratory tract. Small-droplet aerosols do not appear to be an important form of transmission. The survival time of the virus on hands is variable but generally less than an hour. The survival time on other surfaces is also generally short, but RSV can survive for as long as 30 hours on hard, nonporous surfaces when the humidity is high.[43] Shedding of virus by hospitalized infants continues at high levels even after significant clinical improvement, and infants generally continue to shed virus for many days after discharge from the hospital.[44] Thus infants and probably older individuals remain a potential source of infection for a period after resolution of the acute symptoms. Within pediatric units, infected members of the staff are an important source of infection.

DISEASE MECHANISMS AND PATHOLOGY

The RSV is undoubtedly a very successful virus in that it infects extremely large numbers of individuals throughout the world every year and is able to reinfect individuals throughout life. Despite more than 2 decades of research, much still needs to be learned about the virus and the strategies it uses to its promote itself. Despite considerable effort by many workers, a number of separate but possibly overlapping questions remain to be answered. These include the following:

1. How does the virus manage to reinfect individuals so frequently?
2. What aspects of the immune response are important in providing protection?
3. What aspects of the immune response are important in clearing the virus?
4. Do aspects of the immune response play an important role in the causation of symptoms?
5. Why are infants so susceptible to infection?
6. Is the immune response in infants who are developing acute bronchiolitis distinct from that observed in infants who simply develop upper respiratory tract infections? Does it differ only in the magnitude and extent of infection?

Ways that the Virus Frequently Reinfects Individuals

Despite the relatively recent recognition that the virus does display significant heterogeneity, this alone is unlikely to explain its success. It is likely that active immunosuppression by the virus contributes to its success. Both subgroups and their subdivisions cocirculate during most epidemics, and it is possible that the differences are significant enough that individuals regularly encounter new strains. However evidence from experimental inoculation of adults[40] and studies of nosocomial outbreaks suggest that individuals can be reinfected with the same strain shortly after a symptomatic illness. Possible reasons for this susceptibility despite recent infection include the following:

1. Failure of the host immune system to recognize important protective epitopes
2. Impaired induction of an effective memory immune response through the production of an interleukin-1 inhibitor or the infection of macrophages with consequent impairment of their normal antigen-presenting function[45,46]
3. Effective suppression of the secondary immune response by the virus once reinfection has occurred through its ability to infect macrophages and lymphocytes and thus affect their function (see later section); impaired interferon production[47-51]; the induction of interleukin-1 inhibitors[45,46]; suppression of intracellular adhesion molecule-1 and lymphocyte function–associated antigen-1[52]; and blocking of neutralizing antibodies or impairment of cell-to-cell interactions by the large quantities of the soluble form of the G glycoprotein that are released early during infection[53]

It also appears that the infection of monocytes can be enhanced by antibody-dependent mechanisms[54-56]; hence if infection of these cells is important, then the production of nonneutralizing antibodies during one infection may even contribute to subsequent infections.

Which, if any, of these mechanisms proves to be central to the immunosuppression is unclear. As with other aspects of the immune response, certain findings have been extremely difficult to reproduce, whereas other aspects that appear to be well established have recently been challenged. A number of in vitro studies in adults and infants have suggested that the virus is a poor inducer of interferon. However, recent work has suggested that infected macrophages do indeed produce interferon-α (IFN-α) and that this has a suppressive effect on T cell proliferation[57] and hence may play a role in impairing the host response.

Aspects of the Immune Response Important in Providing Protection

High circulating antibody titers are associated with protection from recurrent infection infection,[58] although it has been claimed that protection correlates more closely with levels of mucosal immunoglobulin A (IgA).[59] High maternal and cord antibody levels are associated with protection against developing bronchiolitis,[12,60,61] although the level of protection may be related to the titer of passively acquired neutralizing antibody rather than to the total titer of antibodies directed against RSV because much of this is nonprotective antibody.

A recent multicenter trial appeared to show that intravenous immunoglobulin containing high titers of RSV-specific antibodies protected high-risk infants from significant lower respiratory tract infection,[62] and this was greeted by some as the much-needed breakthrough in the prevention of severe disease in at-risk groups.[63] However, shortly afterward, the Blood Products Advisory Committee of the American Food and Drug Administration (FDA) considered the evidence and recommended that the product should not be granted a license.[64] Further support for the suggestion that there are high levels of protective antibodies within the respiratory tract comes from work using aerosolized immunoglobulin.[65] Animal studies using preparations with high RSV titers[66] also support the belief that high doses of neutralizing antibodies can provide protection and has lead to the belief that bronchiolitis can be prevented by the use of immunoglobulin preparations active against RSV or by the use of monoclonal antibodies against the more highly conserved F protein.[67] To date, no other aspect of the host response has been clearly shown to provide protection.

Aspects of the Immune Response Important in Clearing Virus

Elimination of virus is necessary for recovery from infection, but clinical symptoms improve dramatically before significant falls in the levels of viral shedding occurs. Immunocompromised patients, especially those with defects of cell-mediated immunity, have difficulty eliminating the virus and have a high mortality rate,[68-70] but passively transferred T cells can eradicate persistent RSV infections in athymic nude mice.[71] Hence it seems likely that cell-mediated immunity is important in the recovery from RSV infections.

In addition to providing protection, neutralizing antibodies appear to play a role in clearing the virus. Passively administered antibody given during an infection can reduce viral shedding in infants[72] and experimental animals.[73] Currently underway is a study assessing the potential benefits of a preparation with high RSV antibodies in this situation.[74] Monoclonal antibodies directed against the F protein may also have a role.[75] Recent studies have suggested that the virus is able to remain dormant within cells for prolonged periods.

Role of the Immune Response in Causing Symptoms

A study experimentally infecting adults with the rhinovirus suggested that the virus causes little damage and that only individuals who mount significant neutrophil responses develop symptoms, implying that the response rather than the virus is responsible for causing symptoms.[76] RSV is certainly capable of inducing considerable cytopathology and death in certain human cell lines in the laboratory and presumably is capable of causing considerable damage to the respiratory epithelium during an infection. There is evidence of an intense inflammatory response in the airways of infants with upper respiratory tract symptoms alone or with bronchiolitis. Recent work suggests that the dominant inflammatory cell in the airways of infants with RSV infections is the neutrophil and that this cell, rather than the lymphocyte or mast cell, is probably responsible for much of the pathology associated with this condition.[77,78] These cells release potent stimuli for mucus secretion and damage the respiratory epithelium, contributing to mucosal edema and exudation into the airways. The poor response of neutrophils to chemotactic factors in the first month of life[79,80] may explain why bronchiolitis is rare in this age group. RSV infections do occur in very young infants and can be severe or even fatal,[81] but more often the infection is subclinical, results in nonspecific symptoms, or causes apnea.[81,82]

Histologic examination of the lungs of a small number of infants dying of RSV infections suggested that a lymphocytic infiltrate is characteristic of bronchiolitis,[83] but polymorphonuclear neutrophils traffic rapidly from the circulation into the airways and hence may not be evident in histologic specimens. The RSV is a potent inducer of interleukin-8 production by epithelial cells, macrophages, and neutrophils.[84-86]

These and other studies[87,88] have provided evidence that various cytokines and inflammatory mediators are released in significant quantities; hence the inflammatory response may contribute significantly to the symptoms experienced through the induction of mucus secretion and the transudation of fluid into the airways and airway walls. Such responses likely assist in disseminating the virus through the generation of infectious droplets, which are dispersed by coughing and sneezing.

Susceptibility of Infants to Infection

Very large numbers of individuals are infected by the virus every winter. Hence infants are at risk of infection simply through the opportunities for exposure to the virus during an epidemic. Frequently, the virus is acquired from an older sibling or parent. For infection to occur, protection is inevitably incomplete, and this probably reflects the fact that most mothers do not have adequate immunity themselves for the reasons previously discussed. One possible explanation for the observation that overt clinical infection is uncommon in the first 4 to 6 weeks of life is that passively acquired neutralizing titers are sufficient during this period but later fall and permit infection. Furthermore, preterm infants in whom passively acquired antibody levels are likely to be low are at considerable risk of developing severe disease.

It has also been suggested that the IgG3 subclass is important in providing protection from lower respiratory tract disease because it has relatively strong complement fixing activity[89] and binds more strongly than any of the other subtypes to alveolar macrophages.[90] This subclass has a relatively short half-life; hence passively acquired titers fall rapidly.[91] This has lead to the suggestion that the antibodies of this subtype protect infants from RSV bronchiolitis in the first few weeks of life.[12,92] IgG3 titers in the sera of infants with acute bronchiolitis are low,[92-94] although this is not surprising because after RSV infection in adults, IgG3 titers to the F and G glycoproteins are very low.[95] The importance of IgG3 RSV-specific antibodies in protection remains unclear.

Bronchiolitis and a Specific Immunopathology

Immune Complex Disease

It was originally proposed that bronchiolitis may result from an immune complex reaction between nonneutralizing antibody and virus.[96] This was based on the observation that the illness occurred at an age when passively acquired antibody levels are still generally high and on the results of trials using a formalin-inactivated vaccine in which infants receiving the vaccine had increased morbidity and mortality on subsequent natural exposure to the virus.[97] Several pieces of evidence, including the failure to demonstrate complement consumption and the failure to demonstrate complement within the lungs of a small number of infants crying because of bronchiolitis,[98] led to this hypothesis falling from favor. Furthermore, there is a tendency for high titer levels of maternal antibody to confer some degree of protection, although this does not exclude the possibility that an immune complex reaction occurs in infants whose mothers produce predominantly nonneutralizing antibodies. It is probable that immune complexes do form during infections,[99] and complement activation is likely,[100-102] but RSV bronchiolitis is unlikely to result from an exaggerated immune complex formation.

RSV-Specific IgE Response

The next hypothesis suggested that an IgE response was responsible because very low levels of virus were found in the lungs of a few babies dying as a result of RSV infection.[103] Subsequent epidemiologic studies appear to argue convincingly that prior exposure to the virus is most unlikely; the age distribution of the illness does not change as the epidemic progresses, and the curves representing the incidence of upper respiratory tract illness and that of bronchiolitis are essentially identical.[104] Furthermore, it is well recognized that infants do not demonstrate an accelerated secondary antibody response to the virus during acute illness; indeed, those affected usually have a delayed or an absent response.

Subsequently, another group produced results suggesting that infants acquiring RSV infection may produce an RSV-specific IgE response.[105-110] Their results suggested that such a response was more commonly detected in infants with lower respiratory tract disease and that peak levels tended to correlate both with the severity of the acute illness as determined by the degree of hypoxia and with the prevalence of subsequent symptoms. The response did not appear to be age related. The group also demonstrated elevated histamine levels in the nasal secretions of wheezing infants with RSV infection and cited this as evidence of IgE involvement. It has since been shown that the virus may liberate large amounts of histamine directly from basophils obtained from adults without involving an IgE-mediated process.[111]

Unfortunately, these results implicating a RSV-specific IgE response detected at the mucosal surface have proved difficult to reproduce,[112] although one study has produced similar results correlating serum anti-RSV IgE and IgG4 levels with the likelihood of wheezing.[113]

Several good studies show that atopy is not an important predisposing factor.[12,114-116] If atopy is not an important risk factor for bronchiolitis but an IgE response is, then the virus must specifically influence the host response. What properties of the virus might be responsible and why they appear to operate only in some infants remain obscure. If RSV-specific IgE antibody is produced, the relationship between these antibodies and the acute symptoms needs to be clarified because it is reported that IgE levels do not peak until some time after the acute illness.[106,107] Equally difficult to explain are why the most severe illness occurs during the first exposure to the virus and why subsequent infections are almost always much less severe. A study attempting to find evidence implicating an IgE-mediated mechanism in the causation of acute symptoms failed to find any evidence of significant mast cell degranulation.[78]

Excessive Cytotoxic T Cell Activity

During the past 10 years and based on a the results of a number of animal experiments, considerable efforts have been made to implicate an excessive cytotoxic T cell response in the causation of bronchiolitis. It was proposed that an excessive cell-mediated response was responsible for the increase in severity and mortality in infants to whom the killed vaccine was administered,[117] and animal experiments using mice have indicated that cytotoxic T cells may contribute to lung pathology in a dose-dependent fashion.[71]

RSV-specific cytotoxic T cells have been described in the sera of some adults[118] and infants[119,120] during RSV infections, but their role is unclear. Circulating cytotoxic cells were detected in only 4 of 22 infants with acute bronchiolitis.[120] They were present early in the illness and only in the blood of infants with mild disease. Although circulating cells may not reflect the events within the lungs, this study did not support the notion that cytotoxic T cells are responsible for the inflammation within the lungs. A recent study found no association between HLA class 1 antigens and acute RSV bronchiolitis.[121]

As previously noted, immunocompromised patients, especially those with defects of cell-mediated immunity, have difficulty eliminating the virus and have a high mortality rate, but passively transferred T cells can eradicate persistent RSV infections in athymic nude mice. Hence it seems likely that cytotoxic T cells are important in the recovery from RSV infections rather than are causes of symptoms.

Excessive T-Helper Cell Activity

As with CD8+ cells, it has been shown that CD4+ T-helper (Th) cells can augment lung pathology in experimentally infected animals.[122,123] One group has proposed that a Th2 response to G glycoprotein is responsible for the disease.[124,125] In this rodent model, the lung pathology is characterized by an intense eosinophilic response with these cells, accounting for 20% to 60% of all cells recovered from the lungs by lavage.[125] In contrast, the predominant cell recovered from the lungs of infants with bronchiolitis is the neutrophil, with few if any eosinophils.[77] A recent study in humans suggested that natural RSV infections induces a Th1 rather than a Th2 response.[126] Again the relevance of an animal model of pathogenesis has been brought into question.

Enhanced Infection of Macrophages

In vitro experiments have demonstrated that RSV infects a number of lymphocytes and more frequently, monocytes/macrophages[48,127,128] and productively infects the latter.[48] Circulating mononuclear cells taken from infants with RSV infections and cultured for up to 3 days contained viral antigen, implying that infection of these cells occurs during natural infection[127] and that alveolar macrophages obtained from the lungs of infants with bronchiolitis appear to have been infected.

If infection of monocytes/macrophages with consequent impairment of their function does prove to be important in the immunopathology of acute bronchiolitis, the observation that the entry of virus into macrophages can be facilitated by the presence of antibody[54-56] may explain the following paradox noted more than 20 years ago: Bronchiolitis can still occur in patients with relatively high levels of passively acquired antibody. Again, it is proposed that bronchiolitis develops as neutralizing titers fall below the level necessary for protection. Subsequently, infection of macrophages is enhanced by antibody binding to the virus and facilitating entry into the cell, mediated in part via binding to the Fc receptors.[54] This concept need not be contrary to the observation that high levels of neutralizing antibodies are protective in that the process would only become significant once neutralizing titers fell.

Other factors may also influence the likelihood of infecting mononuclear cells. One study found that monocytes from cord blood were more readily infected than circulating monocytes or alveolar macrophages from adults,[128] whereas another reported that cells cultured for several days were more likely to be infected than fresh monocytes.[48] RSV antigen was more commonly identified in circulating mononuclear cells from the youngest infants with bronchiolitis.[127]

In vitro studies have suggested that the cytopathic effect on monocytes/macrophages is to cause rounding of cells,[48,128] whereas infected lymphocytes develop atypical or lymphoblastoid features[127] accompanied by a rapid fall in CD4+ lymphocytes and a rise in CD8+ cell numbers.[127] Syncytia formation is rare.[48,127]

Suppressed Interferon Production

In vitro experiments have show that the virus appears to be a poor inducer of IFN-α[47,48,129] and indeed appears to inhibit its production in response to other stimuli. The levels of IFN-α detected in the nasal secretion of infants[49,50,51,130] are low compared with those generated by other viruses such as influenza virus, whereas IFN-γ has not been detected in nasal secretions[49,130] or endotracheal tube aspirates.[49] The ability of RSV to suppress interferon production, together with the observation that T cells from infants secrete less IFN-γ than those of adults,[131-133] may explain why infants are relatively more susceptible to severe disease than adults. It appears that IFN-γ may be constantly liberated in the lungs of adults,[134] and it is possible that this may provide some protection because the virus does appear to be sensitive to its effects.[135]

As previously noted, despite the low levels of IFN-α reported in clinical samples, this interferon may be responsible for suppressing T-cell proliferation. It may also have a role in immunosuppression.

Summary

There is little evidence from humans studies that the immunologic process in the airways of infants with acute bronchiolitis is different than that in the airways of infants with only upper respiratory tract symptoms. Only a very small percentage of infected infants develop severe lower respiratory tract symptoms. It is quite possible that the extension of inflammation from the upper to lower respiratory tract is a matter of chance, that it reflects the infecting viral load, or that it simply reflects relatively lower levels of protection in some individuals. The severity of symptoms observed in young infants may also reflect the smaller airways in this age group. However, it is almost certain that some of these observations represent important immunosuppressive strategies that permit the virus to infect individuals of all ages.

Animal Models

Most studies that use an animal model in an attempt to unravel the immune processes contributing to acute RSV bronchiolitis have used rodents. The results obtained in such studies must be interpreted with considerable caution because not only have apparently contradictory results been obtained but also, and perhaps more important, these animals are not the natural host for the virus and they do not develop a clinical significant illness resembling acute bronchiolitis when infected experimentally.[34] Many proposed immunopathologic mechanisms have been supported by at least one rodent model. Rodent models may prove to be more valuable in assessing the potential role of therapeutic interventions such as immunoglobulin preparations.[65,74,136]

A better animal model for determining immunologic responses may prove to be the acute respiratory illness observed in calves caused by the bovine RSV.[137] There are similarities in the clinical picture: Calves develop upper and lower respiratory signs, the youngest calves experience the most severe illness at a time when passively acquired antibodies are present, and only a small number of infected calves experience severe disease. Several studies addressing aspects of the immune response after natural[137-139] and experimental[140] infection of calves have been undertaken. Problems with experimental infection include the cost of rearing the calves and the fact that as with humans, only a relatively low percentage of calves develop severe disease.

ACUTE RSV BRONCHIOLITIS

Differential Diagnosis

In the majority of infants admitted with the clinical syndrome previously described, the causative organism is RSV; indeed, some argue that the definition of *bronchiolitis* should be confined to the typical clinical features and evidence of RSV infection.[141] However, it is generally accepted that the same clinical picture can be produced by other viruses, including parainfluenza viruses, influenza viruses, adenoviruses, and rhinoviruses.

If the illness is severe, unusually prolonged, or otherwise atypical, it is important to consider other primary diagnoses or associated conditions that may be contributing to the severity of the illness. These would include cystic fibrosis, aspiration, congenital lung abnormalities, chlamydial infection, immunodeficiencies, and congenital heart disease, all of which can present with many of the features characteristic of acute bronchiolitis. Likewise, disorders such as interstitial pneumonitis and bronchiolitis obliterans resulting from adenovirus can present with an illness initially suggestive of acute RSV bronchiolitis.

As previously noted, viral pneumonias may present with some of the features of bronchiolitis. The distinction remains essentially a clinical one because 20% of infants with a clinical diagnosis of bronchiolitis have areas of consolidation or subsegmental collapse on the chest radiograph. Hyperinflation on the radiograph is common in bronchiolitis and supports the clinical diagnosis. However, as discussed later, chest radiographs generally add little to the management of the condition.

Diagnosis

The clinical diagnosis of acute viral bronchiolitis can be rapidly supported by identifying or confirming the RSV or other respiratory viruses using immunofluorescent antibody methods or enzyme-linked immunoabsorbent assays.[142,143] Reliable commercial kits are now readily available and widely used; some are designed for use by the clinician at the bedside.[144] Nasopharyngeal aspirates generally provide suitable samples containing a relatively high yield of virus, although nasal lavage is widely used in North America. There appears to be little difference in the quality of samples obtained.[145]

A positive result is valuable in supporting the diagnosis and in isolating infants with the virus. However, it should be remembered that all these methods require good quality samples and that a negative result does not exclude RSV infection.

Most laboratories still confirm RSV infection by culturing the virus in appropriate cell lines and identifying the characteristic cytopathic effects.[34,143] The virus is relatively labile; hence careful handling of samples is required if positive results are to be obtained. A delay of up to a week before confirmation of RSV infection again limits the clinical usefulness of viral culture.

Significant rises in RSV antibody titers are uncommon in young infants. Although enzyme-linked immunoabsorbent assay techniques appear more sensitive, serologic diagnosis is of little value clinically because convalescent sera are required and results are therefore unavailable for many weeks.

Assessment

At present, there is no way of predicting which of the many infants presenting with upper respiratory tract infection during the RSV epidemic will develop acute bronchiolitis. However, certain groups of children are at risk of severe disease if they develop bronchiolitis.

In previously healthy infants, the peak incidence of hospital admissions is in those age 1 to 4 months,[6,9] which is probably because of the low incidence of the condition in younger infants and relatively mild disease in older children, possibly resulting from growth of the airways. For those admitted to the hospital the severity, as judged by the degree of hypoxia,[13] duration of admission,[13,24,146] and need for ventilation,[13,14,24,146] is increased in younger and smaller infants. Maternal smoking is associated with a higher risk of admission to the hospital with acute viral bronchiolitis.

Certain infants are at increased risk of severe disease that may lead to respiratory failure requiring ventilatory support and in a small number, to death. These include infants with congenital cardiac disease, particularly those with pulmonary hypertension; chronic neonatal lung disease with oxygen dependency; immunodeficiencies; and cystic fibrosis. It also includes infants born very prematurely.[17,24,147,148] Hence the development of bronchiolitis in such patients is a cause for concern.

During RSV respiratory infections, the two most serious complications are apnea and respiratory failure.

Apnea

Apnea is the most common symptom in the youngest patients, those born preterm,[15,25,82,148,149] and those with chronic lung disease.[15] Infants may first have apnea and progress to bronchiolitis, show signs of bronchiolitis, and develop apneas or have apnea as the sole sign of RSV infection. RSV infection has been implicated in a number of cases of crib death,[150-152] and its ability to precipitate apnea may be relevant to this observation. A large number of infants with RSV infection requiring assisted ventilation do so because of severe recurrent apneas rather than respiratory failure.[147,152] The mechanisms leading to these apneas is unclear, but they tend to resolve within a few days.[153] The use of apnea monitors is therefore important in young infants, those born preterm, and those with preexisting lung disease.

Respiratory Failure

It is well recognized that the clinical assessment of hypoxia is poor.[154,155] Perhaps the most reliable clinical sign is agitation, which if not relieved by supplemental oxygen, can contribute to exhaustion and respiratory failure. Hypercapnia is of little significance in all but the most severely affected infants[154]; hence with the widespread use of pulse oximetry, blood gas monitoring is usually required only when mechanical ventilation is being considered. Although these monitors have certain limitations, they play a central role in the assessment of hypoxia and subsequent management of oxygen therapy. Two recent studies found that an infant's oxygen saturation, as judged by pulse oximetry, was the best objective predictor of disease severity.[156,157]

Chest Radiographs

No investigations other than chest radiographs are routinely required. Chest radiographs are commonly requested, although there is no evidence that they are of any value in most infants admitted with the clinical diagnosis of RSV bronchiolitis. The chest radiograph typically shows evidence of hyperinflation and frequently demonstrates evidence of collapse and consolidation, especially in the right upper lobe.[158] It has been proposed that most areas of shadowing suggesting subsegmental consolidation are in fact small areas of collapse, and Simpson et al[158] concluded that this appearance should not alter a pediatrician's decision to withhold antibiotics. A recent study found no correlation between the changes on chest radiograph and clinical severity, leading its authors to suggest that this investigation should be limited to those in whom intensive care was being considered, those whose condition deteriorates unexpectedly, and those who have an underlying cardiac or pulmonary disorder.[159] Because secondary bacterial infection is uncommon in RSV bronchiolitis,[160,161] patchy changes on the chest radiograph are not an indication for the use of antibiotics in patients with a typical clinical picture; hence radiography seldom alters management.

One study did find that pulmonary consolidation was a risk factor for increased morbidity,[24] but because the mean age of patients admitted with RSV infection is 9 months, many of these patients are likely to have had RSV pneumonia as previously defined rather than the clinical picture of acute bronchiolitis for which the peak age of admission is 1 to 4 months.

Serum Electrolyte Levels

The syndrome of inappropriate antidiuretic hormone secretion can occur.[162] Electrolyte disturbances are uncommon except in the most severely ill babies; hence there is no indication for the routine assessment of serum electrolytes. Neutrophilia with an excess of immature neutrophils is a frequent finding during RSV infections[154,163]; hence full blood counts are also of little value.

Indications for Hospitalization

Decisions regarding hospital admission are based on age, risk factors, clinical assessment, and oxygen saturation. Most infants in at-risk groups are admitted unless symptoms are very mild; similarly the threshold for admitting infants younger than 6 months of age is relatively low because of the risk of progression to more severe disease and the increased risk of apnea. However, for many infants the illness is mild and can be managed at home. For those not admitted, it is important to alert parents to signs suggesting deterioration, such as poor feeding and agitation, which would justify admission.

Prognosis

The prognosis for the majority of infants who develop acute bronchiolitis is very good, with an overall mortality rate less than 1% in recent reports.[15-17,24] The mortality rate of previously well infants is extremely low, but those in high-risk groups has historically been much higher, with figures as high as 37% reported in infants with congenital heart disease.[164] With improved supportive care, the mortality rate in infants from high-risk groups who develop bronchiolitis is now generally below 4%.[15-17,24,165] The number of infants requiring intensive care, particularly in previously well infants, is generally low.

The long-term morbidity associated with developing bronchiolitis in infancy has been the subject of a number of studies. Some have suggested that as many as 75%[114,141,166-168] of such infants experience recurrent cough and wheeze in subsequent years, although the prevalence declines with age.[166,168] Episodes are usually infrequent, and it is unusual for these symptoms to be severe enough to require readmission.[114,166] Studies have shown that many children with bronchiolitis exhibit increased bronchial responsiveness later in childhood, but there is little correlation between responsiveness and symptoms.[134,141,166,168] Although atopy is not a risk factor for acute bronchiolitis, a personal or family history of atopy appears to play an important role in those with subsequent recurrent symptoms, particularly in those older than 5 years of age.[166-168] At 10 years of age, two thirds of children with recurrent wheeze had IgE levels consistent with personal atopy.[166] Young et al[141] found that infants who developed bronchiolitis in the first year of life had evidence of preexisting small airways, whereas those who developed it in the second year had the asthma and atopy phenotype. The long-term follow-up of the cohort reported by Welliver et al[110] to have high levels of virus-specific IgE found that maternal smoking and recurrent infections were greater risks for ongoing symptoms than atopy and elevated levels of virus-specific IgE. Thus passive smoking is an important risk factor for acute bronchiolitis and subsequent morbidity.

Management

Careful monitoring and good supportive care remain the cornerstones of management. For infants with no underlying immunodeficiency, RSV infections are self-limiting, and management is aimed at providing adequate support until the illness resolves. Monitoring is directed principally at the detection of apnea, hypoxia, and exhaustion. Supportive care is directed at alleviating hypoxia, providing adequate fluids, and preventing exhaustion using minimal handling and respiratory support.

Oxygen

In the early 1960s, Reynolds and Cook[169] noted that "oxygen is vitally important in bronchiolitis and there is little evidence that any other treatment is useful." This is essentially true today. Hypoxia caused by ventilation-perfusion mismatching is frequent,[154,170] although as previously noted, it is difficult to detect clinically. Oxygen (30% to 40%) delivered via a head box is sufficient to correct hypoxia in most cases and rapidly relieves the distress and agitation observed in hypoxic infants.

Fluids

If uncorrected, the poor intake of fluid resulting from respiratory distress and cough can lead to dehydration, and this tendency may be compounded by vomiting associated with the bouts of coughing. Hyponatremia caused by the syndrome of inappropriate antidiuretic hormone can occur,[162] usually in the sickest infants; hence it is sensible to restrict fluids to about two thirds of maintenance.

The route of administration varies among units. Some argue that the risks and disadvantages associated with nasogastric feeding are such that any infants needing supplemental oxygen also require intravenous fluids. The potential problems include increased work of breathing caused by obstruction of the upper airway, increased work of breathing caused by fluid within the stomach, and an increased risk of gastroesophageal reflux and aspiration.[171] Other units find that infants with mild to moderate illness tolerate a nasogastric tube very well and appear more comfortable with frequent small-volume feeds.[172] However, intravenous fluids are recommended in infants more severely affected because occasionally an infant's condition suddenly deteriorates because of aspiration.

Ribavirin

Ribavirin is a broad-spectrum virustatic drug first synthesized in 1972, and its exact mode of action is unclear.[173,174] Since the initial enthusiasm that greeted its launch in 1986, concerns have been raised about its cost, safety, and efficacy. The medication is administered as an aerosol generated by a small-particle aerosol generator. The aerosol is usually delivered into a head box for 12 to 18 hours a day, although a recent small study has used higher doses administered for 2 hours 3 times a day.[175] It can be used in ventilator circuits, although great care must be taken to prevent valves from blocking because of drug crystallizing out on them.[176]

Concerns regarding its safety in both treated infants and their caregivers have been expressed since it was first used, but reported side effects are uncommon. In infants, these have been mainly skin rashes and mild bronchospasm.[177] Ribavirin is apparently not incorporated into host cell ribonucleic acid or deoxyribonucleic acid; hence the potential for unexpected long-term side effects is believed to be low. Although the quantities of ribavirin absorbed by hospital personnel appear to be low, concerns regarding possible teratogenic effects has led some units to use stringent precautions to prevent environmental contamination.[178] The risk to the hospital personnel appears to be low, provided that simple precautions are taken to minimize exposure and that pregnant women are not exposed to the aerosol.[18,179]

In more contention is its role in the management of infants with acute bronchiolitis. The results of early studies led some authors to conclude that its role in treating all but the mildest cases was established beyond doubt and that further studies would be unethical.[180] However, these studies did not show any impact on parameters such as duration of stay or need for intubation, and they were heavily criticized for a number of reasons.[181-183] Years later, there is still no convincing evidence that ribavirin has any role in the treatment of the majority of previously healthy infants. The American Academy of Pediatrics initially recommended that the use of ribavirin should be "considered" in infants at high risk of severe disease, such as those with cardiac disease, chronic lung disease, and cystic fibrosis; in those with an immunodeficiency; in severely ill infants; or in premature infants.[184] They have subsequently recommended that it be used for all hospitalized at-risk patients and for severely ill patients, which includes all those with saturations of less than 90%.[184] These recommendations have attracted further criticism,[185] and there is still much controversy surrounding the use of this medication for treating such patients. Many centers in the United Kingdom and Australia support these criticisms and rarely use ribavirin.[186]

A large, prospective study using ribavirin early in the course of RSV infections in patients with preexisting cardiac and respiratory disease concluded that early ribavirin "may help reduce morbidity."[187] However, none of the infants in either the active treatment or the placebo groups required ventilation or died, a situation very different from that quoted in historical studies.[164] These authors, who support the use of ribavirin, did make the comment that "the early and aggressive medical support and meticulous attention to oxygenation may also have played an important role in decreasing the overall morbidity." The lack of a more impressive effect may have resulted from the fact that only a small number of infants with RSV infections develop severe bronchiolitis but the study treated all RSV infections; hence the numbers treated would obscure any effect in those who do develop bronchiolitis.

A recent retrospective analysis of RSV infection in patients with congenital heart disease found the mortality rate to be much lower than that reported a decade ago and concluded that this was attributable to improvements in management and intensive care rather than to any effect of introducing antiviral therapy.[165] Two other retrospective studies have also found a much lower mortality rate in a range of high-risk groups than the rate reported in previous studies.[17,47] Also, it appeared that improved supportive and intensive care rather than the introduction of antiviral therapy was the major factor. The American Academy also commented that ribavirin may be of greatest benefit in those requiring mechanical ventilation.[18] Again, there is no clear evidence to support this suggestion. One study did show significantly shorter duration of ventilation, supplementary oxygen, and hospital stay in those receiving ribavirin,[188] but this study has been criticized for using distilled water as the placebo, and it has been suggested that this contributed to the unusually long periods of ventilation observed in the placebo group.[47] Another randomized study found no benefit from using ribavirin to treat patients whose lungs are ventilated,[189] and the role of ribavirin, if any, in the intensive care unit has still to be determined.[190]

It would seem reasonable in light of the evidence so far to consider using ribavirin in extremely ill infants because it may hasten the onset of recovery and to have a lower threshold for its use in infants at high risk, particularly those who are immunosuppressed. However, a recent report suggested that RSV infections persisted in a number of immunodeficient patients despite ribavirin treatment.[47] Good supportive care still remains the mainstay of management for all infants.

Assisted Ventilation

Although the number of infants with acute bronchiolitis requiring ventilation can be minimized by good supportive care, a small number admitted to the hospital may require ventilation for either recurrent apnea or respiratory failure. Indications for intubation vary from unit to unit,[27,47,146,191-194] but in general, infants' lungs are intubated for either recurrent apnea with significant oxygen desaturations or respiratory failure with persistent acidosis or hypoxia despite high oxygen use. A rising carbon dioxide level of more than 7 to 8 kPa would be viewed by some as an indication for intubation,[27,33,47] but other infants would tolerate significantly higher levels in the absence of overt exhaustion, acidosis, or uncorrected hypoxia.[146,193] Although high peak pressures are often required, the minimum peak pressures required to achieve acceptable oxygenation with an arterial pH greater than 7.2 should be used.[193] Permissive hypercapnia is preferred to aggressive ventilation designed to normalize carbon dioxide levels.[194] Positive end-expiratory pressure may help and, although frequently used, may in some cases be detrimental.[195] Slow rates with long expiratory times are generally required in infants with respiratory failure.[190-192] Patients should be weaned from the ventilator as rapidly as possible. Occasionally these infants can develop a picture consistent with adult respiratory distress syndrome.[196]

Other Forms of Respiratory Support

Units have reported a reduction in the need for assisted ventilation after the introduction of nasal continuous pressure ventilation (continuous positive airway pressure),[32] and there are anecdotal reports of benefits using continuous negative extrathoracic pressure for the treatment of infants with severe bronchiolitis whose lungs are not ventilated and are using continuous negative extrathoracic pressure and intermittent negative extrathoracic pressure (INEP) for the management of infants with apnea.[197]

A number of infants whose condition continued to deteriorate despite mechanical ventilation have been treated with extracorporeal membrane oxygenation, and preliminary reports are encouraging.[198] A recent case report has suggested that high-frequency ventilation combined with nitric oxide may also be beneficial in infants whose condition does not respond to conventional ventilation.[199] The role of these interventions has still to be clearly determined.

Antibiotics

Secondary bacterial infection appears uncommon in infants with RSV bronchiolitis[47,160,161]; hence antibiotics are rarely indicated even in those with patchy changes on the radiograph suggesting pneumonia. The clinical picture, together with the rapid confirmation of RSV infection, provides reassurance in most mild to moderately unwell infants. Indeed a large prospective study, covering a period of 9 years, found that secondary bacterial infection was more common in those given antibiotics than those who did not receive them. However, dual infections with viruses, *Chlamydia* organisms, and bacteria do occur[161,200,201]; hence it is not unreasonable to start antibiotics in those who are particularly ill or those whose condition has atypical features. It is increasingly recognized that RSV infections can present with an apparent septicemic illness,[27-29] and antibiotics are given to infants with this type of illness and those with apnea.

Although uncommon, it is also important to bear in mind that coincidental infections, such as urinary tract infections or meningitis, do occur in infants with RSV infections, including bronchiolitis.[161]

Bronchodilators

One of the biggest areas for contention in the management of acute bronchiolitis is in the role of bronchodilators. This largely stems from differences in defining the condition. Clinicians who use the label *acute bronchiolitis* as defined in this chapter find no evidence to support the use of β_2-sympathomimetic agents in this illness.[34,202-204] Several studies have failed to show any benefit from the use of β_2-sympathomimetic agents,[205-208] but their use can sometimes have detrimental effects.[209,210] Similarly, there is no convincing evidence that other bronchodilators such as theophylline[211,212] and ipratropium bromide[208,213] are beneficial. These findings are perhaps not surprising in view of the marked mucus production and mucosal inflammation that contribute to the airway obstruction.

Others argue that there is little doubt that bronchodilators are effective in some patients with bronchiolitis,[33] and sympathomimetic agents and theophylline are used extensively.[16,29,214] However, most of the studies cited to support this position use the broader definition of *bronchiolitis,* which includes all wheezy infants.[215-219] These studies generally include many children considerably older than 6 months of age, whereas it is in this younger age group that the infants acutely unwell with acute viral bronchiolitis are seen. Even when this wider definition is used, the efficacy of bronchodilators in infants is still debated.[220] In older infants in whom it may be difficult to distinguish bronchiolitis and other forms of virus-induced wheeze, a trial of bronchodilators is reasonable because the condition of a significant number patients will respond. However, such infants should receive supplementary oxygen and close monitoring because of the potential for exacerbation of ventilation-perfusion mismatching.

Other Therapies

Published studies have consistently failed to show any benefit from the use of systemic[221-224] or inhaled[225] corticosteroids. Despite this, steroids are used extensively in North America to treat these patients. There is also no evidence that "mist therapy" or physiotherapy[226] has any role in the treatment of acute bronchiolitis; indeed the excessive handling associated with physiotherapy can be detrimental.[226] The use of intravenous immunoglobulin in a single study has produced results similar to those obtained when ribavirin is used: The condition of treated patients appeared to have a more rapid improvement in oxygenation with a small effect on viral shedding, but such treatment did not reduce the period of hospitalization.[72] A further study is assessing the role of purified human immunoglobulin with high titers of anti-RSV neutralizing antibodies.[227] Animal work has suggested that less immunoglobulin is required if this is delivered directly to the respiratory tract.[135,225] Human studies using this approach are underway.[66,227]

Studies have shown that monoclonal antibodies used against the relatively highly conserved F glycoprotein are effective in animal models. There is some optimism that such preparations may be valuable in infants.[67,75,227]

As previously noted, RSV appears to be both a poor inducer of interferon and to be sensitive to its effects; it was hoped that the administration of IFN-α would be of benefit in infants with bronchiolitis. However clinical trials have found no significant benefit when it was used to treat infants with bronchiolitis.[228,229]

Prevention

The prevention of acute RSV bronchiolitis remains a major objective for health care. Until recently, the only effective measures available were those designed to prevent nosocomial spread within pediatric wards. Recent studies have indicated that RSV immunoglobulin administered intravenously and intramuscularly can reduce morbidity in high-risk patients.

Cross-Infection

It has been known for many years that the virus spreads rapidly through pediatric wards if precautions are not taken,[230,231] and fatalities among infants acquiring the virus while they are inpatients are well recorded.[164,165] The inhalation of small-droplet aerosols generated by coughing and sneezing does not appear to be an important method of transmission. Infection of the hospital staff is common through self-inoculation from the hands into the eyes or the nose[232]; indeed, infection in members of the staff appears to be a major source of nosocomial spread. The virus is transmitted to infants on the hands of attendant staff or relatives; thus simply isolating infants is inadequate for preventing spread. Careful attention to handwashing[233,234] appears to be the most important aspect in the prevention of cross-infection because it helps reduce both the self-inoculation of staff and the direct transmission of virus to other patients. More extensive precautions have been advocated by some authors who argue that isolation and handwashing are ineffective. These precautions include the use of gowns, gloves, and even goggles.[234-240] Most of these measures principally serve to reduce the infection rate among staff and thus prevent them for passing it to children, but they also heighten appreciation of the need for infection-control measures.

Although severe disease is unusual in neonatal units, it is still very important to try to prevent nosocomial spread in these units because the virus can mimic other forms of sepsis with nonspecific symptoms and may induce significant apneas. During epidemics, it is important to devise specific strategies to prevent spread to inpatients at highest risk.

Vaccines

For over 2 decades, much effort has been devoted to producing a vaccine to prevent much of the respiratory morbidity associated with RSV bronchiolitis. In the 1960s, trials of a formalin-inactivated, alum-precipitated vaccine produced alarming results: Not only did the vaccine fail to protect infants, but there was also excess morbidity and mortality in the immunized children when they subsequently were infected with the virus.[240,241] Despite stimulating fixating and neutralizing antibodies, the vaccine failed to protect infants from infection. This adverse response has yet to be fully explained, but the failure to offer protection despite the generation of high antibody titers is most likely due to the loss of key epitopes on the F and G glycoproteins during the preparation of the vaccine, resulting in the generation of largely nonneutralizing antibodies.[242,243] The neutralizing antibodies produced probably represented only a small fraction of the total antibody response. Whether the enhanced disease severity noted on subsequent exposure to the virus was due to an abnormal response or represented an exaggeration of the natural response is unclear.

Earlier attempts to produce live, attenuated, temperature-sensitive mutants designed to be inoculated into the respiratory tract failed because of inadequate attenuation, overattenuation with failure to replicate, or genetic instability that led to reversion to pathogenic strains.[227] More stable, attenuated, and apparently immunogenic vaccines are being developed and appear to be effective in primate models, but their ability to protect young infants is yet to be tested.

Recent research has included efforts to produce subunit vaccines using recombinant deoxyribonucleic acid technology. These consist of either the F or G antigens in isolation or linked together. Another approach has been to express viral glycoprotein genes on the surface of carrier viruses using recombinant gene technology,[227,244] and a third approach has been to use purified F protein obtained from tissue cultures. Some of the subunit and purified protein preparations have been administered to young children previously infected with the virus and have not caused potentiation of disease severity on subsequent exposure. The level of protection offered is unclear and is of short duration.[227,244-247] Although generally immunogenic in animal models, some of these most recent vaccine preparations have caused enhanced disease in these animal models; hence trials in young infants not previously exposed to the virus are unlikely to commence in the near future.

Debate continues as to whether injection, inoculation into the respiratory tract to produce local immunity, or even administration to the mother would be the most appropriate route if an effective vaccine could be developed. Parenteral administration in young infants with passively acquired antibody is unlikely to generate high neutralizing titers. The use of live, attenuated viruses may prove more valuable in that it will stimulate an immune response at the mucosal surface, but the failure of natural infections to generate effective protection suggests that this may provide at best only partial protection. Immunization of the mother and the resulting passive transfer of antibodies is an alternative approach. Titers will fall with age but may provide protection in the first 6 months when the disease is usually most severe.[248]

Specific Immunoglobulin

The balance of evidence suggests that high levels of passively acquired maternal antibodies are protective,[249,250] and this led to the hope that immunoglobulin preparations would be useful in immunoprophylaxis. One multicenter trial appeared to show that intravenous immunoglobulin containing high titers of RSV-specific antibodies protected high-risk infants from significant lower respiratory tract infection,[61] and this was greeted by some as the much-needed breakthrough in the prevention of severe disease in at-risk groups.[62] Although the study was criticized by the Blood Products Advisory Committee of the American FDA, the results from this and subsequent studies have resulted in the granting of a product license for RSV-specific immunoglobulin intravenous infusions for use in the prevention of severe RSV lower respiratory tract disease in infants and children younger 24 months of age with bronchopulmonary dysplasia and with a history of premature birth (<35 weeks' gestation). The studies and the potential benefits of this form of therapy have been recently reviewed by the American Academy of Pediatrics Committee on Infectious Diseases,[250] and they conclude that it should be considered for infants with bronchopulmonary dysplasia who are receiving or who have received oxygen therapy within the past 6 months and that it should be considered in infants with gestational ages of 32 weeks or less. The committee did point out that the cost of such therapy is considerable. The benefits are far from clear-cut in many children, particularly in view of the need for monthly intravenous infusions.

More recently, work has been undertaken with monoclonal antibodies directed to well-conserved epitopes on the relatively stable F protein. Because of the reduced volume required, these preparations can be given intramuscularly and potentially offer the best prospects for the prevention of severe disease in high-risk groups in the near future.

Conclusions

The prevention of acute RSV bronchiolitis in infancy remains a major challenge. The morbidity associated with this condition is considerable, and the financial strains placed on health services is enormous. With improved supportive care, the mortality rate is now low even in at-risk groups, but the condition still poses a major threat to the health of infants with underlying disease. The basis of treatment remains good supportive care. Antiviral therapy may have a role in a small group of at-risk patients, but it may be replaced in the near future by newer therapies such as RSV-specific immunoglobulin.

REFERENCES

1. Kim HW, Arrabio JO, Brandt CD, Jeffries BC, Pyles G, Reid JL, Chanock RM, Parrott RH: Epidemiology of respiratory syncytial virus infection in Washington DC. I. Importance of the virus in different respiratory tract disease syndromes and temporal distribution of infection, *Am J Epidemiol* 98:216-225, 1973.
2. Martin AJ, Gardner PS, McQuillin J: Epidemiology of respiratory viral infection among paediatric inpatients over a six year period in North East England, *Lancet* 2:1035-1038, 1978.
3. Murphy B, Phelan PD, Jack I, Uren E: Seasonal pattern of respiratory viral infection in children, *Med J Aust* 1:22-24, 1980.
4. Gilchrist S, Torok TJ, Gary HE Jr, Alexander JP, Anderson, LJ: National surveillance for respiratory syncytial virus, United States, 1985-1990, *J Infect Dis* 170:986-990, 1994.
5. Fransen H, Sterner G, Forsgren M, Heigl Z, Wolontis S, Svedmyr A, Tunevall G: Acute lower respiratory illness in elderly patients with respiratory syncytial virus infection, *Acta Med Scand* 182:323-330, 1967.
6. Parrott RH, Kim HW, Arrobio JO, Hodes DS, Murphy BR, Brandt CD, Camargo E, Chanock RM: Epidemiology of respiratory syncytial virus infections in Washington DC. II. Infection and disease with respect to age, immunological status, race and sex, *Am J Epidemiol* 98:289-300, 1973.
7. Hall CB, Geiman JM, Biggar R, Kohok DI, Hogan PM, Douglas GRJ: Respiratory syncytial virus infections within families, *N Engl J Med* 294:414-419, 1976.
8. Hall JW, Hall CB, Speers DM: Respiratory syncytial virus infection in adults, *Ann Intern Med* 88:203-205, 1978.
9. Clarke SKR, Corner BD, Haines C, et al: Respiratory syncytial virus infection: admissions to hospital in industrial, urban and rural areas: report to the MRC Subcommittee on Respiratory Syncytial Virus Vaccines, *Br Med J* 2:796-798, 1978.
10. Glezen WP, Taber LH, Frank AL, Kasel JA: Risk of primary infection and re-infection with respiratory syncytial virus, *Am J Dis Child* 140:543-546, 1986.
11. Henderson FW, Collier AM, Clyde WA, Denny FW: Respiratory syncytial virus infections, reinfections and immunity, *N Engl J Med* 300:530-534, 1979.
12. Glezen WP, Paredes A, Allison JE, Taber LH, Frank AL: Risk of respiratory syncytial virus infection for infants from low income families in relationship to age, sex, ethnic group and maternal antibody level, *J Pediatr* 98:708-715, 1981.
13. Green M, Brayer AF, Schenkman KA, Wald ER: Duration of hospitalisation in previously well infants with respiratory syncytial virus infection, *J Pediatr Infect Dis* 8:601-605, 1989.
14. McMillan JA, Tristram DA, Weiner LB, Higgins AP, Sandstrom C, Brandon R: Prediction of the duration of hospitalization in patients with respiratory syncytial virus infection: use of clinical parameters, *Pediatrics* 81:22-26, 1988.
15. Meert K, Heidemann S, Lieh-Lai M, Sarnaik AP: Clinical characteristics of respiratory syncytial virus infections in healthy versus previously compromised host, *Pediatr Pulmonol* 7:167-170, 1989.
16. Law BJ: Respiratory syncytial virus infections in hospitalized Canadian children: regional differences in patient populations and management practices, *Pediatr Infect Dis J* 12:659-663, 1993.
17. Navas L, Wang E, de Carvalho V: Improved outcome of respiratory syncytial virus infection in a high-risk hospitalized population of Canadian children, *J Pediatr* 121:348-354, 1992.
18. American Academy of Pediatrics Committee on Infectious Disease: Use of ribavirin in the treatment of respiratory syncytial virus infection, *Pediatrics* 92:501-504, 1993.
19. Meissner HC: Economic impact of viral respiratory disease in children, *J Pediatr* 124:S17-S21, 1994.
20. Sly PD, Hibbert HE: Childhood asthma following hospitalization with acute viral bronchiolitis in infancy, *Pediatr Pulmonol* 7:153-158, 1989.
21. Murray M, Webb MS, O'Callaghan C, Swarbrick AS, Milner AD: Respiratory status and allergy after bronchiolitis, *Arch Dis Child* 67: 482-487, 1992.
22. Pullan CR, Hey EW: Wheezing, asthma and pulmonary dysfunction l0 years after infection with respiratory syncytial virus in infancy, *Br Med J* 284:1665-1669, 1982.

Clinical Syndromes

23. Silverman M: Asthma and wheezing in young children, *N Engl J Med* 332:181-182, 1995 (editorial).
24. Wang EE, Law BJ, Stephens D: Pediatric Investigators Collaborative Network on infections in Canada (PICNIC) prospective study of risk factors and outcomes in patients hospitalized with respiratory syncytial viral lower respiratory tract infection, *J Pediatr* 126:212-219, 1995.
25. Church WR, Anas NG, Hall CB, Brooks JG: Respiratory syncytial virus related apnoea in infants, *Am J Dis Child* 138:247-250, 1984.
26. Pickers DL, Schefft GL, Storch GA, Thach BT: Characterisation of prolonged apnoeic episodes associated with respiratory syncytial virus infection, *Pediatr Pulmonol* 6:195-201, 1989.
27. Njoku DB, Kliegman RM: Atypical extrapulmonary presentations of severe RSV infection requiring intensive care, *Clin Pediatr* 32:455-460, 1993.
28. Marks MI: Respiratory syncytial virus infection: the expanded clinical spectrum, *Clin Pediatr* 32:461-462, 1993.
29. La Via WV, Grant SW, Stutman HR, Marks MI: Clinical profile of pediatric patients hospitalised with respiratory syncytial virus infection, *Clin Pediatr* 32:450-454, 1993.
30. Hubble D, Osborn GR: Acute bronchiolitis in children, *Br Med J* 1:107-110, 1941.
31. Henry R, Milner AD, Stokes GM: Bronchiolitis, *Am J Dis Child* 137:805, 1983 (letter).
32. Phelan PD, Olinsky A, Roberton CF: *Respiratory illness in children,* ed 4, Oxford, England, 1994, Blackwell, pp 71-74.
33. Ruuskanen O, Ogra PL: Respiratory syncytial virus, *Current Prob Pediatr* 23:50-79, 1993.

Epidemiology

34. McIntosh K, Chanock RM: Respiratory syncytial virus. In Fields BM, Knipe DM, eds: *Fields' virology,* ed 2, Philadelphia, 1990, Raven, pp 1045-1072.
35. McIntosh K, Fishaut JM: Immunopathologic mechanisms in lower respiratory tract disease of infants due to respiratory syncytial virus, *Prog Med Virol* 26:94-118, 1980.
36. Anderson LJ, Hierholzer JC, Tsou C, Hendry RM, Fernie BF, Stone Y, McIntosh K: Antigenic characterisation of respiratory syncytial virus strains with monoclonal antibodies, *J Infect Dis* 151:626-633, 1985.
37. Anderson LJ, Hendry, RM, Pierik LT, Tsou C, McIntosh K: Multicentre study of strains of respiratory syncytial virus, *J Infect Dis* 163:687-692, 1991.
38. Hendry RM, Talis AL, Godfrey E, Anderson LJ, Fernie BF, McIntosh K: Concurrent circulation of antigenically distinct strains of respiratory syncytial during community outbreaks, *J Infect Dis* 153:291-297, 1986.
39. Garcia O, Martin M, Dopazo J, Arbiza J, Frabasile S, Russ, J, Hortal M, Perez Brena P, Martinez I, Garcia Barreno B: Evolutionary pattern of human respiratory syncytial virus (subgroup A): cocirculating lineages and correlation of genetic and antigenic changes in G glycoprotein, *J Virol* 68:5448-5459, 1994.

40. Hall CB, Walsh EE, Long CE, Schnabel KC: Immunity to and frequency of reinfection with respiratory syncytial virus, *J Infect Dis* 163:693-698, 1991.
41. Fleming DM, Cross KW: Respiratory syncytial virus or influenza, *Lancet* 342:1507-1510, 1993.
42. Hall CB, Douglas RG Jr: Modes of transmission of respiratory syncytial virus, *J Pediatr* 99:100-103, 1981.
43. Hall CB, Geiman JM, Douglas RG Jr: Possible transmission by fomites of respiratory syncytial virus, *J Infect Dis* 141:98-102, 1980.
44. Hall CB, Douglas RG Jr, Geiman JM: Respiratory syncytial virus infections in infants: quantitation and duration of shedding, *J Pediatr* 89:11-15, 1976.

Disease Mechanisms and Pathology

45. Roberts NJ, Prill AH, Mann TN: Interleukin l and interleukin l inhibitor production by human macrophages exposed to influenza virus or respiratory syncytial virus, *J Exp Med* 163:51-59, 1986.
46. Salkind AR, McCarthy DO, Nichols JE, Domurat FM, Walsh EE, Roberts NJ Jr: Interleukin 1–inhibitor activity induced by respiratory syncytial virus: abrogation of virus specific and alternate human lymphocyte proliferative responses, *J Infect Dis* 163:71-77, 1991.
47. Chonmaitree T, Roberts NJ Jr, Douglas RG Jr, Hall CB, Simons RL: Interferon production by human mononuclear leukocytes: differences between respiratory syncytial virus and influenza viruses, *Infect Immunol* 32:300-303, 1981.
48. Krilov LR, Hendry RM, Godfrey E, McIntosh K: Respiratory virus infection of peripheral blood monocytes correlation with ageing of cells and interferon production in-vitro, *J Gen Virol* 68:1749-1753, 1987.
49. Isaacs D: Production of interferon in respiratory syncytial virus bronchiolitis, *Arch Dis Child* 64:92-95, 1989.
50. Taylor CE, Webb MS, Milner AD, Milner PD, Morgan LA, Scott R, Stokes GM, Swarbrick AS, Toms AL: Interferon alpha, infectious virus, virus antigen secretion in respiratory syncytial virus infections of graded severity, *Arch Dis Child* 64:1656-1660, 1989.
51. Nakayama T, Sonoda S, Urano T, Sasaki K, Maehara N, Makino S: Detection of alpha-interferon in nasopharyngeal secretions and sera in children infected with respiratory syncytial virus, *Pediatr Infect Dis J* 12:925-929, 1993.
52. Salkind AR, Nichols JE, Roberts N JJ: Suppressed expression of ICAM-1 and LFA-1 and abrogation of leukocyte collaboration after exposure of human mononuclear leukocytes to respiratory syncytial virus in vitro: comparison with exposure to influenza virus, *J Clin Invest* 88:501-511, 1991.
53. Hendricks DA, Baradaran K, McIntosh, Patterson JL: Appearance of a soluble form of the G protein of respiratory syncytial virus in fluids of infected cells, *J Gen Virol* 68:1750-1754, 1987.
54. Krilov LR, Anderson LJ, Marcoux L, Bonagura VR, Wedgwood JF: Antibody mediated enhancement of respiratory syncytial virus infection in two monocyte/macrophage cell lines, *J Infect Dis* 160:777-782, 1989.
55. Gimenez HB, Keir HM, Cash P: In-vitro enhancement of respiratory syncytial virus infection of U937 cells by human sera, *J Gen Virol* 70:89-96, 1989.
56. Osiowy C, Horne D, Anderson R: Antibody-dependent enhancement of respiratory syncytial virus infection by sera from young infants, *Clin Diag Lab Immunol* 6:670-677, 1994.
57. Preston M: Personal communication.
58. Fernald GW, Almond JR, Henderson F: Cellular and humoral immunity in recurrent respiratory syncytial virus infections, *Pediatr Res* 17:753-758, 1983.
59. Mills JV, Van Kirk JE, Wright PF, Chanock RM: Experimental respiratory syncytial virus infection of adults, *J Immunol* 107:123-130, 1971.
60. Ogilvie MM, Vathenen AS, Radford M, Codd J, Key S: Maternal antibody and respiratory syncytial virus infection in infancy, *J Med Virol* 7:263-271, 1981.
61. Ward KA, Lambden AR, Ogilvie MM, Watt PJ: Antibody to respiratory syncytial virus polypeptides and their significance in human infection, *J Gen Virol* 64:1867-1876, 1983.
62. Groothius JR, Simoes EA, Levin MJ, Hall CB, Long CE, Rodriquez WJ, Arrobio J, Meissner MC, Fulton DR, Welliver RC: Prophylactic administration of respiratory syncytial virus immune globulin to high-risk infants and young children, *N Engl J Med* 329:1524-1530, 1993.
63. McIntosh K: Respiratory syncytial virus: successful immunoprophylaxis at last, *N Engl J Med* 329:1572-1574, 1993.
64. Ellenberg SS, Epstein JS, Fratantoni JC, Scott D, Zoon KC: A trial of RSV immune globulin in infants and young children: the FDA's view, *N Engl J Med* 331:203-204, 1994.
65. Rimensberger PC, Schaad UB: Clinical experience with aerosolized immunoglobulin treatment of respiratory syncytial virus infection in infants, *Pediatr Infect Dis J* 13:328-330, 1994.
66. Siber GR, Leombruno D, Leszczynski J, McIver J, Bodkin D, Aonin R, Thompson CM, Walsh EE, Picdra PA, Hemming VA: Comparison of antibody concentrations and protective activity of respiratory syncytial virus immune globulin and conventional immune globulin, 169:1368-1373, 1994.
67. Taylor G, Stott EJ, Bew M, Bernie BF, Cote PJ: Monoclonal antibodies protect against respiratory syncytial virus, *Lancet* 2:976, 1983.
68. Fishaut M, Tubergen D, McIntosh K: Cellular response to respiratory viruses with particular reference to children with disorders of cell mediated immunity, *J Pediatr* 96:179-186, 1980.
69. Hall CB, Powell KR, MacDonald NE: Respiratory syncytial virus infection in children with compromised immune function, *N Engl J Med* 315:77-81, 1986.
70. Milner ME, de la Monte SM, Hutchins GM: Fatal respiratory syncytial virus infection in severe combined immunodeficiency syndrome, *Am J Dis Child* 139:1111-1114, 1985.
71. Cannon MJ, Openshaw PJ, Askonas BA: Cytotoxic T cells clear virus but augment living pathology in mice infected with respiratory syncytial virus, *J Exp Med* 168:1163-1169, 1988.
72. Hemming VG, Rodriquez W, Kim HW, Brandt CD, Parrott RH, Burch B, Prince GA, Baron PA, Fink RJ, Reaman G: Intravenous immunoglobulin treatment of respiratory syncytial virus infections in infants and young children, *Antimicrob Agents Chemother* 31:1882-1886, 1987.
73. Hemming VG, Prince GA, Horswood RL, London WJ, Murphy BR, Walsh EE, Fischer GW, Weisman LE, Baron PA, Chanock RM: Studies of passive immunotherapy for infections of respiratory syncytial virus in the respiratory tract of a primate model, *J Infect Dis* 12:1083-1087, 1985.
74. Levin MJ: Treatment and prevention options for respiratory syncytial virus infections, *J Pediatr* 124:S22-S27, 1994.
75. Crowe JE Jr, Murphy BR, Chanock RM, Williamson RA, Barbas CF, Burton DR: Recombinant human respiratory syncytial respiratory virus (RSV) monoclonal antibody Fab is effective therapeutically when introduced directly into the lungs of RSV infected mice, *Proc Natl Acad Sci USA* 91:1386-1390, 1994.
76. Turner RB: The role of neutrophils in the pathogenesis of rhinovirus infections, *Pediatr Infect Dis J* 9:832-835, 1990.
77. Everard ML, Swarbrick A, Wrightham M, McIntyre J, Dunkley C, James PD, Sewell HF, Milner AD: Analysis of cells obtained by bronchial lavage of infants with respiratory syncytial virus infection, *Arch Dis Child* 71:428-432, 1994.
78. Everard ML, Fox G, Walls AF, Quint D, Fifield R, Walters C, Swarbrick A, Milner AD: Tryptase and IgE concentrations in the respiratory tract of infants with acute bronchiolitis, *Arch Dis Child* 72:64-69, 1995.
79. Carr R, Pumford D, Davies JM: Neutrophil chemotaxis and adhesion in preterm babies, *Arch Dis Child* 72:64-69, 1992.
80. Dos Santos C, Davidson D: Neutrophil chemotaxis to leukotriene B4 is decreased in the human neonate, *Pediatr Res* 33:242-246, 1993.
81. Hall CB, Kopelman AE, Douglas RG Jr, Geiman JM, Meagher MP: Neonatal respiratory syncytial virus infections, *N Engl J Med* 300:393-396, 1979.
82. Neligan GA, Steiner H, Gardner PS, McQuillan J: Respiratory syncytial virus infection of the newborn, *Br Med J* 3:146-147, 1970.
83. Ahern W, Bird T, Court SDM, Gardner PS, McQuillan J: Pathological changes in virus infections of the lower respiratory tract in children, *J Clin Pathol* 23:7-18, 1970.
84. Becker S, Quay J, Soukup J: Cytokine (tumor necrosis factor, IL-6, IL-8) production by respiratory syncytial virusñinfected human alveolar macrophages, *J Immunol* 147:4307-4312, 1991.
85. Arnold R, Humbert B, Werchau H, Gallati H, Konig W: Interleukin-8, interleukin-6, soluble tumour necrosis factor receptor type 1 release from a human pulmonary epithelial cell line (A549) exposed to respiratory syncytial virus, *Immunology* 82:126-133, 1994.
86. Arnold R, Werner F, Humbert B, Werchau H, Konig W: Effect of respiratory syncytial virus–antibody complexes on cytokine (IL-8, IL-6, TFN-a) release and respiratory burst in human granulocytes, *Immunology* 82:184-191, 1994.

87. Volovitz B, Welliver RC, De Castro G, Krystofik DA, Ogra PL: The release of leukotrienes in the respiratory tract during infection with respiratory syncytial virus: role in obstructive airway disease, *Pediatr Res* 24:504-507, 1988.
88. Villani A, Cirino NM, Baldi E, Kester M, McFadden ER Jr, Panuska JR: Respiratory syncytial virus infection of human macrophages stimulates synthesis of platelet-activating factor, *J Biol Chem* 266:5472-5479, 1991.
89. Spigelberg HL: Biological activities of immunoglobulins of different classes and subclasses, *Adv Immunol* 19:259-294, 1974.
90. Naegel GP, Young KR, Reynolds HY: Receptors for human IgG subclasses on human alveolar macrophages, *Am Rev Respir Dis* 129:413-418, 1984.
91. Schur PH, Rosen F, Norman ME: IgG subclasses in normal children, *Pediatr Res* 13:181-183, 1979.
92. Hornsleth A, Bech-Thomsen N, Friis B: Detection by ELISA of IgG subclass–specific antibodies in primary respiratory syncytial virus infections, *J Med Virol* 16:321-328, 1985.
93. Hornsleth A, Beck Thomson N, Friis B: Detection of RS-virus IgG subclass specific antibodies: variations according to age in infants and small children and diagnostic value in RS virus infected small infants, *J Med Virol* 16:329-335, 1985.
94. Wagner DK, Graham BS, Wright PF, Walsh EE, Kim HW, Reimer CB, Nelson DL, Chanock RM, Murphy BR: Serum immunoglobulin G antibody subclass responses to respiratory syncytial virus F and G glycoproteins after primary infections, *J Clin Microbiol* 24:304-306, 1986.
95. Wagner DK, Nelson DL, Walsh EE, Reimer CB, Henderson FW, Murphy BR: Differential immunoglobulin G subclass antibody titers to respiratory syncytial virus F and G glycoproteins in adults, *J Clin Microbiol* 25:748-750, 1987.
96. Chanock RM, Kapikian AZ, Mills J, Kim HW, Parrott RH: Influence of immunological factors in respiratory syncytial virus disease of the lower respiratory tract, *Arch Environ Health* 21:347-355, 1970.
97. Kim HW, Canchola JG, Brandt CD, Pyles A, Chanock RM, Jensen K, Parrott RH: Respiratory syncytial virus disease in infants despite prior administration of antigenic inactivated vaccine, *Am J Epidemiol* 89:422-434, 1969.
98. Ana PP, Arrobio JO, Kim HW, Brandt CD, Chanock RM, Parrott RN: Serum complement in acute bronchiolitis: *Proc Soc Exp Biol Med* 134:499-503, 1970.
99. Kaul TN, Welliver RC, Faden HS: Respiratory syncytial virus (RSV) specific immune complexes in nasopharyngeal secretions after natural infection with RSV, *J Clin Lab Immunol* 15:187-190, 1984.
100. Smith TF, McIntosh K, Fishaut M, Henson PM: Activation of complement by cells infected with respiratory syncytial virus, *Infect Immunol* 33:43-48, 1981.
101. Edwards KM, Snyder PA, Wright PF: Complement activation by respiratory syncytial virus infected cells, *Arch Virol* 88:49-56, 1986.
102. Kaul TN, Welliver RC, Ogra PL: Appearance of complement components and immunoglobulins on nasopharyngeal epithelial cells following naturally acquired infection with respiratory syncytial virus, *J Med Virol* 9:149-158, 1982.
103. Gardner PS, McQuillin J, Court SDM: Speculation on pathogenesis in death from respiratory syncytial virus infections, *Br Med J* 1:327-330, 1970.
104. Brandt CD, Kim HW, Arrobio JO, Jettries BC, Wood SC, Chanock RM, Parrott RH: Epidemiology of respiratory syncytial virus infections in Washington DC. III. Composite analysis of eleven consecutive yearly epidemics, *Am J Epidemiol* 98:355-364, 1973.
105. Welliver RC, Kaul TN, Ogra PL: The appearance of cell-bound IgE in respiratory tract epithelium after respiratory syncytial virus infection, *N Engl J Med* 303:1198-1202, 1980.
106. Welliver RC, Wong DT, Sun M, Middleton E Jr, Vaughan RS, Ogra PL: The development of respiratory syncytial virus–specific IgE and the release of histamine in nasopharyngeal secretions after infection, *N Engl J Med* 305:841-846, 1981.
107. Welliver RC, Sun M, Rinaldo D, Ogra PL: Respiratory syncytial virus specific IgE responses following infection: evidence for a predominantly mucosal response, *Pediatr Res* 19:420-424, 1985.
108. Welliver RC, Sun M, Rinaldo D, Ogra PL: Predictive valve of respiratory syncytial virus–specific IgE responses for recurrent wheezing following bronchiolitis, *J Pediatr* 109:776-800, 1986.
109. Welliver RC, Sun M, Hildreth SW, Arumugham R, Ogra PL: Respiratory syncytial virus–specific antibody responses in immunoglobulin A and E isotypes to the F and G proteins and to intact virus after natural infection, *J Clin Microbiol* 27:295-299, 1989.
110. Welliver RC, Duffy L: The relationship of RV-specific immunoglobulin E antibody responses in infancy, recurrent wheezing, pulmonary function at age 7-8 years, *Pediatr Pulmonol* 15:19-27, 1993.
111. Sanchez-Legrand F, Smith TF: Interaction of paramyxoviruses with human basophils and their effect on histamine release, *J Allergy Clin Immunol* 84:538-546, 1989.
112. Toms GL, Scott R: Respiratory syncytial virus and the infant's immune response, *Arch Dis Child* 62:544-546, 1987.
113. Bui RHD, Molinaro GA, Kettering JD, Heiner DC, Imagawa DT, St Geme JWJ: Virus specific IgE and IgG4 antibodies in serum of children infected with respiratory syncytial virus, *J Pediatr* 110:87-90, 1987.
114. Sims DG, Downham MAPS, Gardner PS, Webb JK, Weightman D: Study of 8 year old children with a history of respiratory syncytial virus bronchiolitis in infancy, *Br Med J* 1:11-14, 1978.
115. Sims DG, Gardner PS, Weightman D, Turner MW, Soothill JF: Atopy does not predispose to RSV bronchiolitis or post bronchiolitic wheezing, *Br Med J* 282:2086-2088, 1981.
116. Carlsen KH, Larsen S, Bjerve O, Leegaard J: Acute bronchiolitis: predisposing factors and characterisation of infants at risk, *Pediatr Pulmonol* 3:153-160, 1987.
117. Kim HW, Leikin SL, Arrobio J, Brandt CD, Chanock RM, Parrott RH: Cell mediated immunity to respiratory syncytial virus induced by inactivated vaccine or by infection, *Pediatr Res* 10:75-78, 1976.
118. Bangham CRM, McMichael AJ: Specific human cytotoxic T cells recognize B-cell lines persistently infected with respiratory syncytial virus, *Proc Natl Acad Sci USA* 83:9183-9187, 1986.
119. Chiba Y, Higashidate Y, Suga K, Honjo K, Tsutsumi H, Ogra PL: Development of cell mediated cytotoxic immunity to respiratory syncytial virus in human infants following naturally acquired infection, *J Med Virol* 28:133-139, 1989.
120. Isaacs D, Bangham CRM, McMichael AJ: Cell mediated cytotoxic response to respiratory syncytial virus in infants with bronchiolitis, *Lancet* 2:769-771, 1987.
121. Issacs D, Taylor CJ, Ting A, McMichael AJ: HLA class 1 antigens in severe RSV bronchiolitis, *Tissue Antigens* 34:210-222, 1989.
122. Alwan WH, Record FM, Openshaw PJM: CD4+ T cells clear virus but augment disease in mice infected with respiratory syncytial virus: comparison with the effects of CD8+ cells, *Clin Exp Immunol* 88:527-536, 1992.
123. Connors M, Kulkarni AB, Firestone CY, Holmes KL, Morse HC, Sotnikov AV, Murphy BR: Pulmonary histopathology induced by respiratory syncytial virus challenge of formalin-inactivated RSV-immunized BALB/c mice is abrogated by depletion of CD4+ T cells, *J Virol* 66:7444-7451, 1992.
124. Oppenshaw PJM, O'Donnell DR: Asthma and the common cold: can viruses imitate worms? *Thorax* 49:101-103, 1994.
125. Alwan WH, Kozlowski WJ, Openshaw PJM: Distinct types of lung disease caused by functional subsets of antiviral T cells, *J Exp Med* 179:81-89, 1994.
126. Anderson LJ, Tsou C, Potter C, Keyserling HL, Smith TF, Ananaba G, Bangham CR: Cytokine response to respiratory syncytial stimulation of human peripheral blood mononuclear cells, *J Infect Dis* 170:1201-1208, 1994.
127. Domurat F, Roberts NJ, Walsh EE, Dagan R: Respiratory syncytial virus infection of human mononuclear leukocytes in-vitro and in-vivo, *J Infect Dis* 152:895-902, 1985.
128. Midulla F, Huang YT, Gilbert IA, Cirino NA, McFadden ER Jr, Panuska JR: Respiratory syncytial virus infection of human cord and adult blood monocytes and alveolar macrophages, *Am Rev Respir Dis* 140:771-777, 1989.
129. Roberts NJ: Different effects of influenza virus, respiratory syncytial virus and Sendai virus on human lymphocytes and macrophages, *Infect Immunol* 35:1142-1146, 1982.
130. McIntosh K: Interferon in nasal secretions from infants with viral respiratory tract infections, *J Pediatr* 93:33-36, 1987.
131. Taylor S, Bryson YJ: Impaired production of IFN-γ by newborn cells in-vitro is due to a functionally immature macrophage, *J Immunol* 134:1493-1497, 1985.

132. Wakasugi N, Virilezier J-L, Arenzana-Seisdedos F, Rothhut B, Heserta JM, Russo-marie F, Fiers W: Defective IFN-g production in the human neonate: role of increased sensitivity to prostaglandin E, *J Immunol* 134:172-176, 1985.
133. Wilson CB, Westall J, Johnston L, Lewis DB, Dower SK, Alpert AR: Decreased production of IFN-γ by human neonatal cells: intrinsic and regulatory deficiencies, *J Clin Invest* 77:860-867, 1986.
134 Prior C, Haslam PL: Interferon in lungs, *Lancet* 2:1333, 1989.
135. Gardner PS, McGuchin R, Beale AJ, Fernandes R: Interferon and respiratory syncytial virus, *Lancet* 1:574-575, 1970.
136. Piazza FM, Johnson SA, Ottolini MG, Schmidt HJ, Darnell ME, Hemming VG, Prince GA: Immunotherapy of respiratory syncytial virus infection in cotton rats *(Sigmodon fulviventer)* using IgG in a small-particle aerosol, *J Infect Dis* 166:1422-1424, 1992.
137. Sharma R, Woldehiwet Z: Bovine respiratory syncytial virus: a review, *Vet Bull* 61:1117-1131, 1991.
138. Kimman TG, Straver PJ, Zimmer GM: Pathogenesis of naturally acquired bovine respiratory syncytial virus in calves: morphological and serologic findings, *Am J Vet Res* 50:684-693, 1989.
139. Kimman TG, Terpstra GK, Daha MR, Westenbrink F: Pathogenesis of naturally acquired bovine respiratory syncytial virus in calves: evidence for the involvement of complement and mast cell mediators, *Am J Vet Res* 50:694-700, 1989.
140. Stewart RS, Gershwin LJ: Detection of IgE antibodies to bovine respiratory syncytial virus, *Vet Immunol Immunopathol* 20:313-323, 1989.

Acute RSV Bronchiolitis

141. Young S, O'Keeffe PT, Arnott J, Landau LI: Infant lung function airway responsiveness, atopic status and respiratory symptoms before and after bronchiolitis, *Arch Dis Child* 72:16-24, 1995.
142. Chonmaitree T, Bessette-Henderson BJ, Hepler RE, Lucia HL: Comparison of three rapid diagnostic techniques for detection of respiratory syncytial virus from nasal wash specimens, *J Clin Microbiol* 25:746-747, 1987.
143. Hughes JH, Mann DR, Hamparian VV: Detection of respiratory syncytial virus in clinical specimens by viral culture, direct and indirect immunofluorescence and enzyme immunoassay, *J Clin Microbiol* 26:588-591, 1988.
144. Krilov LR, Lipson SM, Barone SR, Kaplan MM, Ciamician Z, Harkness SH: Evaluation of a rapid diagnostic test for respiratory syncytial virus (RSV): potential for bedside diagnosis, *Pediatrics* 93:903-906, 1994.
145. Balfour-Lynn IM, Girdhar DR, Aitken C: Diagnosing respiratory syncytial virus by nasal lavage, *Arch Dis Child* 72:58-59, 1995.
146. Lebel MH, Gauthier M, Lacroix J, Rousseau E, Buithiev M: Respiratory failure and mechanical ventilation in severe bronchiolitis, *Arch Dis Child* 64:1431-1437, 1989.
147. American Academy of Pediatrics: Use of ribavirin in the treatment of respiratory syncytial virus infection, *Pediatrics* 92:501-504, 1993.
148. Stretton M, Ajizian SJ, Mitchell I, Newth CJ: Intensive care course and outcome of patients infected with respiratory syncytial virus, *Pediatr Pulmonol* 13:143-150, 1992.
149. Bruhn FW, Mokrolisky MD, McIntosh K: Apnoea associated with respiratory syncytial virus infection in young infants, *J Pediatr* 90:382-386, 1977.
150. Downham MAPS, Gardner PS, McQuillan J, Ferris JA: Role of respiratory viruses in childhood mortality, *Br Med J* 1:235-239, 1975.
151. Williams AL, Uren EC, Bretherton L: Respiratory viruses and sudden infant death, *Br Med J* 299:1491-1493, 1984.
152. Anderson LJ, Parker RA, Strikas RL: Association between respiratory syncytial virus outbreaks and lower respiratory tract deaths of infants and young children, *J Infect Dis* 161:640-646, 1990.
153. Anas N: The association of apnea and respiratory syncytial virus infections in infants, *J Pediatr* 101:65-68, 1982.
154. Hall CB, Hall WJ, Speers DM: Clinical and physiological manifestations of bronchiolitis and pneumonia, *Am J Dis Child* 133:798-802, 1979.
155. Wang EL, Milner RA, Navas L, Maj H: Observer agreement for respiratory signs and oximetry in infants hospitalized with respiratory infections, *Am Rev Respir Dis* 145:106-109, 1992.
156. Shaw KN, Bell LM, Sherman NH: Outpatient assessment of infants with bronchiolitis, *Am J Dis Child* 145:151-155, 1991.
157. Mulholland EK, Olinski A, Shann FA: Clinical findings and severity of acute bronchiolitis, *Lancet* 335:1259-1261, 1990.
158. Simpson W, Hacking PM, Court SDM, Gardner PS: The radiological findings in respiratory syncytial virus infection in children. II. Correlation of radiological categories with clinical and virological findings, *Pediatr Radiol* 2:155-160, 1974.
159. Dawson KP, Long A, Kennedy J, Mogridge N: The chest radiograph in acute bronchiolitis, *J Paediatr Child Health* 26:209-211, 1990.
160. Friis B, Andersen P, Brenoe E, Hornsleth A, Jensen A, Knudsen FU, Krassilnikov PA, Mordhoust CH, Nielsen S, Uldall P: Antibiotic treatment of pneumonia and bronchiolitis, *Arch Dis Child* 59:1038-1045, 1984.
161. Hall CB, Powell KR, Schnabel K, Gala CL, Pincus PH: The risk of secondary bacterial infection in infants hospitalised with respiratory syncytial virus infection, *J Paediatr* 113:266-271, 1988.
162. van Steensel-Moll HA, Hazelzet JA, van der Voort E, Neijens HJ, Hackeng WH: Excessive secretion of antidiuretic hormone in infections with respiratory syncytial virus, *Arch Dis Child* 65:1237-1239, 1990.
163. Wack RP, Demers DM, Bass JW: Immature neutrophils in the peripheral blood smear of children with viral infections, *Pediatr Infect Dis J* 13:228-230, 1994.
164. MacDonald NE, Hall CB, Suttin SC, Alexson C, Harris PJ, Manning JA: Respiratory syncytial viral infection in infants with congenital heart disease, *N Engl J Med* 307:397-400, 1982.
165. Moler FW, Khan AS, Meliones JN, Custer JR, Palmisano J, Shope TC: Respiratory syncytial virus morbidity and mortality in congenital heart disease patients: a recent experience, *Crit Care Med* 10:1406-1413, 1992.
166. Pullen CR, Hey EN: Wheezing, asthma and pulmonary dysfunction 10 years after infection with respiratory syncytial virus in infancy, *Br Med J* 284:1665-1669, 1982.
167. Carlsen KH, Larsen S, Orstavik I: Acute bronchiolitis: the relationship to later recurrent obstructive airways disease, *Eur J Respir Dis* 70:86-92, 1987.
168. Murray M, Webb MS, O'Callaghan C, Swarbrick AS, Milner AD: Respiratory status and allergy after bronchiolitis, *Arch Dis Child* 67:482-487, 1992.
169. Reynolds EOR, Cook CD: The treatment of bronchiolitis, *J Pediatr* 63:1205-1207, 1963.
170. Reynolds EOR: Arterial blood gas tensions in acute disease of lower respiratory tract in infancy, *Br Med J* 1:1192-1195, 1963.
171. Sporik R: Why block a small hole? *Arch Dis Child* 71:393-394, 1994.
172. Milner AD: Why block a small a small hole? *Arch Dis Child* 71:394, 1994 (commentary).
173. Fernandez H, Banks G, Smith R: Ribavirin: a clinical overview, *Eur J Epidemiol* 2:1-14, 1986.
174. Patterson JL, Fernandez-Larsson R: Molecular mechanisms of action of ribavirin, *Rev Infect Dis* 12:1139-1146, 1990.
175. Englund JA, Piedra PA, Ahn Y-M, Gilbert DC, Hiatt P: High-dose, short-duration ribavirin aerosol therapy compared with standard ribavirin therapy in children with suspected respiratory syncytial virus infection, *J Pediatr* 125:635-641, 1994.
176. Outwater KM, Meissner C, Peterson MB: Ribavirin administration to infants receiving mechanical ventilation, *Am Dis Child* 142:512-515, 1988.
177. Janai HK, Marks MI, Zaleska RN, Stutman HR: Ribavirin: adverse drug reactions, 1986-1988, *Pediatr Infect Dis J* 9:209-211, 1990.
178. Fackler JC, Flannery K, Zipkin M, McIntosh K: Precautions in the use of ribavirin at the Children's Hospital, *N Engl J Med* 322:634, 1990.
179. Infectious Diseases and Immunization Committee, Canadian Paediatric Society: Ribavirin: is there a risk to hospital personnel? *Can Med Assoc J* 144:285-286, 1991.
180. Conrad DA, Christenson JC, Waner JL, Marks MI, Aerosolized ribavirin treatment of respiratory syncytial virus infection in infants hospitalized during an epidemic, *Pediatr Infect Dis* J 6:152-158, 1987.
181. Wald ER, Dashefsky B, Green M: In re ribavirin: a case of premature adjudication? *J Pediatr* 112:154-158, 1988.
182. Issacs D, Moxon ER, Harvey D, Kovar I, Madeley CR, Richardson RJ, Levin M, Whitelaw A, Modi N: Ribavirin in respiratory syncytial virus infection: a double blind placebo controlled trial is needed, *Arch Dis Child* 63:986-990, 1988.
183. Ray CG: Ribavirin: ambivalence about an antiviral agent, *Am J Dis Child* 142:488-489, 1988.

184. American Academy of Pediatrics Committee on Infectious Disease: Ribavirin therapy of respiratory syncytial virus, *Pediatrics* 79:475-478, 1987.
185. Wald ER, Dashefsky B: Ribavirin: Red Book Committee recommendations questioned, *Pediatrics* 93:672-673, 1994.
186. Issac D: Bronchiolitis, *Br Med J* 310:4-5, 1995.
187. Groothuis JR, Woodin KA, Katz R, Robertson AD, McBride TT, Hall CB, McWilliams BC, Lauer BA: Early ribavirin treatment of respiratory syncytial viral infection in high-risk children, *J Pediatr* 117:792-798, 1990.
188. Smith DW, Frankel LR, Mathers LH, Tang AT, Ariagno RL, Prober CG: A controlled trial of aerosol ribavirin in infants receiving mechanical ventilation, *N Engl J Med* 325:24-29, 1991.
189. Meert KL, Sarnaik AP, Gelmini MJ, Lieh Lai MW: Aerosolised ribavirin in mechanically ventilated children with respiratory syncytial virus lower respiratory tract disease: a prospective double blind trial, *Crit Care Med* 22:566-571, 1994.
190. Krafte-Jacobs B, Holbrook PR: Ribavirin in severe respiratory syncytial virus infection, *Crit Care Med* 22:541-543, 1994.
191. Outwater KM, Crone RK: Management of respiratory failure in infants with acute viral bronchiolitis, *Am J Dis Child* 138:1071-1075, 1984.
192. Frankel LR, Lewiston NJ, Smith DW, Stevenson DK: Clinical observations on mechanical ventilation for respiratory failure in bronchiolitis, *Pediatr Pulmonol* 2:307-311, 1986.
193. Rakshi K, Couriel JM: Personal practice: management of acute bronchiolitis, *Arch Dis Child* 71:463-469, 1994.
194. Tuxen DV: Permissive hypercapnic ventilation, *Am Rev Respir Dis* 150:870-874, 1994.
195. Smith PJ, Khatib MF, Carlo W: PEEP does not improve pulmonary mechanics in infants with bronchiolitis, *Am Rev Respir Dis* 147:1295-1298, 1993.
196. Bachmann DCG, Pfenninger J: Respiratory syncytial virus triggered adult respiratory distress syndrome in adults: a report of two cases, *Intensive Care Med* 20:61-63, 1994.
197. Samuels M: Personal communication.
198. Steinhorn RH, Green TP: Use of extracorporeal membrane oxygenation in the treatment of respiratory syncytial virus bronchiolitis: the national experience, 1983-88, *J Pediatr* 116:337-342, 1990.
199. Thompson MW, Bates JN, Klein JM: Treatment of respiratory failure in an infant with bronchopulmonary dysplasia infected with respiratory syncytial virus using inhaled nitric oxide and high frequency ventilation, *Acta Paediatr* 84:100-102, 1995.
200. Tristram DA, Miller RW, McMillan JA, Weiner LB: Simultaneous infection with respiratory syncytial virus and other respiratory pathogens, *Am J Dis Child* 142:834-836, 1988.
201. Ray CG, Minnich LL, Holberg CJ, Shehab ZM, Wright AL, Barton LL, Taussig LM: Respiratory syncytial virus–associated lower respiratory illness: possible influences of other agents, *Pediatr Infect Dis J* 12:15-19, 1993.
202. Milner AD, Murray M: Acute bronchiolitis in infancy: treatment and prognosis, *Thorax* 44:1-5, 1989.
203. Archivist: Salbutamol in bronchiolitis, *Arch Dis Child* 66:1183, 1991.
204. Goodman RT, Chambers TL: Bronchodilators for bronchiolitis? *Lancet* 341:1380, 1993.
205. Phelan PD, Williams HE: Sympathomimetic drugs in acute viral bronchiolitis: their effect on pulmonary resistance, *Paediatrics* 44:493-497, 1969.
206. Rutter N, Milner AD, Hiller EJ: Effect of bronchodilators on respiratory resistance in infants and young children with bronchiolitis and wheezy bronchitis, *Arch Dis Child* 50:719-722, 1975.
207. Sly PD, Lanteri CJ, Raven JM: Do wheezy infants recovering from bronchiolitis respond to inhaled salbutamol? *Pediatr Pulmonol* 10:36-39, 1991.
208. Wang EEL, Milner R, Allen U, Maj H: Bronchodilators for treatment of mild bronchiolitis: a factorial randomised trial, *Arch Dis Child* 67:289-293, 1992.
209. Ho L, Collis G, Landau LI, Le Souëf PN: Effect of salbutamol on oxygen saturation in bronchiolitis, *Arch Dis Child* 66:1061-1064, 1991.
210. Hughes DM, Le Souëf PN, Landau LI: Effect of salbutamol on respiratory mechanics in bronchiolitis, *Pediatr Res* 22:83-86, 1987.
211. Brooks LJ, Cropp GJA: Theophylline therapy in bronchiolitis: a retrospective study, *Am J Dis Child* 135:934-936, 1981.
212. Schena JA, Crone RK, Thompson JE: Theophylline therapy in bronchiolitis, *Crit Care Med* 12:225, 1984.
213. Henry RL, Milner AD, Stokes GM: Ineffectiveness of ipratropium bromide in acute bronchiolitis, *Arch Dis Child* 58:925-926, 1983.
214. Newcombe RW: Use of adrenergic bronchodilators by paediatric allergists and pulmonologists, *Am J Dis Child* 143:481-485, 1989.
215. Sanchez I, De Koster J, Powell RE, Wolstein R, Chernick V: Effect of racemic epinephrine and salbutamol on clinical score and pulmonary mechanics with bronchiolitis, *J Pediatr* 122:145-151, 1993.
216. Schuh S, Canny G, Reisman JJ, Kerem E, Bentur L, Petric M, Levison H: Nebulized albuterol in acute bronchiolitis, *J Pediatr* 117:663-667, 1990.
217. Alario AJ, Leweander WJ, Dennehy P, Seifer R, Mansell AL: The efficacy of nebulised metaproterenol in wheezing infants and young children, *Am J Dis Child* 146:412-418, 1992.
218. Klassen TP, Rowe PC, Sutcliffe T, Ropp LJ, McDowell IW, Li MM: Randomized trial of salbutamol in acute bronchiolitis, *J Pediatr* 118:807-811, 1991.
219. Schweich PJ, Hurt TL, Walkley EI, Mullen N, Archibald CF: The use of nebulized albuterol in wheezing infants, *Pediatr Emerg Care* 8:184-188, 1992.
220. Gadomski AM, Lichenstein R, Horton L, King J, Kenne V, Peranutt T: Efficacy of albuterol in the management of bronchiolitis, *Pediatrics* 93:907-912, 1994.
221. Connolly JH, Field CM, Glasgow JF, Slattery CM, MacLynn DM: A double blind trial of prednisolone in epidemic bronchiolitis due to respiratory syncytial virus, *Acta Paediatr Scand* 58:116, 1969.
222. Leer JA, Green JL, Hemlich EM, et al: Corticosteroid treatment in bronchiolitis: a controlled collaborative study in 272 infants and children, *Am J Dis Child* 117:495-503, 1969.
223. Committee on Drugs: Should steroids be used in treating bronchiolitis? *Pediatrics* 46:640-642, 1970.
224. Springer C, Bar-Yishay E, Uwayyed K, Avital A, Nilozni D, Godfrey S: Corticosteroids do not affect the clinical or physiological status of infants with bronchiolitis, *Pediatr Pulmonol* 9: 181-185, 1990.
225. Sammartino L, Rasiah S, Wale L, Lines D: Budesonide in acute bronchiolitis, *J Paediatr Child Health* 31:61-62, 1995.
226. Webb MSC, Martin GA, Cartlidge PHJ, Ng YK, Wright NA: Chest physiotherapy in acute bronchiolitis, *Arch Dis Child* 60:1078-1079, 1985.
227. Levin MJ: Treatment and prevention options for respiratory syncytial virus infections, *J Pediatr* 124:S22-S27, 1994.
228. Portnoy J, Hicks R, Pacheco F, Olson L: Pilot study of recombinant interferon alpha-2a for treatment of infants with bronchiolitis induced by respiratory syncytial virus, *Antimicrob Agents Chemother* 32:589-591, 1988.
229. Chipps BE, Sullivan WF, Portnoy JM: Alpha 2A interferon for treatment of bronchiolitis caused by respiratory syncytial virus, *Pediatr Infect Dis J* 12:653-658, 1993.
230. Gardner PS, Court SDM, Brocklebank JT, Downham MA, Weightman D: Virus cross infection in paediatric wards, *Br Med J* 2:571-575, 1973.
231. Hall CB, Douglas RG Jr, Geiman JM, Messner MK: Nosocomial respiratory syncytial virus infections, *N Engl J Med* 293:1343-1346, 1975.
232. Hall CB, Douglas RG Jr: Modes of transmission of respiratory syncytial virus, *J Pediatr* 99:100-103, 1981.
233. Issacs D, Dickson H, O'Callaghan CA, Sheaves R, Winter A, Moxon ER: Hand washing and cohorting in prevention of hospital acquired infections with respiratory syncytial virus, *Arch Dis Child* 66:227-231, 1991.
234. O'Callaghan CA: Prevention of nosocomial respiratory syncytial virus infection, *Lancet* 341:182, 1993.
235. Hall CB, Geiman JM, Douglas RG Jr, Meagher MP: Control of nosocomial respiratory syncytial viral infections, *Pediatrics* 62:728-731, 1978.
236. Gala CL, Hall CB, Schnabel KC, Pincus PH, Blossom P, Hildreth SW, Betts RF, Douglas RG Jr: The use of eye-nose goggles to control nosocomial respiratory syncytial virus infection, *JAMA* 256:2706-2708, 1986.
237. Leclair JM, Freeman J, Sullivan BF, Crowley CM, Goldmann DA: Prevention of nosocomial respiratory syncytial virus infections through compliance with glove and gown isolation precautions, *N Engl J Med* 317:329-334, 1987.
238. Agah R, Cherry JD, Garakian AJ, Chapin M: Respiratory syncytial virus (RSV) infection rate in personnel caring for children with RSV infections, *Am J Dis Child* 141:695-697, 1987.

239. Madge P, Paton JY, McColl JH, Mackic PL: Prospective controlled study of four infection-control procedures to prevent nosocomial infection with respiratory syncytial virus, *Lancet* 340:1079-1083, 1992.
240. Kapikian AZ, Mitchell RH, Chanock RM, Shvedott RA, Stewart CE: An epidemiologic study of altered clinical reactivity to respiratory syncytial virus infection in children previously vaccinated with an inactivated RS virus vaccine, *Am J Epidemiol* 89:405-421, 1969.
241. Kim HW, Canchola JG, Brandt CD, Pyles G, Chanock RM, Jensen K, Parrott RH: Respiratory syncytial virus disease in infants despite prior administration of antigenic inactivated vaccine, *Am J Epidemiol* 89: 422-434, 1969.
242. Prince GA, Jenson AB, Hemming VG, Murphy BR, Walsh EE, Horswood RL, Chanock RM: Enhancement of respiratory syncytial virus pulmonary pathology in cotton rats by intramuscular inoculation of formation inactivated virus, *J Virol* 57:721-728, 1986.
243. Murphy BR: Dissociation between serum neutralising and glycoprotein antibody responses of infants and children who received inactivated respiratory syncytial virus vaccine, *J Clin Microbiol* 24:197-202, 1986.
244. Murphy BR, Hall SL, Kulkarni AB, Crowe JE Jr, Collins PL, Connors M, Karron RA, Chanock RM: An update on approaches to the development of respiratory syncytial virus and parainfluenza virus vaccines, *Virus Res* 32:13-36, 1994.
245. Toms GL: Respiratory syncytial virus: how soon will we have a vaccine? *Arch Dis Child* 72:1-5, 1995.
246. Paradiso PR, Hildreth SW, Hogerman DA, Speelman DJ, Lewin EB, Oren J, Smith DH: Safety and immunogenicity of a subunit respiratory syncytial virus vaccine in children 24 to 48 months old, *Pediatr Infect Dis J* 13:792-798, 1994.
247. Tristam DA, Welliver RC, Hogerman DA, Hildreth SW, Paradiso P: Second-year surveillance of recipients of a respiratory syncytial (RSV) F protein subunit vaccine, PFP-1: evaluation of antibody persistence and possible disease enhancement, *Vaccine* 12:551-556, 1994.
248. Englund JA: Passive protection against respiratory syncytial virus disease in infants: the role of maternal antibody, *Pediatr Infect Dis J* 13:449-453, 1994.
249. Everard ML, Milner AD: Respiratory syncytial virus and its role in acute bronchiolitis, *Eur J Pediatr* 151:638-651, 1992.
250. American Academy of Pediatrics: Respiratory syncytial virus immune globulin intravenous infusion: indications for use, *Pediatrics* 99:645-650, 1997.

CHAPTER 39

Bacterial Pneumonia in Neonates and Older Children

Melanie A. Miller, Tamar Ben-Ami, and Robert S. Daum

GENERAL ASPECTS OF BACTERIAL PNEUMONIA

History

The importance of pneumonia has been known at least since the time of Hippocrates, who described *peripneumony* as an acute, febrile illness characterized by unilateral or bilateral pain, painful breathing, cough, scanty "high-colored" urine, and improvement usually by about the seventh day. It was not until around 200 AD, however, that Aretaeus provided a clinical description of this syndrome. In the early 1700s, De Konilfeld offered the first distinction between pleurisy and pneumonia. Later, in 1728, Boerhaave distinguished lobar pneumonia from other syndromes. After the introduction of percussion by Auenbrugger in 1761, Laennec described the signs and symptoms of pleurisy and pneumonia in 1819 and detailed the histopathologic changes for the first time. In 1837, Seiffert introduced the term *bronchopneumonia,* and in 1850, Barthez and Rilliet called attention to the fact that this syndrome also occurred in children.

The modern era of clinical observation regarding pneumonia began in 1880 when Sternberg recognized *Pneumococcus* organisms in the saliva of healthy adults and continued in 1881 with Pasteur's observation of *Pneumococcus* organisms in the saliva of a child with pneumonia. However, not until 1884 did Fraenkel suggest that the organism found by Sternberg and Pasteur (known as the *coccus of sputum septicemia*) was the most common cause of pneumonia. In the early twentieth century, the term *Captain of the Men of Death* was applied to bacterial pneumonia in recognition of its high mortality rate, the term having originally been coined by Bunyan in reference to tuberculosis.[1]

The authors would like to thank the Blowitz-Ridgeway Foundation for its support, Jennifer Scott for her editorial advice, and Abigail Daum for her loss of quality time while this chapter was written.

Epidemiology

Acute childhood respiratory infections are responsible for 4.5 million deaths each year, 70% of which are caused by pneumonia.[2] Results from several studies in the United States indicate that children younger than 5 years of age have an incidence rate of three to four lower respiratory tract infections per 100 children per year.[3,4] Overall, the highest rates have been documented in young children; there has been a gradual decline in the rates in older children, a trend continuing until adolescence.[5,6] Most mortality occurs in developing countries, where a child younger than 5 years of age dies every 7 seconds of an acute respiratory infection. In other words, about 18% to 33% of deaths in children in developing countries are the result of acute respiratory tract infections, mainly pneumonia. Even in developed countries, however, childhood pneumonia is an important cause of morbidity and remains an important reason for the hospitalization of young children.[7,8]

Thus lower respiratory tract infections, particularly pneumonia, constitute a major health problem both in the United States and throughout the world. Bacterial pneumonias make up only a small number of lower respiratory tract infections but have the highest mortality rates. For example, the fatality rates for pneumonia caused by *Streptococcus pneumoniae* and *Haemophilus influenzae* have been more than 50 times higher than those for viral pneumonia. Overall, the mortality rate from bacterial pneumonia is 2.7 times higher than that from presumed viral pneumonia.[2,9]

Several factors have been associated with an increased incidence or an increased severity of pneumonia, particularly in developing countries.[10] These include young age, increasing birth order, low birth weight,[11,12] young maternal age, limited parental education,[2] day-care attendance, exposure to passive tobacco smoke,[13] industrial pollution,[14] urban residence,[15] previous history of pneumonia, chronic heart and lung disease, male gender,[4] and asthma.

In addition, malnutrition has been identified as a risk factor for the incidence and severity of pneumonia. The results of one study found that although the incidence of respiratory infections was similar in nourished and malnourished Costa Rican children, the likelihood of pneumonia was 12 times higher in the malnourished group.[16] A possible explanation for this predisposition is vitamin A deficiency.[17] However, data conflict on this point.[18]

Environmental factors may also affect the incidence of pneumonia. For example, up to 30% of urban households in developing countries use biomass fuels, such as wood, agricultural waste, and manure for cooking and heating, and although a resulting increase in bacterial pneumonia has not been documented,[2] their use has the potential to disrupt physiologic protective mechanisms of the lung. Household crowding may also be a risk factor, presumably because it facilitates the spread of droplets containing relevant pathogens.[2,19]

Many pathogens that cause bacterial pneumonia, such as *S. pneumoniae, H. influenzae* type b, and *Staphylococcus aureus,* are transmitted from person to person by the spread of contaminated droplets during breathing, coughing, or sneezing. Contaminated water and aerosol have been implicated in the spread of some pathogenic bacteria, such as *Legionella pneumophila.* In hospitals and other health care facilities, contaminated equipment used for respiratory support may be involved in outbreaks of nosocomial pneumonia caused by pathogens such as *Klebsiella pneumoniae* or *Pseudomonas aeruginosa.* Some pathogens associated with bacterial pneumonia in children, such as *Francisella tularensis* and *Yersinia pestis,* are zoonoses, animal pathogens that occasionally infect humans.

On contact with a pathogenic organism, many individuals become asymptomatic carriers, whereas others become ill, some in a very short time. Similarly, the time of communicability of the offending pathogen after antibacterial therapy has been initiated is uncertain; this is probably pathogen specific and aided by case-specific clinical features, such as the presence of cough. Many experts consider that communicability is greatly decreased 24 hours after the initiation of therapy, although few explicit data support this view.

Cases of bacterial pneumonia are sporadic and may occur any time throughout the year. However, the results of several studies indicate a peak incidence in winter, which may extend into early spring.[5] This seasonal distribution may partly reflect an association between bacterial pneumonia and certain preceding viral illnesses. In support of this, an increase in the incidence of bacterial pneumonia has been documented during some viral epidemics. For example, *S. aureus* pneumonia has been associated with influenza epidemics.

Epidemics of community-acquired bacterial pneumonia are relatively unusual. In nosocomial settings, such as intensive care units or nurseries, outbreaks of pneumonia caused by *K. pneumoniae,*[20,21] *P. aeruginosa,*[22] and other microorganisms have been described. Typically, the spread of the organism in these settings has implicated contaminated health care delivery materials or local environmental contaminations.

Relatively few causes of bacterial pneumonia in children are preventable by the current universal vaccination programs. An exception is *H. influenzae* type b infection, in which immunization practices in the United States have decreased all invasive infections, including pneumonia, by more than 95%. Currently, several conjugate vaccines designed to prevent *S. pneumoniae* infections are under evaluation; these have the potential for a major impact on the occurrence of bacterial pneumonia in both developed and developing countries.

Certain underlying conditions render a host more susceptible to bacterial pneumonia[23,24] (Box 39-1). These may be divided into those likely to produce pneumonia in a single region of the lung and those likely to produce diffuse or multifocal pneumonia.

Etiology

The etiology of any pneumonia (Box 39-2), including that caused by bacteria, differs according to age of the patient, the clinical setting in which the pneumonia was acquired (e.g., community vs. hospital), relevant local epidemiology (e.g., annual respiratory syncytial virus epidemics and influenza activity), the vaccination status of the child (e.g., *H. influenzae* type b), relevant exposures (e.g., to contaminated water or infected animals), host factors (e.g., the presence of underlying diseases that predispose to pneumonia), and immunologic status. Even with all relevant clinical information, determining the etiology of uncomplicated pneumonia is difficult and infrequently attempted in practice; with the exception of blood cultures, culture material suitable for definitive diagnosis requires invasive procedures not justifiable for mild to moderately ill children. Thus in most cases, the precise etiology is never determined, and the therapeutic approach to the patient is based on generalizations regarding etiology in the relevant clinical setting.[4,25,26] This is particularly true for community-acquired pneumonias, many of which are self-limited diseases for which no specific therapy is available or needed.

In the neonate, the most common causes of bacterial pneumonia are the group B β-hemolytic streptococci (GBS) and gram-negative enteric bacilli, such as *Escherichia coli* and *K. pneumoniae,* the same organisms that cause bacteremia and sepsis. Less frequent etiologic agents include *S. aureus, P. aeruginosa, H. influenzae* (often not serotype b), *Serratia marcescens,* and *Flavobacterium* species.

In children past the neonatal period, viruses are the most frequent etiologic agents, although a viral and bacterial etiology may occur concomitantly.[27-29] In addition, *Chlamydia trachomatis* is an important pathogen in infants who are 3 to 19 weeks of age. Among the bacterial etiologies, *S. pneumoniae* is most frequent.[28,30,31] *H. influenzae* type b was an important cause in the prevaccination era but is now rare. *S. aureus* pneumonia is also infrequent but requires special consideration because it may rapidly progress and because the usual antimicrobial therapy may not provide optimal coverage against this pathogen. Group A β-hemolytic streptococci are an uncommon cause of pneumonia, and their necrotizing nature may prolong its course. In children who chronically aspirate, anaerobic bacteria are important pathogens implicated in pulmonary infections,[32] whereas other bacteria have rarely been implicated as etiologic agents of pneumonia.[31]

BOX 39-1
Conditions Predisposing to Bacterial Pneumonia

Abnormalities usually resulting in pneumonia in a single lung region

- Abnormalities within the airway lumen
  - Foreign body
  - Bronchial tumor
    - Adenomas
    - Mucoepithelial dysplasia
    - Lipoma
    - Papilloma
  - Broncholithiasis
- Abnormalities producing external compression of the airway
  - Lymphadenopathy associated with infections
    - Tuberculosis
    - Histoplasmosis
    - Coccidioidomycosis
    - Blastomycosis
    - Other conditions
  - Lymphadenopathy associated with tumors
  - Structural abnormalities that cause decreased mucus clearance
    - Tracheal bronchus
    - Bronchial stenosis or atresia
    - Localized bronchiectasis
  - Right middle lobe syndrome associated with asthma
  - Bronchogenic cyst
  - Pulmonary sequestration syndrome

Abnormalities usually resulting in pneumonia in one or more contiguous lung regions

- Microaspiration
  - Impaired swallowing
    - Cranial nerve injury
    - Drug-induced injury
    - Seizures
    - Cricopharyngeal incoordination
      - Maturational incoordination
      - Familial dysautonomia
      - Myasthenia gravis
      - Sydenham's chorea
      - Multiple sclerosis
    - Neuromuscular disorders
      - Idiopathic cricopharyngeal
      - Achalasia
      - Myotonic dystrophy

- Microaspiration—cont'd
    - Neuromuscular disorders—cont'd
      - Muscular dystrophy
      - Other conditions
  - Laryngeal cleft
  - Submucosal cleft
  - Obstructive lesions of the tongue or larynx
  - Esophageal obstruction or dysmotility
    - Vascular rings
    - Mediastinal cysts
    - Enteric duplications
    - Esophageal web
    - Esophageal stricture
    - Achalasia
    - Tracheoesophageal fistula before and after repair
  - Gastroesophageal reflux
- Asthma
- Immunodeficiency syndromes
  - Severe combined immunodeficiencies
  - Immunoglobulin deficiencies
  - Wiskott-Aldrich syndrome
  - Ataxia-telangiectasia
  - DiGeorge syndrome
  - Immunodeficiency secondary to other diseases or cytotoxic treatment
  - Complement deficiencies
  - Phagocyte defects
- Acquired immunodeficiency syndrome (AIDS)
- Mucociliary dysfunction
  - Cystic fibrosis
  - Ciliary dyskinesias
  - Tracheobronchomegaly
  - Cartilage deficiency
  - Williams-Campbell syndrome
- Segmental bronchomalacia
- Congenital heart disease
- Bronchopulmonary dysplasia
- Pneumotaxic gases, drugs, and radiation
- Miscellaneous
  - Sickle cell disease
  - Alveolar proteinosis
  - Langerhans' cell histiocytosis
  - Idiopathic pulmonary fibrosis

BOX 39-2
Bacterial Etiology of Pneumonia in Children

Causes of frequent clinical concern

S. pneumoniae
Group B streptococci*
*Escherichia coli**

Causes of occasional clinical concern

S. aureus
Group A streptococci
Anaerobic organisms
H. influenzae†
*K. pneumoniae**

Causes of rare clinical concern

Acinetobacter species
Actinomycosis species
Arcanobacterium haemolyticum
Bacillus anthracis
Bacillus cereus
Bordetella henselae
Bordetella pertussis‡
Brucellosis species
Citrobacter species

Causes of rare clinical concern–cont'd

Coxiella burnetii
Enterobacteriaceae
F. tularensis
Kingella kingae
L. pneumophila
Leptospira interrogans
Listeria monocytogenes
Moraxella catarrhalis
Neisseria meningitidis
Nocardia species
Non–group A and non–group B streptococci
Pasteurella multocida
Proteus species
P. aeruginosa
Pseudomonas cepacia
Pseudomonas pseudomallei
Streptobacillus moniliformis
Salmonella species
Serratia marcescens
Yersinia enterocolitica
Y. pestis

*Designations of *frequent* or *occasional* apply to pneumonia in the neonatal period.
†*H. influenzae* type b vaccine has greatly decreased the number of cases of childhood bacterial pneumonia caused by *H. influenzae*.
‡Pertussis is discussed in Chapter 42.

Viruses are also the most common etiologic agents in school-age children and adolescents, with many of the same considerations as those for preschoolers. For example, *S. pneumoniae* remains the most frequent cause of pneumonia, and *H. influenzae* type b was believed to be less frequent in the prevaccination era. *Mycoplasma pneumoniae* is another important consideration among children in this age group.

In hospital-acquired pneumonia, consideration of the possible etiology requires knowledge of the institution-specific epidemiology of nosocomial infections.[33] Most published data defining the etiology of nosocomially acquired bacterial pneumonia have been gathered from adult populations, and it is likely that the etiologies in children are similar.[34] Gram-negative organisms, such as *K. pneumoniae* and *Pseudomonas* and *Serratia* species, and gram-positive organisms, such as *S. aureus,* appear most frequently. Water-associated organisms, such as *Acinetobacter* and *Flavobacterium* species, are occasionally implicated as well. Nosocomially acquired *Legionella* pneumonia is rare in pediatric populations[35] and has been linked to contaminated aerosols, typically from the water supply or air-conditioning cooling towers.[36]

In developing countries, the bacterial agents frequently responsible for community-acquired pneumonia are not unlike those causing similar disease in developed countries.[2,37] Exceptions include the important role ascribed to nontypeable and non-type b *H. influenzae* isolates in Papua New Guinea, Gambia, and Pakistan[2] as well as an observation of uncertain importance regarding the serologic diagnosis of putative *Moraxella catarrhalis* infection in children with pneumonia in Gambia.[38,39]

Pathophysiology

Most bacterial pneumonia results from inhalation of contaminated air. Bacteria, including pulmonary pathogens, can be found in ambient air, droplets transmitted from person to person, and pharyngeal secretions that may contain up to 10^8 bacteria per milliliter of saliva. Bacteria may gain access to the respiratory tract by inhalation or microaspiration, events occurring daily even in normal children.[40] Whether pneumonia is the result of such bacterial entry depends on the outcome of interactions between the bacterium and the host's respiratory defense system (Fig. 39-1).

Droplet size plays a major role in determining the level of the respiratory system reached by inhaled bacteria. Most inhaled bacteria are enveloped in moisture and therefore acquire aerodynamic and dimensional characteristics that determine their destination. For example, particles larger than 10 μ do not usually traverse the pharynx, whereas those 3 to 10 μ may lodge in the larger airways, and those 0.5 to 3 μ can reach the alveolar surface.[41]

Certain medical interventions or anatomic abnormalities can facilitate bacterial transit toward the alveolus. Examples include tracheostomy, endotracheal intubation, and respiratory therapy. Similarly, direct extension to the pulmonary

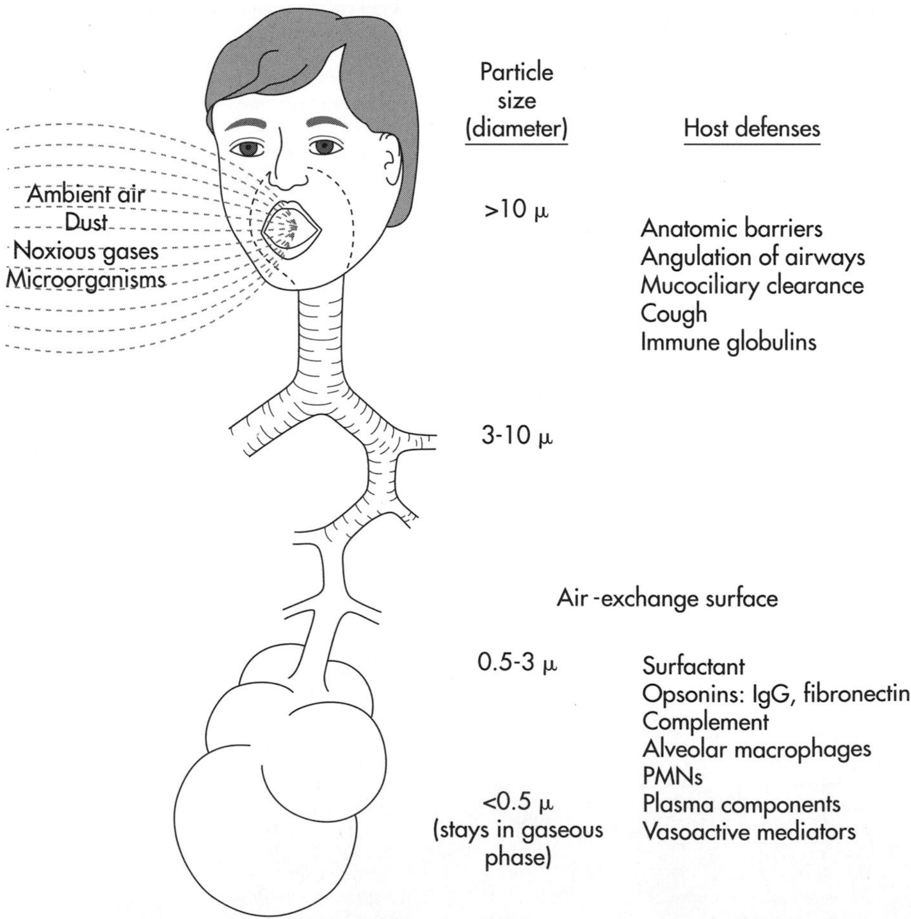

Fig. 39-1. Lung defense system. *IgG,* Immunoglobulin G; *PMNs,* polymorphonuclear neutrophil leukocytes.

parenchyma through a bronchopleural fistula also facilitates bacterial access to the alveolar epithelial surfaces.[42] Bacteria may also reach the lungs via metastatic hematogenous spread from a distant site. It is not known how frequently pneumonia results from such hematogenous seeding of the lung.

Because the usual interaction between bacteria and host has a favorable outcome for the host that effectively limits bacterial access to the lowest regions of the respiratory tract, it is generally believed that the respiratory tract below the major bronchi is sterile or nearly so. However, when a bacterium does gain access to the alveolus, additional host defense mechanisms are called into action. The bacterium makes initial contact with the alveolar wall and is enmeshed in the epithelial lining fluid that contains opsonins and depending on the immunologic experience of the host, specific immunoglobulin G (IgG) antibody. The usual outcome of this interaction is ingestion by alveolar macrophages (alveolar type II cells); an alternative, less common outcome is complement-mediated bacterial lysis. The former mechanism is especially important in dealing with encapsulated bacteria such as *S. pneumoniae.* The process is rapid; in an animal exposed to a bacterial inoculum, whether aerosolized or instilled onto the alveolar surface, bacteria remain free for only 30 minutes before being internalized by a macrophage.[43,44]

When these mechanisms do not destroy alveolar bacteria, polymorphonuclear leukocytes with their phagocytic capability are recruited, and an inflammatory response, presumably mediated by cytokine release, occurs. If continued, this process results in pneumonia with attendant vascular congestion and exuberant edema and has been best characterized for pneumonia caused by pneumococci. In this instance, sheets of pneumococci ride waves of edematous fluid from alveolus to alveolus through the pores of Kohn. This edematous zone of engorgement progresses centrifugally and leaves central areas of erythrocytes and purulent exudate consisting of fibrin, polymorphonuclear leukocytes, and bacteria. This stage is histologically termed *red hepatization.* The pneumococcal cell wall is probably the bacterial component that initiates these events.[45] Pneumococci do not produce a known toxin, and it is thought that bacterial growth and the exudative response to their presence cause consolidation.[45]

The next stage in pathogenesis is termed *grey hepatization.* Events characterizing this stage include the active phagocytosis of pneumococci by polymorphonuclear leukocytes. The release of bacterial cell wall components and pneumolysin by enzymatic degradation leads to increased inflammation and cytotoxic effects on all pulmonary cells. The result is the blurring of cellular elements and the loss of cellular architecture.

Resolution of pneumonic consolidation begins when anticapsular antibody appears and polymorphonuclear leukocytes continue to phagocytose the pneumococci; monocytic cells clean up the debris. The term *zone of resolution* is sometimes applied to such an area.

As long as the reticular structure of the lung remains intact (i.e., involvement of the interstitium is absent), complete parenchymal restoration and healing of the alveolar epithelium occur after successful treatment. Scarring is minimal.[45,46]

Death from bacterial pneumonia is due to respiratory failure, which occurs when the airspaces are filled with edematous fluid or exudate. The residual volume of the lung is markedly expanded by this fluid, which precludes air exchange at the alveolar level. The clinical picture of sepsis may be concomitant; shock may further complicate end-organ perfusion, and a mixed metabolic and respiratory acidosis therefore typically precedes death.[46]

The pathogenesis of other bacteria may vary. For example, tissue necrosis and rapid bacterial spread throughout the alveolar spaces characterize pneumonia caused by *S. aureus* and make full recovery less likely when extensive necrosis occurs.

Clinical Manifestations

In children who are no longer neonates and who have acute pneumonia, no reliable clinical symptoms or signs distinguish the pneumonia caused by bacteria from that caused by other infectious agents. Children with bacterial pneumonia are more likely to appear ill, anxious, or distressed; have a higher incidence of and more severe fever; and have physical signs attributable to respiratory tract infection. However, there is sufficient overlap in the clinical picture to recommend caution in inferring etiology. For bacterial pneumonia of any etiology, cough is usual but not invariable. Sputum production by children younger than about 8 years of age is rare because any sputum produced is swallowed. Abdominal pain and emesis are variable complaints and may be sufficiently severe to misdirect the diagnostic evaluation toward an acute abdominal condition.

Signs localized to the respiratory tract may provide important clues to the diagnosis. Audible expiratory noise or grunting may be present in young children or infants. Cyanosis and hypoxia, flaring of the alae nasi, subcostal and intercostal retractions, and nonspecific signs of dyspnea may also be present. Shallow breathing (splinting) and tachypnea (≥50 to 60 breaths/min in children younger than 12 months of age and ≥40 breaths/min in older children) suggest pneumonia. Pain during respiration, often called *pleuritic pain,* may be present, as may pain appearing to originate from an abdominal process. On auscultation, crackles, evidence of pulmonary consolidation (i.e., decreased breath sounds), bronchophony, increased fremitus, and dullness to percussion are often present. A friction rub suggests pleuritis, a common concomitant condition of bacterial pneumonia.

In the neonate, the clinical picture of bacterial pneumonia may resemble that found in the older child. However, apnea and signs suggestive of a generalized sepsis may be the dominant clinical features. Auscultation of the chest may produce normal results; fever and cough are usually absent.

Diagnosis

Recently formulated guidelines for the diagnosis of pediatric pneumonia were summarized by a group of Canadian pediatricians.[47] Most patients who are no longer neonates and who have bacterial pneumonia have symptoms and signs suggesting an abnormality of the respiratory system; in their absence, bacterial pneumonia is an unlikely diagnostic consideration. An exception may be some children with very high temperature (≥41.1° C) who may have radiographic evidence of pneumonia in the absence of findings attributable to respiratory system infection.[48] In developing countries, where sophisticated diagnostic tools may not be available, it has been suggested by the World Health Organization that tachypnea with indrawing of the respiratory muscles should alert the clinician to a presumptive diagnosis of pneumonia. Although the reliability of this superficial approach is obviously less than optimal, respiratory rates higher than 50 and 40 breaths/min have been used as diagnostic criteria in children younger than 12 months and between 13 months and 5 years of age, respectively,[49-53] particularly when more sophisticated tests are unavailable.

Once a determination is made that pneumonia is likely, defining its etiology poses a clinical challenge. Indeed, for many children with pneumonia, particularly when it is community acquired and mild, clinicians often take an empirical approach and perform little more than a blood culture in the way of investigation. Occasionally, there is no investigation at all; this approach is justified because the procedure required to obtain a specimen is invasive and examination of the specimen is unlikely to accurately provide the etiology. A result of this clinical dilemma is that more than 80% of patients who have "nonbacterial" pneumonia may receive antimicrobial therapy.[54]

In cases of suspected bacterial pneumonia in which precise microbiologic diagnosis is deemed clinically important, a variety of techniques are available to sample respiratory secretions at various levels of the respiratory tract. Many of these procedures use instrumentation, such as a bronchoscope or another suction device, that traverses the pharynx or upper airway.[55] Generally, the easier the specimen is to obtain, the less likely it is useful in providing diagnostic help.

Moffet[56] has divided acute pneumonia culture sources in children into the following categories: conclusive, occasionally conclusive, and dubious. Examples of conclusive culture sources include blood, pleural fluid, and material obtained by open lung biopsy or lung puncture. Occasionally conclusive sources include cultures obtained at bronchoscopy, cultures of tracheostomy secretions, and in older children, cultures of fluid obtained by transtracheal aspiration. Cultures of dubious importance for bacterial pneumonia include nasotracheal aspirates and throat cultures. Potential pathogens may be present as flora at these sites, which may create ambiguity in interpretation. For example, the leading cause of bacterial pneumonia, *S. pneumoniae,* may colonize the nasopharynx in up to 40% of healthy children in the winter.[54]

Therefore the clinician must consider which various diagnostic tests should be used in the evaluation of a patient in whom bacterial pneumonia is likely. Consideration is given as to how the microorganisms obtained from a given site may reflect the theoretic gold standard, the etiologic bacterium in the infected lung.[57]

In a patient presumed to have pneumonia, isolation of a bacterium from the blood,[58] pleural fluid, or lung tissue is considered etiologic. However, bacteremia occurs in only 3% to 12% of cases[54] of presumed bacterial pneumonia, and at least 1 day is required to obtain results from tests. Because phlebotomy is relatively noninvasive and inexpensive, a blood culture is recommended for routine performance when the clinician is evaluating children for possible bacterial pneumonia. When pleural fluid is present, whether ascertained by physical examination or radiography of the chest, sampling it (e.g., by ultrasound-guided needle aspiration) provides a valuable specimen for Gram's staining and culture. Depending on the clinical situation, culture for *Mycobacteria* species, fungi, or bacteria requiring special media may also be relevant. Additional studies commonly performed in the evaluation of such pleural effusions include a leukocyte count (including cytologic analysis when relevant) and measurement of the pH, protein, glucose, and lactate dehydrogenase concentrations. Attempted detection of relevant bacterial antigens (e.g., by latex agglutination) is sometimes performed. In practice, diagnostic pleurocentesis is performed in patients sufficiently ill to require hospitalization for putative bacterial pneumonia, in patients who nosocomially acquire presumed bacterial pneumonia (particularly during a course of antiinfective therapy), or in patients with presumed bacterial pneumonia and pleural effusion who do not respond to initial, empirically chosen therapy.

In children, the examination of sputum by Gram's stain and culture is limited by the difficulty obtaining a satisfactory specimen, especially in children younger than 8 years of age. The quality of the specimen can be interpreted by the paucity of epithelial cells. Material that is produced by cough and that contains excess squamous rather than epithelial cells testifies to an upper tract origin. Clinical laboratories generally do not process specimens submitted as "sputum" with more than 25 squamous cells per low-power field on microscopic examination. Other useful parameters are the presence of polymorphonuclear leukocytes and a monotonous or the relatively monotonous morphologic picture of the bacteria in the specimen. (Upper respiratory tract flora consist of bacteria of diverse morphologic structure.)

Even if a satisfactory specimen can be obtained, its usefulness in the diagnosis of bacterial pneumonia is questionable. Although once considered helpful in defining the etiology, it is now widely accepted that the diagnosis made from organisms recovered from sputum correlates poorly with that made from organisms recovered from more reliable sites, such as blood or pleural fluid, because of contamination of the sputum by the flora in the upper respiratory tract. In adults, these secretions may contain 10^8 to 10^9 bacteria per milliliter. Nevertheless, in the presence of many polymorphonuclear leukocytes and bacteria of a single morphology, Gram's stain and culture of properly collected sputum may provide useful information regarding the etiology of bacterial pneumonia.[59] Identification of acid-fast bacilli or fungi by examination of sputum provides valuable diagnostic information because such microbes are infrequent constituents of the normal flora.

A variety of clinical situations require a more aggressive approach for defining the etiology of a putative bacterial pneumonia. Examples include acute pneumonia when a patient is severely ill or has respiratory failure, the condition fails to respond to therapy, the condition worsens despite initial empiric antimicrobial therapy, or it occurs in a patient with compromised immunologic integrity. In these instances, determining the etiology may be necessary so that more precise therapy can be prescribed and the toxicity of unnecessary agents can be avoided.

Bronchoscopic techniques are sometimes used in the diagnosis of bacterial pneumonia, particularly when there is local expertise in performing the procedure and when the child is sufficiently stable to allow the 1- to 2-day delay required for specimen handling, should the study prove noncontributory. Bronchoalveolar lavage (BAL) fluid obtained during bronchoscopy should be submitted to the appropriate laboratories for histopathologic and microbiologic evaluation. Interpretation of the BAL data is limited by the nonspecificity of the inflammatory cell present (even in large quantities) and the uncertainty regarding the importance of bacteria and yeast present in the specimen, which may represent airway flora or organisms infecting the lung. Aubas et al[60] suggested that two indexes, the simplified bacterial index and the predominant species index obtained from quantitative BAL fluid cultures, were useful in defining the presence and etiology of bacterial pneumonia in adults. However, these indexes are not widely used, and the observations have not yet been extended to children.

To solve the problem of airway contamination, clinicians have used devices such as a protected catheter brush or a telescope-plugged catheter. Cultures obtained by the brush technique correlated well with the isolate obtained from blood in a small number of bacteremic adults with pneumonia.[61] However, the telescope-plugged catheter does not add much to the results obtained from lavage.[62] Few assessments of these bronchoscopy-based techniques have been performed in children, but the available data in adults suggest that quantitative BAL bacterial culture may help in the accurate diagnosis of bacterial pneumonia, particularly when a single or limited number of bacterial species is present in excess of 10^3 colony-forming units per milliliter.

Transtracheal aspirations are generally not performed in young children because of the high rate of complications, particularly in small infants, uncooperative children, and children with bleeding diatheses, severe coughing, severe hypoxemia, and dyspnea. It is uncertain whether the procedure is useful in the accurate diagnosis of bacterial pneumonia. The correlation with organisms obtained by lung puncture[63] is only fair. Lung puncture should be done only by an experienced person.[64]

Obtaining lung tissue for culture can be accomplished by percutaneous lung puncture,[63] transthoracic needle aspiration biopsy (TNAB),[65] or open lung biopsy.[66] These procedures are normally considered in an immunocompromised host and in patients with severe pneumonia, particularly when the condition is nosocomially acquired or when empiric therapy has not produced a clinical response. They are more likely to yield important information regarding etiology when performed early in the clinical course. Percutaneous lung puncture and TNAB are usually performed under radiologic guidance.[65] In both procedures, the pleural space is aspirated to detect an inapparent effusion before entry of the parenchyma proper. The clinician may choose not to continue into the parenchyma when pleural fluid is encountered, reasoning that the pleural fluid may provide sufficient opportunity to recover the pathogen without the increased morbidity of the lung puncture itself. Important complications of these two procedures are hemoptysis and pneumothorax.[64] TNAB has the advantage of providing a core of tissue for histologic examination when a large-bore needle is used, although the results may occasionally be misleading.[67] Dorca et al[65] compared the results of TNAB performed with an ultrathin needle to other microbiologic and serologic criteria frequently used in the diagnosis of nosocomial pneumonia in adults. TNAB results were specific and had a high positive predictive value in this population. However, the relatively low sensitivity (60.9%) and low negative predictive value precluded reliance on this single diagnostic modality.[65]

Open lung biopsy is often considered the gold standard but requires general anesthesia and a skilled support staff. It is usually performed when a variety of microbiologic diagnoses are being considered but seldom performed when bacterial pneumonia is the most likely consideration. Pneumothorax may complicate the postoperative recovery and prolong the ventilator-dependent recovery phase.

A variety of nonspecific laboratory evaluations have been used to support the likelihood of bacterial pneumonia; these include an increased serum concentration of C-reactive protein, an increased erythrocyte sedimentation rate, and an increased blood leukocyte count with a predominance of polymorphonuclear leukocytes.[54] However, all these techniques suffer from poor sensitivity and positive predictive value.[30,68,69]

Bacterial antigen detection in blood and urine has a limited role in the diagnosis of bacterial pneumonia. Several available techniques include counterimmunoelectrophoresis, latex particle agglutination, and staphylococcal coagglutination; the last two are more widely used. Only a limited number of bacterial antigens theoretically useful for the diagnosis of bacterial pneumonia (e.g., *S. pneumoniae, H. influenzae* type b, *N. meningitidis,* group B streptococci) can be detected by commercially available methods; however, false-positive and false-negative results are frequent.[28,30,54,70,71] Furthermore, the meaning of *antigenemia* or *antigenuria* may be difficult to interpret because the patient may have an infection such as pneumonia, be an asymptomatic carrier of an organism such as a pneumococcus, or be colonized by a "cross-reacting" microorganism, such as *S. pneumoniae* type 14, which cross reacts with *H. influenzae* type b. Bacterial antigen detection in other relevant body fluids, such as a pleural effusion, may be useful but has received limited evaluation.

The serologic diagnosis of bacterial pneumonia has received little attention. Reasons include the delayed time frame inherent in the process of gathering sera and performing assays, the paucity of bacterial agents for which reliable antibody assays are available, and the immature immune response often present at the time of infection (e.g., with *H. influenzae* type b) that results in a modest or absent antibody response to infection. Investigators from Finland claimed success in diagnosing pneumonia by performing enzyme immunoassays on "convalescent" sera (obtained as early as 5 days after hospitalization) to detect antibodies directed against *S. pneumoniae* (pneumolysin), *H. influenzae* type b (whole cell), *M. catarrhalis* (whole cell), and *M. pneumoniae* (whole cell).[69] For the reasons already noted, it seems unlikely that this approach will become a widely available, clinically useful tool.

Highly sensitive techniques that detect bacterial nucleic acid sequences, such as in situ hybridization, polymerase chain reaction (PCR), and ligation-mediated PCR, have shown some promise in determining the etiology of bacterial pneumonia. Their value will likely be limited when performed on specimens such as sputum, in which discrimination between a colonizing and an infecting isolate has proved problematic. However, PCR may be a useful diagnostic tool when performed on a normally sterile fluid, such as blood or pleural fluid. For example, streptococcal sequences from an autolysin gene called *lyt* were found in the blood of patients with presumed pneumococcal pneumonia in Gambia.[72] Perhaps the greatest promise of these techniques lies in the relatively rapid diagnosis of infections caused by *Chlamydia, Mycoplasma,* and *Mycobacteria* species; *Bordetella pertussis;* and a variety of viruses. In many of these instances, PCR may be useful on specimens obtained from airway secretions because these microorganisms are not typically among the denizens of the respiratory tract and culturing them requires extra effort and time.

Many patients require evaluation for a variety of pathogens not amenable to detection by standard culture techniques. For example, evaluation of a patient, particularly when severely ill or immunocompromised, includes tests for important viral pathogens. It is important to remember that multiple pathogens may be responsible for pneumonia in a given instance (e.g., when influenza is complicated by bacterial pneumonia). In addition, evaluation of a patient with pneumonia may involve an

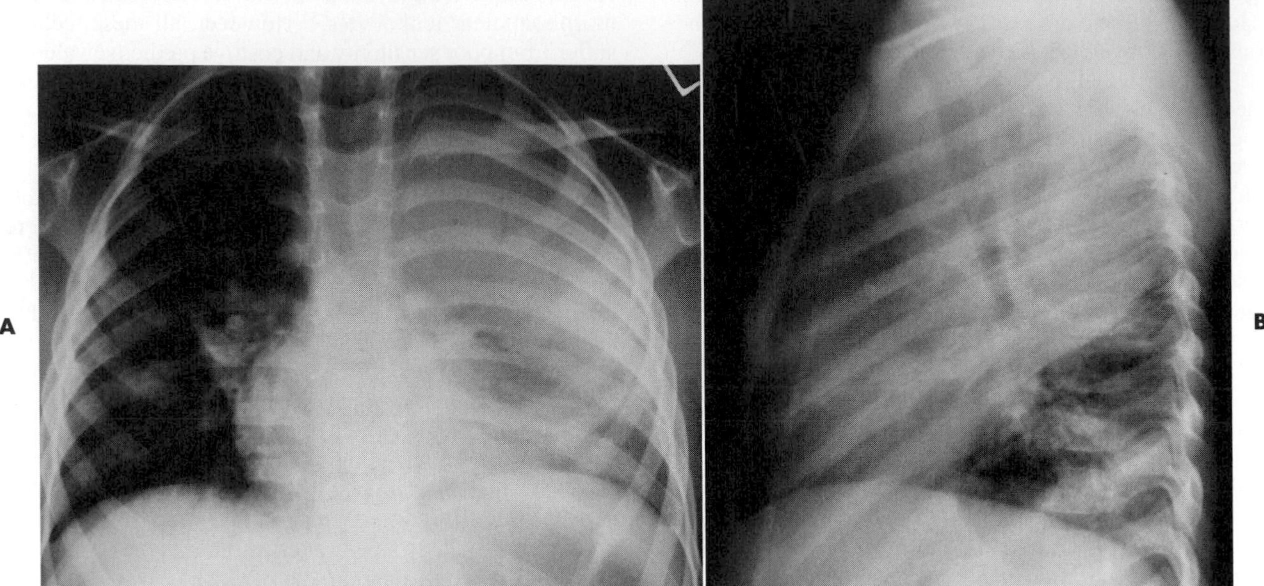

Fig. 39-2. Bulging fissure in a 3-year-old boy with group A streptococcal pneumonia. The chest radiograph demonstrates consolidation in the left upper lobe with expansion of the lobe. The increased volume is manifested as a larger-than-expected infiltrate in the anteroposterior view **(A)** and posterior bulging of the upper portion of the oblique fissure on the lateral view **(B).** Sonography of the same patient on the same day demonstrates areas of early cavitation.

etiologic search for fungi, *Pneumocystis carinii,* mycobacteria, and *Chlamydia* and *Mycoplasma* species.

Imaging Modalities

In the absence of respiratory signs, the recognition of clinically undetected pneumonia by radiography in otherwise healthy young children is unlikely[73]; thus the use of a radiograph as a screening tool should generally be avoided and carefully individualized. In older children, a chest radiograph is usually not indicated in the absence of respiratory signs except as part of an evaluation for prolonged, unexplained fever.

Interpretation of a chest radiograph is seldom performed without clinical data regarding the patient's illness. Even experienced radiologists are biased by this clinical information and incorporate it into an assessment of the radiograph.[74] Indeed, the rate of pneumonia diagnosed when radiologists were aware of the clinical impression was higher than that when radiologist were unaware of the clinical data.[74] Thus despite a tendency to accord a gold standard to the chest radiograph, this potential for "overcall" bias should be borne in mind. Conversely, a negative radiograph does not exclude the diagnosis of bacterial pneumonia, particularly when the illness has been of short duration.

Despite these concerns, the radiograph of the chest remains an important diagnostic tool in the evaluation of a child for bacterial pneumonia.[75] The frontal posteroanterior upright chest view is generally preferred to an anteroposterior view to minimize the cardiac shadow, except in the young child in whom there is no difference in the cardiothoracic ratio between the two positions.[76] In this instance, an anteroposterior supine film is preferred because of the increased likelihood of better inspiration and ease of immobilization. It has been suggested that the frontal posteroanterior chest view (anteroposterior in young children) may often suffice for initial radiographic evaluation. However, the possibility that pneumonia may "hide" behind the dome of the diaphragm or the cardiac silhouette has resulted in the lateral film being routinely obtained at the initial evaluation.

Radiographic findings in children with pneumonia are traditionally divided into interstitial and alveolar/airspace patterns. Bacterial pneumonias are usually alveolar/airspace processes, and interstitial patterns usually reflect other etiologies; however, there is substantial overlap as well as the possibility that one pattern may progress to the other with ongoing disease.[54] Highly suggestive of bacterial pneumonia are a large lobar or diffuse consolidation, a bulging fissure (Fig. 39-2) implying extensive exudate or occult abscess in a lobar pneumonia, and associated pleural effusion[54] in the setting of a clinical pneumonia. Such pleural effusions may occur in about 20%, 40%, and 60% to 80% of children with pneumonia caused by *S. pneumoniae, H. influenzae* type b, and *S. aureus,* respectively.

Swischuk and Hayden[77] suggested that several radiologic patterns help differentiate among possible etiologies of an infective pulmonary infiltrate. A so-called lobar consolidation, whether homogeneous or fluffy, suggests a bacterial or *M. pneumoniae* pneumonia. A diffuse, bilateral, fluffy infiltrate extending into the periphery suggests a bacterial process, whereas a central peribronchial infiltrate with or without atelectasis suggests a viral or *Mycoplasma* infection. A peribronchial infiltrate with peripheral consolidation suggests a viral process but is not inconsistent with a superimposed bacterial infection; a reticulonodular infiltrate restricted to one lobe suggests *Mycoplasma* pneumonia.[77] Although these criteria are helpful in distinguishing bacterial from viral and mycoplasmal pneumonia, the etiology cannot be inferred solely from the chest radiograph because substantial overlap in the observed pattern exists.[54,78-80]

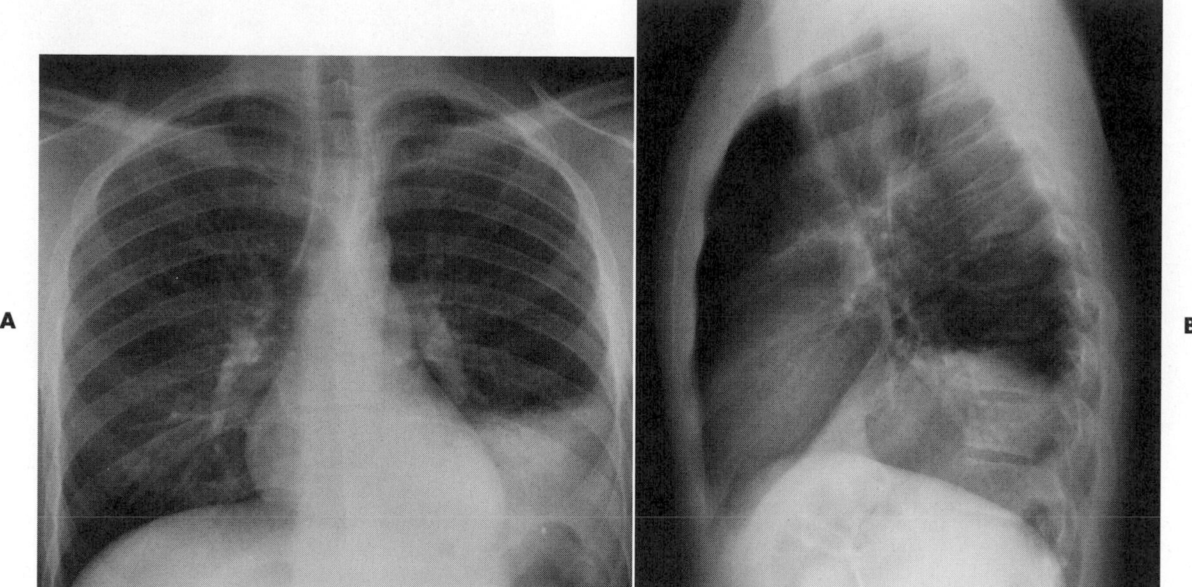

Fig. 39-3. Alveolar pneumonia in the left lower lobe in a 16-year-old boy with fever, chest pain, and cough. Posteroanterior (**A**) and lateral (**B**) radiographs demonstrate the typical characteristics of an alveolar process involving the left lower lobe. The infiltrate stands out against the preserved left cardiac silhouette in the posteroanterior projection. (It is posterior to the heart.) It silhouettes the diaphragm in both the posteroanterior and lateral views.

Bacterial pneumonia is commonly manifested radiographically as an alveolar consolidation whose pattern corresponds to its pathologic characteristics. The basic radiographic unit of the alveolar consolidation is the acinar shadow, which corresponds to a secondary pulmonary lobule in which the air is replaced by fluid. It is 2 to 5 mm in size with an ill-defined margin caused by extension of the exudate into adjacent acini via the canals of Lambert and pores of Kohn. When confluent, acinar nodules produce the typical continuous, homogeneous alveolar infiltrate. The borders are unclear at the interface with uninvolved lung; however, the margins are sharp at the interface with pleural surfaces, such as interlobar fissures. When an alveolar process abuts an adjacent organ (e.g., the heart, another mediastinal structure, the diaphragm), the loss of definition of the margin is called the *silhouette sign* (Fig. 39-3). The larger bronchi frequently remain aerated when the surrounding pulmonary lobules are consolidated. Those bronchi stand out against the opaque background, producing an air bronchogram (Fig. 39-4).

Alveolar consolidative pneumonias have been subclassified into two groups—airspace pneumonia and bronchopneumonia—according to the pattern of distribution of the infiltrate at diagnosis; however, the distinction between them may blur if the process becomes more extensive. Airspace pneumonia is acquired by the inhalation of small particles and starts in the peripheral parenchyma. Typical examples are *S. pneumoniae, Legionella,* and *K. pneumoniae* pneumonia. Consolidation spreads concentrically because of the production of exudate and typically results in a spherical infiltrate (so-called *round pneumonia* [Fig. 39-5]), the most common "mass" lesion of the lung in children. In most patients, this kind of infiltrate has a single focus; however, multiple or bilateral foci also occur, particularly in children with predisposition to pneumococcal infection, such as patients with sickle cell disease. The round

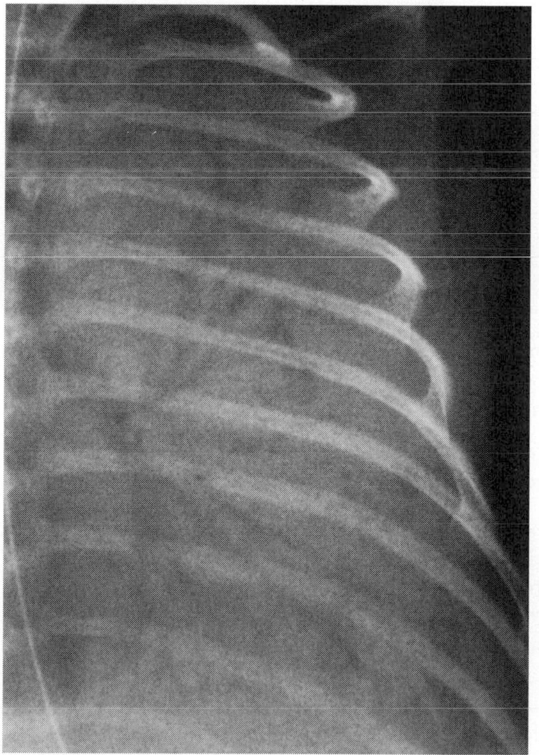

Fig. 39-4. Air bronchogram. The air-filled bronchial tree stands out against the background of consolidated lung. Fatal staphylococcal pneumonia in a 1-month-old infant. Rapid evolution of complete pulmonary consolidation within a few hours caused the entire bronchial tree to be visible on this plain radiograph of the left hemithorax.

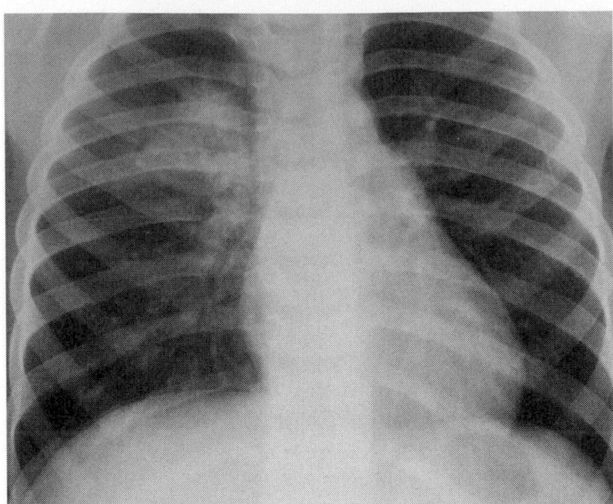

Fig. 39-5. *S. pneumoniae* pneumonia in a 6-year-old boy. A round, masslike infiltrate is present in the right upper lobe. It disappeared at follow-up after treatment.

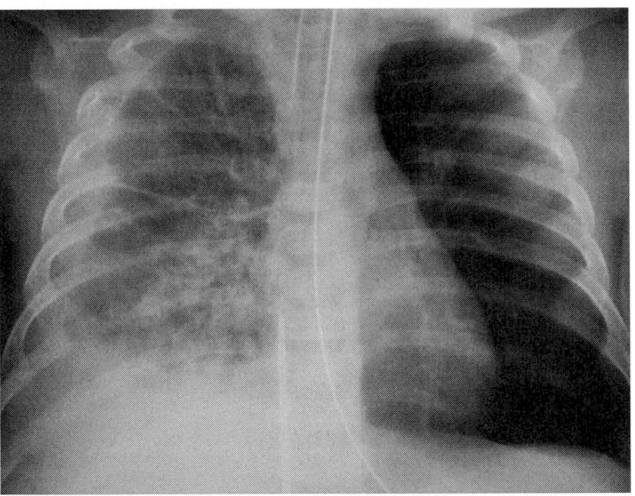

Fig. 39-6. Bronchopneumonia. In this 3-month-old girl, *S. pneumoniae* pneumonia evolves as a typical bronchopneumonia with multiple central patches of segmental and confluent alveolar infiltrates accompanied by a parapneumonic pleural effusion.

configuration may rapidly change to form a more extensive alveolar infiltrate.

Bronchopneumonia (Fig. 39-6) is acquired by the aspiration of larger infective particles and therefore tends to start adjacent to centrally located bronchi. The multiple central segmental infiltrates that are typically produced may become confluent and diffuse. This behavior is typical of pneumonia caused by *S. aureus, Streptococcus pyogenes, H. influenzae,* and enteric gram-negative bacilli. Pathogens associated with bronchopneumonia are more commonly associated with lung necrosis, cavitation, pneumatoceles, and abscesses than those producing airspace pneumonia.

Certain situations (e.g., complete opacification of a hemithorax, differentiation of pleural and parenchymal components of a complex suppurative process) may require resolution between pulmonary and other intrathoracic processes and may exceed the resolution capabilities of a chest radiograph. In these instances, other cross-sectional modalities such as computed tomography (CT) and sonography are useful.

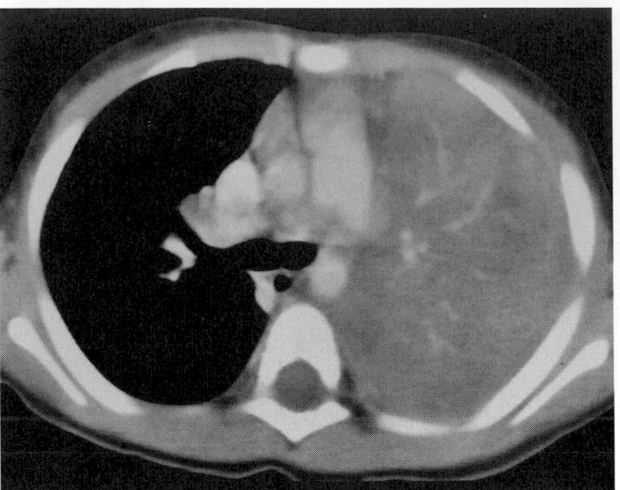

Fig. 39-7. Consolidation without air bronchogram in a 3-year-old boy with extensive pneumonia caused by group A streptococci. CT shows a homogeneous opacification of the entire left chest. The normal branches of the pulmonary vascular system identify the opacity as a pulmonary consolidation.

CT has the advantage of imaging all of the chest anatomic structures, including aerated lung and bony elements. It is not as operator dependent as ultrasound but is better than other modalities at depicting an associated pneumothorax or osteomyelitis of the rib. It is particularly helpful when there are multiple superimposed chest abnormalities involving large areas and more than one anatomic site, such as the lung parenchyma, pleura, and mediastinum. Air bronchograms are more readily seen in pulmonary opacities than in plain radiographs, an observation enabling more confident differentiation of consolidation associated with bacterial pneumonia or any kind of airspace process from other chest opacities. With the administration of intravenous contrast material, the branching pulmonary blood vessels may be visualized within consolidations; this observation may aid in differentiating consolidation associated with bacterial pneumonia from other pulmonary opacities when an air bronchogram is absent[81] (Fig. 39-7).

The value of ultrasonography of the chest varies with the experience of the operator. Modern sonographic equipment has the advantage of superior tissue characterization, real-time acquisition that permits evaluation of tissue motion and adherence, spectral and color Doppler that allows identification of the blood supply, and portability that allows rapid evaluation of critically ill patients in an intensive care unit or emergency department without the need for sedation.[82] This modality is helpful in identifying early cavitation (Fig. 39-8) and in distinguishing a pneumonic process from other intrathoracic events, such as avascular cavities and fluid collections from vascular consolidations. Ultrasonography of the chest requires an acoustic window. Because bone and air interfere with the sound beam, sonography is optimal for lesions that are peripheral without intervening aerated lung (i.e., for processes that abut the chest wall, diaphragm, or both structures). With this modality, the consolidated lung has a liverlike architecture; air bronchograms appear as branching, highly echogenic structures[83,84] (Fig. 39-9). A fluid bronchogram may be seen by sonography but not by CT.[85] In a patient with peripheral le-

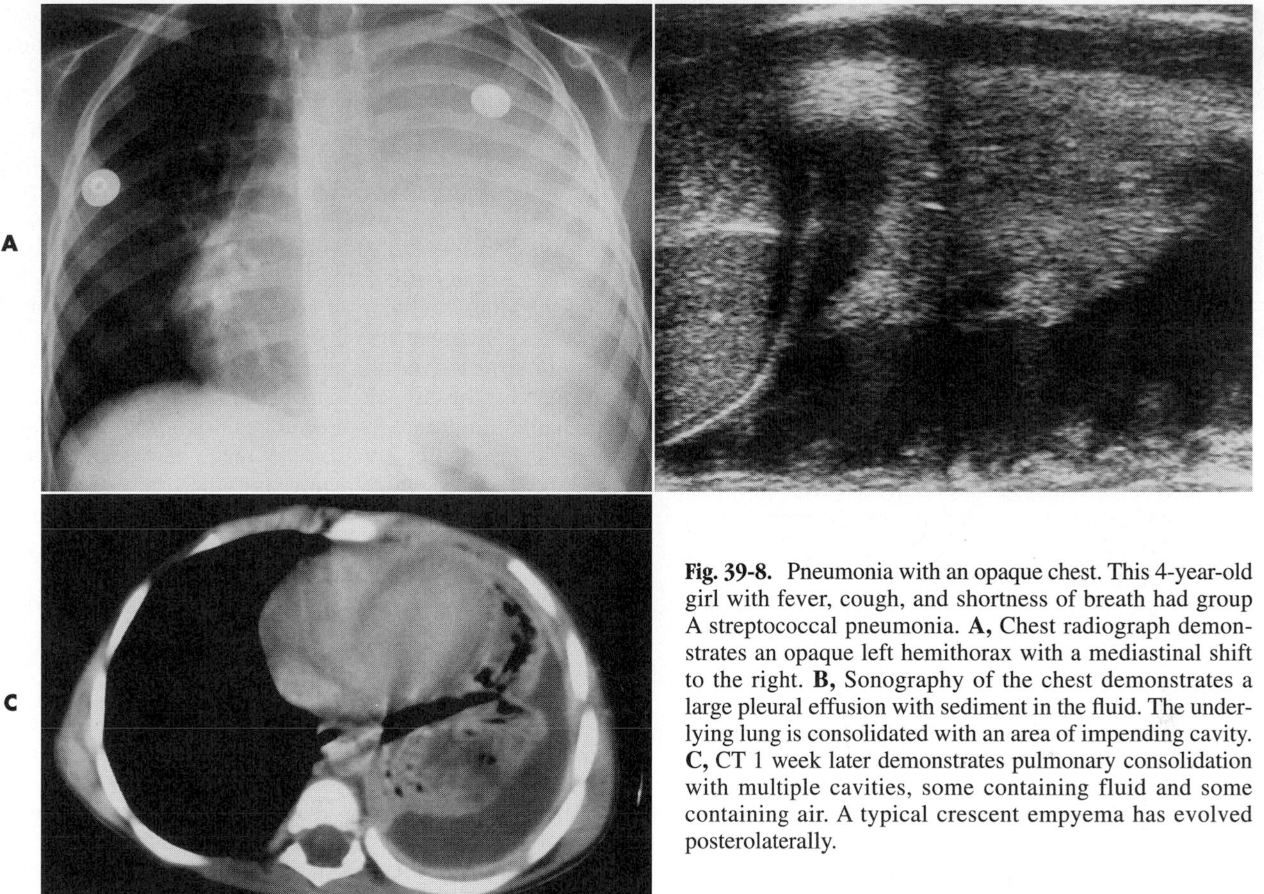

Fig. 39-8. Pneumonia with an opaque chest. This 4-year-old girl with fever, cough, and shortness of breath had group A streptococcal pneumonia. **A,** Chest radiograph demonstrates an opaque left hemithorax with a mediastinal shift to the right. **B,** Sonography of the chest demonstrates a large pleural effusion with sediment in the fluid. The underlying lung is consolidated with an area of impending cavity. **C,** CT 1 week later demonstrates pulmonary consolidation with multiple cavities, some containing fluid and some containing air. A typical crescent empyema has evolved posterolaterally.

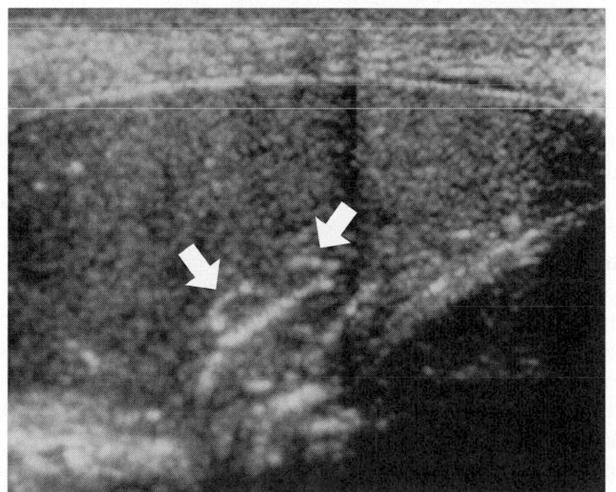

Fig. 39-9. Lung sonography in a 2-year-old girl with *S. pneumoniae* pneumonia. A liverlike pulmonary consolidation (hepatization) can be seen. The air bronchogram appears as branching echogenic stripes radiating from the center of the lobe *(arrows).*

sions, ultrasonography allows differentiation between pulmonary and pleural involvement[86,87] and is also useful for guiding needle aspiration, biopsy, or drainage.

A role for magnetic resonance imaging in imaging pneumonia may be defined in the future. However, to date, the anatomic resolution achievable with this technique in children with bacterial pneumonia has been insufficient to justify its effort and expense.

Management

The approach to management is greatly influenced by the age of the child,[54] the clinical setting in which the illness is acquired (e.g., community or nosocomial), and the immunologic status of the host. For community-acquired pneumonia suspected to be bacterial, hospitalization is the rule for children younger than about 4 to 6 months of age. For older children, the decision to hospitalize should depend on the severity of the clinical picture.

The choice of the antimicrobial regimen for childhood pneumonia is often empirical because of the difficulty in defining the etiology. General guidelines for the initiation of therapy in commonly encountered clinical situations may be found in Table 39-1. These recommendations have been affected by changes in the prevalence of β-lactam resistance in *S. pneumoniae* and *S. aureus* and in ampicillin resistance in *H. influenzae.*

For nosocomially acquired pneumonia suspected to be bacterial, empirical therapy is guided by knowledge of the clinical setting and the underlying disease prompting the hospitalization. Also, the consideration of possible etiologic agents differs from that of community-acquired pneumonias. For example, gram-negative bacilli and *S. aureus* are important causes of nosocomial pneumonia in infants and children, whereas gram-negative bacilli are not an important consideration if the infection is community acquired.

Table 39-1 Approach to Antimicrobial Therapy for Bacterial Pneumonia in Immunocompetent Children

	REGIMEN	
AGE	INPATIENT	OUTPATIENT
Birth-4 wk	Ampicillin and gentamicin*†‡	Not applicable
>4-8 wk	ESC and ampicillin§	Not applicable
>8 wk-1 yr	ESC*‡§	Erythromycin
>1 yr	ESC*‖	Erythromycin

*Add oxacillin, clindamycin, or vancomycin as appropriate if *S. aureus* is suspected.
†ESC (extended-spectrum cephalosporin) and gentamicin if *K. pneumoniae* or another ampicillin-resistant gram-negative bacillus is suspected.
‡Use erythromycin or another macrolide if *B. pertussis* is suspected.
§Use erythromycin if *C. trachomatis* is suspected.
‖Use erythromycin if *M. pneumoniae* is suspected.

In community-acquired or nosocomially acquired pneumonia, antimicrobial therapy is targeted toward the specific bacterium when the etiology is identified. Guidelines for therapy in this instance are detailed in Table 39-2.

Few data exist regarding the duration of antimicrobial therapy for bacterial pneumonia. A 7-day course is usually sufficient for uncomplicated, community-acquired pneumonia in children who are no longer newborns. Pneumonia in the neonate is typically treated for 14 days by the parenteral route. For nosocomial bacterial pneumonia, the duration of therapy (typically 10 to 14 days) is guided by the clinical course and knowledge of the likely causative microorganism. Staphylococcal pneumonia may require treatment for 6 weeks.

Guidelines by the World Health Organization for the therapy of children with pneumonia in developing countries reflect uncertainty regarding the etiology of pneumonia in a given child, the increased likelihood that a clinically relevant pneumonia is bacterial, the cost of antimicrobial agents, the necessity for reliance on clinical signs (e.g., tachypnea) to diagnose pneumonia, and the relatively high mortality rate associated with pneumonia.[2] For outpatient therapy, a 5-day course of amoxicillin, ampicillin, trimethoprim/sulfamethoxazole (TMP/SMX), or procaine penicillin has been recommended. For inpatient therapy, chloramphenicol is often used, particularly in severe cases. In this setting, it may be given intramuscularly,[88] orally, or intravenously per World Health Organization guidelines. In less severe cases requiring hospitalization, penicillin and gentamicin may be used for infants younger than 2 months of age; oxacillin is substituted for penicillin when staphylococcal pneumonia is suspected. Penicillin alone is recommended for other hospitalized children with pneumonia. These antibiotic regimens may be given intramuscularly.[29] The increasing recognition of antimicrobial resistance of *S. pneumoniae, S. aureus,* and *H. influenzae* will prompt ongoing evaluation of these guidelines that will vary according to local resistance patterns and resources available for the purchase of antimicrobials.

Adjuncts to antibiotic therapy for the child with bacterial pneumonia include supplemental oxygen, if needed, and provision of maintenance fluids. Chest physiotherapy has been widely used; however, the modern view is that its efficacy is poor and that it does not hasten resolution.[89] Vitamin A supplementation has not proved to be definitely efficacious.[90]

Long-Term Management and Prognosis

In uncomplicated, community-acquired pneumonia, documentation of a normal chest radiograph is unnecessary.[91] Indications for serial radiography include neonatal pneumonia, severe symptomatology, suspicion of a complication (such as a lung abscess), pleural involvement (such as an effusion or empyema), or an unsatisfactory response to treatment.

The traditional view is that timely administration of antimicrobial therapy renders an excellent outcome in bacterial pneumonia. In developed countries, the mortality rate from uncomplicated cases of pneumonia is less than 1%; lung structure and tissue almost always return to normal, even in patients with empyema or a lung abscess. Some caution regarding this generally bright outlook has come from a recent study, which suggested that a relationship might exist between pneumonia in children younger than 2 years of age and the occurrence of chronic obstructive lung disease later in life[92]; however, no data support this association with bacterial pneumonia.

The mortality rate from acute respiratory illnesses is much higher in developing countries, although the rate of occurrence of acute lower respiratory infections may actually be similar to that for developed countries.[14] This observation suggests that the severity, rather than the incidence, of these infections is responsible for the higher mortality rate.[14]

Recurrent pneumonia, defined as at least two episodes in one year or three or more episodes at any age with radiographic clearing between episodes, requires further investigation.[24] Components of such an evaluation may be found in Box 39-3, but the evaluation of each patient must be individualized. Many of the disorders listed in Box 39-1 are associated with recurrent bacterial pneumonia in children and young adults and should be considered as predisposing to pneumonia in such a patient. These include cystic fibrosis (CF), pulmonary sequestration, bronchiectasis, disorders of normal pulmonary physiology (e.g., immotile cilia syndrome), and a variety of congenital (e.g., severe combined immunodeficiency, immunoglobulin deficiency disorders, Job's syndrome) and acquired (e.g., human immunodeficiency virus [HIV]) immunodeficiency disorders.

Complications and Outcome

Pneumothorax is an uncommon complication of pneumonia and is usually associated with *S. aureus* pneumonia. A cavity containing air may sometimes be associated with bacterial pneumonia. This may represent a pneumatocele, a cavitation, an abscess (see separate section), or rarely, a sequela of massive lung necrosis. A pneumatocele, recognized most commonly in staphylococcal pneumonia, is a thin-walled air collection that can become large and occasionally cause a clinically important mass effect. Its pathogenesis remains controversial. Some argue that a pneumatocele is an enlarged airspace whose walls ruptured after air trapping distal to a bronchus that was occluded by inflammatory exudate and mucosal edema. However, others demonstrated thin-walled, subpleural interstitial blebs that occasionally coalesced and appeared radiographically as a pneumatocele.[93] Although a pneumatocele contains no fluid when it is first formed, an air-fluid level may develop. When this occurs, it may be difficult to differentiate it from a cavity or an abscess, particularly if a surrounding infiltrate prevents accurate evaluation of the lesion wall. A pneumatocele typically appears during convalescence and may either resolve spontaneously within weeks or linger for months before it gradually diminishes and disappears.[94] The earliest radiographic sign of a cavity may be visualized by sonography, before demonstration by CT or plain radiography, as an echolucent focus within the pulmonary consolidation at the hepatization phase. Later, bronchial commu-

Table 39-2 Antimicrobial Therapy When the Etiology Is Known

ORGANISM	REGIMEN OF CHOICE	ALTERNATIVE REGIMENS	REMARKS
S. pneumoniae	Penicillin*	ESC Macrolide† TMP/SMX	Drug is used for pneumonia caused by an isolate with intermediate (MIC <2.0 μg/ml) resistance to penicillin. High-dose penicillin, cefotaxime, or ceftriaxone can also be used. For high-level resistance (MIC ≥2.0 μg/ml), vancomycin can be used.
H. influenzae	Ampicillin/amoxicillin*	ESC Doxycycline Chloramphenicol TMP/SMX	Many strains produce β-lactamase.
S. aureus	Oxacillin/nafcillin*	Cefazolin Macrolide† Vancomycin	Nearly all strains produce β-lactamase.
Group A streptococci	Penicillin	Macrolide†	Nearly all strains produce β-lactamase.
M. catarrhalis	ESC	Macrolide† TMP/SMX	—
Gram-negative enteric bacilli	ESC with or without aminoglycoside	ESC	—
P. aeruginosa	Antipseudomonal β-lactam (e.g., ticarcillin, mezlocillin) and aminoglycoside	Ceftazidime	—
Anaerobes	Clindamycin	Metronidazole Chloramphenicol	—

ESC, Extended-spectrum cephalosporin; *TMP/SMX,* trimethoprim/sulfamethoxazole; *MIC,* minimal inhibitory concentration.
*When susceptible.
†Erythromycin, for example.

BOX 39-3
Evaluation of Children with Recurrent Bacterial Pneumonia

General

A history should be taken, with special attention to high-risk situations for foreign body aspiration, stools consistent with malabsorption, sinusitis, otitis, asthma and atopy, severe pulmonary disease, environmental exposure, prematurity, oxygen exposure, and early deaths in family members.

A physical examination should be done, with special attention to nutritional state, anatomic structures of the upper airway, muscular strength, neurologic functions such as swallowing and gag reflexes, resting respiratory rate, accessory muscle use, inspiratory to expiratory ratio, wheezes, crackles, and cardiovascular system for suggestion of congenital anomalies of the heart or great vessels and the presence of heart failure.

Specific

The chest radiograph should be reviewed by a radiologist.

A complete blood count with differential should be obtained.

A blood culture should be done.

Sputum should be examined for a cell morphologic study if the patient is old enough to comply, Gram's stain, fungal smear, acid-fast smear, and culture for aerobes, fungi, and *Mycobacteria* species.

Fiberoptic bronchoscopy may be needed in some cases to obtain sputum.

BAL fluid should be examined by silver methenamine stain for *Pneumocystis carinii,* fungi, *Mycobacteria* species, and cellular elements (e.g., eosinophils, erythrocytes).

Specific—cont'd

Alveolar macrophages can be stained for hemosiderin for the diagnosis of recurrent pulmonary hemorrhage.

Purified protein derivative analysis should be done.

A sweat chloride test should be obtained.

Further evaluation should be performed as appropriate:
- Chest CT
- Airway fluoroscopy
- Laryngoscopy
- Bronchoscopy
- Endoscopy
- Barium swallow
- Mediastinal magnetic resonance imaging toevaluate vascular structures
- Lung biopsy
- Quantitative serum immunoglobulin assay
- Neutrophil function studies
- T and B cell enumeration, quantitative of subsets' function
- Nasal turbinate or tracheal biopsy for electron microscopy for cilia ultrastructure and phase microscopy for function
- Spirometry without and with β_2-agonist inhalation challenge

nication results in air entering the cavities, rendering them visible first by CT and later by plain radiograph.

PNEUMONIA IN THE FIRST MONTH OF LIFE

Despite having many features in common with pneumonia in older children, certain unique aspects of bacterial pneumonia in the first month of life warrant special consideration. It has been convenient to subdivide neonatal bacterial pneumonia according to the acquisition time of the etiologic microorganism and the onset of clinical manifestations. A classification scheme similar to that proposed by Marks and Klein[95] provides a useful framework. In this scheme, pneumonia occurring in the first month of life is subdivided into congenital or intrauterine pneumonia and neonatal pneumonia.

The term *congenital* or *intrauterine pneumonia* is applied when the bacteria are acquired transplacentally or in utero by the ascending route; the source of the etiologic organism is most often the maternal genitourinary tract. Infants with congenital or intrauterine pneumonia are stillborn or die shortly after birth, usually within 24 hours. The pathogenesis is not completely understood. Identified risk factors, such as prematurity, prolonged rupture of membranes, intrauterine asphyxia, and infection at nonrespiratory tract sites, are similar to those predisposing to neonatal bacteremia. Microorganisms from the maternal genitourinary tract may contaminate the maternal membranes, amniotic fluid, and periumbilical vascular tissues by ascending to them through small, unrecognized defects in the decidua or after premature membrane rupture.

The pulmonary pathology (as defined at autopsy) reflects an inflammatory reaction. Polymorphonuclear leukocytes are evident and are often accompanied by vernix and squamous cells. The interstitial tissue of small bronchioles and the interalveolar septa may be infiltrated by lymphocytes.[96] Alveolar macrophages may also be present and tend to increase in number with the duration of the postnatal illness.[97] The distribution of inflammation is characteristically diffuse. Interestingly, certain features of bacterial pneumonia acquired after birth, such as pleural reaction, alveolar fibrinous exudate, and infiltration or destruction of the bronchopulmonary tissue, rarely occur in congenital or intrauterine pneumonia.

The term *neonatal pneumonia* is used to describe pneumonia in which bacterial acquisition occurs during passage through the maternal genital tract or shortly thereafter; the clinical features are manifested in the first few days to the first month of life.[95] The portal of entry for the etiologic agent may be the lung after the aspiration of infected amniotic fluid and may therefore be a consequence of contact with vaginal or uterine secretions in the birth canal, contaminated water or medical equipment, or contact with caretakers.

The pulmonary pathology in neonatal bacterial pneumonia is similar to that in older children and adults. The lungs may contain regions of exudate with hemorrhage, congestion, and necrosis.[95] Bacteria are often seen in lung sections, a finding absent in the histology of congenital or intrauterine pneumonia. The histopathology depends in part on the microbial etiology. For example, *S. aureus* and *K. pneumoniae* typically cause necrosis of lung tissue, empyema, or microabscesses.[98,99] *S. aureus, E. coli,* and *K. pneumoniae* may be associated with pneumatocele formation.[100] GBS pneumonia has been associated with intraalveolar hyaline membranes in which microorganisms may be visualized.[101] Similar hyaline changes have also been noted with neonatal pneumonia caused by *H. influenzae* and gram-negative enteric bacteria.[102]

The incidence of neonatal pneumonia is difficult to determine because of uncertainty regarding case definitions, rate differences in patient populations, and ascertainment bias. In a study of consecutive live births at a tertiary care center in Oxford, England, *pneumonia* was defined as respiratory distress associated with changes on the chest radiograph that persisted for more than 48 hours. Early onset pneumonia, which occurs in children younger than 48 hours of age, was found in 1.8 per 1000 live births, whereas late-onset pneumonia, which occurs in children older than 48 hours of age (mean, 35 days of age), was found at a rate of 2.0 per 1000 live births.[103] In a review of nine studies describing autopsy findings in stillborn and liveborn neonates, the incidence of pneumonia was 15% to 38% and 20% to 32%, respectively.[95]

Infants from low-income families have a significantly greater incidence of pneumonia than those from higher-income families. At comparable economic levels, however, African-American infants have a higher incidence of newborn pneumonia than Hispanic or white infants, although this racial difference has not yet been reasonably explained.[104,105] Pneumonia in newborns is also found at much higher rates in developing countries.

Epidemics of neonatal pneumonia have occurred. The outbreak is often caused by a single source of infection (e.g., a nursery worker, contaminated equipment or solutions used for patient care). In the 1950s and early 1960s, many nurseries in the United States were plagued by epidemic *S. aureus* pneumonia. The identification of infants colonized with virulent *S. aureus* phage 80/81 was often accompanied by a sharp increase in the incidence of *S. aureus* neonatal pneumonia. For unclear reasons, the frequency of epidemic *S. aureus* pneumonia has greatly decreased since that time, but sporadic cases still occur.[99] Other bacteria, such as *Pseudomonas* species, *Flavobacterium* species, and *S. marcescens,* have also been responsible for nursery epidemics.[95]

When the pathogen is acquired in the maternal genital tract, the most common causes of pneumonia are group B streptococci and gram-negative enteric organisms such as *E. coli, K. pneumoniae,* and *Proteus* and *Enterobacter* species. *Chlamydia* organisms are also believed to be acquired in this manner. Occasionally, pathogens normally associated with respiratory tract spread, such as group A streptococci, *H. influenzae,* and *Neisseria meningitidis,* are found in the maternal genital tract and transmitted vertically to neonates.

After birth, bacteria causing pneumonia are usually acquired from parents, caretakers, or environmental sources. These include *S. aureus* (30% of all cases caused by this organism occur in children younger than 3 months of age)[106] and gram-negative bacilli, such as *Pseudomonas* and *Flavobacterium* species, *Citrobacter diversus,*[107] and *S. marcescens. H. influenzae, M. catarrhalis, L. pneumophila,* and *Bacillus cereus*[108] are infrequently recognized etiologic agents. *S. pneumoniae*[109] pneumonia is infrequent in this age group. It is usually manifested shortly after birth and has a high mortality rate.

Diagnosis is usually based on clinical, microbiologic, and diagnostic imaging data. Because the clinical manifestations are usually nonspecific, especially at the onset, the birth history may provide important clues. Important risk factors in neonates are prolonged rupture of the maternal membranes (particularly longer than 24 hours), prolonged maternal labor, the identification of meconium-stained or malodorous amniotic fluid, and meconium-stained laryngeal or tracheal secretions.

If not stillborn, infants with congenital or intrauterine pneumonia are often very ill at birth. If they are alive, there are usually signs of asphyxia, including the presence of meconium, nuchal cord, apnea, and depressed respirations; the mortality rate within the first 24 hours of life is high. Pneumonia occurring during or shortly after birth is manifested by lethargy and anorexia, both of which are nonspecific signs of a generalized illness. Fever is commonly absent. Signs attributable to the respiratory tract, such as dyspnea, tachypnea, grunting, flaring, coughing, cyanosis, and retractions, either may be initially evident or may develop later. Auscultatory findings of crackles and diminished breath sounds also vary.

The most helpful aid in diagnosing neonatal bacterial pneumonia is a chest radiograph. The so-called typical findings include diffuse or patchy bilateral alveolar infiltrates, streaky densities, confluent opacities, and peribronchial thickening. The presence of these findings is inconsistent, however, and the radiologic diagnosis of pneumonia in the newborn may therefore be difficult.[110] Other causes of respiratory distress in the newborn, such as hyaline membrane disease, retention of fetal fluid, and pulmonary edema, may also be associated with diffuse, bilateral radiographic opacities. Conversely, the chest radiographs may be normal in some infants with pathologically proven bacterial pneumonia.[111] Further complicating this conundrum are the variable radiographic findings when pneumonia is the certain diagnosis. For example, among infants with histologic evidence of pneumonia at autopsy, 77% had diffuse or patchy bilateral alveolar infiltrates. In 17%, however, the radiograph suggested retained fetal fluid consistent with transient tachypnea of the newborn. In 13%, the radiographic picture closely resembled hyaline membrane disease.[111] Indeed, the radiographic picture of this disease may mimic that of pneumonia, particularly when group B streptococcus is the pathogen (Fig. 39-10). The presence of a pleural effusion may aid in differentiation because this finding is not observed in hyaline membrane disease.

The diagnosis of pneumonia in a neonate who is in intensive care and who has underlying chronic lung disease is especially difficult. Infection is suspected in the presence of a suggestive clinical picture (i.e., a sudden increase in the severity of pulmonary abnormalities or another clinical deterioration and a new pleural effusion or an opaque chest radiograph). Pneumonia with pneumatoceles or cavitation may mimic congenital diaphragmatic hernia or a cystic adenomatoid malformation.

CT of the chest with infusion of contrast material is less helpful in the neonate than in the older child but may be of use in localizing a lesion, especially in distinguishing among an abscess, empyema, pneumatoceles, or a bronchopleural fistula. Ultrasonography has been useful in assessing pleural effusions for the presence of loculation or debris, differentiating empyema from lung abscess, and clarifying the components of an opaque chest radiograph. It has also been used to diagnose a case of pneumonia in utero in a fetus of 32 weeks' gestation.[112]

Aspirating pulmonary exudate under radiologic guidance can provide unequivocal information about the causative agent. Bronchoscopy may also be helpful. In addition, open lung biopsy has been useful in newborns when other diagnostic techniques have failed to provide precise information in infants with respiratory failure.[113]

The evaluation of an infant in the first month of life for suspected pneumonia is usually performed in the context of evaluation for a possible systemic infection. Thus many infants with suspected neonatal pneumonia undergo blood, urine, and cerebrospinal fluid (CSF) cultures at the time of initial evaluation. Furthermore, because viruses such as herpes simplex virus and cytomegalovirus may be responsible for pneumonia and even a clinical picture resembling a systemic infectious illness, evaluation of an infant in the first month of life may include consideration of these nonbacterial agents.

A bacterium recovered from blood, urine, or CSF often provides a valuable clue to the etiology of suspected pneumonia. Some researchers have suggested that a tracheal aspirate performed during the first few hours of life may also provide a clue as to the etiology of pneumonia.[114] Antigen-detection techniques such as latex particle agglutination may also provide clues; however, in the neonate, these are limited to detection of group B streptococcal antigens, which have been found in the serum and urine of patients with group B streptococcal pneumonia.

The selection of antimicrobials for the therapy of neonatal pneumonia is also performed in the context of a possible systemic bacterial infection (see Table 39-1). An empiric regimen that includes a β-lactam, such as ampicillin, and an aminoglycoside, such as gentamicin, often constitute initial therapy. Once a bacterium is identified, the regimen may be targeted toward it (Table 39-2). Few explicit data are available to guide the duration of antimicrobial therapy. The decision regarding length of therapy is often guided by treatment response and

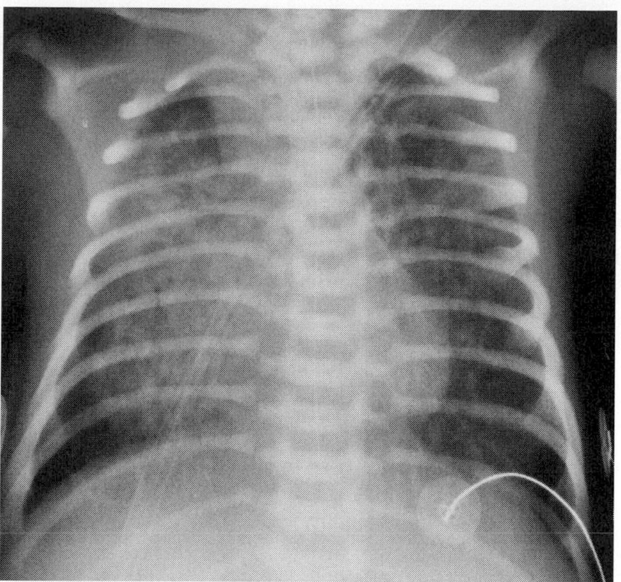

Fig. 39-10. Group B streptococcal pneumonia in a neonate. A full-term male newborn with diffuse bilateral infiltrates, both reticular-linear and confluent.

perhaps by the identified etiology. For example, a 14-day course may suffice when the clinical response has been prompt; however, a course of at least 21 days is often used for pneumonia caused by gram-positive organisms such as *S. aureus* and group B streptococci or that caused by any etiology when the response has been slow.

Supportive care includes the provision of oxygen and mechanical ventilation (when appropriate); maintenance of fluid, electrolyte, and metabolic balance; and drainage of appropriate pleural effusion or abscesses. Such care is essential to optimize chances for a good outcome.

The outcome of therapy depends on many factors. The availability of state-of-the-art neonatal intensive care greatly improves the likelihood of a good outcome; the mortality rates in developing countries lacking these facilities are often high.[115,116] In developed countries, prematurity, underlying diseases, the host response, the aggressiveness and appropriateness of antimicrobial therapy, and supportive care measures all have a great impact on the mortality rates and prognosis.

SPECIFIC CAUSES OF PEDIATRIC PNEUMONIA

Causes of Frequent Clinical Concern

S. Pneumoniae, Pneumococcus

The pneumococcus is the most common cause of bacterial pneumonia in children.[30,117] The observation by Pasteur[118] and Pasteur et al[119] that lancet-shaped pairs of cocci found in human saliva could cause disease in rabbits provided the first notion that these bacteria were important human pathogens. In 1886, Fraenkel[120] named these bacteria *pneumococci* because of their tendency to cause pneumonia, but in 1920, the Society of American Bacteriologists assigned the name *Diplococcus pneumoniae*.[121] However, because pneumococci form chains in liquid media, the name *S. pneumoniae* was assigned to the species in 1974.[122]

The organism is a gram-positive coccus that was among the first bacteria described by the then fledgling technique developed by Gram in 1884.[123] The classic Gram's stain morphology is so-called lancet-shaped, gram-positive diplococci. The organism grows easily in fresh beef heart infusion broth with whole blood or serum, which provides catalase to break down the accumulating hydrogen peroxide. Incubation at 35° to 37° C and an atmosphere containing 5% carbon dioxide improve growth.

Invasive infections caused by pneumococci are a major problem for pediatricians. In Northern California, the age-specific incidence (number of children per 100,000 per year) of invasive pneumococcal infections follows:

Age	Number
≤5 months	103
6-11 months	177
12-17 months	241
18-23 months	139
24-35 months	70
36-47 months	25

This compares to an incidence of 150 per 100,000 per year for invasive *H. influenzae* type b disease in the same population in infants younger than 12 months of age and 63 per 100,000 per year in toddlers before the introduction of vaccination. The problem is not limited to the United States. Among Finnish children, the age-specific incidences of invasive pneumococcal disease were 24.2 and 37 per 100,000 per year in children younger than 5 and 1 year of age, respectively.[124] In Israel, the corresponding estimates were 42 and 104 per 100,000 per year in children younger than 5 and 1 year of age, respectively.[125]

The species *S. pneumoniae* is subdivided into 90 immunologically distinct serotypes. There are two numbering systems: the American system, which numbers serotypes in numerical sequence, and, in wider use, the Danish system, which groups antigens according to immunologic similarity.

The distribution of serotypes responsible for invasive infections has varied with geographic locale, age of the patient (child vs. adult), and clinical syndrome (invasive disease vs. otitis media). For example, in children in Northern California, types 14, 19F, 6B, 23F, and 18C accounted for 95% of all invasive pneumococcal infections. In Connecticut, the same serotypes caused 68.5% of invasive disease in children; the inclusion of types 9V, 6A, 4, and 19A encompassed an additional 20% of cases.[126] The two most common serotypes among Israeli children, types 1 and 5, are rare in Western Europe and North America. Thus an effective pneumococcal conjugate vaccine may need to be formulated for use in different populations.

Asymptomatic nasopharyngeal colonization by the pneumococcus is common; 20% to 40% of healthy children are colonized at any given time.[127] The rate of isolation of pneumococcus from asymptomatic children is also higher in institutional settings. Virtually all infants are carriers at least once when followed longitudinally.[128] Pneumococcal carriage is infrequent in the first 6 months of life, increases thereafter to reach its peak rate among preschool children, and then declines slowly to a nadir among adolescents. The highest rates of colonization have been found from December to April, although carriers can be detected throughout the year among healthy children.[128] The serotypes most commonly associated with asymptomatic carriage—types 6, 14, 19, and 23—are similar to those causing disease.

With respect to invasive disease, male patients are affected more often than female patients. Statistically significant risk factors for invasive disease include attendance at day-care, frequent episodes of otitis media (more than three episodes in 6 months), frequent upper respiratory tract infections (at least three episodes in 6 months), premature birth, and previous hospitalization for respiratory disease. Insignificant trends for increased risk included black race, anemia, asthma, and previous insertion of polyethylene tubes into the tympanic membrane.

Certain populations, such as Alaskan[129] and Apache[130] children, are at higher risk for invasive disease. Indeed, the incidence of pneumococcal infection among the White Mountain Apache population (156 per 100,000 population [1988 U.S. population]) has been the highest reported; the peak incidence was in children 1 to 2 years of age (2396 per 100,000). Some 79% of these invasive pneumococcal infections were pneumonia.[130] Other individuals at increased risk for invasive pneumococcal disease include those with asplenia, those with congenital or acquired immunodeficiency, recipients of cytoreduction or other immunosuppressive therapies, those who have undergone bone marrow transplantation, and those with CSF leaks, chronic pulmonary or renal disease, congestive heart failure, Hodgkin's disease, complement deficiencies, nephrotic syndrome, sickle cell disease, or systemic lupus erythematosus. In addition to their increased risk attributable to sickle cell anemia or low socioeconomic status, African-Americans may generally be at higher risk for invasive disease.[131]

A series of observations early in the twentieth century established the capsule as the critical virulence determinant of pneumococci. After the recognition that the soluble substance found in serum and urine in patients with lobar pneumonia reacts with specific antiserum to pneumococci of identical serotype and that the capsular polysaccharide is the cell wall component responsible for this reaction, Dubos and Avery[132] demonstrated that pneumococci with enzymatically removed capsules were relatively avirulent in mice. Until this time, only proteins were believed to be immunogenic; this was the first demonstration that the immunogenicity of the capsular polysaccharide in mice protected against subsequent pneumococcal challenge.

The mechanism by which the capsule exerts its virulence on the pneumococcus is still not completely understood. The capsular polysaccharide itself is not toxic, but the quantity of elaborated capsular polysaccharide may explain some intraserotypic differences in virulence.[132] Most investigators implicate impaired antibody-mediated, complement-dependent phagocytosis of pneumococci to the capsule to explain its role in virulence, but this traditional explanation may also not be sufficient. For example, a clear relationship between in vitro opsonophagocytosis and protection in an experimental mouse model of pneumococcal disease for serotype 3 exists, but it has not been possible to establish a similar relationship for serotype 1 isolates.[133]

Host defense mechanisms that deal with pneumococcal infection include local respiratory defenses, such as ciliary action, the cough reflex, and the production of mucus. Phagocytosis and the presence of type-specific anticapsule antibody also play crucial roles.

The incubation period varies but can be as short as 1 to 3 days. When invasive disease occurs, it is usually shortly after a new serotype is acquired in the upper respiratory tract. An organism associated with prolonged carriage is an unlikely cause of invasive illness.

Factors influencing transmission of the pneumococcus from person to person have not been thoroughly studied. The recent application of molecular techniques should result in an improved understanding of this problem. For example, despite few reports of clusters of invasive disease in young children, it is now clear that *S. pneumoniae* may occasionally be readily transmitted from child to child in the day-care setting.[134]

The onset of pneumococcal pneumonia may be preceded by a mild upper respiratory tract infection, purulent unilateral conjunctivitis, or otitis media. The clinical manifestations vary somewhat with age. In infants, a sudden rise in temperature may be accompanied by a seizure, and diarrhea or vomiting may be among the earliest manifestations. Restlessness, apprehension, nasal flaring, rapid and shallow respirations, grunting, abdominal distention, perioral cyanosis, tachycardia, and unilateral diminished respiratory excursion (splinting) may variably ensue. Cough may be absent.

In the older child and the adolescent, the clinical features more closely resemble those in adults. Onset is typically abrupt. The patient may appear ill with shaking chills or rigors, fever, headache, dyspnea, pleuritic pain, and cough.[135] Sputum production may be apparent in children older than about 10 years of age. If a viral illness was the predisposing factor, the onset may be more insidious, with coryza and low-grade fever preceding higher fever and possibly sputum production.[136] Pleuritic chest pain reflecting involvement of the visceral pleura may occur. Occasionally, signs and symptoms suggesting bacterial pneumonia may be absent; fever may be the only sign.

Physical examination may elicit splinting on the affected side.[136] Percussion in young children is rarely helpful because pulmonary involvement may be patchy and the chest is small. When dullness is detected, however, the possibility of accompanying empyema should be considered. Auscultation may be misleading. In the infant, the fine crackles audible in older patients may be difficult to hear. Even in the older child, such crackles may be evident only during the resolution phase. A friction rub is rarely heard. Breath sounds may be exaggerated on the healthy side. Pain, when present, may be referred to the abdomen, which may be distended. Occasionally, clinical features of an acute abdominal condition may prompt the mistaken suspicion of acute appendicitis. Symptoms and signs suggestive of meningismus may be present if the upper lobes are involved but, more important, may also reflect concomitant meningitis.

Many patients with pneumococcal pneumonia may have leukocytosis. However, the sensitivity and specificity of the leukocyte count are sufficiently low to preclude reliance on its presence for diagnosis.

The usefulness of sputum as a diagnostic tool in pneumococcal pneumonia falls between "conclusive" and "occasionally conclusive" in terms of clinical importance in properly collected specimens that contain large numbers of polymorphonuclear leukocytes and typical lancet-shaped gram-positive cocci or that yield *S. pneumoniae* on culture. Antigen-detection techniques have been used in the diagnosis of pneumococcal pneumonia. A blood culture may yield the causative pathogen and should therefore be performed during the initial evaluation.

The radiographic changes in acute pneumococcal pneumonia are not pathognomonic. However, pneumococcal pneumonia is frequently associated with the radiographically "classic" acute airspace pneumonia that starts peripherally in the lower lobes or posterior segments of the upper lobes.[136] It then spreads concentrically with no respect for segmental boundaries, unlike bronchopneumonia. This characteristic picture may result in a masslike round infiltrate, the most common pulmonary mass lesion in children. Alternatively, pneumococcal pneumonia may appear radiographically as a patchy or even linear ("interstitial") infiltrate. A radiographically visible pleural effusion occurs in a small percentage of cases and is more common in young children than adults. In infants and young children, pneumococcal pneumonia may occasionally be complicated by pneumatoceles, abscess, and empyema.[137] The resolution of radiographic abnormalities may occur 10 to 14 days after appropriate therapy is initiated but more commonly may persist for weeks or even months after recovery.

Once the diagnosis is suspected, antimicrobial therapy should be started. Characteristically, the fever decreases a few hours later, when the isolate is susceptible. Penicillin has been the drug of choice for pneumococcal infections. Until the late 1970s, penicillin resistance was recognized in only a few, sporadic isolates. An outbreak of disease in South African children in 1978 as a result of penicillin-resistant pneumococci signaled that *S. pneumoniae* would henceforth require routine susceptibility testing by microbiology laboratories. These resistant isolates have now been found in many parts of the world, including the United States.

Penicillin-resistant pneumococci may be relatively (minimum inhibitory concentration of penicillin = 0.1 to 1.0 μg penicillin/ml) or absolutely (minimum inhibitory concentration $\geq$ 2.0 μg/ml) resistant. Resistance is mediated by the production of one or more penicillin-binding proteins with altered affinity for penicillin. Absolute resistance accounts for less than 10% of penicillin-resistant isolates.[138,139] However, dramatic increases in the rate of penicillin resistance have been documented in many parts of the world, including parts of the United States. Susceptibility to extended-spectrum (third-generation) cephalosporins has been assumed until recently, even among penicillin-resistant isolates. However, extended-spectrum cephalosporin resistance has now been documented in association with treatment failure in patients with pneumococcal meningitis. Moreover, these penicillin-resistant pneumococcal isolates are frequently multiply resistant, a fact that further complicates treatment strategies. Serotypes 6, 14, 19, and 23 are most frequently associated with penicillin resistance.

Pneumonia caused by strains with intermediate resistance to penicillin usually responds to high-dose penicillin or to extended-spectrum cephalosporin therapy. Pneumonia caused by absolutely resistant isolates may also respond to high-dose penicillin or extended-spectrum cephalosporin therapy; however, if the isolate is susceptible, clindamycin, vancomycin, or chloramphenicol may provide greater clinical comfort. These compounds may also be appropriate if the child is allergic to penicillin.

Aside from antimicrobial therapy, oxygen and ventilatory support may be necessary. Intensive care may be required, particularly if hypotension is present or hypoxia is severe. Hyponatremia may be present secondary to inappropriate secretion of antidiuretic hormone and may require fluid restriction.

Complications of pneumococcal pneumonia may be "local" (i.e., secondary to the pneumonia itself) or "distant" as a result of a concurrent bacteremia. Empyema is the most common local complication[136] and probably arises when bacteria seed a pleural effusion. Adult respiratory distress syndrome (ARDS) does not commonly occur. Most cases of ARDS are in children; leukopenia during acute pneumonia may be a risk factor.[140] Distant complications include purpura fulminans, meningitis, endocarditis, peritonitis, septic arthritis, and pericarditis.[141]

Clinical features associated with increased morbidity include multilobar involvement with hypoxemia, leukopenia with overwhelming sepsis, bacteremia, and infection caused by serotype 3. Permanent pulmonary sequelae of uncomplicated pneumococcal pneumonia are extremely rare. Slow clinical resolution is usually due to an underlying problem, a mistaken diagnosis, or a superinfection. The mortality rate in those with pneumococcal pneumonia and ARDS may be as high as 50%. Before the introduction of antibiotics, the mortality rate in infants was 20% to 30%; now it is less than 5% in both infants and older children.

Attempts to prevent pneumococcal infection by vaccination began in the early twentieth century with the studies of Wright et al,[142] who used killed whole-cell pneumococcal vaccines in an attempt to prevent pneumonia in South African gold miners. However, no efficacy could be shown with this vaccine. In a study conducted among U.S. Air Force recruits in 1945, MacLeod et al[143] established the efficacy of a pneumococcal vaccine consisting of the capsular polysaccharides of four of the seven serotypes recognized at that time. Subsequently, a hexavalent vaccine manufactured by Squibb and Co. was licensed with separate adult and pediatric formulations, but these vaccines were withdrawn in the early 1950s because penicillin had become firmly entrenched in clinical practice and interest in prevention of these infections had waned. Austrian,[144] however, called attention to the ongoing morbidity and mortality rates from pneumococcal infections and revived interest in developing an efficacious pneumococcal vaccine. Subsequently, Smit et al[145] demonstrated that 6- and 12-valent vaccines were efficacious (vaccine efficacy of 76% and 92%, respectively) in preventing pneumococcal pneumonia in adult South African gold miners. In 1977, these efforts culminated in licensure in the United States of a 14-valent capsular polysaccharide vaccine composed of the serotypes responsible for 70% to 80% of the episodes of bacteremia or meningitis.[145] In 1984, the vaccine was reformulated to become the 23-valent vaccine in current use.

The antigens in the 23-valent vaccines represent the serotypes causing nearly 100% of bacteremia and meningitis cases in children. However, the polysaccharides have limited immunogenicity in children younger than 2 years of age. The Committee on Infectious Diseases of the American Academy of Pediatrics[146] currently recommends the 23-valent vaccine for children older than 2 years of age who have conditions predisposing them to an increased risk of pneumococcal infection. Examples of this are sickle cell disease, functional and anatomic asplenia, nephrotic syndrome, chronic renal failure, conditions associated with immunosuppression, HIV infection and other immunodeficient states, or anatomic CSF leaks. Revaccination after 3 to 5 years should be considered for children remaining in a high-risk group. Passive immunization with intravenous immunoglobulin is recommended for preventing pneumococcal pneumonia in children with certain congenital or acquired immunodeficient states predisposing them to *S. pneumoniae* infection. Examples include hypogammaglobulinemia or agammaglobulinemia, HIV infection, and recurrent serious bacterial infections (including pneumococcal infections) for which these children are unlikely to form specific antibody to common antigens.[146]

The recent success of conjugate vaccines directed against *H. influenzae* type b has promoted the idea that applying similar technologic advances to pneumococcal vaccine development might prevent pneumococcal infection. Investigations are in progress to assess the feasibility of this strategy.

Pneumococcal conjugate vaccines have been produced by several manufacturers and include a 7-valent vaccine linked to an outer membrane protein complex (OMPC) of *Neisseria meningitidis* (Merck and Co.), a 7-valent and a 9-valent vaccine linked to a nontoxic mutant of diphtheria toxin (CRM_{197}) (Wyeth-Lederle Vaccines) and 11-valent vaccines linked to diptheria toxoid (DT) or tetanus toxoid (TT) (Pasteur-Meriéux Connaught). The heptavalent pneumococcal conjuate vaccines contain serotypes 4, 6B, 9V, 14, 18C, 19F, 23F, which account for about 84% of cases of invasive disease in U.S. children. The 9-valent and 11-valent conjugate vaccines include, respectively, 2 and 4 additional serotypes that commonly cause disease in developing countries, consistent with efforts to prevent pneumococcal disease worldwide. Recently, one of these vaccines, the heptavalent vaccine manufactured by Wyeth-Lederle Vaccines and Pediatrics, was demonstrated to have high efficacy (VE = 100%, 95% CI = 75.7%-100%) in infants and children attending Kaiser Permanente Clinics in Northern California.[146a]

S. Aureus

S. aureus and the coagulase-negative species *Staphylococcus epidermidis* are two important human pathogens that may cause pneumonia in children. Pneumonia caused by *S. aureus* is uncommon, but it may be associated with a rapidly progressive course, particularly in children younger than 1 year of age, and antimicrobial regimens commonly used for the therapy of bacterial pneumonia may not provide optimal *S. aureus* coverage. Pneumonia caused by *S. epidermidis* is very rare and occurs almost exclusively in neonates and immunocompromised individuals.

In 1882, Ogston named the family of spherical, cluster-forming microorganisms *Staphylococcus.* Koch had previously described these organisms in the pus obtained from a patient, and Pasteur had cultivated them in liquid medium in 1880. The first attempt at speciation of the staphylococci came in the same year, when Rosenbach defined the species *Staphylococcus pyogenes aureus* and *Staphylococcus pyogenes albus,* distinctions reflecting pigment production by colonies growing on solid media. Today, the detection of coagulase and protein A, compounds produced exclusively by *S. aureus,* is used as the basis of laboratory tests that distinguish the important pathogen *S. aureus* from other so-called coagulase-negative staphylococcal species such as *S. epidermidis.* Morphologically, all staphylococci are gram-positive cocci that resemble clusters of grapes when viewed under the light microscope. Primarily for epidemiologic reasons, a variety of techniques have been used to distinguish clinical isolates of *S. aureus.* In this regard, the pattern of lysis by a "standard" panel of bacteriophages, although historically important, has been replaced by a variety of techniques, the best of which are nucleic acid based. Currently, pulse-field gel electrophoresis is widely used as a first-line tool for distinguishing among isolates, usually for epidemiologic purposes.[147]

Staphylococcal cell walls are composed of teichoic acid, a ribitol phosphate polymer, and peptidoglycan. The cell wall of *S. aureus* also contains protein A, which binds the Fc fragment of IgG and fixes complement in the process. It has been noted that most pathogenic strains of *S. aureus* have a polysaccharide capsule; 8 to 11 types of capsular polysaccharides have been identified in *S. aureus* isolates.[148] Worldwide surveillance in developed countries revealed that capsular polysaccharide types 5 and 8 were identified in 80% of adults with bacteremia.

These data seem to suggest that these capsules play an important role in the pathogenesis of *S. aureus* invasive infections.[149]

A variety of extracellular factors play a role in the virulence and pathogenesis of *S. aureus* infection. Coagulase clots animal plasma and was once thought to be the determinant of virulence. However, *S. aureus* isolates that do not have free or bound coagulase retain their virulence in animal models. Neither does coagulase inhibit polymorphonuclear cell phagocytosis in vivo, nor is there a correlation between circulating anticoagulase antibody and protection from *S. aureus* infection.[150] Leukocidin degranulates and kills human polymorphonuclear cells; patients infected with isolates elaborating leukocidin produce antileukocidin antibody in the convalescent phase. However, among those with invasive infection, leukocidin was detectable in only 25% of isolates. Some have suggested that its importance may lie in the pathophysiology of cutaneous *S. aureus* infections.[151] Other factors produced by *S. aureus* strains that affect virulence include the α-, β-, γ-, and δ-hemolysins; these hemolysins contribute to the virulence of *S. aureus* in addition to their hemolytic activity. For example, α-toxin is toxic to polymorphonuclear leukocytes, macrophages, and platelets and also has dermonecrotic properties.

A family of enterotoxins designated *A* to *G* has also been identified. Members of this family have important roles in the pathophysiology of staphylococcal food poisoning and toxic shock syndrome. Some *S. aureus* isolates elaborate the extracellular toxin exfoliatin, which is important in the pathogenesis of staphylococcal scalded skin syndrome. Others elaborate one or more members of a family of pyrogenic toxins designated *A* to *C* that are analogous to those produced by *S. pyogenes.* Recently, a class of proteins on a variety of gram-positive bacteria surfaces was identified and was believed to play an important role in pathogenicity by allowing bacteria to avoid host defenses and by acting as adhesins.[152] In addition to protein A, the following members of this class have been identified in *S. aureus:* fibronectin-binding protein, collagen-binding protein, and clumping factor. Staphylococci also secrete hyaluronidase, lipases, staphylokinase, and staphylococcal decomplementation antigen, all of which may play a role in the pathogenesis of staphylococcal infections.

S. aureus pneumonia is infrequent in developed countries. Among 102 consecutive cases of pneumonia in children younger than 5 years of age, *S. aureus* was responsible for only one case.[28] Among 1740 children hospitalized with pneumonia in Hong Kong, *S. aureus* was the pathogen (demonstrated by its isolation from blood) in two.[153] Community-acquired *S. aureus* pneumonia typically occurs in very young infants: 30% of cases occur in children younger than 3 months of age, and 70% occur in those younger than 1 year of age. Most cases occur in the colder months, and boys are more frequently affected than girls. A history of an antecedent viral upper respiratory infection, particularly influenza, is common. In years with influenza epidemics, *S. aureus* pneumonia may occur more frequently.[154] The interval between the apparent viral illness and the onset of *S. aureus* pneumonia may be brief.

S. aureus may also cause pneumonia in the nosocomial setting. In fact, epidemics often associated with isolates of phage type 80/81 once plagued neonatal nurseries, but they have largely disappeared for unexplained reasons.

S. aureus pneumonia usually follows inhalation of the infecting organism. Less commonly, *S. aureus* pneumonia may result from seeding of the lung during bacteremia.[155] Predisposing illnesses in this regard include infections of the venous system, intravenous substance abuse, or chronic vascular catheterization for hemodialysis or other purposes. In this instance, the radiographic picture may be that of multiple small, discrete pulmonary infiltrates that may become cavitary within a few days.

On autopsy, few distinctive features (except edema and scattered hemorrhages) are noted in the lungs of patients with *S. aureus* pneumonia. Histopathologically, there is generalized interstitial infiltration with polymorphonuclear and mononuclear cells in both the alveolar walls and septal tissue. There are important differences in the pathology of *S. aureus* pneumonia that depend on the age of the patient and the clinical presentation. In rapidly progressive cases, the large bronchial epithelium may be inflamed, covered with a fibrinous pseudomembrane, or extensively destroyed by infiltration of the underlying walls by polymorphonuclear leukocytes. Necrosis of smaller bronchi leads to pulmonary artery branch thrombosis with septic embolization to the lung parenchyma. The alveoli fill with edematous fluid and contain extravasated blood, polymorphonuclear leukocytes, and hyaline membranes. Destruction of alveoli may lead to the formation of a pneumatocele or tension pneumothorax; unable to escape through a necrosed bronchus, air becomes trapped in an area of necrosed alveoli. A pneumatocele formed in this manner may rupture and produce a pneumothorax or a pyopneumothorax. The pneumatoceles may disappear when the surrounding pneumonia resolves and the trapped area finds an avenue for escape.

In less rapidly progressive cases, the lungs are firm and consolidated beneath the pleural surface; involvement is more patchy and mainly affects the segments of the posterior lower lobe. These segments may coalesce and form small abscess cavities that may communicate with small bronchi and fill them with pus.

In the neonate, the pathology of *S. aureus* pneumonia may resemble both these processes. Alternatively, there may be a more diffuse, nonnecrotizing picture consisting of lobular or lobar areas of hemorrhagic consolidation with a well-structured fibrinous layer that may overlie the pleural surface. Abscess cavities are more common and may also be diffusely distributed.

The severity of the clinical picture varies. Typically, a mild upper respiratory tract infection is followed by fever, cough, grunting, and tachypnea.[156] Occasionally, prostration, cyanosis, dyspnea, shock, or even the toxic shock syndrome[157] may be present, particularly when *S. aureus* pneumonia results from bacteremic seeding of the lung. In neonates, the clinical course of staphylococcal pneumonia is often fulminating and is associated with a high mortality rate shortly after the onset of symptoms. Fever may be absent.

A greatly increased leukocyte count, sometimes called a *leukemoid response,* is said to be classic for *S. aureus* pneumonia but is variably present and nonspecific.[155] Some patients are bacteremic, but the proportion is unknown.

At the onset of clinically manifested *S. aureus* pneumonia, the chest radiograph may be normal.[158] However, the radiographic picture of staphylococcal pneumonia is more commonly bronchopneumonia with a patchy, central alveolar infiltrate. Multiple areas may be involved, but the process is generally unilateral (Fig. 39-11). The infiltrates tend to coalesce rapidly and form large consolidations; cavitations may be present within the infiltrate (Fig. 39-12). Indeed, the rapidity of the radiographic progression to a virtual "whiteout" of the lung may be striking and should raise the possibility of *S. aureus* pneumonia when it occurs. In many patients, a pleural

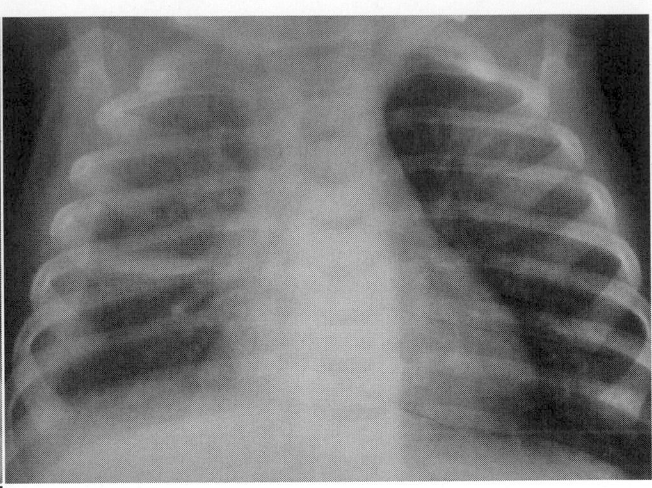

A B C

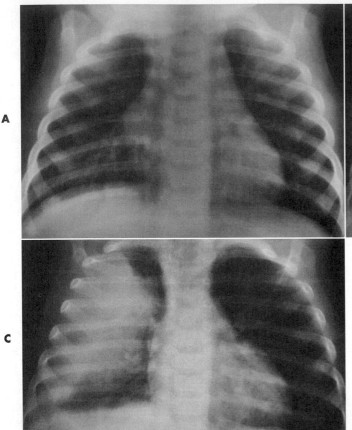

Fig. 39-11. Staphylococcal pneumonia. A 5-month-old boy with clinical pneumonia with fever and cough. **A,** At presentation, the chest radiograph was apparently normal. **B,** On the third day, it showed pneumonia of the right lower lobe with an associated parapneumonic effusion. **C,** On the twelfth day, a typical, fusiform large pleural empyema had evolved.

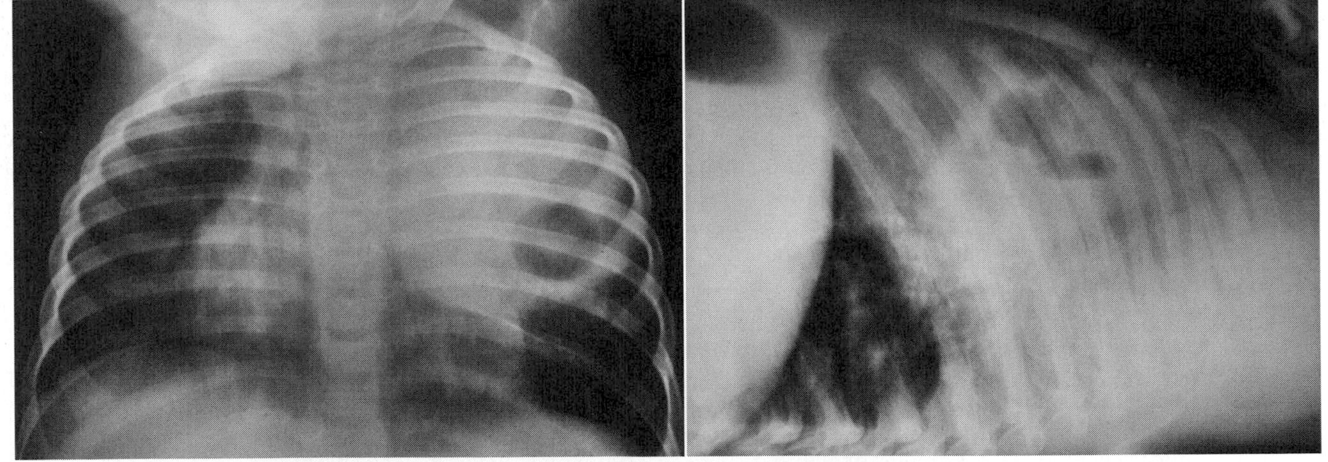

A B

Fig. 39-12. Staphylococcal pneumonia with cavitation. An 11-month-old boy with staphylococcal pneumonia in the left upper lobe. Both radiographs demonstrate the expanded, consolidated left upper lobe, which contains multiple air- and fluid-filled cavities. At 14 years of age, this boy manifests a hyperlucent, hypoperfused left upper lobe with thin-walled clear cavities. **A,** Supine anteroposterior chest radiograph. **B,** Supine horizontal beam lateral chest radiograph.

effusion is not visible on the first radiograph, but an effusion and empyema develops in about 90% of patients. The pleural effusion may be large and therefore may mask the underlying consolidation, the effect being that of an opaque chest. Spontaneous pneumothorax and pyopneumothorax occur in about 25% to 50% of cases. Pneumatoceles occur in more than 50% of cases (Figs. 39-12 and 39-13) and may change hourly in number and size during the acute phase. Occasionally, they are sufficiently large to mimic a tension pneumothorax or to cause mediastinal shift. They may also contain fluid. The finding of a pneumatocele strongly suggests the diagnosis of *S. aureus* pneumonia. The radiographic picture of staphylococcal pneumonia, however, is not pathognomonic. Similar findings, including pneumatoceles, may occur with pneumonia caused by *E. coli, Pseudomonas* or *Klebsiella* species, other gram-negative bacteria, group A streptococci, and occasionally, pneumococci.

Staphylococcal pneumonia should be suspected in hospitalized infants, particularly those in intensive care units, who

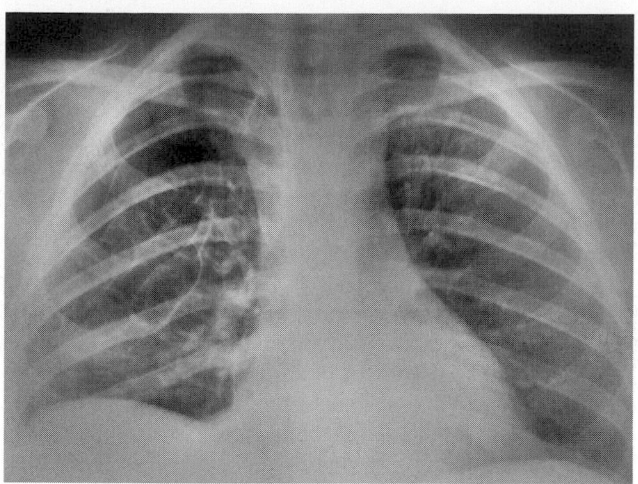

Fig. 39-13. Pneumatocele. Staphylococcal pneumonia in this 17-year-old girl resulted in a very large upper right pneumatocele that imitated a pneumothorax. A multiloculated pyopneumothorax with multiple air-fluid levels was also present.

develop new pleural parenchymal abnormalities or an unexplained opaque chest without volume loss. In the perinatal period, staphylococcal pneumonia with cavities or pneumatoceles may radiographically mimic congenital diaphragmatic hernia or cystic adenomatoid malformation.

When *S. aureus* is a consequence of pulmonary seeding during bacteremia, the chest radiograph may show many small, discrete infiltrates, some of which become cavitary. This entity should be considered in debilitated or young infants in the presence of an effusion or a pneumatocele.

When used for empiric coverage, extended-spectrum cephalosporins provide some coverage against *S. aureus*. Reliance on these agents, however, is suboptimal when *S. aureus* pneumonia is suspected based on clinical evidence.

The production of β-lactamase by nearly all *S. aureus* isolates has rendered ineffective any therapy using compounds hydrolyzed by this enzyme. Thus for many years, the first-line therapy for suspected *S. aureus* infections, including pneumonia, has been the so-called β-lactamase–resistant penicillins, such as methicillin. Although methicillin itself is no longer in use, its modern analogs (i.e., oxacillin cloxacillin, flucloxacillin, nafcillin) or first-generation cephalosporins (e.g., cefazolin) are available. The recognition of *S. aureus* isolates resistant to these agents, generically termed *methicillin-resistant S. aureus (MRSA),* has posed a therapeutic dilemma. By clinical definition, MRSA isolates are considered resistant to all β-lactam and all cephalosporin compounds. MRSA infections that are nosocomially acquired tend to be multiply resistant and have forced reliance on the glycopeptide vancomycin as the agent of choice for serious MRSA infections. Furthermore, community-acquired MRSA infections have recently become an increasing problem. Unlike their nosocomially acquired counterparts, community-acquired MRSA isolates are less likely to be multiply resistant. Clindamycin has been an effective alternative for *S. aureus* infections when the isolate is susceptible to methicillin and the patient is allergic to β-lactams or when the infection is caused by an MRSA isolate susceptible to clindamycin. The duration of antibiotic treatment is usually 2 to 3 weeks unless complications arise, although some would recommend up to 6 weeks to minimize the risk of recrudescence or relapse. Supportive therapy should include oxygen administration, maintenance of hemoglobin levels, and fluid and electrolyte maintenance as indicated. Pneumatoceles may persist for many weeks and require no special therapy.

The most important complications of *S. aureus* pneumonia are empyema and lung abscess.[159] *S. aureus* pneumonia may rarely result in the formation of a bronchopleural fistula, which in turn may lead to the formation of tension pneumothoraxes that are occasionally bilateral. In adults, these have been managed with synchronous independent lung ventilation.[160] Aortobronchial fistulae have also been reported as a complication of *S. aureus* pneumonia.[161] In adults, *S. aureus* pneumonia has also been associated with Pancoast's syndrome.[162]

The prognosis is usually good. Recovery is eventually complete when appropriate therapy is instituted and when complications are identified and treated promptly.

H. Influenzae Type b

Before the introduction of vaccine, *H. influenzae* type b was an important cause of childhood pneumonia. A precise estimate of its incidence has not been available, mainly because of diagnostic difficulties in identifying the etiologic agent, but a recent review concluded that *H. influenzae* type b was responsible for 5% to 18% of cases of bacterial pneumonia.[47] The advent of immunization against this important pediatric pathogen has decreased the occurrence of all invasive *H. influenzae* type b syndromes by more than 95% in many developed countries; presumably this includes pneumonia. The importance of *H. influenzae* type b as a cause of pneumonia was emphasized by a recent vaccine trial completed in Gambia, which suggested that *H. influenzae* type b pneumonia was an important clinical syndrome and accounted for a substantial proportion of presumed bacterial lower respiratory tract infections in children in developing countries.[163]

The first recognition of *H. influenzae* occurred during an influenza outbreak in Europe from 1889 to 1892, when Richard Pfeiffer identified a *Bacillus* species in the sputum of many patients with influenza.[164] Continued belief in associating "Pfeiffer's bacillus" with influenza resulted in the name *H. influenzae,* which was assigned to this bacterium by the Society of American Bacteriologists in the early 1900s. The genus name means "blood loving" in Greek and reflects the bacterium's requirement for the specific growth factors present in blood.

The realization that *H. influenzae* was the cause of several important infectious syndromes in childhood, including pneumonia, and was not the cause of influenza came from the work of Margaret Pittman; in 1931, she also recognized that the serotype b capsule was the major virulence factor among isolates causing invasive disease.[165] Subsequent investigations determined that antibody to polyribosylribitol phosphate (PRP), the serotype b capsular polysaccharide, could protect against invasive disease.[166] This observation spawned efforts to develop immunity by active immunization.

H. influenzae is a fastidious, gram-negative, pleomorphic coccobacillus that requires factors X (hematin, heat stable) and V (phosphopyridine nucleotide, heat labile) for growth. These factors are present within erythrocytes, and the demonstration of their requirement for growth is the basis for speciating *H. influenzae* in the laboratory.

Some *H. influenzae* isolates are surrounded by a polysaccharide capsule. Such isolates can be serotyped into six antigenically and biochemically distinct types, designated *a* to *f*. The most virulent isolates belong to serotype b. Before the introduction of immunization, these were responsible for almost all *H.*

influenzae invasive infections in children, including meningitis, cellulitis, epiglottitis, septic arthritis, osteomyelitis, pericarditis, bacteremia without focality, and a variety of other rare syndromes. Disease caused by other capsular serotypes of *H. influenzae* was rare[167] but is now proportionally more frequent. Nonencapsulated (nontypeable) *H. influenzae* isolates can cause invasive disease in neonates,[168] immunocompromised children,[169] children in certain developing countries,[170] and rarely, children in the United States.[167] Nontypeable isolates are common etiologic agents in certain mucosal infections, such as otitis media and sinusitis.[171,172] They have also been associated with chronic obstructive pulmonary disease in adults. Other *Haemophilus* species are occasional causes of invasive disease, including pneumonia. For example, *Haemophilus parainfluenzae* may cause pneumonia with empyema.

Humans are the only natural hosts for *H. influenzae*. It is not widely appreciated that this species is a constituent of the normal respiratory flora in 60% to 90% of healthy children and is a frequent isolate from the oropharynx. The great majority of these isolates are nontypeable. Colonization by serotype b organisms is infrequent. Before the advent of conjugate vaccine immunization, *H. influenzae* type b could be isolated from the pharynx of 2% to 5% of healthy preschool and school-age children[173,174]; lower rates occurred in infants younger than 1 year of age and in adults. Asymptomatic colonization with *H. influenzae* type b occurs at lower rates in immunized individuals and populations in whom effective vaccine delivery is widespread.

Before the introduction of vaccine, a striking feature of the epidemiology of invasive *H. influenzae* type b infections was its age distribution. In the United States, more than 90% of all infections occurred in children 5 years of age or younger, although a few occurred in older children and adults. Some 69% to 82% of invasive infections occur in children younger than 2 years of age, and about half occur in those younger than 12 months. The peak attack rate occurs at 6 to 12 months of age. Most studies showed a predominance among male patients.

In the era before the availability of *H. influenzae* type b conjugate vaccine in the United States, the annual attack rate of invasive disease was estimated to be 33 to 129 cases per 100,000 children (younger than 5 years of age) per year.[175] In Finland the reported annual incidence was 41 cases per 100,000 children in the prevaccine era; 40% occurred in children older than 2 years of age.[176] Populations identified as having an increased incidence of invasive disease include Alaskan Eskimos, Apache and Navajo Native Americans, and African-Americans.[177] In these populations, the number of cases of invasive disease in children younger than 12 months of age is relatively high. People known to be at an increased risk for invasive disease include those with sickle cell disease, asplenia, congenital and acquired immunodeficiencies, and malignancies. In addition, nonvaccinated infants younger than 12 months of age with previously documented invasive infection are at an increased risk for recurrence.

Socioeconomic risk factors for invasive *H. influenzae* type b disease include day-care outside the home, the presence of either school-age or younger siblings, short duration of breast-feeding, and parental smoking. In addition, previous hospitalization for invasive *H. influenzae* type b disease and a history of otitis media are associated with an increased risk for invasive disease. Much less is known about the epidemiology of *H. influenzae* infections other than serotype b.

For all *H. influenzae* isolates, the most common mode of transmission is by direct contact or by inhalation of respiratory tract droplets containing *H. influenzae*. The incubation period for invasive disease is variable, and the exact period of communicability is unknown. Invasive *H. influenzae* type b colonizes the nasopharynx in the majority of children before the initiation of antimicrobial therapy; 25% to 40% of children were colonized within the first 24 hours of therapy.[178]

Among age-susceptible household contacts who have been exposed to a case of invasive *H. influenzae* type b disease, there is a substantial risk of developing "secondary" invasive disease in the first 30 days (estimated at 0.26%). The attack rate for such disease in household contacts is highest in susceptible children younger than 24 months of age (3.2%) and rare in contacts older than 47 months of age (<0.1%). Unlike in the general population, asymptomatic carriage of *H. influenzae* type b is frequent in household contacts of patients with disease. More than 75% of families have at least one colonized household member in addition to the index patient.[179]

The precise mechanisms that facilitate successful colonization of the respiratory epithelium have yet to be identified. In an organ culture of human nasopharyngeal tissue, both type b and non-b strains of *H. influenzae* organisms attach to nonciliated columnar epithelial cells and subsequently can be seen within those cells and in the intercellular spaces.[180]

The events that result in the entry of serotype b organisms into the intravascular compartment remain unclear. Once there, however, type b strains resist intravascular clearance mechanisms more readily than strains of other serotypes and nonencapsulated organisms. It is uncertain whether the type b PRP capsule itself confers the potential for invasive disease or whether it is another closely linked virulence factor. A yet undeciphered clue may lie in the predilection of genes encoding for PRP to be present in an unusual tandem arrangement on the genome of 98% of clinical isolates.[181]

Once established, *H. influenzae* type b bacteremia is sustained. According to data from both animal models and patients, the magnitude of bacteremia and its duration are independent variables that determine the likelihood of dissemination of bacteria into sites such as the meninges or joints.[182] The bacterial and host mechanisms that determine the magnitude of bacteremia are poorly understood.

Noninvasive *H. influenzae* infections, such as otitis media, sinusitis, and bronchitis, which are usually caused by nontypeable strains, probably gain access to sites such as the middle ear or sinus cavity by direct extension from the pharynx. Serotype b organisms are infrequent causes of these noninvasive infections but probably cause disease by the same mechanism. The factors facilitating spread from the pharynx are not fully understood but include eustachian tube dysfunction and certain antecedent viral infections of the respiratory tract.

In 1933, Fothergill and Wright[183] demonstrated that susceptibility to invasive *H. influenzae* type b disease was related to lack of "bactericidal power" in the blood. It is now known that the bactericidal power of the blood reflects the sum of several elements of host defense, the most important of which is antibody directed against the type b capsular polysaccharide, PRP. It therefore follows that anti-PRP antibody is acquired in an age-related fashion and facilitates clearance of *H. influenzae* type b from blood in experimental animal models[184]; its presence was correlated with protection in several clinical trials that used both active and passive immunization.[166,185]

The mechanism of action of anti-PRP antibody is partly related to its opsonic activity; other antibodies directed against antigens, such as outer membrane proteins or lipopolysaccharides, may also play a role in opsonization. Both the classic and alternative complement pathways are important in the opsonization of *H. influenzae* type b. The macrophages of the reticuloendothelial system aid in the intravascular clearance of *H. influenzae* type b by affecting intracellular killing after opsonization.

Before the introduction of vaccination and then later among recipients of unconjugated PRP vaccines, protection from *H. influenzae* type b infection was presumed to be directly correlated with the concentration of circulating anti-PRP antibody at the time of exposure. A serum antibody concentration of 0.15 to 1.0 μg/ml was considered protective against invasive infection,[186] with the higher concentration in PRP vaccinees possibly predicting maintenance of a level of more than 0.15 μg/ml over time. Most infants lack an anti-PRP antibody concentration of this magnitude and are thus susceptible to disease on exposure to *H. influenzae* type b.

Unlike the PRP unconjugated vaccine, the conjugate vaccines behave as thymus-dependent antigens with the exception of PRP outer membrane protein, which also has thymus-independent type I properties (Table 39-3). That is, they elicit serum antibody responses in young infants although multiple doses may be required, and they prime for memory antibody responses on subsequent encounters with PRP.[187] More important, the concentration of circulating anti-PRP antibody in a child whose immune system has been primed by a conjugate vaccine may not correlate precisely with protection because a memory response may occur rapidly on exposure to PRP and provide protection.[188]

Some have postulated that the anti-PRP antibody response to natural infection and immunization may in part be genetically controlled because certain individuals have a higher relative risk for invasive *H. influenzae* type b disease and may also respond suboptimally to vaccine administration. However, more information is necessary to clarify this interesting possibility.

The signs and symptoms of pneumonia caused by *H. influenzae* type b cannot be distinguished from those caused by pneumonia resulting from many other microorganisms. Associated infectious foci, such as meningitis, are common; pneumonia is frequent in children with acute epiglottitis.[189]

The radiographic manifestations of *H. influenzae* pulmonary infection (Fig. 39-14) vary from a bronchiolitic type of picture with central linear infiltrates and overinflation to bronchopneumonia with patchy consolidation of no lobar predilection. Pleural effusion is present in about a third of patients with *H. influenzae* bronchopneumonia; less commonly, a pericardial effusion may be present and may be seen by plain films when it is large or by sonography when it is smaller. Pneumatoceles are rare but have been reported.[190]

Presumptive identification of *H. influenzae* can be made by direct examination of the collected specimen after Gram's staining. Visualization of *H. influenzae* is sometimes difficult because of its small size, pleomorphism, and poor uptake of stain by some isolates and by the tendency for fluids to have a red background (particularly when proteinaceous); staining with methylene blue may aid in visualization. With this technique, *H. influenzae* organisms appear as a blue-black coccobacilli against a light blue-gray background.

Culture of *H. influenzae* requires prompt transport and processing of specimens because the organism is fastidious. Primary isolation of *H. influenzae* can be accomplished on chocolate agar, *Haemophilus* isolation agar, or blood agar plates. Serotyping of *H. influenzae* is accomplished by slide agglutination with type-specific antisera. Biotyping of *H. influenzae* isolates is seldom performed in clinical laboratories.

Table 39-3 *H. influenzae* Type B Conjugate Vaccines

MANUFACTURER	ABBREVIATION	TRADE NAME	CARRIER PROTEIN
Pasteur-Mérieux-Connaught	PRP-D	ProHIBit	Diphtheria toxoid
Wyeth-Lederle Vaccines and Pediatrics	HbOC	HIBTITER	CRM_{197} (nontoxic mutant diphtheria toxin)
Merck and Co.	PRP-OMP	PedvaxHIB	OMP (outer membrane protein complex of *Neisseria meningitidis*)
Pasteur-Mérieux-Connaught*	PRP-T	ActHIB, OmniHIB	Tetanus toxoid

Modified from American Academy of Pediatrics: *Haemophilus influenzae infections*. In Peter G, ed: *1997 redbook: report of the Committee on Infectious Diseases*, ed 24, Elk Grove Village, Ill, 1997, American Academy of Pediatrics, p 225.
*Distributed in the United States by Connaught Laboratories and by SmithKline Beecham.

The techniques used in the detection of PRP in CSF, serum, urine, or other relevant body fluids are counterimmunoelectrophoresis, latex agglutination, staphylococcal protein A coagglutination, and enzyme immunoassay.[191] Latex agglutination and coagglutination, which use vehicles in suspension that bind antibody to PRP with latex beads and staphylococcal cells, respectively, have been widely used in clinical microbiology laboratories because their sensitivity for detecting PRP is relatively high. Latex agglutination is perhaps the most sensitive, versatile, and accessible method for the direct detection of PRP[191] when the results of culture are not revealing. The use of immunologic methods for detecting type b PRP capsular antigen is most helpful for diagnosing *H. influenzae* type b infections in patients who have received prior antimicrobial therapy.

Children younger than 12 months of age suspected of having *H. influenzae* type b pneumonia should promptly receive parenteral antimicrobial therapy because of their increased risk for bacteremia and its complications. Older children who do not appear severely ill and are therefore unlikely to be bacteremic may be treated with an orally administered antimicrobial; customarily a 7- to 10-day course of parenteral, oral, or combined parenteral-oral therapy is completed.

Diagnostic examination of pleural fluid from an uncomplicated pleural effusion associated with *H. influenzae* type b pneumonia may yield the causative organism. Generally, no special therapeutic intervention is required. However, if clinical evidence of empyema develops, insertion of a chest tube and a more prolonged course of antimicrobial therapy may be necessary.

Before 1974, all *H. influenzae* isolates were presumed to be susceptible to ampicillin. Subsequently, chloramphenicol became the agent of choice for therapy against invasive *H. influenzae* type b disease. Advantages of chloramphenicol have included low cost and good penetration into CSF. In addition, this agent is effective against most isolates of *H. influenzae* type b irrespective of β-lactamase production. The disadvantages of chloramphenicol include the necessity for monitoring serum levels and often emotionally held views re-

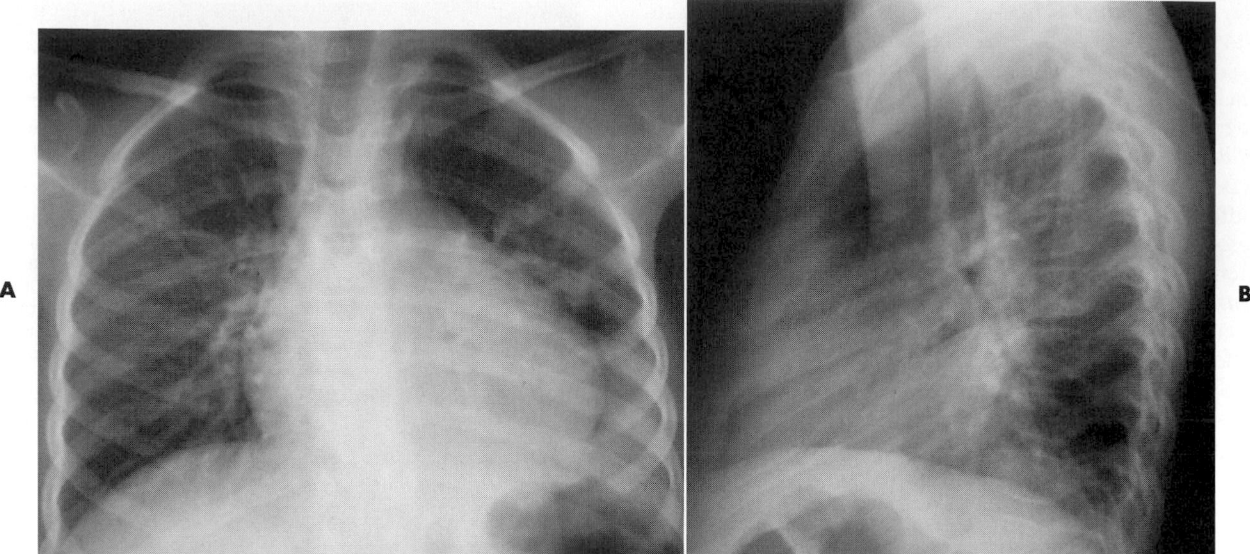

Fig. 39-14. Pneumonia caused by H. influenzae in a 6-year-old girl with cough, fever, and chest pain. **A,** Anteroposterior view. **B,** Lateral chest radiograph reveals an airspace infiltrate in the left lower lobe with an associated small pleural effusion. Cardiomegaly resulted from an associated pericardial effusion.

garding the rare occurrence of idiosyncratic aplastic anemia. Chloramphenicol-resistant isolates of *H. influenzae* type b have been identified but have remained relatively infrequent in the United States and worldwide; however, they are more common in a few locales such as Barcelona and Taiwan.

Isolates resistant to both chloramphenicol and ampicillin have rarely been identified. The most recent worldwide tabulation, done in 1987, identified 39 cases of ampicillin- and chloramphenicol-resistant *H. influenzae* type b meningitis. In the United States, less than 1% of isolates were resistant to both compounds.

Among antimicrobials used for oral therapy of mild *H. influenzae* infections, resistance to TMP/SMX or amoxicillin/clavulanate occurred in less than 1% of clinical isolates in the most recent national survey conducted in the United States from 1987 to 1988. Erythromycin has poor activity against *H. influenzae.*

The initial antibiotic therapy of invasive infections possibly caused by *H. influenzae* type b should be a parenterally administered antimicrobial agent effective in sterilizing all foci of infection. Such therapy should also be effective against ampicillin-resistant strains. Extended-spectrum cephalosporins, such as cefotaxime or ceftriaxone, have achieved popularity because of their relative lack of serious adverse effects and ease of administration. To date, resistance to extended-spectrum cephalosporins has not been documented. Alternatively, chloramphenicol can be used with ampicillin.

Once the antimicrobial susceptibility of the isolate has been determined, an appropriate agent can be selected to complete the therapy. Ampicillin remains the drug of choice against infections caused by susceptible isolates. When the isolate is resistant to ampicillin, extended-spectrum cephalosporins have been widely used. (One of these, ceftriaxone, can be administered to outpatients once a day in selected circumstances.) Chloramphenicol has also received extensive clinical use.

Oral antimicrobial agents are sometimes used to complete a course of therapy initiated by the parenteral route and even as initial therapy for older children with pneumonia who are not very ill. The principles of therapy are the same: When the isolate is susceptible to ampicillin, it or amoxicillin is the compound of choice. When the isolate is resistant to ampicillin, cefixime, amoxicillin/clavulanate, or TMP/SMX may be used. Chloramphenicol is another option that remains popular in some countries because of its low cost.

Before the widespread use of *H. influenzae* type b conjugate vaccines, it was realized that children younger than 48 months of age in close contact with patients with invasive *H. influenzae* type b infections were at an increased risk of invasive infection when exposed to an index case.[178] Many children are now protected against *H. influenzae* type b by prior immunization. Thus with the excellent efficacy associated with conjugate vaccine administration in the United States, the need to offer chemoprophylaxis to household contacts has become infrequent.

In households where one or more children younger than 48 months of age are not fully immunized, rifampin prophylaxis is indicated for all members of the household contact group in whom a case of *H. influenzae* type b disease occurs. This recommendation includes the index patient. Relevant definitions and dosing recommendations have been found in the Report of the Committee of the American Academy of Pediatrics.[146]

Parents of children hospitalized for invasive *H. influenzae* type b disease should be informed about the increased risk for secondary infection caused by this organism in other young, partially immunized children in the same household; parents should be alerted to any signs or symptoms that might indicate such an infection and should be instructed to seek prompt medical attention when such signs appear. Although parents of children exposed to a single case of invasive *H. influenzae* type b disease in a day-care center or nursery school should be similarly warned, there has been disagreement about the use of rifampin for these children. Because the data conflict on the risk of secondary *H. influenzae* type b infection among children who attend group day-care, some experts believe that the risk is too low to justify the effort associated with chemoprophylaxis in this setting. In addition, it would be difficult to institute a uniform policy that would include all the different caretakers and physicians involved. A few general guidelines for chemoprophylaxis that might be useful in evaluating a day-care setting for possible rifampin administration follow:

1. Rifampin prophylaxis may be of benefit in day-care homes resembling households, such as those with children younger than 2 years of age, in whom there is contact at least 25 hours per week.
2. Administration of rifampin to all attendees and supervisory personnel is recommended when two or more cases of invasive disease have occurred within 60 days among attendees, regardless of the size of the day-care.
3. Chemoprophylaxis need not be given if all day-care contacts are older than 2 years of age.

With the development of conjugate vaccines that have proved more immunogenic in younger children than the unconjugated form, the first generation PRP vaccine has been replaced by four licensed *H. influenzae* type b conjugate vaccines that differ in the carrier protein used, the saccharide molecular size, and the method of conjugating the saccharide to the protein[192] (see Table 39-3). The recent introduction of effective immunization against *H. influenzae* type b with the use of the conjugate vaccines has greatly decreased the occurrence of *H. influenzae* type b infections.[193-195]

Streptococcus Agalactiae (GBS)

The designation *group B β-hemolytic streptococci (GBS)* was first applied by Lancefield in 1933[196] to *S. agalactiae,* an important cause of bovine mastitis known to infect cows as early as the 1800s.[197] In the 1960s, GBS became increasingly recognized as a cause of neonatal infection, including pneumonia. Today, GBS are common causes of pneumonia and other invasive infections in neonates.

Group B is distinguished from other streptococcal groups by its distinctive carbohydrate antigen, which is bound to the bacterial cell wall; L-rhamnose is the major antigenic determinant. Several serotypes have been described including Ia, Ib, II, III, IV, V, VI, VII, and VIII.[197a] A surface antigen, protein C is common to all Ib isolates, all isolates formerly designated Ic (now Ia/c), 60% of type II isolates and, occasionally, isolates of serotype IV-VI. Serotypes Ia, III, V, and II cause most disease in young infants.

GBS infections are often classified by the onset time of clinical manifestations. Although this distinction is somewhat artifactual and there is substantial overlap in the comparison of the clinical features of so-called early onset and late-onset disease, differences in pathogenesis, clinical syndromes, and the responsible serotypes have made separation of these syndromes of some use. Early onset disease is manifested in the first week of life, often on the first day. GBS of all serotypes cause this syndrome with roughly equal incidence. Transmission of GBS most likely occurs a short time before birth. Risk factors for early onset disease include prematurity, prolonged rupture of the chorioamnionic membranes before birth, or maternal infection. Late-onset disease is manifested after the first week of life, with most cases occurring in children younger than 1 month of age. GBS disease is extremely rare in toddlers and older children; occasionally, very late-onset GBS disease occurring in older children may be an early manifestation of HIV infection.[198] In late-onset disease, serotype III organisms are almost exclusively responsible for infection. The transmission of GBS in patients with late-onset disease is believed to occur after birth, either during or after the hospital stay. Carriage, once acquired, may persist for many months.

Early onset disease is more frequent than late-onset disease. A prospective study documented the incidence of invasive GBS disease as 3.7 and 1.7 per 1000 live births for early onset and late-onset disease, respectively.[199]

For early onset disease, the clinical picture is one of sepsis.[200] The features may include onset within hours of birth, tachypnea, apnea, and a generally ill appearance. Pneumonia is almost always present. The pulmonary clinical picture may be indistinguishable from the so-called respiratory distress syndrome of prematurity.[201,202]

Late-onset disease is more indolent in its presentation. Fever, bacteremia, and meningitis are commonly but not universally present. GBS with late presentation is not usually associated with pneumonia.[203] If present, the clinical features are characteristic of pneumonia caused by other bacteria. Indeed, an identifiable infectious focus may not be evident. In one series, about one third of infants with GBS disease, most of whom had late-onset disease, did not appear ill or irritable, and about one third had no fever.[203] Occasionally, the clinical picture of early onset disease may be evident, and the chest radiograph may resemble that caused by respiratory distress syndrome.

The diagnosis is made by recovery of the organism from blood or another normally sterile body fluid, such as pleural fluid, CSF, urine, or synovial fluid. Detection of the group B carbohydrate antigen in urine, blood, or CSF (e.g., by latex agglutination)[204] is useful but requires careful interpretation. The sensitivity and specificity of this test are about 90% and 80%, respectively. However, even in a population at relatively high risk for GBS infection, the predictive value of a positive test is only about 60%.[204] Urine testing in particular has been prone to false-positive and false-negative findings; because of this, in March 1997 the Food and Drug Administration issued a safety alert regarding testing of urine specimens.

The treatment for GBS pneumonia in the absence of meningitis involves 200,000 units/kg per day intravenously in three divided doses in the first week of life and 300,000 units/kg per day intravenously in four divided doses thereafter. A 14-day course is usually administered for pneumonia. Higher doses and a 21-day course are often used when meningitis is present. Initial therapy of the β-lactam with an aminoglycoside results in more rapid killing in vitro and may be a useful clinical adjunct.[205] Other options include ampicillin or ceftriaxone. Intravenously administered immune globulin has been used as adjunctive therapy, but data establishing its effectiveness are lacking.

Empyema may complicate group B streptococcal pneumonia. Some have suggested that right diaphragmatic hernia may complicate group B streptococcal pneumonia, but it seems more likely that this association represents a preexisting condition.[206,207] The associations with group B streptococcal pneumonia, group B streptococcal bacteremia, a generalized septic picture, and distant metastatic infectious foci (such as meningitis and skeletal infections) are well described. It is probable that group B streptococcal pneumonia seldom occurs in an infant who is not systemically ill.

Even when appropriate antimicrobial and supportive therapy are initiated in a timely way, the mortality rate from early onset GBS disease is high (about 14%), particularly in cases occurring in the immediate perinatal period and those in small premature infants.[208] Many authors believe that this rate represents a decline from higher rates,[209] possibly as a result of improved supportive care. The mortality rate from late-onset disease is much lower (about 2% to 6%).[203,210]

Some have advocated intravenously administered immune globulin to prevent GBS infections. However, in a prospective trial of 2416 very-low-birth-weight newborns who were randomized to receive either placebo or intravenously administered immune globulin every 2 weeks until the infant weighed 1800 g, no difference was identified between the two groups in the incidence of GBS infection, length of hospitalization, or mortality rates.[211]

Antibiotic administration has been used to interrupt the transmission of GBS from mother to neonate. Antenatal antimicrobial treatment of colonized women aimed at eradicating carriage has not been effective.[212] Moreover, Siegel et al[213] administered penicillin to unselected neonates at birth as prophylaxis against GBS disease but found no associated decrease in mortality rates, an increase in the recovery of penicillin-resistant organisms of other genera, and increased mortality rates from infections caused by these penicillin-resistant isolates; however, intrapartum ampicillin decreased the maternal-fetal transmission of GBS.[214,215] This observation led to recommendations from the Centers for Disease Control and Prevention (CDC)[216] to screen for GBS transmission and assess risk factors to identify a subset of pregnant women who might benefit from intrapartum penicillin therapy aimed at interrupting carriage. Risk factors include a mother previously giving birth to an infant with GBS disease, GBS bacteriuria during the current pregnancy, premature delivery, prolonged rupture of membranes, and intrapartum fever. In the absence of these risk factors, the rectum and vagina are cultured for GBS at 35 to 37 weeks' gestation, and intrapartum penicillin therapy is then offered to women identified as GBS carriers.

Efforts to prevent GBS disease by vaccination are ongoing. Many investigators have advocated immunizing pregnant women in the hope of transferring antibody produced by immunization to the fetus in utero, thereby offering protection in the neonatal period. A tetravalent polysaccharide vaccine produced only a modest response in healthy adults.[217] Conjugate vaccines consisting of the capsular polysaccharide covalently linked to tetanus toxoid have been studied in animals and are currently being evaluated in humans. A novel approach to vaccine development has used Rib and α-proteins on the GBS cell surface as vaccine antigens[218]; however, to date, evaluation of a candidate vaccine consisting of these proteins has been limited to animal models.

Causes of Less Frequent Clinical Concern

Acinetobacter Species

Members of the genus *Acinetobacter*[219] are gram-negative bacilli with variable morphologic pictures depending on the phase of growth in broth culture and environmental conditions. The organism is a strict aerobe that is ubiquitous in water, sewage, and soil. Several species have been described. From clinical specimens, the most common isolates belong to the *A. baumanii–A. calcoaceticus* complex and *A. lwoffi*. *Acinetobacter* species are not members of the resident skin flora but may transiently colonize skin, saliva, or other body secretions. Most often, the organism is a commensal. Invasive infection is associated with a stay in an intensive care unit, immune deficiency, antimicrobial treatment, invasive use of instruments, and prolonged venous catheterization.

Pneumonia caused by *Acinetobacter* species is rare, particularly in children; it has been described only in those with impaired immunity. In adults, *Acinetobacter* pneumonia is usually sporadic, although outbreaks have been described. For example, an outbreak of pneumonia occurred in foundry workers who were presumably exposed to infected metallic dust. Members of *Acinetobacter* species survive well in water; thus the use of respiratory therapy equipment, particularly endotracheal intubation and aerosols, are risk factors for *Acinetobacter* infections. Cases of *Acinetobacter* pneumonia occur more often in the summer than in other seasons.

No unique pathologic or clinical features distinguish *Acinetobacter* pneumonia from other bacterial pneumonias. More than one lobe is involved in most reported cases. Empyema and the formation of intrapulmonary cavitations have been described.

Because this species may colonize asymptomatically, isolation of the organism from pharyngeal secretions is not helpful in the diagnosis of *Acinetobacter* pneumonia. Definitive diagnosis is based on lung aspirate or biopsy or isolation of the organism from blood in the presence of a clinical picture compatible with pneumonia.

Susceptibility testing of clinically relevant isolates aid in antibiotic selection. Therapy usually consists of TMP/SMX, 10 to 12 mg/kg/day (TMP) in two or three doses per day. Meropenem may be of use if TMP/SMX is contraindicated. *Acinetobacter* species are variably susceptible to cephalosporins and aminoglycosides. Synergy between β-lactam and aminoglycoside antibiotics has been reported.

Actinomyces Species

The term *actinomycosis* was first used in 1877 by Bollinger to describe sarcoma-like masses in the jaws of cattle.[220] In the same year, after examining material from such masses under the microscope, Harz described "strahlenpilz," or "ray fungus," in such lesions and named the organism *Actinomycosis bovis*.[221,222] In 1878, Israel discovered the organism in necropsy material in humans.[222] Actinomycosis of the thorax was first described by Ponfick in 1882,[222] and Israel described 38 patients with this disorder 5 years later.[221]

In 1949,[222] the name *Actinomyces bovis* was changed to *Actinomyces israelii* to describe the organism that caused infection in humans, whereas the designation *A. bovis* was reserved for disease occurring in cattle.[223] The current view is that *A. israelii* accounts for the preponderance of cases, but other members of the genus, including *A. naeslundii, A. eriksonii, A. meyeri,* and *A. odontolyticus,* have occasionally been isolated. *Arachnia propionicus,* which was a former member of the genus *Actinomyces,* is an occasional cause of the clinical syndrome of actinomycosis.[224]

Actinomycosis is uncommon in children.[225] About 10% of all cases occur in children younger than 18 years of age.[226] Only six cases were identified in children in the United Kingdom and Ireland in 1971 and 1972.[227] It is more common in immunocompromised children and those with poor oral hygiene. Distribution is worldwide; there is no racial or occupational predisposition. A male predilection has been noted in adults, but studies in children suggest no gender differences.[228] Actinomycosis is not believed to be contagious, and the causative organisms have been isolated only from humans.[226]

The following factors are important in the predisposition to clinical disease: trauma and a favorable anaerobic milieu for the bacterium[229] that may be a saprophytic inhabitant of the normal oral cavity and nasopharynx, particularly at the gum margins and in the presence of dental caries. The organism has also been found in tonsillar crypts, periodontal tissue, paranasal sinuses,[230] and gastric and bronchial secretions.[221] Pulmonary infection is probably initiated when organisms reach lung tissue after ingestion or aspiration.[226] Bates and Cruickshank[222] believed that the tonsillar beds were the most important reservoir for inhalation-acquired pulmonary disease. They further suggested that previous lung injury increases the likelihood of disease when aspiration or inhalation occurs. Because the onset of the disease can occur at any time after colonization is initiated, the incubation time varies from days to years after initial contact with the organism.[231]

Infection occurs by direct tissue invasion[228] without regard for tissue planes.[224] *Actinomyces* organisms are readily phagocytized by host defense cells but, like mycobacteria, are often not killed after the ingestion.[223]

Actinomycosis is classified into the following syndromes: cervicofacial, abdominal, and thoracic. (The last includes pulmonary and extrapulmonary intrathoracic disease.) Overall, about 15% to 20% of patients with actinomycosis have pneumonia.[221] Most have primary pulmonary involvement.[230] Among 48 adults and children with actinomycosis pneumonia, 8 had evidence of bacteremic seeding of the lung or extension from an extrapulmonary site, whereas 40 had lung involvement considered to be primary.[226] In this instance, infection usually arises from aspiration of infected material from the oropharynx[226] and rarely arises after esophageal disruption secondary to nonpenetrating trauma or surgery.

Pulmonary actinomycosis is a chronic, localized inflammatory process.[226] Histologic features include a thick, fibrous wall without necrosis in loculated regions. The finding of so-called sulfur granules (small, lobulated, grainy microcolonies of bacteria 1 to 2 mm in size that are cemented together by a protein-polysaccharide capsular complex) is virtually pathognomonic for actinomycotic infection; the granule may be mineralized with calcium phosphate and may sometimes be visible macroscopically.[232] Necrosis rarely occurs,[226] although focal liquefaction without fibrosis is occasionally present.[226] Large macrophages with foamy cytoplasm accumulate around the purulent center. These may be absent in acute lesions, in which mostly fibrin is found.[227]

Symptoms of pulmonary involvement include low-grade fever and cough productive of purulent or blood-streaked material. Sputum, if present, is usually not malodorous. Dyspnea and orthopnea have been noted.[226] Other symptoms may include malaise, anorexia, weight loss, and localized chest pain.[224] Nonspecific laboratory findings may include moderate leukocytosis and anemia, particularly in more chronic cases.

Physical examination may reveal asymmetric crackles and dullness on percussion. Signs suggesting the presence of a pleural effusion may be apparent. There may be subcutaneous abscesses over the chest wall. Examination of the abdomen may be abnormal and reflect extension of the infectious process through the diaphragm.

A delay in diagnosis is common.[233] The median number of weeks between presentation and diagnosis is 3 to 5 and ranges up to 24 weeks.[233] The initial diagnosis in many cases is malignancy. The presence of chest pain, which is common in actinomycosis but less so in malignancy, may help distinguish this condition from others.[233] For example, a 10-year-old boy with chest pain who had sustained a chest wall injury by falling from his bicycle was treated by a psychiatrist for 12 months for "psychosomatic" chest pain and listlessness before the correct diagnosis of actinomycotic pneumonia was made.[221] Another reason for delay is the lack of a typical picture. Children may be asymptomatic despite the presence of a large pulmonary mass.[230]

The distinctive radiographic characteristics of actinomycosis involving the lung are secondary to its "lack of respect" for the anatomic boundaries of the chest compartments. Pulmonary actinomycosis may appear radiographically as an infiltrate with associated soft tissue, rib, and pleural involvement. Primary pulmonary involvement may start as a patchy, peripheral, airspace infiltrate similar to that occurring in pneumococcal pneumonia and may resolve completely if treated; basal lobe involvement is frequent. If untreated, however, intrapulmonary cavitation or mass lesions may be present; the process may extend peripherally to cause empyema, rib osteomyelitis with the pathognomonic contiguous dense periosteal reaction[220,230] in multiple ribs, or a chest wall abscess.[234] The radiographic "classic triad" of actinomycosis, lung infiltrate, and rib or chest wall involvement as well as empyema[235] are useful in suggesting the correct diagnosis but is infrequently present.[233,235] Occasionally, there is vertebral destruction.[220,230] Parasitization of the blood supply by these lesions from the chest wall circulation may result in systemic to pulmonary shunting.[110]

As with any other complex thoracic process that involves the chest wall as well as intrathoracic structures, CT, preferably contrast enhanced, is the imaging modality of choice. CT is used when chest radiographs do not clarify the findings[236] or when the suspicion of a malignancy is high.

The differential diagnosis includes other infectious processes that tend to disregard tissue boundaries, such as blastomycosis, cryptococcosis, tuberculosis, and rarely, aspergillosis. Rib destruction associated with intrathoracic opacities may be present with pyogenic osteomyelitis, chest wall tumors (particularly Ewing's sarcoma), and primitive neuroectodermal tumors.

Definitive diagnosis is by histopathologic examination.[232] The diagnosis is suggested by the finding of beaded, branched, gram-positive bacilli in pus, and it is strongly endorsed by isolation of the organism; the visualization of typical gram-positive, branching bacilli in histologic sections; or the presence of sulfur granules.

The organism may be isolated from tissue obtained by local resection, lobectomy, transthoracic needle aspiration,[233] or pleural fluid.[237] Resection is most commonly performed because malignancy is incorrectly suspected.[238] *A. israelii,* the most frequent isolate, grows anaerobically and usually requires 4 to 8 days for incubation. *A. meyeri* is occasionally the isolate and has a predilection for the apical region.[239]

Actinomyces species is usually not isolated in pure culture.[230] In about two thirds of cases, another bacterium, often *Actinobacillus actinomycetoconcomitans,* was isolated.[221,229] Some have theorized that the presence of an aerobic bacillus lowers the redox potential of the tissue and thereby promotes the growth of *Actinomyces* species[230] by improving the anaerobic growth conditions.

Both the dosage and duration of penicillin therapy have not been critically evaluated, and clinical experience is therefore anecdotal.[220,230] Most experts recommend an initial course of intravenous penicillin at high dosage (e.g., 250,000 units/kg/day) for 2 to 6 weeks and then oral penicillin (e.g., 125 mg/kg/day) for several months thereafter. One case of thoracic actinomycosis was successfully managed with oral phenoxymethyl penicillin (125 mg/kg/day).[239a]

Actinomyces species is susceptible to penicillin, but prolonged therapy for thoracic actinomycosis is necessary to prevent relapse. Initially a high dosage of penicillin (250,000 units/kg/day in four to six doses given intravenously)[224] is traditionally used.[220] Therapy is given for about 6 weeks and then is continued orally at a lower dosage (50 to 100 mg/kg/day in four divided doses)[224] for an additional 6 to 12 weeks. Some[230] have exclusively advocated oral penicillin V therapy (e.g., 125 mg/kg/day) with reportedly good results. Irrespective of the therapeutic regimen used, the dose and length of penicillin treatment should be related to the amount of induration and fibrosis and the extent of infection at the time of diagnosis.[228,230] Separate therapy directed against concomitantly isolated organisms, such as *A. actinomycetoconcomitans,* is traditionally said not to be necessary. Clindamycin, erythromycin, chloramphenicol, and tetracycline (for children 9 years of age and older) are alternative treatment choices.[237] Serial radiography of the chest is useful in documenting the adequacy of therapy.[224]

The main role of surgery is to drain any abscesses or empyema that may be present. Surgery was once believed necessary to cure actinomycosin. Radical surgery is still sometimes performed, particularly in the presence of extensive fibrosis, or unwittingly as a treatment for a commonly presumed diagnosis of carcinoma.[240] Management in the modern antibiotic era must be individualized; even in the presence of extensive disease, it is reasonable to consider that medical therapy alone warrants consideration.

The mortality rate in untreated or inadequately treated cases has been about 90%.[220,230] Conversely, about 90% of those treated recover.

Complications of actinomycosis pneumonia include the development of parenchymal abscesses or empyema and the formation of draining sinuses. In one review, such sinuses were present in 25% of patients with thoracic actinomycosis.[226] They may connect with the trachea, esophagus, pericardium, heart, or skin.[241] Rib and vertebral destruction may occur by direct extension.[241] Disseminated disease, although rare in children,[242] may complicate thoracic actinomycosis[229,230,242] and may be fatal despite accurate diagnosis and treatment.[226] Good oral hygiene is the best available prevention against actinomycosis.

Anaerobes

Guillemot et al[243] first reported in 1904 that empyema could be caused by bacteria that did not grow under standard, aerobic conditions. It was realized that because similar organisms were also found in the oral cavity, an aspiration event and pneumonia probably preceded the empyema.[244] Subsequently, more than 2000 cases of anaerobic empyema were reported in the preantibiotic era.[245] With the advent of antibiotics, however, interest in anaerobic pneumonias decreased until the 1970s, when a resurgence of interest occurred because of improved techniques for anaerobic culture, organization of anaerobic taxonomy (to lessen confusion), and trials of therapeutic agents that required bacteriologic confirmation.[244]

It is believed that a major role should be ascribed to anaerobic bacteria as a cause of aspiration pneumonia. It follows that patients predisposed to aspiration, such as children with dysphagia, seizures, neurologic disorders (including cerebral palsy), general anesthesia, drug use, gastroesophageal reflux, or compromised consciousness, are at risk. If aspiration occurs when the child is in the upright position, the basal segments of the lower lobes are the most common sites of pneumonia, whereas if the child is recumbent, the posterior segments of the upper lobes or the superior segments of the lower lobes are more likely locations of pneumonia.[244,246]

In the absence of such a predisposition, the role of anaerobes in uncomplicated pneumonia remains uncertain, particularly in children. In adults, some[247,248] have suggested that pneumonitis caused by anaerobes cannot be distinguished from other bacterial pneumonias, and because the microbiologic evaluation of any pneumonia is often difficult and anaerobic cultures are seldom performed, any existing role for anaerobes in uncomplicated pneumonia may not be adequately appreciated.

Few data exist regarding the specific anaerobic organisms that might cause pneumonia in children. Experience in adults suggests that the most frequent isolates are anaerobic streptococci, such as *Peptostreptococcus* species; microaerophilic anaerobic streptococci such as *S. intermedius, S. parvulus, S. constellatus, S. morbillorum* (now reclassified as *Gemella morbillorum*); and other anaerobic organisms such as *Bacteroides melaninogenicus* (now referred to as *Prevotella*), *Porphyromonas* species, and *Fusobacterium nucleatum.*[246] The *Bacteroides fragilis* group includes most of the pathogenic anaerobic organisms.[249]

Treatment of pulmonary infections involving anaerobes usually involves one of three strategies. *Bacteroides* species are usually susceptible to penicillin G, ampicillin, and broad-spectrum penicillins. Some authors believe that penicillin G is the drug of choice for anaerobic pneumonia,[250] whereas others favor clindamycin because it is active against almost all mouth and respiratory tract *Bacteroides* isolates.[146,247] β-Lactamase production has been identified in many non–*B. fragilis* species and in fusobacteria.[249] Susceptibility of non–*B. fragilis Bacteroides* isolates was recently surveyed at 28 U.S. centers, and it was found that 64.7% of *Bacteroides* species and 41.1% of fusobacteria elaborated β-lactamase.[249]Anaerobic susceptibility testing is technically difficult, particularly for slow-growing and fastidious organisms such as *Fusobacteria* and non–*B. fragilis Bacteroides* species.[249] Thus the clinical laboratory seldom provides meaningful guidance in this area.

Complications of anaerobic pneumonia include lung abscess and empyema,[246] entities that are dealt with separately in this chapter.

Arcanobacterium Haemolyticum

A. haemolyticum[251,252] is a rare cause of pneumonia in children. The organism is a gram-positive bacillus, with humans as the primary reservoir. The incubation period is unknown, although long-term pharyngeal carriage has been identified.

The usual manifestation is a skin infection or pharyngitis. However, when this pathogen causes pneumonia, respiratory signs and symptoms, such as tachypnea, fever, and coughing, may be present.

The organism may be isolated from a blood culture. Although serologic antibody tests for *A. haemolyticum* exist, none have been standardized or are commercially available.

The organism is susceptible to penicillin, erythromycin, clindamycin, chloramphenicol, and tetracycline. All these agents appear appropriate for therapy.

Bacillus Anthracis

Anthrax is usually a disease of livestock caused by *B. anthracis,* which are large, aerobic, spore-forming, gram-positive, rod-shaped bacteria. It is found in cattle, sheep and goats.[253] In the United States, it is endemic in the states where livestock is concentrated.[253] Human infection has all but vanished in the United States. When it occurs, it is acquired via the lungs or skin after contact with hides, furs, wool, or other spore-contaminated animal products.[253] With rare exception, finished animal products (e.g., leather coats) are not a source of spores.[253] Anthrax has also been diagnosed in humans living near an animal wool- or hair-processing plant and by human-to-human transmission via shared toilet articles.[253] Transmission has also been identified via insect transport from infected animals.[253]

The virulence of *B. anthracis* is due to its weakly antigenic, antiphagocytic, poly-D-glutamic acid capsule and the production of three exotoxins called *edema factor, lethal factor,* and *protective antigen.* The capsule and toxin genes have been localized to plasmids routinely found in virulent isolates.[254]

There are three clinical forms of anthrax. The majority of cases involve characteristic skin lesions and regional lymphadenopathy. Pulmonary involvement (the so-called inhalational form) is initiated by inhalation.[254] After inhalation, the spores are transported by lung macrophages to mediastinal and hilar nodes.[171,253,255] Either during transport or on arrival at the lymph node, the spore germinates, a process that may result in severe, hemorrhagic lymphangitis with marked adenopathy.[253] The bacilli may then enter the bloodstream and disseminate.[253] The lung may be seeded during this bacteremic phase. Rarely, a patient with anthrax may have clinical features of gastroenteritis.

The hallmark of pulmonary involvement is hemorrhagic edema. Microscopically, there is massive hemorrhage and edema fluid in all involved airspaces. A serofibrinous exudate with many large bacilli and an absence of polymorphonuclear leukocytes is typical. In patients who have survived for a prolonged time, the septa become necrosed, and fibrin thrombi obliterate the pulmonary capillaries.

Clinically, the onset of systemic anthrax is insidious, with malaise, a nonproductive cough lasting many days, and low-grade fever. Stridor may also be present secondary to mediastinal nodal compression of the trachea.[253] When bloodstream invasion occurs, there may be a sudden onset of high fever and shock accompanied by dyspnea and cyanosis. These events usually lead to death within 24 hours.[253]

Obtaining a history of exposure to the infectious agent is important; few cases occur in which such an exposure cannot be identified. The diagnosis of *B. anthracis* infection is made by visualization of the organism after Gram's stain of material obtained from a lesion or discharge, growth in culture, or direct immunofluorescence of tissue or culture material. Several serologic tests are available for the diagnosis of anthrax. Antibodies to the protective antigen and the lethal factor component of the anthrax toxin have been detected by immunoblot. Detection of the antiprotective antigen titer may be more sensitive than detection of antilethal factor antibody.[256] A microhemagglutination test has been used in the past but has been replaced by more modern methodology.[257] Antibody to the poly-D-glutamic acid capsule has also been detected by enzyme-linked immunosorbent assay (ELISA).[256] PCR aimed at detecting a 277–base pair fragment of the *B. anthracis* genome has shown some promise for future clinical application.[258]

The chest radiograph usually demonstrates marked widening of the mediastinum associated with mediastinal and hilar lymphadenopathy, patchy or diffuse confluent infiltrates, and consolidations seen with hemorrhagic pneumonia. Pleural effusions are common, and areas of localized pulmonary edema secondary to lymphatic blockage may occur either unilaterally or bilaterally.[171,253]

High-dose intravenous penicillin is the drug of choice[253] and is given for 5 to 7 days. Tetracycline, chloramphenicol, ciprofloxacin, and erythromycin are also effective and useful for the penicillin-allergic patient. Cutaneous anthrax responds well to therapy, and lesions lack viable bacteria within hours of treatment initiation. The American Academy of Pediatrics[259] suggests using streptomycin in addition to high-dose penicillin for inhalation anthrax, an illness that is usually diagnosed late in the course with near certain mortality. Death from the cutaneous form of anthrax is rare; however, the prognosis is poor for inhalation of anthrax.

Complications of respiratory anthrax include meningitis and gastrointestinal tract involvement. Necrotic intestinal lesions have been found at autopsy.[253]

Patients with anthrax should be isolated until antibiotics have been administered for 72 hours. For individuals at ongoing risk of acquiring anthrax, a killed vaccine is available from the Michigan Department of Public Health. The efficacy of this vaccine has been established in adults. However, no data are available in children, and the vaccine is therefore not licensed for use in them. Development of improved component vaccines is underway.[260]

Other Bacillus Species

Bacillus species are members of the family Bacillaceae, a group of aerobic, saprophytic, sporulating organisms commonly isolated from dust, soil, air, and water. Although they frequently contaminate clinical specimens, members of the genus may cause endophthalmitis, meningitis, and endocarditis; may contaminate hemodialysis equipment; and may cause food poisoning. As a pulmonary pathogen, the species *B. cereus* has received recent attention in immunocompromised hosts[261] and at least occasionally in patients with normal immune systems. Two premature infants who died with evidence of necrotizing pneumonia with *B. cereus* as the causative agent were recently described.[262] At autopsy, one had scattered "tan" areas with well-demarcated areas of necrosis and large numbers of visualized gram-positive rods, and the other had pneumonitis with well-defined areas of necrosis not associated with substantial inflammatory cellular infiltrates. Acquisition of the organism was believed to be nosocomial. Other *Bacillus* species have been implicated even less frequently; pneumonia and empyema were found to be caused by a *Bacillus* species that resembled *B. alvei,*[263] and an adult with chronic asthma had a gelatinous pseudotumor of the lung caused by *B. sphaericus.*[264]

Antimicrobial therapy for infections caused by *B. cereus* is complicated by the realization that members of the species are generally resistant to β-lactams and cephalosporins. However, clindamycin, imipenem, vancomycin, erythromycin, chloramphenicol, and aminoglycosides have been highly active. Other *Bacillus* species are usually susceptible to β-lactams and cephalosporins.[265]

Bartonella Henselae

Cat-scratch disease (CSD) was first described in 1950 by Debre et al.[266] It has now been recognized that the causative organism is usually, if not always, *B. henselae* (formerly known as *Rochalimaea henselae*), a fastidious, slow-growing, gram-negative bacterium. Pneumonia associated with CSD is exceedingly rare and has been described in only a few children.[267]

CSD is a common infection in children[268]; 80% of cases occur in those younger than 20 years of age. Transmission is via contact with a cat or kitten; more than 90% of patients with CSD have a history of feline exposure.

Patients with CSD usually have self-limited regional lymphadenopathy after contact with a cat or more commonly, a kitten.[269] Constitutional symptoms occur in 50% to 70% of cases and are usually limited to fever and less frequently, emesis, seizures, and respiratory distress.[267] Only five cases of pneumonia and pleural effusion were identified in a recent review[267]; all had multisystem involvement. The pathogenesis of CSD pneumonia is uncertain; hematogenous seeding of the lung during bacteremia has been proposed.[267] Pleural effusion is usually present. A recent case report involving a 19-year-old renal transplant recipient called attention to pulmonary nodules thought to be caused by *B. henselae*[270]; interestingly, this patient had frequent contact with cats. Because the association between these nodules and *B. henselae* was established by PCR, it is possible that application of this sensitive technique will expand knowledge of the spectrum of pulmonary infection caused by *B. henselae.*

The diagnosis of CSD is usually made serologically. Immunofluorescent assays and ELISA tests are available for the detection of antibody directed against *B. henselae*. The immunofluorescent assay performed by the CDC[271] has been the gold standard. The newer ELISA assay[272] is more widely available but may be less sensitive than the immunofluorescent assay performed by the CDC.[273]

Detection of *B. henselae* nucleic acid sequences by PCR using primers directed at the citrate synthase gene[274] and the 16S ribosomal ribonucleic acid gene[275] of *B. henselae* was accomplished in bacteremic cats but is not yet available for use in human specimens. Identification of the distinctive morphology of *B. henselae* by Warthin-Starry silver impregnation stain is useful if tissue is available. Culturing *B. henselae* has remained problematic; successful cultivation has been largely limited to the CDC laboratory and is performed there by heart infusion agar with defibrinated rabbit blood in the presence of 5% carbon dioxide for 7 to 14 days at 35° C.[274] Administration of antimicrobials diminishes the likelihood of successfully cultivating the organism or visualizing it by Warthin-Starry staining.

No controlled trials of antimicrobial therapy have been performed for the treatment of CSD, and the few cases of pneumonia described in children provide little help. Clearly, CSD even with pneumonia is a self-limited illness. Thus antibiotics might shorten the clinical course but are unlikely to improve the long-term outcome, which is generally excellent. The choice of antimicrobial agents is another area of uncertainty.[276] Erythromycin and TMP/SMX have been advocated for severe CSD, as has ciprofloxacin alone or in combination with gentamicin, but no data from controlled trials exist. Tetracycline has been found to decrease bartonellemia in cats.[277] Adults with severe *Bartonella* infection have responded to erythromycin, doxycycline alone or in combination with rifampin, or rifampin and gentamicin. Patients with bacillary angiomatosis or parenchymal peliosis, which are unusual and severe manifestations of *Bartonella* infection in patients with HIV infection, have responded to erythromycin, doxycycline, and clarithromycin.

The development of feline vaccines against *B. henselae* might be useful in decreasing the incidence of transmission and infection in human hosts.[277]

Brucella Species

Brucellosis is a rare human disease that may be caused by one of several small, gram-negative rods in the genus *Brucella,* including *B. melitensis, B. abortus,* and *B. suis.*[278] Human infection is caused by direct contact, usually via ingestion of unpasteurized dairy products, accidental laboratory exposure, or contact with diseased swine, cattle, or wild animals (e.g., moose).[253,278] Specific to each organism, *B. melitensis* may be transmitted from goats, their carcasses, or their secretions. *B. abortus* may be transmitted by direct contact with cows, their carcasses, or their secretions, including milk. Pasteurization of milk and milk products is especially important in the prevention of disease in children. The certification of raw milk does not eliminate the risk of transmission of the organism.[146] Humans are also accidental hosts for *B. suis* and contract disease by direct contact with pigs, their carcasses, or their secretions. Rarely has human transmission been thought to occur in family clusters.[278] Infection may also be transmitted by the inhalation of contaminated aerosols. The incubation period varies from less than 1 week to several months; most children are ill within 3 to 4 weeks of exposure.

Brucellosis pneumonia is rare. Histologically, there are fibrinous pleuritis and proliferation of pleural endothelial cells found with a round cell interstitial infiltration. Nodules that resemble a tuberculous granuloma may be found.

Particularly with *B. melitensis,* which is the endemic species, disease can be severe with either an acute or an insidious onset. Although fever is usually present, there are no unique clinical findings, which makes the diagnosis difficult. It has been termed *a disease of mistakes.*[278] Nonspecific complaints, including sweats, weakness, malaise, anorexia, weight loss, arthralgias, myalgias, and backache, abound. Findings on physical examination may include lymphadenopathy and rarely hepatosplenomegaly. Cough is variably present. Chest radiographic findings may include bronchopneumonia, single or multiple nodules, and hilar adenopathy.[253]

Diagnosis is based on the isolation of excised, caseous nodules from the lung. Isolation of the causative organism from the blood is possible, but the yield is low.[279] The laboratory should be alerted that this diagnosis is being considered because the incubation time may be long and the organism may be misidentified by automated identification systems. Serologic testing has been the hallmark of diagnosis. A presumptive diagnosis may be made by showing a high (≥1:160) or rising serum titer of specific antibodies in a child with symptoms consistent with brucellosis. The serum agglutination test is most commonly used and detects antibody to *B. abortus, B. melitensis,* and *B. suis* but not *B. canis.* False-negative results may be related to the prozone effect. Newer serologic tests, including an ELISA for antibodies, are under evaluation but are not yet widely available.[279] Recently, the diagnosis of brucellosis has been accomplished by PCR using primers directed at a 31-kD protein from *B. abortus.*[280]

The standard antigen cross-reacts with all *Brucella* species except *B. canis* but may also react with *Yersinia enterocolitica, Vibrio cholerae,* and *F. tularensis.*[278] When brucellosis is being considered, the laboratory should be notified so that multiple serial dilutions of serum can be performed to exclude the prozone effect.[281] Treatment is with tetracycline, 30 to 40 mg/kg/day in four doses daily (if over 9 years of age), or oral doxycycline, 5 mg/kg/day in two doses, both for 4 to 6 weeks. If the clinical symptoms are severe, streptomycin or gentamicin, in addition to doxycycline or tetracycline, may be administered for the first 7 to 14 days of therapy.[278] In small children, TMP/SMX is usually used.[281] The conditions of most children receiving the appropriate antibiotics respond to treatment.[281]

Complications include lung abscess, pleural effusion, empyema, and atelectasis secondary to large hilar nodes pressing on a bronchus.[253]

Burkholderia (Pseudomonas) Cepacia

B. cepacia is an increasingly recognized cause of nosocomial pneumonia, particularly in children with immunodeficiency. The organism was first described in 1950 as causing a "soft rot" in onions.[282] It is closely related to *Pseudomonas mallei, P. pseudomallei, P. pickettii,* and other *Pseudomonas* species that are plant pathogens. It is only distantly related to *P. aeruginosa.*[282]

The organism is ubiquitous and versatile; it seems to thrive under adverse conditions and can even use penicillin for its "food" supply.[282] The organism is durable and resistant to many disinfectants, antiseptics, and preservatives. Children are thought to acquire the organism in the hospital or via contact with colonized siblings.[282] Strain-specific properties are now being identified that may in part determine which strains are efficient colonizers of susceptible patients, such as those with cystic fibrosis (CF).[283]

The organism is virtually nonpathogenic in the healthy child or adult. In less than 2% of healthy adults the pharynx is colonized.[284] A recent case report documenting community-acquired *B. cepacia* pneumonia in an otherwise normal child[285] attests to the rarity of infection in that clinical setting. In patients with altered host defenses, such as children with CF,[286] burns, and indwelling catheters or other medical devices, serious infection, including pneumonia, endocarditis, meningitis, bacteremia, peritonitis, postoperative and burn wound infections, skeletal infections, and lung abscess, may occur. *B. cepacia* infection may be the first manifestation of chronic granulomatous disease. Children with CF whose respiratory secretions are colonized with *B. cepacia* tend to have more serious lung disease and poorer pulmonary function than those who are not colonized with this organism.

Virulence factors[287] include an extracellular protease,[288] lipase, and siderophore. The genetic regulation of these exoproducts has been the subject of recent attention[289]; extracellular material from broth cultures of *P. aeruginosa* increase the production of protease, lipase, and siderophore in *B. cepacia.* Such interspecies signaling might allow insight into certain bacterial interactions in the lungs of patients with CF.

Histopathologic examination of lungs infected with *B. cepacia* revealed several disease patterns that included severe necrotizing pneumonia[282] and atypical granulomatous lesions in a patient with chronic granulomatous disease. In patients with *B. cepacia* colonization and CF, lobar and peribronchial pneumonia with neutrophilic infiltrates and microabscess formation occurs most commonly without necrotizing pneumonia or vasculitis.[290] A more chronic inflammatory infiltrate with interstitial pneumonitis in the presence of macrophages, lymphocytes, and plasma cells has also been described.

In adults with CF who are colonized with *B. cepacia,* the following clinical patterns have been observed: (1) chronic asymptomatic carriage, (2) progressive deterioration over many months with recurring fever and weight loss, and (3) rapid, usually fatal, deterioration.[291] In other patients, the clinical picture may resemble that of other bacterial pneumonias.

Diagnosis is by isolation of the organism from blood or sputum. Isolation from the latter may pose a problem for the clinical laboratory because other bacteria are likely to be present in the secretions of patients with CF; selective media, such as PC agar or an oxidation-fermentation base, contain antibiotics and other ingredients aimed at suppressing other flora, thereby aiding in the diagnosis.

B. cepacia is resistant to multiple antimicrobials; thus treatment poses a challenge. Previously, the most effective antibiotics were chloramphenicol and TMP/SMX. The child with CF, however, is often resistant to these agents. Ureidopenicillins (e.g., azlocillin, mezlocillin, piperacillin), extended-spectrum (third-generation) cephalosporins, quinolones, minocycline, imipenem, and aztreonam have been variably useful. In vitro susceptibilities may guide the choice of compounds, although ceftazidime has been associated with clinical failure despite in vitro susceptibility.[282] High-dose[292] therapy with the chosen antibiotic may be necessary because the pharmacokinetics of many antibiotics are altered in patients with CF.

There are no definitive measures to prevent *B. cepacia* infections. Cohorting of colonized individuals, education regarding optimal infection-control practices, and careful handwashing all decreased colonization of *B. cepacia* in one large CF center; these measures have been widely adopted.[293]

Citrobacter Species

Citrobacter species are most often associated with neonatal sepsis and meningitis; species members are rare causes of sporadic pneumonia, which occurs almost exclusively in neonates and immunocompromised individuals. *Citrobacter* organisms were first isolated in 1932 by Werkman and Gillen,[294] who proposed the generic term *Citrobacter* and described seven species. A bewildering array of taxonomic changes[295] ended in 1977, when Brenner et al[296] designated the following species: *C. freundii, C. amalonaticus,* and *C. diversus. Citrobacter* organisms are enteric gram-negative rods that are closely related to *Salmonella* organisms. In humans, *Citrobacter* species are most often reported as a cause of meningitis in the neonate.

Most cases are sporadic, although outbreaks have been described. Once introduced into the nursery, *Citrobacter* species colonization may become prevalent. One study in a neonatal nursery identified 11 of 128 infants colonized with *C. diversus.*[297] The umbilicus was the most frequent site of colonization.

The diagnosis is made by identifying the causative bacterium in blood, CSF, or in an older child, sputum. Treatment is with an aminoglycoside or an extended-spectrum cephalosporin. Almost all isolates are ampicillin resistant.

The fatality rate for *Citrobacter* infections in newborns and older immunocompromised patients with *Citrobacter* pneumonia has been said to be high.[295,298] Recent data defining these rates more precisely are not available.

The complications of *Citrobacter* pneumonia include associated bacteremia with metastatic foci, particularly meningitis. *C. diversus* pneumonia may also be associated with abscess formation in the lung[299] and with empyema.

Corynebacterium Species

Members of *Corynebacterium* species are gram-positive bacilli that have rarely been implicated as a cause of pneumonia in either immunologically normal or abnormal hosts. Examples are *C. xerosis,*[300] *C. pseudodiphtheriticum,*[301] and *C. jeikeium.*[302] Most patients have an underlying disorder. Fever is often absent. In vitro, *C. pseudodiphtheriticum* isolates were susceptible to ampicillin and other β-lactams but were often resistant to clindamycin and erythromycin. A report from Spain describing a patient with empyema fluid from which *Corynebacterium* species was isolated suggests that empyema may complicate *Corynebacterium* species pneumonia.[303] The condition of this patient was managed with imipenem and clindamycin.

Coxiella Burnetii

In 1935, the disease caused by the organism *C. burnetii* was given the name *Q fever* by Dr. E.H. Derrick of the Queensland Health Department in Australia because he was unable to diagnosis the disease and therefore referred to it as *Q* for "query" fever. He enlisted the help of Sir MacFarlane Burnet, who pursued the etiology and sent specimens to Dr. Rolla Dyer, then the director of the U.S. National Institutes of Health. Dr. Dyer himself had contracted a similar disease during a site visit to the Rocky Mountain Laboratory in Montana, where two researchers had isolated an organism from a tick that they thought was a rickettsia. There, two U.S. researchers, Dr. Herald Rea Cox and Dr. Gordon Davis, then isolated the same organism from Dr. Dyer's blood and in 1938, demonstrated that the Australian and Montana organisms were the same. In honor of the joint project, the organism was named *C. burnetii* for Drs. Cox and Burnet.[304] The first cases of *C. burnetii* pneumonia were identified in 15 of 153 employees who had contracted the illness in one building of the National Institutes of Health in 1940.[305]

C. burnetii is a gram-negative, pleomorphic coccobacillus that undergoes phase variation. In nature, the organism exists in the phase I state; repeated passage of phase I organisms leads to the isolation of phase II avirulent forms. The morphology of organisms of the two phases is identical, although the biochemistry of the lipopolysaccharide differs.[306] The organism is able to form spores, which allows it to survive for more than 40 months in skim milk at room temperature and more than 1 month on or in meat in cold storage.[304] The six strains follow: Vacca, Rasche, Hamilton, Biotzere, Dod, and Corazon. *C. burnetii* infects many different animal species. Sheep, cattle, and goats are the traditional animal reservoirs, although horses, pigs, cats, and dogs may also be infected.[304] Once infected, animals may shed the organism for several months. For example, cows may shed *C. burnetii* in milk for up to 32 months; after birth, sheep may shed it in feces for 11 to 18 days.[307]

Humans are the only animal in which *C. burnetii* infection usually proceeds to illness. The usual route of infection is by dose-dependent aerosol aspiration.[308] Human-to-human transmission is rare.[304] The organism has been transmitted by a blood transfusion and from human autopsy material.

The illness is commonly limited to a fever lasting 2 to 14 days. Occasionally, pneumonia develops. The incidence of Q fever pneumonia is unknown and varies by geographic region, possibly reflecting strain-specific properties.[304]

The clinical features of Q fever have included fever, fatigue, chills, myalgias, nausea, vomiting, pleuritic chest pain, and cough. Headache may be severe and retroorbital. Signs of Q fever pneumonia vary; clinical evidence of respiratory tract involvement may be absent despite radiographic evidence of pneumonia. Alternatively, a dry, nonproductive cough may be present. Occasionally, the course is rapidly progressive. Physical examination of the chest of the patient with Q fever pneumonia may be normal; alternatively, inspiratory crackles may be present. Some 5% of patients with Q fever pneumonia have splenomegaly.[304]

The radiographic picture of patients with Q fever pneumonia is variable and includes nonsegmental and segmental pleural-based opacities. A pleural effusion is present in about one third. Atelectasis and hilar adenopathy are infrequent findings.

Most laboratories do not have the facilities necessary for the isolation of Q fever. Serologic diagnosis may be made by the detection of antibodies with a variety of techniques, including complement fixation microagglutination, microimmunofluorescence, and ELISA. A fourfold rise in serum antibody titer between the acute and convalescent phases is considered diagnostic.[304]

The best therapy for Q fever pneumonia is doxycycline or a combination of erythromycin and rifampin.[304] Most cases of pneumonia resolve, although death has been reported in one adult.[304]

An inactivated whole-cell Q fever vaccine has been developed but is not yet available.[309] It would presumably be used for high-risk populations, such as animal handlers and abattoirs.

E. Coli

E. coli is an extremely rare cause of childhood pneumonia except in neonates or in those with an underlying disease. *E. coli,* the "colon bacillus," was first isolated in 1885 by T. Escherich from the feces of breast-fed infants.[310] It is a gram-negative, nonencapsulated bacillus that may be either motile or nonmotile. Typing of strains is based on the following antigens: flagellar (H), somatic (O), and capsular (K or B). The ability of *E. coli* to bind to host tissue via specific fimbriae is an important first step in infection. S fimbriae, which bind to sialyl(α-2-3)galactoside, are found on neonatal K1 isolates. Hemolysin is another virulence-associated characteristic of severe *E. coli* infections in children.[311]

E. coli is an important cause of neonatal pneumonia when the causative organism is acquired either shortly before or during delivery.[312] The source of the organism is usually the maternal gastrointestinal tract or aspirated amniotic fluid. The incubation period is variable and ranges from birth to several weeks of age. A study of 34 infants with late neonatal pneumonia (onset of symptoms more than 48 hours after birth) suggested that *E. coli* was the probable etiology in 6%; coliforms accounted for 44% of these episodes.[313] *E. coli* strains with K1 capsular polysaccharide antigen are the most common causes of neonatal *E. coli* meningitis and bacteremia and of the less frequent invasive infections that occur in infants. In children older than 2 years of age, the importance of K1 is diminished[314] because invasive *E. coli* infections usually occur only in association with underlying disease.

Nosocomial acquisition of *E. coli* from nursery personnel and equipment has also been documented. In one intensive care nursery, gram-negative enteric bacilli caused 45.1% of cases of nosocomial pneumonia; *E. coli* was the most frequent of these.[315] Others at increased risk for *E. coli* infections may include neonates with immunologic defects, breakdowns in skin integrity, or asplenia.

E. coli may occur more frequently in malnourished older children in developing countries. In contrast to its rare occurrence in children beyond the neonatal age group in developed countries, a study in Nigeria identified *E. coli* pneumonia by lung aspiration in 8.8% of 99 malnourished children (age, 9 months to 5 years); this organism was the third leading cause of pneumonia in these children.[316] Similarly, 5.3% of malnourished children in Zaire had *E. coli* pneumonia.[317]

E. coli pneumonia may be acquired via inhalation or may result from bacteremic seeding of the lung. The organism is not a usual constituent of normal pharyngeal flora but may be found in the pharynx of ill children or adults, particularly among hospitalized patients. Spread in the hospital is facilitated by hand-to-mouth contact, often with fecal contamination, and by fomites, such as contaminated respiratory equipment.

A study of autopsy findings in neonates with *E. coli* pneumonia identified diffuse inflammation as the most common pathologic finding.[318] In contrast, diffuse bilateral lower lobe bronchopneumonia was found with occasional abscess formation in adults at autopsy. The alveoli were typically filled with fluid in the presence of mononuclear cells. The alveolar cells exhibited cuboidal metaplastic changes with thickened, edematous septa.

The clinical findings of *E. coli* pneumonia are nonspecific[318] and are similar to those of bacterial pneumonia of any etiology in the respective age group. The diagnosis is usually based on recovery of the causative organism from the blood. Because the K1 capsular polysaccharide cross-reacts with group B *N. meningitidis,* using commercially available reagents to detect the capsular polysaccharide of the latter bacterium is theoretically possible for diagnosing K1 infections in the newborn. In practice, however, this strategy has received little critical evaluation, so the clinician should not rely on it.

A pneumatocele has been reported in a neonate with *E. coli* pneumonia[319]; lung abscesses are rare. In general, if the correct diagnosis is made and appropriate treatment is instituted, recovery usually occurs. However, the more serious the underlying etiology, the higher the morbidity and mortality rates.

Childhood *E. coli* pneumonia is usually treated with an aminoglycoside, an extended-spectrum cephalosporin, or the two in combination. Although combination therapy is preferred, few explicit data document its superiority. Ampicillin may be substituted for the cephalosporin when the isolate is susceptible. Amikacin may be substituted for gentamicin if the isolate is resistant. At the University of Chicago Hospitals in 1996, 98% and 99% of *E. coli* isolates were susceptible to gentamicin and extended-spectrum cephalosporins, respectively.

F. Tularensis

The bacterium *F. tularensis* was first identified in 1910 by McCoy and Chapin in Tulare County, California, as the microorganism responsible for the plaguelike disease in ground squirrels (now called *Spermophilus beecheyi*) in that area.[320] The first human infection was identified in 1914 in a 21-year-old meat-cutter with inflammation of the left eye. However, it was not until 1921 that Francis (for whom the microorganism is now named) recognized the transmission pattern and the important role that arthropods play in transmission of the bacterium to humans. Although clinically inapparent pulmonary involvement was identified in a patient with tularemia at necropsy in 1924,[321] the first patient in whom pneumonia was a major clinical manifestation was not described until 1931.[322] The organism in culture is a fastidious, gram-negative coccobacillus.[323] In nature, however, it is a hardy organism that may survive for several weeks in water and mud, particularly around aquatic mammal dwellings.[324] Although it does not form spores, it resists drying and cold and thus may be transmitted as a fomite.[324] Two strains have been distinguished on the basis of biologic rather than serologic differences.[325] The highly virulent type 1 is also called *biovar A (tularensis)* or *Jellison type A,* and the less virulent type 2 is called *biovar* B_1 *(palaearctica)*[326] or *Jellison type B.*

Tularemia is endemic throughout the United States, with the highest number of cases occurring in Arkansas, Missouri, Montana, Oklahoma, Tennessee, Texas, Utah, and Wyoming.[324] Each year, 150 to 300 cases are reported.[325]

Both types 1 and 2 cause disease in the United States. Tularemia is also endemic throughout Europe and Asia,[253] although only type 2 has been identified in these regions.[326,327]

In the United States, transmission occurs mainly in the summer[325] but has been reported in every month of the year.[328] Male patients in rural areas are most commonly infected,[324] although infections are also well documented in urban environments.[329]

Tularemia is primarily a disease of wild animals; human infection is incidental[330] and can be initiated in several ways, including direct contact with or ingestion of infected animals or animal tissues; bites from ticks, flies, or other arthropods; inhalation of dust from contaminated environments[331]; and consumption of contaminated water. There have been no reports of person-to-person spread.

The causative bacterium has been reported in more than 100 species of wild mammals, such as rabbits, squirrels, woodchucks, opossums, and rats.[332] In addition, domestic species such as dogs and cats,[253,332,333] 25 species of birds (such as the chicken hawk), and several species of fish and amphibians,[324] have been implicated. Few of these actually serve as reservoirs, however, and like humans, most are occasional hosts. Species, such as rabbits, that serve as reservoirs do so in that they are frequent carriers but are not often diseased; it has been estimated that 15 to 3% of wild rabbits in the United States serve as a natural reservoir of tularemia[331]; jack, cottontail, and snowshoe varieties have all been implicated.

Tularemia occurring after bites by ticks, especially *Dermacentor andersoni* (wood tick), *Dermacentor variabilis* (dog tick), and *Amblyomma americanum* (Lone Star tick), represents the third most common tick-borne disease in the United States.[334] Tick bites account for about 50% of all cases of tularemia.[325,335] The organism is well-adapted to survive in the tick; it is capable of surviving the winter and of being transmitted from generation to generation. Gnats, mosquitos,[253] deer flies,[332,333] and probably other biting, blood-sucking insects may also serve as vectors for transmission to humans and to other "nonreservoir" animals.

Tularemia has traditionally been classified by its *form,* a term referring to a constellation of the clinical features that are initially recognized. The ulceroglandular form accounts for about 80% of reported cases. As the name implies, an erythematous, punched-out, indurated skin ulcer marks the portal of entry of *F. tularensis.* Tender, localized lymphadenopathy accompanies this lesion. A variant of this is the oculoglandular form, which is infection initiated by inoculation of a conjunctiva, usually by contaminated fingers. The glandular form is said to occur when the entry ulcer cannot be delineated. The oropharyngeal form occurs when the tularemia is characterized by the variable presence of an oral entry point, ulceration, and pseudomembranous tonsillitis. In addition, the following forms reflect the presence of systemic disease, often when the portal of entry is not apparent:

1. The typhoidal form presents a sometimes aggressive, septic clinical picture with high mortality rates. Early diagnosis often depends on whether the clinician considers such an infection.
2. Gastrointestinal tularemia is associated with the ingestion of contaminated food or water.
3. The pneumonic form is said to occur after direct inhalation of infected particles from an animal carcass,[331] a laboratory specimen, or contaminated dust.[324]

Some 6% to 30% of cases of tularemia occur in children,[331] mostly in the second decade of life. In Arkansas, 28% of cases occurred in children 11 to 14 years of age.[336]

Primary tularemia pneumonia can begin after the inhalation of infected particles. Pneumonia may also occur as a consequence of hematogenous spread.[253] In this instance, the organism is inoculated through a break in the surface of the epithelium or through intact skin. After inoculation, lymphatic spread ensues with the development of acute local inflammation, nodal swelling, necrosis, and caseation. The organisms may enter the bloodstream from the lymphatic system and become disseminated. Spontaneous resolution is unlikely once this occurs because *F. tularensis* is able to survive intracellularly, even when entrapped by the reticuloendothelial system.[337] Symptomatic bacteremic seeding of the lungs is manifested as a multifocal lobular or even lobar pneumonia with interstitial involvement. The process may be unilateral or bilateral with segmental, lobar, or patchy infiltrates. Less common manifestations include the formation of multiple small abscesses, cavitation, residual cysts, and a miliary pattern.[253] Microscopically, in patients who die of tularemia with pulmonary involvement, mononuclear cells are found in fibrin-rich alveolar exudate. Thrombosis and necrosis of small and medium-sized arteries and veins are common. A child with tularemic pneumonia and unrecognized chronic granulomatous disease was found to have discrete, round, nodular, well-localized areas of granulomatous inflammation in a subpleural and parenchymal distribution.[338]

Host resistance depends mainly on cell-mediated immunity,[339,340] with the implication that *Francisella*-specific T cells activate macrophages to kill the pathogen; interferon-γ may mediate this effect.[341] Recent evidence has suggested that CD4+ and CD8+ T cell–independent mechanisms may also play a role in host defense: Mice depleted of these cellular elements were still able to control experimental infection with *F. tularensis*.[340] Patients who survive infection are immune. The role of humoral immunity is less clear. Antibodies do not appear until 1 to 2 weeks after the onset of symptom.[339] Passively transferred antibody can confer protection on recipient mice,[342] and specific antibody enhances the rate of clearance of *F. tularensis* from blood.[343]

Tularemic pneumonia may pose a considerable diagnostic dilemma, especially when the portal of infection is not obvious. In an epidemic in Russia, the diagnosis was not initially entertained in 50% of cases.[344] A thorough clinical history, particularly with inquiries about contact with rabbits or other wild animals, provides an aid to diagnosis.[344]

There are no pathognomonic clinical features of tularemic pneumonia. The incubation period is 1 to 14 days.[253] The portal of entry is usually not obvious,[331] and pneumonia may be the sole manifestation of disease. Prodromal symptoms may include malaise, cough, and chest tightness lasting 10 days to 3 weeks. The onset is usually less abrupt than that of pneumococcal pneumonia and may be difficult to pinpoint with certainty. Chills and fever are usual. In Arkansas, 87% of children with pulmonary tularemia had fever.[336] A relative bradycardia may be present; peripheral vascular collapse is rare.

Few laboratory tests contribute valuable diagnostic information. In particular, the leukocyte and platelet count, erythrocyte sedimentation rate, and urinalysis were not found to be helpful.[336]

There is a dissociation between clinical manifestations attributable to pneumonia, which may be minimal or absent, and the chest radiograph, which may be markedly abnormal.[345] This effect may be dramatic when systemic manifestations of tularemia, such as headache, myalgia, and high fever, are apparent.

Hilar adenopathy occurs in about a third to half of cases and pleural effusion in 25% to 30%[346] Radiographs become positive as early as the second day after the onset of symptoms. Most patients have a distinctive pattern of a single (occasionally multiple) oval consolidation that is frequently juxtahilar. Early radiographic changes include peribronchial infiltration with a bronchopneumonia pattern; hilar adenopathy is evident in 32% to 64% of cases[346] and may represent an important clue to the diagnosis. Pleural effusion may occur later and may be the only radiographic abnormality.[347] Cavitary pneumonia is unusual.[348] Fibrosis and calcification changes may occur late.[253]

Care should be taken when cultivation of *F. tularensis* is attempted because inhalation or inoculation with as few as 10 to 50 organisms can produce pneumonia. Many hospital laboratories refer specimens to a reference laboratory or to the CDC for processing.[349] The organism is fastidious but can be recovered on commercially available chocolate agar and from most automated blood culture systems. The laboratory should be notified that *F. tularensis* is suspected because prolonged incubation may be required. Presumptive isolates are identified by agglutination with commercially available antiserum.[323] Immunoelectron microscopy may also be useful for confirming presumptive *F. tularensis* infection.[350]

Serologic diagnosis remains the diagnostic gold standard. The commercially available tube agglutination test is most frequently used. Serologically, tularemia in a patient with a febrile illness is diagnosed when a greater than fourfold rise between acute and chronic serum titers or a single titer of more than 1:160 by agglutination testing occurs.[335] The increase in titer usually occurs during the second week of illness,[349] and in some cases, it is detectable only after therapy is complete.[351] A titer of 1:20 to 1:80 can persist for years. Tularemia may also stimulate antibodies to *Brucella* species and vice versa.[347] Testing for both species usually resolves the dilemma. ELISA using sonicated bacteria can detect antibody earlier than the agglutination test but is not commercially available.[352] In vitro stimulation of lymphocytes has been used[353] but is also not widely available. A skin test was once available, but it was of limited use and is currently not commercially available.

Prompt initiation of antibiotics in patients with tularemic pneumonia (often before agglutinating antibody titer is detectable) may be lifesaving, particularly when the clinical course is severe. Streptomycin was the traditional drug of choice; the response is often dramatic, with symptomatic improvement 12 to 36 hours after the start of therapy. A 7- to 14-day course of parenteral treatment is traditionally given, although few data are available to critically evaluate the duration of therapy.[354] Relapse, which is rare after aminoglycoside therapy but relatively common after therapy with a bacteriostatis agent (such as tetracycline), should be managed with an aminoglycoside.

Today, gentamicin has surpassed streptomycin as the drug of choice.[355] Advantages over streptomycin include broader antibacterial coverage, for example, when an aggressive pneumonia fails to respond to therapy and the clinical diagnosis of tularemic pneumonia is uncertain. Also, the easy availability of assays to measure serum drug concentrations facilitates monitoring and minimizes toxicity. The fever in children treated with gentamicin for 7 days (at a dosage of 6 mg/kg/day divided into every 8 hours)[351] resolved within 24 to 72 hours after the initiation of therapy, and there were no symptoms after 5 days.[351] Chloramphenicol and tetracyclines are second-line bacteriostatic agents; relapses are frequent,[355] often within a few days of the discontinuation of therapy. Initially, the use of cephalosporin antibiotics seemed promising, but treatment failures have occurred.[351] Ciprofloxacin was used successfully in a single patient.[326] In meningitis, combined streptomycin and chloramphenicol were used with success.[349]

Before the availability of streptomycin, the mortality rate from pulmonary tularemia was 47%. With streptomycin or gentamicin therapy, this rate should approach zero, providing that clinicians consider the diagnosis. In adults, serious underlying diseases, such as alcoholism, chronic lung disease, chronic glomerulonephritis, ischemic heart disease, and diabetes mellitus, are associated with a poor outcome, although suboptimal antimicrobial therapy received by many of these patients may have confounded this conclusion.[356] Pulmonary involvement is associated with a poor prognosis.

Lung abscess formation is rare[357] but may be multiple. Pleural effusion, characteristically exudative, is present in tularemic pneumonia[358] in up to 50% of cases.[359] Pericarditis is a rare complication of tularemia. The pathophysiology is unknown. It has been postulated that pericarditis arises by direct extension from adjacent pneumonia, but the occurrence of pericarditis in a few patients with normal chest radiographs suggests that bacteremic seeding of the pericardium may also occur. Meningitis has rarely been identified in patients with tularemic pneumonia.[339] Peripheral neuropathy occurred in one adult.[360] Nonspecific features of severe tularemic pneumonia have included ARDS requiring positive end-expiratory pressure,[361] acute renal insufficiency, and encephalopathy.

Handling of wild animal carcasses while wearing rubber gloves, masks, and protective glasses and taking appropriate precautions to prevent tick bites may decrease exposure to the causative organism. Postexposure chemoprophylaxis has not been recommended.[325] Tularemia is reportable to state or local boards of health.[324]

A live, attenuated vaccine was first developed in the former Soviet Union more than 50 years ago. In the United States in 1960, an attenuated strain was selected and after evaluation, was introduced as the attenuated, live vaccine.[362] Among laboratory workers immunized with this vaccine, the incidence of typhoidal tularemia after vaccination decreased from 5.7 to 0.27 cases per 1000 employee-years, although the rate of ulceroglandular tularemia did not change.[363] For laboratory workers anticipating exposure, this vaccine is available from U.S. Army Medical Research and Development Command at Fort Detrick, Maryland.

Kingella Species

Although rarely reported outside of Israel, *Kingella kingae* infections have been identified as a cause of childhood pneumonia, especially in the very young. The organism, a member of the so-called HACEK group, is a gram-negative coccus with morphologic characteristics similar to those of *Moraxella* species. In a 5-year observational study in Israel, the incidence of invasive *K. kingae* infection was 31.9 per 100,000 children younger than 12 months of age, 27.4 per 100,000 children younger than 2 years of age, and 14.3 per 100,000 children younger than 4 years of age.[364] Of those with invasive disease, 2 of 25 had a lower respiratory infection, and one had a pulmonary infiltrate; both children with respiratory infections recovered fully after antibiotic treatment with ampicillin or cefuroxime.[364]

Empyema with *Kingella* species has also been described. One article described an adult with empyema from which *K. kingae* and *Coccidioides immitis* were isolated from the pleural fluid; the latter organism had previously been isolated from fluid obtained by bronchoscopy performed for the evaluation of a pulmonary nodule.[365] *Kingella denitrificans* was isolated with *Peptostreptococcus* species from the pleural fluid of another adult with bronchogenic carcinoma and empyema.[366]

K. Pneumoniae

Despite its name, *K. pneumoniae* is a rare cause of pneumonia in children. Most cases occur in the neonate or immunocompromised host. In the latter group, it is often nosocomially acquired.

The organism was first identified in 1882 by Carl Friedländer, who recognized it as a cause of lobar pneumonia but incorrectly believed that it was a major cause.[367,368] With the recognition in 1886 that *Diplococcus lanceolatus* (now known as the *pneumococcus*) was the major cause, *K. pneumoniae* (at that time called *Bacillus mucosus capsulatus*) was relegated to the role of a secondary invader[368] or was even ignored. Indeed, in 1912, Osler wrote in the eighth edition of *Principles and Practice of Medicine* that *K. pneumoniae* "is not a cause of genuine lobar pneumonia."

This view of *K. pneumoniae* from the other extreme also proved incorrect as borne out by the well-documented cases of community-acquired pneumonia described by Sisson and Thompson in 1915[369] and by Solomon in 1937.[368] The infrequency of subsequent reporting, however, underscored the infrequency of community-acquired *K. pneumoniae* pneumonia in children and adults. However, although it causes pneumonia infrequently, a role for *Bacillus mucosus capsulatus* as a cause of outbreak-clusters of pneumonia was recognized when 11 cases occurred in temporal proximity in a home where 130 children lived. In addition, a role for *K. pneumoniae* as an occasional cause of neonatal pneumonia was documented in 1896 by Comba, who identified *Bacillus mucosus capsulatus* in pure growth from a postmortem culture of lung exudate and blood from a 6-day-old infant who died of bronchopneumonia.

The genus *Klebsiella* is one of four genera in the tribe Klebsielleae of the family Enterobacteriaceae. There are four species, but *K. pneumoniae,* a gram-negative, encapsulated bacillus, is the most important.[370] Capsular serotypes have been assessed by quellung reaction[371] or indirect immunofluorescence techniques[372]; at least 70 types exist.[371] A clear picture associating certain serotypes with disease has not consistently emerged, however. Cryz et al[373] reviewed 703 *K. pneumoniae* isolates from the blood of hospitalized patients of unspecified age. Serotypes 2, 21, and 55 were most prevalent. More than half of the capsular serotypes had a frequency of more than 0.5% each. Thus many different capsular serotypes can cause human disease, and a capsular polysaccharide-based vaccine will need to be multivalent.[373]

The modern view of *K. pneumoniae* pneumonia can be inferred from the historical information already presented. This infection can be sporadic and occasionally epidemic in several clinical situations. Community-acquired *Klebsiella* pneumonia in children is infrequent. Among 102 children hospitalized for community-acquired pneumonia, *K. pneumoniae* was isolated from a tracheal aspirate of a single child who also had evidence of infection with respiratory syncytial virus.[28] Among adults, the incidence of community-acquired *K. pneumoniae* pneumonia is also low, with less than three bacteremic cases per year at large municipal hospitals.[374]

K. pneumoniae bacteremia is more common than pneumonia. Most children with *K. pneumoniae* bacteremia acquire infection nosocomially and are young; only a small number have pneumonia. For example, among 5156 blood cultures that yielded bacteria in a 10-year period at Children's Hospital of Wisconsin, *K. pneumoniae* was isolated from 60 (1.2%), 8 of whom had pneumonia[375]; 43 of the blood cultures represented infection that was acquired nosocomially, and 38 were obtained from children younger than 1 year of age.

Data to define the incidence of *K. pneumoniae* pneumonia in the neonate are not available; inference is made from data regarding the occurrence of *K. pneumoniae* bacteremia. At Yale from 1966 to 1978, *K. pneumoniae* was responsible for 14% of cases of neonatal bacteremia, the third leading cause after *E. coli* and group B streptococci.[376] The percentage of bacteremic episodes caused by *K. pneumoniae* declined during the study period; from 1979 to 1988, this trend continued.[377] Overall, *K. pneumoniae* accounted for 18 of the 270 bacteremia isolates (6.7%). Risk factors for *K. pneumoniae* neonatal bacteremia included a prior operative procedure, tracheostomy, infected venous cutdown site, and multiple exchange transfusions.[376]

In the hospital, *K. pneumoniae* invasive infection, including pneumonia, has been related to prior colonization,[378] which in turn is related to prior antimicrobial therapy. The rates are high in hospitalized patients, particularly those in postoperative situations or intensive care units. Spread of the organism is facilitated by hand-to-patient contact, and hospital staff can be facilitators. In an intensive care unit, 17% of nursing personnel had *K. pneumoniae* on their hands. Four colonized or infected patients in this unit had organisms of identical serotype.[379] Similar observations have been made in neonatal intensive care units.[380]

Patients receiving immunosuppressive therapy also constitute a group at increased risk,[378] especially in the nosocomial setting. Otherwise healthy children receiving intermittent suppressive therapy, such as those with asthma, may occasionally have *K. pneumoniae pneumonia.*[375] Other factors said to predispose to increased risk include the need for respiratory assistance and invasive procedures.[380]

K. pneumoniae probably reaches the lung most commonly by inhalation. Bacteremic seeding of the pulmonary parenchyma may also occur but has been difficult to document with certainty. Among adults, alcoholics are said to be at high risk; presumably the organism is aspirated during a binge.

K. pneumoniae pneumonia may occur anywhere in the pulmonary parenchyma; multiple lobe involvement is common. In adults in whom alcoholism is the predisposing condition and infection is acquired by aspiration, the most common involvement occurs in the upper lobes, particularly on the right side.[381]

The capsular polysaccharide of *K. pneumoniae* plays an important role in pathogenesis[382] by interfering with opsonization or by preventing complement activation. The amount of capsular polysaccharide produced by an isolate may correlate with virulence; the presence of circulating capsular polysaccharide may predict the severity of illness. In mice, polymorphonuclear cells infiltrated from the circulation played a major role in clearing *K. pneumoniae* from the lungs.[383] This finding may partly explain why neutropenic and immunocompromised individuals are more susceptible to *K. pneumoniae* pneumonia.

Lipopolysaccharide probably also plays a role in the pathogenesis of *K. pneumoniae* infection, most likely by mediating resistance to the lytic activity of normal serum. There are 12 O antigens in *Klebsiella* organisms. Few data are available to document differences among the O serotypes in terms of virulence, although among O1 isolates, certain capsular types were more virulent in a mouse model of *K. pneumoniae* infection. Also, an extracellular complex consisting of purified extracellular lipopolysaccharide and protein elaborated by many strains of *K. pneumoniae* contributed to the virulence in pneumonia in mice, probably by depressing reticuloendothelial system function.[384]

Certain strain-specific factors promote colonization. For example, colonization is promoted by outer membrane proteins that serve both as surface receptors for phage attachment and as mediators of adherence that are inhibitable by mannose[385] and by type II pili.[386] A role for platelet-activating factor, a potent autacoid, in the pathogenesis of *K. pneumoniae* pneumonia in mice was suggested by improved survival rates and decreased numbers of *K. pneumoniae* in the lungs of mice pretreated with an antagonist specific for platelet-activating factor.[383]

Most information regarding the pathology of *K. pneumoniae* pneumonia comes from postmortem data that often predate the antibiotic era and thus represent observations from patients with severe disease. As with pneumococcal pneumonia, the following stages have been described: red hepatization, gray hepatization, and resolution. No single feature histologically distinguishes *K. pneumoniae* pneumonia. In the red hepatization stage, masses of encapsulated organisms may be seen with invasion of the bronchioles and alveoli. Thin fluid containing scanty fibrin and a moderate number of monocytes engulfing the organisms is characteristic. In the gray hepatization stage, polymorphonuclear leukocytes infiltrate the alveolar walls. Blood vessels are engorged. Thrombosis and circulatory impairment follow and terminate in necrosis with sloughing, hemorrhage, and the potential for cavity and abscess formation.[387] Abscesses may be multiple and small, solitary and large, or intermediate between these designations.

The clinical features of *Klebsiella* pneumonia depend on the setting. In the neonate and older child, the clinical features resemble those of bacterial pneumonia of any etiology in the respective age group. Chest pain or discomfort with or without dyspnea may be evident, although the clinical picture in an immunocompromised child may not suggest clear-cut localization to the respiratory tract. *K. pneumoniae* pneumonia may occur with pneumococcal pneumonia, a possibility that should be considered, particularly in an immunocompromised child with an abscess who does not respond to therapy directed against *S. pneumoniae.*[388]

The diagnosis depends on identifying the causative organism in a clinically relevant setting. Sputum, when available (e.g., from older children), may be blood tinged, or "rusty," although this sign was only present in about one third of adults with *Klebsiella* pneumonia. Because asymptomatic colonization may occur, sputum analysis may be misleading,[389] although suspicion should be raised in the presence of monotonous gram-negative rods, a pure or nearly pure culture, or both results.[374]

Isolation of *K. pneumoniae* from the blood during an episode of acute pneumonia is usually accorded diagnostic importance, as is isolation of the organism from pleural fluid.[374] Detection of *Klebsiella* capsular antigens in serum has been attempted, but the procedure is not widely available.[390] More invasive techniques, such as needle aspiration[391,392] and bronchoscopy, may be necessary to make a diagnosis; quantitative cultures of bronchial secretions obtained through a protected catheter have helped distinguish asymptomatic upper airway colonization from pulmonary infection.[393] However, this procedure is limited by small airway size in very young children and is probably most useful in patients who have not received prior antimicrobial therapy.

The so-called classic radiographic findings in adult *K. pneumoniae* pneumonia include a bulging fissure of the involved lobe margin, a sharp infiltrative margin of the pulmonary infiltrate (both occur in about 64% of patients),[394] and a predilection for upper lobes and abscess with cavitation. More important, any or all of these "classic" features may be absent, and the radiographic appearance may not be distinct from that of other airspace pneumonias.[395] Lesions consistent with the radiologic appearance of a pneumatocele in patients with *Klebsiella* pneumonia have also been described.

The treatment of *K. pneumoniae* pneumonia in children usually involves an aminoglycoside, an extended-spectrum cephalosporin, or the two in combination. Combination therapy is preferred, although few explicit data document its superiority. At the University of Chicago Hospitals in 1994, 95% and 97% of *K. pneumoniae* isolates were susceptible to gentamicin and extended-spectrum cephalosporins, respectively. At some institutions, the percentage of *K. pneumoniae* isolates resistant to gentamicin is substantially higher, mostly because of the presence of one of several aminoglycoside-modifying enzymes[396] elaborated by the infecting isolates. The rate of resistance to extended-spectrum cephalosporins is also substantially higher at many institutions, largely because of the presence of extended-spectrum β-lactamases.[397] Resistance may be a particular problem during nosocomial outbreaks.[398] Novel therapeutic modalities using platelet-activating factor antagonists[385] or circulating liposomes to deliver antibiotics to the site of lung infection[399] have received promising experimental evaluation in animal models.

Lung abscess is a frequent complication in children and adults and may occur in a third to half of cases.[394] Surgical treatment may be necessary if medical intervention fails. Percutaneous drainage is usually sufficient.[400] Massive pulmonary gangrene, the rapid total destruction of part of the lung, is an extremely rare complication of *K. pneumoniae* pneumonia. Some have suggested that this entity may represent a synergistic infection caused by *K. pneumoniae* and an undetected anaerobe.[374] The process may resemble a lung abscess initially but reveals itself by its rapid, destructive course; fewer than 20 cases have been reported.[374] Other intrathoracic complications include empyema with residual pleural thickening[368,374] and pneumopericarditis.[401]

"Chronic" *K. pneumoniae* pneumonia, which by definition persists longer than 1 month, is an entity described only in adults, primarily in the older literature. Cavitation may be present (Fig. 39-15), and the clinical picture may resemble that of tuberculosis. Some have suggested that chronic *K. pneumoniae* pneumonia, like massive pulmonary gangrene, may reflect a synergistic infection between *K. pneumoniae* and an anaerobic species.[374]

Because *K. pneumoniae* pneumonia may be associated with bacteremia, the clinical picture of septic shock or distant metastatic seeding may result in an infectious focus, such as meningitis or renal abscess. Some have suggested that *K. pneumoniae* infection may play a role in the pathogenesis of ankylosing spondylitis and Reiter's syndrome.[402] Antibodies directed against *K. pneumoniae* nitrogenase, which is produced during convalescence from *K. pneumoniae* infection, may also recognize cells expressing HLA-B27 and produce an inflammatory response clinically recognized as ankylosing spondylitis[402]; in support of this, IgA antibodies to *K. pneumoniae* were identified in patients with ankylosing spondylitis.[403]

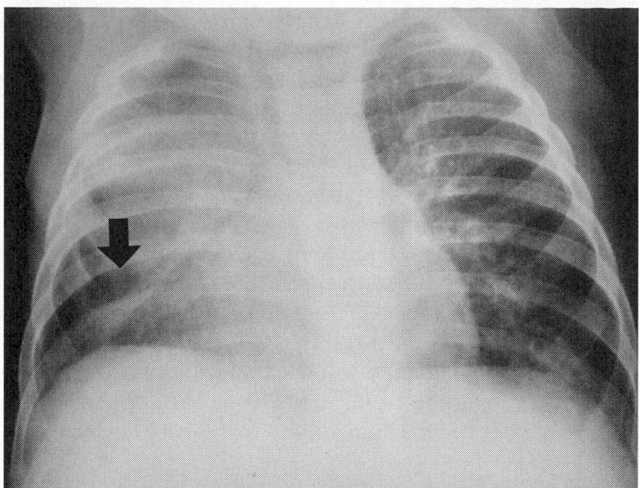

Fig. 39-15. Gram-negative pneumonia with cavitation *(arrow)* in the right upper and middle lobes in a 5-month-old boy.

The mortality rate of *K. pneumoniae* bacteremia in the neonatal period is very high[378] despite appropriate antibiotic therapy. Few specific data exist for older children with uncomplicated *K. pneumoniae* pneumonia and intact host response capability. However, recovery is the rule, providing that appropriate antimicrobial therapy is administered and relevant foci are drained.

To date, a polyvalent polysaccharide vaccine prepared from 24 *Klebsiella* serotypes has been well tolerated and immunogenic among the more than 2000 adults to whom it has been administered. An immune globulin prepared from these individuals enhanced opsonophagocytic killing of bacteria and was more protective in a mouse challenge model than standard intravenously administered immune globulin.[404] Such a preparation would have the potential to prevent 60% to 70% of *Klebsiella* infections if 100% effective. More recently, a vaccine based on O side chains has been evaluated; this approach may prove simpler to implement because a vaccine containing 3 to 7 O serotypes could prevent 60% to 90% of disease in patients.[405]

Leptospira Species

Leptospirosis is a rare cause of childhood pneumonia. The clinical illness was first described by Weil in 1886, and the organism was first seen in 1907. The rat was considered the only animal host until the 1940s, when it became evident that leptospirosis was a zoonosis of worldwide distribution that affected many species of wild and domestic mammals. Worldwide, the rat is the most common source of human infection. In the United States, dogs, livestock, cats, rodents, and wild mammals are the most common sources.

The cause is *Leptospira interrogans,* which is a spirochete. *L. interrogans* is further classified into serogroups and serovars (serotypes). About 19 serogroups and 250 serovars have been recognized. In the United States, disease is caused by over 10 serovars, most commonly *icterohaemorrhagiae* and *canicola. L. interrogans* is pathogenic for both animals and humans.

Transmission of leptospires to humans follows contact with the tissues or body fluid of infected animals or exposure to an environment contaminated by leptospires. The occurrence of flooding (e.g., after a heavy rainfall) facilitates spread of the organism. In 1972, an outbreak of leptospirosis in Missouri was traced to contaminated soil in suburban lawns. Dogs have become an increasingly recognized vector and reservoir of this disease in the United States.[406] In urban environments, rats have been increasingly implicated in the maintenance of the *L. interrogans* reservoir.[407]

After penetration of the skin or mucous membranes, the organisms invade the bloodstream and are spread throughout the body. Although presumed present, leptospires were not demonstrable in the lungs until recently[408]; immunohistochemical techniques using rabbit polyclonal antisera revealed threadlike filaments and granular forms in the lungs of three patients during an outbreak of leptospirosis and pulmonary hemorrhage in Nicaragua.

Pulmonary lesions are usually the result of hemorrhage secondary to the vasculitis that characterizes disseminated leptospirosis rather than acute inflammation. Localized or confluent hemorrhagic pneumonitis may be evident. In addition, petechial and ecchymotic hemorrhages may be found throughout the lungs, pleura, and tracheobronchial tree.[408]

Leptospirosis is usually separated clinically into anicteric and icteric (Weil's syndrome) disease. About 90% of patients have anicteric disease. The traditional view has been that pulmonary manifestations are usually mild and of little clinical importance. A dry, hacking cough, occasionally with blood-stained sputum, may be present. A chest radiograph may show infiltrates that may be diffuse, bilateral, and patchy. Rarely, chest pain, hemoptysis, respiratory distress, and cyanosis may be present.[409] Hemoptysis, if present, usually clears by day 5. Physical examination may reveal crackles on auscultation or a friction rub. In light of reports of severe pulmonary symptoms and pulmonary hemorrhage during outbreaks of leptospirosis in Korea, China, and Nicaragua,[410] the disease spectrum of pulmonary leptospirosis may require expansion.

A blood or CSF culture obtained in the first 7 to 10 days of the illness and plated on special media, such as Fletcher, EMJH, and Tween 80-albumin media, may lead to the diagnosis. The organism may also be isolated from the urine if the specimen has been obtained after about the tenth day of illness. Investigators have suggested that it may be possible to diagnose leptospirosis by using dark-field microscopy to examine BAL specimens.[411] Previously, it was widely held that direct dark-field fluid examination was not recommended because the organisms were present in small numbers and perhaps difficult to distinguish from fibrin filaments.

Several serologic strategies for diagnosis have been used. The macroscopic slide agglutination test using killed antigen is useful for screening. The microscopic agglutination test is the current standard for the serologic diagnosis of leptospirosis and can be arranged at the CDC through referral by state health departments. Indirect hemagglutination, indirect immunofluorescence,[412] ELISA,[413] and dot-ELISA tests have been used well in various circumstances. PCR amplifying a variety of regions from the leptospira genome[414,415] may be useful, particularly in the early days of illness when the diagnosis may not be obvious.

Treatment is with high-dose intravenous penicillin, typically given for 7 days. Although endotoxin has not been demonstrated in the causative bacterium, Jarisch-Herxheimer reactions have been described,[416] as has ARDS. Death from leptospirosis is usually associated with severe jaundice, severe oliguric renal failure, and the recently recognized associated pulmonary hemorrhage. Amoxicillin and doxycycline are alternative treatments.

Leptospirosis is a disease that must be reported to state and local health authorities. While the child is in the hospital, strict universal precautions should be followed. Public health measures include controlling rodents, preventing contact with animal urine, wearing protective clothing when exposure is likely, and avoiding contact with potentially contaminated water. Adult prophylaxis is effective with 200 mg of oral doxycycline once a week in those with occupational exposure. There are no current recommendations for prophylaxis in children.

Listeria Species

Listeria monocytogenes is a gram-positive, facultatively anaerobic rod. It was first recognized as a human pathogen in 1929 and was named after Lord Lister, the British surgeon who developed the technique of antiseptic surgery.[417] The first documentation of infection in infants was published by Burn in the 1930s.[418]

L. monocytogenes accounts for almost all listerial infections in humans, although infections with *L. ivanovii, L. seeligeri,* and *L. welshimeri* have rarely been reported. It is an uncommon cause of neonatal pneumonia.[419] Human groups at risk for infection include pregnant women, immunocompromised patients, and neonates.

Human infection is acquired by contact with domestic or wild birds and animals, meat, milk, vegetables, or contaminated soil.[253] The organism has also been found in the gastrointestinal tract in 1% to 5% of asymptomatic individuals. Neonates may acquire infection transplacentally during passage through an infected birth canal or from maternal bacteremic seeding.[420] Some reports have suggested cross-infection in neonatal nurseries. The organism is distributed worldwide,[253] and although there was a suggestion of geographic differences associated with perinatal listeriosis, surveillance conducted by the CDC did not document a geographic or seasonal pattern.[420]

The pathogenesis of listeriosis involves a complex interaction among the organism, the host immunologic response, and the amount of organism present. Both humoral and cell-mediated immunity are important. Efficient opsonization of *Listeria* species is mediated by IgM and complement, which are at physiologically low concentrations in the neonate; it has been suggested that these physiologic nadirs are what place neonates at particular risk.[421] Remarkably, *Listeria* organisms can mobilize actin filaments and usurp the contractile system of the host cell, which allows cell-to-cell spread. This property accounts for its virulence in individuals with defective cell-mediated immunity; it also accounts for the ability of the organism to invade the gastrointestinal tract without erosive lesions and to invade the placenta and fetus during maternal bacteremia.[422]

Early onset neonatal listeria infections are usually manifested as pneumonia or sepsis.[423] Tachypnea, respiratory distress, or apnea may be present. Others have identified heart failure, cyanosis, seizures, and emesis. Some note the presence of roseoles, or tiny focal cutaneous granulomas. These "listeriomas" are usually present in the posterior pharyngeal wall if dissemination has taken place. In the older literature, a septic-like clinical picture with diffuse granulomas was termed *granulomatosis infantiseptica.* Transmission of the organism is thought to be from mother to infant, with high concordance of recovery of an organism of identical serotype from mothers of infected infants. For late-onset disease, meningitis is more frequent, and there is less likelihood of recovering the infecting organism from the mother.[423]

Careful bacteriologic evaluation of a patient with possible listeriosis is essential because the organism may be mistakenly identified as a *Corynebacterium* species contaminant on Gram's stain. Certainty regarding the diagnosis involves isolation of the organism from a normally sterile site (e.g., blood). The organism will usually grow in culture within 36 hours. Serologic testing is not helpful. PCR coupled with fluorescent antibody reagents and DNA probes may be helpful in the diagnosis, especially when the organism is in a nonsterile environment where isolation from culture may be difficult. Radiographically, *L. monocytogenes* pneumonia may produce diffuse, bilateral infiltrates that may be miliary, patchy, or interstitial.[253]

The most commonly recommended medication for the therapy of listeriosis is ampicillin, either alone or with the addition of an aminoglycoside, such as gentamicin, for synergy. Treatment failures are common with cephalosporins, so their use should be avoided. The optimum length of treatment has not been fully established, but most clinicians treat neonates for 2 to 3 weeks.

The risk of food-borne listeriosis may be decreased if pregnant women and immunosuppressed or immunodeficient patients avoid raw vegetables, unpasteurized dairy products (especially soft cheeses), undercooked meats, or ready-to-eat foods left standing at temperatures at which bacteria may survive and grow. Other measures include avoidance of bovine or ovine contamination of foods meant for human consumption and antimicrobial management of listerial infections diagnosed during pregnancy.

Mortality rates depend on the clinical syndrome. Early onset neonatal infection, especially granulomatosis infantiseptica and listeriosis in immunocompromised hosts, are risk factors for high mortality.

M. Catarrhalis

M. catarrhalis is a gram-negative diplococcus morphologically similar to *Neisseria* species. It was first identified by Frosch and Kolle in 1896 and was given the name *Mikrokokkus catarrhalis;* it was placed in the genus *Neisseria.* In the early 1970s, however, its taxonomy was reconsidered on the basis of DNA base content, fatty acid composition, and genetic transformation, and the organism was then placed in the genus *Branhamella* (named in honor of Dr. Sarah Branham, a *Neisseria* researcher).[424] The correct taxonomic designation for this and related organisms is the subject of current debate,[425,426] but most clinicians have adopted the name *Moraxella catarrhalis.*

It was thought for many years that *M. catarrhalis* was a nonpathogenic inhabitant of the respiratory tract.[427] In Sweden, 17% to 36% of healthy preschool children were found to harbor *M. catarrhalis* in the nasopharynx.[428] It is now clear, however, that this organism is an important cause of otitis media and sinusitis. In addition, it may rarely cause pneumonia[427,428] and a variety of other infections in children.[429]

Establishing a role for *M. catarrhalis* as a pulmonary pathogen has been a complex task because of the frequency with which this organism colonizes the respiratory tract.[429] The following lines of evidence suggest a strong likelihood that *M. catarrhalis* is at least an occasional cause of bacterial pneumonia:

1. It has been occasionally isolated from the pleural fluid of patients with empyema.[429]
2. It was isolated from the lung of a few patients who died from bronchopneumonia.[429]
3. Serologic methods have identified a subset of patients with pneumonia who have increased antibody to *M. catarrhalis* on convalescence.[428]
4. A few children and adults with underlying illnesses have been described with a clinical illness consistent with pneumonia and *M. catarrhalis* bacteremia.[430]

The peak incidence of *M. catarrhalis* infection is believed to occur in the winter.[429] Transmission of the organism may be via person-to-person spread; nosocomial spread in a pediatric intensive care unit may play a role as well.[431] The role of environmental spread remains to be defined, although the organism survives in sputum for weeks.[429] The clinical features of *M. catarrhalis* pneumonia are not specific and resemble pneumonia caused by other bacteria. The diagnosis is made by isolating the organism from a normally sterile site such as blood in a relevant clinical situation. Serologic diagnosis has not been reliable.[432]

Because most strains of *M. catarrhalis* produce β-lactamase, antibiotics useful in the therapy of *M. catarrhalis* infections include amoxicillin/clavulanic acid, erythromycin and other macrolides, TMP/SMX, and extended-spectrum cephalosporins. It has been suggested that the presence of β-lactamase–producing *M. catarrhalis* strains may confound the treatment of pneumonia caused by other β-lactam–susceptible bacteria. For example, in a mouse model of pneumococcal pneumonia, animals inoculated with *S. pneumoniae* and β-lactamase–producing *M. catarrhalis* had a poor outcome when treated with penicillin compared with mice inoculated with *S. pneumoniae* and β-lactamase–negative *M. catarrhalis;* clavulanate therapy ablated this difference.[433]

N. Meningitidis

Meningococcal pneumonia is rare, especially in children.[434] The organism *N. meningitidis* is a gram-negative diplococcus. Members of the species usually produce one of several antigenically and immunologically distinct capsular polysaccharides that are designated *A, B, C, X, Y, Z, 29E, W135, H, I, K,* and *L.*[435] The organism was first identified in 1886 by Anton Weichselbaum in the CSF of a patient who died of purulent meningitis. Meningococcal pneumonia was first recognized by Holm and Davison during the influenza epidemic in 1918 and 1919. Since then, additional cases have been described.

The initial colonization of meningococci is through adherence to the microvilli of nonciliated epithelial cells that line the respiratory mucosa. The mucosal barrier is breached by first entering the apical side of epithelial cells by a process that involves host actin. The bacteria then transcytose through the cell and exocytose at the basolateral side. Once the pathogens are in the subepithelial space, invasion of the bloodstream is likely achieved by entry through endothelial cells lining the blood vessels. M cells in the tonsillar sites of the nasopharynx might also be a portal of entry for invasion. Once bacteremia occurs, overt signs of disease are often present, and meningococci may be spread to target sites for metastatic infection.[436,437] The integrity of the mucosal barrier is the first line of defense against meningococcal infection. Serum specific antibody against meningococcal proteins and capsular polysaccharide causes lysis of bacteria, enhances phagocytosis by monocytes and polymorphonuclear neutrophils, and neutralizes endotoxin. Underscoring the importance of complement in the defense against meningococcal bloodstream invasion is the observation that people with deficiencies in certain complement components, such as C5, C6, C7, C8, and properdin, are more prone to meningococcemia despite the presence of protective antibody. Mucosal IgA may be important in mucosal defense against meningococci. Meningococci also produce an IgA1 protease that cleaves IgA1 into Fab fragments able to bind to specific antigen but lacking the ability to bind complement. It has been postulated that these cleavage fragments may compete with bactericidal IgG and IgM antibodies for binding to epitopes on the bacteria; however, the importance of IgA1 protease in protection against host defenses has not been proved. Recent observations suggest that the IgA1 protease may autocatalytically produce peptides that transport into host cell nuclei, suggesting a means by which meningococci can communicate with host cells.[438]

Several virulence factors are known to allow meningococcal attachment to host cells, invasion, and survival in the human host. The presence of capsule prevents the adherence and invasion of meningococci to host cells unless the bacteria express filamentous structures called *pili.* Also, there is evidence that a protein called *PilC1* localizes to the tips of pili and mediates pilus-associated attachment. Other factors, such as certain proteins belonging to class V meningococcal opacity proteins called *Opc* and *Opa,* are important in mediating attachment when the bacteria are nonpiliated and unencapsulated. Whereas capsule does not prevent pilus-mediated adherence, it does interfere with Opa- and Opc-mediated adherence. Opa and Opc are also used in invading host epithelial and endothelial cells. Factors that protect meningococci against the bactericidal effects of serum are the capsule and lipooligosaccharide (LOS), which is modified by the covalent addition of sialic acid. Capsule and sialic acid-containing LOS may protect the bacteria by shielding surface-exposed epitopes from bactericidal antibodies or complement.[439] Also, serum antibodies against a protein called *Rmp* block the binding of bactericidal antibodies to the major porin protein and LOS. Because Rmp often copurifies with porin, Rmp-blocking antibodies may explain why an effective porin-based vaccine has not been developed.

Scavenging the essential nutrient iron is also an important means by which meningococci may persist in their iron-limited host.[440] Several membrane-associated receptors, including the transferrin- and lactoferrin-binding proteins, are able to scavenge iron from host iron-binding proteins. These iron-scavenging proteins are among a set of proteins whose production increases in response to low iron concentrations. One of these, transferrin-binding protein, is currently being studied as a possible vaccine candidate against serogroup B *N. meningitidis.* Recently a protein belonging to the RTX family of toxins was identified that is also increased in production in low iron concentrations; it remains to be determined whether this protein acts as a toxin.

Although capsule expression and sialylation of LOS interfere with initial stages of colonization, they are nevertheless important in serum resistance and bloodstream invasion. Expression of capsule and sialylation of LOS are both subject to phase variation, possibly keeping them in the off state during the initial phases of infection but then turning them on after entry into the blood.[441]

Infection with the meningococcus results in several clinical entities. The most common is asymptomatic carriage, which results in natural immunity. Humans are the only known reservoirs for transmission.[442] Meningococcemia is a rapidly progressive syndrome with an agressive, downhill course and high mortality. Meningococcal meningitis is a more indolent disease with meningitis clinically resembling that caused by other bacteria. Chronic meningococcemia is a low-grade febrile illness frequently associated with arthritis and rash.

Meningococcal pneumonia may occur as a part of disseminated meningococcal infection variably accompanied by meningitis, arthritis, myocarditis, pericarditis, or endophthalmitis. Systemic illness may be mild. For example, of two infants with meningococcal bacteremia, both had pneumonia and bacteremia (types Y and W135), but neither had meningitis or sepsis.[443]

Meningococcal pneumonia also occurs in the absence of the clinical picture of sepsis. This so-called primary pneumonia is rare in children and adolescents. An association with antecedent viral pneumonia, particularly that caused by influenza and adenovirus, has been described.[444] However, the studies have been small, and the nature of the relationship has been unclear. Others have described a similar association between viral or *M. pneumoniae* infections and bacterial meningitis, but this relationship also requires further study.[442]

The presumed pathogenesis of meningococcal pneumonia begins with inhalation of the organism. Attack rates are highest in infants 6 to 12 months of age. The serotypes of *N. meningitidis* that have been described to cause pneumonia differ from those usually responsible for invasive disease. For example, serotype Y has repeatedly been cited as an important cause of primary meningococcal pneumonia despite its relatively minor role as a cause of septicemia.[445] Serotype W135 has been similarly implicated.[446] The incubation period is 1 to 10 days but is usually less than 4 days. Most cases of *N. meningitidis* pneumonia have been presumed to be community acquired. However, nosocomial pneumonia has also been described.[447] Patients with a variety of complement deficiencies, particularly of a terminal component (C5-9), are at increased risk for invasive and recurrent meningococcal disease.[445]

Macroscopically, meningococcal pneumonia is lobular and rarely, lobar. The pleura is seldom involved. Histologically, affected bronchioles and alveoli are filled with polymorphonuclear cells that contain gram-negative intracellular diplococci.

No distinct clinical features distinguish meningococcal pneumonia from pneumonia caused by other bacteria[448]; adults usually have cough, fever, chest pain, and dyspnea.[253] The diagnosis is based on isolation of the causative microorganism from blood, sputum (when available), or both fluids. Bacteremia is infrequently reported in primary pneumonia but commonly found when pneumonia is part of generalized sepsis. Group-specific meningococcal antigen can sometimes be detected in CSF, serum, and urine, which allows for the possibility of rapid diagnosis; however, false-negative results commonly occur. This diagnostic tool may be particularly helpful if antibiotics have been administered. Detection of a meningococcal insertion sequence IS1106 and ribosomal RNA genes[449] by PCR in CSF is currently available only on a limited basis.[450] Radiographically, patchy or confluent densities in one or both lungs may be present with occasional cavities. A pleural effusion may sometimes be evident.[253]

Meningococcal pneumonia is treated with parenteral penicillin G. Isolates have generally remained susceptible to penicillin. Recently, relatively resistant isolates (minimum inhibitory concentration, 0.1 to 1.28 μg/ml of penicillin) have been reported from several countries,[442] but their clinical importance is currently unknown. In the presence of meningococcemia, meningococcal meningitis, or both conditions, the dosage of penicillin should be high (e.g., 300,000 units/kg/day; maximum, 24 million units/day) and divided into 4 to 6 daily doses. In uncomplicated meningococcal pneumonia, a lower dosage (e.g., 100,000 units/kg/day) will probably suffice. Extended-spectrum cephalosporins such as cefotaxime and ceftriaxone are alternatives but are more expensive. Chloramphenicol remains an excellent alternative and is useful for the child allergic to penicillin. Although specific data are lacking regarding duration of therapy, a 7-day course is usually sufficient.

There are few complications of meningococcal pneumonia when the infection is not disseminated. Empyema may occasionally complicate meningococcal pneumonia.[451]

Respiratory isolation is indicated for 24 hours after the initiation of effective therapy. Control measures also include careful observation of exposed school, household, or child care contacts. If a febrile illness develops in a contact, the person should receive prompt medical evaluation, and if indicated, antimicrobial therapy should be started. Antimicrobial prophylaxis is indicated within 24 hours of illness in the index case for all contacts, including those normally residing in the household of the index patient and day-care and nursery school contacts. Respiratory tract cultures are not helpful in decisions regarding prophylaxis. The drug of choice is rifampin, 10 mg/kg (maximum, 600 mg) every 12 hours; four doses are given in 2 days. If the isolate is known to be sulfonamide susceptible, sulfisoxazole may be used at 500 mg/day for infants younger than 1 year of age, (500 mg every 12 hours for children 1 to 12 years of age and 1 g every 12 hours for children older than 12 years of age and for adults).

In the United States, a serotype-specific quadrivalent meningococcal vaccine is available against groups A, C, Y, and W135 *N. meningitidis.* The duration of protection is not known but is probably less than 3 years against group A infection if the child was immunized when younger than 4 years of age. The vaccine should be given to children older than 2 years of age who are functionally or anatomically asplenic or those with terminal complement component deficiencies, or it should be given as an adjunct to chemoprophylaxis when exposure is ongoing. The vaccine is routinely given to all U.S. military recruits. Adverse reactions are infrequent and usually consist of localized erythema lasting 1 to 2 days. Revaccination after 2 to 3 years is recommended, especially if the first immunization was when the child was younger than 4 years of age. The need for revaccination in older children and adults is not known. Serotype A and C conjugate vaccines are under development. Initial evaluation suggests that, like other conjugate vaccines, these vaccines are well tolerated and immunogenic.

Nocardia Species

The first known recognition of nocardiosis occurred in 1888 when Nocard identified a disease that resembled glanders in cattle on Guadeloupe.[452] The first case in a patient was described in 1890 by Eppinger, who visualized the organism in pus from a brain abscess. In 1904, Stokes recognized that *Nocardia* species could cause pneumonia in children when he reported a case occurring in a 28-day-old infant.

In 1889, it was suggested that the organism be designated *Nocardia,* although it was not until a better classification system for the order Actinomycetales was derived in 1943 that the term was widely used. *Actinomyces* species and *Nocardia* species are microbiologically similar and cause diseases with overlapping clinical and radiographic findings, although the treatments differ.[453]

Nocardia species are bacteria that are distinguished by their filamentous growth with true branching. Members of the genus are acid-fast, gram-positive organisms found in parasitized soil and dust. They are rarely commensals in humans or animals. The most common species causing disease in humans is *N. asteroides;* other human pathogens include *N. brasiliensis, N. otitidis-cavarum (N. caviae),* and *N. farcinica.*

The most frequently isolated pathogen, *N. asteroides,* is found worldwide. Infection caused by this organism has been reported in patients 4 weeks to 70 years of age.[454] A higher percentage of cases occur in male patients.[455] There are no seasonal predilections. *N. asteroides* pneumonia in children is rare[454,456,457] and usually occurs among immunocompromised patients, especially those with HIV infection,[458] chronic granulomatous disease, or other impairments of cell-mediated immunity.[459] Among adults and children, only 500 to 1000 cases were reported in the United States in 1974[460]; 75% were immunocompromised.[455]

The lung is the usual portal of entry; infection begins with inhalation of the organism. The inflammatory response is suppurative and necrotizing with the formation of abscesses filled with neutrophils and inflammatory debris. In chronic infection, the abscesses may be multiple and separated by fibrotic areas. The process is similar to that found in actinomycosis except that the abscesses are less well defined and the fibrinous reaction is sparse.[461] There may be coalescence with cavity formation. A granulomatous reaction that surrounds a central area of caseous necrosis[461] and that forms a nodule similar to the one found in tuberculosis has been described, but sometimes it may represent concomitant tuberculosis.

The clinical presentation is not specific. The child with pulmonary nocardiosis may have fever, cough, anorexia, weight loss, night sweats, fatigue, malaise, chest pain, and dyspnea.[454] Leukocytosis is usual (≤50,000 leukocytes/mm^3).[454] Disease progression may be acute, subacute, or chronic; remissions and exacerbations may occur.[462,463]

The radiographic findings are also not specific.[458] There may be evidence of segmental infiltrates or large lobar consolidations. Pleural involvement is variable. The lower lobes are more frequently affected.[452] One or more lesions typical of a lung abscess may be present, as may small or large cavities with thin walls. Hilar involvement is unusual; bronchiolitis obliterans has been described.[464]

The diagnosis is made by the identification of typical beaded, branched, weakly gram-positive rods in sputum or pus. The organism grows slowly; cultures should be maintained for 7 to 10 days or longer. Although rarely isolated in the absence of infection, recovery of *N. asteroides* from an immunocompromised child should be regarded as proof of active infection until proved otherwise.[463,465] Demonstration of *Nocardia* species in tissue is best done by Brown and Brenn stain or Gomori's methenamine silver stain. The clinical and radiographic picture of pulmonary nocardiosis may mimic malignancy[466] or tuberculosis.

Treatment is with a sulfonamide, usually in combination with TMP.[467] Immunocompetent children are usually treated for 6 to 12 weeks, whereas immunocompromised children or those with hematogenous spread are treated for 6 to 12 months,[468] and those with AIDS may require an even longer course.[469] Treatment failures have been reported.[470] When a patient's condition fails to improve, assessing compliance, measuring serum sulfonamide levels, performing susceptibility tests on the isolate, and draining the abscess may be appropriate. Alternative therapy in this instance may consist of increasing the dose of TMP/SMX; when TMP/SMX is contraindicated, treatment may consist of an alternative agent, such as ampicillin, erythromycin, amikacin, or minocycline. Cefotaxime and ceftriaxone have good in vitro activity, but there has been little clinical experience with these compounds.[471]

Lung abscess and cavity formation may complicate *Nocardia* pneumonia; multiple draining sinus tracts and empyema may be present.[472] Hematogenous spread to the liver, brain, kidney, and other organs occurs in about 30% of cases.[454,461] The central nervous system is the most commonly seeded distant site.[473] Brain abscesses are usually surgically drained. Relapse has been reported years after therapy.[468]

Most children with *Nocardia* pneumonia recover after TMP/SMX therapy. Concomitant corticosteroid or antineoplastic chemotherapy and disseminated disease are associated with increased mortality rates, even when prompt, appropriate treatment is provided.[454,468,474]

Pasteurella Species

The genus *Pasteurella* consists of eight species of small coccobacilli that are animal pathogens. One of these, *P. multocida,* is further divided into the following subspecies: *multocida, septica,* and *gallicida.* Human infections, rarely including pneumonia, are usually caused by *P. multocida* subspecies *multocida* and subspecies *septica.* Other genus members, *P. canis, P. stomatis,* and *P. dagmatis,* are rarely responsible for infections in humans.

P. multocida is a short, ovoid, gram-negative bacillus that may vary to a coccobacillary shape with convex sides and rounded ends. It may appear in pairs, chains, or clusters or may appear as a single organism. It may exhibit bipolar staining and may become increasingly pleomorphic on subculture. Distinguishing *P. multocida* from *H. influenzae* on morphologic grounds is sometimes difficult, but the former does not require X or V factors for growth. The virulence of the organism is believed to be partly related to the presence of a capsule.[475]

P. multocida is found in the oropharyngeal flora of 70% to 90% of cats and 25% to 50% of dogs and in the pharynx and gastrointestinal tract of many other mammals and birds. Human *P. multocida* infections follow dog or, more typically, cat bites or scratches, although infections have been reported with no identifiable animal contact.[476-478] Respiratory spread from animals to humans also may occur. Human-to-human spread has not been documented. One study identified a dog bite-related seasonal variation in human infection, with the highest incidence occurring in the autumn and winter,[479] although others showed no seasonal differences. There is no gender difference in attack rates. The incubation period is usually less than 24 hours.

Patterns of infection in humans with *P. multocida* include local soft tissue infection, chronic respiratory tract infection, and bacteremia.[480-482] Local disease usually occurs within 24 to 48 hours of the animal bite or scratch and may include swelling, tenderness, erythema, and serous or sanguinopurulent discharge. Osteomyelitis and septic arthritis may reflect direct inoculation of the bacterium into a bone or joint. Regional lymphadenopathy, chills, and fever may occur. Pneumonia is most often associated with chronic upper respiratory tract colonization or bacteremia.[483] The former may continue for an undetermined interval before bloodstream invasion or organism spread to contiguous structures (e.g., middle ear, mastoid bone, sinuses, epiglottis, lung) occurs. The bacteremic pattern may be associated with pneumonia, empyema, or septic arthritis.

The diagnosis of *P. multocida* pneumonia can be made definitively by recovering the causative organism from relevant sites. These sites include sputum, pleural fluid, and blood.

The antimicrobial therapy of choice is penicillin, ampicillin, or amoxicillin. These agents in combination with clavulanic acid are often used empirically to manage dog and cat bites in which *P. multocida* and *S. aureus* are potential pathogens. In children allergic to penicillin, appropriate alternatives are TMP/SMX, chloramphenicol, and tetracycline. More important, oral cephalosporins (such as cephalexin), semisynthetic β-lactams (such as oxacillin or nafcillin), and the macrolide erythromycin are unlikely to be effective. The duration of therapy is measured against the clinical course; useful guidelines are 7 to 10 days for local infection and 10 to 14 days for invasive infections.

Reported complications of *P. multocida* pneumonia include several cases of lung abscess,[484] pleural effusion, and empyema.[485]

Proteus Species

Infections by *Proteus* species in children are infrequent and are most often associated with neonatal sepsis and meningitis and with childhood urinary tract infection. Pneumonia has also been described.[486]

Members of the genus *Proteus* are motile, gram-negative, enteric bacilli; the most commonly isolated species is *P. mirabilis.* The organism is found in soil, sewage, and manure. Epidemic spread in a newborn nursery has been described, with multiple cases of invasive *Proteus* infections occurring in a span of several years.

There are no pathognomonic features of *Proteus* pneumonia. In the neonate, the signs and symptoms are the same as those of other causes of neonatal bacterial pneumonia or sepsis. In the older child, the clinical features of *Proteus* pneumonia are also typical of those of any bacterial pneumonia and include fever, chills, chest pain, dyspnea, and cough.

The diagnosis is usually made after isolation of the causative organism from infected pleural fluid, lung abscess material, blood, or another normally sterile site. Radiographic findings of consolidation are common and usually involve an upper lobe (posterior segment) or the superior segment of the right lower lobe.

Most *P. mirabilis* isolates are susceptible to ampicillin; thus this compound is usually the mainstay of treatment. For invasive infections such as pneumonia or meningitis, empiric combination therapy with an aminoglycoside is often used. An extended-spectrum cephalosporin provides an acceptable alternative.

The complications of *Proteus* pneumonia include associated bacteremia with metastatic foci, particularly meningitis. *Proteus* species pneumonia may also be associated with abscess formation in the lung and with empyema.

P. Aeruginosa

P. aeruginosa is a rare, opportunistic cause of community-acquired pneumonia and an occasional cause of nosocomial pneumonia in children. Infection in immunocompetent hosts is unusual. This bacterium is a special problem for patients with CF.

The organism is a usually motile, gram-negative bacillus that lives in soil and water and grows easily on most media. Most strains have a polar flagellum and fimbriae or pili on the cell surface. More than 90% of strains produce the blue-green pigments pyocyanin and pyoverdin. For epidemiologic distinction, strains are sometimes differentiated by serotyping on the basis of immunochemical distinctions of lipopolysaccharides, phage typing, and typing of pyocyanin, a bacteriocin elaborated by many clinical isolates.

P. aeruginosa isolates elaborate a variety of virulence factors,[487] at least some of which are under the control of an autoinducer protein called *LasR*.[488] Pilin and nonpilus adhesins that are enhanced by neuraminidase mediate initial colonization. Exoenzyme S mediates adenosine diphosphate–ribosylation of host cell G proteins, thereby possibly inhibiting phagocytic activity. Exoenzyme A has similar activity to diphtheria toxin: It produces adenosine diphosphate–ribosylation of EF-2 proteins, causes tissue damage, and may also inhibit phagocytic activity. Elastases LasA and LasB damage pulmonary blood vessels and are responsible for the deposition of immune complexes. Other proteases, such as collagenase, elastase, caseinase, gelatinase, lipase, and lecithinase, can necrose lung tissue as well; the elaboration of alginate mediates adherence and prevents phagocytosis. The solubilization and destruction of lecithin by *Pseudomonas* lecithinase may play a role in the atelectasis observed in *P. aeruginosa* pneumonia.

P. aeruginosa can be part of the transient flora of the skin or the gastrointestinal tract. Hospitalization may lead to high rates of colonization on the skin of patients with burns, in the respiratory tract of patients receiving mechanical ventilation, in the gastrointestinal tract of patients receiving cytoreductive chemotherapy, or at any site in people receiving antibiotics. Because it has few nutritional requirements, the organism can be found in swimming pools, hot tubs, contact lens solutions, mop water, and dilute disinfectant solutions.[487]

Childhood infections with *P. aeruginosa* usually occur in patients with neutropenia resulting from chemotherapy for cancer and are associated with prior hospitalization, the receipt of previous antibiotic therapy, disruption of mucocutaneous barriers, and the presence of indwelling central lines. The bacterium may reach the lung by aspiration or by bacteremic seeding. The latter mechanism occurs mainly in patients with malignancies or those who are neutropenic because of chemotherapy for them. Children and adults with HIV may also have serious *P. aeruginosa* infections, which include pneumonia[489] in the absence of neutropenia or prior hospitalization.[490] *P. aeruginosa* is also an important pathogen in the neonate, who may acquire the bacterium in utero[491] or during passage through the maternal genital tract with associated early onset septicemia. *P. aeruginosa* pneumonia in healthy children is rare.

Children with CF constitute a population at unique risk for *P. aeruginosa* lower respiratory infections. The rate of *P. aeruginosa* colonization in patients with CF is related to age. About one fifth of patients are colonized in the first year of life, whereas older patients (in their late twenties) have rates exceeding 80%.[492] The bacteria are present in large numbers in the thick mucus that occupies the intraairway space. The bacteria are often coated with a thick, alginate polysaccharide capsule, which is rarely seen in patients with other disorders.[493] Moreover, the observation that patients with CF rarely develop *P. aeruginosa* bacteremia suggests that these organisms are uniquely adapted for parasitism of the respiratory tract of patients with CF and less effective at survival elsewhere.

P. aeruginosa colonization of the respiratory tracts of patients with CF is also positively correlated with clinical score, extent of pulmonary disease, severity of radiographic changes, and serum immunoglobulin concentrations.[494] Similarly, *P. aeruginosa* has been associated with acute exacerbations and chronic progression of disease. Moreover, there is growing recognition of inflammatory airway disease, the presence of neutrophils, and progressive airway disease in association with the presence of *P. aeruginosa.* These views have caused reassessment of the once prevalent view that *P. aeruginosa* in the lungs of CF patients were harmless commensals.

The persistence of *P. aeruginosa* in the lungs of children with CF has been related to the presence of one or more sputum factors that interfere with bactericidal activity. Blocking IgG antibodies stops the normal bactericidal IgM activity of human sera.[495] During chronic infection with *P. aeruginosa* in the CF population, there may be conversion of the mucoid colony morphology and rough lipopolysaccharide; these mutations occur in global regulators (i.e., alternative σ factors and their accessory elements).[496]

In addition to its important role in the pathogenesis of CF lung disease, *P. aeruginosa* can cause pneumonia in other patients. When pneumonia occurs in this context, it is usually secondary to aspiration of the infecting organism. There are microabscess formation, necrosis of the alveolar septa, and focal hemorrhage. When it results from seeding of the lung during bacteremia, the lesion begins as a small area of necrosis around a medium-sized pulmonary artery; poorly defined hemorrhagic nodular areas that are frequently subpleural may surround the infected vessel. Alveolar necrosis may be present. Because this histopathologic picture usually occurs in severely immunocompromised patients, substantial inflammatory response may be minimal or even absent.[497] Alternatively, a lesion resembling the one caused by intraparenchymal ecthyma gangrenosum may be present. In this instance, bacteria can be seen to invade small muscular arteries and veins with adjacent small, firm, yellow-brown nodules and hemorrhage into the lung parenchyma; microabscess formation may be present with leukocytes and liquefaction necrosis.

P. aeruginosa is an important cause of so-called ventilator-associated pneumonia,[498,499] which is bacterial pneumonia occurring more than 24 hours after the initiation of mechanical ventilation. Ventilator-associated pneumonia is the result of the microaspiration of oropharyngeal bacteria, which occurs in up to 35% of patients whose lungs are mechanically ventilated.[500] The oropharynx of a critically ill patient is often colonized with aerobic gram-negative bacilli, including *P. aeruginosa,*[501] which may originate from contaminated respiratory therapy equipment or the stomach of an ill patient with diminished production of gastric acid.[502]

The clinical features of *P. aeruginosa* pneumonia resemble the age-specific features of other bacterial pneumonias. In the immunocompromised or chronically hospitalized child, signs may include chills, systemic toxicity, apprehension, confusion, and severe dyspnea with progressive cyanosis.

The findings on physical examination of the chest are nonspecific. The chest radiograph may show bilateral bronchopneumonic infiltrates, more often in the lower lobe with a distinctive nodular pattern. The picture of lobar consolidation is unusual. An interstitial pattern may also be present. Small pleural effusions are common; empyema is rare.

P. aeruginosa isolates are often resistant to a variety of antimicrobial agents; thus susceptibility testing of available isolates may be helpful in planning appropriate antimicrobial therapy for suspected or proven *P. aeruginosa* pneumonia. An extended-spectrum cephalosporin with antipseudomonal activity, such as ceftazidime, or an antipseudomonal penicillin, such as mezlocillin, ticarcillin, or piperacillin, is often used with an aminoglycoside, such as gentamicin or tobramycin. Whether such cephalosporin/aminoglycoside or antipseudomonal β-lactam/aminoglycoside combination therapy improves the outcome compared with ceftazidime alone is the subject of some controversy. The preponderance of evidence suggests that routine use of combination therapy is warranted[503] because *P. aeruginosa* pneumonia is often a severe infection and occurs in the clinical setting of an immunocompromised host. Antipseudomonal penicillins should not be used as the sole therapy for *P. aeruginosa* pneumonia; they have not been shown to be effective in this regard, and they may be too vulnerable to hydrolysis by the *P. aeruginosa* β-lactamases for effective therapy. β-lactamase inhibitors, such as clavulanate, do not inhibit *P. aeruginosa* β-lactamases, and thus fixed combinations, such as ticarcillin/clavulanate (Timentin), offer no advantage over, for example, ticarcillin alone. Ciprofloxacin, a quinolone antibiotic, offers good activity against many isolates of *P. aeruginosa.* Although there is concern regarding arthropathies occurring in growing children who receive this antibiotic, accumulating evidence suggests that this concern may be more theoretic than real.[504] Resistance may develop quite rapidly.

High doses of antimicrobials may be needed to achieve a therapeutic effect in patients with CF. Increased nonrenal clearance, decreased tubular reabsorption, and increased renal tubular secretion all play a role in this regard.[505] Thus serum aminoglycoside levels should be monitored to ensure that therapeutic levels of these compounds are achieved.[506] Some investigators have used aerosolized antibiotics with intravenous antibiotics as suppressive therapy in an outpatient setting in patients with CF who are chronically colonized with *P. aeruginosa.* In this regard, therapy with aerosolized aminoglycosides, antipseudomonal penicillins, and ceftazidime has been attempted with some success as measured by improved pulmonary function and decreased need for hospitalization.

The prognosis depends largely on the underlying disease process. Most deaths in children with CF are from progressive pulmonary insufficiency; in almost all of these patients, *P. aeruginosa* is recoverable from the lungs. In other patients, *P. aeruginosa* pneumonia in association with bacteremia may follow an aggressive clinical course, with death ensuing shortly after onset.

Empyema may complicate *P. aeruginosa* pneumonia, with rates reported as high as 22% to 80%. In cases of ventilator-associated pneumonia in which *P. aeruginosa* is the major cause, the duration of intubation is increased a mean threefold; ventilator-associated pneumonia contributes to 60% of infection-related hospital deaths.[498] Reported mortality rates from *P. aeruginosa* pneumonia have varied widely but may be as high as 90%.[507]

P. Pseudomallei

P. pseudomallei[508] is a rare but serious cause of pneumonia. The first cases of human infection were identified in 1910 by Whitmore and Krishnaswami[509] in Rangoon. The etiologic agent is *P. pseudomallei,* a short, gram-negative,[510] aerobic,[511] bipolar-staining bacillus.[510] The organism can grow on MacConkey agar, Sabouraud dextrose medium, or eosin-methylene blue; rough, characteristically wrinkled colonies are usually visible after a 72-hour incubation.[512,513] The organism is a free-living bacterium that is found in surface water and in soil; transmission to humans is thought to be via contaminated food,[510] inhalation, or contamination of wounds.[513]

Acquisition of the causative organism in cases of pneumonia probably results from inhalation of contaminated dust[514] or infected laboratory materials.[515] Although animals (especially sheep and swine) may acquire the causative agent of melioidosis, direct transmission from animal to humans has never been reported.[514]

The endemic region lies in a narrow belt in the tropics within 20 degrees north and south latitude.[511] Subclinical infection is common; 29% of healthy Thai adults had detectable hemagglutinating antibody to *P. pseudomallei*[516]; in Thai children, a trend toward an increasing prevalence of hemagglutinating antibody with increasing age was apparent.

As of 1975, only seven cases of melioidosis (Whitmore's disease) in children 4 days to 10 years of age had been reported.[513,517] Two of these cases, reported in 1975, raise the question of underreporting, because the children were identified in a 3-week period in the same hospital.[513] Thus the true incidence is not known.[513] Cases have been reported from India, Guam, Malaysia, Korea, Madagascar, Australia, Turkey, Central and South America, the Philippines, South Vietnam, and the United States.[513] The mobility of the world's population makes the infection an important consideration for all physicians treating both children living in the endemic regions and those returning from them.[513]

Histologically, the lesions found in pulmonary melioidosis as well as in infection elsewhere begin as a collection of neutrophils surrounded by a zone of congestion, and they progress to disseminated, sharply defined, small, pus-filled abscesses with granulomatous margins and associated with local necrosis. The necrotic regions coalesce with adjacent areas to form a honeycombed lesion.[508] In chronic infections, epithelioid histiocytes, lymphocytes, and multinucleated giant cells surround the abscess, and the lesion becomes granulomatous. Granulomas may become scarred with deposition of dense fibrin; central necrosis of these granulomas may resemble the caseating granulomas found in tuberculosis.[511]

The two clinical patterns are chronic and acute.[518] In both, the lung is the most commonly affected organ.[519] The indolent nature of the pulmonary involvement may simulate a mycotic infection or tuberculosis.[513]

Signs and symptoms of chronic pulmonary melioidosis may be minimal or absent[513] and may render the infection subclinical. Alternatively, fever, malaise, dry cough,[510] weight loss, chest pain, or hemoptysis may be present.[511] The white blood cell count is variable,[508,510,511,513] and neutrophilia is uncommon.[511] Nodlar infiltrates, often with cavitation, are common findings on the chest radiograph.[513] Some 95% of adults with chronic pulmonary melioidosis have upper lobe involvement, either with infiltrates alone or with cavities, usually single, that vary in size.[511] Chronic pulmonary melioidosis may spontaneously resolve without treatment or advance to fulminant sepsis.[519]

The second pattern of melioidosis is more severe. The clinical picture is of generalized sepsis; skin sores resembling boils are widespread, and abscesses are commonly found in the lung, liver, spleen, and bone marrow at autopsy.[510,513] Most cases are accompanied by malnutrition and debilitation.[513] The clinical course may deteriorate quickly[519]; the mortality rate is 60% to 95%.[519]

The most important factor in establishing the diagnosis is a high index of suspicion. For example, melioidosis should be considered[514] in a child who has a travel history or prior or current residence in Southeast Asia and who has a fever and a localized suppurative process. The diagnosis may be confirmed by isolating *P. pseudomallei* from blood or lung tissue obtained by lung aspiration.[513,514] The laboratory should be notified that *P. pseudomallei* is a consideration because the organism may be misidentified as *P. aeruginosa, Klebsiella* or *Enterobacter* species, or another gram-negative bacterium.[519] Several serologic tests, including hemagglutination and complement fixation test, are useful diagnostic tools.[519] The demonstration of a fourfold or higher rise in paired sera is most helpful. Interpretation of a single titer is more difficult. A hemagglutination titer higher than 1:40 or a complement fixation titer higher than 1:8 had 97% sensitivity in culture-proven cases.[520] Antibody may, however, be absent at the time of clinical presentation. High titers are usually present by the third week of illness and may be detectable for more than 9 months.[520] There appears to be no correlation between the magnitude of the initial titer and the prognosis.[511] Lack of antibody as measured by these techniques does not exclude the diagnosis. The specificity of a high antibody level is considered high, although individuals residing in endemic areas may have low-level immunofluorescent assay or CF antibody. Moreover, CF antibody and, rarely, immunofluorescent assay antibody may be found in other bacterial infections, especially those caused by other pseudomonads.[520]

The rapid institution of aggressive antibiotic therapy is important, even when clinical evidence of pulmonary disease is absent because dissemination and overwhelming sepsis may occur quickly.[513] Combination therapy is preferred, with the theoretic goal of minimizing the development of antimicrobial resistance. Antibiotic courses of short duration and the severity of illness at presentation have both been associated with a high rate of relapse after the cessation of therapy.[521] The antibiotic regimen of choice for patients who appear ill (septic form) is ceftazidime and TMP/SMX.[522] A 2- to 4-week course of parenteral antibiotics, followed by a prolonged course (e.g., 6 months) of oral antimicrobial therapy, is recommended.[514,523] For patients who do not appear ill, ampicillin/clavulanate[524] or tetracycline and chloramphenicol[513] have been used, the last two often given in combination with TMP/SMX.[514] A 30-day course is typical.

Until recently, the mortality rate from melioidosis was as high as 95%,[510,514] especially in patients with the septic form of disease, despite prompt antibiotic therapy. The use of ceftazidime has greatly decreased the mortality rate in adults,[523] although specific data in children are lacking. Preliminary evidence with imipenem is encouraging.

Salmonella Species

Bacteria of the genus *Salmonella* are gram-negative, aerobic, enteric organisms. Numerous attempts have been made to order the complex taxonomy of *Salmonella* species. Currently, all *Salmonella* organisms are classified within a single species, *S. choleraesuis.* The species in turn is subdivided into seven subgroups. Subgroup I contains almost all serotypes responsible for human disease. The old serotypes (e.g., A through D) and various species designations (e.g., *paratyphi, dublin, choleraesuis, typhi*) are now incorporated into this system. It is still useful, however, to divide *Salmonella* on clinical grounds into typhoidal and nontyphoidal strains. Typhoid fever continues to be a global health problem, although great progress has been made in controlling this problem in the United States. In contrast, the incidence of invasive nontyphoidal *Salmonella* infections is on the increase in the United States. Transmission to humans from contaminated food, either from animal colonization or during processing, continues to be the most important mode of spread. In addition, the severity of *Salmonella* infections in adults and children with impaired immune systems, particularly as a consequence of HIV infection,[525,526] has been increasing.

Despite the importance of typhoid fever as a childhood health problem in developing countries, *S. typhi* is seldom implicated as a cause of pneumonia,[527] even though a dry cough occurs in many patients with typhoid fever. Indeed, when a pulmonary infiltrate is recognized during the course of typhoid fever, another, supervening bacterium is most often etiologic.[528] On the other hand, nontyphoidal *Salmonella* species rarely cause childhood pneumonia; the pathogenesis is most often believed to be a consequence of seeding of the lung during bacteremia. Gastroenteritis may be absent.[529] No particular *Salmonella* serotype has been implicated in *Salmonella* pneumonia; many, including *S. choleraesuis, S. typhimurium, S. oranienburg, S. paratyphi, S. stanley,* and *S. suipestifer,* have been isolated from lungs and empyema fluid.[254]

Pulmonary involvement by nontyphoidal *Salmonella* species has been manifested as several infectious syndromes. Radiographically, bronchopneumonia, lobar consolidation, miliary lesions, pleural effusion (empyema),[254] lung abscess, and bronchopleural fistula have all been reported.[530] Pulmonary involvement by *Salmonella* species may also reflect transdiaphragmatic spread from a splenic abscess. Pericarditis has also been reported as a complication.[254]

The treatment of *Salmonella* infection, typhoidal and nontyphoidal, has been a subject of controversy. Currently, antimicrobials are not routinely recommended in instances of uncomplicated *Salmonella* gastroenteritis because the disease is self-limited; therapy does not shorten the course, and antimicrobial use may encourage resistance. A possible exception is in young infants in whom extraintestinal complications are relatively common. Antimicrobial therapy is always indicated for typhoid fever or when extraintestinal infection is suspected or proved. Antimicrobial resistance has been a major problem that reflects in part the human-to-animal transmission of many *Salmonella* strains and the use of antibiotics in livestock feed as well as injudicious antibiotic use by physicians and patients. In addition, some compounds to which *Salmonella* species are often susceptible in vitro (such as aminoglycosides) may not perform well in vivo, perhaps because the organisms are pathogens that gain access to the intracellular milieu as an early step in the pathogenesis. Thus selection of an antimicrobial involves a decision as to whether any treatment is necessary as well as knowledge regarding the susceptibility of the infecting isolate. Useful compounds with good therapeutic effectiveness when the isolate is susceptible include ampicillin, chloramphenicol, and extended-spectrum cephalosporins such as ceftriaxone and cefotaxime. A 14-day course is sufficient to manage uncomplicated pneumonia, but empyema and lung abscess may require a longer course.

S. Marcescens

The genus *Serratia* contains many named species, but only one, *S. marcescens,* is associated with human disease. The organism is a gram-negative aerobe and may cause childhood pneumonia, particularly in patients with compromised immunologic integrity in the nosocomial setting.[531] Until the

1950s, *S. marcescens* was considered a harmless saprophyte; a hospital-based review of nosocomial infection identified only three *S. marcescens* infections as late as 1964.[532] *Serratia* organisms are now recognized as important but relatively infrequent causes of hospital-acquired infections, including pneumonia, bacteremia, urinary tract infections, and surgical wound infections. Most are associated with intravenous, intraperitoneal, or urinary tract catheterization and instrumentation of the urinary or respiratory tracts.

The clinical features of *Serratia* pneumonia are not specific. Exceptions are pseudohemoptysis and red sputum secondary to the production of prodigiosin (a red pigment made by some *S. marcescens* strains). This is a dramatic clinical sign but in the authors' experience is seldom present. Radiographically, *S. marcescens* typically appears as confluent or patchy infiltrates; cavitation is usual, although a pleural effusion may be present.[253,531]

S. marcescens may be resistant to a variety of antimicrobials, perhaps because of its hospital habitat. Extended-spectrum cephalosporins (ceftriaxone or cefotaxime) may be useful; these are typically combined with an aminoglycoside.

Local complications include empyema and lung abscess. Concomitant pneumonia and bacteremia caused by *S. marcescens* may lead to distant, infectious complications.

Spirillum Minus and Streptobacillus Moniliformis (Rat-Bite Fever)

Rat-bite fever, a rare, febrile illness, follows a bite from a rat or another small rodent. Although rat-bite fever has been recognized for many centuries, Wilcox[534] published the first account of it in 1839. In 1914, Schottmuller demonstrated the organism causing the disease and named the microbe *Streptothrix muris ratti.* In 1925, Levaditi renamed the organism *Streptobacillus moniliformis.* In Japan during this same period, Futaki identified a separate organism, termed *S. minus,* which caused a similar disease after a rat bite. Although both organisms may be responsible for rat-bite fever, and pleural effusion may rarely occur in infection with *Spirillum minus,* pneumonia is usually only found after infection with *S. moniliformis.*

S. moniliformis is a microaerophilic, gram-negative pleomorphic bacillus transmitted by a bite or scratch from rodents (such as rats, mice, or squirrels) or carnivores that prey on them (such as dogs, pigs, ferrets, cats, or weasels). Oral ingestion by drinking of milk or eating of food products contaminated by an infected animal has been associated with erythema arthriticum epidemicum (Haverhill fever), an illness resembling rat-bite fever. The incubation period ranges from 1 to 22 days but usually lasts less than 10 days.

Clinical manifestations include the bite (which heals quickly), fever, vomiting, severe headache, and chills. A blotchy, irregular, maculopapular rash usually occurs 1 to 8 days after the onset of the fever and can be found over the extensor and lateral surfaces, most prominently over the joints. The rash may last from 1 to 21 days; it may become purpuric and, ultimately desquamate. Migratory arthritis and arthralgias are common. Polyarthritis or true septic arthritis may ensue. The fever spontaneously subsides but may relapse for weeks or months; arthritis may persist for up to 2 years. Focal infections may be manifested as endocarditis, pericarditis, and meningitis.[535,536] Pneumonia is rarely recognized in children or adults, although an interstitial pneumonitis was appreciated at the postmortem examination of a 2-year-old child who died of *S. moniliformis* infection.

Diagnosis is aided by a history of animal contact or other close-contact cases. Direct visualization of typical pleomorphic bacilli by material from an infectious site that is stained with Gram's or Giemsa stain may provide a diagnostic clue. *S. moniliformis* may be isolated by the culture of blood or wound lesion material. Because the organism is fastidious, the laboratory should be notified that *S. moniliformis* is suspected. Rapid identification is possible by gas-liquid chromatography of washed growth from 24-hour broth cultures.[537] Specific agglutinins appear within 10 days of the onset of clinical symptoms and persist for several months. A fourfold rise in the titer or a single titer higher than 1:80 is considered diagnostic. False-positive, nontreponemal tests for syphilis have been described in patients with rat-bite fever.[538]

Treatment is with intravenous penicillin G. A 7- to 14-day course is typical. The last 5 to 7 days can be completed with oral phenoxymethyl penicillin. For penicillin-allergic patients, erythromycin, chloramphenicol, or streptomycin may be substituted. Tetracycline is another alternative for children older than 9 years of age.

Before the advent of penicillin treatment, the mortality rate for *S. moniliformis* rate-bite fever was about 10%. Death is still a possible outcome, particularly if the diagnosis is not considered as a cause of the pneumonia.

S. Pyogenes (Group A Streptococci)

Despite its continued importance as the major cause of bacterial pharyngitis and many other infectious syndromes in children, *S. pyogenes* is a rare cause of pneumonia. The necrotizing nature of pneumonia caused by this organism often makes the clinical course rapidly progressive, severe, and protracted, even when antimicrobial therapy is promptly initiated.

The organism, group A β-hemolytic streptococcus, also called *S. pyogenes,* is gram positive and has a slimy, hyaluronic acid capsule. Among the determinants of virulence are M protein, pyrogenic exotoxins, C5a peptidase, hyaluronidase, streptolysins S and O, and streptokinase. M protein is a major virulence factor, partly because of its antiphagocytic activity. Anti–M antibody is opsonic and contributes to the bactericidal activity of blood. There are more than 80 distinct antigenic M protein types[539]; three types—1, 3, and 18—are more likely to be associated with invasive disease.[540] Lipoteichoic acid is the basic chemical component of hairlike fimbriae that protrude through the hyaluronic acid capsule and mediate the adherence of group A streptococci to epithelial cells.[541]

S. pyogenes makes many extracellular products that are important to its virulence. One such product is streptolysin O, an oxygen-labile hemolysin that targets bronchiolar macrophages and is useful in the diagnosis of group A streptococcal infection because of its immunogenicity. Streptolysin S is a hemolysin that injures the cell membranes of a variety of cells (including those of the myocardium),[542] but it is not immunogenic. In addition, four deoxyribonucleases (DNAses)—A, B, C and D—are elaborated; hyaluronidase, streptokinase, proteinases, amylases, esterases are also produced. These last products facilitate the liquidation of pus and the spread of streptococcus through tissues. In addition, considerable attention has recently been given to a family of molecules produced by group A streptococci called *streptococcal pyrogenic exotoxins.* In the older literature, these have been called *erythrogenic* and *scarlet fever toxins.* Streptococcal pyrogenic exotoxin-A can maximally stimulate the production of tumor necrosis factor-α by peripheral monocytes, which with interleukin-1β, contributes to the pathogenesis of shock and tissue injury.

Before the advent of antibiotics, group A streptococcal pneumonia accounted for 3% to 25% of childhood bacterial pneumonia and had a mortality rate of 75% to 90%.[543] Epidemic pneumonia occurred in military adolescents in the early part of the century[544] and in the 1960s.[545] Many believe that certain antecedent viral illnesses predispose to group A streptococcal pneumonia.[546] Few specific data have been gathered by modern epidemiologic techniques, but the recognition that epidemics of influenza, measles, and varicella have occurred with group A streptococcal outbreaks would seem to support this anecdotal association.[546]

The incidence of streptococcal pneumonia increases after 5 years of age into adolescence.[546] The peak incidence is in winter; most cases occur from late autumn through early spring.

Streptococcal pneumonia is usually acquired by the inhalational route but may also arise from secondary seeding from a bacteremic focus.[547] There are two distribution patterns: Most patients have a patchy, interstitial bronchopneumonia, whereas about one fourth have a lobar pattern.[544] Histologically, the lungs have thickened bronchiolar walls, necrosis of the mucosal lining[546] with formation of ragged ulcers, purulent engorgement of the lymphatic system, and microabscesses that can rupture into the pleura. Pleural effusion is usually present; it is serous initially but may become serosanguinous with rapid progression to fibrinopurulence.

Most children are ill for 2 to 3 days before experiencing an abrupt progression of the symptoms associated with respiratory compromise. Fever, chills, lethargy, myalgia, dyspnea, cough, pleuritic chest pain, and hemoptysis are common presenting complaints.[546] Weight loss is typical and may be profound. About one third of children have an associated streptococcal pharyngitis. Rarely, group A streptococcal pneumonia may be associated with purpura fulminans[548] or streptococcal toxic shock syndrome.[549]

The diagnosis is made by recovery of the causative organism from the lung, pleural fluid, or blood. Suggestive evidence allowing a presumptive diagnosis includes recovery of the organism from the oropharynx or sputum. Serologic diagnosis includes demonstration of a rising titer against a relevant streptococcal antigen. Included in this regard are antistreptolysin-O, antihyaluronidase, and anti-DNAse B. The detection of antibody to streptokinase and anti-DNAase A may also be of use, but these tests are not performed by many laboratories. The Streptozyme test may also be useful for detecting antibodies to streptococcal "extracellular products," but it is less specific. Leukocytosis is variably present; mild to moderate anemia may reflect intrapleural blood loss. Radiographically, group A streptococcal pneumonia is manifested as a patchy bronchopneumonia or lobar pattern with frequent cavitation, parapneumonic effusion, and empyema.[548]

Treatment consists of intravenous penicillin G at a high dose. Resistance has not yet been recognized. A 2- to 4-week course is usual, and the medication may be given orally after satisfactory clinical improvement. Despite the susceptibility of the causative organism to penicillin, the resolution of pneumonia may be slow; fever and pleuritic chest pain may persist for 8 to 10 days.[546]

Pulmonary complications include pneumothorax, pneumatocele, bronchiectasis, persistent atelectasis, and bronchopulmonary fistula.[547] Pleural effusions may be copious in volume and average 100 to 150 ml/day in infants and considerably more in adults.[546] Empyema occurs in a high number of cases.[548] The fluid may be tenacious, and drainage may be difficult[546]; thus surgical drainage or decortication may be required.[550] Pericarditis has been reported in about 10% of children.[546]

Other Streptococcal Species

Pneumonia may occasionally be caused by viridans streptococci, nutritionally deficient streptococci, the *S. intermedius* or *S. milleri* group, or β-hemolytic streptococci groups C and G. The taxonomy of these organisms has been imprecise and controversial. Viridans streptococci possess general characteristics of all streptococci. When cultivated on blood agar, they characteristically produce a zone of greening, so-called α-hemolysis, which is a phenomenon reflecting partial hemolysis. They are distinguished from pneumococci, many enterococci, and nonenterococcal group D streptococci by their resistance to optochin and inhibition of growth in 6.5% sodium chloride. Some viridans streptococci react with Lancefield grouping antisera, but many isolates cannot be grouped. Clinically important species belonging to the viridans group include *S. anginosus, S. constellatus, S. crista, S. gordonii, S. mitis, S. mutans, S. oralis, S. parasanguis, S. salivarius, S. sanguis, S. sobrinus,* and *S. vestibularis.*

The terms *S. intermedius group* and *S. milleri group* are used synonymously as taxonomic designations for a group of organisms that have been described by a variety of other terms. The following species are designated within the group: *S. constellatus, S. anginosus,* and *S. intermedius.* So-called nutritionally variant or deficient streptococci are related to the viridans streptococci but are distinguished by their lack of alkaline phosphatase and inability to hydrolyze arginine or hippurate. The following species have been delineated: *S. adjacens* and *S. defectivus.* Group C streptococci include *S. equisimilis, S. zooepidemicus,* and *S. equi.* This group includes primarily veterinary species, although these organisms can also infect humans. *S. equisimilis* and group G streptococci are occasional constituents of the normal flora of the pharynx, skin, and genital tract.

The viridans streptococci (including the nutritionally deficient streptococci) and the *S. intermedius/S. milleri* group are endogenous flora and are normally carried in the upper respiratory tract, particularly the oropharynx (gingival crevices, dental plaque, teeth surfaces), intestinal tract, female genital tract, and skin. Groups C and G streptococci have been identified as constituents of the normal flora of the nasopharynx, skin, and genital tract. Group C organisms have also been isolated from the umbilical surface of healthy newborns and from vaginal cultures of puerperal women. Group G organisms have also been found in the intestinal tract.

Viridans streptococci are rarely proved to be the cause of pneumonia in adults and children. In a few adults[551-553] and children,[554] they have been isolated from the blood during a clinical illness consistent with bacterial pneumonia. In a Canadian study of 1118 patients with pneumonia, 76 of whom were bacteremic, 7 (9%) of the 76 bacteremic patients had viridans streptococci isolated from the blood.[555] Some of these isolates may, of course, have represented procedural contaminants. More commonly, invasive viridans group infection results in bacteremia or endocarditis. Non–group D α-hemolytic organisms have been implicated as a cause of neonatal sepsis.[556]

Identifying viridans streptococci as a more frequent cause of pneumonia has been difficult, partly because of their presence among the normal flora and because of their susceptibility to many antimicrobials used to treat presumed bacterial pneumonias. It is possible that they have a greater role in the pathogenesis of pneumonias associated with aspiration, but even in this situation, they are usually recovered with other microorganisms, particularly anaerobes. This fact further complicates the understanding of their role. It has even been suggested that the pathogenicity of the *S. intermedius/S. milleri* group in the lung might be related to synergy with an anaerobic organism.[557]

Members of the *S. intermedius/S. milleri* group are also infrequently implicated as etiologic agents in patients with pneumonia. In a review of *S. milleri* infections in 51 adults, no cases of pneumonia were identified, although 8 cases of pleural empyema occurred.[558] Among 186 patients with *S. milleri* infection in New Zealand, 12% of the infections were of pleuropulmonary origin.[559] *S. milleri* has also been reported as a cause of neonatal sepsis.[560,561] In this instance, the organism may be acquired antenatally from the maternal vaginal tract or during the birthing process.[562]

Group C streptococcus is an uncommon cause of pneumonia, but the clinical picture may be severe and may resemble that of pneumonia caused by group A streptococci.[563] The pneumonia is usually lobar, with associated bacteremia occurring in most cases. Group G streptococcus is also a rare cause of pneumonia that occurs in both immunologically normal and immunocompromised patients.

The diagnosis is usually based on recovery of the organism from a culture of blood, sputum, abscess, or pleural fluid. In one review of viridans pneumonia in adults, the chest radiographs were not distinctive: A segmental alveolar opacity was the most common abnormal finding.[154] In a separate report, radiographs of four cases of community-acquired viridans pneumonia in South Africa demonstrated a segmental or subsegmental consolidation, which appeared "mass-like" in two of four patients.[564]

The organisms are usually susceptible to many antibiotics, including penicillins, cephalosporins, clindamycin, and vancomycin. In the neonate, ampicillin and gentamicin are effective. In the child allergic to penicillin, erythromycin may be used.[565] Group C streptococcal pneumonia has been treated with penicillin G; however, because few cases have been well documented, information about the performance of other compounds is limited.

Empyema and lung abscess are common with viridans pneumonia and may require drainage for effective treatment. Complications of group C streptococcal infection include metastatic infectious foci, empyema, and intraparenchymal cavitation.

In adults, the mortality rate reported was 28% in one study[154] and 26% in another.[566] In neonates, the mortality rate from viridans streptococci infection appears to be lower than that from GBS infection.

Yersinia Species

Several species of *Yersinia* organisms—*Y. enterocolitica, Y. pseudotuberculosis,* and *Y. pestis*—can cause disease in humans. The most important species, particularly regarding pneumonia, is *Y. pestis,* the cause of plague. The organism, a gram-negative, nonmotile coccobacillus,[324] was first identified in 1894 by Alexandre Yersin during an epidemic in Hong Kong[567] and was named *Pasteurella pestis* to honor his teacher, Louis Pasteur; it was subsequently renamed *Y. pestis* to honor Dr. Yersin. It is closely related to the relatively benign *Y. pseudotuberculosis.* The disease has played a prominent role in world history since the start of civilization. There are biblical descriptions of outbreaks in 1320 BC, and a pandemic in Europe in AD 542 caused an estimated 100 million deaths.[568] Rat flea-borne plague had a devastating effect in Europe in the Middle Ages, killing 25% of the entire European population[568]; the English plague in 1665 had a similar effect. The plague was first recognized in North America in Pacific and Gulf Coast ports during the pandemic in the first part of the twentieth century.[324] In the United States, however, cases in crowded, urban settings have disappeared, with the last known urban plague occurring in Los Angeles between 1924 and 1925.[324]

Plague occurs worldwide. It has been suggested that there is a decreased incidence of human plague in the past several years,[569] whereas peripatetic plague has increased with travel to areas where human plague is not acquired.[570] Most human cases have been reported in developing countries, especially in South America, Asia, and Africa. In 1987, 33.7% of all cases in the world occurred in Tanzania.[569] Other countries reporting a substantial number of cases include Vietnam, Zaire, Brazil, Madagascar, Peru, Uganda, Burma, Bolivia, and Botswana.

In the United States, human plague is infrequent. Most cases occur in the southwestern states, such as Arizona, Colorado, Utah, and California. New Mexico had the most reported cases in the United States from 1956 to 1987[571]; this state had 53.9% of the 299 cases reported.

A 5- to 8-year periodicity has been evident.[324] From 1908 to 1965, 111 human infections and 64 deaths were reported in the United States,[572] and from 1970 to 1995, 341 were reported. More than half of the cases of plague in the United States occur in children.[573] Human plague is seasonal, and most cases in the United States occur from May to September, with a peak in July,[324] although cases may occur all year. Male patients become ill with plague more often than female patients, except in the oldest and youngest age groups.[324] The youngest reported case was a 5-day-old infant.[573]

Plague is maintained in well-established foci among the wild rodent population, although much is unknown about the transmission cycle.[324] Worldwide, more than 200 species of mammals and 80 species of fleas have been implicated in keeping *Y. pestis* in enzootic foci.[574] The urban and domestic rat, *Rattus rattus* and *R. norvegicus,* are the most important mammals. In the United States, the sciurid rodents (e.g., rock squirrels, California ground squirrels, chipmunks, prairie dogs) are most frequently associated with human cases; cricetid rodents, such as wood rats, are an occasional source.[324] Cases have also occurred after exposure to infected animal carcasses such as those of deer, fox, badger, bobcat, and coyote; these animals are incidentally infected and rarely develop illness.[324] Cats who consume sick or dead plague-infected mammals or who are bitten by infected fleas may sometimes transmit infection to humans by a bite, scratch, or sputum expectoration.[324]

Human plague has also been traced to wild rabbit exposures. Camels and goats in Libya are susceptible to the plague and may pass it to humans.[575]

Worldwide, *Xenopsylla cheopis* is the most efficient flea vector. In the United States, infected rodent fleas important in transmission include *Diamanus montanus* and *Thrassis bacchi.*[324] *Y. pestis* multiplies in the esophagus of the flea and is regurgitated when the flea sucks blood. Once it gains access to the human host, the bacterium may multiply intracellularly and spread from the lesion to the regional lymph nodes, with bacteremia following 5 to 10 days later.

Plague has been classified clinically into the following syndromes: bubonic, septicemic, pneumonic, and meningitic. The terminology can be confusing. Most authors use the term *pneumonic plague* to indicate the presence of pneumonitis. The lung may become infected by two routes. Inhalation of the organism from an infected person or animal, such as a cat,[576] produces so-called primary pneumonia, which is rare. In support of this, no cases of person-to-person spread have been identified in the United States since the 1925 Los Angeles epidemic.[324] Only eight cases of primary inhalational pneumonia from any source were identified from 1970 to 1995 in the United States, and all were believed to be associated with infected animals, cats being implicated in most cases. Indeed, cats who develop pneumonic plague may cough and transmit infectious aerosols to those caring for the sick animal.[324] The method by which cats become infected is unclear, but in one instance, the chipmunk was suggested as a source.

Secondary pneumonic plague, in which the lung is seeded during bacteremia, is more frequent; it usually represents bloodstream invasion from an infected lymph node or bubo.[577] The bubo may be inapparent; when the bubo is absent, the syndrome is termed *septicemic plague.* Such pulmonary seeding during bacteremia is presumed common because 22% of plague cases in the United States from 1975 to 1980 had evidence of pulmonary involvement,[324] whereas from 1970 to 1995, 45 cases of pneumonic plague (primary and secondary) were reported to the CDC; 14 of these patients were up to 18 years of age, and 4 were younger than 10 years of age.

Primary pneumonic plague has a short incubation period (≤3 days) and may quickly spread among close human contacts. Clinical features include cough, chest pain, bloody sputum, high fever, and chills.[578] In addition, nausea, vomiting, diarrhea, and abdominal pain may be present. In children, encephalopathy may be present and is characterized by lethargy, ataxia, and confusion.[577] The course may be fulminant.

The diagnosis is suggested by the demonstration of typical, gram-negative, bipolar, safety pin-shaped coccobacilli in the sputum. When available, sputum is the specimen of highest yield.[569] A smear and culture of a bubo aspirate or other relevant body fluid and a blood culture may be useful. A fluorescent antibody test is available in some laboratories[324] and can be performed directly on clinical specimens. Confirmation by culture should be obtained, but definitive identification may require input from the Plague Branch of the CDC in Fort Collins, Colorado, where a passive hemagglutination serology test is available; a fourfold rise or a single titer higher than 1:16 is diagnostic.[578]

The antimicrobial agent of choice is streptomycin. Other aminoglycosides said to be effective include gentamicin and kanamycin.[324] Tetracycline and sulfadiazine are effective alternatives.[324] TMP/SMX has also been used but is less effective than streptomycin.[579] Chloramphenicol should be used when meningitis or endophthalmitis is present. Resistance has been infrequent, although a virulent streptomycin-resistant strain was isolated in Vietnam in 1965.[580]

A child with plague should be placed into respiratory isolation. If pulmonary involvement is documented, precautions may be discontinued when 4 days of antibiotic therapy have been administered.[324,573,578]

If the condition is untreated, the mortality rate in patients with pulmonary plague is 100%.[578] Survival is rare when treatment is not initiated within 18 to 24 hours after the onset of clinical symptoms. However, with appropriate and timely antibiotic therapy, the condition usually improves within 24 to 48 hours. In reviewed cases of pneumonic plague from 1970 to 1995, the case fatality rate was 40%.

Vaccines against plague have been in development since at least 1897 but were sufficiently reactogenic to produce "local and general reactions to incapacitate a healthy subject for a day or two."[581] Today, a less reactogenic, formalin-killed vaccine is available in the United States and is recommended for laboratory personnel working with *Y. pestis,* people who are exposed to materials or animals with possible infection, isolated park or forest rangers, or wildlife workers. In addition, people traveling to epidemic or hyperendemic areas are possible candidates for immunization.[324] Vaccine-induced immunity is short-lived and probably wanes after 6 months, so reinoculation is recommended.[582] There are no recommendations for the use of this vaccine in children.

Indirect and circumstantial evidence indicates that this vaccine is highly efficacious. It was used in U.S. military personnel in the Vietnam war because human plague was epidemic in Vietnam at that time; the incidence of clinical plague in those Americans was low.[583]

Household contacts and others with intimate exposures to a patient with plague should be instructed to monitor themselves for fever, sore throat, or any respiratory symptoms and to seek immediate medical attention if any symptoms arise.[324] Prophylactic agents should be given to people exposed to a patient who has pneumonic plague.[324] For children younger than 8 years of age, TMP/SMX is usually recommended.[578] For older people, tetracycline or doxycycline is recommended.

When a case of human plague is identified, insecticidal control measures against fleas should be instituted immediately. Areas of human risk should be posted and notices of plague areas announced to the media with the request that all citizens report any sick or dead animals.[324] It has recently been suggested that PCR using a 478–base pair segment of the plasminogen activator gene locus as the amplification target[574] may aid in surveillance. Rodent serologic testing may aid in predicting areas where plague may occur in identified, recently active foci.[584]

Although the inactivated, whole-cell *Y. pestis* vaccine is recommended for individuals with occupational exposure, vaccinated individuals should take precautions identical to those recommended for unvaccinated individuals because the vaccine is unlikely to be 100% efficacious.

Y. enterocolitica is widely distributed in nature and is isolated from animals, particularly pigs, horses, and dogs. It typically causes acute gastroenteritis and enterocolitis[253] and is a rare cause of pneumonia in both immunocompetent and immunocompromised patients.[585] Its epidemiology is obscure. Radiographically, hilar adenopathy may be the only finding,[253] although fluffy infiltrates, consolidations, or nodules may be evident. The organism is susceptible to streptomycin, chloramphenicol, tetracycline,[253] TMP/SMX, aminoglycosides, extended-spectrum cephalosporins, and quinolones.[586] There is no clear therapy of choice. Necrotizing *Y. enterocolitica* pneumonia in an immunocompromised adult was successfully treated with an extended-spectrum cephalosporin for 6 weeks,[587] and a child was treated with cefuroxime followed by TMP/SMX.[586] Complications of *Y. enterocolitica* pneumonia have included lung abscess, empyema,[586] and erythema nodosum as part of a sarcoidlike syndrome with hilar adenopathy.[253]

LUNG ABSCESS

A lung abscess is an accumulation of inflammatory cells, especially polymorphonuclear leukocytes, accompanied by tissue destruction or necrosis that produces one or more large cavities in the lung. It is probably arbitrary to designate larger cavities by the term *lung abscesses,* and smaller, multiple cavities with similar histologic appearance by the term *necrotizing pneumonia.* However, because a lung abscess has distinctive pathophysiologic and clinical features, it will be considered separately here.

Lung abscess is unusual in children. Among 230,325 consecutive admissions to Children's Memorial Hospital in Chicago from 1985 to 1990, only 28 children had a discharge diagnosis of lung abscess, a rate of 1 case per 8226 admissions.[588]

Some authors classify a lung abscess according to whether it occurred in a patient with no underlying disorder (primary) or in a patient with an underlying or predisposing condition (secondary).[589-591] The authors have not found this distinction helpful. Rather, consideration of the pathogenesis of a lung abscess provides a more useful consideration for the approach to diagnosis and therapy.

Pathophysiology

Aspiration is the most important factor predisposing a child to lung abscess. Therefore children who have relevant conditions (e.g., achalasia, chronic neurologic conditions) are at increased risk. Aspiration alone, however, is not sufficient to cause lung abscess because all children and adults aspirate daily to some degree. It is likely that the number of aspirations, the volume of the aspirated material, and any impairment of normal respiratory tract clearance mechanisms of aspirated material contribute to the likelihood of abscess formation. The most common sites of lung abscess formation are the most frequent destinations of aspirated material (i.e., those most dependent in the recumbent position: the right and left upper lobes and the apical segments of both lower lobes). If periodontal disease is present, the potential for lower respiratory tract infections with aspiration is increased because these children have more oropharyngeal organisms.

After a known aspiration event has occurred, it takes several days for an abscess to develop and for signs and symptoms to occur.[592] The localized inflammatory process that constitutes the host response to the aspirated material may paradoxically induce a delay in healing by mechanically obstructing the vascular supply to the area. The result may therefore be an inability to physiologically drain the affected area and to transport other defense mediators to the region. Tissue necrosis may ensue, with the dead tissue forming a spherical cavity bounded by a fibrous wall. Such a walled-off cavity may then lead to a large solitary lung abscess or small regions of necrosis with or without air-fluid levels.

A single abscess is clinically recognized more frequently than multiple abscesses. An abscess may vary from a few millimeters to 5 to 6 cm in diameter. After cavitation has occurred, a putrid oral discharge may be noted in more than 50% of children. This discharge is often copious, fetid, and green-black (hence the name *gangrene of the lung*).[593]

Other predisposing factors may also place a patient at risk for lung abscess. For example, a lung abscess may evolve from untreated pneumonia that progresses to abscess formation or from antecedent bronchiectasis; alternatively, a subdiaphragmatic, intraabdominal infection may extend into the lung or pleural space via the lymphatic system.[592] A lung abscess may also result from airway obstruction by a foreign body, an enlarged mediastinal lymph node, or a neoplastic mass. It may occur with infection in a congenitally abnormal lung (e.g., sequestration, lung cysts). Although rare in children, a lung abscess may result from extension of a parapharyngeal abscess. Seeding of the lung by a septic embolus from bacterial endocarditis (usually right sided in origin), a distant suppurative thrombophlebitis, or seeding of the lung during any bacteremia may also occur. In these instances, multiple small abscess or cavities may be present in the lung, even though the initial lesion may appear to involve only a single lobe. Seeding of other lobes may have occurred but may not become clinically apparent until later.[592]

Clinical Features

The clinical spectrum of illness in children with lung abscess is variable and often indistinct from related pulmonary infectious syndromes such as pneumonia. Tan et al[589] summarized the symptoms and signs of 45 children with lung abscess of varying pathogeneses; only fever (84%) and cough (53%) occurred in the majority of these patients. Other symptoms and signs included dyspnea (35%), chest pain (24%), anorexia (20%), production of "purulent" sputum (18%), rhinorrhea (16%), and malaise and lethargy (11%). Infrequently, diarrhea, vomiting, or irritability may be present. Minor hemoptysis is common in adults but may be life threatening in children.[594] The course of a lung abscess before medical intervention may be surprisingly indolent and may last several weeks. Weight loss may occur. Conversely, the clinical course is occasionally more aggressive; apnea and hypotension may be present.[592]

The physical findings in children with lung abscess resemble those found in early pneumonia and include tachypnea and audible crackles on auscultation. If the abscess persisted for a time before medical intervention, amphoric or cavernous breath sounds may be evident. Digital clubbing is rare.[595]

Laboratory findings are not specific. White blood cell counts range from 14,000 to 23,000/mm^3.[589] Mild anemia may be present.

The diagnosis of lung abscess is usually suggested by a chest radiograph in which an abscess appears as a thick-walled cavity with an air-fluid level (Fig. 39-16). Initially, however, the lung abscess appears as a solid lesion within the parenchyma, most often surrounded by an alveolar infiltrate. At this stage, the chest radiograph may be misleading (Fig. 39-17) because the abscess may appear as a solid mass and may be indistinguishable from the surrounding infiltrate or from a concomitant pleural effusion or an empyema; gas may be absent. Particularly at this stage, an abscess must be distinguished from a loculated empyema and a pneumatocele. The latter have thin walls and do not contain air-fluid levels.[596] Suspicion of an abscess may arise when the "consolidation" is unusually persistent, when "pneumonia" remains persistently round or masslike, or when a bulging fissure representing increased volume of the involved lobe is present.[597]

Gas may be present in an abscess as a result of bacterial metabolism by gas-forming organisms or as a result of a communication with a bronchus. Once gas is present within the abscess cavity, its appearance by radiography is characterized by irregular, thick walls; air-fluid levels may be multiple and are optimally demonstrated when the radiographs are taken with a horizontal beam (upright or decubitus cross-table). Mediastinal adenopathy sometimes accompanies the parenchymal infection and may also be evident on the chest radiograph.[598]

Lung abscesses may occur at any site. A review of several recent series of children with lung abscesses suggested that occurrence in the right lung was more frequent (about 70%) and that although any lobe may be involved, the upper, middle, and lower lobes accounted for about 40%, 20%, and 40%, respectively, of right-sided lung abscess in children.[588,589,591] As noted, the location of a lung abscess may provide a clue as to pathogenesis. For example, abscesses resulting from septic embolic events tend to be multiple and more diffusely situated than the solitary abscess secondary to aspiration, which is often situated in the right upper or lower lobe.

Diagnosis

Contrast-enhanced CT may aid the clinician in localizing an abscess and in distinguishing it from empyema, pneumatocele, bronchopleural fistula, congenital anomalies (such as bronchogenic and duplication cysts), pulmonary sequestration, or rarely, persistent pneumonia[597] (Fig. 39-18). CT is also used to guide diagnostic and therapeutic drainage procedures.[597] The classic findings of a lung abscess by this modality include a thick, ragged wall; central fluid; acute angle with the chest wall; and surrounding parenchymal consolidation. An air-fluid level may be seen even when it is not apparent on the plain radiograph. Helpful features that distinguish abscess from other entities include the well-marginated nature of the abscess mass, distinction between it and the pleura, greater density of the abscess than of water, and contrast enhancement in adjacent tissues. Bolus contrast injection may demonstrate pulmonary vascular branches in the territory of an equivocal lesion and thereby reveals its pulmonary rather than pleural

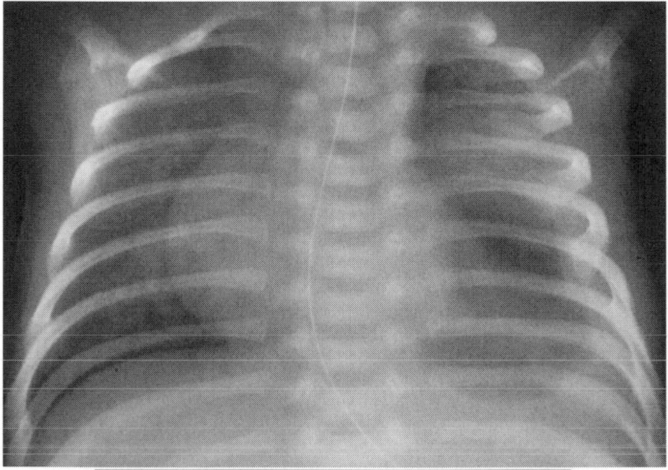

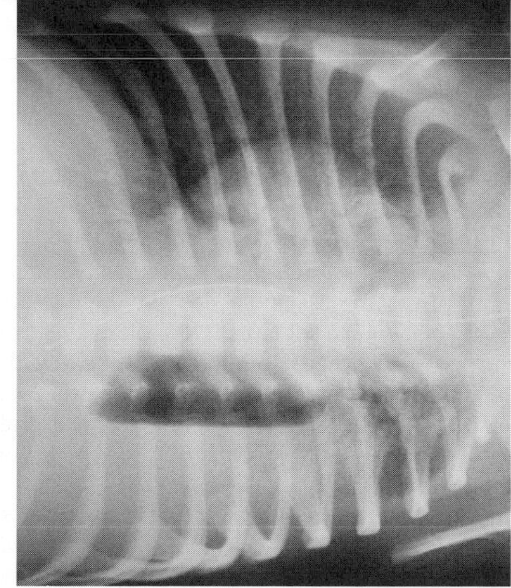

Fig. 39-16. Lung abscess in a 2-week-old boy with a cavitary lesion in the left side of the chest. **A,** Supine anteroposterior chest radiograph demonstrates a large cavity in the left lower lobe, causing a mediastinal shift to the right. **B,** Left side-down decubitus film shows a large air-filled level within the cavity.

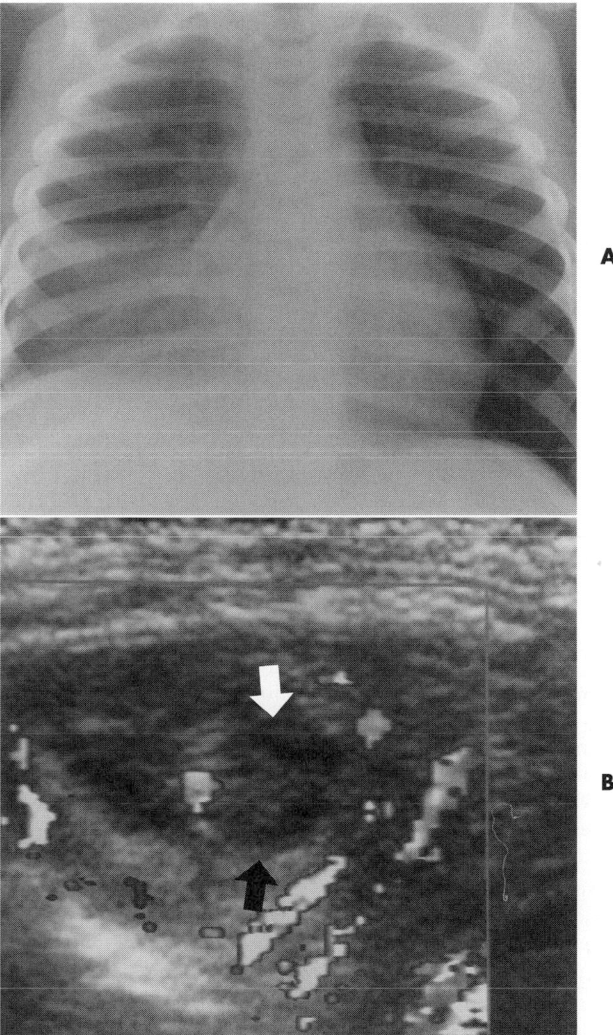

Fig. 39-17. Occult lung abscess. Pneumonia in the right middle lobe in an 18-month-old boy did not respond to antibiotic therapy as expected. **A,** Chest radiograph demonstrates a straightforward pleuropneumonia in the right middle lobe without volume expansion or an air-containing cavity. **B,** Sonography demonstrates a mostly avascular hypoechoic lesion within the consolidation *(arrows).* Black-and-white rendering of a color Doppler examination of the infiltrate demonstrates pulmonary vessels supplying the lung around the abscess and a still-vascular nodule within the abscess.

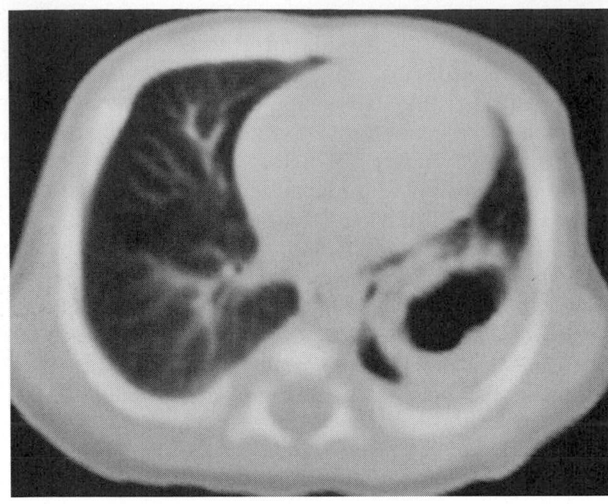

Fig. 39-18. CT of a lung abscess. The cavity has thick, irregular walls and an acute angle with the chest wall, features typical of a lung abscess. A sonographically guided fluid aspiration yielded pus. The lesion healed without further intervention.

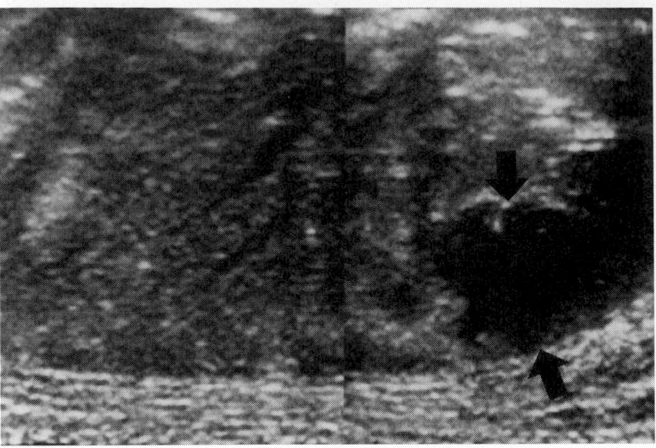

Fig. 39-20. Sonography of lung abscess. An irregular cavity *(arrows)* with irregular walls, an acute angle with the chest wall, a hypoechoic center, and an absence of separation of pleural layers characterize this lung abscess in a 3-year-old girl who developed fever, cough, and a persistent infiltrate in the left lower lobe after trauma.

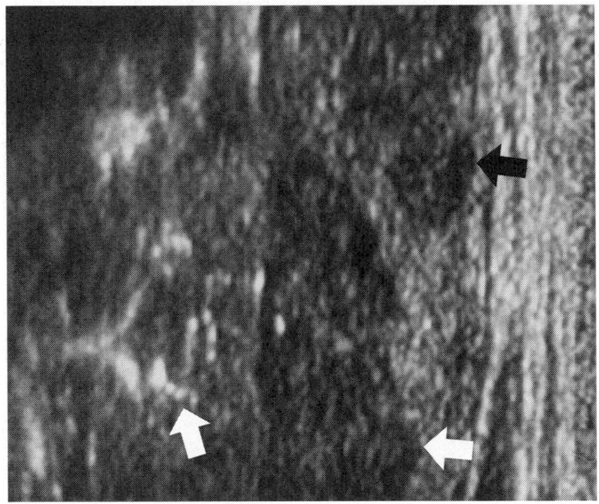

Fig. 39-19. Sonography of early cavitation in a 3-year-old boy with a bulging fissure on the chest radiograph (same patient as in Figs. 39-2 and 39-7; all studies performed within 24 hours of one other). Sonography demonstrates a complete consolidation of the left upper lobe. Discrete areas of decreased echogenicity mark regions of future cavitation *(arrows)*. Those were seen later as air-filled cavities in chest radiographs. This image can be compared with Fig. 39-6, which demonstrates an uncomplicated homogeneous consolidation.

origins.[81] Occasionally, an abscess may rupture into the pleural cavity and result in a combined lesion with CT features of both pleural and pulmonary pathology.

Sonography is also a valuable tool, particularly in patients in emergency situations and in critically ill patients in whom the abscess abuts the chest wall, diaphragm, or mediastinum and thereby provides an acoustic window (Fig. 39-19). With this technique, a lung abscess has a thick, irregular wall with a blurred outer margin and an oval or round shape. It forms an acute angle with the chest wall, and pleural layers are absent.[599] Color and spectral Doppler may allow demonstration of the abscess within the territory supplied by the pulmonary artery. However, any long-standing inflammatory process in the lung, including an abscess, may parasitize the blood supply from the chest wall, and thus the abscess may be supplied by the intercostal and bronchial arteries.[100] A lung abscess may possess an avascular hypoechoic center even before it contains air. If the abscess is adherent to the chest wall, real-time sonography shows absence of gliding against the chest wall (Fig. 39-20).

A lung abscess has also been identified by technetium-99m white blood cell scintigraphy[596] in a patient in whom this diagnosis was not suspected. Therefore a chest radiograph had not been done.

Defining the bacteriologic diagnosis of a lung abscess in children poses some practical problems; bacteremia is infrequent.[600] Material for culture from the abscess cavity itself is usually not obtained because of the procedure's invasive nature. Sputum cannot usually be obtained from young children, and even when available, sputum culture may reflect pharyngeal flora. Diagnostic evaluation of a concomitant pleural effusion associated with a lung abscess may provide an opportunity to isolate the causative organism.

Diagnostic needle aspiration of a lung abscess depends on accessibility of the abscess and a size sufficient to allow procurement of an adequate specimen. It is often performed with ultrasound or CT guidance. Both the sensitivity and the specificity of this procedure are high, although the procedure is not without risk.[601] Among six studies using needle aspiration for diagnosis, 24 complications occurred among 800 children, 2 of which were serious (pneumothorax).[602]

Useful information may be obtained from needle aspiration of a lung abscess when it is performed in appropriately selected cases. Among 35 consecutive patients in Taiwan with lung abscess (31 adults, 3 adolescents, and 1 child), needle aspiration was successfully performed in 33.[603] Two patients developed a pneumothorax of minor clinical importance. One or more microorganisms were recovered from 31 of the 33 patients, many of whom were receiving antibiotics. In contrast, the offending pathogen was recovered from only 3% of blood cultures, 11% of sputum cultures, and 3.1% alveolar lavage fluid cultures.

Transtracheal aspiration, a procedure once commonly used to obtain material in adults for the etiologic diagnosis of lung abscess, is unsuitable in small children for technical reasons and may not yield the offending pathogens. BAL in adults has compared favorably with transtracheal aspiration for identifying aerobic and anaerobic organisms.[604] However, no data are available regarding this modality in the diagnosis of lung abscess in children.

Etiology

For patients with lung abscesses, the techniques required to obtain material for culture are often invasive. As a result, only a subset of patients with lung abscess are subjected to such procedure; therefore published information regarding the etiology may partly reflect selection bias. Nevertheless, it seems reasonable to conclude that the organisms causing lung abscess are generally those normally inhabiting the upper respiratory tract. Thus anaerobes are often implicated in the etiology of lung abscess. Important clues that suggest anaerobic lung infection are observed aspiration, disease in a dependent segment, cavitation or abscess formation with or without empyema, and foul-smelling sputum or another body fluid. Anaerobes, either alone or with aerobes, have been recovered from about 30% of adults with lung abscesses.[605] In one study of children with lung abscess, anaerobes were identified by transtracheal aspiration in all 10.[606] The most common anaerobic isolates were gram-positive cocci, pigmented *Prevotella* species, members of the *Porphyromonas* group, and *Fusobacterium* species. The predominant aerobic bacterial isolates were α-hemolytic streptococci, *E. coli, K. pneumoniae, S. pyogenes, P. aeruginosa,* and *S. pneumoniae. S. aureus* has also been implicated as a cause of lung abscesses, especially when they are multiple or believed to occur as an embolic complication of an intravascular infection, such as endocarditis. In addition, many other bacterial species have occasionally been isolated from lung abscesses. *Mycobacterium fortuitum* may cause lung abscess.[607] *Arcanobacterium hemolyticum* was identified as a cause of lung abscess in a child, and it was also isolated from expectorated sputum and from material obtained from bronchoscopy in an otherwise healthy, immunologically normal adolescent.[608] In immunodeficient patients or those receiving immunosuppressive therapy, *Alcaligenes xylosoxidans*[609] and *Pseudallescheria boydii*[610] have been isolated. *Selenomonas artemidis*[611] was isolated from a patient with lung abscess and tuberculosis. *Lactobacillus casei (L. rhamnosus)*[612] and botryomycosis.[613] *Salmonella* species have been associated with lung abscess, rarely in healthy patients but in a patient with Wegener's granulomatosis.[614]

Lung abscess is rare in neonates[615]; six were found in a review of medical records spanning 20 years at Parkland Memorial Hospital and Children's Medical Center in Dallas. Predisposing factors may include congenital lung cysts or pneumonia. At one time, *S. aureus* pneumonia was an important predisposing factor.[616] However, with the decline in frequency of this bacterium as a cause of pneumonia, its importance as a cause of abscess has diminished as well. Lung abscess in this age group may also be caused by GBS, *E. coli,* and *K. pneumoniae.*[617]

Treatment

Antibiotic therapy is the mainstay of treatment; the length of therapy depends on the rate of abscess resolution, the extent of the abscess, and the severity of illness at presentation. On average, parenteral antibiotic therapy is provided for 2 to 3 weeks. Oral therapy may then be administered for 4 to 8 weeks.[589] Neonates should receive the entire course parenterally.

For the therapy of lung abscess that results from the introduction of pharyngeal flora into the lung (e.g., aspiration), penicillin has long been the front-line agent. However, presumably because of β-lactamase–producing anaerobes, some have preferred metronidazole or clindamycin in addition to penicillin in patients with lung abscesses who are critically ill.[618] Others have suggested ticarcillin/clavulanic acid or piperacillin/tazobactam. Care should be taken to ensure that the chosen antimicrobial regimen includes optimal coverage for *S. aureus* when a lung abscess appears to complicate a preexisting pneumonia or there is metastatic seeding from a distant focus (e.g., endocarditis). In addition to antimicrobials, physiotherapy, particularly postural drainage, is an important mainstay of therapy.

The success of medical treatment with antimicrobials and physiotherapy is related to age. The prognosis for resolution is better in children older than 10 years of age because the child may have a productive cough; thus the abscess can be physiologically drained through the larger airways.

Sometimes surgical intervention is required to provide adequate drainage for a child with a lung abscess. Indications include failure to respond to antimicrobial therapy, especially in neonates, and severity of illness (e.g., critically ill patients).[619] Newer, so-called invasive radiologic techniques aimed at providing drainage generally approach the abscess percutaneously with the guidance of CT, ultrasonography,[597,620,621] or fluoroscopy.[622] Drainage procedures have included needle aspiration or the insertion of small-bore or Malecot or "pigtail" catheters. In many instances, these techniques have replaced more traditional, more invasive procedures. Occasionally, however, the necessity for drainage may still require operative catheter insertion or wedge resection.[623] The need for definitive lobectomy should be infrequent, although in the presence of an underlying immunodeficiency (such as Job's syndrome), elective resection may be the procedure of choice[624] because the involved area may be a nidus for recurring abscesses.

Complications

A lung abscess may rupture into adjacent tissue compartments, an important complication occurring most frequently in abscesses caused by *S. aureus.* Rupture into the pleural space leads to empyema, pyothorax, or pneumothorax. Empyema may sometimes be accompanied by the formation of a bronchopleural fistula. Localized bronchiectasis may also occur as a complication. If the pathogenesis of the lung abscess was associated with bacteremia, distant metastatic foci may also be present.

Prognosis

The prognosis is good if effective therapy and close follow-up are provided and the predisposing causes can be eliminated. Asher et al[591] reported that 9 of 11 patients with "primary" lung abscess (no underlying condition) had normal pulmonary function when assessed approximately 9 years after diagnosis. All these children were growing normally. Radiologic resolution may be delayed and may require more than 6 months for complete resolution.[591]

PLEURAL EMPYEMA

An empyema is the presence of purulent material usually consisting of polymorphonuclear leukocytes and fibrin, in the pleural space. The pleural space is normally a theoretic one between the visceral and parietal pleuras, the former covering the lung parenchyma and the latter lining the interior of the thoracic cavity. The parietal pleura is sometimes said to consist of *costal, mediastinal, and diaphragmatic* parts, descriptive terms referring to the relevant, adjacent anatomic region.[625]

Normally, a small amount of fluid is evenly distributed in the pleural space and lubricates the movement of the visceral pleura on the parietal pleura during respiration. It was believed that this physiologic pleural fluid was a passive transudate from blood; however, important differences between the composition of serum and pleural fluid suggests that this is not the case. Cells (1500 to 2400 cells/mm^3) are normally present in pleural fluid in experimental animals; the majority are mesothelial or mononuclear cells, but some authors report that neutrophils may comprise 2% of the resident leukocyte population.[626]

The lymphatic vessels of the costal pleura drain ventrally to nodes along the internal thoracic artery and dorsally toward the internal intercostal lymph nodes near the insertion of the ribs. The lymphatic system of the mediastinal pleura drains to the tracheobronchial and mediastinal nodes; drainage of the diaphragmatic parietal pleura is to the parasternal, middle phrenic, and posterior mediastinal nodes. The lymphatic vessels communicate with the pleural space by means of stomas 2 to 6 nm in diameter that are found on the mediastinal pleura and intercostal aspects of the costal pleura.

Pathophysiology

Pleural empyema is usually secondary to an infection at another site, frequently pulmonary. Indeed, it occurs most commonly after infection of a parapneumonic pleural effusion, commonly present in bacterial pneumonia. Progression of such an effusion to empyema is said to have a three-stage evolution. The first stage is exudative. Antimicrobial therapy for "pneumonia" is often initiated at this stage and may abort progression.

The second stage is heralded by the arrival of bacteria, most often by pleural invasion from the contiguous pneumonic process. Progression occurs with polymorph accumulation and fibrin deposition; membrane formation occurs, and the developing empyema may become compartmentalized or loculate. With time, the pleural fluid pH and glucose concentration decrease, and the concentration of lactic acid dehydrogenase may increase.

The third stage is characterized by organization; fibroblasts grow into the exudate from the visceral and parietal pleural surfaces. An inelastic membrane called the *pleural peel* is formed and may encase the lung, with the potential to restrict respiration. The thick exudate may drain spontaneously through the chest wall or into the lung and produce either a pleurocutaneous or a bronchopleural fistula.

Less frequently, an empyema may occur in the absence of a parapneumonic process. For example, empyema may complicate a thoracic surgical procedure, especially pneumonectomy.[627] After the pneumonectomy, the space vacated by the procedure fills with serosanguinous fluid. By 2 weeks after surgery the pleural space is about 80% to 90% filled with fluid, and by 2 to 4 months the space is completely filled. As fluid accumulates, the mediastinum also shifts ipsilaterally to fill the vacated space. Failure of this shift to occur or a return to symmetry of the mediastinum may prompt consideration that empyema is present. The infecting bacterium may be introduced during the surgical procedure or may seed the collected fluid during a bacteremia that may be clinically inapparent. The time from surgery to identification of the empyema ranges from 8 days to 7 years, although most are evident within 1 month. Empyema may complicate any invasive intrathoracic procedure, such as thoracentesis, thoracotomy, or esophageal perforation.

Empyema may also be found in association with a bronchopleural fistula. The presence of such a fistula should be suspected when a child with a collection of pleural fluid produces "sputum" only when lying in one position. By radiography, a bronchopleural fistula usually has an air-fluid level in the pleural space in the upright position; CT is valuable in making this diagnosis.

Empyema may also reflect the spread of infection from an adjacent site. Such direct extension was the predisposing factor in 10% of the cases of empyema in one study.[628] Implicated in this regard were periodontal, retropharyngeal, peritonsillar, and subdiaphragmatic abscesses as well as subcutaneous abscesses of the neck.

Clinical Features

The diagnosis of empyema may pose a clinical challenge because the clinical features of empyema (classically heralded by tachypnea, tachycardia, dyspnea, cough, irregular breathing, so-called pleural pain, and possibly cyanosis) resemble those of uncomplicated pneumonia or pneumonia in the presence of an uninfected parapneumonic pleural effusion.[625] So-called pleuritic chest pain is referrable to the parietal pleura, which has pain fibers. Some children with pleural effusion have a dull, aching chest pain rather than pleuritic pain,[629] especially if the underlying process directly involves the parietal pleura (e.g., with a lung abscess). Pleuritic pain that is simultaneously perceived in the ipsilateral shoulder and in the lower chest is highly suggestive of a paradiaphragmatic pleural effusion.

A dry, nonproductive cough may be present. Dyspnea may be associated with a pleural effusion of any etiology. The degree of dyspnea may be out of proportion to the size of the pleural effusion and may reflect splinting caused by pleuritic chest pain. Fever, anorexia, malaise, headache, nausea, vomiting, and prostration are variably present in patients with empyema. In a very young child, signs and symptoms pointing toward an abdominal process may dominate the clinical picture; abdominal distention may be present. The absence of fever and symptomatology involving the chest does not exclude the presence of empyema, especially if the patient is debilitated or receiving immunosuppressive therapy.

The findings on physical examination may reflect the presence of empyema or any pleural effusion and include decreased chest movement, flushed face, nasal flaring, and sternal retractions. On inspection of the chest, a discrepancy in the size of the hemithorax may indicate ipsilateral increased pleural pressure on the larger side. Bulging of the intercostal spaces may be present. Conversely, a relatively small hemithorax may indicate decreased pleural pressure on the same side of the effusion. In this situation, the size of the intercostal spaces may be exaggerated and may retract with inspiratory efforts. Scoliosis may be present; in 44% of children with empyema the curvature of the spine was greater than 5 degrees.[630]

In children with pleural effusion, palpation of the chest may be helpful in determining the extent of the effusion. Tactile fremitus is absent or attenuated in areas of the chest where the pleural fluid separates the chest wall from the lung because the fluid absorbs the lung vibrations. This sign is more reliable than percussion in identifying the upper border of the pleural fluid and the proper location for thoracentesis. Palpation may also be useful in determining whether the cardiac point of maximal impulse is shifted. The trachea should also be palpated because its location indicates the relationship between the pleural pressures in the hemithoraxes.

Percussion over a pleural effusion is flat or dull and maximal at the base of the lung where the fluid is the thickest. If only a thin rim of fluid is present, however, there may be no change in dullness.

On auscultation, breath sounds are decreased or absent over the empyema. Paradoxically, breath sounds may be increased near the upper border of the fluid because of increased sound conductance in the partly atelectatic area under the fluid. A rub may also be present, especially if the effusion is diminishing in size, and may be associated with localized pain on breathing.

Empyema may also become apparent during the resolution of seemingly uncomplicated bacterial pneumonia; thus an apparent "relapse" of bacterial pneumonia should prompt a search for empyema. An empyema may occasionally be chronic; in this instance, symptoms involving the chest may be absent, and therefore only constitutional abnormalities, such as low-grade fever or weight loss, may provide a clinical clue.

Etiology

Historically, the rate of occurrence of empyema has been expressed as a percentage of children hospitalized with pneumonia. In the preantibiotic era, 10% of hospitalized children with pneumonia had empyema; *S. pneumoniae* was the most common pathogen. With the availability of sulfonamide antibiotics, the percentage of hospitalized children with pneumonia diminished greatly but surged in the 1950s to 14% of children hospitalized with pneumonia, with *S. aureus* accounting for 92% of the cases. In the modern antibiotic era, the percentage of children hospitalized with pneumonia that have empyema decreased to about 2%.[631]

Today, most patients develop empyema as a complication of pneumonia. *S. pneumoniae* and *S. aureus* are the most common etiologic agents.[629] *H. influenzae* type b was an important cause[632] in the prevaccination era but is now rare.

Brook[633] called attention to the role of anaerobes in empyemas occurring in children. Anaerobic bacteria (*Bacteroides* species, *Fusobacterium* species, *Peptostreptococcus* species, *Veillonella* species, *Propionibacterium* acnes, and *Clostridium perfringens*) were isolated from blood or pleural fluid in pure culture from 24% of the children studied and in combination with an aerobe in an additional 10%.[633] Foul-smelling pleural fluid was not always present when an anaerobe was isolated.[634] Presumably, anaerobic bacteria associated with empyema originate from a pulmonary process, such as pneumonia or a lung abscess, or an extrapulmonary process, such as a retropharyngeal or lymph node abscess or a paravertebral abscess.

When empyema occurs as a result of external introduction of organisms related to trauma, surgery, or thoracentesis, important causes include *S. aureus* or aerobic gram-negative bacilli.[628] Anaerobes should also be considered in this instance.

Empyema may also complicate a subdiaphragmatic abscess; in this instance, the flora may be mixed and may include enteric gram-negative bacilli, other aerobic intestinal flora, or anaerobes. Other causes of empyema are extremely infrequent. However, it is probable that any bacterium capable of infecting the lung can also be associated with a parapneumonic pleural empyema.

Diagnosis

A parapneumonic pleural effusion and empyema should be considered in the evaluation of any patient for bacterial pneumonia. The presence of an effusion is usually demonstrated by radiography of the chest. However, because uninfected parapneumonic effusions resolve with the resolution of the pneumonia, distinguishing such an uninfected effusion from empyema is of clinical importance and may be challenging. Several distinguishing features may be useful. For example, the rapid loculation of an empyema results in an inability to shift the pleural effusion. Thus demonstration of "layering," a shift in the location of the effusion with change of patient position, suggests that empyema is absent. In practice, this distinction is often made on the basis of lateral decubitus radiographs. Furthermore, a fusiform, pleural-based shadow may be present and is sometimes large enough to obliterate the entire chest and shift the mediastinum contralaterally. Empyema is also more likely when a pulmonary alveolar consolidation is adjacent or when a lung abscess or cavitary pneumonia is present.[635,636] Such an associated cavitation may have eroded into the pleural space.

The occasional complication of a bronchopleural fistula may result in a pyopneumothorax that is manifested radiographically as an air-fluid level within the pleural effusion. Unlike a pulmonary abscess, which has similar length in different projections because of its round nature, the flat geometry of empyema results in an air-fluid level that is long in one projection and much shorter in the perpendicular plane.

CT provides an excellent global view of the abnormality and enables superior evaluation of the extent of pleural involvement (Fig. 39-21). With this modality, an empyema appears with a lentiform shape at an obtuse angle with the chest wall, separation of the two pleural layers, compression of the adjacent lung, and uniform chest wall width with a sharp interface with the lung.[637,638] Contrast enhancement may demonstrate an unexpectedly thick, enhancing rind surrounding an empyema that may fail to resolve after therapy with drainage and antibiotics. Such thick, enhancing walled empyemas may be caused by *S. aureus* or other pathogens[639] and often require surgical decortication.

Sonographic characteristics of pleural empyema are similar to those described for CT (Fig. 39-22). Sonography has the superior ability to assess the quality of the fluid within the pleural space and internal septations that may complicate aspiration and drainage. Doppler sonography may aid in the differentiation of pulmonary and pleural lesions by demonstrating intercostal artery enlargement and increased flow velocities associated with an adjacent empyema.[640]

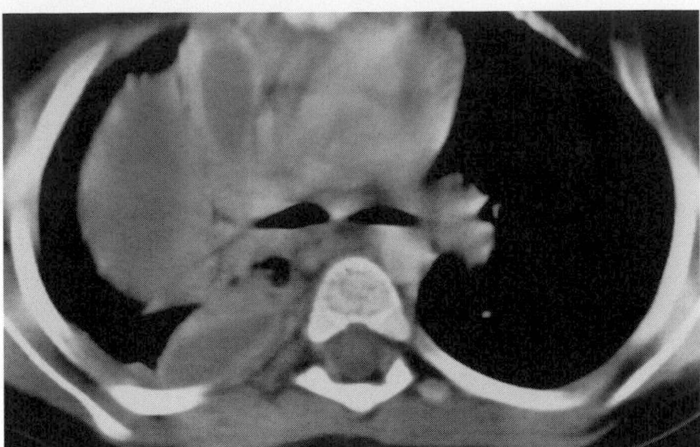

Fig. 39-21. CT of pleural empyema in a 5-year-old boy with extensive right pleuropneumonia *(S. pneumoniae).* CT was performed to clarify the various components of a complex chest radiograph with diffuse opacities. An apical, complex empyema demonstrates the classic characteristics: fusiform shape; smooth, uniform walls; an obtuse angle with the chest wall; and peripheral location (here along the mediastinal, apical, and posterior pleural surface).

Ultimately, diagnostic thoracentesis is necessary to obtain the information that allows distinction between uninfected parapneumonic effusions and empyema. The decision to perform this procedure must be individualized; all parapneumonic pleural effusions do not require diagnostic thoracentesis. However, because the presence of empyema usually necessitates drainage of the infected material, most often via the insertion of a chest tube or serial thoracenteses, the distinction is of clinical importance; therefore thoracentesis should be pursued when empyema is suspected.

The diagnosis of empyema is strongly supported by the presence of thick pus, bacteria demonstrable when the fluid is subjected to Gram's stain, a pH less than 7.3, or a glucose concentration less than 60 mg/dl. In exudative pleural effusions, the protein concentration is rarely less than 3.0 g/dl, and the lactate dehydrogenase concentration is high. The average white blood cell count in empyema fluid is 19,000 cells/mm^3 but may be somewhat lower (about 11,000 cells/mm^3) in a patient with chronic empyema. Culture of the pleural fluid should include procedures appropriate for the growth of aerobic and anaerobic bacteria, fungi, and mycobacteria.

Detection of bacterial antigens in pleural fluid is potentially useful in the diagnosis of empyema.[641] The advantages are the rapidity with which the test can be performed and the possibility that antigen may be present (despite the presence of too few organisms to allow their visualization by Gram's stain or despite a pleural fluid culture rendered sterile by prior antimicrobial therapy). The disadvantages of antigen detection tests lie in the limited availability of reagents for antigen detection for the organisms that commonly cause empyema (only *S. pneumoniae* capsular polysaccharide can be detected with commercially available reagents) and the imperfect sensitivity and specificity of the available tests.

Treatment

The mainstay of therapy in empyema consists of antimicrobial therapy[642] and adequate drainage of infected material in the pleural space. The choice of medications depends on the knowledge of the likely causative microorganisms. An appropriate empiric regimen for empyema presumptively caused by aerobic bacteria usually includes coverage for *S. aureus* and *S. pneumoniae.* A so-called semisynthetic or β-lactamase–resistant penicillin, such as oxacillin, and an extended-spectrum cephalosporin, such as ceftriaxone, are often used together as initial therapy. Most antibiotics diffuse well into the pleural fluid.[642] The duration of therapy has received little critical evaluation, but a 14- to 28-day course of therapy seems appropriate.

Closed chest drainage via a chest tube is often performed after diagnostic thoracentesis when empyema is suspected. Whether it is necessary for the therapy of all patients with empyema has not been established. For serous fluid, such drainage is probably not necessary, although patients with large effusions that cause difficulty in breathing may benefit from drainage. For thick pleural fluid containing frank pus, closed chest drainage is usually performed and may be required for effective therapy. Serial thoracentesis may be necessary to determine the need for a definitive drainage procedure. The chest tube should be positioned in a dependent part of the empyema and should be of sufficient diameter to prevent clogging. The tube should be connected to a drainage system with an underwater seal. Clinical and radiologic improvement should be evident within 24 to 72 hours, and the tube may be removed when the pleural drainage is lower than 50 ml/24 hours and the fluid is clear or yellow.

Despite these measures, the condition in some patients may fail to improve or may have a protracted, acute course; there are many reasons for this. Antibiotics may have a suboptimal antibacterial effect because of previously undetected resistant bacteria, poor penetration into an abscesslike loculation, inactivation of the antibacterial compound (e.g., a β-lactam antibiotic by β-lactamase), suboptimal antibacterial activity in the presence of low pH, or a high degree of protein binding.[643] Alternatively, pleural drainage may be inadequate. The most common explanations are loculation with obstructed communication of empyema fluid or tenacity of the exudate with obstruction of the drainage tube. Ultrasonography or CT may help clarify this situation.

Management of a patients whose condition is unresponsive to standard therapy may include reformulation of the antibacterial regimen or the placement of one or more additional chest tubes. The use of urokinase as a thrombolytic agent instilled into the pleural space via an existing chest tube has been enthusiastically received as a strategy for dissolving fibrinous loculated walls of an empyema before fibroblast collagen production has ensued.[644] This enzyme, produced by the human kidney, is less pyrogenic and is less often associated with the allergic reactions attributed to streptokinase and streptodornase. Typically, it is instilled into the chest tube and left in the pleural space for 2 hours[645] or overnight.[646] The dose instilled should be 10% of the dose used intravenously to lyse clots.[644]

When the response to standard treatment modalities is slow, the timing of further intervention is controversial. Kosloske and Cartwright[647] have argued for the early institution of surgical decortication if "fibrinopurulent" or organizing empyema is present; they intervened in children whose condition failed to improve after only 3 to 5 days of therapy. In contrast, most experts allow additional time before declaring the need for

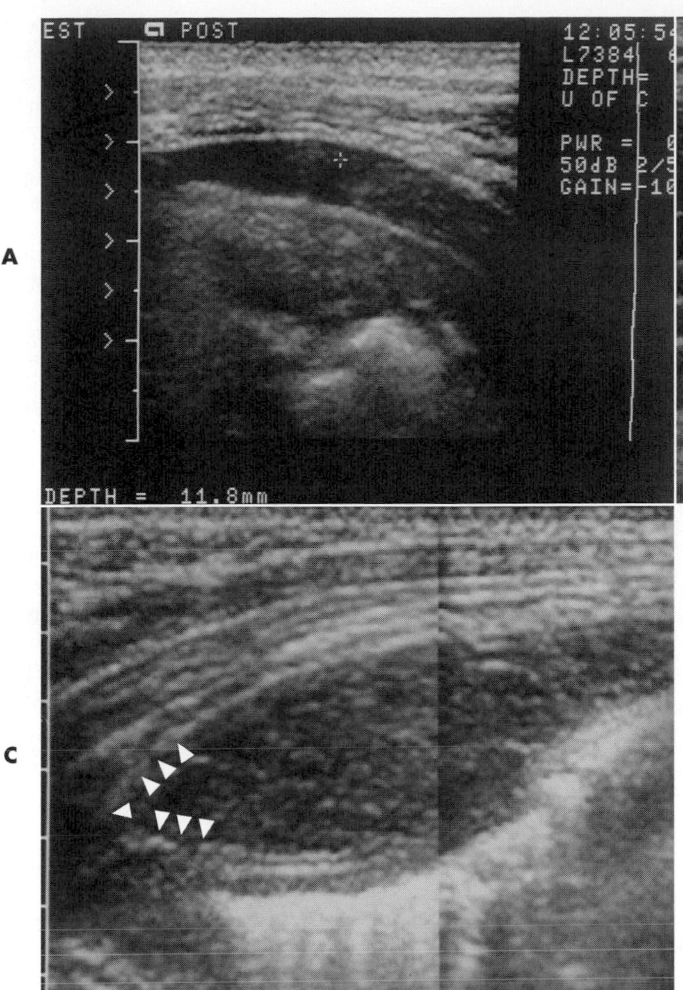

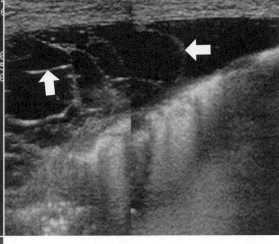

Fig. 39-22. Sonography of pleural empyema in three patients. **A,** In a 3-year-old boy with group A streptococcal pneumonia, an empyema with fluid containing debris (+) separates the chest wall from the consolidated lung. **B,** Empyema with multiple septations in a boy 3 years and 10 months old who has pleuropneumonia. **C,** Typical mature empyema: fusiform shape; thickened, separated pleural layers; uniform wall width; echogenic fluid within the empyema; and obtuse angle with the chest wall.

more aggressive therapy[644]; when necessary, decortication is usually performed 14 to 21 days after the initiation of therapy. Ultrasonographic assessment of the empyema may be useful in making decisions regarding the need for this more aggressive intervention. Surgical intervention performed with evidence of organization detectable by ultrasound was associated with decreased length of hospitalization.[648] CT may also assist decision making in this situation.

The surgical procedure of choice is also controversial. Thoracotomy with decortication (i.e., surgical excision of fibrous tissue and all pus and fluid from the visceral pleura) or drainage through an open chest tube has traditionally been indicated. In a recent review at one institution of children and adults with empyema, this procedure was performed in 56% of patients,[649] although others have indicated a less frequent need.[650] In some instances, video-assisted thoracoscopic surgery has been used in children as an alternative to thoracotomy with decortication. In this procedure, a thoracoscope is introduced into the pleural space; surgical instruments may then be introduced with thoracoscopic guidance, a chest tube may be placed, or both procedures may be done. These procedures have been used to disrupt adhesions in the pleural space, drain loculated effusions, and mechanically lyse intrapleural septations.

After evacuation of the pleural space, it may be inspected for the presence of a "peel," a pleural thickening reflecting accumulation of fibroblasts, collagenous tissue, and other products of organization. Because such a peel may embarrass respiration by restricting normal pulmonary expansion, its presence alone may indicate a thoracotomy for decortication. Such peels have been traditionally scheduled for removal by thoracotomy planned late in the course (>6 weeks), when they are well organized.

Chronic empyema is a vaguely defined term used to refer to a situation in which the patient's condition fails to improve despite therapy and there is evidence of restrictive lung function, increasing fibrosis, and lung fixation.[644,647] Decortication and even rib resection or permanent external drainage have rarely been used to treat the patient in this category. Empyema complicating pneumonectomy may also be refractory to standard therapies and therefore "chronic." In addition to these measures, treatment for postpneumonectomy empyema has included irrigation of the thoracic cavity with antibiotic solutions, open window thoracotomy, and obliteration of the cavities with muscle flaps, although the last is usually a therapeutic effort of last resort.[644]

Complications

In children with a pleural effusion, complications associated with empyema include the creation of a bronchopleural fistula by direct extension of infected pleural fluid into the lung (empyema necessitatis) or the formation of a cutaneous fistula. Other infectious complications include bacteremia and pericarditis by direct extension or bacteremic seeding and pneumothorax.[625]

Prognosis

Morbidity and mortality rates from empyema remain high even in the modern era. Risk factors for bad outcome include inadequate antibiotic therapy (choice of medications, duration of therapy, or poor compliance with a prescribed unsupervised regimen), inadequate surgical management (when indicated), and probably certain underlying conditions that compromise the immune response. An important long-term consequence of untreated empyema relates to the formation of restrictive scar tissue or peel in the pleural space and includes decreased exercise tolerance, chest contour changes, and chronic restrictive pulmonary disease. Some have suggested that scoliosis can complicate empyema.[644]

The mortality rate among patients with empyema has been estimated at 2% to 15%.[644] Risk factors for death include duration of illness, severity of infection, and young age.[644]

REFERENCES

General Aspects of Bacterial Pneumonia

1. Osler W: Lobar pneumonia. In Osler W, ed: *The principles and practice of medicine,* ed 7, New York, 1909, Appleton, pp 164-192.
2. Berman S: Epidemiology of acute respiratory infections in children of developing countries, *Rev Infect Dis* 13(suppl 6):S454-S462, 1991.
3. Foy HM, Cooney MK, Maletzky AJ, Grayston JT: Incidence and etiology of pneumonia, croup and bronchiolitis in preschool children belonging to a prepaid medical care group over a four-year period, *Am J Epidemiol* 97:80-92, 1973.
4. Denny FW, Clyde WA: Acute lower respiratory tract infections in nonhospitalized children, *J Pediatr* 108:635-646, 1986.
5. Glezen WP, Denny FW: Epidemiology of acute lower respiratory disease in children, *N Engl J Med* 288:498-505, 1973.
6. Murphy TH, Henderson FW, Clyde WA, Collier AM, Denny FW: Pneumonia: an eleven-year study in a pediatric practice, *Am J Epidemiol* 113:12-21, 1981.
7. Campbell PW: New developments in pediatric pneumonia and empyema, *Curr Opin Pediatr* 3:278-282, 1995.
8. Garenne M, Ronsmans C, Campbell H: The magnitude of mortality from acute respiratory infections in children under 5 years in developing countries, *World Health Stat Q* 45:180-190, 1992.
9. Denny FW: The replete pediatrician and the etiology of lower respiratory tract infections, *Pediatr Res* 3:464-470, 1969.
10. Tupasi E, Velmonte MA, Sanvictores MEG, Abraham L, De Leon LE, Tan SA, Miguel CA, Saniel MC: Determinants of morbidity and mortality due to acute respiratory infections: implications for intervention, *J Infect Dis* 157:615-623, 1988.
11. Datta N, Kumar V, Kumar L, Singhi S: Application of case management to the control of acute respiratory infections in low-birth-weight infants: a feasibility study, *Bull WHO* 65:77-82, 1987.
12. Lehmann D, Howard P, Heywood P: Nutrition and morbidity: acute lower respiratory tract infections, diarrhoea and malaria, *P N G Med J* 31:109-160, 1988.
13. Jin C, Rossignol AM: Effects of passive smoking on respiratory illness from birth to age eighteen months, in Shanghai, People's Republic of China, *J Pediatr* 123:553-558, 1993.
14. Graham NMH: The epidemiology of acute respiratory infections in children and adults: a global perspective, *Epidemiol Rev* 12:149-178, 1990.
15. Pneumonia in childhood, *Lancet* 1:741-743, 1988.
16. James JW: Longitudinal study of the morbidity of diarrheal and respiratory infections in malnourished children, *Am J Clin Nutr* 25:690-694, 1972.
17. Sommer A, Katz J, Tarwotjo I: Increased risk of respiratory disease and diarrhea in children with preexisting mild vitamin A deficiency, *Am J Clin Nutr* 40:1090-1095, 1984.
18. Coutsoudis A, Adhikari M, Coovadia HM: Serum vitamin A (Retinol) concentrations and association with respiratory disease in premature infants, *J Trop Pediatr* 41:230-233, 1995.
19. Victora GC, Fuchs SC, Flores AC, Fonseca W, Kirkwood B: Risk factors for pneumonia among children in a Brazilian metropolitan area, *Pediatrics* 93:977-985, 1994.
20. Chugh TD, Ghaffoor SA, Kuruvilla AC, Bishbishi EA: Colonization and infections of neonates by *Klebsiella pneumoniae* in an intensive care unit, *J Trop Pediatr* 31:200-203, 1985.
21. Meyer KS, Urban C, Eagan JA, Beraer BJ, Rahal JJ: Nosocomial outbreak of *Klebsiella* infection resistant to late-generation cephalosporins, *Ann Intern Med* 119:353-358, 1993.
22. Light IJ, Sutherland JM, Cochran ML, Sutorius J: Ecological reaction between *Staphylococcus aureus* and *Pseudomonas* in a nursery population, *N Engl J Med* 278:1243-1247, 1968.
23. Regelmann WE: Diagnosing the cause of recurrent and persistent pneumonia in children, *Pediatr Ann* 22:561-568, 1993.
24. Wald ER: Recurrent pneumonia in children, *Adv Pediatr Infect Dis* 5:183-203, 1990.
25. Glezen WP, Loda FA, Clyde WA, Senior RJ, Sheaffer CI, Conley WG, Denny FW: Epidemiologic patterns of acute lower respiratory disease of children in a pediatric group practice, *J Pediatr* 78:397-406, 1971.
26. Korppi M, Heiskanen-Kosma T, Jalonen E, Saikku P, Leinonen M, Halonen P, Makela PH: Aetiology of community-acquired pneumonia in children treated in hospital, *Eur J Pediatr* 152:23-30, 1993.
27. Turner RB, Lande AE, Chase P, Hilton N, Weinbera D: Pneumonia in pediatric outpatients: cause and clinical manifestations, *J Pediatr* 111:194-200, 1987.
28. Paisley JW, Lauer BA, McIntosh KM, Glode MP, Schacter J, Rumack C: Pathogens associated with acute lower respiratory tract infection in young children, *Pediatr Infect Dis J* 3:14-19, 1984.
29. Berman S: Acute respiratory infections, *Infect Dis Clin J* 5:319-336, 1991.
30. Isaacs D: Problems in determining the etiology of community acquired childhood pneumonia, *Pediatr Infect Dis J* 8:143-148, 1989.
31. Schutze GE: Management of community-acquired bacterial pneumonia in hospitalized children, *Pediatr Infect Dis J* 11:160-164, 1992.
32. Brook I, Finegold S: Bacteriology of aspiration pneumonia in children, *Pediatrics* 65:1115-1120, 1980.
33. Jacobs RF: Nosocomial pneumonia in children, *Infection* 19:64-72, 1991.
34. Barzilay Z, Mandel M, Keren G, Davidson S: Nosocomial bacterial pneumonia in ventilated children: clinical significance of culture-positive peripheral bronchial aspirates, *J Pediatr* 112:421-423, 1988.
35. Orenstein WA, Overturf GD, Leedom JM, Alvarado R, Geffner M, Fryer A, Chan L, Haynes V, Starc T, Portnoy B: The frequency of *Legionella* infection prospectively determined in children hospitalized with pneumonia, *J Pediatr* 99:403-406, 1981.
36. Blackmon JA, Chandler FW, Cherry AC, England AC, Feeley JC, Hicklin MD, McKinney RM, Wilkinson HW: Legionellosis, *Am J Path* 103:429-465, 1981.
37. Jiang ZF, Wang JF, Zhaori G, Gu Q, Wang XL, Liu SY: Pneumonia: one of the major health problems of infants and children in China, *Chin Med J* 105:81-86, 1992.
38. Forgie IM, O'Neill KP, Lloyd-Evans N, Leiononen M, Campbell H, Whittle HC, Greenwood BM: Etiology of acute lower respiratory tract infections in Gambian children. I. Acute lower respiratory tract infections in infants presenting at the hospital, *Pediatr Infect Dis J* 10:33-41, 1991.
39. Forgie IM, O'Neill KP, Lloyd-Evans N, Leiononen M, Campbell H, Whittle HC, Greenwood BM: Etiology of acute lower respiratory tract infections in Gambian children. II. Acute lower respiratory tract infections in children ages one to nine years presenting at the hospital, *Pediatr Infect Dis J* 10:42-47, 1991.
40. Laurenzi GA, Potter RT, Kass EH: Bacteriologic flora of the lower respiratory tract, *N Engl J Med* 265:1273-1278, 1961.
41. Reynolds HY: Host defense impairments that may lead to respiratory infections, *Clin Chest Med* 8:339-358, 1987.
42. Wescott JL, Volpe JP: Peripheral bronchopleural fistula: CT evaluation in 20 patients with pneumonia, empyema, or postoperative air leak, *Radiology* 196:175-181, 1995.
43. Green GM, Kass EH: The role of the alveolar macrophage in the clearance of bacteria from the lung, *J Exp Med* 119:167-175, 1964.
44. Jackson AE, Southern PM, Pierce AK, Fallis BD, Sanford JP: Pulmonary clearance of gram negative bacilli, *J Lab Clin Med* 69:833-841, 1967.

45. Tuomanen EI, Austrian R, Masure HR: Pathogenesis of pneumococcal infection, *N Engl J Med* 332:1280-1284, 1995.
46. Anderson VA, Turner T: Histopathology of childhood pneumonia in developing countries, *Rev Infect Dis* 13(suppl 6):S470-S476, 1991.
47. Jadavji T, Law B, Lebel MH, Kennedy WA, Gold R, Wang EEL: A practical guide for the diagnosis and treatment of pediatric pneumonia, *Can Med Assoc J* 156:S703-S711, 1997.
48. Press S: Association of hyperpyrexia with serious disease in children, *Clin Pediatr* 33:19-25, 1994.
49. Harari M: Clinical signs of pneumonia in children, *Lancet* 338:928-930, 1991.
50. Dyke T: Predicting hypoxia in children with acute lower respiratory infection: a study in the Highlands of Papua New Guinea, *J Trop Pediatr* 41:196-201, 1995.
51. Onyango FE, Steinhoff MC, Wafula EM, Wariua S, Musia J, Kitonyi J: Hypoxaemia in young Kenyan children with acute lower respiratory infection, *Br Med J* 306:612-615, 1993.
52. Wang EE, Milner RA, Navas L, Maj H: Observer agreement for respiratory signs and oximetry in infants hospitalized with lower respiratory infections, *Am Rev Respir Dis* 145:106-109, 1992.
53. Simoes EA, McGrath EJ: Recognition of pneumonia by primary health care workers in Swaziland with a simple clinical algorithm, *Lancet* 340:1502-1503, 1992.
54. Overall J: Is it bacterial or viral? Laboratory differentiation, *Pediatr Rev* 14:251-261, 1993.
55. Bartlett JG, Alexander J, Mayhew J, Sullivan-Sigler N, Gorbach SL: Should fiberoptic bronchoscopy aspirates be cultured? *Am Rev Respir Dis* 114:73-78, 1976.
56. Moffet HL: Pneumonia syndromes. In Moffet HL, ed: *Pediatric infectious disease: a problem oriented approach,* ed 3, Philadelphia, 1989, JB Lippincott, pp 146-196.
57. Bromberg K, Hammerschlag MR: Rapid diagnosis of pneumonia in children, *Semin Respir Infect* 2:159-165, 1987.
58. Teele DW, Grant MJ, Hershowitz J, Rosen DJ, Allen CE, Wimmer RS, Klein JO: Bacteremia in febrile children under 2 years of age: results of cultures of blood of 600 consecutive febrile children seen in a "walk-in" clinic, *J Pediatr* 87:227-230, 1975.
59. Rein MF, Gwaltney JM, O'Brien WM, Jennings RH, Mandell GL: Accuracy of Gram's stain in identifying pneumococci in sputum, *JAMA* 239:2671-2673, 1978.
60. Aubas S, Aubas P, Capdevila X, Darbas H, Roustan JP, Du Cailar J: Bronchoalveolar lavage for diagnosing bacterial pneumonia in mechanically ventilated patients, *Am J Respir Crit Care Med* 149:860-866, 1994.
61. Wimberley NW, Bass JB, Boyd BW, Kirkpatrick MB, Serio RA, Pollock HM: Use of a bronchoscopic protected catheter brush for the diagnosis of pulmonary infections, *Chest* 81:556-562, 1982.
62. Jimenez P, Saldias F, Meneses M, Silva ME, Wilson MG, Otth L: Diagnostic fiberoptic bronchoscopy in patients with community acquired pneumonia: comparison between bronchoalveolar lavage and telescoping plugged catheter cultures, *Chest* 103:1023-1027, 1993.
63. Mimica I, Donoso E, Howard JE, Ledermann GW: Lung puncture in the etiological diagnosis of pneumonia, *Am J Dis Child* 122:278-282, 1971.
64. Brook I: Percutaneous transtracheal aspiration in the diagnosis and treatment of aspiration pneumonia in children, *J Pediatr* 96:1000-1002, 1980.
65. Dorca J, Manresa F, Esteban L, Barreiro B, Prats E, Ariza J, Verdaguer R, Guidol F: Efficacy, safety and therapeutic relevance of thoracic aspiration with ultrathin needle in nonventilated nosocomial pneumonia, *Am J Respir Crit Care Med* 151:1491-1496, 1995.
66. Early GL, Williams TE, Kilman JW: Open lung biopsy: its effects on therapy in the pediatric patient, *Chest* 87:467-469, 1985.
67. Michiels E, Demedts M: Pitfalls of transthoracic needle aspiration biopsy, *Acta Clin Belg* 46:359-363, 1991.
68. Nohynek H, Valkeila E, Leinonen M, Eskola J: Erythrocyte sedimentation rate, white blood cell count and serum C-reactive protein in assessing etiologic diagnosis of acute lower respiratory infections in children, *Pediatr Infect Dis J* 14:484-490, 1995.
69. Nohynek H, Eskola J, Kleemola M, Jalonen E, Saikku P, Leinonen M: Bacterial antibody assays in the diagnosis of acute lower respiratory tract infection in children, *Pediatr Infect Dis J* 14:478-484, 1995.
70. Ramsey BW: Use of bacterial antigen detection in the diagnosis of pediatric lower respiratory tract infections, *Pediatrics* 78:1-9, 1986.
71. Korppi M, Koskela M, Jalonen E, Leinonen M: Serologically indicated pneumococcal respiratory infection in children, *Scand J Infect Dis* 24:437-443, 1992.
72. Hassan-King M, Baldeh I, Secka O, Falade A, Greenwood B: Detection of *Streptococcus pneumoniae* DNA in blood cultures by PCR, *J Clin Microbiol* 32:1721-1724, 1994.
73. Heulitt MJ, Ablow RC, Santos CC, O'Shea TM, Hilter CL: Febrile infants less than 3 months old: value of chest radiography, *Radiology* 167:135-137, 1988.
74. Kramer MS: Bias and "overcall" in interpreting chest radiographs in young febrile children, *Pediatrics* 90:11-13, 1992.
75. Grossman LK, Caplan SE: Clinical laboratory and radiological information in the diagnosis of pneumonia in children, *Ann Emerg Med* 17:43-46, 1988.
76. Ablin DS, Newell JD: Diagnostic imaging for evaluation of pediatric chest, *Clin Chest Med* 8:641-660, 1987.
77. Swischuk LE, Hayden CK Jr: Viral vs. bacterial pulmonary infections in children (is roentgenographic differentiation possible?), *Pediatr Radiol* 16:278-284, 1986.
78. Courtoy I, Lande AE, Turner RB: Accuracy of radiographic differentiation of bacterial from nonbacterial pneumonia, *Clin Pediatr* 28:261-264, 1989.
79. Korppi M, Kiekara O, Heiskanen-Kosma T, Soimakallio S: Comparison of radiological findings and microbial aetiology of childhood pneumonia, *Acta Paediatr* 82:360-363, 1993.
80. Kramer, MS: Bias and "overcall" in interpreting chest radiographs in young febrile children, *Pediatrics* 90:11-13, 1992.
81. Bressler EL, Francis IR, Glazer GM, Gross BH: Bolus contrast medium enhancement for distinguishing pleural from parenchymal lung disease: CT features, *J Comput Assist Tomogr* 11:436-440, 1987.
82. Ben-Ami TE, O'Donovan JC, Yousefzadeh DK: Sonography of the chest in children, *Radiol Clin North Am* 31:517-531, 1993.
83. Weinberg B, Diakouakis EE, Kass EG, Seife B, Zvi ZB: The air bronchogram: sonographic demonstration, *Am J Roentgenol* 147:593-595, 1986.
84. Yang PC, Luh KT, Chana DB, Yu CJ, Kuo SH, Wu HD: Ultrasonographic evaluation of pulmonary consolidation, *Am Rev Respir Dis* 146:757-762, 1992.
85. Fataar S: Ultrasound in chest disease. II. Lung and mediastinum *Australas Radiol* 32:302-308, 1988.
86. Doust BD, Baum JK, Maklad NF, Doust VL: Ultrasonic evaluation of pleural opacities, *Radiology* 114:135-140, 1975.
87. Landay MJ, Conrad MR: Lung abscess mimicking empyema on ultrasonography, *Am J Radiol* 133:731-734, 1979.
88. Shann F, Linnemann V, Mackenzie A, Barker J, Gratten M, Crinis N: Absorption of chloramphenicol sodium succinate after intramuscular administration in children, *N Engl J Med* 313:410-414, 1985.
89. Graham WGB, Bradley DA: Efficacy of chest physiotherapy and intermittent positive-pressure breathing in the resolution of pneumonia, *N Engl J Med* 299:624-627, 1978.
90. Kjolhede CL, Chew FJ, Gadomski AM, Marroquin DP: Clinical trial of vitamin A as adjuvant treatment for lower respiratory tract infections, *J Pediatr* 126:807-812, 1995.
91. Gibson NA, Hollman AS, Paton JY: Value of radiological follow up of childhood pneumonia, *Br Med J* 307:1117-1118, 1993.
92. Shaheen SO, Barker DJP, Shiell AW, Crocker FJ, Wield GA, Holgate ST: The relationship between pneumonia in early childhood and impaired lung function in late adult life, *Am J Respir Crit Care Med* 149:616-619, 1994.
93. Boisset GF: Subpleural emphysema complicating staphylococcal and other pneumonias, *J Pediatr* 81:259-266, 1972.
94. Victoria MS, Steiner P, Rao M: Persistent postpneumonic pneumatoceles in children, *Chest* 79:359-361, 1981.
95. Marks MI, Klein JO: Bacterial infections of the respiratory tract. In Remington JS, Klein JO, eds: *Infectious diseases of the fetus & newborn infant,* ed 4, Philadelphia, 1995, WB Saunders, pp 898-905.
96. Anderson G, Green C, Neligan G, Newell D, Russell J: Congenital bacterial pneumonia, *Lancet* 2:585-587, 1962.
97. Alenghat E, Esterly JR: Alveolar macrophages in perinatal infants, *Pediatrics* 74:221-223, 1984.
98. Papageorgiou A, Bauer C, Fletcher B, Stern L: *Klebsiella* pneumonia with pneumatocele formation in a newborn infant, *Can Med Assoc J* 109:1217-1219, 1973.
99. Hendren W, Haggerty R: Staphylococcic pneumonia in infancy and childhood, *JAMA* 168:6-17, 1958.

100. Kuhn J, Lee S: Pneumatoceles associated with *Escherichia coli* pneumonias in the newborn, *Pediatrics* 51:1008-1011, 1973.
101. Katzenstein A, Davis C, Brause A: Pulmonary changes in neonatal sepsis due to group B β-hemolytic streptococcus: relation to hyaline membrane disease, *J Infect Dis* 133:430-435, 1976.
102. Jeffery H, Mitchison R, Wigglesworth JS, Davies PA: Early neonatal bacteraemia: comparison of group B streptococcal, other gram-positive and gram-negative infections, *Arch Dis Child* 52:683-686, 1977.
103. Webber S, Wilkinson A, Lindsell D, Hope P, Dobson S, Isaacs D: Neonatal pneumonia, *Arch Dis Child* 65:207-211, 1990.
104. Naeye RL, Dellinger WS, Blanc WA: Fetal and maternal features of antenatal bacterial infections, *J Pediatr* 79:733-739, 1971.
105. Fujikura T, Froehlich LA: Intrauterine pneumonia in relation to birth weight and race, *Am J Obstet Gynecol* 97:81-84, 1967.
106. Bhalla M, Bhalla JN: Clinical and bacteriological profile of the neonatal infections, *Arch Child Health* 26:13-17, 1981.
107. Shamir R, Horev G, Merlob P, Nutman J: *Citrobacter diversus* lung abscess in a preterm infant, *Pediatr Infect Dis J* 9:221-222, 1990.
108. Jevon GP, Dunne WM Jr, Hicks MJ, Langston C: *Bacillus cereus* pneumonia in premature neonates: a report of two cases, *Pediatr Infect Dis J* 12:251-253, 1993.
109. Moriartey RR, Finer NN: Pneumococcal sepsis and pneumonia in the neonate, *Am J Dis Child* 133:601-602, 1979.
110. Griscom T: Pneumonia in children and some of its variants, *Radiol* 167:297-302, 1988.
111. Haney PJ, Bohlman M, Sun CCJ: Radiographic findings in neonatal pneumonia, *Am J Roentgenol* 143:23-26, 1984.
112. Thomas DB, Anderson JC: Antenatal detection of fetal pleural effusion and neonatal management, *Med J Aust* 2:435-436, 1979.
113. Adeyemi SD, Ein SH, Simpson JS, Turner P: The value of emergency open lung biopsy in infants and children, *J Pediatr Surg* 14:426-427, 1979.
114. Sherman MP, Goetzman BW, Ahlfors CE, Wennbera RP: Tracheal aspiration and its clinical correlates in the diagnosis of congenital pneumonia, *Pediatrics* 65:258-263, 1980.
115. Bang AT, Bang RA, Morankar VP, Sontakke PG, Solanki JM: Pneumonia in neonates: can it be managed in the community? *Arch Dis Child* 68:550-556, 1993.
116. Singhi S, Singhi PD: Clinical signs in neonatal pneumonia, *Lancet* 336:1072-1073, 1990.

Specific Causes of Pediatric Pneumonia

117. Pneumonia in childhood, *Lancet* 1:741-743, 1988.
118. Pasteur L: Note sur la maladie nouvelle provoquee par la salive d'un enfant mort de la rage, *Bull Acad Med (Paris)* [series 2] 10:94-103, 1881.
119. Pasteur L, Chamberland M, Roux M: Sur une maladie nouvelle, provoquee par la salive d'un enfant mort de la rage, *Compt Rend Acad Sci* 92:159-165, 1881.
120. Fraenkel A: Weitere beitrage zur lehre von den mikrococcen der genuinen fibrosieen pneumonia, *Z Klin Med* 11:437-458, 1886.
121. Winslow CEA, Broadhurst J, Buchanen RE, Krumwiede C, Rogers LA, Smith GH: The families and genera of the bacteria: final report of the committee of the Society of American Bacteriologists on the characterization and classification of bacterial types, *J Bacteriol* 5:191-229, 1920.
122. Deibel RH, Seeley HW Jr, Family II: Streptococcaceae Fam. nov. In Buchanan RE, Gibbons NE, eds: *Bergey's manual of determinative bacteriology,* ed 8, Baltimore, 1974, Williams & Wilkins, pp 490-517.
123. Gram C: Ueber die isolierte Farbung der Scizomyceten in Schnitt-und Trockenpraparaten, *Berl Klin Wochenschr* 28:833-835, 1891.
124. Eskola J, Takala AK, Kela E, Pekkanen E, Kalliokoski R, Leinonen M: Epidemiology of invasive pneumococcal infections in children in Finland, *JAMA* 268:3323-3327, 1992.
125. Dagan R, Englehard D, Piccard E: Epidemiology of invasive childhood pneumococcal infections in Israel, *JAMA* 268:3328-3332, 1992.
126. Shapiro ED, Austrian R: Serotypes responsible for invasive *Streptococcus pneumoniae* infections among children in Connecticut, *J Infect Dis* 169:212-214, 1994.
127. Paisley JW, Lauer BA, McIntosh K, Glode MP, Schachter J, Rumack C: Pathogens associated with lower respiratory tract infection in young children, *Pediatr Infect Dis* 3:14-19, 1984.
128. Gray BM, Converse GM, Dillon HC: Epidemiologic studies of *Streptococcus pneumoniae* in infants: acquisition, carriage, and infection during the first 24 months of life, *J Infect Dis* 142:923-933, 1980.
129. Davidson M, Parkinson AJ, Bulkow LR, Fitzgerald MA, Peters HV, Parks DJ: The epidemiology of invasive pneumococcal disease in Alaska, 1986-1990: ethnic differences and opportunities for prevention, *J Infect Dis* 170:368-376, 1994.
130. Cortese MM, Wolff M, Almeido-Hill J, Reid R, Ketcham J, Santosham M: High incidence rates of invasive pneumococcal disease in the White Mountain Apache population, *Arch Intern Med* 152:2277-2282, 1992.
131. Fraser DW, Darby CP, Koehler RE, Jacobs CF, Feldman RA: Risk factors in bacterial meningitis: Charleston County, South Carolina, *J Infect Dis* 127:271-277, 1973.
132. Robbins J, Austrian R, Lee CJ, Rastoui SC, Schiffman G, Henrichsen J, Makela PH, Broome CV, Facklam RR, Tiesjema RH, Parke JC: Considerations for formulating the second-generation pneumococcal capsular polysaccharide vaccine with emphasis on the cross-reactive types within groups, *J Infect Dis* 148:1136-1159, 1983.
133. Fine DP, Kirk JL, Schiffman G, Schweinle JE, Guckian JC: Analysis of humoral and phagocytic defense against *Streptococcus pneumoniae* serotypes 1 and 3, *J Lab Clin Med* 112:487-497, 1988.
134. Barnes DM, Whittier S, Gilliaan PH, Scares S, Tomasz A, Henderson FW: Transmission of multidrug-resistant serotype 23F *S. pneumoniae* in group day care: evidence suggesting capsular transformation of the resistant strain in vivo, *J Infect Dis* 171:890-896, 1995.
135. George WL, Finegold SM: Bacterial infections of the lung, *Chest* 81:502-507, 1982.
136. Musher DM: Infections caused by *Streptococcus pneumoniae:* clinical spectrum, pathogenesis, immunity and treatment, *Clin Infect Dis* 14: 801-809, 1992.
137. Purdy GD, Cullen M, Yedlin S, Bedard MP: An unusual neonatal case presentation: *Streptococcus pneumoniae* pneumonia with abscess and pneumatocele formation, *J Perinatol* 7:378-381, 1987.
138. Friedland IR, McCracken GH: Management of infections caused by antibiotic-resistant *Streptococcus pneumoniae, N Engl J Med* 331:377-382, 1994.
139. Simberkoff MS: Drug-resistant pneumococcal infections in the United States, *JAMA* 271:1875-1876, 1994.
140. Perlino CA, Rimland D: Alcoholism, leukopenia and pneumococcal sepsis, *Am Rev Respir Dis* 132:757-760, 1985.
141. Johnston RB: Pathogenesis of pneumococcal pneumonia, *Rev Infect Dis* 13(suppl 6):S509-S517, 1991.
142. Wright AE, Morgan WP, Cantab MB, Colebrook L, Lend MB, Dodgson RW, Lond MD: On prophylactic inoculation against pneumococcal infections and on the results achieved by it, *Lancet* 1:1-10, 87-95, 1914.
143. MacLeod CM, Hodges RG, Heidelberger M, Bernhard WG: Prevention of pneumococcal pneumonia by immunization with specific capsular polysaccharides, *J Exp Med* 82:445-468, 1948.
144. Austrian R: Pneumococcal infection and pneumococcal vaccine, *N Engl J Med* 297:938-939, 1977.
145. Smit P, Oberholzer D, Hayden-Smith S, Koornhof HJ, Hilleman MR: Protective efficacy of pneumococcal polysaccharide vaccines, *JAMA* 238:2613-2616, 1977.
146. Committee on Infectious Diseases, American Academy of Pediatrics: *1997 redbook: report of the Committee on Infectious Diseases,* ed 24, Elk Grove Village, Ill, 1997, The Academy, pp 417-418.
146a. Black S, Shinefield H, Ray P, Lewis E, Fireman B, the Kaiser Permanente Vaccine Study Group, Ausman R, Siber G, Hackell J, Kohberger R, Chang IH: Efficacy of heptovalent conjugate pneumococcal vaccine (Wyeth-Lederle) in 37,000 infants and children: results of the Northern California Kaiser Permanente efficacy trial. Abstracts of the 38th Interscience Conference on Antimicrobial Agents and Chemotherapy, San Diego, Abstract LB-9, 1998.
147. Tenover FC, Arbeit R, Archer G, Biddle J, Byrne S, Goering R, Hancock G, Hebert GA, Hill B, Hollis R: Comparison of traditional and molecular methods of typing isolates of *Staphylococcus aureus, J Clin Microbiol* 32:407-415, 1994.
148. Karakawa WW, Vann WF: Capsular polysaccharides of *Staphylococcus aureus, Semin Infect Dis* 4:285-293, 1982.

149. Hochkeppel HK, Braun DG, Vischer W, Imm A, Sutter S, Staeubli U, Guggenheim R, Kaplan EL, Boutonnier A, Fournier JM: Serotyping and electron microscopy studies of *Staphylococcus aureus* clinical isolates with monoclonal antibodies to capsular polysaccharide types 5 and 8, *J Clin Microbiol* 25:526-530, 1987.
150. Phonimdaeng P, O'Reilly M, Nowlan P, Bramley AJ, Foster TJ: The coagulase of *Staphylococcus aureus* 8325-4: sequence analysis and virulence of site-specific coagulase-deficient mutants, *Mol Microbiol* 4:393-404, 1990.
151. Cribier B, Prevost G, Couppie P, Finck-Barbancon V, Grosshans E, Piemont Y: *Staphylococcus aureus* leukocidin: a new virulence factor in cutaneous infections? An epidemiological and experimental study, *Dermatology* 185:175-180, 1992.
152. Foster TJ, McDevitt D: Surface-associated proteins of *Staphylococcus aureus:* their possible roles in virulence, *FEMS Microbiol Lett* 118:199-205, 1994.
153. Sung RYT, Cheng AF, Chan RC, Tam JS, Oppenheimer SJ: Epidemiology and etiology of pneumonia in children in Hong Kong, *Clin Infect Dis* 17:894-896, 1993.
154. Marrie TJ: New aspects of old pathogens of pneumonia, *Med Clin North Am* 78:987-995, 1994.
155. Tsao TC, Tsai YH, Lan RS, Shieh WB, Lee CH: Pulmonary manifestations of *Staphylococcus aureus* septicemia, *Chest* 101:574-576, 1992.
156. Chartrand S, McCracken G: Staphylococcal pneumonia in infants and children, *Pediatr Infect Dis* 1:19-23, 1982.
157. Siermann A, Storm W: Toxic shock syndrome in a 6-year-old male, *Monatsschr Kinderheilk* 139:231-234, 1991.
158. Knight GJ, Carman PG: Primary staphylococcal pneumonia in childhood: a review of 69 cases, *J Paediatr Child Health* 28:447450, 1992.
159. George WL, Finegold SM: Bacterial infections of the lung, *Chest* 81:502-507, 1982.
160. Lohse AW, Klein O, Hermann E, Lohr H, Kreitner KF, Steppling H, Meyer zum Buschenfelde KH, Staritz M: Pneumatoceles and pneumothoraces complicating staphylococcal pneumonia: treatment by synchronous independent lung ventilation, *Thorax* 48:578-580, 1993.
161. Rivera CF, Rocha LA, Penaranda JS, Marini M: Massive hemoptysis secondary to an aortobronchial fistula: a rare complication of staphylococcal pneumonia, *Med Clin (Barc)* 95:636, 1990.
162. Silverman MS, MacLeod JP: Pancoast's syndrome due to staphylococcal pneumonia, *Can Med Assoc J* 142:343-345, 1990.
163. Mulholland K: Personal communication, 1997.
164. Pfeiffer R: Vorlaufige mittheilungen uber den erreger der influenza, *Dtsch Med Wochenschr* 18:28, 1892.
165. Pittman M: Variation and type specificity in the bacterial species *H. influenzae, J Exp Med* 58:683-706, 1933.
166. Santosham M, Reid R, Ambrosino DM, Wolff MC, Almeido-Hill J, Priehs C, Aspery KM, Garrett S, Croll L, Foster S, Burge G, Page P, Zacher B, Moxon R, Siber GR: Prevention of *H. influenzae* type b infections in high risk infants treated with bacterial polysaccharide immune globulin, *N Engl J Med* 317:923-929, 1987.
167. Gilsdorf JR: *Haemophilus influenzae* non-type b infections in children, *Am J Dis Child* 141:1063-1065, 1987.
168. Friesen CA, Cho CT: Characteristic features of neonatal sepsis due to *Haemophilus influenzae, Rev Infect Dis* 8:777-780, 1986.
169. Bartlett AV, Zusman J, Daum RS: Unusual presentations of *Haemophilus influenzae* infections in immunocompromised patients, *J Pediatr* 102:55-58, 1983.
170. Weinberg GA, Lehmann D, Tupasi TE, Granoff DM: Diversity of outer membrane protein profiles of nontypeable *Haemophilus intense* isolated from children from Papua New Guinea and the Philippines, *Rev Infect Dis* 12:S1017-S1020, 1991.
171. Klein JO: Role of nontypeable *Haemophilus influenzae* in pediatric respiratory tract infections, *Pediatr Infect Dis J* 16:S5-S8, 1997.
172. St Geme JW III: Nontypeable *Haemophilus influenzae* disease: epidemiology, pathogenesis, and prospects for prevention, *Infect Agents Dis* 2:1-16, 1993.
173. Michaels RH, Pozviak CS, Stonebaker FE, Norden CW: Factors affecting pharyngeal *H. influenzae* type b colonization rates in children, J Clin Microbiol 4:413-417, 1976.
174. Hall DB, Lum MKW, Knutson LR, Heyward WL, Ward JI: Pharyngeal carriage and acquisition of anticapsular antibody to *H. influenzae* type b in a high-risk population in southwestern Alaska, *Am J Epidemiol* 126:1190-1197, 1987.
175. Vadheim CM, Ward JI: Epidemiology in developed countries. In Ellis RW, Granoff DM, eds: *Development and clinical uses of* Haemophilus *b conjugate vaccines,* New York, 1994, Marcel Dekker, pp 231-246.
176. Peltola H, Rod TO, Jonsdottir K, Bottiger M, Coolidge JA: Life threatening *Haemophilus influenzae* infections in Scandinavia: a five-country analysis of the incidence and the main clinical and bacteriologic characteristics, *Rev Infect Dis* 12:708-715, 1990.
177. Shapiro ED, Ward JI: The epidemiology and prevention of disease caused by *Haemophilus influenzae* type b, *Epidemiol Rev* 13:113-142, 1991.
178. Daum RS, Glode MP, Goldmann, DA, Halsey NA, Ambrosino D, Welborn C, Mather F, Willard JE, Sullivan B, Murray M, Johansen T: Rifampin chemoprophylaxis for household contacts of patients with invasive infections due to *Haemophilus influenzae* type b, *J Pediatr* 98:485-491, 1981.
179. Granoff DM, Daum RS: Spread of *Haemophilus influenzae* type b: recent epidemiologic and therapeutic considerations, *J Pediatr* 97:854-860, 1980.
180. St Geme JW, Falkow S: Loss of capsule expression by *Haemophilus influenzae* type b results in enhanced adherence to and invasion of human cells, *Infect Immun* 59:325-333, 1991.
181. Kroll JS: The genetics of encapsulation in *Haemophilus influenzae, J Infect Dis* 165(suppl 1):S93-S96, 1992.
182. Moxon ER: Experimental studies of *Haemophilus influenzae* infection in a rat model. In Sell SH, Wright PF, eds: *Haemophilus influenzae: epidemiology, immunology and prevention of disease,* New York, 1982, Elsevier, pp 59-71.
183. Fothergill FC, Wright J: Influenzal meningitis: the relation of age-incidence to the bactericidal power of the blood against the causative organism, *J Immunol* 24:273-284, 1933.
184. Ambrosino D, Schreiber JR, Daum RS, Siber GR: Efficacy of human hyperimmune globulin in prevention of *Haemophilus influenzae* type b disease in infant rats, *Infect Immun* 39:709-714, 1983.
185. Peltola H, Kayhty H, Virtaneon M, Makela PH: Prevention of *Háemophilus influenzae* type b bacteremic infections with the capsular polysaccharide, *N Engl J Med* 310:1561-1566, 1984.
186. Anderson P: The protective level of serum antibodies to the capsular polysaccharide of *Haemophilus influenzae* type b, *J Infect Dis* 149:1034-1035, 1984.
187. Stein KE: Thymus-independent and thymus-dependent responses to polysaccharide antigens, *J Infect Dis* 165:S49-S52, 1992.
188. Daum RS: The efficacy of the combined diphtheria-tetanus toxoids-pertussis-*Haemophilis influenzae* type b vaccine, *Pediatr Infect Dis J* 14:640-641, 1995.
189. Molteni RA: Epiglottitis: incidence of extraepiglottic infections—report of 72 cases and review of the literature, *Pediatrics* 58:526-531, 1976.
190. Warner JO, Gordon I: Pneumatoceles following *Haemophilus influenzae* pneumonia, *Clin Radiol* 32:99-105, 1981.
191. Kaplan SL: Antigen detection in cerebrospinal fluid: pros and cons, *Am J Med* 75:109-118, 1983.
192. Daum RS, Granoff DM: Lessons from the evaluation of immunogenicity. In Ellis RW, Granoff DM, eds: *Development and clinical uses of* Haemophilus *b conjugate vaccines,* New York, 1994, Marcel Dekker, pp 291-312.
193. Adams WG, Deaver KA, Cochi SL, Plikaytis BD, Zell ER, Broome CV, Wenger JD: Decline of childhood *Haemophilus influenzae* type b (Hib) disease in the Hib vaccine era, *JAMA* 269:221-226, 1993.
194. Broadhurst LE, Erickson RL, Kelley PW: Decreases in invasive *Haemophilus influenzae* diseases in US army children, *JAMA* 269:227-231, 1993.
195. Murphy TV, White KE, Pastor P, Gabriel L, Medley F, Granoff DM, Osterholm MT: Declining incidence of *Haemophilus influenzae* type b disease since the introduction of vaccination, *JAMA* 269:246-248, 1993.
196. Lancefield RC: A serological differentiation of human and other groups of hemolytic streptococci, *J Exp Med* 57:571-595, 1933.
197. Nocard M, Mollereau M: Sur une mammite contagieuse, *Ann Inst Pasteur* 1:109-126, 1887.
197a. Harrison LH, Elliott JA, Dwyer DM, Libonati JP, Ferrieri P, Billmann L, Schuchat A, and the Maryland Emerging Infections Program: Serotype distribution of invasive group B streptococcal isolates in Maryland; complications for vaccine formulation, *J Infect Dis* 177: 998-1002, 1998.

198. Di John D, Krasinski K, Lawrence R, Borkowski W, Johnson JP, Schieken LS, Rennels MB: Very late onset of group B streptococcal disease in infants infected with the human immunodeficiency virus, *Pediatr Infect Dis J* 9:925-928, 1990.
199. Ferrieri P: GBS infections in the newborn infant: diagnosis and treatment, *Antibiot Chemother* 35:211-224, 1985.
200. Yagupsky P, Menegus MA, Powell KR: The changing spectrum of group B streptococcal disease in infants: an eleven-year experience in a tertiary care hospital, *Pediatr Infect Dis J* 10:801808, 1991.
201. Feigin RD: The perinatal group B streptococcal problem: more questions than answers, *N Engl J Med* 294:106-107, 1976.
202. Cochran WD: Hyaline-membrane disease and infection in the newborn, *N Engl J Med* 294:844, 1976.
203. Bonadio WA, Jeruc W, Anderson Y, Smith D: Systemic infection due to group B beta-hemolytic streptococcus in children, *Clin Pediatr* 31:230-233, 1992.
204. Rabalais GP, Bronfin DR, Daum RS: Evaluation of a commercially available latex agglutination test for rapid diagnosis of group B streptococcal infection, *Pediatr Infect Dis* 6:177-181, 1987.
205. Schauf V, Deveikis A, Riff L, Serota A: Antibiotic-killing kinetics of group B streptococci, *J Pediatr* 89:194-198, 1976.
206. Potter B, Philipps AF, Bierny JP, Crowe CP Jr: Neonatal radiology: acquired diaphragmatic hernia with group B streptococcal pneumonia, *J Perinatol* 15:160-162, 1995.
207. Suresh BR, Rios A, Brion LP, Weinberg G, Kresch MJ: Delayed onset right-sided diaphragmatic hernia secondary to group B streptococcal infection, *Pediatr Infect Dis J* 10:166-168, 1991.
208. Weisman LE, Stoll BJ, Cruess DF, Paul RT, Marenstein GB, Hemming VG, Fischer GW: Early-onset group B streptococcal sepsis: a current assessment, *J Pediatr* 1212:428-433, 1992.
209. Payne N, Burke B, Day D: Correlation of clinical and pathologic findings in early-onset neonatal group B streptococcal infection with disease severity and prediction of outcome, *Pediatr Infect Dis J* 7:836-847, 1988.
210. Schuchat A, Oxtoby M, Cochi S: Population-based risk factors for neonatal group B streptococcal disease: results of a cohort study in metropolitan Atlanta, *J Infect Dis* 162:672-677, 1990.
211. Fanaroff AA, Korones SB, Wright LL, Wright EC, Poland RL, Bauer CB, Tyson JE, Philips JB III, Edwards W, Lucey JF, Catz CS, Shankaran S, Ott W, National Institute of Child Health and Human Development Neonatal Research Network: A controlled trial of intravenous immune globulin to reduce nosocomial infections in very-low-birth-weight infants, *N Engl J Med* 330:1107-1113, 1994.
212. Lewin EB, Amstey MS: Natural history of group B streptococcus colonization and its therapy during pregnancy, *Am J Obstet Gynecol* 139: 512-515, 1981.
213. Siegel JD, McCracken GHJ, Threlkeld N, DePasse BM, Rosenfeld CR: Single-dose penicillin prophylaxis against group B streptococcal disease, *N Engl J Med* 303:769-775, 1980.
214. Yow MD, Mason EO, Leeds LJ, Thompson PK, Clark DJ, Gardner SE: Ampicillin prevents intrapartum transmission of group B streptococcus, *JAMA* 241:1245-1247, 1983.
215. Boyer KM, Gotoff SP: Prevention of early onset group B streptococcal disease with selective intrapartum prophylaxis, *N Engl J Med* 314: 1665-1669, 1986.
216. Centers for Disease Control and Prevention: Prevention of perinatal group B streptococcal disease: a public health perspective, *MMWR* 45(No RR-7):1-24, 1996.
217. Kotloff KL, Fattom A, Basham L, Hawwari A, Harkonen S, Edelman R: Safety and immunogenicity of a tetravalent group B streptococcal polysaccharide vaccine in healthy adults, *Vaccine* 14:446-450, 1996.
218. Larsson C: Experimental vaccination against group B streptococcus and encapsulated bacterium with highly purified preparations of cell surface proteins Rib and alpha, *Infect Immun* 64:3518-3523, 1996.
219. Cordes LG, Brink EW, Checko PJ, Lentnek A, Lyons RW, Hayes PS, Wu TC, Tharr DG, Fraser DW: A cluster of *Acinetobacter* pneumonia in foundry workers, *Ann Intern Med* 95:688-693, 1981.
220. Moses J, Bonomo GR, Wenlund DE, Halldorsson TS, Connelly JP: Actinomycosis in childhood: historical review and case presentation, *Clin Pediatr* 6:221-226, 1967.
221. Weese WC, Smith IM: A study of 57 cases of actinomycosis over a 36-year period: a diagnostic "failure" with good prognosis after treatment, *Arch Intern Med* 135:1526-1568, 1975.
222. Bates M, Cruickshank G: Thoracic actinomycosis, *Thorax* 12:99-124, 1957.
223. Bennhoff DF: Actinomycosis: diagnostic and therapeutic considerations and a review of 32 cases, *Laryngoscope* 94:1198-1217, 1984.
224. Lerner PI: Susceptibility of pathogenic actinomycetes to antimicrobial compounds, *Antimicrob Agents Chemother* 5:302-309, 1974.
225. Lockhart GR, Williams GP, Gilbert-Barness E: Thoracic and abdominal actinomycosis, *Am J Dis Child* 147:317-318, 1993.
226. Brown JR: Human actinomycosis: a study of 181 subjects, *Hum Pathol* 4:319-330, 1973.
227. Clinicopathological conference: a case of unsuspected chronic inflammatory disease, *Br Med J* 4:149-154, 1973.
228. Drake DP, Holt RJ: Childhood actinomycosis: report of 3 recent cases, *Arch Dis Child* 51:979-981, 1976.
229. Legum LL, Greer KE, Glessener SF: Disseminated actinomycosis, *South Med J* 71:463-465, 1978.
230. Spinola SM, Bell RA, Henderson FW: Actinomycosis: a cause of pulmonary and mediastinal mass lesions in children, *Am J Dis Child* 135:336-339, 1981.
231. Harvey JC, Cantrell JR, Fisher AM: Actinomycosis: its recognition and treatment, *Ann Intern Med* 46:868-885, 1957.
232. Oddo D, Gonzalez S: Actinomycosis and nocardiosis: a morphologic study of 17 cases, *Pathol Res Pract* 181:320-326, 1986.
233. Kinnear WJM, MacFarlane JT: A survey of thoracic actinomycosis, *Respir Med* 84:57-59, 1990.
234. Snape P: Thoracic actinomycosis: an unusual childhood infection, *South Med J* 86:222-224, 1993.
235. Balikian JP, Cheng TH, Costello P, Herman PG: Pulmonary actinomycosis: a report of three cases, *Radiology* 128:613-616, 1978.
236. Golden N, Cohen H, Weissbrot J, Silverman S: Thoracic actinomycosis in childhood, *Clin Pediatr* 24:646-650, 1985.
237. Lowe RN, Azimi PH, McQuitty J: Acid-fast actinomyces in a child with pulmonary actinomycosis, *J Clin Microbiol* 12:124-126, 1980.
238. Slade PR, Slesser BV, Southgate J: Thoracic actinomycosis, *Thorax* 28:73-85, 1973.
239. Allworth AM, Ghosh HK, Saltos N: A case of *Actinomyces meyeri* pneumonia in a child, *Med J Aust* 145:33, 1986.
239a. Nelson JD, Herman, DW: Oral penicillin therapy for thoracic actinomycosis, *Pediatr Infect Dis J* 5:594-595, 1986.
240. Peabody JW, Seabury JH: Actinomycosis and nocardiosis: a review of basic differences in therapy, *Am J Med* 28:99-115, 1960.
241. Flynn MW, Felson B: The roentgen manifestations of thoracic actinomycosis, *Am J Roentgenol* 110:707-716, 1970.
242. Varkey B, Landis FB, Tang TT, Rose HD: Thoracic actinomycosis: dissemination to skin, subcutaneous tissue, and muscle, *Arch Intern Med* 134:689-693, 1974.
243. Guillemot L, Halle J, Rist E: Recherches bacteriologiques et experimentales sur les pleuresies putrides, *Arch Med Exper P Anat Pathol* 16:571-640, 1904.
244. Bartlett JG: Anaerobic bacterial infections of the lung, *Chest* 91:901-1009, 1987.
245. Bartlett JG, Finegold SM: Anaerobic infections of the lung and pleural space, *Am Rev Respir Dis* 110:56-77, 1974.
246. Bartlett JG: Anaerobic bacterial infections of the lung and pleural space, *Clin Infect Dis* 16:S248-S255, 1993.
247. Bartlett JG, Mundy LM: Community-acquired pneumonia, *N Engl J Med* 333:1618-1624, 1995.
248. Pollock HM, Hawkins EL, Bonner JR, Sparkman T, Bass JB Jr: Diagnosis of bacterial pulmonary infections with quantitative protected catheter cultures obtained during bronchoscopy, *J Clin Microbiol* 17:225-229, 1983.
249. Appelbaum PC, Spangler SK, Jacobs MR: β-Lactamase production and susceptibilities to amoxicillin, amoxicillin-clavulanate, ticarcillin, ticarcillin-clavulanate, cefoxitin, imipenem, and metronidazole of 320 non-*Bacteroides fragilis, Bacteroides* isolates and 129 fusobacteria from 28 U.S. centers, *Antimicrob Agents Chemother* 34:1546-1550, 1990.
250. Bartlett JG, Gorbach, SL: Treatment of aspiration pneumonia and primary lung abscess, *JAMA* 234:935-937, 1975.
251. Waagner DC: *Arcanobacterium haemolyticum:* biology of the organism and diseases in man, *Pediatr Infect Dis J* 10:933-939, 1991.
252. Waller KS, Johnson J, Wood BP: Radiologic case of the month, *Am J Dis Child* 145:209-210, 1991.

253. Berkman YM: Uncommon acute bacterial pneumonias, *Semin Roentgenol* 15:17-24, 1980.
254. LaForce FM: Anthrax, *Clin Infect Dis* 19:1009-1014, 1994.
255. Ross JM: The pathogenesis of anthrax following the administration of spores by the respiratory route, *J Pathol Bacteriol* 73:485-494, 1957.
256. Harrison LH, Ezzell JW, Abshire TG, Kidd S, Kaufmann AF: Evaluation of serologic tests for diagnosis of cutaneous anthrax in Paraguay, *J Infect Dis* 1650:706-710, 1989.
257. Buchanan TM, Feeley JC, Hayes PS, Brachman PS: Anthrax indirect microhemagglutination test, *J Immunol* 197:1631-1636, 1971.
258. Patra G, Sylvestre P, Ramisse V, Therasse J, Guesdon J: Isolation of a chromosomic DNA sequence of *Bacillus anthracis* and its possible use in diagnosis, *FEMS Immunol Mol Microbiol* 15:223231, 1996.
259. American Academy of Pediatrics: Anthrax. In Peter G, ed: *1997 red-book: report of the committee on infectious diseases,* ed 24, Elk Grove Village, Ill, 1997, The Academy, p 136.
260. Farrar WE: Anthrax: virulence and vaccines, *Ann Intern Med* 121:379-380, 1994.
261. Bekemeyer WB, Zimmerman GA: Life threatening complications associated with *Bacillus cereus* pneumonia, *Am Rev Respir Dis* 131:466-469, 1985.
262. Jevon GP, Dunne WM, Hicks MJ, Langston C: *Bacillus cereus* pneumonia in premature infants: report of two cases, *Pediatr Infect Dis J* 12:251-253, 1993.
263. Coudron PE, Payne JM, Markowitz SM: Pneumonia and empyema infection associated with a *Bacillus* species that resembles *B. alvei, J Clin Microbiol* 29:1777-1779, 1991.
264. Isaacson P, Jacobs PH, Mackenzie MR, Mathews AW: Pseudotumour of the lung caused by infection with *Bacillus sphaericus, J Clin Pathol* 29:806-811, 1976.
265. Weber DJ, Saviteer SM, Rutala WA, Thomann CA: In vitro susceptibility of *Bacillus* spp. to selected antimicrobial agents, *Antimicrob Agents Chemother* 32:642-645, 1988.
266. Debre R, Lamy M, Jammet ML, Costil L, Mozziconacci P: La maladie des griffes de chat, *Semin Hop Paris* 26:1895-1901, 1950.
267. Abbasi S, Chesney PJ: Pulmonary manifestations of cat-scratch disease; a case report and review of the literature, *Pediatr Infect Dis J* 14:547-548, 1995.
268. Jackson LA, Perkins BA, Wenger JD: Cat scratch disease in the United States, *Am J Public Health* 83:1707-1711, 1993.
269. Koehler JE, Glaser CA, Tappero JW: *Rochalimaea henselae* infection: a new zoonosis with the domestic cat as reservoir, *JAMA* 271:531-535, 1994.
270. Caniza MA, Granger DL, Wilson KH, Washington MK, Kordick DL, Frush DP, Blitchington RB: *Bartonella henselae:* etiology of pulmonary nodules in a patient with depressed cell-mediated immunity, *Clin Infect Dis* 20:1505-1511, 1995.
271. Regnery RL, Perkins BA, Olson JG, Bibb W: Serological response to *"Rochalimaea henselae"* antigen in suspected cat-scratch disease, *Lancet* 339:1443-1445, 1992.
272. Barka NE, Hadfield T, Patnaik M, Scwartzman WA, Peter JB: EIA for detection of *Rochalimaea henselae*-reactive IgG, IgM, and IgA antibodies in patients with suspected cat-scratch disease, *J Infect Dis* 167:1503-1504, 1993.
273. Szelc-Kelly CM, Goral S, Perez-Perez GI, Perkins BA, Regnery RL, Edwards KM: Serologic responses to *Bartonella* and *Afipia* antigens in patients with cat-scratch disease, *Pediatrics* 96:1137-1142, 1995.
274. Norman AF, Regnery R, Jameson P, Greene C, Krause DC: Differentiation of *Bartonella*-like isolates at the species level by PCR restriction fragment length polymorphism in the citrate synthase gene, *J Clin Microbiol* 33:1797-1803, 1995.
275. Bergmans AMC, Groothedde JW, Schellekens JFP, van Embden JDA, Ossewaarde JM, Schouls LM: Etiology of cat scratch disease: comparison of polymerase chain reaction detection of *Bartonella* (formerly *Rochalimaea*) and *Afipia felis* DNA with serology and skin tests, *J Infect Dis* 171:916-923, 1995.
276. Schwartzman W: *Bartonella (Rochalimaea)* infections: beyond cat scratch, *Ann Rev Med* 47:355-364, 1996.
277. Walker DH, Barbour AG, Oliver JH, Lane RS, Dumler JS, Dennis DT, Persing DH, Azad AF, McSweegan E: Emerging bacterial zoonotic and vector-borne diseases, *JAMA* 275:463-469, 1996.
278. Hines PD, Overturf GD, Hatch D, Kim J: Brucellosis in a California family, *Pediatr Infect Dis J* 5:579-582, 1986.
279. Young EJ: An overview of human brucellosis, *Clin Infect Dis* 21:283-290, 1995.
280. Matar GM, Khneisser IA, Abdelnoor AM: Rapid laboratory confirmation of human brucellosis by PCR analysis of a target sequence on the 31-kilodalton *Brucella* antigen DNA, *J Clin Micro* 34:477-478, 1996.
281. Chusid MJ, Perzigian RW, Dunne WM, Gecht EA: Brucellosis: an unusual cause of a child's fever of unknown origin, *Wisc Med J* 88:11-13, 1989.
282. Goldmann DA, Klinger JD: *Pseudomonas cepacia:* biology, mechanisms of virulence, epidemiology, *J Pediatr* 108:806-812, 1986.
283. Sun L, Jiang RZ, Steinbach S, Holmes A, Campanelli C, Forstner J, Sajjan U, Tan Y, Riley M, Goldstein R: The emergence of a highly transmissible lineage of cbl+ *Pseudomonas (Burkholderia) cepacia* causing CF centre epidemics in North America and Britain, *Nature Med* 1:661-666, 1995.
284. Rosenthal S, Tager IB: Prevalence of gram-negative rods in the normal pharyngeal flora, *Ann Intern Med* 83:355-357, 1975.
285. Pujol M, Corbella X, Carratala J, Gudiol F: Community acquired bacteremic *Pseudomonas cepacia* pneumonia in an immunocompetent host, *Clin Infect Dis* 15:887-888, 1992.
286. Steinbach S, Sun L, Jiang RZ, Flume P, Gilligan P, Egan TM, Goldstein R: Transmissibility of *Pseudomonas cepacia* infection in clinic patients and lung-transplant recipients with cystic fibrosis, *N Engl J Med* 331:981-987, 1994.
287. Nelson JW, Butler SL, Krieg D, Govan JR: Virulence factors of *Burkholderia cepacia, FEMS Immunol Med Microbiol* 8:89-97, 1994.
288. McKevitt AI, Bajaksouzian S, Klinger JD, Woods DE: Purification and characterization of an extracellular protease from *Pseudomonas cepacia, Infect Immun* 57:771-778, 1989.
289. McKenney D, Brown KE, Allison DG: Influence of *Pseudomonas aeruginosa* exoproducts on virulence factor production in *Burkholderia cepacia:* evidence of interspecies communication, *J Bacteriol* 177:6989-6992, 1995.
290. Tomashefski JF, Thomassen MJ, Bruce MC, Goldberg HI, Konstan MW, Stern RC: *Pseudomonas cepacia*–associated pneumonia in cystic fibrosis: relation of clinical features to histopathologic patterns of pneumonia, *Arch Pathol Lab Med* 112:166-172, 1988.
291. Hoiby N: *Hemophilus influenzae, Staphylococcus aureus, Pseudomonas cepacia,* and *Pseudomonas aeruginosa* in patients with cystic fibrosis, *Chest* 94(suppl 2):97S-103S, 1988.
292. Weinstein AJ, Moellering RC Jr, Hopkins CC, Goldblatt A: *Pseudomonas cepacia* pneumonia, *Am J Med Sci* 265:491-494, 1973.
293. Thomassen MJ, Demko CA, Stern RC, Klinger JD: *Pseudomonas cepacia:* decrease in colonization in patients with cystic fibrosis, *Am Rev Respir Dis* 134:669-671, 1986.
294. Werkman CH, Gillen GF: Bacteria producing trimethylene glycol, *J Bacteriol* 23:167-182, 1932.
295. Lipsky BA, Hook EW, Smith AA, Plourde JJ: *Citrobacter* infections in humans: experience at the Seattle Veterans Administration Medical Center and a review of the literature, *Rev Infect Dis* 2:746-760, 1980.
296. Brenner DJ, Farmer JJ, Hickman FW, Asbury MA, Steigerwalt AG: *Taxonomic and nomenclature changes in Enterobacteriaceae,* US Department of Health, Education and Welfare Pub No (CDC) 78-8356, Washington, DC, 1977, The Department, p 7.
297. Parry MF, Hutchinson JH, Brown NA, Wu CH, Estreller L: Gram-negative sepsis in neonates: a nursery outbreak due to hand carriage of *Citrobacter diversus, Pediatrics* 65:1105-1109, 1980.
298. Madrazo A, Geiger J, Lauter CB: *Citrobacter diversus* at Grace Hospital, Detroit, Michigan, *Am J Med Sci* 270:497-501, 1975.
299. Gilman RM, Irwin RS, Garritty FL: Community acquired *Citrobacter diversus* infections, *Respir Care* 25:66-71, 1980.
300. Malik AS, Johari MR: Pneumonia, pericarditis, and endocarditis in a child with *Corynebacterium xerosis* septicemia, *Clin Infect Dis* 20(1):191-192, 1995 (letter).
301. Manzella JP, Kellogg JA, Parsey KS: *Corynebacterium pseudodiphtheriticum:* a respiratory pathogen in adults, *Clin Infect Dis* 20:37-40, 1995.
302. Yoshitomi Y, Kohno S, Koga H, Maesaki S, Higashiyama Y, Matsuda H, Mitsutake K, Miyazaki Y, Yamada H, Hara K, Sugahara K, Kaku M: Fatal pneumonia caused by *Corynebacterium* group JK after treatment of *Staphylococcus aureus* pneumonia, *Intern Med* 31:930-932, 1992.

303. Carrion F, Escoms R, Carretero J, Pedro MV, Prat J: Pleural empyema caused by *Corynebacterium* sp, *Arch Bronconeumol* 31:40-42, 1995.
304. Marrie TJ: *Coxiella burnetii* (Q fever) pneumonia, *Clin Infect Dis* 21(suppl 3):S253-S264, 1995.
305. Hornibrook JW: An institutional outbreak of pneumonitis. I. Epidemiological and clinical studies, *Public Health Rep* 55:1936-1944, 1940.
306. Schramek S, Mayer H: Different sugar composition of lipopolysaccharides isolated from phase I and pure phase II cells of *Coxiella burnetii, Infect Immun* 38:53-57, 1982.
307. Parker RR, Bell EJ, Lackman DB: Experimental studies of Q fever in cattle. I. Observations on four heifers and two milk cows, *Am J Hyg* 48:191-206, 1948.
308. Tigertt WD, Benenson AS: Studies on Q fever in man, *Trans Assoc Am Physicians* 69:98-104, 1956.
309. Izzo AA, Marmion BP, Worswick DA: Markers of cell-mediated immunity after vaccination with an inactivated, whole cell Q fever vaccine, *J Infect Dis* 157:781-789, 1988.
310. Escherich T: Die Darmbacterien des neugeborenen und sauglings, *Fortschr Med* 3:515-522, 1885.
311. Korhonen TK, Valtonen MV, Parkkinen J, Vaisanen-Rhen V, Finne J, Orskov F, Orskov I, Svenson SB, Makela PH: Serotypes, hemolysin production, and receptor recognition of *Escherichia coli* strains associated with neonatal sepsis and meningitis, *Infect Immun* 48:486-491, 1985.
312. Klein JO: Emerging perspectives in management and prevention of infections of the respiratory tract in infants and children, *Am J Med* 78(suppl 6B)38-44, 1985.
313. Webber S, Wilkinson AR, Lindsell D, Hope PL, Dobson SRM, Isaacs D: Neonatal pneumonia, *Arch Dis Child* 65:207-211, 1990.
314. Siitonen A, Takala A, Ratiner YA, Pere A, Makela PH: Invasive *Escherichia coli* infections in children: bacterial characteristics in different age groups and clinical entities, *Pediatr Infect Dis J* 12:606-612, 1993.
315. Hemming VG, McCloskey DW, Hill HR: Pneumonia in the neonate associated with group B streptococcal septicemia, *Am J Dis Child* 130:1231-1233, 1976.
316. Fagbule DO: Bacterial pathogens in malnourished children with pneumonia, *Trop Geogr Med* 45:294-296, 1993.
317. Diallo AA, Siverman M, Egler LJ: Bacteriology of lung puncture aspirates in malnourished children in Zaire, *Nigerian Med J* 9:421-423, 1979.
318. Bernstein J, Wang J: The pathology of neonatal pneumonia, *Am J Dis Child* 101:350-363, 1961.
319. Bermejo VE, Gonzalez ME, Martinez AM, Zubia AA, Nieves GA, Salado MC, Diez OM: Pneumatocele as a complication of *E. coli* pneumonia in a newborn infant: apropos of a case, *An Espanol Pediatr* 37:526-528, 1992.
320. Wherry WB, Lamb BH: Infection of man with *Bacterium tularense,* J Infect Dis 15:331-340, 1914.
321. Verbrycke JR Jr: Tularemia, *JAMA* 82:1577-1581, 1924.
322. Permar HH, MacLachlan WWG: Tularemic pneumonia, *Ann Intern Med* 5:687-698, 1931.
323. Stewart SJ: *Francisella.* In Murray PR, Baron EJ, Pfaller JA, Tenover FC, Yolken RH: *Manual of clinical microbiology,* ed 6, Washington DC, 1995, ASM, pp 545-548.
324. Craven RB, Barnes AM: Plague and tularemia, *Infect Dis Clin North Am* 5:165-175, 1991.
325. Spach DH, Liles WC, Campbell GL, Quick RE, Anderson DE, Fritsche TR: Tick-borne diseases in the United States, *N Engl J Med* 329:936-947, 1993.
326. Scheel O, Reiersen R, Hoel T: Treatment of tularemia with ciprofloxacin, *Eur J Clin Microbiol Infect Dis* 11:447-448, 1992.
327. Summary of notifiable diseases: United States, 1990, *MMWR* 39:55-61, 1991.
328. Byfield GV, Breslow L, Cross RR, Hershey NJ: Tick borne tularemia, *JAMA* 127:191-196, 1945.
329. Halsted C, Kulasinghe H: Tularemia pneumonia in urban children, *Pediatrics* 61:660-662, 1978.
330. Butler T: Plague and tularemia, *Pediatr Clin North Am* 26:355-366, 1979.
331. McCarthy VP, Murphy MD: Lawnmower tularemia, *Pediatr Infect Dis J* 9:298-299, 1990.
332. Avery F, Barnett T: Pulmonary tularemia, *Am Rev Respir Dis* 95:584-591, 1967.
333. Capellan J, Fong IW: Tularemia from a cat bite: case report and review of feline-associated tularemia, *Clin Infect Dis* 16:472-475, 1993.
334. Garver MK, St Geme JW, Siegel MJ: Tularemia presenting with splenic nodules, *Pediatr Infect Dis J* 13:830-831, 1994.
335. Taylor JP, Istre GR, McChesney TC, Satalowich FT, Parker RL, McFarland LM: Epidemiologic characteristics of human tularemia in the Southwest-Central States, 1981-1987, *Am J Epidemiol* 133:1032-1038, 1991.
336. Jacobs R, Condrey Y, Yamauchi T: Tularemia in adults and children: a changing presentation, *Pediatrics* 76:818-822, 1985.
337. Baker CN, Hollis DG, Thornsberry C: Antimicrobial susceptibility of *Francisella tularensis* with a modified Mueller-Hinton broth, *J Clin Microbiol* 22:212-215, 1985.
338. Maranan MC, Schiff D, Johnson DC, Abrahams C, Wylam M, Gerber SI: Pneumonic tularemia in a patient with chronic granulomatous disease, *Clin Infect Dis* 25(3):630-633, 1997.
339. Harper JL, Tso W: Tularemic meningitis in a child with mononuclear pleocytosis, *Pediatr Infect Dis* 5:595-597, 1986.
340. Conlan JW, Sjostedt A, North RJ: CD4+ and CD8+ T-cell-dependent and -independent host defense mechanisms can operate to control and resolve primary and secondary *Francisella tularensis* LSV infection in mice, *Infect Immun* 62:5603-5607, 1994.
341. Leiby DA, Fortier AH, Crawford RM, Schreiber RD, Nacy CA: In vivo modulation of the murine immune response to *Francisella tularensis* LVS by administration of anticytokine antibodies, *Infect Immun* 60:84-89, 1992.
342. Fortier AH, Polsinelli T, Green SJ, Nacy CA: Activation of macrophages for destruction of *Francisella tularensis:* identification of cytokines, effector cells and effector molecules, *Infect Immun* 60:817-825, 1992.
343. Anthony LSD, Kongshavn PAL: Experimental murine tularemia caused by *Francisella tularensis* live vaccine strain: a model of acquired cellular resistance, *Microb Pathog* 2:3-14, 1987.
344. Hughes WT: Tularemia in children, *J Pediatr* 62:495-502, 1963.
345. Cunha BA: The atypical pneumonias: a diagnostic and therapeutic approach, *Postgrad Med* 66:95-102, 1979.
346. Rubin SA: Radiographic spectrum of pleuropulmonary tularemia, *Am J Roentgenol* 131:277-281, 1978.
347. Funk LM, Simpson SQ, Mertz G: Tularemia presenting as an isolated pleural effusion, *West J Med* 15:415-417, 1992.
348. Kozak AJ, Hall WH, Gerding DN: Cavitary pneumonia associated with tularemia, *Chest* 73:426-427, 1978.
349. Alfes JC, Ayers LW: Acute bacterial meningitis caused by *Francisella tularensis, Pediatr Infect Dis J* 9:300-301, 1990.
350. Geisbert TW, Jahrling PB, Ezzell JR: Use of immunoelectron microscopy to demonstrate *Francisella tularensis, J Clin Microbiol* 31:1936-1939, 1993.
351. Cross JT, Jacobs RF: Tularemia: treatment failures with outpatient use of ceftriaxone, *Clin Infect Dis* 17:976-980, 1993.
352. Vilianen MK, Nurmi T, Salminen A: Enzyme-linked immunosorbent assay (ELISA) with bacterial sonicate antigen for IgM, IgA, and IgG antibodies to *Francisella tularensis:* comparison with bacterial agglutination test and ELISA with lipopolysaccharide antigen, *J Infect Dis* 148:715-720, 1983.
353. Syrjala H, Herva E, Ilonen J, Saukkonen K, Salminen A: A whole-blood lymphocyte stimulation test for the diagnosis of human tularemia, *J Infect Dis* 150:912-915, 1984.
354. Evans ME, Gregory DW, Schaffner W, McGee ZA: Tularemia: a 30-year experience with 88 cases, *Medicine* 64:251-269, 1985.
355. Mason WL, Eigelsbach HT, Little SF, Bates JH: Treatment of tularemia, including pulmonary tularemia, with gentamicin, *Am Rev Respir Dis* 121:39-45, 1980.
356. Penn RL: Factors associated with a poor outcome in tularemia, *Arch Intern Med* 147:265-268, 1987.
357. Ray ES, Warren S: Tularemic lung abscess, *Am Rev Tuberc* 65:627-630, 1952.
358. Miller R, Bates J: Pleuropulmonary tularemia: a review of 29 patients, *Am Rev Respir Dis* 99:31-41, 1969.
359. Dennis JM, Boudreau RP: Pleuropulmonary tularemia: its roentgen manifestations, *Radiology* 68:25-30, 1957.

360. Raphael M, Anderson AE: Pleuropulmonary tularemia complicated by peripheral neuritis, *Arch Intern Med* 91:278-280, 1953.
361. Sunderrajan E, Hutton J, Marienfeld D: Adult respiratory distress syndrome secondary to tularemia pneumonia, *Arch Intern Med* 145:1435-1437, 1985.
362. Tarnvik A, Eriksson M, Sandstrom G, Sjostedt A: *Francisella tularensis:* a model for studies of the immune response to intracellular bacteria in man, *Immunology* 76:349-354, 1992.
363. Burke DS: Immunization against tularemia: analysis of the effectiveness of live *Francisella tularensis* vaccine in prevention of laboratory-acquired tularemia, *J Infect Dis* 135:55-60, 1977.
364. Yagupsky P, Dagan R, Howard CB, Einhorn M, Kassis I, Simu A: Clinical features and epidemiology of invasive *Kingella kingae* infections in southern Israel, *Pediatrics* 92:800-804, 1993.
365. Morrison VA, Wagner KF: Clinical manifestations of *Kingella kingae* infections: case report and a review, *Rev Infect Dis* 11:776-782, 1989.
366. Molina R, Baro T, Torne J, Miralles R, Gutierrez J, Solsona JF, Alia C: Empyema caused by *Kingella denitrificans* and *Peptostreptococcus* spp in a patient with bronchogenic carcinoma, *Eur Respir J* 1:870-871, 1988.
367. Friedländer C: Uber die schizomyceten bei der acuten fibrösen pneumonia, *Arch Pathol Anat Physiol Klin Melizen* 87:319-324, 1882.
368. Solomon S: Primary Friedländer pneumonia, *JAMA* 108:937-947, 1937.
369. Sisson WR, Thompson CB: Friedländer bacillus pneumonia with report of cases, *Am J Med Sci* 150:713-727, 1915.
370. Martin W, Yu P, Washington J: Epidemiologic significance of *Klebsiella pneumoniae:* a 3-month study, *Mayo Clin Proc* 46:785-793, 1971.
371. Orskov I, Fife-Asbury M: New *Klebsiella* capsular antigen, K82, and the deletion of five of those previously assigned, *Int J Syst Bacteriol* 27:386-387, 1977.
372. Murcia A, Rubin S: Reproducibility of an indirect immunofluorescent-antibody technique for capsular serotyping of *Klebsiella pneumoniae, J Clin Microbiol* 9:208-213, 1979.
373. Cryz S, Furer E, Germanier R: Immunization against fatal experimental *Klebsiella pneumoniae* pneumonia, *Infect Immun* 54:403-407, 1986.
374. Carpenter J: *Klebsiella* pulmonary infections: occurrence at one medical center and review, *Rev Infect Dis* 12:672-682, 1990.
375. Bonadio W: *Klebsiella pneumoniae* bacteremia in children, *Am J Dis Child* 143:1061-1063, 1989.
376. Freedman R, Ingram D, Gross I, Ehrenkranz R, Warshaw J, Baltimore R: A half century of neonatal sepsis at Yale, *Am J Dis Child* 135:140-144, 1981.
377. Gladstone IM, Ehrenkranz RA, Edberg SC, Baltimore RS: A ten-year review of neonatal sepsis and comparison with the previous fifty-year experience, *Pediatr Infect Dis J* 9:819-825, 1990.
378. Montgomerie JZ, Ota JK: *Klebsiella* bacteremia, *Arch Intern Med* 140:525-527, 1980.
379. Casewell M, Phillips I: Hands as route of transmission for *Klebsiella species, Br Med J* 2:1315-1317, 1977.
380. Chugh T, Ghaffoor S, Juruvilla A, Bishbishi E: Colonization and infections of neonates by *Klebsiella pneumoniae* in an intensive care unit, *J Trop Pediatr* 31:200-203, 1985.
381. Stratton C: Bacterial pneumonias: an overview with emphasis on pathogenesis, diagnosis, and treatment, *Heart Lung* 25:226-244, 1986.
382. Cryz S, Furer E, Germanier R: Safety and immunogenicity of *Klebsiella pneumoniae* Kl capsular polysaccharide vaccine in humans, *J Infect Dis* 151:665-671, 1985.
383. Makristathis A, Stauffer F, Feistauer S, Georgopoulos A: Bacteria induce release of platelet-activating factor (PAF) from polymorphonuclear neutrophil granulocytes: possible role for PAF in pathogenesis of experimentally induced bacterial pneumonia, *Infect Immun* 61:1996-2002, 1993.
384. Straus DC: Production of an extracellular toxic complex by various strains of *Klebsiella pneumoniae, Infect Immun* 55:44-48, 1987.
385. Pruzzo C, Valisena S, Satta G: Laboratory and wild-type *Klebsiella pneumoniae* strains carrying mannose-inhibitable adhesins and receptors for coliphages T3 and T7 are more pathogenic for mice than are strains without such receptors, *Infect Immun* 39:520-527, 1983.
386. Highsmith AK, Jarvis WR: *Klebsiella pneumoniae:* selected virulence factors that contribute to pathogenicity, *Infect Control* 6:75-77, 1985.
387. Sweany H, Stadnichenko A, Henrichsen K: Multiple pulmonary abscesses simulating tuberculosis, *Arch Intern Med* 47:565-582, 1931.
388. Brown R, Sands M, Ryczak M: Community-acquired pneumonia caused by mixed aerobic bacteria, *Chest* 90:810-814, 1986.
389. Palmer D, Davidson M, Lusk R: Needle aspiration of the lung in complex pneumonias, *Chest* 78:16-21, 1980.
390. Guzzetta P, Toews GB, Robertson KJ, Pierce AK: Rapid diagnosis of community-acquired bacterial pneumonia, *Am Rev Respir Dis* 128:461-464, 1983.
391. Bhatt ON, Miller R, Riche JL, King EG: Aspiration biopsy in pulmonary opportunistic infections, *Acta Cytol* 21:206-209, 1977.
392. Hughes J, Sinha D, Cooper M, Shah K, Bose S: Lung tap in childhood, *Pediatrics* 44:477-485, 1969.
393. Pollock H, Hawkins E, Bonner J, Sparkman T, Bass J: Diagnosis of bacterial pulmonary infections with quantitative protected catheter cultures obtained during bronchoscopy, *J Clin Microbiol* 17:255-259, 1983.
394. Felson B, Rosenberg L, Hamburger M: Roentgen findings in acute Friedländer's pneumonia, *Radiology* 46:559-565, 1949.
395. Korvick JA, Hackett AK, Yu VL, Muder RR: *Klebsiella* pneumonia in the modern era: clinicoradiographic correlations, *South Med J* 84:200-204, 1991.
396. Fernandez-Rodriguez A, Canton R, Perez-Diaz JC, Martinez-Beltran J, Picazo J, Baqauero F: Aminoglycoside-modifying enzymes in clinical isolates harboring extended-spectrum β-lactamases, *Antimicrob Agents Chemother* 36:2536-2538, 1992.
397. Philippon A, Arlet G, Lagrange PH: Origin and impact of plasmid-mediated extended-spectrum beta-lactamases, *Eur J Clin Microbiol Infect Dis* 13(suppl 1):S17-S29, 1994.
398. Meyer KA, Urban C, Eagan JA, Berger BJ, Rahal JJ: Nosocomial outbreak of *Klebsiella* infection resistant to late-generation cephalosporins, *Ann Intern Med* 119:353-440, 1993.
399. Bakker-Woudenberg I, Lokerse A, Kate T, Mouton J, Woodle M, Storm G: Liposomes with prolonged blood circulation and selective localization in *Klebsiella pneumoniae*-infected lung tissue, *J Infect Dis* 168:164-171, 1993.
400. Cameron E, Whitton I: Percutaneous drainage in the treatment *of Klebsiella pneumoniae* lung abscess, *Thorax* 32:673-676, 1977.
401. Chugh SN, Mehta LK, Kapoor S, Malhotra KC: Myopericardial involvement in *Klebsiella pneumoniae* infection, *J Assoc Physicians India* 37:354-355, 1989.
402. Schwimmbeck P, Oldstone M: *Klebsiella pneumoniae* and HLA B27-associated diseases of Reiter's syndrome and ankylosing spondylitis, *Curr Top Microbiol Immunol* 145:45-56, 1989.
403. Trull AK, Ebringer R, Panayi G, Colthorpe D, James DC, Ebringer A: IgA antibodies to *K. pneumoniae* in ankylosing spondylitis, *Scand J Rheumatol* 12:249-253, 1983.
404. Cross AS, Sadoff JC, Furer E, Cryz SJ: *Escherichia coli* and *Klebsiella* vaccines and immunotherapy, *Infect Dis Clin North Am* 4:271-281, 1990.
405. Cross A: Personal communication, 1997.
406. Babudieri B: Animal reservoirs of leptospires, *Ann NY Acad Sci* 70:393-413, 1958.
407. Vinetz JM, Glass GE, Flexner CE, Mueller P, Kaslow DC: Sporadic urban leptospirosis, *Ann Intern Med* 125:794-798, 1996.
408. Silverstein CM: Pulmonary manifestations of leptospirosis, *Radiology* 61:327-334, 1953.
409. Centers for Disease Control and Prevention: Outbreak of acute febrile illness and pulmonary hemorrhage: Nicaragua, 1995, *MMWR* 44:839-843, 1995.
410. Teglia OF, Battagliotti C, Villavicencio RL, Cunha BA: Leptospiral pneumonia, *Chest* 108:874-875, 1995.
411. Paganin F, Gauzere BA, Lugagne N, Blanc P, Roblin X: Bronchoalveolar lavage in rapid diagnosis of leptospirosis, *Lancet* 347:1562-1563, 1996.
412. Appassakij H, Silpapojakul K, Wansit R, Woodtayakorn, J: Evaluation of the immunofluorescent antibody test for the diagnosis of human leptospirosis, *Am J Trop Med Hyg* 52:340-343, 1995.
413. Silva MV, Camargo ED, Batista L, Vaz AJ, Brandao AP, Nakamura PM, Negraom JM: Behavior of specific IgM, IgG and IgA class antibodies in human leptospirosis during the acute phase of the disease and during convalescence, *J Trop Med Hyg* 98:268-272, 1995.

414. Merien F, Baranton G, Perolat P: Comparison of polymerase chain reaction with microagglutination test and culture for the diagnosis of leptospirosis, *J Infect Dis* 172:281-285, 1995.
415. Brown PD, Gravekamp C, Carrington DG, Van de Kemp H, Hartskeerl RA, Edwards CN, Everard COR, Terpstra WJ, Levett PN: Evaluation of the polymerase chain reaction for early diagnosis of leptospirosis, *J Med Microbiol* 43:110-114, 1995.
416. Emmanouilides CE, Kohn OF, Garibaldi R: Leptospirosis complicated by a Jarisch-Herxheimer reaction and adult respiratory distress syndrome: case report, *Clin Infect Dis* 18:1004-1006, 1994.
417. Seeliger HPR, Finger H: Listeriosis. In Remington JS, Klein JO, eds: *Infectious diseases of the fetus and newborn infant,* ed 4, Philadelphia, 1995, WB Saunders, p 265.
418. Burn CG: Clinical and pathological features of an infection caused by a new pathogen of the genus *Listerella, Am J Pathol* 12:341-348, 1936.
419. Vawter GF: Perinatal listeriosis, *Perspect Pediatr Pathol* 6:153-166, 1981.
420. Gellin BG, Broome CV: Listeriosis, *JAMA* 261:1313-1320, 1989.
421. Schlech WF III, Lavigne PM, Bortolussi RA, Allen AC, Haldane EV, Wort AJ, Hightower AW, Johnson SE, King SH, Nicholls ES, Broome CV: Epidemic listeriosis: evidence for transmission by food, *N Engl J Med* 308:203-206, 1983.
422. Southwick FS, Purich DL: Intracellular pathogenesis of listeriosis, *N Engl J Med* 334:770-776, 1996.
423. Albritton WL, Wiggins GL, Feeley JC: Neonatal listeriosis: distribution of serotypes in relation to age at onset of disease, *J Pediatr* 88:481-483, 1976.
424. Catlin BW: Transfer of the organism named *Neisseria catarrhalis* to *Branhamella* Gen nov, *Int J Syst Bacteriol* 20:155-159, 1970.
425. Rossau R, Van Landschoot A, Gillis M, De Ley J: Taxonomy of Moraxellaceae Fam. nov., a new bacterial family to accommodate the genera *Moraxella, Acinetobacter,* and *Psychrobacter* and related organisms, *Int J Syst Bacteriol* 41:310-319, 1991.
426. Catlin BW: Branhamaceae fam. nov.: proposed family to accommodate the genera *Branhamella* and *Moraxella, Int J Syst Bacteriol* 41:320-323, 1991.
427. Marchant CD: Spectrum of disease due to *Branhamella catarrhalis* in children with particular reference to acute otitis media, *Am J Med* 88:15S-19S, 1990.
428. Claesson BA, Leinonen M: *Moraxella catarrhalis:* an uncommon cause of community-acquired pneumonia in Swedish children, *Scand J Infect Dis* 26:399-402, 1994.
429. Catlin BW: *Branhamella catarrhalis:* an organism gaining respect as a pathogen, *Clin Microbiol Rev* 3:293-320, 1990.
430. Collazos J, de Miguel J, Ayarza R: *Moraxella catarrhalis* bacteremic pneumonia in adults: two cases and review of the literature, *Eur J Clin Microbiol Infect Dis* 11:237-240, 1992.
431. Cook PP, Hecht DW, Snydman DR: Nosocomial *Branhamella catarrhalis* in a pediatric intensive unit: risk factors for disease, *J Hosp Infect* 13:299-307, 1989.
432. Burman LA, Leionen M, Trollfors B: Use of serology to diagnose pneumonia caused by unencapsulated *Haemophilus influenzae* and *Moraxella catarrhalis, J Infect Dis* 170:220-222, 1994.
433. Hol C, Van Dijke EEM, Verduin CM, Verhoef J, van Dijk H: Experimental evidence for *Moraxella* induced penicillin neutralization in pneumococcal pneumonia, *J Infect Dis* 170:1613-1616, 1994.
434. Goldwater PN, Rice MS: Primary meningococcal pneumonia in a nineteen-month-old child, *Pediatr Infect Dis J* 14:155-156, 1995.
435. Frasch CE: Production and control of *Neisseria meningitides* vaccines. In Mizraki A, ed: *Advances in biotechnical processes: bacterial vaccines,* vol 13, New York, 1990, Wiley-Liss, pp 123-145.
436. Nassif X, So M: Interaction of pathogenic *Neisseriae* with nonphagocytic cells, *Clin Microbiol Rev* 8:376-388, 1995.
437. Stephens DS: Gonococcal and meningococcal pathogenesis as defined by human cell, cell culture, and organ culture assays, *Clin Microbiol Rev* 2:S104-S111, 1989.
438. Pohlner J, Langenberg U, Wolk U, Beck SC, Meyer TF: Uptake and nuclear transport of *Neisseria* IgA1 protease-associated alpha proteins in human cells, *Mol Microbiol* 17:1073-1083, 1995.
439. Hammerschmidt S, Hilse R, vanPutten JPM, Gerardy-Schahn R, Unkmeir A, Frosch M: Modulation of cell surface sialic acid expression in *Neisseria meningitides* via a transposable genetic element, *EMBO J* 15:192-198, 1996.
440. Criado MT, Pintor M, Ferreirós CM: Iron uptake by *Neisseria meningitides, Res Microbiol* 144:77-82, 1993.
441. van Putten JPM, Robertson BD: Molecular mechanisms and implications for infection of lipopolysaccharide variation in *Neisseria, Mol Microbiol* 16:847-853, 1995.
442. Riedo FX, Plakaytis BD, Broome CV: Epidemiology and prevention of meningococcal disease, *Pediatr Infect Dis J* 14:643-657, 1995.
443. Baltimore RS, Hammerschlag M: Meningococcal bacteremia: clinical and serologic studies of infants with mild illness, *Am J Dis Child* 131:1001-1004, 1977.
444. Berkmen YM: Uncommon acute bacterial pneumonias, *Semin Roentgenol* 15:17-24, 1980.
445. Hersh JH, Gold R, Lepow ML: Meningococcal group Y pneumonia in an adolescent female, *Pediatrics* 64:222-224, 1979.
446. Witt D, Olans RN, Bacteremic W-135 meningococcal pneumonia, *Am Rev Respir Dis* 125:255-257, 1982.
447. Rose HD, Lenz IE, Sheth NK: Meningococcal pneumonia: a source of nosocomial infection, *Arch Intern Med* 141:575-577, 1981.
448. Irwin RE, Woelk WK, Coudon WL III: Primary meningococcal pneumonia, *Ann Intern Med* 82:493-498, 1975.
449. Hall LM, Duke B, Urwin G: An approach to the identification of the pathogens of bacterial meningitis by the polymerase chain reaction, *Eur J Clin Microbiol Infect Dis* 14:1090-1094, 1995.
450. Ni H, Knight AI, Cartwright K, Palmer WH, McFadden J: Polymerase chain reaction for diagnosis of meningococcal meningitis, *Lancet* 340:1432-1434, 1992.
451. Sacks HS: Meningococcal pneumonia and empyema, *Am J Med* 80:290-291, 1986.
452. Gundersen GA, Nice CM: Nocardiosis: a case report and brief review of the literature, *Radiology* 68:31-35, 1957.
453. Castleman BJ, McNeely BU: Case records of the Massachusetts General Hospital: case 11-1970, *N Engl J Med* 282:614-619, 1970.
454. Carlile WK, Holley KE, Logan GB: Fatal acute disseminated nocardiosis in a child, *JAMA* 184:477-480, 1963.
455. Holt RIG, Kwan JTC, Sefton AM, Cunningham J: Successful treatment of concomitant pulmonary nocardiosis and aspergillosis in an immunocompromised renal patient, *Eur J Clin Microbiol Infect Dis* 12:110-114, 1993.
456. Law BJ, Marks MI: Pediatric nocardiosis, *Pediatrics* 70:560-565, 1982.
457. Stites DP, Glezen WP: Pulmonary nocardiosis in childhood, *Am J Dis Child* 114:101-105, 1967.
458. Coker RJ, Bignardi G, Horner P, Savage M, Cook T, Tomlinson D, Weber J: *Nocardia* infection in AIDS: a clinical and microbiological challenge, *J Clin Pathol* 45:821-822, 1992.
459. Filice GA, Niewoehner DE: Contribution of neutrophils and cell-mediated immunity to control of *Nocardia asteroides* in murine lungs, *J Infect Dis* 156:113-121, 1987.
460. Smeal WE, Schenfield LA: Nocardiosis in the community hospital, *Postgrad Med* 79:77-82, 1986.
461. Holdaway MD, Kennedy J, Ashcroft T, Kay-Butler JJ: Pulmonary nocardiosis in a 3-year-old child, *Thorax* 22:375-381, 1967.
462. Stropes LS, Bartlett M, White A: Multiple recurrences of nocardial pneumonia, *Am J Med Sci* 280:119-122, 1980.
463. Cornelissen JJ, Bakker LJ, Van der Veen MJ, Rozenberg-Arska M, Bijlsma JWJ: *Nocardia asteroides* pneumonia complicating low dose methotrexate treatment of refractory rheumatoid arthritis, *Ann Rheum Dis* 50:642-644, 1991.
464. Camp M, Mehta JB, Whitson M: Bronchiolitis obliterans and *Nocardia asteroides* infection of the lung, *Chest* 92:1107-1108, 1987.
465. Hoepelman IM, Bakker LJ, Jessurun RF, Rozenberg-Arska M, Verhoef J: Disseminated *Nocardia asteroides* infection complicating renal transplantation, *Neth J Med* 31:175-182, 1987.
466. Henkle JQ, Nair SV: Endobronchial pulmonary nocardiosis, *JAMA* 256:1331-1332, 1986.
467. Wallace RJ, Septimus EJ, Williams TW, Conklin RH, Satterwhite TK, Bushby MB, Hollowell DC: Use of trimethoprim-sulfamethoxazole for treatment of infections due to *Nocardia, Rev Infect Dis* 4:315-325, 1982.
468. King CT, Chapman SW, Butkus DE: Recurrent nocardiosis in a renal transplant recipient, *South Med J* 86:225-228, 1993.
469. Khorrami P, Heffeman EJ: Pneumonia and meningitis due to *Nocardia asteroides* in a patient with AIDS, *Clin Infect Dis* 17:1084-1085, 1993.

470. Stamm AE, McFall DW, Dismukes WE: Failure of sulfonamides and trimethoprim in the treatment of nocardiosis, *Arch Intern Med* 143:383-385, 1983.
471. Gombert ME: Susceptibility of *Nocardia asteroides* to various antibiotics, including β-lactams, trimethoprim-sulfamethoxazole, amikacin and *N*-formidyl thienamycin, *Antimicrob Agents Chemother* 21:1011-1012, 1982.
472. Lajos TZ, Jarzylo SV: Pulmonary nocardiosis and empyema, *NY State J Med* 70:2829-2832, 1970.
473. Weed LA, Andersen HA, Good CA, Baggenstoss AH: Nocardiosis: clinical, bacteriologic and pathological aspects, *N Engl J Med* 253:1137-1143, 1955.
474. Presant CA, Wiernik PH, Serpick AA: Factors affecting survival in nocardiosis, *Am Rev Respir Dis* 108:1444-1448, 1973.
475. Oberhofer TR: Characteristics and biotypes of *Pasteurella multocida* isolated from humans, *J Clin Microbiol* 13:566-577, 1981.
476. Hubbert WJ, Rosen MN: I. *Pasteurella multocida* infection due to animal bite, *Am J Public Health* 60:1103-1108, 1970.
477. Hubbert WJ, Rosen MN: II. *Pasteurella multocida* infection in man unrelated to animal bite, *Am J Public Health* 60:1109-1117, 1970.
478. Johnson RH, Rumans LW: Unusual infections caused by *Pasteurella multocida, JAMA* 237:146-147, 1977.
479. Lee MLH, Buhr AJ: Dog bites and local infection with *Pasteurella septica, Br Med J* 1:169-171, 1960.
480. Strand CL, Helfman L: *Pasteurella multocida* chorioamnionitis associated with premature delivery and neonatal sepsis and death, *Am J Clin Pathol* 55:713-716, 1971.
481. Frutos AA, Levitsky D, Scott EG: A case of septicemia and meningitis in an infant due to *Pasteurella multocida, J Pediatr* 92:853, 1978.
482. Repice JP, Neter E: *Pasteurella multocida* meningitis in an infant with recovery, *J Pediatr* 86:91-93, 1975.
483. Weber DJ, Wolfson JS, Swartz MN, Hooper DC: *Pasteurella multocida* infections: report of 34 cases and review of the literature, *Medicine* 63:133-154, 1991.
484. Rose HD, Mathai G: Acute *Pasteurella multocida* pneumonia, *Br J Dis Chest* 71:123-126, 1977.
485. Schmidt EC, Truitt LV, Koch ML: Pulmonary abscess with empyema caused by *Pasteurella multocida:* report of a fatal case, *Am J Clin Pathol* 54:733-736, 1970.
486. Burke JP, Ingall D, Klein JO, Gezon HM, Finland M: *Proteus mirabilis* infections in a hospital nursery traced to a human carrier, *N Engl J Med* 284:115-121, 1971.
487. Salyers AA, Whitt DD: *Pseudomonas aeruginosa.* In Salyers AA, Whitt DD: *Bacterial pathogenesis, a molecular approach,* Washington, DC, 1994, American Society for Microbiology, pp 260-270.
488. Pearson JP, Gray KM, Passador L, Tucker KD, Eberhard A, Iglewski BH, Greenberg EP: Structure of the autoinducer required for expression of *Pseudomonas aeruginosa* genes, *Proc Natl Acad Sci USA* 91:197-201, 1994.
489. Mendelson MH, Gurtman A, Szabo S, Neibart E, Meyters BR, Policar M, Cheung TW, Lillienfeld D, Hammer G, Reddy S: *Pseudomonas aeruginosa* bacteremia in patients with AIDS, *Clin Infect Dis* 18:886-895, 1994.
490. Roilides E, Butler KM, Husson RN, Mueller BU, Lewis LL, Pizzo PA: *Pseudomonas* infections in children with human immunodeficiency virus infections, *Pediatr Infect Dis J* 11:547-553, 1992.
491. Ruvalo C, Bauer CR: Intrauterinely acquired *Pseudomonas* infection in the neonate, *Clin Pediatr* 21:664-667, 1982.
492. FitzSimmons SC: The changing epidemiology of cystic fibrosis, *J Pediatr* 122:1-9, 1993.
493. Reynolds HY, DiSant'Agnese PA, Zierdt CH: Mucoid *Pseudomonas aeruginosa, JAMA* 236:2190-2192, 1976.
494. Fick RB, Sonoda F, Hornick DB: Emergence and persistence of *P. aeruginosa* in the cystic fibrosis airway, *Semin Respir Infect* 7:168-178, 1991.
495. Penketh AR, Pitt TL, Hodson ME: Bactericidal activity of serum from cystic fibrosis patients for *Pseudomonas aeruginosa, J Med Microbiol* 16:401-408, 1983.
496. Deretic V, Schurr MJ, Yu H: *Pseudomonas aeruginosa,* mucoidy and the chronic infection phenotype in cystic fibrosis, *Trends Microbiol* 3:351-356, 1995.
497. Fetzer AF, Werner AS, Hagstrom JWC: Pathologic features of pseudomonal pneumonia, *Am Rev Respir Dis* 96:1121-1130, 1967.
498. Holt DA, Larkin JA: Continuing issues in ventilator-associated pneumonia, *Infect Med* 12:725-726, 1995.
499. Dunn M, Wunderlink RG: Ventilator-associated pneumonia caused by *Pseudomonas* infection, *Clin Chest Med* 16:95-109, 1995.
500. Metersky ML, Skiest D: Ventilator-associated pneumonia: current concepts, *Infect Med* 12:727-733, 1905.
501. Valenti WM, Trudell RG, Bentley DW: Factors predisposing to oropharyngeal colonization with gram-negative bacilli in the aged, *N Engl J Med* 198:1108-1111, 1978.
502. Heyland D, Mandell LA: Gastric colonization by gram-negative bacilli and nosocomial pneumonia in the intensive care unit patient, *Chest* 101:187-193, 1992.
503. Hilf M, Yu VL, Sharp J, Zuravleff JJ, Korvick JA, Muder RR: Antibiotic therapy for *P. aeruginosa* bacteremia: outcome correlations in a prospective study of 200 patients, *Am J Med* 87:540-546, 1991.
504. Schaad UB, Stoupis, Wedgwood J, Tschaeppeler H, Vock P: Clinical, radiological and magnetic resonance monitoring for skeletal toxicity in pediatric patients with cystic fibrosis receiving a three-month course of ciprofloxacin, *Pediatr Infect Dis J* 10:723-729, 1991.
505. deGroot R, Smith AL: Antibiotic pharmacokinetics in cystic fibrosis: differences and clinical significance, *Clin Pharmacokinet* 13:228-253, 1987.
506. Ramsey BWNL, Dorkin JD, Eisenberg RL, Gibson IR, Harwood RM, Kravitz DV, Schidlow RW, Wilmott SJ, Astley MA, McBurnie K, Wentz A, Smith L: Efficacy of aerosolized tobramycin in patients with cystic fibrosis. *N Engl J Med* 328:1740-1746, 1993.
507. Crane LR, Komshian S: Gram-negative bacillary pneumonias. In Pennington JE, ed: *Respiratory infections: diagnosis and management,* ed 2, New York, 1989, Raven, pp 314-340.
508. Prevatt AL, Hunt JS: Chronic systemic melioidosis, *Am J Med* 23:810-823, 1957.
509. Whitmore A, Krishnaswami CS: An account of the discovery of a hitherto undescribed infective disease occurring among population of Rangoon, *Indian Med Gazette* 47:262-267, 1912.
510. Cox CD, Arbogast JL: Melioidosis, *Am J Clin Pathol* 15:567-570, 1945.
511. Everett ED, Nelson RA: Pulmonary melioidosis, *Am Rev Respir Dis* 112:331-334, 1975.
512. Howe C, Sampath A, Spotnitz M: The pseudomallei group: a review, *J Infect Dis* 124:598-606, 1971.
513. Pattamasukon P, Pichyangkura C, Fischer GW: Melioidosis in childhood, *J Pediatr* 87:133-136, 1975.
514. Koponen MA, Zlock D, Palmer DL, Merlin TL: Melioidosis, *Arch Intern Med* 151:605-608, 1991.
515. Schlech WF, Turchik JB, Westlake RE, Klein GC, Band JD, Weaver RE: Laboratory-acquired infection with *Pseudomonas pseudomallei* (melioidosis), *N Engl J Med* 305:1133-1135, 1981.
516. Nigg C: Serologic studies on subclinical melioidosis, *J Immunol* 91:18-28, 1963.
517. Osteraas GR, Hardman JM, Bass JW, Wilson C: Neonatal melioidosis, *Am J Dis Child* 122:446-448, 1971.
518. Weber DR, Douglass LE, Brundage WG, Stallkamp TC: Acute varieties of melioidosis occurring in US soldiers in Vietnam, *Am J Med* 46:234-244, 1969.
519. Shaefer CF, Trincher RC, Rissing JP: Melioidosis: recrudescence with a strain resistant to multiple antimicrobials, *Am Rev Respir Dis* 128:173-175, 1983.
520. Alexander AD, Huxsoll DL, Warner AR, Sheppler V, Dorsey A: Serological diagnosis of human melioidosis with indirect hemagglutination and complement fixation tests, *Appl Microbiol* 20:825-833, 1970.
521. Chaowagul W, Suputtamonkol Y, Dance DA, RaJchanuvong A, Pattara-arechachai J, White NJ: Relapse in melioidosis: incidence and relapse, *J Infect Dis* 168:1181-1185, 1993.
522. Sookpranee M, Boonma P, Susaengrat W, Bhuripanyo K, Punyagupta S: Multicenter prospective randomized trial comparing ceftazidime with co-trimoxazole with chloramphenicol plus doxycycline and co-trimoxazole for treatment of severe melioidosis, *Antimicrob Agents Chemother* 36:158-162, 1992.

523. White NJ, Chawagul W, Wuthiekanun V, Dance DAB, Wattanagoon Y, Pitakwatchara N: Halving of mortality of severe melioidosis by ceftazidime, *Lancet* 2:698-700, 1989.
524. Chaowagul W, Suputtamongkol Y, Dance DAB, Rajchanuvong A, Pattara-arechachai J, White NJ: Relapse in melioidosis: incidence and risk factors, *J Infect Dis* 168:1181-1185, 1993.
525. Levine WC, Buehler JW, Bean N: Epidemiology of nontyphoidal *Salmonella* bacteremia during the human immunodeficiency virus epidemic, *J Infect Dis* 164:81-87, 1991.
526. Han T, Sokal JE, Neter E: Salmonellosis in disseminated malignant diseases: a seven year review, 1959-1965, *N Engl J Med* 276:1045-1052, 1967.
527. Sharma AM, Sharma OP: Pulmonary manifestations of typhoid fever: two case reports and a review of the literature, *Chest* 101:1144-1166, 1992.
528. Stuart BM, Pullen RL: Typhoid: clinical analysis of 360 cases, *Arch Intern Med* 78:629-661, 1946.
529. Aguado JM, Obeso G, Cabanillas JJ, Fernandez-Guerrero M, Ales J: Pleuropulmonary infections due to nontyphoid strains of *Salmonella, Arch Intern Med* 150:54-56, 1990.
530. Burney DP, Fisher RD, Schaffner W: *Salmonella* empyema: a review, *South Med J* 70:375-377, 1977.
531. Berkmen YM: Uncommon acute bacterial pneumonias, *Semin Roentgenol* 25:17-24, 1980.
532. Yu VL: *Serratia marcescens, N Engl J Med* 300:887-893, 1979.
533. McHenry MC, Hawk WA: Bacteremia caused by gram negative bacilli, *Med Clin North Am* 58:623-638, 1974.
534. Wilcox W: Violent symptoms from the bite of rat, *Am J Med Sci* 26: 245-246, 1839.
535. McHugh TP, Bartlett RL, Raymond JI: Rat bite fever: report of a fatal case, *Ann Emerg Med* 14:1116-1118, 1985.
536. Sens MA, Brown EW, Wilson LR, Crocker TP: Fatal *Streptobacillus moniliformis* infection in a two-month-old infant, *Am J Clin Pathol* 91:612-616, 1989.
537. Rowbotham TJ: Rapid identification of *Streptobacillus moniliformis, Lancet* 2:567, 1983.
538. Raffin BJ, Freemark M: Streptobacillary rat-bite fever: a pediatric problem, *Pediatrics* 64:214-217, 1979.
539. Ferrieri P: Microbiological features of current virulent strains of group A streptococci, *Pediatr Infect Dis J* 10:S20-S24, 1991.
540. Schwartz B, Facklam RR, Breiman RF: Changing epidemiology of group A streptococcal disease in the USA, *Lancet* 336:1167-1171, 1990.
541. Beachey EH, Ofek I: Epithelial cell binding of group A streptococci by lipoteichoic acid on fimbriae denuded of M protein, *J Exp Med* 143:759-771, 1976.
542. Bernheimer AW: Hemolysins of streptococci: characterization and effects on biological membranes. In Wannamaker LW, Matsen JM, eds: *Streptococci and streptococcal diseases: recognition, understanding and management,* New York, 1972, Academic, p 1931.
543. Lyon AB: Bacteriologic studies of 161 cases of pneumonia and post-pneumonia empyema in infants and children, *Am J Dis Child* 23:72-87, 1922.
544. MacCallum WG: *The pathology of pneumonia in the United States Army Camps during the winter of 1917-18,* Monograph 10, New York, 1919, Rockefeller Institute for Medical Research, pp 1-147.
545. Basiliere JL, Bistrong HW, Spence WF: Streptococcal pneumonia: recent outbreaks in military recruit populations, *Am J Med* 44:580-589, 1968.
546. Molteni RA: Group A beta-hemolytic streptococcal pneumonia, *Am J Dis Child* 131:1366-1371, 1977.
547. Duma RJ, Weinberg AN, Medrek TF, Kunz LJ: Streptococcal infections: a bacteriologic and clinical study of bacteremias, *Medicine* 48:87-127, 1969.
548. Kevy SV, Lowe BA: Streptococcal pneumonia and empyema in childhood, *N Engl J Med* 264:738-743, 1961.
549. Hoge CW, Schwartz B, Talkington DF, Breiman RF, MacNeill EM, Englender SJ: The changing epidemiology of invasive group A streptococcal infections and the emergence of streptococcal toxic shock-like syndrome, *JAMA* 269:384-389, 1993.
550. Stiles QR, Lindesmith GG, Tucker BL, Meyer BW, Jones JC: Pleural empyema in children, *Ann Thorac Surg* 10:37-44, 1970.
551. Catto BA, Jacobs MR, Shlaes DM: *Streptococcus mitis:* a cause of serious infection in adults, *Arch Intern Med* 147:885-888, 1987.
552. Pratter MR, Irwin RS: Viridans streptococcal pulmonary parenchymal infections, *JAMA* 243:2515-2517, 1980.
553. Sarkar TK, Murarka RS, Gilardi GL: Primary *Streptococcus viridans* pneumonia, *Chest* 96:831-834, 1989.
554. Gaudreau C, Delage G, Rousseau D, Cantor ED: Bacteremia caused by viridans streptococci in 71 children, *Can Med Assoc J* 125:1246-1249, 1981.
555. Marrie TJ: Bacteremic community-acquired pneumonia due to viridans group streptococci, *Clin Invest Med* 16:38-44, 1993.
556. Broughton RA, Krafka R, Baker CJ: Non-group D alpha-hemolytic streptococci: new neonatal pathogens, *J Pediatr* 99:450-454, 1981.
557. Shinzato T, Saito A: A mechanism of pathogenicity of "*Streptococcus milleri* group" in pulmonary infection: synergy with anaerobe, *J Med Microbiol* 40:118-123, 1994.
558. Molina JM, Leport C, Bure A, Wolff M, Michon C, Vilde JL: Clinical and bacterial features of infections caused by *Streptococcus milleri, Scand J Infect Dis* 23:659-666, 1991.
559. Singh KP, Morris A, Lang SD, MacCulloch DM, Bremner DA: Clinically significant *Streptococcus anginosus (Streptococcus milleri)* infections: a review of 186 cases, *N Z Med J* 101:813-816, 1988.
560. Cox RA, Chen K, Coykendall AL, Wesbecher P, Herson VC: Fatal infection in neonates of 26 weeks' gestation due to *Streptococcus milleri:* report of two cases, *J Clin Pathol* 40:190-193, 1987.
561. Spencer RC, Nanayakarra CS, Coup AJ: Fulminant neonatal sepsis due to *Streptococcus milleri, J Infect* 4:88-89, 1982.
562. Raymond J, Bergeret M, Francoual C, Chavinie J, Gendrel D: Neonatal infection with *Streptococcus milleri, Eur J Clin Microbiol Infect Dis* 14:799-801, 1995.
563. Vartian C: Bacteremic pneumonia due to group C streptococci, *Rev Infect Dis* 13:1029-1030, 1990.
564. Goolam Mahomed A, Feldman C, Smith C, Promnitz DA, Kaka S: Does primary *Streptococcus viridans* pneumonia exist? *South Afr Med J* 82:432-434, 1992.
565. Piscitelli SC, Shwed J, Schreckenberger P, Danziger LH: *Streptococcus milleri* group: renewed interest in an elusive pathogen, *Eur J Clin Microbiol Infect Dis* 11:491-498, 1992.
566. Jacobs JA, Pietersen HG, Stobberingh EE, Soeters PB: Bacteremia involving the *"Streptococcus milleri"* group: analysis of 19 cases, *Clin Infect Dis* 19:704-713, 1994.
567. Howard-Jones N: Was Shibasaburo Kitasato the co-discoverer of the plague bacillus? *Perspect Biol Med* 29:292-307, 1973.
568. Reed WP, Palmer DL, Williams RC, Kisch AL: Bubonic plague in the Southwestern United States: a review of recent experience, *Medicine* 49:465-486, 1970.
569. Lyamuya EF, Myanda P, Mohammedali H, Mhalu FS: Laboratory studies on *Yersinia pestis* during the 1991 outbreak of plaque in Lushoto, Tanzania, *J Trop Med Hyg* 95:335-338, 1992.
570. Mann JM, Schmid GP, Stoesz PA, Skinner MD, Kaufmann AF: Peripatetic plague, *JAMA* 247:47-48, 1982.
571. Human plague, United States, 1988, *MMWR* 37:653-656, 1988.
572. Kartman L, Goldenberg MI, Hubbert WT: Recent observations on the epidemiology of plague in the United States, *Am J Public Health* 56:1554-1569, 1966.
573. White ME, Rosenbaum RJ, Canfield TM, Poland JD: Plague in a neonate, *Am J Dis Child* 135:418-419, 1981.
574. Hinnebusch J, Schwan TG: New method for plague surveillance using polymerase chain reaction to detect *Yersinia pestis* in fleas, *J Clin Microbiol* 31:1511-1514, 1993.
575. Christie AB, Chen TH, Elberg SS: Plague in camels and goats: their role in human epidemics, *J Infect Dis* 141:724-726, 1980.
576. Centers for Disease Control: Pneumonic plague: Arizona, 1992, *JAMA* 268:2146-2147, 1992.
577. White ME, Rosenbaum RJ, Canfield TM, Poland JD: Plague in a neonate, *Am J Dis Child* 135:418-419, 1981.
578. Migden D: Bubonic plague in a child presenting with fever and altered mental status, *Ann Emerg Med* 19:207-209, 1990.
579. Butler T, Levin J, Linh NN, Chan DM, Adickman M, Arnold K: *Yersinia pestis* infection in Vietnam. II. Quantitative blood cultures and detection of endotoxin in the cerebrospinal fluid of patients with meningitis, *J Infect Dis* 133:493-499, 1976.

580. Williams JE, Harrison DN, Quan TJ, Mullins JL, Barnes AM, Cavanaugh DC: Atypical plague bacilli isolated from rodents, fleas, and man, *Am J Public Health* 68:262-264, 1978.
581. Meyer KF, Cavanaugh DC, Bartelloni PJ, Marshall JD: Plague immunization. I. Past and present trends, *J Infect Dis* 129:S13-S25, 1974.
582. Epidemic plague, *JAMA* 205:871, 1968.
583. Cavanaugh DC, Elisberg BL, Llewellyn CH, Marshall JD, Rust JH, Williams JE, Meyer KF: Plague immunization. V. Indirect evidence for the efficacy of plague vaccine, *J Infect Dis* 129:S37-S40, 1974.
584. Almeida CR, Almeida AR, Vieira JB, Guida U, Butler T: Plague in Brazil during two years of bacteriological and serological surveillance, *Bull WHO* 59:591-597, 1981.
585. Berkmen YM: Uncommon acute bacterial pneumonias, *Semin Roentgenol* 15:17-24, 1980.
586. Kane DR, Reuman DD: *Yersinia enterocolitica* causing pneumonia and empyema in a child and a review of the literature, *Pediatr Infect Dis J* 11:591-593, 1992.
587. Greene JN, Herndon P, Nadler JP, Sandin RL: Case report: *Yersinia enterocolitica* in an immunocompromised patient, *Am J Med Sci* 305:171-173, 1993.

Lung Abscess

588. Emanuel B, Shulman ST: Lung abscess in infants and children, *Clin Pediatr* 34:2-6, 1995.
589. Tan TQ, Seilheimer DK, Kaplan SL: Pediatric lung abscess: clinical management and outcome, *Pediatr Infect Dis J* 14:51-55, 1995.
590. McCracken GH: Lung abscess in childhood, *Hosp Pract* 13:35-36, 1978.
591. Asher MI, Spier S, Beland M, Coates AL, Beaudry PH: Primary lung abscess in childhood, *Am J Dis Child* 136:491-494, 1982.
592. Bartlett JG, Finegold SM: Anaerobic infections of the lung and pleural space, *Am Rev Respir Dis* 110:56-77, 1974.
593. Dail DH, Hammar SP: *Pulmonary pathology,* New York, 1988, Springer-Verlag, pp 113-114.
594. Philpott NJ, Woodhead MA, Wilson AG, Millard FJC: Lung abscess: a neglected cause of life threatening haemoptysis, *Thorax* 48:674-675, 1993.
595. Bartlett JG, Gorbach SL, Finegold SM: The bacteriology of aspiration pneumonia, *Am J Med* 56:202-207, 1974.
596. Southee AE, Lee KJ, McLaughlin AF, Borham PW, Bautovich GJ, Morris JG: Tc-99m white cell scintigraphy in suspected acute infection, *Clin Nucl Med* 15:71-75, 1990.
597. Johnson JF, Shields WE, White CB, Williams BD: Concealed pulmonary abscess: diagnosis by computed tomography, *Pediatrics* 78:283-286, 1986.
598. Rohlfing BM, White EA, Webb WR, Goodman PC: Hilar and mediastinal adenopathy caused by bacterial abscess of the lung, *Radiology* 128:289-293, 1978.
599. Wu HD, Yana PC, Lee LN: Differentiation of lung abscess and empyema by ultrasonography, *J Formosan Med Assoc* 90:749-754, 1991.
600. Bartlett JG: Anaerobic bacterial infections of the lung, *Chest* 91:90-99, 1987.
601. Michiels E, Demedts M: Pitfalls of transthoracic needle aspiration biopsy, *Acta Clin Belg* 46:359-363, 1991.
602. Silverman M, Stratton D, Diallo A, Egler LJ: Diagnosis of acute bacterial pneumonia in Nigerian children: value of needle aspiration of lung and counter current immuno-electrophoresis, *Arch Dis Child* 52:925-931, 1977.
603. Yang PC, Luh KT, Lee YC, Chang DB, Yu CJ, Wu HD, Lee LN, Kuo SH: Lung abscesses: US examination and US-guided transthoracic aspiration, *Radiology* 180:171-175, 1991.
604. Henriquez ALT, Mendoza J, Gonzalez PC: Quantitative culture of bronchoalveolar lavage from patients with anaerobic lung abscesses, *J Infect Dis* 164:414-417, 1991.
605. Brook I, Finegold SM: Bacteriology and therapy of lung abscess in children, *J Pediatr* 94:1-12, 1979.
606. Brook I, Feingold SM: Bacteriology of aspiration pneumonia in children, *Pediatrics* 65:1115-1120, 1980.
607. Pacht ER: *Mycobacterium fortuitum* lung abscess: resolution with prolonged trimethoprim/sulfamethoxazole therapy, *Am Rev Respir Dis* 141:1599-1601, 1990.
608. Waller KS, Johnson J, Wood BP: Radiological case of the month, *Am J Dis Child* 145:209-210, 1991.
609. Gradon JD, Mayrer AR, Hayes J: Pulmonary abscess associated with *Alcaligenes xylosoxidans* in a patient with AIDS, *Clin Infect Dis* 17:1071-1072, 1993.
610. Mesnard R, Lamy T, Dauriac C, LePrise PY: Lung abscess due to *Pseudallescheria boydii* in the course of acute leukaemia, *Acta Haematol* 87:78-82, 1992.
611. Bisiaux-Salauze B, Perez C, Sebald M, Petit JC: Bacteremias caused by *Selenomonas artemidis* and *Selenomonas infelix, J Clin Microbiol* 28:140-142, 1990.
612. Namnyak SS, Blair AL, Hughes DF, McElhinney P, Donnelly MR, Corey J: Fatal lung abscess due to *Lactobacillus casei ss rhamnosus, Thorax* 47:666-667, 1992.
613. Paz HL, Little BJ, Ball WC, Winkelstein JA: Primary pulmonary botryomycosis, *Chest* 101:1160-1162, 1992.
614. Chan JC, Raffin TA: *Salmonella* lung abscess complicating Wegener's granulomatosis, *Respir Med* 85:339-341, 1991.
615. Siegel JD, McCracken GH: Neonatal lung abscess: a report of six cases, *Am J Dis Child* 133:947-949, 1979.
616. Sabiston DC, Hopkins EH, Cooke RE, Bennett IL: The surgical management of complications of staphylococcal pneumonia in infancy and childhood, *J Thorac Cardiovasc Surg* 38:421-434, 1959.
617. Klein JO, Marx MI: Bacterial infections of the respiratory tract. In Remington JS, Klein JO, eds: *Infectious diseases of the fetus and newborn infant,* Philadelphia, WB Saunders, ed 4, 1995, pp 899-900.
618. Finegold SM: Aspiration pneumonia, lung abscess, and empyema. In Pennington JE, ed: *Respiratory infections: diagnosis and management,* ed 2, New York, 1988, Raven, pp 270-272.
619. Lee SK, Morris RF, Cramer B: Percutaneous needle aspiration of neonatal lung abscesses, *Pediatr Radiol* 21:254-257, 1991.
620. Ball WS, Bisset GS, Towbin RB: Percutaneous drainage of chest abscess in children, *Radiology* 171:431-434, 1989.
621. Mayer T, Matlak ME, Condon V, Shasha I, Glasgow L: Computed tomographic findings of neonatal lung abscess, *Am J Dis Child* 136:39-41, 1982.
622. Lorenzo RL, Bradford BF, Black J, Smith CD: Lung abscess in children: diagnostic and therapeutic needle aspiration, *Radiology* 157:79-80, 1985.
623. Kosloske AM, Ball WS Jr, Butler CM Nusemech CA: Drainage of pediatric lung abscess by cough, catheter, or complete resection, *J Pediatr Surgery* 21:596-600, 1986.
624. Lui RC, Inculet RI: Job's syndrome: a rare cause of recurrent lung abscess in childhood, *Ann Thorac Surg* 50:992-994, 1990.

Pleural Empyema

625. Freij BJ, Kusmiesz H, Nelson JD, McCracken G: Parapneumonic effusions and effusions and empyema in hospitalized children: a retrospective review of 227 cases, *Pediatr Infect Dis* J 3:578-591, 1984.
626. Wiener-Kronish JP, Broaddus VC: Interrelationships of pleural and pulmonary interstitial liquid, *Annu Rev Physiol* 55:209-226, 1993.
627. Light RW: *Pleural diseases,* ed 3, Baltimore, 1995, Williams and Wilkins, pp 35-36.
628. Brook I: Microbiology of empyema in children and adolescents, *Pediatrics* 85:722-726, 1990.
629. Nelson JD: Pleural empyema, *Pediatr Infect Dis* 4:S31-S33, 1985.
630. Hoff SJ, Neblett WW, Edwards KM Heller RM, Pietsch JB, Holcomb GW Jr, Holcomb GW III: Parapneumonic empyema in children: decortication hastens recovery in patients with severe pleural infections, *Pediatr Infect Dis J* 10:194-199, 1991.
631. Bechamps GJ, Lynn HB, Wenzl JE: Empyema in children: review of Mayo Clinic experience, *Mayo Clin Proc* 45:43-50, 1970.
632. Ginsburg CM, Howard JB, Nelson JD: Report of 65 cases of *Haemophilus influenzae* b pneumonia, *Pediatrics* 64:283-286, 1979.
633. Brook I: Microbiology empyema in children and adolescents, *Pediatrics* 85:722-726, 1990.
634. Bartlett JG, Finegold SM: Anaerobic infections of the lung and pleural space, *Am Rev Respir Dis* 110:56-77, 1974.
635. Purgatch RD, Faling LJ, Robbins AH, Snider GL: Differentiation of pleural and pulmonary lesions using computer tomography, *J Comput Assist Tomogr* 2:601-606, 1978.

636. Stark DD, Federle MP, Goodman PC, Podrasky AE, Webb WR: Differentiating lung abscess and empyema: radiography and computed tomography, *Am J Roentgenol* 141:163-167, 1983.
637. Wu HD, Yang PC, Lee LN: Differentiation of lung abscess and empyema by ultrasonography, *J Formosan Med Assoc* 90:749-754, 1991.
638. Stark DD, Federle MP, Goodman PC, Podrasky AE, Webb WR: Differentiating lung abscess and empyema: radiography and computed tomography, *Am J Roentgenol* 141:163-167, 1983.
639. Cleveland RH, Foglia RD: CT in the evaluation of pleural versus pulmonary disease in children, *Pediatr Radiol* 18:14-19, 1988.
640. Ben-Ami TE, O'Donovan JC, Yousefzadeh DK: Sonography of the chest in children, *Pediatr Chest* 31:517-531, 1993.
641. Lampe RM, Chottipitayasunondh T, Sunakorn P: Detection of bacterial antigen in pleural fluid by counterimmunoelectrophoresis, *J Pediatr* 88:557-560, 1976.
642. Taryle DA, Good JT, Morgan EJ, Reller LB, Sahn SA: Antibiotic concentrations in human parapneumonic effusions, *J Antimicrob Chemother* 7:171-177, 1981.
643. Bartlett JG, Gorbach SL, Finegold SM: The bacteriology of aspiration pneumonia, *Am J Med* 56:202-207, 1974.
644. Bryant RE, Salmon CJ: Pleural empyema, *Clin Infect Dis* 22:747-764, 1996.
645. Moulton JS, Moore PT, Mencini RA: Treatment of loculate pleural effusions with transcatheter intracavitary urokinase, *Am J Roentgenol* 153:941-945, 1989.
646. Robinson LA, Moulton AL, Fleming WH, Alonso A, Galbraith TA: Intrapleural fibrolytic treatment of multiloculated thoracic empyemas, *Ann Thorac Surg* 57:803-814, 1994.
647. Kosloske AM, Cartwright KC: The controversial role of decortication in the management of pediatric empyema, *J Thorac Cardiovasc Surg* 96:166-170, 1988.
648. Ramnath RR, Heller R, Ben-Ami TE, Miller M, Campo P, Neblett W, Holcomb G, Hernandez-Schulman M: Implications of early sonographic evaluation of parapneumonic effusions in children with pneumonia, *Pediatrics* 1998 (in press).
649. Hardie W, Bokulic R, Garcia VF, Reising SF, Christie DC: Pneumococcal pleural empyemas in children, *Clin Infect Dis* 22:1057-1063, 1996.
650. McLaughlin FJ, Goldmann DA, Rosenbaum DM, Harris GBC, Schuster SR, Strieder D: Empyema in children: clinical course and long-term follow-up, *Pediatrics* 73:587-593, 1984.

CHAPTER 40

Respiratory Infections in Immunocompromised Hosts

Dennis C. Stokes

Many noninfectious pulmonary complications occur in immunocompromised pediatric patients, including those with acquired immunodeficiency syndrome (AIDS) and must thus be included in the differential diagnosis of infectious pneumonias. Several excellent reviews cover pulmonary infections in specific immunocompromised populations.[1-15]

HISTORICAL PERSPECTIVE

The use of the term *immunocompromised host* is relatively new. Utz first described the terms *opportunistic pathogens* and *immunodeficiency* in 1962, and in 1967, Ruskin and Remington used the term compromised host.[16,17] During the 1960s, improved therapeutic programs for childhood malignancies, principally acute lymphocytic leukemia, resulted in longer survival times and increased numbers of children at risk for opportunistic infections. Children who no longer died quickly during initial therapy were at risk for pulmonary infections over prolonged remissions while receiving maintenance chemotherapy for at least 5 years. *Pneumocystis carinii,* previously identified as a pathogen primarily in outbreaks in malnourished infants, emerged as a major problem for these children.[18,19] Varicella-zoster pneumonia was also a major problem because of its frequency in childhood and the lack of effective antiviral therapy.[20] During the late 1960s, the first bone marrow transplants were attempted in children with refractory malignancies. Bacterial pneumonias were generally treatable with effective antimicrobial therapy, but fungal pneumonias became a major problem in children with prolonged neutropenia, such as those with aplastic anemia or those receiving intensive chemotherapy. *Aspergillus* pneumonia was a common problem, and the association with hospital construction and other risk factors such as prolonged neutropenia was recognized.[21] In 1976 and 1977, Hughes et al[22,23] described effective treatment and prophylaxis for *P. carinii* pneumonia (PCP) in oncology patients with trimethoprim/sulfamethoxazole (TMP/SMX). This replaced the more toxic medication pentamidine that was available only for biopsy-proven PCP.[22,23] The use of TMP/SMX prophylaxis effectively eliminated PCP as a cause of pneumonia in this population, and the availability of a safer alternative to pentamidine provided a rationale for the empiric treatment of pneumonia in immunocompromised patients.[24] This often delayed more invasive diagnostic studies such as open lung biopsy and generated considerable controversy on the role and timing of open lung biopsy.[25-27] In the late 1970s, pediatric flexible bronchoscopy became increasingly available as an alternative to surgery, providing a specific diagnosis for many opportunistic infections.[28-32] In the 1980s the epidemic of human immunodeficiency virus (HIV) infection and AIDS resulted in a major new group of immunocompromised children, first in those who received contaminated blood transfusions for cancer, hemophilia, or other indications and later in infants of HIV-infected mothers. *P. carinii* reemerged as the major pulmonary pathogen in this group, both as the presenting infection and cause of death.[33] In addition to patients with AIDS, new high-risk groups included patients with acute nonlymphocytic leukemia, lymphoma, and solid tumors (including brain tumors) who were receiving aggressive combined therapy with chemotherapy and radiation therapy.[34] The number of bone marrow and other tissue transplants also continued to expand, and major noninfectious pulmonary complications were described in these populations, including bronchiolitis obliterans in recipients of bone marrow transplants and lymphoid interstitial pneumonia in pediatric patients with AIDS.[35,36] The use of varicella-zoster immune globulin (VZIG) for prophylaxis and acyclovir for treatment significantly reduced the importance of varicella-zoster virus (VZV) as a cause of mortality.[37]

The late 1980s and 1990s have been marked by several early trends. Gram-positive organisms, including *Staphylococcus epidermidis,* methicillin-resistant *Staphylococcus aureus,* streptococci, and *Corynebacterium jeikeium,* have again become major causes of sepsis and bacteremia.[3] Ganciclovir and immunoglobulin have provided some hope for preventing and treating cytomegalovirus (CMV) pneumonitis in high-risk populations.[38-40] Cytokines to accelerate marrow recovery and activate macrophages have helped reduce the risk of bacterial and fungal pathogens in many patients.[41] Fungal pathogens, particularly the rare saprophytic organisms, remain a major problem because of their resistance to antifungal therapy. New diagnostic tests have been added to those previously available, including clinical application of rapid diagnostic tests based on polymerase chain reaction (PCR) and other methods, thoracoscopic biopsy, and computed tomography–guided needle aspiration biopsy.[42-45]

HOST DEFENSE DISORDERS

Many nonimmunologic aspects of pulmonary host defense, including physical barriers, mucociliary clearance, and cough, predispose to pulmonary infections when altered. However, the primary groups of immunocompromised children are those with either congenital or acquired defects in immunologic defenses of the lung. A detailed discussion of pulmonary immunologic defenses is beyond the scope of this chapter but is covered in a recent review.[1] Table 40-1 summarizes the major host defenses of the lung and associated disorders that predispose to pulmonary infections.

Humoral Immunity. Immunoglobulin G (IgG) and IgA are major components of respiratory secretions, with IgA (and secretory IgA) most important in the upper airway. In the lower respiratory tract, IgG provides primary protection against local and systemic infections. Defects of subclasses of IgG, including both IgG2 and IgG4, have been associated with recurrent sinopulmonary infections, although the importance of minor reductions of subclasses in patients with recurrent pneumonias is debated.[46,47] Some individuals with normal levels of total antibody are unable to make IgG to certain important pathogens. Although patients with complement deficiencies are more likely to have systemic infection, some patients with such defects have pneumonias.[48]

Cellular Immunity. Alveolar macrophages are the major phagocytic cells in the lung and are able to handle small numbers of pathogenic organisms. Neutrophils are present in the lung in small numbers but can be rapidly recruited from the vascular compartment via a variety of chemotactic factors produced by complement activation or secreted by macrophages. A reduction in the number of circulating neutrophils is a major cause of pneumonias in immunocompromised hosts. Chronic granulomatous disease, neutrophil motility disorders, and other forms of phagocytic dysfunction also lead to pulmonary infections.

Secretory Factors. Macrophages secrete a number of important cytokines, such as tumor necrosis factor-α and interleukin-1, which have both local immunomodulating effects within the lung and systemic effects such as fever and shock. Nonspecific antibacterial defenses such as lysozyme and surfactant may also be important.

Table 40-1 Host Defense Disorders Leading to Pneumonia

PULMONARY HOST DEFENSE	DEFECTIVE IN:
Upper airway	
Turbinates	Intubation,
Epiglottis	Tracheostomy, aspiration syndromes
Mucociliary clearance	
Cilia	Ciliary dyskinesia syndrome, infections
Mucous blanket	Cystic fibrosis, bronchitis
Cough	Muscle weakness, sedation
Immunoglobulin	
Secretory IgA, IgA	IgA deficiency, IgG subclass deficiency
IgG, including subclasses	Agammaglobulinemia, hypogammaglobulinemia
IgE	Elevated in hyperimmunoglobulinemia E with recurrent infections (Job's syndrome)
Cells	
Alveolar macrophages	Corticosteroids, chemotherapy, chronic granulomatous disease
Polymorphonuclear leukocytes	
Numbers	Chemotherapy, congenital neutropenia
Mobility	Motility disorders
Function	Chronic granulomatous disease
Lymphocytes	
Numbers	AIDS
Function	T cell disorders, including CMC, severe combined immunodeficiency disease, others
Other	
Surfactant	Adult respiratory distress syndrome (?), edema
Fibronectin, lysozyme complement	C3 or C5 deficiency

CLINICAL PRESENTATION

Patterns of Pneumonia

Often the first clue to an abnormal host disorder is the development of recurrent or persistent pneumonia. Patients usually have persistent or recurrent radiologic evidence of pneumonia that is associated with the typical signs of infection such as fever and tachypnea. It is important to note whether these infiltrates clear completely after therapy, whether they involve one lobe or more than one lobe, and whether they are associated with other radiologic findings such as hyperinflation or situs inversus. The differential diagnosis of recurrent or persistent pneumonia is extensive and includes many causes other than immunodeficiency.[49,50]

The condition of a patient with an abnormal ability to deal with infection often has an atypical course when that patient is infected with a "usual" childhood respiratory pathogen. For example, respiratory syncytial virus (RSV) leads to more serious disease in immunocompromised patients.[51-53] Varicella, influenza, parainfluenza, and measles are all potentially devastating pulmonary infections in immunocompromised hosts. Although adenovirus is capable of causing severe pneumonia in any child, it is particularly devastating in immunocompromised hosts and possibly exceeds VZV and *P. carinii* as a cause of fatal pneumonias in high-risk populations such as recipients of bone marrow transplant.[54] Suppurative bronchitis related to *Haemophilus influenzae* and *Streptococcus pneumoniae* infection is common in immunoglobulin deficiency.

The "opportunistic" pathogens are those typically not seen except in the patient with altered host defense. PCP is probably the best example of pulmonary infection caused by an opportunistic pathogen and occurs in a variety of immunocompromised patients, including those with AIDS, T cell disorders, and agammaglobulinemia; pediatric oncology patients; and patients on high doses of corticosteroids.

The clinical course of opportunistic infections varies and may be altered by the degree of residual host immunity. For example, corticosteroid therapy accelerates the resolution of *P. carinii* infection in patients with AIDS, suggesting that the residual host inflammatory response to this organism is important in the pathogenesis of respiratory dysfunction with PCP, even in profoundly immunosuppressed patients.[55-60] Fungal pulmonary infections in patients with chemotherapy-induced neutropenia often result in mild clinical symptoms and radiographic findings until a rise in the neutrophil counts results in significant inflammation, lung destruction and cavitation, and clinical deterioration.

Pathogens and Host Disorder

Another useful way to consider the types of pulmonary infections that occur in immunocompromised hosts is by considering the underlying host disorder. Childhood cancer therapy, bone marrow transplant and organ transplants, primary immunodeficiencies, and AIDS are each associated with specific pathogen groups (Table 40-2).

Childhood Cancer

Patients with childhood cancer are at high risk for respiratory infections for a variety of reasons in addition to the immunosuppressive effects of chemotherapy and radiation (Box 40-1). Among childhood cancer groups, there are differing risks for various pathogens.

The major risk factor for pneumonia in patients with leukemia is chemotherapy-induced neutropenia. Because patients with nonlymphocytic leukemia undergo the most intensive chemotherapy, they are at greatest risk for developing pneumonia. Bacterial pneumonias are most common, but RSV, adenovirus, and enteroviruses are also significant causes of pneumonia in patients with leukemia. Fungal pneumonias oc-

Table 40-2 Typical Pulmonary Pathogens Associated with Immune Disorders

	PATHOGENS		
	BACTERIAL	FUNGAL	VIRAL, PROTOZOAL, OR OTHER
Neutropenia			
Chronic	*H. Influenzae, S. pneumoniae, S. aureus, Klebsiella* species	—	—
Acute	*S. aureus*	—	—
Prolonged hospitalization	Gram-negative organisms, including *Pseudomonas* species	*Candida* species, *Aspergillus* species, *Mucor* species	—
Agammaglobulinemia, hypogammaglobulinemia	*S. pneumoniae, H. influenzae, Pseudomonas* species	*Aspergillus* species	*P. carinii*
Congenital T cell disorders	*Legionella* species, *Nocardia* species, *Listeria* species, *Mycobacteria tuberculosis, Salmonella* species	*Candida* species, *Cryptococcus* species	CMV, *P. carinii,* VZV, HSV
AIDS	*Mycobacteria tuberculosis, Mycobacteria avium-intracellulare*	*Cryptococcus* species	CMV, *P. carinii, Toxoplasma* species
Complement deficiencies	Virulent encapsulated species (e.g., *S. pneumoniae, H. influenzae*)	—	—
Immunosuppressive therapy (e.g., renal, liver, lung transplant)	*S. aureus, Listeria* species, *Mycobacteria tuberculosis*	*Aspergillus* species, *Mucor* species, *Histoplasmosis* species	CMV, *P. carinii,* VZV, *Toxoplasma* species, HSV, *Cryptococcus* species
Bone marrow transplant			
Early <30 days)	*Pseudomonas* species, other gram-negative and gram-positive species	*Candida* species	—
Late (>30 days)	*S. aureus*	*Aspergillus* species	CMV, *Toxoplasma* species, VZV, *P. carinii,* Epstein-Barr virus, Adenovirus
Late (>100 days)	Encapsulated gram-positive *H. influenzae, S. pneumoniae)*	—	VZV

HSV, Herpes simplex virus.

cur in patients with prolonged neutropenia, hospitalization, and broad-spectrum antibiotic therapy. *Aspergillus* species and Zygomycetes (*Mucor, Rhizopus,* and *Cunninghamella* species) are the two most common fungal pulmonary pathogens.[61] *Candida* species frequently cause disseminated fungal infections, but their role in pulmonary disease is difficult to determine because they frequently contaminate sputum and bronchial washes of patients without *Candida* pneumonia and primary isolated *Candida* pneumonia is relatively uncommon.[62] *P. carinii* and varicella-zoster virus were major causes of pneumonia in patients with leukemia in the 1970s, but the use of prophylaxis and effective therapies has reduced their impact as causes of pneumonitis in oncology patients, although both still occur in this population.[63]

Patients with lymphoma are at risk for pneumonia because of neutropenia during therapy and because of a variety of nonspecific immunologic defects, including anergy.[64,65] Patients with Hodgkin's disease are often infected with *Toxoplasma gondii* and fungi such as *Cryptococcus neoformans,* and the mediastinal adenopathy and lung nodules commonly seen in these children at diagnosis often require extensive evaluation to differentiate lymphoma from granulomatous pulmonary infections such as tuberculosis and histoplasmosis.

Tissue Transplantation: Bone Marrow and Solid Organ

The types of pulmonary complications in allogeneic bone marrow transplant vary with the period after transplantation[8,9,66] (Table 40-3). Immediately after transplantation, patients are neutropenic and at risk for bacterial pneumonias caused by *Pseudomonas aeruginosa* and *S. aureus.* As the transplant becomes established and the neutrophil count rises, acute graft-versus-host disease (GVHD) becomes a serious concern. Immunosuppressive therapy for GVHD with corticosteroids or cyclosporin A adds to the risk of pneumonia caused by viral pathogens (CMV, herpes simplex virus [HSV], adenovirus) as well as *P. carinii* and fungi. If engraftment fails and prolonged neutropenia occurs, the risk of fungal pneumonia rises significantly. Idiopathic interstitial pneumonias also occur during this later time, possibly because of radiation or chemotherapy.[67] Late (more than 4 to 6 months after the transplant) causes of pneumonia include *H. influenzae* and *S. pneumoniae* and are associated with persistent humoral immune deficits to these encapsulated organisms. A frequent cause of morbidity in the late transplant period is bronchiolitis obliterans, which is thought to be an immunologic disorder related to chronic GVHD.[35,68,69] The frequency of this complication in pediatric recipients of bone marrow transplants is not clear, and it may be less common than in adult recipients.[70] Infection may play a role in provoking or exacerbating chronic lung damage caused by bronchiolitis obliterans.[71,72]

CMV infection remains a major cause of morbidity and mortality in pediatric recipients of bone marrow transplants. CMV occurs more frequently in allogeneic than recipients of autologous bone marrow transplants (12.4% vs. 3.3%) and in patients who are seropositive before transplant or who receive marrow from seropositive donors.[73] The incidence increases with age and is 1.3% from birth to 9 years of age and 2.1% from 10 to 19 years of age. The mortality rate of CMV pneumonitis was greater than 90% before the use of ganciclovir and immunoglobulin therapy, which must be started early to be effective. In one series, only 10 of 75 recipients of bone marrow transplants with CMV pneumonitis survived for a long time, and of these, 9 were ventilator independent at the initiation of therapy with ganciclovir and immunoglobulin.[74] Studies of risk groups for CMV pneumonitis in a group of 62 allogeneic pediatric and adult recipients of transplants confirmed a low incidence in seronegative recipients who received grafts from seronegative donors and screened blood products. T cell depletion to prevent GVHD in a CMV-seropositive recipient whose tissue was grafted from a nonimmune donor is associated with a high risk of CMV interstitial pneumonia.[75]

Fungal infections, including invasive pulmonary disease, are another major cause of morbidity and mortality in the bone marrow transplant population. Prolonged neutropenia is a major risk factor for the development of fungal infections, and recombinant cytokines to stimulate bone marrow recovery offer promise for reducing the window of vulnerability for fungal

BOX 40-1
Predisposition to Pneumonia in Childhood Malignancy

Granulocytopenia
Mucosal disruption: skin, gut, lung
Cellular immune dysfunction
Humoral defects
Splenectomy
Mechanical catheters
Malnutrition
Radiation
Graft-versus-host disease
Administration of corticosteroids

Table 40-3 Pulmonary Complications After Bone Marrow Transplant

PULMONARY HOST DEFENSE	ASSOCIATION	ORGANISMS	OTHER PULMONARY DISORDERS
Pretransplant	Neutropenia, chemotherapy, prolonged use of antibiotics, iatrogenic procedures	Bacteria, fungi	—
Early posttransplant (<1 month)	Neutropenia, mucositis, use of antibiotics, radiation	Bacteria (particularly gram negative), HSV, RSV, *Candida* species, *Aspergillus* species	Pulmonary edema, ARDS
Late posttransplant (1-4 months)	Acute GVHD, failed engraftment	CMV, adenovirus, PC, *Aspergillus* species, *Mucor* species, HHV-6, EBV	Interstitial pneumonia, lymphoproliferative syndromes
Late posttransplant (<4 months)	Chronic GVHD, poor antibody response	VZV, encapsulated gram-positive bacteria, PC	Bronchiolitis obliterans, BOOP

HSV, Herpes simplex virus; *ARDS,* acute respiratory distress syndrome; *GVHD,* graft-versus-host-disease; *PC, Pneumocystis pneumoniae; HHV-6,* human herpesvirus type 6; *EBV,* Epstein-Barr virus; *BOOP,* bronchiolitis obliterans–organizing pneumonia.

pneumonias. Adult and pediatric recipients of bone marrow transplants who were treated with recombinant human macrophage colony-stimulating factor had greater overall survival rate (27% vs. 5% because of a 50% survival rate in patients with *Candida* infections), although the survival rate in patients who developed *Aspergillus* remained poor.[76]

The development of pulmonary infections after renal and other solid organ transplants is attributable to chronic immunosuppression with cyclosporine A and corticosteroid therapy.[77] CMV is the most significant pulmonary infection in recipients of all transplants, and in recipients of heart-lung transplants, *P. carinii* and *Toxoplasma* infections are also quite common.[78,79] In pediatric recipients of 58 consecutive renal transplants who were followed for up to 72 months, CMV infection occurred in 40% and CMV disease in 15% (1 death).[80] The highest risk for CMV infection occurs in the first 12 weeks after the transplant, and donor CMV seropositivity, regardless of recipient CMV serostatus, is significantly associated with CMV infection.

Gram-negative and fungal infections are the most common pulmonary complications in recipients of liver transplants. They occur primarily in the first month after transplant.[14]

Primary Immunodeficiency

In patients with common variable immunodeficiency and X-linked agammaglobulinemia, repeated bacterial pneumonias are most common, and *P. carinii* is occasionally seen in patients with hypogammaglobulinemia.[81-83] Patients with congenital T cell disorders, including severe combined immunodeficiency, are at risk for most of the same opportunistic pathogens as patients with AIDS, including PCP.[84,85]

Fungi, primarily *Aspergillus* species, and *S. aureus* are the most common lung infections in children with chronic granulomatous disease.[86,87] Extensive lung destruction and hilar adenopathy are common in these patients.

Although persistent and recurrent *Candida albicans* infection of the mucous membranes and skin is associated with this T cell disorder, 50% have recurrent bacterial pneumonias, and they are at risk for infections caused by other opportunistic pathogens, including *P. carinii, Nocardia,* and varicella-zoster virus pneumonias. Pulmonary complications, including bronchiectasis, empyema, and lung abscess, frequently occur.[88]

AIDS

The extensive list of pulmonary infections associated with AIDS includes *P. carinii,* CMV, bacteria, and atypical mycobacteria as major causes of pneumonia in this group[11-13,89,90] (Fig. 40-1).

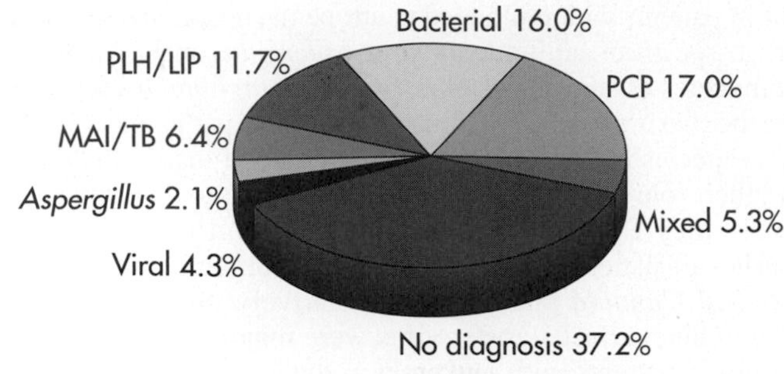

Fig. 40-1. Causes of pneumonia in AIDS. (From Marioda J et al: *Pediatr Pulmonol* 10:231-235, 1991.)

BOX 40-2
Radiologic Presentations

Diffuse interstitial and alveolar
PCP
CMV
C. neoformans
Viruses (e.g., adenovirus)
Aspergillus species (rare)
Candida species (rare)

Lobar or lobular
Bacteria
Nocardia species
C. neoformans
Aspergillus species
Mucor species
Mycobacteria
Viruses
Legionella species

Nodules, cavities, or lung abscess
Bacteria (*S. aureus,* anaerobes)
C. neoformans
Mycobacteria
Nocardia species
Aspergillus species
Legionella species
PCP (rare except in HIV)
Lymphocytic interstitial pneumonitis (reticulonodular)

Radiographic Presentation

Pneumonias in this population can be classified by the general appearance of the radiograph. Findings include diffuse alveolar and interstitial pneumonias, localized alveolar lobar or lobular pneumonias (which may involve more than one lobe), and nodular infiltrates (which may be cavitary or progress to frank lung abscess).[91] The common causes of these general radiographic patterns are listed in Box 40-2, but it must be emphasized that radiographic appearances are often deceptive in immunocompromised hosts and are usually not helpful in making a specific etiologic diagnosis.

P. carinii is the prototypical organism associated with the radiographic pattern of diffuse interstitial and alveolar pneumonias (Fig. 40-2). Although the incidence of *P. carinii* infection has declined significantly in patient populations receiving prophylaxis, PCP remains the major pathogen associated with AIDS, and atypical radiographic appearances of *P. carinii* are common and include normal radiographs; radiographs showing cystic, unilateral, and granulomatous changes; and radiographs showing associated pleural disease.[34,90-95] The use of aerosolized pentamidine for PCP prophylaxis in AIDS may alter the radiographic presentation more toward upper lobe disease. This was thought to occur because of the preferential distribution of the medication to the lower lobes, but studies of drug levels suggest that other factors may be involved because medication levels are similar in both upper and lower lung zones despite larger numbers of organisms in the upper lung zones.[96] CMV is also associated with diffuse pneumonia in immunocompromised patients and is frequently seen in association with other infectious agents. Viral infections, including

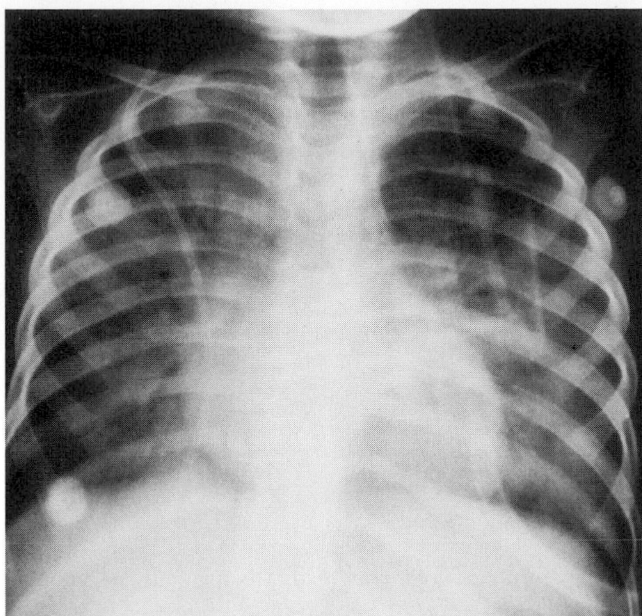

Fig. 40-2. Chest radiograph of PCP.

Table 40-4 Noninfectious Processes Complicating or Simulating Pneumonia

PROCESS	ASSOCIATION
Chemical pneumonitis	Aspiration syndromes, smoke inhalation
Immune-mediated infection	Hypersensitivity pneumonitis, collagen vascular disease
Atelectasis	Reactive airways disease, endobronchial obstruction
Hemorrhage	Hemosiderosis, thrombocytopenia, coagulopathy, *Aspergillus* infection
Pulmonary embolus	Condition secondary to intravascular abnormalities
Pulmonary edema	
Cardiogenic	Anthracycline cardiotoxicity, sepsis, myocarditis
Noncardiogenic	Acute respiratory distress syndrome, pancreatitis, fluid overload
Drug-induced lung injury	Chemotherapy, azathioprine
Radiation pneumonitis	Radiation treatment 6-8 weeks previously
Leukostasis	Hyperleukocytosis, use of amphotericin B, transfusions of white blood cells
Leukemia, lymphoma	Active disease
Lymphocytic interstitial pneumonitis	HIV infection in children
"Idiopathic pneumonitis"	Allogeneic bone marrow transplant
Other	Thymus, sequestration, tumor

adenovirus, and influenza are also important causes of diffuse pneumonia.

Bronchopneumonias and lobar consolidation can occur in immunocompromised patients and are caused by the usual pathogens, such as *S. pneumoniae, H. influenzae,* and *S. aureus.* However, because the radiographic pathology is a product of the host's response to the organism, patients with abnormal host defenses often have an altered initial radiographic pattern.

Solitary pulmonary nodules, either unilateral or bilateral, are less common presentations of infection in most immunocompromised patients but do occur frequently in pediatric oncology patients. Although these most often represent fungal pneumonias, infections of other organisms, including *Nocardia* species, can also present as pulmonary nodules. The development of a lung abscess generally indicates a degree of host immunity sufficient to localize an infection. The most common causes of cavitary lesions in pediatric patients with cancer are fungal infection, especially with *Aspergillus* species. PCP and mycobacterial infections are associated with cavitary disease in patients with AIDS.[93]

COMMON CAUSES OF PNEUMONIA IN THE IMMUNOCOMPROMISED HOST

Noninfectious Pulmonary Disease

Immunocompromised patients are at risk for a variety of noninfectious complications that simulate infection and complicate the diagnostic workup (Table 40-4).

Infectious Pneumonias

Viruses

Herpesviruses. The herpesviruses that cause infectious viral pneumonia are CMV, VZV and HSV, and human herpesvirus type 6 (HHV-6).

CMV. CMV is a herpesvirus that commonly infects both neonates and older immunocompromised children.[97] Whether the virus results in disease depends both on the age and the immune status of the infected individual. The organism can be transmitted through an infected birth canal and via breast milk, saliva, and blood (through infected white cells). Both humoral and cellular immune mechanisms are important in establishing protection against CMV. Individuals who are CMV negative before acquired immunosuppression resulting from organ or marrow transplantation and who acquire the virus by transfusion are particularly at risk for disease. CMV-positive individuals who are then immunosuppressed also run a significant risk for "reactivation" pneumonia.

CMV-infected cells typically contain nuclear inclusions that are deeply basophilic and surrounded by a clear halo, giving the "owl eye" appearance. Typically, inclusions are seen in alveolar cells. The pathologic situation varies from small hemorrhagic nodules scattered throughout the lung and surrounded by relatively normal lung to diffuse alveolar damage or chronic interstitial pneumonitis.

Unless they acquire the virus before birth, most infants infected with CMV are asymptomatic, although occasional cases of protracted pneumonia have been reported. The major risk factors for CMV pneumonia include AIDS, congenital immunodeficiencies, and organ transplants, particularly kidney, bone marrow, and heart-lung. The radiographic pattern of the pneumonia is usually a diffuse reticulonodular pattern that is less alveolar in pattern than PCP. Approximately 50% of patients with aplastic anemia or hematologic malignancy treated by allogenic marrow transplantation develop CMV infection, and CMV pneumonia had a 90% mortality rate in this population before the availability of antiviral therapy. CMV frequently is found as a copathogen with other opportunistic oganisms, including *P. carinii* and *Aspergillus* species, particularly in patients with AIDS.

The diagnosis of CMV pneumonia is usually made by demonstrating typical inclusions in lung tissue. The isolation from the urine is not sufficient evidence that CMV is the cause

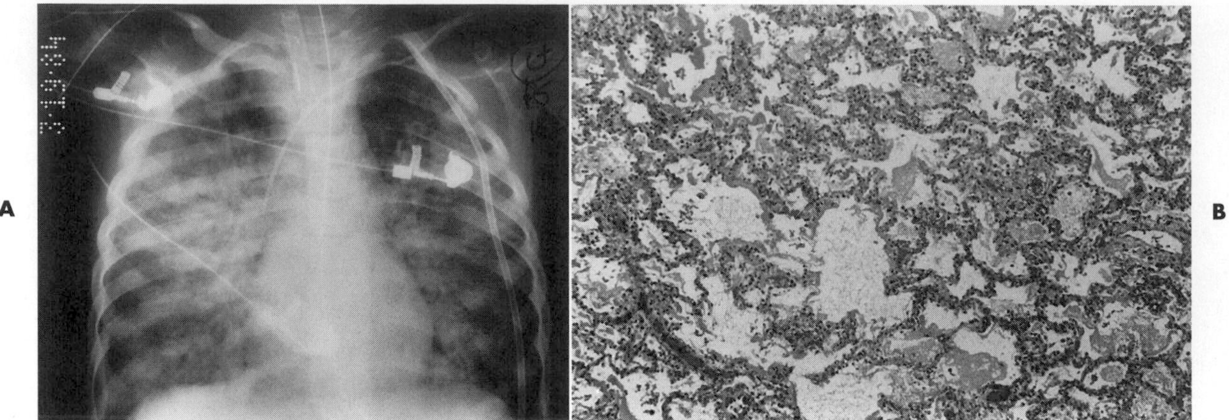

Fig. 40-3. VZV pneumonia. **A,** Chest radiograph. **B,** Histologic section.

of the pneumonia. Recently, immunofluorescence, deoxyribonucleic acid (DNA) hybridization, and shell vial culture have been combined with methods that provide rapid diagnosis of CMV infection from bronchoalveolar lavage fluid.[98-100] Although highly sensitive, the results from such techniques must be interpreted cautiously because CMV can be detected in asymptomatic individuals.

The use of CMV-negative blood products reduces the incidence of CMV pneumonia in seronegative but not seropositive recipients of transplants. PCR for CMV has been used in recipients of bone marrow transplants in an attempt to predict the development of CMV disease. PCR had excellent negative predictive value but a positive predictive value of only 61%. Acute GVHD is associated with CMV disease, as is the development of lymphopenia (predominately CD4+ T cells) starting 49 days after transplant. PCR evidence of viremia and lymphopenia predicted CMV disease 100% of the time.[101] PCR detection precedes culture isolation of CMV by 1 week, and the organism can be detected longer with PCR than with culture. Lack of PCR resolution or a positive culture has a positive predictive value of 60% for the development of CMV disease in recipients of bone marrow transplants.[87] γ-Globulin enriched for anti-CMV activity has been used intravenously for prophylaxis in high-risk populations without clear benefit. However, when CMV-IVIG (intravenous immunoglobulin) was combined with the antiviral medication ganciclovir, the mortality rate in CMV pneumonitis in recipients of bone marrow transplants was reduced.[38,39] At present, ganciclovir and CMV-IVIG are the only effective therapies for CMV pneumonitis in immunocompromised patients.

VZV and HSV. VZV and HSV are DNA viruses that typically cause benign infections of the skin and mucous membranes.[20,37] However, in certain groups (including neonates; patients with cancer, AIDS, and congenital defects of cell-mediated immunity; and recipients of bone marrow transplants), VZV and HSV can lead to visceral dissemination and pneumonia. In patients with cancer, pneumonitis occurs in 85% of cases of visceral dissemination and is the principal cause of death. Before the availability of specific antiviral therapy, the VZV pneumonitis mortality rate was 85%. Pneumonitis is much less common with reactivation of herpes zoster, but it is a potentially serious infection in recipients of bone marrow transplant. HSV is a less common cause of dissemination in oncology patients but is a significant infection in neonates.

The clinical presentation is nonspecific and includes fever, cough, dyspnea, and chest pain. Patients with VZV who have an increasing number of skin lesions, abdominal or back pain, or persistent fevers are at high risk for dissemination and pneumonia. HSV pneumonitis may be more subtle in its presentation, and pneumonitis can occur in the absence of mucocutaneous lesions in newborns and recipients of bone marrow transplants. Chest radiographs of herpesvirus pneumonias typically show ill-defined nodular densities scattered through both lung fields, often beginning at the periphery (Fig. 40-3, *A*). These nodules progress and coalesce into extensive infiltrates. Secondary infections such as staphylococcal pneumonia were more commonly seen in the era before antibiotics. Microscopically the infection involves the alveolar walls, blood vessels, and small bronchioles (Fig. 40-3, *B*). Electron microscopy shows intranuclear inclusions of herpesvirus. Hemorrhage, necrosis, and extensive alveolar edema are seen in severe areas of involvement. The trachea and large bronchi are often involved.

VZIG can modify or prevent varicella in high-risk hosts exposed to the infection if administered within 48 to 72 hours of exposure. Acyclovir and VZIG have been the major factors accounting for the reduced incidence of serious VZV pneumonias in immunocompromised hosts.

HHV-6. HHV-6 is a DNA virus that is the etiologic agent for roseola. It persists in normal hosts and can be isolated from lymphocytes and other sites. In the abnormal host, reactivation can lead to fever, hepatitis, bone marrow suppression, and pneumonia.[102-104]

Cone et al[102] described identification of HHV-6 by PCR in all of 15 lung biopsy specimens from patients with idiopathic pneumonitis after bone marrow transplant; serologic studies also supported its role in pneumonitis after transplant. Further studies are documenting other clinical situations in which HHV-6 causes disease in immunocompromised populations, including renal transplant and AIDS.[103,104] No specific treatment is available.

Adenovirus. Adenovirus is a DNA virus that commonly causes community-acquired lower respiratory disease. Serotypes 1, 2, and 5 are common causes of sporadic respiratory disease, and types 3 and 7 are associated with epidemics of

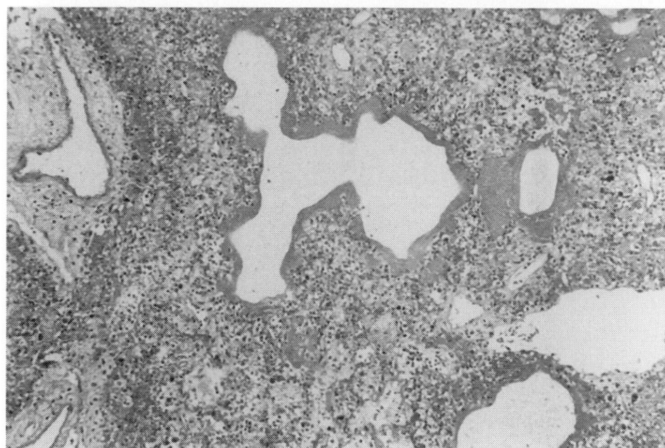

Fig. 40-4. Adenovirus pneumonia: histologic section showing severe interstitial pneumonia in a recipient of a bone marrow transplant.

bronchiolitis and pneumonia in the general population. In immunocompromised patients, adenovirus is one of the most important viral causes of serious morbidity and mortality.[54,105-108] Adenoviral pneumonia acquired by immunocompromised patients often originates as a nosocomial infection from infected members of the hospital staff.

Adenovirus typically causes fever, pharyngitis, cough, and conjunctivitis. Pneumonia is usually mild in normal hosts, but rapid progression can occur in immunocompromised patients with necrotizing bronchitis and bronchiolitis (Fig. 40-4). The radiographic picture is nonspecific and resembles that of other causes of diffuse pneumonia. The diagnosis is usually made by lung biopsy or brushings demonstrating typical adenoviral inclusions or by culture, but the diagnosis may be delayed by the institution of empiric antibiotic and antifungal therapy and a delay in open biopsy. Viral titers may provide a delayed diagnosis. Failure of diffuse pneumonia to respond despite therapy, particularly when there have been epidemics of typical acute respiratory disease in the community or when there is associated renal or liver involvement, should raise the strong possibility of adenovirus.

Unfortunately, there is no specific antiviral therapy for adenovirus infection. Supportive therapy includes the administration of oxygen, treatment of bacterial superinfections, IVIG, and assisted ventilation. The main concern for hospitalized immunocompromised patients is prevention by careful handwashing and other isolation procedures and segregation of staff with respiratory illnesses.

Fungi

***Aspergillus* Species.** *Aspergillus* is a group of ubiquitous fungal organisms found in soil and other settings, including the hospital. *Aspergillus fumigatus* is the most common cause of pneumonia in immunocompromised hosts, but other pathogenic species include *A. niger* and *A. flavus.* In tissue the organisms form septate hyphae with regular 45-degree dichotomous branching, which is best seen with methenamine silver staining (Fig. 40-5).

Aspergillus species causes both acute invasive pulmonary aspergillosis and a more chronic necrotizing form. The former occurs most commonly in patients undergoing cancer therapy as well as other immunocompromised patients such as those with aplastic anemia. *Aspergillus* infection of the lung is often preceded or accompanied by invasion of the nose and paranasal sinuses in susceptible hosts. In a series on invasive *Aspergillus* infection in children (24 definite cases, 15 probable), Walmsley et al[109] confirmed observations in other populations, including those with the major risk factors of prolonged neutropenia, concurrent chemotherapy, and steroid therapy as well as therapy with broad-spectrum antibiotics. The common occurrence of cutaneous aspergillosis in this pediatric series was also noteworthy. A total of 15 of the 16 patients with pulmonary disease in this series died, and premorbid diagnosis was often difficult. In the lungs, *Aspergillus* species can cause tracheobronchitis, pneumonia, abscesses and cavity formation, and diffuse interstitial pneumonia. The organisms often extend along blood vessels, and nodular lesions of necrosis surrounded by air often develop within an area of pneumonia, leading to the typical air crescent sign.

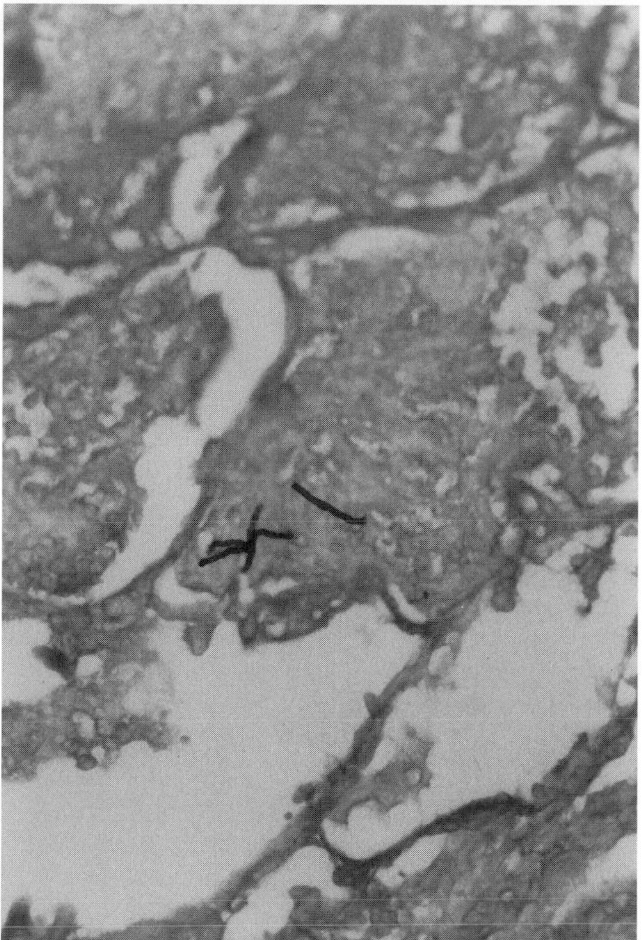

Fig. 40-5. *Aspergillus* species: histologic section. (Grocott-Gomori methenamine-silver nitrate stain.)

Computed tomography of the chest is often very helpful in patients with disseminated fungal disease caused by *Aspergillus* species and other fungal pathogens. In a review of computed tomographic findings from the chests of 14 pediatric patients with malignancy and pulmonary fungal disease caused by *Aspergillus* species, two basic types of involvement were seen: multiple nodules and fluffy masses. Cavitation occurred in 6 of 14 patients.[110] Computed tomography is more sensitive than plain radiographs and can reveal early evidence of cavitation.

Diagnosis of *Aspergillus* pneumonia is generally made by tissue examination. *Aspergillus* organisms can be isolated from

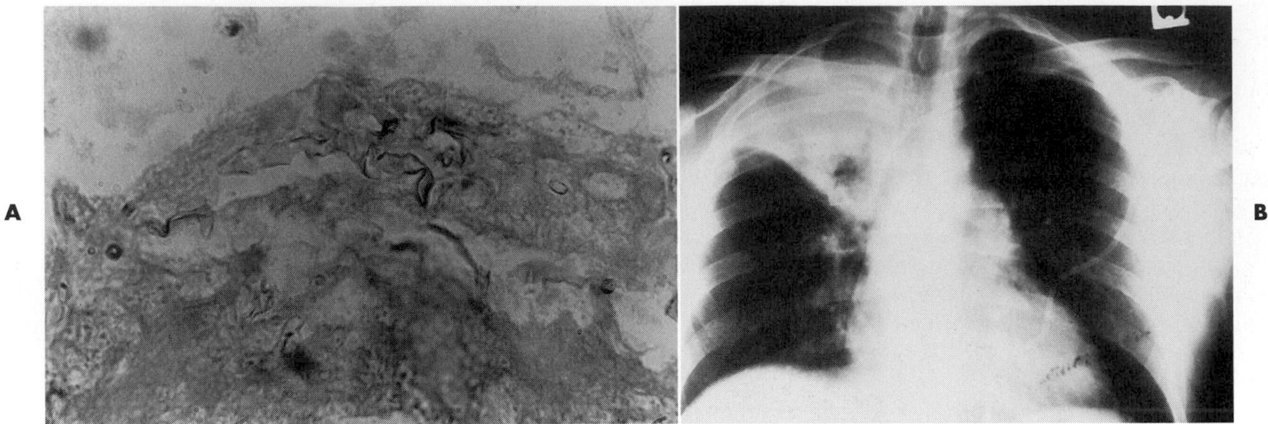

Fig. 40-6. *Mucor* species: **A,** Histologic section. **B,** Chest radiograph showing a cavitary lesion in the right upper lobe.

bronchoalveolar lavage fluid in approximately 50% of cases, and needle aspiration biopsy of suspected lesions can also demonstrate typical fungal lesions. Isolation of the organism from a nasal culture in a patient with typical clinical risk features (i.e., prolonged neutropenia, progressive nodular infiltrates, cavitary lesion) may be helpful, but negative cultures do not exclude *Aspergillus* infection.

The treatment of *Aspergillus* pneumonia includes amphotericin B, given at a dose of 1 to 1.5 mg/kg. Sometimes, flucytosine or rifampin is also administered. The surgical excision of *Aspergillus* lesions is somewhat controversial.[111,112] Invasive pulmonary aspergillosis during treatment of hematologic malignancy is generally considered a contraindication to subsequent bone marrow transplant, but adults treated with amphotericin B and surgery have survived without disease and without reactivation of *Aspergillus* infection after bone marrow transplant.[113] The outcome of *Aspergillus* pneumonia depends primarily on host factors, the degree of immunosuppression, and the return of neutrophil counts to normal levels.

Mucor, Rhizopus,* and *Cunninghamella Species. Mucormycosis includes fungal disease caused by a variety of species in the genera *Rhizopus, Mucor,* and *Cunninghamella.* In tissues, these organisms are differentiated from *Aspergillus* organisms by their broad, nonseptate hyphae that branch at angles up to 90 degrees and that have an appearance of twisted ribbons (Fig. 40-6, *A*). *Rhizopus* organisms cause disease only in patients with underlying disease. In adults, it is associated with chronic acidosis states, such as diabetes mellitus with ketoacidosis. Most pediatric cases of pneumonia occur in the oncology population, in whom the organism is found in the same risk groups as *Aspergillus* species.

Pneumonia caused by *Rhizopus* organisms is usually an insidious segmental pneumonia that is slowly progressive despite antifungal therapy. Persistent fever, chest pain, hemoptysis, and weight loss are typical. Cavitation may occur, and dissemination to the brain and other sites occurs because of the propensity of the organism to invade the blood vessel (Fig. 40-6, *B*). Death may occur suddenly and is caused by massive pulmonary hemorrhage, mediastinitis, or airway obstruction. The specific diagnosis usually depends on demonstration of the organism in open, transbronchial, or needle aspiration lung biopsy specimens.

As with *Aspergillus* organisms, treatment with amphotericin B and possibly surgical resection as early as possible is critical to achieving a cure. Correction of chronic acidosis if present also appears to be important in some forms of this infection.

***Candida* Species.** Although important as a cause of fungal sepsis and secondary hematogenous pulmonary involvement, primary *Candida* pneumonia is unusual.[114,115] *C. albicans* and *Candida tropicalis* are the most important causes of fungal sepsis and secondary pulmonary involvement. Patients with HIV infection, primary immunodeficiencies, and prolonged neutropenia are at greatest risk, but other predisposing conditions include diabetes, corticosteroid administration, treatment with broad-spectrum antibiotics, intravenous hyperalimentation, and venous access devices.

In tissue, silver stains show oval budding yeasts 2 to 6 μ in diameter with pseudohyphae. In one series of 31 patients with primary *Candida* pneumonia, the prominent histologic features included bronchopneumonia, intraalveolar exudates, and hemorrhage.[62]

Amphotericin B is usually the treatment of choice for invasive candidal infections; flucytosine is used if synergism is desired. The imidazole antifungal agents, including ketoconazole, fluconazole, and itraconazole, have activity against *Candida* species and have been used successfully in small series. Use of the imidazole antifungal agents for prophylaxis has helped kill more resistant fungal organisms in high-risk populations.

***Histoplasma* and *Blastomyces* Species.** *Histoplasma capsulatum* and *Blastomyces dermatitidis* are ubiquitous soil fungi endemic to the eastern and southwestern United States. Histoplasmosis, a common infection, it may be asymptomatic or lead to an acute pneumonia with fever, hilar adenopathy, and pulmonary infiltrates. Blastomycosis is a less common, more serious infection. Both can cause chronic granulomatous pulmonary disease as well as disseminated disease.

In the immunocompromised patient, including those with AIDS, the major risk factor is dissemination with pulmonary infiltrates, hepatosplenomegaly, fever, and adenopathy. Histoplasmosis is more common in the immunocompromised host than blastomycosis.

Amphotericin B is indicated for both histoplasmosis and blastomycosis in immunocompromised hosts. Itraconazole is also effective for histoplasmosis and moderate blastomycosis without central nervous system involvement.

C. neoformans. *C. neoformans* is a yeast that causes protean clinical manifestations in immunocompromised patients, particularly those with AIDS. The meninges, endocardium, skin, and lymph nodes are often involved.

The lungs are the portal of entry for *C. neoformans,* and pulmonary involvement may be minimal if dissemination occurs quickly. Pneumonia is typically accompanied by chest pain, fever, and cough. Pulmonary disease with *Cryptococcus* organisms is rarer in pediatric patients with AIDS than in adults. Treatment involves intravenous amphotericin B and oral flucytosine.

Rare Fungi. Several recent trends have been noted in fungal infections caused by rarer fungal pathogens, including saprophytic fungi[3,116] (Box 40-3). These fungi cause skin and soft tissue infections and occasionally invade the lungs and sinuses. They are often difficult to diagnose, and their response to therapy with amphotericin B may be very poor. Non-*Candida* infections after bone marrow transplant were reviewed by Morrison et al.[116] The respiratory tract was involved in 95% of single-organ or site infections and 84% of disseminated infections. Fungal infections that are associated with a high mortality rate included those caused by *Chrysosporium, Fusarium, Mucor,* and *Scopulariopsis* in addition to *Aspergillus* organisms.

Bacteria

The bacterial pathogens associated with pneumonia in immunocompromised hosts include those typically associated with pneumonia in children, including *S. aureus, H. influenzae* type b, and *S. pneumoniae.* They may cause chronic suppurative lung disease and are discussed further in Chapter 58.

Gram-Positive Organisms. *Listeria monocytogenes* is a gram-positive rod that causes primarily septicemia with subsequent pulmonary involvement in immunocompromised patients. Corynebacteria (commonly called *diphtheroids*) are gram-positive bacilli or coccobacilli that exist as saprophytes on the mucous membranes and skin. *C. jeikeium,* a strain from this group, causes sepsis and pneumonia in oncology patients and recipients of bone marrow transplants.[117]

Listeria infection is treated using ampicillin plus an aminoglycoside. Significantly, newer cephalosporins are not active against this species. *C. jeikeium* is resistant to most antibiotics except vancomycin. In most immunocompromised patients with pneumonia, vancomycin should be included in the treatment regimen to cover methicillin-resistant *S. aureus* and *C. jeikeium* when suspected.

Gram-Negative Organisms. *P. aeruginosa* is an important cause of pneumonia in immunocompromised children, particularly hospitalized patients. In a large series of 98 children with bacteremia caused by *P. aeruginosa,* 21% had evidence of pneumonia, and the overall mortality rate from *P. aeruginosa* infection was 27%. Significant risk factors included neutropenia and perineal skin lesions.[118] Other gram-negative organisms that cause pneumonia include *Legionella pneumophila* and *Capnocytophaga* species.

BOX 40-3
Unusual Fungal Infections with Potential Pulmonary Involvement

Aspergillus, Candida, and *Mucor* are the primary pathogens.
Primary *Candida* pneumonia (as opposed to secondary pneumonia after septicemia) is rare.
Infection by *Candida* organisms other than *C. albicans* has become increasingly important (primarily fungemia with secondary pulmonary involvement); species include *C. tropicalis, C. parapsilosis, C. krusei,* and *C. glabrata* (formerly *Torulopsis glabrata*).
Emerging infections and their pathogens follow:
- Phaeohyphomycoses
  - *Curvularia* species: sinusitis
  - *Bipolaris, Exserohilum, Alternaria* species: clinical presentation similar to that of *Aspergillus* species
- Hyalohyphomycoses
  - *Fusarium* species: sinusitis or rhinocerebral disease
  - *Scopulariopsis* species
  - *Pseudallescheria boydii:* sinusitis, pneumonia
- *Trichosporon* infection: risk factors similar to those of *Candida* species (primarily hematogenous)
- *Malassezia furfur:* hematogenous

Mycobacteria

Until recent years, the incidence of pulmonary disease caused by *Mycobacterium tuberculosis* had been declining. With the onset of the AIDS epidemic, however, disease caused by *M. tuberculosis* and atypical strains such as *Mycobacterium avium-intracellulare* have increased. A detailed discussion of mycobacterial infections in patients with AIDS is beyond the scope of this chapter but is covered in Chapters 41 and 43 and in recent reviews.[119]

Parasites and Other Organisms

P. carinii. *P. carinii* has been an organism of uncertain taxonomy and was regarded as a parasite because of its resemblance to cystic spore-forming protozoa.[120-122] More recent studies using DNA hybridization methods place *P. carinii* as a fungus.[123] The organism exists in three forms in tissues: the trophozoite, the sporozoite, and the cyst (Fig. 40-7, *A*). The trophozoites are 2 to 5 μ in diameter and stain best with Giemsa stains but are not visible with Grocott-Gomori methenamine-silver nitrate or toluidine blue O stains, which stain the 5- to 8-μ cyst forms. The cysts are spherical or cup shaped and often appear to contain up to eight 1- to 2-μ sporozoites within the cyst wall (Fig. 40-7, *B*). The organism cannot be cultured from routine clinical specimens and must be identified in tissue, sputum, or alveolar lavage fluid.

The organism is found primarily within the alveoli, although the extrapulmonary occurrence of organisms has been commonly reported in patients with AIDS.[124] The trophozoites appear to attach to type I cells through surface glycoproteins related to lectins and there undergo encystation[125,126] (Fig. 40-8). This interaction directly or through soluble factors leads to cell injury. The alveoli of lungs infected with *P. carinii* are filled with trophozoites and protein-rich debris, and the altered permeability produced by the organism contributes to the development of pulmonary edema and surfactant abnormalities, which lead to stiff lungs.[127,128]

The earliest reports of PCP were in epidemics occurring in severely malnourished infants, a type rarely seen in developed countries. The majority of PCP cases occurs in infants and

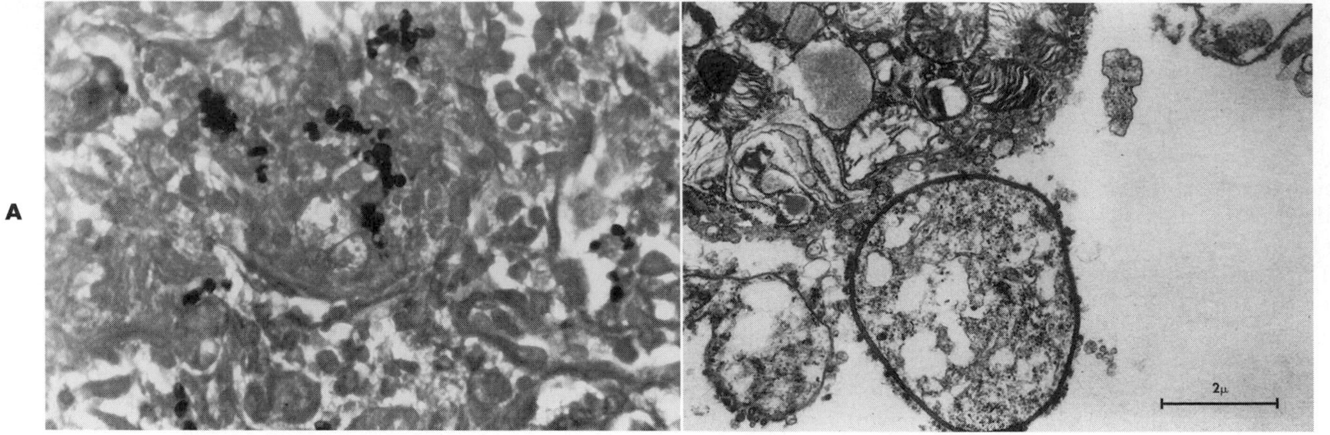

Fig. 40-7. *P. carinii.* **A,** Histologic section. (Grocott-Gomori methenamine-silver nitrate stain.) **B,** Electron microscopy.

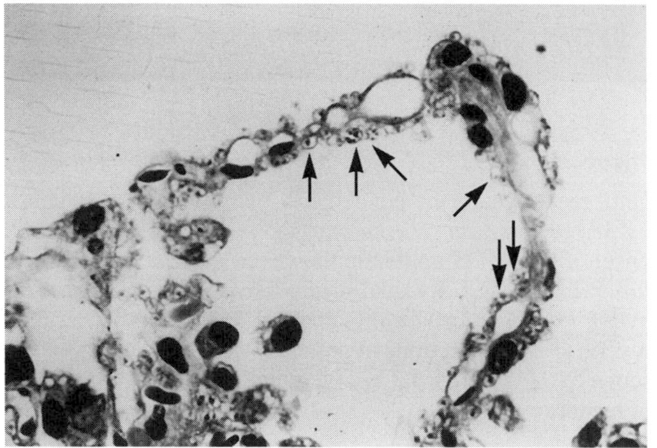

Fig. 40-8. *P. carinii.* Alveolar thin section showing cysts *(arrows)* lining the alveolar wall.

children with congenital or acquired immunodeficiencies. Latent infection with *P. carinii* was thought to be common because serologic studies indicated that 40% of children have antibodies to the organism. Based on this finding, disease was thought to be caused primarily by reactivation of a primary infection, but more recent studies using sensitive PCR and fluorescent antibody tests have failed to demonstrate *P. carinii* in autopsy or BAL fluid specimens from normal lungs. More likely, disease in immunocompromised patients originates from an environmental source, including other infected patients.[129]

In patients with congenital immunodeficiency or malignancy, the clinical features of PCP are nonspecific and include dyspnea, tachypnea, fever, and mild cough. Hypoxemia with a mild respiratory alkalosis is common, but cyanosis occurs later. The most common chest radiographic findings are diffuse bilateral infiltrates commencing in the perihilar regions.

Since 1980, the most common underlying host defect in patients with *P. carinii* is AIDS. The clinical features of PCP in the pediatric AIDS population differs from the pneumonias seen in other populations. In patients with AIDS, the duration of symptoms is typically longer, and the presentation is more insidious. Hypoxemia is less intense. Organisms appear to be abundant in patients with AIDS and can usually be identified in sputum, bronchoalveolar lavage fluid, or even gastric lavage samples. Other superinfections (such as CMV) and pulmonary complications are often present in patients with AIDS, however, and it may be difficult to know what role these infections play in the symptoms. In patients with AIDS, *P. carinii* is more likely to spread to the nodes, spleen, bone marrow, and other sites. These patients are more likely to have atypical radiographic pictures, including lobar pneumonias, unilateral disease, and solitary nodules, although atypical radiographic presentations can also occur in other host disorders.

PCP can be treated using several medications. The earliest medication available for PCP was pentamidine, which appears to work by inhibiting dihydrofolate reductase. Pentamidine was initially given by the intramuscular route, but subsequent studies have shown that dosages of 4.0 mg/kg/day by the intravenous route are as safe as the those given via the intramuscular route, although both are associated with high rates of immediate reaction, such as hypotension, tachycardia, and nausea. Hypoglycemia and nephrotoxicity are the most serious side effects of parenteral pentamidine. Pentamidine is also given by the aerosol route for the treatment of mild to moderate pulmonary disease in patients with AIDS, but its effectiveness is highly dependent on the delivery system used, and the aerosol route may predispose patients to extrapulmonary disease with *P. carinii.* In the early 1970s, Hughes[22,23] described the effectiveness of TMP/SMX for the treatment of PCP in children with malignancies. TMP/SMX is as effective as pentamidine (approximately 70%) with fewer side effects. Some 60% of patients who do not have AIDS and in whom TMP/SMX therapy fails respond to treatment with pentamidine. In addition to pentamidine and TMP/SMX, a number of other medications are effective for the treatment of PCP; these include dapsone and trimetrexate. Patients with AIDS have a high incidence of reactions to many types of medications, including TMP/SMX.

Supportive therapy is a major part of the treatment for PCP. Oxygen, continuous positive airway pressure, continuous negative pressure, and assisted ventilation have all been used effectively in PCP. The role of corticosteroids is controversial. Trials in patients with AIDS indicate that corticosteroid administration during therapy improves outcome.[55-60] Typically, 4 to 6 days pass before improvement occurs with either pentamidine or TMP/SMX, and failure to improve warrants consideration of other infections and a change to another anti-*Pneumocystis* drug.

All patients at known risk for *P. carinii* infection should receive prophylaxis. For pediatric oncology and immunocompromised patients, oral TMP/SMX given 3 days a week is effective. However, if patients or parents are noncompliant, there is a risk of breakthrough pneumonias. For most patients, TMP/SMX remains the drug of choice, but other prophylactic regimens have been used, particularly in patients with AIDS; these include aerosolized and intravenous pentamidine and dapsone. Intravenous pentamidine may be associated with a higher risk of failure.[130] Although there is extensive experience with aerosolized pentamidine in adults, there is less information on its use in infants and children. O'Doherty et al[131] studied lung deposition of nebulized pentamidine in children (50 mg in 6 ml of saline) using the Respirgard II nebulizer and technetium-99m–labeled colloidal albumin as a marker of distribution. Total pentamidine deposition in children 8 to 15 years of age did not differ significantly from that in adults. Overall concentrations were higher than that achieved in adults (2.5% of the nebulizer dose) and were particularly high in the central airways.

***T. gondii* and *Cryptosporidium parvum*.** *T. gondii* and *Cryptosporidium parvum* are both parasites. *T. gondii* infects cats and other animals and secondarily infects man, causing congenital toxoplasmosis during intrauterine infection; primary infection later in life usually causes only lymphadenopathy and mild systemic symptoms. *C. parvum* infects a variety of hosts and often occurs with waterborne outbreaks.

In patients with AIDS, toxoplasma primarily causes central nervous system disease but can cause disseminated disease with secondary pulmonary involvement. *C. parvum* causes severe diarrhea, but disseminated disease with pulmonary involvement can occur.

Treatment of *T. gondii* includes pyrimethamine-sulfadiazine. Treatment of *C. parvum* is with azithromycin.

DIAGNOSTIC STUDIES

General Approach to Immunocompromised Children with Pneumonia

Although clinical factors such as the types of pulmonary pathogens associated with certain at-risk groups and general radiographic patterns may be useful, both approaches have limitations in the immunocompromised patient with pneumonia. Many noninfectious pulmonary processes also occur in this group, and the list of organisms causing pneumonia is extensive. Generally, empiric broad-spectrum antibiotic therapy must be started in patients with known immunodeficiency at the first sign of fever and often before the development of overt pneumonia. This often complicates subsequent diagnostic studies.

Indirect Diagnostic Tests

Sputum Examination and Culture

Sputum samples are difficult to obtain in children younger than 10 years of age and when obtained, must be interpreted cautiously. Analysis of sputum produced by cough induced with the inhalation of hypertonic saline aerosols has been useful in diagnosing infection in older children with AIDS and PCP.[132] Gastric aspirates can be used in the younger child and are particularly helpful when the pathogen being considered is not a usual colonizing organism of the upper airway (e.g., pathogen causing tuberculosis).

Endotracheal Tube Aspirates

If the child requires endotracheal intubation for respiratory distress, endotracheal aspirates are easy to obtain. The diagnostic yield in complex immunocompromised patients is improved by using wax-protected microbiologic brushes or nonbronchoscopic bronchoalveolar lavage.[133,134]

Blood Cultures

Although blood culture should be obtained in all immunocompromised children suspected of having bacterial or fungal pneumonia, positive cultures are unusual, although generally highly specific.

Antigen and Antibody Detection Methods

The ability to detect capsular polysaccharide antigens of bacterial pathogens even after antibiotics have been administered is occasionally helpful in hospitalized patients. Most hospitals can routinely test for group B *Streptococcus, Neisseria meningitidis, S. pneumoniae,* and *H. influenzae* using latex agglutination or counterimmunoelectrophoresis.[135] Concentrated urine samples are superior to serum samples for detecting pathogens. Antibiotic treatment does not affect the sensitivity of the test, which is between 30% and 45% depending on the study. A number of tests for the direct detection of fungal antigens have been described, but none is in widespread clinical use.[136] Direct immunofluorescence used to detect *Legionella* species has a sensitivity of 50% and a specificity of 94%.[137]

The rapid diagnosis of RSV, influenza A virus, parainfluenza virus, and *Chlamydia* infections by enzyme-linked immunosorbent assay and direct immunofluorescence is now available. The sensitivities of these tests depend partly on the adequacy of the sample provided to the laboratory. Viral cultures are generally available, and the shell vial technique for the rapid identification of CMV is very useful. Although *Mycoplasma pneumoniae* can be cultured on enriched media, this usually takes several weeks, and the diagnosis is usually based on serologic conversion. Genetic probes for detecting *Legionella* species, *Mycobacterium* species, and *M. pneumoniae* are now commercially available. The ability of the PCR to amplify specific regions of genomic DNA or ribonucleic acid should allow a broader application of this approach.

Serologic tests demonstrating a fourfold or greater rise in antibody titer to an infectious agent are sensitive and specific ways of documenting an infection in normal hosts. However, they are usually unreliable in the immunocompromised host.

Flexible Bronchoscopy

Flexible bronchoscopy is safe in experienced hands and provides excellent culture material in the immunocompromised child with pneumonia.[32,138-145] Indications in children with pneumonia include (1) failure of the pneumonia or fever to clear with appropriate antibiotic therapy, (2) suspicion of endobronchial obstruction by an infection or a tumor, (3) recurrent pneumonia in a lobe or segment, and (4) suspicion of unusual organisms such as *P. carinii,* fungi, and the pathogens that cause tuberculosis. Although the yield of gastric aspiration is probably superior to that of bronchoscopy for tuberculosis, bronchoscopy can also evaluate for endobronchial disease or bronchial compression.

The bronchoscope suction channel is contaminated by organisms of the upper airway, and simple washings obtained through the bronchoscope channel are generally useless for

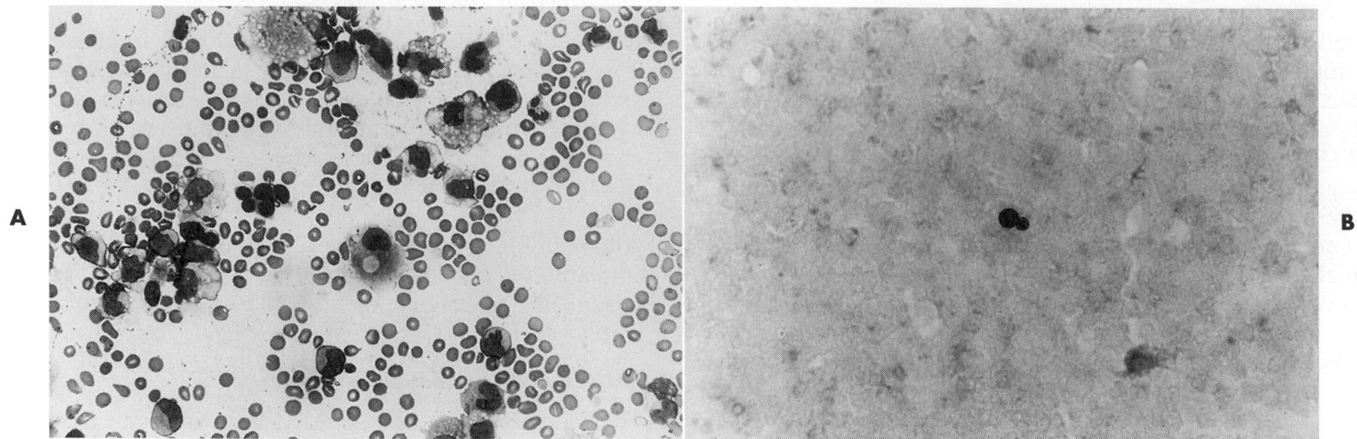

Fig. 40-9. Diagnosis of conditions from specimens obtained from bronchoalveolar lavage. **A,** Monocytic leukemia. **B,** Blastomycosis.

culture. Several techniques, including the use of a double-sheath, wax-protected sterile brush and quantitative cultures of bronchoalveolar lavage fluid, have been developed to avoid this problem. Bronchoalveolar lavage is the most useful technique for diagnosing infection in the immunocompromised host, and a variety of infectious and noninfectious diagnoses, including hemorrhage and pulmonary involvement with leukemia (Fig. 40-9), can be made using it. Bronchoalveolar lavage is generally safe even in patients with reduced numbers of platelets. Brushings obtained through the bronchoscope can be used for cytologic examination and viral cultures, but the yield is usually low.

Although the safety and usefulness of bronchoscopy are well documented in this population, it is important for the clinician to recognize the limitations of bronchoscopy. In patients on empiric broad-spectrum antibiotic therapy, the yield of bacterial pathogens is likely to be low. In oncology patients and other non-AIDS immunocompromised patients, the number of *P. carinii* organisms is usually low compared to the number obtained from patients with AIDS, so the results may be falsely negative. In populations receiving prophylaxis for this infection, the yield for PCP is likely to be low, reducing the overall yield of bronchoscopy for treatable infections. CMV can also be diagnosed rapidly by bronchoscopy, but patients may have other complicating infections, such as those caused by fungi and CMV, that are more easily missed by bronchoscopy. Infections caused by *Aspergillus* and other fungi are often difficult to diagnose by bronchoscopy, particularly early in the infection when therapy is most likely to be effective.

Transbronchial biopsies can also be taken through the bronchoscope. Although safe in older patients, transbronchial lung biopsies yield an unacceptable number of false-negative results in immunosuppressed patients and are most useful when organisms such as *P. carinii* or granulomatous lesions are likely. Reported experience in pediatric patients is limited, but transbronchial biopsy has a significant role in monitoring rejection and infections in the pediatric patient after lung transplant.[146]

Transthoracic Needle Aspiration Biopsy

Needle aspiration of the lung is useful for the diagnosis of PCP in pediatric patients with cancer and for the diagnosis of localized infections in other immunosuppressed patients.[147,148] Pneumothorax was a complication in 37% of the needle aspirates done for PCP, and this risk must be considered. Hemorrhage is more serious but less common. The use of computed tomography or fluoroscopic guidance greatly improves the yield and safety of this procedure, and it is the procedure of choice for many children with suspected peripheral fungal lesions that can safely be aspirated.

Open Lung Biopsy

Open lung biopsy is the standard by which other diagnostic modalities are judged. Because it uses current surgical techniques, open lung biopsy is generally a procedure with a low morbidity that can be done rapidly and allows the surgeon to obtain the optimal tissue for culture and microscopic examination. "Minithoracotomy" and lingular biopsy may be all that are necessary in patients with diffuse pulmonary processes. Biopsy using fiberoptic pleuroscopy may be adequate for pleural-based lesions and reduces the morbidity associated with open biopsy.

In immunocompromised patients, it is difficult to make generalizations about open lung biopsy, and much depends on local factors such as the availability of flexible bronchoscopy, the age of the child, the underlying conditions, complications such as thrombocytopenia and coagulopathies, and prior antibiotic or antifungal therapy. Recent studies have questioned how often the results of open lung biopsy have led to a change in therapy if patients with nonspecific histologic findings and organisms treated by empiric therapy (e.g., *P. carinii*) are excluded. Published results in immunocompromised pediatric patients have indicated yields that range from 36% to 94% for a specific diagnosis.[28]

Although open lung biopsy is the procedure of choice for obtaining definitive diagnostic information in immunosuppressed patients with pulmonary infiltrates, the timing of the biopsy is difficult. The clinician does not want to perform the procedure too early, especially if empirical therapy appears to be working and the patient is in good condition. On the other hand, when therapy is marginally successful, the surgeon does not want to wait so long that the patient's condition deteriorates and the risk of biopsy significantly increases. The author generally suggests relatively early biopsy in immunosuppressed patients with pneumonia (Fig. 40-10). Any patient with a condition not clearly responding to therapy chosen on the ba-

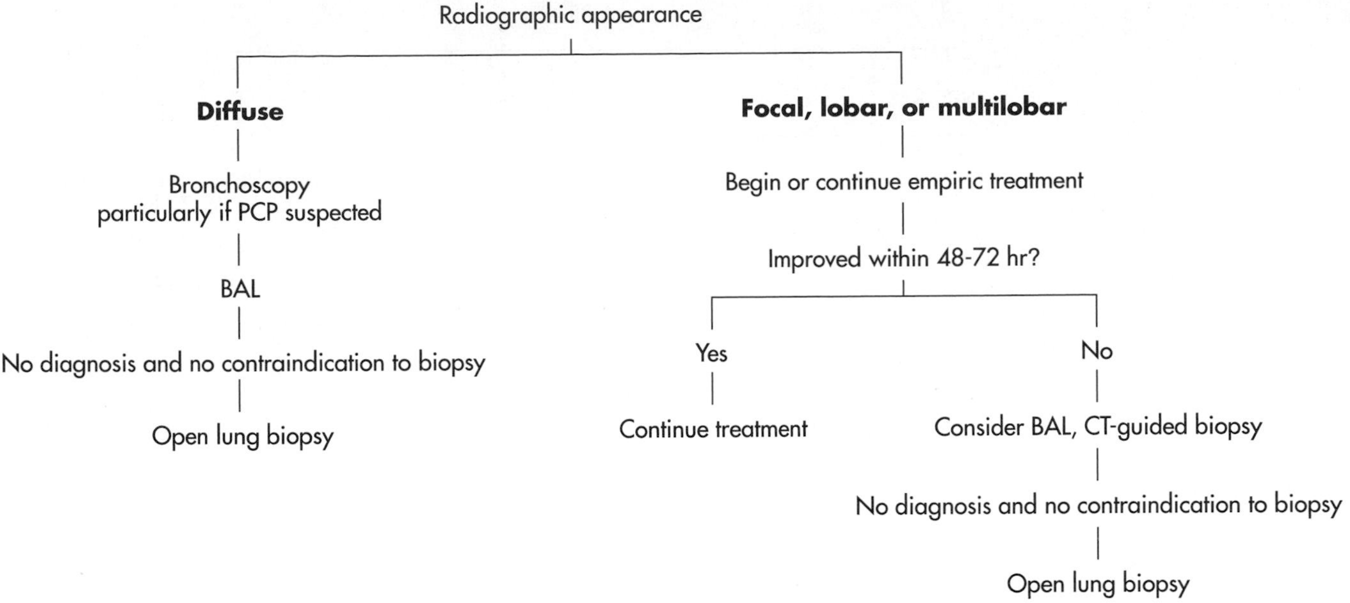

Fig. 40-10. Flow diagram for the diagnosis of pneumonia in immunocompromised hosts. *BAL,* Bronchoalveolar lavage; *CT,* computed tomography.

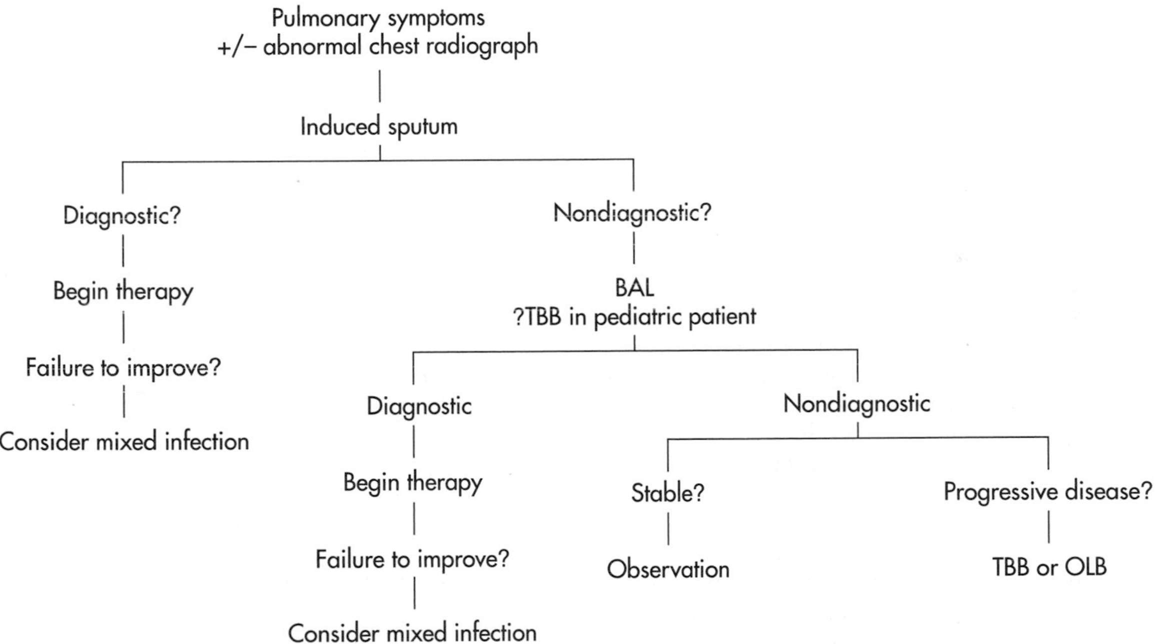

Fig. 40-11. Flow diagram for the diagnosis of pulmonary disease in patients with AIDS. *BAL,* Bronchoalveolar lavage; *TBB,* transbronchial biopsy; *OLB,* open lung biopsy. (From Dichter J et al: *Hematol Oncol Clin North Am* 7:887-912, 1993.)

sis of other diagnostic techniques (including bronchoscopy) or therapy chosen empirically would usually benefit from a specific diagnosis by biopsy. In most medical centers, this is a relatively safe procedure, especially when performed before the patient has the need for respiratory support. The risks increase only when the biopsy is delayed until the patient has become critically ill. When the technique is used for the diagnosis of diffuse disease, only a limited thoracotomy with a superficial subsegmental resection is necessary. In localized disease typical of fungal infections, a more extensive procedure may be required to obtain an adequate specimen.

In specific patient groups such as recipients of bone marrow transplants and patients with AIDS, the use and timing of open biopsy may be different. In patients with AIDS, open lung biopsy is rarely necessary because a specific diagnosis can usually be made by using the results of bronchoalveolar lavage or transbronchial lung biopsy. If the disease progresses despite apparently adequate therapy or bronchoscopy is not diagnostic, open lung biopsy should be considered to rule out other copathogens (Fig. 40-11). In recipients of bone marrow transplants the approach may be modified to allow therapy of common noninfectious complications such as pulmonary

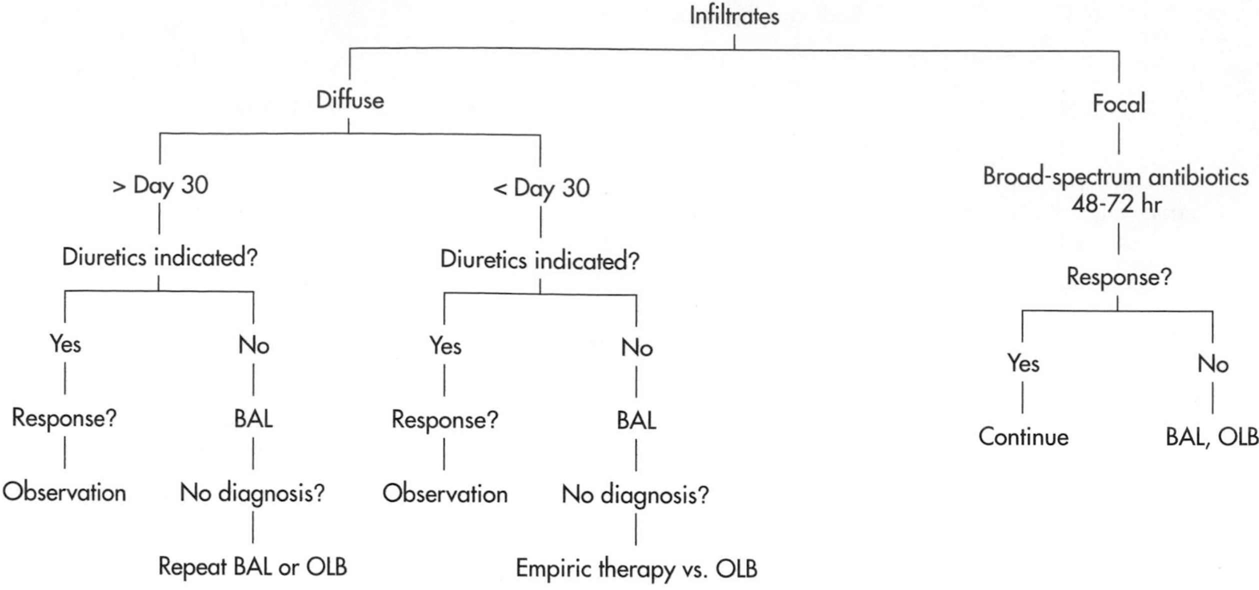

Fig. 40-12. Flow diagram for the diagnosis of pulmonary disease in recipients of bone marrow transplants. *BAL,* Bronchoalveolar lavage; *OLB,* open-liver biopsy. (From Dichter J et al: *Hematol Oncol Clin North Am* 7:887-912, 1993.)

edema before embarking on invasive diagnostic studies (Fig. 40-12).

TREATMENT

Early treatment is necessary for the immunocompromised patient with pneumonia, and empiric antibiotic therapy is generally started at the first sign of clinical pneumonia. In many patients (e.g., the febrile, neutropenic patient), empiric antibiotic therapy may already have started before the pneumonia becomes clinically or radiographically apparent. Antibiotic therapy is typically broad spectrum, aimed at both gram-positive and gram-negative bacterial infections (e.g., vancomycin-aminoglycoside or semisynthetic penicillin, third-generation cephalosporin). If a patient has new diffuse, bilateral pneumonia with respiratory distress and hypoxemia, the clinician must make a rapid decision about whether to proceed to bronchoscopy or open lung biopsy before the patient's condition progresses to respiratory failure and any procedure becomes more hazardous. Empiric therapy is usually guided by the underlying disorder and the radiographic and clinical features of the pneumonia and would usually include TMP/SMX for PCP as well as erythromycin for *Mycoplasma* and *Legionella* infection. Amphotericin B is often started in the febrile neutropenic patient who develops a new pulmonary infiltrate while on antibiotics. Empiric viral therapy with acyclovir for HSV may sometimes be necessary, but the treatment with ganciclovir and immunoglobulin usually requires a histologic diagnosis of CMV pneumonitis. Because of its low morbidity, flexible bronchoscopy should be considered early in the course of the pneumonia. If bronchoscopy is negative, the risks and benefits of open lung biopsy must be weighed in each patient, particularly if the pneumonia progresses despite appropriate antimicrobial therapy. A good response to empiric antibiotic therapy indicates that it should be continued for a minimum of 2 weeks, but in the case of antifungal therapy, treatment may be required for much longer periods.

REFERENCES

1. Patrick CC, ed: *Infections in immunocompromised infants and children,* Edinburgh, 1993, Churchill Livingstone.
2. Infectious complications in the immunocompromised host, *Hematol Oncol Clin North Am,* 2 vol, Oct 1993.
3. Koll BS, Brown AE: Changing patterns of infections in the immunocompromised patient with cancer, *Hematol Oncol Clin North Am* 7:753-769, 1993.
4. Rubin RH, Ferraro MJ: Understanding and diagnosing infectious complications in the immunocompromised host, *Hematol Oncol Clin North Am* 7:795-811, 1993.
5. Dichter JR, Levine SJ, Shelhamer JH: Approach to the immunocompromised host with pulmonary symptoms, *Hematol Oncol Clin North Am* 7:887-912, 1993.
6. Wilson G, Dermody T: Respiratory infections in the immunocompromised host, *Semin Pediatr Infect Dis* 6:156-165, 1995.
7. Stokes DC: Pulmonary complications of tissue transplantation in children, *Curr Opin Pediatr* 6:272-279, 1994.
8. Stokes DC, Bozeman P: Sinopulmonary infections in immunocompromised host. In Patrick CC, ed: *Infections in immunocompromised infants and children,* Edinburgh, 1993, Churchill Livingstone.
9. Robbins RA, Floreani AA, Buchalter SE, Spurzem JR, Sisson JH, Rennard SI: Pulmonary complications of transplantation, *Ann Rev Med* 43:425-435, 1992
10. Sable CA, Donowitz GR: Infections in bone marrow transplant recipients, *Clin Infect Dis* 18:273-284, 1994.
11. Hughes WT: Opportunistic infections in AIDS patients: current management and prevention, *Postgrad Med* 95:81-93, 1994.
12. White DA, Zaman MK: Management of AIDS patients: pulmonary disease, *Med Clin North Am* 76:19-44, 1992.
13. Murray JF, Mills J: Pulmonary infectious complications of human immunodeficiency virus infection, *Am Rev Respir Dis* 141:1356-1372, 1992.
14. Afessa B, Gay PC, Plevak DJ, Swenson SJ, Patel HG, Krowka MJ: Pulmonary complications of orthotopic liver transplantation, *Mayo Clin Proc* 68:427-434, 1993.
15. McLoud TC, Naidich DP: Thoracic disease in the immunocompromised patient, *Radiol Clin North Am* 30:525-554, 1992.

Historical Perspective

16. Armstrong D: History of opportunistic infection in the immunocompromised host, *Clin Infect Dis* 17:S318-S321, 1993.

17. Ruskin J, Remington JS: The compromised host and infection. I. *Pneumocystis carinii* pneumonia, *JAMA* 202:1070-1074, 1967.
18. Hughes WT, Sanyal SK, Price RA: Signs, symptoms, and pathophysiology of *Pneumocystis carinii* pneumonitis, *Natl Cancer Inst Monogr* 4:77-88, 1976.
19. Hughes WT: Intensity of immunosuppressive therapy and the incidence of *Pneumocystis carinii* pneumonitis, *Cancer* 36:2004-2010, 1975.
20. Feldman S, Stokes DC: Varicella zoster and herpes simplex virus pneumonias, *Semin Respir Infect* 2:84-94, 1987.
21. Peterson PK, McGlave P, Ramsay NK, Rhame F, Cohen E, Perry GS, Goldman AI, Kersey J: A prospective study of infectious diseases following bone marrow transplantation: emergence of *Aspergillus* and cytomegalovirus as the major causes of mortality, *Infect Control* 4:81-89, 1983.
22. Hughes WT, Kuhn S, Chaudary S, Feldman S, Verzosa Aur RJ, Pratt C, George SL: Successful chemoprophylaxis for *Pneumocystis carinii* pneumonia, *N Engl J Med* 297:419-426, 1977.
23. Hughes WT: Successful intermittent chemoprophylaxis for *Pneumocystis carinii* pneumonia, *N Engl J Med* 316:1627-1633, 1987.
24. Hughes WT: Five year absence of *Pneumocystic carinii* pneumonitis in a pediatric oncology center, *J Infect Dis* 150:305, 1984.
25. Imoke E, Dudgeon DL, Colombani P, Leventhal B, Buck JR, Haller JA: Open lung biopsy in the immunocompromised pediatric patient, *J Pediatr Surg* 18:816, 1983.
26. Doolin EJ, Luck SR, Sherman JO, Raffensperger JG: Emergency lung biopsy: friend or foe of the immunosuppressed child, *J Pediatr Surg* 21:485, 1986.
27. Shorter NA, Ross AJ III, August C, Schnaufer L, Zeigler M, Templeton JM Jr, Bishop H, O'Neill JA Jr: The usefulness of open lung biopsy in the pediatric bone marrow transplant population, *J Pediatr Surg* 23:533, 1988.
28. Bozeman PM, Stokes DC: Diagnostic methods in pulmonary infections of immunocompromised children: bronchoscopy, needle aspiration, and open biopsy. In Patrick CC, ed: *Infections in immunocompromised infants and children,* Edinburgh, 1992, Churchill Livingstone.
29. Pattishall EN, Noyes BE, Orenstein DM: Use of bronchoalveolar lavage in immunocompromised children with pneumonia, *Pediatr Pulmonol* 5:1-5, 1988.
30. Wood RE: The diagnostic effectiveness of the flexible bronchoscope in children, *Pediatr Pulmonol* 1:188-192, 1985.
31. Wood RE, Leigh MW, Retsch-Bogart G: Diagnosis of pneumonia in immunocompromised patients, *J Pediatr* 116:836-837, 1990.
32. Stokes DC, Shenep JL, Parham D, Bozeman PM, Marienchek W, Mackert PW: Role of flexible bronchoscopy in the diagnosis of pulmonary infiltrates in pediatric patients with cancer, *J Pediatr* 115:561-567, 1989.
33. Jason JM, Stehr-Green J, Solman RC, Evatt BL: Human immunodeficiency virus infection in hemophiliac children, *Pediatrics* 82:565-570, 1988.
34. Stokes DC, Shenep JL, Horowitz ME, Hughes WT: Presentation of *Pneumocystis carinii* pneumonia as unilateral hyperlucent lung, *Chest* 94:201-202, 1988.
35. Johnson FL, Stokes DC, Ruggiero M, Dalla-Pozza L: Chronic obstructive airways disease after bone marrow transplantation, *J Pediatr* 105:370-376, 1984.
36. Joshi VV, Oleske JM, Minneofr AB, Singh R, Bokhari T, Rapkin RH: Pathology of suspected acquired immunodeficiency syndrome in children: a study of eight cases, *Pediatr Pathol* 2:71-87, 1984.
37. Feldman S, Hughes WT, Daniel CB: Varicella in children with cancer: seventy seven cases, *Pediatrics* 56:388-397, 1985.
38. Schmidt GM, Kovacs A, Zaia JA, Horak DA, Blume KG, Nadermanee AP, O'Donnell MR, Snyder DS, Forman SJ: Ganciclovir/immunoglobulin combination therapy for the treatment of human cytomegalovirus-associated interstitial pneumonia in bone marrow allograft recipients, *Transplantation* 46:905, 1988.
39. Goodrich JM, Mori M, Gleaves CA, Dumond C, Cays M, Ebling DF, Buhles WC, DeArmond B, Meyers JD: Early treatment with ganciclovir to prevent cytomegalovirus disease after allogenic bone marrow transplantation *N Engl J Med* 325:1601-1607, 1991.
40. Schmidt GM, Horak DA, Niland JC, Duncan SR, Forman SJ, Zaia JA: A randomized controlled trial of prophylactic ganciclovir for cytomegalovirus pulmonary infection in recipients of bone marrow transplants, *N Engl J Med* 324:1005-1011, 1991.
41. Mathew P, Crist W, Furman W: The use of cytokines in children, *Curr Opin Pediatr* 6:58-67, 1994.
42. Feins RH: The role of thoracoscopy in the AIDS/immunocompromised patient, *Ann Thorac Surg* 56:649-650, 1993.
43. Daniel TM, Kern JA, Tribble CG, Kron IL, Spotnitz WB, Rodgers BM: Thoracoscopic surgery for diseases of the lung and pleura: effectiveness, changing indications, and limitations, *Ann Surg* 217:566-574, 1993.
44. Delvenne P, Arrese JE, Thiry A, Borlee-Hermans G, Pierard GE, Boniver J: Detection of cytomegalovirus, *Pneumocystis carinii,* and *Aspergillus* species in bronchoalveolar lavage fluid: a comparison of techniques, *Am J Clin Pathol* 100:414-418, 1993.
45. Honda J, Hoshino T, Natori H, Tokisawa S, Akiyoshi H, Nakahara S, Oizumi K: Rapid and sensitive diagnosis of cytomegalovirus and *Pneumocystis carinii* pneumonia in patients with hematological neoplasia by using capillary polymerase chain reaction, *Br J Haematol* 86:138-142, 1994.

Host Defense Disorders

46. Oxelius VA, Lavrall AB, Lindquest B, Golebiowska H, Axelsson U, Bjorkander J, Hanson LA: IgG subclasses in selective IgA deficiency: importance of IgG2-IgA deficiency, *N Engl J Med* 306:515, 1981.
47. Smith TF, Morris EC, Bain RP: IgG subclasses in non-allergic children with chronic chest symptoms *J Pediatr* 105:896, 1981.
48. Herrod HG, Gross S, Insel R: Selective antibody deficiency to *Haemophilus influenzae* type B capsular polysaccharide vaccination in children with recurrent respiratory tract infection, *J Clin Immunol* 9:429, 1989.

Clinical Presentation

49. Wald ER: Recurrent pneumonia in children, *Adv Pediatr Infect Dis* 5:183-203, 1990.
50. Rubin BK: The evaluation of the child with recurrent chest infections, *Pediatr Infect Dis* 4:88-98, 1985.
51. Hall CB, Powell KR, MacDonald NE, Gala CL, Menegus ME, Suffrin SC: Respiratory syncytial virus infection in children with compromised immune function, *N Engl J Med* 315:77-81, 1986.
52. Hertz MI, Englund JA, Stover D, Bitterman PB, McGlave PB: Respiratory virus-induced acute lung injury in adult patients with bone marrow transplants: a clinical approach and review of the literature, *Medicine* 68:269, 1989.
53. Parham DM, Bozeman P, Killian C, Murti G, Brenner M, Hanif I: Cytologic diagnosis of respiratory syncytial virus infection in a bronchoalveolar lavage specimen from a bone marrow transplant recipient, *Am J Clin Pathol* 99:588-592, 1993.
54. Flomenberg P, Babbitt J, Drobyski WR, Ash RC, Carrigan DR, Sedmak GV, McAuliffe T, Camitta B, Horowitz MM, Bunin N: Increasing incidence of adenovirus disease in bone marrow transplant recipients, *J Infect Dis* 169:775-781, 1994.
55. Bye MR, Clairs-Bazarian AM, Ewig JM: Markedly reduced mortality associated with corticosteroid therapy of *Pneumocystis carinii* in children with acquired immunodeficiency syndrome, *Arch Pediatr Adolesc Med* 148:638-641, 1994.
56. Sleasman JW, Hemenway C, Klein AS, Barrett DJ: Corticosteroids improve survival of children with AIDS and *Pneumocystis carinii* pneumonia, *Am J Dis Child* 147:30-34, 1993.
57. Rankin JA, Pella JA: Radiographic resolution of *Pneumocystis carinii* pneumonia in response to corticosteroid therapy, *Am Rev Respir Dis* 136:182-183, 1987.
58. Gallacher BP, Gallacher WN, MacFadden DK: Treatment of acute *Pneumocystis carinii* pneumonia with corticosteroids in a patient with acquired immunodeficiency syndrome, *Crit Care Med* 17:104-105, 1989.
59. Bozette SA, Sattler FR, Chiu J, Wu AW, Gluckstein D, Kemper C, Bartok A, Niosi J, Abramson I, Coffman J: A controlled trial of adjunctive treatment with corticosteroids for *Pneumocystis carinii* pneumonia in acquired immunodeficiency syndrome, *N Engl J Med* 323:1451-1457, 1990.
60. NIH Expert Panel for Corticosteroids as Adjunctive Therapy for *Pneumocystis carinii:* Consensus statement on the use of corticosteroids as adjunctive therapy for *Pneumocystis carinii* pneumonia in the acquired immunodeficiency syndrome, *N Engl J Med* 323:1500-1504, 1990.

61. Gold JWM: Opportunistic fungal infections in patients with neoplastic disease, *Am J Med* 76:458-463, 1984.
62. Haron E, Vartivarian S, Anaissie E, Dekmezian R, Bodey GP: Primary *Candida* pneumonia, *Medicine* 72:137-142, 1993.
63. Sapkowitz KA: *Pneumocystis carinii* pneumonia in patients without AIDS, *Clin Infect Dis* 17:S416-S422, 1993.
64. Young RC, Corder MP, Haynes HA, DeVita VT: Delayed hypersensitivity in Hodgkin's disease: a study of 103 untreated patients, *Am J Med* 52:63-72, 1972.
65. Fisher RI, DeVita VT, Bostick F: Persistent immunologic abnormalities in long term survivors of advanced Hodgkin's disease, *Ann Intern Med* 92:595, 1980.
66. Johnson FL, Schofer O: Pulmonary complications of bone marrow transplantation. In Laraya-Cuasay LR, Hughes WT, eds: *Interstitial lung diseases in children,* vol 2, Boca Raton, Fla, 1988, CRC.
67. Clark JG, Hansen JA, Hertz MI, Parkman R, Jensen L, Peavy HH: Idiopathic pneumonia syndrome after bone marrow transplantation, *Am Rev Respir Dis* 147:1601-1606, 1993.
68. Chan CK, Hyland RH, Hucheon MA, Minden MD, Alexander MA, Kosakowska AE, Urbanski SJ, Fyles GM, Fraser IM, Curtis JE: Small-airways disease in recipients of allogenic bone marrow transplants, *Medicine* 66:327-340, 1987.
69. Schwarer AP, Hughes JM, Trotman-Dickenson B, Krausz T, Goldman JM: A chronic pulmonary syndrome associated with graft-versus-host disease after allogeneic marrow transplantation, *Transplantation* 54:1002-1008, 1992.
70. Kaplan EB, Wodell RA, Wilmott RW, Leifer B, Lesser ML, August CS: Chronic graft-versus-host disease and pulmonary function, *Pediatr Pulmonol* 14:141-148, 1992.
71. Clark JG, Schwartz DA, Flournoy N, Sullivan KM, Crawford SW, Thomas ED: Risk factors for airflow obstruction in recipients of bone marrow transplants, *Ann Intern Med* 107:648-656, 1987.
72. Roca J, Granena A, Rodriquez-Roisin R, Alvarez P, Agusti-Vidal A, Rozman C: Fatal airway disease in an adult with chronic graft-versus-host disease, *Thorax* 37:77-78, 1982.
73. Enright H, Haake R, Weisdorf D, Ramsay N, McGlave P, Kersey J, Thomas W, McKenzie D, Miller W: Cytomegalovirus pneumonia after bone marrow transplantation: risk factors and response to therapy, *Transplantation* 55:1339-1346, 1993.
74. Goodrich JM, Bowden RA, Fisher L, Keller C, Schoch G, Meyers JD: Ganciclovir prophylaxis to prevent cytomegalovirus disease after allogenic marrow transplant, *Ann Intern Med* 118:173-178, 1993.
75. Foot ABM, Caul EO, Roome AP, Darville JM, Oakhill A: Cytomegalovirus pneumonitis and bone marrow transplantation: identification of a specific high risk group, *J Clin Pathol* 46:415-419, 1993.
76. Neumanaitis J, Shannon Dorcy, K Appelbaum FR, Meyers J, Owens A, Day R, Ando D, O'Neill C, Buckner D, Singer J: Long-term follow-up of patients with invasive fungal disease who received adjunctive therapy with recombinant human macrophage colony-stimulating factor, *Blood* 82:1422-1427, 1993.
77. Rubin RH: Infectious disease complications of renal transplantation, *Kidney Int* 44:221-236, 1993.
78. Gryzan S, Pardis IL, Zeevi A, Duquesnoy RJ, Dummer JS, Griffin BP, Hardestry RL, Trento A, Nalesnik MA, Dauber JH: Unexpectedly high incidence of *Pneumocystis carinii* infection after lung-heart transplantation: implications for lung defense and allograft survival, *Am Rev Respir Dis* 137:1268-1274, 1988.
79. Hertzler GL, Bryan JA, Perlino C, Kauter KR: Diagnosis of pulmonary toxoplasmosis by bronchoalveolar lavage in cardiac transplant recipients, *Diagn Cytopathol* 9:650-654, 1993.
80. Iragorri S, Pillay D, Scrine M, Trompeter RS, Rees L, Griffiths PD: Prospective cytomegalovirus surveillance in pediatric renal transplant patients, *Pediatr Nephrol* 7:55-60, 1993.
81. Stiehm ER, Chin TW, Haas H, Peerless AG: Infectious complications of the primary immunodeficiencies, *Clin Immunol Immunopathol* 40:69, 1986.
82. Dukes RJ, Rosenow EC III, Hermans PE: Pulmonary manifestations of hypogammaglobulinemia, *Thorax* 33:603-607, 1978.
83. Saulsbury FT, Bernstein MT, Winkelstein JA: *Pneumocystis carinii* pneumonia as the presenting infection in congenital hypogammaglobulinemia, *J Pediatr* 95:559-561, 1979.
84. Conley ME, Park CL, Douglas SD: Childhood common variable immunodeficiency with autoimmune disease, *J Pediatr* 108:915-922, 1986.
85. Leggiadro RJH, Winkelstein JA, Hughes WT: Prevalence of *Pneumocystis carinii* pneumonitis in severe combined immunodeficiency, *J Pediatr* 99:96-98, 1981.
86. Park BH: Chronic granulomatous disease of childhood. In Chernick V, ed: *Kendig's disorders of the respiratory tract in children,* Philadelphia, 1990, WB Saunders.
87. Caldicott WJH, Baehner RL: Chronic granulomatous disease of childhood, *Am J Roentgenol* 103:133-139, 1968.
88. Chipps BE, Saulsbury FT, Hsu SH, Hughes WT, Winkelstein JA: Noncandidal infections in children with chronic mucocutaneous candidiasis, *Johns Hopkins Med J* 144:175-179, 1979.
89. Rubenstein A, Morechi R, Silverman B, Charytan M, Krieger BZ, Andiman W, Ziprkowski MN, Goldman H: Pulmonary disease in children with acquired immune deficiency syndrome and AIDS-related complex, *J Pediatr* 108:498-503, 1986.
90. Goodman PC: Pulmonary disease in children with acquired immunodeficiency syndrome, *J Thorac Imag* 6:60-64, 1991.
91. Infectious disease of the lungs. In Fraser RG, Pare JAP, Pare PD, Fraser RS, Genereux GP, eds: *Diagnosis of diseases of the chest,* vol 2, Philadelphia, 1989, WB Saunders.
92. Gratton-Smith D, Harrison LF, Singleton EB: Radiology of acquired immunodeficiency syndrome in the pediatric patient, *Curr Prob Diagn Radiol* 21:79-109, 1992.
93. Chechani V, Zaman MK, Finch PJP: Chronic cavitary *Pneumocystis carinii* pneumonia in a patient with AIDS, *Chest* 95:1347-1348, 1989.
94. Klein JS, Warnock M, Webb WR, Gamsu G: Cavitating and noncavitating granulomas in AIDS patients with *Pneumocystis pneumonitis, Am J Roentgenol* 152:753-754, 1989.
95. Scannell KA: Atypical presentation of *Pneumocystis carinii* in a patient receiving inhalational pentamidine, *Am J Med* 85:881-884, 1988.
96. O'Riordan TG, Baughman RP, Dohn MN, Smaldone GC: Lobar pentamidine levels and *Pneumocystis carinii* pneumonia following aerosolized pentamidine, *Chest* 105:53-56, 1994.

Common Causes of Pneumonia in Immunocompromised Hosts

97. Demmler GJ: Cytomegalovirus. In Patrick CC, ed: *Infections in immunocompromised infants and children,* Edinburgh, 1993, Churchill Livingstone.
98. Wolf DG, Spector S: Early diagnosis of human cytomegalovirus disease in transplant recipients by DNA amplification in plasma, *Transplantation* 56:330-334, 1993.
99. Storch GA, Ettinger NA, Ockner D, Wick MR, Gandreault-Keener M, Rossiter J, Trulock EP, Cooper JD: Quantitative cultures of the cell fraction and supernatant of bronchoalveolar lavage fluid for the diagnosis of cytomegalovirus pneumonitis in lung transplant recipients, *J Infect Dis* 168:1502-1506, 1993.
100. Crawford SW, Bowden RA, Hackman RC, Gleaves CA, Meyers JD, Clark JG: Rapid detection of cytomegalovirus pulmonary infection by bronchoalveolar lavage, *Ann Intern Med* 108:180-185, 1988.
101. Einsele H, Ehninger G, Steidle M, Fischer I, Bihler S, Gerneth F, Vallbracht A, Schmidt H, Weller HD, Muller CA: Lymphopenia as an unfavorable prognostic factor in patients with cytomegalovirus infection after bone marrow transplantation, *Blood* 82:1672-1678, 1993.
102. Cone RW, Hackman RC, Huang MI, Bowden RA, Meyers JD, Metcalf M, Zeh J, Ashley R, Corey L: Human herpesvirus 6 in lung tissue from patients with pneumonitis after bone marrow transplantation, *N Engl J Med* 329:156-161, 1993.
103. Wilborn F, Brinkman V, Schmidt C, Neipel F, Gelderblom H, Siegert W: Herpesvirus type 6 in patients undergoing bone marrow transplantation: serologic features and detection by PCR, *Blood* 83:3052-3058, 1994.
104. Robinson WS: Human herpes virus 6, *Curr Clin Top Infect Dis* 14:159-169, 1994.
105. Morris DJ, Corbitt G, Bailey AS, Newbould M, Smith E, Picton S, Stevens RF: Fatal disseminated adenovirus type 2 infection after bone marrow transplantation for Hurler's syndrome: a primary infection, *J Infect* 26:181-184, 1993.
106. Shields AF, Hackman RC, Fife KH, Corey L, Meyers JD: Adenovirus infections in patients undergoing bone marrow transplantation, *N Engl J Med* 312:529-533, 1985.
107. Michaels MG, Green M, Wal ER, Starzl TE: Adenovirus infection in pediatric liver transplant recipients, *J Infect Dis* 165:170-174, 1992.
108. Zahradnik JM, Spencer JM, Porter DD: Adenovirus infection in the immunocompromised patient, *Am J Med* 68:725-732, 1980.

109. Walmsley S, Devi S, King S, Schneider R, Richardson S, Ford-Jones L: Invasive *Aspergillus* infections in a pediatric hospital: a ten-year review, *Pediatr Infect Dis J* 12:673-682, 1993.
110. Taccone A, Occhi M, Garaventa A, Manfredini L, Viscoli C: CT of invasive pulmonary aspergillosis in children with cancer, *Cancer* 23:177-180, 1993.
111. Lupinetti FM, Behrendt DM, Giller RH, Trigg ME, deAlarcon P: Pulmonary resection for fungal infection in children undergoing bone marrow transplantation, *J Thorac Cardiovasc Surg* 10:684-687, 1992.
112. Denning DW, Stevens DA: Antifungal and surgical treatment of invasive aspergillosis: review of 2121 published cases, *Rev Infect Dis* 12:1147-1201, 1990.
113. Richard C, Romon I, Baro J, Insunza A, Loyola I, Zurbano F, Tapia M, Iriondo A, Conde E, Zubizarreta A: Invasive pulmonary aspergillosis prior to BMT in acute leukemia patients does not predict a poor outcome, *Bone Marrow Transplant* 12:237-241, 1993.
114. Hughes WT: Systemic candidiasis: a study of 109 fatal cases, *Pediatr Infect Dis* 1:11-18, 1982.
115. Flynn PM, Marina NM, Rivera GK, Hughes WT: *Candida tropicalis* infections in children with leukemia, *Leuk Lymphoma* 10:369-376, 1993.
116. Morrison VA, Haake RJ, Weisdorf DJ: The spectrum of non-*Candida* fungal infections following bone marrow transplantation, *Medicine* 72:78-89, 1993.
117. Water BL: Pathology of culture-proven JK corynebacterium pneumonia: an autopsy case report, *Am J Pathol* 91:616, 1989.
118. Fergie JE, Shema SJ, Lott L, Crawford R, Patrick CC: *Pseudomonas aeruginosa* bacteremia in immunocompromised children: analysis of factors associated with a poor outcome, *Clin Infect Dis* 18:390-394, 1994.
119. Starke JR: Nontuberculous mycobacterial infections in children, *Adv Pediatr Infect Dis* 7:123-159, 1992.
120. Hughes WT: Pneumocystis carinii *pneumonitis,* vol 1 and 2, Boca Raton, Fla, 1987, CRC.
121. Walzer PD: *Pneumocystis carinii:* recent advances in basic biology and their clinical application, *AIDS* 7:1293-1305, 1993.
122. Su TH, Martin WJ: Pathogenesis and host response in *Pneumocystis carinii* pneumonia, *Ann Rev Med* 45:261-272, 1994.
123. Edman J, Kovacs J, Masur H, Santi DV, Elwood HJ, Sogin ML: Ribosomal RNA sequence shows *Pneumocystis carinii* to be a member of the fungi, *Nature* 334:517-522, 1988.
124. Lubat E, Megibow AJ, Bathazar EJ, Goldenberg AS, Birnbaurm BA: Extrapulmonary *Pneumocystis carinii* infection in AIDS: CT findings, *Radiology* 174:157-160, 1990.
125. Pottratz ST, Paulsrud J, Smith JS, Martin WJ *Pneumocystis carinii* attachment to cultured lung cells by *Pneumocystis* gp120, a fibronectin binding protein, *J Clin Invest* 88:403-407, 1991.
126. Wisnioski P, Pasula R, Martin WJ: Isolation of *Pneumocystis carinii* gp120 by fibronectin affinity: evidence for manganese affinity, *Am J Respir Cell Molec Biol* 11:262, 1994.
127. Sheehan PM, Stokes DC, Yeh YY, Hughes WT: Surfactant phospholipid and lavage phospholipase A_2 in experimental *Pneumocystis carinii* pneumonia, *Am Rev Respir Dis* 134:526-531, 1986.
128. Rose RM, Catalon PJ, Koziel H, Furlong ST: Abnormal lipid composition of bronchoalveolar lavage fluid obtained from individuals with AIDS-related lung disease, *Am J Respir Crit Care Med* 149:332-338, 1994.
129. Chen W, Gigliotti F, Harmsen AG: Latency is not an inevitable outcome of infection with *Pneumocystis carinii, Infect Immun* 61:5406-5409, 1993.
130. Schuval SJ, Bonagura VR: Failure of pentamidine as prophylaxis for *Pneumocystis carinii* in HIV-infected children, *Arch Pediatr Adolesc Med* 148:876-879, 1994.
131. O'Doherty MJ, Thomas SHL, Gibb D, Page CJ, Harrington C, Duggan C, Nunan TO, Bateman NT: Lung deposition of nebulized pentamidine in children, *Thorax* 48:220-226, 1993.

Diagnostic Studies

132. Kirsch CM, Jensen WA, Kagawa FT, Azzi RL: Analysis of induced sputum for the diagnosis of recurrent *Pneumocystis pneumonia, Chest* 102:1152-1154, 1992.
133. Rigal E, Roze JC, Villers D, Derriennic M, David-Melon V, Lacroix-Mechinaud F, Mouzard A: Prospective evaluation of the protected specimen brush for the diagnosis of pulmonary infections in ventilated newborns, *Pediatr Pulmonol* 8:268-272, 1990.
134. Koumbourlis AC, Kurland G: Nonbronchoscopic bronchoalveolar lavage in mechanically ventilated infants: technique, efficacy and applications, *Pediatr Pulmonol* 15:257-262, 1993.
135. Ramsey BW, Marcuse EK, Roy HM, Cooney MK, Allan I, Brewer D, Smith AL: Use of bacterial antigen detection in the diagnosis of pediatric lower respiratory tract infections, *Pediatrics* 78:1-9, 1986.
136. Kan VL: Polymerase chain reaction for the diagnosis of candidemia, *J Infect Dis* 168:779-783, 1993.
137. Edelstein PH: The laboratory diagnosis of Legionnaire's disease, *Semin Respir Infect* 2:235-241, 1987.
138. deBlic J, McKelvie P, leBourgeois M, Blanceh S, Benosit MR, Scheinmann P: Value of bronchoalveolar lavage in the management of severe acute pneumonia and interstitial pneumonias in the immunocompromised child, *Thorax* 42:759-765, 1987.
139. Abadco DL, Amaro-Galvez R, Rao M, Steiner F: Experience with flexible bronchoscopy with bronchoalveolar lavage as a diagnostic tool in children with AIDS, *Am J Dis Child* 146:1056-1059, 1992.
140. Mattey JE, Fitzpatrick SB, Josephs SH, Fink RJ: Bronchoalveolar lavage for *Pneumocystis* pneumonia in HIV-infected children, *Ann Allergy* 64:393-397, 1990.
141. Rodriguez de Castro F, Sole Violan J, Lafarga Capuz BM, Caminero Luna J, Gonzalez Rodriguez B, Manzano Alonso JL: Reliability of the bronchoscopic protected catheter brush in the diagnosis of pneumonia in mechanically ventilated patients, *Crit Care Med* 19:171-175, 1991.
142. Grigg J, van den Borre C, Malfroot A, Pierard D, Wang D, Dab I: Bilateral fiberoptic bronchoalveolar lavage in acute unilateral lobar pneumonia, *J Pediatr* 122:606-608, 1993.
143. Birriel JA Jr, Adams JA, Saldana MA, Mavunda K, Goldfinger S, Vernon D, Holzaman B, McKey RM Jr: Role of flexible bronchoscopy and bronchoalveolar lavage in the diagnosis of pediatric acquired immunodeficiency syndrome-related pulmonary disease, *Pediatrics* 87:897-899, 1991.
144. Winthrop AL, Waddell Superina RA: The diagnosis of pneumonia in the immunocompromised child: use of bronchoalveolar lavage, *J Pediatr Surg* 25:878-889, 1990.
145. McCubbin MM, Trigg ME, Hendricker CM, Wagener JS: Bronchoscopy with bronchoalveolar lavage in the evaluation of pulmonary complications of bone marrow transplantation in children, *Pediatr Pulmonol* 12:43-47, 1992.
146. Whitehead B, Scott JP, Helms P, Malone M, Macrae D, Higenbottam TW, Smyth RL, Wallwork J, Elliott M, deLeval M: Technique and use of transbronchial lung biopsy in children and adolescents, *Pediatr Pulmonol* 12:240-246, 1992.
147. Chaudhary S, Hughes WT, Feldman S, Sanyal SK, Coburn T, Ossi M, Cox F: Percutaneous transthoracic needle aspiration of the lung: diagnosing *Pneumocystic carinii* pneumonitis, *Am J Dis Child* 131:902-907, 1977.
148. Sokolowski JW Jr, Burgher LW, Jones FL Jr, Patterson JR, Selecky PA: Guidelines for percutaneous transthoracic needle biopsy, *Am Rev Respir Dis* 140:255-256, 1989.

CHAPTER 41

Human Immunodeficiency Virus Infection

Michael R. Bye

EPIDEMIOLOGY

In 1981 the Centers for Disease Control reported cases of *Pneumocystis carinii* pneumonia (PCP)[1] and Kaposi's sarcoma (KS)[2] in previously well homosexual men. Over the next year an epidemic grew to include patients with hemophilia,[3] transfusion recipients,[4,5] and intravenous drug abusers.[6] In 1987, two groups described children with clinical and laboratory evidence of abnormal immune function similar to those of adults with the acquired immunodeficiency syndrome (AIDS).[7,8] Some of the patients demonstrated clinical manifestations from birth,[7] with 11 of 15 (73%) developing symptoms before the first birthday. The infants had at least one parent in the previously described high-risk groups. By 1983 the caseload had increased to about 50 children; yet there was uncertainty about the diagnosis.[9] The discovery of what is now called the *human immunodeficiency virus (HIV)*[10,11] in 1983 and 1984 allows a definitive diagnosis of AIDS.

As is true in many aspects of medicine, children are not small adults with regard to AIDS. The methods of acquiring HIV are different, the disease may be more fulminant, and organ system involvement is different.

It is estimated that over 85%[12] of affected children are infected by the mother during pregnancy, at delivery, or through breast milk.[13,14] The second largest category of infection is by transfusion, less common since blood supply screening was begun in 1985. Some children are infected through sexual abuse.[15] Early in the epidemic, adolescents were more likely to become infected through blood transfusions, usually secondary to hemophilia or other coagulopathies.[16] Now, however, the adolescent population is similar to adults in how they acquire AIDS: primarily through sexual transmission and less so via sharing of intravenous needles.[17]

When tracking the epidemiology of pediatric AIDS, it is helpful to track the infection in women of child-bearing age, who account for 85% of all HIV-infected women.[18] Early in the course of the epidemic, female patients were infected less frequently than male patients. Among heterosexuals reported in the United States in 1981, the male/female ratio was 4.0:1. Since 1987, that ratio has been 2.4:1. The absolute numbers in both genders have increased since 1987, but the proportion has remained steady. Heterosexually transmitted disease is spreading outside the major urban areas. Of over 1000 women attending a public health clinic for prenatal care in western Palm Beach County, Florida, 5.1% were HIV infected.[19] None reported intravenous drug abuse, and none was from countries where heterosexual contact is the most common method of HIV infection. Infection was associated with crack cocaine use, sexual intercourse with multiple partners, sexual intercourse with a partner known to be in a high-risk category, and positive serologic findings for syphilis.

Studies have looked at the incidence of HIV antibody in newborn blood samples. In Massachusetts[20] the overall incidence was 2.1 per 1000 deliveries, varying from 0.9 per 1000 in suburban and rural hospitals to 8.0 per 1000 in the inner city. In 1988 the rate in New York State was 0.66% but 1.25% in New York City,[21] with rates of 2.4% to 2.5% detected in inner city municipal hospitals.[22,23] In sub-Saharan Africa, rates of 6% to 10% are reported.[24] Disparity in diagnosing HIV infection is seen from a follow-up to the Massachusetts data.[20] By 3 years after the initial anonymous testing, 78 of 223 seropositive infants had been identified, 29 of whom were infected.[25] When hospitals of birth were compared, there was much greater rate of clinical detection in inner city Boston (47% of seropositive infants) than in Boston suburbs or Cape Cod (17%) or other regions of Massachusetts (30%). Because local prevalence rates correlate with the likelihood of clinically detecting the seropositive infant, it is likely that high rates beget awareness and more frequent testing. HIV testing is recommended for all pregnant women in areas of high HIV prevalence.[25,26] Even in areas of low prevalence, aggressive evaluations with subsequent antiretroviral therapy and PCP prophylaxis results in decreased morbidity and mortality rates.[27]

MATERNAL-FETAL TRANSMISSION

The precise timing of the transmission of HIV from mother to the infant or fetus is not known. Transmission occurs in utero as shown by the fact that HIV has been found in 13- to 20-week fetuses[28] and the description of craniofacial anomalies as an AIDS embryopathy.[29,30] Recent data suggest that the majority of transmissions occur at delivery. Data from France show higher transmission rates from mothers with more clinical involvement at the time of delivery.[31] In New York City, transmission rates were significantly higher if the mother had low CD4 counts and if the mother had been hospitalized for pneumonia in the previous year.[32] Kliks et al[33] found that virus from transmitting mothers was more likely to replicate in human peripheral blood mononuclear cells in vitro and that virus from nontransmitting mothers was more likely to be neutralized by autologous serum samples. Further data show increased transmission with greater amounts of maternal viremia at or near the time of delivery. The investigators[34] found a five-fold higher amount of virus in the blood of mothers who transmitted infection to the fetus.

Other data show the possibility of reducing the transmission from mother to child. A nonrandomized, prospective study of infected pregnant women[35] confirmed increased transmission with p24 antigenemia at delivery. Mothers treated with zidovudine during pregnancy or labor and delivery had a significant reduction in transmission rates. Similar data come from the AIDS Clinical Trials Group study 076.[36] This study evaluated HIV-infected pregnant women who did not meet the criteria for antiretroviral treatment. Half were randomized to therapy with oral zidovudine during pregnancy, intravenous zidovudine at delivery, and oral zidovudine for the infant. A control group was treated with placebo. Blood from the infants were cultured for HIV at birth and at 12, 24, and 78 weeks of age. Analysis of the first 364 births showed transmission rates of 25.5% in the placebo group and 8.3% in the treated group. The study was discontinued, and women receiving placebo were offered zidovudine. It is now common practice, in those countries where it is economically feasible, to offer zidovudine to pregnant women during the latter stages of pregnancy, and during labor, and to offer it to their infants.

Because maternal immunoglobulin G (IgG) readily crosses the placenta, its presence in newborn blood does not necessarily reflect infection in the infant. This passively acquired antibody may persist for up to 15 months,[37] making a definitive diagnosis impossible by this common screening method. Infants who lose this antibody, especially without clinical or laboratory manifestations, can be assumed to be uninfected.[38] Three cases of transient seroreversion are reported from Africa.[39] However, these infants were being breast-fed, and transmission of the virus via breast milk cannot be excluded. Attempts have been made to definitively diagnose the condition earlier in infancy so that counseling can be provided and appropriate therapy begun. Early efforts were directed at detection via enzyme-linked immunosorbent assay of the p24 antigen in the infant's serum.[40] Because the amount of p24 antigen in blood varies directly with the virus load,[41] the test is less sensitive in infants tested during the asymptomatic period or early in the course of infection, before the viremic phase.[42] However, recent data in a large cohort of infants[43] showed a high specificity of antigen testing at birth. False-negative p24 tests can occur as a result of immune complexes formed with maternal antibody. An assay has been developed that disrupts these immune complexes in vitro, allowing for 100% specificity and 81% sensitivity in 78 children.[44] Culturing virus from peripheral blood monocytes has been more difficult in young children than in adults with advanced disease.[42] Recent data[43,45] found that 48% of infected infants had a positive culture at birth and 75% were positive at 3 months of age. False-negative cultures may represent a low virus load early in life or infection of the infant during late pregnancy or at delivery, with insufficient time for the viremic stage to occur at the time of testing. Although virus-specific IgM or IgA in newborn serum indicates infection, the low concentrations of these antibodies and the transience of the IgM antibody make them unreliable.[40] Detection of HIV deoxyribonucleic acid via the polymerase chain reaction results in improved test results.[40,46]

The reported transmission rates from mother to child vary. Studies with rates of 21% to 40%[47-49] all evaluated fewer than 100 infants born to seropositive mothers. A study of over 500 infants showed a transmission rate of 23.9%[50] with discordance on one of 18 twin pairs, a 40% infection rate among subsequent infants if the first infant was infected, and an 8.3% rate in infants subsequent to an infant who tested negatively.

AIDS IN THE INFANT

The common clinical manifestations in infancy include poor weight gain,[51] hepatomegaly, lymphadenopathy, recurrent or persistent candidal infection, chronic or recurrent diarrhea, recurrent bacterial infections, and static or progressive encephalopathy. The encephalopathy results in loss of motor function, intellectual abilities, and behavioral abnormalities. Most of the clinical manifestations occur late in infancy[37] with a median age at diagnosis of 9 months.[52] It is helpful to look into the parental history to try to elicit activities indicating risk factors. However, such risk factors may not be obvious. Unless both parents have had only one sexual partner during their entire lives, there is always a possibility of transmission of HIV to a parent and therefore to a fetus.

Infants who develop opportunistic infection or encephalopathy before 25 months of age have lower CD4 counts and a lower age at death than those without these problems early in life.[53] Given the potential benefit from antiretroviral therapy[54,55] and PCP prophylaxis,[56] attempts at finding a reliable, relatively easy, and inexpensive method of detecting HIV infection in infants continue.

When the diagnosis of HIV infection is made, it becomes important to frequently assess the infant for signs of immunologic deterioration.[37,53] Frequent measurement of CD4 lymphocytes[57] is necessary. The onset of PCP is associated with a decreased CD4+ cell count. Infants and young children normally have higher CD4+ counts[58] than adults[59] (see Table 41-1). In a survey of pediatric specialists caring for children with AIDS, 20 of 37 (54%) were using PCP prophylaxis in all infants with symptomatic or documented HIV infection regardless of the CD4+ count.[60] The high morbidity and mortality rates of PCP in infants, combined with a delay in obtaining CD4 cell counts in some areas, and the possibility of developing PCP within 30 days of beginning prophylactic therapy have changed the recommendations by some experts.[61] Many now suggest beginning prophylaxis in any infant born to an HIV-infected mother. Prophylaxis can be discontinued if the infant is found to be definitely HIV negative but continued for the first 1 to 2 years in HIV-infected infants.[61-63]

LUNG DEFENSE

Normal lung defense is discussed in Chapter 6. This section reviews the effects of HIV on lung defense.

The virus is probably first carried to the regional lymph nodes and then disseminated throughout the lymphoid tissues, where it replicates. A massive viral replication results in a viremic stage, clinically manifested by a nonspecific "flu-like" illness. The majority of the HIV remains in the lymphoid tissue, causing growth and malfunction of these tissues. As the lymphoid tissue is disrupted, more virus is released into the bloodstream. This late-phase viremia is often associated with progressive clinical disease. It is not known at what point, or how, in this cycle the lung becomes infected with HIV. Although it is possible that free virus crosses the alveolocapillary membrane, it is more likely that infected circulating cells migrate into the lung.[64] In this "Trojan horse theory," infected peripheral blood mononucleocytes enter the lung and mature into alveolar macrophages (AMs).[65]

Much of the understanding of the abnormal defense derives from data obtained by bronchoalveolar lavage (BAL) in adults. Studies have focused on BAL cell numbers, protein contents, and cell differential and function.[66] Studies of systemic defense have centered on immunoglobulins, lymphocytes, and monocytes/macrophages.

In peripheral blood, HIV infects both CD4 and CD8 lymphocytes. In vitro, CD8 cells can be infected by HIV only in the presence of infected CD4 cells. If infected CD8 cells are stimulated, they can infect CD4 cells.[67] Because CD8 cells resist the cytopathic effects of HIV, they serve as a reservoir for HIV.

CD4 cells not only serve as reservoirs for HIV but are also depleted by the infection.[37] When normal T cells are cultured with infected AMs, the T cells form syncytia.[68] This suggests direct transmission of the virus from the macrophage to the T cell and results in decreased T cell function. The death of the CD4 cells most closely correlates with clinical disease. This can come quickly or after a latency period of years, and the determinants of the progression are unknown. Other factors may lead to immunodeficiency.[69] HIV-specific antibodies destroy infected cells during advanced stages of infection. Cross-reactivity between glycoproteins 120 and 41 of HIV and class II major histocompatibility antigens may inhibit the normal processing and defense against newly presented antigens.[70,71] In addition, glycoprotein 120 on the CD4 cells may prevent the latter from reacting to antigens,[72] resulting in anergy. Superantigens that arise from the virus may render T cells more susceptible to HIV.

The B cell proliferative response is abnormal. Response to T cell–dependent mitogens (such as pokeweed mitogen) and T cell–independent stimuli (such as *Staphylococcus aureus*) are abnormal.[73] Men with AIDS have a tenfold higher number of circulating B cells. These well-differentiated B cells spontaneously secrete immunoglobulin. However, even in the presence of normal T cells, these B cells are unable to produce immunoglobulin specific to pokeweed mitogen.[73] This polyclonal B cell activation may be induced by concomitant viral infection because all subjects had evidence of cytomegalovirus (CMV) and Epstein-Barr virus infection. Increased amounts of interleukin 6[74] (IL-6) from peripheral blood monocytes could be the cause of this B cell gammopathy.

Although up to 58% of AMs are infected,[75,76] very few actively express HIV ribonucleic acid.[77] This is similar to peripheral blood, where there are far more cells infected with HIV than actively creating new viruses.[78] When infected in vitro,[79] AMs remain viable for over 65 days and thus may serve as reservoirs for HIV infection. The viability of the macrophages during an opportunistic infection decreases,[80] although the role of cause and effect has not been determined. As is true in peripheral blood monocytes, AMs produce increased amounts of IL-6.[81] The IL-6 in turn increases HIV expression in infected AMs.[82]

Murray et al[80] isolated AMs from patients with AIDS and controls. The metabolic rates at rest and after stimulation with crude lymphokines were normal. The stimulation with crude lymphokines was blocked by monoclonal antibody against interferon-γ (IFN-γ). This leads to the postulate that a problem in the macrophages is insufficient stimulation by lymphokines and raises the possibility of IFN-γ as a form of therapy. However, in acutely infected peripheral monocytes the production of tumor necrosis factor (TNF) is increased in response to IFN-γ.[83] AMs have high spontaneous TNF production, but those containing p24 antigen (indicating long-standing infection) respond poorly to IFN-γ.[84] TNF release from latently infected AMs is stimulated by opportunistic infections. This TNF-α activates the transcription and release of virions from other latently infected cells, infecting more AMs and worsening the immune response.[64,85,86] Through unknown mechanisms, HIV production by alveolar lymphocytes is increased during acute infection with PCP.[87] This appears to be organ specific because no similar increase was seen in the corresponding blood lymphocytes.

As the number of pulmonary CD4+ cells decreases, the likelihood of pulmonary opportunistic infection increases.[64] This may be from a decreased production of biologic response modifiers (e.g., IL-2) because therapy with such modifiers restores some of the lytic capacity to BAL lymphocytes.[88] There may also be an inappropriate secretion of inhibitory cytokines such as IL-10 and IFN-γ.

Johnson et al[89] performed BAL on 39 asymptomatic seropositive subjects. They found no difference in cell numbers or differentials in the patients regardless of clinical status or CD4 cell count. No organisms other than HIV were recovered in three, all of whom also had HIV viremia. Patients with AIDS and pulmonary infection appear to have normal absolute BAL cell numbers.[90,91] The BAL differentials show fewer macrophages and more polymorphonuclear cells[91] or lymphocytes.[90]

In summary, HIV in the lung first decreases the number of pulmonary CD4+ cells. This causes abnormalities in cytotoxic activity. Pulmonary AMs are recruited and release lymphokines such as TNF-α and IL-6, which activate the local immune system and lead to accumulation of immunocompetent cells such as lymphocytes, polymorphonuclear cells, and monocytes. Because some of the latter are infected, there is additional accumulation of HIV-infected cells.

OPPORTUNISTIC INFECTIONS OF THE LUNG

P. carinii Pneumonia

Clinical Presentation

PCP is described as the most common opportunistic infection in children with AIDS[37] in the United States. The incidence in children is as high as 53%,[52] and a recent review of several studies gave a cumulative incidence of 49%.[92] Data from Africa show a very low incidence of PCP.[93] Although PCP is discussed in Chapter 40, its prominent role in AIDS justifies discussion here.[94] The reader is referred to Chapter 47 for discussion of the microbiology of PCP and its role in disease in other patient populations.

Compared to HIV-infected adults, children with AIDS and PCP are much sicker. In 54 episodes of PCP in children with AIDS, the mean alveolar-arterial oxygen gradient ($P_{AO_2} - Pa_{O_2}$) in 33 patients breathing room air was 56 mm Hg.[61] Of those 54, 34 (63%) developed respiratory failure and required mechanical ventilation, and 17 died during the acute illness. In children with respiratory failure, an 85% mortality rate was found with PCP.[95]

When children develop PCP, the clinical manifestations include tachypnea, dyspnea, and fever. The examination of the chest is unremarkable except for tachypnea and retractions. Asymmetric breath sounds, crackles, and wheezes are all uncommon.[61] The chest radiograph most often reveals diffuse interstitial lung disease, although there are other patterns, including localized infiltrate, "bronchiolitis" (peribronchial cuffing with hyperinflation), noncardiogenic pulmonary edema, and normal findings in 3.7% of cases.[61] A markedly elevated $P_{AO_2} - Pa_{O_2}$ and a high serum lactate dehydrogenase (LDH) level are seen.[61,96,97] The only statistically significant difference between children who require mechanical ventilation and those who did not is the LDH level, which is higher in those with respiratory failure. Other factors, including age and the $P_{AO_2} - Pa_{O_2}$, are not different. In contrast, in adults, both the LDH levels and the $PAO_2 - PaO_2$ are more abnormal in nonsurvivors.[97] An evaluation of immune function in children shows diminished response to phytohemagglutinin in nonsurvivors.[98] No differences are seen in CD4 counts.

Diagnosis

The diagnosis of PCP begins with clinical suspicion. In 34% of patients in one study,[61] there was no initial history to suggest HIV infection, and risk factor activity was elicited only after the diagnosis of PCP was made.

Hughes[92] points out, "PCP is characterized by a tetrad of signs: tachypnea, dyspnea, fever and cough." The same is true of most lower respiratory tract infections and asthma attacks in children. The marked hypoxemia and lack of auscultatory findings in PCP are helpful in suggesting the diagnosis.[61] An elevated LDH level supports the diagnosis. The diagnosis requires demonstration of cysts or organisms in lung secretions or tissue, a process facilitated by improved methods of detection.[99,100] Although open lung biopsy remains the gold standard of diagnosis, BAL[101,102] and induced sputum tests[103] are used successfully to detect the *Pneumocystis* organisms.

Therapy

The most effective specific therapy is trimethoprim/sulfamethoxazole (TMP/SMX) at 20 mg/kg/day of the TMP intravenously.[104] The incidence of significant reaction to TMP/SMX is high, with a 15% reported incidence of neutropenia, severe dermatologic reaction, or both reactions.[61] The second line of therapy is parenteral pentamidine at 4 mg/kg/day. Other therapies under investigation include TMP/dapsone,[105] trimetrexate,[106] clindamycin/primaquine[107] and atovaquoné.[108] Aerosolized pentamidine is used in adults with mild disease but not in children for two reasons: First, the degree of mild disease described (partial pressure of alveolar oxygen >70 mm Hg in room air, $PAO_2 - PaO_2$ <35 mm Hg) is very rare in children,[61] and second, currently available nebulizers may not generate particles small enough to deliver drug to the alveoli of young children.

It may take 4 to 8 days to demonstrate clinical improvement in adults with PCP.[104] Therefore it is prudent to wait that long before considering a change in therapy. Researchers do not know whether failure to respond after this time is due to failure to kill the organisms or other factors. Although it may make sense at this point to consider adding or changing therapy, there is no scientific support for any of the alternatives.

Corticosteroids are helpful adjuncts to specific therapy in adults[109,110] and children.[111,112] Even in the absence of scientific data, many centers use corticosteroids in these patients.[60] These medications do not adversely affect the clinical course of tuberculosis (TB) when given to patients coinfected with PCP.[113] When children free of opportunistic infection were treated with systemic corticosteroids, there was a decrease in the serum p24 concentrations[114] that returned to baseline after the steroids were withdrawn. During steroid therapy, there was no change in the numbers of T cell subsets or the response to mitogens and antigens.

Given the morbidity and mortality rates of PCP in AIDS, greater emphasis is on prophylaxis. Primary prophylaxis is suggested if the CD4+ count is low (Table 41-1). Drugs used for prophylaxis include TMP/SMX at 150 mg/m^2/day of TMP, which may be divided twice a day 3 times a week on consecutive days, once a day 3 times a week on consecutive days, or twice a day 3 times a week on alternate days. If TMP/SMX is not tolerated or cannot be used, alternatives include parenteral pentamidine, 4 mg/kg every 2 to 4 weeks, and if the child is over 5 years of age, aerosolized pentamidine, 300 mg every 4 weeks.[58,115,116] The concerns with using aerosolized pentamidine in younger children deal with safety and efficacy. There are no data on the delivery of medication into the alveoli of young children by the nebulizers currently in use. A study looking at the safety of inhaled pentamidine in young children[117] showed cough, wheeze, or oxygen desaturation in five of seven infants. None of these infants relied on the inhaled pentamidine for prophylaxis, so the authors could not comment on the efficacy of the drug. Oral dapsone, 1 mg/kg/day, has been useful for prophylaxis,[118,119] although higher doses have been suggested.[120] In adults, oral TMP/SMX is the most effective agent available for primary[121] or secondary[122] prophylaxis.

Table 41-1 Indications for PCP Prophylaxis*

AGE	ABSOLUTE CD4+ COUNT	CD4+ %
<11 months	<1500/mm3	<20%
12-23 months	<750/mm^3	<20%
24-71 months	<500/mm^3	<20%
≥72 months	<200/mm3	<20%

From Butler KM et al: *Am J Dis Child* 146:932-936, 1992.
*Secondary prophylaxis is indicated for all children who survive an episode of PCP.

If PCP develops in patients on prophylaxis, the usual procedure is treatment with an alternative drug.[104] However, prophylaxis may fail because of poor compliance or unusual pharmacokinetics as well as drug resistance. Inhaled pentamidine alters the acute infection. Adults in such cases are less likely to require hospitalization for acute PCP than those not on prophylaxis,[123] although there are no differences in other indicators of clinical severity. Patients on inhaled pentamidine are more likely to develop disease localized to the upper lobes, with cyst formation.[124] This is probably related to preferential deposition of the inhaled drug in the lower lobes.[125] If the cysts rupture, the resultant pneumothorax usually requires pleurodesis.[126] Patients in whom acute PCP is suspected and who have been on inhaled pentamidine should have BAL performed in the upper lobes to improve the yield of the procedure.[127]

Tuberculosis

As discussed in Chapter 43, since 1985, there has been a resurgence in TB in the United States and throughout the world. This is especially true in the parts of the world where AIDS is prominent.[128,129] Adults with AIDS are more likely to develop TB disease and to spread the organism. In areas of the world where access to care is limited, multiple factors predispose to increased spread.[130]

From 1985 through 1991 at the Harlem Hospital in New York City, 5 cases of TB disease were found in a population of 369 HIV-infected children.[131] Over a 10-year period ending in December 1990, Khouri et al[132] found 9 cases of TB among 345 children with HIV in Miami. In addition to the lung, the organism was recovered from the blood in two subjects, cerebrospinal fluid in one, stool in two, lymph node in one, and mastoid in one. In Zambia,[133] HIV seroprevalence rates were

37% in 237 children with TB and 10.7% in a control group of 242 children. In those under 12 months of age, the seroprevalence rates were 58.1% in patients with TB and 27.6% in controls. More recent data show the rate of HIV infection among children with TB in Zambia up to 56.7%, and the control population at 9.6%.[134]

In adults with HIV and TB, extrapulmonary disease is common.[135,136] In the data from Harlem,[131] pulmonary TB was the sole manifestation of disease in four of the five children with TB and HIV infection; one child had tuberculous meningitis. In the Zambia data,[133] pulmonary TB was the predominant manifestation of disease in both the HIV and non-HIV groups. There was no increased frequency of extrapulmonary TB in the HIV group. This may result in part from Bacille Calmette-Guérin vaccination; evidence of such vaccination was found in 87% of the group with TB and 90% of the controls.

Multiple drug resistance in TB is being increasingly seen, especially in the inner cities and among AIDS patients.[137,138] In the absence of a known source case and drug susceptibility testing, many now recommend institution of therapy with isoniazid, rifampin, pyrazinamide, and ethambutol until the organism can be detected and tested for drug sensitivity. The 1997 edition of the *Red Book of the American Academy of Pediatrics*[139] suggests three drugs as initial therapy but agrees with the CDC[140] in recommending four drugs in patients at high risk for HIV infection, infections with drug-resistant organisms, or both infections. Children with TB disease are candidates for HIV testing.[139] Pulmonary TB is an AIDS-defining illness in subjects over 13 years of age.[141]

Infection with *Mycobacterium avium-intracellulare*

Pulmonary infection with *Mycobacterium avium-intracellulare* (MAI) is found in elderly patients with preexisting chronic lung disease or in immunocompromised patients. Although reported in apparently immunocompetent children,[142,143] intrathoracic disease is extremely rare.[144]

MAI and other nontuberculous mycobacteria may be detected in the lung in adults with AIDS, but the clinical manifestations are usually due to extrapulmonary disease such as fever and bone marrow suppression.[145,146] This is often the case in children as well. Pulmonary MAI disease is rarely found in children with AIDS, although the organism may be detected in BAL fluid.[101] MAI occurs more commonly in children with transfusion-related AIDS than in children with perinatally acquired infection.[147] In a study of 196 children with AIDS, none of the 22 subjects with MAI had respiratory symptoms.[148] The common symptoms in the MAI-infected children were fever, weight loss, neutropenia, hepatosplenomegaly, and night sweats. Children with MAI had a mean age of 9 years, significantly older than subjects not infected. Children with MAI had mean CD4+ percentages of 2% and mean CD4+ cell counts of 12/mm^3, both significantly lower than the controls without MAI. In this group of children with AIDS, the overall incidence of MAI was 11%, but in those with CD4+ cell counts below 100/mm^3, the incidence rose to 24%. Similar data in children infected with HIV by blood transfusion showed disseminated MAI in those with lower CD4+ counts and greater amounts of p24 antigenemia.[149] Also, pulmonary disease attributable to MAI was not seen. Because the symptoms of disseminated MAI infection are similar to those of advanced HIV disease, the two may be difficult to distinguish on clinical grounds.[148] As drug therapy becomes more effective for MAI,[150-152] this may be an important issue.

Therapy of MAI with standard anti-TB drugs is usually unrewarding. Clarithromycin[153] with the addition of amikacin and/or ciprofloxacin[151] results in clinical improvement but in neither clinical nor microbiologic cure. The author uses rifabutin prophylaxis for patients with low CD4+ counts who are at risk of developing disseminated MAI infection.

Cytomegalovirus Infection

CMV causes diffuse interstitial pneumonia in adults with AIDS. When transbronchial or open lung biopsy is used, the virus is demonstrated in conjunction with intranuclear or intracytoplasmic inclusion bodies.[154] The significance of CMV in BAL fluid is unclear. CMV has been isolated in the BAL fluid of the recipients of bone marrow transplants who have no evidence of pneumonia.[155] In immunosuppressed adults who did not have AIDS, more sensitive methods of detecting CMV in the BAL fluid were not helpful.[156] Both tissue cell culture and spin amplification followed by the use of monoclonal antibody assay to detect the nuclear antigen of CMV were positive in patients without tissue or clinical evidence of CMV pneumonia. In children with AIDS, disseminated CMV is a known opportunistic infection,[37] but pneumonia is rare.[153] When children with PCP and CMV were compared to children with PCP but no evidence of CMV,[157] there was no difference in the severity of disease, need for mechanical ventilation, length of mechanical ventilation, or mortality rates. Infants with CMV pneumonia have been reported,[158] but the method of diagnosis in these subjects is not discussed.

Miscellaneous Viral Infections

Influenza A has been described in adults with AIDS. In one patient, influenza A was clinically indistinguishable from PCP,[159] and the patient did well. Six adults with HIV and influenza were described.[160] Four were infected with influenza B and two with influenza A. The lowest CD4+ cell count was 320/mm^3. All survived, and none developed respiratory failure. Prolonged cough was noted in four, including a subject without preexisting lung disease. HIV-infected children respond to influenza vaccine with antibody production,[161] but their titers are significantly lower than those in children not infected with HIV.

Chandwani et al[162] described 10 HIV-infected children with respiratory syncytial virus infection. Two died, both of whom were coinfected with *Pseudomonas aeruginosa;* one also had PCP. The remaining eight subjects had uncomplicated clinical courses. Three subjects had prolonged shedding (i.e., 25, 23, and 75 days) of respiratory syncytial virus antigen. The last two patients were acutely treated with ribavirin. Prospective data on 102 children confirmed that when HIV-infected children develop respiratory syncytial virus disease, they are less likely to wheeze and more likely to have pneumonia and prolonged shedding of the virus.[163]

Measles caused severe pneumonia in a child with AIDS[164] in whom no rash was seen. The diagnosis was made when the virus grew from lung biopsy specimens. The lung pathologic findings were compatible with those of lymphocytic interstitial pneumonitis (LIP), and the patient's condition improved when corticosteroids were administered before identification of the measles virus.

Bacterial Infections

Despite hypergammaglobulinemia, children with AIDS are at risk for recurrent and severe bacterial infections. Their γ-globulin levels are nonspecific, and they respond poorly to bacterial toxoids.[165] Scott et al[158] reported infection with one or more bacteria in 10 of 14 subjects. Of 46 children with AIDS, 26 (57%) had at least one episode of serious bacterial infection.[166] There were 27 episodes of sepsis, including 5 cases of meningitis. Pneumonia occurred in six, including one with sepsis. In 30 instances, bacteria were recovered from the blood. *Streptococcus pneumoniae* was the most common organism recovered, followed by *Salmonella* species, *Haemophilus influenzae* type b, and *Enterococcus* organisms. Most of the cases of gram-negative sepsis (other than *H. influenzae* or *Salmonella* organisms) occurred in children previously hospitalized. HIV-infected children are at risk for invasive pneumococcal disease.[167] Prospective data on 104 children confirm a greater likelihood of developing invasive bacterial disease[168] after 1 year of age. An HIV-infected child with hemophilia developed acute lower respiratory tract disease caused by *Bordetella pertussis.*[169] This child received his routine pertussis immunizations and had HIV infection from at least age 4 years. The organism was recovered during BAL, which was performed because the child was in respiratory distress.

Marolda et al[170] reviewed 132 admissions to the hospital with pulmonary disease in 50 HIV-infected children over a 6-year period. Not all patients underwent bronchoscopy or lung biopsy, and in 57%, no definitive diagnosis was made. PCP was diagnosed in 12%, bacterial pneumonia in 16%, and pulmonary lymphoid hyperplasia (PLH) and LIP without documented superinfection in 10%. In subjects over 13 years of age, recurrent pneumonia (two or more incidents within 1 year) is an AIDS-defining illness.[141]

NONINFECTIOUS DISORDERS

LIP and PLH

The entities LIP and PLH were both described in the pre-AIDS era. PLH, also referred to as *benign pulmonary lymphoma,* is a generalized hyperplasia of the lymph glands.[171] Enlargement of the subpleural and peribronchial nodes (bronchus-associated lymphoid tissue) is noted. Most cases were asymptomatic, although airway obstruction from the nodes and hemoptysis[171] have occurred. LIP was first described in 1966 by Carrington and Liebow.[172] Spencer[171] considered LIP as part of a continuum with pseudolymphoma and considered both as prelymphomatous disorders. Two siblings with LIP were reported in 1980.[173] They had no evidence of underlying disease and were born before 1970. Three children with hypogammaglobulinemia and LIP were reported in 1981[174]; they had normal T cell numbers and mitogen responses.

In 1986, Rubinstein et al[175] described the differences between PCP and PLH. Subjects with the latter condition had a more gradual onset of disease with a lesser degree of tachypnea, fever, and hypoxemia. On physical examination, they often had diffuse peripheral lymphadenopathy. Digital clubbing was found in all 11 with PLH but none of the patients with PCP. The radiographs of patients with PLH showed diffuse interstitial disease but with a distinctive nodular pattern. The nodules were larger centrally than peripherally (Fig. 41-1). Children with PLH had a lower $P_{AO_2}-Pa_{O_2}$ than patients with PCP, higher serum IgG levels, more modest elevations of LDH, and elevated serum titers to viral capsid antigen of

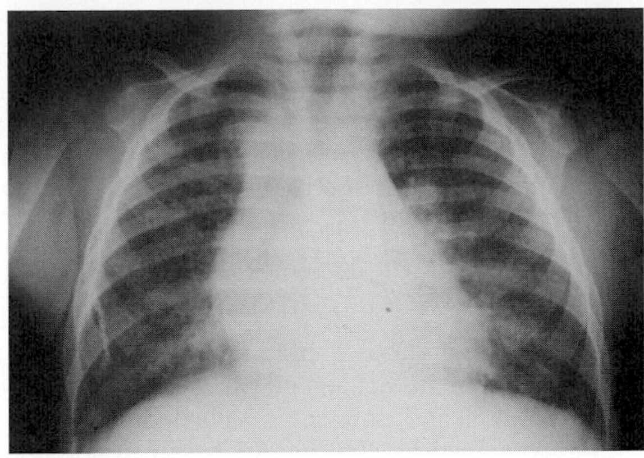

Fig. 41-1. Radiograph of LIP and PLH, revealing multiple nodular densities throughout all lung fields. The nodules are larger centrally than peripherally. Also noted are hilar adenopathy and widening of the mediastinum. (Courtesy Henry Pritzker, Bronx, NY.)

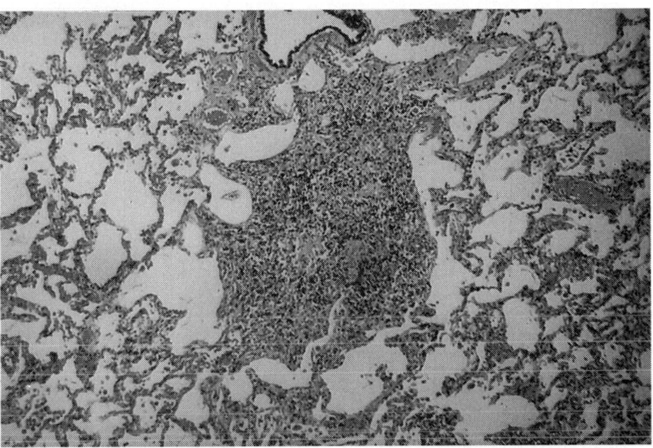

Fig. 41-2. Lung biopsy specimen of a patient with LIP and PLH. There is a diffuse lymphocytic infiltrate present throughout. An aggregate of cells into a germinal center is also seen in the center of the field. (Courtesy Sumi Mitsudo, Bronx, NY.)

Epstein-Barr virus.[176] At biopsy, no child with PLH had PCP. Lung biopsies revealed collections of lymphoid aggregates, often with germinal centers, surrounding the airways. A significant interstitial infiltrate composed primarily of lymphocytes was often seen (Fig. 41-2). Because of the findings compatible with LIP, the entity is occasionally referred to as the *LIP/PLH complex.*

The etiology of LIP/PLH is unknown. Children who develop it have a longer life expectancy than those with PCP.[177] It is rare for children with LIP/PLH to subsequently develop PCP.[175]

The diagnosis of LIP/PLH requires open lung biopsy. Children with PLH have marked BAL lymphocytosis,[178] but the clinician cannot rely on the findings to make a diagnosis because the specificity and sensitivity make the test unreliable for such a purpose. Even in the context of the typical radiographic and clinical findings, the findings from lung tissue are more reliable than BAL results.

LIP/PLH responds to systemic corticosteroids.[179] The author usually reserves treatment for patients who develop significant hypoxemia while awake or asleep. One protocol[179] uses prednisone, 2 mg/kg/day for 2 to 4 weeks, until the partial pressure of oxygen increases by 20 mm Hg. The steroids are then tapered, provided that the partial pressure remains adequate, to 0.5 to 0.75 mg/kg every other day. Further tapering may be possible as long as adequate oxygenation is maintained. No data exist on the use of inhaled corticosteroids at any point in this protocol. The natural course of the lesion is not known.

Kaposi's Sarcoma

KS was one of the diseases found in homosexual males that heralded the onset of this epidemic.[2,180] KS is more common in adults than children and more common in homosexual people than in intravenous drug abusers. KS has been described in young children of Haitian parents in Miami.[181] Although the authors have seen two infants with gastrointestinal bleeding secondary to KS, they have not seen pulmonary KS in young patients. Of 132 people with HIV admitted to the hospital with pulmonary symptoms, none had KS.[170] The author has seen pulmonary KS in two homosexual adolescents with AIDS.

The most common sign is that of violaceous plaques on the skin. The clinical manifestations of pulmonary KS include progressive dyspnea, cough, and fever. Hemoptysis may occur with endobronchial lesions. The degree of hypoxemia is no different from that of adults with opportunistic infections.[176]

Chest radiographs reveal combinations of interstitial, alveolar, and nodular patterns. The finding of poorly marginated discrete lesions on computed tomographic scan may be specific for KS.[182] Enlarged lymph nodes and pleural effusions may be seen. Thoracentesis does not usually help in the definitive diagnosis of KS and reveals an exudate, either serosanguinous or hemorrhagic. The diagnosis is best made by open lung biopsy, although false-negative results occur.[180]

Miscellaneous

Desquamative interstitial pneumonitis, bronchiolitis obliterans, and nonspecific interstitial pneumonitis occur in children with AIDS. The manifestations are progressive dyspnea, hypoxemia, cough, and sometimes fever; radiographs reveal interstitial pneumonitis. The diagnoses are made by open lung biopsy.

Joshi et al[183] described polyclonal polymorphic B cell lymphoproliferative disorder in children with AIDS. In children with this disorder, there is a marked growth of lymphoid tissue throughout the body, including the lungs. Macroscopic examination reveals gross nodules. Microscopic lymphoid infiltrates can be found in any organ. The etiology and history of this lesion are unknown. The lack of cellular atypia, necrosis, or atypical mitoses suggests that this is not truly a malignant lesion. However, the widespread distribution suggests that the lesions may not be completely benign.

Upper Airway Disease

A case of candidal supraglottitis was described[184] with a slowly progressive course and *Candida*-like lesions on the epiglottis, arytenoid cartilages, and aryepiglottic folds. A baby with noninfectious chronic epiglottis had a gradual onset of drooling and difficulty swallowing without respiratory distress.[185] On admission, she was found to have supraglottitis, but no organism was detected. After 33 days, there was no improvement, and a biopsy showed acute and chronic inflammation with granulation tissue and lymphoid follicles in the submucosa.

HIV IN ITS SECOND DECADE

As the HIV epidemic enters its adolescence, the world is starting to see a changing pattern of pulmonary disease.[186] Because of increased awareness and diagnosis of HIV infection, fewer cases of PCP are being seen. With the use of inhaled pentamidine in older children, a different pattern of PCP disease is emerging, with upper lobe predominance, cystic disease, and pneumothorax. Bronchiectasis is seen in older children, usually those who had LIP/PLH earlier in childhood. This is a different pattern of bronchiectasis than clinicians are used to seeing: In children the amount of sputum produced is not large, and *Pseudomonas* infection is rare. Whether the bronchiectasis is part of the new natural history of LIP/PLH or a result of the recurrent infections to which these children are prone is unknown. Finally, pulmonary leiomyomas and leiomyosarcomas are described.[186]

Undoubtedly, as the epidemic continues to grow within the pediatric population and symptomatic therapy allows for improved survival rates, as has happened with CF, new pulmonary manifestations will present as a result of the immunosuppression, the previous infections, and the agents being used to keep the children alive.

REFERENCES

Epidemiology

1. Centers for Disease Control: *Pneumocystis* pneumonia: Los Angeles, *MMWR* 30:250-252, 1981.
2. Centers for Disease Control: Kaposi's sarcoma and *Pneumocystis carinii* pneumonia among homosexual men: New York City and California, *MMWR* 25:305-308, 1981.
3. Centers for Disease Control: *Pneumocystis carinii* pneumonia among persons with hemophilia A, *MMWR* 31:365-367, 1982.
4. Centers for Disease Control: Possible transfusion-associated acquired immune deficiency syndrome: California, *MMWR* 31:652-654, 1982.
5. Ammann AJ, Cowan MJ, Wara DW, Dritz S, Weintrub P, Goldman H, Perkins HA: Acquired immunodeficiency in an infant: possible transmission by means of blood products, *Lancet* 1:956-958, 1983.
6. Schoenbaum EE, Hartel D, Selwyn PA, Klein RS, Davenny K, Rogers M, Feiner C, Friedland G: Risk factors for human immunodeficiency virus infection in intravenous drug users, *N Engl J Med* 321:874-879, 1989.
7. Oleske J, Minnefor A, Cooper R, Thomas K, dela Cruz A, Ahdieh H, Guerrero I, Joshi VV, Desposito F: Immune deficiency syndrome in children, *JAMA* 249:2345-2349, 1983.
8. Rubinstein A, Sicklick M, Gupta A, Bernstein L, Klein N, Rubinstein E, Spigland I, Fruchter L, Litman N, Lee H, Hollander M: Acquired immunodeficiency with reversed T4/T8 ratios in infants born to promiscuous and drug-addicted mothers, *JAMA* 249:2350-2356, 1983.
9. Ammann AJ: Is there an acquired immune deficiency syndrome in infants and children? *Pediatrics* 72:430-432, 1983 (editorial).
10. Barre-Sinoussi F, Chermann JC, Rey F: Isolation of a T-lymphotropic retrovirus from a patient at risk for the acquired immune deficiency syndrome, *Science* 230:868-871, 1983.
11. Gallo RC, Salahuddin SZ, Popovic M: Frequent detection and isolation of cytopathic retroviruses (HTLV-3) from patients with AIDS and at risk for AIDS, *Science* 224:500-503, 1984.
12. Quinn TC, Ruff A, Halsey N: Pediatric acquired immunodeficiency syndrome: special considerations for developing nations, *Pediatr Infect Dis J* 11:558-568, 1992.
13. Rubini NM, Passman LJ: Transmission of human immunodeficiency virus infection from a newly infected mother to her two year old child by breast feeding, *Pediatr Infect Dis J* 11:682-683, 1992.

14. Stiehm ER, Vink P: Transmission of human immunodeficiency virus infection by breast-feeding, *J Pediatr* 118:410-412, 1991.
15. Siegel R, Christie C, Myers M, Duma E, Green L: Incest and *Pneumocystis carinii* pneumonia in a twelve year old girl: a case for early human immunodeficiency virus testing in sexually abused children, *Pediatr Infect Dis J* 11:681-682, 1992.
16. Lindegren ML, Hanson C, Miller K, Byers RH, Onorato I: Epidemiology of human immunodeficiency virus infection in adolescents: United States, *Pediatr Infect Dis J* 13:525-535, 1994.
17. Futterman D, Hein K, Reuben N, Dell R, Shaffer N: Human immunodeficiency virus-infected adolescents: the first 50 patients in a New York City program, *Pediatrics* 91:730-735, 1993.
18. Ellerbrock TV, Bush TJ, Chamberland ME, Oxtoby MJ: Epidemiology of women with AIDS in the United States, 1981 through 1990, *JAMA* 265:2971-2981, 1991.
19. Ellerbrock TV, Lieb S, Harrington PE, Bush TJ, Schoenfisch SA, Oxtoby MJ, Howell JT, Rogers MF, Witte JJ: Heterosexually transmitted human immunodeficiency virus infection among pregnant women in a rural Florida community, *N Engl J Med* 327:1704-1709, 1992.
20. Hoff R, Berardi VP, Weiblen BJ, Mahoney-Trout L, Mitchell ML, Grady GF: Seroprevalence of human immunodeficiency virus among childbearing women, *N Engl J Med* 318:525-530, 1988.
21. Novick LF, Berns D, Stricof R, Stevens R, Pass K, Wethers J: HIV seroprevalence in newborns in New York State, *JAMA* 261:1745-1750, 1989.
22. Landesman S, Minkoff H, Holman S, McCalla S, Sijn O: Serosurvey of human immunodeficiency virus infection in parturients, *JAMA* 258:2701-2703, 1987.
23. Krasinski K, Borkowsky W, Bebenroth D, Moore T: Failure of voluntary testing for human immunodeficiency virus to identify infected parturient women in a high risk population, *N Engl J Med* 318:185, 1988 (letter).
24. Ryder RW, Nsa W, Hassig SE, Behets F, Rayfield M, Ekungola B, Nelson AM, Mulenda U, Francis H, Mwandagalirwa K, Davachi F, Rogers M, Nzilambi N, Greenberg A, Mann J, Quinn TC, Piot P, Curran JW: Perinatal transmission of the human immunodeficiency virus type 1 to infants of seropositive women in Zaire, *N Engl J Med* 320:1637-1642, 1989.
25. Hsu HW, Moye J, Kunches L, Ng P, Shea B, Caldwell B, Demaria A, Mofenson L, Grady GF: Perinatally acquired human immunodeficiency virus infection: extent of clinical recognition in a population-based cohort, *Pediatr Infect Dis J* 11:941-945, 1992.
26. American Academy of Pediatrics: Policy statement, *AAP News* 8:20, 1992.
27. Pratt RD, Hatch R, Dankner WM, Spector SA: Pediatric human immunodeficiency virus infection in a low seroprevalence area, *Pediatr Infect Dis J* 12:304-310, 1993.

Maternal-Fetal Transmission

28. Lapointe N, Michand J, Pekovic D, Chausseau JP, Dupuy J-M: Transplacental transmission of HTLV-III virus, *N Engl J Med* 312:1325-1326, 1985.
29. Marion RW, Wiznia AA, Hutcheon RG, Rubinstein A: Human T-cell lymphotropic virus type III embryopathy: a new dysmorphic syndrome associated with intrauterine HTLV-III infection, *Am J Dis Child* 140:638-640, 1986.
30. Marion RW, Wiznia AA, Hutcheon RG, Rubinstein A: Fetal AIDS syndrome score: correlation between severity of dysmorphism and age at diagnosis of immunodeficiency, *Am J Dis Child* 141:429-431, 1987.
31. Blanche S, Mayaux MUJ, Rouzioux C, Teglas JP, Firtion G, Monpoux F, Cirari-Vigneron N, Meier F, Tricoire J, Courpotin C, Vilmer E, Griscelli C, Delfraissy JF: Relation of the course of HIV infection in children to the severity of the disease in their mothers at delivery, *N Engl J Med* 330:308-312, 1994.
32. Thomas PA, Weeon J, Krasinski K, Abrams E, Shafer N, Matheson P, Bamji M, Kaul A, Hutson D, Grimm KT, Beatrice ST, Rogers M: Maternal predictors of perinatal human immunodeficiency virus transmission, *Pediatr Infect Dis J* 13:489-495, 1994.
33. Kliks SC, Wara DW, Landers DV, Levy JA: Features of HIV-1 that could influence maternal-child transmission, *JAMA* 272:467-474, 1994.
34. Borkowsky W, Krasinski K, Cao Y, Ho D, Pollack H, Moore T, Chen SH, Allen M, Tao PT: Correlation of perinatal transmission of human immunodeficiency virus type 1 with maternal viremia and lymphocyte phenotypes, *J Pediatr* 125:345-351, 1994.
35. Boyer PJ, Dillon M, Navaie M, Deveikis A, Keller M, O'Rourke S, Bryson YJ: Factors predictive of maternal-fetal transmission of HIV-1, *JAMA* 271:1925-1930, 1994.
36. Centers for Disease Control and Prevention: Zidovudine for the prevention of HIV transmission from mother to infant, *MMWR* 43:285-287, 1994.
37. Falloon J, Eddie J, Wiener L, Pizzo PA: Human immunodeficiency virus infection in children, *J Pediatr* 114:1-30, 1989 (review).
38. Jones DS, Abrams E, Ou C-Y, Nesheim S, Connor E, Davenny K, Thomas P, Sawyer M, Krasinski K, Bamji M, Rapier J, Kilbourne B, Rogers M: Lack of detectable human immunodeficiency virus infection in antibody-negative children born to human immunodeficiency virus-infected mothers, *Pediatr Infect Dis J* 12:222-227, 1992.
39. Lepage P, Van de Perre P, Simonon A, Msellati P, Hitimana DG, Dabis F: Transient seroreversion in children born to human immunodeficiency virus 1-infected mothers, *Pediatr Infect Dis J* 11:892-893, 1992.
40. Husson RN, Comeau AM, Hoff R: Diagnosis of human immunodeficiency virus infection in infants and children, *Pediatrics* 86:1-10, 1990.
41. Paul DA, Falk LA, Kessler HA: Correlation of serum HIV antigen and antibody with clinical status in HIV-infected patients, *J Med Virol* 22:357-363, 1987.
42. European Collaborative Study: Mother-to-child transmission of HIV infection, *Lancet* 2:1039-1043, 1988.
43. Burgard M, Mayaux MJ, Blanche S, Ferroni A, Guihard-Moscato ML, Allemon MC, Ciraru-Vigneron N, Firtion G, Floch C, Guillot F, Lachassine E, Vial M, Griscelli C, Rouzioux C: The use of viral culture and p24 antigen testing to diagnose human immunodeficiency virus infection in neonates, *N Engl J Med* 217:1192-1197, 1992.
44. Miles SA, Balden E, Magpantay L, Wei LA, Leiblein A, Hofheinz D, Toedter G, Stiehm ER, Bryson Y: Rapid serologic testing with immune-complex–dissociated HIV p24 antigen for early detection of HIV infection in neonates, *N Engl J Med* 328:297-302, 1993.
45. Kline MW, Hollinger FB, Rosenblatt HM, Bohannon B, Kozinetz CA, Shearer WT: Sensitivity, specificity and predictive value of physical examination, culture and other laboratory studies in the diagnosis during early infancy of vertically acquired human immunodeficiency virus infection, *Pediatr Infect Dis J* 12:33-36, 1993.
46. Krivine A, Yakudima A, LeMay M, Pena-Cruz V, Huang AS, McIntosh K: A comparative study of virus isolation, polymerase chain reaction, and antigen detection in children of mothers infected with human immunodeficiency virus, *J Pediatr* 116:372-376, 1990.
47. Mayers MM, Davenny K, Schoenbaum EE, Feingold AR, Selwyn PA, Robertson V, Ou CY, Rogers MF, Naccarato M: A prospective study of infants of human immunodeficiency virus seropositive and seronegative women with a history of intravenous drug-using sex partners, in the Bronx, New York City, *Pediatrics* 88:1248-1256, 1991.
48. Hutto C, Parks WP, Lai S, Mastrucci MT, Mitchell C, Munoz J, Trapido E, Master IM, Scott GB: A hospital-based prospective study of perinatal infection with human immunodeficiency virus type 1, *J Pediatr* 118:347-353, 1991.
49. Johnson JP, Nair P, Hines SE, Seiden SW, Alger L, Revie DR, O'Neil KM, Hebel R: Natural history and serologic diagnosis of infants born to human immunodeficiency virus-infected women, *Am J Dis Child* 143:1147-1149, 1989.
50. Gabiano C, Tovo PA, deMartino M, Galli L, Giaquinto C, Loy A, Schoeller MC, Giovannini M, Ferranti G, Rancillio L, Caselli D, Segni G, Livadiotti S, Conte A, Rizzi M, Viggiano D, Mazza A, Ferrazzin A, Tozzi A, Cappello N: Mother-to-child transmission of human immunodeficiency virus type 1: risk of infection and correlates of transmission, *Pediatrics* 90:369-374, 1992.

AIDS in the Infant

51. McKinney RE, Robertson JWR: Effect of human immunodeficiency virus infection on the growth of young children, *J Pediatr* 123:579-582, 1993.
52. Rogers MF, Thomas PA, Starcher ET, Noa MC, Bush TJ, Jaffe HW: Acquired immunodeficiency syndrome in children: report of the Centers for Disease Control National Surveillance, 1982 to 1985, *Pediatrics* 79:1008-1014, 1987.
53. Duliege AM, Messiah A, Blanche S, Tardieu M, Griscelli C, Spira A: Natural history of human immunodeficiency virus type 1 infection in children: prognostic value of laboratory tests on the bimodal progression of the disease, *Pediatr Infect Dis J* 11:630-635, 1992.

54. Working Group on Antiretroviral Therapy, National Pediatric HIV Resource Center: Antiretroviral therapy and medical management of the human immunodeficiency virus-infected child, *Pediatr Infect Dis J* 12:513-522, 1993 (review).
55. Hirsch MS, D'Aquila RT: Therapy for human immunodeficiency virus infection, *N Engl J Med* 328:1686-1694, 1993.
56. Rigaud M, Pollack H, Leibovitz E, Kim M, Persaud D, Kaul A, Lawrence R, Di John D, Borkowsky W, Krasinski K: Efficacy of primary chemoprophylaxis against *Pneumocystis carinii* pneumonia during the first year of life in infants infected with human immunodeficiency virus type 1, *J Pediatr* 125:476-480, 1994.
57. Butler KM, Husson RN, Lewis LL, Mueller BU, Venzon D, Pizzo PA: CD4 status and p24 antigenemia: are they useful predictors of survival in HIV-infected children receiving antiretroviral therapy? *Am J Dis Child* 146:932-936, 1992.
58. McKinney RE, Wilfert CM: Lymphocyte subsets in children younger than 2 years old: normal values in a population at risk for human immunodeficiency virus infection and diagnostic and prognostic application to infected children, *Pediatr Infect Dis J* 11:639-644, 1992.
59. Centers for Disease Control: Guidelines for prophylaxis against *Pneumocystis carinii* pneumonia for children infected with human immunodeficiency virus, *MMWR* 40:1-13, 1991.
60. Kline MW, Shearer WT: A national survey on the care of infants and children with human immunodeficiency virus infection, *J Pediatr* 118:817-821, 1991.
61. Simmonds RJ, Lindegren ML, Thomas P, Hanson D, Caldwell B, Scott G, Rogers M: Prophylaxis against *Pneumocystis carinii* pneumonia among children with perinatally acquired human immunodeficiency virus infection in the United States, *N Engl J Med* 332:786-790, 1995.
62. Boucher FD, Modlin JF, Weller S, Ruff AM, Mirochnick M, Pelton S, Wilfert C, Mckinney R, Crain MJ, Elkins MM, Blum MR, Prober CG: Phase 1 evaluation of zidovudine administered to infants exposed at birth to the human immunodeficiency virus, *J Pediatr* 122:137-144, 1993.
63. Husson RN, Mueller BU, Farley M, Woods L, Kovacs A, Goldsmith JC, Ono J, Lewis LL, Balis FM, Brouwers P, Avramis VI, Church JA, Butler KM, Rasheed S, Jarosinski P, Venzon D, Pizzo PA: Zidovudine and didanosine combination therapy in children with human immunodeficiency virus infection, *Pediatrics* 93:316-322, 1994.

Lung Defense

64. Agostini C, Trentin L, Zambello R, Semenzato G: State of the Art: HIV-1 and the lung, *Am Rev Respir Dis* 147:1038-1049, 1993.
65. Garner S, Markovits P, Markovits DM, Kaplan MH, Gallo RC, Popovic M: The role of mononuclear phagocytes in HIV infection, *Science* 232:215-219, 1988.
66. Rankin JA: Pulmonary immunology, *Clin Chest Med* 9:387-394, 1988 (review).
67. DeMaria A, Pantaleo G, Schnittman SM, Greenhouse JE, Baseler M, Orenstein JM, Fauci AS: Infection of CD8 lymphocytes: requirement for interaction with infected CD4 cells and induction of infectious virus from chronically infected CD8 cells, *J Immunol* 146:2220-2226, 1991.
68. Twigg HL, Lipscomb MF, Yoffe B, Barbaro DJ, Weissler JC: Enhanced accessory cell function by alveolar macrophages from patients infected with the human immunodeficiency virus: potential role for depletion of CD4 cells in the lung, *Am J Respir Cell Mol Biol* 1:391-400, 1989.
69. Pantoleo G Graziosi C, Fauci AS: The immunopathogenesis of human immunodeficiency virus infection, *N Engl J Med* 328:327-335, 1993 (review).
70. Golding H, Robey FA, Gates FT: Common epitope in HIV GP41 and human MHC class II beta 1 domain, *J Exp Med* 167:914-923, 1988.
71. Golding H, Shearer GM, Hillman K: Common epitope in HIV GP41 and HLA class II elicits immunosuppressive autoantibodies capable of contributing to immune dysfunction in HIV infected individuals, *J Clin Invest* 83:1430-1435, 1989.
72. Amadori A, deSilvestro G, Zamarchi R: CD4 epitope masking by gp120/antigp120 antibody complexes: a potential mechanism for CD4+ cell function down-regulation in AIDS patients, *J Immunol* 148:2709-2716, 1992.
73. Lane HC, Masur H, Edgar LC: Abnormalities of B-cell activation and immunoregulation in patients with the acquired immunodeficiency syndrome, *N Engl J Med* 309:453-458, 1984.
74. Breen EC, Rezai AR, Nakajima K, Beall GN, Mitsuyasu RT, Hirano T, Kishimoto T, Martinez-Maza O: Infection with HIV is associated with elevated IL-6 levels and production, *J Immunol* 144:480-484, 1990.
75. Autran B, Mayaud C, Raphael M, Plata F, Denis M, Bourguin A, Guillon JM, Debre P, Akoun G: Evidence for a cytotoxic T lymphocyte alveolitis in human immunodeficiency virus-infected patients, *AIDS* 1:179-183, 1988.
76. Plata F, Autran B, Martins LP, Wain-Hobson S, Raphael M, Mayaud C, Denis M, Guillon JM, Debre P: AIDS virus specific cytotoxic T lymphocytes in lung disorders, *Nature* 328:348-351, 1987.
77. Chayt KJ, Harper ME, Marselle LM, Lewin EB, Rose RM, Oleske JM, Epstein LG, Soong-Staal F, Gallo RC: Detection of HIV RNA in lungs of patients with AIDS and pulmonary involvement, *JAMA* 256:2356-2359, 1986.
78. Ho DD, Moudgil T, Alam M: Quantitation of human immunodeficiency virus in the blood of infected persons, *N Engl J Med* 321:1621-1625, 1990.
79. Salahuddin SZ, Rose RM, Groopman JE, Markham PD, Gallo RC: Human T lymphotropic virus type III infection of human alveolar macrophages, *Blood* 68:281-284, 1986.
80. Murray HW, Gellene RA, Libby DM, Rothemel CD, Rubin BY: Activation of tissue macrophages from AIDS patients: in vitro response of AIDS alveolar macrophages to lymphokines and interferon-gamma, *J Immunol* 135:2374-2377, 1987.
81. Trentin L, Garbisa S, Zambello R, Agostini C, Caenazzo C, DiFrancesco C, Cipriani A, Francavilla E, Semenzato G: Spontaneous production of IL-6 by alveolar macrophages of HIV-1 seropositive patients, *J Infect Dis* 116:731-737, 1992.
82. Poli G, Bressler P, Kinter A: Interleukin-6 induced HIV expression in infected monocytic cells alone and in synergy with tumor necrosis alpha by transcriptional and post-transcriptional mechanisms, *J Exp Med* 172:151-158, 1990.
83. Molina JF, Scadden D, Bym R, Dinarello CA, Groopman JE: Production of tumor necrosis factor alpha and interleukin 1beta by monocytic cells infected with human immunodeficiency virus, *J Clin Invest* 84:733-737, 1989.
84. Israel-Biet D, Cadrenel J, Beldjord K, Andrieu JM, Jeffrey A, Even P: Tumor necrosis factor production in HIV-seropositive subjects: relationship with lung opportunistic infections and HIV expression in alveolar macrophages, *J Immunol* 147:490-494, 1991.
85. Poli G, Kinter A, Justement JS: Tumor necrosis factor alpha functions in an autocrine manner in the induction of human immunodeficiency virus expression, *Proc Natl Acad Sci USA* 87:782-785, 1990.
86. Mellors JW, Griffith BP, Ortiz MA, Landry ML, Ryan JL: Tumor necrosis factor alpha/cachectin enhanced replication in primary macrophages, *J Infect Dis* 163:78-82, 1991.
87. Israel-Biet D, Cadranel J, Even P: Human immunodeficiency virus production by alveolar lymphocytes is increased during *Pneumocystis carinii* pneumonia, *Am Rev Respir Dis* 148:1308-1312, 1993.
88. Agostini C, Zembello R, Trentin L, Feruglio C, Masciarelli M, Siviero E, Poletti V, Spiga L, Gritti F, Semenzato G: Cytotoxic events taking place in the lung of patients with HIV-1 infection, *Am Rev Respir Dis* 142:516-522, 1990.
89. Johnson JE, Anders GT, Hawkes CE, LaHatte LJ, Blanton HM: Bronchoalveolar lavage findings in patients seropositive for the human immunodeficiency virus, *Chest* 97:1066-1071, 1990.
90. White DA, Gellene RA, Gupta S, Cunningham-Rundles C, Stover DE: Pulmonary cell populations in the immunosuppressed patient: bronchoalveolar lavage findings during episodes of pneumonitis, *Chest* 88:352-359, 1985.
91. Young KR, Rankin JA, Naegel GP, Paul ES, Reynolds HY: Bronchoalveolar lavage cells and proteins in patients with the acquired immunodeficiency syndrome: an immunologic analysis, *Ann Intern Med* 103:522-533, 1985.

Opportunistic Infections of the Lung

92. Hughes WT: *Pneumocystis carinii* pneumonia: new approaches to diagnosis, treatment and prevention, *Pediatr Infect Dis J* 10:391-399, 1991 (review).
93. Batungwanayo J, Taelman H, Lucas S, Bogaerts J, Alard D, Kagame A, Blanche P, Clerinx J, Van de Perre P, Allen S: Pulmonary disease associated with the human immunodeficiency virus in Kigali, Rwanda, *Am J Respir Crit Care Med* 149:1591-1596, 1994.

94. Bye MR, Bernstein LJ, Glaser J, Kleid D: *Pneumocystis carinii* pneumonia in young children with AIDS, *Pediatr Pulmonol* 9:251-253, 1990.
95. Vernon DD, Holzman BH, Lewis P, Scott GB, Birriel HA, Scott MB: Respiratory failure in children with acquired immunodeficiency syndrome and acquired immunodeficiency syndrome-related complex, *Pediatrics* 82:223-228, 1988.
96. Kagawa FT, Kirsch CM, Yenokida GG, Levine ML: Serum lactate dehydrogenase activity in patients with AIDS and *Pneumocystis carinii* pneumonia, *Chest* 94:1031-1033, 1988.
97. Garay SM, Greene J: Prognostic indicators in the initial presentation of *Pneumocystis carinii* pneumonia, *Chest* 95:769-772, 1989.
98. Bernstein LJ, Bye MR, Rubinstein A: Prognostic factors and life expectancy in children with acquired immunodeficiency syndrome and *Pneumocystis carinii* pneumonia, *Am J Dis Child* 143:775-778, 1989.
99. Gill VJ, Evans G, Stock F, Parrillo JE, Masur H, Kovacs JA: Detection of *Pneumocystis carinii* pneumonia by fluorescent-antibody stain using a combination of three monoclonal antibodies, *J Clin Microbiol* 25:1837-1840, 1987.
100. Tollerud DJ, Wesseler RA, Kim CK, Baughman RP: Use of a rapid differential stain for identifying *Pneumocystis carinii* in bronchoalveolar lavage fluid, *Chest* 95:494-497, 1989.
101. Bye MR, Bernstein L, Shah K, Ellaurie M, Rubinstein A: Diagnostic bronchoalveolar lavage in children with AIDS, *Pediatr Pulmonol* 3:425-428, 1987.
102. Birriel JA, Adams JA, Saldana MA, Mavunda K, Goldfinger S, Vernon D, Holzman B, McKey RM: Role of flexible bronchoscopy and bronchoalveolar lavage in the diagnosis of pediatric acquired immunodeficiency syndrome-related pulmonary disease, *Pediatrics* 87:897-899, 1991.
103. Ognibene GP, Gill VJ, Pizzo PA, Kovacs JA, Godwin C, Suffredini AF, Shelhamer JH, Parrillo JE, Masur H: Induced sputum to diagnose *Pneumocystis carinii* pneumonia in immunosuppressed pediatric patients, *J Pediatr* 115:430-433, 1989.
104. Masur H: Prevention and treatment of *Pneumocystis* pneumonia, *N Engl J Med* 3278:1853-1860, 1992 (review).
105. Lee BL, Medina I, Benowitz NL, Jacob P, Wofsy CB, Mills JV: Dapsone, trimethoprim and sulfamethoxazole plasma levels during treatment of *Pneumocystis* pneumonia in patients with AIDS: evidence of drug interactions, *Ann Intern Med* 110:606-611, 1989.
106. Allegra CJ, Chabner BA, Tuazon CU, Ogata-Arakaki D, Baird B, Drake JC, Simmons JT, Lack EE, Shelhamer JH, Balis F, Walker R, Kovacs JA, Lane HC, Masur H: Trimetrexate for the treatment of *Pneumocystis carinii* pneumonia in patients with the acquired immunodeficiency syndrome, *N Engl J Med* 317:978-985, 1987.
107. Noskin GA, Murphy RL, Black JR, Phair JP: Salvage therapy with clindamycin/primaquine for *Pneumocystis carinii* pneumonia, *Clin Infect Dis* 14:183-188, 1992.
108. Falloon J, Kovacs J, Hughes W, O'Neill D, Polis M, Davey RT, Rogers M, LaFox S, Feuerstein I, Lancaster D, Land M, Tuazon C, Dohn M, Greenberg S, Lane HC, Masur H: A preliminary evaluation of 566C80 for the treatment of *Pneumocystis* pneumonia in patients with the acquired immunodeficiency syndrome, *N Engl J Med* 325:1354-1358, 1991.
109. Gagnon S, Boota AM, Fischl MA, Baier H, Kirksey OW, LaVoie L: Corticosteroids as adjunctive therapy for severe *Pneumocystis carinii* pneumonia in the acquired immunodeficiency syndrome, *N Engl J Med* 323:1444-1450, 1990.
110. Bozzette SA, Sattler FR, Chiu J, Wu AW, Gluckstein D, Kemper C, Bartok A, Niosi J, Abramson I, Coffman J, Hughlett C, Loya R, Cassens B, Akil B, Meng TC, Boylen CT, Nielsen D, Richman DD, Tilles JG, Leedom J, McCutchan JA: A controlled trial of early adjunctive treatment with corticosteroids for *Pneumocystis carinii* pneumonia in the acquired immunodeficiency syndrome, *N Engl J Med* 323:1451-1457, 1990.
111. Bye MR, Carins-Bazarian AM, Ewig JM: Markedly reduced mortality associated with corticosteroid therapy of *Pneumocystis carinii* pneumonia in children with AIDS, *Arch Pediatr Adolesc Med* 148:638-641, 1994.
112. Sleasman JW, Hemenway C, Klein AS, Barrett, DJ: Corticosteroids improve survival of children with AIDS and *Pneumocystis carinii* pneumonia, *Am J Dis Child* 147:30-34, 1993.
113. Jones BE, Taikwel EK, Mercado AL, Sian SU, Barnes PF: Tuberculosis in patients with HIV infection who receive corticosteroids for presumed *Pneumocystis carinii* pneumonia, *Am J Respir Crit Care Med* 149:1686-1688, 1994.
114. Ferdman RM, Church JA: Immunologic and virologic effects of glucocorticoids on human immunodeficiency virus infection in children: a preliminary study, *Pediatr Infect Dis J* 13:212-216, 1994.
115. Connor E: Pediatric HIV infection, *J Respir Dis* 14:75-90, 1993 (review).
116. Orcutt TA, Godwin CR, Pizzo PA, Ognibene FP: Aerosolized pentamidine: a well-tolerated mode of prophylaxis against *Pneumocystis carinii* pneumonia in older children with human immunodeficiency virus infection, *Pediatr Infect Dis J* 11:290-294, 1992.
117. Hand IL, Wiznia AA, Porricolo M, Lambert G, Caspe WB: Aerosolized pentamidine for prophylaxis of *Pneumocystis carinii* pneumonia in infants with human immunodeficiency virus infection, *Pediatr Infect Dis J* 13:100-104, 1994.
118. Stavole JJ, Noel GJ: Efficacy and safety of dapsone prophylaxis against *Pneumocystis carinii* pneumonia in human immunodeficiency virus infected children, *Pediatr Infect Dis J* 12:644-647, 1993.
119. Barnett ED, Pelton SI, Mirochnick M, Cooper ER: Dapsone for prevention of *Pneumocystis* pneumonia in children with acquired immunodeficiency syndrome, *Pediatr Infect Dis J* 13:72-74, 1994.
120. Cruciani M, Concia E, Gatti G, Fioredda F, Bassetti D: Dapsone prophylaxis against *Pneumocystis carinii* pneumonia in human immunodeficiency virus-infected children, *Pediatr Infect Dis J* 13:80-81, 1994.
121. Schneider MME, Hoepelman AIM, Schattenkerk JKME, Nielsen TL, van der Graaf Y, Frissen JPHJ, van der Ende IME, Kolsters AFP, Borleffs JCC: A controlled trial of aerosolized pentamidine or trimethoprim-sulfamethoxazole as primary prophylaxis against *Pneumocystis carinii* pneumonia in patients with human immunodeficiency virus infection, *N Engl J Med* 327:1836-1841, 1992.
122. Hardy WD, Feinberg J, Finkelstein DM, Power ME, He W, Kaczka C, Frame PT, Holmes M, Waskin H, Fass RJ, Powderly WG, Steigbigel RT, Zuger A, Holzman RS: A controlled trial of trimethoprim-sulfamethoxazole or aerosolized pentamidine for secondary prophylaxis of *Pneumocystis carinii* pneumonia in patients with the acquired immunodeficiency syndrome, *N Engl J Med* 327:1842-1848, 1992.
123. Fahy JV, Chin DP, Schnapp LM, Steiger DJ, Schaumberg TH, Geaghan SM, Klein JS, Hopewell PC: Effect of aerosolized pentamidine prophylaxis on the clinical severity and diagnosis of *Pneumocystis carinii* pneumonia, *Am Rev Respir Dis* 146:844-848, 1992.
124. Jules-Elysee KM, Stover DE, Zaman MB, Bernard EM, White DA: Aerosolized pentamidine: effect on diagnosis and presentation of *Pneumocystis carinii* pneumonia, *Ann Intern Med* 112:750-757, 1990.
125. O'Riordan TG, Smaldone GC: Regional deposition and regional ventilation during inhalation of pentamidine, *Chest* 105:395-401, 1994.
126. Read CA, Reddy VD, O'Mara TE, Richardon MSA: Doxycycline pleurodesis for pneumothorax in patients with AIDS, *Chest* 105:823-825, 1994.
127. Read CA, Cerrone F, Busseniers AE, Waldhorn RE, Lavelle JP, Pierce PF: Differential lobe lavage for diagnosis of acute *Pneumocystis carinii* pneumonia in patients receiving prophylactic aerosolized pentamidine therapy, *Chest* 103:1520-1523, 1993.
128. Barnes PF, Bloch AB, Davidson PT, Snider DE: Current concepts: tuberculosis in patients with human immunodeficiency virus infection, *N Engl J Med* 324:1644-1650, 1991.
129. Cantwell MF, Snider DE, Cauthen GM, Onorato IM: Epidemiology of tuberculosis in the United States, 1985 through 1992, *JAMA* 272:535-539, 1994.
130. Villalbi JR, Cayla JA, Iglesias B, Ferrer A, Casanas P: The evolution of tuberculosis infection among schoolchildren in Barcelona and the HIV epidemic, *Tubercle Lung Dis* 75:105-109, 1994.
131. Moss WJ, Dedyo T, Suarez M, Nicholas SW, Abrams E: Tuberculosis in children infected with human immunodeficiency virus: a report of five cases, *Pediatr Infect Dis J* 11:114-120, 1992.
132. Khouri YF, Mastrucci MT, Hutto C, Mitchell CD, Scott GB: *Mycobacterium* tuberculosis in children with human immunodeficiency virus type 1 infection, *Pediatr Infect Dis J* 11:950-955, 1992.
133. Chintu HL, Zumla A: Seroprevalence of human immunodeficiency virus type 1 infection in Zambian children with tuberculosis, *Pediatr Infect Dis J* 12:499-504, 1993.

134. Luo C, Chintu C, Bhat G, Raviglione M, Diwan V, DuPont HL, Zumla A: Human immunodeficiency virus type 1 infection in Zambian children with tuberculosis, *Tubercle Lung Dis* 75:110-115, 1994.
135. Braun MM, Byers RH, Heyward WL: Acquired immunodeficiency syndrome and extrapulmonary tuberculosis in the United States, *Arch Intern Med* 150:1913-1916, 1990.
136. Chaisson RE, Schecter GF, Theuer CP, Rutherford GW, Echenberg DF, Hopewell PC: Tuberculosis in patients with the acquired immunodeficiency syndrome: clinical features, response to therapy and survival, *Am Rev Respir Dis* 136:570-574, 1987.
137. Steiner P, Rao M, Mitchell M, Steiner M: Primary drug-resistant tuberculosis in children, *Am Rev Respir Dis* 134:446-448, 1986.
138. Frieden TR, Sterling T, Pables-Mendez A, Kilburn JO, Cauthen GM, Dooley SW: The emergence of drug-resistant tuberculosis in New York City, *N Engl J Med* 328:521-526, 1993.
139. Committee on Infectious Disease: *Report of the Committee on Infectious Diseases,* American Academy of Pediatrics, 1997, Elk Grove Village, Ill, pp 541-562.
140. Centers for Disease Control and Prevention: Initial therapy for tuberculosis in the era of multidrug resistance: recommendations of the Advisory Council for the Elimination of Tuberculosis, *MMWR* 42:1-8, 1993.
141. Centers for Disease Control and Prevention: 1993 revised classification system for HIV infection and expanded surveillance case definition for AIDS among adolescents and adults, *MMWR* 41:1-19(RR), 1992.
142. Powell DA, Walker DH; Nontuberculous mycobacterial endobronchitis in children, *J Pediatr* 968:268-270, 1980.
143. Kelsey DS, Chambers RT, Hudspeth AS: Nontuberculous mycobacterial infection presenting as a mediastinal mass, *J Pediatr* 98:431-432, 1981.
144. Lincoln EM, Gilbert LA: Disease in children due to mycobacteria other than mycobacterium tuberculosis, *Am Rev Respir Dis* 105:683-714, 1972.
145. Murray JF, Felton CP, Garay SM, Gottlieb MS, Hopewell PC, Stover DE, Teirstein AS: Pulmonary complications of the acquired immunodeficiency syndrome, *N Engl J Med* 310:1682-1688, 1984 (review).
146. Rigsby MO, Curtis AM: Pulmonary disease from nontuberculous mycobacteria in patients with human immunodeficiency virus, *Chest* 106:913-919, 1994.
147. Horsburgh CR, Caldwell B, Simonds RJ: Epidemiology of disseminated nontuberculous mycobacterial disease in children with acquired immunodeficiency syndrome, *Pediatr Infect Dis J* 12:219-222, 1993.
148. Lewis LL, Butler KM, Husson RN, Mueller BU, Fowler CL, Steinberg SM, Pizzo PA: Defining the population of human immunodeficiency virus-infected children at risk for *Mycobacterium avium intracellular* infection, *J Pediatr* 121:677-683, 1992.
149. Gleason-Mogan D, Church JA, Ross LA: A comparative study of transfusion-acquired human immunodeficiency virus-infected children with and without disseminated *Mycobacterium avium complex, Pediatr Infect Dis J* 13:484-488, 1994.
150. Horsburgh CR, Havlik JA, Ellis DA: Survival of patients with acquired immune deficiency syndrome and disseminated *Mycobacterium avium* complex infection with and without antimycobacterial chemotherapy, *Am Rev Respir Dis* 144:557-559, 1991.
151. Hoy J, Mijch A, Sandland M, Grayson L, Lucas R, Dwyer B: Quadruple drug therapy for *Mycobacterium avium intracellulare* bacteremia in AIDS patients, *J Infect Dis* 161:801-805, 1990.
152. Chiu J, Nussbaum J, Bozzette S: Treatment of disseminated *Mycobacterium avium* complex infection in AIDS with amikacin, ethambutol, rifampin and ciprofloxacin, *Ann Intern Med* 113:358-461, 1990.
153. Wallace RJ, Brown BA, Griffith DE, Girard WM, Murphy DT, Onyi GO, Steingrube VA, Mazurek GH: Initial clarithromycin monotherapy for *Mycobacterium avium-intracellulare* complex lung disease, *Am J Respir Crit Care Med* 149:1335-1341, 1994.
154. Mustafa MM: Cytomegalovirus infection and disease in the immunocompromised host, *Pediatr Infect Dis J* 13:249-259, 1994 (review).
155. Ruutu P, Ruutu T, Volin L, Tukiainen P, Ukkonen P, Hovi T: Cytomegalovirus is frequently isolated in bronchoalveolar lavage fluid of bone marrow transplant recipients without pneumonia, *Ann Intern Med* 112:913-916, 1990.
156. Woods GL, Thompson AB, Rennard SL, Linder J: Detection of cytomegalovirus in bronchoalveolar lavage specimens, *Chest* 98:568-575, 1990.
157. Glaser JH, Schuval S, Burstein O, Bye MR: Cytomegalovirus and *Pneumocystis carinii* pneumonia in children with acquired immunodeficiency syndrome, *J Pediatr* 120:929-931, 1992.
158. Scott GB, Buck BE, Peterman JG, Bloom FL, Parks WP: Acquired immunodeficiency syndrome in infants, *N Engl J Med* 310:76-81, 1984.
159. Thurn JR, Henry K: Influenza A pneumonitis in a patient infected with HIV, *Chest* 95:807-810, 1989.
160. Safrin S, Rush JD, Mills J: Influenza in patients with human immunodeficiency virus infection, *Chest* 98:33-37, 1990.
161. Chadwick EG, Chang G, Decker MD, Yogev R, Dimechele D, Edwards KM: Serologic response to standard inactivated influenza vaccine in human immunodeficiency virus-infected children, *Pediatr Infect Dis J* 13:206-211, 1994.
162. Chandwani S, Borkowsky W, Krasinski K, Lawrence R, Welliver R: Respiratory syncytial virus infection in human immunodeficiency virus infected children, *J Pediatr* 117:251-254, 1990.
163. King JC, Burke AR, Clemens JD, Nair P, Farley JJ, Vink PE, Batlas SR, Rao M, Johnson JP: Respiratory syncytial virus illnesses in human immunodeficiency virus and noninfected children, *Pediatr Infect Dis J* 12:733-739, 1993.
164. Park CL, Kirschner BS, Abrahams C: Measles pneumonia in a child with HIV infection, *Pediatr AIDS HIV Infect* 4:83-87, 1993.
165. Borkowsky W, Steele CJ, Grubman S, Moore T, LaRussa P, Krasinski K: Antibody responses to bacterial toxoids in children infected with human immunodeficiency virus, *J Pediatr* 110:563-566, 1987.
166. Bernstein LJ, Krieger BZ, Novick B, Sicklick MJ, Rubinstein A: Bacterial infection in the acquired immunodeficiency syndrome of children, *Pediatr Infect Dis J* 4:472-475, 1985.
167. Farley JJ, King JC, Nair P, Hines SE, Tressler RL, Vink PE: Invasive pneumococcal disease among infected and uninfected children of mothers with human immunodeficiency virus infection, *J Pediatr* 124:853-858, 1994.
168. Andiman WA, Mezger JA, Shapiro E: Invasive bacterial infections in children born to women infected with human immunodeficiency virus type 1, *J Pediatr* 124:846-852, 1994.
169. Adamson PC, Wu TC, Meade BD, Rubin M, Manclark CR, Pizzo PA: Pertussis in a previously immunized child with human immunodeficiency virus infection, *J Pediatr* 115:589-591, 1989.
170. Marolda J, Pace B, Bonforte RJ, Kotin NM, Rabinowitz J, Kattan M: Pulmonary manifestations of HIV infection in children, *Pediatr Pulmonol* 10:231-235, 1991.

Noninfectious Disorders

171. Spencer H: *Pathology of the lung,* Philadelphia, 1977, WB Saunders, pp 937-942.
172. Carrington CB, Liebow AA: Lymphocytic interstitial pneumonia, *Am J Pathol* 48:36a, 1966.
173. O'Brodovich HM, Moser MM, Lu L: Familial lymphoid interstitial pneumonia: a long-term follow-up, *Pediatrics* 65:523-528, 1980.
174. Church JA, Isaacs H, Saxon A, Keens TG, Richards W: Lymphoid interstitial pneumonitis and hypogammaglobulinemia in children, *Am Rev Respir Dis* 124:491-496, 1981.
175. Rubinstein A, Morecki R, Silverman B, Charytan M, Krieger BA, Andiman W, Ziprkowski MN, Goldman H: Pulmonary disease in children with acquired immune deficiency syndrome and AIDS-related complex, *J Pediatr* 108:498-503, 1986.
176. Katz BZ, Berkman AB, Shapiro ED: Serologic evidence of active Epstein-Barr virus infection in Epstein-Barr virus–associated lymphoproliferative disorders of children with acquired immunodeficiency syndrome, *J Pediatr* 120:228-232, 1992.
177. Turner BJ, Denison M, Eppes SC, Houchens R, Fanning T, Markson LE: Survival experience of 789 children with the acquired immunodeficiency syndrome, *Pediatr Infect Dis J* 12:310-320, 1993.
178. deBlic J, Blanche S, Danel C, LeBourgeois M, Caniglia M, Scheinmann P: Bronchoalveolar lavage in HIV infected patients with interstitial pneumonitis, *Arch Dis Child* 64:1246-1250, 1989.
179. Rubinstein A, Bernstein LJ, Charytan M, Krieger BA, Ziprkowski M: Corticosteroid treatment for pulmonary lymphoid hyperplasia in children with the acquired immune deficiency syndrome, *Pediatr Pulmonol* 4:13-17, 1988.
180. Ognibene FP, Shelhamer JH: Kaposi's sarcoma, *Chest Clin North Am* 9:459-465, 1988.

181. Buck BE, Scott GB, Valdes-Dapena M, Parks WP: Kaposi sarcoma in two infants with acquired immune deficiency syndrome, *J Pediatr* 103:911-913, 1983.
182. Naidich DP, Tarras M, Garay SM, Birnbaum B, Rybak BJ, Schinella R: Kaposi's sarcoma: CT-radiographic correlation, *Chest* 96:723-728, 1989.
183. Joshi VV, Kauffman S, Oleske JM, Fikrig S, Denny T, Gadol C, Lee E: Polyclonal polymorphic B-cell lymphoproliferative disorder with prominent pulmonary involvement in children with acquired immune deficiency syndrome, *Cancer* 59:1455-1462, 1987.
184. Bye MR, Palomba A, Bernstein L, Shah K: Clinical *Candida* supraglottitis in an infant with AIDS-related complex, *Pediatr Pulmonol* 3:280-281, 1987.
185. Diamant EP, Dische RM, Barzilai A, Hodes DS, Peters VB: Chronic epiglottitis in a child with acquired immunodeficiency syndrome, *Pediatr Infect Dis J* 11:770-771, 1992.

HIV in Its Second Decade

186. Berdon WE, Mellins RB, Abramson SJ, Ruzal-Shapiro C: Pediatric HIV in its second decade: the changing pattern of lung involvement, *Radiol Clin North Am* 31:453-463, 1993 (review).

CHAPTER 42

Pertussis

Ziad M. Shehab

Pertussis is a serious respiratory illness caused by the bacterium *Bordetella pertussis.* About 60 million cases occur each year worldwide, resulting in 600,000 deaths, mostly among unimmunized children.[1] The original description of the clinical syndrome of pertussis is credited to Guillaume de Baillou's documentation of an epidemic in Paris in 1578.[2] The organism was first identified and cultured at the Pasteur Institute by Jules Bordet and Octave Gengou in 1906.[3] Originally named *Haemophilus pertussis,* it was renamed *Bordetella pertussis* in honor of Bordet. Soon after the description of Bordet and Gengou's culture methods, whole-cell vaccines were developed and used in children, and there was a significant decrease in the incidence of the disease in vaccinated populations. In the United States, mass immunization has decreased the impact of this disease from 115,000 to 270,000 cases with 5000 to 10,000 deaths each year to 1200 to 4000 cases and 5 to 10 deaths yearly.[4]

Whole-cell vaccines that are not too dissimilar to the original vaccines have been used routinely since the 1950s and were the only vaccines used until recently. With a better understanding of the structure and function of the components of the bacterium, new acellular vaccines have been developed; these vaccines are free of some of the products that are not essential for the production of a protective immune response but may be responsible for some of the side effects associated with whole-cell pertussis vaccines.

ETIOLOGY

The genus *Bordetella* comprises four species. *B. pertussis* is the major cause of the pertussis syndrome. *B. parapertussis* can cause a mild pertussis-like illness. Man is the only natural host for both of these agents. *B. bronchiseptica,* a pathogen of cats and rodents can also produce disease in humans. A fourth species, *B. avium* causes respiratory illness in birds.[5]

B. pertussis is a gram-negative, pleomorphic, nonmotile coccobacillus. It is transmitted by the inhalation of aerosols of *B. pertussis* produced by a patient in the catarrhal or paroxysmal phase of the illness. Patients who are past the third week of paroxysmal illness are generally noninfectious. Transmission via fomites is rare.

The organism is fastidious in its growth requirements and is most easily recovered by plating at the bedside on selective media. The usual media used for its isolation include Bordet-Gengou, modified Stainer-Scholte, and Regan-Lowe charcoal agar supplemented with cephalexin. Four phases of growth have been recognized. Freshly recovered organisms belong to a phase I agglutinative group with which virulence is associated. Serial passage in artificial media is associated with changes in phases II, IIIm, and IV and an accompanying loss of virulence. *B. bronchiseptica* and *B. parapertussis* have similar growth requirements and are distinguished primarily by agglutination reactions or fluorescent antibody staining.[6]

In the last 15 years, the understanding of the biology of *B. pertussis* has significantly increased, resulting in better approaches to vaccine development. The organism produces a number of virulence factors that explain some of the clinical manifestations of the disease. The main virulence factors are filamentous hemagglutinin (FHA), lymphocyte-promoting factor (LPF) (also known as *pertussis toxin*), 69-kD protein (pertactin), lipopolysaccharide, heat-labile toxin (also known as *dermonecrotic toxin*), tracheal cytotoxin, adenylate cyclase, and agglutinogens. These antigens are important in the pathogenesis of the disease and in the formulation of the different vaccines and their related side effects.[7,8]

FHA. FHA is a surface cell wall protein of *B. pertussis.*[5] It is an important factor in attachment to respiratory epithelial cells. Antibody to FHA may be important in protecting against respiratory epithelial cell infection and lethal pulmonary infection in the mouse.[9,10]

Pertussis Toxin. Pertussis toxin has many synonyms: LPF, lymphocyte-promoting toxin, LPF-hemagglutinin, leukocytosis-promoting factor, histamine-sensitizing factor, islet-activating protein, heat-labile adjuvant, and pertussinogen. It is an envelope protein antigen with an enzymatically active A subunit and a B oligomer that binds the toxin to receptor molecules on the cell surface. It has multiple biologic functions. It is responsible for the attachment to ciliated respiratory epithelial cells, the leukocytosis and lymphocytosis seen in children with pertussis, the enhancement of the immune response and sensitization of mice to histamine, and a hyperinsulinemic response seen in laboratory animals.[8] Antibodies to pertussis toxin are protective against intracerebral and pulmonary challenge in mice and are thought by some to have a central role in protecting humans.[11]

Pertactin. Pertactin is a 69-kD outer membrane protein produced by all virulent strains of *B. pertussis* and is a component of many vaccines.

Lipopolysaccharide. Lipopolysaccharide is an endotoxin similar to that of other gram-negative bacteria. It is present in all whole-cell vaccines.

Heat-Labile Toxin. Heat-labile toxin, or dermonecrotic toxin, causes skin necrosis in a number of experimental animals.

Tracheal Cytotoxin. Tracheal cytotoxin causes ciliary stasis and cytopathic effects in hamster tracheal organ cultures.

Adenylate Cyclase. Adenylate cyclase interferes with phagocytic functions by the formation of cyclic adenosine monophosphate. It may be a virulence factor.[12]

Agglutinogens. Agglutinogens are protein surface antigens associated with fimbriae, which elicit antibodies that agglutinate *Bordetella* organisms and may play a significant role in protection against disease.

EPIDEMIOLOGY

Pertussis is highly contagious and is worldwide in distribution. It is transmitted from person to person and has an incubation period of about 14 days.[13] Patients are most infectious during the first week of illness, during which time shedding of the organism is at its highest. Shedding declines during the second and third weeks. Transmission occurs by droplet nuclei, and the secondary attack rate in unimmunized populations may be as high as 100% of susceptible household contacts.[14] The risk of transmission is related to the closeness of contact with an index case. Indirect routes of transmission such as fomites are unlikely. Attack rates have ranged from 25% to 50% among unimmunized school contacts to 70% to 100% in households.[7] Natural disease provides almost complete protection during childhood, whereas vaccine-induced immunity is less complete, with an incidence rate of 10% to 20% in fully immunized children and up to 50% in household settings.[15]

Newborns are fully susceptible because of lack of transplacental immunity and are at high risk of severe disease and death.[16] Without immunization, pertussis affects mostly the 2- to 6-year-old age group; approximately half of nonimmunized children develop pertussis by age 5, and essentially all are infected by age 15, with about three fourths experiencing symptomatic infection.

In the prevaccine era, epidemics occurred at 3- to 4-year intervals. Although the size of epidemics has been reduced, the interval between epidemics has not significantly changed since the introduction of the vaccine. Pertussis demonstrates moderate seasonality and has a higher incidence in the summer and autumn. The disease is transmitted through contact with a symptomatic individual typically exhibiting cough or bronchitis. There is little evidence for a symptomless carrier state.[17,18] Silent carriage is infrequent, is transient, and is most likely unimportant in the epidemiology of the disease.[19]

Immunity secondary to natural disease, although persistent, is not complete. In such adults and children, a typical pertussis syndrome may develop, the condition may be asymptomatic, or a short, atypical illness may develop. The rate of infection in adolescents and adults with a history of pertussis or serologic evidence of prior immunity ranges from 5% to 20%.[15,20] These infections may be important in boosting immunity.

Vaccine-related immunity wanes with time. During an epidemic, Lambert[14] demonstrated a household attack rate of 20% in those immunized within 3 years, whereas the attack rate was 95% for those immunized 12 or more years earlier. In another study, Jenkinson showed a decline from a protective efficacy in young infants from 100% in the first year after immunization to 52% 4 years later, highlighting the need for a preschool booster immunization. Asymptomatic infection is now more common in preschoolers than in school-age children, and the attack rate of laboratory-confirmed pertussis increases with the age of children. The protection provided by the vaccine is therefore short lived, and immunization of schoolchildren and adults may be necessary.[21]

The epidemiology of pertussis has been undergoing a change in terms of the affected age groups. There has been a decline in the disease rate in the 1- to 9-year-old age group and a concomitant increase in those under 1 year of age and those older than 15 years. Over a span of 18 years in Dallas, the incidence of whooping cough in children decreased by 50%, but the proportion of cases in infants under 12 weeks of age doubled to 30%.

After a nadir in 1976, the reported incidence of pertussis increased in all age groups, with a disproportionate increase among adolescents and adults; children over 10 years of age and adults now represent 26.9% of the reported cases, up from 15.1% in 1977 to 1979.[22,23] Infants between 1 and 2 months of age are at highest risk for pertussis, and those under 2 months of age have the highest reported rates of hospitalization (82%), pneumonia (25%), seizures (4%), encephalopathy (1%), and death (1%). The rate of these complications is higher among unvaccinated infants compared to those appropriately immunized for age.[24] Recent epidemics have occurred in highly immunized populations of children and were accompanied by a shift in incidence from younger infants to older children. These children were mostly white and in the middle class. In the case of the Cincinnati epidemic of 1993, the majority of children had been appropriately immunized for pertussis, and the disease was not severe.[25] The number of cases reported has continued to rise since 1977, reaching a total of 6586 cases for 1993, the highest since 1967.[23] This number includes 675 (10%) cases in individuals older than 19 years of age. Such cases are often underreported and frequently present with a mild cough.[26] Some 44% of these cases occurred in children under 1 year of age, of whom 79% were under 6 months of age.[23] In addition, less than half the children admitted to the hospital in Toronto had the classical symptoms of pertussis, paroxysmal cough, and whoop.[27]

Health care workers have seroprevalance rates similar to those of other adults not immunized since childhood and may be at risk of acquiring the disease from infected children and adults, with subsequent transmission of the infection to their patients.[28] In addition, Nelson[29] demonstrated that the usual source of infection tends to be adults in the household rather than siblings or other children. This study and others demonstrate that pertussis in adults is often atypical and asymptomatic and occurs in individuals with a history of previous immunization and even prior disease.[30-34] Endemic infection in adults may act as a reservoir from which infection is spread.[35] In community-acquired infections, adolescents are at higher risk than people in other age groups and are likely to introduce the infection into their households.[36] The disease can be transmitted in residential facilities without children.[27] In adults, a persistent cough is a more common presentation of pertussis, although paroxysmal cough, vomiting, and whoop are possible.[37,38] Thus the diagnosis should be considered in a patient of any age who has a chronic cough, especially if pertussis is known to be in the community. Pertussis remains substantially underreported and may have a substantially larger public health impact than reported thus far.[39]

In areas where pertussis vaccination has been discontinued, symptomatic pertussis is common. In Sweden, the discontinuation of pertussis vaccine in 1979 was followed by a gradual increase in the number of pertussis cases, resulting in two outbreaks in 1983 and 1985 that caused significant morbidity and some mortality.[40] A total of 61% of 10-year-old unvaccinated children have had symptomatic disease. Of these, 91% have antibodies against pertussis toxin, as do 64% of those without a history of whooping cough, indicating prior infection.[41] In the United Kingdom, there was a drop in the number of cases of pertussis as vaccine rates increased from 30% in 1978 to 91% in 1992, and most cases occurred in infants younger than 1 year of age.[42] The attack rate is higher in girls than in boys and is associated with an increase in severity and mortality in girls over the age of 5 years.[43]

The disease can be atypical in people infected with the human immunodeficiency virus. In such people it can be manifested by prolonged cough and dyspnea lasting up to 4 months. The results of cultures and direct fluorescent antibody assays of respiratory secretions are positive, illustrating the deficit in cell-mediated immune responses.[44]

CLINICAL MANIFESTATIONS

> It comes only by degrees, and is at first dry, but when it continued ten or twelve days, it turns humid, and the matter which is then coughed up looks ripe; nevertheless it increases more and more, leaving long intervals; the fits return at certain hours, but continue at each time with such violence and for so long a time, that the child grows blue in the face, its eyes look as if they were forced out, and they run besides, and a bleeding of the nose is sometimes brought on; it coughs till it is quite out of breath, that one is in apprehension of its being choaked [sic]; for if the patient now and then is capable of drawing some breath, it is with a sounding which very much indicates with what difficulty the lungs can admit air. The coughing continues, and does not leave off for that time, till the child vomits up a quantity of slime.
>
> **Rosen von Rosenstein (1776)[45]**

The incubation period of pertussis varies from 6 to 20 days but is usually 7 to 10 days.[46] *B. pertussis* invades the mucosa of the nasopharynx, trachea, bronchi, and bronchioles, increasing the secretion of mucus, which is initially thin and later viscid and tenacious. The disease is divided clinically into three stages: catarrhal, paroxysmal, and convalescent.[47,48] The catarrhal phase, which lasts for 1 to 2 weeks, starts with symptoms that are indistinguishable from those of an upper respiratory tract infection and that include rhinorrhea, conjunctival injection, sneezing, anorexia, listlessness, and a hacking nocturnal cough that gradually becomes diurnal. The cough is usually not associated with fever and gradually increases in severity and intensity to become explosive and paroxysmal in the second week after the onset of symptoms. The patient is most infectious during the catarrhal phase, and infectivity decreases during the paroxysmal phase.

The paroxysmal phase persists for 1 to 4 weeks and is dominated by severe coughing that can occur in paroxysms up to 10 or more times a day. Each is characterized by 5 or more short coughs without an inspiration followed by a deep inspiratory effort, which may result in the characteristic whoop. During these episodes, large amounts of mucus are expelled, often causing vomiting and in young infants, choking spells and cyanosis. The child may be exhausted after a paroxysm. The paroxysmal episodes can occur in rapid succession and may be triggered by stimuli such as feeding, sucking, or crying. Apneic spells may occur in young infants under 6 months of age, in whom paroxysmal spells are sometimes not seen. Infants with pertussis have a higher frequency of apneic pauses and hypoxemia along with ventilation-perfusion mismatch, resulting in the rapid onset of hypoxia.[49] Whoops may not be present in atypical cases, in young infants, in immunized individuals, and in children with pneumonia.

The convalescent phase usually starts 4 to 6 weeks after the onset of disease and is characterized by a gradual decrease in the frequency and severity of the episodes. A nonparoxysmal cough may persist for many months. The duration of the illness in uncomplicated cases is 6 to 20 weeks.[45]

Pertussis in the adult may be similar to that in the young infant. Severe disease is unusual in this age group, and the course is less severe; however, the illness is often long lasting.[50] It may also present as an illness with a nonspecific cough, and pertussis should be considered in the differential diagnosis of individuals with paroxysmal cough or with cough persisting longer than 7 days. Indeed, 26% of adults with coughs that persisted 1 week or more during a pertussis outbreak in Chicago had serologic evidence of pertussis.[51] Recurrences of a pertussis-like illness can occur after upper or lower respiratory tract infections. Immunized children can develop subclinical infections.[52]

The white cell count is usually moderately elevated to between 15,000 and 20,000/mm^3 but may be normal or may be as high as 60,000/mm^3, usually with 60% to 80% lymphocytes. Marked leukocytosis with white blood cell counts of more than 25,000/mm^3 is seen in approximately 40% of children. Young infants under 6 months of age are less likely to have marked leukocytosis.[45] The disease caused by *B. parapertussis* resembles that caused by *B. pertussis* except for its milder nature and the absence of lymphocytosis.[53]

Minor complications of pertussis include subconjunctival hemorrhages and epistaxis resulting from the paroxysmal episodes. Major complications are most commonly respiratory in nature, such as asphyxia in infants, bronchopneumonia, atelectasis, bronchiectasis, interstitial and subcutaneous emphysema, and pneumothorax.[45] Central nervous system complications include acute encephalitis that can progress to coma, stupor, or convulsions. Cerebral edema and hemorrhage can be seen. Long-term sequelae include spastic paralysis, mental retardation, and other permanent neurologic sequelae. Central nervous system complications have been reported in up to 14%

of cases.[14] In the recent U.S. experience, isolated seizures occurred in 2.2% of cases and encephalopathy in 0.7%.[24]

Nutritional deficiencies are the direct result of the infants' inability to eat because of the paroxysms associated with feeding. The malnutrition that follows, combined with the disease, can lead to death. The case fatality rate is 1.3% in children younger than 1 month of age and 0.3% in those 2 to 11 months old.[45,54]

After pertussis, there are a decrease in forced expiratory flow at low lung volumes, reflecting obstruction of the more peripheral airways, and a lower mixing index, indicating a maldistribution of ventilation, findings consistent with the diffuse pulmonary inflammation and inspissated mucus seen in this disease. These decreases in pulmonary function persist into later childhood.[55] Other studies failed to show differences in respiratory symptoms or asthma in adolescents with a history of a pertussis-like illness in childhood.[56]

DIAGNOSIS

The disease is difficult to diagnose in the catarrhal stage unless a history of exposure clues the clinician to the diagnosis. The illness is difficult to distinguish from influenza, bronchitis, or other respiratory viral infections. Adenovirus and *Chlamydia trachomatis* infection should be considered because such infection can mimic the pertussis syndrome. The illness in some children may be caused by concomitant infection with respiratory viruses. Only detection of *B. pertussis* and respiratory syncytial virus by culture or fluorescent antibody testing allows the separation of these entities.[57]

Lymphocytosis in which the lymphocyte count equals or is above 70% in an afebrile or a slightly febrile child older than 3 years of age with a suspicious cough suggests pertussis but does not distinguish it from other causes of the pertussis syndrome such as adenoviruses. Cultures of nasopharyngeal specimens for *B. pertussis* are positive in 80% to 90% of cases during the catarrhal and early paroxysmal phases. In a large study, the rate of isolation in those with a cough persisting at least 4 weeks was 59% if the specimen was obtained in the first 2 weeks of cough and increased to 80% if the cough was associated with a whoop.[58] Isolation rates fall markedly after 21 days of cough. The best results are obtained when sterile cotton swabs on a thin metal wire are introduced in the nasopharynx through the nostril. Throat swabs are far less sensitive.[59] Nasopharyngeal secretions can be smeared on slides for fluorescent microscopy examination, and cultures are best inoculated at the bedside on freshly prepared media. Regan-Lowe and Jones-Kendrick media are the optimal transport media. Regan-Lowe or charcoal horse blood agar media supplemented with penicillin or cephalexin to inhibit other flora are optimal for the growth of *B. pertussis.*[60] A positive culture provides positive proof of *B. pertussis* infection.

The fluorescent antibody technique allows for rapid diagnosis but is not as sensitive or specific as cultures. The fluorescent antibody staining sometimes performs well as a screening test for pertussis but requires a substantial commitment of personnel and resources.[60-62] No single serologic test has a high sensitivity and specificity.[63] Because the direct fluorescent antibody assays have false-positive and false-negative results, culture confirmation should be sought for all suspected cases. Multiple reports have indicated that polymerase chain reaction assays are rapid, specific, and sensitive methods for demonstrating *B. pertussis* in nasopharyngeal secretions, especially during the first weeks of the disease.[64-67]

TREATMENT

Treatment with antibiotics does not modify the course of the illness in the paroxysmal phase. Erythromycin treatment during the catarrhal stage may ameliorate the clinical disease. Erythromycin is effective in eradicating the organism within 5 days and results in a decrease in the number of whoops.[68] Its ability to eradicate *B. pertussis* is significantly lower in children up to 2 years of age, in whom the eradication rate may be as low as 39% within 1 week.[69] The agent of choice is erythromycin estolate, which has a lower rate of clinical and bacteriologic relapses and is more effective at lower dose than ethylsuccinate salt in eradicating the organism from the nasopharynx.[70,71] The recommended treatment regimen is 40 to 50 mg/kg/day (maximum, 2 g/day) divided into four doses and given for 14 days. To date, only one instance of erythromycin resistance has been reported.[72] Other macrolides such as roxithromycin, azithromycin, and clarithromycin may be considered. Co-trimoxazole has also shown some efficacy in eradicating the organism and may be an alternative (at a dose of 8 mg/kg of trimethoprim and 40 mg/kg of sulfamethoxazole divided into 2 doses twice a day) in patients unable to tolerate erythromycin. Treatment failures have been described with amoxicillin.[73] One study suggests that the use of a specific high-titer antipertussis toxin immunoglobulin preparation early in the course of the illness significantly decreases the duration of whoops.[74] Specific γ-globulin with high antibody titers against pertussis toxin and FHA has been advocated by some as a therapy based on anecdotal reports.[75] Salbutamol is ineffective in ameliorating the symptoms of pertussis.[76,77] The benefits of the use of steroids have not been established.[78-80] No cough suppressants have proved useful in management. Supportive therapy is a critical component of the care of infants with pertussis. A quiet environment and gentle suctioning of respiratory secretions are important in preventing attacks or paroxysmal coughing. Administration of oxygen may be needed. and careful attention should be paid to hydration and nutrition. Intensive care measures may be needed in severe cases. Infants younger than 6 months of age or those with cyanosis during paroxysms of excessive vomiting may initially be admitted to the hospital.

Respiratory isolation should be instituted and continued until the patient has received erythromycin for 5 days or in the absence of erythromycin therapy, is at least 3 weeks from the onset of paroxysms.[45] Children attending child care facilities should not attend until the disease is evaluated. They can return after the administration of erythromycin for 5 days. Contacts who have immunization delays should be immunized, as should infants under 4 years of age whose last vaccination was given 6 months or longer before the exposure. Erythromycin may be given to household contacts irrespective of immunization status.

PREVENTION

Universal immunization of children younger than 7 years of age is essential for the control of pertussis. Whole-cell pertussis vaccine in combination with tetanus and diphtheria toxoids (DTP) has been recommended and routinely used in the United States for the immunization of infants starting at 2 months of age; it is given in a primary immunization schedule at 2, 4, and 6 months of age, followed at 15 to 18 months and 4 to 6 years of age by boosters of whole-cell or acellular pertussis vaccine combined with tetanus and diphtheria toxoids (diphtheria-tetanus-pertussis [DTP] and diphtheria-tetanus-pertussis with an acellular pertussis component [DtaP]). Because of laws mandating school immunization, almost all children have been immunized by school age.

Ample evidence from many sources is available to indicate the efficacy of this vaccine. In controlled trials, the vaccine provides protection against clinical disease in the majority of recipients and ameliorates the severity of disease of those who are not fully protected,[81-84] although some studies have failed to show such effects.[85,86] Although mortality rates from pertussis were declining before the advent of the pertussis vaccine, it is undeniable that the vaccine has resulted in an impressive decline in the mortality and morbidity rates. Its role in the control of pertussis is further emphasized by the experiences in Japan, Sweden, England, and Wales all of which have experienced major pertussis outbreaks after a decline in immunization rates.[41,87-89] In addition, during epidemics, the reported incidence of the disease in communities varies inversely proportionately with vaccine acceptance. The efficacy of three or more doses of the vaccine is 80% to 95%, with partial protection being offered by incomplete immunization.[98,90] The vaccine is highly effective in preschool children with household exposure. The vaccine efficacy increases with increasing number of doses, from 40% with one dose of DTP to 80% after four or more doses.[90] The reluctance of some practitioners to administer full doses of vaccine or to give the fifth dose scheduled for preschool children may be an important factor in the perpetuation of pertussis.[91] In addition, the different whole-cell vaccines available on the market are not equivalent in their ability to elicit immunologic responses.[93] Herd immunity is thought to play a role in the spacing of epidemics every 3 to 4 years. During epidemics, the vaccine can be given on an accelerated schedule at 2, 3, and 4 months without an increase in the number of unprotected children to any of the three diseases.[93] Pertussis persists in immunized populations, suggesting the potential need to immunize adolescents and adults with the acellular vaccine.[36,94]

In 1981, acellular pertussis vaccines were introduced in Japan. These vaccines fall in two main groups: the B-type vaccines, which contain about equal amounts of FHA and pertussis toxin, and the T-type vaccines, which contain more FHA than pertussis toxin. The efficacy of these vaccines in Japan is estimated to be 78% to 94% in children 2 years of age or older but not in young infants.[95-97] In the United States, two acellular pertussis vaccines combined with tetanus and diphtheria toxoids have been licensed and are recommended for use for the fourth and fifth doses of pertussis immunization.[98] A T-type vaccine licensed by Lederle-Praxis (West Henrietta, NY) contains FHA, pertussis toxin, agglutinogens, and a 69-kD protein, and a B-type vaccine licensed by Pasteur Mérieux Connaught contains FHA and pertussis toxin. The latter vaccine was tested in Sweden in 5- to 11-month-old infants. Its protective efficacy as not as good as anticipated (~70%) when cough with positive culture is used as an endpoint.[99] When given as a booster to 15- to 18-month-old infants and 4- to 6-year-old children who had received DTP as a primary series, DTaP recipients had significantly higher antibody titers to antipertussis toxin and anti-FHA compared to infants whose immune systems were boosted with the whole-cell DTP vaccine.[100] This vaccine results in higher immunoglobulin G antibody levels to pertussis toxin before and after the administration of the 15- to 18-month acellular vaccine (DTaP) booster in infants whose immune systems had been primed with the DTaP compared to infants whose immune systems were primed by the whole-cell (DTP) vaccine.[101] However, this protection does not correlate with the height of the antibody response, and antibody levels cannot therefore predict efficacy. Several studies of acellular vaccines in Europe and Africa are assessing the efficacy of acellular vaccines as well as the protective efficacy of different combinations of antigens in the vaccine preparation. Some monocomponent vaccines have been tested, and the results are variable in young infants.

Monocomponent pertussis toxoid vaccine is immunogenic and most likely confers a high level of protection against pertussis when given to children starting at 3 months of age.[102] In an outbreak of pertussis in a residential facility in Japan, the vaccine was not effective in preventing infection but protected vaccinated children from clinical symptoms.[103] The optimal composition of the acellular pertussis vaccine remains a matter of debate. Some advocate that the vaccine should contain inactivated pertussis toxoid alone because they believe a critical level of antitoxin alone is protective against pertussis.[104] Others believe that monocomponent LPF toxoid or bicomponent LPF toxoid/FHA vaccines are not as effective as vaccines that contain pertactin and fimbrial antigens as well as LPF toxoid and FHA.[105] Although indicating a major role for antibodies to pertussis toxin, the data of different studies could be interpreted to mean that antibodies to the different antigens all contribute to protection against the disease.[106] New additions to the B-type vaccine include the addition of the 69-kD pertactin.[107] Early administration of erythromycin is effective in preventing the secondary spread of pertussis in households. In one retrospective study, the median interval from onset of illness to the initiation of therapy was 11 vs. 21 days for households without and with secondary spread and 16 vs. 22 days for the initiation of prophylaxis among contacts.[108]

Reactions to Pertussis Vaccines

With the disappearance of pertussis as a major public health problem, attention has been directed over the past 20 years to the side effects of the vaccine. These side effects occur commonly within 12 to 24 hours of immunization and consist mostly of localized reactions, including pain, swelling, and redness at the site of injection, and minor systemic reactions, including fever and irritability, which occur in 50% of vaccine recipients. The prophylactic administration of acetaminophen at the time of immunization and for the subsequent 8 to 18 hours decreases the occurrence of febrile reactions and behavioral changes.[109,110] Fewer than 1% of vaccinees develop a temperature of 40.5° C (105° F) or higher. These events are self-limited and of no consequence.[111,112] Local and systemic reactions to acellular pertussis vaccines are considerably less frequent, occurring at a rate of one fourth to two thirds of that seen with the whole-cell vaccine.[104] Most of the information is derived from children 2 years of age or older in Japan.

In addition, seizures or shocklike states were seen after 0.06% of DTP doses. The convulsions are short lived and usually associated with fever. Hypotonic-hyporesponsive episodes are seen at a similar rate. At follow-up 6 to 7 years later, none of the children who exhibited seizures or hypotonic-hyporesponsive episodes had any evidence of neurologic deficit, but 25% had minor neurologic abnormalities.[113] The seizures have clinical features similar to those of febrile seizures, and the episodes of persistent crying seem related to painful local reactions.[114]

Concerns about serious reactions attributed to DTP immunization have resulted in a lower rate of acceptance for these vaccines and in Japan, the discontinuation of the use of the whole-cell pertussis vaccine. The most serious concerns involve the encephalopathy that is attributed to DTP and that often leads to permanent neurologic sequelae. Infantile spasms, sudden infant death syndrome (SIDS), and learning disorders have also raised concerns among the public. Numerous anecdotal reports and uncontrolled series have implicated the use of DTP vaccine in the genesis of encephalopathy. Ström[115] was the first to attempt to quantitate the risk of encephalopathy, which he estimated to be 1 in 170,000 for a three-dose primary immunization series. Later, a carefully designed study in the United Kingdom concluded that the rate of acute encephalopathy with permanent brain damage was 1 per 330,000 doses and the risk of encephalopathy was 1 in 140,000. This was based on seven patients, two of whom had disseminated viral infections and one of whom had Reye's syndrome. In addition, three of the remaining four patients did not appear to be neurologically impaired on follow-up.[116-119] On further analysis, it appears that the increased relative risk observed over the first 7 days is offset over the subsequent 3 weeks.[120]

In the United States, two studies have looked at the possible connection between DTP and encephalopathy. Based on a study of a cohort of 35,581 children receiving care in a health maintenance organization in the Seattle area, a difference with the background rates of initial seizures and other neurologic disorders within 1 month of the receipt of DTP vaccine could not be demonstrated.[121] The rate of febrile seizures was slightly higher in the first 3 days after immunization, with a relative risk of 3.7%. A second study using Tennessee's computerized Medicaid database, which included 38,171 children, failed to show any differences, including rates of febrile seizures.[122] Pertussis vaccine is associated with febrile seizures in children with such a predisposition. A Danish study did not demonstrate a shift in age of onset for epilepsy when the age at immunization was changed in 1970 from 5, 6, and 7 months with a booster at 15 months to 5 and 9 weeks followed by a booster at 10 months.[123] In addition, a pilot project using a case-control methodology in the states of Washington and Oregon prospectively identified cases of neurologic illness by active surveillance over 12 months. A total of 424 cases of neurologic illness was identified in this population of 218,000 1- to 24-month-old children. No statistically significant increase in the risk for serious neurologic illnesses was observed in the 7 days after immunization.[124]

Infantile spasms occur typically in patients younger than 1 year of age, with the majority occurring in the 2- to 8-month age group, the age at which DTP is usually administered. Four studies have demonstrated the lack of association between pertussis vaccine and infantile spasms (hypsarrhythmias).[125-128] The temporal association of SIDS and pertussis vaccine was suggested by two studies.[129,130] Both of these studies were subject to significant recall bias and failed to recognize a decrease in the incidence of SIDS after 2 months of age, a time at which the vaccine is first administered in the United States. Several controlled studies have failed to show an association between SIDS and pertussis immunization.[131-136]

Finally, a committee of the Institute of Medicine was commissioned to conduct a thorough review of the evidence relating to serious adverse effects of pertussis vaccine. The summary of the committee's findings indicated no causal relationship between DTP vaccine and autism, infantile spasms, hypsarrhythmia, Reye's syndrome, or SIDS.[137] The evidence was insufficient to conclude a causal relationship with aseptic meningitis, chronic neurologic damage, erythema multiforme or other rashes, Guillain-Barré syndrome, hemolytic anemia, juvenile diabetes, learning disabilities and attention deficit disorders, peripheral mononeuropathy, and thrombocytopenia. The evidence is consistent with a causal relationship with acute encephalopathy, shock, and "unusual shocklike state." The evidence indicates a relationship with anaphylaxis and protracted, inconsolable crying.[137-139]

Recommended Use of Pertussis Vaccine

In the United States, the vaccine is recommended in a five-dose schedule at 2, 4, 6, and 15 to 18 months and at 4 to 6 years of age.[4,45] The first three doses are recommended as whole-cell vaccine; the acellular vaccine may be substituted for the last two doses. The vaccine is administered as a 0.5-ml intramuscular injection given either as DTP or DTaP. DTP vaccine is not recommended for children 7 years of age or older because the side effects are unpleasant and the risk of severe pertussis is thought to be low. This recommendation may need to be addressed with the advent of acellular vaccines and the significant contribution of adolescents and adults to the spread of pertussis to young infants.

The same vaccine dosage and schedule are recommended for preterm infants. Premature infants are able to mount a satisfactory immune response after the second dose of the vaccine and have a low incidence of side effects.[140,141] Thus immunization should not be delayed beyond 8 weeks of age, and the regular immunization schedule based on chronologic age should be followed.[142] Immunization of preterm infants with half-doses of vaccine results in poor immunologic response without a significant reduction in side effects, which occur less often than in full-term infants.[143]

DTP is given as an intramuscular injection at a dose of 0.5 ml. Split or reduced doses are not recommended. After age 7, the pertussis component is omitted, and diphtheria-tetanus toxoid is given instead.

During epidemics, the schedule can be accelerated, with the first three doses given at 6, 10, and 14 weeks of age. There is some evidence that this accelerated schedule may result in lower immune responses, especially in the presence of high maternal antibody titers.[144]

Adults and adolescents tolerate the acellular pertussis vaccine without undue side effects. Given the important role played by infected adults in the spread of pertussis to high-risk susceptible infants, its role in the interruption of epidemics needs to be carefully evaluated.[145,146]

Contraindications and Precautions

The contraindications and precautions to the DTP vaccine have been considerably modified in recognition of the fact that DTP did not contribute to many of the side effects previously attributed to it.[4,45,147,148] Immunization should not be delayed in children with mild respiratory illnesses or low-grade fever.

Of the six events that were absolute contraindications in the 1985 recommendations, only two are still present in the 1991 version: anaphylaxis and encephalopathy that occurs within 7 days of receipt of a dose of DTP, is defined as a severe acute central nervous system disorder unexplained by another cause, and may be manifested by major alterations of consciousness or by generalized or focal seizures persisting more than a few hours without recovery within 24 hours.[48] Fever up to 40.5° C, hypotonic-hyporesponsive episodes, and persistent or inconsolable crying for 3 or more hours all occurring within 48 hours or convulsions with or without fever occurring within 3 days of immunization are now considered precautions.

Whether to immunize and when to immunize children with neurologic disorders are difficult to determine. In general, children with corrected lesions or with seizure disorders that are under control should be immunized according to schedule. The administration of vaccine to children whose neurologic condition is evolving or changing should be postponed until their situation is clarified. A decision as to whether to proceed with diphtheria-tetanus or DTP should be reached by the children's first birthday. Children with a family history of seizures or SIDS and children who are immunocompromised should receive DTP on the regular schedule. Children should not be given half doses; these only reduce the effective immunity with no reduction in side effects.

REFERENCES

1. Muller AS, Leeuwenburg J, Pratt DS: Pertussis: epidemiology and control, *Bull World Health Organ* 64:321-331, 1986.
2. Linneman CC Jr: Host-parasite interactions in pertussis. In Manclark CR, Hill JC, eds: *International Symposium on Pertussis,* US Department of Health, Education and Welfare, NIH Pub No 79-1830, Washington, DC, 1979, Government Printing Office, pp 3-18.
3. Bordet J, Gengou O: Le microbe de la coqueluche, *Ann Inst Pasteur* 20:731-741, 1906.
4. Diphtheria, tetanus and pertussis: recommendations for vaccine use and other prevention measures—recommendations of the Immunizations Practices Advisory Committee (ACIP), *MMWR* 40(RR10):1-28, 1991.

Etiology

5. Manclark CR, Cowell JL: Pertussis. In Germanier R, ed: *Bacterial vaccines,* New York, 1984, Academic, pp 69-106.
6. Leslie PH, Gardner AD: The phases of *Haemophilus pertussis, J Hyg* 31:423-434, 1931.
7. Cherry JD, Brunell PA, Golden GS, Karzon DT: Report of the task force on pertussis and pertussis immunization: 1988, *Pediatrics* 81:939-984, 1988.
8. Edwards KM: Acellular pertussis vaccines: a solution to the pertussis problem? *J Infect Dis* 168:15-20, 1993.
9. Cowell JL, Oda M, Burstyn DG et al: Prospective protective antigens and animal models for pertussis. In Leive L, Schlessinger D, eds: *Microbiology,* Washington, DC, 1984, American Society for Microbiology, pp 172-175.
10. Redhead K: An assay of *Bordetella pertussis* adhesion to tissue culture cells, *J Med Microbiol* 19:99-108, 1985.
11. Pittman M: The concept of pertussis as a toxin-mediated disease, *Pediatr Infect Dis J* 3:467-486, 1984.
12. Confer DL, Eaton JW: Phagocyte impotence caused by an invasive bacterial adenylate cyclase, *Science* 217:948-950, 1982.

Epidemiology

13. Lawson GM: Epidemiology of whooping cough, *Am J Dis Child* 46:1454-1455, 1933.
14. Lambert HJ: Epidemiology of a small pertussis outbreak in Kent County, Michigan, *Public Health Rep* 80:365-369, 1965.
15. Thomas MG: Epidemiology of pertussis, *Rev Infect Dis* 11:255-262, 1989.
16. Bass JW, Zacher LL: Do newborn infants have passive immunity to pertussis? *Pediatr Infect Dis J* 8:352-353, 1989.
17. Krantz I, Alestig K, Trollfors B, Zackrisson G: The carrier state in pertussis, *Scand J Infect Dis* 18:121-123, 1987.
18. Bass JW: Is there a carrier state in pertussis? *Lancet* 1:96, 1987 (letter).
19. Thomas MG, Lambert HP: From whom do children catch pertussis? *Br Med J* 295:751-752, 1987.
20. Cromer BA, Goydos J, Hackell J, Mezzatesta J, Dekker C, Mortimer EA: Unrecognized pertussis infection in adolescents, *Am J Dis Child* 147:575-577, 1993.
21. He Q, Vijanen MK, Nikkari S, Lyytikainen R, Mertsola J: Outcomes of *Bordetella pertussis* infection in different age groups of an immunized population, *J Infect Dis* 170:873-877, 1994.
22. Davis SF, Strebel PM, Cochi SL, Zell ER, Hadler SC: Pertussis surveillance: United States, 1989-1991, *MMWR* 41(#SS-8):11-19, 1992.
23. Resurgence of pertussis: United States, 1993, *MMWR* 42:952-960, 1993.
24. Farizo KM, Cochi SL, Zell ER, Brink EW, Wassilak SG, Patriarca PA: Epidemiological features of pertussis in the United States, 1980-1989, *Clin Infect Disease* 14:708-719, 1992.
25. Christie CDC, Marx ML, Marchant CD, Reising SF: The 1993 epidemic of pertussis in Cincinnati: resurgence of disease in a highly immunized population of children, *N Engl J Med* 331:16-21, 1994.
26. Transmission of pertussis from adult to infant: Michigan, 1993, *MMWR* 44(4)74-76, 1995.
27. Gordon M, Davies HD, Gold R: Clinical and microbiological features of children presenting with pertussis to a Canadian children's hospital during an eleven-year period, *Pediatr Infect Dis J* 13:617-622, 1994.
28. Wright SW, Edwards KM, Decker MD, Lamberth MM: Pertussis seroprevalence in emergency department staff, *Ann Emerg Med* 24:413-417, 1994.
29. Nelson JD: The changing epidemiology of pertussis in young infants: the role of adults as reservoirs of infection, *Am J Dis Child* 132:371-373, 1978.
30. Trollfors B, Rabo B: Whooping cough in adults, *Br Med J* 1981: 283:696-697, 1987.
31. Mertsola J, Ruuskanen O, Eerola E, Viljanen MK: Intrafamilial spread of pertussis, *J Pediatr* 103:359-363, 1983.
32. Long SS, Welkin CJ, Clark JL: Widespread silent transmission of pertussis in families: antibody correlates of infection and symptomatology, *J Infect Dis* 161:480-486, 1990.
33. Addiss DG, Davis JP, Meade BD, Burstyn DG, Meissner M, Zastrow JA, Berg JL, Drinka A, Phillips R: A pertussis outbreak in a Wisconsin nursing home, *J Infect Dis* 164:704-710, 1991.
34. Mortimer EA Jr: Pertussis and its prevention: a family affair, *J Infect Dis* 161:473-479, 1990.
35. Mink CM, Cherry JD, Christenson A, Lewis K, Pineda E, Shlian DS, Dawson JA, Blumberg DA: A search for *Bordetella pertussis* infection in university students, *Clin Infect Dis* 14:464-471, 1992.
36. Biellik RJ, Patriarca PA, Mullen JR, Rovira EZ, Brink EW, Mitchell P, Hamilton GH, Sullivan BJ, Davis JP: Risk factors for community- and household-acquired pertussis during a large-scale outbreak in Central Wisconsin, *J Infect Dis* 157:1134-1141, 1988.
37. Herwaldt LA: Pertussis in adults, *Arch Intern Med* 151:1510-1512, 1991 (review).
38. Pertussis: adults, infants and herds, *Lancet* 339:526-527, 1992 (editorial).
39. Sutter RW, Cochi SL: Pertussis hospitalizations and mortality in the United States, 1985-1988: evaluation of completeness of national reporting, *JAMA* 267:386-391, 1992.
40. Romanus V, Jonsell R, Bergquist S-O: Pertussis in Sweden after the cessation of general immunization in 1979, *Pediatr Infect Dis J* 6:364-371, 1987.
41. Isacson J, Trollfors B, Taranger J, Zackrisson G, Lagergard T: How common is whooping cough in a nonvaccinating country? *Pediatr Infect Dis J* 12:284-288, 1993.
42. Miller E, Vurdien JE, White JM: The epidemiology of pertussis in England and Wales, *Commun Dis Rep CDR Rev* 2:R152-R154, 1992.
43. Hodder SL, Mortimer EA Jr: Epidemiology of pertussis and reactions to pertussis vaccine, *Epidemiol Rev* 14:243-267, 1992 (review).
44. Doebelling BN, Feilmeier ML, Herwaldt LA: Pertussis in an adult with the human immunodeficiency virus, *J Infect Dis* 161:1286-1298, 1990.

Clinical Manifestations

45. Brooksaler F, Nelson JD: Pertussis: a reappraisal and report of 190 confirmed cases, *Am J Dis Child* 114:389-396, 1967.
46. Committee on Infectious Diseases: Pertussis. In Peter G, ed: *1994 red book: report of the Committee on Infectious Diseases,* ed 23, Elk Grove Village, Ill, 1994, Academy of Pediatrics, pp 355-367.

47. Cherry JD, Barraff LJ, Hewlett E: The past, present, and future of pertussis: the role of adults in epidemiology and future control, *West J Med* 150:319-328, 1989.
48. Mortimer EA: Pertussis vaccine. In Plotkin SA, Mortimer EA, eds: *Vaccines,* ed 2, Philadelphia, 1994, WB Saunders, pp 91-135.
49. Southall DP, Thomas MG, Lambert HP: Severe hypoxaemia in pertussis, *Arch Dis Child* 63:498-605, 1988.
50. Linneman CC Jr, Nasenbeny J: Pertussis in the adult, *Am Rev Med* 28:179-185, 1977.
51. Rosenthal S, Strebel P, Cassiday P, Sanden G, Brusuelas K, Wharton M: Pertussis infection among adults during the 1993 outbreak in Chicago, *J Infect Dis* 171:1650-1652, 1995.
52. Long SS, Lischner HW, Deforest A, Clark JL: Serologic evidence of subclinical pertussis in immunized children, *Pediatr Infect Dis J* 9:700-705, 1990.
53. Heinninger U, Stehr K, Schmitt-Grohé S, Lorenz C, Rost R, Christenson PD, Oberall M, Cherry JD: Clinical characteristics of illness caused by *Bordetella parapertussis* compared with illness caused by *Bordetella pertussis, Pediatr Infect Dis J* 13:306-309, 1994.
54. Cherry JD: "Pertussis vaccine encephalopathy": it is time to recognize it as the myth that it is, *JAMA* 263:1679-1680, 1990.
55. Howenstine M, Eigen H, Tepper R: Pulmonary function in infants after pertussis, *J Pediatr* 118:563-566, 1991.
56. Teculescu DB, Bruant A, Aubry C, Pham QT, Kuntz C, Deschamps JP, Manciaux M: Pertussis in French adolescents: risk factors and respiratory sequels, *Respiration* 58:15-20, 1991.

Diagnosis

57. Nelson WL, Hopkins RS, Roe MH, Glode MP: Simultaneous infection with *Bordetella pertussis* and respiratory syncytial virus in hospitalized children, *Pediatr Infect Dis J* 5:540-544, 1986.
58. Heininger U, Cherry JD, Eckhardt T, Lorenz C, Christenson P, Stehr K: Clinical and laboratory diagnosis of pertussis in the regions of a large vaccine efficacy trial in Germany, *Pediatr Infect Dis J* 12:504-509, 1993.
59. Marcon MJ, Hamoudi AC, Cannon HJ, Hribar MM: Comparison of throat and nasopharyngeal swab specimens for culture diagnosis of *Bordetella pertussis* infection, *J Clin Microbiol* 25:1104-1110, 1987.
60. Friedman RL: Pertussis: the disease and new diagnostic methods, *Clin Microbiol Rev* 1:365-376, 1988 (review).
61. Ewanowich CA, Chui LWL, Paranchych MG, Peppler MS, Marusyk RG, Albritton WL: Major outbreak of pertussis in Northern Alberta, Canada: analysis of discrepant direct fluorescent-antibody and culture results by using polymerase chain reaction methodology, *J Clin Microbiol* 31:1715-1725, 1993.
62. Strebel PM, Cochi SL, Farizo KM, Payne BJ, Hanauer SD, Baughman AL: Pertussis in Missouri: evaluation of nasopharyngeal culture, direct fluorescent antibody testing, and clinical case definitions in the diagnosis of pertussis, *Clin Infect Dis* 16:276-285, 1993.
63. Halperin S: Interpretation of pertussis serologic tests, *Pediatr Infect Dis J* 10:791-792, 1991.
64. He Q, Mertsola J, Soini H, Skurnik M, Ruuskanen O, Viljanen MK: Comparison of a polymerase chain reaction with culture and immunoassay for diagnosis of pertussis, *J Clin Microbiol* 31:642-645, 1993.
65. Birkebaek NH, Heron I, Skojdt K: *Bordetella pertussis* diagnosis by polymerase chain reaction, *APMIS* 102:291-294, 1994.
66. He Q, Mertsola J, Soini H, Viljanen MK: Sensitive and specific polymerase chain reaction assays for the detection of *Bordetella pertussis* in nasopharyngeal specimens, *J Pediatr* 124:421-426, 1994.
67. Li Z, Jansen DL, Finn TM, Halperin SA, Kasina A, O'Connor SP, Aayoma T, Manclark CR, Brennan MJ: Identification of *Bordetella pertussis* infection by shared-primer PCR, *J Clin Microbiol* 32:783-789, 1994.

Treatment

68. Bergquist S-O, Bernander S, Dahnsjö H, Sundelöf B: Erythromycin in the treatment of pertussis: a study of bacteriologic and clinical effects, *Pediatr Infect Dis J* 6:458-461, 1987.
69. Kawai H, Aoyama T, Goto A, Iwai H, Murase Y: Evaluation of pertussis treatment with erythromycin ethylsuccinate and stearate according to age, *J Jpn Assoc Infect Dis* 68:1324-1329, 1994.
70. Bass JW: Erythromycin for treatment and prevention of pertussis, *Pediatr Infect Dis* 5:154-157, 1986.
71. Hoppe JE, The Erythromycin Study Group: Comparison of erythromycin estolate and erythromycin ethylsuccinate for treatment of pertussis, *Pediatr Infect Dis J* 11:189-193, 1992.
72. Erythromycin-resistant *Bordetella pertussis:* Yuma County, Arizona, May-October 1994, *MMWR* 43(44):807-810, 1994.
73. Trollfors B: Effect of erythromycin and amoxicillin on *Bordetella pertussis* in the nasopharynx, *Infection* 6:228-230, 1978.
74. Granstrom M, Olinder-Nielsen AM, Holmblad P, Mark A, Hanngren K: Specific immunoglobulin for treatment of whooping cough, *Lancet* 338:1230-1233, 1991.
75. Ichimaru T, Ohara Y, Hojo M, Miyazaki S, Harano K, Totoki T: Treatment of severe pertussis by administration of specific gamma globulin with high titers anti-toxin antibody, *Acta Paediatr* 82:1076-1078, 1993.
76. Krantz I, Norrby SR, Trollfors B: Salbutamol vs. placebo for treatment of pertussis, *Pediatr Infect Dis* 4:638-640, 1985.
77. Mertsola J, Viljanen MK, Ruuskanen O: Salbutamol in the treatment of whooping cough, *Scand J Infect Dis* 18:593-594, 1986.
78. Zoumboulakis D, Anagnostakis D, Albanis V, Matsaniotis N: Steroids in treatment of pertussis: a controlled clinical trial, *Arch Dis Child* 48:51-54, 1973.
79. Roberts I, Gavin R, Lennon D: Randomized clinical trial of steroids in pertussis, *Pediatr Infect Dis J* 1:982-983, 1992.
80. Torre D, Tambini R, Ferrario G, Bonetta G: Treatment with steroids in children with pertussis, *Pediatr Infect Dis J* 12:419-420, 1993.

Prevention

81. Madsen T: Vaccination against whooping cough, *JAMA* 101:187-288, 1933.
82. Kendrick P, Eldering G: Progress report on pertussis immunization, *Am J Public Health* 26:8-12, 1936.
83. Sauer LW: Whooping cough: new phases of the work of immunization and prophylaxis, *JAMA* 112:305-308, 1939.
84. Medical Research Council: The prevention of whooping-cough by vaccination, *Br Med J* 1:1463-1471, 1951.
85. Doull JA, Shibley GS, McClelland JS: Active immunization against whooping cough: interim report of the Cleveland experience, *Am J Public Health* 26:1097-1105, 1936.
86. Lapin LH: *Whooping cough,* Springfield, Ill, 1943, Charles C Thomas, pp 1-237.
87. Kanai K: Japan's experience in pertussis epidemiology and vaccination in the past thirty years, *Jpn J Sci Biol* 33:107-143, 1980.
88. Cherry JD: The epidemiology of pertussis and pertussis vaccine in the United Kingdom and the United States: a comparative study, *Curr Prob Pediatr* 14(2):1-78, 1984.
89. Storsaeter J, Olin P: Relative efficacy of two acellular pertussis vaccines during three years of passive surveillance, *Vaccine* 10:142-144, 1992.
90. Onorato IM, Wassilak SG, Meade B: Efficacy of whole-cell pertussis vaccine in preschool children in the United States, *JAMA* 267:2745-2749, 1992.
91. Ey JL, Duncan B, Barton LL, Buckett G: The influence of preschool pertussis immunization on an epidemic of pertussis, *Pediatr Infect Dis J* 10:576-578, 1991.
92. Edwards KM, Decker MD, Halsey NA, Koblin BA, Townsend T, Auerbach B, Karzon DT: Differences in antibody response to whole-cell pertussis vaccines, *Pediatrics* 88:1019-1023, 1991.
93. Ramsay ME, Rao M, Begg NT, Redhead K, Attwell AM: Antibody response to accelerated immunization with diphtheria, tetanus, pertussis vaccine, *Lancet* 342:203-205, 1993.
94. Halperin SA, Bortolussi R, MacLean D, Chisholm N: Persistence of pertussis in an immunized population: results of the Nova Scotia enhanced pertussis surveillance program, *J Pediatr* 115:686-693, 1989.
95. Noble GR, Bernier RH, Esber EC, Hardegree MC, Hinman AR, Klein D, Saah AJ: Acellular and whole-cell pertussis vaccine in Japan: report of a visit by U.S. scientists, *JAMA* 257:1351-1356, 1987.
96. Aoyama T, Murase Y, Gonda T, Iwata T: Type-specific efficacy of acellular pertussis vaccine, Am J Dis Child 142:40-42, 1988.
97. Aoyama T, Murase Y, Kato M, Iwai H, Iwata T: Efficacy and immunogenicity of acellular pertussis vaccine by manufacturer and patient age, *Am J Dis Child* 143:655-659, 1989.
98. Pertussis vaccination: acellular pertussis vaccine for reinforcing and booster use—supplementary ACIP statement, *MMWR* 41(#RR-1):1-10, 1992.

99. Ad Hoc Group for the Study of Pertussis Vaccines: Placebo-controlled trial of two acellular pertussis vaccines in Sweden: protective efficacy and adverse events, *Lancet* 1:955-960, 1988.
100. Bernstein DI, Smith VE, Schiff GM, Rathfon HM, Boscia JA: Comparison of acellular pertussis vaccine with whole-cell vaccine as a booster in children 15 to 18 months and 4 to 6 years of age, *Pediatr Infect Dis J* 12:131-135, 1993.
101. Pichichero ME, Francis A, Marsocci SM, Green JL, Disney FA, Meschievitz C: Safety and immunogenicity of an acellular pertussis vaccine booster in 15- to 20-month-old children previously immunized with acellular or whole-cell pertussis vaccine as infants, *Pediatrics* 91:756-760, 1993.
102. Isacson J, Trollfors B, Taranger J, MacDowall I, Johansson J, Lagergard T, Robbins JB: Safety, immunogenicity and an open, retrospective study of efficacy of a monocomponent pertussis toxoid vaccine in infants, *Pediatr Infect Dis J* 13:22-27, 1994.
103. Aoyama T, Iwata T, Iwai H, Murase Y, Saito T, Akamatsu T: Efficacy of acellular pertussis vaccine in young adults, *J Infect Dis* 167:483-486, 1993.
104. Robbins JB, Pittman M: Trollfors B, Lagergard TA, Teranger J: Primum non nocere: a pharmacologically inert pertussis toxoid alone should be the next pertussis vaccine, *Pediatr Infect Dis J* 12:795-807, 1993.
105. Cherry JD: Acellular pertussis vaccines: a solution to the pertussis problem, *J Infect Dis* 168:21-24, 1993.
106. Granstrom M, Granstrom G: Serological correlates in whooping cough, *Vaccine* 11:445-448, 1993.
107. Schmitt HJ, Wagner S: Pertussis vaccines: 1993, *Eur J Pediatr* 152:462-466, 1993 (review).
108. Sprauer MA, Cochi SL, Zell ER, Sutter RW, Mullen JR, Englender SJ, Patriarca PA: Prevention of secondary transmission of pertussis in households with early use of erythromycin, *Am J Dis Child* 146:177-181, 1992.
109. Ipp MM, Gold R, Greenberg S, Goldbach M, Kupfert BB, Lloyd DC, Maresky DC, Saunders N, Wise SA: Acetaminophen prophylaxis of adverse reactions following vaccination of infants with diphtheria-pertussis-tetanus toxoids-polio vaccine, *Pediatr Infect Dis J* 6:721-725, 1987.
110. Lewis K, Cherry JD, Sachs MH, Woo DB, Hamilton RC, Tarle JM, Overturf GD: The effect of prophylactic acetaminophen administration on reactions to DTP vaccination, *Am J Dis Child* 142:62-65, 1988.
111. Mortimer EA Jr, Jones PK: An evaluation of pertussis vaccine, *Rev Infect Dis* 1:927-932, 1979.
112. Cody CL, Baraff LJ, Cherry JD, Marcy SM, Manclark CR: Nature and rates of adverse reactions associated with DTP and DT immunizations in infants and children, *Pediatrics* 68:650-660, 1981.
113. Baraff LJ, Shields WD, Beckwith L, Strome G, Marcy SM, Cherry JD, Manclark CR: Infants and children with convulsions and hypotonic-hyporesponsive episodes following diphtheria-tetanus-pertussis immunization: follow-up evaluation, *Pediatrics* 81:789-794, 1988.
114. Blumberg DA, Lewis K, Mink CM, Christenson PD, Chatfield P, Cherry JD: Severe reactions associated with diphtheria-tetanus-pertussis vaccine: detailed study of children with seizures, hypotonic-hyporesponsive episodes, high fevers, and persistent crying, *Pediatrics* 91:1158-1165, 1993.
115. Ström J: Further experience with reactions, especially of a cerebral nature, in conjunction with triple vaccination: a study based on vaccinations in Sweden, 1959-65, *Br Med J* 2:320-323, 1967.
116. Aldersdale R, Bellman MH, Rawson NSB, Ross EM, Miller DL: The National Childhood Encephalopathy Study: a report of 1000 cases of serious neurological disorders in infants and young children from the NCES research team. In *Whooping cough: reports from the Committee on Safety Of Medicines and the Joint Committee on Vaccination And Immunization,* London, 1981, Department of Health and Social Security, Her Majesty's Stationary Office.
117. Miller D, Ross EM, Alderslade R, Bellman MH, Rawson NS: Pertussis immunization and serious acute neurological illness in children, *Br Med J* 282:1595-1599, 1981.
118. Miller D, Wadsworth J, Diamond J, Ross E: Pertussis vaccine and whooping cough as risk factors for acute neurological illness and death in young children, *Dev Biol Stand* 61:389-394, 1985.
119 Miller D, Madge N, Diamond J, Wadsworth J, Ross E: Pertussis immunization and serious acute neurological illnesses in children, *Br Med J* 307:1171-1176, 1993.
120. MacRae KD: Epidemiology, encephalopathy, and pertussis vaccine. In FEMS-Symposium: Pertussis. Proceedings of the conference organized by the Society for Microbiology and Epidemiology of the GDR, Berlin, April 20-22, 1988, pp 302-311.
121. Walker AM, Jick H, Perera DR, Knauss TA, Thompson RS: Neurologic events following diphtheria-tetanus-pertussis immunization, *Pediatrics* 81:345-349, 1988.
122. Griffin MR, Ray WA, Mortimer EA Jr, Fenichel GM, Schaffner W: Risk of seizures and encephalopathy after immunization with the diphtheria-tetanus-pertussis vaccine, *JAMA* 263:1641-1645, 1990.
123. Shields WD, Nielsen C, Buch D, Jacobsen V, Christenson P, Zachau-Christiansen B, Cherry JD: Relationship of pertussis immunization to the onset of neurologic disorders: a retrospective epidemiologic study, *J Pediatr* 113:801-805, 1988.
124. Gale JL, Thapa PB, Wassilak SGF, Bobo JK, Mendelman PM, Foy HM: Risk of serious acute neurological illness after immunization with diphtheria-tetanus-pertussis vaccine, *JAMA* 271:37-41, 1994.
125. Fukuyama Y, Tomori N, Sugitate M: Critical evaluation of the role of immunization as an etiological factor of infantile spasms, *Neuropediatrie* 8:224-237, 1977.
126. Melchior JC: Infantile spasms and early immunization against whooping cough: Danish survey from 1970 to 1975, *Arch Dis Child* 52:134-137, 1977.
127. Bellman MH, Ross EM, Miller DL: Infantile spasms and pertussis immunization, *Lancet* 1:1031-1034, 1983.
128. Lombroso CR: A prospective study of infantile spasms: clinical and therapeutic correlations, *Epilepsia* 24:135-148, 1983.
129. Bernier RH, Frank JA, Dondero JJ Jr, Turner P: Diphtheria-tetanus toxoids-pertussis vaccination and sudden infant deaths in Tennessee, *J Pediatr* 101:419-421, 1982.
130. Baraff LJ, Ablon WJ, Weiss RC: Possible temporal association between diphtheria-tetanus toxoid-pertussis vaccination and sudden infant death syndrome, *Pediatr Infect Dis* 2:7-11, 1983.
131. Taylor EM, Emery JL: Immunization and cot deaths, *Lancet* 2:721, 1982 (letter).
132. Hoffman HJ, Hunter JC, Damus K, Pakter J, Peterson DR, van Belle G, Hasselmeyer EG: Diphtheria-tetanus-pertussis immunization and sudden infant death: results of the National Institute of Child Health and Human Development cooperative epidemiologic study of sudden infant death syndrome risk factors, *Pediatrics* 79:698-711, 1987.
133. Walker AM, Jick H, Perera DR, Thompson RS, Knauss TA: Diphtheria-tetanus-pertussis immunization and sudden infant death syndrome, *Am J Public Health* 77:945-951, 1987.
134. Wennergren G, Milerad J, Lagercrantz H, Karlberg P, Svenningsen NW, Sedin G, Anderson D, Grogaard J, Bjure J: The epidemiology of sudden infant death syndrome and attacks of listlessness in Sweden, *Acta Pediatr Scand* 76:898-906, 1987.
135. Griffin MR, Ray WA, Livengood JR, Schaffner W: Risk of sudden infant death syndrome (SIDS) after immunization with the diphtheria-tetanus-pertussis vaccine, *N Engl J Med* 319:618-623, 1988.
136. Bouvier-Colle MH, Flahaut A, Messiah A, Jougla E, Hatton F: Sudden infant death and immunization: an extensive epidemiological approach to the problem in France: winter 1986, *Int J Epidemiol* 18:121-126, 1989.
137. Howson CP, Howe CJ, Fineberg HV, eds: *Adverse effects of pertussis and rubella vaccines: a report of the Committee to Review the Adverse Consequences of Pertussis and Rubella Vaccines,* Washington DC, 1991, Division of Health Promotion and Disease Prevention, Institute of Medicine, National Academy Press.
138. Howson CP, Fineberg HV: The ricochet of magic bullets: summary of the Institute of Medicine report, "Adverse effects of pertussis and rubella vaccines," *Pediatrics* 89:318-324, 1992.
139. Cowan LD, Griffin MR, Howson CP, Katz M, Johnston RB Jr, Shaywitz BA, Fineberg HV: Acute encephalopathy and chronic neurological damage after pertussis vaccine, *Vaccine* 11:1371-1379, 1993.
140. Bernbaum JC, Daft A, Anolik R, Samuelson J, Barkin R, Douglas S, Polin R: Response of preterm infants of diphtheria-tetanus-pertussis immunizations, *J Pediatr* 107:184-188, 1985.
141. Koblin BA, Townsend TR, Munoz A, Onorato I, Wilson M, Polk BF: Response of preterm infants to diphtheria-tetanus-pertussis vaccine, *Pediatr Infect Dis J* 7:704-711, 1988.
142. American Academy of Pediatrics, Committee on Infectious Diseases: Acellular pertussis vaccines: recommendations for use as fourth and fifth doses, *Pediatrics* 90:121-123, 1992.

143. Bernbaum J, Daft A, Samuelson J, Polin RA: Half-dose immunization with diphtheria, tetanus, pertussis: response of preterm infants, *Pediatrics* 83:471-476, 1989.
144. Booy R, Aitken SJM, Taylor S, Tudor-Williams G, Macfarlane JA, Moxon ER, Ashworth LA, Mayon-White RT, Griffiths H, Chapel HM: Immunogenicity of combined diphtheria, tetanus and pertussis vaccine given at 2, 3 and 4 months versus 3, 5 and 9 months, *Lancet* 339:507-510, 1992.
145. Edwards KM, Decker MD: Graham BS, Mezzatesta J, Scott J, Hackell J: Adult immunization with acellular pertussis vaccine, *JAMA* 269:53-56, 1993.
146. Shefer A, Dales L, Nelson M, Werner B, Baron R, Jackson R: Use and safety of acellular pertussis vaccine among adult hospital staff during an outbreak of pertussis, *J Infect Dis* 171:1053-1056, 1995.
147. Centers for Disease Control: Diphtheria, tetanus and pertussis: recommendations for vaccine prophylaxis and other preventive measures—recommendations of the Immunization Practices Advisory Committee (ACIP), *MMWR* 34:405-426, 1985.
148. The Australian College of Pediatrics policy statement: Contraindications to immunization against pertussis, *J Paediatr Child Health* 30:310-311, 1994.

CHAPTER 43

Mycobacterial Infections

Max Klein and Michael D. Iseman

Tuberculosis

Max Klein

Tuberculosis (TB) is a chronic bacterial disease caused by infection with the *Mycobacterium tuberculosis* complex (MTC). The MTC comprises *Mycobacterium tuberculosis, Mycobacterium bovis,* and *Mycobacterium africanum.* These three species produce an identical spectrum of clinical disease, although *M. bovis* has a predilection for extrapulmonary spread to bone and is intrinsically resistant to pyrazinamide. Bacille Calmette-Guérin (BCG) is a stable attenuated strain of *M. bovis* that has been used for vaccination since 1921. A fourth member of the MTC, *Mycobacterium microti,* is pathogenic for voles but not humans. Mycobacterium tuberculosis itself is the most important member of the complex and accounts for over 95% of human TB, even in areas of the world where *M. bovis* infection is prevalent.

The disease is named after the tubercle, or small granular nodule, which was first recognized and named by Francis Sylvius in 1671. The essential unity of tuberculosis of different organs was first recognized by Laennec (1781-1826), although its cause remained a mystery. Ancients such as Galen (AD 121-201) considered the exhaled air of consumptive patients dangerous. The term *scrofula,* from the Latin for a breeding sow, reflects fifteenth-century thought linking tuberculous enlargement and ulceration of the cervical lymph nodes to infection from an animal source.[1] Although pigs may be infected with *M. tuberculosis,* it is thought that the principal cause of scrofula at that time was not the sow but the cow—*M. bovis* and bovine TB. However, by the middle of the nineteenth century the prevailing view was that consumption was a constitutional disease and not communicable. In 1865 a French military doctor, Jean-Antoine Villemin (1827-1892), was the first to prove the infectious nature of TB by passing it from humans to cattle and from cattle to rabbits. The modern history of TB starts in 1882 with the discovery by Robert Koch of a staining technique that enabled him to see the microbe. He was able to demonstrate that the bacillus was present consistently in lesions, that it could be isolated from them in pure culture, and that the injection of these pure cultures produced tubercles in healthy animals. The announcement of the discovery came on March 24, 1882, the anniversary of which is now commemorated by the World Health Organization (WHO) as World Tuberculosis Day.

EPIDEMIOLOGY[2-56]

M. tuberculosis is the most lethal bacterial pathogen of all time. The WHO estimates that TB today kills more youth and adults than any other infectious disease, that TB is a bigger killer than malaria and AIDS combined, that it kills more women than all the combined causes of maternal mortality, and that it kills 100,000 children each year. In the century since 1882 when Koch discovered the tubercle bacillus, an estimated 200 million people are thought to have died of the disease.

Conservative WHO estimates indicate that over 8 million new TB cases occur annually. Only 5 million of these persons receive any form of treatment at all, and less than one tenth receive WHO's current global TB control strategy: directly observed treatment, short course (DOTS). It is predicted that if the present rate of increase (approximately 16% per year) is not curbed, nearly 1 billion more people will become infected with *M. tuberculosis* between now and 2020. Of these billion people, 200 million will develop clinical disease, and 70 million will die. In 1993 the WHO took the unprecedented step of declaring TB a global emergency.

Children

Children are the victims of adults and adolescents with TB; child-to-child transmission of *M. tuberculosis* is virtually unknown. Nahmias et al[34] refer to TB as an "adultosis"—a disease inflicted by adults on children and not by children on adults.

The age and gender distributions of TB in the United States are broadly representative of the world at large (Table 43-1). The incidence of TB in childhood is lower than that at older ages. Most children with TB are younger than 5 years of age, and more than 90% of child TB deaths are in this age group. Children 5 to 15 years of age are at lowest risk for TB of any age group. During childhood the genders are equally affected, the 2:1 male preponderance becoming apparent after puberty.

At greatest risk of dying from TB are infants, young children, and the elderly, but the greatest numbers of cases and deaths in absolute terms are in economically active young adults 25 to 44 years of age. Of the 3 million TB deaths worldwide in 1995, an estimated 1 million were women and 100,000 were children.

The fact that "only" 100,000 children die each year from TB, as opposed to millions of adults, creates the illusion that TB is of relatively little importance for children. But the indirect impact of TB on children is immense. As of 1995, an estimated 180 million children younger than 15 years of age were already infected with *M. tuberculosis* and constitute a reservoir from which many adult cases will arise. In addition, the health and lives of millions of children are placed at risk as parents, grandparents, or neighbors become sick with TB and can no longer provide for them. That the majority of women who become sick with TB are mothers in their child-rearing years has especially serious implications for child survival, economic productivity, and family welfare. It is likely that no other infectious disease creates as many orphans as TB, and this problem is set to assume ominous proportions as TB death rates among young people rise as a consequence of human immunodeficiency virus (HIV) coinfection.

Table 43-1 Rates (Total Cases) of Tuberculosis per 100,000 Population, by Gender and Age Group—United States, 1985 and 1992

CHARACTERISTIC	1985	1992	CHANGE IN RATE (%)
Gender			
Male	12.5 (14,496)	14.0 (17,433)	+12.0
Female	6.3 (7704)	7.1 (9236)	+12.7
Age group (years)			
0-4	4.4 (789)	5.5 (1074)	+25.0
5-14	1.4 (472)	1.7 (633)	+21.4
15-24	4.2 (1672)	5.5 (1974)	+31.0
25-44	9.2 (6758)	12.7 (10,444)	+38.0
45-64	13.7 (6138)	13.4 (6487)	−2.1
>65	22.3 (6356)	18.7 (6025)	−16.1

Adapted from CDC: Tuberculosis morbidity—United States, 1992, *MMWR* 42:696-697,703-704, 1993.

Global Trends

The WHO estimates that about 2 billion people—one third of the world's population—are infected with *M. tuberculosis* (Table 43-2), with 3 million TB deaths. Thirteen countries account for nearly 75% of the world's TB cases and about 80% of the deaths: Pakistan, India, Bangladesh, Thailand, Indonesia, Philippines, China, Brazil, Mexico, Russia, Ethiopia, Zaire, and South Africa. But TB is also a problem for developed countries. The dismantling of TB control services in the United States and Eastern Europe during the 1980s triggered a resurgence of the disease and formed a fertile breeding ground for the emergence of drug-resistant TB.

It is estimated that by 2005 the incidence of new TB cases will increase to 12 million per year—an increase of 58% over 1990 (see Table 43-2). This estimate is based primarily on notifications, and because TB cases are generally underreported, the estimate is likely to be conservative. An important contributor to this increase will be the AIDS coepidemic.

The low incidence of TB in the world's most developed countries is somewhat illusory. All have subpopulations at increased risk in whom the incidence of TB equals that of some of the worst-affected countries. In the United Kingdom (UK) the incidence of TB in persons of Indian subcontinent ethnic origin was 120/100,000 in 1988—a rate 25 times that of whites. Although they constitute only 3% of the population, UK Indians account for 40% of all TB cases. In the United States more than two thirds of TB cases occur in racial and ethnic minorities, with Asians 10 times more likely; blacks 8 times more likely; and Hispanics, Native Americans, and Alaskan Natives 5 times more likely than non-Hispanic whites to have TB. Similarly, the aboriginal populations of Canada and Australia have higher rates of TB than persons of European origin. In general TB rates are lower in rural than in urban communities despite the latter usually having access to better medical care.

Table 43-2 Estimated Number of Tuberculosis Cases and Crude Incidence Rates Worldwide—1995, 2000, and 2005

	1995		2000		2005	
REGION	CASES*	RATE†	CASES*	RATE†	CASES*	RATE†
Southeast Asia	3499	241	3952	247	4454	256
Western Pacific ‡	2045	140	2255	144	2469	151
Africa	1467	242	2079	293	2849	345
Eastern Mediterranean	745	168	870	168	987	170
Americas§	606	123	645	120	681	114
Eastern Europe‖	202	47	210	48	218	49
World's most developed countries¶	204	23	211	24	217	24
All regions	8,768	152	10,222	163	11,875	176
Increase since 1990	16.3%		35.6%		57.6%	

Adapted from CDC: Estimates of future global tuberculosis morbidity and mortality, *MMWR* 42:961-964, 1993.
*In thousands.
†Per 100,000 population.
‡Except Japan, Australia, and New Zealand.
§Except the United States and Canada.
‖Includes all independent states of the former Union of Soviet Socialist Republics.
¶Western Europe and the United States, Canada, Japan, Australia, and New Zealand.

U.S. Trends

TB reporting began in the United States in 1944 with more than 126,000 cases recorded. Over the next four decades the incidence declined steadily to reach 22,201 cases in 1985. This was followed by a resurgence, with TB incidence increasing by 14% to 26,673 cases in 1992 with approximately 2000 deaths. Resurgent TB was an urban phenomenon, the incidence of TB in nonurban areas actually falling 3% from 6.7 to 6.5 cases per 100,000 over this period. Rising rates were attributed to a number of causes, including the acquired immunodeficiency syndrome (AIDS) epidemic, a redistribution of funds away from TB programs, and the crowded conditions in inner-city slums, mental institutions, homeless shelters, and prisons. Immigrants from countries where TB is endemic brought the disease with them and accounted for about 25% of new cases. The increased incidence of TB in adults had the expected effect on children; the incidence of TB in children younger than 5 years old increased 25% from 1985 to 1992 (see Table 43-1).

In 1992 a special federal task force was established to address the problem of increasing case rates and outbreaks of drug-resistant TB. Since 1993 there has been a steady drop in the incidence of TB with 11,853 cases reported in 1997—a 38% improvement over 5 years and the lowest incidence ever recorded. The rates in children under 15 years of age are lagging behind the adult trend with a 25% decline over the same period—reflecting prior infection by adult cases during the preceding few years. The remarkable success achieved in this brief period is a dramatic demonstration of the potency of the tools that are available for the control of TB, when properly applied and adequately funded.

Human Immunodeficiency Virus and Tuberculosis

Over the past decade the HIV pandemic has caused a devastating increase in the incidence of TB in adults, with children the secondary victims. For example, it is estimated that one third of TB cases in sub-Saharan Africa after 1985 would not have occurred in the absence of the HIV epidemic. The effect of HIV on the incidence of TB in adults is mainly due to the enormously accelerated rate of reactivation of latent TB infection in HIV-TB–coinfected individuals. Latent infections reactivate at the rate of 10% per year in those coinfected with HIV-TB as opposed to a lifetime risk for reactivation of about 10% in otherwise healthy individuals.

HIV infection adversely affects the outcome of TB in children as assessed by response to treatment and survival. Children with HIV-TB coinfection are commonly anergic to tuberculin testing and more often have clinical evidence of disseminated disease at presentation.

Control of Tuberculosis[57-64]

Principles

> *Poor treatment multiplies the number of surviving, infectious cases in the community and, thus, actually deteriorates the epidemiological situation.*
>
> **Stefan Grzybowski[25]**

The principles of what is needed for the control of TB and its ultimate eradication from the world are simple in concept and easily comprehensible. In the first instance the source of infection must be eliminated. The source of infection is known: almost invariably it is an adult with viable organisms in the sputum. Even in countries where *M. bovis* TB is prevalent in dairy animals, the principal source of tuberculosis is a human with *M. tuberculosis* infection and not milk. The infectiousness of patients who have TB is directly related to the number of tubercle bacilli that they expel into the air. Adults with laryngeal TB or pulmonary cavities have the highest concentrations of bacilli in their sputum and are the most infectious. Children with TB generally have few or no bacilli in the sputum and are thus are not contagious or only feebly so. Children nevertheless are of crucial importance to any control program. A diagnosis of TB in a child is a sentinel event, representing recent transmission of *M. tuberculosis* from an adult who is often in the same home. Because they are such a highly infectious group and pose a danger to everyone in their surroundings, the tracing and treatment of adult sources and contacts of child TB cases deserve the highest priority in any TB control program. High priority should also be given to examining children who are contacts of adult cases, because newly infected children are at high risk for miliary TB and meningitis and require prompt therapy.

Once infectious adult cases are controlled and resources allow, it is appropriate to attempt to find and treat people who have latent *M. tuberculosis* infections instead of waiting for TB to develop. But this is a hugely expensive and complicated undertaking: with the exception of some high-risk groups, including children younger than 5 years of age, only about 10% of individuals who are infected with *M. tuberculosis* will ever develop disease; 90% will thus be treated unnecessarily in such a prevention program. The allocation of resources to the finding and treatment of persons with latent infections before there is control over infectious cases has been a common failure of TB programs worldwide. It accounts in part for the resurgence of TB in the United States during the 1980s, when funding for TB programs was cut and available resources were often misapplied in this direction.

Obstacles

The obstacles in the way of TB control relate to human nature and the lack of political will to fight the disease. There is highly effective therapy for TB that is capable of curing almost all cases, but it is not ideal: medications have to be taken regularly for at least 6 months. The problem is that many people are incapable of adhering to and completing any course of antimicrobial therapy when they feel well, almost regardless of whether it is a 10-day course of penicillin for streptococcal sore throat or a 6-month regimen for TB. Adherence becomes even more problematic for the patient with TB, because the medications often produce unpleasant symptoms such as anorexia or nausea, which frequently are overlooked by physicians. The solution to the adherence problem in TB is to insist that each dose be taken under supervision of a responsible person. This is a core principle of the WHO's DOTS (see below) strategy for dealing with the disease. It is important, however, to appreciate that patients are not the only obstacles. Physicians too have problems with adherence. The implementation of national guidelines remains poor and inconsistent even in developed countries.[58]

DOT and DOTS. There is a fine but important distinction between DOT and DOTS. *DOT* is the acronym for directly observed therapy, whereas *DOTS* is the recommended acronym for WHO's comprehensive strategy of total onslaught against TB: Directly Observed Treatment Short-course. There are five key elements to the DOTS strategy:

1. Resources are first to be **directed** toward identifying sputum smear–positive cases for treatment, because they are the sources of infection.
2. Patients must be **observed** swallowing each dose of their medicines by a health care worker or trained volunteer. There can be flexibility and innovation in observing treatment, provided that the observer is accountable to the health services and accessible to the patient.
3. Tuberculosis patients must be provided complete **treatment** and be monitored to ensure that they are being cured. This includes sputum microscopy for diagnosis and evaluation of treatment, a reporting system to monitor the progress of each TB patient in order to quickly identify districts and communities that are not achieving 85% cure rates, and intervention with additional support and training.
4. **Short-course** chemotherapy with isoniazid, rifampicin, pyrazinamide, and streptomycin or ethambutol for 6 or 8 months and the establishment of a dependable supply of medications to ensure that the treatment of TB patients is never interrupted.
5. Government **support** of the DOTS strategy and a commitment make TB control a high political priority.

The DOTS strategy is ranked by the World Bank as one of the most cost-effective of all health interventions, costing only US $1 to $5 for each year of healthy life saved. A 6-month supply of medicines for DOTS costs only US $11 per patient in some parts of the world, and rarely more than US $40. But even such modest costs are beyond the means of those countries where TB constitutes the major problem. The resources required to control TB in the United States serve to illustrate the gap between the resources that are required and those that are allocated for the control of TB in the world. In 1992 a special federal task force was convened to address the problem. In New York City alone $40 million was made available by 1993 for TB control, the Centers for Disease Control and Prevention (CDC) contributing $28 million. For the United States the direct medical expenditures for TB in 1991 were estimated at $703.1 million. The operating budget of the WHO for its Global Tuberculosis Program for 1996 totaled $9.9 million.

Faced with the stalled or slow progress in many of the 22 countries that account for the vast majority of the world's TB cases, an ad hoc committee convened by the WHO to consider the problem made a desperate call in 1998 on heads of state, parliamentary leaders, and finance, planning, and health ministers to exercise their pivotal roles, accusing them of ignorance of the dimensions and costs of the TB epidemic and of the urgency of controlling it.

PATHOGENESIS[65-152]

Transmission[65-78]

Although many animals may be artificially infected with *M. tuberculosis*, humans are the only species in which *M. tuberculosis* is a self-perpetuating pathogen. The only epidemiologically important mode of transmission is airborne with infection occurring through the inhalation of viable bacilli in an enclosed space: a room, hall, school, hospital, or vehicle (Fig. 43-1). In outside air the bacilli are rapidly killed by ultraviolet light, and viable bacilli are so widely dispersed as to render the inhalation of even a single bacillus extremely improbable. The source of infection is almost invariably an adult or adolescent with cavitatory pulmonary TB. The surface of these cavities may be so heavily populated with bacilli growing at the air-tissue interface that it may appear red to the naked eye when the mycobacteria are stained selectively with an acid-fast stain such as the Ziehl-Neelsen stain. Because the pulmonary cavities are in free communication with the air via the bronchi, such patients are often called "open cases." They are highly infectious, disseminating the infection by generating an aerosol of bacilli when they cough or sneeze, or even during ordinary speech when the sputum is heavily laden with bacilli. For infants and children, the source is often a parent or other adult who lives in the same house or who visits it. Child-to-child transmission is virtually unknown. The closer and the more prolonged the contact with an open case, the more likely the child is to become infected. However, infection may also be acquired by transient contact (e.g., as happened to patients of a pediatrician suffering from infectious pulmonary TB).

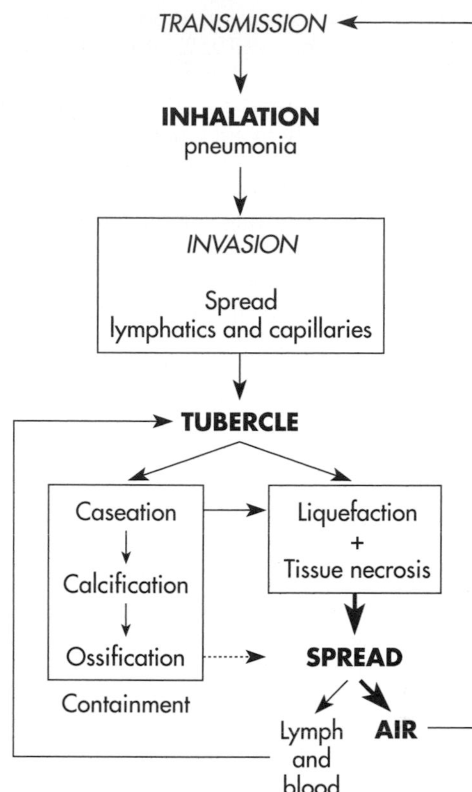

Figure 43-1. Pathogenesis of tuberculosis. Tubercles form when host defenses are unable to eradicate *M. tuberculosis.* Under these circumstances the body adopts a strategy of containment, attempting to permanently entrap bacilli in caseous material. Failure of this mechanism is associated with vigorous bacterial growth, accelerated inflammatory responses, liquefaction, and tissue damage with dissemination of mycobacteria within the body and to the air, initiating the cycle of transmission.

The acquisition of infection through ingestion is of minor importance. Humans may become the incidental hosts of *M. bovis* through drinking contaminated cow's milk. But even where bovine TB is still prevalent, airborne infection with *M. tuberculosis* accounts for over 95% of cases of human TB, including infants.

Aspiration of contaminated material in the birth canal during delivery is a purely hypothetical idea. Transplacental infection is described, but it is a rare curiosity warranting an individual case report, and many such reports are erroneous. Before it was appreciated that inhalational TB was common during the first few months of life in areas of high TB prevalence, it was wrongly assumed that florid TB in children younger than 3 months of age must represent congenital infection.

The aerosol produced by adults and adolescents with infectious pulmonary TB consists of droplets of varying sizes. Droplets larger than 0.1 mm in diameter rapidly settle out of the air because of gravity. If inhaled, these large particles lodge in the nose and upper respiratory tract where infection is unlikely to develop. Droplets smaller than 0.1 mm shrink rapidly by evaporation to form droplet nuclei less than 5 μm in diameter. Droplet nuclei depend primarily on the air for buoyancy, which keeps them suspended for long periods and carries them far. On inhalation, droplet nuclei penetrate the respiratory tract to the level of the alveoli, where a single droplet nucleus containing no more than three bacilli is sufficient to instigate infection.

Molecular Epidemiology

Molecular epidemiology (ME) is the study of the distribution and transmission of disease using molecular methods to identify specific subpopulations of people or strains of microbes. In the case of *M. tuberculosis* ME allows the chain of infection to be tracked, nosocomial infection to be proved, the ratio of reactivation to reinfection TB to be determined for particular communities, and laboratory contamination to be identified. Molecular epidemiology has contributed to an understanding of the origin and spread of multidrug-resistant strains of tuberculosis and the important role of shelters for the homeless in the spread of *M. tuberculosis* in communities. It also has shown that traditional methods of contact tracing do not reliably identify persons infected with the same organism and that measures to reduce TB transmission should focus on locations where persons at high risk of TB congregate in addition to the tracing of personal contacts of infectious cases.

In a feat that ranks in importance with the discovery of the bacillus itself by Koch just over 100 years ago, Cole of the Institut Pasteur in Paris, Barrell of the Sanger Centre in the UK, and 40 colleagues recently reported in *Nature* the complete genomic sequence of *M. tuberculosis* and some of the remarkable insights that this gives into the biology and potentialities of the bacillus.[122] The genome comprises 4,411,529 base pairs, contains around 4000 genes, has a very high guanine-cytosine content, has the capacity for anaerobic metabolism, and differs radically from other bacteria in that a large portion of its coding capacity is devoted to the production of enzymes involved in lipogenesis and lipolysis, presumably concerned with the maintenance of its unique cell wall.[122]

Molecular Tools.[250-266] Fingerprinting of *M. tuberculosis* is usually done by restriction fragment length polymorphism (RFLP) analysis, using Southern blots (after its originator, Edward Southern). RFLP fingerprinting is based on the fact that several copies (commonly 8 to 13, range 0 to >20) of the nucleic acid sequence IS6110 (sixty-one ten) are inserted more or less at random in the genome of *M. tuberculosis*. RFLP analysis is tedious. The bacilli are first grown in culture. The DNA is extracted, amplified using the polymerase chain reaction (PCR), and then split enzymatically into fragments at sites of insertion of IS6110. The DNA fragments are separated electrophoretically and "stained" with a radioactive "probe" specific for IS6110. The fragments appear as distinct bands (the fingerprint) on autoradiographs of the preparation and can be analyzed visually or by computer. The genomic fingerprints were thought to remain stable for years, but it appears that about one third of strains may change within 3 months. Analyses based on an erroneous assumption of genomic stability would underestimate the rate of transmission and of *M. tuberculosis* reinfections in high-prevalence communities and could lead to the misapplication of public health control strategies. Other DNA sequences are often used to subtype IS6110 strains with few insertions (less than 5). Insertion sequences appear to be a fundamental process for generating genomic variation and species diversity in *M. tuberculosis*.

Spacer oligotyping, or spoligotyping, is a more rapid method for typing of *M. tuberculosis* that has recently been developed, based on polymorphism of the chromosomal DR locus.[73] Spoligotyping can be applied directly to clinical samples by PCR and takes a few days, which makes it particularly suitable for the rapid tracing of multidrug-resistant *M. tuberculosis* transmission. For epidemiologic purposes spoligotyping and RFLP fingerprinting provide complementary information.

Immunity[79-116]

Innate Immunity: Invasion

To obtain a foothold in the body, *M. tuberculosis* must first overcome innate defenses that do not require a previous contact with the pathogen. These include the surface epithelia of the respiratory and intestinal tracts and the skin, their secretions and resident flora, and the inflammatory responses that are not antigen specific. Respiratory epithelia are resistant to invasion, and *M. tuberculosis* must penetrate down to the alveoli before it can take root. The defenses of the gastrointestinal tract present an even greater obstacle to invasion with most cases of abdominal TB arising through hematogenous dissemination of pulmonary infection. The intact skin is impregnable to *M. tuberculosis*.

The initial events after the arrival of the droplet nucleus in the alveoli are obscure. The conditions in the alveoli are highly conducive to growth of *M. tuberculosis*, and bacilli probably begin replicating as they alight on the alveolar surface. *M. tuberculosis* is a more aggressive pathogen than was previously imagined. It has at least two strategies for invasion. The relative importance of each is unknown. One involves disruption of the alveolar epithelium. Bacilliary constituents induce alveolar epithelial cells to secrete TNF-α and probably other mediators, which initiate a focal inflammatory reaction in which there is uncoupling of intercellular tight junctions and the recruitment of inflammatory cells to the scene. *M. tuberculosis* is also able to invade, replicate within, and disrupt alveolar epithelial cells directly. How bacilli reach the lung lymph and invade pulmonary capillaries is unknown, because *M. tuberculosis* is immotile.

Another mechanism of invasion is by subverting macrophages to act as Trojan horses and to carry it across the mucosa and beyond: an ingenious solution to the motility problem. In order to enter the macrophage without harming it, *M. tuberculosis* induces phagocytosis, using both opsonic and nonopsonic means to attach to specific receptors on the macrophage wall.

This initiates phagocytosis, and the mycobacteria become internalized within phagosomes. In the case of conventional microbes phagocytosis is followed by fusion of phagosomes with lysosomes and the eradication of the microbe by lysosomal enzymes. *M. tuberculosis* subverts this mechanism and thrives within human macrophages. How it does so is not fully understood, but it has the ability to inhibit phagolysosomal fusion and to escape into the cytosol by disrupting phagosomes.

Adaptive Immune Response

Clonal Expansion and Differentiation. The first macrophages that mycobacteria come into contact with are essentially on sentry duty. They are poorly armed (nonactivated) for killing. The principal task of these macrophages on ingesting *M. tuberculosis* and recognizing it as foreign is to migrate to foci of mucosa-associated lymphoid tissue (MALT) and regional lymph nodes in order to raise the alarm by activating the adaptive immune response (Figure 43-2). Acting as antigen presenting cells (APCs) the macrophages display (present) the foreign antigens prominently by holding them at a distance from their surface at the tips of protruding molecules of the major histocompatibility complex (MHC)—literally as warning flags.

In the lymphoid tissues APCs are brought into contact with migrating naïve (CD4 −, CD8 −) lymphocytes. These recognize the presented antigen and on receipt of a costimulatory signal, to confirm that it is indeed foreign material and not part of self that is being presented, commence clonal expansion and differentiation. Most T cells activated in response to *M. tuberculosis* express the CD4+ phenotype and are divided into TH1 and TH2 subsets depending on the types of cytokines produced.

TH1 and TH2 CD4+ T cell responses. Immunity to TB requires a CD4+ T cell response and a TH1 pattern of cytokine release, dominated by interleukin-2 (IL-2) and interferon gamma (IFN-γ). The *inflammatory* TH1 cells protect against most intracellular infections, including tuberculosis. The helper TH2 subset produces cytokines such as IL-4 and IL-5 that help B cells proliferate and differentiate and is associated

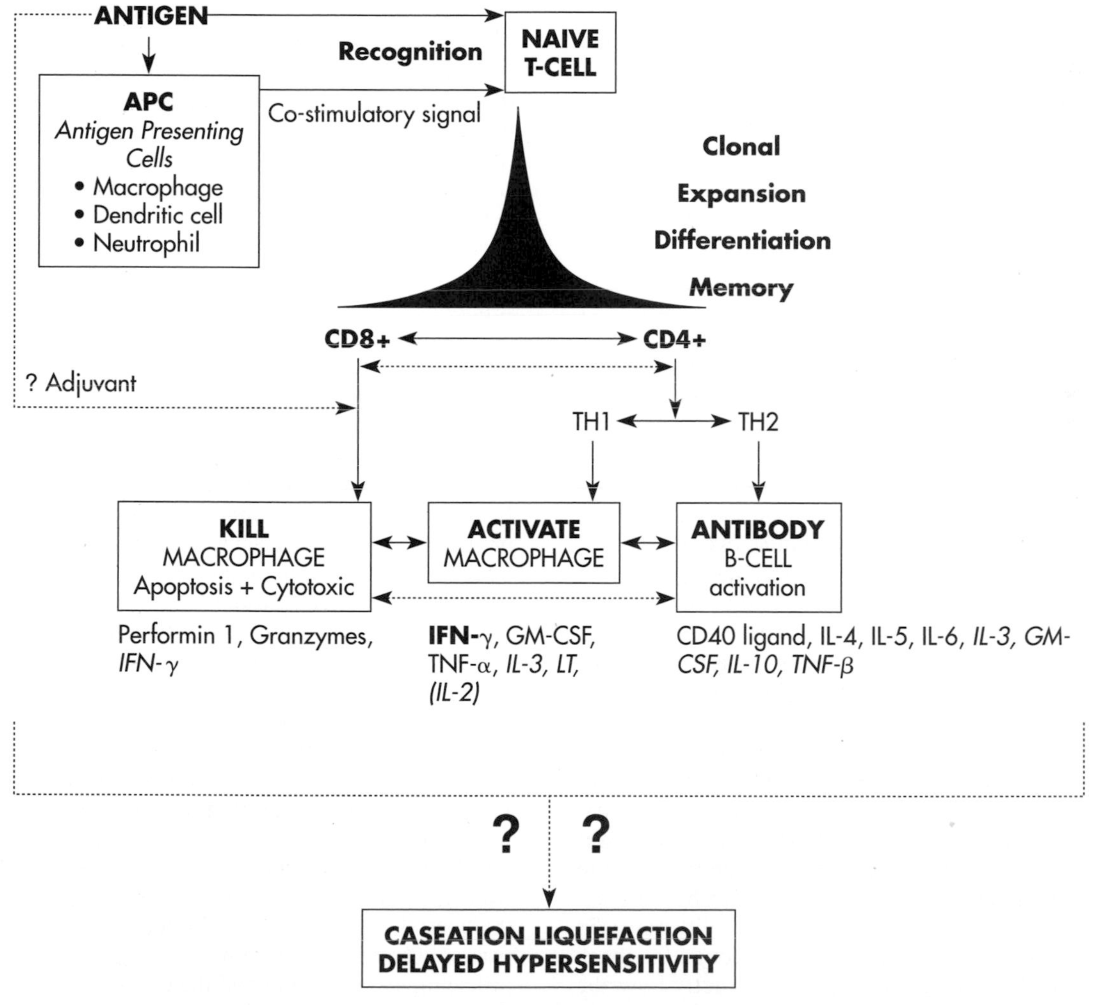

Figure 43-2. Adaptive immune response. The human immune response to *M. tuberculosis* is not well characterized. This representation is extrapolated from experimental work in animals and in vitro. It is widely assumed that a CD4+ T cell response is the fundamental mechanism of protection, with CD8+ T cells playing an uncertain role. Interferon-gamma (IFN-γ) is essential for protective immunity to all mycobacteria. Other cytokines, particularly tumor necrosis factor (TNF), are thought to be responsible for much of the tissue destruction associated with the disease. It is not understood how these immune responses lead to manifestations such as caseation, liquefaction, or cutaneous delayed hypersensitivity to tuberculin.

with humoral-type immune responses. *Killer* CD8+ T cells have the potential to attack and destroy *M. tuberculosis*–containing macrophages by instructing them to die (apoptosis or programmed cell death), by killing them with granzymes (proteases), or by punching holes in their cell walls, but CD8+ T cells appear to play a subsidiary role in the defense against *M. tuberculosis*. TH1 cells activate *M. tuberculosis*–containing macrophages to produce cytotoxins such as nitric oxide (NO) in an attempt to kill the intracellular bacilli. Unlike CD8+ T cells, whose attack is narrowly focused on infected macrophages, the cytotoxic products of TH1 T cell activation are potentially damaging to surrounding tissue cells and may account for collateral tissue damage: anything that is potent enough to kill a microbe can damage normal cells. It should not be thought that the differentiation of T subset function is complete. Most T cells have overlapping effects as evidenced by their cytokine repertoires and interact mutually with one another (see Fig. 43-2, broken arrows) to produce a finely regulated response. Constituents of *M. tuberculosis* are highly immunogenic (adjuvant effect) and may skew the immune response to create conditions favorable to mycobacterial growth and tissue damage.

It is important to appreciate that our understanding of the immunopathogenesis of TB is very limited. Much of our knowledge is extrapolated from animal studies and in vitro work. There are remarkably few critical experimental or clinical data that have defined the immunologic requirements for protection and pathogenesis. It has been questioned whether cell-mediated immunity as manifested by CD4+ cell production of lymphokines and macrophage activation is a sufficient mechanism for protection against *M. tuberculosis* infection.[84] The state of our knowledge may be usefully summarized by substituting "immunology" for "mathematics" in this quotation from Albert Einstein: "As far as the propositions of mathematics refer to reality, they are not certain; and as far as they are certain, they do not refer to reality."

Tubercle[117-120]

Natural History

The visible histologic correlate of the immune events is the tubercle. It is an avascular granuloma—an aggregation of mononuclear cells in response to a continuing presence of *M. tuberculosis* at its center—the evolving appearance of which may be likened to serial aerial photographs of a battle scene. Different cell types are discernible in the defending army, and their origins, hierarchical relationships, and even the fine molecular structure of their walls are known from immunobiology. Diagrams such as Figure 43-2 attempt to extract order from a complex process in which the body's immune and tissue cells, neurohumoral mediators and cytokines, and the microbes and their products are all present and interacting with one another simultaneously. Overall, the system behaves according to the principles of chaos theory: minute differences in the initial conditions are amplified rapidly through feedback to produce markedly divergent effects.[118] Exactly how the unique feature of TB, the tubercle, emerges out of this apparent turmoil is not understood.

Knowledge of the earliest lesions in TB come from studies in experimental animals in which viable *M. tuberculosis* have been injected intravenously. These lodge in pulmonary capillaries, and within a few hours polymorphonuclear neutrophils are seen to be ingesting the bacteria. The initial appearance is the same as in pyogenic infections, but the scene soon becomes dominated by newly arrived macrophages, which proceed to ingest neutrophils containing *M. tuberculosis* and free-lying bacilli. By the end of the second day almost all the organisms are found within the macrophages. The role of neutrophils in the initial response to inhalational infection is unknown. Neutrophils and macrophages are the body's principal machines of defense. How the decision is reached to deploy macrophages in tuberculosis is not understood.

The tubercle starts as a minute cluster of macrophages that by the end of 2 or 3 weeks reaches about 1 mm in diameter and is visible as a small gray point. In the central parts of the cluster adjacent macrophages fuse for unknown reasons and by unknown mechanisms to form multinucleate giant cells. On histology, the cluster of cells has a typical appearance. In the center is a large, multinucleate giant cell, the so-called Langhans' giant cell, which often contains ingested tubercle bacilli in the cytoplasm. Clustered around the giant cell are large numbers of discrete macrophages, most of which have become distorted into slender radiating shapes referred to as *epitheliod.* Last, on the outside of the tubercle and extending into the surrounding tissues there is generally a zone of lymphocytes. The lesion, if not growing rapidly, becomes encapsulated by circumferentially arranged strands of fibrous tissue that tend to restrain the spread of the bacilli.

It is probably rare for the infection to be eradicated before the primary lesion has undergone some degree of necrosis (caseation). It occurs as centrally placed macrophages become further and further separated from the surrounding blood vessels through the crowding in of more and more of them at the periphery, presumably interfering with their oxygen supply. Partly as a result of this anoxia, partly as a result of the substances liberated from the bacilli themselves, these central cells eventually die, releasing contained microorganisms. They do not propagate well within the caseum, which contains relatively few bacilli. Although it is appears homogeneous, the original cellular outlines can be seen within the caseum for some time by special stains. These undergo gradual dissolution with elastic fibers being the last to disappear. Dystrophic calcification follows, which consolidates the entrapment of the bacilli. Calcified lymph nodes may be visible on radiographs within 6 months, but in the majority of instances the lesions are too small or too lightly calcified to be seen radiographically. Revascularization of calcified tubercles may follow years later in the process of ossification. This enables entrapped bacilli to escape and is one of the mechanisms by which disseminated tuberculosis may be produced in apparently immunocompetent adults.

Caseation is a highly effective strategy for the containment of infection and the prevention of dissemination. When caseous containment fails, the necrotic area develops into a viscid liquid pus containing a profusion of growing bacilli. Phagocytosis of these bacilli by marginal macrophages, followed by further giant cell formation, then takes place, so that several satellite giant cell systems now arise at the periphery of the central. These advancing granulomas destroy contiguous tissues. The entire lymph node may become caseous, and the process may extend beyond the capsule to surrounding tissue. Erosion of vessels and airways results in the discharge of the infectious pus into these channels and to hematogenous, bronchial, and airborne dissemination of the disease.

Clinical Significance

That TB is characterized by granuloma formation is of great clinical importance. Being granulomatous means that organ damage is initially limited to small focal areas and that even when the disease is fairly advanced, the bulk of the tissue remains healthy. Consequently organ damage may be far advanced before functional impairment becomes apparent or clinical symptoms occur. It also means that it is possible for TB to resolve on therapy without leaving any permanent disturbance of organ function. Infants and children are at a particular advantage because they have the capacity, which mature adults lack, for compensatory lung growth from the islands of undamaged pulmonary tissue. In the vast majority of infants and young children antimicrobial therapy thus results in complete resolution of pulmonary disease and in full recovery of pulmonary function even when TB is bilateral and widespread in the lungs. With compensatory lung growth damaged foci are diluted and disappear in a sea of normal tissue.

Mycobacterium Tuberculosis

Evolutionary Biology[120-132]

It is thought that *M. tuberculosis* speciated about 15,000 to 20,000 years ago and shares an evolutionary-old common ancestor with *M. bovis*.[130] There is paleontologic evidence of TB of the spine in human remains about 6000 years old. The first written mention of tuberculoses of the lungs occurs in the Indian Rig-Veda (about 1500 BC). TB probably remained an uncommon disease until the Industrial Revolution of the eighteenth and early nineteenth centuries, when it reached epidemic proportions in Western Europe, becoming the single largest cause of death and being notorious as the White Plague:[20]

> Physiological misery and crowding permitted the explosive spread of the disease among the labor classes and from this huge focus the infection spread through society by means of countless unavoidable contacts. . . . The passion for financial gains made acquisitive men blind to the fact that they were part of the same social body as the unfortunates who operated their machines.

In Europe the incidence of TB had begun to decline well before the turn of the century, possibly as the most susceptible were eradicated by disease and the more resistant host survivors reproduced. There is evidence that *M. bovis* was present on the American continent before the age of discovery and colonization, but *M. tuberculosis* was almost certainly introduced from Europe to relatively naïve indigenous populations in the Americas, Africa, and Asia at that time.

Superficially, *M. tuberculosis* would seem to be an unlikely candidate to have become the most lethal bacterial pathogen of all time. By comparison with "major" epidemic diseases such as cholera, diarrhea, typhus, measles, smallpox, malaria, yellow fever, and influenza, *M. tuberculosis* has many disadvantages. It is of relatively low infectivity as compared with diarrheal organisms. It comprises virtually a single clone with remarkably little variation in *M. tuberculosis* complex structural genes, as compared, for example, with enteric organisms and influenza, making it a sitting target for the immune system. It is immotile and replicates very slowly, with a generation time of approximately 18 hours as compared with approximately 20 minutes for diarrheal organisms. It does not produce a toxin, so it must invade the host in order to produce disease. It lacks an efficient animal vector. Although domestic animals, notably the cow, pig, fowl, and cat, are susceptible to infection, they do not constitute an important reservoir for transmission of the disease. Although *M. tuberculosis* is dependent on airborne dissemination, it survives in the atmosphere for only a matter of hours and is readily dispersed by air currents, unlike diarrheal organisms, which propagate actively in the water that distributes them.

However, it possesses three critically important pathogenic factors. The first is its potential to survive and to produce disease throughout the lifetime of its host. The second is its ability to produce pulmonary disease and disseminate itself by provoking the host to cough. The third factor is its ability to produce disease without immobilizing its host and to kill its host only slowly, if at all. Host illness is a potential liability for *M. tuberculosis* because it depends on its host's mobility to reach more hosts. Ineffective therapy that maintains host mobility without achieving disinfection thus aids and abets dissemination of disease. These positive pathogenic attributes are alone not sufficient to account for the astonishing success of *M. tuberculosis* as a pathogen.

Being dependent on virtually direct indoor host-to-host transfer, TB would have remained an uncommon curiosity if not for the propensity of humans to gather in groups and to spend much time indoors. It has been estimated that a social network of 180 to 440 persons is required to achieve the stable host-pathogen relationship necessary for tuberculous infection to become endemic in a community.[129] Population density is a principal determinant of disease. Even in developed countries where TB is uncommon, it is a disease of urban rather than rural communities. The harsh and crowded living conditions of many urban communities facilitate transmission in addition to weakening natural resistance to disease.

Latency. Faced with the body's immune attack, some mycobacteria enter a latent, hibernation-like state within the macrophage. In the absence of active mycobacterial growth the macrophage apparently does not raise a warning flag on its surface, which would mark it for destruction by CD8+ cells or activation by CD4+ cells. It so provides a haven for *M. tuberculosis* where the microbe is invisible to the immune system and free from attack. A sort of living death—the virtual cessation of growth and replication—is the price paid by *M. tuberculosis* for the safe haven that allows it to lurk and await more favorable conditions. In their latent state the mycobacteria are impossible to extract and culture, even though their DNA can be detected and their viability is known from their ability to commence to grow again at any time and produce disease. That latent *M. tuberculosis* organisms are not completely inert is suggested by their vulnerability to antituberculous drugs, if given for several months, and by the fact that they respond to any weakening of host resistance with a resumption in growth.

Nature vs. Nurture

There has long been controversy regarding the relative roles of nature (genetic predisposition) vs. nurture (environment) in the pathogenesis of TB. Socioeconomic influences are so overwhelmingly important that attempts to implicate genetic mechanisms have been viewed as attempts to diminish the political influence of such factors. As with most controversies of this nature, the correct answer lies somewhere in between. Recent studies have not challenged the fact that demographic, environmental, and social factors are the overwhelmingly important determinants of the epidemiology and pathogenesis of the disease. However, they are showing that genetic factors in the host and in the organism play a subsidiary modulating role on the expression of the disease.

Host Factors[133-152]

The terms *susceptibility* and *resistance* are often used interchangeably, but they do in fact refer to different effects. *Susceptibility to infection* refers to the ease with which an infection can be established in the host. Susceptibility reflects the state of innate immune responses. *Resistance to disease* refers to the degree to which the body is able to set up an obstruction that the body offers to the propagation of the organism to disease once infection has been established. Resistance is determined by the adaptive immune response. Predisposition to TB may thus result from increased susceptibility to infection, from reduced resistance to disease, or from a combination of the two. Similarly, reduced susceptibility or increased resistance would be protective.

The 1926 disaster in Lübeck, Germany, provided the first indisputable evidence that certain individuals are more predisposed than others to TB. Of 249 babies mistakenly given the same dose of living virulent TB bacilli instead of BCG, 76 died but 173 survived and were free of clinical disease 12 years later.[20] Further evidence of genetic variability in human predisposition to TB has been difficult to obtain. Several studies have shown TB to be about twice as common in blacks as in whites, but it has not been possible to separate the effects of poverty and deprivation from genetic determinants. A meticulous study of over 25,000 initially tuberculin-negative residents of 165 racially integrated nursing homes in Arkansas found that blacks were twice as susceptible as whites to infection: 13.8% of blacks but only 7.2% of whites developed evidence of a new infection during the study period. However, blacks and whites appear to be equally resistant to the development of disease: Of the newly infected cases, 11.5% of blacks and 10.6% whites developed clinical disease.[149]

A genetic basis for the predisposition of black people to TB has recently been found. In the mouse the gene for natural-resistance–associated macrophage protein 1 (Nramp1)—previously named Bcg—confers protection against intracellular organisms such as leishmania and salmonella, and possibly mycobacteria. A homologue of Nramp1 occurs in humans on chromosome 2, and several polymorphisms in the gene have recently been reported to be associated with TB in black patients in the Gambia.[120] Interestingly, one of the polymorphisms is not found in European populations, providing strong support for the hypothesis that blacks are relatively recent victims of TB as a consequence of exploitation and slavery.[120]

Further evidence that genetic factors affect predisposition to tuberculosis comes from a recent study in Cambodia in which the HLA-DQB1*0503 allele was shown to be significantly associated with TB.[140]

Age and Gender. Unlike immunocompetent adults and adolescents, in whom tuberculous infection is generally contained in the lung with only limited spread to the regional lymph nodes and rarely beyond, the infection in infants and children is rapidly carried by migrating macrophages to regional lymph nodes, which become the predominant site of pathology, with some mycobacteria commonly escaping and establishing themselves elsewhere. The factors that account for these differences in the immune response to *M. tuberculosis* with maturation are not fully understood but include changes in the hormone environment and cross-immunity acquired from exposure to environmental mycobacteria.

The reasons for the 2:1 male predominance after puberty have not been elucidated but almost certainly relate to hormonal influences on immune function.

Comorbid Conditions. Immunocompromise caused by HIV coinfection has decisive effects on resistance to TB and response to treatment.[133-139] HIV-positive children have an up to 8 times higher risk than HIV-negative children of developing TB and have a similarly increased risk of failing standard treatment. However, the largest effect of the HIV epidemic on TB in children is indirect, through an increase in the number of adults with active TB serving as potential sources of TB infection for children. A study in the Bronx, New York, has shown that allowing for the presumed HIV burden in each local community, children living in overcrowded conditions were 5.6-fold more likely to develop TB.[138] Thus, even in the case of HIV-infected children, poverty and household crowding are the most potent determinants of disease.

Children with other causes of immunocompromise, such as malnutrition, severe viral infections (including measles), and malignancies, also are at an increased risk for TB, but the risks have not been well quantified.

DIAGNOSIS[158-273]

Clinical Synopsis[158-184]

The vast majority of infants and children who become infected with *M. tuberculosis* are completely asymptomatic and will never develop TB. Those who do develop the disease demonstrate few symptoms or signs of pulmonary disease at the outset. Fewer than half develop nonspecific symptoms such as fever, anorexia, and weight loss. Most develop cough, and many wheeze. If untreated, symptoms and signs of tuberculous bronchopneumonia and extrapulmonary disease may become apparent.

Tuberculous pleurisy and effusion may develop in association with a subpleural parenchymal focus or after hematogenous spread of tubercle bacilli. The diagnosis is suspected by typical signs of pleural fluid and confirmed radiographically. The protein and cell count of the fluid are increased, and *M. tuberculosis* is rarely detected in smears of the fluid but may grow on culture. Nucleic acid amplification tests may indicate the presence of the bacilli, but a pleural biopsy for histopathologic diagnosis is the investigation of choice, although it is rarely required, because the tuberculin skin test is generally of the order of 15 mm in children with large pleural effusions.

Miliary TB is the result of hematogenous spread, which occurs in the early phase of tuberculous infection. Clinical symptoms are scant early in the course of the disease but rapidly become life threatening.

For the absolute diagnosis of TB the demonstration on culture of *M. tuberculosis* in secretions or tissue of the patient is required. A positive tuberculin skin test shows only that the individual has been infected with *M. tuberculosis* and that the individual has living tubercle bacilli in the body; the tuberculin skin test cannot tell whether the bacilli are living in a quiescent latent state or actively replicating and causing disease. Nucleic acid amplification tests for the diagnosis of TB are limited for the same reason. The presence of living tubercle bacilli in the body as evidenced by a positive tuberculin skin test (or positive nucleic amplification test) thus does not necessarily mean that that individual has the disease TB, or that that individual is infectious to others, or that that individual will ever develop TB. Overall, only about 10% of individuals who are infected with *M. tuberculosis* will develop TB at some time in their lives. The remaining 90%, it is widely believed, will harbor *M. tuberculosis* in their bodies in a latent state throughout life. Because the tuberculin skin test is affected by many factors other than infection with *M. tuberculosis*, a negative tuberculin skin test does not exclude the diagnosis of TB.

When the pathology is virtually confined to the lungs, as is usually the case in adults with pulmonary TB, it is relatively easy to confirm the diagnosis by sputum culture. When the principal focus of infection is the intrathoracic lymph nodes, as often is the situation in infants and young children, the organisms are inaccessible, and it becomes difficult to prove that the person has TB. Compounding the problem is the fact that, by virtue of their size, children produce smaller volumes of sputum than adults, and the sputum that is produced is swallowed. In childhood the sputum also contains fewer organisms as compared with adults because tuberculous pneumonia in childhood takes a caseous "containing" form, as compared with the necrotizing liquefactive process in adults, which generates so many bacilli (see Fig. 43-2).

Because of these factors and the difficulties associated with obtaining adequate samples of swallowed sputum from the stomach, the diagnosis of TB is confirmed bacteriologically in considerably less than half (range 10% to 75%) of infants and young children who are treated for TB. In the majority of cases the diagnosis of TB is based on probability, taking the history, the clinical examination, the radiographic findings, the tuberculin skin test result, and any other appropriate examinations into account. Even in industrialized countries, the triad of a positive tuberculin skin test, an abnormal radiograph, and a history of exposure to an adult with TB remains the most effective method for diagnosing TB in children (Box 43-1). A diagnosis of TB based on probability always errs on the side of overdiagnosis, since underdiagnosis has serious consequences.

Box 43-1
Criteria for the Diagnosis of Pulmonary Tuberculosis

Two or more of the following

- History of close contact with a known or suspected infectious case of TB
- Radiographic finding compatible with TB
- A positive **tuberculin skin test**

  ≥5 mm in children (a) in close contact with known or suspected infectious case of TB; or (b) suspected of having TB on the basis of a chest radiogram; or (c) who have clinical evidence on physical examination or laboratory assessment that would include TB in the working diagnosis (e.g., meningitis, hepatosplenomegaly); or (d) who have immunosupressive conditions, including HIV infection and severe malnutrition; or (e) who are receiving immunosupressive therapy, including immunosupressive therapy, doses of corticosteriods in whom immunosupression or who has HIV infection; or (f) who have features suggestive of HIV infection but are of unknown HIV status.

  ≥10 mm in children at increased risk of dissemination: young age (<4 years) or other medical risk factors including diabetes mellitus, chronic renal failure, or malnutrition.

  ≥15 mm in any child, whether risk factors are present or not.

  Recommendations for considering a Mantoux tuberculin skin test reaction as positive are the same, irrespective of prior BCG vaccination. No reliable method exists for distinguishing tuberculin reactions caused by BCG vaccination from those caused by natural infection.

  Because the interpretation of the TST depends on particular circumstances, both the size of the reaction and the interpretation should be recorded.
- Positive acid-fast stain of sputum or gastric aspirate
- Cough lasting longer than 2 weeks.
- Response to anti-TB therapy (increased by weight by 10% after 2 months, decrease in symptoms)

Modified from Migliori GB et al: *Tuber Lung Dis* 73:145-149,1992; and American Academy of Pediatrics Policy Statement: Update on tuberculosis skin testing of children, *Pediatrics* 97:282-284, 1996.

In the absence of laboratory confirmation the CDC accepts, for purposes of surveillance, a diagnosis of TB that meets the following clinical case definition: a positive tuberculin skin test; other signs and symptoms compatible with TB, such as an abnormal, unstable (worsening or improving) chest radiograph or clinical evidence of current disease; response to treatment with two or more antituberculous medications; and a completed diagnostic evaluation.

Medical History

Presenting Symptoms. In the United States and other developed countries approximately half of children who are infected with *M. tuberculosis* are identified through contact tracing or through screening programs in high-risk communities and can be offered chemoprophylaxis to prevent TB disease. By the time symptoms develop that cause children to be brought for medical attention, the disease is already well established and far advanced. Because TB can affect every organ in the body, the potential symptomatology is protean. In practice over 90% of symptomatic children have complaints related to the respiratory system, and most of these will also have failure to thrive, recent weight loss, or night sweats. In the remaining 10% or so the most common clinical presentation is with neurologic signs of tuberculous meningitis, followed by abdominal TB in frequency: hepatosplenomegaly, tuberculous peritonitis, and protein-losing enteropathy. Of the respiratory symptoms the most common is cough that is insidious in onset and generally has been present for longer than 2 weeks at the time of presentation. Tachypnea and wheeze are common. Presentation is often precipitated by an acute worsening of symptoms, often in conjunction with a concurrent viral respiratory tract infection.

Cough and wheeze are symptomatic of airway irritation and compression by adjacent enlarged and inflamed tracheobronchial lymph nodes (Figs. 43-3 and 43-4) or tuberculous bronchopneumonia. Unless a high index of suspicion for lymphobronchial TB (see p 713) is maintained, such infants and children are at risk of being misdiagnosed as having asthma and being treated with steroids, particularly if there is a positive family history of asthma. As a general rule, children younger than 2 years of age who have wheezing that is not responsive to bronchodilator therapy and that is not clearly related to an antecedent lower respiratory tract infection, or who have a problem such as bronchopulmonary dysplasia, should have other causes of wheezing, such as TB, cystic fibrosis, vascular ring, gastroesophageal reflux, and tracheoesophageal fistula, excluded before being offered a therapeutic trial of corticosteroids.

Family History

Because TB is an "adultosis" and children acquire their *M. tuberculosis* infection from adults,[35] the most important question to ask when taking the history is: Has this child been exposed to an adult who has a chronic cough or TB? All too often, inadequate attention is paid to finding the person who is responsible for infecting the child. An even more important question is, Which children have been in contact with this child? Such children are not at any risk of catching the disease from this child, but they are likely to have been exposed to the same adult(s) and so are also at risk of having been infected.

The social and family history are also worthy of note. Crowding and poverty are the overwhelmingly important determinants of risk for TB, but genetic factors are increasingly being recognized as important contributors to the risk. For ex-

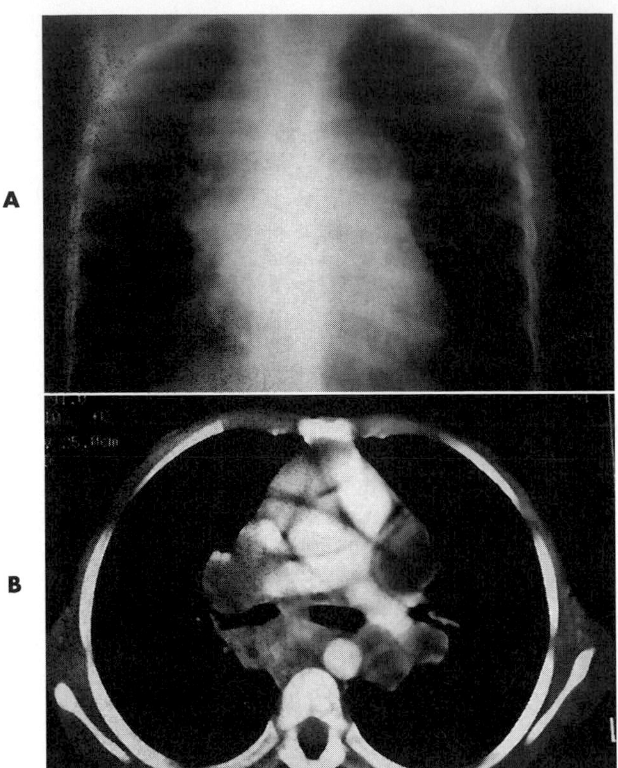

Figure 43-3. **A,** Chest radiograph of a 9-year-old Haitian girl, showing voluminous bilateral paratracheal and hilar lymphadenopathy with obstructive emphysema but without concomitant parenchymal involvement. This radiographic pattern is much more frequent in children than in adults. **B,** Computed tomographic scan from the same child demonstrating central attenuation of the hilar adenopathy. (From Wilson R, ed: *European Respiratory Monograph,* 2:4, July, 1997.)

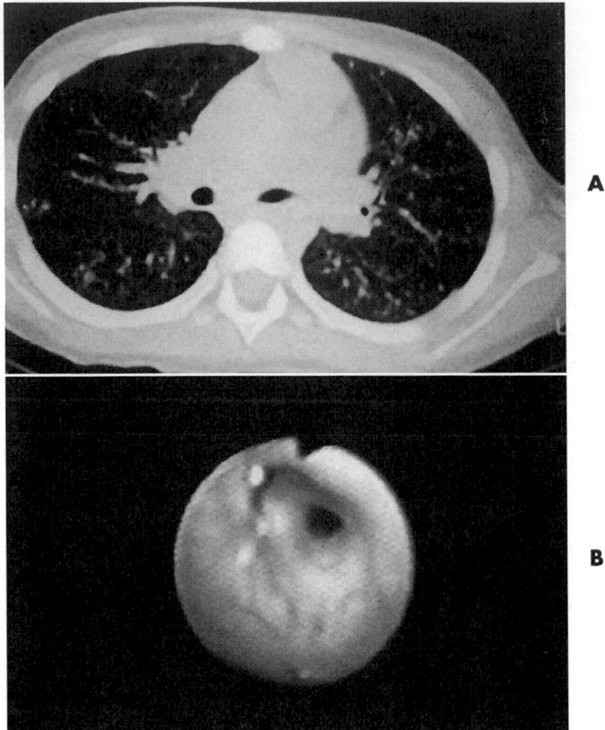

Figure 43-4. **A,** Computed tomographic image of a 4-year-old white girl showing bilateral and discrete micronodular and fine reticulomicronodular opacities, while chest radiograph was not characteristic. **B,** Fibroscopic examination, permitting immediate diagnosis of tuberculosis by showing granulation tissue projecting into the lumen of the right upper bronchus, while bacteriological studies were negative. (From Wilson R, ed: *European Respiratory Monograph,* 2:4, July, 1997.)

ample, black persons are about twice as likely to become infected when exposed to *M. tuberculosis* as those of European extraction, although the risk of progression to disease after infection appears to be the same in both groups.[149] Within groups, familial factors may affect individual predisposition to disease as evidenced by differences in risk according to HLA genotype in Cambodia.[140]

In addition, the physician should determine whether there are medical conditions present, especially HIV infection, that increase the likelihood of TB developing after infection. Patients who have risk factors for HIV infection but who do not know their current HIV status should be offered HIV counseling and testing.

Physical Examination

The only sign on physical examination that is diagnostic of TB is the presence of choroidal tubercles, visible as small, pale areas with indefinite edges adjacent to arterioles in the retina. Approximately one third of children with TB have evidence of failure to thrive or weight loss at presentation. Phlyctenular conjunctivitis and erythema nodosum are sensitivity phenomena that occur with TB and other infections and provide a clue to the possibility of the diagnosis. Generalized lymphadenopathy or clubbing are not features of TB in infants and young children and should alert one to the possibility of HIV infection, among other causes.

Fever greater than 38.5° C may occur from TB but is distinctly unusual in young children with the disease and should raise the possibility of a different or concurrent infection.

Tracheobronchial airway compression is suggested by a harsh Klaxon-like cough and loud wheezing, which is often audible without the aid of a stethoscope. Although tachypneic and recessing, infants with tracheobronchial obstruction often appear remarkably undistressed happy wheezers. This is possibly because of the insidious onset of the disease and its relatively slow progression, which allow the infant to become adapted to it. Tracheobronchial compression that is sufficiently severe to warrant surgical decompression may occur in infants as young as 2 months of age. Marked chest wall retraction in any child is indicative of life-threatening large airway obstruction. In the child with mediastinal adenopathy, marked retractions are indicative of critical tracheobronchial compression and mandate urgent rigid bronchoscopy under general anesthesia with the option to proceed to thoracotomy for surgical relief of airway obstruction if the diagnosis is confirmed.

Percussion often reveals increased resonance over normally dull areas over the heart and upper border of liver caused by bilateral air trapping from peripheral airway obstruction. This probably reflects concurrent lower respiratory tract viral infection, because TB rarely, if ever, produces widespread obstruction of small airways (less than 2 mm in diameter). Dullness on percussion may be caused by underlying consolidation or pleural effusion, but large pleural effusions with stony dullness on percussion are uncommon in children younger than 5 years of age.

Reduced breath sounds over a lung or lobe are a clue to airway obstruction by lymphobronchial TB. Crackles are not a feature of TB and suggest concurrent infection with another pathogen.

TB should always be included in the working diagnosis of children with hepatosplenomegaly and lung disease.

Radiology[185-208]

The radiographic features described below are not mutually exclusive. Often, several patterns coexist, especially in advanced disease.

Lymphobronchial Tuberculosis

Lymph Nodes. The radiographic appearances of TB are diverse, and the disease may mimic virtually every other. However, the hallmark or "footprint" and most constant feature of pulmonary TB in infancy and childhood is mediastinal lymphadenopathy, and most radiologists would be reluctant to consider the diagnosis of TB in its absence (see Fig. 43-3). Adenopathy is usually apparent on conventional anteroposterior (AP) or posteroanterior (PA) views of the chest, the differences between these views being of no practical importance in infants and young children. Lateral views are helpful if there is doubt regarding the anatomic location of intrathoracic masses, helping distinguish thymic shadows (anterior mediastinum) from nodal enlargement (middle mediastinum) or masses in the posterior mediastinum, but enlarged nodes are often difficult to see on lateral views. When there is doubt regarding the presence of nodes, computed tomography (CT) with contrast is generally definitive, showing lymph nodes as ring-enhancing shadows in their expected locations.

Nodal enlargement may be unilateral or bilateral. Hilar lymph node enlargement is usually unilateral and related to pulmonary shadows on the same side. Paratracheal node enlargement is usually unilateral but may be bilateral. Enlarged subcarinal nodes are generally not visible, but their presence may be inferred from narrowing of the left or right main bronchus.

Airways. It is extremely common for tuberculous lymph nodes to involve the adjacent airways by compression from without or by infiltration of the wall and eventual erosion into the lumen. Commonly both mechanisms are operative. Terms applied to the radiographic consequences of this pathology include *endobronchial tuberculosis* (an inaccurate descriptor because most or even all of the pathology may lie outside the lumen), *segmental lesions, right middle lobe syndrome,* and *epituberculosis.* The term *lymphobronchial* has been suggested by Beyers[188] as a unifying term for the spectrum of airway and parenchymal lesions produced by this pathology. Lymphobronchial is apt because it properly reflects the pathology and draws attention to the airways as an integral component of pulmonary TB in childhood.

The trachea and proximal bronchi should be carefully inspected for evidence of narrowing. A mass on one side of the airway tends to displace the airway rather than narrow it. For enlarged lymph nodes to produce extrinsic compression and airway stenosis, they must "grip" the airway circumferentially or, more commonly, on two sides as in a vice (see Fig. 43-3). Circumferential narrowing appears to be due to marked periadenitis enveloping the bronchus. In either case the airway is immobilized in situ. In the case of the trachea, the major vessels may form one side of the vice. In the case of the proximal bronchi, subcarinal lymph node enlargement provides the counterforce to the bronchial lymph nodes. This is the reason why the presence of a subcarinal mass may be inferred when proximal bronchial narrowing is present even though it may not be visible. The vice hypothesis explains why the airways are seldom greatly displaced (see Fig. 43-3), why the angle of the carina is often remarkably well preserved, and why incision and drainage of the subcarinal nodes is generally all that is required to relieve bronchial airway obstruction.

Eroding nodes may cause tracheoesophageal and bronchoesophageal fistula. The usual symptoms are cough, choking, wheezing, and tachypnea on feeding. An air-filled esophagus on chest radiographs of children suspected or known to have TB should suggest the possibility of a fistula. Pneumonia is often severe and is often associated with gastroesophageal reflux and aspiration of acid stomach contents. A diagnostic sign of a fistula between the esophagus and airway in children with severe pneumonia requiring mechanical ventilation is cyclical abdominal distention during each inspiration. A gastrostomy with free communication to the air, gastric drainage to remove acid secretions, and feeding by nasojejunal tube is lifesaving in this situation.

The phrenic nerve must often lie in intimate contact with inflamed tuberculous nodes, yet diaphragmatic paralysis is rare with TB. Phrenic nerve palsy may develop several months after the initiation of therapy for TB, presumably as a consequence of entrapment in healing fibrous tissue.

The often massive mediastinal lymphadenopathy seen in children infected with HIV may be difficult to distinguish from TB. The fact that tuberculous adenopathy commonly is associated with tracheobronchial airway compromise, whereas HIV adenopathy rarely is, is a helpful distinguishing feature.

Lung Fields

TB may present with large mediastinal nodes and clear lung fields, and in rare cases, positive cultures may be obtained from sputum or gastric aspirate in the presence of normal-appearing radiographs. Such inconsistencies are due to the limited power of resolution of the method. CT always shows the disease to be more extensive than can be appreciated on conventional chest films.

Segmental Lesions

The most common changes are inhomogeneous infiltrates with ill-defined borders, a segmental distribution, a base toward the pleura, radiation toward the hila, and often a unilateral presentation. Other varieties of "segmental lesion" include segmental atelectasis with consolidation, segmental consolidation without collapse, lobar or pulmonary hyperinflation, and expansile lobar pneumonia, most commonly of the upper lobes. The foregoing lesions are clearly related in their distribution to the airways with a range of appearances that may reflect varying degrees of airway obstruction.

Cavities

In an attempt to make facts fit the theory, it is still widely taught that cavitation is a feature of "postprimary" adult TB and is rare in childhood. As long as a century ago, however, according to Nauth-Misir,[203] Kuss and D'Avignet found that one in five infants dying of TB in the first year of life showed evidence of cavity formation in the lungs, and contemporary studies have found areas of cavitation in about 15% of infants and young children. The cavities differ from those in adults by having thick walls, being smaller in relation to lung size, and occurring in all zones, not principally the upper lobes.

In the absence of tracheobronchial obstruction, bilateral air trapping (hyperinflation) is suggestive of a concurrent lower respiratory tract viral infection.

Intrapulmonary Bronchial Dissemination

Because the airway mucosa is resistant to invasion, the appearance of "bronchogenic" TB differs from conventional bronchopneumonia in which perihilar infiltrates resulting from airway inflammation are characteristic. The feature of bronchogenic TB is acinar infiltration (acinus: terminal bronchiole and its associated respiratory units) producing widespread 3- to 5-mm rounded shadows with poorly defined margins in the peripheral lung fields. In severe cases a "snowstorm" appearance is produced. As opposed to viral and bacterial bronchopneumonia, respiratory gas exchange often is remarkably well preserved.

Hematogenous Dissemination

Dissemination of bacilli through the pulmonary arterial tree follows contamination of venous blood by infected thoracic duct lymph draining tuberculous lymph nodes. This produces myriads of small disseminated nodular opacities, which are uniformly distributed throughout both lung fields. The appearance is termed *miliary* because of their supposed resemblance to millet seeds, about 1 to 2 mm in diameter. Miliary lesions differ from bronchogenic lesions in being smaller, more numerous, more discrete, and more uniform in appearance during the initial stages of evolution. With more advanced disease the patterns become indistinguishable. CT may reveal several populations of miliary lesions, presumably representing discrete episodes of dissemination.

Acute Respiratory Distress Syndrome

Rarely TB may manifest as a focal intrapulmonary mass or as confluent bilateral consolidation with severe hypoxemic failure that is radiologically indistinguishable from other causes of the acute respiratory distress syndrome (ARDS). An important distinguishing feature of ARDS in TB is that it is responsive to corticosteroid therapy.

Pleura

Small loculated pleural "reactions" (i.e., effusions) are common adjacent to consolidated areas in young children. Chylothorax may occur from lymph node obstruction of the thoracic duct. Large pleural tuberculous effusions requiring treatment in their own right are uncommon in children younger than 5 years of age.

Tuberculin Skin Test[209-233]

The Mantoux test is the standard method for performing tuberculin skin tests (TSTs) and is named after Charles Mantoux (French physician, 1877-1947), who devised it. An intracutaneous injection of 0.1 ml containing five tuberculin units (TU) of a purified protein derivative (PPD) of the bacillus is given into the skin with a fine needle to raise a small bleb on the volar aspect of the forearm. The size of the induration at the site of injection is measured 72 hours later and the greatest diameter recorded in millimeters. The use of multiple-puncture devices for tuberculin testing is strongly discouraged, because the dose of antigen that is injected cannot be quantified. The interpretation of such tests yields even more perplexing problems of interpretation than does the Mantoux test. Reusable testing devices such as the Heaf gun are absolutely contraindicated because of the risk of HIV transmission.

In principle the Mantoux test is simple. Individuals who have been infected with *M. tuberculosis* and who have acquired delayed-type hypersensitivity (DTH) to the bacillus are identified by the fact that they develop induration of the skin at the site of injection. The Mantoux test is a cheap, safe, and efficient tool with which to (1) identify individuals who have been infected with *M. tuberculosis;* (2) screen groups who are at high risk, in order to identify and treat those with TB and to offer the remainder chemoprophylaxis to prevent the progression of infection to disease; and (3) measure the prevalence of *M. tuberculosis* infection. From prevalence data the number of future cases of TB can be estimated and the knowledge used to inform public health policy.[213,214]

In practice the Mantoux test is more complicated, and the result of the test defies simplistic interpretation. First, the antigens employed for testing are not specific for *M. tuberculosis.* Immunization with BCG and exposure to nonpathogenic mycobacteria in the environment induce "nonspecific," generally smaller, "weaker" responses to the Mantoux test. There is no way to tell apart nonspecific reactions from those caused by infection with *M. tuberculosis*. Exposure to nonpathogenic bacteria varies with location: it is minimal in places such as Alaska and heavy in Asia, Africa, parts of the Middle East, and elsewhere. Although nonspecific responses are rarely of concern in young children because of their as yet limited exposure to environmental mycobacteria, nonspecific reactions present a particular problem in population surveys among adults. Second, the same tuberculin and dose are not used globally. The reference standard is 5 TU of PPD-S (Siebert's lot 49608), the preparation employed in the United States. Since 1958 the WHO has recommended the use of 2 TU of PPD-RT (Statens Serum Institut, Copenhagen) for prevalence studies of TB around the world. RT-23-RT is also widely used at the 2 TU dose for diagnostic patient studies. The tuberculin unit is specified in terms of weight of PPD per unit volume. For PPD-23-RT, 2 TU is claimed to be *biologically equivalent* to 5 TU of PPD-S. However, in population surveys RT-23 elicits less cutaneous reactivity when compared with PPD-S, and the manufacturers advise that reactions greater than 6 mm should be regarded as positive. The difference is claimed to be due to greater specificity of RT-23 for *M. tuberculosis* antigen as the result of reduced cross-reactivity to environmental mycobacteria. Differences between products in population studies can generally be factored out by statistical means to render epidemiologic comparisons possible.[230] Whether PPD product differences are of importance in clinical work in pediatrics is not clear. Third, cutaneous DTH may take up to 12 weeks to develop after infection, and the size of the cutaneous reaction is affected by many factors, including the state of the patient's immunity (HIV infection, nutrition, other comorbidity) and technical errors in administration of the PPD. Persons who lack the gene for the major histocompatibility locus HLA-DR3 have diminished responsiveness to tuberculin, probably because of impaired presentation of tubercular antigens by macrophages and other APCs, and may remain persistently tuberculin negative after immunization or infection.[140,181]

Interpretation

The clinical interpretation of Mantoux reactions is clouded in confusion, because of failure to recognize that the cutoff points used in population prevalence studies and in public health TB control programs to categorize patients according to the size of skin induration are not directly applicable to the evaluation of individual patients. The cutoff points that are used in population studies and screening surveys are decided administratively to best meet the objectives of those performing the test.

When the objective is to estimate the prevalence of *M. tuberculosis* infection in a community, the sensitivity of the test is deliberately reduced by selecting a relatively large skin reaction, generally greater than10 mm to 5 TU of PPD-S, as the decision boundary between consequential and inconsequential reactions. This is done to avoid obtaining an overestimate of the number of individuals infected with *M. tuberculosis* by eliminating from the count patients with weaker "nonspecific" reactions resulting from exposure to nonpathogenic environmental mycobacteria and BCG immunization at birth. If, on the other hand, the objective is to screen populations at risk to find *all individuals* who may have infection, a lower cutoff point, say 5 mm, needs to be selected so as to increase the sensitivity of the test and reduce to an absolute minimum the number of individuals with false-negative tests. Increased sensitivity is gained at the cost of a loss of specificity and an increased number of patients with false-positive results who are added to the subsequent intervention program.

For individual patients, a cutaneous response of greater than 15 mm skin induration to 5 TU of PPD-S is universally regarded as proof of infection by *M. tuberculosis*. In the majority of persons with TB, or who are infected with *M. tuberculosis* but are without disease, the induration is less than 15 mm, and the significance of the test must be evaluated in association with other relevant findings (see Box 43-1). This applies to the interpretation of all tests, not only the Mantoux test. The power of a test to correctly predict whether the condition under study is present or not is its predictive value. The higher the positive predictive value of a test, the greater the chance that the abnormality is present. Tests with a high negative predictive value help exclude the condition. What is not intuitively obvious is that the predictive value of a test is not only a function of the test but also of the circumstances under which it is done. An extreme example will make the point: A flat line on the electrocardiogram (ECG) of a patient who is happily conversing with one will immediately raise the thought of a technical error, not of a cardiac arrest. In other words, the risk of the patient having the disease before the test is done, the prior probability of the disease being present, has to be taken into account when interpreting a test result (see Box 43-1).[220] For a test such as the Mantoux with a relatively low sensitivity and specificity, this means that the lower the prevalence rate of TB in a community, the higher the likelihood that a reactive skin test represents a false-positive result. In terms of practical patient management it means that a Mantoux reaction should be regarded as falsely positive in a child from a population that has a low prevalence of TB, who has not been immunized with BCG, who has no known contact with an infections case of pulmonary TB, and who is free of clinical and radiographic signs of the disease. Conversely, even a reaction as small as 1 mm may lend additional support to the diagnosis of TB in a child who is from a population in which TB is prevalent, or who has had contact with a known or suspected case of TB, and who has findings on clinical, radiographic, or laboratory (tuberculous meningitis) examination that are compatible with the disease.

In summary, whether a reaction to the Mantoux tuberculin skin test is classified as positive or negative depends on the size of the induration and the child's risk factors for TB, not on the size of the reaction per se. For this reason both the size of the reaction and the observer's interpretation of the result should always be recorded, not only whether the TST is "positive" or "negative." Someone else may place a different interpretation on the result.

Effects of BCG Vaccination

About 70% of infants worldwide are immunized with BCG in accordance with WHO recommendations. When immunization is given at birth, the DTH that is induced wanes rapidly and generally produces Mantoux responses less than 10 mm when tested after 1 year of age, and reactivity may vanish by about 3 years. When BCG is administered at an older age, DTH may persist for years. The 1996 recommendation of the American Academy of Pediatrics is that BCG immunization status should *not* be taken into account when interpreting the result of a TST.

Screening

There previously was enthusiasm for programs that aimed to establish control over TB by using TSTs to identify patients who were infected with *M. tuberculosis* so that they could be offered preventive therapy (chemoprophylaxis), their latent infection eradicated, progression to TB prevented, and the transmission cycle interrupted. In populations at low risk for TB this is a completely ineffective and very costly form of intervention. For the reasons explained previously, TSTs have a low positive predictive value in persons with a low risk of TB, and most positive tuberculin reactions in persons at low risk will represent false-positive reactions. Even in populations at higher risk, screening coupled with preventive therapy is not a cost-effective solution because only about 10% of individuals who become infected with *M. tuberculosis* will ever develop TB—with the notable exception of patients coinfected with HIV and young children. The vast majority of patients identified as being infected with *M. tuberculosis* in screening programs end up receiving unwarranted therapy.

It now is generally accepted that the most effective TB control programs are based on the finding of all adults with sputum-positive pulmonary TB and their contacts and ensuring that these persons have access to and complete appropriate therapy, rather than on routine skin test screening of large populations.

The American Academy of Pediatrics now recommends screening only under the following circumstances: immediate testing of contacts of a case of known or suspected infectious pulmonary TB, annual testing for HIV-infected children, and testing every 2 to 3 years for children with increased risk of exposure to persons with TB or HIV infection. Elsewhere indications for screening differ, and in most of the world where resources are limited, screening programs have been abandoned in favor of the WHO's more cost-effective DOTS strategy.

The use of TST for screening purposes introduces additional interpretative problems relating to the definition of conversion reactions, booster effects, two-step testing, and anergy testing, which are beyond the scope of this review except to reiterate that the absence of a reaction to the tuberculin test does not rule out the diagnosis of TB.

Diagnostic Microbiology[234-266]

Young children do not expectorate sputum but swallow it. To obtain a specimen of sputum the stomach content is aspirated through a nasogastric tube soon after the child wakes in the morning and before the child has taken any food. The procedure is not standardized. A nasogastric feeding tube is passed and as much gastric juice as possible is gently aspirated by syringe. If no gastric secretions are obtained, lavage should be performed through the tube using about 5 ml/kg body weight of sterile distilled water, because tap water may contain environmental mycobacteria. Some laboratories require specimens to be submitted in containers that contain alkali to neutralize gastric acid. Aspirates should be sent to the laboratory on 3 consecutive days. Gastric aspiration is better than flexible bronchoscopy and bronchoalveolar lavage for diagnosis of TB in childhood. *M. tuberculosis* is isolated from the gastric aspirate in 30% to 40% of infants and young children with a clinical diagnosis of pulmonary TB, but a yield of 75% was achieved in a recent study in infants.[235]

The basic laboratory tools are still microscopy and culture.[238-240] Smears are stained with a fluorescent dye (auramine O or rhodamine). This is faster and more sensitive than the traditional Ziehl-Neelsen carbolfuchsin dye stain for acid-fast bacilli. The lowest concentration of organisms that can be detected by microscopic examination of sputum or gastric aspirate is about 10^4 organisms per milliliter. Acid-fast bacilli are ubiquitous in the environment and may cause false-positive results. If rapid diagnosis is important, *M. tuberculosis* may be positively identified by means of a nucleic acid amplification test.

Regardless of the microscopy result, the specimen should be cultured and the susceptibilities of the organism to antituberculous drugs determined. With radiometric culture methods such as the Bactec system, which employs a ^{14}C-labeled substrate liquid medium that is almost specific for organisms of the *M. tuberculosis* complex, specific identification of *M. tuberculosis* can often be obtained within 1 week. When few bacilli are in the inoculum, identification may take 4 to 6 weeks.

When confirmation of disseminated hematogenous TB (miliary TB) is sought, trephine bone marrow biopsy and culture should be considered.[236]

Many alternative avenues have been explored to expedite the laboratory diagnosis of TB. These include serology and antigen detection,[241-8] high-pressure liquid chromatography,[249] and nucleic acid amplification.[250-266] The possibilities for the new technologies are intriguing, but the results for children have thus far been disappointing.

Differential Diagnosis[267-273]

Because TB can mimic them, the differential diagnosis of pulmonary TB includes asthma, foreign bodies, and virtually all the pulmonary pathogens, including the mycoses, lymphoproliferative diseases, and histiocytosis, in addition to many tumors and diseases of unknown etiology such as sarcoidosis.

In practice the most common diagnostic dilemmas arise in HIV-infected children in whom the reticulonodular infiltrates of lymphocytic interstitial pneumonia closely resemble miliary TB and whose mediastinal adenopathy resembles that of TB but it does not have as great a predilection for airway compression.

PREVENTION[274-304]

The best treatment for TB has always been prevention—and the most efficient form of prevention is to cure those who are suffering from it as fast as possible, so that they stop infecting others.

Sir John Crofton
The Times, London, 1996

BCG Vaccination[277-300]

Koch's discovery of the tubercle bacillus in 1882 led to a search for a vaccine to prevent primary infection. Calmette and Guérin at the Pasteur Institute, France, succeeded, after many years of patient effort, in permanently attenuating an initially virulent strain of *M. bovis* by serial subculture and in demonstrating that, instead of causing progressive fatal disease in cattle, guinea pigs, rabbits, and monkeys, it induced a state of partial resistance that protected these animals against virulent infection. "It must be emphasized, however, that immunity is never absolute, and that guinea pigs, however much vaccine they have received, eventually succumb to virulent infection."[20] In 1921 BCG was first given orally to a newborn in Paris whose mother had died of TB. That child remained free of TB throughout his life. In 1926 Calmette reported a 3.9% mortality rate in 969 BCG-immunized children who were born of tuberculous mothers or who had close tuberculous contacts, as compared with a mortality rate of 32.6% in unimmunized children. In 1927 the League of Nations recommended BCG for widespread use. Many different BCG vaccines are now available, including the Tice strain, which is used in the United States. All come from the original source but vary in their potential to sensitize the skin to tuberculin and in their growth characteristics in culture. The clinical relevance of these differences is not known.

Administration

The preferred method of BCG vaccination is by intradermal injection as a precise dose, but multiple-puncture tools are still used in some countries. Immunization usually leaves a small scar over the deltoid muscle where the vaccine is usually injected. In a study of adolescents, a high proportion of girls found the deltoid scars unacceptable and indicated a preference for sites such as the inner aspect of the arm and the buttock for vaccination.

Efficacy

Recent metanalyses have demonstrated unequivocally that BCG has an overall protective efficacy of about 51% against TB and that it is particularly effective in preventing dissemination of disease, providing greater than 80% protection against meningeal and miliary TB. Rates of protection against cases that are confirmed by laboratory tests, reflecting reduced error in disease classification and consequently more accurate estimates of BCG efficacy, are highest at 83%.

Immunosuppression such as that associated with malnutrition, HIV, and other severe infections may nullify the protective immunity conferred by BCG.

Mechanism: Hypersensitivity vs. Protection

Cutaneous hypersensitivity to tuberculin and protective immunity against *M. tuberculosis* appear to be interrelated but distinct processes. Postvaccinial hypersensitivity (PVH) to tuberculin, as elicited by Mantoux testing, develops in response to BCG immunization and is widely used as an indicator of successful BCG vaccination. PVH does not appear to be essential for the expression of protective immunity after immunization. Over 90% of babies who are immunized with BCG at birth develop PVH to tuberculin; PVH appears to be maximal by about 3 months of age, after which it decays progressively. In contrast, when BCG immunization is performed in children older than 1 year of age, PVH persists for years. Both groups appear to derive equivalent protection from the BCG. The dissociation between PVH and protective immunity in TB is well illustrated by the case histories of two children with severe combined immunodeficiency (SCID) who developed disseminated BCG infections after vaccination.[290] Immunologic reconstitution with bone marrow transplantation and appropriate antimycobacterial therapy resulted in full recovery from BCG infection, implying the development of adequate cell-mediated immunity to BCG, yet their tuberculin skin tests were persistently negative.

Safety

BCG is one of the safest vaccines known. Although local adverse effects such as soreness and swelling are common, serious or long-term complications are rare. For children younger than 1 year old, the incidence of complications after BCG immunization is 387 per million vaccinations for regional lymphadenopathy or local subcutaneous abscess, 0.39 to 0.89 per million for musculoskeletal lesions or multiple lymphadenitis, 0.31 to 0.39 per million for nonfatal disseminated lesions, and 0.19 to 1.56 per million for fatal disseminated lesions. Those vaccinated after 1 year of age have a lesser incidence of complications. The risk of disseminated BCG infections after vaccination at birth appears to parallel the incidence of severe combined immunodeficiency syndromes, cellular immunodeficiency syndromes, and chronic granulomatous disease in the population. Persons who are infected with HIV are probably at greater risk for lymphadenitis and other complications from BCG vaccine than are persons who are not infected with HIV, but the risk appears small.

Recommendations for management of BCG adenitis range from no treatment to surgical drainage, aspiration, administration of anti-TB drugs, or a combination of these. BCG, being a strain of *M. bovis*, is naturally resistant to pyrazinamide. For adherent or fistulated lymph nodes WHO suggests drainage and direct instillation of an anti-TB drug into the lesion. Nonadherent lesions will heal spontaneously without treatment. The skeletal lesions can be treated effectively with anti-TB medications, although surgery also has been necessary in some cases.

Recommendations for BCG Vaccination

Over 80% of babies worldwide are currently immunized with BCG shortly after birth in accordance with the WHO/UNICEF Expanded Program on Immunization (EPI).

Children in the United States are not routinely immunized with BCG, and until recently the policy was to offer BCG only to children who were at high risk for infection with *M. tuberculosis* and for whom other public health measures could not be implemented. In 1996 that policy was revised in light of the metanalyses demonstrating the efficacy of BCG. The current CDC recommendation is that BCG vaccination be considered if the infant or child is continuously exposed to an untreated or ineffectively treated person with infectious pulmonary TB and the child cannot be separated from that person or given long-term primary preventive therapy, or if the patient is suffering from infectious pulmonary TB caused by isoniazid- and rifampicin-resistant strains and it is not possible to remove the child from that environment.

Immunization and HIV Status

BCG is not recommended for anyone with HIV infection or AIDS. In the case of HIV-infected children, action depends on the risk of exposure. In countries with a high prevalence of TB, WHO recommends BCG vaccination for all HIV-infected infants and children according to the standard EPI schedule, the possible benefits of BCG immunization outweighing the possible disadvantages. In low-prevalence areas such as the United States, BCG vaccination is not recommended for HIV-infected children.

Health Care Workers

The CDC now also recommends that health care workers be considered for BCG immunization if they work in settings where they are exposed to patients with isoniazid- and rifampicin-resistant *M. tuberculosis* infections.[280]

Chemoprophylaxis[301-304]

Chemoprophylaxis aims at the prevention of TB through drug therapy. *Primary chemoprophylaxis* refers to drug therapy aimed at preventing infection. *Secondary chemoprophylaxis* refers to drug therapy in persons with latent *M. tuberculosis* infection to prevent reactivation of the infection and its progression to disease. *Preventive therapy* is a generic term covering primary and secondary chemoprophylaxis. In general, a positive TST in the absence of clinical or radiographic signs suggestive of TB is taken as proof of latent infection.

Most cases of children with latent infections are identified through the examination of contacts of adults with infectious pulmonary TB and through the incidental testing of children from communities where TB is prevalent. Without preventive therapy it is estimated that about 1 in 10 infected persons develop TB at some time in their lives. Half do so within 5 years of infection, mainly within the first 2 years. The risk of disease after the initial 5 years becomes less but lasts throughout life (about 0.1% per year). They have roughly a 10% lifetime risk of developing TB as a consequence of reactivation of their latent infections. The probability is not the same the world over and is influenced by many factors. The risk of developing disease is highest in infants and children younger than 4 years of age.

Even if the TST result and chest radiograph do not suggest TB, infants who are close contacts of patients with infectious pulmonary TB should receive preventive therapy because infected infants may be anergic as late as 6 months of age.

The American Academy of Pediatrics currently recommends 6 months of daily therapy with isoniazid (source susceptible) or rifampicin (source isoniazid resistant) or, if daily therapy is not possible, twice-weekly therapy for 9 months. For children with HIV infection, a minimum of 12 months is recommended. However, conditions vary from country to country, and guidelines developed for local conditions should be adhered to.

THERAPY[305-362]

In the absence of chemotherapy, 50% of adult cases die within 5 years, 30% recover spontaneously, and 20% remain sputum positive. Tuberculosis is more malignant in early childhood with over 80% of children probably dying in the absence of treatment. By the mid-1950s it had become possible to cure virtually everyone with TB, but the minimum therapy was for 2 years, and patients required prolonged institutional care to ensure that they took their medicines. When used outside of TB sanatoriums, the success rate fell from nearly 100% to approximately 50% as a result of poor compliance. These regimens were beyond the organizational and financial resources of nearly all developing countries. The imperative to develop affordable and effective regimens for use in developing countries led the British and the East African Medical Research Councils to undertake a series of controlled therapeutic trials in the 1960s and 1970s in Hong Kong and East Africa under the direction of Wallace Fox and underpinned by the scientific laboratory studies of D.A. Mitchison. As a demonstration of the material and social benefits that can accrue from collaborative clinical and laboratory research, these trials are without parallel. By the mid-1970s Fox and Mitchison had devised the highly effective 6-month regimens that are now in current use, had established the scientific basis and efficacy of intermittent therapy, and had recognized the pivotal importance of fully supervised chemotherapy. Recently, public health education and the promotion of the idea of fully supervised therapy have been helped enormously by the appealing acronym DOT (directly observed therapy).

Concepts

Acetylator Status

The rate at which isoniazid is acetylated to microbiologically inactive acetylisoniazid is under the control of a single gene. About 40% of most populations are rapid acetylators and the remainder are slow inactivators. Clinical response to isoniazid appears to be determined by the peak concentration. Rapid acetylators have similar peak isoniazid concentrations as slow acetylators. There appears to be no difference in clinical response to treatment in adults according to acetylator status. Acetylator status may have implications for the treatment of tuberculous meningitis but probably is not of significance for other forms of TB.

Bactericidal Activity

The early bactericidal activity (EBA) and sterilizing activity are important characteristics of antituberculous drugs or their combinations. The EBA is the rate of kill during the first 2 days of therapy and determines the speed with which the disease is brought under control and the patient rendered noninfectious. The sterilizing activity is a function of the time to kill the last surviving slowly growing or dormant organism, and it determines how effective the drug will be in shortening the period of therapy. Isoniazid has powerful EBA, killing 90% of the total population of bacilli during the first few days of treatment. Pyrazinamide and rifampicin have the most potent sterilizing activity (Table 43-3).

Table 43-3 Comparison of Early Bactericidal and Sterilizing Activities of Commonly Used Drugs

DRUG	EARLY BACTERICIDAL ACTIVITY	STERILIZING ACTIVITY
Isoniazid	+++	+
Pyrazinamide	+	+++
Rifampicin	++	+++
Ethambutol	++	0
Streptomycin	+	±

Modified from Mitchison DA: *J Antimicrob Chemother* 29:477-493, 1992.

Drug Resistance

The current definition of resistance is 1% or more of the bacilli in the clinical specimen. Primary drug resistance is the presence of drug-resistant organisms in a person who has received no treatment for TB. Acquired resistance is the presence of drug-resistant strains in someone who has had antituberculous therapy.

M. tuberculosis becomes drug resistant through random, spontaneous genetic mutations at a fixed rate, which ranges from $1/10^8$ for rifampicin to $1/10^6$ for isoniazid and $1/10^4$ for ethambutol (Table 43-4). Thus spontaneous mutations causing isoniazid resistance occur approximately 100 times more frequently in *M. tuberculosis* than mutations causing rifampicin resistance. In patients coinfected with HIV the mutation rate for rifampicin resistance appears to be increased, and patients may develop rifampicin resistance in the absence of isoniazid resistance. Because adults with cavitary pulmonary TB typically have bacillary loads of the order of 10^9 organisms, there inevitably will be organisms resistant to one antituberculous drug present. The probability of an organism spontaneously developing resistance to more than one drug is remote: it is the product of the probabilities for each individual drug. For example, the probability of isoniazid and rifampicin resistance occurring together is of the order of $1/10^{14}$ ($1/10^8$ times $1/10^6$), 100,000 times less than the number of organisms present in a heavily infected adult.

Multiple drug resistance caused by spontaneously occurring mutations is thus virtually impossible. This is the reason for always using at least two drugs in combination to treat TB. Multiple drug resistance can develop only with the assistance of inadequate antibiotic therapy. If a large bacterial population is exposed to a single drug, because of poor compliance or for some other reason, the growth of susceptible bacilli will be suppressed and singly resistant organisms will multiply and become predominant. Once the population size of the singly resistant strain has grown to approach the natural mutation rate, another resistant organism is likely to evolve.

Failure to supervise therapy and ensure completion of treatment has resulted in multidrug-resistant TB emerging as a major problem in certain adult populations. Exposure to these individuals places not only children but also health care workers at risk for infection with lethal organisms that, in some cases, are unresponsive to all known therapeutic agents.

Postantibiotic Effect[326-328]

Postantibiotic effect describes the suppression of bacterial growth that occurs after short exposure of organisms to antimicrobials. The mechanism is unknown. Isoniazid, rifampicin, ethambutol, ethionamide, and streptomycin all have a prolonged postantibiotic effect on *M. tuberculosis*. Growth of *M. tuberculosis* is suppressed for about 4 days by isoniazid and for 1 week or longer by the other drugs, rendering intermittent therapy possible.[326-328] In guinea pigs isoniazid and rifampicin

Table 43-4 Drugs Used in the Treatment of Tuberculosis

DRUG	YEAR INTRODUCED	PHYSIOLOGIC EFFECT	MOLECULAR TARGET	GENES ASSOCIATED WITH RESISTANCE	MUTATION RATE	WILD-TYPE RESISTANCE
First-line drugs						
Isoniazid	1952	Cell wall mycolic acid synthesis NAD metabolism? Active oxygen species (hydroxyl radical)?	Enoylacyl carrier protein reductase	*inhA, kat6*	10^{-8}	1 in 10^6
Rifampicin (Rifabutin, Rifapentine)	1965	RNA transcription	Prokaryotic DNA-dependent RNA polymerases	*rpo*B	10^{-10}	1 in 10^8
Pyrazinamide	1970	Unknown	Direct pH effect	*pnc*A	10^{-3}	1 in 10^6
Streptomycin	1944	Protein synthesis	Ribosomal post-translational to pretranslational transition	*RpoL, rrs, str*A, *S*12	10^{-8}	1 in 10^7
Ethambutol	1968	Cell wall arabinoglycan synthesis	Unknown	*Emb* A, B & C	10^{-7}	1 in 10^5
Second-line drugs					10	
Ethionamide	1966	Cell wall mycolic acid synthesis	Enoylacyl carrier protein reductase	*inhA*	10^{-3}	?
Kanamycin/Amikin	1957	Ribosomal proteins			10^{-6}	?
Cycloserine	1955	Cell wall synthesis	D-Alanylalanine synthetase, alanine racemase, D-alanine permease	Unknown	10^{-10}	?
						?
Capreomycin	1967				10^{-3}	?
Thioacetazone	1950				10^{-3}	?
P-Aminosalicylic acid (PAS)	1946	Folic acid synthesis Salicylic acid metabolism	Unknown	Unknown	10^{-8}	?
Quinolones: Ofloxacin, sparfloxacin, and levofloxacin	1987	DNA synthesis, RNA transcription	DNA gyrase (topoisomerase II)	*Gyr*A & B	?	
Other						?
Macrolides		Protein synthesis	Ribosome peptidyltransferase	23S rRNA	?	?
Metronidazole		Nitrite radical production as metronidazole is decomposed by electrons of ferredoxin electron transfer protein?			?	

Modified from Inderlied CB, Nash KA: Antimycobacterial agents: in vitro susceptibility testing, spectra of activity, mechanisms of action and resistance, and assays for activity in biologic fluids. In Lorian V, ed: *Antibiotics in laboratory medicine,* ed 4, New York, 1996, Williams & Wilkins, pp 127-175. Updated from WHO/IUATLD Global Project on Anti-Tuberculosis Drug Resistance Surveillance 1994-1997: Anti-Tuberculosis Drug Resistance in the World—TB97.229.

are more effective when given intermittently than when given daily.[328] The efficacy of intermittent ethambutol is not proven.

Special Populations Hypothesis

To explain the observed actions of the main antibacterial drugs, Mitchison[326] postulated the presence of four bacterial populations in human lesions and differential effects of drugs on these (Table 43-5).

Isoniazid is mainly responsible for rapid killing of the bulk of rapidly growing organisms during the first days of treatment, but all of the drugs help in the slower killing of less active growers that then occurs. Pyrazinamide is active only at an acid pH and appears to act principally on bacilli multiplying in an extracellular acidic environment, but the precise anatomic location of this is unknown. It was at first thought that pyrazinamide also acts on bacteria in phagosomes in macrophages, but it is now known that the *M. tuberculosis*–containing phagosomes are not acidic. Rifampicin kills very rapidly and is postulated to selectively kill organisms that are usually dormant but have short periods of active metabolism or growth.

Definitions

Exposed or Contact

Being exposed or being a contact means that the child has had recent and substantial contact with an adult or adolescent with suspected or confirmed contagious pulmonary TB. Substantial contact means having spent enough time and being close enough to an infectious person with TB to be at real risk of having become infected. For a child, this may mean spending only minutes with someone who may have coughed directly in the child's face, some hours in a closed room or vehicle, or some days in the same house or classroom.

Infected

A child is infected if, having taken all the pertinent circumstances into account, the TST is interpreted as positive.

Table 43-5 Mitchison's Special Populations Hypothesis for the Action of Antibacterial Drugs on Different Parts of the Bacterial Population in Human Lesions[326,328]

POPULATION	RATE OF GROWTH AND RELATIVE SIZE	ANTIBACTERIAL DRUG
A. Continuous growth with rates that vary from very fast to slow	++++	INH kills rapid growers but requires alkaline medium and relatively long exposure for effect; ineffective with slow growers (RMP, SM)
B. Slowly growing organisms in acid medium	++	PZA activity increases as growth rate of organism goes down
C. Usually dormant with spurts of rapid growth undergoing a growth spurt	++	RMP kills rapidly (15-20 min) so likely to "catch" organisms
D. Dormant	+	Metronidazole?

INH, Isoniazid; *RMP,* rifampicin; *SM,* streptomycin; *PZA,* pyrazinamide.

Table 43-6 International Classification System for Tuberculosis

CLASS/GROUP	TYPE	DESCRIPTION
0	No TB exposure, not infected	No history of exposure, negative reaction to tuberculin skin test
1	TB exposure, no evidence of infection	History of exposure, negative reaction to tuberculin skin test
2	TB infection, no disease	Positive reaction to tuberculin skin test, negative bacteriologic studies (if done), no clinical or radiographic evidence of TB
3	Current TB disease	*M. tuberculosis* cultured *or* positive reaction to tuberculin skin test *and* clinical or radiographic evidence of current disease
4	Previous TB disease	History of prior episode(s) of TB or abnormal but stable radiographic findings; positive reaction to the tuberculin skin test; negative bacteriologic studies (if done) and no clinical or radiographic evidence of current disease
5	TB suspected, diagnosis pending	Suspected on the basis of clinical or radiographic signs, but negative tuberculin skin test and negative or unknown result of cultures

From CDC: *Core curriculum on tuberculosis,* ed 3, 1994. http://www.cdc.gov/nchstp/tb/pubs/corecurr.html.

Disease

Disease is the presence of clinical or radiographic signs that are compatible with the diagnosis of TB. Symptoms are not necessarily present.

Prevalence

The prevalence of TB is the proportion of patients with the disease in a population at any time. Because this number is hardly ever known, the prevalence of TB is defined in terms of its incidence: the number of new cases that are recognized per year. For practical purposes a high prevalence is defined as a community in which the incidence of TB is more than 100 new cases of TB per 100,000 population per year.

Classification of Patients

The international system for classifying individuals according to their TB status has evolved from a system devised by the American Thoracic Society in 1974. Although it is intended for epidemiologic purposes, it provides an extremely useful framework within which to consider the management of children. When referring to the status of individual patients, it is preferable to use the verbal descriptors rather than the class numerals (Table 43-6).

Guidelines for treating and controlling TB continue to evolve and differ according to prevailing local circumstances. Nothing described here should be applied in the management of individual patients without ensuring that it conforms to local practice guidelines.

Group 0: No Exposure to Tuberculosis, Not Infected

This group includes children with no history of exposure to TB, such as babies at the time of birth and older children with no history of exposure and who are TST negative.

Management. Where the prevalence of TB is high the WHO recommends BCG immunization for all children in this group *unless there are symptoms of HIV disease or AIDS present.* In high-prevalence countries BCG is thus given at birth whether the child is infected with HIV or not. Under these circumstances the risk of disseminated BCG following vaccination of an HIV-infected (but not HIV-diseased) child appears to be small in relation to the protection that BCG confers.

In the United States the administration of BCG vaccine has been cautiously encouraged since 1996 for infants and tuberculin-negative children from groups with a high prevalence of TB, for children who are exposed to persons with infectious pulmonary TB and who cannot be separated from them or placed on long-term preventive therapy, and for children exposed to persons infected with isoniazid- and rifampicin-resistant organisms.

Group I: Exposed to Tuberculosis, No Evidence of Infection

This group includes infants and children who are contacts of an infectious case of pulmonary TB, but have no clinical disease, have a normal chest radiograph, and have a negative tuberculin skin test.

Caution. The TST may not become positive for up to 2 months after infection, and infants may be anergic to tuberculin, although rarely, up to the age of 6 months.

Management. Because the TST cannot be relied on under the previously mentioned circumstances, all infants and children with recent exposure should be assumed to be infected and offered preventive therapy as for group III. The TST should be repeated 8 to 12 weeks later. If the skin test is still negative and the child is well and is no longer exposed, the child may be assumed to be free of infection and preventive therapy ended. In infants exposed before 6 months of age it may be wiser to continue preventive therapy for a full 6 months.

All infants and children who are tuberculin negative when preventive therapy is terminated should be offered BCG immunization according to the criteria for Group 0.

Group II: Infected with M. Tuberculosis*, No Disease*

This group includes children who have latent infections, are clinically well and have a normal chest radiograph, but have a positive TST. Children in this category are usually identified by health care workers during contact tracing of newly identified adults and adolescents with infectious pulmonary TB.

TB is one of the few instances in medicine in which the risk of developing the disease after infection has been directly measured. Innate herd resistance to *M. tuberculosis* is well developed in populations of European origin through selective evolutionary pressure as a consequence of their prolonged interaction with *M. tuberculosis*. For populations that have experienced TB only since the era of European colonization, the risks are much greater.

In general, the risk of TB developing after infection is greatest in the first 2 years after becoming infected and in children younger than 5 years of age, with up to 50% of infants younger than 2 years of age developing the disease.

Management. The mycobacterial load is small in patients with infection but no clinical radiographic evidence of disease. The probability of a resistant organism to even a single drug being present is therefore very low. Monotherapy with isoniazid alone for 6 to 9 months is thus possible, and this reduces the risk of TB by over 90%.

In the case of contact with a patient whose sputum has been proven microbiologically to contain isoniazid-resistant organisms, rifampicin given for 9 months is recommended.

Group III: Disease—Current Tuberculosis

This group includes children in whom *M. tuberculosis* has been cultured from sputum or gastric aspirate and children who have a negative or unknown culture result with a positive TST in association with clinical or radiographic features of current disease, particularly hilar adenopathy in childhood.

Management. The aim of treatment is to provide the safest and most effective therapy in the shortest period of time. Given adequate treatment all children will recover and thereafter remain well. Regimens for the treatment of TB must contain multiple drugs to which the organisms are susceptible to prevent the outgrowth of resistant organisms.

For drug-susceptible pulmonary TB, the American Academy of Pediatrics (AAP) recommends as standard therapy a 6-month regimen using isoniazid, rifampicin, and pyrazinamide daily for 2 months, followed by isoniazid and rifampicin given daily or twice weekly for 4 months (see Table 43-4). If for any reason pyrazinamide cannot be used, an alternative 9-month regimen is described using only isoniazid and rifampicin. The AAP recommends that if intermittent twice-weekly drug therapy is used, a health care professional must be present when the medication is administered. However, the WHO suggests that any responsible person be allowed to supervise therapy, provided that the person is accountable to a health care professional.

If drug resistance is possible or has been proved in the source case, an additional drug (ethambutol or streptomycin) should be added to the initial therapy until drug susceptibility is determined.

A strong emotional prejudice exists in favor of giving medicines daily, and most regimens still incorporate daily therapy during the initial 2 months of treatment. This may well be justifiable in children hospitalized with severe disease. However, conversion to a 2 or 3 times a week dose schedule should be considered as soon as there has been definite improvement, provided that the administration of the drugs can be fully supervised. All first-line antimycobacterial drugs have a pronounced postantibiotic effect, with suppression of bacterial growth for 4 days (isoniazid) to 7 days (pyrazinamide, rifampicin) after a single dose. Because mycobacteria are susceptible to these agents only when actively growing, it is wasteful to give drugs more often than required. Intermittent therapy may also reduce the already low incidence of side effects in childhood, of which life-threatening acute hepatic failure is the most serious. Hepatic failure does not yet appear to have been described in children undergoing intermittent therapy, but that may be because relatively few children are on intermittent regimens.

Special Situations

HIV coinfection. Children with HIV coinfection are treated by the same regimens as non–HIV-infected children. However, because of the increased risk of rifampicin resistance developing while on therapy, it is recommended that three first-line drugs always be included in the initial phase of therapy and that therapy treatment be continued for at least 9 months. HIV testing is not routinely recommended for infants and children with TB.

Pregnancy. Streptomycin may cause congenital deafness and is the only anti-TB drug with known harmful effects on the fetus. Routine use of pyrazinamide also is not recommended during pregnancy because the risk of teratogenicity has not been determined. Because the small concentrations of anti-TB drugs in breast milk do not produce toxicity in the nursing newborn, breast feeding should be encouraged if the mother's health permits. All infants of tuberculous mothers require preventive therapy (group I). Because drug levels are low in breast milk, conventional doses of antituberculous drugs are used without downward adjustment in breast-fed babies (Table 43-7).

Group IV: Previous Tuberculosis

There are two subgroups in this category: The first comprises children who have completed a full course of chemotherapy for TB. The second is a relatively uncommon group comprising children who are not known to have had TB but are found to have a positive TST, are free of symptoms suggestive of pulmonary TB, and have chest radiographs that show evidence of healed TB such as calcified mediastinal lymph nodes with or without parenchymal scars.

Management. Children who have responded to and completed a full course of chemotherapy should be discharged. Relapse is rare. The vast majority of relapses occur in adolescents and adults and occur within the first 6 months of cessation of

Table 43-7 Dosage Recommendation for the Initial Treatment of Tuberculosis Among Children Younger Than 12 Years of Age

DRUG	DAILY	TWO TIMES PER WEEK	THREE TIMES PER WEEK
Isoniazid	10-20 mg/kg Max. 300 mg	20-40 mg/kg Max. 900 mg	20-40 mg/kg Max. 900 mg
Rifampicin	10-20 mg/kg Max. 600 mg	10-20 mg/kg Max. 600 mg	10-20 mg/kg Max. 600 mg
Pyrazinamide	15-30 mg/kg Max. 2 g	50-70 mg/kg Max. 4 g	50-70 mg/kg Max. 3 g
Ethambutol	15-25 mg/kg Max. 2.5 g	50 mg/kg Max. 2.5 g	25-30 mg/kg Max. 2.5 g
Streptomycin	20-30 mg/kg Max. 1 g	25-30 mg/kg Max. 1.5 g	25-30 mg/kg Max. 1 g

Modified from CDC: Initial therapy for tuberculosis in the era of multidrug resistance. Recommendations of the Advisory Council for the Elimination of Tuberculosis, *MMWR* 42(no. RR-7):3, 1993.

therapy. Routine follow-up examination of children who have completed their treatment is thus rarely indicated.

The optimal management of children who have evidence of healed but previously untreated TB is unclear. It is currently suggested that they be treated as for current disease (group III).

Group V: Tuberculosis Suspected, Diagnosis Pending

This group includes patients in whom TB is suspected on the basis of clinical or radiographic signs, but the TST is negative and the result of cultures is negative or unknown.

This is a very large group in the spectrum of childhood TB. Proof of infection by culture is obtained in only about 30% of children with TB under the best of circumstances, and in many parts of the world the isolation rate is even lower. The TST may be persistently negative in up to 5% of culture-positive cases.

Management. Treatment is commenced as for current disease (group III). The diagnosis should be reviewed if the child's clinical condition does not show definite improvement within 10 to 14 days. Radiographic resolution generally lags behind. The TST is repeated after 4 to 6 weeks. If the test is still negative, the diagnosis of TB should be reviewed and causes of comorbidity such as HIV infection sought.

OTHER THERAPIES

Corticosteroids[342-347]

Corticosteroid therapy, in conjunction with antituberculous drug therapy, is indicated for all patients with tuberculous meningitis or pericarditis but is not used in the routine management of pulmonary TB. It is indicated, however, in infants and children who have symptomatic airway obstruction caused by TB. The usual cause of this is tracheobronchial obstruction by tuberculous lymph nodes, rarely tuberculous laryngitis. Corticosteroids should be considered for all infants and children who have tachypnea with stridor or bronchodilator-nonresponsive wheezing in association with radiographic signs of tracheobronchial compression. Corticosteroids may also accelerate resolution in tuberculous laryngitis. In the case of the large serous tuberculous pleural effusions that occur in older children and adults, corticosteroids should be considered if the patient is uncomfortable in order to accelerate the resorption of fluid.

For the relief of airway obstruction, oral prednisolone 2 mg/kg/day (maximum 40 mg/day), or equivalent, as a single daily dose is used. Clinical response, if it does occur, is apparent within 2 to 3 days. If there is not a definite improvement by 7 days, steroids are discontinued. In children who show a response, the steroid dosage is reduced at 1 week to alternate-day treatment with the same daily dose. This is gradually reduced and discontinued at 1 month. There is no benefit of more prolonged corticosteroid therapy. Initially, improvement in airway obstruction is not accompanied by a perceptible reduction in the radiographic size of the mediastinal lymph nodes. This is probably because the lymph nodes causing tracheobronchial compression are caseous, and only the periadenitis—the noncaseous surrounding inflammation—is responsive to steroids.

Adrenal insufficiency requiring replacement steroid therapy is a rare late complication of TB in adults but has not been reported in childhood. Similarly, debilitating tuberculous fever in adults that sometimes requires suppression with corticosteroids is also not a feature of childhood TB. Local corticosteroid therapy may be useful for BCG-related keloid reactions or for reactions to tuberculin that are painful or threatening to ulcerate.

Surgery[348-351]

Approximately 15 per 1000 infants and children with acute pulmonary TB have complications of mediastinal tuberculous lymphadenitis requiring surgical intervention for relief of airway obstruction. Airway compromise may result from extrinsic tracheobronchial compression (see Figs. 43-3 and 43-4) or from intraluminal obstruction by eroding tuberculous lymph nodes (see Fig. 43-4) or associated granulation tissue. Rarely, erosion may result in tracheoesophageal and bronchoesophageal fistulae. Bronchiectasis requiring lobectomy or pneumonectomy may follow bronchial obstruction. Uncommon surgical complications of thoracic TB in the pediatric age group are large pulmonary cysts, fibrothorax following tuberculous empyema, bronchopleural fistula, tuberculous osteitis of the ribs, and unilateral diaphragmatic paralysis. Additional indications for surgery in adolescents and adults include massive hemoptysis, pulmonary aspergilloma, and resection of lung tissue infected with multiresistant organisms.

Children who have radiographic evidence of marked lower tracheal or bilateral main bronchial obstruction require urgent surgical decompression of subcarinal and other affected nodes if they have tachypnea, marked recession, and a $P_{CO_2} \geq 40$ mm Hg (5.3 kPa) or desaturation in 40% inspired oxygen. The nodes should be decompressed only by incision and curettage. Attempts to excise affected nodes are associated with increased complications. Children with less severe bilateral bronchial obstruction may respond to corticosteroids as discussed previously. Those who fail to progress on treatment or who at 1 month still have clinical evidence of tracheobronchial obstruction should be reevaluated with a view to surgery.

Emerging Therapies

Immunotherapy: Mycobacterium Vaccae[352-360]

Reported results of clinical studies have included only adults to date. These are encouraging and suggest that a single dose of vaccine containing 10^9 radiation-killed *M. vaccae,* when given as an adjunct with modern short-course chemotherapy, may reduce treatment failures and deaths. *M. vaccae* is an environmental saprophyte that only rarely has been associated with human disease. The selection of *M. vaccae* for evaluation as a

TABLE 43-8 Clinical Manifestations of Common Pathogenic Nontuberculous Mycobacteria

	DISEASE					
SPECIES	LYMPHADENITIS—CHILD	CHRONIC PULMONARY DISEASE: ADULT*	DISSEMINATED DISEASE IN AIDS	DISSEMINATED DISEASE, *NOT* AIDS	SKIN AND SOFT TISSUE	BONES, JOINTS, BURSAE, AND TENDONS
M. avium-intracellulare-scrofulaceum complex	+++†	+++	+++	PUO		++
M. kansasii		++		Skin		+
M. marinum				Skin	+++	++
M. fortuitum		+		Skin	++	+
M. chelonei		+		Skin	++	+
Other	*M. haemophilum*	*M. xenopi, M. malmoense, M. szulgai, M. simiae*		*M. haemophilum*	*M. ulcerans*	

+, Relative frequency of occurrence.
*Differs radiographically from TB in adults: thin-walled cavities, more contiguous disease and less bronchogenic spread, preference for apical anterior segments of upper lobes, marked pleurisy contiguous to pneumonic infiltrate is common. Pleural effusion is rare.
†A disease of children <5 years old. Cervical lymphadenitis (scrofula) at older ages is a manifestation of tuberculosis, more commonly *M. bovis* than other *M.tb* complex species.

vaccine for immunotherapy of TB is based on its being a potent source of antigens that are common to *M. tuberculosis*, BCG, and *Mycobacterium leprae.* Patients with mycobacterial disease develop delayed-type hypersensitivity responses to their species-specific antigens but not to these antigens, which are common to the group. Because BCG vaccination is protective against TB and leprosy, it was postulated that the group antigens confer the protection and that the administration of group antigens as a vaccine may be of benefit to patients with TB. There are hopes that combined immunochemotherapy will enable therapeutic regimens to be reduced in duration, facilitating adherence and cure of infection, and that it may be of benefit in the treatment of patients coinfected with HIV and in those with multidrug-resistant TB. Whether these hopes will be realized is too early to tell.

Metronidazole[361,362]

The prolonged treatment that is required to eradicate dormant tubercle bacilli and sterilize the patient is the single most important impediment to the control and eradication of the disease. A recent in vitro study reported that metronidazole, a drug that is specific for anaerobes, killed dormant *M. tuberculosis* under anaerobic conditions but had no effect on actively growing cultures.[362] That this finding may have clinical relevance is suggested by a preceding 1989 report from India that described remarkable therapeutic benefits from the use of metronidazole in conjunction with conventional therapy in adult patients with advanced pulmonary TB.[361] That *M. tuberculosis* may be susceptible to attack by already available drugs in its dormant state is of enormous importance.

MYCOBACTERIA OTHER THAN TUBERCULOSIS[363-371]

The principal mycobacterial pathogens of humans are *M. leprae* (leprosy, Hansen's bacillus, 1878) and *M. tuberculosis* (Koch's bacillus, 1882). Other potentially pathogenic mycobacteria are known as *MOTTs* (mycobacteria other than TB) or as NTM (nontuberculous mycobacteria) because they do not cause TB. NTM are widely distributed in the environment. A large reservoir appears to be growing fodder plants. In Southern Africa, for example, population surveys have shown MOTTs to be present in the mouths or sputum of 3% to 4% of rural adults with about half the isolates belonging to the *Mycobacterium avium-intracellulare-scrofulaceum* (MAIS) complex.

Pulmonary infections with MOTTs have not been described in immunocompetent children (Table 43-8). NTM infections in children most commonly manifest as cervical lymphadenitis, and NTM account for roughly 90% of cases of mycobacterial cervical lymphadenitis in developed countries. Elsewhere, where TB is prevalent, *M. tuberculosis* is the predominant cause. It is important to differentiate nontuberculous mycobacterial lymphadenitis from tuberculous lymphadenitis because the treatment is different. Clinical features may help but are not entirely reliable. With NTM the child is generally younger than 10 years old with no history of contact with TB. Constitutional symptoms are absent, the affected nodes are unilateral and confined to the neck, a cold abscess may have formed, the chest radiograph is normal, and the Mantoux test is negative (<5 mm). Skin testing with purified NTM antigens may be useful in the diagnostic evaluation but are not generally available.

The vast majority of cases of NTM lymphadenitis are caused by organisms of the MAIS group. These are highly resistant to first-line antituberculous drugs, and treatment of NTM cervical adenitis is surgical excision.

Disseminated NTM infections are associated with AIDS in adults but have been rarely reported in children with the disease.[145]

Cervical lymphadenitis (scrofula) at older ages is a manifestation of TB, more commonly *M. bovis* than other *M. tuberculosis*–complex species.

ACKNOWLEDGMENT

In writing this chapter I have quoted extensively from the copies of manuals, guidelines, and reports that have most generously been made freely available to the entire world on the Internet pages of the CDC, WHO, American Academy of Pediatrics, and New York Department of Health. The Medline searches, which are now also provided free of charge by the National Library of Medicine, have been of inestimable help. The provision of health-related information of remarkable quality, free of charge on the Internet by agencies of the U.S. government and nongovernmental U.S. institutions in particular, is an altruistic endeavor in pursuit of health for all humankind to which the health of future generations will attest.

BIBLIOGRAPHY

International Guidelines

Tuberculosis in children. Guidelines for diagnosis, prevention and treatment (a statement of the Scientific Committees of the IUATLD), *Bull Int Union Tuberc Lung Dis* 66:61-67, 1991.

Ormerod LP: Chemotherapy and management of Tuberculosis in the United Kingdom: recommendations of the Joint Tuberculosis Committee of the British Thoracic Society, *Thorax* 45:403-408, 1990.

Monographs and Reviews

Bloom BR, ed: *Tuberculosis: pathogenesis, protection, and control,* Washington, DC, 1994, ASM Press.

Cremin BJ, Jamieson DH, eds: *Childhood tuberculosis: modern imaging and clinical aspects,* London, 1995, Springer-Verlag.

Crofton J, Horne N, Miller F: *Clinical tuberculosis,* New York, 1992, Macmillan.

Knudsin RB, ed: Airborne contagion, *Ann NY Acad Sci* 353:1-341, 1980.

Miller FW: *Tuberculosis in children,* Edinburgh, 1982, Churchill Livingstone.

Patel AM, Abrahams EW: Pulmonary tuberculosis. In Ratledge C, Stanford J, Grange JM, eds: *The biology of the mycobacteria,* vol 3, *Clinical aspects of mycobacterial disease,* London, 1989, Academic Press, pp 179-243.

Reichman LB, Hershfield ES, eds: *Tuberculosis: a comprehensive international approach,* New York, 1993, Marcel Dekker.

Committee on Postgraduate Medical Education of the ACCP: Tuberculosis supplement, *Chest* 76:737-817, 1979.

INTERNET RESOURCES

Medline

National Library of Medicine
http://www4.ncbi.nlm.nih.gov/Entrez/medline.html

http://www.ncbi.nlm.nih.gov/PubMed/

HealthGate
http://www.healthgate.com/HealthGate/MEDLINE/search-adv.shtml
Also access to other health-related news and articles.

American Academy of Pediatrics

http://www.aap.org/policy/pprgtoc.html
Full text of policy statements on diagnosis and treatment of tuberculosis in childhood.

CDC Division of Tuberculosis Elimination

http://www.cdc.gov/nchstp/tb/dtbe.html

CDC Core Curriculum on Tuberculosis
http://www.cdc.gov/nchstp/tb/pubs/corecurr.html
What the clinician should know.

CDC TB-related *MMWR*s and Reports
http://www.cdc.gov/nchstp/tb/pubs/tbmmwr.html

New York City Department of Health

http://www.cpmc.columbia.edu/tbcpp/cover.html
A manual of the clinical policies and practice of the New York City Department of Health. Also available are electronic pamphlets for the public that describe what a layperson needs to know about the detection, prevention, and cure of tuberculosis.
WHO Global Tuberculosis Programme
http://www.who.ch/programmes/gtb/

Guidelines for national programmes, ed 2, 1997, WHO/TB/97.
Contents: global TB burden; framework for effective TB control; standardized treatment regimens according to TB case definitions and categories; monitoring of individual patients and ensuring of adherence to treatment; treatment of HIV-infected TB patients; and anti-TB drug supply in the context of national pharmaceutical policies and essential drug programs
http://www.who.ch/programmes/gtb/publications/

TB/HIV—a clinical manual. *A comprehensive 118-page manual on the diagnosis and management of tuberculosis, with and without HIV infection.*
http://www.who.ch/programmes/gtb/publications/tb
hiv/index.html

Crofton J, Chaulet P, Maher D: *Guidelines for the management of tuberculosis—drug resistance,* WHO—TB96.210.
http://www.who.ch/programmes/gtb/publications/gmdrt/index.html

Anti-tuberculosis drug resistance in the world, TB97.229.
http://www.who.ch/programmes/gtb/publications/gmdrt/index.html
WHO report on the tuberculosis epidemic 1996: groups at risk.
http://www.who.ch/programmes/gtb/publications/tbrep_96/index.html

WHO-integrated management of the sick child.
http://www.who.ch/chd/pub/sickchi/sickchi3.html

Emerging Infectious Diseases (EID) Journal
http://www.cdc.gov/ncidod/EID/eidtext.htm
Complete text of the printed version of the EID *Journal.*

Listing of Internet Tuberculosis Resources
http://www.cpmc.columbia.edu/tbcpp/extres.html
List of other web sites that have information about tuberculosis. The resources have been categorized by the type of information they have.

The International Journal of Tuberculosis and Lung Disease
http://iuatld.vjf.inserm.fr/IUATLD/publication.html#Contents

American Thoracic Society
http://www.thoracic.org/statemnt.html
Abstracts only of *Am J Respir Crit Care Med* and lists of statements and position papers but not contents.

Centers for Disease Control and Prevention

Centers for Disease Control and Prevention, Advisory Committee for the Elimination of Tuberculosis: Screening for tuberculosis and tuberculosis infection in high-risk populations; and the use of preventive therapy for tuberculosis infection in the United States, *MMWR* 39(RR-8):1-12, 1990.

Centers for Disease Control: Guidelines for preventing the transmission of *Mycobacterium tuberculosis* in health-care facilities, *MMWR* 43(RR-12), 1994.

Centers for Disease Control: Management of persons exposed to multidrug-resistant tuberculosis, *MMWR* 41(RR-1):59-71, 1992.

Centers for Disease Control: National action plan to combat multidrug-resistant tuberculosis, *MMWR* 41(RR-11), 1992.

Centers for Disease Control: Purified protein derivative (PPD)–tuberculin anergy and HIV infection: guidelines for anergy testing and management of anergic persons at risk of tuberculosis, *MMWR* 40(RR-5):27-32, 1991.

Centers for Disease Control: Tuberculosis and human immunodeficiency virus infection: recommendations of the Advisory Committee for Elimination of Tuberculosis, *MMWR* 38:236-239, 243-250, 1989.

Centers for Disease Control: Use of BCG vaccines in the control of tuberculosis: a joint statement by the Immunization Practices Advisory Committee and the Advisory Committee for Elimination of Tuberculosis, *MMWR* 37:663-664, 669-675, 1988.

Centers for Disease Control and Prevention: Approaches to improving adherence to antituberculosis therapy, *MMWR* 42:74-75, 1993.

Centers for Disease Control and Prevention: Expanded tuberculosis surveillance and tuberculosis morbidity—United States, 1993, *MMWR* 43(RR-20):361-366, 1994.

Centers for Disease Control and Prevention: Initial therapy for tuberculosis in the era of multidrug resistance, *MMWR* 42(RR-7):1-8, 1993.

Centers for Disease Control, National Institute for Occupational Safety and Health: *Recommended guidelines for personal respiratory protection of workers in health care facilities potentially exposed to tuberculosis,* Washington, DC, 1992, Department of Health and Human Services.

Selected Bibliography

General US Congress, Office of Technology Assessment: *The continuing challenge of tuberculosis,* Washington, DC, 1993, US Government Printing Office.

Snider DE, Hutton MD: *Improving patient compliance in tuberculosis treatment programs,* Atlanta, 1989, Centers for Disease Control.

American Thoracic Society

American Thoracic Society: Treatment of tuberculosis and tuberculosis infection in adults and children, *Am J Respir Crit Care Med* 149:1359-1374, 1994.

American Thoracic Society and Centers for Disease Control: Control of tuberculosis in the United States, *Am Rev Respir Dis* 146:1623-1633, 1992.

American Thoracic Society and Centers for Disease Control: Diagnostic standards and classification of tuberculosis, *Am Rev Respir Dis* 142:725-735, 1990.

REFERENCES

1. Ayvazian LF: History of tuberculosis. In Reichman LB, Hershfield ES, eds: *Tuberculosis: a comprehensive international approach,* New York, 1993, Marcel Dekker, pp 1-20.

Epidemiology

2. Abrahams EW: Tuberculosis in indigenous Australians, *Med J Aust* 24(suppl):23-27, 1975.
3. Abughali N, van der Kuyp F, Annable W, Kumar ML: Congenital tuberculosis, *Pediatr Infect Dis J* 13:738-741, 1994.
4. Advisory Committee for the Elimination of Tuberculosis: A strategic plan for the elimination of tuberculosis in the United States, *MMWR* 38(suppl S-3), 1989.
5. Braun MM, Byers RH, Heyward WL, Ciesielski CA, Bloch AB, Berkelman RL, Snider DE: Acquired immunodeficiency syndrome and extrapulmonary tuberculosis in the United States, *Arch Intern Med* 150:1913-1916, 1990.
6. Braun MM, Cote TR, Robkin CS: Trends in death with tuberculosis during the AIDS era, *JAMA* 269(22):2865-2868, 1993.
7. Brown RE, Miller B, Taylor WR, Palmer C, Bosco L, Nicola RM, Zelinger J, Simpson K: Health-care expenditures for tuberculosis in the United States, *Arch Intern Med* 155:1595-1600, 1995.
8. Brudney K, Dobkin J: Resurgent tuberculosis in New York City: human immunodeficiency virus, homelessness and the decline of tuberculosis control programs, *Am Rev Respir Dis* 144:745-749, 1991.
9. Cantwell MF, Snider DE, Cauthen GM, Onorato I: Epidemiology of tuberculosis in the United States, 1985 through 1992, *JAMA* 272:535-539, 1994.
10. Centers for Disease Control and Prevention: National action plan to combat multidrug-resistant tuberculosis; meeting the challenge of multidrug-resistant tuberculosis: summary of a conference; management of persons exposed to multidrug-resistant tuberculosis, *MMWR* 41:5-50, 1992.
11. Centers for Disease Control and Prevention: 1994 revised classification system for human immunodeficiency virus infection in children less than 13 years of age; official authorized addenda: human immunodeficiency virus infection codes and official guidelines for coding and reporting ICD-9-CM, *MMWR* 43(no. RR-12), 1994.
12. Centers for Disease Control and Prevention. A strategic plan for the elimination of tuberculosis in the United States, *MMWR* 38(S-3), 1989.
13. Centers for Disease Control and Prevention: Tuberculosis—Western Europe, 1974-1991, *MMWR* 42:628-631, 1993.
14. Centers for Disease Control and Prevention: Tuberculosis morbidity—United States, 1997, *MMWR* 47:253-257, 1998.
15. Chawla PK, Klapper PJ, Kamholz SL, Pollack AH, Heurich AE: Drug-resistant in an urban population including patients at risk for human immunodeficiency virus infection, *Am Rev Respir Dis* 146:280-284, 1992.
16. Comstock GW: The International Tuberculosis Campaign: a pioneering venture in mass vaccination and research, *Clin Infect Dis* 19:528-540, 1994.
17. Cosivi O, Grange JM, Daborn CJ, Raviglione MC, Fujikura T, Cousins D, Robinson RA, Huchzermeyer HFAK, de Kantor I, Meslin FX: Zoonotic tuberculosis due to *Mycobacterium bovis* in developing countries, *Emerg Infect Dis* 4:59-70, 1998.
18. Dannenberg AM: Transmission and pathogenesis delayed-type hypersensitivity and cell-mediated immunity in the pathogenesis of tuberculosis, *Immunol Today* 12:228-233, 1991.
19. Dolin PJ, Raviglione MC, Kochi A: Global tuberculosis incidence and mortality during 1990-2000, *Bull WHO* 72:213-220, 1994.
20. Dubos R, Dubos J: *The white plague: tuberculosis, man and society,* New Brunswick, NJ, 1987, Rutgers University Press.
21. Edlin BR, Tokars JI, Grieco MH, Crawford JT, Williams J, Sordillo EM, Ong KR, Kilburn JO, Dooley SW, Castro KG, et al: An outbreak of multidrug-resistant tuberculosis among hospitalized patients with the acquired immunodeficiency syndrome, *N Engl J Med* 326:1514-1521, 1992.
22. Enarson DA, Grzybowski S: Incidence of active tuberculosis in the native population of Canada, *Can Med Assoc J* 134:1149-1152, 1986.
23. Feldberg GD: *Disease and class: tuberculosis and the shaping of modern North American society,* New Brunswick, NJ, 1995, Rutgers University Press.
24. Fitzgerald JM, Grzybowski S, Allen EA: The impact of human immunodeficiency virus infection on tuberculosis and its control, *Chest* 100(1):191-200, 1991.
25. Grzybowski S: Natural history of tuberculosis: epidemiology, *Bull Int Union Tuberc Lung Dis* 66:193-194, 1991.
26. Huebner RE, Schein MF, Bass JB: The tuberculin skin test, *Clin Infect Dis* 17:968-975, 1993.
27. Huebner RE, Villarino ME, Snider DE: Tuberculin skin testing and the HIV epidemic, *JAMA* 267(3):409-410, 1992.
28. Jereb JA, Kelly GD, Dooley SW Jr, Cauthen GM, Snider DE Jr: Tuberculosis morbidity in the United States: final data, 1990, *MMWR* 40(SS-3):23-27, 1991.
29. Jereb JA, Kelly GD, Porterfield DS: The epidemiology of tuberculosis in children, *Semin Pediatr Infect Dis J* 4(4):220-231, 1993.
30. Jones DS, Malecki JM, Bigler WJ, Witte JJ, Oxtoby MJ: Pediatric tuberculosis and human immunodeficiency virus infection in Palm Beach County, Florida, *Am J Dis Child* 146:1166-1170, 1992.
31. Lange WR, Warnock-Eckhart E, Bean ME: *Mycobacterium tuberculosis* infection in foreign born adoptees, *Pediatr Infect Dis J* 8:625-629, 1989.
32. Malasky C, Jordan T, Potulski F, Reichman LB: Occupational tuberculous infection among pulmonary physicians in training, *Am Rev Respir Dis* 142:505-507, 1990.
33. McCray E, Weinbaum CM, Braden CR, Onorato IM: The epidemiology of tuberculosis in the United States, *Clin Chest Med* 18(1):99-113, 1997.
34. Nahmias AJ, de Sousa A, Freiji R, Lee FK: Older and newer challenges of tuberculosis in children, *Pediatr Pulmonol Suppl* 11:28-29, 1995.
35. Onorato IM, McCray E: Prevalence of human immunodeficiency virus infection among patients attending tuberculosis clinics in the United States, *J Infect Dis* 165:87-92, 1992.
36. Raviglione MC, Snider D, Kochi A: Global epidemiology of tuberculosis. Morbidity and mortality of a worldwide epidemic, *JAMA* 273:220-226, 1995.
37. Rieder HL, Kelly GD, Bloch AB, Cauthen GM, Snider DE Jr: Tuberculosis diagnosed at death in the United States, *Chest* 100:678-681, 1991.
38. Reider HL, Snider DE, Cauthen GM: Extrapulmonary tuberculosis in the United States, *Am Rev Respir Dis* 141:347-351, 1990.
39. Rodrigues LC, Smith PG: Tuberculosis in developing countries and methods for its control, *Trans R Soc Trop Med Hyg* 84:739-744, 1990.
40. Rosenberg T, Manfreda J, Hershfield ES: Two-step tuberculin testing in staff and residents of a nursing home, *Am Rev Respir Dis* 148:1537-1540, 1993.
41. Ryan F: *The forgotten plague: how the battle against tuberculosis was won—and lost,* Boston, 1992, Little, Brown.
42. Graham NMH, Nelson KE, Solomon L, Bonds M, Rizzo RT, Scavotto J, Astemborski J, Vlahov D: Prevalence of tuberculin positivity and skin test anergy in HIV-1-seropositive and seronegative intravenous drug users, *JAMA* 267(3):369-373, 1992.
43. Selwyn PA, Hartel D, Lewis VA, Schoenbaum EE, Vermund SH, Klein RS, Walker AT, Friedland GH: A prospective study of the risk of tuberculosis among intravenous drug users with human immunodeficiency virus infection, *N Engl J Med* 320:545-550, 1989.
44. Selwyn PA, Sckell BM, Alcabes P, Friedland GH, Klein RS, Schoenbaum EE: High risk of active tuberculosis in HIV-infected drug users with cutaneous anergy, *JAMA* 268(4):504-509, 1992.
45. Snider DE, Seggerson JJ, Hutton MD: Tuberculosis and migrant farm workers, *JAMA* 265(13):1732, 1991.

46. Starke JR, Jacobs RF, Jereb J: Resurgence of tuberculosis in children, *J Pediatr* 120(6):839-855, 1992.
47. Steele RW: Tuberculosis in children: a growing concern, *Infect Med* 12:442-453, 1995.
48. Torres RA, Mani S, Altholz J, Brickner PW: Human immunodeficiency virus infection among homeless men in a New York City shelter: association with *Mycobacterium tuberculosis* infection, *Arch Intern Med* 150:2030-2036, 1990.
49. WHO report on the tuberculosis epidemic 1996: *Groups at risk,* WHO/TB/96-198.
50. Wilson ME: Travel and the emergence of infectious diseases, *Emerg Infect Dis* 1:39-46, 1995.
51. Barnes PF, Bloch AB, Davidson PT, Snider DE Jr: Tuberculosis in patients with human immunodeficiency virus infection, *N Engl J Med* 324:1644-1650, 1991.
52. Busillo CP, Lessnau KD, Sanjana V: Multidrug resistant *Mycobacterium tuberculosis* in patients with human immunodeficiency virus infection, *Chest* 102:797-801, 1992.
52a. Hoernle EH, Reid TE: Human immunodeficiency virus infection in children, *Am J Health Syst Pharm* 52:961-979, 1995.
53. Cantwell MF, Binkin NJ: Impact of HIV on tuberculosis in sub-Saharan Africa: a regional perspective, *Int J Tuberc Lung Dis* 1:205-214, 1997.
54. Khouri YF, Mastrucci MT, Hutto C, Mitchell CD, Scott GB: *Mycobacterium tuberculosis* in children with human immunodeficiency virus type 1 infection, *Pediatr Infect Dis J,* 11:950-955, 1992.
55. McSherry GD: Human immunodeficiency virus–related pulmonary infections in children, *Semin Respir Infect* 11:173-183, 1996.
56. Centers for Disease Control and Prevention: Essential components of a tuberculosis prevention and control program; and screening for tuberculosis and tuberculosis infection in high-risk populations: recommendations of the Advisory Council for the Elimination of Tuberculosis, *MMWR* 44(no. RR-11):1-34, 1995.
57. Mathew V, Alfaham M, Evans MR, Adams H, Jones RV, Campbell I, Jenkins T: Management of tuberculosis in Wales: 1986-92, *Arch Dis Child* 78:349-353, 1998.
58. Raviglione MC, Dye C, Schmidt SA: Assessment of worldwide tuberculosis control, *Lancet* 350:624-629, 1997.
59. Raviglione MC, Snider DE, Kochi A: Global epidemiology of tuberculosis. Morbidity and mortality of a worldwide epidemic, *JAMA* 273:220-226, 1995.
60. Rubel AJ, Garro LC: Social and cultural factors in the successful control of tuberculosis, *Public Health Rep* 107:626-636, 1992.
61. Squire SB, Wilkinson D: Strengthening "DOTS" through community care for tuberculosis. Observation alone isn't the key, *BMJ* 315:1395-1396, 1997.
62. Styblo K, Rouillon A: Tuberculosis in developing countries: burden, intervention and cost, *Bull Int Union Tuberc Lung Dis* 65:6-24, 1990.
63. World Health Organization: *Treatment of tuberculosis: guidelines for national programmes,* ed 2, 1997.
64. Binkin NJ, Ghersi G, Boeri V, Lo Monaco R, Salamina G: An epidemic of tuberculosis in an elementary school, Sanremo, Italy, 1993, *Rev Epidemiol Sante Publique* 42:138-143, 1994.

Pathogenesis

65. Askew GL, Finelli L, Hutton M, Laraque F, Porterfield D, Shilkret K, Valway SE, Onorato I, Spitalny K: *Mycobacterium tuberculosis* transmission from a pediatrician to patients, *Pediatrics* 100:19-23, 1997.
66. Barnes PF, Yang Z, Preston-Martin S, Pogoda JM, Jones BE, Otaya M, Eisenach KD, Knowles L, Harvey S, Cave MD: Patterns of tuberculosis transmission in central Los Angeles, *JAMA* 278:1159-1163, 1997.
67. Centers for Disease Control and Prevention: Guidelines for preventing the transmission of *Mycobacterium tuberculosis* in health-care facilities, 1994, *MMWR* 43(no. RR-13):1-132, 1994.
68. Cohn DL, O'Brien RJ. The use of restriction fragment length polymorphism (RFLP) analysis for epidemiological studies of tuberculosis in developing countries, *Int J Tuberc Lung Dis* 2:16-26, 1998.
69. Das S, Paramasivan CN, Lowrie DB, Prabhakar R, Narayanan PR: IS6110 restriction fragment length polymorphism typing of clinical isolates of *Mycobacterium tuberculosis* from patients with pulmonary tuberculosis in Madras, South India, *Tuber Lung Dis* 76:550-554, 1995.
70. Frew AJ, Mayon-White RT, Benson MK: An outbreak of tuberculosis in an Oxfordshire school, *Br J Dis Chest* 81:293-295, 1987.
71. Genewein A, Telenti A, Bernasconi C, Mordasini C, Weiss S, Maurer AM, Rieder HL, Schopfer K, Bodmer T: Molecular approach to identifying route of transmission of tuberculosis in the community, *Lancet* 342:841-844, 1993.
72. Kamerbeek J, Schouls L, Kolk A, van Agterveld M, van Soolingen D, Kuijper S, Bunschoten A, Molhuizen H, Shaw R, Goyal M, van Embden J: Simultaneous detection and strain differentiation of *Mycobacterium tuberculosis* for diagnosis and epidemiology, *J Clin Microbiol* 35:907-914, 1997.
73. Lutfey M, Della-Latta P, Kapur V, Palumbo LA, Gurner D, Stotzky G, Brudney K, Dobkin J, Moss A, Musser JM, Kreiswirth BN: Independent origin of mono-rifampin-resistant *Mycobacterium tuberculosis* in patients with AIDS, *Am J Respir Crit Care Med* 153:837-840, 1996.
74. Riley RL: Historical background, *Ann N Y Acad Sci* 353:3-9, 1980.
75. Riley RL: Transmission and environmental control of tuberculosis. In Reichman LB, Hershfield ES, eds: *Tuberculosis: a comprehensive international approach,* New York, 1993, Marcel Dekker.
76. Warren R, Hauman J, Beyers JN, Richardson M, Schaaf HS, Donald P, van Helden P: Unexpectedly high strain diversity of *Mycobacterium tuberculosis* in a high-incidence community, *S Afr Med J* 86:45-49, 1996.
77. Yeh RW, Ponce de Leon A, Agasino CB, Hahn JA, Daley CL, Hopewell PC, Small PM: Stability of *Mycobacterium tuberculosis* DNA genotypes, *J Infect Dis* 177:1107-1111, 1998.
78. Arruda S, Bomfim G, Knights R, Huima-Byron T, Riley LW: Cloning of an *M. tuberculosis* DNA fragment associated with entry and survival inside cells, *Science* 261:1454-1457, 1993.
79. Bach EA, Aguet M, Schreiber RD: The IFN gamma receptor: a paradigm for cytokine receptor signaling, *Annu Rev Immunol* 15:563-591, 1997.
80. Baker R, Rook GA, Zumla A: Adrenal function and the hypothalamo-pituitary adrenal axis in immunodeficiency virus-associated tuberculosis, *Int J Tuberc Lung Dis* 1:289-290, 1997.
81. Barnes PF, Modlin RL: Human cellular immune responses to *Mycobacterium tuberculosis, Curr Top Microbiol Immunol* 215:197-219, 1996.
82. Bermudez LE, Goodman J: *Mycobacterium tuberculosis* invades and replicates within type II alveolar cells, *Infect Immun* 64:1400-1406, 1996.
83. Bloom BR, Flynn J, McDonough K, Kress Y, Chan J: Experimental approaches to mechanisms of protection and pathogenesis in *M. tuberculosis* infection, *Immunobiology* 191:526-536, 1994.
84. Bolin CA, Whipple DL, Khanna KV, Risdahl JM, Peterson PK, Molitor TW: Infection of swine with *Mycobacterium bovis* as a model of human tuberculosis, *J Infect Dis* 176:1559-1566, 1997.
85. Constant SL, Bottomly K: Induction of TH1 and TH2 CD4+ T cell responses. The alternative approaches, *Annu Rev Immunol* 15:297-322, 1997.
86. Cooper AM, D'Souza C, Frank AA, Orme IM: The course of *Mycobacterium tuberculosis* infection in the lungs of mice lacking expression of either perforin- or granzyme-mediated cytolytic mechanisms, *Infect Immun* 65:1317-1320, 1997.
87. Costello AM, Kumar A, Narayan V, Akbar MS, Ahmed S, Abou-Zeid C, Rook GA, Stanford J, Moreno C: Does antibody to mycobacterial antigens, including lipoarabinomannan, limit dissemination in childhood tuberculosis? *Trans R Soc Trop Med Hyg* 86:686-692, 1992.
88. Cywes C, Hoppe HC, Daffé M, Ehlers MRW: Nonopsonic binding of *Mycobacterium tuberculosis* to complement receptor type 3 is mediated by capsular polysaccharides and is strain dependent, *Infect Immun* 65:4258-4266, 1997.
89. Dannenberg AM, Rook GAW: Pathogenesis of pulmonary tuberculosis: an interplay of tissue-damaging and macrophage activating immune responses—dual mechanisms that control bacillary multiplication. In Bloom BR, ed: *Tuberculosis: pathogenesis, protection, and control,* Washington, DC, 1994, ASM Press, pp 459-483.
90. Ehlers MRW: Biology of *Mycobacterium tuberculosis* and the host-parasite relationship. In Cremin BJ, Jamieson DH, eds: *Childhood tuberculosis: modern imaging and clinical aspects,* London, 1995, Springer-Verlag, pp 7-18.
91. Ehlers MRW: The wolf at the door: some thoughts on the biochemistry of the tubercle bacillus, *S Afr Med J* 83:900-903, 1993.
92. Finlay BB, Falcow S: Common themes in microbial pathogenicity, *Microbiol Rev* 53:210-230, 1989.

93. Hernandez-Pando R, Rook GA: The role of TNF-alpha in T-cell-mediated inflammation depends on the Th1/Th2 cytokine balance, *Immunology* 82:591-595, 1994.
94. Ivanyi J, Sharp K: Control by H-2 genes of murine antibody responses to protein antigens of *Mycobacterium tuberculosis*, *Immunology* 59:329-332, 1986.
95. Kisielow P, von Boehmer H: Development and selection of T cells: facts and puzzles, *Adv Immunol* 58:87-209, 1995.
96. Leake ES, Myrvik QN, Wright MJ: Phagosomal membranes of *Mycobacterium bovis* BCG-immune alveolar macrophages are resistant to disruption by *Mycobacterium tuberculosis* H37RV, *Infect Immunol* 45:443-446, 1984.
97. Lipscomb MF, Bice DE, Lyons CR, Schuyler MR, Wilkes D: The regulation of pulmonary immunity, *Adv Immunol* 59:369-455, 1995.
98. Lukacs NW, Ward PA: Inflammatory mediators, cytokines, and adhesion molecules in pulmonary inflammation and injury, *Adv Immunol* 62:257-304, 1996.
99. MacMicking J, Xie Q, Nathan C: Nitric oxide and macrophage function, *Annu Rev Immunol* 15:323-350, 1997.
100. McDonough KA, Kress Y, Bloom BR: Pathogenesis of tuberculosis: interaction of *Mycobacterium tuberculosis* with macrophages, *Infect Immunol* 61:2763-2773, 1993.
101. McDonough KA, Kress Y: Cytotoxicity for lung epithelial cells is a virulence-associated phenotype of *Mycobacterium tuberculosis*, *Infect Immunol* 63:4802-4811, 1995.
102. Mustafa AS, Oftung F: Cytokine production and cytotoxicity mediated by CD4+ T cells from healthy subjects vaccinated with *Mycobacterium bovis* BCG and from pulmonary tuberculosis patients, *Nutrition* 11:698-701, 1995.
103. Newport MJ,Huxley CM, Huston S, Hawrylowicz CM, Oostra BA, Williamson R, Levin M: A mutation in the interferon-γ-receptor gene and susceptibility to mycobacterial infection, *N Engl J Med* 335:1941-1949, 1996.
104. North RJ: *Mycobacterium tuberculosis* is strikingly more virulent for mice when given via the respiratory than via the intravenous route, *J Infect Dis* 172:1550-1553, 1995.
105. Orme IM, Andersen P, Boom WH: T cell response to *Mycobacterium tuberculosis*, *J Infect Dis* 167:1481-1497, 1993.
106. Quinn FD, Newman GW, King CH: Virulence determinants of *Mycobacterium tuberculosis*, *Curr Top Microbiol Immunol* 215:131-156, 1996.
107. Rook GA, Hernandez-Pando R: The pathogenesis of tuberculosis, *Annu Rev Microbiol* 50:259-284, 1996.
108. Salyers AA, Whitt DD: *Bacterial pathogenesis: a molecular approach,* Washington, DC, 1994, ASM Press, pp 307-321.
109. Skinner MA, Yuan S, Prestidge R, Chuk D, Watson JD, Tan PLJ: Immunization with heat-killed *Mycobacterium vaccae* stimulates CD8+ cytotoxic T cells specific for macrophages infected with *Mycobacterium tuberculosis, Infection* 65:4525-4530, 1997.
110. Smith S, Jacobs RF, Wilson CB: Immunobiology of childhood tuberculosis: a window on the ontogeny of cellular immunity, *J Pediatr* 131:16-26, 1997.
111. Stanford JL: Immunologically important constituents of mycobacteria: antigens. In Ratledge C, Stanford J, eds: *The biology of the mycobacteria,* vol 2, *Immunological and environmental aspects,* London, 1983, Academic Press, pp 85-126.
112. Stewart-Tull DES: Immunologically important constituents of mycobacteria: adjuvants. In Ratledge C, Stanford J, eds: *The biology of the mycobacteria,* vol 2, *Immunological and environmental aspects,* London, 1983, Academic Press, pp 4-58.
113. Sweany HC: Studies on the pathogenesis of primary tuberculous infection. I. The regressive lesions, *Am Rev Tuberc* 27:559-574, 1933.
114. Zhang M, Kim KJ, Iyer D, Lin YG, Belisle J, McEnery K, Crandall ED, Barnes PF: Effects of *Mycobacterium tuberculosis* on the bioelectric properties of the alveolar epithelium, *Infect* 65:692-698, 1997.
115. Zimmerli S, Edwards S, Ernst JD: Selective receptor blockade during phagocytosis does not alter the survival and growth of *Mycobacterium tuberculosis* in human macrophages, *Am J Respir Cell Mol Biol* 15:760-770, 1996.
116. Beck JS, Gibbs JH, Potts RC, Kardjito T, Grange JM, Jawad ES, Spence VA: Histometric studies on biopsies of tuberculin skin tests showing evidence of ischaemia and necrosis, *J Pathol* 159:317-322, 1989.
117. Hall N, ed: *The* New Scientist *guide to chaos,* London, 1992, Penguin Books, pp 7-10.
118. Ridley DS: The histopathological spectrum of the mycobacterioses. In Ratledge C, Stanford J, Grange JM, eds: *The biology of the mycobacteria,* vol 3, *Clinical aspects of mycobacterial disease,* London, 1989, Academic Press, pp 129-143.
119. Wright GP: *An introduction to pathology,* ed 3, London, 1958 Longmans Green, pp 243-261.
120. Ayvazian LF: History of tuberculosis. In Reichman LB, Hershfield ES, eds: *Tuberculosis: a comprehensive international approach,* New York, 1993, Marcel Dekker, pp 1-20.
121. Bloom BR, Small PM: The evolving relation between humans and *Mycobacterium tuberculosis*, *N Engl J Med* 338:677-678, 1998.
122. Cole ST, Brosch R, Parkhill J, Garnier T, Churcher C, Harris D, Gordon SV, Eiglmeier K, Gas S, Barry III CE, Tekaia F, Badcock K, Basham D, Brown D, Chillingworth T, Connor R, Davies R, Devlin K, Feltwell T, Gentles S, Hamlin N, Holroyd S, Hornsby T, Jagels K, Krogh A, McLean J, Moule S, Murphy L, Oliver K, Osborne J, Quail MA, Rajandream MA, Rogers J, Rutter S, Seeger K, Skelton J, Squares R, Squares S, Sulston JE, Taylor K, Whitehead S, Barrell BG: Deciphering the biology of *Mycobacterium tuberculosis* from the complete genome sequence, *Nature* 393:537-544, 1998.
123. Collins TFB: The history of southern Africa's first tuberculosis epidemic, *S Afr Med J* 62:780-788, 1982.
124. Daniel TM, Downes KA, Bates JH: Early history of tuberculosis. In Bloom BR, ed: *Tuberculosis: pathogenesis, protection, and control,* Washington, DC, 1994, ASM Press, pp 13-24.
125. Dubos R, Dubos J: *The white plague: tuberculosis, man and society,* New Brunswick, NJ, 1987, Rutgers University Press.
126. Ewald PW: Guarding against the most dangerous emerging pathogens: insights from evolutionary biology, *Emerg Infect Dis* 2:245-256, 1996.
127. Gale AH: *Epidemic diseases,* Harmondsworth, 1959, Penguin, pp 123-131.
128. Lederberg J: Infectious disease as an evolutionary paradigm, *Emerg Infect Dis* 3:417-423, 1997.
129. McGrath, JW: Social networks of disease spread in the lower Illinois valley: a simulation approach, *Am J Phys Anthropol* 77:483-496, 1988.
130. Sreevatsan S, Pan X, Stockbauer KE, Connell ND, Kreiswirth BN, Whittam TS, Musser JM: Restricted structural gene polymorphism in the *Mycobacterium tuberculosis* complex indicates evolutionarily recent global dissemination, *Proc Natl Acad Sci USA* 94:9869-9874, 1997.
131. Sumartojo E: When tuberculosis treatment fails. A social behavioural account of patient adherence, *Am Rev Respir Dis* 147:1311-1320, 1993.
132. Valway SE, Sanchez MP, Shinnick TF, Orme I, Agerton T, Hoy D, Jones JS, Westmoreland H, Onorato IM: An outbreak involving extensive transmission of a virulent strain of *Mycobacterium tuberculosis*, *N Engl J Med* 338:633-639, 1998.
133. Bakshi SS, Alvarez D, Hilfer CL, Sordillo EM, Grover R, Kairam R: Tuberculosis in human immunodeficiency virus–infected children. A family infection, *Am J Dis Child* 147:320-324, 1993.
134. Bhat GJ, Diwan VK, Chintu C, Kabika M, Masona J: HIV, BCG and TB in children: a case control study in Lusaka, Zambia, *J Trop Pediatr* 39:219-223, 1993.
135. Braun MM, Cauthen G: Relationship of the human immunodeficiency virus epidemic to pediatric tuberculosis and bacillus Calmette-Guérin immunization, *Pediatr Infect Dis J* 11:220-227, 1992.
136. Chan SP, Birnbaum J, Rao M, Steiner P: Clinical manifestation and outcome of tuberculosis in children with acquired immunodeficiency syndrome, *Pediatr Infect Dis J* 15:443-447, 1996.
137. Chintu C, Bhat G, Luo C, Raviglione M, Diwan V, Dupont HL, Zumla A: Seroprevalence of human immunodeficiency virus type 1 infection in Zambian children with tuberculosis, *Pediatr Infect Dis J* 12:499-504, 1993.
138. Drucker E, Alcabes P, Bosworth W, Sckell B: Childhood tuberculosis in the Bronx, New York, *Lancet* 343:1482-1485, 1994.
139. Espinal MA, Reingold AL, Perez G, Camilo E, Soto S, Cruz E, Matos N, Gonzalez G: Human immunodeficiency virus infection in children with tuberculosis in Santo Domingo, Dominican Republic: prevalence, clinical findings, and response to antituberculosis treatment, *J Acquir Immune Defic Syndr Hum Retrovirol* 13:155-159, 1996.
140. Goldfeld AE, Delgado JC, Thim S, Bozon MV, Uglialoro AM, Turbay D, Cohen C, Yunis EJ: Association of an HLA-DQ allele with clinical tuberculosis, *JAMA* 279:226-228, 1998.

141. Gonzalez B, Moreno S, Burdach R, Valenzuela MT, Henriquez A, Ramos MI, Sorensen RU: Clinical presentation of bacillus Calmette-Guérin infections in patients with immunodeficiency syndromes, *Pediatr Infect Dis J* 8:201-206, 1989.
142. Gutman LT, Moye J, Zimmer B, Tian C: Tuberculosis in human immunodeficiency virus–exposed or –infected United States children, *Pediatr Infect Dis J* 13:963-968, 1994.
143. Jeena PM, Mitha T, Bamber S, Wesley A, Coutsoudis A, Coovadia HM: Effects of the human immunodeficiency virus on tuberculosis in children, *Tuber Lung Dis* 77:437-443, 1996.
144. Jones DS, Malecki JM, Bigler WJ, Witte JJ, Oxtoby MJ: Pediatric tuberculosis and human immunodeficiency virus infection in Palm Beach County, Florida, *Am J Dis Child* 146:1166-1170, 1992.
145. Joshi VV, Oleske JM, Saad S, Connor EM, Rapkin RH, Minnefor AB: Pathology of opportunistic infections in children with acquired immune deficiency syndrome, *Pediatr Pathol* 6:145-150, 1986.
146. Khouri YF, Mastrucci MT, Hutto C, Mitchell CD, Scott GB: *Mycobacterium tuberculosis* in children with human immunodeficiency virus type 1 infection, *Pediatr Infect Dis J* 11:950-955, 1992.
147. Maher D: Tuberculosis is important problem in children with HIV infection in sub-Saharan Africa, *BMJ* 313:562-563, 1996 (letter, comment).
148. Sifford M, Bates JH: Host determinants of susceptibility to *Mycobacterium tuberculosis*, *Semin Respir Infect* 6:44-50, 1991.
149. Stead WW, Senner JW, Reddick WT, Lofgren JP: Racial differences in susceptibility to infection by *Mycobacterium tuberculosis*, *N Engl J Med* 322:422-427, 1990.
150. van der Merwe PL, Kalis N, Schaaf HS, Nel EH, Gie RP: Risk of pulmonary tuberculosis in children with congenital heart disease, *Pediatr Cardiol* 16:172-175, 1995.
151. Vijayakumar M, Bhaskaram P, Hemalatha P: Malnutrition and childhood tuberculosis, *J Trop Pediatr* 36:294-298, 1990.
152. Wessels G, Hesseling PB, Gie RP, Nel E: The increased risk of developing tuberculosis in children with malignancy, *Ann Trop Paediatr* 12:277-281, 1992.

Diagnosis

153. Bates JH: Diagnosis of tuberculosis, *Chest* 76:757-763, 1979.
154. Centers for Disease Control and Prevention: Case definitions for public health surveillance, *MMWR* 39(no. RR-13):41-42, 1990.
155. Inselman LS: Tuberculosis in children: an update, *Pediatr Pulmonol* 21:101-120, 1996.
156. Khan EA, Starke JR: Diagnosis of tuberculosis in children: increased need for better methods, *Emerg Infect Dis* 1:115-123, 1995.
157. Vallejo JG, Ong LT, Starke JR: Clinical features, diagnosis and treatment of tuberculosis in infants, *Pediatrics* 94:1-7, 1994.
158. American Thoracic Society and Centers for Disease Control: Diagnostic standards and classification of tuberculosis, *Am Rev Respir Dis* 142:725-735, 1990.
159. Anuntaseree W, Suntornlohanakul S, Mitarnun W: Disseminated tuberculosis in a 2-month-old infant, *Pediatr Pulmonol* 13:255-258, 1992.
160. Cundall DB: The diagnosis of pulmonary tuberculosis in malnourished Kenyan children, *Ann Trop Paed* 6:249-255, 1986.
161. de Blic J, Azevedo I, Burren CP, Le Bourgeois M, Lallemand D, Scheinmann P: The value of flexible bronchoscopy in childhood pulmonary tuberculosis, *Chest* 100:688-692, 1991.
162. Glidey Y, Hable D: Tuberculosis in childhood: an analysis of 412 cases, *Ethiop Med J* 21:161-167, 1983.
163. Gogus S, Umer H, Akcoren Z, Sanal O, Osmanlioglu G, Cimbis M: Neonatal tuberculosis, *Pediatr Pathol* 13:299-304, 1993.
164. Hennink MJ, Skibbe A, Donald PJ: Failure to gain weight prior to the diagnosis of pulmonary tuberculosis, *J Trop Paed* 34:108-109, 1988.
165. Hershfield E: Tuberculosis in children. Guidelines for diagnosis, prevention and treatment. A Statement of the Scientific Committees of the IUATLD, *Bull Int Union Tuberc Lung Dis* 66:61-67, 1991.
166. Hsu KHK: Contact investigation: a practical approach to tuberculosis eradication, *Am J Public Health* 53:1761-1769, 1963.
167. Hugo-Hamman CT, Scher H, de Moor MMA: Tuberculous pericarditis in children: a review of 44 cases, *Pediatr Infect Dis J* 13:13-18, 1994.
168. Hussey G, Chisholm T, Kibel M: Miliary tuberculosis in children: a review of 94 cases, *Pediatr Infect Dis J* 10:832-836, 1991.
169. Kennedy DH: Extrapulmonary tuberculosis. In Ratledge C, Stanford J, Grange JM, eds: *The biology of the mycobacteria,* vol 3, *Clinical aspects of mycobacterial disease,* London, 1989, Academic Press, pp 246-285.
170. Kitai IC, Sanders DM, Manungo J: Tuberculosis presenting as corticosteroid responsive wheezing in infancy, *Trop Geogr Med* 41:274-276, 1989.
171. Lorber J: The long-term prognosis of generalised miliary tuberculosis in children, *Lancet* ii:1447-1449, 1966.
172. Martinez-Azagra A, Serrano A, Casado-Flores J: Adult respiratory distress syndrome in children, associated with miliary tuberculosis, *J Pediatr* 126:678-679, 1995 (letter, comment).
173. Migliori GB, Borghesi A, Rossanigo P, Adriko C, Neri M, Santini S, Bartoloni A, Paradisi F, Acocella G: Proposal for an improved score method for the diagnosis of pulmonary tuberculosis in childhood in developing countries, *Tuber Lung Dis* 73:145-149, 1992.
174. Rahajoe NN: Miliary tuberculosis in children. A clinical review, *Paediatr Indones* 30:233-240, 1990.
175. Rosen EN: The problems of diagnosis and treatment of childhood pulmonary tuberculosis in developing countries, *S Afr Med J* 62:26-28, 1982.
176. Roux P, Delport SV, Klein M: Clinical presentation and diagnosis of childhood pulmonary tuberculosis (in press).
177. Schaaf HS, Beyers N, Gie RP, Nel ED, Smuts NA, Scott FE, Donald PR, Fourie PB: Respiratory tuberculosis in childhood: the diagnostic value of clinical features and special investigations, *Pediatr Infect Dis J* 14:189-194, 1995.
178. Schaaf HS, Gie RP, Beyers N, Smuts N, Donald PR: Tuberculosis in infants less than 3 months of age, *Arch Dis Child* 69:371-374, 1993.
179. Schuit KE: Miliary tuberculosis in children. Clinical and laboratory manifestation in 19 patients, *Am J Dis Child* 133:583-585, 1979.
180. Schuster A, Duffau G, Nicholls E, Pino M: Lung aspirate puncture as a diagnostic aid in pulmonary tuberculosis in childhood. A preliminary study, *Pediatrics* 42:647-650, 1968.
181. Steiner P, Rao M, Victoria MS, Jabbar H, Steiner M: Persistently negative tuberculin reactions: their presence among children with culture positive for *Mycobacterium tuberculosis* (tuberculin-negative tuberculosis), *Am J Dis Child* 134:747-750, 1980.
182. Stoltz AP, Donald PR, Strebel PM, Talent JM: Criteria for the notification of childhood tuberculosis in a high-incidence area of the western Cape Province, *S Afr Med J* 77:385-386, 1990.
183. Wallgren A: The time table of tuberculosis, *Tubercle* 29:245-251, 1948.
184. Williams DJ, York EL, Sproule BJ: Endobronchial tuberculosis presenting as asthma, *Chest* 93:836-838, 1988.
185. Aderele WI: Radiological patterns of pulmonary tuberculosis in Nigerian children, *Tubercle* 61:157-163, 1980.
186. Agrons GA, Markowitz RI, Kramer SS: Pulmonary tuberculosis in children, *Semin Roentgenol* 28:158-172, 1993.
187. Amodio J, Abramson S, Berdon W: Primary pulmonary tuberculosis in infancy: a resurgent disease in the urban United States, *Pediatr Radiol* 16:185-189, 1986.
188. Beyers JA: Radiographic manifestations. In Coovadia HM, Benatar SR, eds: *A century of tuberculosis,* Cape Town, 1991, Oxford University Press, pp 203-223.
189. Bhatia R, Mitra DK, Mukherjee S, Berry M: Bronchoesophageal fistula of tuberculous origin in a child, *Pediatr Radiol* 22:154, 1992.
190. Bui HD, Keller MA, Jayich SA, Nelson RJ, Harley DP, Lachman RS, Young LW: Radiological case of the month. Asymptomatic calcified pulmonary tuberculosis, *Am J Dis Child* 138:91-93, 1984.
191. Chanoine JP, Toppet M, Dab I, Toppet V, Tondeur M, Ham H, Piepsz A: Unusual ventilation-perfusion patterns in primary lung tuberculosis, *Pediatr Pulmonol* 5:51-54, 1988.
192. Cremin BJ, Jamieson DH, eds: *Childhood tuberculosis: modern imaging and clinical aspects,* London, 1995, Springer-Verlag.
193. Delacourt C, Mani TM, Bonnerot V, de Blic J, Sayeg N, Lallemand D, Scheinmann P: Computed tomography with normal chest radiograph in tuberculous infection, *Arch Dis Child* 69:430-432, 1993.
194. Donald PR, Ball JB, Burger PJ: Bacteriologically confirmed pulmonary tuberculosis in childhood: clinical and radiological features, *S Afr Med J* 67:588-590, 1985.
195. Freiman I, Geefhuysen J, Solomon A: The radiological presentation of pulmonary tuberculosis in children, *S Afr Med J* 49:1703-1706, 1975.
196. Gie R, Kling S, Schaaf HS, Beyers N, Moore S, Schneider J: Tuberculous bronchopleural fistula in children: a description of two cases, *Pediatr Pulmonol* 25:285-288, 1998.
197. Gupta RK, Sharma BK, Jena A, Pant K, Prakash R, Talukdar B: Primary mediastinal tuberculous abscess: demonstration with MR, *Pediatr Radiol* 19:330-332, 1989.

198. Haller JO, Cohen HL: Pediatric HIV infection: an imaging update, *Pediatr Radiol* 24:224-230, 1994.
199. Lamont AC, Cremin BJ, Pelteret RM: Radiological patterns of pulmonary tuberculosis in the pediatric age group, *Pediatr Radiol* 16:2-7, 1986.
200. Leung AN, Muller NL, Pineda PR, FitzGerald JM: Primary tuberculosis in childhood: radiographic manifestations, *Radiology* 182:87-91, 1992.
201. Lincoln EM, Harris LC, Bovornkitti S, Carretero RW: Endobronchial tuberculosis in children, *Am Rev Tuberc* 77:39-61, 1958.
202. Lucaya J, Sole S, Badosa J, Manzanares R: Bronchial perforation and bronchoesophageal fistulas: tuberculous origin in children, *Am J Roentgenol* 135:525-528, 1980.
203. Nauth-Misir TN: Tuberculous cavitation of the lungs in infancy with the report of a case, *Tubercle* 29:277-283, 1948.
204. Parisi MT, Jensen MC, Wood BP: Pictorial review of the usual and unusual roentgen manifestations of childhood tuberculosis, *Clin Imag* 18:149-154, 1994.
205. Reed MH, Pagtakhan RD, Zylak CJ, Berg TJ: Radiologic features of miliary tuberculosis in children and adults, *J Can Assoc Radiol* 28:175-181, 1977.
206. Schaaf HS, Donald PR, Scott F: Maternal chest radiography as supporting evidence for the diagnosis of tuberculosis in childhood, *J Trop Pediatr* 37:223-225, 1991.
207. Strouse PJ, Dessner DA, Watson WJ, Blane CE: *Mycobacterium tuberculosis* infection in immunocompetent children, *Pediatr Radiol* 26:134-140, 1996.
208. Vijayasekaran D, Selvakumar P, Balachandran A, Elizabeth J, Subramanyam L, Somu N: Pulmonary cavitatory tuberculosis in children, *Indian Pediatr* 31:1075-1078, 1994.
209. American Academy of Pediatrics Committee on Infectious Diseases: Update on tuberculosis skin testing of children, *Pediatrics* 97:282-284, 1996.
210. American Thoracic Society and Centers for Disease Control: Diagnostic standards and classification of tuberculosis, *Am Rev Respir Dis* 142:725-735, 1990.
211. Beck JS, Morley SM, Lowe JG, Brown RA, Grange JM, Gibbs JH, Potts RC, Kardjito T: Diversity in migration of CD4 and CD8 lymphocytes in different microanatomical compartments of the skin in the tuberculin reaction in man, *Br J Exp Pathol* 69:771-780, 1988.
212. Black S, Humphrey JH, Niven JSF: Inhibition of Mantoux reaction by direct suggestion under hypnosis, *BMJ* 2:1649, 1963.
213. Bleiker MA, Styblo K: Estimated and observed risk of tuberculous infection in the Netherlands, 1967 to 1975, *Scand J Respir Dis Suppl* 102:228-229, 1978.
214. Bleiker MA, Sutherland I, Styblo K, ten Dam HG, Misljenovic O: Guidelines for estimating the risks of tuberculous infection from tuberculin test results in a representative sample of children, *Bull Int Union Tuberc Lung Dis* 64:7-12, 1989.
215. Canadian Pediatric Society: Childhood tuberculosis: current concepts in diagnosis, *Can J Pediatr* 1:97-100, 1994.
216. Carr DT, Karlson AG, Stillwell AA: A comparison of cultures of induced sputum and gastric washings in the diagnosis of tuberculosis, *Mayo Clinic Proc* 42:23-25, 1967.
217. Centers for Disease Control and Prevention: Essential components of a tuberculosis prevention and control program; and screening for tuberculosis and tuberculosis infection in high-risk populations: recommendations of the Advisory Council for the Elimination of Tuberculosis, *MMWR* 44(no. RR-11):1-34, 1995.
218. Chan S, Abadco DL, Steiner P: Role of flexible fiberoptic bronchoscopy in the diagnosis of childhood endobronchial tuberculosis, *Pediatr Infect Dis J* 13:506-509, 1994.
219. Dawodu AH: Tuberculin conversion following BCG vaccination in preterm infants, *Acta Paediatr Scand* 74:564-567, 1985.
220. Fletcher RH, Fletcher SW, Wagner EH: *Clinical epidemiology,* ed 2, Baltimore, 1988, Williams & Wilkins, pp 42-75.
221. Gibbs JH, Grange JM, Beck JS, Jawad E, Potts RC, Bothamley GH, Kardjito T: Early delayed hypersensitivity responses in tuberculin skin tests after heavy occupational exposure to tuberculosis, *J Clin Pathol* 44:919-923, 1991.
222. Gocmen A, Kiper N, Ertan U, Kalayci O, Ozcelik U: Is the BCG test of diagnostic value in tuberculosis? *Tuber Lung Dis* 75:54-57, 1994.
223. Huebner RE, Schein MF, Bass JB Jr: The tuberculin skin test, *Clin Infect Dis* 17:968-975, 1993.
224. Joncas JH, Robitaille R, Gauthier T: Interpretation of the PPD skin test in BCG-vaccinated children, *Can Med Assoc J* 113:127-128, 1975.
225. Jordan TJ, Lewit EM, Reichman LB: Isoniazid preventive therapy for tuberculosis: decision analysis considering ethnicity and gender, *Am Rev Respir Dis* 144:1357-1360, 1991.
226. Kardjito T, Grange JM, Beck JS: Cooperative studies on the immunology of tuberculosis at Airlangga University, Surabaya, Indonesia, *Asian Pac J Allergy Immunol* 8:141-146, 1990.
227. Menzies R, Vissandjee B: Effect of bacille Calmette-Guérin vaccination on tuberculin reactivity, *Am Rev Respir Dis* 141:621-655, 1992.
228. Molina-Gamboa JD, Ponce-de-Leon-Rosales S, Rivera-Morales I, Romero C, Baez R, Huertas M, Osornio G: Evaluation of the sensitivity of RT-23 purified protein derivative for determining tuberculin reactivity in a group of health care workers, *Clin Infect Dis* 19:784-786, 1994.
229. Pust RE, Erickson P: Determining *Mycobacterium tuberculosis* infection in high prevalence groups: a comparative study among Nigerian adults, *Tubercle* 65:263-278, 1984.
230. Reichman LB: Tuberculin skin testing: state of the art, *Chest* 76:764-770, 1979.
231. Sbarbaro JA: Tuberculin test: a re-emphasis on clinical judgement, *Am Rev Respir Dis* 132:177-178, 1985.
232. Sepulveda RL, Burr C, Ferrer X, Sorensen RU: Booster effect of tuberculin testing in healthy 6-year-old school children vaccinated with bacille Calmette-Guérin at birth in Santiago, Chile, *Pediatr Infect Dis J* 7:578-582, 1988.
233. Snider DE: Bacille Calmette-Guérin vaccinations and tuberculin skin tests, *JAMA* 253:3438-3439, 1985.
234. Abadco DL, Steiner P: Gastric lavage is better than bronchoalveolar lavage for isolation of *Mycobacterium tuberculosis* in childhood tuberculosis, *Pediatr Infect Dis J* 11:735-738, 1992.
235. Pomputius WF, Rost J, Dennehy PH, Carter EJ: Standardization of gastric aspirate technique improves yield in the diagnosis of tuberculosis in children, *Pediatr Infect Dis J* 16:222-226, 1997.
236. Riley UBG, Crawford S, Barrett SP, Abdalla SH: Detection of mycobacteria in bone marrow biopsy specimens taken to investigate pyrexia of unknown origin, *J Clin Pathol* 48:706-770, 1995.
237. Somu N, Swaminathan S, Paramasivan CN, Vijayasekaran D, Chandrabhooshanam A, Vijayan VK, Prabhakar R: Value of bronchoalveolar lavage and gastric lavage in the diagnosis of pulmonary tuberculosis in children, *Tuber Lung Dis* 76(4):295-299, 1995.
238. Lipsky BA, Bates J, Tenover FC, Plorde JJ: Factors affecting the clinical value of microscopy for acid-fast bacilli, *Rev Infect Dis* 6:214-222, 1984.
239. Strumpf IJ, Tsang AY, Syre JW: Reevaluation of sputum staining for the diagnosis of pulmonary tuberculosis, *Am Rev Respir Dis* 119:599-602, 1979.
240. Heifets LB: Rapid automated methods (BACTEC system) in clinical microbiology, *Semin Respir Infect* 1:242-249, 1986.
241. Barrera L, Miceli I, Ritacco V, Torrea G, Broglia B, Botta R, Maldonado CP, Ferrero N, Pinasco A, Cutillo I, et al: Detection of circulating antibodies to purified protein derivative by enzyme-linked immunosorbent assay: its potential for the rapid diagnosis of tuberculosis, *Pediatr Infect Dis J* 8:763-767, 1989.
242. Delacourt C, Gobin J, Gaillard JL, de Blic J, Veran M, Scheinmann P: Value of ELISA using antigen 60 for the diagnosis of tuberculosis in children, *Chest* 104:393-398, 1993.
243. Dhand R, Ganguly NK, Vaishnavi C, Gilhotra R, Malik SK: False-positive reactions with enzyme-linked immunosorbent assay of *Mycobacterium tuberculosis* antigens in pleural fluid, *J Med Microbiol* 26:241-243, 1988.
244. Fadda G, Grillo R, Ginesu F, Santoru L, Zanetti S, Dettori G: Serodiagnosis and follow up of patients with pulmonary tuberculosis by enzyme-linked immunosorbent assay, *Eur J Epidemiol* 8(1):81-87, 1992.
245. Hussey G, Kibel M, Dempster W: The serodiagnosis of tuberculosis in children: an evaluation of an ELISA test using IgG antibodies to *M. tuberculosis,* strain H37RV, *Ann Trop Paediatr* 11:113-118, 1991.
246. Rosen EU: The diagnostic value of an enzyme-linked immunosorbent assay using adsorbed mycobacterial sonicates in children, *Tubercle* 71:127-130, 1990.
247. Sada E, Aguilar D, Torres M, Herrera T: Detection of lipoarabinomannan as a diagnostic test for tuberculosis, *J Clin Microbiol* 30:2415-2418, 1992.

248. Turneer M, Nerom EV, Nyabenda J, Waelbroeck A, Duvivier A, Toppet M: Determination of humoral immunoglobulins M and G directed against mycobacterial antigen 60 failed to diagnose primary tuberculosis and mycobacterial adenitis in children, *Am J Respir Crit Care Med* 150:1508-1512, 1994.
249. Butler WR, Kilburn JO: Identification of major slowly growing pathogenic mycobacteria and *Mycobacterium gordonae* by high-performance liquid chromatography of their mycolic acids, *J Clin Microbiol* 26:50-53, 1988.
250. Brisson-Noel A, Aznar C, Chureau C, Nguyen S, Pierre C, Bartoli M, Bonete R, Pialoux G, Gicquel G, Garrigue G: Diagnosis of tuberculosis by DNA amplification in clinical practice evaluation, *Lancet* 338:364-366, 1991.
251. Broomfield A, Bourn D: Basic techniques in molecular genetics, *J Laryngol Otol* 112:230-234, 1998.
252. Centers for Disease Control and Prevention: Nucleic acid amplification tests for tuberculosis, *MMWR* 45:950-952, 1996.
253. Daniel TM: The rapid diagnosis of tuberculosis: a selective review, *J Lab Clin Med 1*16:277-282, 1990.
254. Delacourt C, Poveda JD, Chureau C, Beydon N, Mahut B, de Blic J, Scheinmann P, Garrigue G: Use of polymerase chain reaction for improved diagnosis of tuberculosis in children, *J Pediatr* 126:703-709, 1995.
255. Eisenach KD, Sifford MD, Cane MD, Bates JH, Crawford JT: Detection of *Mycobacterium tuberculosis* in sputum samples using a polymerase chain reaction, *Am Rev Respir Dis* 144:1160-1163, 1991.
256. Ellner PD, Kiehn TE, Cammarata R, Hosmer M: Rapid detection and identification of pathogenic mycobacteria by combining radiometric and nucleic probe methods, *J Clin Microbiol* 26(7):1349-1352, 1988.
257. Gamboa F, Manterola JM, Lonca J, Viñado B, Matas L, Giménez M, Ruiz Manzano J, Rodrigo C, Cardona PJ, Padilla E, Dominguez J, Ausina V: Rapid detection of *Mycobacterium tuberculosis* in respiratory specimens, blood and other non-respiratory specimens by amplification of rRNA, *Int J Tuberc Lung Dis* 1:542-555, 1997.
258. Jacobs WR Jr, Barletta RG, Udani R, Chan J, Kalkut G, Sosne G, Kieser T, Sarkis GJ, Hatfull GF, Bloom BR: Rapid assessment of drug susceptibilities of *Mycobacterium tuberculosis* by means of luciferase reporter pages, *Science* 260:819-822, 1993.
259. Noordhock A, Kolk A, Bjune G, Catty D, Dale JW, Fine PE, Godfrey-Faussett P, Cho SN, Shinnick T, Svenson SB, et al: Sensitivity and specificity of polymerase chain reaction for detection of *Mycobacterium tuberculosis*: a blind comparison study among seven laboratories, *J Clin Microbiol* 32:277-284, 1994.
260. Pierre C, Oliver C, Lecossier D, Bousssougant Y, Yemi P, Hance AJ: Diagnosis of primary tuberculosis in children by amplification and detection of mycobacterial DNA, *Am Rev Respir Dis* 147:420-424, 1993.
261. Radhakrishnan VV, Sehgal S, Mathai A: Correlation between culture of *Mycobacterium tuberculosis* and detection of mycobacterial antigens in cerebrospinal fluid of patients with tuberculous meningitis, *J Med Microbiol* 33:223-226, 1990.
262. Sada E, Ruiz-Palacios GM, Lopez-Vidal Y, Ponce de Leon S: Detection of mycobacterial antigens in cerebrospinal fluid of patients with tuberculous meningitis by enzyme-linked immunosorbent assay, *Lancet* 2:651-652, 1983.
263. Shankar P, Manjunath N, Lakshmi R, Aditi B, Seth P, Shriniwas A: Identification of *Mycobacterium tuberculosis* by polymerase chain reaction, *Lancet* 335:423, 1990.
264. Shoemaker SA, Fisher JH, Jones WD, Scoggin CH: Restriction fragment analysis of chromosomal DNA defines different strains of *Mycobacterium tuberculosis*, *Am Rev Respir Dis* 134:210-213, 1986.
265. Starke JR, Ong LT, Eisenach KD, et al: Detection of *M. tuberculosis* in gastric aspirate samples from children using polymerase chain reaction, *Am Rev Respir Dis* 147(suppl):A801, 1993.
266. Thierry D, Chureau C, Aznar C, Guesdon JL: The detection of *Mycobacterium tuberculosis* in uncultured clinical specimens using the polymerase chain reaction and a non-radioactive DNA probe, *Mol Cell Probes* 6:181-191, 1992.
267. al-Eissa YA: Unusual suppurative complications of brucellosis in children, *Acta Paediatr* 82:987-992, 1993.
268. Allworth AM, Ghosh HK, Saltos N: A case of *Actinomyces meyeri* pneumonia in a child, *Med J Aust* 145:33, 1986.
269. Burton K, Yogev R, London N, Boyer K, Shulman ST: Pulmonary paragonimiasis in Laotian refugee children, *Pediatrics* 70:246-248, 1982.
270. Butler JC, Heller R, Wright PF: Histoplasmosis during childhood, *South Med J* 87:476-480, 1994.
271. Kendig EL Jr: The clinical picture of sarcoidosis in children, *Pediatrics* 54:289-292, 1974.
272. Kim OH, Yang HR, Bahk YW: Pulmonary nocardiosis manifested as miliary nodules in a neonate—a case report, *Pediatr Radiol* 22:229-230, 1992.
273. Loos T: Differences between intrathoracic sarcoidosis and pulmonary tuberculosis in childhood, *Scand J Respir Dis Suppl* 102:191-193, 1978.

Prevention

274. Martinez-Azagra A, Serrano A, Casado-Flores J: Adult respiratory distress syndrome in children, associated with miliary tuberculosis, *J Pediatr* 126:678-679, 1995.
275. Ng KK, Cheng YF, Ko SF, Ng SH, Pai SC, Tsai CC: CT findings of pediatric thoracic actinomycosis: report of four cases, *J Formos Med Assoc* 91(3):346-350, 1992.
276. Usuda K, Saito Y, Imai T, Ota S, Sato M, Fujimura S, Tanahashi N: Inflammatory pseudotumor of the lung diagnosed as granulomatous lesion by preoperative brushing cytology. A case report, *Acta Cytol* 34:685-689, 1990.
277. Banani SA, Alborzi A: Needle aspiration for suppurative post-BCG adenitis, *Arch Dis Child* 71:446-447, 1994.
278. Bass JB: Tuberculin test, preventive therapy, and elimination of tuberculosis, *Am Rev Respir Dis* 141:812-813, 1990.
279. Besnard M, Sauvion S, Offredo C, Gaudelus J, Gaillard JL, Veber F, Blanche S: Bacillus Calmette-Guérin infection after vaccination of human immunodeficiency virus–infected children, *Pediatr Infect Dis J* 12:993-997, 1993.
280. Centers for Disease Control and Prevention: The role of BCG vaccine in the prevention and control of tuberculosis in the United States: a joint statement by the Advisory Council for the Elimination of Tuberculosis and the Advisory Committee on Immunization Practices, *MMWR* 45(no. RR-4), 1996.
281. Centers for Disease Control and Prevention: The role of BCG vaccine in the prevention and control of tuberculosis in the United States: a joint statement by the Advisory Council for the Elimination of Tuberculosis and the Advisory Committee on Immunization Practices, *MMWR* 45(no. RR-4):1-18, 1996.
282. Cheng SH, Walker L, Poole J, Aber VR, Walker KB, Mitchison DA, Lowrie DB: Demonstration of increased anti-mycobacterial activity in peripheral blood monocytes after BCG vaccination in British school children, *Clin Exp Immunol* 74:20-25, 1988.
283. Chhatwal J, Verma M, Thaper N, Aneja R: Waning of post vaccinial allergy after neonatal BCG vaccination, *Indian Pediatr* 31:1529-1533, 1994.
284. Colditz GA, Berkey CS, Mosteller F, Brewer TF, Wilson ME, Burdick E, Fineberg HV: The efficacy of bacillus Calmette-Guérin vaccination of newborns and infants in the prevention of tuberculosis: meta-analyses of the published literature, *Pediatrics* 96:29-35, 1995.
285. Colditz GA, Berkey CS, Mosteller F, Brewer TF, Wilson ME, Burdick E, Fineberg HV: The efficacy of bacillus Calmette-Guérin vaccination of newborns and infants in the prevention of tuberculosis: meta-analyses of the published literature, *Pediatrics* 96:29-35, 1995.
286. Eddy DM: Principles for making difficult decisions in difficult times, *JAMA* 27:1792-1798, 1994.
287. Fine PE, Sterne JA, Ponnighaus JM, Rees RJ: Delayed-type hypersensitivity, mycobacterial vaccines and protective immunity, *Lancet* 344:1245-1249, 1994.
288. Goh TE, Low M, Chen CH, Tan TH: A comparative study of Japanese and British BCG vaccine strains in newborn infants, *Asia Pac J Public Health* 3:32-40, 1989.
289. Greenberg PD, Lax KG, Schechter CB: Tuberculosis in house staff: a decision analysis comparing the tuberculin strategy with the BCG vaccination, *Am Rev Respir Dis* 143:490-495, 1991.
290. Heyderman RS, Morgan G, Levinsky RJ, Strobel S: Successful bone marrow transplantation and treatment of BCG infection in two patients with severe combined immunodeficiency, *Eur J Pediatr* 150:477-480, 1991.

291. Irwig L, Tosteson ANA, Gatsonis C, Lau J, Colditz G, Chalmers TC, Mosteller F: Guidelines for meta-analyses evaluating diagnostic tests, *Ann Intern Med* 120:667-676, 1994.
292. Jouanguy E, Altare F, Lamhamedi S, Revy P, Emile J, Newport M, Levin M, Blanche S, Seboun E, Fischer A, Casanova J: Brief report: interferon-gamma-receptor deficiency in an infant with fatal bacille Calmette-Guérin infection, *N Engl J Med* 335:1956-1961, 1996.
293. Lallemant-Le Coeur S, Lallemant M, Cheynier D, Nzingoula S, Drucker J, Larouze B: Bacillus Calmette-Guérin immunization in infants born to HIV-1-seropositive mothers, *AIDS* 5:195-199, 1991.
294. Lotte A, Wasz-Hockert O, Poisson N, Engbaek H, Landmann H, Quast U, Andrasofszky B, Lugosi L, Vadasz, I, Mihailescu P, et al: Second IUATLD study on complications induced by intradermal BCG-vaccination, *Bull Int Union Tuberc* 63:47-59, 1988.
295. Lugosi L: Trends in childhood tuberculosis in Hungary 1953-1983: quantitative methods for evaluation of BCG policy, *Int J Epidemiol* 14:304-312, 1985.
296. Mahairas GG, Sabo PJ, Hickey MJ, Singh DC, Stover CK: Molecular analysis of genetic differences between *Mycobacterium bovis* BCG and virulent *M. bovis, J Bacteriol* 178:1274-1282, 1996.
297. McMurray DN, Carlomagno MA, Mintzer CL, Tetzlaff CL: *Mycobacterium bovis* BCG vaccine fails to protect protein-deficient guinea pigs against respiratory challenge with virulent *Mycobacterium tuberculosis, Infect Immun* 50:555-559, 1985.
298. Quinn TC: Interactions of the human immunodeficiency virus and tuberculosis and the implications for BCG vaccination. *Rev Infect Dis* (suppl 2):S379-S384, 1989.
299. Rodrigues LC, Diwan VK, Wheeler JG: Protective effect of BCG against tuberculous meningitis and miliary tuberculosis: a meta-analysis, *Int J Epidemiol* 22:1154-1158, 1993.
300. Sorensen RU: Clinical presentation of bacillus Calmette-Guérin infections in patients with immunodeficiency syndromes, *Pediatr Infect Dis J* 8:201-206, 1989.
301. Fitzgerald JM, Gafni A: A cost-effectiveness analysis of the routine use of isoniazid prophylaxis in patients with a positive Mantoux skin test, *Am Rev Respir Dis* 142:848-853, 1990.
302. Koplan JP, Farer LS: Choice of preventive treatment for isoniazid-resistant tuberculous infection: use of decision analysis and the delphi technique, *JAMA* 244:2736-2740, 1980.
303. Nazar-Stewart V, Nolan CM: Results of a directly observed intermittent isoniazid preventive therapy program in a shelter for homeless men, *Am Rev Respir Dis* 146:57-60, 1992.
304. Passanante MR, Restifo RA, Reichman LB: Preventive therapy for the patient with both universal indication and contraindication for isoniazid, *Chest* 103:825-831, 1993.

Therapy

305. American Academy of Pediatrics, Committee on Infectious Diseases: Policy statement: chemotherapy for tuberculosis in infants and children, *Pediatrics* 89:161-165, 1992.
306. American Academy of Pediatrics: Tuberculosis. In Peter G, ed: *1997 red book: report of the Committee on Infectious Diseases,* ed 24, Elk Grove Village, Ill, 1997, The Academy, pp 551-555.
307. Bass JB Jr, Farer LS, Hopewell PC, O'Brien R, Jacobs RF, Ruben F, Snide DE Jr, Thornton G: Treatment of tuberculosis and tuberculosis infection in adults and children, *Am J Respir Crit Care Med* 149:1359-1374, 1994.
308. Bayer R, Wilkinson D: Directly observed therapy for tuberculosis: history of an idea, *Lancet* 345:1545-1548, 1995.
309. Centers for Disease Control and Prevention: Clinical update: impact of HIV protease inhibitors on the treatment of HIV-infected tuberculosis patients with rifampin, *MMWR* 45:921-926, 1996.
310. Centers for Disease Control and Prevention: The use of preventive therapy for tuberculous infection in the United States: recommendations of the Advisory Committee for Elimination of Tuberculosis, *MMWR* 39(no.RR-8):9-12, 1990.
311. China Tuberculosis Control Collaboration: Results of directly observed short-course chemotherapy in 112,842 Chinese patients with smear-positive tuberculosis, *Lancet* 347:358-362, 1996.
312. Cohn DL, Catlin BJ, Peterson KL, Judson FN, Sbarbaro JA: A 62-dose, 6-month therapy for pulmonary and extrapulmonary tuberculosis, *Ann Intern Med* 112:407-415, 1990.
313. Combs DL, Geiter LJ, O'Brien RJ: The USPHS tuberculosis short-course chemotherapy trial 21: effectiveness, toxicity and acceptability: the report of final results, *Ann Intern Med* 112:397-406, 1990.
314. East African/British Medical Research Council Co-operative Investigation: Controlled clinical trial of short course (6-month) regimens of chemotherapy for treatment of pulmonary tuberculosis. Second report, *Lancet* 1:133-139, 1973.
315. Fischl MA, Daikos GL, Uttamchandani RB, Poblete RB, Moreno JN, Reyes RR, Boota AM, Thompson LM, Cleary TJ, Oldham SA: Clinical presentation and outcome of patients with HIV infection and tuberculosis caused by multiple-drug-resistant bacilli, *Ann Intern Med* 117:184-190, 1992.
316. Fox W: Philip Ellman lecture. The modern management and therapy of pulmonary tuberculosis, *Proc R Soc Med* 70:4-15, 1977.
317. Fox W: The chemotherapy of pulmonary tuberculosis: a review, *Chest* 76:785-796, 1979.
318. Fox W: Compliance of patients and physicians: experience and lessons from tuberculosis, *BMJ* 287:33-35, 101-105, 1983.
319. Frieden TR, Sterling T, Pablos-Mendez A, Kilburn JO, Cauthen GM, Dooley SW: The emergence of drug-resistant tuberculosis in New York City, *N Engl J Med* 328(8):521-526, 1993.
320. Goble M, Iseman MD, Madsen LA, Waite D, Ackerson L, Horsburgh CR Jr: Treatment of 171 patients with pulmonary tuberculosis resistant to isoniazid and rifampin, *N Engl J Med* 328(8):527-532, 1993.
321. Hong Kong Chest Service/British Medical Research Council: Controlled trial of 4 three-times-weekly regimens and a daily regimen given for 6 months for pulmonary TB. Second report: the results of final results up to 24 months, *Tubercle* 63:89, 1982.
322. Iseman MD, Cohn DL, Sbarbaro JA: Directly observed treatment of tuberculosis—we can't afford not to try it, *N Engl J Med* 328:576, 1993.
323. Kendig EL Jr: Evolution of short-course antimicrobial treatment of tuberculosis in children, 1951-1984, *Pediatrics* 75:684-686, 1985.
324. Mahmoudi A, Iseman MD: Pitfalls in the care of patients with tuberculosis: common errors and their association with the acquisition of drug resistance, *JAMA* 270(1)65-68, 1993.
325. McDonald RJ, Memon AM, Reichman LB: Successful supervised ambulatory management of tuberculosis treatment failures, *Ann Intern Med* 96:297-303, 1982.
326. Mitchison DA: Basic mechanisms of chemotherapy, *Chest* 76:771-781, 1979.
327. Mitchison DA: Drug resistance in mycobacteria, *Br Med Bull* 40:84-90, 1984.
328. Mitchison DA: The Garrod lecture. Understanding the chemotherapy of tuberculosis—current problems, *J Antimicrob Chemother* 29:477-493, 1992.
329. Nolan CM, Williams DL, Cave MD, Eisenach KD, el-Hajj H, Hooton TM, Thompson RL, Goldberg SV: Evolution of rifampin resistance in human immunodeficiency virus–associated tuberculosis, *Am J Respir Crit Care Med* 152:1067-1071, 1995.
330. Schluger NW, Lawrence RM, McGuiness G, Park M, Rom WN: Multidrug-resistant tuberculosis in children: two cases and a review of the literature, *Pediatr Pulmonol* 21:138-142, 1996.
331. Seifart HI, Parkin DP, Donald PR: Stability of isoniazid, rifampin and pyrazinamide in suspensions used for the treatment of tuberculosis in children, *Pediatr Infect Dis J* 10:827-831, 1991.
332. Small PM, Schecter GF, Goodman PC, Sande MA, Chaisson RE, Hopewell PC: Treatment of tuberculosis in patients with advanced human immunodeficiency virus infection, *N Engl J Med* 324:289-294, 1991.
333. Smith MHS: What about short course and intermittent chemotherapy for tuberculosis in children? *Pediatr Infect Dis J* 1:298-303, 1982.
334. Snider DE, Caras GJ: Isoniazid-associated hepatitis deaths: a review of available information, *Am Rev Respir Dis* 145:494-497, 1992.
335. Snider DE: Pregnancy and tuberculosis, *Chest* 86S:10S-13S, 1984.
336. Starke JR, Correa AG: Management of mycobacterial infection and disease in children, *Pediatr Infect Dis J* 14:455-470, 1995.
337. Steiner P, Rao M, Mitchell M, Steiner M: Primary drug-resistant tuberculosis in children. Emergence of primary drug-resistant strains of *M. tuberculosis* to rifampin, *Am Rev Respir Dis* 134:446-448, 1986.
338. Trébucq A: Should ethambutol be recommended for routine treatment of tuberculosis in children? A review of the literature, *Int J Tuberc Lung Dis* 1:12-15, 1997.
339. Volmink J, Garner P: Systematic review of randomised controlled trials of strategies to promote adherence to tuberculosis treatment, *BMJ* 315:1403-1406, 1997.

340. Weis SE, Slocum PC, Blais FX, King B, Nunn M, Matney GB, Gomez E, Foresman BH: The effect of directly observed therapy on the rates of drug resistance and relapse in tuberculosis, *N Engl J Med* 330:1179-1184, 1994.
341. Young DB, Duncan K: Prospects for new interventions in the treatment and prevention of mycobacterial disease, *Annu Rev Microbiol* 49:641-673, 1995.

Drugs

342. Alzeer AH, Fitzgerald JM: Corticosteroids and tuberculosis: risks and use as adjunct therapy, *Tuber Lung Dis* 74:6-11, 1993.
343. du Plessis A, Hussey G: Laryngeal tuberculosis in childhood, *Pediatr Infect Dis J* 6:678-681, 1987.
344. Gerbeaux J, Baculard A, Couvreur J: Primary tuberculosis in childhood. Indications and contraindications for corticosteroid therapy, *Am J Dis Child* 110:507-518, 1965.
345. Kitai IC, Sanders DM, Manungo J: Tuberculosis presenting as corticosteroid responsive wheezing in infancy, *Trop Geogr Med* 41:274-276, 1989.
346. Nemir RL, Cardona J, Vaziri F, Toledo R: Prednisone as an adjunct in the chemotherapy of lymph node–bronchial tuberculosis in childhood: a double-blind study. II. Further term observation, *Am Rev Respir Dis* 95:402-410, 1967.
347. Toppet M, Malfroot A, Derde MP, Toppet V, Spehl M, Dab I: Corticosteroids in primary tuberculosis with bronchial obstruction, *Arch Dis Child* 65:1222-1226, 1990.
348. Feltis JM Jr, Campbell D: Changing role of surgery in the treatment of pulmonary tuberculosis in children, *Chest* 61:101-103, 1972.
349. Hewitson JP, Von Oppell UO: Role of thoracic surgery for childhood tuberculosis, *World J Surg* 21:468-474, 1997.
350. Nakvi AJ, Nohl-Oser HC: Surgical treatment of bronchial obstruction in primary tuberculosis in children: report of seven cases, *Thorax* 34:464-469, 1979.
351. Worthington MG, Brink JG, Odell JA, Buckels J, de Groot MK, Klein M, Gunning AJ: Surgical relief of acute airway obstruction due to primary tuberculosis, *Ann Thorac Surg* 56:1054-1062, 1993.
352. Bahr GM, Shaaban MA, Gabriel M, al-Shimali B, Siddiqui Z, Chugh TD, Denath FM, Shahin A, Behbehani K, Chedid L, Rook GAW, Stanford JL: Improved immunotherapy for pulmonary tuberculosis with *Mycobacterium vaccae*, *Tubercle* 71:259-266, 1990.
353. Corlan E, Marica C, Macavei C, Stanford JL, Stanford CA: Immunotherapy with *Mycobacterium vaccae* in the treatment of tuberculosis in Romania. II. Chronic or relapsed disease, *Respir Med* 91:21-29, 1997.
354. Grange JM: Immunotherapy of tuberculosis, *Tubercle* 71:237-239, 1990.
355. Marsh BJ, Fordham von Reyn C, Arbeit RD, Morin P: Immunization of HIV-infected adults with a three-dose series of inactivated *Mycobacterium vaccae, Am J Med Sci* 313:377-383, 1997.
356. Onyebujoh PC, Abdulmumini T, Robinson S, Rook GA, Stanford JL: Immunotherapy with *Mycobacterium vaccae* as an addition to chemotherapy for the treatment of pulmonary tuberculosis under difficult conditions in Africa, *Respir Med* 89:199-207, 1995.
357. Prior JG, Khan AA, Cartwright KA, Jenkins PA, Stanford JL: Immunotherapy with *Mycobacterium vaccae* combined with second line chemotherapy in drug-resistant abdominal tuberculosis, *J Infect* 31:59-61, 1995.
358. Stanford JL: Immunotherapy for mycobacterial disease. In Ratledge C, Stanford J, Grange JM, eds: *The biology of the mycobacteria,* vol 3, *Clinical aspects of mycobacterial disease,* London, 1989, Academic Press, pp 568-593.
359. Stanford JL, Stanford CA: Immunotherapy of tuberculosis with *Mycobacterium vaccae* NCTC 11659, *Immunobiology* 191:555-563, 1994.
360. Stanford JL, Stanford CA: Immunotherapy with *Mycobacterium vaccae* in the treatment of tuberculosis in Romania. II. Chronic or relapsed disease, *Respir Med* 91:21-29, 1997.
361. Desai CR, Heera S, Patel A, Babrekar AB, Mahashur AA, Kamat SR: Role of metronidazole in improving response and specific drug sensitivity in advanced pulmonary tuberculosis, *J Assoc Physicians India* 37: 694-697, 1989.
362. Wayne LG, Sramek HA: Metronidazole is bactericidal to dormant cells of *Mycobacterium tuberculosis, Antimicrob Agents Chemother* 38:2054-2058, 1994.

Mycobacteria Other than Tuberculosis

363. American Thoracic Society: Diagnosis and treatment of disease caused by nontuberculous mycobacteria, *Am Rev Respir Dis* 142:940-953, 1990.
364. Lincoln EM, Gilbert LA: Disease in children due to mycobacteria other than *Mycobacterium tuberculosis, Am Rev Respir Dis* 105:683-714, 1972.
365. Margileth AM: Management of nontuberculous (atypical) mycobacterial infections in children and adolescents, *Pediatr Infect Dis* 4:119-121, 1985.
366. O'Brien RJ: The epidemiology of nontuberculous mycobacterial disease, *Clin Chest Med* 10:407-418, 1989.
367. Pang SC: Mycobacterial lymphadenitis in Western Australia, *Tuber Lung Dis* 73:362-367, 1992.
368. Pitchenik AE, Fertel D: Tuberculosis and nontuberculous mycobacterial disease, *Med Clin North Am* 76(1):121-171, 1992.
369. Proust AJ, Wiles H: Pulmonary disease in a child caused by atypical mycobacteria, *Med J Aust* 141:242-243, 1984.
370. Schaad UB, Votteler TP, McCracken GH, Nelson JD: Management of atypical mycobacterial lymphadenitis in childhood: review based on 380 cases, *J Pediatr* 95:356-360, 1979.
371. Wolinsky E: Mycobacterial diseases other than tuberculosis, *Clin Infect Dis* 15:1-10, 1992.

Nontuberculous Mycobacterial Infections

Michael D. Iseman

"Nontuberculous" mycobacteria (NTM) include species of the genus *Mycobacterium* that are associated with human infection and disease (excluding *M. tuberculosis, M. bovis,* and *M. leprae*). Semantically, this terminology may not be wholly accurate because these mycobacteria do produce "tuberculosis" (TB) lesions. However, the usage NTM has gained preference over other references such as mycobacteria other than tuberculosis (MOTT), "atypical," or "environmental" mycobacteria.

The NTM are variably but widely distributed in nature. Considerable evidence suggests that potable or environmental water may be contaminated with and the source of many NTM infections.[1] The rapid-growing mycobacteria (in group IV, discussed later) are quite resistant to sterilization procedures, and they have been commonly reported to cause nosocomial infections as a result of contamination of fluids or devices in hospitals. The presence of NTMs in nonsterile spaces or tissues of the human body, including the lungs, may represent a colonizing or saprophytic status; this is in contrast to TB, in which recovery of the organism is tantamount to diagnosis. Hence disease refers to cases in which there are not only significant numbers of mycobacteria in the tissues, but the tissues are sufficiently inflamed or damaged to be characterized as disease.[2,3]

PATHOGENIC SPECIES OF NTM

The mycobacteria have been grouped historically by the Runyon classification, which organizes the species according to basic biologic or laboratory traits. The groupings do not necessarily indicate commonality for epidemiologic, pathogenic, or therapeutic purposes.

Group I

Photochromogenic mycobacteria, when grown in the dark, have cream- or buff-colored colonial pigment; however, after exposure to light they rapidly become yellow or orange—the property of photochromogenicity. *M. kansasii* is the most common pathogen in this group and is most commonly distributed in the central and south central United States. *M. simiae* is reported in small but apparently increasing numbers, particularly in the south and southwest United States. *M. marinum* is common in coastal waters or may be involved with fish-tank cutaneous infections. Pulmonary disease has not been reported.

Group II

Scotochromogenic mycobacteria, whether grown in the light or dark, produce yellow or orange pigmented colonies. *M. scrofulaceum* is the prototype of this group and formerly was a common cause of lymphadenitis in children and pulmonary disease in adults. However, for reasons unclear, it has receded as a human pathogen in the United States and now is only reported episodically. *M. gordonae* is a common contaminant of laboratory specimens. However, there have been occasional reports of pulmonary disease associated with this microbe. *M. szulgai* is an uncommon pathogen in this group. Overall, these scotochromogenic bacteria are the least common human pathogens.

Group III

Nonchromogenic mycobacteria are the most significant cluster of NTM producing human disease. Two closely related species, *M. avium* and *M. intracellulare,* have been grouped taxonomically as *M. avium* complex (MAC). These organisms historically were associated with disease mainly in the southeastern United States. However, over the past quarter century MAC cases have been seen in apparently increasing numbers from all of the continental states, Alaska, and Hawaii. Less frequent pathogens of this group include *M. xenopi* and *M. malmoense.*

Group IV

Rapid-growing mycobacteria (RGM) are emerging as a relatively more common form of NTM disease following MAC and *M. kansasii* in prevalence.[1,4] *M. abscessus,* formerly designated as a subspecies of *M. chelonae,* is now the commonest cause of pulmonary disease among the RGM. Other RGMs such as *M. chelonae* and *M. fortuitum* may produce pulmonary infections, but significantly less often than *M. abscessus.* RGM pulmonary disease is associated with achalasia or esophageal dysmotility in some cases.

FORMS OF PULMONARY DISEASE

The NTM can involve human lung tissue in either a primary invasive capacity or as a secondary invader of previously damaged or abnormal lung parenchyma. These cases may present as air-space filling processes or "pneumonia," as obstructing endobronchial lesions, or as a compressive peribronchial lymphadenitis. Intrathoracic lymphadentitis without airway involvement also has been described. Compared with adults, infants and children are far more likely to manifest disease associated with exuberant lymphadenitis and less likely to experience focal, destructive parenchymal disease. This is closely analogous to the situation with *M. tuberculosis.* Pleural disease in children caused by the NTM, as with adults, is quite uncommon.

In some cases, the NTM secondarily invade regions of bronchiectasis caused by other disorders. NTM may also be the primary cause of bronchiectasis.

The tissue response typically has granulomatous features. To various degrees noncaseating granulomas, necrotizing granulomas, or, less commonly, caseation necrosis may be present. The rapid growing mycobacteria may elicit a dimorphic response with both granulomatous and pyogenic features.

HOST RISK FACTORS ASSOCIATED WITH PEDIATRIC NTM LUNG DISEASE

As with adult NTM disease most pediatric pulmonary cases occur in children who have some underlying disorder that makes them more susceptible. These conditions may be regarded generally as a pulmonary structural abnormality, an immunologic disorder, or a combination of both.

Normal Hosts

In some cases, no discernible underlying abnormalities may be found. Many of these cases appear to be primarily forms of lymphadenitis.[5-9] These patients probably had a very large inoculum that produced hypertrophic lymphadenopathy. Alternatively, these individuals may be genetically disposed to an exaggerated lymphadenitis.

Underlying Lung Disorders

Given the wide distribution of NTM in the environment,[1] exposure must be nearly universal. Thus persons with conditions that result in impaired, nonimmunologic defenses seem predisposed to colonization and, in some cases, invasion by the NTM. Among the conditions reported in association with pulmonary NTM disease are cystic fibrosis,[10-13] tracheobronchomegaly,[14-16] recurrent aspiration,[17] lipoid pneumonia,[18] and ciliary dyskinesia.[19] Early necrotizing lung infections may also result in bronchiectasis and NTM infections.[20]

Immune Deficiency States

Inherited disorders such as common-variable immunodeficiency (CVID),[20] selective IgA deficiency,[21] IgG subclass deficiency,[22] intestinal lymphangiectasia, and deficient receptors for interferon-gamma[23,24] or interleukin-12[25,26] have been noted in association with NTM lung disease. In the immunoglobulin deficiencies it is presumed that recurrent pyogenic infections result in bronchciectasis and heightened vulnerability to the NTM.

Patients with impaired cellular immunity caused by inherited disorders commonly present with bizarre, multifocal or disseminated NTM disease as well as diffuse or miliary lung involvement.[27]

Other conditions associated with impaired cellular immunity and NTM risk include acquired disturbances such as HIV infection or AIDS,[2] cancer with or without chemotherapy,[28] and organ transplantation.[29] AIDS is most commonly seen in association with disseminated NTM infection, particularly with MAC. Pulmonary disease may be seen independently or in association with disseminated infection.

DIAGNOSIS

Diagnosis is often problematic because of the wide distribution of the NTM in the environment.[2-4] Thus, establishing a specific pulmonary diagnosis typically entails these elements: (1) characteristic signs and/or symptoms; (2) representative radiographic abnormalities; (3) isolation, preferably repeatedly, of the mycobacteria from secretions or tissues; (4) granulomatous features on histopathology, if tissue is available; (5) absence of evidence for other potential pathogens; and (6) inferential evidence including plausible histories of exposure, skin test reactivity, and occasionally responses to therapeutic trials. In some cases, one might reasonably conclude that an intrathoracic process, lymphatic or parenchymal, was the result of an NTM if biopsy of a lymph node in the cervical region demonstrated the mycobacteria.

Cystic fibrosis (CF) patients constitute a particularly vexing set of cases in which to diagnose NTM lung disease. In large measure, this reflects the fact that CF itself causes many symptoms, signs, and radiographic abnormalities, which are also seen with NTM lung diseases. Because CF patients have retained secretions, they appear prone to become colonized with environmental microbes including the NTM. Surveys in CF clinics suggest that patients with NTM in their respiratory secretions tend to be older[10-14]; however, this range includes individuals in the pediatric age group. Rapid progression of symptoms and radiographic deterioration coupled with large numbers of mycobacteria in sputum strongly suggest disease.

Skin testing for NTM infection is difficult to interpret because of the lack of sensitivity and specificity of available antigens. The only currently available agent now is tuberculin. This is an antigen prepared from *M. tuberculosis.* It is available in the United States for the Mantoux intradermal technique in the form of PPD-T Tubersol and Aplisol. Multipuncture devices or tine tests employ a less refined extract, old tuberculin, and are available as Mono-Vacc or Tuberculin Old Time Test. The Mantoux technique is most advantageous when attempting to discriminate between TB and NTM infection because of more quantitative readings. However, even this may be confounded by antigenic cross-reactivity. It has been said that NTM infections tend to produce intermediate reactions, 3 to 9 mm of induration. A recent report on reactivity to PPD-T (or the earlier product, PPD-S) among children with NTM cervical lymphadenitis indicates the limitations of this logic: among the 91 patients, 35% had reactions of 10 mm or more.[30]

Clinicians formerly used two antigens for comparative skin testing, typically PPD-T and PPD-B, the so-called Battey antigen prepared from *M. avium* complex.[9] Most patients with NTM disease reportedly had greater induration to PPD-B. But this antigen and other NTM sensitins were withdrawn from the market in the 1970s because of lack of standardized human testing. However, a new *M. avium* sensitin is being tested and appears promising in terms of its potential to discriminate NTM from TB.[31]

TB or not TB?

For many youngsters with pulmonary manifestations just described, the differential diagnosis initially involves signs and symptoms, radiography, microscopy, histopathology, and skin testing reactivity. Even with this evaluation, clinicians rarely can provide early assurance that a case does not represent TB. Therefore, one may need to initiate treatment on the presumption of TB.[32] This is particularly true in the cases of infants or young children in whom TB may rapidly progress to life threatening or disabling forms of TB, including miliary, meningeal, or spinal disease. For seriously ill patients, empirical therapy with a regimen adequate to cover both TB and most NTM infections may be indicated.

PRINCIPLES OF CHEMOTHERAPY

In vitro susceptibility testing is an integral part in selecting drug agents for NTM infections. Although the relationship between in vitro susceptibility and response to therapy is not as straightforward as it is in TB, the limited evidence available indicates that careful, quantitative in vitro susceptibility testing is an appropriate guideline in choosing drugs.[3]

The basic pharmacologic principles of antimicrobial therapy intuitively should be applicable in NTM disease.[3] At the simplest level, this means that the maximum achievable serum level of any drug should substantially exceed the minimum inhibitory concentration established in vitro. This relationship does not necessarily mean that the drug will be effective, but the converse—failure to achieve inhibition or killing at achievable serum concentrations—is quite likely to predict lack of efficacy. In addition, dosing intervals should be established in relationship to growth rates of bacilli. Thus schedules less frequent than commonly employed for conventional pathogenic bacteria appear to be appropriate.

Combination therapy to prevent acquired drug resistance is an essential component of the treatment of TB and should almost certainly be applied to the NTM as well. Single drugs, no matter how efficacious, are subject to selection of drug-resistant variants, leading to clinical resistance to the individual agent. The principle that drug A kills bacilli resistant to drug B and drug B kills bacilli resistant to drug A mandates that in virtually all cases, multiple drugs be used for active disease.

Similar to TB, treatment must generally be extended well beyond the time of initial bacteriologic and clinical improvement. This is necessary to prevent recurrence by eliminating persistent, slow-growing, or semidormant bacilli that may reactivate if chemotherapy is prematurely terminated.

RECOMMENDED MANAGEMENT

Recommended drugs and drug regimens for the common NTM diseases are outlined in Tables 43-9 and 43-10. It should be emphasized that these represent generally uncontrolled experience with use of individual agents or regimens.[3,33] In many cases, treating individuals with deep invasive disease entails aggressive long-term management and probably should be conducted by specialists.

Issues specific to psychiatric patients apply to some of the medications used against NTM infections in adults. Ethambutol has been problematic because of difficulty monitoring vision in infants and children; however, two recent publications indicate that optic neuritis has not been described in these younger patients.[32,34] Based on animal studies, concern has been expressed about the potential for fluoroquinolones to interfere with cartilage growth and development. And tetracyclines, including doxycyclines and minocycline, may cause discolored teeth. Hence the decisions to treat and the choices of agents must be considered with special concern.

Among pediatric cases, the role of chemotherapy is less well defined than for adult patients. As noted above, a substantial portion of pulmonary disease reflects the effects of exuberant lymphadenitis rather than primary parenchymal destruction. In these lymphadenitis cases, the mycobacterial

Table 43-9 Suggested Medical Regimens for Common NTM Pulmonary Disease

	REGIMEN	ADDITIONAL OR ALTERNATIVE AGENTS	COMMENTS
GROUP I			
M. kansasii	RIF, EMB, IHN, [AK or SM]	CLARI, CIP, TM/S	Usual duration: 12 to 18 months. AK may be used initially for 2-4 months for more extensive disease.
GROUP II			
M. scrofulaceum	CLARI, EMB, AK±CFZ	AZI, RIF, CIP	Usual duration: up to 24 months. RIF lowers bioavailability of CLARI.
GROUP III			
M. avium complex (MAC)	CLARI, EMB AK, ±CFZ	AZI, RIF, CIP	Usual duration: up to 24 months. RIF lowers bioavailability of CLARI.
GROUP IV			
M. abscessus	CEFOX, AK	CLARI, MINO or DOXY, CIP	Usual duration: 6 to 12 weeks for palliation course. Most strains are resistant to oral meds; Rx is rarely curative.
M. chelonae	CLARI, AK, [CEFOX]*	TOB, IMI, DOXY, CIP	Usual duration: 6 to 12 weeks for palliation.
M. fortuitum	CLARI, DOXI, CIP	SMX, IMI, AK	Usual duration: 4 to 6 months, attempting cure.

*Some regard resistance to CEF as a distinguishing feature of *M. chelonae,* but at National Jewish, the great majority of strains we identified as *M. chelonae* are susceptible.

Table 43-10 Information on NTM Medications for Pediatric Usage

DRUG	ORAL	IV	ORAL DOSES SUPPLIED	USUAL DOSES SCHEDULE(S)
Clarithromycin (Biaxin) (CLARI)	Y	N	250, 500, 750 mg	7.5 mg/kg, BID.
Azithromycin (Zithromax) (AZI)	Y	Y	250 gm, 600 mg tabs 100 and 200 mg/5 ml susp	10 mg/kg for day 1, then 5 mg/kg/d or 3x wk for mycobacterial disease; max = 500 mg.
Rifampin (Rifadin) (RIF)	Y	Y	150, 300 mg	10-20 mg/kg/d po, single doses; max = 600 mg.
Ethambutol (Myambutol) (EMB)	Y	N/A	100, 400 mg	5 mg/kg/d po single dose; may use 25 mg/kg/d for 2 mos for serious infection. Safety: see text.
Ciprofloxacin (Cipro) (CIP)	Y	Y	250, 500, 750 mg	250 to 750 mg 2x daily. (Caution for use in growing children; see Mosby's GenRx.)
Isoniazid (IHH)	Y	Y	100, 300 mg	10-20 mg/kg po, single dose; max = 300 mg. Liquid suspension poorly tolerated.
Trimethoprim/Sulfamethoxasole (Bactrim) (TMP/SMX)	Y	Y	TMP 40 mg/5 ml, SMX 200 mg/5 ml; 80 mg TMP/400 mg SMX; 160 mg TMP/800 mg SMX	7.5-8.0 mg/kg TM in 2 doses (Q12 hr); max = 960 mg TM.
Sulfamethoxasole (SMX)	Y	N	500 mg	50-60 mg/kg dose 1, followed by 25-30 mg/kg BID or 1-2 g/m^2 dose 1, followed by 0.6 g/m^2 BID; max = 75 mg/kg/day.
Doxycyline (Vibramycin) (DOXY)	Y	Y	100 mg	2-4 mg/kg po in 2 doses; max 200 mg. (Caution: dental issues; see Mosby's GenRx.)
Minocycline (Minocin) (MINO)	Y	Y	50, 100 mg, 50 mg/5 ml susp, 100 mg IV	For child >8 yr, 4 mg/kg dose 1, followed by 2 mg/kg Q12 hr. (Caution: dental issues; see Mosby's GenRx.)
Clofazimine (Lamprene) (CFZ)	Y	N	50 mg	50-100 mg/d; max = 100 mg. Note: transient skin pigmentation.
Amikacin (Amikin) (AK)	N	Y	—	15 mg/kg IV (or IM) daily; less frequently in continuation phase. Note: hearing, balance, renal toxicities.
Streptomycin (SM)	N	Y	—	15 mg/kg IV (or IM) daily; less frequently in continuation phase. Note: hearing, balance, renal toxicities.
Tobramycin (Nebcin) (TOB)	N	Y	—	3 mg/kg/day in 3-4 equally divided doses. Adjust according to concs. Note: hearing, balance, renal toxicities.
Cefoxitin (Mefoxin) (CEFOX)	N	Y	—	100-200 mg/kg IV q8h; max = 12 g/day. Note: *C. difficile* colitis risk.
Imipenem (Primaxin) (IMI)	N	Y	—	80-160 mg/kg/d in 3-5 equally divided doses; max = 12 g/day.

burden is relatively small, the host is generating an apparently active immune response, and the literature showing the necessity and utility of drug therapy is marginal.[5,6] In fact, in most reported pediatric lymphadenitis cases, rather minimal drug therapy is given for relatively short periods, about 3 to 12 months.[5,6]

ADJUNCT TREATMENT

Surgical treatment for NTM disease may be useful, including resection of localized and refractory pulmonary disease associated with irreversible damage to the airways or lung parenchyma. Endobronchial disease in adults has been approached by sharp dissection or laser surgery to relieve obstruction; however, pediatric experience with these modalities is minimal and therefore problematic.

Immunologic interventions may be appropriate in selected instances. In some cases where NTM disease has evolved as a result of immunosuppressive therapy given for other disorders, it is desirable to stop or minimize the predisposing immunosuppressive treatments. Despite aggressive drug therapy, cures are seldom achieved if the hosts' immune systems are substantially inhibited. Alternatively, positive immunotherapy can be considered using selective agents to enhance the host's immune response, particularly in cases with either an underlying or an acquired defect of cellular immune capacity. Recent studies have documented the efficacy of IFN-γ in selected patients with disseminated NTM disease, many of whom had non–HIV-related abnormalities of T cell and/or macrophage function.

Corticosteroids may be given in cases in which hypertrophic lympadenitis is obstructing or compressing airways. Glucocorticoids have been shown to reduce inflammation and swelling in meningeal tuberculosis,[34] and clinicians have reasoned that shrinking these inflamed nodes may provide for the long-term relief from obstruction. Although anecdotal experience suggests the efficacy of this approach, no systematic observations have confirmed or quantitated the benefit.[35] In any case, this may be a logical intervention if antimicrobial coverage is provided and the duration of steroids is not protracted.

REFERENCES

1. Falkinham JO: Epidemiology of infection by nontuberculous mycobacteria, *Clin Microbiol Rev J* 9(2):177-215, 1996.
2. Wallace RJ Jr., Brown BA, Griffith DE, et al: Diagnosis and treatment of disease caused by nontuberculous mycobacteria, *Am J Respir Crit Care Med* 156:Sl-S25, 1997.
3. Iseman M: Nontuberculous mycobacterial infections. In Gorbach S, Bartlett J, Blacklow N, eds: *Infectious diseases,* ed 2, Philadelphia, 1992, WB Saunders, pp 1246-1256.

Pathogenic Species of NTM

4. Griffith D, Girard W, Wallace R Jr: Clinical features of pulmonary disease caused by rapidly growing mycobacteria. An analysis of 154 patients, *Am Rev Respir Dis* 147:1271-1278, 1993.

Host Risk Factors Associated with Pediatric NTM Lung Disease

5. Margileth AM: Management of nontuberculosis (atypical) mycobacterial infections in children and adolescents, *Pediatr Infect Dis* 4(2):119-121, 1985.
6. Powell DA, Walker DA: Nontuberculosis mycobacterial endobronchitis in children, *J Pediatr* 96:268-270, 1980.
7. Lincoln EM, Gilbert LA: Disease in children due to mycobacteria other than *M. tuberculosis, Am Rev Respir Dis* 105:683-713, 1972.
8. Fergie JE, Milligan T, Henderson BM, Stafford WW: Intrathoracic *M. avium* complex infection in immunocompetent children: case report and review, *Clin Infect Dis* 24:250-253, 1997.
9. Hsu K: Atypical mycobacterial infections in children, *Rev Infect Dis* 3(5):1075-1080, 1981.
10. Smith MJ, Efthimiou J, Hodson M, Batten JC: Mycobacterial isolations in young adults with cystic fibrosis, *Thorax* 39:369-375, 1984.
11. Hjelte L, Petrini B, Kallenius G, Strandvick B: Prospective study of mycobacterial infections in patients with cystic fibrosis, *Thorax* 45:397-400, 1990.
12. Kilby JM, Gilligan PH, Yankaskas JR, et al: Nontuberculosis mycobacteria in adult patients with cystic fibrosis, *Chest* 102:70-75, 1992.
13. Aitken ML, Burke WB, McDonald G, et al: Nontuberculosis mycobacterial disease in adult cystic fibrosis patients, *Chest* 103:1096-1099, 1993.
14. Shin MS, Jackson RM, Ho KJ: Tracheobronchomegaly (Mounier-Kuhn syndrome): CT diagnosis, *Am J Roentgenol* 150(4):777-779, 1988.
15. Woodring JE, Howard II RS, Rehm SR: Congenital tracheobronchomegaly (Mounier-Kuhn syndrome): a report of 10 cases and review of the literature, *J Thorac Imag* 6(2):1-10, 1991.
16. Schwartz M, Rossoff L: Tracheobronchomegaly, *Chest* 106:1589-1590, 1994.
17. Bagarazzi ML, Watson B, Kim IK, et al: Pulmonary *M. gordonae* infection in a two-year-old child: case report, *Clin Infect Dis* 22:1124-1125, 1996.
18. Cox EG, Heil SA, Kleiman MB: Lipoid pneumonia and *M. smegmatihs, Pediatr Infect Dis J* 13(5):414-415, 1994.
19. Charlotte F, Rayner J, Rutman A, Dewar A et al: Ciliary disorientation in patients with chronic upper respiratory tract inflammation, *Am J Respir Crit Care Med* 151:800-804, 1995.
20. Barker AF, Bardana EJ: Bronchiectasis: update of an orphan disease, *Am Rev Respir Dis* 137:969-978, 1988.
21. Chipps BE, Talamo RC, Winkelstein JA: IgA deficiency, recurrent pneumonias, and bronchiectasis, *Chest* 73:519-526, 1978.
22. De Gracia PD, Rodrigo MJ, Morell F et al: IgG subclass deficiencies associated with bronchiectasis, *Am J Respir Crit Care Med* 153:650-655, 1996.
23. Jouanguy E, Altare F, Lamhamedi S, et al: Interferon-γ-receptor deficiency in an infant with fatal bacille Calmette-Guerin infection, *N Engl J Med* 335:1956-1961, 1996.
24. Pierre-Audigier C, Jouanguy E, Lamhamedi S et al: Fatal dissemination *M. smegmatis* infection in a child with inherited interferon-γ receptor deficiency, *Clin Infect Dis* 24:982-984, 1997.
25. Levin M, Newport MJ, D'Souza S et al: Familial disseminated (atypical) mycobacterial infection in childhood: a human mycobacterial susceptibility gene? *Lancet* 345:79-83, 1995.
26. De Jong R, Altare F, Haagen IA et al: Severe mycobacterial and salmonella infections in interleukin-12 receptor-deficient patients, *Science* 280:1435-1438, 1998.
27. Holland S, Eisenstein E, Kuhns D, et al: Treatment of refractory disseminated nontuberculous mycobacterial infection with interferon gamma, *N Engl J Med* 330:1348-1355, 1994.
28. Stone AB, Schelonka RL, Drehner DM: Disseminated *M. avium* complex in non-human immunodeficiency virus infected pediatric patients, *Pediatr Infect Dis J* 11:960-964, 1992.
29. Patel R, Roberts GD, Keating MR, et al: Infections due to nontuberculosis mycobacteria in kidney, heart, and liver transplant recipients, *Clin Infect Dis* 19:263-73, 1994.

Diagnosis

30. Wolinsky E: Mycobacterial lymphadenitis in children: a prospective study of 105 nontuberculosis cases with long-term follow-up, *Clin Infect Dis* 20:954-963, 1995.
31. Pinto-Powell R, Olivier KN, Marsh B, Donaldson S et al: Skin testing with *M. avium* sensitin to identify infection with *M. avium* complex in patients with cyctic fibrosis, *Clin Infect Dis* 22:560-562, 1996.
32. Starke JR: Nontuberculosis mycobacterial infections in children, *Adv Pediatr Infect Dis* 7:123-159, 1992.

Recommended Management

33. Wallace RJ Jr: Treatment of infections caused by rapidly growing mycobacteria in the era of newer macrolides, *Res Microbiol* 147:30-35, 1996.

Adjunct Treatment

34. Trebucq A: Should ethambutol be recommended for routine treatment of tuberculosis in children? A review of the literature, *Int J Tuberc Lung Dis* 1(1):12-15, 1997.
35. Alzeer AH, Fitzgerald JM: Corticosteriods and tuberculosis: risk and use of adjunctive therapy, *Tubercle Lung Dis* 74:6-11, 1993.

CHAPTER 44

Mycoplasma Infections

Ziad M. Shehab

Numerous species of mycoplasmas colonize man and animals. The main species associated with disease in man are *Mycoplasma pneumoniae*, which is most commonly involved in respiratory infections in humans, and the genital mycoplasmas, which include *Mycoplasma hominis* and *Ureaplasma urealyticum*.[1]

In 1944, Eaton et al[2] isolated a filtrable organism from patients ill with primary atypical pneumonia. This group of nonclassic bacterial pneumonias was rarely fatal and did not respond to antibiotics.[3] In 1961, Eaton's agent was recognized to have morphologic similarities to pleuropneumonia–like organisms isolated from a variety of animal species. In 1963, it was cultivated on cell-free agar medium, placed in the genus *Mycoplasma,* and given the name *M. pneumoniae* to underscore its relationship to pneumonias.[4]

Mycoplasmas are the smallest organisms that are able to live outside the host cell. Because they have no cell wall, they are pleomorphic, do not stain well with the usual bacteriologic stains, and are not killed by cell wall–active agents such as penicillins and cephalosporins. Like bacteria, they multiply by binary fission.[5]

M. PNEUMONIAE INFECTIONS

Epidemiology

Understanding of the epidemiology of mycoplasmal infections results from population studies undertaken in the 1960s and 1970s. Infections occur endemically in urban settings, although epidemics occur periodically at irregular intervals of about 4 years. Although these outbreaks can occur at any time of the year, they are more commonly seen in the autumn, and they last several months.[6-11] These infections occur throughout life and are particularly apparent in older children and adolescents.

Infection and disease with *M. pneumoniae* are common. Among healthy school-age children enrolled in a health care plan in Seattle, Foy et al[6] found infection rates ranging from 2% in endemic years to 35% during epidemics. In the day-care center study by Fernald et al,[12] the yearly risk of infection was estimated to be 12%, the ages of infected children ranged from 2 months to 8 years, and most infections were asymptomatic (74%) or mildly symptomatic, manifesting with coryza and cough. In subjectively healthy individuals, the isolation rate of *M. pneumoniae* ranged from 4.6% to 13.5%.[13]

Seroepidemiologic studies show antibody prevalence rates rising from 28% in 7- to 12-month-old infants to 55% in 13- to 24-month-old infants, 67% in 25- to 60-month-old infants, and 97% in people over the age of 17 years.[14] The prevalence of complement fixation antibody was 40% in 6- to 11-month-old children and about 66% in those 1 to 9 years old.[15]

The clinical manifestations of *M. pneumoniae* disease are related to the prevalence of the organism in the community as well as the age of the child. The disease manifests mostly in those 5 to 9 years of age, followed by those 10 to 14 years of age. Infection results in clinical disease more commonly in this age group than in adolescents.[6] The rate of infection in children under 5 years of age and in adolescents is half that of children 5 to 9 years of age and about twice that of adults; most of the infections in children under 5 years of age occur in 2 to 4 year olds, with very few infections occurring in patients under 6 months of age, presumably because of transplacentally derived immunity.[16]

Pneumonia in preschool children is most commonly related to viral infections, which obscure mycoplasmal infections; with increasing age, as viral pneumonia becomes less common, the proportion of episodes related to mycoplasmal infection increases to 9% to 16% in the early school-age group and 16% to 21% in older children. Some 30% to 50% of episodes of pneumonia are related to mycoplasmal infection among college students and military recruits. Symptomatic infection is rare after age 40.[9,17]

The incubation period is 1 to 2 weeks in volunteer studies and up to 3 weeks in community or family outbreaks, presumably because of the potentially higher inocula encountered in volunteer studies.[18-20] In the family setting, infection spreads slowly but extensively. Intrafamilial spread occurs in 65% of families, with 84% of children and 41% of adults being infected.[20,21] Of the secondary cases, 71% had lower respiratory tract involvement, 14% had otitis media, 10% had pharyngitis, and 15% were asymptomatic. Communicability in the school setting is limited.[22] The progression of the disease in communities is slow, although rapid epidemics can occur. Recurrent infections are usual.[13,14,23]

Pathogenesis of Pulmonary Infection

Infections with *M. pneumoniae* are acquired via the respiratory route from small-particle aerosols or more likely from large droplets.[24] The organism attaches to a receptor on respiratory epithelia via a terminal structure containing an electron-dense core. This attachment factor has been identified as the P1 protein.[25,26] Once adherence occurs, the organism remains extracellular. Cellular damage occurs primarily in the epithelium of the bronchi and bronchioles.[27,28] Injury to the cell is accompanied by ciliostasis.[29]

Specific serum antibody develops after infection, as does secretory antibody in respiratory secretions. The responses tend to be milder in children than in adults, and infection may recur.[12,30] Specific cell-mediated immune responses increase with age and are likely the result of repeated infections.[12] It has been postulated that primary infection may sensitize the young infant so that more severe disease develops on reinfection. Only 11% of children younger 4 years of age with documented prior infection had specific cell-mediated immunity compared to 58% of children older than 4 years and 87% of adults.[12] In a study of infants and young children, Foy et al[6] demonstrated partial protective immunity when infection was acquired early in life, especially when manifested with pneumonia as opposed to milder symptoms.

Clinical Manifestations

Respiratory Disease

Pneumonia. Mycoplasmal pneumonia is a common form of community-acquired pneumonia that occurs after only 3% to 10% of infections[1] and accounts for 20% of episodes of pneumonia in the general population.[7,31] The illness typically presents with a gradual onset of malaise, headache, and fever to 100° to 103° F (38° to 39° C) occurring over several days to 1 week.[32] Cough presents 3 to 5 days after the onset of symptoms and is initially nonproductive but may become productive of mucoid or mucopurulent sputum that can sometimes be blood tinged.[33] Associated symptoms may include chills, hoarseness, sore throat, chest pain, nausea, vomiting, and diarrhea. Coryza is an unusual finding except in young children, and its presence as a prodrome suggests a different diagnosis.[34]

Findings on physical examination are relatively minimal and include crackles in 78% of patients, wheezes on auscultation in 32%, and bronchial breathing in 27%.[34] However, early in the course of the illness, there may be no findings on chest examination. Audible wheezing was described in up to 40% of children, including patients who did not have asthma.[35] Colonization rates are higher in individuals with than without asthma (24.7% vs. 5.7%).[36] Nonexudative pharyngitis, cervical lymphadenopathy, conjunctivitis, otitis media, and rash have also been noted.[37] The severity of the clinical symptoms often exceeds that of the physical signs detected.[7]

Recovery is the rule in *M. pneumoniae* pneumonia. Although the clinical course is quite variable, the illness usually resolves within 3 to 4 weeks.[7,33] Pulmonary function abnormalities may persist up to 3 years. In a noncontrolled study of children without asthma, the mean forced vital capacity, 1-second forced expiratory volume, and forced expiratory flow were significantly reduced.[35]

Severe pneumonia is uncommon and may occur in healthy children and adults of all ages,[34,38-42] especially in those with sickle cell disease,[43,44] immunodeficiency,[45] drug-induced immunosuppression,[46] and preexisting cardiopulmonary dysfunction.[47] Massive lobar consolidation, pleural effusions,[38,41,44] pneumatoceles, lung abscesses,[48,49] adult respiratory distress syndrome,[50,51] and the evolution of obliterative bronchiolitis and diffuse interstitial fibrosis[52] have all been observed but are rare.

The radiologic findings are usually unilateral (87%) and involve the lower lobes, the midlung fields (less frequent), and the upper lobes (least frequent).[53] In the early stages, the pattern is reticular and interstitial; patchy and segmental areas of consolidation are noted later. Lobar involvement is occasionally seen. Hilar adenopathy occurs in 34% of patients, and effusions are seen in 20% when lateral decubitus films are used.[54] A hallmark of *M. pneumoniae* infections is the often poor correlation among the degree of clinical symptoms, pulmonary physical findings, and findings on chest radiographs.[6,32,37]

The differential diagnosis of community-acquired pneumonia includes that of the viral pneumonias (caused by the influenza virus, parainfluenza virus, respiratory syncytial virus, and adenovirus) as well as infection caused by *Chlamydia pneumoniae* and *Legionella pneumophila.* Some of the characteristics that help identify mycoplasmal pneumonia is the generally mild course of the illness, which has a progressive onset. The fever tends to be low grade, and constitutional symptoms are prominent. Ear, throat, and skin involvement are common, but coryza is not. Adenoviral and mycoplasmal pneumonia share clinical and radiologic features and may not be separable clinically.[10] Hoarseness is more likely to occur with *C. pneumoniae* infections than with mycoplasmal pneumonias.[55]

Respiratory Disease Other than Pneumonia. *M. pneumoniae* infections have been associated with a variety of clinical syndromes. Pharyngitis was present in 32% of children with lower respiratory infection in one series,[34] but was not a major manifestation of the infection. Glezen et al[56] found that only 3% of children and adolescents with pharyngitis had *M. pneumoniae* infections, with a peak incidence in the 12- to 14-year age group. Serologic evidence of infection was demonstrated in 11% of adults with pharyngitis.[57]

Otitis media was noted in 27% of children in the series by Stevens et al[34]; however, no attempt was made to establish the etiology of the otitis. The body of evidence would suggest a minimal role for *Mycoplasma* organisms in the etiology of otitis or bullous myringitis.[58] Radiographic evidence for sinusitis is commonly detected, but attempts at isolating the organism from middle ears and sinuses have largely been unsuccessful. Approximately 2% of cases of laryngotracheobronchitis,[6,59,60] 10% to 20% of cases of acute bronchitis,[6,9,10] 4% to 5% of cases of bronchiolitis,[6,60,61] and 2% to 5% of cases of nonspecific upper respiratory infection[6,62] are due to *M. pneumoniae.*

Nonrespiratory Disease

A variety of extrapulmonary complications have been described. Such complications commonly occur 1 to 21 days after the onset of respiratory illness, although concomitant respiratory symptoms have not been noted in some patients.[1] Most of the diagnoses have been based on the results of serologic testing, mostly fourfold rises in complement fixation titers rather than on culture confirmation.

Neurologic Manifestations. The incidence of neurologic disease has been estimated at 0.1%[63]; in selected populations such as hospitalized patients, it may be as high as 7%.[64] Onset occurs 3 to 23 days after respiratory illness, which itself was demonstrated in 79% of patients.[65] A variety of syndromes has been described, the most frequent of which is meningoencephalitis. Others include transverse myelitis, cranial neuropathy, myeloradiculopathy, a poliomyelitis-like syndrome, cerebellar ataxia, a brain-stem syndrome, psychosis, cerebral infarction, focal encephalitis, and Guillain-Barré syndrome. The prognosis has been variable, and the mortality rate is estimated at about 10%. Recovery is slow and is often associated with permanent sequelae.[37]

Dermatologic Manifestations. Erythematous maculopapular or vesicular exanthems are the most common cutaneous manifestations of *M. pneumoniae* infection, although vesiculopustular, bullous, urticarial, and petechial lesions occur. The most serious manifestations are erythema multiforme and Stevens-Johnson syndrome.[66,67] In the series by Cherry et al,[66] 95% of patients were between 4 and 20 years of age, and 90% had clinical or radiographic evidence of pneumonia. The duration of the rash typically exceeds 1 week.

Cardiac Manifestations. Cardiac involvement may occur in up to 4.5% of patients.[68] Pericarditis and myocarditis are most frequent; congestive heart failure, heart block, and infarction have also occurred.[37]

Gastrointestinal Manifestations. Nonspecific gastrointestinal complaints often accompany *M. pneumoniae* infections.[33] Occasionally, hepatic dysfunction and rarely jaundice develop with increases in enzyme levels.[39,69,70]

Hematologic Manifestations. Hemolytic anemia is a common manifestation of infection.[71] The results of the direct Coombs' test are usually positive. Other reported manifestations include bone marrow suppression, thrombocytopenia, and disseminated intravascular coagulation.[37]

Musculoskeletal Manifestations. Myalgias and arthralgias occur in 15% to 45% of patients.[39,72] These manifestations have generally been transient and have resolved during the acute phase of the illness. Occasionally, frank arthritis may be severe and may last up to 18 months.

Genitourinary Manifestations. Both glomerulonephritis and interstitial tubulonephritis have been described.[37]

Immunologic Manifestations. Transient depression of immune function has been reported during and after mycoplasmal infections.[37]

Diagnosis

Culture

M. pneumoniae can be cultured from the throat or nasopharynx of infected individuals. The specimens need to be transported and inoculated in special media. The introduction of SP4 media has markedly enhanced the isolation of *M. pneumoniae.* These culture systems are not widely available and require 2 to 3 weeks before identification can be accomplished. In a study of Japanese children with lower respiratory tract infections, the isolation rate was 22% in children with pneumonia and 11% in those without pneumonia.[73] The isolation rate was similar in children under 4 years of age irrespective of the presence of fever or wheezing. In older patients, the organism was frequently isolated from febrile children who were not wheezing. *M. pneumoniae* has rarely been isolated from pleural or cerebrospinal fluid.[74]

Antigen Detection

An enzyme immunoassay has been evaluated for the detection of *M. pneumoniae* antigens in young adults with respiratory infections. When sputa are used, the sensitivity of the this assay ranges from 40% to 80%, and its specificity is 64% to 100%. The assay has a poor sensitivity when nasopharyngeal aspirates are used.[75]

Serology

Serologic assays are the mainstay for diagnosing mycoplasmal infections because cultures and direct detection methods such as hybridization techniques or polymerase chain reaction are not widely available.

Cold Agglutinin Identification. Cold agglutinins usually appear by the end of the first week or the beginning of the second week of illness and disappear by 2 to 3 months. Cold agglutinin responses are nonspecific and consist mostly of immunoglobulin M (IgM). The test requires an overnight incubation step. The likelihood that a particular illness is related to *M. pneumoniae* is proportional to the height of the titer.[5] A bedside cold agglutinin screening test is available but lacks specificity and sensitivity, being negative in 50% to 70% of those tested. In addition, a low positive antibody titer may result from a number of respiratory or collagen vascular diseases.

Specific Serologic Tests. The most widely available serologic assay is the complement fixation test, which has been used as the standard. Sera from patients in the acute and convalescent stages are run in pairs, and a fourfold rise or fall in the antibody titer is diagnostic of infection. A titer greater than 1:32 in a single serum sample is also considered diagnostic. The test measures primarily IgM antibodies and to a lesser extent IgG. Therefore a negative test does not exclude reinfection. The glycolipid antigen used in the assay cross-reacts with other plant and human antigens and has been reported to cross-react in patients with legionnaires' disease in some investigations. A recent 12-year study of pneumonia indicated the sensitivity and specificity of this test to be 90% and 94%, respectively.[76] In this study, the geometric mean titer of sera from a patient in the acute stage was 1:2.9 compared to 1:62 in sera from a patient in the convalescent stage.

Immunofluorescent and enzyme-linked immunoassays have been described for the detection of IgG and IgM to *M. pneumoniae.*[77,78] The diagnosis of primary infection may be separated from that of reinfection by the presence of IgM; IgG levels remain elevated for several weeks and are not useful diagnostically.[79] A major limitation of serologic methods is that antibody responses may not be apparent in immunocompromised children or in infants under 12 months of age.[80] For enzyme immunoassays,[81] the use of combined IgG and IgM measurements yields a high degree of sensitivity and specificity compared to the complement fixation assay. Whereas children and adolescents show primarily an IgM response, patients older than 40 years often do not. Thus the absence of an IgM response does not necessarily indicate the absence of infection, especially in adults. Specific IgM antibodies are detectable in 80% of sera sampled 9 days or more after the onset of symptoms, whereas only 40% of sera have detectable IgM antibodies 7 to 8 days after the onset of symptoms, and rarely a sample has IgM when tested earlier.[82] The response peaks at 10 to 30 days and falls to undetectable levels in 12 to 26 weeks. This response appears somewhat earlier than that seen with the complement fixation assay.[83]

Molecular Probes

Nucleic acid hybridization using radioiodinated deoxyribonucleic acid probes have been developed for the diagnosis of *M. pneumoniae* infections. One such commercial test (Gen-Probe) is quite sensitive and specific when compared to culture and serologic tests if sputum samples are used. Its usefulness with throat swabs is limited.[84]

Polymerase Chain Reaction

The polymerase chain reaction has been used in the detection of *M. pneumoniae* from clinical specimens.[85] The optimal specimen is a throat swab because nasopharyngeal specimens have nonspecific inhibitors.[86] The technique can also be used for the diagnosis of central nervous system infections when cerebrospinal fluid is examined.[87]

Nonspecific Laboratory Data

The white blood cell count is usually normal, and there is an absolute neutrophilia. The erythrocyte sedimentation rate is commonly elevated, and the direct Coombs' test may be positive, as may serologic tests for syphilis and antinuclear antibody tests.

Therapy

M. pneumoniae is sensitive to erythromycin and tetracycline. Because it has no cell wall, it is resistant to penicillins, cephalosporins, and other cell wall–active agents. Both erythromycin and tetracycline are given in a dose of 30 to 50 mg/kg/day (maximum, 1 to 2 g/day) for 7 to 10 days. The treatment is most effective when initiated within 4 days of the onset of symptoms.[88] With therapy, most patients become afebrile within 48 hours.[87] The treatment does not appreciably affect the culture positivity.[87] Prophylactic use of oxytetracycline for 10 days to prevent pneumonia in family contacts has been effective. There are no good data on the benefit of steroids in the treatment of severe pulmonary or extrapulmonary infections. Newer macrolides such as azithromycin have shown efficacy when used for a 3-day course.[89] In experimental and in vitro models, azithromycin is the most active of the macrolides.[90]

U. Urealyticum and *M. Hominis* Infection

U. urealyticum is a very common isolate from the lower genital tract, being recovered in 40% to 80% of such cultures.[91] Infection of the chorioamnion is less common and is associated with chorioamnionitis, premature birth, and perinatal morbidity and mortality.[92] The rate of vertical transmission ranges from 18% to 55% in full-term newborns to 29% to 55% in preterm neonates. The transmission is more efficient in the presence of chorioamnionitis and is not affected by the mode of delivery.[93] Identification of the maternal and neonatal isolates and hence vertical transmission have been confirmed by polymerase chain reaction.[94]

U. urealyticum is the most common organism isolated from the lower respiratory tract of newborns, particularly those born prematurely. It has been isolated in pure culture from pleural fluid, lung biopsy samples, and lung tissue at autopsy. Systemic neonatal infections, including bloodstream infections, meningitis, and congenital and neonatal pneumonias, have been documented.[95] Rare case reports have implicated *U. urealyticum* in the etiology of neonatal persistent pulmonary hypertension,[96] neonatal meningitis,[97] and osteomyelitis or soft tissue abscesses.[98] Multiple studies have now associated lower respiratory tract infection with the development of chronic lung disease, primarily in low-birth-weight infants. In addition, a systemic reaction can be demonstrated in colonized neonates with elevated white cell counts and increased numbers of neutrophils at 2 or 3 days of age[99]; this raises the possibility that an elevated neutrophil count in the preterm infant may be a marker for infection.

M. hominis is isolated from 10% to 55% of vaginal cultures of sexually active adult women. This high rate of colonization is associated with positive cultures from the amniotic fluid in 66% of mothers and in 26% of their offspring.[95] Prolonged rupture of membranes correlated with detection of *M. hominis* but not *U. urealyticum* in this study. *M. hominis* has also been isolated from soft tissue abscesses, lymph nodes, and the cerebrospinal fluid of neonates.[101] Its role in neonatal pneumonia and chronic lung disease is not clear.

Congenital Pneumonia

U. urealyticum is a cause of amnionitis and has been isolated from the lung in the absence of other pathogens. Congenital pneumonia, or pneumonia acquired during the birth process, is accompanied almost invariably by chorioamnionitis. Isolation of the organism in the first 7 days of life has been associated with a significantly higher rate of radiologic indicators of pneumonia as well as evidence of early bronchopulmonary dysplasia independent of prematurity.[102] In one report, it has been associated with fatal neonatal pneumonia.[103] Inoculation of experimental animals with human isolates also produces pneumonia.

Chronic Lung Disease and Death of the Newborn

Four independent studies have linked *U. urealyticum* to chronic lung disease. They indicate a significant association between colonization of the respiratory tract at 24 to 72 hours of age and the development of chronic lung disease in the very-low-birth-weight infant. The magnitude of the relative risk in infants weighing less than 1250 g has been estimated to be 2.04 to 2.78 compared to that in uninfected newborns. The increased risk seems to disappear in infants who weigh more than 1250 g.[104] The organism can be found in pure culture in tracheal aspirates in up to 85% of infants and can also be found in the bloodstream in 26%. *U. urealyticum* has been cultured in 4 of 8 infants with chronic lung disease who have undergone open lung biopsy, and its recovery was not associated with specific pathologic changes.[105]

U. urealyticum may not be the primary cause of the chronic lung disease, but it produces pneumonia that goes undetected and untreated and results in increased oxygen requirements and subsequently chronic lung disease as a result of oxygen toxicity. Such findings have been corroborated in neonatal mice.

Pneumonia during Infancy

No prospective studies address the role of *U. urealyticum* in lower respiratory tract infections beyond the neonatal period. In light of the differences in susceptibility of very-low-birth-weight infants compared to full-term infants, it is unlikely that *U. urealyticum* is a major cause of respiratory disease in otherwise healthy infants after the first month of life.[92]

REFERENCES

1. Cassell GH, Cole BC: Mycoplasmas as agents of human disease, *N Engl J Med* 304:80-89, 1981.
2. Eaton MD, Mieklejohn G, van Herick W: Studies on the etiology of primary atypical pneumonia: a filtrable agent transmissible to cotton rats, hamsters, and chick embryos, *J Exp Med* 79:649-668, 1944.
3. Dingle JH, Finland M: Virus pneumonias. II. Primary atypical pneumonias of unknown etiology, *N Engl J Med* 227:378-385, 1942.
4. Chanock RM, Hayflick L, Barile MF: *Mycoplasma pneumoniae*: proposed nomenclature for atypical pneumonia organism (Eaton agent), *Science* 140:662, 1963.
5. Chanock RM: Mycoplasma infections in man, *N Engl J Med* 273:1199-1206, 1965.

M. Pneumoniae Infection

6. Foy HM, Kenny GE, Cooney MK, Allan ID: Long-term epidemiology of infections with *Mycoplasma pneumoniae*, *J Infect Dis* 139:681-687, 1979.
7. Denny FW, Clyde WA Jr, Glezen WP: *Mycoplasma pneumoniae* disease: clinical spectrum, pathophysiology, epidemiology and control, *J Infect Dis* 123:74-92, 1971 (review).
8. Monto AS, Bryan ER, Rhoads LM: The Tecumseh study of respiratory illnesses. VII. Further observations on the occurrence of respiratory syncytial virus and *Mycoplasma pneumoniae* infections, *Am J Epidemiol* 100:458-468, 1975.
9. Evans AS, Allen V, Sueltmann S: *Mycoplasma pneumoniae* infections in University of Wisconsin students, *Am Rev Respir Dis* 96:237-244, 1967.

10. Mogabgab WJ: *Mycoplasma pneumoniae* and adenovirus respiratory illnesses in military and university personnel, 1959-1966, *Am Rev Respir Dis* 97:345-358, 1968.
11. Clyde WA Jr: Clinical overview of typical *Mycoplasma pneumoniae* infections, *Clin Infect Dis* 17(suppl 1):S32-S36, 1993.
12. Fernald GW, Collier AM, Clyde WA Jr: Respiratory infections due to *Mycoplasma pneumoniae* in infants and children, *Pediatrics* 55:327-335, 1975.
13. Gnarpe J, Lundback A, Sundelof B, Gnarpe H: Prevalence of *Mycoplasma pneumoniae* in subjectively healthy individuals, Scand *J Infect Dis* 24:161-164, 1992.
14. Brunner H, Prescott B, Greenberg H, James WD, Horsewood RL, Channock RM: Unexpectedly high frequency of antibody to *Mycoplasma pneumoniae* in human sera as measured by sensitive techniques, *J Infect Dis* 135:524-530, 1977.
15. Hornsleth A: Mycoplasma pneumonia infection in infants and children in Copenhagen, 1963-65: incidence of complement-fixing antibodies in age groups 0-9 years, *Acta Pathol Microbiol Scand* 69:304-311, 1967.
16. Weiser OL, Higaki HH, Nolte LB: *Mycoplasma pneumoniae*: complement fixing antibody titers at birth, *Am J Clin Pathol* 47:641-642, 1967.
17. Chanock RM, Fox HH, James WD, Gutekunst RR, White RJ, Senterfit LB: Epidemiology of *M. pneumoniae* infection in military recruits, *Ann NY Acad Sci* 143:484-496, 1967.
18. Rifkind D, Chanock R, Kravetz HM, et al: Ear involvement (myringitis) and primary atypical pneumonia following inoculation of volunteers with Eaton agent, *Am Rev Respir Dis* 85:479-489, 1962.
19. Evatt BL, Dowdle WR, Johnson M Jr, Heath CW Jr: Epidemic *Mycoplasma* pneumonia, *N Engl J Med* 285:374-377, 1971.
20. Foy HM, Grayston JT, Kenny GE, Alexander ER, McMahan R: Epidemiology of *Mycoplasma pneumoniae* infections in families, JAMA 197:859-866, 1966.
21. Biberfeld G, Sterner G: A study of *Mycoplasma pneumoniae* infections in families, Scand *J Infect Dis* 1:39-46, 1969.
22. Foy HM, Alexander ER: *Mycoplasma pneumoniae* infections in childhood, Adv Pediatr 16:301-323, 1969 (review).
23. Foy HM, Kenny GE, Sefi R, Ochs HD, Allan ID: Second attacks of pneumonia due to *Mycoplasma pneumoniae*, *J Infect Dis* 135:673-677, 1977.
24. Foy HM, Kenny GE, McMahan R, Kaiser G, Grayston JT: *Mycoplasma pneumoniae* in the community, *Am J Epidemiol* 93:55-67, 1970.
25. Carson JL, Collier AM: Host-pathogen interactions in experimental *Mycoplasma pneumoniae* disease studied by the freeze-fracture technique, *Rev Infect Dis* 4:S185-S192, 1982.
26. Layh-Schmitt G, Herrmann R: Spatial arrangement of gene products of the P1 operon in the membrane of *Mycoplasma pneumoniae*, *Infect Immun* 62:974-979, 1994.
27. Parker F, Joliffe LS, Finland M: Primary atypical pneumonia: report of eight cases with autopsies, *Arch Pathol* 44:581-608, 1947.
28. Maisel JC, Babbitt LH, John TJ: Fatal *Mycoplasma pneumoniae* infection with isolation of the organism from the lung, *JAMA* 202:287-290, 1967.
29. Carson JL, Collier AM, Clyde W: Ciliary membrane alterations occurring in experimental *Mycoplasma pneumoniae* infection, *Science* 206:349-351, 1979.
30. Brunner H, James WD, Horswod RL, Chanock RM: Measurement of *Mycoplasma pneumoniae* mycoplasmacidal antibody in human serum, *J Immunol* 108:1491-1498, 1972.
31. Foy HM, Kenny GE, McMahan R, Mansy AM, Grayston JT: *Mycoplasma pneumoniae* pneumonia in an urban area: five years of surveillance, *JAMA* 214:1666-1672, 1970.
32. Copps SC, Allen VD, Sueltmann S, Evans AS: A community outbreak of *Mycoplasma* pneumonia, *JAMA* 204:123-128, 1968.
33. Cherry JD, Welliver RC: *Mycoplasma pneumoniae* infections of adults and children, West J Med 125:47-55, 1976.
34. Stevens D, Swift PGF, Johnston PGB, Kearney PJ, Corner BD, Burman D: *Mycoplasma pneumoniae* infections in children, *Arch Dis Child* 53:38-42, 1978.
35. Sabato AR, Martin AJ, Marmion BP, Kok TW, Cooper DM: *Mycoplasma pneumoniae*: acute illness, antibiotics and subsequent pulmonary function, *Arch Dis Child* 59:1034-1037, 1984.
36. Gil JC, Cedillo RL, Mayagoitia BG, Paz MD: Isolation of *Mycoplasma pneumoniae* from asthmatic patients, *Ann Allergy* 70:23-25, 1993.
37. Broughton RA: Infections with *Mycoplasma pneumoniae* in childhood, *Pediatr Infect Dis J* 5:71-86, 1986 (review).
38. Singer JI, DeVoe WM: Severe *Mycoplasma pneumoniae* infection in otherwise healthy siblings, *J Pediatr* 95:999-1001, 1979.
39. Grix A, Giammona ST: Pneumonitis with pleural effusion in children due to *Mycoplasma pneumoniae*, *Am Rev Respir Dis* 109:665-671, 1974.
40. Levine DP, Lerner AM: The clinical spectrum of *Mycoplasma pneumoniae* infections, *Med Clin North Am* 62:961-978, 1978.
41. Linz DH, Tolle SW, Elliot DL: *Mycoplasma pneumoniae* pneumonia: experience at a referral center, *West J Med* 140:895-900, 1984.
42. Murray HW, Masur H, Senterfit LB, Roberts RB: The protean manifestations of *Mycoplasma pneumoniae* infections in adults, *Am J Med* 58:229-242, 1975.
43. Shulman ST, Bartlett J, Clyde WA Jr, Ayoub EM: The unusual severity of mycoplasmal pneumonia in children with sickle cell disease, *N Engl J Med* 287:164-167, 1972.
44. Solanki KL, Berdoff RL: Severe *Mycoplasma* pneumonia with severe pleural effusions in a patient with sickle cell-hemoglobin C (SC) disease: case report and review of the literature, *Am J Med* 66:707-710, 1979.
45. Foy HM, Ochs H, Davis SD: *Mycoplasma pneumoniae* infections in patients with immunodeficiency syndromes: report of four cases, *J Infect Dis* 127:388-393, 1973.
46. Ganick DJ, Wolfson J, Gilbert EF, Joo P: *Mycoplasma* infection in the immunosuppressed leukemic patient, *Arch Pathol Lab Med* 104:535-536, 1980.
47. Meyers BR, Hirschman SZ: Fatal infections associated with *Mycoplasma pneumoniae*: discussion of three cases with necropsy findings, *Mt Sinai J Med (NY)* 39:358-364, 1972.
48. Lewis JE, Sheptin C: Mycoplasmal pneumonia associated with abscess of the lung, *Calif Med* 117:69-72, 1972.
49. Siegler DIM: Lung abscess associated with *Mycoplasma pneumoniae* infection, *Br J Dis Chest* 67:123-127, 1973.
50. Fischman RA, Marschall KE, Kislak JW, Greenbaum DM: Adult respiratory distress syndrome caused by *Mycoplasma pneumoniae, Chest* 74:471-473, 1978.
51. Jastremski MS: Adult respiratory distress syndrome due to *Mycoplasma pneumoniae*, *Chest* 75:529, 1979 (letter).
52. Kaufman JM, Cuvelier CA, Van Der Streten M: *Mycoplasma* pneumonia with fulminant evolution into diffuse interstitial fibrosis, *Thorax* 35:140-144, 1980.
53. Niitu Y: *M. pneumoniae* respiratory disease: clinical features—children, *Yale J Biol Med* 56:493-503, 1983 (review).
54. Fine NL, Smith LR, Sheedy PF: Frequency of pleural effusions in *Mycoplasma* and viral pneumonias, *N Engl J Med* 283:790-793, 1970.
55. Grayston JT, Campbell LA, Kuo CC, Mordhorst CT, Saikku P, Thom DH, Wang SP: A new respiratory tract pathogen: *Chlamydia trachomatis strain* TWAR, *J Infect Dis* 161:618-625, 1990.
56. Glezen WP, Clyde WA Jr, Senior RJ, Shaeffer CI, Denny FW: Group A streptococci, mycoplasmas, and viruses associated with acute pharyngitis, *JAMA* 202:455-460, 1967.
57. Komaroff AL, Aronson MD, Pass TM, Ervin CT, Brauch JT Jr, Schachter J: Serologic evidence of chlamydial and *Mycoplasma* pharyngitis in adults, *Science* 222:927-928, 1983.
58. Roberts DB: The etiology of bullous myringitis and the role of mycoplasmas in ear disease: a review, *Pediatrics* 65:761-766, 1980.
59. Glezen WP, Loda FA, Clyde WA Jr, Senior RJ, Sheaffer CI, Conley WG, Denny FW: Epidemiologic patterns of acute lower respiratory disease of children in a pediatric group practice, *J Pediatr* 78:397-406, 1971.
60. Foy HM, Cooney MK, Maletzky AJ, Grayston JT: Incidence and etiology of pneumonia, croup and bronchiolitis in preschool children belonging to a prepaid medical care group over a four-year period, *Am J Epidemiol* 97:80-92, 1973.
61. Loda FA, Clyde WA Jr, Glezen WP, Senior RJ, Shaeffer CI, Denny FW Jr: Studies on the role of viruses, bacteria, and *M. pneumoniae* as causes of lower respiratory tract infections in children, *J Pediatr* 72:161-176, 1968.
62. Loda FA, Glezen WP, Clyde WA: Respiratory disease in group day care, *Pediatrics* 49:428-437, 1972.
63. Ogata S, Kitamoto D: Clinical complications of *Mycoplasma pneumoniae* disease: central nervous system, *Yale J Biol Med* 56:481-486, 1983.
64. Sterner G, Biberfeld G: Central nervous system complications of *M. pneumoniae* infection, Scand *J Infect Dis* 1:203-208, 1969.

65. Lerer RJ, Kalavsky SM: Central nervous system disease associated with *Mycoplasma pneumoniae* infection: report of five cases and review of the literature, *Pediatrics* 52:658-668, 1973.
66. Cherry JD, Hurwitz ES, Welliver RC: *Mycoplasma pneumoniae* infections and exanthems, *J Pediatr* 87:369-373, 1975.
67. Teisch JA, Shapiro L, Walzer RA: Vesiculopustular eruption with *Mycoplasma pneumoniae, JAMA* 211:1694-1697, 1970.
68. Pönka A: Carditis associated with *Mycoplasma pneumoniae* infection, *Acta Med Scand* 206:77-86, 1979.
69. Suzuyama Y, Iwasaki H, Izumikawa K, Hara K: Other organs, *Yale J Biol Med* 56:487-491, 1983.
70. Arav-Boger R, Assia A, Spirer Z, Bujanover Y, Reif S: Cholestatic hepatitis as a main manifestation of *Mycoplasma pneumoniae* infection, *J Pediatr Gastroenterol Nutr* 21:450-460, 1995.
71. Feizi T: Cold agglutinins, the direct Coombs' test and serum immunoglobulins in *Mycoplasma pneumoniae* infection, *Ann NY Acad Sci* 143:801-812, 1967.
72. Hernandez LA, Urqhart GED, Dick WC: *Mycoplasma pneumoniae* infection and arthritis in man, *Br Med* J 2:14-16, 1977.
73. Nagayama Y, Sakurai N, Yamamoto K, Honda A, Makuta M, Suzuki R: Isolation of *Mycoplasma pneumoniae* from children with lower-respiratory-tract infections, *J Infect Dis* 157:911-917, 1988.
74. Nagayama Y, Sakurai N, Tamai K, Niwa A, Yamamoto K: Isolation of *Mycoplasma pneumoniae* from pleural and/or cerebrospinal fluid: report of four cases, Scand *J Infect Dis* 19:521-524, 1987.
75. Kleemola M, Raty R, Karjalainen J, Schuy W, Gerstenecker B, Jacobs E: Evaluation of an antigen-capture immunoassay for rapid diagnosis of *Mycoplasma pneumoniae* infection, *Eur J Clin Microbiol Infect Dis* 12:872-875, 1993.
76. Kenny GE, Kaiser GG, Cooney MK, Foy HM: Diagnosis of *Mycoplasma pneumoniae* pneumonia: sensitivities and specificities of serology with lipid antigen and isolation of the organism on soy peptone medium for identification of infections, *J Clin Microbiol* 28:2087-2093, 1990.
77. Smith TF: *Mycoplasma pneumoniae* infections: diagnosis based on immunofluorescence titer of IgG and IgM antibodies, *Mayo Clin Proc* 61:830-831, 1986.
78. Shearman MJ, Cubie HA, Inglis JM: *Mycoplasma pneumoniae* infection: early diagnosis by detection of specific IgM by immunofluorescence, *Br J Biomed Sci* 50:305-308, 1993.
79. Sillis M: The limitations of IgM assays in the serological diagnosis of *Mycoplasma pneumoniae* infections, *J Med Microbiol* 33:253-258, 1990.
80. Skakni L, Sardet A, Just J, Landman-Parker J, Costil J, Moniot-Ville N, Bricout F, Garbarg-Chenon A: Detection of *Mycoplasma pneumoniae* in clinical samples from pediatric patients by polymerase chain reaction, *J Clin Microbiol* 30:2638-2643, 1992.
81. Uldum SA, Jensen JS, Sondergard-Andersen J, Lind K: Enzyme immunoassay for detection of immunoglobulin M (IgM) and IgG antibodies to *Mycoplasma pneumoniae, J Clin Microbiol* 30:1198-1204, 1992.
82. Vikerfors T, Brodin G, Grandien M, Hirschberg L, Krook A, Pettersson CA: Detection of specific IgM antibodies for the diagnosis of *Mycoplasma pneumoniae* infections: a clinical evaluation, *Scand J Infect Dis* 20:601-610, 1988.
83. Moule JH, Caul EO, Wreghitt TG: The specific IgM response to *Mycoplasma pneumoniae* infection: interpretation and application to early diagnosis, *Epidemiol Infect* 99:685-692, 1987.
84. Kleemola M, Karjalainen JE, Raty RK: Rapid diagnosis of *Mycoplasma pneumoniae* infection: clinical evaluation of a commercial probe test, *J Infect Dis* 162:70-75, 1990.
85. Blackmore TK, Reznikov M, Gordon DL: Clinical utility of the polymerase chain reaction to diagnose *Mycoplasma pneumoniae* infection, *Pathology* 27:177-181, 1995.
86. Reznikov M, Blackmore TK, Finlay-Jones JJ, Gordon DL: Comparison of nasopharyngeal aspirates and throat swab specimens in a polymerase chain reaction–based test for *Mycoplasma pneumoniae, Eur J Clin Microbiol Infect Dis* 14:58-61, 1995.
87. Narita M, Matsuzono Y, Togashi T, Kajii N: DNA diagnosis of central nervous system infection by *Mycoplasma pneumoniae, Pediatrics* 90:250-253, 1992.
88. McCracken GH: Current status of antibiotic treatment for *Mycoplasma pneumoniae* infections, *Pediatr Infect Dis J* 5:167-171, 1986.
89. Schonwald S, Barsic B, Kinar I, Gunjaca M: Three-day azithromycin compared with ten-day roxithromycin treatment of atypical pneumonia, Scand *J Infect Dis* 26:706-710, 1994.
90. Ishida K, Kaku M, Irifune K, Mizukane R, Takemura H, Yoshida R: In vitro and in vivo activities of macrolides against *Mycoplasma pneumoniae, Antimicrob Agents Chemother* 38:790-798, 1994.

***U. Urealyticium* and *M. Hominis* Infection**

91. Carey JC, Blackwelder WC, Nugent RP, Matteson MA, Rao AV, Eschenbach DA, Lee ML, Rettig PJ, Regan JA, Geromanis KL: Antepartum cultures for *Ureaplasma urealyticum* are not useful in predicting pregnancy outcome, *Am J Obstet Gynecol* 164:728-733, 1991.
92. Cassell GH, Waites KB, Watson HL, Crouse DT, Harasawa R: *Ureaplasma urealyticum* intrauterine infection: role in prematurity and disease in newborns, *Clin Microbiol Rev* 6:69-87, 1993.
93. Sánchez PJ: Perinatal transmission of *Ureaplasma urealyticum*: current concepts based on review of the literature, *Clin Infect Dis* 17(suppl 1):S107-S111, 1993.
94. Grattard F, Soleihac B, Barbeyrac B, Bebear C, Seffert P, Pozetto P: Epidemiologic and molecular investigations of genital mycoplasmas from women and neonates at delivery, *Pediatr Infect Dis J* 14:853-858, 1995.
95. Waites KB, Crouse DT, Cassell GH: Systemic neonatal infection due to *Ureaplasma urealyticum, Clin Infect Dis* 17(suppl 1):S131-S135, 1993.
96. Waites KB, Crouse DT, Philips JB III, Canupp KC, Cassell GH: Ureaplasmal pneumonia and sepsis associated with persistent pulmonary hypertension of the newborn, *Pediatrics* 83:79-85, 1989.
97. Heggie AD, Jacobs MR, Butler VT, Baley JE, Boxerbaum B: Frequency of isolation of *Ureaplasma urealyticum* and *Mycoplasma hominis* from cerebrospinal fluid and tracheal aspirate specimens from low birth weight infants, *J Pediatr* 124:956-961, 1994.
98. Hamrick HJ, Mangum ME, Katz VL: *Ureaplasma urealyticum* abscess at site of an internal fetal heart rate monitor, *Pediatr Infect Dis J* 12:410-411, 1993.
99. Ohlsson A, Wang E, Vearncombe M: Leukocyte counts and colonization with *Ureaplasma urealyticum* in preterm neonates, *Clin Infect Dis* 17(suppl 1):S144-S147, 1993.
100. Dinsmoor MJ, Ramamurthy RS, Gibbs RS: Transmission of genital mycoplasmas from mother to neonate in women with prolonged membrane rupture, *Pediatr Infect Dis J* 8:483-487, 1989.
101. Waites KB, Duffy LB, Crouse DT, Dworsky ME, Strange MJ, Nelson KG, Cassell GH: Mycoplasmal infections of cerebrospinal fluid in newborn infants from a community hospital population, *Pediatr Infect Dis J* 9:241-245, 1990.
102. Crouse DT, Odrezin GT, Cutter GR, Reese JM, Hamrick WB, Waites KB, Cassell GH: Radiographic changes associated with tracheal isolation of *Ureaplasma urealyticum* from neonates, *Clin Infect Dis* 17(suppl 1):S122-S130, 1993.
103. Quinn PA, Gillian JE, Markestad T, St John MA, Daneman A, Lie KI, Li HCS, Czegledy-Nagy E, Klein M: Intrauterine infection with *Ureaplasma urealyticum* as a cause of fatal neonatal pneumonia, *Pediatr Infect Dis J* 4:538-543, 1985.
104. Wang EEL, Cassell GH, Sánchez PJ, Regan JA, Payne NR, Liu PP: *Ureaplasma urealyticum* and chronic lung disease of prematurity: critical appraisal of the literature on causation, *Clin Infect Dis* 17(suppl 1):S112-S116, 1993.
105. Walsh WF, Stanley S, Lally KP, Stribley RE, Treece DP, McCleskey F, Null DM: *Ureaplasma urealyticum* demonstrated by open lung biopsy in newborns with chronic lung disease, *Pediatr Infect Dis J* 10:823-827, 1991.

CHAPTER 45

Chlamydial Infections

Gwendolyn L. Gilbert

In 1907, intraepithelial inclusions were seen in the conjunctival scrapings of orangutans inoculated with material from patients with trachoma.[1] Subsequently, similar inclusions were seen in epithelial cells from the conjunctivas of infants with nongonococcal ophthalmia (inclusion conjunctivitis) and from genital specimens of the parents of infected infants.[1] They were described (somewhat fancifully) as being draped around the cell nucleus like a cloak and because of their size, were thought to be protozoa. Thus the organism was named *Chlamydozoaceae* (mantled animals; *chlamys*, "a cloak"). It first was isolated in embryonated hens' eggs in 1957 and in cell culture in 1965.[2] Human psittacosis was first described in the late nineteenth century as an unusual pneumonia that followed exposure to tropical birds (*psittakos*, Greek, "parrot").[3] It was recognized more commonly in Europe during the 1930s, when importation of South American birds became fashionable.[3] The causative organism was isolated by Bedson from avian and animal tissue in 1930 during an investigation of an outbreak in the London zoo.[4] Both of these agents were initially thought to be viruses but are now recognized as unique bacteria that contain both ribonucleic acid and deoxyribonucleic acid (DNA) and are susceptible to some antibiotics. *Chlamydia trachomatis* is a human pathogen, whereas *C. psittaci* affects primarily birds and a variety of wild and domestic animals and is a rare, accidental human pathogen.

The third member of the genus *Chlamydia* was first isolated in 1965 from the eye of a Taiwanese child thought to have trachoma and was later isolated from the respiratory tract of an American student with an upper respiratory tract infection. The organism was initially called *TWAR* (Taiwan, acute respiratory) and thought to be a variant of *C. psittaci* but later given a separate species as *C. pneumoniae*.[5,6]

MICROBIOLOGY AND *CHLAMYDIA*-CELL INTERACTIONS

Chlamydiae have a unique life cycle with two morphologic forms. Elementary bodies (EBs) are small, spherical (or pear-shaped in the case of *C. pneumoniae*) particles (0.3 μ diameter) that are relatively hardy and capable of extracellular survival but that do not replicate. Reticulate bodies (RBs) are the intracellular, replicative, metabolically active form of chlamydiae that multiply by binary fission within the cell. Chlamydiae are unable to synthesize energy-rich compounds such as adenosine triphosphate and instead use the compounds of the host cell; they are therefore obligate intracellular "energy" parasites (Fig. 45-1). They have a cell wall, which consists of inner and outer cytoplasmic membranes and lipopolysaccharide and is similar to that of a gram-negative bacterium except that it lacks peptidoglycan. The rigidity of the EB cell wall is due to disulfide cross-linking between cysteine-rich proteins. The lipopolysaccharide is specific to the genus *Chlamydia* and is structurally similar to the core lipopolysaccharide of the rough mutants of Enterobacteriaceae. Several envelope proteins are apparently involved in the attachment of chlamydiae to host cells; these include the serovar-specific major outer membrane protein and 18- and 32-kD eukaryotic cell–binding proteins.[7]

EBs infect susceptible epithelial cells, presumably after attachment to a specific receptor by one or more specific adhesins. No specific host cell receptor has yet been identified. EBs enter the cell by a process that apparently shares features of both phagocytosis and receptor-mediated pinocytosis and may depend on the type of cell and the organism's mode of presentation. Within the cell, *Chlamydia*-dependent modification of the endocytic membrane prevents its fusion with the cell's lysosome. EBs change into RBs, which replicate by binary fission to form the intracellular inclusion body.[7]

As the inclusion matures, RBs are converted to EBs and are released by the rupture of the inclusion. This process normally takes 48 to 72 hours but can be slowed to the point where multiplication virtually ceases and viable organisms persist within cells for long periods in a "latent" state. This nonproductive infection is induced in vitro through the limitation of concentrations of certain nutrients and through the actions of cytokines (including tumor necrosis factor and interferon-γ) and macrophages.[8] Thus the host immune response may be microbistatic (rather than microbicidal) and contribute to persistence of the chlamydial infection.

C. TRACHOMATIS INFECTIONS

C. trachomatis is a human pathogen, of which there are 2 biovars and 15 serovars. The trachoma biovar includes 12 serovars (A, B, Ba, and C through K) of which A to C usually cause the blinding eye disease trachoma and D to K usually cause sexually transmissible genital infection in men and women and neonatal infection in infants of infected women. The serovar distribution within these two groups is partly determined by geographic distribution; it is less distinct in communities where both trachoma and sexually transmitted chlamydial infections are endemic.[9,10] *C. trachomatis* serovars L1 to L3 (LGV biovar) cause lymphogranuloma venereum, a sexually transmissible disease with a limited geographic distribution in Africa, Asia, and South America. It is characterized by a mild, self-limited genital ulceration followed by regional lymphadenopathy associated with systemic symptoms. Complications in about 5% of cases are related to scarring and fibrosis of affected tissues, leading to the development of fistulas or lymphatic obstruction that causes lymphedema.

Transmission and Epidemiology

It is difficult to obtain accurate prevalence data for chlamydial genital infection because it is often asymptomatic and the diagnosis often is not confirmed by laboratory tests. The preva-

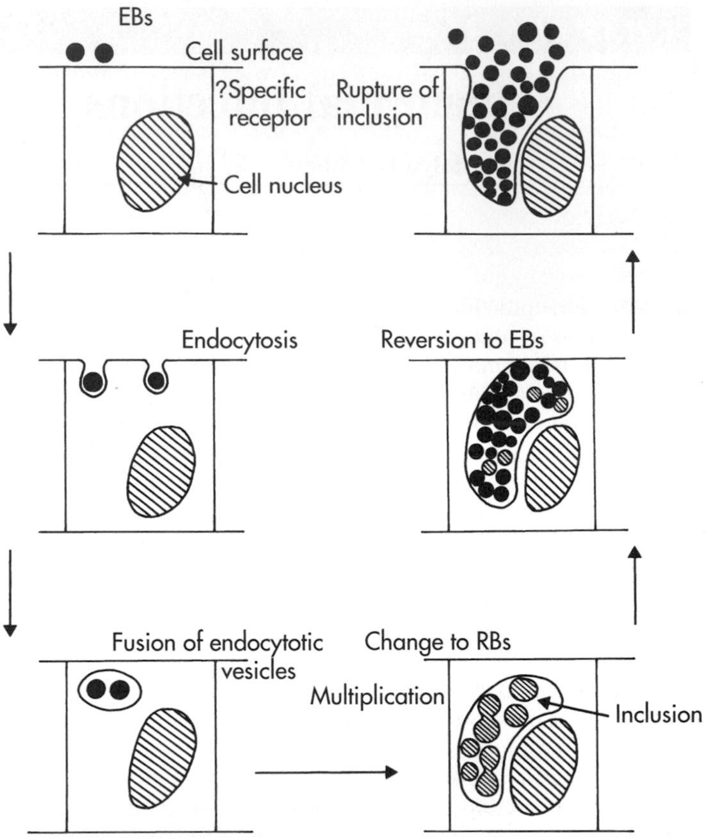

Figure 45-1. Life cycle of *C. trachomatis* in epithelial cells. (From Gilbert GL: *Infectious diseases in pregnancy and the newborn infant,* Amsterdam, 1991, Harwood Academic, p 249.)

lence among asymptomatic women in the United States varies from 2% to 40%; overall, it is about 5%.[11,12] It is generally similar in women of childbearing age in urban centers in other Western countries[12,13] but recently has fallen significantly in some places; for example, in Sydney, it has fallen from 20% to less than 5% in women attending a large sexual health clinic[14] and is now rare in pregnant women. In contrast, chlamydial infection was found in 20% to 40% of pregnant Aboriginal women in Darwin, Australia,[15] and 29% of pregnant women in Nairobi,[16] and the prevalence is likely to be similar in other developing countries.

Clinical Manifestations

Adults

The major clinical manifestations of chlamydial infections are similar to those of gonorrhea but are generally milder. Asymptomatic infection is common. *C. trachomatis* is the most common cause of nongonococcal and postgonococcal urethritis in men and epididymoorchitis in young men. The latter is usually unilateral, and chlamydial infection is not a significant cause of male infertility. In women, the usual symptoms, if any, are abnormal vaginal discharge caused by mucopurulent cervicitis, lower abdominal pain and abnormal uterine bleeding caused by endometritis, and frequency, dysuria, and sterile pyuria caused by urethritis.[11,17-19] Inclusion conjunctivitis and Reiter's syndrome (urethritis, uveitis, and arthritis) are uncommon complications of genital infection in both genders. The most important complication of chlamydial infection in women is salpingitis, which is estimated to occur in 10% to 20% of women with untreated chlamydial infection. It is associated with a high incidence of serious sequelae, including infertility and ectopic pregnancy, which can occur after apparently mild or even asymptomatic infection.[20]

Studies of chlamydial infection during pregnancy have led to conflicting results; some suggest that it does not affect the outcome, whereas others have demonstrated an increased risk of premature delivery and perinatal complications.[21,22] A prospective study of more than 11,500 pregnant women showed that 21% had chlamydial cervical infection in the first trimester.[23] Approximately half the infected women were treated. Premature rupture of the membranes, low birth weight, and perinatal death were significantly more frequent in infected women who were not treated than in those who were uninfected or those whose condition had been treated. Other studies have shown that the patients who are most at risk are women with chlamydial infection associated with serum chlamydial immunoglobulin M (IgM), suggesting recently acquired or more active infection.[21,24]

Neonates

Neonatal chlamydial infection is usually acquired during delivery. There are anecdotal reports of intrauterine chlamydial infections causing fetal death[25] or pneumonia in infants delivered by cesarean section or with symptoms at birth.[26-28] Approximately 60% of infants exposed at birth have cultural or serologic evidence of infection, and a third have clinical manifestations.[29] In a prospective study of infants of women with chlamydial genital infection at delivery, 18% developed conjunctivitis and 16% developed pneumonia caused by *C. trachomatis;* 14% were asymptomatically colonized.[30] In a population in whom the prevalence of chlamydial infection in pregnancy was 5%, nearly 1% of infants (or 15% to 20% of infants of mothers with chlamydial infection) developed chlamydial pneumonia.

Chlamydial conjunctivitis presents from 2 days to 1 month of age. It is responsible for 10% to 30% of cases of conjunctivitis in infants in the first month of life but is uncommon after this age.[31] It can be severe and protracted but is eventually self-limited, even without treatment. It is characterized by mucopurulent discharge, pseudomembrane formation, edema, and papillary atrophy. Because of the paucity of lymphoid tissue in neonates, conjunctival follicles—a feature of trachoma—are rare. Micropannus formation and corneal scarring can occur but rarely cause visual impairment. Without treatment, about half of infants who have conjunctivitis later develop pneumonia. Nasal congestion, typically without rhinorrhea, often precedes chlamydial pneumonia. Otitis media has been reported to be more common in infants exposed to chlamydia at birth than in controls, but a role for *C. trachomatis* in acute or chronic otitis media has not been proved.[32]

Chlamydial pneumonia was probably first described in 1941 by Botszejn[33] as an "interstitial pertussoid eosinophilic pneumonia of the infant." In 1975, an infant was described who had chlamydial conjunctivitis and in whom a dry cough, tachypnea, and pulmonary infiltrates had developed at 7 weeks of age;[34] *C. trachomatis* was isolated from the upper respiratory tract. Two years later, a syndrome was described that is now recognized as characteristic of chlamydial pneumonia. Typically, the symptoms begin insidiously at 2 to 8 weeks of age; there is a history of conjunctivitis in about 50% of cases, and nasal obstruction is common. The main symptoms are respiratory distress, tachypnea, a paroxysmal cough (often mistaken for whooping cough) associated with vomiting and weight loss, and periods of apnea and cyanosis; fever and toxicity are mild.[34] Clinical examination often shows few abnormalities apart from generalized crackles; middle ear abnormalities (dullness and bulging of the tympanic membrane) occur in about 50% of infants. Symptoms have usually been present for about 2 weeks at the time of presentation.

Chest radiographs show generalized hyperinflation, diffuse interstitial changes, and areas of atelectasis with or without a mild pleural reaction; the partial pressure of arterial oxygen is often reduced. Peripheral blood eosinophilia and hypergammaglobulinemia (especially IgM) are common abnormal laboratory findings. The diagnosis is confirmed by isolation of *C. trachomatis* from the nasopharynx, demonstration of specific IgM in serum, or both methods (see later section).[29]

The disease is usually mild, but resolution of symptoms can take several weeks. Less commonly, severe and occasionally fatal symptoms occur within the first month of life, especially in premature infants.[27,35] *C. trachomatis* has been implicated in up to one third of cases of pneumonia in hospitalized infants younger than 6 months of age.[36] Chlamydial pneumonia may be indistinguishable clinically from bronchiolitis, and apnea occurs in about the same proportion of infants infected with *C. trachomatis* (20%) as those with respiratory syncytial virus infection.[37] Many other respiratory pathogens, including respiratory syncytial virus, cytomegalovirus, *Ureaplasma urealyticum,* and *Pneumocystis carinii*, have been detected in association with *C. trachomatis* in respiratory tract specimens from infants with pneumonia, and mixed infection may be clinically more severe than isolated chlamydial pneumonia.[36] Long-term follow-up of children who have had chlamydial pneumonia indicates that they are more likely than controls or children who have had neonatal pneumonia from other causes to have abnormal respiratory function and chronic symptoms at 5 to 8 years of age.[38]

The pathologic manifestations have not been studied extensively because chlamydial pneumonia is rarely fatal. A recent review of published cases described a wide range of histologic changes, including diffuse interstitial and intraalveolar infiltrates of histiocytes, lymphocytes, plasma cells, eosinophils, and neutrophils; necrotizing bronchiolitis; and alveolitis.[39] Chlamydial inclusions have been demonstrated in epithelial cells by immunofluorescence and electron microscopy (Fig. 45-2).

Disease Mechanisms

C. trachomatis infection is usually confined to susceptible mucous membranes of the genital tract, conjunctivas, or respiratory tract. Disseminated infection rarely, if ever, occurs. Initial episodes of chlamydial infection (e.g., trachoma, cervicitis) are often mild and self-limited. There is a short period of serovar-specific protective immunity after infection, which is attributable to neutralizing mucosal antibody. However, subsequent infections can cause severe disease. Blinding trachoma is associated with repeated episodes of infection and increasingly severe inflammation and scarring.[40] In pig-tailed macaques, a single intratubal inoculation of *C. trachomatis* causes self-limited acute salpingitis with mild clinical signs and minimal histologic evidence of inflammation.[41] However, in a previously infected animal, tubal inoculation causes chronic salpingitis with scarring and adhesions, which is not prevented by high levels of circulating chlamydial antibodies.[42] Similar immunopathologic changes underlie the development of tubal scarring and infertility resulting from chlamydial salpingitis in women.

The pathogenesis of infant chlamydial pneumonia is less well defined. Upper respiratory colonization occurs at birth, usually in the presence of maternal chlamydial IgG antibody. It is not clear whether the relatively long incubation period represents the time required for the protective effect of maternal antibody to disappear, whether it represents the time required for the infant's own cell-mediated immune response to develop, or whether both explanations are correct. Most reported cases of severe, early onset chlamydial pneumonia have usually been in premature infants; in one, maternal IgG antibody was not present.[27] Maternal antibody may have some protective effect but clearly does not prevent infection, and chlamydial pneumonia persists despite a strong humoral immune response by the infant. The fact that irreversible pulmonary damage can occur is indicated by the increased incidence of chronic symptoms and impaired pulmonary function after chlamydial pneumonia in infancy.[38]

Only a minority of individuals infected with *C. trachomatis* develop an exaggerated, potentially damaging immune response. A 57- to 60-kD chlamydial heat shock protein (hsp60), which is one of a widely conserved family of bacterial and eucaryotic stress-response proteins, is the target for this response. It stimulates an intense, local, delayed-type hypersensitivity response in immune animals—analogous to severe trachoma—and the presence of antibody correlates with chronic tubal disease and ectopic pregnancy in seropositive women and with the development of Reiter's syndrome.[43] The existence of related heat shock proteins in mammalian cells suggests that chlamydial hsp60 may provoke an autoimmune response. In experimental infection in mice, there is evidence of genetic

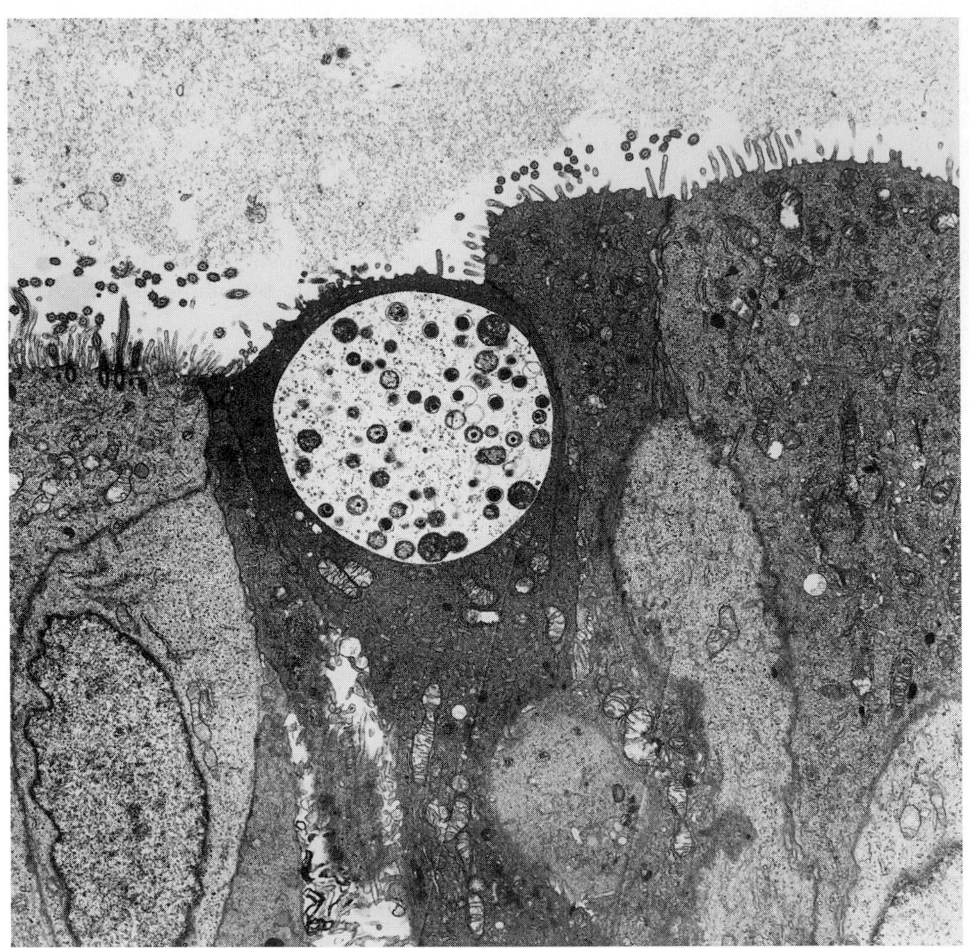

Figure 45-2. Electron micrograph of a *C. trachomatis* inclusion in bronchial epithelium from a lung biopsy of an infant with severe chlamydial pneumonia.

control of immune responses to hsp60, which could explain differences in individual responses.[44]

Laboratory Diagnosis

The diagnosis of *C. trachomatis* infection can be confirmed by culture, by detection of specific antigen or DNA, or by serologic techniques. Culture is currently the "gold standard" but requires cell culture, which is available only in larger laboratories and is time consuming and expensive. The sensitivity of a single culture is not 100% and is reduced by the suboptimal collection, transport, and storage of specimens. Specific chlamydial antigen can be detected in clinical specimens by immunofluorescence or enzyme immunoassay. In patients with symptoms consistent with chlamydial infection, antigen tests have a high sensitivity and specificity and can be performed rapidly by most laboratories. Specimens from the cervix, urethra, conjunctiva, and nasopharynx (in infants) are suitable and must be carefully collected to obtain epithelial cells, not just purulent secretions. Antigen tests are less sensitive than culture for detecting asymptomatic chlamydial infection, and false-positive results can occur. These tests should not be used for screening in populations in whom the prevalence of infection is low or for cases in which there are potential medicolegal implications (e.g., in cases of suspected sexual abuse).[45] Because of the limitations of antigen tests and the cost of culture, routine antenatal screening for maternal chlamydial infection is recommended only in populations in whom the prevalence is relatively high (>5%).

Recently commercial polymerase chain reaction kits have become available for detecting *C. trachomatis* DNA. This method is more sensitive than antigen tests and culture, the specificity and costs are comparable to those of culture, and a greater range of specimens, including urine, can be used.[46] This is likely to replace culture as the gold standard for diagnosis.

Serologic tests for serum antibody to *C. trachomatis* are of limited value in the diagnosis of infection. The standard method is microimmunofluorescence to detect serovar-specific antibody. Various modifications have been described in which pooled or cross-reacting antigens are used, and enzyme immunoassay kits are commercially available. However, the diagnosis of acute infection requires demonstration of seroconversion, which is usually not possible. The detection of specific IgG usually indicates past infection, but its absence does not exclude it. Low-level IgG antibody can result from previous infection with more invasive chlamydiae, including *C. pneumoniae*. This apparently explains the steady increase in the prevalence of low-level chlamydial antibody in children after the neonatal period. Nevertheless, tests for IgG are useful for seroepidemiologic studies.

The only circumstance in which serologic techniques are widely used for diagnosis is in neonatal pneumonia, in which the presence of specific IgM in a titer of more than 1:64 in the serum of an infant with pneumonia strongly suggests that *C. trachomatis* infection is the cause. Lower titers may be present in infants with infection confined to the conjunctivas or nasopharynx.[47]

Antibiotic Susceptibility and Management

C. trachomatis is susceptible to tetracycline, erythromycin, and rifampin (rifampicin). Reduced susceptibility to erythromycin has been reported, but its clinical significance is unknown. Tetracycline resistance has not been reported. Although it lacks a cell wall, *C. trachomatis* is inhibited by ampicillin in vitro and to some extent in vivo. Clindamycin, sulfonamides, chloramphenicol, and the fluoroquinolones have some activity, but the cephalosporins, aminoglycosides, metronidazole, and trimethoprim are inactive against *C. trachomatis* in vitro.[48]

Doxycycline, 200 mg daily for 7 days, is the treatment of choice for uncomplicated chlamydial infection in adults; treatment failure is rare if compliance is good. During pregnancy, erythromycin is used. Sexual partners should be investigated (if possible) and treated.[49] Neonatal chlamydial infection is treated with erythromycin (50 mg/kg/day) given orally for 2 weeks for conjunctivitis and at least 3 weeks for pneumonia. Topical antibiotic therapy (tetracycline or erythromycin) can be used as additional therapy for conjunctivitis but is inadequate alone. The parents of infants with chlamydial infection should be assumed to be infected, investigated, and treated accordingly.

Attempts to prevent neonatal chlamydial infection with topical eye preparations have had mixed results. Silver nitrate, which has been used extensively to prevent gonococcal ophthalmia, is not active against *C. trachomatis.* Early studies suggested that topical erythromycin could prevent chlamydial conjunctivitis, but it was subsequently shown to be ineffective,[50] presumably because it does not affect nasopharyngeal colonization.

C. PNEUMONIAE INFECTIONS

C. pneumoniae is a human pathogen that has been classified as a separate species on the bases of differences in EB ultrastructure and the fact that there is less than 10% DNA homology between it and the other *Chlamydia* species but at least 94% between strains of *C. pneumoniae* from several countries.[51] It is not clear how many different antigenic types exist, but there is probably more than one.[52]

Epidemiology

Seroepidemiologic studies suggest that infection with *C. pneumoniae* has been prevalent but unrecognized for many years. About 50% of adults in Western countries have serologic evidence of past infection. It is uncommon in preschool children, but seroprevalence rates increase 6% to 9% per annum in the 5- to 14-year age group, falling to about 2% per annum during adolescence and early adult life.[6,52] Most people are apparently infected during childhood, and infection in adults is usually reinfection. *C. pneumoniae* infection may be more common in developing countries and may contribute to life-threatening acute respiratory infection. The first reported isolate of *C. pneumoniae* (in Australia) was from an Aboriginal infant with otitis media,[53] and there is evidence of a high seroprevalence in Aboriginal children.

In the relatively short time since the discovery of *C. pneumoniae,* it has been recognized as a common cause of respiratory infection. Infection in children is usually asymptomatic, and the incidence and severity of symptomatic infection increase with age. In one study of community-acquired pneumonia in a defined population, *Mycoplasma pneumoniae* was implicated in 17% and *C. pneumoniae* in 10% of cases overall. *M. pneumoniae* pneumonia was most common in older children and required admission to the hospital in only 4.5% of cases, whereas *C. pneumoniae* pneumonia was more common in the elderly, and 11.4% of patients were admitted to the hospital.[51]

Infection also occurs sporadically and in epidemics at 2- to 3-year intervals. Epidemics have been reported among groups of young people, such as military recruits.[54] It is assumed that the organism is spread via the respiratory route with variable but relatively low efficiency by both symptomatic and asymptomatic carriers; the case-to-case interval is about 30 days.

Clinical Manifestations

The onset of symptomatic infection is usually subacute and the course protracted. Pharyngitis often precedes the onset of cough by several days, and fever occurs early but usually does not persist. The disease is similar to other types of atypical pneumonia. Clinical findings and chest radiographic changes are nonspecific. Sinus tenderness is often present, the peripheral blood white cell count is usually normal, and the erythrocyte sedimentation rate is elevated. The disease is generally mild in otherwise healthy individuals, but symptoms can be protracted, even with appropriate therapy. More severe and occasionally fatal disease can occur in the elderly. Possible complications include pericarditis, myocarditis, endocarditis, and erythema nodosum. Seroepidemiologic studies suggest a link with coronary artery disease and atherosclerosis; chlamydiae have been demonstrated in atheromatous plaques via immunocytochemical staining and polymerase chain reaction. The role of this agent in the pathogenesis of atherosclerosis requires further study.[6]

Laboratory Diagnosis

Laboratory diagnosis of *C. pneumoniae* is difficult. It grows relatively poorly in cell lines that support the growth of *C. trachomatis.* Culture is therefore not widely available and is at best successful in only 50% to 75% of cases in which there is serologic evidence of recent infection. Detection of *C. pneumoniae* in throat swabs can be increased by the use of polymerase chain reaction. However, the diagnosis usually depends on serologic testing. Microimmunofluorescence is the most sensitive and specific method. The diagnosis is made by the demonstration of seroconversion, a fourfold increase in the IgG titer, or the presence of IgM. Chlamydia complement fixing antibody can be detected in primary infection but often not during reinfections. It can be distinguished from *C. psittaci* antibody only by clinical and epidemiologic criteria.[51]

Treatment

C. pneumoniae is treated with tetracycline or erythromycin for 10 to 14 days. Treatment failures occur, especially with erythromycin; retreatment with tetracycline or doxycycline may succeed. New macrolide antibiotics such as roxithromycin, azithromycin or clarithromycin will probably replace erythromycin and may be more effective than tetracycline.[6]

C. PSITTACI INFECTIONS

C. psittaci is only an incidental human pathogen. It can infect most types of birds, causing effects varying from subclinical infection to rapidly fatal disease. It is responsible for a variety of diseases in domestic and wild animals, including feline pneumonitis, bovine and ovine abortion,[4] and genital and ocular infections in koalas. Most human infection results from contact with infected captive birds but has been described in poultry-processing plants or after contact with infected animals (e.g., aborting sheep).[12] There is wide variation in the incidence in different parts of the world. Most cases occur in adults, presumably because they are more likely to have close contact with birds, have more severe symptoms than children, or both reasons. In a large series of cases in Melbourne, the youngest patient was 17 years old.[55]

Pneumonia is the predominant clinical manifestation of psittacosis. The onset is usually abrupt; fever, rigors, and myalgia may precede the onset of respiratory symptoms by several days. Severe headache is common and may be the predominant symptom. In one series, lumbar puncture was performed in 33% of patients who were subsequently shown to have psittacosis; an elevated protein level in cerebrospinal fluid was found in nearly 50% of cases.[55] *C. psittaci* is more invasive than other chlamydiae, and rare cases of endocarditis have been reported.[56] Human abortion caused by *C. psittaci* after patient contact with aborting ewes has been described.[12,57] In one reported case, the diagnosis was confirmed by isolation of *C. psittaci* from the placenta and fetus; isolates were identical to ovine isolates by DNA fingerprinting.[58]

Diagnosis

C. psittaci is relatively easy to isolate in cell culture but is dangerous to handle, so culture should be attempted only in laboratories with appropriate containment facilities. The diagnosis of human psittacosis is usually made serologically by complement fixing texts, ideally by showing a fourfold or greater increase in titer between paired sera. A high titer (>1:128) in association with a compatible clinical illness and history of exposure suggests recent psittacosis. If possible, *C. pneumoniae* infection should be excluded by microimmunofluorescence testing.

Treatment

Tetracyclines are the agents of choice for treating psittacosis.[59] There is usually a prompt clinical response, but therapy should be continued for an additional 10 to 14 days to reduce the chance of relapse.[55]

CONCLUSION

Of the three species of chlamydiae, *C. trachomatis* is the most important. In developing countries, trachoma is the most common preventable cause of blindness; sexually transmissible genital and vertically transmissible neonatal infections are common worldwide and cause significant morbidity, especially infertility. A great deal is known of the molecular basis of pathogenicity and immune responses to chlamydiae, and the development of recombinant, subunit vaccines is in progress. Whether these vaccines will be able to induce protective immunity without damaging immunopathology remains to be seen.

REFERENCES

1. Thygeson P, Stone W: Epidemiology of inclusion conjunctivitis, *Arch Ophthalmol* 27:91-122, 1942.
2. Schachter J: Chlamydial infections, *N Engl J Med* 298:428-435, 490-495, 540-549, 1978.
3. Harris RL, Williams TW: "Contributions to the question of pneumotyphus": a discussion of the original article by J Ritter in 1880, *Rev Infect Dis* 7:119-122, 1985.
4. Schaffner W: *Chlamydia psittaci* (psittacosis). In Mandell GL, Douglas RG, Bennett JE, eds: *Principles and practice of infectious diseases,* ed 3, New York, 1990, Churchill Livingstone, pp 1440-1443
5. Grayston JT, Kuo CC, Wang SP, Altman J: A new *Chlamydia psittaci* strains called TWAR from acute respiratory tract infections, *N Engl J Med* 315:161-168, 1986.
6. Grayston JT: Infections caused by *Chlamydia pneumoniae* strain TWAR, *Clin Infect Dis* 15:757-763, 1992.

Microbiology and *Chlamydia*-Cell Interactions

7. Ward ME, Clark IN: New perspectives in chlamydial biology and development. In Bowie WR, Caldwell HD, Jones RP, Ridgway EL, Schachter J, Stamm E, Ward ME, eds: *Chlamydial infections. Proceedings of the Seventh International Symposium on Human Chlamydial Infections,* Cambridge, England, 1990, Cambridge University Press, pp 3-14.
8. Ward ME: The chlamydial developmental cycle. In Barron A, ed: *The microbiology of Chlamydia,* Boca Raton, Fla, 1988, CRC, pp 71-97.

***C. trachomatis* Infections**

9. Mabey DCW, Whittle HC: Genital and neonatal chlamydial infections in a trachoma-endemic area, *Lancet* 2:300-301, 1982.
10. Asche LV, Hutton SI: Serovars of *C. trachomatis* in northern Australia. In Bowie WR, Caldwell HD, Jones RP, Ridgway EL, Schachter J, Stamm E, Ward ME, eds: *Chlamydial infections. Proceedings of the Seventh International Symposium on Human Chlamydial Infections,* Cambridge, England, 1990, Cambridge University Press, pp 555-558.
11. Fraiz J, Jones RB: Chlamydial infections, *Ann Rev Med* 39:357-370, 1988.
12. Smith JR, Taylor-Robinson D: Infection due to *Chlamydia trachomatis* in pregnancy and the newborn, *Bailliere Clin Obstet Gynaecol* 7:237-255, 1993.
13. Kovacs GT, Westcott M, Rusden J, Asche V, King H, Haynes SE, Moore EK, Ketelbey JW: The prevalence of *Chlamydia trachomatis* in a young, sexually-active population, *Med J Aust* 147:550-552, 1987.
14. Packham D: Personal communication, 1995.
15. Douglas FP, Bidawid-Woodsoffe S, McDonnell J, Hyne SG, Mathews JD: Genital infection with *Chlamydia trachomatis* in Aboriginal women in Northern Australia. In Oriel D, Ridgway G, Schachter J, Taylor-Robinson D, Ward M, eds: *Chlamydial infections. Proceedings of the Sixth International Symposium on Human Chlamydial Infections,* Cambridge, England, 1986, Cambridge University Press, pp 237-240.
16. Laga M, Plummer FA, Nzanze H, Namarra W, Brunham RC, Ndinya-Achola JO, Maitha G, Ronald AR, D'Costa LJD, Bhullar VB, Mait JK, Fransen L, Cheang M, Piot P: Epidemiology of ophthalmia neonatorum in Kenya, *Lancet* 2:1145-1149, 1986.
17. Faro S: *Chlamydia trachomatis* infection in women, *J Reprod Med* 30(suppl 3):273-278, 1985.
18. Jones RB, Mammel JB, Shepard MK, Fisher RR: Recovery of *Chlamydia trachomatis* from the endometrium of women at risk for chlamydial infection, *Am J Obstet Gynecol* 155:35-39, 1986.
19. Stamm WE, Wagner KF, Ansel R, Alexander ER, Turck M, Counti CG, Holmes KK: Etiology of the acute urethral syndrome in women, *N Engl J Med* 303:409-415, 1980.
20. Gilbert GL, Weisberg E: Infertility as an infectious disease: epidemiology and prevention, *Bailliere Clin Obstet Gynaecol* 7:159-182, 1993.
21. Harrison HR, Alexander ER, Weinstein L, Lewis M, Nash M, Sim DA: Cervical *Chlamydia trachomatis* and mycoplasmal infections in pregnancy, *JAMA* 250:1721-1727, 1983.

22. Gravett MG, Nelson P, Critchlow C, Eschenbach DA, Holmes KK: Independent associations of bacterial vaginosis and *Chlamydia trachomatis* infection with adverse pregnancy outcome, *JAMA* 256:1899-1903, 1986.
23. Ryan GM, Abdella TN, McNeeley SG, Baselski VS, Drummond DE: *Chlamydia trachomatis* infection in pregnancy and effect of treatment on outcome, *Am J Obstet Gynecol* 162:34-39, 1990.
24. Sweet RL, Landers DV, Walker C, Schachten J: *Chlamydia trachomatis* infection and pregnancy outcome, *Am J Obstet Gynecol* 156:824-833, 1987.
25. Thorp JM, Katz VL, Fowler LJ, Kurtzmann JT, Bowes WA: Fetal death from chlamydial infection across intact amniotic membranes, *Am J Obstet Gynecol* 161:1245-1247, 1989.
26. Givner LB, Rennels MB, Woodward CL, Huang S-W: *Chlamydia trachomatis* infection in an infant delivered by Caesarean section, *Pediatrics* 68:420-421, 1981.
27. Märdh P-A, Johansson PJH, Svenningsen N: Intrauterine lung infection with *Chlamydia trachomatis* in a premature infant, *Acta Paediatr Scand* 73:569-572, 1984.
28. Attenburrow AA, Barker CM: Chlamydial pneumonia in the low birth weight infant, *Arch Dis Child* 60:1169-1171, 1985.
29. Gilbert GL: Gonococcal and chlamydial infections. In Gilbert GL: *Infectious disease in pregnancy and the newborn infant*, Amsterdam, 1992, Harwood Academic, pp 241-271.
30. Schachter J, Grossman M, Sweet RL, Hold J, Jordan C, Bishop E: Prospective study of perinatal transmission of *Chlamydia trachomatis, JAMA* 255:3374-3377, 1986.
31. Sandstrom KI, Bell TA, Chandler JW, Kuo C-C, Wang S-P, Grayston TT, Foy HM, Stamm WE, Cooney MK, Smith AL, Holmes KK: Microbial cause of neonatal conjunctivitis, *J Pediatr* 105:706-711, 1984.
32. Schaefer C, Harrison HR, Boyce WT, Laois M: Illness in infants born to women with *Chlamydia trachomatis* infection, *Am J Dis Child* 139:127-133, 1985.
33. Botszejn A: Die pertussoide, eosinophile Pneumoniaw des Sauglings, *Ann Pediatr (Basel)* 157:28-46, 1941.
34. Beem MO, Saxon EM: Respiratory tract colonization and a distinctive pneumonia syndrome in infants with *Chlamydia trachomatis, N Engl J Med* 296:306-310, 1977.
35. Sagy M, Barzilay Z, Yahav J, Ginsberg R, Sompolinsky D: Severe neonatal chlamydial pneumonia, *Am J Dis Child* 134:89-91, 1980.
36. Stagno S, Brasfield DM, Brown MB, Cassell GH, Pifer LL, Whitley RJ, Tiller RE: Infant pneumonitis associated with cytomegalovirus, *Chlamydia, Pneumocystis* and *Ureaplasma:* a prospective study, *Pediatrics* 68:322-329, 1981.
37. Brayden RM, Paisley JW, Lauer BA: Apnoea in infants with *Chlamydia trachomatis* pneumonia, *Pediatr Infect Dis J* 6:423-425, 1987.
38. Weiss SG, Newcomb RW, Beem MO: Pulmonary assessment of children after chlamydial pneumonia in infancy, *J Pediatr* 108:659-664, 1986.
39. Griffin M, Pushpanathan C, Andrews W: *Chlamydia trachomatis* pneumonitis: a case study and literature review, *Pediatr Pathol* 10:843-852, 1990.
40. Grayston JT, Wang S-P, Yeh L-J, Kuo C-C: Importance of reinfection in the pathogenesis of trachoma, *Rev Infect Dis* 7:717-725, 1985.
41. Patton DL: Immunology and histopathology of experimental chlamydial salpingitis, *Rev Infect Dis* 7:745-753, 1985.
42. Patton DL, Wolner-Hanssen P, Cosgrove ST, Holmes KK: The effects of *Chlamydia trachomatis* on the female reproductive tract of the *Macaca nemestrina* after a single tubal challenge following repeated cervical inoculations, *Obstet Gynecol* 76:643-650, 1990.
43. Morrison RP: Immune responses to *Chlamydia* are protective and pathogenic. In Bowie WR, Caldwell HD, Jones RP, Ridgway EL, Schachter J, Stamm E, Ward ME, eds: *Chlamydial infections. Proceedings of the Seventh International Symposium on Human Chlamydial Infections,* Cambridge, England, 1990, Cambridge University Press, pp 163-172.
44. Zhong G, Brunham RC: Antibody responses to the chlamydial heat shock proteins hsp60 and hsp70 are H-2 linked, *Infect Immun* 60:3143-3149, 1992.
45. Taylor-Robinson D, Thomas BJ: Laboratory techniques for the diagnosis of chlamydial infection, *Genitourin Med* 67:256-266, 1991.
46. Jaschek G, Gaydos CA, Welsh LE, Quinn TC: Direct detection of *Chlamydia trachomatis* in urine specimens from symptomatic and asymptomatic men by using a rapid polymerase chain reaction assay, *J Clin Microbiol* 31:1209-1212, 1993.
47. Mahoney JB, Chernesky MA, Bromberg K, Schachter J: Accuracy of immunoglobulin M immunoassay for diagnosis of chlamydial infection in infants and adults, *J Clin Microbiol* 24:731-735, 1986.
48. Gilbert GL: Treatment of chlamydial and mycoplasmal infections, *Med J Aust* 146:205-258, 1987.
49. Bell TA, Grayston JT: Centers for Disease Control guidelines for prevention and control of *Chlamydial trachomatis* infections, *Ann Intern Med* 104:524-532, 1986.
50. Hammerschlag MR, Cummings C, Roblin PM, Williams TH, Delke I: Efficacy of neonatal ocular prophylaxis for the prevention of gonococcal and chlamydial conjunctivitis, *N Engl J Med* 320:769-772, 1989.

C. Pneumoniae Infections

51. Grayston JT: *Chlamydia pneumoniae,* strain TWAR, *Chest* 95:664-669, 1989.
52. Black CM, Johnson JE, Farshy CE, Brown TM, Berdal BP: Antigenic variation among strains of *Chlamydia pneumoniae, J Clin Microbiol* 29:1312-1316, 1991.
53. Hutton S, Dodd H, Asche V: *C. pneumoniae* successfully isolated, *Todays Life Sci* 2:42-43, 1993.
54. Kleemola M, Saikku P, Visakorpi R, Wang S-P, Grayston JT: Epidemics of pneumonia caused by TWAR, a new *Chlamydia* organism, in military trainees in Finland, *J Infect Dis* 157:230-236, 1988.

C. Psittaci Infections

55. Yung AP, Grayson ML: Psittacosis: a review of 135 cases, *Med J Aust* 148:228-233, 1988.
56. Ettienne J, Ory D, Thourenot D, Eb F, Raoult D, Loire R, Delahaye JP, Beaune J: Chlamydial endocarditis: a report on ten cases, *Eur Heart J* 13:1422-1426, 1992.
57. Johnson FWA, Matheson BA, Williams H, Laing AG, Jandial V, Davidson-Lamb R, Halliday GJ, Hobson D, Wong SY, Hadley KM, Moffat MAJ, Postlethwaite R: Abortion due to *Chlamydia psittaci* in a sheep farmer's wife, *Br Med J* 290:592-594, 1985.
58. Herring AJ, Anderson IE, McLenaghan M, Inglis NF, Williams H, Matheson BA, West CP: Restriction endonuclease analysis of DNA from two isolated of *Chlamydia psittaci* obtained from human abortions, *Br Med J* 295:1239, 1987.
59. Yung AP, Newton-John HF, Stanley PA: Atypical pneumonia: recognition and treatment, *Med J Aust* 147:132-136, 1987.

CHAPTER 46

Other Fungal Infections

Behnoosh Afghani and Melvin I. Marks

COCCIDIOIDOMYCOSIS

Coccidioides immitis, the etiologic agent of coccidioidomycosis, is a dimorphic fungus that usually produces a self-limited pulmonary infection in otherwise healthy people. Some 60% of infections are asymptomatic, and about 40% of patients develop an influenza-like illness. Extrathoracic dissemination is common in infants or immunocompromised patients and rare in normal hosts.[1] Because of its variable clinical course, coccidioidomycosis presents a challenge in diagnosis and treatment.

The disease was first described in Argentina in 1892. It was known as *Coccidia,* a form of skin tumor. Years later, in 1936, primary and secondary forms of the disease were described. The primary form has been known as *San Joaquin* or *valley fever.*[2]

Coccidioidomycosis is endemic to the southwestern United States. However, increased numbers of cases have been reported in nonendemic areas.[3]

Microbiology

Coccidioides immitis is a dimorphic fungus that exists as a mycelium in nature or the laboratory environment and as a spherule containing endospores in host tissues at 37° C. This appears to be an adaptation of the organism to the elevated temperatures of the host tissues or a response to the host immune cells.

In culture, *C. immitis* produces white to tan-brown colonies at 25° C. Purple and black colonies have also been reported. After about 1 week, the mycelia fragment into arthroconidia (Fig. 46-1). In the laboratory, extreme caution should be used when cultures of suspected *C. immitis* are handled because this fungus is one of the most infectious. At 37° to 40° C, it begins its parasitic life cycle, producing spherules. These round structures measure 20 to 200 μm in diameter.[4] On rupture, they can release up to 10^5 endospores into the surrounding tissues (Fig. 46-2).

Tissue histopathologic features are characterized by caseating necrosis and a granulomatous reaction. Spherules can be identified freely or within macrophages.

Disease Mechanisms

A history of dust exposure in endemic areas is of particular significance. During windstorms, construction work, or farming, the arthroconidia break from the parent mycelium in the soil and become airborne. Because of the ease that an arthroconidia can become airborne, they pose a great danger to laboratory personnel. Even a single fungal spore and brief exposure can result in an infection. When arthroconidia are inhaled, primary pulmonary infection occurs. In most healthy people, infection remains confined to the respiratory tract. However, in immunocompromised patients and rarely in healthy people, extrapulmonary dissemination can occur. As the spherule grows in the lung, it becomes filled with endospores, and a polymorphonuclear reaction occurs around it. This is probably mediated via chemotactic factors and complement activation. There is some evidence that virulence of *C. immitis* might be linked to the proteinases that it produces. These enzymes may be responsible for the rupture of spherules, leading to the release of endospores.[5] Disease is self-limited in people with good T cell responses and progressive in those with poor lymphocyte reactivity.[6]

Epidemiology

C. immitis naturally occurs in the soil and air of the southwestern United States, Central America, Argentina, and parts of northwestern Mexico. The climate in these areas is arid to semiarid with low annual rainfalls. In the United States, where 50,000 people are infected annually, the disease is endemic in certain parts of Arizona, California, Nevada, New Mexico, Texas, and Utah. In California, there has been a threefold to tenfold increase in the number of cases in 1991 and 1992 compared to 1990 (Fig. 46-3). It is postulated that weather changes—the prolonged drought followed by heavy rains—may be responsible.[3] Recently, an outbreak of coccidioidomycosis was reported in California after the Northridge earthquake.[7] Sporadic, nonendemic cases are reported each year as a result of travel through endemic areas, inhalation of contaminated fomites, or laboratory exposure.

The incubation period is 7 to 21 days depending on the quantity of arthroconidia inhaled. In patients infected with the human immunodeficiency virus (HIV), reactivation of primary infection can occur months to years later.[8]

Estimates based on repeated skin testing indicate that the annual risk of infection in endemic areas is about 3%. Although primary coccidioidomycosis affects all age groups and races equally, the probability of dissemination is higher in certain groups. These include the very young and very old, Filipinos, Hispanics, and blacks. Immunocompromised patients and women in the last trimester of pregnancy are also at higher risk of developing disseminated disease.[7] No special isolation precautions are recommended for a person with coccidioidomycosis. The spherule form of the fungus has very low rate of infectivity, and the infective arthroconidia are generally not expelled in high numbers, even in patients with cavitary disease.[9]

Clinical Manifestations

Pulmonary

About 60% of children develop an influenza-like illness with headache, fever, and cough. More than 90% of such infections

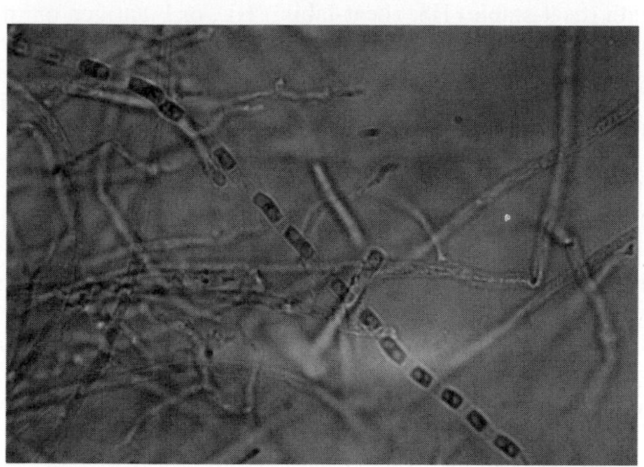

Figure 46-1. Mycelial form of *C. immitis* showing arthroconidia at 25° C. (×400.)

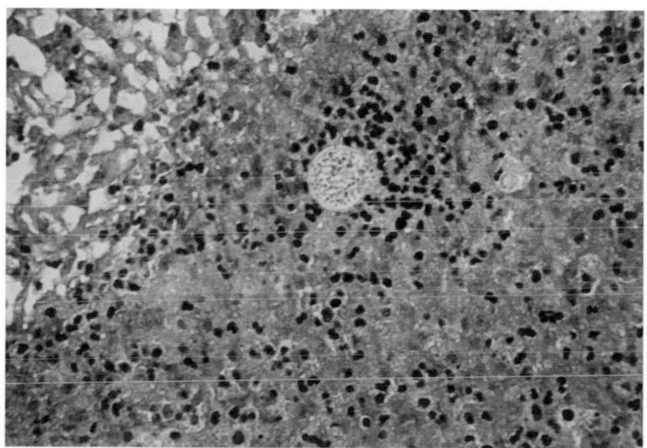

Figure 46-2. Tissue form of *C. immitis* showing a spherule filled with endospores. (×100.)

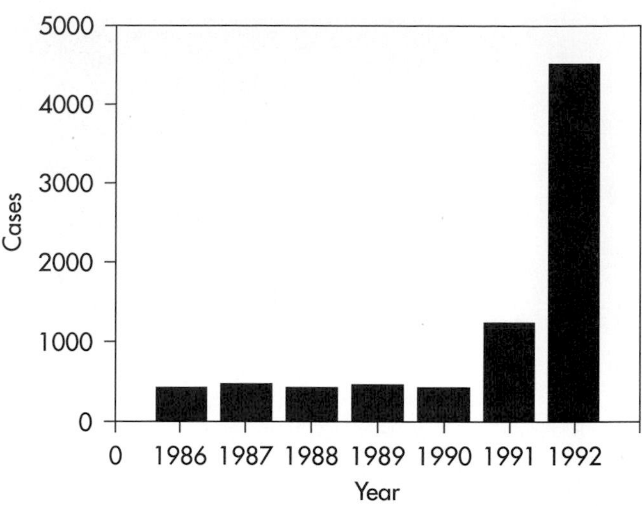

Figure 46-3. Reported cases of coccidioidomycosis by year in California from 1986 to 1992. (From *MMWR* 42(2):21-24, 1993.)

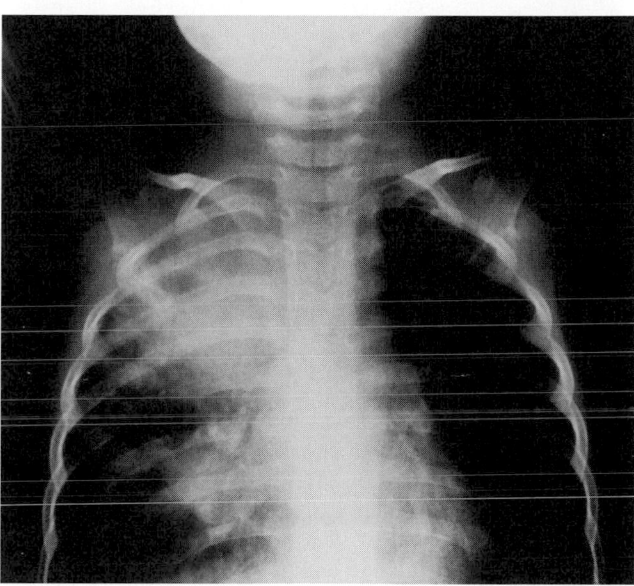

Figure 46-4. Chest radiograph of a 4-year-old girl with disseminated coccidioidomycosis.

resolve spontaneously. In infants, coccidioidomycosis can present as stridor because of involvement of the subglottic area. Chest pain can occur; however, hemoptysis with cavitary coccidioidomycosis is rare in children. Although dissemination or severe pulmonary disease is seen mostly in immunocompromised patients, there has been reports of severe respiratory disease leading to respiratory failure in immunocompetent children.[10]

In patients with acute pulmonary infections, lobar or segmental consolidation is frequent (Fig. 46-4). Hilar and mediastinal adenopathy may be present in 20% of cases; cavities are rare in children. They have distinctive thin walls, and in more than half of patients, these close spontaneously within 2 years. Rarely, however, they can rupture and produce a pyopneumothorax. Approximately 5% of adults and older children with pulmonary disease are left with chronic residual lesions such as nodules, calcifications, adenopathy, cavities, fibrosis, and bronchiectasis. In about 0.5% of cases the disease spreads beyond the respiratory tract. The chest radiograph in these fungemic cases demonstrates a miliary or reticuloendothelial pattern and mediastinal adenopathy.[11]

Extrapulmonary

Dissemination in immunocompetent children is rare; however, a few cases in infants have been reported (Fig. 46-5). Most of these infants acquired the infection after birth.[12] Although coccidioidomycosis can be severe later in pregnancy, vertical transmission is very rare.[13] Few cases of perinatal transmission have been reported. In these cases, the mother had cervical and endometrial involvement.[14]

The most common site of dissemination is the skin, where verrucous, papular, and nodular lesions occur. These can form sinuses and abscesses. The next frequent site of spread is the skeletal system. The bones most commonly involved are the vertebrae, skull, ribs, and long bones. Joint arthritis occurs most frequently in the knees, ankles, and elbows. Meningitis is the most serious form of disseminated coccidioidomycosis; although transient remissions occur, it is fatal if not treated.

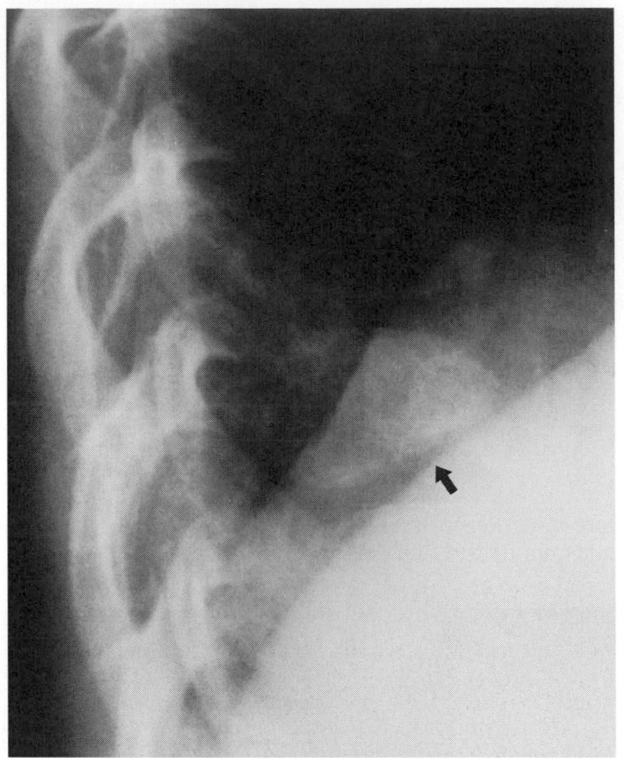

Figure 46-5. Disseminated coccidioidomycosis in a 4-year-old girl involving the T11 vertebra *(arrow).*

Diagnosis

Clinical Observation

A history of travel to endemic areas is helpful in establishing the diagnosis. However, cases of fomite transmission have been reported in nonendemic areas. A travel history in HIV patients years before active disease might be of significance because in these patients there can be a reactivation of prior dormant infection.[1] Laboratory data associated but nonspecific for coccidioidomycosis include leukocytosis, an increased erythrocyte sedimentation rate, and eosinophilia.

Skin Test

The skin test is performed by intradermal injection of either 2.8 μg of spherulin, the mycelial phase, or a 1:100 dilution of coccidioidin, the mycelial phase. Spherulin appears to be more sensitive in diagnosing infection. A transverse diameter of more than 5 mm of induration is considered positive. Skin testing is not very helpful in the diagnosis of acute disease because a positive skin test does not differentiate between an acute and a remote infection and because a negative skin test does not rule out disease.

Culture

Demonstration of *C. immitis* in tissues indicates infection. Stains most commonly used are periodic acid–Schiff and methenamine silver. If they become airborne, cultures of *C. immitis* pose a risk to laboratory personnel. When *C. immitis* cultures are being handled, all laboratory activities should be performed at biosafety level three. Final identification is based on demonstration of the spherule phase by animal inoculation, by deoxyribonucleic acid (DNA) probe, or by use of the exoantigen test. With this test a positive precipitin band with (heat-stable) HS, (heat-labile) HL, or F antigen on immunodiffusion agar plate confirms the diagnosis. In vitro conversion of *C. immitis* is of little use and is not recommended.[4] DNA probes have been developed for the rapid diagnosis of coccidioidomycosis.[15]

Serology

Serologic testing provides a rapid means of diagnosing coccidioidomycosis because isolation of the organism can be difficult and final identification can take up to several weeks. The serologic tests routinely used are tube precipitin, complement fixation, and double diffusion. Precipitating antibody detected by the tube precipitin test is of the immunoglobulin M (IgM) type and usually indicates acute infection. It appears between the first and second week after the start of clinical symptoms and lasts 3 to 4 months.[16]

Complement fixation and double diffusion tests use a heat-labile antigen isolated from the spherule phase of *C. immitis.* The antibody measured is primarily IgG. Usually, these antibodies are detected 1 to 2 months after the infection.[16] The correlation between the results of complement fixation and those of the immunodiffusion test is greater than 95%. They both provide diagnostic and prognostic information. Titers greater than 1:16 by complement fixation are associated with severe pulmonary disease or dissemination. There have been reports of negative tests in HIV patients with dissemination.[17] Low or negative titers in immunocompromised patients should be interpreted with caution.

New diagnostic serologic tests, such as circulating antigen and antibody detection by enzyme-linked immunosorbent assay, are under evaluation. These methods might provide more sensitive means of diagnosing coccidioidomycosis in the immunocompromised host or of diagnosing early disease.[18,19]

Management

Primary coccidioidomycosis usually resolves spontaneously in healthy children and adults. Hence there are no studies on antifungal treatment and the prevention of late complications. Patients who might benefit from treatment are those in whom symptoms persist for several weeks and those who have disseminated disease or are at high risk for dissemination. Treatment is also indicated for patients with enlarging or spreading infiltrates.

Cure rates with different antifungal medications are difficult to evaluate because the criteria used for improvement by different investigators have varied. Because of extended experience with amphotericin B, it is the medication of choice for the treatment of pulmonary coccidioidomycosis. The role of azoles has been explored because they are well tolerated and are easy to administer.[20,21] In adults, itraconazole, 100 to 400 mg/day for the treatment of pulmonary and extrapulmonary coccidioidomycosis, has been associated with response rates of 60% to 70%, and the relapse rate of 15% to 20% is similar to that of amphotericin B. Ketoconazole and fluconazole have been associated with relapse rates of 30% to 50%.22 Itraconazole, 100 to 400 mg/kg, is less toxic than amphotericin B. At higher doses (400 to 800 mg/day), however, itraconazole was less well tolerated and was associated with edema, hypertension, and elevated liver enzymes.[20] Fluconazole might have a role in the treatment of coccidioidal meningitis because of its high penetration of cerebrospinal fluid. The use of imidazoles in pediatric patients is limited, and no dosage recommendations have yet been established.

Another medication under investigation is liposomal amphotericin B, which is a form of amphotericin B encapsulated in unilamellar membranes. Although it is feasible that this medication can be given at much higher doses with fewer toxicities compared to free amphotericin B, controlled trials comparing the toxicity and efficacy of the two medications have not been completed.

Because of lack of comparative studies, there are no definite guidelines for the treatment of coccidioidomycosis. Amphotericin B, 1 mg/kg/day, should be used initially for severe or progressive disease to ensure absorption through the parenteral route and rapid onset of action. It can be used for a few weeks until the infection is stabilized. This can be followed by an oral azole (fluconazole or itraconazole) for 4 to 8 months after the stabilization of infection. It is reasonable to continue suppressive therapy with fluconazole or itraconazole for immunocompromised patients for lifetime. However, suppressive therapy with oral azoles has not been 100% effective in preventing relapses, and its cost-effectiveness needs further evaluation.

Surgical intervention may be required for symptomatic patients with persistent cavities or with parapneumonic processes.

HISTOPLASMOSIS

Histoplasmosis is the most common mycosis in the United States, although only a small number of individuals infected with *Histoplasma capsulatum* become symptomatic. Infants with immature immune systems and immunocompromised patients are among those most likely to develop disseminated histoplasmosis.

H. capsulatum was first described by Samuel Darling in 1906 at the autopsy of a patient with disseminated disease.[23] For many years, histoplasmosis was described as a rare and uniformly fatal disease. In 1946, it was demonstrated that a large number of pulmonary calcifications resulted from infection with *H. capsulatum*.[24]

Epidemiology

Histoplasmosis is endemic to the midwestern United States, particularly the Ohio and Mississippi Valleys. Outbreaks have been reported in pigeon or chicken breeders, explorers of caves with bats, and in populations living close to construction that causes the fungus to become airborne. Multiple outbreaks of histoplasmosis have occurred in Indianapolis since 1978. In the most recent outbreak in 1988, 50% of culture-positive cases were in patients with acquired immunodeficiency syndrome (AIDS).[25] Although construction had recently occurred in these areas, no fungus was isolated from the soil, and the cause of these outbreaks remains undetermined.

In recent years, cases of histoplasmosis have also been reported in nonendemic areas such as Minnesota, New York, and California. Most of these cases were in patients with AIDS.

The natural habitat of *H. capsulatum* is soil, particularly that contaminated by bat or bird droppings, which creates an environment of high nitrogen content. Infection occurs by the inhalation of spores. The incubation period is variable but is usually no more than a few weeks from exposure. Person-to-person or animal to person transmission does not occur, and no isolation precautions are needed.

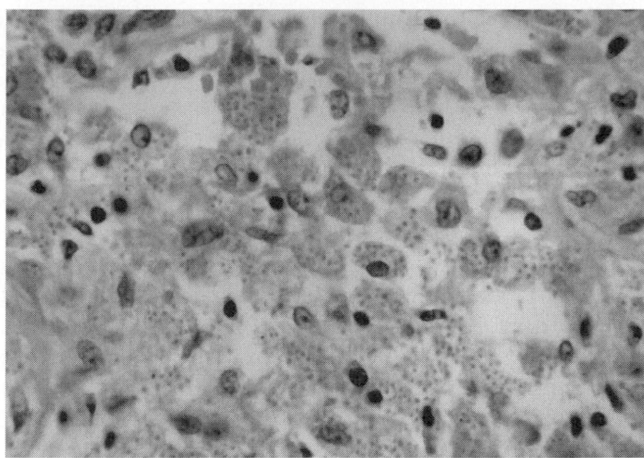

Figure 46-6. Tissue form of *H. capsulatum* at 37° C. (×100.)

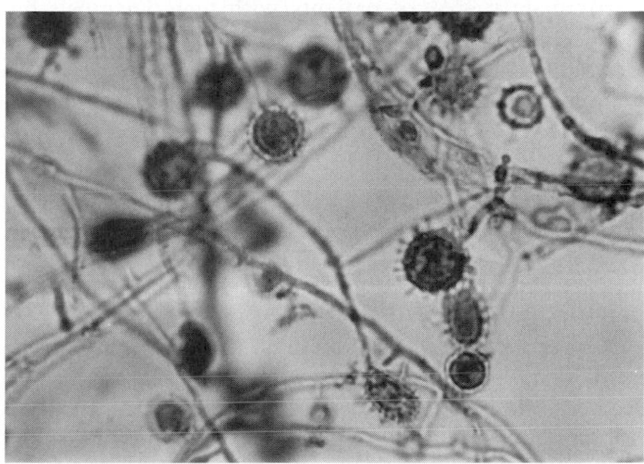

Figure 46-7. Tuberculate macroconidia of *H. capsulatum*. (×400.)

Microbiology

H. capsulatum is a dimorphic fungus that exists in mycelial form in the environment at 25° C and in yeast form in tissues at 37° C (Fig. 46-6). The organism is slow growing, requiring 2 to 4 weeks for colonies to appear. However, isolates have been identified in less than 7 days when a large number of infecting cells have been present. Most isolates initially appear as pinkish, and with age, they turn mycelial and buff to brownish.

The hyphae are 1 to 2 μm in diameter with characteristic macroconidia and microconidia. The tuberculate macroconidia are spherical with spikelike projections and measure 8 to 14 μm in diameter (Fig. 46-7). The yeast forms measure 2 to 5 μm and are found in mononuclear cells.[4]

Disease Mechanisms

Once the microconidia or mycelial fragments of *H. capsulatum* are inhaled, they undergo transition to a yeast phase in the lower respiratory tract. The ability of the organism to cause clinical symptoms depends on the host's immune status and the size of the inhaled inoculum. T cell immunity plays an important role in this process.[26] Decreased lymphocyte activity or numbers can enhance dissemination in immunocompromised patients. T cell activity develops 10 to 21 days after infection. The number of T-suppressor cells decreases, whereas the number of T-helper cells rises at this time, resulting in a delayed-type hypersensitivity reaction. *H. capsulatum* yeast cells are phagocytosed by human macrophages, but killing does not occur. The yeast cells replicate inside macrophages and spread via the lymphatic or hematogenous route. New foci of infection develop at these sites. These lesions eventually develop caseating necrosis or heal with fibrosis and calcification.

Grocott-Gomori methenamine–silver nitrate and periodic acid–Schiff stains are the most useful in visualizing *Histoplasma* organisms in tissues. Areas of caseous necrosis with a surrounding fibrous capsule that prevents the spread of the organism are characteristic. *H. capsulatum* may also be seen in tissues inside macrophages.

Clinical Manifestations

Approximately 95% of patients with histoplasmosis have asymptomatic disease. Symptoms develop in 50% to 100% of individuals after heavy inoculum exposure. Some 80% of symptomatic patients develop an influenza-like syndrome with headache, fever, and cough. Another 10% to 20% of patients with symptomatic disease develop pericarditis, arthritis, or erythema nodosum. These are usually self-limited manifestations and resolve after a few weeks without antifungal therapy.

Chest radiography in acute pulmonary histoplasmosis is characterized by enlarged hilar or mediastinal lymph nodes and lobar infiltrates. Pulmonary effusion occurs in about 10% of adults and less than 5% of children with acute histoplasmosis.[27] Chronic histoplasmosis resembles chronic tuberculosis. Calcified lesions, fibrosis, cavitation, and nodules usually develop in patients with chronic obstructive lung disease or in immunocompromised patients. Other complications of chronic histoplasmosis include mediastinal granuloma and fibrosing mediastinitis. These patients have superior vena caval, tracheobronchial, or esophageal obstruction. Pulmonary artery obstruction is rare but has the worst prognosis; these patients usually die of chronic pulmonary hypertension.[28]

Progressive dissemination or cavitary disease develops after heavy exposure to *H. capsulatum* in about 1 of 2000 infected individuals. Risk factors for dissemination include an old and a very young age, chronic debilitating disease, and impaired cellular immunity. The incidence of dissemination in patients with AIDS is 5% to 10% in endemic areas.[29] Active disease can develop shortly after primary infection or years later as a result of reactivation.

Patients with disseminated histoplasmosis usually have prolonged fever, malaise, cough, and weight loss. Hepatosplenomegaly is found in 30% of adults and 89% of infants.[30] Patients may have disseminated intravascular coagulation, adult respiratory distress syndrome, renal failure, endocarditis, or Addison's disease.[28] Thrombocytopenia and bone marrow suppression that leads to anemia are common laboratory findings. Chest radiographs are characterized by lobar or diffuse infiltrates, cavitation, hilar adenopathy, or any combination thereof. However, 40% to 50% of immunocompromised patients with disseminated histoplasmosis have been reported to have a normal chest radiograph.[29,30]

Diagnosis

Isolation of *H. capsulatum* on culture is the most definitive method for diagnosis. However, an incubation period of 2 to 4 weeks is required before the organism is identified. Moreover, cultures of sputum are positive in only two thirds of patients with cavitary disease and in less than one third of patients with chronic or noncavitary disease.[28] Blood and bone marrow specimens are especially useful for the diagnosis of disseminated histoplasmosis. Examination of the peripheral blood smear, especially the buffy coat, using Grocott-Gomori methenamine–silver nitrate stain yields positive findings in more than 50% of cases of disseminated histoplasmosis. Bone marrow and blood cultures done by lysis centrifugation are positive in 80% to 90% of AIDS patients with disseminated histoplasmosis.[29,31]

An in vitro conversion of mold to a yeast form or an exoantigen test establishes the final diagnosis. The exoantigen test relies on the presence of mycelial antigens obtained from cultured isolates that react with serum known to contain antibodies directed against *H. capsulatum.* The presence of an H or M precipitin band (or both) on immunodiffusion agar plate confirms the diagnosis. DNA probes on clinical isolates are also being used by many centers to confirm the diagnosis.[32]

Immunodiffusion and complement fixation are the most commonly used methods for serologic diagnosis (Fig. 46-8). About 1% to 3% of residents from endemic areas are seropositive for histoplasmosis. These people usually have borderline titers of 1:8 to 1:16 by complement fixation. Serologic tests are positive in 90% of patients with symptomatic disease. The complement fixation and immunodiffusion tests become positive at 4 to 6 weeks and peak 2 to 3 months after infection. They decline over a 2- to 5-year period.[25] The sensitivity of serologic testing is increased by performing both complement fixation and immunodiffusion. Although complement fixation is more sensitive than immunodiffusion, especially early in disease, the immunodiffusion test remains positive longer and is more specific than complement fixation. Complement fixation titers of greater than 1:8 and fourfold increases in the titer provide the best evidence of acute infection. However, the height of the titer does not correlate with the severity of infection. Immunocompromised patients with disseminated disease may in particular have low or negative titers. There are other pitfalls of serologic tests. False-positive results occur in patients with other diseases, such as blastomycosis, coccidioidomycosis, paracoccidioidomycosis, and tuberculosis.[33] Moreover, patients with a past history of histoplasmosis who have other illnesses may also have borderline titers.[25]

Skin testing is not helpful in the diagnosis of acute infection because the skin test is positive in 80% to 90% of people without evidence of active disease in endemic areas. Conversely, up to 50% of immunocompromised patients with disseminated disease have negative skin test results. In addition, administration of the histoplasmin skin test can falsely elevate antibody titers in 15% to 25% of patients.[34] False-positive skin tests have been seen with blastomycosis and coccidioidomycosis.

H. capsulatum antigen detection by radioimmunoassay provides a rapid means of diagnosing histoplasmosis. Antigen appears 2 to 3 weeks after exposure,[35] and hemagglutinin can be found in the urine or blood of 50% to 80% of patients with disseminated histoplasmosis and in the bronchoalveolar lavage fluid of 70% of AIDS patients with pulmonary histoplasmosis.[36] False-positive results have been reported in patients with blastomycosis, paracoccidioidomycosis, and coccidioidomycosis. Hemagglutinin levels decline in response to treatment and may provide a useful tool for the follow-up of patients with histoplasmosis.[37]

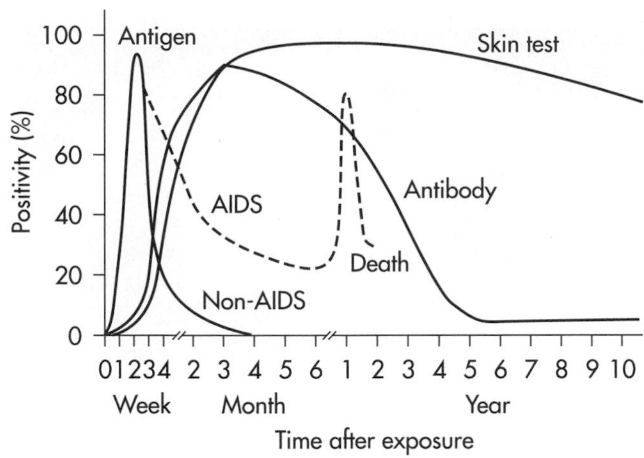

Figure 46-8. Time course of serologic and skin test findings for the diagnosis of histoplasmosis. (From Wheat LJ: *Eur J Clin Microbiol Infect Dis* 8:480-490, 1989.)

Management

In a majority of individuals with pulmonary histoplasmosis, the disease is self-limited, and therapy is not required. No controlled trials have been performed to evaluate the effect of antifungal therapy on the course of disease for patients with nonprogressive pulmonary disease. Pericarditis and rheumatologic manifestations typically do not require therapy because they are probably caused by an immune reaction to *H. capsulatum* infection. Treatment is recommended for patients with progressive pulmonary disease, dissemination, symptoms persisting more than 2 to 4 weeks, and acute pulmonary disease complicated with adult respiratory distress syndrome or obstruction.

The mainstay of therapy for progressive disease is amphotericin B at a minimum total dose of 30 mg/kg.[38] Shorter durations of therapy have been associated with higher relapse rates. Because of high relapse rates in AIDS patients with disseminated histoplasmosis, an initial induction treatment of amphotericin B, 15 mg/kg, total dose, followed by weekly or biweekly suppressive treatment, 1 to 1.5 mg/kg/dose for an indefinite period, has been used. This regimen has been successful in preventing relapses in about 90% of patients.[30] A recent trial using itraconazole, 200 mg twice daily, as suppressive therapy was also safe and effective in preventing relapses in adults with AIDS.[39]

Several studies have been done using ketoconazole, another imidazole, for the treatment of histoplasmosis. Ketoconazole has been associated with response rates of 44% to 92% in immunocompetent patients with pulmonary histoplasmosis. A daily dose of 400 mg was better tolerated than a daily dose of 800 mg and was associated with better response rates. Higher response rates were also seen in the group receiving therapy for more than 6 months.[40] The recommended dosage for pediatric patients is up to 6 mg/kg/day. The rate of response to ketoconazole is slower than that of amphotericin B, and its efficacy is limited in immunocompromised patients.[40,41] Suppressive therapy with ketoconazole has been associated with relapse rates of 40% to 50%. Ketoconazole should be used with caution in patients receiving H_2 blockers because its absorption is decreased in the achlorhydric state. Ketoconazole also interferes with the metabolism of other medications used concomitantly, such as isoniazid, rifampin, phenytoin, and cyclosporine. Rifampin and phenytoin can markedly reduce ketoconazole levels.

Fluconazole is efficacious in a murine model of histoplasmosis[42]; however, studies in humans are still in progress. Itraconazole, a newer triazole antifungal, shows more activity in vitro than ketoconazole against *H. capsulatum.* In a study of patients with nonmeningeal, non–life-threatening histoplasmosis, success was documented in 81% of patients treated with 200 to 400 mg daily, and there was minimal toxicity. Treatment failure was seen in a few patients with chronic cavitary pulmonary disease.[43] Other studies have reported a response rate of 90% in patients with pulmonary or disseminated histoplasmosis treated with itraconazole.[44,45] The efficacy of itraconazole is comparable to that of amphotericin B with less toxicity, although the data on itraconazole therapy are limited in immunocompromised patients, those with chronic cavitary pulmonary disease, and those with central nervous system involvement.

Liposomal amphotericin may have a promising role because it delivers higher doses of amphotericin B with less toxicity. However, studies on its efficacy have not been completed.

Amphotericin B, at a total minimum dosage of 30 mg/kg, should be used in patients with life-threatening, progressive disease or those with chronic cavitary histoplasmosis. In immunocompromised patients with disseminated histoplasmosis, initial induction therapy should be used until the disease is stabilized. This can be followed by indefinite weekly or biweekly suppressive treatment with amphotericin B or itraconazole. Trials with fluconazole suppressive therapy in patients with AIDS are in progress. It is reasonable to use itraconazole or ketoconazole as primary therapy in immunocompetent patients with mild disease for 3 to 6 months. Itraconazole appears to be better tolerated than ketoconazole. The role of fluconazole has not been established in patients with histoplasmosis.

Corticosteroids may be helpful with antifungal therapy in patients with pulmonary histoplasmosis complicated by obstruction or adult respiratory distress syndrome.[46,47]

PULMONARY ASPERGILLOSIS

Pulmonary aspergillosis is manifested by aspergillomas, allergic bronchopulmonary aspergillosis, and invasive pulmonary aspergillosis. Invasive pulmonary aspergillosis has become a major cause of morbidity and mortality in patients with hematologic malignancies and those undergoing organ transplantation.

More than 250 species of *Aspergillus* have been recognized. Most infections are caused by *A. fumigatus* and *A. flavus. A. terreus* and *A. niger* are also emerging as significant pathogens in immunocompromised patients.

Aspergilli are ubiquitous in the environment and are primarily acquired through the respiratory route. They are found in high concentrations in damp cellars, potted plants, and dusty environments, especially during construction.

Aspergillus organisms rarely cause disease in the normal host unless they are inhaled at high concentrations. Bronchopulmonary colonization occurs most frequently in patients with asthma, bronchiectasis, cystic fibrosis, and primary ciliary dyskinesia syndrome.[48]

Macrophages and neutrophils are involved mainly in preventing *Aspergillus* infections. In patients with impaired macrophage function, such as those treated with cortico-

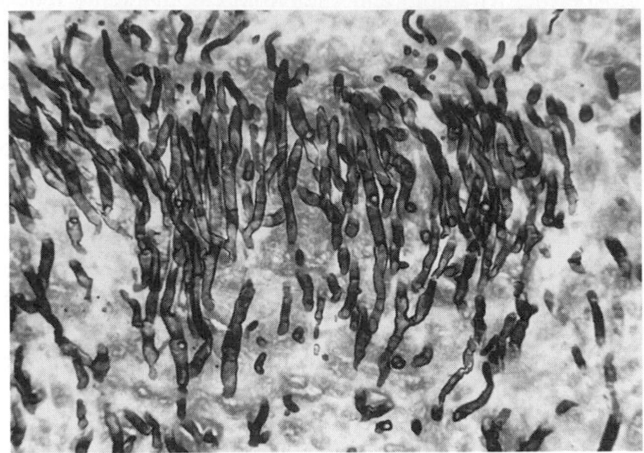

Figure 46-9. *Aspergillus* species isolated from a patient with chemotherapy-induced granulocytopenia. (×400.)

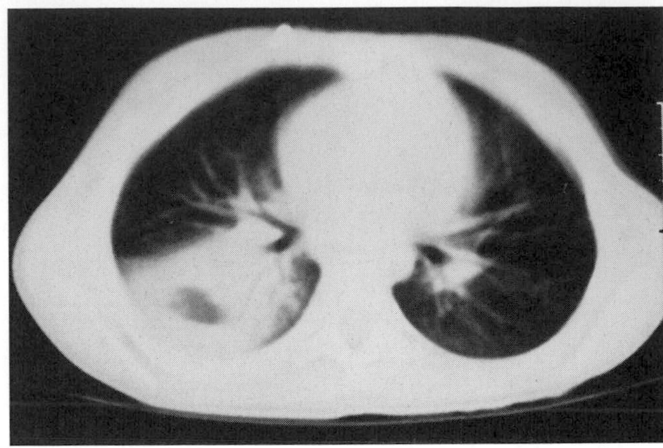

Figure 46-10. Computed tomographic scan of the chest in a 6-year-old child with acute nonlymphocytic leukemia and aspergillosis in the right lower lobe.

steroids more than 1 week or transplant recipients, inhaled *Aspergillus* conidia can germinate and lead to invasive aspergillosis. Patients with prolonged granulocytopenia are also at risk of developing pulmonary aspergillosis. In a study of patients with chemotherapy-induced granulocytopenia (Fig. 46-9), the rate of infection increased progressively after the sixth day of neutropenia.[49]

Aspergillomas occur most frequently in patients with old cavities, congenital pulmonary cysts, or chronic lung disease. The most common symptom is hemoptysis, which results from the propensity of *Aspergillus* organisms to invade blood vessels. The chest radiograph is characterized by an ovoid opacity surrounded by a halo that usually involves the upper lobes or a superior segment of a lower lobe.

Allergic bronchopulmonary aspergillosis results from a hypersensitivity reaction to the fungus. With few exceptions, it occurs mainly in patients with a history of chronic asthma or cystic fibrosis. Patients have wheezing, fever, chest pain, and cough with blood-streaked sputum. In chronic disease, bronchiectasis develops, and patients expectorate mucus plugs containing eosinophils. Other laboratory findings include, eosinophilia, positive serum precipitins to *A. fumigatus,* elevated total serum IgE levels, and elevated levels of serum IgE and IgG to *A. fumigatus.* The chest radiograph findings are variable. In acute disease the upper lobes are usually involved, and in the chronic form, central bronchiectasis is frequently seen.

Invasive aspergillosis is frequently a nosocomial disease, and outbreaks have been reported among immunocompromised patients after hospital construction.[50] Reactivation of an endogenous organism has also been reported to cause disease. Patients with hematologic malignancies and those undergoing organ transplants are at highest risk of developing invasive disease. Invasive aspergillosis has also been increasing in frequency in patients with advanced HIV infection.[51]

The diagnosis of invasive pulmonary aspergillosis can be difficult because clinical signs are nonspecific. Patients usually have fever and respiratory distress. Hemoptysis is sometimes present. Chest radiographs are characterized by patchy infiltrates in any lobe of the lungs. As the disease progresses, pulmonary infarction occurs, and wedge-shaped densities with the crescent sign are seen on the chest radiographs (Figs. 46-10 and 46-11). The chest radiograph can be normal because of severe immunosuppression and lack of inflammatory response.

Another clinical entity that is caused by *Aspergillus* species and that has recently been recognized is ulcerative tracheobronchitis, most frequently seen in patients with AIDS or patients after lung transplantation. This condition is characterized by superficial ulcers with mucosal and cartilage invasion by *Aspergillus* organisms.

For a definite diagnosis, demonstration of tissue invasion on histologic examination or isolation of the organism by culture from biopsy specimens is essential. However, the risks of invasive procedures in immunocompromised patients should be weighed against the benefits. Although *Aspergillus* can be simply a colonizer of the respiratory tract, its isolation from sputum or bronchoalveolar lavage fluid in an immunocompromised patient is highly suggestive of invasive disease, particularly if a single species of *Aspergillus* is isolated.

Serologic tests have also been developed for diagnosing aspergillosis, although they are still not widely available. Antibody tests are insensitive in the diagnosis of early invasive aspergillosis because the antibodies appear late in the course of illness,[52] when the patient's immune function starts to recover. A number of investigators have evaluated methods for detecting an antigen called *galactomannan,* which is a component of the *Aspergillus* cell wall.[53] This antigen is present in serum transiently and at low concentrations and requires serial sampling for diagnosis, which can be expensive and time consuming. Polymerase chain reaction has become available as a rapid means of diagnosis of *A. fumigatus.*[54]

Amphotericin B at a high dose, 1 to 1.5 mg/kg/day, should be used in patients with invasive pulmonary aspergillosis. The duration of treatment depends on the patient's clinical and radiographic improvement and the resolution of neutropenia. For documented disease amphotericin B at minimum total dosage, 30 mg/kg, should be used.

The concurrent use of flucytosine with amphotericin B remains controversial.[55,56] Flucytosine, 100 to 150 mg/kg/day in four divided doses, can be added to the antifungal regimen of patients who are critically ill, those who cannot tolerate a high daily dose of amphotericin B because of nephrotoxicity, or those who are not responding to amphotericin B monotherapy. Prophylactic therapy with or without flucytosine should be

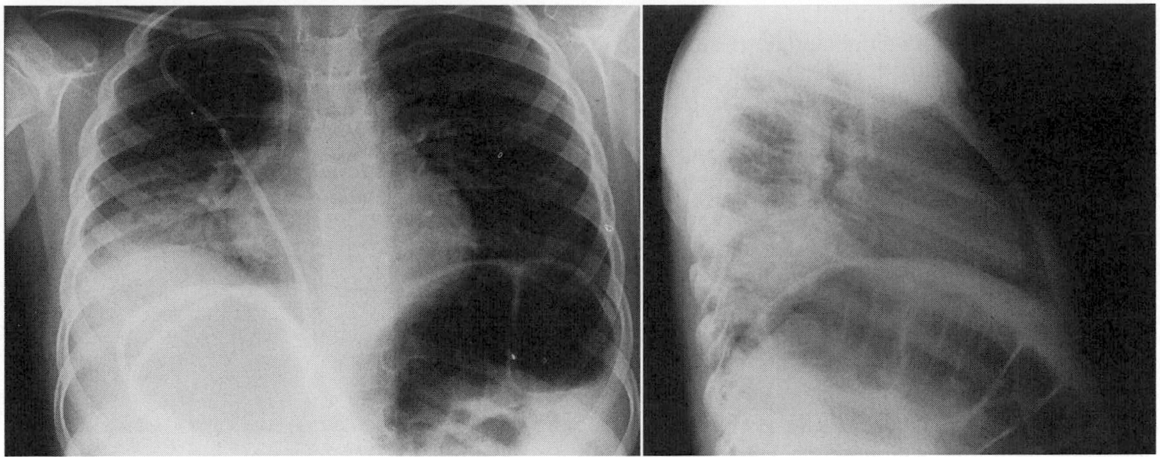

Figure 46-11. Chest radiographs of a 6-year-old child with acute nonlymphocytic leukemia and aspergillosis.

used in patients with a history of invasive aspergillosis who become neutropenic as a result of chemotherapy.[57] Flucytosine with amphotericin B can be used for the duration of therapy unless there is evidence of myelotoxicity, the main side effect of flucytosine.

Liposomal amphotericin, an investigational medication, might have a role in delivering higher doses of amphotericin with less toxicity. Studies on its efficacy are in progress.

Among the azoles, itraconazole has shown good activity against *Aspergillus* organisms in vitro. Clinical studies comparing itraconazole and amphotericin are in progress.

The role of surgical intervention in critically ill patients with invasive pulmonary aspergillosis is limited. Surgical resection should be considered in patients with well-defined lesions or those with an aspergilloma that does not respond to conventional antifungal therapy.

PULMONARY CANDIDIASIS

Over the past few years, *Candida albicans* and its related species have become major causes of morbidity and mortality. There are over 250 different species of *Candida,* but *C. albicans* accounts for approximately 80% of clinical isolates. *Candida* species are ubiquitous in soil, food, and the hospital environment; they are a commensal flora of the gastrointestinal tract, vagina, and mucous membranes of healthy individuals. Person-to-person transmission can occur; however, most infections are endogenous in origin.

Pulmonary candidiasis as a primary disease is rare. However, it is frequently encountered in invasive candidiasis in immunocompromised patients, those on chronic steroids or prolonged antibiotics, and those with indwelling catheters.

Microscopically, *Candida* organisms appear as gram-positive, thin-walled, budding yeasts. In vitro the colonies are creamy white and have a smooth appearance. Germ tube formation distinguishes *C. albicans* from other species of *Candida.* Further speciation is often important and is done by metabolic tests. *C. tropicalis* is more pathogenic than other species of *Candida* in patients with hematologic malignancies.[58] *C. lusitaniae* is known for its resistance to amphotericin B and to the azoles. There have been a few case reports of amphotericin B resistance among *C. albicans, C. tropicalis,* and *C. parapsilosis.*[59,60] This resistance has been mainly among immunosuppressed patients. The frequency of azole resistance among *C. krusei*[61] and *Torulopsis glabrata*[62] has also been increasing.

Polymorphonucleocytes and humoral immunity are important in the defense against invasive candidiasis. T cell dysfunction can predispose to mucosal or cutaneous candidiasis; however, it does not seem to play a major role in primary protection against invasive candidiasis.[63] The preservation of normal gastrointestinal flora is associated with decreased colonization of *Candida* species because these species compete with bacterial flora for nutrients and adherence sites in the gastrointestinal tract. An interplay between the host's immune status and factors such as chronic antibiotic use and prolonged use of a central venous catheter determine the risk for dissemination.

Patients with pulmonary candidiasis can appear septic with various degrees of dyspnea. The chest radiograph is characterized by interstitial or lobar disease. Pleural effusion along with other radiographic findings occurs in about 20% of cases.[64]

Pulmonary disease is usually due to septicemia or dissemination from other organs. Isolation of *Candida* species from the sputum or bronchoalveolar lavage fluid can be difficult to interpret because it may simply represent colonization. However, in an ill-appearing patient with an abnormal chest radiograph not explained by other etiologies or in a patient with concomitant candidemia, isolation of *Candida* organisms from the respiratory tract suggests candidal pneumonia.

Amphotericin B at a minimum total dosage of 25 to 30 mg/kg remains the cornerstone of therapy for patients with pulmonary or invasive candidiasis. In neutropenic patients with candidiasis, amphotericin B should be continued at least for the duration of neutropenia. Fluconazole can be used in patients intolerant to amphotericin B or in patients whose condition has stabilized after a short course of amphotericin B. However, fluconazole should not be used for the treatment of *C. krusei* or *T. glabrata* infections because of an increasing number of resistant strains. In addition to antifungal therapy, it is also important to remove indwelling lines infected with *Candida* organisms.

Although there are no clinical studies comparing flucytosine and amphotericin B combination therapy to amphotericin B monotherapy, flucytosine has been shown to be synergistic with amphotericin B in vitro against certain *Candida* species. Hence combination therapy using amphotericin B and flucytosine is recommended in critically ill patients or in those with evidence of organ invasion (i.e., meningitis,[65] endocarditis, ophthalmitis, pneumonitis, renal candidiasis).

BLASTOMYCOSIS

Blastomycosis is a chronic granulomatous and suppurative disease that occurs primarily in men between 20 and 50 years of age in the south central and midwestern United States. Blastomycosis was once thought to be restricted to North America; however, the disease has now been described in Africa, South America, Asia, and Europe.

The etiologic agent of blastomycosis is the dimorphic fungus *Blastomyces dermatitidis,* which exists in yeast form at 37° C and a mycelial form at room temperature. Microscopically, the mycelial form is characterized by pyriform conidia produced on long to short conidiophores that resemble lollipops. The yeast form is thick walled and usually produces a single bud with a broad base (Figs. 46-12 and 46-13). The definitive diagnosis is based on the in vitro conversion of the mold to the yeast form by demonstration of the A exoantigen or by DNA probe.[4]

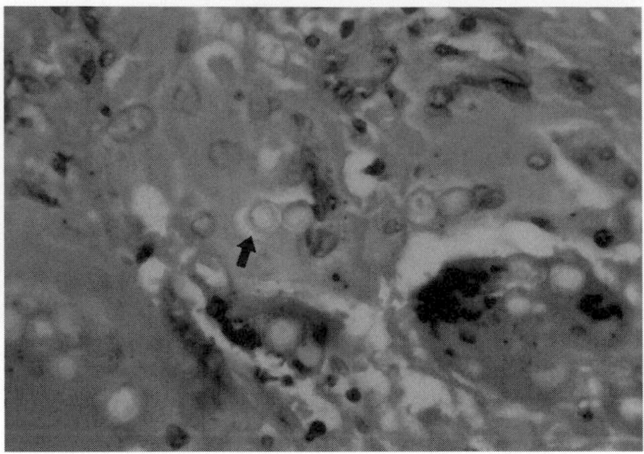

Figure 46-12. Thick-walled spherical yeast form of *B. dermatitidis (arrow).* (×400.)

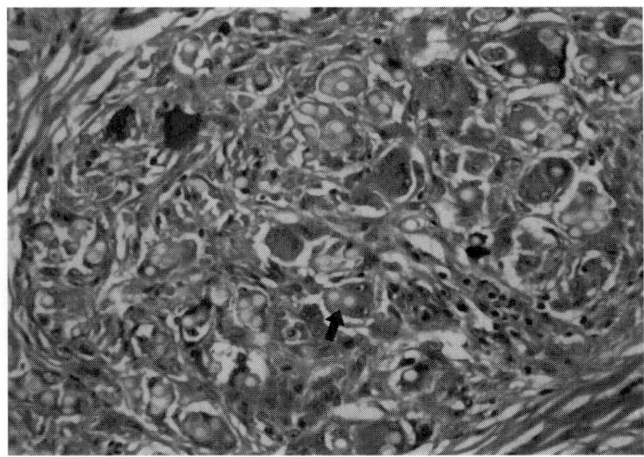

Figure 46-13. Cutaneous blastomycoses illustrating tissue form at 37° C. (×100.)

The ecologic niche inhabited by *B. dermatitidis* remains a mystery. It has been postulated that blastomycosis results from inhalation of conidia residing in the soil. However, it has been very difficult to isolate the organism from the environment, possibly because of its short life span. The fungus has been isolated on a few occasions from the soil, decaying organic material, and bird dropping.[66,67]

After *B. dermatitidis* conidia are inhaled by the host, those that escape ingestion by alveolar macrophages undergo conversion to the yeast phase. A granuloma forms as a result of an inflammatory response consisting principally of macrophages and neutrophils. The fungus may then spread to other organs by the hematogenous route. Unlike other dimorphic fungi, blastomycosis is rare in patients with cellular immunodeficiency.

The two most common forms of blastomycosis are pulmonary and chronic cutaneous blastomycosis. Patients with primary pulmonary blastomycosis usually have the nonspecific symptoms of cough, fever, and fatigue. The primary pulmonary form can result in resolution, dissemination to other organs, or chronic pulmonary disease. The chest radiograph in acute pulmonary disease is characterized by infiltrates, which usually involve the lower lobes. Nodular infiltrates can be confused with pulmonary carcinomas. Chronic pulmonary disease is characterized by cavitation or fibronodular lesions predominantly of the upper lobes. A diffuse miliary or reticulonodular pattern can occur in patients with the chronic form or in neonates.[68,69] Dissemination often follows pulmonary blastomycosis.

Cutaneous blastomycosis is the most common form of extrapulmonary disease. Subcutaneous nodules are seen and eventually ulcerate. They occur most frequently on exposed peripheral areas such as the face, hands, wrists, and lower extremities.

Identification of the organism through light microscopy in tissues and culture is relatively easy and is the most reliable method of diagnosis. Serologic methods such as complement fixation and immunodiffusion are not helpful because of their low sensitivity and specificity. Up to 80% of patients with blastomycosis develop precipitins to antigen A of *B. dermatitidis.* Enzyme immunoassay is more sensitive than immunodiffusion (77% vs. 28%) in detecting antibodies to antigen A, especially in localized disease.[70]

Blastomycosis in immunocompetent patients is usually self-limited. Amphotericin B, for a total minimum dosage of 25 to 30 mg/kg, remains the drug of choice for the treatment of progressive disease, disseminated blastomycosis, or central nervous system disease. Ketoconazole, 400 to 800 mg/day, or itraconazole, 200 to 400 mg/day, can be used in nonprogressive blastomycosis for at least 6 months.[71,72] It is also reasonable to change to oral imidazole therapy after progressive disease has been stabilized with amphotericin B therapy. Experience with fluconazole is limited in the treatment of blastomycosis.

CRYPTOCOCCOSIS

Cryptococcus neoformans is an encapsulated yeast with a worldwide distribution. It is commonly found in soil contaminated with bird droppings, especially those of pigeons. The disease is acquired through the inhalation of airborne particles containing the yeast. Infection is typically subclinical or is limited to the lungs. However, dissemination to other organs, such as the central nervous system, bones, and skin, can occur, mostly in immunocompromised patients. Although cryptococcosis is a frequent opportunistic infection in adults with AIDS, it is rare in pediatric patients with AIDS.

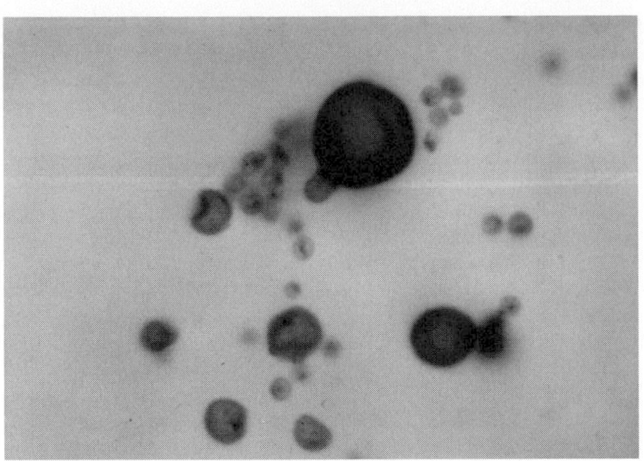

Figure 46-14. *C. neoformans* isolated from cerebrospinal fluid. (×400.)

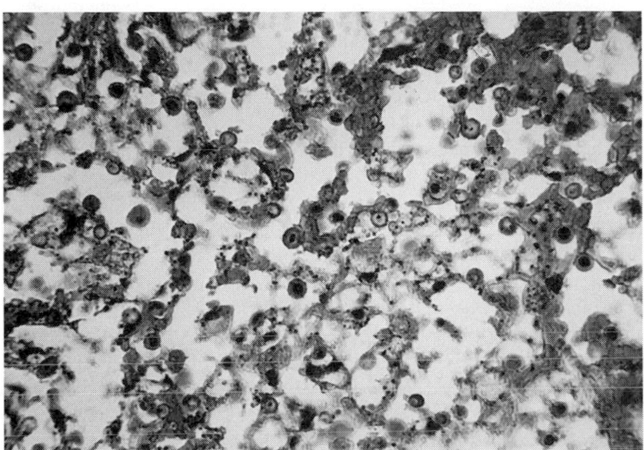

Figure 46-15. Pulmonary cryptococcosis. (×100.)

Less than 50% of patients with pulmonary cryptococcosis have symptomatic disease. These patients have headache, fever, chest pain, and cough. The chest radiograph is characterized by nodules, cavities, or diffuse infiltrates usually involving the lower lung fields.

The diagnosis of cryptococcosis is often made by the demonstration of budding, encapsulated yeast in India ink or wet-mount preparations of clinical specimens (Figs. 46-14 and 46-15). The latex agglutination test for the detection of cryptococcal capsular antigen remains highly sensitive and specific, especially in patients with meningitis or disseminated forms of cryptococcosis.[73]

Amphotericin B, 0.5 to 1 mg/kg/day for 6 to 8 weeks, remains the mainstay of therapy in patients with symptomatic pulmonary cryptococcosis. However, in cryptococcal meningitis, which occurs in 80% to 90% of AIDS patients with cryptococcal infection, amphotericin B, 1 mg/kg, is necessary because of high relapse rates. Flucytosine and amphotericin B combination therapy remains controversial.[74,75] Flucytosine should be used with amphotericin B in patients with progressive disease who cannot tolerate high doses of amphotericin B. After 4 to 6 weeks, if a repeat examination of the cerebrospinal fluid is negative, fluconazole, 200 mg/day (3 to 6 mg/kg/day for children), is used for lifetime maintenance therapy.[76]

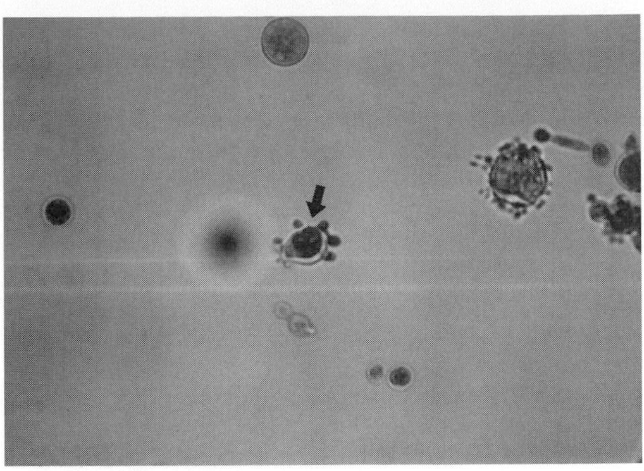

Figure 46-16. *Paracoccidioides* organisms isolated from bronchial wash, illustrating multiple budding yeast *(arrow)*. (×400.)

PARACOCCIDIOIDOMYCOSIS

Paracoccidioidomycosis is caused by the dimorphic fungus *Paracoccidioides brasiliensis.* The disease is endemic to Latin America, mostly Brazil, Colombia, and Venezuela.

Paracoccidioidomycosis is classified into an acute type and a chronic type. The acute form occurs in children and young adults; most commonly, it involves the reticuloendothelial and skeletal systems. The chronic form is more common, occurs in adults, and can be limited to the lungs or can disseminate to other organs. The chest radiograph in pulmonary paracoccidioidomycosis is characterized by nodules, cavities, and lobar or diffuse infiltrates.

P. brasiliensis grows as a yeast at 37° C and as a mold at 25° C. Direct examination of a clinical specimen is the best method of establishing the diagnosis. The yeast form frequently has a pilot-wheel appearance with multiple buds (Fig. 46-16). Serologic tests are of both diagnostic and prognostic value. Agar gel immunodiffusion, tube precipitation, and complement fixation are the most widely used serologic tests. Tube precipitation test is positive in the majority of patients with active disease, whereas complement fixation and immunodiffusion antibodies appear 1 to 2 months after infection but persist for long periods and tend to rise with relapses.[77]

Amphotericin B, 0.5 to 1 mg/kg/day for 3 to 4 months, remains the therapy of choice for disseminated or progressive disease. Among the imidazoles, ketoconazole, 200 mg/day for 6 to 12 months, and itraconazole, 100 mg/day for 3 to 6 months, have been studied in adults and are associated with high response rates (85% to 95%).[78,79] They can be used in patients with progressive disease who cannot tolerate amphotericin B, in patients with mild disease, or in patients whose condition has been stabilized after a few weeks of amphotericin B therapy.

UNCOMMON PULMONARY MYCOSES

Pulmonary Mucormycoses

Mucormycosis most commonly occurs in immunocompromised patients, such as those with malignancies, those receiving immunosuppressive therapy or long-term corticosteroids, or those with diabetes mellitus. The clinical picture is similar to that of aspergillosis. Patients usually have fever and hemoptysis. Histologic demonstration of the nonseptate, ribbonlike hyphal forms in tissues establishes the diagnosis. The mainstay of treatment is stabilization of the underlying disease, such as correction of hyperglycemia in diabetic ketoacidosis. Amphotericin B, 1 to 1.5 mg/kg, remains the drug of choice for the treatment of pulmonary mucormycosis, although surgical resection is of value in patients with well-localized pulmonary disease. In vitro synergism against *Rhizopus* species has also been shown between amphotericin B and rifampin.[80]

Pulmonary Sporotrichosis

Pulmonary sporotrichosis is probably underdiagnosed because its radiographic and clinical courses are similar to those of other granulomatous infections of the lungs and because it is difficult to diagnose. Pulmonary sporotrichosis can occur as a primary infection or can occur secondary to disseminated sporotrichosis. The most reliable method of diagnosis is by culturing the organism from infected tissues. Amphotericin B, 1 mg/kg/day, is given for a total minimum dosage of 30 mg/kg. Surgical resection is important in well-localized disease.

Pulmonary Pseudallescheriasis

Isolation of *Pseudallescheria boydii* from the respiratory tract usually represents colonization in patients with chronic pulmonary disease. A few cases with pulmonary fungal balls or cavities have been described. *P. boydii* is known for its resistance to amphotericin B. Miconazole and other imidazoles, with or without surgery, have been successful in some cases of pulmonary pseudoallescheriasis.[81,82]

REFERENCES

Coccidioidomycosis

1. Galgiani JN, Ampel NM: Coccidioidomycosis in human immunodeficiency virus–infected patients, *J Infect Dis* 162:1165-1169, 1990.
2. Gifford MA, Bass WC, Douds RJ: *Summary of a special study of available data on coccidioides fungus infection, Kern County, 1900-1936,* Kern County, Calif, Department of Public Health, Annual Report, 1936-1937, pp 39-54.
3. Coccidioidomycosis, United States, 1991-1992, *MMWR* 42(2):21-24, 1993.
4. Baron EJ, Finegold SM: Systemic mycoses. In Baron EJ, Finegold SM: *Bailey and Scott's diagnostic microbiology,* St Louis, 1990, Mosby, p 730-740.
5. Yuan L, Cole GT: Possible role of a proteinase in endosporulation of *Coccidioides immitis, Infect Immun* 55:1970-1978, 1987.
6. Vartivarian SE: Virulence properties and nonimmune pathogenic mechanisms of fungi, *Clin Infect Dis* 14(suppl 1):S30-S36, 1992.
7. Coccidioidomycosis following the Northridge earthquake: California, 1994, *MMWR* 43(10):194-195, 1994.
8. Einstein HE, Johnson RH: Coccidioidomycosis: new aspects of epidemiology and therapy, *Clin Infect Dis* 16:349-356, 1993.
9. Fiese MJ, Cheu S, Sorensen RH: Mycelial forms of *Coccidioides immitis* in sputum and tissues of human host, *Ann Intern Med* 43:255-270, 1955.
10. Gururaj VJ, Marsh WW, Aiyar SR: Fulminant pulmonary Coccidioidomycosis in association with coxsackie B4 infection, *Clin Pediatr* 24(7):406-408, 1984.
11. Batra P: Pulmonary coccidioidomycosis, *J Thorac Imaging* 7(4):29-38, 1992.
12. Cohen R: Coccidiodomycosis: case studies in children, *Arch Pediatr* 66:241-265, 1949.
13. Wack EE, Ampel NM, Galgiani JN, Bronnimann DA: Coccidioidomycosis during pregnancy: an analysis of the cases among 47,120 pregnancies, *Chest* 94(2):376-379, 1988.
14. Beard JS, Benson PM, Skillman L: Rapid diagnosis of coccidioidomycosis with a DNA probe to ribosomal RNA, *Arch Dermatol* 129:1589-1593, 1993.
15. Bernstein DI, Tipton JR, Schott SF, Cherry JD: Coccidioidomycosis in a neonate; maternal-infant transmission, *J Pediatr* 99:752-754, 1981.
16. Pappagianis D, Zimmer BL: Serology of coccidioidomycosis, *Clin Microbiol Rev* 3:247-268, 1990.
17. Fish DG, Ampel NM, Galgiani JN, Dols CL, Kelly PC, Johnson CH, Pappagianis D, Edwards JE, Wasserman R, Clark RJ, Antoniskis D, Larsen RA, Englender SJ, Petersen EA: Coccidioidomycosis during human immunodeficiency virus infection: a review of 77 patients, *Medicine (Baltimore)* 69:384-391, 1990.
18. Galgiani JN: Coccidioidomycosis: changes in clinical expression, serological diagnosis, and therapeutic options, *Clin Infect Dis* 14(suppl 1)S100-S105, 1992.
19. Galgiani JN, Grace GM, Lundergan LL: New serologic tests for early detection of coccidioidomycosis, *J Infect Dis* 163:671-674, 1991.
20. Graybill JR, Stevens DA, Galgiani JN, Dismukes WE, Cloud G: Itraconazole treatment of coccidioidomycosis, *Am J Med* 89:282-290, 1990.
21. Tucker RM, Williams PL, Arathoon EG, Stevens DA: Treatment of mycosis with itraconazole, *Ann NY Acad Sci* 544:451-470, 1988.
22. Catanzaro A, Fierer J, Friedman P: Fluconazole in the treatment of persistent coccidioidomycosis, *Chest* 97:661-669, 1990.

Histoplasmosis

23. Darling ST: A protozoan general infection producing pseudotubercles in the lungs and focal necrosis in the liver, spleen, and lymph nodes, *JAMA* 46:1283, 1906.
24. Christie A, Peterson JC: Pulmonary calcifications in negative reactors to tuberculin, *Am J Public Health* 35:1131, 1945.
25. Wheat LJ: Histoplasmosis in Indianapolis, *Clin Infect Dis* 14(suppl): S91-S99, 1992.
26. Taylor ML, Diaz S, Gonzales PA, Sosa AC, Toriello C: Relationship between pathogenesis and immune regulation mechanisms in histoplasmosis: a hypothetical approach, *Rev Infect Dis* 6:775-782, 1984.
27. Quasney MW, Leggiadro RJ: Pleural effusion associated with histoplasmosis, *Pediatr Infect Dis J* 12(5):415-417, 1993.
28. Wheat LJ: Histoplasmosis, *Infect Dis Clin North Am* 2(4):841-859, 1988.
29. Wheat LJ, Connolly-Stringfield PA, Baker RL, Curfman MF, Eads ME, Israel KS, Norris SA, Webb DH, Zeckel ML: Disseminated histoplasmosis in the acquired immunodeficiency syndrome: clinical finding, diagnosis and treatment, and review of literature, *Medicine* 69:361-374, 1990.
30. Leggiadro RJ, Barrett FF, Hughes WT: Disseminated histoplasmosis of infancy, *Pediatr Infect Dis J* 7:799-805, 1988.
31. Zarabi CM, Thomas R, Adesokan A: Diagnosis of systemic histoplasmosis in patients with AIDS, *South Med J* 85(12):1172-1175, 1992.
32. Huffnagle KE, Gander RM: Evaluation of Gen-Probe's *Histoplasma capsulatum* and *Cryptococcus neoformans* AccuProbes, *J Clin Microbiol* 31(2):419-421, 1993.
33. Wheat LJ, French MLV, Kamel S: Evaluation of cross reactions in Histoplasma capsulatum serologic tests, *J Clin Microbiol* 23:493-499, 1986.
34. Heusinkveld R, Tosh F, Newberry W: Antibody response to the histoplasma skin test, *Am Rev Respir Dis* 96:1069-1071, 1967.
35. Wheat LJ, Kohler RB, Tewari RP: Diagnosis of disseminated histoplasmosis by detection of *Histoplasma capsulatum* in serum and urine specimens, *N Engl J Med* 314:83-88, 1986.
36. Wheat LJ, Connolly-Stringfield P, Williams B, Connolly K, Bair R, Bartlett M, Durkin M: Diagnosis of histoplasmosis in patients with the acquired immunodeficiency syndrome by detection of *Histoplasma capsulatum* polysaccharide antigen in bronchoalveolar lavage fluid, *Am Rev Respir Dis* 145(6):1421-1424, 1992.
37. Wheat LJ, Connolly-Stringfield P, Blair R, Connolly K, Garringer T, Katz BP, Gupta M: Effect of successful treatment with amphotericin B on *Histoplasma capsulatum* polysaccharide antigen levels in patients with AIDS and histoplasmosis, *Am J Med* 92(2):153-160, 1992.
38. Hughes WT: Hematogenous histoplasmosis in the immunocompromised child, *J Pediatr* 105:569-575, 1984.
39. The National Institute of Allergy and Infectious Diseases Clinical Trials and Mycoses Study Group Collaborators: Prevention of relapse of histoplasmosis with itraconazole in patients with the acquired immunodeficiency syndrome, *Ann Intern Med* 118(8):610-616, 1993.
40. The National Institute of Allergy and Infectious Disease Mycoses Study Group: Treatment of blastomycosis and histoplasmosis with ketoconazole, *Ann Intern Med* 103:861-872, 1985.

41. Slama TG: Treatment of disseminated and progressive cavitary histoplasmosis with ketoconazole, *Am J Med* 74(suppl 10):70-73, 1983.
42. Kobayashi GS, Travis SJ, Medoff G: Comparison of fluconazole with amphotericin B in treatment of histoplasmosis in normal and immunosuppressed mice, *Rev Infect Dis* 12(suppl 3):S291-S293, 1990.
43. Dismukes WE, Bradsher RW Jr, Cloud GC, Kauffman CA, Chapman SW, George RB, Stevens DA, Girard WM, Saag MS, Bowles-Patton C: Itraconazole therapy for blastomycosis and histoplasmosis: NIAID Mycoses Study Group, *Am J Med* 93(5):89-97, 1992.
44. Negroni R, Robles AM, Arechavala A, Taborda A: Itraconazole in human histoplasmosis, *Mycoses* 32:123-130, 1989.
45. Negroni R, Taborda A, Robies AM, Archevala A: Itraconazole in the treatment of histoplasmosis associated with AIDS, *Mycoses* 35(11-12):281-287, 1992.
46. Wynne JW, Olsen GN: Acute histoplasmosis presenting as the adult respiratory distress syndrome, *Chest* 66:158-161, 1974.
47. Greenwood MF, Holland P: Tracheal obstruction secondary to *Histoplasma* mediastinal granuloma, *Chest* 62:642-645, 1972.

Pulmonary Aspergillosis

48. Bardana E Jr: The clinical spectrum of aspergillosis. II. Classification and description of saprophytic, allergic, and invasive variants of human disease, *Crit Rev Clin Lab Sci* 13:85-159, 1981.
49. Gerson SL, Talbot GH, Hurwitz S, Strom BL, Lusk EJ, Cassileth PA: Prolonged granulocytopenia: the major risk factor for invasive pulmonary aspergillosis in patients with acute leukemia, *Ann Intern Med* 100:345-351, 1984.
50. Sarubbi FA, Kopf HB, Wilson MB, McGinnis MR, Rutala WA: Increased recovery of *Aspergillus flavus* from respiratory specimens during hospital construction, *Am Rev Respir Dis* 125:33-38, 1982.
51. Denning DW: Pulmonary aspergillosis in the acquired immunodeficiency syndrome, *N Engl J Med* 324:654-662, 1991.
52. deRepentigny L: Serological techniques for diagnosis of fungal infection, *Eur J Clin Microbiol Infect Dis* 8:362-875, 1989.
53. Haynes KA, Latge J-P, Rogers TR: Detection of *Aspergillus* antigens associated with invasive disease, *J Clin Microbiol* 28:2040-2044, 1990.
54. Spreadbury O, Holden D, Anfauvre-Brown A, Brainbridge B, Cohen J: Detection of *Aspergillus fumigatus* by polymerase chain reaction, *J Clin Microbiol* 31:615-621, 1993.
55. Lauer BA, Reller LB, Schroter GP: Susceptibility of *Aspergillus* to 5-fluorocytosine and amphotericin B alone and in combination, *J Antimicrobial Chemother* 4:375-380, 1978.
56. Saral R: *Candida* and *Aspergillus* infections in immunocompromised patients, *Rev Infect Dis* 13:487-492, 1991.
57. Karp JE, Burch PA, Merz WG: An approach to invasive antileukemia therapy in patients with previous invasive aspergillosis, *Am J Med* 85:203-206, 1988.

Pulmonary Candidiasis

58. Komshian SV, Uwaydah AK, Sobel JD, Crane LR: Fungemia caused by *Candida* species and *Torulopsis glabrata* in the hospitalized patient: frequency, characteristics, and evaluation of factors influencing outcome, *Rev Infect Dis* 11:379-390, 1989.
59. Powderly WG, Kobayashi GS, Herzig GP, Medoff G: Amphotericin B resistant yeast infection in severely immunocompromised patients, *Am J Med* 84:826-832, 1988.
60. Christenson JC, Guruswany A, Mukwaya G, Rettig PJ: *Candida lusitaniae:* an emerging human pathogen, *Pediatr Infect Dis J* 6:755-757, 1987.
61. Wingard JR, Merz WG, Rinaldi MG: Increase in *Candida krusei* infection among patients with bone marrow transplantation and neutropenia treated prophylactically with fluconazole, *N Engl J Med* 325:1274-1277, 1991.
62. Warnock DW, Burke J, Cope NJ, Johnson EM, von Fraunhofer NA, Williams EW: Fluconazole resistance in *Candida glabrata, Lancet* 2:1310, 1988.
63. Denning DW: Epidemiology and pathogenesis of systemic fungal infections in the immunocompromised host, *J Antimicrob Chem* 28(suppl B):1-16, 1991.
64. Buff SJ, McLelland R, Gallis HA, Matthay R, Putman CE: *Candida albicans* pneumonia: radiographic appearance, *Am J Radiol* 138:645-648, 1982.
65. Smego RA, Perfect JR, Dwack DT: Combined therapy with amphotericin B and 5-flucytosine for *Candida* meningitis, *Rev Infect Dis* 6:791-801, 1984.

Blastomycosis

66. Denton JF, Disalvo AF: Isolation of *Blastomyces dermatitidis* from natural sites in Augusta, Georgia, *Am J Trop Med Hyg* 13:716-722, 1964.
67. Sarosi GA, Serstock DS: Isolation of *Blastomyces dermatitidis* from pigeon manure, *Am Rev Respir Dis* 114:1179-1183, 1976.
68. Bradsher RW, Rice DC, Abernathy RS: Ketoconazole therapy of endemic blastomycosis, *Ann Intern Med* 103:872-879, 1985.
69. Maxon S, Miller SF, Tryka AF, Shutze GE: Perinatal blastomycosis: a review, *Pediatr Infect Dis J* 11:760-763, 1992.
70. Klein BS, Kuritsky JN, Chappell WA: Comparison of the enzyme immunoassay, immunodiffusion, and complement fixation tests in detecting antibody in human serum to the A antigen of *Blastomyces dermatitidis, Am Rev Respir Dis* 133:144-148, 1986.
71. National Institute of Allergy and Infectious Disease Mycoses Study Group: Treatment of blastomycosis and histoplasmosis with ketoconazole, *Ann Intern Med* 103:861-872, 1985.
72. National Institute of Allergy and Infectious Disease Mycoses Study Group: Itraconazole therapy for blastomycosis and histoplasmosis, *Am J Med* 93:489-497, 1992.

Cryptococcosis

73. Bhattacharjee AK, Bennett JE, Glaudemans CPJ: Capsular polysaccharides of *Cryptococcus neoformans, Rev Infect Dis* 6:619-624, 1984.
74. The National Institute of Allergy and Infectious Diseases Mycoses Study Group: Treatment of cryptococcal meningitis with combination amphotericin B and flucytosine for four as compared with six weeks, *N Engl J Med* 317:334-341, 1987.
75. Chuck SL, Sande MA: Infections with *Cryptococcus neoformans* in the acquired immunodeficiency syndrome, *N Engl J Med* 321:794-799, 1989.
76. The National Institute of Allergy and Infectious Disease AIDS Clinical Trials Group and The National Institute of Allergy and Infectious Disease Mycoses Study Group: A controlled trial of fluconazole and amphotericin B to prevent relapse of cryptococcal meningitis in patients with the acquired immunodeficiency syndrome, *N Engl J Med* 326:793-798, 1992.

Paracoccidioidomycosis

77. Brummer E, Castaneda E, Restrepo A: Paracoccidioidomycosis: an update, *Clin Microbiol Rev* 6(2):89-117, 1993.
78. Restrepo A, Gomez I, Cano LE, Arango MD, Gutierrez F, Sanin AS, Robledo MA: Treatment of paracoccidioidomycosis with ketoconazole: a 3 year experience, *Am J Med* 78:48-52, 1985.
79. Naranjo MS, Trujillo M, Munera MI, Restrepo P, Gomez I, Restrepo A: Treatment of paracoccidioidomycosis with itraconazole, *J Med Vet Mycol* 28:67-76, 1990.

Uncommon Pulmonary Mycoses

80. Christenson JC, Shalit I, Welch DF, Guruswamy A, Marks MI: Synergistic action of amphotericin B and rifampin against *Rhizopus* species, *Antimicrob Agents Chemother* 31:1775-1778, 1987.
81. Walsh M, White L, Atkinson K, Enno A: Fungal *Pseudallescheria boydii* lung infiltrates unresponsive to amphotericin B in leukaemic patients, *Aust NZ J Med* 22(3):265-268, 1992.
82. Gumbart CH: *Pseudallescheria boydii* infection after bone marrow transplantation, *Ann Intern Med* 99:193-194, 1983.

CHAPTER 47

Other Infectious Agents

Geoffrey A. Weinberg, Mobeen H. Rathore, and A. Clinton White, Jr.

A number of infectious agents of several types (beyond those discussed in other chapters of this textbook) can cause infections of the lung in childhood. Perhaps the most commonly considered unusual infectious etiologies for pediatric pneumonia in children in the developed world are *Pneumocystis carinii* and *Legionella pneumophila.* Less commonly, pulmonary infections caused by *Toxoplasma gondii, Ascaris lumbricoides, Toxocara,* hookworms, filaria, *Strongyloides stercoralis, Echinococcus, Paragonimus westermani, Trichinella, Schistosoma, Cryptosporidium, Entamoeba,* or *Plasmodium* might be encountered. It is beyond the scope of this chapter to include full sections on each of these unusual pediatric pulmonary pathogens, but *P. carinii* and *L. pneumophila* are addressed in detail, and salient features of several of the parasitic causes of pneumonia are summarized.

PNEUMOCYSTIS CARINII

Pneumocystis carinii is one of the most common causes of pneumonia in the immunocompromised host, whether the immunocompromise results from a congenital defect (e.g., severe combined immunodeficiency syndrome), an acquired defect (e.g., human immunodeficiency virus [HIV] infection), or an iatrogenic cause (e.g., immune suppression associated with therapy of malignancy or prevention of organ transplant rejection) (reviewed in references 1 through 9). The occurrence of several consecutive cases of *P. carinii* pneumonia among apparently healthy young men in Los Angeles and New York City led to the rapid recognition of acquired immunodeficiency syndrome (AIDS) as a new diagnostic entity in the early 1980s. With the spread of the HIV pandemic, the importance of accurate diagnosis of and effective therapy for *P. carinii* disease has greatly increased.

Disease Mechanisms

Organism. *Pneumocystis carinii* is an extracellular eukaryotic pathogen whose taxonomic classification has been a matter of controversy ever since its description in 1909. Chagas originally thought that the organism was a variant form of *Trypanosoma cruzi* infecting animals, but by 1912 this assignment was shown to be incorrect.[1,6] In the 1950s the organism was found to be the cause of interstitial plasma cell pneumonia in infants and children, most of whom were malnourished residents of orphanages and foundling homes following World War II.[1,6] Over the next 30 years, some investigators classified the pathogen as a protozoan because of its morphologic structural properties and susceptibility to antiprotozoal agents.[1] Other investigators preferred to classify *P. carinii* as a fungus because of its subcellular organelle structure, cell wall biochemistry, and staining characteristics.[1] Recently, many investigators have applied molecular biology techniques to *P. carinii* and have found that the organism's genome exhibits greater homology with fungal gene sequences than with protozoal gene sequences at a number of loci (ribosomal RNA, β-tubulin, folate metabolism pathway, and mitochondrial enzyme genes, among others); thus the organism is probably best classified as an unusual fungus that infects both humans and animals, yet retains many biologic features more typical of protozoa (reviewed in references 1, 6, 8, 9, and 10). Recent attempts at synthesizing both phenotypic and genotypic data have led to a trinomial system of names to distinguish among *P. carinii* from human and animal hosts;[11] for the sake of simplicity, this chapter will refer to all *P. carinii* organisms with the older binomial system.

Three developmental stages of *P. carinii* have been identified: trophozoites, cysts, and precysts (the terminology reflects the old protozoal nomenclature; some have suggested the use of the terms *trophic form, spore case,* and *sporocyte,* respectively).[1,2,8] Trophozoites are small (1 to 5 μm), are pleomorphic, and commonly exist in large clusters in lung tissue or respiratory secretions. This form is identified on Giemsa stain, rapid Giemsa stain variants such as the Diff-Quik stain, or Wright stain, by its dotlike reddish nucleus with surrounding blue cytoplasm (Fig. 47-1).[1,6] It is thought that trophozoites reproduce by binary fission. The cyst wall will not be visualized with Giemsa stain, but up to eight round or spindle-shaped intracystic bodies may be seen, surrounded by a clear halo. The cyst wall is readily stained by the Gomori methenamine silver nitrate procedure (Fig. 47-2), the more rapid Grocott silver stain, or other cell wall stains such as toluidine blue O, cresyl echt violet, or calcofluor white.[1,6] Cysts appear as spherical or crescent-shaped structures about 5 μm in size, often with a fold that gives them a parentheses-like or cup-shaped appearance. The precyst is an intermediate stage of reproduction, about 4 to 6 μm in size, which may represent a parent cell undergoing encystment.

A few laboratories have successfully propagated *P. carinii* from infected rats for 1 to 2 weeks in cell culture using epithelial or fibroblast cells such as HEL and WI-38 cells.[1,12] Attempts at long-term or continuous cultures of rat *P. carinii,* or short-term culture of *P. carinii* from humans, have not been successful.

Epidemiology. Many questions about the natural habitat, modes of transmission, and attack rates of *P. carinii* remain unanswered. It is well established that *P. carinii* infects a wide variety of wild, domestic, and laboratory animals, as well as humans, in a worldwide distribution.[2] Airborne transmission of infection has been shown to occur among infected rats in the laboratory,[13,14] and recently *P. carinii* DNA has been amplified by the polymerase chain reaction (PCR) from filtered air samples taken from country orchards.[15] Thus circumstantial evidence indicates that *P. carinii* might be an opportunistic zoonosis in humans. However, no firm evidence of animal-to-human transmission has been found, and recent discoveries of substantial chromosomal and DNA sequence diversity among *P. carinii* recovered from humans, rats, mice, and

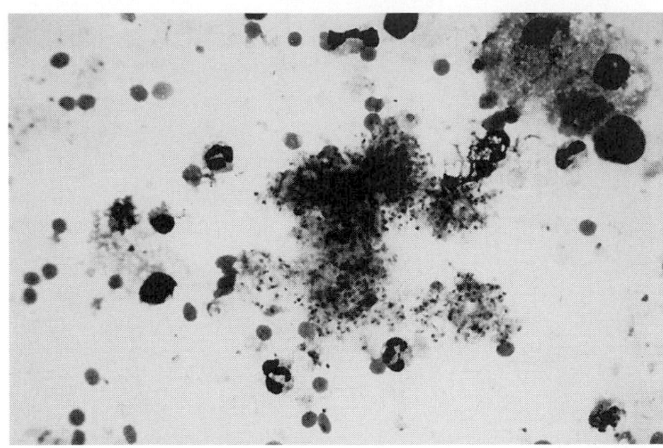

Fig. 47-1. *Pneumocystis carinii* trophozoites in bronchoalveolar lavage fluid as stained by Giemsa stain. (×1000.)

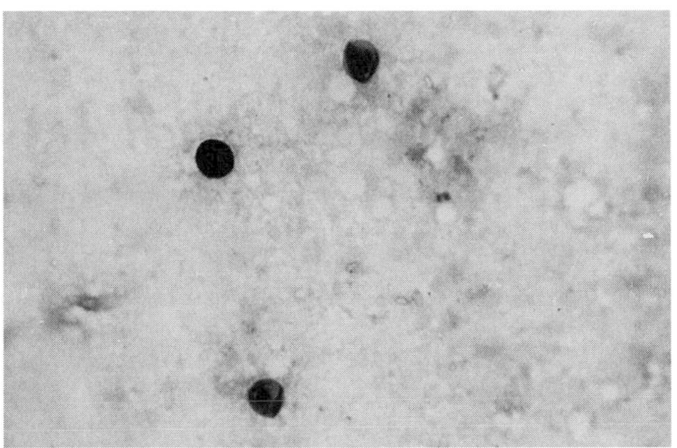

Fig. 47-2. *Pneumocystis carinii* cysts in bronchoalveolar lavage fluid as stained by modified Gomori methenamine silver stain. (×1000.)

ferrets would make zoonotic transmission seem unlikely.[16,17] In addition, attempts to produce experimental infections between different mammalian species have been unsuccessful.[18] Thus several *P. carinii* lineages (perhaps distinct species of the genus *Pneumocystis*) appear to infect different mammals, perhaps with transmission only to homologous hosts.

It is generally accepted that most children and adults have been asymptomatically infected with *P. carinii,* based on seropositivity rates of 75% in children and 90% in adults.[1,2] Reactivation of latent organisms when the host becomes immunosuppressed would then explain disease appearance.[3] It is difficult to prove or disprove this accepted hypothesis. Autopsy surveys have shown *P. carinii* organisms as incidental lung findings in 5% to 8% of immunocompromised children and adults, but in otherwise healthy individuals the detection rate of organisms has been much less, even when more sensitive techniques such as immunologic staining or PCR amplification are used.[4] On the other hand, person-to-person spread of new (nonreactivated) infection has been suggested by the occurrence of apparent outbreaks of *P. carinii* pneumonia in some (but not all) nurseries and orphanages in Central and Eastern Europe after World War II, in some children's hospitals in the United States, and in outpatient clinics for immunocompromised patients in Europe.[6] In addition, animal experiments suggest that latency does not occur in the absence of immunologic abnormalities.[19] Until more firm evidence suggesting horizontal spread of disease is found, and the precise roles of reactivation vs. acquisition of new infection are determined, isolation policies for patients with *P. carinii* pneumonia will be difficult to construct; some authorities favor respiratory isolation procedures for patients with *P. carinii* disease, but others stress that it would be sufficient to separate patients with *P. carinii* disease only from other patients with immune compromise.

Whether disease is manifested after reactivation of latent infection or after acquisition of new infection, it is clear that *P. carinii* disease is opportunistic, occurring in patients with immunodeficiency disorders. Before the beginning of the HIV pandemic, the disease was rare and was found almost exclusively in hosts with malnourishment, malignancy, or primary immunodeficiency disorders or those undergoing immunosuppressive therapy for malignancies, connective tissue disease, or organ transplantation.[20] Without chemoprophylaxis, *P. carinii* pneumonia will affect about 75% of adults with AIDS and at least 50% of children with AIDS.[3,4] Interestingly, *P. carinii* pneumonia appears to be much less common in patients with AIDS in Central Africa than in North America and Europe;[6] whether patients die first from other, more common, infections (such as tuberculosis or measles); whether the diagnosis is missed in the absence of sophisticated medical services; or whether there are true geographic differences in the prevalence of the microorganism remains uncertain.

Pathology and Pathogenesis. After the presumed airborne acquisition of organisms, *P. carinii* adheres to type I alveolar cells via binding to fibronectin, vitronectin, or other host components.[21,22] Reproduction of the organisms takes place in the alveolus. Malnutrition, hypogammaglobulinemia, and severe combined immunodeficiency (SCID) have all been associated with *P. carinii* disease, although T lymphocyte immune defects seem to be important in the pathogenesis of *P. carinii* pneumonia as manifested by its prominent occurrence in patients with AIDS. The central role of T cells is borne out by the resolution of *P. carinii* pneumonia in nude mice and SCID mice after adoptive transfer of splenic helper T cells from normal heterozygote mice.[1,19] However, the humoral immune system does seem to play a role in protection against *P. carinii,* because the disease has been found in hypogammaglobulinemic children, and experimental animal studies show that passive protection can be afforded by monoclonal antibodies and also that CD4+ T cells alone are not required for protection in previously immunized animals.[1,23]

Alterations in both amount and distribution of pulmonary surfactant occur during *P. carinii* pneumonia.[4,9] Surfactant protein A binds to *P. carinii* surface glycoproteins, which could possibly enhance attachment of the organisms to the alveolus and retard phagocytosis by alveolar macrophages. The alteration in surfactant phospholipids might contribute to ventilation-perfusion mismatches and altered lung compliance.[1,4,9,24]

Interstitial plasma cell pneumonitis is seen in the epidemic form of pneumocystosis among malnourished children.[1] In other patients, the classic histopathologic appearance is characterized more by a prominent eosinophilic foamy intralveolar exudate with a mild interstitial pneumonitis (Fig. 47-3).[1] On staining with Giemsa or silver stains, organisms are seen within the exudate. Organizing diffuse alveolar damage with interstitial fibrosis is commonly seen (63%) in HIV-infected patients with *P. carinii* pneumonia. Less common findings include absence of foamy exudate (20% of patients with AIDS, nearly 50% in those without AIDS), granuloma formation (5%

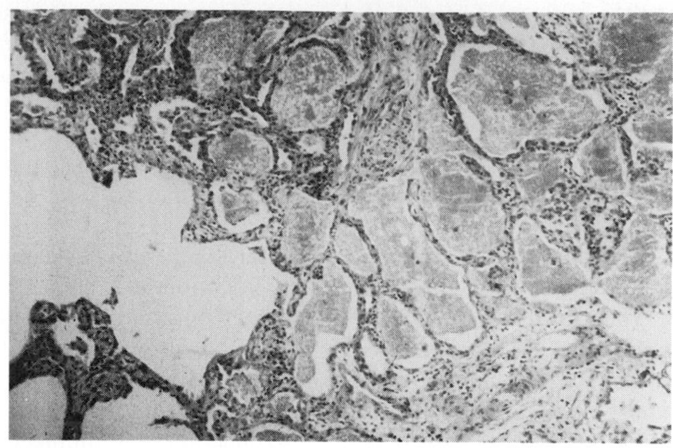

Fig. 47-3. Foamy alveolar exudate and mild interstitial fibrosis characteristic of *P. carinii* pneumonia. (hematoxylin and eosin stain, ×450.)

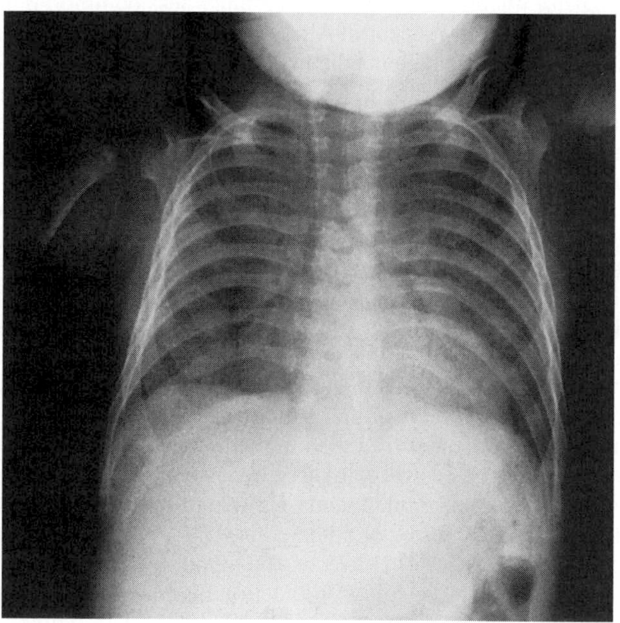

Fig. 47-4. Chest radiograph showing diffuse interstitial infiltrates in a 7-month-old child with AIDS.

to 10%), calcification (2%), and cyst formation (2%).[1] Extrapulmonary disease is uncommon (1% to 3%) but well described in adults with AIDS; dissemination in pediatric AIDS patients and in non-AIDS patients appears to be much more rare.[1,25]

Clinical Manifestations

Pneumocystis carinii pneumonia is characterized by tachypnea, dyspnea, fever, and nonproductive cough.[1] The course of the disease is variable, however, and symptoms distressing enough to bring the patient to medical attention may not occur until late in the infection. This is particularly true in patients with AIDS, in which the onset of disease is more insidious (over several weeks) than in the pediatric cancer patient (in whom fever and respiratory distress occurs over a period of days).[26,27] Crackles are conspicuously absent in most cases (60% to 70%) of *P. carinii* pneumonia; few abnormalities on physical examination are evident beyond tachypnea and respiratory distress.[3,4,26]

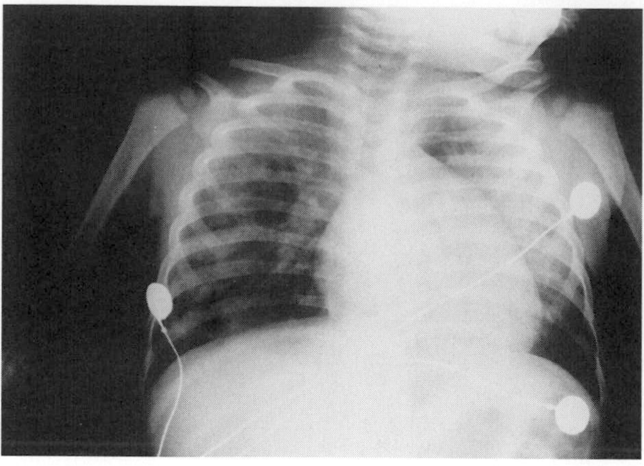

Fig. 47-5. Chest radiograph showing right lung interstitial infiltrates and left lung consolidation in an 18-month-old child with AIDS.

The mortality of *P. carinii* pneumonia among immunosuppressed patients approaches 100% without therapy.[3] Most infants with perinatally acquired HIV infection have onset of *P. carinii* pneumonia between 3 and 6 months of age.[28,29]

Epidemic plasma cell pneumonia in malnourished babies, now a rarely recognized condition, was associated with an even more insidious onset, often following weight loss and chronic diarrhea. Fever was less prominent to absent; the mortality rate was at least 50%.[1]

Radiology. Chest radiographs typically show interstitial infiltrates, beginning in the perihilar regions and spreading to the periphery (Fig. 47-4).[1] The apices are usually spared until late in the disease. Less commonly, atypical lesions are found, such as asymmetric lobar or segmental consolidation (Fig. 47-5), cavitary, nodular, or upper lobe disease (the latter is especially noted in patients receiving aerosolized pentamidine chemoprophylaxis).[1]

Computed tomography (CT) scans of the chest have shown diffuse alveolar consolidation in some cases in which chest radiographs appeared normal, but CT has limited diagnostic value in most children. Similarly, gallium nuclear imaging has been suggested to be of value in the diagnosis of *P. carinii* in adults with AIDS, but the sensitivity and specificity of the test have varied between 50% and 90%, and the test takes up to 72 hours to perform. In addition, data among pediatric populations (who might suffer from other conditions yielding abnormal gallium uptake, such as lymphoid interstitial pneumonia) are limited, making gallium imaging much less useful.[3]

Laboratory Diagnosis. The most important indirect marker of *P. carinii* pneumonia is hypoxemia (i.e., a PaO_2 in room air of <80 mm Hg or an alveolar-arterial oxygen gradient of >35 mm Hg).[4] Although more difficult to measure, carbon monoxide diffusion capacity is below 70% of predicted values in nearly all patients with *P. carinii* disease. Serum lactate dehydrogenase (LDH) levels are elevated in both children and adults with AIDS and *P. carinii,* but the finding has limited specificity (75%).[3,4] Serum antibody tests for *P. carinii* are useful in epidemiologic work but not for diagnosis, because low antibody titers are found in normal hosts, and the immunosuppressed host may not be competent enough to show antibody increases.[2] Serum antigen tests were studied at one time but were prohibitively nonspecific.[2] It is possible that serum (or sputum) *P. carinii* DNA, which has been detected by PCR amplification in several laboratories, may someday be a useful diagnostic technique.[30-32]

When an immunocompromised child has tachypnea, cough, dyspnea, fever, and diffuse interstitial infiltrates on chest radiographs, *P. carinii* disease must be considered, along with a number of other etiologies, including cytomegalovirus, *Mycobacterium tuberculosis, Mycobacterium avium-intracellulare, Histoplasma capsulatum,* and lymphoid interstitial pneumonitis. Thus effective therapy depends on definitive tissue diagnosis, which in turn currently depends on demonstration of organisms in lower respiratory secretions or lung tissue.

A staged approach is useful to maximize diagnostic information and minimize patient risk. Techniques that have been advocated include sputum induction, bronchial biopsy, bronchial wash, bronchoalveolar lavage (BAL), and open lung biopsy.[1,3,4] Sputum induced by ultrasonic nebulization and then subjected to Giemsa staining, silver staining, and immunologic staining has been useful for adults with AIDS at medical centers familiar with the technique. However, the procedure is labor intensive when done correctly, and the predictive values have ranged widely (between 40% and 90%). Experience with children has been limited. Bronchial washes (suctioning secretions through the bronchoscope) increase sensitivity somewhat, and transbronchial biopsy can be very sensitive if 20 to 25 alveoli are obtained without crushing; however, the risk of bleeding and pneumothorax approaches 10%.

The cornerstone of diagnostic procedures in adults, and one that is rapidly being adapted for children, is the BAL.[3,4] In this procedure, aliquots of sterile nonpreservative saline are instilled in a peripheral nondependent airway (e.g., right middle lobe) after the bronchoscope is wedged. After a few seconds, the saline is aspirated and the procedure repeated several times. The yield of BAL is often 85% to 95%. Some success has been achieved with nonbronchoscopic lavage via a small feeding tube placed through the endotracheal tube in patients already undergoing mechanical ventilation.

When the BAL is nondiagnostic, when controlled hemostasis is desirable because of bleeding disorders, or when diffuse nodular infiltrates are present that may not yield a diagnosis by BAL, the open lung biopsy is performed. This procedure remains the gold standard diagnostic procedure, being the most sensitive and specific, but it involves the most risk, requiring general anesthesia and the risk of some impairment of pulmonary function. It is possible that open lung biopsy might be superior to BAL for the non-AIDS patient, because the organism load is lower than that seen in the AIDS patient.

Once BAL fluid or lung tissue is obtained for diagnosis, the material should be examined by experienced personnel using two or more staining techniques, preferably one that stains cysts and another trophozoites.[1,3,4,6] The Gomori or Grocott methenamine silver stain for cysts is widely used. It has sensitivity and specificity exceeding 95%, and the cysts are relatively easy to see.[1,4] Disadvantages include a more intensive procedure, which can take 6 to 24 hours to perform. However, several rapid modifications exist that can cut down the preparation time to a few hours and utilize a microwave oven rather than boiling water baths. Other cyst stains used less widely include toluidine blue O, crystal echt violet, and calcofluor white.[1,4]

Trophozoites are stained by the Giemsa stain and its derivatives such as Diff-Quik. The cost of these stains is minimal, and they require only a few minutes to an hour to perform. However, the sensitivity and specificity are slightly less than silver stains (perhaps 85% to 90% each), and more experience is needed to recognize the trophozoites among the stained host cells and debris.[1,4] Papanicolau stain can be useful but is more labor intensive and slightly less sensitive in detecting trophozoites.

Immunologic stains (direct and indirect immunofluorescent antibodies) are now commercially available and may be a reasonable choice for some laboratories. The diagnostic sensitivity exceeds 90% in BAL fluid, and these stains may be useful for induced sputum as well. However, the kits are costly and require considerable experience to discern false positives from true positives.[1,4] Molecular techniques (PCR amplification and oligonucleotide probing) may someday be validated as clinical tests; they have the potential to have exquisite sensitivity, but possibly at the cost of decreased specificity.[30-32]

BOX 47-1

Conventional and Experimental Agents Used or Under Investigation for Prophylaxis and Therapy of *P. carinii* Pneumonia*

Conventional

First-line agents
Trimethoprim-sulfamethoxazole
Pentamidine

Second-line agents
Trimetrexate
Dapsone
Atovaquone
Clindamycin and primaquine

Experimental

New dihydrofolate reductase inhibitors
New pentamidine analogues
Echinocandins
Miscellaneous growth inhibitors
8-Aminoquinolines
Iron chelators

*Conventional refers to accepted drugs licensed for use in the United States; experimental refers to compounds or classes of compounds that show promising activity in in vitro or animal models, but for which few if any human data exist. Note that most of the conventional agents have been used mainly in adults, not children; see text for details.

Management

Antimicrobial Therapy. A number of agents are currently in use or under active investigation for the therapy of *P. carinii* pneumonia (Box 47-1).[1-4, 33-38] Most of the conventional agents have been tested only in adults with *P. carinii* disease, and substantially fewer controlled data are available to provide guidelines for appropriate pediatric use. Thus the published pediatric experience primarily concerns trimethoprim-sulfamethoxazole (TMP-SMX), pentamidine, and to a lesser extent dapsone.

The mortality rate of *P. carinii* pneumonia has been strongly correlated (in adults) with the degree of hypoxemia at presentation. Patients with either Pao_2 values less than 70 or alveolar-arterial (A-a) gradients greater than 35 while inspiring room air experience 20% to 30% mortality rates even with rapid, aggressive therapy, whereas those who have less severe hypoxemia experience a 5% or less mortality rate. Thus many authorities differentiate moderate to severe disease (room air Pao_2 <70 or A-a gradient >35) from mild to moderate disease (room air Pa_{O_2} >70 or A-a gradient <35) in planning therapy.[4]

For the initial therapy of moderate to severe disease, parenteral TMP-SMX remains the drug of first choice, and parenteral pentamidine is the most suitable alternative for those intolerant of or not responding to TMP-SMX.[3,4,33] For initial therapy of mild to moderate disease in adults and older adolescents, a number of alternatives exist, including oral or intravenous TMP-SMX, oral TMP-dapsone, oral atovaquone, and intravenous or oral clindamycin with oral primaquine.[4,33] Experience with therapy of mild disease in younger children and infants is limited to TMP-SMX for the most part.[3]

It is often noted that response to therapy can be delayed for 4 to 8 days, and that patients may in fact worsen initially (presumably from pulmonary inflammation incited by dying organisms). Thus determining whether a patient has failed initial therapy or is simply slow to respond is difficult, and further therapeutic options ("salvage therapy") are controversial.[33] For those patients failing TMP-SMX, intravenous pentamidine is generally added or used as a single replacement agent. For those given pentamidine initially, TMP-SMX is used if tolerated. For those patients failing or intolerant to both TMP-SMX and pentamidine, the next best studied agent is parenteral trimetrexate in combination with leucovorin rescue; the combination of clindamycin and primaquine may also have a role in salvage therapy.[4,33] It is unclear whether adding high-dose corticosteroids serves a useful role in salvage therapy, although steroids are often advocated as adjuncts to initial therapy.

Therapy for *P. carinii* pneumonia in patients with HIV infection is given for 21 days. In non–HIV-infected individuals, 14 days of therapy generally will suffice.

Specific agents. Trimethoprim-sulfamethoxazole remains the preferred drug for all patients (children and adults) who can tolerate it, because it is the most effective agent, is generally safe, is inexpensive, and is available in both oral and intravenous formulations.[4,33,39] The drug combination inhibits two sequential steps in *P. carinii* folate metabolism; TMP inhibits the enzyme dihydrofolate reductase and SMX inhibits dihydropteroate synthetase. The usual dose for children and adults is 15 to 20 mg/kg/day of the TMP component (75 to 100 mg/kg/day of the SMX component), given in four divided doses. Therapy is given intravenously at the onset for all but very mild disease; oral therapy can be used to finish a course of parenteral therapy for those who have responded well. The intravenous infusion should be infused over at least 60 minutes, and the dose must be adjusted for renal failure. It is possible (but not established) that holding the dose to 15 mg/kg/day (to provide trough serum levels of 5 to 8 μg/ml of TMP and 100 to 150 μg/ml of SMX) may reduce toxicity while providing efficacy.[4,33] Trimethoprim-sulfamethoxazole is generally well tolerated, although adult patients with HIV infection (and to a lesser extent children with HIV infection) have a much higher rate of adverse effects than do other patients.[3,4] Many of the adverse effects are thought to be due to the SMX component or its metabolites; desensitization of individuals with a history of adverse reactions has been advocated by some authorities but has not been studied in a controlled manner.[3,4,33] Mild adverse effects are not necessarily contraindications for further therapy, because they can be managed with antihistamines or antipyretics, or may even resolve and not recurr if the drug is temporarily withdrawn.[4,34,35] Such side effects include transient maculopapular rashes, itching, nausea, and fever; neutropenia can also occur. Urticaria, the Stevens-Johnson syndrome, or hepatitis may contraindicate further therapy.

Pentamidine isethionate is the most commonly used alternative to TMP-SMX.[3,4,33] It is an antiparasitic agent whose mechanism of action is not well established. For moderate to severe *P. carinii* disease in children or adults, pentamidine is best administered once daily as a slow (60 to 120 minutes) intravenous infusion of 4 mg/kg. In the past, intramuscular injections were used, but these led to the development of painful sterile abscesses. Pentamidine is a toxic drug in both patients with and without coexisting HIV infection. Nephrotoxicity, pancreatitis, hypotension, and hypoglycemia can develop during therapy or even days to weeks later. Azotemia and hypoglycemia tend to occur in the second and third weeks of therapy; the latter is thought to be due to pancreatic injury with subsequent release of insulin. Some patients develop insulin deficiency resulting in hyperglycemia. An aerosolized form of pentamidine was developed in an attempt to deliver medication to the lung while reducing toxicity. Aerosolized pentamidine is an effective agent for prophylaxis but is less effective for therapy of established disease than intravenous pentamidine or TMP-SMX, and thus it can be used for therapy of only very mild disease.[4,33] Aerosolized pentamidine has rarely been associated with pancreatitis, nephrotoxicity, and hypoglycemia, but it is commonly associated with cough due to bronchospasm.

Trimetrexate is a powerful inhibitor of dihydrofolate reductase. It is perhaps 1500 times more avid in binding the enzyme than TMP, but TMP is more selective for the *P. carinii* protein instead of the mammalian protein.[4] Thus trimetrexate must be given with leucovorin (folinic acid, which *P. carinii* cannot use as an extrinsic source for folate metabolism) to attenuate potentially severe trimetrexate-induced hematologic toxicity. When careful attention is paid to adjustment of the trimetrexate dosing and leucovorin dosing depending on observed hematologic toxicities, trimetrexate can serve as a better tolerated (but somewhat less effective) agent for severe *P. carinii* pneumonia than TMP-SMX.[40] Suggested starting points for dosing in adults are trimetrexate, 45 mg/m^2 given once daily intravenously over 60 to 90 minutes, and leucovorin, 80 $mg/m^2/day$ in four divided doses intravenously or orally. It is critical to extend the leucovorin administration for 3 days beyond the last administered dose of trimetrexate. A few children have been treated using this protocol as well, but data are limited.

Dapsone, like SMX, is a dihydropteroate synthetase inhibitor that is reportedly somewhat better tolerated than SMX. The drug is potentially useful because it is orally bioavailable, is inexpensive, and has a long half-life. However, it is not clear whether dapsone's efficacy when administered with TMP equals that of TMP-SMX or whether it is indeed less toxic.[4,33] Dapsone can cause methemoglobinemia (almost uniformly, but rarely to a treatment-limiting degree), anemia (especially if glucose-6-phosphate dehydrogenase deficiency is present), rash, and vomiting. Dapsone, 100 mg/day, has been used in adults as daily therapy for mild *P. carinii* pneumonia in combination with daily TMP (dapsone is not acceptable as single-agent therapy).[4] Perhaps a better role for dapsone is as a prophylactic agent (see discussion later in this chapter).

Atovaquone (formerly BW566C80) is an antimalarial hydroxynaphthoquinone. It inhibits protozoan mitochondrial electron transport, but the mechanism of action against *P. carinii* is unknown. The drug has a long serum half-life and is bioavailable orally (especially if ingested with fat-rich food and if no diarrhea or gastrointestinal disease is present), lending itself to use in mild to moderate *P. carinii* pneumonia. In a randomized, double-blind study of oral atovaquone, 750 mg tablets three times daily, vs. oral TMP-SMX, 320 mg to 1600 mg three times daily, conducted in 322 adults with mild to moderate *P. carinii* pneumonia, there were more therapeutic failures with atovaquone (20% vs. 7%, $p = 0.002$), but fewer patients required change of therapy because of treatment-limiting side effects (7% vs. 20%, $p = 0.001$).[41] Overall success rates were similar between the two groups. Thus atovaquone might serve as an alternative agent for mild *P. carinii* pneumonia in those patients who cannot tolerate TMP-SMX. Limited pharmacokinetic data in children suggest that 30 mg/kg/day of the suspension yields serum concentrations comparable with those found in adults given 750 mg twice daily, but controlled efficacy studies have not been completed in children as of this writing (June 1998). Palatability of the suspension has been problematic for some children and adults.

The combination of clindamycin and primaquine shows excellent activity in cell culture and experimental animal models of *P. carinii* infection, although neither agent is effective if used alone.[42] This regimen is attractive because of the relative inexpense of the drugs, their oral bioavailability, and the fact that each appears to concentrate in lung tissue. Several studies have been performed in adults using clindamycin-primaquine as either salvage therapy for patients not responding to or intolerant of conventional agents (TMP-SMX or pentamidine) and as primary therapy in mild to moderate *P. carinii* disease.[4] In one prospective noncomparative study, 20 (91%) of 22 patients given intravenous clindamycin, 900 mg every 8 hours, and oral primaquine, 30 mg/day for 10 days, followed by oral clindamycin, 450 mg every 6 hours, and primaquine, 30 mg/day, responded to therapy, and 16 (73%) completed therapy.[43] In a follow-up trial, 38 adults were treated for the entire course with oral medication (clindamycin, 600 mg every 8 hours, and primaquine, 30 mg/day);[43] 92% responded and 79% completed therapy. In these and other studies, the primary toxicity was a macular or maculopapular erythematous rash developing in about 60% of patients around day 10 of therapy, which often subsequently regressed, rarely necessitating limitation of therapy. About 10% of patients experienced diarrhea; because clindamycin has been associated with pseudomembranous colitis, therapy may need to be altered if severe diarrhea occurs. Like dapsone, primaquine causes methemoglobinemia (40% incidence in the previously mentioned study, but none requiring treatment or with serum methemoglobin >20%), and it can cause hemolytic anemia in patients with glucose-6-phosphate dehydrogenase deficiency. The combination of clindamycin-primaquine thus seems promising for therapy of mild to moderate *P. carinii* pneumonia in adults.[4,43] Although there is no theoretic reason why the combination should not also be effective in children, few data are available to guide its use.

Several classes of experimental therapeutic agents for *P. carinii* are listed in Box 47-1. New inhibitors of dihydrofolate reductase under investigation include the TMP analog RO 11-8958[44] and the biguanide antimalarial PS-15.[45] A number of novel pentamidine analogs are under active investigation as well, some of which are orally bioavailable and perhaps less toxic than parenteral pentamidine.[46] Members of the echinocandin class of compounds have both antifungal and anti–*P. carinii* activity, via inhibition of β-1,3 glucan synthetase.[1,47] Other inhibitors of enzymes or proteins required for *P. carinii* growth include topoisomerase inhibitors and β-tubulin antagonists.[10,48,49] Several antimalarial 8-aminoquinolines show promising activity in experimental animal models of *P. carinii* pneumonia prophylaxis and therapy; early trials of their use in human malaria are already under way.[48,50]

Finally, iron chelators, most prominently the licensed parenteral agent deferoxamine, show excellent activity in experimental models of *P. carinii* infection and have already demonstrated good adjunctive activity in clinical trials of malaria therapy in children and adults.[51-53]

Adjunct Therapy. Anti–*P. carinii* therapy is often associated with a decline in $Pa{O_2}$ of 10 to 30 mm Hg during the first few days, especially in patients with AIDS. Such a decline may be tolerated in those with mild disease, but it can be harmful in moderate to severely ill patients who already have $Pa{O_2}$ values below 70 mm Hg. It is not certain whether the decline in oxygenation is part of the natural progression of *P. carinii* pneumonia or whether dying organisms incite further pulmonary inflammation. The possibility that pulmonary inflammation might significantly contribute to lung damage in *P. carinii* pneumonia, along with the observation that *P. carinii* pneumonia in cancer patients often developed while corticosteroids were being tapered, suggested that corticosteroid therapy could serve as a useful adjunct to antimicrobial therapy.

Five recent controlled trials assessing the efficacy of adjunctive corticosteroid therapy in reducing pulmonary morbidity and mortality in adults with moderate to severe *P. carinii* pneumonia have been reviewed by a National Institutes of Health–University of California Expert Panel.[54] All four trials in which steroids were begun within 72 hours of anti–*P. carinii* therapy showed improved outcome, as documented by (in various combinations) prevention of initial decline in oxygenation, reduced need for mechanical ventilation, and reduced mortality rate (from 22% to 11% overall mortality rate in the largest trial).[54]

Adverse effects of steroid therapy included an excess of oral thrush and development of mucocutaneous herpes; there was no observed increase in Kaposi's sarcoma or life-threatening opportunistic fungal or mycobacterial infections. However, the threat of these complications mandates that the diagnosis of *P. carinii* pneumonia be made as definitively as possible, so as not to lead to adjunctive corticosteroid treatment of a process initially mimicking *Pneumocystis* disease that will worsen with therapy. Other adverse effects, such as gastrointestinal hemorrhage and metabolic disturbances, may occur as well.

The Expert Panel consensus was that for adults and adolescents over 13 years of age with moderate to severe *P. carinii* pneumonia, as defined by $Pa{O_2}$ below 70 mm Hg or A-a gradient above 35 mm Hg, adjunctive corticosteroid therapy should be begun as soon as possible after anti–*P. carinii* therapy is instituted.[54] The dosage regimen recommended was that used by the largest published study, as follows: on days 1 through 5 of therapy, 40 mg of oral prednisone twice daily; on days 6 through 10, 40 mg of prednisone once daily; and on days 11 through 21, 20 mg of oral prednisone once daily.[54]

Left unanswered by the Expert Panel, because of lack of available data, was whether adjunctive corticosteroid therapy would benefit patients with mild *P. carinii* pneumonia, *P. carinii*-infected pregnant women with HIV infection, *P. carinii* pneumonia patients with other forms of immunocompromise besides HIV infection, or children younger than 13 years of age with *P. carinii* pneumonia.[54]

Four recent reports have described the use of steroids in children with *P. carinii* pneumonia to be beneficial, but each study has been an open, nonrandomized trial without concurrent controls, using different dosages of medications among a combined study population of less than 50 children.[55-58] Despite these statistical limitations, it seems reasonable to consider using steroids as adjunctive therapy for children with moderate to severe *P. carinii* pneumonia, pending further data from controlled trials.

Antimicrobial Prophylaxis. Antimicrobial prophylaxis is highly effective in preventing the development of *P. carinii* pneumonia and is indicated for any group of patients with a high incidence of the disease resulting from immunosuppressive therapy or primary immune dysfunction.[2-4,33-36] Such groups include children with T lymphocyte dysfunction, such as those with acute lymphocytic leukemia, those with severe combined immunodeficiency syndromes, children undergoing intensive chemotherapy for lymphomas or solid tumors, and recipients of solid organ and bone marrow transplants.[2,20,33] A few children with humoral immune defects have also developed *P. carinii* pneumonia and may warrant prophylaxis, as have children with diseases such as rheumatoid arthritis or systemic lupus erythematosis who are undergoing high-dose corticosteroid therapy.[2,20] Finally, the most important group of immunodeficient patients recently recognized is the HIV-infected population, who require lifelong prophylaxis against *P. carinii* pneumonia.[34-36] Primary prophylaxis refers to the use of medication to prevent the initial episode of *P. carinii* pneumonia; secondary prophylaxis refers to the use of medication to prevent recurrences of disease.

Seminal controlled studies by Hughes et al[59] in 1977 showed that the incidence of *P. carinii* pneumonia in children with acute lymphocytic leukemia undergoing chemotherapy could be reduced from 21% to 0% by daily oral administration of TMP-SMX (150 mg/m^2 TMP and 750 mg/m^2 SMX divided in two daily doses). Subsequent studies by the same workers showed that TMP-SMX could be given on three consecutive days per week rather than daily, with equivalent efficacy.[60] These results now have been generalized to other groups of patients. Although controlled studies are lacking in other groups of patients, a number of retrospective analyses and a large body of clinical experience have indicated that a number of different dosage regimens of TMP-SMX (once or twice daily, 3 or 7 days per week) effectively prevent the development (primary prophylaxis) and recurrence (secondary prophylaxis) of *P. carinii* pneumonia in children and adults with both primary and acquired immunodeficiency, including those with HIV infection.[3,4,33-36]

Prophylaxis with TMP-SMX is simple, safe, inexpensive, and highly effective in patients with immunosuppression of any cause. Unfortunately, in the HIV-infected individual, the incidence of adverse effects is much higher than in other immunocompromised patients, especially in the HIV-infected adult.[3,4] Thus many adults and some children cannot tolerate TMP-SMX because of the development of substantial pruritis, rash, leukopenia, transaminase elevation, and nausea. For these individuals, the development of aerosolized pentamidine was an important advance. Aerosolized pentamidine delivered by the Respirgard II nebulizer at a monthly dose of 300 mg was shown to be effective in two controlled trials in adults with HIV infection (one trial was a primary prophylaxis study and the other a secondary prophylaxis study).[4,34,35] Two other controlled trials in Canada also demonstrated the effectiveness of aerosolized pentamidine, 60 mg every 2 weeks delivered by the Fisoneb ultrasonic nebulizer (a product not currently available in the United States).[4,34,35] The toxicity of aerosolized pentamidine is primarily limited to bad taste and bronchospasm and coughing. The latter complications can be reduced by administration of β-agonists such as albuterol, but they are of concern because of the possibility of coughing increasing the transmission of other coinfecting opportunistic pathogens (such as *M. tuberculosis*). Systemic toxicity of aerosolized pentamidine is rare, but it has been described. In addition, atypical *P. carinii* disease has developed in aerosolized pentamidine recipients (upper lobe pneumonia, extrapulmonary disease, etc.), complicating diagnosis and management. Finally, the medication is expensive and requires a source of compressed air.

Two recent controlled trials in adults with AIDS has shown that aerosolized pentamidine is less effective than TMP-SMX for primary and secondary prophylaxis.[61,62] Thus, when TMP-SMX is tolerated, it is the first choice for both children and adults. A third, recently reported randomized controlled trial of TMP-SMX, aerosolized pentamidine, and oral dapsone as primary prophylaxis in adults with advanced HIV infection showed that all three regimens were similarly effective for patients with 100 to 200 CD4+ lymphocytes/μl, but that aerosolized pentamidine was inferior for those patients with fewer than 100 CD4+ lymphocytes/μl.[50] Aerosolized pentamidine was better tolerated than systemic therapy.[63] If TMP-SMX, pentamidine, and dapsone are not tolerated, many theoretic options exist, but few have been subjected to large controlled trials. Dapsone with pyrimethamine, dapsone with TMP, sulfadoxine with pyrimethamine, and intermittent parenteral pentamidine also have all been tried in adults with HIV infection.[4] Limited data exist on the use of dapsone in children. Atovaquone and clindamycin-primaquine have theoretic attractiveness for children, but no data allow firm conclusions about their use in primary or secondary prophylaxis.

On the basis of the previously discussed considerations and other data, recent guidelines have been issued by the U.S. Public Health Service Task Force on Antipneumocystis Prophylaxis for Patients with HIV Infection for adults and adolescents over the age of 13,[35] and by the Working Group on *P. carinii* Prophylaxis for Children younger than 13 years of age.[36] In addition, the U.S. Public Health Service/Infectious Diseases Society of America Prevention of Opportunistic Infections Working Group has issued comprehensive guidelines on prevention of opportunistic infections, including those caused by *P. carinii,* in adults and children with HIV infection.[37,38] These important documents (and any future publications from the groups) should be consulted for detailed recommendations on prophylactic agents, choice of regimens, monitoring of patients, and treatment of breakthrough *P. carinii* disease. A summary of the guidelines is presented next.[35-38]

In the HIV-infected adolescent and adult, the CD4+ lymphocyte count below 200 cells/μl or the previous occurrence of *P. carinii* disease indicates high susceptibility to infection and mandates prophylaxis.[35,37,38] The preferred regimen for both primary and secondary prophylaxis is TMP-SMX for those who can tolerate it.[35,37,38] It is given for the lifetime of the patient, at a dose of one double-strength tablet (160 mg

TMP and 800 mg SMX) daily, 7 days a week.[35,37,38] Intermittent TMP-SMX regimens (2 or 3 days a week) have been effective in smaller, open-label trials, but the data have not been sufficient for the Task Force to recommend their routine use.[35,37,38] For those intolerant to TMP-SMX, dapsone (100 mg daily in one or two divided doses), dapsone plus pyrimethamine plus leucovorin (either 50 mg/day dapsone plus 50 mg/week pyrimethamine plus 25 mg/week leucovorin or 200 mg dapsone, 75 mg pyrimethamine, and 25 mg leucovorin all administered weekly), or aerosolized pentamidine (300 mg monthly by the Respirgard II nebulizer) is recommended.[37,38] Evaluation for tuberculosis is suggested before aerosolized pentamidine prophylaxis is instituted.[35] In the unusual situation in which TMP-SMX, dapsone, and aerosolized pentamidine all are not tolerated, other agents may need to be considered (e.g., atovaquone, clindamycin plus primaquine, parenteral pentamidine, or, in countries where available, 60 mg of aerosolized pentamidine every 2 weeks by the Fisoneb ultrasonic nebulizer).[35,37,38]

For HIV-infected children younger than 13 years of age, CD4+ lymphocyte counts have been used in the past to identify susceptibility to infection, but they must be interpreted carefully based on age-adjusted normal ranges.[36] A complicating factor is that because the normal counts are greater earlier in life, the numerical thresholds for prophylaxis used in adolescents and adults are not applicable to young children; 90% of HIV-infected infants with *P. carinii* pneumonia have CD4+ T lymphocyte counts below 1500 cells/μl, while in adults, a similar proportion have counts below 200 cells/μl.[36] Moreover, CD4+ lymphocyte counts can drop rapidly in infants in the days to weeks preceding diagnosis of *P. carinii* pneumonia. Finally, a recent study of HIV-infected children diagnosed with *P. carinii* pneumonia in the United States during 1991 through 1993 showed that most of the children who had not received prophylaxis had not yet even been identified as HIV exposed soon enough for CD4+ lymphocyte–based prophylaxis. For these reasons, the Working Group on *P. carinii* Prophylaxis for Children has released revised guidelines for prophylaxis against *P. carinii* pneumonia for children infected with or perinatally exposed to HIV (Fig. 47-6).[36] The recommendations include universal prophylaxis for HIV-exposed infants until such time that HIV infection is reasonably excluded (see Fig. 47-6). The preferred regimen is TMP-SMX in two divided doses, three times weekly; acceptable alternatives include once-daily TMP-SMX three times a week or twice-daily TMP-SMX seven times a week (see Fig. 47-6).[36] Aerosolized pentamidine, oral dapsone, and (least desirable) intravenous pentamidine are suggested alternatives for TMP-SMX-intolerant patients.[36]

Because of the recognized advantages of TMP-SMX (efficacy against pulmonary and extrapulmonary *P. carinii,* low cost, cross-protection against toxoplasmosis and bacterial infections), the guidelines call for consideration of rechallenge with TMP-SMX in case of non–life-threatening adverse effects, because many patients seem to tolerate rechallenge and can thus be continued on TMP-SMX.[35,37,38] Preliminary data suggest that TMP-SMX is better tolerated by HIV-infected children than adults, and that TMP-SMX prophylaxis is better tolerated than therapy.[3]

The prophylactic drug regimens shown in Fig. 47-6 may be used for the primary prophylaxis of *P. carinii* disease in children with non–HIV-related immunocompromise (e.g., cancer and cancer chemotherapy, congenital immunodeficiency, transplant recipients) as well. All children and adults with a previous episode of *P. carinii* disease require secondary prophylaxis, whether or not HIV infection is present.

LEGIONELLA PNEUMOPHILA

A number of species of genus *Legionella* of the family *Legionellaceae* are responsible for causing infection in humans.[64] *Legionella pneumophila,* the cause of legionnaires' disease, was the first species to be associated with fatal pneumonia and is the one most commonly implicated in human legionellosis.[65] Legionnaires' disease is uncommon in children. The illness is often grouped with the "atypical pneumonias" caused by *Chlamydia* or *Mycoplasma,* but this classification is unsatisfactory because the clinical features of legionellosis are much more variable.

Disease Mechanisms

Organism. *Legionella* organisms are pleomorphic gram-negative rods that are aerobic, motile, and nutritionally fastidious. On Gram's stain they may appear as small, faintly gram-negative coccobacilli or filamentous organisms. Growth of *Legionella* depends on the presence of L-cysteine and iron in specialized growth media, which often results in unsuccessful bacterial isolation unless the laboratory is forewarned that *Legionella* infection is suspected. The lack of growth on media routinely used in microbiology laboratories most likely plays a role in the underdiagnosis of *Legionella* infection. Similar to other gram-negative rods, the outer membrane of *Legionella* is primarily lipopolysaccharide, and the serogroup-specific antigen of the lipopolysaccharide is used for serotyping of the organism. *Legionella* species are saprophytic aquatic microorganisms that rarely become human pathogens. Most cases of *Legionella* infection are caused by only a few of the 50 or so serogroups among the 30 or more known species. The *L. pneumophila* serogroup 1 is responsible for up to 95% of *Legionella* infection in healthy individuals, and serogroups 4 and 6 are responsible for much of the rest.

Epidemiology. *Legionella* organisms are most commonly found in water sources; the natural reservoir may be freshwater amoebae.[66] The organism has been isolated both from natural (freshwater streams and lakes, water reservoirs) and artificial (cooling towers, potable-water distribution systems) aquatic habitats. The optimal temperature for growth is between 28° C and 40° C, a range present in both natural and artificial habitats.

In the initial period after the recognition of *Legionella* as a cause of pulmonary disease, the infection was most often identified in point-source epidemics. Sporadic individual infections often went unrecognized. However, more recent data from studies performed in adults suggest that *Legionella* may be responsible for up to 15% of community-acquired pneumonias and 40% of nosocomial pneumonias in some areas.[67-70] Immunodeficiency, corticosteroid and other immunosuppressive therapy, old age, chronic obstructive pulmonary disease, and cigarette smoking have been considered risks for *Legionella* infection in adults. Surgery also appears to be a risk factor in nosocomial infection,[71,72] and transplant patients are among the patients at the highest risk for *Legionella* infection.[73-75]

Recommendations for PCP prophylaxis and CD4+ monitoring for HIV-exposed infants and HIV-infected children, by age and HIV-infection status

Age/HIV-infection status	PCP prophylaxis	CD4+ monitoring
Birth to 4-6 wk HIV exposed	No prophylaxis	1 mo
4-6 wk to 4 mo HIV exposed	Prophylaxis	3 mo
4-12 mo		
HIV infected or indeterminate	Prophylaxis	6, 9, and 12 mo
HIV infection reasonably excluded*	No prophylaxis	None
1-5 yr, HIV infected	Prophylaxis if: CD4+ count is <500 cells/μL or CD4+ percentage is <15%‡§	Every 3-4 mo†
6-12 yr, HIV infected	Prophylaxis if: CD4+ count is <200 cells/μL or CD4+ percentage is <15%§	Every 3-4 mo†

*HIV infection can be reasonably excluded among children who have had two or more negative HIV diagnostic tests (i.e., HIV culture or PCR), both of which are performed at ≥1 month of age and one of which is performed at ≥4 months of age, or two or more negative HIV IgG antibody tests performed at >6 months of age among children who have no clinical evidence of HIV disease.
†More frequent monitoring (e.g., monthly) is recommended for children whose CD4+ counts or percentages are approaching the threshold at which prophylaxis is recommended.
‡Children 1-2 years of age who were receiving PCP prophylaxis and had a CD4+ count of <750 cells/μL or percentage of <15% at <12 months of age should continue prophylaxis.
§Prophylaxis should be considered on a case-by-case basis for children who might otherwise be at risk for PCP, such as children with rapidly declining CD4+ counts or percentages or children with Category C conditions. Children who have had PCP should receive lifelong PCP prophylaxis.

Drug regimens for PCP prophylaxis for children ≥4 weeks of age

Recommended regimen:

Trimethoprim/sulfamethoxazole (TMP-SMX) 150 mg TMP/m²/day with 750 mg SMX/M²/day administered orally in divided doses twice a day (bid) 3 times per week on consecutive days (e.g., Monday-Tuesday-Wednesday).

Acceptable alternative TMP-SMX dosage schedules:

- 150 mg TMP/m²/day with 750 mg SMX/m²/day administered orally as a **single daily dose** 3 times per week on consecutive days (e.g., Monday-Tuesday-Wednesday).
- 150 mg TMP/m²/day with 750 mg SMX/m²/day orally divided bid and **administered 7 days per week.**
- 150 mg TMP/m²/day with 750 mg SMX/m²/day administered orally divided bid and administered 3 times per week on **alternate days** (e.g., Monday-Wednesday-Friday).

Alternative regimens if TMP-SMX is not tolerated:

- **Dapsone***

  2 mg/kg (not to exceed 100 mg) administered orally once daily.
- **Aerosolized pentamidine*** (children ≥5 years of age)

  300 mg administered via Respirgard II inhaler monthly.

*If neither dapsone nor aerosolized pentamidine is tolerated, some clinicians use intravenous pentamidine (4 mg/kg) administered every 2 or 4 weeks.

Fig. 47-6. Recommendations for initiation of *P. carinii* pneumonia prophylaxis for HIV-exposed infants and HIV-infected children, by age and HIV infection status. (From Centers for Disease Control and Prevention: 1995 revised guidelines for prophylaxis against *Pneumocystis carinii* pneumonia for children infected with or perinatally exposed to human immunodeficiency virus, *MMWR Morbid Mortal Wkly Rep* 44(RR-4):1-11, 1995.)

BOX 47-2
Risk Factors for *Legionella* Infection

Immunocompromise

Human immunodeficiency virus infection
Severe combined immunodeficiency
Chronic granulomatous disease
Leukemia
Post transplantation
Steroid use
Hypogammaglobulinemia
Systemic lupus erythematosus
Wegener's granulomatosis

Pulmonary compromise

Severe asthma
Aspiration pneumonitis
Viral pneumonia
Chronic pulmonary disease (e.g., BPD)

Miscellaneous

Chronic underlying disease (Neurodegenerative disease)
Trisomy 21

In children, immunologic and pulmonary compromise have also been considered risks for *Legionella* infection (Box 47-2), but sound data regarding the actual incidence of pediatric *Legionella* are lacking. Most of the information has been obtained by serologic surveys of specific groups of patients under medical care and therefore may be biased. In one study from Iceland, 14% of children showed serologic evidence of previous *Legionella* infection.[76] Legionnaires' disease has been documented in children with immunosuppression, but large studies of this population have not been completed.[77-81] Nevertheless, as in adults, immunosuppression must be considered one of the most important factors assumed to increase the risk of *Legionella* infection in childhood.

The literature suggests that *Legionella* infection in children is uncommon. *Legionella* appeared to be responsible for only about 1% of cases of pneumonia in seven surveys involving a total of 742 children (range 0% to 6% in individual studies).[82-88] A number of reports of nosocomial transmission of *Legionella* infection in children have been published.[89-91] These reports have most often been linked to contaminated water supplies, and aerosol-generating respiratory equipment has been implicated in outbreaks. Person-to-person transmission probably does not play a role in the nosocomial spread of *Legionella.*

Pathology and Pathogenesis. *Legionella* organisms are facultative intracellular pathogens that cause an acute fibrinopurulent pneumonia with alveolitis and bronchiolitis. Histologically, organisms can be seen both intracellularly and extracellularly along with inflammatory cells in the purulent exudate. Besides the lungs, *Legionella* has also been found in the lymph nodes, brain, kidney, liver, spleen, bone marrow, and myocardium.[92] *Legionella* is cleared from the upper respiratory tract by the mucociliary action. Therefore, any process that compromises mucociliary clearance (such as tobacco smoke) will increase the risk of legionellosis. It is phagocytosed by local pulmonary macrophages but is not actively killed, and macrophages may actually support the growth of *Legionella* (thereby allowing the organism to evade one of the first lines of pulmonary host defense). *Legionella* multiplies intracellularly and kills infected macrophages, and then spreads to infect other macrophages. Cell-mediated immunity appears to be the primary host defense mechanism against this intracellular pathogen, although the roles of neutrophils and humoral immunity have not yet been well characterized. The mode of acquisition of original infection in humans is uncertain but is likely to be airborne inhalation of contaminated aerosols, or perhaps aspiration of contaminated water or oropharyngeal secretions.

Clinical Manifestations

Most of the information regarding the classic clinical features of *Legionella* infection is from studies of adults, because of the rarity of documented pediatric legionellosis. *Legionella* infection in adults has a wide spectrum of clinical manifestations ranging from serious and fatal pneumonia to a self-limiting viral-like illness, but typically the infection manifests as one of two clinical syndromes: Pontiac fever or legionnaires' disease.

Pontiac fever is a viral-like illness with high fever, headache, malaise, and myalgias. The illness is self-limiting, with a short incubation period (24 to 48 hours) and recovery in 7 to 10 days, usually without sequelae. Pneumonia is not usually a part of Pontiac fever, although nonproductive cough may be present. Antibiotic therapy is not necessarily required.

Legionnaires' disease is a multisystem disease that primarily affects lungs. The onset of illness may be acute or insidious. Although pneumonia is the predominant feature of this disease, respiratory symptoms may be absent initially. After an incubation period (which can be as short as 48 hours or as long as 10 days) patients have weakness, lethargy, fatigability, myalgia, and malaise. High fevers (greater than 40° C) and chills are not uncommon. Almost all patients are febrile, although initially fever may be absent or low grade.[64] Relative bradycardia may be present in febrile patients. A dry cough is present in almost all patients. Most adults develop purulent sputum and sometimes hemoptysis. Patients may complain of pleuritic chest pain and shaking chills. Neurologic and gastrointestinal symptoms may also be prominent in some patients. Neurologic complaints may include headache, lethargy, confusion, cerebellar ataxia, agitation, mental status changes, and encephalopathy. Although isolation of *Legionella* from the cerebrospinal fluid (CSF) has not been successful, CSF pleocytosis and elevated protein concentration is seen.[93] Diarrhea is often the most prominent gastrointestinal symptom, with stools being watery and nonbloody. Anorexia may be present, and some patients may complain of abdominal cramps.[72] Hyponatremia and elevated serum transaminase levels are seen more commonly with *Legionella* than pneumonias caused by other organisms. A number of extrapulmonary sites of *Legionella* infection occur as a result of bacteremic dissemination.

In short, the triad of confusion, diarrhea, and pneumonia, especially if accompanied by hyponatremia and elevated serum transaminase levels, should raise the suspicion of legionnaires' disease. Unfortunately, several prospective studies have noted that it is not possible to distinguish between legionnaires' disease and other causes of pneumonia on the basis of one or more of these findings alone.

Radiographic findings of legionellosis are variable and nonspecific, from patchy alveolar infiltration to a consolidated pneumonia (Fig. 47-7). Pleural effusions may be seen, and cavitary lesions develop occasionally.[94] The usual progression is from patchy areas or nodules to multilobar, almost homoge-

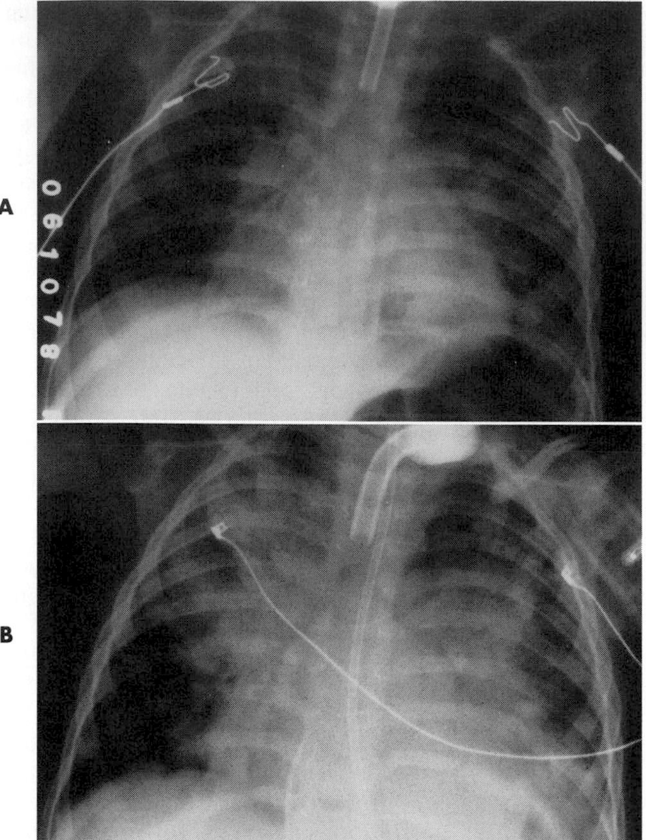

Fig. 47-7. Serial radiographs of a 19-month-old who developed lipoid-like pneumonia after the ingestion of oil of cloves, followed by induced emesis and aspiration. Subsequently this child required a tracheostomy, steroid therapy, and multiple antimicrobial agents. One month after the aspiration the patient died from respiratory failure secondary to *Legionella pneumophila* serogroup 6 pneumonia. **A,** Chest x-ray 26 days after aspiration and 1 day after onset of fever and increasing respiratory distress. **B,** Chest x-ray 2 days later, showing increasing infiltrates. One day later the child died. (Radiographs courtesy Leland L. Fan, MD, National Jewish Center for Immunology and Respiratory Medicine and Department of Pathology, Children's Hospital, Denver, Colo.)

neous infiltrates. A somewhat typical feature is the centripetal progression of *L. pneumophila* pneumonia. Initially the pneumonia is present in the peripheral lung regions and then becomes sublobar and finally lobar, involving contiguous lobes on the same side.[95-97] This progression may be complicated by adenopathy, abscess, or atelectasis.[98,99] The majority of patients with legionnaires' disease develop radiographic evidence of pneumonia.[94]

Patients who are healthy before the infection will most likely recover in 7 to 10 days. Immunocompromised or debilitated patients may develop multiorgan failure and die of respiratory failure. Some patients may have other complications of one of the organ systems involved (such as colitis or peritonitis) that may take weeks to resolve.

Laboratory Diagnosis. Various methods are available for laboratory diagnosis of *Legionella* infection. Culture is currently considered the gold standard but requires special media, such as buffered charcoal yeast extract agar with L-cysteine and ferric ions to support growth. Selective media that contain antibacterial and antifungal agents to suppress the growth of other organisms may increase the yield. When *Legionella* is suspected, the clinical laboratory may also "decontaminate" the specimen with a brief acid treatment before inoculation of the specialized growth medium, again to reduce the overgrowth of other organisms. Even with these specialized techniques, it may take up to 5 days to isolate the slow-growing *Legionella.*

Direct fluorescent antibody (DFA) staining for *Legionella* is a rapid test requiring as few as 2 to 4 hours for results. This test is highly specific for diagnosis; very rarely, there may be cross-reaction with *Pseudomonas* species. However, the sensitivity of DFA can vary with the experience of the technician and quality of the specimen. Therefore, a negative DFA does not exclude *Legionella* infection. A monoclonal antibody "cocktail" for the eight *L. pneumophila* serotypes is more specific than the polyclonal anti-*Legionella* antibody preparations for diagnosis of *Legionella.*

Specimens for culture and DFA stain commonly must be obtained by bronchoscopy, because sputum specimens are usually not available from children. Even if available, sputum is not the optimum specimen. Bronchoalveolar lavage is the method of choice, because bronchial washings are not very useful. A pleural fluid specimen, if available, is also useful for culture and DFA stain for diagnosis of *Legionella* infection.

Serologic assays for *Legionella* antibodies are not generally useful in clinical decision making. The antibody detected by indirect immunofluorescence tests is produced against the lipopolysaccharides in the outer membrane of *Legionella.* Diagnosis is based on a fourfold or greater rise in antibody titer, between acute and convalescent serum specimens, to at least 1:128. This seroconversion may take up to 4 to 8 weeks to develop. In epidemics, a single titer of 1:256 or greater, with supporting clinical illness, has been considered sufficient to make a presumptive diagnosis of legionellosis,[100] but this definition has been questioned recently.[101] The antibody titers are often difficult to interpret because they may remain elevated for months after an infection, there may be cross-reactions with other gram-negative organisms, and some patients altogether fail to mount an antibody response to *Legionella.*

Commercially available DNA probes and urinary antigen tests for the diagnosis of *Legionella* infection are not yet as commonly used in clinical practice but may offer a rapid turnaround time with relatively high sensitivity and specificity. These diagnostic techniques may become more prominent in the near future.[101] Although the urinary antigen test reacts only with serogroup 1 *Legionella,* this limited cross-reactivity is less of a problem clinically because serogroup 1 organisms are the cause of most clinical disease.

The diagnosis of *Legionella* infection cannot be excluded on the basis of any single test. These tests can be complementary, and more than one test may need to be performed for the diagnosis of *Legionella* infection.

Management

Many antibiotics inhibit the growth of *Legionella* in vitro, but only those that concentrate well inside cells are clinically useful to combat this intracellular pathogen.[102] Thus only erythromycin, doxycycline, rifampin, possibly TMP-SMX, and perhaps the fluoroquinolones should even be considered as therapeutic agents; β-lactams and aminoglycosides will not be clinically effective, despite in vitro activity.

Erythromycin (40 to 50 mg/kg/day in children, 2 to 4 g/day in adults) is the antibiotic of choice for *Legionella* infection.

This choice is not based on carefully controlled clinical trials, but rather on clinical experience in isolated legionellosis, nosocomial infections, and outbreaks of legionnaires' disease.[102] The newer macrolides (azithromycin and clarithromycin) show good in vitro and animal model activity against *Legionella,* and would be expected to work well, but clinical experience is limited.[102]

Doxycycline is also effective, although experience with the drug is limited, and it is not suitable for therapy of children younger than 7 to 9 years of age. Rifampin may be beneficial in some patients with severe legionellosis in combination with erythromycin.[102] Trimethoprim-sulfamethoxazole also has been reported to successfully treat *Legionella* infections, as have newer fluoroquinolones such as ciprofloxacin.[102] However, the experience with TMP-SMX is meager. It is recommended not to use ciprofloxacin and other quinolones in young children, but these agents may be the most useful for adolescents and adults.[102]

The initial antibiotic therapy of severe *Legionella* infection should be given intravenously, and when clinical improvement occurs antibiotic administration may be changed to the oral route to complete at least 14 days of therapy. Unfortunately, high-dose intravenous erythromycin can cause painful phlebitis and also gastrointestinal upset; oral high-dose erythromycin can be irritating to the gastrointestinal tract as well. It is possible that the newer macrolides (azithromycin and clarithromycin), or, for older patients, doxycycline or a fluoroquinolone (ciprofloxacin, ofloxacin), would be more appropriate for erythromycin-intolerant patients. Immunosuppressed patients and patients with lung abscess may require longer courses of antibiotic therapy, perhaps erythromycin and rifampin for the first 5 days and then erythromycin alone for 2 to 3 weeks. Length of the antibiotic therapy should not be gauged solely by radiologic manifestations, because the radiograph may show progression, even when the patient is receiving adequate antibiotic therapy (similar to what occurs during the therapy of pneumococcal pneumonia).

PROTOZOAN INFECTIONS

Protozoan infections are common worldwide, but pulmonary complications are relatively rare. This section reviews notable pulmonary disease caused by protozoa; helminthic pulmonary infections will be discussed individually.

Amebiasis is endemic worldwide, but the prevalence of disease is highest in areas with poorer sanitation systems, including nearly all developing countries. Although a large number of species infect humans, most human disease is associated with *Entamoeba histolytica.* Recent evidence suggests that even most organisms identified as *E. histolytica* are not actually pathogenic; rather, a minority of strains that contain a number of virulence genes cause nearly all clinical disease. Cysts are shed in the stools of individuals with intestinal infection (either symptomatic or asymptomatic) and are ingested by others via contaminated food or water. Direct person-to-person transmission can also occur. Although intestinal disease causes dysentery, most patients with extraintestinal disease do not have dysentery. The most common extraintestinal manifestation is amebic liver abscess, which typically causes fever, abdominal pain or tenderness, and leukocytosis.

Pleuropulmonary involvement is seen in only 0.1% of cases of amebiasis and usually represents a complication of amebic liver abscess.[103] An inflammatory reaction may develop adjacent to an abscess in the liver or subphrenic space, causing pleural effusion or pneumonitis. Hepatic abscesses can also rupture into the pleural space and cause localized empyema, pneumonitis, or lung abscess.[103,104] Erosion into the airways may lead to chocolate-colored sputum or even to a bronchobiliary fistula. Pericardial involvement is rarely noted. Only rarely are *E. histolytica* trophozoites identified in aspirated or expectorated material. Thus diagnosis is usually based on demonstration of serum antibodies. Extraintestinal amebiasis usually responds to treatment with antiparasitic agents such as metronidazole, followed by therapy with an agent directed at cysts such as paromomycin or iodoquinol to clear intestinal cyst carriage. Surgical drainage may be used as an adjunct to therapy in some cases of hepatic abscesses.

Malaria is a common infection worldwide, with 270 million persons infected and 1 to 2 million deaths per year. Uncomplicated malaria is characterized by fever, chills, and hemolysis. Malaria can be complicated by involvement of the central nervous system, kidneys, or lungs. Pulmonary involvement is thought to result from a combination of cytokine-associated damage and perhaps localized ischemia caused by vessels occluded with adherent parasitized erythrocytes.[105] The clinical picture of bilateral infiltrates and hypoxia resembles that seen in other causes of noncardiac pulmonary edema, such as the adult respiratory distress syndrome. Management involves aggressive therapy for the parasitemia with chemotherapeutic agents and possibly exchange transfusion. In addition, ventilatory support is often required.

Leishmania donovani and *Cryptosporidium parvum* have been identified in pleuropulmonary infections in a few cases.[103] Most of these patients had depressed immunity, most often from AIDS.

Toxoplasma gondii can cause clinically and radiologically discernible pneumonia, or it can be found as a silent component in patients with clinical toxoplasmosis of other organ systems.[106] Pulmonary toxoplasmosis is rare among infections in immunocompetent hosts (probably much less than 1%), but it is increasingly reported among immunosuppressed adults with malignancy or AIDS.[106,107] The symptoms, signs, and radiographic findings provide few clues to the diagnosis and may easily be confused with those of *P. carinii* or cytomegalovirus disease (dyspnea, cough, fever, rales, and interstitial infiltrates). Serologic diagnosis can be difficult in immunocompromised hosts who may not produce antibody, and thus BAL or lung biopsy may be required. Pyrimethamine combined with sulfadiazine is the standard therapeutic regimen for severe toxoplasmosis, as summarized elsewhere.[108-110] Both the mortality rate and the relapse rate among survivors have been reported to be high,[106] although the lack of prospective contemporary data may have biased these estimates.

Echinococcosis

Echinococcosis, also known as hydatid disease, is caused by the cestode parasites of the genus *Echinococcus.* The three species that infect humans, *Echinococcus granulosus, Echinococcus multilocularis,* and *Echinococcus vogeli,* differ in geographic location, host specificity, and disease manifestations.

Echinococcus granulosus has separate domestic and sylvatic life cycles, which roughly correlate with disease manifestations. In the domestic cycle, the definitive host (i.e., the host harboring the intestinal tapeworm form) is the domestic dog. The most common intermediate host (i.e., the host harboring the tissue cyst) is sheep. Other intermediate hosts include goats, swine, cattle, buffalo, horses, and camels. In the sylvatic cycle, wild carnivores, such as wolves, coyotes, jackals, and dingos, are the normal definitive hosts. The intermediate hosts include moose, elk, and deer. Sylvatic hydatid disease is usually acquired from domestic dogs, which are in turn infected by ingestion of contaminated game.

Human disease caused by *E. granulosus* is termed *cystic hydatid disease.* Cystic hydatid disease has a wide geographic distribution and is endemic in most areas where sheep are raised. Highly endemic areas include eastern and southern Europe, the Middle East, North Africa, Australia, and southern portions of South America. There are also endemic foci in North America. The domestic cycle has been described in sheep-raising areas of the American Southwest, including among Navajo and Zuni Indians in Arizona and New Mexico, among Mormons in Utah, and among Basque shepherds in California. The sylvatic cycle occurs in Alaska and Canada.

Human disease caused by *E. multilocularis* is termed *alveolar hydatid disease. Echinococcus multilocularis* is limited to colder portions of the Northern Hemisphere, including most of the arctic and subarctic regions, the alpine regions of central Europe, and much of Russia and central Asia. In North America, endemic areas include the subarctic tundra and scattered areas in the north central plains. The usual definitive hosts are foxes. Dogs and cats can serve as definitive hosts as well. The most important intermediate hosts are small rodents such as mice and voles.

Human disease caused by *E. vogeli* is termed *multicystic hydatid disease. Echinococcus vogeli* is limited to parts of lower Central America and upper South America. The normal definitive host is the bush dog, and the intermediate host is the paca.

Disease Mechanisms

The most common pattern of *E. granulosus* infection is for the parasites to cycle between sheep (or cattle) and dogs. Dogs (definitive hosts) harbor the intestinal tapeworms, which shed segments containing eggs into the environment. Sheep (intermediate hosts) are infected by ingestion of the tapeworm eggs. The eggs hatch in the sheep intestine and migrate via the portal veins to the liver and lung, where they mature into cysts. The cysts contain germinal membranes and protoscolices, which can form daughter cysts if the cyst ruptures. To complete the life cycle, dogs must have access to the viscera of the slaughtered intermediate host. Thus when dogs eat infected mutton or lamb (or beef) they become infected with the echinococcal cysts, which then mature into the intestinal tapeworm form, completing the life cycle.

People are infected by exposure to parasite eggs from infected dogs. The eggs hatch in the intestines, and the larvae penetrate the intestinal mucosa into the portal veins and lodge in the liver, or in some cases the lung. The cysts do not cause symptoms until they have enlarged to several centimeters in diameter. Symptoms usually result from mass effects of the expanding cyst. The rate of cyst expansion is determined in part by the tissue infected. Cysts in the liver typically expand at a rate of 1 to 5 cm in diameter per year and require decades before causing symptoms. Lung tissue offers less resistance than liver, such that pulmonary cysts may expand more rapidly and cause clinical symptoms earlier in life. In one recent series, one third of patients with pulmonary cysts were 20 years of age or younger.[111] Cyst rupture is associated with localized inflammation, allergic manifestations, and the formation of daughter cysts. Bacterial superinfection of the cyst may lead to symptoms suggestive of bacterial infections, such as fever and leukocytosis.

Clinical Manifestations

The majority of patients with intact pulmonary hydatid cysts are asymptomatic and are discovered incidentally at autopsy or by radiographic studies. Signs and symptoms vary with the location, number, and size of cysts. Domestic cycle cystic hydatid disease causes single cysts in 80% of cases. About 25% of single cysts are located in the lungs, about 60% to 70% are in the liver, and fewer than 5% are in other organs, including muscle, spleen, brain, and bone. Isolated pulmonary disease, however, appears to be more common in children and in adults with sylvatic disease.[112,113] Cough, hemoptysis, and chest pain are the most common symptoms in patients with hydatid disease of the lungs. In the case of cyst rupture, patients may note abrupt onset of cough and expectoration of cyst fluid, parasite membranes (described as "grape skins"), or even scolices. Cyst rupture may also be associated with allergic manifestations, including urticaria, pruritis, and anaphylactic shock, and may lead to pneumothorax or empyema. Secondary bacterial infection is common and causes fever and purulent sputum. The less common sylvatic echinococcal disease is typically mild and is often self-limited. Allergic manifestations and other complications of rupture are rare.[113]

One fourth of patients with pulmonary hydatid cysts also have liver involvement. Symptoms of liver disease include epigastric pain, bloating, and indigestion, and signs include hepatomegaly and obstructive jaundice. If cysts are secondarily infected, patients may have signs and symptoms of liver abscess.

Alveolar hydatid disease (caused by *E. multilocularis*) invariably involves the liver; pulmonary disease, when present, is due to metastatic lesions. Clinical disease is limited to adults.[114] Similarly, multicystic hydatid disease *(E. vogeli)* typically causes hepatic disease in middle-aged adults.

Radiographic Features. Cysts are single in 80% and bilateral in 20% of cases. There is a predilection for the lower lobes and the right lung over the left. Intact cysts appear as well-defined, rounded masses on chest x-ray (Fig. 47-8). Cysts adjacent to the pleura may conform to the shape of adjoining structures. On CT scan the cyst fluid is at water density, and the cyst wall may vary in thickness. Daughter cysts are occasionally seen within the cyst. If the cysts have eroded into bronchioles, air can be introduced between the pericyst and the parasite membrane, resulting in the appearance of a thin lucent crescent in the upper portion of the cyst: the "air meniscus" or "crescent" sign.[115] When the cyst has collapsed, the collapsed endocyst membrane may appear floating freely in the remaining fluid, producing an irregular air-fluid level ("water lilly sign") (see Fig. 47-8). Ruptured cysts may be associated with surrounding broncho-pneumonia or may be secondarily infected, appearing as a lung abscess with thickened walls and an air-fluid level. Collapsed or detached endocysts or daughter cysts are more readily visualized by CT scan.[116] The role of magnetic resonance imaging (MRI) in pulmonary hydatid disease is as yet undefined.

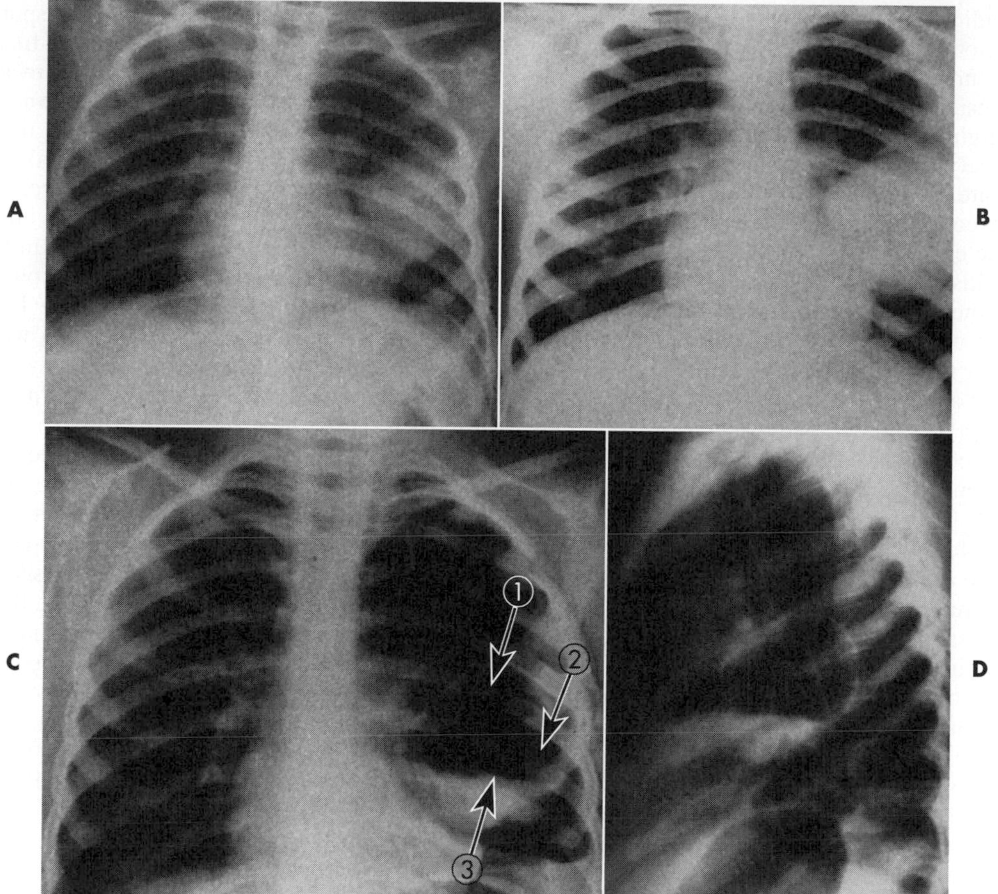

Fig. 47-8. Serial chest radiographs of a 4-year-old girl with cystic hydatid disease caused by *Echinococcus granulosus.* **A,** Chest x-ray taken during asymptomatic period reveals large solitary left-lung lesion. **B,** Subsequent film taken 1 year later shows growth of cyst. **C,** The cyst has now ruptured, producing a left hydropneumothorax; the characteristic "air meniscus" or "crescent" sign is seen when air is introduced between the cyst and the host adventitia *(arrow 1).* The remnants of the cyst *(arrow 2)* appear inside the pericyst, and the irregular air-fluid level caused by the floating collapsed endocyst membrane ("water-lilly sign") is also seen *(arrow 3).* **D,** Lateral view of the chest corresponding to panel **C.** (Figure reproduced from Reeder MM, Palmer PES, eds: *The radiology of tropical diseases with epidemiological, pathological, and clinical correlation,* Baltimore, 1981, Williams & Wilkins.)

Laboratory Diagnosis. Laboratory findings in all forms of hydatid disease are nonspecific. Only 30% or less of patients manifest eosinophilia. Serologic tests can be used to confirm a clinical diagnosis of hydatid disease. Indirect hemagglutination and enzyme-linked immunosorbent assay (ELISA) techniques are about 90% sensitive.[117] The sensitivity of these assays is lower for isolated pulmonary disease.[117] Specificity can be improved by employing either immunoprecipitation or enzyme-linked immunotransfer blot for confirmation. Antibodies to cyst antigens are not always present, especially in patients with unruptured cysts. For *E. multilocularis* and *E. vogeli* infection, assays employing semipurified antigens from *E. multilocularis* (e.g., Em2 ELISA) are more sensitive than tests employing *E. granulosus* antigens.

In the setting of a ruptured pulmonary cyst, parasite membranes or hooks may be visualized on sputum examination. The hooks stain well with the Ziehl-Neelsen acid-fast stain. The laminated membranes stain with periodic acid-Schiff stain. Cyst aspiration should be avoided in most cases of hydatid disease because of the potential risks of metastatic infection and anaphylactic reactions. For sylvatic disease, however, there are no documented cases of spread of cysts or of anaphylactic reactions with rupture of cysts. Thus cyst aspiration for sylvatic pulmonary disease and perhaps for hepatic hydatid disease can probably be used safely as a diagnostic technique.[113,118] In some patients, a definitive diagnosis may be possible only at surgery.

Management

Surgical resection is the best established therapy for domestic cystic hydatid disease when treatment is necessary. Until recently, all cases were believed to require radical surgery to avoid spillage of cyst contents and associated risk of anaphylaxis or the development of metastatic cysts. However, many authorities are now using a combined approach to therapy involving surgery, chemotherapy, or even careful monitoring with time alone depending on the *Echinococcus* organism type (domestic or sylvatic), the number and location of lesions, symptomatology, and underlying health of the patient.

If surgery is indicated (either at the onset of therapy or after a trial of chemotherapy to reduce worm viability), care is taken to avoid rupture and release of cyst contents. For pulmonary cysts, the usual approach is to remove the entire cyst, pericyst, and a margin of normal lung. Scolicidal agents such as 0.1% to 0.5% cetyltrimethylammonium bromide (Cetrimide), silver nitrate, or hypertonic saline can be instilled within cysts before completing resection. The use of scolicidal agents with hepatic cysts, however, has been associated with sclerosing cholangitis or hypernatremia. Preoperative and perioperative chemotherapy with antiparasitic agents (e.g., albendazole) may be used to kill the scolices and prevent intraoperative spread from spillage of cyst contents.[119] Percutaneous drainage and instillation of scolicidal agents has been useful for hepatic cysts.[120] At present, however, there are too few data to comment on the safety or efficacy of this treatment with pulmonary cysts, and this procedure is not recommended.[120]

The benzimidazole antiparasitic drugs mebendazole and albendazole are active against *Echinococcus,* but initial clinical studies gave conflicting results. The consensus of recent studies, however, suggests that most patients will respond to antiparasitic agents, although many of the responses are only partial (i.e., reduction in size of the cysts rather than disappearance).[121-123] The response rate with albendazole is usually better than with mebendazole; some experts think that pulmonary cysts respond more often than hepatic cysts. Albendazole therapy is indicated as an adjunct to surgery, or as sole therapy for those patients with inoperable, widespread, or numerous cysts, as well as for those patients who are judged to be unsuitable for surgery because of complicated medical problems.[119] Albendazole was recently approved for use in the United States. The suggested dose is 15 mg/kg per day orally divided twice daily (up to 400 mg twice daily) for 28 days, followed by a "drug-free holiday" of 2 weeks, with repetition of the 28-day course twice more (three cycles of 28-day therapy each separated by 14-day drug-free intervals).

Sylvatic cystic hydatid disease is usually self-limited. Symptomatic treatment of associated bacterial infections may be required. In general, however, patients do not require either operative intervention or antiparasitic agents.

Alveolar hydatid disease caused by *E. multilocularis* is probably best managed by prolonged chemotherapy, because only a minority of cases of this metastatic infection can be cured surgically.[114,119]

Too few data exist to guide therapy for multicystic *E. vogeli* disease; preliminary reports suggest that albendazole therapy may be effective.[119]

Paragonimiasis

Human paragonimiasis is caused by infection with trematode lung flukes of the genus *Paragonimus,* most commonly *P. westermani.* Infection is acquired by ingesting undercooked crustaceans. Eastern Asia is the primary endemic region, but there are also foci in western Africa and, less commonly, in Latin America.[124] In endemic areas, paragonimiasis is a common cause of bronchitis and hemoptysis, and it must be differentiated from tuberculosis, which may cause similar clinical and radiographic findings.

Disease Mechanisms

The adult parasites live within cystic lesions in the lung parenchyma.[124] The eggs are passed via tunnels into the bronchi and are either expectorated in sputum or swallowed and eventually passed in the stools. In fresh water, the eggs embryonate, hatch into miracidia, and invade snails (the first intermediate host). After a cycle of asexual reproduction, the cercarial form can either emerge from the snail and invade freshwater crabs (or sometimes crayfish) or be ingested with the snail by the crab. Infectious metacercariae form in the tissues of the crabs. Mammalian hosts are infected by ingesting raw or undercooked crab (or crayfish). In humans, the metacercariae excyst and penetrate the duodenum and, after a period of further development in the liver, penetrate the diaphragm into the lung. Over 5 to 6 weeks the parasites mature into adults, which can begin to lay eggs as early as 8 to 10 weeks after infection. The adult worms may persist in the lungs for up to 20 years.

In the lung, the parasite cysts are 1 to 4 cm nodules, typically located within a few centimeters of the pleura, adjacent to bronchi or bronchioles. The cysts consist of a pseudocapsule of host granulation tissue and contain one or two adult worms (7 to 12 mm by 4 to 7 mm). Parasite eggs and Charcot-Leyden crystals are also present within the cyst. Associated pathology may include bronchopneumonia, bronchitis and bronchiectasis, fibrosis, or angiitis. There are often tunnels, egg granulomas, and calcified eggs in the vicinity of the cysts.

Each of the three endemic regions for paragonimiasis is associated with different species of parasite and minor differences in epidemiology and clinical manifestations. The major factors necessary for transmission include the presence of large numbers of the snail and crustacean intermediate hosts and local customs in which raw or lightly cooked crustaceans are ingested. The prevalence of infection has been estimated to range from 15% to 45% in endemic regions in China and 0.3% to 78% in Korea. A number of recent reports have stressed the prevalence of this infection in newly arrived Southeast Asian refugees in the United States.

Clinical Manifestations

Acute infection is typically asymptomatic, but it may be associated with abdominal pain, diarrhea, urticaria, cough, fever, or chest pain.[124] Chronic pulmonary infection usually follows an incubation period of about 6 months. Mild infections may be asymptomatic or associated with symptoms of bronchitis (cough, sputum production, and chest discomfort). Many patients will complain of dyspnea and wheezing. Pleuritic chest pain and production of rusty brown ("golden flake") sputum or even frank hemoptysis are typically present. Mild fever may be present also. Symptoms are usually episodic and are frequently associated with exertion. Some patients primarily manifest with pleural disease. Pleural effusions are exudative, frequently contain numerous eosinophils, and may be quite large. Ectopic worms sometimes can be found in the brain and abdominal cavity.

Radiographic Features. Up to 20% of patients with pulmonary paragonimiasis will have normal chest radiographs.[103] One third of patients have patchy infiltrates and one third have well-defined homogeneous densities. Many of the chest radiographs show either cystic lesions or streaks within the infiltrates, depending on the stage of the infection. Early in infection when the larvae first arrive in the lung, poorly defined cottonwool shadows are seen. Later, when the mature worms produce eggs, characteristic ring shadows with a corona (thin-walled cysts with crescent-shaped opacities along one edge) are noted (Fig. 47-9).[125] Linear worm burrows may be seen adjacent to the cysts (see Fig. 47-9). Pleural abnormalities are

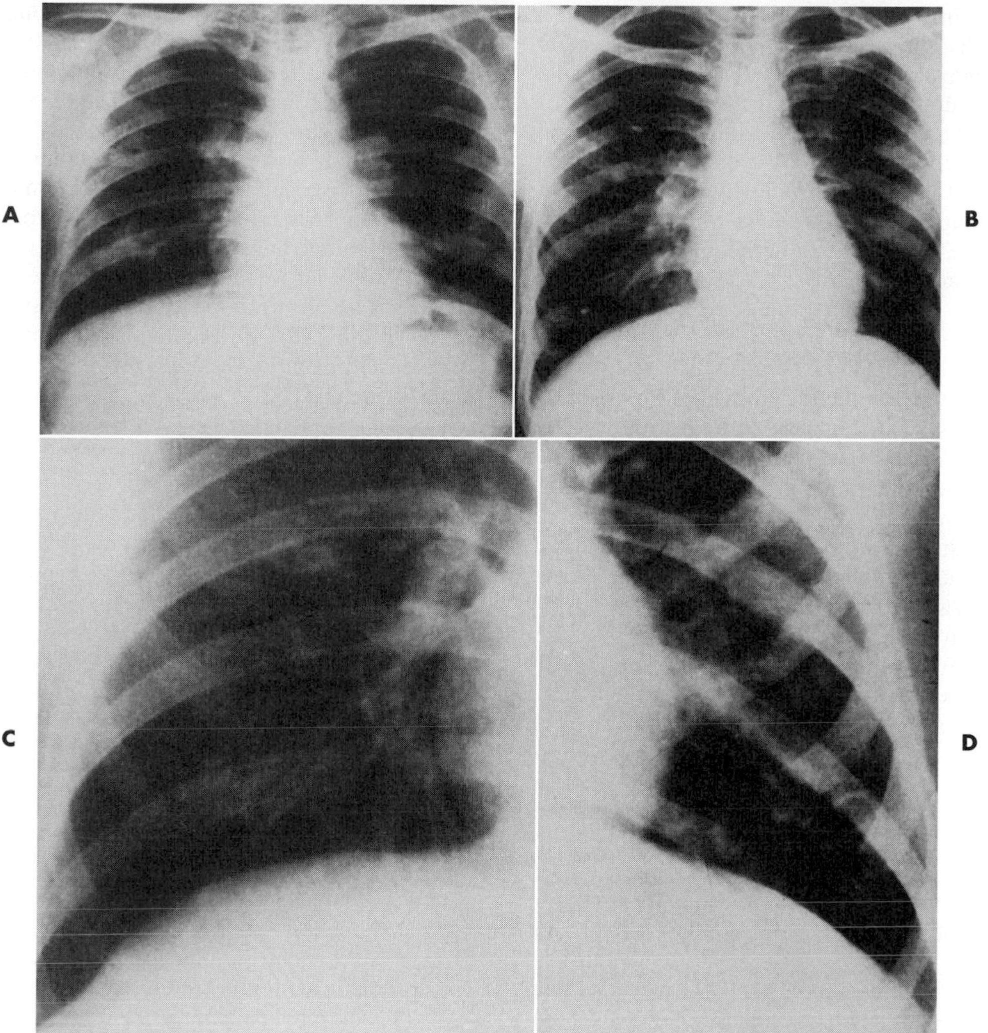

Fig. 47-9. Chest radiographs from four different Korean adults with *Paragonimus westermani* infection. **A,** Multiple cystic cavities of 1 to 2 cm are seen in the right midlung and lower lung. **B,** Aggregates of 5 mm ringlike cysts appear in the right midlung, right base, and left upper lobe (especially under the left clavicle). Older calcified lesions appear in the right lung also. **C,** A single ring shadow with medial corona is seen in the right midlung. **D,** Numerous cystic cavities, some of which show coronas as well as adjacent linear tracts representing worm burrows. (Figure reproduced from Reeder MM, Palmer PES, eds: *The radiology of tropical diseases with epidemiological, pathological, and clinical correlation,* Baltimore, 1981, Williams & Wilkins.)

noted in up to half of all cases and may occasionally be the only abnormality.[125,126] Late in the infection after the death of the parasite, cysts often become calcified, simulating the radiographic appearance of tuberculosis (see Fig. 47-9).

Laboratory Diagnosis. Laboratory tests often reveal eosinophilia. Sputum examination may reveal ova, necrotic tissue, erythrocytes, leukocytes, or Charcot-Leyden crystals. Definitive diagnosis requires demonstration of the operculated eggs in sputum or stools. The eggs may be visualized directly or with the Papanicolaou stain. Because the eggs are shed intermittently, multiple specimens or 24-hour collections are often required to demonstrate the eggs. Body fluids from involved sites, such as cerebrospinal fluid or pleural fluid, may occasionally contain eggs, but demonstration of eggs is usually not possible. A number of serologic assays have been employed and may be required to make a firm diagnosis in cases in which eggs cannot be identified, such as in extrapulmonary disease.

Treatment

Praziquantel is the drug of choice for treating paragonimiasis. At a dose of 75 mg/kg per day in three divided doses for 2 to 3 days, cure rates approach 100%.[127] Symptoms improve rapidly, and eggs typically clear from the sputum in a matter of weeks. Radiographic clearing may be slower. Side effects such as drowsiness and headaches are noted occasionally but are typically mild. Bithionol is available from the Centers for Disease Control and Prevention as an alternative treatment, but it is associated with more frequent and severe side effects.

Strongyloidiasis

Strongyloides stercoralis is the cause of human strongyloidiasis. *Strongyloides* has a wide geographic distribution, including most of the developing world, parts of Europe, and scattered foci in the United States, especially in the Appalachian region.[128] The clinical presentation of strongyloidiasis can vary from asymptomatic infection and mild intestinal disease to fatal disseminated disease with multiple organ involvement. Unlike other nematode parasites, *Strongyloides* larvae can mature into free-living adults in the soil; furthermore, the worms also can multiply in humans without passing through the soil or any other host via an autoinfectious cycle. Recently, many authors have reported the *Strongyloides* hyperinfection syndrome in immunosuppressed older adults who were infected decades earlier as a result of serving in the military in the Far East during World War II.

Disease Mechanisms

The *Strongyloides* life cycle is more complex than that of other nematodes. It begins when infective filariform larvae in the soil penetrate intact skin. After passive migration (via the bloodstream) to the lungs, the parasites exit the capillaries into the alveoli. After further maturation in the lung, the larvae migrate up the trachea and are swallowed. The adult females attach to the small intestine and produce eggs, which are laid in the lamina propria. The eggs hatch within the lumen of the gut, and rhabditiform larvae are excreted into the soil, where they either molt into infective filariform larvae or mature into free-living adults. The free-living adults, unique among the pathogenic nematodes, can lay eggs in the soil that will hatch into rhabditiform larvae; these larvae will subsequently molt into infective filariform larvae. The autoinfective cycle of *Strongyloides* arises when some of the rhabditiform larvae in the intestines or perianal area molt into filariform larvae before reaching the soil. These filariform larvae can directly reinfect the host by penetrating either the colonic mucosa or the perianal skin. It is the autoinfective cycle that is thought to be responsible for chronic infection, which can last virtually indefinitely (for at least 40 years).

Strongyloidiasis is primarily acquired by skin contact with contaminated soil. There is no clear evidence of direct person-to-person transmission. Fecal-oral spread is thought to occur rarely.[129]

In most cases, strongyloidiasis is only mildly symptomatic. Intestinal infection is associated with congestion and mononuclear cell infiltration. There are descriptions of rare cases with spruelike malabsorption. Migration of the larvae through the lungs may stimulate a hypersensitivity response presenting as asthma and eosinophilia (Loeffler's pneumonia).

In uncomplicated cases of chronic infection, low numbers of parasites are in equilibrium with the host. Disease is primarily abdominal and cutaneous in nature; respiratory complaints are distinctly unusual, but asthma and chronic obstructive lung disease have been reported.

The symptomatic hyperinfection syndrome occurs primarily in compromised hosts. Although hyperinfection has been associated with various malignancies, renal disease, asthma, and autoimmune diseases, the vast majority of cases are associated with corticosteroid treatment.[130] In the past, it was thought that hyperinfection resulted from failure of the host response to kill migratory larvae. More recently, it has been hypothesized that hyperinfection may result from a direct effect of corticosteroids on larvae via acceleration of molting, rather than the immunocompromised state itself.[130] This theory would explain why patients with HIV infection–induced immunocompromise living in endemic areas for strongyloidiasis do not commonly develop the *Strongyloides* hyperinfection syndrome.[130]

Patients with the *Strongyloides* hyperinfection syndrome have massive worm burdens, with hundreds of thousands of adult parasites in the intestines.[129] The lung is the primary extraintestinal organ involved. Damage to the lung is in part mechanical. Passage of larvae from the bloodstream to the alveoli causes microhemorrhages. When there are low numbers of larvae the microhemorrhages are of little consequence. With dissemination, however, innumerable microhemorrhages may lead to massive pulmonary hemorrhage, manifested as hemoptysis, pulmonary infiltrates, and respiratory distress. Because alveolar hemorrhage may occur after treatment, some have speculated that immunologic mechanisms may also be involved. Larval migration from the intestines may be associated with invasion of the bloodstream by bacteria, either because of breaks in the mucosa or in association with the parasite cuticle.

Clinical Manifestations

Chronic strongyloidiasis may be asymptomatic. When symptoms are present, they are often nonspecific: abdominal pain, bloating, heartburn, diarrhea, constipation, and chronic urticaria.[129,131] When the filariform larvae migrate through the skin, serpiginous urticarial lesions termed *larva currens* may be noted. These lesions appear to reflect both direct parasite migration and an associated hypersensitivity response. Cough, dyspnea, wheezing, and fleeting pulmonary infiltrates have been described in association with larval migration also. Asthma and chronic obstructive lung disease have been reported in strongyloidiasis. Although the role the parasite plays in the pathogenesis is not clear, strongyloidiasis should be considered in patients with asthma and significant eosinophilia.

The *Strongyloides* hyperinfection syndrome, which may occur days to months after the initiation of immunosuppression, primarily causes gastrointestinal and pulmonary manifestations.[129,131] In contrast to uncomplicated disease, most patients with hyperinfection do not have eosinophilia. In addition to severe abdominal pain, nausea, vomiting, and diarrhea, hyperinfection may progress to intestinal obstruction, paralytic ileus, gastrointestinal bleeding, protein-losing enteropathy, peritonitis, and shock. The pulmonary symptoms of hyperinfection are nonspecific. A minority of patients will have only bronchospasm, but most patients will have pulmonary infiltrates (which may be focal or diffuse), opacities with or without cavitation, or consolidation. Common symptoms include cough productive of sputum, hemoptysis, dyspnea, and wheezing. Respiratory failure may develop in severe cases. In nearly one third of cases, hyperinfection is accompanied by severe bacterial infections.[129] These infections include pneumonia, lung abscess, sepsis, meningitis, and brain abscess. The most common bacterial isolates are enteric gram-negative bacilli and group D streptococci (including *Enterococcus*). The source of enteric bacteria may be damaged intestinal mucosa, organisms associated with the surface of the filariform larvae, or even organisms from the parasites' intestinal tracts. Other systems commonly affected include skin, liver, and biliary tract.

Radiographic Features. The results of intestinal x-rays are typically nondiagnostic but may show gastritis, duodenitis, and mucosal thickening, spasm, and transverse folds in the duodenum. In hyperinfection, there may be disruption of the mucosa, ulcerations, or ileus.[129]

Chest radiographs are usually normal in uncomplicated disease. In contrast, hyperinfection is usually accompanied by changes on chest radiographs.[129] Pulmonary infiltrates are typically diffuse but may be focal. Lobar consolidation may occur with or without accompanying bacterial superinfection. Some patients have localized nodules. Cavitation and abscess formation have been associated with both infiltrates and nodules.

Laboratory Diagnosis. Uncomplicated strongyloidiasis is usually diagnosed by examination of three separate stool specimens for rhabditiform larvae. Because the burden of organisms is low, larvae may be difficult to detect, however, and a positive diagnosis cannot always be obtained even with multiple specimens.[129] Additional methods of diagnosing infection include sampling of duodenal fluid for larvae (string test), duodenal biopsy, and serologic assays for antibody. ELISA titers are available from the Centers for Disease Control and Prevention.

For patients with hyperinfection, demonstration of parasites is less difficult. The key is to consider the diagnosis of strongyloidiasis in immunocompromised hosts with nonspecific symptoms. The burden of parasites in the stool is high.

Management

Both thiabendazole and ivermectin are approved in the United States for use in the treatment of strongyloidiasis. Thiabendazole therapy consists of 50 mg/kg per day orally in two divided doses for periods of 2 days for acute uncomplicated disease or 5 to 10 days for complicated disease. The duration should be determined by following clinical response and parasite burden. Thiabendazole therapy is frequently complicated by side effects, including nausea, vomiting, and dizziness. Treatment failures have been noted in 15% of uncomplicated cases, and fatality in hyperinfected patients may occur despite chemotherapy. No parenteral formulation is available; patients with intestinal obstruction or ileus must be treated with intermittent therapy via nasogastric tube.

Recent trials with ivermectin have shown response rates at least as good as thiabendazole with fewer side effects,[130-133] and this drug is now approved for use in the United States. For nondisseminated strongyloidiasis, a single dose of 200 μg/kg by mouth is given. For disseminated strongyloidiasis (hyperinfection syndrome), repeated courses of single-dose therapy may be required at 2-week intervals; data are lacking to determine the optimal regimen. Albendazole, a broad-spectrum benzimidazole antiparasitic agent, also appears to be at least as effective as thiabendazole (although perhaps less so than ivermectin) but with fewer side effects.[131,132] It is used elsewhere in the world but is not approved for this use in the United States.

Visceral Larva Migrans

Migration of larvae of several nematode species through the liver, lung, and central nervous system can give rise to the syndrome of visceral larva migrans, causing pulmonary manifestations such as asthma and eosinophilic pneumonitis. Although most of the infections are due to *Toxocara canis,* the canine roundworm, a similar clinical picture can be seen with *Toxocara cati,* the cat roundworm, *Ascaris suum,* a pig roundworm, and, rarely, *Baylisascaris procyonis,* a raccoon ascarid.

Toxocara is endemic worldwide, and human toxocariasis has been recognized in nearly every country. In the United States, most of the 52 million domestic dogs are infected with *Toxocara,* usually from perinatal exposure.[134] Up to one third of puppies and dogs at any one time pass *Toxocara* ova into the soil. The eggs can withstand a wide variety of environmental conditions and remain infective for years. *Toxocara* eggs can be recovered from yards of homes, parks, and playgrounds frequented by children. The seroprevalence of antibodies to *Toxocara* in the United States is 2.8%, with rates of 4.6% to 7.3% in children ages 1 to 11 years old.[135] In contrast, seroprevalence rates in developing countries are typically 50% to 80%.[134] Infection is associated with pica and geophagia.

Disease Mechanisms

The life cycle of *T. canis* in dogs is similar to that of *Ascaris* in humans. After ingestion of the ova, the larvae hatch, migrate through the lungs, are swallowed, and develop into adult worms in the canine intestines. Ova are shed in the stool but must embryonate in the soil over a period of weeks before they are infectious. Humans are infected after ingesting embryonated eggs from the soil. The *Toxocara* ova hatch in the intestines and penetrate the intestinal wall. Humans are an abnormal host, however, and the larvae are unable to complete their migration and maturation into adult worms. Instead, the larvae continue to migrate through the tissues of the liver, lung, and to a lesser extent the eye and the central nervous system. The larvae can continue to migrate for years within the human viscera.

Migratory larvae and their excretory products induce a strong inflammatory response, with eosinophils as the predominant cell. Most patients also have a prominent peripheral eosinophilia. Hemorrhages may be noted at sites where the larvae exit the host venules. Asthma and urticaria are associated with an elevated IgE response. When the larvae become trapped in the host tissues, they typically induce an eosinophilic granulomatous response, which may subsequently lead to fibrosis and calcification. Thus disease is related to both parasite migration and host inflammation.

The pathogenesis of *Toxocara* infections is thought to be related to the number of infecting organisms.[136] Thus infections with low numbers of organisms evoke only a minimal immune response. In these cases, disease may not be apparent until the larvae migrate to the eye (causing the ocular larva migrans syndrome). Heavier infections elicit a stronger host response, with larvae trapped and destroyed in the liver and lungs causing symptoms of visceral larva migrans. Rarely, as the numbers of larvae increase still further (e.g., a large inoculum in a very young child), the host is unable to trap the migratory larvae, and patients may have both visceral and ocular larva migrans.

Clinical Manifestations

The clinical presentation of visceral larva migrans varies with the number of larvae and the organs infected. Most infected patients are asymptomatic, but some have pulmonary symptoms and signs.[134,136-138] Cough is the most common symptom, and wheezing is reported in over half of cases. Examination may reveal wheezes, crepitations, or signs of consolidation. One third to one half of patients have pulmonary infiltrates. Visceral larva migrans should be considered in children with asthma of unknown cause, especially with a history of pica. Eosinophilia is usually present and may be pronounced. However, recent descriptions note normal eosinophil counts in up to 27% of patients with elevated *Toxocara* titers.[137] Other common clinical manifestations of visceral larva migrans relate to involvement of the abdomen: abdominal pain, hepatomegaly, anorexia, nausea, and vomiting. Lethargy and sleep and behavior disturbances are also common. Only a minority of patients have cervical lymphadenopathy or fever.

Ocular larva migrans is generally distinct from visceral larva migrans, and takes the form of leukocoria and posterior granulomas (mimicking retinoblastoma), chronic endophthalmitis, retinal detachment, and uveitis. It is distinctly unusual to see any visceral signs or symptoms in children with ocular disease, and such patients are generally older (mean age 8 years vs. 2 years for visceral disease) and have normal eosinophil counts and lower antibody titers.

Occasional involvement of the nervous system may take the form of seizures, eosinophilic meningitis, or one of a variety of focal neurologic symptoms.[138]

Radiographic Features. The chest radiograph will be abnormal in 30% to 50% of cases of visceral larva migrans. Abnormalities are described as alveolar, interstitial, or miliary. The infiltrates may be unilateral or bilateral, patchy or diffuse. Infiltrates are often migratory. Hilar adenopathy may be present.

Laboratory Diagnosis. It is difficult to make a definitive specific diagnosis of visceral larva migrans. Definitive diagnosis requires the demonstration of larvae in biopsy specimens, especially from the liver. A presumptive diagnosis, however, can be made based on a consistent clinical picture in a child with a history of soil, grass, or feces pica. Because the human host does not allow the worms to mature, *no* ova are found in the stool.

Eosinophilia, hyperglobulinemia (IgG, IgM, and IgE), and elevated isohemagglutinin titers (due to worm surface components that cross-react serologically with blood-group antigens) are often found in children with visceral larva migrans. Anti-*Toxocara* antibody tests also aid in diagnosis. An ELISA assay employing *Toxocara* larval excretory-secretory antigens has been shown to be a specific indicator of *Toxocara* infection (using a cutoff of 1:32, sensitivity in visceral larva migrans of 73% to 78%, and specificity greater than 90%).[136] Many of the "negative" specimens nonetheless showed low but detectable titers of antibody (1:8 to 1:16). There are some cross-reactions to other species of ascarids. A positive ELISA does not ensure that a patient's illness is due to *Toxocara,* because a small percentage of normals will also have antibody titers.

Management

The symptoms usually regress spontaneously over a period of months to years such that mild disease may not require specific treatment. Treatments include measures aimed at decreasing the host inflammatory response in addition to antihelminthic drugs. Antihistamines have been used to diminish symptoms in some cases. Corticosteroids may dramatically reduce pulmonary inflammation and are indicated in life-threatening infection, including severe bronchospasm and disease of the myocardium or central nervous system.

The precise role of antihelminthic drugs in visceral larva migrans is unclear. Thiabendazole treatment was associated with improvement in clinical symptoms in case series at doses of 50 mg/kg per day orally in two divided doses for 3 days to 1 month. Treatment is associated with a transient rise in eosinophil count (thought to be due to release of antigen by dying larvae) followed by resolution of symptoms and of the eosinophilia. In a double-blind controlled trial in asymptomatic cases, however, treatment with thiabendazole was no more effective than placebo at lowering eosinophil counts or antibody titers.[139]

Diethylcarbamazine has also been reported as effective in human and experimental studies. In a controlled trial, patients treated with diethylcarbamazine had a significant decrease in eosinophilia and parasite-specific IgE compared with untreated controls.[140] The clinical response is also thought to be superior to that seen with thiabendazole. Diethylcarbamazine should be started at a dose of 3 mg/kg per day orally in three divided doses and increased as tolerated to 6 mg/kg per day in three divided doses for 5 to 10 days. The drug is not approved for general use in the United States but can be obtained from the manufacturer on compassionate use protocols.

Other Helminthic Infections

Tropical pulmonary eosinophilia is one of the causes of the syndrome of pulmonary infiltrates with eosinophilia.[103,141] The disease is thought to represent an unusual immunologic reaction to the microfilariae of parasites more commonly associated with lymphatic filariasis (*Wuchereria bancrofti* and *Brugia malayi*). The clinical presentation includes cough, wheezing, and peripheral blood eosinophilia. Patients have a gradual onset of cough and paroxysms of wheezing and breathlessness mimicking asthmatic attacks. Systemic complaints can include fever, weight loss, and fatigue. Chest radiographs show increased vascular markings, diffuse interstitial nodular lesions, and mottled opacities. Pulmonary function tests usually show restrictive defects, although obstructive defects are also noted. Antifilarial antibodies are present and can be used to confirm the diagnosis. Patients usually respond to treatment with diethylcarbamazine 6 mg/kg per day in three divided doses given for 3 weeks, although several courses may be required. *Dirofilaria,* the dog heartworm, is endemic in the United States and can cause pulmonary nodules.[103] This syndome has been described only in adults.

Pulmonary symptoms can also be identified during larval migration through the lungs for *Ascaris lumbricoides,* hookworm, and other roundworms.[103] The symptoms and pathogenesis are similar to those seen with *Toxocara* infection. However, because the larvae are able to complete their normal migration, symptoms are self-limited (i.e., there is no chronic larva migrans stage), and ova later appear in the stool. *Ascaris* infections with low numbers of organisms are usually asymptomatic. Symptoms may develop 9 to 12 days after ingestion of large numbers of ova and include cough, chest discomfort, wheezing, and hemoptysis. Some patients have urticaria or pruritic skin lesion. Low-grade fever is common. On examination, there may be wheezing and crepitations, but signs of consolidation are absent. Chest radiographs may reveal oval infiltrates, which are migratory. Eosinophilia is characteristic. Symptoms resolve spontaneously in 5 to 10 days. Diagnosis at the time of chest symptomatology requires demonstration of the larvae in sputum or gastric aspirate, because ova passed in the stool are not produced until weeks after pulmonary symptoms resolve. Therapy is given with mebendazole, 100 mg orally twice daily for 3 days (same dose for all ages), or pyrantel pamoate, 11 mg/kg orally once. With therapy, some migrating worms may be expelled orally.

Schistosomiasis is caused by infection with the blood flukes *Schistosoma mansoni, S. japonicum, S. hematobium, S. mekongi,* and *S. intercalatum.*[103] Approximately 200 million people are infected worldwide, with endemic areas in Asia, the Middle East, Africa, and Latin America. Human infection is acquired by penetration of the skin by cercaria released from freshwater snails. The adult worms live in the mesenteric (most species) or vesical *(S. hematobium)* venules. Disease results from a granulomatous reaction to the eggs resulting in portal hypertension or fibrosis of the urinary tract. Eggs may also migrate to the lungs, where they may cause an obliterative arteriolitis that may result in pulmonary hypertension. Schistosomiasis is treated with praziquantel.

REFERENCES

Pneumocystis Carinii

1. Walzer PD, ed: Pneumocystis carinii *pneumonia,* ed 2, New York, 1994, Marcel Dekker.
2. Hughes WT, Anderson DC: *Pneumocystis carinii* pneumonia. In Fiegin RD, Cherry JD, eds: *Textbook of pediatric infectious diseases,* ed 4, Philadelphia, 1998, WB Saunders, pp 2490-2499.
3. Hughes WT: *Pneumocystis carinii* pneumonia. In Pizzo PA, Wilfert CM, eds: *Pediatric AIDS: the challenge of HIV infection in infants, children, and adolescents,* ed 2, Baltimore, 1994, Williams & Wilkins, pp 405-418.
4. Sattler FR: *Pneumocystis carinii* pneumonia. In Broder S, Merigan TC Jr, Bolognesi D, eds: *Textbook of AIDS medicine,* Baltimore, 1994, Williams & Wilkins, pp 193-221.
5. Walzer PD: *Pneumocystis carinii.* In Mandell GL, Bennett JE, Dolin R, eds: *Mandell, Douglas and Bennett's principles and practice of infectious diseases,* ed 4, New York, 1995, Churchill Livingstone, pp 2475-2487.
6. Bartlett MS, Smith JW: *Pneumocystis carinii,* an opportunist in immunocompromised patients, *Clin Microbiol Rev* 4:137-149, 1991.
7. Hughes WT: *Pneumocystis carinii* pneumonia: new approaches to diagnosis, treatment, and prevention, *Pediatr Infect Dis J* 10:391-399, 1991.
8. Smulian AG, Walzer PD: The biology of *Pneumocystis carinii, Crit Rev Microbiol* 18:191-216, 1992.
9. Walzer PD: *Pneumocystis carinii:* recent advances in basic biology and their clinical application, *AIDS* 7:1293-1305, 1993.
10. Edlind TD, Bartlett MS, Weinberg GA, Prah GN, Smith JW: The β-tubulin gene from rat and human isolates of *Pneumocystis carinii, Mol Microbiol* 6:3365-3373, 1992.
11. Bartlett M, Cushion MT, Fishman JA, Kaneshiro ES, Lee CH, Leibowitz MJ, Lu JJ, Lundgren B, Peters SE, Smith JW, Smulian AG, Staben C, Stringer, JR, Stringer, SL, Wakefield AE, Walzer PD, Weinberg, GA, for the *Pneumocystis* Workshop: Revised nomenclature for *Pneumocystis carinii, J Eukaryotic Microbiol* 41:121S-122S, 1994.
12. Sloand E, Laughon B, Armstrong M, Bartlett MS, Blumenfeld W, Cushion M, Kalica A, Kovacs JA, Martin W, Pitt E, Pesanti EL, Richards F, Rose R, Walzer P: The challenge of *Pneumocystis carinii* culture, *J Eukaryotic Microbiol* 40:188-195, 1993.
13. Hughes WT: Natural mode of acquisition for de novo infection with *Pneumocystis carinii, J Infect Dis* 145:842-848, 1982.
14. Hughes WT, Bartley DL, Smith BM: A natural source of infection due to *Pneumocystis carinii, J Infect Dis* 147:595, 1983.
15. Wakefield AE: Detection of DNA sequences identical to *Pneumocystis carinii* in samples of ambient air, *J Eukaryotic Microbiol* 41:116S, 1994.
16. Weinberg GA, Durant PJ: Genetic diversity of *Pneumocystis carinii* derived from infected rats, mice, ferrets, and cell cultures, *J Eukaryotic Microbiol* 41:223-228, 1994.
17. Weinberg GA, Edlind TD, Lu JJ, Lee CH, Bauer NL, Durant PJ: Genetic diversity of *Pneumocystis carinii* from different host species at the β-tubulin gene locus and at the internal transcribed spacer regions of the rRNA gene cluster, *J Eukaryotic Microbiol* 41:118S, 1994.
18. Gigliotti F, Harmsen AG, Haidaris CG, Haidaris PJ: *Pneumocystis carinii* is not universally transmissable between mammalian species, *Infect Immun* 61:2886-2890, 1993.
19. Chen W, Gigliotti F, Harmsen AG: Latency is not an inevitable outcome of infection with *Pneumocystis carinii, Infect Immun* 61:5406-5409, 1993.
20. Sepkowitz KA: *Pneumocystis carinii* pneumonia in patients without AIDS, *Clin Infect Dis* 17(suppl 2):S416-S422, 1993.
21. Martin WJ II: Pathogenesis of *Pneumocystis carinii* pneumonia, *Am J Respir Cell Mol Biol* 8:356-357, 1993.
22. Limper AH: Adhesive glycoproteins in the pathogenesis of *Pneumocystis carinii* pneumonia: host defense or microbial offense? *J Lab Clin Med* 125:12-13, 1995.
23. Harmsen AG, Chen W, Gigliotti F: Active immunity to *Pneumocystis carinii* reinfection in T-cell-depleted mice, *Infect Immun* 63:2391-2395, 1995.
24. Su TH, Martin WJ II: Pathogenesis and host response in *Pneumocystis carinii* pneumonia, *Annu Rev Med* 45:61-72, 1994.
25. Raviglione MC: Extrapulmonary pneumocystosis: the first 50 cases, *Rev Infect Dis* 12:1127-1138, 1990.
26. Kovacs JA, Hiemenz JW, Macher AM, Stover D, Murray HW, Shellhamer J, Lane HC, Urmacher C, Honig C, Longo DL, Parker MM, Natanson C, Parrillo JE, Fauci AS, Pizzo PA, Masur H: *Pneumocystis carinii* pneumonia: a comparison between patients with the acquired immunodeficiency syndrome and patients with other immunodeficiencies, *Ann Intern Med* 100:663-671, 1984.
27. Limper AH, Offord KD, Smith TF, Martin WJ II: *Pneumocystis carinii* pneumonia. Differences in lung parasite number and inflammation in patients with and without AIDS, *Am Rev Respir Dis* 140:1204-1209, 1989.
28. Simonds RJ, Oxtoby MJ, Caldwell B, Gwinn ML, Rogers MF: *Pneumocystis carinii* pneumonia among US children with perinatally acquired HIV infection, *JAMA* 270:470-473, 1993.
29. Simonds RJ, Lindegren ML, Thomas P, Hanson D, Caldwell B, Scott G, Rogers MF: Prophylaxis against *Pneumocystis carinii* pneumonia among children with perinatally acquired human immunodeficiency virus infection in the United States, *N Engl J Med* 332:786-790, 1995.
30. Wakefield AE, Guiver L, Miller RF, Hopkin JM: DNA-amplification on induced sputum samples for diagnosis of *Pneumocystis carinii* pneumonia, *Lancet* 337:1378-1379, 1991.
31. Lu JJ, Chen CH, Bartlett MS, Smith JW, Lee CH: Comparison of six different PCR methods for detection of *Pneumocystis carinii, J Clin Microbiol* 33:2785-2788, 1995.
32. Atzori C, Lu JJ, Jiang B, Bartlett MS, Orlando G, Queener, SF, Smith JW, Cargnel A, Lee CH: Diagnosis of *Pneumocystis carinii* pneumonia in AIDS patients by using polymerase chain reactions on serum specimens, *J Infect Dis* 172:1623-1626, 1995.
33. Masur H: Prevention and treatment of *Pneumocystis* pneumonia, *N Engl J Med* 327:1853-1860, 1992.
34. Kovacs JA, Masur H: Prophylaxis for *Pneumocystis carinii* pneumonia in patients infected with human immunodeficiency virus, *Clin Infect Dis* 14:1005-1009, 1992.
35. Centers for Disease Control: Recommendations for prophylaxis against *Pneumocystis carinii* pneumonia for adults and adolescents infected with human immunodeficiency virus, *MMWR Morbid Mortal Wkly Rep* 41(RR-4):1-11, 1992.
36. Centers for Disease Control: 1995 revised guidelines for prophylaxis against *Pneumocystis carinii* pneumonia for children infected with or perinatally exposed to human immunodeficiency virus, *MMWR Morbid Mortal Wkly Rep* 44(RR-4):1-11, 1995.
37. Centers for Disease Control and Prevention: USPHS/IDSA guidelines for the prevention of opportunitistic infections in persons infected with human immunodeficiency virus: a summary, *MMWR Morbid Mortal Wkly Rep* 46(RR-12):1-46, 1997.
38. Kaplan JE, Masur, H, Holmes KK, eds: Prevention of opportunistic infections in persons infected with human immunodeficiency virus, *Clin Infect Dis* 25(suppl 3):S299-S335, 1997.
39. Sattler FR, Cowan R, Nielson DM, Ruskin J: Trimethoprim-sulfamethoxazole compared with pentamidine for treatment of *Pneumocystis carinii* pneumonia in the acquired immunodeficiency syndrome: a prospective noncrossover study, *Ann Intern Med* 109:280-287, 1988.
40. Sattler FR, Frame P, Davis R, Nichols L, Shelton B, Akil B, Baughman R, Hughlett C, Weins W, Boylen CT, van der Horst C, Black J, Powderly W, Steigbigel RT, Leedon JM, Masur H, Feinberg J, and the AIDS Clinical Trials Group 029/031 Research Team: Trimetrexate with leucovorin versus trimethoprim-sulfamethoxazole for moderate to severe episodes of *Pneumocystis carinii* pneumonia in patients with AIDS: a prospective controlled multicenter investigation of the AIDS Clinical Trials Group Protocol 029/031, *J Infect Dis* 170:165-172, 1994.
41. Hughes W, Leoung G, Kramer F, Bozette SA, Safrin S, Frame P, Clumeck N, Masur H, Lancaster D, Chan C, Lavelle J, Rosenstock J, Falloon J, Feinberg J, LaFon, S, Rogers M, Sattler F: Comparison of atovaquone (566C80) with trimethoprim-sulfamethoxazole to treat *Pneumocystis carinii* pneumonia in patients with AIDS, *N Engl J Med* 328:1521-1527, 1993.
42. Queener SF, Bartlett MS, Richardson JD, Durkin MM, Jay MA, Smith JW: Activity of clindamycin with primaquine against *Pneumocystis carinii* in vitro and in vivo, *Antimicrobial Agents Chemother* 32:807-813, 1988.

43. Black JR, Feinberg J, Murphy RL, Fass RJ, Finkelstein D, Akil B, Safrin S, Carey JT, Stansell J, Plouffe JF, He W, Shelton B, Sattler FR: Clindamycin and primaquine therapy for mild-to-moderate episodes of *Pneumocystis carinii* pneumonia in patients with AIDS: AIDS Clinical Trials Group 044, *Clin Infect Dis* 18:905-913, 1994.
44. Walzer PD, Foy J, Steele P, White M: Synergistic combinations of Ro 11-8958 and other dihydrofolate reductase inhibitors for therapy of experimental pneumocystosis, *Antimicrobial Agents Chemother* 37:1436-1443, 1993.
45. Hughes WT, Jacobus DP, Canfield C, Killmar J: Anti–*Pneumocystis carinii* activity of PS-15, a new biguanide folate antagonist, *Antimicrobial Agents Chemother* 37:1417-1419, 1993.
46. Jones SK, Hall JH, Allen MA, Morrison SD, Ohemeng KA, Reddy V, Geratz D, Tidwell RR: Novel pentamidine analogs in the treatment of experimental *Pneumocystis carinii* pneumonia, *Antimicrobial Agents Chemother* 34:1026-1030, 1990.
47. Schmatz DM, Romancheck MA, Pittarelli LA, Schwartz RE, Fromtling RA, Nollstadt KH, Van Middlesworth FL, Wilson KE, Turner MJ: Treatment of *Pneumocystis carinii* pneumonia with 1,3-β-glucan synthesis inhibitors, *Proc Natl Acad Sci USA* 87:5950-5954, 1990.
48. Queener SF: New drug developments for opportunitistic infections in immunosuppresed patients: *Pneumocystis carinii, J Med Chem* 38: 4739-4759, 1995.
49. Bartlett MS, Edlind TD, Durkin MM, Shaw MM, Queener SF, Smith JW: Antimicrotubule benzimidazoles inhibit in vitro growth of *Pneumocystis carinii, Antimicrobial Agents Chemother* 36:779-782, 1992.
50. Bartlett MS, Queener SF, Tidwell RR, Milhous WK, Berman JD, Ellis WY, Smith JW: 8-Aminoquinolines from Walter Reed Army Institute for Research for treatment and prophylaxis of *Pneumocystis* pneumonia in rat models, *Antimicrobial Agents Chemother* 35:277-282, 1991.
51. Weinberg GA: Iron chelators as therapeutic agents against *Pneumocystis carinii, Antimicrobial Agents Chemother* 38:997-1003, 1994.
52. Weinberg GA: Multiple iron chelators of diverse chemical classes are active against *Pneumocystis carinii, Pediatr Res* 39:188A, 1996.
53. Merali S, Chin K, Grady RW, Clarkson AB Jr: Trophozoite elimination in a rate model of *Pneumocystis carinii* pneumonia by clinically achievable plasma deferoxamine concentrations, *Antimicrobial Agents Chemother* 40:1298-1300, 1996.
54. National Institutes of Health–University of California Expert Panel for Corticosteroids as Adjunctive Therapy for *Pneumocystis* Pneumonia: Consensus statement on the use of corticosteroids as adjunctive therapy for *Pneumocystis* pneumonia in the acquired immunodeficiency syndrome, *N Engl J Med* 323:1500-1504, 1990.
55. Sleasman JW, Hemenway C, Klein AS, Barrett DJ: Corticosteroids improve survival of children with AIDS and *Pneumocystis carinii* pneumonia, *Am J Dis Child* 147:30-34, 1993.
56. Bye MR, Cairns-Bazarian AM, Ewig JM: Markedly reduced mortality associated with corticosterioid therapy of *Pneumocystis carinii* pneumonia in children with acquired immunodeficiency syndrome, *Arch Pediatr Adolesc Med* 148:638-641, 1994.
57. Barone SR, Aiuto LT, Krilov LR: Increased survival of young infants with *Pneumocystis carinii* pneumonia and acute respiratory failure with early steroid administration, *Clin Infect Dis* 19:212-213, 1994.
58. McLaughlin GE, Virdee SS, Schleien CL, Holzman BH, Scott GB: Effect of corticosteroid on survival of children with acquired immunodeficiency syndrome and *Pneumocystis carinii*–related respiratory failure, *J Pediatr* 126:821-824, 1995.
59. Hughes WT, Kuhn S, Chaudhary S, Feldman S, Verzosa M, Aur RJ, Pratt C, George SL: Successful chemoprophylaxis for *Pneumocystis carinii* pneumonitis, *N Engl J Med* 297:1419-1426, 1977.
60. Hughes WT, Rivera GF, Schell MJ, Thornton D, Lott L: Successful intermittent chemoprophylaxis for *Pneumocystis carinii* pneumonitis, *N Engl J Med* 316:1627-1632, 1987.
61. Hardy DW, Feinberg J, Finkelstein DM, Power ME, He W, Kaczka C, Frame PT, Holmes M, Waskin H, Fass RJ, Powderly WG, Steigbigel RT, Zuger A, Holzman RS, for the AIDS Clinical Trials Group: A controlled trial of trimethoprim-sulfamethoxazole or aerosolized pentamidine for secondary prophylaxis of *Pneumocystis carinii* pneumonia in patients with the acquired immunodeficiency syndrome. AIDS Clinical Trials Group Protocol 021, *N Engl J Med* 327:1842-1848, 1992.
62. Schneider ME, Hopelman AIM, Eeftinck Schattenkerk JKM, Nielsen TL, van der Graaf Y, Frissen JPHJ, van der Ende IME, Kolsters AFP, Borleffs JCC, and the Dutch AIDS Treatment Group: A controlled trial of aerosolized pentamidine or trimethoprim-sulfamethoxazole as primary prophylaxis against *Pneumocystis carinii* pneumonia in patients with human immunodeficiency virus infection, *N Engl J Med* 327: 1836-1841, 1992.
63. Bozzette SA, Finkelstein DM, Spector SA, Frame P, Powderly WG, He W, Phillips L, Craven D, van der Horst C, Feinberg J, for the NIAID AIDS Clinical Trials Group: A randomized trial of three antipneumocystis agents in patients with advanced human immunodeficiency virus infection, *N Engl J Med* 332:696-699, 1995.

Legionella Pneumophila

64. Fang GD, Yu VL, Vickers RM: Disease due to the *Legionellaceae* (other than *Legionella pneumophila*), *Medicine* 68:116-132, 1989.
65. McDade J, Shepard C, Fraser D, Tsai TR, Redus MA, Dowdle WR, and the Laboratory Investigation Team: Legionnaires' disease: isolation of a bacterium and demonstration of its role in other respiratory disease, *N Engl J Med* 297:1197-1203, 1977.
66. Fields BS, Sander GN, Barbaree JM, Morrill WE, Wadowsky RM, White EH, Feeley JC: Intracellular multiplication of *Legionella pneumophila* in amoebae isolated from hospital hot water tanks, *Curr Microbiol* 18: 131-137, 1989.
67. McFarlane JT, Finch RG, Ward, MJ, Macrae AD: Hospital study of adult community-acquired pneumonia, *Lancet* 2:255-258, 1982.
68. Friss-Moller A, Rechnitzer C, Black F, Collins MT, Lind K, Aalund O: Prevalence of legionnaires' disease in pneumonia patients admitted to a Danish department of infectious diseases, *Scand J Infect Dis* 18:321-328, 1986.
69. Ruf B, Schurmann D, Horbach I, Fehrenbach FJ, Pohle HD: The incidence of *Legionella* pneumonia: A 1-year prospective study in a large community hospital, *Lung* 167:11-22, 1989.
70. Muder RR, Yu VL, McClure J, Kroboth FJ, Kominos SD, Lumish RM: Nosocomial legionnaires' disease uncovered in a prospective pneumonia study: implications for underdiagnosis, *JAMA* 249:3184-3188, 1983.
71. Korvick J, Yu VL: Legionnaires' disease: an emerging surgical problem, *Ann Thoracic Surg* 43:341-347, 1987.
72. Yu VL, Kroboth FJ, Shonnard J, Brown A, McDearman S, Magnussen M: Legionnaires' disease: new clinical perspective from a prospective pneumonia study, *Am J Med* 73:357-361, 1982.
73. Block B, Edelstein P, Snyder K, Hatayama CM, Lewis RP, Kirby BD, George Wl, Owens ML, Haley CE, Meyer RD, Finegold SM: Legionnaires' disease in renal transplant recipients, *Lancet* 1:410-413, 1978.
74. Hofflin JM, Potasman I, Baldwin JC, Oyer PE, Stinson EB, Remington JS: Infectious complications in heart transplant recipients receiving cyclosporine and corticosteroids, *Ann Intern Med* 106:209-216, 1987.
75. Schwebke J, Hackman R, Bowden R: *Legionella micdadei* in bone marrow transplant recipients, *Rev Infect Dis* 12:824-828, 1990.
76. Haraldsson A, Rechnitzer C, Friis-Moller A, Briem H: Prevalence of IgM antibodies to nine *Legionella* species in Icelandic children, *Scand J Infect Dis* 22:445-449, 1990.
77. Peeters M, Cornu G, DeMeyer R: Legionnaires' disease in an immunosupporessed child, *Acta Paediatr Belg* 33:189-193, 1980.
78. Kovatch AL, Jardine DS, Dowling JN, Yee RB, Pasculle AW: Legionellosis in children with leukemia in relapse, *Pediatrics* 73:811-815, 1984.
79. Cutz E, Thorner PS, Rao CP, Toma S, Gold R, Gelfand EW: Disseminated *Legionella pneumophila* infection in an infant with severe combined immunodeficiency, *J Pediatr* 100:760-762, 1982.
80. Peerless AG, Liebhaber M, Anderson S, Lehrer RI, Stiehm ER: *Legionella* pneumonia in chronic granulomatous disease, *J Pediatr* 106:783-785, 1985.
81. Ephros M, Engelhard D, Maayan S, Bercovier H, Avital A, Yatsiv I: *Legionella gormanii* pneumonia in a child with chronic granulomatous disease, *Pediatr Infect Dis J* 8:726-727, 1989.
82. Foy HM, Hayes PS, Cooney K, Brome CV, Allan I, Tobe R: Legionnaires' disease in a prepaid medical care group in Seattle, 1963-1975, *Lancet* 1:767-770, 1979.
83. Andersen RD, Lauer BA, Fraser DW, Hayes PS, McIntosh K: Infections with *Legionella pneumophila* in children, *J Infect Dis* 143:386-390, 1981.
84. Renner ED, Helms CM, Hierholzer WJ, Hall N, Wong YW, Viner JP, Johnson W, Hausler WJ: Legionnaires' disease in pneumonia patients in Iowa: a retrospective seroepidemiologic study, 1972-1977, *Ann Intern Med* 90:603-606, 1979.

85. Ryan ME, Feldman S, Pruitt B, Fraser DW: Legionnaires' disease in a child with cancer, *Pediatrics* 64:951-953, 1979.

86. Orenstein WA, Overturf GD, Leedom JM, Alvarado R, Geffner M, Fryer A, Chan L, Haynes V, Stare T, Portnoy B: The frequency of *Legionella* infection prospectively determined in children hospitalized with pneumonia, *J Pediatr* 99:403-406, 1981.

87. Muldoon RL, Jaecker MS, Kiefer HK: Legionnaires' disease in children, *Pediatrics* 67:329-332, 1981.

88. Claesson BA, Trollfors B, Brolin I, Granstrom M, Henrichsen J, Jodal U, Juto P, Kallings I, Kanclerski K, Lagergard T, Steinwall L, Strannegard O: Etiology of community-acquired pneumonia in children based on antibody responses to bacterial and viral antigens, *Pediatr Infect Dis J* 8:856-862, 1989.

89. Verissimo A, Vesey G, Rocha GM, Marrao G, Colbourne J, Dennis PJ, da Costa MS: A hot water supply as the source of *Legionella pneumophila* in incubators of a neonatology unit, *J Hosp Infect* 15:255-263, 1990.

90. Aubert G, Bornstein N, Rayet I, Pozzetto B, Lenormand PH: Nosocomial infection with *Legionella pneumophila* serogroup 1 and 8 in a neonate, *Scand J Infect Dis* 22:367-376, 1990.

91. Brady MT: Nosocomial legionnaires' disease in a children's hospital, *J Pediatr* 115:46-50, 1989.

92. Monforte R, Maro F, Estruch R, Campo E: Multiple organ involvement of *L. pneumophila* in a fatal case of legionnaires' disease, *J Infect Dis* 159:809, 1989.

93. Johnson JD, Raff M, Van Arsdall J: Neurologic manifestations of legionnaires' disease, *Medicine* 63:303-310, 1984.

94. Taguchi Y, Nakahama C, Inamatsu T, Arakawa M, Saito A, Hara K, Ezaki T, Yabuchi E, Ueda Y: Analysis of chest radiographs of culture-positive *Legionella* pneumonia in Japan, 1980-1990, *J Japanese Assoc Infect Dis (Kansenshogaku Zasshi)* 66:1580-1586, 1991.

95. Kroboth FJ, Yu VL, Reddy SC, Yu AC: Clinicoradiographic correlation with the extent of legionnaires' disease, *AJR Am J Roentgenol* 141:263-268, 1983.

96. Storch GA, Sagel SS, Baine WB: The chest roentgenogram in sporadic cases of legionnaires' disease, *JAMA* 245:587-590, 1981.

97. Dietrich PA, Johnson RD, Fairbank JT, Walke JS: The chest radiograph in legionnaires' disease, *Radiology* 127:577-582, 1978.

98. MacFarlane J, Miller AC, Roderick SWH, Morris AH, Rose DH: Comparative radiographic features of community acquired legionnaires' disease, pneumococcal pneumonia, mycoplasma pneumonia and psittacosis, *Thorax* 39:28-33, 1984.

99. Felman AH: Bacterial infections. In Felman AH, ed: *Radiology of the pediatric chest: clinical and pathological correlations,* New York, 1987, McGraw-Hill.

100. Davis GS, Winn WC, Beaty HN: Legionnaires' disease: infections caused by *Legionella pneumophila* and *Legionella*-like organisms, *Clin Chest Med* 2:145-166, 1981.

101. Plouffe JF, File TM Jr, Breiman RF, Hackman BA, Salstrom SJ, Marston BJ, Field BS, and the Community Based Pneumonia Incidence Study Group: Reevaluation of the definition of legionnaire's disease: use of the urinary antigen assay, *Clin Infect Dis* 20:1286-1291, 1995.

102. Edelstein PH: Antimicrobial chemotherapy for legionnaire's disease: a review, *Clin Infect Dis* 21(suppl 3):S265-S276, 1995.

Protozoan Infections

103. Fraser RG, Paré JAP, Paré PD, Fraser RS, Genereux GP: Parasitic infestation of the lung. In Fraser RG, Paré JAP, Paré PD, Fraser RS, Genereux GP, eds: *Diagnosis of diseases of the chest,* ed 3, Philadelphia, 1989, WB Saunders, pp 1081-1176.

104. Ibarra-Peréz C: Thoracic complications of amebic abscess of the liver: report of 501 cases, *Chest* 79:672-677, 1981.

105. Charoenpan P, Indraprasit S, Kiatboonsri S, Suvachittanont O, Tanomsup S: Pulmonary edema in severe falciparum malaria, *Chest* 97:1190-1197, 1990.

106. Pomeroy C, Filice GA: Pulmonary toxoplasmosis: a review, *Clin Infect Dis* 14:863-870, 1992.

107. Israelski DM, Remington JS: Toxoplasmosis in patients with cancer, *Clin Infect Dis* 17(suppl 2):S423-S435, 1993.

108. Remington JS, McLeod R, Desmonts G: Toxoplasmosis. In Remington JS, Klein JO, eds: *Infectious diseases of the fetus and newborn infant,* ed 4, Philadelphia, 1995, WB Saunders, pp 140-267.

109. Wilson CB, Remington JS: Toxoplasmosis. In Feigin RD, Cherry JD, eds: *Textbook of pediatric infectious diseases,* ed 3, Philadelphia, 1992, WB Saunders, pp 2057-2069.

110. McAuley J, Boyer KM, Patel D, Mets M, Swisher C, Roizen N, Wolters C, Stein L, Stein M, Schey W, Remington J, Meier P, Johnson D, Heydeman P, Holfels E, Withers S, Mack D, Brown C, Patton D, McLeod R: Early and longitudinal evaluations of treated infants and children and untreated historical patients with congenital toxoplasmosis: the Chicago Collaborative Treatment Trial, *Clin Infect Dis* 18:38-72, 1994.

111. Jerray M, Benzarti M, Garrouche A, Klabi N, Hayouni A: Hydatid disease of the lungs: a study of 386 cases, *Am Rev Respir Dis* 146:185-189, 1992.

112. Katz R, Murphy S, Kosloske A: Pulmonary echinococcosis: a pediatric disease of the southwestern United States, *Pediatrics* 65:1003-1006, 1980.

113. Finlay JC, Speert DP: Sylvatic hydatid disease in children: case reports and review of endemic *Echinococcus granulosus* infection in Canada and Alaska, *Pediatr Infect Dis J* 11:322-326, 1992.

114. Wilson JF, Rausch RL, McMahon BJ, Schantz PM: Parasiticidal effect of chemotherapy in alveolar hydatid disease: review of experience with mebendazole and albendazole in Alaskan eskimos, *Clin Infect Dis* 15:234-239, 1992.

115. Beggs I: The radiology of hydatid disease, *AJR Am J Roentgenol* 145:639-648, 1985.

116. Saksouk FA, Fahl MH, Rizk GK: Computer tomography of pulmonary hydatid disase, *J Computer Assist Tomogr* 10:226-232, 1986.

117. Force L, Torres JM, Carrillo A, Busca J: Evaluation of eight serological tests in the diagnosis of human echinococcosis and follow-up, *Clin Infect Dis* 15:473-480, 1992.

118. Salama H, Abdel-Wahab MF, Strickland GT: Diagnosis and treatment of hepatic hydatid cysts with the aid of echo-guided percutaneous cyst puncture, *Clin Infect Dis* 21:1372-1376, 1995.

119. Liu LX, Weller, PF: Antiparasitic drugs, *N Engl J Med* 334:1178-1184, 1996.

120. WHO Informal Working Group on Echinococcosis: Guidelines for treatment of cystic and alveolar echinococcosis in humans, *Bull WHO* 74:231-242, 1996.

121. Davis A, Pawlowski ZS, Dixon H: Multicentre clinical trials of benzimidazolecarbamates in human echinococcosis, *Bull WHO* 64:383-388, 1986.

122. Horton RJ: Chemotherapy of Echinococcus infection in man with albendazole, *Trans R Soc Trop Med Hyg* 83:97-102, 1989.

123. Todorov T, Vutova K, Mechkov G, Petkov D, Nedelkov G, Tonchev Z: Evaluation of response to chemotherapy of human cystic echinococcosis, *Br J Radiol* 63:523-531, 1990.

124. Goldsmith R, Bunnag D, Bunnag T: Lung fluke infections: paragonimiasis. In Strickland GT, ed: *Hunter's tropical medicine,* ed 7, Philadelphia, 1991, WB Saunders, pp 827-831.

125. Johnson RJ, Johnson JR: Paragonimiasis in Indochinese refugees: roentgenographic findings with clinical correlations, *Am Rev Respir Dis* 128:534-538, 1983.

126. Im JG, Whang HY, Han MC, Shim YS, Cho SY: Pleuropulmonary paragonimiasis: radiologic findings in 71 patients, *AJR Am J Roentgenol* 159:39-43, 1992.

127. Johnson RJ, Jong EC, Dunning SB, Carberry WL, Minshew BH: Paragonimiasis: diagnosis and the use of praziquantel in treatment, *Rev Infect Dis* 7:200-206, 1985.

128. Genta RM: Global prevalence of strongyloidiasis: critical review with epidemiologic insights into the prevention of disseminated disease, *Rev Infect Dis* 11:755-767, 1989.

129. Genta RM, Walzer PD: Strongyloidiasis. In Walzer PD, Genta RM, eds: *Parasitic infections in the compromised host,* New York, 1989, Marcel Dekker, pp 463-525.

130. Genta RM: Dysregulation of strongyloidiasis: a new hypothesis, *Clin Microbiol Rev* 5:345-355, 1992.

131. Liu LX, Weller PF: Strongyloidiasis and other intestinal nematode infections, *Infect Dis Clin North Am* 7:655-682, 1993.

132. Mahmoud AAF: Strongyloidiasis, *Clin Infect Dis* 23:949-953, 1996.

133. Salazar SA, Berk SH, Howe D, Berk SL: Ivermectin vs. thiabendazole in the treatment of strongyloidiasis, *Infect Med* 11:50-54, 59, 1994.

134. Anderson DC: *Toxocara* pneumonia. In Feigin RD, Cherry JD, eds: *Textbook of pediatric infectious diseases,* ed 3, Philadelphia, 1992, WB Saunders, pp 297-299.
135. Herman N, Glickman LT, Schantz PM: Seroprevalence of zoonotic toxocariasis in the United States, *Am J Epidemiol* 122:890-896, 1985.
136. Schantz PM: *Toxocara* larva migrans now, *Am J Trop Med Hyg* 41(suppl 3):21-34, 1989.
137. Taylor MRH, Keane CT, O'Connor P, Mulvihill E, Holland C: The expanded spectrum of toxocaral disease, *Lancet* 1:692-695, 1988.
138. Glickman LT, Magnaval JF: Zoonotic roundworm infections, *Infect Dis Clin North Am* 7:717-732, 1993.
139. Bass JL, Mehta KA, Glickman LT, Blocker R, Eppes BM: Asymptomatic toxocariasis in children: a prospective study and treatment trial, *Clin Pediatr* 26:441-446, 1987.
140. Magnaval JF, Fabre R, Maurieres P, Charlet JP, deLarrard B: Evaluation of an immunoenzymatic assay detecting anti-*Toxocara* immunoglobulin E for diagnosis and posttreatment follow-up of human toxocariasis, *J Clin Microbiol* 30:2269-2274, 1992.
141. Ottesen EA, Nutman TB: Tropical pulmonary eosinophilia, *Annu Rev Med* 43:417-424, 1992.

SUGGESTED READINGS

Anonymous: Drugs for parasitic infections, *Med Lett* 40:1-12, 1998.
Edelstein PH: Antimicrobial chemotherapy for legionnaires' disease: a review, *Clin Infect Dis* 21(suppl 3):S265-S276, 1995.
Edelstein PH: Legionnaires' disease, *Clin Infect Dis* 16:741-749, 1993.
Edlestein PH: Legionnaires' disease, Pontiac fever, and related illnesses. In Feigen RD, Cherry JD, eds: *Textbook of pediatric infection diseases,* ed 4, Philadelphia, 1998, WB Saunders, pp 1499-1508.
Feigin RD, Cherry JD, eds: *Textbook of pediatric infectious diseases,* ed 4, Philadelphia, 1998, WB Saunders.
Hughes WT: *Pneumocystis carinii* pneumonia. In Pizzo PA, Wilfert CM, eds: *Pediatrics AIDS: the challenge of HIV infection in infants, children, and adolescents,* ed 2, Baltimore, 1994, Williams & Wilkins, pp 405-418.
Hughes WT, Anderson DC: *Pneumocystis carinii* pneumonia. In Feigin RD, Cherry JD, eds: *Textbook of pediatric infectious diseases,* ed 4, Philadelphia, 1998, WB Saunders, pp 2490-2499.
Liu LX, Weller PF: Antiparasitic drugs, *N Engl J Med* 334:1178-1184, 1996.
Mandell GL, Bennett JE, Dolin R, eds: *Mandell, Douglas and Bennett's principles and practice of infectious diseases,* ed 4, New York, 1995, Churchill Livingstone.
Reeder MM, Palmer PES, eds: *The radiology of tropical diseases with epidemiological, pathological, and clinical correlation,* Baltimore, 1981, Williams & Wilkins.
Sattler FR: *Pneumocystis carinii* pneumonia. In Broder S, Merigan TC Jr, Bolognesi D, eds: *Textbook of AIDS medicine,* Baltimore, 1994, Williams & Wilkins, pp 193-221.
Strickland GT, ed: *Hunter's tropical medicine,* ed 7, Philadelphia, 1991, WB Saunders.
Walzer PD: *Pneumocystis carinii.* In Mandell GL, Bennett JE, Dolin R, eds: *Mandell, Douglas and Bennett's principles and practice of infectious diseases,* ed 4, New York, 1995, Churchill Livingstone, pp 2475-2487.
Walzer PD, ed: *Pneumocystis carinii* pneumonia, ed 2, New York, 1994, Marcel Dekker.
Warren KS, Mahmoud AAF, eds: *Tropical and geographical medicine,* ed 2, New York, 1990, McGraw-Hill.

CHAPTER 48

Bronchiectasis and Bronchiolitis Obliterans

Thomas William Ferkol, Jr., and Pamela B. Davis

Although alveoli perform the major function of the lung, gas exchange, the conducting airways are critical for communication between these terminal respiratory units and the atmosphere. These structures ensure the access of gas to the alveoli and protect the delicate alveoli from noxious agents in the environment by trapping and expelling infectious and polluting particles in the airstream. The breakdown of any of these functions has serious and even fatal consequences.

Bronchiectasis is a disorder of the segmental and subsegmental bronchi that is typically associated with abnormal dilation of the affected airways and recurrent infections. Bronchiolitis obliterans is a disorder of the distal respiratory tract that arises from an intense inflammatory reaction secondary to infectious, chemical, or immunologic injury. Both disorders often arise from airway obstruction. Both may have a variable course, progress after the initiating stimulus is removed, and may remain static for long periods. Both conditions may be fatal. In bronchiectasis, the postinfectious etiology in the normal host is becoming distinctly uncommon, and most patients with the disorder have an underlying systemic illness. In bronchiolitis obliterans, the burgeoning number of pediatric transplant recipients has produced more children with this disorder, thus changing the epidemiology of the disease.

BRONCHIECTASIS

Disease Mechanisms

Initially described by Laennec in 1819,[1] *bronchiectasis* is defined as an abnormal dilation of the subsegmental airways. It is a pathophysiologic entity, not a discrete disease. Thus it may be the consequence of antecedent events or a pulmonary manifestation of a systemic disorder, especially one that confers vulnerability to bacterial infection (Box 48-1). Although in most cases, bronchiectasis develops as a result of airway obstruction or inflammation in response to chronic or repeated infection, congenital forms of bronchiectasis with abnormal formation of the tracheobronchial cartilage have also been described. Mounier-Kuhn[2] reported a rare condition of tracheobronchomegaly characterized by a markedly dilated intrathoracic trachea and bronchi. Dilation of the proximal airways is caused by enlargement of the cartilaginous tracheal rings and membranous trachea. The original cases of Mounier-

BOX 48-1
Causes of Bronchiectasis

Bacterial pneumonia
Bordetella pertussis tracheobronchitis
Adenovirus pneumonia
Measles pneumonitis
Influenza pneumonitis
Mycobacteria tuberculosis endobronchitis
Hypogammaglobinemia
- Severe combined immunodeficiency
- Common variable hypogammaglobinemia
- Immunoglobulin G subclass deficiency
- Immunoglobulin A deficiency

Neutrophil deficiencies
- Schwachman-Diamond syndrome
- Chronic granulomatous disease
- Chédiak-Higashi syndrome
- Job's syndrome

Complement deficiency
Dyskinetic cilia syndrome (Kartagener's syndrome)
Cystic fibrosis
Young's syndrome
α_1-Antitrypsin deficiency
Allergic bronchopulmonary aspergillosis
Foreign body aspiration
Aspiration of gastric or oropharyngeal contents
Bronchogenic carcinoma
Autoimmune disorders (rheumatoid arthritis)
Williams-Campbell syndrome
Mounier-Kuhn syndrome
Ehlers-Danlos syndrome
Marfan syndrome
Yellow nail syndrome

Kuhn syndrome were described in adults, although many of the patients had chronic respiratory symptoms beginning in early childhood; young children with this condition have been described.[3] Furthermore, acquired tracheomegaly has been described in premature infants after prolonged mechanical ventilatory support, presumably as a result of barotrauma.[4] Otherwise, the etiology of tracheobronchomegaly is unclear. Patients with tracheobronchomegaly are predisposed to recurrent pneumonias, and hemoptysis and pneumothorax have been described in these individuals. Williams and Campbell[5] described five patients who had recurrent lower respiratory infections, fever, failure to thrive, and a persistent, productive cough. Although the trachea and segmental bronchi appears normal on bronchoscopic examination, bronchography reveals dilation of the bronchi in the second and third divisions. Postmortem examination of the airways of patients with Williams-Campbell syndrome has shown that the involved segmental bronchi are devoid of normal cartilage. The abnormal airways are hyperdynamic, greatly expanding and collapsing during inspiration and expiration, respectively. Familial forms of this unusual disorder have been reported.[6] Other congenital syndromes associated with cartilage abnormalities, such as Ehlers-Danlos[7] and Marfan syndrome,[8] have been associated with bronchiectasis. These congenital syndromes, which are related to defective cartilage or connective tissue, suggest that enlargement or increased compliance of the bronchi can cause disease without antecedent infection and inflammation. They also imply that once structural abnormalities of the bronchi (congenital or acquired) are present, even control of infection and inflammation may not be sufficient to arrest the progression of the disease.

Transient bronchial dilation has been observed after acute pneumonia and airway obstruction,[9,10] so observation of cylindric bronchial dilation at a single point in time may not provide a diagnosis of bronchiectasis. To some extent, cylindric bronchiectasis must be reversible. However, in some patients, repeated infection and plugging of airways lead to a permanent pathologic condition. Affected bronchial segments are pliant and frequently distorted because of the destruction of the muscular and elastic components of the airway walls. Dilation of the bronchus is believed to result from atelectasis caused by the accumulation of purulent secretions and obstruction of the peripheral airway.[11] The atelectasis generates negative intrapleural pressure,[11] which is exerted on the wall of the bronchus already weakened by lytic enzymes,[12] such as elastase, collagenase, and cathepsin, released from the neutrophils in the purulent material in the airway. The combination of traction on the airway wall and internal digestion of its structural proteins results in distention of the airway. The involved bronchi are edematous and infiltrated with inflammatory cells, and areas of fibrosis and ulceration of the endobronchial epithelium may also be evident. Such ulcerations may erode into an underlying blood vessel, resulting in hemoptysis. Squamous metaplasia of the respiratory epithelium is also frequent. Chronic inflammation may eventually destroy the bronchial cartilage, leading to bronchomalacia. The lumen of the bronchiectatic airway is often obstructed by exudates, and the peripheral airways may be similarly inflamed and filled with secretions.[13] Persistent obstruction can lead to obliteration of the smaller airways and pulmonary fibrosis, and the peribronchial alveoli may also be damaged. Prolonged bronchial dilation stimulates contraction of the surrounding smooth muscle, which can cause hypertrophy of the musculature. The bronchial arteries supplying the diseased lobe or lobes are often dilated and form anastomoses with pulmonary arteries.[14] This enlargement of the bronchial arteries is generally attributed to the increased blood flow related to chronic inflammation (Fig. 48-1). Alveolar hypoxia in patients with bronchiectasis can result in pulmonary hypertension and cor pulmonale.[15] The systemic-pulmonary arterial connections result in a left-to-right shunt, which may further increase the workload of the right ventricle.

Several systems have been introduced to classify the various forms of bronchiectasis; they are based on the anatomic changes observed at autopsy or during bronchography. Reid[16] correlated the pathologic and bronchographic findings in lungs removed from patients during autopsy. Three general types of bronchiectasis were described: cylindric, varicose, and saccular (or cystic). In cylindric bronchiectasis, the bronchial outlines are regular and diffusely dilated, and the distal portion of the involved airway terminates abruptly because of plugging of the smaller airways by mucus. Focal constrictions and sacculations are present in varicose bronchiectasis, producing an irregular bronchial outline. In the saccular form, cystic dilation of the affected airway increases toward the lung periphery and is characterized by a ballooning of the bronchus (Fig. 48-2). Although the Reid clasification has been useful in the radiographic description of bronchiectasis, no association between the type of bronchiectasis and the patient's clinical condition, prognosis, or underlying pathophysiology has been established.

Local obstruction and inflammation of an airway can produce bronchiectasis in any lobe. Diffuse bronchiectasis is common in patients who have impaired clearance from the airways

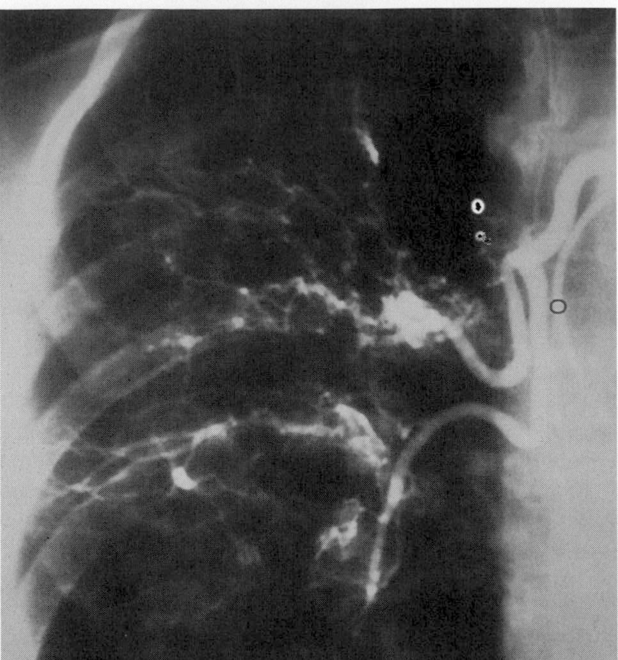

Fig. 48-1. Selective bronchial arteriography, which demonstrates dilated bronchial arteries that supply the bronchiectatic lobe or lobes and extravasation of contrast material in the lung parenchyma.

(cystic fibrosis[17-19] and dyskinetic cilia syndrome[20-22]), immunodeficiency states (including acquired immunodeficiency syndrome),[23-25] chronic airway diseases,[26] and allergic bronchopulmonary aspergillosis.[27,28] In cystic fibrosis, the upper lobes are often affected before the lower lobes. The occurrence of bronchiectasis in the upper lobe is unusual outside of cystic fibrosis, and if present the bronchiectasis is most often a sequela of the aspiration of milk or another foreign body, allergic bronchopulmonary aspergillosis, or tuberculous endobronchitis. In other forms of bronchiectasis, the left lower lobe and lingula are most frequently affected, probably because the left mainstem bronchus is smaller in diameter, lacks gravitational drainage, and may be more readily compromised than the right mainstem bronchus.[16,29] Bilateral lower lobe disease occurs in approximately one third of cases. Bronchiectasis involving the right side is predominant when the affected airway is obstructed by a tuberculous lesion or a foreign body. Chronic atelectasis of the right middle lobe is often clinically silent, may thus be unrecognized, and may lead to bronchiectasis. In the right middle lobe syndrome, the affected bronchus is postulated to have been compressed extrinsically by enlarged regional lymph nodes.[30] These nodes drain lymph from the right lower lobe bronchus and distal esophagus as well as the right middle lobe. Compression of the bronchus results in impaired bronchial drainage and recurrent suppurative infections. However, doubt was cast on this theory after investigators found that several patients with right middle lobe syndrome had a normal bronchus that was completely patent by bronchography and bronchoscopy.[31] An alternative explanation is that the collateral ventilation of the right middle lobe is less effective.[32]

Epidemiology

The incidence of bronchiectasis in children is unknown because in many cases the diagnosis is not considered. Bronchiectasis develops in nearly all patients with cystic fibrosis, the incidence of which is estimated at 1 in 2500 white live births. It may also accompany the ciliary dyskinesia syndrome, which is estimated to occur in 1 in 16,000 births, or various types of immunoglobulin deficiencies, which occur with variable frequency. Bronchiectasis unassociated with an underlying disease is now considered to be rare. Ruberman et al[33] in 1957 identified 29 cases of bronchiectasis in 1711 children who had acute pneumonia, and the annual incidence of bronchiectasis in Great Britain was estimated to be 1.1 per 10,000 children.[34] Both of these studies were performed 3 decades ago, and the incidence of bronchiectasis has significantly decreased since then for several reasons. The frequency and severity of two common antecedent infections, measles and pertussis, have diminished greatly after the institution of preventive immunization programs. The incidence of pulmonary tuberculosis, which often leads to extrinsic bronchial obstruction and secondary bacterial infection of the affected airways in children and infants, has also declined. Finally, improved social circumstances, the development of broad-spectrum antibiotics, and the effective treatment of bacterial pneumonia and suppurative bronchitis have contributed to the decreased incidence of bronchiectasis.[10] Nevertheless, bron-

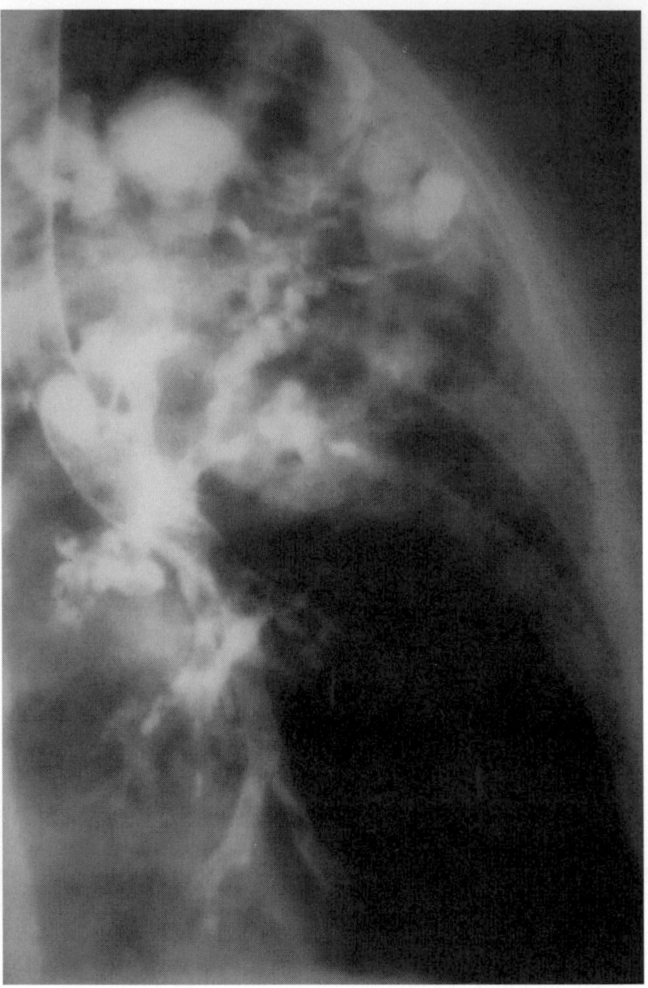

Fig. 48-2. Contrast bronchogram showing cystic dilation and ballooning of several of the subsegmental bronchi in the left upper lobe, which are consistent with saccular bronchiectasis. There are also regular, diffusely dilated bronchial outlines in the left lower lobe that end abruptly because of the plugging of the smaller airways by mucus. These findings are typical of the cylindric form of bronchiectasis.

Table 48-1 Conditions Associated with Bronchiolitis Obliterans

DIAGNOSIS	CLINICAL FEATURES	LABORATORY STUDIES
Cystic fibrosis	Pancreatic insufficiency Chronic sinusitis *Pseudomonas* bronchitis Infertility	Sweat chloride concentration
Dyskinetic cilia syndrome	Chronic otitis media Chronic sinusitis Recurrent pneumonias Infertility	Electron microscopy of cilia Ciliary motility studies
Humoral immunodeficiency	Recurrent infections Atopy	Quantitative serum immunoglobulin measurements Immunoglobulin G subclass determination
Neutrophil abnormalities	Recurrent infections Pancreatic insufficiency Thrombocytopenia Anemia	Complete blood count with leukocyte differential Nitroblue tetrazolium reductase assay
Complement deficiency	Recurrent infections	Hemolytic complement (CH_{50}) determination Serum C3 measurement
Allergic bronchopulmonary aspergillosis	Bronchial hyperreactivity Pulmonary infiltrates Emphysema	Serum immunoglobulin E measurement Blood eosinophil count Cutaneous reactivity to antigen Specific immunoglobulin E against *Aspergillus* species
α_1-Antitrypsin deficiency	Cholestatic disease Cirrhosis	α_1-Antitrypsin determination P_i typing
Gastroesophageal reflux	Recurrent emesis Recurrent pneumonias Failure to thrive	Esophageal pH monitoring
Foreign body aspiration	Persistent pneumonia Unilateral lung hyperinflation	Bronchoscopy

Modified from Davis PB et al: *J Pediatr* 102:177-185, 1983.
P_i, Protease inhibitor.

chiectasis may be more common than suspected. As computed tomography has become more widely used for the evaluation of lung disease, milder forms of bronchiectasis have been recognized in patients who have minimal findings on physical examination and chest radiographs.[35]

Although postinfectious bronchiectasis has become an uncommon condition in most people in the United States, it continues to be a problem in Native Americans. The annual incidence of postinfectious bronchiectasis in this population has been calculated to be approximately 4.0 per 10,000,[36] and this number probably is an underestimation. Bronchiectasis remains a relatively frequent complication of lower respiratory tract infections in children from developing countries.[37,38]

Clinical Presentation

Patients with bronchiectasis typically have chronic cough, purulent sputum, fever, and weight loss. Breathlessness and dyspnea have also been reported but may be related to concomitant bronchitis or emphysema. Recurrent or persistent pulmonary infections are common. Although the hemoptysis is a frequent symptom in adults with bronchiectasis, occurring in 92% of patients in one series,[39] it is relatively uncommon in children. The bleeding is generally mild, consisting of the expectoration of purulent secretions streaked with blood. Hemoptysis is rarely the cause of death in patients with bronchiectasis, although hemoptysis can be massive because the bleeding may arise from systemic-pulmonary arterial anastomoses. Because hypoxemia is usually mild, cor pulmonale is generally believed to be an infrequent complication. However, Konietzko et al[15] identified cor pulmonale in 37% of adults with bronchiectasis evaluated over 12 years. Other complications associated with bronchiectasis include empyema, lung abscess, and pneumothorax.

Not surprisingly, the findings on physical examination are nonspecific for bronchiectasis. Various adventitious sounds are often encountered on auscultation of the lungs. Crackles over the affected region of lung are common. Wheeze on auscultation may also be appreciated, particularly if bacterial superinfection and endobronchial secretions are present. Foul-smelling sputum or breath may be noted. Clubbing of the digits is an inconsistent finding but is found in many patients with bronchiectasis. Furthermore, the presence of clubbing may not correlate with the severity of pulmonary involvement.[40]

Diagnosis

Bronchiectasis may be considered on the basis of the clinical history and physical findings[41] (Table 48-1). Recurrent pulmonary infections and persistent productive cough are the historic hallmarks of the disease. The family history is especially important, as is the presence or absence of associated disease involving the gastrointestinal tract (suggestive of cystic fibrosis or immunoglobulin A [IgA] deficiency), sinuses (suggestive of cystic fibrosis, ciliary dyskinesia syndrome, or immunodeficiency), middle ear (ciliary dyskinesia syndrome or immunodeficiency), genital tract (cystic fibrosis or Young's syndrome), liver (α_1-antitrypsin deficiency), or skin (pyogenic infections suggestive of immunodeficiency). A previous history of asthma may suggest evaluation for allergic bronchopulmonary aspergillosis. Dextrocardia may suggest Kartagener's syndrome and congenital ciliary dyskinesia.[42,43]

Establishing an anatomic diagnosis of bronchiectasis requires bronchography, which is considered the definitive study modality, but as noted later, this study has some risk and is rarely performed today unless surgery is being considered. High-resolution computed tomographic scanning has replaced bronchography as the diagnostic procedure of choice. Plain chest radiographs are rarely definitive, but the plain film in the context of the clinical history, response to therapy, and clinical course may be sufficient for determining the diagnosis.

Initial evaluation of the patient should include a search for familial and treatable causes. Serum immunoglobulin levels are valuable: IgG deficiency is a treatable cause of bronchiectasis. If IgA levels are low, measurements of IgG subclasses should be obtained because many patients with IgA deficiency and chronic respiratory infection have a concomitant deficiency of IgG_2 or IgG_4. Sweat chloride concentration should be measured to evaluate for cystic fibrosis. Although the pulmonary manifestations of α_1-antitrypsin deficiency seldom present during childhood and bronchiectasis is an unusual complication, measurement of serum concentrations of α_1-antitrypsin can be diagnostic. Neutrophil counts and serum complement concentrations may be valuable. Assays of mucociliary clearance or ciliary biopsy are required to establish a diagnosis of ciliary dyskinesia syndrome.

Laboratory evaluation may reveal the consequences of bronchiectasis. Immunoglobulin levels are often elevated, reflecting the chronic stimulation from persistent or repeated infections. Hypoxemia and an increased alveolar-arterial difference in the partial pressures of oxygen secondary to ventilation-perfusion inequalities are often present in patients with bronchiectasis, and chronic respiratory insufficiency and persistent hypercapnia are ominous findings. The results of the complete blood count are often nonspecific, with either no abnormality or peripheral blood leukocytosis. Polycythemia may be present in patients who have chronic hypoxia, or anemia may occur in the setting of unremitting suppurative lung disease.

Sputum cultures frequently yield bacteria that are present as constituents of normal oropharyngeal flora; these include *Streptococcus pneumoniae, Staphylococcus aureus,* and nontypeable *Haemophilus influenzae. Escherichia coli* and *Pseudomonas aeruginosa* may be found in the sputum of individuals with bronchiectasis, including patients who do not have cystic fibrosis,[44] but mucoid phenotypes of *P. aeruginosa* should prompt an evaluation for cystic fibrosis. The presence of *Aspergillus* species may be suggestive but not diagnostic of allergic bronchopulmonary aspergillosis. Stains and cultures for *Mycobacterium tuberculosis* and a tuberculin test should also be performed. Bronchiectasis has been described as a sequela of various viral,[45,46] *Bordetella pertussis,*[47] and *Mycoplasma pneumoniae* infections.[48] However, because bronchiectasis is usually a late complication of the infection, the organism is seldom recovered.

Most patients with bronchiectasis have some abnormality of pulmonary function, but some individuals have entirely normal tests. Often, the maximal breathing capacity is abnormal. Spirometry demonstrates a predominantly obstructive pattern, although the degree of abnormality does not correlate with the type of bronchiectasis. The forced expiratory volume in 1 second and the forced vital capacity are often reduced.[49,50] In advanced disease, combined obstructive and restrictive pulmonary defects may be present as a result of destruction of the lung parenchyma.

Patients with bronchiectasis seldom have normal plain chest radiographs. The typical radiographic findings include increased bronchopulmonary markings and opacification of the affected area. Other nonspecific findings (i.e., localized atelectasis or consolidation) have also been described. In advanced cylindric or varicose bronchiectasis, characteristic linear radiolucencies and parallel markings radiating from the hilum (tram tracks or toothpaste lines) may be found. Isolated or multiple cysts (honeycombing) may be evident on chest radiographs of patients with the cystic form of the disease. None of these findings is specific for bronchiectasis, and the chest radiograph has generally been unreliable in establishing the location and distribution of the bronchiectatic airways.[35]

Contrast bronchography has been and remains the most sensitive method for determining the presence and exact anatomic distribution of bronchiectasis (see Fig. 48-2). First described in 1922, bronchography was the imaging modality of choice before the advent of computed tomography. The procedure is performed with the introduction of a radiopaque contrast medium via a catheter positioned by either a rigid or flexible fiberoptic bronchoscope. Although bronchography permits the imaging of the affected airway or airways and is usually safe, the technique is not without potential risks. Certain contrast materials, such as iodized oil (Lipiodol), are viscous and can obstruct segmental bronchi and bronchioles, which may further compromise ventilation in patients who already have respiratory embarrassment. Bronchography should not be performed in patients during acute exacerbations of bronchiectasis. These viscid contrast materials may not completely fill the airways, so an inadequate examination may be obtained. Allergic reactions to the contrast material, although infrequent, can also occur.[51] For these reasons, bronchography is now limited to determining the extent of lung involvement before resection and is rarely performed today.

Computed tomography of the chest has become the method of choice for detecting bronchiectasis, partly because of the relative ease and safety of the technique (Fig. 48-3). Dilated, thickened bronchi are often found extending into the lung periphery and may be accompanied by the associated pulmonary artery, which produces a signet-ring appearance. Unfortunately, this method is less sensitive (63% to 100%) and less specific (92% to 100%) than bronchography. The recognition of bronchiectasis by computed tomography depends on the characteristics of the affected airway and the technique used to acquire the images. The sensitivity is greatest when thin,

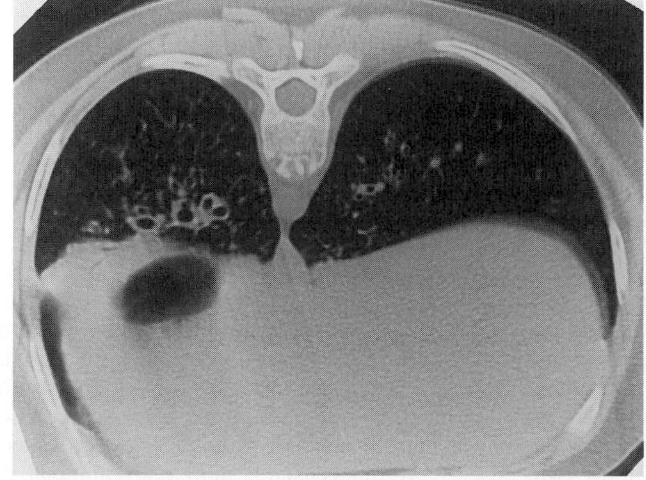

Fig. 48-3. Computed tomographic image demonstrating dilated bronchi with thickened walls in both lower lobes. Note the bronchiectatic airways and associated branches of the pulmonary arteries, which produce the characteristic signet-ring appearance.

contiguous sections are obtained, particularly when smaller airways are examined.[33,51-53]

Flexible fiberoptic bronchoscopy cannot determine the diagnosis of bronchiectasis but may be useful in elucidating the origin of the disease. Bronchoscopy is indicated for the detection of persistent segmental atelectasis refractory to chest physiotherapy and of lesions obstructing the airway (e.g., endobronchial foreign bodies). Bacterial and fungal cultures of bronchoalveolar lavage fluid or bronchial washings may also be useful in guiding antimicrobial therapy. Bronchial biopsy in which cilia are recovered for electron microscopy may demonstrate abnormalities of ciliary ultrastructure. Otherwise, the findings on bronchoscopy are usually nonspecific (i.e., mucosal inflammation and edema), so its use is limited.

Management and Prognosis

The natural history of bronchiectasis depends on the precipitating event or events. In bronchiectasis caused by cystic fibrosis, a fatal outcome is the rule, whereas in ciliary dyskinesia or postinfectious bronchiectasis, the patient has a normal life expectancy. Bronchiectasis is often not progressive, and patients may remain asymptomatic for extended periods. In these cases or at the other extreme when the pulmonary disease is widespread and progressive, medical treatment is preferred. Chest physiotherapy and postural drainage assist in the mobilization of endobronchial secretions and are mainstays of treatment. The use of mucolytic agents has generally been disappointing, although aerosolized recombinant human deoxyribonuclease shows some promise in the treatment of bronchiectasis in patients with cystic fibrosis, in whom the inflammatory response is especially intense.[54] Bronchodilators may be of benefit but should be used with monitoring of pulmonary function. Much of the impairment in bronchiectasis is irreversible and may not be improved by bronchodilators. In some cases, reduction in bronchomotor tone may impair the cough reflex and promote pooling of secretions, worsening pulmonary function.[55] Prompt and vigorous antibiotic therapy during exacerbations is the cornerstone of management. The antimicrobial agent should be determined by bacterial cultures of respiratory secretions and antibiotic sensitivities of the organisms isolated. *S. pneumoniae* and nontypeable *H. influenzae* are frequently found in the sputum of patients with bronchiectasis. The isolation of *P. aeruginosa,* particularly mucoid strains, from respiratory secretions suggests cystic fibrosis. Prophylactic antibiotics have not generally been recommended, although in a study 30 years ago, continuous therapy with tetracycline in adults reduced the frequency and severity of exacerbations but did not prevent the decline of pulmonary function. More recently, investigations have shown that regular treatment with nebulized tobramycin reduces the progress of lung disease in cystic fibrosis. Thus, such therapy may have a role in the treatment of bronchiectasis.[56] Despite the prominent role of inflammatory mediators in the development of bronchiectasis, the use of antiinflammatory agents in the treatment of bronchiectasis has not been established. Other therapies directed against the underlying cause of the pulmonary involvement may be beneficial in the management of bronchiectasis; for example, intravenous infusions of γ-globulin may arrest the progression of pulmonary disease in patients with hypogammaglobulinemia.

Surgical resection of the bronchiectatic section of lung is considered only if the patient's condition is symptomatic and is not based on the diagnosis or extent of disease alone. If symptoms cannot be controlled by antibiotic therapy and postural drainage and disease is progressive and localized, resection may be indicated.[57,58] If disease is widespread, however, resection has little advantage. Other indications for surgical intervention include an irretrievable foreign body and repeated or intractable hemorrhage from the affected lobe.

BRONCHIOLITIS OBLITERANS

Epidemiology and Disease Mechanisms

Initially reported by Lange in 1901,[59] bronchiolitis obliterans is a rare consequence of epithelial injury of the lower respiratory tract and is characterized by the obstruction and destruction of the distal airways. Hardy et al[60] reviewed the autopsies of almost 3000 pediatric patients performed during a 25-year period and identified 7 cases of bronchiolitis obliterans. In contrast, LaDue,[61] found only 1 case of bronchiolitis obliterans after review of the autopsies of 42,000 adults. The histologic examination of the lungs may reveal nonspecific findings but typically demonstrates concentric fibrosis of the small airways, masses of granulation tissue that occlude the peripheral bronchi, and bronchioles that may extend into the alveoli, resulting in an organizing pneumonia. Obstruction of the airway results in overinflation with areas of atelectasis, impaired mobilization of secretions, bronchiectasis, and fibrosis. In addition, hyperlucent lung syndrome is considered a postobstructive complication of bronchiolitis obliterans and is due to marked air trapping, secondary reduction in pulmonary blood flow, and atrophy of the affected lung. First reported by Swyer and James[62] as well as by McLeod[63] in 1953, this type of postobstructive hyperinflation has been described as a chronic sequela of adenovirus infection. Idiopathic forms of bronchiolitis obliterans have been reported and are more common in adults.

The origins of bronchiolitis obliterans may be divided into three broad categories: chemical injury, infectious injury, and immunologic injury (Box 48-2). With the advent of organ and tissue transplantation, the last category has assumed a more prominent role in pediatric populations.

Chemical Injury

Exposures to noxious gases or aerosolized chemicals (i.e., nitrogen dioxide, hydrochloric acid, sulfur dioxide, carbonic dichloride [phosgene]) have been reported as causes of bronchiolitis obliterans in adults. The inhalation of toxic fumes can result in acute respiratory compromise, but a few patients develop irreversible obstruction of the airways, usually within 3 weeks of the insult. The level of respiratory impairment caused by exposure to toxic fumes depends on the severity and extent of the inhalation injury. Other inhaled irritants, such as talc, have also produced profound pulmonary disease and obliterative bronchiolitis.

Recurrent pulmonary aspiration of gastric and oropharyngeal contents has been described as a precipitant of bronchiolitis obliterans in both pediatric and adult patients, an association that has been generally neglected in the literature. Of the 19 pediatric patients with bronchiolitis obliterans reported by Hardy et al,[60] 4 had documented or suspected gastroesophageal reflux. Two other patients in this series had underlying neurologic or cardiovascular disease and had pulmonary aspiration based on the presence of lipid-laden alveolar macrophages in autopsy specimens. Bronchiolitis obliterans

BOX 48-2
Conditions Associated with Bronchiolitis Obliterans

Inhalation of toxins
- Ammonia
- Hydrochloric acid
- Dichlorodiethyl sulfide (mustard gas)
- Nitric acid
- Nitrogen dioxide (silo filler's disease)
- Carbonic dichloride (phosgene)
- Sulfuric acid
- Talcum powder
- Zinc chloride

Aspiration
- Gastroesophageal reflux
- Foreign body aspiration
- Lipids

Infections
- Adenovirus infection
- Influenza
- Measles
- *B. pertussis* infection
- *M. pneumoniae* infection

Immunologic disease or transplantation
- Autoimmune hemolytic anemia
- Rheumatoid arthritis
- Scleroderma
- Sjögren's syndrome
- Bone marrow transplantation
- Heart and lung transplantation

Miscellaneous
- Penicillamine administration
- Sulfasalazine administration
- Alveolar proteinosis
- Bronchopulmonary dysplasia

Idiopathic conditions

Modified from Hardy KA et al: *Chest* 93:460-466, 1988.

has been experimentally induced by the instillation of hydrochloric acid into the tracheas of dogs.[64] Although the aspiration of gastric contents has been assumed to cause chemical damage to the bronchioles, infectious damage may also be possible by this mechanism.

Infectious Injury

In children, bronchiolitis obliterans has most frequently been associated with preceding infection with viral pathogens, including the influenza virus, the measles virus, and especially adenoviruses. Although many patients completely recover, chronic pulmonary disease is detected in the majority of children who had preceding adenovirus bronchiolitis and pneumonia.[65] Although hyperlucent lung syndrome may be secondary to a number of pulmonary insults, it has also been attributed to adenovirus infection, especially of serotypes 7 and 21.[66] Bronchiectasis has also been described as a sequela of adenovirus infections. *M. pneumoniae* is another infectious agent associated with the development of bronchiolitis obliterans.[67] Patients typically have tachypnea, dyspnea, fever, and persistent, nonproductive cough several days after the initial infection. On physical examination, wheezes and crackles are present. The disease may persist several weeks or months after the insult and is often accompanied by repeated atelectasis and pneumonias.

Immunologic Injury

Bronchiolitis obliterans has been reported as a form of pulmonary involvement in adults with various rheumatologic diseases (i.e., rheumatoid arthritis[68] and systemic lupus erythematosus[69]). Although its actual incidence is unclear, bronchiolitis obliterans may be a relatively frequent complication of these disorders and is probably due to the same inflammatory process that characterizes this group of diseases. To confound matters, the administration of penicillamine, an anti-inflammatory agent occasionally used in the treatment of rheumatoid arthritis, has been associated with the development of obliterative bronchiolitis.[70] Similar pulmonary complications have been described in patients receiving sulfasalazine for the treatment of ulcerative colitis.[71]

Obliterative bronchiolitis has been recognized as a postoperative sequela of graft-versus-host disease in transplant patients and is an increasingly frequent form of the disease.[72,73] Initially reported in a 22-year-old man who underwent allogenic bone marrow transplantation for aplastic anemia,[74] bronchiolitis obliterans has been described in 10% of all patients who develop chronic graft-versus-host disease after bone marrow transplantation. The respiratory signs and symptoms (cough, fever, and progressive dyspnea) develop approximately 6 months after transplantation. Other manifestations of chronic graft-versus-host disease, such as mucositis and sicca syndrome, often precede the pulmonary complications. Furthermore, bronchiolitis obliterans has been described in patients who have received lung and heart-lung transplants.[75] Burke et al[76] reviewed their experience with heart-lung transplantation and associated airway disease. Bronchiolitis obliterans developed in 50% of 20 survivors, and 4 patients subsequently died. Adjusting or increasing immunosuppressive therapy may delay the progression of this complication, although these reports are largely anecdotal. Nevertheless, the majority of affected patients still experience unrelenting deterioration in their clinical status, leading to death or retransplantation.

Diagnosis

Chest radiographs are universally abnormal. The findings are initially nonspecific, but diffuse interstitial infiltrates, atelectasis, and patchy reticulonodular densities are often present. In addition, lung volumes may be decreased. Bronchial wall thickening, air-space consolidation, and small nodules are frequently demonstrated on computed tomography.[53] Pulmonary function studies typically reveal a restrictive pulmonary defect and diminished diffusion capacity. Radioisotope scans can show either a matched decrease or an ineqality in ventilation and perfusion,[77] particularly in patients with hyperlucent lung syndrome. Bronchoscopy is generally not useful in establishing the diagnosis of bronchiolitis obliterans. When performed, bronchography usually demonstrates bronchial dilation and a characteristic pruned-tree appearance of the airways.

The diagnosis is confirmed by histologic examination of the involved lung tissue. However, because of the irregular distribution of airway involvement, lung biopsy does not always establish the diagnosis. Concentric fibrosis of the small airways and masses of granulation tissue that occlude peripheral bronchi and bronchioles are classic histologic findings. However, during the acute phase of the disease, scarring often is not evident. Tissue destruction and necrosis in the affected areas of the lung may be complete, and the affected bronchioles may not be recognizable. Emphysematous changes secondary to airway obstruction may also be present in the involved portion of the lung.

Table 48-2 Clinical Spectrum, Prognosis, and Treatment of Bronchiolotis Obliterans

CATEGORY	PROGNOSIS	TREATMENT
Toxic fume exposure	Poor-good	Corticosteroids
Postinfection effects	Fair-good	Corticosteroids
Autoimmune infection	Poor-good	Corticosteroids
Localized infection	Good	Resection
Idiopathic infection	Fair-good	Corticosteroids

Modified from Epler GR, Colby TV: *Chest* 83:161-162, 1983.

Management and Prognosis

The treatment and prognosis of bronchiolitis obliterans greatly depend on the associated disease. Graft-versus-host disease may be progressive and fatal, whereas damage caused by the inhalation of toxic fumes may not progress. Although corticosteroids retard the acute fibroblastic response in the damaged airways of experimental animals,[74] the clinical response of patients with bronchiolitis obliterans to systemic corticosteroids is variable[75] (Table 48-2). Other immunosuppressive agents and antibiotics have not been proved to be beneficial in the treatment of patients during the acute phase of the lung injury. Resection of the affected segments of lung in patients who have localized disease may be necessary.

REFERENCES

Bronchiectasis

1. Laennec RTH: *De l'auscultation médiate, un traite du diagnostie des maladies des poumons et de coeur: fondé principaliment sur ce nouveau moyen d'exploration,* Paris, 1819, Brosson et Chaudé.
2. Mounier-Kuhn P: Dilation de la trachée constatations radiographiques et bronchoscopiques, *Lyon Med* 150:106-109, 1932.
3. On an 18 month old child, *Am J* 123:687-680, 1995.
4. Bhutani VK, Ritchie WG, Schaffer TH: Acquired tracheomegaly in very preterm neonates, *Am J Dis Child* 140:449-452, 1986.
5. Williams H, Campbell P: Generalized bronchiectasis associated with deficiency of cartilage in the bronchial tree, *Arch Dis Child* 35:182-191, 1960.
6. Wayne KS, Taussig LM: Probable familial congenital bronchiectasis due to cartilage deficiency (Williams-Campbell syndrome), *Am Rev Respir Dis* 114:15-22, 1976.
7. Robitaille GA: Ehlers-Danlos syndrome and recurrent hemoptysis, *Ann Intern Med* 61:716-721, 1964.
8. Foster ME, Foster DE: Bronchiectasis and Marfan's syndrome, *Postgrad Med J* 56:718-719, 1980.
9. Lander FPL: Bronchiectasis and atelectasis: temporary and permanent changes, *Thorax* 1:198-210, 1946.
10. Nemir RL: Bronchiectasis. In Kendig EL, Chernick V, eds: *Disorders of the respiratory tract in children,* ed 4, Philadelphia, 1983, WB Saunders, pp 348-368.
11. Barker AF, Bardana EJ: Bronchiectasis: update of an orphan disease, *Am Rev Respir Dis* 137:969-978, 1988 (review).
12. Fahy JV, Schuster A, Ueki I, Boushey HA, Nadel JA: Mucus hypersecretion in bronchiectasis: the role of neutrophil proteases, *Am Rev Respir Dis* 146:1430-1433, 1992.
13. Cole PJ: Inflammation: a two-edged sword—the model of bronchiectasis, *Eur J Respir Dis* 69(suppl):6-15, 1986.
14. Liebow AA, Hales MR, Lindskog GE: Enlargement of the bronchial arteries and their anastomoses with the pulmonary arteries in bronchiectasis, *Am J Pathol* 25:211-231, 1949.
15. Konietzko NFJ, Carton RW, Leroy EP: Causes of death in patients with bronchiectasis, *Am Rev Respir Dis* 100:852-858, 1969.
16. Reid LM: Reduction in bronchial subdivisions in bronchiectasis, *Thorax* 5:233-247, 1950.
17. Shwachman H, Kowalski M, Khaw KT: Cystic fibrosis: a new outlook—seventy patients above 25 years of age, *Medicine (Baltimore)* 56:129-149, 1977.
18. di Sant'agnese PA, Davis PB: Cystic fibrosis in adults: seventy-five cases and a review of 232 cases in the literature, *Am J Med* 66:121-132, 1979.
19. Wood RE, Wanner A, Hirsch J, Farrell PM: Tracheal mucociliary transport in patients with cystic fibrosis and its stimulation of terbutaline, *Am Rev Respir Dis* 111:733-738, 1975.
20. Eliasson R, Mossberg B, Camner P, Afzelius BA: The immotile cilia syndrome: a congenital ciliary abnormality as an etiologic factor in chronic airway infections and male sterility, *New Engl J Med* 297:1-6, 1977.
21. Turner JAP, Corkey CWB, Lee JYC, Levison H, Sturgess J: Clinical expressions of immotile cilia syndrome, *Pediatrics* 67:805-810, 1981.
22. Corbeel L, Cornillie F, Lauweryns J, Boel M, van den Berghe G: Ultrastructural abnormalities of bronchial cilia in children with recurrent airway infections and bronchiectasis, *Arch Dis Child* 56:929-933, 1981.
23. Lischner HW, Huang NN: Respiratory complications of primary hypogammaglobulinemia, *Pediatr Ann* 6:514-525, 1977 (review).
24. Chipps BE, Talamo RL, Windelstern JA: IgA deficiency, recurrent pneumonias, and bronchiectasis, *Chest* 73:519-526, 1978.
25. Hilton AM, Doyle L: Immunologic abnormalities in bronchiectasis with chronic bronchial suppuration, *Br J Dis Chest* 72:207-216, 1978.
26. Longstreth GF, Weitzman SA, Browning RJ, Lieberman J: Bronchiectasis and homozygous $alpha_1$-antitrypsin deficiency, *Chest* 67:233-235, 1975.
27. Hinson KFW, Moon AJ, Plummer NS: Bronchopulmonary aspergillosis: a review and a report of eight new cases, *Thorax* 7:317-333, 1952.
28. Rosenberg M, Patterson R, Mintzer R, Cooper BJ, Roberts M, Harris KE: Clinical and immunologic criteria for the diagnosis of allergic bronchopulmonary aspergillosis, *Ann Intern Med* 86:405-414, 1977.
29. Moll HH: A clinical and pathological study of bronchiectasis, *Q J Med* 25:457-469, 1932.
30. Graham EA, Burford TH, Mayer JH: Middle lobe syndrome, *Postgrad Med* 4:29-34, 1948.
31. Culiner MM: The right middle lobe syndrome: a non-obstructive complex, *Dis Chest* 50:57-66, 1966.
32. Inners CR, Terry PB, Traystman RJ, Menkes HA: Collateral ventilation and the right middle lobe syndrome, *Am Rev Respir Dis* 118:305-310, 1978.
33. Ruberman W, Shauffer I, Biondo T: Bronchiectasis and acute pneumonia, *Am Rev Tuberc* 76:761-769, 1957.
34. Clark NS: Bronchiectasis in childhood, *Br Med J* 1:80-88, 1963.
35. Westcott JL: Bronchiectasis, *Radiol Clin North Am* 29:1031-1042, 1991 (review).
36. Fleshman MD, Wilson JF, Cohen JJ: Bronchiectasis in Alaska native children, *Arch Environ Health* 17:517-523, 1968.
37. Adebonojo SA, Grillo IA, Osinowo O, Adebo OA: Suppurative diseases of the lung and pleura: a continuing challenge in developing countries, *Ann Thorac Surg* 33:40-47, 1982.
38. Luce JM: Bronchiectasis. In Murray JF, Nadel JA, eds: *Textbook of respiratory medicine,* Philadelphia, 1988, WB Saunders, pp 1107-1125.
39. Baum GL, Racz I, Bubis JJ, Molho M, Shapiro BL: Cystic disease of the lung: a report of eighty-eight cases, with an ethnologic relationship, *Am J Med* 40:578-602, 1966.
40. Whitwell F: A study of the pathology and pathogenesis of bronchiectasis, *Thorax* 7:213-239, 1952.
41. Davis PB, Hubbard VS, McCoy K, Taussig LM: Familial bronchiectasis, *J Pediatr* 102:177-185, 1983 (review).
42. Siewert AK, Ueber einen Fall von Bronchiectasis bei einem: patienten mit Situs inversus vicerum, *Berlin München Tieraertzl Wschr* 2:139-141, 1904.
43. Kartagener M: Zur Pathologenese der Bronchiektasien: Bronchiektasien bei Situs Viscerum Inversus, *Beitr Klin Erforsch Tuberk Lungenkr* 83:489-501, 1933.
44. Rivera M, Nicotra MB: *Pseudomonas aeruginosa* mucoid strain: its significance in adult chest disease, *Am Rev Respir Dis* 126:833-836, 1982.
45. Lang WR, Howden CW, Laws J, Burton LF: Bronchopneumonia with serious sequelae in children with evidence of adenovirus type 21 infection, *Br Med J* 1:73-79, 1969.
46. Fawcett J, Parry HE: Lung changes in pertussis and measles in childhood: a review of 1894 cases with a follow-up study of the pulmonary complications, *Br J Radiol*30:76-82, 1957.
47. Lees AW: Atelectasis and bronchiectasis in pertussis, *Br Med J* 2:1138-1141, 1950.
48. Goudie BM, Kerr MR, Johnson RN: *Mycoplasma* pneumonia complicated by bronchiectasis, *J Infect* 7:151-152, 1983.

49. Cherniak N, Vosti KL, Saxton GA, Lepper MH, Dowling HF: Pulmonary function tests in fifty patients with bronchiectasis, *J Lab Clin Med* 53:693-707, 1959.
50. Cherniak N, Carton RW: Factors associated with respiratory insufficiency in bronchiectasis, *Am J Med* 41:562-571, 1966.
51. Stanford W, Galvin JR: The diagnosis of bronchiectasis, *Clin Chest Med* 9:691-699, 1988 (review).
52. Grenier P, Maurice F, Musset D, Menu Y, Nahum H: Bronchiectasis: assessment by thin-section CT, *Radiology* 161:95-99, 1986.
53. Lynch DA, Brasch RC, Hardy KA, Webb WR: Pediatric pulmonary disease: assessment with high resolution ultrafast CT, *Radiology* 176:243-248, 1990.
54. Hubbard RC, McElvony NG, Bierre P, Jolley C, Wu M: A pulmonary *N Engl J Med* 326:812-815, 1992.
55. Shapiro GG, Bamman J, Kanarek P, Bierman CW: The paradoxical effect of adrenergic and methylxanthine drugs in cystic fibrosis, *Pediatrics* 58:740-743, 1976.
56. BW, Dorhine HL, Haiwood IR, Achedlow DV, Wentz K: Efficacy in patients with cystic fibrosis. *N Engl J Med* 328:1740-1746, 1993.
57. Annest LS, Kratz JM, Crawford FA: Current results of treatment of bronchiectasis, *J Thorac Cardiovasc Surg* 83:546-550, 1982.
58. Wilson JF, Decker AM: The surgical management of childhood bronchiectasis: a review of 96 consecutive pulmonary resections in children with nontuberculous bronchiectasis, *Ann Surg* 195:354-363, 1982.

Bronchiolitis Obliterans

59. Lange W: Über eine eigentumliche Erkrankung der klemen: Branchen und Branchiolen (Bronchitis et Bronchiolitis obliterans), *Deutsch Arch Klin Med* 70:342-364, 1901.
60. Hardy KA, Schidlow DV, Zaeri N: Obliterative bronchiolitis in children, *Chest* 93:460-466, 1988.
61. LaDue JS: Bronchiolitis fibrosa obliterans, *Arch Intern Med* 68:663-673, 1941.
62. Swyer P, James G: Case of unilateral pulmonary emphysema, *Thorax* 8:133-136, 1953.
63. Macleod WM: Abnormal transradiancy of one lung. Thorax 9:147-153, 1954.
64. Moran TJ: Experimental aspiration pneumonia. IV. Inflammatory and reparative changes produced by intratracheal injections of autologous gastric juice and hydrochloric acid, *Arch Pathol* 60:122-129, 1955.
65. Chernick V, Macpherson RI: Respiratory syncytial and adenovirus infections of the lower respiratory tract in infancy, *Clin Notes Respir Dis* 10:3-7, 1971.
66. Wohl MEB, Chernick V: Bronchiolitis, *Am Rev Respir Dis* 118:759-781, 1978 (review).
67. Isles AF, Masel J, O'Duffy J: Obliterative bronchiolitis due to *Mycoplasma pneumoniae* infection in a child, *Pediatr Radiol* 17:109-111, 1987.
68. Herzog CA, Miller RR, Hoidal JR: Bronchiolitis and rheumatoid arthritis, *Am Rev Respir Dis* 124:636-639, 1981.
69. Kinney WW, Angelillo VA: Bronchiolitis in systemic lupus erythematosus, *Chest* 82:646-649, 1982.
70. Epler GR, Snider GL, Gaensler EA, Cathcart ES, FitzGerald MX, Carrington CB: Bronchiolitis and bronchitis in connective tissue disease: a possible relationship to the use of penicillamine, *JAMA* 242:528-532, 1979.
71. Williams T, Eidur L, Thomas P: Bronchiolitis obliterans, and therapy. *Chest* 81:766-768, 1982.
72. Epler GR: Bronchiolitis obliterans and airways obstruction associated with graft-versus-host disease, *Clin Chest Med* 9:551-556, 1988 (review).
73. Burke CM, Theodore J, Dawkins KD: Post-transplant obliterative bronchiolitis and other late lung sequelae in human heart-lung transplantation, *Chest* 86:824-829, 1984.
74. Roca J, Granenea A, Rodriguez-Roisin R: Fatal airway disease in an adult with chronic graft-versus-host disease, *Thorax* 37:77-78, 1982.
75. Burke CM, Glanville AR, Theodore J, Robin ED: Lung immunogenicity, rejection, and obliterative bronchiolitis, *Chest* 92:547-549, 1987.
76. Burke CM, Baldwin JC, Morris AJ: Twenty-eight cases of human heart-lung transplantation, *Lancet* 1:517-519, 1986.
77. Palmer J, Harcke T, Deforest A, Schidlow D, Cuasay L, Huang N: Matched ventilation-perfusion defects in the lung scans of children with obliterative bronchiolitis and long term clinical follow-up, *Am Rev Respir Dis* 119:280, 1979 (abstract).
78. Moran TJ, Hellstrom NR: Bronchiolitis obliterans, *Arch Pathol* 66:691-707, 1958.
79. Epler GR, Colby TV: The spectrum of bronchiolitis obliterans, *Chest* 83:161-162, 1983.

PART EIGHT

Disorders with Known or Suspected Immunologic Abnormalities

CHAPTER 49

Idiopathic Pulmonary Fibrosis and Lymphocytic Interstitial Pneumonia

Gregory J. Redding and Leland L. Fan

Chronic interstitial lung diseases (ILDs) are uncommon compared with other chronic pulmonary conditions of childhood. Of 184 children with chronic pulmonary complaints evaluated at a tertiary-level medical center, none had interstitial pneumonitis.[1] The largest series, reported by Fan et al,[2] included 48 patients over a 12-year period. As a group, these disorders are defined by histologic alterations in alveolar structures, predominantly alveolitis, tissue remodeling, fibrosis, or a combination thereof. The immune processes producing these abnormalities cause functional changes that can include restrictive lung mechanics; loss of lung volume; arterial hypoxemia, initially only with exercise but later at rest; cor pulmonale; and death.

Although chronic ILDs may result from infections such as chlamydial and cytomegaloviral pneumonias,[3] this chapter deals only with noninfectious chronic ILDs in children. Even with this narrowed focus, the differential diagnosis of chronic ILD is broad. The general categories of etiologies producing this clinical picture are listed in Box 49-1. Hypersensitivity pneumonitis, sarcoidosis, hemosiderosis, alveolar proteinosis, and lung disease associated with collagen vascular disease are the subjects of Chapters 50 and 52 through 55. Diseases producing diffuse lung injury and subsequent chronic fibrosis, such as recurrent aspiration syndromes and adult respiratory distress syndrome, are covered in Chapters 25 and 28.

This chapter addresses the diagnosis and management of the child in whom the cause of ILD is neither readily apparent by history (e.g., radiation, drug, or antigen exposure) nor associated with systemic diseases (e.g., autoimmune or storage diseases) and whose findings are localized to the lung. These diseases have been combined under the term *chronic interstitial pneumonitis* but also divided into more specific histologic descriptions, including desquamative interstitial pneumonitis (DIP), usual interstitial pneumonitis (UIP), and lymphocytic interstitial pneumonitis (LIP).[4] UIP and DIP have been combined by some authors to represent a single entity known as *cryptogenic fibrosing alveolitis* or *idiopathic pulmonary fibrosis (IPF).*[5,6] It is unclear whether IPF represents a continuum of lung responses to alveolar injury or whether UIP and DIP are distinct diseases.[7] Multiple lung biopsies from different sites at a single time in the same patient have yielded combinations of these histologic diagnoses.[6,8] Similarly, biopsies from the lungs of patients at different times have demonstrated a transition from an active interstitial pneumonitis to predominantly interstitial fibrosis.[5] To the extent that the different interstitial pneumonitides portend a different prognosis, response to therapy, or concern about an underlying disease, they are discussed separately.

BOX 49-1
Etiologies of ILDs

Inflammatory etiologies

- Infections: viruses, *Chlamydia* species, *Mycoplasma pneumoniae, Pneumocystis carinii, Aspergillus fumigatus*
- Hypersensitivity syndromes: medication (nitrofurantoin, carbamazepine), inhaled organic dusts
- Aspiration syndromes: thesaurosis, gastric contents, lipoid aspiration
- Fibrosing alveolitis: usual interstitial pneumonitis, desquamative interstitial pneumonitis, lymphoid interstitial pneumonitis
- Collagen vascular diseases: lupus erythematosus, systemic sclerosis, rheumatoid lung, polyarteritis nodosa
- Sarcoidosis
- Toxicologic effects of radiation or medications (bleomycin, busulfan, methotrexate)

Noninflammatory etiologies

- Hemosiderosis
- Alveolar proteinosis
- Idiopathic pulmonary fibrosis
- Storage diseases: Gaucher's disease, Hermansky-Pudlak syndrome, Niemann-Pick disease
- Oncologic disease
- Leukemic infiltrates

PREVALENCE

ILDs account for 15% of all disorders of patients managed by adult pulmonologists.[9] IPF accounts for up to 30% of all chronic ILDs in adults.[10] In a review of 40% of all inpatient records in the United States in 1977, 89,000 cases were estimated to be chronic interstitial fibrosis.[11] In two pediatric series, 14 of 65 patients (22%) with chronic noninfectious ILD had IPF.[2,12] This compared with 10 cases of LIP in these same series, suggesting that LIP is almost as common as IPF in children. LIP is most often encountered in children infected with human immunodeficiency virus and represents one of the criteria set forth by the Centers for Disease Control for the diagnosis of acquired immunodeficiency syndrome.[13] Between 28% and 40% of symptomatic human immunodeficiency virus–positive children with chronic interstitial pulmonary infiltrates have biopsy-proven LIP.[14,15] LIP is also more common among children with autoimmune disorders and primary immunodeficiency diseases.[16] In five of the largest series reporting on DIP and IPF in children,[2,17-20] 101 cases were reported from a cumulative 54 years of records, demonstrating the infrequent occurrence of the disorder. The current prevalences of ILD and more specifically IPF in children are unknown because of the lack of systematic reporting of cases.

Children younger than 4 months of age have developed IPF and LIP; other cases have been diagnosed in adolescence. Although some studies have indicated that most cases of DIP and IPF are diagnosed within the first year of life[17,18] (Fig. 49-1), one study reported 14 cases of IPF that were initially diagnosed at 6 to 16 years of age.[19] Unlike the male predominance of IPF among adults, there is no apparent gender predisposition for IPF or LIP in children.[17-19,21] A heritable form has been suggested from reports of family clustering within and across generations.[22-24] DIP, LIP, and IPF have all been described in multiple family members.[23-26] The familial form of IPF is thought to be inherited as an autosomal dominant trait with variable penetrance, which may account for 5% of cases.[24,27]

Although IPF and LIP occur as idiopathic lung diseases unrelated to other conditions, both entities have been described as part of multisystem inflammatory or autoimmune conditions. These conditions are listed in Box 49-2. The variety of organ systems involved supports the notion that IPF and LIP are both undefined pulmonary manifestations of immune processes.

DISEASE MECHANISMS AND HISTOPATHOLOGY

The pathogenic process in chronic interstitial pneumonitis begins with an immune-mediated alveolitis that produces injury to alveolar, capillary, and interstitial structures and leads to subsequent tissue repair and fibrosis. The inciting event may be an occult infection, as has been suggested for some cases of LIP in response to Epstein-Barr virus.[28] Most often, however, no infection or evidence of past infection has been identified by serologic tests or cultures. Polymerase chain reaction is currently being used to restudy this question. Circulating immune complexes have been detected in some patients with IPF, as have immune deposits localized histochemically to alveolar epithelial surfaces and capillary walls.[29,30] However, the antigens within these immune complexes have not yet been identified. In most cases of IPF, the inciting agent and route of exposure are unknown.

The histologic patterns of UIP and DIP suggest that the alveolitis can exist as a homogeneous stage of inflammation or as a spatially and temporally heterogeneous process. UIP is characterized by a patchy distribution of inflammation that is in various stages of injury and repair at any one time. UIP produces a pattern of normal lung regions juxtaposed next to regions of active inflammation with increased numbers of lymphocytes, plasma cells, and macrophages. Lung regions with extensive fibrosis, producing a "honeycomb lung," coexist with areas of active inflammation. In contrast, DIP is defined by a diffuse but uniform pattern with type II alveolar cell hyperplasia, septal hypertrophy, abundant intraalveolar macrophages, and interstitial accumulation of lymphocytes and plasma cells. Histiocytes and eosinophils may also be present. There is little evidence of fibrosis despite widespread inflammation. The condition of patients diagnosed with DIP by lung biopsy can nonetheless proceed to fatal pulmonary fibrosis.[31] Up to 20% of lung biopsies from children with chronic interstitial pneumonitis have a spectrum of histologic abnormalities that do not neatly fit with a definitive diagnosis.[2] A report of five infants with interstitial pneumonitis and an accumulation of histiocytes raises questions as to whether some variants from UIP and DIP represent additional distinct forms of chronic ILD.[32]

The pathogenesis of the disease may also reflect the immune response of a particularly susceptible host and the unusual tendency for persistent inflammation and progressive lung fibrosis. The numbers and activities of T cells, alveolar macrophages, and neutrophils are increased in patients with IPF. These cell types are all found in increased numbers in bronchoalveolar lavage (BAL) fluid and in lung tissue on biopsy, albeit in different proportions in various patients at different stages of disease.[33,34] Increased lymphocyte proportions in BAL correlate with minimal progression of IPF during steroid therapy, suggesting that the inflammatory process may be T cell driven and responsive to therapy at the stage when lymphocytes predominate.[34-37] Alveolar macrophages proliferate faster than normal in patients with IPF and produce increased levels of oxidants in both the activated and baseline states when harvested in BAL fluid from children with ILD compared with children without lung disease.[38] Both T cells and macrophages produce cytokines that amplify inflammation via neutrophil and monocyte recruitment and activation.[39] Increased numbers of neutrophils in the BAL fluid of patients with ILD portend a poor response to steroid therapy, suggesting that neutrophil-induced lung injury may herald an irreversible component of interstitial inflammation and fibrosis.[34,40] Alveolar macrophages also produce fibrogenic cytokines (tumor necrosis factor-α and interleukin-1) and growth factors (transforming growth factor-β and platelet-derived growth factor) that stimulate fibroblast activity.[41,42] The BAL fluid from patients with IPF contains increased amounts of type III procollagen peptides, suggesting an ongo-

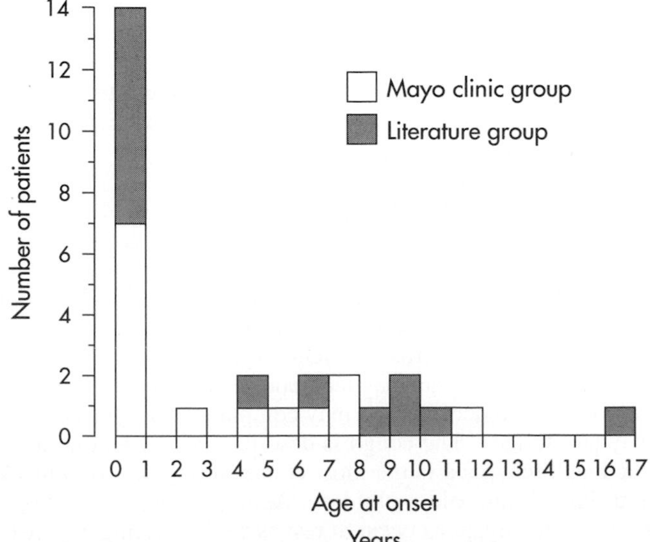

Fig. 49-1. Distribution of ages of children with DIP at the onset of disease. (From Stillwell PC et al: *Chest* 77:165-171, 1980.)

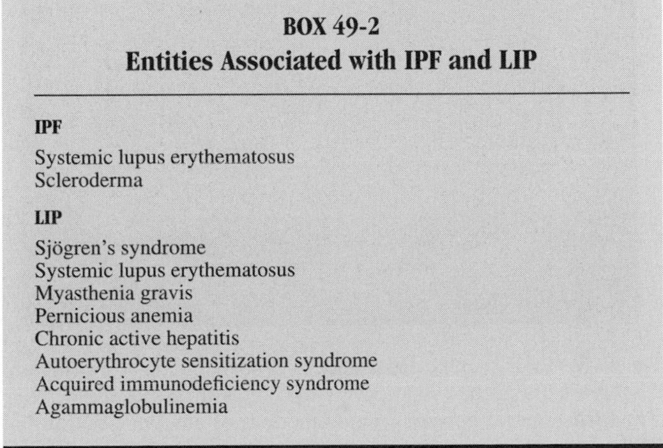

BOX 49-2
Entities Associated with IPF and LIP

IPF

Systemic lupus erythematosus
Scleroderma

LIP

Sjögren's syndrome
Systemic lupus erythematosus
Myasthenia gravis
Pernicious anemia
Chronic active hepatitis
Autoerythrocyte sensitization syndrome
Acquired immunodeficiency syndrome
Agammaglobulinemia

ing and perhaps overexuberant degree of fibroblast activity.[43] The normal lung parenchyma is approximately one-third type III collagen and two-thirds type I collagen, the latter being a less distensible form. The lungs of patients with IPF contain only 12% to 24% type III collagen and increased amounts of type I collagen, suggesting a change in the metabolic pathways of fibroblasts in this disease.[44] Currently, the pulmonary cell-cell interactions and the mechanisms that specifically produce the persistent and progressive lung inflammation, injury, and fibrosis of IPF are poorly understood.

It has been suggested that the consequences of immunologic injury to the alveolar-capillary region include the loss of alveolar type I cells and repopulation along the denuded basement membrane with proliferating type II pneumocytes.[45] Before reepithelialization, proteinaceous exudate from the inflamed interstitium activates both inflammatory cells and fibroblasts to phagocytose the debris and also to produce collagen and elastin to repair defects in the alveolar-capillary basement membrane. Reepithelialization of this repaired structure leads to the histologic picture of thickened alveolar septa, a hallmark of ILD.

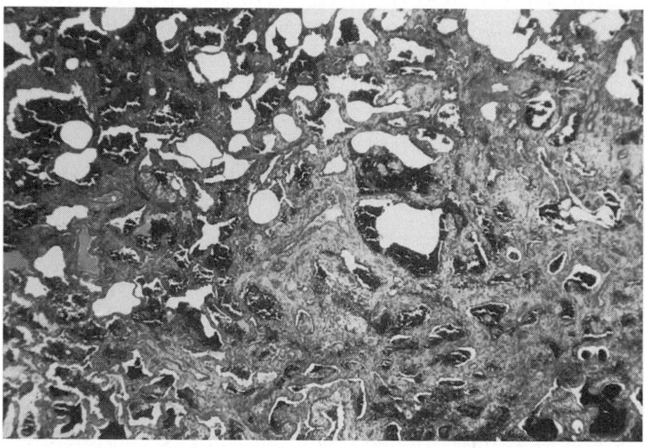

Fig. 49-2. Histopathologic appearance of honeycombing from a lung biopsy of a boy with IPF. The tissue demonstrates the extensive fibrosis and multiple small cysts that are characteristic of advanced ILD.

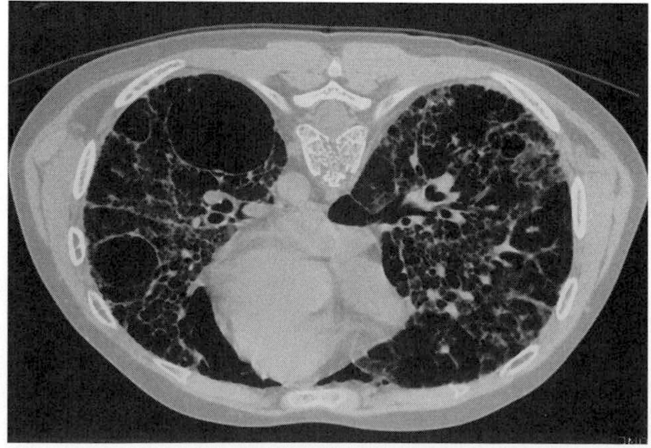

Fig. 49-3. Radiographic appearance of honeycombing on a computed tomogram of the chest in a 12-year-old boy with advanced IPF. Note the diffuse cystic appearance and the loss of anatomic definitions of the lung.

The interstitial and alveolar inflammation and fibrosis may also involve neighboring bronchiolar and vascular structures. Vasculitis per se is not a feature of IPF; however, vascular injury and fibrosis occur secondary to nearby interstitial inflammation. Obliterative bronchiolitis, bronchiolectasis, and pulmonary vascular involvement resulting from interstitial involvement can lead to peripheral airway obstruction, pulmonary hypertension, and cor pulmonale. Approximately one third of reported cases of IPF in children have objective evidence of cor pulmonale.[17,18] Approximately half of the children who have IPF and who have been tested with maximum expiratory flow-volume loops demonstrate reduced flow in the small airways.[46]

It is unclear how the duration and severity of inflammation predispose to progressive pulmonary fibrosis. Some patients have active inflammation without fibrosis; others develop a rapidly progressive fibrosis (e.g., Hamman-Rich syndrome).[27] In severe chronic cases, continual loss of epithelial integrity and intact basement membrane scaffolding during the inflammatory process lead to disorganized tissue repair with irreversible fibrosis that obliterates the alveolar airspaces. The end stage of this fibrotic and obliterative process is a honeycomb lung, which is characteristic of but not specific for IPF. Histologically, honeycomb lung consists of matrix reorganization, alveolar and vascular obliteration, and bronchiolectasis (Fig. 49-2). A computed tomogram of the chest of a child with honeycomb lung illustrates the macroscopic appearance of these structural changes (Fig. 49-3).

The histologic appearance of LIP differs from that of IPF, suggesting a different pathogenic process. LIP is defined by sheets of polytypic mature lymphocytes within the interstitium and alveolar spaces and along lymphatic pathways. Predominant lymphocyte cell types differ among patients with LIP and include B cells, CD8 T-suppressor cells, and CD4 T-helper cells.[16] Plasma cells and macrophages are also encountered but in smaller numbers. Additional features include noncaseating granulomas composed of mononuclear and giant cells and micronodules with lymphoid germinal centers. The histology of LIP is similar to that of primary pulmonary lymphomas but differs insofar as LIP produces no tissue necrosis and spares the airways, lung vessels, and lymph nodes.[47] Unlike IPF, the association of LIP with Epstein-Barr virus in children with acquired immunodeficiency syndrome raises a stronger potential relationship between the viruses and a pulmonary immune response.[14,28] However, like IPF, LIP can progress to produce life-threatening pulmonary fibrosis.[25,47] The mechanisms by which this happens are unknown.

CLINICAL MANIFESTATIONS

Signs and Symptoms

The most common symptoms and signs of IPF compiled from four series of pediatric cases are listed in Table 49-1. The initial symptoms may differ in infants compared with older children. Younger patients may feed poorly and present with failure to thrive; older children may complain of dyspnea during play and fatigue. The cough is described as dry and nonproductive. Tachypnea is the most common physical finding in both infants and older children. As the disease progresses, cyanosis and dyspnea occur at rest as well as during exercise. Crackles are initially heard only at the end of a full inspiration but become more prominent and are heard throughout inspiration as the disease progresses. Less common symptoms and signs include anorexia, chest pain, fever, rhonchi, chest deformities, retractions, and signs of pulmonary hypertension. The initial presentation can be an apparently spontaneous pneumothorax.[17,48] These clinical findings do not differ from those described in children with other forms of ILD[2,12] nor from those described in adults with IPF,[49,50] suggesting little specificity with regard to the type of interstitial disease or the age of the patient. LIP in children has a similar presentation.[16,25] The duration of symptoms is often difficult to determine because the onset of tachypnea may be unnoticed and exertional dyspnea may progress insidiously. In many cases the physical findings of clubbing and cyanosis reflect the advanced nature of the disease at the time of diagnosis. As with adults, delays in diagnosis may last months to years because of the subtle nature of the early clinical manifestations.[17,19]

Radiographic Features

Radiographic abnormalities are present initially in the majority of children with chronic ILD. However, normal chest radiographs in the presence of symptoms and abnormal physical findings have been described in both adults and children.[19,51,52] There are five radiographic patterns associated with ILDs: ground glass, reticular, nodular, reticulonodular, and honeycomb. The reticular pattern of IPF in childhood is illustrated in Fig. 49-4. None of these patterns is specific for IPF. In adults, initial interstitial radiographic changes are noted in the lung bases and become more diffuse as the disease progresses.[22] This distribution has not been reported in children. The ground-glass appearance is found early in the disease and corresponds to active alveolitis on lung biopsy. The radiographic honeycomb pattern correlates well with histologic honeycombing and severe fibrosis. Most children with IPF have the reticulonodular radiographic pattern and a combination of both interstitial and alveolar radiographic changes.[17-20] Although the correlations have not been made in children, the radiographic appearance in adults with ILD correlates poorly with severity of symptoms, pulmonary function abnormalities, and degree of inflammation on lung biopsy.[53-55] The radiographic appearance also correlates poorly with response to therapy and with progression of disease until honeycombing develops.[53]

The development of high-resolution computed tomography (HRCT) has provided a more precise, sensitive, and noninvasive means of detecting and describing the extent and distribution of pulmonary changes associated with ILD. HRCT differs from conventional computed tomography because it reconstructs cross-sectional images from only 1- to 2-mm sections of tissue with high-frequency algorithms, thereby enhancing the spatial resolution of parenchymal features. HRCT has detected abnormalities in the lungs of patients with chronic ILD who had normal chest radiographs.[56] HRCT has also helped to determine the best site to obtain a lung biopsy specimen by locating areas of active inflammation and avoiding areas of honeycombing and extensive fibrosis.[57] IPF in particular produces a characteristic appearance of patchy reticular densities in the subpleural peripheral lung regions and lung bases. Some authors believe that this pattern is specific enough for IPF to obviate the need for tissue diagnosis.[57] Whether this is true of children will require a multicenter prospective study. HRCT also has potential as a device for monitoring disease progression; it can document the development of new areas of active alveolitis and subpleural honeycombing more clearly than chest radiographs.

Table 49-1 Common Symptoms and Signs in Children with IPF*

SYMPTOM OR SIGN	INCIDENCE
Dyspnea	57/62 (92%)
Growth retardation	38/52 (73%)
Cough	50/62 (81%)
Crackles	28/34 (82%)
Tachypnea	37/52 (71%)
Cyanosis	30/62 (40%)
Clubbing	22/62 (35%)

Data from Hewitt CJ et al: *Arch Dis Child* 52:22-37, 1977; Stillwell PC et al: *Chest* 77:165-171, 1980; Steinkamp G et al: *Acta Paediatr Scand* 79:823-831, 1990; and Chetty A et al: *Ann Allergy* 58:336-340, 1987.
*Based on 62 infants and children.

Pulmonary Function

Pulmonary function abnormalities in most ILDs reflect restrictive changes with reduced lung volume and reduced lung compliance. Airway involvement occurs in a variable minority of patients as documented by air trapping via plethysmography and reduced flow in the small airways. Children with IPF have lung function changes similar to those observed in adults.[46,49] Three reports have measured lung function in 34 children with biopsy-proven IPF.[19,20,46] Vital capacity and total lung capacity were diminished in virtually everyone; vital capacity was more severely reduced than total lung capacity. Thoracic gas volume at functional residual capacity was re-

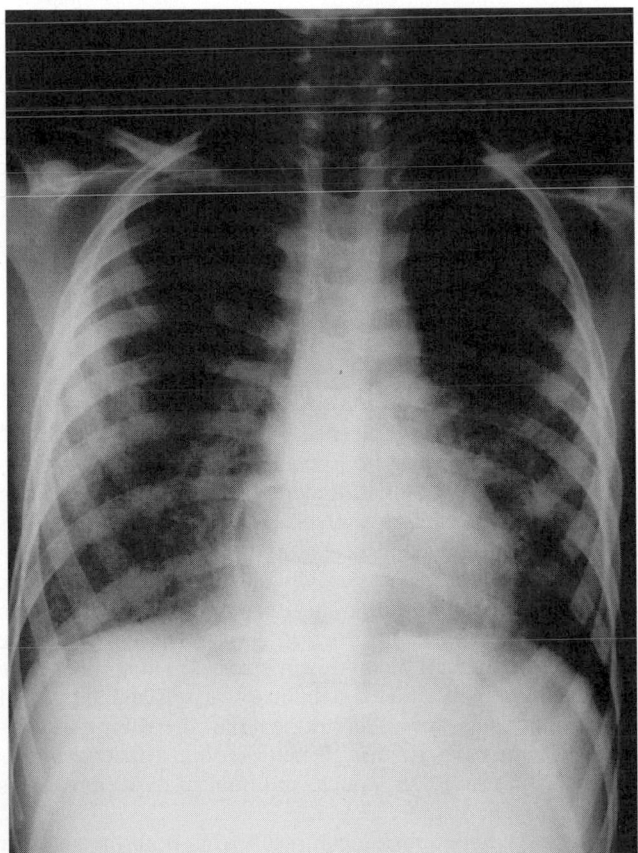

Fig. 49-4. Chest radiograph from a child with IPF, demonstrating the bilateral reticular densities characteristic of ILD.

duced in 7 and increased in 14 of 28 cases tested. Air trapping as measured by increased functional residual capacity/total lung capacity or residual volume/total lung capacity via body plethysmography was also detected. These increased ratios in part reflect reductions in total lung capacity and vital capacity. It is unclear how much they also reflect peripheral airway narrowing, gas trapped within cystic lung regions, or both effects. The 1-second forced expiratory volume and airway conductance were normal when corrected for lung volume, suggesting that large airway obstruction is not present. However, maximum expiratory flows at 60% of total lung capacity were reduced in 5 of 15 cases, perhaps related to inflammation and fibrosis involving the small airways as well as the interstitium. The prevalence of bronchial hyperreactivity in these patients has not been described. Both static and dynamic specific lung compliances are reduced in the majority of cases of IPF in both infants and older children.[48]

Lung diffusion capacity when corrected for lung volume is normal in many children with IPF.[20,46] These findings conflict with those in adults, in whom this value is often reduced before the lung volume is reduced and is therefore used to quantitate early functional changes in patients with IPF.[58] Normal values in children with IPF also contrast with reports of children with other forms of ILD, in whom almost half of patients have reduced diffusing capacities.[59] This suggests that the lung diffusion capacity may be a more informative variable for monitoring in other pediatric ILDs.

Arterial hypoxemia resulting from ventilation-perfusion mismatching is a cardinal feature of ILDs in both adults and children.[2,59,60] Reduced arterial oxygen tension and reduced lung compliance correlate somewhat in children with ILD.[59] In adults with IPF, hypoxemia correlates with the severity of pulmonary hypertension, severity of fibrosis, and survival.[61,62] Similar correlates have not yet been made in children. Patients with IPF have variable degrees of hypoxemia when awake at rest; the hypoxemia can worsen dramatically during exercise and sleep.[63] In mild and moderate disease, patients have mild respiratory alkalosis; only late in the disease does hypercapnia occur.

Pulmonary Hemodynamics

Pulmonary hypertension and cor pulmonale exist in the majority of children with IPF. Of 59 patients reported in two series, 30 had evidence of cor pulmonale by electrocardiography, echocardiography, or cardiac catheterization.[17,18] In 5 other children, the condition presented clinically with right-sided heart failure.[17] This incidence is only slightly greater than the 42% of children with chronic interstitial conditions that have cor pulmonale, suggesting that pulmonary hypertension is related to the severity of disease more than the specific type of ILD.[2] In adults with mild IPF, pulmonary hypertension is absent at rest but manifests during exercise, when cardiac output and pulmonary blood flow increase.[64] This is due to the indistensibility of remodeled pulmonary vessels and the lack of normal pulmonary vessel recruitment during exercise as a result of capillary destruction. When the vital capacity is less than 50% of predicted values, pulmonary hypertension is likely to exist at rest.[65]

Pulmonary hypertension can result from both the alveolar hypoxia that is associated with chronic parenchymal disease and the vascular obliteration that results from inflammation and fibrosis of the neighboring interstitium. To the extent that hypoxia produces pulmonary vasoconstriction and vascular remodeling, the use of supplemental oxygen may forestall progression of pulmonary hypertension and cor pulmonale. The pulmonary vascular response to oxygen and other pulmonary vasodilators in children with ILD has not been reported. In adults with other forms of pulmonary hypertension, an improved cardiac output or a reduction in pulmonary vascular resistance in response to pulmonary vasodilators portends a longer survival than in nonresponders.[66] Whether this is the case in children with ILD and specifically with IPF remains to be determined.

Serology

The serologic results in both children and adults with IPF are often abnormal but nonspecific. Elevations in serum levels of immunoglobulins, a positive rheumatoid factor, and increased titers for antinuclear antibodies have all been described in subgroups of patients.[19,53,61,67] Reports of these findings in children have not been sufficiently standardized to know the numbers of patients with these abnormalities, and serial evaluations of these changes have not been described. Serum immune complexes have been detected in patients with idiopathic interstitial pneumonias; these abnormalities in blood have been associated with active inflammation and increased cellularity on lung biopsy and indicate a higher likelihood of response to steroid therapy than in patients with fibrotic IPF.[68]

DIAGNOSIS AND STAGING

The diagnosis of chronic interstitial pneumonitis usually requires histopathologic examination of lung tissue obtained from an open lung biopsy. This is particularly true because therapy for IPF and LIP includes long-term immunosuppressive agents with potentially serious side effects. In certain types of ILD, a diagnosis can be successfully inferred from the history, as with radiation pneumonitis, or by serologic studies, as with hypersensitivity pneumonitis to birds. If a patient with diffuse interstitial infiltrates is immunocompromised, infection may be identified by several techniques, including immunofluorescence of nasopharyngeal cells, BAL, or open lung biopsy. However, for most noninfectious etiologies of ILD in the absence of extrapulmonary manifestations of disease, a tissue diagnosis is necessary. There are several exceptions when BAL can retrieve cell types or material that is diagnostic. Iron-laden macrophages reflect pulmonary hemorrhage, suggesting vasculitis or hemosiderosis. Histiocytosis X can be diagnosed with the retrieval of Langerhans' cells, which stain positively with the monoclonal antibody OKT6.[69] Alveolar proteinosis can be diagnosed from BAL fluid based on the material staining positively with periodic acid-Schiff and minimally with Alcian blue.[70] In a recent series of immunocompetent children with chronic interstitial pneumonitis, a specific diagnosis was established in 80% (24 of 30) of cases by open lung biopsy in contrast to 30% (6 of 20) by BAL.[2]

The yield from an open lung biopsy improves if HRCT of the chest is performed to identify the distribution of disease. Biopsy of an abnormal area that does not demonstrate cystic changes or honeycombing increases the identification of alveolitis instead of fibrosis and hence the type of interstitial pneumonitis present.[71] Enough of the sample must be resected that portions can be preserved in formalin and in glutaraldehyde for electron microscopy and touch preparations. It is unclear whether multiple biopsy sites are necessary to maximize the likelihood of a definitive diagnosis. In view of the infrequency of IPF and LIP, the histology should ideally be interpreted by a pathologist who has expertise in ILDs. Reported complications in children from the open biopsy procedure range between 10% and 27% for minor complications and 1% and 2% for serious problems.[72,73]

Transbronchial biopsies are increasingly used in children after lung transplantation and may eventually emerge as a tenable alternative to open lung biopsy for children with ILD.[74,75] However, multiple specimens are necessary, and the small tissue specimens obtained make histologic interpretation less definitive than with open lung biopsy.[76]

Lung biopsy is the gold standard not only for diagnosing the type of interstitial pneumonitis but also for staging the degree of inflammatory cellular activity and fibrosis in a patient with IPF. The premise behind staging procedures is that patients with active inflammation have more potential to respond to antiinflammatory therapies and hence live longer than patients with fibrosis, as suggested in several studies in adults with IPF.[6,21,77]

The first problem with staging is the lack of standardized means that can be used by many pathologists to quantitate the degree of inflammation and fibrosis and thus provide consistent conclusions. Several scoring systems have been developed for this purpose.[78,79] The most recent one by Cherniack et al[78] is depicted in Table 49-2. In 50 patients in whom a diagnosis of IPF had been made, four pathologists using this scoring system reached uniform agreement about the degree of cellularity and the degree of fibrosis in 54% and 64% of cases, respectively. The authors recommended that a panel of pathologists be used to stage lung biopsies of patients with IPF to minimize interpretation errors.

The additional challenge for clinicians is to identify a noninvasive means of serially reevaluating the staging of ILD as the disease progresses or abates in response to therapy. Multiple investigators have used lung functions, imaging techniques, gallium scans, serologic tests, and BAL to prognosticate about the response to therapy and hence survival. There is minimal information in children regarding this issue; thus the relevance of adult data to children is unclear.

Among the variety of lung function tests studied, few are able to distinguish whether functional abnormalities are due to fibrosis or to active alveolitis. Both pathologic events produce restrictive lung mechanics and abnormal gas exchange. In adults, changes in the partial pressure of arterial oxygen per liter of oxygen consumed during exercise seem to correlate with pulmonary fibrosis.[80] In the only study evaluating lung function as a means of staging disease in older children with IPF, a reduced specific dynamic lung compliance (dynamic lung compliance/functional residual capacity) correlated with fibrosis on lung biopsy.[19] Spirometry and blood gas analysis at rest are helpful in monitoring the clinical course of disease but not in staging the inflammatory activity of the disease.

Chest radiographs correlate poorly with lung function, clinical symptoms, and the appearance of lung biopsies.[21,53] Chest films are more useful in identifying complications such as intercurrent infections and pneumothoraces. In contrast, HRCT has been successfully used to predict cellularity vs. fibrosis in the lung biopsies of adults with mild and advanced IPF.[81] Alveolar opacifications correlate with histologic alveolitis, whereas reticular densities interspersed with small cysts correlate with fibrosis and early honeycombing. HRCT has significant potential for both initial staging and serial evaluations for progression to resolution. No experience using HRCT for staging IPF in children has been reported.

Gallium lung scans have been used to assess disease activity in adults with IPF.[54] Increased gallium uptake in the lungs is not specific for IPF and is seen in other ILDs.[53] Although positive gallium scans have correlated with cellularity in the lung biopsies of patients with IPF, enthusiasm for this technique has waned over the last decade because of difficulties correlating amount of gallium uptake (i.e., degree of positivity) with degree of disease activity in a serial fashion.[49,50] No literature exists regarding its use in children with ILD.

BAL has received considerable attention as a means of retrieving lung cells representative of the interstitium on a serial basis in patients with IPF. The results have been used for staging IPF and prognosticating about the response to antiinflammatory therapy. In contrast to the adult experience, BAL results for children suffer from lack of substantial data in normal children and lack of standardized techniques for the instillation of fluid and the handling of the sequential aliquots retrieved. Normal reference values from two published reports and one recent abstract are listed in Table 49-3 and provide a range of results reflecting both patient selection and lavage technique.[38,82,83] Use of BAL analysis in pediatric patients with known IPF should be considered a research tool at this time.

The BAL fluid from adults with IPF has multiple differences compared with adult norms (Table 49-4). The counts of all cell types, including macrophages, neutrophils, eosinophils,

Table 49-2 Scoring of Open Lung Biopsies in IPF

	VARIABLE SCORE GRADE (% TISSUE INVOLVEMENT)*: 0-5
Overall assessment	
Cellularity (inflammatory cells)	
Fibrosis	
Inflammatory/exudative changes	
Alveolar wall	
Cell infiltrate, extent	
Cell infiltrate, severity	
Cell metaplasia	
Lymphoid aggregates, total number	
Alveolar space, including alveolar duct, respiratory bronchioles	
Cellularity, extent	
Cellularity, severity	
Granulation tissue, degree: Absent, present, or marked	
Fibrotic/reparative changes	
Alveolar wall	
Interstitial young connective tissue	
Interstitial fibrosis, five alveolar walls, including honeycombing	
Honeycombing alone, %	
Smooth muscle, % low power	
Vessel myointimal changes	
Airways, including respiratory and terminal bronchioles	
Absent, present, or marked	
Mural inflammation, degree	
Luminal granulation tissue, degree	
Mural fibrosis	

From Cherniack RM et al: *Am Rev Respir Dis* 144:892-900, 1991.
*Whichever is appropriate for the individual parameter.

Table 49-3 BAL Values in Normal Children

N	VOLUME	ALIQUOT	% RETURN	CELL NO. ($\times 10^5$)	AM (%)	LYM (%)	PMN (%)
11	10% FRC	5	60-70	2.6 ± 0.4	90 ± 2	9 ± 2	<3
13	2-4 cc/kg	1	50 ± 3	8 ± 8	84 ± 8	10 ± 6	6 ± 6
14	20 cc	2	60 ± 1	8 ± 3	87 ± 3	9 ± 4	3 ± 2

Data from Clement A et al: *Am Rev Respir Dis* 136:1424-1428, 1987; Ronchetti R et al: *Am Rev Respir Dis* 145:556A, 1992; and Midulla F et al: *Pediatr Pulmonol* 20(2):112-118, 1995.
AM, Alveolar macrophage; *LYM,* lymphocyte; *PMN,* polymorphonuclear neutrophils; *FRC,* functional residual capacity

Table 49-4 BAL Fluid in Normal Adults and Adults with IPF

FEATURE	NORMALS	IPF
Total cells ($\times 10^6$)	32 ± 3	37 ± 7
Alveolar macrophages (%)	88 ± 1.0	75 ± 3
Lymphocytes (%)	10 ± 1	11 ± 2
Neutrophils (%)	2 ± 1	9 ± 2
Eosinophils (%)	<1	4 ± 1
Protein (μ/ml)	90 ± 3.0	174 ± 18
Immunoglobulin G (μ/ml)	8 ± 0.5	30 ± 4

Data from the BAL Cooperative Group Steering Committee: *Am Rev Respir Dis* 141:5169-5201, 1990.

and lymphocytes, are increased. The ratio of cell types is also abnormal, with an increased percentage of lymphocytes, neutrophils, and eosinophils and a reduced percentage of macrophages. In one study, 97% of patients with IPF had BAL fluid abnormalities involving at least one cell type.[34] The number of neutrophils was increased in 81% of these cases, eosinophils in 66%, and lymphocytes in 25%. Concentrations of soluble BAL constituents are also abnormal and include increased levels of serum proteins, immunoglobulins, procollagen peptides, and complement fragments and reduced levels of surfactant phospholipids and surfactant apoproteins.[49] In addition, the metabolic activities of alveolar macrophages retrieved in BAL fluid from patients with IPF demonstrate increased production of interleukin-8, leukotriene B_4, platelet-derived growth factor, interferon-γ, and oxygen radicals.[38,49]

Multiple reports have correlated BAL abnormalities in patients with IPF to cellularity and fibrosis on lung histology, positive responses to therapy, and survival. Most studies have correlated the BAL at the time of biopsy to the subsequent clinical response rather than serial changes in BAL over time. Increased proportions of lymphocytes and ratios of phosphatidylglycerol to phosphatidylinositol in BAL both correlate with interstitial and alveolar cellularity on lung biopsies,[34,36,84,85] whereas increased proportions of neutrophils and eosinophils do not.[34,84] Lymphocytosis in which the lymphocyte count in BAL fluid is more than 11% portends a positive response to steroid therapy; a neutrophil count of more than 4% and an eosinophil count of more than 3% in the absence of lymphocytosis in BAL fluid portend a minimal response to therapy.[34,40] Mild as opposed to severe reductions in phospholipid content in BAL fluid correlate with improvement during therapy.[85] Reduced levels of surfactant apoprotein A, normalized total phospholipid content, and increased levels of procollagen III N-peptides in BAL fluid correlate with poor clinical outcomes.[86,87] No studies have combined BAL fluid abnormalities to determine whether multiple factors better predict response to therapy or subsequent clinical outcome.

Turner-Warwick and Haslam[34] evaluated serial changes in BAL fluid from adults with IPF during treatment with either steroids or cyclophosphamide over a median of 4 years. Patients whose conditions clinically responded to treatment experienced a reduction in BAL cell proportions toward normal values. Patients whose conditions were clinically stable and did not change during therapy had elevated neutrophil and eosinophil counts throughout follow-up. The condition of 10 of 12 (83%) patients with increased neutrophils in BAL fluid improved during steroid therapy. In contrast, the condition of patients with increased levels of eosinophils in BAL fluid responded to cyclophosphamide. This contrasts with another study using serial BAL analysis to evaluate response to therapy: O'Donnell et al[40] performed BAL at baseline and at 3 and 6 months after the onset of therapy with either steroids or cyclophosphamide in patients with IPF who had neutrophilia (neutrophil count >10%) in BAL fluid before treatment. Neutrophil counts did not change in patients treated with steroids but fell substantially at 3 and 6 months in the cyclophosphamide-treated group. These studies suggest that BAL analysis is helpful in monitoring pulmonary cellular responses to different therapies or changes in therapy.

Treatment

Once children have been diagnosed with IPF, treatment should be initiated with appropriate supportive care and antiinflammatory agents. Supportive measures include aggressive treatment of superimposed respiratory infections, adequate nutrition by a route that minimizes respiratory complications, and minimization of environmental irritants that may exacerbate the inflammatory process. In adults with IPF, active smoking has a deleterious effect on the clinical course and response to therapy.[88] Whether exposure to passive smoke in children with IPF is similarly harmful is unknown. Oxygen therapy can improve sleep quality in patients whose hypoxemia during sleep produces frequent arousals and sleep fragmentation.[63] Oxygen also improves exercise tolerance and may forestall the progression of pulmonary hypertension caused by alveolar hypoxia.

Unlike occasional adult cases,[31] no untreated children with IPF have experienced spontaneous remissions. Most are treated with one or more antiinflammatory agents. Medications that have been used for IPF are listed in Box 49-3. No control trials of therapy in children with ILD have been reported, so which agent or combination of agents is most effective is unknown. Traditionally, glucocorticoids have been the drug of choice in children based on the early experience in adults with IPF that demonstrated longer survival times in patients responding to steroids.[6,21,31] The majority of children reported with IPF have received steroid therapy.[17,18,20] Chloroquine and hydroxychloroquine have been reported anecdotally as alternative medications in children and more commonly as drugs of choice when steroids are ineffective.[25,48,89-91] Of the remaining agents, cyclophosphamide and azathioprine have been used

BOX 49-3
Drug Therapy for IPF

Steroids
Steroid pulse therapy
Chloroquine
Hydroxychloroquine
Cyclophosphamide
Azathioprine
Chlorambucil
Methotrexate
D-Penicillamine
Cyclosporine

sporadically in children with poor responses to steroids.[23,92,93] LIP responds to these same agents.[25,48]

It is unclear whether there is a threshold dose at which steroid treatment becomes effective. It is clear, however, that as doses are tapered in children with IPF who initially respond to the drug, symptoms reappear, sometimes with subsequent death.[17] For this reason, the initial dosage should be 2 mg/kg/day or more for 6 to 8 weeks. In three studies that described initial responses to steroids, 28 of 34 (88%) of children with IPF improved during the first 3 months of treatment.[17,19,20] The rate of improvement varies; clinical improvement may be noticed as early as 1 week after the initiation of therapy. Children younger than 1 year of age improve less often than older children.[17,19] In older children, the most pronounced improvement in lung function occurs within the first 3 months of treatment, but maximum lung function values may be achieved after 9 to 24 months (Fig. 49-5). In several cases, particularly in infants, the initial improvement was not sustained.[17] This was ascribed in some to rapid tapering of the initial steroid dose and in others to the progressive nature of the interstitial disease.

Clinical improvement can manifest as a reduction in symptoms, radiographic improvement, and improved lung function with increased lung compliance in infants; larger vital capacities in older children; and reduced oxygen requirements in all children.[17,19] Often, only one of these parameters improves. For example, a patient may have symptomatic relief with less dyspnea without changes in lung function or the appearance of the chest radiograph. For this reason, clinical scoring systems based on multiple indexes have been used in adults to quantitate the degree of response.[79] These scoring systems rely on lung function tests and cardiopulmonary responses to exercise and are not applicable to younger children. Some authors believe that a reduction in inflammatory markers within BAL fluid should be monitored[94]; others are content with improvement in clinical parameters.

The goal of therapy is to maximize pulmonary improvement but avoid side effects. Cautious tapering of the initial dose is recommended with the goal of reaching an alternate-day steroid regimen that produces continued improvement or maintains maximal improvement. If there is no improvement within 3 months on high-dose therapy, the dose should be tapered to minimize side effects while an alternative agent is initiated. If the child or infant with IPF or LIP is seriously ill with minimal cardiopulmonary reserve and the condition is not responding to single-agent therapy, combination therapy is advisable.

An alternative regimen designed to minimize steroid-induced side effects is periodic high-dose glucocorticoid treatment ("pulse" therapy). This has been used for rheumatologic diseases in children and for IPF in adults.[95,96] A daily intravenous dose of 30 mg/kg of methylprednisolone for 3 days each month has been used in children. There are no data on the relative efficacy of this approach compared with daily steroids in the treatment of pediatric IPF.

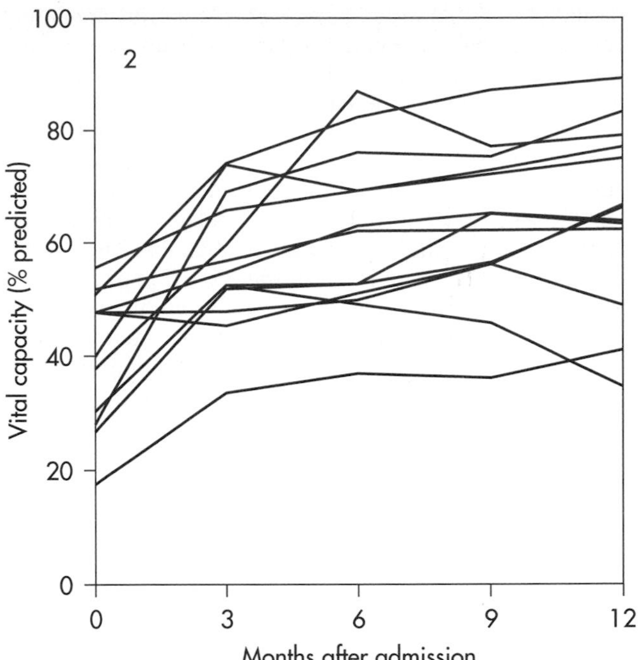

Fig. 49-5. Time course of vital capacity expressed as percentages of predicted norms in 13 children with fibrosing alveolitis during the first year after initial diagnosis and subsequent treatment. (From Steinkamp G et al: *Acta Pediatr Scand* 79:823-831, 1990.)

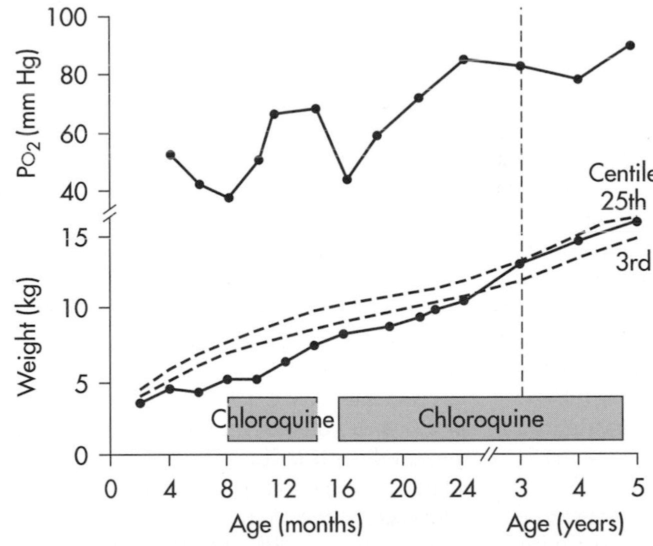

Fig. 49-6. Changes in weight and arterial oxygen tension in a child with DIP during a first and second course of treatment with chloroquine. Po_2, Partial pressure of oxygen. (From Springer C et al: *Arch Dis Child* 62:76-77, 1987.)

Chloroquine and hydroxychloroquine have been used in a small number of children with IPF, particularly when steroids were no longer efficacious. The responses have been variable but at times dramatic (Fig. 49-6). Hydroxychloroquine is preferred to chloroquine because it causes less retinopathy.[97] These drugs have multiple antiinflammatory effects, providing a rationale for their use in chronic inflammatory lung diseases such as IPF and LIP.[98] In some case reports, hydroxychloroquine has been initiated during steroid therapy and maintained after steroids were completely withdrawn.[89,91] The side effects are primarily ocular in nature and include corneal deposition of the drug and macular degeneration.[99,100] The former problem is dose related and improves with reduction or withdrawal of the medication. The latter is usually irreversible. The initial dosage is 10 mg/kg/day. As with steroids, a reduction in dose or a discontinuation of hydroxychloroquine can precipitate worsening interstitial pulmonary disease.[89,90] It is useful to think of any antiinflammatory medication therapy as suppressing an ongoing disease rather than curing the condition. Antiinflammatory therapy for IPF may be necessary for years.

When therapy fails in children who have a confirmed diagnosis of IPF but whose conditions slowly decline, lung transplant may be an option. IPF is one indication for single or double lung transplantation in adults.[101] Pediatric lung transplantation is occurring in increasing numbers with good outcomes in many children. There is currently too little experience with this therapeutic modality to know its efficacy for IPF relative to other chronic life-threatening pulmonary conditions in children.

Survival

The mortality rate for children with IPF, which includes both UIP and DIP, was 45 of 104 (43%) reported cases.[2,17-20,23,48] This contrasts with the mortality rate for children with all types of chronic ILD, which is estimated to be 11% (7 of 65 cases from two series).[2,12] IPF in children is therefore a greater life-threatening condition compared with other forms of pediatric ILD. To the extent that DIP was distinguished from UIP in published reports, 15 of 36 (42%) children with DIP died compared with 30 of 60 (44%) children with UIP or cryptogenic fibrosing alveolitis.[17-20,23,48,89] These numbers must be interpreted with caution because the number of years of follow-up for each study varies from 1 to 10 years. The similarity of mortality rates in children with DIP and IPF contrasts with those in the adult literature, which suggests that the mortality rate for DIP (4.8% for 5 years and 30.4% for 10 years) is lower than in UIP or IPF (57% at 5 years and 74% at 10 years).[31] In addition, the mortality rate for children younger than 1 year of age was 28 of 45 (62%) compared with children older than a year (13 of 53 [25%]), suggesting that age of onset influences the outcome more than the specific histologic diagnosis.[17-20,23,48,89] Children with the familial form of IPF appear to have a very high mortality rate; among 13 reported infants with familial IPF, 11 died despite therapy.[11,23,42,62]

CONCLUSION

IPF and lymphoid interstitial pneumonitis are rare but serious and often progressive lung diseases in children and require chronic antiinflammatory therapy. The etiologies, predictive indexes, and optimal therapies for these pediatric disorders are unknown. To advance knowledge in this area, large multicenter studies and an international registry are needed. Such a registry has been recommended by members of a National Heart, Lung, and Blood Institute workshop on IPF in adults.[102] A similarly organized effort has not been implemented for children with chronic ILD.

REFERENCES

1. Fernald GW, Denny FW, Fairclough DL, Helms RW, Volberg FM: Chronic lung disease in children referred to a teaching hospital, *Pediatr Pulmonol* 2:27-34, 1986.
2. Fan LL, Mullen ALW, Brugman SM, Inscore SC, Parks DP, White CW: Clinical spectrum in chronic interstitial lung disease in children, *J Pediatr* 121:867-872, 1987.
3. Stagno S, Brasfield DM, Brown MB, Cassell GH, Pifer LL, Whitley RJ, Tiller RE: Infant pneumonitis associated with cytomegalovirus, *Chlamydia, Pneumocystic,* and *Ureaplasma:* a prospective study, *Pediatrics* 68:322-329, 1981.
4. Liebow AA: Definition and classification of interstitial pneumonias in human pathology, *Acta Paediatr* 8:1-33, 1975.
5. Patchefsky AS, Israel HL, Hoch WS, Gordon G: Desquamative interstitial pneumonia: relationship to interstitial fibrosis, *Thorax* 28:680-693, 1973.
6. Scadding JG, Hinson KFW: Diffuse fibrosing alveolitis (diffuse interstitial fibrosis of the lungs): correlation of histology at biopsy with prognosis, *Thorax* 22:291-304, 1967.
7. Fishman AP: UIP, DIP, and all that, *N Engl J Med* 298(15):843-845, 1978 (editorial).
8. Winterbauer RH, Hammar SP, Hallman KO, Hayes JE, Pardee NE, Morgan EH, Allen JD, Moores KD, Bush W, Walker JH: Diffuse interstitial pneumonitis: clinicopathologic correlations in 20 patients treated with prednisone/azathioprine, *Am J Med* 65:661-672, 1978.

Prevalence

9. Respiratory Diseases Task Force: Report on problems, research, approaches, and needs, DHEW Pub No 76-432, *Am J Med* 1972.
10. Schwartz MI: Idiopathic pulmonary fibrosis, *West J Med* 149:199-203, 1988.
11. Commission on Professional and Hospital Activities: *The hospital record study,* Ambler, Penn, 1977, IMS American.
12. Diaz RP, Bowman CM: Childhood interstitial lung disease, *Semin Respir Med* 11:253-268, 1990.
13. Centers for Disease Control: Revision of the case definition of AIDS for national reporting: United States, *Ann Intern Med* 103:402-403, 1985.
14. Rubinstein A, Morecki R, Silverman B, Charytan M, Krieger BZ, Andiman W, Ziprkowski MN, Goldman H: Pulmonary disease in children with acquired immune deficiency syndrome and AIDS-related complex, *J Pediatr* 108:498-503, 1986.
15. Pahwa S, Kaplan M, Fikrig S, Pahwa R, Sarngadharan MG, Popvic M, Gallo RC: Spectrum of human T-cell lymphotropic virus type III infection in children, *JAMA* 255:2296-2305, 1986.
16. Pitt J: Lymphotic interstitial pneumonia, *Pediatr Clin North Am* 38:89-94, 1991.
17. Hewitt CJ, Hull D, Keeling JW: Fibrosing alveolitis in infancy and childhood, *Arch Dis Child* 52:22-37, 1977.
18. Stillwell PC, Norris DG, O'Connell EJ, Rosenow EC, Weiland LH, Harrison EG: Desquamative interstitial pneumonitis in children, *Chest* 77:165-171, 1980.
19. Steinkamp G, Muller KM, Schirg E, Von Der Hardt H: Fibrosing alveolitis in childhood, *Acta Paediatr Scand* 79:823-831, 1990.
20. Chetty A, Bhuyan UN, Mitra DK, Roy S, Deoarari A: Cryptogenic fibrosing alveolitis in children, *Ann Allergy* 58:336-340, 1987.
21. Turner-Warwick M, Burrows B, Johnson A: Cryptogenic fibrosing alveolitis: clinical features and their influence on survival, *Thorax* 35:171-180, 1980.
22. Farrell PM, Gilbert EF, Zimmerman JJ, Warner TF, Saari TN: Familial lung disease associated with proliferation and desquamation of type II pneumonocytes, *Am J Dis Child* 140:262-266, 1986.
23. Tal A, Maor E, Bar-Aiz J, Gorodischer R: Fatal desquamative interstitial pneumonia in three infant siblings, *J Pediatr* 104:873-876, 1984.
24. Solliday NH, Williams JA, Gaensler EA, Coutu RE, Carrington CB: Familial chronic interstitial pneumonia, *Am Rev Respir Dis* 108:193-204, 1973.
25. O'Brodovich HM, Moser MM: Familial lymphoid interstitial pneumonia: a long-term follow-up, *Pediatrics* 65:523-528, 1980.
26. Swaye P, Van Ordstrand HS, McCormack LJ, Wolpaw SE: Familial Hamman-Rich syndrome, *Dis Chest* 55:7-12, 1969.
27. Thurlbeck WM, Fleetham JA: Usual interstitial pneumonia (cryptogenic or idiopathic fibrosing alveolitis). In Chernick V, Kendig EL, eds: *Kendig's disorders of the respiratory tract in children,* Philadelphia, 1990, WB Saunders, pp 480-484.

Disease Mechanisms and Histopathology

28. Katz BZ, Berkman AB, Shapiro ED: Serologic evidence of active Epstein-Barr virus infection in Epstein-Barr virus–associated lymphoproliferative disorders of children with acquired immunodeficiency syndrome, *J Pediatr* 120:228-232, 1992.
29. Dreisin RB, Schwarz MI, Theofilopoulos AN, Stanford RE: Circulating immune complexes in the idiopathic interstitial pneumonias, *N Engl J Med* 298:353-357, 1978.
30. Schwarz MI, Dreisin RB, Pratt DS, Stanford RE: Immunofluorescent patterns in the idiopathic interstitial pneumonias, *J Clin Lab Med* 91:929-938, 1978.
31. Carrington CB, Gaensler EA, Coutu RE, Fitzgerald MX, Gupta RG: Natural history and treated course of usual and desquamative interstitial pneumonia, *N Engl J Med* 298:801-809, 1978.
32. Schroeder SA, Shannon DC, Mark EJ: Cellular interstitial pneumonitis in infants: a clinicopathologic study, *Chest* 101:1065-1069, 1992.
33. BAL Cooperative Group Steering Committee: Bronchoalveolar lavage constituents in healthy individuals, idiopathic pulmonary fibrosis and selected comparison groups, *Am Rev Respir Dis* 141:S169-S201, 1990.
34. Turner-Warwick M, Haslam PL: The value of serial bronchoalveolar lavages in assessing the clinical progress of patients with cryptogenic fibrosing alveolitis, *Am Rev Respir Dis* 135:26-34, 1987.
35. Hunninghake GW, Gade JE, Lawley JJ, Crystal RG: Mechanism of neutrophil accumulation in the lungs of patients with idiopathic pulmonary fibrosis, *J Clin Invest* 68:259-269, 1981.
36. Rudd RM, Haslam PL, Turner-Warwick M: Cryptogenic fibrosing alveolitis: relationships of pulmonary physiology and bronchoalveolar lavage to response to treatment and prognosis, *Am Rev Respir Dis* 124:1-8, 1981.
37. Haslam PL, Turton CW, Heard B, Lukoszek A, Collins JV, Salsbury AJ, Turner-Warwick M: Bronchoalveolar lavage in pulmonary fibrosis: comparison of cells obtained with lung biopsy and clinical features, *Thorax* 35(1):9-18, 1980.
38. Clement A, Chadelat K, Masliah J, Housset B, Sardet A, Grimfeld A, Tournier G: A controlled study of oxygen metabolite release by alveolar macrophages from children with interstitial lung disease, *Am Rev Respir Dis* 136:1424-1428, 1987.
39. Rochemonteix-Galve B, Dayer JM, Junod AF: Fibroblast-alveolar cell interactions in sarcoidosis and idiopathic pulmonary fibrosis: evidence for stimulatory and inhibitory cytokine production by alveolar cells, *Eur Respir J* 3:653-664, 1990.
40. O'Donnell K, Brendan K, Cantin A, Crystal RG: Pharmacologic suppression of the neutrophil component of the alveolitis in idiopathic pulmonary fibrosis, *Am Rev Respir Dis* 136:288-292, 1987.
41. Bitterman PB, Rennard SI, Hunninghake GW, Crystal RG: Human alveolar macrophage growth factor for fibroblasts, regulation, and partial characterization, *J Clin Invest* 70:806-822, 1982.
42. Martinenet Y, Rom WN, Grotendorst GR, Martin GR, Crystal RG: Exaggerated spontaneous release of platelet-derived growth factor by alveolar macrophages from patients with idiopathic pulmonary fibrosis, *N Engl J Med* 317:202-209, 1987.
43. Bjermer L, Lundgren R, Hallgren R: Hyaluronan and type III procollagen peptide concentrations in bronchoalveolar lavage fluid in idiopathic pulmonary fibrosis, *Thorax* 44:126-131, 1989.
44. Seyer JM, Hutcheson ET, Kang AH: Collagen polymorphism in idiopathic chronic pulmonary fibrosis, *J Clin Invest* 57:1498-1507, 1976.
45. Crouch E: Pathology of pulmonary fibrosis, *Am J Physiol* 259(4):L159-L184, 1990.
46. Zapletal A, Houstek J, Samanek M, Copova M, Paul T: Lung function in children and adolescents with idiopathic interstitial pulmonary fibrosis, *Pediatr Pulmonol* 1:154-166, 1985.
47. Teirstein AS, Rosen MJ: Lymphocytic interstitial pneumonia, *Clin Chest Med* 9(3):467-471, 1988.

Clinical Manifestations

48. Kerem E, Bentur L, England S, Reisman J, O'Brodovich H, Bryan AC, Levison H: Sequential pulmonary function measurements during treatment of infantile chronic interstitial pneumonitis, *J Pediatr* 116:61-67, 1990.
49. Davis GS: Idiopathic pulmonary fibrosis: current concepts and management. In Simmons DH, ed: *Current pulmonology,* St Louis, 1993, Mosby, pp 321-355.
50. King TE Jr: Idiopathic pulmonary fibrosis. In Schwarz MI, King TE Jr, eds: *Interstitial lung disease,* St Louis, 1993, Mosby, pp 367-404.
51. Epler GR, McLeod TC, Gaensler EA, Mikeus JP, Carrington CB: Normal chest roentgenograms in chronic diffuse infiltrative lung disease, *N Engl J Med* 298:934-939, 1978.
52. Vlagopoulos B, Chung HT, Fitzmaurice FM, Campbell JC, Villacorte GV: Desquamative interstitial pneumonia associated with granulomatous lymphadenopathy, *Chest* 72:780-781, 1977.
53. Crystal RG, Fulmer JD, Roberts WC, Moss ML, Line BR, Reynolds HY: Idiopathic pulmonary fibrosis: clinical, histologic, radiographic, physiologic, scintigraphic, cytologic, and biochemical aspects, *Ann Intern Med* 85:769-788, 1976.
54. Crystal RG, Gadek JE, Ferrans VJ, Fulmer JD, Line BR, Hunninghake GW: Interstitial lung disease: current concepts of pathogenesis, staging and therapy, *Am J Med* 70:542-568, 1981.
55. Staples CA, Müller NL, Vedal S, Abboud R, Ostrow D, Miller RR: Usual interstitial pneumonia: correlation of CT with clinical, functional, and radiologic findings, *Radiology* 162:377-381, 1987.
56. Müller NL, Ostrow DN: High-resolution computed tomography of chronic interstitial lung disease, *Clin Chest Med* 12:97-114, 1991.
57. Müller NL, Miller RR, Webb WR, Evans KG, Ostrow DN: Fibrosing alveolitis: CT-pathologic correlation, *Radiology* 160:585-588, 1986.
58. Englert M, Yernault JC, de Coster A, Clumeck N: Diffusing properties and elastic properties in interstitial diseases of the lung, *Prog Respir Res* 8:177-185, 1975.
59. Gaulteri CI, Chaussain M, Boule M, Buvry A, Allaire Y, Perret L, Girard F: Lung function in interstitial lung diseases in children, *Bull Eur Physiopathol Respir* 16:57-66, 1980.
60. Fulmer JD: An introduction to the interstitial lung diseases, *Clin Chest Med* 3(3):457-473, 1982.
61. Stack BHR, Choo-Kang YFJ, Heard BE: The prognosis of cryptogenic fibrosing alveolitis, *Thorax* 27:535-542, 1972.
62. Strumpf IJ, Feld MK, Cornelius MJ, Keogh BA, Crystal RG: Safety of fiberoptic bronchoalveolar lavage in evaluation of interstitial lung disease, *Chest* 80(3):268-271, 1981.
63. Perez-Padilla R, West R, Lertzman M, Kryger MH: Breathing during sleep in patients with interstitial lung disease, *Am Rev Respir Dis* 132:224-229, 1985.
64. Hawrylkiewicz I, Izadebska-Makosa Z, Grebska E, Zielinski J: Pulmonary haemodynamics at rest and on exercise in patients with idiopathic pulmonary fibrosis, *Bull Eur Physiopathol Respir* 18(3):403-410, 1982.
65. Campbell EJ, Harris B, Avioli LV: Idiopathic pulmonary fibrosis, *Arch Intern Med* 141:771-774, 1981.
66. Reeves JT, Groves BM, Turkevich D: The case for treatment of selected patients with primary pulmonary hypertension, *Am Rev Respir Dis* 134:342-346, 1986.
67. Haslam PL, Thompson B, Mohammed I, Townsend PJ, Hodson ME, Holborow EJ, Turner-Warwick M: Circulating immune complexes in patients with cryptogenic fibrosing alveolitis, *Clin Exp Immunol* 37(3):381-390, 1979.
68. Franchi LM, Chin TW, Nussbaum E, Riker J, Robert M, Talbert WM: Familial pulmonary nodular lymphoid hyperplasia, *J Pediatr* 121:89-92, 1992.

Diagnosis and Staging

69. Chollet S, Soler P, Dournovo P, Richard MS, Forrans VJ, Basset F: Diagnosis of pulmonary histiocytosis X by immunodetection of Langerhans cells in bronchoalveolar lavage fluid, *Am J Pathol* 115:225-232, 1984.
70. Martin RJ, Coalson JJ, Rogers RM, Horton FO, Manous LE: Pulmonary alveolar proteinosis: the diagnosis by segmental lavage, *Am Rev Respir Dis* 121:819-825, 1980.
71. Gaensler EA, Carrington CB: Open biopsy for chronic diffuse infiltrative lung disease: clinical, roentgenographic, and physiological correlations in 502 patients, *Ann Thorac Surg* 30:411-425, 1980.
72. Prober CG, Whyte H, Smith CR: Open lung biopsy in immunocompromised children with pulmonary infiltrates, *Am J Dis Child* 138:60-63, 1984.
73. Leijala M, Louhimo I, Lindfors EL: Open lung biopsy in children with diffuse lung disease, *Acta Paediatr Scand* 71:717-720, 1982.
74. Whitehead B, Scott JP, Helms P, Malone M, Macrae D, Higenbottam TW, Smyth RL, Wallwork J, Elliott M, de Leval M: Technique and use of transbronchial biopsy in children and adolescents, *Pediatr Pulmonol* 12:240-246, 1992.

75. Fitzpatrick SB, Stokes DC, Marsh B, Wang K: Transbronchial lung biopsy in pediatric and adolescent patients, *Am J Dis Child* 139:46-49, 1985.
76. Wall CP, Gaensler EA, Carrington CB, Hayes JA: Comparison of transbronchial and open biopsies in chronic infiltrative lung diseases, *Am Rev Respir Dis* 123:280-285, 1981.
77. Wright PH, Heard BE, Steel SJ, Turner-Warwick M: Cryptogenic fibrosing alveolitis: assessment by graded trephine lung biopsy histology compared with clinical, radiographic, and physiological features, *Br J Dis Chest* 75:61-70, 1981.
78. Cherniack RM, Colby TV, Flint A, Thurlbeck WM, Waldron J, Ackerson L, King TE, BAL Cooperative Group Steering Committee: Quantitative assessment of lung pathology in idiopathic pulmonary fibrosis, *Am Rev Respir Dis* 144:892-900, 1991.
79. Waters LC, King TE, Schwarz MI, Waldron JA, Stanford RE, Cherniack RM: A clinical, radiographic, and physiologic scoring system for the longitudinal assessment of patients with idiopathic pulmonary fibrosis, *Am Rev Respir Dis* 133:97-103, 1986.
80. Keogh BA, Lakatos E, Price D, Crystal RG: Importance of the lower respiratory tract in oxygen transfer: exercise testing in patients with interstitial and destructive lung disease, *Am Rev Respir Dis* 129(suppl):S76-S80, 1984.
81. Müller NL, Staples CA, Miller RR, Vedal S, Thurlbeck WM, Ostrow DN: Disease activity in idiopathic pulmonary fibrosis: CT and pathologic correlation, *Radiology* 165:731-734, 1987.
82. Ronchetti R, Villani A, Dotta A, Signoretti F, Rognone F, Manganaro M, Ricci R, Rota R, Midulla F: Pediatric bronchoalveolar lavage: reference values, *Am Rev Respir Dis* 145:556A, 1992 (abstract).
83. Midulla F, Villani A, Merolla R, Bjermer L, Sandstrom T, Ronchetti R: Bronchoalveolar lavage studies in children without parenchymal lung disease: cellular constituents and protein levels, *Pediatr Pumonol* 20(2):112-118, 1995.
84. Watters LC, Schwarz MI, Cherniack RM, Waldron JA, Dunn TL, Stanford RE, King TE: Idiopathic pulmonary fibrosis: pretreatment bronchoalveolar lavage cellular constituents and their relationship with lung histopathology and clinical response to therapy, *Am Rev Respir Dis* 135:696-704, 1987.
85. Robinson PC, Watters LC, King TE, Mason RJ: Idiopathic pulmonary fibrosis: abnormalities in bronchoalveolar lavage fluid phospholipids, *Am Rev Respir Dis* 137:585-591, 1988.
86. McCormack FX, King TE, Voelker DR, Robinson PC, Mason RJ: Idiopathic pulmonary fibrosis: abnormalities in the bronchoalveolar lavage content of surfactant protein A, *Am Rev Respir Dis* 144:160-166, 1991.
87. Low RB, Giancola MS, King TE Jr, Chapitis J, Vacek P, Davis GS: Serum and bronchoalveolar lavage of N-terminal type III procollagen peptides in idiopathic pulmonary fibrosis, *Am Rev Respir Dis* 146:701-706, 1992.
88. de Cremous H, Bernaudin JF, Laurent P, Brochard P, Bignon J: Interactions between cigarette smoking and the natural history of idiopathic pulmonary fibrosis, *Chest* 98(1):71-76, 1990.
89. Leahy F, Pasterkamp H, Tal A: Desquamative interstitial pneumonia responsive to chloroquine, *Clin Pediatr* 24:230-232, 1985.
90. Springer C, Maayan C, Katzir Z, Ariel I, Godfrey S: Chloroquine treatment in desquamative interstitial pneumonia, *Arch Dis Child* 62:76-77, 1987.
91. Waters KA, Bale P, Isaacs D, Mellis C: Successful chloroquine therapy in a child with lymphoid interstitial pneumonitis, *J Pediatr* 119:989-991, 1991.
92. Howatt WF, Heidelberger KP, LeGlovan DP, Schnitzer B: Desquamative interstitial pneumonia, *Am J Dis Child* 126:346-348, 1973.
93. Barnes SE, Godfrey S, Millward-Sadler GH, Roberton NRC: Desquamative fibrosing alveolitis unresponsive to steroid or cytotoxic therapy, *Arch Dis Child* 50:324-327, 1975.
94. Wheeler WB, Kurachek SC, Lobas JG, Einzig MJ: Acute hypoxemic respiratory failure caused by *Chlamydia trachomatis* and diagnosed by flexible bronchoscopy, *Am Rev Respir Dis* 142:471-473, 1990.
95. Miller JJ: Prolonged use of large intravenous steroid pulses in the rheumatic diseases of children, *Pediatrics* 65:989-994, 1980.
96. Keogh BA, Bernardo J, Hunninghake GW, Line BR, Price DL, Crystal RG: Effect of intermittent high dose parenteral corticosteroids on the alveolitis of idiopathic pulmonary fibrosis, *Am Rev Respir Dis* 127:18-22, 1983.
97. Maksymowich W, Russel AS: Antimalarials in rheumatology: efficacy and safety, *Semin Arthritis Rheum* 16:206-221, 1987.
98. Salmeron G, Lipsky PE: Immunosuppressive potential of antimalarials, *Am J Med* 75:S19-S24, 1983.
99. Laaksonen AL, Koskiahde V, Juva K: Dosage of antimalarial drugs for children with juvenile rheumatoid arthritis and systemic lupus erythematosus, *Scand J Rheumatol* 3:103-108, 1974.
100. Johnson MW, Vine AK: Hydroxychloroquine therapy in massive total doses without retinopathy, *Am J Ophthalmol* 104:139-144, 1987.
101. Grossman RF, Frost A, Zamel N, Patterson GA, Cooper JD, Myron PR, Dear CL, Maurer J: Results of single-lung transplantation for bilateral pulmonary fibrosis, *N Engl J Med* 322:727-733, 1990.

Conclusion

102. Cherniack RM, Crystal RG, Kalica AR: NHLBI Workshop summary: current concepts in IPF—a road map for the future, *Am Rev Respir Dis* 143:680-683, 1991.

CHAPTER 50

Eosinophilic Lung Disorders and Hypersensitivity Pneumonitis

John L. Carroll and Laura M. Sterni

PULMONARY INFILTRATES WITH EOSINOPHILIA

For the clinical evaluation of a child with pulmonary infiltrates, peripheral blood eosinophilia can be a valuable diagnostic guide. Eosinophilia focuses the differential diagnosis on several specific respiratory diseases grouped under the term *pulmonary infiltrates with eosinophilia (PIE).* PIE was first described by Crofton et al in 1952 at a time when specific etiologies for the conditions included in the syndrome were not well defined. In 1981, knowledge of PIE or conditions leading to PIE had progressed to the point that Schatz et al[1,2] were able to propose a new classification based on an etiology or on clearly definable clinical syndromes. A modified version of this classification is shown in Table 50-1.

The terms *pulmonary eosinophilia, eosinophilic pneumonia,* and *pulmonary infiltrates with eosinophilia*should not be used interchangeably.[2] Although in most of the PIE illnesses,

Table 50-1 Clinical Classification of PIE

GROUP	TYPE OF ILLNESS	EXAMPLES
Illnesses in which PIE is a major component	Allergic bronchopulmonary aspergillosis	—
	Chronic eosinophilic pneumonia	—
	Medication reaction	Reactions to nitrofurantoin, nonsteroidal antiinflammatory drugs, and others
	Hypereosinophilic syndrome	—
	Allergic bronchopulmonary helminthiasis	Tropical pulmonary eosinophilia
	Polyarteritis nodosa	Churg-Strauss syndrome
	Toxic oil poisoning	Oil-associated pneumonic paralytic eosinophilic syndrome
Illnesses in which PIE occurs infrequently and is a minor component	Infection	Bacterial (tuberculosis, brucellosis), fungal (histoplasmosis coccidiomycosis), chlamydial, and viral infection
	Neoplasm	Hodgkin's disease and others
	Immunologic disorders	Rheumatoid lung disease, sarcoidosis
PIE without features of the other groups	Unknown	—

Modified from Schatz M et al: *Arch Intern Med* 142:1515-1519, 1982; and Schatz M et al: *Med Clin North Am* 65:1055-1071, 1981.

the number of eosinophils is elevated in the blood and eosinophils are seen in the pulmonary lesions, there are respiratory diseases, such as pulmonary eosinophilic granuloma, in which peripheral blood eosinophilia is absent.[2] The old term *Löffler's syndrome* (migratory, transient pulmonary infiltrates and eosinophilia with minimal or no respiratory symptoms) is no longer used because most of these patients probably had undiagnosed allergic bronchopulmonary helminthiasis (ABPH), medication reactions, or allergic bronchopulmonary aspergillosis (ABPA). Last, asthma is not included in the PIE classification because many patients previously thought to have eosinophilia with asthma probably had ABPA and because irreversible wheezing ("asthma") may occur in virtually any of the diseases included under the PIE syndrome.[3] Eosinophilia is associated with a variety of lung diseases (see Chapters 30, 46, 47, and 51).

Eosinophils in the lung are thought to have two major beneficial functions: (1) modulating mast cell reactions by degrading mast cell mediators and phagocytosing mast cell granules and immunoglobulin E (IgE) antigen complexes and (2) causing antibody- or complement-dependent damage to the larval to tissue stages of helminths by releasing several toxic substances.[1] However, these "beneficial" effects can also cause the severe mucosal, parenchymal, and interstitial pulmonary damage associated with states of hypereosinophilia.[1,4] For example, major basic protein released by the eosinophil is helminthotoxic but also induces dose-dependent epithelial damage in tracheal explants and can kill several cell lines in tissue culture.[2] Damage caused by major basic protein may be augmented by numerous other eosinophil products. Glucocorticoids are important in the therapy of many PIE illnesses, perhaps partly because of their ability to induce eosinopenia. A detailed discussion of the eosinophil and its effects on the lung is found in Chapter 6.

Chronic Eosinophilic Pneumonia

Chronic eosinophilic pneumonia is rare in children, usually occurring in women between 20 and 30 years of age[2,4]; a case of biopsy-confirmed chronic eosinophilic pneumonia occurring in a 1-year-old boy has been reported.[5] Common clinical features are cough, malaise, dyspnea, night sweats, fever, and weight loss. Asthma, usually of recent onset, and hemoptysis may be present.[2] Common pulmonary function findings include a decreased diffusing capacity and a pattern of restrictive lung disease. Peripheral nonlobar, nonsegmental infiltrates with ill-defined margins are characteristic of the chest radiograph in these patients,[2] although the radiograph's appearance may be normal.[6] The characteristic radiographic picture has been described as "the photographic negative of pulmonary edema."[7,8] Other unique features are the propensity of the infiltrates to have a similar size, shape, and location on chest radiograph and subsequent relapses.[7] Laboratory findings include anemia, a markedly elevated erythrocyte sedimentation rate, and peripheral blood eosinophilia, although the eosinophilia may be absent in up to a third of cases.[2,7] Lung biopsy reveals intraalveolar and interstitial infiltration with mainly eosinophils and macrophages and some plasma cells and lymphocytes.[2,4] The etiology and immunopathogenesis are unknown. A type I immune mechanism (IgE mediated) has been suggested, but results from several studies are conflicting.[9-11] The clinical features are so characteristic in adults that a trial of corticosteroid therapy can be undertaken without confirmation of the diagnosis by lung biopsy.[2] However, because steroid therapy may be needed for years in some cases, biopsy may be useful for confirmation. Steroid therapy usually results in rapid improvement, and the dose can be tapered when the chest radiograph becomes normal.[2] Corticosteroid therapy can eventually be discontinued in most patients, although years of therapy may be required.[2] In the 1-year-old patient, prednisone was successfully discontinued 1 year after the initial diagnosis.[5]

Medication Reactions

A variety of medications can cause the PIE syndrome (Box 50-1). The clinical laboratory features of pulmonary medication reactions are discussed in Chapter 18. Nitrofurantoin-induced PIE produces a well-defined and studied syndrome. Histologic examination of the lung after nitrofurantoin administration reveals histiocytic and eosinophilic infiltrates and proteinaceous fluid within the alveolar spaces. Interstitial inflammation, vasculitis, and granuloma formation have also been seen. The pathologic findings in PIE caused by other medications are largely unknown.[2] The immunopathogenesis of medication-induced PIE syndrome is unknown for most medications. Type IV (cell-mediated) immunologic reactions may be the mechanism in cases of acute reaction to nitrofurantoin in the lung.[2] The diagnosis depends on a high index of suspicion, and one of the best diagnostic tools is a trial withdrawal of the potentially responsible medication.[2] Discontin-

BOX 50-1
Medications Associated with Eosinophilia and Pulmonary Infiltrates

Nitrofurantoin
Sulfonamides
Penicillin
Aspirin
Mephenesin
Imipramine
Methylphenidate
p-Aminosalicylic acid and aminosalicylic acid
Cromolyn
Beclomethasone
Tetracycline
Carbamazepine
Chlorpromazine
Chlorpropamide

Modified from Schatz M et al: *Med Clin North Am* 65:1055-1071, 1981.

uation is also the most effective therapy, although steroids may be necessary for the treatment of severe symptoms. The prognosis is excellent.

Recently, a pulmonary syndrome was described in four of eight 5- to 23-year-old patients who had β-thalassemia major and were receiving intravenous deferoxamine.[12] Respiratory symptoms and signs occurred suddenly and included cough, tachypnea, hypoxemia, a restrictive pattern on pulmonary function tests, and diffuse interstitial infiltrates on chest radiographs.[12] Lung biopsy in one patient revealed interstitial fibrosis and inflammatory infiltrates consisting of eosinophils, lymphocytes, and mast cells. Peripheral blood eosinophil counts were not reported.[12]

Hypereosinophilic Syndrome and Eosinophilic Leukemia

Hypereosinophilic syndrome is characterized by a peripheral blood eosinophilia (≥1500 eosinophils/mm^3) that persists longer than 6 months, a lack of evidence for other causes of eosinophilia, and evidence of eosinophilic infiltration of the organs. The clinical presentation is related to the involved organ systems and can include congestive heart failure, endocarditis, a new heart murmur, hepatosplenomegaly, central nervous system abnormalities, diarrhea, rashes, anemia, fever, and weight loss. Pulmonary involvement may present as a nonproductive cough, interstitial infiltrates on the chest radiograph, and pleural effusion.[13,14] It is mainly a disease of middle-aged men but has been reported in children as young as 1 year of age.[13,15] Respiratory symptoms in 19 cases of childhood hypereosinophilic syndrome consisted of cough, pulmonary infiltrates, dyspnea, pleural effusion, and pulmonary edema.[15] Postmortem pulmonary findings vary, but eosinophilic lung infiltration is a common feature. Cardiovascular involvement is a prominent feature and is responsible for the high morbidity and mortality rates.[13-15] Treatment regimens designed to lower eosinophil counts include the administration of corticosteroids, cytotoxic agents, or both; these medications have improved the prognosis.[13,15]

Neither Chusid et al[13] nor Alfaham et al[15] clearly distinguished idiopathic hypereosinophilic syndrome from eosinophilic leukemia; 54% of the patients of Chusid et al and 42% of the patients of Alfaham et al showed markers or signs suggestive of leukemia. Both these groups considered hypereosinophilic syndrome to be a continuum with mild disease at one end and eosinophilic leukemia at the other. Eosinophilic gastroenteritis may also be a part of this spectrum.[15] A total of 9 of 14 cases of hypereosinophilia associated with acute lymphoblastic leukemia in children ranging from 2 to 17 years of age exhibited pulmonary infiltrates on chest radiographs.[16] A 4-year-old boy with fever, cough, tachypnea, nodular pulmonary opacities on chest radiography, and extreme eosinophilia (90% of white blood cells) has been reported.[17] Although no cause for the eosinophilia could be initially found (including no evidence of malignancy on bone marrow examination), within 6 months the full picture of lymphosarcoma with bone marrow involvement emerged. Given the heterogeneity of the hypereosinophilic syndromes, it is not surprising that the immunopathogenesis is unclear and that the response to steroid and cytotoxic therapy varies.

Eosinophilia and Nonparasitic Infection

In 1941, Botsztejn[18] described a syndrome of interstitial pneumonia with eosinophilia occurring in very young infants; it was termed *interstitial pertussoid eosinophilic pneumonia.* During the 1960s and 1970s, there were more reports of young infants 3 weeks to 4 months of age who had staccato dry cough, tachypnea, minimal or no fever, peripheral eosinophilia (as high as 4000 cells/mm^3), elevated IgG and IgM levels, and bilateral interstitial infiltrates on chest radiographs.[19,20] In 1976 and 1977, researchers[21-23] described the clinical features of a distinctive pneumonia syndrome in infants infected with *Chlamydia trachomatis;* this picture was essentially identical to that of pertussoid eosinophilic pneumonia. Since then, hundreds of cases have been reported, and chlamydial pneumonia is now a well-characterized syndrome[24] (see Chapter 45). Although original reports indicated peripheral blood eosinophil counts in the thousands per cubic millimeter, the mean absolute count in infants with chlamydial pneumonia is about 870 cells/mm^3.[24] Although eosinophilia is not a characteristic of bronchiolitis caused by respiratory syncytial virus, a recent report suggests that the inflammatory mediators released by eosinophils (eosinophil cationic protein) may be important in the pathogenesis of pulmonary damage caused by this virus.[25] Peripheral eosinophilia or pulmonary eosinophilic infiltration may be a minor feature of a variety of other infections (see Table 50-1).

Allergic Bronchopulmonary Helminthiasis

Immunologic hyperresponsiveness to parasitic infection leading to PIE syndrome has been termed *allergic bronchopulmonary helminthiasis.*[26] In these syndromes, some of the manifestations are due directly to infection with the parasite, whereas others are due to the immunologic hyperresponsiveness and the resulting accumulation of eosinophils in the lung. ABPH may be caused by many parasitic infections, including those of the *Ascaris, Toxocara,* and *Strongyloides* species.[2] In fact, *Ascaris* infestation was likely the etiology in many of the original cases of Löffler's syndrome.[4] Toxocariasis is relatively common in children (~5% to 15% prevalence of seropositivity in Europe and the United States) and is associated with cough, wheezing, pneumonia, pharyngitis, abdominal pain, and other systemic symptoms.[27] About 73% of children with elevated *Toxocara* titers have eosinophilia.[27] Parasitic respiratory diseases are discussed in depth in Chapter 47.

One of the most common and severe ABPH syndromes is caused by infestation by the filariae *Wuchereria bancrofti* and *Brugia malayi* and is called *tropical pulmonary eosinophilia syndrome*. This eosinophilia is common in men during the third and fourth decades of life and begins with extreme peripheral blood eosinophilia (>3000 cells/mm^3) accompanied by minimal symptoms.[26] Progression to a predominately nocturnal cough and wheeze, dyspnea, chest pain, fatigue, low-grade fever, and weight loss soon follows.[26] Chest radiographs show mottled opacities or diffuse 1- to 3-mm interstitial lesions in the middle and basilar regions without hilar adenopathy or pleural effusion.[26] A high IgE level (>2000 ng/ml) may be seen.[2] Lung biopsy reveals infiltration with eosinophils and histiocytes; eosinophils predominate early, and histiocytes predominate later. Progressive fibrosis occurs within 6 months after symptoms begin.[26] Pulmonary function tests reveal a pattern of restrictive lung disease in most patients and an abnormal diffusing capacity.[2,26] Available information on the pathogenesis indicates that adult parasites living in the lymphatic system release microfilariae into the circulation, where they are opsonized with antifilarial antibody and trapped in the pulmonary vascular bed. There the microfilariae degenerate, causing a marked eosinophilic inflammatory reaction involving the release of damaging granule proteins (e.g., major basic protein, eosinophil cationic protein, eosinophil-derived neurotoxin), which are thought to play a major role in the lung injury that ensues.[26] The treatment of tropical pulmonary eosinophilia with diethylcarbamazine is usually but not always effective.[26]

Pulmonary Vasculitis

In 1939, Rackemann and Greene[28] described a subset of patients with polyarteritis nodosa who also had allergic rhinitis, asthma, episodes of pneumonia, and blood eosinophilia.[29] The histopathology of this syndrome was defined by Churg and Strauss in 1951, and since then it has been called *allergic granulomatous angiitis* or *Churg-Strauss syndrome*.[29] Churg-Strauss syndrome is still considered a variant of polyarteritis nodosa set apart from other such syndromes by the prominent pulmonary involvement. The allergic rhinitis, reactive airway disease, pulmonary infiltrates, and marked eosinophilia may precede the development of systemic vasculitis by many years.[30] In the prodromal stage, the histologic picture is one of eosinophilic infiltration; later, granulomas and necrotizing vasculitis involving primarily the small arteries and veins predominate.[28,30] The immunopathogenesis of Churg-Strauss syndrome is unknown. Treatment usually involves high-dose corticosteroids and cytotoxic agents.[2,28]

As classically described, Churg-Strauss syndrome usually begins in the third decade of life, proceeding to vasculitis by the end of the fourth decade.[28] However, it has been described in a 16-year-old boy[30] and a 9-year-old girl with interstitial pneumonia, systemic eosinophilic vasculitis, and marked eosinophilia.[31] Lung biopsy from the latter patient showed interstitial infiltrates containing eosinophils, necrotizing vasculitis, and deposition of extracellular major basic protein in alveolar hyaline membranes.[31] Although the authors were reluctant to diagnose this patient as having Churg-Strauss syndrome (mainly because of her young age, her gender, and the absence of severe asthma), the clinical and pathologic features were very similar.[31]

ABPA and Pulmonary Aspergillosis

Peripheral blood eosinophilia and eosinophilic pulmonary infiltrates are common during exacerbations of ABPA[32] (see Chapter 51). Of special note is the report of a previously healthy 11-year-old boy with "acute eosinophilic pneumonia" characterized by fever, cough, shortness of breath, bilateral diffuse interstitial infiltrates on the chest radiograph, and peripheral blood eosinophilia (absolute count, 1224 cells/mm^3).[33] The white blood cell count from bronchoalveolar lavage fluid showed 27% eosinophils but did not show *Aspergillus fumigatus* fungal forms. Precipitating antibodies and skin tests for *A. fumigatus* were negative. After improvement on corticosteroids, the symptoms recurred, leading to respiratory failure and death from invasive aspergillosis and *Pseudomonas cepacia sepsis*.[33] It should be pointed out that invasive pulmonary aspergillosis is extremely rare in immunocompetent children; this case is discussed here because of the initial (false) clinical presentation of acute eosinophilic pneumonia.

Oil-Associated Pneumonic Paralytic Eosinophilic Syndrome

In 1981, an outbreak of a previously unknown syndrome began in Madrid; it consisted of cough, shortness of breath, fever, headaches, severe neuromuscular symptoms, and eosinophilia.[34,35] Chest radiographs showed a diffuse interstitial pattern of infiltrates, and hypoxemia was characteristic. Within 6 to 7 months, 327 patients had died, including children, and at least 18,000 people were affected.[35] Pulmonary pathologic study revealed nonnecrotizing vasculitis.[35] After a search lasting several months, the illness was linked to the consumption of adulterated "cooking oil" that was sold as "pure olive oil" but was actually a mixture of rapeseed oil, other oils, and aniline.[34-36] The mechanisms of injury or the reasons for the eosinophilia in these patients are unknown. A similar outbreak caused by ingestion of contaminated margarine, also characterized by systemic symptoms and eosinophilia, has been reported.[36]

HYPERSENSITIVITY PNEUMONITIS

Prolonged or intense exposure to inhaled organic dusts can produce an immunologic interstitial and alveolar-filling pulmonary disease that is termed *hypersensitivity pneumonitis* or *extrinsic allergic alveolitis*.[37,38] Although hypersensitivity pneumonitis was first described in 1713 by Ramazzini,[39] it was over 200 years later before farmer's lung was described in the modern medical literature and 1965 before specific etiologic agents were identified.[40] Inhalation of nearly any organic dust can cause hypersensitivity pneumonitis (Table 50-2). Many cases are related to occupational exposures and are therefore not likely to occur in children. In pediatrics, most cases are caused by animal protein antigens or molds and dusts found in households or on farms.[41-60] Hypersensitivity pneumonitis caused by fungal antigens has been reported in a child 10 months of age.[60]

Clinical Manifestations

There are different patterns of illness depending on the magnitude and duration of exposure, the size of dust particles, and the individual's immune response.[37,38,61-63] Symptoms mimicking an influenza-like illness, such as high fever, chills, dry

Table 50-2 Etiologic Agents in Hypersensitivity Pneumonitis

ANTIGEN	ANTIGEN SOURCE	TYPICAL DISORDER
Animal products		
Avian serum proteins: pigeon, dove, parrot, cockatiel, parakeet	Droppings	Bird-breeder's lung, pigeon breeder's lung, etc.
Duck proteins	Feathers	Duck fever
Turkey proteins	Turkey products	Turkey handler's disease
Chicken proteins	Chicken products	Chicken plucker's disease
Bovine and porcine proteins	Pituitary snuff	Pituitary snuff taker's disease
Rat serum proteins	Rat urine and droppings	Rat lung, laboratory animal worker's lung
Actinomycetes- and fungus-laden vegetable products		
Thermophilic actinomycetes *(Micromonosporo faeni, Thermoactinomyces vulgaris), Aspergillus* species	Moldy hay	Farmer's lung
Thermophilic actinomycetes *(Thermoactinomyces sacchari, T. vulgaris)*	Moldy pressed sugar cane	Bagassosis
Thermophilic actinomycetes *(M. faeni, T. vulgaris)*	Moldy compost	Mushroom worker's disease
Penicillium frequentans	Moldy cork	Suberosis
Aspergillus clavatus	Contaminated barley	Malt worker's lung
Cryptostroma corticale	Contaminated maple logs	Maple bark disease
Alternaria species	Contaminated wood pulp	Wood worker's lung
Thermophilic actinomycetes *(Thermoactinomyces candidus, T. vulgaris), Penicillium* species, *Cephalosporium* species, amebas	Contaminated humidifiers, dehumidifiers, and air conditioners	Humidifier lung
Bacillus subtilis	Contaminated wood dust in walls	Familial hypersensitivity pneumonitis
Penicillium casei, P. roqueforti	Cheese casings (mold)	Cheese washer's lung, cheese handler's lung
Rhizopus species, *Mucor* species	Contaminated wood trimmings	Wood trimmer's disease
Saccharomonospora viridis	Dried grasses and leaves	Thatched roof disease
Streptomyces albus	Contaminated fertilizer	*Streptomyces* hypersensitivity pneumonitis
Cephalosporium species	Contaminated basement (sewage)	*Cephalosporium* hypersensitivity
Pullularia species	Sauna water	Sauna taker's disease
B. subtilis enzymes	Detergent	Detergent worker's disease
Mucor stolonifa	Paprika dust	Paprika splitter's disease
Insect products		
Acarus siro (mite)	Dust	—
Sitophilus granarius (wheat weevil)	Contaminated grain	Miller's lung (wheat weevil disease)
Chemicals		
Altered proteins or hapten protein conjugates	Toluene diisocyanate	TDI hypersensitivity pneumonitis
	Trimellitic anhydride	TMA hypersensitivity pneumonitis
	Diphenylmethane diisocyanate	MDI hypersensitivity pneumonitis
	Heated epoxy resin	Epoxy resin lung
Other agents		
Coffee dust	?	Coffee worker's lung
Hair dust	Animal proteins	Furrier's lung

Modified from Salvaggio JE: *J Allergy Clin Immunol* 79:558-571, 1987; and Fink JN: *J Allergy Clin Immunol* 74:1-10, 1984.

cough, shortness of breath, and malaise, begin about 4 to 8 hours after acute inhalational contact (e.g., cleaning out a pigeon coop). These intense symptoms diminish over the next 12 to 24 hours, assuming that there is no additional exposure. Wheezing (bronchospasm) during or after acute hypersensitivity pneumonitis is uncommon in patients who do not have asthma. With each exposure symptoms recur; frequent reexposure can lead to progressive shortness of breath, chronic cough, anorexia, and weight loss. Physical examination reveals a dyspneic, ill-appearing patient with bilateral basilar crackles. Chest radiographs may reveal several patterns, including bilateral basilar infiltrates, fine parenchymal nodulations and reticulations, soft and patchy parenchymal densities, and diffuse or localized interstitial and alveolar pulmonary infiltrates. The chest radiograph may be normal if sufficient time has passed after the last insult. In the patient with multiple exposure-related exacerbations, early fibrosis may be evident. Chest radiographs usually do not show pleural effusions, calcification, atelectasis, cavitation, coin lesions, or hilar adenopathy. Pulmonary function tests during the acute phase reveal significant hypoxemia, a reduced forced vital capacity and a proportionally reduced 1-second forced expiratory volume, decreased dynamic lung compliance, and a reduced carbon monoxide diffusing capacity. Pulmonary function abnormalities are transient in the acute phase and parallel pulmonary and systemic symptoms.

If exposure to the offending antigen is low grade and long term, an insidious, progressive lung disease can develop. This chronic form of hypersensitivity pneumonitis is characterized by a chronic cough that may be mucopurulent, shortness of breath, weight loss, and anorexia. The influenza-like systemic symptoms found in the acute form of this disease are absent unless patients are exposed to large amounts of the offending antigen. Early in the condition, chest radiographs show nonspecific findings of interstitial lung disease, later progressing to a reticulonodular pattern with honeycombing. Pulmonary function testing in patients with chronic, severe disease can demonstrate both obstructive and restrictive patterns, reduced carbon monoxide diffusing capacity, hypoxemia, and decreased exercise tolerance. Routine laboratory findings include leukocytosis with a left shift and eosinophilia (eosinophil

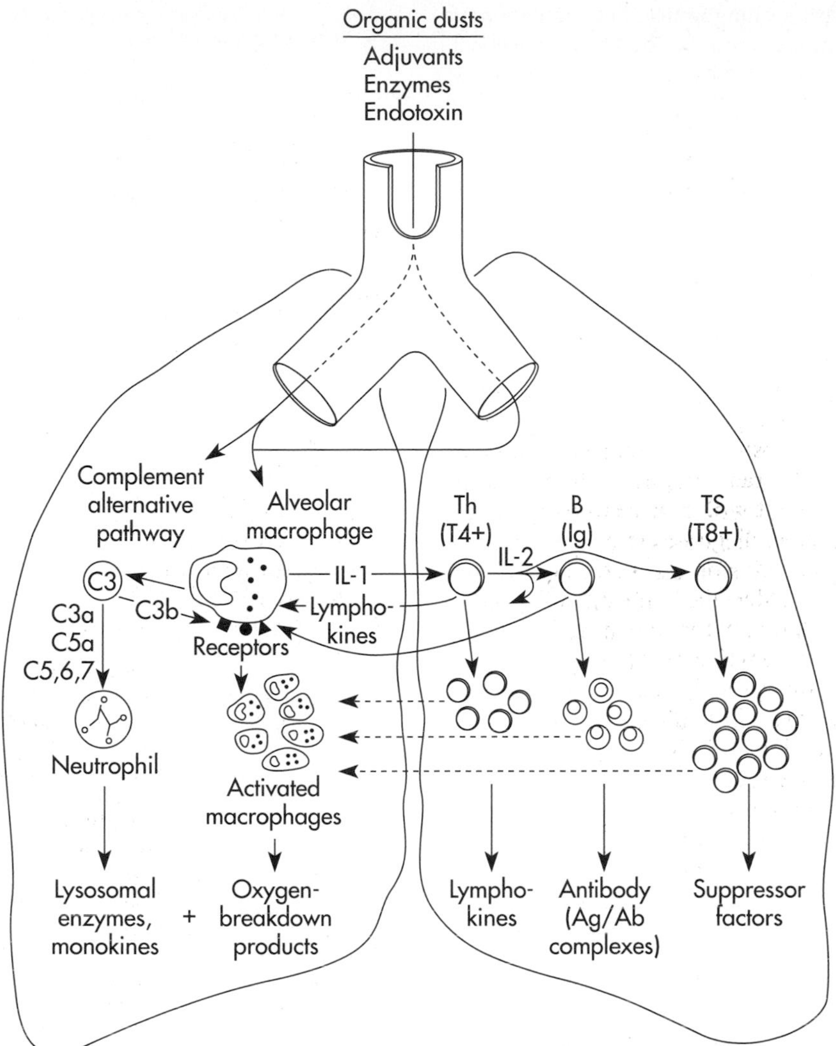

Fig. 50-1. Proposed pathophysiologic processes involved in hypersensitivity pneumonitis to organic dusts. *Th,* T helper (cell); *TS,* T suppressor (cell); *IL,* interleukin. (From Toxic Epidemic Study Group: *Lancet* 2:697-702, 1982.)

count of up to 10%), which may persist for months after cessation of antigen exposure. IgE levels are not increased in hypersensitivity pneumonitis, although other immunoglobulin levels may be elevated.

Disease Mechanisms

Pathologic examination reveals interstitial and alveolar mononuclear cell lung infiltrates.[38] Other organs are generally not involved, and vasculitis is not a prominent feature. Pulmonary infiltrates consist mainly of T cells and activated alveolar macrophages. Noncaseating granulomas are often seen, especially in more chronic cases.[38] Bronchial wall narrowing leading to bronchiolitis obliterans may occur. Over time, the granulomatous lesions may disappear, and the mononuclear infiltrates may subside (even with continued exposure); after long exposure, fibrosis may become prominent.[38,64]

The pathogenesis of hypersensitivity pneumonitis is still not well understood, but evidence is mounting that it is mainly a result of cell-mediated (type IV) hypersensitivity.[38] Type I (immediate) hypersensitivity is thought to play little or no role. Type II (antibody-mediated) hypersensitivity was thought to be important for many years because of the presence of precipitating (IgG) antibodies in the serum of patients. However, it is now known that antigen-exposed individuals with asymptomatic disease also have high levels of precipitating antibody. Therefore precipitating antibody appears to reflect exposure and not disease.[38,64] The lack of vasculitis and normal serum complement levels suggest that type III immune mechanisms (immune complex deposition) are also not important in this disease. Fig. 50-1 shows the probable mechanisms by which exposure to organic dusts leads to lung injury. The inhalation of organic dust leads to activation of the alternative complement pathway, which increases vascular permeability, recruits neutrophils, and activates alveolar macrophages. The macrophages release enzymes, interleukin-1, other monokines, and oxygen metabolites, which leads to acute tissue injury and lymphocyte infiltration. Local B cell production of antibody may lead to the local formation of immune complexes, which bind complement and continue to activate alveolar macrophages. Intense T cell–mediated hypersensitivity results from repeated exposure.[38] Sensitized T cells release interleukin-2, which increases the size of the lymphocyte population, and lymphokines, which continue to activate macrophages, leading to further lung injury. The regulation of this complex immune response is not yet understood. Recent studies point to a genetically determined immunoregulatory imbalance that results in local hypersensitivity, distinguishing exposed ill from exposed asymptomatic individuals. Proposed immunoregulatory abnormalities and insights gained from animal models of hypersensitivity pneumonitis are reviewed elsewhere.[61,64,65]

Diagnosis and Management

The diagnosis of hypersensitivity pneumonitis is based largely on the clinical presentation. In children, a high level of suspicion is required. Guidelines for clinical evaluation have recently been published.[63] A thorough history, inquiring about possible sources of antigen exposure, is extremely important. Physical examination and chest radiographs are important in the search for findings consistent with hypersensitivity pneumonitis or those suggesting other diagnoses (e.g., wheezing on physical examination, pleural effusion on chest radiograph). Measuring serum precipitins against the likely offending antigen or antigens is important but only for demonstrating exposure. False-positive and false-negative results may occur, so precipitin results must be interpreted with caution. Eosinophilia, if present, is suggestive of the diagnosis, but the absence of peripheral blood eosinophilia is not. Skin testing is impractical and is not recommended because antigens are not commercially available. Inhalation challenge with the suspected antigen is also not routinely recommended. However, if reexposure to the offending antigen is necessary to confirm the diagnosis, intentional exposure in the natural environment may be preferable to laboratory exposure. The patient's respiratory and systemic symptoms, vital signs, leukocyte count, and pulmonary function tests should be closely monitored within the first 24 hours after exposure. Until more information is available concerning the clinical usefulness of the findings, bronchoalveolar lavage is also not recommended unless it is necessary to rule out another disorder. Similarly, lung biopsy should be performed only when the diagnosis cannot be made by other means. Biopsy is useful for ruling out other diseases because pathologic findings are not pathognomonic. Open lung biopsy is more likely to yield useful information than transbronchial biopsy, especially in children. Probably the most useful "test" for hypersensitivity pneumonitis is to separate the patient from the suspected causative agent.[63]

Removal of the offending agent from the patient's environment, or vice versa, is the most effective therapy for hypersensitivity pneumonitis.[40,63,64] The administration of corticosteroids can result in rapid improvement of symptoms but is generally unnecessary. Opponents of the use of corticosteroids in this setting point out that these agents are nonspecific and may be hazardous if the diagnosis is incorrect and the cause is infectious.[63]

REFERENCES

Pulmonary Infiltrates with Eosinophilia

1. Schatz M, Wasserman S, Patterson R: The eosinophil and the lung, *Arch Intern Med* 142:1515-1519, 1982.
2. Schatz M, Wasserman S, Patterson R: Eosinophils and immunologic lung disease, *Med Clin North Am* 65:1055-1071, 1981.
3. Leitch AG: Pulmonary eosinophilia, *Basics Respir Dis* 7:1-6, 1979.
4. Weller PF: Eosinophilia, *J Allergy Clin Immunol* 73:1-14, 1984.
5. Rao M, Steiner P, Rose JS, Kassner EG, Kottmeier P, Steiner M: Chronic eosinophilic pneumonia in a one-year-old child, *Chest* 68:118-120, 1975.
6. Dejaegher P, Derveaux L, Dubois P, Demedts M: Eosinophilic pneumonia without radiographic infiltrates, *Chest* 84:637-638, 1983.
7. Carrington CB, Addington WW, Goff AM, Madoff IM, Marks A, Schwaber JR, Gaensler EA: Chronic eosinophilic pneumonia, *N Engl J Med* 298:801-809, 1969.
8. Gaensler EA, Carrington CB: Peripheral opacities in chronic eosinophilic pneumonia: the photographic negative of pulmonary edema, *Am J Roentgen* 128:1, 1977.
9. McCarthy DS, Pepys J: Cryptogenic pulmonary eosinophilias, *Clin Allergy* 3:339-351, 1973.
10. Turner-Warwick M, Assem ESK, Lockwood M: Cryptogenic pulmonary eosinophilia, *Clin Allergy* 6:135, 1976.
11. McEvoy JDS: Immunoglobulin levels and electron microscopy in eosinophilic pneumonia, *Am J Med* 64:529, 1978.
12. Freedman MH, Grisaru D, Olivieri N, MacLusky I, Thorner PS: Pulmonary syndrome in patients with thalassemia major receiving intravenous deferoxamine infusions, *Am J Dis Child* 144:565-569, 1990.
13. Chusid MJ, Dale DC, West BC, Wolff SM: The hypereosinophilic syndrome: analysis of fourteen cases with review of the literature, *Medicine (Baltimore)* 54:1-27, 1975.
14. Fauci AS, Harley JB, Roberts WC, Ferran VJ, Gralnick HR, Bjornson BH: The idiopathic hypereosinophilic syndrome: clinical, pathophysiologic and therapeutic considerations, *Ann Intern Med* 97:78-92, 1982.
15. Alfaham MA, Ferguson SD, Sihra B, Davies J: The idiopathic hypereosinophilic syndrome, *Arch Dis Child* 62:601-613, 1987.
16. Gaynon PS, Gonzalez-Crussi F: Exaggerated eosinophilia and acute lymphoid leukemia, *Am J Pediatr Hematol Oncol* 6:334-337, 1984.
17. Bailey CC, Campbell RH: Lymphosarcoma presenting as Löffler's syndrome, *Br Med J* 1:460-461, 1973.
18. Botsztejn A: Die pertussoide, eosinophile Pneumonie des Sauglings, *Ann Paediatr (Basel)* 157:28-46, 1941.
19. Oetgen WJ: Pertussoid eosinophilic pneumonia: pulmonary infiltrates with eosinophilia in very young infants, *Chest* 71:492-496, 1977.
20. Biro Z: Twelve more cases of interstitial pertussoid eosinophilic pneumonia in infants, *Helv Paediatr Acta* 15:135, 1960.
21. Tipple MA, Beem MO, Saxon EM: Clinical characteristics of the afebrile pneumonia associated with *Chlamydia trachomatis* infection in infants less than 6 months of age, *Pediatrics* 63:192-197, 1979.
22. Beem MO, Saxon E: Pneumonia in infants infected with *Chlamydia trachomatis, Pediatr Res* 10:395, 1976.
23. Beem MO, Saxon EM: Respiratory-tract colonization and a distinctive pneumonia syndrome in infants infected with *Chlamydia trachomatis, N Engl J Med* 296:306-310, 1977.
24. Schaad UB, Rossi E: Infantile chlamydial pneumonia: a review based on 115 cases, *Eur J Pediatr* 138:105-109, 1982.
25. Garofalo R, Kimpen JL, Welliver RC, Ogra PL: Eosinophil degranulation in the respiratory tract during naturally acquired respiratory syncytial virus infection, *J Pediatr* 120:28-32, 1992.
26. Ottesen EA, Nutman TB: Tropical pulmonary eosinophilia, *Annu Rev Med* 43:417-424, 1992.
27. Taylor MR, Keane CT, OConnor P, Mulvihill E, Holland C: The expanded spectrum of toxocaral disease, *Lancet* 1:692-695, 1988.
28. Rackemann FM, Greene EJ: Periarteritis nodosa and asthma, *Trans Assoc Am Physicians* 54:112, 1939.
29. Lanham JG, Elkon KB, Pusey CD, Hughes GR: Systemic vasculitis with asthma and eosinophilia: a clinical approach to the Churg-Strauss syndrome, *Medicine (Baltimore)* 63:65-81, 1984.
30. Wishnick MM, Valensi Q, Doyle EF, Balian A, Genieser NB, Chrousos G: Churg-Strauss syndrome: development of cardiomyopathy during corticosteroid treatment, *Am J Dis Child* 136:339-344, 1982.
31. Fischer TJ, Daugherty C, Gushurst C, Kephart GM, Gleich GJ: Systemic vasculitis associated with eosinophilia and marked degranulation of tissue eosinophils, *Pediatrics* 82:69-75, 1988.

32. Bosken CH, Myers JL, Greenberger PA, Katzenstein AL: Pathologic features of allergic bronchopulmonary aspergillosis, *Am J Surg Pathol* 12:216-222, 1988.
33. Ricker DH, Taylor SR, Gartner JC Jr, Kurland G: Fatal pulmonary aspergillosis presenting as acute eosinophilic pneumonia in a previously healthy child, *Chest* 100:875-877, 1991.
34. Tabuenca JM: Toxic-allergic syndrome caused by ingestion of rapeseed oil denatured with aniline, *Lancet* 2:567-568, 1981.
35. Toxic Epidemic Study Group: Toxic epidemic syndrome: Spain, 1981, *Lancet* 2:697-702, 1982.
36. Rigau-Perez JG, Perez-Alvarez L, Duenas-Castro S, Choi K, Thacker SB, Germain JL, Gonzalez-de-Andres G, Canada-Royo L, Perez-Gallardo F: Epidemiologic investigation of an oil-associated pneumonic paralytic eosinophilic syndrome in Spain, *Am J Epidemiol* 119:250-260, 1984.

Hypersensitivity Pneumonitis

37. Fink JN: Hypersensitivity pneumonitis, *J Allergy Clin Immunol* 74:1-10, 1984.
38. Salvaggio JE, deShazo RD: Pathogenesis of hypersensitivity pneumonitis, *Chest* 89:190S-193S, 1986.
39. Ramazzini B: *De morbus artificum diatriba,* Chicago, 1713, University of Chicago Press.
40. Levy MB, Fink JN: Hypersensitivity pneumonitis, *Ann Allergy* 54:167-171, 1985.
41. El-Hefney A, Ekladious EM, El-Sharkawy S, El-Ghadban H, El-Heneidy F, Frankland AW: Extrinsic allergic bronchiolo-alveolitis in children, *Clin Allergy* 10:651-658, 1980.
42. Grammer LC, Roberts M, Lerner C, Patterson R: Clinical and serologic follow-up of four children and five adults with bird-fancier's lung, *J Allergy Clin Immunol* 85:655-660, 1990.
43. Swingler GH: Summer-type hypersensitivity pneumonitis in southern Africa: a report of 5 cases in one family, *S Afr Med J* 77:104-107, 1990.
44. Saltos N, Saunders NA, Bhagwandeen SB, Jarvie B: Hypersensitivity pneumonitis in a mouldy house, *Med J Aust* 2:244-246, 1982.
45. Shannon DC, Andrews JL, Recavarren S, Kazemi H: Pigeon breeder's lung disease and interstitial pulmonary fibrosis, *Am J Dis Child* 117:504-510, 1969.
46. Chandra S, Jones HE: Pigeon fancier's lung in children, *Arch Dis Child* 47:716-718, 1972.
47. Purtilo DT, Brem J, Ceccaci L, Cassel C, Fitzpatrick AJ: A family study of pigeon breeder's disease, *J Pediatr* 86:569-571, 1975.
48. Stiehm ER, Reed CE, Tooley WH: Pigeon breeder's lung in children, *Pediatrics* 39:904-915, 1967.
49. Hodges GR, Fink JN, Schlueter DP: Hypersensitivity pneumonitis caused by a contaminated cool-mist vaporizer, *Ann Intern Med* 80:501-504, 1974.
50. Allen DH, Basten A, Williams GV, Woolcock AJ: Familial hypersensitivity pneumonitis, *Am J Med* 59:505-514, 1975.
51. Cunningham AS, Fink JN, Schlueter DP: Childhood hypersensitivity pneumonitis due to dove antigens, *Pediatrics* 58:436-442, 1976.
52. Wolf SJ, Stillerman A, Weinberger M, Smith W: Chronic interstitial pneumonitis in a 3-year-old child with hypersensitivity to dove antigens, *Pediatrics* 79:1027-1029, 1987.
53. Yee WF, Castile RG, Cooper A, Roberts M, Patterson R: Diagnosing bird fancier's disease in children, *Pediatrics* 85:848-852, 1990.
54. Grimfeld A, Gaultier C, Baculard A, Le-Moing G, Tournier G, Gerbeaux J: Hypersensitivity pneumonitis in children: a study of 5 cases, *Sem Hop* 57:1267-1272, 1981 (translated by author).
55. Barker PM, Warner JO: 'Atypical pneumonia' due to parakeet sensitivity: bird fancier's lung in a 10-year-old girl, *Br J Dis Chest* 78:404-407, 1984.
56. Keith HH, Holsclaw DS Jr, Dunsky EH: Pigeon breeder's disease in children: a family study, *Chest* 79:107-110, 1981.
57. Balasubramaniam SK, O'Connell EJ, Yunginger JW, McDougall JC, Sachs MI: Hypersensitivity pneumonitis due to dove antigens in an adolescent, *Clin Pediatr (Phila)* 26:174-176, 1987.
58. Schatz M, Patterson R, Fink J, Moore V, Rodey G, Cunningham A, Roberts M, Harris K: Pigeon breeders disease. III. A study of a family exposed to doves, *Clin Exp Immunol* 24:33-41, 1976.
59. Reiss JS, Weiss NS, Payette KM, Strimas J: Childhood pigeon breeder's disease, *Ann Allergy* 32:208-212, 1974.
60. Eisenberg JD, Montanero A, Lee RG: Hypersensitivity pneumonitis in an infant, *Pediatr Pulmonol* 12:186-190, 1992.
61. Salvaggio JE: Robert A. Cooke memorial lecture: hypersensitivity pneumonitis, *J Allergy Clin Immunol* 79:558-571, 1987.
62. Stankus RP, Salvaggio JE: Hypersensitivity pneumonitis, *Clin Chest Med* 4:55-62, 1983.
63. Richerson HB, Bernstein IL, Fink JN, Hunninghake GW, Novey HS, Reed CE, Salvaggio JE, Schuyler MR, Schwartz HJ, Stechschulte DJ: Guidelines for the clinical evaluation of hypersensitivity pneumonitis: report of the Subcommittee on Hypersensitivity Pneumonitis, *J Allergy Clin Immunol* 84:839-844, 1989.
64. Fink JN: Hypersensitivity pneumonitis, *Clin Chest Med* 13:303-309, 1992.
65. Salvaggio JE: Current concepts in the pathogenesis of occupationally induced allergic pneumonitis, *Int Arch Allergy Appl Immunol* 82:424-434, 1987.

CHAPTER 51

Allergic Bronchopulmonary Aspergillosis

Fleming Carswell

Allergic bronchopulmonary aspergillosis (ABPA) has been defined as "an acute, subacute chronic or recurrent bronchial and pulmonary inflammatory disease due to various immunologic reactants directed against and interacting with antigens of *Aspergillus fumigatus* growing in the bronchi of asthmatic patients."[1] This chapter documents ABPA but does not specifically address invasive aspergillosis, distant complications of aspergillosis such as secondary amyloidosis (which has been reported in three patients with ABPA[2]), or pulmonary disease produced by other fungi.[3,4]

ABPA was first described by Hinson et al[5] in 1952, when three of their eight reported cases of bronchopulmonary aspergillosis had a characteristic syndrome with transient, often extensive shadows on the chest radiograph; cough; and sputum that contained hyphae of *A. fumigatus.* Each patient had considerable eosinophilia; one who did not have asthma before the onset of illness died during status asthmaticus, and two had recurrent pyrexial attacks and saccular bronchiectasis. The authors suggested that the fungus could be acting as a saprophytic, allergic, or septicemic agent in different subjects.

Although this is the first clear description of ABPA, these authors reported papers documenting cases of *Aspergillus* isolation from diseased lungs as early as 1842. A series of papers documented the presence of *Aspergillus* precipitins in the serum and the nature of the pathophysiologic reaction in the skin, nose, and lungs of patients with ABPA.[6-8] Meanwhile, in 1965, transient pulmonary infiltrations were described in two children with cystic fibrosis.[9] Again, transient lung shadows were found on chest radiograph, *A. fumigatus* was isolated from the sputum, precipitins against the fungus were found in the blood, and immediate skin hypersensitivity to a fungal extract was demonstrated.

DIAGNOSIS

In the 40 years since the first clear description of the syndrome,[5] increasing numbers of patients have been reported. Diagnoses that may require exclusion are listed in Box 51-1. ABPA needs to be distinguished from other forms of lung disease produced by *A. fumigatus,* including invasive or septicemic aspergillosis, aspergilloma, and atopic asthma provoked by *Aspergillus* antigen inhalation.

Aspergillus organisms are found all year round in the air, although higher counts have been reported in the autumn. It tends, as a saprophyte, to be found in decaying vegetation in the garden and especially in compost heaps but has a very wide distribution in the house and in areas near water.

The clinical symptoms include anorexia, fever, night sweats, wheezing, and a productive cough, sometimes including the classic brown plugs. Wheeze may be heard over parts of the chest, particularly the upper lobes, and there is usually a profound eosinophilia (>1000 cells/mm^3).

The criteria developed by Rosenberg et al[10] for diagnosing ABPA are listed in Box 51-2. These authors suggest that all the primary findings are required for the confirmed diagnosis; the presence of the first six without the seventh (central bronchiectasis) makes the diagnosis probable.

The only change in diagnostic criteria from the original description[5] involves immunologic measurements, and this modest change dates from the descriptions and investigations of the precipitin reaction of serum to *Aspergillus* antigens.[6-8] One study[11] reaffirmed the supportive role of *Aspergillus* precipitins in making the diagnosis and found no additional diagnostic benefit in the routine enzyme-linked immunosorbent assays of serum immunoglobulin E (IgE) or IgG. Rosenberg et al[10] found the secondary characteristics of comparatively little value because, for instance, only 1 in 20 of the described cases produced the brown plugs of sputum. This classic paper,[10] however, gives a description of ABPA in asthmatic adults in whom the syndrome is more obvious than in patients with cystic fibrosis in whom the fungus often has a simple saprophytic rather than an allergic or invasive role. The diagnosis of ABPA is also more difficult when cystic fibrosis is present because the patients tend to produce more sputum and changes in chest radiograph other than ABPA are more common.

ABPA is described in asthmatics in the pediatric age group.[12,13] The early diagnosis of ABPA in children is made difficult[12] by the insensitivity of computed tomographic scans in detecting central bronchiectasis, the lack of current chest radiographic infiltrates in remission, the lack of peripheral blood eosinophilia and precipitins, and weakly reactive skin tests. Despite this, the infection has been reported in patients as young as 14 months of age.[14] Its persistence from childhood has often been inferred in adults.

The nature of the immune reaction and any consequent pathophysiologic reaction may be different in cystic fibrosis than in asthma. Thus the episodic reversible bronchial obstruction or bronchial lability in cystic fibrosis has a different pattern from that in asthma; for instance, the increase in the peak flow rate during exercise is greater and the decrease after exercise smaller than in asthma.[15] The incidence of positive cultures from sputum[16] is tenfold greater in patients with cystic fibrosis than in patients with other sputum-producing diseases, which may mean either that such patients are particularly liable to ABPA or that the lung conditions favor saprophytic growth of *Aspergillus* species. The *Aspergillus* hyphae isolated from the sputum[16] or bronchial aspirates[5] in both cystic fibrosis and asthma tend to be short with only occasional branching, and there is little suggestion of invasion of the underlying bronchial epithelium. The paper by Rosenberg et al[10] is based on American adults with asthma, but the reported diagnostic pattern of ABPA is similar elsewhere,[17-21] even in children with cystic fibrosis. In children, it is commonly difficult to make a definitive diagnosis because the central bronchiectasis required for the diagnosis[10] occurs later in the disease.[22]

It is apparent that diagnostic rigor reduces the apparent prevalence of "proven" cases. Thus a minor reduction in the severity of the criteria—for instance the extent of the eosinophilia (more than 1000 cells/mm^3 in the paper by Hinson et al[5] and more than 400 cells/mm^3 in that of Simmonds et al[19])—partly explains the reported wide variation in preva-

BOX 51-1
Differential Diagnosis of ABPA

Mucoid impaction and bronchiectasis in poorly controlled asthma
Infective chest diseases, including viral or bacterial pneumonitis, tuberculosis, and other immune-mediated diseases such as Churg-Strauss vasculitis, hypersensitivity pneumonitis, and drug- and toxin-mediated pneumonitis
Parasitism, such as tropical pulmonary eosinophilia produced by *Wuchereria bancrofti*
Saprophytic or allergic invasion by other fungi, including *Candida, Penicillium, Stemphyllium, Geotrichum, Curvularia,* and *Drechslera* species

BOX 51-2
Criteria for the Diagnosis of ABPA

Primary
Episodic bronchial obstruction (asthma)
Peripheral blood eosinophilia
Immediate skin reactivity to *Aspergillus* antigen
Precipitating antibodies against *Aspergillus* antigen
Elevated serum immunoglobulin E concentrations
History of pulmonary infiltrates (transient or fixed)
Central bronchiectasis

Secondary
A. fumigatus in sputum (by repeated culture or microscopic examination)
History of expectoration of brown plugs or flecks
Arthus reaction (late skin reactivity) to *Aspergillus* antigen

From Rosenberg M et al: *Ann Intern Med* 86:404-415, 1977.

lence. Despite the rigor of the 1977 paper by Rosenberg et al,[10] the same group emphasized in 1989 that positive precipitins do not establish a diagnosis and negative precipitins do not necessarily exclude the diagnosis.[1] In that paper, they quote four cases in which the correct diagnosis was eventually made only because of the physician's reaction to the pattern of illness rather than the incongruous test result. They now expect a consistent serologic response in ABPA to include a total serum IgE level greater than 1000 ng/ml, positive precipitins for *Aspergillus* species, and demonstration of specific IgE and IgG antibody against *Aspergillus* species.[1]

Obviously the transient pulmonary infiltrates, which are often asymptomatic, are more likely to be found if physicians order chest radiographs frequently.[19] Regarding the secondary diagnostic criterion of *Aspergillus* isolation, it is important to remember that the saprophyte *A. fumigatus* has been found very extensively in dead organic material and is frequently recovered during autopsy from the lungs of patients not apparently suffering from ABPA.[23] Spores may readily "contaminate" sputum during collection or examination. Accordingly, two or more isolations of *A. fumigatus,* a suggestion that culture was rapid and easy because of multiple spores, and preferably, the observation of branching fungal hyphae are required before the clinician can assume the fungi came from the lung.

Before therapeutic intervention can be justified, the clinician needs to weight the extent of the pathologic involvement of *A. fumigatus* against the severity of the infection in a particular patient. This is illustrated in one study that documents the wide range of responses to *A. fumigatus* in individuals with cystic fibrosis.[24] Thus 8 of 75 patients (10.7%) had ABPA as shown by immediate cutaneous reactivity to *Aspergillus* species, peripheral blood eosinophilia, elevated serum total IgE levels, elevated levels of specific IgE or IgG against *A. fumigatus,* and specific precipitating antibody. The results from some of these tests were positive in 50 patients (67%); only 17 (23%) had no detectable immune response. The pattern of *Aspergillus* sensitivity measured in an individual may also fluctuate.[25] The diagnosis of ABPA can be confused with other conditions, particularly hypersensitivity pneumonitis, but Table 51-1 lists the significant differences.

Appearance of Chest Radiograph

In 1970, the first chest radiographs of ABPA had normal appearances in only 14% of 111 well-documented cases[26]; 71% showed massive consolidation as indicated by homogeneous shadows without fissure displacement. Commonly, only very minor clinical upset accompanied extensive pulmonary consolidation, a pattern very different from the usual manifestations of a bacterial pneumonia with a similar area of consolidation. Parallel lines or ring shadows also occurred in 79% of patients. These included tramline shadows with parallel hairline shadows extending from the hilum in the direction of the bronchi; the width of the transradiant zone between the lines was that of a normal bronchus (Fig. 51-1, *A*). Similar parallel line shadows in which the bronchus appears dilated were described as permanent and presumably show irreversible bronchiectasis (Fig. 51-1, *B*). Similarly the ring shadow represented a cross-sectional view of a dilated bronchus. Bandlike or toothpaste shadows representing secretions in dilated bronchi were described, and the transition from a toothpaste to a tubular shadow was noted after the patient coughed up a sputum plug. Glove-finger shadows tended to be more from the hila, with the expanded round distal end of the dilated bronchi giving the characteristic finger appearance. Line shadows, nodular shadows, atelectasis of a lobe or lung, and local emphysema were also described, but the more characteristic and also uncommon appearance of permanent lobar shrinkage with the lobe still aerated was a feature of only 36% of these adults with asthma (Fig. 51-2).

Bronchographic appearances were also characteristic, with dilation and occlusion of some of the proximal bronchi being common; however, often in central lesions with a similar degree of dilation of the proximal bronchi, the contrast media flowed into bronchi of normal caliber. That particular appearance is specific to ABPA. Circular dilations were also sometimes noted on bronchography. The series by McCarthy et al[26] was predominantly of adults, but because the central bronchiectasis develops with age, the bronchiectasis and even the dilated bronchi may commonly be absent or at an early stage in pediatric patients. Robinson and Campbell[27] agree

Table 51-1 Differential Diagnosis of Hypersensitivity Pneumonitis and ABPA

DIAGNOSTIC FEATURES	HYPERSENSITIVITY PNEUMONITIS	ABPA
Nature of patient	Nonatopic (nonallergic)	Atopic (allergic)
Symptoms and physical findings	Cough, dyspnea, fever, no wheezing, weight loss, crackles at lung bases	Asthma, fever, +/− hemoptysis, chest pain
Skin tests	+/− (positive immediate and late reactions in some cases of pigeon breeder's lung)	+ (immediate and late responses)
Blood count	Normal or lymphopenia	Eosinophilia
Immunoglobulins	Elevated IgG and IgA, IgG precipitating antibodies	Elevated IgE, IgG-precipitating antibodies
Sputum	Normal	Eosinophilia, mycelia
Chest radiograph	Pulmonary interstitial infiltrates	Pulmonary lobar infiltrates
Complications	Pulmonary fibrosis	Atelectasis, proximal bronchiectasis, fibrosis (late)
Pulmonary function tests	Restrictive	Obstructive (restrictive late)
Inhalation challenge tests	Late restriction (+/− immediate/late obstruction) (positive immediate and late reactions in some cases of pigeon breeder's lung)	Immediate and late obstruction
Immune mechanism	Immune complexes and delayed hypersensitivity	Immediate hypersensitivity and delayed hypersensitivity
Treatment	Avoidance, corticosteroids	Bronchodilators, corticosteroids

From Slavin RG: *Clin Rev Allergy* 3:167-182, 1985.

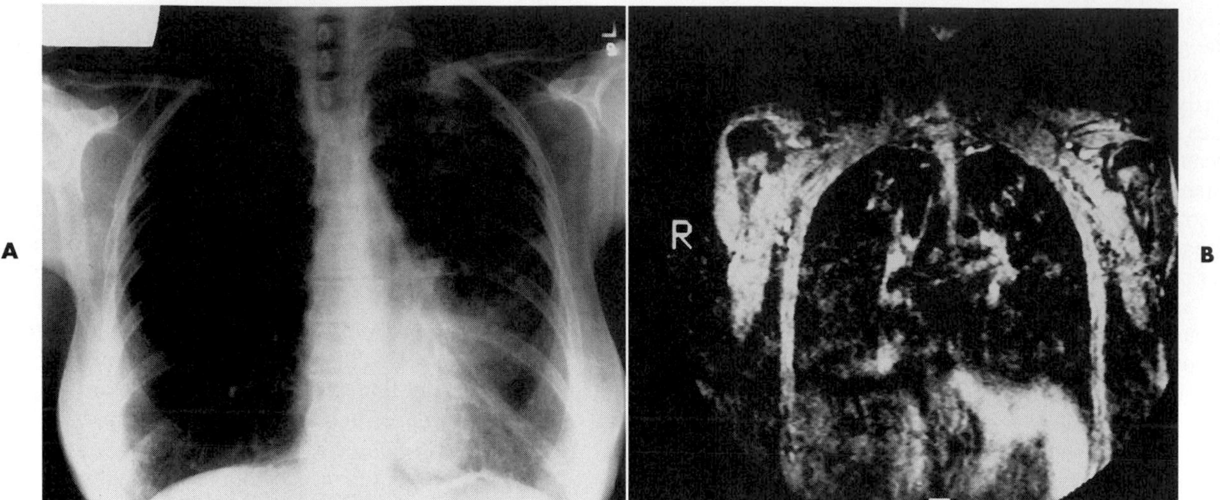

Fig. 51-1. ABPA in patients with asthma. **A,** Collapse and wedge-shaped lesion commonly found in ABPA. **B,** Computed tomographic scan showing the central bronchial dilation typical of ABPA. (Courtesy J Catterall and G Lazlo, Bristol.)

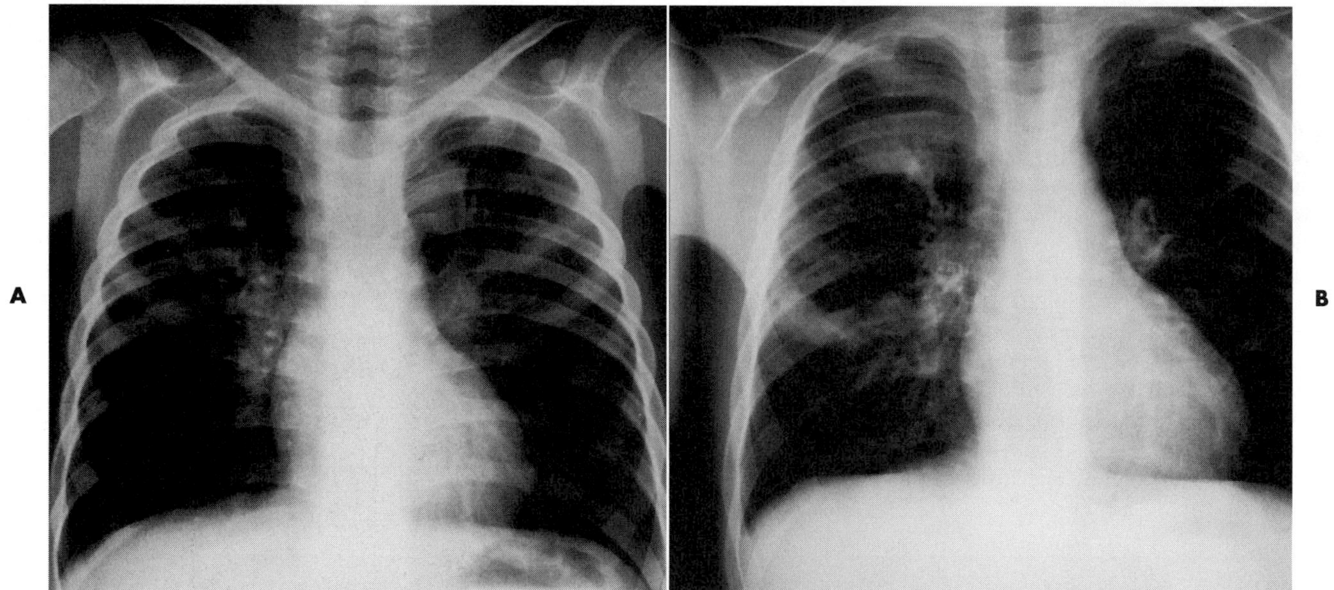

Fig. 51-2. ABPA in a patient with cystic fibrosis. **A,** Aspergilloma. **B,** Areas of atelectasis (Courtesy M Alfaham, Caroiff.)

with the substance of these changes. Computed tomography has virtually replaced bronchography in the diagnosis of bronchiectasis. Narrow-section computed tomography may be particularly helpful; in fact, Currie et al[28] found that it detected significantly more cases of bronchiectasis and ABPA than plain chest radiographs (see Fig. 51-1, *B*). The importance of magnetic resonance imaging and other newer diagnostic methods is likely to be considerably greater in the future because they can detail the individual lesions of ABPA and can help the clinician make the diagnosis.

Laboratory Results

The blood of patients with ABPA has eosinophilia, elevated total and *Aspergillus*-specific IgE levels, and multiple precipitins to *Aspergillus* antigens. The eosinophils and IgE are also found in the sputum, as may be fungal hyphae, and *Aspergillus* organisms may be found on culture.

Respiratory function changes are those of airway obstruction, which is not responsive to bronchodilators, but it may be severe and associated with hyperinflation (increased total lung capacity) and decreased carbon monoxide diffusing capacity.[29] In one series, the condition of a third of all patients with recurrent consolidations was asymptomatic.[29] In many cases in untreated patients, there was a chronic relapsing course with recurrent obstruction and consolidation and often severe lung destruction; in other patients, recurrences occurred for many years and produced no functional deterioration. In another series of six patients who had exacerbations of ABPA (diagnosed by eosinophilia and changes on the appearance of the chest radiograph), the total lung capacity, vital capacity, 1-second forced expiratory volume, and carbon monoxide diffusing capacity were reduced but uniformly returned to baseline values during steroid therapy.[30] Although a minority of patients had reduced function in interval measurements (3 of 16 in the 1-second forced expiratory volume, 2 of 16 in vital capacity, none of 10 for carbon monoxide diffusing capacity), there was no relationship between the duration of ABPA or asthma and respiratory function change.

Precipitin tests using a variety of different techniques reveal IgG-precipitating antibodies to multiple *Aspergillus* antigens.[31] In exacerbations, more precipitins tend to be found, and these are also found in invasive aspergillosis. The raised total serum IgE level is probably the best single discriminator of ABPA from the other forms of aspergillosis, but raised levels of IgA and C3 can help the clinician make the diagnosis.[31] An increase in the total serum IgE level often precedes or accompanies symptoms, but such an association is not seen in acute asthma.[32] Inhalation challenge with carefully quantified concentrations of antigens[8] has provided useful information on pathogenesis but is no longer used in routine clinical practice.

PROGNOSIS

Despite many follow-up studies, the prognosis cannot be accurately predicted because of the various diagnostic criteria in different centers and because of the condition's varying natural progression. The underlying chest condition predisposing toward the induction of infection by *Aspergillus* organisms can range from normal health to asthma, cystic fibrosis, and variable immunodeficiency to the severe defects of granulomatous disease. Markedly variable exposure also occurs. Genetic variables are likely to produce differences in disease progression.[33] Mendelson et al[13] have characterized five stages in adult ABPA: (1) the acute stage, (2) remission, (3) exacerbation, (4) corticosteroid-dependent asthma, and (5) pulmonary fibrosis. In stage I, during which classically acute symptoms are present with modest chest infiltrates, the symptoms may not actually correlate with the presence of chest infiltrates. Total serum IgE levels do correlate with the appearance on the radiographs.[34] Statements from several studies[29,35,36] imply either a very indolent process or a highly successful treatment for ABPA. Various authors[18,19,36] claimed good prognoses because of their treatment, for example, in childhood cystic fibrosis. Brueton et al[17] administered steroids to only two of seven patients with ABPA and found that these two had as good a prognosis as the rest of the patients at the clinic. In an 11-year follow-up of 47 patients with cystic fibrosis, Hamilton and Carswell[37] failed to show any relationship between a positive skin prick test for *A. fumigatus* and a decline in respiratory function. It is possible that these patients had mainly saprophytic involvement with *A. fumigatus* without direct bronchial damage. Such allergic reactivity without apparent disease has been described.[38,39]

PATHOGENESIS

Pathologic Changes

Bronchiectasis involving segmental bronchi, particularly in the upper lobes with minimal involvement of the periphery, is the most characteristic lesion of ABPA. The fundamental lesion is an inflammatory hypersecretory bronchial obstruction syndrome[40] that can be differentiated from the bronchiectasis of asthma without aspergillosis by seeking the normal peripheral tapering of the bronchi in ABPA.[27] The sputum may contain inspissated mucus, Curschmann's spirals, Charcot-Leyden crystals, eosinophils, and mononuclear cells. Fungal hyphae may be seen, and *A. fumigatus* may be cultured from the luminal fluid. The fungus commonly has shorter and fewer branching hyphae than in invasive aspergillosis or in culture in vitro. There is no invasion of the bronchial walls. A granulomatous bronchiolitis is commonly present, and the pathologic appearances, which are influenced by the nature of the predisposition to ABPA, may include microabscesses with overt *A. fumigatus;* pneumonia, which can be eosinophilic, lipid, lymphocytic, desquamative, or interstitial, may be also present. Fibrosis, bronchiolitis obliterans, and bronchocentric granulomatosis are also reported. In one report, all 18 cases of ABPA showed bronchocentric granulomatosis, mucoid impaction, or both effects.[41] The exudative bronchiolitis was distal to the bronchocentric granulomatosis and was present in 13 of the 18 cases. In these lungs, there was marked filling of the bronchial lumens with necrotic neutrophils and eosinophils in a mucinous exudate. A total of 13 patients had eosinophilic pneumonia, and in 14, it was possible to stain noninvasive fungal hyphae. The pattern has been suggested to be typical of a hypersecretory bronchial obstruction syndrome,[40] which can be produced by fungi other than *A. fumigatus* and indeed can be produced by nonfungal agents. The presence of *A. fumigatus* by itself is not conclusive evidence of the etiologic importance of the fungi in that process, particularly in view of the high isolation rate of *A. fumigatus* from postmortem lung specimens.[23] Although involvement of other fungi in this syndrome is not commonly described, the pattern of increased immediate reactivity to many fungi on skin prick testing[15] implies that they can produce similar syndromes.

Disease Process

The elicitable reaction on challenge of sensitive subjects can be related to the presence and nature of the antibodies.[6-8] These studies emphasized the importance of precipitins to *A. fumigatus* because the precipitins seemed most closely associated with the development of ABPA. The presence of precipitins is also related to the occurrence of the late reaction, which occurs 3 to 12 hours after an inhaled challenge in sensitive subjects. The productive cough, wheezing, dyspnea, influenza-like symptoms, and objective evidence of airway obstruction are the hallmarks of this reaction. The presence of precipitins in the serum and the late reaction on bronchial challenge correlate well with the diagnosis of ABPA. Extracts of *A. fumigatus* elicited dual skin test reactions on skin challenge, and pulmonary infiltrations appeared after inhaled challenge in monkeys passively sensitized with sera from patients with ABPA if the sera had precipitins against *Aspergillus* species but not if the sera had specific IgE but no precipitins.[42] Studies[11] confirm that *Aspergillus* precipitins are commonly of considerable diagnostic usefulness.

The production of precipitins is not entirely genetic; in some monozygotic twins, only one developed precipitins.[43] Part of the mechanism of producing the syndrome may just be excessive dose because in some situations,[5] subjects who apparently did not even have asthma developed ABPA when they were constantly exposed to *Aspergillus*-rich material. Even invasive aspergillosis has been described in nonimmunocompromised hosts.[44] The small spore size[3] (2 μ) makes it readily inhalable into the lung. Some clustering of cases has been reported: Maguire et al[45] described five acute cases of ABPA seen over 4 months in a single center. This could be explained by high exposure to *Aspergillus* organisms resulting either from external environmental reasons or from contamination of medical equipment.

Study of bronchoalveolar lavage fluid[35] in patients with infection indicates highly significant elevations of both IgE- and IgA-specific antibodies against *A. fumigatus* when compared with controls. There was a 48-fold greater concentration of specific IgE in the bronchoalveolar lavage fluid and a 96-fold greater concentration of IgA antibody specific for *A. fumigatus* than in serum, implying that locally produced specific antibodies are relevant in the disease. Although this is true of the specific antibody response, the nonspecific stimulatory effect of the fungal infection on the total serum IgE concentration does not seem to be entirely mediated from the local reaction because the ratio of total IgE to albumin in the serum approximately equalled that found in the bronchoalveolar lavage fluid. Total serum IgE and *Aspergillus*-specific IgE levels are useful measurements of disease activity, although some suggest that the total serum IgE level is a more significant marker of disease activity if it is elevated. However, Forsyth et al[46] found that 35 of 50 patients with cystic fibrosis had IgG antibodies to *Aspergillus* species. The progressive fall in the 1-second forced expiratory volume in their series was associated with a rise in the level of IgG antibodies, as was increasing age. In that series, there was no relationship between total IgE levels and disease progression; only 19% of patients had IgE antibodies to *Aspergillus* species in the serum, and only 24% had raised total serum IgE levels. No relationship was found between specific IgE antibodies and the progression of lung disease in cystic fibrosis.[46] IgE and IgG have been reported to be cytophilic for human basophils.[3,31]

The levels of IgA antibodies specific for *A. fumigatus* are markedly elevated in the serum and bronchoalveolar fluid in acute disease, during exacerbations, and during the fibrotic stage of ABPA; these antibodies could be involved in the pathogenesis of the infection.[47] Another diagnostic method includes the immunoprint pattern of the serum of patients with ABPA.[48] This technique showed strong IgE responses against more *A. fumigatus* components in acute exacerbation and sometimes in the fibrotic stage. The IgE antibody pattern was less complex and less strong when the patient was receiving corticosteroid treatment or when the condition was in natural remission. The pattern of IgG antibodies was said to resemble that of the IgE antibodies but did not as clearly allow discrimination between the different disease stages.

The best method for testing serum precipitins to permit a rapid serodiagnosis of ABPA was examined by Chaturvedi et al.[49] Counterimmunoelectrophoresis seemed more efficacious than Wadsworth's gel diffusion or Auchterlony's double diffusion, assuming that IgE and precipitating antibodies are the immunopathologic mediators of the reaction that occurs principally in the lumen and on the surface of epithelial cells. In fact, *A. fumigatus* could directly produce damage without immune mediation. For instance, the major *Aspergillus* allergen, Asp f I, is a potent inhibitor of eukaryotic protein synthesis,[50] and this could selectively modify antibody synthesis. An *A. fumigatus* proteinase can directly induce human epithelial cell detachment.[51] Schonheyder[20] finds antibodies to the catalase of the *A. fumigatus* even in patients with asymptomatic cystic fibrosis. It is probable that these or other enzymes directly produce some component of the damage of ABPA.

MANAGEMENT

Corticosteroids (prednisolone) remain the treatment of choice with suggested courses of 0.5 mg/kg daily in the morning for 2 weeks reduced to 0.5 mg/kg on alternate days.[10,35] There is debate about the necessary duration of therapy in both adult and pediatric patients. Capewell et al[36] found that 186 episodes of pulmonary eosinophilia in 65 patients treated with short-course steroids for a mean follow-up of 12 years showed that 65% had complete clearing of the lungs. Despite a total follow-up of 897 patients years, this report suggested that prospective studies were urgently needed. There is no doubt that episodes of chest infiltrates may occur without symptoms, but exacerbations are said to be diagnosable via the identification of elevated total serum IgE levels.[35] The decline in total IgE levels and in eosinophilia after the oral administration of steroids can be used as an indication to taper treatment.[32] Those who receive continuous steroid therapy have significantly fewer (asymptomatic) recurrences than those who do not.[29] Even in adult practice the need for steroid therapy is debated; for instance, five patients followed for a total of 83 years from the time of diagnosis each required less than one self-administered oral steroid course per year, perhaps because of the regularly administered inhaled corticosteroids.[52]

In pediatric practice, the debate is more intense; in a follow-up of seven patients with ABPA complicating cystic fibrosis, the morbidity rate was no greater in those with ABPA than in the rest of the population, although only two of the seven received oral corticosteroid treatment.[17] In an 11-year prospective follow-up of 46 pediatric patients with cystic fibrosis who were not treated with oral corticosteroids, there was no relationship between the decline in respiratory function and immediate cutaneous hypersensitivity to *A. fumigatus*.[37] It has also been reported that oral corticosteroids are of overall benefit in children with cystic fibrosis without reference to the presence or absence of ABPA[53]; indeed short courses of corticosteroids have been reported to be of benefit in children with cystic fibrosis who specifically did not have the airway reactivity regarded as essential for the diagnosis of ABPA.[54] It would be reasonable to follow the schedule suggested by Rosenberg et al[10] as subsequently modified by Wang et al[32] until the lung lesions no longer appear on the chest radiograph. That paper[32] states that the occurrence of asthma symptoms did not correlate well with exacerbations of ABPA proved on radiograph. The recommended regimen is illustrated in Box 51-3.

The administration of beclomethasone dipropionate via inhalation did not apparently reduce the frequency of the ABPA attacks.[32] A total of 12 of 25 patients followed for an average of 2.6 years had a recurrence. Seaton[52] quoted a similar recurrence rate for patients with ABPA who were treated with inhaled steroids. Nevertheless, a prospective follow-up of children in New Zealand found that a positive skin prick test for *Aspergillus* species was an independent significant risk factor for asthma attacks.[39] Safirstein et al[29] also suggested that daily doses of at least 7.5 mg of prednisone are required to prevent fresh infiltrations and that disodium cromoglycate had no effect. Clinicians generally watch for relapse by monitoring total serum IgE levels and chest radiographs. A total of 6 months of steroid therapy on this regimen[32] does not convert a positive precipitin test to a negative one.[1]

The well-described complications of oral corticosteroid therapy may occur in ABPA. In a study of 15 patients with cystic fibrosis and ABPA who were treated with oral prednisolone, subcapsular cataracts developed in two.[55] The researchers could not identify any significant risk factors for this complication, but a prednisone dosage higher than 40 mg/day for longer than 2 months in young patients appeared to be relevant. This suggests that the more modest maximum dosage of the regi-

BOX 51-3
Suggested Protocol for Managing ABPA

Initial therapy after diagnosis

Prednisone, 0.5 mg/kg, is administered as a single daily dose for 2 weeks and then every other day. (Occasionally, longer daily dose therapy is required for complete clearing of chest radiographs.)

Prednisone is continued at 0.5 mg/kg every other day for 3 months and then is tapered and discontinued during a 3-month period.

After initial clearing of lung lesions as determined by radiograph, repeated chest films are obtained every 4 months for 2 years, then every 6 months for 2 years, and then annually if no exacerbations occur.

A total serum IgE concentration is obtained monthly. A decrease in the IgE concentration appears in 1 to 2 months, and a plateau occurs after 6 months. A significant increase in the total IgE level suggests the presence of asymptomatic infiltrates or a subsequent recurrence of infiltrates and is thus an indication for the resumption of prednisone therapy, even in the absence of symptoms.

After 2 years of observation without evidence of recurrences, a total serum IgE concentration is obtained every 2 months.

Determinations of pulmonary function are made at every visit for at least a year.

Recurrence of ABPA involves resumption of this regimen at the beginning.

Modified from Wang JLF et al: *Am Rev Respir Dis* 120:87-92, 1979.

men of Wang et al[32] (0.5 mg/kg for 2 weeks initially) should be followed.

Regimens for invasive aspergillosis might seem logical, but they are toxic. Thus intravenous amphotericin B remains the standard treatment for invasive bronchopulmonary aspergillosis but is very toxic. Other triazole compounds such as fluconazole, itraconazole, and 5-fluorocytosine, which are being trailed for invasive aspergillosis, may eventually generate suitable compounds for the treatment of ABPA. Natamycin and nystatin, which are also thought to have some value in the therapy for invasive aspergillosis, could likewise lead to a new treatment. A potentially useful method of delivery is likely to be by liposomal intravenous administration, and itraconazole has been successfully used in this way in an animal model.[56] Ketoconazole has efficacy in the treatment of ABPA because it reduced the concentrations of specific serum IgG and the severity symptoms in a double-blind, placebo-controlled trial.[57] Bronchoscopic clearance may occasionally be required and should be particularly effective in the presence of bronchocentric granulomatosis.[4]

REFERENCES

1. Patterson R, Greenberger PA, Castile RG, Yee WFH, Roberts M: Diagnostic problems in hypersensitivity lung disease, *Allergy Proc* 10:141-147, 1989.
2. Winter JH, Milroy R, Stevenson RD, Hunter J: Secondary amyloidosis in association with *Aspergillus* lung disease, *Br J Dis Chest* 80:400-403, 1986.
3. Citron KM: Respiratory fungus allergy and infection, *Proc Roy Soc Med* 68:587-591, 1975.
4. Geddes DC: Pulmonary eosinophilia, *J Roy Coll Phys* 20:139-145, 1986.
5. Hinson KFW, Moon AJ, Plummer NJ: Bronchopulmonary aspergillosis: a review and a report of eight new cases, *Thorax* 7:317-333, 1952.
6. Pepys J, Riddell RW, Citron KM, Clayton YM, Syort EM: Clinical and immunological significance of *Aspergillus fumigatus* in the sputum, *Am Rev Respir Dis* 80:167-180, 1959.
7. Longbottom JL, Pepys J: Pulmonary aspergillosis: diagnostic and immunological significance of antigens and C-substance in *Aspergillus fumigatus, J Pathol Bact* 88:141-151, 1964.
8. McCarthy DS, Pepys J: Allergic bronchopulmonary aspergillosis, *J Clin Allergy* 1:415-432, 1971.
9. Mearns M, Young W, Batten J: Transient pulmonary infiltrations in cystic fibrosis due to allergic aspergillosis, *Thorax* 20:385-392, 1965.

Diagnosis

10. Rosenberg M, Patterson R, Mintzer MD, Cooper BJ, Roberts M, Harris KE: Clinical and immunological criteria for the diagnosis of allergic bronchopulmonary aspergillosis, *Ann Intern Med* 86:404-415, 1977.
11. Faux JA, Shale DJ, Lane DJ: Precipitins and specific IgE antibody to *Aspergillus fumigatus* in a chest unit population, *Thorax* 47:48-52, 1992.
12. Turner ES, Greenberger PA, Sider L: Complexities of establishing an early diagnosis of allergic bronchopulmonary aspergillosis in children, *Allergy Proc* 10:63-69, 1989.
13. Mendelson EB, Fisher MR, Mintzer RA, Halwig JM, Greenberger PA: Roentgenographic and clinical staging of allergic bronchopulmonary aspergillosis, *Chest* 87:334-339, 1985.
14. Katz R, Kniker WT: Infantile hypersensitivity pneumonitis as a reaction to organic antigens, *N Engl J Med* 28:233-237, 1973.
15. Silverman M, Hobbs FDR, Gordon IRS, Carswell F: Cystic fibrosis, atopy and airways lability, *Arch Dis Child* 53:873-877, 1978.
16. Nelson LA, Callerame ML, Schwartz R: Aspergillosis and atopy in cystic fibrosis, *Am Rev Respir Dis* 120:863-873, 1979.
17. Brueton MJ, Ormerod LP, Shah KJ, Anderson CM: Allergic bronchopulmonary aspergillosis complicating cystic fibrosis in childhood, *Arch Dis Child* 55:348-355, 1980.
18. Hiller EJ: Pathogenesis and management of aspergillosis in cystic fibrosis, *Arch Dis Child* 65(4):397-398, 1990.
19. Simmonds EJ, Littlewood JM, Evans EGV: Cystic fibrosis and allergic bronchopulmonary aspergillosis, *Arch Dis Child* 65(5):507-511, 1990.
20. Schonheyder H: Clinical and serological survey of pulmonary aspergillosis in patients with cystic fibrosis, *Int Arch Allergy Appl Immunol* 85:474-477, 1988.
21. Chetty A, Bhargava S, Jain RK: Allergic bronchopulmonary aspergillosis in Indian children with bronchial asthma, *Ann Allergy* 54:46-49, 1985.
22. Patterson R, Greenberger PA, Halwig JM, Liotta JL, Roberts M: Allergic bronchopulmonary aspergillosis: natural history and classification of early disease by serologic and roentgenographic studies, *Arch Intern Med* 146:916-918, 1986.
23. Seaton A, Robertson MD: *Aspergillus,* asthma and amoeba, *Lancet* 1:893-894, 1989.
24. Zeaske R, Bruns WT, Fink JN, Greenberger PA, Colby H, Liotta JL, Roberts M: Immune responses to *Aspergillus* in cystic fibrosis, *J Allergy Clin Immunol* 82:73-77, 1988.
25. Hutcheson PS, Rejent AJ, Slavin RG: Variability in parameters of allergic bronchopulmonary aspergillosis in patients with cystic fibrosis, *J Allergy Clin Immunol* 88:390-394, 1991.
26. McCarthy S, Simon G, Hargreave FE: The radiological appearances in allergic bronchopulmonary aspergillosis, *Clin Radiol* 21:366-375, 1970.
27. Robinson AE, Campbell JB: Bronchography in childhood asthma, *Am J Radiol* 116:559-566, 1972.
28. Currie DC, Goldman JM, Cole PJ, Strickland B: Comparison of narrow section computed tomography and plain chest radiography in chronic allergic bronchopulmonary aspergillosis, *Clin Radiol* 38:593-596, 1987.
29. Safirstein BH, D'Souza MF, Simon G, Tai EH-C, Pepys J: Five year follow-up of allergic bronchopulmonary aspergillosis, *Am Rev Respir Dis* 108:450-459, 1973.
30. Nichols D, Dopico GA, Braun S, Imbeau S, Peters ME, Rankin J: Acute and chronic pulmonary function changes in allergic bronchopulmonary aspergillosis, *Am J Med* 67:631-637, 1979.
31. Bardana EJ Jr, Gerber JD, Craig S, Cianciulli FD: The general and specific humoral immune response to pulmonary aspergillosis, *Am Rev Respir Dis* 112:797-805, 1975.
32. Wang JLF, Patterson R, Roberts M, Ghory AC: The management of allergic bronchopulmonary aspergillosis, *Am Rev Respir Dis* 120:87-92, 1979.

Prognosis

33. Marsh DG, Meyers DA, Bias WB: The epidemiology and genetics of atopic allergy, *N Engl J Med* 305(26):1551-1559, 1981.
34. Imbeau SA, Nichols D, Flaherty D, Dickie H, Reed C: Relationships between prednisone therapy, disease activity, and the total serum IgE level in allergic bronchopulmonary aspergillosis, *J Allergy Clin Immunol* 62:91-95, 1978.

35. Greenberger PA: Allergic bronchopulmonary aspergillosis and fungoses, *Clin Chest Med* 9:599-608, 1988.
36. Capewell S, Chapman BJ, Alexander F, Greening AP, Crompton GK: Corticosteroid treatment and prognosis in pulmonary eosinophilia, *Thorax* 44:925-929, 1989.
37. Hamilton A, Carswell F: The prevalence of cutaneous hypersensitivity and its relationship to *Pseudomonas* colonisation and outcome in cystic fibrosis, *Clin Exp Allergy* 20:415-420, 1990.
38. Slavin RG: Allergic bronchopulmonary aspergillosis, *Clin Rev Allergy* 3:167-182, 1985.
39. Sears MR, Herbison GP, Holdaway MD, Hewitt CJ, Flannery EM, Silva PA: The relative risks of sensitivity to grass pollen, house dust mite and cat dander in the development of childhood asthma, *Clin Exp Allergy* 19:419-424, 1989.

Pathogenesis

40. Sulavik SB: Bronchocentric granulomatosis and allergic bronchopulmonary aspergillosis, *Clin Chest Med* 9:609-621, 1988.
41. Bosken CH, Myers JL, Greenberger PA, Katzenstein AL: Pathologic features of allergic bronchopulmonary aspergillosis, *Am J Surg Pathol* 12:216-222, 1988.
42. Goldbert TM, Patterson R: Pulmonary allergic aspergillosis, *Ann Intern Med* 72:395-403, 1970.
43. Starke ID: Asthma and allergic aspergillosis in monozygotic twins, *Br J Dis Chest* 79:295-300, 1985.
44. Karam GH, Griffin FM: Invasive pulmonary aspergillosis in non-immunocompromised, non-neutrophilic hosts, *Rev Infect Dis* 8:357-363, 1988.
45. Maguire S, Moriarty P, Tempany E, Fitzgerald M: Unusual clustering of allergic bronchopulmonary aspergillosis and cystic fibrosis, *Pediatrics* 82:835-839, 1988.
46. Forsyth KD, Hohmann AW, Martin AJ, Bradley J: IgG antibodies to *Aspergillus fumigatus* in cystic fibrosis: a laboratory correlate of disease activity, *Arch Dis Child* 63:953-957, 1988.
47. Gutt L, Greenberger PA, Liotta JL: Serum IgA antibodies to *Aspergillus fumigatus* in various stages of allergic bronchopulmonary aspergillosis, *J Allergy Clin Immunol* 78:98-101, 1986.
48. Baur X, Weiss W, Jarusch B, Menz G, Schoch C, Schmitz-Schumann M, Virchow C: Immunoprint pattern in patients with allergic bronchopulmonary aspergillosis in different stages, *J Allergy Clin Immunol* 83:839-844, 1989.
49. Chaturvedi VP, Chaturvedi S, Khan ZU, Rhandhawa HS: Efficacy of immunoprecipitation methods for rapid serodiagnosis of allergic bronchopulmonary aspergillosis, *Mycoses* 32:136-138, 1989.
50. Arruda LK, Platts-Mills TAE, Longbottom JL, El-Dahr JM, Chapman MD: *Aspergillus fumigatus:* identification of 16, 18, and 45 kd antigens recognised by human IgG and IgE antibodies and murine monoclonal antibodies, *J Allergy Clin Immunol* 89:1166-1176, 1992.
51. Robinson BWS, Venaille TJ, Mendis AHW, McAleer R: Allergens as proteases: an *Aspergillus fumigatus* proteinase directly induces human epithelial cell detachment, *J Allergy Clin Immunol* 86(5):726-731, 1990.

Management

52. Seaton A: How progressive is bronchopulmonary aspergillosis? *Thorax* 47:854, 1992 (abstract).
53. Auerbach HS, Williams M, Kirkpatrick JA, Colten HR: Alternate-day prednisolone reduces morbidity and improves pulmonary function in cystic fibrosis, *Lancet* 2:686-688, 1985.
54. Greally P, Sampson AP, Piper PJ, Price JF: *Prednisolone reduces airways constriction in children with cystic fibrosis.* Paper presented at the International Cystic Fibrosis Congress, Dublin, 1992, p TS12.
55. Majure M, Mroueh S, Spock A: Risk factors for the development of posterior subcapsular cataracts in patients with cystic fibrosis and allergic bronchopulmonary aspergillosis treated with corticosteroids, *Paediatr Pulmonol* 6:260-262, 1989.
56. Conte PL, Joly V, Saint-Julien L, Gillardin J-M, Carbon C, Yeni P: Tissue distribution and antifungal effect of liposomal itraconazole in experimental cryptococcosis and pulmonary aspergillosis, *Am Rev Respir Dis* 145:424-429, 1992.
57. Shale DJ, Faux JA, Lane DJ: Trial of ketoconazole in non-invasive pulmonary aspergillosis, *Thorax* 42:26-31, 1987.

CHAPTER 52

Collagen Vascular Disorders

Jeff S. Wagener, J. Roger Hollister, and Thomas C. Hay

Collagen vascular diseases (CVDs) include many illnesses that have autoimmune bases.[1] Although no separation is ideal, for the purpose of this chapter, these diseases are divided into the rheumatic diseases (Box 52-1), vasculitic diseases (Box 52-2), and other inflammatory diseases (Reiter's syndrome and inflammatory bowel disease). Expression of these diseases is rarely seen in a familial pattern, and they are all felt to represent an abnormal reaction by the immune system toward a variety of yet unidentified environmental factors.

DISEASE MECHANISMS

Pulmonary abnormalities in patients with CVDs can be divided into three groups. First, patients with CVDs are at an increased risk for infections, both because of their primary disease and because of disease secondary to immunosuppressive therapy.[2,3] Opportunistic infections must always be considered first when a CVD patient has respiratory symptoms. Cough and sputum production are particularly important signs that suggest infection. Although all potential infecting organisms should be considered, particular attention should be paid to cytomegalovirus, *E. coli,* α-hemolytic streptococci, *Klebsiella* and *Aerobacter* species, *Legionella pneumophila, Candida albicans, Aspergillus* species, and *Pneumocystis carinii.*[2-5]

Second, pulmonary disease as a complication of potent pharmacotherapies often must be considered. In addition to general immunosuppression, many of the medications used to treat CVDs have selective harmful effects on the lung. Both penicillamine and gold can produce hypersensitivity pneumonitis and occasionally, bronchiolitis obliterans.[5-9] In addition, penicillamine has been associated with acute pulmonary hemorrhage, alveolar and interstitial fibrosis, and a pulmonary and renal syndrome similar to Goodpasture's.[10] Methotrexate can produce an acute pneumonitis as well as pulmonary fibro-

BOX 52-1
Pediatric Rheumatic Diseases Affecting the Pulmonary System

Juvenile rheumatoid arthritis
Systemic lupus erythematosus
Progressive systemic sclerosis (scleroderma)
Polymyositis and dermatomyositis
Mixed connective tissue disease
Ankylosing spondylitis
Sjögren's syndrome

BOX 52-2
Pediatric Vasculitic Diseases Affecting the Pulmonary System

- Granulomatous vasculitis
  - Wegener's granulomatosis
  - Churg-Strauss syndrome (allergic granulomatosis)
  - Lymphomatoid granulomatosis
- Leukocytoclastic vasculitis
  - Henoch-Schönlein purpura (anaphylactoid purpura)
  - Hypersensitivity vasculitis
- Polyarteritis
  - Kawasaki disease
  - Polyarteritis nodosa
- Giant cell arteritis
  - Takayasu's arteritis
- Other
  - Behçet's disease
  - Erythema nodosum

Table 52-1 Pulmonary Manifestations of CVDs in Childhood

DISEASE	CW	DD	PPE	ILD	LIP	VAS	PHTN	AIP	DAH	BO	AW	OTHER
Rheumatic diseases												
Juvenile rheumatoid arthritis	+	−	++	±	w/SS		±	+	±	−	±	+
Systemic lupus erythematosus	−	++	++	++	w/SS	+	+	+++	++	±	−	
Progressive systemic sclerosis	±	−	+	+++	w/SS	++	+	−	−	+	−	
Dermatomyositis/polymyositis	++	+	−	+	−	−	+	+	−	+	+	+++
Mixed connective tissue disease	−	±	++	+	−	±	++	±	+	±	−	
Ankylosing spondylitis		++	−	±	+	−	−	−	−	−	−	−
Sjögren's syndrome	−	−	+	+	++	−	−	−	−	−		
Vasculitic diseases												
Wegener's granulomatosis	−	−	+	−	−	++	−	−	++	−	+	+
Churg-Strauss syndrome	−	−	−	−	−	++	−	−	−	−	+++	+
Henoch-Schönlein purpura	−	−	−	−	−	+	−	−	+	−	−	
Kawasaki disease	−	−	+	+	−	++	−	−	−	−	−	
Polyarteritis nodosa	±	−	−	−	−	+	−	−	−	−	−	+
Behçet's disease	−	−	−	−	−	+	−	−	+	−	−	+

CW, Chest wall disease; *DD,* diaphragm dysfunction; *PPE,* pleuritis and/or pleural effusion; *VAS,* vasculitis; *PHTN,* pulmonary arterial hypertension; *AIP,* acute immunologic pneumonia; *DAH,* diffuse alveolar hemorrhage; *BO,* bronchiolitis obliterans; *AW,* airway disease; *other,* aspiration, atelectasis, granulomas, thrombosis; *w/SS,* with Sjögren's syndrome.

sis.[11-13] In sensitive individuals, salicylates and nonsteroidal antiinflammatory drugs produce bronchoconstriction. Typically, affected patients have moderate to severe asthma and nasal polyps or sinusitis.[14] Antiinflammatory drugs have also been related to acute noncardiogenic pulmonary edema and hypersensitivity pneumonitis, although this is rare.[11,12]

Third, all CVDs manifest a degree of chronic systemic inflammation. Tissue damage can result from numerous products of inflammation, including hydrolases, collagenases, neutral proteases, and elastase. Because the lungs have a rich vascular supply and are constantly exposed to environmental stimuli over a large surface area, they are vulnerable to systemic diseases involving circulating immune complexes, biochemical mediators, and local tissue responses to antigens. Most of the severe pulmonary complications of CVDs have been described primarily in adults.[5] However, pediatric patients may occasionally be affected, and more important, some of the more insidious processes may begin in childhood.[2] Whether early identification of these complications might prevent their progression is unknown.

Lung disease in patients with CVD can involve virtually every part of the respiratory system, including the chest wall, diaphragm, pleura and pleural space, interstitium, pulmonary vasculature, alveoli, and airways (Table 52-1). Chest wall disease is usually related to muscle weakness, as occurs with polymyositis,[15] or to skeletal rigidity, as with ankylosing spondylitis.[16] These complications are rare in children. Muscle weakness may also represent a complication of steroid therapy.[17]

Diaphragm dysfunction and basilar lung atelectasis occur with systemic lupus erythematosus (SLE) in both adults and children.[18-21] This "shrinking lung" syndrome is rarely disabling or progressive if the primary disease is adequately treated. Studies of lung mechanics demonstrate inspiratory and expiratory muscle weakness with decreased transdiaphragmatic pressures.[20]

Pleurisy and pleural effusions are particular problems in patients with SLE but also occur in children with rheumatoid arthritis.[21-23] Pleural effusions are usually bilateral exudates, although a unilateral exudate can occur (Fig. 52-1) and result from a localized intrapleural immunologic reaction. When effusions present acutely, they should always be evaluated for a possible infectious etiology. If the effusions are due to CVD, then antiinflammatory treatment for the primary disease results in resolution without any resulting fibrosis or restrictive changes.

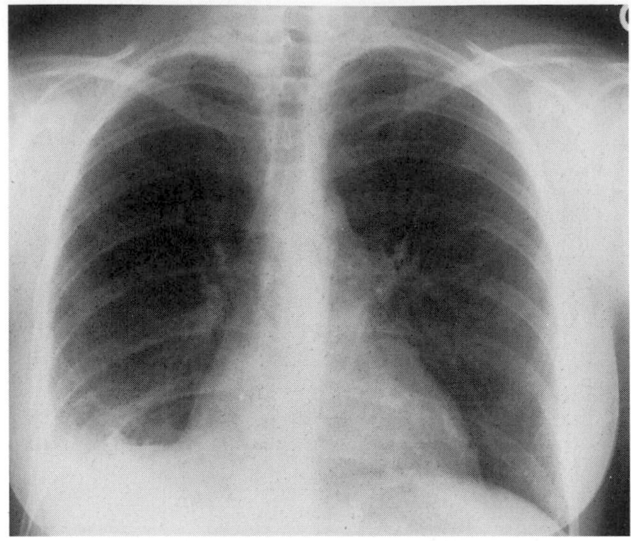

Fig. 52-1. Patient with SLE, right pleural effusion, and blunting of the right costophrenic sulcus plus partial right lower lobe atelectasis.

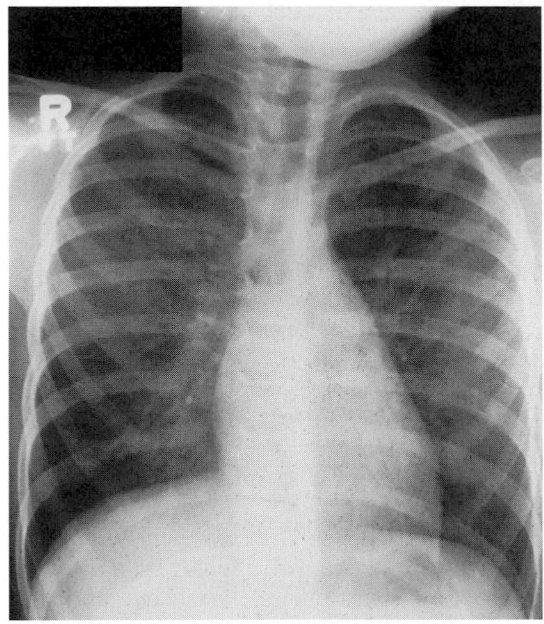

Fig. 52-2. Patient with Wegener's granulomatosis and a poorly defined diffuse reticular nodular infiltrate, which probably represents distal airspace as well as interstitial disease. The initial presentation in this young child was felt to be "idiopathic" pulmonary hemosiderosis.

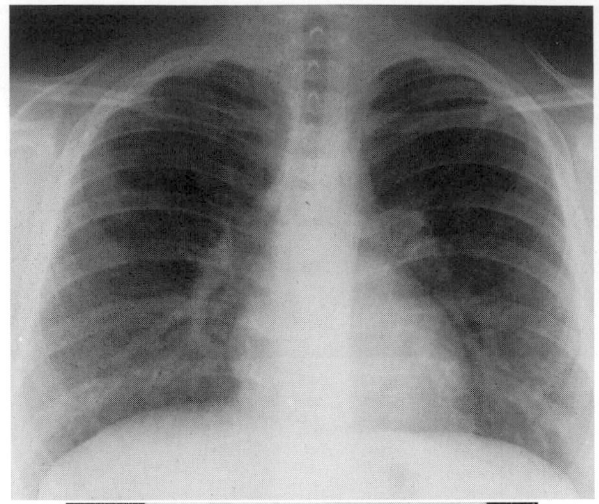

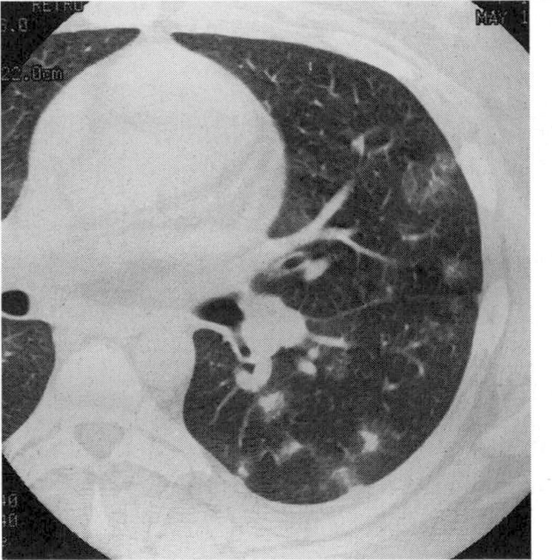

Fig. 52-3. Churg-Strauss syndrome. **A,** Minimal changes on chest radiograph. **B,** High-resolution computed tomogram provides a clearer demonstration of the multiple poorly defined, patchy areas of consolidation caused by hemorrhage and vascular exudate.

Interstitial lung disease (ILD) can complicate any of the CVDs (Fig. 52-2). This interstitial pneumonitis begins early in the disease process, when the terminal airways and alveolar walls are infiltrated with inflammatory cells (mononuclear cells with occasional neutrophils and eosinophils),[24] probably because of immune complex deposition and alveolar macrophage activation. With progressive disease, cytokines, particularly transforming growth factor-β, are released and activate gene expression, resulting in collagen deposition.[25] The result, which is rarely seen in children, is extensive fibrosis and honeycomb lung. A different pathologic picture seen in Sjögren's syndrome is lymphocytic interstitial pneumonitis (LIP).[26] With LIP, there is a dense infiltrate of lymphoplasmacytic cells that are within the alveolar walls and that fill the alveolar spaces. The interstitial infiltrates in LIP do not show the heterogeneous cell types seen with the more common interstitial pneumonitis. LIP can have associated amyloid deposition, lymphoid follicles, and giant cells.

Vasculitis is the identifying pathologic finding of the various vasculitides and is also seen in SLE. The primary disease process of most vasculitides is the deposition of intermediate-size immune complexes (type III immunologic reaction) in vessel walls.[27] Neutrophils adhere to the endothelium, producing a microangiitis of the arterioles and small muscular arteries. Vessel wall disruption can then occur from the release of neutrophil enzymes, leading to patchy alveolar hemorrhage and adjacent lung necrosis (Fig. 52-3). Capillaritis can also develop from neutrophil infiltration of the adjacent alveolar walls. This can result in necrosis of the alveolar wall and capillaries, resulting in diffuse alveolar hemorrhage.[24]

Pulmonary arterial hypertension can occur either as a problem secondary to hypoxic vasoconstriction related to pulmonary fibrosis or as a primary problem, most commonly progressive systemic sclerosis (PSS, "scleroderma") and its variants, mixed

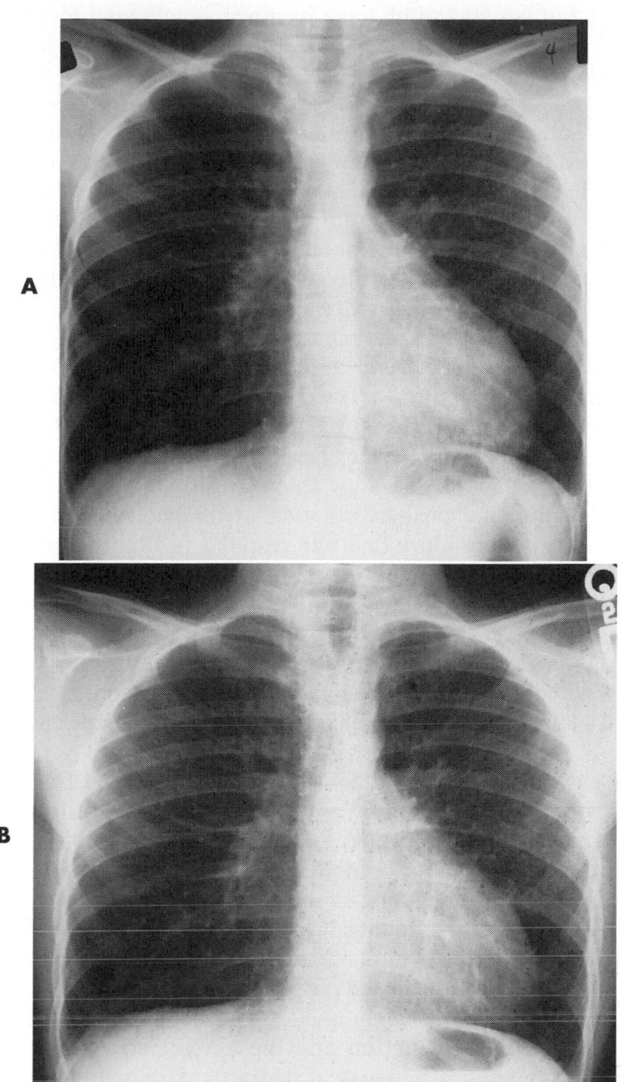

Fig. 52-4. SLE. **A,** Immunologic pneumonia with infiltrate in the retrocardiac left lower lobe. A small pleural effusion is present. This pneumonia is indistinguishable from acute infectious pneumonia. **B,** Rapid resolution of pneumonia with steroid therapy. Lupus pneumonitis is usually basilar, patchy, and lobar, consisting of poorly defined nodules.

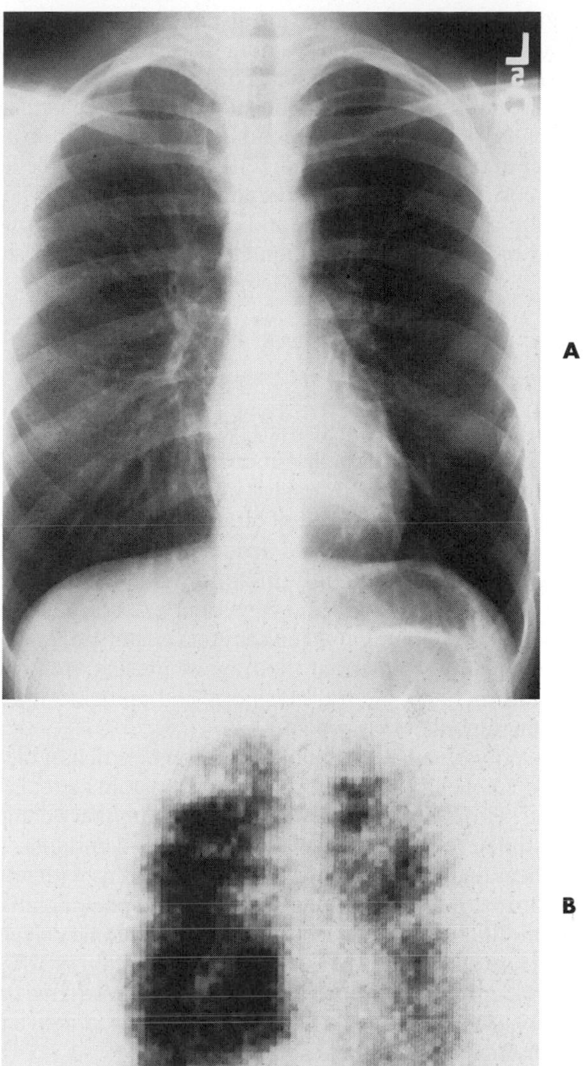

Fig. 52-5. Juvenile rheumatoid arthritis. **A,** Chest radiograph demonstrating a hyperlucent left lung with a paucity of pulmonary vasculature. **B,** Perfusion scintigraph showing a marked decrease in perfusion of the left lung and patchy perfusion of both lungs. This finding is consistent with bronchiolitis obliterans, although additional considerations include vasculitis and multiple pulmonary emboli.

connective tissue disease and the CREST syndrome (calcinosis, Raynaud's phenomenon, esophageal dysfunction, sclerodactyly, and telangiectasias). Pulmonary hypertension related to CVD is a primary plexogenic arteriopathy and is characterized by onion-skin proliferation of the intima with medial thickening of the arterioles and small muscular arteries of the lung. Eventually, luminal obliteration occurs. Inflammation and vessel wall necrosis are not present. Pulmonary arterial hypertension may also be related to pulmonary arteriolar thrombosis caused by circulating anticoagulants or increased pulmonary vasoreactivity.[29]

Acute immunologic pneumonia is occasionally the presenting problem in CVDs and is most common in SLE[19,21] (Fig. 52-4). Pathologically, there is diffuse alveolar damage with mixed interstitial inflammatory cellular deposits, interstitial edema, and fibrin deposition. Red blood cells and hyaline membranes are present in the alveoli.[30]

Diffuse alveolar hemorrhage is seen in SLE and is a possible, but rare, complication of any of the vasculitic diseases.[31] Unlike acute immunologic pneumonia, diffuse alveolar hemorrhage is most likely a complication in an already diagnosed condition and does not usually occur with pleural or pericardial disease. Pathologic findings vary from diffuse microangiitis and capillaritis to hemorrhage without vasculitis. Diagnosis is based on the clinical presentation of an acute infiltrate and a dropping hematocrit.

Bronchiolitis obliterans usually occurs in adults with rheumatoid arthritis and other CVDs[32] but may begin in childhood (Fig. 52-5). This is a progressive obstructive airway disease that follows inflammation and produces fibrous proliferation of the terminal bronchiolar walls. At the end, there is total obliteration of the airway lumina. Bronchiolitis obliterans with organizing pneumonia is a distinctly different condition that is seen primarily in adults.[24] Patients with this condition have histologic findings of inflammatory polyps produced by proliferating collagen bundles and acute and chronic inflammatory cells in the terminal and respiratory bronchioles. This organizing process extends into the alveolar spaces and produces a clinical picture of restrictive lung disease; the onset is often acute. This clinical presentation is distinctly different from that of bronchiolitis obliterans, which is chronic and obstructive.

Finally, airway disease occurs in a higher-than-expected number of patients with certain CVDs. Asthma may be related to the eosinophilic infiltrates seen in Churg-Strauss syndrome (allergic granulomatosis),[33] and endobronchial obstruction caused by granuloma formation can occur in other vasculitic diseases.[34]

CLINICAL MANIFESTATIONS

Rheumatic Diseases

Juvenile rheumatoid arthritis (JRA) is the most common CVD in children; although minor pulmonary complications are common, severe pulmonary involvement is rare.[23] JRA can present with four different clinical patterns, all of which have different prognoses and sequelae. Systemic-onset disease occurs most frequently in children under the age of 4 years and includes fever, an evanescent macular rash, arthritis, hepatosplenomegaly, leukocytosis, and polyserositis. Pulmonary involvement at the time of presentation is common and includes pleural effusions and an acute immunologic pneumonia.

The polyarticular pattern of JRA resembles that of the adult disease, frequently having a positive rheumatoid factor in older patients. However, clinically significant pulmonary complications similar to those seen in adults are rare in children. These complications include recurrent pleurisy with or without pleural effusion, pulmonary nodules, interstitial pneumonitis, and bronchiolitis obliterans (see Fig. 52-5). Pulmonary hypertension is rare and usually represents a complication of ILD. Pulmonary function abnormalities, including a restrictive pattern with abnormal diffusing capacity, were identified in two thirds of pediatric patients in one small study.[35]

Pauciarticular disease is characterized by chronic arthritis of only a few, usually large joints. Antinuclear antibodies are often present with negative rheumatoid factor. Systemic symptoms, except iridocyclitis, are uncommon. Although symptomatic pulmonary complications have not been described in children with this form of disease, abnormal carbon monoxide diffusion and small airway obstructive changes have been noted on pulmonary function evaluation.[35]

The fourth pattern of disease occurs in late childhood and is most common in HLA-B27–positive male patients. The presentation of this disease is similar to that of pauciarticular disease, but the condition progresses to include spinal and sacroiliac joint disease. Restrictive lung disease from chest wall complications and upper lobe infiltrates may occur.[2]

SLE is less common than JRA but is more likely to manifest as pulmonary disease in children.[19,36] This multisystem inflammatory disease is diagnosed by the presence of antinuclear antibodies during active or untreated disease. Life-threatening acute immunologic pneumonia can be the presenting manifestation of SLE. This is often difficult to distinguish from an infectious pneumonia; this separation is essential, however, because lupus immunologic pneumonia usually responds to corticosteroids (see Fig. 52-4). When steroids are not effective, other immunosuppressive medications or plasmapheresis may be needed.[37-39]

Pleuritis with or without effusion is relatively common in children with SLE[21] (see Fig. 52-1). Effusions are typically small, but patients often have dyspnea, cough, and fever in addition to pleuritic pain.[22] The painful nature of SLE-related pleuritis separates these pleural effusions from those caused by SLE-related renal disease. Pleural fluid usually has a normal glucose level and pH, helping to separate this condition from bacterial infection and JRA (which usually have low lupus erythematosus (LE) glucose).[40] A positive LE preparation in the pleural fluid is diagnostic, and high concentrations of anti-nuclear antibody are suggestive of SLE. Although double-stranded deoxyribonucleic acid in serum is specific for SLE, its presence in pleural fluid has been described in tuberculosis and pleural malignancies.[41]

ILD has been reported in children with SLE from both clinical and autopsy studies.[3,19] The clinical signs and symptoms of dyspnea, cough, and chest discomfort may be present, although the appearance of the chest radiograph may be normal. Pulmonary function tests may show a restrictive pattern with reduced diffusing capacity.[42] Patients with evidence of active inflammation are more likely to respond favorably to corticosteroid therapy than those with fibrosis.[5,42]

Alveolar hemorrhage may mimic acute immunologic pneumonia but typically occurs in patients with an already established diagnosis of SLE.[31] Separating this complication from an acute infectious pneumonia is important. An abrupt fall in hemoglobin values in combination with a new infiltrate and an increased diffusing capacity is highly suggestive.[43]

The most insidious pulmonary complication of SLE is the development of pulmonary arterial hypertension. Mild pulmonary arterial hypertension is common in adults and is associated with Raynaud's phenomenon and positive serum factors, including rheumatoid factor and the lupus anticoagulant.[44] Clinical signs include dyspnea at rest or with exertion. Echocardiography should be used to evaluate the pulmonary artery size and the estimated pulmonary artery pressure in the patient whose SLE is symptomatic.

Diaphragm dysfunction and the associated "shrinking lung" have been described in pediatric SLE patients.[19-21] Small airway obstruction has also been described, although no clinical correlate was noted.[5] Finally, SLE patients may experience upper airway obstruction caused by laryngeal involvement.[45,46]

PSS, also known as *scleroderma,* is a rare disease in pediatrics. Pulmonary and cardiac complications are common once the disease develops and occasionally can be responsible for death during childhood.[1] Although the pathogenesis is unclear, the clinical diagnosis is based on a skin disease that progresses from an edematous phase to an atrophic, taut, immobile dermis, plus a systemic disease, including arthralgias, renal disease, Raynaud's phenomenon, and pulmonary fibrosis.

Some 50% to 90% of adults with PSS develop ILD, eventually leading to death.[47] Patients have dyspnea on exertion and bibasilar crackles on examination. Radiographic changes include a diffuse reticulonodular interstitial infiltrate (Fig. 52-6) with progression to cystic changes and honeycomb lung.[48] Vasculitis progressing to pulmonary arterial hypertension has also been described in children with PSS.[28] Cor pulmonale can develop rapidly or can have a more insidious onset secondary to pulmonary fibrosis. Patients with the CREST syndrome are at greater risk of developing primary pulmonary vascular disease and should be monitored closely for signs of pulmonary arterial hypertension. Pulmonary function testing, including lung volumes, carbon monoxide diffusing capacity,

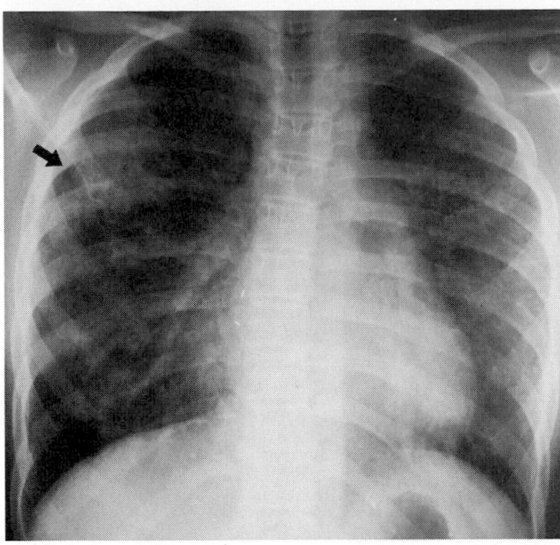

Fig. 52-6. Patient with PSS and a diffuse reticular nodular infiltrate. The spontaneous pneumothorax *(arrow)* is a known complication of this disease.

and the degree of oxygen desaturation with exercise, may be particularly helpful in detecting and monitoring the early effects of pulmonary restrictive and vascular complications.[49]

Polymyositis and dermatomyositis are characterized by a chronic myopathy with vasculitis involving the skin and muscles. The diagnosis requires the characteristic skin rash, symmetric proximal muscle weakness, elevated serum levels of muscle enzymes, a myopathic electromyogram, and in cases difficult to diagnose, a consistent muscle biopsy. The vasculitis seen in childhood dermatomyositis involves the small arteries and veins and differs pathologically from that seen in adult disease. Symptoms are uniquely responsive to corticosteroid therapy, and resolution is more frequent in children. This probably accounts for the relative lack of pulmonary complications in children.

Difficulty in swallowing related to the weakness of pharyngeal muscles and the resulting aspiration of food and saliva are the most worrisome complications.[50] Recurrent atelectasis may be present on chest radiographs. Patients also may develop progressive respiratory muscle weakness, leading to decreased cough efficiency and eventually ventilatory insufficiency.[15] Monitoring vital capacity and respiratory muscle strength may be beneficial.

Adults develop ILD associated with dermatomyositis. Most of these patients respond to corticosteroid therapy if fibrosis is absent on lung biopsy. How frequently this complication occurs in childhood dermatomyositis and whether early therapy can prevent fibrosis are unknown. The few reports of ILD occurring in childhood dermatomyositis suggest that the onset can be either acute or insidious, and usually there are clinical symptoms, including dyspnea, dry cough, and rarely, fever.[51,52] Chest radiographs may show diffuse infiltrates (Fig. 52-7), and the pulmonary disease may be complicated by pneumothoraces. One interesting pediatric case of pulmonary alveolar proteinosis complicating dermatomyositis has also been reported.[53]

Mixed connective tissue disease is a clinical syndrome with features similar to those of SLE, dermatomyositis, and PSS; it is associated with a circulating hemagglutinating antibody spe-

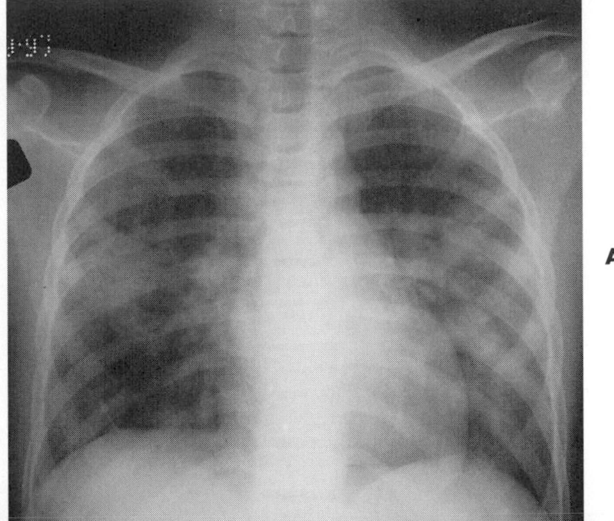

A

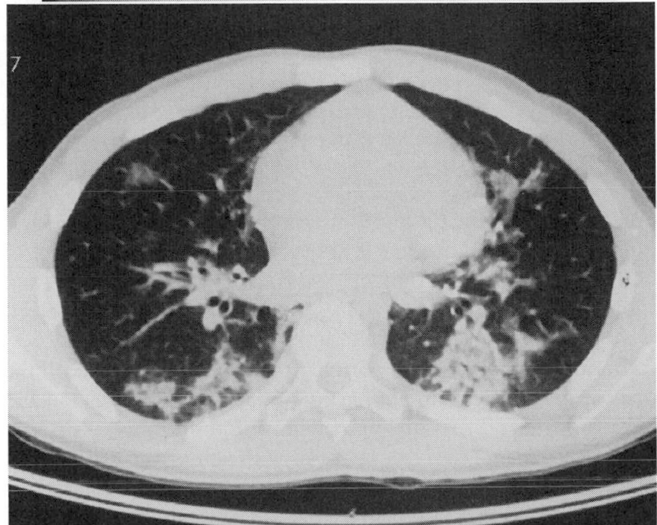

B

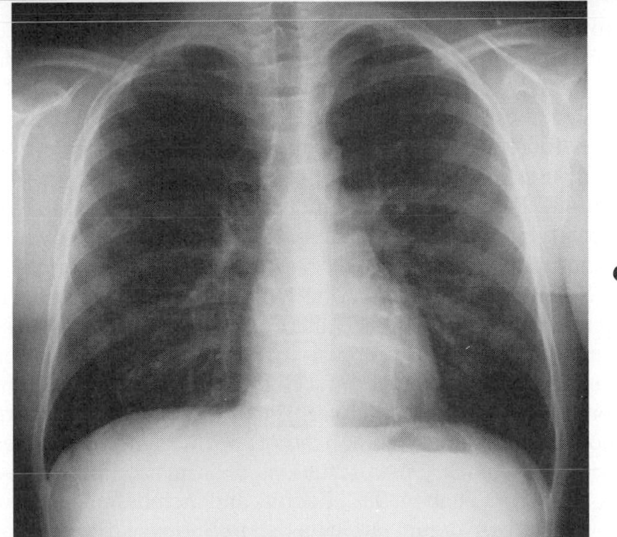

C

Fig. 52-7. Polymyositis and dermatomyositis. **A,** Diffuse, patchy alveolar infiltrates on chest radiograph. Organizing pneumonia was diagnosed by lung biopsy. **B,** High-resolution computed tomogram demonstrates the peripheral patchy nature of this infiltrate, which is consistent with organizing pneumonia. **C,** Complete resolution of pneumonia after steroid therapy.

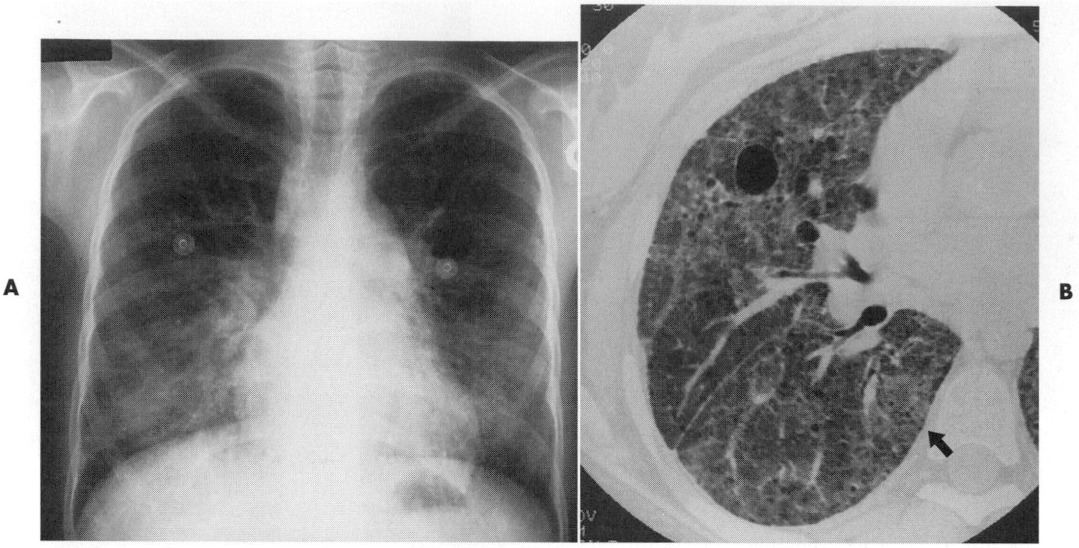

Fig. 52-8. Mixed connective tissue disease. **A,** Diffuse reticular nodular infiltrate on chest radiograph in a 16-year-old patient. **B,** High-resolution computed tomogram demonstrates diffuse ground-glass opacity with cystic and fibrotic changes. Bronchiolectasis is noted peripherally *(arrow)* and is better defined than on plain chest radiography.

cific for the ribonucleoprotein component of extractable nuclear antigen.[54] Pulmonary disease is a common finding in children with mixed connective tissue disease (Fig. 52-8) and includes pleural effusions, restrictive pulmonary function changes resulting from ILD, and pulmonary hypertension.[55] Pulmonary involvement is often clinically inapparent until the disease is relatively far advanced, and it is variably responsive to corticosteroid therapy.[56,57] Because the pulmonary disease can be severe and rapidly progressive in adults, the early use of cytotoxic agents is recommended in patients not responding adequately to corticosteroids.[58]

Ankylosing spondylitis is an inflammatory joint disease involving the spine and sacroiliac joints. Although pulmonary disease has not been reported in children, adults with ankylosing spondylitis may experience restrictive changes caused by limited chest wall expansion and upper lobe fibrobullous disease. Infection may complicate the clinical course of upper lobe bullae. Clinical symptoms are rare in the absence of infection.[5] Pulmonary function changes include a reduced vital capacity and total lung capacity with evidence of normal lung compliance.[16]

Sjögren's syndrome is often associated with other CVDs, including JRA, SLE, PSS, and dermatomyositis. The classic symptoms of keratoconjunctivitis sicca (dry eyes) and xerostomia (dry mouth) are produced by a lymphocytic inflammation of the exocrine glandular tissue. Little has been reported about the pulmonary complications of this syndrome in pediatrics.[59] Pulmonary manifestations of primary Sjögren's syndrome occurs in about 9% of adults and includes pleurisy with or without effusion, atelectasis, pulmonary fibrosis, and LIP.[26,60] Diffuse airway dryness ("xerotrachea") may be responsible for the dry cough and recurrent respiratory infections experienced by many of these patients.[5] Radiographic changes include diffuse reticular or reticulonodular infiltrates and bronchiectasis. LIP is a pathologic finding not seen with other CVDs in the absence of Sjögren's syndrome. The natural history of this process is variable and may be related to more malignant lymphoproliferative diseases in the lungs of adults with Sjögren's syndrome.[5,61]

Vasculitic Diseases

Wegener's granulomatosis is a diffuse, small-vessel vasculitis producing necrotizing granulomas, particularly in the respiratory and renal systems. Pediatric patients of all ages can be affected. Presenting symptoms include cough, fever, chronic sinusitis, epistaxis, arthralgias, vasculitic rash, hemoptysis, and hematuria or proteinuria.[62,63] Pulmonary disease may predate systemic symptoms and delay eventual diagnosis, particularly in patients with hemoptysis or "idiopathic" pulmonary hemosiderosis (see Fig. 52-2). Radiographic changes typically include bilateral nodular infiltrates, often with cavitation (Fig. 52-9). Other findings include pleural effusions, pleural thickening, migratory acute infiltrates, pneumothorax, and endobronchial granulomas producing atelectasis.[34] Diagnosis is confirmed with the identification of positive antineutrophil cytoplasmic antibodies, and rising titers may precede relapses.[64] Early initiation of vigorous therapy, including corticosteroids and cyclophosphamide, is important to reduce the major complication of focal glomerulonephritis and chronic renal failure.[65]

Churg-Strauss syndrome, or allergic angiitis and granulomatosis, is characterized by eosinophilia, fever, vasculitis, and asthma. The most common pulmonary manifestation is asthma, which usually predates the vasculitis. Patchy, nodular infiltrates (see Fig. 52-4) can occur in the lungs with rare cavitation[33] (Fig. 52-10). Histologic findings include eosinophilic pneumonia, necrotizing vasculitis, and granuloma formation.[66]

Henoch-Schönlein purpura, or anaphylactoid purpura, is one of the most common vasculitides in childhood. Henoch-Schönlein purpura is most common during the winter and is frequently preceded by an infection of the upper respiratory tract. There may also be a relationship with heterozygous C2 deficiency. Characteristic signs and symptoms include arthritis, arthralgia, abdominal pain, nephritis, and nonthrombocytopenic purpura. Pulmonary complications are rare, but a few cases of fatal alveolar hemorrhage have been reported.[67,68]

Kawasaki disease is a necrotizing arteritis seen most commonly in children. An infectious etiology is suspected, but no single organism has been identified. Presenting symptoms in-

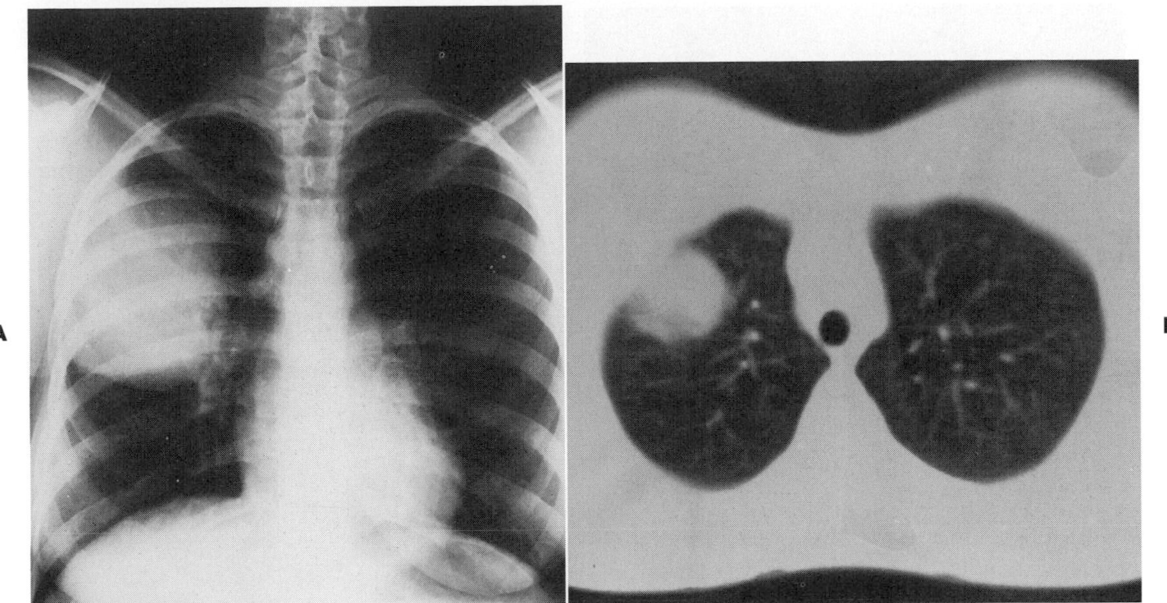

Fig. 52-9. Wegener's granulomatosis. **A,** Large mass in the right upper lobe extending from the hilum to the pleural surface. **B,** Chest computed tomogram showing the homogenous nature of the mass. Differential considerations included lobar pneumonia, inflammatory pseudotumor, and a mass of the chest wall. Wegener's granulomatosis was diagnosed on biopsy.

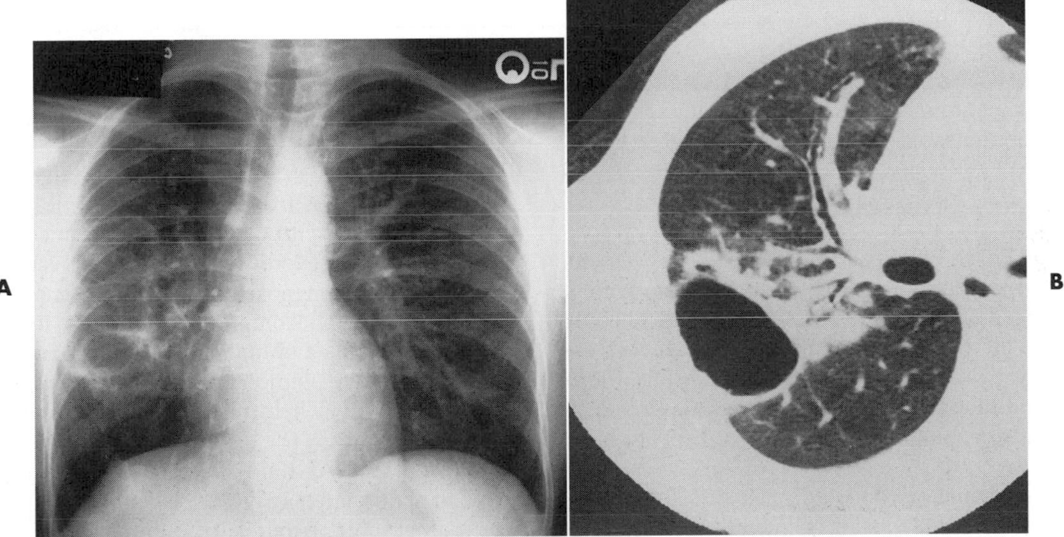

Fig. 52-10. Churg-Strauss syndrome. **A,** Large cavitary lesion in the peripheral lung with adjacent pleural thickening and volume loss of the right lung. **B,** Chest computed tomogram demonstrating bronchiectasis of the right middle lobe in addition to the cavitary lesion.

clude fever, conjunctivitis, lymph node enlargement, rash, "strawberry" tongue, and erythema of the palms or soles. Cough and respiratory distress have been occasionally reported,[69,70] and a review of chest radiographs demonstrated 15% with abnormalities, including reticulogranular infiltrates, peribronchial cuffing, pleural effusion, atelectasis, and air trapping.[71] In addition, cardiac involvement is frequent, with the most serious chronic complication being coronary artery aneurysm. Pulmonary edema secondary to heart failure can occur. Pathologic examination of the lungs often reveals interstitial pneumonia and pulmonary arteritis in fatal cases.

Polyarteritis nodosa is a multiorgan necrotizing vasculitis involving small to medium-sized muscular arteries.[72] Pulmonary manifestations are uncommon in children and include vasculitis, local thrombosis, and pulmonary edema secondary to cardiac and renal involvement.[73,74] The clinical onset of disease is usually insidious with unexplained fever and weight loss. Abdominal pain, central nervous system disease, arthritis, myalgia, and skin lesions eventually develop in most patients. Vascular thrombosis, necrosis, and aneurysms are seen in the kidneys, heart, and lungs.[72]

Behçet's disease is characterized by oral aphthous and genital ulcers plus relapsing iritis. The onset of disease can be insidious and prolonged. One patient only 2 months old has been described.[75] Pulmonary involvement has not been described in children. In adults, pulmonary complications can be serious and include pleural effusion, hemorrhage, vasculitis, aneurysms, and emboli.[76]

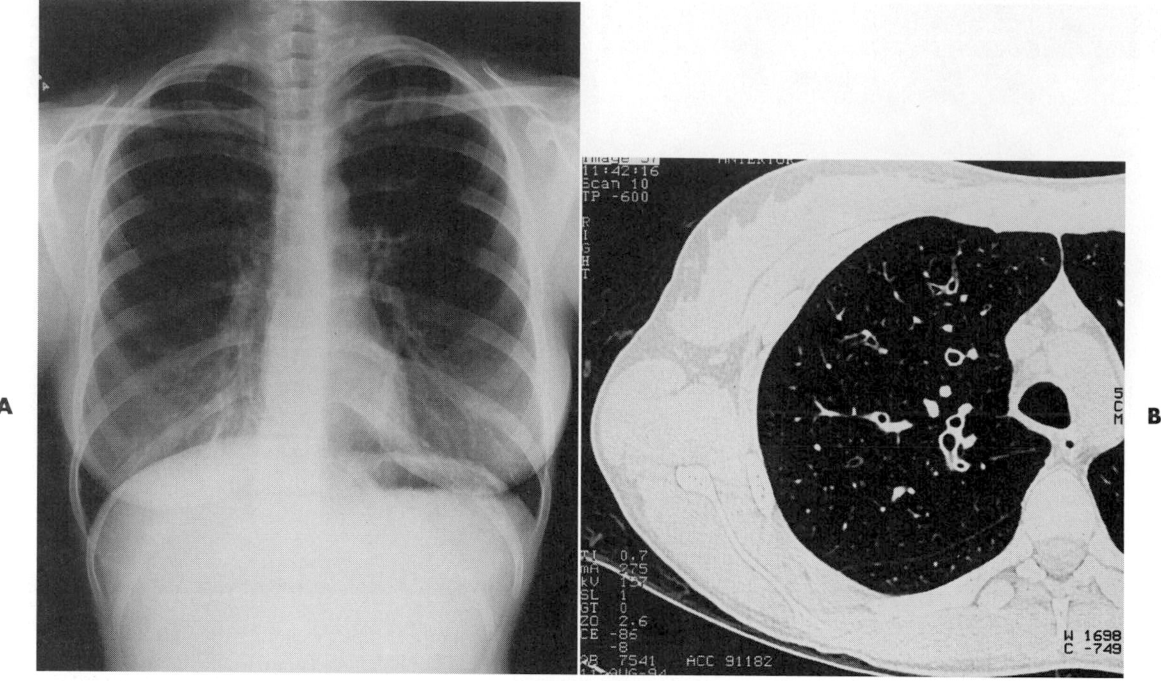

Fig. 52-11. Inflammatory bowel disease. **A,** Diffuse peribronchial thickening suggests bronchiectasis in an adolescent with ulcerative colitis. **B,** High-resolution computed tomogram confirms the presence of bronchiectasis and quantitates the extent of disease. Bronchiectasis typically develops after colectomy.

Other vasculitides occur in both children and adults (see Box 52-2). Reports of respiratory complications in adults with other vasculitic syndromes have recently been summarized.[77,78]

Other Inflammatory Diseases

Reiter's syndrome describes a triad of inflammatory lesions that includes arthritis, conjunctivitis, and urethritis. This is almost certainly a postinfectious or reactive arthritis. There is a high frequency of HLA-B27–positive male patients affected, a rate similar to that of ankylosing spondylitis. Pleuritic chest pain and pleural effusion have been described in acute Reiter's syndrome, although no follow-up studies have been reported.[79]

Patients with inflammatory bowel disease develop arthropathies similar to JRA and ankylosing spondylitis in 8% to 21% of cases. In addition to the symptoms of arthritis, other systemic manifestations of inflammatory bowel disease include erythema nodosum, pyoderma gangrenosum, and pulmonary disease. Most frequently the pulmonary disease is an ILD, although vasculitis, bronchiectasis (Fig. 52-11), granulomas, pleuritis, and pleural effusion may occur in both adults and children.[80-84] These complications are seen in both ulcerative colitis and regional enteritis (Crohn's disease).[80,81] In at least one case, the ILD improved with therapy for ulcerative colitis.[85]

MANAGEMENT

The main challenge in managing pulmonary manifestations of CVDs is determining whether pulmonary symptoms represent a complication of the primary illness, an infectious complication, or a complication related to ongoing therapy. Because of the importance of this separation, invasive diagnostic techniques, such as bronchoalveolar lavage (BAL), are frequently necessary. Therapy includes treating infectious complications, reducing the exposure to toxic medications, or improving the pharmacologic management of the primary CVD (Table 52-2).

BAL is the most valuable invasive diagnostic test used to separate infectious from noninfectious etiologies of lung disease in children with CVDs. Although this procedure entails some risk in the severely ill patient, BAL is both sensitive and specific for the diagnosis of infectious complications, particularly in the immunocompromised host.[86,87] It may also be helpful in diagnosing a pulmonary complication of the CVD, particularly if acute pulmonary hemorrhage is suspected. Finally, BAL cellularity is helpful for the early detection of ILD complications with CVDs[88,89] (Table 52-3). The presence of neutrophils in the BAL fluid of patients with CVD indicates an active alveolitis and may be seen even in patients without clinical or radiographic evidence of pulmonary involvement.[90] The neutrophilic alveolitis in adults treated with corticosteroids was improved at the 1-year follow-up compared with the alveolitis in untreated patients. Lymphocytosis or occasionally eosinophilia may be seen early in CVD, before clinical symptoms of ILD develop.[89-91]

High-resolution computed tomographic scanning is becoming the standard for diagnosis, determination of the best location for lung biopsy, and follow-up of the therapy for pulmonary complications related to CVDs (see Figs. 52-3, *B*; 52-7, *B*; and 52-8, *B*). In addition to disease in the airways, diffuse or focal peripheral lung disease is detected by high-resolution computed tomography[92,93] (Fig. 52-12). Parenchymal involvement in CVDs is usually more peripheral and subpleurally distributed than with other ILDs. Bronchiolitis obliterans is probably the best studied of the small airway diseases, and both early and late changes have been described.[94]

Magnetic resonance imaging may be helpful when vasculitis and pulmonary hemorrhage are suspected. This has been shown recently in patients with SLE.[95]

Table 52-2 Treatments for Pulmonary Manifestations of CVDs in Childhood

DISEASE	ANTIGEN REMOVAL	CORTICOSTEROIDS	CYTOTOXIC THERAPY	IVIG	NSAIDs
Rheumatic diseases					
JRA	–	++	++		+
SLE	–	+++	++		+
PSS	–	++	+		+
Dermatomyositis/polymyositis	–	+	–		+
Mixed connective tissue disease	–	+	++		
Ankylosing spondylitis	–	+	–	–	++
Sjögren's syndrome	+	+	+		
Vasculitic diseases					
Wegener's granulomatosis	–	++	++	–	–
Churg-Strauss syndrome	–	++	+	–	–
Henoch-Schönlein purpura	?	+	–	–	++
Kawasaki disease	–	–	–	+++	++
Polyarteritis nodosa	–	++	+	+	–
Behçet's disease	–	–	–	–	–

IVIG, Intravenous immunoglobulin; *NSAIDs,* nonsteroidal antiinflammatory drugs.

Table 52-3 BAL Findings in CVDs

DISEASE	BAL FINDINGS
Rheumatoid arthritis	Increased numbers of macrophages and neutrophils in patients with pulmonary symptoms Increased numbers of lymphocytes in patients without pulmonary symptoms Increased histamine levels Increased levels of procollagen and collagenase Increased levels of superoxide anion, fibronectin, and neutrophil chemotactic factor Increased levels of tumor necrosis factor-α Increased immune complex/albumin ratio
SLE	Reduced CD4/CD8 ratio Hemosiderin-laden macrophages 48 hours after pulmonary hemorrhage Free red blood cells in patients with acute pulmonary hemorrhage
PSS	Hypercellularity of all cell types Lymphocytosis before or soon after development of pulmonary complications Lipid-laden macrophages if there is chronic aspiration Eosinophilia (occasionally)
Polymyositis and dermatomyositis	Lipid-laden macrophages if there is chronic aspiration
Sjögren's syndrome	Mixed hypercellularity Increased numbers of lymphocytes Reduced CD4/CD8 ratio in pulmonary disease
Mixed connective tissue disease	Increased numbers of neutrophils
Vasculitic diseases	Hemosiderin-laden macrophages

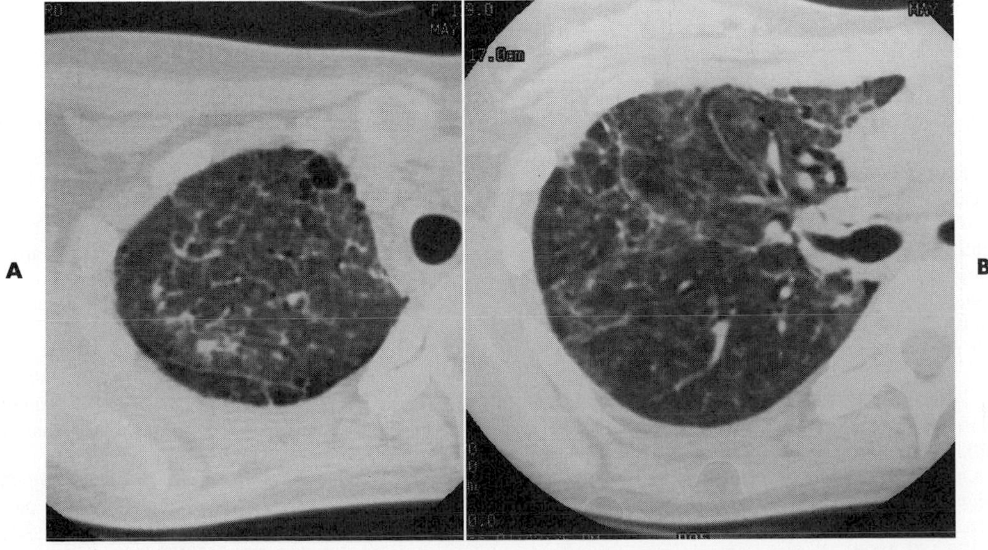

Fig. 52-12. PSS. High-resolution computed tomogram showing fibrotic changes with subpleural blebs, septal thickening, and bronchiolectasis in **A,** the apex, and **B,** midlung fields. Multiple poorly defined nodular densities are seen; they were not appreciated on chest radiograph 4 days earlier (see Fig. 52-8).

Pulmonary function testing is of value in explaining respiratory symptoms in patients with CVDs.[35,96,97] Airway disease may be missed clinically because the clinician is more likely to expect restrictive disease or only acute complications. When airway obstructive changes are present, it is important for the clinician to determine reversibility with bronchodilators because these findings may represent undiagnosed asthma instead of a complication of the primary CVD.

Therapy is selective to the complication and in general is supportive; it includes antibiotics for infections and alternative medications if an adverse drug effect is suspected. When the pulmonary symptoms are thought to be secondary to CVD, then enhancement of pharmacologic management is indicated. Examples of therapies for different CVDs are listed in Table 52-2.

CONCLUSION

Acute pulmonary complications in a patient with CVD can be life threatening and often require invasive techniques to obtain an early diagnosis. Infection- or medication-related complications need to be separated from pulmonary disease related to the CVD. Because all CVDs have possible pulmonary complications, the clinician must diagnose these problems and treat them early. Although the incidence of pulmonary complications is reduced during childhood, the identification of early changes in the lung may be valuable in preventing progressive, irreversible complications in adulthood.

REFERENCES

1. Cassidy JT, Petty RE: *Textbook of pediatric rheumatology,* New York, 1990, Churchill Livingstone.

Disease Mechanisms

2. Singsen BH, Platzker ACG: Pulmonary involvement in the rheumatic disorders of childhood. In Chernick V, Kendig EL, eds: *Disorders of the respiratory tract in children,* Philadelphia, 1990, WB Saunders.
3. Nadorra RL, Landing BH: Pulmonary lesions in childhood onset systemic lupus erythematosus: analysis of 26 cases and summary of the literature, *Pediatr Pathol* 7:1-18, 1987.
4. Hellmann DB, Petri M, Whiting-O'Keefe Q: Fatal infections in systemic lupus erythematosus: the role of opportunistic organisms, *Medicine* 66:341-348, 1987.
5. Wiedeman HP, Matthay RA: Pulmonary manifestations of the collagen vascular diseases, *Clin Chest Med* 10:677-722, 1989.
6. Stein HB, Patterson AC, Offer RC, Atkins CJH, Teufel A, Robinson HS: Adverse effects of D-penicillamine in rheumatoid arthritis, *Ann Intern Med* 92:24-29, 1980.
7. Howard-Lock HE, Lock CJ, Mewa A, Kean WF: D-Penicillamine: chemistry and clinical use in rheumatic disease, *Semin Arthritis Rheum* 15:261-281, 1986.
8. Evans RB, Ettensohn DB, Fawaz-Estrup F, Lally EV, Kaplan SR: Gold lung: recent developments in pathogenesis, diagnosis, and therapy, *Semin Arthritis Rheum* 16:196-205, 1987.
9. O'Duffy JD, Luthra HS, Unni KK, Hyatt RE: Bronchiolitis in a rheumatoid arthritis patient receiving auranofin, *Arthritis Rheum* 29:556-559, 1986.
10. Peces R, Riera JR, Arboleya LR, Lopez-Larrea C, Alvarez J: Goodpasture's syndrome in a patient receiving penicillamine and carbimazole, *Nephron* 45:316-320, 1987.
11. Cannon GW: Pulmonary complications of antirheumatic drug therapy, *Semin Arthritis Rheum* 19:353-364, 1990.
12. Zitnik RJ, Cooper JAD: Pulmonary disease due to antirheumatic agents, *Clin Chest Med* 11:139-150, 1990.
13. Carson CW, Cannon GW, Egger MJ, Ward JR, Clegg DO: Pulmonary disease during the treatment of rheumatoid arthritis with low dose pulse methotrexate, *Semin Arthritis Rheum* 16:186-195, 1987.
14. Samter M, Beers RF Jr: Intolerance to aspirin, *Ann Intern Med* 68:975-983, 1968.
15. DeVere R, Bradley WG: Polymyositis: its presentation, morbidity and mortality, *Brain* 98:637-666, 1975.
16. Feltelius N, Hedenstrom H, Hillerdal G, Hallgren R: Pulmonary involvement in ankylosing spondylitis, *Ann Rheum Dis* 45:736-740, 1986.
17. Bowyer S, LaMothe MP, Hollister JR: Steroid myopathy: incidence and detection in an asthmatic population, *J Allergy Clin Immunol* 76:234-242, 1985.
18. Gibson GJ, Edminds JP, Hughs GRV: Diaphragm function and lung involvement in systemic lupus erythematosus, *Am J Med* 63:926-932, 1977.
19. DeJongste JC, Neijens HJ, Duiverman EJ, Gogaard JM, Kerrebijn KF: Respiratory tract disease in systemic lupus erythematosus, *Arch Dis Child* 61:478-483, 1986.
20. Stevens WM, Burdon JG, Clemens LE, Webb J: The "shrinking lungs syndrome," an infrequently recognised feature of systemic lupus erythematosus, *Aust NZ J Med* 20:67-70, 1990.
21. Delgado EA, Malleson PN, Pirie GE, Petty RE: The pulmonary manifestations of childhood onset systemic lupus erythematosus, *Semin Arthritis Rheum* 19:285-293, 1990.
22. Good JT, King TE, Antony VB, Sahn SA: Lupus pleuritis: clinical factors and pleural fluid characteristics with special reference to pleural fluid antinuclear antibodies, *Chest* 84:714-718, 1983.
23. Athreya BH, Doughty RA, Bookspan M, Schumacher HR, Sewell EM, Cahtten J: Pulmonary manifestations of juvenile rheumatoid arthritis: a report of eight cases and review, *Clin Chest Med* 1:361-374, 1980.
24. Schwarz MI: Pulmonary manifestations of the collagen-vascular diseases. In Bone RC, ed: *Pulmonary and critical care medicine,* St Louis, 1993, Mosby.
25. McDonald JA, Kuhn C: Fibroblast and collagen deposition in interstitial lung disease. In Schwarz MI, King TE, eds: *Interstitial lung disease,* St Louis, 1993, Mosby.
26. Strimlan CV, Rosenow EC, Divertie MB, Harrison EG: Pulmonary manifestations of Sjögren's syndrome, *Chest* 70:354-361, 1976.
27. Myers JL, Datzenstein AL: Microangiitis in lupus-induced pulmonary hemorrhage, *Am J Clin Pathol* 85:552-556, 1986.
28. Bulkley GH, Ridolfi RL, Salyer WR, Hutchins GM: Myocardial lesions of progressive systemic sclerosis: a cause of cardiac dysfunction, *Circulation* 53:483-490, 1976.
29. Simonson JS, Schiller NB, Petri M, Hellman DB: Pulmonary hypertension in systemic lupus erythematosus, *J Rheumatol* 16:918-925, 1989.
30. Matthay RA, Schwarz MI, Petty TL, Stanford RE, Gupta RC, Sahn SA, Steigerwald JC: Pulmonary manifestations of systemic lupus erythematosus: review of 12 cases of acute lupus pneumonitis, *Medicine* 54:397-409, 1975.
31. Miller RW, Salcedo JR, Fink RJ, Murphy TM, Magilavy DB: Pulmonary hemorrhage in pediatric patients with systemic lupus erythematosus, *J Pediatr* 108:576-579, 1986.
32. Herzog CA, Miller RA, Hoidar JR: Bronchiolitis and rheumatoid arthritis, *Am Rev Respir Dis* 124:636-639, 1981.
33. Lanham JC, Elkon KB, Pusey CD, Hughes GR: Systemic vasculitis with asthma and eosinophilia: a clinical approach to Churg-Strauss syndrome, *Medicine* 63:65-81, 1984.
34. Landman S, Burgener F: Pulmonary manifestations in Wegener's granulomatosis, *Am J Roentgenol Radium Ther Nucl Med* 122:750-757, 1974.

Clinical Manifestations

35. Wagener JS, Taussig LM, DeBenedetti C, Lemen RJ, Loughlin GM: Pulmonary function in juvenile rheumatoid arthritis, *J Pediatr* 99:108-110, 1981.
36. Emery H: Clinical aspects of systemic lupus erythematosus in childhood, *Pediatr Clin North Am* 33:1177-1190, 1986.
37. Brasington RD, Furst DE: Pulmonary disease in systemic lupus erythematosus, *Clin Exp Rheumatol* 3:269-276, 1985.
38. Howe HS, Boey ML, Fong KY, Feng PH: Pulmonary haemorrhage, pulmonary infarction, and the lupus anticoagulant, *Ann Rheum Dis* 47:869-872, 1988.
39. Fukuda M, Kamiyama Y, Kawahara K, Kawamura K, Mori T, Honda M: The favourable effect of cyclophosphamide pulse therapy in the treatment of massive pulmonary haemorrhage in systemic lupus erythematosus, *Eur J Pediatr* 153:167-170, 1994.
40. Halla JT, Schrohenloher RE, Volanakis JE: Immune complexes and other laboratory features of pleural effusions: a comparison of rheumatoid arthritis, systemic lupus erythematosus, and other diseases, *Ann Intern Med* 92:748-752, 1980.

41. Riska H, Fyhrquiest F, Selander RK, Hellstrom PE: Systemic lupus erythematosus and DNA antibodies in pleural effusion, *Scand J Rheumatol* 7:159-160, 1978.
42. Eisenberg H: The interstitial lung diseases associated with the collagen vascular disorders, *Clin Chest Med* 3:565-578, 1982.
43. Greening AP, Hughs JMB: Serial estimations of carbon monoxide diffusing capacity in intrapulmonary haemorrhage, *Clin Sci* 60:507-512, 1981.
44. Asherson RA, Oakley CM: Pulmonary hypertension and systemic lupus erythematosus, *J Rheumatol* 13:1-5, 1986.
45. Smith GA, Ward PH: Laryngeal involvement in systemic lupus erythematosus, *Trans Am Acad Ophthalmol Otolaryngol* 84:124-128, 1977.
46. Chan CN, Li E, Lai FM, Pang JA: An unusual case of systemic lupus erythematosus with isolated hypoglossal nerve palsy, fulminant acute pneumonitis, and pulmonary amyloidosis, *Ann Rheum Dis* 48:236-239, 1989.
47. Silver RM, Miller KS: Lung involvement in systemic sclerosis, *Rheum Dis Clin North Am* 16:199-216, 1990.
48. McCarthy DS, Baragar FD, Dhingra S, Sigurdson M, Sutherland JB, Rigby M, Martin L: The lungs in systemic sclerosis: a review and new information, *Semin Arthritis Rheum* 17:271-283, 1988.
49. Bagg LR, Hughes DT: Serial pulmonary function tests in progressive systemic sclerosis, *Thorax* 34:224-228, 1979.
50. Bitnum S, Daeschner CWJ, Travis LB, Dodge WF, Hopps HC: Dermatomyositis, *J Pediatr* 64:101-131, 1964.
51. Park S, Nyhan WL: Fatal pulmonary involvement in dermatomyositis, *Am J Dis Child* 129:723-736, 1975.
52. Singsen BH, Tedford JC, Platzker ACG, Hanson V: Spontaneous pneumothorax: a complication of juvenile dermatomyositis, *J Pediatr* 92:771-774, 1978.
53. Samuels MP, Warner JO: Pulmonary alveolar lipoproteinosis complicating juvenile dermatomyositis, *Thorax* 43:939-940, 1988.
54. Sharp GC, Irvin WS, Tan EM, Gould RG, Homan HR: Mixed connective tissue disease: an apparently distinct rheumatic disease syndrome associated with a specific antibody to an extractable nuclear antigen, *Am J Med* 52:148-159, 1972.
55. Singsen BH, Bernstein BH, Kornreich HK, King KK, Hanson V, Tan EM: Mixed connective tissue disease in childhood, *J Pediatr* 90:893-900, 1977.
56. Prakash UB: Lungs in mixed connective tissue disease, *J Thorac Imaging* 7:55-61, 1992.
57. Sullivan WD, Hurst DJ, Harmon CE, Esther JH, Agia GA, Maltby JD, Lillard SB, Held CN, Wolfe JF, Sunlesrajan EV: A prospective evaluation emphasizing pulmonary involvement in patients with mixed connective tissue disease, *Medicine* 63:92-107, 1984.
58. Wiener-Kronish JP, Solinger AM, Warnock ML, Churg A, Ordoñez N, Golden JA: Severe pulmonary involvement in mixed connective tissue disease, *Am Rev Respir Dis* 124:499-503, 1981.
59. Athreya BH, Horman ME, Myers AR, South MA: Sjögren's syndrome in children, *Pediatrics* 59:931-938, 1977.
60. Kelly C, Gardiner P, Pal B, Griffiths I: Lung function in primary Sjögren's syndrome: a cross sectional and longitudinal study, *Thorax* 46:180-183, 1991.
61. Anderson LG, Talal N: The spectrum of benign to malignant lymphoproliferation in Sjögren's syndrome, *Clin Exp Immunol* 10:199-221, 1972.
62. Wolff SM, Fauci AS, Horn RG, Dale DC: Wegener's granulomatosis, *Ann Intern Med* 81:513-525, 1974.
63. Hall SL, Miller LC, Duggan E, Mauer SM, Beatty EC, Hellerstein S: Wegener's granulomatosis in pediatric patients, *J Pediatr* 106:739-744, 1985.
64. Specks U, Wheatley CL, McDonald TJ, Rohrbach MS, DeRemee RA: Anticytoplasmic antibodies in the diagnosis and follow-up of Wegener's granulomatosis, *Mayo Clin Proc* 64:28-36, 1989.
65. Fauci AS, Haynes B, Katz P, Wolff S: Wegener's granulomatosis: prospective clinical and therapeutic experience with 85 patients for 21 years, *Ann Intern Med* 98:76-85, 1983.
66. Koss MN, Antonovych T, Hochholzer L: Allergic granulomatosis (Churg-Strauss syndrome): pulmonary and renal morphologic findings, *Am J Surg Pathol* 5:21-28, 1981.
67. Weiss VF, Naidu S: Fatal pulmonary hemorrhage in Henoch-Schönlein purpura, *Cutis* 23:687-688, 1979.
68. Kathuria S, Cheifec G: Fatal pulmonary Henoch-Schönlein syndrome, *Chest* 82:654-656, 1982.
69. Meade RH III, Brandt L: Manifestations of Kawasaki disease in the New England outbreak of 1980, *J Pediatr* 100:558-562, 1982.
70. Byard RW, Edmonds JF, Silverman E, Silver MM: Respiratory distress and fever in a 2-month-old child, *J Pediatr* 118:306-313, 1991.
71. Umezawa T, Saji T, Matsuo N, Odagiri K: Chest x-ray findings in the acute phase of Kawasaki disease, *Pediatr Radiol* 20:48-51, 1989.
72. Zeek PM: Periarteritis nodosa and other forms of necrotizing angiitis, *N Engl J Med* 18:764-772, 1953.
73. Reimold EW, Weinberg AG, Fink CW, Battles ND: Polyarteritis in children, *Am J Dis Child* 130:534-541, 1976.
74. Ettlinger RE, Nelson AM, Burke EC, Lie JT: Polyarteritis nodosa in childhood: a clinical pathologic study, *Arthritis Rheum* 22:820-825, 1979.
75. Ammann AJ, Johnson A, Fyfe GA, Leonards R, Wara DW, Cowan M: Behçet syndrome, *J Pediatr* 107:41-43, 1985.
76. Raz I, Okon E, Chajek-Shaul T: Pulmonary manifestations in Behçet's syndrome, *Chest* 95:585-589, 1989.
77. Leavitt RY, Fauci AS: Pulmonary vasculitis, *Am Rev Respir Dis* 134:149-166, 1986.
78. Kennedy JI, Fulmer JD: Pulmonary vasculitis. In Schwarz MI, King TE, eds: *Interstitial lung disease,* St Louis, 1993, Mosby.
79. Rosenberg AM, Petty RE: Reiter's disease in children, *Am J Dis Child* 133:394-398, 1979.
80. Camus P, Piard F, Ashcroft T, Gal AA, Colby TV: The lung in inflammatory bowel disease, *Medicine* 72:151-183, 1993.
81. Bonniere P, Wallaert B, Cortot A, Marchandise X, Riou Y, Tonnel AB, Colombel JF, Voisin C, Paris JC: Latent pulmonary involvement in Crohn's disease: biological, functional, bronchoalveolar lavage and scintigraphic studies, *Gut* 27:919-925, 1986.
82. Collins WJ, Bendig DW, Taylor WF: Pulmonary vasculitis complicating childhood ulcerative colitis, *Gastroenterology* 77:1091-1093, 1979.
83. Puntis JW, Tarlow MJ, Raafat F, Booth IW: Crohn's disease of the lung, *Arch Dis Child* 65:1270-1271, 1990.
84. Calder CJ, Lacy D, Raafat F, Weller PH, Booth IW: Crohn's disease with pulmonary involvement in a 3 year old boy, *Gut* 34:1636-1638, 1993.
85. Mazer B, Eigen H, Gelfand E, Brugman S: Revision of interstitial lung disease following therapy of associated ulcerative colitis, *Pediatr Pulmonol* 15:55-59, 1993.

Management

86. deBlic J, Mckelvie P, Le Bourgeois M, Blanche S, Benoist MR, Scheinmann P: Value of bronchoalveolar lavage in the management of severe acute pneumonia and interstitial pneumonitis in the immunocompromised child, *Thorax* 42:759-765, 1987.
87. Pattishall EN, Noyes BE, Orenstein DM: Use of bronchoalveolar lavage in immunocompromised children with pneumonia, *Pediatr Pulmonol* 5:1-5, 1988.
88. Wallaert B, Rossi GA, Sibille Y: Collagen-vascular diseases, *Eur Respir J* 3:942-943, 1990.
89. King TE: Connective tissue disease. In Schwarz MI, King TE, eds: *Interstitial lung disease,* St Louis, 1993, Mosby.
90. Wallaert B, Hatron P, Grosbois J, Tonnel A, Devulder G, Voisin C: Subclinical pulmonary involvement in collagen-vascular diseases assessed by bronchoalveolar lavage, *Am Rev Respir Dis* 133:574-590, 1986.
91. Klech HH, Pohl WW: Use of bronchoalveolar lavage in interstitial lung disease. In Bone RC, ed: *Pulmonary and critical care medicine,* St Louis, 1993, Mosby.
92. Nakata H, Kimoto T, Nakayama T, Kido M, Miyazaki N, Harada S: Diffuse peripheral lung disease: evaluation by high-resolution computed tomography, *Radiology* 157:181-185, 1985.
93. Makino Y, Ogawa M, Ueda S, Ohto M: CT appearance of diffuse alveolar hemorrhage in a patient with systemic lupus erythematosus, *Acta Radiol* 34:634-635, 1993.
94. Lynch DA, Brasch RC, Hardy KA, Webb WR: Pediatric pulmonary disease: assessment with high-resolution ultrafast CT, *Radiology* 176:243-248, 1990.
95. Hsu BY, Edwards DK, Trambert MA: Pulmonary hemorrhage complicating systemic lupus erythematosus: role of MR imaging in diagnosis, *Am J Roentgenol* 158:519-520, 1992.
96. Cerveri I, Bruschi C, Ravelli A, Zoia MC, Fanfulla F, Zonta L, Pellegrini G, Martini A: Pulmonary function in childhood connective tissue diseases, *Eur Respir J* 5:733-738, 1992.
97. Vitali C, Viegi G, Tassoni S, Tavoni A, Paoletti P, Bibolotti E, Ferri C, Bombardieri S: Lung function abnormalities in different connective tissue diseases, *Clin Rheumatol* 5:181-188, 1986.

CHAPTER 53

Alveolar Proteinosis

Jeff S. Wagener and Robin R. Deterding

Alveolar proteinosis was originally described in 1958 by Rosen et al[1] as a new disease with an unknown etiology. Although the majority of patients diagnosed with alveolar proteinosis are adults, two review articles[2,3] included several children and adolescents with this disease. Although many etiologies have been proposed, the cause of this disease in older children and adults remains unknown. Recently, a congenital form of alveolar proteinosis has been recognized as a cause of fatal neonatal respiratory distress and linked to a genetic deficiency of surfactant protein B (SP-B).[4,5] The discovery of genetic markers for SP-B deficiency may increase our understanding of the incidence and pathogenesis of alveolar proteinosis in all age groups.[4,6-9]

Numerous therapeutic interventions have been tried, including systemic steroids, inhaled heparin, acetylcysteine, trypsin, surfactant, and whole lung lavage. Pharmacologic therapies have not proven efficacious, partially because spontaneous remission can occur in the older patient population and partially because of the toxicities of these agents. Current therapy is supportive and centered primarily around removing the proteinaceous material from the lung using whole lung lavage.[10] With or without treatment, in 20% to 30% of older patients the disease will "burn out," and most patients will recover near-normal lung function.[11] In hereditary SP-B deficiency, replacement therapy with commercially available surfactant has been unsuccessful and lung transplantation is the only viable treatment option.[12]

DISEASE MECHANISMS

Alveolar proteinosis is diagnosed histologically by the presence of periodic acid-Schiff (PAS)–positive, amorphous, granular material deposited diffusely in the alveolar spaces.[1] The material is rich in phospholipids (surfactant like), and although this finding on bronchoalveolar lavage (BAL) is highly suggestive of the diagnosis,[13] an open lung or transbronchial biopsy is needed to confirm the diagnosis. Airway abnormalities are not seen, but hyperplasia of the alveolar epithelium, especially type II pneumocytes, is usually present. It is significant that alveolar septal fibrosis and inflammation are absent. If inflammation is present, an additional precipitating disease, such as infection or malignancy, should be suspected. Large macrophages are commonly found in the midst of this insoluble, diastase-resistant material. These macrophages have PAS-positive cytoplasm, presumably resulting from phagocytosis and failure to digest the surrounding material. As a result, these distended macrophages have decreased function, contributing to an increased risk of infectious complications, especially in the untreated subject.

Material obtained via lung lavage has a creamy, beige appearance and separates into a precipitate and a soluble fraction when allowed to sit for a brief time. The sediment contains glycoproteins and phospholipid, often in the form of lamellar bodies, and resists degradation by trypsin, acetylcysteine, and heparin, all of which have been tried therapeutically. The soluble component contains serum and apoproteins with elevated concentrations of immunoglobulin G (IgG) and reduced amounts of α_2-macroglobulin. Rarely an infectious agent, such as *Pneumocystis carinii,* causes BAL findings that mimic alveolar proteinosis. Thus, special stains for *P. carinii,* fungi, cytomegalovirus (CMV), bacteria, and acid-fast bacilli should be obtained before making the diagnosis of primary alveolar proteinosis.

The pathogenesis for alveolar proteinosis remains unclear in those patients who develop the disease after the newborn period; however, many hypotheses have been advanced. Mechanisms can be divided functionally into five possible lesions: (1) overproduction of normal or abnormal alveolar substances (including phospholipids and lamellar bodies),[14] (2) abnormal alveolar clearance of normal or abnormal lipoproteins,[15,16] (3) imbalance between production and removal of alveolar phospholipids,[17] (4) impaired catabolic capacity of alveolar macrophages to clear ingested lamellar bodies,[18] and (5) excessive proliferation and destruction of alveolar type II cells.[19]

The similarity between surfactant and the proteinaceous material in alveolar proteinosis suggests that this material might result from an overproduction of surfactant.[14] Patient lavage material has been studied extensively, and although it is similar to naturally occurring surfactant, several differences have been identified. Unlike the absence of SP-B in congenital alveolar proteinosis, surfactant proteins A, B, and C have all been identified in the lavage fluid of older patients with alveolar proteinosis. However, significant structural modifications in these proteins are present.[20] Surfactant protein A, the most abundant surfactant protein, functions in tubular myelin formation, phospholipid secretion, and surfactant reuptake by the alveolar type II cells.[21-23] Surfactant proteins A and B enhance monolayer formation at the air-liquid interface and contribute to lowering surface tension.[24] Thus structural modification of these proteins may lead to altered surfactant function and metabolism.

In addition to type II pneumocytes, alveolar macrophages are also responsible for clearance of surfactant. The apparent inability of macrophages to detoxify the alveolar material of alveolar proteinosis results in macrophage death and filling of the alveolus with cell debris.[25] Additionally, these macrophages have abnormal migration and phagocytic function, possibly explaining the increased risk for opportunistic infections in patients with alveolar proteinosis. After whole lung lavage, macrophage function returns to normal.[26] This may explain the absence of infectious complications in patients regularly treated with lavage.

Rosen et al[1] originally proposed that this condition was a result of excessive alveolar cell death. A moderate amount of cell debris is present in the alveolar material, and histologically there is often hyperplasia of type II pneumocytes.

Several reports have described pathologic findings of alveolar proteinosis in humans and animals after exposure to toxins such as silica, aluminum dust, fiberglass, and volcanic ash.[27-31] A variety of infections (e.g., *Pneumocystis, Nocardia*) and malignancies may also produce findings similar to alveolar proteinosis, and one case has been reported of alveolar proteinosis in a 9-year-old boy with juvenile dermatomyositis.[32] These findings have led some investigators to separate disease into primary or secondary alveolar proteinosis based on the presence of a coexisting diagnosis. The usual lack of any environmental exposure or pathogen in children makes this classification less valuable in pediatric patients. A careful review of the patient's history, physical examination, and pathology, including special staining, can usually identify patients with a possible precipitating cause for disease.

Alveolar proteinosis in pediatric patients is best categorized by age because neonates have a distinctly different prognosis and probably different pathogenesis from older patients. By analyzing BAL fluid and SP-B genetic transcripts in infants afflicted with congenital alveolar proteinosis, it has been determined[4,5] that these newborns have a marked deficiency of SP-B secondary to autosomal recessive mutations of the SP-B gene.[4,5,33] Experimental inhibition of SP-B with monoclonal antibodies in rabbits results in severe hyaline membrane disease.[34] Also, homozygous SP-B gene abnormalities are lethal in transgenic mice. Heterozygous transgenic mice survive, but develop decreased lung compliance and gas trapping.[35] The lethal absence of SP-B in congenital alveolar proteinosis and in some newborns with fatal respiratory distress syndrome points to the importance of SP-B in normal alveolar function.

In the young child who becomes ill after the neonatal period, alveolar proteinosis may represent a variation in the genetic abnormality described for congenital alveolar proteinosis or may be more closely related to the form seen in older patients. To date there have been no published reports of SP-B deficiency occurring outside the immediate newborn period. Distinguishing the absence of SP-B from secondary causes such as malignancy, immunodeficiency, infection, and autoimmune disease in pediatric patients with alveolar proteinosis is essential to guide therapy and predict prognosis.

In summary, the appearance of the lung, as well as the lavage fluid, provides insight into the pathogenesis of alveolar proteinosis. Some cases of congenital alveolar proteinosis may result from a genetic deficiency in SP-B. The presentation in older patients may result from an inappropriate response to a pulmonary insult. This insult may include (1) infection; (2) an immunodeficiency state, including neoplastic disease; or (3) inhaled toxic agents, or it may be idiopathic. Ultimately, an abnormality in surfactant turnover by type II cells and alveolar macrophages, with either overproduction, underabsorption, or cell destruction, appears to be the final pathway by which numerous initiating events contribute to this interesting disease.

CLINICAL MANIFESTATIONS

Exercise intolerance is the most common initial symptom in older children and adults with alveolar proteinosis.[36] If the diagnosis is delayed, dyspnea, nonproductive cough, and occasionally chest pain may be the chief complaints. In young children and infants, respiratory symptoms are often insidious in onset, and failure to thrive, gastrointestinal symptoms, and bacterial infections are more common.[6] The persistence of pneumonia and diffuse infiltrates on chest radiographs may be another sign that eventually leads to the diagnosis. In contrast, newborns with congenital alveolar proteinosis have respiratory distress and chest radiographs consistent with respiratory distress syndrome.[4,6,37,38] Rarely, concomitant illnesses such as acquired immunodeficiency syndrome (AIDS), malignancies, or infections complicate the diagnosis because chills, weight loss, and hemoptysis can occur either primarily with alveolar proteinosis or with these underlying diseases.

Physical examination is characterized by the presence of diffuse crackles and occasional tachypnea. Digital clubbing is present in nearly one third of adults, although this has not been commented on in pediatric cases. Early in the time course of the disease the examination may be entirely normal, and late in the disease there may be cyanosis. Fever should not be present unless there is a complicating infection.

Chest radiographic findings (Fig. 53-1) include bilateral, symmetric alveolar filling defects in over 50% of cases. This "bat-wing" appearance is due to the perihilar nature of the infiltrate and the sparing of disease in the costophrenic angles. Computed tomography (CT) (Fig. 53-2) usually discloses a far more extensive pattern of diffuse involvement of alveolar spaces. The presence of localized disease on the CT scan should raise concern for another diagnosis. Heart size should be normal, and the pleural space should be free of effusion. Additionally, the mediastinum is not involved and lymphadenopathy should not be seen.[39] Magnetic resonance imaging and radionucleotide lung scans have little to add to the diagnosis or management of alveolar proteinosis.

In patients old enough to perform pulmonary function testing, there is a typical restrictive pattern with a decreased total lung capacity and found vital capacity plus proportionately decreased airflows. Diffusing capacity is decreased; how-

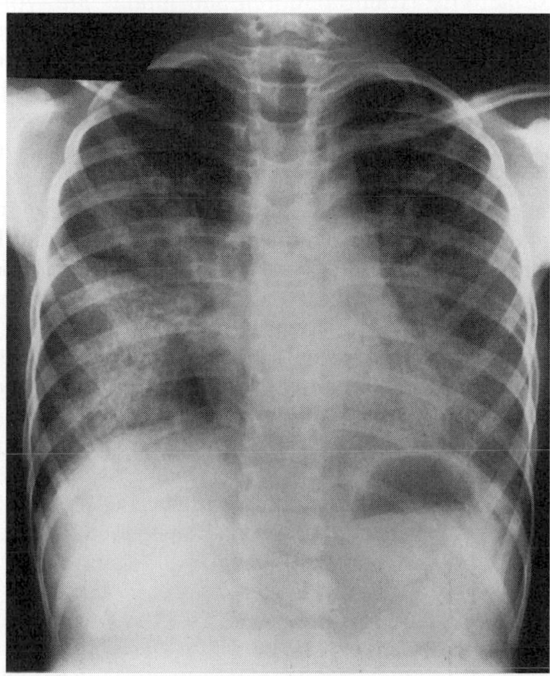

Fig. 53-1. Chest radiograph of a 9-year-old at the time of pulmonary alveolar proteinosis.

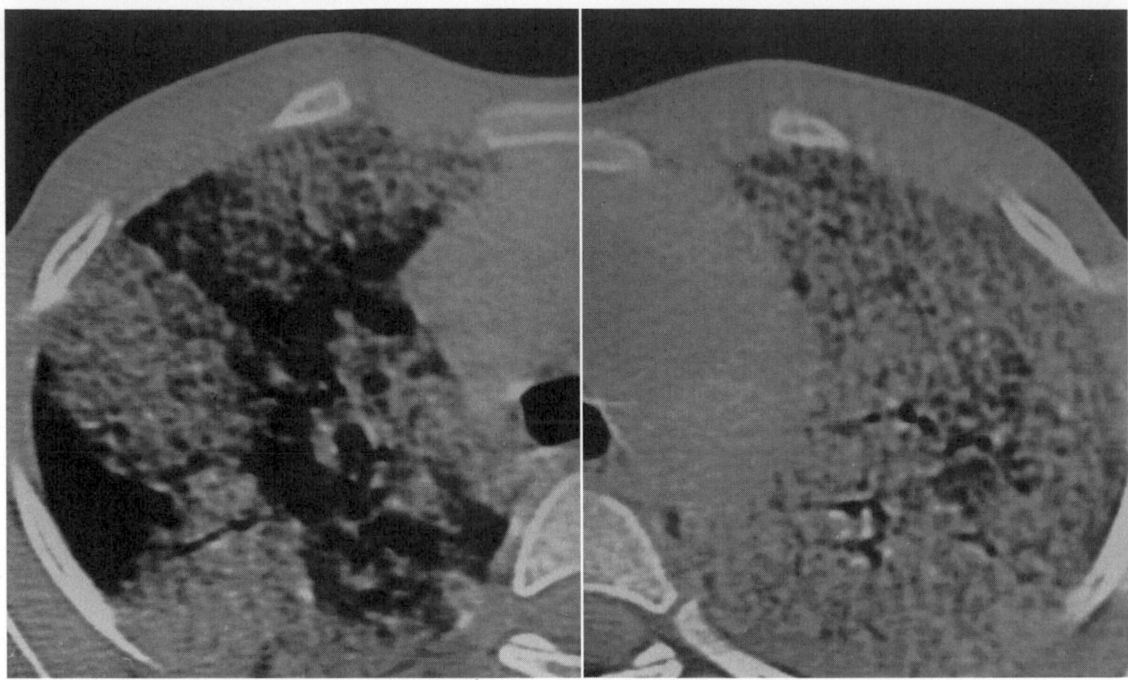

Fig. 53-2. Chest computed tomography in the 9-year-old with alveolar proteinosis whose chest radiograph is shown in Fig. 53-1.

ever, this is primarily related to the restrictive pattern, and diffusing capacity corrected for alveolar volume is commonly normal. Blood gases at rest are usually normal in older patients, but with exercise, oxygenation worsens, often dramatically. Exercise-related desaturation is one of the most sensitive measures of disease activity and progression. We have noted that longitudinal quantitation of the level of exercise at which a patient develops desaturation commonly falls sooner than other pulmonary function measurements and signifies increased disease activity. Young children and infants are typically tachypneic and may have desaturation at the time of initial treatment. Newborns with congenital alveolar proteinosis develop severe respiratory distress within the first 24 hours of birth.

Laboratory tests have little value in making the diagnosis of alveolar proteinosis. Serum lactic dehydrogenase (LDH) may be elevated,[40] but this can also occur with *P. carinii* pneumonia and with various malignancies. Whether serial LDH levels can be used to follow the progress of disease is debatable because serial exercise and pulmonary function testing are so valuable.

Definitive diagnosis usually requires lung biopsy. In small children this usually requires open or thoracoscopic biopsy. Transbronchial biopsy in older patients may be diagnostic, especially if guided by chest CT to ensure that tissue from the most affected area is obtained. In newborns suspected of having SP-B deficiency, lung lavage can be analyzed for SP-B and blood from the patient or parents can be used for mutation analysis.[41]

MANAGEMENT

Although the etiology for alveolar proteinosis is not known, symptomatic therapy for the older patient has proven fairly successful. Young children with this disease have been treated similar to adults, but either because of a different etiology or because of technical difficulties, the success rate for disease control in this group has been poor.

Therapeutic whole lung lavage was introduced in 1965[10] and is indicated primarily to manage symptoms. Lavage may also decrease the likelihood of opportunistic infections, and a trial of lavage therapy is usually indicated at the time of diagnosis. Results are often immediate and dramatic, with the patient's exercise tolerance improving most remarkably.

Whole lung lavage requires an experienced team of individuals, including nurses, respiratory therapists, anesthesiologists, and pulmonologists experienced in bronchoscopy and in managing infants and children. The procedure is performed under general anesthesia. A double-lumen endotracheal tube is inserted with bronchoscopic guidance, ensuring that the tip of the tube is in the mainstem bronchus and the balloon, when inflated, is just below the carina and occludes the mainstem bronchus without occluding the upper lobe bronchus. Double-lumen endotracheal tubes are generally not available for children who weigh less than 25 kg. A more limited lavage of individual lung segments must be performed in younger patients.[42] Two infants (1 month and 7 months old) treated of age were successfully treated with whole lung lavage in a hyperbaric oxygen chamber.[43] Additionally, cardiopulmonary by-pass may be used to perform whole lung lavage through a single-lumen endotracheal tube.[44,45]

Once the patient is appropriately intubated with both lungs isolated using the double-lumen endotracheal tube, the lung with the more severe disease is lavaged. The choice of lung can be based on the CT scan or intraoperatively by isolated ventilation and determining the oxygen uptake from each lung. After ventilation with 100% oxygen, one lung is deflated by occluding the tube going to the side to be lavaged, and the patient is placed with this side down. After approximately 5 minutes to allow for degassing of the dependent, nonventilated lung, body temperature lavage fluid (normal saline with or without 0.1 U/ml heparin) is instilled, first using 3 to 5 ml/kg to ensure that no fluid leaks into the ventilated side. Once it is established that no leak exists, larger amounts of fluid can be instilled. After approximately 12 to 15 ml/kg have been instilled, the inflow tube is clamped; chest percussion, which increases the yield of proteinaceous material, is performed for 1 minute; and then the inflow tube is unclamped, allowing effluent to leave the lung.[46] Initially this fluid is milky and yellow to brown in color. This procedure is repeated numerous times (average 10 to 15) until the effluent is clear. The volume of all fluid instilled and all effluent should be recorded. Patients commonly retain 20 to 30 ml/kg because of alveolar filling and fluid absorption. If greater amounts of fluid are retained, a fluid leak into the contralateral side must be suspected. Oxygen saturation must be monitored closely during the procedure to prevent complications and as an indicator if the procedure should be terminated. Usually only one side is lavaged at a single procedure (Fig. 53-3), with a repeat procedure scheduled for the next day. Bilateral lavages can be completed on the same day if, after 10 minutes of recovery, the lavaged lung is able to maintain adequate ventilation and oxygenation when the unlavaged lung is degassed.

After lavage, both lungs are ventilated. Usually a moderate amount of foamy fluid continues to be suctioned from the lavaged lung before normal lung compliance returns. Pressure-volume measurements can be made for each lung to ensure that improved compliance has been achieved. This usually occurs 15 to 30 minutes after completion of lavage and can be enhanced by occasional large tidal volumes to distend the lung. Positive end-expiratory pressure is not necessary and has been implicated as the cause of a pneumothorax in one patient. Complications are rare; however, serum electrolytes should be monitored after the procedure because fluid can be absorbed from the lavaged lung, resulting in hyperchloremia and hypokalemia.

In older patients and adults, lavaging both lungs once may be all that is necessary to attain long-term remission. The experience in infants has been less promising because of difficulties lavaging an entire lung[42,44,45,47] and also because of differences in disease pathophysiology. Repeated procedures are indicated for worsening oxygenation because complications of hypoxia are the usual cause for demise in these patients. Active or recurrent infection may also justify lavage because alveolar macrophage function is reported to improve after lavage. Although infants usually die before age 2 from their disease, older children and adults usually recover, and death from alveolar proteinosis is uncommon for patients treated with lavage. Rarely, adults experience long-term complications of pulmonary fibrosis or emphysematous bullae.[48,49] These complications have not been reported in children with pulmonary alveolar proteinosis.

The management of congenital alveolar proteinosis requires the confirmation of SP-B deficiency, which can be done by analysis of BAL fluid combined with genetic analysis of lung tissue or blood from the patient or genetic analysis of blood from both parents.[5] This diagnosis has significant genetic implications for the family and prognostic implications for the patient. Currently, pediatric lung transplantation is the therapeutic intervention of choice. With continued advancement in our understanding of this disease, SP-B gene replacement may be the ultimate therapy in the future.

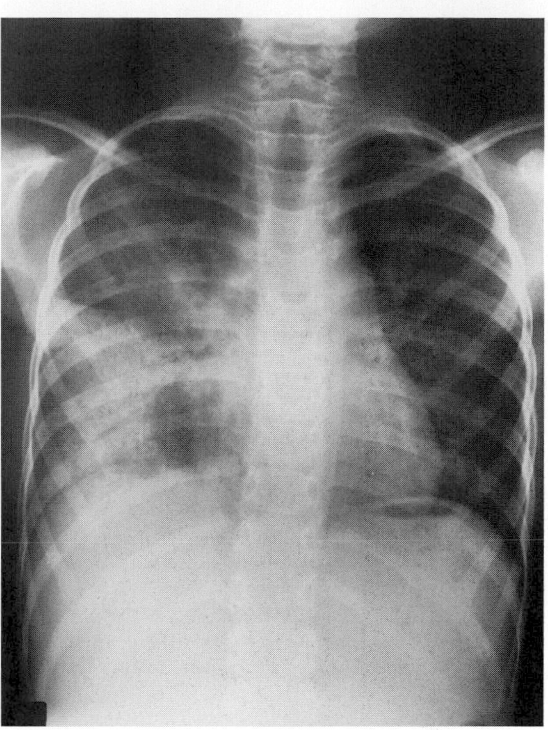

Fig. 53-3. Chest radiograph after unilateral (left) lung lavage. Prelavage chest radiograph is shown in Fig. 53-1.

REFERENCES

1. Rosen SH, Castleman B, Liebow AA: Pulmonary alveolar proteinosis, *N Engl J Med* 258:1123-1142, 1958.
2. Davidson JM, Macleod WM: Pulmonary alveolar proteinosis, *Br J Dis Chest* 63:13-28, 1969 (review).
3. Bedrossian CWM, Luna MA, Conklin RH, Miller WC: Alveolar proteinosis as a consequence of immunosuppression: a hypothesis based on clinical and pathologic observations, *Hum Pathol* 11:527-535, 1980 (review).
4. Nogee LM, de Mello DE, Dehner LP, Colten HR: Deficiency of pulmonary surfactant protein B in congenital alveolar proteinosis, *N Engl J Med* 328:406-410, 1993.
5. Nogee LM, Gamler G, Dietz HC, Singer L, Murphy AM, deMello DE, Colten HR: A mutation in the surfactant protein B gene for fatal neonatal respiratory disease in multiple kindreds, *J Clin Invest* 93:1860-1863, 1994.
6. Schumacher RE, Marrogi AJ, Heidelberger KP: Pulmonary alveolar proteinosis in a newborn, *Pediatr Pulmonol* 7:178-182, 1989.
7. Wilkinson RH, Blanc WA, Hagstrom JWC: Pulmonary alveolar proteinosis in three infants, *Pediatrics* 41:510-515, 1968.
8. Webster JR, Batifora H, Furey C,: Pulmonary alveolar proteinosis in two siblings with decreased immunoglobulin A, *Am J Med* 69:786-789, 1980.
9. Teja K, Cooper PH, Squires JE, Schnatterly PT: Pulmonary alveolar proteinosis in four siblings, *N Engl J Med* 305:1390-1392, 1981.
10. Ramirez-R J, Kieffer RF, Ball D: Bronchopulmonary lavage in man, *Ann Intern Med* 63:819-828, 1965.
11. Prakash UBS, Barham SS, Carpenter HA, Dines DE, Marsh HM: Pulmonary alveolar phospholipoproteinosis: experience with 34 cases and a review, *Mayo Clin Proc* 62:499-518, 1987 (review).
12. Hamvas A, Nogee LM, Mallory GB, Spray TL, Huddleston CB, August A, Dehner LP, de Mello DE, Moxley M, Nelson R, Cole FS, Colten HR: Lung transplantation for treatment of infants with surfactant protein B deficiency. *J Pediatr* 130:231-239, 1997.

Disease Mechanisms

13. Martin RJ, Coalson JJ, Rogers RM, Horton FO, Manous LE: Pulmonary alveolar proteinosis: the diagnosis by segmental lavage, *Am Rev Respir Dis* 121:819-825, 1980.
14. Larson RK, Gordinier R: Pulmonary alveolar proteinosis: report of six cases, review of the literature, and formulation of a new theory, *Ann Intern Med* 62:292-312, 1965 (review).
15. Duhn C, Gyorkey F, Levine BE, Ramirez-Rivera J: Pulmonary alveolar proteinosis: a study using enzyme histochemistry, electron microscopy, and surface tension measurement, *Lab Invest* 15:492-509, 1966.
16. Ramirez-RJ, Harlan WR: Pulmonary alveolar proteinosis, *Am J Med* 45:502-512, 1968.
17. Heppleston AG, Fletcher K, Wyatt I: Changes in the composition of lung lipids and the "turnover" of dipalmitoyl lecithin in experimental alveolar lipoproteinosis induced by inhaled quartz, *Br J Exp Pathol* 55:384-395, 1974.
18. Schober R, Bensch KG, Kosek JC, Northway WH: On the origin of the membranous intra-alveolar material in pulmonary alveolar proteinosis, *Exp Mol Pathol* 21:246-258, 1974.
19. Bhagwat AG, Wentworth P, Conen PE: Observations on the relationship of desquamative interstitial pneumonia and pulmonary alveolar proteinosis in childhood: a pathologic and experimental study, *Chest* 58:26-32, 1970.
20. Voss T, Schafer KP, Nielsen PF, Schafer A, Maier C, Hannappel E, MaaBen J, Landis B, Klemm K, Przybylski M: Primary structure differences of human surfactant–associated proteins isolated from normal and proteinosis lung, *Biochim Biophys Acta* 1138:261-267, 1992.
21. Benson BJ, Williams MC, Sueishi K, Goerke R, Sargeant T: Role of calcium ions in the structure and function of pulmonary surfactant, *Biochim Biophys Acta* 793:18-27, 1984.
22. Dobbs LG, Wright JR, Hawgood S, Gonzales R, Venstrom K, Nellenbogen J: Pulmonary surfactant and its components inhibit secretion of phosphatidylcholine from cultured rat alveolar type II cells, *Proc Natl Acad Sci* 84:1010-1014, 1987.
23. Corbet A, Bedi H, Owens M, Taeusch W: Surfactant protein-A inhibits lavage induced surfactant secretion in newborn rabbits, *Am J Med Sci* 304:264-251, 1992.
24. Revak SD, Merritt TA, Degryse E, Stefani L, Courtney M, Hallman M, Cochrane CG: Use of human surfactant low molecular weight apoproteins in the reconstitution of surfactant biologic activity, *J Clin Invest* 81:826-833, 1988.
25. Gonzalez-Rothi RJ, Harris JO: Pulmonary alveolar proteinosis: further evaluation of abnormal alveolar macrophages, *Chest* 90:656-661, 1986.
26. Hoffman RM, Dauber JH, Rogers RM: Improvements in alveolar macrophage migration after therapeutic whole lung lavage in pulmonary alveolar proteinosis, *Am Rev Respir Dis* 139:1030-1032, 1989.
27. Heppleston AG, Wright NA, Stewart JA: Experimental alveolar lipoproteinosis following the inhalation of silica, *J Pathol* 101:293-307, 1970.
28. Buechner HA, Ansari A: Acute silico-proteinosis: a new pathologic variant of acute silicosis in sandblasters, characterized by histologic features resembling alveolar proteinosis, *Dis Chest* 55:274-284, 1969.
29. Miller RR, Churg AM, Hutcheon M, Lam S: Pulmonary alveolar proteinosis and aluminum dust exposure, *Am Rev Respir Dis* 130:312-315, 1984.
30. Lee KP, Barras CE, Griffith FD, Waritz RS: Pulmonary response to glass fiber by inhalation exposure, *Lab Invest* 40:123-133, 1979.
31. Martin TR, Wehner AP, Butler J: Pulmonary toxicity of Mt. St. Helens volcanic ash: a review of experimental studies, *Am Rev Respir Dis* 128:158-162, 1983.
32. Samuels MP, Warner J: Pulmonary alveolar lipoproteinosis complicating juvenile dermatomyositis, *Thorax* 43:939-940, 1988.
33. Ballard PL, Nogee LM, Beers MF, Ballard RA, Planner BC, Polk L, de Mello DE, Moxley MA, Longmore WJ: Partial deficiency of surfactant protein B in an infant with chronic lung disease, *Pediatrics* 96:1046-1052, 1995.
34. Robertson B, Kobayashi T, Ganzuka M, Grossman G, LiW, Suzuki Y: Experimental neonatal respiratory failure induced by a monoclonal antibody to the hydrophobic surfactant-associated protein SP-B, *Pediatr Res* 30:239-243, 1991.
35. Clark JC, Weaver TE, Iwamoto HS, Ikegami M, Jobe AH, Hull WM, Whitsett JA: Decreased lung compliance and air trapping in heterozygous SP-B deficient mice, *Am J Resp Cell Mil Biol* 16:46-52, 1997.

Clinical Manifestations

36. Claypool WD, Rogers RM, Matuschak GM: Update on the clinical diagnosis, management, and pathogenesis of pulmonary alveolar proteinosis, *Chest* 85:550-558, 1984.
37. Coleman M, Dehner LP, Sibley RK, Burke BA, L'Heureux PR, Thompson TR: Pulmonary alveolar proteinosis: an uncommon cause of chronic neonatal respiratory distress, *Am Rev Respir Dis* 121:583-586, 1980.
38. Knight DP, Knight JA: Pulmonary alveolar proteinosis in the newborn, *Arch Pathol Lab Med* 109:529-531, 1985.
39. Murch CR, Carr DH: Computed tomography appearance of pulmonary alveolar proteinosis, *Clin Radiol* 40:240-243, 1989.
40. Martin RJ, Rogers RM, Myers NM: Pulmonary alveolar proteinosis: shunt fraction and lactic acid dehydrogenase concentration as aids to diagnosis, *Am Rev Respir Dis* 117:1059-1062, 1978.
41. Ballard PL: Neonatal respiratory disease due to surfactant protein B deficiency, *J Perinatology* 16:528-533, 1996.

Management

42. Mahut B, de Blic J, Le Bourgeois M, Beringer A, Chevalier JY, Scheinmann P: Partial and massive lung lavages in an infant with severe pulmonary alveolar proteinosis, *Pediatr Pulmonol* 13:50-53, 1992.
43. Spock A: Treatment of congenital alveolar proteinosis, *J Pediatr* 123:495, 1993 (letter).
44. Hiratzka LF, Swan DM, Rose EF, Ahrens RC: Bilateral simultaneous lung lavage utilizing membrane oxygenator for pulmonary alveolar proteinosis in an 8-month-old infant, *Ann Thorac Surg* 35:313-317, 1983.
45. Moulton SL, Krous HF, Merritt TA, Odell RM, Gangitano E, Cornish JD: Congenital pulmonary alveolar proteinosis: failure of treatment with extracorporeal life support, *J Pediatr* 120:297-302, 1992.
46. Hammon WE, McCaffree R, Cuchiara AJ: A comparison of manual to mechanical chest percussion for clearance of alveolar material in patients with pulmonary alveolar proteinosis, *Chest* 103:1409-1412, 1993.
47. Mazyck EM, Bonner JT, Herd HM, Symbas PN: Pulmonary lavage for childhood pulmonary alveolar proteinosis, *J Pediatr* 80:839-842, 1972.
48. Hudson AR, Halprin GM, Miller JA, Kilburn KH: Pulmonary interstitial fibrosis following alveolar proteinosis, *Chest* 55:700-702, 1974.
49. Anton HC, Gray B: Pulmonary alveolar proteinosis presenting with pneumothorax, *Clin Radiol* 18:428-431, 1967.

SUGGESTED READINGS

Claypool WD, Rogers RM, Mtuschak GM: Update on the clinical diagnosis, management, and pathogenesis of pulmonary alveolar proteinosis, *Chest* 85:550-558, 1984.

Nogee LM, de Mello DE, Dehner LP, Colten HR: Deficiency of pulmonary surfactant protein B in congenital alveolar proteinosis, *N Engl J Med* 328:406-410, 1993.

Prakash UBS, Barham SS, Carpenter HA, Dines DE, Marsh HM: Pulmonary alveolar phospholipoproteinosis: experience with 34 cases and a review, *Mayo Clin Proc* 62:499-518, 1987 (review).

CHAPTER 54

Hemosiderosis

Karen S. McCoy

After bleeding occurs in the alveoli, airways, or lung parenchyma, hemoglobin is ingested by macrophages and converted to hemosiderin by lysosomal degradation. Characteristic hemosiderin-laden macrophages may be seen in the bronchoalveolar lavage fluid or biopsy specimen, whether the blood is aspirated from the upper airway or is pulmonary in origin. Expectorated blood may not originate from the respiratory tract but may be gastrointestinal in origin.

The syndrome of pulmonary hemosiderosis (PH) is characterized by pulmonary infiltrates, iron deficiency anemia, and hemoptysis.[1] In children, hemoptysis may or may not be present, even though pulmonary hemorrhage sufficiently large to be life threatening has occurred. Three variants of primary PH are recognized: (1) idiopathic PH,[1] (2) PH associated with cow's milk allergy,[2] and (3) PH associated with antibody to basement membrane of the lung and kidney, (Goodpasture's syndrome).[3] The three (or possibly four) general variants of secondary hemosiderosis are (1) pulmonary venoocclusive disease associated with ventricular failure, mitral stenosis, and pulmonary hypertension[4]; (2) generalized vasculitides such as those associated with systemic lupus erythematosus[5] and immune-complex–mediated glomerulonephritis[6]; and (3) generalized hemorrhagic disorders, including purpuric syndromes[7,8] and coagulopathies associated with sepsis. A syndrome of PH associated with other, more variable diagnoses may represent a fourth group. These include ingestion or exposure to certain drugs and chemicals,[7] pancreatitis, myocarditis,[9] diabetic vascular disease,[10] and inflammatory bowel disease[11] and are hard to fit exactly into any of these categories, but probably are related to associated vasculitis. The diagnosis of isolated or idiopathic pulmonary hemosiderosis (IPH) is a diagnosis of exclusion, requiring thorough review and elimination of other causes of primary and secondary hemosiderosis.

PREVALENCE

Primary pulmonary hemosiderosis (PPH) is an uncommon yet well-recognized disorder characterized by episodic pulmonary hemorrhage and iron deficiency anemia. Hemoptysis may not always be evident, especially in infants. The disease is generally seen in children and young adults, but it has also been reported in very young infants and older individuals.[1,12] Most often diagnosis occurs between 1 year and 7 years of age, but 15% of patients are over 16 years of age at the time of diagnosis.[1] Male-female distribution is equal in children under 10 years, but males predominate 2:1 above this age.[1] Familial recurrence has been reported, but is rare.[13,14] Exact figures regarding prevalence are lacking. Children with PPH may be followed by pediatric hematologists because of the anemia, and the pulmonary manifestations may be unrecognized or not clinically apparent. In one study, pulmonary symptoms were absent in 50% of patients.[15]

The high likelihood of serious morbidity and even mortality in children with PPH necessitates early recognition and initiation of appropriate therapy. The clinical manifestations of PPH are extremely variable.[16] This variability, combined with the relative infrequency of this disorder, often causes a long delay in diagnosis. Therefore clinical suspicion regarding the possibility of PPH in a suggestive clinical situation is extremely important.

PATHOLOGIC MECHANISMS

In Goodpasture's syndrome, serum antibodies directed against alveolar basement membrane are found. Immunofluorescent staining is positive in linear arrangements along basement membranes of lung and kidney. These deposits consist of immunoglobulins (IgG, IgM) and complement, along the alveolar septa in the lungs.[17-19] Renal deposits are similar, with basement membrane deposits of IgA, IgG, IgM, and complement.[20] Electron microscopy shows fragmentation of basement membranes and interruption of vascular endothelium. These changes are presumed to be responsible for loss of vascular integrity, allowing rupture of red blood cells into the alveoli. Many of the findings are believed to be compatible with a cytotoxic type of immune response. Pulmonary hemorrhage is known to occur, at times, before evidence of renal disease is present.[21]

Pulmonary hemorrhage associated with immune-complex–mediated glomerulonephritis (PHIMG) may appear very similar to Goodpasture's syndrome. Differentiating these entities requires identification of granular or lumpy deposits of immunoglobulins by immunofluorescence along basement membranes and mesangium of the kidney. These lesions are similar to the renal lesions in systemic lupus erythematosus. Such deposits may not always be found in lung tissue.[6] Characteristics differentiating PHIMG from Goodpasture's syndrome are the absence of circulating antinuclear antibodies and the pattern of immunofluorescent deposits in PHIMG.

Heiner's syndrome, or PH associated with allergy to cow's milk, occurs with serum-precipitating antibodies to cow's milk proteins and varying but usually multiple symptoms of milk intolerance. Among these symptoms may be failure to thrive, vomiting, diarrhea, gastrointestinal blood loss, rhinitis, and nasopharyngeal congestion. Serum IgE[22,23] and, at times, milk-specific IgD are elevated.[24] Certain children with Heiner's syndrome have also been found to have such profound nasopharyngeal obstruction from adenotonsillar hypertrophy that cor pulmonale has developed because of chronic upper airway obstruction; this is relieved after the elimination of milk protein from the diet.[23] Controversy still exists regarding the role of milk in causing the pulmonary hemorrhage.

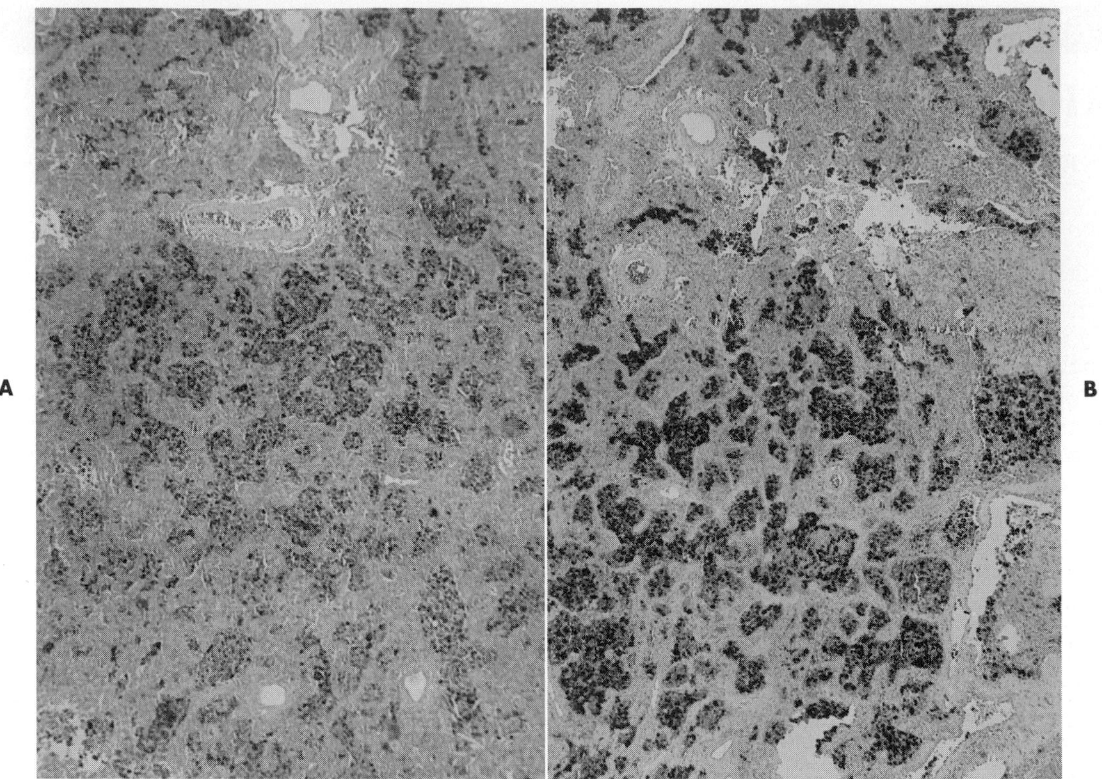

Fig. 54-1. A, Lung biopsy specimen from case 1. Hematoxylin and eosin stain. (Magnification 50 ×.) **B,** Lung biopsy, same patient. Iron stain. (50 ×.)

It remains unclear whether milk sensitivity is the primary cause or if the presence of milk-precipitating anti-bodies is secondary to a derangement in gastrointestinal absorption of milk.

In IPH no evidence for an immune mechanism has been found. The finding of pulmonary hemorrhage and iron deficiency anemia in the absence of circulating antibodies to basement membrane or renal involvement constitutes the basis for this diagnosis. The primary lesions appear to be damage to the capillary endothelium and the basement membrane and are detectable by transmission electron microscopy.[25,26]

Secondary forms of hemosiderosis are highly varied. There are numerous examples of reported autoimmune associations, including immune-complex–mediated nephritis,[10] poly-arteritis nodosa,[27] Wegener's granulomatosis,[28] rheumatoid arthritis,[29] systemic lupus erythematosus,[6] and mixed connective tissue disease.[30] PH has been reported in association with anaphylactoid purpura,[7] thrombocytopenic purpura,[8] microangioipathic hemolytic anemia,[12] and sepsis-related coagulopathies. Cardiac disease with associated pulmonary vascular disease, ventricular failure, mitral stenosis with pulmonary venous obstruction, and possibly myocarditis[9] have been reported to occur with PH. Primary or secondary pulmonary hypertension may precipitate PH. PH and intestinal villous atrophy, suggestive of celiac disease, have been described to coexist in the same individual.[11]

PATHOLOGY

Hemosiderin-laden macrophages are seen in both alveolar and interstitial areas within 72 hours of diffuse pulmonary hemorrhage. Alveoli are filled with phagocytes and cellular debris, and alveolar septa may be thickened by responsive inflammatory cell infiltration.[21] Focal areas of consolidation are common because of massive accumulations of hemosiderin-laden macrophages, which obliterate alveolar spaces and precipitate interstitial fibrosis (Fig. 54-1).[31] These findings may be present in varying stages in different areas of the lungs, which may make interpretation of biopsies more difficult. Macrophages containing hemosiderin can also be found in interstitial or alveolar areas in infection, bleeding disorders, chronic heart failure, and pulmonary hypertension and should therefore be considered a somewhat nonspecific finding.

Bronchoalveolar lavage (BAL) often reveals hemosiderin-laden macrophages in large numbers. Improved specificity and sensitivity are achieved by quantitating hemosiderin-containing macrophages in BAL specimens.[32] Hemosiderin clearance after acute hemorrhage occurs within 1 to 2 weeks of an isolated episode of bleeding.

Anemia that is microcytic is seen in nearly all cases. Bone marrow examination demonstrates reactive erythroid hyperplasia. Serum iron and bone marrow iron stores are usually reduced, and iron binding capacity is elevated. Hemolytic anemia has occasionally been erroneously diagnosed early in the presentation of children with PH, when elevated reticulocyte counts are seen.[33]

CLINICAL PRESENTATION AND DIAGNOSIS

The clinical history may reveal a variable combination of pallor, shortness of breath at rest or with exercise, tachypnea, cough, wheezing, or even color change. Complaints of chronic fatigue, severe exercise limitation, and growth failure may accompany more long-standing PH.

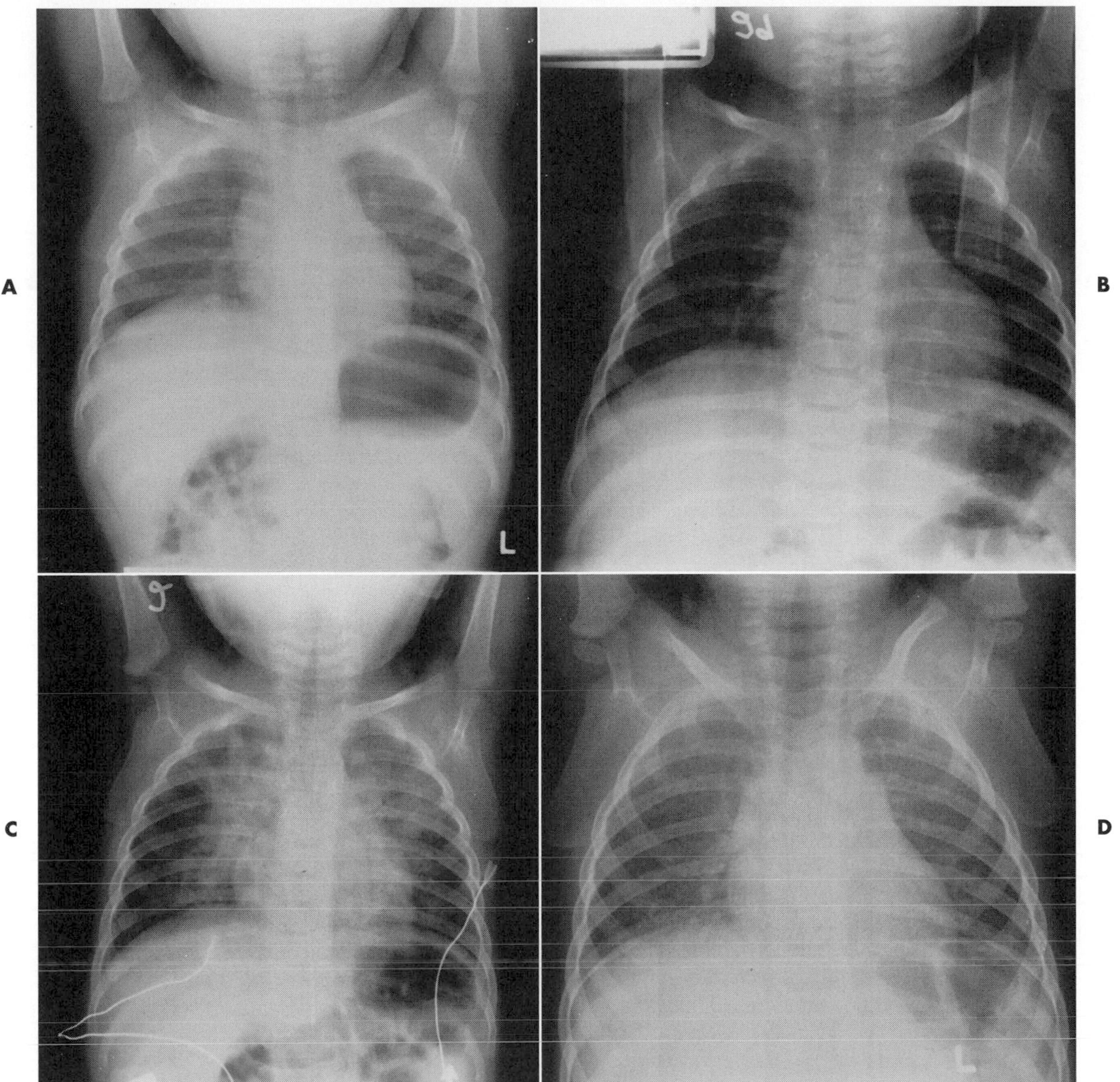

Fig. 54-2. **A,** Radiograph of case 2 at the time of initial diagnosis by BAL at 4 weeks of age. **B,** Chest radiograph, case 2, at 5 months of age. **C,** Radiographic changes seen in case 2 after an acute bleeding episode at 7 months of age. **D,** Follow-up chest radiograph of case 2 at age 2 years while asymptomatic.

Immediately after an acute hemorrhage, there is irritation from the blood and the inflammatory cell influx, resulting in edema, bronchospasm, increased mucus secretion, and airflow obstruction. Gas exchange is hampered by these alterations, and arterial oxygen tension and oxygen saturation are reduced. Carbon dioxide retention is not usually observed with acute hemorrhage. Pulmonary function testing demonstrates decreased compliance and airflow obstruction. Immediately after a bleeding episode, the diffusing capacity for carbon monoxide (CO) is increased, due to increased hemoglobin uptake of CO by sequestered red blood cells in the lungs. In the absence of acute hemorrhage, but with progressive pulmonary changes, diffusing capacity is reduced and pulmonary function testing demonstrates a restrictive pattern.

On physical examination, cough, pallor, tachypnea, dyspnea, fever, tachycardia, crackles or wheezes, cyanosis, and clubbing are compatible with the diagnosis but may not be present in any individual patient or if the disease is quiescent. Cough may be dry or productive, but it may be absent for periods of time during disease inactivity.

Radiographic manifestations usually vary with disease activity and the degree of chronicity. Infiltrates are usually alveolar and tend to be bilateral with an acute episode (Fig. 54-2). However, unilateral disease, small or patchy infiltrates, an interstitial pattern, and perihilar densities are also consistent with the diagnosis. Hilar and mediastinal adenopathy have also been described.[16] With chronicity and fibrosis, a more coarse, generalized interstitial pattern may persist, despite remission of episodic hemorrhages (Fig. 54-3); this may be the initial radiographic pattern in a few children whose diagnosis is made late in the course of the disease.

Because of the extreme variability of clinical manifestations in PH, clinical suspicion and the recognition of the simultaneous occurrence of pulmonary symptoms and iron deficiency anemia are essential for a timely diagnosis. The importance of early diagnosis cannot be overemphasized, because delay may

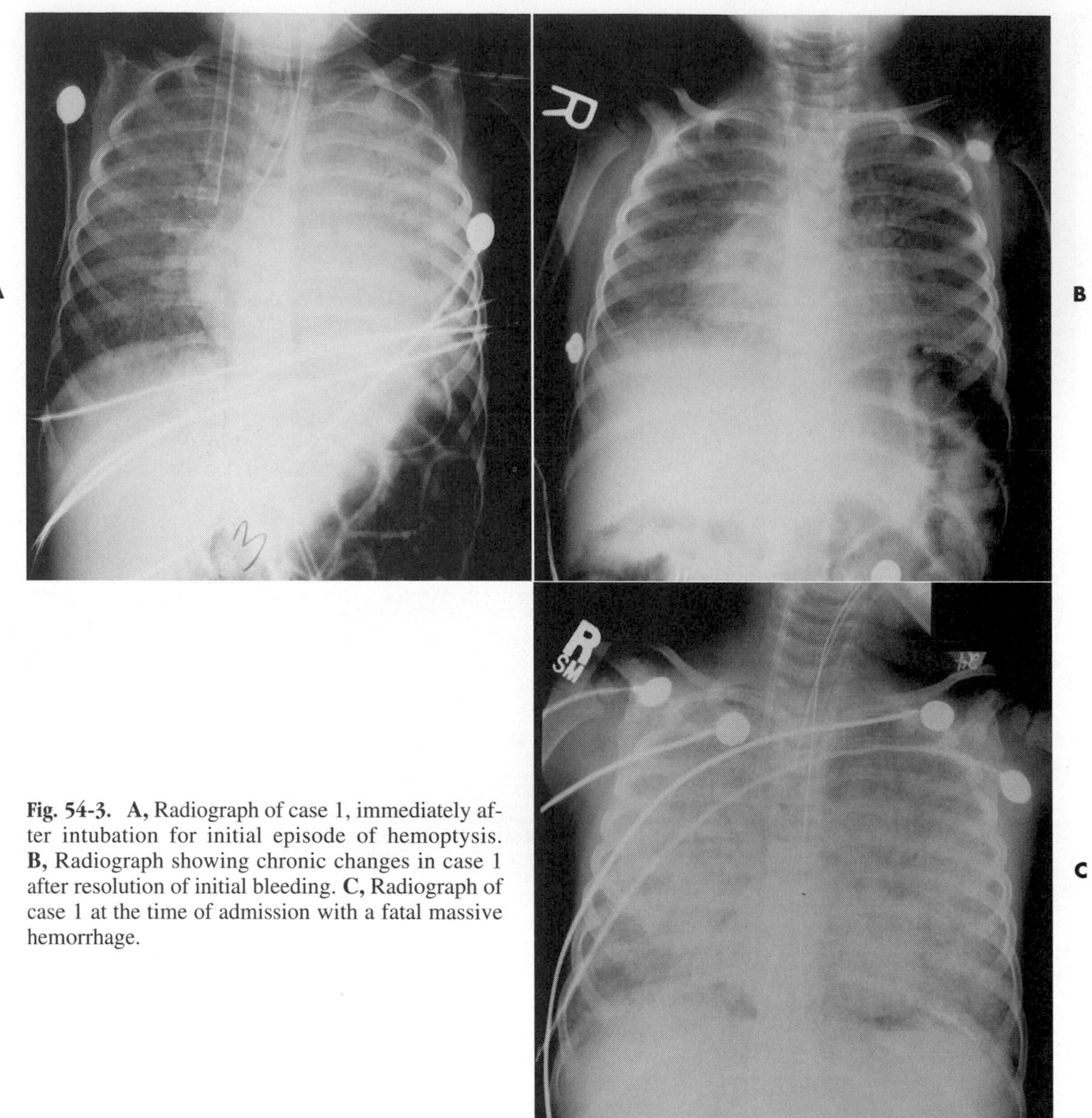

Fig. 54-3. **A,** Radiograph of case 1, immediately after intubation for initial episode of hemoptysis. **B,** Radiograph showing chronic changes in case 1 after resolution of initial bleeding. **C,** Radiograph of case 1 at the time of admission with a fatal massive hemorrhage.

result in irreversible lung damage or death. Iron deficiency is a common occurrence in childhood and usually is thought to be dietary. If a dietary cause is not found, attention often is next focused on the gastrointestinal tract. The pulmonary symptoms may be vague, subacute, and nonspecific. Even when there is a prominent respiratory component, a respiratory infection is often initially thought to be the cause. Severe bleeding may result in hemoptysis, but this finding is absent in many patients, especially infants. The amount of hemoptysis, when present, may lead one to underestimate the amount of actual bleeding.

The differential diagnosis of PH usually includes acute infectious pneumonia, cystic fibrosis, aspiration, and other, more unusual causes of interstitial lung diseases in the pediatric age-group. Because infection is a common cause of pneumonia, and because of the rising incidence of acquired immunodeficiency syndrome, an infectious agent is often sought first. The presence of hemoptysis, anemia, or coexistent renal disease strongly suggests PH. Bronchoalveolar lavage is diagnostic, revealing large numbers of hemosiderin-laden macrophages (Fig. 54-4) and negative cultures and stains. The timing of BAL after an episode may be problematic. In some patients who are acutely ill and require oxygen or ventilatory support, BAL may be delayed until the patient recovers sufficiently to undergo the procedure more safely. A negative BAL after a small acute bleed may be misleading if the procedure is performed less than 72 hours after the bleed, because hemosiderin may not yet have been incorporated into macrophages. In the absence of BAL, chromium labeling of red blood cells may lead to localization of the labeled cells to the lungs and may suggest the correct diagnosis of PH.[33] Lung biopsy is rarely needed if an adequate specimen can be obtained from BAL or sputum expectoration. In certain circumstances, however, lung biopsy may be the diagnostic procedure of choice.

Because IPH is a diagnosis of exclusion, evidence to suggest an immunopathogenic association with the pulmonary hemorrhages must be sought before arriving at this diagnosis. Appropriate testing should be done for anti–basement membrane antibodies, antinuclear antibodies, sedimentation rate, rheumatoid factor, complement, serum precipitins to cow's

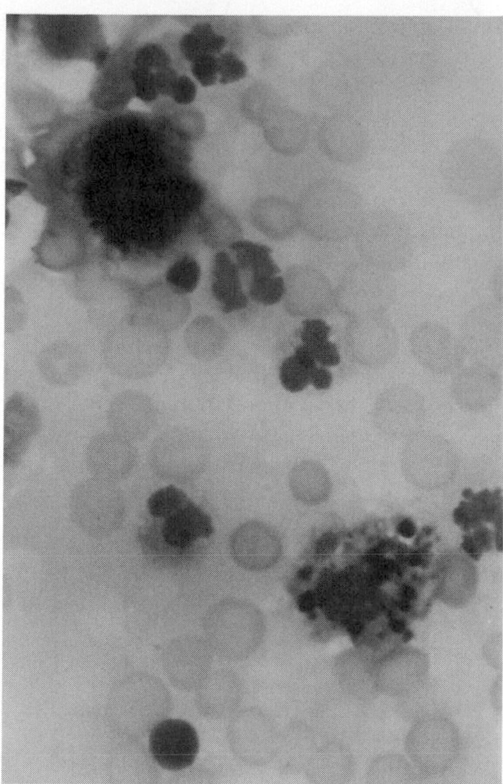

Fig. 54-4. BAL specimen from case 2 showing iron staining of macrophages. (200 ×.)

milk (which should include evaluation of antibodies of different immunoglobulin classes), anemia, and renal function. Evaluation for the degree and type of anemia and for renal function should be performed. Serial determinations of renal function or, in certain circumstances, renal biopsy may be required. Immunofluorescence and electron microscopy of lung or kidney tissue may differentiate IPH from Goodpasture's syndrome, immune-complex–mediated nephritis, and lung disease. An elevated IgE level and peripheral eosinophilia may indicate milk-associated pulmonary hemorrhage. Confirmation is by identification of multiple serum precipitins to cow's milk. A search for possible causes of secondary hemosiderosis is required before making the diagnosis of IPH. It should be remembered that both systemic lupus erythematosus and Goodpasture's syndrome may cause pulmonary hemorrhage years before serologic and immunologic changes and clinically detectable renal disease.[5,21]

More extensive thoracic imaging may be helpful if intrapulmonary vascular malformations, focal pulmonary causes, or endobronchial lesions are suspected.[34]

MANAGEMENT

General stabilization measures, including oxygen supplementation, ventilation, transfusion, and supportive respiratory therapy for excessive secretions and bronchospasm, are provided appropriate to the level of impairment. Immediately after the establishment of the diagnosis, initiation of high-dose corticosteroids is the treatment of choice. A dose of prednisone, 2 to 5 mg/kg per day, or the equivalent dosage of an intravenous preparation should be used. For IPH, steroid usage at high dosage should continue until at least 7 days after substantial bleeding has subsided, and the dosage should then be tapered over several weeks. Some children tolerate complete weaning from steroids in this fashion, but others demonstrate the need for more chronic usage. If, after weaning or discontinuing steroids, bleeding recurs and higher doses are again required, vigorous attempts should be made to reduce the dosage to the lowest amount that appears to prevent recurrence. Failure to respond adequately to steroids alone or unacceptable steroid side effects may be indications for using other forms of immunosuppression, such as azathioprine, chloroquine, or cyclophosphamide.[35-37]

After the acute episode of IPH is under adequate control, children should be followed closely. Specific monitoring should include periodic evaluation of growth, oxygen saturation, hemogram, chest radiograph, and pulmonary function. Early and periodic evaluations of renal function are appropriate. For children whose steroid weaning is complicated by recurrence of bleeding, the use of chronic steroids requires frequent attention to possible steroid side effects. In spite of chronic immune suppression therapy, massive acute bleeding may occur at any time and may be fatal. Severe acute hemorrhage does not usually result from steroid weaning, although bleeding usually is responsive to acute intensification of this therapy or the addition of one of the other immunosuppressive agents.

Controversy continues regarding the need for and usefulness of chronic immunosuppressive therapy in managing hemosiderosis. In a single limited series, there appears to be no prognostic advantage to chronic medication.[38] However, many clinicians have found that individual patients tend to have recurrent hemorrhages after reduction or discontinuation of these drugs. At the present time there are no definitive recommendations about the duration of immunosuppressive therapy.

The main treatment for milk-associated PH is cessation of milk and milk products. The treatment of secondary PH is usually the therapy used for the primary disease process.

COURSE AND PROGNOSIS

It is difficult to determine the prognosis for all of the PH syndromes because of the infrequency of the diagnosis and the variability among cases. Clinical differences between cases are also related to the degree of established pulmonary damage at diagnosis and the impact of immune-associated forms of the disease. Furthermore, there exists no national database monitoring children with PH.

Focusing on IPH allows a better understanding of course and prognosis. Early reports suggested a short period of approximately 2 years between diagnosis and death.[1] Improved survival in IPH is likely with aggressive management; this is also true for the immune-associated forms of the disease. In the individual case, awareness of potential complications, vigilant surveillance for infection, and close monitoring provide an improved outlook. Another significant factor in establishing case severity is the tendency toward massive hemorrhage. It is virtually impossible to predict which patients will have this potentially fatal occurrence with the disease. In IPH, in the absence of life-threatening acute hemorrhage or significant established lung disease, with close follow-up and aggressive surveillance for infection or other complications of immunosuppression, a favorable outcome may be achieved. In certain cases, permanent remission apparently occurs, usually during or after puberty.

The prognosis in other forms of PH can still be grim and tends to be so especially in immune-mediated forms or in cases in which organ damage is severe. In PH associated with milk protein allergy, avoidance of the antigen is usually associated with a good prognosis.

Evaluation of drug therapy regimens is clouded by the inherent clinical variability in PH syndromes and apparently spontaneous remissions and exacerbations while patients are on therapy.

CASE REPORTS

Case 1

A 3½-year-old girl had been followed by the pediatric hematology division for about 1 year for poorly differentiated hemolytic anemia. She had required multiple transfusions and was described as frail and always breathing hard, but she was not diagnosed with IPH until she experienced a severe pulmonary hemorrhage. She required intubation and aggressive ventilation. Her examination was remarkable for an emaciated, pale-appearing child with coarse breath sounds on the ventilator and definite clubbing. There was difficulty in oxygenating the patient consistently above 80% saturation, despite an FIO_2 of 1.0. Diffuse bilateral chest infiltrates were present on the radiographs (see Fig. 54-3, *A*). At the time of this admission, the patient underwent lung biopsy, demonstrating interstitial fibrosis and abundant hemosiderin-laden macrophages (see Fig. 54-1). Findings of evaluation for antinuclear antibodies, sweat chloride determination, anti–basement membrane antibodies, milk precipitins, evidence of renal dysfunction, rheumatoid factor, and human immunodeficiency virus infection were all normal or negative; cultures were negative. Serum iron was reduced.

After initiation of steroids, dramatic weaning from the ventilator was accomplished. The patient was subsequently extubated and weaned from oxygen supplementation. Milk products were withheld. After discharge, she was seen frequently and gradually weaned to an alternate-day steroid regimen. Her appetite improved, her growth progressed, and her anemia resolved. Because milk precipitins were not present, the patient was cautiously returned to the use of milk products 4 months after the initial severe hemorrhage. She remained on alternate-day prednisone therapy. Radiographic resolution was incomplete (see Fig. 54-3, *B*). Approximately 5 months after diagnosis, she suddenly deteriorated, despite continuedalternate-day steroids. She suffered a massive pulmonary hemorrhage and died within 24 hours of hospitalization. Radiographs taken at the time of that admission are shown (see Fig. 54-3, *C*).

Case 2

A 4-week-old boy was seen 1 week after his parents witnessed bright red blood coming from the nose and mouth. A bloody stool was described on the night after the expectorated blood. He had been clinically well. The parents' concern was increased because an older male sibling had previously died with a clinical diagnosis of PH before full diagnostic studies could be performed. Diagnostic studies on this infant were negative except for a BAL positive for hemosiderin-laden macrophages in large numbers (see Fig. 54-2, *B*). The hemoglobin level and radiographs were normal. The patient was placed on prednisone and trimethoprim-sulfamethoxazole, and close follow-up was begun. He remained symptom free with respect to bleeding for several months. He was hospitalized again for investigation of apnea at 5 months of age. The chest radiograph was again normal, but a pH probe revealed severe gastroesophageal reflux. He was placed on ranitidine and metoclopramide. At 6 months of age, he was reduced to alternate-day steroid therapy. Approximately 1 month later, he experienced a sudden deterioration, with expectorated blood, a respiratory rate of 80, need for oxygen supplementation to maintain adequate saturation, a decrease in hemoglobin from 12 to 8.1 g/dl, and significant bilateral infiltrates on the chest radiograph (see Fig. 54-2, *C*). After stabilization, a BAL was done, which demonstrated large numbers of hemosiderin-laden macrophages and numerous lipid-laden macrophages. Subsequently the patient underwent fundoplication, after which he continued to do well. His prednisone dose was tapered to every other day, and radiographs (see Fig. 54-2, *D*), oxygen saturation, and pulmonary function returned to normal. Approximately 3 years after diagnosis, he remained symptom free on prednisone, 1 mg every other day.

REFERENCES

1. Soergel KH, Sommers SC: Idiopathic pulmonary hemosiderosis and related syndromes, *Am J Med* 32:499-511, 1962.
2. Heiner DC, Sears JW, Kniker WT: Multiple precipitins to cow's milk in chronic respiratory disease, *Am J Dis Child* 103:634-654, 1962.
3. Beniot FL, Rulon DB, Thiel GB, Doolan PD, Whatten RH: Goodpasture's syndrome, *Am J Med* 37:424-444, 1964.
4. Levy J, Wilmott RW: Pulmonary hemosiderosis, *Pediatr Pulmonol* 2:384-391, 1986.
5. Ramirez RE, Glasier C, Kirks D, Shackleford GD, Locey M: Pulmonary hemorrhage associated with systemic lupus erythematosus in children, *Radiology* 152:409-412, 1984.
6. Loughlin GM, Taussig LM, Murphy SA, Strunk RC, Kohenen PW: Immune-complex–mediated glomerulonephritis and pulmonary hemorrhage simulating Goodpasture syndrome, *J Pediatr* 93:181-184, 1978.
7. Kendig EL, Chernick V: *Disorders of the respiratory tract in children,* ed 4, Philadelphia, 1983, WB Saunders.
8. Buchanon GR, Moore GC: Pulmonary hemosiderosis and immune thrombocytopenia, initial manifestations of collagen-vascular disease, *JAMA* 246:861-864, 1981.
9. Gaum WE, Alterman K: Complete left bundle branch block in idiopathic pulmonary hemosiderosis, *J Pediatr* 85:633-638, 1974.
10. Yodiaken RE, Pardo V: Diabetic capillaritis, *Human Pathol* 6:455-465, 1975.
11. Wright PH, Mengies IS, Punder RE, Keeling PWN: Adult idiopathic pulmonary hemosiderosis and celiac disease, *Q J Med* 197:95-102, 1981.

Prevalence

12. Morgan PGM, Turner-Warwick M: Pulmonary hemosiderosis and pulmonary hemorrhage, *Br J Dis Chest* 75:225-242, 1981.
13. Thaell JF, Greipp PR, Stubbs SE, Siegal GP: Idiopathic pulmonary hemosiderosis: two cases in a family, *Mayo Clin Proc* 53:113-118, 1978.
14. Beckerman RC, Taussig LM, Pinnas JL: Familial idiopathic hemosiderosis, *Am J Dis Child* 133:609-611, 1979.
15. Kjellman B, Elinder AG, Garwicz S, Swan H: Idiopathic pulmonary hemosiderosis in Swedish children, *Acta Pediatr Scand* 73:584-588, 1984.
16. Case records of the Massachusetts General Hospital (Case 30-1988), *N Engl J Med* 319:227-237, 1988.

Pathologic Mechanisms

17. Poskitt TR: Immunologic and electron microscopic studies in Goodpasture's syndrome, *Am J Med* 49:250-257, 1970.
18. Sturgill BC, Westervelt FB: Immunofluorescent studies in a case of Goodpasture's syndrome, *JAMA* 194:172-174, 1965.
19. Beirne GJ, Octaviano GN, Koop WL, Burns RD: Immunohistology of the lung in Goodpasture's syndrome, *Ann Intern Med* 69:1207-1212, 1968.
20. Donald KJ, Edwards RL, McEroy JDS: Alveolar capillary basement membrane lesions in Goodpasture's syndrome, *Am J Med* 59:642-649, 1975.
21. Boat TF: Pulmonary hemosiderosis. In Nussbaum E, Galant S, eds: *Pediatric respiratory disorders: clinical approaches,* New York, 1984, Grune & Stratton, pp 59-65.

22. Heiner DC, Rose B: Elevated levels of YE (IgE) in conditions other than classical allergy, *J Allergy* 45:30-42, 1970.
23. Boat TF, Polmar SH, Whitman V, Kleinerman JI, Stern RC, Coershuk CF: Hyperactivity to cow milk in young children with pulmonary hemosiderosis and cor pulmonale secondary to nasopharyngeal obstruction, *J Pediatr* 87:23-29, 1975.
24. Gallant S, Nussbaum E, Wittner R, DeWeck AL, Heiner DC: Increased IgD mild antibody responses in a patient with Down's syndrome, pulmonary hemosiderosis and cor-pulmonale, *Ann Allergy* 51:446-449, 1983.
25. Yeager H, Powell D, Weinberg RM, Bauer H, Bellanti JA, Katz S: Idiopathic pulmonary hemosiderosis, *Arch Intern Med* 136:1145-1149, 1976.
26. Hyatt RW, Adelstein ER, Halozun JF, Lukens JN: Ultrastructure of lung in idiopathic pulmonary hemosiderosis, *Am J Med* 52:822-829, 1972.
27. Leaker B, Cambridge G, du Bois RM, Neild GH: Idiopathic pulmonary haemosiderosis: a form of microscopic polyarteritis? *Thorax* 47:988-990, 1992.
28. Kincaid-Smith P, D'arice AJF: Plasmapheresis in rapidly progressive glomulonephritis, *Am J Med* 65:564-566, 1978.
29. Smith BS: Idiopathic pulmonary hemosiderosis and rheumatoid arthritis, *Br Med J* 1:1403-1404, 1966.
30. O'Donohue WJ: Idiopathic pulmonary hemosiderosis with manifestations with multiple connective tissue and immune disorders, *Am Rev Resp Dis* 109:473-479, 1974.

Pathology

31. Stocker JT: The respiratory tract. In Stocker JT, Dehner LD, eds: *Pediatric pathology,* Philadelphia, 1992, JB Lippincott.
32. Perez-Arellano JL, Garcia JL, Macias MCG, Gomez FG, Lopez AJ, de Castro S: Hemosiderin-laden macrophages in bronchoalveolar lavage fluid, *Acta Cytolog* 36:26-30, 1992.
33. Kurzweil PR, Miller DR, Freeman JE, Reiman RE, Mayer K: Use of sodium chromate Cr 51 in diagnosing childhood idiopathic pulmonary hemosiderosis, *Am J Dis Child* 138:746-748, 1984.

Clinical Presentation and Diagnosis

34. Haponik EF, Britt EJ, Smith PL, Bleecker ER: Computed chest tomography in the evaluation of hemoptysis: impact on diagnosis and treatment, *Chest* 91:80-85, 1987.

Management

35. Rossi GA, Balsano E, Battistini E, Oddera S, Marchese P, Acquila M, Fregonese B, Mori PG: Long term prednisone and azathioprine treatment of a patient with idiopathic pulmonary hemosiderosis, *Pediatr Pulmonol* 13:176-180, 1992.
36. Bush A, Sheppard MN, Warner JO: Chloroquine in idiopathic pulmonary hemosiderosis, *Archiv Dis Child* 67:625-627, 1992.
37. Colombo JL, Stolz SM: Treatment of life-threatening primary pulmonary hemosiderosis with cyclophosphamide, *Chest* 102:959-960, 1992.
38. Chryssanthopoulos C, Cassimos C, Panagiotidou C: Prognostic criteria in idiopathic pulmonary hemosiderosis in children, *Eur J Pediatr* 140: 123-125, 1983.

CHAPTER 55

Sarcoidosis

Edward N. Pattishall, Edwin L. Kendig, Jr., and Floyd W. Denny, Jr.

Sarcoidosis, a chronic, multisystem, granulomatous disorder of unknown etiology, is rarely diagnosed in children. It affects young adults most commonly and usually manifests with bilateral hilar lymphadenopathy, pulmonary infiltrates, and skin or eye lesions. In infants and young children it often involves the skin, joints, and eyes, without typical lung involvement. Sarcoidosis is a diagnosis by exclusion and is established when clinical features are supported by histologic evidence of noncaseating granuloma. Corticosteroids are the mainstay of therapy, but other antiinflammatory agents occasionally have been used. Although spontaneous resolution occurs in most children, a significant number have residual organ system damage or progressive disease.

EPIDEMIOLOGY

The incidence and prevalence of sarcoidosis in children are unknown because of the lack of symptoms in a significant proportion of patients and lack of diagnostic accuracy. Recognized cases are predominantly symptomatic, whereas a number of asymptomatic cases are identified by routine radiographic screening.[1,2] Thus the number of cases is probably underestimated. Sarcoidosis is recognized less commonly in children than in adults, in whom sarcoidosis is most often recognized between 20 and 40 years of age.[3] In the pediatric age group, sarcoidosis is most commonly recognized in adolescents, although the youngest patient reported is a 2-month-old infant.[1]

Although sarcoidosis has a worldwide distribution, it has been reported most frequently in certain geographic locations. In the United States, there is a high incidence of reported sarcoidosis in the South Atlantic and Gulf states, particularly in the coastal plain (Fig. 55-1).[4] Most of the previously reported cases of childhood sarcoidosis in the United States are from these areas. Sweden has the highest reported incidence of sarcoidosis in Europe, ranging from 64 per 100,000 population using mass radiographic screening to 641 per 100,000 population using autopsy studies.[5] In the United Kingdom, nine radiographic surveys of 3,232,910 individuals revealed an incidence of 20 per 100,000 population.

In the United States, blacks are affected more commonly than whites, and the previous reports in children reflect this race predominance.[6] Outside the United States, sarcoidosis appears most often in the predominant race of that particular country. Thus, in Scandinavia, most patients are white, and in Japan, most patients are Asian.

Sarcoidosis in children affects both male and females in equal proportion.[6] Although some reports of adults indicate a

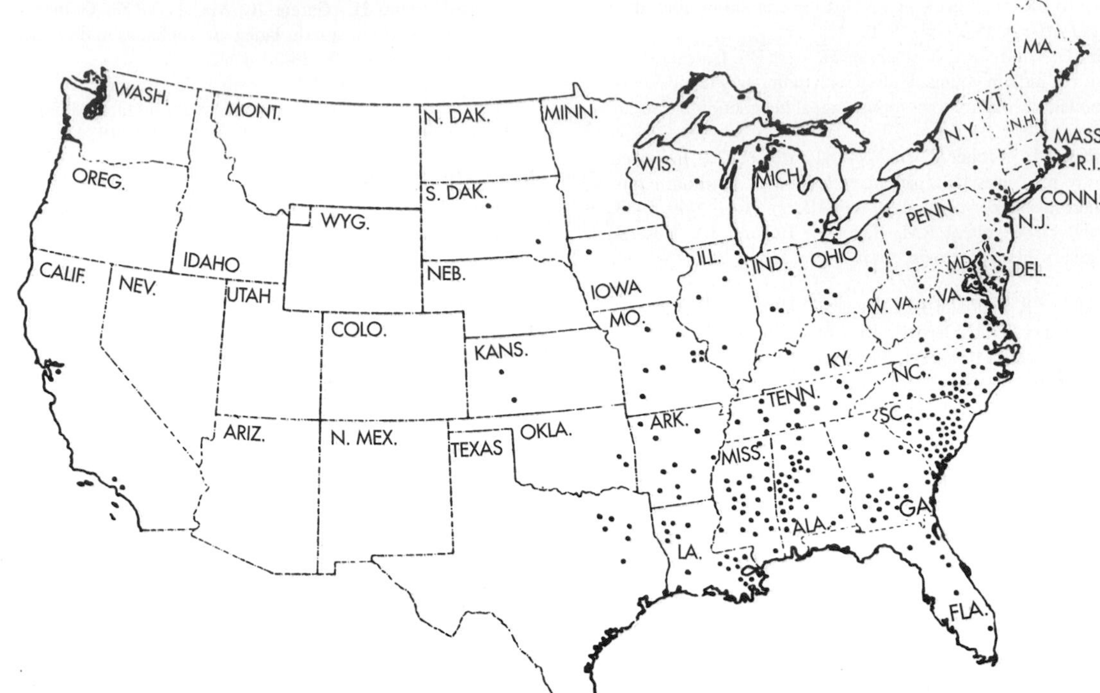

Fig. 55-1. Birthplaces of patients with sarcoidosis. (From Cooch JW: *Am Rev Respir Dis* 84:103-108, 1961.)

higher proportion of females with sarcoidosis, other reports do not support a difference in gender.[5]

ETIOLOGY

The cause of sarcoidosis in unknown. Investigations of the cause have focused on a combination of environmental agents and host factors. The most commonly cited etiology is from one or more environmental agents in a susceptible host.[1]

Primarily because of the geographic clustering of cases, some investigations have concentrated on environmental agents, such as soil types, plants, and specific occupations or behaviors common in these regions. No clear relationship has been found with any of these factors. Similarly, no infectious agent has been identified as a cause of sarcoidosis, although the association with tuberculosis remains controversial.[7,8] Studies have documented an association in the prevalences of sarcoidosis and mycobacteria, the presence of antibody titers to atypical mycobacteria in many patients with sarcoidosis, and the presence of mycobacteria from tissues in patients with sarcoidosis in a higher frequency than in other patients.[5] Although one study found mycobacterial DNA in 10 out of 20 samples of patients with sarcoidosis using the polymerase chain reaction,[8] others have not been able to substantiate this finding, and the association between mycobacteria and sarcoidosis remains uncertain.[9]

Host factors have been evaluated because of reports of familial association and the high prevalence of sarcoidosis in certain racial and ethnic groups. Familial associations are being recognized with increased frequency, the most common being a sibling-sibling relationship, followed by a parent-child relationship.[5] In addition to the increased prevalence in blacks in the United States, increased prevalences of sarcoidosis in other ethnic groups also exist. For example, the prevalence rate of sarcoidosis in north London is 27 per 100,000 in British-born persons, 155 per 100,000 among Irish immigrants, and 183 per 100,000 among those of West Indian origin.[7] These associations indicate that host factors are likely to affect the etiology of sarcoidosis. Although associations with specific human lymphocyte antigen have been reported, the data are not consistent.[1,5]

PATHOLOGY AND PATHOGENESIS

The hallmark of sarcoidosis is a well-defined, noncaseating granuloma of compact, radially arranged, epithelioid cells with pale-staining nuclei, some multinucleate giant cells, and a rim of lymphocytes (Fig. 55-2).[2,3] The giant cells are usually of the Langhans' type, in which the nuclei are arranged in an arc around a central granular zone. Granulomas can be present in almost any organ of the body. Unfortunately, granulomas are not diagnostic, and similar pathology can be found in other diseases (see Diagnosis and Differential Diagnosis, later in this chapter).

It has been suggested that there is an immune response to an unknown antigen that initiates a cascade of events that result in granuloma formation.[10] In sarcoidosis, the ratio of helper to suppressor T cells is reduced in the blood but is increased at the site of inflammation. Activated T lymphocytes and macrophages recruit blood monocytes that differentiate into macrophages, which produce an alveolitis. Thus, although lymphopenia may exist in the blood, there is an increase in the number of helper T cells at the site of inflammation. Once formed, the granulomas may resolve spontaneously or, if they persist, become hyalinized and eventually fibrotic, with tissue scarring as the final outcome.

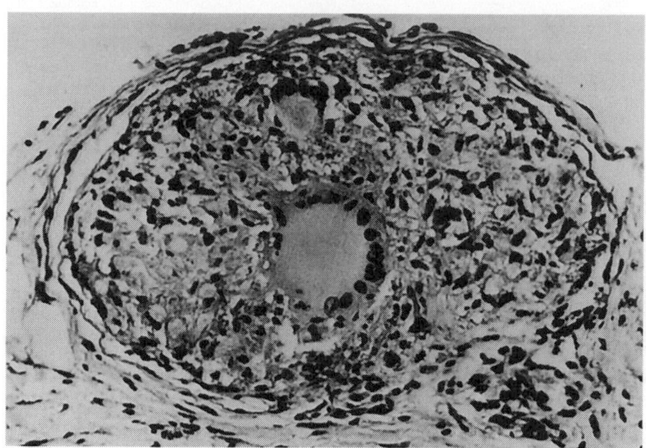

Fig. 55-2. Typical noncaseating granuloma. (From James DG, Williams WJ: *Sarcoidosis and other granulomatous diseases,* Philadelphia, 1985, WB Saunders, p 22.)

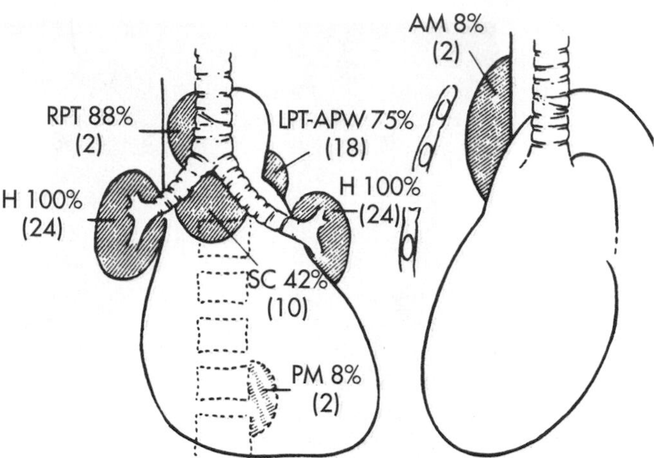

Fig. 55-3. Lymph node involvement in 24 pediatric cases of pulmonary sarcoidosis. *H,* hilar; *RPT,* right paratracheal; *LPT-APW,* left paratracheal–aortic pulmonic window; *SC,* subcarinal; *AM,* anterior mediastinal; *PM,* posterior mediastinal. (From Merten DF, Kirks DR, Grossman H: *Am J Roentgenol* 135:673-679, 1980.)

CLINICAL FEATURES

Although sarcoid lesions can occur in almost any organ of the body, lesions commonly involve the lungs, lymph nodes, eyes, skin, liver, and spleen. More than one system is usually involved, and in one report, 75% of children had five or more different areas of involvement.[6] Symptoms and physical findings largely depend on the organ system involved and are due primarily to local tissue infiltration and injury by pressure or displacement. Thus patients can have a variety of symptoms and physical findings.

Symptoms

Approximately 90% of children diagnosed with sarcoidosis have symptoms.[6,11] In areas where mass chest radiographic screening is performed, a larger proportion of asymptomatic children is reported. The symptoms may be nonspecific and include weight loss, fatigue, lethargy, anorexia, headache, and, less commonly, fever. Other symptoms relate to the organ system involved and commonly include symptoms related to the lungs (cough, dyspnea, and sometimes chest pain), eyes (visual disturbances), joints (arthritis and arthralgias), and peripheral lymphadenitis. Although skin lesions are common, they do not usually cause patients to seek treatment. Less common symptoms include parotid gland enlargement, abdominal pain, and nausea.

Physical Findings

The most common physical findings include peripheral lymphadenopathy, eye changes, skin lesions, and liver or spleen enlargement.[6,12] Physical findings in the chest are not common. The peripheral lymphadenopathy typically consists of firm, movable, nontender nodes. Although almost any eye involvement may occur, most often there is iritis, uveitis, and conjunctival granulomas.[13] Skin lesions are common and varied, including papules, plaques, nodules, hyperpigmented lesions, hypopigmented lesions, and changes in old scars.[14] In contrast to adults, erythema nodosum is rare in children.

Less common physical findings include respiratory findings, musculoskeletal changes, parotid enlargement, cardiovascular changes, and neurologic abnormalities.[2,5,6] Respiratory findings may include rales, rhonchi, wheezing, and decreased breath sounds. Obstruction of the airways can occur from endobronchial granulomas or compression from lymph nodes. Musculoskeletal changes include joint effusions, joint pain, or, less commonly, bone abnormalities. Cardiovascular abnormalities include conduction and rhythm disturbances caused by granuloma infiltration of the heart. Clinically recognizable heart involvement is uncommon; however, at autopsy, granulomas are present in the heart in as many as 27% of adults.[5] Neurologic abnormalities are rare but may include signs of obstructive hydrocephalus and seventh nerve palsy.[15] Optic nerve involvement, meningitis, and seizures have also been reported.

Radiographic, Pulmonary Function, and Laboratory Findings

The most helpful laboratory finding is a chest radiograph. In one large series of 60 children, only 3 had normal chest radiographs; all 3 of these children had eye involvement.[6] The radiograph often appears to show more involvement than would be predicted based on symptoms. The most common chest radiographic finding in children is bilateral hilar lymph node enlargement, with or without parenchymal involvement (Figs. 55-3 through 55-5).[16] Although hilar adenopathy is most common, paratracheal adenopathy is often present. The parenchymal involvement is most often a small, irregular, interstitial pattern; however, alveolar, small nodular, and fibrotic patterns are also described. Uncommonly, chest radiographs may reveal pleural effusions, pneumothorax, pleural thickening, calcifications, or atelectasis.

There are several classifications for the radiographic features seen at presentation. Commonly, a normal chest radiograph is stage 0, bilateral hilar lymphadenopathy alone is stage I, bilateral hilar lymphadenopathy with pulmonary infiltrates is stage II, and parenchymal infiltrates without hilar adenopathy is stage III.[3] Some physicians have added a stage IV, which represents a worsening of stage III, including fibrosis and emphysema with formation of bullae.[5]

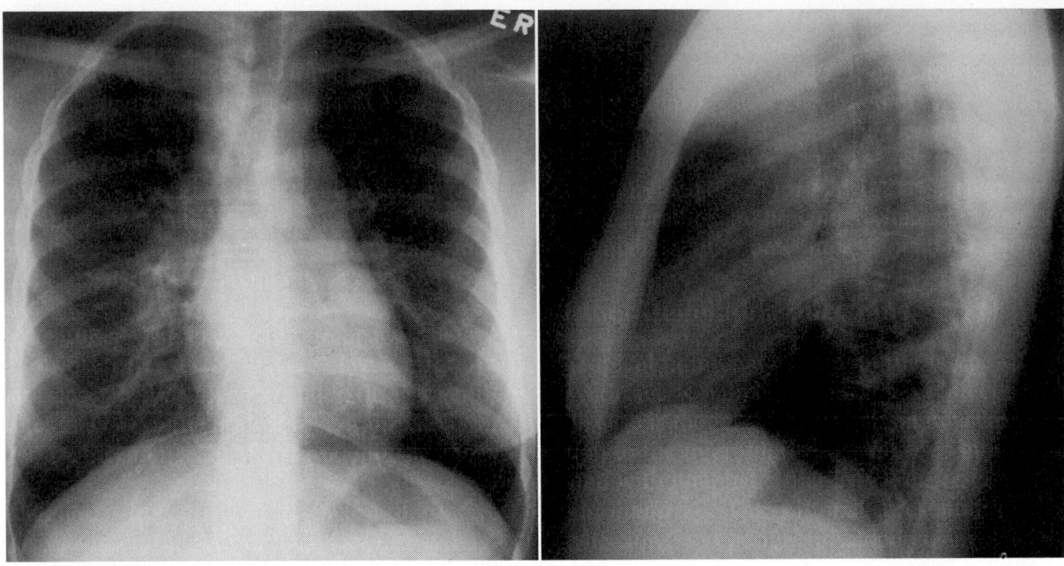

Fig. 55-4. Typical chest radiograph from a 14-year-old black female with sarcoidosis. The chest radiograph reveals bilateral hilar and paratracheal adenopathy and no parenchymal infiltrates. (Courtesy David Merten, University of North Carolina, Chapel Hill.)

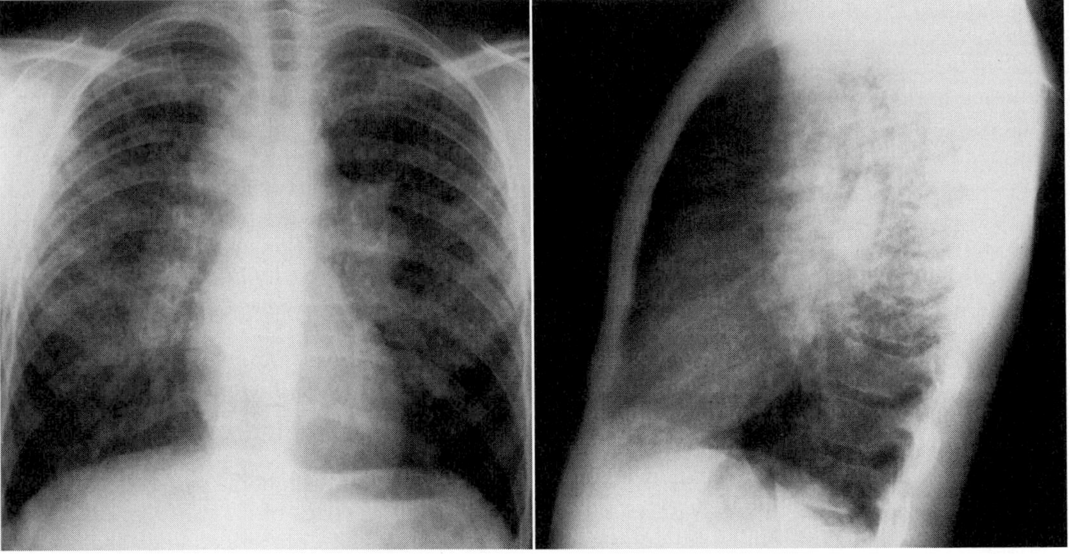

Fig. 55-5. Chest radiograph from a 12-year-old black male with sarcoidosis. The chest radiograph reveals diffuse miliary nodules in addition to the typical mediastinal and bilateral hilar adenopathy. (Courtesy David Merten, University of North Carolina, Chapel Hill.)

Although radiographs of the chest or extremities occasionally detect lytic bone lesions, such lesions are less common now than a few decades ago.

Although pulmonary function test results are not well documented in children, approximately 50% of children have the characteristic functional changes of restrictive lung disease, including reductions in forced vital capacity, total lung capacity, and functional residual capacity.[6,17] These changes appear to be secondary to the early alveolitis progressing to fibrosis. Changes consistent with obstructive changes are seen in 15% of children. Obstruction may be secondary to reactive airway disease, lymph node compression, or intrabronchial sarcoid granuloma.

A variety of blood and urine tests may be abnormal in sarcoidosis, and, although none are diagnostic, some may be helpful in the management or detection of disease activity. An elevated erythrocyte sedimentation rate (ESR), high immunoglobulin levels, and increased serum proteins are common and presumably are the result of the acute inflammatory phase of the disease. Hypercalcemia and hypercalciuria are also common abnormalities and are thought to result from vitamin D secretion from sarcoid granulomas. Other abnormalities may include leukopenia, eosinophilia, and hepatic and renal dysfunction. The renal and hepatic dysfunction are most commonly related to local infiltration of sarcoid granulomas; however, renal disease can also result from hypercalciuria

BOX 55-1
Differential Diagnosis of Chest Radiographic Findings of Sarcoidosis

Hilar adenopathy

Lymphoma
Tuberculosis
Metastases
Enlarged pulmonary arteries
Leukemia
Infectious mononucleosis
Berylliosis
Coccidioidomycosis
Histoplasmosis

Hilar adenopathy and pulmonary infiltrates

Tuberculosis
Pneumoconiosis
Cartinoma
Idiopathic hemosiderosis
Pulmonary eosinophilia
Histiocytosis X

Diffuse pulmonary infiltrates
Same as above, plus the following:
Honeycomb lung
Rheumatoid lung
Progressive systemic sclerosis
Fibrosing alveolitis
Hemosiderosis
Extrinsic allergic alveolitis

Adapted from James DG, Williams WJ: *Sarcoidosis and other granulomatous diseases of the lung,* New York, 1983, Marcel Dekker; and Saboor SA: *Br J Hosp Med* 48:293-302, 1992.

Table 55-1 Differential Diagnosis of Nonscaseating Granulomas

Bacteria	Brucellosis
	Yersinia
Mycobacteria	*Mycobactrium tuberculosis*
	Atypical mycobacteria
Fungi	Histoplasmosis
	Coccidioidomycosis
	Blastomycocis
	Cryptococcosis
Spirochetes	Tertiary syphilis
Protozoa	Toxoplasmosis
	Leishmaniasis
Chemicals	Beryllium
	Zirconium
	Silica
	Starch
Neoplasms	Seminoma
	Carcinoma
Allergen	Extrinsic allergic alveolitis
Other	Sarcoidosis
	Chronic granulomatous disease of childhood
	Crohn's disease
	Primary biliary cirrhosis
	Granulomatous hepatitis
	Whipple's disease
	Wegener's granulomatosis
	Lymphatoid granulomatosis
	Churg-Strauss allergic granulomatosis
	Giant cell arteritis
	Polyarteritis
	Systemic lupus erythematosus
	Hypogammaglobulinemia
	Histiocytosis X
	Peyronie's disease

Adapted from Fanburg BL: *Sarcoidosis and other granulomatous diseases of the lung,* New York, 1983, Marcel Dekker; James DG, Williams WJ: Sarcoidosis and other granulomatous diseases, Philadelphia, 1985, WB Saunders; and Sharma OP: *Dis Monthly* 9:471-535, 1990.

or circulating antibodies to an unknown antigen. The most common urine abnormalities include hematuria, pyuria, and proteinuria.

DIAGNOSIS AND DIFFERENTIAL DIAGNOSIS

A consistent clinical history and compatible chest radiograph and tissue histology establish the diagnosis in the majority of cases. Although the clinical picture can be variable, most patients have vague, generalized symptoms and physical findings consistent with involvement of the lungs, eyes, or skin. A chest radiograph, which typically reveals hilar adenopathy, is one of the most helpful noninvasive test to support the diagnosis. However, other diseases can also manifest with hilar lymphadenopathy or other radiographic findings similar to sarcoidosis (Box 55-1).[3,7]

A tissue biopsy confirmation was demonstrated in 90% of children previously reported.[6,11] Potential sites to obtain tissue in general order of increased invasiveness include cutaneous lesions, conjunctival nodules, enlarged lacrimal or parotid glands, peripheral lymph nodes, liver, lung tissue by transbronchial biopsy, mediastinal lymph nodes by mediastinoscopy, and lung tissue by open lung biopsy. If conjunctival or skin lesions or enlarged lacrimal or parotid glands are absent, palpable peripheral lymph nodes are the most preferable tissue; 37 of 41 children in one series had positive findings.[6] Biopsies were obtained from lymph nodes in all sites, and the location did not alter the success rate. If liver enlargement or abnormal liver function tests exist, a liver biopsy can also be helpful; 8 of 10 children had positive findings. Because of the size of bronchoscope necessary for transbronchial biopsies, this procedure has thus far been used primarily in adults, although the technique should be technically feasible in most adolescents. Mediastinal lymph node biopsy has been regarded as the standard for obtaining tissue and almost always produces positive results. Open lung biopsies are rarely needed and should be considered only if parenchymal involvement exists, there are no palpable peripheral lymph nodes, and mediastinoscopy cannot be performed. Although there are other diseases with noncaseating granulomas, most can be distinguished from sarcoidosis by clinical presentation or laboratory studies (Table 55-1).[5,7]

In many cases, a serum angiotensin-converting enzyme (ACE) is helpful in supporting the diagnosis.[18] ACE is produced from the epithelioid cells of the granulomas, and an elevated level indicates a large number of active granulomas. ACE is elevated in up to 80% of children and in 60% of adults.[5,18] However, the diagnostic value of the serum ACE is limited because in adults there is a false-negative rate of 40% and a false-positive rate of 10% (Table 55-2).[19] In addition, normal values for children are higher than those in adults, most laboratories do not have standardized values for children, and various methods are used.[18,20] Table 55-3 shows the percentage difference in ACE values in children compared with adults using two different methods. The test is most useful in monitoring the course of the disease. Other blood studies (e.g., ESR, serum proteins) are nonspecific and in general are not helpful in supporting the diagnosis.

Gallium uptake is increased in the lungs of patients with active sarcoidosis; however, this study is not specific, and increased uptake can occur in a variety of disorders, including tuberculosis, various other interstitial diseases, and pulmonary tumors.[7] Bronchoscopy with bronchoalveolar lavage (BAL) has also been used to obtain specimens for bacteriology, cytology, and lymphocytes for study. An increase in T lymphocytes is commonly seen in sarcoidosis; however, the same results are seen in other interstitial lung diseases.[21] Thus BAL and gallium scans may be useful as research tools; however, as diagnostic tools, their usefulness is limited. They may be more useful as an index of disease activity once the diagnosis is established.

The Kveim test is not widely used today. In this test, sarcoid tissue homogenate is injected intracutaneously, and, if a reaction develops, a biopsy is performed at 24 to 42 days to identify sarcoid granuloma. The test is not generally used because wide ranges of sensitivity and specificity have been reported and a standardized reagent is not widely available. In addition, injection of a tissue homogenate of unknown nature may be hazardous.

Table 55-2 Differential Diagnosis of Elevated ACE

DISEASE	% WITH ELEVATED ACE
Asbestosis	*
Berylliosis	*
Cirrhosis of the liver	*
Diabetes mellitus	13
Gaucher's disease	*
Granulomatous hepatitis	*
Hypersensitivity pneumonitis	*
Inflammatory bowel disease	5
Leprosy	11
Lymphoma	11
Primary biliary cirrhosis	29
Pulmonary neoplasm	13
Respiratory distress syndrome	*
Sarcoidosis (active)	87
Sarcoidosis (inactive)	9
Silicosis	*
Tuberculosis	24

Adapted from Fanburg BL: *Sarcoidosis and other granulomatous diseases of the lung,* New York, 1983, Marcell Dekker; James DG, Williams WJ: *Sarcoidosis and other granulomatous diseases,* Philadelphia, 1985, WB Saunders, Sharma OP: *Dis Monthly* 9:471-535, 1990; and Saboor SA: *Br J Hosp Med* 48:293-302, 1992.
*Not systematically evaluated.

A consistent clinical history, chest radiographic findings, and tissue biopsy are most useful in the diagnosis of sarcoidosis. Other granulomatous disorders that must be excluded are listed in Box 55-1 and Tables 55-1 and 55-2. Most of these other diagnoses can be eliminated relatively easily by history, physical examination, or clinical tests. The most important differential diagnosis is between sarcoidosis and tuberculosis or lymphoma.

Sarcoidosis in Very Young Children

Sarcoidosis in adolescents is similar to that in adults; however, sarcoidosis in very young children appears to be distinct. In the young child, sarcoidosis is manifested primarily in the skin, joints, and eyes and uncommonly in the lungs. In children under 4 years of age, a maculopapular, erythematous rash was present in 76%, uveitis in 58%, and arthritis in 58%; pulmonary involvement was present in only 22%.[22] Distinction of sarcoidosis from juvenile rheumatoid arthritis (JRA) in young children may be difficult, especially when the arthropathy precedes other features.[23-25] However, JRA has tendinous and articular synovitis with joint limitation, whereas in sarcoidosis there is tenosynovitis of the dorsal tendon sheaths of the wrists and ankles without limitation of movement. In addition, the anterior uveitis in JRA usually has less nodule formation than sarcoidosis, and corneal deposits are generally more diffuse and centrally located. Although sarcoidosis can cause a variety of skin lesions, the typical exanthem of JRA (evanescent salmon-colored macules and urticarial papules) is not common in sarcoidosis. Noncaseating granuloma are not present in JRA.

Noncaseating granuloma may be present in familial granulomatous arteritis of juvenile onset, a syndrome with many features common to early-onset sarcoidosis, including a rash, uveitis, and granulomatous synovitis. These patients usually develop hypertension and vasculitis. It has been suggested that noncaseating granuloma be grouped under the syndrome of juvenile systemic granulomatosis; this may be indistinguishable from sarcoidosis in the very young.[26]

MANAGEMENT AND TREATMENT

Once the diagnosis is established, all organ systems, especially the lungs, eyes, and calcium metabolism, must be evaluated and reevaluated to assess their degree of involvement. In addition to a complete history and physical examination, which should reveal most organ systems involved, other tests or examinations may be useful. The lungs are easily assessed with

Table 55-3 Percentage Increase in Serum ACE of Healthy Children Compared with Adults

AGE (YR)	INCREASE FROM ADULT VALUE*	AGE (YR)	INCREASE FROM ADULT VALUE†
0.5-2	9%	0-3	43%
2-4	0%	3-6	50%
4-9	24%	5-9	45%
9-13	38%	9-12	43%
13-18	26%	12-15	46%
Males Females	2%	12-18	21%
All children (<18)	18%	All children (<18)	45%

*Serum ACE in adults (>18 years old) 100 ± 35 U/L. (Adapted from Benetequ-Burnat B, Baudin B, Morgant G, Baumann FC, Giboudeau J: *Clin Chem* 35:344-346, 1990.)
†Serum ACE in adults (>18 years old) 32.1 ± 8.53 nM/min/ml. (Adapted from Rodriguez GE, Shin BC, Abernathy RS, Kendig EL: *J Pediatr* 99:68-72, 1981.)

chest radiograph and pulmonary function tests. The eyes should be routinely evaluated by an ophthalmologist using a slit-lamp examination, and hypercalcemia and hypercalciuria should be evaluated by blood calcium levels and urinary calcium excretion. Under usual dietary conditions, the normal urinary excretion of calcium in healthy children is less than 4 mg (0.1 mmol) per kilogram of body weight per day.[27] An elevated ACE, although not diagnostic, is useful in following disease activity and the effects of therapy in children.[18] Although general tests, such as the ESR, serum proteins, and eosinophil count, may be elevated, other tests, including liver and renal function tests, are more specific for certain organ involvement. Once an organ system is found to be involved, it should be followed closely because this is often the best way to indicate disease activity.

Treatment is indicated when there are significant symptoms or there is evidence of progressive damage to involved organs. Corticosteroids are the treatment of choice, and the responses may be dramatic. Extrapulmonary sarcoidosis, such as ocular, neurologic, and cardiac involvement, usually requires large doses of corticosteroids. Glandular involvement, splenic enlargement, parotid swelling, and skin lesions usually respond to modest doses of corticosteroids. Aysmptomatic hepatic involvement usually requires no therapy, unless progressive impairment of liver function is evident.

For pulmonary sarcoidosis alone, corticosteroids are effective for symptomatic treatment and acute decreases in pulmonary function.[28,29] Several controlled trials have documented the short-term (6 month) efficacy of steroids. The long-term effectiveness of corticosteroids in averting pulmonary fibrosis and chronic impairment of pulmonary function is unclear. Patients who are asymptomatic with bilateral hilar adenopathy without parenchymal lung disease generally are not treated. When troublesome symptoms or progressive laboratory derangements develop, corticosteroids are introduced.

Prednisone or prednisolone is usually initiated at 1 mg/kg per day. A gradual reduction in the dose is initiated when clinical manifestations of the disease disappear. A maintenance dose of 0.25 mg/kg per day of prednisone every other day is usually required for at least a 6-month course of treatment. If a relapse occurs, the dose is increased to control the disease and then gradually reduced to a maintenance dose, which is usually higher than the dose at which the elapse occurred.

In selected cases with no extrapulmonary involvement, inhalational corticosteroids have been reported to be useful in adults, although controlled data are not available.[28] When adult patients do not respond to or suffer severe side effects from corticosteroids, other drugs may be used.[5,29]

In selected cases with no extrapulmonary involvement, inhalational corticosteroids have been reported to be useful in adults, although controlled data are not available.[28] When adult patients do not respond to or suffer severe side effects from corticosteroids, other drugs may be used.[5,29] Chlorambucil, 2 mg 4 times daily; methotrexate, 20 mg twice weekly; and chloroquine, 500 mg daily for 2 weeks followed by 250 mg daily for 6 months, have been used successfully in adults. Results with levamisole, azathioprine, colchicine, oxyphenbutazone, and cyclosporine have been variable.

PROGNOSIS

In approximately 60% of adult patients with thoracic sarcoidosis, spontaneous resolution occurs within 2 years, 20% resolve with steroid treatment, and in 10% to 20% resolution is unlikely.[8] Chronic extrathoracic involvement, especially neurologic involvement, has a poor response.

Overall, the prognosis of childhood sarcoidosis is good with considerable improvement in clinical manifestations, chest radiographs, and pulmonary function tests in most children.[5,30,31] The resolution of chest radiographic abnormalities appears to be approximately 60% to 70%. Most patients also show improvement in pulmonary function. Results from 16 patients with childhood sarcoidosis 4 years after diagnosis indicated improvement of the forced vital capacity from 80.3% ± 16.4% predicted at presentation to 97.1% ± 18.8%.[17] A larger proportion of patients with pulmonary dysfunction was noted in another series with a longer period of follow-up.[31] In general, a poorer prognosis is predicted by severity of involvement at presentation. Asymptomatic patients with hilar adenopathy have a good prognosis, whereas patients with stage IV disease have a poorer prognosis. Although most children with parenchymal involvement do improve, most patients with progressive lung disease have parenchymal involvement at presentation.[31]

Some children have sequelae or progressive disease. In one study, 5 of 28 children had severe sequelae.[30] In another series, 4 of 61 patients had long-term pulmonary morbidity; in addition, 1 of the 4 and 4 others had nonpulmonary sequelae.[31] Progressive lung disease and fibrosis can occur. Eye involvement, if appropriately treated with corticosteroids, usually resolves; however, blindness in children has resulted from sarcoidosis. The hypercalciuria of sarcoidosis may be followed by nephrolithiasis; 5 of 50 children in one series developed nephrolithiasis.[6] Any organ involvement may produce sequelae, and the prognosis of sarcoidosis in children does not appear to be significantly different from that in adults.

REFERENCES

Epidemiology

1. Bresnitz EA, Strom BL: Epidemiology of sarcoidosis, *Epidemiol Rev* 5:124-156, 1983.
2. Fanburg BL: *Sarcoidosis and other granulomatous diseases of the lung,* New York, 1983, Marcel Dekker.
3. James DG, Williams WJ: *Sarcoidosis and other granulomatous diseases,* Philadelphia, 1985, WB Saunders.
4. Cooch JW: Sarcoidosis in the United States Army, 1952 through 1956, *Am Rev Respir Dis* 84:103-108, 1961.
5. Sharma OP: Sarcoidosis, *Dis Monthly* 9:471-535, 1990.
6. Pattishall EN, Strope GL, Spinola SM, Denny FW: Childhood sarcoidosis, *Pediatr* 108:169-177, 1986.

Etiology

7. Saboor SA: Sarcoidosis, *Br J Hosp Med* 48:293-302, 1992.
8. Saboor SA, Johnson NM, McFadden JJ: Detection of mycobacterial DNA I sarcoidosis and tuberculosis with polymerase chain reaction, *Lancet* 339:1012-1015, 1992.
9. Bocart D. De Lecossier A, Valeyre DK, Battesti J, Hance AJ: A search for mycobacterial DNA in granulomatous tissues from patients with sarcoidosis using the polymerase chain reaction, *Am Rev Respir Dis* 145:1142-1148, 1992.

Pathology and Pathogenesis

10. Crystal RG, Bitterman PB, Rennard SI, Hance AJ, Keogh BA: Interstitial lung diseases of unknown cause: disorders characterized by chronic inflammation of the lower respiratory tract [second of two parts], *N Engl J Med* 310:235-244, 1983.

Clinical Features

11. Kendig EL: The clinical picture of sarcoidosis in children, *Pediatrics* 54:289-292, 1974.

12. James DG, Kendig EL: Childhood sarcoidosis, *Sarcoidosis* 5:57-59, 1988.
13. Kataria S, Trevathan GE, Holland JE, Kataria YP: Ocular presentation of sarcoidosis in children, *Clin Pediatr* 22:793-797, 1983.
14. Elgart ML: Cutaneous sarcoidosis: definitions and types of lesions, *Clin Dermatol* 4:35-45, 1986.
15. Weinberg S, Bennett H: Central nervous system manifestations of sarcoidosis in children, *Clin Pediatr* 22:477-481, 1983.
16. Merten DF, Kirks DR, Grossman H: Pulmonary sarcoidosis in childhood, *Am J Roentgenol* 135:673-679, 1980.
17. Pattishall EN, Strope GL, Denny FW: Pulmonary function in children with sarcoidosis, *Am Rev Respir Dis* 133:94-96, 1986.

Diagnosis and Differential Diagnosis

18. Rodriguez GE, Shin BC, Abernathy RS, Kendig EL: Serum angiotension-converting enzyme activity in normal children and in those with sarcoidosis, *J Pediatr* 99:68-72, 1981.
19. Allen RKA: A review of angiotensin converting enzyme in health and disease, *Sarcoidosis* 8:95-100, 1991.
20. Beneteau-Burnat B, Baudin B, Morgant G, Baumann FC, Giboudeau J: Serum angiotensin-converting enzyme in healthy and sarcoidotic children: comparison with the reference interval for adults, *Clin Chem* 36:344-346, 1990.
21. Arnoux A, Danel C, Chretien J: Is bronchoalveolar lavage a mirror of granulomas in the lungs? *Sarcoidosis* 6:10-11, 1989.
22. Hetherington S: Sarcoidosis in young children, *Am J Dis Child* 136:13-15, 1982.
23. North AF, Fink CW, Gibson WM, Levison JE, Schichter SL, Howard WK, Johnson NH, Harris C: Sarcoid arthritis in children, *Am J Med* 48:449-455, 1970.
24. Mallory SB, Paller AS, Ginsburg BC, McCrossin ID, Abernathy R: Sarcoidosis in children: differentiation from juvenile rheumatoid arthritis, *Pediatr Dermatol* 4:313-319, 1987.
25. Sahn EE, Hampton MT, Garen PD, Warrick J, Smith D, Silver RM: Preschool sarcoidosis masquerading as juvenile rheumatoid arthritis: two case reports and a review of the literature, *Pediatr Dermatol* 7:208-213, 1990.
26. Miller JJ: Early-onset "sarcoidosis" and "familial granulomatous arthritis (arteritis)": the same disease, *J Pediatr* 108:387-388, 1986.

Management and Treatment

27. Stapleton FB, McKay CP, Noe HN: Urolithiasis in children: the role of hypercalciuria, *Pediatr Ann* 16:980-992, 1987.
28. Sharma OP: Pulmonary sarcoidosis and corticosteroids, *Am Rev Respir Dis* 147:1598-1600, 1993.
29. Muthiah MM, Macfarlane JT: Current concepts in the management of sarcoidosis, *Drugs* 40:231-237, 1990.

Prognosis

30. Kendig EL, Brummer DL: The prognosis of sarcoidosis in children, *Chest* 70:351-353, 1976.
31. Marcille R, McCarthy M, Barton JW, Merten DG, Spock A: Long-term outcome of pediatric sarcoidosis with emphasis on pulmonary status, *Chest* 102:1444-1449, 1992.

CHAPTER 56

Congenital Immune Deficiency Syndromes

Andrew S. Kemp

There are approximately 100 primary immunodeficiency disorders.[1] This chapter will discuss disorders that may have significant respiratory tract symptoms. These are considered in 4 groups:

1. Disorders of antibody function
2. Disorders of T cells
3. Disorders of phagocytes
4. Miscellaneous

DISORDERS OF ANTIBODY FUNCTION

IgA Deficiency

Selective IgA deficiency has been defined as a serum IgA level less than 0.05 g/L with normal IgG and IgM levels.[1] As serum IgA levels increase significantly throughout childhood there is no clear definition of selective IgA deficiency in infants. IgA deficiency is diagnosed by measurement of serum IgA, and virtually all subjects who lack IgA in their sera will also lack it in their secretions. Rare cases with lack of secretory IgA, with normal serum IgA levels, have been described; however, these cases did not have significant respiratory problems. Acquired IgA, deficiency has been observed associated with the use of phenytoin, penicillamine, sulfasalazine, and captopril. IgA deficiency may be associated with abnormalities of chromosomes 18 and 22 in developmentally delayed children. An incidence of selective IgA deficiency of the order of 1 in 500 subjects has been reported in normal blood donors.[2] Two subclasses of IgA, IgA1 and IgA2, can be distinguished serologically. A family with two subjects with IgA2 deficiency has been reported; respiratory symptoms were not observed.[3] Human IgA genes are found on chromosome 14 in association with genes for immunoglobulin subclasses and IgE, which may explain the occurrence of IgA deficiency with IgG subclass deficiency. The molecular basis for IgA deficiency is unclear but appears to involve impairment in the switching from IgM to IgA production.[4]

IgA deficiency may be transient, and children with levels indicative of selective IgA deficiency (<0.05 g/L) have subsequently had serum IgA detected. The measurement of salivary IgA is a useful way of distinguishing subjects with low but potentially transient IgA deficiency from those with a true selective IgA deficiency that will persist throughout life. Salivary IgA levels reach normal adult levels by 6 months of age.[5] The significance of an IgA level below the limit of normal but above 0.05 g/L is uncertain. These children should not be classified as having selective IgA deficiency. In at least half of these subjects IgA levels will increase into the normal range.[6] As compared with selective IgA deficiency these children have a lower incidence of significant lower respiratory tract infections.[6] In fact, it is uncertain whether these subjects have a greater incidence or severity of respiratory infections than normal children.

Approximately one third of subjects with selective IgA deficiency develop symptoms. The major symptoms are recurrent respiratory tract infection with bronchitis and otitis media.[7,8] More severe lower respiratory tract infections are uncommon and symptoms frequently improve over 5 to 10 years. In symptomatic cases, other immunoglobulins in the secretions may compensate for the lack of IgA. In some cases where suppurative disease of the upper or lower respiratory tract is present this is the result of an associated IgG2 subclass deficiency.[9,10] One study of 40 children with IgA levels less than 0.05 g/L and absent secretory IgA reported an incidence of pneumonia of 30%.[6] Whether any of these children had an associated IgG subclass deficiency was not determined.

The longer term sequelae of IgA deficiency are unclear. The incidence of apparently asymptomatic subjects with IgA deficiency in the normal population indicates that IgA deficiency does not necessarily predispose to significant disease. Lower respiratory tract suppuration with bronchiectasis is more common in IgA-deficient adults when the deficiency is associated with abnormalities of other subclasses.[11] Common variable hypogammaglobulinemia can present initially as selective IgA deficiency with IgG and IgM levels subsequently declining over a number of years. This condition should be considered in any case of selective IgA deficiency who subsequently develops serious bacterial infections, in particular recurrent pneumonia or meningitis.

Immunoglobulin therapy is not indicated for patients with isolated IgA deficiency. If an IgG subclass deficiency is associated with a defective specific antibody response, immunoglobulin therapy may be indicated. Anaphylactoid reactions are possible in subjects with selective IgA deficiency given immunoglobulin because of the presence of IgG anti-IgA antibodies, which are found in about 25% of subjects.[12] Commercial preparations of intravenous IgG that are low in IgA have been used in these patients without problem but the risk of anaphylaxis is not completely eliminated.[12] IgA-depleted intravenous immunoglobulin has been used with success in subjects with high titers of anti-IgA antibodies and severe infusion reactions to normal immunoglobulin infusions.[13]

X-Linked Agammaglobulinemia

This disorder is caused by the failure of pre–B cells to develop into mature circulating B cells. Affected males have a normal number of pre–B cells in their bone marrow with an absence of mature B cells in the circulating lymphocyte population. The defect has been shown to involve the gene that encodes a protein tyrosine-kinase expressed in B cells.[14] Although the precise function of the protein tyrosine-kinase is not known, it appears to be required for normal B cell development.

Most subjects remain healthy for the first 6 to 9 months of life. In association with the normal decline in maternally transferred immunoglobulin they develop upper and lower respiratory tract infections with common respiratory tract organisms, in particular pneumococci and *Haemophilus influenzae B.*[15] *Staphylococcus aureus* may also be isolated from the sputum.[15] Some subjects are susceptible to *Mycoplasma pneumoniae* infection, which can present as pneumonitis, sinusitis, or arthritis.[16] Nearly all subjects will develop symptoms by 18 months of age, and the diagnosis is usually made within the first 3 years of life.[15] The majority of patients suffer infections at more than one anatomic site (Table 56-1). Common manifestations are discharging ears and sinusitis. Recurrent pneumonia that usually affects dependent lobes is a common presentation.[17] In contrast to pneumonia in immunocompetent infants resolution is often incomplete or slow. There may be persistent collapse of affected lobes. With delayed diagnosis, bronchiectasis develops. Repeated infection may result in pulmonary fibrosis, cor pulmonale, and eventually respiratory failure, which develops in about half the patients and is the most common cause of death. Early treatment will minimize complications, and high dose intravenous gammaglobulin appears to reduce chronic lung disease. Death can also occur from severe and widely disseminated enterovirus infections.[15] In contrast to conditions associated with defects of antibody and cell-mediated immunity, pneumonia caused by *Pneumocystis carinii* rarely occurs in X-linked agammaglobulinemia.[15] Severe viral pneumonitis is also very uncommon. In addition to upper and lower respiratory tract symptoms, mono- or oligoarticular arthritis, which can mimic juvenile rheumatoid arthritis, is a presenting feature in approximately 20% of patients. Septic arthritis caused by *Haemophilus influenzae b* or pneumococcus occurs as well as arthritis from infection with mycoplasma and ureaplasma. Chronic or recurrent conjunctivitis is common, probably related to deficiency of secretory antibodies.

Table 56-1 The Incidence of Infections in Patients with X-linked Agammaglobulinemia at Diagnosis and the Incidence of Chronic Infections

At diagnosis
Upper respiratory tract 75%
Lower respiratory tract 65%
Gastrointestinal tract 35%
Skin 28%
Central nervous system 10%
Chronic
Otitis media 44%
Lower respiratory tract 39%
Sinusitis 39%
Conjunctivitis 19%
Pyoderma 13%
Gastroenteritis 10%

(From Lederman HM, Winkelstein JA: *Medicine* 64:145-146, 1985.)

The diagnosis can be established by demonstrating reduced concentrations of IgG, IgA, and IgM and usually an absence of B cells in the peripheral circulation. There will be no specific antibody response to common antigens such as tetanus and diphtheria. The diagnosis may be suspected in the newborn male with a family history by demonstrating lack of B cells in the cord blood. This can allow institution of therapy (intravenous immunoglobulin) before the development of infection. Transient neutropenia is often associated with acute infections.[15] Pulmonary function tests demonstrate an obstructive pattern with progressive disease. The incidence of pulmonary complications in X-linked agammaglobulinemia is less than in patients with common variable immunodeficiency.[18] This may partly relate to the T cell defects found in the latter condition, which may predispose subjects to a more severe and a wider range of infections.

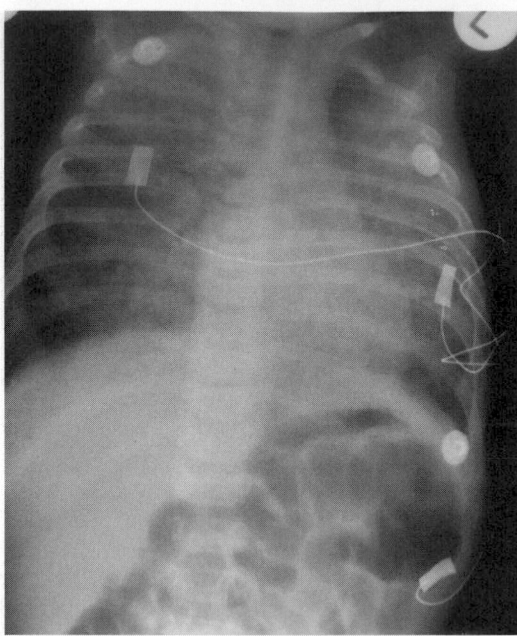

Fig. 56-1. Pneumocystis pneumonitis in a 6-month-old male infant with immunodeficiency and elevated IgM.

Immunodeficiency with Elevated IgM

This immunodeficiency is functionally similar to X-linked hypogammaglobulinemia. It is the result of a defective ability of B cells to switch from IgM to IgG and IgA production. This disorder is caused by a defect in CD40 ligand, a cell surface structure required for antibody switching.[19,20] The disease is usually X-linked although non–X-linked forms have been described.

Children present with suppurative infections of the upper and lower respiratory tract in the first or second year of life. In contrast to other types of hypogammaglobulinemia, pneumocystis pneumonia is a common presentation[21] (Fig. 56-1). This disorder is associated with neutropenia, which may be either cyclic or persistent. Mouth ulcers or ulcers elsewhere in the upper gastrointestinal tract occur. Hemolytic anemia, thrombocytopenia, nephritis, and arthritis are also observed.[21] The diagnosis is suggested by low IgA and IgG levels with a normal or elevated IgM, which is polyclonal. Subjects have normal numbers of circulating B cells, which express IgM or IgD or both but not other immunoglobulins. Primary and secondary antibody responses are diminished and limited to IgM; isoagglutinin titers are low or absent. T cell numbers and function are usually normal.

Treatment is similar to other forms of agammaglobulinemia with regular intravenous immunoglobulin therapy. Prophylaxis for pneumocystis infection with trimethoprim-sulfamethoxazole should be given. In some cases, the neutropenia may resolve after immunoglobulin therapy. In severe cases of neutropenia, granulocyte-macrophage colony–stimulating factor has been used with beneficial results.

Common Variable Immunodeficiency

Common variable immunodeficiency is also known as acquired hypogammaglobulinemia. In contrast to X-linked agammaglobulinemia, the disease usually has a later onset and the symptoms of infections may be more insidious.[22] Although cases of common variable immunodeficiency present most often in the second or third decade of life, symptoms may begin in the first years of life usually as diarrhea and respiratory tract infection. More than 95% of cases present after the age of 6 years.[23] The disease is associated with autoimmune disorders, particularly hemolytic anemia, thrombocytopenia, and autoimmune neutropenia.[22] The diagnosis is made by finding abnormal levels of immunoglobulins, a variable T cell defect, and either normal or reduced B cells. The ratio of T helper (CD4) cells to T suppressor (CD8) cells is often increased, which is not seen in patients with X-linked agammaglobulinemia.[24] This disorder may be caused by a defect on chromosome 6 in the major histocompatibility complex region, which results in arrested B-cell differentiation. This produces a spectrum of immune deficiencies ranging from IgA deficiency to common variable immunodeficiency.[25] IgA deficiency may evolve into common variable immunodeficiency.

The spectrum of respiratory infections is similar to that observed in X-linked agammaglobulinemia. Episodes of pneumococcal or *Haemophilus influenzae* pneumonia are common.[26] *Candida albicans* has been isolated from bronchial secretions. On rare occasions pneumonia has been associated with a *Pseudomonas aeruginosa* or *Pneumocystis carinii.*

Another complication is lymphoid interstitial pneumonitis which presents with cough, dyspnea, weight loss and an interstitial infiltrate, particularly at the lung bases on the chest radiograph.[27] The pulmonary function tests will usually show a restrictive pattern, and lung biopsy may be necessary to make a definitive diagnosis. Lymphoid interstitial pneumonitis may progress to pulmonary fibrosis. Improvement has been noted following the institution of gammaglobulin therapy.

In addition to the symptoms of recurrent upper and lower respiratory infections caused by the lack of antibodies, noncaseating granulomas of the lungs, spleen, skin, and liver occur.[22] Splenomegaly may be prominent. Gastrointestinal disease with diarrhea associated with *Campylobacter jejeuni* and *Giardia lamblia* and hepatitis are common complications.[22] In adult subjects the incidence of lymphoma is increased. Atypical lymphoid hyperplasia, which may be confused with malignant lymphoma, can develop.[28] The occurrence of splenomegaly, granulomatous and autoimmune phenomena differs from X-linked agammaglobulinemia.[22]

Management is with intravenous gammaglobulin but may be complicated by autoimmune hemolytic anemia, thrombocytopenia, or neutropenia, which often requires corticosteroid therapy. The associated T cell defects, which may worsen with age,[23] may predispose patients to more severe pulmonary disease than is seen in X-linked agammaglobulinemia.[29] Despite apparently adequate immunoglobulin replacement, chronic respiratory symptoms are common.

IgG Subclass Deficiency

Four subclasses of IgG contribute to the total IgG level. IgG1 contributes 65%, IgG2 25%, IgG3 7%, and IgG4 less than 5%. Thus a deficiency of IgG2, 3, or 4 can exist with a normal total IgG level.[30] IgG1 and IgG3 are immunoglobulins that develop against protein antigens and bind complement. IgG2 is predominantly active against polysaccharide antigens although IgG1 and IgG3 antibodies can also react with polysaccharide antigens. IgG2 does not bind complement effectively. The role of IgG4 is unclear, but is increased in atopic dermatitis and asthma. IgG4 may be important for secretory immunity because an increased number of IgG4 committed B cells exist at mucosal sites. Only IgG1 and IgG3 cross the placenta; thus IgG2 and IgG4 are not present in the newborn. The genes for IgG2 and IgG4 are linked with the genes for IgA on chromosome 14.

The establishment of normal ranges for immunoglobulin subclasses throughout childhood has proved difficult. Levels change substantially with age and lower levels have been observed in healthy black as compared with white children.[31] The assays have technical difficulties and the reliability of commercial kits has been questioned.[32] Healthy blood donors may have low levels of subclasses.[33] A normal total serum IgG level with one or more subclasses greater than 2 standard deviations below the mean may also occur. Thus the criteria for diagnosis of a deficiency are uncertain. Of more importance than the level is the functional ability of the antibodies. Healthy children with low serum concentrations of IgG2 may have normal antibody response to polysaccharide vaccine antigens, whereas symptomatic children with similar levels of IgG2 have a defective antibody response.[33] In attempting to establish whether a low subclass antibody titer is contributing to respiratory tract infections, it is important to document that specific antibody responses to polysaccharide antigens, such as HiB or pneumococcal vaccine, are defective. The conjugated HiB vaccine used for infant immunization will generate antibody responses in the IgG1 subclass and is not suitable for evaluating specific defects in IgG2 antigen response. Low subclass levels in children do not necessarily correlate with defective antibody production.[34] Furthermore young children under 2 years have a defective antibody to polysaccharide antigens, which increases the difficulty in determining the significance of a subclass deficiency in this group. In adults with subclass deficiency and respiratory tract infections, the response to conjugated HiB vaccine did not appear to predict the severity of the respiratory infections.[35]

Normal individuals may have low or undetectable antibody subclasses.[36] The incidence of IgG2 deficiency in over 500 healthy children was found to be 2%.[33] All these children were found to have normal responses to polysaccharide antigens and normal in vitro production of IgG2. IgG2 deficiency may also be transient in healthy individuals, and resolution over a period of 3 or 4 years has been documented. Because of the insensitivity of the assay, up to 20% of the population may appear to be deficient in IgG4; to establish IgG4 deficiency, radioimmunoassay is required.[37]

Immunoglobulin subclass deficiency may be multiple or single. Symptoms, which may result from subclass deficiency, are recurrent otitis media, recurrent sinusitis, mastoiditis, and suppurative lower respiratory tract disease with bronchitis and bronchiectasis.[38,39] Radiologic abnormalities include consolidation and atelectasis.[39] A history of recurrent bronchitis, particularly if associated with purulent sputum production, recurrent pneumonia, and persisting chest radiographic abnormalities, suggests the possibility of a subclass deficiency. The most commonly detected deficiencies are IgG2, IgG3, and IgG4; IgG1 deficiency is uncommon.[10] Low levels of IgG1 may predispose infants to acute bronchiolitis.[40] Pre-school age children are commonly found to have subclass deficiency, which may relate to the lower levels of IgG subclasses often observed in young children, the difficulties in distinguishing normal from abnormal, and a transient immaturity of the immune system.[41]

Immunoglobulin subclass deficiency has been found in children evaluated for chronic sinusitis. In one study of the children with sinusitis, half the patients were shown to have either low immunoglobulin subclasses or poor response to polysaccharide antigens. IgG3 subclass deficiency was the most common abnormality.[42]

The significance of isolated IgG4 subclass deficiency is controversial. Much confusion has arisen because of the varying sensitivity of the assays used. With a sensitive radioimmunoassay, IgG4 deficiency has been detected in individuals with so-called idiopathic bronchiectasis, or chronic sinusitis and recurrent otitis media.[38,43] Individuals with isolated IgG4 deficiency have demonstrated a normal antibody response to polysaccharide antigens.[43] There are anecdotal reports of symptomatic improvement following the administration of immunoglobulin in subjects with isolated IgG4 deficiency.

Regimens for management of subclass deficiencies with proven defective specific antibody responses are not well established. Trials comparing regular use of prophylactic broad spectrum antibiotics and gammaglobulin have not been carried out. Some patients will improve with regular or liberal use of a broad spectrum antibiotic. Immunoglobulin therapy should only be instituted on the basis of a proven defect in specific antibody responses and suppurative respiratory tract disease. The dosage of gammaglobulin is uncertain but in general the dosages used for hypogammaglobulinemia (200 to 600 mg/kg) on a monthly basis have been used. It is possible that dosages of intravenous gammaglobulin lower than those recommended for more severe immunoglobulin deficiencies will be effective. A trial of monthly intravenous immunoglobulin in children with IgG3 subclass deficiency reduced hospitalizations and antibiotic use.[44] If immunoglobulin therapy is instituted it is important to have a measurable end point such as diminution in episodes of otitis media with drainage, reduction in cough and purulent sputum, or reduction in episodes of documented lower respiratory tract infection. In children with subclass deficiency, the appropriate duration of immunoglobulin therapy is not clear. As children are more prone than adults to viral respiratory infections, which may initiate secondary bacterial infections, the need for immunoglobulin therapy can diminish with increasing age; however, bronchiectasis has been detected in subclass-deficient adults.

The relationship between IgG subclass deficiency and asthma is uncertain. IgG subclass levels in asthmatic children appear to be similar to healthy controls.[45] Low IgG subclasses have been found in children with endoscopically proven chronic bronchitis.[46] Some children with recurrent wheezing, normal IgE levels, and negative immediate hypersensitivity skin tests have low IgG subclass levels.[47] Immunoglobulin infusions have been reported to improve severe chronic asthma with associated subclass deficiency.[48] It is an unproven possibility that subclass deficiency may contribute to more persistent viral infections or secondary bacterial infections, worsening asthmatic symptoms.

Immunoglobulin Therapy

Immunoglobulin is usually administered intravenously. Dosage ranges from 200 to 600 mg/kg administered every 3 to 4 weeks.[49,50] This is based on a half-life of IgG in normal individuals of 18 to 24 days. Catabolism of intravenous immunoglobulin varies in different patients, and dosages may need to be individualized. Criteria for dosage are uncertain but a reasonable aim is to keep the IgG level within the normal range for age. One study maintained a trough level above an arbitrary 5 g/L.[51] Patients given high dose intravenous immunoglobulin therapy develop less complications than those who have been treated with intramuscular therapy, which provides significantly less gammaglobulin.[52] Meticulous attention should be paid to the episodes of lower respiratory tract suppuration. Prophylactic antibiotics are not generally required but any occurrence of infection, as indicated by purulent sputum, should be treated vigorously with a broad spectrum antibiotic. If symptoms do not resolve a chest radiograph is usually necessary to determine the extent of infection and the need for hospital admission for intravenous antibiotic therapy and physiotherapy. Progress of respiratory disease should be monitored by yearly pulmonary function tests. Because of the change from intramuscular to high-dose intravenous immunoglobulin therapy, the long-term results of high-dose therapy are not fully defined. Initial studies indicate that the incidence of recurrent respiratory infection and complications such as pulmonary fibrosis and bronchiectasis is reduced.[52,53]

With improved methods of preparation and minimization of aggregate formation, reactions to intravenous infusions are uncommon. A rare complication of intravenous gammaglobulin therapy is acquisition of non-A, non-B hepatitis which is thought to be a result of deficiencies in preparation of the product.[54] Thus subjects on regular immunoglobulin therapy should have liver function tests performed 3 to 4 times a year. Another rare complication is aseptic meningitis.[55]

In older children, home administration of intravenous gammaglobulin can often be accomplished. Another route of administration is the subcutaneous route, which can also be administered at home. The duration of therapy is generally lifelong. With appropriate therapy, subjects may have minimal upper and lower respiratory tract symptoms. Other symptoms such as recurrent conjunctivitis and recurrent diarrhea associated with giardiasis are not necessarily eliminated by intravenous therapy because such treatment does not replace defects in secretory IgA function.

Transient Hypogammaglobulinemia of Infancy

Transient hypogammaglobulinemia of infancy usually presents in the second 6 months of life and has an incidence similar to that for symptomatic IgA deficiency.[59] Most children do not have a significant incidence of serious infections.[56,57,58,59] The IgG is low but comes into the normal range usually within the first 2 years of life. This disorder is often associated with IgA deficiency, which may persist. Low immunoglobulin levels may be found when investigating infants for recurrent respiratory tract infections, but it is not clear whether children with transient hypogammaglobulinemia have an increased incidence of infections as compared with normal children. The incidence of atopic disease is increased, particularly food hypersensitivity, atopic dermatitis, and asthma, in these infants.[59,60]

This disorder can be distinguished from other forms of hypogammaglobulinemia by demonstration of a normal specific antibody response to antigens such as tetanus and diphtheria toxoids.[56] Intravenous immunoglobulin therapy is not required. The mechanism of the transient hypogammaglobulinemia is unknown. It has been suggested that subclinical protein loss in atopic individuals resulting from an enteropathy may contribute to the disorder in some cases.[59] The importance of the disorder lies in distinguishing it from more severe causes of hypogammaglobulinemia. By analogy with selective IgA deficiency, transient hypogammaglobulinemia may not necessarily give rise to significant symptoms, and there is probably a significant group of asymptomatic infants with undetected transient hypogammaglobulinemia.

DISORDERS OF T CELLS

Severe Combined Immunodeficiency

Severe combined immunodeficiency results in a deficiency of both B and T cell function. A number of variants[61] exist: X-linked severe combined immunodeficiency, autosomal recessive combined immunodeficiency caused by adenosine deaminase deficiency (ADA),[62] and the bare lymphocyte syndrome associated with defective expression of class 1[63] and/or class 2[64] HLA antigens. X-linked severe combined immunodeficiency is caused by mutations in the gene for the interleukin 2 receptor.[65] Severe combined immunodeficiency is associated with a profound deficiency of T cells, lack of immunoglobulins and generally presents within the first 6 months of life with diarrhea, lower respiratory tract infections, and failure to thrive.[1,4] The less severe forms (an X-linked form[66] and Nezelof syndrome[67]) may present later in childhood but often have a history of symptoms beginning in the first year of life.

More than half the children present with pneumocystis pneumonia.[61] Early presentation within the first 2 months of life with pneumonitis is particularly likely in patients with ADA deficiency. Pneumocystis infection may often be insidious with a history of cough that progresses over several weeks to marked pulmonary involvement. In addition to pneumocystis these children often have cytomegalovirus pneumonitis. A common accompaniment to the respiratory infections is failure to thrive, diarrhea, and candidiasis, particularly of the oral mucosa. Skin rashes are common, in particular a sebhorreic dermatitis-like rash of the scalp. The finding of erythroderma and eosinophilia suggests either the occurrence of the Ommen syndrome variant[68] or graft versus host disease as a result of maternal lymphocytes that have crossed the placenta.[61] The presence of hepatomegaly and ascites suggests the occurrence of venoocclusive disease of the liver.[69] Recurrent pneumonias can occur with cytomegalovirus, respiratory syncytial virus, pneumocystis, *Candida,* and gram-positive and gram-negative bacteria.[61] In the absence of marrow transplan-

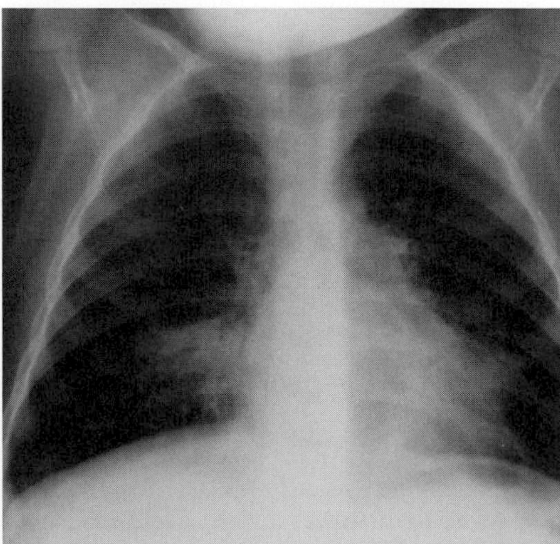

Fig. 56-2. Chronic bilateral changes in a 4-year-old male with an X-linked combined immunodeficiency. Lung biopsy showed a non-specific infiltrate with mononuclear and polymorphonuclear cells.

tation, death is usual in the pre-school years often from an overwhelming viral infection. Lung biopsy of children with chronic respiratory symptoms may show a nonspecific chronic inflammatory infiltrate with lymphoid or histiocytic cells (Fig. 56-2). Chest radiographs often show a diffuse bilateral disease that is alveolar and/or interstitial in nature. The lower respiratory tract disease is often resistant to therapy and may progress despite antimicrobial therapy and immunoglobulin.

Combined immunodeficiency should be suspected in any infant who presents with pneumocystis pneumonia. Other clues of the diagnosis are lymphopenia and low levels of immunoglobulins G, A, and M. The number of T cells is markedly reduced, proliferative response of T cells to mitogens is low or absent, and specific antibody responses are lacking. Treatment involves specific antimicrobial therapy and administration of intravenous immunoglobulin. The definitive therapy is bone marrow transplantation. Transplantation from an HLA-identical sibling has a more than 90% success rate if performed early in life before the onset of significant infections.[70] In the absence of an HLA-identical donor, a T cell-depleted bone marrow transplant from a parent, family relative, or unrelated donor is used. The overall success rate with a non–HLA-identical marrow graft is less, with a 50% to 70% long-term survival.[71] If mismatched marrow transplants are used in the absence of conditioning, restoration of T cell function without B cell function may occur. Conditioning with intense immunosuppression before transplantation is more likely to result in eventual restoration of B cell function but has a higher risk in the immediate posttransplant period of death from either sepsis or hemorrhage. Lung infection before transplantation is associated with a worse outcome. Prophylactic therapy against pneumocystis should be given to all patients following diagnosis. Live virus vaccines should be avoided and, before transplantation, patients should be isolated to prevent life-threatening infections with viruses such as measles, chicken pox, and influenza.

A complication of combined immunodeficiency is lymphoproliferative disease, which is often caused by Epstein-Barr virus (EBV) infection.[72,73] The abnormal lymphocyte proliferation is usually of B cell origin and may be associated with abnormal paraproteins. Lung infiltrates and pleural effusions occur. Histology shows infiltration of immunoblasts in multiple organs including the lung. T cell cytokine imbalance, with increased IL4 secretion favoring B cell proliferation, may be a factor in the development of this abnormal lymphoproliferation.[73] These B cell proliferative disorders can also occur following marrow transplantation. In addition, abnormal oligoclonal T cell proliferation with hepatosplenomegaly and interstitial pulmonary disease has been described.

Di George Anomalad

The Di George anomalad consists of varying degrees of thymic and parathyroid hypoplasia and cardiac outflow anomalies, especially truncus arteriosus and interrupted aortic arch, type B.[74,75] The disorder is the result of abnormal embryogenesis of the pharyngeal arches and pouches resulting from defective innervation.[76] The majority of cases results from deletions within chromosome 22q11.[77] Any of the structures derived from the first to the sixth pharyngeal arches and pouches can be affected.

Affected infants usually present because of the cardiac problem and the Di George anomalad is diagnosed during investigation of the cardiac lesion. Hypocalcemia may be found or an absent thymus noted at operation. The immunologic defect is variable.[78-80] The more severe cases are associated with marked reductions in T cell numbers. A T helper cell count of less than 500 has been associated with a greater incidence of subsequent immunologic problems.[80] Lesser degrees of immunologic abnormality are not always associated with any clinical problems.

More severely affected cases have an increased susceptibility to viral infections of the respiratory tract. The combination of cardiac disease and reduced T cell activity may lead to more severe respiratory syncytial virus infections with prolonged shedding of respiratory syncytial virus. Pneumocystis pneumonia may occur in cases with marked T cell deficiency. A complicating factor is the occurrence of tracheo- or bronchomalacia, often caused by compression by abnormal vessels. This may complicate management and predispose to more severe lower respiratory tract symptoms (Fig. 56-3). Abnor-

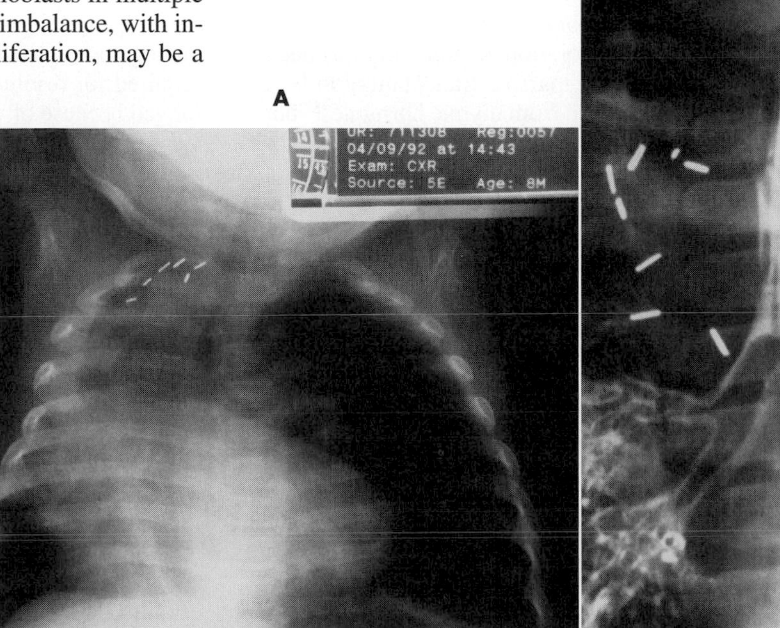

Fig. 56-3. A, Right upper lobe collapse in an 8-month-old male infant with Di George anomalad. **B,** Bronchogram showing malacia in the left main stem bronchus and narrowing at the origin of the right upper lobe bronchus.

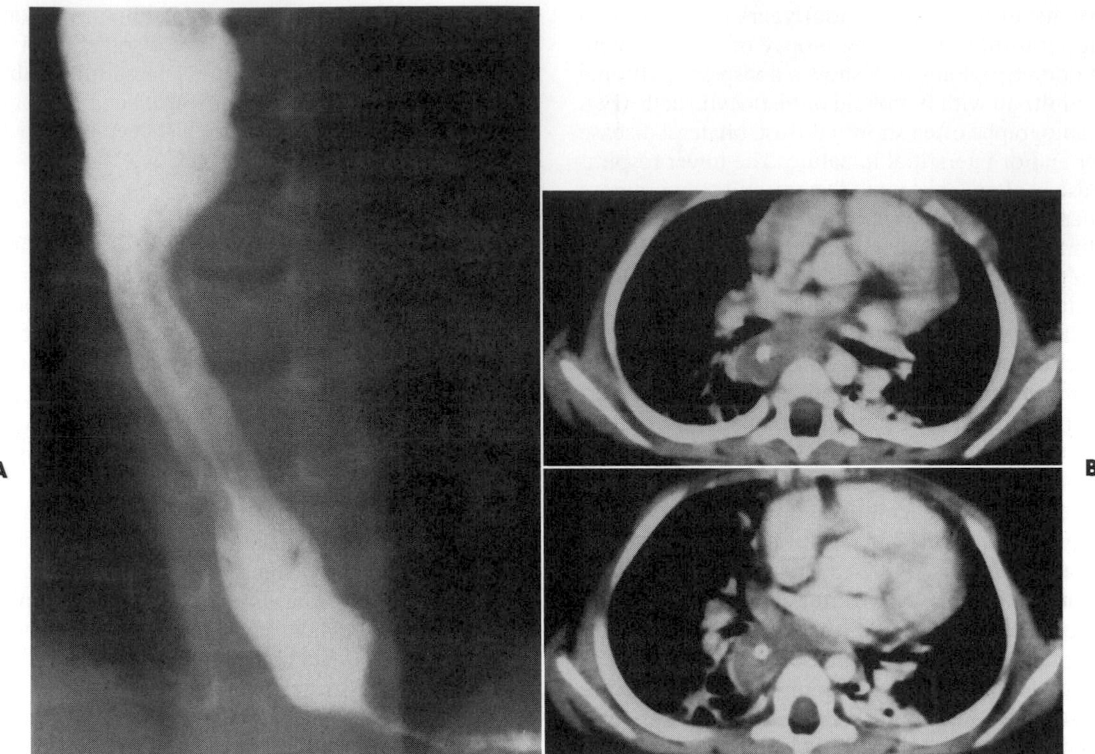

Fig. 56-4. **A,** Esophageal obstruction caused by an inflammatory granulomatous mass in a 3-year-old male with chronic granulomatous disease. **B,** CT scan showing mass surrounding the esophagus.

mal airway development during embryogenesis may also contribute to the malacia. This is suggested by the observation of defective tracheal ring formation in the Di George anomalad.[81]

The natural history is variable and in some subjects immune function can improve with time. Subjects with T cell counts less than 500 and abnormal lymphocyte mitogenic responses should be given prophylactic trimethoprim-sulfamethoxazole. If a defective antibody response to common antigens, such as tetanus and diphtheria, is present, immunoglobulin therapy is indicated. Definitive cure of the immune defect has been difficult. Thymic transplantation has been tried but because of the variability in the natural history of the disorder, the efficacy of this treatment is uncertain. Restoration of immunity has been achieved in rare cases by bone marrow transplantation.[82] A variable benefit has been obtained from thymic hormones[83] but the long-term benefits of this mode of therapy have also not been established.

DISORDERS OF PHAGOCYTES

Chronic Granulomatous Disease

Chronic granulomatous disease is a disorder of oxidative metabolism of phagocytic cells. Phagocytes can ingest microorganisms normally, but killing is defective. This disorder stems from defects in cytochrome B or cytosolic proteins required for oxidative activity. Two thirds of the cases are inherited in an X-linked manner and one third by autosomal recessive pattern.[84] The autosomal recessive disorder may have less severe clinical manifestations than the X-linked form.[85]

Patients develop recurrent infections with staphylococci; gram-negative enteric bacteria;[86,87] fungi, especially *Aspergillus;*[88] and unusual pathogens such as *Pseudomonas cepacia,*[89] *Nocardia,* and botryomycosis.[90] The lung is the most common site of infection.[86] Infections often begin early in life and include lymphadenitis, cutaneous infections, and obstructive lesions of the genitourinary and gastrointestinal tract (Fig. 56-4). Pneumonia is seen in most patients. Pulmonary lesions can vary from a patchy bronchopneumonia to extensive consolidation of a lobe or entire lung. Pneumonias may begin as a unilateral or bilateral hilar consolidation and persist for months or progress slowly to involve an entire lobe despite antibiotic treatment; an usual "encapsulated" pneumonia with hilar lymphadenopathy that progresses despite therapy may occur. Lung biopsy shows granuloma but not necessarily any pathogenic organisms. Often lobectomy or segmentectomy is required for resolution[87,91,92] and hospitalization is often prolonged because of wound infection and breakdown. Direct invasion of the chest may occur with associated osteomyelitis of ribs and vertebral bodies; this is often caused by *Aspergillus.*[93] Lung abscesses, empyema, and pleural effusion are uncommon. In a prospective study approximately one third of patients required admission to a hospital for treatment of pulmonary infection over a period of 9 months.[94] Another pulmonary manifestation of chronic granulomatous disease is a widespread nodular infiltrate. Histology shows multiple small granulomata. These lesions are often asymptomatic but can progress to pulmonary insufficiency and death.

In addition to standard antimicrobial therapies, which are often required in high dosage for long periods of time, additional measures that may be used to treat chronic granulomatous disease include white cell transfusions and use of the cytokine gamma interferon. Although gamma interferon has been shown to be effective when given prophylactically, its use in established infections is less certain. In a controlled trial there was no significant benefit from gamma interferon therapy for established lymphadenitis and subcutaneous abscesses.[94] There are individual case reports of resolution or improvement in infection following a combination of gamma interferon with antimicrobial therapy.[95,96]

Long-term prophylactic therapy with trimethoprim-sulfamethoxazole has been used in chronic granulomatous disease at a dosage of 15 mg sulfamethoxazole and 3 mg trimethoprim per kg body weight per day.[97] It has been difficult to study prophylactic therapy because the number of patients with chronic granulomatous disease at any center is small. Long-term prophylaxis appears to result in a significant reduction in dermatitis and lymphadenitis; however, it is less clear whether such prophylaxis reduces the incidence of lower respiratory tract infections. Prophylaxis has no effect on the occurrence of *Candida* and *Aspergillus* infections but does not appear to increase the incidence of fungal infections.[98]

Subcutaneous gamma interferon significantly reduced serious infections in a prospective controlled multicenter trial.[94] The dosage was 50 μg/m^2 (body surface area >0.5 m^2 or 1.5 μg/kg body surface area <0.5 m^2), subcutaneously 3 days per week for a mean period of 9 months. In addition to a reduction in lymphadenitis, prophylactic gamma interferon reduced episodes of lower respiratory tract infection, including fungal disease. Although gamma interferon has been shown to increase the oxidative metabolic activity of phagocytes from some, but not all, patients with chronic granulomatous disease in vivo and in vitro, its mode of action when used prophylactically is uncertain. It is possible that the beneficial effects result from nonspecific activation of the immune system rather than restoration of the metabolic defect in granulocytes. The beneficial effects of interferon are more marked in subjects under 10 years of age and in those with the X-linked form of the disease.[94] There are many unknowns concerning interferon therapy, in particular the side effects of prolonged treatment and which patients are most likely to benefit. Gamma interferon activates the immune system and induction of autoimmune diseases has been reported.

Cell Adhesion Molecule Deficiency

These subjects have deficiency of the beta chain subunit of the cell adhesion molecules that occur on lymphocytes, natural killer cells, and hematopoietic cells. The failure to express adhesion molecules leads to deficient cellular interactions and cellular motility. Moderate and severe phenotypes of the disease exist, which relate to the degree of expression of the cell adhesion molecules.[99] The more severe forms of this condition are usually fatal within the first 5 years of life.

Affected children have delayed separation of the umbilical cord, profound gingivitis, and otitis media. Viral respiratory tract infections may lead to severe secondary bacterial infections of the trachea and bronchial tree[99]; pneumonia has been reported in only a minority of subjects.[100] Pyoderma gangrenosum–like skin lesions are common and occur in virtually all patients. Delayed wound healing is common.

These subjects often have extremely high levels of circulating neutrophils (20 to 60 $\times$ 10^9/L), but they fail to form pus because of defective neutrophil migration into the tissues. The diagnosis is established by demonstrating deficiency of cell adhesion molecules on neutrophils with monoclonal antibodies, anti-Mac-1, OKM1, or Leu15. Definitive treatment is bone marrow transplantation.

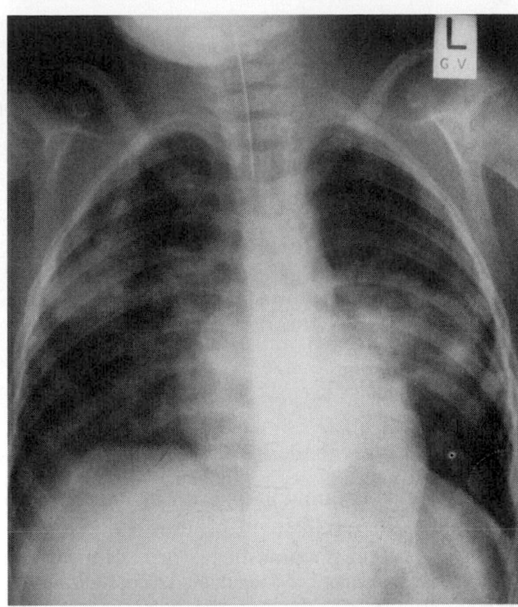

Fig. 56-5. Varicella pneumonitis in a 5-year-old male with natural killer cell deficiency and defective alpha interferon release. This was associated with extensive cutaneous lesions.

MISCELLANEOUS DISORDERS

Natural Killer Cell Deficiency

Several patients with a defect in natural killer cells have been described.[101-103] This defect has been observed in association with Fanconi anemia.[102,103] In childhood, the presentation has been with severe overwhelming varicella infection.[101] Children present with extensive varicella lesions on the skin and mucous membranes together with lung involvement and, occasionally, secondary sepsis (Fig. 56-5). This disorder can be suspected by finding an absence of natural killer cells in peripheral blood. Some cases have a deficiency of circulating B cells although specific antibody function is present.[103] Because only a few cases have been described, the long-term outlook for this disorder is unknown. It is uncertain whether patients have a defective immune response to other herpes virus infections. One patient developed a CMV interstitial pneumonia 4 years after the initial presentation with severe varicella.[103] Another had a defect in interferon release, which might contribute to the overwhelming viral infection. Varicella should be treated with intravenous acyclovir. In view of defective interferon release, alpha interferon might be helpful.

Hyper IgE Syndrome

Hyper IgE syndrome was described in 1972.[104] It presents in infancy with coarse facies, nonspecific eczematous dermatitis, peripheral blood eosinophilia, and cutaneous *Candida* infection. A vesicular eruption associated with eosinophilia may occur in infancy.[105] The cutaneous changes in infancy are followed by lower respiratory tract infections and marked elevation in serum IgE. Familial occurrences are described but the genetic defect is not known. An autosomal dominant inheritance with incomplete penetrance is considered most likely.[106] Subcutaneous cold abscesses and lower respiratory tract suppurative disease caused by organisms such as *Staphylococcus, Haemophilus influenzae,* and *Pseudomonas pyo-*

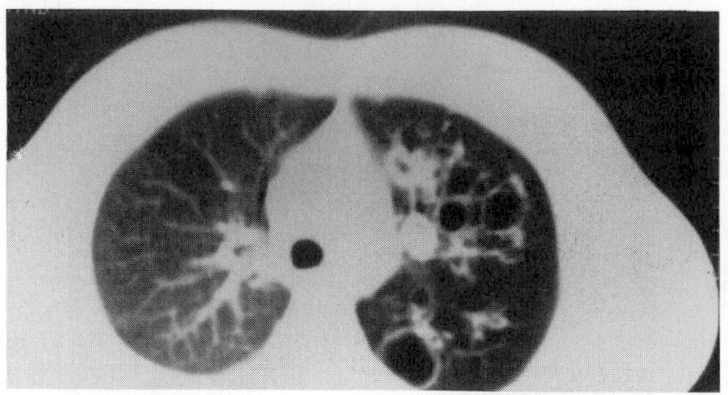

Fig. 56-6. Pneumatoceles in a 12-year-old male with hyper IgE syndrome.

cyanea often occur. Pneumonia and empyema develop in the first years of life. Pneumatoceles, pulmonary abscesses, bronchopleural fistula, and pneumothorax are common. Pneumatoceles are best demonstrated by CT scan (Fig. 56-6)[107]; they and pulmonary abscesses do not resolve spontaneously and lobectomy or pneumonectomy may be required.[108] Rarely spontaneous regression of pneumatoceles has been observed. The reason for the predilection for infection to occur in the upper lobes is unclear.

The immunologic defect is unknown. IgE levels are extremely high (often >10,000 U/ml). There are variable defects in neutrophil chemotaxis.[109,110] Specific IgE antibodies against *Staphylococcus aureus* and *Candida albicans* are found in the majority of patients. How these contribute to the pathogenesis is unclear.[111] Some subjects have a defective antibody response to polysaccharide antigens despite having normal immunoglobulin and immunoglobulin subclass levels.[112] This observation suggests that immunoglobulin therapy may be useful.

Management consists of long-term antistaphylococcal antibiotic prophylaxis which may act to limit the severity of both the cutaneous involvement and the lung disease. Sputum should be cultured regularly as the detection of *Pseudomonas* may require changes in therapy. The role of immunoglobulin and gamma interferon[113] is unclear. Despite regular medical attention, deterioration often occurs and respiratory failure eventually results.

Mucocutaneous Candidiasis

Mucocutaneous candidiasis is characterized by *Candida* infections of the skin, mucous membrane, and nails. Many, but not all cases, have defects in cell-mediated immunity to *Candida* antigens when measured by delayed hypersensitivity skin tests or in vitro techniques. Some patients have an increased susceptibility to bacterial infections, and develop pneumonia caused by *Staphylococcus aureus, Streptococcus pneumoniae,* or *Haemophilus influenzae b.*[114] Fungal or viral pneumonias occur less commonly. A long-term multicenter follow-up study of patients with chronic mucocutaneous candidiasis showed that 14% of these subjects had bronchiectasis and another 40% had either obstructive or restrictive lung disease.[114] Lung disease has been associated with IgG2 and IgG4 subclass deficiency.[115]

The assessment of patients with chronic mucocutaneous candidiasis and lower respiratory tract disease should include measurement of immunoglobulins, immunoglobulin subclasses, and evaluation of specific antibody responses to polysaccharides such as *Haemophilus influenzae b* and pneumococcus. Management is particularly difficult as the use of broad-spectrum antibiotics for lower respiratory tract symptoms exacerbates the candidiasis despite concurrent use of antifungal agents. The therapeutic effect of intravenous gammaglobulin in chronic mucocutaneous candidiasis with associated lung disease is not clear. It is likely that subjects with an ineffective response to polysaccharide antigen will benefit from such therapy with a reduction in episodes of acute pneumonia. The effect of immunoglobulin therapy on the development of bronchiectasis is unknown.

Wiskott-Aldrich Syndrome

This X-linked disorder is associated with a defective expression of sialoglycoprotein CD43 on circulating leucocytes and platelets. Infants usually present with refractory atopic dermatitis and thrombocytopenic purpura. A defective antibody response to polysaccharide antigens is universal,[116,117] and infection by encapsulated bacteria with associated otitis media or pneumonia is common, particularly after the first year of life. The immune defect is variable and some cases in infancy are indistinguishable from isolated thrombocytopenia.[118] In addition to a defective antibody response, there is a variable T cell defect and infections with pneumocystis[118] and herpes viruses can occur in later life. Often the major morbidity is bleeding caused by the thrombocytopenia.

The diagnosis can be established by sizing the platelets, which are smaller than usual.[119] The disorder is usually associated with a high IgA and low or normal IgG and IgM levels. There is a variable degree of reduction in T cell number and T cell response to mitogens. A defective expression to the sialoglyco-protein CD43 on T cells can sometimes be demonstrated after culturing cells in vitro.[120]

Treatment consists of intravenous gammaglobulin when significant antibody defects have been demonstrated. If bleeding has been a problem, splenectomy has been used, but this increases the risk of serious infection with encapsulated organisms.[122] Definitive treatment is by bone marrow transplantation, which can be successful if a matched donor is available. In the absence of a matched sibling donor, the success of bone marrow transplantation is considerably reduced and rejection of the graft is common.[122]

Ataxia Telangiectasis

Ataxia telangiectasis is a complex autosomal recessive disorder with neurologic, endocrinologic, immunologic, and cutaneous abnormalities. The gene for the disorder has been localized to chromosome 11 and appears to facilitate DNA recombination. T cell chromosomal rearrangements involving chromosomes 7 and 14 are common. Most cases present with ataxia in infancy or early childhood. Subsequently, telangiectasias on the skin and eyes and hyperpigmented and depigmented patches become prominent. Approximately half the patients develop significant sinopulmonary infections, in particular recurrent sinusitis and lower respiratory tract suppurative disease,[123,124] which may progress to bronchiectasis. IgA deficiency is found in approximately 50% of cases. When IgA deficiency is found, this is usually associated with an IgG2 subclass deficiency. IgG2 subclass deficiency does not always correlate with the development of suppurative lower respiratory tract disease.[125] IgE is often absent. More severe respiratory tract disease appears to be associated with more severe neurologic abnormalities. However, cases with relatively minor neurologic defects may demonstrate severe pulmonary disease. With progressive disease, aspiration may worsen the pulmonary problems and a major cause of death is pneumonia. Fungal infections are rare.

Immunologic investigation reveals variable defects in cell-mediated immunity with reduced numbers of circulating T cells and a diminished response to mitogens. Total IgG levels can be normal. The most common serologic abnormality is a raised alpha-fetoprotein, which is present in virtually all cases[126] and can be helpful in making the diagnosis. The defects in DNA repair lead to an increased incidence of chromosome breaks in cytogenetic studies. The management is similar to other cases of antibody or immunoglobulin subclass deficiency with intravenous immunoglobulin and antibiotics. Immunoglobulin is indicated if a significant antibody defect is demonstrated. The course is complicated by a high incidence of malignancy of the lymphoreticular system.

Nijmegen Breakage Syndrome

The Nijmegen breakage syndrome is an autosomal recessive disorder with defects in DNA repair and similar immunologic, cytogenetic, and cell biological abnormalities as seen in ataxia telangiectasis. In contrast to ataxia telangiectasia, alpha-fetoprotein levels are normal. The affected children have microcephaly, abnormal facies, and suffer from recurrent lower respiratory tract infections.[127]

REFERENCES

Disorders of Antibody Function

1. Hong R, Amman AJ: In *Immunologic disorders in infants and children,* ed 3, Philadelphia, 1989, WB Saunders, p 329.
2. Frommai D, Moullec J, Lambin P, Fine JM: Selective serum IgA deficiency. Frequency among 15,200 French donors, *Vox Sang* 25:513-518, 1973.
3. Van Loghem E, Zegers BJ, Bast EJ, Kater L: Selective deficiency of immunoglobulin A2, *J Clin Invest* 72:1918-1923, 1983.
4. Islam KB, Bakin B, Nilsson G, Hammarstrom L, Sideras P, Smith CI: Molecular analysis of IgA deficiency. Evidence for impaired switching to IgA, *J Immunol* 152:1242-1252, 1994.
5. Gleeson M, Cripps AW, Clancy RL, Husband AJ, Hensley MJ, Leeder SR: Ontogeny of the secretory immune system in man, *Aust NZ J Med* 12:256-258, 1982.
6. Plebani A, Ugazio AG, Monafo V, Burgio GR: Clinical heterogeneity and reversibility of selective immunoglobulin A deficiency in 80 children, *Lancet* 1:829-831, 1986.
7. Hanson LA, Bjorkander J, Carlsson B, Roberton D, Soderstrom T: The heterogeneity of IgA deficiency, *J Clin Immunol* 8:159-162, 1988.
8. De Laat PCJ, Weemaes CMR, Gonera R, Van Munster PJJ, Bakkeren JAJ, Stoelinga GBA: Clinical manifestations in selective IgA deficiency in childhood, *Acta Paediatr Scand* 80:798-804, 1991.
9. Oxelius VA, Laurell AB, Lindquist B, Golebiowska H, Axelsson U, Bjorkander J, Hanson LA: IgG subclasses in selective IgA deficiency, *N Engl J Med* 304:1476-1477, 1981.
10. Beard LJ, Ferrante A: IgG4 deficiency in IgA-deficient patients, *Pediatr Infect Dis J* 8:705-709, 1989.
11. Bjorkander J, Bake B, Oxelius VA, Hanson LA: Impaired lung function in patients with IgA deficiency and low levels of IgG2 or IgG3, *N Engl J Med* 313:720-4, 1985.
12. Bjorkander J, Hammarstrom L, Edvard Smith CI, Buckley RH, Cunningham-Rundles C, Hanson LA: Immunoglobulin prophylaxis in patients with antibody deficiency syndromes and anti-IgA antibodies, *J Clin Immunol* 7:8-15, 1987.
13. Cunningham-Rundles C, Zhou Z, Mankarious S, Courter S: Long term use of IgA-depleted intravenous immunoglobulin in immunodeficient subjects with anti-IgA antibodies, *J Clin Immunol* 13:272-278, 1993.
14. Vetrie D, Vorechovsky I, Sideras P, Holland J, Davies A, Flinter F, Hammarstrom L, Kinnon C, Levinsky R, Bobrow M, Smith CIE, Bentley DR: The gene involved in X-linked agammaglobulinaemia is a member of the src family of protein-tyrosine kinases, *Nature* 361:1226-233, 1993.
15. Lederman HM, Winkelstein JA: X-linked agammaglobulinaemia an analysis of 96 patients, *Medicine* 64:145-156, 1985.
16. Gelfand EW: Unique susceptibility of patients with antibody deficiency to mycoplasma infection, *Clin Infect Dis* 17:S250-253, 1993.
17. Phelan PD, Laudau LI, Williams HE: Lung disease associated with infantile agammaglobulinaemia, *Aust Paediatr* J 9:147-151, 1973.
18. Sweinberg SK, Wodell RA, Grodofsky MP, Greene JM, Conley ME: Retrospective analysis of the incidence of pulmonary disease in hypogammaglobulinaemia, *J Allergy Clin Immunol* 88:96-104, 1991.
19. Aruffo A, Farrington M, Hollenbaugh D, Milatovich A, Nonoyama S, Bajorath J, Grosmaire LS, Stenkamp R, Neubauer M: The CD40 ligand, gp39, is defective in activated T cells from patients with X-linked hyper-IgM syndrome, *Cell* 72:291-300, 1993.
20. Allen RC, Armitage RJ, Conley ME, Rosenblatt H, Jenkins NA, Copeland NG, Bedell MA, Edelhoff S, Disteche CM, Simoneaux DK, Fanslow WC, Belmont J, Spriggs MK: CD40 ligand gene defects responsible for x-linked hyper-IgM syndrome, *Science* 259:990-993, 1993.
21. Notarangelo LD, Duse M, Ugazio AG: Immunodeficiency with hyper-IgM (HIM), *Immunodefic Rev* 3:101-122, 1992.
22. Hermaszewski RA, Webster ADB: Primary hypogammaglobulinaemia: a survey of clinical manifestations and complications, *Q J Med* 86:31-42, 1993.
23. Hausser C, Virelizier JL, Buriot D, Griscelli C: Common variable hypogammaglobulinaemia in children, *Am J Dis Child* 137:833-837, 1983.
24. Conley ME, Park CL, Douglas SD: Childhood common variable immunodeficiency with autoimmune disease, *J Pediatr* 108:915-922, 1986.
25. Schaffer FM, Palermos J, Zhu B, Burger BO, Cooper MD: Individuals with IgA deficiency and common variable immunodeficiency share polymorphisms of major histocompatibility complex class III genes, *Proc Natl Acad Sci USA* 86:8015-8019, 1989.
26. Cunningham-Rundles C: Clinical and immunological analyses of 103 patients with common variable immunodeficiency, *J Clin Immunol* 9:22-33, 1989.
27. Strimlan CV, Rosenow EC, Weiland LH, Brown LR: Lymphocytic interstitial pneumonitis, *Ann Intern Med* 88:616-621, 1978.
28. Sander CA, Medeiros LJ, Weiss LM, Yano T, Sneller MC, Jaffe ES: Lymphoproliferative lesions in patients with common variable immunodeficiency syndrome, *Am J Surg Pathol* 16:1170-1182, 1992.
29. Sweinberg K, Wodell RA, Grodofsky MP, Greene JM, Conley ME: Retrospective analysis of pulmonary disease in hypogammaglobulinaemia, *J Allergy Clin Immunol* 88:96-104, 1991.
30. Morgan G, Levinsky RJ: Clinical significance of IgG subclass deficiency, *Arch Dis Child* 63:771-773, 1988.
31. Ambrosino DM, Black CM, Plikaytis BD, Reimer CB, Lee MC, Evatt BL, Carlone GM: Immunoglobulin G subclass values in healthy black and white children, *J Pediatr* 119:875-9, 1991.
32. Aucouturier P, Mariault M, Lacombe C, Preud'homme JL: Frequency of selective IgG subclass deficiency: a reappraisal, *Clin Immunol Immunopathol* 63:289-291, 1992.
33. Shackelford PG, Granoff DM, Madassery JV, Scott MG, Nahm MH: Clinical and immunologic characteristics of healthy children with subnormal serum concentrations of IgG2, *Pediatr Res* 27:16-21, 1990.
34. Gross S, Blaiss MS, Herrod HG: Role of immunoglobulin subclasses and specific antibody determinations in the evaluation of recurrent infection in children, *J Pediatr* 121:516-522, 1992.
35. Avanzini MA, Bjorkander J, Soderstrom R, Soderstrom T, Schneerson R, Robbins JB, Hanson LA: Qualitative and quantitative analyses of the antibody response elicited by *Haemophilus influenzae* type b capsular polysaccharide-tetanus toxoid conjugates in adults with IgG subclass deficiencies and frequent infections, *Clin Exp Immunol* 96:54-58, 1994.
36. Nahm MH, Macke K, Oh-Hun Kwon, Madassery JV, Sherman LA, Scott MG: Immunologic and clinical status of blood donors with subnormal levels of IgG2, *J Allergy Clin Immunol* 85:769-777, 1990.

37. Beck CS, Heiner DC: Selective immunoglobulin G4 deficiency and recurrent infections of the respiratory tract, *Am Rev Resp Dis* 124:94-96, 1981.
38. Umetsu DT, Ambrosino DM, Quinti I, Siber GR, Geha RS: Recurrent sinopulmonary infection and impaired antibody response to bacterial capsular polysaccharide antigen in children with selective IgG-subclass deficiency, *N Engl J Med* 313:1247-1251, 1985.
39. De Baets F, Kint J, Pauwels R, Leroy J: IgG subclass deficiency in children with recurrent bronchitis, *Eur J Pediatr* 151:274-278, 1992.
40. Carlsen KH, Mellbye OJ, Fuglerud P, Johansen B, Solheim AB, Belsnes D, Danielsen A, Henrichson L: Serum immunoglobulin G subclasses and serum immunoglobulin A in acute bronchiolitis in infants, *Pediatr Allergy Immunol* 4:20-25, 1993.
41. Shackelford PG, Granoff DM, Polmar SH, Scott MG, Goskowicz MC, Madassery JV, Nahm MH: Subnormal serum concentrations of IgG2 in children with frequent infections associated with varied patterns of immunologic dysfunction, *J Pediatr* 116:529-538, 1990.
42. Shapiro GG, Virant FS, Furukawa CT, Pierson WE, Bierman CW: Immunologic defects in patients with refractory sinusitis, *Pediatrics* 87:311-316, 1991.
43. Moss RB, Carmack MA, Esrig S: Deficiency of IgG4 in children: association of isolated IgG4 deficiency with recurrent respiratory tract infection, *J Pediatr* 120:16-21, 1992.
44. Bernatowska-Mauszkiewicz E, Pac M, Skopcynska H, Pum M, Eibl MM: Clinical efficacy of intravenous immunoglobulin in patients with severe inflammatory chest disease and IgG3 subclass deficiency, *Clin Exp Immunol* 85:193-197, 1991.
45. Hoeger PH, Niggemann B, Haeuser G: Age related IgG subclass concentrations in asthma, *Arch Dis Child* 70:179-182, 1994.
46. Smith TF, Ireland TA, Zaatari GS, Gay BB, Zwiren GT, Andrews HG: Characteristics of children with endoscopically proved chronic bronchitis, *Am J Dis Child* 139:1039-1044, 1985.
47. Smith TF, Morris EC, Bain RP: IgG subclasses in nonallergic children with chronic chest symptoms, *J Pediatr* 105:896-899, 1984.
48. Page R, Friday G, Stillwagon P, Skoner D, Caliguiri L, Fireman P: Asthma and selective immunoglobulin subclass deficiency. Improvement of asthma after immunoglobulin replacement therapy, *J Pediatr* 112:127-130, 1988.
49. Haeney M: Intravenous immune globulin in primary immunodeficiency, *Clin Exp Immunol* 97:11-15, 1994.
50. Chapel HM: Consensus panel for the diagnosis and management of primary antibody deficiencies. Consensus on diagnosis and management of primary antibody deficiencies, *BMJ* 308:581-585, 1994.
51. Roifman CM, Levison H, Gelfand EW: High-dose versus low-dose intravenous immunoglobulin in hypogammaglobulinaemia and chronic lung disease, *Lancet* i:1075-1077, 1987.
52. Nolte MT, Pirofsky B, Ferritz GA, Golding B: Intravenous immunoglobulin therapy for antibody deficiency, *Clin Exp Immunol* 36:237-243, 1979.
53. Hermaszewski RA, Webster ADB: Primary hypogammaglobulinaemia: a survey of clinical manifestations and complications, *Quart J Med* 86:31-42, 1993.
54. Lever AML, Webster ADB, Brown D, Thomas HC: Non-A, non-B hepatitis occurring in agammaglobulinaemia patients after intravenous immunoglobulin, *Lancet* ii:1062-1064, 1984.
55. Casteels-Van Daele M, Wijndaele L, Hunninck K, Gillis P: Intravenous immune globulin and acute aseptic meningitis, *N Engl J Med* 323:614-615, 1990.
56. Tiller TL, Buckley RH: Transient hypogammaglobulinaemia of infancy: review of literature, clinical and immunologic features of 11 new cases, and long term follow up, *J Pediatr* 92:347-353, 1978.
57. McGready SJ: Transient hypogammaglobulinaemia of infancy: need to reconsider name and definition, *J Pediatr* 110:47-50, 1987.
58. Dressler F, Peter HH, Muller W, Reiger CHL: Transient hypogammaglobulinaemia of infancy. Five new cases, review of literature, and definition, *Acta Paediatr Scand* 78:767-774, 1989.
59. Walker AM, Kemp AS, Hill DJ: Features of transient hypogammaglobulinaemia in infants screened for immunological abnormalities, *Arch Dis Child* 70:183-186, 1994.
60. Fineman SM, Rosen FS, Geha RS: Transient hypogammaglobulinaemia, elevated immunoglobulin E levels, and food allergy, *J Allergy Clin Immunol* 64:216-222, 1979.

Disorders of T Cells

61. Stephan JL, Vlekova V, Le Deist F, Blanche S, Donadieu J, De Saint-Basile G, Durandy A, Griscelli C, Fischer A: Severe combined immunodeficiency: a retrospective single-center study of clinical presentation and outcome in 117 patients, *J Pediatr* 123:574-572, 1993.
62. Hirschhorn R: Overview of biochemical abnormalities and molecular genetics of adenosine diaminase deficiency, *Pediatr Res* (Suppl):S35-S41, 1991.
63. Rouraine JL: The bare lymphocyte syndrome: report on the registry, *Lancet* i:319-321, 1981.
64. Klein C, Lisowska-Grospierre B, LeDeist F, Fischer A, Griscelli C: Major histocompatibility complex II deficiency: clinical manifestations, immunologic features and outcome, *J Pediatr* 123:921-928, 1993.
65. Noguchi M, Huafang Y, Rosenblatt H, Filipovitch A, Adelstein S, Modi W, McBride W, Leonard W: Interluekin-2 receptor gamma chain mutation results in x-linked severe combined immunodeficiency in humans, *Cell* 73:147-157, 1993.
66. de Saint-Basile G, Le Deist F, Caniglia M, Lebranchu Y, Giscelli C, Fischer A: Genetic study of a new x-linked recessive immunodeficiency syndrome, *J Clin Invest* 89:861-866, 1992.
67. Lawlor GJ, Ammann AJ, Wright WC, La Franchi SH, Bilstrom D, Stiehm ER: The syndrome of cellular immunodeficiency with immunoglobulins, *J Pediatr* 84:183-192, 1974.
68. Omenn GS: Familial reticuloendotheliosis with eosinophilia, *N Engl J Med* 273:427-432, 1965.
69. Etzioni A, Benderly A, Rosenthal E, Shehadah V, Auslander L, Lahat N, Plllack S: Defective humoral and cellular immune functions associated with veno-occlusive disease of the liver, *J Pediatr* 110:549-554, 1987.
70. Fischer A, Landais P, Friedrich W, Morgan G, Gerritsen B, Fasth A, Porta F, Griscelli C, Goldman SF, Levinsky R, Vossen J: European experience of bone-marrow transplantation for severe combined immunodeficiency, *Lancet* 336:850-854, 1990.
71. Dror Y, Gallagher R, Wara DW, Colome BW, Merino A, Benkerrou M, Cowan MJ: Immune reconstitution in severe combined immunodeficiency disease after lectin-treated, T-cell-depleted haplocompatible bone marrow transplantation, *Blood* 81:2021, 1993.
72. Shearer T, Ritz J, Finegold MJ, Guerra IC, Rosenblatt HM, Lewis DE, Pollack MS, Taber LH, Sumaya CV, Grumet FC, Cleary ML, Wanke R, Sklar J: Epstein-Barr virus-associated B-cell proliferations of diverse clonal origins after bone marrow transplantation in a 12-year-old patient with severe combined immunodeficiency, *N Engl J Med* 312:1151-1159, 1985.
73. Filipovich AH, Mathur A, Kamat D, Shapiro RS: Primary immunodeficiencies: genetic risk factors for lymphoma, *Cancer Res* 52:5465S-5467S, 1992.
74. Thomas RA, Landing BH, Wells TR: Embryologic and other developmental considerations of thirty-eight possible variants of the Di George anomaly, *Am J Med Genet Suppl* 3:43-66, 1987.
75. Hong R: The Di George anomaly, *Immunodeficiency Rev* 3:1-14, 1991.
76. Bockman DE, Kirby ML: Dependence of thymus development on derivatives of the neural crest, *Science* 223:498-500, 1984.
77. Driscoll AD, Budarf MI, Emanuel BS: A genetic etiology for Di George syndrome: consistent deletions and microdeletions of 22q II, *Am J Hum Genet* 50:924-933, 1992.
78. Muller W, Peter HH, Kallfelz HC, Franz A, Rieger CHL: The Di George syndrome II. Immunologic findings in partial and complete forms of the disorder, *Eur J Pediatr* 149:96-103, 1989.
79. Barrett DJ, Amman AJ, Wara DW, Cowan MJ, Fisher TJ, Stiehm ER: Clinical and immunologic spectrum of the Di George syndrome, *J Clin Lab Immunol* 6:1-6, 1981.
80. Bastian J, Law S, Volger L, et al: Prediction of persistent immunodeficiency in the Di George anomaly, *J Pediatr* 115:391-396, 1989.
81. Sein K, Wells TR, Landing BH, Chow CR: Short trachea with reduced number of cartilage rings—A hitherto unrecognised feature of Di George syndrome, *Pediatr Pathol* 4:81-88, 1985.
82. Goldsobel AB, Haas A, Stiehm ER: Bone marrow transplantation in Di George syndrome, *J Pediatr* 111:40-44, 1987.
83. Businco L, Ruballelli FF, Paganelli R, Galli E, Ensoli B, Betti P, Aiuti F: Results in 2 infants with Di George syndrome—Effects of long-term TP5, *Clin Immunol Immunopathol* 39:22-30, 1986.

Disorders of Phagocytes

84. Smith RM, Curnutte JT: Molecular basis of chronic granulomatous disease, *Blood* 77:673-686, 1991.
85. Weening RS, Adriaansz LH, Weemaes CMR, Lutter R, Roos D: Clinical differences in chronic granulomatous disease in patients with cytochrome b-negative or cytochrome b-positive neutrophils, *J Pediatr* 107:102-104, 1985.
86. Gallin JI, Buescher FS, Seligmann BE, Nath J, Gaiather TE, Katz P: Recent advances in chronic granulomatous disease, *Ann Intern Med* 99:647-674, 1983.
87. Curnette JI: *Haematology of infancy and childhood,* ed 4, Philadelphia, 1993, WB Saunders, p 923.
88. Cohen MS, Isturiz RE, Malech HL, Root RK, Wilfert CM, Gutman L, Buckley RH: Fungal infection in chronic granulomatous disease. The importance of the phagocyte in defense against fungi, *Am J Med* 71:59-66, 1981.
89. O'Neil KM, Herman JH, Modkin JF, Moxon ER, Winkelstein JA: *Pseudomonas cepacia:* an emerging pathogen in chronic granulomatous disease, *J Pediatr* 108:940-942, 1986.
90. Paz HL, Little BJ, Ball WC, Winkelstein JA: Primary pulmonary botryomycosis. A manifestation of chronic granulomatous disease, *Chest* 101:1160-1162, 1992.
91. Pegrebniak HW, Gallin JI, Malech HL, Baker AR, Moskaluk CA, Tavis WD, Pass HI: Surgical management of pulmonary infections in chronic granulomatous disease of childhood, *Ann Thorac Surg* 55:844-849, 1993.
92. Roback SA, Weintraub WH, Good RA, Lindsay WG, Quie PG, Park B, Leonard S: Chronic granulomatous disease of childhood: surgical considerations, *J Paediatr Surg* 6:601-611, 1971.
93. Kawashima A, Kuhlman JE, Fishman EK, Tempany CM, Magid D, Lederman HM, Windelstein JA, Zerhouni EA: Pulmonary *Aspergillus* chest wall involvement in chronic granulomatous disease: CT and MRI findings, *Skeletal Radiol* 20:487-493, 1991.
94. The International Chronic Granulomatous Disease Co-Operative Study Group: A controlled trial of interferon gamma to prevent infection in chronic granulomatous disease, *N Engl J Med* 324:509-516, 1991.
95. Hague KA, Eastham EJ, Lee RE, Cant AJ: Resolution of hepatic abscess after interferon gamma in chronic granulomatous disease, *Arch Dis Child* 69:443-445, 1993.
96. Bernhisel-Broadbent J, Camargo EE, Jaffe HS, Lederman HM: Recombinant human interferon gamma as adjunct therapy for *Aspergillus* in a patient with chronic granulomatous disease, *J Infect Dis* 163:908-911, 1991.
97. Weening RS, Kabel P, Pijman P, Roos D: Continuous therapy with sulfamethoxazole-trimethoprim in patients with chronic granulomatous disease, *J Pediatr* 103:127-130, 1983.
98. Margolis DM, Melnick DA, Alling DW, Gallin JI: Trimethoprim-sulfamethoxazole prophylaxis in the management of chronic granulomatous disease, *J Infect Dis* 162:723-726, 1990.
99. Anderson DC, Schmalsteig FC, Finegold MJ, Hughes BJ, Rothlein R, Miller LJ, Kohl S, Tsoi M, Jacobs RL, Waldrop TC, Goldman AS, Shearer WT, Springer TA: The severe and moderate phenotypes of heritable Mac-1-LFA-1 deficiency: their quantitative definition and relation to leukocyte dysfunction and clinical features, *J Infect Dis* 152: 668-689, 1985.
100. Schmalstieg FC: Leukocyte adherence defect, *Pediatr Infect Dis J* 7:867-872, 1988.

Miscellaneous Disorders

101. Biron CA, Byron KS, Sullivan JL: Severe herpes virus infection in an adolescent without natural killer cells, *N Engl J Med* 320:1731-35, 1989.
102. Hersey P, Edwards A, Lewis R, Singh S, Kemp AS, Mcinnes A: Deficient natural killer cell activity in a patient with Fanconi's anaemia and squamous cell carcinoma. Association with a defect in interferon release, *Clin Exp Immunol* 4:205-212, 1982.
103. Ballas ZK, Turner JM, Turner DA, Guetzman EA, Kemp JD: A patient with simultaneous absence of "classical" natural killer cells (CD3-, CD 16+, CD5, NKH 1+) and expansion of CD3+, CD4-, CD8-, NKH1 + subset, *J Allergy Clin Immunol* 85:453-59, 1990.
104. Buckley RH, Wray BB, Belmake EZ: Extreme hyperimmunoglobulinemia E and undue susceptibility to infection, *Pediatr* 49:59-70, 1972.
105. Kamei R, Honig PJ: Neonatal Job's syndrome featuring a vesicular eruption, *Pediatr Derm* 2:75-82, 1988.
106. Buckley RH, Becker WG: Abnormalities in the regulation of human IgE synthesis, *Immunol Rev* 41:288-314, 1978.
107. Fitch SJ, Magill HL, Herrod HG, Moinuddin M: Hyperimmunoglobulinemia E syndrome: pulmonary imaging considerations, *Pediatr Radiol* 16:285-288, 1986.
108. Donabedian H, Gallin JI: The hyperimmunoglobulin E recurrent infection syndrome; a review of the NIH experience and the literature, *Medicine* 62:195-208, 1983.
109. Schopfer K, Baerlocher K, Price P, Krech U, Quie PG, Douglas SD: Staphylococcal IgE antibodies, hyperimmunoglobulinemia E and *Staphylococcus aureus* infection, *N Engl J Med* 300:835-838, 1979.
110. Jeppson JD, Jaffe HS, Hill HR: Use of recombinant human interferon gamma to enhance entrophil chemotactic responses in Job syndrome of hyperimmunoglobulinemia E and recurrent infections, *J Pediatr* 118:383-387, 1991.
111. Berger M, Kirkpatrick CH, Goldsmith PK, Gallin JI: IgE antibodies to *Staphylococcus aureus* and *Candida albicans* in patients with the syndrome of hyperimmunoglobulin E and recurrent infections, *J Immunol* 125:2437-2443, 1980.
112. Leung DYM, Ambrosino DM, Arbeit RD, Newton JL, Geha RS: Impaired antibody responses in the hypergammaglobulinemia E syndrome, *J Allergy Clin Immunol* 81:1082-1087, 1988.
113. Pung YH, Vetro SW, Bellanti JA: Use of interferons in atopic (IgE mediated) diseases, *Ann Allergy* 71:234-238, 1993.
114. Herrod HG: Chronic mucocutaneous candidiasis in childhood and complications of non-*Candida* infection: a report of the Pediatric Immunodeficiency Collaborative Study Group, *J Pediatr* 116:377-382, 1990.
115. Bentur L, Nisbet-Brown E, Levison H, Roifman CM: Lung disease associated with IgG subclass deficiency in chronic mucocutaneous candidiasis, *J Pediatr* 118:82-86, 1991.
116. Blaese RM, Strober W, Brown RS, Waldmann TA: The Wiskott-Aldrich syndrome: a disorder with possible defect in antigen processing or recognition, *Lancet* i:1056-1061, 1968.
117. Cooper MD, Chase HP, Lowman JT, Krivit W, Good RA: Wiskott-Aldrich syndrome: an immunologic deficiency disease involving the afferent limb of immunity, *Am J Med* 44:499-513, 1968.
118. Puck JM, Siminovitch KA, Poncz M: Atypical presentation of the Wiskott-Alrich syndrome: diagnosis in two unrelated males based on studies on maternal T cell activation, *Blood* 75:2369-2374, 1990.
119. Ochs HD, Slichter SJ, Harker LA, Von Behrens WE, Clark RA, Wedgwood RJ: The Wiskott-Aldrich syndrome: studies of lymphocytes, granulocytes and platelets, *Blood* 55:243-252, 1980.
120. Remold-O'Donnell E, Kenney DM, Parkman R, Cairns L, Savage B, Rosen FS: Characterisation of a human lymphocyte surface sialoglycoprotein that is defective in Wiskott-Aldrich syndrome, *J Exp Med* 159:1705-1723, 1984.
121. Lum LG, Tubergen DG, Corash L, Blaese RM: Splenectomy in the management of the thrombocytopenia of the Wiskott-Aldrich syndrome, *N Engl J Med* 302:892-896, 1980.
122. Mullen CA, Anderson KD, Blaese RM: Splenectomy and/or bone marrow transplantation in the management of the Wiskott-Aldrich syndrome: long term follow up of 62 cases, *Blood* 82:2961-2966, 1993.
123. McFarlin DE, Strober W, Waldmann TA: Ataxia-telangiectasis, *Medicine* 51:281-314, 1972.
124. Gatti RA, Boder E, Vinters HV, Sparkes RS, Norman A, Lange K: Ataxia-telangiectasia: an interdisciplinary approach to pathogenesis, *Medicie* 70:99-117, 1991.
125. Aucouturier P, Bremard-Oury C, Griscelli C, Berthier M, Preud'Home JL: Serum IgG subclass deficiency in ataxis-telangiectasis, *Clin Exp Immunol* 68:392-396, 1987.
126. Jason JM, Gelfand EW: Diagnostic considerations in ataxia-telangiectasia, *Arch Dis Child* 54:682-686, 1979.
127. Weemaes CM, Smeets DF, Horstink M, Haraldsson A, Bakkeren JA: Variants of Nijmegen breakage syndrome and ataxia telangiectasis, *Immunodeficiency* 4:109-111, 1993.

SUGGESTED READING

Stiehm ER: New and old immunodeficiencies, *Pediatr Res* 33(suppl):S2-S8, 1993.

PART NINE

Cardiopulmonary and Pulmonary Vascular Disorders

CHAPTER 57

Fluid Balance in the Developing Lung

Richard D. Bland and David P. Carlton

Pulmonary edema is a common cause of respiratory distress in infants and children. Because their primary function is respiratory gas exchange, the lungs are especially vulnerable to the adverse effects of excess water accumulation. Normally, protein-rich liquid flows continuously out of the bloodstream into the interstitium of the lungs and returns to the circulation either directly across the microvascular endothelium or through an extensive network of pulmonary lymphatics that drain into the systemic venous system. The lungs become edematous when the net outward flow of fluid from the pulmonary vasculature exceeds the clearance capacity of the lymphatics and microcirculation. If the epithelial barrier is intact, excessive fluid is contained within the lung interstitium, with little or no effect on respiratory gas exchange. If the epithelial barrier becomes permeable to solutes of large molecular weight, such as plasma proteins, the airspaces rapidly fill with liquid, thereby impairing the respiratory function of the lungs. During the past two decades, a large body of evidence has appeared in the literature demonstrating that the alveolar epithelium of the mature lung is endowed with important ion transport mechanisms that serve to keep *the airspaces* relatively dry. In some cases, however, lung injury may either impair or overwhelm both the normal barrier function and the ion transport mechanisms of the epithelium, with resultant alveolar edema and associated respiratory failure.

The purpose of this chapter is to describe the normal physiology of lung fluid balance during development and the abnormal conditions that sometimes disrupt this balance to cause pulmonary edema. Much of our knowledge about the pathogenesis of pulmonary edema in infants and children derives from experiments performed with animals at various stages of development. This chapter addresses much of this experimental work. Because respiratory distress in newborn infants often has a prenatal origin, and because the immature lungs contain more water at birth than mature lungs do, a discussion of fetal lung liquid and its removal before, during, and after birth is included in this chapter. Important gaps in our knowledge of the processes that regulate fluid balance in the developing lung are noted, with the expectation that further research will provide important new information on which to base improved treatment or perhaps prevention of pulmonary edema in infants and children.

FETAL LUNG LIQUID

Secretion of Liquid in the Fetal Lung

During fetal development, the lungs are secretory organs that make breathing-like movements but have no role in respiratory gas exchange, which before birth is a function of the placenta. In utero the lungs are filled with liquid and receive less than 10% of the combined ventricular output of blood from the heart.[1] In fetal sheep, however, this relatively modest blood supply is sufficient to deliver the substrate needed by the pulmonary epithelium to make surfactant and secrete into the lung lumen as much as 500 ml of liquid daily during the last third of gestation.[2,3] At least one published report indicated that liquid production by the bronchopulmonary epithelium of human fetuses may occur as early as the sixth week of gestation, with resultant expansion of the lung lumen.[4] The presence of an appropriate volume of secreted liquid within the fetal respiratory tract is essential for normal lung growth and development before birth.[5-7] Conditions that interfere with normal lung liquid production, such as pulmonary artery occlusion,[8,9] diaphragmatic hernia,[10,11] and uterine compression of the fetal chest from chronic leakage of amniotic liquid,[12,13] also inhibit lung growth. These observations underscore the importance of liquid expansion of potential airspaces in the development of normal lung structure before birth, which in turn may influence lung function after birth.

Fig. 57-1 is a schematic diagram of the fluid compartments of the fetal lung, in which potential airspaces are filled with a liquid that is rich in Cl (approximately150 mEq/L) and almost free of protein (less than 0.03 mg/ml).[3,14,15] Strang et al[16-21] did extensive studies of water and solute exchange across the epithelium and endothelium of the fetal lung. They sampled liquid from the trachea, lung lymphatics, and bloodstream of fetal lambs and followed the movement of radioactive tracers between the three fluid compartments. These studies demonstrated that the pulmonary epithelium has openings of less than 0.6 nm,[19,20] thereby providing an effective barrier to macromolecules, whereas the vascular endothelium has much wider gaps that allow passage of even large proteins.[17,19] Thus liquid in the interstitial space, which in fetal sheep is sampled by collecting lung lymph, has a protein concentration that is about 100 times greater than the protein concentration of liquid obtained from the lung lumen.[22] Despite this large transepithelial protein difference, which presumably inhibits water entry into potential airspaces, active transport of Cl ions across the fetal pulmonary epithelium generates an electrical potential difference that averages about -5 mV, luminal side negative.[21] The osmotic force generated by this process causes liquid to flow from the pulmonary microcirculation through the interstitium into potential airspaces.

During fetal development, the pulmonary epithelium actively transports Cl in the direction of the lung lumen as early as mid-gestation.[23,24] This secretory process can be inhibited by diuretics that block Na-K-2C1 cotransport.[25-27] This observation supports the concept that the driving force for transepithelial movement of Cl in the fetal lung is similar to the mechanism described for Cl transport across other epithelia.[28,29] According to this view, Cl enters the epithelial cell across its basal membrane linked to Na and to K (Na-K-2C1). Na enters the cell down its electrochemical gradient and is subsequently extruded in exchange for K (3 Na ions exchanged

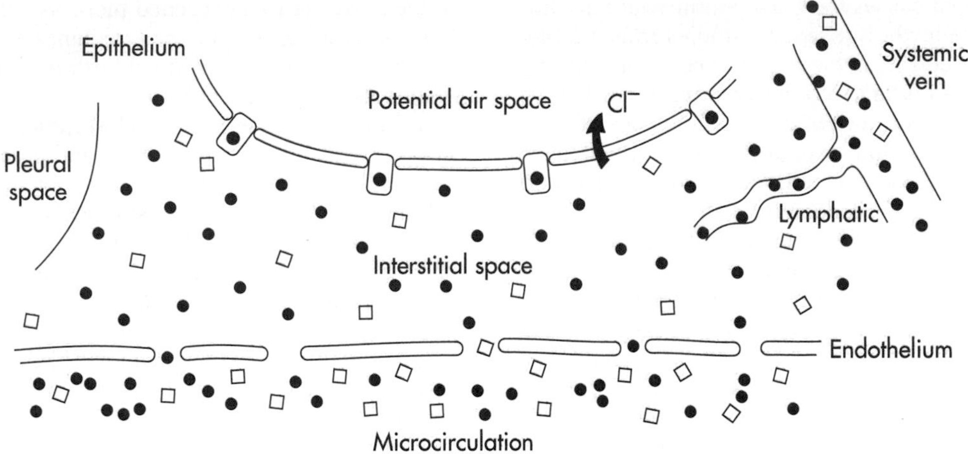

Fig. 57-1. Schematic diagram of the fluid compartments in the fetal lung, showing the tight epithelial barrier to protein and the more permeable vascular endothelium, which restricts passage of globulins *(open squares)* more than it restricts albumin *(solid circles)*. In the fetal mammalian lung, chloride secretion is responsible for luminal liquid production. (From Bland RD: *Adv Pediatr* 34:175-222, 1989.)

for 2 K ions) by the action of Na-K-ATPase located on the basolateral surface of the cell. This energy-dependent process increases the concentration of Cl within the cell so that it exceeds its electrochemical equilibrium. As a result, Cl passively exits the epithelial cell through channels that are located on the apical membrane.[30-33] Although there is strong evidence supporting this mechanism for Cl secretion across the airway epithelium,[29] additional studies are needed to establish whether this sequence of events is responsible for Cl secretion across the distal epithelium of the fetal lung.

The Na concentration of fetal lung liquid is virtually identical to that of plasma.[14,15] The concentration of bicarbonate in the luminal liquid of fetal sheep is less than 3 mEq/L. This observation led to the notion that the pulmonary epithelium of fetal sheep may actively transport bicarbonate out of the lung lumen.[175] The finding that acetazolamide, a carbonic anhydrase inhibitor, slows secretion of lung liquid in fetal sheep supports this view.[34] Both physiologic and immunohistochemical studies have shown that H^+-ATPases are present on the respiratory epithelium of fetal sheep, where they likely provide an important mechanism for acidification of liquid within the lung lumen during development.[34a,34b] In fetal dogs and monkeys, however, the bicarbonate concentration of lung luminal liquid is not significantly different from that of fetal plasma.[35,36] Thus the importance of lung liquid pH and acidification mechanisms during fetal development remains unclear. The concentration of K in luminal liquid exceeds that of plasma and increases further at the end of gestation as lung epithelial cells release surfactant into potential airspaces.[3]

The volume of liquid within the lung lumen of fetal lambs increases from 4 to 6 ml/kg body weight at mid-gestation[23] to more than 20 ml/kg near term.[18-20] The hourly flow rate of tracheal liquid increases from approximately 2 ml/kg body weight at mid-gestation[23] to about 5 ml/kg body weight at term.[2,3,37] This increased production of luminal liquid during development probably reflects an increase in pulmonary microvascular and epithelial surface area, associated with proliferation and growth of lung capillaries and respiratory units.[23,38] The observation that unilateral pulmonary artery occlusion reduces tracheal liquid production in fetal lambs by at least 50%[39] indicates that the pulmonary circulation, rather than the bronchial circulation, is the major source of this liquid. Intravenous infusion of isotonic saline at a rate sufficient to increase lung microvascular pressure and lung lymph flow in fetal lambs has no effect on the flow of liquid across the pulmonary epithelium.[40,41] Thus transepithelial Cl secretion appears to be the major driving force responsible for the production of luminal liquid in the fetal lung. In vitro studies of epithelial ion transport across the fetal trachea indicate that the epithelium of the upper respiratory tract secretes Cl and thereby contributes to liquid production.[35,42-45] Most of the luminal liquid, however, forms in distal portions of the fetal lung, where the total surface area is many times greater than it is in the conducting airways.

Decrease in Lung Liquid Before Birth

Several studies have shown that both the rate of liquid formation and the liquid volume within the lumen of the fetal lung normally decrease before birth.[22,37,46-48] Thus lung water content is about 25% greater after preterm delivery than it is at term, and newborn animals that are delivered by cesarean section without prior labor have significantly more liquid in their lungs than do animals that are delivered vaginally or by cesarean section after the onset of labor.[22,49] In studies performed with fetal lambs, extravascular lung water was 45% less in mature fetuses that were killed during labor than it was in fetuses that had no labor, and there was a further 38% reduction in extravascular lung water measured in lambs that were studied 6 hours after birth.[22] Morphometric analysis of sections of frozen lung obtained from fetal lambs with and without prior labor showed that the reduction in lung water content that occurs before birth is the result of a decrease in the volume of liquid in potential airspaces relative to the volume in the interstitium. These studies showed that diminished secretion, and perhaps absorption, of luminal liquid before birth decreases lung water by approximately 15 ml/kg body weight, leaving a residual volume of about 6 ml/kg,[22] which must be removed from potential airspaces soon after birth to permit effective pulmonary gas exchange.

It is unknown what causes the reduction in fetal lung liquid secretion before birth, but several studies indicate that hormonal changes occurring in the fetus just before and during labor may have an important role in triggering this adaptive process. Several studies have examined the influence of catecholamines on the formation of fetal lung liquid. One such study demonstrated that injection of β-adrenergic agonists into pregnant rabbits reduced the amount of water in the lungs of their pups.[51] Studies performed with fetal lambs late in gestation showed that intravenous infusion of epinephrine or isoproterenol, but not norepinephrine, caused reabsorption of liquid from potential airspaces, an effect that β-adrenergic blockade with propranolol prevented.[52,53] A subsequent report showed that intraluminal administration of amiloride, a Na-transport inhibitor, blocked the effect of epinephrine on fetal lung liquid absorption.[54] This finding suggests that β-adrenergic agonists stimulate Na uptake by the lung epithelium, which in turn drives liquid from the lung lumen into the interstitium, where it can be absorbed into the bloodstream.

Tracheal instillation of dibutyryl cAMP (db-cAMP) also causes absorption of lung liquid in fetal lambs late in gestation.[55] The inhibitory effects of both intrapulmonary db-cAMP and intravenous epinephrine on net production of lung luminal liquid in fetal sheep increase with advancing gestational age, and both responses are attenuated by prior removal of the thyroid gland.[56] Replacement therapy with triiodothyronine after thyroidectomy restored the inhibitory effect of epinephrine on lung liquid formation in fetal sheep.[57] Moreover, treatment of preterm fetal sheep with triiodothyronine and hydrocortisone, given together, may stimulate early maturation of epinephrine-induced absorption of lung liquid.[58] Other studies showed that there is a synergistic effect of terbutaline, a β-adrenergic agonist, and aminophylline, a phosphodiesterase inhibitor, in switching lung liquid secretion to absorption in fetal lambs.[59] In these studies, addition of amiloride to the lung liquid prevented its absorption. These findings support the notion that as birth approaches, conditions that stimulate the release of cAMP in the lung may trigger absorption of luminal liquid through a Na-dependent epithelial transport process.

The decrease in fetal lung liquid production that occurs in sheep before birth might be related in some cases to a rise in plasma epinephrine concentration late in labor.[46] However, lung water content in fetal sheep often decreases before there is any detectable release of catecholamines.[22,47] Several investigators have reported that the concentration of β-adrenergic receptors in lung tissue increases late in gestation,[60-62] which may make the lungs more responsive to the effects of epinephrine during labor.[46]

Other reports have indicated that lung liquid absorption near birth does not depend on epinephrine. Studies performed with fetal rabbits showed that irreversible blockade of adrenergic receptors did not prevent the normal decrease in lung water that occurs during parturition,[63] and studies conducted with fetal lambs late in labor showed that inhibition of β-adrenergic activity with propranolol did not prevent absorption of lung liquid.[47]

A number of other hormones have been shown to inhibit production of fetal lung liquid. Several studies have shown that intravenous infusion of arginine vasopressin reduces lung liquid formation in fetal goats and sheep.[64-69] It is noteworthy, however, that the dose of vasopressin needed to cause lung liquid absorption in these studies produced plasma concentrations of the hormone that exceeded those usually found during labor.[65] Nevertheless, there is evidence that release of both epinephrine and vasopressin at birth may be additive in stimulating lung liquid absorption.[68]

Intravenous infusions of aldosterone,[70] epidermal growth factor,[71] atrial natriuretic factor,[72] and prostaglandin E_2[73] also reduced lung liquid production in fetal lambs late in gestation. Inhibition of prostaglandin synthesis with meclofenamate, however, did not block the decrease in lung liquid secretion observed in sheep during the 2 to 3 days before birth.[74] Thus the importance of epinephrine, prostaglandins, vasopressin, and other hormones in regulating the formation and removal of lung liquid during, before, and after birth remains uncertain.

Recent observations indicate that nitric oxide and surfactant, which are important modulators of lung function during and soon after birth, may inhibit lung liquid production by apparently different mechanisms that are yet to be defined.[75,76] Whereas the Na-transport inhibitor amiloride partially blocks the decrease in lung liquid production that occurs with bovine surfactant administration in immature fetal sheep,[75] amiloride had no such effect on the decrease in lung liquid production associated with nitric oxide administration.[76] It is possible that these and other biologically active substances that are released in the lungs around the time of birth may have important effects on the shift of liquid from the lung lumen into the interstitium during and after birth.

Postnatal Clearance of Fetal Lung Liquid

The process by which liquid in potential airspaces drains from the lungs during and after birth has two components: transepithelial flow into the interstitium, followed by flow of liquid into the bloodstream, either directly into the pulmonary circulation or through lymphatics that empty into the systemic venous system. Development of effective respiratory gas exchange and lung volume soon after birth makes it likely that the shift of liquid from airspaces into the interstitium occurs quickly, after which there is slower uptake into the pulmonary circulation or lung lymphatics.[22,77,78] In sheep, absorption of liquid from the lung lumen often begins during labor and accelerates immediately after birth.[46,47]

Several conditions may contribute to this liquid absorption, including a decrease in net Cl secretion and a corresponding increase in Na uptake by the respiratory tract epithelium around the time of birth. The fact that Na-transport inhibitors reverse lung liquid absorption in fetal sheep during labor[46,47] and slow the rate of lung liquid clearance in newborn guinea pigs[79,80] underscores the importance of this change in epithelial Na uptake in facilitating liquid removal from the lung lumen near birth.

Studies done with fetal lambs at the start of breathing demonstrated a transient postnatal increase in hydraulic conductivity and small solute permeability of the pulmonary epithelium, which may contribute to an increase in bulk flow of liquid from potential airspaces into the interstitium.[81] Air inflation also decreases hydraulic pressure in the pulmonary interstitium, which may help to siphon liquid out of the lung lumen into the tissue.[82,83] Moreover, it is possible that biophysical changes that occur soon after birth, such as somatic nerve stimulation[84] and modest decreases in body temperature,[85] may hasten removal of liquid from the lung lumen. As plasma protein concentration increases during the few days be-

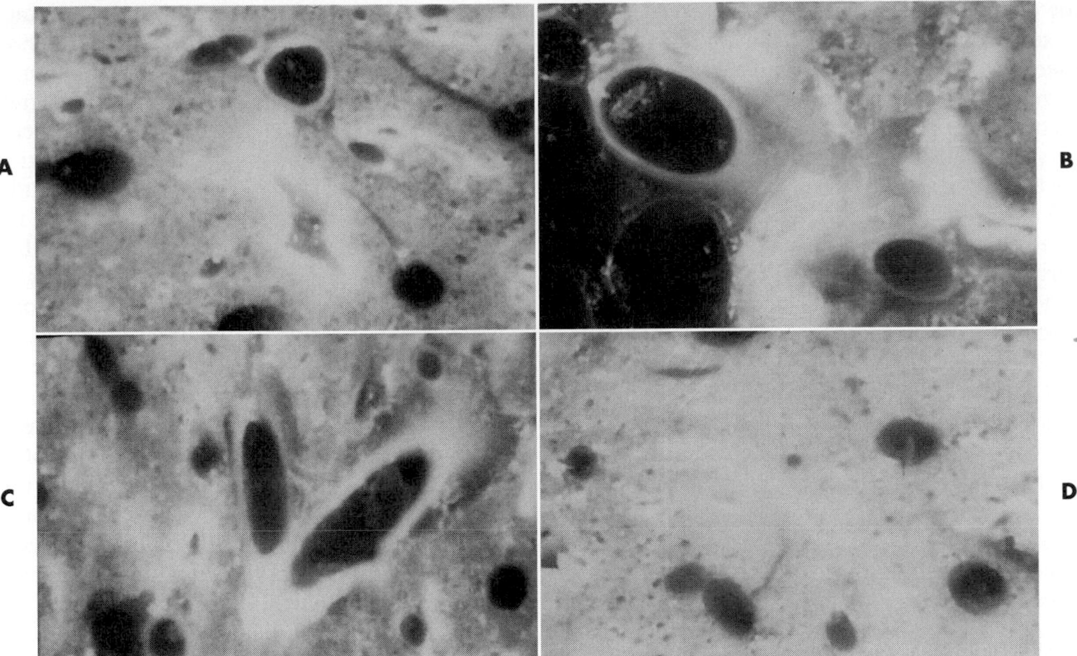

Fig. 57-2. Representative photographs (magnification ×8) of sections of lung taken from vaginally delivered rabbits that were killed before breathing **(A),** 30 minutes after birth **(B),** 1 hour after birth **(C),** and 6 hours after birth **(D).** Before birth, airways are filled with fluid, and there are small cuffs of fluid surrounding pulmonary arteries. By 30 minutes of age, perivascular and peribronchial cuffs are large, and airways appear compressed in the absence of distending pressure. At 60 minutes of age, fluid cuffs are smaller, and several hours later they are virtually absent. (From Bland RD, McMillan DD, Bressack MA, Dong LA: *J Appl Physiol* 49:171-177, 1980.)

fore spontaneous birth,[49,22] the resultant increase in protein osmotic pressure of plasma may help to draw liquid into the pulmonary circulation.

Removal of liquid from the lungs continues for several hours after birth. Studies performed with fetal and newborn rabbits showed that pulmonary blood volume increases with the onset of breathing, whereas lung water content does not begin to decrease postnatally until about 30 to 60 minutes after birth.[86] When breathing begins, air inflation shifts residual liquid from the lumen into distensible perivascular spaces around large pulmonary blood vessels and airways (Fig. 57-2). Accumulation of liquid in these connective tissue spaces, which are distant from sites of respiratory gas exchange, allows time for small blood vessels and lymphatics to remove the displaced liquid, with little or no impairment of lung function. In rabbits delivered at term gestation, perivascular cuffs of liquid are of maximal size 30 minutes after birth, at which time they may store up to 75% of the total amount of extravascular water in the lungs.[86] These fluid cuffs normally disappear by about 6 hours after birth.

The pattern of lung liquid clearance near birth is similar in sheep.[22] As liquid production decreases before birth, lung luminal volume also decreases, with a corresponding reduction in the caliber of potential airspaces. After breathing begins, residual liquid flows into the interstitium and collects around large pulmonary blood vessels and airways. Perivascular fluid cuffs are smaller after premature birth than they are after birth at term gestation.[87] These perivascular cuffs progressively decrease in size as aeration of terminal respiratory units improves postnatally. Thus clearance of fetal lung liquid in lambs is complete by about 6 hours after normal vaginal delivery. The process is slower in preterm lambs,[88,89] as it is in preterm rabbits.[49]

Changes in Lung Epithelial Cell Ion Transport at Birth

The stimulus for lung liquid absorption near birth remains unclear, but studies performed with sheep[54,90,91] and with isolated perfused rat lungs[92-95] indicate that active Na transport across the mature pulmonary epithelium drives liquid from the lung lumen into the interstitium, with subsequent absorption into the vasculature. Thus the lung epithelium switches from a predominantly Cl-secreting membrane before birth to a predominantly Na-absorbing membrane after birth. In support of this concept, at least two reports have demonstrated that intrapulmonary delivery of amiloride, a Na-transport inhibitor, inhibits absorption of lung luminal liquid during labor and after birth.[47,80] Other studies have shown that the characteristic Cl secretion of fetal airway epithelium switches to net Na absorption during the immediate postnatal period.[35]

In vitro studies of ion transport and the bioelectric properties of cultured alveolar epithelial cells harvested from fetal and adult rats have shown that the same cells that secrete surfactant into the airspaces also may pump Na in the opposite direction, thereby generating the driving force for absorption of liquid from the lung lumen.[96-101] These studies have demonstrated that monolayers of cultured distal lung epithelial cells (type II cells), when mounted in an Ussing-type chamber, maintain a transepithelial electrical potential difference (luminal side negative) that increases in response to β-adrenergic stimulation with terbutaline and decreases in response to luminal amiloride or abluminal ouabain. Although type II cells occupy only a small portion of the surface area of terminal airspaces, numerous microvilli on the luminal aspect of these cells greatly increase their absorptive surface area.[102] In addition, morphometric studies indicate that there are almost three times as many type II cells per unit tissue mass lining the interior of the newborn lung as there are lining the interior of the adult lung.[103] Thus it is reasonable to postulate that Na transport by type II cells might be important in liquid clearance during and after birth. It is also possible that Na-pump activity in type I lung epithelial cells might have a role in liquid removal from the airspaces. Electron microscopic studies, however, showed little or no Na-K-ATPase on type I cells of adult rat lungs, whereas it was present on the basolateral surface of type II cells.[104] More definitive assessment of the possible contribution of type I cells to the formation and clearance of fetal lung liquid awaits improved methods to isolate these cells in sufficient purity and number to permit in vitro study of their ion transport properties.

Several studies have shown that Na-K-ATPase of distal lung epithelial cells increases around the time of birth.[105-109] Studies using freshly isolated distal lung epithelial cells from fetal, newborn, and adult rabbits showed that Na-pump turnover number increased fourfold during labor, followed by a threefold increase in Na-pump number between the newborn and adult stages of lung development.[105,106] Turnover number, an index of Na-K-ATPase activity, was not significantly different in newborn and adult cells. Thus Na-pump activity in distal lung epithelium of rabbits increases at birth, whereas the number of Na pumps increases after birth. In related studies, Na-pump activity was similar in cells harvested from fetal rabbits and from newborn pups that had respiratory distress after premature birth.[105] These findings indicate that the stress of premature birth and subsequent respiratory failure do not increase lung epithelial cell cation flux, an observation that may help to explain the lung liquid retention often associated with premature birth.[110]

Other investigators have shown that mRNA abundance for the α_1 and β_1 isoforms of Na-K-ATPase in fetal rat lungs increases just before birth.[108,109] These changes are associated with parallel increases in the expression of epithelial Na and water channels in perinatal rat lung.[111,112] Other studies suggest that glucocorticoids may increase mRNA abundance for the α_1 and β_1 isoforms of Na-K-ATPase in rat lungs during early development,[113] and recently it was shown that glucocorticoids also may help to regulate the expression of Na channels and of aquaporins in the developing rat lung.[114,115] Thus hormones that are released into the circulation around the time of birth may have important effects on lung epithelial ion transport and related removal of liquid from the lungs during and immediately after birth. Recent reports also indicate that the increase in pulmonary oxygen tension that occurs around the time of birth may play an important role in signaling the switch from Cl secretion to Na absorption in the respiratory epithelium near birth.[116,117]

Pathways for Removal of Fetal Lung Liquid

Potential routes for removal of lung luminal liquid at birth include pulmonary lymphatics, the circulation, the pleural space, the mediastinum, and the upper airway. Studies performed with chronically catheterized fetal and newborn lambs demonstrated that the postnatal increase in lung lymph flow is transient and small, accounting for no more than about 15% of the amount of excess liquid that drains from the lungs postnatally.[22,77,78] These studies showed that lymph protein concentration decreases with the start of ventilation, as protein-poor luminal liquid enters the interstitium and decreases the protein concentration of lung lymph. With subsequent uptake of this liquid into the bloodstream, the concentration of protein in lymph returns to its baseline level. These studies showed that lung lymphatics normally drain only a small fraction of liquid in potential airspaces. In preterm lambs with respiratory distress, the postnatal increase in lung lymph flow lasts for several hours and is accompanied by a substantial increase in protein clearance, indicative of abnormal lung vascular protein permeability.[88] Other studies conducted in the same laboratory showed that either elevated left-atrial pressure or a reduction of plasma protein concentration slows the rate at which liquid from potential airspaces leaves the lungs of healthy, mature lambs.[22,77,78] These findings support the view that the pulmonary circulation absorbs at least some, and perhaps most, of the residual liquid present in potential airspaces at birth. It is also possible that some liquid enters the bloodstream through the mediastinum and pleural cavity, although other studies indicate that in normal lambs very little luminal liquid drains by way of the pleural space.

How important is the upper airway as a pathway for liquid drainage from the lung lumen at birth? Karlberg et al[118] measured changes in thoracic pressure and volume in human infants during birth and concluded that chest compression associated with vaginal delivery drives liquid from the lungs into the oropharynx. Other studies, however, indicate that thoracic squeeze during spontaneous birth may have little effect on clearance of fetal lung liquid. As noted above, animals in labor that are delivered by cesarean section after tracheal ligation have no more water in their lungs than do animals that are born vaginally.[22,50] Moreover, studies of lung liquid dynamics in near-term fetal lambs have shown that late in labor, as luminal liquid is absorbed across the epithelium, the upper airway functions as a one-way valve, inhibiting entry of amniotic liquid into the lung lumen, but allowing outward flow of pulmonary liquid into the oropharynx.[46] Thus, although the conducting airways may serve as an escape route for lung liquid during delivery without prior labor, they probably play a minor role in liquid clearance during the normal birth process.

Summary

Fig. 57-3 is a schematic diagram of the liquid compartments of the fetal lung and the forces that contribute to liquid clearance. As noted previously, luminal liquid in the fetal lung contains less than 0.3 mg of protein/ml, whereas pulmonary interstitial liquid has a protein concentration of approximately 30 mg/ml.[15,22,119] This transepithelial difference in protein concentration generates an osmotic pressure difference of greater than 10 cm H_2O, which draws liquid from the lumen into the interstitium, as Cl secretion decreases.[120] Epithelial Na pumps and transpulmonary pressure associated with lung inflation also drive liquid from potential airspaces into the interstitium, thereby increasing the protein osmotic pressure difference between plasma and interstitial fluid. Air entry into the lungs not only displaces liquid, but also decreases hydraulic pressure in the pulmonary circulation and increases pulmonary blood flow,[121] which in turn increases lung blood volume and effective vascular surface area for fluid uptake.[122] These circulatory changes facilitate absorption of liquid into the pulmonary vascular bed. About 10% of the luminal liquid leaves the lungs

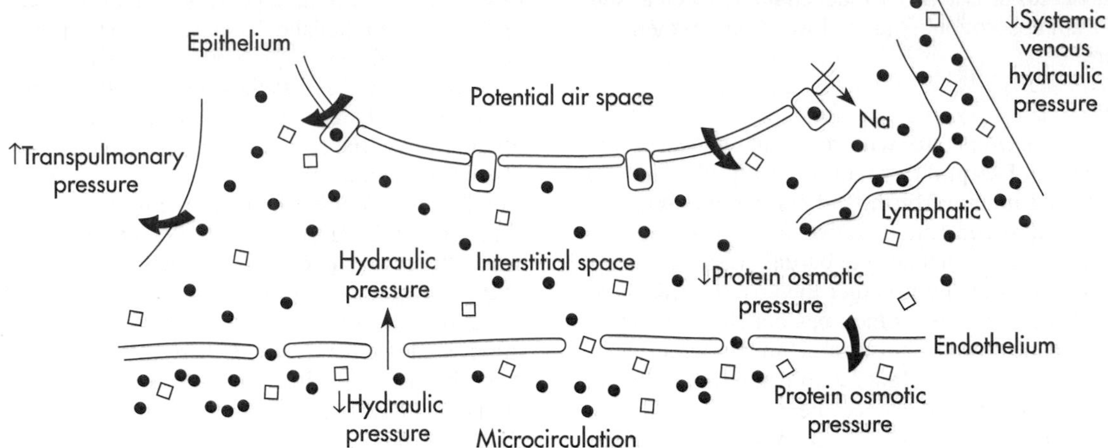

Fig. 57-3. Schematic diagram of the fluid compartments in the fetal lung illustrating the forces that influence removal of liquid near birth. *Solid circles* represent albumin molecules; *squares* represent globulins. (From Bland RD: *Adv Pediatr* 34:175-222, 1987.)

through lymphatics, which drain via the thoracic duct into the superior vena cava. With spontaneous breathing, the postnatal reduction of intrathoracic pressure decreases systemic venous pressure, which may hasten lymphatic drainage, but most of the displaced luminal liquid enters the pulmonary microcirculation or seeps into the mediastinum, with subsequent absorption into the bloodstream.

Persistent Postnatal Pulmonary Edema

Liquid contained within the lung lumen during normal fetal development must be displaced from potential airspaces and absorbed into the bloodstream soon after birth to permit successful pulmonary gas exchange. This essential adaptive process occurs rapidly in most infants, but sometimes the process is delayed, yielding the clinical and radiographic features of a condition that has been called transient tachypnea of the newborn, or the syndrome of retained fetal lung liquid. Because tachypnea is not a consistent finding in this condition, and because some of the liquid may enter the lungs postnatally from the pulmonary circulation, a more appropriate term for this mild form of respiratory dysfunction is *persistent postnatal pulmonary edema.*

Clinical Features

Three decades have passed since the initial description of the clinical and radiographic features of transient neonatal tachypnea were first described.[123] The condition was attributed to delayed absorption of fetal lung liquid. The report described eight infants, all of whom were born at term gestation, and only one of whom was delivered by cesarean section. Subsequent reports have noted an association with premature birth, operative delivery, and excessive intravenous fluids administered to the mother during labor. Persistent postnatal pulmonary edema is more common in males than it is in females. The disorder typically begins soon after birth with a rapid respiratory rate, ranging from 60 to 160 breaths/minute, sometimes with sternal and subcostal retractions of the chest wall, grunting during expiration, and occasionally mild cyanosis that disappears with delivery of supplemental oxygen. In some cases, postnatal depression from birth asphyxia or from drugs administered to the mother during labor may obscure the underlying pathologic condition, causing hypoventilation and even apnea, rather than rapid breathing.

On physical examination, breath sounds are usually clear, without rales or rhonchi, except during the first hour after birth, when residual liquid is often present within the airspaces. Signs and symptoms usually resolve within 3 to 4 days after birth. Many infants with this condition have generalized edema and hypoproteinemia, supporting the notion that low intravascular protein osmotic pressure may contribute to the delay in absorption of lung liquid after birth.

Studies of pulmonary function in babies with this type of mild respiratory distress have shown increased total ventilation, low tidal volumes, normal or increased functional residual capacity, reduced dynamic compliance, and relatively uniform gas distribution in the lungs. Echocardiographic assessment sometimes shows evidence of mild left-ventricular dysfunction in babies who are presumed to have persistent postnatal pulmonary edema.

The differential diagnosis includes respiratory distress from surfactant deficiency, extrapulmonary air leaks (pneumomediastinum and pneumothorax), congestive heart failure, meconium aspiration, bacterial or viral pneumonia, airway obstruction, and diaphragmatic hernia with associated pulmonary hypoplasia. The radiographic features and greater severity of respiratory distress usually distinguish these conditions from persistent postnatal pulmonary edema.

Radiographic findings include prominent pulmonary vascular markings, particularly in the perihilar region, hyperaeration, flattening and depression of the diaphragm, widening of the interlobar fissures, and a cardiac silhouette slightly greater than normal. In addition, there may be fluid within the pleural space. Rapid clinical improvement usually parallels resolution of these radiographic abnormalities.

Transient tachypnea from persistent postnatal pulmonary edema often occurs in infants who are delivered prematurely, especially in the absence of prior labor.[124,125] Premature birth is associated with several conditions that may contribute to delayed removal of fetal lung liquid, including impaired Na-pump activity in lung epithelial cells,[106] high filtration pressure in the pulmonary circulation,[88] often with persistent patency of the ductus arteriosus,[126] reduced microvascular surface area for fluid absorption,[127] and a low plasma protein osmotic pressure.[128]

Management

Unless the lungs are immature, with resultant atelectasis and respiratory failure, absorption of fetal lung liquid is usually complete within 24 hours of birth, and symptoms disappear accordingly. An increased concentration of inspired oxygen may be required to maintain a normal partial pressure of oxygen in arterial blood. Usually no other therapy is needed. Infants with respiratory distress sometimes benefit from being managed in the prone, head-up position. Until symptoms subside, fluid and salt intake of infants with persistent postnatal pulmonary edema should not exceed their insensible losses. Diuretics offer little or no benefit and may produce complicating abnormalities of serum electrolytes.

FLUID BALANCE IN THE NEWBORN LUNG

Fig. 57-4 shows the fluid compartments of the normal newborn lung and the major forces that regulate filtration in the pulmonary microcirculation. The epithelium, consisting of surfactant producing columnar, type II cells and flattened type I cells bound together by tight junctions, separates airspaces from interstitium and is virtually impermeable to protein.[19,20] Epithelial protein leaks may occur when transpulmonary pressure exceeds 35 to 40 cm H_2O,[81] as it often does after premature birth, when surface tension at the air-liquid interface renders the lungs stiff and vulnerable to injury. The endothelium, which divides the microcirculation from the interstitium, allows macromolecules to pass through it, but it restricts passage of large molecules more than it restricts small ones.[17] Thus the concentration of albumin in the interstitium of the newborn lung averages 75% to 80% of the concentration of albumin in plasma, whereas the concentration of globulins in interstitial fluid averages 50% to 55% of the concentration of globulins in plasma.[129] These tissue proteins generate an osmotic pressure of greater than 10 cm H_2O which inhibits the flow of water into the airspaces. In addition, active Na transport by lung epithelial cells may help to keep the airspaces free of excess fluid.[47,79,80,105,106,108,111]

Flow of liquid across the microvascular membrane depends largely on the balance between differences in (1) intravascular and extravascular hydraulic pressures, and (2) intravascular and extravascular protein osmotic pressures (see Fig. 57-4). Conditions that either increase the transmural hydraulic pressure difference, or decrease the transmural difference in protein osmotic pressure tend to hasten liquid flow into the interstitium, whereas conditions that decrease the sum of these filtration forces tend to reduce fluid movement, thereby inhibiting edema formation. Other variables that influence lung water balance are microvascular surface area, endothelial and epithelial permeability to protein, and the capacity of the pulmonary lymphatics to pump fluid out of the lungs into the bloodstream.

Assessment of Lung Fluid Balance

Measurement of pulmonary lymph flow under steady-state conditions is a useful means of assessing lung fluid balance over time in living animals.[17-20,131] Staub et al[132,133] demonstrated the feasibility of measuring lymph flow as an index of lung fluid filtration in awake sheep. This experimental approach provides a sensitive and reproducible way of detecting lung endothelial injury early, even in the absence of fluid accumulation.[134] Some investigators suggested that contamination by systemic lymph might be a problem with this experimental technique,[135] but subsequent studies showed that such contamination is not a major issue if appropriate preventive measures are taken.[136-138] Thus the chronic lymph fistula preparation has been used to examine the relationship between normal lung development and lung fluid balance in lambs and to study the variables that influence edema formation in the newborn lung.[22,40,88,129,139-142] Lung histology and measurement of extravascular lung water have helped to define the degree of fluid accumulation under the various experimental conditions. These studies have furnished the basis for our current under-

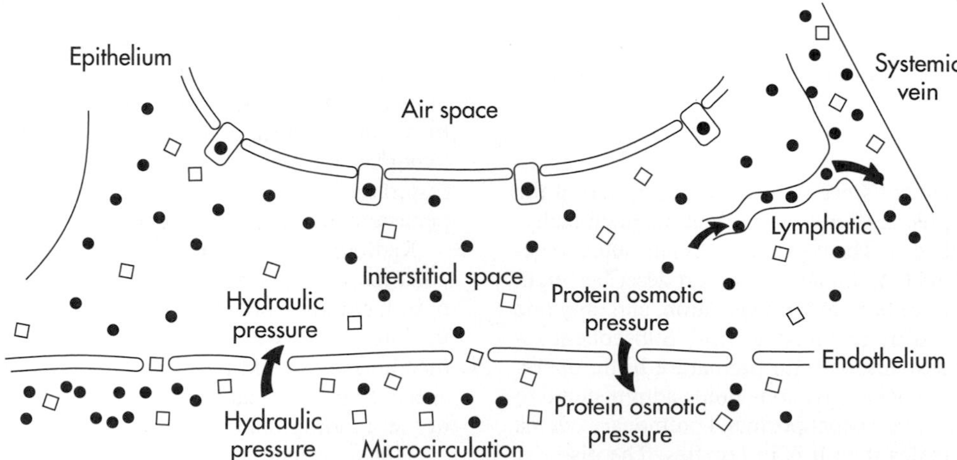

Fig. 57-4. Schematic drawing of the fluid compartments in the newborn lung and the variables that affect filtration in the pulmonary microcirculation. *Dots* represent albumin molecules, *open squares* indicate globulin molecules. (From Bland RD: *Clin Perinatol* 19:593-611, 1982.)

standing of normal and abnormal fluid balance in the newborn lung, and they also have provided some insight regarding the vulnerability to pulmonary edema and associated respiratory distress after premature birth.

FACTORS AFFECTING LUNG FLUID FILTRATION IN NEWBORN LAMBS

Hemodynamic Influences

Fluid filtration pressure and microvascular surface area per unit lung mass are greater in the newborn lung than in the adult lung.[129,139,143] These developmental differences in the pulmonary circulation may reflect the fact that blood flow per unit lung mass is considerably greater in newborn lungs than it is in adult lungs.[144] Moreover, because the neonatal lung is about one-quarter the size of the mature lung,[129] it is likely that left-atrial pressure exceeds alveolar pressure (West zone III[145]) throughout a greater fraction of the pulmonary circulation in the newborn lung. Measurements of alveolar liquid pressure in excised lungs of newborn and adult animals have provided evidence that hydraulic pressure in the pulmonary interstitium may be less soon after birth than it is later in life.[82,83] In addition, plasma protein concentration of newborn animals is significantly less than it is in adult animals, so that the difference in protein osmotic pressure between plasma and lung interstitial fluid is less in the younger animals.[141] It is not surprising, therefore, that net lung fluid filtration is greater per unit lung mass in newborn lambs than it is in mature sheep.[129,139]

To see whether protein permeability of the pulmonary microcirculation might change during normal postnatal lung development, our group measured pulmonary vascular pressures and lung lymph flow in newborn and adult sheep with increased pulmonary microvascular pressure produced by saline filling a balloon catheter in the left atrium.[139] This maneuver establishes patency of most, if not all, of the vessels in the pulmonary microcirculation, and it should accentuate differences in lymph flow that occur as a result of increased protein permeability.[146] Results of studies performed with eight unanesthetized lambs that were 2 to 3 weeks old were compared with results of similar studies done with adult sheep. In all cases, increased pulmonary microvascular pressure caused a persistent increase in lung lymph flow and a corresponding reduction in lymph protein concentration. When lymph flow increases in response to increased vascular filtration pressure, the concentration of protein in lymph decreases as a result of macromolecular sieving across the microvascular membrane.[141,147] Fig. 57-5 shows the relationship between lymph/plasma protein concentration ratio and lung lymph flow before and during persistent left-atrial hypertension in newborn and adult sheep. Left-atrial pressure increased by an average of 12 mm Hg in both groups of animals. The lymph/plasma protein concentration ratio is less in lambs than it is sheep because net filtration pressure is greater in the younger animals, but there is no significant difference in the slopes of the two lines. These data provide strong evidence that permeability to plasma proteins in the pulmonary microcirculation is not appreciably different in newborn and adult sheep.

Elevation of lung microvascular pressure, as described previously, reduces cardiac output because the saline-filled balloon in the left atrium partially occludes the mitral valve. In contrast, blood flow to the lungs often increases in clinical conditions associated with pulmonary edema, such as acute in-

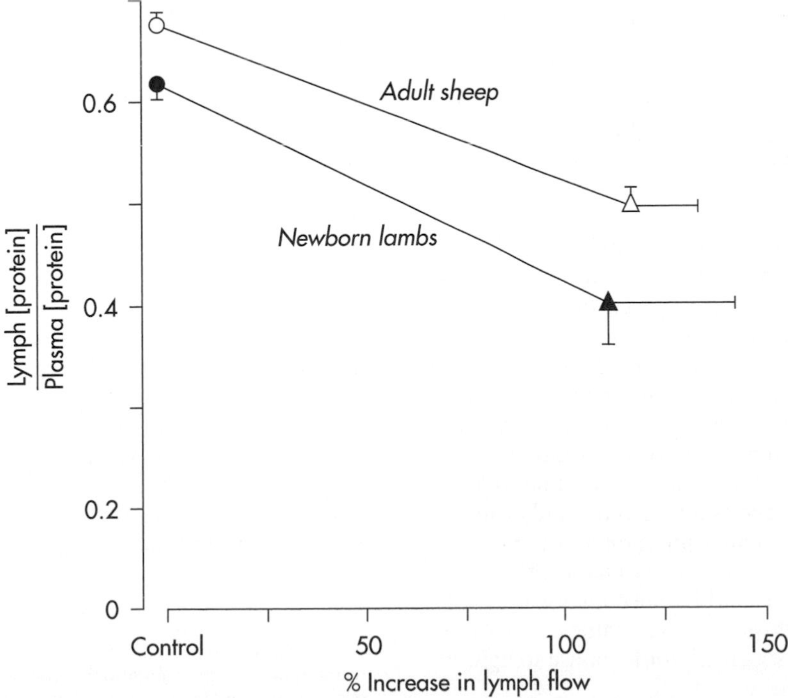

Fig. 57-5. Effect of left-atrial pressure elevation on lung lymph flow and the ratio of lymph total protein concentration/plasma total protein concentration (mean ± SD) in 8 newborn lambs and 25 adult sheep studied before *(circles)* and after *(triangles)* distention of a balloon in the left atrium. Increase in lymph flow after pressure elevation is expressed as percent change relative to lymph flow measured during the control period when left-atrial pressure was normal. (From Hazinski TA, Bland RD, Hansen TN, Sedin EG, Goldberg RB: *J Appl Physiol* 61:1139-1148, 1986.)

travascular volume overload or shunting of blood from the aorta into the pulmonary artery through a patent ductus arteriosus. To study the effects of increased pulmonary perfusion on fluid balance in the newborn lung, lambs were chronically catheterized for measurement of pulmonary arterial and left-atrial pressures, cardiac output, lung lymph flow, and concentrations of protein in lymph and plasma during a 2-hour control period, followed by 3 to 4 hours of increased cardiac output produced by an external shunt between the carotid artery and jugular vein.[142] Cardiac output increased by 21%, and pulmonary arterial pressure increased by 2 mm Hg during the period in which the shunt was open. These changes were associated with a 46% increase in lung lymph flow without a significant change in the lymph/plasma protein concentration ratio. These findings indicate that in normal lambs increased pulmonary blood flow also increases lung fluid filtration, probably by expanding the perfused surface area of the pulmonary microcirculation. In related experiments performed with lambs during left-atrial hypertension, increasing pulmonary perfusion did not change lung lymph flow or lymph protein concentration. These results suggest that when the entire lung microvascular bed is patent, as it is during left-atrial hypertension, superimposed increases in lung blood flow do not affect filtration of fluid from the pulmonary microcirculation into the interstitium, provided vascular pressures do not increase. In a related study, lung lymph flow almost doubled and lymph protein concentration decreased significantly in newborn lambs subjected to a 35% aortopulmonary shunt, which produced a 2 to 4 mm Hg increase in lung microvascular pressure.[148]

In studies designed to examine the effect of a patent ductus arteriosus on pulmonary hemodynamics and lung lymph flow in preterm lambs that were mechanically ventilated for several hours after birth, ductal patency doubled pulmonary blood flow and increased lung vascular pressures. As a result of these hemodynamic changes, lung lymph flow was about 70% greater and the lymph/plasma protein concentration ratio was significantly less when the ductus arteriosus was open.[126] These findings may help to explain why some infants who are born prematurely experience respiratory failure in the presence of a large left-to-right shunt through a patent ductus arteriosus.

Other conditions that increase filtration pressure in the pulmonary circulation may contribute to edema formation in the newborn lung. When the lung vascular bed fails to develop normally before birth, as in cases of pulmonary hypoplasia, or when the lung's circulation is reduced in size because of fibrosis or partial lung resection, an increase in pulmonary perfusion is likely to elevate microvascular pressure and cause edema. Excessive intravascular infusions of fluid also may overload the pulmonary circulation and cause fluid to accumulate in the lungs.[130] Intravenous infusion of lipid emulsion increases pulmonary microvascular pressure and transvascular filtration of fluid in the lungs of newborn lambs.[149] This effect most likely is the result of lipid-induced release of arachidonic acid metabolites, as thromboxane synthesis inhibitors prevented the pulmonary vasoconstrictor response to lipid infusion in the lambs.

When pulmonary microvascular pressure increases, net filtration of fluid into the lungs increases, and the concentration of protein in interstitial fluid decreases (see Fig. 57-5). Resultant increases in lymph flow and in the protein osmotic pressure difference between plasma and tissue fluid (lymph) protect the lungs from edema until the drainage capacity of lymphatics is overwhelmed by the increased rate of fluid filtration.

Hypoproteinemia

Several studies have demonstrated that a reduction in plasma protein osmotic pressure may have a substantial effect on fluid filtration in the pulmonary circulation of adult animals of several species.[150-153] Newborn animals have lower concentrations of protein in their plasma than mature animals do. Studies of plasma protein reduction in chronically catheterized, awake lambs showed that a 50% reduction in intravascular protein osmotic pressure led to an increase in lung lymph flow that averaged 53%.[141] With development of hypoproteinemia, the average difference in plasma protein osmotic pressure between plasma and lymph decreased by about 2 mm Hg at normal left-atrial pressure and by approximately 5 mm Hg in the presence of left-atrial hypertension.

When applied to the Starling equation governing microvascular fluid filtration,* these changes in liquid driving pressure were sufficient to account for the observed increases in lung fluid filtration. Thus small changes in transvascular protein osmotic pressure have a substantial effect on the flow of fluid from the microcirculation into the interstitium of the lungs. Reduction of plasma protein concentration caused no significant change in calculated filtration coefficient. Protein loss did not affect net protein clearance from the lungs, nor did it accentuate the increase in lymph flow associated with left-atrial pressure elevation. Tracer studies performed with radiolabeled albumin injected intravenously before and after protein drainage confirmed the absence of a change in lung vascular protein permeability. Pulmonary edema did not develop in hypoproteinemic lambs, even when their left-atrial pressure was increased to 16 $\pm$ 1 mm Hg for 4 hours, demonstrating the capacity of lymphatics to keep pace with transvascular fluid filtration and thereby inhibit edema formation.

In another series of experiments, pulmonary edema did develop in newborn lambs that received rapid intravenous infusion of isotonic saline. In addition to increasing lung microvascular pressure and decreasing plasma protein osmotic pressure, acute fluid overload also enhances pulmonary blood flow and elevates systemic venous pressure, which may impair lymphatic drainage from the lungs.[154,155] This may help to explain why pulmonary edema occurred in lambs that received excessive intravascular fluid, whereas it did not occur in hypoproteinemic lambs with mechanically induced left-atrial hypertension. Impaired lymphatic drainage may contribute to lung edema in some cases of right-sided heart failure, or when there is blockage of the superior vena cava, such that lung lymphatics must pump against an exceedingly high central venous pressure. Following lymphatic obstruction, edema persists until new channels form or until the damaged lymphatics heal.[156]

---

*$\dot{Q}f = K_f[(Pmv\text{-}Ppmv) - \sigma(\pi mv - \pi pmv)]$, where $\dot{Q}f$ equals total lung lymph flow; K_f is the fluid filtration coefficient, which varies as a function of microvascular surface area and hydraulic conductance between fluid exchange vessels and lung lymphatics; *Pmv* and *Ppmv* are microvascular and perimicrovascular hydraulic pressures; πmv and πpmv are microvascular and perimicrovascular protein osmotic pressures; and σ is the average osmotic reflection coefficient for plasma proteins, a term that indicates the effectiveness of the microvascular membrane as a barrier to protein flow relative to water flow (σ of 1 represents total impermeability to protein, σ of 0 indicates free flow of protein through the membrane).

Hypoxia

In adult sheep, hypoxia causes pulmonary hypertension without affecting lung lymph flow or lymph protein concentration, indicating that hypoxia has no significant effect on net fluid filtration in the adult lung.[159] In lambs, however, pulmonary vasoconstriction from hypoxia increases lung lymph flow, with an associated reduction in lymph protein concentration.[139,144,158] These changes in lymph flow and lymph protein concentration are similar to those that occur when a balloon catheter in the left atrium is filled with saline to raise lung microvascular pressure in lambs (see Fig. 57-5). Thus hypoxia in newborn sheep appears to constrict lung vessels distal to sites of fluid exchange. Alternatively, neonatal hypoxia may cause intense pulmonary vasoconstriction, redirecting the increased blood flow that occurs during hypoxia to fewer lung vessels and thereby transmitting to fluid exchange sites a greater fraction of the pressure in the pulmonary artery.

Different studies have provided evidence supporting both of these explanations. Direct micropuncture measurement of microvascular pressures in isolated, perfused lungs of newborn lambs showed an increase in pulmonary venular as well as arterial pressure during hypoxia.[159] Other studies performed with newborn lambs before and during hypoxia showed that hypoxia shifts blood flow from the lower to the upper portions of the newborn lung.[160] This observation supports the hypothesis that redistribution of perfusion in young animals with high pulmonary blood flow may account for the increase in lung fluid filtration that occurs in hypoxic lambs. Other investigators found a significant increase in lung lymph flow and a decrease in lymph protein concentration in adult sheep after extensive lung resection, also suggesting a threshold of pulmonary blood flow per unit lung mass above which lung fluid filtration increases even in the mature lung.[161] There is no evidence that hypoxia alters lung microvascular protein permeability in either newborn or adult sheep.[139,157,158,162-164]

Hyperoxia

Lung edema sometimes occurs as a result of pulmonary microvascular injury, in which damage of the endothelial membrane allows protein-rich liquid to leak at an increased rate from the microcirculation into the interstitium of the lungs. If there is coexisting epithelial injury, proteinaceous liquid enters air spaces and interferes with respiratory gas exchange. One source of neonatal lung microvascular injury is prolonged oxygen breathing. Studies of lung fluid balance in unanesthetized lambs showed increased pulmonary microvascular protein permeability within 3 to 4 days of sustained hyperoxia.[165] In these studies, lung lymph flow began to increase on the third day of hyperoxia, and the concentration of protein in lymph increased progressively from the third to the fifth day of oxygen breathing, with no appreciable change in lung vascular pressures. These changes in pulmonary lymph flow and lymph protein concentration are indicative of abnormal lung vascular protein permeability. Radioactive protein tracer studies in these animals also demonstrated an increase in permeability within 5 days, when all of the lambs were suffering respiratory failure from oxygen toxicity. Extravascular lung water content and histology confirmed the presence of severe pulmonary edema (Fig. 57-6). In a subsequent study, lambs pretreated with large doses of vitamin E, an antioxidant, acquired the same degree of oxygen-induced lung endothelial injury as did lambs that did not receive vitamin E.[166]

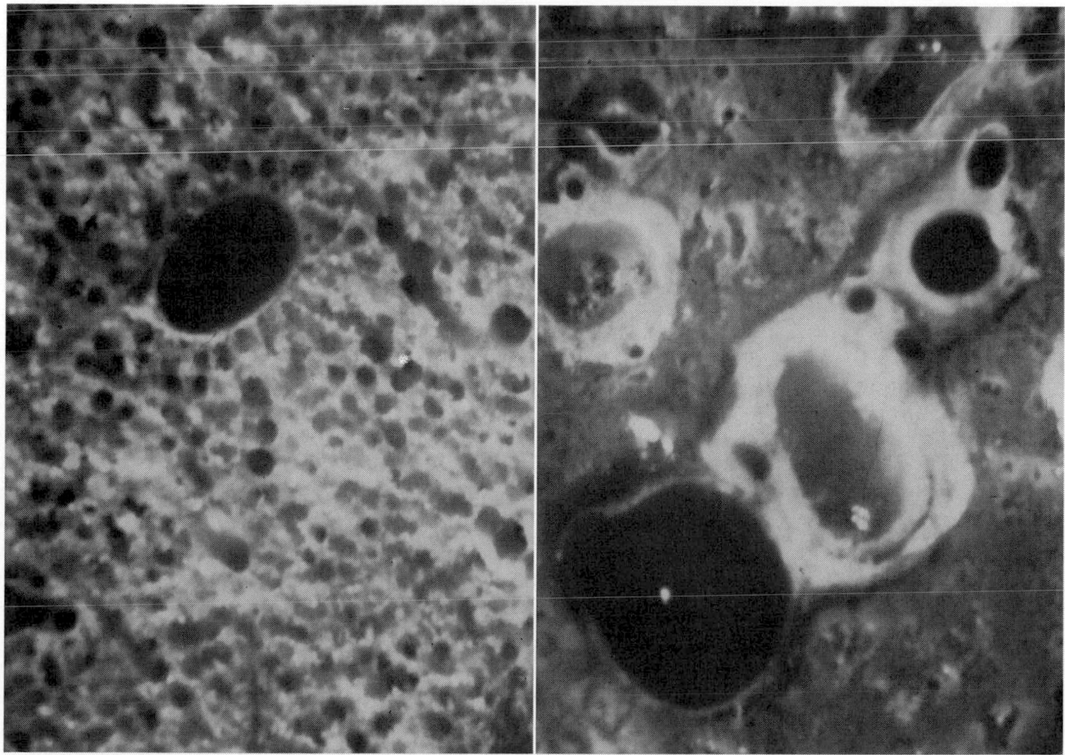

Fig. 57-6. Sections of lung, frozen in liquid nitrogen at an inflation pressure of 25 cm H_2O. Normal lamb *(left)* and lamb killed after 5 days in 100% oxygen *(right)*. The injured lung contains fluid in air spaces, as well as the perivascular tissue spaces around large blood vessels and airways. Original magnification, ×8.5. (From Bland RD: *Clin Perinatol* 9:593-611, 1982.)

Several reports have shown that granulocytes may contribute to the development of various types of lung microvascular injury,[167-170] including endothelial damage and edema from prolonged oxygen breathing.[171,172] In studies designed to assess the importance of neutrophils as possible mediators of pulmonary oxygen toxicity, rabbits and lambs were rendered neutropenic by treatment with nitrogen mustard or hydroxyurea before they were placed in 100% oxygen for several days.[173] Neutrophil depletion had no effect on survival time or on lung water content of either adult rabbits or newborn lambs that continuously breathed pure oxygen at one atmosphere of pressure. Neutropenia also had no influence on lung lymph protein clearance in lambs with sustained hyperoxia. Thus polymorphonuclear leukocytes are not essential for the development of oxygen-induced lung microvascular injury. Other cells within the lung, including alveolar macrophages[174,175] and other pulmonary parenchymal cells,[176] are capable of generating toxic oxygen metabolites which may contribute to the development of lung injury, particularly if endogenous antioxidant enzymes are lacking, as they may be following premature birth.[177]

A number of experimental approaches have been used to try to prevent or lessen the severity of oxygen-induced lung vascular injury in newborn animals. One study showed that intraperitoneal injection of liposomes containing superoxide dismutase and catalase decreased mortality among neonatal rats that were placed in 100% oxygen.[178] Although the rate of survival was greater among rats that received antioxidant enzymes, there was no indication that this treatment reduced the severity of lung injury. Other investigators have shown that a single dose of bacterial endotoxin prolongs survival and reduces lung injury in hyperoxic adult rats, a response that seems to be related to increased pulmonary antioxidant enzyme activity following injection of endotoxin.[179] Low doses of endotoxin have been shown to partially protect newborn sheep from the toxic pulmonary effects of prolonged hyperoxia.[180] Lambs that received endotoxin before oxygen exposure had delayed onset of lung vascular protein leakage and pulmonary edema, and these lambs survived longer in oxygen than did lambs that received no endotoxin. Unlike the studies with adult rats, however, treatment of lambs with endotoxin did not increase lung antioxidant enzyme activity. These findings, coupled with a higher ratio of reduced/oxidized glutathione in the lungs of endotoxin-treated lambs, led the authors to speculate that endotoxin pretreatment may reduce the oxidant stress of prolonged hyperoxia by inhibiting production of toxic oxygen metabolites within the lung, possibly by blocking the activity of cytochrome P-450.[180] In a subsequent report, the same group of investigators[181] showed that treatment of newborn lambs with cimetidine, a noncompetitive inhibitor of cytochrome P-450 activity, slowed the progression of oxygen-induced lung microvascular injury and increased the ratio of reduced/oxidized glutathione in the lung. Cimetidine also inhibited the increase in pulmonary microsomal P-450 activity that was associated with prolonged oxygen breathing. These observations indicate that improved understanding of the mechanisms responsible for oxygen-induced lung injury may provide the basis for effective treatment, or possibly prevention, of this and other conditions that cause neonatal respiratory failure.

At least two groups of investigators have examined the influence of dietary fat on oxygen-induced lung injury in newborn animals. In one study, there was less lung vascular protein leak and longer survival in hyperoxic lambs whose milk feedings were supplemented with sunflower oil (rich in polyunsaturated fatty acids) compared with lambs that received milk alone.[182] Other investigators reported a protective effect of unsaturated fatty acids in the diet of newborn rats exposed continuously to pure oxygen.[183] The specific mechanism by which these dietary modifications alter susceptibility to pulmonary oxygen toxicity remains to be determined.

Group B Streptococcal Sepsis

Neonatal infection with group B, β-hemolytic Streptococcus often leads to respiratory failure from pulmonary edema associated with lung microvascular injury. An elegant series of studies conducted with newborn sheep demonstrated the pathophysiology of this condition.[184-187] Intravenous infusion of live bacteria (group B, β-hemolytic streptococci, type III) or their polysaccharide toxin caused a biphasic reaction, with an initial period of fever, shaking, and tachypnea, accompanied by pulmonary hypertension, granulocytopenia, and increased flow of protein-poor lymph, followed by a period of increased lymph protein clearance, indicative of lung endothelial injury.[184] Pretreatment with indomethacin prevented the initial phase of pulmonary hypertension and fever, but it did not modify the granulocytopenia or the apparent increase in lung vascular protein permeability that occurred between 2 and 6 hours after the infusion of bacteria or toxin.[186] Lung morphology showed dilated capillaries with disrupted and fragmented basement membranes, numerous granulocytes both within and around the pulmonary microcirculation, and extensive interstitial edema.[185] Treatment with large doses of methylprednisolone before and after injection of the bacterial toxin did not prevent the early febrile response or pulmonary hypertension, but it completely blocked the granulocytopenia and the increase in lung vascular permeability to protein. A subsequent study by the same group showed that the pulmonary vascular response to group B Streptococcus toxin was virtually the same in young lambs as it was in older sheep.[188] Increased total lung resistance and decreased lung compliance during the early phase of toxemia coincided with increased concentrations of thromboxane B_2 measured in lung lymph. These observations support the notion that both lipid mediators and granulocyte products probably contribute to the lung vascular response and injury that often develop in infants with systemic bacterial infection. Similar observations of pulmonary hypertension and protein-rich pulmonary edema have been reported in adult sheep infected with *Pseudomonas aeruginosa*[134] or with *E. coli* endotoxin.[169]

Pulmonary Microembolism

Pulmonary microembolism, a common cause of respiratory failure and lung edema in adults, is considered a rare event in infants and children. In the presence of deep vein thrombosis, notably after trauma or major surgery, embolization may lead to acute pulmonary hypertension and rapid accumulation of protein-rich fluid in the lungs. These life-threatening complications can also occur as a result of air microembolism associated with open-heart surgery or with inadvertent delivery of air through intravenous infusion of fluid. The frequency with which these mishaps occur is unknown, but they may be more common than appreciated in infants and children who are managed in intensive care units.

Continuous intravenous infusion of air in adult sheep causes reproducible and reversible injury of the pulmonary microcirculation, leading to increased flow of protein-rich lung lymph, sometimes progressing to interstitial pulmonary edema.[189] Air microemboli lodge in small pulmonary arteries, with accumulation of neutrophils at the air-liquid interface. When neutrophils are activated, as they may be in the presence of circulating complement or when exposed to platelet-activating factor, they may produce acute endothelial injury, either by secretion of proteolytic enzymes or by production of toxic oxygen metabolites, or both.[167,190] Electron microscopy shows gaps between endothelial cells, through which neutrophils migrate into the interstitium, with disruption of the basal lamina.[191] Granulocyte depletion attenuates this injury,[168] implying that inflammatory cells have an important role in the development of the increased lung vascular protein permeability that occurs during air microembolism.

In studies performed with mature newborn lambs, continuous intravenous infusion of tiny air bubbles for 8 hours led to a sustained increase in pulmonary arterial pressure, as left-atrial pressure and lung blood flow did not change significantly.[192] Lung lymph flow and lymph protein clearance nearly tripled during these studies, despite the fact that surface area for liquid filtration probably decreased because of mechanical obstruction of the vascular bed by the air bubbles. These findings are consistent with a change in pulmonary microvascular permeability to protein, during which there was a significant reduction in arterial oxygenation that probably resulted from a mismatch of ventilation and perfusion, perhaps from bronchoconstriction and nonuniform distribution of blood flow within the lungs, which typically occur in pulmonary microembolism.[193,194] These experimental observations may provide an explanation for the respiratory deterioration that sometimes accompanies inadvertent injection of air in infants receiving intravenous fluids, and the apparent benefit of diuretics in reducing lung dysfunction associated with abnormal lung vascular protein leaks.

Furosemide

Diuretics are the mainstay in the management of infants and children with pulmonary edema. Effective diuresis decreases pulmonary microvascular pressure and increases protein osmotic pressure in plasma. These two changes inhibit fluid filtration into the lungs and hasten the entry of water into the pulmonary microcirculation from the interstitium.

In studies carried out with newborn lambs, intravenous furosemide caused an increase in plasma protein concentration and a decrease in pulmonary vascular pressures, with resultant reduction in lung fluid filtration, indicated by a decrease in lung lymph flow.[195] These changes occurred both in the presence and absence of lung microvascular injury.[192,195] Furosemide also has an effect on lung fluid balance that is independent of the drug's diuretic action: in lambs without kidneys, intravenous infusion of furosemide consistently led to a small decrease in lymph flow without any change in pulmonary vascular pressure or plasma protein concentration. This nondiuretic influence of furosemide may derive from increased apacitance of peripheral systemic veins,[196] with diminished pulmonary blood flow and resultant reduction in lung microvascular surface area for fluid exchange.[189] The depressant effect of furosemide on cardiac output probably limits its usefulness in the early postnatal management of respiratory distress in preterm infants.[197-200]

Lung Overinflation

The lung epithelium normally forms a tight barrier against protein movement between the interstitium and air spaces, but epithelial leaks and alveolar edema may occur when excessive transpulmonary pressure overinflates the lungs.[81] In studies performed with mechanically ventilated lambs that were delivered prematurely, a direct relationship was noted between the peak airway pressure used to inflate the lungs during the first 3 hours after birth and subsequent epithelial protein leak.[201] These changes in epithelial protein permeability probably reflect overexpansion of at least some areas of the lung, with distortion of intercellular junctions and resultant transudation of protein from the interstitium into the air spaces.[202] Lung immaturity appears to increase the vulnerability of the pulmonary epithelium to protein leaks associated with lung overinflation.[203] The presence of plasma-derived fibrin in the terminal air sacs of infants with respiratory distress syndrome[204] is indicative of epithelial injury.

Several studies have shown that lung overinflation causes vascular injury and edema in lungs of adult animals.[205-207] One report showed that application of positive end-expiratory pressure decreased diffuse alveolar damage in adult rats that were mechanically ventilated with high-volume ventilation for a period of 20 minutes.[206] Studies performed with isolated lungs from young rabbits showed that positive pressure ventilation for 1 hour with peak inflation pressures of up to 45 cm H_2O also increased lung vascular filtration coefficient.[208] In these experiments, restriction of chest wall movement with a plaster cast inhibited the increase in filtration coefficient.

In vivo studies of lung overinflation in chronically catheterized newborn lambs showed that high inflation pressure, coupled with lung overexpansion, on average caused a sevenfold increase in lung lymph flow and lymph protein flow, indicative of increased pulmonary microvascular permeability to protein.[140] In a related series of experiments, high pressure without lung overexpansion did not increase either lymph flow or protein flow. These observations may have important implications regarding the clinical management of patients with respiratory failure. For example, in the presence of nonuniform lung inflation, which is common in many types of newborn and adult respiratory disease, overexpansion of relatively normal regions of lung might contribute to the development of endothelial injury and edema.

Mechanical stress and release of vasoactive substances and oxygen radicals within the lung probably play an important role in the pathogenesis of this type of pulmonary injury. Proteolytic enzymes released from inflammatory and lung parenchymal cells also may contribute to the development of neonatal pulmonary edema. Newborn infants with respiratory distress, especially those who are born prematurely, are deficient in protease inhibitors, both in their plasma[209-213] and in their lungs.[214] At least three groups of investigators have demonstrated an increase in the number of neutrophils, macrophages, and neutrophil-derived elastase activity in liquid suctioned from the airways of infants with respiratory distress.[214-216] These investigators also showed that both elastase inhibitory capacity and α_1-proteinase inhibitor activity were reduced in infants with chronic lung disease following acute neonatal lung injury. There is also evidence that these early inflammatory changes may contribute to the development of chronic lung disease of early infancy, often referred to as bronchopulmonary dysplasia.[217]

Mechanical Ventilation After Premature Birth

Lambs that are delivered prematurely often die of respiratory failure from a condition that mimics the clinical, physiologic, and histologic features observed in human infants with hyaline membrane disease.[88,218-220] Studies performed with chronically catheterized lambs that were delivered prematurely by

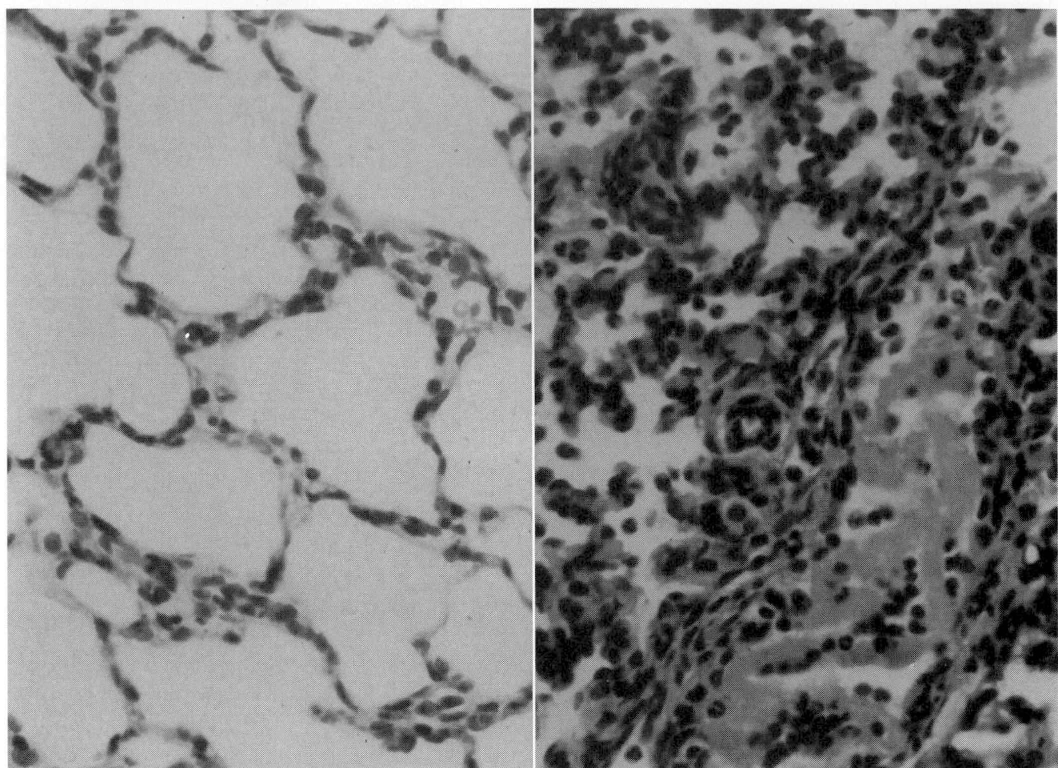

Fig. 57-7. Photographs of lung tissue from lambs with *(right)* and without *(left)* severe respiratory failure after premature birth and mechanical ventilation for 8 hours. Atelectasis, inflammatory cells, and protein-rich fluid within the airspaces are characteristic of the increased microvascular and epithelial permeability that occur in this type of neonatal lung injury.

cesarean section at about 130 days' gestation (term = 147 days) showed that severe respiratory failure developed in 6 of 10 lambs that were mechanically ventilated with 100% oxygen for 8 hours after birth.[88] These 6 lambs required peak inflation pressures that averaged over 50 cm H_2O between 4 and 8 hours after birth. They had severe hypoxemia and pulmonary hypertension, with a progressive increase in hematocrit and a reduction in plasma protein concentration secondary to generalized protein loss from the circulation. In contrast to previous studies performed with more mature lambs,[22] lymph flow and lymph protein flow remained high for the entire study. The postnatal tripling of lymph flow and lymph protein flow clearly showed that lung vascular permeability to protein increased in these preterm lambs with severe respiratory distress. Lung histology and postmortem measurement of lung water content confirmed the presence of severe pulmonary edema (Fig. 57-7). In the 4 lambs that did not have respiratory distress, lung lymph flow and protein clearance decreased to values that were not greater than prenatal measurements, and their postmortem lung water measurements were significantly less than the lambs that had respiratory distress. Thus abnormal leakage of protein-rich liquid from the lung microcirculation into the interstitium constitutes a major component in the pathogenesis of neonatal respiratory distress in preterm lambs.[88] Subsequent studies showed that this lung vascular injury can be inhibited by surfactant administration at birth,[221] probably by reducing the need for high inflation pressures to achieve adequate ventilation and oxygenation and by yielding uniform inflation of distal respiratory units in the immature lung.[222]

It is noteworthy that lambs with severe respiratory failure after premature birth and mechanical ventilation had a significant decrease in circulating neutrophils within 30 minutes of birth and that this was associated with accumulation of neutrophils within the lungs. The magnitude of the early postnatal decrease in circulating neutrophils correlated with the degree of lung vascular protein leak and pulmonary edema.[223] When lambs were rendered neutropenic from prenatal treatment with nitrogen mustard, lung vascular injury and edema did not occur postnatally. These and earlier observations of neutrophil abundance in airway secretions of infants with severe respiratory distress indicate that circulating neutrophils and their secretory products, specifically proteolytic enzymes and toxic oxygen metabolites, may play an important role in the pathogenesis of acute lung vascular protein leak and edema formation in hyaline membrane disease.[214,215,223,224] The mechanisms by which neutrophils are recruited into the lungs after premature birth and mechanical ventilation are unclear, but it is likely that a variety of chemoattractants, including interleukin-8,[225] are released in response to the pulmonary stresses associated with increased blood flow and pressures within the lung circulation, and increased gas flow and pressures within the airways and distal airspaces. Sustained mechanical ventilation for 3 to 4 weeks after premature birth of lambs leads to a chronic form of lung injury that closely mimics the pathophysiology and histopathology of bronchopulmonary dysplasia, including pulmonary vascular dysfunction and edema[226,227]

NEONATAL PULMONARY EDEMA

Predisposing Conditions

Most cases of pulmonary edema in the newborn period result from increased lung microvascular pressure. This may occur when the heart fails and left-atrial pressure increases, as it does in cases of left-ventricular outflow obstruction. Pressure in the pulmonary microcirculation also may increase because of myocardial dysfunction from infection, metabolic abnormalities, insufficient myocardial blood flow because of an aberrant coronary artery, exposure to toxic drugs, or severe asphyxia. Large placental transfusions of blood at birth or excessive intravascular infusions of fluid after birth may overload the lung circulation and lead to pulmonary edema. Increased blood flow to the lungs, associated with large left-to-right shunts, fever, hypoxia, noxious stimuli, or other stressful conditions may increase pulmonary microvascular pressure and thereby cause fluid to accumulate in the lungs. This probably is the source of respiratory distress in babies who are born prematurely and have large systemic-to-pulmonary shunts through a ductus arteriosus. When the lung vascular bed is reduced in size, as it is in pulmonary hypoplasia, fibrosis, or following lung resection, any increase in blood flow to the lungs is likely to elevate microvascular pressure and lead to edema. Intravenous infusions of lipid increase pulmonary arterial pressure and transvascular filtration of fluid in the lungs of lambs, an observation that may help to explain the lung dysfunction that sometimes occurs in infants who receive large intravenous infusions of lipid.

Almost half a century ago, the discovery of surfactant and its role in keeping the lungs inflated after birth prompted speculation that an abnormally high surface tension at the air-liquid interface of terminal respiratory units might be expected to lower lung interstitial hydraulic pressure, resulting in extravasation of liquid and protein from the vascular space.[228,229] This concept, which was supported by micropuncture studies of alveolar liquid pressures in lungs of preterm rabbits,[83] could help to explain the presence of pulmonary edema in hyaline membrane disease. A similar explanation has been invoked to explain the pulmonary edema that sometimes accompanies upper airway obstruction, in which substantial increases in transpulmonary pressure may lower interstitial hydraulic pressure and thereby increase liquid and protein movement out of the circulation.[230] The precise mechanism by which upper airway obstruction may lead to pulmonary edema, however, is uncertain because animal studies have shown that a decrease in interstitial pressure resulting from inspiratory airway obstruction is offset by a corresponding decrease in microvascular hydraulic pressure, so that net fluid filtration remains unchanged.[231] Hypoxia might contribute to the lung edema that is associated with airway obstruction; several studies have documented increased lung vascular filtration pressure during hypoxia in newborn animals.[139,158,162,163]

Another condition that facilitates edema formation in the neonatal lung is decreased intravascular protein osmotic pressure. Hypoproteinemia typically exists in babies who are born prematurely, and large intravascular infusions of protein-free liquids may further depress the concentration of protein in plasma, thus predisposing such infants to pulmonary edema. Hypoproteinemia also occurs in cases of fetal hydrops, and it may develop as a consequence of protein loss through the kidneys or intestinal tract, or from inadequate nutrition.

Impaired lymphatic drainage is a less commonly recognized cause of lung liquid accumulation. Pulmonary edema sometimes accompanies interstitial emphysema and fibrosis, in which air bubbles or scar tissue block lymphatic flow. Experimental studies with sheep indicate that lymphatic outflow obstruction may reduce drainage of lung interstitial fluid.[154] Thus pulmonary edema may ensue if lymphatics must pump against an exceedingly high central venous pressure, particularly if this pressure is sustained for a prolonged period. This may be the source of lung edema in some cases of right-sided heart failure or blockage of the superior vena cava.

Lung edema sometimes develops as a result of microvascular injury, in which disruption of the endothelial membrane allows protein-rich liquid to leak at an increased rate from the lung microcirculation into the interstitium. If there is coexisting epithelial injury, proteinaceous fluid enters the air spaces and interferes with respiratory gas exchange. As noted, studies of lung fluid balance in preterm lambs have demonstrated that lung vascular protein permeability may increase after birth when the lungs are not fully developed and respiratory failure occurs.[88,223] The combination of a high lung vascular filtration pressure and leaky vessels in these preterm lambs caused protein-rich pulmonary edema and pleural effusions. Bacteremia, endotoxemia, pulmonary emboli (including inadvertent air emboli delivered via intravenous fluid infusion), and lung overinflation, as well as breathing high concentrations of oxygen for prolonged periods also may damage the pulmonary microcirculation and cause lung edema. Although hypoxia increases filtration pressure in the neonatal pulmonary microcirculation, there is no evidence that hypoxia adversely affects lung endothelial permeability to protein.[157,162]

Infants who are born prematurely have a high incidence of respiratory distress associated with pulmonary edema.[232,233] Filtration pressure in their pulmonary circulation is greater than normal,[234] particularly if they experience hypoxia or if they have increased pulmonary blood flow from persistent patency of the ductus arteriosus. Protein osmotic pressure in their plasma is low,[128,235] especially if they receive too much fluid. Because the air spaces of their lungs are often unstable from too little surfactant, a large transpulmonary pressure often develops, with considerable heterogeneity of lung expansion. Chemoattractants in the lung draw neutrophils from the pulmonary circulation into the airspaces, with subsequent release of inflammatory mediators.[216,224,225] These developments may cause leaks in the epithelium[236] and endothelium[88] and reduce interstitial pressure around extra-alveolar vessels,[82] which may contribute to edema formation.[228,237]

The early postnatal inflammatory changes that accompany acute respiratory failure after premature birth and positive-pressure ventilation may be associated with increased accumulation of hyaluronan in the lungs.[238] The hydrophilic nature of this large extracellular matrix proteoglycans may contribute to water retention in the lungs of infants with acute respiratory distress syndrome. Infants with respiratory distress often require mechanical ventilation with high concentrations of inspired oxygen, which may injure the lungs, cause release of toxic oxygen metabolites and proteolytic enzymes, and possibly interfere with lymphatic drainage, particularly in the presence of interstitial emphysema or fibrosis. As Fig. 57-6 illustrates, these events may cause fluid accumulation and an abnormal distribution of protein in the lungs, with impaired respiratory gas exchange.

Pathology

During the initial stage of edema formation, liquid accumulates in the loose connective tissue of the pulmonary interstitium, beneath the pleura, between lobes, and around large vessels and airways. Most of this extravascular liquid flows to the dependent portions of the lung, where intravascular hydraulic pressure is greatest. When fluid accumulation exceeds the capacity of the interstitium, protein-rich liquid enters the air spaces across the normally solute-restrictive respiratory tract epithelium. The locus of this fluid and protein leak is diffuse, involving the epithelium of respiratory bronchioles, as well as terminal air sacs. The lungs become boggy and congested, fluid distends the lymphatics, lung compliance and vital capacity decrease, and gas exchange is impaired.

Clinical Features

The usual clinical manifestations of lung edema in infancy are tachypnea, chest wall retractions, flaring of the nostrils, grunting, oxygen dependence (cyanosis), and feeding intolerance. Rales are usually present, although they may be absent if the edema is confined to the lung interstitium. Compression of small airways by tissue fluid may produce expiratory wheezing. Tachycardia, peripheral edema, and hepatomegaly are inconsistent findings. Progressive decompensation leads to gasping respirations, apnea, peripheral vasoconstriction, and bradycardia. With alveolar flooding, there may be blood-tinged or grossly bloody orotracheal secretions, as well as rales. Ventilatory failure, with insufficient oxygen delivery to tissues, results in combined metabolic and respiratory acidemia.

Diagnosis

Pulmonary edema is usually difficult to diagnose before the onset of overt physical signs of respiratory distress. Generalized fluid retention, with an abrupt or insidious weight gain, may signal the development of pulmonary edema. The diagnosis should be considered in all babies with cardiovascular abnormalities and associated respiratory distress.

Chest radiographs usually show diffuse, bilateral infiltrates, particularly in the peripheral and basilar areas of the lungs, together with prominent vascularity and cardiomegaly. Fluid in the interlobar fissures and pleural space also may be present. If alveolar flooding occurs, the picture may progress to a diffuse, bilateral haziness with air bronchograms and obliteration of the cardiac silhouette.

When there is severe alveolar edema, the diagnosis may be confirmed by analysis of lung effluent collected from the airway. This liquid usually has a high protein concentration (at least one half that of plasma), and when pulmonary vascular permeability is increased, the protein concentration in this liquid may approach that of plasma. Moreover, the albumin:globulin ratio in liquid collected from the airways of infants with severe pulmonary edema is greater than the albumin:globulin ratio in plasma. This finding reflects the fact that the vascular endothelium restricts passage of large molecules (globulins, fibrinogen) more than it restricts albumin.

Management

Effective treatment of lung edema includes measures designed to reduce hydraulic pressure in the pulmonary microcirculation and to increase intravascular protein osmotic pressure. When edema results from increased microvascular protein permeability, supportive therapy should be provided, thus allowing time for the pulmonary endothelium to heal, with resolution of edema.

Whatever the cause of the edema, fluid and salt intake should not exceed insensible losses. In cases of cardiogenic edema, treatment with digitalis is often useful. Morphine sulfate, given intramuscularly in a dose of 0.1 to 0.2 mg/kg body weight, may be useful for treating acute pulmonary edema, but it must be administered cautiously because of its potential depressant effect on ventilation.

Diuretics are the mainstay of therapy for lung edema. In cases of severe edema, furosemide may be given intravenously in a dose of 1 to 2 mg/kg body weight. This usually produces an abrupt diuresis, which decreases pulmonary microvascular pressure and increases the concentration of protein in plasma.[195] These two changes inhibit fluid filtration into the lungs and hasten the entry of water into the pulmonary microcirculation from the interstitium. Continued therapy with furosemide, sometimes in conjunction with other diuretics, such as spironolactone and thiazides, may help to control the degree of lung edema. Patients who require prolonged treatment with diuretics often lose a considerable amount of potassium chloride in their urine. Depletion of these electrolytes usually can be prevented by treatment with supplemental potassium chloride, 3 to 5 mEq/kg body weight daily.

Although hypoproteinemia may predispose patients to pulmonary edema, infusions of albumin or plasma usually do not benefit infants and children with severe pulmonary edema. Such infusions tend to increase pulmonary microvascular pressure, and this offsets the effect of increased intravascular protein osmotic pressure. Furthermore, the infused protein leaks into the interstitium of the lungs within a short period of time, and this often aggravates the edema.

If there is cyanosis or arterial oxygen desaturation, supplemental oxygen should be provided to maintain a normal partial pressure of oxygen in arterial blood. If anemia and severe pulmonary edema coexist, a partial exchange transfusion with packed red blood cells may be safer and offer more benefit than a simple transfusion. Conditions that impair myocardial performance, such as hypoglycemia, hypocalcemia, or infection, require specific therapy, which usually restores normal myocardial contractility. Conditions that increase pulmonary blood flow, such as hypoxia, pain, and fever, should be avoided or treated promptly. Environmental conditions should be adjusted to minimize oxygen consumption. A semi-upright, prone position sometimes lessens respiratory distress in infants with pulmonary edema.

If these measures are not successful in reducing edema, ventilatory support with positive end-expiratory pressure is often beneficial. Positive end-expiratory pressure does not reduce lung water content, but it does redistribute fluid in the air spaces and improve respiratory gas exchange. Ventilation also spares energy reserves by reducing the work of breathing. If ventilatory assistance becomes necessary, sedation may further decrease oxygen consumption and thereby facilitate recovery. When intractable lung edema complicates the course of infants and children with congenital abnormalities of the heart, diagnostic procedures such as echocardiography and cardiac catheterization should be performed to determine the potential benefit of surgical intervention.

REFERENCES

1. Rudolph AM, Heymann MA: Circulatory changes during growth in the fetal lamb, *Circ Res* 26:289-299, 1970.
2. Adamson TM, Brodecky V, Lambert TF, Maloney JE, Ritchie BC, Walker AM: Lung liquid production and composition in the "in utero" foetal lamb, *Aust J Exp Biol Med Sci* 53:65-75, 1975.
3. Mescher EJ, Platzker ACG, Ballard PL, Kitterman JA, Clements JA, Tooley WH: Ontogeny of tracheal fluid, pulmonary surfactant, and plasma corticoids in the fetal lamb, *J Appl Physiol* 39:1017-1021, 1975.

4. McCray PB Jr, Bettencourt JD, Bastacky J: Developing bronchopulmonary epithelium of the human fetus secretes fluid, *Am J Physiol* 262:L270-L279, 1992.
5. Alcorn D, Adamson TM, Lambert TF, Maloney JE, Ritchie BC, Robinson PM: Morphological effects of chronic tracheal ligation and drainage in the fetal lamb lung, *J Anat* 123:649-660, 1977.
6. Harding R, Hooper SB: Regulation of lung expansion and lung growth before birth, *J Appl Physiol* 81:209-224, 1996.
7. Moessinger AC, Harding R, Adamson TM, Singh M, Kiu GT: Role of lung fluid volume in growth and maturation of the fetal sheep lung, *J Clin Invest* 86:1270-1277, 1990.
8. Wallen LD, Kulisz E, Maloney JE: Main pulmonary artery ligation reduces lung fluid production in fetal sheep, *J Dev Physiol* 16:173-179, 1991.
9. Wallen LD, Perry SF, Alston JT, Maloney JE: Morphometric study of the role of pulmonary arterial flow in fetal lung growth in sheep, *Pediatr Res* 27:122-127, 1990.
10. Harrison MR, Bressack MA, Churg AM, de Lorimier AA: Correction of congenital diaphragmatic hernia in utero. II. Simulated correction permits fetal lung growth survival at birth, *Surgery* 88:260-268, 1980.
11. Pringle KC, Turner JW, Schofield JC, Soper RT: Creation and repair of diaphragmatic hernia in fetal lamb: lung development and morphology, *J Pediatr Surg* 19:131-140, 1984.
12. Adzick NS, Harrison MR, Glick PL, Villa RL, Finkbeiner W: Experimental pulmonary hypoplasia and oligohydramnios: relative contributions of lung fluid and fetal breathing movements, *J Pediatr Res* 19:658-665, 1984.
13. Dickson KA, Harding R: Decline in lung liquid volume and secretion rate during oligohydramnios in fetal sheep, *J Appl Physiol* 67:2401-2407, 1989.
14. Adams FH, Fujiwara T, Rowshan G: The nature and origin of the fluid in the fetal lamb lung, *J Pediatr* 63:881-888, 1963.
15. Adamson TM, Boyd RDH, Platt HS, Strang LB: Composition of alveolar liquid in the foetal lamb, *J Physiol* 204:159-163, 1969.
16. Boston RW, Humphreys PW, Reynolds EOR, Strang LB: Lymph flow and clearance of liquid from the lungs of the fetal lamb, *Lancet* ii:473-474, 1965.
17. Boyd RDH, Hill JR, Humphreys PW, Normand ICS, Reynolds EOR, Strang LB: Permeability of lung capillaries to macromolecules in fetal and newborn lambs and sheep, *J Physiol* 201:567-588, 1969.
18. Humphreys PW, Normand ICS, Reynolds EOR, Strang LB: Pulmonary lymph flow and the uptake of liquid from the lungs of the lamb at the start of breathing, *J Physiol* 193:1-29, 1967.
19. Normand ICS, Olver RE, Reynolds EOR, Strang LB: Permeability of lung capillaries and alveoli to non-electrolytes in the foetal lamb, *J Physiol* 219:303-330, 1971.
20. Normand ICS, Reynolds EOR, Strang LB: Passage of macromolecules between alveolar and interstitial spaces in foetal and newly ventilated lungs of the lamb, *J Physiol* 210:151-164, 1970.
21. Olver RE, Strang LB: Ion fluxes across the pulmonary epithelium and the secretion of lung liquid in the foetal lamb, *J Physiol* 241:327-357, 1974.
22. Bland RD, Hansen TN, Haberkern CM, Bressack MA, Hazinski TA, Raj JU, Goldberg RB: Lung fluid balance in lambs before and after birth, *J Appl Physiol* 53:992-1004, 1982.
23. Olver RE, Schneeberger EE, Walters DV: Epithelial solute permeability, ion transport and tight junction morphology in the developing lung of the fetal lamb, *J Physiol* 315:395-412, 1981.
24. Schneeberger EE, Walters DV, Olver RE: Development of intercellular junctions in the pulmonary epithelium of the foetal lamb, *J Cell Sci* 32:307-324, 1978.
25. Carlton DP, Cummings JJ, Chapman DL, Poulain FR, Bland RD: Ion transport regulation of lung liquid secretion in foetal lambs, *J Dev Physiol* 17:99-107, 1992.
26. Cassin S, Gause G, Perks AM: The effects of bumetanide and furosemide on lung liquid secretion in fetal sheep, *Proc Soc Exp Biol Med* 181:427-431, 1986.
27. Thom J, Perks AM: The effects of furosemide and bumetanide on lung liquid production by in vitro lungs from fetal guinea pigs, *Can J Physiol Pharmacol* 68:1131-1135, 1990.
28. Frizzell RA, Field M, Schultz SG: Sodium-coupled chloride transport by epithelial tissues, *Am J Physiol* 236:Fl-F8, 1979.
29. Welsh MJ: Electrolyte transport by airway epithelia, *Physiol Rev* 67:1143-1184, 1987.
30. McCray PB, Reenstra WW, Louie E, Johnson J, Bettencourt JD, Bastacky J: Expression of CFTR and presence of cAMP-mediated fluid secretion in human fetal lung, *Am J Physiol* 262:L472-L481, 1992.
31. McGrath SA, Basu A, Zeitlin PL: Cystic fibrosis gene and protein expression during fetal lung development, *Am J Respir Cell Mol Biol* 8:201-208, 1993.
32. Murray CB, Morales NM, Flotte TR, McGrath-Morrow SA, Guggino WB, Zeitlin PL: ClC-2: A developmentally dependent chloride channel expressed in the fetal lung and downregulated after birth, *Am J Respir Cell Mol Biol* 12:597-604, 1995.
33. Tizzano EF, O'Brodovich H, Chitayat D, Benichou JC, Buchwald M: Regional expression of CFTR in developing human respiratory tissues, *Am J Respir Cell Mol Biol* 10:355-362, 1994.
34. Adamson TM, Waxman BP: Carbonate dehydratase (carbonic anydrase) and the fetal lung, Ciba Symposium, *Lung Liquids,* Amsterdam, 1976, Elsevier/North-Holland, pp 221-233.
34a. Chapman DL, Nielson DW, Bland RD: Acidification of lung luminal liquid in fetal lambs, *Am Rev Respir Dis* 147:A1007, 1993.
34b. Albertine KH, Nelson R, Chapman DL, Nielson DW, Bland RD: H^+-ATPase on the respiratory epithelium helps to regulate acidification of lung liquid during fetal development, *Pediatr Res* 40:40A, 1997.
35. Cotton CU, Boucher RC, Gatzy JC: Bioelectric properties and ion transport across excised canine fetal and neonatal airways, *J Appl Physiol* 65:2367-2375, 1988.
36. O'Brodovich H, Merritt TA: Bicarbonate concentration in Rhesus monkey and guinea pig fetal lung liquid, *Am Rev Respir Dis* 146:1613-1614, 1992.
37. Kitterman JA, Ballard PL, Clements JA, Mescher EJ, Tooley WH: Tracheal fluid in fetal lambs: spontaneous decrease prior to birth, *J Appl Physiol* 47:985-989, 1979.
38. Schneeberger EE: Plasmalemmal vesicles in pulmonary capillary endothelium of developing fetal lamb lungs, *Microvasc Res* 25:40-55, 1983.
39. Shermeta DW, Oesch I: Characteristics of fetal lung fluid production, *J Pediatr Surg* 16:943-946, 1981.
40. Carlton DP, Cummings JJ, Poulain FR, Bland RD: Increased pulmonary vascular filtration pressure does not alter lung liquid secretion in fetal sheep, *J Appl Physiol* 72:650-655, 1992.
41. Olver RE: Fetal lung liquids, *Fed Proc* 36:2669-2675, 1977.
42. Cotton CU, Boucher RC, Gatzy JT: Paths of ion transport across canine fetal tracheal epithelium, *J Appl Physiol* 65:2376-2382, 1988.
43. Cotton CU, Lawson EE, Boucher RC, Gatzy JT: Bioelectric properties and ion transport of airways excised from adult and fetal sheep, *J Appl Physiol* 55:1542-1549, 1983.
44. Krochmal EM, Ballard ST, Yankaskas JR, Boucher RC, Gatzy JT: Volume and ion transport by fetal rat alveolar and tracheal epithelia in submersion culture, *Am J Physiol* 256:F397-F407, 1989.
45. Zeitlin PL, Loughlin GM, Guggino WB: Ion transport in cultured fetal and adult rabbit tracheal epithelia, *Am J Physiol* 254:C691-C698, 1988.
46. Brown MJ, Olver RE, Ramsden CA, Strang LB, Walters DV: Effects of adrenaline and of spontaneous labour on the secretion and absorption of lung liquid in the fetal lamb, *J Physiol* 344:137-152, 1983.
47. Chapman DL, Carlton DP, Nielson DW, Cummings JJ, Poulain FR, Bland RD: Changes in lung liquid during spontaneous labor in fetal sheep, *J Appl Physiol* 76:523-530, 1994.
48. Dickson KA, Maloney JE, Berger PJ: Decline in lung liquid volume before labor in fetal lambs, *J Appl Physiol* 61:2266-2272, 1986.
49. Bland RD: Dynamics of pulmonary water before and after birth, *Acta Paediatr Scand* Suppl 305:12-20, 1983.
50. Bland RD, Bressack MA, McMillan DD: Labor decreases the lung water content of newborn rabbits, *Am J Obstet Gynecol* 135:364-367, 1979.
51. Enhoming G, Chamberlain D, Contreras C, Burgoyne R, Robertson B: Isoxsuprine-induced release of pulmonary surfactant in the rabbit fetus, *Am J Obstet Gynecol* 129:197-202, 1977.
52. Lawson EE, Brown ER, Torday JS, Madansky DL, Taeusch HW Jr: The effect of epinephrine on tracheal fluid flow and surfactant efflux in fetal sheep, *Am Rev Respir Dis* 118:1023-1026, 1978.
53. Walters DV, Olver RE: The role of catecholamines in lung liquid absorption at birth, *Pediatr Res* 12:239-242, 1978.

54. Olver RE, Ramsden CA, Strang LB, Walters DV: The role of amiloride-blockable sodium transport in adrenaline-induced lung liquid reabsorption in the fetal lamb, *J Physiol* 376:321-340, 1986.
55. Walters DV, Ramsden CA, Olver RE: Dibutyryl cyclic AMP induces a gestation-dependent absorption of fetal lung liquid, *J Appl Physiol* 68:2054-2059, 1990.
56. Barker PM, Brown MJ, Ramsden CA, Strang LB, Walters DV: The effect of thyroidectomy in the fetal sheep on lung liquid reabsorption induced by adrenaline or cyclic AMP, *J Physiol* 407:373-383, 1988.
57. Barker PM, Walters DV, Strang LB: The role of thyroid hormones in maturation of the adrenaline-sensitive lung-liquid reabsorption mechanism in the fetal sheep, *J Physiol* 424:473-485, 1990.
58. Barker PM, Walters DV, Markiewicz M, Strang LB: Development of the lung liquid reabsorptive mechanism in fetal sheep; synergism of triiodothyronine and hydrocortisone, *J Physiol* 433:435-449, 1991.
59. Chapman DL, Carlton DP, Cummings JJ, Poulain FR, Bland RD: Intrapulmonary terbutaline and aminophylline decrease lung liquid in fetal lambs, *Pediatr Res* 29:357-361, 1991.
60. Cheng JB, Goldfein A, Ballard PL, Roberts JM: Glucocorticoids increase pulmonary adrenergic receptors in fetal rabbit, *Endocrinology* 107:1646-1648, 1980.
61. Warburton DL, Parton L, Buckley S, Cosico L, Saluna T: β-Receptors and surface active material flux in fetal lamb lung: female advantage, *J Appl Physiol* 63:828-833, 1987.
62. Whitsett JA, Manton MA, Carovec-Beckerman C, Adams KG, Moore JJ: β-Adrenergic receptors in the developing rabbit lung, *Am J Physiol* 240:E351-E357, 1981.
63. McDonald JV, Gonzales LW, Ballard PL, Pitha J, Roberts JM: Lung β-adrenergic blockade affects perinatal surfactant release but not lung water, *J Appl Physiol* 60:1727-1733, 1986.
64. Cassin S, Perks AM: Amiloride inhibits arginine vasopressin-induced decrease in fetal lung liquid secretion, *J Appl Physiol* 75:1925-1929, 1993.
65. Cummings JJ, Carlton DP, Poulain FR, Fike CD, Keil LC, Bland RD: Vasopressin effects on lung liquid volume in fetal sheep, *Pediatr Res* 38:30-35, 1995.
66. Perks AM, Cassin S: The effects of arginine vasopressin and other factors on the production of lung liquid in fetal goats, *Chest* 81:63S-65S, 1982.
67. Perks AM, Cassin S: The rate of production of lung liquid in fetal goats, and the effect of expansion of the lungs, *J Dev Physiol* 7:149-160, 1985.
68. Perks AM, Cassin S: The effects of arginine vasopressin and epinephrine on lung liquid production in fetal goats, *Can J Physiol Pharmacol* 67:491-499, 1989.
69. Wallace MJ, Hooper SB, Harding R: Regulation of lung liquid secretion by arginine vasopressin in fetal sheep, *Am J Physiol* 258:R104-R111, 1990.
70. Kullama L, Davis P, Packham K, Godfrey B, Ericksen M, Bland R: Effects of aldosterone on net lung liquid production in fetal sheep, *FASEB J* 9:A568, 1995.
71. Kennedy KA, Wilton P, Mellander M, Rojas J, Sundell H: Effect of epidermal growth factor on lung liquid secretion in fetal sheep, *J Dev Physiol* 8:421-433, 1986.
72. Castro R, Ervin MG, Ross MG, Sherman DJ, Leake RD, Fisher DA: Ovine fetal lung response to atrial natriuretic factor, *Am J Obstet Gynecol* 161:1337-1343, 1989.
73. Kitterman JA: Fetal lung development, *J Dev Physiol* 6:67-82, 1984.
74. Wallen LD, Murai DT, Clyman RI, Lee CH, Mauray FE, Ballard PL, Kitterman JA: Meclofenamate does not affect lung development in fetal sheep, *J Dev Physiol* 12:109-115, 1989.
75. Carlton DP, Davis PL, Gismondi PA, Kullama LK, Larsen GY, Bland RD: Surfactant alters lung liquid production and epithelial ion transport in fetal sheep, *Pediatr Res* 39:327A, 1996.
76. Cummings JJ, Wang H: Nitric oxide induced reduction in fetal lung liquid production does not depend on Na^+ resorption, *Pediatr Res* 37: 329A, 1995.
77. Cummings JJ, Carlton DP, Poulain FR, Raj JU, Bland RD: Hypoproteinemia slows lung liquid clearance in young lambs, *J Appl Physiol* 74:153-160, 1993.
78. Raj JU, Bland RD: Lung luminal liquid clearance in newborn lambs, *Am Rev Respir Dis* 134:305-310, 1986.
79. O'Brodovich H, Hannam V, Rafii B: Sodium channel but neither Na^+-H^+ nor Na-glucose symport inhibitors slow neonatal lung water clearance, *Am J Respir Cell Mol Biol* 5:377-384, 1991.
80. O'Brodovich H, Hannam V, Spear M, Mullen JBM: Amiloride impairs lung liquid clearance in newborn guinea pigs, *J Appl Physiol* 68:1758-1762, 1990.
81. Egan EA, Olver RE, Strang LB: Changes in non-electrolyte permeability of alveoli and the absorption of lung liquid at the start of breathing in the lamb, *J Physiol* 244:161-179, 1975.
82. Fike CD, Lai-Fook SJ, Bland RD: Alveolar liquid pressures in newborn and adult rabbit lungs, *J Appl Physiol* 64:1629-1635, 1988.
83. Raj JU: Alveolar liquid pressure measured by micropuncture in isolated lungs of mature and immature fetal rabbits, *J Clin Invest* 79:1579-1588, 1987.
84. Scarpelli EM, Condorelli S, Cosmi EV: Lamb fetal pulmonary fluid. I. Validation and significance of method for determination of volume and volume change, *Pediatr Res* 9:190-195, 1975.
85. Garrad P, Perks AM: The effects of temperature change on lung liquid production by in vitro lungs from fetal guinea pigs, *J Dev Physiol* 14:109-114, 1990.
86. Bland RD, McMillan DD, Bressack MA, Dong LA: Clearance of liquid from lungs of newborn rabbits, *J Appl Physiol* 49:171-177, 1980.
87. Hall J, Haberkern C, Callaway P, Hansen T, Bland R: Lung blood and water content of preterm and term rabbits, *Clin Res* 28:122A, 1980.
88. Bland RD, Carlton DP, Scheerer RG, Cummings JJ, Chapman DL: Lung fluid balance in lambs before and after premature birth, *J Clin Invest* 84:568-576, 1989.
89. Egan EA, Dillon WP, Zorn S: Fetal lung liquid absorption and alveolar epithelial solute permeability in surfactant deficient, breathing fetal lambs, *Pediatr Res* 18:566-570, 1984.
90. Matthay MA, Berthiaume Y, Staub NC: Long-term clearance of liquid and protein from the lungs of unanesthetized sheep, *J Appl Physiol* 59:928-934, 1985.
91. Matthay MA, Landolt CC, Staub NC: Differential liquid and protein clearance from the alveoli of anesthetized sheep, *J Appl Physiol* 53:96-104, 1982.
92. Basset G, Crone C, Saumon G: Fluid absorption by the rat lung in situ: pathways for sodium entry in the luminal membrane of alveolar epithelium, *J Physiol* 384:325-345, 1987.
93. Basset G, Crone C, Saumon G: Significance of active ion transport in transalveolar water absorption: a study on isolated rat lung, *J Physiol* 384:311-324, 1987.
94. Crandall ED, Heming TA, Palombo RL, Goodman BE: Effects of terbutaline on sodium transport in isolated perfused rat lung, *J Appl Physiol* 60:289-294, 1986.
95. Goodman BE, Kim KJ, Crandall ED: Evidence for active sodium transport across alveolar epithelium of isolated rat lung, *J Appl Physiol* 62:2460-2466, 1987.
96. Barker PM, Stiles AD, Boucher RC, Gatzy JT: Bioelectric properties of cultured epithelial monolayers from distal lung of 18-day fetal rat, *Am J Physiol* 262:L628-L636, 1992.
97. Cheek JM, Kim KI, Crandall ED: Tight monolayers of rat alveolar epithelial cells: bioelectric properties and active sodium transport, *Am J Physiol* 256:C688-C693, 1989.
98. Mason RJ, Williams MC, Widdicombe JH, Sanders MJ, Misfeldt DS, Berry LG Jr: Transepithelial transport by pulmonary alveolar type II cells in primary culture, *Proc Natl Acad Sci USA* 79:6033-6037, 1982.
99. O'Brodovich H, Rafii B, Post M: Bioelectric properties of fetal alveolar epithelial monolayers, *Am J Physiol* 258:L201-L206, 1990.
100. Pitkänen OM, Tanswell AK, O'Brodovich HM: Fetal lung cell-derived matrix alters distal lung epithelial ion transport, *Am J Physiol* 268: L762-L771, 1995.
101. Rao AK, Cott GR: Ontogeny of ion transport across fetal pulmonary epithelial cells in monolayer culture, *Am J Physiol* 261:L178-L187, 1991.
102. Weibel ER, Gehr P, Haies D, Gil J, Bachofen M: The cell population of the normal lung. In Bouhuys A, ed: *Lung cells in disease,* Amsterdam, 1976, Elsevier/North-Holland, pp 3-16.
103. Randell SH, Silbajoris R, Young SL: Ontogeny of rat lung type II cells correlated with surfactant lipid and surfactant apoprotein expression, *Am J Physiol* 266:L562-L570, 1991.
104. Schneeberger EE, McCarthy KM: Cytochemical localization of Na-K-ATPase in rat type II pneumocytes, *J Appl Physiol* 60:1584-1589, 1986.
105. Bland RD, Boyd CAR: Cation transport in lung epithelial cells derived from fetal, newborn and adult rabbits. Influence of birth, labor and postnatal development, *J Appl Physiol* 62:507-515, 1986.

106. Chapman DL, Widdicombe JH, Bland RD: Developmental differences in rabbit lung epithelial cell Na-K-ATPase, *Am J Physiol* 259:L481-L487,1990.
107. Crump RG, Askew GR, Wert SE, Lingrel JB, Joiner CH: In situ localization of sodium potassium ATPase mRNA in developing mouse lung epithelium, *Am J Physiol* 269:L299-L308, 1995.
108. Ingbar DH, Weeks CB, Gilmore-Hebert M, Jacobsen E, Duvick S, Dowin R, Savik SK, Jamieson JD: Developmental regulation of Na,K-ATPase in rat lung, *Am J Physiol* 270:L619-L629, 1996.
109. O'Brodovich H, Staub O, Rossier BC, Geering K, Kraehenbuhl JP: Ontogeny of α_1- and β_1-isoforms of Na^+-K^+-ATPase in fetal distal rat lung epithelium, *Am J Physiol* 264:C1137-C1143, 1993.
110. Bland RD: Pathogenesis of pulmonary edema after premature birth, *Adv Pediatr* 34:175-222, 1987.
111. O'Brodovich H, Cannessa C, Ueda J, Rafii B, Rossier BC, Edelson J: Expression of the epithelial Na^+ channel in the developing rat lung, *Am J Physiol* 265:C491-C496, 1993.
112. Umenishi F, Carter EP, Yang B, Oliver B, Matthay MA, Verkman AS: Sharp increase in rat lung water channel expression in the perinatal period, *Am J Respir Cell Mol Biol* 15:673-679, 1996.
113. Celsi G, Wang ZM, Akusjarvi G, Aperia A: Sensitive periods for glucocorticoids' regulation of Na,K-ATPase mRNA in the developing lung and kidney, *Pediatr Res* 33:5-9, 1993.
114. King LS, Nielsen S, Agre P: Aquaporin-1 water channel protein in lung, *J Clin Invest* 97:2183-2191, 1996.
115. Tchepichev S, Ueda J, Canessa C, Rossier BC, O'Brodovich H: Lung epithelial Na channel subunits are differentially regulated during development and by steroids, *Am J Physiol* 269:C805-C812, 1995.
116. Barker PM, Gatzy JT: Effect of gas composition on liquid secretion by explants of distal lung of fetal rat in submersion culture, *Am J Physiol* 265:L512-L517, 1993.
117. Pitkänen O, Tanswell AK, Downey G, O'Brodovich H: Increased PO_2 alters the bioelectric properties of fetal distal lung epithelium, *Am J Physiol* 270:L1060-L1066, 1996.
118. Karlberg P, Adams FH, Beubelle F, Wallgren G: Alteration of the infant's thorax during vaginal delivery, *Acta Obstet Gynecol Scand* 41: 223-229, 1962.
119. Humphreys PW, Normand ICS, Reynolds EOR, Strang LB: Lymph flow and clearance of liquid from the lungs of the lamb at the start of breathing, *J Physiol* 193:1-29, 1967.
120. Nielson DW: Changes in the pulmonary alveolar subphase at birth in term and premature lambs, *Pediatr Res* 23:418-422, 1988.
121. Dawes GS, Mott JC, Widdicombe JG, Wyatt DG: Changes in the lungs of the newborn lamb, *J Physiol* 121:141-162, 1953.
122. Walker AM, Alcom DG, Cannata JC, Maloney JE, Ritchie BC: Effect of ventilation of pulmonary blood volume of the fetal lamb, *J Appl Physiol* 39:969-975, 1975.
123. Avery ME, Gatewood OB, Brumley G: Transient tachypnea of newborn. Possible delayed resorption of fluid at birth, *Am J Dis Child* 111: 380-385, 1966.
124. Malan AF: Neonatal tachypnoea, *Aust Paediatr J* 3:159-164, 1966.
125. Sundell H, Garrott J, Blankenship WJ, Shephard FM, Stahlman MT: Studies on infants with type II respiratory distress syndrome, *J Pediatr* 78:754-764, 1971.
126. Alpan G, Scheerer R, Bland R, Clyman R: Patent ductus arteriosus increases lung fluid filtration in preterm lambs, *Pediatr Res* 30:616-621, 1991.
127. Sundell HW, Harris TR, Cannon JR, Lindstrom DP, Green R, Rojas J, Brigham KL: Lung water and vascular permeability-surface area in premature newborn lambs with hyaline membrane disease, *Circ Res* 60:923-932, 1987.
128. Bland RD: Cord-blood total protein level as a screening aid for the idiopathic respiratory distress syndrome, *N Engl J Med* 287:9-13, 1972.
129. Bland RD, McMillan DD: Lung fluid dynamics in awake newborn lambs, *J Clin Invest* 60:1107-1115, 1977.
130. Bland RD, Bressack MA: Lung fluid balance in awake newborn lambs with pulmonary edema from rapid intravenous infusion of isotonic saline, *Pediatr Res* 13:1037-1042, 1979.
131. Warren MF, Drinker CK: The flow of lymph from the lungs of the dog, *Am J Physiol* 136:207-221, 1941.
132. Staub N: Steady-state pulmonary transvascular water filtration in unanesthetized sheep, *Circ Res* 28/29 (suppl 1):135-139, 1971.
133. Staub NC, Bland RD, Brigham KL, Demling R, Erdmann AJ III, Woolverton WC: Preparation of chronic lung lymph fistulas in sheep, *J Surg Res* 19:315-320, 1975.
134. Brigham KL, Woolverton WC, Blake LH, Staub NC: Increased sheep lung vascular permeability caused by pseudomonas bacteremia, *J Clin Invest* 54:792-804, 1974.
135. Drake R, Adair T, Traber D, Gabel J: Contamination of caudal mediastinal node efferent lymph in the sheep, *Am J Physiol* 241:H354-H357, 1981.
136. Chanana AD, Joel DD: Contamination of lung lymph following standard and modified procedures in sheep, *J Appl Physiol* 60:809-816, 1986.
137. Drake RE, Laine GA, Allen SJ, Katz J, Gabel JC: Overestimation of sheep lung lymph contamination, *J Appl Physiol* 61:1590-1592, 1986.
138. Roos PJ, Wierner-Kronish JP, Albertine KH, Staub NC: Removal of abdominal sources of caudal mediastinal node lymph in anesthetized sheep, *J Appl Physiol* 55:996-1001, 1983.
139. Bland RD, Hansen TN, Hazinski TA, Haberkern CM, Bressack MA: Studies of lung fluid balance in newborn lambs, *Ann NY Acad Sci* 384:126-145, 1982.
140. Carlton DP, Cummings JJ, Scheerer RG, Poulain FR, Bland RD: Lung overexpansion increases pulmonary microvascular protein permeability in young lambs, *J Appl Physiol* 69:577-583, 1990.
141. Hazinski TA, Bland RD, Hansen TN, Sedin EG, Goldberg RB: Effect of hypoproteinemia on lung fluid balance in awake newborn lambs, *J Appl Physiol* 61:1139-1148, 1986.
142. Teague WG, Bemer ME, Bland RD: Effect of pulmonary perfusion on lung fluid filtration in young lambs, *Am J Physiol* 255:H1336-Hl341, 1988.
143. Sundell HW, Brigham KL, Harris TR, Lindstrom DP, Catterton WZ, Green R, Rojas J, Stahlman MT: Lung water and vascular permeability-surface area in newborn lambs delivered by cesarean section compared with the 3-5-day-old lamb and adult sheep, *J Dev Physiol* 2:191-204, 1980.
144. Bland RD, Bressack MA, Haberkem CM, Hansen TN: Lung fluid balance in hypoxic, awake newborn lambs and mature sheep, *Biol Neonate* 38:221-228, 1980.
145. West JB, Dollery CT, Naimark A: Distribution of blood flow in isolated lung: relation to vascular and alveolar pressures, *J Appl Physiol* 19:713-724, 1964.
146. Staub NC: Pulmonary edema, *Physiol Rev* 54:678-811, 1974.
147. Erdmann AJ III, Vaughan TR Jr, Brigham KL, Woolverton WC, Staub NC: Effect of increased vascular pressure on lung fluid balance in unanesthetized sheep, *Circ Res* 37:271-285, 1975.
148. Feltes TF, Hansen TH: Effects of an aorticopulmonary shunt on lung fluid balance in the young lamb, *Pediatr Res* 26:94-97, 1989.
149. Teague WG, Raj JU, Braun D, Berner ME, Clyman RI, Bland RD: Lung vascular effects of lipid infusion in awake lambs, *Pediatr Res* 22:714-719, 1987.
150. Guyton AC, Lindsey AW: Effect of elevated left atrial pressure and decreased plasma protein concentration on the development of pulmonary edema, *Circ Res* 7:649-657, 1959.
151. Kramer G, Harmes B, Gunther R, Renkin E, Demling R: The effects of hypoproteinemia on blood-to-lymph fluid transport in sheep lung, *Circ Res* 49:1173-1180, 1981.
152. Kramer GC, Harms BA, Bodai BI, Renkin EM, Demling RH: Effects of hypoproteinemia and increased vascular pressure on lung fluid balance in sheep, *J Appl Physiol* 55:1514-1522, 1983.
153. Zarins CK, Rice CL, Peters RM, Virgilio RW: Lymph and pulmonary response to isobaric reduction in plasma oncotic pressure in baboons, *Circ Res* 43:925-930, 1978.
154. Drake R, Giesler M, Laine G, Gabel J, Hansen T: Effect of outflow pressure on lung lymph flow in unanesthetized sheep, *J Appl Physiol* 58:70-76, 1985.
155. Laine GA, Allen SJ, Katz J, Gabel JC, Drake RE: Effect of systemic venous pressure elevation on lymph flow and lung edema formation, *J Appl Physiol* 61:1634-1638, 1986.
156. Cowan GSM Jr, Staub NC, Edmunds LG Jr: Changes in the fluid compartments and dry weights of reimplanted dog lungs, *J Appl Physiol* 40:962-970, 1976.
157. Bland RD, Demling RH, Selinger SL, Staub NC: Effects of alveolar hypoxia on lung fluid and protein transport in unanesthetized sheep, *Circ Res* 40:269-274, 1977.

158. Bressack MA, Bland RD: Alveolar hypoxia increases lung fluid filtration in unanesthetized newborn lambs, *Circ Res* 46:111-116, 1980.
159. Raj JU, Chen P: Micropuncture measurements of microvascular pressures in isolated lamb lungs during hypoxia, *Circ Res* 59:398-404, 1986.
160. Hansen TN, LeBlanc AL, Gest AL: Hypoxia and angiotensin II infusion redistribute lung blood flow in lambs, *J Appl Physiol* 58:812-818, 1985.
161. Landolt CC, Matthay MA, Albertine KH, Roos PJ, Weiner-Kronish JP, Staub NC: Overperfusion, hypoxia and increased pressure cause only hydrostatic pulmonary edema in anesthetized sheep, *Circ Res* 52:335-341, 1986.
162. Hansen TN, Hazinski TA, Bland RD: Effects of asphyxia on lung fluid balance in baby lambs, *J Clin Invest* 74:370-376, 1984.
163. Hansen TN, Hazinski TA, Bland RD: Effects of hypoxia on transvascular fluid filtration in newborn lambs, *Pediatr Res* 18:434-440, 1984.
164. Raj JU, Hazinski TA, Bland RD: Effect of hypoxia on lung lymph flow in newborn lambs with left atrial hypertension, *Am J Physiol* 254:H487-H493, 1988.
165. Bressack MA, McMillan DD, Bland RD: Pulmonary oxygen toxicity: increased microvascular permeability to protein in unanesthetized lambs, *Lymphology* 12:133-139, 1979.
166. Hansen TN, Hazinski TA, Bland RD: Vitamin E does not prevent oxygen-induced lung injury in newborn lambs, *Pediatr Res* 16:583-587, 1982.
167. Craddock PR, Fehr J, Brigham KL, Kronenberg RS, Jacob HS: Complement and leukocyte-mediated pulmonary dysfunction in hemodialysis, *New Engl J Med* 296:769-774, 1977.
168. Flick M, Perel A, Staub N: Leukocytes are required for increased lung microvascular permeability after microembolization in sheep, *Circ Res* 48:344-351, 1981.
169. Heflin AC, Brigham KL: Prevention by granulocyte depletion of increased vascular permeability of sheep lung following endotoxemia, *J Clin Invest* 68:1253-1260, 1981.
170. Johnson A, Malik AB: Pulmonary edema after glass bead microembolization: Protective effect of granulocytopenia, *J Appl Physiol* 52: 155-161, 1982.
171. Fox RB, Hoidal JR, Brown DM, Repine JE: Pulmonary inflammation due to oxygen toxicity: Involvement of chemotactic factors and polymorphonuclear leukocytes, *Am Rev Respir Dis* 123:521-523, 1981.
172. Shasby DM, Fox RB, Harada RN, Repine JE: Reduction of the edema of acute hyperoxic lung injury by granulocyte depletion, *J Appl Physiol* 52:1237-1244, 1982.
173. Raj JU, Hazinski TA, Bland RD: Oxygen-induced lung microvascular injury in neutropenic rabbits and lambs, *J Appl Physiol* 58:921-927, 1985.
174. Clement A, Chadelat K, Sardet A, Grimfeld A, Tournier G: Alveolar macrophage status in bronchopulmonary dysplasia, *Pediatr Res* 23: 470-473, 1988.
175. Hoidal JR, Beall GD, Repine JE: Production of hydroxyl radical by human alveolar macrophages, *Infect Immunol* 26:1088-1092, 1979.
176. Freeman BA, Crapo JD: Hyperoxia increases oxygen radical production in rat lungs and lung mitochondria, *J Biol Chem* 256:10986-10992, 1981.
177. Frank L, Sosenko IRS: Prenatal development of lung antioxidant enzymes in four species, *J Pediatr* 110:106-110, 1987
178. Tanswell AK, Freeman BA: Liposome-entrapped antioxidant enzymes prevent lethal O_2 toxicity in the newborn rat, *J Appl Physiol* 63:347-352, 1987.
179. Frank L, Summerville J, Massaro D: Protection from oxygen toxicity with endotoxin, *J Clin Invest* 65:1104-1110, 1980.
180. Hazinski TA, Kennedy KA, France ML, Hansen TM: Pulmonary O_2 toxicity in lambs: physiological and biochemical effects of endotoxin infusion, *J Appl Physiol* 65:1579-1585, 1988.
181. Hazinski TA, France ML, Kennedy KA: Cimetidine reduces hyperoxic lung injury in lambs, *J Appl Physiol* 67:1586-1592, 1989.
182. McMillan DD, Boyd GN: The role of antioxidants and diet in the prevention or treatment of oxygen-induced lung microvascular injury, *Ann NY Acad Sci* 384:535-543, 1982.
183. Sosenko IRS, Innis SM, Frank L: Polyunsaturated fatty acids and protection of newborn rats from oxygen toxicity, *J Pediatr* 112:630-637, 1988.
184. Rojas J, Green RS, Hellerqvist CG, Olegard R, Brigham KL, Stahlman MT: Studies on group B β-hemolytic Streptococcus. II. Effects on pulmonary hemodynamics and vascular permeability in unanesthetized sheep, *Pediatr Res* 15:899-904, 1981.
185. Rojas J, Larsson LE, Hellerqvist CG, Brigham KL, Gray ME, Stahlman MT: Pulmonary hemodynamic and ultrastructural changes associated with group B streptococcal toxemia in adult sheep and newborn lambs, *Pediatr Res* 17:1002-1008, 1983.
186. Rojas J, Larsson LE, Ogletree ML, Brigham KL, Stahlman M: Effects of cyclooxygenase inhibition on the response to group B streptococcal toxin in sheep, *Pediatr Res* 17:107-110, 1983.
187. Rojas J, Palme C, Ogletree ML, Hellerqvist CG, Brigham KL, Stahlman MT: Effects of methylprednisolone on the response to group B streptococcal toxin in sheep, *Pediatr Res* 18:1141-1144, 1984.
188. Sandberg,K, Engelhardt B, Hellerqvist C, Sundell H: Pulmonary response to group β-streptococcal toxin in young lambs, *J Appl Physiol* 63:2024-2030, 1987.
189. Ohkuda K, Nakahara K, Binder A, Staub N: Venous air emboli in sheep: Reversible increase in lung microvascular permeability, *J Appl Physiol* 51:887-894, 1981.
190. Henson PM, McArthy K, Larsen GL, Webster RO, Gidas PC, Dreisin RB, King TE, Shaw JO: Complement fragments, alveolar macrophages and alveolitis, *Am J Pathol* 97:93-110, 1979.
191. Albertine KH, Wiener-Kronish JP, Koike K, Staub NC: Quantification of damage by air emboli to lung microvessels in anesthetized sheep, *J Appl Physiol* 57:1360-1368, 1984.
192. Berner ME, Teague WG Jr, Scheerer RG, Bland RD: Furosemide reduces lung fluid filtration in lambs with lung microvascular injury from air emboli, *J Appl Physiol* 67:1990-1996, 1989.
193. Malik AB: Pulmonary microembolism, *Physiol Rev* 63:1114-1207, 1983.
194. Nadel JA, Colebatch HJH, Olsen CR: Location and mechanism of airway constriction after barium sulfate microembolism, *J Appl Physiol* 19:387-394, 1964.
195. Bland RD, McMillan DD, Bressack MA: Decreased pulmonary transvascular fluid filtration in awake newborn lambs after intravenous furosemide, *J Clin Invest* 62:601-609, 1978.
196. Dikshit K, Vyden JK, Forrester JS: Renal and extrarenal hemodynamic effects of furosemide in congestive heart failure after acute myocardial infarction, *N Engl J Med* 288:1087-1090, 1978.
197. Green TP, Johnson DE, Bass JL, Landrum BG, Ferrara B, Thompson TR: Prophylactic furosemide in severe respiratory distress syndrome: blinded prospective study, *J Pediatr* 112:605-612, 1988.
198. Green TP, Thompson TR, Johnson DE, Lock JE: Diuresis and pulmonary function in premature infants with respiratory distress syndrome, *J Pediatr* 103:618-623, 1983.
199. Marks KH, Berman W, Friedman Z, Whitman Y, Lee C, Maisels MJ: Furosemide in hyaline membrane disease, *Pediatrics* 62:785-788, 1978.
200. Savage MO, Wilkinson AR, Baum JD, Roberton NR: Furosemide in respiratory distress syndrome, *Arch Dis Child* 50:709-713, 1975.
201. Jobe A, Ikegami M, Jacobs H, Jones S, Conaway D: Permeability of premature lamb lungs to protein and the effect of surfactant on that permeability, *J Appl Physiol* 55:169-176, 1983.
202. Nilsson R, Grossman G, Robertson B: Lung surfactant and the pathogenesis of neonatal bronchiolar lesions induced by artificial ventilation, *Pediatr Res* 12:249-255, 1978.
203. Jobe A, Jacobs H, Ikegami M, Berry D: Lung protein leaks in ventilated lambs: effect of gestational age, *J Appl Physiol* 58:1246-1251, 1985.
204. Gitlin D, Craig JM: The nature of the hyaline membrane in asphyxia of the newborn, *Pediatrics* 17:64-71, 1956.
205. Dreyfuss D, Basset G, Soler P, Saumon G: Intermittent positive-pressure hyperventilation with high inflation pressures produces pulmonary microvascular injury in rats, *Am Rev Respir Dis* 132:880-884, 1985.
206. Dreyfuss D, Soler P, Basset G, Saumon G: High inflation pressure pulmonary edema. Respective effects of high airway pressure, high tidal volume, and positive end-expiratory pressure, *Am Rev Respir Dis* 137: 1159-1164, 1988.
207. Parker JC, Townsley MI, Rippe B, Taylor AE, Thigpen J: Increased microvascular permeability in dog lungs due to high peak airway pressures, *J Appl Physiol* 57:1809-1816, 1984.
208. Hernandez LA, Peevy KJ, Moise AA, Parker JC: Chest wall restriction limits high airway pressure-induced lung injury in young rabbits, *J Appl Physiol* 66:2364-2368, 1989.
209. Evans HE, Keller S, Mandl I: Serum trypsin inhibitory capacity and the idiopathic respiratory distress syndrome, *J Pediatr* 81:588-592, 1982.
210. Evans HE, Levi M, Mandl I: Serum enzyme inhibitor concentrations in the respiratory distress syndrome, *Am Rev Respir Dis* 101:359-363, 1970.

211. Kotas RV, Fazen LE, Moore TE: Umbilical cord serum trypsin inhibitor capacity and the idiopathic respiratory distress syndrome, *J Pediatr* 81:593-599, 1982.
212. Makram WE, Johnson AM: Serum proteinase inhibitors in infants with hyaline membrane disease, *J Pediatr* 81:579-587, 1972.
213. Mathis RK, Freier EF, Hunt CE, Krivit W, Sharp HL: Alpha$_1$-antitrypsin in the respiratory distress syndrome, *N Engl J Med* 288:59-64, 1973.
214. Merritt TA, Cochrane CG, Holcomb K, Bohl B, Hallman M, Strayer D, Edwards DK, Gluck L: Elastase and α-proteinase inhibitor activity in tracheal aspirates during respiratory distress syndrome, *J Clin Invest* 72:656-666, 1983.
215. Ogden BE, Murphy SA, Saunders GC, Pathak D, Johnson JD: Neonatal lung neutrophils and elastase/proteinase inhibitor imbalance, *Am Rev Respir Dis* 130:817-821, 1984.
216. Speed CP, Ruess D, Harms K, Herting E, Gefeller O: Neutrophil elastase and acute pulmonary damage in neonates with severe respiratory distress syndrome, *Pediatrics* 91:794-799, 1993.
217. Groneck P, Gotze-Speer B, Oppermann M, Eiffert H, Speed CP: Association of pulmonary inflammation and increased microvascular permeability during the development of bronchopulmonary dysplasia: a sequential analysis of inflammatory mediators in respiratory fluid of high-risk preterm neonates, *Pediatrics* 93:712-718, 1994.
218. Normand ICS, Reynolds EOR, Strang LB, Wigglesworth JS: Flow and protein concentration of lymph from lungs of lambs developing hyaline membrane disease, *Arch Dis Child* 43:334-339, 1968.
219. Reynolds EOR, Jacobson HN, Motoyama EK, Kikkawa Y, Craig JM, Orzalesi MM, Cook CD: The effect of immaturity and prenatal asphyxia on the lungs and pulmonary function of newborn lambs: the experimental production of respiratory distress, *Pediatrics* 35:382-392, 1965.
220. Stahlman M, LeQuire VS, Young WC, Merrill RE, Birmingham RT, Payne GA, Gray J: Pathophysiology of respiratory distress in newborn lambs, *Am J Dis Child* 108:375-393, 1964.
221. Carlton DP, Cho SC, Davis P, Lont M, Bland RD: Surfactant treatment at birth reduces lung vascular injury and edema in preterm lambs, *Pediatr Res* 37:265-270, 1995.
222. Carlton DP, Cho SC, Davis P, Bland RD: Inflation pressure and lung vascular injury in preterm lambs, *Chest* 105:115S-116S, 1994.
223. Carlton DP, Albertine KH, Cho SC, Davis PL, Long M, Bland RD: Role of neutrophils in lung vascular injury and edema after premature birth in lambs, *J Appl Physiol* 83:1307-1317, 1997.
224. Jackson JC, Chi EY, Wilson CB, Truog WE, Teh EC, Hodson WA: Sequence of inflammatory cell migration into lung during recovery from hyaline membrane disease in premature newborn monkeys, *Am Rev Respir Dis* 135:937-940, 1987.
225. Jones CA, Cayabyab RG, Kwong KY, Stotts C, Wong B, Hamdan H, Minoo P, DeLemos RA: Undetectable interleukin (IL)-10 and persistent IL-8 expression early in hyaline membrane disease: a possible developmental basis for the predisposition to chronic lung inflammation in preterm newborns, *Pediatr Res* 39:966-975, 1996.
226. Albertine KH, Carlton DP, Cho S, Davis PL, Bland RD: Histopathology of chronic lung injury in preterm lambs, *FASEB* 9:A275, 1995.
227. Bland RD, Cho SC, Carlton D, Albertine K, Davis P: Chronic lung injury in mechanically ventilated preterm lambs, *FASEB J* 9:A275, 1995.
228. Clements, JA: Pulmonary edema and permeability of alveolar membranes, *Arch Environ Health* 2:280-283, 1961.
229. Pattle RE: Properties, function and origin of the alveolar lining layer, *Proc R Soc Lond* Ser B 148:217-240, 1958.
230. Mellins RB, Levine OR, Skalak R, Fishman AP: Interstitial pressure of the lung, *Circ Res* 24:197-212, 1969.
231. Hansen TN, Gest AL, Landers S: Inspiratory airway obstruction does not affect lung fluid balance in lambs, *J Appl Physiol* 58:1314-1318, 1985.
232. DeSa DJ: Pulmonary fluid content in infants with respiratory distress, *J Pathol* 97:469-479, 1969.
233. Lauweryns JM: Hyaline membrane disease: a pathological study of 55 infants, *Arch Dis Child* 40:618-625, 1965.
234. Rudolph AM, Drorbaugh JE, Auld PAM, Rudolph AJ, Nadas AS, Smith CA, Hubbell JP: Studies on the circulation in the neonatal period. The circulation in the respiratory distress syndrome, *Pediatrics* 27:551-566, 1961.
235. Wu PYK: Colloid oncotic pressure: Current status and clinical applications in neonatal medicine, *Clin Perinatol* 9:645-657, 1982.
236. Jefferies AL, Coates G, O'Brodovich H: Pulmonary epithelial permeability in hyaline-membrane disease, *N Engl J Med* 311:1075-1080, 1984.
237. Albert RK, Lakshminarayan S, Hildebrandt J, Kirk W: Increased surface tension favors pulmonary edema formation in anesthetized dogs' lungs, *J Clin Invest* 63:1015-1018, 1979.
238. Juul SE, Kinsella MG, Jackson JC, Truog WE, Standaert TA, Hodson WA: Changes in hyaluronan deposition during early respiratory distress syndrome in premature monkeys, *Pediatr Res* 35:238-243, 1994.

CHAPTER 58

Cor Pulmonale and Pulmonary Complications of Cardiac Abnormalities

Steven H. Abman

Abnormalities of the pulmonary circulation contribute significantly to morbidity and mortality in many cardiac and pulmonary diseases of childhood. The pulmonary circulation can be altered by primary aberrations of lung growth or development (such as lung hypoplasia, pulmonary hemangiomatosis, arteriovenous fistula, anomalous pulmonary venous return, pulmonary venoocclusive disease, and others), or secondary injury associated with acute respiratory failure, chronic lung disease, chronic hypoventilation, and congenital heart disease. Whereas the impact of pulmonary hypertension on the clinical course of children with congenital heart disease, persistent pulmonary hypertension of the newborn, and primary pulmonary hypertension are most clearly appreciated, the contribution of pulmonary hypertension to the course and ultimate outcome of children with lung disease is often overlooked or underestimated. Pulmonary hypertension is too often a "silent" contributor to morbidity and mortality of many chronic lung disorders in pediatrics, including chronic neonatal lung disease (CNLD), cystic fibrosis (CF), sickle cell anemia, and various interstitial lung diseases.[1-9] For example, 42% of pediatric patients with interstitial lung disease have evidence of pulmonary hypertension early in their clinical course.[8] Progressive pul-

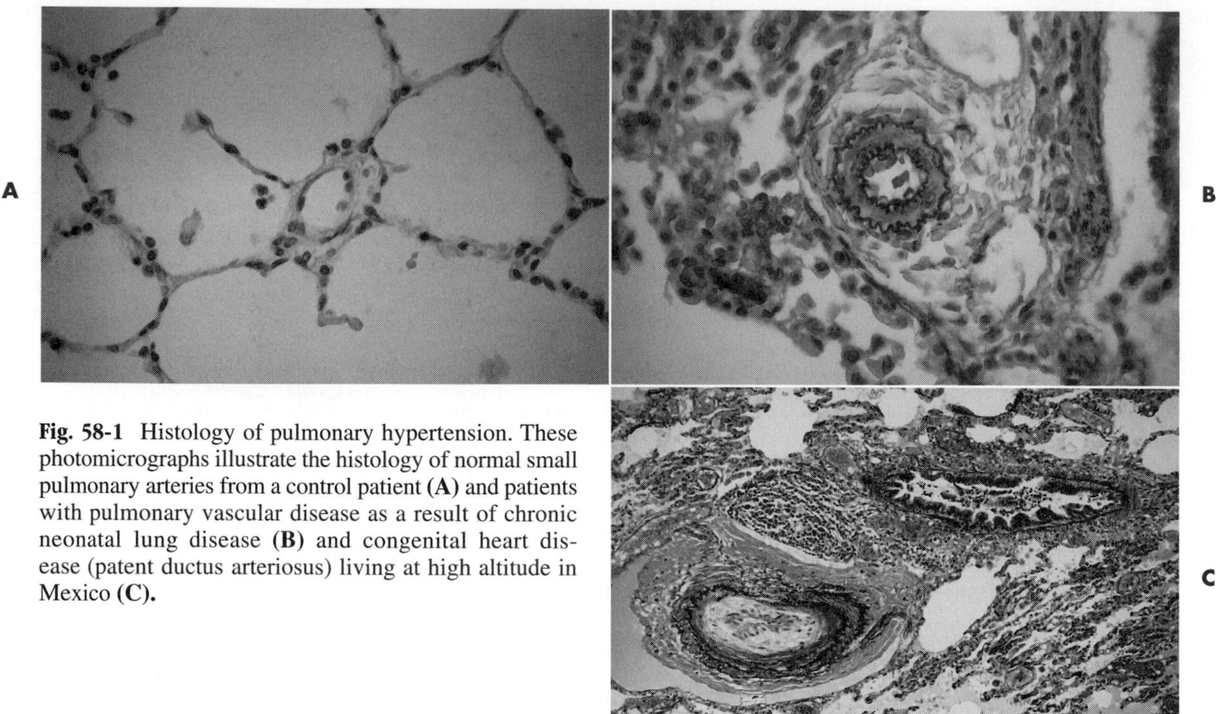

Fig. 58-1 Histology of pulmonary hypertension. These photomicrographs illustrate the histology of normal small pulmonary arteries from a control patient **(A)** and patients with pulmonary vascular disease as a result of chronic neonatal lung disease **(B)** and congenital heart disease (patent ductus arteriosus) living at high altitude in Mexico **(C).**

monary hypertension and cor pulmonale, beginning in the pediatric age range, is a common cause of death in chronic diseases such as sickle cell anemia.[7] In general, clinical strategies that anticipate the development of pulmonary hypertension may allow earlier recognition, more aggressive therapy, and may slow the development of pulmonary hypertension and related cardiac sequelae in many chronic lung diseases.

Although some disease mechanisms and the clinical management of pulmonary hypertension in pediatric patients are similar to adults with pulmonary hypertension, many aspects of pulmonary vascular disease in children are quite unique. In contrast to pulmonary vascular disease in adults, pediatric pulmonary hypertension is intrinsically linked to issues of lung growth and development, including many prenatal, perinatal, and later postnatal events. First, the development of pulmonary hypertension in the neonate and young infant reflects the interplay between the normal transition of the pulmonary circulation from fetal to postnatal life. Second, the timing of pulmonary vascular injury is an important determinant of the subsequent response of the developing lung to such adverse stimuli as hypoxia, hypertension, high flow, inflammation, and others.[10] Third, just as the proliferative response of the pulmonary vasculature may be more pronounced in the young lung,[10] it is possible that the developing lung may also have more potential for recovery over time after removal of an adverse stimulus.[11] However, the impact of pulmonary hypertension on long-term outcome is strikingly different among various pediatric cardiac and respiratory disorders. For example, pulmonary hypertension in infants with CNLD is often present early but frequently resolves with therapy over time[1,12]; in contrast, pulmonary hypertension develops late in patients with CF and accompanies the steady decline in lung function.[5,6] Thus in young children and infants with chronic lung disease, changes in the pulmonary circulation and the right side of the heart represent an interplay between normal developmental changes and superimposed cardiovascular and pulmonary stresses (Fig. 58-1).

The purpose of this chapter is to provide a brief overview of the disease mechanisms, evaluation, and treatment of pulmonary hypertension and cor pulmonale associated with acute and chronic lung diseases in pediatric patients. In addition, related cardiopulmonary interactions, including respiratory complications of cardiac abnormalities, are briefly reviewed. Pulmonary hypertension caused by congenital heart disease, vascular rings and slings, vascular anomalies (such as associated with pulmonary sequestration or lung agenesis), and primary pulmonary hypertension are discussed in other chapters.

DEFINITIONS OF COR PULMONALE AND PULMONARY HYPERTENSION

Cor pulmonale is synonymous with *pulmonary heart disease,* and represents the adaptive response of the right ventricle to increased afterload caused by pulmonary hypertension.[13] Historically, cor pulmonale has been defined as "*hypertrophy* of the right ventricle resulting from diseases affecting the function and/or structure of the lung except where the pulmonary alterations are the result of diseases that primarily affect the left side of the heart or of congenital heart disease."[14] Right-ventricular (RV) hypertrophy occurs in response to chronic increases in RV afterload. Although the term *cor pulmonale* has often been reserved for patients with overt signs of RV failure, such signs are generally present very late in the clinical course of pulmonary heart disease. Furthermore, clinical signs of overt right-sided heart failure can easily be masked by signs of severe chronic respiratory disease. A more clinically useful definition of cor pulmonale is the involvement of the right ventricle (either hypertrophy, dilation, or failure), as detected by clinical signs, chest radiograph, electrocardiogram (ECG), echocardiogram, cardiac catheterization, or autopsy, which is caused by altered pulmonary structure and function, provided that the changes are not the result of diseases primarily involving the left or right side of the heart. This is a more expansive definition because signs of advanced right-sided heart failure need not be present.[15]

Although the actual incidence of pulmonary hypertension and cor pulmonale in pediatric patients is uncertain, their impact on the clinical course of many children with severe lung disease is clear. The definition of pulmonary hypertension depends on age and altitude of residence. When directly measured by pulmonary artery catheterization, a mean pulmonary artery pressure (PAP) greater than 20 mm Hg is considered abnormal beyond infancy. During the early neonatal period, mean PAP gradually falls from systemic levels immediately at birth to adult values by 3 to 4 months. Functionally, PAP is often considered to be clinically significant at a ratio or proportion of mean systemic arterial pressure greater than 50% systemic arterial pressure. ECG and echocardiogram criteria for pulmonary hypertension are discussed in the following section.

CLINICAL SETTINGS ASSOCIATED WITH PULMONARY HYPERTENSION

Pulmonary hypertension can occur as part of an acute or chronic cardiorespiratory process (Box 58-1). For example, high-altitude pulmonary edema (HAPE) or acute hypoxemic respiratory failure in a previously healthy child can cause moderate elevations of PAP as well as increased vascular permeability and altered vasoreactivity. The severity of pulmonary hypertension in response to acute respiratory disease depends in part on age, the presence of underlying cardiac or respiratory disease, genetic makeup, and other factors (discussed in a later section). For example, neonates with acute respiratory failure often have striking elevations in PAP, which may cause right-to-left shunting across the patent ductus arteriosus or foramen ovale, causing more marked hypoxemia. More commonly, pulmonary hypertension and cor pulmonale are recognized in association with chronic lung, neuromuscular, or cardiac diseases. Disorders commonly associated with chronic hypoxia can be divided into those associated with intrinsic lung disease or with hypoventilation caused by neurologic or muscular impairment. Although chronic hypoxia contributes to the development and progression of pulmonary hypertension, pulmonary hypertension often occurs in settings where chronic inflammation and other stimuli are important etiologic factors as well (discussed later). The severity of pulmonary hypertension and degree of RV hypertrophy are likely related to the timing of injury (e.g., interruption of the normal decline in right ventricular predominance during early infancy), duration of pulmonary hypertension, and the presence or absence of left-sided congenital heart disease. Pulmonary venous obstruction, due to venoocclusive disease or abnormal pulmonary venous return, can masquerade as interstitial lung disease.[8,16] Pulmonary hypertension is associated with high mortality in many chronic lung diseases, including BPD, CF, and interstitial lung disease. It clearly remains a leading cause of death in BPD, but in many settings, it is unclear whether RV hypertrophy serves as an important marker of advanced disease or an actual cause of death. Similarly, cor pulmonale is present in more than 70% of patients dying with CF,[5] but whether aggressive treatment of pulmonary hypertension will alter outcome is unknown.

BOX 58-1
Diseases Associated with Pulmonary Hypertension in Pediatrics

Pulmonary vascular diseases

Persistent pulmonary hypertension of the newborn (PPHN), idiopathic
Primary, or "unexplained" pulmonary hypertension
Abnormalities of pulmonary vascular growth, including:
- lung hypoplasia, congenital diaphragmatic hernia
- alveolar-capillary dysplasia
- pulmonary venoocclusive disease
- pulmonary hemangiomatosis, lymphangiectasia
- peripheral pulmonary arterial stenosis

Secondary causes of pediatric pulmonary hypertension

Associated with neonatal lung diseases:
- hyaline membrane disease, meconium aspiration, pneumonia, sepsis, congenital diaphragmatic hernia, others

Congenital heart disease
Acute hypoxemic respiratory failure
High-altitude pulmonary edema
Chronic lung disease:
- CNLD, CF, interstitial lung diseases

Chronic upper airway obstruction
Chronic hypoventilation:
- neuromuscular disease, abnormal chest wall or diaphragm function
- central hypoventilation syndromes

Sickle cell anemia, hematologic disorders, vasculitis
Drug- or toxin-induced (toxic oil syndrome, aminorex) portal hypertension
Thromboembolic diseases:
- protein C and protein S deficiencies, lupus anticoagulant, antithrombin III deficiency

Lung transplantation
Tuberculosis, schistosomiasis
Cardiomyopathy, left-sided cardiovascular obstruction:
- TAPVR, cor triatriatum, mitral valve stenosis, severe LV failure

DEVELOPMENTAL PHYSIOLOGY OF THE PULMONARY CIRCULATION

Insight into pulmonary hypertension in infants and young children must begin with an understanding of normal growth and development of the perinatal lung, mechanisms that contribute to the normal postnatal adaptation of the pulmonary circulation after birth and during infancy, and unique responses of the developing lung circulation to injury.

Fetal Pulmonary Circulation

Development of the pulmonary circulation in utero is characterized by early growth of large central arteries with the subsequent development of the microcirculation later in gestation.[17] By the 16th week of gestation, all bronchial airway generations have formed along with their accompanying conducting pulmonary arteries. During the third trimester, pulmonary vascular surface area increases tenfold with the concomitant development of the distal airway, alveolar ducts, and saccules. In addition to increases in pulmonary artery number, changes in pulmonary vascular structure also occur with development. In the normal fetus, small pulmonary arteries associated with the respiratory bronchioles, alveolar ducts, and saccules have minimal smooth muscle (Fig. 58-2).[18] As the pulmonary circulation develops, pulmonary arteries acquire a

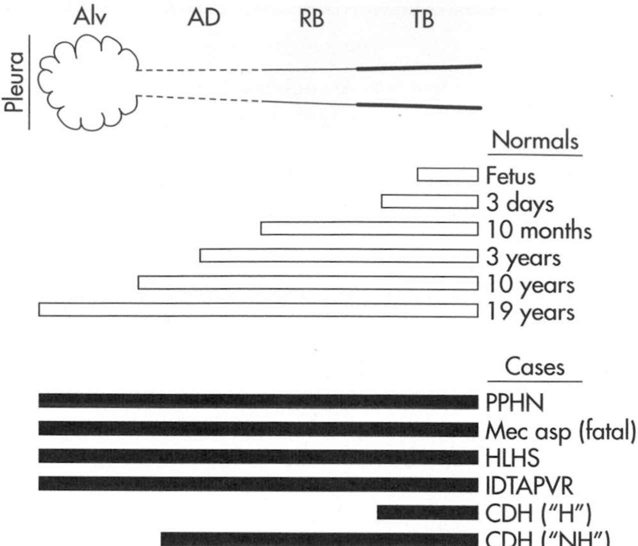

Fig. 58-2 Maturational changes in the distribution of smooth muscle in the fetal and postnatal pulmonary circulation. Small pulmonary arteries that accompany the respiratory bronchioles (*RB*), alveolar ducts (*AD*), and alveoli (*Alv*) lack muscularization during fetal life, and extension of smooth muscle occurs throughout childhood. Neonates dying with persistent pulmonary hypertension (*PPHN*), meconium aspiration (*Mec asp*), hypoplastic left heart syndrome (*HLHS*), infradiaphragmatic total anomalous pulmonary venous return (*IDTAPVR*), and congenital diaphragmatic hernia (*CDH*) without a 'honeymoon' period ("NH") demonstrate increased muscularization of small preacinar and acinar vessels, suggesting altered intrauterine growth. (From Reid L, Fried R, Geggel R, Langleben D: Anatomy of pulmonary hypertensive states. In Bergofsky EF, ed: *Abnormal pulmonary circulation,* New York, 1986, Churchill Livingstone, p 227.)

muscle coat, whose thickness is proportionate to vessel size. At birth, few intraacinar arteries are muscularized, and vascular smooth muscle cells differentiate in distal arteries with normal postnatal growth. Larger arteries (>200 μ) are muscularized early, and intermediate pulmonary arteries have variable medial coats, appearing either fully, partially, or nonmuscularized.[18] The apparent lack of extension of smooth muscle in small pulmonary arteries has been misinterpreted to suggest that the pulmonary circulation after premature delivery lacks the ability to vasoconstrict and that pulmonary vasospasm plays a little role in premature infants with respiratory failure. More recent studies have demonstrated that high pulmonary vascular resistance (PVR) in premature neonates can be the result of active vasoconstriction, suggesting a role for vasodilator therapy in some newborns with severe hyaline membrane disease.[20]

The fetal pulmonary circulation receives less than 8% of combined ventricular output as a result of its high basal PVR, causing most of the RV output to cross the ductus arteriosus to the aorta, bypassing the lung.[21] Despite the apparent low level of pulmonary blood flow, it remains essential for providing adequate substrate to allow lung growth, as pulmonary artery ligation in the late-gestation fetal lamb causes lung hypoplasia.[22] During late gestation, pulmonary blood flow increases in proportion to lung weight and increased vascular cross-sectional area, as the number of blood vessels increase more than tenfold. Although flow increases with advancing gestation, mean PAP increases as well, and when corrected for lung weight, PVR increases with gestational age. Mechanisms maintaining high fetal PVR include physical stimuli, such as the lack of a gas-liquid interface and rhythmic distention of the lung. In addition, low oxygen tension (normal fetal Pa_{O_2} is 20 to 25 mm Hg), low basal production of endogenous dilator products (such as prostacyclin and nitric oxide [NO][23-26]), and increased production of vasoconstrictor substances (including endothelin-1[27-29] and leukotrienes[30]) also contribute to high PVR in utero.

In addition to the structural changes previously described, marked changes in pulmonary vascular tone and reactivity also occur with development.[31] For example, experimental studies of maturational changes of pulmonary vasoregulation suggest that endogenous NO production modulates basal fetal PVR and that the fetal smooth muscle is responsive to vasodilators, such as NO or NO-donors, quite early in gestation.[32-34] Maturational changes in endothelial and smooth muscle function contribute to the regulation of vascular tone in fetal life (Fig. 58-3).

The distal lung develops extensively during the third trimester, including a dramatic increase in small pulmonary arteries, which continues during the first few years after birth.[35] With premature birth, the normal sequence of lung growth and development is disrupted, and at least in children requiring mechanical ventilation because of hyaline membrane disease, lung growth may be severely impaired by hyperoxia, barotrauma, and inflammation, causing CNLD.[36] In older patients dying with CNLD, lung septation and capillary surface area are markedly decreased.[37,38] As a result, premature birth, respiratory distress, and sequelae of its treatment remain major causes of pulmonary hypertension in infancy (as discussed later).

During late gestation, intrauterine stimuli, such as systemic or pulmonary hypertension, can alter vascular growth in response, leading to striking hypertensive remodeling or decreased vessel number. Although exact mechanisms causing vascular remodeling are incompletely understood, experimental studies suggest that intrauterine hypertension may be more critical than chronic hypoxia in the pathogenesis of structural and functional impairment during the transition at birth.[39-42] Partial compression or early closure of the ductus arteriosus in fetal lambs alters vascular reactivity and lung structure, leading to the failure of postnatal adaptation at delivery, providing an experimental model of persistent pulmonary hypertension of the newborn (PPHN).[39,40]

Transitional Pulmonary Circulation

At birth, the pulmonary circulation undergoes a dramatic transition, as pulmonary blood flow rapidly increases eightfold and PAP decrease to levels approximately 50% of systemic arterial pressure.[21] Mechanisms causing this fall in PVR include establishment of an air-liquid interface, rhythmic lung distention with respiration, increased oxygen tension, and altered production of vasoactive substances.[31] Marked stimulation of endogenous NO, primarily the result of increased oxygen and shear stress, contributes substantially to the fall in PVR.[27,43] Similarly, prostacyclin, largely released from increased lung ventilation and shear stress, but not increased oxygen, also contributes to postnatal adaptation.[44,45] Decreased production or responsiveness to local vasoconstrictors, such as leukotrienes or endothelin-1, may also contribute to the normal fall in PVR.[29] A concomitant structural reorganization of small pulmonary arteries occurs, as the vascular endothelium is flattened with high flow, and vascular dimensions change

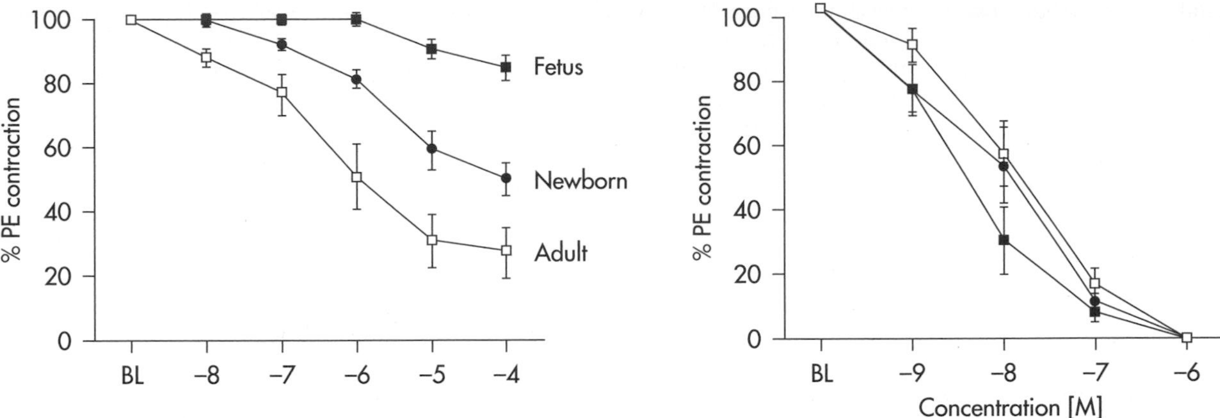

Fig. 58-3 Maturation-related changes in pulmonary vasodilation to endothelium dependent and independent stimuli. In comparison with neonatal and adult pulmonary arteries, pulmonary arteries isolated from late-gestation fetal lambs have diminished relaxation to acetylcholine (*ACH*), an endothelium-dependent agonist (*left*). In contrast, the relaxation to sodium nitroprusside (*SNP*), an agent that directly stimulates smooth muscle cell relaxation, causes marked relaxation at each age (*right*). These findings suggest that maturational changes occur in endothelial function but that vascular smooth muscle is able to respond to vasodilator stimuli early in development. (From Abman SH, Chatfield BA, Rodman DM, Hall SL, McMurty IF: *Am J Physiol* 260:L280-L285, 1991.)

rapidly with birth.[46] Progressive pulmonary vascular dilation, recruitment, and structural adaptations are reflected by further decreases in resistance during late infancy, when adult values of PVR are achieved.

The pulmonary circulation during this transitional period (at birth and during early infancy) may be particularly sensitive to injury. Not only is this a time period of rapid vessel growth, but functional changes in vascular tone and reactivity occur with age as well. Such developmental aspects of the pulmonary circulation not only are important in regard to PPHN, congenital heart disease, and CNLD, but also have clinical ramifications in other settings of pediatric pulmonary hypertension. As suggested in two experimental models of chronic pulmonary hypertension, the immature or infant lung circulation may not only be more susceptible to injury, but it may also be uniquely capable of recovering more readily than adult circulation.[10,11] Insight into responses of the developing lung to growth factors, vasoactive mediators, and related stimuli are likely to provide novel approaches toward the management of pediatric pulmonary hypertension.

Normal Postnatal Anatomy

Blood flow in the lung has two sources, including the pulmonary and bronchial circulations, which behave differently in health and disease states.[47] The pulmonary circulation includes the RV outflow tract, main pulmonary artery and its major branches to left and right lung, lobar branches, intrapulmonary arteries, arterioles, capillaries, venules, and large pulmonary veins. Normally, the right pulmonary artery divides into a lower branch, which supplies the right middle and lower lobes, and a smaller upper branch to the right upper lobe. The left pulmonary artery lies above the left mainstem bronchus until the first branch, then travels behind the bronchus. Some variability exists with the distribution of smaller arterial branches. There are striking differences in vascular growth and function of vessels throughout the pulmonary circulation, at least partly dependent on their size and location, which may be related to chronic exposure to different hemodynamic forces (discussed in a later section). There are three types of arteries. First, elastic pulmonary arteries (>1000 μm external diameter) consist of distinctive layers of elastic fibers in a coat of smooth muscle cells in central pulmonary arteries and extralobular pulmonary arteries. Second, muscular pulmonary arteries (100 to 1000 μm external diameter) have a thin medial layer of muscle between internal and external elastic laminae, which is usually less than 5% of the vessel's external diameter. Muscular arteries accompany bronchioles within lobules. Normal muscle layer remains. Third, pulmonary arterioles (<100 μm external diameter) are the terminal branches of the pulmonary arterial tree and, at their origin from muscular arteries, contain a partial layer of muscle that gradually disappears. Pulmonary arterioles supply alveolar ducts and alveoli.

Two types of small pulmonary artery branches have been described, including "conventional" branches, which accompany airways, and "supernumerary" branches, which travel alone and are usually smaller. Conventional arteries branch from main arterial channels and extend to the periphery, at the end of the respiratory bronchioles. Supernumerary vessels outnumber the conventional branches, constituting 25% of the total cross-sectional area of the pulmonary arterial bed near the hilum and about 40% at the periphery. Supernumerary arteries are present at birth and can participate in gas exchange. Extensive growth of conventional and supernumerary branches accompanies the development of new alveolar ducts and alveoli and contributes to the progressive increase in surface area during the first few years of life.[35] After 18 months, the number of conventional arteries is fixed, but supernumerary arteries continue to increase with septation and formation of new alveoli (up to 3 to 7 years of age).

The microcirculation consists of small capillaries that form an extensive network in interalveolar septae. Capillaries are mostly composed of cytoplasmic extensions of endothelial cells, which, by their contiguous arrangement, form a thin vascular tube. Both the endothelium and the neighboring alveolar epithelium lie on separate basement membranes. Fusion of endothelial and epithelial basement membranes cover half of the capillary border, forming the thin portion of the alveolar-capillary membrane, which provides the site for gas exchange. For the other half of the capillary perimeter, these basement membranes remain separated by an interstitial space and are sites for liquid and solute exchange.

Arterial and venous blood supplies of pulmonary lobules differ anatomically. A lobule consists of a cluster of three to five terminal bronchioles, and neighboring lobules are partly contained by connective tissue septae. Branches of pulmonary arteries and small bronchi travel together, supplying terminal respiratory units within a single lobule. In contrast, pulmonary veins drain blood from several different lobules. Normal veins have less muscularity and much thinner walls than arteries, but like arteries, veins are either conventional or supernumerary. Small intrapulmonary venules successively fuse to form increasingly larger veins until a lobar vein emerges from each lobe. The right upper and middle lobe veins usually combine; thus there are superior and inferior pulmonary veins from each lung. Although the branching pattern of the airways increases the cross-sectional area of the bronchial tree longitudinally, the cross-sectional area of the vascular bed gets smaller from the central vessels to the arterioles or venules. Most of the blood in the pulmonary circulation is contained in large, not small, vessels. Velocity of blood flow in arteries decreases as vessels get smaller, but the decrease is not as marked as with airways.

Although the bronchial circulation normally receives only 1% to 2% of the total cardiac output, it provides flow, which is essential for maintaining normal lung growth and function.[48] The bronchial circulation is the principal source of nutrient blood and oxygen to airways (large and small), pulmonary nerves and ganglia, walls of elastic and some muscular pulmonary arteries and veins, lymph nodes and connective tissue septae, and the pleura. Bronchial blood flow may increase substantially with pathologic conditions, such as in diseases associated with chronic inflammation and injury (such as CF, CNLD, and bronchiectasis).[49,50] Acute increases in bronchial flow may also contribute to lung edema with acute lung injury.[50] There is marked variability of bronchial branching patterns; 40% of children have one bronchial artery to each lung. Bronchial blood returns to the heart via bronchial veins, from branches perfusing the lobar and segmental bronchi and from branches from the pleura near the hilus. Bronchial venous blood empties into the azygos, hemiazygos, or intercostal veins and then flows into the right atrium. Veins that originate from bronchial capillaries within the lung unite to form tributaries that join pulmonary veins (bronchopulmonary veins). Blood leaving the capillary bed near terminal bronchioles flows through anastomoses with the alveolar capillaries, and the mixture of blood returns to the left atrium through pulmonary veins. About one fourth to one third of blood goes to the right atrium via bronchial veins; the remainder flows to the left atrium via pulmonary veins.

Normal Postnatal Physiology

Although the lungs normally receive the entire cardiac output, PAP remains low because of the low basal vascular resistance. The distribution of pulmonary flow within the lung is nonuniform and depends partly on relationships among gravity, alveolar pressure, PAP, and pulmonary venous or left-atrial pressure.[47,51] Three zones have been proposed to explain regional variations in flow (Fig. 58-4). In zone 1, normal PAP is insufficient to perfuse the uppermost regions of the lung, and pulmonary capillaries are collapsed because alveolar pressure exceeds pulmonary arterial and venous pressures. Pulmonary blood flow begins at the top of zone 2, as PAP exceeds alveolar pressure, and continues to increase with increased PAP. As alveolar pressure is greater than pulmonary venous pressure, flow is determined by the difference between pulmonary artery and alveolar pressures. In zone 3, both pulmonary artery and venous pressures exceed alveolar pressure; therefore, driving pressure is determined by the difference between inflow and outflow vascular pressures. In the normal upright adult, most of the lung is in zone 3 conditions. Passive changes in PVR, that is, changes in vessel caliber not caused by active vasoconstriction or vasodilation, are affected by differences between pressures within and surrounding pulmonary blood vessels, shifts of blood into and out of the lungs, and alterations in whole blood viscosity. Changing hydrostatic pressures relative to the height of the lung affects distribution of pulmonary blood flow (for example, distribution of flow is more even while supine than in the upright position). Increased pulmonary artery or left-atrial pressure acutely increases flow, causing a drop in PVR. The longitudinal distribution of PVR in the normal lung using micropipette techniques demonstrated that under zone 3 conditions, the largest contribution to resistance lies in the capillaries of the alveolar septum, with most of the remaining resistance in arterioles, and little contribution from venules to veins (Fig. 58-5).[52]

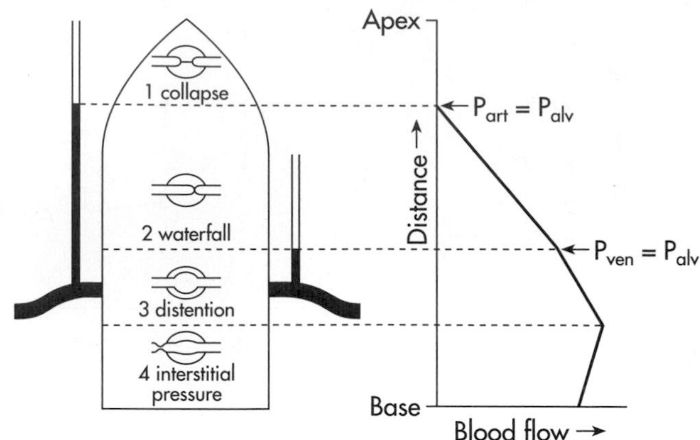

Fig. 58-4 Effects of alveolar, arterial, and venous pressures on regional distribution of blood flow in the pulmonary circulation. (From Murray JF: *The normal lung,* Philadelphia, 1986, WB Saunders, pp 139-150.)

Multiple mechanisms contribute to regulation of vascular tone and distribution of blood flow within the lung. Active and passive changes in PVR during exercise and the regional effects of hypoxia illustrate how the lung can alter distribu-tion of blood flow to sustain gas exchange. Because of its low basal PVR and high compliance, the normal pulmonary circulation tolerates marked increases in flow during exercise, with only small increases in pressure and decreases in PVR. Pulmonary artery and capillary wedge pressures rise, increasing flow to the upper lobes and making overall perfusion more uniform. With high flow with exercise, low PVR is maintained by passive vascular distention,

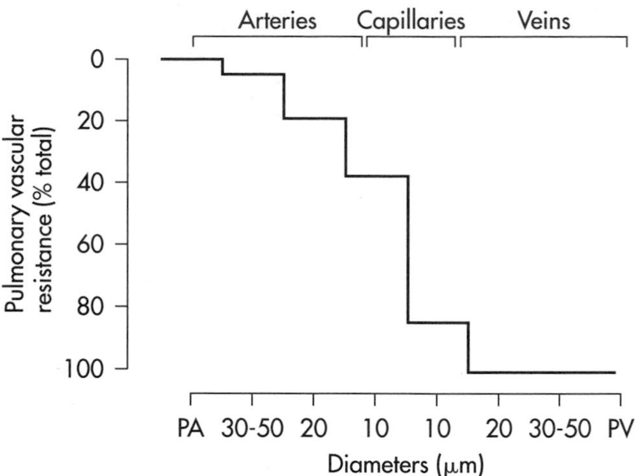

Fig. 58-5 Distribution of resistance in pulmonary circulation from isolated perfused dog lung. (From West JB, Dollery CT, Naimark A: *J Appl Physiol* 19:713-724, 1964.)

recruitment of small pulmonary arteries, and vasodilation. Patients with chronic lung disease can have larger than normal increases in PAP with the increase in pulmonary blood flow during exercise, even with normal resting hemodynamics.

As first described by von Euler,[53] the unique ability of pulmonary arteries to constrict with exposure to low oxygen tension plays a central role in controlling the distribution of blood flow through the lung. Although many vasoactive substances modulate the degree of hypoxic vasoconstriction, hypoxia causes contraction by direct effects on vascular smooth muscle.[54] Regional vasoconstriction redirects blood flow to lung regions with better aeration, allowing for enhanced ventilation-perfusion matching.

In addition to its gas exchange function, the pulmonary circulation also provides nutritional and metabolic support for the lung and is the site for synthesis, storage, and metabolism of various circulating and local vasoactive substances.[55,56] Although past studies primarily emphasized its barrier function, the endothelial cell releases multiple vasoactive products that regulate vascular tone, smooth muscle growth, angiogenesis, liquid and solute transport, thrombosis, synthesis or clearance of circulating hormones, and others. Clinical and experimental studies suggest that vascular metabolic functions are altered with pulmonary vascular injury, contributing to hemodynamic and structural abnormalities in chronic pulmonary hypertension.

DISEASE MECHANISMS

As with pulmonary hypertension in adults, numerous factors contribute to disease severity in pediatric patients, including high basal tone, abnormal vasoreactivity, thrombosis, inflammation, and vascular remodeling. Although pulmonary hypertension occurs in diverse clinical settings, several features are common regardless of the specific disease associated with pulmonary hypertension. First, pulmonary vascular disease is generally associated with changes in both structure and function, and the relative contribution of remodeling with changes in vascular tone is variable even within diseases. Second, pulmonary vascular disorders are commonly associated with altered vascular reactivity, not only high basal pulmonary vacular tone, and exaggerated vasoconstriction to certain stimuli (especially acute hypoxia) are often central pathophysiologic features. For example, altered pulmonary vasoreactivity leads to the vasolability or "flip-flopping" in patients with PPHN,[57] recurrent cyanotic episodes in apparently normal children,[58] recurrent HAPE,[59] sudden death or "dying spells" in CNLD, and other disorders. Mechanisms contributing to heightened pulmonary vasoreactivity are poorly understood, but may include alterations in endothelial-smooth muscle cell interactions. Various factors determine the development and severity of pulmonary hypertension in animal models, including age.[11]

Recent developments in vascular biology have demonstrated that the endothelial cell produces a wide variety of vasoactive compounds, including dilators such as prostacyclin (PgI2), NO, and endothelium-derived hyperpolarizing factor (EDHF).[53,56] In addition, vascular endothelium is further capable of producing potent vasoconstrictors, including endothelin-1, thromboxane, and other endothelium-derived contracting factors. Vascular injury from hemodynamic stresses (high flow, high pressure, shear stress, or stretch), hypoxia, or inflammation may alter endothelial production of these products, creating an imbalance between vasodilators and vasoconstrictors, which favor increased basal tone or heightened vasoreactivity.[60,61] Pulmonary vascular production and responsiveness to many of these products change with normal maturation and postnatal age.[31-33] The effects of vascular injury production of or response to vasoactive agents are currently under active investigation. However, recent in vitro studies of human pulmonary arteries suggest that impaired endogenous NO activity is likely to contribute to heightened pulmonary vasoconstriction in patients with pulmonary hypertension associated with several chronic lung diseases, including CF and chronic obstructive pulmonary disease (COPD) (Fig. 58-6).[62] In addition, increased immunoreactivity and gene expression of endothelin-l is present in lung tissue from adults with severe pulmonary hypertension, suggesting that enhanced endothelin production may also contribute to heightened vasoreactivity and hypertensive vascular remodeling in chronic pulmonary hypertension.[63]

Unlike the pulmonary vascular response to acute hypoxia, prolonged exposure to hypoxia causes sustained elevations of PAP that do not totally improve with return to normal oxygenation. In addition to hypoxia, other mechanisms that contribute to the development of chronic pulmonary hypertension include hemodynamic stresses (increased pressure, flow, shear, stretch, and wall tension), sustained release of vasoactive products and growth factors (inflammatory, autocoids, paracrine mediators, or neurohumoral stimuli), and combinations of these stimuli. Pulmonary vascular responses to these stimuli are also dependent on the strength and duration of the stimulus, the patient's age, genetic factors, infection, inflammation, and others. Whereas the short-term responses to these agonists generally alter vascular tone and reactivity, long-term exposure to the same stimuli is likely to contribute to altered vascular growth and remodeling. Persistent elevation of PAP can be due to at least three general causes, including vasoconstriction, vessel wall proliferation and remodeling, and altered vessel number or surface area.

Pulmonary hypertension is commonly defined as mean pulmonary artery pressure above 25 mm Hg, with normal values reported between 10 and 16 mm Hg. As discussed previously, mean pulmonary artery pressure is roughly 50% of systemic

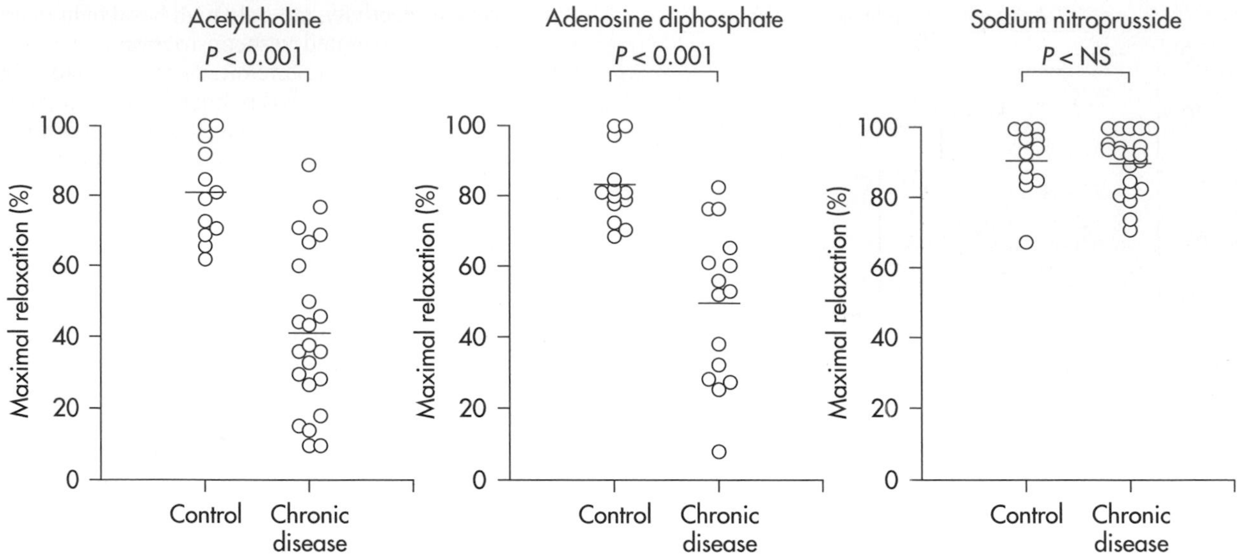

Fig. 58-6 Loss of endothelium-dependent vasorelaxation in pulmonary artery rings from patients with pulmonary hypertension associated with chronic lung disease. (From Battacharya J, Staub NC: *Science* 210:327-328, 1980.)

arterial pressure at the end of the first day of life and gradually decreases during early infancy.[64] Determinants of pulmonary artery pressure include cardiac output (CO), pulmonary vascular resistance, and pulmonary capillary wedge or venous pressure.

$$PVR = \frac{PAP - PCWP}{CO}$$

As CO varies with body size, pulmonary vascular resistance is often indexed according to surface area (PVRI). PVR is often expressed as resistance units (mm Hg/L/min) or as dynes/sec/cm^{-5} (multiply PVRI by 80).

Diverse mechanisms may contribute to high PAP, including high PVR caused by vascular remodeling, vasoconstriction, vascular occlusion (from thromboemboli), or compression of small pulmonary arteries (for example, at high or low lung volumes during mechanical ventilation). In addition, elevated PCWP resulting from left-ventricular failure, pulmonary venous obstruction or constriction, mitral valve disease, and others can also increase PAP without marked changes in PVR. For example, assessments of transpulmonary artery pressure gradient are important in the setting of high PCWP to directly assess pulmonary vascular disease in potential candidates for cardiac transplantation due to severe cardiomyopathy. PAP may be elevated in the absence of high PVR with anatomic cardiac lesions with large left-to-right shunting. Long-standing pulmonary venous obstruction or high-flow lesions are associated with high PVR resulting from upstream pulmonary vascular disease from remodeling or vasoconstriction. Hyperviscosity and intrathoracic pressure can also influence pulmonary vascular resistance in the presence of marked polycythemia associated with chronic hypoxia or during mechanical ventilation, respectively. Positive end-expiratory pressure (PEEP) influences lung volume, depending on its effects on lung volume and intrathoracic pressure.[65] Whereas low lung volumes may elevate PVR because of the loss of the "tethering" effect of normal distention of neighboring parenchyma, hyperinflation may cause mechanical compression of intraacinar vessels.

The earliest clinical signs of pulmonary hypertension first become apparent during exercise, even in the presence of normal or minimal increases in baseline PAP.[66,67] The normal physiologic response to exercise includes a marked increase in CO with small increases in PAP and PCWP, decreasing PVR by 60% to 70% from baseline. Increased pulmonary blood flow would markedly increase PAP if there was not a concomitant decrease in pulmonary vascular tone and increase in vascular distention and recruitment. With early pulmonary vascular disease, increased CO during exercise markedly increases PAP as a result of high blood flow through a restricted vascular bed and its inability to distend or dilate because of altered vascular structure and reactivity. With severe pulmonary hypertension, exercise is extremely limited because CO is unable to increase, predisposing patients to fatigue, dyspnea on exertion, and with advanced disease, syncope or sudden death. In the absence of shunt lesions, right- and left-ventricular outputs are the same.

As PVR is normally about 20% of systemic vascular resistance, the right ventricle has a thinner wall and a greater volume and surface area than the left ventricle. This configuration is better suited to ejecting large volumes of blood with minimal myocardial shortening, providing a highly compliant chamber that better accommodates increases in filling pressure, as with normal exercise. Unfortunately, the right ventricle is poorly designed to handle rapid increases in wall tension and high systolic ejection pressure, such that an abrupt rise in RV afterload markedly increases RV end-diastolic pressure, decreasing ejection fraction, and RV output. A sudden rise in PVR rapidly dilates the right ventricle, as it attempts to improve function according to the Frank-Starling curve. Mean PAP near 50 mm Hg is poorly tolerated, leading to acute right-sided heart failure.[68] For example, although cardiac transplant patients may have tolerated moderate pulmonary vascular disease before surgery, rapid deterioration of function in the right side of the heart can occur after surgery because of the lack of adaptation of the "new" right ventricle. Interestingly, the failing right ventricle may not be able to generate enough CO to sustain elevated PAP despite high PVR, causing overt clinical signs of right-sided heart failure in some patients with only mild or moderate elevations of PAP. Reduced right coronary artery perfusion pressure, especially during systole, decreases oxygen delivery and causes subendocardial ischemia, further contributing to right ventricular dysfunction.

Experimental studies suggest that even small increases in PAP result in rapid reduction of RV stroke volume. With the gradual development of pulmonary hypertension that occurs with chronic lung disease, the right ventricle is able to adapt to increased afterload by muscle hypertrophy. Acute pulmonary hypertension does not develop until there is a 60% reduction in functional surface area.[69,70] With chronic pulmonary hypertension, smaller degrees of obstruction or loss of vascular bed increases PAP and causes RV hypertrophy. Hypertrophy represents an adaptive response, which reduces ventricular compliance and increases RV end-diastolic and right-atrial pressure. High right-atrial pressure is an important marker of advanced RV failure because CO falls with right-atrial pressure above 8 to 10 mm Hg in adults.[70] Systemic venous distention, hepatomegaly, peripheral edema, and other clinical signs of right-sided heart failure can develop with acute elevations of PAP in patients with chronic mild-to-moderate pulmonary hypertension, as with respiratory syncytial virus infections in patients with CNLD and congenital heart disease.[71]

Left-ventricular function is generally well preserved in most patients with chronic lung disease despite pulmonary hypertension and suboptimal RV function.[72] However, high PVR can impair CO, especially with exercise, and in some patients, poor left-ventricular function is present, further aggravating lung mechanics and gas exchange.[73,74] High PVR causes left-ventricular dysfunction by decreasing preload and causing paradoxical interventricular septal motion (ventricular interdependence).[75] Increased RV dilation mechanically distorts the left ventricle, impedes left-ventricular filling, and decreases CO in proportion to the severity of RV failure. Histologic studies suggest remodeling of left-ventricular myocytes and interstitium, suggesting that along with functional changes in left- and right-ventricular interactions, structural remodeling may also account for changes in myocardial compliance or function.[76] Left-ventricular hypertrophy may represent an adaptive response to increased septal wall tension and is not uncommon in infants with CNLD and pulmonary hypertension.[1] Mechanisms leading to the development of left-ventricular hypertrophy in CNLD or other chronic lung diseases are unclear, but they may be related to systemic hypertension, β-agonist therapy, or other stimuli. Low CO is an important marker of severe pulmonary hypertension and poor long-term outcome. Decreased CO increases fluid and salt retention as a result of increased antidiuretic hormone and aldosterone release, which may account for worsening peripheral edema and other signs of congestive heart failure.[77]

Pulmonary hypertension can alter lung mechanics and gas exchange, causing mild decreases in lung compliance and volume.[78] The direct effects of pulmonary hypertension on gas exchange are difficult to distinguish from signs and symptoms of chronic lung disease. However, patients with primary pulmonary hypertension have only mild abnormalities in ventilation-perfusion ($\dot{V}/\dot{Q}$) matching.[79] Pulmonary hypertension with chronic lung disease may impair lung function and gas exchange by increasing pulmonary edema formation as well as by altering reactivity.

ASSESSMENT AND DIAGNOSIS

Because pulmonary hypertension is not a single disease, but rather is a hemodynamic abnormality common to many different cardiac and respiratory abnormalities, its diagnosis, evaluation, and management require a methodical approach. Increased awareness of at-risk patient populations with chronic lung disease and other disorders associated with pulmonary hypertension may allow for earlier diagnosis and a greater likelihood for successful intervention. Too often, pulmonary hypertension is not recognized until overt RV dysfunction is already present. Clinically, RV dysfunction may occur at lower PAP in chronic lung disease than with primary pulmonary hypertension, making diagnosis and assessments of its contribution to the clinical picture in those with chronic lung disease difficult. Whereas adults with primary pulmonary hypertension may tolerate mean PAPs of about 60 mm Hg, those with chronic obstructive lung disease often have RV dysfunction at 40 mm Hg.[80]

Once recognized, assessment and treatment of clinical factors that potentially contribute to progressive pulmonary vascular disease becomes critical. For example, causes of intermittent or chronic hypoxemia, such as obstructive sleep apnea, chronic aspiration, unrecognized airway lesions, unsuspected anatomic cardiac disease, and others can potentiate pulmonary vascular injury associated with any primary etiology. As with adult pulmonary hypertension, clinical symptoms and signs commonly associated with pediatric pulmonary hypertension include dyspnea, fatigue, exercise intolerance, syncope, cyanosis, chest pain, palpitations, intermittent dry cough, or vomiting. Unexplained seizures, especially in children living at or visiting high altitudes, can be a presenting sign of severe reactive pulmonary hypertension. Primary pulmonary hypertension may appear to be unexplained "portal hypertension" caused by hepatomegaly,[81] recurrent cyanotic episodes, or seizures. Young infants often have feeding difficulties, such as cyanosis, choking, sweating, decreased intake as a result of fatigue, and failure to thrive. Evaluations should seek a history of snoring and obstructive sleep apnea (even in the presence of underlying chronic lung disease), including inquiries regarding daytime somnolence, enuresis, and systemic hypertension.

Signs and symptoms of pulmonary hypertension in children with cor pulmonale can be nonspecific and are often difficult to distinguish from progression of the underlying respiratory problem. Such signs include dyspnea, fatigue, exercise intolerance, recurrent cyanotic or breath-holding spells, poor growth, diaphoresis, chest pain, syncope, and palpitations. Infants and young children often have poor feeding associated with choking, sweating, and cyanosis. In selected cases, unexplained seizures can be a presenting sign, especially in children with primary pulmonary hypertension. As pulmonary hypertension worsens and contributes to the underlying lung disease, progressive dyspnea, fatigue, and other signs are often attributed to exacerbations of the primary lung disease. Similarly, physical findings of pulmonary hypertension are often subtle early; neck vein distention, peripheral edema, hepatomegaly, syncope, and other problems present late in the course. Signs of worsening exercise intolerance or fatigue in the absence of proportionate declines in airflow limitation or lung mechanics by formal pulmonary function testing raise the possibility that pulmonary hypertension and cardiacdysfunction may be contributing factors (discussed later). Physical examination may disclose signs of associated multisystem diseases that can cause pulmonary hypertension, such as cirrhosis, collagen vascular disorders, hematologic abnormalities, and others.

Common findings on physical examination in patients with moderate pulmonary hypertension include tachypnea, tachycardia, an increased second heart sound with narrow or fixed splitting, and a systolic ejection murmur at the left upper sternal border. Signs of advanced RV failure include RV heave, increased jugular venous distention (prominent "a" wave), hepatomegaly and hepatic tenderness, and peripheral edema. In patients with chronic lung disease, signs and symptoms of pulmonary hypertension are often difficult to distinguish from progressive respiratory deterioration. Fluid retention, increasing hepatomegaly, hepatic tenderness, and peripheral edema should heighten suspicion of RV failure in this setting. Although differentiating signs and symptoms from the primary lung disease vs. pulmonary hypertension is difficult, awareness of the risk for pulmonary hypertension and early evaluation may lead to the diagnosis. For example, CF patients with progressive dyspnea or exercise intolerance that seems discordant with the degree of decline in pulmonary function or persists despite aggressive antimicrobial and antiinflammatory therapy may suggest a significant clinical contribution of pulmonary hypertension and cor pulmonale. Similarly, infants with CNLD and unexplained poor growth, persistent or increased oxygen requirements, recurrent cyanotic episodes, or the lack of resolution of RV hypertrophy by ECG warrants more thorough investigation.[82]

The clinical evaluation depends on whether the evolution of pulmonary hypertension is for patients with recognized lung disease or in patients with an unknown etiology. The role of laboratory studies is to identify the presence and severity of pulmonary hypertension, to identify pathogenetic mechanisms that may contribute to its severity, and to assess response to therapeutic intervention. Although ECG, echocardiogram, and cardiac catheterization are direct assessments of pulmonary hypertension, studies such as chest radiographic examinations, chest computed tomography (CT), $\dot{V}/\dot{Q}$ scans, and pulmonary angiogram provide important clinical information in many settings. Initial evaluation includes arterial blood gases (to assess chronic hypoventilation), chest radiograph, ECG, echocardiogram, $\dot{V}/\dot{Q}$ scan, sleep study, exercise testing, and others (Box 58-2). In addition to excluding the presence of parenchymal disease in patients with unexplained pulmonary hypertension, a basic laboratory workup may include hematologic, liver function tests, clotting studies, screening for collagen vascular disease, and others.

Chest radiograph findings suggestive of pulmonary hypertension in chronic lung disease include RV enlargement with prominent appearance of dilated central pulmonary arteries. In older patients a descending right pulmonary artery diameter greater than 20 mm and an increased hilar thoracic index are highly suggestive of pulmonary hypertension.[83] Vascular markings may appear reduced in the lung periphery, coinciding with the appearance of "pruning" detectable by angiography. Pulmonary venoocclusive disease can appear as a reticular or reticulonodular infiltrates, masquerading as interstitial lung disease. Obstruction and infiltrates may be unilateral. Irregular or marginated densities may be suggestive of pulmonary vasculitis. One of the major problems in the evaluation of pulmonary hypertension with underlying chronic lung disease is that hyperinflation masks cardiomegaly. Also interstitial infiltrates of patchy large densities can obscure vessels. Absence of changes by chest x-ray should not limit further evaluation. Chest CT scans may help evaluate lung parenchyma for signs of early interstitial lung disease and help image pulmonary arteries. Magnetic resonance imaging (MRI) may provide an additional noninvasive method for evaluating pulmonary hypertension by assessing right-ventricular wall thickness (RVWT) and the ratio of RVWT to left-ventricular posterior wall thickness, and RV end-systolic and diastolic volume indexes.[84]

Perfusion studies using radiolabeled albumin are helpful for identifying pulmonary vascular abnormalities, such as arteriovenous malformations and intrapulmonary shunting in cirrhotics (discussed later). $\dot{V}/\dot{Q}$ scans aid in differentiating thromboembolic disease from other causes of pulmonary hypertension because thrombosis produces large perfusion defects in contrast with the small "moth-eaten" peripheral defects found with advanced pulmonary hypertension from other mechanisms. Pulmonary arterial angiography provides a more precise approach to the identification of vascular obstruction, the presence of structural lesions such as hemangiomatosis and arteriovenous malformations, as well as assessments of vascular pruning. Unfortunately, the degree of pruning, or distal vascular narrowing and small vessel filling, is not a sensitive method of distinguishing severe pulmonary hypertension caused by vascular remodeling vs. vasoconstriction.

Detection and assessment of pulmonary hypertension and its severity primarily requires serial ECG and echocardiogram studies. Although ECG findings of RV hypertrophy or strain are diagnostically useful for patients with pulmonary hyper-

BOX 58-2

Diagnostic Evaluation of Pulmonary Hypertension

The following tests may be useful depending on the clinical features.

Arterial blood gas
Pulse oximetry studies (awake, asleep, exercise)
Hematocrit, platelet count
Bleeding time, coagulation profile, antiphospholipid antibody
Liver function tests (liver enzymes, albumin, clotting studies)
Collagen vascular disease evaluation: ESR, ANA, ANCA
Pilocarpine iontophoresis (sweat test)
Chest radiographs
Barium swallow
Sleep study
Flexible laryngoscopy/bronchoscopy with lavage
Lung biopsy
Esophageal pH study
Pulmonary function testing with exercise testing
ECG
Echocardiogram
Cardiac catheterization
$\dot{V}/\dot{Q}$ scan
Chest CT scan

BOX 58-3
ECG Criteria for Right-Ventricular Hypertrophy

Right-axis deviation
Right-atrial hypertrophy: (p-pulmonale: P waves >3 mm)
Increased rightward and anterior ORS vector
R in Vl, V2, or aVR > ULN for age
S in I and V6> ULN for age
Abnormal R:S ratio in favor of RV (in absence of bundle branch block)
R:S ratio in Vl and V2> ULN for age
R:S ratio in V6 <1 after 1 month of age
Upright T in Vl (in patients >3 days of age)
q wave in Vl (qR or qRs patterns)

Newborn:

Pure R wave in Vl >10 mm
R in Vl >25 mm, or R in aVR >8 mm
qR pattern in Vl
Upright T in Vl in neonates more than 3 days of age
RAD >180 degrees

tension, signs are usually less pronounced with chronic lung disease. This may be due to the effects of hyperinflation or the presence of milder levels of pulmonary hypertension commonly associated with lung disease. ECG findings of RV hypertrophy are present in 28% to 75% of patients with cor pulmonale.[85] Because the developmental shift from RV predominance normally occurs during infancy, diagnostic evaluations with ECG and echocardiography must take into account normal age-related changes in right-axis deviation, indexes of RV hypertrophy, and other physiologic changes (Box 58-3).

Advances in Doppler and two-dimensional echocardiography have markedly improved noninvasive assessments of pulmonary hypertension. A major problem, however, is the technical difficulty of obtaining interpretable information in severe obstructive lung diseases, because marked hyperinflation and marked swings in intrathoracic pressures with respiratory efforts reduce the windows through which the right ventricle and valves can be imaged. Echocardiographic signs of pulmonary hypertension include increased RVWT, chamber size, flattening or paradoxic motion of the interventricular septum, early closure of the pulmonic valve, and incomplete tricuspid valve closure. Increased RV anterior wall thickness and interventricular septal wall thickness reflect RV hypertrophy. Paradoxical septal wall motion is a sign of impending RV failure. Quantitative assessments of pulmonary hypertension include measurements of right ventricular systolic time interval (RVSTI) and tricuspid regurgitation. RVSTI is the ratio of measurements of RV preejection period (PEP) to ejection time (ET). The PEP is the duration of time after electrical activation of the ventricle to the onset of ejection during systole. RV ET is measured from the time of opening to closure of the pulmonic valve during systole. Pulmonary hypertension delays pulmonic valve opening (because the valve does not open until RV systolic pressure exceeds PAP), causing prolongation of PEP and shortening ET. RVSTI increases the sensitivity of the echocardiogram and provides a noninvasive quantitative assessment for serial comparisons with subsequent clinic visits. Although several past publications used measurements of RVSTI to reflect acute changes in PAP during exposure to oxygen or vasodilators,[86] variability and lack of sensitivity makes this measurement unreliable for routine assessments of reactivity. Perhaps a more sensitive assessment of pulmonary hypertension is the measurement of peak pulmonary artery systolic pressure obtained form continuous-wave Doppler measurements of the tricuspid jet.[87] The tricuspid insufficiency jet, as measured by pulsed Doppler echocardiography, reflects the pressure difference between the right ventricle and the right atrium. By using the Bernoulli principle (Pressure $= 4V^2$, where V is the peak systolic velocity in m/sec), the sum of this measurement with estimated or measured right-atrial pressure provides a fairly accurate assessment of RV systolic pressure.[88] As with other echocardiographic assessments of pulmonary hypertension, imaging the tricuspid regurgitant jet can be difficult with chronic lung disease, leading to a low success rate (24%) in adults with COPD.[89]

Although serial studies with ECG or echocardiogram are useful during long-term follow-up, cardiac catheterization may be necessary to better define the role of pulmonary vascular disease in the clinical course. Cardiac catheterization serves to quantitate the severity of pulmonary hypertension; to rule out anatomic cardiac lesions, structural pulmonary vascular lesions, thromboemboli, or significant hypertrophy of bronchial collaterals; to define optimal treatment levels for supplemental oxygen; to assess pulmonary vasoreactivity; and to test potential pharmacologic agents for long-term therapy. Delays in performing cardiac catheterization in patients with chronic lung disease are common, however, potentially contributing to delays in diagnosis or therapy. Probe-patent foramen ovale may be present in many young children, suggesting that intracardiac shunt may contribute to the severity of hypoxemia in patients with pulmonary hypertension more often than expected. Cardiac catheterization should include angiography to avoid missing structural lesions, such as pulmonary arterial stenosis, pulmonary venoocclusive disease, enlarged bronchial collateral vessels with chronic lung disease, diffuse pulmonary hemangiomatosis or arteriovenous shunts, and other diagnoses. Although concerns persist regarding the potential risks of angiography in precipitating pulmonary hypertensive crises or dysrhythmias in severe pulmonary hypertension, the use of newer contrast material seems to have decreased these risks. Undersedation and subsequent agitation may also increase the risk for precipitating a pulmonary hypertensive crisis.

Assessment of pulmonary vasoreactivity is an essential part of the evaluation, but it is too often not included with basal hemodynamic measurements. For example, exaggerated vasoconstrictor responses to acute hypoxia in patients with only mild baseline pulmonary hypertension may help explain episodic cyanosis or progressive pulmonary hypertension in children with recurrent cyanosis, HAPE, CNLD, or other diseases (Fig. 58-7).[58,59,90] The use of anesthesia and inadvertent oversedation, hypoventilation or hyperventilation, and hypoxia can alter basal PAP and reactivity during cardiac catheterization, potentially limiting the usefulness of clinical information. On the other hand, controlled hypoxic and hypercarbic challenges during catheterization may provide critical insight into pulmonary vascular hyperreactivity. For example, some patients require higher target oxygen saturations to maintain maximal decreases in pulmonary vascular resistance and to lower the risk of intermittent spikes in PAP. Whereas the vasodilator response while breathing 100% oxygen is commonly

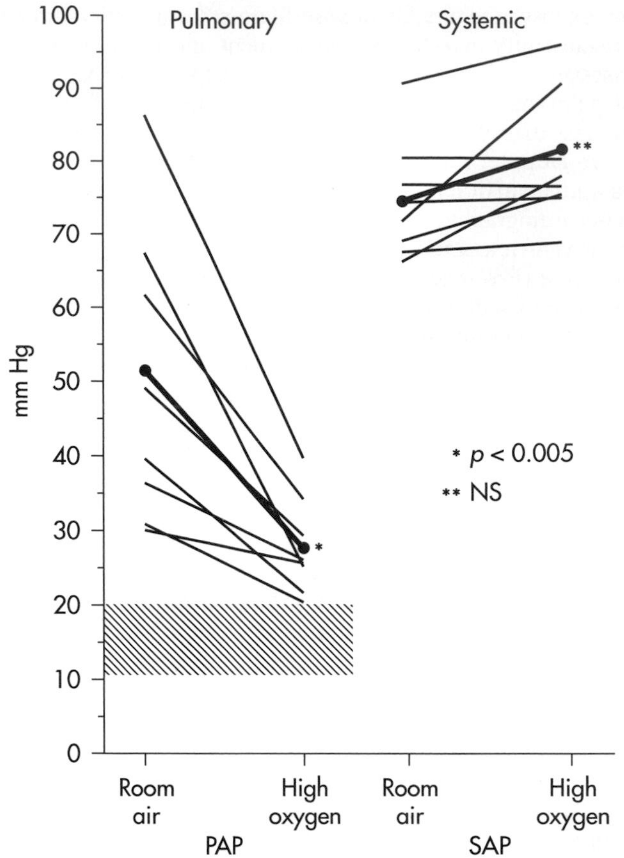

Fig. 58-7 Exaggerated hypoxic pulmonary vasoconstrictor response during brief expose to hypoxia in children with CNLD. Responses to mean pulmonary artery pressures and systemic arterial pressures to high levels of inspired oxygen (FiO_2 >0.80). (From Abman SH, Wolfe RR, Accurso FJ. Koops BL, Bowman CM, Wiggins JW: *Pediatrics* 75:80-84, 1985.)

used to assess potential reversibility of pulmonary hypertension, correlation between the dilator response to oxygen and outcome is unclear. Measurement of acute hemodynamic responses while breathing high concentrations of supplemental oxygen is useful to assess vasoreactivity because of its selective pulmonary vasodilation and because it allows adjustment of oxygen therapy. However, hyperoxia alone is not a very potent vasodilator beyond its ability to reverse hypoxic vasoconstriction, and this response is often used to prognosticate on reversibility of pulmonary hypertension and outcome. Long-term therapy with supplemental oxygen to correct hypoxia-induced pulmonary vasoconstriction will decrease the adverse effects of chronic or intermittent hypoxia and often improve clinical outcome. However, the response to high oxygen concentration may not be sufficient for determining the relative contributions of vasoconstriction vs. structural remodeling to basal pulmonary hypertension. For example, it is not uncommon that pharmacologic vasodilators (such as prostacyclin, sodium nitroprusside, hydralazine, calcium channel blockers, and others) or inhaled NO can often cause further vasodilation than high concentrations of inspired oxygen alone. Although it remains unclear which vasodilator should be used to assess pulmonary vascular tone, inhaled NO may be a good choice because of its short half-life, selectivity for the pulmonary circulation (less risk for systemic hypotension, fatal dysrhythmia), and its ability to improve gas exchange, rather than worsen oxygenation, with lung disease.

Links between acute pulmonary vasoreactivity and long-term outcome require further study. Clinical decision making is often based on data from small numbers of patients with congenital heart disease because of the lack of data from patients with chronic lung disease. Conclusions regarding the relative contribution of vasoconstriction vs. vascular remodeling to the severity of pulmonary hypertension presume that the degree of pulmonary hypertension remaining after administration of a vasodilator must be due to structural remodeling. This is not always true and may partially depend on the selection and relative potency of the vasodilator. Similarly, the acute response may not predict the potential for reversal of pulmonary hypertension with time. Lung biopsies are used to assess the severity of structural changes in some cases and for further diagnostic evaluation (to rule out interstitial lung disease, venoocclusive disease, and others). The biopsy allows grading of vascular lesions, but tissue should be obtained from multiple sites to allow for heterogeneity. In general, the histology of patients with secondary pulmonary hypertension lacks the severe intimal changes present in patients with primary pulmonary hypertension or congenital heart disease. Uncertainty exists regarding the potential reversibility of pulmonary vascular structural lesions, and further studies are needed to examine the relationships between vascular reactivity, remodeling, and outcome.

MANAGEMENT

Acute management of severe right-sided heart failure requires rapid lowering of PAP to reduce RV afterload to maintain CO, systemic blood pressure, and tissue oxygen delivery. Dramatic elevations of PAP are more common in patients with primary pulmonary hypertension, PPHN, and postoperative congenital heart disease than with pulmonary hypertension associated with acute respiratory failure or chronic lung disease. Patients with life-threatening acute episodes of pulmonary hypertension are managed by sedation, paralysis, hyperventilation, alkalosis, and high inspired concentrations of oxygen. Pharmacologic vasodilator therapy is reserved for RV failure unresponsive to oxygen and standard therapy, or in the setting of marked pulmonary "vasolability." Pulmonary artery catheters provide close monitoring of PAP and PCWP, CO, systemic vascular resistance, and related hemodynamic measurements during acute therapeutic interventions. Whereas pharmacologic therapy may rapidly decrease PAP, vasodilators can markedly impair gas exchange with severe lung disease, causing worsening hypoxemia. Inhaled NO may provide selective pulmonary vasodilation without adverse effects on gas exchange in children with hypoxemic respiratory failure or primary pulmonary hypertension.

The primary approach to the long-term treatment of pulmonary hypertension in patients with chronic lung disease is to optimize lung function and gas exchange. In addition to managing right-sided heart failure, the long-term goal is to avoid the adverse effects of sustained pulmonary hypertension on progressive vascular remodeling. Mechanisms leading to reversibility of pulmonary hypertension and vascular remodeling are poorly understood but partly depend on the severity of vascular remodeling at diagnosis and recognition of complicating factors that contribute to its progression. Thus early anticipation and recognition of pulmonary hypertension in at-risk patients may improve outcome in many cases. Therapy generally targets three areas: (1) optimal management of underlying lung disease (for example, lung inflammation and infection in CF, mechanical ventilation with hypoventilation and neuromuscular weakness, and others); (2) diagnosis and treatment of complicating or "unsuspected" cardiopulmonary abnormalities (such as aspiration, upper airway obstruction or anatomic cardiac defects in CNLD, and others); and (3) treatment of the pulmonary hypertension with oxygen and pharmacologic agents.

Because the most common cause of progressive pulmonary hypertension in chronic lung disease is hypoxia, supplemental oxygen is the mainstay of therapy. Oxygen therapy is the only treatment that has been shown to improve the clinical course of patients with pulmonary hypertension and chronic lung disease.[91,92] The British Medical Research Council study and the NIH Nocturnal Oxygen Therapy Trial (NOTT) demonstrated that adults with COPD who use supplemental oxygen for the greatest period of time each day (19 vs. 12 hr/day) derive the greatest advantage in survival, and that oxygen therapy prevents further increases in PAP. Whether patients who decrease PAP during acute administration of supplemental oxygen have a better survival than nonresponders is unproven, but it has been suggested in a small clinical trial.[93] Mortality was significantly decreased in adults with COPD and slowed progression of pulmonary hypertension; these responses were directly related to the duration of daily use. Long-term oxygen therapy may enhance oxygen delivery in addition to its effects on pulmonary vasodilation and may partially explain improved clinical outcome. In addition, long-term oxygen therapy counters the adverse effects of episodic hypoxia on intermittent elevations of PAP with sleep or activity and may influence smooth muscle cell growth or production of extracellular matrix independent of its effects on lowering pressure.[94,95] We recommend an aggressive approach toward maintaining adequate oxygenation (oxygen saturations above 94% while awake, while asleep, and with activity).

Infants with chronic lung disease require frequent noninvasive assessments of oxygenation and serial ECGs or echocardiograms while receiving supplemental oxygen, especially if signs of RV hypertrophy persist despite therapy. Monitoring of oxygenation to avoid even intermittent hypoxemia will enhance recovery or slow progression of pulmonary hypertension in children with pulmonary hypertension of many etiologies. Perhaps the clearest illustration of this strategy is in infants with CNLD.[1] Chronic intermittent or persistent hypoxia blocks recovery and accelerates progression of pulmonary vascular disease. Infants with CNLD are often undertreated because of fear of oxygen toxicity during the chronic stages of disease despite the presence of pulmonary hypertension. Once persistent signs of pulmonary hypertension have been identified in older CNLD infants, even mild levels of hypoxia should not be tolerated. Reversal of hypoxia with supplemental oxygen in patients with chronic lung disease will acutely lower PVR in many patients and avoid intermittent episodes of hypoxic pulmonary vasoconstriction. Although increasing FiO_2 improves systemic oxygenation and lowers pulmonary vascular resistance, regional alveolar hypoxia may persist in some lung units, perhaps allowing for continued vascular injury despite therapy.[96]

Progression of pulmonary hypertension in association with any disease should lead to investigation of potential contributing factors, including obstructive sleep apnea, chronic aspiration, structural airway lesions, and other problems. For example, children with Down syndrome with or without anatomic heart disease often have more severe pulmonary hypertension than other children, which is often partly due to chronic pharyngeal collapse with sleep, tracheomalacia, or other structural lesions. Evaluations should include sleep studies, imaging of the upper airway by flexible laryngoscopy and bronchoscopy, radiologic studies (such as barium swallow and isovue bronchograms), pulmonary function testing, and lung biopsy in selected cases. In addition to correction of hypoxemia, acidosis and hypercarbia may contribute to progressive pulmonary hypertension. Although hypercarbia is commonly tolerated with chronic lung disease, we recommend more aggressive ventilator therapy in patients with chronic lung disease and concomitant pulmonary hypertension.

Diuretics and digoxin are commonly prescribed in patients with chronic lung disease and cor pulmonale. Although diuretics may acutely improve gas exchange in chronic lung diseases such as CNLD,[97] mechanisms underlying this response are more likely related to relief of pulmonary edema than direct improvement of pulmonary hypertension. When administered for treatment of right-sided heart failure, diuresis can acutely decrease fluid retention, especially in patients with hepatomegaly, peripheral edema, and signs of systemic venous congestion. Frequent use of diuretics in the presence of high pulmonary vascular resistance may markedly decrease RV preload, thereby decreasing pulmonary blood flow and CO. In addition, electrolyte imbalance with chloride depletion and elevated serum bicarbonate may cause metabolic alkalosis and hypoventilation. Digoxin use in cor pulmonale remains controversial. Although it may improve myocardial performance and CO in patients with impaired left-ventricular function, most patients have little clinical benefit. Furthermore, digoxin may increase pulmonary hypertension in some settings.[98]

Several pharmacologic agents are used for short-term therapy of pulmonary hypertension, including prostaglandins E_1 and I_2, sodium nitroprusside, isoproterenol, tolazoline, hydralazine, phentolamine, and others. Adenosine is a promising new drug, as early studies suggest relative selectivity for the pulmonary circulation.[99] Whereas various agents may be effective in acutely lowering PAP, pulmonary vasodilation in the setting of parenchymal lung disease can cause severe hypoxemia by worsening $\dot{V}/\dot{Q}$ mismatch, limiting their usefulness in the presence of lung disease.[100]

The benefits of pharmacologic vasodilator therapy in the long-term management of pulmonary hypertension secondary to chronic lung disease remain unproven. Long-term therapy of severe pulmonary hypertension includes calcium channel blockers (diltiazem and nifedipine) and antiplatelet agents or anticoagulants (coumadin, heparin, or dipyridamole).[101-103] Long-term PgI2 therapy in young children and infants with unexplained or primary pulmonary hypertension is promising, but experience has been limited.[104] Unfortunately, there is little clinical experience with long-term PgI2 therapy in pediatric patients with other lesions, especially Eisenmenger syndrome, where in the absence of parenchymal lung disease, the use of PgI2 should not be limited by adverse effects on oxygenation (discussed later). Selective patients with primary pulmonary hypertension have demonstrated sustained clinical benefits from long-term therapy with a calcium channel blocker, diltiazem, especially in combination with an anticoagulant.[101] Responses were variable, however, and most patients failed to respond. The rationale for vasodilator therapy is that pulmonary vasoconstriction, and not simply advanced structural vascular disease, contributes to pulmonary hypertension; however, although the acute hemodynamic response to vasodilators is an encouraging sign, it does not always translate to long-term effectiveness or prolonged survival. Whether long-term drug therapy will improve morbidity and mortality or slow the progression of cardiopulmonary disease in pediatric chronic lung disease is largely unstudied. Short-term studies of calcium channel antagonists have demonstrated some decrease in pulmonary vascular resistance in adults with COPD. However, long-term studies suggest that patients deteriorate clinically despite hemodynamic improvement.[105] Because long-term benefits are unclear, vasodilator use must be individualized. Improved exercise tolerance has been reported in some patients with CF.[106,107] Long-term use of calcium channel blockers has not been studied in infants with CNLD (discussed later).

In addition to long-term vasodilator therapy, many patients with severe pulmonary hypertension are treated with anticoagulant or antiplatelet therapy. The rationale for these agents is to decrease the development of thrombosis in situ in small pulmonary arteries.[101] Combining Coumadin with diltiazem therapy may provide a better long-term clinical response than diltiazem without anticoagulant therapy. Future therapies directed toward inhibition of vascular remodeling will provide novel approaches distinct from vasodilator therapy. Lung transplantation is currently offered by many centers for patients with advanced cor pulmonale associated with progressive lung disorders as well as primary pulmonary hypertension, but continued problems with unavailability of donors and the high risk of bronchiolitis obliterans (up to 50% in some centers) remains problematic.

SPECIFIC DISEASES ASSOCIATED WITH PULMONARY HYPERTENSION

Persistent Pulmonary Hypertension of the Newborn

PPHN represents the failure of the pulmonary circulation to achieve or sustain the normal decrease in PVR at birth.[57,108] High PVR in the neonate causes marked hypoxemia as a result of right-to-left shunting of blood across the patent ductus arteriosus or foramen ovale. The diagnosis of PPHN has replaced the older term *persistent fetal circulation*, and refers to a clinical *syndrome* of a wide variety of cardiovascular and pulmonary disorders, such as meconium aspiration syndrome, sepsis, pneumonia, congenital diaphragmatic hernia, or respiratory distress syndrome, or can be idiopathic. Idiopathic PPHN is characterized by severe cyanosis with tachypnea and respiratory distress in term or postdate newborns with chest radiograph findings of clear lung fields and a normal cardiothymic silhouette. Although often associated with perinatal stress (for example, maternal bleeding or asphyxia), specific etiologies are rarely identified in idiopathic PPHN. When associated with asphyxia or marked stress, meconium aspiration may be present, further complicating the clinical course. Most patients with asphyxia, intrauterine growth retardation, or meconium aspiration, however, do not develop PPHN. Etiologic mechanisms leading to the failure of postnatal adaptation are incompletely understood, but intrauterine stimuli, such as chronic hypertension or closure of the ductus arteriosus, may contribute to the characteristic alterations of pulmonary vasoreactivity and structure that are present at birth.[39-42] Mechanisms underlying PPHN may include failure to release sufficient vasodilators (such as endogenous NO[26] or prostacyclin[44]); increased vasoconstrictor production (endothelin,[28,29] leukotrienes,[30] and thromboxane); altered smooth muscle cell responsiveness to vasoactive stimuli; or altered vascular growth (smooth muscle hypertrophy and increased extracellular matrix production). Evidence supporting the hypothesis that chronic prenatal events may lead to PPHN include data from experimental animal models as well as autopsy data demonstrating extensive vascular remodeling in neonates dying with PPHN within the first days of life.[109]

Although the diagnosis of PPHN requires echocardiographic confirmation of right-to-left shunting at the ductus arteriosus or foramen ovale in the absence of anatomic heart disease, several clinical features are highly suggestive: (1) marked or "labile" hypoxemia; (2) differences in preductal and postductal PaO_2 of at least 5 to 10 mm Hg (not present if shunting is predominantly at the foramen ovale); and (3) clinical improvement with hyperventilation.[57] Treatment includes high FiO_2, hyperventilation, and infusions of sodium bicarbonate (for alkalosis) and cardiotonic agents (dopamine, dobutamine) for cardiovascular support. Optimal lung inflation is essential for aggressive treatment of parenchymal lung disease that contributes to high PVR as a result of mechanical vascular compression and marked intrapulmonary shunting at low lung volumes. Pharmacologic vasodilators, such as tolazoline, prostaglandins (PgI_2 or PgE_1), and sodium nitroprusside, have been used with success in some cases. Intravenous vasodilator therapy has been limited, however, by adverse side effects, including systemic hypotension because of the lack of selectivity for the pulmonary circulation and aggravation of right-to-left shunting, and by worsening of $\dot{V}/\dot{Q}$ mismatch in patients with parenchymal lung disease. Patients failing conventional therapy often require extracorporeal membrane oxygenation (ECMO) therapy. Although lifesaving in many cases, ECMO is costly and associated with significant complications, such as intracranial hemorrhage or systemic bleeding from heparinization, and requires carotid artery ligation, which may contribute to adverse neurologic sequelae. ECMO centers are now using venovenous ECMO in patients with stable cardiac function to avoid carotid artery cannulation. However, unrecognized or late development of myocardial dysfunction may lead to failure of venovenous ECMO, requiring conversion to a venoarterial approach. More recent studies have suggested that adjuvant therapies such as inhaled NO,[110-112] high frequency oscillatory ventilation, and surfactant may provide effective interventions in various conditions associated with PPHN and may decrease the need for ECMO in selected patients.[112] Combined modalities, such as inhaled NO with HFOV, may provide more effective therapy in some patients with parenchymal lung disease and pulmonary hypertension[112] because responsiveness to inhaled NO appears to partly depend on adequate lung inflation for delivery of NO to resistance vessels in the distal lung. PPHN survivors are at risk for chronic lung disease, including BPD or airways hyperreactivity, as well as neurodevelopmental sequelae.

Chronic Neonatal Lung Disease

CNLD is the chronic lung disease of infancy that follows ventilator and oxygen therapy for neonatal respiratory distress. Since the earliest descriptions of CNLD, pulmonary hypertension and cor pulmonale have been recognized as being associated with high mortality.[1] Mortality in CNLD patients with persistent echocardiographic findings of pulmonary hypertension beyond 4 months of age has been reported as 50%.[113] Recent studies have reported similar mortality in selected populations of older CNLD infants with persistent pulmonary hypertension.[3] Clinically, CNLD infants with severe pulmonary hypertension are prone to recurrent pulmonary edema, frequent respiratory exacerbations, congestive heart failure, and late morbidity from viral infections or sudden death.[1,114] Related cardiovascular sequelae include left-ventricular hypertrophy, systemic hypertension, and hypertrophied systemic-to-pulmonary collaterals.[1] Pulmonary vascular disease in CNLD reflects the direct effects of ventilator and hyperoxia-induced lung injury, but chronic inflammation, hypoxia, neurohumoral stimuli, and altered production of vasoactive substances contribute to the severity or persistence of pulmonary hypertension. Physiologically, the pulmonary circulation in CNLD is characterized by heightened pulmonary vasoreactivity, hypertensive vascular remodeling (increased muscularization with adventitial thickening), and decreased arterial number as a result of altered surface area caused by lung injury and decreased septation ("alveolar simplification").[44,115] Altered metabolic lung function, as assessed by decreased uptake of circulating nor-epinephrine, has been described in CNLD infants with pulmonary hypertension.[116]

As described previously, clinical management of pulmonary hypertension in CNLD revolves around vigilant monitoring and aggressive use of supplemental oxygen therapy.[12] Although oxygen saturations below 90% may be well tolerated in normal children recovering from viral respiratory infections, CNLD infants require better oxygenation to minimize the adverse effects of chronic hypoxic pulmonary vasoconstriction.[90] Based on clinical studies, oxygen saturations above 94% while awake, while asleep, and during feeding are often recommended for infants with CNLD and pulmonary hypertension.[1]

Resolution of pulmonary hypertension by ECG or echocardiographic criteria is often found with appropriate therapy over time.[12] Children with persistent RV hypertrophy require more aggressive measures to evaluate potential mechanisms complicating their recovery. These include reassessment of oxygenation levels during prolonged pulse oximetry studies; formal sleep studies; and assessment for unsuspected cardiac or lung problems contributing to the severity of the clinical course (such as aspiration, upper airway obstruction, anatomic heart disease, large bronchial collaterals causing pulmonary edema, and others).[1,82] Early identification and treatment of left-to-right shunt cardiovascular lesions may enhance long-term outcome in selected CNLD patients, decreasing progressive pulmonary vascular injury in a lung circulation that is already limited by decreased surface area, vascular remodeling, and vasoconstriction.

Hemodynamic improvement in CNLD infants with pulmonary hypertension has been reported after brief vasodilator therapy with prostacyclin[4] and nifedipine[117] during cardiac catheterization. However, prostacyclin increased CO but did not lower PAP, and although PVR fell by 23%, systemic vascular resistance decreased by 39%.[4] Similarly, the drop in mean PAP achieved during acute nifedipine treatment was similar to the response to supplemental oxygen alone.[117] Because nifedipine increased CO, however, PVR was lower after nifedipine administration than after oxygen therapy. Whether the combination of supplemental oxygen with chronic calcium channel blockers will enhance long-term outcome in selected CNLD patients with pulmonary hypertension has not been studied. Assessment of the acute response to pulmonary vasodilator therapy during cardiac catheterization is necessary to optimize treatment dose and to avoid potential adverse effects, as observed in severe CNLD with pulmonary hypertension with hydralazine. Goodman et al[3] reported that CNLD patients with severe pulmonary hypertension developed marked hypercarbia with acute pulmonary edema after hydralazine infusion, perhaps as a result of increased left-to-right shunting across enlarged bronchial collaterals. These observations support the need for careful assessment of the effects of vasodilator therapy on gas exchange and hemodynamic measurements before initiating long-term therapy.

Thus management of pulmonary hypertension in CNLD remains largely supportive, with careful attention to the avoidance of the adverse effects of episodic hypoxia and hypercarbia on lung vascular remodeling and reactivity. In selected cases, long-term therapy with calcium channel blockers or other agents with oxygen therapy may be indicated, but patient selection would require careful initial assessment with cardiac catheterization and close follow-up.

Cystic Fibrosis

Although pulmonary hypertension was first recognized as a significant clinical problem in CF almost 50 years ago,[118] detection and management of pulmonary hypertension in CF remains an ongoing challenge. Despite dramatic advances in our understanding of the genetics and pathophysiology of CF, little progress has been made regarding the contribution of pulmonary hypertension to mortality and morbidity in CF or its treatment.[5,6,118-121] In 1951, Royce et al[119] reported that 70% of patients dying with CF had marked RV hypertrophy at autopsy. In 1980, Stern et al[5] found that 46% of CF patients who died after 15 years of age had clinical signs of right-sided heart failure for at least 2 weeks before death and that mean survival was only 8 months after the onset of RV failure. Whether pulmonary hypertension and RV dysfunction are markers of disease severity or directly contribute to mortality are unclear. Similarly, whether aggressive management of pulmonary hypertension could improve morbidity and long-term outcome is unknown.

Mechanisms leading to the development of pulmonary hypertension in CF include chronic hypoxia caused by severe $\dot{V}/\dot{Q}$ mismatch from severe lung disease with airways obstruction and chronic infection and inflammation. Although chronic hypoxia contributes significantly to the progression of pulmonary hypertension in CF, it is unlikely that hypoxia is the sole factor in its pathogenesis. Chronic hypercarbia with acidosis may cause intermittent spikes in PAP, leading to vascular remodeling. Exaggerated respiratory efforts can increase intrathoracic pressure, which may increase RV afterload. In addition, severe bronchiectasis with progressive interstitial disease decreases alveolar-capillary surface area, further promoting the development of pulmonary hypertension. Chronic infection and inflammation caused by increased release of vasoactive bacterial products and mediators from inflammatory cells (cytokines, lipid mediators, others) can also directly alter pulmonary vascular reactivity and structure.[122] In its early stages, active vasoconstriction contributes to high PAP resistance in CF, which appears to predate subsequent development of hypertensive vascular remodeling found in older patients with CF. The role of vasoconstriction was first clinically demonstrated with studies of the acute pulmonary vasodilator response to supplemental oxygen and tolazoline treatment.[118-121,123] Although structural pulmonary vascular lesions contribute to cor pulmonale over time, recent in vitro studies of conduit pulmonary arteries from CF patients undergoing lung transplantation have suggested that impaired release of endothelium-derived relaxing factor (EDRF) contributes to increased vasoconstriction and high PVR with advanced lung disease.[124] These findings suggest that altered pulmonary vasoreactivity persists late in the clinical course of CF and that this is in part due to endothelial dysfunction.

Recognition of clinical signs of cor pulmonale generally occurs late. Clinical predictors of cor pulmonale in CF include Pa_{O_2} less than 50 mm Hg, Pa_{CO_2} greater than 45 mm Hg, forced vital P4 capacity less than 60% of predicted, and right-axis deviation by ECG.[121] The degree of hypoxia while breathing room air is inversely correlated with severity of PAP. The diagnosis of cor pulmonale in CF by clinical evaluation can be masked by severe CF lung disease. Signs that are usually ascribed to right-sided heart failure, such as tachypnea, hepatomegaly, hepatic tenderness, and cyanosis, may be results of underlying lung or liver disease. Increased second heart sounds, murmurs, and gallop rhythms may not be heard during auscultation because of loud adventitious breath sounds. Peripheral edema is rarely detected, even with cor pulmonale, and is usually caused by poor nutrition with low oncotic pressure from hypoalbuminemia. Chest radiograph findings may include dilated central pulmonary arteries; heart size may appear normal as a result of hyperinflation or infiltrates. ECGs are not sensitive because RV hypertrophy may be absent by ECG even when moderate pulmonary hypertension is found with cardiac catheterization.[125-130] Echocardiographic estimates of pulmonary hypertension, such as RV systolic time intervals, appear to correlate well with PAP directly measured at cardiac catheterization and RVWT at autopsy. Although echocardiograms increase the diagnostic yield of pulmonary hypertension, cardiac imaging can be difficult because of severe hyperinflation. For example, complete assessments of RV function were obtained in less than 50% of CF patients. However, longitudinal studies have reported RV wall thickening and dilation, even in some cases of mild CF lung disease. Exercise stress testing with echocardiography may further increase the diagnostic yield and may be present in patients with relatively mild CF lung disease. Radionuclide measurements of RV ejection fraction are more sensitive than echocardiogram or ECG studies of RV function.

Left-ventricular dysfunction has been identified in some patients with CF, but its role in clinical disease is unclear. Left-ventricular free wall weight can be increased at autopsy and areas of myocardial fibrosis have been reported. Echocardiography can demonstrate flattening or compression of the left ventricle along its minor dimension by a massively dilated right ventricle. RV enlargement could produce left-ventricular dysfunction in severe CF.[130] Left-ventricular compression and abnormal interventricular septal motion can cause dyskinetic contraction and relaxation, which could contribute to diminished stroke volume.

Therapy includes liberal use of supplemental oxygen while continuing aggressive management of the underlying lung disease. In theory, improved lung function will enhance gas exchange, decrease regional hypoxia, and slow the progression of pulmonary hypertension. Similarly, relief of airways obstruction and reduction of lung infection and inflammation should decrease lung injury and alter production of vasoactive mediators or growth factors that contribute to pulmonary vasoconstriction, structural remodeling, and loss of vascular surface area. Supplemental oxygen therapy should be administered to avoid episodic or persistent hypoxemia; target Pa_{O_2} is generally recommended to be maintained above 60 to 65 mm Hg, or oxygen saturations by pulse oximetry greater than 94% during sleep and while awake. Oxygen therapy may further attenuate increases in PAP during acute or subacute respiratory deteriorations. Serial evaluations of CF patients with ECG and echocardiogram should be performed regularly to monitor for early signs of RV hypertrophy, especially with moderate lung disease, even in the absence of overt signs of cor pulmonale. Sleep-associated hypoxemia should be sought and treated in CF patients with early morning headaches, signs of obstructive sleep apnea, or in the presence of RV hypertrophy. Recent changes in ECG or echocardiogram, excessive fatigue, poor exercise tolerance, cardiac signs on examination, hepatomegaly, right upper quadrant tenderness, and declines in pulmonary function may warrant further evaluations, such as cardiac catheterization.

Most recommendations for the use of supplemental oxygen therapy in CF are based on clinical observations or data from studies of other chronic lung diseases. There are no published studies that demonstrate benefits from early and long-term oxygen therapy in CF. One study that examined the effects of nocturnal oxygen therapy on the short-term (6-month) course of CF patients with advanced lung disease reported no improvement.[131] In this study, however, patients were treated only with nocturnal oxygen despite having hypoxia (room air Pa_{O_2} less than 65 mm Hg) while awake. In addition, no documentation of sleep-associated hypoxemia or its resolution with therapy was present, and ECG and echocardiographic assessments of pulmonary hypertension were not included. Whether early and aggressive use of supplemental oxygen improves clinical outcome, reduces pulmonary hypertension, and enhances the quality of life in CF patients remains speculative.

Data on the role of drug therapy are also limited. Acute diuretic therapy improves signs of systemic venous congestion in CF patients with severe cor pulmonale, decreasing mean PAP without changing CO.[132] Whether long-term diuretic therapy sustains clinical improvement is unclear. Aggressive diuresis could potentially worsen hemodynamic status by dropping RV preload, further decreasing pulmonary blood flow and systemic CO. If diuretics are used, careful monitoring of fluid and electrolyte status are important to avoid the dangers of marked hypokalemic, hypochloremic metabolic alkalosis, and aggravation of chronic CO_2 retention. Digoxin has been used in some patients with severe right-sided heart failure and may be of benefit in selected patients with signs of left-ventricular dysfunction.

Several studies have examined acute hemodynamic responses to vasodilators.[106,107,133] Although there are reports of favorable hemodynamic responses to tolazoline and calcium channel blockers, supplemental oxygen therapy more consistently improves PAP. Davidson et al[133] compared the acute effects of supplemental oxygen and calcium channel blockers in eight CF patients with mild clinical disease. Increased FiO_2 lowered mean PAP by 23%, and PVR by 21%; nifedipine did not alter PAP but lowered PVR by increasing cardiac index by 30%. Diltiazem lowered mean PAP by 24% without changing cardiac index. The degree of oxygen-induced pulmonary vasodilation was not predictive of responses to calcium channel blockers. In some cases, supplemental oxygen lowered mean PAP to normal values, reflecting the relative lack of structural remodeling in early disease. Geggel et al[106] also reported a favorable acute hemodynamic response to oxygen but no improvement with calcium-channel blockers. Sustained improvement in exercise tolerance has been reported in some CF patients[106,107]; however, whether chronic pharmacologic intervention will improve long-term outcome in most CF patients with cor pulmonale is not known.

Pulmonary Hypertension and High Altitude

Studies of physiologic adaptations to acute and chronic exposure to high altitude provide unique insights into mechanisms of human diseases associated with hypoxia.[134] In most clinical settings, chronic hypoxia accompanies severe lung disease, making it difficult to differentiate the effects of hypoxia itself on lung function. To determine the direct cardiopulmonary effects of severe hypoxia, extensive studies of adult volunteers were performed before and during exposure to hypobaric hypoxia by simulating altitude of 8848 meters.[135] These investigators demonstrated that high altitude increased PAP (from 15 to 33 mm Hg); decreased forced vital capacity, which was interpreted as reflecting a restrictive defect caused by increased central blood volume and edema; altered $\dot{V}/\dot{Q}$ mismatch caused by continued perfusion of poorly ventilated regions; and normal cardiac function at rest and with exercise. These findings demonstrate that chronic hypoxia, in the absence of underlying lung disease, markedly impairs respiratory function.

In children living at altitude, the normal postnatal decline in PAP is delayed.[136] For example, infants living above 14,000 feet in Peru have higher mean PAP (45 mm Hg at 1 to 5 years; 28 mm Hg at 6 to 14 years) than do children at lower altitudes. Children living at high altitude have persistence of RV predominance by ECG; increased RV weight; increased muscularization of small pulmonary arteries; and increased incidence of patent ductus arteriosus. However, there is marked individual variability in basal PAP in long-term residents of high altitude.[137-140]

Although acute hypoxia generally increases mean PAP from 13 to 17 mm Hg in normal adults, the pulmonary vasoconstrictor response is markedly heightened in some individuals, even in the absence of underlying cardiopulmonary disease. For example, some children develop severe symptomatic pulmonary hypertension while living at altitude. Khoury and Hawes[36] described 11 infants (less than 2 years old) residing above 10,000 feet in Leadville, Colorado. Symptoms included cyanosis, dyspnea, poor growth, cough, sleeplessness, oliguria, seizure, syncope, and cyanotic spells. Cardiac catheterization revealed suprasystemic or near systemic levels of pulmonary hypertension. At autopsy, advanced hypertensive pulmonary vascular lesions (Heath-Edwards Grade 3-6) were common. To determine mechanisms that may contribute to severe pulmonary hypertension, a subsequent study examined pulmonary vascular responses to acute hypoxia in a similar study group from Leadville.[59] Although mean PAP was only mildly elevated while breathing room air (mean, 24 mm Hg), PAP increased dramatically (to 81 mm Hg) while the group was exposed to an hypoxic gas mixture (16% FiO_2). Marked pulmonary vascular hyperreactivity has been observed in children with chronic lung disease and early in the course of primary pulmonary hypertension. This exaggerated responsiveness is likely to contribute to progressive pulmonary vascular injury associated with these diseases and may be present in occasional cases of children with unexplained cyanotic spells.[58] High altitude can have dramatic effects on pulmonary vascular disease in chronic heart and lung disease. For example, more advanced pulmonary vascular disease in patients with anatomic shunt lesions such as ventricular septal defect or patent ductus arteriosus at altitude, suggesting that the combined effects of hypoxia with high flow may accelerate vascular injury.

Mechanisms causing altered pulmonary vasoreactivity to hypoxia in patients without underlying cardiopulmonary disease are unknown. Pulmonary vascular responses to high altitude depend on multiple factors, including age, genetics, severity of elevation, duration of exposure to high altitude, presence of triggering factors (for example, viral infection), and the presence of underlying chronic cardiovascular or lung disease. Although acute hypoxic pulmonary vasoconstriction is primarily due to direct effects of low oxygen tension on the vascular smooth muscle, various mechanisms play a vital role in modulating vascular tone and reactivity (discussed previously). Local mediators (such as NO, prostacyclin, endothelin, endothelium-derived contracting factors, and lipid mediators) and various neurohumoral stimuli modulate the degree of pulmonary vasoconstriction. For example, an inability to produce increased NO to attenuate the severity of pulmonary vasoconstriction may lead to more sustained, severe pulmonary hypertension during acute hypoxia. The contribution of genetics to exaggerated pulmonary vasoreactivity and increased susceptibility to hypoxic pulmonary hypertension has been suggested by animal and clinical studies. Grover et al[139] identified increased severity of hypoxic pulmonary hypertension ("brisket disease") in some cattle strains. Similarly, human infants who are born at sea level but later moved to high altitude (3600 meters) in Lhasa, Tibet, develop severe pulmonary hypertension and right-sided heart failure within weeks to months. Massive RV hypertrophy and hypertensive pulmonary vascular remodeling is present at autopsy. This disease (called subacute infantile mountain sickness) represents the failure of lowlanders of Han origin to adapt to hypobaric hypoxia.[140] Interestingly, other Hans have lived in Lhasa for generations but are apparently well-adapted to high altitude, demonstrating biologic variability.

HAPE primarily occurs in previously healthy individuals ascending to altitudes, usually above 8000 feet. Typically, patients have made a rapid ascent from sea level. Additional risk factors include poor conditioning, increased activity at altitude, underlying viral illness, lack of progressive adaptation to altitude by gradually increasing altitude, sleep apnea, and alcohol intake. HAPE often occurs in patients who have previously tolerated altitude and with reascent of some long-term altitude residents after travel for a few days at a lower altitude. The incidence of HAPE is unclear, but severe disease occurs in less than 0.1% of visitors to Summit County, Colorado; however, mild disease is unlikely to lead to medical attention. Clinical signs include severe dyspnea, fatigue, weakness, dry cough, and anxiety or restlessness. Some patients develop hemoptysis. A viral illness is often initially suspected in young children with HAPE because of such nonspecific signs as anorexia, vomiting, and low-grade fever. The differential diagnosis also includes congestive heart failure, pneumonia, pulmonary embolus, alcohol, viral syndrome, severe exhaustion, or carbon monoxide poisoning. On examination, patients have tachypnea, tachycardia, cyanosis, and diffuse crackles. Chest radiographs generally show fluffy densities, which may appear unilateral early, along with pulmonary artery enlargement, normal heart size, and progressive alveolar infiltrates. ECG studies often show tachycardia, peaked P waves, right-axis deviation, ST-T changes, and perhaps RV hypertrophy. Arterial blood gas tensions show severe hypoxia with low CO_2 (early). If cardiac catheterization is performed, marked pulmonary hypertension with normal PCWP and normal left-sided heart function is often found. Follow-up studies generally report normal or mildly elevated baseline PVR, which increases dramatically with acute hypoxia.[59,137]

Detection of high concentrations of albumin in bronchoalveolar lavage fluid confirms that HAPE is characterized by permeability edema[141,142] and is associated with increased inflammation, as reflected by increased inflammatory cells and products, including leukotrienes.[143] Mechanisms that disrupt the alveolar-capillary barrier leading to increased permeability are unclear but may be related to the direct effects of hypoxia on endothelium through altered cyclic adenosine monophosphate (cAMP) activity.[144] Although pulmonary edema in HAPE may not be primarily caused by pulmonary hypertension per se, elevation of microvascular pressure contributes to the severity of edema formation in the presence of increased permeability. Patients with a history of HAPE have marked hypoxic pulmonary vasoconstriction, which is likely to accelerate edema formation. Thus the sequence of events contributing to the pathophysiology of HAPE may be as follows: at altitude, alveolar hypoxia disrupts the alveolar-capillary barrier, promotes lung inflammation, causes intense vasoconstriction, and worsens $\dot{V}/\dot{Q}$ mismatch. Overperfusion of some nonconstricted capillaries may cause stress failure, worsening vascular injury and increasing interstitial and alveolar edema formation. Etiologic factors contributing to HAPE include exposure to altitude, nonspecific triggers (such as viral illness), and genetics. Because a marked individual variability in susceptibility and recurrence risks for HAPE exists, the role of genetic factors has been suggested.[139] Hypoxic ventilatory drive is often diminished in individuals with recurrent HAPE, perhaps because of altered nocturnal respiratory patterns. Nocturnal hypoxia caused by hypoventilation may contribute to the development of acute mountain sickness and HAPE.

Treatment of HAPE includes early recognition of its signs and symptoms, rapid descent to lower altitude, administration of supplemental oxygen, cautious use of diuretics, and bed rest. There is no role for digoxin or antibiotics. Although treatment is simple, mortality is high if untreated; early treatment should lead to full recovery. With severe symptoms, nifedipine may lower PAP and hasten recovery[145]; it also provides effective prophylaxis in HAPE-susceptible individuals. In anticipation of ascent to high altitude, gradual increases in altitude with limited activity is recommended.

Chronic Upper Airway Obstruction

Pulmonary hypertension develops in children with upper airway obstruction or obstructive sleep apnea caused by repeated episodes of marked hypoxia. Diverse etiologies of upper airway obstruction share common pathophysiologic features of episodic hypoxia, causing intermittent elevations of PAP, which can eventually lead to sustained pulmonary hypertension and RV hypertrophy. Although airway obstruction can lead to striking cor pulmonale in otherwise healthy children, it can accelerate pulmonary hypertension associated with chronic lung and heart disease. Every child with significant pulmonary hypertension should be evaluated for upper airway obstruction and obstructive sleep apnea. Clinical signs include noisy breathing, snoring, restless sleep with frequent arousal, appearance of air hunger, and retractions with sleep. Other signs include excessive daytime somnolence, deteriorating school performance, behavioral changes, enuresis, systemic hypertension, and morning headache. Failure to thrive is not uncommon, with growth improving with therapy. Similarly, correction of hypoxia can improve neurodevelopmental delays in children with chronic obstruction, as in infants with Pierre-Robin syndrome. Diagnostic evaluations include pulse oximetry and arterial or capillary blood gas tension (to evaluate $Pa{CO_2}$), sleep studies, flexible bronchoscopy, barium swallow, and other studies as indicated. Management depends on the cause and severity of obstruction, whether hypoxia is easily corrected with supplemental oxygen, and the severity of pulmonary hypertension. The roles of tonsillectomy with adenoidectomy, oxygen therapy, repeat sleep studies, nasal CPAP or BiPAP ventilation, tracheostomy, and other strategies are discussed elsewhere. Because pulmonary hypertension from upper airway obstruction can be severe at presentation, diagnosis and therapy usually lead to complete resolution with time.

Pulmonary Circulation in Liver Disease

Pulmonary vascular disease associated with chronic liver disease includes two strikingly different clinical abnormalities, including (1) low-resistance vascular lesions with marked hypoxemia and (2) high PVR, often with extensive structural remodeling (often with "onionskinning").[146] Hypoxemia with chronic liver disease may be due to lung disease, including decreased lung volumes, pleural effusions, atelectasis, or pulmonary edema. However, up to one third of patients with chronic liver disease have hypoxemia without underlying cardiac or lung disease. Patients with hepatopulmonary syndrome have severe dyspnea on exertion, shortness of breath, clubbing, cyanosis, and cutaneous spider nevi. Hypoxemia is often severe and is aggravated in the upright position (orthodeoxia) and with exercise. Hypoxemia may precede the onset of severe liver disease, and there is little correlation between the degree of hypoxemia and severity of hepatic function. Chest radiographs may be normal or show increased interstitial markings with more prominence in the bases. Pulmonary function tests may demonstrate restrictive or mixed abnormalities. Diffusing capacity for carbon monoxide (DLCO) is abnormal. Chest CT shows increased central and peripheral vascularity without interstitial abnormalities. Diagnosis is confirmed by perfusion lung scans using technetium Tc 99m-labeled macroaggregated albumin, in which radiolabeled albumin particles, 20 to 60 microns, are injected intravenously. With normal pulmonary capillaries, which are 8 to 15 microns in diameter, the particles are trapped in the pulmonary microcirculation and do not pass to the systemic circulation. Increased activity in extrapulmonary sites as detected by scanning over the kidneys or brain implies the presence of marked right-to-left cardiac or intrapulmonary shunting. Echocardiography rules out intracardiac shunting. Pulmonary angiography is usually not necessary for diagnosis but would show a diffuse (spongy) arterial phase or discrete focal arteriovenous communications.

Hypoxemia and exercise intolerance in the hepatopulmonary syndrome is partly due to low $\dot{V}/\dot{Q}$ zones at the lung bases from airway closure during tidal volume breathing. Impaired hypoxic pulmonary vasoconstriction has been demonstrated in patients with cirrhosis, suggesting that an inability to redistribute blood flow to match ventilation further contributes to $\dot{V}/\dot{Q}$ inequality.[147] Lack of marked improvement while breathing 100% oxygen in these patients, however, implies that $\dot{V}/\dot{Q}$ alone does not account for severe hypoxemia. Intrapulmonary shunting through dramatically enlarged or dilated vessels in the microcirculation causes refractory hypoxemia The marked increase in vessel diameter increases diffusion distance for oxygen from the alveolus to capillary blood; equilibrium may not be achieved, especially with exercise. Alternatively, the low resistance in these vessels may decrease perfusion of distal microcirculation within the lung periphery. Pulmonary vascular lesions are associated with spider angiomas on the skin and pleura, suggesting that an unknown systemic factor contributes to altered vascular function or growth. Past unsuccessful medical therapies have included drug treatment with estrogens, β blockers, cyclooxygenase inhibitors, and somatostatin. Almitrine, a drug that augments hypoxic pulmonary vasoconstriction, has little effect in these patients. Although in the past hypoxemia was considered a contraindication for liver transplantation, recent evidence has suggested that hypoxemia, clubbing, and related signs of hepatopulmonary syndrome improve after transplantation.

In contrast with the low-resistance shunt vessels in the lung microcirculation, some patients have severe unexplained pulmonary hypertension. The presence of portal hypertension may be a critical factor among cirrhotic patients who develop pulmonary hypertension, as pulmonary hypertension has complicated portal hypertension in the absence of underlying liver disease. Pulmonary hypertension is not restricted to specific types of liver disease and can be present in the absence of portal hypertension. The pathogenesis is unknown, but it has been speculated to be related to an autoimmune process or related to circulating mediators with potent vasoconstrictor or growth-stimulating effects that may be produced in excess or not cleared by the diseased liver. Clinically, patient evaluation should include a workup for portal vein thrombosis and hypercoagulability. Moderate pulmonary hypertension may serve as a contraindication for liver transplantation because of the risks of graft dysfunction from severe postoperative right-sided heart failure as well as the difficult hemodynamic management of these patients in the immediate perioperative period. Preoperative evaluation may be aided by assessing pulmonary vasoreactivity in these patients; however, whether the acute hemodynamic response to vasodilators predicts a favorable outcome is unproven.

Acute Respiratory Distress Syndrome

Current treatment of acute hypoxemic respiratory failure, including acute respiratory distress syndrome (ARDS), is often unsuccessful, with mortality at 50% to 75%. Although death is commonly associated with multiple organ failure, progressive respiratory failure contributes to poor outcome. Injury to the pulmonary circulation during acute respiratory failure leads to increased permeability, leading to pulmonary edema with surfactant inactivation, low lung compliance, and decreased gas exchange. In addition, the pathophysiology of ARDS is characterized by pulmonary hypertension and altered pulmonary vasoreactivity, which worsens $\dot{V}/\dot{Q}$ mismatch, accelerates pulmonary edema formation, and may cause RV dysfunction. Despite the presence of pulmonary hypertension, vasodilator therapy has been limited by the inability to selectively lower PAP without causing systemic hypotension or worsening gas exchange by increasing perfusion of underventilated lung regions. The contribution of pulmonary vasoconstriction to the pathophysiology of ARDS has been recently demonstrated in studies examining the response to inhaled NO.[148-150] Inhaled NO selectively lowers PAP and improves gas exchange in selected patients. Whether inhaled NO treatment will improve outcome in ARDS is currently under study.

RESPIRATORY COMPLICATIONS OF CARDIAC DISEASE

As chronic lung disease contributes to pulmonary hypertension, altered cardiac function can also adversely affect lung function. Many respiratory complications accompany cardiac disorders, complicating acute management following surgical repair of anatomic heart disease as well as long-term outcome. Three general categories of cardiovascular lesions cause concomitant abnormalities in lung function: first, vascular anomalies that obstruct large airways; second, high pulmonary blood flow caused by large volume left-to-right shunts; and third, inflow or outflow obstruction to the left (systemic) ventricle. Central airways obstruction resulting from vascular compression can be caused by structural lesions such as double aortic arch, right-sided aortic arch, aberrant right subclavian artery, anomalous innominate artery, and pulmonary artery sling. These can accompany congenital cardiac lesions and should be sought in clinical settings of stridor, recurrent or persistent wheezing, cough, apnea, and feeding difficulties. In addition, structural abnormalities of the central airways can also be associated with cardiac lesions, such as complete tracheal rings and narrowing (with agenesis of right lung or pulmonary sling). Structural abnormalities of small airways may also accompany some cardiac lesions. Small airway obstruction with heart disease is commonly caused by mechanical compression by small pulmonary arteries, pulmonary edema, bronchial edema, or bronchoconstriction (discussed later).

Increased pulmonary blood flow occurs with large left-to-right anatomic shunts, such as with ventricular septal defects, patent ductus arteriosus, atrioventricular canals, single ventricle, aortopulmonary window, or truncus arteriosus. High pulmonary blood flow distends small pulmonary arteries and increases PAP. High flow also increases left-ventricular end-diastolic volume and pressure, which raises left-atrial and pulmonary venous pressures. Increased blood flow with elevated pulmonary arterial and venous pressures contribute to peribronchial and interstitial edema, causing small airway obstruction, causing "cardiac asthma," which is characterized by clinical signs of high airway resistance as a result of small airway obstruction. Airway edema causes mechanical obstruction of small airways as a result of peribronchial and mucosal swelling. Distended pulmonary arteries cause extrinsic compression of small airways, which can occur with high flow even in the absence of overt heart failure. Bronchoconstriction and altered bronchial reactivity may further contribute to small airways narrowing.[151] Chronic elevation of pulmonary blood flow may also be associated with increased peribronchial wall thickening caused by smooth muscle hypertrophy and increased extracellular matrix production.

Along with increased airways resistance, high pulmonary blood flow decreases lung compliance and increases work of breathing, especially when associated with mean PAP above 25 mm Hg.[152,153] Marked left-atrial enlargement can compress the left or right mainstem bronchi, causing airflow obstruction and hyperinflation. Clinical findings include tachypnea with shallow breathing, which may increase physiologic dead space. Other signs are retractions, rhonchi, and wheezing. Chest radiograph findings include hyperinflation or, in some cases, lobar emphysema or atelectasis. Therapy includes medical management of pulmonary edema and failure (diuresis, digoxin), and acute assessment for clinical improvement after an inhaled bronchodilator. These patients are at marked risk for severe respiratory failure with superimposed lower respiratory infections, including respiratory syncytial virus bronchiolitis. Surgical correction of the underlying lesion should improve respiratory signs, but in some cases, airways obstruction persists.

Inflow or outflow obstruction to the left (or systemic) ventricle, from pulmonary venoocclusive disease, total anomalous pulmonary venous return, mitral stenosis, cor triatriatum, and left-ventricular obstruction caused by coarctation of the aorta, interrupted arch, aortic stenosis, or atresia and cardiomyopathy, can also impair lung function. Pulmonary venous obstruction or hypertension initially increases pulmonary blood volume and interstitial edema, causing many of the effects on lung mechanics discussed previously. Clinically, children can present with clinical signs of airways obstruction, but more commonly, they present as "interstitial lung disease," with marked tachypnea, cyanosis, and rales. Chest radiograph usually shows a normal cardiac silhouette with increased venous or interstitial markings. Asymmetry may suggest unilateral venous obstruction. Prolonged pulmonary venous hypertension over time can subsequently lead to striking structural venous and arterial changes, contributing to severe pulmonary hypertension.

NEW THERAPEUTIC APPROACHES TO PEDIATRIC PULMONARY HYPERTENSION

Among recent discoveries in basic vascular biology were reports that the endothelium produces a substance with potent vasodilator properties (EDRF)[23] and that EDRF is a gas (NO).[24,25] Based on past experience studying inhaled NO as a potential clinical test for lung diffusion capacity, Higenbottam et al[154] first recognized its potential clinical application as an inhalational therapy for pulmonary hypertension (Fig. 58-8). Brief exposure to inhaled NO acutely lowered PVR in adults with primary pulmonary hypertension without adverse effects on systemic hemodynamics. Subsequent work demonstrated that inhaled NO acutely lowered PVR and improved oxygenation in newborns with severe pulmonary hypertension[110,111] and that prolonged low-dose NO therapy may provide sustained improvement in PPHN, decreasing the need for extracorporeal membrane oxygenation (Fig. 58-9).[112] Inhaled NO acutely lowers PVR in children with congenital heart disease[155,156] and adults and children with severe ARDS.[148-150] Although pharmacologic vasodilators, such as prostacyclin and sodium nitroprusside, can lower PAP in ARDS, these agents often worsen $\dot{V}/\dot{Q}$ mismatch, decreasing gas-exchange and lowering Pa_{O_2}.[148] In contrast, inhaled NO redistributes pulmonary blood flow to better ventilated regions of lung, increasing oxygenation in many patients. Thus unlike most therapeutic agents, inhaled NO has the unique ability not only to selectively lower PAP without affecting systemic pressure, but also to enhance $\dot{V}/\dot{Q}$ matching in the presence of parenchymal lung disease.

Similar findings have been observed in children with acute hypoxemic respiratory failure, including CNLD infants with influenza or respiratory syncytial virus pneumonitis, both of which can be major causes of prolonged morbidity or death.[150] Further clinical experience with inhaled NO suggests efficacy in selected cases of postoperative pulmonary hypertension associated with congenital heart disease, and after heart and lung transplantation. Some patients have little response to inhaled NO; whether this reflects severe structural remodeling of small pulmonary arteries, functional impairment of the soluble guanylate cyclase system in hypertensive smooth muscle cells, or other mechanisms requires further study. Despite current enthusiasm for the therapeutic role of inhaled NO, many concerns exist regarding potential toxicities (such as lung inflammation, decreased surfactant production or activity, and others).[157] However, recent studies have suggested that very low dosages of inhaled NO may provide effective vasodilation in PPHN and ARDS, and in many cases, clinical improvement can be sustained without tachyphylaxis at these dosages. Whether low dosages of inhaled NO can be safely used for prolonged therapy requires further study. Several multicenter clinical trials are under way, examining its safety and efficacy in PPHN, ARDS, congenital heart disease, and other acute settings. The long-term response and its potential role in treating chronic pulmonary hypertension with or without severe lung disease is unknown; however, recent studies have suggested that chronic NO administration attenuates the severity of pulmonary hypertension and pulmonary vascular remodeling.[158]

In addition to inhaled NO, new alternative pharmacologic approaches are likely to evolve from recent findings regarding the role of ion flux in pulmonary vascular tone and growth. Additional therapies for treating chronic pulmonary hypertension will most likely target mechanisms contributing to vascular remodeling with long-standing pulmonary hypertension, using heparin-related compounds, chronic endothelin blockade, elastase inhibition,[159] angiotensin-converting enzyme inhibition,[160] or selective blockers of extracellular matrix proteins. With rapid developments in strategies for gene therapy or the use of antisense oligonucleotides, the interface between

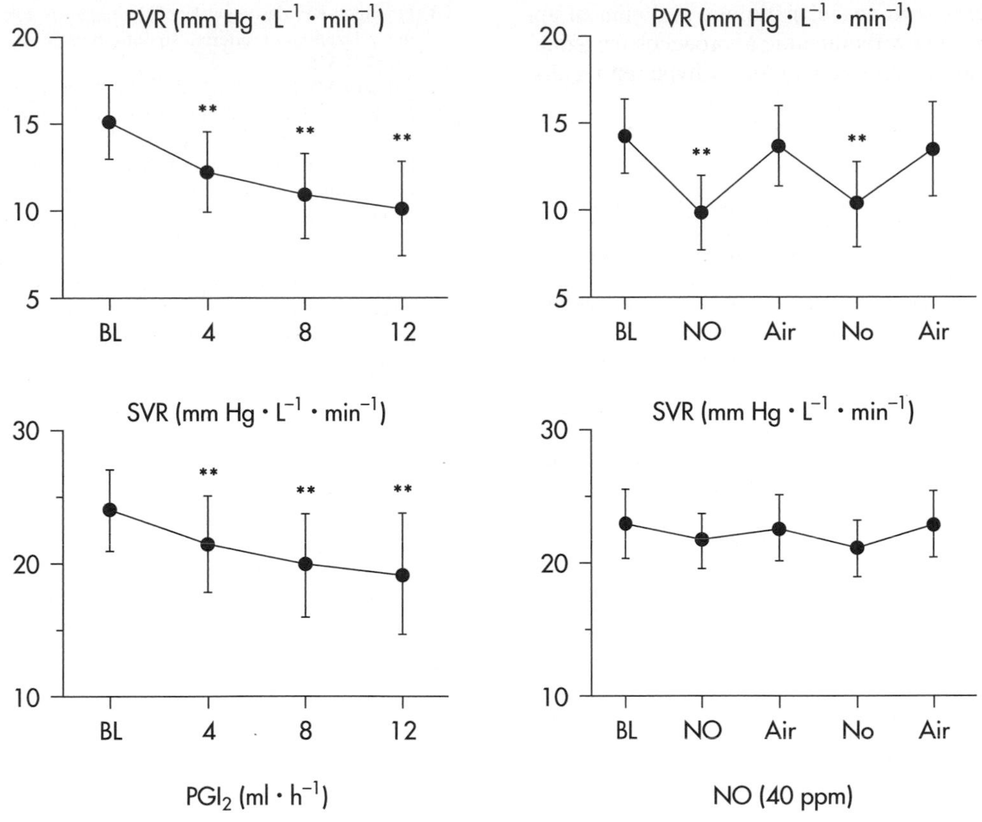

Fig. 58-8 Selective pulmonary vasodilator response to inhaled NO in adults with primary pulmonary hypertension. Unlike the drop in systemic vascular resistance *(SVR)* -Z with infusions of the vasodilator, prostacyclin (Pg_2), inhaled NO lowered pulmonary vascular resistance *(PVR)* without affecting SVR. (From Pepke-Zaba J, Higgenbottam TW, Dinh Xuan T, Stone D, Wallwork J: *Lancet* 338:1173-1174, 1991.)

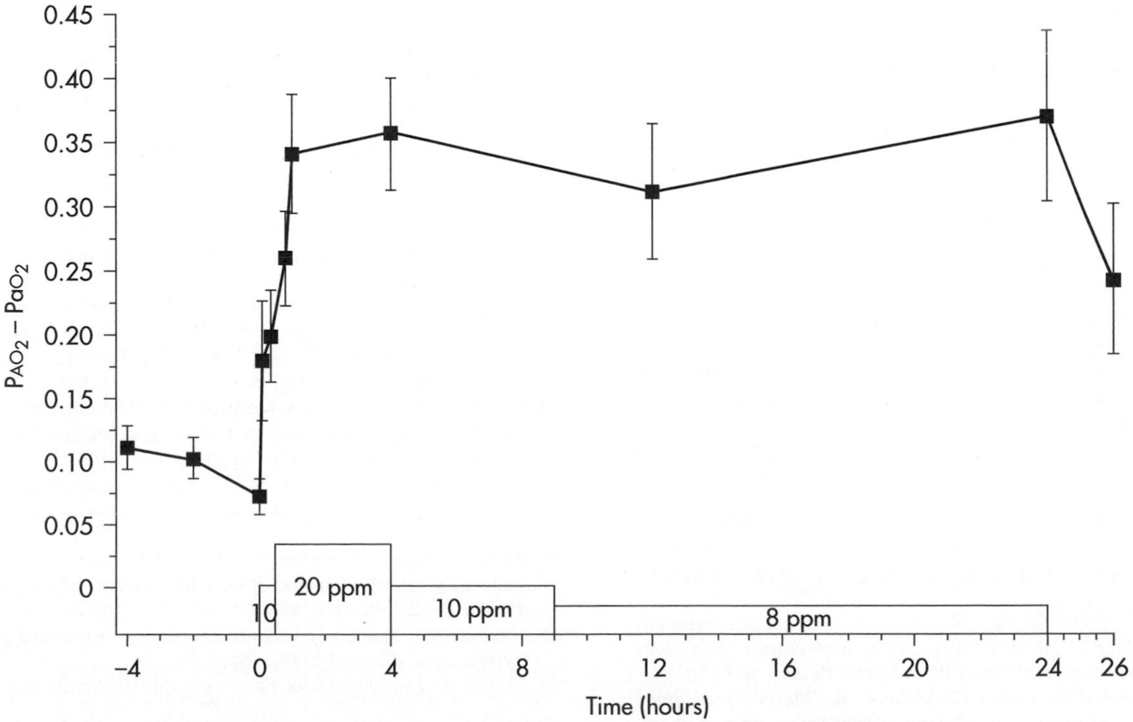

Fig. 58-9 Sustained improvement in oxygenation in neonates with severe PPHN during treatment with inhaled NO. (From Kinsella JP, Neish SR, Shaffer E, Abman SH: *Lancet* 340:819-820, 1992.)

basic *scientific* advances in vascular biology and clinical applications will provide new therapeutic approaches for reducing the morbidity and mortality of pulmonary hypertensive disorders in pediatrics.

REFERENCES

1. Abman SH, Sondheimer HM: Pulmonary circulation and cardiovascular sequelae of BPD. In Weir EK, Archer SL, Reeves JT, eds: *Diagnosis and treatment of pulmonary hypertension,* Mount Kisco, NY, 1992, Futura Publishing, pp l55-180.
2. Berman W, Yabek SM, Dillon T, et al: Evaluation of infants with BPD using cardiac catheterization, *Pediatrics* 70:708-712, 1982.
3. Goodman G, Perkin RM, Anas NG, et al: Pulmonary hypertension in infants with BPD, *J Pediatr* 112:67-72, 1988.
4. Bush A, Busst CM, Knight WB, et al: Changes in pulmonary circulation in severe BPD, *Arch Dis Child* 65:739-745, 1990.
5. Stern RC, Borket G, Hirschfield SS, et al: Heart failure in CF: treatment and prognosis of cor pulmonale with failure of the right side of the heart, *Am J Dis Child* 134:267, 1980.
6. Ryland D, Reid L: The pulmonary circulation in CF, *Thorax* 30:285-292, 1975.
7. Moser KM, Shea JG: The relationship between pulmonary infarction, cor pulmonale and the sickle states, *Am J Med* 22:561-579, 1957.
8. Fan LL, Mullen ALW, Brugman SM, Inscore SC, Parks DP, White CW: Clinical spectrum of chronic interstitial lung disease in children, *J Pediatr* 121:867-872, 1993.
9. Fayemi AO: Pulmonary vascular disease in systemic lupus erythematosus, *Am J Clin Pathol* 65:284, 1976.
10. Stenmark KR, Orton EC, Reeves JT, et al: Vascular remodeling in neonatal pulmonary hypertension: role of the smooth muscle cell, *Chest* 93:127S-133S, 1988.
11. Todd L, Mullen M, Olley P, et al: Pulmonary toxicity of monocrotaline differs at critical periods of lung development, *Pediatr Res* 1:731-737, 1985.
12. Abman SH, Accurso FJ, Koops BL: Experience with home oxygen in the management of infants with BPD, *Clin Pediatr* 23:471-476, 1984.

Definitions of Cor Pulmonale and Pulmonary Hypertension

13. Fishman AP: Chronic cor pulmonale, *Am Rev Respir Dis* 114:775-794, 1976.
14. World Health Organization: Chronic cor pulmonale. A report of the expert committee, *Circulation* 27:594-615, 1963.
15. Bhargava RK: *Cor pulmonale (pulmonary heart disease),* Mount Kisco, NY, 1973, Futura.

Clinical Settings Associated with Pulmonary Hypertension

16. Justo RN, Dare AD, Whight CM, Radford DJ: Pulmonary veno-occlusive disease: diagnosis during life in four patients, *Arch Dis Child* 68:97-100, 1993.

Developmental Physiology of the Pulmonary Circulation

17. Hislop A, Reid L: Formation of the pulmonary vasculature: development of the lung. In Hodson WA, Lenfant C, eds: *Lung biology in health and disease,* New York, 1977, Marcel Dekker, pp 3-35.
18. Reid L, Fried R, Geggel R, Langleben D: Anatomy of pulmonary hypertensive states. In Bergofsky EF, ed: *Abnormal pulmonary circulation,* New York, 1986, Churchill Livingstone, p 227.
19. Levin DL, Hyman AL, Heymann MA, Rudolph AM: Fetal hypertension and the development of increased pulmonary vascular smooth muscle: a possible mechanism for PPHN, *J Pediatr* 92:265-269, 1978.
20. Abman SH, Kinsella JP, Schaffer MS, Wilkening RB: Inhaled nitric oxide therapy in the management of a premature newborn with severe respiratory distress and pulmonary hypertension, *Pediatrics* 92:606-609, 1993.
21. Heymann MA, Soifer SJ: Control of fetal and neonatal pulmonary circulation. In Weir EK, Reeves JT, eds: *Pulmonary vascular physiology and pathophysiology,* New York, 1989, Marcel Dekker, pp 33-50.
22. Wallen LD, Perry SF, Alston JT, Maloney JE: Morphometric study of the role of pulmonary arterial flow in fetal lung growth in sheep, *Pediatr Res* 27: l22-127, 1990.
23. Furchgott RF, Zawadski JV: The obligatory role of endothelial cells in the relaxation of arterial smooth muscle by acetylcholine, *Nature* 288:373-376, 1980.
24. Palmer RMJ, Ferrige AG, Moncado S: NO release accounts for the biological activity of endothelium-derived relaxing factor, *Nature* 327:524-526, 1987.
25. Ignarro LJ, Buga GM, Woods KS, et al: Endothelium-derived relaxing factor produced and released from artery and vein is NO, *Proc Natl Acad Sci USA* 84:9265-9269, 1987.
26. Abman SH, Chatfield BA, Hall SL, McMurtry IF: Role of endothelium-derived relaxing factor during transition of pulmonary circulation at birth, *Am J Physiol* 259:Hl921-H1927, 1990.
27. Yanagasawa M, Kurihara S, Kimura S, Tomobe Y, Kobayashi M, Mitsui Y, Yazaki Y, Goto K, Masaki T: A novel potent vasoconstrictor peptide produced by vascular endothelial cells, *Nature* 332:411-415, 1988.
28. Ivy DD, Kinsella JP, Abman SH: Physiologic characterization of endothelin A and B receptor activity in the ovine fetal pulmonary circulation, *J Clin Invest* 93:2141-2148, 1994.
29. Rosenberg AA, Kennaugh J, Koppenhafer SL, Loomis ML, Chatfield BA, Agman SH: Elevated immunoreactive endothelin-1 levels in newborns with persistent pulmonary hypertension of the newborn, *J Pediatr* 123:109-114, 1993.
30. Soifer S, Loitz RD, Roman C, Heymann MA: Leukotriene end organ antagonists increase pulmonary blood flow in fetal lambs, *Am J Physiol* 249:H570-H576, 1985.
31. Tod ML, Cassin S: Fetal and neonatal pulmonary circulation. In Crystal RG, West JB, eds: *The lung: scientific foundations,* New York, 1991, Raven Press, pp 1687-1698.
32. Abman SH, Chatfield BA, Rodman DM, Hall SL, McMurtry IF: Maturation-related changes in endothelium-dependent relaxation of ovine pulmonary arteries, *Am J Physiol* 260: L280-L285, 1991.
33. Shaul P, Farrar MA, Zellers TM: Oxygen modulates endothelium-derived relaxing factor production in fetal pulmonary arteries, *Am J Physiol* 262:H355-H364, 1992.
34. Kinsella JP, McQueston JA, Rosenberg AA, Abman SH: Effects of inhaled nitric oxide on the ovine transitional pulmonary circulation, *Am J Physiol* 263:H875-H880, 1992.
35. Langston C, Kida K, Reed M, Thuribeck WM: Human lung growth in late gestation and in the neonate, *Am Rev Respir Dis* 129:607-613, 1984.
36. O'Brodovich HM, Mellins RB: Bronchopulmonary dysplasia, *Am Rev Respir Dis* 132:694-709, 1985.
37. Sobonya RE, Logvinoff MM, Taussig LM, et al: Morphometric analysis of the lung in prolonged BPD, *Pediatr Res* 16:969-972, 1982.
38. Tomashefski JF, Opperman HC, Vawter GF, et al: BPD: A morphometric study with emphasis on pulmonary vasculature, *Pediatr Pathol* 2:469-487, 1984.
39. Abman SH, Shanley PF, Accurso FJ: Failure of postnatal adaptation of the pulmonary circulation after chronic intrauterine pulmonary hypertension in fetal lambs, *J Clin Invest* 83:1849-1858, 1989.
40. Wild LM, Nickerson PA, Morin FC: Ligating the ductus arteriosus before birth remodels the pulmonary vasculature of the lamb, *Pediatr Res* 25:251-258, 1989.
41. Geggel RL, Aronovitz MJ, Reid LM: Effects of chronic in utero hypoxia on rat neonatal pulmonary artery structure, *J Pediatr* 108:756, 1986.
42. Murphy JD, Aronovitz MJ, Reid LM: Effects of chronic in utero hypoxia in the newborn guinea pig, *Pediatr Res* 20:292, 1986.
43. Cornfield DN, Chaffield BA, McQueston JA, McMurtry lF, Abman SH: Effects of birth-related stimuli on L-arginine dependent vasodilation in the ovine fetal lung, *Am J Physiol* 262:H1474-H1481, 1992.
44. Leffler CW, Tyler TL, Cassin S: Effect of indomethacin on pulmonary vascular response to ventilation of fetal goats, *Am J Physiol* 235:346, 1978.
45. Morin FC, Egan EA, Norfleet WT: Indomethacin does not diminish the pulmonary vascular response of the fetus to increased oxygen tension, *Pediatr Res* 24:696-700, 1988.
46. Haworth SG: Pulmonary vascular remodeling in neonatal pulmonary hypertension, *Chest* 93:133S-138S, 1988.
47. Murray JF: *The normal lung,* Philadelphia, 1986, WB Saunders, pp 139-150.
48. Deffebach ME, Widdicombe J: The bronchial circulation. In Crystal RG, West JB, eds: *The lung: scientific foundations,* New York, 1991, Raven Press, pp 741-757.

49. Moss AJ: Cardiovascular system in CF, *Pediatrics* 70:728-741, 1982.
50. Abdi S, Herndon DN, Traber LD, Ashley KD, Stothert JC, Maguire J, Butler R, Traber DL: Lung edema formation following inhalation injury: role of the bronchial blood flow, *J Appl Physiol* 71:727-734, 1991.
51. West JB, Dollery CT, Naimark A: Distribution of blood flow in isolated lung: relation to vascular and alveolar pressures, *J Appl Physiol* 19:713-724, 1964.
52. Battacharya J, Staub NC: Direct measurements of microvascular pressures in the isolated perfused dog lung, *Science* 210:327-328, 1980.
53. Von Euler US, Liljestrand G: Observations on the pulmonary arterial blood pressure in the cat, *Acta Physiol Scand* 12:301-320, 1947.
54. Voelkel NF: Mechanisms of hypoxic pulmonary vasoconstriction, *Am Rev Respir Dis* 133:1186-1195, 1986.
55. Ryan US, Rubanyi GM: *Endothelial regulation of vascular tone,* New York, 1992, Marcel Dekker.
56. Vane JR, Anggard EE, Bofting RM: Regulatory functions of the vascular endothelium, *N Engl J Med* 323:27-36, 1990.

Disease Mechanisms

57. Fox WW, Duara S: Persistent pulmonary hypertension of the newborn: diagnosis and management, *J Pediatr* 103:505-514, 1993.
58. Southall DP, Samuels MP, Talbert DG: Recurrent cyanotic episodes with severe arterial hypoxemia and intrapulmonary shunting: a mechanism for sudden death, *Arch Dis Child* 65:953-961, 1990.
59. Fasules JW, Wiggins JW, Wolfe RR: Increased lung vasoreactivity in children from Leadville, Colorado, after recovery from high attitude pulmonary edema, *Circulation* 72:957-962, 1985.
60. Peach MJ, Johns RA, Rose CE: Potential role of interactions between endothelium and smooth muscle in pulmonary vascular physiology and pathophysiology. In Weir EK, Reeves JT, eds: *Pulmonary vascular physiology and pathophysiology,* New York, 1985, Marcel Dekker, pp 643-697.
61. Christman BW, McPherson CD, Newman JH, et al: An imbalance between the excretion of thromboxane and prostacyclin metabolites in pulmonary hypertension, *N Engl J Med* 327:70-75, 1992.
62. Dinh Xuan AT, Higenbottam TW, Cleland CA, et al: Impairment of endothelium-dependent pulmonary artery relaxation in chronic obstructive lung disease, *N Engl J Med* 324:1539-1542, 1991.
63. Giaid A, Yanagasawa M, Langleben D, Michel R, Levy R, Shennib H, Kimura S, Masaki T, Duguid WP, Stewart DJ: Expression of endothelin-1 in the lungs of patients with pulmonary hypertension, *N Engl J Med* 328:1732-1739, 1993.
64. Rowe RD, James LS: The normal pulmonary arterial pressure during the first year of life, *J Pediatr* 51:1-4, 1957.
65. Howell JBL, Permutt S, Proctor DF, Riley RL: Effect of inflation of the lung on different parts of pulmonary vascular bed, *J Appl Physiol* 16:71-76, 1961.
66. Reeves JT, Dempsey JA, Grover RF: Pulmonary circulation during exercise. In Weir EK, Reeves JT, eds: *Pulmonary vascular physiology and pathophysiology,* New York, 1985, Marcel Dekker, pp 107-135.
67. Jezek V, Schrijen F, Sadoul P: Right ventricular function and pulmonary hemodynamics during exercise in patients with COPD, *Cardiology* 58:20-31, 1973.
68. Burrows B, Keffel LJ, Niden AH, et al: Patterns of cardiovascular dysfunction in chronic obstructive lung disease, *N Engl J Med* 286:912-918, 1972.
69. Guyton AC, Linsey AW, Gilluly JJ: The limits of right ventricular compensation following acute increase in pulmonary circulatory resistance, *Circ Res* 2:326-332, 1954.
70. Reeves JT, Groves BM, Turkevich D, Morrison DA, Trapp JA: Right ventricular function in pulmonary hypertension. In Weir EK, Reeves JT, eds: *Pulmonary vascular physiology and pathophysiology,* New York, 1985, Marcel Dekker, pp 325-354.
71. MacDonald N, Hall C, Suffin S, et al: RSV infection in infants with congenital heart disease, *N Engl J Med* 307:397-400, 1982.
72. Janicki JS, Weber KT: Altered left ventricular function in pulmonary hypertension. In Weir EK, Archer SL, Reeves JT, eds: *The diagnosis and treatment of pulmonary hypertension,* Mount Kisco, NY, 1992, Futura, pp 61-78.
73. Khaia F, Parker JO: Right and left ventricular performance in COLD, *Am Heart J* 82:319-327, 1971.
74. Mathay RA, Berger HJ, Davies R, et al: Right and left ventricular exercise performance in COPD. Radionuclide assessment, *Ann Intern Med* 93:234-239, 1980.
75. Matthay RA, Niederman MS, Wiedemann HP: Cardiovascular-pulmonary interaction in COPD with special reference to the pathogenesis and management of cor pulmonale, *Med Clin North Am* 74:571-618, 1990.
76. Buccino RA, Harris E, Spann JF, et al: Response of myocardial connective tissue to development of experimetal hypertrophy, *Am J Physiol* 216:425-428, 1969.
77. Weitzenblum E, Apprill M, Oswald M, Chaout A, Imbs J-L: Pulmonary hemodynamics in patients with COPD before and during an epsiode of peripheral edema, *Chest* 105:1377-1382, 1994.
78. Wagner PD, Rodriquez-Roisin R: Clinical advances in pulmonary gas exchange, *Am Rev Respir Dis* 143:883-888, 1991.
79. Agusti AGN, Rodriguez-Roisin R: Effect of pulmonary hypertension on gas exchange, *Eur Resp J* 6:1371-1377, 1993.

Assessment and Diagnosis

80. Klinger JR, Hill NS: Right ventricular dysfunction in chronic obstructive pulmonary disease. Evaluation and management, *Chest* 99:715-723, 1991.
81. Levine OR, Harris RC, Blanc WA, Mellins RB: Progressive pulmonary hypertension in children with portal hypertension, *J Pediatr* 83:964-972, 1973.
82. Abman SH, Accurso FJ, Bowman CM: Unsuspected cardiopulmonary abnormalities in infants with BPD, *Arch Dis Child* 59:966-970, 1984.
83. Matthay RA, Schwarz Ml, Ellis JH, Steele PP, Siebert PE, Durrance JR, et al: Pulmonary artery hypertension in COPD: chest radiographic assessment, *Invest Radiol* 16:95-100, 1981.
84. Saito H, Dambara T, Aiba M, Suzuki T, Kira S: Evaluation of cor pulmonale on a modified short-axis section of the heart by magnetic resonance imaging, *Am Rev Respir Dis* 146:1576-1581, 1992.
85. Chipps BE, Alderson PPO, Roland JM, et al: Non-invasive evaluation of ventricular function in CF, *J Pediatr* 95:379-384, 1979.
86. Halliday HL, Dumpit FM, Brady JP: Effects of inspired oxygen on echocardiographic assessment of pulmonary vascular resistance and myocardial contractility in BPD, *Pediatrics* 65:536-540, 1980.
87. Berger M, Haimowitz A, Van Tosh A, Berdoff RL, Goldberg E: Quantitative assessment of pulmonary hypertension in patients with tricuspid regurgitation using continuous wave Doppler ultrasound, *J Am Coll Cardiol* 19:1508-1515, 1992.
88. Hatle L, Angelsen BA, Tromsdal A: Non-invasive estimation of pulmonary artery systolic pressure with Doppler ultrasound, *Br Heart J* 45:157-165, 1981.
89. Torbicki A, Skwarski K, Hawrylkiewicz I, Pasierski T, Miskiewicz Z, Zielinski J: Attempts at measuring pulmonary artery pressure by means of Doppler echocardiography in patients with chronic lung disease, *Eur Respir J* 2:856-860, 1989.
90. Abman SH, Wolfe RR, Accurso FJ, Koops BL, Bowman CM, Wiggins JW: Pulmonary vascular response to oxygen in infants with severe BPD, *Pediatrics* 75:80-84, 1985.

Management

91. British Medical Research Council Party: Long term domiciliary oxygen therapy in hypoxic cor pulmonale complicating bronchitis and emphysema, *Lancet* i:681-685, 1981.
92. Nocturnal Oxygen Therapy Trial Group: Continuous or nocturnal oxygen therapy in hypoxemic chronic obstructive lung disease, *Ann Intern Med* 102:29-36, 1980.
93. Ashutosh K, Mead J, Dunsky M: Early effect of oxygen administration and prognosis in COPD and cor pulmonale, *Am Rev Respir Dis* 127: 399-404, 1983.
94. Vender RL: Chronic hypoxic pulmonary hypertension: cell biology to pathophysiology, *Chest* 106:236-243, 1994.
95. Gibbons GH, Dzau VJ: Emerging concept of vascular remodeling, *N Engl J Med* 330:1431-1438, 1994.
96. Wagner PD, Dantzker DR, Dueck R, et al: Ventilation-perfusion inequality in COPD, *J Clin Invest* 59:203-216, 1977.
97. Rush MG, Hazinski TA: Current therapy of BPD, *Clin Perinatol* 19: 563-590, 1992.
98. Kim YS, Aviado DM: Digitalis and the pulmonary circulation, *Am Heart J* 62:680-686, 1961.

99. Morgan JM, McCormack DG, Griffiths MJD, et al: Adenosine as a vasodilator in primary pulmonary hypertension, *Circulation* 84:1145-1149, 1991.
100. Melot C, Hallemans R, Naeije R, Mols P, Lejeune P: Deleterious effect of nifedipine on pulmonary gas exchange in COPD, *Am Rev Respir Dis* 130:612-616, 1984.
101. Rich S, Kaufmann E, Levy PS: Effect of high doses of calcium channel blockers on survival in primary pulmonary hypertension, *N Engl J Med* 327:76-81, 1992.
102. McMurtry IF, Davidson AB, Reeves JT, Grover RF: Inhibition of hypoxic pulmonary vasoconstriction by calcium antagonist in isolated rat lungs, *Circ Res* 38:99-104, 1976.
103. Simonneau G, Escourrou P, Duroux P, Lockhart A: Inhibition of hypoxic pulmonary vasoconstriction by nifedipine, *N Engl J Med* 304:1582-1585, 1981.
104. Barst RJ, Hall JC, Stalcup SA: Responses to prostacyclin predicts response to subsequent vasodilator therapy in children and young adults with primary pulmonary hypertension. In Doyle EF, ed: *Pediatric cardiology.* Proceedings of the second world congress, New York, 1986, Springer, pp 952-953.
105. Sturin C, Bassein L, Schiavina M, Gunelia G: Oral nifedipine in chronic cor pulmonale secondary to severe chronic obstructive pulmonary disease: short and long term hemodynamic effects, *Chest* 84:135-142, 1983.
106. Michael JR, Kennedy TP, Fitzpatrick S, et al: Nifedipine inhibits hypoxic pulmonary vasoconstriction during rest and exercise in patients with CF and cor pulmonale, *Am Rev Respir Dis* 130:516-519, 1984.
107. Geggel RL, Dozor AJ, Fyler DC, et al: Effect of vasodilators at rest and during exercise in young adults with CF and cor pulmonale, *Am Rev Respir Dis* 131:531-536, 1985.

Specific Diseases Associated with Pulmonary Hypertension

108. Long WA: PPHN. In Long WA, ed: *Fetal and neonatal cardiology,* Philadelphia, 1989, Saunders, pp 627-655.
109. Haworth SG, Reid L: Persistent fetal circulation. Newly recognized structural features, *J Pediatr* 88:614-620, 1976.
110. Roberts JD, Polaner DM, Lang P, Zapol WM: Inhaled NO in PPHN, *Lancet* 340:818-819, 1992.
111. Kinsella JP, Neish SR, Shaffer E, Abman SH: Low dose inhalational NO therapy in PPHN, *Lancet* 340:819-820, 1992.
112. Kinsella JP, Neish SR, Ivy DD, et al: Clinical responses to prolonged treatment of PPHN with low dose inhaled NO, *J Pediatr* 123:103-108, 1993.
113. Fouron JC, LeGuennec JC, Villemont D, et al: Value of echocardiography in assesing the outcome of BPD, *Pediatrics* 65:529-535, 1980.
114. Abman SH, Burchell MF, Schaffer MS, et al: Late sudden unexpected deaths in hospitalized infants with BPD, *Am J Dis Child* 143:815-819, 1989.
115. Stocker JT: Pathology of long-standing "healed" BPD, *Hum Pathol* 17: 943-961, 1986.
116. Abman SH, Schaffer MS, Wiggins JW, et al: Pulmonary vascular extraction of circulating norepinephrine in infants with BPD, *Pediatr Pulmonol* 3:386-391, 1987.
117. Brownlee JR, Beekman RH, Rosenthal A: Acute hemodynamic effects of nifedipine in infants with BPD and pulmonary hypertension, *Pediatr Res* 24:186-190, 1988.
118. Wigglesworth FW: Fibrocystic disease of the pancreas, *Am J Med Sci* 212:351, 1946.
119. Royce SW: Cor pulmonale in infancy and early childhood. Report on 34 patients with special reference to the occurence of pulmonary heart disease in CF of the pancreas, *Pediatrics* 8:225, 1951.
120. Goldring RM, Fishman AP, Turino GM, Cohen HI, Denning CR, Andersen: Pulmonary hypertension and cor pulmonale in CF of the pancreas, *J Pediatr* 65:501-524, 1964.
121. Siassi B, Moss AJ, Dooley RR: Clinical recognition of cor pulmonale in CF, *J Pediatr* 78:794-805, 1971.
122. Graham LM, Vasil A, Vasil ML, et al: Pulmonary vascular effects of chronic Pseudomonas aeruginosa pneumonia—potential roles of exotoxin phospholipase C, *Am Rev Respir Dis* 142:221-229, 1990.
123. Kelminson LL, Cotton EK, Vogel JHK: The reversibility of pulmonary hypertension in patients with CF, *Pediatrics* 39:24-35, 1967.
124. Dinh-Xuan AT, Higenbottam TW, Pepke-Zaba J, Clelland CA, Wallwork J: Reduced endothelium-dependent relaxation of CF pulmonary arteries, *Eur J Pharmacol* 163:401-403, 1989.
125. Allen HD, Taussig LM, Gaines JA, Sahn DJ, Goldberg SJ: Echocardiographic profiles of the long-term cardiac changes in CF, *Chest* 75:428-433, 1979.
126. Rosenthal A, Tucker CR, Williams RG, Khaw KT, Strieder D, Schwachman H: Echocardiographic assessment of cor pulmonale in CF, *Pediatr Clin North Am* 23:327-344, 1976.
127. Gewitz M, Eshaghpour E, Holsclaw DS, Miller HA, Kawai N: Echocardiography in CF, *Am J Dis Child* 131:275-280,1977.
128. Moskowitz WB, Gewitz MH, Heyman S, Ruddy RM, Scanlin TF: Cardiac involvement in CF: early noninvasive detection and vasodilator therapy, *Pediatr Pharmacol* 5:139-148, 1985.
129. Bowden DH, Fischer VW, Wyatt JP: Cor pulmonale in CF: a morphometric analysis, *Am J Med* 38:226, 1965.
130. Jacobstein MD, Hirschfield SS, Winnie G, Doershuk C, Liebman J: Ventricular interdependence in severe CF, *Chest* 80:399-403, 1981.
131. Zinman R, Corey M, Coates AL, Canny GJ, Connolly J, Levison H, Beaudry PH: Nocturnal home oxygen in the treatment of hypoxemic CF patients, *J Pediatr* 114:368-377, 1989.
132. Whitman V, Stern RC, Bellet P, Doershuk CF, Liebman J, Boat TF, Borkat G, Matthews LW: Studies on cor pulmonale in CF: 1. Effects of diuresis, *Pediatrics* 55: 83-85, 1975.
133. Davidson A, Bossuyt A, Dab I: Acute effects of oxygen, nifedipine, and diltiazem in patients with CF and mild pulmonary hypertension, *Pediatr Pulmonol* 6:53-59, 1989.
134. West JB: High altitude pulmonary edema. In Ward MP, Milledge JS, West JB, eds: *High altitude medicine and physiology,* London, 1989, Chapman and Hall Medical, pp 383-398.
135. Reeves JT, Welsh CH, Wagner PD: The heart and lungs at extreme attitude, *Therapy* 49:631-633, 1994.
136. Khoury GH, Hawes CR: Primary pulmonary hypertension in children living at high altitude, *J Pediatr* 62:177-185, 1963.
137. Hultgren HN, Grover RF, Hartley LH: Abnormal circulatory responses to high altitude in subjects with previous history of high altitude pulmonary edema, *Circulation* 44:759, 1971.
138. Kawashima A, Kubo K, Koboyashi T, et al: Hemodynamic responses to acute hypoxia, hypobaria, and exercise in subjects susceptible to high altitude pulmonary edema, *J Appl Physiol* 67:1982-1989, 1989.
139. Grover RF, Will DH, Reeves JT, Weir EK, McMurtry IF, Alexander AF: Genetic transmission of susceptibility to hypoxic pulmonary hypertension, *Prog Resp Res* 9:112-117, 1975.
140. Sui GJ, Liu YH, Cheng XS, et al: Subacute infantile mountain sickness, *J Pathol* 155:161-170, 1988.
141. Hackett PH, Bertman, Rodriguez G: Pulmonary edema fluid protein in high altitude pulmonary edema, *JAMA* 256:36, 1986.
142. West JB, Tsukimoto BK, Mathieu-Costello O, Prediletto R: Stress failure in pulmonary capillaries, *J Appl Physiol* 70:1731-1742, 1991.
143. Schoene RB, Swenson ER, Pizzo CJ, et al: The lung at high altitude: bronchoalveolar lavage in acute mountain sickness and pulmonary edema, *J Appl Physiol* 64:2605-2613, 1988.
144. Stelzner TJ, O'Brien RF, Sato K, et al: Hypoxia induced increases in pulmonary transvascular protein in rats. Modulation by glucocorticoids, *J Clin Invest* 82:1840-1847, 1988.
145. Bartsch P, Maggiorini M, Ritter M, et al: Prevention of high altitude pulmonary edema by nifedipine, *N Engl J Med* 325:1284-1289, 1991.
146. Krowka MJ, Cortese DA: Hepatopulmonary syndrome. Current concepts in diagnostic and therapeutic considerations, *Chest* 105:1528-1537, 1994.
147. Daoud FS, Reeves JT, Schaefer JW: Failure of hypoxic vasoconstriction in patients with liver cirrhosis, *J Clin Invest* 51:1076-1080, 1972.
148. Rossaint R, Falke KJ, Lopez F, et al: Inhaled NO for adult respiratory distress syndrome, *N Engl J Med* 328:399-405, 1993.
149. Gerlach H, Rossaint R, Pappert D, Falke KJ: Time-course and dose-response of NO inhalation for systemic oxygenation and pulmonary hypertension in patients with adult respiratory distress syndrome, *Eur J Clin Invest* 23: 499-502, 1993.
150. Abman SH, Griebel JL, Parker DK, et al: Acute effects of inhaled NO in severe hypoxemic respiratory failure, *J Pediatr* 124:881-888, 1994.

Respiratory Complications of Cardiac Disease

151. Snashall PD, Chung KF: Airway obstruction and bronchial hyperresponsiveness in left ventricular failure and mitral stenosis, *Am Rev Respir Dis* 144:945-956, 1991.
152. Bancalari E, Jesse MJ, Gelband H, et al: Lung mechanics in congenital heart disease with increased and decreased pulmonary blood flow, *J Pediatr* 90:192, 1977.
153. DeTroyer A, Yernault JC, Englert M: Mechanics of breathing in patients with atria septal defect, *Am Rev Respir Dis* 115:413, 1977.

New Therapeutic Approaches to Pediatric Pulmonary Hypertension

154. Pepke-Zaba J, Higenbottam TW, Dinh Xuan AT, et al: Inhaled NO as a clause of selective pulmonary vasodilation in pulmonary hypertension, *Lancet* 338: 1173-1174, 1991.
155. Roberts JD, Lang P, Bigatello LM, et al: Inhaled NO in congenital heart disease, *Circulation* 87:447-453, 1993.
156. Wessel DL, Adatia L, Giglia TM, et al: Use of inhaled NO and acetylcholine in the evaluation of pulmonary hypertension and endothelial function after cardiopulmonary bypass, *Circulation* 88:2128-2138, 1993.
157. Beckman JS, Beckman TW, Chen J, et al: Apparent hydroxyl radical production by peroxynitrite: Implications for endothelial injury from NO and superoxide, *Proc Natl Acad Sci USA* 87:1620-1624, 1990.
158. Kouyamdjian C, Adnot S, Levame M, Eddahibi S, Bousbaa H, Raffestin B: Continuous inhalation of NO protects against development of pulmonary hypertension in chronically hypoxic rats, *J Clin Invest* 94:578-584, 1994.
159. Zhu L, Wigle D, Hinek A, Kobayashi J, Ye C, Zuker M, Dodo H, Keeley FW, Rabinovitch M: Endogenous vascular elastase that governs development and progression of monocrotaline-induced pulmonary hypertension in rats is a novel enzyme related to the serine proteinase adipsin, *J Clin Invest* 94:1163-1171, 1994.
160. Morishita R, Gibbons G, Ellison K, Lee W, Zhang L, Yu H, Kaneda Y, Ogihara T, Dzau V: Evidence for direct local effect of angiotensin in vascular hypertrophy, *J Clin Invest* 94:978-984, 1994.

CHAPTER 59

Primary Pulmonary Hypertension

Stanley J. Goldberg

Pulmonary hypertension exists early in the natural evolutionary process of lung maturation in the newborn. Pulmonary pressures are at systemic levels in the fetus and fall in the hours after birth to reach the final lower levels within days to weeks following birth. Persistence of hypertension beyond this period occurs in many conditions. Perhaps one of the more commonly encountered etiologies of pulmonary hypertension in humans and animals is that associated with high altitude. A variable pulmonary pressure increase occurs during residence at high altitude as a result of decreased Po_2.[1] Those with high-altitude pulmonary hypertension usually experience a decrease in pulmonary artery pressure when residing at lower altitudes.[2] Children with certain forms of congenital cardiac disease constitute another population with pulmonary hypertension. Usually pulmonary hypertension in this group is associated with left-to-right shunting lesions with elevated pulmonary blood flow, high left-atrial pressures, or nonavailable portions of the lung circulation, causing all pulmonary flow to divert to the remaining portions of the lung circulation. Another important cause of pulmonary hypertension in children is loss of lung tissue as a result of surgery or various diseases.

The diagnosis of primary pulmonary hypertension is one of exclusion of the just-mentioned and other causes of pulmonary hypertension. Primary pulmonary hypertension is a rare disease of obscure etiology. The occurrence rate of primary pulmonary hypertension in children is far lower than in adults, and reports in children often refer to only one or two patients. Fujinami et al[3] reported that only two children with primary pulmonary hypertension were registered among the 45,000 patients treated at the Heart Institute of Japan over a 23-year span, whereas approximately 20 times as many adults with primary pulmonary hypertension were registered over the same time period. The greatest probability is that primary pulmonary hypertension is not a single disease entity but rather a final common pathway of a number of entities.

DISEASE MECHANISMS

The etiology of primary pulmonary hypertension is unknown. Various causes have been postulated, but it is probable that the cause of primary pulmonary hypertension is multifactorial, possibly because the disease is a final common pathway of a number of entities. The possibility that it could be due to multiple small pulmonary embolisms has neither been substantiated nor totally rejected.[4] In adults an association of connective tissue disease, Raynaud phenomenon, and primary pulmonary hypertension has been recognized.[5-7] In scleroderma patients, similar vascular changes occur in digital and pulmonary arteries[6] and patients with lupus may have apparent nonembolic pulmonary hypertension.[7] Recently, Barst et al[8] provided evidence relating unexplained pulmonary hypertension (but not pulmonary hypertension associated with cardiac lesions) and major histocompatibility complexes, thus suggesting immune mediation of primary pulmonary hypertension. Rabinovitch, however, cautioned that even pulmonary hypertension associated with cardiac lesions could have an immunologic basis.[9]

PATHOLOGY

Wagenvoort and Wagenvoort studied pathologic material of 156 patients who were diagnosed with primary pulmonary hypertension and found different diseases in 46.[10] In the remaining 110, they made the observation that the younger patients had mainly medial hypertrophy and less intimal fibrosis and little or no plexiform lesions. In older patients the reverse was true. Heath and Edwards[11] and Roberts[12] demonstrated that the pulmonary trunk elastic pattern in patients with pulmonary hypertension beginning in infancy resembled that of the aorta, whereas in acquired pulmonary hypertension the histology was more similar to the adult pattern.

CLINICAL MANIFESTATIONS

History in primary pulmonary hypertension usually indicates gradual onset of exercise fatigue and breathlessness. Palpitation, syncope (or dizziness), and exertional chest pain also occur. Usually symptoms have not been present for long durations. Familial occurrence and presence of collagen disease are not unusual.[13]

The physical examination is not specific for primary pulmonary hypertension. The child may or may not exhibit mild cyanosis and clubbing as a result of intrapulmonary shunting. Large A waves may be present in the jugular veins, but because many young children have short, thick necks, these waves may be difficult to observe. An increased right-ventricular impulse is usually palpable. Often, pulmonary valve closure, as palpated at the upper left precordium, is increased. During the auscultatory examination, a pulmonary click, which results from the dilated pulmonary artery, can be heard. The pulmonary component of the second heart sound usually has an increased intensity and is narrowly split from the aortic component. A fourth sound may also be present. Some patients may have a low-intensity systolic ejection murmur of uncertain etiology. More commonly, a murmur of pulmonary regurgitation can be heard at the upper left sternal border. This murmur is caused by the high diastolic pulmonary artery pressure, and the duration and intensity mirror the instantaneous difference in diastolic pressure between the pulmonary artery and right ventricle. Signs of right-ventricular failure are often present, and these usually consist of hepatomegaly and occasionally, in the later stages, peripheral edema. Ascites is common.

ASSESSMENT AND DIAGNOSIS

Electrocardiogram

The electrocardiogram usually shows evidence of right-ventricular and right-atrial hypertrophy. ST- and T-wave changes may be present in the anterior and lateral precordium. Because these patients may die of arrhythmias, Holter monitoring may also be useful.

Chest Radiograph

The chest radiograph is usually abnormal, but the degree of abnormality may be subtle. The heart may or may not be enlarged early in the course of the disease, but later, right-atrial and right-ventricular enlargement are the rule rather than the exception. Pulmonary artery enlargement is often an early finding. Increased size of large pulmonary arteries and decreased peripheral lung vasculature are characteristics of the condition, but findings may be quite subtle.

Echocardiogram

The echocardiogram is probably the most useful of the noninvasive diagnostic tests for investigating a patient with suspected diagnosis of primary pulmonary hypertension. Perhaps one of the most important features of the echocardiogram is the confirmation of normal cardiac structure, which excludes congenital cardiac disease as an etiologic factor for the pulmonary hypertension. Once all aspects of congenital cardiac malformations are excluded, the main features of the echocardiogram are those of generic pulmonary vascular obstructive disease. The M-mode examination is useful to demonstrate right-ventricular anterior wall hypertrophy. Normal children and adolescents do not exceed a thickness of 3 mm at end diastole for the right-ventricular anterior wall,[14] whereas children with significant pulmonary hypertension usually have right-ventricular anterior walls of 5 mm or more. The right-ventricular cavity dimension, measured at end diastole, is usually enlarged beyond that for age.[15] The septum may be hypertrophied out of proportion to the left-ventricular posterior free wall dimension as a result of right-ventricular hypertrophy.[16] Septal dimensional increased thickness may be the only evidence of hypertrophy if imaging of the right-ventricular anterior wall is difficult. Paradoxical septal motion is often present. The M-mode tracing of the pulmonary valve demonstrates the "flying W" configuration, which is not specific for primary pulmonary hypertension but is specific for generic pulmonary vascular obstructive disease.[17] This finding, which also has a Doppler counterpart,[18] has a hemodynamic origin. Blood initially flows into the available pulmonary artery space, but because this vascular space is quite limited in pulmonary vascular obstructive disease, pressure rises quickly and the flow reflects off of the limited vascular bed, causing early termination of forward flow. However, as systole proceeds, some of the initial blood passes through the available pulmonary circulation, making room for additional flow. This subsequent flow causes a second velocity wave form during the same systole (Fig. 59-1).

Doppler findings in primary pulmonary hypertension include a pulmonary wave form similar to that found in the pulmonary valve M-mode (see Fig. 59-1), a rapid time to peak for the pulmonary velocity, elevated regurgitation velocities from the pulmonary and tricuspid valves, abnormal tricuspid inflow velocities, and abnormal hepatic vein and superior venal velocities. Time to peak velocity beyond infancy is usually longer than 90 ms.[19] Shorter times indicate a high probability of pulmonary hypertension. Although a significant inverse relationship exists between time to peak pulmonary velocity and pulmonary artery pressure, exact prediction of pulmonary artery pressure is not warranted. Nonetheless, time to peak pulmonary velocity will be less than 90 ms in patients with true primary pulmonary hypertension. Most normal individuals and most patients with pulmonary hypertension have pulmonary and tricuspid regurgitation. More exact peak right-ventricular pressure can be estimated from the tricuspid regurgitation velocity by the following formula: $P_1 - P_2 = 4(V_2^2)$, where P_1 = peak right-ventricular pressure, P_2 = right atrial pressure, 4 = an approximate factor to take into account the transfer of velocity into mm Hg, V_2 = the peak velocity in milliseconds of the tricuspid regurgitation. Addition of peak $P_1 - P_2$ to the central venous pressure will approximate right-ventricular pressure.[20] In a similar manner, instantaneous diastolic pulmonary artery pressure can be estimated from the magnitude of the pulmonary regurgitation jet. Finally, inflow velocities for the right atrium and right ventricle are usually abnormal in patients

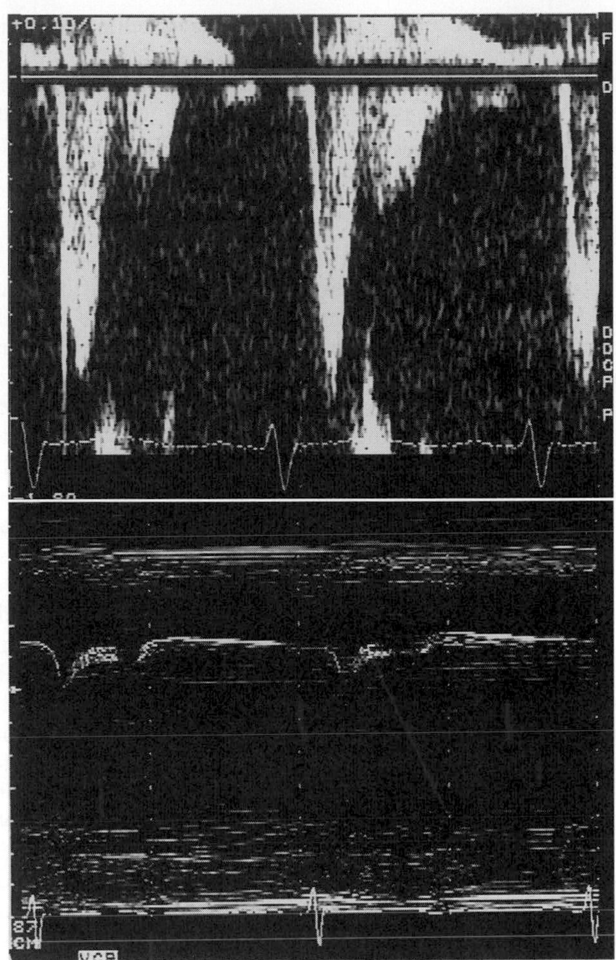

Fig. 59-1. Examples of the "flying W" formation in pulmonary hypertension. The upper panel depicts a velocity tracing with the "flying W" complex. Note the very rapid increase in velocity following the ECG QRS complex and the very rapid deceleration so that velocity returns almost to baseline early in systole, then a second forward velocity of lesser magnitude later in systole occurs. The lower panel demonstrates the "flying W" formation in the M-mode pulmonary valve motion. Although the traces are from the same patient, the R-to-R times are not matched. Nonetheless, it is possible to see that the secondary deflection of the pulmonary valve requires approximately the same time as the secondary velocity noted for the upper trace.

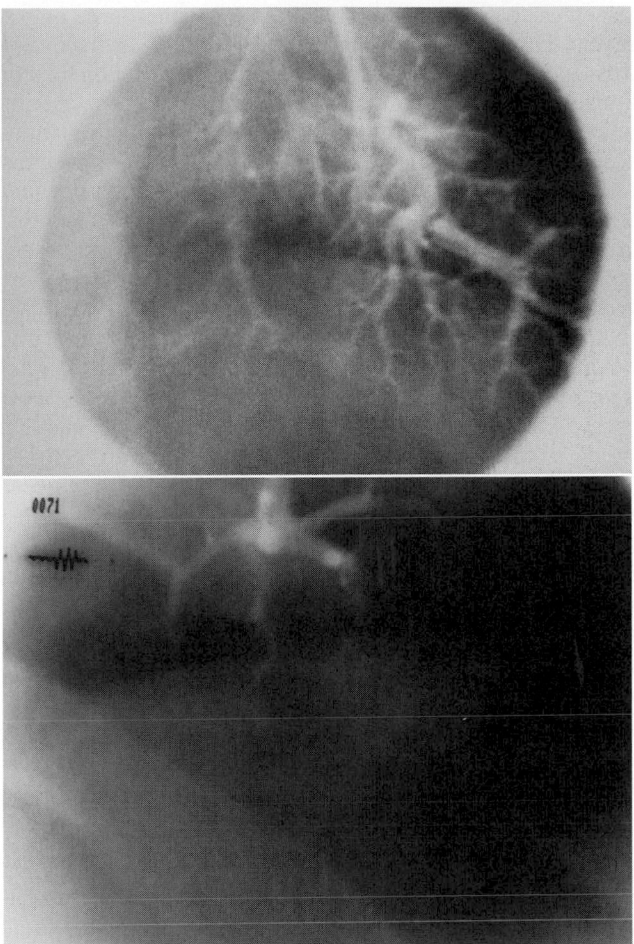

Fig. 59-2. The upper trace demonstrates a pulmonary artery wedge injection in a normal patient. The catheter can be seen extending from the top of the cine frame to approximately the middle of the image. Note the rich branching of the vessels in this frame. The lower panel demonstrates a similar injection in a patient with severe pulmonary hypertension. Note the absence of branching of the remaining vessels. It is clear from the lower wedge angiogram that some vessels have disappeared and that the lower branches are no longer visualized.

with primary pulmonary hypertension and have wave forms that suggest decreased right-ventricular compliance.

The major utility of two-dimensional echocardiography and color-coded Doppler is exclusion of congenital cardiac disease. Two-dimensional echocardiography demonstrates the dilated, thickened right ventricle; paradoxical septal motion; and the dilated pulmonary artery. Beyond visual display of these structures, no new information is added beyond the M-mode examination for confirmation of a diagnosis of primary pulmonary hypertension. Color-coded Doppler improves the ease of Doppler sample volume placement, but it adds little more in confirmation of a diagnosis of primary pulmonary hypertension.

Cardiac Catheterization

Cardiac catheterization in the past was the principal method of eliminating the diagnosis of cardiac lesions and establishing a stronger probability of primary pulmonary hypertension. Currently, this role has been assumed mainly by Doppler echocardiography. Cardiac catheterization, however, still allows direct study of small pulmonary arteries and their branching pattern via pulmonary artery wedge angiography.[21] This test is performed by wedging a small (5- or 6-French) catheter in distal pulmonary arteries. Although the usual method is to use an end-hole catheter, we have better results with a side-hole catheter. Use of an end-hole catheter with an occluding balloon placed more proximally in the pulmonary artery than the wedge usually, in our hands, provides inferior results compared with a true wedge injection. The normal wedge injection displays a profusely branched small pulmonary artery system, whereas pulmonary hypertension from any cause demonstrates that vessels are of smaller-than-normal size because of deeper extension of the media and thicker media. Moreover, loss of vessels is usually very striking (Fig. 59-2).

Cardiac catheterization also allows direct measurement of pressures, oxygen saturations, and angiography. We prefer to study these patients, if possible, with local anesthesia only to prevent the possibility of medication[22] or alveolar hypoventilation-induced pulmonary hypertension. Qualification for a diagnosis of primary pulmonary hypertension requires that the patient have no evidence of cardiac structural malformations, no other pulmonary disease, and a pulmonary artery pressure of at least 70% of systemic while breathing air with a Po_2 equivalent to sea level. Left-atrial saturation will usually be normal, but loss of pulmonary vessels may lead to a low saturation as a result of the equivalent of an arteriovenous fistula. Furthermore, patients with a patent foramen ovale may develop a right-to-left atrial shunt. Left-ventricular end-diastolic pressure should be normal, but regional wall studies for function may demonstrate abnormal septal motion as a result of paradoxical septal motion. Cardiac angiography will cause a transient increase in circulating blood volume, and this could cause difficulty for some patients with severe forms of primary pulmonary hypertension. If pulmonary embolism has been ruled out by nuclear studies, the risk of a pulmonary artery angiogram may be decided on an individual basis. Pulmonary artery wedge angiography usually does not provoke the problems of a full angiogram. We routinely perform pulmonary artery wedge angiography with approximately 2-ml injections of contrast material in these patients and have not yet experienced significant difficulty as a result of this type of angiography.

Ventilation/Perfusion Scan

The major use of the ventilation/perfusion scan is to detect the patient with pulmonary embolism; in this stance large perfusion defects are found. Most perfusion and ventilation scans in patients with primary pulmonary hypertension are normal, but a few may show minor perfusion defects.[23]

MANAGEMENT

Treatment of primary pulmonary hypertension is presently changing, and it is unclear which will become the treatment of choice by the time this book is published. Early the main treatment was aimed only at control of congestive cardiac failure.[24] A number of vasodilators were used with varying results,[25] including tolazoline,[26] phentolamine,[27,28] isoproterenol,[29,30] and diazoxide.[31-33] In 1980 De Feyter et al reported sustained beneficial effects of oral nifedipine in a patient with primary pulmonary hypertension.[34] This report and a nearly simultaneous one by Camerini et al[35] was followed by others that indicated the beneficial and adverse effects of calcium channel blockers in primary pulmonary hypertension.[36-39] Later beneficial results of continuous epoprostenol infusion have been published by Rubin and coworkers.[40] Still more recently, nitric oxide, administered by ventilation, has been used as a specific pulmonary vasodilator.[41] Endogenous nitric oxide is an endothelial-derived relaxation factor, but it can also be administered therapeutically to achieve approximately the same effect. A major advantage of nitric oxide is that it acts almost exclusively on the pulmonary circulation. Because inhaled nitric oxide acts in the areas of ventilation, where it is delivered, it has the effect of matching areas of ventilation and perfusion more exactly than drugs delivered via the circulation. More experience will be necessary to evaluate this new therapy, which is under investigational use only at the time of writing.

Lung transplantation is another treatment for primary pulmonary hypertension. Timing and perhaps need for lung transplantation may be altered by therapy with vasodilators. Lung transplantation carries substantial risk and morbidity. Furthermore, if the patient has a collagen vascular disease, or if the primary pulmonary hypertension was caused by other immunologic factors, it is possible that the graft will suffer consequences similar to the native lung.

OUTCOME

In his original report of primary pulmonary hypertension, Paul Wood indicated a median survival of 2 years.[42] One nonpulmonary factor that influences survival is low cardiac output. Thus any treatment or condition that causes reduced systemic pressure without an increase in cardiac output leads to a decreased survival. An example of this effect is that patients with a patent foramen ovale have a better prognosis, presumably because the right-to-left atrial shunt increases systemic cardiac output and decreases the volume the right side of the heart has to pump. Creation of an ASD has been used to increase systemic cardiac output and permit longer survival.[43]

The natural history before vasodilator therapy was studied by Rozkovek et al in a Hammersmith Hospital patient population, ages 5 to 28 years at entry.[13] This group was uniformly treated with anticoagulants. Results of this study showed no relationship between age at diagnosis and mean survival. They divided their groups rather arbitrarily into those who survived less than 5 years (52%), those who survived longer than 5 years (35%), and those who showed evidence of disease regression (12%). For those who survived less than 5 years, the average survival was 2.7 years. For those surviving longer than 5 years, the average survival was 9.7 years. Average survival for the group whose findings regressed was 18.7 years. Cardiac output was directly and pulmonary vascular resistance was indirectly related to longer survival. Presence of right-sided heart failure was associated with a poor prognosis.

The influence of vasodilator therapy on outcome has only recently been addressed.[43] One multicenter study attempted to evaluate results of a large cohort of patients diagnosed with primary pulmonary hypertension between 1981 and 1985 and followed until 1988. Many of these patients were receiving vasodilator therapy. In this study survival data were judged from the date of catheterization. During follow-up 56% of patients (106 of 194) died; 26% experienced sudden, unexpected death; and 47% died of right-ventricular failure. Untreated patients had a mean survival of 2.9 years, and treated patients had a significantly longer survival of 3.8 years. Significant risk factors for death included Raynaud phenomenon (odd ratio 2.11), increased right-atrial pressure (odd ratio 1.99), and increasing pulmonary artery pressure (odd ratio 1.16). Accordingly, in this study presence of right-sided heart failure, as previously reported by Rozkovek et al,[13] and low cardiac output were associated with a poor prognosis.

Although the prognosis, in terms of duration of survival, does not appear to be much different over the course of the years since the disease was first reported, increased knowledge of the response and physiology of small pulmonary vessels may lead to improved treatment in the future.

REFERENCES

1. Grover RF, Reeves JT, Will DH, Blout SG: Pulmonary vasoconstriction in steers at high altitude, *J Physiol* 18:567-574, 1963.
2. Fishman AP: Respiratory gases in the regulation of the pulmonary circulation, *Physiol Rev* 41:214-280, 1961.

3. Fujinami M, Nishikawa T, Kajita A, Takao A: Primary pulmonary hypertension in infancy: report of two autopsy cases, *Acta Cardiol* 44:19-28, 1989.

Disease Mechanisms

4. Fuster V, Steele PM, Edwards WD, Gersh BS, McGoon MD, Frye RL: Primary pulmonary hypertension: natural history and importance of thrombosis, *Circulation* 70:580-587, 1984.
5. Wagenvoort CA, Wagenvoort N: Primary pulmonary hypertension: a pathologic study of the lung vessels in 156 clinically diagnosed cases, *Circulation* 42:1163-1184, 1970.
6. Rodnan GP, Myerowitz RL, Justh GO: Morphologic progressive systemic sclerosis (scleroderma) and Raynaud phenomenon, *Medicine* 59: 393-408, 1980.
7. Asherson RA, Machworth-Young CG, Boey ML, et al: Pulmonary hypertension in systemic lupus erythematosus, *Br Med J* 287:1024-1025, 1983.
8. Barst RJ, Flaster ER, Menon A, Fotino M, Morse JH: Evidence for the association of unexplained pulmonary hypertension in children with the major histocompatibility complex, *Circulation* 85:249-258, 1992.
9. Rabinovitch M: Autoimmune disease and unexplained pulmonary hypertension, *Circulation* 85:380-381, 1992.

Pathology

10. Wagenvoort CA, Wagenvoort N: Primary pulmonary hypertension, *Circulation* 42:1163-1181, 1970.
11. Heath D, Edwards JE: Configuration of elastic tissue of the pulmonary trunk in idiopathic pulmonary hypertension, *Circulation* 21:59-62, 1960.
12. Roberts WC: The histologic structure of the pulmonary trunk in patients with "primary" pulmonary hypertension, *Br Heart J* 55:449-458, 1986.
13. Rozkovec A, Montanes P, Oakley CM: Factors that influence outcome of primary pulmonary hypertension, *Br Heart J* 55:449-458, 1986.

Assessment and Diagnosis

14. Epstein M, Goldberg SJ, Allen HD, Konecke L, Wood J: Great vessel, cardiac chamber and wall growth pattern in normal children, *Circulation* 51:1124-1129, 1975.
15. Goldberg SJ, Allen HD, Sahn DJ: *Pediatric and adolescent echocardiography: a handbook,* ed 2, Chicago, 1980, Year Book Medical Publishers.
16. Larter WE, Allen HD, Sahn DJ, Goldberg SJ: The asymmetrically hypertrophied septum, *Circulation* 53:19-27, 1976.
17. Weyman AE: Pulmonary valve echo motion in clinical practice, *Am J Med* 62:843-855, 1977.
18. Goldberg SJ, Allen HD, Marx GR, Donnerstein RL: *Doppler echocardiography,* ed 2, Philadelphia, 1988, Lea & Febiger.
19. Kosturakis D, Allen HD, Goldberg SJ, Sahn DJ, Valdes-Cruz LM: Noninvasive quantification of stenotic semilunar valve areas by Doppler echocardiography, *J Am Coll Cardiol* 3:1256-1262, 1984.
20. Yock PG, Popp RL: Noninvasive estimation of right ventricular systolic pressure by Doppler ultrasound in patients with tricuspid regurgitation, *Circulation* 70:657-662, 1984.
21. Nihill MR, McNamara DG: Magnification pulmonary wedge angiography in the evaluation of children with congenital cardiac disease and pulmonary hypertension, *Circulation* 58:1094-1106, 1978.
22. Goldberg SJ, Linde L: Effects of sedation on the controlled pulmonary circulation, *Life Sci* 14:751-768, 1974.
23. Wilson AG, Harris CN, Lavender JP, Oakley CM: Perfusion lung scanning in obliterative pulmonary hypertension, *Br Heart J* 35:917-930, 1973.

Management

24. Kaplan S, in Vaughn VC, McKay J, Behrman RE, eds: *Textbook of pediatrics,* Philadelphia, 1979, WB Saunders, p 1325.
25. Wood P: Pulmonary hypertension with special reference to the vasoconstrictive factor, *Br Heart J* 20:557-570, 1958.
26. Rudolph AM, Paul MH, Sommer LS, Nadas AS: Effects of tolazoline hydrochloride (priscoline) on circulatory dynamics of patients with pulmonary hypertension, *Am Heart J* 55:424-432, 1958.
27. Ruskin JN, Hutter AM Jr: Primary pulmonary hypertension treated with oral phentolamine, *Ann Intern Med* 90:772-774, 1979.
28. Cohen ML, Krozon I: Adverse hemodynamic effects of phentolamine in primary pulmonary hypertension, *Ann Intern Med* 95:591-592, 1981.
29. Daoud FS, Reeves JT, Kelly DB: Isoproterenol as a potential pulmonary vasodilator in primary pulmonary hypertension, *Am J Cardiol* 42:817-822, 1978.
30. Shettigar UR, Hultgren HN, Specter M, Martin R, Davies DH: Primary pulmonary hypertension: favourable effect of isoproterenol, *N Engl J Med* 295:1414-1415, 1976.
31. Wang SWS, Pohl JEF, Rowlands DJ, Wade EG: Diazoxide in treatment of primary pulmonary hypertension, *Br Heart J* 40:572-574, 1978.
32. Honey M, Cotter L, Daview N, Denison D: Clinical and haemodynamic effects of diazoxide in primary pulmonary hypertension, *Thorax* 35:269-276, 1980.
33. Klinke WP, Gilbert JAL: Diazoxide in primary pulmonary hypertension, *N Engl J Med* 302:91-92, 1980.
34. De Feyter PJ, Kerkkamp HJJ, de Jong JP: Sustained beneficial effect of nifedipine in primary pulmonary hypertension, *Am Heart J* 105:333-334, 1980.
35. Camerini F, Alberti E, Klugmann S, Salvi A: Primary pulmonary hypertension: effects of nifedipine, *Br Heart J* 44:352-356, 1980.
36. Wise JR Jr: Nifedipine in the treatment of primary pulmonary hypertension, *Am Heart J* 105:693-694;1983.
37. Kambara H, Fujimoto K, Wakabayashi A, Kawai C: Primary pulmonary hypertension: beneficial therapy with diltiazem, *Am Heart J* 101:230-231, 1981.
38. Wood BA, Tortoledo F, Luck JC, Fennell WH: Rapid attenuation of response to nifedipine in primary pulmonary hypertension, *Chest* 82:793-794, 1982.
39. Farber HW, Karlinsky JB, Faling LJ: Fatal outcome following nifedipine for pulmonary hypertension, *Chest* 83:708-709, 1983.
40. Rubin LJ, Mendoza J, Hoof M, McGoon M, Barst R, Williams WB, et al: Treatment of primary pulmonary hypertension with continuous intravenous prostacylcin (epoprostenol). Results of a randomized trial, *Ann Intern Med* 112:485-491, 1990.
41. Pepke-Zaba J, Higenbottam TW, Dinh-Xuan AT, Stone D, Wallwork J: Inhaled nitric oxide as a cause of selective pulmonary vasodilation in pulmonary hypertension, *Lancet* 338:1173-1774, 1991.

Outcome

42. Wood P: Pulmonary hypertension, *Br Med Bull* 8:348-352, 1952.
43. D'Alonzo GE, Barst RJ, Ayres SM, Bergofsky EH, Brundage BH, et al: Survival inpatients with primary pulmonary hypertension: results from a national prospective registry, *Ann Intern Med* 115:343-349, 1991.

CHAPTER 60

Pulmonary Embolism

Richard L. Donnerstein and Robert A. Berg

EPIDEMIOLOGY

Although it has been more than 130 years since Löschner described a case of a pulmonary thromboembolism in a 9-year-old child,[1] pulmonary embolism is rarely clinically diagnosed or treated in children.[2-4] Although pulmonary emboli may be caused by air, fat, amniotic fluid, tumors, infected masses, or foreign bodies,[5,6] as well as thrombus, this chapter refers primarily to thromboemboli. In adults acute pulmonary embolism is a major cause of morbidity and is one of the most common causes of death in the United States.[3,7,8] Autopsy series have suggested that the incidence of pulmonary embolism is as high as 1 per 1000 hospital admissions in the pediatric and adolescent age groups,[3,4] with about 25% of these being clinically significant.[3] Although approximately 3% of fatal pulmonary emboli occur in patients under 19 years of age,[1] sudden, unexpected death in children directly attributable to massive pulmonary thromboembolus is unusual (less than 0.05% in large retrospective autopsy series).[4,9] However, in unselected pediatric autopsy series the incidence of pulmonary embolism was estimated to be as high as 4%,[3,10,11] and most of the clinically significant pulmonary emboli were not recognized before death.[3]

Virchow noted in 1856 that the risk of thrombosis is increased with stasis of blood flow, injury to the vessel wall, and hypercoagulability of blood.[3,12,13] Known causes for these conditions in adults include recent surgery, immobility, deep vein thrombophlebitis, collagen vascular disease,[4,12] malignancies,[14] congestive heart failure, infections, pregnancy, oral contraceptive use,[1,2,10,12] and underlying hypercoagulable states.[5,12,13,15,16] Diseases such as Guillain-Barré syndrome,[17,18] Duchenne muscular dystrophy,[19] systemic lupus erythematosus (SLE) and other collagen vascular diseases,[12,15] homocystinuria,[20] and nephrotic syndrome[13] have been specifically associated with pulmonary emboli.

All of the disease states in adults that increase the risk of thromboembolism occur in children and adolescents and may place them at increased risk as well. However, specific processes in younger patients that result in stasis, vascular injury, or hypercoagulability may differ from those in adults.[7] High-risk factors in children and adolescents include trauma, immobility, elective termination of pregnancy, nephrotic syndrome,[7,16,21] ventriculoatrial shunts for hydrocephalus, central venous catheters, congenital coagulation disorders, dilated cardiomyopathies,[19,22] and other cardiac diseases.[2-4,10] The risk of pulmonary embolism in children with neoplasms appears to be greater with solid tumors than with lymphomas or leukemias.[3] However, significant pulmonary thrombosis has been noted in children with leukemia.[23] Recent studies have suggested a decreasing risk of pulmonary embolism associated with oral contraceptive use, possibly because of the trend toward the use of a lower estrogen content in these drugs.[7] A substantial portion of young patients with pulmonary emboli may have no identifiable risk factor.[7] In newborns the risk of venous thrombosis and subsequent pulmonary embolism is increased with birth trauma, dehydration, sepsis, recent surgery, and heart disease or in the presence of maternal risk factors such as diabetes, hydramnios, and toxemia.[24,25] Pulmonary thrombi have been found in infants with a patent ductus arteriosus[26] or nonpatent ductus arteriosus aneurysm.[27]

Children and infants in intensive care settings are at particular risk for thromboembolism because of the high incidence of immobility, central venous catheterization, and recent operations.[2,28] Central venous and pulmonary artery catheters are increasingly used in children despite the potential for pulmonary thromboembolism and air embolism. Sleeve thrombi have been demonstrated around most indwelling central venous catheters.[29] Extensive thrombosis may occur from vascular injury caused by the catheter tip or stasis caused by blockage of a vessel.[28] The incidence of thrombosis increases as the duration of catheterization increases.[10,29-31] Pulmonary embolism may occur while the catheter is in place, during catheter removal (if there is a clot on the catheter), or days or weeks after catheter removal.[30] Small asymptomatic pulmonary emboli are probably released during the removal of most central venous catheters. Hyperosmolality, caused by either treatment (for control of cerebral edema) or disease state (diabetes insipidus), occurs often in intensive care units and increases the risk of thromboembolism.[2]

Multiple defects in the hemostatic system have been associated with thromboembolism.[13] Inherited deficiencies of the endogenous anticoagulants protein C, protein S, and antithrombin III[13] have been observed in some patients with thromboembolism. The incidence of antithrombin III deficiency is estimated at 1 in 2000.[13] Congenital protein C deficiency may account for up to 6% to 10% of all adults with venous thrombosis or pulmonary embolism.[13] Numerous other, relatively uncommon, congenital defects of the coagulation system have also been identified.[13] Lupus anticoagulants, immunoglobulins that prolong phospholipid-dependent coagulation tests (such as the prothrombin time and partial thromboplastin time), paradoxically are associated with thromboembolism. Thrombosis occurs in 25% to 50% of systemic lupus patients who have lupus anticoagulants.[13] Although initially noted in patients with SLE, the lupus anticoagulant and anticardiolipin antibody are found in patients with other diseases (such as other autoimmune diseases and neoplasms), as well as in otherwise normal individuals, and may account for 6% to 10% of thromboses in otherwise normal adults.[12,13,32] Certain medications have also been associated with the development of these antibodies.[32] In addition to the lupus anticoagulant, many other defects in the coagulation system, including deficiencies of proteins C and S and antithrombin III, may be acquired.[5,13,14,21]

The anatomic site of venous thrombi associated with pulmonary emboli in children differ from those in adults.[3] Similar to adults, the child described by Löschner in 1861 had a symptomatic thrombus of a lower extremity.[1] However, when compared with thrombi in adults, venous thrombi in children are often asymptomatic and are less likely to involve the veins of the pelvis or lower extremities[3,31] and more likely to involve cranial or abdominal veins.[1,31] Venous thrombi are commonly within or adjacent to areas of infection or trauma.[1]

DISEASE MECHANISMS

An acute increase in pulmonary vascular resistance associated with right-ventricular failure and shock is the principal cause of death after pulmonary embolism.[33] In the absence of preexisting lung disease, mean pulmonary pressure increases approximately in proportion to the degree of obstruction of the pulmonary arteries.[34] Because of the limited ability of the normal right ventricle to respond to an acute increase in afterload, a right-ventricular systolic pressure greater than 60 mm Hg, or a mean pulmonary artery pressure of 30 to 40 mm Hg, represents severe pulmonary artery hypertension.[34-36] However, patients with underlying chronic pulmonary hypertension may generate right-ventricular pressures near or greater than systemic pressures.[35] Although vasoactive substances and baroreceptor reflexes may affect pulmonary vascular resistance after pulmonary embolism, vascular obstruction by the embolus is probably the major cause of the pulmonary hypertension.[34]

Acute changes in ventilation and perfusion result in abnormalities of gas exchange.[37] Following a pulmonary embolus there is a redistribution of blood flow from obstructed to nonobstructed lung units.[37] An increase in alveolar dead space, resulting from a ventilated but poorly perfused lung, can affect CO_2 elimination.[34,37] However, except for the most severe pulmonary embolism, hyperventilation compensates for this increased dead space, and most patients are hypocarbic.[34,37] This hyperventilation and resulting hypocapnia are rarely eliminated by the correction of hypoxemia with supplemental oxygen, suggesting that it is a reflex response of proprioceptors or chemoreceptors to stimuli other than oxygen or carbon dioxide.[34] Abnormalities of ventilation and perfusion, right-to-left shunting through a patent foramen ovale due to right-ventricular failure, and decreased mixed venous saturation caused by a low cardiac output may all contribute to an abnormally low Pao_2.[34,37,38] When resulting atelectasis and pulmonary edema contribute to hypoxemia caused by a pulmonary embolus,[37-39] supplemental oxygen or positive airway pressure may help alleviate the hypoxemia.[39] It is important to ascertain the etiology of right-to-left shunting (for instance, by using echocardiography) because positive airway pressure could worsen an intracardiac right-to-left shunt.[39] Arterial blood gas abnormalities such as hypoxemia or hypocarbia may not be as prominent in adolescents and young adults as they are in older adults.[7] This is probably because of the more intact pulmonary bed and cardiopulmonary reserve in most younger patients.[7]

Because of multiple sources of oxygen supply to the lung tissue, pulmonary infarction is an unusual sequela to a pulmonary embolus.[34,40] When infarction does occur, it may be due to obstruction of distal pulmonary arteries and hemorrhage into the airways.[34,40]

CLINICAL MANIFESTATIONS

Most small pulmonary emboli are asymptomatic. The presentation of a symptomatic pulmonary embolus may often be subtle, and this is probably especially true for younger patients.[7] Pulmonary embolism should be considered in the evaluation of unexplained pulmonary hypertension, respiratory insufficiency, and disseminated intravascular coagulation in children.[10] Arterial hypoxemia or need for increasing inspired oxygen suggests the possibility of pulmonary embolism.[2] The most common symptoms of pulmonary embolism, such as chest pain (pleuritic or nonpleuritic), shortness of breath, cough, and diaphoresis, are nonspecific and may occur in a variety of disease states, including acute respiratory infections.[4,7,11] Moreover, the diagnosis of pulmonary embolism is often masked by the underlying disease, or concomitant sedation, muscle relaxation, or artificial ventilation. Hemoptysis is reported to occur only in a minority of adolescents and young adults with pulmonary emboli.[4,7] Signs of pulmonary or cardiac dysfunction appear to be less common in younger patients than in adults.[7] Because of the nonspecificity of the signs and symptoms, it is hazardous to make a diagnosis of pulmonary embolism solely on clinical grounds.[4]

DIAGNOSIS

Although prompt diagnosis and therapy can significantly reduce mortality, the diagnosis of pulmonary embolism is often not considered in children.[7] Unfortunately, symptoms are nonspecific, and clinical diagnosis is not reliable.[41] Although most patients will have some degree of hypoxemia (Pao_2 less than 80 mm Hg), a significant proportion will have a normal Pao_2.[4,42] Because hyperventilation and resulting hypocapnia may blunt abnormalities of Pao_2, the alveolar-arterial oxygen tension difference, $P(A\text{-}a)o_2$, is a more sensitive indicator of abnormalities of gas exchange.[7,34,42]

Chest radiographs and electrocardiograms are often normal in young patients with a pulmonary embolus.[4,7] In the presence of obstructed pulmonary vessels caused by pulmonary embolism, ventilation and perfusion radionuclide studies would be expected to show a mismatched defect with areas of absent or abnormal pulmonary perfusion associated with normal ventilation[2,43] (Fig. 60-1). Ventilation studies are usually performed with xenon-133 and perfusion studies with technetium-99m macroaggregated albumin.[43] Ventilation/perfusion ($\dot{V}/\dot{Q}$) scans for diagnosing pulmonary emboli are usually classified as "high probability," "intermediate probability (indeterminate)," "moderate probability," "low probability," or "normal."[43-45] Although a high-probability scan strongly suggests pulmonary embolism, only a minority of adult patients with proven pulmonary embolism will have a high-probability $\dot{V}/\dot{Q}$ scan.[43] Patients with normal $\dot{V}/\dot{Q}$ scans rarely have a clinically significant pulmonary embolus.[41,43,46,47] Although a matched defect (abnormal ventilation and perfusion) suggests other pulmonary disease,[2,43] a pulmonary embolus cannot be excluded.[45,48] If a ventilation scan is not available, a relatively normal chest radiograph in the presence of multiple perfusion abnormalities suggests pulmonary emboli.[2,4,48] Nonetheless, in studies of adults with suspected pulmonary embolism, a significant portion of patients with a high-probability $\dot{V}/\dot{Q}$ scan and a normal chest radiograph did not have evidence of a pulmonary embolus on angiography.[43,46]

Although $\dot{V}/\dot{Q}$ studies may be highly suggestive of the diagnosis,[8] noninvasive methods are often not definitive for the

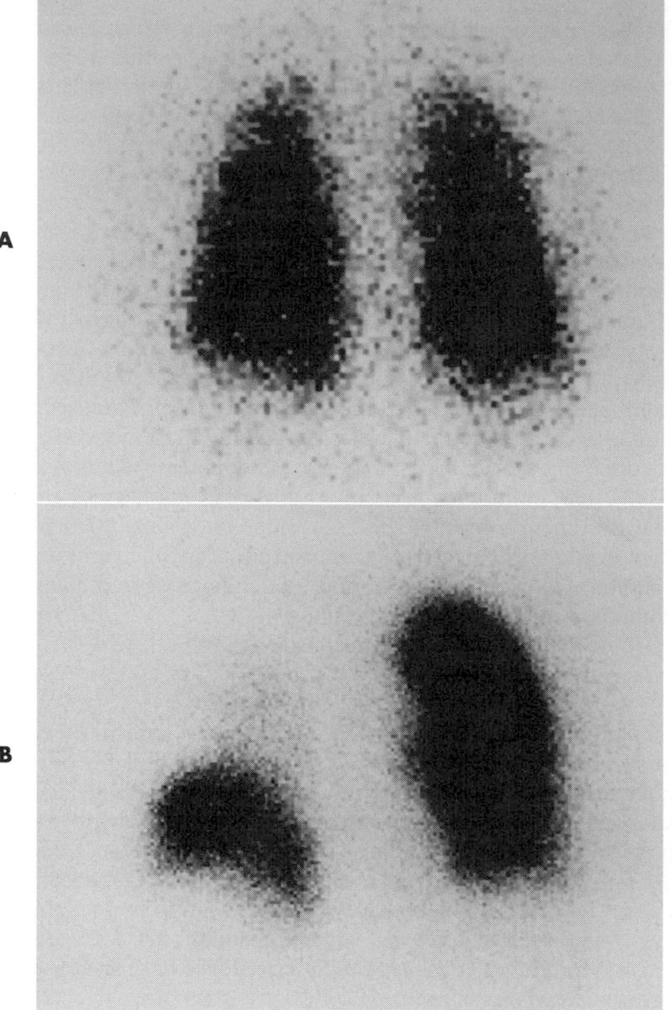

Fig. 60-1. Ventilation and perfusion scans from a patient with pulmonary embolism. **A,** Posterior view of the ventilation scan shows normal xenon-133 distribution in both lungs. **B,** Posterior view of the perfusion scan demonstrates markedly decreased perfusion of the left upper lobe with smaller filling defects of the right lung.

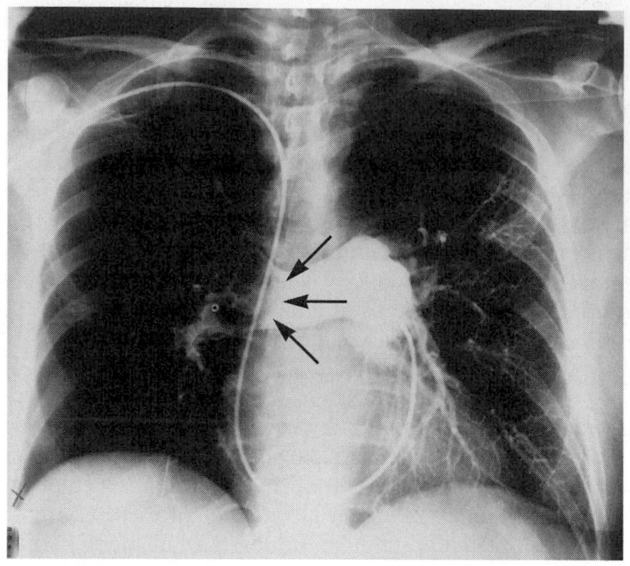

Fig. 60-2. Pulmonary angiography in a patient with pulmonary embolism. A large filling defect is seen in the proximal right pulmonary artery *(arrows).* Smaller filling defects are seen in branches of the left pulmonary artery.

diagnosis of pulmonary embolism. The relatively low incidence of pulmonary embolism and problems of long-term anticoagulation in the pediatric age group make accurate diagnosis essential. Magnetic resonance imaging and computed tomography may detect large emboli in the central pulmonary arteries.[49] However, pulmonary angiography should be considered in most children and adolescents with a suspected pulmonary embolus.[4,41,47] Moderate probability or indeterminate scans may also warrant further investigation with angiography because clinical signs and symptoms in these patients are often ambiguous.[44] Angiographic visualization of a constant intraluminal filling defect in the pulmonary artery seen in several projections is currently the most reliable method to diagnose a pulmonary embolus[8] (Fig. 60-2). Angiography should generally be performed early in the course of pulmonary embolism because its reliability decreases over time.[4]

Echocardiography is useful for detecting signs of acute right-ventricular overload or failure, and many patients with a significant pulmonary embolus will have detectable echocardiographic abnormalities.[35,36] In adults, significant hemodynamic changes generally require obliteration of 30% to 40% of the pulmonary arterial bed.[35,36] When right-ventricular afterload is excessive, right-ventricular failure will ensue with passive venous congestion and a decrease in forward cardiac output.[36] Echocardiography may help identify those patients with significant hemodynamic compromise before the onset of clinically apparent cardiogenic shock.[36] Two-dimensional echocardiographic findings that suggest a pulmonary embolus include dilation of the right ventricle or pulmonary artery, abnormal ventricular septal motion, or decreased left-ventricular diastolic size.[35,36] Thrombi within the right-sided cardiac structures such as the right atrium, right ventricle, or proximal pulmonary arteries, as well as the vena cavae, can be detected.[35] Patients with mobile right-atrial thrombi are at particularly high risk for pulmonary emboli and should receive aggressive treatment without the need for pulmonary angiography.[8,35] Echocardiographic visualization of thrombi within the proximal pulmonary arteries may also obviate the need for pulmonary angiography.[8]

Doppler echocardiography can accurately estimate pulmonary pressures in the presence of tricuspid or pulmonary regurgitation.[35,36,50] Many normal individuals and most patients with acute pulmonary embolism and right-ventricular failure will have some degree of tricuspid regurgitation.[35,36] In the absence of structural heart abnormalities, flow velocities of tricuspid regurgitation can be used to estimate systolic right-ventricular, and therefore, systolic pulmonary artery pressures, whereas pulmonary regurgitation flow velocities can be used to estimate diastolic pulmonary artery pressures.[36,50] In adults, there is a good correlation between estimated pulmonary artery systolic pressures and the percentage of vascular obstruction.[36]

Because pulmonary emboli are unusual in children and adolescents, patients without clear risk factors should be investigated for the possibility of SLE, homocystinuria,[20] or congenital or acquired coagulopathies associated with spontaneous thromboses.[13,15] In particular, these patients should be screened for the presence of the lupus anticoagulant, anticardiolipin antibodies, and deficiencies of protein C, protein S, or antithrombin III.[13] In some cases further investigations to detect rarer forms of defects causing hypercoagulation may be indicated.[13]

MANAGEMENT

Ideally, drugs used to treat pulmonary embolism should be easy and safe to administer with minimal need for laboratory monitoring, should demonstrate rapid improvement in clinical status, and should produce good long-term results.[51,52] As yet, no single regimen has been shown to meet all of these objectives.[51] Various new approaches to thrombolytic therapy are presently being evaluated in adults, and therefore, the following recommendations regarding therapy in both adults and children may soon be outdated. As new therapeutic regimens are developed, perhaps further studies in children will result in improved pediatric protocols. However, definitive protocols for treatment of pulmonary emboli in children will almost certainly lag behind those of adults because of the scarcity of pediatric patients diagnosed and treated for pulmonary embolism.

Because a major objective of treatment for pulmonary embolism is to prevent clot extension and recurrent emboli, anticoagulation is used in most patients.[33] Patients with a diagnosis of pulmonary embolism are generally treated with intravenous heparin at a dosage of 500 to 750 U/kg/24 hours, which is adjusted to maintain an activated partial thromboplastin time of approximately twice the control value.[2,8] If not contraindicated, oral therapy with warfarin is subsequently started and is generally continued to at least 6 weeks and possibly longer under some circumstances.[2,53] Warfarin therapy is most appropriately titrated by using the international normalized ratio (INR), which should be approximately 2.0 to 3.0.[8] Heparin and warfarin therapy should overlap for a least 4 days.[8] Heparin alone will result in only minimal changes in the amount of obstruction within the first few days after a pulmonary embolism, and it may take several weeks before there is evidence of significant improvement.[54]

Although still investigational for pediatric patients, both urokinase and streptokinase have been used to dissolve vascular clots and pulmonary emboli in children.[16,21,23,25,30] For urokinase a recommended loading dose is 4400 U/kg followed by a continuous infusion of 2000 to 4400 U/kg/hr for up to 36 hours.[23,25] Newborns may be relatively unresponsive to thrombolytic therapy because of inadequate fibrinogen activity.[25] Relatively high dosages of urokinase may be necessary in infants (up to 8000 U/kg/hr) when compared with dosages used in older patients.[30] For streptokinase, a loading dose of 3500 to 4000 U/kg is followed by a continuous infusion of 1000 to 1500 U/kg/hr.[25] Short-term results using urokinase in children and adults may be dramatic with rapid dissolution of the embolus.[30,51,55] However, studies in adults did not find a significant long-term difference between the outcome of patients treated with urokinase or heparin for pulmonary embolism.[51,55,56] Moreover, bleeding complications were more common with urokinase therapy than with heparin use.[51,56] There did not appear to be any significant difference in the efficacy or complication rate when using a 12-hour urokinase infusion, a 24-hour urokinase infusion or a 24-hour streptokinase infusion.[55] Except for severe pulmonary embolism with hemodynamic compromise, these results have discouraged the use of these agents for routine therapy in patients with pulmonary emboli.[55,56] If thrombolytic therapy is used, the diagnosis should be confirmed by angiography.[2,33]

Studies in adults with pulmonary emboli have demonstrated significant angiographic improvement in most patients after treatment with human recombinant tissue plasminogen activator (rt-PA).[51,52] Pyles et al used catheter-directed local infusion of rt-PA at a dosage of 0.1 mg/kg/hr for 11 hours with significant improvement in pulmonary perfusion in a 19-month-old child.[10] This dosage was chosen to be approximately equivalent to the total rt-PA dosage of 50 to 100 mg used in adults, which has been associated with a relatively low risk of hemorrhagic complications.[10,51,57] Recent studies have suggested that short-duration thrombolytic therapy may be more successful and have less complications than long-term infusions.[56,58] Directed thrombolytic therapy through a pulmonary artery catheter appears to be neither safer nor more effective than delivery through a peripheral vein.[8,52,58]

Inotropic support should be used in the presence of right-sided heart failure or shock caused by a pulmonary embolus[8,49] and surgical embolectomy[26,27,60] or aggressive thrombolytic therapy[58,59] should be considered. The relative merits of surgical embolectomy and thrombolytic therapy in this situation are debatable.[60] However, when thrombolytic therapy is contraindicated, when severe hemodynamic compromise limits the time for response to thrombolytic therapy, or when the patient shows hemodynamic deterioration despite thrombolytic therapy, embolectomy must be considered.[60] Transvenous catheter embolectomy[61] or clot fragmentation[62] and simultaneous pharmacologic thrombolysis have been used to provide a rapid increase in cardiac output and a decrease in right-ventricular pressure in young adults with massive pulmonary embolism. There is usually immediate improvement in hemodynamics when sufficient clot is removed.[61]

Various regimens using low-dose or low-molecular-weight heparin have been proposed for the prophylaxis of deep venous thrombosis or pulmonary thromboembolism in high-risk patients.[3,8,17] However, antithrombotic therapy with aspirin, disopyramide, or low-dose subcutaneous heparin was not adequate for preventing pulmonary emboli in a group of children awaiting cardiac transplantation because of dilated cardiomyopathy.[22] Warfarin has been recommended to prevent thrombus formation in this group of patients.[22] In general, patients should receive warfarin for at least 1 month if risk factors persist.[53] A significant portion of patients with pulmonary embolism and anticardiolipin antibody have been shown to fail warfarin therapy, and it has been suggested that these patients be treated with heparin for at least 4 to 6 months after the antibody has been demonstrated to be absent.[15] Some patients with protein C or protein S deficiency may develop skin necrosis early in the course of warfarin therapy.[13,16]

OUTCOME

Because of the effective fibrinolytic system in the lung, most pulmonary emboli will spontaneously resolve.[54,60] Because of their better underlying cardiopulmonary fitness, when properly diagnosed and treated, the mortality from pulmonary embolism in younger individuals appears to be significantly lower than in older adults.[7]

REFERENCES

Epidemiology

1. Stevenson GF, Stevenson FL: Pulmonary embolism in childhood, *J Pediatr* 34:62-69, 1949.
2. Matthew DJ, Levin M: Pulmonary thromboembolism in children, *Intensive Care Med* 12:404-406, 1986.
3. Buck JR, Connors RH, Coon WW, Weintraub WH, Wesley JR, Coran AG: Pulmonary embolism in children, *J Pediatr Surg* 16:385-391, 1981.
4. Bernstein D, Coupey S, Schonberg SK: Pulmonary embolism in adolescents, *Am J Dis Child* 140:667-671, 1986.
5. Sternberg TL, Bailey MK, Lazarchick J, Brahen NH: Protein C deficiency as a cause of pulmonary embolism in the perioperative period, *Anesthesiology* 74:364-366, 1991.
6. Berg RA, Stein JM: Medical management of fungal suppurative thrombosis of great central veins in a child, *Pediatr Infect Dis J* 8:469-470, 1989.
7. Green RM, Meyer TJ, Dunn M, Glassroth J: Pulmonary embolism in younger adults, *Chest* 101:1507-1511, 1992.
8. Goldhaber SZ, Morpurgo M, for the WHO/ISFC Task Force on Pulmonary Embolism: Diagnosis, treatment, and prevention of pulmonary embolism, *JAMA* 268:1727-1733, 1992.
9. Byard RW, Cutz E: Sudden and unexpected death in infancy and childhood due to pulmonary thromboembolism, *Arch Pathol Lab Med* 114: 142-144, 1990.
10. Pyles LA, Pierpont MEM, Steiner ME, Hesslein PS, Smith CM II: Fibrinolysis by tissue plasminogen activator in a child with pulmonary embolism, *J Pediatr* 116:801-808, 1990.
11. Emery JL: Pulmonary embolism in children, *Arch Dis Child* 37:591-595, 1962.
12. Bick RL, Baker WF: Anticardiolipin antibodies and thrombosis, *Hematol Oncol Clin North Am* 6:1287-1299, 1992.
13. Bick RL, Ucar K: Hypercoagulability and thrombosis, *Hematol Oncol Clin North Am* 6:1421-1431, 1992.
14. Cheruku R, Tapazoglou E, Ensley J, Kish JA, Cummings GD, Al-Sarraf M: The incidence and significance of thromboembolic complications in patients with high-grade gliomas, *Cancer* 68:2621-2624, 1991.
15. Montes de Oca MA, Babron MC, Blétry O, et al: Thombosis in systemic lupus erythematosus: a French collaborative study, *Arch Dis Child* 66: 713-717, 1991.
16. Garbrecht F, Gardner S, Johnson V, Grabowski E: Deep venous thrombosis in a child with nephrotic syndrome associated with a circulating anticoagulant and acquired protein S deficiency, *Am J Pediatr Hematol Oncol* 13:330-333, 1991.
17. Zwerdling RG, Brown J: Pulmonary embolism in children: risks and prevention, *JAMA* 265:2888, 1991.
18. Raman TK, Blake JA, Harris TM: Pulmonary embolism in Landry-Guillain-Barré-Strohl syndrome, *Chest* 60:555-557, 1971.
19. Riggs T: Cardiomyopathy and pulmonary emboli in terminal Duchenne's muscular dystrophy, *Am Heart J* 119:690-693, 1990.
20. Mudd SH, Skovby F, Levy HL, et al: The natural history of homocystinuria due to cystathionine b-synthase deficiency, *Am J Hum Genet* 37:1-31, 1985.
21. Jones CL, Hébert D: Pulmonary thrombo-embolism in the nephrotic syndrome, *Pediatr Nephrol* 5:56-58, 1991.
22. Hsu DT, Addonizio LJ, Hordof AJ, Gersony WM: Acute pulmonary embolism in pediatric patients awaiting heart transplantation, *J Am Coll Cardiol* 17:1621-1625, 1991.
23. Marraro G, Uderzo C, Marchi P, Castagnini G, Vaj PL, Masera G: Acute respiratory failure and pulmonary thrombosis in leukemic children, *Cancer* 67:696-702, 1991.
24. Oppenheimer EH, Esterly JR: Thrombosis in the newborn: comparison between infants of diabetic and nondiabetic mothers, *J Pediatr* 67:549-556, 1965.
25. Corrigan JJ Jr: Neonatal thrombosis and the thrombolytic system: pathophysiology and therapy, *Am J Pediatr Hematol Oncol* 10:83-91, 1988.
26. Clapp S, Bedard M, Farooki ZQ, Arcinegas E: Pulmonary artery thrombus associated with the ductus arteriosus, *Am Heart J* 111:796-797, 1986.
27. Fripp RR, Whitman V, Waldhausen JA, Boal DK: Ductus arteriosus aneurysm presenting as pulmonary artery obstruction: diagnosis and management, *J Am Coll Cardiol* 6:234-236, 1985.
28. Wigger HJ, Bransilver BR, Blanc WA: Thromboses due to catheterization in infants and children, *J Pediatr* 76:1-11, 1970.
29. Brismar B, Hardstedt C, Jacobson S: Diagnosis of thrombosis by catheter phlebography after prolonged central venous catheterization, *Ann Surg* 194:779-783, 1981.
30. Zureikat GY, Martin GR, Silverman NH, Newth CJL: Urokinase therapy for a catheter-related right atrial thrombus and pulmonary embolism in a 2-month-old infant, *Pediatr Pulmonol* 2:303-306, 1986.
31. Jones DRB, Macintye IMC: Venous thromboembolism in infancy and childhood, *Arch Dis Child* 50:153-155, 1975.
32. Mueh JR, Herbst KD, Rapaport SI: Thrombosis in patients with the lupus anticoagulant, *Ann Intern Med* 92:156-159, 1980.

Disease Mechanisms

33. Dalen JE: The case against fibrinolytic therapy, *J Cardiovasc Med* 5:799-807, 1980.
34. Elliot CG: Pulmonary physiology during pulmonary embolism, *Chest* 101:163S-171S, 1992.
35. Torbicki A, Tramarin R, Morpurgo M: Role of echo/Doppler in the diagnosis of pulmonary embolism, *Clin Cardiol* 15:805-810, 1992.
36. Come PC: Echocardiographic evaluation of pulmonary embolism and its response to therapeutic interventions, *Chest* 101:151S-162S, 1992.
37. Dantzker DR, Bower JS: Clinical significance of pulmonary function tests: alterations in gas exchange following pulmonary thromboembolism, *Chest* 81:495-501, 1982.
38. D'Alonze GE, Bower JS, DeHart P, Dantzker DR: The mechanisms of abnormal gas exchange in acute massive pulmonary embolism, *Am Rev Respir Dis* 128:170-172, 1983.
39. Herve P, Petitpretz P, Simonneau G, Salmeron S, Laine JF, Duroux P: The mechanisms of abnormal gas exchange in acute massive pulmonary embolism (letter), *Am Rev Respir Dis* 128:1101-1102, 1983.
40. Dalen JE, Haffajee CI, Alpert JS, Howe JP III, Ockene IS, Paraskos JA: Pulmonary embolism, pulmonary hemorrhage and pulmonary infarction, *N Engl J Med* 296:1431-1435, 1977.

Assessment and Diagnosis

41. Sors H, Safran D, Stern M, Reynaud P, Bons J, Even P: An analysis of the diagnostic methods for acute pulmonary embolism, *Intensive Care Med* 10:81-84, 1984.
42. Cvitanic O, Marino PL: Improved use of arterial blood gas analysis in suspected pulmonary embolism, *Chest* 95:48-51, 1989.
43. The PIOPED Investigators: Value of the ventilation/perfusion scan in acute pulmonary embolism: results of the Prospective Investigation of Pulmonary Embolism Diagnosis (PIOPED), *JAMA* 263:2753-2759, 1990.
44. Dawley D, Goldhaber SZ: Impact of lung scanning on the management of suspected pulmonary embolism, *Am Heart J* 114:669-671, 1987.
45. Biello DR, Mattar AG, McKnight RC, Siegel BA: Ventilation-perfusion studies in suspected pulmonary embolism, *Am J Roentgenol* 133:1033-1037, 1979.
46. Stein PD, Alavi A, Gottschalk A, Hales CA, Saltzman HA, Vreim CE, Weg JG: Usefulness of noninvasive diagnostic tools for diagnosis of acute pulmonary embolism in patients with a normal chest radiograph, *Am J Cardiol* 67:1117-1120, 1991.
47. Robin ED: Overdiagnosis and overtreatment of pulmonary embolism: the emperor may have no clothes, *Ann Intern Med* 87:775-781, 1977.
48. Hull RD, Hirsh J, Carter CJ, et al: Pulmonary angiography, ventilation lung scanning, and venography for clinically suspected pulmonary embolism with abnormal perfusion lung scan, *Ann Intern Med* 98:891-899, 1983.
49. Shah HR, Buckner CB, Purnell GL, Walker GW: Computed tomography and magnetic resonance imaging in the diagnosis of pulmonary thromboembolic disease, *J Thorac Imaging* 4:58-61, 1989.
50. Goldberg SJ, Allen HD, Marx GR, Donerstein RL: *Doppler echocardiography,* ed 2, Philadelphia, 1988, Lea & Febiger.

Management

51. Goldhaber SZ, Meyerovitz MF, Markis JE, et al: Thrombolytic therapy of acute pulmonary embolism: current status and future potential, *J Am Coll Cardiol* 10:96B-104B, 1987.
52. Verstraete M, Miller GAH, Bounameaux H, et al: Intravenous and intrapulmonary recombinant tissue-type plasminogen activator in the treatment of acute massive pulmonary embolism, *Circulation* 77:353-360, 1988.

53. Research Committee of the British Thoracic Society: Optimum duration of anticoagulation for deep-vein thrombosis and pulmonary embolism, *Lancet* 340:873-876, 1992.
54. Dalen JE, Banas JS Jr, Brooks HL, Evans GL, Paraskos JA, Dexter L: Resolution rate of acute pulmonary embolism in man, *N Engl J Med* 280:1194-1199, 1969.
55. The Urokinase Pulmonary Embolism Trial Study Group: Urokinase-streptokinase embolism trial: phase 2 results, *JAMA* 229:1606-1613, 1974.
56. Agnelli G, Parise P: Bolus thrombolysis in venous thromboembolism, *Chest* 101:172S-182S, 1992.
57. Sobel BE: Safety and efficacy of tissue-type plasminogen activator produced by recombinant DNA technology, *J Am Coll Cardiol* 10(suppl):40B-44B, 1987.
58. Goldhaber SZ: Evolving concepts in thrombolytic therapy for pulmonary embolism, *Chest* 101:183S-185S, 1992.
59. Prewitt RM: Hemodynamic management in pulmonary embolism and acute hypoxemic respiratory failure, *Crit Care Med* 18:S61-S69, 1990.
60. Gray HH, Morgan JM, Paneth M, Miller GAH: Pulmonary embolectomy for acute massive pulmonary embolism: an analysis of 71 cases, *Br Heart J* 60:196-200, 1988.
61. Moore JH Jr, Koolpe HA, Carabasi A, Yang SL, Jarrell BE: Transvenous catheter pulmonary embolectomy, *Arch Surg* 120:1372-1375, 1985.
62. Essop MR, Middlemost S, Skoularigis J, Sareli P: Simultaneous mechanical clot fragmentation and pharmacologic thrombolysis in acute massive pulmonary embolism, *Am J Cardiol* 69:427-430, 1992.

PART TEN

Asthma

CHAPTER 61

Mechanisms of Disease in Childhood Asthma

Renato T. Stein and Fernando D. Martinez

Significant advances have been made in the last few years in our understanding of the disease mechanisms in chronic asthma. For decades, asthma had been regarded as a classical type I hypersensitivity reaction of Gell and Coombs, with IgE-triggered release of mast cell mediators leading to the intermittent bronchoconstriction that characterizes the disease. It is now acknowledged that these mechanisms play a very important role in the inflammatory response present in chronic asthma but that they do not explain many recently described biological and clinical features of the disease. Postmortem studies of patients dying from asthma have identified a cell infiltration in the bronchial mucosa[1,2] that is mainly characterized by the presence of mononuclear cells and eosinophils. Bronchoalveolar lavage studies of moderately severe asthmatics even during periods of apparent clinical remission have clearly demonstrated that chronic inflammatory changes may persist for months, with a large array of cells and mediators being released into the airways.[3-5]

The factors responsible for these chronic changes are not well understood. It is likely that different pathogenetic mechanisms may be present in different patients, and alterations of a large number of cells and tissues have been intensely explored. It is now widely believed that asthma is a heterogeneous disease, with different phenotypes and clinical expressions that depend on age, gender, genetic background, and environmental exposures. There is also convincing evidence suggesting that, if left untreated, asthma associated with chronic inflammation may induce important structural changes in the asthmatic airway leading to irreversible abnormalities in lung function and to enhanced clinical expression of the disease. This new concept of asthma has led to a very significant change in the treatment strategy for the disease. Inhaled antiinflammatory therapy is now considered first-line treatment for those asthmatic patients in whom the clinical expression of the disease is compatible with chronic inflammation of the airways.

HETEROGENEITY OF ASTHMALIKE SYMPTOMS

The presence of different conditions that may be associated with lower airway obstruction during childhood complicates our understanding of the pathogenesis of the disease. Most asthmatic children present with recurrent episodes of wheezing and dyspnea, which may be triggered by viral infections or by exposure to environmental stimuli such as allergens, cold air, and tobacco smoke, among many others. Wheezing, however, is simply the expression of a mechanical restriction to airflow in airways that, when obstructed, elicit the characteristic high pitch, polyphonic "whistling" sound. The factors that provoke the changes associated with intermittent airway narrowing during childhood are numerous. Because asthma is rarely lethal in children and because invasive airway studies have only recently become available in this age group, our knowledge about the pathologic changes occurring in the airways of young asthmatics is very limited. The very concept of asthma as an inflammatory disease was developed in adults, and there are very few direct demonstrations of the validity of this concept in children. However, longitudinal studies have convincingly shown that most cases of asthma begin in childhood,[6] and many asthmatic children have symptoms and risk factors that are analogous to those of adults. It is thus reasonable to surmise that a significant proportion of children with asthma have a condition that is similar to that of adults.

The possibility that different wheezing phenotypes may coexist during childhood has been suggested by recent longitudinal studies.[7] Although these wheezing phenotypes may overlap at this age, they seem to be associated with different risk factors. Diminished airway function assessed during infancy has been found to predispose to wheezing during lower respiratory illnesses (LRIs) during the first years of life, independently of a relation with increased serum IgE levels.[7] There is also increasing evidence suggesting that IgE-related asthma in older children coexists with an alternate form of recurrent airway obstruction usually associated with abnormal responses to one main form of environmental insult, namely viral infections. This form of recurrent airway obstruction usually occurs during the preschool years, may be less persistent in time than classical IgE-mediated asthma, and is apparently not associated with bronchial hyperresponsiveness to methacholine.[8] Children with chronic symptoms of asthma also have altered reactivity to viruses,[9] but it is not known if the same abnormality in immune reaction to viruses is present in these two clinically different forms of childhood asthma.

As explained earlier, epidemiologic evidence suggests that, in many cases of chronic asthma, the disease may start during early childhood. Incidence of asthma is highest during the first 3 to 4 years of life,[6] with more than 80% of cases starting before 4 years of age. During these first years of life, both the immune system and the respiratory system go through a profound process of growth and maturation. This process determines the pattern of subsequent response to environmental exposures in both systems. It is thus plausible to consider childhood asthma as a developmental disease, that is, as a condition in which the basic abnormality consists of an altered development of the patterns of immune and airway response to external stimuli, an abnormality that probably persists for life. This more persistent form of the disease coexists with milder forms, in which it is likely that other inflammatory mechanisms, perhaps associated with altered responses to viral infections described earlier, are involved.

GENE-ENVIRONMENT INTERACTIONS IN ASTHMA

Important determinants of the heterogeneity of the clinical expressions of childhood asthma are the complex interactions between genetic predisposition and environmental influences. There is now good evidence suggesting that asthma has a strong genetic component. Twin studies have shown that approximately half of the susceptibility to developing asthma is determined by genetic influences.[10] However, segregation analysis has shown that asthma is a polygenic condition,[11] and only very weak, if any, major genes determine the disease. In other words, a large number of genes may cause asthma at different ages and in association with different environmental exposures.

Most studies that have addressed the genetics of asthma have dealt with intermediate phenotypes for asthma, that is, quantitative or qualitative phenotypes that are associated with asthma and that are more easily amenable to genetic analysis. One such phenotype is total serum IgE levels. Epidemiologic studies have recently shown a strong association between total serum IgE levels and the prevalence of asthma in large community samples.[12,13] Moreover, no cases of asthma were reported among subjects with very low levels of serum IgE.[12,13] Total serum IgE levels are known to aggregate in families,[14] and recent data from the Tucson Children's Respiratory Study have shown that serum IgE may be controlled by a major codominant gene.[15] These results confirmed work done by others, although the exact hereditary mechanism has not been elucidated.

Marsh et al[16] and Meyers et al[17] recently reported an inverse correlation of the square of the difference in serum IgE levels between siblings to the proportion of alleles shared identically by descent at different markers in chromosome 5q. However, whereas the highest correlation coefficient observed by Marsh et al[16] was on a marker located within the interleukin-4 (IL-4) gene, Meyers et al[17] reported that their highest correlation coefficient was with the marker D5S436, which is located at least 10 million bases away from the IL-4 gene cluster. These results suggest that there may be more than one locus in chromosome 5q that participates in the regulation of total serum IgE level in humans but that the mechanisms of inheritance and the exact location of the locus or loci linked to these markers remain to be determined.

Other atopic markers have also been used in genetic analysis of asthma. Cookson et al[18] reported that an elaborate atopic phenotype was linked to markers on chromosome 11q. Initially, it was thought that this linkage signal was due to the presence of the gene for the high affinity receptor for IgE in chromosome 11q.[19] More recent evidence suggests that, although polymorphisms in the gene for the high affinity receptor for IgE may explain in part the linkage signal observed in chromosome 11q, other genes must be present in the area that are associated with the atopic status.[20] This more recent evidence also suggests that many genes may determine bronchial hyperresponsiveness, high levels of serum IgE, and sensitization to allergens, all of which are phenotypes that are known to be strongly associated with asthma.[20] It is thus likely that elucidating the genetic bases for asthma will be a very complex task, which will be rendered even more complex by the different interactions of these genes with different exposures occurring at different times during life (see also Chapter 2 on Environmental Factors and Chapter 3 on Molecular Genetics).

CHILDHOOD ASTHMA: VIRUSES AND ATOPY

Two main pathogenetic mechanisms are responsible for recurrent wheezing during childhood: altered reactivity to viral infections and allergic airway inflammation. These mechanisms are discussed in the next paragraphs.

Virus-Induced Wheezing During Childhood

Wheezing with viral infections is a very common occurrence during childhood. One fifth of all children have at least one episode of LRI with wheezing in the first year of life, and up to 70% of these cases are associated with documented viral infections.[21] Up to 30% of all children have one or more episodes of wheezing during LRIs.[7] Such episodes are mainly caused by respiratory syncytial virus (RSV), parainfluenza viruses, and to a lesser extent, adenoviruses and influenza virus.[21] In older children it is mainly rhinoviruses that have been associated with respiratory infections with wheezing.[22] This suggests that the mechanisms through which viral infections induce airway obstruction may be different in children of different ages. Certain factors, however, are common to all forms of virus-associated childhood wheezing. In general, male children tend to develop wheezing more commonly than female children,[23] as do children of lower socioeconomic status and of less educated and younger mothers.[24] Children who spend several hours each day in settings where several other children are taken care of also tend to develop more wheezing illnesses than other children.[25] Therefore both factors that increase the likelihood of becoming infected with viruses and factors associated with the nature of the response to the virus tend to increase the likelihood of wheezing.

Mechanisms of Viral-Induced Airway Obstruction

Considerable advances have been made in the last few years in our understanding of the alterations that may be associated with bronchial obstruction during viral infections in childhood. Two main areas of knowledge have been extensively explored: the possibility that intrinsic characteristics of the lungs may enhance airway obstruction during viral infections and the possibility that altered immune reactions to the virus itself may enhance bronchial obstruction in certain children.

Role of Lung Function and Bronchial Responsiveness. It is now apparent that infants and young children whose airway function is in the lower percentiles of the population distribution are at increased risk of developing wheezing during lower respiratory tract illnesses.[26,27] If not associated with other risk factors for asthma, this condition is transitory and not characterized by persistence of symptoms beyond the preschool years. For this reason it has been called transient early wheezing.[7]

For years it had been known that children hospitalized with bronchiolitis showed persistent reductions in lung function.[28] Several studies have found that these children had lower flow rates, increased inspiratory or expiratory resistance, or increased gas volume months or years after the initial event.[28,29] Until recently, it was not known if these lower levels of lung function were the consequence or the cause of these wheezing illnesses. Several studies have now demonstrated that children who will go on to wheeze during the first 3 years of life have diminished levels of lung function that precede the development of the wheezing illnesses.[26,27,30] It has thus been suggested that these lower levels of lung function are a predisposing factor for airway obstruction during viral infections. The nature of the alteration in airway dynamics present in these "transient infant wheezers" is not known. It is possible that diminished airway function may be associated with narrower airway diameter for a given airway generation.[27] The internal diameter of an intrapulmonary airway is determined by the balance between pressures that tend to keep it open (airway resistive pressure, elastic recoil pressure of the airway, and alveolar pressure) and the elastic recoil pressure of the lung, which tethers the airway.[31] Because of its immaturity, the infant's lung has a low content of elastin and collagen.[32] Also, the chest wall is quite compliant during the first years of life.[33] These two factors contribute to a lower elastic recoil pressure of the lung in this age group when compared with adults.[34] The infant is thus particularly vulnerable to airway closure during tidal breathing.[35] Genetic factors or environmental exposures such as maternal smoking during pregnancy[36] may further decrease elastic recoil pressure of the lung and resting airway diameter. It is also possible that some infants may have particularly compliant intrapulmonary airways because of lack of adequate development of airway cartilage, thus representing a form of bronchomalacia. In children with any of these alterations, mucus deposition and airway edema occurring during viral infections may cause sufficient narrowing to allow the airways to reach a critical diameter. This may predispose these children to airway obstruction and wheezing. Interestingly, although these children tend to outgrow their symptoms with age, their mean levels of lung function remain lower than those of children without any history of wheezing.[7]

There are alternative scenarios to the hypothetical pathogenetic mechanism just proposed to explain transient infant wheezing. Diminished airway function could be explained, for example, by an increase in basal airway tone, caused by either an impairment of autonomic control or an increase in airway responsiveness. Assessment of asymptomatic infants 6 months after they had bronchiolitis showed they had increased airway responsiveness compared with age-matched controls.[37] However, infants with a history of recurrent wheezing were not found to have increased airway responsiveness.[30,38] Infants with bronchiolitis have lower baseline airway function than controls. The relation between baseline lung function and bronchial challenge has, so far, not been evaluated in infants. Both in vitro studies and animal studies have shown that viral-induced changes in lung function could be partially explained by an altered β-adrenergic function.[39,40] Granulocytes taken from asthmatic subjects did not respond well to β-adrenergic stimulation when compared with those taken from normal subjects, and this abnormality was enhanced when viral infections occurred.[39] It has also been shown that the cell receptors for certain viruses have structural similarities with β-adrenergic receptors,[40] and this may explain impaired β-adrenergic function during viral infection. Unfortunately, there are no published studies assessing reversibility of the diminished levels of airway function observed in transient infant wheezers. However, several studies have shown that children who would fit into the category of transient infant wheezers do not have increased airway responsiveness when compared with children with no history of wheezing.[31,38,41]

Defense Mechanisms Against Viral Infections. The data presently available suggest that both children and adults show diminished levels of lung function[42] during apparently asymptomatic viral infections. It is thus possible that some form of involvement of the lower airways may be present even in mild forms of viral respiratory infection. Because viral infections induce clinically relevant airway obstruction in only a minority of infected children, the mechanism responsible for these overt cases probably lies in the specific immune response to respiratory viruses by the lungs. These response mechanisms are reviewed in the following paragraphs.

Epithelial cells. Epithelial cells are an important part of the defense against viral infections. The epithelium has a role that goes beyond that of a simple mechanical barrier. Early studies of the pathology of RSV infection showed that RSV mainly infects respiratory epithelial cells, causing proliferation and necrosis of the epithelium. Recent data[43] demonstrated that, when exposed to RSV, a human bronchial epithelial cell line produced IL-8 shortly after infection and that IL-6 and granulocyte/macrophage colony-stimulating factor (GM-CSF) were also produced. IL-8 is a strong chemoattractant and activator of neutrophils. It is thus possible that this cytokine may be a crucial inflammatory mediator, contributing to the airway obstruction often observed during RSV infections. Work in experimental animals has also shown that airway damage caused by influenza virus can elicit bronchoconstriction by reducing the enzymatic action of enkephalinase, a neutral endopeptidase that normally degrades substance P. Substance P is a neuropeptide that induces airway smooth muscle contraction and airway narrowing (discussed later).[44,45] Damage to the epithelium can also activate sensory nerves, causing release of tachykinins, a group of neuropeptides that can produce acute inflammatory responses by stimulating mucus secretion, increasing vascular permeability, and causing neutrophils to adhere to the vascular endothelium. Piedimonte et al[46] observed that Sendai virus infection made the rat trachea particularly susceptible to neurogenic inflammation, as manifested by a large increase in vascular permeability and an exaggerated influx of neutrophils in response to sensory nerve stimulation with capsaicin. It is thus possible that disruption of the epithelium by viruses may not only elicit neurogenic inflammation, but also potentiate the effects of its mediators.

IgG antibodies. The low incidence of viral LRIs during the first few weeks of life has suggested that high titers of maternal antibodies against viruses can be protective against LRIs. Epidemiologic studies have shown that maternal neutralizing antibodies do not prevent infection, but higher antibody titers are associated with less severe clinical symptoms.[47] Studies of association between maternal RSV antibodies in the serum of young infants and subsequent severity of RSV infection have yielded contradictory results. When challenged by RSV, infants were able to mount a response through the diffusion of maternal IgG able to form immune complexes into the airway lumen.[48] Once phagocytized, these immune complexes have been shown to stimulate release of inflammatory mediators by neutrophils, which could contribute to the disease process.[49] In contrast, other studies have suggested that maternal antibodies may have some active protective role. Infants with high titers of transplacentally acquired RSV-specific IgG had less severe RSV pneumonia and fewer respiratory infections than those with lower titers.[50,51] At this time there is no good explanation for the inconsistency of these findings or for the failure of maternal antibodies to completely protect against RSV infections in their children.

IgG-virus interactions associated with high levels of IgG are probably not responsible for the pathogenesis of RSV-LRIs. This is further supported by the description of strong effects of RSV immunoglobulin in protecting high-risk infants against RSV- LRIs. In a recent study,[52] children who received intravenous administration of large doses of RSV hyperimmunoglobulin presented decreased incidence of lower respiratory tract illnesses, fewer days of hospitalization, and fewer days in the intensive care unit compared with adequately matched controls who did not receive RSV immunoglobulin.

Some studies have focused on the role of IgG subclass deficiencies related to infant wheezing[53,54] but have shown contradictory results. Another study showed that serum concentration of virus specific IgG-4 was significantly higher in infants who wheezed with RSV compared with those with upper respiratory tract infections.[55]

IgE antibodies against viruses. Previously, Welliver et al[56] had described the development of RSV-specific IgE in nasal secretions of hospitalized children who had documented RSV-LRIs before 12 months of age. They observed that RSV titers were higher in patients with wheezing LRIs than in those with nonwheezing LRIs. There was also a strong correlation between the lower arterial Po_2 measured during hospitalization and the peak RSV-titer in nasal secretions. Concentrations of histamine (a potent bronchoconstrictor) measured in nasal secretions were also correlated with the degree of hypoxia, but this correlation was not particularly strong. These results suggested that mediators other than histamine could be released by an IgE-related mechanism during viral infections and be important in determining the severity of the illness. Indeed, this same group of investigators subsequently showed that patients with RSV-LRI were twice more likely to have detectable levels of leukotriene C_4 (LTC_4) in the respiratory tract than infants with upper respiratory infections.[57] Moreover, LTC_4 production seemed to be a RSV-IgE-dependent mechanism, because detectable levels of LTC_4 were found in 83% of infants who developed RSV-IGE compared with only 29% of infants who did not develop an RSV-IgE response. Detectable levels of leukotriene D_4 (LTD_4) and leukotriene B_4 (LTB_4) were found in 30% of infants with RSV-LRIs. Leukotrienes are mast-cell derived metabolites of arachidonic acid, with LTC_4 being capable of causing bronchoconstriction, whereas LTB_4 is a chemoattractant for neutrophils and eosinophils. LTC_4 levels were significantly higher in wheezing subjects than in nonwheezing subjects. It has also been recently shown that concentrations of eosinophilic cationic protein are higher in nasopharyngeal secretions of children with RSV-LRIs than in those with RSV upper respiratory illnesses and that RSV can prime eosinophils to release various inflammatory mediators including LTC_4 when subsequently stimulated with chemical activators.[58] These studies identified an asthmalike, IgE-mediated mechanism by which viral infections could cause wheezing in certain apparently predisposed infants. In this scenario, direct viral damage would work in concert with toxic damage by eosinophil products and with edema and bronchoconstriction provoked by LTC_4, and this would bring about the airway obstruction seen in wheezing viral infections. Furthermore, a similar relation between severity of symptoms and virus specific IgE has been described for LRIs caused by parainfluenza virus.[59] All these results were based on studies of highly selected populations, and therefore, it was not possible to assess the proportion of all infants with wheezing LRIs who develop RSV-specific IgE. However, the data suggest that there is a group of infants with LRIs who are more prone to developing virus-specific IgE and to have persistent wheeze in the first few years of life.

Cell-mediated immunity. In children with impaired cell-mediated immunity, RSV is still detected 3 to 4 months after the initial insult, compared with a mean of 7 days in normal children.[60] Virus-specific cellular cytotoxic activity was found within a week of infection with RSV in infants.[61] This activity was age dependent, with the response being more significant in infants under 6 months of age, compared with those over 6 months,[62] which can account for more severe disease in the younger age group. Apparently, a prompt cell-mediated immune response to RSV is associated with increased likelihood of wheezing[63]; in contrast, infants who develop upper respiratory tract illness or pneumonia have a more gradual cell-mediated response.

Viruses-Receptor Interactions. In initiating an immune response, respiratory viruses bind to the surface of the host cells through specific receptors present in the surface of these cells. This binding triggers an intracellular mechanism by which the viruses are processed and both viral antigens and HLA proteins are expressed by the cell. The final result of this activity is binding of T lymphocytes to the target cell surface through nonspecific adhesion molecules such as lymphocyte-function associated antigen-1 (LFA-1). These adhesion molecules attach to ligands in the target cells; intracellular adhesion molecule 1 (ICAM-1) is an example of such ligands. Some viruses (rhinoviruses and Coxsackie viruses) attach to ICAM-1 and could block adhesion of the T lymphocyte to the antigen-presenting cell, thus delaying the immune response to the virus. Furthermore, interaction between viruses and lymphocytes activates T cells and promotes the release of cytokines such as interferon-γ (IFN-γ) and tumor necrosis factor (TNF). These cytokines and some proteins derived from eosinophils[64] up-regulate ICAM-1 receptors, thus increasing the potential spread of the infection and the immunologic inflammatory response. Recent studies by Salkind[65] have demonstrated that RSV infections can block the early events necessary for cellular collaboration in response to infection.

Viruses and the Selection of Th-Cell Responses. The factors that determine the nature of the immune reaction elicited by respiratory viruses are not well understood. In a recent report, Anderson et al[66] assessed cytokine responses by peripheral blood mononuclear cells to identify the type of T-helper cell responses elicited by RSV. They showed that cells exposed to RSV presented primarily increases in IL-2 and IFN-γ production, consistent with a Th-1-like response.

Viruses have also been implicated in determining the type of T-helper cell reaction that is selected in early life in susceptible subjects. For some time, circumstantial evidence seemed to implicate viral infections in predisposing to the development of allergies, thus suggesting that viral infections could enhance the selection of Th-2-like clones in early life. This concept has been recently challenged by epidemiologic data suggesting an inverse relationship between incidence of infection and development of allergies in large population samples.[67] The experimental data supporting either hypothesis are quite scanty. Kudlacz and Knippenberg[68] studied the effects of parainfluenza virus type-3 (PI-3) infection on the respiratory response of sensitized guinea pigs to allergen challenge. They found that after the antigen challenge, sensitized animals had significantly increased numbers of eosinophils in the bronchoalveolar lavage (BAL) fluid than did nonsensitized animals and exhibited airway hyperresponsiveness to methacholine by aerosol. When sensitization was initiated 7 days after inoculation with PI-3, it did not promote airway hyperresponsiveness, increased eosinophils in the BAL fluid, or histamine release from the infected lung tissue. These results thus suggest that early respiratory infections do not predispose for the development of allergic responses. Moreover, it appears that viral respiratory infections may impair antigen sensitization or mast cell mediator release, resulting in attenuation of the respiratory effects associated with antigen challenge in sensitized animals.

Studies performed in Tucson, Arizona, support the hypothesis that certain infections may enhance the development of Th-1-like responses, thus blocking the establishment of Th-2-like responses.[69] Total serum IgE levels were measured at birth, 9 months, and 6 years of age, and IFN-γ production by blood mononuclear cells was measured at birth and 9 months in children with no history of viral LRIs and in those with a history of wheezing LRIs (WLRI) and nonwheezing LRIs (NWLRI) assessed in the first 3 years of life. The results showed that children with NWLRIs had significantly higher IFN-γ production at 9 months when compared with the no LRI or WLRI groups. Children who had NWLRIs early in life had significantly lower IgE levels at 9 months and at 6 years compared with either children who had WLRIs or with children with no LRIs. It is thus possible that children with certain types of respiratory infections in early life may show significant, subsequent enhancement of Th-1-like responses with associated suppression of IgE production and allergic sensitization.

It is not possible to determine with our present knowledge why certain children develop a Th-2-like response to viral infection with subsequent increased risk of allergic sensitization and asthma, whereas others seem to have the exactly opposite pattern of reaction, with enhancement of Th-1-like responses and persistently decreased serum IgE levels. Genetic factors seem to play an important role, because children of atopic parents have less IFN-γ-producing cells in circulation than children of nonatopic parents.[69] Environmental factors may also exert their influence as IFN-γ is produced in high quantities during certain infections.[67] We can speculate that repeated viral infections, particularly during early life, may selectively enhance the development of Th-1-type cells, thus inhibiting the proliferation of Th-2 clones and the development of allergic sensitization. Conversely, in susceptible subjects less exposed to respiratory infections, Th-2-like clones would be preferentially activated, with increased production of specific IgE against aeroallergens and increased prevalence of asthmatic symptoms.

Conclusions

The mechanisms by which viral infections induce lower airway obstruction are complex and involve altered airway reactivity, diminished airway caliber, and enhanced immune response to the viral insult. These multifactorial elements of the airway response to viruses in wheezing children are summarized in Fig. 61-1.

Wheezing Associated with Allergic Airway Inflammation

The great majority of school-age children with recurrent wheezing have high levels of circulating specific IgE against common aeroallergens.[70] At the same time, recurrent wheezing is associated with bronchial hyperresponsiveness. These two fundamental abnormalities of asthma are not easy to separate from each other, and it is therefore possible that inflammatory mediators may themselves induce, for example, increased airway responsiveness to physical stimuli. Also, these abnormalities are present to a different extent in different patients, thus contributing to the marked heterogeneity of the disease. There is convincing evidence suggesting that in the most troublesome forms of childhood asthma, usually characterized by early onset, persistent symptoms, and deterioration of lung function, chronic inflammation and persistent bronchial hyperresponsiveness are almost invariable features. In the next paragraphs the present knowledge of the alterations in immune and airway responsiveness in IgE-related asthma are reviewed, with special reference to the developmental aspects of these alterations.

Mechanisms of IgE-related Asthma

Airway Inflammatory Response. In the last decade our understanding of the characteristics of airway inflammation in chronic asthma has been considerably enhanced by the availability of BAL and bronchial biopsies. These bronchoscopic

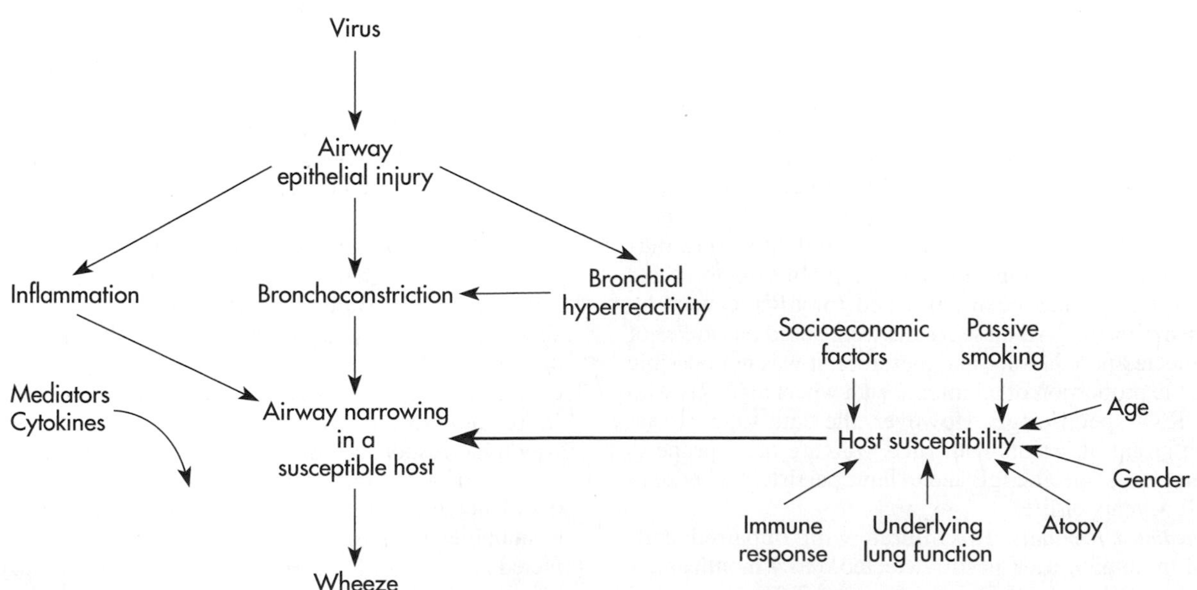

Fig. 61-1. Viral respiratory infections and wheezing: mechanisms of association. (From Balfour-Lynn: *Arch Dis Child* 74:257, 1996.)

techniques have provided new insights into the dynamics and complexity of the inflammatory changes occurring in asthma. Various studies have consistently shown the presence of increased numbers of ciliated epithelial cells often in clumps, mast cells, and eosinophils,[71-73] whereas others have revealed increase in lymphocytes[74,75] and epithelial cells[76,77] in the BAL of asthmatic patients. In mild asthmatics, numbers of T lymphocytes (CD3) and their subclasses (CD4 helper, CD8 suppressor/cytotoxic) are not increased, although using activation markers there is accumulating evidence of T-cell activation. Macrophage and neutrophil function are also enhanced; even in mild disease, macrophages have been shown to respond to allergen by generating cytokines such as IL-8 and IL-1B, and this may reflect an important change in the phenotype of these cells in asthmatics. Both mast cells and eosinophils are also present in airway secretions. A variety of different mediators from many cell types have been described, but some of the most important are: histamine, prostaglandin D_2 (and other prostanoids), 15-hydroxyeicosatetraenoic acid (15-HETE), leukotrienes B_4, C_4, D_4, and E_4, lysosomal enzymes, and a number of basic proteins from the eosinophil. Many of these mediators originate from activated mast cells and eosinophils, but platelets, macrophages, and monocytes also contribute to the autacoid pool.

Some aspects of the inflammatory response in asthma can be represented in the form of early and late asthmatic reactions (EAR, LAR)[78] (Fig. 61-2). After bronchial provocation with an allergen to which the subject is sensitized, a rapid bronchoconstriction usually occurs, which lasts for about 1 hour (EAR). This is often followed by a more prolonged phase of airway narrowing (LAR) that starts 2 to 3 hours after exposure, reaches a maximal airway response by 4 to 8 hours, and resolves in 12 to 24 hours. LAR has been shown to occur in parallel with an increase in airway hyperresponsiveness to bronchoconstrictor agents such as methacholine and histamine, and this hyperresponsiveness may persist for days after the LAR has resolved.

The EAR is mostly characterized by activation and degranulation of the mast cell with release of mediators. After inhalation of challenging allergens there is airway smooth muscle contraction following the release, among others, of the lipid-derived mediators prostaglandin PGD_2, $9\alpha11\beta P\text{-}PGF_2$, thromboxane, leukotriene LTC_4 and 15-HETE, and kinins,[79] as well as proteases, lysosomal hydrolases, and proteoglycans that will, in a later phase, act on tissue damage and repair.

The LAR expresses itself in the airways with an important edema component and BAL fluid during this phase contains increased numbers of eosinophils.[80] Some studies have shown increased numbers of neutrophils and lymphocytes after anti-

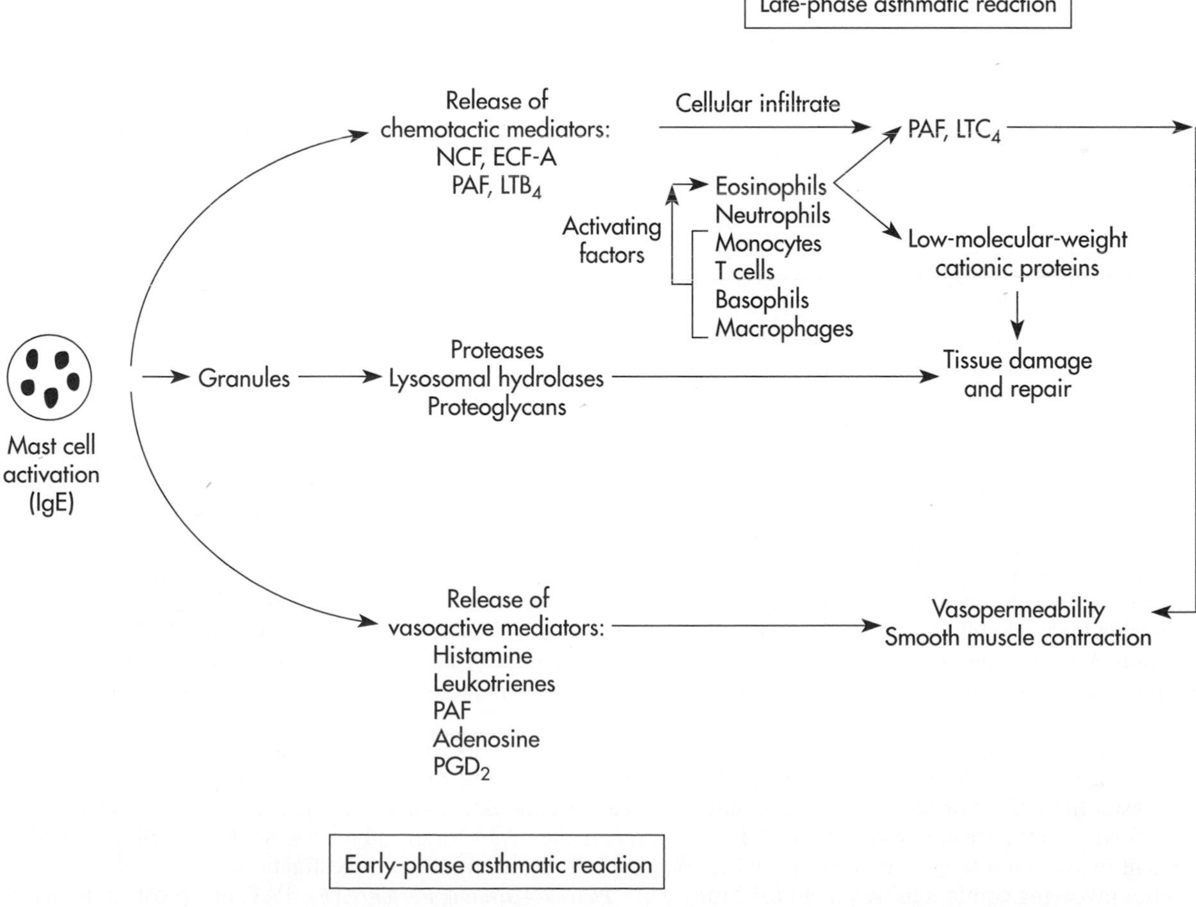

Fig. 61-2. Early- and late-phase asthmatic reaction (EAR, LAR) model. *ECF,* Neutrophil chemotactic factor; *ECF-A,* eosinophilic chemotatic factor of anaphylaxis; *PAF,* platelet-activating factor; *LT,* leukotriene; *PG,* prostaglandin. (From Malo JL, Cartier A: Late asthmatic reactions. In Weiss EB, Stein M (eds): *Bronchial asthma: mechanisms and therapeutics,* ed 3, Boston, 1993, Little, Brown, p 140.)

gen challenge; these changes were not seen in subjects with an EAR only.[79,81] Patients who demonstrate both EAR and LAR show increased levels of eosinophil-derived major basic protein (MBP) and neurotoxin (EDN), but LTC_4 is seen only in patients who have a LAR. The second inflammatory "wave" represented by LAR may be important in asthma, because it may lead to proliferative and repair responses, including the targeted destruction of the bronchial epithelium, the expansion and activation of fibroblasts, hypertrophy and hyperplasia of the smooth muscle, and proliferation of neuropeptide-containing nerves.

It is clear from the preceding description that many inflammatory mediators and cells are involved in the disease process in chronic asthma. The model of EAR and LAR has been very useful in expanding an understanding of the immunopathology of hyperreactive airways. However, consensus has been reached today that there is overlap between the two responses. Interaction among cells and mediators in the airway inflammatory response could be responsible for airway bronchial hyperresponsiveness. Because of the various, overlapping actions of a large array of mediators, it was until recently considered unlikely that antagonizing a single family of mediators would have a major clinical impact on the treatment of asthma. The promising results recently suggested by studies with leukotriene antagonists seem to challenge this concept,[82] although the role of this set of drugs in the treatment of asthma has not yet been elucidated (discussed in a later section).

The biology and possible role of the most important mediators and cells involved in the airway inflammatory process are briefly discussed in the next section.

Inflammatory Mediators in IgE-related Asthma

Histamine. Histamine is probably one of the most widely studied inflammatory mediators in asthma. A rise in plasma histamine concentrations is seen minutes after allergen inhalation,[83-85] and the subsequent increase in urinary *N*-methylhistamine[86] indicates that histamine is responsible at least in part for the early asthmatic response. Mast cells are the main source of this mediator,[77] as demonstrated by the increased levels of histamine seen in BALs from stable asthmatics, together with increased mast-cell activation.

Three types of histamine receptors are known to be present in the airway[87]: H_1, H_2, and H_3. H_1 receptors mediate histamine-induced bronchospasm in asthmatics as well as in normal subjects in higher concentrations. Histamine also elicits activation of sensory reflexes, vasoconstriction, and vasodilation of bronchial vessels through H_1 receptors.[87] H_2 receptors mediate mucus secretion and vasodilation, whereas H_3 receptors are responsible for the regulation of cholinergic and sensory nerve function. Most histamine receptors also mediate feedback inhibitory mechanisms for histamine secretion by mast cells.

Although there is evidence indicating that histamine contributes to the EAR, a direct role for histamine in the LAR has not been well established.[88] Antihistamines have not proven to be very effective in the treatment of asthma.[89] Despite the improvement in symptom scores and airway caliber measurements, studies involving continuous treatment for 2 to 7 weeks with antihistamines have not shown any significant change in airway responsiveness when assessed by methacholine inhalation challenge.[90,91] This may be related to the limited role of histamine in the chronic inflammation present in asthma.

Prostaglandins. Prostaglandins or prostanoids are one of a group of local mediators believed to play a role in the asthmatic inflammatory process. After immunologic or nonimmunologic stimulation, cytosolic phospholipase A_2 (PLA_2) is activated, causing cleavage of arachidonic acid from the cell membrane phospholipid. Arachidonic acid is then metabolized in either of two pathways: the cyclooxygenase pathway, leading to the formation of prostaglandins, thromboxane, and prostacyclin and, the 5-lipoxygenase enzyme system pathway, to form leukotrienes. To become active, this PLA_2 enzyme requires the action of another protein called 5-lipoxygenase activating protein (FLAP).[92]

Alveolar macrophages also generate various prostaglandins (PG_2, PGE_2, and PGF_2-B_5) and thromboxanes. In humans, prostanoids (except those of the E series) contract airway muscle.[93,94] PGF_2-B_5 causes increased airway secretions with the production of glycoproteins.[94] Prostaglandins cause contraction of airway smooth muscle by activating the thromboxane receptor.

The role of thromboxane and prostaglandins in chronic asthma is not well understood. Cyclooxygenase inhibitors do not appear to have a beneficial effect in clinical asthma.[95]

Leukotrienes. The leukotrienes are biologically active fatty acids derived from the oxidative metabolism of arachidonic acid[96] and can be produced by mast cells (cysteinyl leukotrienes and LTB_4), eosinophils (cysteinyl leukotrienes), and neutrophils (LTB_4). Epithelial cells and macrophages have also been shown to produce leukotrienes. Drugs binding to FLAP block the path to leukotriene production. In the continuation of the cascade of leukotriene production, leukotriene A_4 is formed, and then converted to leukotriene B_4 (LTB_4). This leads to the formation of cysteinyl leukotrienes LTC_4, LTD_4, and LTE_4, which are potent constrictors of human airways.

Immunoreactive LTC_4 has been recovered from the plasma of children with severe asthma; the amounts recovered are significantly greater than those recovered from the plasma of normal children.[97] In addition, treatment of asthma is related to a decrease in the amount of immunoreactive LTC_4 recovered from plasma. LTC_4 is detectable in significant amounts in the BAL fluid of patients with chronic stable asthma in the absence of a specific challenge.[98] Both LTD_4 and LTE_4 have been reported to increase airway hyperresponsiveness[89,99] and may play an important role in asthma. LTB_4 is a potent chemokine: it acts at accumulating and activating inflammatory cells (mostly neutrophils and eosinophils).[100] Although it has been found in BAL of asthmatic subjects,[85] the role of LTB_4 in asthma remains unclear. LTC_4, LTD_4, and LTE_4 bind to the same receptor (LT_1) on the bronchial smooth muscle. Most leukotriene antagonist drugs that have been developed block this receptor.[101]

Effective leukotriene antagonists such as ICI-204,219 (Zafirlukast) and MK-571 or ONO 1078 (Prankulast) have been recently developed by the pharmaceutical industry. Their role in the treatment of asthma has not been well evaluated yet but is a matter of intense investigation.[102]

Platelet-Activating Factor (PAF). PAF, like prostaglandins and leukotrienes, is formed by the action of phospholipase A_2 on membrane phospholipids and may be produced by several of the inflammatory cells implicated in asthma (i.e., macrophages, eosinophils, and neutrophils). Inhaled PAF causes bronchoconstriction and a small increase in airway hyperreactivity[103] in normal subjects. Once PAF is rapidly inactivated in vivo, it apparently triggers a chain of inflammatory events that lead to increased bronchial responsiveness. Release of PAF is apparently associated with increased accumulation of eosinophils in the lungs[104] and skin of atopic subjects.[105] PAF makes eosinophils adhere more easily to endothelial surfaces, a property that may be involved in the recruitment of eosinophils into tissues.[106] Because eosinophils are a source of PAF, they can attract more eosinophils and perpetuate an inflammatory reaction. PAF stimulates eosinophils to release basic proteins, which are known to cause tissue damage. PAF also causes an increased expression of low-affinity IgE receptors on monocytes.[107] In addition, PAF induces microvascular leakage[108] and increases airway secretions and epithelial permeability.

Most prophylactic asthma drugs, such as glucocorticosteroids, methylxanthines, chromoglycate, and nedocromil sodium, impair various components of PAF-induced bronchopulmonary alterations, cell activation, and cell migration into the airways in various species, including humans.[109] This suggests that this phospholipid mediator may play an important role in allergic hypersensitivity reactions like asthma. However, results of different trials with anti-PAF compounds have not yet shown encouraging results.

Bradykinin. Bradykinin is derived from kininogens in the plasma by the action of kininogenases (including kallikrein and tryptase from mast cells). Inhaled bradykinin causes bronchoconstriction in asthmatics but not in normal subjects,[110,111] inducing a sensation of dyspnea and coughing spells similar to those observed during asthmatic attack. This supports the idea that bradykinin acts as an activator of sensory nerves in the airways.[112] Mucus hypersecretion and airway edema are main features of asthma. Bradykinins could contribute to both these phenomena by dilating blood vessels, increasing vascular permeability, and stimulating ion transport. Kinins can also activate inflammatory cells and amplify the release or production of other putative mediators in asthma, notably histamine, lipid-derived mediators, and neuropeptides.[113] Bradykinin may also contribute to bronchial obstruction by mechanisms other than spasmogenesis. Bradykinin increases mucus production[114] and elicits airway edema with microvascular leakage.[115] The presence of kinins, tissue kallikrein, and kininogen in the airways at the time of either provoked or naturally occurring asthmatic attacks has been documented.[116] Recent studies have suggested that bronchial responses to bradykinin are strongly correlated with airway eosinophilic inflammation,[117] perhaps explained by damage to the airway epithelium.[118,119] It has been suggested that eosinophils may damage the airway epithelium, thus impairing the production of two major bronchial peptides, neutral endopeptidase (NEP) and kinase II.[120] These peptides are mainly produced by the airway epithelium, and they degrade bradykinin thus limiting its bronchoconstrictive effects.[116,119-121] Prostaglandin E_2 is also released by the airway epithelium, and it has a strong bronchodilating effect that also balances the effect of bradykinin.[121]

Oxygen-derived free radicals. Many inflammatory cells produce oxygen-derived free radicals such as superoxide anions. They can have an important role in asthmatic inflammation and may contribute to epithelial damage.[122] Activated neutrophils, eosinophils, monocytes, mast cells, and alveolar macrophages release oxyradicals, which in turn provoke bronchoconstriction[123] and changes in receptor function, which could influence airway reactivity.

Neutrophil and eosinophil generation of superoxide anion have been studied and compared extensively, with somewhat conflicting results.[122-127] Contradictions and differences among studies may be the result of selection bias, parameters of the assay, or the agonist used. Despite these contradictions, there is now good evidence suggesting that superoxide anion generation may be an important factor in eosinophil participation in both host defense and inflammation and that the presence of an eosinophil infiltrate in the airway of asthmatic patients can provide a potent mechanism for tissue damage.

Cytokines. Cytokines are peptide mediators released from different inflammatory cells that have a function in cell-cell communications and may determine type and duration of an inflammatory response. Whereas histamine, PAF, and leukotrienes play a role in the acute and subacute inflammatory response, cytokines are involved in the chronic inflammatory process. Cytokines such as IL-5, GM-CSF, and IL-3 are found in a biologically active state in the circulation of asthmatic subjects.[127] Elevated levels of these cytokines, which are able to prolong eosinophil survival in vitro, have been found in serum as well as in supernatants from purified and cultured peripheral blood T cells of asthmatic subjects compared with normal individuals. Overtly atopic ("extrinsic") and apparently nonatopic ("intrinsic") patients with asthma have been shown to have different cytokine production patterns.[128] Table 61-1 summarizes the functions and cell origin(s) of some of the most important cytokines involved in the airway inflammation in asthmatic subjects.

A different group of cytokines called chemokines has a specific leukocyte-selective chemotactic activity, and they are divided into two subfamilies. IL-8 is a CXC chemokine and is a chemotactic factor for neutrophils and T lymphocytes, and under some conditions for eosinophils. Other members of the CXC subfamily are MGSA/Gro-α, CTAP-III, and NAP-2, and they have similar chemotactic activities. The CC subfamily has proteins that are chemotactic for monocytes, but not neutrophils. One such cytokine is RANTES, which has been shown to be a chemoattractant for memory T cells.[129] RANTES also stimulates the migration of eosinophils across IL-1-stimulated endothelium.[130] This suggests that RANTES has an important role as a selective chemoattractant pathway for eosinophils and memory T cells in asthma.

Many cells participate in the orchestrated process leading to airway inflammation in asthma. The role of these cells and their interaction with mediators produced by other cells are reviewed below.

Inflammatory Cells in the Asthmatic Airways

Eosinophils. The importance of eosinophils in the pathogenesis of asthma is related to its central role in the airway inflammatory process.[131,132] To stress this role, some authors have described asthma as "chronic eosinophilic bronchitis," a concept that perhaps underestimates the importance of the contribution of many other, interconnected cells in the development and persistence of asthma. An increase in eosinophil counts is found in sputum,[133] BAL fluid,[134,135] airway epithelium and submucosa,[136,137] and commonly in blood[138] of asthmatic subjects. Although both lymphocytes and eosinophils often infiltrate the airway mucosa of asthmatics, eosinophils seem to play a major role. Eosinophils are now believed to

Table 61-1 Cytokines and Their Role in Airway Inflammation Reaction in Asthmatics

CYTOKINE	CELL SOURCE	FUNCTIONS
Interleukin-2 (IL-2)	T cells	T cell growth factor Eosinophil chemoattractant
Interleukin-3 (IL-3)	T cells Mast cells Eosinophils	Granulocyte (eosinophil and neutrophil) differentation activation in vitro survival enhancement primary chemotaxis (eosinophil)
Interleukin-4 (IL-4)	T cells Mast cells	Essential for IgE synthesis (isotype switch of B cells) Inhibition of IFN-γ-mediated responses T cell growth factor Inhibits macrophage-activated inflammatory cytokines Survival enhancement (eosinophils)
Interleukin-5 (IL-5)	T cells Mast cells Eosinophils	Eosinophil differentiation and maturation activation transmigration endothelial adhesion chemotaxis (eosinophilis) survival enhancement Basophil differentiation priming Cofactor for IgE synthesis
Interleukin-1 (IL-1a and b) Tumor necrosis factor (TNF-α) Interleukin-6 (IL-6)	Many cell types	Increased endothelial adhesion molecule expression T cell activation costimuli Macrophage activators Eosinophil activators
Granulocyte/macrophage colony-stimulating factor (GM-CSF)	T cells Mast cells Macrophages Epithelial cells Eosinophils	Granulocyte (eosinophil and neutrophil) differentiation activation in vitro survival chemotaxis (eosinphils)
Interferon-γ (IFN-γ)	T cells	Inhibition IgE isotype switch Inhibition of Th-2 cell growth Eosinphil activation (late acting) Macrophage activation
Interleukin-8 (IL-8)	Monocytes T cells Fibroblasts	Neutrophil and T cell chemoattractant Neutrophil activator Inhibition of IgE synthesis Primes for eosinphil chemotaxis
RANTES	T cells Platelets	Memory T cell and eosinophil chemoattractant
Interleukin-10: human (IL-10)	T cells Monocytes Macrophages	Inhibition of Th-2 and Th-1 cytokine production Inhibition of macrophage-activated inflammatory cytokines Inhibition of eosinphil survival Inhibition of IgE synthesis
Interleukin-12 (IL-12)	T cells	Natural killer cell, T cell growth Inhibition of IgE synthesis
Interleukin-13 (IL-13)	T cells Mast cells	Induces isotype B cell switch to IgE Inhibition of macrophage-activated inflammatory cytokines
Platelet-derived growth factor b (PGDF-b)	Monocytes Macrophages	Fibrosis Th-2 cytokine inhibition
Transforming growth factor b (TGF-b)	Monocytes Macrophages	Fibrosis Th-2 cytokine inhibition

Modified from Robinson DS et al: *Thorax* 48(8):845-853, 1993.

be the cells responsible for the development of many features of asthma, such as damage and desquamation of the respiratory epithelium,[139] allergen-induced LAR,[140] and airway hyperresponsiveness.[77]

Eosinophils are derived from bone marrow precursors. After allergen challenge, eosinophils appear in BAL fluid during the LAR,[134] and this is associated with a decrease in peripheral eosinophil counts and with the appearance of eosinophil progenitors in the circulation.[140] This signal for eosinophil recruitment probably originates in the inflamed airway. The recruitment initially involves adhesion of eosinophils to vascular endothelial cells in the airway circulation, their migration into the submucosa, and their subsequent activation. This process involves interactions between specific adhesion molecules expressed in the endothelium and their complementary ligands expressed in the leukocytes. These adhesion molecules are classified into families of related molecules: one of these families is that of the selectins.[141] E-selectin is present in cell surface glycoproteins and glycolipids of many leukocytes, including eosinophils, neutrophils, monocytes, and some lymphocytes; P-selectin[142] responds to the stimuli of histamine; L-selectin[143] is present in lymphocytes and also in eosinophils and neutrophils. There are two other large families: the immunoglobulin gene superfamily[144] and the integrins. ICAM-1[145] belongs to the immunoglobulin gene superfamily and is expressed in the vascular endothelium. It binds to two integrins that are expressed in many types of leukocytes. VCAM-1 (vascular cell adhesion molecule-1)[146] is also a member of the same family and mediates leukocyte adhesion via an integrin present on eosinophils, monocytes, and basophils. The selectins mediate central contact between the eosinophils and the endothelium, whereas the integrins and their ligands ensure a stable adhesion, following which the eosinophils transmigrate into the submucosa.

IL-1 and TNF-α increase the expression of HUVEC (human umbilical vein endothelial cells), ICAM-1 and VCAM-1, whereas IL-4 is selective for VCAM-1 and IFN-γ for ICAM-1.[147,148] Although both ICAM-1 and E-selectin appear to be involved in the process of eosinophil adhesion, the specific upregulation of VCAM-1 by IL-4 may play a crucial role in this process. The role of individual cytokines and mediators in coordinating these responses is not yet fully understood. Eosinophils can respond to cytokines but are also able to produce cytokines themselves.[149,150] Attention has also been focused recently on the production of growth factors by eosinophils. TGF-α mRNA has been detected in eosinophils of patients with high eosinophil counts.[151] If these findings are confirmed in bronchial tissue from asthmatics, they would suggest that TGF-α and also TGF-β[152] may be important in the epithelial regeneration, myofibroblast proliferation, and subepithelial collagen deposition that are characteristic of chronic asthma.

Eosinophils can be activated in a number of different ways, including by allergen exposure, PAF, and cytokines such as GM-CSF and IL-5. Eosinophils release a variety of mediators, including LTC_4, PAF, 15-HETE, and oxygen-derived free radicals. Eosinophils also release four basic proteins that are toxic to the airway epithelium: MBP, eosinophil cationic protein (ECP), eosinophil-derived neurotoxin, and eosinophil peroxidase.[132,153] These basic proteins are involved in such actions as bronchoconstriction, mucus hypersecretion, increased vascular permeability, and epithelial desquamation, causing damage to the respiratory epithelium, which ultimately leads to the clinical features of asthma.

A number of tissue leukocyte-induced eosinophil surface proteins act to regulate airway eosinophilic inflammation. ICAM-1 was demonstrated on the surface of eosinophils in sputum. Blood eosinophils also show ICAM-1 after incubation with TNF-α and eosinophil survival factors. By these and other pathways, the eosinophil is able to maintain eosinophil-lymphocyte and eosinophil-eosinophil interactions to directly influence its own accumulation and activity and that of other inflammatory cells.[154] The same cytokines that are responsible for eosinophil production also have an important role in the priming of eosinophils.

Even though it is well recognized that the resolution of eosinophilic inflammation is associated with clinical improvement of asthma, mechanisms explaining how eosinophils are removed from the airway remain obscure. A recent study in humans[155] described eosinophil apoptosis occurring during the resolution of eosinophilic inflammation, typical of acute asthma. Apoptosis is a form of programmed cell death, with eosinophils possibly being phagocytosed as intact cells by macrophages in the airways.[156]

Mast cells. Mast cells are widely distributed in the body and are part of its defense against harmful agents. They can also be found in the connective tissue of the lamina propria in the airways. Mast cells release a variety of preformed and newly synthesized mediators that could be responsible for many of the clinical expressions of asthma.[77] Moreover, mast cells are one of the only cell types carrying the high-affinity receptor for IgE (FcGRl), suggesting that this cell plays an important role in signaling the presence of antigen in its vicinity. An important feature in asthmatic patients is the presence, density, and degranulation of mast cells within the epithelium. Once activated, mast cells release a number of mediators. Histamine, neutral proteases, and proteoglycans are preformed and stored in granules, whereas the lipid mediators, PGD_2, LTC_4, and PAF are all newly synthesized. As discussed earlier, histamine is a bronchoconstrictor that may also mediate vasodilation, increase vascular permeability, and increase mucus secretion. PGD_2 is a potent bronchoconstrictor; LTC_4 and its metabolites also contract smooth muscle and increase vascular permeability. Many findings support the conclusion that mast cell degranulation causes the early asthmatic response.[83-85,87]

It has been recently demonstrated that mast cells are also able to synthesize and release cytokines.[157] Murine cell lines when activated have been shown to secrete a large number of cytokines: GM-CSF,[158,159] IL-3,[159] IL-4,[160] IL-5, and IL-6.[161] Lately, the range of cytokines produced by murine cell lines when activated has been extended to include IL-1, IL-2, IFN-γ, and four members of the chemokine family. It is also known that human mast cells release TNF-α when activated.[162] This molecule is believed to play an important part in the recruitment of inflammatory cells from the peripheral circulation, and the proportion of mast cells expressing this cytokine has been found to be increased in asthmatics.[163] Human mast cells also produce IL-4, and the proportion of mast cells expressing IL-4 has also been found to be increased in asthmatics.[163] These observations help identify a broader role for mast cells in the inflammatory process in the airways. Previously it was commonly believed that the main source of cytokine production was T lymphocytes, in particular those of a Th-2-like type (discussed later). The studies quoted previously raise the possibility that cytokine production by mast cells could contribute to the induction and maintenance of the inflammatory infiltrate.

Macrophages. Macrophages can be activated by allergen via a low-affinity IgE receptor (FcGR1).[164] They are derived from blood monocytes and are the cells found in largest numbers in the BAL fluid. Macrophages are found in increased numbers after allergen challenge in asthmatic patients.[164] Macrophages from asthmatic subjects release increased amounts of oxygen-derived free radicals,[165] indicating that they have been activated by some endogenous mechanisms.

Macrophages produce a great number of mediators, with more than 100 secretory products identified.[166] One important feature of the macrophage is to help determine the characteristics of the inflammatory response. Thus after allergen exposure alveolar macrophages release a number of inflammatory mediators (LTB_4, PGF_{22}, thromboxane B_2, and PAF).[167,168] They are also able to release a great number of cytokines.[169] These cytokines include IL-1, IL-8, IL-10, GM-CSF, histamine-releasing factors, and TNF-α.[170,171]

Macrophages normally have a suppressive role on lymphocyte function, but this function may be impaired in asthma after allergen exposure.[172,173] Dendritic cells, which are specialized macrophages in the airway epithelium, are very effective antigen-presenting cells[174] and probably have a very important role in the initiation of allergen-induced responses.

Neutrophils. The role of neutrophils in asthma is uncertain. Studies have shown an influx of these cells in experimental allergen challenge in humans, but the functional consequences of this influx are still unknown. However, neutrophils may have a role in asthma because they contain many destructive proteases, are able to secrete arachidonic acid metabolites and leukotrienes, and can produce active oxygen metabolites and cytokines such as IL-8 and IL-1. Several studies have failed to find any difference in baseline neutrophil numbers between asthmatic and nonasthmatic subjects in BAL fluid.[175,176] Unless it can be established that neutrophils in tissues are increased in either number or degree of activation, studies on peripheral blood must be interpreted cautiously.[177] An exception is occupational asthma, where there seems to be stronger evidence of an early and sustained BAL fluid neutrophilia after inhalation challenge with toluene diisocyanate.[178]

Epithelial cells. As explained earlier, recent evidence has demonstrated that the airway epithelium may play an important regulatory role in the inflammatory mechanism of asthma. In addition to its function as a barrier to the outside environment, the epithelial lining of airways has a number of metabolic functions. These include regulation of fluid and ion transport, production, secretion, and movement of mucus, and presentation of antigen and foreign substances to immunologic cells within the airway. It has been recently proposed that the epithelium also regulates airway caliber by secreting substances that alter smooth-muscle reactivity.

Injury caused by environmental insults or other stimuli inhibit the ability of the epithelium to produce mediators that regulate airway responsiveness and caliber. After an acute asthmatic exacerbation, cells and mediators of airway inflammation persist within the airway and submucosa, providing a continued stimulus to the epithelium both to produce factors that may enhance reactivity and to disrupt the production of factors that could normally downregulate reactivity. Epithelial cells are also able to produce the cyclooxygenase products PGE_2 and $PGF_{2\alpha}$, influencing bronchial smooth muscle tone in either direction, depending on their relative levels of production, which may in turn be influenced by other factors such as bradykinin, histamine, and PAF.[179]

Ozone is another environmental agent that may alter airway responsiveness by damaging the epithelium, causing bronchial hyperreactivity[178] or increased permeability.[179] There are also some data suggesting that the airway epithelium might secrete contractile factors that modulate smooth-muscle reactivity. Experiments removing epithelium from the airways[180] showed that this procedure also removed a factor that had tonically relaxed the smooth muscle, the "epithelium-derived relaxing factor" (EpDRF). The identity of EpDRF has not been confirmed,[181] and experiments have demonstrated that it is not similar to the relaxing factors produced by endothelial cells (for example nitric oxide [NO]).[182] Even if EpDRF exists, the potential physiologic significance of this epithelium-derived molecule is unclear.

In addition to interactions with antigens and secretion of arachidonic mediators, the epithelium also produces cytokine mediators that may both up-regulate and perpetuate the inflammatory state in asthma. As discussed earlier, eosinophils and epithelial cells may interact through intercellular adhesion molecules. Epithelial cells are able to generate lipid mediators such as PGE_1 and PGE_2[185] and 15-HETE by the expression of the enzyme neutral endopeptidase and by the production of cytokines. Production of GM-CSF by epithelial cells after stimulation by IL-1 has been well documented.[186] BAL of asthmatic patients have shown higher levels of IL-1 than those observed in controls, and it is thus possible that the IL-1 GM-CSF interaction may be of biological significance in asthma. Synthesis and release of IL-6 and IL-8 are also mediated by IL-1 and TNF-α. The recruitment of inflammatory cells to sites of injury is then possibly affected by epithelial cell cytokine production. Epithelial cells also produce a potent vasoconstrictor and bronchoconstrictor peptide amino acid, endothelin-1 (ET-1) that is increased in the airways of asthmatic patients.[187] Increased immunoreactivity for ET-1 has also been described in the bronchial epithelium of asthmatics compared with normal subjects. This suggests that endothelin can act as a bronchoconstrictor as well as an inducer of airway fibrosis, because one of its functions is to stimulate fibroblast production.[188]

Lymphocytes. T lymphocytes play a central role in the regulation and coordination of immune responses. Their most important function is to recognize and respond to processed antigens. CD4+ T-helper cells, after activation by specific antigens, have the propensity to orchestrate the influx of granulocytes and other cells into chronic inflammatory reactions in the presence or absence of antibodies. It is likely, therefore, that CD4+ T lymphocytes play a role in all inflammatory responses that are antigen-driven, including those that characterize most cases of chronic asthma.[189]

The reaction of the CD4+ T cells to the antigen presented by the antigen-presenting cells determines the type of immune response to that particular antigen and, specifically, whether that response will include the production of IgE, which is strongly associated with childhood asthma. The regulation of IgE synthesis by lymphocytes is mediated through the specific cytokines produced by the different types of T-helper cells. IL-4 plays a pivotal role, being involved in the isotype switching of B cells from synthesis of IgD and IgM to IgE through a sequence of intracellular events.[190] Switching of B cells to IgE synthesis is potently inhibited by IFN-γ.[191] A great number of cytokines are implicated in the control of IgE synthesis by B cells.[191] IgE production depends on IL-4 and is enhanced by IL-5,[192] IL-6, and IL-13,[193] whereas IFN-γ, IL-8, and IL-12 are inhibitory.[194] These cytokines act with an array of cell surface signals to activate or regress gene splicing, which results in the production of IgE mRNA transcript (Fig. 61-3).

In mice models, two types of Th clones can be clearly distinguished: Th-1 clones secrete among others IL-2, IFN-γ, and TNF-β, whereas Th-2 clones secrete among others IL-4, IL-5, IL-6, and IL-10. Th-1 cytokines suppress the Th-2 cell expansion,[194] and when in a dominant status, Th-1 type of response may protect against the development of Th-2-dependent allergic disease.[192] Although Th-1-like and Th-2-like T-cell clones are also described in humans,[195] it is not clear if most T cells fall into this strict dichotomy. It is thus more accurate to consider Th-1-like and Th-2-like cells as two developmental T-helper cell poles that coexist in humans with many intermediate, less well-polarized cells both in tissues and in circulation.

The selection of the appropriate T-cell population is an antigen-driven process that probably occurs during the early stages of the immune response in the host, even before birth.[196] If T-cell selection favors the growth of Th-1 cells, which secrete IL-2 and IFN-γ, low-grade nonpathogenic IgA and IgG responses follow. However, the emergence of Th-2 cells, secreting IL-4 and IL-5, can lead to IgE production, eosinophilia, and atopic disease.[197]

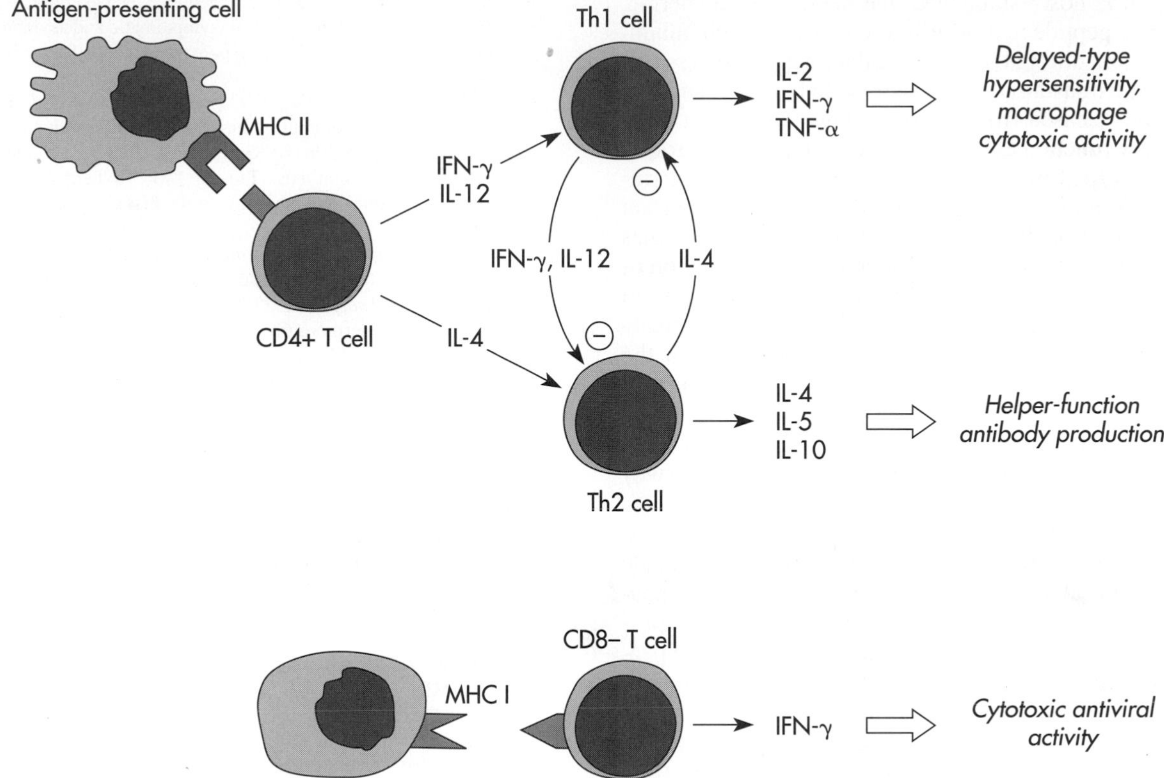

Fig. 61-3. CD4+ T cells recognize foreign antigen presented by major histocompatibility complex class II molecules (MHC II) on the surface of specialized antigen-presenting cells. Under the influence of soluble cytokines, CD4+ T cells adopt distinct function phenotypes termed Th-1 and Th-2 cells. By contrast, CD8+ T cells recognize the antigens of intracellular parasites or virus presented by MHC class I molecules (MHC I). *IFN-γ*, Interferon-γ; *IL*, interleukin; *TFN-α*, tumor necrosis factor α. (From Anderson GP, Coyle AJ: *Trends in Pharmacological Sciences* 15:327, 1994.)

Holt[198] has suggested that early childhood is the period when specific T-cell responses to environmental antigens are determined. He has also hypothesized that this would also be the perfect time to modify the development of normal anti-allergen immunity in unsensitized children. Development of immune tolerance to allergens, which is a normal pattern of response to these antigens, functions poorly in the preweaning period. Therefore, allergen exposure in the very early phase of infancy may prime for subsequent T-cell reactivity.[198,199] This phenomenon would be consistent with the existence of an early window of high risk for allergic sensitization, presumably because of delayed postnatal maturation of one or more key elements of mucosal immune function that are rate-limiting in inducing tolerance.[200,201] It is thus possible that, once a certain pattern of immune response has been selected and a preferential Th-2-like response has been established early in life, this same pattern of response may persist without the development of tolerance in predisposed individuals.

Recent studies involving peripheral blood mononuclear cells (PBMC) in infants have provided strong evidence suggesting that early selection of Th-1-like or Th-2-like clones may play a decisive role in determining susceptibility to sensitization to asthma-related allergens. Martinez et al[202] have shown that children who would subsequently become sensitized to aeroallergens had significantly reduced IFN-γ production by PBMC when compared with children who would not become sensitized to these same aeroallergens.

The factors that determine preferential selection of Th-1-like or Th-2-like clones in early life are not well understood. Genetic influences seem to play an important role. It has been recently shown that parents who are themselves allergic to aeroallergens have children who have lower production of IFN-γ by PBMC than nonallergic parents.[202] As stated earlier, certain infections associated with nonwheezing LRIs in early life may also be associated with preferential selection of Th-1-clones, persistently diminished serum IgE levels, and decreased incidence of sensitization to aeroallergens later in life.[67] It is possible that infections themselves may be responsible for these effects, but it is also possible that some unknown factor may predispose both to nonwheezing LRIs and to the immune changes associated with them. This is a very important issue to elucidate because if it were possible to mimic by noninfectious means possible effects of certain infections on the immune system, primary prevention of allergic sensitization might be an achievable goal.

Interaction Between Airway Inflammation and Neural Responses in Asthma

The fact that neural mechanisms are involved in the regulation of airway tone convinced many researchers in the past that neural abnormalities could be involved in the pathogenesis of asthma. This idea has been all but abandoned, but there is now significant evidence that points to important interactions between neural and immunologic mechanisms of inflammation.

Specifically, it is now established that neural nonadrenergic, noncholinergic peptide neurotransmitters interact with inflammatory mediators during the airway inflammatory process that is characteristic of asthma.[203] These peptide neurotransmitters are stored and released from nerve endings that have a more classic primary function as cholinergic or adrenergic neurones.

Two main types of NANC neurotransmitters exist: inhibitory and excitatory. NO appears to be the most important inhibitory neurotransmitter in the airways. Several enzymes (NO synthases) contribute to its production, and inhibition of these enzymes blocks the neural bronchodilator response in vitro. However, NO may have the undesired effect of increasing airway inflammation by increasing blood flow to the airway, with consequent plasma leakage. Other neurotransmitters such as vasoactive intestinal polypeptide (VIP) and peptide histidine isoleucine (PHI) are also very abundant in the lung but seem not to have a physiologic role in airway bronchodilation.[204,205]

The excitatory NANC neurotransmitters are colocalized at the nerve endings of afferent nerves, or C-fibers, and include tachykinins—substance P (SP), neurokinin A (NKA), and neurokinin B (NKB)—named as such because of their rapid spasmogenic effect on smooth muscle; calcitonin gene-related peptide (CGRP), and gastrin-releasing peptide. An increased population of SP-containing nerves may be identified in the airways of subjects who died with severe asthma, suggesting a neural tropism is concomitant with chronic inflammation. Once released, the effects of these neuropeptides are regulated, in part, by distinct peptidases, such as NEP and angiotensin-converting enzyme.[204] Disruption of the airway epithelium (either mechanically or by viral infection) increases the bronchoconstrictor effect of tachykinins, presumably by limiting its degradation.[207]

Although the role of tachykinins in the human airway is still uncertain,[204] their inhibition has potential therapeutic properties. Tachykinin antagonists are under development. A number of compounds can potentially reduce neuropeptide release, including opioids, furosemide, γ-aminobutyric acid, nedocromil, α_2 agonists, and histamine H_3 receptor agonists.

Conclusions

During the last 20 years, extensive studies of airway lability in asthma have allowed a much better understanding of the different mediators and cells involved in the pathogenesis of this chronic condition. The picture that emerges is one of complex and redundant disease pathways, which may affect different subjects at different times. In children the chronic inflammatory process itself may be responsible for irreversible changes in airway structure and function, which may further enhance clinical expression of the disease.

REFERENCES

1. Dunill MS: The pathology of asthma, with special reference to changes in the bronchial mucosa, *Clin J Pathol* 13:27-33, 1960.
2. Dunill MS, Massarela, GR, Anderson JA: A comparison of the quantitative anatomy of the bronchi in normal subjects, in status asthmaticus, chronic bronchitis and in emphysema, *Thorax* 24:176-179, 1969.
3. Wardlaw AJ, Dunnette S, Gleish GJ, O'Byrne PM: Bronchoalveolar cell profiles of asthmatic and nonasthmatic subjects, *Am Rev Respir Dis* 136:379-383, 1987.
4. Ferguson AC, Whitelaw M, Brown H: Correlation of bronchial eosinophils and mast cell activation with bronchial hyperresponsiveness in children with asthma, *J Allergy Clin Immunol* 90:609-613, 1992.
5. Pin I, Radford S, Kolendowicz R, Jennings B, Demburg JA, Hargreave FE, et al: Airway inflammation in symptomatic and asymptomatic children with methacholine hyperresponsiveness, *Eur Resp J* 6:1249-1256, 1993.
6. Yunginger JW, Reed CE, O'Connel EJ, Melton J, O'Fallon WM, Silverstein MD: A community-based study of the epidemiology of asthma. Incidence rates, 1964-1983, *Am Rev Respir Dis* 146:888-894, 1992.
7. Martinez FD, Wright AL, Taussig LM, Holberg CJ, Halonen M, Morgan W: Asthma and wheezing in the first six years of life, *N Engl J Med* 332:133-138, 1995.
8. Wilson NM, Bridge P, Silverman M: Bronchial responsiveness and symptoms in 5-6 year old children: a comparison of a direct and indirect challenge, *Thorax* 50:339-345, 1995.
9. Johnston SL, Pattermore PK, Sanderson G, Smith S, Lampe F, Josephs L, Symington P, O'Toole B, Myint SH, Tyrrel DA, et al: Community study of the role of viral infections in exacerbations of asthma in 9-11 year old children, *Br Med J* 310:69-89, 1995.
10. Duffy DL, Martin NG, Battistutta D, Hopper JL, Mathews JD: Genetics of asthma and hay fever in Australian twins, *Am Rev Respir Dis* 142: 1351-1358, 1990.
11. Holberg CJ, Elston RC, Halonen M, Wright AL, Taussig LM, Morgan WJ, Martinez FD: Segregation analysis of physician-diagnosed asthma in hispanic and non-hispanic white families: a recessive component? *Am J Respir Crit Care Med* 154:144-150, 1996.
12. Burrows B, Martinez FD, Halonen M, Barbee RA, Cline MG: Association of asthma with serum IgE levels and skin test reactivity to allergens, *N Engl J Med* 320:272-277, 1989.
13. Sears MR, Burrows B, Flannery EM, Herbison GP, Hewitt CJ, Holdaway MD: Relation between airway responsiveness and serum IgE in children with asthma and in apparently normal children, *N Engl J Med* 325:1067-1071, 1991.
14. Blumenthal MN, Namboodiri KK, Mendel NR, Gleich GJ, Elston RC, Yunis EJ: Genetic transmission of serum IgE levels, *Am J Med Genet* 10:219-228, 1981.
15. Martinez FD, Holberg CJ, Halonen M, Morgan WJ, Wright AL, Taussig LM: Evidence for mendelian inheritance of serum IgE levels in Hispanic and non-Hispanic White families, *Am J Hum Genet* 5:555-565, 1994.
16. Marsh DG, Neely JD, Breazeale DR, Ghosh B, Freidhoff LR, Ehrlish-Kantsky E, Schon C, Krishnaswarny G, Beaty TM: Linkage analysis of IL-4 and other chromosome 5q 31.1 markers and total serum IgE concentrations, *Science* 264:1152-1156, 1994.
17. Meyers DA, Postma DS, Panhuysen Cl, Xu J, Amelung PJ, Levitt RC, Bleecker ER: Evidence for a locus regulating total serum IgE levels mapping to chromosome 5q, *Genomics* 23:464-470, 1994.
18. Cookson WOCM, Sharp PA, Faux JA, Hopkin JM: Linkage between immunoglobulin E responses underlying asthma and rhinitis and chromosome 11 q, *Lancet* i:1292-1295, 1989.
19. Shirikawa T, Hashimoto T, Furuvama J, Takeshita T, Morimoto K: Linkage between severe atopy and chromosome 11 q 13 in Japanese families, *Clin Genet* 46:228-232, 1994.
20. Daniels SE, Battacharryas S, James A, Leaves NI, Young A, Hill MR, Faux JA, Ryan GF, le Souef PN, Lathrop GM, Musk AW, Cookson WO: A genome-wide search for quantitative trait loci underlying asthma, *Nature* 386 (6597):247-250, 1996.
21. Wright AL, Taussig LM, Ray CG, Harrison HR, Holberg CJ: The Tucson Children's respiratory study, II: Lower respiratory tract illnesses in the first year of life, *Am J Epidemiol* 129:1232-46, 1989.
22. Duff AL, Pomeranz ES, Gelber LE, Price GW, Farris H, Hayden FG, Platts-Mills TA, Heymann PW: Risk factors for acute wheezing in infants and children: viruses, passive smoke, and IgE antibodies to inhalant allergens, *Pediatrics* 92(4):535-540, 1993.
23. Tepper RS, Morgan WJ, Cota W, Wright AL, Taussig LM: Physiologic growth and development of the lung during the first year of life, *Am Rev Respir Dis* 134:513-519, 1986.
24. Holberg CJ, Wright AL, Martinez FD, Ray CG, Taussig LM, Lebowitz MD: Risk factors for respiratory syncytial virus-associated lower respiratory illnesses in the first year of life, *Am J Epidemiol* 133:1135-1151, 1991.
25. Holberg CJ, Wright AL, Martinez FD, Morgan WJ, Taussig LM: Child day care, smoking by caregivers, and lower respiratory tract illness in the first three years of life, *Pediatrics* 91:885-892, 1993.

26. Tager IB, Hanrahan JP, Tosteson TD, et al: Lung function, pre- and post-natal smoke exposure, and wheezing in the first year of life, *Am Rev Respir Dis* 147:811-817, 1993.
27. Martinez FD, Morgan WJ, Wright AL, Holberg CJ, Taussig LM, GHMA personnel: Diminished lung function as a predisposing factor for wheezing respiratory illness in infants, *N Engl J Med* 319:1112-1117, 1988.
28. Henderson FW, Stewart PW, Burchinal MR, Voter KZ, Strope GL, lrvins SS, et al: Respiratory allergy and the relationship between early childhood lower respiratory illness and subsequent lung function, *Am Rev Respir Dis* 145:283-290, 1992.
29. Pullan CR, Hey EN: Wheezing, asthma, and pulmonary dysfunction 10 years after infection with respiratory syncytial virus in infancy, *Br Med J* 284:1655-1669, 1982.
30. Clarke JR, Reese A, Silverman M: Bronchial responsiveness and lung function in infants with lower respiratory tract illness over the first six months of life, *Arch Dis Child* 67:1454-1457, 1992.
31. Martinez FD: Sudden infant death syndrome and small airway occlusion: facts and a hypothesis, *Pediatrics* 87(2):190-198, 1991.
32. Hislop A, Muir DCF, Jacobsen M, Simon G, Reid L: Post-natal growth and function of pre-acinar airways, *Thorax* 27:265-273, 1972.
33. Gerhardt T, Bancalari E: Chest wall compliance in full term and premature infants, *Acta Pediatr Scand* 69:359-364, 1980.
34. Helms P, Beardsmore CS, Stocks J: Absolute intraesophageal pressure at functional residual capacity in infancy, *J Appl Physiol* 51:270-275, 1981.
35. Mansell A, Bryan C, Levison H: Airways closure in children, *J Appl Physiol* 33:711-714, 1972.
36. Neddenriep D, Martinez FD, Morgan WJ: Increased specific lung compliance in newborns whose mothers smoked during pregnancy, *Am Rev Respir Dis* 140(4):A282, 1990.
37. Tepper RS, Rosemberg D, Eigen H: Airway responsiveness in infants following bronchiolitis, *Pediatr Pulmonol* 13:6-10, 1992.
38. Stick SM, Arnott J, Turner DJ, Young S, Landau LI, Le Souef P: Bronchial responsiveness and lung function in recurrently wheezy infants, *Am Rev Respir Dis* 144:1012-1015, 1991.
39. Busse WW: Decreased granulocyte response to isoproterenol in asthma during upper respiratory infections, *Am Rev Respir Dis* 115:783-791, 1977.
40. Co MS, Gaulton GN, Tominaga A, Homcy CJ, Fields BN, Greene MI: Structural similarities between the mammalian beta-adrenergic and rheovirus type 3 receptors, *Proc Natl Acad Sci USA* 82:5315-5318, 1985.
41. Voter KZ, Henry MM, Stewart PW, Henderson FW: Lower respiratory illness in early childhood and lung function and bronchial reactivity in adolescent males, *Am Rev Respir Dis* 137:302-307, 1988.
42. Martinez FD, Taussig LM, Morgan WJ: Infants with upper respiratory illnesses have significant reductions in maximal expiratory flows, *Pediatr Pulmonol* 9:91-95, 1990.
43. Noah T, Becker S: Respiratory syncitial virus-induced cytokine production by a human bronchial epithelial cell line, *Am J Physiol* 265: L472-478, 1993.
44. Jacoby DB, Tamaoki J, Borson DB, Nadel JA: Influenza infection causes airway hyperresponsiveness by decreasing enkephalinase, *J Appl Physiol* 64:2653-2658, 1988.
45. Dusser D, Jacoby D, et al: Virus induces airway hyperresponsiveness to tachikinins: role of neural endopeptidase, *J Appl Physiol* 67(4):1504-1511, 1989.
46. Piedmonte G, Nadel J, Umeno E, et al: Sendai virus infection potentiates neurogenic inflammation in the rat trachea, *J Appl Physiol* 68(2): 754-760, 1990.
47. Lamprecht C, Krause H, Mufson M: Role of maternal antibody in pneumonia and bronchiolitis due to respiratory syncytial virus, *J Infect Dis* 134(3):211-217, 1976.
48. Nadal D, Ogra PL: Development of local immunity: role in mechanisms of protection against or pathogenesis of respiratory syncitial viral infections, *Lung* 168(suppl):3379-3387, 1990.
49. Kaul TN, Faden H, Ogra PL: Effect of respiratory syncitial virus and virus antibody complexes in the oxidative metabolism of human neutrophiles, *Infect Immun* 32:649-654, 1981.
50. Djukanovic R, Wilson JW, Britten KM, Wilson SJ, Walls AF, Roche WR, Howarth PH, Holgate ST: Quantitation of mast cells and eosinophils in the bronchial mucosa of symptomatic atopic asthmatic and healthy control subjects using immunohistochemistry, *Am Rev Respir Dis* 142:863-871, 1990.
51. Balfour-Lynn IM: Why do viruses make infants wheeze? *Arch Dis Child* 74:251-259, 1996.
52. Groothuis J, Simoes E, Levin, et al: Prophylactic administration of respiratory syncytial virus immune globulin to high-risk infants and young children. The respiratory syncytial virus, *N Engl J Med* 329(21):1572-1574, 1993.
53. Carlsen KH, Mellbye OJ, Flugerud P, et al: Serum immunoglobulin G subclasses and serum immuniglobulin A in acute bronchiolitis in infants, *Pediatr Allergy Immunol* 4:20-25, 1993.
54. Tissing WJE, van Steensel-Moll HA, Offringa M: Severity of respiratory syncitial virus infections and immunoglobulin concentrations, *Arch Dis Child* 69:156-157, 1993.
55. Oxelius VA: IgG subclasses and human disease, *Am J Med* 76(suppl 3a):7-18, 1984.
56. Welliver R, Wong D, Sum M, et al: The development of respiratory syncytial virus specific IgE and the release of histamine in nasopharyngeal secretions after infection, *N Engl J Med* 305(15):841-846, 1981.
57. Garofalo R, Welliver R, Ogra P: Concentrations of LTB4, LTC4, and LTE4 in bronchiolitis due to respiratory syncytial virus, *Pediatr Allergy Immunol* 2:30-32, 1991.
58. Kimpen J, Garofalo R, Welliver R, et al: Activation of human eosinophils in vitro by respiratory syncytial virus, *Pediatr Res* 32(2):160-164, 1992.
59. Welliver R, Wong D, Sun M, et al: Parainfluenza virus bronchiolitis. Epidemiology and pathogenesis, *Am J Dis Child* 140(l):34-40, 1986.
60. Fishault M, Tubergen D, McIntosh K: Cellular response to respiratory viruses with particular reference to children with disorders of cell-mediated immunity, *J Pediatr* 96:179-186, 1980.
61. Isaacs D, Bangham CRM, McMichael AJ: Cell-mediated cytotoxic response to respiratory syncitial virus in infants with bronchiolitis, *Lancet* ii:769-771, 1987.
62. Scott R, Kaul A, Scott M, Chiba Y, Ogra PL: Development of in vitro correlates of cell-mediated immunity to respiratory syncitial virus infections in humans, *J Infect Dis* 137:810-817, 1978.
63. Welliver RC, Kaul A, Ogra PL: Cell mediated immune response to respiratory syncitial virus infectin: relationship to the developments of rective airways disease, *J Pediatr* 94:370-375, 1979.
64. Altman L, Ayars G, Baker C, et al: Cytokines and eosinophil-derived cationic proteins upregulate, *J Allergy Clin Immunol* 92(4):527-536, 1993.
65. Salkind A, Nichols J, Roberts N: Suppressed expression of ICAM-1 and LFA-1 and abrogation of leukocyte collaboration after exposure of human mononuclear leukocytes to respiratory syncytial virus in vitro. Comparison with exposure to influenza virus, *J Allergy Clin Immunol* 81:505-511, 1991.
66. Anderson LJ, Tsou C, Potter C, Keyserling HL, Smith TF, Anababa G, Bangha CR: Cytokine response to respiratory syncytial virus stimulation of human peripheral blood mononuclear cells, *J Infect Dis* 170:1201-1208, 1994.
67. Martinez FD: Role of viral infections in the inception of asthma and allergies during childhood: could they be proctective? *Thorax* 49(12): 1189-1191, 1995.
68. Kudlacz EM, Knippenberg RW: Parainfluenza virus type-3 infection attenuates the respiratory effects of antigen challenge in sensitized guinea pigs, *Inflam Res* 44:105-110, 1995.
69. Martinez FD, Stern DA, Wrigt AL, Taussig LM, Halonen M: Association of nonwheezing lower respiratory tract illnesses in early life with persistently diminished serum IgE levels, *Thorax* 50:1067-1072, 1995.
70. Burrows B, Sears MR, Flannery EM, Herbison GP, Holdaway MD: Relations of bronchial responsiveness to allergy skin test reactivity, lung function, respiratory symptoms, and diagnoses in thirteen-year-old New Zealand children, *J Allergy Clin Immunol* 95(2):548-556, 1995.
71. Flint KC, et al: Bronchoalveolar mast cells in extrinsic asthma: a mechanism for the initiation of antigen specific bronchoconstriction, *Br Med J* 291:923, 1985.
72. Kirby JG, et al: Bronchoalveolar lavage profiles of asthmatic and nonasthmatic subjects, *Am Rev Respir Dis* 1 36:379, 1987.

73. Wardlaw AJ, et al: Platelet activating factor. A potent chemostactic and chemokinetic factor from human eosinophils, *J Clin Invest* 78:1701, 1986.
74. Godard P, et al: Functional assessment of alveolar macrophages: comparison of cells from asthmatics and normal subjects, *J Allergy Clin Immunol* 70:88, 1982.
75. Kelly CA, et al: Numbers and activity of cells obtained at bronchoalveolar lavage in asthma, and their relationship to airway responsiveness, *Thorax* 43:684, 1988.
76. Hogg JC: The pathology of asthma. In Weiss EB, Segal MS, Stein M, eds: *Bronchial asthma: mechanisms and therapeutics,* Boston, 1985, Little, Brown, pp 209-217.
77. Wardlaw A, Dunnette L, Gleish G, Collins J, Kay AB: Eosinophils and mast cells in bronchoalveolar lavage in subjects with mild asthma, *Am Rev Respir Dis* 137:62-69, 1988.
78. Lemanske Jr RF, Kaliner M: Late phase allergic reactions. In Middleton E, Reed C, Ellis E, Adkinson F, Yunginger J, Busse W, eds: *Allergy, principles and practice,* ed 4, St Louis, 1993, Mosby, pp 320-361.
79. Liu MC, Hubbard WC, Proud D, et al: Immediate and late inflammatory responses to ragweed antigen challenge of the peripheral airways in allergic asthmatics, *Am Rev Respir Dis* 144:51-58, 1991.
80. Djukanovic R, Roche WR, Wilson JW, et al: State of the art: Mucosal inflammation in asthma, *Am Rev Respir Dis* 142:434-457, 1990.
81. Metzger WJ, Zavala D, Richerson HB, et al: Local allergen challenge and bronchoalveolar lavage of allergic asthmatic lungs, *Am Rev Respir Dis* 135:433-440, 1987.
82. Barnes NC, Kuitert LM: Drugs affecting the leukotriene pathway in asthma, *Brit J Clin Practice* 49(5):262-266, 1995.
83. Howarth P, Durham S, Lee T, Kay B, Church M, Holgate S: Influence of albuterol, cromolyn sodium and ipratropium bromide on the airway and circulating mediator responses to allergen bronchial provocation in asthma, *Am Rev Respir Dis* 132:986-992, 1985.
84. Busse W, Swenson C: The relationship between plasma histamine concentrations and bronchial obstruction to antigen challenge in allergic rhinitis, *J Allergy Clin Immunol* 84:658-666, 1989.
85. Phillips G, Ng W, Church M, Holgate ST: The response of plasma histamine to bronchoprovocation with methacholine, adenosine 5′′-monophosphate and allergen in atopic nonasthmatic subjects, *Am Rev Respir Dis* 1419-1413, 1990.
86. De Monchy J, Keyzer J, Kauffmann H, Beaumont, De Vries K: Histamine in late asthmatic reactions following house-dust mite inhalation, *Agents Actions* 16:252-255, 1985.
87. Barnes PJ: Histamine receptors in airways, *Agents Actions* (suppl) 33:103, 1991.
88. Rafferty P, Ng W, Phillips G, Clough J, Church M, Holgate S: The inhibitory actions of azelastine hydrochloride on the early and late bronchoconstrictor responses to inhaled allergen in atopic asthma, *J Allergy Clin Immunol* 84:649-657, 1989.
89. Holgate ST, Finnerty JP: Antihistamines in asthma, *J Allergy Clin Immunol* 83:537, 1989.
90. Rafferty P, Jackson L, Smith R, Holgate S: Terfenadine, a potent histamine Hl receptor antagonist in the treatment of grass pollen sensitive asthma, *Br J Clin Pharmacol* 30:229-235, 1990.
91. Finnerty J, Holgate S, Rihoux J-P: The effect of two weeks treatment with cetirizine on bronchial reactivity to methacholine in asthma, *Br J Clin Pharmacol* 29:79-84, 1990.
92. Dixon RA, Diehl RE, Opas E, et al: Requirements of a 5-lipoxygenase activating protein for leukotriene synthesis, *Nature* 343:282-284, 1990.
93. Hardy CC, et al: The bronchoconstrictor effect of inhaled PGD2 in normal and asthmatic men, *N Engl J Med* 311:209, 1984.
94. Henderson WR: Eicosanoids and lung inflammation, *Am Rev Respir Dis* 143:586, 1991.
95. Lopez-Vidreiro MI, et al: Bronchial secretion from normal human airways after inhalation of PGF-Alpha-2, methacholine, histamine and citric acid, *Thorax* 32:734, 1977.
96. Kaiser E, Chiba P, Zaky K: Phospholipases in biology and medicine, *Clin Biochem* 23:3645-3651, 1990.
97. Okubo T, Takahashi H, Sumitomo M, Shindoh K, Suzuki S: Plasma levels of leukotrienes C4 and D4 during wheezing attacks in asthmatic patients, *Intl Arch Allergy Appl Immunol* 84:19-26, 1987.
98. Wardlaw AJ, Hay H, Cromwell O, Collins JV, Kay AB: Leukotrienes LTC4 and LTB4 in bronchoalveolar lavage in bronchial asthma and other respiratory diseases, *J Allergy Clin Immunol* 84:19-26, 1989.
99. Caughey GH: Roles of mast cell tryptase and chymase in airway function, *Am J Physiol* 257:L39, 1989.
100. Smith MJH, Ford-Hutcingson AW, Bray MA: Leukotriene B: a potential mediator of inflammation, *J Pharm* 52:51-78, 1980.
101. Gardiner PJ, Abrams TS, Tudhope SR, et al: Leukotriene receptors and their selective antagonists, Av in Prostaglandin, *Tromboxane Review* 22:49-61, 1994.
102. O'Shaughenessy TC, Georgiou P, Howland K, Barnes NC: The effect of Prankulast, an oral leukotriene antagonist on leukotriene D4 (LTD4): challenges in normal subjects, *Am J Respir Crit Care Med* 151:4 (suppl):A378, 1995.
103. Cuss FM, Dixon CMS, Barnes PJ: Effects of inhaled platelet activated factor on pulmonary function and bronchial responsiveness in man, *Lancet* ii:189, 1986.
104. Denjean A, Arnoux B, Benveniste J: Long-lasting effect of intratracheal administration of PAF-acether in baboons, *Am Rev Respir Dis* 137:283, 1988.
105. Sonjar S, et al: Pre-treatment with rh-GMCSF, but not rh-IL3, enhances PAF-induced eosinophil accumulation in guinea-pig airways, *Br J Pharmacol* 100:399, 1990.
106. Henog E, Vargraftig BB: Skin eosinophils in atopic patients, *J Allergy Clin Immunol* 81:691, 1988.
107. Mogbel R, et al: The effect of platelet-activating factor on IgE binding to, and IgE dependent biological properties of human eosinophils, *Immunology* 70:251, 1990.
108. Paul-Eujene N, et al: Influence of interleukin-4 and platelet activating factor on the fce RIT/CD 23 expression on human monocytes, *J Lipid Mediat* 2:95, 1990.
109. Bel EH, De Smet M, Rossing Th, Immers MC, Dijkman JH, Sterk PJ: The effect of a specificoral PAF-antagonist, MK-287, on antigen-induced early and late asthmatic reactions in man, *Am Rev Respir Dis* 143:A811, 1991.
110. Rodgers DF, et al: Effect of platelet activating factor on formation and composition of airway fluid in the guinea pig trachea, *J Physiol* 437: 643, 1991.
111. Simonsson BG, Skoog BE, Bergh NP, Anderson P, Sudmyr N: In vivo and in vitro effect of bradykinin on bronchial motor tome in normal subjects and in patients with airway obstruction, *Respiration* 30:378, 1973.
112. Fuller RW, Dixon CMS, Cuss FMC, Barnes PJ: Bradykinin-induced bronchoconstriction in man: mode of action, *Am Rev Respir Dis* 135: 176, 1987.
113. Proud D, Kaplan AP: Kinin formation: mechanisms and role in inflammatory disorders, *Annu Rev Immunol* 6:49-83, 1988.
114. Boraniuk JN, Lundgren JD, Mizogushi H, Peden D, Gawin A, Meridam, Shelhamer JH, Kaliner MA: Bradykinin and respiratory mucous membranes. Analysis of bradykinin binding site distribution and secretary responses in vitro and in vivo, *Am Rev Resp Crit Care Med* 141:706-14, 1990.
115. Ichinose M, Barnes PJ: Bradykinin-induced airway microvascular leakage and bronchoconstriction are mediated via a bradykinin beta-2 receptor, *Am Rev Respir Dis* 142:1104-1107, 1990.
116. Barnes PJ: Bradykinin and asthma, *Thorax* 47(11), 979-983, 1992.
117. Roisman GL, Lacronique JG, Deumazes-Dufeu N, Carr C, Le Cae A, Dusser DJ: Airway responsiveness to bradykinin is related to eosinophilic inflammation in asthma, *Am J Resp Crit Care Med* 153: 381-390, 1996.
118. Barnes PJ: Asthma as an axon reflex, *Lancet* 1:242-244, 1986.
119. Frossard N, Stretton CD, Barnes PJ: Modulation of bradykinin responses in airway smooth muscle by epithelial enzymes, *Agents Actions* 31:204-209, 1990.
120. Dusser DJ, Nadel JA, Sekizawa K, Graf PD, Borson DB: Neutral endopeptidases and angiotensin converting enzyme inhibitors potentiate kinininduced contraction of ferret trachea, *J Pharmacol Exp Ther* 244:531-536, 1988.
121. Branley AM, Samhourn MN, Piper PJ: The role of epitheliium in modulating the response of guinea pig trachea induced by bradykinin in vitro, *Br J Pharmacol* 90:762-766, 1990.

122. Barnes PJ: Reactive oxygen species and airway inflammation, *Free Radicals Biol Med* 9:235, 1990.
123. De Chatelet LR, Shirley PS, Mc Phail LC, Huntley CC, Muss HB, Bass DA: Oxidative metabolism of the human eosinophil, *Blood* 50:525-535, 1977.
124. Shult PA, Graziano FM, Wallow IH, Busse WW: Comparison of superoxide generation and luminol-dependent cheminulescence with eosinophils and neutrophils from normal individuals, *J Lab Clin Med* 106:638-645, 1985.
125. Zoratti EM, Sedgewick JB, Vrtis RF, Busse WW: The effect of platlet activating factor on the generation of superoxide anion in human eosinophils and neutrophils, *J Allergy Clin Immunol* 81:749-758, 1991.
126. Corrigan CJ, Kay AB: The lymphocyte in asthma. In Busse WW, Holgate S, eds: *Asthma and rhinitis,* Oxford, 1995, Blackwell Scientific Publications, ch 34.
127. Rhoden KJ, Barnes PJ: Effect of oxygen-derived free radicals on responses of guinea-pig tracheal smooth muscle in vitro, *Br J Pharmacol* 98:325, 1989.
128. Walker C, Virchow J-C, Bruijnzeel PLB, Blaser K: T cell subsets and their soluble products regulate eosinophilia in allergic and non allergic asthma, *J Immunol* 146:1829-1835, 1991.
129. Kameyoshi Y, Dorschner A, Mallet AL, et al: RANTES released by thrombinstimulated platlets is a potent chemoattractant for human eosinophils, *J Exp Med* 176:587-592, 1992.
130. Ebisawa M, Yamada T, Klunk D, et al: Regulation of eosinophil and neutrophil transendothelial migration by cytokines and chemokines (abstract), *J Allergy Clin Immunol* 91:313, 1993.
131. Azzawi M, Bradley B, Jeffery PK, et al: Identification of activated T lymphocytes and eosinophils in bronchial biopsies in stable atopic asthma, *Am Rev Respir Dis* 142:1407-1413, 1990.
132. Gleich GJ: The eosinophil and bronchial asthma: current understanding, *J Allergy Clin Immunol* 85:422-436, 1990.
133. Frigas E, Loegering DA, Solley GO, Farrow GM, Gleich GJ: Elevated levels of eosinophil granule major basic protein in the sputum of patients with bronchial asthma, *Mayo Clin Proc* 56:345-353, 1981.
134. DeMonchy JGR, et al: Bronchoalveolar eosinophilia during allergen-induced late asthmatic reactions, *Am Rev Respir Dis* 131:373, 1985.
135. Metzger WJ, et al: Local allergen challenge and bronchoalveolar lavage of allergic asthmatic lungs, *Am Rev Respir Dis* 135:433, 1987.
136. Laitinen LA, Laitinen A, Hahtela T: A comparative study of the effects of an inhaled corticosteroid, budesonide, and a beta-2 agonist, terbutaline, on airway inflammation in newly diagnosed asthma: a randomized, double-blind, paralel group controlled trial, *J Allergy Clin Immunol* 90:32-42, 1992.
137. Beasley R, Roche WR, Roberts JA, Holgate ST: Cellular events in the bronchi in mild asthma and after bronchial provocation, *Am Rev Respir Dis* 139:806-817, 1989.
138. Horn BR, Robin ED, Theodore J, Van Kessel A: Total eosinophil counts in the management of bronchial asthma, *N Engl J Med* 242-255, 1975.
139. Dahl R, Venge P, Fredens K: Eosinophils. In Barnes P, Rodger IW, Thomson NC, eds: *Asthma: basic mechanisms and clinical management,* San Diego, 1988, Academic Press, pp 115-129.
140. Gibson PG, et al: Allergen-induced asthmatic responses: relationship between increases in airway responsiveness and increases in circulating eosinophils, basophils and their progenitors, *Am Rev Respir Dis* 143: 331, 1991.
141. Rosen SD: The LEC-CAMS: an emerging family of cell-cell adhesion receptors based upon carbohydrate recognition, *Am J Respir Cell Mol Biol* 3:397-402, 1990.
142. Johnston GI, Cook RG, McEver RP: Cloning of GMP-140, a granule membrane protein of platiets and endothelium: sequence similarity to proteins involved in cell adhesion and inflammation, *Cell* 56:1033-1044, 1989.
143. Bowen BR, Nguyen T, Lasky LA: Characterization of a human homologue of murine peripheral lymph node homing receptor, *J Cell Biol* 109:421-427, 1989.
144. Williams AF, Barclay AN: The immunoglobulin super-family domains for cell-surface recognition, *Annu Rev Immunol* 6:381-405, 1988.
145. Rothlein R, Dustin ML, Martin SD, Springer TA: A human intercellular adhesion molecule (ICAM-1) distinct from LFA-1, *J Immunol* 137:1270-1274, 1986.
146. Osborn L, Hession C, Tizard R, et al: Direct expression and cloning of vascular cell adhesion molecule 1, a cytokine induced endothelial protein that binds to lymphocytes, *Cell* 59:1203-1211, 1989.
147. Thornhill MH, Haskard DO: IL-4 regulates endothelial cell activation by IL-1, tumor necrosis factor, or IFN-gamma, *J Immunol* 145:865-872, 1990.
148. Pober JS, Bevilacqua MP, Mendrick DL, et al: Two distinct monokines, interleukin 1 and tumor necrosis factor, each independently induce biosynthesis of the same antigen on the surface of cultured human vascular endothelial cells, *J Immunol* 136:1680-1687, 1986.
149. Corrigan CJ, Kay AB: T cells and eosinophils in the pathogenesis of asthma, *Immunology Today* 13:501-517, 1992.
150. Owen WF: Cytokine regulation of eosinophil inflammatory disease, *Allergy Clin Immunol News* 3:85-89, 1991.
151. Wong DTW, Weller PF, Galli SJ, et al: Human eosinophils express transforming growth factor alpha, *J Exper Med* 172:673-681, 1990.
152. Wong DTW, Elovic A, Matossian K, et al: Eosinophils from patients with blood eosinophilia express transforming growth factor Beta-1, *Blood* 78:2702-2707, 1991.
153. Motojima S, et al: Toxicity of eosinophil cationic proteins for guinea pig tracheal epithelium in vitro, *Am Rev Respir Dis* 139:801, 1989.
154. Wooley KL, Gibson PG, Carty K, Wilson AJ, Twaddell SH, Wooley MJ: Eosinophil apoptosis and the resolution of airway inflammation in asthma, *Am J Respir Crit Care Med* 154:237-243, 1996.
155. Stern M, Meagher L, Savill J, Haslett C: Apoptosis in human eosinphils: programmed cell death in the eosinophils leads to phagocytosis by macrophages and is modulated by IL-5, *J Immunol* 148:3543-3549, 1992.
156. Hansel TT, Walker C: The migration of eosinophils into the sputum of asthmatics: the role of adhesion molecules, *Clin Exp Allergy* 22:345-356, 1992.
157. Redington AE, Bradding P, Holgate ST: The role of cytokines in the pathogenesis of allergic asthma, *Reg Immunol* 5:174-200, 1993.
158. Chung SW, Wong PMC, Shen-ONg G, et al: Production of granulocyte-macrophage colony-stimulating factor by Abelson virus-induced tumorigenic mast cell lines, *Blood* 68:1074-1081, 1986.
159. Humphries RK, Abraham S, Krystal G, et al: Activation of multiple hematopoietic growth factor genes in Abelson virus-transformed myeloid cells, *Exp Hematol* 16:774-781, 1988.
160. Brown MA, Pierce JH, Watson CJ, et al: B cell stimulatory factor-1 interleukin-4 mRNA is expressed by normal and transformed mast cells, *Cell* 50:809-818, 1987.
161. Plaut M, Pierce JH, Watson CJ, et al: Mast cell lines produce lymphokines in response to cross linkage of FceRI or to calcium ionophoresis, *Nature* 339:64-67, 1989.
162. Beynon RC, Bissonette EY, Befus D: Tumor necrosis factor-alpha dependent cytotoxicity of human skin mast cells is enhanced by anti-IgE antibodies, *J Immunol* 147:2253-2258, 1991.
163. Bradding P, Roberts JA, Britten KM, et al: Interleukins (IL-4), -5,-6 and TNF-alpha in normal and asthamatic airways: evidence for human mast cells as an important source of these cytokines, *Am J Resp Cell Biol* 10(5):471-480, 1994.
164. Joseph M, et al: Involvement of immunoglobulin E in the secretory process of alveolar macrophages from asthmatic patients, *J Clin Invest* 71:221, 1983.
165. Kelly CA, et al: Numbers and activity of cells obtained at bronchoalveolar lavage in asthma, and their relationship to airway responsiveness, *Thorax* 43:684, 1988.
166. Nathan CF: Secretory products of macrophages, *J Clin Invest* 79:319, 1987.
167. Arnoux B, et al: Antigenic release of PAF-aceter and beta-glucuronidase from alveolar macrophages of asthmatics, *Bull Eur Physiopathol Respir* 23:119, 1987.
168. MacDermot J, Fuller RW: Macrophages. In Barnes PJ, Rodger IW, Thompson NC, eds: *Asthma: basic mechanisms and clinical management,* London, 1988, Academic, pp 97-114.
169. Kelley J: Cytokines of the lung, *Am Rev Respir Dis* 141:765, 1990.
170. Bousquet J, Chavez P, Michel FB: Inflammation in chronic asthma, *ACI News* 3:170-174, 1991.
171. Lee TH, Lane SJ: The role of macrophages in the mechanisms of airway inflammation in asthma, *Am Rev Respir Dis* 145:527-530, 1992.

172. Aubus P, et al: Decreased suppressor cell activity of alveolar macrophages in bronchial asthma, *Am Rev Respir Dis* 130:875, 1984.
173. Spiter MA, et al: Alveolar macrophage-induced suppressor of T-cell hyperresponsiveness in asthma is reversed following allergen exposure in vitro, *Am Rev Respir Dis* 143:A821, 1992.
174. Holt PG, Shon-Hegrad MA, Phillips MJ: Positive dendritic cells form a tightly meshed network within the human airway epithelium, *Clin Exp Allergy* 19:597, 1989.
175. Beasley R, Roche WR, Roberts JA, Holgate ST: Cellular events in the bronchi in mild asthma and after bronchial provocation, *Am Rev Respir Dis* 139:806-817, 1989.
176. Bousquet J, Chanez P, Lacost JY, et al: Eosinophilic inflammation in asthma, *N Engl J Med* 323:1033-1039, 1990.
177. Kirby JG, Hargreave FE, Gleich GJ, O'Byrne PM: Bronchoalveolar cell profiles of asthmatic and non asthmatic subjects, *Am Rev Respir Dis* 136:379-383, 1987.
178. Fabbri LM, Boschetto P, Zocca E, et al: Bronchoalveolar neutrophilia during late asthmatic reactions induced by Toluene diisocyanate, *Am Rev Respir Dis* 136:36-42, 1987.
179. Proud D: The epithelial cell as target and effector cell in airway inflammation. In Holgate ST, Austen KF, Lichtenstein LM, Kay AB, eds: *Asthma: physiology, immunopharmacology and treatment,* Fourth International Symposium, London, 1993, Academic Press.
180. Holtzman MJ, Cunningham JH, Sheller JR, Irsigler GB, Nadel JA, Bouchey HA: Effect of ozone on bronchial reactivity in atopic and non atopic subjects, *Am Rev Respir Dis* 120:1059-1067, 1979.
181. Koren HS, Deulin RB, Graham DE, et al: Ozone-induced inflammation of the lower airways of human subjects, *Am Rev Respir Dis* 139:407-415, 1989.
182. O'Byrne DM, Walters EH, Gold BD, et al: Neutrophil depletion inhibits airway responsiveness induced by ozone exposure, *Am Rev Respir Dis* 130:214-219, 1984.
183. Fernandes LB, Patterson JW, Goldic RG: Co-axial bioassay of a smooth muscle relaxant factor released from guinea-pig tracheal epithelium, *Br J Pharmacol* 96:117-124, 1989.
184. Munataka M, Masaki Y, Sakuma I, et al, Pharmacological differentiation of pithelium-derived relaxing factor from nitric oxide, *J Appl Physiol* 69:665-670, 1990.
185. Churchil L, Chilton FH, Resau JH, et al: Cyclooxygenase metabolism of endogenous arachidonic acid by cultured human tracheal epithelial cells, *Am Rev Respir Dis* 140:449-459, 1989.
186. Marini M, Soloperto M, Mazetti M, et al: Interleukin-1 binds to specific receptors on human bronchial epithelial cells and upregulates granulocyte/macrophage colony-stimulating factor synthesis and release, *Am Rev Respir Dis* 4:519-524, 1991.
187. Gajewski TF, Fitch FW: Anti-proliferative effect of IFN-Gamma in immune regulation: IFN-Gamma inhibits the proliferation of Th2 but not Thl murine helper T lymphocyte clones, *J Immunol* 140:4245-4252, 1988.
188. Takawa N, Takuwa Y, Yanagisawa M, et al: A novel vasoactive peptide endothelin stimulates mitogenesis through inositol lipid turnover in Swiss 3T3 fibroblasts, *J Biol Chem* 264:7856-7861, 1989.
189. Robinson DR, Hamid Q, Ying S Tsicopoulos A, Barkans J, Bentley AM, Corrigan C, Durham SR, Kay AB: Predominant Th2-like bronchoalveolar T-lymphocyte population in atopic asthma, *N Engl J Med* 326:298-304, 1992.
190. Del Prete GF, Maggi E, Parronchi P, et al: IL-4 is an essential factor for the IgE synthesis induced in vitro by human T-cell clones and their supernatants, *J Immunol* 140:4193-4198, 1988.
191. Geha RS: Regulation of IgE synthesis in humans, *J Allergy Clin Immunol* 90(2):143-150, 1992.
192. Pene J, Rousset F, Briere F, et al: IgE production by normal human B cells induced by alloreactive T cells clones is mediated by IL-4 and suppressed by IFN-Y, *J Immunol* 141:1218-1224, 1988.
193. Punnonen J: Interleukin 13, a T-cell derived cytokine that regulates B cell stimulatory factor-l reciprocally regulates Ig isotope production, *Science* 236(4804):944-947, 1987.
194. Mosman TR, Coffman RL: Thl and TH2 cells: different functional properties, *Annu Rev Immunol* 7:145-173, 1989.
195. Romagnani S: Human TH1 and TH2: doubt no more, *Immunology Today* 12:256-257, 1991.
196. Godfrey KM, Barker DJP, Osmond C: Disproportionate fetal growth and raised IgE concentration in adult life, *Clin Exp Allergy* 24:641-648, 1994.
197. Holt PG: A potential vaccine strategy for asthma and allied atopic diseases during early childhood, *Lancet* 344:456-458, 1994.
198. Holt PG, McMenamin C, Nelson D: Primary sensitization to inhalant allergens during infancy, *Pediatr Allergy Immunol* 1:3-13, 1990.
199. Nelson D, McMenamin C, Wildes L, Holt PG: Postnatal development of respiratory mucosal immune function in the rat. Regulation of IgE responses to inhaled allergens, *Pediatr Allergy Immunol* 4:170-177, 1991.
200. Hanson DG: Ontogeny to orally induced tolerance to soluble proteins in mice: I primary and tolerance in newborns, *J Immunol* 127:1518-1524, 1981.
201. Strobel S, Ferguson H: Immune responses to fed protein antigens in mice: a systemic tolerance or priming is related to age at which antigen is first encountered, *Pediatr Res* 18:588-594, 1984.
202. Martinez FD, Stern DA, Wright AL, Holberg CJ, Taussig LM, Halonen M: Association of interleukin-2 and interferon-gamma production by blood mononuclear cells in infancy with parental allergy skin tests and subsequent development of atopy, *J Allergy Clin Immunol* 96(5):652-660, 1995.
203. Danielle RP, Barnes PJ, Goetz EJ, et al: Neuroimmune interactions in the lung, *Am Rev Respir Dis* 145:1230-1235, 1992.
204. Barnes PJ, Baraniuk JN, Belvisi MG: Neuropeptides in the respiratory tract, *Am Rev Respir Dis* 144:1187-1198, 1991.
205. Barnes PJ: Neural mechanisms in asthma. In Holgate ST, Austen KF, Lichtenstein LM, Kay AB, eds: *Asthma: physiology, immunopharmacology, and treatment,* Fourth International Symposium, London, 1993, Academic Press.
206. Erdos EG, Skidgel RA: Neutral endopeptidase 24.11 (enkephalinase) and related regulators of peptide hormones, *FASEB J* 3:145-151, 1989.
207. Nadel J: Regulation of neurogenic inflammation by neutral endopeptidase, *Am Rev Respir Dis* 145:S48-S52, 1992.

CHAPTER 62

Asthma: Prognosis

Louis I. Landau

Opinions about the natural history of asthma from childhood to adult life vary considerably. Population-based prospective epidemiologic studies are now beginning to provide valuable information towards a better understanding of the patterns of asthma seen through childhood. Asthma may commence in the first year of life, but about 60% will start to wheeze between 2 and 5 years. Most demonstrate an improvement with cessation or amelioration of wheezing through late childhood and adolescence. The degree of improvement and suggested risk factors for continuing wheeze have differed. This partly relates to the different cohorts investigated, the age of entry into the studies, and the retrospective nature of data recorded in many of these mostly cross-sectional studies. Much of the initial information came from hospital-based or practice-based cohorts providing information on those with more severe childhood asthma. Longitudinal studies of community-based cohorts who have reached adulthood in recent years are now providing a more accurate description of the natural history across the total spectrum of childhood asthma. Many of the studies commenced at school age, so information regarding symptoms in the early years would have been limited by recall bias. Many infants wheeze in the first 2 years. More than half cease, whereas others continue. Yet others start wheezing after 2 years of age. Recall of infant wheezing in those recruited in early school years will be different, with those who have continued being more likely to remember these early problems.

Changing diagnostic criteria over the past two decades will have influenced data analysis. Up until the early 1970s, more than half the asthmatics would not have been identified, and the entity of wheezy bronchitis included many asthmatics who were undiagnosed and undertreated. Toward the end of the 1980s the recognition of asthma was promoted, and the word *wheeze* was used for almost any noisy breathing. Some studies then probably overestimated the prevalence of asthma. Symptom-based questionnaires have allowed more accurate documentation of community prevalence of conditions likely to be asthma. However, the lack of specific diagnostic criteria because of inadequate understanding of the basic abnormality continues to cause difficulties, especially when comparing studies from different countries and different ethnic groups within a country.

PREVALENCE

Approximately 30% of infants will wheeze during the first year of life. Most have preexisting evidence of abnormal airway function, cease to wheeze by year 3, and do not have subsequent evidence of asthma.[1] About 25% to 50% are atopic and do continue to have typical childhood asthma,[2] and these include some of those with more severe asthma. The rest of the childhood asthma population will start to wheeze from the second year, most by 5 years but up to 10% starting later.

The prevalence of asthma is increasing worldwide within populations[3] and in association with migration to different environments.[4,5] The exact reason for this increase is not known. Diagnostic transfer as a result of greater recognition because of lack of a specific definition of asthma and increased awareness of the varying patterns of asthma in childhood certainly accounts for some of the increase,[6] but much is real and associated with a similar increase in other manifestations of atopy such as hayfever and eczema.[7] Genetic drift would not account for such a rapid change, suggesting that there has been a change in host response to the environment.

PROGNOSTIC FACTORS

Data indicate that the response to allergens in utero as reflected by the variation in cord IgE levels, interferon-γ levels, and T-cell responses, followed by postnatal responses to ingested allergens[8] and later to aeroallergens,[9] may be important. Cord blood IgE levels are somewhat predictive of atopy in early life and asthma later in childhood, but not early lower respiratory symptoms.[10] Antibody responses to ingested allergens start around 4 months, peak about 12 months, and return to baseline by 2 years, except in a few very atopic infants; whereas responses to aeroallergens start around 12 months and plateau between 2 and 5 years at high or low levels.[9] An elevated and persistent atopic response is associated with continuing asthma, bronchial hyperresponsiveness, and hayfever through childhood[11] and persistence into adult life.[12,13]

Bronchial hyperresponsiveness in childhood associated with asthma symptoms and atopy is predictive of bronchial hyperresponsiveness in adults, but less so when the bronchial hyperresponsiveness is found in isolation.[12,14] Persistent bronchial hyperresponsiveness through childhood, especially associated with atopy, is strongly associated with continuing asthma, whereas variable bronchial hyperresponsivenes is less consistently associated with continuing asthma.

Reports of death from asthma have increased, although there were fluctuations and peaks over the past 30 years that have been claimed to be associated with excessive β agonist use. Although it is likely that the inappropriate use of β agonists may have contributed to some deaths, a causal relationship for most deaths has not been confirmed. Fortunately death from asthma is rare in early childhood. It remains a major problem in teenagers at a time of denial and rebellion when acceptance and compliance with treatment is compromised. Undertreatment remains the major preventable cause of death.

It is claimed that some of the increase in deaths could be the result of increased prevalence and increased severity, as well as undertreatment. But some studies suggest that severity may be decreasing with reduced school absence and less restriction of physical activity.[15]

Most childhood asthmatics improve and many cease to wheeze, but the predisposition persists so other manifestations of atopy become more common, and up to one third of ex-wheezers relapse.[16] This improvement generally occurs during the second decade, and few stop wheezing subsequently.[17] Approximately one in ten will start to wheeze after childhood.[18]

Generalizing from the major longitudinal studies, it can be suggested that more than half of mild infrequent episodic childhood asthmatics will cease to wheeze in late childhood.[19-26] Park et al[27] reported that only 8% of those with one wheezing attack before 5 years of age was still wheezing at 10. Only 30% of those with frequent episodic asthma ceased to wheeze before adult life,[22,28,29] and less than 10% of those with severe chronic asthma ceased wheezing[22] (Table 62-1).

It is impossible to predict the outcome in an individual child with a high probability, although some factors do appear to be consistently significant. Age of onset in itself does not appear significant. In some studies the prognosis is worse for those under 2 years of age, whereas in others it is worse for those older than 2 years of age. As discussed, many infants with wheeze will cease to wheeze by 2 years and others will continue to have asthma—this group including the severe end of the spectrum. If all wheezing infants under 2 years are considered, they will have a good prognosis, but if only those who go on to have asthma are considered, the prognosis will be worse than those who start wheezing after 2 years. Early onset of severe frequent symptoms does appear to be a poorer prognostic sign for continuing asthma in adult life. Although boys have more severe asthma during childhood, girls do less well subsequently, with fewer improving during adolescence.[18,22,29] Atopy was not found to be a significant prognostic factor by Broder et al,[26] but atopy, particularly eczema in later childhood, was significant in studies by Jenkins et al,[18] Blair,[28] Martin et al,[30] and Kelly et al.[31] Sears and Burrows[32] showed atopy was an important predictor for persistence of airway responsiveness from 9 to 15 years of age.

Most longitudinal studies have demonstrated a decrease in airway responsiveness to various challenges with age. Gerritsen et al[33] found 83% of children but only 58% of adults with current asthma had increased responsiveness to histamine. It is not clear whether this decrease in responsiveness is a real change in the functional response of the airway or a change in dose and deposition of aerosol with growth. Irrespective of this, those with continuing symptoms remain more responsive than others of the same age,[34,35] and this responsiveness correlates with the presence of atopy manifested by positive skin allergen tests.[32]

Lung function remains abnormal in many children even following cessation of symptoms. Up to 20% will continue to have an abnormally low FEV_1 and more than 40% a reduced FEF_{25-75}.[34] Bronchial hyperresponsiveness is associated with a less satisfactory rate of growth of FEF_{25-75}. Roorda et al[29] noted that persisting abnormal lung function and increased airway hyperresponsiveness predicted a worse outcome. Weiss et al[36] found that young women had a greater decrease in lung function following childhood asthma.

An elevated total lung capacity has been documented[34,37] in adolescents who have had childhood asthma. This could not be correlated with degree of airway obstruction, and there was no physiologic evidence of tissue destruction or emphysema. It appeared to be a specific effect of the condition on lung growth and to some extent correlated with delayed puberty. By the time young adulthood was reached, these lung volumes had returned to the normal range (Table 62-2).

By 28 years of age, most of those with childhood asthma were demonstrating other forms of atopic disease. Of those who had severe asthma, 67% also had hayfever at 28 years compared with 25% of controls.[31] Most had positive skin test

Table 62-1 Asthma at 21 Years According to Clinical Pattern at 14 Years

		PATTERN AT 21 YEARS			
		CEASED	INFREQUENT EPISODIC ASTHMA	FREQUENT EPISODIC ASTHMA	CHRONIC ASTHMA
PATTERN AT 14 YEARS	INFREQUENT EPISODIC ASTHMA	54%	26%	15%	5%
	FREQUENT EPISODIC ASTHMA	20%	20%	35%	25%
	CHRONIC ASTHMA	5%	14%	26%	55%

Adapted from Martin AJ, McLennan LA, Landau LI, Phelan PD: *Br Med J* 280:1397-1400, 1980.

Table 62-2 Lung Function at 21 Years in Controls and Four Groups of Subjects Who Had Wheezed in Childhood

	CONTROL SUBJECTS	CEASED WHEEZING	INFREQUENT EPISODIC ASTHMA	FREQUENT EPISODIC ASTHMA	CHRONIC ASTHMA
FEV_1	100.5	99.0	96.8	92.4*	80.3*
(% predicted)	±12.4	±22.2	±13.0	±16.2	±27.8
FEF_{25-75}	102.0	98.9	91.5*	78.7*	61.6*
(% predicted)	±19.0	±25.3	±26.6	±25.8	±28.5
$\dot{V}max50$	101.2	103.7	97.2	75.7*	57.1*
(% predicted)	±29.2	±40.8	±32.9	±25.8	±34.5
TLC	100.7	99.1	99.5	102.4	105.1*
(% predicted)	±9.8	±16.1	±14.6	±12.5	±12.6
RV/TLC	101.5	101.3	106.4	117.7*	126.6*
(% predicted)	±22.1	±23.7	±25.0	±27.1	±34.3

*Statistically significant difference from controls.

responses to common allergens. Eosinophil counts decreased with age, but were still elevated in those with more severe symptoms.

Somatic growth was delayed between 10 and 14 years in those with severe asthma.[38,39] Growth retardation is associated with delayed puberty. Although it is more likely in those with severe asthma, it is also seen in some with severe atopy without troublesome asthma. Suggested mechanisms include reduced growth hormone, reduced thyroxine, hypoxia, decreased appetite, and increased energy demands. In spite of the growth retardation and delay in puberty during adolescence, almost all children with asthma reach predicted normal adult height.[22,39,40] Corticosteroids may contribute to growth retardation. However, corticosteroids administered to those with troublesome asthma may lead to improved growth as a result of control of the asthma. Inhaled corticosteroids have been demonstrated to have systemic effects on growth and bone metabolism, but their long-term effects have not yet been adequately documented. At present it appears that corticosteroids by any route given when they are not justified may cause growth retardation, but when given to those with troublesome asthma, they may contribute to normalization in growth.

Surveys of young adults following childhood asthma show that continued treatment in those with ongoing symptoms is often poor.[22] Many were not accepting that symptoms related to asthma were not being adequately treated and limiting their lifestyle. Roorda et al[29] found that only 19% of those with symptoms will have adequately supervised care.

Martin et al[30] could find no evidence that ongoing, consistent drug treatment resulted in a better prognosis, although the design of the study was not appropriate to make definite conclusions. VanEssen-Zandvleit et al[41] reported improvement in symptoms and bronchial responsiveness with long-term corticosteroids, but this improvement did not persist after cessation of those steroids. Johnstone[42] reported improved prognosis with hyposensitization in childhood, but this has not been confirmed by well-controlled double-blind trials. Smoking remains unacceptably high with approximately one third of young adults who had childhood asthma continuing to smoke.[22,29]

Martin et al[22] documented limitations of lifestyle in those with troublesome childhood asthma, but Ross et al[43] found that wheeze in childhood did not affect education, employment, or social class in a 25-year follow-up.

CONCLUSIONS

Asthma improves through adolescence, and many cease to have symptoms, but abnormalities of airway function and other manifestations of atopy often persist. It is not yet known whether these risks predispose to irreversible airway obstruction and chronic obstructive airway disease in later life. The ability to ensure a relatively normal lifestyle with appropriate treatment through childhood and the generally good prognosis of infrequent episodic asthma means that most childhood asthmatics reach adult life without continuing symptons or significant disability.

REFERENCES

Prevalence

1. Martinez FD, Wright AL, Taussig LM, Holberg CJ, Halonen M, Morgan WJ: Asthma and wheezing in the first six years of life, *N Engl J Med* 332:133-138, 1995.
2. Sporik R, Holgate ST, Cogswell JJ: Natural history of asthma in childhood—a birth cohort study, *Arch Dis Child* 66:1050-1053, 1991.
3. Burr ML, Butland BK, King S, Vaughan-Williams E:Changes in asthma prevalence: two surveys 15 years apart, *Arch Dis Child* 64:1452-1456, 1989.
4. Van Niekerk CH, Weinberg EG, Short SC, Heese H de V, Van Schalkulcy DJ: Prevalence of asthma: a comparison of urban and rural Xhosa children, *Clin Allergy* 9:319-324, 1979.
5. Waite DA, Eyles EF, Tonkin SL, Eyles EF, Tonkin SL, O'Donnell TV: Asthma prevalence in Tokolauan children in 2 environments, *Clin Allergy* 10:71-75, 1980.
6. Carman PG, Landau LI: Increased paediatric asthma admissions in Western Australia. Is it a problem of diagnosis? *Med J Aust* 152:23-26, 1980.
7. Ninan TK, Russell G: Respiratory symptoms and atopy in Aberdeen school children. Evidence from 2 surveys 25 years apart, *Br Med J* 304: 873-875, 1992.

Prognostic Factors

8. VanAsperen PP, Kemp AS: The natural history of IgE sensitisation and atopic disease in early childhood, *Acta Paediatr Scand* 78:239-245, 1989.
9. Sporik R, Holgate ST, Platts-Mills TAE, Cogswell JJ: Exposure to house dust mite allergen (Der p) and the development of asthma in childhood, *N Engl J Med* 323:502-507, 1990.
10. Halonen M, Stern D, Taussig LM, Wright A, Ray CG, Martinez FD: The predictive relationship between serum IgE levels at birth and subsequent incidences of lower respiratory illness and eczema in infants, *Am Rev Respir Dis* 146:866-870, 1992.
11. Peat JK, Salome CM, Woolcock AJ: Longitudinal changes in atopy during a 4 year period: relation to bronchial hyper-responsiveness and respiratory symptoms in a population sample of Australian school children, *J Allergy Clin Immunol* 85:65-74, 1990.
12. De Grooijer A, Brand PLP, Gerritsen J, Koeter GH, Postma DS, Knol K: Changes in respiratory symptoms and airway hyper-responsiveness after 27 years in a population based sample of school children, *Eur Respir J* 6:848-854, 1993.
13. Burrows B, Martinez FD, Halonen M, Barbee RA, Cline MG: Association of asthma with serum IgE levels and skin test reactivity to allergens, *N Engl J Med* 320:271-276, 1989.
14. Roorda RJ, Gerritsen J, Van Aalderen WMC, Schouten JP, Veltman JC, Weiss ST, Knol K: Follow up of asthma from childhood to adulthood, *J Allergy Clin Immunol* 93:575-584, 1994.
15. Anderson HR, Butland BK, Strachan DP: Trends in prevalence and severity of childhood asthma, *Br Med J* 308:1600-1604, 1994.
16. Kelly WJW, Hudson I, Phelan PD, Pain MCF, Olinsky A: Childhood asthma in adult life: a further study at 28 years of age, *Br Med J* 294: 1059-1062, 1987.
17. Oswald H, Phelan PD, Lanigan A, Hibbert M, Bowes G, Olinsky S: Outcome of childhood asthma in mid-adult life, *Br Med J* 309:95-96, 1994.
18. Jenkins MA, Hopper JL, Bowes E, Carlin JB, Flander LB, Giles GG: Factors in childhood as predictors of asthma to adult life, *Br Med J* 309: 90-93, 1994.
19. Williams HE, McNicol KN: Prevalence, natural history, and relationship of wheezy bronchitis and asthma in children: an epidemiological study, *Br Med J* 4:321-325, 1969.
20. McNicol KN, Williams HE: Spectrum of asthma in children. I. Clinical and physiological components, *Br Med J* 4:7-11, 1973.
21. McNicol KN, Williams HE: Spectrum of asthma in children. II. Allergic components, *Br Med J* 4:12-416, 1973.
22. Martin AJ, McLennan LA, Landau LI, Phelan PD: The natural history of childhood asthma to adult life, *Br Med J* 280:1397-1400, 1980.
23. Martin AJ, Landau LI, Phelan PD: Natural history of allergy in asthmatic children followed to adult life, *Med J Aust* 2:470-474, 1981.
24. Anderson HR, Bland JM, Patel S, Peckham C: The natural history of asthma in childhood, *J Epidemiol Community Health* 40:121-129, 1986.
25. Giles GG, Gibson HB, Lickiss N, Shaw K: Respiratory symptoms in Tasmanian adolescents: a follow-up of the 1961 birth cohort, *Aust NZ J Med* 14:631-637, 1984.
26. Broder I, Higgins MW, Mathews KP, Keller JB: Epidemiology of asthma and allergic rhinitis in a total community, Tecumseh, Michigan: IV natural history, *J Allergy Clin Immunol* 54:100-110, 1974.
27. Park ES, Golding J, Carswell F, Stewart-Brown S: Preschool wheezing and prognosis at 10, *Arch Dis Child* 61:642-646, 1986.
28. Blair H: Natural history of childhood asthma: 20 year follow-up, *Arch Dis Child* 52:613-619, 1977.
29. Roorda RJ, Gerritsen J, Van Aalderen WMC, Schouten JP, Veltman JC, Weiss ST, Knol K: Risk factors for the persistence of respiratory symptoms in childhood asthma, *Am Rev Respir Dis* 148:1490-1495, 1993.

30. Martin AJ, Landau LI, Phelan PD: Predicting the course of asthma in children, *Aust Paediatr J* 18:84-87, 1982.
31. Kelly WJW, Hudson I, Phelan PD, Pain MCF, Olinsky A: Atopy in subjects with asthma followed to the age of 28 years, *J Allergy Clin Immunol* 85:548-557, 1990.
32. Burrows B, Sears MR, Flannery ED, Herbison GP, Holdaway MD, Silva PA: Relation of the course of bronchial responsiveness from age 9 to age 15 to allergy, *Am J Respir Crit Care Med* 152:1302-1306, 1995.
33. Gerritsen J, Koeter GH, Postma DS, Schouten JP, Knol K: Prognosis of asthma from childhood to adulthood, *Am Rev Respir Dis* 140:1325-1330, 1989.
34. Martin AJ, Landau LI, Phelan PD: Lung function in young adults who had asthma in childhood, *Am Rev Respir Dis* 122:609-616, 1980.
35. Kelly WJW, Hudson I, Raven J, Phelan PD, Pain MCF, Olinsky A: Childhood asthma and adult lung function, *Am Rev Respir Dis* 138:26-30, 1988.
36. Weiss ST, Tosteson TD, Segal MR, Tager IB, Redline I, Speizer FE: Effects of asthma on pulmonary function in children, *Am Rev Respir Dis* 145:58-63, 1992.
37. Merkus PJFM, Van Essen-Zandvleit EEM, Kouwenberg JM, Duiverman EJ, Van Houlingen HG, Kerrïbijn KF, Quanjer PH: Large lungs after childhood asthma. A case control study, *Am Rev Respir Dis* 148:1484-1489, 1993.
38. Nassif E, Weinberger M, Sherman B, Brown K: Extrapulmonary effects of maintenance corticosteroid therapy with alternate-day prednisolone and inhaled beclomethasone in children with chronic asthma, *J Allergy Clin Immunol* 80:518-528, 1987.
39. Russell G: Asthma and growth, *Arch Dis Child* 69:695-698, 1993.
40. Balfour-Lynn L: Growth and childhood asthma, *Arch Dis Child* 61:1049-1055, 1986.
41. Van Essen-Zandvleit EE, Hughes MD, Waalkens HJ, Duiverman EJ, Kerrïbijn: Remission of childhood asthma after long-term treatment with an inhaled corticosteroid (budesonide): can it be achieved? *Eur Respir J* 7:63-68, 1994.
42. Johnstone DE: Some aspects of the natural history of asthma, *Ann Allergy* 49:257-264, 1982.
43. Ross S, Godden D, McMurray D, Douglas A, Oldman D, Friend J, Legge J, Douglas G: Social effects of wheeze in childhood: a 25 year follow-up, *Br Med J* 305:545-548, 1992.

CHAPTER 63

Clinical Presentation and Ongoing Clinical and Physiologic Assessment of Asthma in Children

Sandra D. Anderson and Craig M. Mellis

CLINICAL PRESENTATION AND CLINICAL ASSESSMENT OF ASTHMA

The major clinical decision in children with cough, wheeze, or difficulty breathing is whether or not the diagnosis is asthma (Box 63-1). The distinction between the mild end of the asthma spectrum and the child with simple recurrent viral bronchitis can be difficult.[1,2] Indeed, the clinical constellation of lower respiratory symptoms (cough, wheeze, and shortness of breath) is likely to be a continuum from persistent asthma, frequent episodic asthma, infrequent episodic asthma, recurrent viral bronchitis, through to normal. Clearly these clinical distinctions are arbitrary. The role of physiologic measures as an aid in this process and to eliminate the possibility of rare, more serious causes of cough, wheeze, and shortness of breath is discussed later in this chapter.

Persistent asthma should now be considered a chronic inflammatory disorder of the airways,[3,4] best managed with long-term disease modifying aerosol medications, such as cromoglycate or inhaled corticosteroids.[5,6] However, most children with asthma (75% of the total) have trivial asthma or mild, infrequent symptoms.[7-11] Fortunately, these children, with infrequent episodic (mild/trivial) asthma, require no treatment apart from occasional bronchodilators when symptomatic.[9,10] Thus an important clinical objective is to distinguish between the infrequent episodic and the more severe categories, which require long-term preventive therapy.

Similarities have been drawn between persistent asthma and other chronic inflammatory disease, especially arthritis. Indeed, asthma has been referred to as arthritis of the lung, and analogies have also been drawn between the assessment and management of asthma and arthritis,[12] in particular the arbitrary grading of severity of both asthma and rheumatoid arthritis (based on symptoms, physical findings, and investigations), which then dictates initial treatment.[9,10,13]

Assessing severity of asthma in the infant and preschool child is entirely clinical and includes a comprehensive history (from the parents) and physical examination because no standard lung function measurements are possible. When there is no doubt about the diagnosis, the only routine investigations that may be of value are a plain chest radiograph and allergen skin prick testing (to likely food or airborne allergens).[14-16] Clearly, however, other investigations may be warranted if clinical findings cast doubt on the provisional diagnosis of asthma. Rarer airway disorders (Box 63-2) such as cystic fibrosis, pulmonary aspiration, foreign body aspiration, and chronic suppuration may need to be ruled out by specific diagnostic tests. However, in the young patient with mild infrequent asthma or atypical asthma symptoms (especially those with predominantly cough), the major difficulty is distinguishing this from the child with simple recurrent acute viral bronchitis.

During the initial clinical assessment the primary objectives are to (1) confirm the diagnosis of asthma (see Box 63-1), (2) assign a clinical level of disease severity to enable rational initial management (Table 63-1), and (3) identify (on history) any trigger factors of exacerbations, particularly those that are potentially avoidable (Box 63-3). The major objectives of ongoing clinical assessments are (1) to ensure the disease is being optimally controlled, (2) to ensure that the child does not have any adverse effects from therapy, and (3) to observe whether those receiving aerosol therapy have satisfactory inhalation technique (see Box 63-1). Other ongoing management issues include assessing compliance with therapy, reviewing written action plans, observing technique for measuring peak flow, and continuing education of parents and children about asthma.

Key Questions in History Taking

In the very young the history will not be directly from the child but from a parent, usually the mother (Box 63-4). Because this is less than ideal, as soon as the child is old enough (from age 5 to 6 years onward), it is essential to obtain at least some of this information directly from the child.

The major information to gain from the history is whether symptoms are persistent or interval. This immediately allows differentiation between "episodic" and "persistent" (or chronic) asthma. Further inquiries about frequency of exacerbations, triggers, and severity of episodes should allow differentiation between "infrequent episodic" and "frequent episodic" asthma.[8]

Although no valid instrument is currently available for measuring quality of life in children with asthma, Christie et al[17] have identified major domains of this important measure (Box 63-5). It is clear from Box 63-5 that many of the features of asthma that concern children are nonmedical and could easily be overlooked by the physician and the parents. From the child's perspective, however, there is little doubt that these nonmedical aspects of childhood asthma are of critical importance. It seems likely that in the near future we will be able to measure quality of life in childhood asthma with valid age-specific instruments.[18] Thus improvement in the child's quality of life could become a major goal of asthma management and a major outcome measure in clinical research trials in childhood asthma.[19]

BOX 63-1
Clinical Assessment of Childhood Asthma

A. Initial assessment

1. Diagnosis
   Consider other possible explanations for the cough, wheeze, or breathing difficulties, especially in infants.
2. Assess severity
   Assign the most suitable category to describe disease severity to enable rational initial medical therapy.
3. Trigger factors
   Are there any identifiable triggers (and any available strategies to reduce or avoid these triggers)?

B. Ongoing assessment

1. Response to treatment
   Has there been an optimal response to initial therapy?
   (If not, question compliance and inhalation technique, and consider altering treatment.)
2. Compliance
   Inquire about compliance (and if suboptimal, identify barriers to compliance).
3. Continuing asthma education
   This should include both factual information on all aspects of asthma, and a thorough check of techniques with aerosol devices (and peak flow meters). Also ensure the written action plan is up-to-date, and well understood by parents (and child).

BOX 63-2
Conditions That Can Mimic Asthma

A. Predominant small airways obstruction

1. Pulmonary aspiration
   - During swallowing or secondary to gastroesophageal reflux
2. Chronic neonatal lung disease
3. Acute viral bronchiolitis
4. Cystic fibrosis

B. Predominant large airways obstruction

1. Foreign body inhalation/ingestion
   - Especially in toddlers
   - Airway vs. esophageal foreign bodies
   - Acute vs. retained foreign bodies
2. Congenital malformations of lungs/airways
   - Lung (e.g., congenital lobar emphysema, cystic malformations)
   - Airways (e.g., tracheomalacia/bronchomalacia, tracheal or bronchial stenosis)
3. Cardiac disease
   - Large left-to-right shunts (e.g., VSD)
   - Myocarditis/cardiomyopathy
4. Endobronchial tumors
   (Rare, e.g., bronchial adenoma, carcinoid; postinflammatory pseudotumor)
5. Extrabronchial obstruction
   - Enlarged hilar nodes (especially due to primary TB); medastinal cysts or tumors, vascular rings (especially double aortic arch)
6. Supraglottic obstruction
   - Tonsillar/adenoid hypertrophy (and possible obstructive sleep apnea)
   - Acute tonsillar enlargement (e.g., Epstein-Barr virus infection; Group A and hemolytic streptococcus)
   - Acute epiglottitis/supraglottitis (*Haemophilus influenzae*, type B)
7. Hysterical symptoms
   - Including psychogenic cough, fictitious asthma/laryngeal wheeze, hyperventilation syndrome

Table 63-1 Arbitrary Grading of the Severity of Childhood Asthma

CATEGORY (AND SYNONYM)	FREQUENCY AND SEVERITY OF EPISODES	INTERVAL SYMPTOMS	PERCENTAGE OF TOTAL CHILDHOOD ASTHMA
Infrequent episodic (mild/trivial asthma)	Not more than once every 4-6 weeks Usually mild episodes	Nil	75%
Frequent episodic (moderate asthma)	More than once every 4-6 weeks Can be severe episodes	X2-X3/week	20%
Persistent (severe/chronic asthma)	Wheeze (or cough) most days or nights Often severe episodes	Every day (or every night)	5%

BOX 63-3
Trigger Factors for Episodes (from History)

1. Respiratory viruses
2. Exercise
3. Inhaled
   i) Allergens
      House dust mite
      Grass pollen
      Animal dander
   ii) Nonallergens
      Dust
      Cigarette smoke
      Air pollution
4. Ingested
   Drugs (aspirin, β blockers)
   Nuts (especially peanuts)
   Food additives (especially metabisulfate)
5. Meteorologic
   Sudden weather changes (temperature and barometric pressure)
6. Emotional
   Laughter/overexcitement
   Family or peer conflict or other chronic stress (especially school/home)

BOX 63-4
Key Questions in History

A. Interval symptoms

1. Cough—day vs. night, dry vs. moist, persistent vs. episodic, triggers
2. Wheeze—day vs. night, on waking only, with exercise only, frequency and severity of wheeze (particularly, responsiveness to bronchodilator treatment)
3. Shortness of breath—difficulty breathing or chest "pain/tightness," only with exercise (light, medium, or heavy exercise), during the night, on waking in morning
4. Exercise tolerance/exercise induced asthma (EIA)—wheeze only with prolonged running vs. wheeze with normal activities; is the child "restricted" by EIA?
5. Frequency of bronchodilator use—preexercise or postexercise only; day vs. night

B. Frequency and severity of acute exacerbations (see Table 63-1)

1. More or less than every 4-6 weeks (on average)
2. Treatment required during exacerbations (frequency, of bronchodilators, duration of effect, need for oral corticosteroids) and duration of exacerbations (time to return to "normal" status)

C. "Hard" morbidity secondary to asthma

1. School absenteeism
2. Unscheduled doctor visits
3. Hospital A&E attendances
4. Hospitalization

D. Quality of life ("soft" morbidity) (see Box 63-5)

BOX 63-5
Domains of Quality of Life in Childhood Asthma

A. Medical factors

1. Interval asthma symptoms
2. Asthma episodes (frequency/severity) and trigger factors for episodes
3. Medication needs
4. "Hard" morbidity (see Box 63-4)

B. Nonmedical factors

1. Psychologic—including fears/anxieties about asthma, attitudes to asthma, and self-esteem
2. Home and social—including any limitation of social activities or inability to have pets at home; peer and family interaction
3. Educational—including school academic performance, school absenteeism, limitation of sports/games/physical activities, or excursions/camps

Modified from Christie MJ, French D, Weatherstone L, West A: *Psychotherapy and Psychosomatics* 56:197-203, 1991.

BOX 63-6
Key Information from the Clinical Examination

1. Growth and nutrition
   - Height and weight percentiles
   - Delayed puberty (especially in males)
2. Chest deformity
   - Hyperinflation/pectus carinatum
   - Harrison's sulcus
3. Auscultation
   - Crackles vs. wheeze; differential breath sounds/air entry
   - Generalized wheeze even when "well" between attacks
4. Clinical provocation of bronchoconstriction
   - Auscultation of chest before and after "cough" or "simple exercise"
5. Other atopic disease
   - Allergic rhinitis (perennial vs. seasonal)
   - Eczema (especially chronic flexural)
6. Other upper airway pathology
   - Clinical evidence of chronic paranasal sinusitis/tonsillar or adenoid hypertrophy
7. Any evidence of treatment side effects
   - Especially inhaled corticosteroids (local vs. systemic)
8. Any finger clubbing
   - Indicates a cause other than asthma for chest symptoms
9. Abnormal cardiovascular signs
   - Especially large left-to-right shunts (ASD, VSD) masquerading as asthma

From the history, any likely trigger factors for exacerbations should be identified (see Box 63-3), and this may be supported by specific allergen skin prick testing.[14-16] However, respiratory viruses are the major identifiable trigger and are extremely difficult to avoid or reduce.[20]

Key Information from the Clinical Examination

Physical examination should be comprehensive (Box 63-6) to ensure that the asthmalike symptoms are not due to another cause (see Box 63-2). Another major issue is whether there is physical evidence of chronic airflow obstruction, indicating persistent or chronic asthma. Namely, hyperinflation of the thoracic cage, lower rib retraction (Harrison's sulcus), diffuse wheeze on auscultation (when well), underweight, or growth retardation. Identification and appropriate management of other atopic disease, especially perennial upper airway allergic rhinitis, is mandatory because appropriate management of allergic rhinitis can substantially improve overall asthma control.[21,22] Nasal patency must be checked, and if not present, the cause determined.

A simple clinical or office-based bronchial provocation test can be useful even in very young children. Namely, the chest should be ausculated, and if clear, the child should be asked to cough forcefully several times, then the chest should be reexamined. The acute development of widespread expiratory wheezes indicates an abnormal degree of bronchial hyperresponsiveness, highly suggestive of asthma. An alternate test is to run the child "on the spot" or up and down a suitable corridor for several minutes, listening for the acute appearance of diffuse wheeze on auscultation. This can be particularly useful in the very young child who is unable to do any form of measured lung function. A positive response to these simple tests would strongly support the presence of underlying asthma; however, a negative test does not rule out asthma.

Assessing Asthma Severity

Three arbitrary grades of asthma severity can be used to describe most children with typical asthma (see Table 63-1).[7-9] Although various descriptive terms are used, there is a broad dichotomy between episodic (95% of all children with asthma) and persistent (5%) asthma. The latter category will have symptoms most days (and/or nights) of either cough or wheeze, and a history of needing frequent (usually at least once daily) bronchodilators for relief. Within the much more common episodic group, two arbitrary categories are described, depending on frequency and severity of the episodes as shown in Table 63-1.[8] These categories are infrequent episodic (75% of all children with asthma) and frequent episodic asthma (20%). Other terms used to describe these three categories of childhood asthma are *mild* (or *trivial*), *moderate,* and *severe,* corresponding to *infrequent episodic, frequent episodic,* and *persistent* (*chronic*), respectively.[7] Clearly, however, these categories are arbitrary and serve only as a guide to severity and initial management, including bronchodilators as required, regular cromoglycate, and regular inhaled cortico-steroids for categories with infrequent episodic, frequent episodic, and persistent, respectively.[7-9]

Despite these clinical descriptions, if in the past 12 months the child has had a severe, apparently life-threatening episode of asthma (e.g., needed intensive care; been unconscious, syncopal, or cyanotic; or had a respiratory arrest with an episode), then the child must be considered to have severe or persistent asthma and treated accordingly.

Clinical Presentation of Asthma

The many different clinical presentations of childhood asthma are listed in Box 63-7. Infants and young children often have atypical features—particularly cough only.[11,23] This cough may be either a chronic symptom, especially at night[24] or recurrent bouts of cough with "rattliness" of the chest (caused by excessive bronchial secretions).[11,25] Wheeze is either absent or a minor feature and often overlooked by the parents because the cough is usually very striking (persistent, irritating, and frustratingly unresponsive to medical therapy). However, the age group of greatest concern are infants, who are discussed in the next section.

Specific Age-Related Issues

The pediatric age group encompasses a very wide range of growth and development and there are many issues specific to certain age groups (Box 63-8). A principal concern is the extensive differential diagnosis of wheeze and cough in infants (see Box 63-2). Furthermore, many normal infants wheeze for "physiologic" reasons unique to this age group, specifically, relatively low numbers of small peripheral airways with consequent relatively high resistance to air flow and soft, floppy, medium, and large airways. Such wheeze is probably not related to asthma and generally disappears by age 12 months.[26] In children between 1 and 5 years (preschool/toddler age group), common, atypical forms of asthma are "recurrent bronchitis" and "recurrent pneumonia" caused by hypersecretory asthma. This form of asthma is often complicated by persistent or recurrent atelectasis (especially of the right middle lobe).[11,27] In the adolescent, hysterical symptoms that can mimic all aspects of asthma must be considered. These include hysterical cough,[28] laryngeal wheeze,[29] and the hyperventilation syndrome.[30] In the adolescent with a long history of troublesome asthma, delayed puberty and delayed growth spurt are

BOX 63-7
Clinical Presentations of Asthma in Children

1. Classical episodic asthma
   Usual presentation; typical episodes of cough, wheeze, shortness of breath—well in the interval between episodes (see Table 63-1)
2. Persistent asthma
   Constant, daily (or every night) symptoms, plus acute exacerbations (often severe) (see Table 63-1)
3. Cough only
   Especially persistent, dry night cough
4. Recurrent cough/bronchitis
   "Hypersecretory" asthma; prolonged bouts of cough and/or "rattliness" in chest after respiratory viruses; common in infants and preschoolers
5. Recurrent "pneumonia"
   Persistent/recurrent atelectasis (especially right middle lobe); common in preschoolers; considerable overlap with number 4 (above).
6. Exercise-induced asthma
   Wheeze or cough during or immediately after exercise only, few other symptoms
7. Severe episodic asthma
   Infrequent but "explosive" episodes, which are often extremely severe and life-threatening—surprisingly well in the interval between episodes
8. Persistent infant wheeze
   Usually without respiratory distress or other morbidity (e.g., troublesome cough or disturbed sleep); in many cases the wheeze probably not due to asthma ("physiologic" wheeze); also known as Fat Happy Wheezer, Transient Infant Wheeze, and Transient Early Wheeze

BOX 63-8
Key Issues Specific to Age Groups

1. Infants (age 0-1 yr)
   - Complete extensive differential diagnosis.
   - Exclude congenital malformations (airways, lungs, mediastinum, and cardiovascular).
   - Consider "physiologic" wheeze (nonasthma).
2. Toddlers/preschoolers (age 1-5 yrs)
   - High proportion have atypical presentation (especially chronic and recurrent cough).
   - Exclude inhaled/ingested foreign body.
   - Difficult to differentiate atypical asthma from recurrent viral bronchitis.
   - Viruses are major trigger factor.
3. School age
   a) Dependent (age 5-10 yr)
      - Consider impact of asthma on school performance.
      - Look for problems with exercise.
      - Allergic and viral triggers are seen.
   b) Independent (age 10-14 yr)
      - Expect poor compliance, risk-taking, cigarette smoking.
      - Consider endobronchial tumors and possible hysterical symptoms.
      - Allergic triggers are seen.

common, especially in boys.[31] Counseling and repeated reassurances that ultimate height will be as per predicted from parental heights is crucial.[32] Poor compliance, denial of disease, and risk-taking behavior are other potential problems in this difficult age group.[33]

THE ROLE OF PEAK FLOW METERS IN CHILDHOOD ASTHMA

Asthma is characterized by variable airflow obstruction, and unfortunately the child's perception of this obstruction is often poor.[34] Therefore airway caliber should be measured regularly, ideally in the subject's own home. Peak flow (PF) meters are a simple and inexpensive method of accomplishing such measurements.[35] In theory, then it could be argued that all children with asthma should have a PF meter and furthermore that they should measure their PF regularly. However, in practice their role is limited.[36] Although home monitoring of PF can be highly advantageous in selected patients, there are major limitations to their widespread use (Box 63-9).

More than 75% of children with asthma have trivial or mild episodic asthma, and it would be inappropriate to inflict the burden of regular PF measurements (which would be always virtually normal) on such children. Very few children under the age of 4 to 5 years are capable of reproducible PF readings, and this nonrepeatability is worse at times of airflow obstruction or respiratory symptoms. PF recordings are highly effort dependent, and because there is no visual display to indicate adequacy of effort, it is extremely difficult for parents (and physicians) to differentiate poor effort from genuine airflow obstruction. Some children can produce artificially high or low readings by using trick maneuvers such as coughing or partially adducting their vocal cords, resulting in potentially gross misinterpretation of the true airway status. PF is an insensitive measure that mainly reflects the caliber of the large central airways, especially the trachea.[37] Thus a "normal" value does not rule out significant small airway narrowing—the usual site of persistent obstruction in asthma.[38] As well as these limitations, compliance with regular PF measurements is generally poor.[39]

Therefore, in practice, only a small minority of children with asthma should be asked to monitor PF regularly,[40] namely those over the age of 5 to 6 years with unstable, severe chronic asthma, and particularly those with frequent and/or severe exacerbations and/or those who are poor perceivers of airflow obstruction during their exacerbations. However, intermittent use—say twice daily for 2 to 3 weeks—can be of considerable value in many clinical situations (discussed under Applications of PF Monitoring).

BOX 63-9
The Advantages and Disadvantages of PF Monitoring

A. Advantages

1. Permits early detection and treatment of acute exacerbations
2. Provides objective evidence for diagnosis of asthma
3. Identifies trigger factors
4. Monitors response to therapy (and changes in therapy)
5. Improves the child's perception of asthma/airflow obstruction

B. Disadvantages

1. Age (generally not reproducible under 4-5 years)
2. Highly effort dependent (and high inherent variability)
3. Predominantly reflects caliber of large airways rather than small ones therefore insensitive
4. Wide range in predicted normal values
5. Measurement is an additional burden on child/family
6. Generally poor compliance
7. Possibility of fictitious results, which may be deliberate

The Technique for Measuring Peak Flow

The technique for measuring PF has great potential for error. Thus it is mandatory to give both child and parents explicit instructions (including written instructions) on the correct use of PF meters. The child must be taken through the following steps by both demonstration and then participation.

1. With the child standing, reset the indicator to zero and ask the child to hold the meter horizontal, taking care to ensure that the fingers do not obstruct the indicator.
2. Have the child take a maximal inhalation to total lung capacity (but not via the PF meter).
3. Immediately place his or her lips tightly around the mouthpiece to ensure no leakage.
4. Instruct the child to blow out as hard and as fast as possible. Because it is only the instant of maximal flow that is being recorded, there is no need for the child to exhale fully (to residual volume). Therefore the technique is far easier than spirometry.

The physician, nurse, or laboratory technician should demonstrate the technique several times before asking the child to use the PF meter.

The importance of repeatability of performance must be stressed so that the child and parents understand that before recording a PF in a diary, the procedure is repeated at least 3 times. The best (maximal) value should be noted. Unfortunately, however, some children may need up to six blows to reach their maximum value.[41] If numerous blows are required each time PF is recorded, it becomes too tedious for the child and compliance will be poor.

Interpreting the Results of Peak Flow

1. Comparing PF with predicted normal: There is a very wide range of predicted normal values according to the child's sex and height. Although this limits the value of PF as a standard measure of normality of lung function, it does not limit its value as a measure of change over time in a given individual.
2. Comparing PF to "personal best" (PB): For the child who is to undertake home PF monitoring, it is essential to establish the PB. After several days practice the target (or PB) should be established, and all subsequent measures compared with this (as a percentage of PB). With linear growth and better asthma control, this PB will progressively increase. Occasional outlying high values should be discarded because these usually represent flow transients from coughing into the PF meter. If the values are less than 80% of the child's PB, a bronchodilator aerosol should be given and the PF recorded 5 to 10 minutes later. Both the prebronchodilator and postbronchodilator values should be recorded.
3. Establishing diurnal variability: To measure diurnal variation of PF, the measures must be done at the same time each morning and evening. There is a normal circadian (24-hour period) rhythm of PF, it being higher during the day than

at night. Although there are a number of methods of analyzing PF recordings, the best discriminating index between asthma and normality is called "amplitude % mean."[42] This is calculated by the following formula:

$$= \frac{\text{Highest PF} - \text{Lowest PF}}{\text{Mean PF}} \times 100 \quad (1)$$

A simpler method is the ratio of maximum to minimum PF, expressed as a percentage.[43] The arbitrary values for "normal" PF diurnal variability are 15% to 20% for adults (over 15 years) and 25% to 30% for children (age 6 to 14 years).[43] However, because PF has a continuous distribution, the arbitrary nature of these cutoffs should be recognized.

Clinical Applications of Peak Flow Monitoring

For Diagnostic Purposes

Confirming a clinical suspicion of asthma is possible with PF monitoring (Box 63-10). Simply showing an abnormally high level (over 25% to 30%) of diurnal variability supplies strong objective evidence to support a diagnosis of asthma in children with atypical symptoms of asthma (e.g., recurrent or persistent cough). An adequate duration of monitoring is 2 to 3 weeks, with measurements taken morning and evening throughout. There is an imperfect but significant correlation between diurnal variability of PF and measured bronchial hyperresponsiveness.[44] Other diagnostic uses of PF monitoring include measuring prebronchodilator and postbronchodilator PF at home over several weeks to establish whether there is acute bronchodilator responsiveness (>15% increase), and therefore a very high likelihood of underlying asthma. Measuring PF before and after vigorous exercise and demonstrating a significant (>15%) decrease in PF adds strong objective evidence to support a diagnosis of asthma. This is particularly useful in children with atypical exercise-induced asthma (e.g., cough only or chest discomfort or "pain") rather than wheeze, or inappropriate shortness of breath.

Similarly, suspected asthma trigger factors can be evaluated objectively in the child's own environment. Such measurements can be just as valuable in excluding possible triggers (e.g., suspected food allergies) as well as identifying genuine triggers (e.g., contact with domestic pets).

BOX 63-10

Clinical Application of PF Monitoring

A. Diagnostic uses (for 2-3 weeks, AM and PM)

Children aged >4-5 years and reliable/repeatable
- To measure airway response to bronchodilators
- To monitor diurnal variation
- To document the effect of triggers (e.g., viral URTI, allergens)
- To quantify effect of exercise (to detect EIA)

B. Monitoring progress

1. Continuously (AM and PM)
   Limited application
   - Age >4-5 years and
   - Reliable PF technique and
   - Poor patient perception of airflow obstruction and
   - Severe, persistent asthma or
   - Unstable asthma (e.g., frequent severe exacerbation)
2. Intermittently (for 2-3 weeks, AM and PM)
   Children aged >4-5 years and reliable PF technique
   - At times of major treatment changes
   - To validate "asymptomatic" child is well controlled
   - During viral URTIs or other asthma-likely triggers

Monitoring Asthma Control

Occasional periods of 2 to 3 weeks of PF monitoring (twice daily) can be useful to ensure the asymptomatic child on regular prophylaxis has normal (or near-normal) diurnal variation of PF, which indicates good asthma control. This is particularly relevant when substantial changes are being made to the child's treatment regimen (e.g., reducing the dosage of inhaled corticosteroids or switching from inhaled corticosteroids to cromoglycate).

More prolonged periods of PF monitoring are justified in those children (aged >5 years) whose asthma is unstable and severe, especially if the child has poor perception of airflow obstruction. Regular measurement of PF can assist some children to appreciate their airway function better, and in this case, the PF meter acts as a training device.[45]

Not surprisingly, many parents have a poor perception of the extent of their child's airflow limitation, and therefore PF monitoring can be invaluable for enabling parents to detect impending severe exacerbations. Unfortunately, however, there appears to be minimal "training effect" in terms of parents improving their ability to detect airflow limitation in their children following a period of PF monitoring.[34]

Self-Management (Action/Crisis) Plans

A logical use of PF monitoring is to establish an objective stepwise plan of action for early detection (and treatment) of exacerbations.[46] These plans are generally based on three color zones for simplicity.[13] The "green" zone is when PF is within 80% of PB, and no additional treatment is indicated. "Amber" zone indicates caution, when PF is between 50% and 75% of PB. Treatment is stepped up by adding regular bronchodilators and either increasing the dosage of inhaled corticosteroids or commencing oral corticosteroids. "Red" signals a crisis and is indicated by PF below 50% of PB. If this persists despite bronchodilators, immediate medical attention (preferably in a hospital emergency setting) is indicated.

Parents generally find PF monitoring useful for assessing the severity of acute exacerbations.[47] However, a randomized trial in children and adults found symptom-based action plans were as effective as PF-based in reducing morbidity.[48]

Accuracy of Peak Flow Meters

The currently available, mass produced, and relatively inexpensive PF meters have reasonable accuracy. A study of eight common brands of these devices, using a standardized flow generator, found all were highly repeatable to within the limits of accuracy of reading the indicator by eye.[49] Unfortunately most of the devices overestimated flow in the mid to high range (300 to 500 L/min).

SPIROMETRY AND FLOW RATES

The measurement of spirometry and the recording of an artifact-free flow-volume curve for permanent record is the single most valuable test to perform on the asthmatic child. A record of flow volume before and after a bronchodilator or a bronchoconstricting agent, can be useful to confirm the presence of airflow limitation, its acute reversibility, and bronchial

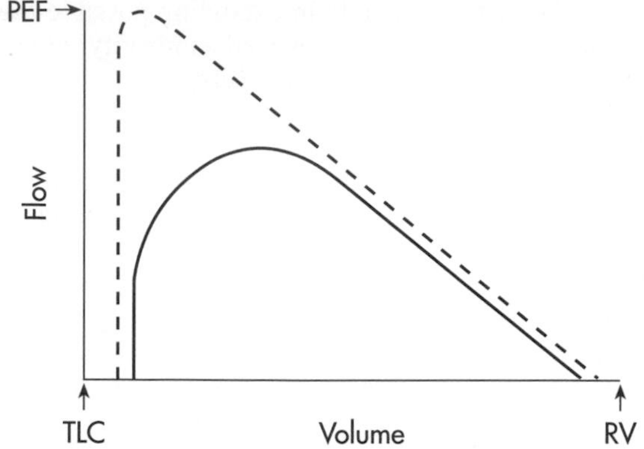

Fig. 63-1. *Dashed curve* illustrates the normal shaped flow-volume curve with a sharp rise to peak flow and a progressive fall in flow rates throughout the vital capacity until residual volume is reached. *Unbroken curve* shows poor effort at the beginning of the forced maneuver and therefore a fictitiously low peak flow, but flow rates in the mid and low portion of the vital capacity are normal.

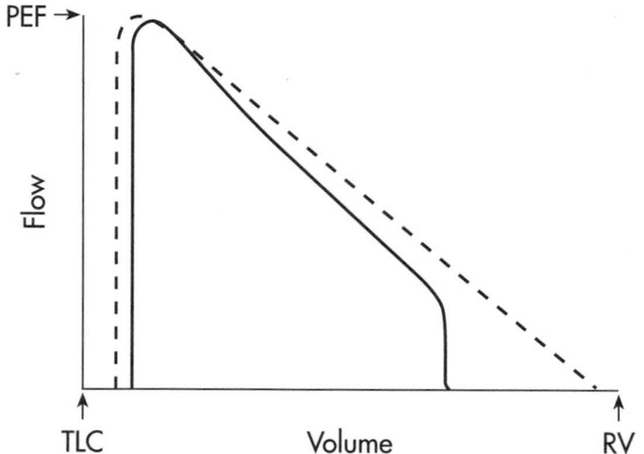

Fig. 63-2. *Dashed curve* illustrates the normal shaped flow volume curve with a sharp rise to peak flow and a progressive fall in flow rates throughout the vital capacity until residual volume is reached. *Unbroken curve* shows the typical shape of a child who takes a good inspiratory volume, makes a good forced expiration in the initial phases of the vital capacity, but does not prolong the effort to residual volume; there is a sudden drop in flow rate to zero.

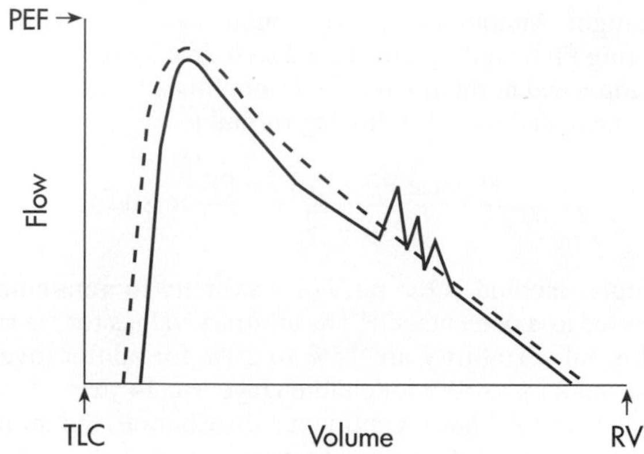

Fig. 63-3. *Dashed curve* illustrates the normal shaped flow-volume curve with a sharp rise to peak flow and a steady drop in flow rates until residual volume is reached. *Unbroken curve* is the typical picture of a child coughing during performance of the flow-volume maneuver.

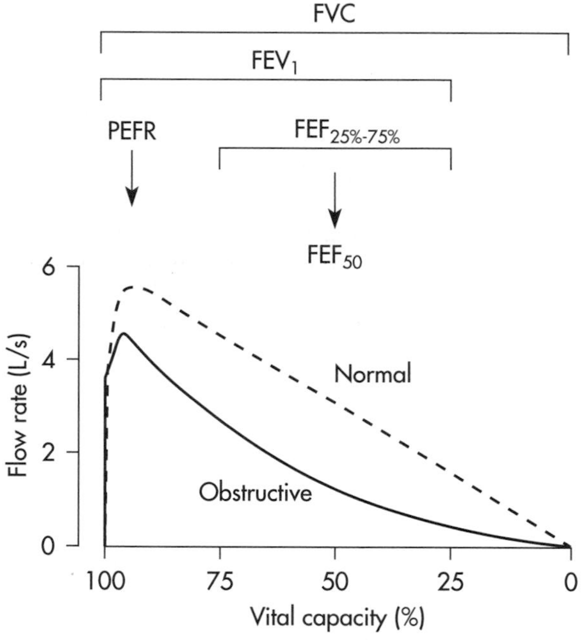

Fig. 63-4. Expiratory flow rate in relation to vital capacity in a normal subject and one with obstructive lung disease. The peak expiratory flow rate represents only the peak of the flow. The FEV_1 encompasses about 90% of the flow-volume curve. The flow rates through the middle portion of the vital capacity are shown as $FEF_{25\text{-}75}$.

hyperresponsiveness. Because these tests of flow and volume may be measured on many occasions over months or years, it is essential that the reproducibility of the test on each occasion is good. The best test will be performed with willing parents, cooperative children, and experienced laboratory personnel.

The aim of spirometry is to obtain the highest flow rate possible and to obtain the greatest emptying of the lungs in the shortest possible time.[50] The accurate documentation of a flow-volume or time-volume curve is obtained only if the forced expiratory maneuver to residual volume follows a maximal inspiration to total lung capacity and no leaks occur during expiration. These tests are entirely effort dependent. The recording of flow and volume or time and volume instantaneously and simultaneously allows the operator to judge whether a maximum effort has been made on inspiration and expiration. A permanent recording for filing is advisable for comparison with future tests after treatment. Examples of flow-volumes curves obtained at different levels of effort are illustrated in Figs. 63-1 to 63-3.

The flow-volume curve includes the measurement of peak flow so that home monitored values can be compared with those in the laboratory. However, the PF is often lower when performed during spirometry. Because the PF represents only one point on the curve and usually occurs within the first 200 ms, other indexes such as the forced expiratory volume in one second (FEV_1), forced vital capacity (FVC), and forced expiratory flow through the midportion of the FVC ($FEF_{25\text{-}75}$) are more informative. The FVC encompasses the entire flow-volume history, whereas the FEV_1 usually represents 90% of the curve in a normal subject (Fig. 63-4). The $FEF_{25\text{-}75}$, also known as the maximum midexpiratory flow (MMEF, or $V_{25\text{-}75}$), is sensitive to small changes in airway caliber and provides useful additional information. When a value for total lung capacity (TLC) is available, the flow can be related to this volume. The reproducibility of the FVC and FEV_1 is better than $FEF_{25\text{-}75}$, with a coefficient of variation being approximately 5%, 5%, and 8%, respectively.[51] The normal predicted values for $FEF_{25\text{-}75}$ are

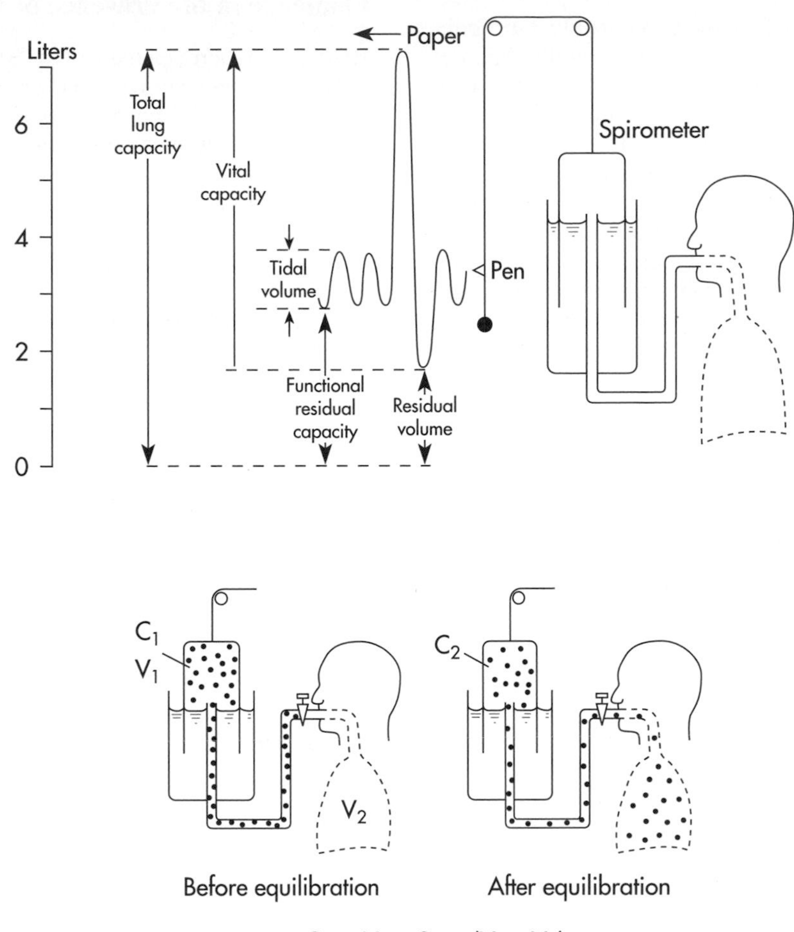

Fig. 63-5. Reproduced with permission from West JB: *Respiratory physiology—the essentials,* Baltimore, 1974, Williams & Wilkins.[54]

also more variable compared with FVC and FEV_1. The $FEF_{25\text{-}75}$ is usually taken from the best vital capacity measurement. Measurement of PF is commonly used for measuring responses to exercise, and the changes in PF correlate well with the changes in FEV_1 and $FEF_{25\text{-}75}$ after exercise in children.[52] A change of 10% in FEV_1 or PF is equivalent to a change of about 30% in $FEF_{25\text{-}75}$. In asthmatics, repeated measurements occasionally provoke a reduction in flow and volume, and this is an indication of hyperresponsive airways. By contrast others will improve their flow and volume with repeated blows.

Lung function correlates well with height, so it is essential that height is measured at regular intervals and that the predicted values used are appropriate for the healthy population being studied and the ethnic origin of the subject.[53]

TOTAL LUNG CAPACITY AND FUNCTIONAL RESIDUAL CAPACITY

Functional residual capacity (FRC) is the volume of gas present in the airways at the end of tidal respiration and can be measured to within 50 ml. Its accurate measurement is important as most other values for lung capacity are derived from it. For example, the TLC is the summation of the measured inspiratory capacity and FRC. The measurement of FRC (using helium dilution or thoracic gas volume in a whole body plethysmograph) can be useful in an asthmatic child, provided he or she is able to perform the tests properly. A measurement of these volumes determines whether the child has hyperinflation of the lungs, that is, increase in TLC or FRC. An increase in these volumes is a consequence of airway narrowing and can occur over minutes (as with exercise) or weeks (following an infection). This hyperinflation is protective because the increase in volume provides greater traction for the airways, and thus they are restrained from narrowing further. As lung volume increases, the resistance to flow in the airways falls, thus the mechanism of hyperinflation is known as nature's bronchodilator. Chronic or repeated hyperinflation in childhood leads to a chest wall deformity (pectus carinatum). Attaining good lung function in asthma is achieving a normal TLC and FRC as well as a normal FEV_1.

The body plethysmography provides a rapid technique for measuring thoracic gas volume (FRC plus the panting volume) and has the advantage that airways resistance can be measured at the same time, thus allowing correction of resistance for volume (specific airways resistance and specific conductance). However, measurements of volume and resistance require the child to sit in an enclosed box with a volume of 450 to 650 L and to pant gently against a closed shutter with an open glottis. Thus acquisition of this information requires some considerable level of cooperation and intelligence on the part of the child and skill by the operator. For this reason the closed circuit helium dilution method for measuring FRC remains popular, and TLC can be determined simply by measuring inspiratory capacity at the same time and adding this value to the FRC (Fig. 63-5).[54] In severe airflow limitation, equilibration of helium may take longer than the usual time as there will be uneven distribution of ventilation within the lung. Usually only 3 to 5 minutes of steady-state rebreathing is required for equilibration of helium in children. During this time the initial concentration of helium (C_1) in the known volume (V_1) is reduced by the unknown volume (V_2), the FRC, and the value for the FRC can be calculated (see Fig. 63-5).[54] The carbon dioxide produced is absorbed from the system and oxygen added in order to maintain the original volume. This technique for measuring FRC gives a value for the volume of the lungs, which is communicating freely with the ambient air and thus taking part in gas exchange. By contrast the volume measured by the whole body plethysmograph technique includes all air in the thorax including that trapped in bullae or in the stomach.

BRONCHIAL RESPONSIVENESS IN THE ASTHMATIC CHILD

After measurements of spirometry and lung volumes and skin tests for allergy, a physician may choose to carry out a measurement of BR. There has been considerable debate as to the diagnostic value of a measurement of BR in the child suspected of having asthma or its value in assessing response to treatment. Many pediatricians argue that diagnosis and treatment of asthma can be based on history and symptoms alone. Further, it would be impossible to have every child suspected of having asthma referred to a laboratory for assessment of BR. For physicians who do choose to have BR measured, the protocols for a variety of challenge tests and their advantages and disadvantages are given below. These protocols include the so-called direct challenge tests, such as pharmacologic challenges by which the administered substance, usually histamine or methacholine, has a specific receptor-mediated action on bronchial smooth muscle, causing it to contract. They also cover the indirect challenges, including exercise, hyperventilation, hypertonic saline, and distilled water, which stimulate release of endogenous substances that cause the airways to narrow. These endogenous substances are present as a result of airway inflammation. Thus the severity of the airway response to indirect challenges is thought to provide indirect evidence that inflammation is present.

DIRECT OR PHARMACOLOGIC CHALLENGES: HISTAMINE OR METHACHOLINE

Argument continues as to whether there are benefits in performing direct challenge tests with histamine or methacholine to identify asthma in children. One epidemiologic study reported that 48% of children with diagnosed asthma and 42% of those with a diagnosis and symptoms of asthma did not have hyperresponsiveness to histamine,[55] and other studies have made similar findings.[56,57] This has led some investigators to conclude that symptoms and BR are independent.[58,59] Another argument is that challenge with pharmacologic agents is unable to distinguish between chronic obstructive lung disease and asthma.[60,61]

Measuring severity of BR to histamine and methacholine does not help in choosing the appropriate medication or its dose. Some of these problems occur because poor lung function is associated with BR to these agents and paradoxically BR can be present for years after lung function has returned to normal. There are other difficulties with these challenge tests and these relate to accuracy in measuring the delivered dose of aerosol and defining the cutoff dose for abnormality.

Challenge in the Presence of Airflow Limitation

Bronchial hyperresponsiveness (BHR) to histamine or methacholine has been shown to be associated with low FEV_1:vital capacity ratios.[56,62] For this reason a challenge test performed when lung function is poor is unlikely to provide useful information. When lung function is poor it is better to have the child's response to a bronchodilator measured. A positive response to a bronchodilator is considered as a 15% or more rise in FEV_1 and demonstrates BHR.

To exclude airway caliber as a contributing factor to BHR, a challenge should be performed only when lung function is normal or at its best. A challenge 7 to 14 days after starting treatment with aerosol steroids is appropriate because airway edema will be reduced by steroids, and lung function is likely to be close to its usual value by this time. Under these conditions airway narrowing to a pharmacologic agent is more likely to reflect true hyperresponsiveness of the bronchial smooth muscle in the absence of the amplifying effect of edema.

Because recent viral and upper respiratory tract infections and exposure to allergens or irritants can alter airway caliber, at least 4 weeks should elapse before measurements of BR are made following these events.[63] It is also important that the child is not symptomatic at the time of study.

Challenge When There Is No Airflow Limitation

It is well known that improvement in lung function and symptoms precede by months, and often years, the resolution of BHR to histamine or methacholine, even though some reduction in BHR usually occurs within weeks.[64,65] Steinbrugger et al[66] recently reported that, in a group of 128 pediatric and adolescent asthma patients, all but 5 had a positive response to histamine, even though they had been symptom free for 18 months and medication free for 12 months. Airway narrowing was present in 52 of the children, provoked by the inhalation of cold air for 4 minutes, and there was only a poor relationship between responses to histamine and cold air ($r = 0.54$). Similarly Wilson et al[67] found 14 of 15 children symptom and medication free for 3 months, with a positive response to methacholine, but only 5 of the 15 had a positive response to hypertonic saline.

Studies in random populations of children have shown histamine and methacholine to have a low specificity (<50%) and in some studies a low sensitivity for detecting clinically recognized asthma.[55-57,68] Thus many children demonstrate BHR to histamine or methacholine in the absence of either symptoms or a history of asthma. In this regard, a challenge with histamine or methacholine may not be superior to exercise or other indirect challenges in the field in identifying currently active asthma.[57,69,70] It would seem wise, however, to inform subjects with BHR to pharmacologic agents, particularly those teenagers who are atopic, that they may be at risk of subsequently getting asthma. A positive response to a pharmacologic challenge could be an indication of asthma in the past or it could be predictive for asthma.[71]

By contrast, negative responses to histamine or methacholine may occur in children positive to indirect challenges such as exercise and cold air. A recent epidemiologic field study found that 15% of children negative to histamine were positive to exercise challenge,[72] confirming similar observations made earlier.[73,74] If it is accepted that responses to exercise and cold air are consistent with asthma,[63] then the widely held opinion that the sensitivity and the negative predictive value of these pharmacologic challenges for identifying BHR is high, is in question. There is now sufficient evidence from studies using both a direct and indirect challenge to suggest that it would be useful to perform both to exclude BHR.

Dose of Agent

It is impossible to measure accurately the delivered dose of a provoking agent to any child, particularly when a face mask is used or in small children and infants.[75] Provided that breathing is by mouth and air is entrained while inhaling the test aerosol, the delivered dose can be used as an estimate of the inhaled dose. The dose will be lower if inhalation occurs by nose. Children over the age of 1 year will normally entrain air so that the whole dose is inhaled.[75] Peat et al[76] recently recommended adjusting airway hyperresponsiveness, as measured by PD_{20} and response:dose ratio, for lung size and airway calibre for estimating prevalence in epidemiologic studies.

What Constitutes Abnormal Responsiveness to Histamine or Methacholine

The arbitrary nature of the choice of dose defined for abnormality and the large "gray area" is considered by some to render the measurement of borderline BHR using pharmacologic agents as uninterpretable. This attitude is understandable if there is difficulty in measuring accurately the dose because dose defines abnormality. A positive test result is taken if the provoking dose required to induce a 20% decrease in $FEV_1(PD_{20})$ is less than 3.6 micromols using the Yan technique,[77] although some investigators use a cutoff point of less than 8.0 micromols. For the Cockcroft technique[78] a positive response is taken if the provoking concentration to induce a 20% decrease in FEV_1 occurs at less than 16 mg/ml (PC_{20}). A PD_{20} of 8 micromols is approximately equivalent to a PC_{20} of 16 mg/ml and a PD_{20} of 4 micromols to a PC_{20} of 8 mg/ml. For the technique of Chai[79] a PC_{20} of up to 32 mg/ml is considered positive. These values are those used to define abnormality in adults. It has been suggested that these values should be corrected for size or age in children.[76] However, for short-term studies, when a child is his or her own control, it is unnecessary to apply a correction to the PD_{20} or PC_{20} to account for size.[76]

Reproducibility of Bronchial Hyperresponsiveness

Challenge testing using pharmacologic challenges has also been criticized because BHR may not be recorded on all occasions in children with symptoms of asthma. However, variability in BR between occasions may itself be diagnostic of asthma.[58] The lack of association between exacerbations of asthma and increase in BHR for some individuals[58] may be explained, in part, by changes in their baseline lung function. When lung function is low because of an exacerbation of asthma, BHR may be paradoxically reduced because the airways are maximally narrowed.[80] In this situation measuring responsiveness to a bronchodilator is preferable to using a bronchoconstricting agent.

Although many of the shortcomings of using histamine or methacholine as the provocative agents can be overcome, it may be preferable to choose an indirect challenge test as an alternative.

INDIRECT CHALLENGES

Indirect challenge tests include exercise, hyperventilation, and the inhalation of nonisotonic aerosols such as hypertonic saline or distilled water. A compelling argument for using an indirect challenge test is that a positive response indicates that the child's asthma is active and an attack can be provoked by a common stimulus such as exercise or inhalation of cold air. Further, the type and dose of therapy or a reduction in therapy can be determined by measuring responsiveness to an indirect challenge before and after acute and chronic treatment. With adequate treatment BR to indirect challenges diminishes to normal so that a child will no longer have an attack of asthma provoked by exercise.

Exercise and Hyperventilation

Exercise testing in asthmatic children became popular in the 1970s after the description by Jones et al[81] that vigorous exercise provoked an attack of asthma. Godfrey et al[82] identified many of the factors that determined the severity of the airway narrowing provoked by exercise in asthmatic children, including nature, intensity, and duration of exercise. The physiologic responses to exercise were also described at that time, and it was shown that hyperinflation and hypoxemia were associated with airway narrowing.[83-85] Later it was found that exercise itself was not necessary for the asthmatic response, and it was the rate of ventilation reached and the time for which this rate was sustained that determined the severity of EIA.[86] This observation led to the use of voluntary eucapnic hyperventilation with 5% CO_2 as a challenge test for EIA.[87] Water and heat content of the inspired air were identified as important determinants of the response to hyper-pnea.[88-92] The drier the air the greater the rate of water loss by evaporation, and the greater the asthmatic response. It has been proposed that the stimulus whereby hyperpnea with dry air provokes airway narrowing is the osmotic[91,93] and the thermal effects[94,95] resulting from water lost in bringing large volumes of air to alveolar conditions of water and temperature in a short time. The identification of these important factors determining the severity of the airway response to hyperpnea allowed the standardization of protocols for exercise and hyperventilation. Dry air hyperpnea at 60% to 75% of the maximum voluntary ventilation rate for 4 to 8 minutes has become the standard stimulus for identifying patients with exercise-induced attacks of asthma in the pulmonary function laboratory.[63]

The advantages of using hyperpnea as the stimulus for detecting BHR are many. The stimulus is natural and encountered daily by physically active children. There is no relationship between baseline lung function and response to exercise.[96] Hyperpnea with dry air has the advantage of provoking cough as well as airway narrowing. If a child has a cough, it is possible to ascertain, using hyperpnea as a stimulus, whether this is or is not accompanied by airway narrowing.[97] Although cough and bronchoconstriction provoked by dry air hyperpnea probably share a common mechanism, bronchoconstriction occurs only in a child who has asthma.

In terms of the dose of the stimulus, the protocols designed for exercise and hyperventilation have attempted to maximize the airway response by optimizing the conditions for hyperpnea. Although some children will find maximum effort difficult, most do not. In those children, in whom the diagnosis is in doubt, a hyperventilation challenge using progressively increasing levels of ventilation rate (30%, 60%, and 90% of

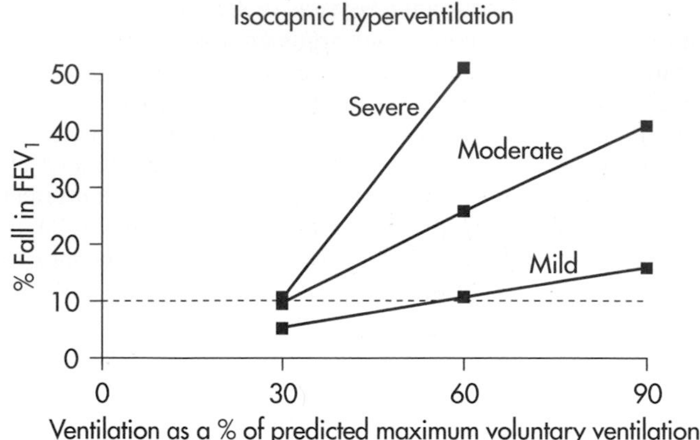

Fig. 63-6. Percent decline in forced expiratory volume (FEV_1) in three subjects who performed hyperventilation with dry air containing 4.9% carbon dioxide at different ventilation levels. The ventilation level is expressed as a percentage of the predicted maximum voluntary ventilation (FEV_1 x 35). The technique is described in detail in Phillips YY, Jaeger JJ, Laube BL, Rosenthal RR: *Am Rev Respir Dis* 131:31-35, 1985.

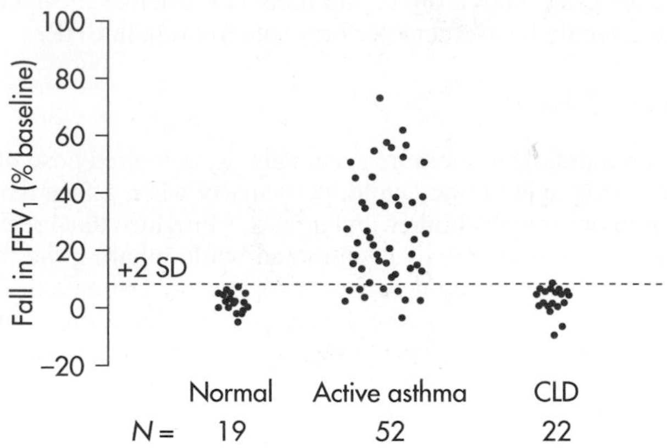

Fig. 63-7. Individual values for the change in forced expiratory volume in one second (ΔFEV_1) after exercise in normal children and those with asthma and chronic lung disease. The horizontal dashed line shows the upper limit of normal as the mean + SD derived from the normal group. (From Godfrey S, Springer C, Noviski N, Maayan CH, Avital A: *Thorax* 46:488-492, 1991.)

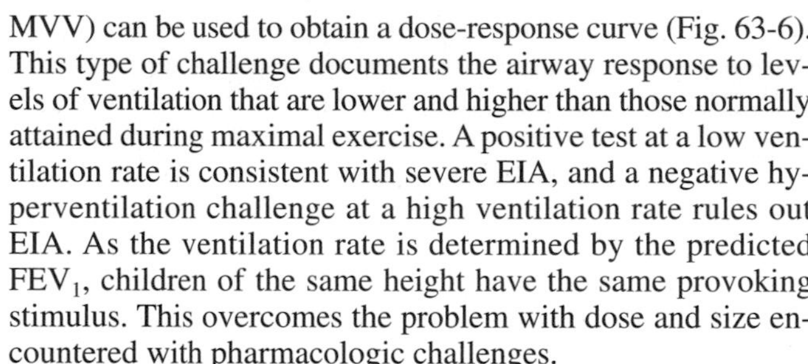

MVV) can be used to obtain a dose-response curve (Fig. 63-6). This type of challenge documents the airway response to levels of ventilation that are lower and higher than those normally attained during maximal exercise. A positive test at a low ventilation rate is consistent with severe EIA, and a negative hyperventilation challenge at a high ventilation rate rules out EIA. As the ventilation rate is determined by the predicted FEV_1, children of the same height have the same provoking stimulus. This overcomes the problem with dose and size encountered with pharmacologic challenges.

One of the great advantages of hyperpnea as a challenge test is that healthy subjects have very little airway response even at the highest level of ventilation. There is a normal distribution for the percent decrease in the healthy population of children.[2] The mean decrease (+2 SD of the decrease) in PF or FEV_1 is less than 10%, and for this reason a decrease of 10% or more has been selected as abnormal.[63] Less than 5% of normal subjects will have a decrease of more than 10% and only 0.3% will have one more than 13%. In epidemiologic studies in the field a value of 15% or more has been more commonly taken.[72,98-102] A positive response to exercise is in keeping with a diagnosis of asthma,[60] whereas a negative response to exercise does not rule out asthma. Therefore, challenge by exercise has a high positive predictive value but a low negative predictive value (Fig. 63-7). However, children who are clinically recognized as having asthma, but in whom maximum exercise does not provoke an attack, are unlikely to require long-term treatment for asthma,[103] particularly if their lung function is normal as is likely to be the case.[104]

One of the major advantages of using exercise as a challenge test to identify BR in children is that it can be performed in the school playgrounds and by most children. During epidemiologic surveys using exercise, investigators have been surprised by the number of positive test results in children who do not report symptoms and do not have positive responses to histamine.[72,74] There are many possible reasons for this. Breathlessness often accompanies vigorous exercise in children. EIA usually comes on after exercise, at least in mild to moderate cases, and breathlessness following exercise may be simply thought of as a normal response to exercise. In addition refractoriness to exercise occurs in 50% of asthmatic children,[105] so EIA may be intermittent and not perceived by the child as a respiratory problem related to exercise. Further, a diagnosis of EIA is made when the decrease in PF or FEV_1 is greater than 10% or 15%, yet few children complain of symptoms of asthma until the FEV_1 has fallen by 25% or more. Similarly wheeze may not be audible until the FEV_1 has fallen by 30%.[67]

In the study of Haby et al,[106] 40% of the 152 children found to have EIA had no symptoms or doctor diagnosis of asthma. Similarly 50% of the positive responses to cold air hyperventilation or exercise reported by Weiss et al[73] and Backer and Ulrik[74] did not have a diagnosis of asthma. This finding supports the argument that exercise tests for asthma should be carried out routinely, and there are now several exercise protocols that have been designed specifically for use in schools (Fig. 63-8).[106,107] A recent study that took climatic conditions and intensity of exercise into account found a prevalence of EIA in school children of 18.9%.[106] The most likely reason that this value is higher than that found in previous studies[74,100] is that the important factors that determine severity (intensity of exercise, inspired water content) were taken into account. Few pediatricians would choose to ignore EIA and would advise treatment immediately before exercise, even if the child did not have symptoms. For this reason exercise testing in schools would be of value.

The International Pediatric Asthma Consensus Group[13] states, "The goal of treatment should be to allow children to be involved with normal activity, including full participation in exercise and sport." There are many benefits from exercise and it is important that children are not excluded from strenuous activity because of their asthma. Further, it is important to note

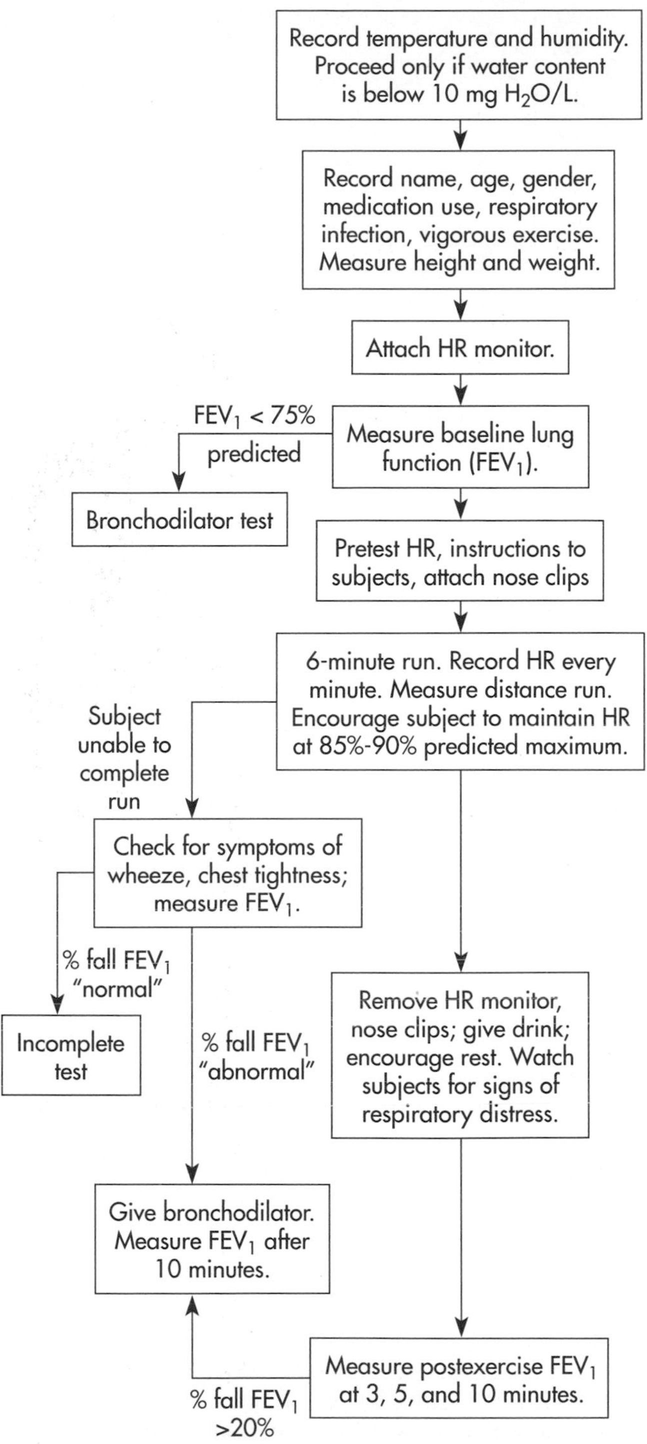

Fig. 63-8. Field procedure for exercise challenge. Based on the protocol from Haby MM, Anderson SD, Peat JK, Mellis CM, Toelle BG, Woolcock AJ: *Eur Respir J* 7:43-49, 1994.

that medication must be used and nonpharmacologic techniques such as physical training do not generally improve EIA.[108] Physical training in an unfit child is likely to increase the threshold at which EIA occurs and can have other cardiopulmonary benefits.[109] Because EIA is likely to result from airway inflammation, failure to treat may contribute to a more rapid decline in cardiopulmonary function in the long term.

Exercise-induced Asthma and Its Modification by Drugs

Exercise testing has long been used as an objective measure to assess both the acute and long-term effects of drugs used to treat asthma.[52,80,84,110,111] The pioneering studies of Godfrey et al and those that followed demonstrated the efficacy of sodium cromoglycate, nedocromil sodium, and the β_2-adrenoceptor agonists, given as aerosols, in preventing EIA (Figs. 63-9 and 63-10). Theophylline or β agonists given orally or anticholinergic agents, given by aerosol, have been shown to have little effect on the postexercise decrease in lung function, even though they improve baseline lung function (Fig. 63-11).[52,112-114]

The biggest change in treatment of asthma in children in the last 10 years has been the use of high dosages of aerosol corticosteroids. This treatment regimen has had an important outcome on children with EIA. For example, 400 μg of budesonide daily can reduce the severity of EIA[115,116] and the amount of bronchodilator medication required to prevent it.[115] Although EIA can be completely inhibited by long-term (8 weeks or more) use of inhaled steroids in some subjects, this is not always the case. A study in 116 asthmatic children receiving budesonide daily showed that 55% of the children still had EIA.[116] Thus a child with no daily symptoms of asthma and normal preexercise lung function, taking inhaled steroids, may still require medication such as sodium cromoglycate or nedocromil sodium for prevention of EIA. In children with more severe EIA a β_2 agonist may also be required. However, daily use of albuterol (8 inhalations) for 1 week has been reported to make EIA more severe.[117]

In most children a marked reduction in severity of EIA is achieved with the standard dosage of medication. Total inhibition of EIA, however, often requires higher dosages of medication. In today's competitive environment the athletic asthmatic child often demands normal lung function to compete successfully against nonasthmatics. For these children β agonists are used in combination with standard or double the standard dose of nedocromil sodium or sodium cromoglycate immediately before exercise.

The long-acting β agonists (salmeterol and formoterol) are often prescribed for EIA, particularly for children exercising many times a day. The advantage of long-acting β agonists is that in mild EIA (less than 25% decrease in FEV_1) the protective effect can last for up to 12 hours.[118] However, for moderate to severe EIA the protective effect may only last 4 to 6 hours.[119] The disadvantages of the long-acting β agonist salmeterol are that the onset of their protective effect is slower than the short-acting β agonists, and optimal protection against EIA occurs 2.5 hours after medication.[119] The slow onset of action also means that salmetrol is not recommended as rescue medication for EIA. Another problem with the long-acting β agonists is a reduction in their protective effect against EIA when taken daily.[120]

One of the proposed mechanisms whereby exercise and hyperventilation cause the airways to narrow is an increase in osmolarity of the airways as a result of evaporative water loss.[91,93] A hyperosmolar environment is thought to be ideal for the release of mast cell mediators and possibly neuropeptides from sensory nerves.[121,122] The reason that high dosages of aerosol steroids reduce severity of EIA is likely due to their action in reducing the number of mast cells[123,124] and increasing the concentration of neural endopeptidase, the enzyme that breaks down neuropeptides.[125] Short-term treatment (less

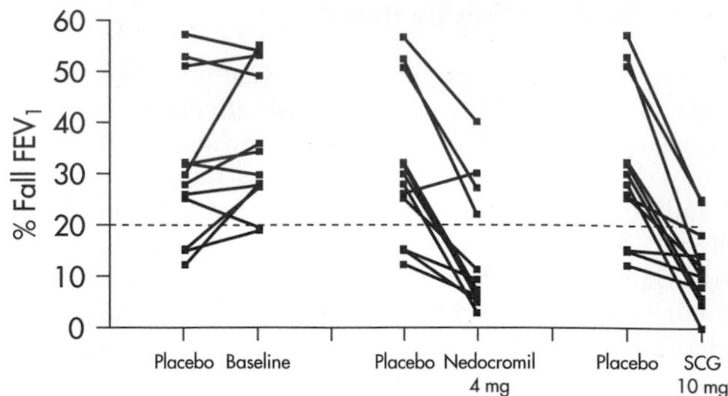

Fig. 63-9. Percentage fall in FEV_1 in 12 asthmatic children after the control exercise test and after treatment with nedocromil sodium (NS) 4 mg, sodium cromoglycate (SCG) 10 mg, or placebo administered with a metered-dose inhaler (MDI) without or with the spacer (Fisonair). Exercise was performed 30 minutes after the aerosol had been taken. Based on the data given by Comis A, Valletta EA, Sette L, Andreoli A, Boner AL: *Eur Respir J* 6:523-526, 1993.

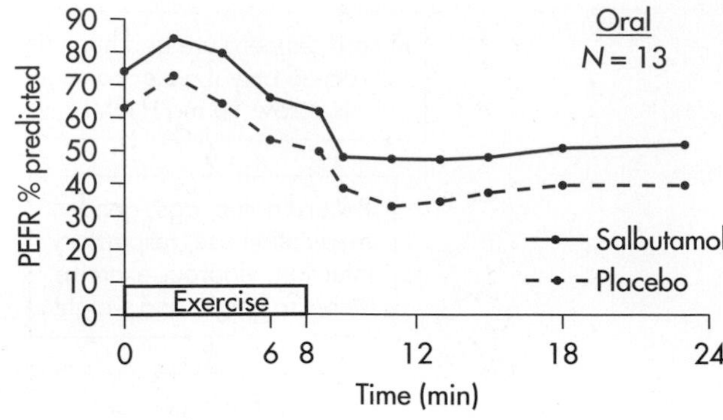

Fig. 63-11. The peak expiratory flow (PEFR) expressed as a percentage of the predicted normal value at rest and during and after exercise in 13 children with asthma. The preexercise values were taken 90 minutes after the administration of 4 mg of salbutamol given by tablet. Data from Anderson SD, Seale JP, Rozea P, Bandler L, Theobald G, Lindsay DA: *Am Rev Respir Dis* 114:493-500, 1976.

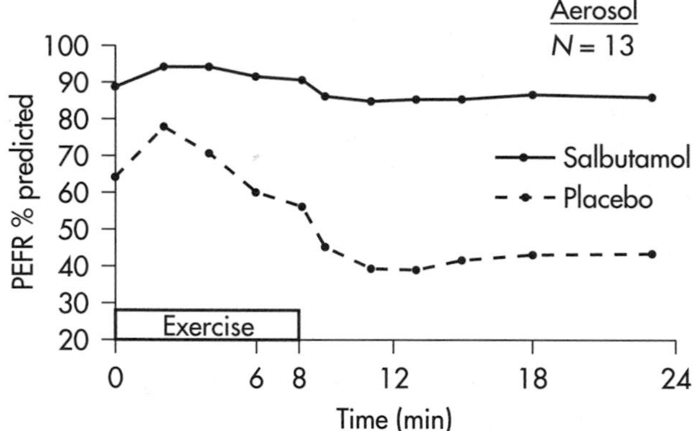

Fig. 63-10. The peak expiratory flow rate (PEFR) expressed as a percentage of the predicted normal value at rest and during and after exercise in 13 children with asthma. The preexercise values were taken 15 minutes after 200 μg of salbutamol. Data from Anderson SD, Seale JP, Rozea P, Bandler L, Theobald G, Lindsay DA: *Am Rev Respir Dis* 114:493-500, 1976.

than 2 weeks) with steroids usually improves lung function, but a longer time is required to reduce severity of EIA.[101] Repeating an exercise challenge 4 to 8 weeks after commencement of treatment with budesonide is likely to reveal a marked reduction in severity of EIA.[64,116]

The mechanism of action of sodium cromoglycate and nedocromil sodium in the prevention of EIA is not precisely understood but may relate to their ability to block chloride ion channels on mast cells, sensory nerves, and epithelial cells.[126-128] Nedocromil sodium and sodium cromoglycate, although very effective, have a relatively short duration of action (often less than 2 hours). Providing these drugs are given in an adequate dose, even severe EIA may be prevented in some, although not all, children.[129-131] The combination of sodium cromoglycate and steroids, or nedocromil sodium and steroids, has been shown to be extremely effective against a hyperosmolar stimulus.[132-133] On the basis of this finding it has been suggested that nedocromil sodium and sodium cromoglycate may be more effective against severe EIA in patients taking aerosol steroids regularly.[134]

In summary, the measurement of BR using dry air hyperpnea as the provoking stimulus appears to have a number of advantages over challenge with pharmacologic stimuli. Thus the ambivalence toward performing challenge tests in children may be overcome if exercise or hyperventilation, rather than histamine or methacholine, is used.

There are, however, some disadvantages to bronchial provocation testing by hyperpnea. These include the level of cooperation required by the child to exercise and the need for the FEV_1 to be greater than 1.5 L for the hyperventilation test to be performed adequately. These disadvantages have led to a surrogate challenge to predict EIA—using hypertonic saline.

Challenge with Hypertonic Saline

The identification of hyperosmolarity as a potent trigger for an attack of asthma,[135] the subsequent development and standardization of the challenge tests with hypertonic saline,[136-138] and the modification of responses after acute and long-term treatment with asthma drugs[132,136,139] has led to the increased use of this challenge to identify people with asthma[140-142] (Box 63-11). Many studies have demonstrated the efficacy of using hypertonic saline challenge to identify asthma in children.[70,143-145] The safety of this challenge has been established both in the laboratory and field.[70,138,144,146] A child who responds to 4.5% saline is also likely to have EIA.[70]

The mechanism for hyperosmolarity provoking airway narrowing is the same as that described for hyperpnea, that is, mast cell release of mediators and neuropeptides from sensory nerves. Many other similarities occur in the airway response to hyperpnea of dry air and hypertonic saline: There is cross refractoriness between the two challenges,[147] the time course of the response is similar,[148] the release of neutrophil chemotactic factor,[149] the provocation of cough,[150] the sensitivity and specificity of the response to both stimuli,[143] and the response to drugs. In the study of Riedler et al[70] the factors most strongly associated with a positive response to 4.5% saline

BOX 63-11

Method for Sputum Induction with Hypertonic Saline

Protocol

1. Assemble equipment and calibrate spirometer. Place 180 ml of 4.5% hypertonic saline into the well of the nebuliser, attach the tubing (which connects to the mouthpiece), and weigh 2 decimal places. Record the same.
2. Ascertain that the participant has withheld bronchodilator medication for the specified time.
3. Document the type, amount, and time of last medication.
4. Explain to the participant the purpose of the test, how it is to be conducted, and possible side effects (e.g., coughing, dry mouth, gagging, chest tightness, wheezing, dyspnea, nausea, and excess salivation).
5. Instruct and demonstrate how to obtain sputum from the lungs by coughing and clearing the throat.
6. Measure the baseline FEV_1 and FVC as per ATS guidelines.
7. Calculate a 20% fall of the highest FEV_1 and record ($FEV_1 \times 0.8 = 20\%$).
8. Ask the participant to rinse her or his mouth to eliminate spuamous cell contamination of the specimen.
9. Ask the participant to put on the gown and to apply the nose clips. The mouthpiece is inserted into the mouth in a similar manner to a snorkel.
10. When the participant is comfortable, turn on the nebuliser and begin the stopwatch. Record the 24-hour starting time. Instruct the participant to breathe "normally" (tidal breathing) through the mouthpiece. Turn the machine off after 30 seconds have elapsed.
11. Place the mouthpiece, opening down, on the absorbent sheet so that any excess residue can be drained. This prevents a potential backwash of pooled secretions through the one-way valve.
12. It is necessary to wait 1 minute after each nebulization episode to record maximal bronchoconstriction. During this period the participant may wish to rinse his or her mouth.
13. FEV_1 is recorded at the end of 1 minute. The nebulization resumes immediately the percentage of the FEV_1 fall has been calculated. [(Baseline FEV_1 - FEV_1) / baseline FEV_1] $\times$ 100.
14. Repeat steps 10-11, increasing the nebulization time by doubling the time period: 1 minute, 2 minutes, 4 minutes. A 4-minute period is the maximum time for continuous nebulization. Continue up to a cumulative nebulization time of 20 minutes.
15. Between each period there is a 1-minute break. Use this time to encourage the participant to produce sputum. Ask the participant to clear his or her throat and deposit all or any oral contents into the specimen container.
16. It usually takes a cumulative nebulization time of 11 minutes to produce an adequate specimen. Listen for a moist cough as a sign the participant is ready to produce sputum.
17. If the FEV_1 falls by 20% and there is not enough sputum produced, instruct the participant to inhale a β_2 agonist and wait 10 minutes, or until the FEV_1 has risen to within 10% of the baseline measurement.
18. Recommence the nebulization of 4.5% hypertonic saline, delivered in 4-minute doses, until sputum is obtained or a cumulative nebulization time of 20 minutes is reached. The nebulization time is counted at 2-minute intervals if the participant demonstrates severe airway hyperresponsiveness to 4.5% saline (PD_{20} saline, 2 ml).
19. Once an adequate specimen has been obtained, refrigerate and process it within a maximum of 4 hours.
20. Stop the nebulisation immediately if the following occur:
    i) An adequate specimen has been produced and the FEV_1 has dropped 20%.
    ii) An adequate specimen has been produced and the cumulative nebulization time is 20 minutes.
    iii) The participant requests the nebulization to stop.
21. Ensure the participant's FEV_1 has returned to 10% of the baseline measurement and that he or she is experiencing minimal discomfort before being allowed to leave a supervised area.

Medications

Medications that are used to achieve bronchodilation inhibit the response of the airways to nebulized 4.5% hypertonic saline and should not be used before the test. Examples of some of those medications are as follows:

1. Inhaled β_2 agagonists (not long acting) 6 hours (e.g., Ventolin, Bricanyl, Respolin, Berotec, Alupent, Asmol)
2. Inhaled β_2 agonists (long acting) 36 hours (e.g., Serevent)
3. Oral β_2 agonists (not long acting) 12 hours (e.g., Ventolin syrup)
4. Inhaled anticholinergics 12 hours (e.g., Atropine)
5. Theophylline 24 hours (e.g., Brondecon, Choledyl, Elixophylline, Cardohylline, Somophyline, Nuelin, Quibron)
6. Slow-release Theophylline 48 hours (e.g., Theo-dur, Nuelin-SR)
7. Antihistamines 5 days (e.g., Aller G, Andrumin, Avil, Avil Retard, Benadryl, Clarityne, Demazin, Disolyn, Dramamine, Hismanal [6 weeks], Panadol Sinus, Panquil, Periactin, Phenergan, Polaramine, Sinutab, Sudagesic, Teldane, Vallergan, Zadine for 5 days before the test)

Modified from Wilson A, Gibson P: Protocol. Airway Research Centre, Respiratory Unit, John Hunter Hospital, Oct. 1994.

were a history of current wheeze (odds ratio 6.96) and a positive response to exercise (odds ratio 4.26).

The advantages of challenging with hypertonic saline include the fact that little cooperation is required from the patient to perform the challenge and that the equipment is readily available and cheap, relative to exercise. Sodium chloride (dialysis grade) is approved for use in humans. A dose-response curve is obtained, and the response is reproducible.[144] Airway narrowing to 4.5% saline occurs during challenge, with the maximum effect usually observed within 60 seconds of the end of the exposure period.[148] This contrasts to challenge with hyperpnea when the response may occur as long as 5 to 10 minutes after challenge.

There now seems to be sufficient evidence to suggest that the severity of the airway response to hypertonic saline aerosol reflects the presence of inflammatory cells and their mediators in the airways. The responsiveness to 4.5% saline has been shown in asthmatics to correlate with numbers of mast cells[151] and numbers and activity of eosinophils[152] obtained from bronchial brushings and biopsies. A major advantage to using hypertonic saline as a challenge test is that responsiveness can be measured at the same time as sputum is induced and collected.[145] With improvements in collection and analysis of cells, particularly eosinophils, sputum collection and analysis may give a noninvasive guide to the degree of airway inflammation (Box 63-11).[153]

Thus in addition to demonstrating the capacity of the airways to narrow in response to the endogenous release of inflammatory mediators, challenges with hypertonic saline and sputum analysis, followed over time, could be useful in evaluating both the acute and the long-term effect of medications used in the treatment of airway inflammation.

A new hypertonic challenge has recently been developed.[154] This involves inhaling progressively increasing doses of a dry powder of mannitol from capsules through a dry powder device. The test is potentially disposable and could be performed in an office.

Challenge with Distilled Water

The challenge with distilled water was originally described by Allegra and Bianco.[155] Patients with asthma were shown to be reactive to inhaling distilled water delivered as an aerosol by an ultrasonic nebulizer. This challenge protocol was later modified by Anderson et al,[136] Hopp et al,[156] and Groot et al.[157] It has been used in epidemiology[156] to assess the effect of asthma drugs,[157,159] to determine whether BHR increases following exposure to allergen,[160] and for identifying drugs with possible benefits for treating asthma.[161]

Challenge using water in children was pioneered by Levison's group,[162] and in epidemiology it was taken up by Hopp et al.[156] It has been shown to be less sensitive than other provocation tests for identifying asthma in children.[156] A good relationship between BR to exercise and to distilled water has been reported,[163] but children are less sensitive to water. The reason for children being less sensitive to water compared with exercise or saline is not known. It may relate to cough provoked by the inhalation of water, an effect that would result in less deposition of particles in the respiratory tract. It could relate to a more rapid compensation for hypoosmolarity than hyperosmolarity on the airway surface.

PROTOCOLS FOR CHALLENGE TESTS

Exercise: Experimental Set-up

In the laboratory, exercise is usually performed on either a bicycle ergometer or a motor-driven treadmill. There are practical advantages in using a bicycle in that it is easy to deliver dry air and collect expired air because the head is stable during exercise. Further, it is easy to predict the workload required to achieve the target ventilation when bicycle exercise is used because there is a close relationship between the workload and ventilation rate. By contrast, running at the same speed and slope does not provoke the same ventilation because the work performed depends on body weight.

The time of exercise should be 6 to 8 minutes, and ventilation rate in liters per minute should be measured, at least during the last 4 minutes of exercise. Heart rate should be monitored continuously to confirm the intensity of the exercise and should be greater than 175 beats/min in the last 2 minutes of exercise.

The water content of air inspired during exercise should be as low as possible and less than 10 mg/L (relative humidity less than 50% between 20 and 25° C). This can easily be achieved in the laboratory by having the subject inspire compressed medical air via a demand valve and regulator. For most children there is no need to have expensive equipment to condition the inspired air to low or subfreezing temperatures. Providing the inspired air is dry, air at room temperature can be used. Under these conditions simply increasing the time of exercise will usually increase the severity of the airway response to that observed with cold air.[63]

Before proceeding to an exercise challenge it is important to ensure that the child has adequate lung function (FEV_1 greater than 74% of the predicted normal) and has been the appropriate time without medication. These are as follows: antihistamines, 48 hours; sustained-release preparations of theophylline and β adrenoceptor agonists or long-acting β agonists by aerosol, 24 hours; for ordinary preparations, 12 hours; sodium cromoglycate, nedocromil sodium, and short-acting bronchodilators 6 hours; corticosteroids, either aerosol or oral, are withheld on the morning of the study. For research studies the dosage and type of medication should remain stable for 4 weeks before and throughout the study. Measurements of FEV_1 should be made repeatedly at rest to demonstrate the stability and reproducibility of the baseline value. The best values should not vary by more than 10%, and the absolute value should be within 80% of the child's usual value and preferably better than 74% of the predicted value for FEV_1.

Changes in airway caliber are best measured by making multiple measurements of FEV_1 or PF before and after exercise. Although PF is easier to measure, it is limited by the fact that it measures only one point on the flow-volume curve. By contrast the FEV_1 is a value representing 80% or more of the flow-volume curve (see Fig. 63-4).

Protocol

The highest of the FEV_1 measurements taken immediately before exercise is recorded and used to measure EIA. The work intensity is selected for the child to achieve between 45% and 60% of their predicted maximum voluntary ventilation (which can be taken as FEV_1 predicted × 35) during the last 4 minutes of exercise.

The oxygen consumption to achieve this ventilation in children and the workload to achieve this ventilation is graphically shown in Figs. 63-12 and 63-13.[164] For the first minute the workload is set to 60% of the target load. This is increased to 75% in the second minute, 90% in the third minute, and 100% in the fourth minute. When the child has achieved the target level of ventilation or reached his or her ventilatory or working capacity, the workload is sustained for 4 minutes. For younger children a single load for 6 minutes may be preferable. Minor adjustments may need to be made to this workload. Undoubtedly it will be difficult for some children to achieve and sustain the target workload on the bicycle, and running on a treadmill may be easier.

To select a workload for running on a treadmill it is necessary to know the weight of the child. It is usual to aim for a speed and slope on the treadmill that will induce 30 to 45 ml of oxygen consumption per kilogram. For most children, running at 5 to 9 km/hr (3 to 5 mph) up a 10% incline is usually sufficient work to obtain this oxygen consumption. Once the target ventilation is achieved it should be sustained for 4 minutes if possible. The child must have his or her nose clipped to ensure mouth breathing. The measurements of FEV_1 are made, in duplicate, after exercise at 1, 3, 5, 7, 10, and 15 minutes and the highest at each time recorded.

Expression of the Response

The percent fall index is used to express the severity of EIA. It is calculated by subtracting the lowest value of the measurement of FEV_1 recorded in the 15 minutes after exercise from the preexercise level and expressing it as a percentage of the value recorded immediately before exercise (Fig. 63-14). A fall in FEV_1 of 10% or more of the preexercise value is abnormal when the test is performed using a standardized protocol in the laboratory under controlled conditions. If measurements are made during exercise (this is now unusual) the percent rise index can be calculated (see Fig. 63-14). This is calculated by subtracting the value recorded immediately before exercise from the highest value measured during exercise and express-

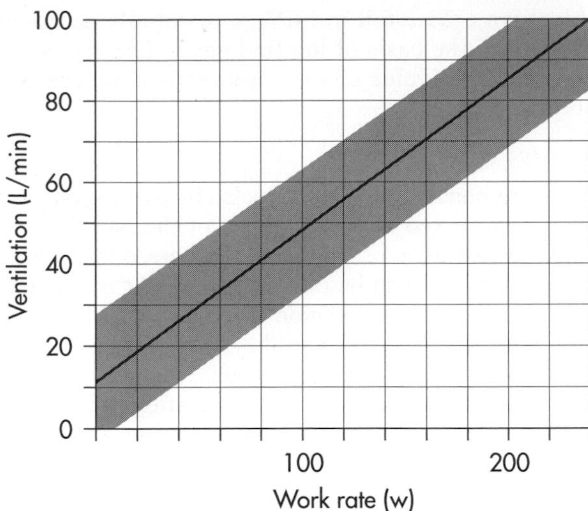

Fig. 63-12. Relationship between ventilation and power output during simple progressive exercise in children. The shaded area in this and subsequent illustrations indicates the approximate 95% confidence limit. (From Godfrey S: *Exercise testing in children. applications in health and disease,* London, 1974, WB Saunders, p 70.)

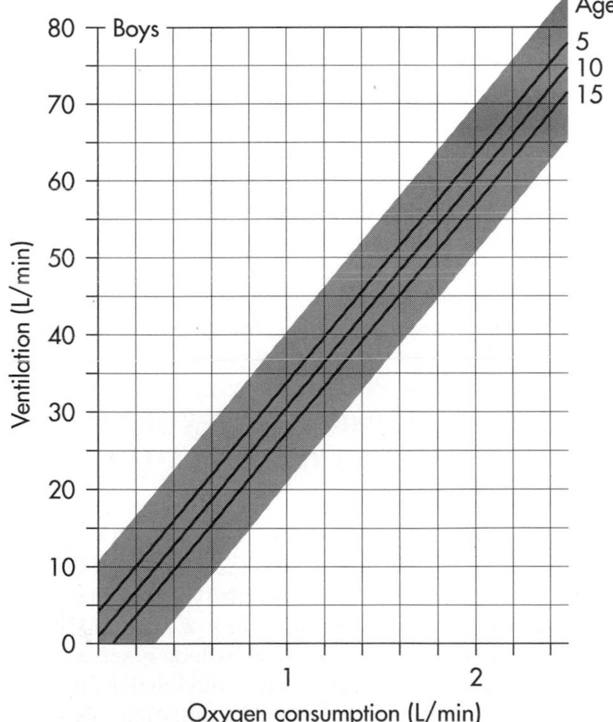

Fig. 63-13. Relationship between steady-state ventilation and O_2 consumption in boys. The effect of age on the mean line is indicated. The shaded area indicates the approximate 95% confidence limits for the line representing 10-year-old children. (From Godfrey S: *Exercise testing in children. applications in health and disease,* London, 1974, WB Saunders, p 86.)

ing it as a percentage of the value measured before exercise. The exercise lability index is the sum of the percent fall and the percent rise and is an excellent index for characterizing BR to exercise.[165] A value of 22% or more is abnormal.

For the clinical significance of the exercise response to be appreciated it is recommended that the preexercise value for

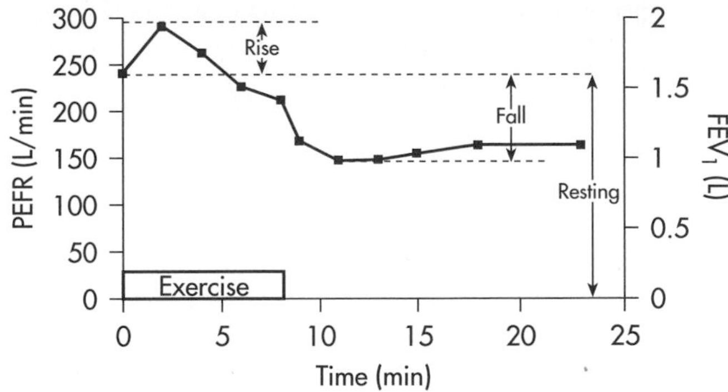

Fig. 63-14. Changes in peak expiratory flow (PEFR) and forced expiratory volume in 1 second (FEV_1) recorded during and after running exercise in 12 asthmatic children who had some airflow limitation at rest. The highest, lowest, and resting values are used to assess the % rise and % fall and are shown by the broken lines. The % rise and % fall are calculated as follows:

$$\% \text{ Rise} = \frac{\text{Rise}}{\text{Resting}} \times 100$$

$$\% \text{ Fall} = \frac{\text{Fall}}{\text{Resting}} \times 100$$

FEV_1 and the lowest value after exercise be reported in percent predicted, in addition to the percent fall index. This information will provide a better guide to the choice of medication.

The ventilation rate required to induce the percent fall in FEV_1 is useful for predicting the intensity of exercise that will provoke EIA. The ventilation should be reported together with the temperature and water content of the air inspired during exercise. Giving values for total respiratory heat loss is of no significance.

Challenge with Hypotonic and Hypertonic Aerosols

Solutions

Distilled water and 4.5% saline have been the most widely used.[67,70,143-146,163] A concentration of 2.7% saline is often used in patients with severe asthma. A dose-response curve is obtained by doubling the exposure time (or volume of aerosol inhaled) to the same aerosol. The exposure time can be kept the same and the concentration of sodium chloride increased (0.9, 1.8, 3.6, 7.2, 14.4%), but this method is not very practical. A single concentration of 4.5% saline is recommended (Fig. 63-15) because the test is shorter compared with using a lower concentration, and 80% of clinically recognized asthmatics have a 15% fall in FEV_1 after inhaling this aerosol for 15 minutes or less.

Aerosol Generation and Delivery

Ultrasonic nebulizers (Mistogen, Timeter, Penn; DeVilbiss, Somerset, Penn; Monaghans, Plattsburg, NY) are used for generation of nonisotonic aerosols because they produce aerosols that are more dense than conventional jet nebulizers. The range in the droplet size is usually between 2 and 10 microns, and this is reduced to less than 5 microns after impaction of the large droplets occur on the breathing circuit. For reasons of safety, as well as estimating delivered dosage, we recommend the use of a two-way valve, not a face mask, for challenge with nonisotonic aerosols. The reason for this is that the valve acts to reduce the volume of aerosol. However, excessive impaction of particles on the valve is not wanted, so a larger rather than smaller valve is best. The Hans Rudolf 2700 is rec-

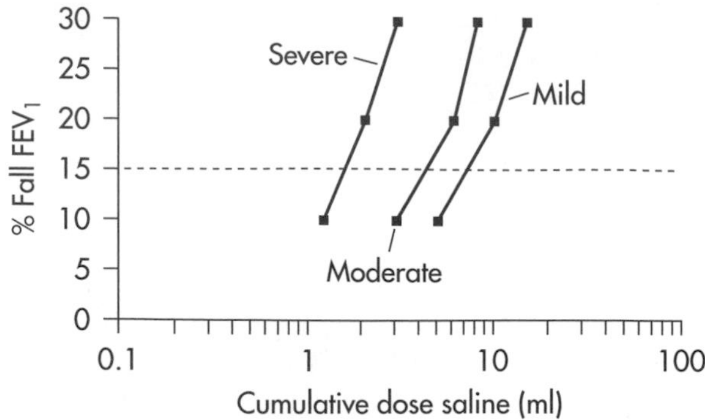

Fig. 63-15. The fall in FEV_1, expressed as a percentage of prechallenge value, in relation to the cumulative dose of 4.5% saline aerosol in three asthmatic subjects. (From Anderson SD, Smith CM, Rodwell LT, du Toit JI: The use of non-isotonic aerosols for evaluating bronchial hyperresponsiveness. In Spector S, ed: *Provocation challenge procedures,* New York, 1995, Marcel Dekker, pp 249-278.)

ommended for adults and older children,[138] but the dead space may be too large for young children, and the smaller valve Hans Rudolf No 1410, which has been well characterized,[146] may be preferable. There is the potential for the aerosol delivery to be markedly reduced with some small valves, and it is mandatory for this to be checked.

The nebulizer should have a stable output and be able to deliver at least 1.2 ml/min, preferably 1.5 ml/min, to the inspiratory port of the two-way valve with the breathing circuit attached. Higher output, as occurs with a face mask, can cause cough and a more rapid onset of bronchoconstriction.

The temperature of the solution is important and should be at least 23° C in order for the nebulizer to have the appropriate output. It is also important that the nebulizer bowl or canister be easily detached for weighing. The valve is not included as salivation occurs during challenge. The same volume fill for each subject and the same setting for the nebulizer output is used for each child. Using a canister with a volume capacity of 100 to 200 ml minimizes temperature changes and provides a more consistent output of aerosol. The dosage is obtained by measuring the change in weight of the canister and tubing, but not the valve.[138]

Protocol

We recommend that the dosage of aerosol be increased by increasing the length of each challenge interval. This can be done using time or volume. Although the nebulizer output could be increased to achieve a higher dosage, this may cause cough and can be distressing to the patient. In the routine laboratory it is more practical to use a single concentration and increase the time of exposure. We recommend distilled water or 0.03% saline for hypotonic challenge and 4.5% saline for hypertonic challenge.

Measurements of FEV_1 or specific resistance are made in duplicate or triplicate before and between 60 and 90 seconds after each exposure to the aerosol. The exposure times are doubled as follows: 30 seconds, 1, 2, 4, and 8 minutes. If volume is used, 3, 5, 10, 20, 40, 80, and 160 L is used.[136] If the fall in FEV_1 is greater than 10% of baseline, the previous exposure time or volume is repeated rather than increased. The challenge is stopped after 23 ml of aerosol is delivered or when there is a 15% or 20% reduction in FEV_1 or a 100% to 200% increase in sRaw.

Although a 20% fall in FEV_1 was initially accepted as abnormal, on the basis of the findings in healthy nonasthmatic subjects, a value of 15% or more is now regarded as abnormal.[70,138]

Expression of the Response

The dose-response curve is constructed by plotting the change in FEV_1, expressed as a percentage of the baseline value, against the dose of aerosol delivered expressed in ml. A value for PD_{15} and PD_{20} can be obtained by linear interpolation. Within the asthmatic population the values for PD_{20} or PD_{15} are log normally distributed so they are log transformed before a statistical analysis is carried out.

To assess changes in responsiveness after an intervention the values for PD_{20} or PD_{15} are compared using a paired t-test after log transformation.[166] For an individual the fold-change in PD_{15} or PD_{20} after an intervention can also be calculated after log transformation.[166] Because baseline lung function can be altered by treatment or change spontaneously over time, a reactivity index can be calculated. This is defined as the change in FEV_1, expressed as a percentage of the predicted value, per unit dose of aerosol.[139] To compare the responses after an intervention, particularly steroids, the index can also be calculated over the same values of percent predicted FEV_1.[139]

For children who do not record a 15% or 20% decrease in FEV_1, we report the maximum percent fall in FEV_1 and the dose of aerosol delivered. By dividing one by the other, a response:dose ratio is obtained.[166] A mean value and 95% confidence intervals of 0.15% (0.10% to 0.21%) fall in FEV_1/ml of 4.5% saline delivered has been found in 55 healthy young adults with normal lung function in our laboratory.[166] The normal range for response:dose ratio provides an end-point to gauge the success of treatment with steroids.[166]

Equipment

Equipment required for the challenge includes spirometer, ultrasonic nebulizer, large two-way valve, nose clip, smooth bore tubing, stopwatch, and balance for weighing.

ISOCAPNIC OR EUCAPNIC HYPERVENTILATION WITH DRY AIR AT AMBIENT TEMPERATURE

Experimental Set-up

Hyperventilation of a dry gas containing 4.9% CO_2, 21% O_2, balance N_2 is used, thus overcoming the problem of having to add CO_2 to the inspired air. The gas is delivered from the cylinder by a demand valve, via a rotameter to a meteorologic balloon. The flow rate of the gas into the balloon is set at the flow required for the child to breathe. The child inhales the dry gas via a two-way valve, and the expired ventilation rate is measured. The rotameter is used as a guide. Because voluntary hyperventilation is not natural it can be difficult for some children to perform.

Protocol

Measurements of FEV_1 are made at rest, and challenge proceeds if this is greater than 74% of predicted. The predicted maximum voluntary ventilation (MVV) is taken as the predicted value for $FEV_1 \times 35$. The predicted value for FEV_1 is used because it is likely to be achieved after treatment and the lung function change can be compared at the same ventilation rate. The ventilation rates used are commonly 30%, 60%, and 90% of MVV and MVV itself (see Fig. 63-6). Each level of ventilation is sustained for 3 minutes, and the FEV_1 measured 3 minutes after challenge. The ventilation rate is increased until there is a positive response or until MVV has been attained and sustained for 3 minutes.[111]

Hyperventilation is a very potent challenge, and severe responses can occur quite unexpectedly even in a child with normal baseline lung function. For this reason the use of a progressive challenge at 30%, 60%, and 90% MVV for a patient with clinically recognized asthma is advised. Although a 4- or 6-minute challenge at 60% MVV is faster and useful for epidemiologic studies,[66,167] acute severe responses can occur to hyperventilation. As for all challenges, it is necessary to have resuscitation equipment available.

Expression of the Response

The severity of the response to hyperventilation can be expressed in different ways. A positive response is a 10% reduction in FEV_1.[168] The ventilation rate that resulted in a 10%, 15%, or 20% fall in FEV_1 (PVE_{10}, PVE_{15}, PVE_{20}) or the percent fall in FEV_1 after each level of ventilation can be reported.

If a positive response is recorded at 90% MVV, it is classified as a mild response, whereas if it is recorded at 60% MVV, it is moderate. A positive response occurring after 30% MVV is severe.

The superiority of hyperventilation over exercise is the ability to obtain a dose-response curve. This allows a better comparison of values before and after treatment or over time.[166]

Hyperventilation challenge using dry air at 20° C has been found to be very potent and is the challenge recommended by the U.S. defense forces for identifying EIA.[111,148,166,167,169,170] Unless the symptoms only occur with cold air inhalation, it is only necessary to inhale dry air.

Hyperventilation with Cold Air

Cold air hyperventilation challenge has been carried out in children using 4 minutes of a single level of ventilation ($FEV_1 \times 22$)[171,172] and multiple 1-minute exposures at one level of ventilation.[173] These respective protocols are probably most useful in the field or in children with severe responses. A fall in FEV_1 of 9% or more is taken as above the 95th percentile for healthy children.[167] The test has been shown to have a specificity of 88% and sensitivity of 30.7%.

Conditioning the inspired air to low temperatures can increase substantially the cost of challenge because for most systems the amount of gas required is increased. Further, the low sensitivity of the cold air challenge may be explained in part by the inhibitory effect of cooling on airway responses to hyperpnea with dry air.[174] Another reason for the reported low sensitivity is that, in some field studies, medication has not been withdrawn, and many asthmatics are no longer responsive to cold air after long-term treatment with aerosol steroids or acute treatment with β agonists, nedocromil sodium, sodium cromoglycate, or leukotriene antagonists.

HISTAMINE AND METHACHOLINE DIRECT CHALLENGE TESTS

Many techniques have been described for using these pharmacologic agents to measure BR. The techniques used to deliver the aerosol all use jet nebulizers, but the method of delivery and inhalation is different for each technique. For the technique of Chai[79] the aerosol is delivered by a dosimeter

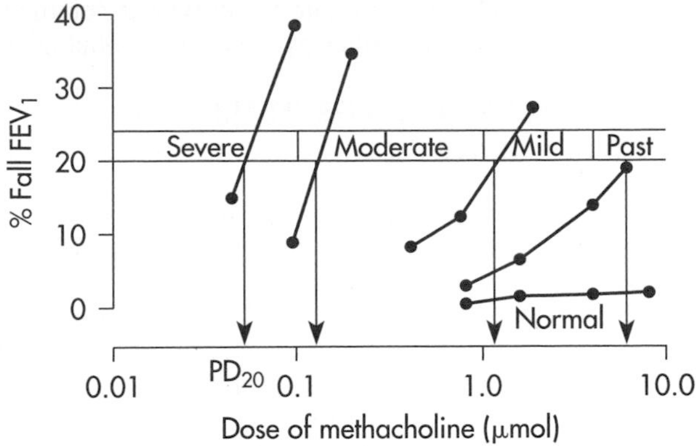

Fig. 63-16. Typical dose-response curves to methacholine in patients with severe, moderate, and mild asthma. The response curve of a patient with a history of asthma and of a normal patient are also illustrated. The arrows indicate the values for the dose of methacholine required to induce a 20% fall in FEV_1.

controlled by an electrical valve system over five consecutive breaths from FRC to TLC. For the technique of Cockcroft[78] tidal-breathing is used, and for the technique of Yan[77] a hand-operated nebulizer is used to deliver a bolus. The rapid protocol and technique described by Yan[77] is the most practical for children and for epidemiology. This technique does, however, require coordination between activation and inhalation of the aerosol, which is not necessary with the tidal breathing technique. The outcome appears unaffected by the use of a bolus or tidal breathing technique.[175] The Yan technique compares favorably with other published techniques[176] and has been widely used in children.[55,56,60,101,177]

The method for preparing the solutions of histamine diphosphate and acetyl-β-methylcholine chloride are given in detail by Sterk et al.[63] The responses to the two pharmacologic agents are comparable.[177] It is essential that the output of the jet nebulizers is measured and is known to be consistent.

For the bolus methods (dosimeter and Yan method) the dose of aerosol required to provoke a 20% reduction in FEV_1 is used (PD_{20}) (Fig. 63-16). The dose for each inhalation is determined by the nebulizer weight loss per actuation. For the tidal breathing technique the concentration required to produce a 20% reduction is used (PC_{20}), and the usual output for the nebulizer used (Wright) is 0.15 ml/min at a driving flow rate of 8 L/min.[178] The details of two techniques to deliver these aerosols are given in the following paragraphs for the methods of Yan et al[77] and Cockcroft et al.[78]

The Yan technique, often referred to as the rapid method, uses hand-operated nebulizers (DeVilbiss No. 40 or No. 45) that deliver between 1.6 and 3.8 μl per squeeze. The concentrations of methacholine or histamine used are 0.3%, 0.6%, 1.25%, 2.5%, and 5.0%. An inhalation of normal saline is often given before challenge. The inhalation of the aerosols is taken from FRC to TLC and is held for about 3 to 10 seconds. The doses are delivered in a progressive manner (approximately 0.03 to 2.0 μmoles), and the FEV_1 is measured 60 seconds after each dose has been administered. The cumulative dose is used to calculate the PD_{20}. The technique described by Chai[79] is similar and the concentration of aerosol varies from 0.03 to 32 mg/ml.

It may be preferable for younger children to breathe quietly from a mouthpiece of a nebulizer, and the Cockcroft technique permits this. Serial dilution of histamine acid phosphate is made up with phosphate-buffered saline in the doubling concentrations from 0.03 to 8 mg per ml. A Wright nebulizer is used to deliver the aerosol either by mask or by mouthpiece.

INDIRECT TECHNIQUES FOR DETECTION OF AIRWAY NARROWING

To measure BR in children unable to perform spirometry, Godfrey et al investigated the relationship between the provoking concentration of methacholine required to cause a 20% reduction in FEV_1 ($PC_{20}FEV_1$) and that required to cause audible wheeze (PC_W). They identified wheeze by listening with a stethoscope positioned over the trachea.[179,180] To have an objective test, the concept of audible wheeze was extended by Beck et al[181] to record lung sounds. Recording the sounds allowed the airway responses to be detected at a concentration of histamine 25% to 50% lower than that required to produce symptoms. In a similar study comparing PC_W, using computer analysis of breath sounds and comparing responses to methacholine PC_{20}, Sanchez et al[182] found a good relationship between the two indexes. They concluded, however, that detection of wheeze could not replace spirometry in bronchial provocation testing.

One of the uses of PC_W has been in assessing the benefits of drugs and the devices used to deliver them in very young children. For example, the efficacy of the delivery of albuterol through a Babyhaler device was established by challenging the child with methacholine and measuring PC_W in the presence of albuterol and its placebo.[183]

Recently there has been some criticism of PC_W in that it was not found to be as sensitive as measuring a reduction in transcutaneous oxygen tension ($Ptco_2$).[184] In only 3 of 21 children aged 5 was wheeze detectable by auscultation at a time when the fall in $Ptco_2$ was deemed positive. Wilson et al[184] considered that the differences between their study and the original one of Avital[179] may relate to the higher output of the nebulizer, used by Avital, resulting in differences in particle size generated and subsequent site of aerosol deposition. Wilson concluded that relying on auscultation was "not a reliable or safe method for assessing bronchoconstriction" because large reductions in FEV_1 can occur before wheezing is heard and there can be a significant decrease in $Ptco_2$.

TRANSCUTANEOUS OXYGEN

The advent of skin electrodes for the measurement of $Ptco_2$ and carbon dioxide has provided an indirect measure of BHR. Indeed some authors suggest a measurement of change in arterial oxygen tension as diagnostic of BHR in response to an inhalational challenge.[185-188] A fall in $Ptco_2$ of 10% to 15% is regarded as diagnostic. Changes in $Ptco_2$ appear to be more sensitive for picking up BHR compared with other indirect measures.[184,189] It is also useful in young subjects who may have difficulty in performing forced expiratory maneuvers but no difficulty in breathing normally and inhaling the test aerosol. One problem with this technique is that the magnitude of the reduction in $Ptco_2$ in response to methacholine inhalation varies with age both in asthmatic subjects and in controls. The variation with age, however, occurred with the same pattern in mild, moderate, and severe asthmatics.[188] Because the equipment for measuring gases transcutaneously is expensive, its use is probably confined to hospital respiratory laboratories.

CONCLUSION

Measurement of lung function in a laboratory can be important in assessing the asthmatic child. Home monitoring of flow rates can also be useful, but only as a guide. A challenge test for bronchial responsiveness can provide valuable information about severity of asthma and the need for medication or a change in medication. In selecting the provoking stimulus for challenge, it is important that the factors that can influence the airway response are taken into account. One of the most important factors is baseline lung function. If this is reduced, documenting the response to a bronchodilator is probably the most useful test. When lung function is within normal limits, a provocation test can be selected. A positive response to a pharmacologic challenge, although indicating hyperresponsiveness, is not necessarily useful for evaluating either the type or dose of medication required for treatment or the effect of treatment itself. There is also a possibility that a pharmacologic challenge test will be negative in a child who is recognized by a doctor as having asthma. A negative test to an indirect challenge in a child with asthma is consistent only with mild asthma. A positive response to an indirect challenge is consistent with current asthma and permits appropriate medication to be identified.

An important question arising from epidemiologic studies is what action should be taken when the level of BHR measured is consistent with asthma, but the child has no symptoms or history of asthma. One could argue that the patient with chronic airflow limitation of tomorrow is the asymptomatic child with BHR today. For some children symptoms may be an excellent indicator of current BHR, but for other children significant BHR as demonstrated by EIA may occur without any symptoms. Recognition of those with EIA and no symptoms may be very important for reducing the risk of poor lung function in the long term.

REFERENCES

Clinical Presentation and Clinical Assessment of Asthma

1. Kamei R: Chronic cough in children, *Pediatr Clin North Am* 38:593-615, 1991.
2. Wilson N: Wheezy bronchitis revisited, *Arch Dis Child* 64:1194-1199, 1989.
3. Kay AB: Asthma and inflammation, *J Allergy Clin Immunol* 87:893-910, 1991.
4. Mellis C, Woolcock A: Asthma/airway hyper-responsiveness, *Curr Opin Pediatr* 4:401-409, 1992.
5. Barnes P: A new approach to the treatment of asthma, *N Engl J Med* 321:1517, 1989.
6. McFadden E, Gilbert I: Asthma, *N Engl J Med* 327:1928-1937, 1992.
7. Larsen GL: Asthma in children, *New Engl J Med* 326:1540-1545, 1992.
8. Isles A, Robertson C: Position statement: treatment of asthma in children and adolescents: the need for a different approach, *Med J Aust* 158:761-763, 1993.
9. Warner JO, Gotz M, Landau L: Management of asthma: a consensus statement, *Arch Dis Child* 64:1065-1079, 1989.
10. Warner JO, Neijens H, Landau L: Asthma: a follow up statement of an international paediatric asthma consensus group, *Arch Dis Child* 67: 240-248, 1992.
11. McNicol K, Williams H: Spectrum of asthma in children-l, Clinical and physiological considerations, *Br Med J* 4:7-11, 1973.
12. Stempel D, Szefler S: Management of chronic asthma, *Pediatr Clin North Am* 39:1293-1310, 1992.
13. National Heart, Lung & Blood Institutes: International consensus report on diagnosis and treatment of asthma, *Eur Respir J* 5:601-641, 1992.
14. Barbee RA, Lebowitz MD, Thompson HC, Burrows B: Immediate skin-test negativity in a general population sample, *Ann Intern Med* 84:129-133, 1976.

15. Godfrey R, Griffiths M: The prevalence of immediate positive skin tests to Dermatophagoides pteronyssinus and grass pollen in school children, *Clin Allergy* 6:79-82, 1976.
16. David TJ: Conventional allergy tests, *Arch Dis Child* 65:281-282, 1990.
17. Christie MJ, French D, Weatherstone L, West A: The patients' perceptions of chronic disease and its management: psychosomatics, holism and quality of life in contemporary management of childhood asthma, *Psychother Psychosom* 56:197-203, 1991.
18. Rosenbaum P, Cadman D, Kirpalani H: Pediatrics: assessing quality of life. In Spilker B, ed: *Quality of life assessments in clinical trials,* New York, 1990, Raven Press, pp 205-215.
19. Juniper E, Guyatt G, Ferrie P, Griffith L: Measuring quality of life in asthma, *Am Rev Respir Dis* 147:832-838, 1993.
20. Bardin P, Johnston S, Pattemore P: Viruses as precipitants of asthma symptoms II. Physiology and mechanisms, *Clin Exp Allergy* 22:809-822, 1992.
21. Henricksen J, Wenzel A: Effect of an intranasally administered corticosteroid (budesonide) on nasal obstruction, mouth breathing, and asthma, *Am Rev Respir Dis* 130:1014-1018, 1984.
22. Welsh P, Stricker W, Chu C: Efficacy of beclomethasone nasal solution, flunisolide, and cromolyn in relieving symptoms of ragweed allergy, *Mayo Clin Proc* 62:125-134, 1987.
23. Lewis H, Haeney M, Jeacock J, Thomas H: Chronic cough in a hospital population; its relationship to atopy and defects in host defense, *Arch Dis Child* 64:1593-1598, 1989.
24. Thomson A, Pratt C, Simpson H: Nocturnal cough in asthma, *Arch Dis Child* 62:1001-1004, 1987.
25. Cloutier M, Loughlin G: Chronic cough in children: a manifestation of airway hyperreactivity, *Pediatrics* 67:6-12, 1981.
26. Phelan P, Landau L, Olinsky A: *Respiratory illness in children,* ed 3, Oxford, 1990, Blackwell Scientific Publications, ch 7.
27. Eigen H, Laughlin J, Homrighausen R: Recurrent pneumonia in children and its relationship to bronchial hyperreactivity, *Pediatrics* 70:698-704, 1982.
28. Milner A: Psychogenic cough in childhood, *Br Med J* 290:1847-1848, 1985.
29. Christopher K, Wood R, Eckert C, Blager F, Raney R, Souhrada J: Vocal-cord dysfunction presenting as asthma, *N Engl J Med* 308:1566-1570, 1983.
30. Demeter S, Cordasco E: Hyperventilation syndrome and asthma, *Am J Med* 81:989-994, 1986.
31. Balfour-Lynn L: Growth and childhood asthma, *Arch Dis Child* 61: 1049-1055, 1986.
32. Martin AJ, Landau LI, Phelan PD: The effects on growth of childhood asthma, *Acta Paediatr Scand* 70:683-688, 1981.
33. Mellins R, Zimmerman B, Clark N: Patient compliance. Are we wasting our time and don't know it? *Am Rev Respir Dis* 146:1376-1377, 1992.

The Role of Peak Flow Meters in Childhood Asthma

34. Sly P, Landau L, Weymouth R: Home recording of peak expiratory flow rates and perception of asthma, *Am J Dis Child* 139:479-482, 1985.
35. Lebowitz MD: The use of peak expiratory flow rate measurements in respiratory disease, *Pediatr Pulmonol* 11:166-174, 1991.
36. Clark NE, Evans D, Mellins R: Patient use of peak flow monitoring, *Am Rev Respir Dis* 145:722-725, 1992.
37. Osmanliev D, Bowley N, Hunter DM, Pride NB: Relation between tracheal size and FEV_1 in young men, *Am Rev Respir Dis* 126:179-182, 1982.
38. Ferguson A: Persisting airway obstruction in asymptomatic children with asthma with normal peak flow rates, *J Allergy Clin Immunol* 82:19-22, 1988.
39. Hyland M, Kenyon C, Allen R, Howarth P: Diary keeping in asthma: comparison of written and electronic methods, *Br Med J* 306:487-489, 1993.
40. Cross D, Nelson H: The role of the peak flow meter in the diagnosis and management of asthma, *J Allergy Clin Immunol* 87:120-128, 1991.
41. Greenough A, Everett L, Price J: Are we recording peak flows properly in young children? *Eur Respir J* 3:1193-1196, 1990.
42. Higgens B, Britton J, Chinn S, Jones TD, Jenkinson D, Burney PGJ, Tattersfield AE: The distribution of peak expiratory flow variability in a population sample, *Am Rev Respir Dis* 140:1368-1372, 1989.
43. Quackenboss J, Lebowitz M, Krzyzanowski M: The normal range of diurnal changes in peak expiratory flow rates. Relationship to symptoms and respiratory disease, *Am Respir Dis* 143:323-330, 1991.
44. Higgens BG, Britton JR, Chinn S, Cooper S, Burney PGJ, Tattersfield AE: Comparison of bronchial reactivity and peak expiratory flow variability measurements for epidemiological studies, *Am Rev Respir Dis* 145:588-593, 1992.
45. Reeder K, Dolce J, Duke L, Raczynski J, Bailey W: Peak flow meters: are they monitoring tools or training devices? *J Asthma* 27:219-227, 1990.
46. Beasley R, Cushley M, Holgate S: A self management plan in the treatment of adult asthma, *Thorax* 44:200-204, 1989.
47. Lloyd B, Ali M: How useful do parents find home peak flow monitoring for children with asthma? *Br Med J* 305:1128-1129, 1992.
48. Charlton I, Charlton G, Broomfield J, Mullee MA: Evaluation of peak flow and symptoms only self management plans for control of asthma in general practice, *Br Med J* 301:1355-1359, 1990.
49. Miller M, Dickson S, Hitchings D: The accuracy of portable peak flow meters, *Thorax* 47:904-909, 1992.

Spirometry and Flow Rates

50. Damato S: Volume, flow and resistance assessment in asthma. In Allegra L, Braga PC, Dal Negro R, eds: *Methods in asthmology,* London, 1993, Springer-Verlag, pp 89-125.
51. Silverman M: Respiratory function testing in infancy and childhood. In Laszlo G, Sudlow MF, eds: *Measurement in clinical respiratory physiology,* London, 1993, Academic Press, ch 14, pp 293-328.
52. Anderson SD, Seale JP, Rozea P, Bandler L, Theobald G, Lindsay DA: Inhaled and oral salbutamol in exercise-induced asthma, *Am Rev Respir Dis* 114:493-500, 1976.
53. Quanjer PH, Stocks J, Polgar G, Wise M, Karlberg J, Borsboom G: Compilation of reference values for lung function measurement in children, *Eur Respir J* 2(suppl 4):184-261, 1989.

Total Lung Capacity (TLC) and Functional Residual Capacity (FRC)

54. West JB: *Respiratory physiology-the essentials,* Baltimore, 1974, Williams & Wilkins.

"Direct" or Pharmacological Challenges: Histamine or Methacholine

55. Pattemore PK, Asher MI, Harrison AC, Mitchell EA, Rea HH, Stewart AW: The interrelationship among bronchial hyperresponsiveness, the diagnosis of asthma, and asthma symptoms, *Am Rev Respir Dis* 142: 549-554, 1990.
56. Sears MR, Jones DT, Holdaway MD, Hewitt CJ, Flannery EM, Herbison GP, Silva PA: Prevalence of bronchial reactivity to inhaled methacholine in New Zealand children, *Thorax* 41:283-289, 1986.
57. Salome CM, Peat JK, Britton WJ, Woolcock AJ: Bronchial hyperresponsiveness in two populations of Australian schoolchildren. 1. Relation to respiratory symptoms and diagnosed asthma, *Clin Allergy* 17:271-281, 1987.
58. Josephs LK, Gregg I, Mullee MA, Holgate ST: Non-specific bronchial reactivity and its relationship to the clinical expression of asthma: a longitudinal study, *Am Rev Respir Dis* 140:350-357, 1989.
59. Peat JK, Gray EJ, Mellis CM, Leeder SR, Woolcock AJ: Differences in airway responsiveness between children and adults in the same environment: an epidemilogical study in two regions of New South Wales, *Eur Respir J* 7:1805-1813, 1994.
60. Godfrey S, Springer C, Noviski N, Maayan Ch, Avital A: Exercise but not methacholine differentiates asthma from chronic lung disease in children, *Thorax* 46:488-492, 1991.
61. Avital A, Springer C, Bar-Yishay E, Godfrey S: Adenosine, methacholine, and exercise challenges in children with asthma or paediatric chronic obstructive pulmonary disease, *Thorax* 50:511-516, 1995.
62. Holgate ST, Pattermore PK: Asthma in childhood. In Page CP, Gardiner PJ, eds: *Airway hyperresponsiveness: is it really important for asthma?* London, 1993, Blackwell Scientific Publications, pp 55-78.
63. Sterk PJ, Fabbri LM, Quanjer PhH, Cockcroft DW, O'Byrne PM, Anderson SD, Juniper EF, Malo J-L: Airway responsiveness: standardized challenge testing with pharmacological, physical and sensitizing stimuli in adults, *Eur Respir J* 6(suppl 16):53-83, 1993.
64. Vathenen AS, Knox AJ, Wisniewski A, Tattersfield AE: Effect of inhaled budesonide on bronchial reactivity to histamine, exercise, and eucapnic dry air hyperventilation in patients with asthma, *Thorax* 46:811-816, 1991.

65. Van Essen-Zandvliet EE, Hughes MD, Waalkens HJ, Duiverman EJ, Pocock SJ, Kerrebijn KF, and the Dutch Chronic Non-Specific Lung Disease Study Group: Effects of 22 months of treatment with inhaled corticosteroids and/or beta-2-agonists on lung function, airway responsiveness, and symptoms in children with asthma, *Am Rev Respir Dis* 146:547-554, 1992.
66. Steinbrugger B, Eber E, Modl M, Weinhandl E, Zach MS: A comparison of a single-step cold-dry air challenge and a routine histamine provocation for the assessment of bronchial responsiveness in children and adolescents, *Chest* 108:741-745, 1995.
67. Wilson NM, Bridge P, Silverman M: Bronchial responsiveness and symptoms in 5-6 year old children: a comparison of a direct and indirect challenge, *Thorax* 50:339-345, 1995.
68. Cockcroft DW, Murdock KY, Berscheid BA, Gore BP: Sensitivity and specificity of histamine PC_{20} determination in a random selection of young college students, *J Allergy Clin Immunol* 89:23-30, 1992.
69. Backer V, Groth S, Dirksen A, Bach-Mortensen N, Hanseb KK, Laursen EM, Wendelboe D: Sensitivity and specificity of the histamine challenge test for the diagnosis of asthma in an unselected sample of children and adolescents, *Eur Respir J* 4:1093-1100, 1991.
70. Riedler J, Reade T, Dalton M, Holst D, Robertson CF: Hypertonic saline challenge in an epidemiological survey of asthma in children, *Am J Respir Crit Care Med* 150:1632-1639, 1994.
71. Ulrik CS, Backer V, Hesse B, Dirksen A: Risk factors for development of asthma in children and adolescents: findings from a longitudinal population study, *Respir Med* 90:623-630, 1996.
72. Haby MM, Peat JK, Mellis CM, Anderson SD, Woolcock AJ: An exercise challenge for epidemiological studies of childhood asthma; validity and repeatability, *Eur Respir J* 8:729-736, 1995.
73. Weiss ST, Tager IB, Weiss JW, Munoz A, Speizer FE, Ingram RH: Airways responsiveness in a population sample of adults and children, *Am Rev Respir Dis* 129:898-902, 1984.
74. Backer V, Ulrik CS: Bronchial responsiveness to exercise in a random sample of 494 children and adolescents from Copenhagen, *Clin Exp Allergy* 22:741-747, 1992.
75. Collis GG, Cole CH, Le Souef PN: Dilution of nebulised aerosols by air entrainment in children, *Lancet* 336:341-343, 1990.
76. Peat JK, Salome CM, Xuan W: On adjusting measurements of airway responsiveness for lung size and airway caliber, *Am J Respir Crit Care Med* 154:870-875, 1996.
77. Yan K, Salome C, Woolcock AJ: Rapid method for measurement of bronchial responsiveness, *Thorax* 38:760-765, 1983.
78. Cockcroft DW, Killian DN, Mellon JJA, Hargreave FE: Bronchial reactivity to inhaled histamine: a method and clinical survey, *Clin Allergy* 7:235-243, 1977.
79. Chai H, Farr RS, Froehlich LA, et al: Standardisation of bronchial inhalation procedures, *J Allergy Clin Immunol* 56:323-327, 1975.
80. Jones RS, Wharton MJ, Buston MH: The place of physical exercise and bronchodilator drugs in the assessment of the asthmatic child, *Arch Dis Child* 38:539-545, 1963.

"Indirect" Challenges

81. Jones RS, Buston MH, Wharton MJ: The effect of exercise on ventilatory function in the child with asthma, *Br J Dis Chest* 56:78-86, 1962.
82. Anderson SD, Silverman M, Konig P, Godfrey S: Exercise-induced asthma. A review, *Br J Dis Chest* 69:1-39, 1975.
83. Anderson SD, Silverman M, Walker SR: Metabolic and ventilatory changes in asthmatic patients during and after exercise, *Thorax* 27:718-725, 1972.
84. Anderson SD, Mc Evoy JDS, Bianco S: Changes in lung volumes and airway resistance after exercise in asthmatic subjects, *Am Rev Respir Dis* 106:30-37, 1972.
85. Freychuss U, Hedlin G, Hedenstierna G: Ventilation-perfusion relationships during exercise-induced asthma in children, *Am Rev Respir Dis* 130:888-894, 1984.
86. Deal EC, McFadden ER, Ingram RH, Jaeger JJ: Hyperpnea and heat flux: initial reaction sequence in exercise-induced asthma, *J Appl Physiol: Respir, Environ Exercis Physiol* 46:476-483, 1979.
87. Phillips YY, Jaeger JJ, Laube BL, Rosenthal RR: Eucapnic voluntary hyperventilation of compressed gas mixture. A simple system for bronchial challenge by respiratory heat loss, *Am Rev Respir Dis* 131:31-35, 1985.
88. Chen WY, Horton DJ: Heat and water loss from the airways and exercise-induced asthma, *Respiration* 34:305-313, 1977.
89. Bar-Or O, Neuman I, Dotan R: Effects of dry and humid climates on exercise-induced asthma in children and preadolescents, *J Allergy Clin Immunol* 60:163-168, 1977.
90. Strauss RH, McFadden ER, Ingram RH, Deal CE: Influence of heat and humidity on the airway obstruction induced by exercise in asthma, *J Clin Invest* 61:433-440, 1978.
91. Anderson SD, Schoeffel RE, Follet R, Perry CP, Daviskas E, Kendall M: Sensitivity to heat and water loss at rest and during exercise in asthmatic patients, *Eur J Respir Dis* 63:459-471, 1982.
92. Hahn A, Anderson SD, Morton AR, Black JL, Fitch KD: A re-interpretation of the effect of temperature and water content of the inspired air in exercise-induced asthma, *Am Rev Respir Dis* 130:575-579, 1984.
93. Anderson SD, Daviskas E: The airway microvasculature in exercise-induced asthma, *Thorax* 47:748-752, 1992.
94. McFadden ER, Lenner KA, Strohl KP: Postexertional airway rewarming and thermally induced asthma, *J Clin Invest* 78:18-25, 1986.
95. Gilbert IA, McFadden ER: Airway cooling and rewarming. The second reaction sequence in exercise-induced asthma, *J Clin Invest* 90:699-704, 1992.
96. Anderson SD: Current concepts of exercise-induced asthma, a review, *Allergy* 38:289-302, 1983.
97. Banner AS, Green J, O'Connor M: Relation of respiratory water loss to coughing after exercise, *N Engl J Med* 311:883-886, 1984.
98. Burr ML, Eldridge BA, Borysiewicz LK: Peak expiratory flow rates before and after exercise in schoolchildren, *Arch Dis Child* 49:923-926, 1974.
99. Burr ML, Butland BK, King S, Vaughan-Williams E: Changes in asthma prevalence: two surveys 15 years apart, *Arch Dis Child* 64:1452-1456, 1989.
100. Keeley DJ, Neill P, Gallivan S: Comparison of the prevalence of reversible airways obstruction in rural and urban Zimbabwean children, *Thorax* 46:549-553, 1991.
101. Clough JB, Hutchinson SA, Williams JD, Holgate ST: Airway response to exercise and methacholine in children with respiratory symptoms, *Arch Dis Child* 66:579-583, 1991.
102. Barry DMJ, Burr ML, Limb ES: Prevalence of asthma among 12 year old children in New Zealand and South Wales: a comparative survey, *Thorax* 46:405-409, 1991.
103. Balfour-Lynn L, Tooley M, Godfrey S: A study comparing the relationship of exercise-induced asthma to clinical asthma in childhood, *Arch Dis Child* 56:450-454, 1980.
104. Anderson SD, Schoeffel RE: The importance of standardizing exercise tests in the evaluation of asthmatic children. In Oseid S, Edwards A, eds: *The asthmatic child in play and sport,* U.K, 1983, Pitman Medical, pp 145-158.
105. Anderson SD: Asthma provoked by exercise, hyperventilation, and the inhalation of non-isotonic aerosols. In Barnes PJ, Rodger IW, Thomson NC, eds: *Asthma: basic mechanisms and clinical management:* ed 2, London, 1992, Academic Press, pp 473-490.
106. Haby MM, Anderson SD, Peat JK, Mellis CM, Toelle BG, Woolcock AJ: An exercise challenge protocol for epidemiological studies of asthma in children: comparison with histamine challenge, *Eur Respir J* 7:43-49, 1994.
107. Freeman W, Weir DC, Sapiano SB, Whitehead JE, Burge PS, Cayton RM: The twenty-metre shuttle-running test: a combined test for maximal oxygen uptake and exercise-induced asthma? *Respir Med* 84:31-35, 1990.
108. Fitch KD, Blitvich JD, Morton AR: The effect of running training on exercise-induced asthma, *Ann Allergy* 57:90-94, 1986.
109. Varray A, Mercier J, Savy-Pacaux A-M, Préfaut C: Cardiac role in exercise limitation in asthmatic subjects with special reference to disease severity, *Eur Respir J* 6:1011-1017, 1993.
110. Godfrey S, Konig P: Inhibition of exercise-induced asthma by different pharmacological pathways, *Thorax* 31:137-143, 1976.
111. Anderson SD: Exercise-induced asthma. In Kay AB, ed: *Allergy and allergic diseases,* vol 1, Oxford, 1997, Blackwell Science, pp 692-711.
112. Laursen LC, Johannesson N, Weeke B: Effects of enprofylline and theophylline on exercise-induced asthma, *Allergy* 40:506-509, 1985.

113. Fuglsang G, Hertz B, Holm E-B: No protection by oral terbutaline against exercise-induced asthma in children: a dose-response study, *Eur Respir J* 6:527-530, 1993.
114. Wilson NM, Barnes PJ, Vickers H, Silverman M: Hyperventilation-induced asthma: evidence for two mechanisms, *Thorax* 37:65-66, 1982.
115. Henriksen JM, Dahl R: Effects of inhaled budesonide alone and in combination with low-dose terbutaline in children with exercise-induced asthma, *Am Rev Respir Dis* 128:993-997,1983.
116. Waalkens HJ, van Essen-Zandvliet EEM, Gerritsen J, Duiverman EJ, Kerrebijn KF, Knol K: The effect of an inhaled corticosteroid (budesonide) on exercise-induced asthma in children, *Eur Respir J* 6:652-656, 1993.
117. Inman MD, O'Byrne P: The effect of regular inhaled albuterol on exercise-induced bronchoconstriction, *Am J Respir Crit Care Med* 153:65-69, 1996.
118. Kemp JP, Dockhorn RJ, Busse WW, Bleecker ER, Van As A: Prolonged effect of inhaled salmeterol against exercise-induced bronchospasm, *Am J Respir Crit Care Med* 150:1612-1615, 1994.
119. Anderson SD, Rodwell LT, Du Toit J, Young IH: Duration of protection of inhaled salmeterol in exercise-induced asthma, *Chest* 100:1254-1260, 1991.
120. Ramage L, Lipworth BJ, Ingram CG, Cree IA, Dhillon DP: Reduced protection against exercise induced bronchoconstriction after chronic dosing with salmeterol, *Resp Med* 88:363-368, 1994.
121. Anderson SD: Issues in exercise-induced asthma, *J Allergy Clin Immunol* 76:763-772, 1985.
122. Solway J, Leff AR: Sensory neuropeptides and airway function, a review, *J Appl Physiol* 71:2077-2087, 1991.
123. Djukanovic R, Wilson JW, Britten KM, Wilson SJ, Walls AF, Roche WR, Howarth PH, Holgate ST: Effect of an inhaled corticosteroid on airway inflammation and symptoms in asthma, *Am Rev Respir Dis* 145: 669-674, 1992.
124. Jeffrey PK, Godfrey RW, Adelroth E, Nelson F, Rogers A, Johansson S-A: Effect of treatment on airway inflammation and thickening of basement membrane reticular collagen in asthma. A quantitative light and electron study, *Am Rev Respir Dis* 145:890-899, 1992.
125. Borson DB, Gruenart DC: Glucocorticoids induce neutral endopeptidase in transformed human tracheal epithelial cells, *Am J Physiol* 260 (Lung Cell Mol Physiol):L83-L89, 1991.
126. Alton EWFW, Kingsleigh-Smith DJ, Munkonge FM, Norris A, Geddes DM, Williams AJ: Asthma prophylaxis agents alter the function of an airway epithelial chloride channel, *Am J Respir Cell Mol Biol* 14:380-387, 1996.
127. Jackson DM, Pollard CE, Roberts SM: The effect of nedocromil sodium on the isolated rabbit vagus nerve, *Eur J Pharmacol* 221:175-177, 1992.
128. Anderson SD, Rodwell LT, Daviskas E, Spring JF, du Toit J: The protective effect of nedocromil sodium and other drugs on airway narrowing provoked by hyperosmolar stimuli: role of the epithelium, *J Allergy Clin Immunol* 98:S124-S134, 1996.
129. Silverman M, Turner-Warwick M: Exercise induced asthma: response to disodium cromoglycate in skin-test positive and skin-test negative subjects, *Clin Allergy* 2:137-142, 1972.
130. Novembre E, Frongia GF, Veneruso G, Vierucci A: Inhibition of exercise induced asthma (EIA) by nedocromil sodium and sodium cromoglycate in children, *Pediatr Allergy Immunol* 5:107-110, 1994.
131. Comis A, Valletta EA, Sette L, Andreoli A, Boner AL: Comparison of nedocromil sodium and sodium cromoglycate administered by pressurized aerosol, with and without a spacer device in exercise-induced asthma in children, *Eur Respir J* 6:523-526, 1993.
132. Rodwell LT, Anderson SD, du Toit J, Seale JP: Nedocromil sodium inhibits the airway response to hyperosmolar challenge in patients with asthma, *Am Rev Respir Dis* 146:1149-1155, 1993.
133. Anderson SD, du Toit JI, Rodwell LT, Jenkins CR: Acute effect of sodium cromoglycate on airway narrowing induced by 4.5% saline aerosol. Outcome before and during treatment with aerosol corticosteroids in patients with asthma, *Chest* 105:673-680, 1994.
134. Anderson SD: Drugs and the control of exercise-induced asthma. Editorial, *Eur Respir J* 6:1090-1092, 1993.
135. Schoeffel RE, Anderson SD, Altounyan RE: Bronchial hyperreactivity in response to inhalation of ultrasonically nebulised solutions of distilled water and saline, *Br Med J* 283:1285-1287, 1981.
136. Smith CM, Anderson SD: Inhalation provocation tests using non-isotonic aerosols, *J Allergy Clin Immunol* 4:781-790, 1989.
137. Anderson SD, Smith CM, Rodwell LT, du Toit JI, Riedler J, Robertson CF: The use of non-isotonic aerosols for evaluating bronchial hyperresponsiveness. In Spector S, ed: *Provocation challenge procedures,* New York, 1995, Marcel Dekker, pp 249-278.
138. Anderson SD, Gibson P: Use of aerosols of hypertonic saline and distilled water (fog). In Barnes PJ, Grunstein MM, Leff AR, Woolcock AJ, eds: *Asthma,* Philadelphia, 1997, Lippincott-Raven, pp 1135-1149.
139. Rodwell LT, Anderson SD, Seale JP: Inhaled steroids modify bronchial responses to hyperosmolar saline, *Eur Respir J* 5:953-962, 1992.
140. Boulet LP, Legris C, Thibault L, Turcotte H: Comparative bronchial responses to hyperosmolar saline and methacholine in asthma, *Thorax* 42:953-958, 1987.
141. Belcher NG, Lee TH, Rees PJ: Airway responses to hypertonic saline, exercise and histamine challenges in bronchial asthma, *Eur Respir J* 2:44-248, 1989.
142. Finnerty JP, Wilmot C, Holgate ST: Inhibition of hypertonic saline-induced bronchoconstriction by terfenadine and flurbiprofen. Evidence for the predominant role of histamine, *Am Rev Respir Dis* 140:593-597, 1989.
143. Araki H, Sly PD: Inhalation of hypertonic saline as a bronchial challenge in children with mild asthma and normal children, *J Allergy Clin Immunol* 84:99-107, 1989.
144. Riedler J, Reade T, Robertson CF: Repeatability of the response to 4.5% NaCl challenge in children with mild to severe asthma, *Pediatr Pulmonol* 18:330-336, 1994.
145. Gibson PG, Wlodarczyk J, Hensley MJ: Induced sputum eosinophils and mast cells in a birth cohort, *Am J Resp Crit Care Med* 151:A37, 1995.
146. Riedler J, Robertson CF: Effect of tidal volume on the output and particle size distribution of hypertonic saline from an ultrasonic nebulizer, *Eur Respir J* 7:998-1002, 1994.
147. Belcher NG, Rees PJ, Clark TJH, Lee TH: A comparison of the refractory periods induced by hypertonic airway challenge and exercise in bronchial asthma, *Am Rev Resir Dis* 135:822-825, 1987.
148. Smith CM, Anderson SD: A comparison between the airway response to isocapnic hyperventilation and hypertonic saline in subjects with asthma, *Eur Respir J* 2:36-43, 1989.
149. Belcher NG, Murdoch RD, Dalton N, House FR, Clark TJH, Rees PJ, Lee TH: A comparison of mediator and catecholamine release between exercise- and hypertonic saline-induced asthma, *Am Rev Respir Dis* 137:1026-1032, 1988.
150. Higgenbottam T: Cough induced by changes of ionic composition of airway surface liquid, *Bull Eur Physiopathol Resp* 20:553-562, 1984.
151. Gibson PG, Salton N, Hopkins YJ, Borgas T, Saunders NA: Repair of airway inflammation in asthma: the role of mast cells in persisting airway hyperresponsiveness, *Am Rev Respir Dis* 145:A19, 1992.
152. Sont JK, Willems LNA, van Krieken JHJM, Sterk PJ: The determinants of airway hyperresponsiveness to hypertonic saline and methacholine in bronchial biopsy specimens from atopic asthmatics, *Am Rev Respir Dis* 147:A825, 1993.
153. Gibson PG, Girgis Gabaroo A, Morris MM, Mattoli S, Kay JM, Dolovich J, Denburg JA, Hargreave FE: Cellular characteristic of sputum from patients with asthma and chronic bronchitis, *Thorax* 44:693-699, 1989.
154. Anderson SD, Brannan J, Spring J, Spalding N, Rodwell LT, Chan K, Gonda I, Walsh A, Clark A: A new method for bronchial provocation testing in asthmatic subjects using a dry powder of mannitol, *Am J Respir Crit Care Med* 156:3, 1997.
155. Allegra L, Bianco S: Non-specific broncho-reactivity obtained with an ultrasonic aerosol of distilled water, *Eur J Respir Dis* 61(suppl 106):41-49, 1980.
156. Hopp RJ, Christy J, Bewtra AK, Nair NK, Townley RG: Incorporation and analysis of ultrasonically nebulized distilled water challenges in an epidemiological study of asthma and bronchial reactivity, *Ann Allergy* 60:129-133, 1990.
157. Groot C: Refractoriness to distilled water after histamine, *J Appl Physiol* 70:1011-1015, 1991.
158. Bianco S, Robushi M, Damonte C: Drug effect on bronchial response to $PGF_{2\alpha}$ and water inhalation, *Eur J Respir Dis* 64:213-221, 1983.
159. Anderson SD: Bronchial challenge by ultrasonically nebulized aerosols, *Clin Rev Allergy* 3:427-439, 1985.

160. Mormile F, Mattoli S, Rosati G, Di Marzo A, Ciappi G: Allergen-induced increases in non-allergic bronchial responsiveness to ultrasonic mist, *Prog Resp Res* 19:256-265, 1985.
161. Robuschi M, Gambaro G, Spagnotto S, Vaghi A, Bianco S: Inhaled furosemide is highly effective in preventing ultrasonically nebulised water bronchoconstriction, *Pulm Pharmacol* 1:187-191, 1989.
162. Galdes-Sebalt M, McLaughlin FJ, Levison H: Comparison of cold air, ultrasonic mist and methacholine inhalations as tests of bronchial reactivity in normal and asthmatic children, *J Pediatr* 107:526-530, 1985.
163. Obata T, Iikura Y: Comparison of bronchial reactivity to ultrasonically nebulized distilled water, exercise and methacholine challenge test in asthmatic children, *Ann Allergy* 72:167-172, 1994.

Protocols for Challenge Tests

164. Godfrey S: *Exercise testing in children. Applications in health and disease,* London, 1974, WB Saunders.
165. Silverman M, Anderson SD: Standardization of exercise tests in asthmatic children, *Arch Dis Child* 47:882-889, 1972.
166. du Toit JI, Anderson SD, Jenkins CR, Woolcock AJ, Rodwell LT: Airway responsiveness in asthma: bronchial challenge with histamine and 4.5% sodium chloride before and after budesonide, *Allergy Proc* 18:7-14, 1997.
167. Nicolai T, von Mutius E, Reitmeir P, Wjst M: Reactivity to cold-air hyperventilation in normal and in asthmatic children in a survey of 5,697 schoolchildren in Southern Bavaria, *Am Rev Respir Dis* 147:565-572, 1993.
168. Asoufi BK, Dalley MB, Newman-Taylor AJ, Denison DM: Cold air test. A simplified standard method for airway reactivity, *Bull Eur Physiopathol Respir* 22:349-357, 1986.
169. Smith CM, Anderson SD: Inhalational challenge using hypertonic saline in asthmatic subjects: a comparison with responses to hyperpnoea, methacholine, and water, *Eur Respir J* 3:144-151, 1989.
170. Eliasson AH, Phillips YY, Rajagopal KR: Sensitivity and specificity of bronchial provocation testing. An evaluation of four techniques in exercise-induced bronchospasm, *Chest* 1992.
171. Reisman J, Mappa L, De Benedictis F, McLaughlin J, Levison M: Cold air challenge in children with asthma, *Pediatr Pulmonol* 3:251-254, 1987.
172. Weiss JW, Rossing TH, McFadden ER, Ingram RH: Relationship between bronchial responsiveness to hyperventilation with cold and methacholine in asthma, *J Allergy Clin Immunol* 72:140-144, 1983.
173. Zach M, Polgar G, Kump H, Kroisel P: Cold air challenge of airway hyperreactivity in children: practical application and theoretical aspects, *Pediatr Res* 18:469-478, 1984.
174. Freed AN, Stream CE: Airway cooling: stimulus specific modulation of airway responsiveness in the canine lung periphery, *Eur Respir J* 4:568-574, 1991.
175. Birnie D, thoe Schwartzenberg GWS, Hop WCJ, van Essen-Zandvliet EEM, Kerrebijn KF: Does the outcome of the tidal breathing and dosimeter methods of assessing bronchial responsiveness in children with asthma depend on age? *Thorax* 45:199-202, 1990.
176. Britton J, Mortagy A, Tattersfield A: Histamine challenge testing: comparison of three methods, *Thorax* 41:128-132, 1986.
177. Peat JK, Salome CM, Bauman A, Toelle BG, Wachinger SL, Woolcock AJ: Repeatability of histamine bronchial challenge and comparability with methacholine bronchial challenge in a population of Australian schoolchildren, *Am Rev Respir Dis* 144:338-343, 1991.
178. Dolovich MB: Technical factor influencing response to challenge aerosols. In Hargreave FE, Woolcock AJ, eds: *Airway responsiveness. Measurement and interpretation,* Ontario, 1985, Astra Pharmaceuticals Canada, ch 9.
179. Avital A, Bar-Yishay E, Springer C, Godfrey S: Bronchial provocation tests in young children using tracheal auscultation, *J Pediatr* 112:591-594, 1988.

Indirect Techniques for Detection of Airway Narrowing

180. Noviski N, Cohen L, Springer C, Bar-Yishay E, Avital A, Godfrey S: Bronchial provocation determined by breath sounds compared with lung function, *Arch Dis Child* 66:952-955, 1991.
181. Beck R, Dickson U, Montgomery MD, Mitchell I: Histamine challenge in young children using computerized lung sounds analysis, *Chest* 102:759-763, 1992.
182. Sanchez I, Avital A, Wong I, Tal A, Pasterkamp H: Acoustic vs. spirometric assessment of bronchial responsiveness to methacholine in children, *Pediatr Pulmonol* 15:28-35, 1993.
183. Avital A, Godfrey S, Schachter J, Springer C: Protective effect of albuterol delivered via a spacer device (Babyhaler) against methacholine induced bronchoconstriction in young wheezy children, *Pediatr Pulmonol* 17:281-284, 1994.
184. Wilson NM, Bridge P, Phagoo SB, Silverman M: The measurement of methacholine responsiveness in 5 year old children: three methods compared, *Eur Respir J* 8:364-370, 1995.

Transcutaneous Oxygen

185. Mochizuki M, Mitsuhashi K, Tokuyama K, Tajima A, Morikawa A, Kuroume T: A new method of estimating bronchial hyperresponsiveness in younger children, *Ann Allergy* 55:162-166, 1985.
186. Mochizuki M, Mitsuhashi K, Tokuyama K, Tajima A, Morikawa A, Kuroume T: Bronchial hyperresponsiveness in younger children with asthma, *Ann Allergy* 60:103-106, 1988.
187. Eber E, Varga E-M, Zach MS: Cold air challenge of airway reactivity in children: a correlation of transcutaneously measured oxygen tension and conventional lung functions, *Pediatr Pulmonol* 10:273-277, 1991.
188. Mochizuki H, Shigeta M, Kato M, Maed S, Shimizu T, Morikawa A: Age-related changes in bronchial hyperreactivity to methacholine in asthmatic children, *Am J Crit Care Med* 152:906-910, 1995.
189. Phagoo SB, Wilson NM, Silverman M: Repeatability of methacholine challenge in asthmatic children measured by change in transcutaneous oxygen tension, *Thorax* 47:804-808, 1992.

CHAPTER 64

Asthma Treatment

Louis I. Landau

DIAGNOSIS

Appropriate treatment is initially dependent on the correct diagnosis being made. As described in the previous section, this is primarily determined by evaluation of accurate and appropriate historical information. Physical examination may help support the diagnosis, define severity, and exclude alternative diagnoses. Diagnostic tests are of limited value in most children with asthma. Lung function measurements will be of value in older children, particularly when historical events are not clear and objective measures of the degree of airway obstruction with response to bronchodilator is helpful. Most children who are old enough should have spirometry performed at least once. In those with severe disease, spirometry will be repeated at each visit. In others, peak flow measures may be adequate. A small group with troublesome asthma may require peak flow monitoring at home, some for a short period until symptoms are controlled, whereas others with persisting unstable asthma may continue regular peak flow monitoring to document early deterioration and the need for increasing medication.

A chest radiograph may be helpful for very young infants in whom alternative diagnoses are more common, for those with severe disease, and for those with localizing signs on physical examination. However, chest radiographs are not necessary for all children with mild asthma.

Skin allergy testing, RAST testing, and total IgE measurements may be useful additional tests to document atopy in those with an uncertain diagnosis. Rarely will they provide additional information to identify specific environmental allergens responsible for symptoms. Children with such reactions usually have a clear history. One can predict that most children will show a skin and RAST response to house dust mites in those areas where it is prevalent, grass and tree pollens, molds, and cat fur. Some will respond to various food agents, but this need not necessarily indicate clinically significant allergy to that substance. Production of IgE is a normal phase in the development of tolerance to many foods. More than 90% of those with respiratory symptoms caused by food allergens will also have a skin disorder. Occasionally these tests may be helpful in convincing the parents that the child is not allergic to a particular substance and does not require elimination of that substance from the diet.

The assessment of asthma is usually based on the pattern of wheeze and breathlessness. Cough is usually associated with these symptoms. Some have argued that asthmatics may present with cough alone and have called this entity cough variant asthma. Evidence would suggest that it is reasonably uncommon.[1] Those children with cough alone are less atopic and less responsive to challenges with cold dry air, exercise, or methacholine and more responsive to capsaicin, suggesting that they have what could be called a hypersensitive cough receptor syndrome, which is not particularly responsive to asthma medication.

Some children present with recurrent atelectasis incorrectly diagnosed on chest radiograph as recurrent pneumonia.[2] This appears to be related to increased mucus production-forming eosinophil and mucous plugs or casts of the airways. This pattern is sometimes called hypersecretory asthma.

The diagnosis of asthma is particularly difficult during the first year of life. Wheezing associated with lower respiratory illness occurs in more than 30% of infants during this period. Uncommonly, it may be due to conditions such as cystic fibrosis, milk aspiration, or congenital structural abnormalities. In many cases it may relate to smaller airway caliber as a result of factors, including a familial predisposition, male gender, or maternal smoking during pregnancy. In approximately one third of infants the wheezing will represent the early onset of asthma. It is often difficult to differentiate those with smaller airways from those with early-onset asthma.

SEVERITY

The asthma severity of each child should be assessed so that treatment can be individualized. Most of the information can be obtained from an accurate history of symptoms, although some cases will require supporting objective evidence with lung function measurements. Children must be asked specifically if they have a cough or wheeze and whether this occurs regularly or intermittently. This can often be determined by asking (1) whether the child wakes at night because of cough or wheeze; (2) whether he or she has cough or wheeze on waking first thing in the morning requiring urgent bronchodilator therapy; (3) whether the child's sport or physical activity is limited by cough, wheeze, or tightness in the chest; (4) how frequently the child require bronchodilator for symptom relief; (5) whether a metered-dose inhaler lasts at least 1 to 2 months; and (6) whether school attendance has been affected by symptoms. Information regarding the use of medication should be sought because inappropriate medications such as antibiotics, antihistamines, and nonprescription medications may be given for symptoms that are actually caused by asthma.

Poorly controlled asthma will be recognized by the presence of these symptoms, excessive use of reliever medication, inadequate length of response to reliever medication, and supporting evidence of abnormal lung function.

Treatment will be based on the pattern of symptoms, which can be classified as infrequent episodic (75% of childhood asthmatics), frequent episodic (20%), and persistent (5%). The latter can be defined as mild persistent, moderate persistent, or severe persistent. Criteria for this classification are shown in Table 64-1.

Table 64-1 Severity of Asthma

PATTERN	INFREQUENT EPISODIC	FREQUENT EPISODIC	PERSISTENT
Wheeze, tightness, cough infection or exercise	Occasional (e.g., with viral)	Most days	Every day
Nocturnal asthma	Usually absent	<once per 4-6 weeks	>once per week
Asthma on waking	Usually absent	<once per 4-6 weeks	>once per week
Hospital admission in past year	Absent	Usually not	Usually
Previous life-threatening attack	Absent	Usually not	May have a history
Bronchodilator use	Infrequent	Needed most weeks	Needed most days
FEV_1 (%predicted)	Normal	Normal/low	Usually low
Mean peak flow variability over 2 weeks	10%-20%	20%-30%	>30%

$$\text{Mean Peak Flow Variability \%} = \frac{(\text{Highest} - \text{Lowest})}{\text{Highest}} \times 100$$

High-risk patients for life-threatening asthma may be recognized by (1) repeated visits to the doctor or emergency department or admissions to a hospital, especially the intensive care unit; (2) previous life-threatening attacks; (3) poor compliance with treatment, especially in teenagers and young adults; (4) poor perception of symptoms; (5) persistently abnormal lung function measurements; (6) denial of asthma; and (7) overt psychosocial problems. However, it must be recognized that there is a risk of dying from asthma in every child with asthma, and every child should be carefully assessed and appropriately managed to minimize that risk.

PRINCIPLES OF MANAGEMENT

Although asthma is now clearly recognized as a disease associated with airway inflammation and characterized by hyperresponsiveness of the airways with reversible airway obstruction, there are many differences between children and adults. About 30% of children will have respiratory symptoms consistent with asthma during childhood, and many will cease to wheeze. Because two-thirds do have mild symptoms that can be easily controlled and are not necessarily associated with increasing morbidity in adult life, aggressive treatment with early introduction of steroids cannot be justified at this time in this group. In those with moderate to severe symptoms, there is certainly sufficient evidence that better control of symptoms with inhaled corticosteroids can be supported.

Most children who wheeze are young and are not able to coordinate well enough to use metered-dose inhalers (MDIs) or dry powder inhalers (DPIs) effectively. However, spacer devices and other aids ensure that children from the first year of life can still be treated with aerosol medications provided the method of delivery is suited for the age of the patient.

There appears to be an age-related difference in response to medications with younger children less responsive to β agonists. This should be taken into account when planning treatment regimens so that unnecessary excessive doses of medication that would cause side effects without benefit are avoided.

An extensive education program involving the child, the parents, other health professionals, and the physician in comanagement is vital to ensure complete understanding of the natural history of the disease and the roles of particular medications. Without this understanding, adherence will be severely compromised. It is also important that the health professionals address real concerns of the parents that may not be related purely to the symptoms presented at consultation. Written material in the form of action plans with detailed personalized information as illustrated in Fig. 64-1 is necessary to improve adherence. Peak flow meters may be of additional value for those with troublesome asthma and poor perception of symptoms. However, peak flow meters are not necessary to improve control of symptoms in the vast majority of children.[3] Support groups can help with information and encouragement. A detailed discussion of important components of the education program is found in Chapter 65.

The immediate aims of treatment are (1) to make the correct diagnosis; (2) to abolish symptoms; and (3) to maximize lung function. In the long term, one should aim for the following:

1. Maintain the child symptom free.
2. Maintain best lung function at all times. Those with persistent asthma will have spirometry at each consultation. Those with troublesome symptoms may have a peak flow meter at home. The aim is to ensure lung function remains within normal limits for each individual child and that diurnal variation in peak flow is less than 10%.
3. Avoid need for extra bronchodilators.
4. Prevent the restriction of normal childhood activities.
5. Prevent the development of irreversible airway obstruction.
6. Reduce risk of death from acute attacks of asthma.
7. Avoid unnecessary side effects from medications.

TRIGGER FACTORS

Continued exposure to allergens and other trigger factors may be associated with worsening of asthma. Avoidance of trigger factors should be considered at all times to maximize potential for improvement of the asthma.

The role of sensitization in utero is uncertain. Some studies suggest that restriction of cow's milk, soy protein, and eggs during pregnancy may help. However, most studies do not show any benefit from restrictive diets during pregnancy, and severe restriction can be detrimental with impaired nutrition to the mother and the fetus. At present, there are no proven strategies for prenatal avoidance.

Some avoidance measures may be justified after birth in those at high risk. It is not easy to accurately identify those at risk. Although cord blood IgE levels have been found by some to be elevated, albeit at very low levels, in those with a risk of asthma and atopy, many who become asthmatic do not have high levels, so this is not a clinically useful test for prediction of atopic disease. At present, the family history is the most useful criterion, with increasing probability of atopy when one parent, and especially two parents, or siblings have such a history.[4] The season of birth has been associated with increased airway responsiveness, especially in Finns exposed to birch pollen allergen.[5] Exposure to high levels of house dust mites in the first year

ASTHMA MANAGEMENT PLAN FOR YOUNG PEOPLE

NAME:____________________ DATE:__________ BEST PEAK FLOW__________
(6 years and over)

WHEN WELL **PEAK FLOW**

Take preventer (if prescribed):____________________ ABOVE:

Dose:____________________ How often:__________

Take reliever:____________________ Dose:__________ __________

(Take only when necessary for relief of symptoms)

Before exercise, take:____________________

WHEN NOT WELL **PEAK FLOW**

At the first sign of a cold or if asthma symptoms get worse:

Take reliever:____________________ BETWEEN:

Dose:____________________ How often:__________ __________

Take preventer if prescribed:____________________ AND

Dose:____________________ How often:__________ __________

When your symptoms get better, return to the treatment when well.

IF SYMPTOMS GET WORSE **PEAK FLOW**

Extra steps to take:

- ____________________ LESS THAN
- ____________________
- ____________________ __________
- Emergency medication:____________________ Dose:__________

  Take:____________________

  ____

  ____

If you follow this plan but your symptoms get worse, see a doctor immediately or call an ambulance.

AMBULANCE **DOCTOR** **HOSPITAL**

Fig. 64-1. Asthma management plan for young people.

of life has been reported to be associated with troublesome asthma symptoms over the next 8 years.[6]

Some foods and additives may trigger attacks of asthma. There are no foods that affect all asthmatics, therefore their role needs to be considered individually in each patient. A common trigger is the preservative sodium metabisulfite, commonly present in dried fruits, sausages, wines, and other drinks, which releases sulfur dioxide, especially in the presence of acid drinks. Cold drinks may lead to increased airway responsiveness, especially in Asian children. There are anecdotal reports of asthma attacks caused by monosodium glutamate and tartrazine, but no consistent observations. Occasionally foods such as nuts, shellfish, strawberries, eggs, and cow's milk will produce an acute response, but this is usually associated with generalized anaphylaxis and is obviously recognized. If uncertain, double-blind challenge may be necessary.

Attempts have been made to influence the induction of asthma in early childhood by dietary modification. Maternal restriction of cow's milk, eggs, and nuts during pregnancy and postnatally with subsequent breastfeeding followed by soy supplements and a restrictive infant diet without cow's milk, eggs, or fish has been reported to be associated with a decrease in eczema and gastrointestinal symptoms[7] and on one occasion a decrease in asthma.[8] Wheeze has been noted to be less with breastfeeding in the first few months,[9] but even more so in nonatopics,[10] possibly related to reduced respiratory infections. The effect on asthma is not consistent, and the observations have been associated with multiple changes in the environment, and these need to be sorted out before restrictive diets can be recommended. There is little evidence that soya replacement is significantly better than cow's milk formula. At present, one could suggest that those infants born to parents with a strong family history of atopy should be breastfed during the first year of life and that in the latter half of the first year of life foods be introduced carefully one at a time with a particular preference for less allergenic foods such as rice, vegetables, and noncitrus fruits and avoidance of eggs and nuts.

Aeroallergens are the agents to which most asthmatics develop long-term sensitization, and this sensitization is associated with persistence of symptoms. A direct causal relationship is not always clear, and further studies must be done to clarify this association between sensitization and symptoms. From present knowledge it does seem reasonable to exclude furry pets, particularly cats whose fur is often coated with saliva with enzymes that assist passage across the epithelial surfaces. It may take many months for the environment to clear of cat fur allergens.[11] There is no evidence that particular dogs are nonallergenic. If it is not possible to exclude pets, then they should be kept out of the child's bedroom.

Even though house dust mite sensitization is one of the more common associations with continuing asthma,[12] avoidance measures have not always proved successful. Extreme measures such as admitting subjects to a hospital or living in alpine environments does appear to be associated with a decrease in sensitization and improvement in symptoms and lung function. Less extreme measures do not often work. Murray and Ferguson[13] have shown benefit with pillows encased or replaced regularly, mattresses encased with thick plastic, bedding warm washed, and humidity kept at less than 50%. Pulling up carpets, high-grade filters, acaricides, and special vacuum cleaners have not consistently shown significant benefit.

Pollens, particularly in some environments, have been shown to be important allergens, but it is difficult to do much that will influence exposure. Molds, particularly alternaria, are again important inducers of sensitization, but they are outdoor allergens, and little can be done except ensuring that the humidity in the house is decreased. Cockroach allergens may also be important, and cockroach eradication may be helpful.

Exposure to environmental tobacco smoke is associated with increased asthma, and maternal smoking has been documented to be associated with increased symptoms, decreased lung function, and increased airway responsiveness, and to be responsible for up to 20% of acute attacks of asthma and for an increase in emergency room visits.[14-16] An improvement has been documented with cessation of parental smoking.[17] However, avoidance of exposure to environmental tobacco smoke has not been shown to be associated with a reduced prevalence of asthma. Active smoking becomes an important trigger for progression of symptoms and should be considered in all children from the age of 10 years.

Although external pollution is an important cause of lower respiratory symptoms, particularly bronchitis, and for the triggering of asthma symptoms, it has not been shown to be a major factor associated with an increased prevalence of asthma.[18] Pollutants can be associated with increased atopy and airway responsiveness and may initiate attacks of asthma in those with the disease. Ozone[19] and traffic pollutants[20] have been reported to be associated with increased airway responsiveness and atopy to local allergens. Public health measures to reduce pollution will be of benefit. Filters and ionizers have not been found to have any clinically significant benefit.

Drugs are not a common cause of asthma attacks in children. Aspirin and other nonsteroidal antiinflammatory drugs rarely cause symptoms in younger children. β Blockers, either orally or as eyedrops, should be avoided or used with caution because these can certainly cause severe asthma in children.[21] Paints and other fumes can usually be avoided. Gastroesophageal reflux has been reported to be associated with exacerbations of asthma, but this has not been found to be common in children. Obstructive sleep apnea and rhinitis have also been associated with increased asthma symptoms, but this does not seem to be a particularly common association in children.

It is recommended that children with chronic asthma receive influenza vaccination. The benefits for this in children with asthma have not been documented.

Exercise is an important trigger of asthma but should not be avoided. With appropriate warm-up sprints so that tachyphylaxis can be induced and premedication with β_2 agonists or sodium cromoglycate if necessary, a more sustained period of exercise will not cause significant symptoms. Approximately 30-second sprints every 2 minutes for 10 to 20 minutes have been shown to be a useful warm-up.[22]

Physiotherapy is used in asthma for specific purposes. Those with mucous plugging and subsequent atelectasis will benefit with physiotherapy as well as adequate treatment of their asthma. This group often needs steroids to reduce the mucus hypersecretion. Physiotherapists have an important role as part of the health care team in educating the children in use of their aerosol devices.

DRUG TREATMENT

Current concepts on the use of drugs in asthma are based on the treatment of the underlying inflammatory disease as well as prevention and treatment of acute attacks of asthma associated with environmental triggers.[23] These attacks of asthma will be treated with reliever medications such as β_2 agonists, ipratropium bromide, and theophylline. The underlying disease process is generally controlled with sodium cromoglycate, nedocromil, inhaled and oral corticosteroids, and possibly oral theophylline.

In children the initial treatment for those with mild episodes less than every 2 months and free of symptoms in between attacks is with intermittent short-acting aerosol β_2 agonists such as salbutamol (albuterol) or terbutaline.

β_2 Agonists

β_2 Agonists act through the β_2 receptor, which is a G protein–linked receptor in the cell membrane. Stimulation causes activation of adenylcyclase, which opens K+ channels and catalyzes the production of cyclic adenosine monophosphate (cAMP).

β_2 Agonists relax smooth muscle, decrease vascular permeability, increase mucociliary clearance, and decrease mucus secretion. They may modulate mediator release from mast cells. There appears to be an age effect, with these agents having little effect in normal infants under the age of 12 months and increasing effect from 1 to 5 years.[24] They have a greater effect in infants born preterm in the first year of life, and this may be related to the greater amount of smooth muscle seen more peripherally in the airways of these infants. Receptors are certainly present, and β_2 agonists in the early months of life can block the response to mediator challenge.[25] The drugs are safe and effective. They produce acute bronchodilation and prevent exercise-induced bronchoconstriction. They should almost always be used by aerosol. Once again, there may well be significant differences in deposition with age, although these have not been defined. Inhalation of agents through the nose and breathing patterns of infants lead to reduced deposition in younger infants. However, a lack of response rarely justifies increasing the dosage in infants because it is unlikely that they will respond to the higher dosages. It is important to use the minimum dosage needed to produce the beneficial effect without side effects.

Salbutamol (albuterol) and terbutaline have similar β_2 selectivity, although fenoterol may be a little less selective. Duration of action is normally up to 4 to 6 hours, with maximum effect for 1 to 2 hours, and an onset of action between 3 and 10 minutes.

Inhaler Devices

Inhaler devices will be used with MDIs with or without spacer, DPIs, or nebulizers in children (Table 64-2). Clear instructions are essential. Children must be observed repeatedly using these devices to ensure that technique is satisfactory because they will often revert to bad habits despite detailed instructions. Most children over the age of 7 years can use an MDI, a DPI, or the breath-activated autohaler. Some may be helped with a large volume (750 ml) spacer, which will improve deposition and may, in some cases, allow larger doses to be given to have an effect similar to a nebulizer during an acute attack. Some children will need a nebulizer if they have severe acute attacks of asthma or troublesome chronic asthma.

Children from 4 to 7 years can use an MDI with the large volume spacer. This can be inhaled through the mouth as a single breath or with panting tidal maneuvers, both being equally effective. Only 1 to 2 actuations at a time should be used because any larger number significantly reduces the available respirable particles.[26] Spacers should be washed with detergent and left to dry, not wiped, to reduce electrostatic forces that cause increased aerosol fallout. Some can use the DPI, but deposition is unreliable in those less than 5 years old,[27] especially during symptomatic periods when inspiratory flow rates are low. A rate of at least 30 L/min is required for optimal deaggregation and appropriate deposition of particles. It is not clear whether the breath-actuated autohaler is of significant benefit in this age group.

Table 64-2 Medication Delivery for Young Children

ROUTE ADMINISTRATION	LESS THAN 4 YEARS	4-6 YEARS	7 YEARS AND OLDER
Nebulizer	Yes	Yes	Yes
MDI/small volume spacer/mask	Yes		
MDI/large volume spacer		Yes	Yes
DPI		Sometimes	Yes
MDI			Yes

Always assess compliance and delivery technique when symptom control or response to medication is poor.
MDI, Metered dose inhaler; *DPI,* dry powder inhaler.

Below 4 years of age, MDIs with a small volume spacer and face mask can provide adequate deposition and similar therapeutic response to that seen with nebulizers.[28,29]

In some societies, access to and cost of these devices are a particular problem, and a large plastic coffee cup or half of a 1-liter plastic Coke bottle may be modified to produce a reasonable spacer device.

Nebulizers are effective because large doses can be administered and breathing pattern does not have as significant an effect on deposition, but they are bulky and expensive and not necessary for most asthmatics. An MDI and spacer with 6 to 10 puffs of β_2 agonist will produce almost the same result as a nebulizer. Nebulizers with a venturi design to drive air through the fluid and with a separate expiratory valve provide a better dose of drug.

MDIs are available as salbutamol 100 μg and terbutaline 250 μg. One to two puffs are usually used in normal symptomatic periods, but six to ten puffs in a spacer may be used during a severe acute attack. DPIs usually contain the equivalent of two puffs. Nebulizing solutions contain the equivalent of 2.5 μg or 5 μg of salbutamol, or 10 μg of terbutaline per ml and approximately 0.02 to 0.03 ml/kg of these solutions is usually used.

Common side effects of the β_2 agonists include tremor,[30] tachycardia headache, and hyperactivity. Large doses may be associated with hypokalemia and alteration of the ST segment on electrocardiograms. In vitro tolerance or tachyphylaxis to β_2 agonists is seen with long-term use. Tolerance to both side effects such as tremor and protection against inhalational challenge is also shown with regular use. The clinical significance is not clear, especially because the bronchodilator response does not appear to be significantly affected. Some epidemiologic studies have documented an association with long-term use more than 4 times daily and increased morbidity and mortality,[31,32] but this relationship is not consistent and has not been proven to be causal, clinically significant, or a particular problem in children. However, increased airway responsiveness has been shown with withdrawal of β_2 agonist after long-term use,[33] and this observation in association with the metabolic and cardiac effects that can be seen with these agents provide biologic plausibility for a potential risk. Thus it appears reasonable to attempt to maintain minimal use of β_2 agonists that will control symptoms. It must be remembered that some children will still require β_2 agonists long term and that in these situations the benefit outweighs the potential risks.

Preventive Agents

Preventive agents are used to prevent exacerbations and are thought to control the inflammatory process. Sodium cromoglycate or nedocromil are generally used in those with mild to moderate asthma, even though their long-term effect on the inflammatory process is not clear. Inhaled corticosteroids are used in those with severe asthma or those who fail to respond to sodium cromoglycate and nedocromil. Indications for the introduction of preventive agents are not clear-cut, but most would agree that symptoms or the need for β agonists more than twice weekly, attacks of asthma more than every 2 months, any life-threatening attacks of asthma, abnormal lung function in the interval phase especially with increased diurnal variation of peak flows, and interference of normal lifestyle because of symptoms would justify the introduction of preventive agents. There is argument whether to use a low dosage of inhaled corticosteroids and increase if necessary or to start with a high dosage to gain maximum control and an effective baseline and then reduce the dosage while maintaining the effect. Both are probably appropriate—those with moderate symptoms could start at a low dosage ICS because it is unlikely that any increase will be required; those with severe disease should be bought under best control with a high dosage then weaned to the minimum required.

Sodium Cromoglycate

Sodium cromoglycate has been shown to be an effective preventive agent in some children and is good particularly for preventing the bronchoconstriction associated with exercise. It also decreases both the immediate and late response following an allergen challenge. It is a mast cell stabilizer but stronger mast cell stabilizers such as β agonists do not block the late allergen response. It may influence cytokine production and release, and it appears to have some effect on nonadrenergic, noncholinergic nerve endings and neuropeptides. Long-term treatment may lead to reduced airway responsiveness, but this is not consistently found. It must be used by aerosol and is usually given as two puffs of 5 mg per puff MDI 2 or 3 times daily or in a nebulizer solution with 20 mg of sodium cromoglycate for wheezy infants.[34] In some countries only a 1 mg per puff MDI is available. It is a very useful drug in those 25% to 50% that do respond. It is generally free of side effects, although some complain of the taste and develop cough following inhalation.

Nedocromil Sodium

Nedocromil sodium is a novel antiinflammatory agent that appears to have a similar place to sodium cromoglycate. Further trials are needed to see whether it has a further or different role in children than that so far described in adults.[35] Children usually cease sodium cromoglycate or nedocromil sodium when they have failed to work and inhaled corticosteroids have been started. Some suggest that they may be continued in this situation for their corticosteroid sparing effect. This has not been consistently noted.[36] Therefore a combination is not justified as a routine but is worth considering in those requiring high-dose inhaled corticosteroids.

Inhaled Corticosteroids

Inhaled corticosteroids are used in those who have severe symptoms or those who have failed to respond to sodium cromoglycate or nedocromil sodium.[37] They are antiinflammatory agents that exert their effect after binding to a glucocorticoid receptor in the cytoplasm, which then moves into the nuclear compartment where it regulates the transcription of target genes, leading to many actions including the modification of arachidonic acid metabolism, synthesis of prostaglandins and leukotrienes, as well as decreasing vascular leakage, inhibiting cytokines, preventing activation and migration of inflammatory cells, and augmenting β_2-receptor responsiveness. They are associated with decreased airway responsiveness to histamine and the late reaction to allergens, but they do not alter the early allergen response and do not induce permanent cure as these responses return after cessation of inhaled corticosteroids even when used for many years.[38,39] Inhaled corticosteroids are available as beclomethasone, budesonide, fluticasone, and triamcinolone in doses of 50, 100, 250, 400, and 500 μg per puff. Rapid topical biotransformation reduces the amount of active metabolite absorbed. Budesonide and fluticasone are more potent and lipophilic than the others, and this is associated with increased activity, decreased absorption, and first pass hepatic cytochrome P-450 metabolism. This tends to allow improved effect with smaller doses and decreased side effects.[40] In childhood, most physicians aim to obtain an effect at less than 400 μg/day because the maximum improvement is seen between 100 and 400 μg and this dosage minimizes any potential for side effects. Above 800 μg the dose-response curve flattens with less improvement for the same increase in dosage and greater risk of side effects. The agents are administered as MDIs, PDIs, and nebulizers. A large volume spacer with an MDI will decrease side effects as a result of raining out of larger particles, which are then not swallowed or deposited in the mouth.[41] A mouth rinse following PDIs will decrease absorption and side effects. Some have documented increased deposition with PDIs and recommend a reduction in dosage when changing to this form of administration.[42] Budesonide is available as a nebulizer solution. This is rarely needed, although it may be helpful in some infants with troublesome symptoms. In this case goggles and face cream should be used and/or face wash washed after administration to decrease topical side effects. If possible, attempts are made to administer these drugs in young infants through MDI, small volume spacer, and face mask.

Some would introduce inhaled corticosteroids at the lowest possible dosage and increase as required. Others recommend maximal steroid dosage, as oral steroid or high-dose inhaled corticosteroid, to produce the optimal response, then weaning the dosage. It is likely that each has its place. In those with frequent episodic asthma not controlled with sodium cromoglycate, a low dosage of inhaled corticosteroid is likely to be effective. However, those with persistent symptoms and abnormal lung function would be more suitable for an initial high dosage regimen and weaning down to a level that maintains the improvement obtained.

Some studies have suggested that a greater improvement in lung function is achieved if steroids are introduced sooner after a diagnosis of asthma is made, suggesting prevention of irreversible changes. Selection bias cannot be ruled out in these studies, and confirmation is needed before earlier introduction of steroids can be justified in children.

Side effects have been reported with all dosages, although they appear to be clinically insignificant below 400 μg/day. Suppression of the hypothalamic-pituitary-adrenal (HPA) axis with reduced cortisol levels[43] have been reported, but few studies show a significant effect below 800 μg. Cushingoid appearance can be seen in some children following the use of inhaled corticosteroids, but there appears to be significant individual variation. The effects on bone turnover and growth are inconsistent. The problem is confounded by the fact that asthma itself will have an effect on growth and pubertal development and it becomes difficult to separate the two. Some have not documented any effect on growth, serum calcium and phosphorus, bone density, or osteocalcin levels,[44] but others have shown delayed puberty with subsequent catch-up,[45] some have found reduced osteocalcin levels,[46] and some documented decreased growth measured by knemometry,[47] at dosages above 400 μg/day.[48] A significant effect on growth has been demonstrated in mild asthmatics given 400 μg/day. This is evidence of a systemic effect, but this does not correlate with long-term growth. Linear growth was not affected in young children at 200 μg/day, but was reduced at 400 and especially 800 μg/day. Hoarseness, oral thrush, and cough are relatively common and can usually be minimized by using spacers. Purpura, bruising, psychological disturbances, and posterior subcapsular cataracts have all been occasionally reported.

Corticosteroids are usually given twice daily, although some have documented benefit when used once daily[49] and others would suggest that they should be given around 3 PM because this has been documented to produce maximum effect with oral corticosteroid medications.[50] One should aim to reduce the dosage to the minimum needed with occasional increases for intercurrent exacerbations. Consideration of reduction in dosage should be given every 6 months if the patient is symptom free.

Other Medications

If there is no response to a regular dosage of inhaled corticosteroids, a variety of options are available, none of which has been consistently proven to be superior.[51] Some would add long-acting β_2 agonists. Others would consider leukotriene-receptor antagonists or theophylline as appropriate. It is usually reasonable to increase the dosage of inhaled corticosteroid, but further benefit with dosages above 1 mg/day is difficult to demonstrate. It may be preferable to use a more powerful locally acting corticosteroid. Troleandomycin (TAO) has been suggested to be steroid sparing. It does increase the half-life,[52] but it also increases the side effects.[53] Some children appear to be steroid resistant. The mechanism is uncertain, although changes in receptor binding have been suggested. It is important to recognize this phenomenon to avoid unnecessary side effects with overuse when the drug is not likely to be effective.

Oral Steroids

Oral prednisolone or methylprednisolone may be used in a very small group of children as a trial to diagnose asthma, for acute management of a severe attack, and in some with troublesome chronic asthma for long-term treatment. High dosages of 1 to 2 mg/kg will be necessary to achieve control, but it should then be used in the lowest possible dosage, and this may be as low as 1 to 2 mg/day. Some children can be managed on alternate day regimens, although this is not a consistent finding. Most will use oral prednisolone intermittently for episodes of acute deterioration. Long-term treatment can be associated with reduced growth, HPA axis suppression, hypertension, posterior subcapsular cataracts, and psychological changes.

Nonsteroidal Antiinflammatory Agents

Many other antiinflammatory agents have been tried in those not responding to moderate dosages of steroids. Methotrexate appears to help some but is not uniformly effective.[54] Gammaglobulins have been used, but consistent benefit has not been confirmed.[55] It has been noted that gold may have a steroid-sparing effect.[56] Nifedipine has been associated with a reduction in circadian peak flow variation.[57] PAF antagonists[58] and inhaled diuretics are being tried experimentally, but as yet have no clinical application.

Theophylline

Theophyllines have been widely used in the past. They are bronchodilators with considerable extrapulmonary effects. Some have argued that they have an effect on late response to allergen challenge and that they have antiinflammatory activity as a result of more selective phosphodiesterase inhibition in small doses.[59] They produce some muscle relaxation, increase mucociliary clearance, inhibit mediator release, suppress edema, stimulate ventilation, and reduce diaphragmatic fatigue. With long-term use they do not lead to a reduction in the inflammatory infiltrate or nonspecific airway hyperresponsiveness. They may be useful in acute attacks by reducing diaphragm fatigue and by central nervous system stimulation. They are available orally in slow-release preparations and remain useful in some children with troublesome nocturnal symptoms. Absorption may be erratic and leads to considerable variation in serum levels. They are usually given at dosages of approximately 5 mg/kg of regular theophylline up to six hourly, or 7 to 8 mg/kg of the slow-release preparation every 12 hours. The dosage may be increased if a therapeutic response is not obtained with an aim to a serum level of 55 to 110 mmol/L (10 to 20 mg/L). The drug has a narrow therapeutic index, with side effects often seen even at therapeutic dosages. Some are due to direct irritation of the gastrointestinal tract, such as nausea and vomiting, whereas others are associated with increased serum levels. These side effects include vomiting, hematemesis, tachycardia, and dysrhythmia. With long-term use, headache, learning difficulties, sleep disturbance, and behavioral problems[60] have been reported, but theophyllines are more likely to exacerbate these symptoms in those predisposed. Uncommonly, convulsions and death may develop. These drugs may also aggravate gastroesophageal reflux. Serum levels must be monitored in those taking high-dose theophylline or those experiencing side effects. Levels also should be monitored with conditions that alter theophylline metabolism, such as fever, liver disease, and concomitant use of drugs like cimetidine and macrolide antibiotics. Currently theophyllines are being considered as an added option for those needing high-dose inhaled corticosteroids in an attempt to allow reduction in steroid dosage.

Anticholinergic Agents

The anticholinergic agent ipratropium bromide will block the postganglionic efferent vagal pathways leading to bronchodilation associated with decreased vagal tone.[61] It blocks the reflex bronchoconstriction to irritants but has no effect on the early or late response to antigen challenge or on the inflammatory response. Some would suggest that these agents have an additive effect to β_2 agonists with acute attacks of asthma and should be used for anyone with moderately severe symptoms, and some would consider that they be used occasionally for long-term management. They are certainly useful for those who have significant side effects such as tremor with high-dose β_2 agonists. They are administered as an MDI using two to four puffs of 20 μg/puff, or as a nebulizer with 250 μg/dose. They have a slow onset of action, with maximum effect at 30 to 60 minutes. They have few systemic side effects, although paradoxical bronchoconstriction has been reported and may be due to the effect on M1 and M2 receptors, which may cause increased acetylcholine release as well as the block of M1 receptors at the neuromuscular junction and of M3 receptors on smooth muscle and mucous glands. High dosages given frequently to young infants cause significant skin vascular dilation. Currently, they are used in some centers in association with β_2 agonists for the acute management of asthma.[62] They may be used in those requiring high-dose corticosteroids or those who experience significant side effects with β_2 agonists. Some consider that they may be more effective in those with postviral cough or cough-variant asthma, although this needs further study. Some reported better response in infants under 18 months of age although this has not proven to be consistent.[63] Some consider that they may be effective in infants with chronic lung disease of prematurity.

Long-Acting β_2 Agonists

Long-acting β_2 agonists such as salmeterol, formoterol, and bambuterol have lipophilic side chains, which ensure tighter binding to receptor sites and action up to 12 hours. They have a slightly slower onset of action than short-acting β_2 agonists, hence short-acting agents are necessary for bronchodilation during acute episodes and for protection against challenges.[64] Some antiinflammatory activity is argued, although this has not been confirmed. They are available as MDIs, and salmeterol has 25 μg/puff and is usually administered as two puffs twice daily. Side effects are the same as for short-acting β_2 agonists.[65] There have been concerns regarding the risk of long-acting β_2 agonists in view of the studies regarding regular short-acting β_2 agonist use. No clinically significant tachyphylaxis has been observed, but it is recommended that they be used in association with inhaled corticosteroids. Some early reports suggest that the combination of the long-acting β_2 agonist and regular dose inhaled corticosteroid may be more effective than high-dose inhaled corticosteroids, and they are currently used for long-term management in that situation.

Leukotriene Modifiers

The recent availability of leukotriene-receptor antagonists (Zafirlukast, Montelukast) and leukotriene-synthesis inhibitors (Zileuton) provide new mediator-specific therapy for asthma. Their specific role is not yet clear. They have been shown to block airway response to challenge and, in chronic asthma, to lead to improved lung function, reduced symptoms, and some steroid sparing. Few comparative studies have been done, but they appear less effective than steroids. Therefore specific recommendations cannot yet be made, but they may prove useful in mild asthma if an oral preparation is required and in those where steroid reduction is sought.

Other Agents

Ketotifen is a potent oral H_1-antagonist that has been shown to increase β_2 receptor density on lymphocytes with reduced levels, and it has been suggested that this agent is a useful preventive agent in asthma.[66] This benefit has not been consistently reported,[67] and most studies have shown minimal benefit compared with placebo, nor is there any evidence of any significant long-term benefit. One trial of ketotifen in infants with dermatitis demonstrated a decrease in the prevalence of subsequent asthma symptoms,[68] but this observation was associated with many confounders and must be confirmed. Drowsiness, dry mouth, and abnormal weight gain can be seen with long-term use.

Antihistamines may be used for many of the associated symptoms that occur in asthmatics such as rhinitis, eczema, and conjunctivitis but currently have no role in the management of the asthma. Cough suppressants and demulcents should not be used in the treatment of asthma. Antibiotics are rarely needed because bacterial infections, except for mycoplasma, Chlamydia, and pertussis, do not cause asthmatic wheezing and secondary infections are uncommon in children.

ALTERNATIVE THERAPIES

Many resort to alternative health therapies in asthma.[69] Most have failed to be shown to be effective where appropriate trials have been undertaken. Ionizers[70] and acupuncture[71] were shown to be ineffective in controlled trials. Most studies of homeopathy, yoga, and hypnosis have also been disappointing, although suggesting some individuals may benefit.

IMMUNOTHERAPY

The role of immunotherapy in asthma is continuing to be evaluated. At present, avoidance and pharmacotherapy are more appropriate initial approaches to management because they give good control without significant side effects. This makes immunotherapy with its moderate benefit and significant side effects less justified as an early intervention. Efficacy has been documented,[72] but the effect is mild and less than that obtained with antiinflammatory agents and associated with more side effects. It will be considered occasionally in highly selected children who are sensitive to a specific single allergen such as grass pollen, mites, or alternaria and when it can be done under specialist supervision and safe conditions. Usually it must be given for at least 3 years.

ONGOING TREATMENT

Specialist referral should be considered in anyone who has a life-threatening attack of asthma, frequent hospital admission, poor parental management, uncertainty of diagnosis, and poor response to regular treatment and regular doses.

The natural history of childhood asthma is for improvement, and a decrease in drug treatment and cessation of therapy should be considered every 6 months.

MANAGEMENT OF ACUTE ATTACKS

In spite of the availability of good preventive treatment, acute attacks still occur and are responsible for considerable hospital admissions and missed school days.

Assessment of Severity

Good management will be based on accurate assessment of each attack. Historical information is vital with clear documentation of the duration of symptoms, cause of the exacerbation, severity of symptoms, current medication, prior hospitalization, and past history of events such as syncopal fits. Physical examination for tachycardia, tachypnea, cyanosis, changes in demeanor, silent chest, use of accessory muscles, subcutaneous emphysema, and pulsus paradoxus of greater than 20 mm Hg should be undertaken to categorize severity as mild, moderate, or severe (Table 64-3). Attempts to develop reliable and predictive asthma scores have not been successful. Few extra investigations are needed. A chest radiograph is not routinely done but should be considered with differential chest signs that may indicate a complication such as lung collapse or pneumothorax. It may also be justified with unexplained deterioration or failure to respond to treatment. Peak flow or spirometric measurements can be made in older children without severe distress and should be performed when possible. Oximetry has proved to be a good predictor of subsequent progress.[73] Those with oxygen saturation of greater than 95% are likely to respond rapidly and be discharged. Those at 91% or less are very likely to require admission to a hospital. Those between 92% and 94% should be given aggressive therapy to achieve a satisfactory response.

Each acute attack of asthma is a failure of prophylaxis and prophylactic treatment does need to be reviewed.

Treatment

Treatment will usually be initiated at home with regular β-agonist treatment. Repeated β_2 agonists should be given for an acute attack of asthma not responding to standard treatment at home while seeking medical attention. Failure to respond should lead to a visit to the emergency room or doctor's office where β_2 agonist would be given through a nebulizer with oxygen (Table 64-4). Mild to moderate episodes can be treated with an MDI and spacer using 6 to 10 puffs, which can be given with 30 seconds between each actuation or some would give 2 actuations every 5 minutes. Some centers would use additional ipratropium bromide, suggesting that this results in a 10% increase in response and a greater duration of response.[74] If the child responds to this treatment, he or she should be observed for 1 to 4 hours and then sent home with continuing treatment. If the child does not respond optimally, steroids will be added.[75] Hydrocortisone in a dose of 4 mg/kg or prednisolone or methylprednisolone in doses of 1 to 2 mg/kg will generally be used. Although there has been controversy regarding the effects of steroids, their benefit in moderately ill patients has been documented.[76] The optimal dose is not known. Response can usually be documented between 4 and 12 hours. Some have recommended a single dose of corticosteroids in the emergency department,[77] but others have not shown that this significantly alters the natural history.[78] It does appear that if the child needs corticosteroids for an acute attack of asthma, then a short course should be given. Very large doses may be associated with side effects such as peptic ulceration, hypertension, behavioral disorder, and myopathy.

Table 64-3 Initial Assessment of Severity of Acute Asthma in Children

SYMPTOMS	MILD	MODERATE	SEVERE
	Probably manage at home	**May need hospital admission**	**Admission required**
Altered consciousness	No	No	Yes
Physical exhaustion	No	No	Yes
Talks in	Sentences	Phrases	Words
Pulsus paradoxus	Not palpable	May be palpable	Present
Central cyanosis	Absent	Absent	Present
Wheeze on auscultation	Present	Present	Present
Use of accessory muscles	Absent	Moderate	Marked
Sternal retraction (in young children)	Absent	Moderate	Marked
Initial PF or FEV_1 (% predicted or % child's best)	>60%	40%-60%	<40%
Oximetry on presentation before treatment (Sao_2)	>95%	92%-94%	<91%

Table 64-4 Initial Management of Acute Asthma in Children

TREATMENT	MILD	MODERATE	SEVERE
	Probably manage at home	**May need hospital admission**	**Admission required**
Nebulized short-acting β agonist	Single dose	3 doses at 20-min intervals	Continuous initially then hourly; when stable, decrease to second hourly
Oxygen	No	Up to 8 L/min by face mask to achieve Sao_2>93%	Up to 8 L/min by face mask to achieve Sao_2 >93%
Nebulized ipratropium with β agonist	No	Optional	250 μg/4 hr may be used (1 ml of 0.025%)
Corticosteroid	No	Consider	Yes; oral or IV
Aminophylline	No	No	Possible
Observation	For 1 hour, if improvement maintained—home	1 hour after last dose, if improvement maintained—home; if not, admit	Continuous and admit

Those not responding to treatment over 1 to 4 hours will require admission to a hospital. Admission criteria are based on severity of clinical signs, peak flow, Sao_2, and lack of response to bronchodilator, but admission is often influenced by social circumstances. The mainstay of treatment is repeated β_2 agonist (Table 64-5) in various dosing regimens, depending on response. Addition of ipratropium bromide will be considered in those with severe attacks because the data are inconsistent. Some, but not all, show benefit. Therefore in most centers it is still used in those who do not show a good response to β_2 agonist and steroids.

Careful clinical monitoring is essential with peak flow measurements in those able to perform the maneuver and Sao_2 in those with moderate to severe disease. If there is a continued deterioration or failure to respond, blood gases may be justified to document the level of $Paco_2$. Supplemental oxygen should be given to maintain Sao_2 above 93%.

Inadequate response to these regimens will warrant admission to the intensive care unit and may justify the addition of IV aminophylline. This is usually given as a single dose of 6 mg/kg over 30 minutes followed by 1 mg/kg/hr to maintain serum levels in the therapeutic range. The loading dose may be reduced or omitted if the child is on theophylline. The effects of aminophylline are not clear, although apart from bronchodilation it may help by stimulating ventilation and decreasing diaphragmatic fatigue. Aminophylline has been required less frequently because regular or even constant β_2 agonist inhalation has been used. In fact, some argue that it increases the toxicity without significant benefit.[79,80] Continuous nebulized β_2 agonists[81] or IV β_2 agonists will generally be used.[82] Experience with continuous nebulized β_2 agonists has been encouraging with reduced need for other interventions. Sedation or antibiotics are rarely required. Repeated assessment is important, and occasionally the child may require intubation and ventilation[83] if the $Paco_2$ continues to rise and the child tires. Intubation and ventilation should be performed by experienced pediatric practitioners because children with severe acute asthma can be very difficult to manage during induction and maintenance. Air leaks and hypoxic ischemic encephalopathy may occur. Administration of β agonists into the ventilator circuit can be difficult.

LONG TERM MANAGEMENT

Successful long-term management is achieved by adherence to a treatment strategy by the family, health care providers, and temporary caregivers such as teachers. Recently published guidelines provide algorithms that recommend currently agreed-upon good clinical practice (Tables 64-6 through 6-8). However, treatment must be individualized, and the ideal for each child will differ; choice provides an opportunity to find the most suitable regimen based on initial assessment and to then move up or down the protocol depending on the response.

Infrequent Episodic Asthma

Children with infrequent episodic asthma will usually require only intermittent inhaled short-acting β_2 agonists. The parents should be aware of signs such as runny nose, itchy throat, or cough for early recognition of an attack so that treatment can be instituted early. Treatment is usually continued until free of symptoms for at least 48 hours.

Table 64-5 Recommended Dosages for Bronchodilators for Acute Exacerbations

TREATMENT	FORMULATION	DOSAGE	COMMENT
Albuterol/salbutamol	Metered-dose inhaler (MDI) (90 μg/actuation or 100 μg/actuation)	2 actuations inhaled, may be repeated every 5 min for a total of 12 actuations if necessary. Then repeat between 20 min and 4 hr as required.	Monitor response via peak flows or spirometry, if possible. If improved, decrease frequency of administration, if not improved, switch to nebulizer.
	Nebulizer solution 0.5% (5 mg/ml)	0.10-0.15 mg/kg/dose up to 5 mg inhaled via nebulizer every 20 min for 1-2 hr if required. 0.5 mg/kg/hr by continuous nebulization.	If improved, decrease to 1 treatment every 1-4 hr, if not improved, use continuous inhalation. Maximum 15 mg/hr
Terbutaline	MDI (200 μg/actuation or 250 μg/actuation)	2 actuations inhaled, may be repeated every 5 min for total of 12 actuations if necessary. Then repeat 20 min and 4 hr as required.	
	Nebulizer solution (2 mg/2 ml)	0.2 mg/kg/dose to a maximum of 2 ml/4 hr as required.	
	Injectable solution 0.1 mg/ml in 0.9% sodium chloride or 0.5 mg/ml	0.01 mg/kg up to 0.3 mg injected subcutaneously every 2-6 hr as needed. 10 μg IV over 10 min as loading dose, then 0.4 μg/kg/min increased as needed by 0.2 μg/kg/min.	Inhaled bronchodilator preferred. Should expect to use 3-6 μg/kg/min for final maintenance dose.
Epinephrine/adrenaline	Injectable solution: 1:1000 (1 mg/ml)	0.01 ml/kg up to 0.3 ml injected subcutaneously every 20 min for a total of 3 doses.	Inhaled bronchodilator preferred.
Metaproterenol	MDI (650 μg/actuation or 750 μg/actuation)	2 actuations inhaled.	Frequent high-dose administration has not been evaluated, not interchangeable with albuterol or terbutaline.
	Nebulizer solution 5% (50 mg/ml)	0.1-0.3 ml (5-15 mg) inhaled via nebulizer.	Do not exceed 15 mg.
Ipratropium bromine	Nebulizer solution (250 μg/ml)	1 ml up to 4 times/day in older children. 0.5 ml up to 4 times/day in younger children.	

Table 64-6 Maintenance Medication for Children

CLASSIFICATION OF SEVERITY	COMMON FEATURES	MAINTENANCE THERAPY
Infrequent episode	Episodes more than 6-8 weeks apart. Attacks generally not severe. Physical examination and spirometry between attacks normal.	Nil preventive treatment; prn use of short-acting β agonist.
Frequent episode	Attacks <6-8 weeks apart. Attacks more troublesome. Increasing symptoms between attacks. Abnormal spirometry when symptomatic.	Begin with sodium cromoglycate/nedocrimil sodium. If not effective, use inhaled corticosteroids in minimum effective dose. Plus prn use of short-acting β agonists.
Persistent	Symptoms most days. Nocturnal asthma >3/week. Attacks <6-8 weeks apart. Daily use of short-acting β agonist. Abnormal lung function. History of A&E visits or hospital admissions.	Inhaled corticosteroid using minimum effective. If high dosages of inhaled steroids are required long term, consider specialist referral. Consider other drugs to minimize corticosteroid dosage (e.g., theophylline, cromoglycate, nedocromil, ipratropium, long-acting β agonists, or leukotriene-receptor antagonists).

Table 64-7 Recommended Dosages for Bronchodilators for Long-Term Care

DRUG	FORMULATION	DOSAGE
Albuterol/salmeterol	Metered-dose inhaler (MDI) (90 μg/actuation) (100 μg/actuation)	2 actuations inhaled up to every 4-6 hr.
	Dry powder inhaler (DPI) (200 μg/capsule)	Contents of 1 capsule inhaled every 4-6 hr.
	Nebulizer solution 0.5% (5 mg/ml)	0.10-0.15 mg/kg up to 5 mg in 2 ml sodium chloride inhaled via nebulizer every 4-6 hr.
	Oral syrup	0.1-0.2 mg/kg orally every 6-8 hr under 6 years (maximum 24 mg/day) from 6-14 years. Rarely needed. 2-4 mg orally every 6-8 hr (maximum 32 mg/day) over 14 years.
	Oral tablet, plain (2 mg)	2 mg orally every 6-8 hr (maximum 24 mg/day) from 6-14 years. 2-4 mg orally every 6-8 hr (maximum 32 mg/day) over 14 years.
	Oral tablet, extended release (4-8 mg)	4-8 mg orally every 6-8 hr (maximum 32 mg/day) over 12 years.
Biolterol	MDI (370 μg/actuation)	2 actuations inhaled every 8 hr (maximum 2 treatments in 4 hr or 3 treatments in 6 hr).
	Nebulizer solution 0.2% (2 mg/ml)	0.5-0.75 ml (1.0-1.5 mg) inhaled via nebulizer every 4-6 hr (maximum 8 mg/day).
Pirbuterol	MDI (200 μg/actuation)	2 actuations inhaled every 4-6 hr (maximum 12 actuations/day).
Terbutaline	MDI (200 μg/actuation or 250 μg/actuation)	2 actuations up to every 4-6 hr.
	Oral tablet (2.5 mg, 5mg)	2.5 mg orally every 8 hr from 12-15 years (maximum 7.5 mg/day).
	Oral syrup (1.5 mg/5ml)	2.5-5.0 ml orally every 6 hr, over 15 years (maximum 15 ml/day).
	DPI (500 μg/actuation)	1 actuation inhaled up to every 4-6 hr.
Metaproterenol	MDI (650 μg/actuation)	2-3 actuations inhaled up to 6-8 hr.
	Nebulizer solution 5% (50 mg/ml)	0.2-0.3 ml (10-15 mg) in 2.5 ml 0.9% sodium chloride inhaled via nebulizer every 6-8 hr.
	Oral syrup	1.3-2.6 mg/kg/day orally divided every 6-8 hr under 6 years. 10 mg orally every 6-8 hr from 6-10 years. 20 mg orally every 6-8 hr over 10 years.
Ipratropium bromide	MDI (18 μg/actuation) (20 μg/actuation)	2 actuations inhaled up to 4 times daily (maximum 12 actuations/day).
	Nebulizer solution (250 μg/ml)	1 ml up to 4 times/day in older children. 0.5 ml up to 4 times/day in younger children.
Salmeterol xinafoate	MDI (25 μg/actuation)	2 actuations twice daily.
	DPI (50 μg/actuation)	1 actuation twice daily.

Table 64-8 Recommended Dosages for Inhaled Glucocorticoids

DRUG	FORMULATION	DOSAGE
Beclomethasone dipropionate	Metered-dose inhaler (MDI) (42, 50, 100, 250 μg/actuation) Dry powder inhaler (DPI) (100 μg/actuation)	1-2 actuations inhaled twice daily. Dose dependent on severity of asthma and previous response.
Flunisolide	MDI (250 μg/actuation)	2 actuations inhaled every 12 hr up to 15 years. 4 actuations inhaled every 12 hr if required over 15 years.
Triamcinolone acetonide	MDI (100 μg/actuation with spacer included)	1-2 actuations inhaled twice daily and increased if needed.
Fluticasone	MDI (50, 250 μg/actuation) DPI (100, 500 μg/actuation)	1-2 actuations twice daily.
Budesonide	MDI (50, 100, 200 μg/actuation)	1-2 actuations twice daily; dose dependent on severity of asthma and previous response.
	DPI (100, 200 μg/actuation)	1 actuation twice daily.
Budesonide	Nebulizer suspension (250 μg/ml, 500 μg/ml)	250 or 500 μg twice daily for severe chronic asthma where an MDI with spacer or PDI not effective.

Frequent Episodic Asthma

Children with symptoms at least every month but with clear periods in between should be given a regular preventive agent. This will usually be sodium cromoglycate or nedocromil sodium, but if frequent bronchodilator is still required or peak flow diurnal variation continues to be at least 20%, then low-dose inhaled corticosteroids may be needed.

Persistent Asthma

Children with troublesome symptoms on most days will require inhaled corticosteroids once or twice daily with added bronchodilator as required. The starting dosage of inhaled steroids will depend on asthma severity. If symptoms are not well controlled, then regular peak flow measurements may be needed to monitor response to additional treatments that could be higher-dose inhaled corticosteroids, long-acting β_2 agonist, theophylline, ipratropium bromide, oral steroids, leukotriene-receptor antagonists, or other preventive agents. A spacer device should be used with inhaled corticosteroid used by an MDI or mouth rinsing and spitting out with dry powder devices.

The family must be aware of action to take if the child does not respond to the regular bronchodilator or if the response does not last 3 to 4 hours. This may require introduction of oral prednisolone (1 to 2 mg/kg) at home or attendance at a doctor's office or emergency room. Because asthma is often worse at night because of the normal circadian rhythm, the family must be comfortable that they can cope at that time. The reason for decreased peak flow and increased symptoms at night is not certain, but factors that may contribute include reduced catecholamines, reduced cortisone, increased vagal tone, cold dry air, allergens such as house dust mites, gastroesophageal reflux, and sleep state. Asthma has a tendency to interfere with activities at school, and efforts should be made to minimize any disruption. Teachers must be informed about asthma symptoms and how to respond. Schools should have a policy regarding administration of drugs. The family should provide the teacher with details of treatment that may be required at school.

In the past special schools and residential units were required for troublesome asthmatics. This is rarely necessary because children can be managed in a mainstream school program and can achieve excellence in study and sport and not be held back by their asthma.

SPECIFIC PROBLEMS

Infants

The wheezing infant is more difficult to manage because the diagnosis is often uncertain and response to therapy is decreased. Some may have a transient wheezy illness associated with viral infections, which settles over the first 1 to 2 years and is not associated with risk factors considered to be important for the development of asthma. Many will have other diagnoses such as viral bronchiolitis, cystic fibrosis, milk inhalation, and congenital abnormalities. Others will have chronic lung disease of prematurity or bronchopulmonary dysplasia. Some of these may be associated with asthma, and some may require the same treatment, although each must be considered individually.

The pathophysiology of wheezing in this age group is associated with smaller absolute size of the airways, decreased collateral channels, more peripheral airway smooth muscle, decreased static elastic recoil, and a mechanically disadvantaged chest wall so that wheezing is noted with milder degrees of airway obstruction. Hyperinflation occurs more readily, and carbon dioxide rises earlier in the course of the disease, so artificial ventilation will not be required at levels that may justify ventilation in older children. Lung function measurements are not easy in this age group. Arterial oxygen saturation may help, but decisions regarding the progress of the disease are generally dependent on clinical observation of alertness, feeding, cry, chest movement, and signs of hypoxia.

β_2 Agonists will generally be used, although response will be decreased. In the first year of life there is a negligible response in most infants, although some may respond, and a therapeutic trial may be justified, especially in the second 6 months. Some will show a significant decrease in Sao_2 that may be related to shunting by vascular dilation or bronchoconstriction to the tonicity or acidity of the aerosol. Anticholinergic agents are favored by some, although considerable benefit has not been documented. Inhaled corticosteroids and sodium cromoglycate have been used in some with chronic lung disease. The metabolism of theophylline is decreased in this age group and dosage adjustments need to be made.

Adolescents

Adherence with treatment during adolescence as a result of perceptions related to drug taking, body image, and being seen to be different is a problem, and this is associated with a significantly higher death rate from asthma in this age group. Smoking is common in those with asthma, and unfortunately the number is no less than in the general community in spite of the potential for significant deleterious effects on subsequent lung health. It appears to be part of the risk taking behavior that is normal in this age group. It is an important time for establishing rapport, improving educational techniques, and providing guidelines for better care.

CESSATION OF TREATMENT

Because asthma symptoms subside in 60% of childhood asthmatics, cessation of treatment should be regularly considered. Every 6 months, weaning could be considered if the child has remained asymptomatic. This should be gradual and with the assistance of lung function measurements.

FUTURE MANAGEMENT

The future in the management of asthma will be the prevention of the disease. Asthma prevalence has increased in the last 25 years, so it should certainly be possible to reduce the prevalence by at least half. Environmental manipulation may help; however, it is likely that it will be more important to identify those at risk and consider early intervention with avoidance measures, antiinflammatory agents, or vaccination during the critical period in early infancy when the predisposition to asthma appears to be set.

Although asthma cannot be cured at present, the increasing understanding of the development of asthma symptoms in early childhood may mean that early intervention in the future will lead to a cure.

REFERENCES

Diagnosis

1. Wright AL, Holberg C, Morgan WJ: Recurrent cough in childhood and its relation to asthma, *Am Respir Crit Care Med* 153:1259-1263, 1996.
2. Eigen H, Loughlin JL, Homrighausen J: Recurrent pneumonia in children and its relationship to bronchial hyper-reactivity, *Pediatrics,* 70: 689-692, 1982.

Principles of Management

3. Grampian Asthma Study of Integrated Care: Effectiveness of routine self-montioring of peak flow in patients with asthma, *Br Med J* 308:564-567, 1994.

Trigger Factors

4. Bergmann KL, Bergmann RL, Schulz J, Grass T, Wahr W: Prediction of atopic disease in the newborn: methodological aspects, *Clin Exp Allergy* 20:21-26, 1990.
5. Bjorksten B, Kjellman NIM: Perinatal environmental factors influencing the development of allergy, *Clin Exp Allergy* 20:3-8, 1990.
6. Sporik R, Holgate ST, Platts-Mills TAE, Cogswell JJ: Exposure to house-dust mite allergen Der P1 and the development of asthma in childhood—a prospective study, *N Engl J Med* 323:502-507, 1990.
7. Zeiger RS, Heller S, Mellon MH, Forsythe AB, O'Connor RD, Hamburger AN, Schatz M: Effect of combined maternal and infant food allergen avoidance on development of atopy in early infancy: a randomized study, *J Allergy Clin Immunol* 84:72-89, 1989.
8. Ashad SH, Matthews S, Gant C, Hide DW: Effect of allergen avoidance on development of allergic disorders in infancy, *Lancet* 339:1493-1497, 1992.
9. Wright AL, Taussig LM, Ray GC, Harrison HR, Holberg CJ: The Tucson Children's respiratory study. Lower respiratory tract illness in the first year of life, *Am J Epidemiol* 129:1232-1246, 1989.
10. Burr ML, Limb ES, Maguire MJ, Amarah L, Eldridge BA, Layzell JC, Merrett TG: Infant feeding, wheezing and allergy, *Arch Dis Child* 68: 724-728, 1993.
11. Woods RA, Chapman MD, Adkinson FN Jr, Eggleston PA: The effect of cat removal on allergen content in household dust samples, *J Allergy Clin Immunol* 83:730-734, 1989.
12. Platts-Mills TAE, deWeck AL: Dust mite allergens and asthma—worldwide problem, *J Allergy Clin Immunol* 83:416-426, 1989.
13. Murray AB, Ferguson AC: Dust-free bedrooms in the treatment of asthmatic children with house dust mite or house dust mite allergy: a controlled trial, *Pediatrics* 71:418-422, 1983.
14. Gortmaker SL, Walker DK, Jacobs FH, Ruch-Ross H: Parental smoking and the risk of childhood asthma, *Am J Public Health* 72:574-579, 1982.
15. Murray AD, Morrison BJ: The effect of cigarette smoke from the mother on bronchial responsiveness and severity of symptoms in children with asthma, *J Allergy Clin Immunol* 77:575-581, 1986.
16. Evans D, Levison MJ, Feldman CH, Clark NM, Wasilesky V, Levin B, Mellins RB: The impact of passive smoking on emergency room visits of urban children with asthma, *Am Rev Respir Dis* 135:567-572, 1987.
17. Murray AB, Morrison BJ: The decrease in severity of asthma in children of parents who smoke since the parents have been exposing them to less cigarette smoke, *J Allergy Clin Immunol* 91:102-110, 1993.
18. vonMutius E, Fritzsch C, Weiland KW, Roll G, Magnussen H: Prevalence of asthma and allergic disorders among children in United Germany: a descriptive comparison, *Br Med J* 305:1395-1399, 1992.
19. Molfino NA, Wright SC, Katz I, Tarlo S, Silverman F, McLean PA, Szala JP, Raizene M, Slutsky AS, Zamel N: Effect of low concentrations of ozone on inhaled allergen responses in asthmatic subjects, *Lancet* 338: 199-203, 1991.
20. Ishizaki T, Koizuma K, Ikemori R, Ishiyama Y, Kushibiki E: Studies of prevalence of Japanese cedar pollinosis among the residents in a densely cultivated area, *Ann Allergy* 58:265-270, 1987.
21. Meeker DP, Wiedemann HP: Drug-induced bronchospasm, *Am Chest Med* 11:163-177, 1990.
22. Schnall R, Landau LI: The protective effect of repeated short sprints in exercise induced asthma, *Thorax* 35:828-832, 1980.

Drug Treatment

23. Barnes PJ: A new approach to the treatment of asthma, *N Engl J Med* 321:1517-1527, 1989.
24. Turner DJ, Landau LI, LeSouef PN: The effect of age on bronchodilator responsiveness in children, *Pediatr Pulmonol* 15:98-104, 1993.
25. Prendiville A, Green S, Silverman M: Airway responsiveness in wheezy infants: evidence for functional β-adrenoreceptors, *Thorax* 42:100-104, 1987.
26. Barry PW, O'Callaghan C: Multiple acutations of salbutamol MDI into a spacer device reduce the amount of drug recovered into the respirable range, *Eur Respir J* 7:1707-1709, 1994.
27. Bisgaard H, Pederson S, Nikander K: Use of budesonide turbuhaler in young children suspected of asthma, *Eur Respir J* 7:740-742, 1994.
28. Kerem E, Levison H, Schuh S, O'Brodovich H, Reisman J, Bentus L, Carry GJ: Efficacy of albuterol administered by nebulizer versus spacer device in children with acute asthma, *J Pediatr* 123:313-317, 1993.
29. Connor WT, Dolovich MB, Frame RA, Newhouse MT: Reliable salbutamol administration in 6 to 36 month old children by means of a metered dose inhaler and aerochamber with mask, *Pediatr Pulmonol* 6:263-267, 1989.
30. Mazer B, Figueroa-Rosario W, Bender B: The effect of albuterol aerosol on fine-motor performance in children with chronic asthma, *J Allergy Clin Immunol* 86:243-248, 1990.
31. Crane J, Pearce N, Flatt A, Burgess C, Jackson A, Kwong T, Ball M, Beasley R: Prescribed fenoterol and death from asthma in New Zealand, *Lancet* 917-922, 1989.
32. Ernst P, Habbick B, Suissa S, Hemmelgarn B, Cockroft D, Brist AS, Horwitz RS, McNutt M, Spitzer WO: Is the association between inhaled β agonist use and life threatening asthma because of confounding by severity? *Am Rev Respir Dis* 148:75-79, 1993.
33. Vatheren AS, Knox AJ, Higgins BG, Britton JR, Tattersfield AE: Rebound increase in bronchial responsiveness after treatment with inhaled terbutaline, *Lancet* i:554-558, 1988.
34. Cogswell JJ, Simpkins MJ: Nebulized sodium cromoglycate in recurrently wheezy preschool children, *Arch Dis Child* 60:736-738, 1986.
35. Wasserman SI: A review of some recent clinical studies with nodocromil sodium, *J Allergy Clin Immunol* 92:210-215, 1993.
36. Svendsen VG, Jorgensen H: Inhaled nedocromil sodium as additional treatment to high dose inhaled corticosteroids in the management of bronchial asthma, *Eur Respir J* 4:992-999, 1991.
37. VanAsperen PP, Mellis CM, Sly PD: The role of corticosteroids in the management of childhood asthma, *Med J Aust* 156:48-56, 1992.
38. DeBaets FM, Goeteyn M, Kerribijn KF: The effect of 2 months treatment with inhaled budesonide on bronchial responsiveness to histamine and house dust mite antigen in asthmatic children, *Am Rev Respir Dis* 142:581-586, 1990.
39. Waalkens HJ, Van Essen-Zandvliet EE, Hughes MD, et al: Cessation of long-term treatment with inhaled corticosteroid (Budesonide) in children with asthma results in deterioration, *Am Rev Respir Dis* 148:1252-1257, 1993.
40. Fabbri L, Burge PS, Croonenborgh L, Warlies F, Weeke B, Ciaccia A, Parker C: Comparison of Fluticasone propionate with beclomethasone dipropionate in moderate to severe asthma treated for one year, *Thorax* 48:817-823, 1993.
41. Brown PH, Blundell G, Greening AP, Crompton GK: Do large volume spacer devices reduce the systemic effects of high dose inhaled corticosteroids? *Thorax* 45:736-739, 1990.
42. Agertoft L, Persersen S: Importance of the inhalation device on the effect of budesonide, *Arch Dis Child* 69:130-133, 1993.
43. Law CM, Marchant JL, Honour JW, Preece MA, Warner JO: Nocturnal adrenal suppression in asthmatic children takeing inhaled beclomethasone dipropionate, *Lancet* i:942-944, 1986.
44. Balfour-Lynn L: Growth and childhood asthma, *Arch Dis Child* 61:1049-1055, 1986.
45. Merkus PJFM, Van Essen-Zandvliet EE, Duiverman EJ, van Houwelingen HC, Kerribijn KF, Quanjer PF: Long-term effect of inhaled corticosteroids on growth rate in adolescents with asthma, *Pediatrics* 91:1121-1126, 1993.
46. Pouw EM, Prummel MF, Dosting H, Roos CM, Endert E: Beclomethasone inhalation decreases serum osteocalcium concentrations, *Br Med J* 302:677-678, 1991.
47. Wolthers OD, Pedersen S: Controlled study of linear growth in asthmatic children during treatment with inhaled glucocorticoids, *Pediatrics* 89:839-842, 1992.

48. Doull IJ, Freezer NJ, Holgate ST: Growth of prepubertal children with mild asthma treated with inhaled beclomethasone dipropionate, *Am J Respir Crit Care Med* 151:1715-1719, 1995.
49. Jones AH, Langdon CG, Lee PS, Lingham SA, Mankani JP, Follows RM, Tollemar V, Richardson PD: Pulmicort turbuhaler once daily as initial prophylactic therapy for asthma, *Respir Med* 88:293-299, 1994.
50. Beam WR, Weiner DE, Martin RJ: Timing of prednisolone and alterations of airway inflammation in nocturnal asthma, *Am Rev Respir Dis* 146:1524-1530, 1992.
51. Sears MR, Taylor R, Print CG, Lake DC, Herbison GP, Flannery EM: Increased inhaled bronchodilator vs increased inhaled corticosteroid in the control of moderate asthma, *Chest* 102:1709-1715, 1992.
52. Ball BD, Hill MR, Brenner M, Sauks R, Szefler SJ: Effect of low dose troleandomycin on glucocorticoid pharmacokinetics and airway hyperresponsiveness in severely asthmatic children, *Ann Allergy* 65:37-45, 1990.
53. Flolte TR, Loughlin EM: Benefits and complications of Troleandomycin (TAO) in young children with steroid dependent asthma, *Pediatr Pulmonol* 10:178-182, 1991.
54. Erzurum SC, Leff JA, Cochran JE, Ackerson LM, Szefler SJ, Martin RG, Colt GR: Lack of benefit of methotrexate in severe steroid dependent asthma: a double blind placebo controlled trial, *Ann Intern Med* 114:353-360, 1991.
55. Mazer BD, Gelfand EW: Open-label study of high dose intravenous immunoglobulin in severe childhood asthma, *J Allergy Clin Immunol* 87: 976-983, 1991.
56. Bernstein DI, Bernstein IL, Bodenheimer SS, Pietrusko RG: An open study of avranofin in the treatment of steroid dependent asthma, *J Allergy Clin Immunol* 81:6-16, 1988.
57. Patakors D, Vlachoianni E, Tsara V, Louridas G, Argiropoulou P: Nifedipine in bronchial asthma, *J Allergy Clin Immunol* 72:269-273, 1983.
58. Chung KF, Barnes PJ: PAF antagonists: their potential therapeutic role in asthma, *Drugs* 35:93-99, 1988.
59. Pavwels RA: New aspects of the therapeutic potential of theophylline in asthma, *J Allergy Clin Immunol* 83:548-553, 1989.
60. Rachelefsky GS, Adelson J, Mickey MR, Mickey MR, Spector SL, Katz AM, Siegel SC, Rohr AS: Behavioural abnormalities and poor school performance due to oral theophylline use, *Pediatrics* 78:1133-1138, 1986.
61. Gross NJ: Ipratropium bromide, *N Engl J Med* 319:486-494, 1988.
62. Schuh S, Johnson DW, Callahan S, Canny G, Levison H: Efficacy of frequent nebulized ipratropium bromide added to frequent high dose albuterol therapy in severe childhood asthma, *J Pediatr* 126:639-645, 1995.
63. Henry RL, Hiller EJ, Milner AD, Hodges IGC, Stokes GM: Nebulized ipratropium bromide and sodium cromoglycate in the first 2 years of life, *Arch Dis Child* 59:54-57, 1984.
64. Ramsdale EH, Otis J, Kline PA, Gontornick LS, Hargreave FE, O'Byrne PM: Prolonged protection against methacholine induced bronchoconstriction by the inhaled β-2-agonist formterol, *Am Rev Respir Dis* 143: 998-1001, 1991.
65. Bennett JA, Smith ET, Pavord ID, Wilding PJ, Tattersfield AE: Systemic effects of salbutamol and salmeterol in patients with asthma, *Thorax* 49: 771-774, 1994.
66. Tinkelman DG, Moss BA, Bukantz SC, Sheffer AL, Dobken JH, Chodosh S, Cohen BM, Rosenthal RR, Rappaport I, Buckley CE: Multicenter trial of the prophylactic effect of ketotifen, theophylline and placebo in atopic asthma, *J Allergy Clin Immunol* 76:487-497, 1985.
67. Loftus BG, Price JF: Long term, placebo controlled trial of ketotifen in the management of preschool children with asthma, *J Allergy Clin Immunol* 79:350-355, 1987.
68. Iikura Y, Naspitz CK, Mikawa H, et al: Prevention of asthma by ketotifen in infants with atopic dermatitis, *Ann Allergy* 68:233-236, 1992.

Alternative Therapies

69. Lane DJ: Editorial: Alternative and complementary medicine for asthma, *Thorax* 46:787-797, 1991.
70. Nogrady SG, Furnass SB: Ionizers in the management of bronchial asthma, *Thorax* 38:919-922, 1983.
71. Tandon MK, Soh PFT, Wood AT: Acupuncture for bronchial asthma, *Med J Aust* 154:409-412, 1991.

Immunotherapy

72. Bousquet J, Hejjaove A, Michel FB: Specific immunotherapy in asthma, *J Allergy Clin Immunol* 86:292-306, 1990.

Management of Acute Attacks

73. Geelhoed GC, Landau LI, LeSouef PN: Predictive value of oxygen saturation in emergency evaluation of asthmatic children, *Br Med J* 297: 395-396, 1988.
74. Reisman J, Galdes-Sebalt M, Kazim F, Canny G, Levison H: Frequent administration by inhalation of salbutamol and ipratropium bromide in the initial management of severe acute asthma in children, *J Allergy Clin Immunol* 81:16-20, 1988.
75. Littenberg B, Gluck EH: A controlled trial with methylprednisone in the emergency treatment of asthma, *N Engl J Med* 314:150-152, 1986.
76. Scarfone RJ, Fuchs SM, Nager AL, Shand SA: Controlled trial of oral prednisolone in the emergency department treatment of children with acute asthma, *Pediatrics* 92:512-518, 1993.
77. Storr J, Barry W. Berrell E, Lenny W: Effect of single dose of oral prednisolone in acute childhood asthma, *Lancet* i:879-881, 1987.
78. Ho L, Landau LI, LeSouef PN: Lack of efficacy of single dose prednisolone in moderately severe asthma, *Med J Aust* 160:701-704, 1994.
79. Fanta CH, Rossing TH, McFadden ER: Treatment of acute asthma: is combining therapy with sympathomimetics and methylxanthines indicated? *Am J Med* 80:5-10, 1986.
80. Siegel D, Sheppard D, Gells A, Weinberg PF: Aminophylline increases the toxicity but not the efficacy of an inhaled β adrenergic agonist in the treatment of acute exacerbations of asthma, *Am Rev Respir Dis* 132:283-286, 1985.
81. Kelly HW, McWilliam BC, Katz R, Murphy S: Safety of frequent high dose nebulized terbutaline in children with acute severe asthma, *Ann Allergy* 64:229-233, 1990.
82. Bohn D, Kalloghlian A, Jenkins J, Edmonds J, Barker G: Intravenous salbutamol in the treatment of status asthmaticus in children, *Crit Care Med* 12:392-396, 1984.
83. Dworkin G, Kattan M: Mechanical ventilation for status asthmaticus in children, *J Pediatr* 114:545-549, 1989.

CHAPTER 65

The Role of Health Education in the Management of Asthma

Robert B. Mellins and David Evans

The recent increase in prevalence of asthma displays some very disturbing trends.[1-4] One paradox is that our understanding of the pathogenesis and treatment of asthma has increased, and yet the morbidity and mortality for asthma appears to have increased worldwide. There has also been a disturbing trend toward increase in hospitalization, particularly in the group under 5 years of age. A second paradox is that our understanding of the steps that can be taken to prevent severe asthma has increased, and yet emergency visits and hospitalizations for asthma have also increased worldwide. Recent surveys in British schools show that 50% of children with symptoms of asthma are underdiagnosed or undertreated.[5] Several deductions naturally follow from these observations: (1) patients and families are not recognizing the symptoms, (2) physicians are not making the diagnosis, and (3) either physicians are not providing state-of-the-art care, or if they are, patients are not adhering to the recommended programs. This in turn leads us to several conclusions: (1) the public must be educated to recognize asthma symptoms and seek informed medical care, (2) the medical profession must be educated to provide state-of-the-art medical care, and (3) patients must be educated to manage asthma effectively so that they can live active and unrestricted lives.

This chapter will emphasize that (1) good control of *frequent* asthma symptoms requires daily use of antiinflammatory medicine; (2) to be able to respond to changing conditions promptly, families must be able to adjust medications at home according to a *long-term plan* worked out jointly with them; (3) effective control of asthma requires changing both patient and physician behavior; (4) physicians must assume the role of teachers developing a complete plan with active participation by patients (physician-patient partnership); and finally (5) this has to be achieved within the conventional time allotted for a patient visit.

PATIENT ADHERENCE

Recent studies have shown that less than 50% of patients adhere to daily prescribed medication.[6] Physicians cannot predict better than chance which of their patients will comply; they think they can, but studies demonstrate that they cannot.[7,8] So it is prudent to assume that every patient needs help to follow the therapeutic plan. Being sure patients are willing and able to follow the treatment plan worked out with them enhances their compliance. A corollary to this stresses the importance of making it possible for patients or families to express their true feelings. If clinicians do not make it possible for patients to tell them what they are and are not willing to do, more than likely clinicians are wasting their time writing prescriptions.[9]

PHYSICIAN-PATIENT INTERACTION: AN EQUAL PARTNERSHIP

From the very beginning of a patient visit, the tone should promote a physician-patient partnership and an equal partnership at that. Good or effective communication and health education are critical to the success of the physician-patient interaction and both should begin at the start of the visit. With respect to the history, it is worth emphasizing that the chief complaint is rarely the patient's chief concern. Before proceeding beyond the physical examination, it is important to identify and deal with major concerns. A direct question (which cannot be answered with just a "yes" or "no") like "What really concerns you?" is one way of giving parents or families permission to tell their concerns even though often they are embarrassed to do so. Most doctors are reluctant to do this because they think patients will take up a lot of valuable time to unburden themselves. Most of the time this turns out not to be the case. Usually what follows is something like "I thought she might die in the middle of the night," if it is a child. Asking what the patient's concerns or feelings are about the medicines is also important because many patients are concerned about harmful side effects. It is critical to allay their apprehension by giving some reassurance before proceeding. If the physician does not deal satisfactorily with patient or family concerns, anxiety may be so distracting as to prevent the patient from remembering what transpires during the rest of the visit, including the details of the therapeutic plan. As June Osborne has recently said, "Care, compassion and dignity are the common currency of medicine."

Other than obtaining some objective measure of lung function, extensive laboratory testing is necessary only if there are atypical or worrisome features to the history or physical examination, or if the diagnosis is unclear. Obviously, all that wheezes is not asthma, and if the clinical presentation has atypical features, or if one thinks there is a foreign body, cystic fibrosis, vascular ring, or gastroesophageal reflux, one must proceed with the appropriate diagnostic tests. On the other hand, if the history and physical findings are classical, it may be appropriate to begin with a reasonable treatment plan with the provision that if the patient does not respond favorably, it may still be necessary to pursue diagnostic tests. This is one way to cut down on unnecessary expenses while putting patients on notice that, if there is not a good response, they need to return promptly for further studies.

Having completed the history and physical examination and having dealt with the patient's concerns and ordered laboratory tests, everything else in the visit is part of patient education and is key to successful management of asthma.[10] What is patient education? First, begin with a description of the pathogenesis of asthma in plain language, emphasizing how airway inflammation, mucus production, and bronchoconstriction can each contribute to airway obstruction. One approach we use, which patients find intuitively easy to grasp, is to point out that the airways (the trachea and the bronchial tubes) are lined with a membrane that is very much like the inside of the nose. When the membrane lining the airways becomes irritated, the nerves in the walls are stimulated, producing cough. Also, when the membrane becomes irritated it may become inflamed, swell, and form mucus much like the nose does during a cold, leading to clogging, difficulty with air moving through the airways, and wheezing. This emphasizes how inflammation can lead to airway obstruction. We also point out that the muscles around the airways may constrict (bronchospasm) to narrow the airway diameter, also making it harder to move air in and out. By producing obstruction to air flow, both airway inflammation/clogging or bronchospasm can lead to wheezing, chest retractions, and difficulty breathing. It is important to communicate the essence of the pathogenesis without using medical jargon. Patients are confused by the multiple terms used to describe asthma, including *bronchitis, asthmatic bronchitis, wheezy bronchitis, reactive airways disease,* and *hyperreactive airways disease.* What patients and families really want to know is, will this condition impair or interfere with a normal active life, but they rarely ask the question directly. Emphasizing that there is a wide spectrum of severity in children and adults with asthma but that most are able to lead active and productive lives sets the right tone and provides motivation for the patient to play an active role in controlling and managing asthma. It is always worthwhile to point out that there are Olympic athletes with asthma who manage to win gold medals.

ENVIRONMENTAL CONTROLS

Once the pathogenesis has been explained in plain language, it is useful to review the potential environmental triggers and to see whether any practical steps can be taken to minimize exposure; for example, encasing the mattress and pillows in plastic to avoid dust mites or eliminating cockroaches and damp areas that predispose to the growth of molds. Other important steps include eliminating smoking or other airborne irritants in the home and identifying and removing other allergens such as fur-bearing pets, which may provoke asthma symptoms.

Asking patients and families to keep a diary that relates activities or locations to symptoms or peak flow may help identify environmental triggers.

SETTING LONG- AND SHORT-TERM GOALS

Before proceeding with the drug regimen recommended, it may be useful to set some short-term and long-term therapeutic goals for the families. To identify a short-term goal, ask the patient what bothers him or her most about asthma. Usually, the answer will be something like "coughing all the time," or "waking at night wheezing," or "not being able to play a sport without having symptoms or needing to rest." Then, tell the patient, "Let's make eliminating this problem our short-term goal. If you follow the plan outlined faithfully, we should be able to eliminate or reduce the problem in the next few weeks."

By linking treatment to control of a problem the patient has identified, you provide incentive for following a preventive treatment plan, and some criteria for measuring success of treatment. Patients are far more motivated by their own goals than those of the physician.

Setting long-term goals for preventive therapy is also important. Many families do not like the idea of giving their child medicine over a long period, particularly if the child seems well. It is important to set the goal of gradually reducing inflammation and, once good control is established, to try to reduce the amount of medication needed to maintain the child in that state. Thus parents can be encouraged to take all practical environmental control measures as a way of reducing the need for medication. It is important to establish criteria, such as experiencing a cold without asthma symptoms, that let parents know how to assess how well controlled their children's airways are.

PHARMACOLOGIC THERAPY

With respect to drug therapy, it is important to be explicit about how the medicines work; how to take the medicines correctly, including the use of spacers; and the potentially harmful effects of drugs. The latter is essential to cover whether the patient or family express concern. Most patients are very concerned about drug toxicity whether or not they articulate this concern. Some confuse muscle-building or anabolic steroids with antiinflammatory steroids. Others have seen patients with considerable facial swelling following systemic doses of corticosteroids and may be terribly worried about their use. They need to be reassured that in the conventional inhalation doses currently recommended, the risks of serious asthma far outweigh the side effects of the medication, including inhibition of growth, and that the regimen that is being recommended represents the most favorable risk:benefit ratio. Following an extensive meta-analysis, Allen et al[11] concluded that children treated with inhaled beclomethasone were more likely to reach predicted or normal heights than children whose asthma was not treated with preventive medication. Since that report there have been disquieting studies in adults indicating increased incidence of cataracts in those receiving *inhaled* corticosteroids.[12] Because there is still considerable controversy about the possibility that inhaled steroids may inhibit growth even when used in conventional doses, it is reassuring for patients to know that once the asthma is brought under *good* control, the dosage of inhaled steroids will be reduced. It also helps for patients and families to understand that poorly controlled asthma can lead to impaired growth as well and that risks and benefits have been weighed carefully in developing the treatment plan. The physician's task is to recommend a regimen that maximizes prevention and the use of the least medication over the long haul consistent with good control of asthma.

THE NEED FOR A LONG-TERM PLAN

Patients, and in the case of children, families, need to have a *long-term plan.* They need to know how to respond to colds because we know that whether one is atopic or not, whether one has allergic asthma or not, viral infections are still very common triggers in children.[13] They need to know how to respond to mild and severe exacerbations and how to respond to exercise-induced asthma. They need guidelines for home management, including criteria for increasing or decreasing the medication and criteria for seeking emergency care.

RATIONALE FOR THE THERAPEUTIC PLAN

Although there are several possible ways to define severity of illness in asthma, we have chosen a definition in the young child that depends on frequent vs. infrequent asthma because this will separate those patients who need continuous medication from those who need only intermittent therapy.[14,15] We have chosen to focus on exacerbations complicating respiratory infections, not because that is necessarily the most important trigger,[13] although in the very early years of life, it often is, but first because viral respiratory illnesses are common triggers, second because they may increase airway hyperresponsiveness, and third, airway inflammation and any concomitant epithelial injury from respiratory infections can last 6 to 8 weeks at both the functional and the microscopic level.[16-19] By this definition of severity, infrequent episodes occur less often than every 2 months, and for these, treatment only as necessary, with a β agonist may be all that is required. But if one is having frequent attacks, that is, more often than every 2 months, continuous treatment involving the use of other drugs, especially those with primarily antiinflammatory effects, is going to be important.

There are, of course, exceptions. For example, some patients have infrequent asthma by this definition, but when their asthma flares, it may progress very rapidly and become extremely severe requiring intensive care. These patients may benefit from continuous therapy. Conversely, some children may have mild wheezing or cough much of the time, but rarely have severe attacks. These children may also benefit from continuous therapy.

For the child beyond the first few years of life, the definition of severity as provided by the revised guidelines of the National Asthma Education and Prevention Program[22] are also useful and are keyed to a stepped down therapeutic plan.

GOALS AND THERAPY

The goals of therapy are shown in Box 65-1. The patient should maintain near-normal pulmonary function and near-normal physical activity levels, including exercise. This may not be feasible until the asthma is brought under good control. We would like to prevent chronic and troublesome symptoms; coughing and breathlessness at night or in the early hours of the morning is a particularly important and common symptom with which to deal. We would like to prevent recurrent exacerbations of asthma, and most important, we would also like to avoid adverse effects from the medications.

BOX 65-1
Goals of Therapy

1. Maintain near-normal pulmonary function.
2. Maintain near-normal physical activity.
3. Prevent nighttime cough or wheeze.
4. Prevent exacerbations of asthma.
5. Avoid adverse effects of medication.

WRITTEN PLAN FOR COMMUNICATING THE THERAPEUTIC PLAN

Tables 65-1 and 65-2 present a schema of how to *communicate* a long-term medical plan that patients with frequent asthma and their families have found very helpful.[14,15] Before presenting the actual drug regimens being recommended, it is worth stressing that once families understand how the chart is constructed, they can easily follow the clinician's directions for changing dosages or medications in response to a variety of conditions that are likely to occur. Although the actual drug regimen will no doubt change with newer and presumably more effective therapeutic or preventive agents, the *method* of communicating or writing out the recommendations is what we wish to emphasize here. The format presented in the tables can be adapted for use by clinicians who may wish to use other drug regimens as part of a long-term treatment plan.

In the example given in Table 65-1 for infrequent asthma (exacerbations less often than every 2 months), the medications we wish to use, a short-acting β_2 agonist, and the number of times a day, are listed on the vertical axis. Some important clinical conditions or endpoints are listed across the top. At the first sign of a cold (because it is such a common trigger), we have recommended 2 puffs of the short-acting β_2 agonist 3 times a day. When indicating the first sign of a cold, it is important to emphasize that we are referring to the *earliest* signs, such as a little scratchy throat, not waiting until there are full blown signs and symptoms, such as thick nasal mucoid discharge, prominent cough, or wheeze. Once there is cough or wheeze, the treatment is given 4 times a day or every 4 hours. When there is no cough or wheeze for 1 week, the medication can be discontinued.

In Table 65-2 we present the plan for frequent asthma (exacerbations more often than every 2 months). In this example, for someone with a history of frequent asthma, we are recommending 2 puffs of a short-acting β_2 agonist as a reliever and 2 to 4 puffs of a corticosteroid or a nonsteroid, 4 times per day, or if necessary, every 4 hours. If the patient worsens in spite of this program, for example development of chest retractions and breathlessness, then we recommend adding oral corticosteroids. However, if oral steroids are necessary, we always indicate that it is also essential that patients be checked by their physician as well to confirm the assessment and to make sure that some infection is not overlooked.

Now for the average patient, this may be sufficient for an initial visit. After a period of observation for approximately 2 to 4 weeks, the clinical course can be reevaluated and questions by the patient can be addressed. Once there is no cough or wheeze for 2 weeks, even with running, it is not likely there is much in the way of bronchospasm, and the β agonist can be discontinued. Because, as discussed previously, it is likely that airway inflammation could persist for 6 to 8 weeks, it is reasonable to recommend maintaining antiinflammatory medication. If the patient is free of symptoms for a minimum of 2 months, one can be reasonably certain that there is not much active inflammation, and it may therefore be reasonable in some patients to eliminate the inhaled corticosteroids, maintaining the inhaled nonsteroid alone 3 times a day; as the patients improve, twice a day may be sufficient. Of course, if a cold develops, the patient should return to the treatment plan in the first column. It is worth emphasizing to the patient that when a flare-up of symptoms begins or can be anticipated, the earlier the in-

Table 65-1 Long-Term Treatment Plan for Infrequent Asthma*

MEDICATION NAME OF SPACER	AT THE FIRST SIGN OF A COLD OR EXPOSURE TO KNOWN TRIGGER	IF COUGH OR WHEEZE IS PRESENT	WHEN THERE IS NO COUGH OR WHEEZE FOR 1 WEEK
Inhaled short-acting β_2 agonist	2 puffs	2 puffs	0
Times per day	3	4 (every 4 hr)	0

*Infrequent asthma = exacerbations less often than every 2 months.

Table 65-2 Long-Term Treatment Plan for Frequent Asthma*

SPACER	AT THE FIRST SIGN OF A COLD OR IF COUGH OR WHEEZE IS PRESENT	IF COUGH OR WHEEZE WORSENS	AS SOON AS COUGH AND WHEEZE HAVE STOPPED	WHEN THERE IS NO COUGH OR WHEEZE FOR 2 MONTHS	FOR COUGH OR WHEEZE WITH EXERCISE	FOR RAPIDLY WORSENING ASTHMA (SEVERE ATTACK)
MEDICATION	Peak flow is between 60% and 80% of personal best	Peak flow is below 60% of personal best	Peak flow is above 80% of personal best	Peak flow is above 80% of personal best for 2 months		Peak flow is below 50% of personal best
Reliever						
Inhaled short-acting β_2 agonist	2 puffs	2-4 puffs	0	0	2 puffs	4-8 puffs every 20 minutes for 3 doses†
Controller inhaled						
1) Steroid or 2) Nonsteroid	2-4 puffs	2-4 puffs	2 puffs	2 puffs		
Times per day	4 (or very 4 hr)	4 (or every 4 hr)	2	2	5-10 minutes before exercise	
Oral corticosteroid	0	Begin with 2 mg/kg/day (3-11 day course) NOTIFY MD	0	0		Begin with 2 mg/kg/day (3-11 day course) NOTIFY MD

*Frequent asthma = exacerbations more frequently than every 2 months
†If there is not a good response, seek emergency care immediately. If there is a good response, return to the second column.

tensive program begins, the quicker the symptoms can be brought under control and the dosage of medicines reduced.

The basic strategy for this plan is to eliminate the symptoms of asthma quickly with an intensive regimen and then to decrease the number or dosage of medications. From a psychological point of view, patients are more motivated to adhere to a regimen if they believe they are improving. Furthermore, they are much more encouraged to follow the regimen if they believe they are making progress. This is reinforced if they see that some medications are either being reduced or discontinued. Finally, it is easier for patients to follow a set routine. Some compromise in this optimal regimen may be needed if cost of medication or compliance is an important issue.

Although the long-term plan in Table 65-2 is given with symptoms as the guide because this is most useful for very young children, we have also indicated in this table how peak flow can be used as a guide. For example, if peak flow is between 50% and 80% of personal best, 2 puffs of a short-acting β_2 agonist and 2 to 4 puffs of a steroid or nonsteroid 4 times a day is recommended. If peak flow is below 50% of personal best, oral corticosteroids are also recommended.

Additional columns in Table 65-2 are provided for rapidly worsening asthma and for exercise-induced asthma. It may also be that some patients have marked symptoms not only with exercise but at other times as well. When their asthma is brought under good control, they may only need a β agonist just before exercise. Once a family has been taken through this table a couple of times, it enhances their whole level of communication. But more importantly, this chart can be put in some convenient place such as on the refrigerator door or family bulletin board so it can be used and easily followed.

With new patients of any age, it is essential to use spacers so that there is no doubt that the patient is actually getting the medication. If inhaled steroids are used, the use of spacers minimizes the need for patients to rinse the month to reduce systemic absorption and avoid the development of oral fungal infection or hoarseness. Once patients are doing well, if they are old enough to use inhalers directly or can use breath-activated devices, these may be substituted. For the very young and the aged in whom mouth control or cooperation is lacking, spacers with face masks may be essential.

Developing a long-term plan and teaching a patient or a family to follow it will probably require several visits. These visits will be necessary to get patient feedback, provide the additional health education, adjust the pharmacologic regimen, and also correct any misunderstandings.

In applying the regimens as outlined, we strive to make the patient as symptom free and as physically active as possible. With respect to inhaled corticosteroids, the strategy of aggressively treating asthma early including inhaled steroids for suppressing inflammation and then decreasing the medication may in fact lead to less use of medication long term. If the patient delays, the inflammation may become more severe, and it may then be necessary to use oral steroids for some time to get the asthma under control.

PLAN FOR RAPIDLY WORSENING ASTHMA

An important part of health education is instructing the patient how to recognize and manage asthma that is rapidly worsening at home in spite of the long-term treatment plan shown in Table 65-2. Following the recommendations of the Expert Panel Report Guidelines for the Diagnosis and Management of Asthma,[22] we have used an increasing respiratory rate, breathlessness, use of accessory respiratory muscles, alertness, and change in color (cyanosis) to assess severity and have recommended a short-acting β_2 agonist by nebulizer (0.1 mg/kg/dose) or 4 to 8 puffs by metered-dose inhaler in a spacer, every 20 minutes up to 1 hour (Table 65-2). If there is no response, emergency care must be sought immediately.

TAILORING THE THERAPEUTIC PLAN

Tailoring the therapeutic plan to the family's routine or lifestyle is essential to encourage adherence to the therapeutic programs. For example, for children who have a long school day and find it difficult to take the medication at school, it may be preferable to use nedocromil and salmeterol, which are longer acting than cromolyn or albuterol, twice a day. The effect of salmeterol, which has only been approved in the United States for children over 12 years of age, persists for 12 hours. Because the onset of action of salmeterol may take 20 minutes, patients must be cautioned not to assess its effectiveness by the speed of the response. If the patient has a flare-up of symptoms and requires more β agonist than salmeterol twice a day, the salmeterol will have to be discontinued and albuterol begun every 4 hours. We will need further studies before we will know how safe it is to give 2 puffs of a short-acting β_2 agonist just before sports for individuals who are already receiving salmeterol.

IMAGES AND METAPHORS

We have previously used the image of a clogged nose as a way of communicating how airway inflammation, swelling, and mucus lead to airway clogging or obstruction. Persuading families to start or increase treatment early is key to successful management. Many families treat asthma like a headache; if it is mild, ignore it and hope it will disappear. It is important to teach them a better metaphor: treat asthma like a fire. If you saw smoke in your kitchen, would you sit down and say, "Let's see what develops"? This question usually elicits a smile, indicating that patients and families get the message.

PEAK FLOW MONITORING

Peak flow measurements are simple and practical for assessing lung function, especially in the home. However, without health education, peak flow is of limited value.[20] Peak flow with health education is especially valuable for (1) detecting early deterioration in lung function, (2) managing asthma in patients who have difficulty sensing the changes in severity of airway obstruction, and (3) managing patients whose asthma severity changes very rapidly. Reliable peak flow measurements are often not feasible in the very young or the aged. For some patients and families, clinical signs and symptoms coupled with effective health education are sufficient to manage asthma; for others, monitoring peak flow is very important. Nevertheless, objective measurements of pulmonary functions over time is important in guiding the long term management plan.

NEGOTIATION BY EQUAL PARTNERS

In some ways the physician-patient interaction is a negotiation between equal partners. Part of that negotiation is to (1) afford patients the opportunity to make certain that they have been heard and that their concerns have been addressed; (2) enable the physician to develop the therapeutic plan, explain the underlying rationale, and weigh the risks and benefits, and (3) enable patients to indicate their degree of comfort with the therapeutic program and their willingness and ability to adhere to it. If they have concerns with the therapeutic program, such as fear of the side effects of steroids, it may be necessary, at least at the beginning, to modify the regimen so that their comfort level will allow them to adhere to a reasonable program. Sometimes this requires prescribing regimens that are acceptable but not optimal. Under these circumstances part of the negotiation is to require patients to return quickly for a more intensive regimen if they are not doing well. Engaging in this type of negotiation is an effective way to improve adherence to a program of preventive therapy and increase patient satisfaction.

We have emphasized health education delivered by the clinician on a one-to-one basis because if done well it will have a major impact on families and children. Nevertheless, the individual health education programs can be supplemented and amplified by group sessions and we have recently reviewed a number that have been developed and shown to be effective.[21] Some of the materials developed by these programs can also be adapted for individual practitioner use.

REFERENCES

1. Woolcock, AJ: Worldwide trends in asthma morbidity and mortality. Explanation of trends, *Bull IUATLD* 66:85-89, 1991.
2. Sly RM: Mortality from asthma, 1974-1984, *J Allergy Clin Immunol* 82: 705-717, 1988.
3. Weiss DB, Wagener DK: Changing patterns of asthma mortality: identifying target populations at high risk, *JAMA* 264:1683-1687, 1990.
4. Gergen PH, Weiss KB: Changing patterns of asthma hospitalization among children, 1979 to 1987, *JAMA* 264:1688-1692, 1990.
5. Speight ANP, Lee DA, Hey EN: Underdiagnosis and undertreatment of asthma in childhood, *Br Med J* 286:1253-1256, 1983.

Patient Adherence

6. Ley P: *Communicating with patients: improving communication, satisfaction and compliance,* New York, 1988, Chapman and Hall, pp 61-63.
7. Charney E, Bynum R, Eldredge D, Frank D, MacWhinney JB, McNabb N, Scheiner A, Sumpeter E, Iher H: How well do patients take oral penicillin? A collaborative study in private practice, *Pediatrics* 40:180-195, 1967.
8. Mushlin AL, Appel FA: Diagnosing potential noncompliance: physicians' ability in a behavioral dimension of medical care, *Arch Intern Med* 37:318-321, 1977.
9. Mellins RB, Evans D, Zimmerman B, Clark NM: Patient compliance: are we wasting our time and don't know it? *Am Rev Respir Dis* 146: 1376-1377, 1992.

Physician-Patient Interaction: An Equal Partnership

10. Mellins RB: Patient education is key to successful clinical management of asthma, *J Respir Dis* suppl S47-52, 1989.

Pharmacologic Therapy

11. Allen DB, Mullen ML, Mullen B: A meta-analysis of the effect of oral and inhaled corticosteroids on growth, *J Allergy Clin Immunol* 93:967-976, 1994.
12. Cumming RG, Mitchell P, Leeder SR: Use of inhaled corticosteroids and the risk of cataracts, *N Engl J Med* 337:8-14, 1997.

The Need for a Long Term Plan

13. Clough JB, Holgate ST: Episodes of respiratory morbidity in children with cough and wheeze, *Am J Respir Crit Care Med* 150:48-53, 1994.

Rationale for the Therapeutic Plan

14. Mellins RB: Developing a therapeutic plan for asthma in a primary-care setting. *City Health Information* (CHI) 15:4-6, 1996.
15. Evans D, Mellins RB, Lobach K, Ramos-Bonoam C, Pinkett-Heller M, Wiesemann S, Klein I, Donahue C, Burke D, Levison M, Levin B, Zimmerman B, Clark N: Improving care for minority children with asthma: professional education in public health clinics, *Pediatrics* 99:157-164, 1997.
16. Empey DW, Lartinen LA, Jacobs L, Gold WM, Nadel JA: Mechanism of bronchial hyperactivity in normal subjects after upper respiratory tract infection, *Am Rev Respir Dis* 113:131-139, 1976.
17. Little JW, Hall WJ, Douglas RG Jr, Mudholkar GS, Spears DM, Patel K: Airway hyperactivity and peripheral airway dysfunction in Influenza A infection, *Am Rev Respir Dis* 118:295-303, 1978.
18. Lemanske RF, Dick EC, Swenson CA, Vrtis RF, Busse WW: Rhinovirus upper respiratory infection increases airway hyperactivity and late asthmatic reactions, *J Clin Invest* 83:1-10, 1989.
19. Fraenkel DJ, Bardin PG, Sanderson G, Lampe F, Johnston SL, Holgate ST: Lower airway inflammation during rhinovirus colds in normal and in asthmatic subjects, *Am J Respir Crit Care Med* 151:879-886, 1995.

Peak Flow Monitoring

20. Clark NM, Evans D, Mellins RB: Pulmonary perspective: patient use of peak flow monitoring, *Am Rev Respir Dis* 145:711-725, 1992.

Negotiation by Equal Partners

21. Evans D, Mellins RB: Educational programs for children with asthma, *Pediatrician* 18:317-323, 1991.

Clinical Practice Guidelines

22. Guidelines for the diagnosis and management of asthma: expert panel report 2: NIH publication no. 97-4051, April 1997.

PART ELEVEN

Cystic Fibrosis

CHAPTER 66

Cystic Fibrosis: General Overview

Benjamin S. Wilfond and Lynn M. Taussig

Cystic fibrosis (CF) is a chronic, multisystem, life-shortening disorder resulting from defective epithelial ion transport with primary manifestations in the respiratory, digestive, and reproductive systems. The predominant morbidity for people with CF is from progressive obstructive lung disease, but additional problems include pancreatic malabsorption, chronic sinusitis, elevated sweat electrolytes, infertility, and less commonly, diabetes, cirrhosis, pancreatitis, and nasal polyps. There is a wide variability in the severity of symptoms and the rate of decline in pulmonary function.

In 1996, 20,886 individuals with CF were seen in one of 113 designated CF centers in the United States and for whom clinical information is maintained in the Cystic Fibrosis Patient Registry maintained by the U.S. Cystic Fibrosis Foundation. Although a few children still die in infancy, others live into the 40s and 50s and beyond with minimal dysfunction. The median survival age for individuals with cystic fibrosis in the United States is approximately 31 years,[1] but it is difficult to predict the life expectancy of children born with CF in 1998 because of the time delay of the impact of changes in therapy on life expectancy. Currently in the United States, 36% of people with CF are over 18 years of age, of which 90% have a high school diploma/equivalent and 30% have a 4-year college degree. Approximately 34% have been married and close to 80% are either in school or employed. These statistics challenge the classic image of CF as a fatal childhood disease.

CF is inherited in an autosomal recessive pattern, with both parents being asymptomatic carriers. For this reason, there is a family history of CF in only 16% of newly diagnosed individuals (Table 66-1). The incidence of CF in the United States is approximately 1 in 4000, with a corresponding carrier frequency of 1 in 32. These numbers vary by race, and there is a lower incidence in Hispanics of 1 in 9500 (carrier rate 1 in 49) (Table 66-2).[2] The relatively high gene frequency may be related to the observation that the heterozygote state may protect against the secretory diarrhea in cholera.[3]

HISTORICAL OVERVIEW

Occasional references have been made to children with clinical symptoms suggestive of CF for centuries,[4] but the first comprehensive description of CF was published in 1936 by Fanconi.[5] In 1938, Andersen described the characteristic pathologic finding as *cystic fibrosis of the pancreas,* and thus was responsible for the current English name for this disease.[6] In 1944, Farber hypothesized that CF was the result of inspisated mucus from exocrine glands and suggested the term *mucoviscidosis.*[7] The difficulty in pronouncing these names may have been what led some young children to refer to themselves as having *65 roses.*

In the 1940s, antibiotics were first used to treat lung infections in patients with cystic fibrosis,[8] and in the 1950s, pancreatic enzyme supplementation began to be utilized.[9] In 1965, Matthews et al in Cleveland described a comprehensive treatment approach for CF.[10] Although many of the specific treatments are no longer used, including initial 2 to 3 week hospitalizations for education, nocturnal mist tents, IPPB, phenylephrine, and low fat diets, the comprehensive multidisciplinary approach that emphasizes prevention of progression of the disease and the coordinated treatment of pulmonary, nutritional, gastrointestinal, and psychosocial issues, is still the foundation for the care of CF patients.

After a severe heat wave in New York resulted in dehydration in many children with CF, di Sant'Agnese hypothesized that CF was associated with sweat electrolyte abnormalities.[11] This led to the development of the sweat test by pilocarpine electrophoresis by Gibson and Cooke in 1959 as the foundation of the laboratory diagnosis of cystic fibrosis.[12]

Between 1966 and 1996, the median survival of people with CF increased from 10 years to 31 years. Many advances have been made in therapy, including the development of antipseudomonal antibiotics such as aminoglycosides and fluroquinolones, more efficacious approaches to airway clearance, and the use of a high fat/high calorie diet and nutritional supplements.

In the early 1980s, a series of observations were made suggesting that the basic defect in CF was related to decreased chloride conductance (transport) in exocrine glands,[13] which could be physiologically measured by nasal electric potential differences. Shortly thereafter, in 1985, the gene associated with CF was linked to chromosome 7. In 1989, after an extensive search using positional cloning techniques, the gene was cloned.[14] This gene codes for a protein, named the cystic fibrosis transmembrane conductance regulator protein (CFTR), which is a cAMP-regulated chloride channel that may also affect sodium transport and certain intercellular functions.[15]

Some CFTR mutations affect mRNA processing, whereas others cause abnormal intracellular processing of the protein or affect the functioning of the final protein product.[15] However, there is a large gap in understanding how the alterations in function of CFTR cause variation in disease expression. Although genotype/phenotype correlations are not very strong, one notable exception is that individuals with some genotypes, especially homozygous ΔF508, can be predicted to have pancreatic insufficiency.[16] However, individuals with the same genotype can have widely discrepant pulmonary status. Other modifier genes and environmental influences appear to influence the course of CF, especially the pulmonary involvement, in a given patient.

Although the functions of CFTR continue to be investigated, patients with CF have limited chloride secretion and

Table 66-1 Symptoms Present in 900 Newly Diagnosed Patients*

SIGN/SYMPTOM	N	%
Acute or persistent respiratory symptoms	452	50.2
Nasal polyps/sinus disease	29	3.2
Failure to thrive/malnutrition	306	34.0
Steatorrhea/abnormal stools	235	26.1
Rectal prolapse	27	3.0
Liver problems	21	2.3
Meconium ileus/intestinal obstruction	181	20.1
Family history	140	15.6
Genotype	52	5.8
Electrolyte imbalance	31	3.4
Newborn screening	56	6.2
Prenatal screening	26	2.9

From Cystic Fibrosis Foundation: Patient Registry, 1996. Annual Data Report, 1997.
*Not mutually exclusive.

Table 66-2 Incidence of Cystic Fibrosis Based on Race

	ESTIMATED INCIDENCE (1:)	CALCULATED CARRIER RATE (1:)
White	3,200	28
African-American	15,000	61
Native American	10,900	52
Asian-American	31,000	88
Total	4,000	31

From Hamosh A, FitzSimmons SC, Macek M, Knowles MR, Rosenstein BJ, Cutting GR: *J Pediatr* 132:255-259, 1997.

possibly increased sodium absorption in airway epithelia, which alters the physiochemical properties of airway secretions.[17] This results in impaired mucociliary clearance and mucus plugging of small airways. The CFTR defect may also enhance bacterial adherence to epithelial cells. All of this results in patients becoming colonized with bacteria, such as *Pseudomonas aeruginosa* (60%), *Staphylococcus aureus* (38%), *Haemophilus influenzae* (15%), and less commonly *Stenotrophomonas maltophilia* (4%) and *Burkholderia cepacia* (4%) (Table 66-3). The *Pseudomonas* organizm frequently adapts by developing mucoid variants, which are more resistant to antibiotics.[18] The result of the persistent infection is a sustained inflammatory response that culminates in progressive bronchiectasis.[19]

In the past five years, progress has been made in the development of new therapies for the pulmonary involvement in CF. In 1994, dornase alpha, which improves the viscosity of sputum in CF patients by the degradation of DNA, was approved for inhalation therapy.[20] Therapies directed at affecting ion transport that remain investigational include amiloride, which blocks sodium resorption, and uridine triphosphate (UTP), which activates cAMP independent chloride channels to increase chloride secretion.[21] Potential treatments that alter the inflammatory response to infection include ibuprofen,[22] corticosteriods,[23] pentoxifylline,[24] α-1-antitrypsin,[25] and secretory leukoprotease inhibitor.[26] The development of gene transfer to improve pulmonary function remains the holy grail of CF therapeutics. Because significant technical[27] and regulatory[28] hurdles remain, the routine clinical use of gene therapy appears to be years away.

Table 66-3 Results of Respiratory Tract Cultures in 17,620 Patients

ORGANISM*	N	%
Pseudomonas aeruginosa	10,551	59.9
Staphylococcus aureus	6,607	37.5
Haemophilus influenzae	2,721	15.4
Aspergillus species	1,258	7.1
Other gram-negative bacteria	1,201	6.8
Stenotrophomonas maltophilia	683	3.9
Burkholderia cepacia	627	3.6
Other *Pseudomonas* species	450	2.6
Escherichia coli	360	2.0
Multiple-resistant *S. aureus*	357	2.0
Alkaligenes xylosoxidans	334	1.9
Klebsiella (any species)	240	1.4
Nontuberculous *Mycobacterium* species	130	0.7
Normal flora	2,126	11.2
Sterile culture	291	1.7

From Cystic Fibrosis Foundation: Patient Registry, 1996. Annual Data Report, 1997.
*Not mutually exclusive.

DIAGNOSIS

Presenting Symptoms

Each year in the United States, 800 to 1000 individuals are diagnosed with CF and reported to the CF Registry. The median age of diagnosis is 6 months.[1] The most common presentations are pulmonary or gastrointestinal symptoms (Box 66-1). Although some children will have both respiratory and gastrointestinal symptoms, the symptoms in others may be less protean.

Because respiratory symptoms such as cough are so common among infants, a high index of suspicion is necessary to distinguish the infant with CF. Most likely there will not be a family history, and gastrointestinal symptoms may not be readily apparent. Persistent wheezing or coughing, recurrent pneumonia, or chest radiographic changes are reasons to consider a diagnosis of CF in an infant.

The most common gastrointestinal symptoms include frequent loose, foul-smelling, and greasy stools; a voracious appetite; and failure to thrive. However, the gastrointestinal symptoms may also be more subtle, and many infants are labeled as having formula intolerance or are treated for gastroesophageal reflux before the diagnosis.

Toddlers and older children with CF, whose primary symptoms are pulmonary, may be labeled as having asthma before the correct diagnosis. In fact, one value of obtaining a baseline chest radiograph and spirometry in patients with asthma is to look for other causes of coughing or wheezing. Fixed airway obstruction, even with a reversible component, or chest radiograph changes may be indicative of CF. Additionally, clubbing of the nailbeds in a child diagnosed with asthma suggests the presence of bronchiectasis and warrants a further evaluation for CF.

CF may also have more uncommon clinical presentations. These include nasal polyposis, rectal prolapse, focal billiary cirrhosis, appendicitis, gallbladder disease, hypochloremic metabolic alkalosis, hypoproteinemia and edema, skin rash due to fatty acid deficiency, and fat-soluble vitamin deficiency involving vitamins A, E, and K (Table 66-4). Because cystic fibrosis is a significant cause of any of these conditions, evaluation for cystic fibrosis, including a sweat test, should be part of the assessment of a child presenting with any of these problems.

BOX 66-1
Phenotypic Features Consistent with a Diagnosis of Cystic Fibrosis

1. Chronic sinopulmonary disease manifested by the following:
   a. Persistent colonization/infection with typical CF pathogens including *Staphylococcus aureus*, nontypeable *Haemophilus influenzae*, mucoid and nonmucoid *Pseudomonas aeruginosa*, and *Burkholderia cepacia*.
   b. Chronic cough and sputum production.
   c. Persistent radiograph abnormalities (e.g. bronchiectasis, atelectasis, infiltrates, hyperinflation).
   d. Airway obstruction manifested by wheezing and air trapping.
   e. Nasal polyps; radiographic or CT abnormalities of the paranasal sinuses.
   f. Digital clubbing.
2. Gastrointestinal and nutritional abnormalities, including the following:
   a. *Intestinal:* meconium ileus; distal intestinal obstruction syndrome (DIOS); rectal prolapse.
   b. *Pancreatic:* pancreatic insufficiency; recurrent pancreatitis.
   c. *Hepatic:* chronic hepatic disease manifested by clinical or histologic evidence of focal biliary cirrhosis or multilobular cirrhosis.
   d. *Nutritional:* failure to thrive (protein-calorie malnutrition; hypoproteinemia and edema; complications secondary to fat-soluble vitamin deficiency).
3. Salt loss syndromes: acute salt depletion; chronic metabolic alkalosis.
4. Positive family history defined as a sibling with CF.
5. Male urogenital abnormalities resulting in obstructive azoospermia.

From *Diagnosis of cystic fibrosis: a consensus statement, 1997.*

Occasionally, the diagnosis of CF is not made until adulthood. Such individuals have usually been diagnosed with asthma, bronchitis, or bronchiectasis and generally have less overt gastrointestinal symptoms, but males will usually be infertile. Thus it is important to consider CF in the differential diagnosis of adults with chronic pulmonary symptoms or bronchiectasis.

A recent consensus conference on the diagnosis of CF suggested that the diagnosis be based on laboratory evidence of the CFTR abnormality, including an elevated sweat chloride concentration, or identification of two CFTR mutations, or evidence of characteristic patterns of ion transport across nasal epithelia.[29] In addition, there must either be clinical evidence of typical phenotypic findings or, in the absence of such features, an increased probability of having CF based on a the presence of CF in a sibling or a positive newborn screening result.

Sweat Test

In the presence of clinical symptoms, the diagnosis of CF is confirmed by a quantitative pilocarpine iontophoresis sweat test.[30] Sweat chloride levels between 60 mEq/L and 165 mEq/L are considered diagnostic for CF in children. Because normal adults may have slightly elevated sweat chloride levels, a threshold level of 70 mEq/L is often used. Generally, individuals without CF have sweat chloride levels below 40 mEq/L, and commonly below 20 mEq/L. The borderline range between 40 and 60 mEq includes individuals with and without cystic fibrosis. In this situation, the diagnosis must be supported by either clinical symptoms or other evidence of CFTR dysfunction.

False-negative and false-positive sweat tests results can occur because of complexities in the methodologies of collecting the sweat. Typically, the skin is stimulated with pilocarpine and a small electrical current for 5 minutes and then the sweat is collected on a 2 × 2 gauze pad or filter paper for 30 minutes. The weight of the sample and the concentration of chloride are measured. Special care must be taken to make sure adequate sweat is collected. According to published guidelines, 75 mg of sweat must be collected in 30 minutes to insure an adequate sweat rate.[31] An inadequate sweat rate may produce false-negative results, and evaporation can cause false-positive results. It may be difficult to collect sweat from infants during the first month or two of life. Edema, which can be a presenting sign of CF, can also cause a false-negative result.

A number of other medical conditions can produce elevated sweat chloride levels in children without CF,[32] including adrenal insufficiency, hypothyroidism, hypoparathyroidism, nephrogenic diabetes insipidus, pseudohypoaldosteronism, mauriac syndrome, ectodermal dysplasia, fucosidosis, mucopolysaccharidoses, glucose-6-phosphatase deficiency, and malnutrition.

Mutation Analysis

The first mutation identified in the CFTR gene was a deletion of a nucleotide sequence that coded for one phenylalanine residue in the amino acid sequence of CFTR. This mutation, called ΔF508, is found in approximately 70% of CF chromosomes in patients from North America.[33] Because each patient has two CF genes, approximately 50% of patients will have two ΔF508 mutations, 40% have only one, and less that 10% have two other mutations.

Over 700 mutations have been identified. Generally, 32 to 70 mutations can be identified through commercially available screening tests. This can detect from 60% of mutations in African-Americans to 97% among Ashkenazi Jews. In descendants from Northern Europe with CF in whom the detection rate is 90% of mutations, 81% will have two mutations identifiable, 18% will have one identifiable mutation, and 1% will have no mutations identified.

Some adult males will have abnormal CFTR alleles, but the only clinical expression is congenital bilateral absence of the vas deferens (CBAVD).[34] The recommendation by the recent consensus statement to broaden the definition of CF, by including people whose only expression of CFTR mutations is CBAVD, is controversial.[29] It will increase the number of people with CF and increase the described variability of the expression of CF. These features may decrease the stigma of CF patients as a group. However, this definition may cause confusion and pose risks of stigmatization or discrimination by labeling such people as having CF. The identification of people with CFTR mutations but without typical pulmonary or gastrointestinal symptoms has raised questions about the definition and diagnosis of CF. There are other examples of mutations in the same gene being categorized by contrasting phenotypic characteristics and defined as different diseases. One example is sickle cell anemia and thalassemia, which are both caused by mutations in the hemoglobin gene. The definition and categorization of disease is arbitrary, and the social implications of definitions must be considered.

Nasal Potential Differences

Mutation analysis may have a limited role in diagnosis because children with borderline sweat tests are less likely to have more common identifiable mutant alleles.[35] Some patients with

Table 66-4 Nutritional Status, Respiratory Microbial Colonization, Health Care Utilization Stratified by Pulmonary Severity in 14,707 Patients

FEV_1% PREDICTED	N	%	MEAN OFFICE VISITS	MEAN ACUTE EXACERBATIONS*	MEAN HOSPITAL STAY (DAYS)	% CULTURED + *P. AERUGINOSA*	% CULTURED + *B. CEPACIA*	% NCHS WEIGHT <5%
Normal ≥90%	4,346	32%	3.7	0.3	7.3	44.9%	1.3%	9.5%
Mild 70%-89%	3,884	24%	4.5	0.6	8.8	64.1%	3.0%	14.4%
Moderate 40%-69%	4,182	28%	5.7	1.5	9.6	80.9%	5.6%	31.3%
Severe <40%	2,295	16%	6.3	2.9	11.9	87.3%	8.4%	61.2%
Total	14,707	100%	4.9	1.1	9.8	67.2%	4.2%	25.1%

*Acute exacerbations include total hospitalizations and total home-IV episodes.
From Cystic Fibrosis Foundation. Patient Registry, 1996. Annual Data Report, 1997.

borderline sweat tests, or even with chloride values below 40 mEq/L, may be identified by the assessment of nasal potential differences, which are characteristically altered in CF. These differences include an elevated basal potential difference, an exaggerated inhibition of the potential difference in response to amiloride, and no change in potential difference in response to a chloride-free solution in conjunction with isoproterenol.[29]

NEWBORN SCREENING

Since the early 1980s a number of programs have been developed for the early identification of neonates with CF through newborn screening.[36] These programs are often linked to existing programs for phenylketonuria and hypothyrodism. One difference between these diseases and CF is that it has been difficult to determine if there is a medical benefit from presymptomtic detection of CF.[37] When newborn screening programs began in the 1980s in the United Kingdom,[38] United States,[39] Australia,[40] and Europe,[41] the studies used historical controls. Thus it was not clear if observed improvement was related to changes in therapy that were provided to the younger cohort. One randomized controlled trial of CF newborn screening has been conducted in Wisconsin from 1985 to 1994.[42] Although this study has not yet published any evidence of pulmonary benefit from newborn screening, it has demonstrated improved nutritional status during the first 5 years of life. 40% of unscreened infants were below the 10th percentile in weight by age 5 in contrast to 10% in the screened group.

Although a number of approaches to newborn screening for CF have been tried, the most common involves the measurement of immunoreactive trypsinogen (IRT) from a Guthrie card. An additional IRT level may be used as a second tier screen.[39] Alternatively, a second tier evaluation can be based on detection of the ΔF508 allele on mutation analysis.[42] These two approaches have similar sensitivity, but differ in the detection of false-positive infants. The advantage of the DNA approach is that only one blood sample is needed, which minimizes the number of false-positive families contacted. However, the families with a positive screening test have their child identified as a carrier, which may cause confusion and complicate the explanation to such families.[43]

CF newborn screening is not yet done routinely in most countries. With increasing evidence of benefit from early diagnosis, such programs are likely to increase once there is further refinement of the delivery program. Current problems include developing the resources for reliable sweat tests, genetic counseling for false-positive families, and the availability of follow-up services.[44]

PRENATAL DIAGNOSIS

CF can be detected prenatally by DNA analysis using amniocentesis at 16 to 18 weeks' gestation or by chorionic villus sampling in couples who both have identifiable CFTR mutations. This could include couples with a previous child with CF, a family history of CF, or those who have been detected in general population carrier screening programs. For couples who have had a previous child with CF, even if one of the mutations in the child is not identifiable, haplotype analyses of the child, parents, and fetus can be used to make a diagnosis.[33] However, this approach will be limited by misattributed biologic paternity.

In couples who are both carriers, 75% of fetuses will not have CF, and prenatal diagnosis can provide reassurance. Some parents who have a fetus with CF choose abortion, whereas others continue the pregnancy. Even if the couple is not considering abortion, prenatal diagnosis can facilitate perinatal management, particularly if the infant has symptoms of intestinal obstruction. The parents may also have the opportunity to prepare emotionally.

Because of the complexity of information and the emotional issues involved in such decisions, many families are refered to genetic counselors when they are considering pregnancies. The proportion of families who choose prenatal diagnosis is variable. A recent study of 33 families from Wisconsin demonstrated only a 26% use of prenatal diagnosis services.[43] Factors that may influence a family's decision include attitudes about CF, attitudes about abortion, availability of medical care, and financial and emotional support. One of the roles of the CF clinician is to provide a balanced account of what is involved in raising a child with CF and to explain the variability of CF. Some families with young healthy children may not appreciate the potential severity of symptoms, or those who have or know a child who has had certain complications at a young age may not realize that this is not common.

CARRIER SCREENING

Once the CFTR gene was identified in 1989, calls were made for general population carrier screening.[45] However, there were concerns about the confusion that might be caused by the limited sensitivity of the tests and the need to develop mechanisms to provide such information to large populations. In the early 1990s several statements were made by professional groups proposing clinical trials to address these issues.[46,47] These studies showed that there was less confusion and fewer concerns about anxiety and stigmatization than anticipated.[48] However, interest in the test was very low (4% to 25%) when presented to healthy adults.[49,50] In the prenatal setting, the rate of interest in screening increased to 50% to 75%.[51,52]

This variable interest seems to be influenced not only by pregnancy but also by the method of presentation of information.[53] Thus one of the current controversies involves how and when to present information about CF. Furthermore, there is wide variablity in what information is presented,[54] and current approaches need further refinement. A 1997 NIH Consensus Development Conference recommended routinely offering carrier testing in the prenatal setting,[55] but no professional organizations have adopted this recommendation yet,[56] because of uncertainties about the availability of appropriate education and counseling services.

Siblings of people with CF have a 67% chance of being a carrier. However, many of these siblings have a misunderstanding about their own carrier status and risk of having a child with CF.[57] There may also be psychologic and delivery system barriers that make it even more difficult to obtain genetic counseling.[58] Thus if a person has a sibling with CF, reproductive issues should be discussed and opportunities for genetic counseling be made available.

EPIDEMIOLOGY

There is a broad range of expression of disease in people with CF. FEV_1 is commonly used to categorize the severity of pulmonary disease (Table 66-4). Decline in any individual's lung function cannot be predicted, although lower lung function is associated with older age, presence of *P. aeruginosa* and *B. cepacia,* and weight below the 5th percentile. A few individuals will have an FEV_1 below 40% before 10 years of age whereas others may have an FEV_1 greater than 60% at age 40. Lung function and quality of life are not always correlated. Some people with an FEV_1 of 60% may work full time, whereas others are unable to do so. One plausible explanation for this discrepancy is the variable coping strategies of people with CF. Some adults may have spent their childhood being told that they would not live until adulthood and may not have developed skills of independent living.

FEV_1 has been used to predict mortality. Once the FEV_1 falls below 30%, the 2-year survival rate is 50%.[59] Because this is similar to the survival after lung transplantation, an FEV_1 between 30% and 40% is often used as one criterion for consideration for transplantation. However, some patients may have a rapid deterioration and die after several months even when the FEV_1 is greater than 30%, whereas others maintain an FEV_1 below 30% for more than 10 years.

As seen in Table 66-4, people with lower lung function are more likely to have an exacerbation of pulmonary symptoms. Table 66-5 shows the frequency of hospitalizations reported to the U.S. Cystic Fibrosis Patient Registry in 1996. The majority of hospitalizations occur in less than 15% of the patients.

The frequency of complications reported to the U.S. Cystic Fibrosis Patient Registry in 1996 is described in Table 66-6; 77% have no complications. Most complications are more common in older patients. However, distal intestinal obstruction syndrome (DIOS) occurs with similar frequency in all age groups, and rectal prolapse occurs primarily in young children. CF-related diabetes is the most common complication. Although less than 1% of CF patients younger than 10 years have diabetes, in the second decade the prevalence is 4%. It occurs in approximately 10% of patients in their 20s, and approaches 20% in patients who are older than 30.[1] Although cancer occurs infrequently, there may be an increased risk of digestive tract cancers in adults with CF.[60]

Table 66-7 shows the distributions of height and weight as reported to the U.S. Cystic Fibrosis Patient Registry in 1996. More than 20% of all people with CF are below the 5th percentile for weight. The cause and effect relationship between nutritional status and lung disease remains unclear. Lung disease may be associated with increased caloric needs and decreased intake secondary to anorexia. Poor nutritional status may contribute to the progression of lung disease.

Table 66-5 Frequency of Hospitalizations in 19,064 Patients

TOTAL HOSPITALIZATIONS		PERCENT OF ALL PATIENTS	N = 6,872 PERCENT OF ALL PATIENTS HOSPITALIZED
0	12,192	64.0	—
1	3,662	19.2	53.3
2	1,507	7.9	21.9
3	740	3.9	10.8
4	438	2.3	6.4
5	240	1.3	3.5
6	124	0.7	1.8
7-14	161	0.8	2.4
TOTAL	19,064	100%	100%

From Cystic Fibrosis Foundation: Patient Registry, 1996, Annual Data Report, 1997.

Table 66-6 Reported Complications in 19,064 Patients Reported to the CFF Patient Data Registry in 1996

COMPLICATION*	N	%
Nasal polyp requiring surgery	477	2.5
Allergic bronchopulmonary aspergillosis (ABPA)	368	1.9
Massive hemoptysis (240 ml in 24 hr or transfused)	182	1.0
Pneumothorax requiring chest tube	136	0.7
Diabetes requiring insulin	1,099	5.8
Distal intestinal obstruction syndrome (DIOS)	486	2.5
Elevated liver enzyme level	459	2.4
Liver disease requiring GI consult	379	2.0
Cirrhosis with portal hypertension	186	1.0
Rectal prolapse	98	0.5
Pancreatitis	90	0.5
Gallbladder disease requiring surgery	51	0.3
Fibrosing colonopathy requiring surgery	4	
Peptic ulcer	48	0.3
Arthropathy/arthritis	179	0.9
Hypertension requiring treatment	122	0.6
Cancer	20	0.1
None	14,679	77.0

From Cystic Fibrosis Foundation: Patient Registry, 1996, Annual Data Report, 1997.
*Not mutually exclusive.

Table 66-7 Height and Weight Percentile Groups by Age Group

	CHILDREN				ADULTS			
	HEIGHT		WEIGHT		HEIGHT		WEIGHT	
PERCENTILE	N	%	N	%	N	%	N	%
<5th	2,815	22.4	2,446	19.4	933	14.7	2,174	34.2
5th-9.99th	1,096	8.7	1,014	8.1	497	7.8	721	11.3
10th-24.99th	2,762	22.1	2,748	21.8	1,319	20.8	1,305	20.5
25th-49.99th	2,919	23.2	3,016	24.0	1,454	22.9	1,161	18.3
50th-74.99th	1,800	14.3	2,032	16.2	1,236	19.5	653	10.3
75th-89.99th	757	6.0	814	6.5	570	9.0	252	4.0
90th-95.00th	204	1.6	287	2.3	162	2.6	43	0.7
>95th	194	1.5	224	1.8	165	2.6	44	0.7
	Mean 30.5 (SD 25.9)		Mean 32.8 (SD 26.5)		Mean 37.5 (SD 27.9)		Mean 23.1 (SD 23.1)	

From Cystic Fibrosis Foundation: Patient Registry, 1996, Annual Data Report, 1997.

ETHICAL ISSUES

In the following chapters, there will be further discussion of the pulmonary and gastrointestinal manifestations of CF and their treatment. The approach to management includes an emphasis on airway clearance, pancreatic enzyme supplementation, high-fat diets, vitamins, and quarterly clinical evaluations to determine if changes in interventions are necessary and to address psychosocial issues. The clinician may face a number of ethical issues during the provision of these routine services, as well as those related to end-of-life decisions. Additional ethical issues are posed by the development of new technologies, including genetic testing, prenatal diagnosis, and transplants. Finally, there are the issues raised by the participation of individuals in clinical trials. The purpose of this section is to provide a framework for the clinician to consider these issues and to offer some practical suggestions for addressing them with patients.

One of the central goals of the profession of medicine is to help people use medical information and technologies to improve the quality of their lives. All the ethical issues listed in the previous paragraph involve a judgment about the value of a particular intervention. One reason some patients may not adhere to recommendations by their physician is that they do not prioritize the importance of their health in the same way. Or, they may have different views about the impact of certain interventions on their health. For example, a person with CF may believe that daily chest physiotherapy will not extend his or her life, or he or she may believe that it would but that the benefit is not worth the time and effort. Thus a central theme in medical ethics is to establish guidelines for decision making that balance respect for autonomy and promote patients' well-being (beneficence).

Respect for patient autonomy in decision making is embodied in the doctrine of informed consent. Informed consent has four components: (1) patients must have the decision-making capacity, (2) adequate information must be disclosed, (3) the information must be understood, and (4) the decision must be voluntary.[61]

Decision-making capacity is a function of the patient, not the decision. It requires that the patient have the capacity to understand the choices and consequences of the choices, and that the choice be related to a stable set of values.[62] Decision-making capacity increases with age, and there is an emerging consensus that children should participate in medical decisions, including end-of-life decisions, provided that they have adequate decision-making capacity.[63-65]

The physician has a responsibility to determine that the patient has decision-making capacity, and also to disclose information in an understandable manner. Although it is not controversial that adequate information must be disclosed, there may be some disagreement about how to present information. Physicians are generally in a position of authority, and how medical options are framed by the physician may have some impact on what patients end up doing.[66] However, the principles of both autonomy and beneficence each suggest that physicians should be careful not to influence inappropriately their patients' decisions. This caution is consistent with a view of autonomy advocating that people should be facilitated in making decisions in line with their own values. But an appeal to beneficence might also justify a similar respect: patient values should be supported because it fosters a more collaborative physician-patient relationship. The maintenance of a positive and respectful physician-patient relationship is central to the goal of using the profession of medicine to improve the quality of the patient's life.

Adherence to Treatment

In chronic conditions such as CF, people do not always follow the recommendations of physicians. Examples might include diet, enzymes, airway clearance, and decisions about hospitalizations. The medical literature describing this situation has shifted from the term *compliance* to *adherence,* reflecting an emerging acknowledgment that a person's choices deserve a greater degree of respect.[67,68] This does not mean that physicians should not attempt to develop strategies to improve adherence, but respect of an individual's autonomy is important and may influence how recommendations are conveyed. Information may be presented neutrally, or with varying degrees of persuasion or coercion. The decision of how to present the information is not just based on the appreciation of different values, but other factors as well, such as the likelihood of harm if the recommendation is not followed, the likelihood of preventing harm if the recommendation is followed, and the presence of other alternatives.

These issues become more complex when parents are making decisions for their children. Although parents' decisions should be respected generally, as the potential for harm increases, so does the responsibility of the physician to advocate for the child.[64] In the case of children, there may even be extreme circumstances when coercion or use of social service agencies to force parents to provide certain types of care are justified. If a parent refused to provide pancreatic enzymes to an infant with failure to thrive, it would be justified to have the child removed from the home because that harm is immediate and profound and the treatment is effective. However, it would be harder to justify such an intervention in a 5-year-old whose parents refused to provide airway clearance, because the harm is less immediate and the impact of the therapy has not been well defined. Yet a greater degree of persuasion may still be justified in contrast to the approach with a 35-year-old patient.

Death and Dying

Many groups, committees, and organizations have developed recommendations for the care of the dying.[69-71] There is an established consensus that patients have a right to refuse life-saving treatment. This includes CPR, ventilatory support, and artificial nutrition and hydration. Furthermore, there are recommendations that physicians discuss end-of-life care with patients to explain the options and ascertain the patient's preferences.[72] These decisions are generally referred to as "advance directives," and include DNAR (do not attempt resuscitation) orders, living wills, and the designation of surrogate decision makers. One approach to this issue is to make such conversations part of routine care. This has several advantages in contrast to waiting for a life-threatening situation. First, it is often psychologically easier for both the physician and the patient to have this discussion when the decision to withdraw or withhold support is not imminent. Second, it decreases the chance that the patient will lose decision-making capacity before the discussion occurs.

Although some people with CF may have close friends with CF who have died, they may still not know what to expect. Thus descriptions of the dying process from chronic lung disease may be helpful, including what may be done to ease pain and suffering. One central issue is the use of ventilatory support for people with end-stage lung disease. It is helpful to discuss options such as nonintubation or withdrawal from a ventilator to ascertain patient preference. There has also been an emerging use of noninvasive positive pressure ventilation (NIPPV) because this may ease discomfort and fatigue without the morbidity of endotracheal intubation.

One approach to discussing these issues is to clarify that the issue is not whether the patient with end-stage lung disease will die, but with how and where this should occur. Whereas some may prefer to die at home, others may prefer to die in the hospital, and still others in the ICU. The patient will need detailed information about each of these situations, such as, for example, the availability of home hospice support and how pain will be controlled. If a patient wishes not to die in a hospital and not to be intubated, it may be necessary to discuss alternatives to calling an ambulance if there is an acute event at home.

In the last 10 years, it has been suggested that futile care can be withheld, even against the wishes of the family.[73-75] For example, consider a patient who has not expressed his wishes and is on a ventilator, with renal failure and cardiovascular collapse. Although the physician may believe that continued treatment has a low likelihood of achieving meaningful survival, the family may wish for it to be continued. However, a judgment of futility trumps further discussion with family.[76-78] When such disagreements occur, ethics committees can help the physician and family to reach a consensus. Sometimes all that is necessary is a forum to listen to the concerns of the involved parties.

Transplantation

The advent of transplantation has changed the nature of choices that people with end-stage lung disease must consider. Prior to deciding about such issues as withholding of ventilator support, patients will need to decide if they want to be listed for a transplant. This adds a new dimension for patients who are dying with CF. They will either have to decide not to pursue a transplant or their physician will have to decide not to refer them. Thus decisions about end-of-life care will need to address transplant issues.

With the current 5-year survival of 48%, lung transplantation for CF can at best be considered a modest life-prolonging procedure.[79] This situation may be perceived by some patients as an exciting opportunity, whereas others may perceive this as just trading one disease for another. A number of factors may influence patient decisions, in addition to the perception of the value of transplantation, such as personal views about control. Because the transplant process is highly regimented, there may be less opportunity for negotiated decisions. Others may be uncomfortable with the tension between accepting the dying process and the hope of identifying a donor. The goal of informed consent is for patients to have a clear understanding of the potential benefits and risks, and this may be dependent on how information is presented.

Just as the option of transplantions has required new choices for patients, the option of living related lung donors has created new choices for family members.[80] This may address the problem of finding a suitable donor, yet also poses risks to the other family members. Because of the potential problems of coercion, such discussion should be conducted sensitively and with explicit disclosure of the risks.

Participation of Patients in Research

The ethical principles that guide human subjects research around the world include protecting subjects from harm and ensuring that subjects are adequately informed and volunteer to participate.[81,82] Most countries have regulations that require review of most research to ensure that it fulfills these criteria.

The consent process should include disclosures of risks and benefits, alternatives to participation, and explicit statements about voluntariness. Yet there may be some barriers to achieving these goals in practice. When the investigator also provides clinical care for patients, some patients may perceive the need to participate to please the investigator/clinician. This concern can be minimized by explicit statements to the contrary and also by having the request for participation be presented by someone not directly involved in clinical care. A different concern is that some patients may assume that research is intended to provide direct benefits. It is important to explain the role of placebos in research and that many studies are either not designed to provide benefits (phase 1 trials), may not be found to have adequate benefits (phase II), or may include placebos (phase III).

Because most children are incapable of providing consent, the permission of their parents is obtained. A higher standard of minimizing potential harm before the approval of studies involving children is required.[83] Further, to the extent possible, the assent of the child should also be obtained.[84]

Carrier Testing and Prenatal Diagnosis

These issues are complex because they touch on the profoundly personal issues of whether it is morally justified to terminate pregnancy because of CF. Less than 20% of CF families are opposed to abortion for any reason, but more than 70% of families believe it should be available even if they would not choose this option.[85] Even physicians who believe that people should make these choices for themselves may also have specific views. One of the principles of contemporary genetic counseling is a nondirective approach in the reproductive setting. However, this approach has been criticized as not being achievable.[48] It may be better for physicians to acknowledge their biases when having discussions with patients about such issues and for them to strive to present balanced information in spite of personal feelings.

REFERENCES

1. Cystic Fibrosis Foundation: Patient Registry 1996 annual data report, 1997.
2. Hamosh A, FitzSimmons SC, Macek M, Knowles MR, Rosenstein BJ, Cutting GR: Comparison of the clinical manifestations of cystic fibrosis in black and white patients, *J Pediatr* 132:255-259, 1997.
3. Gabriel SE, Brigman KN, Koller BH, Boucher RC, Stutts MJ: Cystic fibrosis heterozygote resistance to cholera toxin in the cystic fibrosis mouse model, *Science* 266:107-109, 1994.

Historical Overview

4. Taussig LM: Cystic fibrosis: an overview. In Taussig LM, ed: *Cystic fibrosis,* New York, 1984, Thieme-Stratton, pp 1-9.
5. Fanconi G, Uehlinger E, Knauer C: Das coeliakiesyndrom bei angeborener zysticher pankreasfibromatose und brochiektasien, *Wein Med Wochenschr* 86:753-756, 1936.
6. Andersen DH: Cystic fibrosis of the pancreas and its relation to celiac disease: a clinical and pathological study, *Am J Dis Child* 56:344-399, 1938.
7. Farber S: Some organic digestive disturbances in early life, *J Mich Med Soc* 44:587-590, 1945.
8. di Sant'Agnese PA, Andersen DH: Celiac syndrome. IV. Chemotherapy in infections of the respiratory tract associated with cystic fibrosis of the pancreas; observations with penicillin and drugs of the sulfonamide group with special reference to penicillin aerosol, *Am J Dis Child* 72:17-61, 1946.
9. Harris R, Norman AP, Payne WW: The effect of pancreatin therapy on fat absorption and nitrogen retention in children with fibrocystic disease of the pancreas, *Arch Dis Child* 30:424, 1955.
10. Matthews LW: Doershuk CF, Wise M, Eddy G, Nudelman H, Spector S: A therapeutic regimen for patients with cystic fibrosis, *J Pediatr* 63:558-575, 1964.
11. di Sant'Agnese PA, Darling RC, Perera GA, Shea E: Sweat electorlyte disturbances associated with childhood pancreatic disease, *Am J Med* 15:777-784, 1953.
12. Gibson LE, Cooke RE: A test for concentration of electrolytes in sweat in cystic fibrosis of the pancreas utilizing pilocarpine by iontophoresis, *Pediatrics* 23:545-549, 1959.
13. Knowles M, Gatzy J, Boucher R: Increased bioelectric potential difference across respiratory epithelia in cystic fibrosis, *N Engl J Med* 305: 1489-1495, 1981.
14. Kerem BS, Rommans JM, Buchanan JA, Markiewicz D, Cox TK, Chakravarti A, Buchwald M, Tsui LC: Identification of the cystic fibrosis gene: genetic analysis, *Science* 245i:1073-1080, 1989.
15. Welsh MJ, Smith AE: Molecular mechanisms of CFTR chloride channel dysfunction in cystic fibrosis, *Cell* 73:1251-1254, 1993.
16. Kristidis P, Bozon D, Corey M, Markiewicz D, Rommens J, Tsui LC, Durie P: Genetic determination of exocrine pancreatic function in cystic fibrosis, *Am J Hum Genet* 50(6):1178-1184, 1992.
17. Davis PB, Drumm M, Konstan MW: Cystic fibrosis, *Am J Respir Crit Care Med* 154:1229-1256, 1996.
18. Hoiby N: Prevalence of mucoid strains of *Pseudomonas aeruginosa* in bacterial specimens from patients with other diseases, *Acta Pathol Microbiol Scand* 83:2190-2192, 1975.
19. Konstan MW, Berger M: Infection and inflammation of the lung in cystic fibrosis. In Davis PB, ed: *Cystic fibrosis,* New York, 1993, Marcel Dekker, pp 219-276.
20. Fuchs HJ, Borowitz DS, Christiansen DH, Morris EM, Nash ML, Ramsey BW, Rosenstein BR, Smith AL, Wohl ME: Effect of aerosolized recombinant human DNAse on exacerbations of respiratory symptoms and on pulmonary function in patients with cystic fibrosis, *N Engl J Med* 331:637-642, 1994.
21. Knowles MR, Clarke LL, Boucher RC: Activation by extracellular nucleotides of chloride secretion in the airways of epithelia of patients with cystic fibrosis, *N Engl J Med* 325:533-538, 1991.
22. Konstan MK, Byard PJ, Hoppel CH, Davis PB: Effect of high-dose ibuprofen in patients with cystic fibrosis, *N Engl J Med* 332:848-854, 1995.
23. Eigen H, Rosenstein BJ, FitzSimmons S, Schidlow DV: A multicenter study of alternate-day prednisone therapy in patients with cystic fibrosis, *J Pediatr* 126:15-23, 1995.
24. Aronoff SC, Quinn FJ, Carpenter LS, Novick WJ: Effects of pentoxifylline on sputum neutrophil elastase and pulmonary function in patients with cystic fibrosis: preliminary observations, *J Pediatr* 125:992-997, 1994.
25. McElvaney NG, Hubbard RC, Birrer P, Chernick MS, Caplan DB, Frank MM, Crystal RG: Aerosol alpha-1-antitrypsin treatment for cystic fibrosis, *Lancet* 337:392-394, 1991.
26. McElvaney NG, Doujaiji B, Moan MJ, Burnham MR, Wu MC, Crystal RG: Pharmacokinetics of recombinant secretory leukoprotease inhibitor aerosolized to normals and individuals with cystic fibrosis, *Am Rev Respir Dis* 148:1056-1060, 1993.
27. Rosenfeld MA, Collins FS: Gene therapy for cystic fibrosis, *Chest* 109: 241-252, 1996.
28. Kessler DA, Siegel JP, Noguchi PC, Zoon KC, Feiden KL, Woodcock J: Regulation of somatic-cell therapy and gene therapy by the Food and Drug Administration, *N Engl J Med* 329:1169-1173, 1993.

Diagnosis

29. Boat TF, Cantin AM, Cutting GR, Dorkin HL, Durie P, FitzSimmons S, Knowles M, Rosenstein BJ, Saiman L, Tullis E: *The diagnosis of cystic fibrosis,* Bethesda, 1998, Cystic Fibrosis Foundation.
30. LeGrys VA: Sweat testing for the diagnosis of cystic fibrosis: practical considerations, *J Pediatr* 129:892-897, 1996.
31. National Committee for Clinical Laboratory Standards: *Sweat testing: sample collection and quantitative analysis—approved guideline,* Wayne, Penn, 1994, The Committee.
32. Wood RE, Boat TF, Doershuk CF: Cystic fibrosis, *Am Rev Respir Dis* 113:833-838, 1976.
33. Lemna WK, Feldman GL, Kerem BS, Fernbach SD, Zevokovich EP, O'Brien WE, Riordan JR, Collins FS, Tsui LC, Beadet AL: Mutation analysis for heterozygote detection and the prenatal diagnosis of cystic fibrosis, *N Engl J Med* 332:291-296, 1990.
34. Chillon M, Casals T, Marcier B, Bassas L, Lissens W, Silber S, Romey MC, Ruiz-Romero J, Verlingue C, Claustres M: Mutations in the cystic fibrosis gene in patients with congenital absence of the vas deferens, *N Engl J Med* 332:1475-1480, 1995.
35. Strong TV, Smit LS, Hon CT, Markiewicz D, Petty TL, Craig MW, Rosenow EC, Tsui L-C, Iannuzi MC, Knowles MR, Collins FS: Cystic fibrosis gene mutation in two sisters with mild disease and normal sweat electrolyte levels, *N Engl J Med* 325:1630-1634, 1991.

Newborn Screening

36. Wilcken B: Newborn screening for cystic fibrosis: its evolution and a review of the current situation, *Screening* 2:43-62, 1993.
37. Wilfond BS: Screening policy for cystic fibrosis: the role of evidence, *Hastings Cent Rep* 25:S21-S23, 1995.
38. Chatfield S, Owen G, Ryley HC: Neonatal screening for cystic fibrosis in Wales and the West Midlands: clinical assessment after five years of screening, *Arch Dis Child* 66:29-33, 1991.
39. Hammond KB, Abman SH, Sokol RJ, Accurso FJ: Efficacy of statewide neonatal screening for cystic fibrosis by assay of trypsinogen concentrations, *N Engl J Med* 325:769-774, 1991.

40. Balnaves ME, Bonacquisto L, Francis I, Glazner J, Forrest S: The impact of newborn screening on cystic fibrosis testing in Victoria, Australia, *J Med Genet* 32:537-542, 1995.
41. Dankert Roelse JE, te Meerman GJ: Long term prognosis of patients with cystic fibrosis in relation to early detection by neonatal screening and treatment in a cystic fibrosis centre, *Thorax* 50:712-718, 1995.
42. Farrell PM, Kosorok MR, Laxova A, Shen G, Koscik RE, Bruns T, Splaingard M, Mischler EH: Nutritional benefits of neonatal screening for cystic fibrosis, *New Engl J Med* 337:963-969, 1997.
43. Mischler EH, Wilfond BS, Fost N, Laxova A, Reiser C, Sauer CM, Makholm LM, Shen G, Feenan L, McCarthy C, Farrell PM: Cystic fibrosis newborn screening: impact on reproductive behavior and implications for genetic counseling, *Pediatrics* I02:44-52, 1998.
44. Centers for Disease Control and Prevention: Newborn screening for cystic fibrosis: a paradigm for public health genetics policy development. Proceedings of a 1997 workshop, *MMWR* 46:1-24, 1997.

Carrier Screening

45. Wilfond BS, Fost N: The cystic fibrosis gene: medical and social implications for heterozygote detection, *JAMA* 263:2777-2783, 1990.
46. Caskey CT, Kaback MM, Beaudet AL: The American Society of Human Genetics statement on cystic fibrosis, *Am J Hum Genet* 46:393-390, 1990.
47. Workshop on population screening for the cystic fibrosis gene: Statement from the National Institutes of Health workshop on population screening for the cystic fibrosis gene, *N Engl J Med* 323:70-71, 1990.
48. Marteau TM, Croylke RT: Psychological response to genetic testing, *Brit Med J* 316:693-696, 1998.
49. Tambor ES, Bernhardt BA, Chase GA, Faden RR, Geller G, Hofman KJ, Holtzman NA: Offering cystic fibrosis carrier screening to an HMO population: factors associated with utilization, *Am J Hum Genet* 55:626-637, 1994.
50. Clayton EW, Hannig VL, Pfotenhauer JP, Parker RA, Campbell PW, Phillips JA: Lack of interest by nonpregnant couples in population-based cystic fibrosis carrier screening, *Am J Hum Genet* 58:617-627, 1996.
51. Grody WW, Dunkel-Schetter C, Tatsugawa ZH, Fox MA, Fang CY, Cantor RM, Novak JM, Bass HN, Crandall BF: PCR-based screening for cystic fibrosis carrier mutations in an ethnically diverse pregnant population, *Am J Hum Genet* 60:935-947, 1997.
52. Loader S, Caldwell P, Kozyra A, Levenkron JC, Boehm CD, Kazazian HH Jr, Rowley PT: Cystic fibrosis carrier population screening in the primary care setting, *Am J Hum Genet* 59:234-247, 1996.
53. Bekker H, Modell M, Denniss G, Silver A, Mathew C, Bobrow M, Marteau T: Uptake of cystic fibrosis testing in primary care: supply push or demand pull? *Br Med J* 306:1584-1586, 1993.
54. Loeben GL, Marteau TM, Wilfond BS: Mixed messages: presentation of information on cystic fibrosis screening pamphlets, *Am J Hum Genet* 1998, in press.
55. Statement of the Consensus Development Conference on Genetic Testing for Cystic Fibrosis, Bethesda, 1997, National Institutes of Health.
56. American College of Medical Genetics Board of Directors: Statement on genetic testing for cystic fibrosis, Bethesda, 1997.
57. Fanos JH, Johnson JP: Perception of carrier status by cystic fibrosis siblings, *Am J Hum Genet* 57:431-438, 1995.
58. Fanos JH, Johnson JP: Barriers to carrier testing for adult cystic fibrosis sibs: the importance of not knowing, *Am J Med Genet* 59:85-91, 1995.

Epidemiology

59. Kerem E, Reisman J, Corey M, Canny G, Levision H: Prediction of mortality in patients with cystic fibrosis, *N Engl J Med* 326:1187-1191, 1992.
60. Neglia JP, Maisonneuve P: The risk of cancer among patients with cystic fibrosis, *N Engl J Med* 332:494-499, 1995.

Ethical Issues

61. Faden RR, Beauchamp TL: *A history and theory of informed consent,* New York, 1986, Oxford University Press.
62. Buchanan AE, Brock DW: *Deciding for others: the ethics of surrogate decision making,* Cambridge, 1989, Cambridge University Press.
63. Leikin S: A proposal concerning decisions to forgo life-sustaining treatment for young people, *J Pediatr* 115:17-22, 1989.
64. American Academy of Pediatrics Committee on Bioethics: Informed consent, parental permission, and assent in pediatric practice, *Pediatrics* 95:314-317, 1995.
65. American Academy of Pediatrics Committee on Bioethics: Guidelines for foregoing life-sustaining medical treatment, *Pediatrics* 93:532-536, 1994.
66. McNeil BJ, Pauker SG, Sox HC, Tversky A: On the selection of preferences for alternative therapies, *N Engl J Med* 306:1259-1262, 1982.
67. Conway SP, Pond MN, Hammett T, Watson A: Compliance with treatment in adult patients with cystic fibrosis, *Thorax* 51:29-33, 1996.
68. Abbot J, Dodd M, Webb AK: Health perceptions and treatment adherence in adults with cystic fibrosis, *Thorax* 51:1233-1238, 1996.
69. *Guidelines on the termination of life-sustaining treatment and the care of the dying,* Briarcliff Manor, NY, 1987, The Hastings Center.
70. President's Commission for the Study of Ethical Problems in Medicine and Biomedical and Behavioral Research: *Deciding to forego life-sustaining treatment: a report on the ethical, medical, and legal issues in treatment decisions,* Washington DC, 1983.
71. American College of Physicians: Ethics Manual, Part 2: The physician and society; research; life-sustaining treatment; other issues, *Ann Intern Med* 111:327-335, 1989.
72. Wolf SM, Boyle P, Callahan D, Fins J, Jennings B, Nelson JL, Brock DW: Sources of concern about the Patient Self-Determination Act, *N Engl J Med* 325:1666-1671, 1991.
73. Committee SoCCMsE: Consensus statement of the Society of Critical Care Medicine's Ethics Committee regarding futile and other possibly inadvisable treatments, *Crit Care Med* 25:887-891, 1997.
74. Asch DA, Hansen-Flaschen J, Lanken PN: Decisions to limit or continue life-sustaining treatment by critical care physicians in the United States: conflicts between physicians' practices and patients' wishes, *Am J Respir Crit Care Med* 151:288-292, 1995.
75. Curtis JR, Park DR, Krone MR, Pearlmen RA: Use of the medical futility rationale in do-not-attempt-resuscitation orders, *JAMA* 273:124-128, 1995.
76. Caplan AL: Odds and ends: trust and the debate over medical futility, *Ann Intern Med* 125:688-689, 1996.
77. Quill TE, Brody H: Physician recommendations and patient autonomy: finding a balance between physician power and patient choice, *Ann Intern Med* 125:763-769, 1996.
78. Schneiderman LJ, Jecker NS, Jonsen AR: Medical futility: response to critiques, *Ann Intern Med* 125:669-674, 1996.
79. Yankaskas JR, Mallory GB: *Lung transplantation in cystic fibrosis:* consensus conference statement, Bethesda, 1997, Cystic Fibrosis Foundation.
80. Starnes VA, Barr M, Cohen R: Living donor lobar lung transplantation experience: intermediate results, *J Thorac Cardiovasc Surg* 112:1284-1291, 1996.
81. Levine RJ: Ethics and regulation of clinical research, New Haven, 1986, Yale University Press.
82. Lederer SE, Grodin MA: Historical overview: pediatric experimentation. In Grodin MA, Glantz LH, eds: *Children as research subjects: science, ethics & law,* New York, 1994, Oxford University Press.
83. Freedman B, Fuks A, Weijer C: In loco parentis. Minimal risk as an ethical threshold for research upon children, *Hastings Cent Rep* 23:13-19, 1993.
84. Grodin MA, Alpert JJ: Children as participants in medical research, *Pediatr Clin North Am* 35:1389-1401, 1988.
85. Wertz DC, Rosenfeld JM, Janes SR, Erbe RW: Attitudes towards abortion among parents of children with cystic fibrosis, *Am J Public Health* 81:992-996, 1991.

CHAPTER 67

Cystic Fibrosis: Genetics and Disease Mechanisms

Margaret W. Leigh, Michael R. Knowles, and Richard C. Boucher

Identification of the cystic fibrosis (CF) gene that encodes the cystic fibrosis transmembrane regulator (CFTR) in 1989[1] was a major milestone in our journey toward understanding the pathogenesis of CF.

CFTR PROTEIN

The CF gene codes for a relatively large, single chain polypeptide of 1480 amino acids. A putative two-dimensional model of this protein is shown in Figure 67-1.[1] The polypeptide contains 12 hydrophobic regions, which are thought to represent individual transmembrane spanning regions of this protein. Thus the polypeptide is pictured as being embedded in a lipid membrane. A variety of functional and morphologic studies have shown the plasma membrane of epithelial cells to be a predominant site for its lipid membrane localization. Another general feature of this protein is that it contains two regions that, based on homology to other proteins, are thought to be nucleotide binding folds (NBFs). These domains in other similar proteins bind and hydrolyze ATP and appear to have similar activity in CFTR. Finally, a large (more than 400 amino acid) hydrophilic region, containing 17 putative cAMP-dependent protein kinase and protein kinase C phosphorylation targets, is known as the regulatory (R) domain. The sequence of the R domain appears unique to CFTR. The overall structure of six transmembrane spanning domains followed by a nucleotide binding fold, with the motif repeated, is consistent with CFTR being a member of a family of proteins called the ATP-binding cassette (ABC) proteins. In general, these proteins have been associated with functions that involve ATP hydrolysis–mediated solute transport.

A number of studies have been performed to identify expression of CFTR in the various organs of the body. This task has proved to be relatively difficult because of the generally low level of expression of CFTR protein per cell. Within the lung, the protein is generally below the level of detection in the superficial airway epithelium of the adult airways. In situ hybridization studies, sensitive for detecting mRNA for CFTR, have been able to identify low-level expression of the CFTR gene in this region.[2] The resolution of this technique, however, does not allow assignment of CFTR expression to individual cell types within the superficial epithelium, that is, ciliated, goblet, or basal cells.

CFTR expression, however, has been detected by in situ hybridization and immunocytochemical techniques in the glands of the airways.[2] In particular, it appears that the serous cells of the gland acinus and intercalated cells in the gland duct express high levels of CFTR. There is at present no general agreement (discussed later) about whether or not the pathophysiologic consequences of mutations in CFTR reflect the low level of expression of CFTR in superficial airways epithelium or the relatively high level of expression in the proximal airway glands, or both.

Studies of other organs have been able to identify CFTR expression and localize it to not only individual cell types but specific regions of cells. Perhaps the most definitive studies are those of the pancreas, in which CFTR has been localized to the apical membrane of the intralobular pancreatic duct.[3] Other studies have identified a predominant localization of CFTR in apical membranes of sweat ductal epithelia, with some evidence for a lower level of expression in the basolateral membrane.[4] Studies from rodents have localized CFTR expression in the uterine epithelium, and expression in this region appears to be menstrual cycle-dependent.[5] In general, the studies of protein localization have detected CFTR primarily in epithelia and have pinpointed the cellular location to the apical membrane of cells.

A number of studies have begun to characterize the cellular metabolism of the CFTR protein.[6-8] Like many other membrane proteins, CFTR is translated and processed in the endoplasmic reticulum but does not have a classic leader sequence. Although the exact details of the interactions of the nascent polypeptide and the endoplasmic reticulum lipid membrane are not known, it appears that a core glycosylated polypeptide embedded in a lipid membrane translocates from the endoplasmic reticulum to the Golgi apparatus. In the Golgi apparatus, depending on tissues and species, the CFTR protein is further glycosylated and ultimately routed from this compartment to the plasma membrane, typically at the apical pole of the cell. Because of the influence of mutations on this metabolic processing, an intense interest has focused on the "chaperone" proteins that interact with the CFTR protein in the endoplasmic reticulum and the steps that lead to the translocation of the polypeptide from the endoplasmic reticulum to the Golgi apparatus. After the CFTR protein is embedded in the apical plasma membrane, it may have one of two fates. In the gut, there may be a recycling pathway from the plasma membrane to submembrane vesicles that may then recycle back into the plasma membrane under the control of hormones that influence cell cAMP levels.[9,10] In other organs, the polypeptide, after a period of function, is removed from the plasma membrane and degraded. Studies of the plasma membrane half-life of the CFTR protein have only been performed in heterologous expression systems, and these estimates are for a short (4 to 6 hour) half-life. Accurate data describing turnover of CFTR in the plasma membrane will be important for an understanding of the overall biology of the system and ultimately for estimates of dosage intervals should protein therapy become feasible.

FUNCTION OF THE CFTR PROTEIN

Like many cellular proteins, CFTR may exhibit more than one function. It appears likely that CFTR can act both as a cAMP-regulated Cl^- ion channel and as a regulator of other ion channels, whereas no data have yet been produced that suggest CFTR may act as an ATP-hydrolyzing solute-transporting pump.

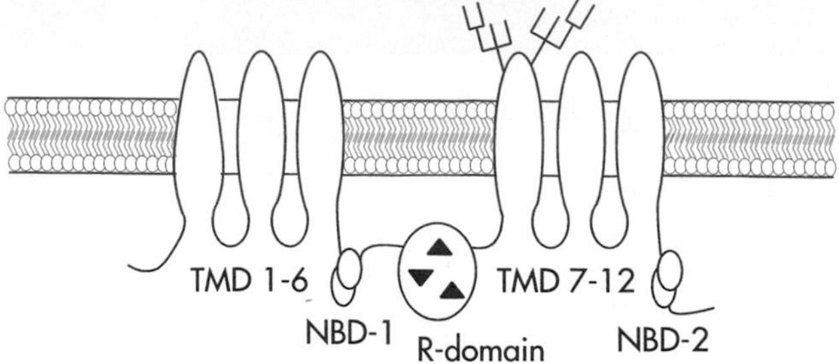

Fig. 67-1. Topographic depiction of the CFTR protein. The polypeptide spans the plasma membrane 12 times. The first 6 transmembrane domains (TMD 1-6) are followed by a nucleotide binding domain (NBD-1) that is a site for ATP binding/hydrolysis. The regulatory (R) domain follows NBD-1 and is the site for protein kinase A- and C-dependent phosphorylation and consequently regulation of protein activity. These domains are followed by a second grouping of 6 TMDs (the seventh is glycosylated as indicated by the pitchforks) and NBD-2, which also may bind ATP.

Characterization of CFTR Cl^- Channel Function

A large number of studies have been reported that are consistent with CFTR being a cAMP-regulated Cl^- channel. First, studies in which the cDNA for CFTR is expressed in "foreign" (heterologous) cells demonstrate increased cAMP-regulated Cl^- channel activity.[11,12] Second, mutagenesis studies have shown that mutations in specific regions of the CFTR protein (discussed in a following section) appear to confer quantitatable changes in the features of cAMP-regulated protein Cl^- channel activity.[13] Third, and most compelling, expression of high concentrations of the CFTR protein in heterologous cells, followed by purification of CFTR to biochemical homogeneity, and reconstitution of protein into artificial lipid bilayers have demonstrated that this protein can exhibit cAMP-regulated Cl^- channel activity in this system.[14]

The CFTR channel has several distinguishing characteristics. The channel under "physiologic" conditions conducts anions far better than cations (ratio >10:1). The single channel conductance, a measure of the ability of the channel to permit passage of ions per unit time, is ~8 pS. In addition, the channel conducts Cl^- ions equally well in both directions; that is, it does not rectify ionic current. Finally, the activity of the channel, quantitated as the open probability (P_0), is regulated by cell cAMP levels.

Mutagenesis studies have been performed to correlate the biochemical functions of different domains of the CFTR molecule with their functional role in a cAMP-regulated Cl^- channel activity. Mutations in the transmembrane spanning regions appear generally to affect the ion permeation properties of the CFTR molecule.[13] Mutations in this region thus may affect the ability of the molecule to conduct ions at a high rate, which is reflected in the "conductance" of the channel to ion movement, and/or ion selectivity (anion vs. cations; Cl^- versus other anions).

It has been known for some time that an active cellular metabolic rate is required to initiate Cl^- secretion in epithelia.[15,16] It appears from a wide number of studies that the nucleotide binding folds are the regions that couple cellular metabolism to cAMP-regulated Cl^- ion channel function. Mutations in the NBF regions have been made that suggest that ATP is important in permitting activation of CFTR via interactions at these sites, and indeed that the functions of NBF_1 and NBF_2 may differ in this regard.[17] However, it is not yet clear whether ATP hydrolysis or binding is required for activation and whether other nucleotides, such as pyridine nucleotides, may also be important in this activity.[18]

A hallmark of the CFTR Cl^- channel is its ability to be regulated by cell cAMP levels. The intracellular actions of cAMP are mediated by interactions with protein kinase A (PKA). The large, approximately 400 amino acid, hydrophilic region between the first NBF and the second set of six transmembrane spanners is thought to be the site of the majority of PKA regulation of CFTR and CFTR function.[1] This region contains 10 consensus amino acid sequences that are targets for PKA-mediated phosphorylation. In addition, another protein kinase activated by cell surface receptors, protein kinase C (PKC), has also been shown to regulate Cl^- secretion,[19,20] and seven potential PKC phosphorylation sites are also located in this region. Hence this region is called the regulatory or "R" domain. Mutagenesis studies have shown that replacement of all 17 potential PKA/PKC phosphorylation sites greatly decreases the capacity of the CFTR molecule to be activated as a Cl^- channel.[21] A hierarchy seems to exist such that at least four amino acids (serines at positions 668, 737, 795, and 813), the "quad 4,"[8] appear to account for approximately half of the capacity to activate CFTR whereas the rest of the amino acids that function in this role are more diverse, possibly including some outside the R domain.

Finally, when CFTR Cl^- channels are expressed in heterologous systems or when studied in tissues that natively express high levels of CFTR, CFTR Cl^- channels appear to express coordinated behavior; that is, they appear to interact with one another to produce multiple active channels. As yet, there is no satisfactory explanation for this behavior. This type of behavior, however, does imply that the CFTR channels are topographically co-localized with one another and can interact positively with one another when one is activated to promote activation of neighboring CFTR molecules. The potential roles of the cytoskeletal components, particularly actins and G proteins, in this type of behavior are unknown but are under investigation.

CFTR as a Regulator of Other Channels

The CFTR protein, as the original name implies, has the capacity to regulate molecularly distinct proteins. The best-documented example of this type of behavior is the interaction between CFTR and an anion channel identified in patch clamp studies as the outward rectifying Cl^- channel (ORCC). The ORCC was the original channel that was identified in patch clamp studies as being abnormal in CF airway epithelia; that is, it could not be activated by PKA and ATP, whereas ORCC identified in normal airway epithelia could.[22,23] Thus this channel was a candidate channel for the CFTR channel. In subsequent studies it became apparent (as discussed earlier) that the CFTR channel was a smaller (8 pS) channel than ORCC and exhibited no rectifying properties. The resolution of the apparent discrepancy was made when it was observed in both (1) human CF airway epithelial cells that were "corrected" by introduction of the normal CFTR cDNA[24] and (2) mouse CF airway epithelia as compared with control mice that an intact functioning CFTR molecule could confer PKC/ATP regulation on the ORCC.[25] The precise mechanism and its physiologic function are unknown at present. As reviewed later in this chapter, the hallmark of the CF phenotype in proximal airway epithelia is increased Na^+ transport rates, which at the single channel level reflects an increased activation (open probability) of the Na^+ channel.[26] Thus interactions between the CFTR protein and apical membrane Na^+ channels represent another site for a regulatory action of CFTR on an independent ion channel. In summary, the demonstration that CFTR can regulate independent ion channels broadens the scope of possible outcomes of abnormal CFTR function on normal cellular activities.

CFTR Solute Transport Activity

The possibility that CFTR may exhibit activities of an ATP-hydrolyzing solute-transporting "pump" was raised by the homology of the CFTR molecule to members of the ABC family of proteins.[27] As a group, these proteins transport a wide variety of solutes, ranging from amino acids to long single-chain hydrophobic peptides, across lipid membranes. Whereas this hypothetical function of CFTR provides provocative mechanisms to account for certain CF phenotypes, as yet there has been no demonstration of high ATPase activity of CFTR or transport of solutes.

CELLULAR FUNCTIONS OF CFTR

The CFTR protein is expressed at different levels in different organs and appears to have different functions in different organ epithelia. Indeed, in the lung the CFTR protein may have different functions in different regions of the pulmonary epithelia. Thus a review of CFTR cellular functions must define these functions with reference to individual epithelia.

Pulmonary Epithelia

Proximal Airway Epithelium

Maintenance of electrolyte and water balance on proximal airway epithelial surfaces is a complex process that reflects the addition of fluid to proximal airway surfaces via the axial flow from distal airway surfaces via the mucociliary system, the ion transport activities of the superficial airway epithelia that line the proximal airways, and the activities of the glands that are located in the submucosal space of the cartilaginous airway epithelia. Most is known about the electrolyte transport properties of CFTR in the superficial epithelium of the proximal airways because of the accessibility of tissues from this region.

A schematic of the functional activities of the superficial airway epithelial cell is shown in Figure 67-2. Shown on the left panel are net electrolyte transport movements (represented as vectors) and the transepithelial and cellular membrane potentials associated with active electrolyte transport. On the right panel are shown the cellular elements that participate in active salt transport. A number of studies have demonstrated that net Na^+ absorption is the major tonic active ion transport process of superficial airway epithelium.[28,29] The electrochemical gradients for Na^+ to enter the cell are generated by a basolaterally located Na^+-K^+-ATPase, and Na^+ enters the cell from the airway lumen into the cell via an amiloride-sensitive epithelial Na^+ channel (ENaC). To maintain electrical neutrality, it appears that Cl^- moves via the paracellular path and water moves via both cellular and paracellular paths in response to the gradients generated by net salt transport.

Also located in the apical (airway lumen facing) cell membrane are two Cl^- channels. The first channel is the CFTR Cl^- channel, which exhibits a basal activity that is about twofold higher than the resting activity of Na^+ channels.[30-32] A second channel, called the alternative Cl^- channel (Cl^-_a), is regulated

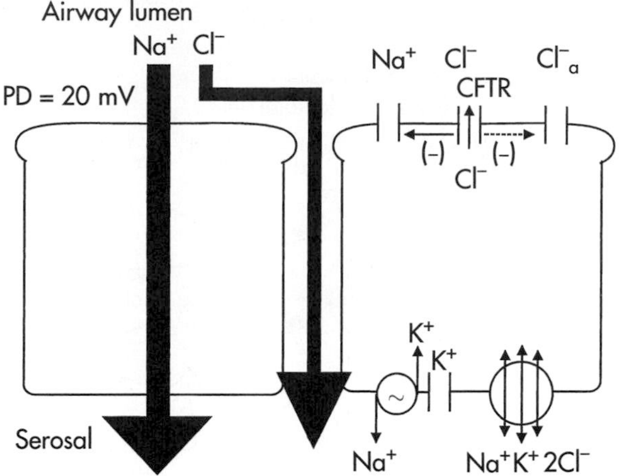

Fig. 67-2. Ion transport properties of normal airway epithelium. The vectors *(left)* describe routes and magnitudes of Na^+ and Cl^- transport. The normal basal pattern for ion transport is absorption of Na^+ via a transcellular route, whereas Cl^- follows to preserve electroneutrality via the paracellular route. The right panel depicts the proteins that mediate these ion transport processes. The motive force for ion transport is generated by a serosally located Na^+-K^+-ATPase. Under basal conditions, Na^+ enters across the apical membrane via the epithelial Na^+ channel (ENaC). Under conditions that inhibit Na^+ absorption, such as amiloride administration, a net entry of Cl^- into the cell via a basolaterally located Na^+-K^+-Cl^- co-transporter is triggered and Cl^- is secreted into the lumen via either the cAMP-regulated CFTR Cl^- channel or a Ca^{2+}-regulated "alternative" Cl^- channel (Cl^-_a). The solid arrow indicates that CFTR functions as an inhibitory regulator of Na^+ channels, thereby functioning as a coordinator of net cellular Na^+ absorption vs. Cl^- secretion. The dashed arrow describes a reciprocal relationship between cAMP-mediated and Ca^{2+}-mediated Cl^- secretion. The dashed motif indicates that the mechanism (protein-protein vs. mRNA expression) is not known.

by intracellular Ca^{2+}.[33] Interestingly, there appears to be little basal net Cl^- absorption or secretion across these two Cl^- channels, raising the question of their role in superficial airway physiology. Two putative roles have been suggested. First, the channels may be available to secrete Cl^- under conditions that can block the apical Na^+ permeability. Whether such conditions occur in vivo is not yet known. The second putative function may be that the CFTR Cl^- channel buffers the apical membrane electrical potential, thereby modulating the rate of Na^+ absorption.[28] With respect to Cl^-_a, it is likely that this channel is poised to respond with Cl^- secretion to the actions of acute extracellular mediators that may raise intracellular Ca^{2+} levels. Thus a major goal still remaining in airway epithelial physiology is to understand the regulation of net ion transport activities in vivo and hopefully then define a role for the CFTR Cl^- channel.

Immunocytochemical studies have identified that the highest levels of CFTR expression in the lung are in the serous cells of the submucosal glands of the proximal airways.[2] A diagram of the electrolyte transport activities of the gland and serous cell are shown in Figure 67-3. The current model is that the serous cell secretes salt and water, and because it is located in the pole of the gland, the secreted liquid flushes mucins from the mucin-secreting cells to the gland orifice and hence to the airway surface. Glandular epithelial cells are somewhat simpler with respect to electrolyte transport than are proximal superficial airway epithelial cells. There is little absorptive activity, and the main secretory activity is Cl^- secretion. The

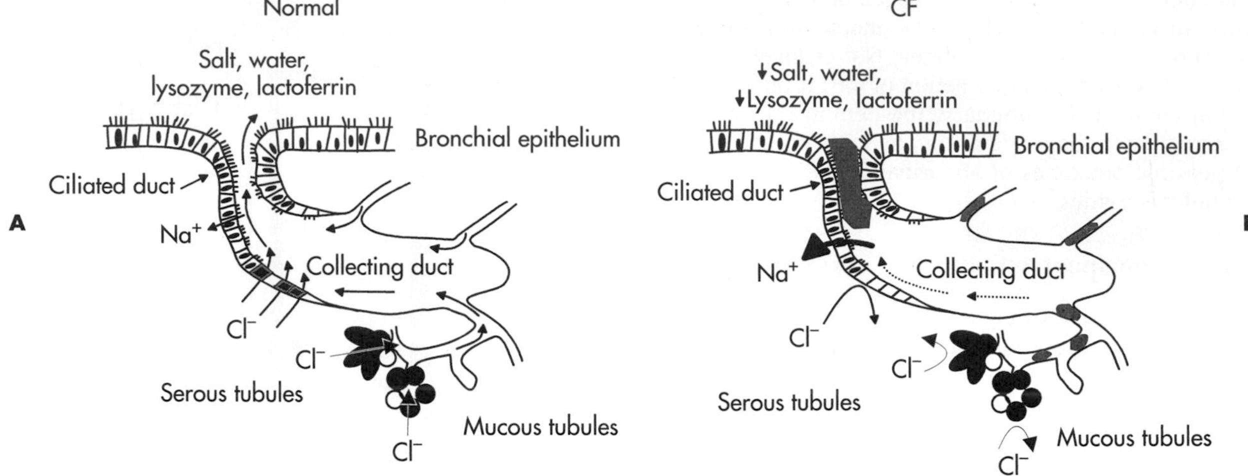

Fig. 67-3. Electrolyte transport activities of submucosal glands. The primary volume secretion by the normal gland **(A)** occurs in serous tubules and reflects predominantly CFTR-mediated Cl^- secretion. This fluid secretion serves to "flush" mucus derived from mucous tubules into the airway lumen. The presence of CFTR-expressing cells, as well as epithelial Na^+ channels, in duct cells suggests that the duct may modify the volume and composition of the primary serous tubular secretion. In CF **(B)**, there is a failure to secrete adequate fluid in the serous tubule because of the absence of CFTR function. Abnormalities of ductal modification of fluid also may occur. The net effect is the release of desiccated mucus onto airway surfaces and/or obstruction of ductal lumens.

mechanism for Cl^- secretion reflects activities of the following elements: (1) a basolaterally located Na^+-K^+-ATPase that generates gradients, principally for Na^+, that drive cotransporter activity; (2) a basolaterally located membrane Na^+, K^+, $2Cl^-$ loop diuretic-sensitive cotransporter that moves Cl^- into the cell above its electrochemical equilibrium; and (3) an apical membrane Cl^- channel, principally CFTR, that permits Cl^- to exit the cell across the apical membrane, into the acinar lumen.[34] In this model, Na^+ follows Cl^- into the lumen through the paracellular path, and water again moves through and around the cell. The rate of Cl^- secretion is in part proportional to PKA/PKC activation of CFTR. However, a more important mode of regulation of gland secretion rates may involve activation of basolateral membrane K^+ channels that, when activated, raise the intracellular electric potential, and consequently increase the electrochemical driving force for Cl^- exit across the apical membrane. These basolateral membrane K^+ channels are activated by regulatory agents, such as acetylcholine, released from efferent nerve terminals that raise intracellular Ca^{2+}, and hence activate K^+ channels. What distinguishes CFTR cellular function in the serous cell from its function in the superficial airway epithelium is the fact that it is the only Cl^- channel in this cell type.

Distal Airway and Alveolar Epithelium

Relatively little is known about the ion transport functions of the epithelium that lines the small airways. Because there are no glands in the region, the superficial epithelium alone must maintain salt and water balance on these airway surfaces. A few studies have been reported utilizing in vivo and in vitro techniques suggesting that the distal airway epithelium is primarily absorptive.[35,36] Indeed, relatively little secretory activity has been identified in studies that measure the aggregate activity of this epithelium. In situ hybridization and immunocytochemical studies have localized an uncommon cell type within the distal epithelium that expresses high levels of CFTR.[37] The identification of this cell type and the function of CFTR in it are as yet unknown. Because many of the early changes in CF children appear to reside in the bronchiolar region, that is, bronchiolitis, it is important to understand electrolyte transport in this region.

Finally, little CFTR appears to be expressed in the adult alveolar epithelium. No convincing in situ or immunocytochemical data are available that suggest a high level of expression of CFTR in either type I or type II cells. Perhaps this is not surprising because CF appears to have little impact on the alveolar, as compared with airways, regions of the lung.

Fetal Pulmonary Epithelium

CFTR appears to be expressed at levels that vary with gestational age in the fetal pulmonary epithelium.[38,39] The precise functions of the expressed CFTR in the fetal lung are as yet unknown. In situ hybridization and immunocytochemical data indicate that CFTR is expressed at high levels in both rodent and human lungs during mid-gestation. At this stage, CFTR is expressed primarily in airway epithelial cells and alveolar progenitor cells at the distal ends of branching airways. The level of expression is high throughout the late third trimester, and slowly evolves into the pattern of the adult lung, with low-level expression in the superficial airway epithelium, a high level of expression in the gland, and little alveolar expression over the early neonatal period.

The major question with regard to CFTR expression in the fetal lung is the functional role of this protein. Fetal lung liquid secretion generates a positive intrapulmonary pressure, which appears to be a major stimulus for lung growth. Based on the normal pulmonary function and morphology of CF patients at birth, it has been speculated that fetal lung liquid metabolism, that is, Cl^- secretory rates, is indeed normal in the CF lung in the intrauterine period. Preliminary experiments from cultured fetal airway cells, both from human and from mouse models, indicate that there may be alternative pathways for maintaining Cl^- secretion rates that can account for normal rates of lung liquid secretion and consequently normal lung growth.[40,41] Hence the paradox is that an alternative Cl^- channel may regulate fetal lung liquid secretion, accounting for the absence of disease in CF fetal lung, yet CFTR is expressed at high levels in the fetal lung, implying function.

Other Sites

Pancreas

In situ hybridization and immunocytochemical studies show that CFTR is primarily expressed in the pancreatic ducts.[3] It is believed that the pancreatic ductal epithelium is responsible for secreting a liquid rich in sodium bicarbonate (Na^+ HCO_3^-), which flushes pancreatic enzymes from the pancreas into the duodenum. It is likely that the CFTR protein in the duct is expressed in the apical cell membrane in parallel with a Cl^--HCO_3^- exchange pathway. Current models suggest that Cl^- is primarily secreted across the ductal epithelium, entering the cell via a loop diuretic-sensitive triple cotransporter energized by a basolateral membrane Na^+-K^+-ATPase, and exiting the cell across the apical membrane via the CFTR Cl^- channel. Cl^- thus secreted into the lumen is then exchanged for bicarbonate by the apical Cl^--HCO_3^- exchanger. The net transport then is for bicarbonate secretion, and again, as in the airway gland, Na^+ follows through the paracellular path. Thus by an indirect mechanism, the CFTR Cl^- protein is limiting for the rate of Na^+ bicarbonate and water secretion by pancreatic ducts.

Intestinal Epithelium

The defects in intestinal function are widespread. In general, the defects appear to lead to dehydration of fecal contents, leading to intestinal obstruction. The intestinal electrolyte defects are complicated by the superimposed dysfunction of pancreatic insufficiency.

The fundamental defect in the intestine (both large and small) is the defective capacity to secrete Cl^- ions via a cAMP-regulated mechanism. The mechanism of Cl^- secretion, that is, entry of Cl^- via a basolateral co-transporter energized by the Na^+-K^+-ATPase and exit via the CFTR Cl^- channel, is similar to that described previously. The site of Cl^- secretion in the intestine is the crypt region, which lies at the base of the intestinal microvillus. This is a site of intestinal mucus secretion as well. The failure to secrete Cl^-, and presumably Na^+ and water, leads to obstruction of the crypt region, which can extend into the intestinal lumen. This pattern of dysfunction leads to distal intestinal obstruction. Recently it has been speculated that the high prevalence of intestinal disease reflects the absence of expression of the Ca^{2+} regulated, "alternative" Cl^- channel in intestinal epithelia.

However, the intestinal epithelial dysfunction in CF may be more complex than solely dysfunction of electrogenic Cl^- secretion. For example, reports have appeared that suggest the rate of electroneutral NaCl absorption is increased in CF intestines.[42,43] This dysfunction would be expected to exacerbate the problem of dehydration of lumenal contents. The mechanism for this dysfunction is not known. However, a possible mechanism would involve abnormal CFTR-mediated regulation of one of the antiporters involved in electroneutral NaCl absorption, that is, a Na^+-H^+ or Cl^--HCO_3^- exchanger.

Sweat Gland

The sweat gland is a complex structure with an acinar region that secretes an isotonic liquid and a ductal region that is functionally designed to absorb salt but not water.[44] The net effect is to deposit a dilute watery solution on the skin surface for evaporative water loss and cooling. CFTR is expressed at a low level in the gland acinar secretory cells and, unlike the situation in airway gland serous cells, an alternative Cl^- channel likely is the principal Cl^- secretory channel in this cell type. The function of the CFTR Cl^- channel can be detected in the acinus, for example, in studies that block activation of the alternative channel with cholinergic antagonists and raise cellular cAMP with β-agonists.[45] Injection of such a mixture of agents initiates small rates of Cl^- secretion in normal but not CF subjects.

Sodium chloride, but not water, absorption occurs in the sweat duct. Sodium is absorbed through a mechanism much like that in the superficial airway epithelial cell. Na^+ enters the cell via an amiloride-sensitive Na^+ channel in the lumenal membrane and is exported from the cell via a basolaterally located Na^+-K^+-ATPase. However, unlike airway epithelial cells, the sweat duct epithelium uses apical membrane and basolateral Cl^- conductances to absorb Cl^- transcellularly. This mechanism is necessary because a leaky paracellular path would not be able to selectively permit salt, but not water, movement. It appears likely that the Cl^- conductance in the luminal membrane is CFTR.[16] Less is known about the identity and regulation of the basolateral channel, including whether or not it is CFTR.

Epididymis and Oviduct

The function of CFTR functionally in human epididymis and oviduct has not been directly measured. However, based on studies in several animal species, it appears that CFTR is expressed in the apical membrane of both reproductive ductal epithelia and functions in these Cl^- secretory epithelia to provide sufficient liquid secretion to "lubricate" sperm or eggs during their migration through these epithelial ducts.[46,47]

Other Epithelia

Although the kidney has the highest content of epithelia of any organ in the body, and the kidney expresses CFTR, it has been difficult to pinpoint specific CFTR-related defects in renal epithelial function. Abnormalities in free water clearance[48,49] and abnormal renal drug metabolism have been speculated to reflect abnormal CFTR renal function.

Obstructive liver failure is believed to reflect abnormal biliary duct CFTR function. CFTR has been localized to biliary ducts by immunocytochemical studies, but its function has not been directly described, nor has the ratio of CFTR versus alternative Cl^- channel contribution to hepatic duct secretion been quantitated.

CFTR MUTATIONS

Molecular and Cellular Mechanisms

More than 700 mutations in the CFTR gene have been reported that are thought to cause disease. Despite the identification of this large number of mutations, approximately 7% to 8% of CF mutations are still not identified at the molecular level, suggesting that mutations in noncoding regions, such as promoter regions, may be found.

A simple classification of CFTR mutations, their mechanisms, and their projected outcomes with regard to production of protein and routing of CFTR protein to relevant plasma membrane site is shown in Figure 67-4.[17] In this schema, there are three major types of mutations. Type I mutations reflect abnormalities in initiation of transcription (promoters) and problems in splicing the mature transcript from the 27 exons that

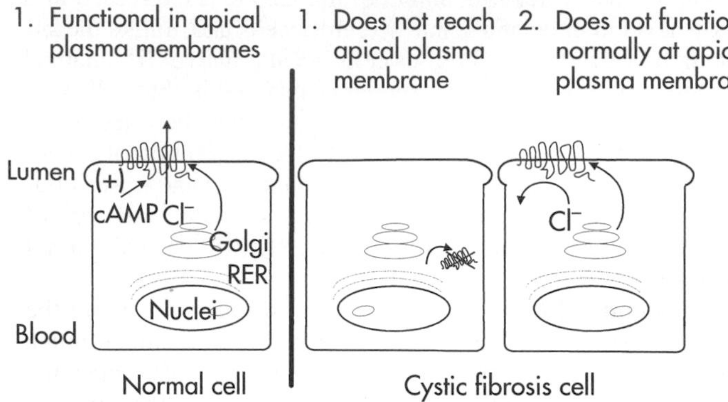

Fig. 67-4. Cellular metabolism of the CFTR protein. In a normal cell *(left)*, CFTR is synthesized in the rough endoplasmic reticulum *(RER)*, glycosylated in the Golgi apparatus, and functions as a Cl^- channel and regulator of other ion channels after insertion into the plasma membrane. Two possible outcomes of mutations in the CF gene are shown *(right)*. (1) If a mutation disturbs protein folding, for example, the ΔF508 mutation, CFTR is degraded intracellularly so that no protein is transported to the plasma membrane. (2) With other mutations, the abnormal protein is processed and traffics to the plasma membrane but functions abnormally at that site.

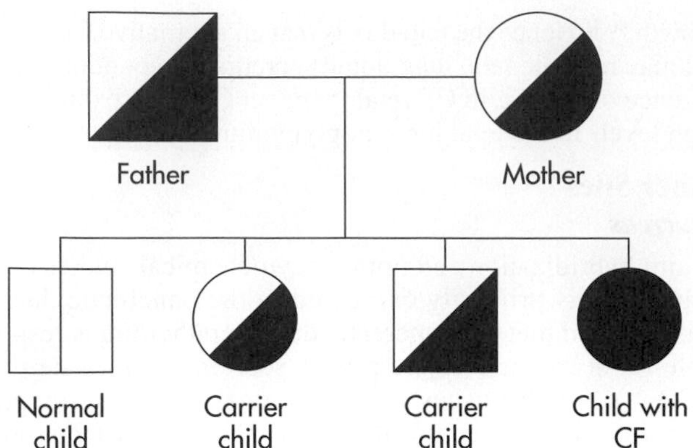

Fig. 67-5. Pattern of inheritance of CF from two carrier parents (◪, father; ◒, mother). The predicted probability is that one in four children is normal (□), two of four children are carriers (◒, ◪), and one in four children inherits a mutated CFTR gene from each parent and has cystic fibrosis (●).

characterize the CF gene. Type II mutations reflect problems in CFTR protein processing, primarily in the endoplasmic reticulum (ER), which ultimately lead to proteins being recognized as abnormal by specific chaperone proteins, resulting in their being catabolized rather than being inserted into plasma membranes. This type of mutation includes the most common mutation in CF, the ΔF508 mutation. Types III and IV mutations reflect abnormalities in the mature CFTR protein that has successfully transited from the ER via the Golgi apparatus to the plasma membrane. These mutations typically reflect abnormalities in activating the CFTR via intracellular messengers, and mutations of this type are often clustered in the nucleotide binding folds or the R domain, and mutations in the transmembrane spanning regions that produce abnormalities in the conduction properties of the CFTR protein that has been properly localized to the plasma membrane. An immense effort has been made to develop genotype and phenotype correlations based on identification of these mutations, elucidation of the molecular consequences of these mutations, and the functional outcome on an organ. As reviewed later in the chapter, these types of correlations appear to be better made with pancreatic function than with pulmonary function.

GENETIC DEFECT

CF is an autosomal recessive disease reflecting mutations in the CFTR gene.[1,50-52] Heterozygotes who carry a normal CFTR allele and a mutated CFTR allele are clinically asymptomatic, and are called *carriers*.[53] The child of two carriers has one chance in four of inheriting a normal CFTR allele from each parent, or two chances in four of inheriting one normal and one mutated CFTR allele and becoming a carrier, or one chance in four of inheriting the mutated CFTR allele from each parent and having the clinical disease, CF (Fig. 67-5). More than 700 mutations in CFTR have been reported, and disease expression relates, in part, to the genotype, that is, the type of mutation in CFTR[54,55] (see following discussion).

The frequency of a mutated CFTR gene and the disease varies among ethnic groups. The frequency is highest in people of Northern European extraction; approximately 5% of such individuals are carriers, and 1 in 2500 newborns is affected.[52,56] Mutations in CFTR are common (5% in whites), perhaps because heterozygosity confers a selective advantage.[57] It has been suggested that gene carriers may be partially protected against life-threatening childhood diarrheal syndromes mediated through the CFTR Cl^- channel secretory pathway.[58-60] It has been suggested that the most common CF mutation, ΔF508, occurred more than 52,000 years ago and spread through Europe in a heterogeneous time frame.[57] CF is slightly less common in individuals of Southern European extraction, but occurs with much less frequency in African-American (1:17,000) and Asian (<1:100,000) populations.[56] There is also ethnic-related diversity in the types of mutations in CFTR (discussed later).

MUTATIONS IN THE *CFTR* GENE

The CFTR gene was cloned in 1989, after it was mapped to the long arm of chromosome 7 by linkage analysis of affected individuals using polymorphic DNA markers.[1,50,51] The gene is large (~250,000 base pairs containing 27 exons), and its messenger RNA transcript (~6500 base pairs) encodes a protein of 1480 amino acids. The rapid accumulation and integration of information about mutations in this genetic disease has occurred with unprecedented rapidity. This has been facilitated by the CF Genetic Analysis consortium, organized by Lap-Chee Tsui. More than 90 laboratories worldwide have submitted new findings to the consortium for dissemination to participating investigators.[61,62]

The most common mutation in CFTR is a three base-pair deletion in exon 10, which results in deletion of a phenylalanine at position 508, which is termed ΔF508. The ΔF508 mutation occurs on about 70% of chromosomes reported worldwide, although it occurs with less frequency in individuals of Southern European extraction (50% of chromosomes), Ashkenazi Jewish extraction (30% of chromosomes),[56,63,64] African-Americans (45% of chromosomes),[65] and Native Americans (<5% of chromosomes).[66]

In addition to the deletion of an amino acid, such as occurs in ΔF508, four other general types of mutations may occur in CFTR. Missense mutations involve a change in a single base

Table 67-1 Frequency of Common Mutations in CFTR Worldwide

NAME	%	REFERENCE*
ΔF508	67.2	51
G542X	2.4	167
G551D	1.8	168
W1282X	1.5	169
N1303K	1.2	170
R553X	1.0	168
3849+10 kb C to T; 621+1 G to T	0.9	77, 171
1717-1 G to A; 1078 del T	0.8	167, 172
1898+1 G to A; R1162X; 711+1 G to T	0.7	54, 64, 169
2789 + 5 G to A; R117H	0.6	54, 173

Adapted from Tsui L: *Trends Genet* 8(11):392-398, 1992; and Kazazian HH: *Hum Mutat* 4(3):167-177, 1994.
*Reference to original description of the mutation.

in the coding sequence, which leads to substitution of an amino acid in the CFTR protein; for example, G551D indicates a base change has led to a substitution of aspartic acid (D) for glycine (G) at position 551 of the CFTR protein. Nonsense mutations involve a base substitution leading to a stop codon, which results in a truncated, and presumably nonfunctional, CFTR protein; for example, G542X indicates a stop codon "X" is substituted for glycine (G) at position 542. Frameshift mutations reflect deletions, or insertions, of a base (or bases), which alters the reading frame and results in deletion or addition of amino acids (for example, 3659 del C and 3905 ins T), and alteration of protein function, or a truncated protein. Mutations in splice sites, usually involving a base change at an exon/intron border, alter RNA splicing (discussed later).

In addition to ΔF508, about 15 mutations occur in common among whites, and account for up to 15% of the CF alleles, depending on the ethnic origin of patients.[67] Many of these mutations occur in most ethnic groups (Table 67-1). The rest of the mutations are rare and occur on only one or a few chromosomes. Some mutations are clustered in specific ethnic populations.[56,67] The most striking example is in the Ashkenazi Jewish population, in whom the W1282X mutation accounts for 50% of the mutations in CFTR.[68]

GENOTYPE AND PHENOTYPE

Studies of the relationship between CFTR genotype and clinical phenotype have been complicated by variables that may modify the clinical expression of the disease, including genetic factors other than CFTR, environmental and infectious influences, and differences in medical treatment.[69-71] Early studies of CFTR structure and function focused on the type of mutation and the locus of the mutation in the CFTR protein, such as transmembrane domain, nucleotide binding fold, or the regulatory (R) domain.[52,61,62,72]

Information quickly emerged from individual investigators and the CF consortium to indicate that complete loss of CFTR function as a Cl^- channel results in a clinical phenotype of pancreatic exocrine insufficiency at birth or an early age, elevated sweat Cl^- values, a high risk of meconium ileus, absence of the vas deferens in males, and pulmonary disease of variable severity[17,54,61,62,67,73-75] (Table 67-2). The loss of CFTR function as a Cl^- channel may be the result of nonsense mutations (for example, G542X), abnormal processing of CFTR to the plasma membrane (for example, ΔF508), or totally defective function of CFTR protein as a Cl^- channel, even when properly processed to the cell membrane (for example, G551D).[17] Such mutations have been termed "severe," although the designation correlates with loss of pancreatic exocrine function rather than pulmonary disease status.

CF patients homozygous for the ΔF508 mutation have been the most extensively studied group with a severe mutation.[73-75] These studies clearly established the link between genotype and pancreatic exocrine function; 99% of these patients have pancreatic exocrine insufficiency, although a few had adequate pancreatic exocrine function to prevent malabsorption in early childhood. About 15% were born with meconium ileus. These patients uniformly have diagnostically raised sweat Cl^- values (when performed in a qualified laboratory), and more than 99% of the adult males are infertile with obstructive azoospermia. However, there is a broad range of pulmonary functional status for ΔF508 homozygotes. Many patients develop end-stage lung disease within a decade of birth, whereas other patients have normal airflow mechanics (FEV_1) after several decades of life. The variability in pulmonary disease severity likely reflects multiple factors, including genetic factors other than CFTR, environmental and infectious events, and perhaps differences in medical treatment. A specific definition of the determinants of pulmonary outcome in CF patients is the focus of ongoing research.

Subsequent studies have demonstrated that genetic heterozygotes bearing two severe mutations (for example, ΔF508 and G542X) have pancreatic exocrine insufficiency, raised sweat Cl^- values, and other clinical features that are indistinguishable from ΔF508 homozygotes, including variability of pulmonary disease.[55] Thus the combination of any two severe mutations produces a similar clinical phenotype.

Preservation of some function of CFTR as a Cl^- channel, whether the result of partial function of a defective channel (usually mutations in the transmembrane region, which allows some partial Cl^- channel conductance), or of low levels of normal CFTR from splice-mutations, is associated with a modified clinical phenotype[13,17,44,55,68,74-84] (see Table 67-2). This altered phenotype is correlated strongly with pancreatic exocrine sufficiency, although these mutations sometimes also have a different effect on sweat gland function or pulmonary status (see details in later section).

Landmark observations evolved from two studies from Toronto, which demonstrated that some non-ΔF508 mutations (genotypes) were associated with pancreatic exocrine sufficiency, lower sweat Cl^- values, and later age of diagnosis.[73,74] These and subsequent studies also clearly demonstrated that patients with pancreatic exocrine insufficiency were carrying two copies of severe mutations, whereas patients carrying one mild mutation and one severe mutation (or two mild mutations) typically had preservation of pancreatic exocrine function.[68,75-77,80,81] Pancreatic exocrine insufficiency was always associated with single amino acid deletions or nonsense or frameshift mutations, whereas missense mutations and splice mutations could be associated with either pancreatic exocrine insufficiency or sufficiency, depending on whether mutations caused total or partial loss of CFTR function.[55]

Although there is a firm relationship between mild mutations and preservation of pancreatic exocrine function, these relationships were less obvious regarding the status of pulmonary disease. The overlapping range of pulmonary disease severity for mild and severe mutations has not allowed clear correlation of milder pulmonary disease with the mutations associated with pancreatic exocrine sufficiency.[75,77,80] One study reports that

Table 67-2 Clinical Phenotype and CFTR Mutations*

LUNG DISEASE AND PANCREATIC EXOCRINE INSUFFICIENCY "SEVERE"	LUNG DISEASE AND PANCREATIC EXOCRINE SUFFICIENCY "MILD"	LUNG DISEASE, PANCREATIC EXOCRINE SUFFICIENCY AND BORDERLINE OR NORMAL SWEAT CHLORIDES	NO LUNG DISEASE AND CONGENITAL BILATERAL ABSENCE OF THE VAS DEFERENS
ΔF508	R117H	R117H	R117H
G542X	3849+10 kb C to T	3849+10 kb C to T	D1152H
G551D	2789+5 G to A	G551S	D1270N
R553X	R334W	D1152H	P67L
W1282X	G85E		
N1303K	R347P		
3905 ins T	R347H		
1078 del T	R347L		
621+1 G to T	A455E		
1717-1 G to A	Y563N		
ΔI507	P574H		
R560T	S945L		
S549N	L1065P		
3659 del C	D1152H		
G480C	F1286S		
V520F	Q1291H		

*Not inclusive; adapted from references 17, 51, 52, 55, 68, and 73-81.

colonization with *Pseudomonas aeruginosa* is delayed in CF patients with pancreatic sufficiency.[85] It has been suggested that black patients with CF may have milder respiratory disease than whites with CF.[65] Studies regarding pulmonary functional status have involved small numbers of patients, and a world-wide survey is underway to further study the relationship between genotype and pulmonary disease.

Several interesting observations about genotype and phenotype have recently emerged, which suggests that better understanding of molecular mechanisms of disease will allow more rigorous definition of the relationship between genotype and pulmonary phenotype. As a group, patients carrying the R117H mutation have lower sweat Cl^- values and are older when the diagnosis of CF was initially made, whereas pulmonary disease severity is not different as compared with ΔF508 homozygotes.[75] However, we now recognize that the range of disease expression associated with the R117H mutation is striking (see Table 67-2). The clinical phenotype ranges from patients with diagnostically-elevated sweat Cl^- levels, and pulmonary disease of varying severity, to men who have no pulmonary disease, normal (or borderline) sweat Cl^- values, and congenital absence of the vas deferens (CBAVD).[76,78,79] This diverse clinical phenotype reflects, at least in part, varying degrees of splice-out of exon 9, which yields a CFTR protein with no Cl^- channel activity.[86,87a] Thus the partial Cl^- channel function of full-length CFTR with the R117H mutation may be further decreased by splice-out of exon 9 in some transcripts. Specifically, the haplotype with frequent splice-out of exon 9 (5T polypyrimidine sequence in intron 8) is seen in CF patients with lung disease, whereas the most common haplotype (associated with the 7T haplotype, and less splice-out of exon 9) occurs in the normal population and in men with CBAVD but no pulmonary disease.[76] Population screening studies show that the R117H mutation is more than 10 times more common than expected in the general population, and a small number of females have been identified by carrier screening tests who have no pulmonary disease and are otherwise asymptomatic (R117H/ΔF508).[55] Thus individuals with the R117H mutation in association with little splice-out of exon 9 may have adequate CFTR function to cause only CBAVD in some men or no disease. These observations are compatible with the R117H mutation occurring at least two times in CFTR genes with different chromosomal backgrounds,[76] and future studies will include such considerations in characterizing the relationship between genotype and phenotype.

Mutations that create novel splice sites have provided other insights into the relationship between CFTR genotype and-phenotype. A point mutation in intron 19 of the CFTR gene, termed 3849+10 kb C to T, leads to creation of a partially active splice site in intron 19, and insertion into most CFTR transcripts of a segment containing an inframe stop codon, between exons 19 and 20.[77] This mutation is associated with some normally spliced CFTR transcripts and presumably low levels of normal CFTR protein. Patients with this mutation usually have preservation of pancreatic exocrine function, and-many have normal (or borderline) sweat Cl^- values.[77,80] Thus disease expression associated with this mutation may reflect the level of tissue-specific splicing.

It has recently been recognized that a group of men who have CBAVD may have mutations in CFTR, but have no lung or pancreatic dysfunction and a range of sweat Cl^- values.[78,79] This observation suggests that the levels of CFTR function maintained in the lung and pancreas of these men are sufficient to preclude the development of disease, at least for several decades. There is ongoing debate as to whether or not these men should be said to have CF.

An intriguing concept introduced by recent studies in CFTR-deficient mice suggests that modulation of disease severity may be genetically determined by modifier genes.[87b] Specifically, CFTR-deficient mice displaying a genetic background with an alternative (non-CFTR) Cl^- conductance channel were less likely to develop intestinal obstruction than those without this genetic background. Research is underway to characterize other potential modifier genes that influence the heterogeneous phenotypic expression in CF.

GENETIC TESTING

The use of genotyping is particularly important for pursuing the diagnosis of CF in clinical situations when the diagnosis is unclear, that is, atypical pulmonary disease and/or normal pancreatic exocrine function and nondiagnostic or normal sweat Cl^- tests. If disease-associated mutations can be defined on each allele of CFTR, the diagnosis of CF is confirmed.

However, it is important to recognize that the diagnosis of CF cannot be ruled out on the basis of negative genetic tests, because not all mutations are known, and a mutation in any individual may be rare, or unique. Another clinical value of genotype information is to predict the status of pancreatic exocrine function. It must be emphasized that prognostic counseling cannot be undertaken on the basis of genetic data alone at the current time.

The high risk (1 in 4) that a couple who both carry a mutation in CFTR will have a child affected with CF makes carrier testing and prenatal diagnosis very important in at-risk families. Genetic testing for specific CFTR mutations offers definitive information in the vast majority of circumstances. Appropriate education and counseling would then offer the opportunity for couples to prospectively examine their reproductive options, including not having biological children, or using egg or sperm donors with low risk of transmitting a CF mutation, or attempting to conceive, with perhaps prenatal testing being subsequently undertaken. A recent alternative to in vivo prenatal testing is in vitro fertilization and diagnosis before implantation.[88] Prenatal testing allows parents to consider possible termination of the pregnancy, although many couples do not consider selective abortion of an affected fetus as an acceptable approach.[89]

CF patients and carriers of a CF mutation should be encouraged to inform blood relatives of the potential risk for this genetic disease so that they can consider carrier testing. The testing requires appropriate education and counseling, and should be offered in parallel to the genetic analyses.

Population Carrier Screening and Neonatal Screening

Although there is general agreement that carrier testing should be offered to people with a family history of CF or a relative known to be a carrier of a mutation in CFTR (discussed earlier), population-based screening is not recommended for individuals with a negative family history.[90-93] The heterogeneity of mutations that is present in most populations precludes accurate definition of more than 85% to 90% of carriers, which means that about 1 in 15 white couples will be at modest risk (1 in 1000) of having a child with CF.[94] The educational and counseling requisites of that circumstance are beyond current capabilities. In certain ethnic groups with less mutational heterogeneity, screening can identify the great majority of carriers; for example, 97% of carriers can be detected by screening for only 5 mutations in the Ashkenazi Jewish population of Israel.[68] Thus carrier screening in such a population may be feasible.

It is undecided whether CF should be added to the list of diseases routinely screened in neonates. There is some evidence that early diagnosis of CF improves clinical outcome,[95,96] but long-term benefits have yet to be defined.

DISEASE MECHANISMS

CF involves several organ systems, including the lungs, pancreas, intestines, hepatobiliary tract, genitourinary tract, and sweat duct. A common physiologic feature of these organs is CFTR-mediated alteration in electrolyte and water transport across the surface epithelium as discussed previously. Presumably, altered function of CFTR is the basic defect common to each of these organs. Despite the recent advances in our knowledge of the basic defect in CF, considerable gaps persist in our understanding of how CFTR dysfunction leads to dysfunction in each of the organs.

Lung Disease

Pathology

Progressive obstructive airway disease leading to bronchiectasis and respiratory failure accounts for the majority of severe morbidity and mortality from CF. The typical features of CF lung disease are mucus plugging of the airways, hypertrophy and hyperplasia of the secretory elements, and chronic infection, primarily with *Pseudomonas aeruginosa* and *Staphylococcus aureus.* Interestingly, the airways of CF infants who die in the first days of life appear normal, with no evidence of infection, inflammation, or mucus plugging.[97] At birth, both sources of mucus secretions, goblet cells and submucosal glands, appear normal in size, number, and distribution. One of the earliest detectable abnormalities is dilation of the submucosal gland ducts in the absence of inflammation,[97] suggesting that alterations in gland secretions occur before infection and inflammation. Presumably, this dilation results from either increased gland secretion or "plugging" of the gland duct by viscous mucus secretions. The earliest evidence of airway obstruction is thought to occur at the level of the bronchioles with mucus plugging and inflammation consistent with bronchiolitis.[98] The mucus plugging and inflammation extends from the bronchioles to progressively larger airways; pathologic features include inflammatory cell infiltration of the airways, goblet cell hyperplasia, submucosal gland hypertrophy, and regions of squamous metaplasia of the airway epithelium. Chronic infection and inflammation of the airways leads to bronchiectasis, then peribronchial fibrosis. It is not clear whether these pathologic features are direct results of the basic defect or secondary to chronic infection and inflammation.

Cellular Defects

In the proximal airways, the effects of mutations in CFTR on airway epithelial physiology appear to be multiple. In the superficial epithelium (Fig. 67-6), the absence of CFTR function has at least three major consequences. First, the absence of the CFTR Cl^- channel limits the ability of the tissue to respond to cAMP agonists with activation of Cl^- and presumably water secretion.[44] The precise functional consequences of this missing activity are not yet known. Second, and perhaps more important, the absence of CFTR protein function leads to up-regulation of the apical membrane Na^+ influx pathway. The up-regulation of the Na^+ absorptive pathway appears to be at the Na^+ channel level and is reflected in increased open probability (i.e., activation) of this channel.[99] This increased activation (P_0) is sufficient to increase the rate of transepithelial NaCl absorption by the CF airway epithelium by a factor of approximately 3 over normals.[100] The recognition of this abnormality led to the hypothesis that treating CF airways with Na^+ channel blockers, such as amiloride, would be therapeutically beneficial. The CF airways epithelium appears to compensate for this increased Na^+ influx by increasing the numbers of Na^+-K^+-ATPase pump proteins per cell and increasing the rate of energy (ATP) production by the cell, as reflected in O_2 consumption measurements. Third, it appears that the functional activity of Cl^-_a is increased in CF.[101] The predicted effect is to compensate the loss of airway Cl^- secretory capacity. It is not yet known whether this phenomenon reflects increased activation ($\uparrow P_0$) of Cl^-_a or an increased number of Cl^-_a proteins.

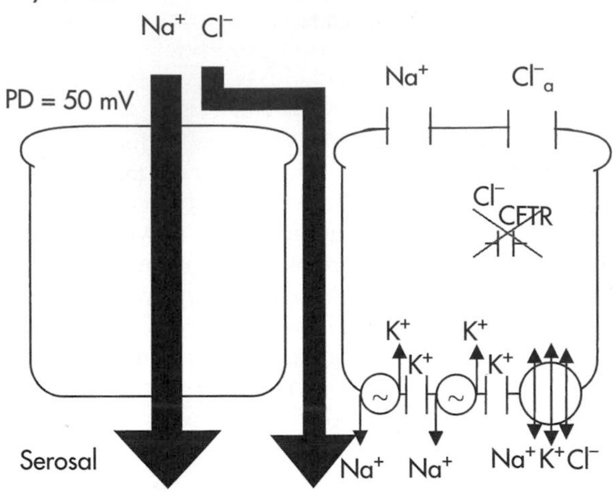

Fig. 67-6. Schema describing abnormal electrolyte transport in CF airway epithelia. The vectors *(left)* depict the raised Na^+ (and Cl^-) absorption in proximal airway epithelia in CF. The right panel depicts the ion transport elements in CF airway epithelia. The Cl^-_{CFTR} in the middle of the cell depicts "mutated" and degraded CFTR. The increased width of the Na^+ channel depicts the increased activity of ENaC without the inhibitory regulation by CFTR. The increase in Na^+-K^+-ATPase molecules on the serosal membrane likely reflects compensation for the increased Na^+ influx. The increased width of the Cl^-_a channel reflects the increased capacity of this channel to mediate Cl^- secretion in CF. Under basal (non-stimulated) conditions, this channel appears to be inactive.

Altered Airway Secretions

The airway surface, from the nose to the terminal bronchioles, is lined with a thin layer of fluid that is thought to be divided into a periciliary fluid phase through which cilia beat freely and an overlying mucus gel phase that entraps particles and is transported cephalad by coordinated ciliary movement. The efficiency of mucociliary clearance may be impaired by changes in airway secretions, including decreased hydration, increased volume, or altered physicochemical properties. All three of these alterations may occur in CF.

Water and Electrolyte Composition of Airway Secretions. Studies as early as 1959 demonstrated that the relative water content of expectorated secretions and bronchoscopic aspirates from CF patients was less than that in normal subjects and in patients with bronchiectasis of non-CF etiology.[102,103] These studies were performed in CF patients with advanced lung disease. It is unclear whether a similar decrease in water content is apparent in the early stages of CF lung disease. This relative dehydration of CF secretions could reflect decreased water content or increased solid content of the secretions.

The electrolyte composition of airway surface fluid from normal and CF airways has been a recent subject for debate. Precise measurement of the electrolyte composition of airway surface liquid is difficult. The small volume of the airway-lining fluid layer in normal subjects limits the ability to selectively sample and analyze surface fluid composition, and current approaches to sampling lower airways may be complicated by artifactual alterations. Presently, there are two competing hypotheses: one proposes isotonic airway surface liquid and the other proposes hypotoic airway surface liquid in normal airways. According to the isotonic hypothesis, based on observations by Kilburn, isotonic volume absorption occurs across normal airway surface epithelia, as the volume of airway surface liquid is moved by mucociliary clearnace from distal (large surface area) to proximal airways (much smaller surface area).[28-29,104,105a-c] In CF, excessive isotonic volume absorption, driven by accelerated Na^+ transport, limits the volume of airway surface liquid available to hydrate airway mucus, and leads to concentration of secreted macromolecules, poor clearance of impacted secretions and chronic bacterial infection. The hypotonic hypothesis, based on concepts by Quinton and reports from Smith et al, suggests that normal airways maintain ion concentration gradients, that is, absorb ions but not volume, and generate hypotonic surface liquid, which implies the epithelium is either water impermeable or other forces (capillarity) retain water on airway surfaces.[105d-e] In CF, the inability to absorb NaCl results in airway surface liquid with a higher salt concentration than in normal airway surface fluid, leading to inhibition of salt-sensitive antimicrobial activity and chronic bacterial infection.[105e-f] Further studies are needed to definitively characterize electrolyte composition of CF airway surface liquid and its influence on early pathogenesis of CF lung disease.

The major secretory structures in the airways are goblet cells and submucosal glands that secrete mucin-type glycoproteins and other high molecular weight glycoconjugates. Typically, goblet cells account for up to 15% of the cells in surface epithelium, but an increased prevalence occurs with airway disease. Two typical pathologic findings in CF airways are goblet cell hyperplasia (increase in goblet cell prevalence) and goblet cell metaplasia (extension of goblet cells into bronchioles, where they usually do not occur). This increased number of goblet cells could account for an increase in baseline secretion assuming that the basal regulation is unchanged. Studies of nasal and tracheobronchial tissues have shown that baseline degranulation of single goblet cells from CF subjects is not different from those obtained from non-CF subjects.[106] Likewise, regulation of goblet cell secretion by ATP in CF airway tissues does not differ from non-CF tissues.[106] However, inflamed CF airways contain a number of factors, such as neutrophil elastase, cathepsin G, bacterial proteases, and serum proteins, that are known to enhance goblet cell secretion. The combination of increased prevalence of goblet cells and mediators that stimulate goblet cell secretion in CF airways could result in a substantial increase in secretions derived from goblet cells.

Similarly, submucosal gland secretions may be increased in CF. Submucosal glands are complex tubuloacinar structures found in the cartilaginous airways, typically located in the submucosal space between the surface epithelium and underlying cartilage. These glands contain multiple acini opening into tubules that drain into a collecting duct that opens to the airway surface.[107] The secretory cell types in submucosal glands are mucous cells that secrete mucin-type glycoproteins and serous cells that secrete lysozyme, lactoferrin, bronchial antileukoprotease, proline-rich proteins, and proteoglycans.[108] A hallmark of CF is hypertrophy of the submucosal glands,[109,110] suggesting increased secretory capacity of these structures. Even though submucosal gland hypertrophy is one of the earliest pathologic features of CF,[109] submucosal gland size is normal in newborns with CF,[97,111] suggesting the stimuli promoting gland growth are not present during the fetal period but are activated early in the disease process. Processes involved in submucosal gland growth and hypertrophy include gland cell proliferation and invasion into the submucosal matrix. Proliferating cells are more prevalent in bronchial submucosal glands from CF patients with advanced lung disease than in glands from non-CF subjects.[112] Recent studies suggest that metalloproteinases and plasminogen activators degrade the extracellular matrix, enabling enlarging glands to invade the submucosal region,[113,114] although their specific role in CF has not been defined. Presumably, inflammatory mediators and cytokines promote cell proliferation and expression of the matrix-degrading enzymes to promote gland hypertrophy in chronically infected CF airways.

One characteristic feature of CF submucosal glands that is apparent even before hypertrophy is dilation of the gland lumina.[97] This dilation could result from an increased rate of secretion by the mucous and serous cells and/or from plugging of the lumina by abnormally thick mucus secretions. Recent studies provide indirect evidence for the latter explanation. Studies by Engelhardt et al demonstrated that the predominant site of CFTR in non-CF bronchi is the submucosal gland, particularly at the apical surface of cells in ducts and serous tubules; however, in airways from CF patients with the ΔF508/ΔF508 mutation, no CFTR protein was detectable in either ducts or serous cells.[2] These observations have emphasized the relative importance of the submucosal gland and provide another link between the basic defect in CFTR and alterations in airway secretions. Submucosal gland cells in culture exhibit active Cl^- ion secretion, which may be important for hydration of their secretions; active Cl^- secretion is limited in CF gland cells.[115,116] This reduced chloride ion secretion by CF gland cells could lead to dehydrated, viscous secretions that could obstruct gland ducts.

The hypertrophied submucosal glands in CF may have an increased secretory capacity that contributes to the increased secretions and sputum production seen in CF. Modulation of submucosal gland secretion involves neural pathways. The most completely studied mechanism for regulation of submucosal gland secretion is the cholinergic neural pathway. Postganglionic parasympathetic efferent nerve endings are apparent in submucosal glands.[117] Submucosal gland secretion is increased by direct stimulation of the vagus nerve or its branches.[118,119] In addition, parasympathomimetic agents such as acetylcholine and methacholine stimulate gland secretion, but cholinergic antagonists, such as atropine, block gland secretion in response to vagal stimulation or cholinergic agonists. Although cholinergic fibers are most prevalent, submucosal glands also contain adrenergic and nonadrenergic, noncholinergic (NANC) nerve fibers.[120,121] The role of these neural pathways in regulation of CF submucosal gland secretion is undefined. It is not clear whether the inflammatory cell mediators and bacterial products in CF airways have a specific role in the regulation of gland secretion by either direct stimulation of glands or indirectly through activation of one of the neural pathways. Some studies suggest that neutrophil proteases can stimulate gland secretion.[122,123]

Altered Physicochemical Properties of Airway Secretions. One of the early names for CF was "mucoviscidosis," reflecting the abnormally thick and viscous sputum found in these patients. For several decades, investigators have focused on characterizing differences in CF secretions that may explain the altered viscosity of CF sputum and contribute to the pathogenesis of the disease. Indeed, some studies suggest that increased sputum viscosity correlates with degree of infection and severity of lung disease.[124,125]

Mucous glycoproteins (mucins) are high molecular weight, highly glycosylated glycoproteins thought to be the major determinants of the viscoelastic properties of airway mucus. These heterogeneous, polydisperse glycoproteins consist of a peptide core and multiple sugar side chains, typically attached by O-glycosidic linkages between *N*-acetylgalactosamine in the sugar chain and serine or threonine in the peptide core. The sugar chains contain negatively charged moieties, sialic acid and sulfate; repulsion of negative charges in adjacent sugar chains is thought to influence molecular structure, resulting in a rigid, "rodlike" conformation of mucin molecules[126,127] (Fig. 67-7, *A*). The overall composition is 70% to 80% carbohydrate, 20% amino acids, and 2% to 7% sulfate. The central portion of the peptide core is composed of tandem repeats of amino acid sequences rich in potential glycosylation sites, serine, and threonine.[128] The varying size of mucin molecules is attributable in part to the varying number of tandem repeats in the central portion. The unique sequences that flank the tandem repeats contain cysteine residues that are thought to link the large, rigid mucin molecules through disulfide bonds. These intermolecular bonds are key influences on the rigidity of the mucus gel.

The oligosaccharide chains of mucin molecules are composed of five sugars: L-fucose, D-*N*-acetylgalactosamine, D-*N*-acetylglucosamine, galactose, and sialic acid, with little to no mannose (prevalent in serum and membrane glycoproteins but not mucous glycoproteins). The final structure and length of the oligosaccharide chains are variable. Some of the oligosaccharide chains are sulfated, particularly those that are relatively long, containing seven or more sugars.[129]

The variability in mucin peptide length and in sugar side chain length, structure, and sulfation complicates analyses to characterize differences in CF mucins. Early studies suggested a number of compositional differences, including increased fucose content and decreased sialic acid content[130,131]; however, subsequent studies identified no alterations in the fucose and sialic acid content.[132,133] One alteration that has been demonstrated by a variety of approaches is increased sulfation of CF respiratory mucins.[129,134-136] Studies of expectorated sputum from CF patients demonstrated that the level of mucin sulfation increased with severity of disease,[137] suggesting that chronic infection and inflammation influence sulfation. However, when isolated from inflammatory influences, primary cultures of CF nasal epithelial cells continue to secrete mucins that are more highly sulfated than those from non-CF nasal cells,[136] suggesting that altered sulfation may result from the basic defect in CF. Recent studies suggest that sulfate uptake and distribution in airway epithelial cells may be linked to that of chloride via a heteroexchanger.[136] This linkage of sulfate and chloride distribution could ultimately interrelate the increased sulfation of mucins with the basic defect in chloride secretion.

Analysis of sulfated oligosaccharides purified from sputum of a CF patient have identified long, branched chains with up to 160 to 200 sugar residues; many of these side chains contain varying amounts of a repeating oligosaccharide sequence with sulfate linked to the 6 position of galactose and possibly *N*-acetylglucosamine residues.[139] Presumably, these long sugar side chains with negatively charged sulfate increase the rigidity of the mucin molecule, and likewise, increase the rigidity of the gel that incorporates these mucin molecules.

A number of other factors influence the viscosity of CF sputum, including content of other large, highly charged mole-

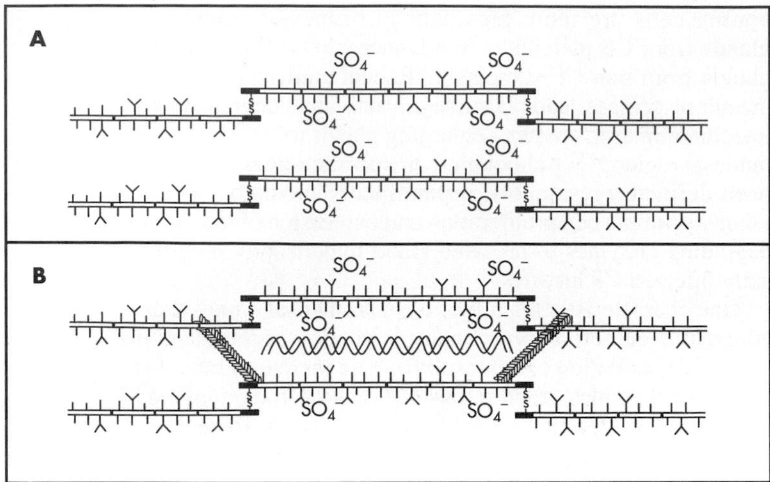

Fig. 67-7. **A,** Mucin molecule interactions in non-inflamed mucin secretions. Each mucin molecule is composed of a peptide core with numerous sugar side chains. The entire peptide core is heavily glycosylated except for the "naked" regions at the ends. The negatively charged sugar chains tend to repel each other, adding rigidity to the molecule. Adjacent mucin molecules may interact through disulfide bonds between cysteine residues in the naked region to form a loose network of these rigid molecules. **B,** Interaction between macromolecules in inflamed airway secretions. Degradation of neutrophils in inflamed airways releases DNA *(helix)* and filamentous actin *(linear aggregates of leaflets)* that interact and interweave with mucin molecules to form a more rigid gel. The polyanionic DNA interacts with the sugar chains of the mucin molecule to form a dense network that entraps long actin strands and forms a solid gel.

cules such as DNA and actin. Purulent airway secretions from CF patients contain high concentrations of extracellular DNA[140] thought to arise from degenerating polymorphonuclear neutrophils. Large, polymerized, polyanionic DNA molecules interact with mucin molecules and increase the viscosity of the mucus gel (Fig. 67-7, *B*). Enzymatic depolymerization of DNA by recombinant human DNase I reduces the viscosity of purulent CF sputum.[141] Another sputum component thought to arise from degenerating neutrophils is filamentous actin (F-actin), which forms long, protease-resistant filaments (Fig. 67-7, *B*). Recent studies of CF sputum have identified varying amounts of F-actin; addition of human gelsolin, a protein that severs actin filaments, reduces viscosity of purulent CF sputum,[142] suggesting that actin influences sputum viscosity.

Mucociliary Clearance

Over the past two decades, mucociliary clearance has been assessed in CF patients by a variety of methods. The results have been variable from markedly impaired clearance to normal clearance. Reasons for the variable results include variable deposition of labeled particles because of mucus plugging, failure to control for cough clearance, incomplete characterization of disease severity, and lack of age-matched controls. In a recent study, Regnis et al[143] systematically evaluated clearance of technetium (^{99}Tc)-sulphur colloid administered by aerosol to subjects instructed to perform a controlled breathing pattern to ensure a central deposition that matched that in CF patients. Patients were grouped according to disease severity and were compared with age-matched controls. Rate of clearance varied according to the severity of lung disease (Fig. 67-8); patients with severe lung disease had essentially no clearance, whereas patients with very mild lung disease and normal lung function had more rapid clearance; two of these patients had clearance within the normal range (Fig. 67-8). Patients with mild to moderate disease had a clearance rate that fell between that for patients with severe lung disease and those with normal lung function. The impaired clearance is thought to be attributable to the abnormal physicochemical properties and excessive volume of airway secretions. Cilia appear to be unaffected in CF. Cilia from CF patients have normal ultrastructure and normal ciliary beat frequency;[144,145] however, chronic inflammation may promote goblet cell hyperplasia and squamous cell metaplasia, and consequently loss of ciliated cells. This loss of cilia could further impair mucociliary clearance.

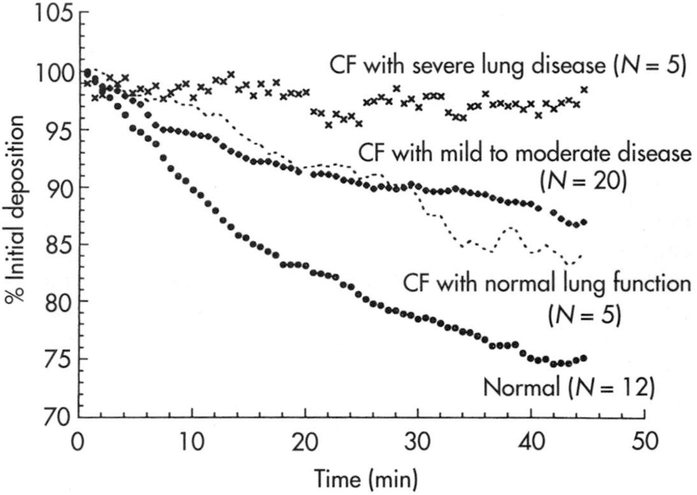

Fig. 67-8. Relationship of mucociliary clearance to severity of cystic fibrosis lung disease. Mucociliary clearance of deposited 99 Tc-sulfur colloid from the whole right lung was calculated from gamma camera images obtained at different times at initial deposition. The mean clearance curves are shown for normal subjects and for CF patients grouped by severity of lung disease. (From Regnis et al: *Am J Respir Crit Care Med* 150:66-71, 1994.)

Bacterial Adherence

One of the intriguing mysteries about CF is the predisposition to colonization and chronic infection with *P. aeruginosa* and *S. aureus.* A number of pathogenic mechanisms may be involved, including increased adherence of these organisms to CF airway epithelial cells and/or CF airway mucins, as well as adaptive modifications of these organisms in the CF airway microenvironment resulting in acquisition of characteristics that interfere with clearance. The most extensively investigated mechanism is bacterial adherence. Several *Pseudomonas* adhesins have been defined, but the adhesin that mediates initial colonization of CF airways is not known.[146] Receptors for *P. aeruginosa* attachment are roughly 2 times more prevalent on CF airway epithelial cells than on non-CF epithelial cells,[147] suggesting that CFTR mutations influence expression of *Pseudomonas* receptors, either directly or indirectly. It is unlikely that mutated CFTR itself is a *Pseudomonas* receptor, because the mutations that are common in CF are not located in the extracellular regions. Conceivably, CFTR may influence post-translational modification of glycolipids and glycoproteins that serve as *Pseudomonas* receptors, as proposed by Barasch.[148] *Pseudomonas* pili bind to the asialoganglioside (asialoGM1) that contains the GalNAcβ1-4 Gal sequence but not to the sialylated form of this ganglioside. AsioloGM1 is more prevalent on the surface of CF airway epithelial cells.[149] It has been speculated that decreased sialylation of this ganglioside may reflect increased acidification of the Golgi apparatus as the result of an absence of CFTR Cl^- channels; the enzyme that sialylates this ganglioside (sialyl transferase) is less efficient at a lower pH and hence sialylation is impaired.[148] Alternatively, decreased sialylation may reflect enzymatic removal of sialic acid by *Pseudomonas* neuraminidase; expression of this enzyme may be increased by the hyperosmolar conditions postulated to exist in CF airways.[150]

Another area of investigation is binding of bacteria with airway mucus components. In normal airways, inhaled particles and bacteria are entrapped in the mucus layer and cleared by mucociliary clearance. In CF airways, bacteria may be entrapped in a similar fashion but not cleared efficiently because of impaired mucociliary clearance as a result of increased, viscous secretions. In addition, there may be bacterial receptors in airway mucus. A likely location for *Pseudomonas* receptors is on the highly glycosylated mucin molecules. Despite extensive studies, no *P. aeruginosa* receptors have been identified in mucins purified from CF patients, as reviewed in detail elsewhere.[146] Interestingly, some strains of *Burkholderia cepacia* (formerly *Pseudomonas cepacia)* bind specifically to mucin components by a *B. cepacia* mucin binding adhesin.[151,152] Further study in this area is needed.

In addition to host factors favoring bacterial adherence to CF airways, there is evidence for bacterial factors that promote chronic colonization. One of the distinctive features of CF lung disease is the prevalence of mucoid strains of *P. aeruginosa.* Typically, CF airways are colonized initially with nonmucoid strains, but later, mucoid strains are isolated. Presumably, the microenvironment in CF airways contains factors that promote the transition to a mucoid phenotype; this mucoid phenotype is rarely isolated from patients with other conditions associated with chronic *P. aeruginosa* lung infections. Mucoid colonies produce a distinctive capsular slime that is known as *mucoid exopolysaccaride (MEP).* Several studies suggest that MEP interferes with phagocytosis of *P. aeruginosa,*[153,154] thereby allowing chronic colonization.

Less is known about adherence of *S. aureus* to airway epithelial cells. A recent study demonstrated that *S. aureus* strains isolated from CF patients bound to bronchial epithelial cell lines, epithelial cells from CF airways, and epithelial cells from non-CF airways more avidly than *S. aureus* strains isolated from non-CF patients.[155a] It is not clear whether the greater adherence expressed by isolation from CF patients reflects selection of adherent strains in the CF airway environment or up-regulation of *S. aureus* adhesins by factors in CF airway secretions.

Airway Inflammation

Infiltration of inflammatory cells into the airways is a classic pathologic feature of CF, even in early lung disease. Presumably, the chronic bacterial infection in the bronchi and bronchioles results in chronic inflammation of these airways. However, there is some evidence that airway inflammation may occur even before chronic infection with *S. aureus* or *P. aeruginosa.* Bronchoalveolar lavage (BAL) of some CF infants yields mucus plugs and increased prevalence of neutrophils without significant bacterial infection. It is not clear whether this early inflammatory response is precipitated by a respiratory viral infection or other insult.

Recent studies suggest that inflammatory responsiveness is enhanced in CF. Interleukin 10 (IL-10), a potent regulatory cytokine that decreases inflammatory responses, is constituitively produced by bronchial epithelial cells from healthy control subjects; however, IL-10 production appears to be down regulated in CF patients[155b] leading to enhanced airway inflammation that may occur even in the absence of infection. It is not clear whether this altered production of IL-10 is directly linked with the basic CFTR defect.

Neutrophils and their proteolytic enzymes are thought to be important mediators of airway destruction in CF lung disease. Abundant neutrophils and neutrophil elastase are present in the airways of CF patients. Even in patients with stable, clinically mild lung disease, the number of neutrophils in bronchoalveolar lavage fluids is approximately 400-fold greater than in control subjects.[156] The major proteolytic enzyme released by neutrophils is neutrophil elastase. The two antiproteases in the airways, α-1 protease inhibitor and secretory leukoprotease inhibitor (SLPI), bind and inactivate this proteolytic enzyme. However, in CF airways, the abundance of neutrophil elastase exceeds the capacity of these antiproteases, resulting in abundant active elastase activity. BAL fluid from CF patients with stable, mild lung disease has abundant active elastase despite a threefold elevation of α1 protease inhibitor.[156] This imbalance between neutrophil elastase and antineutrophil elastase molecules develops as early as 1 year of age[157] and is thought to play a central role in the pathogenesis of CF lung disease.

Some studies suggest that neutrophil elastase may induce production of interleukin-8 (IL-8), a cytokine that attracts and activates neutrophils. Both CF epithelial lining fluid and purified neutrophil elastase induce IL-8 production by bronchial epithelial cells.[158] Therefore, neutrophil elastase may mediate a self-perpetuating inflammatory response in CF airways by inducing the epithelium to secrete IL-8, which in turn recruits more neutrophils to the airway. Administration of aerosolized recombinant secretory leukoprotease inhibitor (rSLPI) to CF patients results in a decrease in active neutrophil elastase and a decrease in IL-8 expression, suggesting that antiprotease therapy could break the cycle of inflammation in CF airways.[159]

Neutrophil elastase may mediate a variety of other processes, including tissue damage, interference with opsonophagocytic defense, increased mucus secretion, and impaired ciliary beat (Fig. 67-9). In α-l antitrypsin deficiency, neutrophil elastase is thought to mediate the destructive changes that result in emphysema. This proteolytic enzyme may well mediate the destruction of airway structural proteins leading to bronchiectasis in CF. Evidence for proteolytic destruction of lung tissue in vivo was demonstrated by Bruce et al, who showed that urinary excretion of desmosines (breakdown products of elastin) was increased in CF patients; urinary desmosine concentrations correlated with severity of CF lung disease.[160]

Somewhat paradoxically, neutrophil elastase may interfere with opsonization and phagocytosis of bacteria such as *P. aeruginosa.* Neutrophil elastase is capable of destroying complement receptors and complement components, specifically the CRb receptor on neutrophils[161] and the C3bi opsonin on *P. aeruginosa.*[162] In addition, neutrophil elastase cleaves IgG antibodies to *P. aeruginosa* so that they bind to *P. aeruginosa,* but lack the Fc recognition signal for macrophages.[163] Therefore, neutrophil elastase is capable of impairing both neutrophil and macrophage phagocytosis of *P. aeruginosa.*

In addition, neutrophil elastase may have a direct influence on airway epithelial cells, particularly secretory cells. Admin-

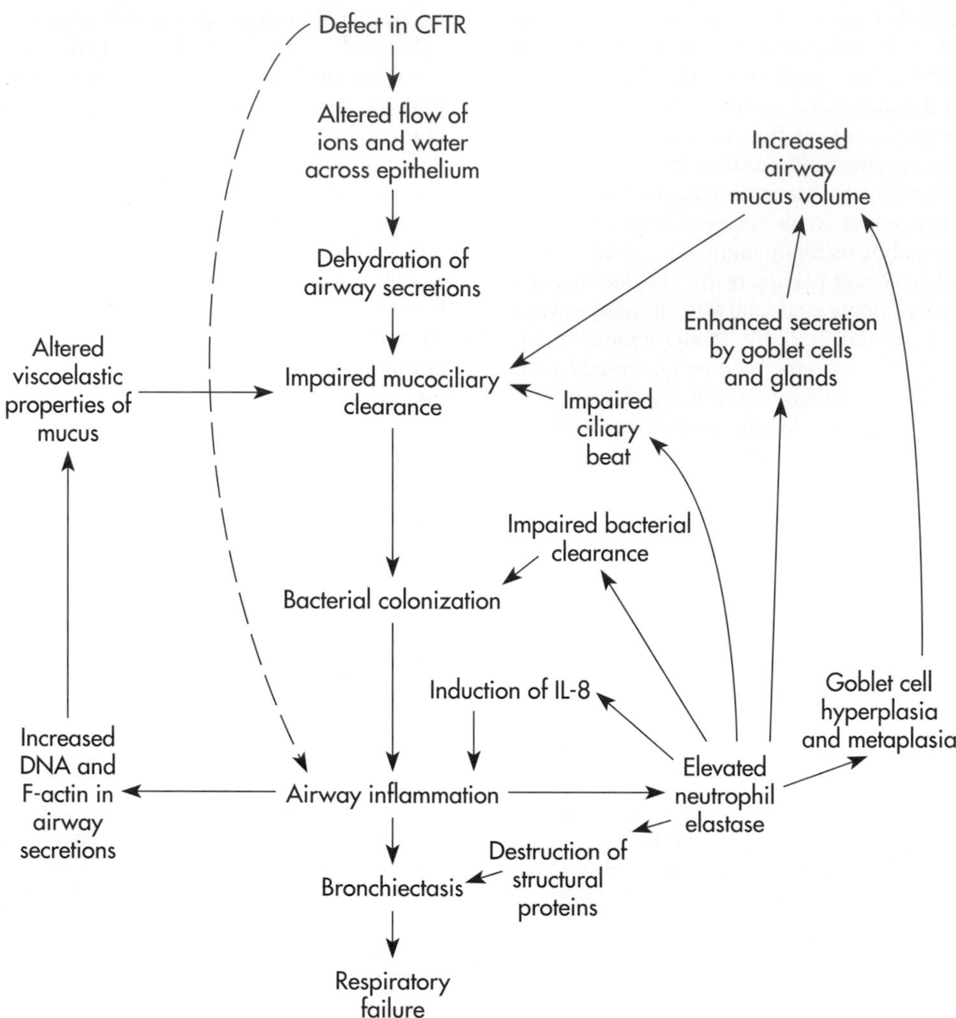

Fig. 67-9. Pathogenesis of cystic fibrosis lung disease, detailing the influence of airway inflammation.

istration of neutrophil elastase to hamsters produces secretory cell metaplasia; this effect can be blocked by administration of rSLPI.[164] Conceivably, neutrophil elastase may contribute to the goblet cell metaplasia seen in CF. In addition, neutrophil elastase is a potent secretagogue,[122,123] suggesting that neutrophil elastase may mediate mucus hypersecretion in CF. Finally, there is some evidence that neutrophil elastase may inhibit beating of respiratory cilia.[165,166] Taken together, neutrophil elastase may mediate many of the pathologic features in CF airways, as shown in Figure 67-9.

Other inflammatory cell products and mediators can influence the pathogenesis of CF lung disease. DNA and actin released by degrading neutrophils in the airways interweave with mucins in the airway mucus (see Fig. 67-7) to increase the viscosity of the mucus gel and further impair mucociliary clearance. Cathepsin G, transudated serum proteins, and arachidonic acid metabolites may stimulate secretion by goblet cells or glands.

Pathophysiology of Other Organs

Pancreas

The pancreas is severely affected in most patients with CF. At the time of birth, pancreatic ducts and ductules are obstructed with inspissated secretions. Later, the ducts and acini are dilated to form cysts and increasing fibrosis occurs. It is thought that the abnormalities in the pancreas in CF patients reflect the inability to secrete pancreatic ductal fluid in normal quantities with an alkaline pH, so that pancreatic enzymes cannot be delivered from the acinar region of the pancreas to the gut. Retention of enzymes in the ductal region results in enzymatic activation and autodigestion, inflammation, and finally, scarring of the pancreas. The typical early consequence of pancreatic destruction is pancreatic insufficiency, reflecting inadequate release of pancreatic enzymes into the intestine and consequent failure to digest and absorb intestinal nutrients. A late consequence of pancreatic insufficiency is destruction of sufficient islet cells, which leads to diabetes.

Sweat Gland

The consequences of CF in the sweat gland principally relate to failure of ductal function. The problem of ductal regulation of the NaCl concentration in sweat leads to the delivery of large quantities of salt onto the skin surface and, under conditions of heat stress, volume depletion and dehydration. The secretory problem in the sweat gland acinar region appears to be quantitatively small and of little clinical significance. Typically, children and adults increase their salt intake in response to their salt losses in sweat. Occasionally, infants limited to low-salt formula and baby foods develop hypochloremic, metabolic alkalosis from uncompensated loss of salt in sweat.

Intestine

Intestinal obstruction is fairly common in CF patients. Approximately 10% to 15% of CF infants present with meconium ileus in the newborn period. Typically, the distal ileus is obstructed with inspissated, tenacious meconium. Older patients are also prone to intestinal obstruction, a process called *distal intestinal obstruction syndrome*. In these older patients, the distal intestine is dilated and filled with large fecal masses. For both meconium ileus and distal intestinal syndrome, the most likely mechanism is dehydration of intestinal contents from impaired secretion of salt and water across the intestinal epithelium.

Reproductive Organs

With few exceptions, CF males are sterile with obstructive azoospermia. The anatomic defect is absence, atrophy, or obstruction of the vas deferens as well as the tail and body of the epididymis. The pathophysiologic basis for these changes is unclear. One proposed mechanism for atrophy of the vas deferens and epididymis is prenatal failure of the CF epididymis epithelium to secrete ions and water that dilate the lumens of these structures. Alternatively, CFTR itself may be important for maturation of the epididymis.

Females also have decreased fertility. Cervical mucus in CF women is thickened. Typically, cervical submucosal glands and the endocervical canal are dilated and obstructed by mucus plugs. This viscous cervical mucus impedes sperm migration, leading to decreased fertility. Another potential mechanism is altered salt and water secretion by the oviduct epithelium. The resulting dehydration of oviduct fluid may impair migration of sperm and eggs through the oviduct.

REFERENCES

1. Riordan JR, Rommens JM, Kerem B, Alon N, Rozmahel R, Grzelczak Z, Zielenski J, Lok S, Plavsic N, Chou J, Drumm ML, Iannuzzi MC, Collins FS, Tsui L: Identification of the cystic fibrosis gene: Cloning and characterization of complementary DNA, *Science* 245(4922):1066-1073, 1989.

CFTR Protein

2. Engelhardt JF, Yankaskas JR, Ernst SA, Yang Y, Marino CR, Boucher RC, Cohn JA, Wilson JM: Submucosal glands are the predominant site of CFTR expression in human bronchus, *Nat Genet* 2(3):240-247, 1992.
3. Marino CR, Matovcik LM, Gorelick FS, Cohn JA: Localization of the Cystic Fibrosis Transmembrane Conductance Regulator in pancreas, *J Clin Invest* 88(2):712-716, 1991.
4. Kartner N, Augustinas O, Jensen TJ, Naismith AL, Riordan JR: Mislocalization of DF508 CFTR in cystic fibrosis sweat gland, *Nat Genet* 1(5):321-327, 1992.
5. Trezise AEO, Buchwald M: In vivo cell-specific expression of the cystic fibrosis transmembrane conductance regulator, *Nature* 353(6343): 434-437, 1991.
6. Cheng SH, Gregory RJ, Marshall J, Paul S, Souza DW, White GA, O'Riordan C, Smith AE: Defective intracellular transport and processing of CFTR is the molecular basis of most cystic fibrosis, *Cell* 63(4):827-834, 1990.
7. Anderson MP, Berger HA, Rich DP, Gregory RJ, Smith AE, Welsh MJ: Nucleoside triphosphates are required to open the CFTR chloride channel, *Cell* 67(4):775-784, 1991.
8. Cheng SH, Rich DP, Marshall J, Gregory RJ, Welsh MJ, Smith AE: Phosphorylation of the R domain by cAMP-dependent protein kinase regulates the CFTR chloride channel, *Cell* 66(5):1027-1036, 1991.
9. Bradbury NA, Jilling T, Berta G, Sorscher EJ, Bridges RJ, Kirk KL: Regulation of plasma membrane recycling by CFTR, *Science* 256 (5056):530-532, 1992.
10. Bubien JK, Kirk KL, Rado TA, Frizzell RA: Cell cycle dependence of chloride permeability in normal and cystic fibrosis lymphocytes, *Science* 248(4961):1416-1419, 1990.

Function of the CFTR Protein

11. Anderson MP, Rich DP, Gregory RJ, Smith AE, Welsh MJ: Generation of cAMP-activated chloride currents by expression of CFTR, *Science* 251(4994):679-682, 1991.
12. Anderson MP, Gregory RJ, Thompson S, Souza DW, Paul S, Mulligan RC, Smith AE, Welsh MJ: Demonstration that CFTR is a chloride channel by alteration of its anion selectivity, *Science* 253(5016):202-205, 1991.
13. Sheppard DN, Rich DP, Ostedgaard LS, Gregory RJ, Smith AE, Welsh MJ: Mutations in CFTR associated with mild-disease-form Cl^- channels with altered pore properties, *Nature* 362(6416):160-164, 1993.
14. Bear CE, Li C, Kartner N, Bridges RJ, Jensen TJ, Ramjeesingh M, Riordan JR: Purification and functional reconstitution of the cystic fibrosis transmembrane conductance regulator (CFTR), *Cell* 68(4): 809-818, 1992.
15. Stutts MJ, Gatzy JT, Boucher RC: Effects of metabolic inhibition on ion transport by dog bronchial epithelium, *J Appl Physiol* 64(1):253-258, 1988.
16. Quinton PM, Reddy MM: Control of CFTR chloride conductance by ATP levels through non-hydrolytic binding, *Nature* 360(6399):79-81, 1992.
17. Welsh MJ, Smith AE: Molecular mechanisms of CFTR chloride channel dysfunction in cystic fibrosis, *Cell* 73(7):1251-1254, 1993.
18. Stutts MJ, Gabriel SE, Price EM, Sarkadi B, Olsen JC, Boucher RC: Pyridine nucleotide redox potential modulates cystic fibrosis transmembrane conductance regulator Cl^- conductance, *J Biol Chem* 269 (12):8667-8674, 1994.
19. Tabcharani JA, Chang XB, Riordan JR, Hanrahan JW: Phosphorylation-regulated Cl^- channel in CHO cells stably expressing the cystic fibrosis gene, *Nature* 352(6336):628-631, 1991.
20. Boucher RC, Cheng EHC, Paradiso AM, Stutts MJ, Knowles MR, Earp HS: Chloride secretory response of cystic fibrosis human airway epithelia: preservation of calcium but not protein kinase C- and A-dependent mechanisms, *J Clin Invest* 84(5):1424-1431, 1989.
21. Chang X, Tabcharani JA, Hou Y, Jensen TJ, Kartner N, Alon N, Hanrahan JW, Riordan JR: Protein kinase A (PKA) still activates CFTR chloride channel after mutagenesis of all 10 PKA consensus phosphorylation sites, *J Biol Chem* 268(15):11304-11311, 1993.
22. Welsh MJ, Liedtke CM: Chloride and potassium channels in cystic fibrosis airway epithelia, *Nature* 322(6078):467-470, 1986.
23. Schoumacher RA, Shoemaker RL, Halm DR, Tallant EA, Wallace RW, Frizzell RA: Phosphorylation fails to activate chloride channels from cystic fibrosis airway cells, *Nature* 330(6150):752-754, 1987.
24. Egan M, Flotte T, Afione S, Solow R, Zeitlin PL, Carter BJ, Guggino WB: Defective regulation of outwardly rectifying Cl^- channels by protein kinase A corrected by insertion of CFTR, *Nature* 358(6387):581-584, 1992.
25. Gabriel SE, Clarke LL, Boucher RC, Stutts MJ: CFTR and outward rectifying chloride channels are distinct proteins with a regulatory relationship, *Nature* 363(6426):263-268, 1993.
26. Chinet TC, Fullton JM, Yankaskas JR, Boucher RC, Stutts MJ: Sodium-permeable channels in the apical membrane of human nasal epithelial cells, *Am J Physiol* 265(4 Pt 1):C1050-C1060, 1993.
27. Hyde SC, Emsley P, Hartshorn MJ, Mimmack MM, Gileadi U, Pearce SR, Gallagher MP, Gill DR, Hubbard RE, Higgins CF: Structural model of ATP-binding proteins associated with cystic fibrosis, multidrug resistance and bacterial transport, *Nature* 346(6282):362-365, 1990 (comments).

Cellular Functions of CFTR

28. Boucher RC: Human airway ion transport (part 1), *Am J Respir Crit Care Med* 150(1):271-281, 1994.
29. Boucher RC: Human airway ion transport (part 2), *Am J Respir Crit Care Med* 150(2):581-593, 1994.
30. Willumsen NJ, Davis CW, Boucher RC: Cellular Cl^- transport in cultured cystic fibrosis airway epithelium, *Am J Physiol* 256(5 Pt 1): C1045-C1053, 1989.
31. Willumsen NJ, Davis CW, Boucher RC: Intracellular Cl^- activity and cellular Cl^- pathways in cultured human airway epithelium, *Am J Physiol* 256(5 Pt 1):C1033-C1044, 1989.
32. Willumsen NJ, Boucher RC: Shunt resistance and ion permeabilities in normal and cystic fibrosis airway epithelium, *Am J Physiol* 256(5 Pt 1): C1054-C1063, 1989.

33. Clarke LL, Grubb BR, Yankaskas JR, Cotton CU, McKenzie A, Boucher RC: Relationship of a non-CFTR mediated chloride conductance to organ-level disease in *cftr(-/-)* mice, *Proc Natl Acad Sci USA* 91(2):479-483, 1994.
34. Finkbeiner WE, Shen B, Widdicombe JH: Chloride secretion and function of serous and mucous cells of human airway glands, *Am J Physiol* 267(2 Pt 1):L206-L210, 1994.
35. Ballard ST, Taylor AE: Bioelectric properties of proximal bronchiolar epithelium, *Am J Physiol* 267(1 Pt 1):L79-L84, 1994.
36. Van Scott MR, Hester S, Boucher RC: Ion transport by rabbit nonciliated bronchiolar epithelial cells (Clara cells) in culture, *Proc Natl Acad Sci USA* 84(15):5496-5500, 1987.
37. Engelhardt JF, Zepeda M, Cohn JA, Yankaskas JR, Wilson JM: Expression of the cystic fibrosis gene in adult human lung, *J Clin Invest* 93(2):737-749, 1994.
38. McCray PB Jr, Bettencourt JD, Bastacky J, Denning GM, Welsh MJ: Expression of CFTR and a cAMP-stimulated chloride secretory current in cultured human fetal alveolar epithelial cells, *Am J Respir Cell Mol Biol* 9(6):578-585, 1993.
39. Tizzano EF, O'Brodovich H, Chitayat D, Benichou JC, Buchwald M: Regional expression of CFTR in developing human respiratory tissues, *Am J Respir Cell Mol Biol* 10(4):355-362, 1994.
40. Barker PM, Boucher RC, Yankaskas JR: Bioelectric properties of cultured monolayers from epithelium of distal human fetal lung, *Am J Physiol* 268(2 Pt 1):L270-L277, 1995.
41. Barker PM, Brigman KK, Paradiso AM, Boucher RC, Gatzy JT: Cl^- secretion by trachea of CFTR(+/-) and (-/-) fetal mouse. *Am J Respir Cell Mol Biol* 13(3):307-313, 1995.
42. Baxter P, Goldhill J, Hardcastle J, Hardcastle PT, Taylor CJ: Enhanced intestinal glucose and alanine transport in cystic fibrosis, *Gut* 31(7): 817-820, 1990.
43. Berschneider HM, Knowles MR, Azizkhan RG, Boucher RC, Tobey NA, Orlando RC, Powell DW: Altered intestinal chloride transport in cystic fibrosis, *FASEB J* 2(10):2625-2629, 1988.
44. Quinton PM: Cystic fibrosis: a disease in electrolyte transport, *FASEB J* 4(10):2709-2717, 1990.
45. Sato K, Sato F: Defective beta adrenergic response of cystic fibrosis sweat glands in vivo and in vitro, *J Clin Invest* 73(6):1763-1771, 1984.
46. Leung AH, Wong PYD, Gabriel SE, Yankaskas JR, Boucher RC: cAMP- but not Ca^{2+}-regulated Cl^- conductance in the oviduct is defective in a mouse model of cystic fibrosis, *Am J Physiol* 268(3 Pt 1): C708-C712, 1995.
47. Leung AYH, Wong PYD, Yankaskas JR, Boucher RC: cAMP-regulated but not Ca^{2+}-regulated Cl^- conductance in the epididymes and seminal vesicles is defective in a mouse model of cystic fibrosis (unpublished), 1994.
48. Robson AM, Tateishi S, Ingelfinger JR, Strominger DB, Klahr S: Renal function in cystic fibrosis, *J Pediatr* 79(1):42-50, 1971.
49. Stenvinkel P, Hjelte L, Alvan G, Hedman A, Hultman E, Strandvik B: Decreased renal clearance of sodium in cystic fibrosis, *Acta Paediatr Scand* 80(2):194-198, 1991.

Genetic Defect

50. Rommens JM, Iannuzzi MC, Kerem B, Drumm ML, Melmer G, Dean M, Rozmahel R, Cole JL, Kennedy D, Hidaka N, Zsiga M, Buchwald M, Riordan JR, Tsui L, Collins FS: Identification of the cystic fibrosis gene: chromosome walking and jumping, *Science* 245(4922):1059-1065, 1989.
51. Kerem B, Rommens JM, Buchanan JA, Markiewicz D, Cox TK, Chakravarti A, Buchwald M, Tsui L: Identification of the cystic fibrosis gene: genetic analysis, *Science* 245(4922):1073-1080, 1989.
52. Collins FS: Cystic fibrosis: molecular biology and therapeutic implications, *Science* 256(5058):774-779, 1992.
53. Boat TF, Welsh MJ, Beaudet AL: Cystic fibrosis. In Scriver CR, Beaudet AL, Sly WS et al, eds: *The metabolic basis of inherited disease,* ed 6, New York, 1989, McGraw-Hill, pp 2649-2680.
54. Tsui L: The spectrum of cystic fibrosis mutations, *Trends Genet* 8(11):392-398, 1992.
55. Cutting GR: Genotype defect: its effect on cellular function and phenotypic expression, *Semin Respir Crit Care Med* 15(5):356-363, 1994.
56. Kazazian HH Jr: Population variation of common cystic fibrosis mutations. The Cystic Fibrosis Genetic Analysis Consortium, *Hum Mutat* 4(3):167-177, 1994.
57. Morral N, Bertranpetit J, Estivill X, Nunes V, Casals T, Gimenez J, Reis A, Varon-Mateeva R, Macek M, Jr., Kalaydjieva L, Angelicheva D, Dancheva R, Romeo G, Russo MP, Garnerone S, Restagno G, Ferrari M, Magnani C, Claustres M, Desgeorges M, Schwartz M, Schwarz M, Dallapiccola B, Novelli G, Ferec C, de Arce M, Nemeti M, Kere J, Anvret M, Dahl N et al: The origin of the major cystic fibrosis mutation (DeltaF508) in European populations, *Nat Genet* 7(2):169-175, 1994.
58. Quinton PM: Abnormalities in electrolyte secretion in cystic fibrosis sweat glands due to decreased anion permeability. In Quinton PM, Martinez RJ, Hopfer U, eds: *Fluid and electrolyte abnormalities in exocrine glands in cystic fibrosis,* San Francisco, 1982, San Francisco Press, pp 53-76.
59. Quinton PM: What is good about cystic fibrosis? *Curr Biol* 4(8):742-743, 1994.
60. Gabriel SE, Brigman KN, Koller BH, Boucher RC, Stutts MJ: Cystic fibrosis heterozygote resistance to cholera toxin in the cystic fibrosis mouse model, *Science* 266(5182):107-109, 1994.

Mutations in the CFTR Gene

61. Worldwide survey of the delta F508 mutation—report from the cystic fibrosis genetic analysis consortium, *Am J Hum Genet* 47(2):354-359, 1990.
62. Tsui L: Mutations and sequence variations detected in the cystic fibrosis transmembrane conductance regulator (CFTR) gene: a report from the Cystic Fibrosis Genetic Analysis Consortium, *Hum Mutat* 1(3):197-203, 1992.
63. Gasparini P, Pignatti PF, Novelli G, Dallapiccola B, Nunes V, Casals T, Estivill X, Fernandez E, Balassopoulou A, Loukopoulos D, Lavinha J, Simova L, Komel R: Mutation analysis in cystic fibrosis [letter], *N Engl J Med* 323(1):62-63, 1990.
64. Gasparini P, Nunes V, Savoia A, Dognini M, Morral N, Gaona A, Bonizzato A, Chillon M, Sangiuolo F, Novelli G, Dallapiccola B, Pignatti PF, Estivill X: The search for South European cystic fibrosis mutations: identification of two new mutations, four variants, and intronic sequences, *Genomics* 10(1):193-200, 1991.
65. McColley SA, Rosenstein BJ, Cutting GR: Differences in expression of cystic fibrosis in blacks and whites, *Am J Dis Child* 145(1):94-97, 1991.
66. Mercier B, Raguenes O, Estivill X, Morral N, Kaplan GC, McClure M, Grebe TA, Kessler D, Pignatti PF, Marigo C, Bombieri C, Audrezet MP, Verlingue C, Ferec C: Complete detection of mutations in cystic fibrosis patients of Native American origin, *Hum Genet* 94(6):629-632, 1994.
67. Cutting GR, Curristin SM, Nash E, Rosenstein BJ, Lerer I, Abeliovich D, Hill A, Graham C: Analysis of four diverse population groups indicates that a subset of cystic fibrosis mutations occur in common among Caucasians, *Am J Hum Genet* 50(6):1185-1194, 1992.
68. Abeliovich D, Lavon IP, Lerer I, Cohen T, Springer C, Avital A, Cutting GR: Screening for five mutations detects 97% of cystic fibrosis (CF) chromosomes and predicts a carrier frequency of 1:29 in the Jewish Ashkenazi population, *Am J Hum Genet* 51(5):951-956, 1992.

Genotype and Phenotype

69. McIntosh I, Cutting GR: Cystic fibrosis transmembrane conductance regulator and the etiology and pathogenesis of cystic fibrosis, *FASEB J* 6(10):2775-2782, 1992.
70. Dean M, Santis G: Heterogeneity in the severity of cystic fibrosis and the role of CFTR gene mutations, *Hum Genet* 93(4):364-368, 1994.
71. Rosenstein BJ: Genotype-phenotype correlations in cystic fibrosis, *Lancet* 343(8900):746-747, 1994.
72. Davis PB: Molecular and cell biology of cystic fibrosis, *J Appl Physiol* 70(5):2331-2333, 1991.
73. Kerem E, Corey M, Kerem B, Rommens J, Markiewicz D, Levison H, Tsui L, Durie P: The relation between genotype and phenotype in cystic fibrosis-analysis of the most common mutation (DF_{508}), *N Engl J Med* 323(22):1517-1522, 1990.
74. Kristidis P, Bozon D, Corey M, Markiewicz D, Rommens J, Tsui L, Durie P: Genetic determination of exocrine pancreatic function in cystic fibrosis, *Am J Hum Genet* 50(6):1178-1184, 1992.
75. Hamosh A, Corey M: Correlation between genotype and phenotype in patients with cystic fibrosis. The Cystic Fibrosis Genotype-Phenotype Consortium, *N Engl J Med* 329(18):1308-1313, 1993.
76. Kiesewetter S, Macek M Jr, Davis C, Curristin SM, Chu CS, Graham C, Shrimpton AE, Cashman SM, Tsui L, Mickle J et al: A mutation in CFTR produces different phenotypes depending on chromosomal background, *Nat Genet* 5(3):274-278, 1993.

77. Highsmith WE, Burch LH, Zhou Z, Olsen JC, Boat TE, Spock A, Gorvoy JD, Quittell L, Friedman KJ, Silverman LM, Boucher RC, Knowles MR: A novel mutation in the cystic fibrosis gene in patients with pulmonary disease but normal sweat chloride concentrations, *N Engl J Med* 331(15):974-980, 1994.
78. Anguiano A, Oates RD, Amos JA, Dean M, Gerrard B, Stewart C, Maher TA, White WB, Milunsky A: Congenital bilateral absence of the vas deferens. A primarily genital form of cystic fibrosis, *JAMA* 267(13):1794-1797, 1992.
79. Osborne LR, Lynch M, Middleton PG, Alton EWFW, Geddes DM, Pryor JP, Hodson ME, Santis GK: Nasal epithelial ion transport and genetic analysis of infertile men with congenital bilateral absence of the vas deferens, *Hum Mol Genet* 2(10):1605-1609, 1993.
80. Augarten A, Kerem B, Yahav Y, Noiman S, Rivlin Y, Tal A, Blau H, Ben-Tur L, Szeinburg A, Kerem E, Gazit E: Mild cystic fibrosis and normal or borderline sweat test in patients with the 3849+10 kb C to T mutation, *Lancet* 342(8862):25-26, 1993.
81. Strong TV, Smit LS, Turpin SV, Cole JL, Hon CT, Markiewicz D, Craig MW, Rosenow EC III, Petty TL, Tsui L, Iannuzzi MC, Knowles MR, Collins FS: Cystic fibrosis gene mutation in two sisters with mild disease and normal sweat electrolyte levels, *N Engl J Med* 325(23):1630-1634, 1991.
82. Drumm ML, Wilkinson DJ, Smith LS, Worrell RT, Strong TV, Frizzell RA, Dawson DC, Collins FS: Chloride conductance expressed by delta F508 and other mutant CFTRs in *Xenopus* oocytes, *Science* 254(5039):1797-1799, 1991.
83. Anderson MP, Welsh MJ: Regulation by ATP and ADP of CFTR chloride channels that contain mutant nucleotide-binding domains, *Science* 257(5077):1701-1704, 1992.
84. Welsh MJ, Anderson MP, Rich DP, Berger HA, Denning GM, Ostedgaard LS, Sheppard DN, Cheng SH, Gregory RJ, Smith AE: Cystic fibrosis transmembrane conductance regulator: a chloride channel with novel regulation, *Neuron* 8(5):821-829, 1992.
85. Kubesch P, Doerk T, Wulbrand U, Kaelin N, Neumann T, Wulf B, Geerlings H, Weissbrodt H, von der Hardt H, Tuemmler B: Genetic determinants of airways' colonisation with *Pseudomonas aeruginosa* in cystic fibrosis, *Lancet* 341(8839):189-193, 1993.
86. Chu C, Trapnell BC, Curristin SM, Cutting GR, Crystal RG: Extensive posttranscriptional deletion of the coding sequences for part of nucleotide-binding fold 1 in respiratory epithelial mRNA transcripts of the cystic fibrosis transmembrane regulator gene is not associated with the clinical manifestations of cystic fibrosis, *J Clin Invest* 90(3):785-790, 1992.
87a. Strong TV, Wilkinson DJ, Mansoura MK, Devor DC, Henze K, Yang Y, Wilson JM, Cohn JA, Dawson DC, Frizzell RA, et al. Expression of an abundant alternatively spliced form of the cystic fibrosis transmembrane conductance regulator (CFTR) gene is not associated with a cAMP-activated chloride conductance, *Hum Mol Genet* 2(3):225-230, 1993.
87b. Rozmahel R, Wilschanski M, Matin A, Plyte S, Oliver M, Auerbach W, Moore A, Forstner J, Durie P, Nadeau J, Bear C, Tsui LC: Modulation of disease severity in cystic fibrosis transmembrane conductance regulator deficient mice by a secondary genetic factor, *Nat Genet* 12(3):280-287, 1996.

Genetic Testing

88. Simpson JL: Preimplantation genetics and recovery of fetal cells from maternal blood, *Curr Opin Obstet Gynecol* 4(2):295-301, 1992.
89. Wertz DC, Janes SR, Rosenfield JM, Erbe RW: Attitudes toward the prenatal diagnosis of cystic fibrosis: factors in decision making among affected families, *Am J Hum Genet* 50(5):1077-1085, 1992.
90. Caskey CT, Kaback MM, Beaudet AL, Cavalli-Sforza LL: The American Society of Human Genetics statement on cystic fibrosis screening, *Am J Hum Genet* 46(2):393, 1990.
91. Statement from the National Institututes of Health Workshop on Population Screening for the Cystic Fibrosis Gene: Workshop on population screening for the cystic fibrosis gene, *N Engl J Med* 323(1):70-71, 1990.
92. Biesecker L, Bowles-Biesecker B, Collins F, Kaback M, Wilfond B: General population screening for cystic fibrosis is premature, *Am J Hum Genet* 50(2):438-439, 1992.
93. Statement of the American Society of Human Genetics on cystic fibrosis carrier screening: ASHG Ad Hoc Committee on cystic fibrosis carrier screening, *Am J Hum Genet* 51(6):1443-1444, 1992.
94. Lemna WK, Feldman GL, Kerem B, Fernbach SD, Zevkovich EP, O'Brien WE, Riordan JR, Collins FS, Tsui L, Beaudet AL: Mutation analysis for heterozygote detection and the prenatal diagnosis of cystic fibrosis, *N Engl J Med* 322(5):291-296, 1990.
95. Wilcken B, Chalmers G: Reduced morbidity in patients with cystic fibrosis detected by neonatal screening, *Lancet* ii(8468):1319-1321, 1985.
96. Bowling F, Cleghorn G, Chester A, Curran J, Griffin B, Prado J, Francis P, Shepherd R: Neonatal screening for cystic fibrosis, *Arch Dis Child* 63(2):196-198, 1988.

Disease Mechanisms

97. Sturgess J, Imrie J: Quantitative evaluation of the development of tracheal submucosal glands in infants with cystic fibrosis and control infants, *Am J Pathol* 106(3):303-311, 1982.
98. Zuelzer WW, Newton WA Jr: The pathogenesis of fibrocystic disease of the pancreas. A study of 36 cases with special reference to the pulmonary lesions, *Pediatrics* 4(1):53-69, 1949.
99. Chinet TC, Fullton JM, Yankaskas JR, Boucher RC, Stutts MJ: Mechanism of sodium hyperabsorption in cultured cystic fibrosis nasal epithelium: a patch clamp study, *Am J Physiol* 266(4 Pt 1):C1061-C1068, 1994.
100. Boucher RC, Stutts MJ, Knowles MR, Cantley L, Gatzy JT: Na^+ transport in cystic fibrosis respiratory epithelia. Abnormal basal rate and response to adenylate cyclase activation, *J Clin Invest* 78(5):1245-1252, 1986.
101. Johnson LG, Boyles SE, Wilson J, Boucher RC: Normalization of raised sodium absorption and raised calcium-mediated chloride secretion by adenovirus-mediated expression of cystic fibrosis transmembrane conductance regulator in primary human cystic fibrosis airway epithelial cells, *J Clin Invest* 95(3):1377-1382, 1995.
102. Chernick WS, Barbero GJ: Composition of tracheobronchial secretions in cystic fibrosis of the pancreas and bronchiectasis, *Pediatrics* 24(5 Pt 1):739-745, 1959.
103. Matthews LW, Spector S, Lemm J, Potter JL: Studies on pulmonary secretions. I. The over-all chemical composition of pulmonary secretions from patients with cystic fibrosis, bronchiectasis, and laryngectomy, *Am Rev Respir Dis* 88(2):199-204, 1963.
104. Wanner A, Salathe M, O'Riordan TG: Mucociliary clearance in the airways, *Am J Respir Crit Care Med* 154:1868-1902, 1996 (State of the Art).
105a. Widdicombe JH, Widdicombe JG: Regulation of human airway surface liquid, *Respir Physiol* 99:3-12, 1995.
105b. Sleigh MA, Blake JR, Liron N: The propulsion of mucus by cilia, *Am Rev Respir Dis* 137:726-741, 1988.
105c. Kilburn KH: A hypothesis for pulmonary clearance and its implications, *Am Rev Respir Dis* 98:449-463, 1968.
105d. Quinton PM: Viscosity versus composition in airway pathology, *Am J Respir Crit Care Med* 149:6-7, 1994 (editorial).
105e. Smith JJ, Travis SM, Greenberg EP, Welsh MJ: Cystic fibrosis airway epithelia fail to kill bacteria because of abnormal airway surface fluid, *Cell* 85:229-236, 1996.
105f. Goldman MJ, Anderson GM, Stolzenberg ED, Dari UP, Zasloff M, and Wilson JM: Human beta-defensin-1 is a salt-sensitive antibiotic that is inactivated in cystic fibrosis, *Cell* 88:553-560, 1997.
106. Lethem MI, Dowell ML, Van Scott M, Yankaskas JR, Egan T, Boucher RC, Davis CW: Nucleotide regulation of goblet cells in human airway epithelial explants: normal exocytosis in cystic fibrosis, *Am J Respir Cell Mol Biol* 9(3):315-322, 1993.
107. Meyrick B, Sturgess JM, Reid L: A reconstruction of the duct system and secretory tubules of the human bronchial submucosal gland, *Thorax* 24(6):729-736, 1969.
108. Basbaum CB, Jany B, Finkbeiner WE: The serous cell, *Annu Rev Physiol* 52:97-113, 1990.
109. Bedrossian CWM, Greenberg SD, Singer DB, Hansen JJ, Rosenberg HS: The lung in cystic fibrosis. A quantitative study including prevalence of pathologic findings among different age groups, *Hum Pathol* 7(2):195-204, 1976.
110. Lamb D, Reid L: The tracheobronchial submucosal glands in cystic fibrosis: a qualitative and quantitative histochemical study, *Br J Dis Chest* 66(4):239-247, 1972.

111. Chow CW, Landau LI, Taussig LM: Bronchial mucous glands in the newborn with cystic fibrosis, *Eur J Pediatr* 139(4):240-243, 1982.
112. Leigh MW, Kylander JE, Yankaskas JR, Boucher RC: Cell proliferation in bronchial epithelium and submucosal glands of cystic fibrosis patients, *Am J Respir Cell Mol Biol* 12:605-612, 1995.
113. Infeld MD, Brennan JA, Davis PB: Human fetal lung fibroblasts promote invasion of extracellular matrix by normal human tracheobronchial epithelial cells in vitro: a model of early airway gland development, *Am J Respir Cell Mol Biol* 8(1):69-76, 1993.
114. Lim M, Bowden J, McDonald D, Basbaum C: Analysis of metalloproteinases and plasminogen activators in tracheal submucosal gland development and hypertrophy, *Pediatr Pulmonol* suppl 9:252, 1993 (abstract).
115. Yamaya M, Finkbeiner WE, Widdicombe JH: Altered ion transport by tracheal glands in cystic fibrosis, *Am J Physiol* 261(6 Pt 1):L491-L494, 1991.
116. Becq F, Merten MD, Voelckel MA, Gola M, Figarella C: Characterization of cAMP dependent CFTR-chloride channels in human tracheal gland cells, *FEBS Lett* 321(1):73-78, 1993.
117. Meyrick B, Reid L: Ultrastructure of cells in the human bronchial submucosal glands, *J Anat* 107(2):281-299, 1970.
118. Davis B, Marin M, Fischer S, Graf P, Widdicombe J, Nadel J: New method for study of canine mucous gland secretion in vivo cholinergic regulation, *Am Rev Respir Dis* 113(4):257, 1976 (abstract).
119. Ueki I, German VF, Nadel JA: Micropipette measurement of airway submucosal gland secretion: autonomic effects, *Am Rev Respir Dis* 121(2):351-357, 1980.
120. Laitinen A, Partanen M, Hervonen A, Laitinen LA: Electron microscopic study on the innervation of the human lower respiratory tract: evidence of adrenergic nerves, *Eur J Respir Dis* 67(3):209-215, 1985.
121. Dey RD, Shannon WA Jr, Said SI: Localization of VIP-immunoreactive nerves in airways and pulmonary vessels of dogs, cats and human subjects, *Cell Tissue Res* 220(2):231-238, 1981.
122. Fahy JV, Schuster A, Ueki I, Boushey HA, Nadel JA: Mucus hypersecretion in bronchiectasis. The role of neutrophil proteases, *Am Rev Respir Dis* 146(6):1430-1433, 1992.
123. Schuster A, Ueki I, Nadel JA: Neutrophil elastase stimulates tracheal submucosal gland secretion that is inhibited by ICI 200, 355, *Am J Physiol* 262(1 Pt 1):L86-L91, 1992.
124. Feather EA, Russell G: Sputum viscosity and pulmonary function in cystic fibrosis, *Arch Dis Child* 45(244):807-808, 1970.
125. Puchelle E, Jacquot J, Beck G, Zahm JM, Galabert C: Rheological and transport properties of airway secretions in cystic fibrosis—relationships with the degree of infection and severity of the disease, *Eur J Clin Invest* 15(6):389-394, 1985.
126. Lamblin G, Lhermitte M, Degand P, Roussel P, Slayter HS: Chemical and physical properties of human bronchial mucus glycoproteins, *Biochimie* 61(1):23-43, 1979.
127. Rose MC, Voter WA, Brown CF, Kaufman B: Structural features of human tracheobronchial mucus glycoprotein, *Biochem J* 222(2):371-377, 1984.
128. Gum JR, Jr. Mucin genes and the proteins they encode: structure, diversity and regulation, *Am J Respir Cell Mol Biol* 7(6):557-564, 1992.
129. Roussel P, Lamblin G, Degand P, Walker-Nasir E, Jeanloz RW: Heterogeneity of the carbohydrate chains of sulfated bronchial glycoproteins isolated from a patient suffering from cystic fibrosis, *J Biol Chem* 250(6):2114-2122, 1975.
130. Dische Z, di Sant'Agnese P, Pallavicini C, Youlos J: Composition of mucoprotein fractions from duodenal fluid of patients with cystic fibrosis of the pancreas and from controls, *Pediatrics* 24(1):74-91, 1959.
131. Chernick WS, Berbero GJ: Studies on human tracheobronchial and submaxillary secretions in normal and pathophysiological conditions, *Ann NY Acad Sci* 106(2):698-708, 1963.
132. Menguy R, Masters YF, Desbaillets L: Salivary mucins of patients with cystic fibrosis: composition and susceptibility to degradation by salivary glycosidases, *Gastroenterology* 59(2):257-264, 1970.
133. Boat TF, Cheng PW, Wood RE: Tracheobronchial mucus secretion in vivo and in vitro by epithelial tissues from cystic fibrosis and control subjects. In Forstner GG, ed: *Mucus secretions and cystic fibrosis,* Basel, Switzerland, 1977, S Karger, pp 141-152.
134. Boat TF, Cheng P, Iyer RN, Carlson DM, Polony I: Human respiratory tract secretions. Mucous glycoproteins of nonpurulent tracheobronchial secretions, and sputum of patients with bronchitis and cystic fibrosis, *Arch Biochem Biophys* 177(1):95-104, 1976.
135. Frates RC Jr, Kaizu TT, Last JA: Mucus glycoproteins secreted by respiratory epithelial tissue from cystic fibrosis patients, *Pediatr Res* 17(1):30-34, 1983.
136. Cheng P, Boat TF, Cranfill K, Yankaskas JR, Boucher RC: Increased sulfation of glycoconjugates by cultured nasal epithelial cells from patients with cystic fibrosis, *J Clin Invest* 84(1):68-72, 1989.
137. Chace KV, Leahy DS, Martin R, Carubelli R, Flux M, Sachdev GP: Respiratory mucous secretions in patients with cystic fibrosis: relationship between levels of highly sulfated mucin component and severity of the disease, *Clin Chim Acta* 132(2):143-155, 1983.
138. Mohapatra NK, Cheng P, Parker JC, Paradiso AM, Yankaskas JR, Boucher RC, Boat TF: Sulfate concentrations and transport in human bronchial epithelial cells, *Am J Physiol* 264(5 Pt 1):C1229-C1237, 1993.
139. Sangadala S, Bhat UR, Mendicino J: Structures of sulfated oligosaccharides in human trachea mucin glycoproteins, *Mol Cell Biochem* 126(1):37-47, 1993.
140. Potter JL, Spector S, Matthews LW, Lemm J: Studies on pulmonary secretions. III. The nucleic acids in whole pulmonary secretions from patients with cystic fibrosis, bronchiectasis, and laryngectomy, *Am Rev Respir Dis* 99(6):909-916, 1969.
141. Shak S, Capon DJ, Hellmiss R, Marsters SA, Baker CL: Recombinant human DNase I reduces the viscosity of cystic fibrosis sputum, *Proc Natl Acad Sci USA* 87(23):9188-9192, 1990.
142. Vasconcellos CA, Allen PG, Wohl ME, Drazen JM, Janmey PA, Stossel TP: Reduction in viscosity of cystic fibrosis sputum by gelsolin, *Science* 263(5149):969-971, 1994.
143. Regnis JA, Robinson M, Bailey DL, Cook P, Hooper P, Chan HK, Gonda I, Bautovich G, Bye PT: Mucociliary clearance in patients with cystic fibrosis and in normal subjects, *Am J Respir Crit Care Med* 150(1):66-71, 1994.
144. Katz SM, Holsclaw DS Jr: Ultrastructural features of respiratory cilia in cystic fibrosis, *Am J Clin Pathol* 73(5):682-685, 1980.
145. Rutland J, Cole PJ: Nasal mucociliary clearance and ciliary beat frequency in cystic fibrosis compared with sinusitis and bronchiectasis, *Thorax* 36(9):654-658, 1981.
146. Prince A: Adhesins and receptors of *Pseudomonas aeruginosa* associated with infection of the respiratory tract, *Microb Pathol* 13(4):251-260, 1992.
147. Saiman L, Cacalano G, Gruenert D, Prince A: Comparison of adherence of *Pseudomonas aeruginosa* to respiratory epithelial cells from cystic fibrosis patients and healthy subjects, *Infect Immun* 60(7):2808-2814, 1992.
148. Barasch J, Kiss B, Prince A, Saiman L, Gruenert D, Al-Awqati Q: Defective acidification of intracellular organelles in cystic fibrosis, *Nature* 352(6330):70-73, 1991.
149. Saiman L, Prince A: *Pseudomonas aeruginosa* pili bind to asioloGM1 which is increased on the surface of cystic fibrosis epithelial cells, *J Clin Invest* 92(4):1875-1880, 1993.
150. Cacalano G, Kays M, Saiman L, Prince A: Production of the *Pseudomonas aeruginosa* neuraminidase is increased under hyperosmolar conditions and is regulated by genes involved in alginate expression, *J Clin Invest* 89(6):1866-1874, 1992.
151. Sajjan US, Corey M, Karmali MA, Forstner JF: Binding of *Pseudomonas cepacia* to normal human intestinal mucin and respiratory mucin from patients with cystic fibrosis, *J Clin Invest* 89(2):648-656, 1992.
152. Sajjan US, Forstner JF: Identification of the mucin-binding adhesin of *Pseudomonas cepacia* isolated from patients with cystic fibrosis, *Infect Immun* 60(4):1434-1440, 1992.
153. Pier GB, Saunders JM, Ames P, Edwards MS, Auerbach H, Goldfarb J, Speert DP, Hurwitch S: Opsonophagocytic killing antibody to *Pseudomonas aeruginosa* mucoid exopolysaccharide in older noncolonized patients with cystic fibrosis, *N Engl J Med* 317(13):793-798, 1987.
154. Cabral DA, Loh BA, Speert DP: Mucoid *Pseudomonas aeruginosa* resists nonopsonic phagocytosis by human neutrophils and macrophages, *Pediatr Res* 22(4):429-431, 1987.
155a. Schwab UE, Wold AE, Carson JL, Leigh MW, Cheng P, Gilligan PH, Boat TF: Increased adherence of *Staphylococcus aureus* from cystic fibrosis lungs to airway epithelial cells, *Am Rev Respir Dis* 148(2):365-369, 1993.
155b. Bonfield TL, Konstan MW, Burfeind P, Panuska JR, Hilliard JB, Berger M: Normal bronchial epithelial cells constitutively produce the anti-inflammatory cytokine interleukin-10, which is downregulated in cystic fibrosis, *Am J Respir Cell Mol Biol* 13(3):257-261, 1995.

156. Konstan MW, Hilliard KA, Norvell TM, Berger M: Bronchoalveolar lavage findings in cystic fibrosis patients with stable, clinical mild lung disease suggest ongoing infection and inflammation, *Am J Respir Crit Care Med* 150(2):448-454, 1994.
157. Birrer P, McElvaney NG, Rudeberg A, Sommer CW, Liechti-Gallati S, Kraemer R, Hubbard R, Crystal RG: Protease-antiprotease imbalance in the lungs of children with cystic fibrosis, *Am J Respir Crit Care Med* 150(1):207-213, 1994.
158. Nakamura H, Yoshimura K, McElvaney NG, Crystal RG: Neutrophil elastase in respiratory epithelial lining fluid of individuals with cystic fibrosis induces interleukin-8 gene expression in a human bronchial epithelial cell line, *J Clin Invest* 89(5):1478-1484, 1992.
159. McElvaney NG, Nakamura H, Birrer P, Hebert CA, Wong WL, Alphonso M, Baker JB, Catalano MA, Crystal RG: Modulation of airway inflammation in cystic fibrosis. In vivo suppression of interleukin-8 levels on the respiratory epithelial surface by aerosolization of recombinant secretory leukoprotease inhibitor, *J Clin Invest* 90(4):1296-1301, 1992.
160. Frizzell RA, Rechkemmer G, Shoemaker RL: Altered regulation of airway epithelial cell chloride channels in cystic fibrosis, *Science* 233:558-560, 1986.
161. Berger M, Sorensen RU, Tosi MF, Dearborn DG, Doering G: Complement receptor expression on neutrophils at an inflammatory site, the *Pseudomonas*-infected lung in cystic fibrosis, *J Clin Invest* 84(4):1302-1313, 1989.
162. Tosi MF, Zakem H, Berger M: Neutrophil elastase cleaves C3bi on opsonized *Pseudomonas* as well as CR1 on neutrophils to create a functionally important opsonin receptor mismatch, *J Clin Invest* 86(1):300-308, 1990.
163. Fick RB Jr, Naegel GP, Squier SU, Wood RE, Gee BL, Reynolds HY: Proteins of the cystic fibrosis respiratory tract: fragmented G opsonic antibody causing defective opsonophagocytosis, *J Clin Invest* 74(1): 236-248, 1984.
164. Lucey EC, Stone PJ, Ciccolella DE, Breuer R, Christensen TG, Thompson RC, Snider GL: Recombinant human secretory leukocyte-protease inhibitor: in vitro properties, and amelioration of human neutrophil elastase-induced emphysema and secretory cell metaplasia in the hamster, *J Lab Clin Med* 115(2):224-232, 1990.
165. Tegner H, Ohlsson K, Toremalm NG, von Mecklenburg C: Effect of human leukocyte enzymes on tracheal mucosa and its mucociliary activity, *Rhinology* 17(3):199-206, 1979.
166. Smallman LA, Hill SL, Stockley RA: Reduction of ciliary beat frequency in vitro by sputum from patients with bronchiectasis: a serine proteinase effect, *Thorax* 39(9):663-667, 1984.
167. Kerem B, Zielenski J, Markiewicz D, Bozon D, Gazit E, Yahaf J, Kennedy D, Riordan JR, Collins FS, Rommens JM, Tsui L: Identification of mutations in regions corresponding to the two putative nucleotide (ATP)-binding folds of the cystic fibrosis gene, *Proc Natl Acad Sci USA* 87(21):8447-8451, 1990.
168. Cutting GR, Kasch LM, Rosenstein BJ, Zielenski J, Tsui L, Antonarakis SE, Kazazian HH Jr: A cluster of cystic fibrosis mutations in the first nucleotide-binding fold of the cystic fibrosis conductance regulator protein, *Nature* 346(6282):366-369, 1990.
169. Vidaud M, Fanen P, Martin J, Ghanem N, Nicolas S, Goossens M: Three point mutations in the CFTR gene in French cystic fibrosis patients: identification by denaturing gradient gel electrophoresis, *Hum Genet* 85(4):446-449, 1990.
170. Osborne L, Knight R, Santis G, Hodson M: A mutation in the second nucleotide binding fold of the cystic fibrosis gene, *Am J Hum Genet* 48(3):608-612, 1991.
171. Zielenski J, Bozon D, Kerem B, Markiewicz D, Durie P, Rommens JM, Tsui L: Identification of mutations in exons 1 through 8 of the cystic fibrosis transmembrane conductance regulator (CFTR) gene, *Genomics* 10(1):229-235, 1991.
172. Claustres M, Gerrard B, White MB, Desgeorges M, Kjellberg P, Rollin B, Dean M: A new mutation (1078delT) in exon 7 of the CFTR gene in a southern French adult with cystic fibrosis, *Genomics* 13(3):907-908, 1992.
173. Dean M, White MB, Amos J, Gerrard B, Stewart C, Khaw KT, Leppert M: Multiple mutations in highly conserved residues are found in mildly affected cystic fibrosis patients, *Cell* 61(5):863-870, 1990.

CHAPTER 68

Cystic Fibrosis: Respiratory Manifestations

Moira L. Aitken, Stanley B. Fiel, and Robert C. Stern

CLINICAL RESPIRATORY MANIFESTATIONS

The median survival of cystic fibrosis (CF) patients continues to increase. In 1996 the median survival of the 20,886 CF patients reported to the registry was 28.3 years for men and 31.8 years for women.[1] Although there is multiorgan involvement in CF, pulmonary disease is the cause of premature death in more than 95% of cases. The initial histopathologic appearance is mucus obstruction. This is followed by infection and leads to bronchiolectasis, bronchitis, and later, bronchiectasis. The most prevalent organisms that chronically infect the airway are *Haemophilus influenzae, Staphylococcus aureus,* and *Pseudomonas aeruginosa.* Pulmonary function testing initially shows airflow obstruction, but as disease progresses, a restrictive and obstructive pattern is seen. The chest radiograph initially shows hyperinflation secondary to air trapping. Later, mucus plugging and peribronchial thickening is seen with predominance of disease in the upper lobes, but over time, fibrosis and bronchiectasis are found in all lung fields. Pulmonary disease may be complicated by hyperresponsive airways, hemoptysis, pneumothorax, and allergic bronchopulmonary aspergillosis. The chronic pulmonary disease is treated with chest physical therapy, antibiotics, bronchodilators and optimizing the nutritional status of the patient.

PATHOPHYSIOLOGY

CF is caused by mutations in the cystic fibrosis transmembrane conductance regulator (CFTR), a membrane glycoprotein that forms or influences chloride ion channels and influences sodium channels.[2] The ion channels involved in airway epithelium are complex. Three different Cl^- ion channels have been described on the apical surface of the airway epithelial cell. In CF, one of these Cl^- ion channels is either absent or does not open under the appropriate stimuli. The apical membrane of the airway epithelial cells also shows an abnormality in Na^+ ion absorption. CFTR functions as a regulator of sodium channels and may interact with sodium channels directly through cytoskeletal elements, regulatory proteins, or soluble extracellular mediators released by CFTR.[2,3] Despite the ion channel abnormalities of the airway epithelial cells being well characterized, the adverse effects of these channel defects have not yet been described at a cellular level. The pathophysiologic mechanism by which these ion channel defects leads to the organ disease state is unknown. Increased sodium absorption and decreased chloride secretion reduce the water content of the periciliary fluid. The hyperosmolar periciliary fluid may lead to thick unhydrated mucins[4] and increased mucus viscosity. Increasing the viscosity of mucus slows ciliary beat frequency[5] in vitro. However, in vivo measurements of mucociliary transport suggest that it is variable in CF.[6,7] Slowing mucociliary transport per se is probably not the only process involved because diseases such as primary ciliary dyskinesia, in which there may be no ciliary movement, have a more benign clinical course than in CF.[8]

Other mechanisms by which CFTR may produce lung disease have been postulated.[10] CFTR may be expressed in the intracellular organelles. If the intracellular organelles have pH-dependent enzymes, then many abnormal proteins may be produced, such as epithelial cell receptors, which may have a predilection for *Pseudomonas* attachment. Alternatively, there may be increased sulfation of CF mucins,[11] which, in turn, may lead to increased viscosity of mucus or may increase bacterial adherence to these altered mucins.[12] Many other intracellular functions could be affected through this potential mechanism of action of CFTR.

It has recently been suggested that defensins in the airway surface fluid are important in killing bacterial pathogens and that the high NaC1 concentration of CF airway fluid may impair bacterial killing.[9]

PATHOPHYSIOLOGY OF PULMONARY DISEASE

The prognosis for meconium ileus and other life-threatening problems in young infants with CF has markedly improved and, consequently, the absolute number of autopsies performed on infants is decreasing. Therefore, the pathology published shortly after the disease was first described is still important for our understanding of the initial pathologic events that occur in the lungs.

The ion transport abnormalities caused by defective CFTR apparently have little functional adverse effect on unventilated fetal airways. Many investigators have confirmed that the lung is histologically normal at birth and may remain normal for the first several weeks of extrauterine life.[13-17] The earliest pathologic change is plugging of submucosal gland ducts in the large airways. This can be detected in very young infants.[18] This duct obstruction is probably responsible for the dilation of submucosal gland acini, although the overall size of the mucus glands is probably normal.[13] These pathologic changes appear to precede infection and subsequent inflammation.[17]

Recent studies of bronchoalveolar lavage (BAL) fluid from infants suggest that airway inflammation is present in those as young as 4 weeks,[19] possibly before infection. Thereafter, infection plays a more major role, and it becomes more difficult to distinguish primary from secondary pathologic changes. Pulmonary disease can progress rapidly, and some degree of bronchiectasis can almost always be demonstrated by age 6 to 24 months,[20] even in the few patients with clinically mild pulmonary disease who come to autopsy. This strongly suggests that some infection has already begun in these patients. These observations suggest that the chronic inflammation of CF can lead relatively rapidly to bronchiectasis. In patients who seem to have a milder phenotype, the same pathologic processes are seen in their lungs, but are found at an older age.[21]

Persistent and worsening infection results in squamous epithelial metaplasia and increasingly severe neutrophilic infiltration of the bronchial and peribronchial tissue (with purulent rather than just mucoid secretions in the airways), producing bronchitis and bronchiolitis. There is progressive thickening of the airway walls. Eventually, after progressive destruction of airway wall components, bronchiolectasis and saccular bronchiectasis develop. Erosion and subsequent healing within the airway may lead to constrictive scars that could aggravate hyperinflation and further impede drainage of purulent secretions.[22]

Inspection of the thoracic cavity at autopsy of patients who died of respiratory failure often reveals pleural adhesions, especially in those patients with a history of pneumothorax, recurrent pleurisy, or chest surgery. These adhesions are of variable density and strength. The lungs show extreme overinflation and are paler than normal, except for areas of hemorrhagic pneumonia. Bullae, which may be partially filled with purulent secretions, may be present, particularly in the upper lobes (Fig. 68-1). Lymphoid hypertrophy is often found with enlargement of the hilar and peribronchial nodes. The bronchial arteries are enlarged, occasionally contain aneurysms, and often follow a very tortuous course (Fig. 68-2). Erosion of branches of these systemic pressure vessels within the submucosa is probably the cause of bleeding in patients with massive hemoptysis. Patients with severe pulmonary hypertension may manifest obvious dilation of the main pulmonary arteries. Cor pulmonale and heart failure are not uncommon terminal complications, and cardiac dilation and right-sided hypertrophy are then found. Small amounts of nonpurulent pericardial fluid may be present.

Initial sectioning of the lung at autopsy reveals extensive bronchiectasis extending into the small airways. Green purulent pus oozes from virtually all airways. There are usually scattered pneumonic consolidations, occasionally with areas of hemorrhage. Mucoid impaction of airways with resultant segmental or lobar collapse is not an uncommon event during life and is occasionally seen at autopsy.[23,24] Similarly, large lung abscesses and pus-filled cysts, recognized during life, are noted at autopsy.

On microscopic examination of patients who die of respiratory failure, there is extensive neutrophilic infiltration of the peribronchial parenchyma with some extension into the perialveolar region (Fig. 68-3). Bronchiolectasis is widespread, and few normal or near-normal airways are found. The alveoli may show some neutrophilic infiltration, but mononuclear cells often predominate. Alveoli appear reduced in number, perhaps partially resulting from fusion in the wake of previous organizing pneumonia. However, se-

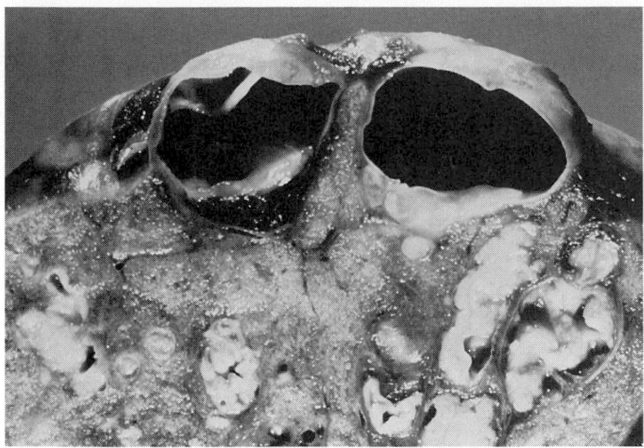

Fig. 68-1. Gross pathologic section from a patient who died from cystic fibrosis. Bullae are seen at the lung surface. Extensive bronchiectasis is seen with thick purulent secretions within the airways.

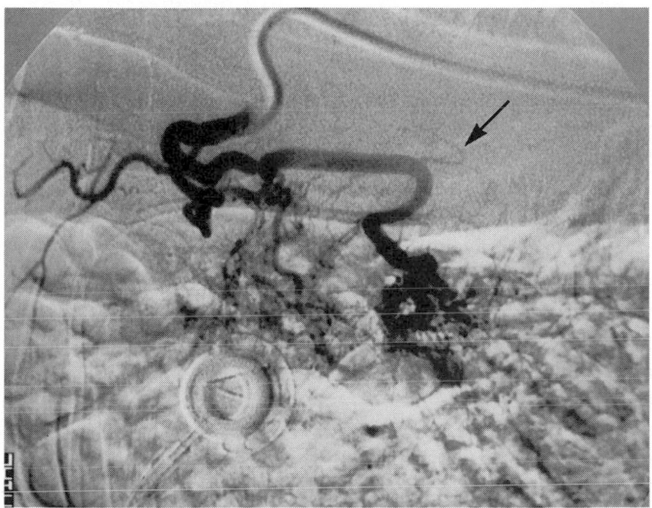

Fig. 68-2. Bronchial arteriogram of a 21-year-old man with cystic fibrosis who had massive hemoptysis. An anterior spinal artery (*arrow*) originates from the right bronchial artery which is prominent and tortuous.

vere bronchiolitis may also have led to alveolar hypoplasia. The alveolar shape is often distorted, and there may be some true emphysema with rupture of alveolar septae, particularly in adult patients. Microscopic areas of atelectasis are very common. Some patients may also show evidence of an interstitial pneumonia.[25] The extent of interstitial pneumonia at autopsy may be of sufficient severity to suggest that it was clinically important.

There may be enormous variation in severity between the two lungs, from lobe to lobe, from segment to segment, and even between adjacent airways. Parenchymal disease occurs later, and the related pathologic findings should really be considered secondary complications of the initial airway infection. Some complications such as true anatomic emphysema (as opposed to simple and presumably reversible overinflation) may never occur to any significant extent. Other possible, but not inevitable, complications include parenchymal hemorrhage, hemorrhagic pneumonia, and lobar or segmental atelectasis.

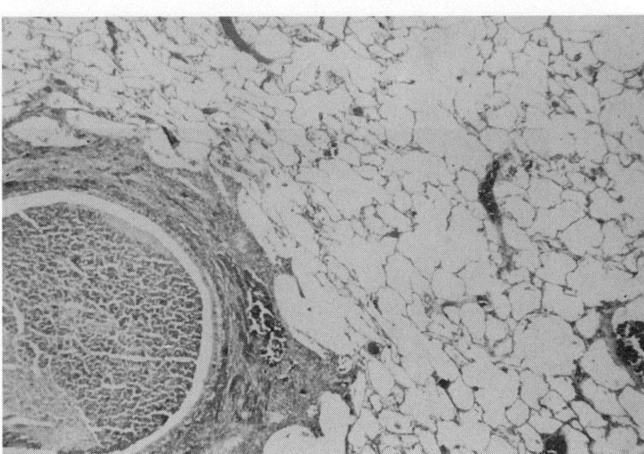

Fig. 68-3. Histologic section from the lung of a patient with cystic fibrosis. An airway in cross section is filled with mucopurulent material. There is fibrosis around the airway with relative sparing of the lung parenchyma.

Although the severity of pathologic changes often varies greatly within each lobe or segment, the upper lobes (and particularly the right upper lobe) tend to be the earliest and most severely affected,[26-29] confirming radiographic studies.[30] No anatomic basis (for example, congenital airway stenosis) for this predilection for the upper lobes has been demonstrated (aspiration during infancy has been proposed). In addition to overall severity, some complications (such as lung cysts[31] and mucoid impaction[32]) occur much more often in the upper lobes. Atelectasis also occurs predominantly in the upper lobes, at least in childhood.[23,24] The fact that lobectomy for localized severe disease most commonly targets an upper lobe[33] is additional indirect evidence of the increased susceptibility of this lobe to severe involvement.

The intrapulmonary blood vessels show a variety of abnormalities. Intraacinar vessels are decreased in number because chronic infection and/or pulmonary hypertension impeded their development or because they were secondarily destroyed. The remaining vessels are also small. Whatever the cause, these pathologic changes increase pulmonary vascular resistance and contribute to pulmonary hypertension, which can approach systemic pressure levels and cause death from cardiac failure.

PATHOPHYSIOLOGY OF SINUS DISEASE

The initiating event that leads to sinus disease in CF is felt to be alteration in the mucus, impaired mucociliary transport, and mechanical obstruction of the sinus ostia.[34] Obstruction is followed by bacterial infection (*P. aeruginosa, H. influenzae,* streptococci, and *S. aureus*).[35] Panopacification of the paranasal sinuses is present on the sinus radiographs in 90% to 100% of patients older than 8 months[36] (Fig. 68-4). The frontal sinuses rarely develop in CF patients. It is believed that the early onset of sinusitis prevents pneumatization. Nasal polyposis is found in 10% to 32% of patients and is more commonly seen in the pediatric age group. The histologic features of CF nasal polyps are similar to allergic polyps except that CF polyps contain few eosinophils.[37]

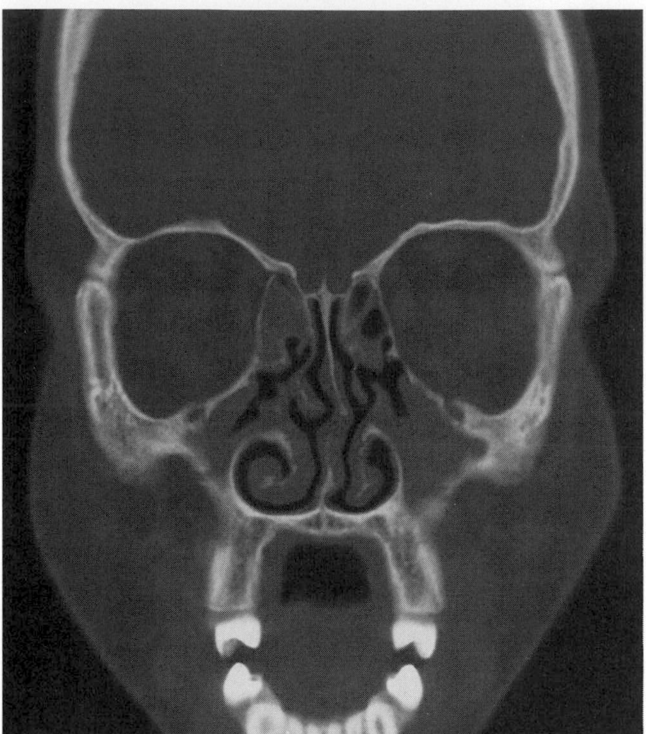

Fig. 68-4. This is a sinus CT scan of a 21-year-old man with cystic fibrosis. There is mucosal thickening of the maxillary and ethmoid sinuses and turbinates. The frontal sinuses are hypoplastic. There are small air fluid levels in the left maxillary sinus.

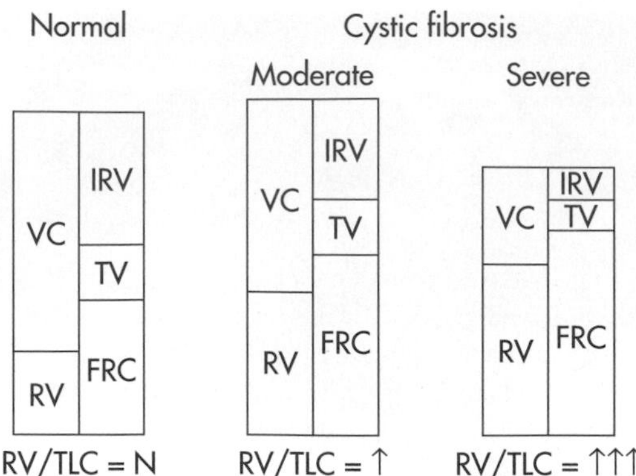

Fig. 68-5. Change in lung volumes in cystic fibrosis. Early in the course of the disease, residual volume increases considerably, whereas total lung capacity only increases a small amount. With advanced disease, a restrictive process may be superimposed on the obstructive disease and the RV/TLC ratio is greatly increased. (From Taussig L: *Cystic fibrosis,* New York, 1984, Thieme-Stratton.)

LUNG FUNCTION

The majority of patients with CF develop pulmonary involvement during infancy or early childhood, periods of time when it is difficult to assess lung function objectively. During early infancy, tests performed during quiet breathing, such as the measurement of respiratory resistance, are possible.[38] Forced expiratory flow rates can be measured in young infants with CF by the chest compression technique,[39,40] as can functional residual capacity. In older children (4 to 6 years of age), peak expiratory flow rates can often be obtained,[41] but such flows do not reflect changes in the small peripheral airways where it is thought the early disease in CF occurs. Total respiratory resistance by the forced oscillation method has been used with young children as well as partial expiratory flow volume curves.[42]

The newborn with CF probably has normal pulmonary function until peripheral airways become obstructed.[39,40] Infant CF patients with respiratory symptoms often demonstrate increased total respiratory resistance and decreased expiratory flows. As the CF child grows, airway resistance may become "normal" because, with lung growth, the relative distribution of resistance between central and peripheral airways changes and peripheral resistance may decrease. As lung disease progresses, airways become further obstructed and air trapping increases; measurements of air flow (FVC, FEV_1, FEF_{25-75}, and peak flow) become abnormal.[43-45]

Dynamic compliance decreases early in the course of the lung disease, reflecting peripheral airway obstruction.[46] Initially, static compliance is normal. Because the pulmonary disease is inhomogeneous, no single pulmonary function test is most sensitive for detection of early lung disease.[47] Pulmonary function tests reported as sensitive indices of pathologic abnormalities in older children include reduced maximum expiratory flow rates,[48] an elevated slope of phase III of nitrogen washout,[46] elevated dead space,[49] and an increased A-a difference.[50] RV/TLC ratios and Po_2 values may also be sensitive indicators of early disease.[51] The closing volume has not been found to be a sensitive detector of early peripheral airway obstruction.

Lung Volumes

Lung volume measurements in CF should be performed using a body plethysmograph, as air-trapping in CF will lead to underestimation of lung volumes using helium or nitrogen washout techniques. Air trapping leads to an increase in residual volume, and vital capacity is decreased. Total lung capacity remains within normal values until there is widespread fibrosis, when it may decrease. An increase in RV/TLC is seen (Fig. 68-5) and this is felt by some clinicians to be a sensitive indicator of disease.

Spirometry

As disease in CF progresses, FEV_1, FVC, and FEF_{25-75} decrease. The FEV_1/VC ratio also decreases early in the course of the lung disease, but as the disease progresses and a restrictive pattern develops, the FEV_1/VC ratio may rise again although not to normal values, while the absolute values of FEV_1 and FVC are both declining.

Airway Resistance

Airway resistance and conductance reflect changes in the large airways or extensive small airway disease. Small infants may have an increase in airway resistance as their small airways may contribute proportionally more to airway resistance than occurs in larger people.

Maximum Expiratory Flow Volume Curve

Maximum expiratory flow volume (MEFV) curves can be useful in detecting early changes in disease. The shape of the curve gives an indication of airway obstruction because convexity of the curve in relation to the volume axis is suggestive of airflow obstruction.[43]

ARTERIAL BLOOD GASES

Arterial blood gases show progressive widening of the A-a difference with disease progression, and the presence of CO_2 retention is an ominous sign.[52] Patients with Pco_2 values greater than 50 torr had a 2-year survival of approximately 50%; a Pco_2 of greater than 55 torr had a 2-year survival of less than 20%.[52] Arterialized capillary blood gas measurements can be used for patient assessment.[53]

PROGNOSIS AND PULMONARY FUNCTION TESTS

Clinical scoring systems of disease severity often include pulmonary function measurements.[54] The largest study to date to determine prognosis using pulmonary function results involved 673 patients and demonstrated that FEV_1 correlated best with mortality risk.[52] A FEV_1 of less than 30% predicted normal had a 45% 2-year mortality risk.

Airway hyperreactivity, defined by a positive methacholine challenge test, is present in 50% to 60% of patients with CF.[55,56] The presence of airway hyperreactivity, without apparent pulmonary exacerbation, correlates with a more rapid decline in pulmonary function.[56] There is a high rate of within-subject variability in spirometric testing at any point in time in the CF population, which may contribute to the high rate of airway hyperresponsiveness in these patients.[57,58] One study demonstrated a significant response to β agonists in 19 of 20 (95%) CF patients, age range 7 to 25 years, at some time during a 12-month period.[59] In this study, there was an increased incidence of reactivity during acute exacerbations of the disease. Some of the airway hyperreactivity may be caused by secretions and edema in the airway wall rather than smooth muscle hyperresponsiveness per se. It has not been determined for the CF population whether bronchial reactivity is more common in males or more common with increasing age.

Recently Eggleston et al[56] felt that a subpopulation of CF patients could be selected to have a response to bronchodilators on the basis of a positive methacholine challenge test at least 4 weeks following their last exacerbation (at a time when they were clinically stable). In a double-blind cross-over study in selected patients (mean age 15 years) over a 4-week period, these investigators showed that β agonists did improve peak expiratory flow rates in 14 of 15 patients with a positive methacholine challenge, but in only 1 of 8 with a negative methacholine challenge. No significant changes were seen in FEV_1 or FVC with β agonists in these patients. Tobin et al[60] found no correlation between atopy and bronchial hyperreactivity in their study of 25 patients, 88% of whom were atopic and 35% of whom had airway hyperreactivity as defined by a positive histamine challenge test. However, with such a large percentage of the CF population being atopic and with such a high propensity to bronchial reactivity (up to 95% in some studies), a large study is required to determine whether atopy is associated with bronchial hyperreactivity.

NUTRITION AND PULMONARY FUNCTION TESTS

Retrospective cross-sectional studies have documented a correlation between good nutrition and improved lung function and survival.[61,62] Patients are at risk for nutritional deficiencies because of malabsorption, decreased food intake, and increased metabolic requirements secondary to their disease. CF patients often have poor weight gain, growth retardation, delayed puberty, muscle wasting, and vitamin, mineral, essential fatty acid, and taurine deficiencies. Improvement in nutrition should enhance respiratory muscle strength and immunity, and may have important long-term effects on the state of the lungs and ultimately on prognosis. Improved nutrition has been associated with a slower deterioration, or with improvement, in lung function and improved expiratory muscle strength.[63-66]

PREGNANCY AND PULMONARY FUNCTION

In 1994, 135 CF women were reported to the CF registry as having conceived. This represents 3.7% of all CF women aged 15 to 41 years.[1] Pregnancy occurred in women with all levels of pulmonary function.[67] The distribution of pulmonary impairment among the pregnant women was not significantly different from that seen in the nonpregnant population. The highest level of pulmonary function was seen in those women who delivered at term. Women who delivered prematurely, and those who chose or were possibly counseled to undertake therapeutic abortion had more severe pulmonary function testing. An important question is whether pregnancy adversely affects the course of the disease in the mother. Preliminary evidence suggests that it does not.[68] Those women with mild disease, indicated by a Shwachman score in the mid 70s, relatively mild airflow obstruction, and good nutritional status should tolerate pregnancy well.[69] For women with more severe, but stable disease, pregnancy may be endorsed, but with the understanding that close medical observation will be essential and therapeutic abortion may be necessary if pregnancy leads to life-threatening medical deterioration.

GASTROESOPHAGEAL REFLUX

The incidence of clinically apparent gastroesophageal reflux was 57 of 412 (14%) in a large series by Stringer et al.[70] The predominant reflux mechanism in these patients is a transient inappropriate relaxation of the lower esophageal sphincter rather than a decreased steady-state lower esophageal sphincter pressure. It has been postulated that the presence of gastroesophageal reflux may correlate with poor pulmonary function because of recurrent aspiration. In Stringer's series, 18 patients with demonstrable reflux had significantly reduced forced expiratory volume and forced vital capacity. CF patients respond well to cisapride and antireflux therapy[71-73] and are not good candidates for surgical intervention.[70]

MICROBIOLOGY AND IMMUNOLOGY

Infection plays a major role in the progression of the obstructive pulmonary disease, which causes over 95% of the mortality from CF.

S. aureus, H. influenzae, or both are often recovered from respiratory secretions of infants and young children with CF.[74] Generally, *S. aureus* infection precedes *H. influenzae. H. influenzae* is usually found only intermittently on culture[75] and is rarely present in later childhood, particularly after the patient is colonized with gram-negative organisms. However, *S. aureus* may persist in the presence of gram negative organisms, including *P. aeruginosa. P. aeruginosa* eventually becomes the dominant organism in the majority of CF patients.[74,76] In a recent CF Foundation yearly report, over 75% of CF adults had been reported to be culture positive for *P. aeruginosa* during the preceding year (Cystic Fibrosis Foundation Registry 1991). Once *P. aeruginosa* is firmly established, *S. aureus* becomes an inconstant culture finding and often disappears. *Pseudomonas cepacia* is not an inevitable colonizer, but in some patients it can become the dominant pathogen, replacing all others, including *P. aeruginosa.* These four organisms are discussed in more detail in the following section.

SPECIFIC PATHOGENS

Haemophilus Influenzae

Cross sectional studies indicate that from 10% to 15% of CF patients harbor *H. influenzae* at any one time.[74,75] Unlike *S. aureus, P. aeruginosa,* and *P. cepacia, H. influenzae* rarely establishes long term colonization and infection as the dominant organism. Thus the percentage of patients who harbor this organism at some time in their disease course has not been specifically investigated, but presumably is considerably higher, perhaps approaching 100%. Furthermore, isolation of the organism is not always easy (anaerobic culture techniques and/or the use of inhibitory agents to suppress *P. aeruginosa* such as pyocins may be useful).[75] This also affects the accuracy of incidence statistics. Organisms recovered from CF patients are not encapsulated and are usually biotype 1[77] (which is usually associated with virulence[78]), but are often untypable and β-lactamase negative (usually associated with relative lack of pathogenicity).

H. influenzae has been recovered from the periphery of the lung at thoracotomy[79] and has been associated with pulmonary exacerbations.[80] The lack of definitive evidence that *H. influenzae* is a major pathogen in patients with moderate or severe pulmonary disease does not exclude the possibility that it (acting alone, or more likely after or in concert with colonization by *S. aureus*) may be an important pathogen much earlier, perhaps by injuring the airway epithelium and allowing gram-negative organisms such as *P. aeruginosa* to colonize the lung.

We have encountered two patients with *H. influenzae* empyema (unpublished data). Although this complication is rare, it does serve to emphasize the potential role for this organism as a pulmonary pathogen in CF. Patients in whom pulmonary exacerbations seem associated with *H. influenzae* recovery in the sputum improve with antihemophilus treatment.[81] Furthermore, a large statistical study of risk factors (for death within 5 years) indicted that the presence of *H. influenzae* in sputum was an important negative predictor, suggesting (but not proving) a pathogenic role for the organism.[82]

Staphylococcus Aureus

Unlike *H. influenzae,* for which only scant hard data have been accumulated over 50 years to support a pathogenic role in CF, *S. aureus* has been known to be capable of causing progressive pulmonary disease and death since the early descriptions of CF.[83] Acute staphylococcal pneumonia (including empyema[80]) has been frequently reported in CF patients, and is now considered an indication for sweat testing. The organism has also been associated with less acute progression of disease and, albeit infrequently in recent years, is occasionally the only pathogen found in the lungs of CF patients who die of respiratory insufficiency.

The pathology of acute staphylococcal pneumonia is no different in CF patients than it is in previously healthy children. The pathology of chronic staphylococcal infection in CF is not known to be different from that caused by *P. aeruginosa.*

In one study of strains of *S. aureus* obtained from 107 CF patients, the organism was always susceptible to vancomycin and netilmicin.[84] In this series, 11.7% of the isolates were methicillin resistant; these organisms were always resistant to rifampicin as well. Drugs that are effective in achievable concentrations against methicillin-susceptible *S. aureus* (MSSA) include cephalexin, ciprofloxacin, and rifampicin.

The epidemiology of *S. aureus* (outside of CF) includes person-to-person spread by direct contact and, less commonly, by respiratory droplets or aerosol. In CF, the source of the original colonizing organisms is usually unknown, at least in part because the organism is so often found in the upper respiratory tract of normal persons.

Many hospitals isolate CF patients who harbor MRSA, but this is not universal, and the exact risk of MRSA-colonized CF patients mingling with uncolonized patients is unknown. In one study, the MRSA-positive patients at a large center had a great variety of antibiograms, evidence against a common source.[85]

The need for treatment of CF patients for *S. aureus* is unequivocal for acute staphylococcal pneumonia, but the decision to treat is not always obvious in other patients who are known to harbor the organism but who either are not symptomatic or have one or more other potential pathogens recovered on culture. The acquisition of MRSA does not have obvious clinical impact.[85] Furthermore, antibiotic treatment of *S. aureus* seems to facilitate colonization by *P. aeruginosa.*[86] Prophylactic continuous antistaphylococcal therapy (especially for young children) has been proposed. In a 5-year, placebo-controlled, double-blind, multicenter cephalexin study, patients were given cephalexin (90 to 100 mg/kg/day) or placebo. The entry criteria for that study were that patients had to be less than 2 years old and have no sign of clinical disease. Of 209 patients who were enrolled, 119 completed the study. Preliminary data suggested no differences in clinical variables examined. Specifically, there was no difference in growth, number of acute exacerbations, hospitalizations or hospital days, Brasfield scores (a chest radiograph score), or pulmonary function testing. Patients treated with cephalexin had less infection with *S. aureus* but had more colonization with *P. aeruginosa.* In short, this well designed and well-conducted study showed that an antistaphylococcal antibiotic had no positive outcome, and indeed may have a negative outcome in that it promoted earlier colonization with *P. aeruginosa.* On the other hand, Frederiksen et al[87] reported a high survival rate in their single Danish center since 1976 and attributed this increased survival rate in large part to more frequent and to more aggressive antibiotic regimens. Another recent study[88] demonstrated that infants treated with continuous antistaphylococcal antibiotics, starting in the neonatal period, had fewer hospitalizations and milder respiratory symptoms.

The short-term prognosis for CF patients with acute staphylococcal empyema and pneumonia is quite good with appropriate antibiotic treatment. Eradication of the organism from the upper respiratory tract or the sputum in chronically colonized patients is occasionally accomplished, but this does not always correlate with clinical improvement.

Pseudomonas Aeruginosa

P. aeruginosa was the first gram-negative organism reported to be an important pathogen in CF.[89] Its prevalence has steadily increased as the prognosis for the disease has improved and the CF patient population has become older. *P. aeruginosa* replaced *S. aureus* as the dominant pulmonary pathogen beginning in about 1950.

Colonization of the respiratory tract with *P. aeruginosa* almost always begins with the morphologically "classic" (nonmucoid) strain. Onset of *P. aeruginosa* colonization often begins while *S. aureus* is still present. A variety of morphologic variants can occasionally be detected thereafter, but eventually a "smooth" mucoid strain appears,[90] and it is this strain that ultimately dominates or totally replaces the other *P. aeruginosa* variants and often all other pathogens as well.

The mucoid variant, although very common in CF patients, is rarely found in non-CF lung disease, even among patients who do have chronic *P. aeruginosa* infection. Considerable, and for the most part unsuccessful, effort has been directed at clarifying the specific reasons for this unique association. However, there is substantial evidence that the mucoid organism is more virulent and that the mucoid material itself contributes to the vicious cycles that perpetuate and worsen inflammation.[91] This is supported by the observation in one study that older patients who are culture negative for *P. aeruginosa* all make antibodies to its mucoexopolysaccharide.[92]

P. aeruginosa is almost always susceptible to the polymyxins and is usually susceptible to the aminoglycosides, ceftazidime, thienamycin/cilastatin, piperacillin/mezlocillin, aztreonam, and the newer quinolone derivatives, including ciprofloxacin and norfloxacin. They are occasionally susceptible to chloramphenicol, trimethoprim sulfa, and tetracycline.

The primary environmental source(s) of the *P. aeruginosa* that initially colonizes the CF patient is unknown. Non-CF family members virtually never harbor *P. aeruginosa* in the respiratory tract.[93] For many years, patient-to-patient transmission of *P. aeruginosa* strains was also thought to be rare or nonexistent. Early studies had failed to demonstrate transmission in summer camps or among siblings.[94-96] However, the possibility of direct or indirect transmission among CF patients has been reconsidered recently. This reconsideration has been sparked by the following: (1) the demonstration of isolated instances of nosocomial spread[97,98]; (2) the demonstration of an increased prevalence of *P. aeruginosa* colonization among patients treated at a CF center, compared with those not attending a center (even allowing for the indication for referral for center care)[99]; (3) the occasional suggestive evidence indicating transmission at summer camps[100]; and (4) the recent strong evidence favoring nosocomial spread of *P. cepacia.*

P. aeruginosa is rarely seen outside the upper and lower respiratory tract (lungs, airways, nose, and sinuses) in CF patients, despite very severe airway infection, including widespread microabscesses. Empyema is very rare, as are positive blood cultures.

The acquisition of *P. aeruginosa* is associated with a mild but statistically demonstrable worsening in pulmonary function,[101] but unlike *P. cepacia* acquisition, no acute catastrophic deterioration has been observed.

Antimicrobial Treatment

Early reports of *P. aeruginosa* colonization and infection in CF noted that bacteriologic "cure" could not be effected with antimicrobial treatment.[90,102] Nonetheless, treatment with appropriate antibiotics usually resulted in clinical improvement. Although decreased numbers of organisms on quantitative sputum cultures do occur with therapy, the magnitude of the change does not always correlate with the degree of clinical improvement.

Considerable effort has been invested in developing a clinically useful *Pseudomonas* vaccine. Preliminary studies have shown them to be safe, but efficacy has not been shown.[103,104] However, the observation that antimucopolysaccharide antibody may be protective is intriguing.[92]

With conventional treatment, *P. aeruginosa* colonization is permanent once firmly established (defined as three consecutive position sputum cultures). Patients in whom *P. aeruginosa* colonization is replaced by *P. cepacia* colonization are the rare exceptions. Recent reports from Europe[106] suggest that the organism can be eradicated if treated very aggressively soon after colonization, but how much impact this will have on the course of the disease is not known.

Pseudomonas Cepacia

Early reports of *P. cepacia* colonization[107] and clinical disease[108] in CF patients were uncommon and involved only isolated patients. Understandably, these reports did not suggest much cause for general alarm. However, the rapid rise in prevalence of this organism at some of the largest CF centers in North America has allowed clarification of the course of patients once they have acquired this organism[109] and has generated considerable debate about its epidemiology.

P. cepacia was first described as a cause of soft rot in onions.[110] It is remarkably versatile in its nutrition requirements (capable, for example, of using penicillin as its only fuel and source of carbon).[111] It is also remarkably hardy and is able to survive in distilled water[112] and some iodinated disinfectants.

P. cepacia is a very rare pathogen in healthy immunocompetent humans, unable to cause sustained infection even with a huge inoculum.[113] However, in the presence of a foreign body or medical prosthesis (such as an artificial heart valve), serious infection can occur.[114] *P. cepacia* binds to normal (and CF) intestinal and respiratory mucin. The intensity of the binding may be correlated to the severity of clinical disease. Mucus binding may be a protective mechanism in normal persons (by preventing attachment to cells), but in areas where there is stagnation of secretions, mucus binding to cells may occur, which permits infection.[115] This binding could not be demonstrated with *P. aeruginosa.*[116]

A variety of other characteristics, including production of various enzymes (such as catalase and alginase), have been statistically associated with colonization in CF patients, but none have yet been shown to confer increased pathogenicity.[117]

Antimicrobial Susceptibility

Unlike *P. aeruginosa, P. cepacia* is always resistant to aminoglycosides (a characteristic that is useful in identifying the organism and preparing selective media for culture[118]) and may be resistant to all known antimicrobial agents. However, ceftazidime, piperacillin, Imipenem, novobiocin, chloramphenicol, ciprofloxacin, and trimethoprim sulfa may be effective in vitro.

Most of the pathology evident in lungs obtained at autopsy from *P. cepacia* colonized and infected CF patients is indistinguishable from the pathology associated with *P. aeruginosa* colonization and infection. However, some data suggest that *P. cepacia* is more likely to cause an acute necrotizing pneumonia with microabscess formation. In one study, this pathologic finding was more common in patients who experienced the most rapid decline.[119] Contiguous bronchiolocentric abscesses were found in 54% of these patients, compared with 10% in other *P. cepacia* or any *P. aeruginosa* CF patients. Lungs from the patients who had died following rapid deterioration were also heavier than those from *P. aeruginosa* patients, probably as a result of inflammatory infiltrate and edema fluid. This finding of contiguous bronchiolocentric abscesses has not been reported in non-CF patients. Four patients who had *P. cepacia* bacteremia had evidence of diffuse alveolar damage consistent with septic shock.

The suggestion that the rapid rise in the prevalence of *P. cepacia* in some CF centers was caused by a nosocomial epidemic was met at first with considerable skepticism.[120] Other explanations for the sudden rise in the prevalence of *P. cepacia* in CF patients and the poor prognosis after its acquisition included that the organism: (1) was simply a "marker" of severe disease,[120,121] (2) was the result of "antibiotic pressure,"[121] (3) was the result of the gradually increasing age of patients, and (4) was endemic (as opposed to epidemic).[121] Many studies failed to demonstrate the organism in the hospitalized patients' immediate environment.

The possibility that person-to-person transmission (either directly or indirectly) plays an important role has gained much wider acceptance in recent years.[122,123] The evidence upon which this conclusion is based includes: (1) the frequency and rapidity with which the organism is acquired by siblings of the index patient,[108] (2) the decrease in new acquisitions following the start of cohorting at a large center,[124] (3) The North American Camp Study,[125] (4) the tendency for each CF center that has multiple colonized patients to have a single *P. cepacia* ribotype account for the great majority of its colonized patients,[126] (5) the unequivocal demonstration of person-to-person transmission,[127] and (6) scattered reports of outbreaks suggesting social transmission.[128,129] Identification of specific strains by ribotyping, as utilized in numbers 4 and 5, is probably more useful than other methods (such as antibiograms) for epidemiologic studies.[126,127]

Despite substantial evidence of patient-to-patient transmission, a few series, usually with a relatively small number of patients and with very short follow-up, purport to show the lack of contagion risk.[130] This has fostered an aura of "continuing controversy." Other workers have documented the possibility of indirect person-to-person transmission but still conclude that segregation is "controversial."[131]

P. cepacia contamination could not be demonstrated in one study of home inhalation equipment used by patients with CF, although some evidence of contamination by *P. aeruginosa* was shown.[132] However, hospital pulmonary function test equipment was shown to be contaminated by *P. cepacia* in one study.[133]

Following acquisition of *P. cepacia,* CF patients follow one of three clinical pathways.[124,133]

1. No discernible clinical effect[124,133] (about 60% of all newly colonized patients).[124] These patients show no obvious clinical decline within 1 year of acquisition of the organism. Patients in this group may have had mild, moderate, or severe lung disease prior to acquisition of *P. cepacia.*
2. Definite decline in pulmonary status[124,133] (about 22% of all newly colonized patients).[124] These patients with previously moderate or severe disease experience an accelerated decline after acquisition of the organism.
3. Unexpectedly rapid decline in pulmonary status[124,133,134] (about 18% of all newly colonized patients).[124] These patients, with previously mild or moderate pulmonary disease, begin a rapid and usually fatal decline after acquisition of the organism. Approximately 20% to 25% of these patients (almost always women) become septic, with *P. cepacia* recovered from multiple blood cultures despite ongoing antimicrobial treatment.

P. cepacia is characteristically extremely resistant to antimicrobials. Occasional strains are susceptible in vitro to trimethoprim, ceftazidime, piperacillin, chloramphenicol, ciprofloxacin, and novobiocin. They are rarely if ever susceptible to aminoglycosides and are always resistant to colistin. Organisms susceptible to piperacillin (and presumably other synthetic penicillins) have low baseline b-lactamase production.[135] In any case, in vitro susceptibility does not guarantee clinical effectiveness,[124,133,136] and in vitro resistance does not preclude in vivo effectiveness.[137] Furthermore, in vivo failure with one apparently effective agent does not preclude subsequent in vivo success with another agent. The most widely used antimicrobial for severe exacerbation or life-threatening disease is ceftazidime. For outpatients, oral trimethoprim, chloramphenicol, or novobiocin may be useful. Ceftazidime can also be given by the aerosol route.

In addition to standard supportive treatment for advancing pulmonary disease (such as supplemental oxygen, diuretic treatment of cor pulmonale with right heart failure, or others), corticosteroids are often used and may induce some clinical improvement at least temporarily. The efficacy of intravenous gammaglobulin (IVIG) has not been reported, but this may be worth trying when conventional treatment has failed, particularly for those patients in whom rapid deterioration is associated with sepsis.

The possibility of catastrophic deterioration following acquisition of *P. cepacia* and the growing evidence that the organism can be acquired from another CF patient have led to a variety of recommendations concerning isolation. These recommendations are still evolving, but the main thrust is to eliminate exposure of uncolonized patients to colonized patients.

At some hospitals, total segregation of colonized patients (for example, on different hospital floors) may be possible; otherwise, segregation by room may be the best that is achievable. Social interactions including summer camp, educational meetings, and dating all pose some risk, and promoters and sponsors of such activities may wish to consult the CF Foundation for advice. Center directors and CF physicians should educate all CF patients and their families about *P. cepacia.* This should include specific advice about the risks of contagion. As with any infectious agent that can cause nosocomial epidemics, it is reasonable to propose that careful handwashing is important in infection control. However, transmission of *P. cepacia* from one CF patient to another by the contaminated hands of a medical worker (or anyone else) has not actually been demonstrated.

The overall prognosis for survival is worse after acquisition of *P. cepacia* (discussed previously), but some patients are remarkably unaffected, at least in the short term (occasionally up to 10 years). However, the longest survival after acquisition is now only about 15 years, and these patients are quite rare. Whether really long-term survival is possible is unknown.

Other Gram-Negative Pathogens

Several species of *Pseudomonas* (including *Pseudomonas gladioli*[138] and *Pseudomonas fluorescens*), *Xanthomonas mal-*

tophilia, Proteus mirabilis, Escherichia coli, and *Klebsiella* sp, including mucoid strains,[139,140] are also encountered fairly often. The mucoid material obtained from non-*Pseudomonas* gram-negative pathogens is not the same material produced by mucoid *P. aeruginosa. Klebsiella* organisms can cause acute life-threatening disease in infancy. *X. maltophilia* tends to be extremely resistant to antibiotics, but is not obviously more aggressive than other colonizers.

Mycobacterium Tuberculosis

There are only scattered reports of tuberculosis in CF patients[141-143] and it is therefore not possible to draw general conclusions about CF patient susceptibility or to make sweeping recommendations about treatment and prognosis. However, unlike the nontuberculous mycobacteria, *Mycobacterium tuberculosis* does not colonize the human as a saprophyte. All positive cultures should be interpreted as active infection. Pending in vitro susceptibility studies on the specific organism recovered, treatment should be instituted according to recommendations of the American Thoracic Society.[144] Cultures for mycobacteria should be part of the routine workup of any CF patient who develops an exacerbation requiring intravenous antibiotic treatment. Overgrowth of cultures by *P. aeruginosa* can be minimized by treating the specimen with *N*-acetyl-*L*-cysteine (0.25%)/sodium hydroxide (1%) and then 5% oxalic acid.[145]

Other Mycobacteria

Colonization of respiratory secretions with nontuberculous mycobacteria has been reported with increasing frequency recently. Organisms reported include *Mycobacterium fortuitum,*[84,141,146-148] *Mycobacterium chelonei,*[84,141,146,148] *Mycobacterium avium,*[143,146,148,149] *Mycobacterium terrae,*[149] *Mycobacterium kansasii,*[143,150] and *Mycobacterium gordonae.*[143] Surveys of CF patients in Washington State and North Carolina found colonization with nontuberculous mycobacteria in 8 of 64 (13%) and 17 of 87 (20%), respectively.[146,148]

In rare patients,[85,149] there is excellent documentation of invasive mycobacterial disease that required therapeutic intervention. However, for the majority of patients, there is not yet conclusive evidence that these organisms are anything more than colonizers. Nonetheless, their presence adds uncertainty to the patient's management, and may prove more important if the organisms persist after bilateral pneumonectomy in the then immunosuppressed posttransplant patient. Furthermore, because atypical mycobacteria are usually "rapid growers," the laboratory may be unable (or simply may not think it necessary) to continue the search for *M. tuberculosis* on the same specimen. If *M. tuberculosis* is suspected and another (rapid-grower) mycobacterium is recovered, the laboratory director should be consulted.

Streptococcus Pneumoniae

Although some CF patients develop typical lobar pneumococcal pneumonia, the vast majority do not. *Streptococcus pneumoniae* may be isolated from occasional sputum and throat cultures,[151] but its significance is unknown. Pneumococcal vaccine is not recommended for routine use in CF.

Fungi

Because recovery of fungi from CF sputum samples may be hampered by the presence of huge numbers of bacteria, appropriate antibiotics may have to be added to the culture media.[150] Serologic studies may be useful.[153]

Aspergillus Species

Aspergillus organisms, usually *Aspergillus fumigatus,* are often recovered from CF respiratory secretions in some centers.[152,154] Although invasive aspergillosis has been reported in CF,[155] it is quite rare. Allergic bronchopulmonary aspergillosis (ABPA), however, appears to occur in approximately 2% of patients[1,152,154] (Fig. 68-6). The organism can be recovered on media used for routine bacterial cultures, but if ABPA is suspected, specialized fungal cultures should also be done.

Yeast is recovered very often from routine CF respiratory cultures, particularly from patients who have been treated with potent wide-spectrum antimicrobial agents. Its clinical signif-

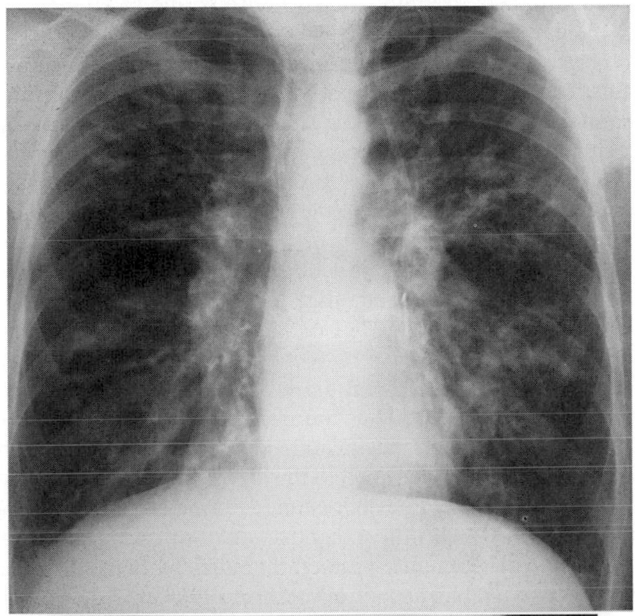

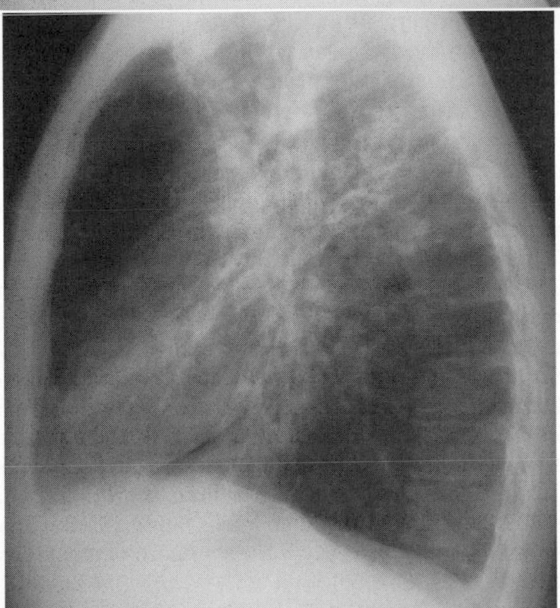

Fig. 68-6 Chest radiograph of a 24-year-old man with cystic fibrosis with allergic bronchopulmonary aspergillosis. There is widespread bronchiectasis and numerous mucus plugs, which are not distinctive in appearance from patients without allergic bronchopulmonary aspergillosis. There is consolidation in the medial basalar segment of the right lower lobe.

icance is not clear. Pulmonary candidiasis has been suspected in CF,[156] but it does not appear to be common. Hypersensitivity pneumonitis caused by Candida antigen has not been reported in CF. Candidal sepsis has occurred in CF patients who have implanted central venous access devices.[157]

Viruses

Although patients and clinicians have long "known" that minor viral upper respiratory illnesses often result in pulmonary exacerbations, such an association has not been documented often. However, there are sufficient data now to link pulmonary deterioration with some common respiratory viruses, particularly RSV.[158] Influenza[159] and measles are also widely accepted to be capable of precipitating CF pulmonary exacerbations. Measles is included in the routine immunization series, but influenza requires yearly boosters (indicated for most CF patients).

The role of viral infection in CF is intrinsically difficult to assess because it is usually not obvious which of the patient's symptoms or laboratory findings are results of the underlying CF-related bacterial infection and which are caused by the virus. Furthermore, CF secretions are thought to interfere with the recovery of viruses.[160] Serology can be useful in establishing acute infection.

Despite this overwhelming body of information, four clinical observations have been raised by those skeptical of the importance of infection in CF. First, as noted since the original description of the disease,[161] there is characteristically little histologic evidence of local tissue invasion by the proposed pulmonary pathogens. Thus the pulmonary infection, with a central clinical importance assumed by virtually all CF physicians, appears to be confined to the airway. Second, the respiratory microbiology does not change during periods of exacerbation. Third, with the exception of fulminant *P. cepacia* infection, extrapulmonary infection, either by hematogenous spread (for example, hepatic abscess) or direct extension (such as empyema or pericarditis), is extremely rare.[80] Fourth, patients with pulmonary exacerbations may improve during hospitalizations even if antibiotic use is not guided by in vitro susceptibility studies to *P. aeruginosa.*[162]

On the other hand, treatment of infection, beginning with the introduction of sulfonamides, penicillin, and tetracycline in the 1940s,[163] has clearly been a very important component of the comprehensive treatment programs that have so dramatically altered the prognosis for the disease. Even in recent times, the introduction of new classes of potent antimicrobial agents with gram-negative coverage (carbenicillin and other penicillins, ceftazidime, and the new systemic quinolones) has been associated with improvement in short-term prognosis. Furthermore, in some situations (such as acute staphylococcal pneumonia[80] in infants and fulminating *P. cepacia* infection in young women[109,133]) the role of infection is unequivocal. Finally, the occasional patients who do not harbor respiratory pathogens even in adulthood and their benign course provide additional suggestive evidence of the important role played by chronic infection.

PULMONARY IMMUNOLOGY AND INFLAMMATION

Inflammation is clearly severe in advanced CF pulmonary disease and has long been thought to play a pathophysiologic role in end-stage disease by interfering with host defense and therapeutic measures directed at suppressing infection. More recently, however, the importance of chemical mediators of inflammation as the major cause of tissue injury has become increasingly clear.

Immunology

During the 50 years since the relationship between CF and pulmonary infection has been recognized, the fundamental components of the immune system have been identified and considerable understanding of their interactions have emerged. Every new finding has been rigorously investigated in CF patients, but no consistent pattern of abnormality that would suggest a primary defect of CF has been uncovered. This is not unexpected in view of the great rarity of extrapulmonary infections in this disease. A tendency toward hypogammaglobulinemia has been reported in younger (healthier) patients,[164] but this has not been convincingly confirmed. Increasing serum gammaglobulin levels with advancing age probably represents nonspecific reactions to chronic infection.

Some qualitative immune defects have been reported in patients with severe lung disease,[165] but the global function of T cells, B cells, complement, polymorphonuclear cells, and others is normal in patients who do not have advanced lung disease. The qualitative abnormalities, although they may contribute to a pathophysiologic cascade that increases the rate with which severe disease progresses, do not appear to be primary defects (that is, directly related to the gene product). Some may be induced by bacterial toxins.[166]

A fundamental explanation of the predisposition to infection by *P. aeruginosa* remains elusive. However, the recent suggestion that the CFTR abnormality may affect organelle ionic transport as well as cell membrane ionic transport may be important.[9,10] Intracellular abnormalities could lead to abnormalities in cell products (for example, by altering local pH or ion concentration, during the synthesis of various proteins), and these molecules may facilitate bacterial adhesion.

Inflammation

Intense bronchocentric inflammation, easily demonstrable histologically at postmortem and reflected by the extraordinary number of neutrophils found on BAL analyses,[167] is virtually universal in CF patients. The fact that the *P. aeruginosa* pulmonary colonization and infection in CF, once firmly established, is almost always permanent indicates that the inflammatory response is unable to eradicate the organisms. There is increasing evidence that the inflammatory reaction eventually establishes its own momentum and is responsible in large part for the destruction of lung parenchyma, which eventually leads to the patient's death from respiratory failure.

The central event in the establishment of a self-perpetuating destructive inflammatory reaction in the CF lung is the chronic presence of potent neutrophil chemoattractants. A wide spectrum of mediators with chemoattractant activity have been demonstrated in sputum and BAL.[19,168] The interplay of inflammatory mediators that attract neutrophils to the airway is a challenging area of current investigation. Once neutrophils are present in large numbers, they become active participants in their own recruitment, both directly by the release of chemoattractants such as LTB_4[169] and indirectly through the release of elastase and other cell constituents. Neutrophil elastase cleaves C5 (producing chemoattractant peptides) and stimulates production of IL-8 by both bronchial epithelial cells and macrophages. Neutrophil elastase also cleaves IgG and abolishes its ability to interact with the Fc receptor. Neutrophil elastase may inactivate γ-interferon, a major stimulant for macrophage phagocytosis. It also interferes with the complement system by inactivating two of its opsonin-receptor pairs by its effect on one opsonin (C3bi) and the receptor for another (CR1), creating an "opsonin-receptor mismatch."[91] Elastase also rapidly inactivates fibronectin, a protein that promotes phagocytosis of many bacteria. These and other adverse consequences of excess amounts of neutrophil elastase (and other host and bacterial proteases) illustrate how the inflammatory reaction in CF airways, in addition to being self-perpetuating, also interferes with host efforts to reduce or eliminate the invading pathogens.

Bacterial (mostly *Pseudomonas*) elastase is also present in the CF lung, but neutrophil products, including elastase and toxic forms of oxygen (such as singlet oxygen, hydroxyl radicals, and hydrogen peroxide), are probably the principal agents of tissue destruction. Although these oxygen species can kill bacteria and are useful in the defense against ordinary bacterial lung infections in normal persons, intracellular killing of *P. aeruginosa* appears defective in CF. Whereas naturally occurring inhibitors can "mop up" a small amount of "leftover" proteolytic enzymes after infection resolves in normal persons, they are totally inadequate to cope with the continuous deluge of destructive proteases produced by the chronic infection and inflammation in CF airways. Unopposed proteases can then cause tissue injury.

ANTIINFLAMMATORIES

In an attempt to prevent pulmonary fibrosis, antiinflammatory agents, including corticosteroids, ibuprofen, and antiproteases, are under clinical trial. In one 4-year, multicenter trial of systemic corticosteroids, 285 patients were enrolled.[170] Patients were given 1 mg/kg, 2 mg/kg, or placebo every other day. The 2 mg/kg arm was stopped because of steroid side effects. The 1 mg/kg arm showed that the FEV 1% predicted in the treated patients was greater than in the untreated patients and declined more slowly. There was significant growth retardation, however, in the 1 mg/kg treated group. Thus the potential benefit of systemic corticosteroids has to be balanced against growth retardation and the possibility of increased susceptibility to osteoporosis, which was not evaluated in this study.

Konstan et al gave ibuprofen at a dose of 20 to 30 mg/kg or placebo to 85 primarily pediatric patients for 4 years.[171] The annual rate of change in FEV_1 was greater in the placebo group than in the treated group (-3.60% vs. -2.17%), and body weight was better maintained in the treated group. In this small study, no gastrointestinal problems or nephrotoxicity were reported.

Three specific antiproteases are currently being studied: α-1 antitrypsin, secretary leukocyte protease inhibitor (SLPI), and ICI 200,880. McElvaney[172] nebulized α-1 antitrypsin to 12 CF patients for a week and examined their BAL for the presence of α-1 antitrypsin and also looked for interference of neutrophil killing of *Pseudomonas* and showed that following α-1 antitrypsin inhalation, the lavage of patients had a greater ability to kill *Pseudomonas*. McElvaney et al[173] aerosolized rhSLPI to 20 CF patients and demonstrated decreased neutrophil, decreased neutrophil elastase, and decreased IL-8 levels in the BAL fluid of these patients.

RADIOLOGY

Standard Chest Radiograph

The standard (anteroposterior and lateral) radiograph of the chest yields considerable information and is the most often used radiologic examination for evaluation and follow-up of CF pulmonary disease.

CF clinical scoring systems also incorporate standard chest films as part of the score of disease severity.[54] The major radiologic systems for assessing chronic pulmonary disease provide criteria for "deductions" from a starting "normal" score of 25 points.[174-176] The deductions are based mainly on severity of overinflation and infiltrates. For Brasfield scoring,[174] good correlation between standard chest film scoring and pulmonary function tests has been demonstrated for both children and adults.[177,178]

Overinflation, the hallmark of the disease, is usually the earliest radiologic manifestation. CF should be considered in any pediatric patient who manifests radiologic evidence of severe overinflation, even if typical digestive symptoms are not present.

Interpretation of plain chest radiographs in CF patients includes analysis of overinflation, peribronchial cuffing, infiltrates, atelectasis, and fibrosis.[179] Uncomplicated overinflation results in lowering or flattening of the diaphragm and hyperlucency (which at first may appear to be the result of "overexposure"). The lateral films may show an increased anteroposterior distance, kyphosis, and hyperlucency (air) in front of the heart.

Peribronchial cuffing (indicating airway inflammation) is another early change (Fig. 68-7). The differentiation of infiltrates and cuffing from fibrosis may be difficult on any one film, but resolution after treatment helps confirms that it was not fibrosis. Worsening of hyperinflation by making the entire film appear darker may lead to underestimation of the severity of infiltrates and fibrosis. Similarly, rapid improvement with hospital treatment may result in decreased overinflation and a false impression of worsening infiltrates as previously present infiltrates and fibrosis become more apparent. With disease progression, there is bronchiectasis and diffuse fibrosis most marked in the upper lobes, leading to scarring and upward retraction of the hila (Fig. 68-8).

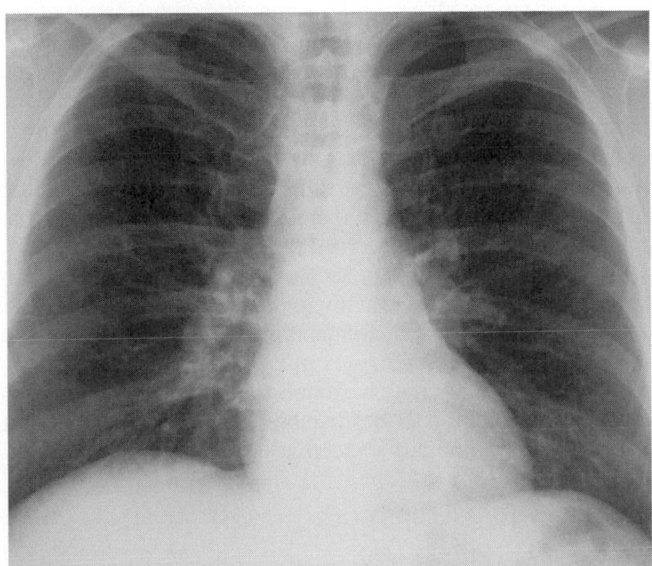

Fig. 68-7. Chest radiograph of a 52-year-old man with CF with normal spirometry. There is mild peribronchial thickening in the upper lobes.

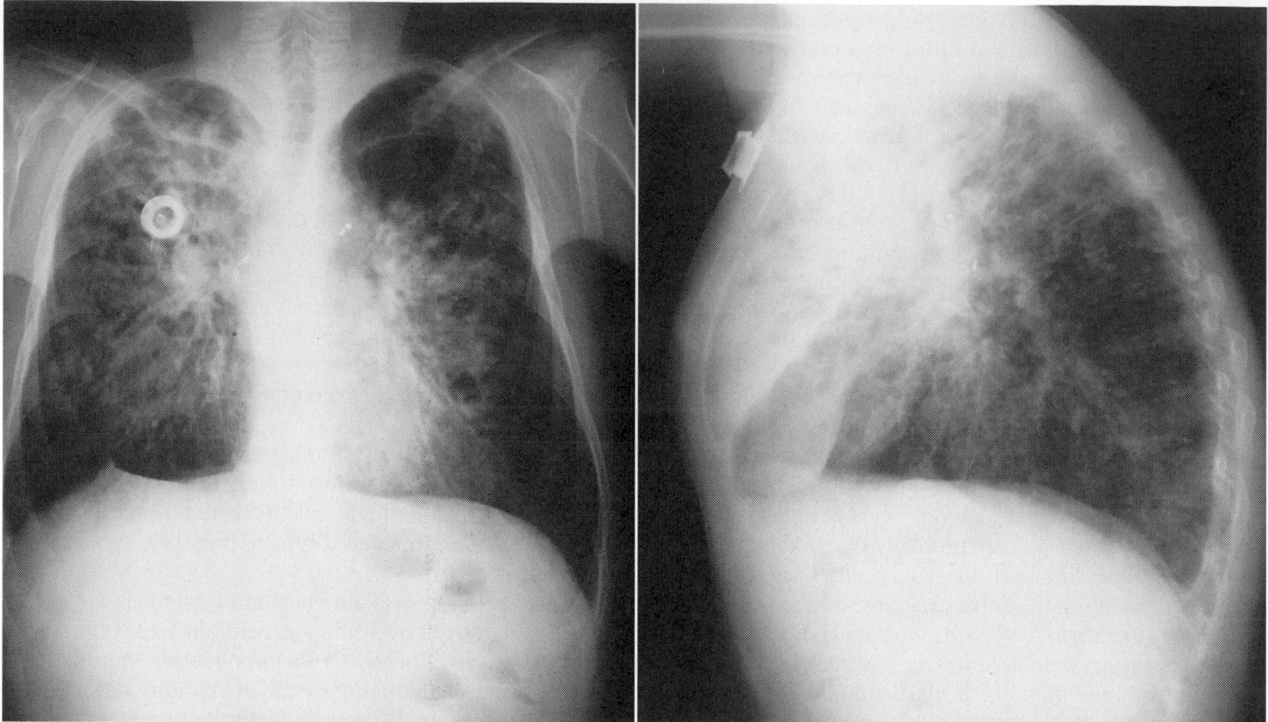

Fig. 68-8. Chest radiograph of a 21-year-old man with cystic fibrosis and extensive bilateral bronchiectasis concentrated in the upper lobes. A Port-a-Cath, accessed with a Huber needle, is in place. There are coils from a previous episode of bronchial artery embolization to control massive hemoptysis. There is scarring of the right apex. Lucency in the left apex is dilated bronchi and bullae. The tenting of the right hemidiaphragm reflects upper lobe volume loss.

Large lung lesions, including pneumothorax, pneumomediastinum (and subcutaneous emphysema), lobar and segmental atelectasis, pleural fluid, and large cysts/blebs (occasionally fluid filled) are rarely subtle. Occasionally, however, expiratory films are needed to rule out a small pneumothorax, and decubitus films (and/or ultrasound) are needed to confirm a small pleural effusion and establish whether it is loculated. Mucoid-impacted bronchi can occasionally present as pulmonary nodules.

Chest films are also useful for nonparenchymal evaluation. There is often hilar adenopathy, usually more clearly seen on CT scan. The pulmonary arteries are enlarged later in the course of the disease. The transverse cardiac diameter may be enlarged in terminal disease. Rib fracture secondary to paroxysmal forceful coughing can occur, and the ribs should be examined carefully when chest films are obtained as part of an evaluation for chest pain. The fracture may not be detectable until callus has formed several days later.

Inconsistent changes are seen on the chest roentgenogram when CF patients present with an acute exacerbation of their disease.[179] An acute parenchymal infiltrate is unusual, but more subtle findings such as mucus plugging and increased peribronchial thickening may be found. These findings are insensitive and nonspecific as they can be seen when patients do not have an acute pulmonary exacerbation.[179]

Computed Tomography

Computed Tomography (CT) scanning detects pulmonary complications with greater sensitivity than standard chest films.[180] CT can show disease in patients when it is absent on standard chest films, and bronchiectasis can be seen at a much earlier stage. Concerns about the use of chest CT for evaluation of infants and small children with CF have included the need for cooperation (breath holding) to minimize motion, the radiation dosage, and the relatively high cost of the procedure. Imaging often requires sedation or even anesthesia in infants and young children. These additional risks makes chest CT scans impractical for routine use.

Airway structures can be demonstrated on CT scans to the level of the segmental and subsegmental bronchi. Changes in pulmonary parenchyma are easily detected and reflect the status of the peripheral airways. Bronchial wall thickness, bronchiectasis, and mucus plugging can be objectively evaluated. In one study,[180] bronchial wall thickening (occasionally occurring in the absence of obvious hyperinflation) was the earliest radiographic change in adult patients whose usually mild disease had not progressed over a long period of follow-up. Few patients had nonvascular linear or nodular lesions.

In a series of adult CF patients with severe disease, bronchiectasis was easily seen on plain radiographs, but when studied with high-resolution CT, the lesions were found to be more severe and extensive (Fig. 68-9).[181]In another series of 39 patients with mild to severe disease, high-resolution CT improved the localization of the disease processes within the secondary pulmonary lobule.[182] High-resolution CT is also sensitive for small cysts (3 mm), bullae, fibrosis, and early infiltrates. An expiration study may be additionally revealing in patients whose findings on inspiration are suggestive, but not conclusive.[183]

CF bronchiectasis as visualized by CT appears different than that of ABPA or postpneumonic bronchiectasis. In CF, bronchiectasis is seen predominantly in the upper lobes and is associated with proximal bronchial wall thickening.[180] This is

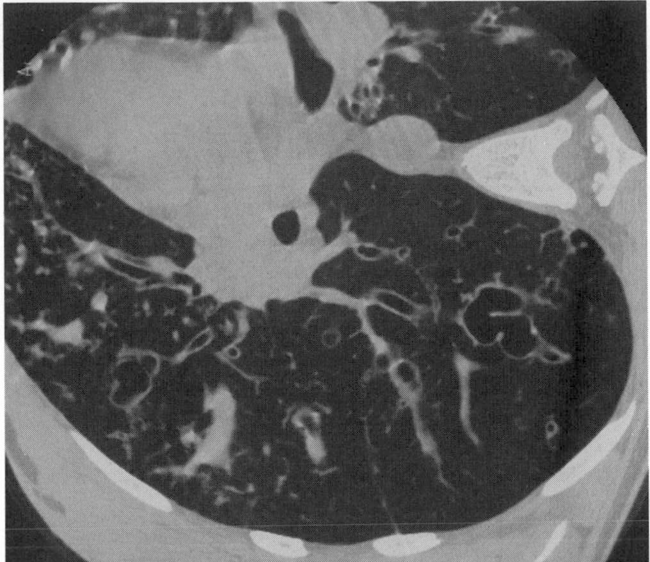

Fig. 68-9. Chest CT scan of a 23-year-old woman with cystic fibrosis. There is extensive bronchiectasis and mucus plugging.

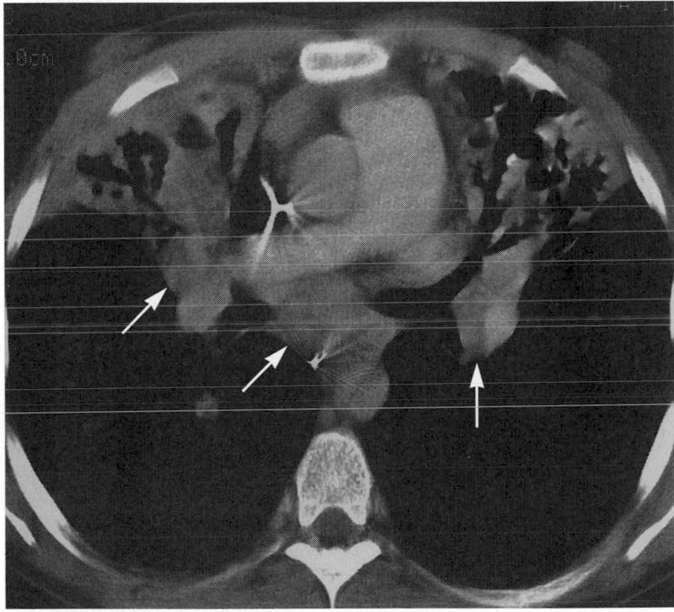

Fig. 68-10. Chest CT scan of a 2l-year-old man with cystic fibrosis. There is lymphadenopathy in the mediastinum and in the hila (*arrows*). Usually adenopathy in cystic fibrosis is l to 2 cm in diameter. In this example the subcarinal lymph node mass measured 4 cm in diameter. The upper lobes are densely consolidated and fibrosed. The bronchiectasis extends to the pleural surface.

unlike postinfectious bronchiectasis, which usually involves the periphery of the lower lobes early, and allergic bronchopulmonary aspergillosis in which airway dilation is relatively more prominent.

Preliminary attempts have been made to develop scoring systems for chest CT scans in CF.[180,184,185]

Nuclear Magnetic Resonance

Nuclear magnetic resonance (NMR) scans are more accurate than plain chest radiography in identifying and in assessing hilar lymphadenopathy.[185] Enlarged lymph nodes are easily differentiated from pulmonary vessels by the absence of the signal void indicative of flowing blood. Mucoid-impacted bronchi, identified as high-signal branching structures, are more easily compared with the standard chest radiograph if coronal images are obtained. Fiel et al[18] compared the image produced by a NMR with a chest radiograph and found that NMR was superior in detecting hilar and mediastinal adenopathy and in the evaluation of bronchiectasis (Fig. 68-10). The chest film was superior for infiltrates, hyperinflation, sternal bowing, volume loss, and hilar retraction. The lack of ionizing radiation is an advantage of NMR if the patient needs sequential radiologic reevaluation.

Bronchograms

Although bronchograms remain the gold standard to assess airway anatomy, they have been largely replaced by the less invasive technique of thin-cut high-resolution CT scanning.[187] Bronchograms were occasionally used to document the severity and distribution of bronchiectasis. This was most commonly done prior to lobectomy in patients with localized severe disease and systemic symptoms. The demonstration of normal or near-normal airways in all areas other than the lobe to be removed supports the decision to proceed to surgery.

Ultrasound

The principal use of noncardiac thoracic ultrasound in CF patients is to establish the presence of a pleural effusion and whether it is loculated, thus helping to decide if multiple chest tubes will be necessary and aiding in the selection of the best site(s) for thoracentesis or chest tube placement. Sonography is also useful in evaluating fatty infiltration of the pancreas, hepatosplenomegaly, portal hypertension, and gallbladder involvement.

Arteriography

Arteriography in CF patients is used to delineate the anatomy of the bronchial vasculature during embolization procedures for hemoptysis.[188,189] Spinal arteries may arise from bronchial arteries and must not be embolized. If bleeding recurs months or years after embolization, repeat arteriography may demonstrate that neovascularization has occurred and repeat embolization is necessary.

Ventilation-Perfusion Scans

Quantitative ventilation-perfusion scans (using technetium or xenon) are helpful if a CF patient is being evaluated for possible lobectomy or pneumonectomy. If the scan shows markedly reduced perfusion to the area that has been proposed for removal (and no other areas have distinctly low perfusion), the case for removal has been strengthened and the probability of severe postoperative problems is reduced.

In more advanced disease, the characteristic pattern of ventilation is central deposition of the radionucleotide particles secondary to severe peripheral airway obstruction.

COMPLICATIONS AND TREATMENT

Infection

This is discussed in a previous section.

Table 68-1 Bacteria Associated with Exacerbations of Pulmonary Infection in Patients with Cystic Fibrosis and Approporiate Intravenous Treatments

	FIRST CHOICE			ALTERNATIVE		
		DOSAGE[1]			DOSAGE[1]	
PREVALENT BACTERIA	ANTIBIOTIC	CHILD	ADULT	ANTIBIOTIC	CHILD	ADULT
S. aureus	Cephalothin	25-50 mg/kg every 6 hr	1 g every 6 hr	Vancomycin[2]	15 mg/kg every 6 hr	500 mg every 6 hr
	Nafcillin[3]	25-50 mg/kg every 6 hr	1 g every 6 hr			
H. influenzae and *S. aureus*	Ticarcillin-clavulanate[4]	100 mg of ticarcillin/kg and 3.3 mg of clavulanate/kg every 6 hr	3 g of ticarcillin and 0.1 g of clavulanate every 6 hr	Nafcillin[3] *plus* gentamicin[5]	25-50 mg/kg every 6 hr 3 mg/kg every 8 hr	1 g every 6 hr 3 mg/kg every 8 hr
	plus gentamicin[5]	3 mg every 8 hr	3 mg/kg every 8 hr			
S. aureus and *P. aeruginosa*	Ticarcillin-clavulanate[4]	100 mg of ticarcillin/kg and 3.3 mg of clavulanate/kg every 6 hr	3 g of ticarcillin and 0.1 g of clavulanate every 6 hr			
	plus tobramycin[5]	3 mg/kg every 8 hr	3 mg/kg every 8 hr			
P. aeruginosa only	Ticarcillin[4]	100 mg/kg every 6 hr	3 g every 6 hr	Tobramycin[5] *plus* ceftazidime, piperacillin, *or* imipenem[6]	3 mg/kg every 8 hr 50 mg/kg every 8 hr 100 mg/kg every 6 hr 15-25 mg/kg every 6 hr 50 mg/kg every 6 hr	3 mg/kg every 8 hr 2 g every 8 hr 3 g every 6 hr 500 mg-1 g every 6 hr 2 g every 8 hr 5-7.5 mg/kg every 8 hr
	plus tobramycin[5]	3 mg/kg every 8 hr	3 mg/kg every 8 hr			
				Aztreonam[7] *plus* amikacin[8]	5-7.5 mg/kg every 8 hr	
P. aeruginosa and *P. cepacia*[7]	Ceftazidime *plus* ciprofloxacin	50-75 mg/kg every 8 hr	2 g every 8 hr	Ceftazidime	50-75 mg/kg every 8 hr	2 g every 8 hr
				plus chloramphenicol[9]	15-20 mg/kg every 6 hr	15-20 mg/kg every 6 hr
		15 mg/kg every 12 hr	400 mg every 12 hr IV	*or* trimethoprim-sulfamethoxazole	5 mg of trimethoprim/kg IV and 25 mg of sulfamethoxazole/kg every	5 mg of trimethoprim/ kg IV and 25 mg of sulfamethoxazole/kg every 6 hr
P. cepacia only	Chloramphenicol[8] *or* trimethoprim-sulfamethoxazole *or both*	15-20 mg/kg every 6 hr 5 mg of trimethoprim/kg and 25 mg of sulfamethoxazole/kg every 6 hr	15-20 mg/kg every 6 hr 5 mg of trimethoprim/kg and 25 mg of sulfamethoxazole/kg every 6 hr			

From Ramsey BW: *N Engl J Med* 335(3):179-188, 1996.
[1]Most doses are expressed as mg/kg of body weight. The dose given to children should not exceed that for adults. IV denotes intravenous.
[2]Vancomycin should be infused slowly to avoid histamine release. Serum concentrations should be monitored; the peak concentration ranges from 20 to 30 μg/ml, and the trough from 5 to 10 μg/ml.
[3]To minimize phlebitis, nafcillin should be diluted to a concentration of less than 20 mg/ml.
[4]Ticarcillin may be associated with occasional platelet dysfunction. Its use is limited by concern about the possibility of selection for resistant organisms such as *Stenotrophomonas maltophilia* and *P. cepacia.*
[5]Serum concentrations should be monitored; the peak concentration ranges from 8 to 12 μg/ml, and the trough concentration is less than 2 μg/ml.
((This drug is for patients with sensitivity to cephalosporin or multidrug-resistant organisms.
[7]Frequent antibiotic susceptibility testing is recommended to ensure treatment with the optimal combination of antibiotics.
[8]Serum concentrations should be monitored; the peak concentration ranges from 15 to 25 μg/ml, and the trough concentration is less than 5 μg/ml.
[9]Serum concentrations should be monitored; the peak concentration ranges from 10 to 25 μg/ml, and the trough from 5 to 10 μg/ml.

Antibiotics

The mainstay of treatment for pulmonary disease in CF has been chest physical therapy[136] and antibiotics.[190,191] At the present time, it is generally agreed that antibiotics should be used for exacerbations of the disease, although it has been considered unethical to conduct randomized studies of this problem.[192] Unfortunately, to date, there is no clear definition of a CF pulmonary exacerbation. In the majority of the pediatric population there is no fever and no rise in peripheral white count with an exacerbation of respiratory symptoms.[193] A diagnosis of acute exacerbation is usually made on subjective symptoms. Fever and leukocytosis may be seen more commonly in the adult population.[179] A more ob-

Table 68-2 Oral Antibiotics Commonly Used to Suppress Respiratory Pathogens in Patients with Cystic Fibrosis*

PATHOGEN	ANTIBIOTIC	DOSAGE: CHILD	DOSAGE: ADULT
S. aureus	Dicloxacillin	6.25 mg/kg every hr	250-500 mg every 6 hr
	Cephalexin	12.5 mg/kg every 6 hr	500 mg every 6 hr
	Amoxicillin-clavulanate†	10-15 mg of amoxicillin/kg and 2.5-3.75 mg of clavulanate/kg every 8 hr	250-500 mg of amoxicillin and 125 mg of clavulanate every 8 hr
	Erythromycin	15 mg/kg every 8 hr	250 mg every 8 hr
	Clarithromycin	7.5 mg/kg every 12 hr	500 mg every 12 hr
H. influenzae	Cefaclor	10-15 mg/kg every 8 hr	250-500 mg every 8 hr
	Amoxicillin	20-40 mg/kg every 8 hr	500 mg every 8 hr
S. aureus and *H. influenzae*	Cefixime	8 mg/kg/day	400 mg/day
	Amoxicillin-clavulanate†	10-15 mg of amoxicillin/kg and 2.5 -3.75 mg of clavulanate/kg every 8 hr	250-500 mg of amoxicillin and 125 mg of clavulanate every 8 hr
	Trimethoprim-sulfamethoxazole	4 mg of trimethoprim/kg and 20 mg of sulfamethoxazole/kg every 12 hr	160 mg of trimethoprim and 800 mg of sulfamethoxaxole every 12 hr
	Cefpodoxime	5 mg/kg every 12 hr	200 mg every 12 hr
	Cefuroxime	20 mg/kg every 12 hr	250-500 mg every 12 hr
P. aeruginosa	Ciprofloxacin‡	Not approved	500-750 mg every 12 hr
	Ofloxacin‡	Not approved	400 mg every 12 hr
P. cepacia	Trimethoprim-sulfamethoxazole	4 mg of trimethoprim/kg and 20 mg of sulfamethoxazole/kg every 12 hr	160 mg of trimethoprim and 800 mg of sulfamethoxazole every 12 hr

From Ramsey BW: *New Engl J Med,* 335(3):179-188, 1996.
*The list is not intended to be exhaustive. The dose given to children should not exceed that for adults.
†Higher doses of clavulanate are frequently associated with diarrhea.
‡Ciprofloxacin and ofloxacin have not been approved for use in patients under 18 years of age.

jective way to assess an exacerbation is by the decline in pulmonary function seen during an exacerbation that improves with treatment.[194] Acute exacerbation may also be associated with poor appetite, increased calorie requirements, and weight loss. Another objective means of assessing exacerbation is to measure sputum quantitative cultures and DNA concentration.[193] DNA is derived from the dead leukocytes and may be a quantitative marker of inflammation.[193] Bacteria are present in CF sputum in as many as 10^8 colony-forming units per gram of sputum. As a patient group, the quantitative cultures improve after a treatment course of antibiotics and aggressive chest physical therapy, but this is unhelpful in assessing the individual patient.[193]

Antibiotics are usually given for at least 2 weeks, although no trials have been conducted to ascertain the optimum duration of treatment.[190] The bacterial pathogens are rarely irradiated from the airway. The value of in vitro sensitivities in guiding antimicrobial therapy has not been established. In 58 exacerbations of CF in a pediatric population, Smith[195] found no difference in pulmonary function or clinical improvement in the 19 patients whose *P. aeruginosa* was resistant to the chosen antipseudomonal antibiotic regimen vs. the 36 patients whose *P. aeruginosa* was sensitive. Smith concluded that the conventional criteria of defining sensitive and resistant organisms in the CF population may require re-definition.[195] It should be noted that CF patients require very high aminoglycoside doses to achieve therapeutic levels. Aminoglycosides bind covalently to abundant DNA in CF sputum, and the volume of distribution of the drug is increased. The antibiotic regimens often used for exacerbation of pulmonary infection and to suppress respiratory pathogens are shown in Tables 68-1 and 68-2.[191]

Several studies have shown that home intravenous antibiotic therapy may be as effective as hospitalization.[196] The advantages of home intravenous therapy include cost savings and less psychosocial disruption. The advantage of hospitalized treatment may be more intensive chest physical therapy, more rest, and a constant supply of food for patients who may not have a "nourishing" home environment.

Although there is consensus that exacerbations of CF should be treated with antibiotics, no such consensus exists with respect to the use of prophylactic and suppressive oral antibiotics to retard lung damage from chronic infection or to prevent acute exacerbations. Frequent antibiotic treatments in some studies have been shown to improve survival.[197,198] Valerius et al[106] reported on 26 patients who had never received antipseudomonal therapy and who were randomized to receive placebo or a 3-week antibiotic regimen whenever *P. aeruginosa* was isolated from the sputum over a 27-month period. The patients who received antibiotics were less likely to be chronically infected, and there were fewer pseudomonal isolates on culture.

Aerosolized penicillin was used to treat CF patients in the 1940s. Aerosol administration of antibiotics is an attractive approach because it offers the possibility of delivering these drugs directly to the site of infection and preventing potential systemic side effects, especially from aminoglycosides. Hodson et al[199] showed that in 17 patients treated with aerosolized carbenicillin and gentamicin, spirometric measurements were higher and hospital admissions reduced during the 6-month treatment arm. In the most recent study, 300 mg of tobramycin was delivered twice daily by jet nebulizer. A total of 520 subjects were randomized to drug or placebo for 28 days, followed by 28 days of study drug for 24 weeks. Patients in the tobramycin group had an average increase in FEV_1 of 10% and were less likely to have an acute exacerbation of their pulmonary disease.[200] Other antibiotics have also been used by inhalation in the CF population including colistin, neomycin, and ceftazidime. In summary, inhaled antibiotics in CF have been shown to decrease the number of acute exacerbations, decrease pseudomonal load, improve lung function, but increase antibiotic resistance.[201] Whether aerosol antibiotics should be used for deteriorating patients and patients requiring frequent intravenous medication or whether aerosol antibiotics should be used in patients with less severe disease is not clear.[200]

Chest Physical Therapy

Conventional treatment of CF includes removal of the purulent secretions from the lung.[202] Pulmonary function tests improve with treatment of an exacerbation with or without antibiotic therapy,[162] illustrating the importance of pulmonary toilet. Postural drainage usually accompanied by percussion, deep breathing exercises, directed cough, forced expiration,[203] and exercise all have been used in clinical practice.[204] The "optimal" chest physical therapy is somewhat controversial. Rossman et al[205] demonstrated that cough was as good as chest physical therapy in the clearance of radiolabeled albumin (large airway clearance). De Boeck et al[206] also showed cough to be equivalent to chest physical therapy, although they did find better flow rates with chest physical therapy. Postural drainage alone can be of benefit in CF patients.[207] Desmond et al[202] examined the immediate and long term effects of chest physiotherapy in eight pediatric patients. They showed that there was only a small immediate effect on peak flow in patients who had been performing regular chest physical therapy. However, if chest physical therapy was discontinued, there was a fall in spirometric measurements, which would be regained during long-term (3 weeks) physical therapy. More recently, attention has been given to the use of positive expiratory pressure (PEP). Hodson et al[208] found no increase in sputum production with the addition of PEP in 18 patients. Falk et al,[209] studying 14 patients, came to the opposite conclusion. More recent studies have shown PEP to be an effective chest PT and more acceptable to patients.[210] PEP does not improve mucociliary clearance.[211] Autogenic drainage has recently been advocated for CF, but there are no trials to demonstrate its advantage over other forms of chest physical therapy. Two chest physical therapy "vests" have recently been introduced, one of which is currently available, but at a very high cost.[212-215] The advantage of these, as with PEP and autogenic drainage, is that the patient can perform therapy unaided. Both vests have been shown to be efficacious in removing secretions.

There have been two trials of the Flutter device (a hand-held instrument, exhalation through which results in oscillation of airflow and vibration of the airways) with opposite results. Konstan et al measured the weight of sputum obtained with this device compared with postural drainage with cough and with cough alone over a 15-minute interval. The mean weights of sputum expectorated with the Flutter device were 8.2 g to 11.0 g compared with cough at 1.7 g to 2.7 g and with postural drainage and cough at 1.6 g to 2.2 g.[216] Pryor et al compared the Flutter device with active cycle of breathing techniques over a 24-hour period. Outcomes measured were spirometry, oximetry, and sputum weight.[217] Pulmonary function and oximetry did not change. The mean net weight of sputum with the Flutter device with each treatment was 16.6 g and over 24 hours was 66.0 g compared with 21.2 g and 66.4 g without the device. It is not obvious how to explain the conflicting results. The time of each treatment was similar (15 minutes vs. average of 23.7 minutes); the number of patients (18 vs. 20) and age range (8 to 38 years vs. 16 to 36 years) of the subjects were similar in both studies. Perhaps the Flutter device is helpful if patient compliance is improved with this simple device, but the Flutter does not appear to be any more effective than traditional methods of chest physical therapy.

In summary, a variety of chest physical therapy maneuvers appear to be efficacious in CF. Choosing a therapy with which the patient will be compliant is the most important factor in determining which method to use.

Exercise

Some physicians believe that regular exercise may be a substitute for chest physical therapy.[218] Orenstein et al[219] demonstrated that regular exercise increases physical fitness in CF patients. Keens et al[220] demonstrated that upper body exercises increase respiratory muscle endurance. There is no evidence that a regular exercise program improves pulmonary function or reduces morbidity or mortality. However, exercise programs do improve maximum oxygen consumption, exercise tolerance, and psychological well-being. Anecdotally, we have observed that adult patients who exercise regularly appear to have fewer exacerbations than those with similar pulmonary function who do not.

β Agonists

Airway hyperreactivity is present in 50% to 60% of CF patients.[55,56] In addition to having a direct effect on smooth muscle relaxation, β agonists also increase ciliary beat frequency in vitro.[221] However, the increased viscosity of CF sputum may overcome this potential benefit,[5] and it is not surprising that in-vivo measurements of mucociliary clearance in CF patients with β agonists are variable.[7,222]

It would seem reasonable to advocate β agonists in those patients who are clinically wheezy, demonstrate a significant bronchodilator response to β agonists, or have a positive methacholine challenge. Routine methacholine challenge testing cannot be recommended, however. It could be argued, setting aside such factors as cost, inconvenience, and patient compliance, all CF patients should receive β agonists. Recent controversial studies of longer acting β agonists in asthmatics might suggest that β agonists have a deleterious effect, perhaps allowing greater distal penetration of toxic environmental substances and not suppressing the inflammatory response in the airway.[223,224]

Theophylline

There have been variable reports on the benefit of theophylline on pulmonary function in CF patients.[225,226] Shapiro et al[227] performed a study in 12 CF patients, mean age 10 years, over 4 weeks with a 4-week crossover with placebo. Two of 12 had an increase in FVC, one an increase in FEV_1 and two a decrease in FEV_1 while on theophylline. Many patients seem symptomatically improved on theophylline preparations, and this may be an effect of improving diaphragmatic contractility in patients with air trapping and hyperexpansion. Avital et al demonstrated less nocturnal desaturation in patients with severe disease while on the drug, but sleep efficiency also decreased.[228]

Cromolyn

Small studies suggest cromolyn sodium is not an effective treatment in CF. This appears counterintuitive as atopy may be present in up to 75% of CF patients and 50% of patients demonstrate airway hyperreactivity. Sivan et al in a double-blind crossover study of 14 CF patients with demonstrable hyperreactivity with a methacholine challenge showed no improvement after 8 weeks of treatment with cromolyn.[229] As this study had a small sample size, a therapeutic trial of cromolyn may seem reasonable in an atopic person with airflow obstruction.

Anticholinergics

There are theoretical problems with the use of anticholinergic agents in patients with CF, primarily gastrointestinal (GI) motility and alteration in mucus production and viscosity. Studies examining the usefulness of anticholinergic agents have all been done with small numbers of CF patients. Larsen et al administered atropine by inhalation to 10 CF patients. $\dot{V}_{max}$ 60 improved in all patients. The authors concluded that the side effects of atropine (dry mouth and possible decreased GI motility in one patient) prohibited clinical usefulness.[230]

There are no reported side effects with ipratropium bromide in patients with CF. No changes in the rheologic properties of sputum from patients with chronic bronchitis were found with this medication.[231] The bronchodilatory effects of anticholinergic agents vary (20% to 100%), but appear equally or more efficacious than β agonists. In one study, ipratropium bromide caused an improvement in pulmonary function in 4 of 20 patients and a decrease in pulmonary function in 2 of 20.[232] However, another study showed significant improvement in 7 of 10 adult CF patients.[233] Tobin et al demonstrated a significant change in peak flows in 7 of 25 patients.[60] It would appear that ipratropium bromide is a useful bronchodilator in CF.

Inhaled Corticosteroids

In a small study of 12 patients with CF, van Haren et al showed that there was an improvement in methacholine challenge testing and in cough and dyspnea following a 6 week trial of budesonide.[234] In a nonblinded study, Nikolaizik and Schonl showed statistical improvement in lung volumes and diffusion capacity of carbon monoxide in 25 patients taking inhaled corticosteroids for a month.[235] A large multicenter trial is required to demonstrate efficacy in the CF population.

Mucolytic Agents

Sputum in CF is more abundant and has increased viscosity because of increased glycoprotein sulfation and the presence of DNA released from dead leukocytes in a concentration of 3 to 14 mg/ml.[193,236,237] With the exception of rhDNase, mucolytic agents are not effective in CF. The results of oral *N*-Acetylcysteine are controversial.[238] *N*-Acetylcysteine by inhalation may cause bronchospasm. Iodinated therapy may have some usefulness in asthma and COPD,[239,240] but is unproved in CF. Glyceryl guaiacolate is not believed to have a place in the management of CF.

Recombinant DNase 1 reduces the viscosity of purulent sputum[237,241] by randomly cutting up the DNA into fragments. The phase 3 study of rhDNase[242] involved 968 CF patients over a 6 month period and showed that there were 1.4 days less of antibiotic use and that spirometric values improved by approximately 5%. Less than 5% of patients developed antibodies to rhDNase. The development of antibody appeared to be without clinical side effects. Voice alteration was noted in up to 16% of patients taking the medications, which resolved when the medication was discontinued. Patients taking inhaled corticosteroids for a month required to demonstrate efficacy in the CF patients whose FVC is less than 40% predicted have not shown improvement in spirometric values nor has it been shown to be effective in acute pulmonary exacerbations.[243] Whether rhDNase will have an effect on longevity is yet to be determined.

In 1994, Vasconcellos et al reported that gelsolin, a protein that severs actin filaments, rapidly decreased the viscosity of CF sputum samples in vitro.[244] These investigators found that gelsolin was more efficient in reducing sputum viscosity than DNase 1. Clinical data are not yet available.

Recently some investigators have proposed inhalation of a hypertonic saline solution following premedication with a β agonist to enhance mucociliary clearance.[245] Advocation of such a practice should be with extreme caution as hypertonic solutions cause bronchoconstriction in patients with hyperresponsive airways.[246]

Hemoptysis

Blood streaking of the sputum is very common in patients over 10 years of age, but massive hemoptysis is relatively unusual, occurring in less than 10% of adults.[247] It is estimated that 1% of patients die from massive hemoptysis. Mild streaking hemoptysis is presumably caused by mucosal irritation in the airways. Streaking hemoptysis is often associated with an acute pulmonary exacerbation. With disease progression, bronchiectasis and infection persist in the airways, accompanied by hypertrophy of the bronchial circulation. Massive hemoptysis is believed to be caused by bleeding from the high systemic pressure of the bronchial circulation. It is unclear whether the symptom of massive hemoptysis adversely affects prognosis in CF per se.[189,248] Patients with massive hemoptysis tend to have poor pulmonary function.

All CF patients should be warned of the potential of massive hemoptysis and to seek emergency treatment if it occurs. Sometimes the bleeding can be controlled with bedrest, discontinuation of chest physiotherapy, cough suppressants, and antibiotics. Often an untreated exacerbation of the disease has triggered the hemoptysis, but sometimes there is no obvious precipitating event. If hemoptysis persists, embolization of the bronchial artery may be indicated.[188,189] Although previously it was felt that the site of the bleeding should be localized with either rigid or fiberoptic bronchoscopy, it is now believed that this procedure in itself may increase coughing and exacerbate the hemoptysis. Most large centers proceed directly to embolization. Bronchial artery embolization is not without hazard. Rarely, embolization of the anterior spinal artery with subsequent paraplegia can occur as the take-off of the anterior spinal artery is not constant (Fig. 68-2). The procedure should be performed by experienced interventional radiologists. In studies by Sweeney et al and Cohen et al,[188,189] acute bleeding stopped in 21 of 25 and 19 of 20 patients, respectively. Sweeney et al[189] followed 18 of 25 patients who had undergone bronchial artery embolization for at least 20 months. Compared with controls matched for age, gender, and pulmonary function, the patients with massive hemoptysis had a higher mortality rate, and 13 of 18 had recurrent severe hemoptysis. There are no data supporting prophylactic bronchial artery embolization. Indeed the recurrent hemoptysis in Sweeney's study[189] suggests that it is not helpful.

An immediate temporizing measure for massive hemoptysis is to stabilize the patient with intubation and control bleeding to one lung or one lobe with Fogarty balloon tamponade. If hemoptysis persists or the patient is unable to undergo bronchial artery embolization, it may be necessary to proceed to pulmonary resection. As pulmonary function is often severely impaired in patients with massive hemoptysis, pulmonary resection may risk leaving the patient a pulmonary cripple or ventilator dependent.

Pneumothorax

Pneumothorax occurs in 8% to 23% of older CF patients with more severe pulmonary disease.[249,250] The incidence in males and females is equal and is as common on the right as the left. It is felt that the incidence of pneumothorax may be rising as the age of the CF population is increasing. Historically, the presence of pneumothorax was associated with a worsened prognosis (20% mortality),[251] but other studies do not suggest a negative outcome from pneumothorax per se,[252] with a mortality rate of 1 of 27 patients (4%).[253] In Spector's study,[250] of 144 pneumothoraces in 99 patients dating back to 1959, the median survival following pneumothorax was 29.9 months. There were no age, gender, or pulmonary function matched controls.

Subpleural blebs are a part of the pathology of longstanding pulmonary disease, and rupture of these blebs may lead to a pneumothorax. There is a 50% to 70% chance of recurrence with pneumothoraces.[249,250] Because of the high incidence of recurrence, the treatment of choice is obliteration of the pleural space. The procedure of choice depends on whether the patient may be a candidate for lung transplantation in the future. Partial pleurectomy has the best success rate, at 95%.[250] However, if the patient is a lung transplant candidate, intercostal drainage, chemical pleurodesis, ligation of bullae, or limited surgical pleurodesis should be performed in preference to pleurectomy.[253] It should also be noted that the majority of CF patients who never have had a clinical pneumothorax have pleural scarring possibly because of air or bacterial leakage into the pleural space. Adult CF patients occasionally complain of acute pleuritic pain when neither an acute infiltrate nor a pneumothorax is present.

Clubbing and Hypertrophic Osteoarthropathy

Clubbing of the fingers is eventually a universal finding in patients with pulmonary disease, but the severity is extremely variable and not related to pulmonary function testing. Hypertrophic osteoarthropathy is seen in approximately 4% of older CF patients.[254]

Respiratory Failure and Cor Pulmonale

Hypertrophy of the right ventricle from CF pulmonary disease is not uncommon in the later stages of disease. Overt right heart failure was seen in 55 of 170 of patients (32%) who died in one retrospective study.[255] This study dated back to 1960. Cardiac catheterization was performed in 30 patients, some of whom had high wedge pressures and were severely hypoxemic, suggesting possible left ventricular dysfunction. ECHO data were not available. The mean survival time for the patients who were clinically thought to have right heart failure was 8 months.

The question of oxygen therapy remains controversial in CF.[256] Many centers treating CF have tended to extrapolate the recommendations for oxygen therapy in adults with chronic obstructive pulmonary disease to young adults with CF. In COPD, the Nocturnal Oxygen Therapy Trial group results suggested that oxygen reduced mortality, preserved exercise capacity, and improved neuropsychological function. In 1989, Zinman et al[257] showed no improvement in these parameters in CF patients, but the CF group receiving oxygen had a better quality of life in that they had an increased ability to work or go to school.

Intubation and Ventilator Therapy

As with all end-stage pulmonary disease patients, intubation and mechanical ventilation is considered to be a futile procedure, unless there is an acute reversible problem, and mechanical ventilation can be successfully removed. A handful of CF patients have successfully undergone lung transplantation from mechanical ventilation, although this makes them suboptimal candidates for surgery. Patients can be supported with nasal mechanical ventilation while awaiting transplantation.[258] Some end-stage patients are placed on BiPAP in an attempt to reduce work of breathing and to give symptomatic relief, sometimes with improvement in arterial blood gases.

Lung Transplantation

A final therapeutic option for a few CF patients may be lung transplantation.[259] Since 1985, more than 750 CF Patients have undergone lung transplantation. Nationally, the 2-year survival rate is 60%.[260] The survival rate of CF patients is no different than for non-CF patients who undergo heart-lung or double lung transplantation.[261] This is perhaps surprising as the CF patients may be in a poor nutritional state or have diabetes mellitus, pleural adhesions or pleurodeses, and sinuses colonized with antibiotic-resistant bacteria.

Postoperatively, the metabolism of cyclosporin is increased,[262,263] and trying to obtain a constant therapeutic level is challenging in patients with malabsorption, abnormal hepatic function,[264] and inconsistent bowel transit times. The transepithelial potential difference in the transplanted lung is normal, demonstrating that the stem cell of the airway epithelium is transplanted[265] and there is no CF pulmonary disease recurrence. This has not yet been confirmed by genetic testing of airway epithelial cells. The possibility of lung transplantation poses certain psychologic stresses for CF patients, their families, and their physicians as only a small minority are selected to undergo surgery and not all candidates survive until surgery.

Multidrug-resistant bacteria infecting the airway prior to transplantation is a problem in the CF population. The Toronto lung transplant group published their experience with *P. cepacia*.[266] They reported 24 double lung transplantations in 22 CF patients.[266] Patients who had *P. cepacia* either before or following transplantation had an increased mortality over those who did not. In one series, 4 of 6 deaths in CF patients were thought to be secondary to *P. cepacia* infection.[267] Currently, some lung transplantation centers will not accept patients with *P. cepacia* or patients with multiresistant *P. aeruginosa*.

Living related donors have been used as a method of lung transplantation in CF.[268] The procedure involves removing a lower lobe from the left or the right lung of each living related donor, usually the patient's parents, and transplanting the left lower lobe and the right lower lobe into each respective hemithorax of the CF recipient. The long term follow-up of this procedure is not known. There is continued ethical debate about whether this procedure should be offered to patients because lobectomy carries considerable morbidity and possible mortality for the donors, the survival of double lung transplantation is 60% at 2 years, and it is unclear that this procedure will enhance the posttransplantation survival rate.

Amiloride

In the CF airway epithelium, there is excessive absorption of sodium as well as defective chloride secretion.[6] Amiloride is a sodium channel blocker, although another mechanism of action may be inhibition of protein tyrosine kinase.[269] Knowles et al[270] undertook a crossover study of inhaled amiloride to determine whether this treatment would, by changing the rheologic properties of mucus, improve clinical outcome. In a preliminary trial with 14 patients, the decline in forced vital capacity over the 25 weeks of study was less than in the placebo period. Graham et al published their pilot study of nebulized amiloride over a 6-month period.[271] Of the 23 patients enrolled in the study, 14 completed the study. Unlike the earlier U.S. pilot study,[270] inhaled amiloride did not produce any difference in spirometric values. Although the British and U.S. trials were similar in design, the patients participating in the British study were given all existing medication and treatment for infective exacerbations in the usual way, whereas in the U.S. study antibiotics and bronchodilators were discontinued. A large multicenter trial is underway in the U.S. More recently Knowles et al[272] administered ATP and UTP to the nasal mucosa in CF patients. ATP and UTP induce chloride secretion through apical-membrane purinergic receptors. The authors postulated that an ATP analog or UTP in addition to amiloride may be considered a therapeutic option as it can increase mucociliary clearance.[273]

Sinus Complications

Radiographic evidence of sinusitis is found in over 90% of CF patients.[36,274] Normal sinus films suggest a diagnosis other than CF. Acute symptoms of sinusitis are far less common than the radiologic appearance. The etiology of the sinusitis is thought to be abnormal mucus occluding the ducts and preventing mucus drainage. The maxillary and ethmoid sinuses are most commonly involved (Fig. 68-4). Treatment is with antibiotics; surgery is rarely performed. Whether the organisms giving rise to the sinusitis are the same as those in the sputum remains controversial,[35,275] but they appear not to correlate. It is controversial whether a sinus drainage procedure should be performed in patients who are to undergo lung transplantation. Some transplant centers believe that the incidence of postoperative bacterial infection is reduced in patients who have had a drainage procedure, but there are no data to support this. It also is controversial whether surgery will help chronic facial pain or whether this is a symptom of chronic anxiety in some CF patients.

Nasal polyps occur in 10% to 25% of CF patients, most commonly in the older child and adolescent. The etiology of the polyposis is unknown. Surgical removal of polyps is associated with a 50% to 90% recurrence rate. In uncontrolled trials, topical steroids, cromolyn, and sinus irrigation appeared to be helpful in some patients.[276]

REFERENCES

Clinical Respiratory Manifestations

1. Cystic Fibrosis Foundation: Patient Registry 1994, Annual Data Report, Bethesda, Md, 1995.

Pathophysiology

2. Al-Awqati Q: Regulation of ion channels by ABC transporters that secrete ATP, *Science* 269:805-806, 1995.
3. Stutts M, Canessa C, Olsen J, Hamrick M, Cohn J, Rossier B, Boucher R: CFTR as a cAMP-dependent regulator of sodium channels, *Science* 269:847-850, 1995.
4. Verdugo P: Hydration kinetics of exocytosed mucins in cultured secretary cells of the rabbit trachea: a new model, *Ciba Found Symp* 212-225, 1984.
5. Johnson N, Royce F, Villalon M, Hard R, Verdugo P: Autoregulation of beat frequency in respiratory cells: demonstration by viscous load, *Am J Respir Dis* 144:1091-1094, 1991.
6. Knowles M, Stutts M, Yankaskas J, Gatzy J, Boucher R: Abnormal respiratory epithelial ion transport in cystic fibrosis, *Clin Chest Med* 7:285-297, 1986.
7. Wood R, Wanner A, Hirsch J, Farrell P: Tracheal mucociliary transport in patients with cystic fibrosis and its stimulation by terbutaline, *Am Rev Respir Dis* 111:733-738, 1975.
8. Yeates D, Sturgess J, Kahn S, Levison H, Aspin N: Mucociliary transport in trachea of patients with cystic fibrosis, *Arch Dis Child* 51:28-33, 1976.
9. Smith J, Travis S, Greenberg E, Welsh M: Cystic fibrosis airway epithelia fail to kill bacteria because of abnormal surface fluid, *Cell* 85:229-236, 1996.
10. Barasch J, Kiss B, Prince A, Saiman L, Gruenert D, Al-Awqati Q: Defective acidification of intracellular organelles in cystic fibrosis, *Nature* 325:70-73, 1991.
11. Kollberg H, Mossberg B, Afzelius B, Philipson K, Camner P: Cystic fibrosis compared with the immotile-cilia syndrome, *Scand J Respir Dis* 59:297-306, 1978.
12. Lambin G, Roussel P: Airway mucins and their role in defence against microorganisms, *Respir Med* 87:421-426, 1993.

Pathophysiology of Pulmonary Disease

13. Chow C, Landau L, Taussig L: Bronchial mucous glands in the newborn with cystic fibrosis, *Eur J Pediatr* 139:240-243, 1982.
14. Claireaux A: Fibrocystic disease of the pancreas in the newborn, *Arch Dis Child* 31:22-27, 1956.
15. Nash F, Smith J: Fibrocystic disease of the pancreas with meconium peritonitis at birth, *Arch Dis Child* 27:73-78, 1952.
16. Reid L, Haller RD: The bronchial mucous glands: their hypertrophy and changes in intracellular mucus. In Grindelwald Rossi E, Stoll E, eds: *Clinical investigations on cystic fibrosis,* 4th International conference on cystic fibrosis of the pancreas, Berne, 1966.
17. Zuelzer W, Newton W: The pathogenesis of fibrocystic disease of the pancreas. A study of 36 cases with special reference to the pulmonary lesions, *Pediatrics* 4:53-69, 1949.
18. Lamb D, Reid L: The tracheobronchial submucosal glands in cystic fibrosis: a qualitative and quantitative histochemical study, *Br J Dis Chest* 66:240-247, 1972.
19. Khan T, Wagener J, Bost T, Martinez J, Accurso F, Riches D: Early pulmonary inflammation in infants with cystic fibrosis, *Am J Respir Crit Care Med* 151:1075-1082, 1995.
20. Bedrossian C, Greenberg S, Singer D, Hansen J, Rosenberg H: The lung in cystic fibrosis: a quantitative study including prevalence of pathologic findings among different age groups, *Hum Pathol* 7:195-204, 1976.
21. Guidotti T, Line B, Luetzeler J: Cystic fibrosis related lung disease in young adults with minimal impairment, *Respiration* 44:351-359, 1983.
22. Sobonya R, Taussig L: Quantitative aspects of lung pathology in cystic fibrosis, *Am Rev Respir Dis* 134:290-295, 1986.
23. Stern R, Boat T, Orenstein D, Wood R, Matthews L, Doershuk C: Treatment and prognosis of lobar and segmental atelectasis in cystic fibrosis, *Am Rev Respir Dis* 118:821-826, 1978.
24. diSant'Agnese P: Bronchial obstruction with lobar atelectasis and emphysema in cystic fibrosis of the pancreas, *Pediatrics* 12:178-190, 1953.
25. Tomashefski J Jr, Konstan M, Bruce M, Abramowski C: The pathologic characteristics of interstitial pneumonia in cystic fibrosis, *Am J Clin Pathol* 91:522-530, 1989.
26. Tomashefski J Jr, Bruce M, Goldberg H, Dearborn D: Regional distribution of macroscopic lung disease in cystic fibrosis, *Am Rev Respir Dis* 133:535-540, 1986.
27. Tomashefski J, Christoforidis A, Abdullah A: Cystic fibrosis in young adults, an overlooked diagnosis with emphasis on pulmonary function and radiological patterns, *Chest* 57:28-36, 1970.
28. Friedman P, Harwood I, Ellenbogen P: Pulmonary cystic fibrosis in the adult: early and late radiologic findings with pathologic correlations, *Am J Roentgenology* 136:1131-1134, 1981.
29. Coates E Jr: Characteristics of cystic fibrosis in adults. A report of seven patients, *Dis Chest* 49:195-204, 1966.

30. Gyepes M, Bennett L, Hassakis P: Regional pulmonary blood flow in cystic fibrosis, *Am J Roentgenol Radium Ther Nucl Med* 106:567-575, 1969.
31. Tomashefski J Jr, Bruce M, Stern R, Dearborn D, Dahms B: Pulmonary air cysts in cystic fibrosis: relation of pathologic features to radiologic findings and history of pneumothorax, *Hum Pathol* 16:253-261, 1985.
32. Waring W, Brunt C, Hilman B: Mucoid impaction of the bronchi in cystic fibrosis, *Pediatrics* 39:166-175, 1967.
33. Mearns M, Hodson C, Jackson A, Haworth E, Sellors T, Sturridge M, France N, Reid L: Pulmonary resection in cystic fibrosis, results in 23 cases, 1957-1970, *Arch Dis Child* 47:499-508, 1972.

Pathophysiology of Sinus Disease

34. Ramsey B, Richardson M: Impact of sinusitis in cystic fibrosis, *J Allergy Clin Immunol* 90:547-552, 1992.
35. Shapiro E, Milmoe G, Ward E, Rodman J, Bowen A: Bacteriology of the maxillary sinuses in patients with cystic fibrosis, *J Infect Dis* 146:589-593, 1982.
36. Neely J, Harrison G, Jerger J, Greenberger S, Presberg H: The otolaryngolic aspects of cystic fibrosis, *Trans Am Acad Ophthal Otolaryngol* 76:313-324, 1972.
37. Oppenheimer E, Rosenstein B: Differential pathology of nasal polyps in cystic fibrosis and atopy, *Lab Invest* 40:455-459, 1979.

Lung Function

38. Taussig L, Lemen R: Interpretation of pulmonary function tests in children. In Sackner MA, ed: New York, 1980, Basel Dekker, pp 427-472.
39. Beardsmore CS, Bar-Yishay E, Maayan C et al: Lung function in infants with cystic fibrosis, *Thorax* 43:545-551, 1988.
40. Tepper RS, Hiatt P, Eigen HJ: Infants with cystic fibrosis: pulmonary function at diagnosis, *Pediatr Pulmonol* 5:15-18, 1988.
41. Milner A, Ingram D: Peak expiratory flow rates in children under 5 years of age, *Arch Dis Child* 45:780-782, 1970.
42. Taussig LM: Maximal expiratory flows at functional residual capacity: a test of lung function for young children, *Am Rev Respir Dis* 116:1031-1038, 1977.
43. Doershuk C, Fisher B, Mathews L: Specific airway resistance from perinatal period into adulthood, *Am Rev Respir Dis* 109:452-457, 1974.
44. Godfrey S, Bar-Yishay E, Arad I, Landau L, Taussig L: Flow-volume curves in infants with lung disease, *Pediatrics* 72:517-522, 1983.
45. Phelan P, Gracey M, Williams H et al: Ventilatory function in infants with cystic fibrosis, *Arch Dis Child* 44:393-400, 1969.
46. Landau L, Phelan P: The spectrum of cystic fibrosis. A study of pulmonary mechanics in 46 patients, *Am Rev Respir Dis* 108:593-602, 1973.
47. Landau L, Mellis C, Phelan P, Bristone B, McLennan L: Small airways disease in children: no test is best, *Thorax* 34:217-223, 1979.
48. Zapletal A, Motoyama E, Gibson L, Bouhuys A: Pulmonary mechanics in asthma and cystic fibrosis, *Pediatrics* 48:64-72, 1971.
49. Featherby E, Weng T, Crozier D, Duic A, Reilly B, Levison H: Dynamic and static lung volumes, gas tensions and diffusing capacity in patients with cystic fibrosis, *Am Rev Respir Dis* 102:737-749, 1970.
50. Lamarre A, Reilly B, Byran A, Levison H: Early detection of pulmonary function abnormalities in cystic fibrosis, *Pediatrics* 50:291-298, 1972.
51. Levison H, Godfrey S: Cystic fibrosis: projections into the future. In Mangos JA, Talamo RE, eds: *Pulmonary aspects,* New York, 1976, Stratton Intercontinental Medical.

Arterial Blood Gases

52. Kerem E, Reisman J, Corey M, Canny G, Levison H: Prediction of mortality in patients with cystic fibrosis, *N Engl J Med* 326:1187-1191, 1992.
53. Canny G, Levison H: The accuracy of arterialized capillary blood for the measurement of blood gas tensions in patients with lung disease, *Pediatr Pulmonol* 2:313-314, 1986.

Prognosis and Pulmonary Function Tests

54. Taussig L, Kattwinkel J, Friedewald W, di Sant'Agnese P: A new prognostic score and clinical evaluation system for cystic fibrosis, *J Pediatr* 82:380-390, 1973.
55. Davis P: Airway responsiveness and atopy in cystic fibrosis. Airway responsiveness and atopy in the development of chronic lung disease. In Weiss S, Sparrow D, eds: New York, 1989, Raven Press, pp 293-313.
56. Eggleston P, Rosenstein B, Stackhouse C, Alexander M: Airway hyperreactivity in cystic fibrosis: clinical correlates and possible effects on the course of the disease, *Chest* 94:360-365, 1988.
57. Cooper P, Robertson C, Hudson I, Phelan P: Variability of pulmonary function teats in cystic fibrosis, *Pediatr Pulmonol* 8:16-22, 1990.
58. Nickerson B, Lemen R, Gerdes C, Wegmann M, Robertson G: Within-subject variability and percent change for significance of spirometry in normal subjects and in patients with cystic fibrosis, *Am Rev Respir Dis* 122:859-866, 1980.
59. Hordvik N, Konig P, Morris D, Kreutz C, Barbero G: A longitudinal study of bronchodilator responsiveness in cystic fibrosis, *Am Rev Respir Dis* 131:889-893, 1985.
60. Tobin M, Maguire O, Reed D, Tempany E, Fitzgerald M: Atopy and bronchial reactivity in older patients with cystic fibrosis, *Thorax* 35:807-813, 1980.

Nutrition and Pulmonary Function Tests

61. Ramsey B, Farrell P, Pencharz P, Consensus Committee: Nutritional assessment and management in cystic fibrosis: a consensus report, *Am J Clin Nutr* 55:108-116, 1992.
62. Gaskin K, Gurwitz D, Durie P, Corey M, Levison H, Forstner G: Improved respiratory prognosis in patients with cystic fibrosis with normal fat absorption, *J Pediatr* 100:857-862, 1982.
63. Boland M, Stoski D, MacDonald N, Soucy P, Patrick J: Chronic jejunostomy feeding with a non-elemental formula in undernourished patients with cystic fibrosis, *Lancet* 1:232-234, 1986.
64. Drury D, Pianosi P, Kopelman H, Charge D, Coates A: The effect of nutritional status on respiratory muscle strength and work capacity in cystic fibrosis, *Pediatr Res* 104A, 1990.
65. Levy L, Durie P, Pencharz P, Corey M: Effects of long term nutritional rehabilitation on body composition and clinical status in malnourished children and adolescents with cystic fibrosis, *J Pediatr* 107:225-230, 1985.
66. Steitikamp G, Hardt H: Improvement of nutritional status and lung function after long-term nocturnal gastrostomy feedings in cystic fibrosis, *J Pediatr* 124:244-249, 1994.

Pregnancy and Pulmonary Function

67. Hilman B, Aitken M, Constantinescu M: Pregnancy in patients with cystic fibrosis, *Clin Obstet Gynecol* 39:70-86, 1996.
68. Kotloff R, Fitzsimmons S, Fiel S: Fertility and pregnancy in patients with cystic fibrosis, *Clin Chest Med* 13:623-635, 1992.
69. Canny G, Corey M, Livingstone R, Carpenter S, Green L, Levison H: Pregnancy and cystic fibrosis, *Obstet Gynecol* 77:850-862, 1991.

Gastroesophageal Reflux

70. Stringer DA, Sprigg A, Juodis E, Corey M, Daneman A, Levison HJ, Durie PR: The association of cystic fibrosis, gastroesophageal reflux, and reduced pulmonary function, *Can Assoc Radiol J* 39:100-102, 1988.
71. Dab I, Malfroot A: Gastroesophageal reflux: a primary defect in cystic fibrosis? *Scand J Gastroenterol* 143:125-131, (suppl) 1988.
72. Malfroot A, Dab I: New insight on gastro-oesophageal reflux in cystic fibrosis by longitudinal follow up, *Arch Dis Child* 66:1339-1345, 1991.
73. Vigneri S, Termini R, Leandro G, Badlamenti S, Pantalena M, Savarino V, DiMario F, Battaglia G, Mela G, Pilotto A, Plebani M, Davi G: A comparison of five maintenance therapies for reflux esophagitis, *N Engl J Med* 333:1106-1110, 1995.

Microbiology and Immunology

74. Hoiby N: Microbiology of lung infections in cystic fibrosis patients, *Acta Paediatr Scand* 301 (suppl C):33-54, 1982.
75. Bauernfeind A, Rotter K, Weisslein-Pfister C: Selective procedure to isolate *Haemophilus influenzae* from sputa with large quantities of *Pseudomonas aeruginosa, Infection* 15:278-280, 1987.
76. diSantAgnese P, Davis P: Research in cystic fibrosis, *N Engl J Med* 295:597-602, 1979.

Specific Pathogens

77. Watson K, Kerr E, Hinks C: Distribution of biotypes of *Hemophilus influenzae* and *H. parainfluenzae* in patients with cystic fibrosis, *J Clin Pathol* 38:750-753, 1985.
78. Long S, Teter M, Gilligan P: Biotype of *Haemophilus influenzae:* correlation with virulence and ampicillin resistance, *J Infect Dis* 147:800-806, 1983.

79. Thomassen M, Klinger J, Badger S, Heeckeren DV, Stern R: Cultures of thoracotomy specimens confirm usefulness of sputum cultures in cystic fibrosis, *J Pediatr* 104:352-356, 1984.
80. Taussig L, Belmonte M, Beaudry P: *Staphylococcus aureus* empyema in cystic fibrosis, *J Pediatr* 84:724-727, 1974.
81. Pressler T, Szaff M, Hoiby N: Antibiotic treatment of *Haemophilus influenzae* and *Haemophilus parainfluenzae* infections in patients with cystic fibrosis, *Acta Paediatr Scand* 73:541-547, 1984.
82. Knoke J, St Knoern R, Doershuk C, Boat T, Matthews L: Cystic fibrosis: the prognosis for five-year survival, *Pediatr Res* 12:676-679, 1978.
83. Anderson D: Therapy and prognosis of fibrocystic disease of the pancreas, *Pediatrics* 3:406-417, 1949.
84. Bauernfeind A, Przyklenk B, Matthias C, Jungwirth R, Bertele R, Harms K: Staphylococcal aspects of cystic fibrosis, *Infection* 18: 68/126-72/130, 1990.
85. Boxerbaum B, Jacobs M, Cechner R: Prevalence and significance of methicillin-resistant *Staphylococcus aureus* in patients with cystic fibrosis, *Pediatr Pulmonol* 4:159-163, 1988.
86. Bauernfeind A, Horl G, Przyklenk B: Microbiologic and therapeutic aspects of *Staphylococcus aureus* in cystic fibrosis patients, *Scand J Gastroenterol* 23(suppl 143):99-102, 1988.
87. Frederiksen B, Lanngg S, Koch C, Hoiby N: Improved survival in the Danish center-treated cystic fibrosis patients: results of aggressive treatment, *Pediatr Pulmonol* 21:153-158, 1996.
88. Weaver LT, Green MR, Nicholson K et al: Prognosis in cystic fibrosis treated with continuous flucloxacillin from the neonatal period, *Arch Dis Child* 70:84-89, 1994.
89. Huang N, Hoon EV, Sheng K: The flora of the respiratory tract of patients with cystic fibrosis, *J Pediatr* 59:512-521, 1961.
90. Doggett R, Harrison G, Stillwell R, Wallis E: An atypical *Pseudomonas aeruginosa* associated with cystic fibrosis of the pancreas, *J Pediatr* 68:215-221, 1966.
91. Berger M, Sorensen R, Tosi M, Dearborn D, Doring G: Complement receptor expression on neutrophils at an inflammatory site, the *Pseudomonas*-infected lung in cystic fibrosis, *J Clin Invest* 84:1302-1313, 1989.
92. Pier G, Saunders J, Ames P, Edwards M, Auerbach H, Goldfarb J, Speert D, Hurwitch S: Opsonophagocytic killing antibody of *Pseudomonas aeruginosa* mucoid exopolysaccharide in older non-colonized patients with cystic fibrosis, *N Engl J Med* 317:793-798, 1987.
93. Laraya-Cuasay L, Cundy K, Huang N: *Pseudomonas* carrier rates of patients with cystic fibrosis and of members of their families, *J Pediatr* 89:23-26, 1976.
94. Speert D, Lawton D, Damm S: Communicability of *Pseudomonas aeruginosa* in a cystic fibrosis summer camp, *J Pediatr* 101:227-229, 1982.
95. Kelly N, Fitzgerald M, Tempany E, O'Boyle C, Falkiner F, Keane C: Does *Pseudomonas* cross-infection occur between cystic fibrosis patients? *Lancet* ii:688-690, 1982.
96. Thomassen M, Demko C, Doershuk C, Root J: *Pseudomonas aeruginosa* isolates: comparisons of isolates from campers and from sibling pairs with cystic fibrosis, *Pediatr Pulmonol* 1:40-45, 1985.
97. Pedersen S, Koch C, Hoiby N, Rosendal K: An epidemic spread of multiresistant *Pseudomonas aeruginosa* in a cystic fibrosis centre, *J Antimicrob Chemother* 17:505-510, 1986.
98. Tummler B, Koopman U, Grothues D, Weissbrodt H, Steinkamp G, Hardt Hvd: Nosocomial acquisition of *Pseudomonas aeruginosa* by cystic fibrosis patients, *J Clin Microbiol* 29:1265-1267, 1991.
99. Pedersen S, Jensen T, Pressler T, Hoiby N, Rosendal K: Does centralized treatment of cystic fibrosis increase the risk of *Pseudomonas aeruginosa* infection? *Acta Paediatr Scand* 75:840-845, 1986.
100. Hoogkamp-Korstanje J, Laag Jvd: Incidence and risk of cross-colonization in cystic fibrosis holiday camps, *Antonie Van Leeuwenhoek* 46:100-101, 1980.
101. Kerem E, Corey M, Gold R, Levinson H: Pulmonary function and clinical course in patients with cystic fibrosis after pulmonary colonization with *Pseudomonas aeruginosa, J Pediatr* 116: 714-719, 1990.
102. Kulczycki L, Murphy T, Bellanti J: *Pseudomonas* colonization in cystic fibrosis, *JAMA* 240:30-34, 1978.
103. Cryz S Jr, Wedgewood J, Lang A, Ruedeberg A, Que J, Furer E, Schaad U: Immunization of noncolonized cystic fibrosis patients against *Pseudomonas aeruginosa, J Infect Dis* 169:1159-1162, 1994.
104. Lang A, Schaad U, Rudeberg A, Wedgwood J, Que J, Furer E, Cryz S: Effect of high-affinity anti-*Pseudomonas aeruginosa* lipopolysaccharide antibodies induced by immunization on the rate of *Pseudomonas aeruginosa* infection in patients with cystic fibrosis, *J Pediatr* 127:711-717, 1995.
105. Sharma G, Tosi M, Stern R, Davis P: Progression of lung disease despite apparent eradication of *Pseudomonas aeruginosa* from the lower airways of three previously colonized cystic fibrosis patients, *Pediatr Pulmonol* 9S:234 1993, (abstract).
106. Valerius N, Koch C, Hoiby N: Prevention of chronic *Pseudomonas aeruginosa* colonisation in cystic fibrosis by early treatment, *Lancet* 338:725-726, 1991.
107. Ederer G, JM: Colonization and infection with *Pseudomonas cepacia, J Infect Dis* 125:613-618, 1972.
108. Rosenstein B, Hall D: Pneumonia and septicemia due to *Pseudomonas cepacia* in a patient with cystic fibrosis, *Johns Hopkins Med J* 147:188-189, 1980.
109. Thomassen M, Demko C, Klinger J, Stern R: *Pseudomonas cepacia* colonization among cystic fibrosis patients: a new opportunist, *Am Rev Respir Dis* 131:791-796, 1985.
110. Burkholder W: Sour skin, a bacterial rot of onion bulbs, *Phytopathology* 40:115-117, 1950.
111. Beckman W, Lessie T: Response of *Pseudomonas cepacia* to b-lactam antibiotics: utilization of penicillin G as the carbon source, *J Bacteriol* 140:1126-1128, 1979.
112. Carson L, Favero M, Bond W, Peterson N: Morphological, biochemical, and growth characteristics of *Pseudomonas cepacia* from distilled water, *Appl Microbiol* 25:476-483, 1973.
113. Schaffner W, Reisig G, Verrall R: Outbreak of *Pseudomonas cepacia* infection due to contaminated anaesthetics, *Lancet* I:1050-1051, 1973.
114. Phillips I, Eykyn S, Curtis M, Snell J: *Pseudomonas cepacia* (mulfivorans) septicemia in an intensive care unit, *Lancet* I:375-377, 1971.
115. Sajjan U, Corey M, Karmali M, Forstner J: Binding of *Pseudomonas cepacia* to normal human intestinal mucin and respiratory mucin from patients with cystic fibrosis, *J Clin Invest* 89:648-656, 1992.
116. Sajjan U, Reisman J, Doig P, Irvin R, Forstner G, Forstner J: Binding of nonmucoid *Pseudomonas aeruginosa* to normal intestinal mucin and respiratory mucin from patients with cystic fibrosis, *J Clin Invest* 89:657-665, 1992.
117. Gessner A, Mortensen J: Pathogenic factors of *Pseudomonas cepacia* isolates from patients with cystic fibrosis, *J Med Microbiol* 33:115-120, 1990.
118. Gilligan P, Gage P, Bradshaw L, Schidlow D, DeCicco B: Isolation medium for the recovery of *Pseudomonas cepacia* from respiratory secretions of patients with cystic fibrosis, *J Clin Microbiol* 22:5-8, 1985.
119. Tomashefski J, Jr, Thomassen M, Bruce M, Goldberg H, Konstan M, Stern R: *Pseudomonas cepacia* associated pneumonia in cystic fibrosis, *Arch Pathol Lab Med* 112:106-172, 1988.
120. Hardy K, McGowan K, Fisher M, Schidlow D: *Pseudomonas cepacia* in the hospital setting: lack of transmission between cystic fibrosis patients, *J Pediatr* 109:51-55, 1986.
121. Tablan O, Chorba T, Schidlow D, White J, Hardy K, Gilligan P, Morgan W, Carson L, Martone W, Jason J, Jarvis W: *Pseudomonas cepacia* colonization in patients with cystic fibrosis: risk factors and clinical outcome, *J Pediatr* 107:382-387, 1985.
122. *Lancet: Pseudomonas cepacia*—more than a harmless commensal? (Editorial). *Lancet* 339:1385-1386, 1992.
123. Prince A: *Pseudomonas cepacia* in cystic fibrosis patients, *Am Rev Respir Dis* 134:644-645, 1986.
124. Thomassen M, Demko C, Doershuk C, Stern R, Klinger J: *Pseudomonas cepacia:* decrease in colonization in patients with cystic fibrosis, *Am Rev Respir Dis* 134:669-671, 1986.
125. Pegues D, Carson L, Roman S, Fitzsimmons S, Tablan O, and the CF study group: Acquisition of *Pseudomonas cepacia* at cystic fibrosis summer camps, *Pediatr Pulmonol* 6(suppl):326A, 1991.
126. LiPuma J, Mortensen J, Dasen S, Edlind T, Schidlow D, Burns J, Stull T: Ribotype analysis of *Pseudomonas cepacia* from cystic fibrosis treatment centers, *J Pediatr* 113:859-862, 1988.
127. LiPuma J, Dasen S, Nielson D, Stern R, Stull T: Person-to-person transmission of *Pseudomonas cepacia* between patients with cystic fibrosis, *Lancet* 336:1094-1096, 1990.
128. Smith D, Smith E, Gumery L, Stableforth D: *Pseudomonas cepacia* infection in cystic fibrosis, *Lancet* 339:252, 1992 (letter).

129. Gowan J, Doherty C, Nelson J, Brown P, Greening A: Transmission of *Pseudomonas cepacia* in cystic fibrosis patients, XI International Cystic Fibrosis Conference, Dublin, Ireland 1992, abstract.
130. Kaplan T, McKey Jr RM, Toraya N, Moccia G: Impact of CF summer camp, *Clin Pediatr* 31:161-167, 1992.
131. Nelson J, Doherty C, Brown P, Greening A, Kaufmann M, Gowan J: *Pseudomonas cepacia* in inpatients with cystic fibrosis, *Lancet* 338:152-155, 1991 (letter).
132. Pitchford K, Corey M, Highsmith A, Perlman R, Bannatyne R, Gold R, Levison H, Ford-Jones E: *Pseudomonas* species contamination of cystic fibrosis patients' home inhalation equipment, *J Pediatr* 111:212-216, 1987.
133. Isles A, Maclusky L, Corey M, Gold R, Prober C, Fleming P, Levison H: *Pseudomonas cepacia* infection in cystic fibrosis: an emerging problem, *J Pediatr* 104:206-210, 1984.
134. Simmonds E, Conway S, Ghoneim A, Ross H, Littlewood J: *Pseudomonas cepacia:* a new pathogen in patients with cystic fibrosis referred to a large centre in the United Kingdom, *Arch Dis Child* 65:874-877, 1990.
135. Chiesa C, Labrozzi P, Aronoff S: Decreased baseline b-lactamase production and inducibility associated with increased piperacillin susceptibility of *Pseudomonas cepacia* isolated from children with cystic fibrosis, *Pediatr Res* 20:1174-1177, 1986.
136. Gold R, Jin E, Levison H, Isles A, Fleming P: Ceftazidime alone and in combination in patients with cystic fibrosis: lack of efficacy in treatment of severe respiratory infections caused by *Pseudomonas cepacia, J Antimicrob Chemother* 12(suppl A):331-336, 1983.
137. Taylor R, Gaya H, Hodson M: Temocillin and cystic fibrosis: outcome of intravenous administration in patients infected with *Pseudomonas cepacia, J Antimicrob Chemother* 3:341-344, 1992.
138. Christenson J, Welch D, Mukwaya G, Muszynski M, Weaver R, Brenner D: Recovery of *Pseudomonas gladioli* from respiratory tract specimens of patients with cystic fibrosis, *J Clin Microbiol* 27:270-273, 1989.
139. Kelly N, Falkiner F, Keane C, Fitzgerald M, Tampany E: Mucoid gram-negative bacilli in cystic fibrosis, *Lancet* i:705, 1983.
140. Macone A, Pier G, Pennington J, Matthewws Jr W, Goldmann D: Mucoid *Escherichia coli* in cystic fibrosis, *N Engl J Med* 304:1445-1449, 1981.
141. Smith M, Efthimiou J, Hodson M, Batten J: Mycobacterial isolations in young adults with cystic fibrosis, *Thorax* 39:369-375, 1984.
142. Wood R, Boat T, Doershuk C: State of the art: cystic fibrosis, *Am Rev Respir Dis* 113:833-878, 1976.
143. Hjelte L, Petrini B, Kallenius G, Strandvik B: Prospective study of mycobacterial infections in patients with cystic fibrosis, *Thorax* 45:397-400, 1990.
144. American Thoracic Society: Control of tuberculosis in the United States, *Am Rev Respir Dis* 146:1623-1633, 1992.
145. Whittier S, Hopfer R, Knowles M, Gilligan P: Improved recovery of mycobacteria from respiratory secretions of patients with cystic fibrosis, *J Clin Microbiol* 31:861-864, 1993.
146. Kilby J, Gilligan P, Yankaskas J, Highsmith Jr W, Edwards L, Knowles M: Non tuberculous mycobacteria in adult patients with cystic fibrosis, *Chest* 102:70-75, 1992.
147. Efthimiou J, Smith M, Hodson M, Batten J: Fatal pulmonary infection with *Mycobacterium fortuitum* in cystic fibrosis, *Brit J Dis Chest* 78:299-302, 1984.
148. Aitken M, Burke W, McDonald G, Wallis C, Ramsey B, Nolan C: Nontuberculous mycobacterial disease in adult cystic fibrosis patients, *Chest* 104:1096-1099, 1993.
149. Kinney J, Little B, Yolken R, Rosenstein B: *Mycobacterium avium* complex in a patient with cystic fibrosis: disease vs. colonization, *Pediatr Infect Dis* 8:393-396, 1989.
150. Stern R: Pulmonary complications of cystic fibrosis. In Davis PB, ed: *Cystic fibrosis,* New York, 1993, Marcel Dekker.
151. Hoiby N, Hoff G, Jenson K, Lund E: Serological types of *Diplococcus pneumoniae* isolated from the respiratory tract of children with cystic fibrosis and children with other disease, *Scand J Respir Dis* 57:37-40, 1976.
152. Nelson L, Callerame M, Schwartz R: Aspergillosis and atopy in cystic fibrosis, *Am Rev Respir Dis* 120:863-873, 1979.
153. Schwartz R, Johnstone D, Holsclaw D, Dooley R: Serum precipitins to *Aspergillus fumigatus* in cystic fibrosis, *Am J Dis Child* 120:432-433, 1970.
154. Becker J, Burke W, McDonald G, Greenberger P, Henderson W, Aitken M: Prevalence of allergic bronchopulmonary aspergillosis and atopy in adult patients with cystic fibrosis, *Chest* 109:1536-1540, 1996.
155. Guidotti T, Luetzeler J, Sant'Agnese PD, Escaro D: Fatal disseminated aspergillosis in a previously well young adult with cystic fibrosis, *Am J Med Sci* 283:157-160, 1982.
156. Jenner B, Landau L, Phelan P: Pulmonary candidiasis in cystic fibrosis, *Arch Dis Child* 1979: 54:555-556.
157. Fahy J, Keoghan M, Crummy E, FitzGerald M: Bacteraemia and fungaemia in adults with cystic fibrosis, *J Infection* 22:241-245, 1991.
158. Abman S, Ogle J, Butler-Siinon N, Rumack C, Accurso F: Role of respiratory syncytial virus in early hospitalizations for respiratory distress of young infants with cystic fibrosis, *J Pediatr* 113:826-830, 1988.
159. Conway S, Simmonds E, Littlewood J: Acute severe deterioration in cystic fibrosis associated with influenza A virus infection, *Thorax* 47:112-114, 1992.
160. Wang E, Prober C, Manson B, Corey M, Levison H: Association of respiratory viral infections with pulmonary deterioration in patients with cystic fibrosis, *N Engl J Med* 311:1653-1658, 1984.
161. Andersen D: Cystic fibrosis of the pancreas and its relation to celiac disease, *Am J Dis Child* 56:344-399, 1938.
162. Gold R, Carpenter S, Heurter H, Corey M, Levison H: Randomized trial of ceftazidime versus placebo in the management of acute respiratory exacerbations in patients with cystic fibrosis, *J Pediatr* 111:907-913, 1987.
163. diSantAgnese P, Anderson D: Celiac syndrome IV. Chemotherapy in infections of the respiratory tract associated with cystic fibrosis of the pancreas: observations with penicillin and drugs of the sulfonamide group, with special reference to penicillin aerosol, *Am J Dis Child* 72:17-61, 1946.

Pulmonary Immunology and Inflammation

164. Matthews W Jr, Williams M, Oliphint B, Geha R, Colten H: Hypogammaglobulinemia in patients with cystic fibrosis, *N Engl J Med* 302:245-249, 1980.
165. Sorensen R, Stern R, Polmar S: Lymphocyte responsiveness to *Pseudomonas aeruginosa* in cystic fibrosis: relationship to status of pulmonary disease in sibling pairs, *J Pediatrics* 93:201-205, 1978.
166. Sorensen R, Klinger J, Cash H, Chase P, Dearborn D: In vitro inhibition of lymphocyte proliferation by *Pseudomonas aeruginosa* phenazine pigments, *Infect Immun* 41:321-330, 1983.
167. Konstan M, Norvell T, Hilliard K, Shiratsuchi H, Berger M: Serial bronchoalveolar lavage to evaluate inflammation in cystic fibrosis (CF) lung disease, *Pediatr Pulmonol* 5(suppl):273, 1990.
168. Konstan M, Berger M: Infection and inflammation of the lung in cystic fibrosis. In Davis PB, ed: *Cystic fibrosis,* New York, 1993, Marcel Dekker.
169. Konstan M, Walenga R, Hilliard K, Hilliard J: Leukotriene B_4 is markedly elevated in the epithelial lining fluid of patients with cystic fibrosis, *Am Rev Respir Dis* 148:896-901, 1993.

Antiinflammatories

170. Eigen H, Rosenstein B, FitzSimmons S, Schidlow D, CF Foundation Prednisone Trial Group: A multicenter study of alternate-day prednisone therapy in patients with cystic fibrosis, *J Pediatr* 126:515-523, 1995.
171. Konstan M, Byard P, Hoppel C, Davis P: Effect of high-dose ibuprofen in patients with cystic fibrosis, *N Engl J Med* 332:848-854, 1995.
172. McElvaney N, Hubbard R, Birrer P, Chernick M, Caplan D, Frank M, Crystal R: Aerosol al-antitrypsin treatment for cystic fibrosis, *Lancet* 337:392-394, 1991.
173. McElvaney N, Nakamura H, Birrer P, H'ebert C, Wong W, Alphonso M, Baker J, Catalano M, Crystal R: Modulation of airway inflammation in cystic fibrosis. In vivo suppression of interleukin-8 levels on the respiratory epithelial surface by aerosolization of recombinant secretory leukoprotease inhibitor, *J Clin Invest* 90(4):296-301, 1992.

Radiology

174. Brasfield D, Hicks G, Soong S, Tiller R: The chest roentgenogram in cystic fibrosis: a new scoring system, *Pediatrics* 63:24-101, 1979.
175. Brasfield D, Hicks G, Soong S, Peters J, Tiller R: Evaluation of scoring system of the chest radiograph in cystic fibrosis: a collaborative study, *Am J Radiol* 134:1195-1198, 1980.
176. Chrispin A, Norman A: The systemic evaluation of the chest radiograph in cystic fibrosis, *Pediatr Radiol* 2:101-106, 1974.

177. Coates A, Boyce P, Shaw D, Godfrey S, Mearns M: Relationship between the chest radiograph, regional lung function studies, exercise tolerance, and clinical condition in cystic fibrosis, *Arch Dis Child* 56:106-111, 1981.
178. Rosenberg S, Howatt W, Grum C: Spirometry and chest roentgenographic appearance in adults with cystic fibrosis, *Chest* 101:961-964, 1992.
179. Greene K, Takasugi J, Godwin J, Richardson M, Burke W, Aitken M: Radiographic changes seen in acute exacerbations of cystic fibrosis in adults: a pilot study, *Am J Radiol* 163:557-562, 1994.
180. Santis G, Hodson M, Strickland B: High-resolution computed tomography in adult cystic fibrosis patients with mild lung disease, *Clin Radiol* 44:20-22, 1991.
181. Hansell D, Strickland B: High resolution computed tomography in pulmonary cystic fibrosis, *Brit J Clin Radiology* 62:1-5, 1989.
182. Taccone A, Romano L, Marzoli A, Girosi D, Dell'Acqua A, Romano C: High resolution computed tomography in cystic fibrosis, *Eur J Radiology* 15:125-129, 1992.
183. Wilson J, Saunders A: Narrow section computed tomography in diffuse lung disease, *Radiography* 53:122-124, 1987.
184. Nathanson I, Conboy K, Murphy S et al: Ultrafast computerized tomography of the chest in cystic fibrosis: a new scoring system, *Pediatr Pulmonol* 11:81-86, 1991.
185. Bhalla M, Turcios N, Aponte V, Jenkins M, Leitman B, McCauley D, Naidich D: Cystic fibrosis: scoring system with thin-section CT, *Radiology* 179:783-788, 1991.
186. Fiel S, Friedman A, Caroline D, Radecki P, Faerber E, Grumbach K: Magnetic resonance imaging in young adults with cystic fibrosis, *Chest* 91:181-194, 1987.
187. Grenier P, Maurice F, Musset D, Menu Y, Nahum H: Bronchiectasis: assessment by thin-section CT, *Radiology* 161:95-99, 1986.
188. Cohen A, Doershuk C, Stem R: Bronchial artery embolization to control hemoptysis in cystic fibrosis, *Radiology* 175:401-405, 1990.
189. Sweeney N, Fellows K: Bronchial artery embolization for severe hemoptysis in cystic fibrosis, *Chest* 97:1322-1326, 1990.

Complications and Treatment

190. Kerrebijn K, Michel M, Horrevorts A: Pulmonary infection and antibiotic treatment in cystic fibrosis, *Chest* 94(2):97S-169S, 1988.
191. Ramsey B: Management of pulmonary disease in patients with cystic fibrosis, *N Engl J Med* 335:179-188, 1996.
192. Smith A: Antibiotic therapy in cystic fibrosis: evaluation of clinical trials, *J Pediatr* 108:866-870, 1986.
193. Smith A, Redding G, Doershuk C, Goldmann D, Gore E, Hilman B, Marks M, Moss R, Ramsey B, Rubio T, Schwartz R, Thomassen M, Williams-Warren J, Weber A, Wilmott R, Wilson H, Yogev R: Sputum changes associated with therapy for endobronchial exacerbation in cystic fibrosis, *J Pediatr* 112:547-554, 1988.
194. Redding G, Restuccia R, Cotton E, Brooks J: Serial changes in pulmonary functions in children hospitalized with cystic fibrosis, *Am Rev Respir Dis* 126:31, 1982.
195. Smith A: Antibiotic resistance is not relevant in infections in cystic fibrosis, *Pediatr Pulmonol* 5(suppl):93, 1990.
196. Donati M, Guenett G, Anerbach H: Prospective controlled study of home and hospital therapy for cystic fibrosis pulmonary disease, *J Pediatr* 111:28-33, 1987.
197. Doershuk C, Matthews L, Tucker A, Spector S: Evaluation of a prophylactic and therapeutic program for patients with cystic fibrosis, *Pediatrics* 36:675-688, 1965.
198. Pedersen S, Jensen T, Hoiby N, Koch C, Flensborg E: Management of *Pseudomonas aeruginosa* lung infection in Danish cystic fibrosis patients, *Acta Pediatr Scand* 76:955-961, 1987.
199. Hodson M, Penreth A, Batten J: Aerosol carbenicillin and gentamicin treatment of *Pseudomonas aeruginosa* infection in patients with cystic fibrosis, *Lancet* 1137-1139, 1981.
200. Ramsey B, Pepe M, Otto K, Quan J, Montgomery A, Williams-Warren J, Vasiljev-K M, Borowitz D, Bowman C, Marshall B, Marshall S, Smith A: *N Engl J Med.* In press.
201. Mukhopadhyay S, Singh M, Cater J, Ogston S, Franklin M, Olver R: Nebulised antipseudomonal antibiotic therapy in cystic fibrosis: a meta-analysis of benefits and risks, *Thorax* 51:364-368, 1995.
202. Desmond K, Schwenk W, Thomas E, Beaudry P, Coates A: Immediate and long term effects of chest physiotherapy in patients with cystic fibrosis, *J Pediatr* 103:538-542, 1983.
203. Pryor J, Webber B, Hodson M, Batten J: Evaluation of the forced expiration technique as an adjunct to postural drainage in the treatment of cystic fibrosis, *Br Med J* 2:417-418, 1979.
204. Zach M, Oberwaldner B, Hauser F: Cystic fibrosis: physical exercise versus chest physiotherapy, *Arch Dis Child* 57:587-589, 1982.
205. Rossman C, Waldes R, Sampson D, Newhouse M: Effect of chest physiotherapy on the removal of mucus in patients with cystic fibrosis, *Am Rev Respir Dis* 126:131-135, 1982.
206. deBoeck C, Zinman R: Cough versus chest physiotherapy: a comparison of the acute effects on pulmonary function in patients with cystic fibrosis, *Am Rev Respir Dis* 129:182-184, 1984.
207. Wong J, Keens T, Wannamaker E, Crozier D, Levison H, Aspin N: Effects of gravity on tracheal transport rates in normal subjects and in patients with cystic fibrosis, *Pediatrics* 60:146-152, 1977.
208. Hofmyer J, Webber B, Hodson M: Evaluation of positive expiratory pressure as an adjunct to chest physiotherapy in the treatment of cystic fibrosis, *Thorax* 41:951-954, 1986.
209. Falk M, Kelstrup M, Andersen J, Kinoshita T, Falk P, Stovring S, Gothgen I: Improving the ketchup bottle method with positive pressure expiratory pressure, PEP, in cystic fibrosis, *Eur J Respir Dis* 65:423-432, 1984.
210. Stern H, Redmond A, O'Neill D, Beattie F: Evaluation of the PEP mask in cystic fibrosis, *Acta Pediatr Scand* 80:51-56, 1991.
211. vanderSchans C, vanderMark T, deVries G, Piers D, Beekhuis H, Dankert-Roelse J, Postma D, Koeter G: Effect of positive expiratory pressure breathing in patients with cystic fibrosis, *Thorax* 46:252-256, 1991.
212. Ohnsorg F: A cost analysis of high-frequency chest wall oscillation in cystic fibrosis, *Am Rev Respir Dis* 149:A669, 1994.
213. Burnett M, Taikis C, Hoffmeyer B, Patil S, Pichurko B: Comparative efficacy of manual chest physiotherapy and a high frequency chest compression vest in inpatient treatment of cystic fibrosis, *Am Rev Respir Dis* 147:A30, 1993.
214. Hansen L, Warwick W: High-frequency chest compression system to aid in clearance of mucus from the lung, *Biomed Instrumen Tech* July/August issue, 289-294, 1990.
215. Warwick W, Hansen L: The long-term effect of high-frequency chest compression therapy on pulmonary complications of cystic fibrosis, *Pediatr Pulmonol* 11:265-271, 1991.
216. Konstan M, Stern R, Doershuk C: Efficacy of the Flutter device for airway mucus clearance in patients with cystic fibrosis, *J Pediatr* 124:689-693, 1994.
217. Pryor J, Webber B, Hodson M, Warner J: The Flutter VRPI as an adjunct to chest physiotherapy in cystic fibrosis, *Respir Med* 88:677-681, 1994.
218. Zach M, Purrer B, Oberwaldner B: Effect of swimming on forced expiration and sputum clearance in cystic fibrosis, *Lancet* 2:1201-1203, 1981.
219. Orenstein D, Franklin B, Doershuk C, Hellerstein H, Germann K, Horwitz J, Stern R: Exercise conditioning and cardiopulmonary fitness in cystic fibrosis, *Chest* 80:392-398, 1981.
220. Keens T, Krastins I, Wannamaker E, Levison H, Crozier D, Bryan A: Ventilatory muscle endurance in normal subjects and patients with cystic fibrosis, *Am Rev Respir Dis* 117:853-860, 1977.
221. Verdugo P, Johnson N, Tam P: Beta-adrenergic stimulation of respiratory ciliary activity, *J Appl Physiol* 48:868-871, 1980.
222. Wanner A: Clinical aspects of mucociliary transport, *Am Rev Respir Dis* 116(1):73-125, 1977.
223. Sears M, Taylor D, Print C, Lake D et al: Regular inhaled beta-agonist treatment in bronchial asthma, *Lancet,* 336:1391-1396, 1990.
224. Spitzer W, Suissa S, Ernst P, Horwitz R, Habbick B, Cockcroft D, Boivin J-F, McNutt M, Buist A, Rebuck A: The use of b-agonists and the risk of death and near death from asthma, *N Engl J Med* 326:501-506, 1992.
225. Eber E, Oberwaldner B, Zach M: Airway obstruction and airway wall instability in cystic fibrosis: the isolated and combined effect of theophylline and sympathomimetics, *Pediatr Pulmonol* 4:205-212, 1988.
226. Larsen G, Barron R, Landy R, Cotton E, Gonzalez M, Brooks J: Intravenous aminophylline in patients with cystic fibrosis. Pharmacokinetics and effect on pulmonary function, *Am J Dis Child* 134:1143-1148, 1980.
227. Shapiro G, Bamman J, Kanarele P, Bierman C: The paradoxical effect of adrenergic and methylxanthine drugs in cystic fibrosis, 58:740-743, 1976.

228. Avital A, Sanchez I, Holbrow J, Kryger M, Chernick V: Effect of theophylline on lung function tests, sleep quality, and nighttime SaO_2 in children with cystic fibrosis, *Am Rev Respir Dis* 144:1245-1249, 1991.
229. Sivan Y, Arce P, Eigen H, Nickerson B, Newth C: A double-blind, randomized study of sodium cromoglycate versus placebo in patients with cystic fibrosis and bronchial hyperreactivity, *J Allergy Clin Immunol* 85:649-654, 1990.
230. Larsen G, Barron R, Cotton E, Brooks J: A comparative study of inhaled atropine sulfate and isoproterenol hydrochloride in cystic fibrosis, *Am Rev Respir Dis* 119:399-407, 1979.
231. Ghafouri M, Patil K, Kass I: Sputum changes associated with the use of ipratropium bromide, *Chest* 86:387-393, 1984.
232. Kattan M, Mansell A, Levison H, Corey M, Krastins I: Response to aerosol salbutamol. SCH 1000, and placebo in cystic fibrosis, *Thorax* 35:531-535, 1980.
233. Weintraum S, Eschenbacher W: The inhaled bronchodilators ipratropium bromide and metaproterenol in adults with CF, *Chest* 95:861-864, 1989.
234. vanHaren E, Lammers J, Festen J, Heijerman H, Groot C, Herwaarden CV: The effects of inhaled corticosteroid budesonide on lung function and bronchial hyperresponsiveness in adult patients with cystic fibrosis, *Am Rev Respir Dis* 149:A667, 1994.
235. Nikolaizik W, Schonl M: Pilot study to assess the effect of inhaled corticosteroids on lung function in patients with cystic fibrosis, *J Pediatr* 128:271-274, 1996.
236. Cheng P-W, Boat T, Cranfill K, Yankaskas J, Boucher R: Increased sulfation of glycoconjugates by cultured nasal epithelial cells from patients with cystic fibrosis, *J Clin Invest* 84:68-72, 1989.
237. Shak S, Baker C, Capon D, Hellmiss R, Marsters S: Recombinant human DNase 1 (rh Dnase) greatly reduces the viscosity of cystic fibrosis sputum, *Pediatr Pulmonol* 5(suppl):173, 1990.
238. Stafanger G, Garne S, Howitz P, Morkassel E, Koch C: The clinical effect and the effect on the ciliary motility of oraI N-acetylcysteine in patients with cystic fibrosis and primary ciliary dyskinesia, *Eur Respir J* 1:161-167, 1988.
239. Falliers C, McCann W, Chai H, Ellis E, Yazdi N: Controlled study of iodotherapy for childhood asthma, *J Allergy* 38:183-192, 1966.
240. Petty T: The national mucolytic study. Results of a randomized, double-blind, placebo-controlled study of iodinated glycerol in chronic obstructive bronchitis, *Chest* 97:75-83, 1990.
241. Ramsey B, Astley S, Aitken M, Burke W, Dorkin H, Eisenberg J, Gibson R, Harwood I, Schidlow D, Wilmot R, Wohl M, Meyerson L, Fuchs H, Shak S, Smity A: Efficacy and safety of aerosolized recombinant human deoxyribose nuclease in patients with cystic fibrosis, *Am Rev Respir Dis* 148:145-151, 1993.
242. Fuchs H, Borowitz D, Christiansen D, Morris E, Nash M, Ramsey B, Rosenstein B, Smith A, Wohl M: Effect of aerosolized recombinant DNase on exacerbations of respiratory symptoms and on pulmonary function in patients with cystic fibrosis, *N Engl J Med* 331:637-642, 1994.
243. Wilmott R, Amin R, Colin A, DeVault A, Dozer A, Eigen H, Johnson C, Lester L, McCoy K, McKean L, Moss R, Nash M, PagelJue C, Regelmann W, Stokes D, Fuchs H: Aerosolized recombinant human DNase in hospitalized cystic fibrosis patients with acute pulmonary exacerbation, *Am J Respir Crit Care Med* 153:1914-1917, 1996.
244. Vasconcellos C, Allen P, Wohl M, Drazen J, Janmey P, Stossel T: Reduction in viscosity of cystic fibrosis sputum in vitro by gelsolin, *Science* 263:969-971, 1994.
245. Robinson M, Regnis J, Bailey D, King M, Bautovich G, Bye P: Effect of hypertonic saline, amiloride and cough on mucociliary clearance in patients with cystic fibrosis, *Am J Respir Crit Care Med* 153:1503-1509, 1996.
246. Eschenbacher W, Boushey H, Sheppard D: Alteration in osmolarity of inhaled aerosol cause bronchoconstriction and cough, but absence of a permeant anion causes cough alone, *Am Rev Respir Dis* 129:211-215, 1984.
247. diSant'Agnese P, Davis P: Adults with cystic fibrosis: 75 cases and a review of 232 cases in the literature, *Am J Med* 66:121-132, 1979.
248. Stern R, Wood R, Boat T et al: Treatment and prognosis of massive hemoptysis in cystic fibrosis, *Am Rev Respir Dis* 117:825-828, 1978.
249. Knight R, Batten J: Pneumothorax in cystic fibrosis: In Sturgess J, ed: *Perspectives in cystic fibrosis,* Mississauga, Ontario, 1980, Imperial Press, pp 376-381.
250. Spector M, Stern R: Pneumothorax in cystic fibrosis: a 26-year experience, *Ann Thorac Surg* 47:204-207, 1989.
251. Davis P, diSant'Agnese P: Diagnosis and treatment of cystic fibrosis: an update, *Chest* 85:802-809, 1984.
252. McLaughlin F, Mathews W, Strieder D, Khaw K, Schuster S, Shwachman H: Pneumothorax in cystic fibrosis: management and outcome, *J Pediatr* 100:863-869, 1982.
253. Seddon D, Hodson M: Surgical management of pneumothorax in cystic fibrosis. *Thorax* 43:739-740, 1988.
254. Dixey J, Redington A, Butler R, Smith M, Batchelor J, Woodrow D, Hodson M, Batten J, Brewerton D: The arthropathy of cystic fibrosis, *Ann Rheum Dis* 47:218-223, 1988.
255. Stern R, Borkat G, Hirschfeld S, Boat T, Matthews L, Liebman J, Doershuk C: Heart failure in cystic fibrosis, *Am J Dis Child* 134:267-272, 1980.
256. Coates A: Oxygen therapy, exercise, and cystic fibrosis, *Chest* 101:2-4, 1992.
257. Zinman R, Corey M, Coates A, Canny G, Connolly J, Levison H, Beaudry P: Nocturnal home oxygen in the treatment of hypoxemic cystic fibrosis patients, *J Pediatr* 114:368-377, 1989.
258. Hodson M, Madden M, Steven V, Tsang V, Yacoub M: Non-invasive mechanical ventilation for cystic fibrosis patients—a potential bridge to transplantation, *Eur Respir J* 4:524-527, 1991.
259. Fiel S: Heart-lung transplantation for patients with cystic fibrosis. A test of clinical wisdom, *Arch Intern Med* 151:870-872, 1991.
260. St. Louis International Lung Transplant Registry: April report, 1995.
261. Caine N, Sharples L, Smyth R, Scott J, Hathaway T, Higgenbottam T, Wallwork J: Survival and quality of life of cystic fibrosis patients before and after heart-lung transplantation, *Transplant Proc* 23:1203-1204, 1991.
262. Cooney G, Fiel S, Shaw L, Cavarocchi N: Cyclosporine availability in heart-lung transplant candidates with cystic fibrosis, *Transplantation* 49:821-823, 1990.
263. Tan K, Hue K, Strickland S, Hull A, Smyth R, Scott J, Kelman A, Whiting B, Higenbottam T, Wallwork J: Altered pharmacokinetics of cyclosporin in heart-lung transplant recipients with cystic fibrosis, *Ther Drug Monitor* 12:520-524, 1990.
264. Klima L, Kowdley K, Lewis S, Wood D, Aitken M: Successful lung transplantation despite cystic fibrosis associated liver disease: a case series, *J Heart Lung Transplant* 16:934-938, 1997.
265. Alton E, Khagani A, Taylor R, Logan-Sinclair R, Yacoub M, Geddes D: Effect of heart-lung transplantation on airway potential difference in patients with and without cystic fibrosis, *Eur Respir J* 4:5-9, 1991.
266. Snell G, Hoyos AD, Krajden M, Winton T, Maurer J: *Pseudomonas cepacia* in lung transplant recipients with cystic fibrosis, *Chest* 103:466-471, 1993.
267. Ramirez J, Patterson G, Winton T, deHoyos A, Miller J, Maurer J: Bilateral lung transplantation for cystic fibrosis, *J Thorac Cardiovasc Surg* 103:287-294, 1992.
268. Starnes V, Barr M, Cohen R: Lobar transplantation: indications, technique and outcome, *J Thorac Cardiovasc Surg* 108:403-410, 1994.
269. Presek P, Reuter C: Amiloride inhibits the protein tyrosine kinases associated with the cellular and the transforming SRC-gene products, *Biochem Pharmacol* 36:2821-2826, 1987.
270. Knowles M, Church N, Waltner W, Yankaskas J, Gilligan P, King M, Edwards L, Helms R, Boucher R: A pilot study of aerosolized amiloride for the treatment of lung disease in cystic fibrosis, *N Engl J Med* 322:1189-1194, 1990.
271. Graham A, Hasani A, Alton E, Martin G, Marriott C, Hodson M, Clarke S, Geddes D: No added benefit from nebulized amiloride in patients with cystic fibrosis, *Eur Respir J* 6:1243-1248, 1993.
272. Knowles M, Clarke L, Boucher R: Activation by extracellular nucleotides of chloride secretion in the airway epithelia of patients with cystic fibrosis, *N Engl J Med* 325:533-538, 1991.
273. Bennett W, Olivier K, Zeman K, Hohneker K, Boucher R, Knowles M: Effect of uridine 5'-triphosphate plus ameloride on mucociliary clearance in adult cystic fibrosis, *Am J Respir Crit Care Med* 153:1796-1801, 1996.
274. Shwachman H, Kukychi 1, Mueller H, Flake C: Nasal polyps in patients with cystic fibrosis, *Pediatrics* 30:389-401, 1962.
275. Drake-Lee A, Morgan D: Nasal polyps and sinusitis in children with cystic fibrosis, *J Laryngol Otol* 103:753-755, 1989.
276. Donaldson J, Gillespie C: Observations on the efficacy of intranasal beclomethasone dipropionate in cystic fibrosis patients, *J Otolaryngol* 17:43-45, 1988.

CHAPTER 69

Cystic Fibrosis: Other Clinical Manifestations

Beryl J. Rosenstein

PANCREATIC EXOCRINE INSUFFICIENCY

Pathophysiology

Among patients with cystic fibrosis (CF), 85% to 90% will have exocrine pancreatic insufficiency.[1] Pancreatic function status is genetically determined by specific CF mutations. There is striking concordance for pancreatic status among CF families[2] and CF genotype is strongly predictive of pancreatic status.[3] Mutations can be classified as mild (predictive of pancreatic sufficiency) or severe (predictive of pancreatic insufficiency). Patients carrying one or two mild mutations are almost always pancreatic sufficient.[3] Among patients homozygous for the common ΔF508 mutation, 99% will be pancreatic insufficient.[3,4] Mutations associated with pancreatic sufficiency are generally class IV or V cystic fibrosis transmembrane conductance regulator (CFTR) defects, and include R117H, R334W, R347P, A455E, and P574H.[3] In patients with pancreatic insufficiency, the pancreas is shrunken and shows marked fibrosis, fatty replacement, and cyst formation.[5,6] Stenosis[7] and atresia[8] of large pancreatic ducts have been reported but, in general, pancreatic lesions are caused by obstruction of small ducts by inspissated secretions. Hypoplasia and eventually necrosis of ductular and centroacinar cells, together with inspissated secretions, block pancreatic ductules and can cause atrophy of the lining epithelium.[6,9] Cystic spaces filled with eosinophilic concretions are embedded in a fibrous stroma. A mild inflammatory reaction may be present around obliterated acini, and progressive fibrosis gradually separates and replaces the pancreatic lobules.[6]

Ultrasonography of the pancreas shows a small and echodense pancreatic body and a large pancreatic head.[10] Multiple diffuse granular calcifications may be present inside pancreatic ducts and can be detected by radiography (with gastric insufflation) and computed tomography.[11] Rarely, multiple macroscopic cysts of the pancreas have been diagnosed at autopsy[9] or antemortem by computed tomography, ultrasound, and radionuclide imaging.[12]

It is postulated that abnormal CFTR processing leads to a defect in epithelial electrolyte permeability within the pancreatic ducts.[3] This leads to reduced ductular flow and hyperconcentrated proteinaceous secretions that precipitate and block pancreatic ductules.[13-15] Eventually there is acinar atrophy. Secondary to ductular obstruction, volume and bicarbonate secretion (ductular activity) are greatly reduced irrespective of pancreatic enzyme output.[16] This leads to a consistently lower fasting and postprandial duodenal pH.[17,18] In patients with steatorrhea, enzyme secretion (acinar activity) is virtually absent.[16] Only 1% to 2% of residual colipase and lipase secretion is required to prevent steatorrhea.[19] Pancreatic function can decline progressively with advancing age.[20,21] Among infants found to have CF in a neonatal screening program, 37% were found to have substantial preservation of pancreatic function, but 21% of these patients developed pancreatic failure by 3 years of age.[20] The majority of older pancreatic-sufficient patients with enzyme secretion within the normal range show no deterioration of function over an extended time period.[21] However, a small percentage of older pancreatic-sufficient patients, especially those with reduced enzyme, fluid, and electrolyte secretion, are at risk of progression to pancreatic failure.[21]

Pancreatic Function Testing

Assessment of pancreatic function is useful in newly diagnosed clients to determine whether malabsorption is present. When the diagnosis of CF is in doubt, specific tests of pancreatic function may be of value in supporting a diagnosis.[22] Direct testing of pancreatic function involves exogenous hormonal (secretin/cholecystokinin) or endogenous nutrient (Lundh test meal) pancreatic stimulation, collection of pancreatic secretions via duodenal intubation, and analysis of enzyme (lipase, colipase) output.[22] This is the best method for accurately measuring pancreatic exocrine function over its entire range, but it is invasive, expensive, and difficult to perform.

As an alternative, a number of noninvasive indirect tests of pancreatic function are available. Random stool samples can be examined for the presence of fat globules or trypsin, chymotrypsin, or pancreatic elastase 1 concentrations.[23-26] Of these tests, an enzyme-linked immunosorbent assay (ELISA) for pancreatic elastase 1 appears to be the most sensitive and specific assay for exocrine pancreatic function.[25,26] A 72-hour stool collection for measurement of fat output is cumbersome but is probably the most commonly used test of pancreatic function in patients with CF. Normally, stool fat output is <7% of fat intake (coefficient of fat absorption >93%).

Several tests of pancreatic function involve the oral administration of a measurable tracer bound to a peptide specifically cleaved by one of the pancreatic enzymes. The synthetic peptide N-benzoyl-l-tyrosyl-p-aminobenzoic acid (bentiromide) is cleaved by chymotrypsin. The liberated *p*-aminobenzoic acid (PABA) is absorbed and excreted in the urine. Accordingly, PABA recovery reflects intraluminal chymotrypsin activity.[27] The sensitivity and specificity of the test can be improved by measuring PABA in plasma 90 minutes after the administration of a large (500 mg) dose of bentiromide[28] or by administration of a test meal to stimulate enzyme secretion.[28,29]

The pancreolauryl test consists of the administration of fluorescein dilaurate.[30] The substrate is hydrolyzed by cholesterol ester hydrolase of pancreatic origin in the upper small intestine and releases fluorescein which is absorbed and excreted in the urine, where it can be quantitated. Stimulation of enzyme secretion with a test meal and measurement of plasma fluorescein have been used to increase the sensitivity and specificity of the test.[31] Pancreolauryl and bentiromide test results correlate well with other measures of pancreatic exocrine function, but abnormal results are also seen in patients with malabsorption unrelated to CF.

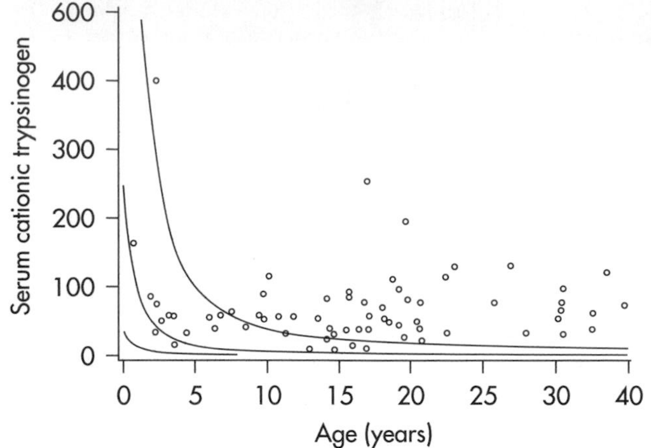

Fig. 69-1. Individual serum trypsinogen values (mg/L) plotted against age for 67 patients with pancreatic sufficiency, superimposed on a mathematically derived equation for CF patients with pancreatic insufficiency. After 7 years of age only 6 patients with pancreatic sufficiency had values within the 95% confidence limits of the values for those with pancreatic insufficiency. (From Durie PR et al: *Pediatr Res* 20:209, 1986.)

Several methods directly measure various pancreatic enzymes in serum or plasma. Patients with CF have low serum concentrations of pancreas-specific isoenzymes of amylase (isoamylases),[32-34] immunoreactive cationic trypsinogen,[35-37] and pancreatic lipase.[36] In infants less than 2 years of age, serum trypsinogen and pancreatic lipase values are *elevated* secondary to pancreatic ductular obstruction and reflux of pancreatic enzymes into the circulation.[35,36] With advancing age, however, serum levels of these enzymes decline progressively, and after the age of 7 years most patients with pancreatic insufficiency have undetectable or low levels.[35,36] Enzyme assays are of value in discriminating older CF patients with or without pancreatic insufficiency[37] (Fig. 69-1) and for monitoring longitudinal changes in pancreatic function, particularly in patients with pancreatic sufficiency.[36,37] Between 2 and 7 years of age, serum enzyme assays are of little diagnostic value unless levels are markedly low.

Clinical Manifestations

Exocrine pancreatic insufficiency leads to intestinal malabsorption of fats and proteins and, to a lesser extent, carbohydrates. Steatorrhea and azotorrhea can be pronounced[38] (Fig. 69-2). Clinical consequences include poor or absent weight gain; abdominal distention; deficiency of subcutaneous fat and muscle tissue; frequent passage of pale, bulky, malodorous, and often oily stools; and rectal prolapse. Patients with preservation of exocrine pancreatic function (pancreatic sufficiency) are clinically distinguishable in that they are diagnosed at a later age, have lower mean sweat chloride values, maintain better pulmonary function with age, are less likely to be colonized by *Pseudomonas aeruginosa* and have a better prognosis.[1] However, patients with residual acinar function are at risk of developing episodes of acute pancreatitis.[39]

Nutrition

Chronic undernutrition with significant weight retardation and linear growth failure is a major problem in patients with CF.[40-42] Nutritional deficiencies such as decreased body fat stores and decreased serum levels of essential fatty acids, prealbumin, albumin, cholesterol, retinol, 25-hydroxyvitamin

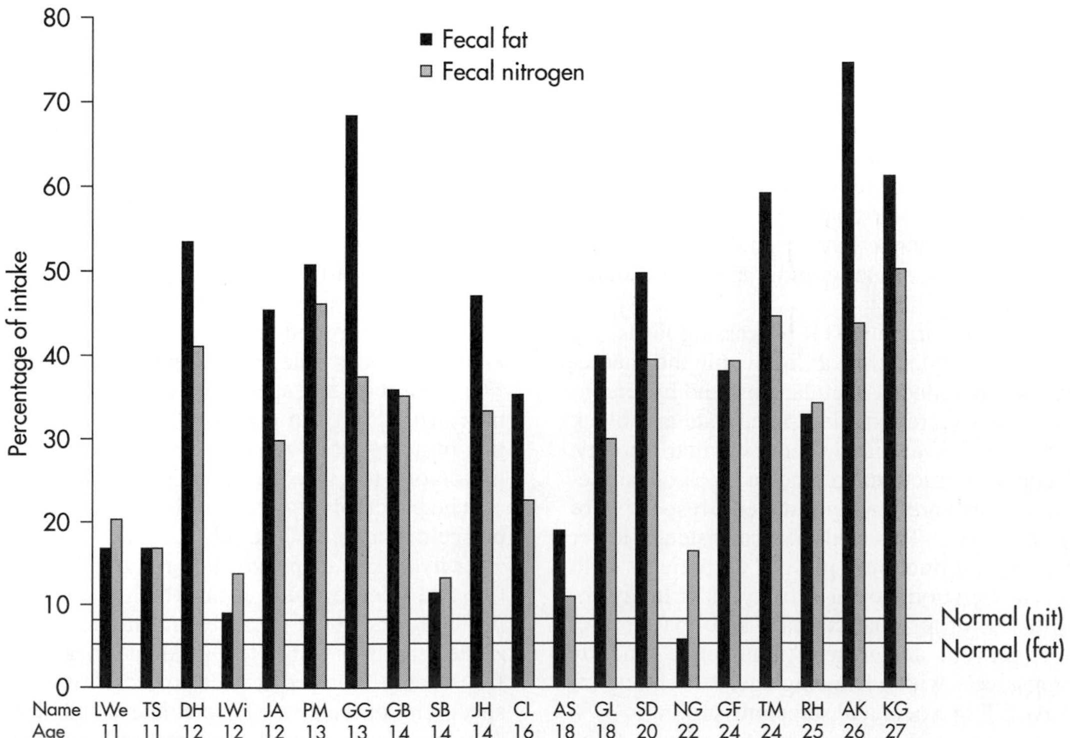

Fig. 69-2. Fecal fat and nitrogen excretion in 20 patients with CF not receiving pancreatic supplements. (From Lapey A, et al: *J Pediatr* 84:328, 1974.)

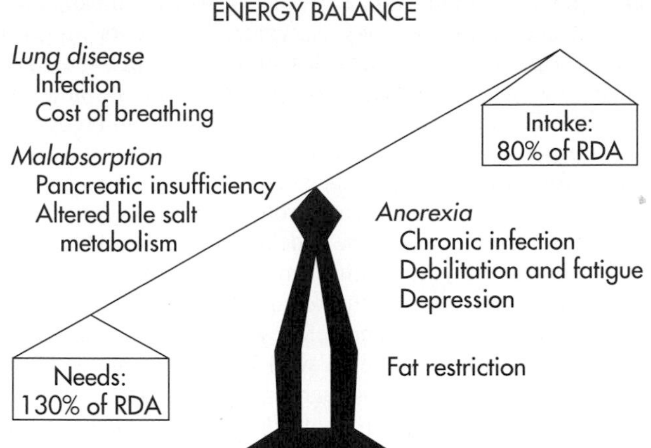

Fig. 69-3. Factors leading to energy imbalance in patients with CF. (From Roy C, et al: *J Pediatr Gastroenterol Nutr* 3:(suppl)154, 1985.)

D, and α-tocopherol have been well documented and may be evident as early as 2 months of age in presymptomatic infants with CF detected by newborn screening.[43,44] Growth retardation and wasting often accelerate before and during adolescence and patients often fail to achieve their genetic growth potential.[45] There is a correlation among degree of malnutrition, pulmonary function, clinical status, and survival.[46]

Most growth problems in patients with CF are caused by unfavorable energy balance rather than an inherent factor of the disease itself. Energy imbalance is related to the combination of increased energy losses, suboptimal energy intake, and increased energy expenditure in patients who are recommended to receive 120% to 140% of daily energy requirements[42,47] (Fig. 69-3). Increased energy loss is primarily the result of pancreatic exocrine insufficiency but reduced bile salt pool and increased intestinal mucus may play a role.

Despite anecdotal reports of a voracious appetite in patients with CF, it is now recognized that energy intake is often 80% to 100% of recommended daily allowances (RDA) for age, weight, and sex.[48-51] Appetite and oral intake may be limited by esophagitis, postprandial abdominal pain, depression, fatigue, and acute and chronic respiratory tract infection.[42,47] Some data suggest that there is an increased rate of resting energy expenditure and total energy expenditure in patients with CF.[52-56] These increases appear to be independent of the degree of pulmonary disease but may be related to genotype.[55,56]

Edema and Hypoproteinemia

Secondary to proteolytic enzyme deficiency and malabsorption, infants with CF may develop severe protein-calorie malnutrition and edema, often as the presenting manifestation of their disease.[57-62] Features include severe hypoalbuminemia, advanced pulmonary symptoms, hepatomegaly, elevation of liver enzyme values, anemia, and a characteristic dermatitis[62] secondary to deficiencies of protein, zinc, and essential fatty acids. Infants fed breast milk or soy-protein–based formula may be at increased risk for this syndrome.[57,59] A false-negative sweat test result may occur in the presence of edema, probably secondary to a low sweat secretory rate.[63] Infants with this syndrome need intensive nutritional therapy, including adequate calories, essential fatty acids, protein, zinc, and vitamins, along with pancreatic enzyme supplementation. A prolonged course of parenteral nutrition or enteral supplementation often is required. Patients with this syndrome have been shown to be at high risk for early pulmonary complications, prolonged hospitalization, and a high mortality rate.[61,64]

Vitamins and Trace Metals

Water-Soluble Vitamins

All water-soluble vitamins except vitamin B_{12} appear to be well absorbed and there is no evidence of clinically significant deficiency in well-nourished patients.[48] With pancreatic enzyme supplementation, vitamin B absorption normalizes and supplementation is not necessary.[65,66]

Fat-Soluble Vitamins

Biochemical deficiencies of vitamins A, D, E, and K have been demonstrated repeatedly in patients with CF at the time of diagnosis.[42-44,48] Serum vitamin levels may be low even in patients receiving pancreatic enzyme and vitamin supplementation.[67]

Vitamin A

Serum concentrations of vitamin A (retinol) are often low[68,69] despite of apparently adequate supplementation[67] and significantly increased hepatic stores of vitamin A.[68] Decreased serum vitamin A levels correlate with decreased levels of retinol-binding protein.[70] These abnormalities may be caused by a marked decrease in vitamin A absorption from the digestive tract,[71] defective synthesis of retinol-binding protein, or defective release of vitamin A stores from the liver.[68] Signs of vitamin A deficiency are uncommon. Infants may rarely present with a bulging fontanel secondary to increased intracranial pressure.[72] Conjunctival xerosis and night blindness (decreased dark adaptation) have been found to be surprisingly common in adolescents and young adults,[69,73] especially those with liver disease and noncompliance with enzyme supplementation.[73]

Vitamin D

Although full-blown rickets is rare in patients with CF,[74] they often have a significant reduction in vitamin D activity manifested by secondary hyperparathyroidism,[75-77] reduced bone mineral content,[78-82] delayed bone maturation,[80] and an increased risk of atraumatic fractures (especially in vertebrae). The degree of demineralization correlates with disease severity.[78,82]

Vitamin E

Biochemical evidence of vitamin E deficiency is present in virtually all untreated patients with CF who have pancreatic exocrine insufficiency.[83] Erythrocyte survival is shortened[83] and may lead to hemolytic anemia in infancy.[84,85] Other manifestations include ophthalmoplegia, diminished deep tendon reflexes, decreased vibratory and proprioceptive sensation, ataxia, and muscle weakness.[86,87] Axonal dystrophy and degenerative changes within the posterior columns have been demonstrated postmortem.[88]

Vitamin K

Although severe bleeding in association with hypoprothrombinemia and deficiency of clotting factors II, VII, IX, and X may occur in infants secondary to vitamin K deficiency,[89,90] in patients who receive adequate pancreatic enzyme supplementation, vitamin K deficiency is very uncommon.[91] Patients with liver disease and those on prolonged antibiotic therapy appear to be at greatest risk.[89,90]

Trace Metals

Plasma zinc levels are low in patients with CF who are moderately to severely malnourished.[92] There is no recognized defect in zinc absorption or metabolism. Plasma levels of copper and ceruloplasmin may be elevated, possibly because ceruloplasmin is an acute-phase reactant.[92] Plasma or whole-blood selenium levels may be low[93,94] and are probably related to geography and selenium levels in the soil.[93] There is no evidence that selenium deficiency is clinically significant. Chronic hypomagnesemia may occur, usually in the absence of symptoms. Symptomatic hypomagnesemia (paresthesias, weakness, tremulousness, muscle cramps, carpopedal spasm) has been reported in patients treated with repeated courses of intravenous aminoglycoside therapy[95] and in those treated for the distal intestinal obstruction syndrome (DIOS) with N-acetylcysteine or sodium diatrizoate orally or by enema.[96] Malabsorption may also play a role.[97] Magnesium replacement is indicated in symptomatic patients. Iron deficiency anemia occurs in 33% to 66% of patients[98-101] and is probably related to inadequate dietary iron intake, blood loss, iron malabsorption, and chronic infection.

Patients with CF should receive daily supplementation with a water-soluble vitamin-mineral preparation that includes B vitamins, vitamin C, vitamin A 5000 units, vitamin D 400 units, zinc, and iron.[48] Patients should also receive a water-soluble preparation of vitamin E (α-tocopherol) at a dosage of 5 to 10 units/kg/day (maximum 400 units). Vitamin K supplementation at a dosage of 5 mg twice weekly is indicated for patients with liver disease or abnormal clotting study results and those on prolonged antibiotic therapy. Routine supplementation with vitamin K is not recommended.[91] Documented vitamin A deficiency is treated with 25,000 units vitamin A daily for 1 week followed by supplementation with 5000 to 10,000 units/day.

Essential Fatty Acids

In CF patients with pancreatic insufficiency, all four plasma lipid factors (triglycerides, phospholipids, free fatty acids, and cholesterol esters) are abnormal.[102] In the plasma, linoleic acid is decreased, whereas palmitoleic and oleic acids are increased.[102-105] Linoleic acid levels are decreased in various tissues.[102] Deficiency of fatty acids is primarily related to malabsorption because essential fatty acid levels are normal in CF patients with pancreatic sufficiency.[102,106] Untreated infants with CF may have dermatitis, growth failure, and thrombocytopenia secondary to linoleic acid deficiency,[48] but in older patients clinical manifestations of fatty acid deficiency are rare.[102] Plasma fatty acid profiles can be normalized by the oral (corn oil, safflower oil) or intravenous (Intralipid) administration of fatty acids,[104,105,107-109] but there is no evidence that this results in any major clinical benefit.[102,104,109] Fatty acid deficiency might lead to a subtle alteration in cellular metabolism or in the composition of membranes that could lead to cellular dysfunction.[102,103]

Pancreatic Enzyme Therapy

Patients with exocrine pancreatic insufficiency require long-term replacement therapy with pancreatic enzyme supplements. In young infants this is given as a powdered pancreatic extract. Beyond early infancy, enzyme supplements are given in the form of gelatin capsules containing pH-sensitive, enteric-coated microspheres or microtablets of pancrelipase.[110-112] The capsule can be swallowed or it can be opened and the microspheres or microtablets placed in a soft, non-alkaline food such as applesauce. These preparations are formulated so that the enzymes are protected against gastric acid inactivation; release of enzyme is delayed until the pH is above 5.5. In infants, enzyme dosing can be based on food intake, starting with 2000 to 4000 lipase units per 120 ml formula or per breast feeding.[113] Beyond infancy, weight-based dosing is more practical. It should begin with 1000 lipase units/kg per meal for children less than 4 years and 500 lipase units/kg for those older than 4 years.[113] Enzyme dosage expressed as lipase units/kg per meal should be decreased in older patients because they tend to ingest less fat per kilogram of body weight. Usually, half the standard dose is given with snacks. There is great interindividual variation in response to enzymes, so a range of dosages is recommended, based on stool pattern and weight gain. Dosages greater than 2500 lipase units/kg per meal or 10,000 lipase units/kg per day should be used with caution[113,114] and only if they are documented to be effective by 3-day fecal fat measure.[113] Dosages greater than 6000 lipase units/kg per meal have been associated with the development of fibrosing colonopathy in patients less than 12 years old regardless of enzyme strength or brand. After initiation of enzyme therapy, there should be almost immediate reduction in stool frequency and degree of steatorrhea, improvement in abdominal symptoms, and decrease in appetite. Most patients are able to achieve a coefficient of fat absorption greater than 85%.

Variations in enzyme requirements and patient response may be related to endogenous enzyme output, type of diet, microsphere size,[112] gastric emptying time of microspheres,[112] postprandial duodenal pH,[18] and bile salt concentration. Failure of enzyme release secondary to a low postprandial duodenal pH is probably the major factor leading to inefficient enzyme function.[18] In patients who have persistent steatorrhea[3] (>10% fecal fat loss) despite apparently adequate enzyme dosage, addition of an acid-reducing agent such as cimetidine,[115] famotidine,[116] misoprostol,[18,117] or omeprazole[118] may lead to significant enhancement of fat absorption. Some patients on high-dose enzyme therapy have ongoing abdominal symptoms unrelated to exocrine pancreatic deficiency.[119] In such cases, 72-hour fecal fat measure and evaluation for concurrent gastrointestinal disorders (lactose malabsorption, giardiasis, bacterial overgrowth, celiac disease, Crohn disease) are indicated.

The development of constipation in a patient who is taking enzymes may be an indication for *more* enzymes. A misguided reduction in enzyme dosage in this situation may precipitate an episode of DIOS.

The most significant complication of pancreatic enzymes is fibrosing colonopathy,[114,120-122] a condition associated with the use of high daily doses of enzyme. This diagnosis should be considered in patients who have symptoms of obstruction, bloody diarrhea, chylous ascites, or the combination of abdominal pain with ongoing diarrhea or poor weight gain.[121] Patients at highest risk are those who are less than 12 years old have taken more than 6000 lipase units/kg per meal for more than 6 months, or have a history of gastrointestinal surgery or complications.[114] Most cases involve the ascending colon, but pancolonic involvement can occur.[121] A barium enema is the most reliable diagnostic measure. Colonic shortening, focal or extensive narrowing, and a lack of distensibility are highly suggestive. Diagnosis is confirmed by biopsy. Bowel wall thickening, which may be a precursor of stricture formation, may be detected by ultrasonography.[122] Most cases of fibrosing colonopathy require hemicolectomy.[120]

Skin and mucous membrane irritation secondary to pancreatic extract may be seen in infants. Before the advent of enteric-coated microsphere preparations, hyperuricosemia[123] and hyperuricosuria[124] resulted from the high purine content of powdered preparations. Immunoglobulin E–mediated nasal and bronchial immediate hypersensitivity reactions and anaphylaxis may occur in individuals exposed to powdered pancreatic extracts,[125-127] but clinical hypersensitivity is extremely rare in patients themselves.[125]

NUTRITIONAL MANAGEMENT

The nutritional support of patients with CF should be an integral part of overall care and requires close clinical evaluation, monitoring of growth rates and nutritional status, and appropriate dietary counseling.[42,47] This is best accomplished in collaboration with an experienced dietitian. The goal is to promote normal growth and nutrition. The diet should be tailored to meet individual caloric needs and should be consistent with food preferences and lifestyle. It should provide 130% to 140% of the recommended daily allowance for calories. This usually can be achieved by a well-balanced diet with increased fat as a source of energy.[42,128] Complex carbohydrates are well tolerated and are another good energy source. *Fat restriction is not recommended.*

Infants can be breast fed but they require pancreatic enzyme supplements, sodium chloride supplementation (⅛ to ¼ tsp table salt/day), especially during summer, and close monitoring of nutritional status. Most infants show adequate growth on standard formula feedings. Predigested formulas containing medium-chain triglycerides (MCT) may be advantageous in infants with liver involvement, persistent steatorrhea, or short gut syndrome; soy-based formulas are not recommended. In older patients, caloric intake can be boosted by encouraging the use of nutrient-dense foods, homemade oral supplements, or commercially available high-energy liquid dietary supplements. This approach, however, may be hard to maintain over an extended period of time.

In patients who have inadequate caloric intake and poor growth despite nutritional counseling and attempts at oral supplementation, enteral feeding techniques may be useful.[129-135] This is accomplished by the nocturnal infusion of a high-calorie elemental or semielemental formula via a nasogastric, gastrostomy, or jejunostomy tube. This approach, when carried out over an extended period, can improve growth velocity,[129-133,135] body composition,[130,133,134] and patient well-being,[133] and may stabilize or even improve pulmonary function[129,130,135] (Fig. 69-4). Parenteral nutritional support may be indicated for short-term use in patients with specific problems such as short gut syndrome and pancreatitis, and in the postoperative period. Long-term use is not indicated because of cost, inconvenience, and potential complications. It is doubtful that any form of aggressive nutritional therapy has any impact during the terminal stage of a patient's course.[42] Artificial means of nutritional support should be discouraged at this time.

There is no evidence to support strongly the use of artificial elemental diets or supplements with essential fatty acids.[102,104,109] Results are somewhat conflicting, but taurine supplementation may improve fat absorption in patients with poorly controlled steatorrhea.[136-138] The effect on overall growth is questionable.[138]

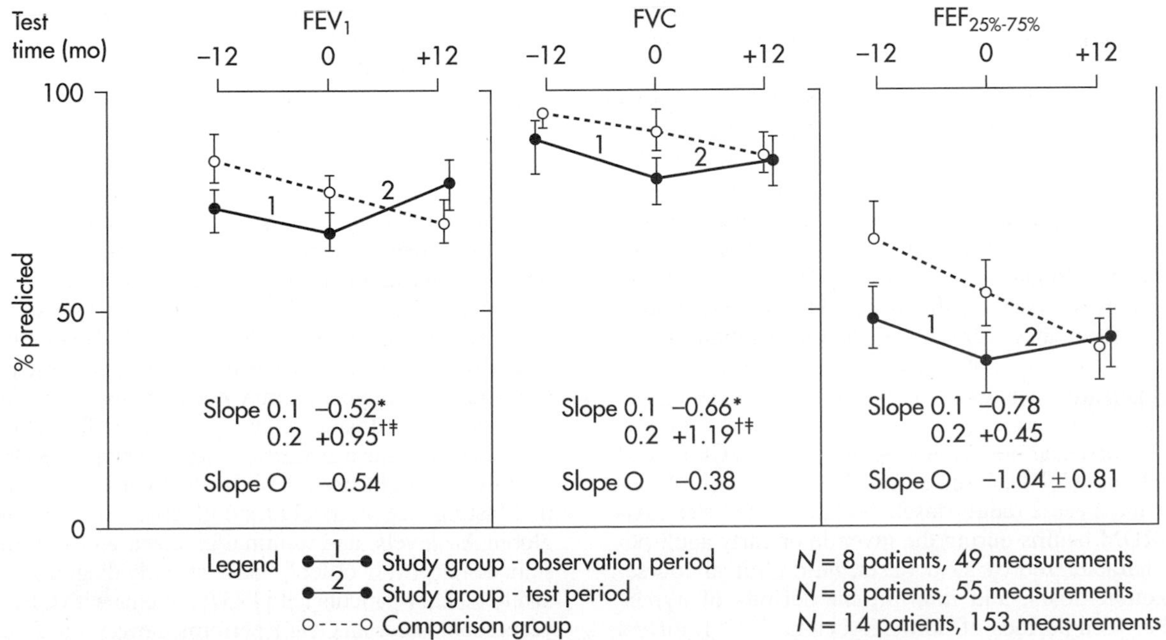

Fig. 69-4. Serial tests of pulmonary function in a study group of patients with CF before (-12 to 0 months) and after (0 to 12 months) aggressive nutritional supplementation and in a comparison group of matched patients with CF receiving conventional therapy. (From Shepherd RW et al: *J Pediatr* 109:788, 1986.)

PANCREATITIS

Recurrent episodes of acute pancreatitis have been reported in 15% of pancreatic-sufficient patients with CF.[139] Most cases occur in older patients[39] but pancreatitis has been reported as early as 1 year of age.[139] In some patients, pancreatitis is the initial or only feature suggesting the diagnosis of CF.[139,140] Detection of CF mutations may be diagnostically helpful in such cases. Presumably, hyperconcentration of pancreatic secretions leads to obstruction of the pancreatic ducts, which provokes autodigestion of the pancreas by activated pancreatic proteolytic enzymes.[141] Patients manifest severe abdominal pain, usually with vomiting, midepigastric tenderness, and elevated levels of serum and urinary amylase and serum lipase.[139] Ultrasonography may demonstrate increased echogenicity of the pancreas.[139] Serum amylase values may remain elevated for 4 to 6 months after resolution of symptoms.[39] Attacks may be precipitated by ingestion of a fatty meal, alcohol, or tetracycline.[39] Patients with pancreatitis may develop abdominal pain and hyperamylasemia in response to the intravenous administration of secretin and pancreozymin.[39] Treatment consists of intravenous fluids, analgesics, antacids and H_2 blockers, and nutritional support. There is some evidence that administration of pancreatic enzymes may inhibit pancreatic exocrine function, thus decreasing pancreatic autodigestion and pain.[142] Pancreatic-sufficient patients who develop pancreatitis should be closely monitored for progression to pancreatic insufficiency.

PANCREATIC ENDOCRINE DEFICIENCY

Pathology

With advancing age, there is acinar atrophy, fatty infiltration, fibrosis of the pancreas, and a decrease in the number of pancreatic islets in CF patients with and without diabetes mellitus (DM).[143,144] Pancreatic neoislet formation (nesidioblastosis) is present and may be protective against DM.[143,145] The proportions of glucagon-secreting α cells and insulin-secreting β cells are significantly decreased (although with marked variation), and somatostatin-containing cells are moderately increased.[143,144,146] The decrease in the proportion of β cells is more pronounced in patients with DM.[143,146] Secondary to a decrease in the proportion of β cells and reduction in total pancreatic mass, the number of β cells may be decreased by 90% or more.[144] Because somatostatin inhibits both insulin and glucagon release, it is postulated that both decreased insulin production and increased somatostatin production contribute to DM in patients with CF.[144] In contrast to Type 1 DM, however, in CF patients with DM there is relative insulin preservation and decreased glucagon secretion.

Pathophysiology

The clinical course and metabolic responses seen in CF-related diabetes mellitus (CFRDM) differ from both Type 1 (juvenile-onset DM) and Type 2 (adult-onset, nonketotic diabetes). Although CFRDM begins during the juvenile or early adult period, it is characterized by slow onset, mild clinical course, rarity of ketoacidosis, and intermittent periods of hyperglycemia between periods of normoglycemia.[147-149] It differs from Type 2 DM in that it is associated with underweight, hypoinsulinemia, and onset in early life.[147-149] The HLA-related genes that confer susceptibility to Type 1 DM are not necessary for the development of glucose intolerance in patients with CF.[150,151] Unlike Type 1 DM, CFRDM is not an autoimmune process, but islet-cell antibodies may play a role in some patients.[151] Patients are modestly resistant to insulin,[152] probably as a result of hyperglycemia.

From a biochemical standpoint, CFRDM is characterized by (1) reduction in serum levels of insulin, glucagon, and pancreatic polypeptide;[153-155] (2) normal levels of gastric inhibitory polypeptide (GIP);[154] (3) diminished GIP and pancreatic polypeptide responses after ingestion of a meal;[156] (4) reduction and delay in insulin secretion in response to oral or IV glucose, IV arginine, and IV tolbutamide;[153,155] and (5) impaired glucagon release following an arginine infusion.[157] Insulin and GIP responses may be improved after an elemental meal, suggesting that insulin deficiency may arise via deficient GIP release secondary to malabsorption.[156] The loss of carbohydrate tolerance in patients with CF, like that seen with classic chronic pancreatitis, parallels the loss of pancreatic exocrine function.[158] There is evidence of some loss of pancreatic endocrine and exocrine reserve in CF heterozygotes.[159]

Clinical Features

CFRDM is associated with a variety of adverse consequences, including loss of calories secondary to glycosuria, muscle wasting, fatigue, impaired ability to respond to infection, and renal insufficiency.[160,161] Retinopathy, nephropathy, and neuropathy probably occur as often in CFRDM as in other forms of diabetes.[161-164] Other potential adverse metabolic effects relate to the role of insulin as an anabolic hormone involved in cellular amino acid uptake and as a stimulator of other growth factors.[165] There is evidence that when DM develops in patients with CF, an insidious decline in overall clinical status is observed for years before its diagnosis.[166] Body weight and body mass index begin to deviate about 4 years before the diagnosis of DM, whereas deviation in pulmonary function appears 1 to 3 years before the diagnosis of DM.[166]

The milder clinical course of DM in patients with CF may be accounted for by relative insulin preservation,[163] impaired glucagon secretion,[153,157] and enhanced sensitivity of peripheral tissues to insulin.[167] There are conflicting data on the effect of CFRDM on survival.[168-170]

Diagnosis

The spectrum of glucose tolerance in CF ranges from normal to varying degrees of impaired tolerance and overt diabetes. Patients can be classified based on the results of fasting blood glucose and oral glucose tolerance test (OGTT) results[171] (Table 69-1). It is not clear whether patients with diabetic glucose tolerance (DGT) should be labeled as diabetic because progression to fasting hyperglycemia may occur in less than 40% of such patients.[171] There is no reliable way to predict which patients with abnormal glucose tolerance will develop CFRDM. Patients with impaired glucose tolerance (IGT) or DGT may have normal fasting and premeal blood glucose levels, normal hemoglobin A_{1c} levels, and minimal glucosuria despite relative insulin deficiency. In order to make an early diagnosis of CFRDM and to identify patients with DGT, patients with CF over age 10 years should have an OGTT performed every 1 to 2 years. Those with DGT should be monitored with home blood glucose testing for the development of CFRDM. Monitoring should be intensified at times of stress (infection, glucocorticoid therapy, pregnancy, and enteral or parenteral feedings). Measurement of hemoglobin A_{1c} is not a useful screening procedure.[169,171,172]

Table 69-1 Glucose Tolerance Categories in CF

CATEGORY	FASTING BLOOD GLUCOSE (MG/DL)	ORAL GLUCOSE TOLERANCE TEST (MG/DL AT 2 H)
Normal glucose tolerance (NGT)	<126	<140
Impaired glucose tolerance (IGT)	<126	140-200 or 1 h glucose ≥200
Diabetic glucose tolerance (DGT)	<126	≥200
CF-related diabetes mellitus (CFRDM)*	≥126	OGTT not necessary

*CFRDM may be chronic or intermittent, depending on whether fasting hyperglycemia is present at all times or only during periods of stress. (From Moran A: *New Insights into Cystic Fibrosis* 5:1, 1997.)

Although CFRDM can occur at any age, it is rare in young children; average age of onset is between 18 and 21 years.[168-171] Approximately 5% of patients with CF require chronic insulin therapy, 5% require intermittent insulin during periods of stress, and 30% have a DGT profile.[171] After 20 years of age, 25% have a DGT profile and 15% have CFRDM.[171]

Management

The goal of treatment is to achieve glucose homeostasis and good nutritional status with minimal hypoglycemia. Blood glucose goals include levels of 80 to 120 mg/dl before meals and levels of 100 to 140 mg/dl at bedtime. In most patients this can be achieved with split-dose NPH/regular insulin, or regular insulin before meals with or without nighttime NPH. Oral hypoglycemic agents have not been found to be helpful in CFRDM. Patients may develop hypoglycemia on low-dose sulfonylurea therapy while still experiencing postprandial hyperglycemia.[171] Hyperglycemia seen in association with parenteral nutrition can be managed by adding regular insulin to the total parenteral nutrition (TPN) solution or into the infusion line. Patients with hyperglycemia secondary to nighttime enteral supplementation should receive regular and NPH insulin before the start of feedings.[173] Short-term insulin therapy is recommended for patients with IGT or DGT at times of stress-induced hyperglycemia.

Nutritional management of CFRDM should focus on consistent timing and carbohydrate content of meals and snacks. Fat is emphasized as an important energy source. Simple carbohydrates are not limited, but patients are discouraged from ingesting highly absorbable sugars such as those in cola drinks. Caloric restriction is not an appropriate method of controlling blood glucose levels. Patients and families should be instructed in the use of sucrose for mild hypoglycemia and glucagon for severe hypoglycemia.

HEPATOBILIARY DISEASE

Liver Pathology

Nonspecific hepatic lesions consisting of periportal inflammation, fibrosis, bile duct proliferation, and cholestasis are present in approximately one third of infants with CF[174] (Fig. 69-5). In approximately 10% of young infants and 20% of older patients, focal biliary fibrosis is present, characterized by inspissation of granular eosinophilic material in the portal

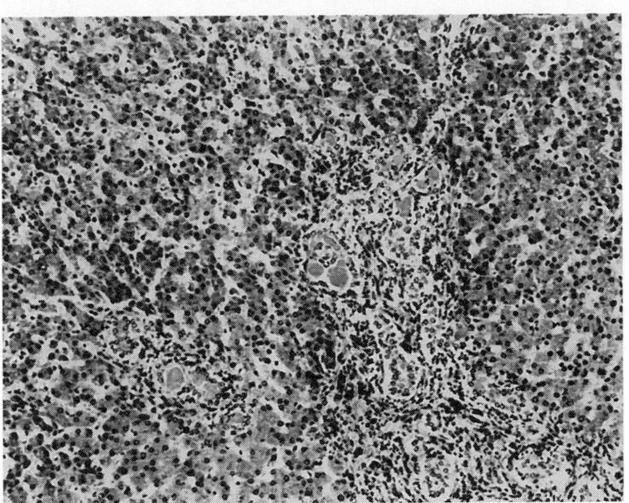

Fig. 69-5. Typical focal biliary cirrhosis in the liver of a 2-month-old infant with CF. Dilated bile ducts are filled with solid secretions. The proliferated ducts are in a sparse stroma containing a few mononuclear inflammatory cells.

ducts, bile duct proliferation, chronic inflammatory infiltration, and a variable degree of fibrosis.[5] This lesion is considered pathognomonic of CF. With increasing age, the percentage of cases with excessive intrahepatic mucus decreases; cholestasis is not a prominent feature in older patients.[174,175] In approximately 2% to 5% of patients, periportal fibrosis progresses to a destructive type of multilobular biliary cirrhosis with concretions, in which there are large irregular nodules with regenerative microscopic nodules, massive foci of fibrosis, and bile duct proliferation adjacent to preserved hepatic lobular architecture.[176-178]

Clinically, patients may manifest prolonged neonatal jaundice, steatosis (fatty liver), cirrhosis with portal hypertension, or hepatocellular failure.

Prolonged Neonatal Jaundice

Neonates with CF may present with prolonged obstructive jaundice, presumably secondary to obstruction of extrahepatic bile ducts by thick bile along with intrahepatic bile stasis (inspissated bile syndrome).[179-184] In most cases, liver histology shows features compatible with bile obstruction.[184] The liver is usually enlarged and firm. Approximately 50% of cases occur in association with meconium ileus (MI) or delayed passage of meconium. The prognosis for patients with neonatal cholestasis is generally good. However, elevated bilirubin values may persist for up to 7 months[185] and early-onset liver failure or cirrhosis may develop.[184] In some patients the biliary obstruction can be relieved by intraoperative irrigation of the biliary tree with saline and *N*-acetylcysteine.[186,187]

Other reported causes of prolonged jaundice in neonates and young infants with CF include extrinsic biliary obstruction,[188] extrahepatic atresia or obstruction of bile ducts,[189] giant-cell hepatitis,[190] intrauterine cytomegalovirus infection,[191] and paucity of intralobular bile ducts.[192]

Fatty Replacement of the Liver

Massive hepatomegaly with steatosis (fatty replacement) has been reported in infants with CF, possibly related to protein-calorie malnutrition or essential fatty acid deficiency.[193,194] In one such case, there was evidence that carnitine deficiency may have been a contributory factor.[194]

Cirrhosis and Portal Hypertension

Clinically apparent liver disease is present in 2% to 4% of patients with CF.[195,196] At times liver disease can be the predominant, and in some instances, the presenting manifestation of CF.[195] There is a progressive rise in prevalence from 0.3% in patients 0 to 5 years to a peak of 8.7% among patients 16 to 20 years.[196] The male:female ratio of affected patients is 2 to 3:1.[196] There are conflicting data as to familial concordance.[196,197] Almost all patients with liver disease have evidence of pancreatic exocrine deficiency.[198,199] There is no association between specific CF mutations and the development of liver disease.[199] The pathogenesis of cirrhosis in CF is not well understood. Initially, it was thought that cholestasis was an important predisposing factor,[200] but more recent evidence suggests "toxic" liver injury perhaps related to the accumulation of potentially cytotoxic bile acids such as lithocholic and chenodeoxycholic acids.[175] Metabolic and nutritional deficiencies may play a role. Hypoproteinemia in infancy[185] and MI or its equivalent[199] have been implicated as predictors of subsequent liver disease.

The diagnosis of liver disease is based on enlargement of the liver or spleen, abnormal liver enzyme values, abnormal hepatobiliary scintigraphy, portal hypertension and esophageal varices, and liver histology.[185,189,195,200] Among patients with liver disease, at least 20% have esophageal varices.[196] Splenomegaly indicates risk for variceal bleeding.[196] Physical examination is as effective as any biochemical parameter in demonstrating significant hepatic involvement.[196,201] There is an inconsistent relationship between hepatosplenomegaly and liver enzyme activity; 10% to 20% of patients have elevated liver enzyme values in the absence of other evidence of liver disease, whereas patients with hepatomegaly may have normal enzyme values.[195,196,201] In patients with elevated enzyme values, there may be no detectable biochemical progression of liver disease over long periods of time.[200] Hepatocellular failure occurs but is uncommon.[195,196]

Liver and spleen scans,[202] computed tomography,[203] and ultrasonography[204,205] demonstrate abnormalities in a high percentage of patients but the findings do not always correlate with clinically apparent liver disease.[202] Liver biopsy is the definitive procedure to document cirrhosis but its routine use is not indicated. In a study of 50 CF patients with hepatomegaly or abnormal liver function test results, hepatobiliary scanning showed evidence of a stricture of the distal common bile duct in 96% of cases.[206] However, this observation was not confirmed in two other large studies in which the incidence of common bile duct stenosis was 1%[207] and 13%.[208]

Patients with liver disease should have close monitoring of their nutritional status to optimize caloric intake and correct or prevent deficiencies of vitamins, minerals, carnitine, and essential fatty acids. Vitamin K supplementation should be given and the patient's clotting status followed closely. Aspirin-containing medications should be avoided[201] and nonsteroidal antiinflammatory agents used with caution. Control of variceal bleeding can be achieved with sclerotherapy or endoscopic esophageal variceal ligation.[201,209] Prophylactic sclerotherapy is not indicated. The transjugular intrahepatic portacaval shunt (TIPS) procedure can be used for short-term decompression in patients awaiting liver transplantation.[209] Surgical decompression of the portal venous system by portosystemic shunting (distal splenorenal shunt) should be considered for long-term management of patients who continue to bleed following endoscopic procedures and who are poor candidates for liver transplantation.[195,197,209] Patients who have recurrent episodes of variceal bleeding or hepatocellular failure in the presence of good pulmonary status are candidates for liver transplantation.[210,211] The results are similar to those obtained in patients without CF.[211]

The hydrophilic bile acid ursodeoxycholate (UDCA), which has potent choleretic properties, is used in CF patients with liver disease[212-215] and has a beneficial effect on liver function profiles,[212-214] nutritional status,[212] lipid profiles, and retinol status.[215] However, there is no beneficial effect on fat absorption.[212-214] After administration of UDCA for 2 months to 1 year, there is enrichment of the bile acid pool in UDCA and a reduction in chenodeoxycholic acid; UDCA becomes the principal fecal bile acid excreted.[213] Although these results are promising, the abililty of UDCA to halt progression of hepatobiliary disease or improve survival has not yet been demonstrated.

Gallbladder

Anatomic abnormalities of the gallbladder are present in approximately one third of patients with CF.[216,217] The gallbladder is often hypoplastic (microgallbladder) and filled with thick, colorless bile. There may be atresia and stricture of the cystic duct. Histologically, there are numerous multiloculated mucus-containing cysts in and beneath the mucosa.[216,217]

A variety of gallbladder abnormalities occur in patients with CF.[218-221] These include nonvisualization of the gallbladder on oral (31% to 33%) or IV cholecystography (12% to 23%), cholecystitis (5% to 10%), radiolucent gallstones (12% to 33%), and biliary sludge (6%). The incidence of these abnormalities increases with patient age. There are isolated reports of atonic gallbladder,[221] sclerosing cholangitis,[222] and cholangiocarcinoma of the gallbladder.[223] The high incidence of gallstones has been related to biliary stasis, increased bile viscosity secondary to the underlying defect in fluid and electrolyte transport, the presence of mucin glycoproteins that act as a "nucleating" factor,[224] and abnormalities of bile salt metabolism.[225-228] In CF there is interruption of enterohepatic circulation of bile, leading to a reduction in the size of the bile salt pool and to an increased proportion of glycine conjugates (lithogenic bile). Early reports of an increase in the cholesterol saturation of bile[225] have not been confirmed.[229,230] The gallstones are composed of calcium bilirubinate, protein, and other unidentified materials.[231]

Most CF patients with gallbladder abnormalities are asymptomatic.[218-221] In the largest reported series, only 24 (3.6%) of 670 patients developed symptomatic disease.[221] All but one of these patients had exocrine pancreatic deficiency and all but one were above age 12 years. In patients with typical biliary colic, cholecystectomy leads to total cessation of symptoms.[221] In patients with atypical symptoms, the results of cholecystectomy are often equivocal.[221] Laparoscopic cholecystectomy under continuous epidural anesthesia is preferred, especially in patients with severe pulmonary disease.[232] Anecdotally, administration of UDCA led to the dissolution of symptomatic gallstones in several patients with CF.[233]

GASTROESOPHAGEAL REFLUX

Although the exact prevalence of gastroesophageal reflux (GER) in patients with CF is not known, a number of reports suggest that it occurs with considerable frequency.[234-239] Heartburn and regurgitation are reported by more than 20% of patients with CF.[237] Gastroesophageal reflux has been documented in approximately 80% of unselected patients with CF under 5 years of age[239] and 75% of symptomatic patients over the age of 4 years.[235]

The mechanism leading to GER in patients with CF is not well understood. It is postulated that recurrent/chronic cough, chest hyperinflation, and an increased thoracoabdominal pressure gradient may be contributory factors.[240] Reflux has also been documented during chest physiotherapy.[241,242] The frequency and severity of GER are correlated with the severity of the underlying pulmonary disease.[235] It is known from esophageal manometry studies in patients with CF that resting lower esophageal sphincter pressure is normal.[237] However, transient, inappropriate episodes of lower esophageal sphincter relaxation occur along with abnormal distal esophageal motility.[237,238] It is likely that in some patients, underlying pulmonary disease facilitates GER which, in turn, contributes to the progression of pulmonary disease. However, there is evidence that in young infants with CF, GER may precede significant pulmonary disease.[239] A relationship between GER and use of methylxanthines has not been documented in patients with CF.[237]

Patients with GER may have upper abdominal pain, epigastric or substernal burning, vomiting, hematemesis, dysphagia, failure to thrive, or pulmonary disease that does not respond to usual therapy.[235,238] Esophageal strictures may develop secondary to chronic esophagitis.[236] Infants with reflux or esophagitis may manifest irritability, vomiting, regurgitation, poor oral intake, and growth failure. There have been several reports in which GER has dominated the clinical picture and has been the presenting manifestation of CF.[243,244] The diagnosis is suspected on the basis of symptoms and then confirmed by prolonged intraesophageal pH monitoring, upper gastrointestinal endoscopy, and esophageal biopsy. An upper gastrointestinal series should be done to exclude an anatomic lesion.

Treatment must be tailored to the individual patient, but may include frequent small meals, avoidance of caffeine and theophylline, positioning, antacids, H_2 blockers, and avoidance of head downtilting during chest physiotherapy.[242] Because of underlying pulmonary disease, the use of bethanechol is not recommended. The prokinetic agent cisapride, which increases the tone of the lower esophageal sphincter, has been shown to be effective in young CF patients with GER.[239] In older patients, the results have not been as impressive.[238] Beyond infancy, GER often follows a relapsing course and may necessitate repeated or chronic courses of therapy. When medical management fails, a Nissen fundoplication may be indicated.

PEPTIC ULCER DISEASE

Patients with CF appear to be at increased risk for the development of peptic ulcer disease (PUD). They show hypersecretion of gastric acid in response to pentagastrin stimulation,[245] and bicarbonate secretion from the pancreas is greatly reduced.[16] The result is a duodenal content pH range of 5.5 to 6.5, compared with a normal pH of about 7.0.[17,18] Also, a marked increase in the incidence of PUD has been reported in adults with chronic obstructive pulmonary disease[246] and in patients with chronic pancreatitis and pancreatic insufficiency.[247] However, an increased antemortem incidence of PUD has not been documented in patients with CF,[248-250] with the exception of an unexplained cluster of cases in black adolescents.[251] In a review of the pathologic findings in 146 CF cases, there were 12 instances (8%) of peptic ulcerations involving the stomach and duodenum.[252] However, these may have represented an agonal feature of CF and its complications.

In the patient with symptoms suggestive of PUD, endoscopy is the diagnostic procedure of choice.[253] Contrast radiography is not useful because of the underlying radiographic abnormalities of the duodenum seen in almost all patients with CF.[249,254]

DUODENAL ABNORMALITIES

Radiographically demonstrable abnormalities of the duodenum are present in approximately 85% of patients with CF at all ages.[249,254] These consist of thickened and coarse mucosal folds, nodular indentations along the duodenal wall, smudging or poor definition of the normal mucosal pattern, and a redundant and distorted duodenal contour (Fig. 69-6). These findings are most prevalent in the first and second portions of the duodenum. There is no apparent relationship between the radiographic findings and symptomatology. However, they can be confused with other diagnoses and this may interfere with the usefulness of radiographic studies in the diagnosis of PUD.[253] The cause of these abnormalities is unknown. It has been postulated that Brunner's gland hyperplasia, goblet cell hypertrophy, adherent mucus, and contraction of the underlying circular muscle may play a role.

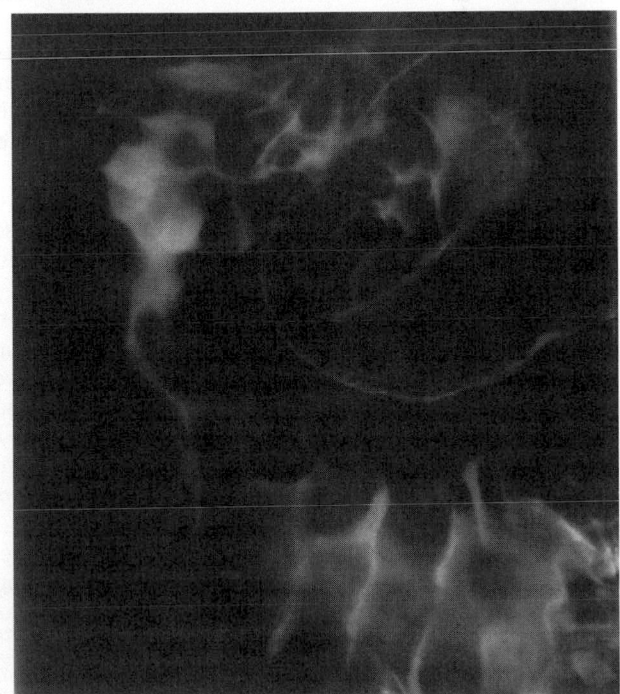

Fig. 69-6. Contrast material outlines thickened mucosal folds and nodular indentations along the duodenal wall. (Courtesy John Dorst, MD.)

DISTAL INTESTINAL OBSTRUCTION SYNDROME

DIOS, also called meconium ileus (MI) equivalent, is a common cause of partial small bowel obstruction in patients with CF.[255-258] It is caused by the impaction of mucofeculent material in the distal ileum, cecum, and proximal colon, and with rare exception is seen only in patients with pancreatic exocrine insufficiency.[259] Contributing factors include abnormal intestinal mucins, undigested food residues, prolonged intestinal transit time, low dietary fiber content, bowel dilation, and abnormal intestinal electrolyte and water transport.[258,260] There may be a higher incidence among patients who had MI in the newborn period.[258,261] There is often no identifiable precipitating event, but dehydration, inadequate enzyme supplementation, and change in diet have been implicated. The exact incidence is unknown but DIOS has been reported in 9% to 40% of patients.[258] It has been described in patients of all ages but the incidence is probably higher in adolescents and adults.[262]

Clinical manifestations include crampy lower abdominal pain, distention, vomiting, anorexia, abdominal tenderness, and palpable masses in the right lower quadrant. Episodes may occur within a normal stooling pattern, even during symptomatic periods. There may be progression to complete obstruction, volvulus, or intussusception. Patients may have isolated episodes with long symptom-free periods or chronic symptoms with intermittent exacerbations.

In evaluating a CF patient with abdominal pain, one should consider a wide range of possibilities, including DIOS, intussusception, volvulus, appendiceal disease, esophagitis, peptic ulcer disease, gallbladder disease, pancreatitis, and other conditions that may be unrelated to CF. In most cases, the diagnosis of DIOS is suspected on the basis of the history and physical findings. Abdominal radiographs show a bubbly, granular appearance in the area of the ileum and cecum consistent with retained stool;[263] there may be air-fluid levels (Fig. 69-7). An enema using an isoosmolar water-soluble contrast material may be both diagnostic and therapeutic. Hyperosmolar contrast agents are irritating to the colon and may cause large fluid and electrolyte shifts. Careful monitoring is essential if they are used. The most specific radiologic finding is the presence of inspissated material demonstrated on reflux of contrast into the terminal ileum.

In the absence of complete obstruction, the treatment of choice is the administration of a balanced intestinal lavage solution (GoLYTELY) orally or by nasogastric tube at a dosage of 20 to 40 ml/kg/hr, with a maximum of 1200 ml/hr.[259,264] Effective therapy may take 4 to 6 hours. The endpoint of therapy is determined by passage of stool, resolution of symptoms, and disappearance of a previously palpated right lower quadrant mass. Clear effluent by itself is not an adequate endpoint.[259] Follow-up abdominal radiographs can be helpful in documenting the resolution of DIOS. Balanced electrolyte solutions have largely replaced *N*-acetylcysteine enemas and other previously reported methods.

In the absence of peritoneal irritation, nonoperative therapy is almost always successful, although full resolution of symptoms may take several days. If there is complete obstruction or peritoneal irritation, surgical intervention is indicated.[265] Following an acute episode of DIOS, a variety of preventive measures can be instituted, including increased fluid intake, optimization of pancreatic enzyme supplementation, lactulose, laxatives, and a prokinetic agent such as cisapride.[266,267]

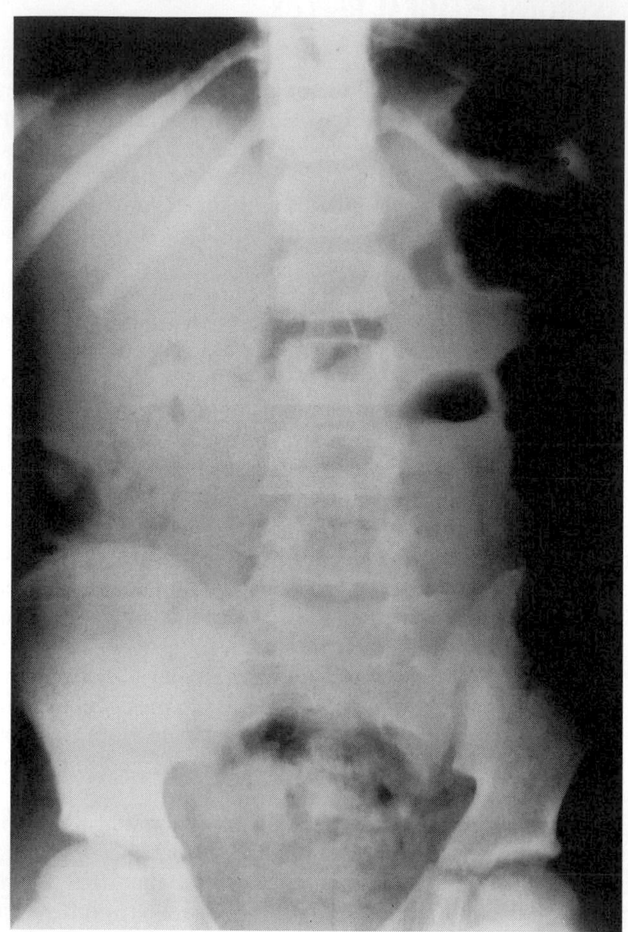

Fig. 69-7. Abdominal radiograph in a patient with DIOS. The diffuse granular appearance is consistent with retained stool, along with scattered air-fluid levels.

INTUSSUSCEPTION

Secondary to the accumulation of inspissated puttylike material in the cecum, terminal ileum, and ascending colon, CF patients with pancreatic insufficiency are at increased risk for the development of intussusception.[268,269] Episodes tend to occur in older patients (4 to 16 years), may be recurrent, and occasionally precede the diagnosis of CF.[268] It is probably part of the spectrum of the DIOS. Patients usually present with the acute onset of intermittent crampy abdominal pain often accompanied by vomiting. Other manifestations include a palpable abdominal mass, rectal bleeding, and decreased or absent bowel movements. Atypical or chronic symptoms occur in 25% of patients with intussusception.[268] Most episodes are ileocolic, but ileoileal, ileocecal, colocolic, and even appendiceal locations have been reported.[270]

Intussusception may be difficult to distinguish from uncomplicated DIOS. It should be suspected in the patient with a presumptive diagnosis of DIOS who does not to respond to usual therapy. Plain radiographs of the abdomen and abdominal ultrasound may not be helpful in identifying an intussusception. The diagnosis is usually confirmed by contrast enema but in some cases is made only at laparotomy.[268,269] Hydrostatic reduction may be successful but most cases require surgical correction.[268,269]

APPENDICEAL DISEASE

In patients with CF, there are typical histologic findings in the appendix.[5,271] The number of goblet cells is increased and they are often markedly distended with mucus secretions. The crypts are dilated and appear wider, and at times deeper, because of distention of the lumen by accumulated secretions. Eosinophilic casts of the crypts may extrude into the lumen of the appendix. Inspissated secretions may extrude through the orifice of the appendix to form a local cecal mass. There is little or no cellular infiltration and the muscularis layer is not affected. The diagnosis of CF has been suggested by the histologic appearance of an appendix removed from some patients with acute[272] or recurrent/chronic abdominal pain.[273] An asymptomatic right lower quadrant mass secondary to mucoid impaction of the appendix has been described as a presenting manifestation of CF.[274]

The reported incidence of acute appendicitis in patients with CF is only 1% to 2%, compared with a rate of 7% in the general population.[275,276] This may be accounted for by the long-term use of antibiotics in many patients with CF. Patients with CF who have acute appendicitis may present with classic symptoms,[277] but the diagnosis is often delayed because of an atypical or "subacute" presentation and confusion with DIOS.[276] At laparotomy, a high percentage of patients show appendiceal perforation and periappendiceal abscess formation.[275,277]

Clinically, CF patients with acute appendicitis have right lower quadrant pain, nausea, and anorexia. Fever and change in stool frequency may or may not be present.[276] The initial diagnosis is usually DIOS. Abdominal ultrasound, computed tomography, and gallium scans generally are not helpful in establishing a diagnosis.[276] A contrast enema may be helpful if it shows extrinsic cecal compression or appendiceal filling. However, failure to visualize (fill) the appendix before or after evacuation of contrast material cannot be used as a sign of appendicitis in patients with CF.[278] Failure of visualization is most often related to mucus plugging of the appendiceal lumen.

The possibility of an appendiceal abscess should be considered when a patient with CF presents with pain, a mass, or drainage from the right flank; prolonged fever; a limp; or failure of suspected DIOS to respond to appropriate therapy.[279] In patients with DIOS, abdominal radiographs usually show extensive stool accumulation and the white blood cell count is normal or only mildly elevated. Abdominal computed tomography may be a useful diagnostic tool.[279] Treatment usually involves surgical drainage and intravenous antibiotics followed by an elective appendectomy.

MECONIUM ABNORMALITIES

In newborns with CF, the mineral and water content of meconium is decreased[280]; undigested serum proteins, especially albumin, are increased[281,282]; and disaccharidases, lactase, and β-D-fucosidase are increased.[283] Increased albumin concentration, abnormal salt and water transport, and excessive mucus production by intestinal goblet cells are thought to be responsible for inspissation of meconium and several clinical complications, including delayed passage of meconium, MI, and meconium plug syndrome (MPS).

Meconium Ileus

MI, in which intraluminal intestinal obstruction is secondary to inspissation of tenacious meconium in the terminal ileum, occurs in approximately 18% of newborns with CF.[284] With rare exception,[282-287] almost all full-term infants with MI eventually have a confirmed diagnosis of CF. There is a strong familial trend for the occurrence of MI, with a recurrence rate of 29% to 39% in subsequent CF-affected siblings.[288-289] There is evidence that MI is, in part, genetically determined. There is a decreased risk in patients who carry R117H, A455E, or other mild mutations that confer pancreatic sufficiency,[261,290] and an increased risk in patients who carry certain severe mutations.[261]

Affected infants present within the first 48 hours of life with abdominal distention, bilious vomiting, and failure to pass meconium.[291-293] There may be a maternal history of polyhydramnios.[294] Approximately 50% of cases are complicated by volvulus, atresia, perforation, ischemic necrosis, meconium peritonitis, or pseudocyst formation.[217,292,293] The diagnosis of MI is supported by abdominal radiography which shows distended loops of bowel, usually without air-fluid levels, and a granular ground-glass appearance in the area of the terminal ileum, indicating the mixture of air bubbles with meconium (soap-bubble sign).[295] Contrast enema shows an unused microcolon (Fig. 69-8). In the presence of meconium peritonitis, there may be flecks of intraperitoneal calcium throughout the abdomen. Intramural jejunal calcification has been reported in a newborn with CF who had MI complicated by jejunal atresia.[296] The presence of abdominal calcification, however, is usually associated with non-CF causes of meconium peritonitis[294]; conversely, the absence of calcification favors CF as the cause of meconium peritonitis.[294] Male infants with in utero meconium peritonitis may present with scrotal calcification.[297] The diagnosis of MI and meconium peritonitis can be made prenatally by ultrasonography.[294] In several cases, the obstruction has been relieved by intrauterine amniography with urografin.[298]

In the absence of complications, up to 50% of cases can be treated successfully by the administration of hyperosmolar (Gastrografin) or isoosmolar contrast enemas under fluoroscopic control.[293] With this therapy, the patient's fluid and electrolyte status must be monitored closely to prevent hypovolemia. Repeated attempts to evacuate meconium may be required. If the patient's condition remains stable without change in abdominal findings, therapeutic enemas can be repeated over several days. The procedure may be complicated by intestinal perforation in up to 15% of cases.[299] Patients who have complications of MI or do not respond to nonoperative therapy require surgical intervention. In some instances, the inspissated meconium can be cleared by intraoperative irrigation with acetylcysteine,[300,301] hyperosmolar contrast,[301] or saline.[298] If irrigation is unsuccessful or if there are complications, patients are managed by resection of the involved bowel followed by primary anastomosis or a temporary double-barrel (side-by-side) enterostomy.[293] After surgery, patients will require a period of total parenteral nutrition followed by intensive enteral nutritional support. In patients with a history of MI, there is earlier acquisition of *P. aeruginosa*,

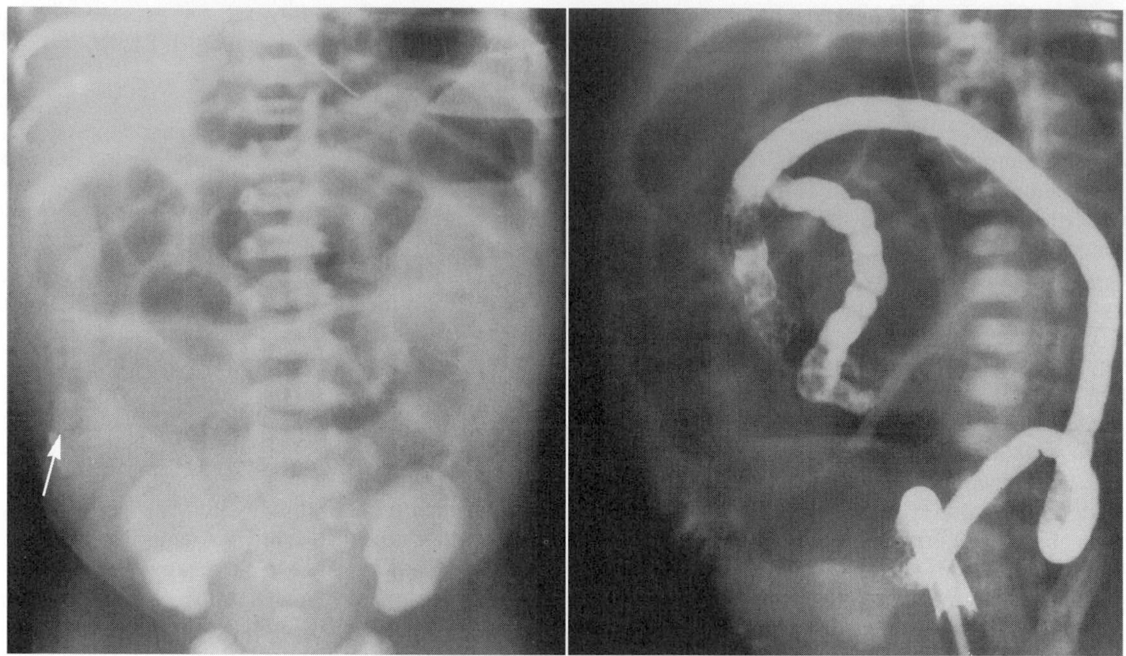

Fig. 69-8. Radiographic findings in a newborn infant with MI. The area of the terminal ileum *(arrow)* has a granular ground-glass appearance and a contrast enema shows an unused microcolon.

but at ages 8 and 13 years pulmonary function is similar in patients with and without MI.[288] Long-term survival among males and females with MI is similar to that of females without MI but significantly shorter than that of males without MI.[288]

Meconium Plug Syndrome

Meconium plug syndrome (MPS) is a well-recognized cause of low intestinal obstruction in newborn infants secondary to inspissated meconium.[302,303] It is manifested by progressive abdominal distention, vomiting that is often bilious, and failure to pass meconium. There may be visible and palpable loops of tense bowel. Rectal examination may be normal or the leading edge of the meconium may be felt. With a contrast enema, contrast material may mix with large pieces of meconium to produce radiolucent filling defects or it may outline a long, continuous meconium cast filling the colon. The caliber of the colon is normal.

MPS occurs in association with prematurity, hypotonia, and hypermagnesemia, and as the earliest manifestation of Hirschsprung disease. It is well recognized that MPS may also occur as the presenting manifestation of CF. In one series, MPS occurred in 12 of 87 newborns with CF in the absence of MI[304] and in another series, 6 of 25 newborns who presented with MPS eventually had a diagnosis of CF.[303] It is likely that MPS and MI represent gradations of the same underlying abnormality, differing only in degree of severity and site of obstruction. In general, MPS is a benign condition usually relieved following anal stimulation, administration of enemas, or a diagnostic contrast enema. The success of nonoperative treatment is probably a result of the lower site and significantly easier removal of the obstructing meconium in infants with MPS as compared with those with MI.

RECTAL PROLAPSE

Rectal prolapse occurs in approximately 20% of patients with CF,[305,306] usually between 6 months and 3 years of age and often preceding the diagnosis of CF.[306] Onset after age 5 years is unusual. The incidence is very low (2%) in patients treated before 3 months of age.[307] In the United States, severe constipation is the most common cause of rectal prolapse,[308] but a sweat test is probably indicated in every child with this complication. In patients with CF, episodes of prolapse are often recurrent and may range from a simple mucosal prolapse to prolapse of all layers of the ano-rectum (procidentia). The occurrence of prolapse is probably related to malnutrition, poor muscle tone, and the passage of voluminous stools. Episodes may be precipitated by paroxysmal cough.

Following the initiation of pancreatic enzyme therapy, there is a marked reduction in the frequency of prolapse.[305,306] Recurrences may indicate a need for increased pancreatic enzyme dosage. The prolapse can almost always be easily reduced manually by a parent. Older patients learn to prevent or reduce prolapses by voluntary muscle action.[306] In the rare instances in which recurrent episodes of prolapse are accompanied by pain, bleeding, or incontinence, an anal sling procedure[309] or submucosal injection of a sclerosing agent[310] may be beneficial.

MISCELLANEOUS AND ASSOCIATED INTESTINAL ABNORMALITIES

Cancer

A number of case reports[223,311,312] and one cohort study[313] have suggested that adult patients with CF may have an increased risk of cancer, particularly digestive tract tumors and leukemia. A large retrospective cohort study of U.S., Canadian, and European patients[314] found that the overall cancer risk in patients with CF was similar to the general population, but did confirm a marked elevation in the risk ratio for digestive tract tumors (esophagus, small and large intestine, pancreas) for the age group 20 to 29 years. A case control study[314] did not identify any characteristics associated with an increased risk. The increased risk of digestive tract cancers may be related to differential localization and expression of the CFTR gene,[315] persistent pathologic alterations in digestive tract organs leading to increased cell turnover,[316] and antioxidant deficiency.[83]

Celiac Disease

In several patients, celiac disease (or a celiac-like syndrome), manifested by persistence of bulky stools, irritability, and growth failure and documented by intestinal biopsy findings and response to a gluten-free diet has been reported to coexist with CF.[317] This may represent a chance association of these two conditions. Alternatively, increased intestinal permeability and impaired protein digestion secondary to lack of proteases could lead to a high antigen load to the small intestinal mucosa.[318]

Clostridium Difficile

Clostridium difficile colonization was reported in 22% of 107 patients with CF who had a history of frequent antibiotic use.[319] Two thirds of colonized patients also had cytotoxin recovered from their stools. However, the majority of the colonized patients, including those with cytotoxin, had no evidence of diarrheal disease. Patients with CF and neonates[320] are the only populations reported in which *C. difficile* cytotoxin is frequently recovered from asymptomatic individuals. The mechanism by which colonized patients with CF are protected from diarrheal disease is not known. However, in the evaluation of the CF patient who has prolonged diarrhea, one needs to consider the possibility of *C. difficile*–induced disease.

Crohn Disease

Based on a number of case reports, it has recently been recognized that there is more than a coincidental association between CF and Crohn disease.[318,321-323] Such patients usually manifest significant weight loss, intestinal fistula formation, and perianal disease. There is evidence that patients with CF operated on for MI may be at increased risk for the development of inflammatory bowel disease.[318]

Giardiasis

Patients with CF have a significantly higher risk of giardiasis than controls, possibly because of abnormal bile composition.[324]

Intestinal Permeability, Transit Time, and Absorption

In patients with CF there is evidence of increased small intestinal permeability, probably because of the leakage of large molecules (disaccharides) through paracellular pathways.[325-328] This increased intestinal permeability is probably related to underlying pancreatic dysfunction.[327] The passive transcellular uptake of small molecules is preserved.[325,328] Orocecal transit time has been shown to be prolonged in both children and adults with CF.[328,329]

In general, small intestine biopsies from patients with CF show normal histology[330]; however, there may be a thick mucus cover over the brush border membrane. Enhanced intestinal active transport of glucose has been demonstrated,[331] possibly related to a decreased intestinal diffusion barrier. Enzyme-depleted small intestinal villi are present in some patients.[332] This may be a result of impaired maturation secondary to nutritional deficiencies[332] or failure of enterocytes to increase their brush border enzymes secondary to impaired absorption of nutrients.[333]

Pneumatosis Intestinalis

Pneumatosis intestinalis is characterized by the presence of gaseous cysts in the wall of the bowel. It is often associated with mechanical intestinal obstruction or chronic lung disease,[334,335] but is usually an incidental finding at laparotomy or autopsy. It has been reported only rarely in patients with CF.[336,337] Clinically, abdominal distention and palpable crepitant abdominal masses are present. Contrast enema demonstrates numerous cystic collections of air within the bowel wall. Complications such as intestinal obstruction, volvulus, perforation, pneumoperitoneum, rectal prolapse,[336] and intussusception[335] may occur. On pathologic examination, the intestinal mucosa appears to be stretched over a solid matting of air-filled blebs in the mucosa and submucosa surrounded by dense fibrous connective tissue.[336] The pathogenesis is not known, but it has been postulated that it may represent dissection of air from the alveoli to the gut via the mediastinum and retroperitoneal space.[338] The natural history is variable. Lesions may spontaneously disappear or persist for many years.[335] In the absence of complications, treatment is not indicated.

CARDIOVASCULAR COMPLICATIONS

Cor pulmonale secondary to chronic hypoxemia is a common complication in CF patients with advanced pulmonary disease and remains a significant cause of morbidity and mortality. In addition, a number of other cardiovascular complications have been documented.

Evaluation of Cardiac Status

Physical Examination

The early clinical recognition of cor pulmonale may be difficult in patients with CF.[339] Tachypnea, tachycardia, and hepatomegaly are common secondary to underlying pulmonary disease. However, an enlarged tender liver is often an early clue to right ventricular failure.[340] An accentuated second heart sound in the pulmonic area may be a helpful sign but is often blunted by an anterior chest wall deformity and air trapping. Patients may develop a tricuspid insufficiency murmur, either during or shortly after the onset of cardiac enlargement.[340] Peripheral edema is not a common finding and when present, appears late in the clinical course. In patients with heart failure, weight loss is as common as weight gain.[340]

Laboratory Findings

The degree of hypoxemia and pulmonary artery pressure are closely correlated. A Pa_{O_2} below 50 mm Hg and Pc_{O_2} above 45 mm Hg are consistently associated with severe cor pulmonale.[341,342] Hypoalbuminemia secondary to expansion of plasma volume may be a helpful early clue to right ventricular failure.[343]

Chest Radiograph

Because of severe air trapping in patients with CF, it is often difficult to assess heart size[339]; in general, there is poor correlation between echocardiographic findings and cardiothoracic ratio.[344] Cardiomegaly may be obvious only in patients with overt right heart failure. There may be enlargement of the main pulmonary arteries, but this is often obscured by striking hilar adenopathy and parenchymal disease.

Electrocardiogram

The electrocardiogram (ECG) is not generally helpful in the diagnosis of cor pulmonale in patients with CF.[339,344-346] The majority of patients with confirmed right ventricular hypertrophy have a normal ECG.[339,344-346] In some patients, however, especially those with heart failure, the ECG may show evidence of right ventricular hypertrophy, right atrial hypertrophy, left ventricular hypertrophy, ST and T wave abnormalities, and low voltage.[340]

Echocardiogram

Echocardiography is the most useful noninvasive clinical tool for the early diagnosis and longitudinal assessment of cor pulmonale in patients with CF.[344,346-350] Even in patients with clinically mild disease, there is thickening of the anterior wall of the right ventricle, which progresses to enlargement (dilation) of the right ventricular cavity and right ventricular outflow tract, along with abnormal right ventricular systolic time intervals.[346] Patients with advanced disease may show left ventricular wall hypertrophy, decrease in the size of the left ventricular cavity, and abnormal septal motion (flattened or reversed).[346,349] Echocardiographic changes correlate with clinical score, chest radiograph score, pulmonary function, and postmortem cardiac findings.[344,346,349] A composite echocardiogram scoring system has been proposed and has been shown to correlate with clinical score, chest radiograph score, pulmonary function, and prognosis.[347]

Radionuclide Scans

Quantitative radionuclide angiography is a reproducible technique to assess biventricular function.[348,351-353] Using this technique to measure ejection fractions, right ventricular dysfunction at rest has been demonstrated in 41% to 72% of patients,[348,351,353] and a significant percentage of patients exhibit an abnormal right ventricular response to exercise.[348,352] Abnormal left ventricular function at rest is present in up to 25% of patients[348,351,352] with a variable response to exercise.[352] Radionuclide studies suggest that in CF, abnormal right ventricular function may occur before clinically significant disease is present and that the stress of exercise may uncover latent dysfunction.[348,351,352] Thallium myocardial perfusion scans can be used to assess right ventricular hypertrophy, but in patients with CF this technique offers no advantage over echocardiography.[354]

Cardiac Catheterization

Right heart catheterization with direct measurement of pulmonary artery pressure remains the gold standard for evaluation of pulmonary hypertension.[341,342,345] Although this procedure is too invasive for the routine assessment of cor pulmonale, it can be used to monitor the response to various therapeutic interventions.

Cor Pulmonale

Secondary to alveolar hypoventilation, chronic hypoxemia, and pulmonary vasoconstriction, up to 70% of patients eventually develop pulmonary hypertension and hypertrophy of the right ventricle (cor pulmonale).[339] A clear relationship has been demonstrated between the degree of hypoxemia and pulmonary artery pressure.[339,341,342,345] Airflow obstruction and wide ranges in intrathoracic pressure may augment venous return to the right heart, with resultant increase in pulmonary artery flow and aggravation of an already increased right ventricle afterload.[339] In patients with CF, there is probably slowly progressive hypertrophy and dilation of the right ventricle over a period of years. At one extreme, pulmonary hypertension may be only mild, with minimal right ventricular hypertrophy, whereas at the other extreme right ventricular overload may be severe, with overt right-sided heart failure.

In the absence of obvious heart failure, the diagnosis of cor pulmonale by clinical findings usually is not possible.[339] Echocardiography is the most sensitive noninvasive technique for the early recognition and monitoring of cor pulmonale.[344,347-350] For practical purposes, cor pulmonale is assumed to be present when one or more of the following is present: right ventricular hypertrophy by ECG, Pa_{O_2} <50 mm Hg, signs of heart failure; radiographic evidence of enlarged pulmonary arteries, and forced vital capacity <60% predicted.[346]

Approximately one third of patients with CF have right-sided failure during the terminal phase of their illness.[340] Clinical features include enlargement and tenderness of the liver (90%), peripheral edema (64%), and weight gain (37%).[340] Such patients usually have markedly abnormal pulmonary function, severe hypoxemia, ECG evidence of right ventricular hypertrophy, and abnormal echocardiograms. At catheterization, pulmonary artery pressure is elevated but the range of values is considerable.[340]

Treatment of heart failure consists of oxygen, lowered salt intake, diuretics, and aggressive treatment of underlying pulmonary obstruction and infection.[339,340,355] There is no demonstrated benefit to the use of digitalis.[340] Tolazoline transiently reduces pulmonary artery pressure[356] but has not been shown to be of long-term benefit.[340] Other pulmonary vasodilators, including phentolamine, hydralazine, and nifedipine, have not reduced pulmonary artery pressure in patients with CF and prior episodes of right heart failure.[357] After the onset of right-sided failure, most patients are significantly disabled and mean survival is 8 months (range 1 to 63 months).[340] Although some data support a role for chronic oxygen therapy in adults with COPD, a similar benefit has not been demonstrated in a small trial carried out in patients with CF.[358] However, supplemental oxygen has been shown to minimize oxyhemoglobin desaturation in patients with CF who desaturate during exercise in room air.[359] Acute administration of aminophylline and digoxin has not been shown to improve cardiac function in patients with CF, either at rest or during exercise.[353,360]

Myocardial Lesions

There have been several reports of focal areas of myocardial necrosis and fibrosis in patients with CF before age 3 years.[361,362] Lesions involve mainly the left ventricle and spare the endocardium, pericardium, atria, and coronary vessels. Microscopically, the lesions consist of connective tissue or fibrosis in the absence of an inflammatory reaction. Patients have had the sudden onset of congestive heart failure or asystole preceded by episodes of dyspnea, pallor, and tachycardia. Radiographs may be normal or show cardiomegaly. Metabolic and nutritional factors have been postulated, but the cause of these lesions remains unknown.

Arrhythmias

Recurrent episodes of supraventricular tachycardia (SVT) have been observed in a small number of patients with CF.[363] Patients have baseline tachycardia but there is no correlation between severity of pulmonary disease and frequency of SVT. The etiology of the arrhythmia is unclear, but possible causes include myocardial fibrosis and necrosis, stimulation of pressure receptors in a distended right atrium, intracardiac autonomic imbalance, or reaction to combination bronchodilator therapy. Acute management consists of vagal maneuvers or intravenous verapamil. Long-term management consists of digoxin or verapamil. Bronchodilator therapy should be reduced as clinically indicated.

There is a single report of an adolescent with CF who showed first degree AV block, ventricular trigeminy, and multiple premature ventricular contractions.[364] Echocardiogram and thallium scan were suggestive of an infiltrative process in the anteroseptal region.

Atherosclerosis

Postmortem studies of the aorta in patients with CF demonstrate that both fatty streaks[365,366] and late fibromusculoelastic lesions (atherosclerotic precursor lesions)[366] are less common than in age-matched controls. It has been postulated that the decreased incidence of these lesions is secondary to impaired fat absorption and low serum lipid levels.

ENDOCRINE AND METABOLIC COMPLICATIONS

Parathyroid Gland

In some patients with CF, there is evidence of secondary hyperparathyroidism, evidenced by elevated levels of immunoreactive parathyroid hormone.[75-77] Results are conflicting as to whether the elevated levels correlate with low serum concentrations of 25-hydroxyvitamin D and degree of bone demineralization.[76,77] The absence of secondary hyperparathyroidism in the majority of patients, in the presence of subnormal 25-hydroxyvitamin D concentrations, is probably explained by normal serum concentrations of 1, 25-dihydroxyvitamin D_3. Gastrointestinal absorption of calcium is normal and end-organ responsiveness to parathyroid extract is normal.[75]

Pituitary Gland

In patients with CF, there is retardation of physical growth in all age groups[40,284] and an average delay of 2 years in pubertal development.[367,368] Skeletal maturation is delayed in approximately 40% of patients.[40,368] There is a significant correlation among growth retardation, severity of pulmonary disease,[40] and survival.[369] The hypothalamic-pituitary-gonadal axis is intact, but there is a substantial delay in the normal pubertal rise of gonadotropins and testicular androgens.[370] Plasma growth hormone[371] and somatomedin C levels are normal.[372] Short-course testosterone therapy has been shown to be a safe and effective means of improving the growth rate in male adolescents with CF and pubertal delay.[373] Isolated growth hormone deficiency has been reported in several patients with CF, probably as a chance coincidence of the two disorders.[374] Among nine prepubertal endocrinologically normal CF patients, a 12-month trial of biosynthetic recombinant human growth hormone resulted in a significant anabolic effect, as shown[375] by increased growth velocity, somatomedin C values, and protein stores. However, a long-term benefit from such therapy has not been demonstrated.

Thyroid Gland

At autopsy the thyroid gland of older patients with CF contains excessive quantities of lipofuscin (ceroid) pigment in follicular epithelial cells,[376] possibly related to the autooxidation of cellular lipids secondary to chronic vitamin E deficiency. The development of a goiter with or without hypothyroidism has been well documented in patients with CF following chronic administration of iodide.[377,378] In several patients treated with iodide, hypothyroidism occurred in the absence of a goiter.[377,379] Studies of thyroid metabolism in patients with CF have failed to explain the apparently enhanced sensitivity of the thyroid gland to the inhibitory action of iodides on hormone synthesis. Although serum T_4 concentrations are within the normal range, T_3 concentrations may be low suggesting a defect in the peripheral deiodination of T_4 to T_3.[378] In a study using an iodide-perchlorate discharge test, there was no defect in thyroidal iodide organification. Thyroid stimulating hormone (TSH) reserve was normal and response to endogenous TSH stimulation was normal.[380] Dysgenetic congenital hypothyroidism has been recognized in association with CF.[381] There is evidence that gastrointestinal absorption of L-thyroxine may be reduced in such patients.[381]

Adrenal Gland

Cortex

Hyperplasia of the zona glomerulosa (site of aldosterone production) in the adrenal cortex has been demonstrated on autopsy in children with CF.[382] The other zones are normal and no other characteristic histologic changes are found in the adrenal gland. Older nonstressed patients show normal to slightly elevated urinary aldosterone excretion, plasma aldosterone levels, and aldosterone secretion rates.[383] These results are consistent with a state of secondary hyperaldosteronism, probably related to excessive loss of sodium in sweat. Young CF patients with dehydration, hypoelectrolytemia, and metabolic alkalosis have elevated plasma renin activity, hyperaldosteronemia, and hyperaldo-steronuria secondary to sodium depletion and intravascular volume contraction[384]; plasma and urinary levels of mineralocorticoids are elevated. All values return to normal upon restoration of fluid and electrolyte balance and maintenance on a high-sodium diet.[384]

Medulla

There is histologic evidence of adrenal medullary hyperplasia in patients with CF.[385] Studies of circulating plasma catecholamines, their precursors, metabolites, and major urinary products have yielded conflicting results.[386,387] Plasma norepinephrine levels have been reported to be normal[387] or slightly elevated.[386] Free plasma dopamine levels have been reported to be significantly elevated,[386] but in this group of patients there was no concomitant increase in urinary levels of dopamine or homovanillic acid, the final breakdown product of dopamine. The significance of these findings and their relationship to autonomic dysfunction[388] and clinical outcomes in patients with CF is not clear.

RENAL ABNORMALITIES

Although renal involvement is not a major clinical concern in CF, a number of conditions are present, including immune-complex deposition, heavy exposure to aminoglycosides, DM, steatorrhea, and cor pulmonale, which place patients at increased risk of renal injury.[389] Histologic abnormalities, described largely in autopsy material, include glomerular alterations[389,390] (glomerulomegaly, amyloid deposition,[391,392] glomerulosclerosis, mesangial proliferation, and mesangial deposits of immunoglobulin M (IgM) and C3) suggestive of immune-complex–mediated injuries, tubulointerstitial lesions[389,393] (tubular lysosomal proliferation, lymphoplasmocytic infiltration, fibrosis, and tubular atrophy) suggestive of chronic aminoglycoside injury, and microscopic nephrocalcinosis.[394] Changes consistent with diabetic nephropathy have also been described.[160,163]

Patients may manifest proteinuria, nephrotic syndrome, renal colic and hematuria, severe nephropathy with progressive renal insufficiency, or end-stage renal disease.[389,391-393] These may be related to renal amyloidosis, immunoglobulin A (IgA) nephropathy, aminoglycoside nephrotoxicity,[395] diabetic nephropathy, or nephro-lithiasis.[396] The occurrence of renal stones in patients with CF is probably related to steatorrhea and hyperoxaluria.[397] Patients with secondary amyloidosis may have proteinuria which rapidly progresses to nephrotic syndrome and then end-stage renal disease.[391,392] Proteinuria greater than 1 g/24 hours is uncommon in patients with CF and warrants further investigation. Nephrotic syndrome may occur coincidentally with CF, unrelated to amyloidosis.[398] In such patients, unlike those with amyloidosis, response to glucocorticoid therapy has been good.

Renal physiology studies in patients with CF reveal that the glomerular filtration rate is slightly decreased,[399] normal,[400-402] or slightly increased,[403] probably depending on experimental conditions of salt and water balance. Effective renal plasma flow is normal.[400,403] Patients are capable of lowering urinary excretion of sodium when placed on a moderately reduced sodium intake,[401] and renal tubular anion secreting mechanisms are intact.[400,403] There is evidence, however, of decreased free water clearance[401,403] and impaired ability to excrete sodium in response to an oral or intravenous sodium load. These findings are consistent with increased sodium reabsorption in the renal proximal tubule and decreased delivery of sodium to more distal segments of the nephron.[400,403] The finding of microscopic nephrocalcinosis in a high percentage of patients, including those under 1 year of age, suggests that a primary renal defect may be present in CF.[394]

ELECTROLYTE ABNORMALITIES

Secondary to increased electrolyte loss in sweat, patients with CF may manifest a salty taste to the skin or salt crystals on the skin, either of which may be the initial clue to the diagnosis.

Metabolic Alkalosis

Increased electrolyte loss in the sweat over a prolonged period of time may lead to electrolyte depletion and chronic metabolic alkalosis as the initial presentation or as a complication of CF.[404-411] Contributory factors include increased gastrointestinal losses,[411] acute intercurrent illness, thermal stress, and limited electrolyte intake.[410] Although current feeding recommendations satisfy sodium requirements for growth of healthy infants, they are inadequate to compensate for the increased electrolyte losses present in infants with CF.[410] During a period of profuse sweating, an infant with CF may lose 80 mEq sodium, 100 mEq chloride, and 40 mEq potassium per day, depending on body surface area and sweating rate.[407,408] The incidence of this complication in arid climates may be higher,[409] but there have been reports of cases in the absence of environmental or endogenous thermal stress.[405,406]

Patients present with anorexia, irritability, vomiting, and failure to thrive, usually in the absence of dehydration or cardiovascular instability.[404-413] Laboratory abnormalities include elevation of blood pH and P_{CO_2}, bicarbonate and base excess, and low serum concentrations of sodium, chloride, and potassium. Urinary excretion of sodium and chloride is markedly decreased, probably related to secondary hyperaldosteronism.[406-408] Preventive measures include avoidance of thermal stress and provision of adequate salt in the diet. This can be accomplished by adding ¼ teaspoon table salt (23 mEq sodium) to each liter of infant formula or liberal amounts of salt to solid foods.[410] Treatment consists of the replacement of calculated fluid and electrolyte losses.

Acute Salt Depletion

In 1951 it was first reported that patients with CF are susceptible to dehydration and vasomotor collapse during periods of environmental thermal stress.[412] This observation led di Sant'Agnese et al to elucidate the sweat gland defect in such patients.[413] Subsequently, there have been a number of reports of acute hypoelectrolytemia and dehydration as a presenting manifestation or complication of CF.[414-418] Patients have with anorexia, decreased oral intake, lethargy, and signs of dehydration. Laboratory findings include low serum electrolyte concentrations and metabolic (contraction) alkalosis. Serum chloride concentrations can be strikingly low (40 to 50 mEq/L).[418] Episodes may be precipitated by acute intercurrent illness, gastrointestinal losses, fever, decreased oral intake, and environmental thermal stress. However, a number of cases have been reported in the absence of thermal stress.[414,416]

It is important to consider the possibility of CF in any child with dehydration and severe hypoelectrolytemia, especially in the absence of obvious gastrointestinal losses. Management consists of replacement of fluid and electrolyte losses. Preventive measures include avoidance of thermal stress along with maintenance of adequate fluid and electrolyte intake during periods of stress. Salt needs should be met through increased dietary salt intake. Supplementation with salt tablets is not generally recommended.

Heat Acclimation

Patients with CF have normal thermal, renal, and cardiac responses to exercise and heat and can heat acclimate.[419,420] In response to salt and fluid losses, they maintain normal sweat volumes and show the expected increase in renin and aldosterone with normal renal salt conservation. However, during exposure to exercise and heat stress, patients with CF lose significantly more electrolyte in sweat than controls, with a concomitant fall in serum sodium and chloride concentrations and serum osmolality.[419,420] During extended exposure to heat and exercise, patients may underestimate their fluid needs and place themselves at risk of dehydration.[421] This probably results from absence of hyperosmolality of body fluids as a stimulus to thirst. During vigorous exercise, patients should be encouraged to drink electrolyte-containing solutions at regular intervals.

FEMALE REPRODUCTIVE TRACT

Genital Abnormalities

Excess of cytoplasmic and extracellular cervical mucus is present in patients with CF in the absence of inflammation or other obvious contributory factors.[422] This is a consistent finding in newborns and although it decreases in frequency, it remains a common finding throughout infancy and childhood.[422] The submucosal glands, uterine cavity, and cervical os may also be filled with mucin-rich material. In one third of adult patients, multicystic ovaries and reduced uterine size are demonstrated on ultrasonography, especially in patients with amenorrhea or irregular menstrual cycles.[423] The histologic appearance of the endometrium, fallopian tubes, and ovaries is otherwise normal.[422]

Analysis of cervical mucus reveals that it is scanty and dehydrated, usually containing less than 80% water.[424] This is below the minimum critical water level of 93% to 95% believed to be essential for sperm migration.[425] Moreover, the typical midcycle increase in water content and the accompanying thinning of cervical mucus that occur in normal subjects are not seen in patients with CF.[424] This may result in the formation of a tenacious mucus plug in the os that impedes sperm penetration. The electrolyte pattern of the cervical mucus is noncyclic; the average sodium concentration in the dry residue is only one tenth of normal during the critical midcycle period.[424]

Pubertal Delay

In girls with CF, age at menarche is delayed by an average of 2 years (14.5 to 14.9 years).[367,423,426] The finding of delayed puberty, increases of serum gonadotropin, and sex steroid levels suggests late maturation of the reproductive endocrine system.[370] Generally, appropriate levels of these hormones are finally attained in most patients by the late teenage years. There is evidence that the neuroendocrine mechanism controlling onset of puberty can be modified by various factors, including inadequate fat reserve. In patients with CF, pubertal development may be related to the severity of disease and nutritional status,[367] but pubertal delay also occurs in patients with good clinical and nutritional status.[426] In these patients, genotype, maternal menarchal age, and abnormal glucose tolerance may influence timing of puberty.[426]

Menstrual Abnormalities

Among adolescent and adult patients with CF, primary and secondary amenorrhea and irregular cycles (missed periods, prolonged cycle lengths) are common.[423]

Fertility

Despite reduced fertility in patients with CF, the potential for pregnancy exists and is likely to increase in association with improved survival. It is essential that all patients wishing to avoid pregnancy use adequate methods of contraception. Barrier methods are safe and highly effective in the well-motivated patient but are associated with unacceptably high failure rates in adolescents. The use of oral contraceptives has been somewhat controversial because of potential CF-related side effects such as diabetes, cholelithiasis, hepatic dysfunction, and bronchial mucus obstruction. There is one report of atypical polypoid endocervical hyperplasia in CF patients using combination birth control pills.[427] However, in a prospective study of women with moderate to severe pulmonary disease, use of a combination contraceptive pill was not associated with cervical changes or decline in pulmonary function.[428]

Pregnancy

In recent years, there has been a dramatic increase in the number of pregnancies reported among women with CF. In 1996, 145 pregnancies were reported to the Cystic Fibrosis Foundation Patient Registry, compared with 52 pregnancies in 1986. Normal physiologic adaptations seen during pregnancy, such as increase in minute ventilation, alterations in gas exchange, decrease in residual volume and functional residual capacity, and increase in blood volume and cardiac output, place the patient with CF at risk for respiratory failure and right ventricular decompensation.[429] In addition, the increased nutritional demands during pregnancy may be unattainable.

Early reports of pregnancy outcomes among patients with CF suggested a significant risk, both for the mother and fetus, including decline in pulmonary status and increased rates of stillbirth and prematurity.[430,431] It is not clear, however, whether pregnancy per se was responsible for the clinical decline or whether this was the natural history of disease in patients of this age and severity. More recently it has been shown that pregnancy in patients with mild disease is well tolerated, with little decline in pulmonary and nutritional status 1 year postpregnancy.[432-434] Prepregnancy pulmonary function is the most useful predictive measure.[429,432-435] A prepregnancy forced expiratory volume in 1 second (FEV_1) greater than 60% generally predicts a good outcome, whereas a significant decline in FEV_1 during pregnancy is associated with significant postpregnancy mortality.[433] Approximately one fourth of CF pregnancies result in preterm labor and delivery.[429,433,434] Duration of pregnancy and birth weight correlate most closely with prepregnancy pulmonary function.[429,433,434]

Patients contemplating pregnancy require counseling regarding the advisability and potential risks of pregnancy. Patients who become pregnant require close supervision by an obstetrician skilled in high-risk obstetrics and a pulmonologist, dietitian, and respiratory therapist. Pulmonary exacerbations require aggressive management, including intravenous antipseudomonal penicillins and cephalosporins. The use of intravenous aminoglycosides is generally discouraged because of concerns of fetal ototoxicity. In patients with severe exacerbations, however, the benefit of their use may outweigh the potential risk. The use of tetracyclines, fluoroquinolones, and trimethoprim-sulfamethoxazole should be avoided. The safety of dornase alfa (pulmozyme) has not been established. The decision to terminate a pregnancy should be weighed in favor of protecting the immediate health of the mother. Indications for pregnancy termination include marked and sustained decline in pulmonary function, development of right-sided failure, refractory hypoxemia, and progressive hypercapnia and respiratory acidosis.[429]

Genetic counseling and mutation screening of the prospective father should be offered to all couples contemplating a pregnancy. All offspring will be obligate carriers of a CF mutation. For a woman with CF whose partner does not carry a common CF mutation, the risk of an affected infant is 1:160. Couples also must be counseled as to nonmedical issues including the additional demands of child-rearing, financial aspects of parenting, and the potential premature loss of a parent.[436]

Breast-Feeding

Mothers with CF can successfully breast-feed,[437-441] but they and their infants need careful nutrition monitoring. Studies of CF breast milk composition indicate a normal electrolyte composition,[438-440] increased protein content,[438] and a slight decrease in lipid levels.[438-440] The lipid pattern of CF breast milk (decreased content of linoleic and arachidonic acid) reflects the blood lipid pattern of patients with CF.[437]

MALE REPRODUCTIVE TRACT

Genital Abnormalities

The external genitalia are grossly normal. The testes are usually normal in size and contour[442,443] but may be reduced in size in the presence of advanced disease or malnutrition. There are, however, abnormalities of Wolffian duct–derived structures. The epididymis is not palpable or reduced in size, soft, and poorly formed.[443] In almost all patients, there is bilateral atresia or absence of the vas deferens.[442-445] Pathologic studies reveal absence of epididymal ducts and vas deferens and atrophy and fibrosis of the epididymis.[442,446] The presence of normal ureters and kidneys (metanephroi) indicates that the Wolffian duct was present in early embryonic life but disappeared during development.[446] Studies suggest that the observed genital tract lesions may be secondary to intraluminal obstruction by abnormally viscous secretions and subsequent atrophy.[447] There is an increased incidence of abnormalities associated with testicular descent, including inguinal hernia, hydrocele, and undescended testicle.[443] Testicular function and male sexual activity are otherwise normal, but serum testosterone levels are low in 20% of men.

Pubertal Delay

Linear growth and onset of puberty are often retarded in male patients with CF.[40,284,368] The hypothalamic-pituitary-gonadal axis is intact, but the normal pubertal rise of gonadotropins and testicular androgens is substantially delayed.[370] Generally, this is accompanied by retardation of skeletal maturation, reflected in delayed bone age and short stature. Maximal growth velocity is shifted from age 13 years in normal subjects to age 15 years in patients with CF.[373] Short-term treatment with testosterone enanthate, 200 mg intramuscularly every 3 weeks for a total of four injections, has been associated with significantly increased growth velocity and objective and subjective improvement in self-image.[373]

Azoospermia

Almost all postpubescent male patients with CF demonstrate obstructive azoospermia.[442,443,445] Characteristically, the ejaculate is of low volume (0.5 to 1.0 ml) and acidic (pH <7.2) compared with controls (volume 3.0 to 5.0 ml; pH 7.2 to 8.0).[442,443,445] The concentration of fructose, which is of seminal vesicle origin, is diminished, whereas the concentration of citric acid and the activity of acid phosphatase, both of which are of prostatic origin, are increased.[442,443,445] Microscopic examination of the testes shows active meiosis and spermatogenesis but a reduction in the number of mature spermatozoa produced, with up to 50% abnormal forms.[442] In male patients with azoospermia and chronic sinopulmonary infection, the differential diagnosis includes CF, Young syndrome, and ciliary dyskinesia (immotile cilia syndrome).[448] Testicular biopsy, electron microscopy of bronchial mucosal biopsy specimens, sweat testing, measurement of transepithelial potential differences, and genotype analysis may be required to arrive at a conclusive diagnosis.

Of particular interest are otherwise healthy men who present with obstructive azoospermia secondary to bilateral absence or atresia of the vas deferens.[449-454] Most have no pulmonary or gastrointestinal manifestations. Among such cases, 50% to 65% have one detectable CF mutation or an incompletely penetrant mutation (5T) on a noncoding region of CFTR and 10% to 15% are compound heterozygotes.[449-454] Sweat electrolyte levels are usually normal but may be intermediate or elevated. Such patients should be assigned a CF diagnosis only if an abnormality of CFTR function can be demonstrated by sweat test, nasal potential difference measurement, or mutation analysis. The prognosis for such patients appears to be excellent,[454] but they should be monitored for the development of CF-related complications and genetic counseling should be offered to their relatives.

Fertility

Although the overwhelming majority of male patients with CF are infertile secondary to obstructive azoospermia, fertility has been documented in 2% to 3% of male patients, usually those with mild pulmonary disease[455-457] or specific mutations.[458] For purposes of reproductive counseling, semen analysis should be offered to all postpubescent male patients. The finding on testicular biopsy of active spermatogenesis in patients with CF has raised the possibility of microscopic sperm aspiration from the epididymal remnant combined with in vitro fertilization and tubal embryo transfer.[459,460] In such cases, including men with the syndrome of congenital bilateral absence or atresia of the vas deferens, it is important to test the partner for CF mutations in order to evaluate the risk of CF in their offspring.

HEMATOLOGIC ABNORMALITIES

In patients with CF there is an inverse relationship between Pa_{O_2} levels and hemoglobin and hematocrit,[98] but the degree of compensatory polycythemia is less than expected.[461,462] Although there is a blunted compensatory increase in erythropoietin relative to the degree of underlying anemia and hypoxemia,[99,462] red blood cell (RBC) mass in hypoxic patients with CF increases similarly to that of healthy individuals living at high altitude.[462] The lack of polycythemia is more related to a disproportionate rise in plasma volume relative to RBC mass.

Iron deficiency anemia is present in 33% to 66% of patients with CF.[98-100,463] The etiology is probably multifactorial, including inadequate dietary iron intake, blood loss, iron malabsorption, and chronic infection. In vitro and in vivo studies suggest that iron absorption is increased with exocrine pancreatic insufficiency[464,465] and that the administration of pancreatic enzymes may impair oral iron absorption.[98,466,467] The mechanism by which pancreatic enzymes impair iron absorption is not clear. The iron status of patients should be routinely monitored; a low serum ferritin level is a useful measure of decreased total body iron stores. If supplemental iron is given, it should not be in close proximity to the administration of pancreatic enzyme supplements.[467]

Beyond infancy, there is no evidence of increased hepatic iron stores in patients with CF.[468] An early report of hemosiderosis in patients with CF[469] is probably explained by the persistence of fetal iron in the livers of young infants.

Thrombocytopenia in patients with CF is almost always related to hypersplenism secondary to cirrhosis and portal hypertension.

CENTRAL NERVOUS SYSTEM COMPLICATIONS

Brain Abscess

Brain abscess has been reported in a small number of adolescents and adults with CF,[470-473] usually in association with advanced pulmonary disease. In most cases, there have been multiple abscesses remote from the paranasal sinuses. The responsible organisms are aerobic and anaerobic mouth bacteria of low virulence. This suggests hematogenous spread, probably from a site other than the lungs. The possibility of brain abscess should be pursued vigorously in patients with CF and a compatible clinical history.

Increased Intracranial Pressure

Increased intracranial pressure manifested by a bulging fontanel, irritability, and rapid head growth has been documented in malnourished infants with CF shortly after initiation of nutritional therapy.[474-477] There are usually no associated neurologic abnormalities. On lumbar puncture, cerebrospinal fluid pressure may be increased; computed tomography is normal. The fontanel gradually returns to normal over a period of several days to several months. In such patients, vitamin A deficiency must be considered in the differential diagnosis. The cause of the increased intracranial pressure is unclear. It has been suggested that it may be secondary to intrathoracic obstruction to venous return.[475] The rapidity of onset and resolution suggests a mechanism other than catch-up brain growth.

Neurologic Dysfunction Related to Vitamin E Deficiency

Neuropathologic changes and a spinocerebellar syndrome have been described in patients with CF in association with vitamin E deficiency.[86,478-480] Patients with liver disease and decreased intraluminal bile salt concentrations may be at particular risk.[86,478,479] Neuropathologic studies have demonstrated a high incidence of axonal degeneration in the rostral parts of the posterior columns in the spinal cords of patients with CF, a lesion characteristic of vitamin E deficiency.[481,482] The incidence of this finding increases with age in untreated patients.[482] Among 89 patients who died after the age of 5 years, 17 (19%) had evidence at autopsy of posterior column degeneration.[483] Most often, there was bilateral degeneration limited to the fasciculus gracilis extending from thoracic through cervical segments. The lesions involve both axons and myelin and the site of degeneration is marked by cellular and fibrillary astrogliosis.

Patients may manifest ophthalmoplegia, peripheral and truncal ataxia, peripheral neuropathy, proximal muscle weakness, areflexia, and decreased vibratory and proprioceptive sensation.[478,480] In vitamin E–deficient patients, sural nerve conduction latency is increased and action potential amplitude is decreased.[480] Somatosensory and visual evoked potentials are abnormal.[479] Although the relationship between vitamin E deficiency and neurologic dysfunction is not clear-cut, significant clinical improvement or stabilization of neurologic status has been documented following vitamin E supplementation.[86,478,479]

OCULAR COMPLICATIONS

Ocular abnormalities in CF include visual field defects, venous engorgement, tortuosity, hyperemia and blurring of the optic nerve head, abnormal pupillary responses, and decreased contrast sensitivity.[484-486] Examination of the ocular surface shows an increase in fluorescein staining and clinical blepharitis, as well as decreased Schirmer testing and tear lysozyme. Conjunctival epithelial cell morphology is normal.[487] Adolescents and young adults with vitamin A deficiency may manifest conjunctival xerosis and night blindness (decreased dark adaptation).[69,73] In patients with hyperglycemia there is evidence of breakdown of the blood-retinal barrier; this is considered to represent a functional abnormality that is a precursor to diabetic microangiopathy.[162] Proliferative diabetic retinopathy with blurred vision, neovascularization, vitreous hemorrhages, and cataract formation occurs in CF patients with long-standing diabetes.[161,163] Patients with CFRDM should have an annual ophthalmologic evaluation. Acute hemorrhagic retinopathy may occur at high altitude.[488] Optic atrophy and neuropathy with decreased contrast sensitivity and visual acuity have been observed in patients treated with chloramphenicol.[486,489,490]

SALIVARY GLANDS

In patients with CF, there are characteristic histologic abnormalities of the salivary glands. In the submaxillary glands, there are dilated mucus acini and ductules filled with inspissated mucus secretions.[5] In the labial (mucus) glands there are dilated ducts with inspissated mucus, atrophy and cyst-like dilation of acini, and metaplasia of the ductule epithelium.[491] Enlargement of the submaxillary glands has been observed in 90% of patients of all ages[492] (Fig. 69-9). Parotid gland enlargement is rare and there is no evidence of sialoangiectasis.[493]

Studies of flow rates and constituent composition of the various salivary glands have yielded somewhat conflicting data, probably related to differences in methods of salivary gland stimulation and saliva collection. In the parotid gland (serous) there is an increased flow rate[494-496] and increases in the concentrations of urea nitrogen and uric acid. Amylase activity[494-496] and sodium concentration[495,497] are normal. In the submaxillary gland (seromucoid), flow rate is normal to slightly

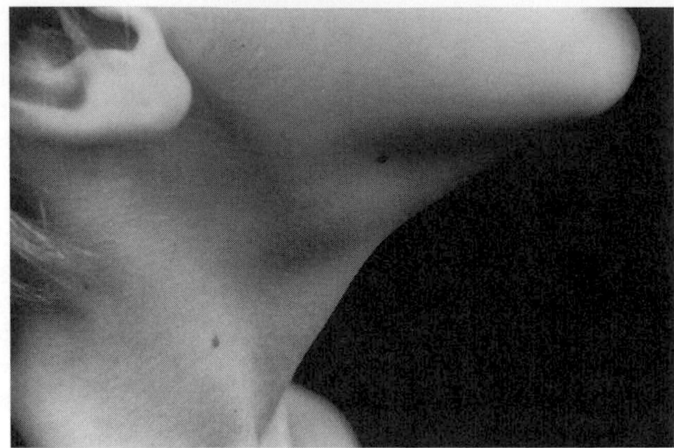

Fig. 69-9. Enlarged submaxillary glands in a patient with CF.

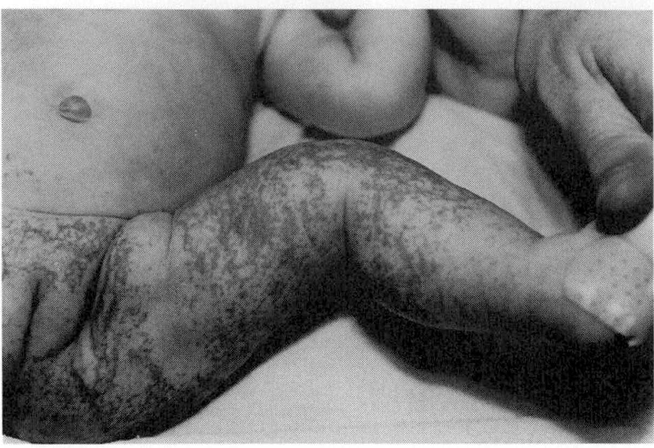

Fig. 69-10. 6-month-old infant with CF who initially had extensive dry, scaling, fissured erythematous plaques and papules involving the diaper region, extremities, shoulders, and perioral area. Clinically, it closely resembled acrodermatitis enteropathica.

decreased[496,498,499] and concentrations of calcium, amylase, total protein, acid and alkaline ribonuclease, lysozyme, and immunoglobulin A are increased.[496,499,500] Sodium and chloride concentrations are normal.[496,500,501] Turbidity of submaxillary gland saliva is increased,[498-500] probably because of the formation of high-molecular-weight calcium and glycoprotein precipitates. In the small salivary glands (mixed type) there is a moderately decreased flow rate and a markedly increased sodium concentration.[502] This is the only exocrine gland (apart from the eccrine sweat glands) that consistently exhibits the sodium abnormality characteristic of CF. The increased sodium concentration observed in mixed mouth saliva[494] is probably caused by the sodium contribution by the small salivary glands.[502]

SKIN MANIFESTATIONS

Skin manifestations occur in patients with CF secondary to nutritional deficiencies and vasculitis. Patients with vasculitis may develop sudden onset of raised, palpable, petechial lesions over the lower extremities.[503-505] The rash is often associated with pruritus, a burning sensation, slight edema of the feet, and concomitant arthritis.[504,505] It fades spontaneously in 3 to 7 days but is followed by multiple recurrences and eventually a diffuse purple-brown pigmentation of the affected areas.[505] Skin biopsy shows vasculitis and perivascular infiltrates.[505] Most of these patients have evidence of advanced pulmonary disease, elevated serum immunoglobulin G (IgG) levels, and circulating immune complexes.[505] There is usually no response to antiinflammatory agents.

Infants with CF may present with a periorofacial dermatitis that closely resembles acrodermatitis enteropathica[62,506,507] (Fig. 69-10). The rash consists of extensive dry, scaling, fissured, erythematous plaques and papules involving the diaper region, extremities, shoulders, and perioral area. It may be pruritic, with extensive excoriation. Mucous membranes and nails are not affected. There may be mild diffuse alopecia. The rash is usually seen in association with failure to thrive, hypoalbuminemia, anemia, and hepatomegaly. Although the pathogenesis of the rash is not entirely clear, it is probably related to deficiencies of zinc, protein, and essential fatty acids, along with altered prostaglandin metabolism.[62,506] It responds rapidly to nutritional therapy including protein, essential fatty acids, zinc, and pancreatic enzyme supplementation.

MUSCULOSKELETAL ABNORMALITIES

Digital Clubbing

Digital clubbing is an almost universal finding in patients with CF. In most instances, both fingers and toes are involved. The diagnosis is based on bulbous enlargement of the distal segment of the digit, change in the angle between the nail and the proximal skin to >180°, sponginess of the nail bed when pressure is applied, and increased nail curvature.[508] It can be assessed by placing the dorsal surfaces of the terminal phalanges of both long fingers together and observing the "angle" and "window" signs.[509] The degree of clubbing is related to the severity of the patient's pulmonary disease,[510] but the correlation is often poor; the relative importance of hypoxemia and lung suppuration has not been determined. It has been hypothesized that the increased digital blood flow observed in clubbed digits[511] may be caused by increased plasma levels of prostaglandin E or other vasoactive substances.[510]

Pulmonary Hypertrophic Osteoarthropathy

Pulmonary hypertrophic osteoarthropathy (PHOA) occurs in 5% to 15% of patients with CF,[512-514] usually in those over age 12 years and with advanced suppurative lung disease. It manifests as bilateral painful swelling of the distal third of affected bones (Fig. 69-11). Most commonly involved are the femur, tibia, fibula, radius, ulna, and humerus. Metacarpals and metatarsals are less commonly involved. There may be arthralgia, stiffness, joint swelling, and effusion. Radiographic findings are diagnostic and include periostitis and subperiosteal new bone formation. Periarticular manifestations may precede radiographic findings by months.[514] The arthropathy is usually chronic, with intermittent exacerbations at times of pulmonary exacerbations. Pathologically, there is edematous thickening of the periosteum, inflammatory periostitis, and subperiosteal new bone formation.[515] Synovial biopsy shows cellular infiltration, hyperplasia of synovial cells, and fibrosis. The pathogenesis of PHOA is obscure. Treatment with nonsteroidal antiinflammatory agents usually produces symptomatic improvement.

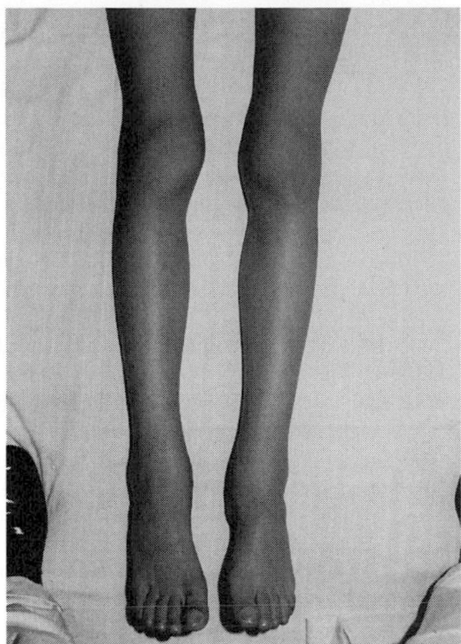

Fig. 69-11. Adolescent with CF and PHOA, manifested as painful swelling of the distal ends of the long bones.

Episodic Arthritis

Transient episodic seronegative arthritis has been described in 1.5% to 5% of patients with CF[504,505,516,517] and in up to 8.5% of adult patients.[518] The most commonly affected joints in decreasing order of frequency are the knees, ankles, wrists, proximal interphalangeal joints of the hands, shoulders, elbows, and hips. The pattern may be monarticular, pauciarticular, or polyarticular. Episodes last from 1 to 10 days and recur at intervals ranging from several weeks to several months. Marked joint stiffness and deformity are rare. Episodes may be accompanied by low-grade fever, generalized or localized erythematous maculopapular rash, painful erythematous nodules over the anterior tibia (erythema nodosum), or vascular purpura over the lower extremities. In general, there is no relationship between the episodes of arthritis and the severity of the underlying pulmonary disease.[504,505,518,519] There are reports, however, in which episodes of arthritis occurred in association with infectious respiratory exacerbations and improved with antibiotic therapy for the lung infection.[516,517,520]

Positive laboratory findings include a moderately elevated sedimentation rate, detectable circulating immune complexes, and elevated IgG levels.[517-519] These latter findings suggest an immune-mediated basis for the arthritis. Rheumatoid factor and antinuclear antibodies are not present. Radiographic studies are normal except for joint effusions and soft tissue swelling. Synovial biopsy shows nonspecific sub-acute synovitis[519]; on immunofluorescent staining there may be deposits of IgM, IgG, and complement components. Episodes usually respond to nonsteroidal antiinflammatory agents, although in some cases a short course of glucocorticoids may be required.

Seropositive Rheumatoid Arthritis

Seropositive rheumatoid arthritis has been reported in several patients with CF, probably as a coincidental finding.[517,519,521] The arthritis is progressive, sustained, and not associated with rash.

Back Pain and Spinal Deformity

Recurring back pain is eventually present in most patients with CF and relates to the severity of the underlying pulmonary disease.[522] Pain varies in intensity from mild to severe and it affects both the mid and lower back. Episodes often occur in association with paroxysms of cough, position, and respiratory infection. Associated findings include decreased range of motion and muscle strength. Patients with CF often assume a kyphotic, hunched-over posture secondary to abdominal flexion, shoulder protraction, and increased anterior-posterior chest diameter. Among patients over age 15 years, kyphosis is present in three fourths of females and one third of males.[523] Radiographs of the spine may show apical vertebral wedging, probably related to underlying osteopenia.[524] Postural abnormalities may be improved by appropriate exercises and postural counseling.

Fractures

Episodes of severe low back pain may occur secondary to vertebral compression fractures. These are usually seen in association with osteopenia and prolonged administration of glucocorticoids. A higher than normal fracture rate has been reported in female patients 6 to 16 years of age.[523]

Spontaneous fracture of the sternum has been reported in an adolescent with CF, probably related to underlying osteopenia.[524]

PSYCHOSOCIAL CONCERNS

Impact on Family

Cystic fibrosis is accompanied by a series of psychologic crises from the time of diagnosis to the patient's death.[525,526] The impact on the family is related to severity of the disease, rate of progression, stability and mental health of the family before diagnosis, and availability of support systems. Initially, parents may be frustrated and angry by medical delays in making the diagnosis of CF. After the diagnosis is confirmed, there is shock and disbelief, accompanied by the guilt associated with the transmission of a genetic disease. Eventually there is acceptance of the diagnosis, but denial is used as the overriding defense mechanism. If adaptive, denial enables families to cope; if maladaptive it can lead to denial of the diagnosis by the patient and noncompliance with the treatment program. The impact on family functioning is usually significant. Hardest to accept by families is the concept of intensive, long-term care carried out with no guarantee of success. There is often a breakdown in intrafamilial communication and withdrawal from the community. Psychosomatic complaints and depression are common.[527] Siblings are often resentful of the extra care and time required by the patient with CF, but in general, they function quite well.[528] The occupational goals of the parents may have to be modified and the financial burden can be considerable.

Impact on Patient

The reaction of the patient to the diagnosis of CF is variable, depending on age and parental response. There is often denial of symptoms, with maladaptive use of fantasy, repression, and regression. Feelings of anxiety and depression can lead to psychosomatic complaints and problems with discipline and academic achievement. The well-adjusted child is not embarrassed about having CF, discusses it openly with friends, and readily takes medications and treatments in front of others. Adolescence is a critical period during which psychologic problems are prominent. Patients are dissatisfied with their appearance and have to cope with a delay in physical development and maturation. They may be forced to compromise academic and vocational goals. The extended dependency caused by CF interferes with the normal process of separation from parents. Conflicts during adolescence are often manifested by social withdrawal, noncompliance with medical regimens, and risk-taking behavior.

The Terminally Ill Patient

In the terminally ill patient, the response to impending death varies greatly depending on age, developmental level, family support systems, and openness of communication.[529] In younger patients there may be loneliness and fear of abandonment, whereas older patients usually experience feelings of anxiety and depression. Open communication has been shown to decrease feelings of isolation, alienation, and the perception that the dying process is too terrible to talk about. Death is often a lingering process with repeated "final episodes" from which the patient rebounds. The accompanying anger, confusion, and guilt challenge the coping abilities of most families.

Management

Psychosocial support for the patient and other family members is especially important at the time of diagnosis, with exacerbations, and during the terminal phase of the disease. As with any chronic illness, consistency of medical care providers is essential. Members of the health care team should be willing to allow patients to develop close relationships with them and to provide ongoing support throughout life. It is important to know the entire family medically and psychosocially and to be sensitive to individual needs and coping mechanisms. Open communication is essential from the time of diagnosis. Questions should be answered honestly and directly but within a framework of guarded optimism.

Part of every visit should be devoted to a discussion of psychosocial issues. Parents should be encouraged to be open about CF rather than acting as though it did not exist. The involvement and support of extended family members should be encouraged. Parents constantly need to be encouraged to treat their child normally and to avoid overprotection. Special treatment and privileges should be discouraged. It is important to work with adolescents to promote independence and to encourage realistic academic and vocational goals. Families can be helped in a number of ways, including introduction to a CF family that is coping well, informational and support groups, respite care services, and counseling. It is the responsibility of the health care team to make appropriate referrals to and interact with mental health consultants, interact with the patient's teachers, ensure that the family is using all appropriate community and financial resources, arrange for vocational counseling, and, in the case of adolescents, plan for a smooth transition to adult care. With appropriate support, most patients are able to make an age-appropriate adjustment at home and school.

REFERENCES

Pancreatic Exocrine Insufficiency

1. Gaskin K, Gurwitz D, Durie P, Corey M, Levison H, Forstner G: Improved respiratory prognosis in patients with cystic fibrosis with normal fat absorption, *J Pediatr* 100:857-862, 1982.
2. Corey M, Durie P, Moore D, Forstner G, Levison H: Familial concordance of pancreatic function in cystic fibrosis, *J Pediatr* 115:273-277, 1989.
3. Kristidis P, Bozon D, Corey M, Markiewicz D, Rommens J, Tsui L-C, Durie P: Genetic determination of exocrine pancreatic function in cystic fibrosis, *Am J Hum Genet* 50:1178-1184, 1992.
4. Kerem E, Corey M, Kerem B, Rommens J, Markiewicz D, Levison H, Tsui L-C, Durie P: The relation between genotype and phenotype in cystic fibrosis—analysis of the most common mutation δF508, *N Engl J Med* 323:1517-1522, 1990.
5. Bodian M: *Fibrocystic disease of the pancreas: a congenital disorder of mucus production*, New York, 1953, Grune & Stratton.
6. Park RW, Grand RJ: Gastrointestinal manifestations of cystic fibrosis: a review, *Gastroenterology* 81:1143-1161, 1981.
7. Snyder WH, Cleland RS: Stenosis of the pancreatic ducts in fibrocystic disease: a study of the ducts by vinyl acetate technique, *Pediatrics* 29: 636-642, 1962.
8. Oppenheimer EH: Congenital atresia of the pancreatic duct with cystic fibrosis of the pancreas, *Arch Pathol* 29:790-795, 1940.
9. Grand RJ, Schwartz RH, di Sant'Agnese PA, Gelderman AH: Macroscopic cysts of the pancreas in a case of cystic fibrosis, *J Pediatr* 69:393-398, 1966.
10. Van Haren EHJ, Hopman WPM, Rosenbusch G, Jansen JBMJ, Van Herwaarden CLA: Pancreatic morphology and function in adult patients with cystic fibrosis, *Scand J Gastroenterol* 27:695-698, 1992.
11. Iannaccone G, Antonelli M: Calcification of the pancreas in cystic fibrosis, *Pediatr Radiol* 9:85-89, 1980.
12. Churchill RJ, Cunningham DG, Henkin RE, Reynes CJ: Macroscopic cysts of the pancreas in cystic fibrosis demonstrated by multiple radiological modalities, *JAMA* 245:72-74, 1981.
13. Imrie JR, Fagan OG, Sturgess JM: Structural and developmental abnormalities of the exocrine pancreas in cystic fibrosis, *Am J Pathol* 95:697-707, 1979.
14. Kopelman H, Durie P, Gaskin K, Weizman Z, Forstner G: Pancreatic fluid secretion and protein hyperconcentration in cystic fibrosis, *N Engl J Med* 312:329-334, 1985.
15. Kopelman H, Corey M, Gaskin K, Durie P, Weizman Z, Forstner G: Impaired chloride secretion, as well as bicarbonate secretion, underlies the fluid secretory defect in the cystic fibrosis pancreas, *Gastroenterology* 95:349-355, 1988.
16. Hadorn B, Zoppi G, Shmerling DH, Prader A, McIntyre I, Anderson CM: Quantitative assessment of exocrine pancreatic function in infants and children, *J Pediatr* 73:39-50, 1968.
17. Youngberg CA, Berardi RR, Howatt WF, Hyneck ML, Amidon GL, Meyer JH, Dressman JB: Comparison of gastrointestinal pH in cystic fibrosis and healthy subjects, *Dig Dis Sci* 32:472-480, 1987.
18. Robinson PJ, Smith AL, Sly PD: Duodenal pH in cystic fibrosis and its relationship to fat malabsorption, *Dig Dis Sci* 35:1299-1304, 1990.
19. Gaskin KJ, Durie PR, Lee L, Hill R, Forstner GG: Colipase and lipase secretion in childhood onset pancreatic insufficiency: delineation of patients with steatorrhea secondary to relative colipase deficiency, *Gastroenterology* 86:1-7, 1984.
20. Waters DL, Dorney SFA, Gaskin KJ, Gruca MA, O'Halloran M, Wilcken B: Pancreatic function in infants identified as having cystic fibrosis in a neonatal screening program, *N Engl J Med* 322:303-308, 1990.
21. Couper RTL, Corey M, Moore DJ, Fisher LJ, Forstner GG, Durie PR: Decline of exocrine pancreatic function in cystic fibrosis patients with pancreatic sufficiency, *Pediatr Res* 32:179-182, 1992.
22. Durie PR, Gaskin KJ, Corey M, Kopelman H, Weizman Z, Gorstner GG: Pancreatic function testing in cystic fibrosis, *J Pediatr Gastroenterol Nutr* 3(suppl 1):S89-S98, 1984.
23. Barbero GJ, Sibinga MS, Marino JM, Seibel R: Stool trypsin and chymotrypsin, *Am J Dis Child* 112:536-540, 1966.
24. Brown GA, Halliday RB, Turner PJ, Smalley CA: Faecal chymotrypsin concentrations in neonates with cystic fibrosis and healthy controls, *Arch Dis Child* 63:1229-1233, 1988.

25. Stein J, Jung M, Sziegoleit A, Zeuzem S, Lembcke B, Caspary WF, Lembcke B: Immunoreactive elastase 1: clinical evaluation of a new noninvasive test of pancreatic function, *Clin Chem* 42:222-226, 1996.
26. Dominguez-Munoz JE, Hieronymus C, Sauerbruch T, Malfertheiner P: Fecal elastase test: evaluation of a new noninvasive pancreatic function test, *Am J Gastroenterol* 90:1834-1837, 1995.
27. Nousia-Arvanitakis S, Arvanitakis C, Desai N, Greenberger NJ: Diagnosis of exocrine pancreatic insufficiency in cystic fibrosis by the synthetic peptide *N*-benzoyl-*L*-tyrosyl-p-aminobenzoic acid, *J Pediatr* 92:734-737, 1978.
28. Lang C, Gyr K, Tonko I, Conen D, Stalder GA: Value of serum PABA as a pancreatic function test, *Gut* 25:508, 1984.
29. Malis F, Fric P, Kasafirek E, Jodl J, Vavrova V, Slaby J: A peroral test of pancreatic insufficiency with 4-(*N*-acetyl-*L*-tyrosyl) aminobenzoic acid in children with cystic fibrosis, *J Pediatr* 94:942-944, 1979.
30. Dalzell AM, Heaf DP: Fluorescein dilaurate test of exocrine pancreatic function in cystic fibrosis, *Arch Dis Child* 65:788-789, 1990.
31. Goldberg DM: Biochemical tests in the diagnosis of chronic pancreatic enzyme insufficiency, *Clin Biochem Rev* 5:110, 1985.
32. Taussig LM, Wolf RO, Woods RE, Deckelbaum RJ: Use of serum amylase isoenzymes in evaluation of pancreatic function, *Pediatrics* 54: 229-235, 1974.
33. Skude G, Kollberg H: Serum isoamylases in cystic fibrosis, *Acta Paediatr Scand* 65:145-149, 1976.
34. Gillard BK, Cox KL, Pollack PA, Geffner ME: Cystic fibrosis serum pancreatic amylase, *Am J Dis Child* 138:577-580, 1984.
35. Durie PR, Largman C, Brodrick JW, Johnson JH, Gaskin KJ, Forstner GG, Geokas MC: Plasma immunoreactive pancreatic cationic trypsinogen in cystic fibrosis: a sensitive indicator of exocrine pancreatic dysfunction, *Pediatr Res* 15:1351-1355, 1981.
36. Durie PR, Forstner GG, Gaskin KJ, Moore DJ, Cleghorn GJ, Wong SS, Corey ML: Age-related alterations of immunoreactive pancreatic cationic trypsinogen in sera from cystic fibrosis patients with and without pancreatic insufficiency, *Pediatr Res* 20:209-213, 1986.
37. Cleghorn G, Benjamin L, Corey M, Forstner G, Dati F, Durie P: Serum immunoreactive pancreatic lipase and cationic trypsinogen for the assessment of exocrine pancreatic function in older patients with cystic fibrosis, *Pediatrics* 77:301-306, 1986.
38. Lapey A, Kattwinkel J, di Sant'Agnese PA, Lester L: Steatorrhea and azotorrhea and their relation to growth and nutrition in adolescents and young adults with cystic fibrosis, *J Pediatr* 84:328-334, 1974.
39. Shwachman H, Lebenthal E, Khaw K: Recurrent acute pancreatitis in patients with cystic fibrosis with normal pancreatic enzymes, *Pediatrics* 55:86-95, 1975.
40. Sproul A, Huang N: Growth patterns in children with cystic fibrosis, *J Pediatr* 65:664-676, 1964.
41. Miller M, Ward L, Thomas BJ, Cooksley WGC, Shepherd RW: Altered body composition and muscle protein degradation in nutritionally growth-retarded children with cystic fibrosis, *Am J Clin Nutr* 36:492-499, 1982.
42. Durie PR, Pencharz PB: A rational approach to the nutritional care of patients with cystic fibrosis, *J Soc Med* 82:11-20, 1989.
43. Reardon MC, Hammond KB, Accurso FJ, Fisher CD, McCabe ERB, Cotton EK, Bowman CM: Nutritional deficits exist before 2 months of age in some infants with cystic fibrosis identified by screening test, *J Pediatr* 105:271-274, 1984.
44. Sokol FJ, Reardon MC, Accurso FJ, Stall C, Narkewicz M, Abman SH, Hammond KB: Fat-soluble-vitamin status during the first year of life in infants with cystic fibrosis identified by screening of newborns, *Am J Clin Nutr* 50:1064-1071, 1989.
45. Soutter VL, Kristidis P, Gruca MA, Gaskin KJ: Chronic undernutrition/growth retardation in cystic fibrosis, *Clin Gastroenterol* 15:137-155, 1986.
46. Kraemer R, Rudeberg A, Hadorn B, Rossi E: Relative underweight in cystic fibrosis and its prognostic value, *Acta Paediatr Scand* 67:33-37, 1978.
47. Roy CC, Darling P, Weber AM: A rational approach to meeting macro- and micronutrient needs in cystic fibrosis, *J Pediatr Gastroenterol Nutr* 3(suppl 1):S154-S162, 1985.
48. Chase HP, Long MA, Lavin MH: Cystic fibrosis and malnutrition, *J Pediatr* 95:337-347, 1979.
49. Kindstedt-Arfwidson K, Strandvik B: Food intake in patients with cystic fibrosis on an ordinary diet, *Scand J Gastroenterol* 23(suppl 143):160-162, 1988.
50. Daniels L, Davidson GP, Cooper DM: Assessment of nutrient intake of patients with cystic fibrosis compared with healthy children, *Appl Nutr* 41A:151-159, 1987.
51. Kawchak DA, Zhao H, Scanlin TF, Tomezsko JL, Chaan A, Stallings VA: Longitudinal, prospecive analysis of dietary intake in children with cystic fibrosis, *J Pediatr* 129:119-129, 1996.
52. Pencharz P, Hill R, Archibald E, Levy L, Newth C: Energy needs and nutritional rehabilitation in undernourished adolescents and adults with CF, *J Pediatr Gastroenterol Nutr* 3(suppl 1):S147-S153, 1984.
53. Vaisman N, Pencharz PB, Corey M, Canny GJ, Hahn E: Energy expenditure of patients with cystic fibrosis, *J Pediatr* 111:496-500, 1987.
54. Buchdahl RM, Cox M, Fulleylove C: Increased resting energy expenditure in cystic fibrosis, *J Appl Physiol* 64:1810-1816, 1988.
55. O'Rawe A, McIntosh I, Dodge JA, Brock DJ, Redmond AOB, Ward R, MacPherson AJS: Increased energy expenditure in cystic fibrosis is associated with specific mutations, *Clin Sci* 82:71-76, 1992.
56. Tomezsko JL, Stallings VA, Kawchak DA, Goin JE, Diamond G, Scanlin TF: Energy expenditure and genotype of children with cystic fibrosis, *Pediatr Res* 35:451-460, 1994.
57. Fleisher DS, DiGeorge AM, Barness LA, Cornfeld D: Hypoproteinemia and edema in infants with cystic fibrosis of the pancreas, *J Pediatr* 64:341-348, 1964.
58. Dolan TF, Rowe DS, Gibson LE: Edema and hypoproteinemia in infants with cystic fibrosis, *Clin Pediatr* 9:295-297, 1970.
59. Lee PA, Roloff DW, Howatt WF: Hypoproteinemia and anemia in infants with cystic fibrosis, *JAMA* 228:585-588, 1974.
60. Gunn T, Belmonte MM, Colle E, Dupont C: Edema as the presenting symptom of cystic fibrosis: difficulties in diagnosis, *Am J Dis Child* 132:317-318, 1978.
61. Abman SH, Accurso FJ, Bowman CM: Persistent morbidity and mortality of protein calorie malnutrition in young infants with CF, *J Pediatr Gastroenterol Nutr* 5:393-396, 1986.
62. Darmstadt GL, Schmidt CP, Wechsler DS, Tunnessen WW, Rosenstein BJ: Dermatitis as a presenting sign of cystic fibrosis, *Arch Dermatol* 128:1358-1364, 1992.
63. MacLean WC, Tripp RW: Cystic fibrosis with edema and falsely negative sweat test, *J Pediatr* 83:86-88, 1973.
64. Abman SH, Reardon MC, Accurso FJ, Hammond KB, Sokol RJ: Hypoalbuminemia at diagnosis as a marker for severe respiratory course in infants with cystic fibrosis identified by newborn screening, *J Pediatr* 107:933-935, 1985.
65. Deren JJ, Arora B, Toskes PP, Hansel J, Sibinga MS: Malabsorption of crystalline vitamin B12 in cystic fibrosis, *N Engl J Med* 288:949-950, 1973.
66. Lindemans J, Neijens HJ, Kerrebijn KF, Abaels J: Vitamin B_{12} absorption in cystic fibrosis, *Acta Paediatr Scand* 73:537-540, 1984.
67. Congden PJ, Bruce G, Rothburn MM, Clarke PCN, Littlewood JM, Kelleher J, Losowsky MS: Vitamin status in treated patients with cystic fibrosis, *Arch Dis Child* 56:708-714, 1981.
68. Underwood BA, Denning CR: Blood and liver concentrations of vitamins A and E in children with cystic fibrosis of the pancreas, *Pediatr Res* 6:26-31, 1972.
69. Petersen RA, Petersen VS, Robb RM: Vitamin A deficiency with xerophthalmia and night blindness in cystic fibrosis, *Am J Dis Child* 116:662-665, 1968.
70. Smith FR, Underwood BA, Denning CR, Varma A, Goodman DS: Depressed plasma retinol binding protein levels in cystic fibrosis, *J Lab Clin Med* 80:423-433, 1972.
71. Ahmed F, Ellis J, Murphy J, Wootton S, Jackson AA: Excessive faecal losses of vitamin A (retinol) in cystic fibrosis, *Arch Dis Child* 65:589-593, 1990.
72. Abernathy RS: Bulging fontanelle as a presenting sign in cystic fibrosis: vitamin A metabolism and effect on CSF pressure, *Am J Dis Child* 130:1360-1362, 1976.
73. Rayner RJ, Tyrrell JC, Hiller EJ, Marenah C, Neugebauer MA, Vernon SA, Brimlow G: Night blindness and conjunctival xerosis caused by vitamin A deficiency in patients with cystic fibrosis, *Arch Dis Child* 64:1151-1156, 1989.
74. Scott J, Elias E, Moult PJA, Barnes S, Wills MR: Rickets in adult cystic fibrosis with myopathy, pancreatic insufficiency and proximal renal tubular dysfunction, *Am J Med* 63:488-492, 1977.
75. Simopoulos AP, Taussig LM, Murad F, Arnaud CD, di Sant'Agnese PA, Kattwinkel J, Barter FC: Parathyroid function in patients with cystic fibrosis, *Pediatr Res* 6:95(abstract), 1972.

76. Hahn TJ, Squires AE, Halstead LR, Strominger DB: Reduced serum 25-hydroxyvitamin D concentration and disordered mineral metabolism in patients with cystic fibrosis, *J Pediatr* 94:38-42, 1979.
77. Stead RJ, Houlder S, Agnew J, Thomas M, Hodson ME, Batten JC, Dandona P: Vitamin D and parathyroid hormone and bone mineralisation in adults with cystic fibrosis, *Thorax* 43:190-194, 1988.
78. Mischler EH, Chesney J, Chesney RW, Mazess RB: Demineralization in cystic fibrosis, *Am J Dis Child* 133:632-635, 1979.
79. Reiter EO, Brugman SM, Pike JW, Pitt M, Dokoh S, Haussler MR, Gerstle RS, Taussig LM: Vitamin D metabolites in adolescents and young adults with cystic fibrosis: effects of sun and season, *J Pediatr* 106:21-26, 1985.
80. Hanly JG, McKenna MJ, Quigley C, Freaney R, Muldowney FP, Fitzgerald MX: Hypovitaminosis D and response to supplementation in older patients with cystic fibrosis, *Q J Med* 219:377-385, 1985.
81. Gibbens DT, Gilsanz V, Boechat MI, Dufer D, Carlson ME, Wang CI: Osteoporosis in cystic fibrosis, *J Pediatr* 113:295-300, 1988.
82. Henderson RC, Madsen CD: Bone density in children and adolescents with cystic fibrosis, *J Pediatr* 128:28-34, 1996.
83. Farrell PM, Bieri JG, Frantantoni JF, Wood RE, di Sant'Agnese PA: The occurrence and effects of human vitamin E deficiency, *J Clin Invest* 60:233-241, 1977.
84. Dolan TF: Hemolytic anemia and edema as the initial signs in infants with cystic fibrosis, *Clin Pediatr* 15:597-600, 1976.
85. Wilfond BS, Farrell PM, Laxova A, Mischler E: Severe hemolytic anemia associated with vitamin E deficiency in infants with cystic fibrosis, *Clin Pediatr* 33:2-7, 1994.
86. Elias E, Muller DPR, Scott J: Association of spinocerebellar disorders with cystic fibrosis or chronic childhood cholestasis and low serum vitamin E, *Lancet* 2:1319-1321,1981.
87. Sitrin MD, Lieberman F, Jensen WE: Vitamin E deficiency and neurologic disease in adults with cystic fibrosis, *Ann Intern Med* 107:51-54, 1987.
88. Sung JH: Neuroaxonal dystrophy in mucoviscidosis, *J Neuropathol Exp Neurol* 23:567-583, 1964.
89. Tortenson OL, Humphrey GB, Edson JR, Warwick WJ: Cystic fibrosis presenting with severe hemorrhage due to vitamin K malabsorption: a report of three cases, *Pediatrics* 45:857-860, 1970.
90. Walters TR, Koch HF: Hemorrhagic diathesis and cystic fibrosis in infancy, *Am J Dis Child* 124:641-642, 1972.
91. Cornelissen EAM, van Lieburg AF, Motohara K, van Oostrom CG: Vitamin K status in cystic fibrosis, *Acta Paediatr* 81:658-661, 1992.
92. Solomons NW, Wagonfield JB, Rieger C: Some biochemical indices of nutrition in treated patients with cystic fibrosis, *Am J Clin Nutr* 34:462-474, 1981.
93. Lloyd-Still JD, Ganther HE: Selenium and glutathione peroxidase levels in cystic fibrosis, *Pediatrics* 65:1010-1012, 1980.
94. Stead RJ, Redington AN, Hinks LJ, Clayton BE, Hodson ME, Batten JC: Selenium deficiency and possible increased risks of carcinoma in adults with cystic fibrosis, *Lancet* 2:862-863, 1985.
95. Green CG, Doershuk CF, Stern RC: Symptomatic hypomagnesemia in cystic fibrosis, *J Pediatr* 107:425-428, 1985.
96. Godson C, Ryan MP, Brady HR, Bourke S, Fitzgerald MX: Acute hypomagnesaemia complicating the treatment of meconium ileus equivalent in cystic fibrosis, *Scand J Gastroenterol* 23(suppl 143):148-150, 1988.
97. Both CC, Babouris N, Hanna S, MacIntyre I: Incidence of hypomagnesemia in intestinal malabsorption, *Br Med J* 3:141-144, 1963.
98. Caplan A, Gross S: Hematologic and serologic studies in cystic fibrosis, *J Pediatr* 73:540-547, 1968.
99. Vichinsky EP, Pennathur-Das R, Nickerson B: Inadequate erythroid response to hypoxia in cystic fibrosis, *J Pediatr* 105:15-21, 1984.
100. Ater JL, Herbst JJ, Landaw SA, O'Brien RT: Relative anemia and iron deficiency in cystic fibrosis, *Pediatrics* 71:810-814, 1983.
101. Ehrhardt P, Miller MG, Littlewood JM: Iron deficiency in cystic fibrosis, *Arch Dis Child* 62:185-187, 1987.
102. Farrell PM, Mischler EH, Engle MJ, Brown J, Lau S-M: Fatty acid abnormalities in cystic fibrosis, *Pediatr Res* 19:104-109, 1985.
103. Campbell IM, Crozier DN, Caton RB: Abnormal fatty acid composition and impaired oxygen supply in cystic fibrosis patients, *Pediatrics* 57: 480-486, 1976.
104. Rosenlund ML, Selekman JA, Kim HK, Kritchevsky D: Dietary essential fatty acids in cystic fibrosis, *Pediatrics* 59:428-432, 1977.
105. Landon C, Kerner JA, Castillo R, Adams L, Whalen R, Lewiston NJ: Oral correction of essential fatty acid deficiency in cystic fibrosis, *J Parenter Enter Nutr* 5:501-504, 1981.
106. Hubbard VS, Dunn GD, Di Sant'Agnese PA: Abnormal fatty acid composition of plasma lipids in cystic fibrosis: a primary or secondary defect, *Lancet* 2:1302, 1977.
107. Elliott RB: A therapeutic trial of fatty acid supplementation in cystic fibrosis, *Pediatrics* 57:474-479, 1976.
108. Chase HP, Cotton EK, Elliott RB: Intravenous linoleic acid supplementation in children with cystic fibrosis, *Pediatrics* 64:207-213, 1979.
109. Lloyd-Still JD, Simon SH, Wessel HU, Gibson LE: Negative effects of oral fatty acid supplementation on sweat chloride in cystic fibrosis, *Pediatrics* 64:50-52, 1979.
110. Petersen W, Heilmann C, Garne S: Pancreatic enzyme supplementation as acid-resistant microspheres versus enteric-coated granules in cystic fibrosis, *Acta Paediatr Scand* 76:66-69, 1967.
111. Beverley DW, Kelleher J, MacDonald A, Littlewood JM, Robinson T, Walters MP: Comparison of four pancreatic extracts in cystic fibrosis, *Arch Dis Child* 62:564-568, 1987.
112. Meyer JH, Elashoff J, Porter-Fink V, Dressman J, Amidon GL: Human postprandial gastric emptying of 1-3 millimeter spheres, *Gastroenterol* 94:1315-1325, 1988.
113. Borowitz DS, Grand RJ, Durie PR, Consensus Committee: Use of pancreatic enzyme supplements for patients with cystic fibrosis in the context of fibrosing colonopathy, *J Pediatr* 127:681-684, 1995.
114. Fitzsimmons SC, Burkhart GA, Borowitz D, Grand RJ, Hammerstom T, Durie PR, Lloyd-Still JD, Lowenfels AB: High-dose pancreatic-enzyme supplements and fibrosing colonopathy in children with cystic fibrosis, *N Engl J Med* 336:1283-1289, 1997.
115. Cox KL, Isenberg JN, Osher AB, Dooley RR: The effect of cimetidine on maldigestion in cystic fibrosis, *J Pediatr* 94:448-492, 1979.
116. Carroccio A, Pardo F, Montalto G, Lapichino L, Soresi M, Averna MR, Iacono G, Notarbartola A: Use of famotidine in severe exocrine pancreatic insufficiency with persistent maldigestion on enzymatic replacement therapy: a long-term study in cystic fibrosis, *Dig Dis Sci* 37:1441-1446, 1992.
117. Robinson P, Sly PD: Placebo-controlled trial of misoprostol in cystic fibrosis, *J Pediatr Gastroenterol Nutr* 11:37-40, 1990.
118. Heijerman HG, Lamers CB, Baker W: Omeprazole enhances the efficacy of pancreatin (pancrease) in cystic fibrosis, *Ann Intern Med* 114:200-201, 1991.
119. Robinson PJ, Sly PD: High dose pancreatic enzymes in cystic fibrosis, *Arch Dis Child* 65:311-312, 1990.
120. Smyth RL, Van Velzen D, Smyth AR, Lloyd DA, Heaf DP: Strictures of the ascending colon in cystic fibrosis and high-strength pancreatic enzymes, *Lancet* 343:85-86, 1994.
121. Pettei MJ, Leonidas JC, Levine JJ, Gorvoy JD: Pancolonic disease in cystic fibrosis and high-dose pancreatic enzyme therapy, *J Pediatr* 125: 587-589, 1994.
122. MacSweeney E, Oades PJ, Buchdahl RM, Phelan M, Bush A: Relationship betweeen ultrasonic colonic thickening and pancreatic enzymes, *Pediatr Pulmonol* 10(suppl):274, 1994.
123. Davidson GP, Hassel FM, Crozier D, Corey M, Forstner GG: Iatrogenic hyperuricemia in children with cystic fibrosis, *J Pediatr* 93:976-978, 1978.
124. Stapleton FB, Kennedy J, Nousia-Arvanitakis S, Linshaw MA: Hyperuricosuria due to high-dose pancreatic extract therapy in cystic fibrosis, *N Engl J Med* 295:246-248, 1976.
125. Twarog FJ, Weinstein SF, Khaw KT, Strieder DJ, Colten HR: Hypersensitivity to pancreatic extracts in parents of patients with cystic fibrosis, *J Allergy Clin Immunol* 59:35-40, 1977.
126. Askula A: Bronchial asthma due to allergy to pancreatic extract: a hazard in the treatment of cystic fibrosis, *Br J Dis Chest* 71:295-299, 1977.
127. Ganier M, Lieberman P: IgE mediated hypersensitivity to pancreatic extract (PE) in parents of cystic fibrosis (CF) children, *Clin Allergy* 9:125-132, 1979.

Nutritional Management

128. Luder E, Kattan M, Thornton JC, Koehler KM, Bonforte RJ: Efficacy of a nonrestricted fat diet in patients with cystic fibrosis, *Am J Dis Child* 143:458-464, 1989.
129. Levy LD, Durie PR, Pencharz PB, Corey ML: Effects of long-term nutritional rehabilitation on body composition and clinical status in malnourished children and adolescents with cystic fibrosis, *J Pediatr* 107:225-230, 1985.

130. Shepherd RW, Holt TL, Thomas BJ, Kay L, Isles A, Francis PJ, Ward LC: Nutritional rehabilitation in cystic fibrosis: controlled studies of effects on nutritional growth retardation, body protein turnover, and course of pulmonary disease, *J Pediatr* 109:788-794, 1986.
131. Boland MP, Stoski DS, MacDonald NE, Soucy P: Chronic jejunostomy feeding with a non-elemental formula in under-nourished patients with cystic fibrosis, *Lancet* 1:232-234, 1986.
132. Moore MC, Greene HL, Donald WD, Dunn GD: Enteral-tube feeding as adjunct therapy in malnourished patients with cystic fibrosis: a clinical study and literature review, *Am J Clin Nutr* 44:33-41, 1986.
133. O'Loughlin E, Forbes D, Parsons H, Scott B, Cooper D, Gall G: Nutritional rehabilitation of malnourished patients with cystic fibrosis, *Am J Clin Nutr* 43:732-737, 1986.
134. Shepherd RW, Holt TL, Cleghorn G, Ward LC, Isles A, Francis P: Short-term nutritional supplementation during management of pulmonary exacerbations in cystic fibrosis: a controlled study, including effects of protein turnover, *Am J Clin Nutr* 48:235-239, 1988.
135. Steinkamp G, von der Hardt H: Improvement of nutritional status and lung function after long-term nocturnal gastrostomy feedings in cystic fibrosis, *J Pediatr* 124:244-249, 1994.
136. Belli DC, Levy E, Darling P, Leroy C, Lepage G, Giguere R, Roy CC: Taurine improves the absorption of a fat meal in patients with cystic fibrosis, *Pediatrics* 80:517-523, 1987.
137. Darling PB, Lepage G, Leroy C, Masson P, Roy CC: Effect of taurine supplements on fat absorption in cystic fibrosis, *Pediatr Res* 19:578-582, 1985.
138. Thompson GN, Robb TA, Davidson GP: Taurine supplementation, fat absorption, and growth in cystic fibrosis, *J Pediatr* 111:501-506, 1987.

Pancreatitis

139. Atlas AB, Orenstein SR, Orenstein DM: Pancreatitis in young children with cystic fibrosis, *J Pediatr* 120:756-759, 1992.
140. Masaryk TJ, Achkar E: Pancreatitis as initial presentation of cystic fibrosis in young adults: a report of two cases, *Dig Dis Sci* 28:874-878, 1983.
141. Shepard RW, Cleghorn GJ: The pancreas: clinical aspects and investigation of pancreatic function. In Shepherd RW, Cleghorn GJ, eds: *Cystic fibrosis: nutritional and intestinal disorders,* Boca Raton, Fla, 1989, CRC Press, pp 87-90.
142. Slaff J, Jacobson D, Tillman CR, Curington C, Toskes P: Protease-specific suppression of pancreatic exocrine secretion, *Gastroenterology* 87:44-52, 1984.

Pancreatic Endocrine Deficiency

143. Iannucci A, Mukai K, Johnson D, Burke B: Endocrine pancreas in cystic fibrosis: an immunohistochemical study, *Hum Pathol* 15:278-284, 1984.
144. Soejima K, Landing BH: Pancreatic islets in older patients with cystic fibrosis with and without diabetes mellitus: morphometric and immunocytologic studies, *Pediatr Pathol* 6:25-46, 1986.
145. Brown RE, Madge GE: Cystic fibrosis and nesidioblastosis, *Arch Pathol* 92:53-57, 1971.
146. Abdul-Karim FW, Dahms BB, Velasco ME, Rodman HM: Islets of Langerhans in adolescents and adults with cystic fibrosis, *Arch Pathol Lab Med* 110:602-606, 1986.
147. Schwartz RH, Milner MR: Other manifestations and organ involvement. In Taussig LN, ed: *Cystic fibrosis,* New York, 1984, Thieme-Stratton.
148. Geffner ME, Lippe BM, MacLaren NK, Riley WJ: Role of autoimmunity in insulinopenia and carbohydrate derangements associated with cystic fibrosis, *J Pediatr* 112:419-420, 1988.
149. Knowles MR: Diabetes and cystic fibrosis: new questions emerging from increased longevity, *J Pediatr* 112:415-416, 1988.
150. Schwarz HP, Bonnard GD, Neri TM, Braga S, Zuppinger KA: Histocompatibility antigens in patients with cystic fibrosis and diabetes mellitus, *J Pediatr* 104:799-800, 1984.
151. Stutchfield PR, O'Halloran SM, Smith CS, Woodrow JC, Bottazzo GF, Heaf D: HLA type, islet cell antibodies, and glucose intolerance in cystic fibrosis, *Arch Dis Child* 63:1234-1239, 1988.
152. Geffner ME, Lippe BM, Itami RM, Kaplan SA, Billard BK, Levin SR, Taylor IL: Insulin resistance in a young man with cystic fibrosis, *Am J Dis Child* 138:677-680, 1984.
153. Milner AD: Blood glucose and serum insulin levels in children with cystic fibrosis, *Arch Dis Child* 44:351-355, 1969.
154. Buchanan KD, Kerr JI, Johnston CF, Redmond AO, Craig BG: The diffuse endocrine system in cystic fibrosis, *Scand J Gastroenterol* (suppl)82:155-163, 1983.
155. Moran A, Diem P, Klein DJ, Levitt MD, Robertson RP: Pancreatic endocrine function in cystic fibrosis, *J Pediatr* 118:15-23, 1991.
156. Adrian TE, McKieran J, Johnstone DI, Hiller EJ, Sarson DL, Bloom SR: Hormonal abnormalities of the pancreas and gut in cystic fibrosis, *Gastroenterology* 79:460-465, 1980.
157. Stahl M, Girard J, Rutishauser M, Nars PW, Zuppinger K: Endocrine function of the pancreas in cystic fibrosis: evidence for an impaired glucagon and insulin response following arginine infusion, *J Pediatr* 84:821-824, 1974.
158. Geffner ME, Lippe BM, Kaplan SA, Itami RM, Gillard BK, Levin SR, Taylor IL: Carbohydrate tolerance in cystic fibrosis is closely linked to pancreatic exocrine function, *Pediatr Res* 18:1107-1111, 1984.
159. Dandone P, Hodson ME, Batten JC: β cell reserve in cystic fibrosis patients and heterozygotes, *J Clin Pathol* 36:790-792, 1983.
160. Allen JL: Progressive nephropathy in a patient with cystic fibrosis and diabetes, *N Engl J Med* 315:764, 1986.
161. Sullivan MM, Denning CR: Diabetic microangiopathy in cystic fibrosis, *Pediatrics* 84:642-647, 1989.
162. Rodman HM, Waltman SR, Krupin T, Lee AT, Frank KE, Matthews LW: Quantitative vitreous fluorophotometry in insulin-treated cystic fibrosis patients, *Diabetes* 32:505-508, 1983.
163. Dolan TF: Microangiopathy in a young adult with cystic fibrosis and diabetes mellitus, *N Engl J Med* 314:991-992, 1986.
164. Lanng S, Thorsteinsson B, Lund-Andersen C, Nerup J, Schiotz PO, Koch C: Diabetes mellitus in Danish cystic fibrosis patients: prevalence and late diabetic complications, *Acta Paediatr Scand* 83:72-77, 1994.
165. Van Yuk JJ, Underwood LE, Hintz RL, Clemmans DR, Viona SJ, Weaver RP: The somatomedins: a family of insulin-like hormones under growth hormone control, *Rec Prog Horm Res* 30:259-318, 1974.
166. Lanng S, Thorsteinsson B, Nerup J, Koch C: Influence of the development of diabetes mellitus on clinical status in patients with cystic fibrosis, *Eur J Pediatr* 151:684-687, 1992.
167. Lippe BM, Kaplan SA, Neufeld ND, Smith A, Scott M: Insulin receptors in cystic fibrosis: increased receptor number and altered affinity, *Pediatrics* 65:1018-1022, 1980.
168. Rodman HM, Doershuk CF, Roland JM: The interaction of 2 diseases: diabetes mellitus and cystic fibrosis, *Medicine* (Baltimore) 65:389-397, 1986.
169. Finkelstein SM, Wielinski CL, Elliot GR, Warwick WJ, Barbosa J, Wu S-C, Klein DJ: Diabetes mellitus associated with cystic fibrosis, *J Pediatr* 112:373-377, 1988.
170. Reisman J, Corey M, Canny G, Levison H: Diabetes mellitus in patients with cystic fibrosis: effect on survival, *Pediatrics* 86:374-377, 1990.
171. Moran A: Diabetes and glucose intolerance in cystic fibrosis, *New Insights into Cystic Fibrosis* 5:1-6, 1997.
172. Lanng S, Hansen A, Thorsteinsson B, Nerup J, Koch C: Glucose tolerance in patients with cystic fibrosis: five years propsective study, *Br Med J* 311:655-659, 1995.
173. Kane RE, Black P: Glucose intolerance with low-, medium-, and high-carbohydrate formulas during nighttime enteral feedings in cystic fibrosis patients, *J Pediatr Gastroenterol Nutr* 8:321-326, 1989.

Hepatobiliary Disease

174. Oppenheimer EH, Esterly JR: Hepatic changes in young infants with cystic fibrosis: possible relation to focal biliary cirrhosis, *J Pediatr* 86:683-689, 1975.
175. Lindblad A, Hultcrantz R, Strandvik B: Bile-duct destruction and collagen deposition: a prominent ultrastructural feature of the liver in cystic fibrosis, *Hepatology* 16:372-381, 1992.
176. Webster R, Williams H: Hepatic cirrhosis associated with fibrocystic disease of the pancreas, *Arch Dis Child* 28:343-350, 1953.
177. di Sant'Agnese PA, Blanc WA: A distinctive type of biliary cirrhosis of the liver associated with cystic fibrosis of the pancreas, *Pediatrics* 18:387-409, 1956.
178. Craig JM, Haddad H, Shwachman H: The pathological changes in the liver in cystic fibrosis of the pancreas, *Am J Dis Child* 93:357-369, 1957.
179. Gatzimos CD, Jowitt RH: Jaundice in mucoviscidosis (fibrocystic disease of pancreas), *Am J Dis Child* 89:182-186, 1955.
180. Talamo RC, Hendren WH: Prolonged obstructive jaundice, *Am J Dis Child* 115:74-79, 1968.

181. Perkins WG, Klein GL, Beckerman RC: Cystic fibrosis mistaken for idiopathic biliary atresia, *Clin Pediatr* 24:107-109, 1985.
182. Taylor WF, Qaqundah BY: Neonatal jaundice associated with cystic fibrosis, *Am J Dis Child* 123:161-162, 1972.
183. Valman HB, France NE, Wallis PG: Prolonged neonatal jaundice in cystic fibrosis, *Arch Dis Child* 46:805-809, 1971.
184. Lykavieris P, Bernard O, Hadchove I: Neonatal cholestasis as the presenting feature in cystic fibrosis, *Arch Dis Child* 75:67-70, 1996.
185. Lloyd-Still JD, Crussi F: Hepatic complications in cystic fibrosis (CF): clinical and pathological features, *CF Club Abstracts* 25:163, 1984.
186. Kulczycki LL: In quarterly annotated references to Cystic Fibrosis, Vol VI, p. 2. National Cystic Fibrosis Research Foundation, 1967, New York (editorial).
187. Evans JS, George DE, Mollit D: Infusion therapy in the inspissated bile syndrome of cystic fibrosis, *J Pediatr Gastroenterol Nutr* 12:131-135, 1991.
188. Vitullo BB, Rochon L, Seemayer TA, Beardmore H, de Belle RC: Intrapancreatic compression of the common bile duct in cystic fibrosis, *J Pediatr* 93:1060-1061, 1978.
189. Schwarz HP, Kraemer R, Thurnheer U, Rossi E: Liver involvement in cystic fibrosis, *Helv Paediat Acta* 33:351-364, 1978.
190. Rosenstein BJ, Oppenheimer EH: Prolonged obstructive jaundice and giant cell hepatitis in an infant with cystic fibrosis, *J Pediatr* 91:1022-1023, 1977.
191. Oppenheimer EH, Esterly JR: Congenital cytomegalovirus infection and bile duct obstruction in newborn infant with cystic fibrosis of pancreas, *Lancet* 2:1031-1032, 1973.
192. Furuya KN, Roberts EA, Canny GJ, Phillips MJ: Neonatal hepatitis syndrome with paucity of interlobular bile ducts in cystic fibrosis, *J Pediatr Gastroenterol Nutr* 12:127-130, 1991.
193. Wilroy RS, Crawford SE, Johnson WW: Cystic fibrosis with extensive fat replacement of the liver, *J Pediatr* 68:67-73, 1966.
194. Treem WR, Stanley CA: Massive hepatomegaly, steatosis, and secondary plasma carnitine deficiency in an infant with cystic fibrosis, *Pediatrics* 83:993-997, 1989.
195. Stern RC, Stevens DP, Boat TF, Doershuk CF, Izant RJ, Matthews LW: Symptomatic hepatic disease in cystic fibrosis: incidence, course, and outcome of portal systemic shunting, *Gastroenterology* 70:645-649, 1976.
196. Scott-Jupp R, Lama M, Tanner MS: Prevalance of liver disease in cystic fibrosis, *Arch Dis Child* 66:698-701, 1991.
197. Shuster SR, Shwachman H, Toyama WM, Rubino A, Khaw K-T: The management of portal hypertension in cystic fibrosis, *J Pediatr Surg* 12:201-206, 1977.
198. Quattrucci S, Dallapiccola B, Leoni G, Zanda M, Romano L, Devoto M: Cystic fibrosis patients with liver disease are not genetically distinct, *Am J Hum Genet* 48:815-816, 1991.
199. Colombo C, Apostolo MG, Ferrari M, Seia M, Genoni S, Guinta A, Sereni LP: Analysis of risk factors for the development of liver disease associated with cystic fibrosis, *J Pediatr* 124:393-399, 1994.
200. Sinaasappel M: Hepatobiliary pathology in patients with cystic fibrosis, *Acta Paediatr Scand* 363(suppl):45-51, 1989.
201. Psacharopoulos HT, Howard ER, Portmann B, Mowat AP: Hepatic complications of cystic fibrosis, *Lancet* 2:78-80, 1981.
202. Goodchild MC, Banks AJ, Drolc Z, Anderson CM: Liver scans in cystic fibrosis, *Arch Dis Child* 50:813-815, 1975.
203. Cunningham DG, Churchill RJ, Reynes CJ: Computed tomography in the evaluation of liver disease in cystic fibrosis patients, *J Comp Assist Tomography* 4:151-154, 1980.
204. Willi UV, Reddish JM, Telle RL: Cystic fibrosis: its characteristic appearance on abdominal ultrasonography, *Am J Radiol* 134:1005-1010, 1980.
205. Wilson-Sharp RC, Irving HC, Brown RC, Chalmers DM, Littlewood JM: Ultrasonography of the pancreas, liver and biliary system in cystic fibrosis, *Arch Dis Child* 59:923-926, 1984.
206. Gaskin KJ, Waters DLM, Howman-Giles R, De Silva M, Earl JW, Martin HCO, Kan AE, Brown JM, Dorney SFA: Liver disease and common-bile-duct stenosis in cystic fibrosis, *N Engl J Med* 318:340-346, 1988.
207. Roy CC, Lenaerts C, Garel L, Patriquin H, Weber AM: Biliary disease in cystic fibrosis, *N Engl J Med* 319:312-313, 1988.
208. Nagel RA, Javaid A, Meire HB, Wise A, Westaby D, Kavani J, Lombard MG, Williams R: Liver disease and bile duct abnormalities in adults with cystic fibrosis, *Lancet* 2:1422-1425, 1989.
209. Bern EM, Grand RJ: Management of therapy for hepatobiliary disease in cyctic fibrosis, *New Insights into Cystic Fibrosis* 4:4-8, 1996.
210. Cox KL, Ward RE, Furgiuele TL, Cannon RA, Sanders KD, Kurland G: Orthotopic liver transplantation in patients with cystic fibrosis, *Pediatrics* 80:571-574, 1987.
211. Mieles LA, Orenstein D, Teperman L, Podesta L, Koneu B, Starzl TE: Liver transplantation in cystic fibrosis, *Lancet* 1:1073, 1989.
212. Cotting J, Lentze MJ, Reichen J: Effects of ursodeoxycholic acid treatment on nutrition and liver function in patients with cystic fibrosis and longstanding cholestasis, *Gut* 31:918-921, 1990.
213. Colombo C, Setchell KDR, Podda M, Crosignani A, Ruda A, Curcio L, Ronchi M, Giunta A: Effects of urso-deoxycholic acid therapy for liver disease associated with cystic fibrosis, *J Pediatr* 117:482-489, 1990.
214. Galabert C, Montet JC, Lengrand D, Lecuire A, Sotta C, Figarella C, Chazalette JP: Effects of ursodeoxycholic acid on liver function in patients with cystic fibrosis and chronic cholestasis, *J Pediatr* 121:138-141, 1992.
215. LePage G, Paradis K, Lacaille F, Senechal L, Ronco N, Champagne J, Lenaerts C, Roy CC, Rasquin-Weber A: Ursodeoxycholic acid improves the hepatic metabolism of essential fatty acids and retinol in children with cystic fibrosis, *J Pediatr* 130:52-58, 1997.
216. Esterly JR, Oppenheimer EH: Observations in cystic fibrosis of the pancreas. I. The gallbladder. *Bull Johns Hopkins Hosp* 110:247-254, 1962.
217. Oppenheimer EH, Esterly JR: Pathology of cystic fibrosis: review of the literature and comparison with 146 autopsied cases, *Perspec Pediatr Pathol* 2:241-278, 1975.
218. Isenberg JN, L'Heureux PR, Warwick WJ, Sharp HL: Clinical observations on the biliary system in cystic fibrosis, *Am J Gastroenterol* 65:134-141, 1976.
219. L'Heureux, Isenberg JN, Sharp HL, Warwick WJ: Gallbladder disease in cystic fibrosis, *Am J Roentgenol* 128:953-956, 1977.
220. Wilson-Sharp RC, Irving HC, Brown RC, Chalmers DM, Littlewood JM: Ultrasonography of the pancreas, liver, and biliary system in cystic fibrosis, *Arch Dis Child* 59:923-926, 1984.
221. Stern RC, Rothstein FC, Doershuk CF: Treatment and prognosis of symptomatic gallbladder disease in patients with cystic fibrosis, *J Pediatr Gastroenterol Nutr* 5:35-40, 1986.
222. Strandvik B, Hjelte L, Gabrielsson N, Glaumann H: Sclerosing cholangitis in cystic fibrosis, *Scand J Gastroenterol* 23(suppl 143):121-124, 1988.
223. Abdul-Karim FW, King TA, Dahms BB, Gauderer MWL, Boat TF: Carcinoma of extrahepatic biliary system in an adult with cystic fibrosis, *Gastroenterology* 82:758-762, 1982.
224. Forstner J, Wesley A, Mantle M, Kopelman H, Man D, Forstner GG: Abnormal mucus: nominated but not yet elected, *J Pediatr Gastroenterol Nutr* 3(suppl):567-673, 1984.
225. Roy CC, Weber AM, Morin CL, Combes JC, Nussle D, Megevand A, Lasalle R: Abnormal biliary lipid composition in cystic fibrosis, *N Engl J Med* 297:1301-1305, 1977.
226. Weber AM, Roy CC, Morin CL, LaSalle R: Malabsorption of bile acids in children with cystic fibrosis *N Engl J Med* 289:1001-1005, 1973.
227. Goodchild MC, Murphy GM, Howell AM, Nutter SA, Anderson CM: Aspects of bile acid metabolism in cystic fibrosis, *Arch Dis Child* 50:769-778, 1975.
228. Watkins JB, Tercyak AM, Szczepanik P, Klein PD: Bile salt kinetics in cystic fibrosis (CF), *Gastroenterology* 67:835A, 1974.
229. Weizman Z, Durie PR, Kopelman HR, Vesley SM, Forstner GG: Bile acid secretion in cystic fibrosis: evidence of a defect unrelated to fat malabsorption, *Gut* 27:1043-1048, 1986.
230. Becker M, Stabb D, Leiss O, von Bergman K: Biliary acid composition in patients with cystic fibrosis, *J Pediatr Gastroenterol Nutr* 8:308-312,1989.
231. Angelico M, Gandin C, Canuzzi P, Bertasi S, Cantafora A, DeSantis A, Quattrucci S, Antonelli M: Gallstones in cystic fibrosis: a critical reappraisal, *Hepatology* 14:768-775, 1991.
232. Edelman DS: Laparoscopic cholecystectomy under continuous epidural anesthesia in patients with cystic fibrosis, *Am J Dis Child* 145:723-724, 1991.
233. Salh B, Howat J, Webb K: Ursodeoxycholic acid dissolution of gallstones in cystic fibrosis, *Thorax* 43:490-491, 1988.

Gastroesophageal Reflux

234. Fiegelson J, Girault F, Pecau Y: Gastro-oesophageal reflux and esophagitis in cystic fibrosis, *Acta Paediatr Scand* 76:989-990, 1987.

235. Gustafsson PM, Gransson S-G, Kjellman N-IM, Tibbling L: Gastro-oesophageal reflux and severity of pulmonary disease in cystic fibrosis, *Scand J Gastroenterol* 26:449-456, 1991.
236. Bendig DW, Seilheimer DK, Wagner ML, Ferry GD, Harrison GM: Complications of gastroesophageal reflux in patients with cystic fibrosis, *J Pediatr* 100:536-540, 1982.
237. Scott RB, O'Loughlin EV, Gall DG: Gastroesophageal reflux in patients with cystic fibrosis, *J Pediatr* 106:223-227, 1985.
238. Cucchiara S, Santamarie F, Andreotti MR, Minella R, Erocolini P, Oggero V, de Ritis G: Mechanisms of gastro-oesophageal reflux in cystic fibrosis, *Arch Dis Child* 66:617-622, 1991.
239. Malfroot A, Dab I: New insights on gastro-oesophageal reflux in cystic fibrosis by longitudinal follow up, *Arch Dis Child* 66:1339-1345, 1991.
240. Orenstein SR, Orenstein DM: Gastroesophageal reflux and respiratory disease in children, *J Pediatr* 112:847-858, 1988.
241. Vandenplas Y, Diericx A, Blecker U, et al: Esophageal pH monitoring data during chest physiotherapy, *Gastroenterol Nutr* 13:23-26, 1991.
242. Button BM, Heine RG, Catto-Smith AG, Phelan PD, Olinsky A: Postural drainage and gastro-oesophageal reflux in infants with cystic fibrosis, *Arch Dis Child* 76:148-150, 1997.
243. Thomas D, Rothberg RM, Lester LA: Cystic fibrosis and gastro-esophageal reflux in infancy, *Am J Dis Child* 139:66-67, 1985.
244. Frates RC, Cox KL: Cystic fibrosis mistaken for gastro-esophageal reflux with aspiration, *Am J Dis Child* 135:719-720, 1981.

Peptic Ulcer Disease

245. Cox K, Isenberg JN, Ament NE: Gastric acid hypersecretion in cystic fibrosis, *J Pediatr Gastroenterol Nutr* 1:559-565, 1982.
246. Zasly L, Baum GL, Rumball JM: The incidence of peptic ulceration in chronic obstructive pulmonary emphysema, *Chest* 37:400-405, 1960.
247. Dreiling DA, Naqvi MA: Peptic ulcer diathesis in patients with chronic pancreatitis, *Am J Gastroenterol* 51:503-510, 1969.
248. Shwachman H: Gastrointestinal manifestations of cystic fibrosis, *Pediatr Clin North Am* 22:787-805, 1975.
249. Taussig LM, Saldino RM, di Sant'Agnese PA: Radiographic abnormalities of the duodenum and small bowel in cystic fibrosis of the pancreas, *Radiology* 106:369-376, 1973.
250. di Sant'Agnese PA, Davis PB: Cystic fibrosis in adults, *Am J Med* 66:121-132, 1979.
251. Rosenstein BJ, Perman JA, Kramer SS: Peptic ulcer disease in cystic fibrosis: an unusual occurrence in black adolescents, *Am J Dis Child* 140:966-969, 1986.
252. Oppenheimer EH, Esterly JR: Pathology of cystic fibrosis: review of the literature and comparison with 146 autopsied cases, *Perspect Pediatr Pathol* 2:241-278, 1975.

Duodenal Abnormalities

253. Fiedorek SC, Shulman RJ, Klish WJ: Endoscopic detection of peptic ulcer disease in cystic fibrosis, *Clin Pediatr* 25:243-246, 1986.
254. Phelan MS, Fine DR, Zentler-Munro PH, Hodson ME, Batten JC, Kerr IH: Radiographic abnormalities of the duodenum in cystic fibrosis, *Clin Radiol* 34:573-577, 1983.

Distal Intestinal Obstruction Syndrome

255. Mullins F, Talamo R, di Sant'Agnese PA: Late intestinal complications of cystic fibrosis, *JAMA* 192:741-746, 1965.
256. Hodson ME, Mearns MB, Batten JC: Meconium ileus equivalent in adults with cystic fibrosis of pancreas: a report of six cases, *Br Med J* 2:790-791, 1976.
257. Matseshe JW, Go VLW, DiMagno EP: Meconium ileus equivalent complicating cystic fibrosis in postneonatal children and young adults, *Gastroenterology* 72:732-736, 1977.
258. Rubenstein S, Moss R, Lewiston N: Constipation and meconium ileus equivalent in patients with cystic fibrosis, *Pediatrics* 78:473-479, 1986.
259. Koletzko S, Stringer DA, Cleghorn GJ, Durie PR: Lavage treatment of distal intestinal obstruction syndrome in children with cystic fibrosis, *Pediatrics* 83:727-733, 1989.
260. Gavin J, Ellis J, Dewar AL, Rolles CJ, Connett GJ: Dietary fibre and the occurrence of gut symptoms in cystic fibrosis, *Arch Dis Child* 76:35-37, 1997.
261. DeBraekeleer M, Allard C, LeBlanc J-P, Aubin G, Simard F: Is meconium ileus genetically determined or associated with a more severe evolution of cystic fibrosis? *J Med Genet* 35:262-263, 1998.
262. Andersen HO, Hjelt K, Waever E, Overgaard K: The age-related incidence of meconium ileus equivalent in a cystic fibrosis population: the impact of high-energy intake, *J Pediatr Gastroenterol Nutr* 11:356-360, 1990.
263. Dilling DW, Steiner GM: The radiology of meconium ileus equivalent, *Br J Radiol* 54:562-565, 1981.
264. Cleghorn GJ, Stringer DA, Forstner GG, Durie PR: Treatment of distal intestinal obstruction syndrome in cystic fibrosis with a balanced intestinal lavage solution, *Lancet* 1:8-11, 1986.
265. Apelgren KN, Yuen JC: Distal colonic impaction requiring laparotomy in an adult with cystic fibrosis, *J Clin Gastroenterol* 11:687-690, 1989.
266. Prinsen JE, Thomas M: Cisapride in cystic fibrosis, *Lancet* 1:512-513, 1985.
267. Koletzko S, Corey M, Ellis L, Spino M, Stringer DS, Durie PR: Effects of cisapride in patients with cystic fibrosis and distal intestinal obstruction syndrome, *J Pediatr* 117:815-822, 1990.

Intussusception

268. Holsclaw DS, Rocmans C, Shwachman H: Intussusception in patients with cystic fibrosis, *Pediatrics* 48:51-58, 1971.
269. Holmes M, Murphy V, Taylor M, Denham B: Intussusception in cystic fibrosis, *Arch Dis Child* 66:726-727, 1991.

Appendiceal Disease

270. McIntosh JC, Mroczek EC, Baldwin C, Mestre J: Intussusception of the appendix in a patient with cystic fibrosis, *J Pediatr Gastroenterol Nutr* 110:542-544,1990.
271. Andersen DH: Pathology of cystic fibrosis, *Ann NY Acad Sci* 93:500-517, 1962.
272. Oestreich AE, Adelstein EH: Appendicitis as the presenting complaint in cystic fibrosis, *J Pediatr Surg* 17:191-194, 1982.
273. Shwachman H, Holsclaw D: Examination of the appendix at laparotomy as a diagnostic clue in cystic fibrosis, *N Engl J Med* 286:1300-1301, 1972.
274. Dolan TF, Meyers A: Mild cystic fibrosis presenting as an asymptomatic distended appendiceal mass: a case report, *Clin Pediatr* 9:862-863, 1975.
275. McCarthy VP, Mischler EH, Hubbard VS, Chernick MS, di Sant' Agnese PA: Appendiceal abscess in cystic fibrosis: a diagnostic challenge, *Gastroenterol* 86:564-568, 1984.
276. Shields MD, Levison H, Reisman JJ, Durie PR, Canny GJ: Appendicitis in cystic fibrosis, *Arch Dis Child* 65:307-310, 1991.
277. Coughlin JP, Gauderer MWL, Stern RC, Doershuk CF, Izant RJ, Zollinger RM: The spectrum of appendiceal disease in cystic fibrosis, *J Pediatr Surg* 25:835-839, 1990.
278. Fletcher BD, Abramowksy CR: Contrast enemas in cystic fibrosis: implications of appendiceal nonfilling, *Am J Radiol* 137:323-326, 1981.
279. Allen ED, Pfaff JK, Taussig LM, McCoy KS: The clinical spectrum of chronic appendiceal abscess in cystic fibrosis, *Am J Dis Child* 146: 1190-1193, 1992.

Meconium Abnormalities

280. Kopito L, Shwachman H: Mineral composition of meconium, *J Pediatr* 68:313-314, 1966.
281. Green MN, Shwachman H: Presumptive tests for cystic fibrosis based on serum protein in meconium, *Pediatrics* 41:989-992, 1968.
282. Ryley HC, Neale L, Brogan TD, Bray PT: Plasma proteins in meconium from normal infants and from babies with cystic fibrosis, *Arch Dis Child* 49:901-904, 1974.
283. Shwachman H, Antonowicz I, Mahmoodian A, Ishida S: Studies in meconium: an approach to screening tests to detect cystic fibrosis, *Am J Dis Child* 132:1112-1114, 1978.
284. FitzSimmons SC: The changing epidemiology of cystic fibrosis, *J Pediatr* 122:1-9, 1993.
285. Dolan TF, Touloukian RJ: Familial meconium ileus not associated with cystic fibrosis, *J Pediatr Surg* 9:821-824, 1974.
286. Shigemoto H, Endo S, Isomoto T, Sano K, Taguchi K: Neonatal meconium obstruction in the ileum without mucoviscidosis, *J Pediatr Surg* 13:475-479, 1978.
287. Wilcox DT, Borowitz DS, Stovroff MC, Glick PL: Chronic intestinal pseudo-obstruction with meconium ileus at onset, *J Pediatr* 123:751-752, 1993.

288. Kerem E, Corey M, Kerem B, Durie P, Tsui L-C: Clinical and genetic comparisons of patients with cystic fibrosis, with or without meconium ileus, *J Pediatr* 114:767-773, 1989.
289. Allan JL, Robbie M, Phelan PD, Danks DM: Familial occurrence of meconium ileus, *Eur J Pediatr* 135:291-292, 1981.
290. The cystic fibrosis genotype-phenotype consortium: Correlation between genotype and phenotype in patients with cystic fibrosis, *N Engl J Med* 329:1308-1313, 1993.
291. Rescorla FJ, Grosfeld JL: Contemporary management of mecunium ileus, *World J Surg* 17:318-325, 1993.
292. Donnison AB, Shwachman H, Gross RE: A review of 164 children with meconium ileus seen at the Children's Medical Center, Boston, *Pediatrics* 37:833-850, 1966.
293. Rescorla FJ, Grosfeld JL, West KJ, Vane DW: Changing patterns of treatment and survival in neonates with meconium ileus, *Arch Surg* 142:837-840, 1989.
294. Foster MA, Nyberg DA, Mahony BS, Mack LA, Marks WM, Raabe RD: Meconium peritonitis: prenatal sonographic findings and their clinical significance, *Radiology* 165:661-665, 1987.
295. Neuhauser EBD: Roentgen changes associated with pancreatic insufficiency in early life, *Radiology* 46:319-328, 1946.
296. VanBuskirk RW, Kurlander GJ, Samter TG: Intramural jejunal calcification in a newborn, *Am J Dis Child* 110:329-332, 1965.
297. Berdon WE, Baker DH, Becker J, De Sanctis P: Scrotal masses in healed meconium peritonitis, *N Engl J Med* 277:585-587, 1967.
298. Samuel N, Dicker D, Landman J, Feldberg D, Goldman JA: Early diagnosis and intrauterine therapy of meconium plug syndrome in the fetus: risks and benefits, *J Ultrasound Med* 5:425-428, 1986.
299. Ein SH, Shandling B, Reilly BJ, Stephens CA: Bowel perforation in the nonoperative treatment of meconium ileus, *J Pediatr Surg* 22:146-147, 1987.
300. Meeker IA, Kincannon WN: Acetylcysteine used to liquefy inspissated meconium causing intestinal obstruction in the newborn, *Surgery* 56: 419-425, 1964.
301. Caniano DA, Beaver BL: Meconium ileus: a fifteen year experience with forty-two neonates, *Surgery* 102:699-703, 1987.
302. Rosenstein BJ: Cystic fibrosis presenting with the meconium plug syndrome, *Am J Dis Child* 231:167-169, 1978.
303. Olsen MM, Luck SR, Lloyd-Still J, Raffensperger JG: The spectrum of meconium disease in infancy, *J Pediatr Surg* 17:479-481, 1982.
304. Rosenstein BJ, Langbaum TS: Incidence of meconium abnormalities in newborn infants with cystic fibrosis, *Am J Dis Child* 134:72-73, 1980.

Rectal Prolapse

305. Kulczycki LL, Shwachman H: Studies in cystic fibrosis of the pancreas: occurrence of rectal prolapse, *N Engl J Med* 259:409-412, 1958.
306. Stern RC, Izant RJ, Boat TF, Wood RE, Matthews LW, Doershuk CF: Treatment and prognosis of rectal prolapse in cystic fibrosis, *Gastroenterology* 82:707-710, 1982.
307. Barbero GJ, Shwachman H, Grand R, Woodruff C: Gastrointestinal and nutritional manifestations of cystic fibrosis. In Mangos JA, Talamo RC, eds: *Cystic fibrosis: projections into the future,* Miami, 1976, Symposia Specialist Medical Books, pp 83-111.
308. Zempsky WT, Rosenstein BJ: The cause of rectal prolapse in children, *Am J Dis Child* 142:338-339, 1988.
309. Ashcraft KW, Amoury RA, Holder TM: Levator repair and posterior suspension for rectal prolapse, *J Pediatr Surg* 12:241-245, 1977.
310. Wyllie GG: The injection treatment of rectal prolapse, *J Pediatr Surg* 14:62-64, 1979.

Miscellaneous and Associated Intestinal Abnormalities

311. Siraganian PA, Miller RW, Swender PT: Cystic fibrosis and ileal carcinoma, *Lancet* 2:1158, 1987.
312. McIntosh JC, Schoumacher RA, Tiler RE: Pancreatic adenocarcinoma in a patient with cystic fibrosis, *Am J Med* 85:592, 1988.
313. Sheldon CD, Hodson ME, Carpenter LM, Swerdlow AJ: A cohort study of cystic fibrosis and malignancy, *Br J Cancer* 68:1025-1028, 1993.
314. Neglia JP, Fitzsimmons SC, Maisonneuve P, Schoni MH, Schoni-Affolter F, Corey M, Lowenfels AB, Cystic Fibrosis and Cancer Study Group: The risk of cancer among patients with cystic fibrosis, *N Engl J Med* 332:494-499, 1995.
315. Tizzano EF, Chitayat D, Buchwald M: Cell-specific localization of CFTR mRNA shows developmentally regulated expression in human fetal tissues, *Hum Mol Genet* 2:219-224, 1993.
316. Hassall E, Isreal DM, Davidson AGF, Wong LTK: Barrett's esophagus in children with cystic fibrosis: not a coincidental association, *Am J Gastroenterol* 88:1934-1938, 1993.
317. Taylor B, Sokol G: Cystic fibrosis and coeliac disease: report of two cases, *Arch Dis Child* 48:692-696, 1973.
318. Lloyd-Still JD: Cystic fibrosis, Crohn's disease, biliary abnormalities and cancer, *J Pediatr Gastroenterol Nutr* 11:434-437, 1990.
319. Welkon CJ, Long SS, Thompson M, Gilligan PH: *Clostridium difficile* in patients with cystic fibrosis, *Am J Dis Child* 139:805-808, 1985.
320. Sheretz RJ, Saruba FA: The prevalence of *Clostridium difficile* and toxin in a nursery population: a comparison between patients with necrotizing enterocolitis and an asymptomatic group, *J Pediatr* 100:435-439, 1982.
321. Feigelson J, Girault F, Faure C: Late and unusual intestinal features in cystic fibrosis. Presented at 16th annual meeting of the European Working Group for Cystic Fibrosis, Prague, June 6-9, 1989, p 71.
322. O'Connor J, Lawson J: Fibrocystic disease of pancreas and Crohn's disease, *Br Med J* 4:610, 1972.
323. Lerner A, Gal N, Mares AJ, Maor E, Iancu TC: Pitfall in diagnosis of Crohn's disease in a cystic fibrosis patient, *J Pediatr Gastroenterol Nutr* 12:369-371, 1991.
324. Roberts DM, Craft JC, Mather FJ, Davis SH: Prevalence of giardiasis in patients with cystic fibrosis, *Pediatrics* 112:555-559, 1988.
325. Leclercq-Foucart J, Forget PP, Van Cutsem JL: Lactulose-rhamnose intestinal permeability in children with cystic fibrosis, *J Pediatr Gastroenterol Nutr* 6:66-70, 1987.
326. Penny DJ, Ingall CB, Boulton P, Walker-Smith JA, Basheer SM: Intestinal malabsorption in cystic fibrosis, *Arch Dis Child* 61:1127-1128, 1986.
327. Mack DR, Flick JA, Durie PR, Rosenstein BJ, Ellis LE, Perman JA: Correlation of intestinal lactulose permeability with exocrine pancreatic dysfunction, *J Pediatr* 5:696-701, 1992.
328. Dalzell AM, Freestone NS, Billington D, Heaf DP: Small intestinal permeability and orocaecal transit time in cystic fibrosis, *Arch Dis Child* 65:585-588, 1990.
329. Bali A, Stableforth D, Asquith P: Prolonged small-intestinal transit time in cystic fibrosis, *Br Med J* 287:1011-1013, 1983.
330. Frey HB, Kurtz SM, Spock A, Capp MP: Light and electron microscopic examination of the small bowel of children with cystic fibrosis, *Pediatrics* 64:575-579, 1964.
331. Frase LL, Strickland AD, Kachel GW, Krets GJ: Enhanced glucose absorption in the jejunum of patients with cystic fibrosis, *Gastroenterology* 88:478-484, 1985.
332. Eggermont E, De Boeck K: Small-intestinal abnormalities in cystic fibrosis patients, *Eur J Pediatr* 150:824-828, 1991.
333. Eggermont E: The role of the small intestine in cystic fibrosis patients, *Acta Paediatr Scand* (suppl) 317:16-21, 1985.
334. Ecker JA, Williams RG, Clay KL: Pneumatosis cytoides intestinalis: bullous emphysema of the intestine, *Am J Gastroenterol* 56:125-136, 1971.
335. Koss LG: Abdominal gas cysts (pneumatosis cytoides intestinorum hominis): an analysis with a report of a case and a critical review of the literature, *Arch Pathol* 53:523-549, 1952.
336. Wood RE, Herman CJ, Johnson KW, di Sant'Agnese PA: Pneumatosis coli in cystic fibrosis, *Am J Dis Child* 129:246-248, 1975.
337. White H, Rowley WF: Cystic fibrosis of the pancreas: clinical and roentgenographic manifestations, *Radiol Clin North Am* 1:1539-1556, 1963.
338. Keyting WS, McCarver RR, Kovarik JL, et al: Pneumatosis intestinalis: a new concept, *Radiology* 76:733-741, 1961.

Cardiovascular Complications

339. Moss AJ: The cardiovascular system in cystic fibrosis, *Pediatrics* 70:728-741, 1982.
340. Stern RC, Borkat G, Hirschfeld SS, Boat TF, Matthews LW, Liebman J, Doershuk CF: Heart failure in cystic fibrosis, *Am J Dis Child* 134:267-272, 1980.
341. Siassi B, Moss AJ, Dooley RR: Clinical recognition of cor pulmonale in cystic fibrosis, *J Pediatr* 78:794-805, 1971.
342. Goldring RM, Fishman AP, Turino IM, Cohen HI, Denning CR, Andersen DN: Pulmonary hypertension and cor pulmonale in cystic fibrosis of the pancreas, *J Pediatr* 65:501-524, 1964.
343. Pittman FE, Denning CR, Barker HG: Albumin metabolism in cystic fibrosis, *Am J Dis Child* 108:360-365, 1964.

344. Gewitz M, Eshaghpour E, Holsclaw DS, Miller HA, Kawai N: Echocardiography in cystic fibrosis, *Am J Dis Child* 131:275-280, 1977.
345. Moss AJ, Harper WH, Dooley RR, Murray JF, Mack JF: Cor pulmonale in cystic fibrosis of the pancreas, *J Pediatr* 67:797-807, 1965.
346. Rosenthal A, Tucker CR, Williams RG, Khaw KT, Strieder D, Shwachman H: Echocardiographic assessment of cor pulmonale in cystic fibrosis, *Pediatr Clin North Am* 23:327-344, 1976.
347. Lester LA, Egge AC, Hubbard VS, Camerini-Otero CS, Fink RJ: Echocardiography in cystic fibrosis: a proposed scoring system, *J Pediatr* 97:742-748, 1980.
348. Chipps BE, Alderson PO, Roland J-MA, Yang S, van Aswegen A, Martinez CR, Rosenstein BJ: Noninvasive evaluation of ventricular function in cystic fibrosis, *J Pediatr* 95:379-384, 1979.
349. Allen HD, Taussig LM, Gaines JA, Sahn DJ, Goldberg SJ: Echocardiographic profiles of the long-term cardiac changes in cystic fibrosis, *Chest* 75:428-433, 1979.
350. Ryssing E: Assessment of cor pulmonale in cystic fibrosis by echocardiography, *Acta Paediatr Scand* 66:753-756, 1977.
351. Matthay RA, Berger HJ, Loke J, Dolan TF, Fagenholz SA, Gottschalk A, Zaret BL: Right and left ventricular performance in ambulatory young adults with cystic fibrosis, *Br Heart J* 43:474-480, 1980.
352. Benson LN, Newth CJL, Desouza M, Lobraico R, Kartodihardjo W, Corkey C, Gilday D, Olley PM: Radionuclide assessment of right and left ventricular function during bicycle exercise in young patients with cystic fibrosis, *Am Rev Respir Dis* 130:987-992, 1984.
353. Canny GJ, de Souza ME, Gilday DL, Newth CJL: Radionuclide assessment of cardiac performance in cystic fibrosis, *Am Rev Respir Dis* 130:822-826, 1984.
354. Newth CJL, Corey ML, Fowler RS, Gilday DL, Gross D, Mitchell I: Thallium myocardial perfusion scans for the assessment of right ventricular hypertrophy in patients with cystic fibrosis, *Am Rev Respir Dis* 124:463-468, 1981.
355. Whitman V, Stern RC, Bellet P, Doershuk CF, Liebman J, Boat TF, Borkat G, Matthews LW: Studies on cor pulmonale in cystic fibrosis: I. Effects of diuresis, *Pediatrics* 55:83-85, 1975.
356. Kelminson LL, Cotton EK, Vogel JHK: The reversibility of pulmonary hypertension in patients with cystic fibrosis: observations on the effects of tolazoline hydrochloride, *Pediatrics* 39:24-34, 1967.
357. Geggel RL, Dozor AJ, Fyler DC, Reid LM: Effect of vasodilators at rest and during exercise in young adults with cystic fibrosis and chronic cor pulmonale, *Am Rev Respir Dis* 131:531-536, 1985.
358. Zinman R, Corey M, Coates AL, Canny GJ, Connolly J, Levison H, Beaudry PH: Nocturnal home oxygen in the treatment of hypoxemic cystic fibrosis patients, *J Pediatr* 114:368-377, 1989.
359. Nixon PA, Orenstein DM, Curtis SE, Ross EA: Oxygen supplementation during exercise in cystic fibrosis, *Am Rev Respir Dis* 142:807-811, 1990.
360. Coates AL, Desmond K, Asher MI, Hortop J, Beaudry PH: The effect of digoxin on exercise capacity and exercising cardiac function in cystic fibrosis, *Chest* 82:543-547, 1982.
361. Barnes GL, Gwynne JF, Watt JM: Myocardial fibrosis in cystic fibrosis of the pancreas, *Aust Paediatr J* 6:81-87, 1970.
362. Nezelof C, LeSec G: Multifocal myocardial necrosis and fibrosis in pancreatic diseases of children, *Pediatrics* 63:361-368, 1979.
363. Sullivan MM, Moss RB, Hindi RD, Lewiston NJ: Supra-ventricular tachycardia in patients with cystic fibrosis, *Chest* 90:239-242, 1986.
364. Cheron G, Paradis K, Steru D, Demay G, Lenoir G: Cardiac involvement in cystic fibrosis revealed by a ventricular arrhythmia, *Acta Paediatr Scand* 73:697-700, 1984.
365. Holman RL, Blanc WA, Andersen D: Decreased aortic atherosclerosis in cystic fibrosis of the pancreas, *Pediatrics* 24:34-39, 1959.
366. Moss TJ, Austin GE, Moss AJ: Preatherosclerotic aortic lesions in cystic fibrosis, *J Pediatr* 94:32-37, 1979.

Endocrine-Metabolic

367. Moshang T, Holsclaw DS: Mernarchal determinants in cystic fibrosis, *Am J Dis Child* 134:1139-1142, 1980.
368. Mitchell-Heggs P, Mearns M, Batten JC: Cystic fibrosis in adolescents and adults, *Q J Med* 179:479-504, 1976.
369. Kerem E, Reisman J, Corey M, Canny GJ, Levison H: Prediction of mortality in patients with cystic fibrosis, *N Engl J Med* 326:1187-1191, 1992.
370. Reiter EO, Stern RC, Root AW: The reproductive endocrine system in cystic fibrosis: I. Basal gonado-tropin and sex steroid levels, *Am J Dis Child* 135:422-426, 1981.
371. Biswas S, Norman AP, Baffoe G, Graves L: Prolactin, growth hormone and alpha-fetoprotein in children with cystic fibrosis, *Clin Chim Acta* 69:541-542, 1976.
372. Rosenfeld RG, Landon C, Lewiston N, Nagashima R, Hintz RL: Demonstration of normal plasma somatomedin concentration in cystic fibrosis, *J Pediatr* 99:252-254, 1981.
373. Landon C, Rosenfeld RG: Short stature and pubertal delay in male adolescents with cystic fibrosis, *Am J Dis Child* 138:388-391, 1984.
374. Hubbard VS, Davis PB, di Sant'Agnese PA, Gordon P, Schwartz RH: Isolated growth hormone deficiency and cystic fibrosis: a report of two cases, *Am J Dis Child* 134:317-318, 1980.
375. Huseman CA, Colombo JL, Brooks MA, Smay JR, Greger NG, Sammut PH, Bier DM: Anabolic effect of biosynthetic growth hormone in cystic fibrosis patients, *Pediatr Pulmonol* 22:90-95, 1996.
376. Borel DM, Reddy JK: Excessive lipofuscin accumulation in the thyroid gland in mucoviscidosis, *Arch Pathol* 96:269-271, 1973.
377. Dolan TF, Gibson LE: Complications of iodide therapy in patients with cystic fibrosis, *J Pediatr* 79:684-687, 1971.
378. Azizi F, Bentley D, Vagenakis A, Portnay G, Bush JE, Shwachman H, Ingbar SH, Bravermen LE: Abnormal thyroid function and response to iodides in patients with cystic fibrosis, *Trans Assoc Am Phys* 87:111-119, 1974.
379. Rosenstein BJ, Plotnick LP, Blasco PA: Iodide-induced hypothyroidism without a goiter in an infant with cystic fibrosis, *J Pediatr* 93:261-262, 1978.
380. Segall-Blank M, Vagenakis AG, Treves S, Shwachman H, Ingbar SH, Braverman LE: Evaluation of thyroid function and pituitary TSH reserve in patients with cystic fibrosis, *Cystic Fibrosis Club Abstracts,* Atlanta, 1977, Cystic Fibrosis Foundation, p 21.
381. Depasse C, Chanoine JP, Casimir G, Van Vliet G: Congenital hypothyroidism and cystic fibrosis, *Acta Paediatr Scand* 80:981-983, 1991.
382. Hawkins E, Singer DS: The adrenal cortex in cystic fibrosis of the pancreas, *Am J Clin Pathol* 66:710-714, 1976.
383. Simopoulos AP, Lapey A, Boat TF, di Sant'Agnese PA, Bartter FC: The renin-angiotensin-aldosterone system in patients with cystic fibrosis of the pancreas, *Pediatr Res* 5:626-632, 1971.
384. Rapaport R, Levine LS, Petrovic M, Wilson T, Draznin M, Bejar RL, Johanson A, New MI: The renin-aldosterone system in cystic fibrosis, *J Pediatr* 98:768-771, 1981.
385. Bongiovanni AM, Yakovac WC, Steiker DD: Study of adrenal glands in childhood: hormonal content correlated with morphologic characteristics, *Lab Invest* 10:956-967, 1961.
386. Schoni MH, Turler K, Kaser H, Kraemer R: Plasma and urinary catecholamines in patients with cystic fibrosis, *Pediatr Res* 19:47-52, 1985.
387. Lake CR, Davis PB, Ziegler M, Kopin IJ: Electrolytes and norepinephrine levels in blood of patients with cystic fibrosis, *Clin Chim Acta* 92:141-146, 1979.
388. Davis PB, Kaliner M: Autonomic nervous system abnormalities in cystic fibrosis, *J Chronic Dis* 36:269-278, 1983.

Renal Abnormalities

389. Abramowsky CR, Swinehart GL: The nephropathy of cystic fibrosis: a human model of chronic nephrotoxicity, *Hum Pathol* 13:934-939, 1982.
390. Oppenheimer EH: Glomerular lesions in cystic fibrosis: possible relation to diabetes mellitus, acquired cyanotic heart disease and cirrhosis of the liver, *Johns Hopkins Med J* 131:351-366, 1972.
391. Castile R, Shwachman H, Travis W, Hadley CA, Warwick W, Missmahl HP: Amyloidosis as a complication of cystic fibrosis, *Am J Dis Child* 139:728-732, 1985.
392. Melzi ML, Costantini D, Giani M, Appiani AC, Giunta AM: Severe nephropathy in three adolescents with cystic fibrosis, *Arch Dis Child* 66:144-147, 1991.
393. Rotellar C, Mazzoni MJ, Austin HA, Sabnis SH, Kulczycki L, Rakowski TA, Mackow RC, Winchester JF: Chronic dialysis in a patient with cystic fibrosis, *Nephron* 52:178-182, 1989.
394. Katz SM, Krueger LJ, Falkner B: Microscopic nephrocalcinosis in cystic fibrosis, *N Engl J Med* 319:263-266, 1988.
395. Samaniego-Picota MD, Whelton A: Aminoglycoside-induced nephrotoxicity in cystic fibrosis: a case presentation and review of the literature, *Am J Ther* 3:248-257, 1996.

396. Strandvik B, Hjeltel L: Nephrolithiasis in cystic fibrosis, *Acta Paediatr* 82:306-307, 1993.
397. Dobbins JW, Binder HJ: Importance of the colon in enteric hyperoxaluria, *N Engl J Med* 296:298-301, 1997.
398. Roussey M, Dabadie A, Lennon A, Gie S, Legall E, Le Marec B: Nephrotic syndrome in a child with cystic fibrosis, *Acta Paediatr Scand* 77:920-921, 1988.
399. Aladjem M, Lotan D, Boichis H, Orda S, Katznelson D: Renal function in patients with cystic fibrosis, *Nephron* 34:84-88, 1983.
400. Spino M, Chai RP, Isles AF, Balfe JW, Brown RG, Thiessen JJ, MacLoed SM: Assessment of glomerular filtration rate and effective renal plasma flow in cystic fibrosis, *J Pediatr* 107:64-70, 1985.
401. Robson AM, Tateishi S, Ingelfinger JR, Strominger DB, Klahr S: Renal function in patients with cystic fibrosis, *J Pediatr* 79:42-50, 1971.
402. Levy J, Smith AL, Koup JR, Williams-Warren J, Ramsey B: Disposition of tobramycin in patients with cystic fibrosis: a prospective controlled study, *J Pediatr* 105:117-124, 1984.
403. Berg U, Kusoffksy E, Strandvik B: Renal function in cystic fibrosis with special reference to the renal sodium handling, *Acta Paediatr Scand* 71:833-838, 1982.

Electrolyte Abnormalities

404. Nussbaum E, Boat TF, Wood RE, Doershuk CF: Cystic fibrosis with acute hypoelectrolytemia and metabolic alkalosis in infancy, *Am J Dis Child* 133:465-966, 1979.
405. Eigenmann P, Deleze G, Kuchler H: Chronic metabolic alkalosis in an infant with cystic fibrosis, *Eur J Pediatr* 150:669-670, 1991.
406. Kennedy JD, Dinwiddie R, Daman-Willems C, Dillon MJ, Matthew DJ: Pseudo-Bartter's syndrome in cystic fibrosis, *Arch Dis Child* 65:786-787, 1990.
407. Gottlieb RP: Metabolic alkalosis in cystic fibrosis, *J Pediatr* 79:930-936, 1971.
408. Arvanitakis SN, Lobeck CC: Metabolic alkalosis and salt depletion in cystic fibrosis, *J Pediatr* 82:535-536,1973.
409. Beckerman RC, Taussig LM: Hypoelectrolytemia and metabolic alkalosis in infants with cystic fibrosis, *Pediatrics* 63:580-583, 1979.
410. Laughlin JJ, Brady MS, Eigen H: Changing feeding trends as a cause of electrolyte depletion in infants with cystic fibrosis, *Pediatrics* 68:203-207, 1981.
411. Hochman HI, Feins NR, Rubin R, Gould J: Chloride losing diarrhea and metabolic alkalosis in an infant with cystic fibrosis, *Arch Dis Child* 51:390-391, 1976.
412. Kessler WR, Andersen DH: Heat prostration in fibrocystic disease of the pancreas and other conditions, *Pediatrics* 8:648-655, 1951.
413. di Sant'Agnese PA, Darling RC, Perera GA, Shea E: Abnormal electrolyte composition of sweat in cystic fibrosis of the pancreas, *Pediatrics* 12:549-562, 1953.
414. Nussbaum E, Boat TF, Wood RE, Doershuk CF: Cystic fibrosis with acute hypoelectrolytemia and metabolic alkalosis in infancy, *Am J Dis Child* 133:965-966, 1979.
415. Finberg L, Bernstein J: Acute hyponatremic dehydration, *J Pediatr* 79:499-503, 1971.
416. di Sant'Agnese PA: Salt depletion in cold weather in infants with cystic fibrosis of the pancreas, *JAMA* 172:84-91, 1960.
417. Williams AJ, McKiernan J, Harris F: Heat prostration in children with cystic fibrosis, *Br Med J* 2:297, 1976.
418. Ruddy R, Anolik R, Scanlin TF: Hypoelectrolytemia as a presentation and complication of cystic fibrosis, *Clin Pediatr* 21:367-369, 1982.
419. Orenstein DM, Henke KG, Costill DL, Doershuk CF, Lemon PJ, Stern RC: Exercise and heat stress in cystic fibrosis patients, *Pediatr Res* 17: 267-269, 1983.
420. Orenstein DM, Henke KG, Green CG: Heat acclimation in cystic fibrosis, *J Appl Physiol* 57:408-412, 1984.
421. Bar-Or O, Blimkie CJR, Hay JA, MacDougall JD, Ward DS, Wilson WM: Voluntary dehydration and heat intolerance in cystic fibrosis, *Lancet* 339:696-699, 1992.

Female Reproductive Tract

422. Oppenheimer EH, Esterly JR: Observations on cystic fibrosis of the pancreas. VI. The uterine cervix, *J Pediatr* 77:991-995, 1970.
423. Stead RJ, Hodson ME, Batten JC, Adams J, Jacobs HS: Amenorrhoea in cystic fibrosis, *Clin Endocrin* 26:187-195, 1987.
424. Kopito LE, Kosasky JH, Shwachman H: Water and electrolytes in cervical mucus from patients with cystic fibrosis, *Fertil Steril* 24:512-516, 1973.
425. Bergman P: The cervical cycle, *Acta Obstet Gynecol Scand* 29(suppl):74, 1950.
426. Johannesson M, Gottlieb C, Hjelte L: Delayed puberty in girls with cystic fibrosis despite good clinical status, *Pediatrics* 99:29-34, 1997.
427. Dooley RR, Braunstein H, Osher AB: Polypoid cervicitis in cystic fibrosis patients receiving oral contraceptives, *Am J Obstet Gynecol* 118:971-974, 1974.
428. Fitzpatrick SH, Stokes DC, Rosenstein BJ, Terry P, Hubbard VS: Use of oral contraceptives in women with cystic fibrosis, *Chest* 86:863-867, 1984.
429. Kotloff RM, FitzSimmons SC, Fiel SB: Fertility and pregnancy in patients with cystic fibrosis, *Clin Chest Med* 13:623-635, 1992.
430. Grand RJ, Talamo RC, di Sant'Agnese PA, Schwartz RH: Pregnancy in cystic fibrosis of the pancreas, *JAMA* 195:993-1000, 1966.
431. Cohen LF, di Sant'Agnese PA, Friedlander J: Cystic fibrosis and pregnancy: a national survey, *Lancet* 2:842-844, 1980.
430. Canny GJ, Corey M, Livingstone RA, Carpenter S, Green L, Levison H: Pregnancy and cystic fibrosis, *Obstet Gynecol* 77:850-853, 1991.
433. Edenborough FP, Stableforth DE, Webb AK, MacKenzie WE, Smith DL: Outcome of pregnancy in women with cysytic fibrosis, *Thorax* 50:170-174, 1995.
434. Kent NE, Farquharson DF: Cystic fibrosis in pregnancy, *Can Med Assoc J* 149:809-813, 1993.
435. Palmer J, Dillon-Baker C, Tecklin JS, Wolfson B, Rosenberg B, Burroughs B, Holsclaw DS, Scanlin TF, Huang NN, Sewell EM: Pregnancy in patients with cystic fibrosis, *Ann Intern Med* 99:596-600, 1983.
436. Davis PB: Reproductive complications of cystic fibrosis, *Semin Resp Med* 6:314-318, 1985.
437. Whitelaw A, Butterfield A: High breast-milk sodium in cystic fibrosis, *Lancet* 2:1288, 1977.
438. Welch MJ, Phelps DL, Osher AB: Breast-feeding by a mother with cystic fibrosis, *Pediatrics* 67:664-666, 1981.
439. Shiffman ML, Seale TW, Flux M, et al: Breast milk composition in women with cystic fibrosis: report of two cases and a review of the literature, *Am J Clin Nutr* 49:612-617, 1989.
440. Bitman J, Hamosh M, Wood KL, Freed LM, Hamosh P: Lipid composition of milk from mothers with cystic fibrosis, *Pediatrics* 80:927-932, 1987.
441. Luder E, Kattan M, Tanzer-Torres G, Bonforte RJ: Current recommendations for breast-feeding in cystic fibrosis centers, *Am J Dis Child* 144:1153-1156, 1990.

Male Reproductive Tract

442. Denning CR, Sommers SC, Quigley HJ: Infertility in male patients with cystic fibrosis, *Pediatrics* 41:7-17, 1968.
443. Holsclaw DS, Perlmutter AD, Jockin H, Shwachman H: Genital abnormalities in male patients with cystic fibrosis, *J Urology* 106:568-574, 1971.
444. Heaton ND, Pryor JP: Vasa aplasia and cystic fibrosis, *Br J Urol* 66:538-540, 1990.
445. Kaplan E, Shwachman H, Perlmutter AD, et al: Reproductive failure in males with cystic fibrosis, *N Engl J Med* 279:65-69, 1968.
446. Landing BH, Wells TR, Wang C-I: Abnormality of the epididymis and vas deferens in cystic fibrosis, *Arch Pathol* 88:569-580, 1969.
447. Oppenheimer EH, Esterly JR: Observations on cystic fibrosis of the pancreas V. Developmental changes in the male genital system, *J Pediatr* 75:806-811, 1969.
448. Handelsman DJ, Conway AJ, Boylan LM, Turtle JR: Young's syndrome: obstructive azoospermia and chronic sinopulmonary infections, *N Engl J Med* 310:3-9, 1984.
449. Anguiano A, Oates RD, Amos JA, Dean M, Gerrard B, Stewart C, Maher TA, White MB, Milunsky A: Congenital bilateral absence of the vas deferens, *JAMA* 267:1794-1797, 1992.
450. Chillon M, Casals T, Mercier B, Bassas L, Lissens W, Silber S, Romey MC, Ruiz-Romero J, Verlingue C, Claustres M, Nunes V, Fergc C, Estivill X: Mutations in the cystic fibrosis gene in patients with congenital absence of the vas deferens, *N Engl J Med* 332:1475-1480, 1995.

451. Patrizio P, Asch RH, Handelin B, Silber SJ: Aetiology of congenital absence of vas deferens: genetic study of three generations, *Hum Reprod* 8:215-220, 1993.
452. Jarvi K, Zielenski J, Wilschanski M, Durie P, Buckspan M, Tullis E, Markiewicz D, Tsui L-C: Cystic fibrosis transmembrane conductance regulator and obstructive azoospermia, *Lancet* 344:1578, 1995.
453. Osborne LR, Lynch M, Middleton PG, Alton E, Geddes DM, Pryor JP, Hodson ME, Santis GK: Nasal epithelial ion transport and genetic analysis of infertile men with congenital bilateral absence of the vas deferens, *Hum Mol Genet* 2:1605-1609, 1993.
454. Colin AA, Sawyer SM, Mickle JE, Oates RD, Milunsky A, Amos JA: Pulmonary function and clinical observations in men with congenital bilateral absence of the vas deferens, *Chest* 110:440-445, 1996.
455. Taussig LM, Lobeck CC, di Sant'Agnese PA, Ackerman DR, Kattwinkel J: Fertility in males with cystic fibrosis, *N Engl J Med* 287: 586-589, 1972.
456. Blanck RR, Mendoza EM: Fertility in a man with cystic fibrosis, *JAMA* 235:1364, 1976.
457. Feigelson J, Pecau Y, Shwachman H: A propos d'une paternite chez un malade atteint de mucoviscidose: etudes des fonctions genitales et de la filiation, *Arch Fr Pediatr* 26:937-944, 1969.
458. Dreyfus DH, Bethel R, Gelfand EW: Cystic fibrosis 3849+10kbC>T mutation associated with severe pulmonary disease and male ferility, *Am J Respir Crit Care Med* 153:858-860, 1996.
459. Silber SJ, Ord T, Balmaceda J, Patrizio P, Asch RH: Congenital absence of the vas deferens—the fertilizing capacity of human epididymal sperm, *N Engl J Med* 323:1788-1792, 1990.
460. Oates RD, Honig S, Berger MJ, Harris D: Microscopic epididymal sperm aspiration (MESA): a new option for treatment of the obstructive azoospermia associated with cystic fibrosis, *J Assisted Reprod Genet* 9:36-40, 1992.

Hematologic Abnormalities

461. Rosenthal A, Button LN, Khaw KT: Blood volume changes in patients with cystic fibrosis, *Pediatrics* 59:588-594, 1977.
462. Wagener JS, Corrigan JJ, McNeil GC, Lemen R, Taussig LM: Ferrokinetic and hematologic studies in cystic fibrosis patients, *Am J Ped Hematol Oncol* 5:153-159, 1083.
463. Ehrhardt P, Miller MG, Littlewood JM: Iron deficiency in cystic fibrosis, *Arch Dis Child* 62:185-187, 1987.
464. Davis AE, Biggs JC: The pancreas and iron absorption, *Gut* 6:140-142, 1965.
465. Tonz O, Weiss S, Strahm HW, Rossi E: Iron absorption in cystic fibrosis, *Lancet* 2:1097-1099, 1965.
466. Smith RS: Iron absorption in cystic fibrosis, *Br Med J* 1:608-609, 1964.
467. Zempsky WT, Rosenstein BJ, Carroll JA, Oski FA: Effect of pancreatic enzyme supplements on iron absorption, *Am J Dis Child* 143:969-972, 1989.
468. Longnecker DS: Hepatic iron stores in patients with cystic fibrosis, *Arch Pathol* 80:148-152, 1965.
469. Anderson DH: Cystic fibrosis of pancreas and its relations to celiac disease, *Am J Dis Child* 56:344-399, 1938.

Central Nervous System Complications

470. Fischer EG, Shwachman H, Wepsie JG: Brain abscess and cystic fibrosis, *J Pediatr* 95:385-388, 1979.
471. Duffner PK, Cohen ME: Cystic fibrosis with brain abscess, *Arch Neurol* 36:27-28, 1979.
472. Ayres J, Kinsella H: Multiple cerebral abscesses in an adult with cystic fibrosis, *Br J Dis Chest* 76:99-100, 1982.
473. Kline MW: Brain abscess in a patient with cystic fibrosis, *Pediatr Infect Dis* 4:72-73, 1985.
474. Bray PF, Herbst JJ: Pseudotumor cerebri as a sign of "catch-up" growth in cystic fibrosis, *Am J Dis Child* 126:78-79, 1973.
475. Katznelson D: Increased intracranial pressure in cystic fibrosis, *Acta Paediatr Scand* 67:607-609, 1978.
476. Roach ES, Sinal SH: Increased intracranial pressure following treatment of cystic fibrosis, *Pediatrics* 66:622-623, 1980.
477. Roach ES, Sinal SH: Initial treatment of cystic fibrosis: frequency of transient bulging fontanel, *Clin Pediatr* 28:371-373, 1989.
478. Bye AME, Muller DPR, Wilson J, Wright VM, Mearns MB: Symptomatic vitamin E deficiency in cystic fibrosis, *Arch Dis Child* 60: 162-164, 1985.
479. Willison JH, Muller DPR, Matthews S, Jones S, Kriss A, Stead RJ, Hodson ME, Harding AE: A study of the relationship between neurological function and serum vitamin E concentrations in patients with cystic fibrosis, *J Neurol Neurosurg Psych* 48:1097-1102, 1985.
480. Cynamon HA, Milov DE, Valenstein E, Wagner M: Effect of vitamin E deficiency on neurologic function in patients with cystic fibrosis, *J Pediatr* 113:637-640, 1988.
481. Sung JH, Park SH, Mastri AR, Warwick WJ: Axonal dystrophy in the gracile nucleus in congenital biliary atresia and cystic fibrosis (mucoviscidosis): beneficial effect of vitamin E therapy, *J Neuropathol Exp Neurol* 39:584-597, 1980.
482. Cavalier SJ, Gambetti P: Dystrophic axons and spinal cord demyelination in cystic fibrosis, *Neurology* (NY) 31:714-718, 1981.
483. Geller A, Gilles F, Shwachman H: Degeneration of fasciculus gracilis in cystic fibrosis, *Neurology* 27:185-187, 1977.

Ocular Complications

484. Bruce GM, Denning CR, Spalter HF: Ocular findings in cystic fibrosis of the pancreas, *Arch Ophthalmol* 63:391-401, 1960.
485. Chazan BI, Balodimos MC, Holsclaw DS, Shwachman H: Microcirculation in young adults with cystic fibrosis: retinal and microvascular changes in relation to diabetes, *J Pediatr* 77:86-92, 1970.
486. Spaide RF, Diamond G, D'Amico RA, Gaerlan PF, Bisberg DS: Ocular findings in cystic fibrosis, *Am J Ophthalmol* 103:204-210, 1987.
487. Sheppard JD, Orenstein DM, Chao C-C, Butala S, Kowalski RP: The ocular surface in cystic fibrosis, *Ophthalmology* 96:1624-1630, 1989.
488. Rimsza ME, Hernied LS, Kaplan AM: Hemorrhagic retinopathy in a patient with cystic fibrosis, *Pediatrics* 62:336-338, 1978.
489. Lietman PS, di Sant'Agnese PA, Wong V: Optic neuritis in cystic fibrosis of the pancreas: role of chloramphenicol therapy, *JAMA* 189:924-927, 1964.
490. Huang NH, Harley RD, Promadhattavedi V, Sproul A: Visual disturbances in cystic fibrosis following chloramphenicol administration, *J Pediatr* 68:32-44, 1966.

Salivary Glands

491. Warwick WJ, Bernard B, Meskin LH: The involvement of the labial mucous salivary gland in patients with cystic fibrosis, *Pediatrics* 34:621-628, 1964.
492. Barbero GJ, Sibinga MS: Enlargement of the submaxillary salivary glands in cystic fibrosis, *Pediatrics* 29:788-793, 1962.
493. Leake D, Khaw K-T, Shwachman H: Parotid gland sialograms in cystic fibrosis, *J Pediatr* 76:301-304, 1970.
494. di Sant'Agnese PA, Grossman H, Darling RC, Denning CR: Saliva, tears and duodenal contents in cystic fibrosis of the pancreas, *Pediatrics* 22:507-514, 1958.
495. Marmar J, Barbero GJ, Sibinga MS: The pattern of parotid gland secretion in cystic fibrosis of the pancreas, *Gastroenterol* 50:551-556, 1966.
496. Mandel ID, Kutscher A, Denning CR, Thompson RH, Zegarelli EV: Salivary studies in cystic fibrosis, *Am J Dis Child* 113:431-438, 1967.
497. Wiesmann UN, Boat TF, di Sant'Agnese PA: Sodium concentration in unstimulated parotid saliva and on oral mucosa in normal subjects and in patients with cystic fibrosis, *J Pediatr* 76:444-448, 1970.
498. Chernick WS, Barbero GJ, Parkins FM: Studies on submaxillary saliva in cystic fibrosis, *J Pediatr* 59:890-898, 1961.
499. Blomfield J, Warton K, Brown JM: Flow rate and inorganic components of submandibular saliva in cystic fibrosis, *Arch Dis Child* 48:267-274, 1973.
500. Gugler E, Pallavicini JC, Swerdlow H, Zipkin I, di Sant'Agnese PA: Immunological studies of submaxillary saliva from patients with cystic fibrosis and from normal children, *J Pediatr* 73:548-559, 1968.
501. di Sant'Agnese PA, Talamo RC: Pathogenesis and physio-pathology of cystic fibrosis of the pancreas, *N Engl J Med* 277:1287, 1967.
502. Wiesman UN, Boat TF, di Sant'Agnese PA: Flow-rates and electrolytes in minor-salivary-gland saliva in normal subjects and patients with cystic fibrosis, *Lancet* 2:510-512, 1972.

Skin Manifestations

503. Soter NA, Mihm MC Jr, Colten HR: Cutaneous necrotizing venulitis in patients with cystic fibrosis, *J Pediatr* 95:197-201, 1979.
504. Newman AJ, Ansell BM: Episodic arthritis in children with cystic fibrosis, *J Pediatr* 95:594-596, 1979.

505. Schidlow DV, Panitch HB, Zaeri N, Zenel J, Alpert BE: Purpuric rashes in cystic fibrosis, *Am J Dis Child* 143:1030-1032, 1989.
506. Hansen RC, Lemen R, Revsin B: Cystic fibrosis manifesting with acrodermatitis enteropathica-like eruption: association with essential fatty acid and zinc deficiencies, *Arch Dermatol* 119:51-55, 1983.
507. Rosenblum JL, Schweitzer J, Kissane JM, Cooper TW: Failure to thrive presenting with an unusual skin rash, *J Pediatr* 107:149-153, 1985.

Musculoskeletal Abnormalities

508. Alberts WM, Moser KM: Objective criteria to define and monitor changes: a clinician's guide to clubbing, *J Respir Dis* 2:17-21, 1981.
509. Lampe RM, Kagan A: Detection of clubbing—Schamroth's sign, *Clin Pediatr* 22:125, 1983.
510. Lemen RJ, Gates AJ, Mathe AA, Waring WW, Hyman AL, Kadowitz PD: Relationships among digital clubbing, disease severity, and serum prostaglandins F2a and E concentrations in cystic fibrosis patients, *Am Rev Respir Dis* 117:639-645, 1978.
511. Fara EF, Baughman RP: A study of capillary morphology in the digits of patients with acquired clubbing, *Am Rev Respir Dis* 140:1063-1066, 1989.
512. Grossman H, Denning CR, Baker DH: Hypertrophic osteoarthropathy in cystic fibrosis, *Am J Dis Child* 107:1-6, 1964.
513. Nathanson I, Riddlesberger MM Jr.: Pulmonary hypertrophic osteoarthropathy in cystic fibrosis, *Radiology* 135:649-651, 1980.
514. Cohen AM, Yulish BS, Wasser KB, Vignos PJ, Jones PK, Sorin SB: Evaluation of pulmonary hypertrophic osteoarthropathy in cystic fibrosis, *Am J Dis Child* 140:74-77, 1986.
515. Gall EA, Bennett GA, Bauer W: Generalized hypertrophic osteoarthropathy: a pathological study of seven cases, *Am J Pathol* 27: 349-367, 1951.
516. Pertuiset E, Menkes CJ, Lenoir G, Jehanne M, Douchain F, Guillot M: Cystic fibrosis arthritis. A report of five cases, *Br J Rheumatol* 31:535-538, 1992.
517. Wulffraat NM, de Graeff-Meeder ER, Rijkers GT, van der Laag H, Kuis W: Prevalence of circulating immune complexes in patients with cystic fibrosis and arthritis, *J Pediatr* 125:374-378, 1994.
518. Bourke S, Rooney M, Fitzgerald M, Bresnihan B: Episodic arthropathy in adult cystic fibrosis, *Q J Med* 244:651-659, 1987.
519. Phillips BM, David TJ: Pathogenesis and management of arthropathy in cystic fibrosis, *J R Soc Med* 79:44-49, 1986.
520. Bowler IM, Littlewood JM: Episodic arthritis in cystic fibrosis, *Lancet* 340:244, 1992.
521. Sagransky DM, Greenwald RA, Gorvoy JD: Seropositive rheumatoid arthritis in a patient with cystic fibrosis, *Am J Dis Child* 134:319-320, 1980.
522. Rose J, Gamble J, Schultz A, Lewiston N: Back pain and spinal deformity in cystic fibrosis, *Am J Dis Child* 141:1313-1316, 1987.
523. Henderson RC, Specter BB: Kyphosis and fractures in children and young adults with cystic fibrosis, *J Pediatr* 125:208-212, 1994.
524. Mitchell EA, Elliott RB: Spontaneous fracture of the sternum in a youth with cystic fibrosis, *J Pediatr* 97:789-790, 1980.

Psychosocial

525. Lewiston NJ: Psychosocial impact of cystic fibrosis, *Semin Respir Med* 6:321-333, 1985.
526. Denning CR, Gluckson MM: Psychosocial aspects of cystic fibrosis, In Taussig LM, ed: *Cystic fibrosis.* New York, 1984, Thieme-Stratton, pp 461-492.
527. Walker LS, Ford MB, Donald WD: Cystic fibrosis and family stress: effects of age and severity of illness, *Pediatrics* 79:239-246, 1987.
528. Gayton WF, Friedman SB, Tavormina JF, Tucker F: Children with cystic fibrosis: I. Psychological test findings of patients, siblings, and parents, *Pediatrics* 59:888-894, 1977.
529. Spinetta J, Deasey-Spinetta P: Talking with children with a life-threatening illness: a handbook for health care professionals, *Cystic Fibrosis Foundation,* Rockville, MD, 1980.

CHAPTER 70

Cystic Fibrosis: Prognosis

Ian B. MacLusky, Mary Corey, and Henry Levison

The prognosis for patients with cystic fibrosis (CF) has changed drastically over the last 40 years. In the decade following the initial description by Andersen et al,[1] life expectancy of patients with CF was under 10 years. However, by 1969 the median survival for patients with CF in the United States was 14 years, by 1978 it was 21 years and by 1996 it was 31.3 years.[2] Similar improvements have been seen worldwide.[3] In Canada, the median survival is currently 36.2 years for men, 28.6 for women.[4] Moreover, the life expectancy still appears to be rising, with increasing numbers of individuals surviving into adulthood (Fig. 70-1). This increasing survival has had a number of consequences.

First, the number of individuals with CF is continuing to increase. The number of affected individuals in the United States rose from around 8000 in 1969 to over 20,886 in 1996.[2] As these individuals enter adulthood, they require increasing autonomy and more resources to support their education and careers. Counseling regarding sexuality and fertility issues also becomes of increasing importance. Because these areas are not usually well covered in pediatric clinics, increasing numbers of adult clinics have been established to address these specific needs.

Second, the increasing age of patients with CF is associated with a change in the spectrum of clinical disease. Concurrent with increasing age, patients tend to present with the more serious complications of the disease, such as hemoptysis, pneumothorax, progressive gastrointestinal complications (cirrhosis, distal intestinal obstruction syndrome), and diabetes mellitus.[2]

CF is a remarkably heterogeneous disease, with marked variability in clinical presentation and rate of progress. Despite the increasing survival of patients with CF, there are still patients with early onset of pulmonary disease who die, despite intensive therapy, in the first decade of life. At the opposite extreme, occasional patients have no evidence of clinical disease until adulthood and survive into their third and fourth decades of life with minimal, if any, therapy.[5]

Although CF is a multisystem disease, the respiratory disease remains the major cause of morbidity, with progressive respiratory failure the principal cause of death in 95% of pa-

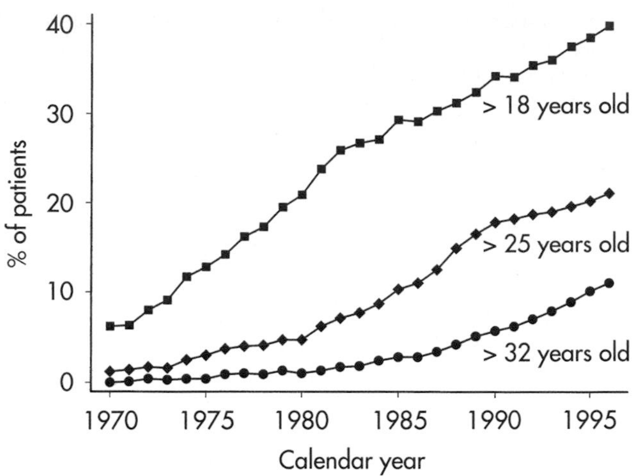

Fig. 70-1. Proportion of patients over age 18, 25, and 32 years old, respectively, expressed as a percentage of the total annual national registered patient population with Cystic Fibrosis in Canada. (Data obtained from the *Report of the Canadian Cystic Fibrosis Patient Registry,* 1996, with permission of the Canadian Cystic Fibrosis Foundation, Toronto, Canada, 1998.)

BOX 70-1
Factors Involved in the Changing Survival of Patients with CF

Influencing population survival patterns

I. Improved diagnosis
  1. Recognition of clinical spectrum
  2. Improved diagnostic techniques
  3. Population screening
II. Improved treatment
  1. Antibiotics
  2. Nutrition
  3. Regional center care

Affecting individual rate of disease progression

I. Pattern of disease
  1. Meconium ileus
  2. Postnatal gastrointestinal disease
  3. Nutritional status
  4. Respiratory involvement
II. Individual genotype
  1. Specific genetic mutation
  2. Gender
  3. Race
III. Other factors
  1. Family functioning
  2. Social class
  3. Parental smoking

Indicators of poor prognosis in individuals

I. Respiratory
  1. Pulmonary function
  2. Exercise testing
  3. Blood gases
II. Cardiac function
III. Clinical signs

tients surviving the neonatal period. Although a number of factors have been identified that seem to correlate with subsequent survival, we still know little about what influences disease progression and what occurs purely as a consequence of deteriorating clinical status. This chapter discusses the current state of knowledge regarding factors that:

- are implicated in the changing patterns in overall population survival.
- appear to influence the rate of progression of disease in individual patients.
- are reliable indicators of poor prognosis in individual patients though not directly influencing disease progression (Box 70-1).

FACTORS IMPLICATED IN CHANGE IN OVERALL POPULATION SURVIVAL

Diagnosis

A number of improvements in diagnosis are presumed to have influenced the overall survival of patients with CF.

Appreciation of the Range and Spectrum of Clinical Disease

The appreciation of the wide range of clinical disease in patients with CF has led to the diagnosis of previously undiagnosed patients with milder disease. One evident example is pancreatic-sufficient patients, some of whom may not be diagnosed until adulthood.[6] Inclusion of these patients into the CF population will obviously raise the overall survival statistics.

Improved Diagnostic Techniques

In the early days of CF, diagnosis was based primarily on the clinical picture, the only reliable in vivo diagnostic test being assay of duodenal secretions, with confirmation based largely on postmortem findings.[7] This almost certainly resulted in underdiagnosis of CF, with only the more severe cases being clinically recognized.[8] The identification by di Sant'Agnese of the sweat chloride abnormality[7] and the subsequent development of the pilocarpine iontophoresis sweat test allowed the easy and accurate diagnosis of CF. The resulting diagnosis of milder cases, associated with the growing appreciation of the spectrum of disease, may have been a significant factor in the marked improvement in survival curves described in the following two decades. Until recently, however, diagnosis still depended on physician acumen in recognizing the early signs of CF, with confirmation by sweat testing. Even in the best hands, this still leads to delays and inaccuracies in diagnosis.[9] Following discovery of the CF gene,[10] direct analysis of DNA for known mutations can be useful to confirm the diagnosis of CF. However, the large number of CF mutations, and the likelihood that a patient with mild symptoms will carry an obscure mutation, limits the usefulness of DNA analysis in diagnosing CF.

Population Screening

Currently, 15% of patients with CF present in the neonatal period with meconium ileus. In the absence of neonatal screening, 70% of patients are diagnosed within the first year of life, largely because of the presence of clinical disease, 80% by 4 years of age, and 90% by 12 years of age.[2] This still leaves 10% who are not diagnosed until the second or even third decade of life. Of the earlier techniques suggested as a screening test for CF, none proved sufficiently accurate or practicable to be used for screening of the general population.[11] Newer techniques, such as neonatal screening using serum immunoreactive trypsinogen (IRT) assay, alone or in combination with DNA analysis, or genetic testing of fertile adults for carrier detection, present the possibility for earlier and more accurate diagnosis.[12] However, population screening of newborns for CF, or of fertile adults for carrier status based on genetic tests alone is not possible at this time because of the large number of CF mutations and the inability of most programs to test for more than a few.[13]

The major justification for a screening program is that early diagnosis significantly affects overall survival. In the absence of definitive therapy, it is unclear whether this is actually the case in CF. In families with an affected child, subsequent children, diagnosed before the onset of symptoms, tend to have better pulmonary status, at the same age, than the children who were diagnosed because of the presence of clinical disease,[14] suggesting that early diagnosis is of benefit. Neonatal screening, using blood assay for IRT, has been available for almost 10 years. It is, however, not widely used, largely because of debate over whether its clinical benefits outweigh the problems associated with erroneous results.[12] A nonrandomized study[15] documented better clinical status and improved survival to 9 years of age in patients diagnosed by neonatal screening compared with a control group whose diagnosis was based on clinical indications. There was, however, no significant difference in pulmonary function between the two groups of survivors. In addition, the unscreened group had an unusually high mortality rate (40% by 11 years of age, with two of the nine deaths being caused by liver failure). The applicability of these data to the general CF population is therefore questionable. In contrast, Chatfield et al[16a] have been performing neonatal testing only on alternate weeks, hence providing a randomized, clinically diagnosed control cohort. At 5 year follow-up, there was no significant difference in clinical status, growth, or chest radiograph score between patients diagnosed by neonatal screening and the control group of patients. This compares to data from the Wisconsin Cystic Fibrosis Neonatal Screening Study, in which all neonates were screened, but only those born on alternate weeks informed of the results. This study has documented better nutritional status in children diagnosed by neonatal screening than in children diagnosed consequent to overt clinical disease or family history. This advantage not only was present at time of initial diagnosis, but persisted, although to a lesser extent, through 10 years of age.[16b] Whether early diagnosis has an equivalent effect on pulmonary status has, however, yet to be determined.

The precise value of early diagnosis is therefore still unresolved. Once gene or somatic therapy becomes available, it will presumably be most effective if initiated early in the disease, before the onset of significant pulmonary involvement. At that point, early diagnosis should logically have a marked effect on prognosis.

Treatment

It is tempting to attribute the improvement in survival over the years to improved therapy; however, treatment of patients with CF has, at least until recently, been largely empirically derived. It has therefore often been difficult to determine which facets of established therapy are truly effective and which are ineffective, or even deleterious. One area in which treatment has clearly affected overall survival is in the treatment of meconium ileus. Apart from this exception, significant differences in therapeutic approaches continue between many clinics,[17] with a paucity of data to determine which is the optimum approach.

Antibiotics

Because chronic endobronchial infection is a primary feature of the pulmonary disease in CF, antibiotic therapy has long been a mainstay of therapy.[18,19] Although it seems logical to suppose that at least some of the improvement in survival of individuals with CF is the result of improved antibacterial therapy, objective evidence is surprisingly limited.

Short Term. Patients with CF often have episodes of acute exacerbation of their chest disease; these episodes become more prominent as the disease progresses. The standard approach to treatment of these episodes is short-term courses of antibiotics, either orally if an effective oral agent is available or intravenously (usually, but not necessarily, in hospital) if no effective oral agent is available. Although significant improvements in both clinical status and pulmonary functions are usually achieved, this improvement is often temporary; long-term eradication of the infecting organisms is rare.[20,21] Moreover, few randomized controlled trials document whether antibiotics are the primary cause of this improvement in clinical status. In two trials, improvement similar to that seen in the treatment group was observed in the control population, who received ineffective[22] or no[23] antibiotic therapy. This contrasts sharply with the Danish experience in which frequent, short-term antipseudomonal therapy was associated with both reduction in *Pseudomonas aeruginosa* colonization[24] and an overall improvement in patient survival.[25] It should be noted that the Danish survival studies used historical controls. In addition, similar survival statistics have been achieved by clinics using a much less aggressive antibiotic regimen.[26] Thus the exact influence of short-term antibiotic therapy on long-term survival is still questionable.

Long Term. There is even more controversy regarding the effectiveness of long-term antibiotic therapy on prognosis in patients with CF.

Long-term oral antistaphylococcal agents are used by many clinics. Although this has been routine care for many years, there are few objective data to document its effectiveness. Over the years, there has been a significant reduction in the severity of staphylococcal disease in patients with CF. However, how much of this is the result of improved nutrition and how much of "prophylactic" anti-staphylococcal antibiotics is unclear. Many patients (often the healthiest) are still chronically colonized with *Streptococcus aureus,* despite being on long-term antistaphylococcal antibiotics. In addition, the long-term use of these agents has been implicated in the subsequent acquisition of *P. aeruginosa.*[27] Thus there are concerns as to whether antistaphylococcal antibiotics may actually be detrimental.

Long-term antipseudomonal therapy has only recently been studied, largely because of the prior lack of any effective oral agents. However, several studies have documented an apparent beneficial effect on disease progression of chronically inhaled aminoglycosides,[28,29] although the exact mode of action is unclear. It is questionable whether bactericidal levels of antibiotics are achieved within the airways, yet therapeutic effectiveness seems to be achieved despite the persistence of endobronchial infection. The improvement in pulmonary status may therefore arise as a result of suppression of bacterial exotoxin production, rather than any antibacterial effect.

Nutrition

It has long been recognized that poor nutritional status is associated with a worse prognosis, malnutrition being common in the presence of deteriorating pulmonary disease. As a consequence, aggressive nutritional support has become one of the mainstays of the current management of CF.[30,31] With this approach, the majority of patients with CF can achieve normal, or near normal, growth patterns.[4] However, how much of a role poor nutrition plays in influencing pulmonary disease, and, as a corollary, how much maintenance of good nutrition helps in preventing clinical deterioration, has not been clarified.

Evidence of the Role of Nutrition. Before the advent of pancreatic enzyme supplementation, patients with CF tended to develop progressive malnutrition, with fulminant staphylococcal pulmonary infection occurring as the terminal event. With the advent of pancreatic enzyme supplements, patients with CF can now achieve nearly, if not completely, normal growth. The coincidence in timing (availability of pancreatic enzyme supplements, the resulting improvements in nutritional status of patients, and the marked improvements in reported survival) suggest that improved nutrition may be one of the major factors delaying pulmonary deterioration. Certainly there is good evidence that malnutrition has a deleterious effect on both humoral and cell-mediated immunity, with associated decreased resistance to a wide variety of infectious agents.[32] It is therefore tempting to speculate that the improved nutrition may at least partly explain both the apparent reduction in severity of staphylococcal disease and improved survival of patients with CF.

The Toronto clinic has for many years reported one of the highest survival rates for patients with CF. In a study comparing the Toronto and Boston clinics, both of which are large, tertiary center–based clinics with very similar patient populations in terms of numbers, age, and gender distribution, and ethnic and social backgrounds, there were significant differences in survival patterns between the clinics.[26] This was particularly pronounced for male patients, with those at the Toronto clinic having the highest overall survival. Although the age-specific pulmonary function was not different between the two clinics (similar age and sex patients having similar pulmonary function), Toronto patients were significantly taller than their Boston counterparts, whereas the Toronto male (though not female) patients were also significantly better nourished. In general, both clinics had similar treatment approaches, with the exception that the Boston clinic had historically used a low-fat, low–pancreatic-enzyme supplement approach, whereas the Toronto clinic used a high-fat, high-calorie diet, with more individualized pancreatic enzyme supplementation. The conclusion from this study was that this difference in approach explained the difference in apparent nutrition between the two clinics and perhaps the difference in survival rates.

Although improved nutrition may delay pulmonary deterioration, its effect on already existing pulmonary disease is less clear. A number of programs have used aggressive nutritional rehabilitation in patients with malnutrition and advanced pulmonary disease. Although these techniques are usually successful in improving overall nutritional status, there is little evidence that they significantly improve the pulmonary status, at least in the short term,[33,34] although they may have a beneficial effect on the rate of further pulmonary deterioration.[35-37]

Regional Center Care

Over the last three decades, care of patients with CF has evolved away from small groups of patients being followed by local community physicians into large, regional centers, with the availability of multidisciplinary expertise to cover the wide range of problems to which patients with CF are prone. Although this is not without attendant risks, particularly in relation to nosocomial spread of pathogens,[38,39] the available evidence is that care of patients with CF by larger, regional centers has resulted in improved survival.[40,41]

FACTORS AFFECTING INDIVIDUAL PROGNOSIS

Pattern of Clinical Disease

Of the different modes of presentation and subsequent clinical problems, several have been suggested as influencing, or at least correlating with, subsequent prognosis in any individual patient.

Meconium Ileus

Approximately 15% of patients with CF present in the neonatal period with meconium ileus (MI). Before 1961, MI was associated with an immediate mortality of close to 70%, with a less than 15% survival at 1 year,[42] most dying because of postoperative complications. However, improvements in operative care, medical management of MI, and general neonatal care have resulted in a marked decrease in mortality rate. Consequently the survival rate at 1 year, which was almost 55% before 1972, is now approximately 96%.[43] Patients born with MI have lower birth weights and earlier colonization with *P. aeruginosa,*[44] but the rate of progression of their pulmonary disease and subsequent survival is similar to that of female patients without MI.[43] It was initially suggested that patients with MI formed a genetically different subpopulation,[45] but this has not been supported by a subsequent report.[43]

Gastrointestinal Involvement

Pancreatic Exocrine Function. Of patients with CF, 15% have sufficient residual pancreatic function for normal digestion, and hence do not have steatorrhea. Pancreatic-sufficient (PS) patients therefore have normal digestion and growth. Although in an initial report there did not appear to be an improved survival rate for PS patients compared with pancreatic-insufficient (PI) patients,[46] a subsequent long-term study[47] did demonstrate a survival advantage for PS patients. The improved survival was attributed to either better nutrition (although in this study male PI patients maintained normal growth) or to a difference in genetic factors. The identification of the multiplicity of mutations that may cause CF suggest that any survival differences between PS and PI patients might indeed arise as a result of the varying severity of expression of different mutations. Indeed, PS patients as a group tend to have lower sweat chloride levels than PI patients (although there is no demonstrable correlation between the sweat chloride level at diagnosis and subsequent prognosis).[48]

Pancreatic Endocrine Function. With increasing age, abnormal glucose tolerance is found in an increasing percentage of patients. As a consequence, around 35% of adult patients have abnormal glucose tolerance tests, with 5% to 15% developing frank diabetes mellitus.[49] Diabetes mellitus in patients with CF is rarely a major therapeutic problem usually easily managed by insulin supplementation, with diabetic ketoacidosis being a rare complication. An early report documented a significantly worse prognosis in patients with diabetes.[50] This, however, appeared to be a consequence of an unusually high survival rate in the control population.[51] Subsequent reports failed to demonstrate any significant effect of diabetes on patient survival.[49,52] Patients with CF are, however, now living long enough for diabetes-related vascular complications to be reported,[53] which, by themselves, may eventually have a significant effect on patient survival.

Liver Disease. Overt liver disease occurs in approximately 4% of patients with CF,[54] the peak incidence being in late adolescence. Although liver disease is, if anything, underdiagnosed, it is not usually of major clinical import, with death from liver disease being rare. The severity of liver disease seldom has significant influence on subsequent survival.[55]

Nutritional Status

At Diagnosis. Evidence of protein-calorie malnutrition (PCM) is a common finding in the 85% of children with pancreatic insufficiency, and may occur surprisingly early.[56] This is not usually of major clinical import; the majority of children show significant catch-up in growth when treated with pancreatic enzyme supplementation and a high-calorie, high-fat diet.[57] There is, however, evidence that this early malnutrition does adversely affect subsequent survival. The rare patient who presents with severe PCM, sufficient to result in hypoproteinemia, edema, and anemia, has a poor prognosis, associated with early onset of pulmonary disease. In 1964, Fleisher et al reviewed the 26 cases reported to that time with PCM.[58] Eighteen (70%) of these patients had died within the first 2 years of life, the majority apparently from progressive pulmonary disease. Subsequent reports have confirmed the poor prognosis in these patients.[59] This suggests that early severe malnutrition may adversely affect the early onset of pulmonary disease, which does not seem to be completely corrected by nutritional rehabilitation. Obviously, this could equally reflect severe clinical expression generally, rather than a direct effect of malnutrition on the pulmonary course. However, even in patients diagnosed with CF by neonatal screening, who have hypoalbuminemia alone with otherwise normal growth and no other signs of PCM, there still seems to be an increased risk of early-onset pulmonary disease.[60]

Subsequent Course. As the pulmonary disease progresses, there is both increased caloric expenditure, from the increased work of breathing,[61] and decreased caloric intake because of the anorexia associated with chronic pulmonary infection. In one study, patients with weight for height ratio below 70% had more than a 50% risk of dying within the next 2 years (over 70% in patients 18 years and over).[62] Thus deteriorating nutritional status, expressed as a decrease in weight for height ratio, clearly correlates with a deteriorating prognosis.[63]

Respiratory Disease

Age of Onset of Pulmonary Disease. The rate of progress of respiratory disease is the major determinant of subsequent survival. Thus it is not surprising that patients presenting early with evidence of pulmonary disease have a worse prognosis than patients either presenting with just gastrointestinal symptoms[64] or diagnosed purely because of family history.[14]

Pulmonary Infection. Patients with CF have normal lungs at birth. The subsequent chronic endobronchial infection and the associated host immune response, that cause the chronic inflammatory changes within the airways, resulting in progressive airway destruction. The influence of the various organisms associated with this endobronchial disease has therefore been under intense scrutiny.[17]

Bacteria. Patients with CF acquire infection with a specific yet disparate group of organisms.[4] The precise influence of each organism on the progression of the lung disease is complicated by the fact that most patients develop concurrent endobronchial infection by a variety of organisms. It is therefore often difficult, in any one individual, to be sure which of the organisms is actually the primary pathogen.

Staphylococcus aureus. *S. aureus* is isolated from approximately 25% to 30% of patients with CF.[2,4] The incidence falls with increasing age of the patient population. As previously noted, before the advent of pancreatic enzyme supplements, patients with CF tended to develop fulminant staphylococcal pulmonary disease. Coincident with the development of pancreatic enzyme supplements and the resulting improved nutrition, staphylococcal disease has become both less common and of reduced severity. Thus *S. aureus* infection is not regarded as having as marked an influence on survival as previously thought, with some of the mildest affected patients being colonized for many years. *S. aureus* infection, however, commonly precedes *P. aeruginosa* infection, and concern remains as to whether *S. aureus* infection initiates the epithelial damage that facilitates *P. aeruginosa* adhesion and subsequent colonization.[65]

Pseudomonas aeruginosa. *P. aeruginosa* is the most commonly isolated organism in patients with CF, being found in 50% to 80% of patients.[2,4] The incidence of *P. aeruginosa* infection rises with increasing age of the patients, with approximately 20% of patients under 1 year of age being colonized, compared with around 80% of those over 20 years of age.[2] There seems to be little doubt that *P. aeruginosa* is the primary pathogen in CF. Once infection with *P. aeruginosa* has occurred, eradication rarely, if ever, occurs. The resulting chronic endobronchial infection causes progressive airway destruction, both as a consequence of the release of bacterial endotoxins and as a result of immune-mediated damage of the airway epithelium secondary to the ineffectual immune response to the chronic infection.[66] However, it is unclear how much of a role *P. aeruginosa* plays in influencing the rate of deterioration in pulmonary disease. *P. aeruginosa* infection is clearly associated with more severe pulmonary disease; the early acquisition of *P. aeruginosa,*[67] especially mucoid strains,[68] and the development of elevated levels of anti-pseudomonal antibodies[69] are both associated with a worse prognosis. Obviously, this may be because patients with inherently more severe disease are more likely to become colonized earlier with *P. aeruginosa.* Initial reports suggested that acquisition of *P. aeruginosa* infection was indeed associated with a significant deterioration in the pulmonary disease.[70] A more recent report,[71] however, although finding that patients with *P. aeruginosa* infection did have consistently worse pulmonary function than patients of the same age without *P. aeruginosa* infection, failed to demonstrate any direct influence by *P. aeruginosa* infection on the rate of progression of the pulmonary disease. In this study, the rate of deterioration following infection with *P. aeruginosa* was no different from that seen during the 2 years before onset of the infection or that found in patients not yet infected by *P. aeruginosa.* Thus although *P. aeruginosa* infection is clearly associated with pulmonary deterioration in patients with CF, how directly it influences disease progression, as opposed to merely being an opportunistic agent in patients with inherently more severe disease, is unknown.

Pseudomonas cepacia (Burkholderia cepacia). The overall incidence of *P. cepacia* infection in CF is around 10% in Canada[4] and 5% in the United States.[2] As with *P. aeruginosa,* the incidence of *P. cepacia* infection increases with the increasing age of the patient population.[2] In addition, the incidence of *P. cepacia* varies markedly between different clinics and across differing geographic regions, with some clinics never reporting its isolation and other regions reporting an incidence as high as 22%.[4] *P. cepacia* infection has been of particular concern for several reasons.

First, the frequency of isolation of *P. cepacia* rises with increasing severity of pulmonary damage[72]; thus the organism is more closely associated with advanced pulmonary disease.[63]

Second, several reports have linked it to a syndrome of rapidly progressive pulmonary disease characterized by fever, malaise, anorexia, nausea, elevated white cell count, and erythrocyte sedimentation rate, with death within 3 months ("the *cepacia* syndrome").[73,74] *P. cepacia* is therefore generally believed to result in more aggressive pulmonary disease.

Finally, prior colonization with *P. cepacia* is associated with a poor postoperative course in patients receiving lung transplantation.[75] *P. cepacia* is, however, ordinarily nonpathogenic in immunocompetent individuals. Some patients with CF may harbor endobronchial infection for many years without apparent adverse consequences on their pulmonary disease, whereas the "cepacia syndrome" occurs only in a small subgroup of individuals.[74] To date no researcher has identified the factors that initiate the fulminant pulmonary infection in this subgroup of patients. It is therefore possible that *P. cepacia* does not itself cause aggressive pulmonary disease, but is merely an opportunistic colonizer of damaged airways in patients with more severe disease. However, when compared with a control group with equivalent age and pulmonary function, patients colonized with *P. cepacia* seem to have a more rapid rate of progression in their pulmonary disease and a worse overall prognosis,[72] suggesting that, at least in older patients, *P. cepacia* does indeed result in a more aggressive pulmonary infection.

Viruses/mycoplasma. The course of the pulmonary disease in CF is often marked by episodes of acute exacerbation, characterized by increased cough, deterioration in pulmonary function, and malaise, with or without fever. Although patients with CF appear no more likely than the general population to develop viral infections,[76] probably at least 30% of acute exacerbations are precipitated by infection with respiratory viruses or mycoplasma.[76,77] These episodes may be associated with marked deterioration in clinical status,[78] although there is generally a return to baseline status following therapy. There is, however, evidence that viral or mycoplasma infections may adversely affect overall prognosis of patients with CF. It is well documented that viral respiratory tract infections predispose any host to opportunistic bacterial infections. In patients with CF, viral-mediated damage to the respiratory epithelium may promote bacterial adherence and help initiate colonization by *P. aeruginosa*.[79] This is supported by the seasonal variability in onset of *P. aeruginosa* infection, the peak incidence for initial colonization being during the winter, coincident with the peak period for viral respiratory tract infections.[80] This may explain the association between the number of viral infections and the rate of deterioration of clinical disease,[81] patients with the highest number of such infections having the greatest rate of deterioration. Antiviral therapy[82] and immunizations[83] may therefore have a role in delaying the progression of the pulmonary disease in CF.

Fungal infection. Endobronchial colonization by various fungi is common with advancing disease. The two most common colonizing agents are *Candida* and *Aspergillus fumigatus* (each being isolated in 3% to 4.5% of patients).[2] Despite the frequency with which fungi are isolated from the sputum of patients with CF, surprisingly little is known about how much these fungi contribute to disease progression.[84] In some patients, endobronchial colonization by *Aspergillus* may induce an allergic response,[85] resulting in a hyperimmune response (allergic bronchopulmonary aspergillosis) that, if untreated, may lead to proximal bronchiectasis, thereby clearly contributing to the disease process. In the remaining patients with fungal colonization, it appears that the fungi are primarily innocent commensals and do not actually lead to significant pulmonary damage.

Airway Obstruction. Recurrent wheezing is a common symptom in young children with CF, with as many as 25% of children with CF having physician-documented wheezing during the first 2 years of life[86] (median age of onset being 5 months). Although recurrent episodes of wheezing were common in these children, 50% had stopped wheezing by 2 years and 75% by 4 years of age. The cause of this wheezing is unclear. Nearly 50% of children with CF who wheezed had a family history of atopy.[86] Some of these children clearly had a significant element of hyperactive airway disease, usually triggered by respiratory viruses and responsive to inhaled bronchodilators or, if necessary, systemic steroids. One study[87] reported 17 infants, under 1 year of age, admitted over a 5-year period with respiratory distress, in whom CF was subsequently diagnosed. These children had early onset of endobronchial infection (*P. aeruginosa* in 11, *Klebsiella pneumoniae* in 11, *Escherichia coli* in 8, and *S. aureus* in 5), with 10 children (60% of the group) dying during the first year of life. In this group of children, wheezing in infancy was a very ominous finding. However, in a recent report from this institution,[86] no statistical difference could be demonstrated in survival or age of onset of colonization of *P. aeruginosa* between children with a history of wheezing during the first 2 years of life (25% of the population) and those without such a history. At age 13, however, children with a history of early wheezing had significantly worse pulmonary function; thus with larger numbers, a difference in survival may become apparent. In general, wheezing in infancy does not appear to carry as severe a prognosis as was previously thought.

Genotype

Genetic Mutation

At the time of writing, over 700 different mutations have been described within the CF locus, with the majority causing disease.[88] However, around 85% of cases of CF are caused by only one of four or five common mutations (ΔF_{508} being the most common in patients of Celtic and French descent). There is both a growing understanding of the specific function of the CF transmembrane conductance regulator (CFTR)[88] and an increasing knowledge of precisely how the various mutations within the CFTR gene affect the structure and function of the protein product.[89] Depending on the specific mutation, CF arises as a consequence of one of four broad categories of defect in intracellular processing or functioning of the CFTR (Fig. 70-2). Differences in severity of clinical disease might therefore be explained by differing phenotypic expressions of the different mutations, as a result of their respective effects on the presence or functioning of CFTR within the apical membrane. Since the identification of the ΔF_{508} mutation, a plethora of papers have attempted to correlate different mutations with clinical outcome.[90-94] These papers have, in general, been limited both by the paucity of patients with non-ΔF_{508}

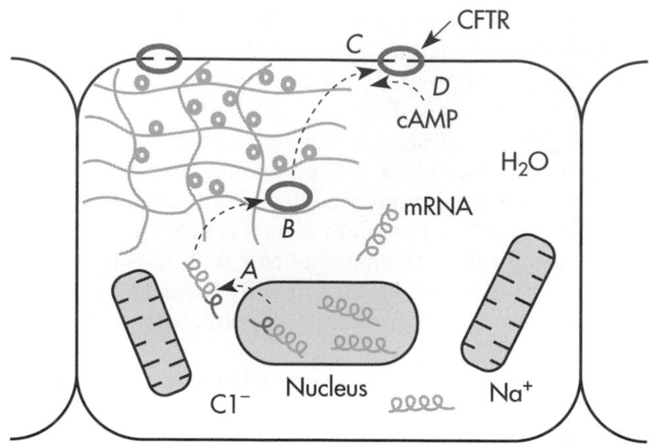

Fig. 70-2. The effect of differing classes of mutation on intracellular processing of CFTR. *A,* Nonsense mutations, which result in no effective messenger RNA or a nonfunctional protein product. *B,* Mutations that result in production of a protein product by the endoplasmic reticulum that, if incorporated into the cellular membrane, would produce a functioning chloride channel. However, the mutation results in failed intracellular glycosylation of the CFTR, which therefore does not undergo secondary maturation on the Golgi apparatus, and hence fails to be incorporated into the apical membrane of the cell. As a result, no functioning CFTR channels are present within the cell membrane (ΔF_{508} being the most common cause of this variant). *C,* Mutations that result in production of a protein that is glycosylated, and hence incorporated into the apical membrane. The mutation, however, results in abnormalities (usually within the membrane-spanning portions of the CFTR) that result in a reduced chloride permeability of the CFTR. Thus although functioning chloride channels are present within the cellular membrane, they show reduced chloride transport (such as the R117H mutation). *D,* Mutations, usually within the regulatory domain, that result in a functioning protein, which is again incorporated into the cellular membrane, but this time the resulting chloride channels are poorly responsive to intracellular regulation by cyclic AMP.

mutations and the marked interpatient variability in pulmonary disease. However, a pattern of clinical disease has been identified as being associated with some specific genotypes. In an initial report,[95] patients homozygous for ΔF_{508} (52% of the population) were compared with both those heterozygous for ΔF_{508} and one other mutation (40% of the population) and those with a non-ΔF_{508}/non-ΔF_{508} genotype (8% of the population). Patients whose genotype contained a non-ΔF_{508} mutation were more likely to be PS (53% vs. 1%) and to be diagnosed at older ages. In all three genotype groups, PI patients had similar pulmonary function for a given age, but PS patients had significantly better pulmonary function than age-matched PS patients. A subsequent study in the same group of patients identified many of the specific mutations associated with pancreatic sufficiency that appear to confer milder pulmonary disease.[96] A recent multicenter study[97] compared 399 patients homozygous for ΔF_{508} with 399 age-matched controls whose genotype contained one of six other common CF mutations. There was no significant difference in any clinical parameter between patients homozygous for ΔF_{508} and patients whose genotype contained any of the five other mutations. However, 87% of patients whose genotype contained the R117H mutation were PS, compared with around 1% of patients homozygous for ΔF_{508}. R117H is a missense mutation in which arginine is replaced by histidine at residue 117, affecting the first membrane-spanning sequence of CFTR. Compared with ΔF_{508}, which results in defective intracellular processing of CFTR within the cells, and hence no measurable chloride channel within the apical membrane, R117H results in a CFTR molecule that is incorporated into the apical membrane but has reduced chloride conductance.[98] Although the various genetic mutations result in differing severity of the chloride channel defect and are associated with varying severity of pancreatic involvement, there is such a wide range of pulmonary disease within each of the differing genotypes studied that no statistical difference in pulmonary prognosis has been associated with any particular genotype.[97a] Therefore, at this point, genetic factors, associated with differing severity in the chloride channel defect, may explain the varying levels of pancreatic involvement seen between patients. Other, nongenetic factors, such as age of acquisition and type of endobronchial infection, nutritional status, and compliance with therapy, seem to have roles at least as important, if not more so, in determining the rate of progression of the pulmonary disease. However, data from the CF mouse model suggest the presence of modifier genes, distinct from the CFTR locus, that may serve, via calcium-activated chloride channels, to ameliorate the ion transport abnormalities caused by absence of CFTR function.[97b] The presence of these modifier genes may therefore explain some of the phenotypic variability seen in patients with CF.

Gender

CF is unusual in that a significant difference in survival rates between the sexes has been reported by many authors,[2,41,99] with female patients having a consistently worse prognosis than their male counterparts (Fig. 70-3). Although this has been a common, if not universal, finding,[14] the explanation for this difference is still unclear. It is notable, however, that the major difference in mortality rates between the sexes seems to occur primarily under the age of 18 years, the surviving women who reach adulthood having a subsequent prognosis equivalent to that of men.[63]

Poor compliance with therapy, or the effects of hormones on endobronchial mucus (either a beneficial effect of androgens or a detrimental effect of progestogens or estrogens) have all been suggested as causes for this poorer survival of female patients. However, few objective data support any of these theories. Of note, girls with CF generally have a worse growth pattern than boys. This is particularly apparent in adolescence,[4] when girls often demonstrate a significant fall-off in growth. Patients with the greatest fall-off in weight show the worst prognosis. This might simply be the result of endocrine effects on disease status, but may also reflect the societal pressures placed on adolescent girls, who find that they can readily (by reducing caloric or pancreatic enzyme intake) achieve a certain appearance, to the detriment of their health.

Race

Several papers have attempted to look at the influence of race on disease severity.[100,101] The varying geographic incidence of the various mutations[102] and the very low incidence of CF in nonwhite individuals, resulting in small numbers in any population study, make it difficult to ascertain whether there is any real difference in survival between races and, if so, how much of this difference is the result of a racial effect and how much is the influence of differing mutations.[100]

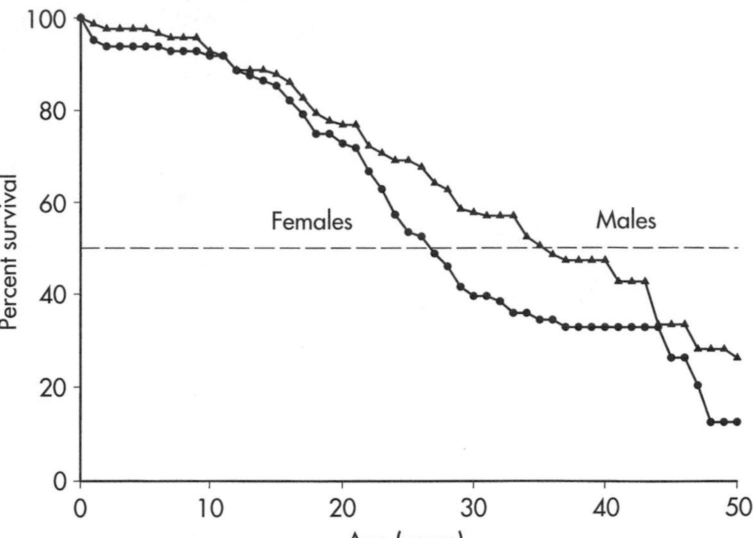

Fig. 70-3. Percent survival against age of patients followed at the Cystic Fibrosis clinic, the Hospital for Sick Children, Toronto, based on age specific death rates during the period from 1987 to 1996.

Other Factors

There is evidence that childhood environment can have an influence on the survival of patients with CF.

Family Functioning

Like any chronic, ultimately fatal disease, CF would be expected to be associated with significant psychosocial effects on the child and the immediate family. This has, however, received little, and somewhat contradictory, study. Various studies have reported increased marital conflicts, parental depression,[103] behavioral problems in siblings,[104] and even improved psychosocial functioning,[105] these observations being attributed to the consequences of living with a chronic disease.[106] A recent study evaluated 91 families with CF children.[107] Measurements of family compliance with therapy, family resources, and coping techniques were all made at the start of the study and the children were followed prospectively (92% being followed for 5 years, 80% for 10 years). Over the subsequent 10-year period, 33% of the variance in pulmonary function could be explained by three factors; emphasis on personal growth in the family, family coping skills, and compliance score. The conclusion was that the subsequent rate of deterioration in pulmonary function could be predicted by indices of family coping at outset, the inference being that psychosocial factors may play a significant role in determining subsequent clinical course.

Social Class

Although obviously influenced by many confounding factors, one paper from England implicated social class as a significant, independent determinant on survival,[99] with children whose parents were manual laborers having significantly worse survival than those whose parents fell into the professional class. This is consistent with the general observation that poorer health is associated with lower social class and/or poverty, whatever the disease.

Environment

Increasing exposure to second-hand cigarette smoke also seems to adversely affect survival.[108] This is of note because a variant of the "healthy smoker effect" (where parents of healthy children are less likely to quit smoking compared with parents of children with advanced pulmonary disease) would be expected to obscure any association between parental smoking and the health of the child.[109] Because of the differing incidence of parental smoking between various social classes, it is difficult to distinguish the effects of second-hand smoke from the influence of social class.

FACTORS INDICATIVE OF POOR SURVIVAL

There are several factors which, although not directly influencing the overall outcome, reflect deteriorating clinical status.

Respiratory

Progressive respiratory failure, as a result of chronic suppurative endobronchial disease, is the cause of death in 95% of patients. Thus evidence of diminishing respiratory reserve is one of the primary indicators of worsening prognosis.

Pulmonary Function

A recent retrospective review[62] studied the prior history of 673 patients followed at the Toronto clinic, 190 (28%) of whom died over the previous 12-year period, to evaluate factors that predicted mortality. They found that patients with forced vital capacities (FVC) between 51% and 60% predicted had a less than 4% risk of death within 1 year, and around 10% by 2 years (Fig. 70-4). This compared with 50% and 34% 1- and 2-year survival rates, respectively, for patients with FVCs below 30% predicted. Similarly, patients with forced 1-second expiratory volumes (FEV_1) between 51% and 60% had over 96% survival to 1 year and 90% survival at 2 years, whereas patients with FEV_1s less than 20% had a 50% survival to 1 year and 40% at 2 years. These factors were significantly influenced by age and sex, in that for any given pulmonary function female and younger patients had a significantly worse prognosis compared with male and older patients (Fig. 70-5). Sequential pulmonary function testing is therefore one of the most reliable indicators of individual prognosis.

Exercise Testing

The level of aerobic fitness (as measured using formal graded exercise testing) also seems to have a direct relationship with subsequent survival, with patients whose VO_{2max} was more

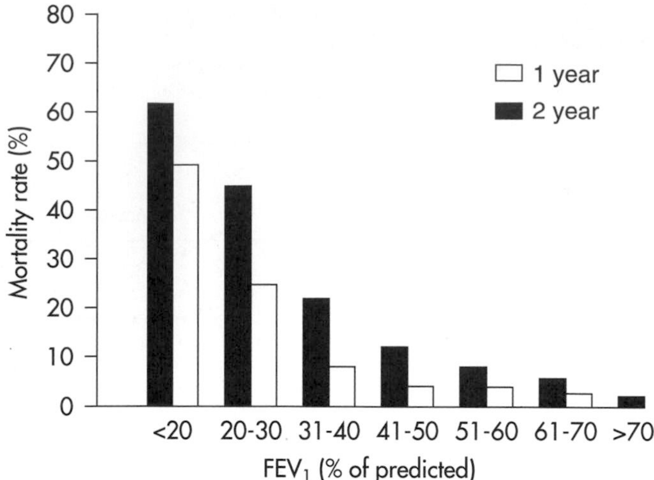

Fig. 70-4. 1- and 2-year mortality rates among patients with CF, according to FEV$_1$. Values were calculated from pooled measurements. (From Kerem E, Reisman J, Corey M, Canny GJ, Levison H: *N Engl J Med* 326:1187-1191, 1992.)

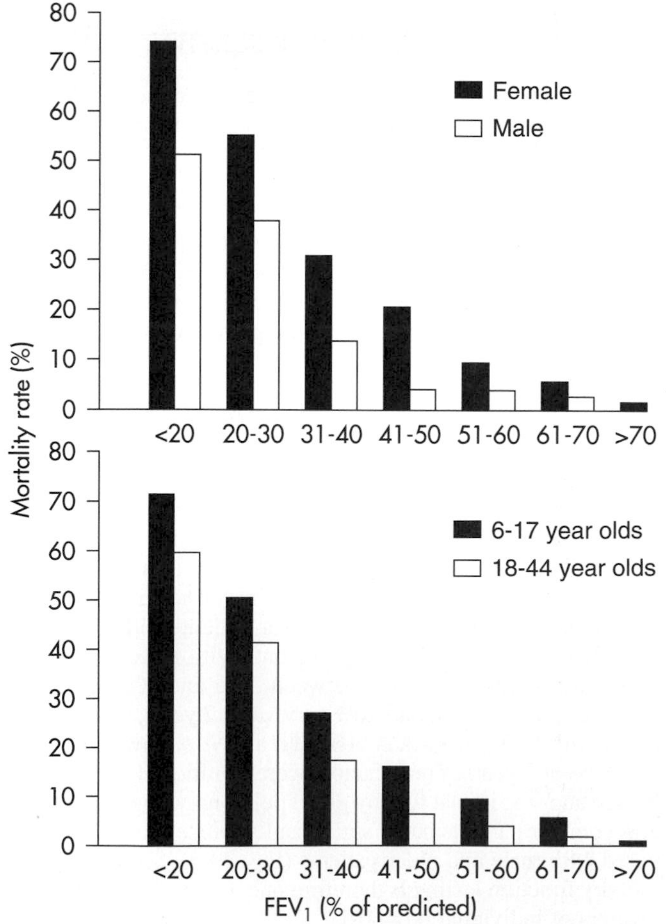

Fig. 70-5. 2-year mortality rates among patients with CF, according to FEV$_1$ and sex *(top panel)* and age *(bottom panel)*. Values were calculated from pooled measurements. (From Kerem E, Reisman J, Corey M, Canny GJ, Levison H: *N Engl J Med* 326:1187-1191, 1992.)

than 80% predicted having a threefold lower mortality rate compared with those with a VO_{2max} of less than 60% predicted.[110] Although this might simply reflect the severity of their pulmonary function abnormalities, exercise testing appeared to be an independent predictor of subsequent prognosis, suggesting that maintenance of overall fitness may improve subsequent prognosis.

Blood Gases

As the pulmonary disease progresses, increasing ventilation-perfusion mismatching results in progressive hypoxemia. By maintaining relative hyperventilation, arterial carbon dioxide tension (CO_2) remains normal until late in the disease process. However, ultimately the pulmonary damage progresses to the point that the patient is unable to maintain a normal arterial CO_2 and the level rises. The influence of hypoxemia and carbon dioxide retention on subsequent survival has recently been studied.[62] A significant association between blood gas tensions and survival was found, with patients whose arterial Pao_2 was less than 55 mm Hg or arterial Pco_2 greater than 50 mm Hg having only a 50% chance of surviving 2 years. However, multivariate analysis indicated that, although subsequent survival was associated with blood gas values, the primary determinant was the severity of the pulmonary disease, as documented by pulmonary function tests, with the blood gas abnormalities arising as a consequence, rather than being independent predictors of prognosis. Once blood gas status has deteriorated to the point of requiring artificial ventilation, the prognosis is poor, with less than 30% of patients improving to the point of extubation, and only 6% actually living for more than another year[111] (0% in patients with chronic, progressive CO_2 retention).

Cardiac Function

Progressive pulmonary destruction, and the resulting hypoxemia, results in progressive elevation of the pulmonary artery pressure, with cor pulmonale being present in 70% of patients dying from CF.[112] Overt right-sided cardiac failure is therefore indicative of advanced pulmonary disease and carries a poor prognosis (mean survival after onset of overt heart failure 8 months).[113] Treatment of the cardiac failure is usually ineffectual; the only effective therapy is correction of the underlying pulmonary disease (that is, lung transplantation).

Clinical Signs

Finger clubbing, pneumothorax, and hemoptysis all occur as a consequence of the progressive pulmonary disease, their presence therefore correlating, to a degree, with the overall prognosis.[114]

FUTURE CHANGES IN SURVIVAL

The prospects for the future obviously depend largely on whether a more specific therapy becomes available, either in terms of gene therapy or pharmacologic replacement or modulation of the chloride channel. Even without these therapies, the survival of patients with CF continues to rise. Can this be expected to continue? The sequelae of diabetes mellitus, the problems associated with progressive hepatic cirrhosis, and, most importantly, the increasing prevalence of resistant organisms all assume increasing significance with advancing patient age. Because of the limited availability of donor organs, the high costs of the technique, and the ongoing problems of immunosuppression and chronic rejection, lung transplantation will probably remain a limited option for patients with end-stage pulmonary disease. Thus using conventional therapy, we suspect that a maximum survival may be reached, with patients living until their late 30s or early 40s before succumbing to the consequences of chronic endobronchial infection with resistant organisms. This has certainly been the experience at our clinic, where the median survival for patients with CF is in the late 20s for women, early 30s for men (Fig. 70-3); this has not changed significantly over the last decade compared with previously reported data.[26] At the same time, the prognosis for patients now being diagnosed with CF is the brightest it has been at any time during the history of the disease. The genetic structure of the most common mutations causing CF has been elucidated, along with an increasing knowledge of exactly how these mutations affect both intracellular processing and function of CFTR. Moreover, developments in gene therapy, specifically in techniques of incorporation of genetic material into functioning, mature cells, opens up the potential for modulation or replacement of CFTR into airway cells of patients with CF. These novel therapies are expected to be of most benefit to children who have not developed irreversible pulmonary damage. Correcting the underlying defect may arrest the progress of the disease, but, once endobronchial infection has progressed to saccular bronchiectasis, chronic endobronchial infection is liable to persist, resulting in ongoing pulmonary damage. Thus even with the development of a definitive therapy, there will probably remain a cohort of individuals with CF who continue to demonstrate the progressive pulmonary disease characteristic of CF.

REFERENCES

1. Andersen DH: Cystic fibrosis of the pancreas and its relation to celiac disease, a clinical and pathological study, *Am J Dis Child* 56:344-348, 1938.
2. FitzSimmons SC: The changing epidemiology of cystic fibrosis, *J Pediatr* 122:1-9, 1993.
3. Dinwiddie R: Cystic fibrosis: yesterday, today and tomorrow, *J R Soc Med* 84 suppl 18:36-39, 1991 [review].
4. Report of the Canadian Cystic Fibrosis Patient Data Registry, 1991. Toronto, 1993, Canadian Cystic Fibrosis Foundation.
5. Strong TV, Smit LS, Turpin SV, Cole JL, Hon CT, Markiewicz MS, Petty TL, Craig MW, Rosenow EC, Tsui LC, Ianuzzi MC, Knowles MR, Collins FS: Cystic fibrosis gene mutation in two sisters with mild disease and normal sweat electrolyte levels, *N Engl J Med* 325:1630-1634, 1991.

Factors Implicated in Change in Overall Population Survival

6. Hunt B, Geddes DM: Newly diagnosed cystic fibrosis in middle and later life, *Thorax* 40:23-26, 1985.
7. di Sant'Agnese PA, Darling RC, Perera GA, Shea A: Abnormal electrolyte composition of sweat in cystic fibrosis of the pancreas, *Pediatrics* 12:549-563, 1953.
8. Matheson WJ: Fibrocystic disease of the pancreas, *Br Med J* 2:204-209, 1949.
9. LeGrys VA, Wood RE: Incidence and implications of false-negative sweat test reports in patients with cystic fibrosis, *Pediatr Pulmonol* 4:169-172, 1988.
10. Kerem BS, Rommens JM, Buchanan JA, Markiewicz D, Cox TK, Chakravarti A, Buchwald M, Tsui LC: Identification of the cystic fibrosis gene: genetic analysis, *Science* 245:1073-1080, 1989.
11. Heeley AF, Watson D: Cystic fibrosis—its biochemical detection, *Clin Chem* 29:2011-2018, 1983 [review].
12. Holtzman NA: What drives neonatal screening programs? *N Engl J Med* 325:802-804, 1991.
13. Anonymous: Statement from the National Institutes of Health workshop on population screening for the cystic fibrosis gene, *N Engl J Med* 323:70-71, 1990.
14. Hodson I, Phelan PD: Are sex, age at diagnosis, or mode of presentation prognostic factors for cystic fibrosis? *Pediatr Pulmonol* 3:288-297, 1987.
15. Dankert-Roelse JE, te Meerman GJ, Martijn A, Ten Kate LP, Knol K: Survival and clinical outcome in patients with cystic fibrosis, with or without neonatal screening, *J Pediatr* 114:362-367, 1989.

16a. Chatfield S, Owen G, Ryley HC, Williams J, Alfaham M, Goodchild MC, Weller P: Neonatal screening for cystic fibrosis in Wales and the West Midlands: clinical assessment after five years of screening, *Arch Dis Child* 66:29-33, 1991.

16b. Farrell PM, Kosorok MR, Laxova A, Shen G, Koscik RE, Bruns WT, Splaingard M, Mischler EH: Nutritional benefits of neonatal screening for cystic fibrosis. Wisconsin Cystic Fibrosis Neonatal Screening Study Group, *N Engl J Med* 337:963-969, 1997.

17. Thomassen MJ, Demko CA, Doershuk CF: Cystic fibrosis: a review of pulmonary infections and interventions, *Pediatr Pulmonol* 3:334-351, 1987 [review].
18. Boxerbaum B: The art and science of the use of antibiotics in cystic fibrosis, *Pediatr Infect Dis* 1:381-383, 1982 [review].
19. Phillips BM, David TJ: Management of the chest in cystic fibrosis, *J R Soc Med* 80 (suppl 15):30-37, 1987 [review].
20. Padoan R, Cambisano W, Constantini D, Crossignani RM, Danza ML, Trezzi G, Giunta A: Ceftazidime monotherapy vs. combined therapy in *Pseudomonas* pulmonary infections in cystic fibrosis, *Pediatr Infect Dis* 6:648-653, 1987.
21. British Thoracic Society Research Committee: Ceftazidime compared with gentamycin and carbenicillin in patients with cystic fibrosis, pulmonary *Pseudomonas* infection, and an exacerbation of respiratory symptoms, *Thorax* 40:358-363, 1985.
22. Beaudry PH, Marks MI, McDougall D, Desmond K, Rangel R: Is anti-pseudomonas therapy warranted in acute exacerbations in children with cystic fibrosis? *J Pediatr* 97:144-147, 1980.
23. Gold R, Carpenter S, Heurter H, Corey M, Levison H: Randomized trial of ceftazidime versus placebo in the management of acute respiratory exacerbations in patients with cystic fibrosis, *J Pediatr* 111:907-913, 1987.
24. Valerius NH, Koch C, Hoiby N: Prevention of chronic *Pseudomonas aeruginosa* colonisation in cystic fibrosis by early treatment, *Lancet* 338:725-726, 1991.
25. Pedersen SS, Jensen T, Hoiby N, Koch C, Flensborg EW: Management of *Pseudomonas aeruginosa* lung infection in Danish cystic fibrosis patients, *Acta Paediatr Scand* 76:955-961, 1987.
26. Corey M, McLaughlin FJ, Williams M, Levison H: A comparison of survival, growth, and pulmonary function in patients with cystic fibrosis in Boston and Toronto, *J Clin Epidemiol* 41:583-591, 1988.
27. Bauernfeind A, Emminger G, Horl G, Lorbeer B, Pryzklenk B, Weisslein-Pfister C: Selective pressures of antistaphylococcal chemotherapeutics in favour of *Pseudomonas aeruginosa* in cystic fibrosis, *Infection* 15:469-470, 1987.
28. MacLusky IB, Gold R, Corey M, Levison H: Long-term effects of inhaled tobramycin in patients with cystic fibrosis colonized with *Pseudomonas aeruginosa, Pediatr Pulmonol* 7:42-48, 1989.
29. Steinkamp G, Tummler B, Gappa M, Albus A, Potel J, Doring G, von der Hardt H: Long-term tobramycin aerosol therapy in cystic fibrosis, *Pediatr Pulmonol* 6:91-98, 1989.
30. Dodge JA: Nutrition in cystic fibrosis: a historical overview, *Proc Nutr Soc* 51:225-235, 1992 [review].
31. Ramsey BW, Farrell PM, Pencharz P: Nutritional assessment and management in cystic fibrosis: a consensus report. The Consensus Committee, *Am J Clin Nutr* 55:108-116, 1992.
32. Martin TR: The relationship between malnutrition and lung infections, *Clin Chest Med* 8(3):359-372, 1987 [review].
33. Mansell AL, Andersen JC, Muttart CR, Ores CN, Loeff DS, Levy JS, Heird WC: Short-term pulmonary effects of total parenteral nutrition in children with cystic fibrosis, *J Pediatr* 104:700-705, 1984.

34. Bertrand JM, Morin CL, Lasalle R, Patrick J, Coates AL: Short-term clinical, nutritional, and functional effects of continuous elemental enteral alimentation in children with cystic fibrosis, *J Pediatr* 104:41-46, 1984.
35. Levy LD, Durie PR, Pencharz PB, Corey ML: Effects of long-term nutritional rehabilitation on body composition and clinical status in malnourished children and adolescents with cystic fibrosis, *J Pediatr* 107:225-230, 1985.
36. Shepherd RW, Holt TL, Thomas BJ, Kay L, Isles A, Francis PJ, Ward LC: Nutritional rehabilitation in cystic fibrosis: controlled studies of effects on nutritional growth retardation, body protein turnover, and course of pulmonary disease, *J Pediatr* 109:788-794, 1986.
37. Dalzell AM, Shepherd RW, Dean B, Cleghorn GJ, Holt TL, Francis PJ: Nutritional rehabilitation in cystic fibrosis: a 5 year follow-up study, *J Pediatr Gastroenterol Nutr* 15:141-145, 1992.
38. Tummler B, Koopmann U, Grothues D, Weissbrodt H, Steinkamp G, von der Hardt H: Nosocomial acquisition of *Pseudomonas aeruginosa* by cystic fibrosis patients, *J Clin Microbiol* 29:1265-1267, 1991.
39. Hoiby N, Pedersen SS: Estimated risk of cross infection with *Pseudomonas aeruginosa* in Danish cystic fibrosis patients, *Acta Paediatr Scand* 78:395-404, 1989.
40. Warwick WJ: Prognosis for survival with cystic fibrosis: the effects of early diagnosis and cystic fibrosis center care, *Acta Paediatr Scand* suppl 301:27-31, 1982.
41. British Paediatric Association Working Party on Cystic Fibrosis: Cystic fibrosis in the United Kingdom 1977-85: an improving picture, *Br Med J* 297:1599-1602, 1988.

Factors Affecting Individual Prognosis

42. McPartlin JF, Dickson JAS, Swain VA: Meconium ileus: immediate and long-term survival, *Arch Dis Child* 47:207-210, 1972.
43. Kerem E, Corey M, Kerem B, Durie P, Tsui LC, Levison L: Clinical and genetic comparisons of patients with cystic fibrosis, with or without meconium ileus, *J Pediatr* 114:767-773, 1989.
44. Kerem E, Corey M, Stein R, Gold R, Levison H: Risk factors for *Pseudomonas aeruginosa* colonization in cystic fibrosis patients, *Pediatr Infect Dis J* 9:494-498, 1990.
45. Mornet E, Serre JL, Farrall M, Boue J, Simon-Bouy B, Estivill X, Williamson R, Boue A: Genetic differences between cystic fibrosis with and without meconium ileus, *Lancet* 1:376-378, 1988.
46. Shwachman H, Dooley RR, Guilmette F, Patterson PR, Weil C, Leubner H: Cystic fibrosis of the pancreas with varying degrees of pancreatic insufficiency, *Am J Dis Child* 92:347-368, 1956.
47. Gaskin K, Gurwitz D, Durie P, Corey M, Levison H, Forstner G: Improved respiratory prognosis in patients with cystic fibrosis with normal fat absorption, *J Pediatr* 100:857-862, 1982.
48. Corkey CWB, Corey M, Gaskin K, Levison H: Prognostic value of sweat-chloride levels in cystic fibrosis: a negative report, *Eur J Respir Dis* 6:434-436, 1983.
49. Reisman J, Corey M, Canny G, Levison H: Diabetes mellitus in patients with cystic fibrosis: effect on survival [see comments], *Pediatrics* 86:374-377, 1990.
50. Finkelstein SM, Wielinski CL, Elliott GR, Warwick WJ, Barbosa J, Wu S, Klein DJ: Diabetes mellitus associated with cystic fibrosis, *J Pediatr* 112:373-377, 1988.
51. Knowles MR: Diabetes and cystic fibrosis: new questions emerging from increased longevity, *J Pediatr* 112:415-416, 1988.
52. Rodman HM, Doershuk CF, Roland JM: The interaction of 2 diseases: diabetes mellitus and cystic fibrosis, *Medicine (Baltimore)* 65:389-397, 1986.
53. Pfeifer T: Diabetes in cystic fibrosis, *Clin Pediatr (Phila)* 31:682-687, 1992.
54. Scott Jupp R, Lama M, Tanner MS: Prevalence of liver disease in cystic fibrosis, *Arch Dis Child* 66:698-701, 1991.
55. Tanner MS: Liver and biliary problems in cystic fibrosis, *J R Soc Med* 85(suppl 19):20-24, 1992 [review].
56. Reardon MC, Hammond KB, Accurso FJ, Fisher CD, McCabe ERB, Cotton EK, Bowman CM: Nutritional deficits exist before 2 months of age in some infants with cystic fibrosis identified by screening test, *J Pediatr* 105:271-274, 1984.
57. Marcus MS, Sondel SA, Farrell PM, Laxova A, Carey PM, Langhough R, Mischler EH: Nutritional status of infants with cystic fibrosis associated with early diagnosis and intervention, *Am J Clin Nutr* 54:578-585, 1991.
58. Fleisher DS, DiGeorge AM, Barness LA, Cornfeld D: Hypoproteinemia and edema in infants with cystic fibrosis of the pancreas, *J Pediatr* 64:341-348, 1994.
59. Abman SH, Accurso FJ, Bowman CM: Persistent morbidity and mortality of protein calorie malnutrition in young infants with CF, *J Pediatr Gastroenterol Nutr* 5:393-396, 1986.
60. Abman SH, Reardon MC, Accurso FJ, Hammond KB, Sokol R: Hypoalbuminemia at diagnosis as a marker for severe respiratory course in infants with cystic fibrosis identified by newborn screening, *J Pediatr* 107:933-935, 1985.
61. Spicher V, Roulet M, Schutz Y: Assessment of total energy expenditure in free-living patients with cystic fibrosis, *J Pediatr* 118:865-872, 1991.
62. Kerem E, Reisman J, Corey M, Canny GJ, Levison H: Prediction of mortality in patients with cystic fibrosis, *N Engl J Med* 326:1187-1191, 1992.
63. Huang NN, Schidlow DV, Szatrowski TH, Palmer J, Laraya-Cuasay LR, Yeung W, Hardy K, Quitell L, Fiel S: Clinical features, survival rate, and prognostic factors in young adults with cystic fibrosis, *Am J Med* 82:871-879, 1987.
64. Katz JN, Horwitz RI, Dolan TF, Shapiro ED: Clinical features as predictors of functional status in children with cystic fibrosis, *J Pediatr* 108:352-358, 1986.
65. Marks MI: Clinical significance of *Staphylococcus aureus* in cystic fibrosis, *Infection* 18:53-56, 1990.
66. Grimwood K: The pathogenesis of *Pseudomonas aeruginosa* lung infections in cystic fibrosis, *J Paediatr Child Health* 28:4-11, 1992 [review].
67. Wilmott RW, Tyson SL, Mathew DJ: Cystic fibrosis survival rates: The influences of allergy and *Pseudomonas aeruginosa, Am J Dis Child* 139:669-671, 1985.
68. Henry RL, Mellis CM, Petrovic L: Mucoid *Pseudomonas aeruginosa* is a marker of poor survival in cystic fibrosis, *Pediatr Pulmonol* 12:158-161, 1992.
69. Dasgupta MK, Lam J, Doring G, Harley FL, Zuberbuhler P, Lam K, Reichert A, Costerton JW, Dossetor JB: Prognostic implications of circulating immune complexes and *Pseudomonas aeruginosa*-specific antibodies in cystic fibrosis, *J Clin Lab Immunol* 23:25-30, 1987.
70. Hoiby N: Microbiology of lung infections in cystic fibrosis patients, *Acta Paediatr Scand* 301(suppl):33-54, 1982 [review].
71. Kerem E, Corey M, Gold R, Levison H: Pulmonary function and clinical course in patients with cystic fibrosis after pulmonary colonization with *Pseudomonas aeruginosa, J Pediatr* 116:714-719, 1990.
72. Tablan OC, Martone WJ, Doershuk CF, Stern RC, Thomassen MJ, Klinger JD, White JW, Carson LA, Jarvis WR: Colonization of the respiratory tract with *Pseudomonas cepacia* in cystic fibrosis. Risk factors and outcomes, *Chest* 91:527-532, 1987.
73. Isles A, MacLusky IB, Corey M, Gold R, Prober C, Fleming P, Levison H: *Pseudomonas cepacia* infection in cystic fibrosis: an emerging problem, *J Pediatr* 206:206-210, 1984.
74. Anonymous: *Pseudomonas cepacia* colonization among patients with cystic fibrosis. A new opportunist, *Am Rev Respir Dis* 131:791-796, 1985.
75. Snell GI, de Hoyos A, Krajden M, Winton T, Maurer JR: *Pseudomonas cepacia* in lung transplant recipients with cystic fibrosis, *Chest* 103:466-471, 1993.
76. Deforest H, Grosz H, Larayu-Cussay L, Gregory JB, Satz J, Huang HH: The association of viral and mycoplasma infections with lower respiratory tract disease in patients with cystic fibrosis, *Pediatr Res* 6:388 1973.
77. Stroobant J: Viral infection in cystic fibrosis, *J R Soc Med* 79:S19-S22, 1986 [review].
78. Conway SP, Simmonds EJ, Littlewood JM: Acute severe deterioration in cystic fibrosis associated with influenza A virus infection, *Thorax* 47:112-114, 1992.
79. Ramphal R, Small PM, Shands JW, Fischweiger W, Small PA: Adherence of *Pseudomonas aeruginosa* to tracheal cells injured by influenza infection or by endotracheal intubation, *Infect Immun* 27:614-619, 1980.
80. Johansen HK, Hoiby N: Seasonal onset of initial colonisation and chronic infection with *Pseudomonas aeruginosa* in patients with cystic fibrosis in Denmark, *Thorax* 47:109-111, 1992.
81. Wang EL, Prober C, Manson B, Corey M, Levison H: Association of respiratory viral infections with pulmonary deterioration in patients with cystic fibrosis, *N Engl J Med* 311:1653-1658, 1984.

82. Wright PF, Khaw KT, Oxman MN, Shwachman H: Evaluation of the safety of amantadine HCl and the role of respiratory viral infections in cystic fibrosis, *J Infect Dis* 134:144-149, 1976.
83. Ong EL, Bilton D, Abbott J, Webb AK, McCartney RA, Caul EO: Influenza vaccination in adults with cystic fibrosis, *Br Med J* 303:557 1991.
84. Bhargava V, Tomashefski JF Jr, Stern RC, Abramowsky CR: The pathology of fungal infection and colonization in patients with cystic fibrosis, *Hum Pathol* 20:977-986, 1989.
85. Hiller EJ: Pathogenesis and management of aspergillosis in cystic fibrosis, *Arch Dis Child* 65:397-398, 1990.
86. Kerem E, Reisman J, Corey M, Bentur L, Canny G, Levison H: Wheezing in infants with cystic fibrosis: clinical course, pulmonary function, and survival analysis, *Pediatrics* 90:703-706, 1992.
87. Lloyd-Still JD, Khaw K, Shwachman H: Severe respiratory disease in infants with cystic fibrosis, *Pediatrics* 53:678-682, 1974.
88. Tizzano EF, Buchwald M: Recent advances in cystic fibrosis research, *J Pediatr* 122:985-988, 1993 [review].
89. Collins FS: Cystic fibrosis: molecular biology and therapeutic implications, *Science* 256:774-779, 1992 [review].
90. Santis G, Osborne L, Knight RA, Hodson ME: Independent genetic determinants of pancreatic and pulmonary status in cystic fibrosis, *Lancet* 336:1081-1084, 1990.
91. Campbell PW, Phillips JA, Krishnamani MR, Maness KJ, Hazinski TA: Cystic fibrosis: relationship between clinical status and F508 deletion, *J Pediatr* 118:239-241, 1991.
92. Curtis A, Nelson R, Porteous M, Burn J, Bhattacharya SS: Association of less common cystic fibrosis mutations with a mild phenotype, *J Med Genet* 28:34-37, 1991.
93. Johansen HK, Nir M, Hoiby N, Koch C, Schwartz M: Severity of cystic fibrosis in patients homozygous and heterozygous for ΔF508 mutation, *Lancet* 337:631-634, 1991.
94. al-Jader LN, Meredith AL, Ryley HC, Cheadle JP, Maguire S, Owen G, Goodchild MC, Harper PS: Severity of chest disease in cystic fibrosis patients in relation to their genotypes, *J Med Genet* 29:883-887, 1992.
95. Kerem E, Corey M, Kerem BS, Rommens J, Markiewicz D, Levison H, Tsui LC, Durie P: The relation between genotype and phenotype in cystic fibrosis—analysis of the most common mutation (ΔF508), *N Engl J Med* 323:1517-1522, 1990.
96. Kristidis P, Bozon D, Corey M, Markiewicz D, Rommens J, Tsui LC, Durie P: Genetic determination of exocrine pancreatic function in cystic fibrosis, *Am J Hum Genet* 50:1178-1184, 1992.
97a. The Cystic Fibrosis Genotype-Phenotype Consortium: Correlation between genotype and phenotype in patients with cystic fibrosis, *N Engl J Med* 329:1308-1313, 1993.
97b. Rozmahel R, Wilschanski M, Matin A, Plyte S, Oliver M, Auerbach W, Moore A, Forstner J, Durie P, Nadeau J, Bear C, Tsui L-C: Modulation of disease severity in cystic fibrosis transmembrane conductance regulator deficient mice by a secondary genetic factor, *Nat Genet* 12:280-287, 1996.
98. Sheppard DN, Rich DP, Ostedgaard LS, Gregory RJ, Smith AE, Welsh MJ: Mutations in CFTR associated with mild-disease-form Cl^- channels with altered pore properties [see comments], *Nature* 362:160-164, 1993.
99. Britton JR: Effects of social class, sex, and region of residence on age at death fom cystic fibrosis, *Br Med J* 298:483-487, 1989.
100. McColley SA, Rosenstein BJ, Cutting GR: Differences in expression of cystic fibrosis in blacks and whites, *Am J Dis Child* 145:94-97, 1991.
101. Bowler IM, Estlin EJ, Littlewood JM: Cystic fibrosis in Asians, *Arch Dis Child* 68:120-122, 1993.
102. Lucotte G, Hazout S, Loirat F: North-west/south-east gradient in ΔF508 frequency in Europe, *Lancet* 338:882-883, 1991.
103. Walker LS, Ford MB, Donald WD: Cystic fibrosis and family stress: effects of age and severity of illness, *Pediatrics* 79:239-246, 1987.
104. Cowen L, Mok J, Corey M, MacMillan H, Simmons R, Levison H: Psychologic adjustment of the family with a member who has cystic fibrosis, *Pediatrics* 77:745-753, 1986.
105. Simmons RJ, Corey M, Cowen L, Keenan N, Levison H: Emotional adjustment of early adolescents with cystic fibrosis, *Psychosom Med* 47:111-122, 1985.
106. Eigen H, Clark NM, Wolle JM: Clinical-behavioural aspects of cystic fibrosis: Directions for future research, *Am Rev Respir Dis* 136:1509-1513, 1987.
107. Patterson JM, Budd J, Goetz D, Warwick WJ: Family correlates of a 10-year pulmonary health trend in cystic fibrosis, *Pediatrics* 91:383-389, 1993.
108. Campbell PW, Parker RA, Roberts BT, Krishnamani MR, Phillips JA: Association of poor clinical status and heavy exposure to tobacco smoke in patients with cystic fibrosis who are homozygous for the F508 deletion, *J Pediatr* 120:261-264, 1992.
109. Kovesi T, Corey M, Levison H: Passive smoking and lung function in cystic fibrosis, *Am Rev Respir Dis* 148:1266-1271, 1993.

Factors Indicative of Poor Survival

110. Nixon PA, Orenstein DM, Kelsey SF, Doershuk CF: The prognostic value of exercise testing in patients with cystic fibrosis, *N Engl J Med* 327:1785-1788, 1992.
111. Davis PB, di Sant'Agnese PA: Assisted ventilation for patients with cystic fibrosis, *JAMA* 239:1851-1854, 1978.
112. Moss AJ: The cardiovascular system in cystic fibrosis, *Pediatrics* 70:728-741, 1982 [review].
113. Stern RC, Borkat G, Hirschfield SS, Boat TF, Mathews LW, Liebman J, Doershuk CF: Heart failure in cystic fibrosis: treatment and prognosis of cor pulmonale with failure of the right side of the heart, *Am J Dis Child* 134:267-272, 1980.
114. Pitts-Tucker TJ, Miller MG, Littlewood JM: Finger clubbing in cystic fibrosis, *Arch Dis Child* 61:576-579, 1986.

SUGGESTED READINGS

Dinwiddie R: Cystic fibrosis: yesterday, today and tomorrow, *J R Soc Med* 84 Suppl 18:36-39, 1991.

FitzSimmons SC: The changing epidemiology of cystic fibrosis, *J Pediatr* 122:1-9, 1991.

Karem E, Reisman J, Corey M, Canny GJ, Levison H: Prediction of mortality in patients with cystic fibrosis, *N Engl J Med* 326:1187-1191, 1992.

Tizzano EF, Buchwald M: Recent advances in cystic fibrosis research, *J Pediatr* 122:985-988, 1993.

PART TWELVE

SIDS

CHAPTER 71

Sudden Infant Death Syndrome and Apparent Life-Threatening Events

Christian F. Poets and David P. Southhall

Sudden and unexpected infant deaths have been recognized since biblical times (I Kings 3:19: "And this woman's child died in the night; because she overlaid it"). As in the Bible, these deaths were believed to be caused by the parents accidentally or intentionally overlaying their children. For example, a law issued in mediaeval Germany in 1291 forbade parents to take children younger than 3 years of age into their bed[1]; a very similar law still existed in Prussia in 1791.[2] In 1834, Fearn was the first who argued against overlaying as the cause of death. He used the term "sudden and unexplained death" in his description of two infants "who, without having been previously indisposed, were found dead in bed" and in whom he could not discover any "lesions . . . sufficient to produce death."[3]

One of the first scientific attempts to explain sudden and unexpected infant deaths was made by Paltauf, an Austrian pathologist, in 1889. He observed an enlarged thymus, a narrowing of the aorta, and an overdevelopment of the lymphatic system in infants who had died suddenly and unexpectedly and introduced the concept of "status thymico-lymphaticus."[4] Despite good evidence against it, this concept persisted into the first half of this century, leading to the prophylactic irradiation of the thymus, with subsequent malignancy of the thyroid, in the 1920s. With the decline of this theory in the 1930s, voices accusing the parents of having killed or neglected their babies grew again, and it was only in the 1950s and 1960s that doctors became aware that these deaths might form a distinct entity of unexplained natural deaths.

In 1970, Bergman et al[5] coined the term *sudden infant death syndrome* (SIDS), which they defined as the "sudden death of an infant or young child, which is unexpected by history, and in which a thorough postmortem examination fails to demonstrate an adequate cause for death." This definition clearly has its weaknesses, which mainly relate to the fact that it defines a syndrome by exclusion.[6] Nevertheless, it helped a great deal with transmitting to the public that the vast majority of sudden unexpected deaths in infants have a natural cause.

This chapter will summarize current knowledge concerning the epidemiology, pathology, and pathophysiology of SIDS, discuss some prevention strategies, and then focus on the clinical management of infants at risk of SIDS, with particular emphasis on the management of infants with a history of an apparent life-threatening event (ALTE).

TERMINOLOGY

In the following, the term *SIDS* will be used as defined by Bergman et al in 1970.[5] That this definition is still valid was confirmed only recently by an expert panel at the Third SIDS International Conference in Stavanger, Norway, in August 1994.

An apparent life-threatening event (ALTE) has been defined as "an episode that is frightening to the observer and that is characterized by some combination of apnea (central or occasionally obstructive), color change (usually cyanotic or pallid but occasionally erythematous or plethoric), marked change in muscle tone (usually marked limpness), choking, or gagging."[7] In clinical practice, the term *ALTE* has been restricted to events that fulfill the above criteria, but also involve vigorous stimulation or resuscitation. This somewhat narrower definition will also be used in this chapter.

No consistent definition exists for apneas. In this chapter, we will use the term *apneic pause* to describe spontaneous interruptions in breathing movements and nasal airflow, lasting for 4 to 20 seconds, and *prolonged apneic pause* for apneic pauses that last for more than 20 seconds. The term *periodic apnea* will describe a pattern during which 3 or more apneic pauses, each followed by less than 20 breaths, occur in sequence. An obstructive apnea is characterized as an episode of continuous breathing movements but absent airflow, presumed to be caused by an intermittent closure of the upper airway, and a mixed apnea is a combination of an obstructive event and an apneic pause of any length.

EPIDEMIOLOGY

Incidence

In contrast to previous centuries, when sudden unexpected deaths accounted for only a small proportion of total infant mortality, SIDS is now the leading cause of postperinatal mortality in developed countries, accounting for approximately 3000 deaths per year in the United States.[8] In the late 1980s, several studies reported an alarming trend toward an increase in SIDS rates over the preceding 10 to 20 years, leading to a doubling of the SIDS incidence in Norway[9] and a threefold increase in Denmark and the Netherlands (Fig. 71-1).[10,11] This increase was paralleled by an increase in total postneonatal mortality; that is, it was not the result of changes in diagnostic fashions. The reasons for this increase are unclear, but it has been related to changes in child care practice. For example, in the Netherlands SIDS rates began to increase shortly after general advice had been given that babies should be put to sleep in the prone position, and recent data from this and other countries have shown that SIDS rates decreased dramatically after this advice was reversed.[12-14] The implications of these observations with regard to the relationship between SIDS and child care practices will be discussed later.

SIDS rates vary considerably between countries and between different ethnic groups within a country[9,15-22] (Table 71-1). These differences may be related to both socioeconomic and genetic factors. For example, Black et al concluded that the differences in SIDS rates between American blacks and

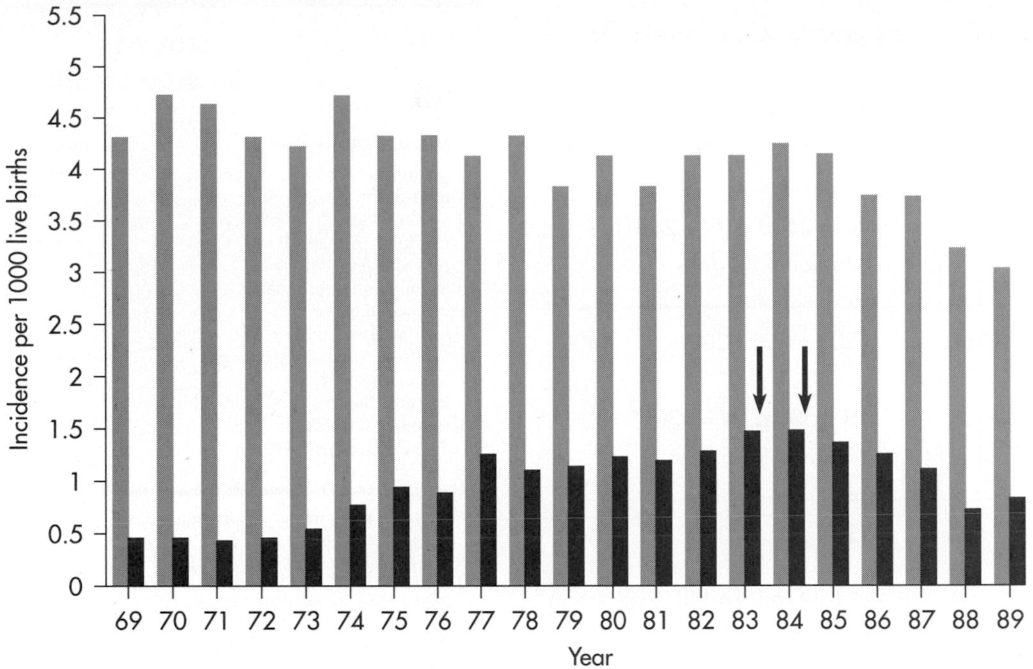

Fig. 71-1. Changing trends in postperinatal infant mortality *(gray bars)* and sudden unexpected deaths *(black bars)* in the Netherlands 1969-89. *Arrows* indicate years when sudden death incidence was not corrected for autopsy data; the given incidences during these 2 years are therefore estimated as being 10% too high. The prone sleeping position was publicly recommended in 1972. A campaign aimed at avoiding the prone sleeping position was started in October 1987. (From Engelberts AC, de Jonge GA, Kostense PJ: *J Paediatr Child Health* 27:329-333, 1991.)

Table 71-1 SIDS Incidence in Different Countries and Ethnic Groups

COUNTRY / ETHNIC GROUP	YEAR	RATE (DEATHS/ 1000 LIVE BIRTHS)	REFERENCE
Finland	1969-80	0.4	Rintahaka
Cook County, USA	1975-80	2.7	Black et al
- Blacks		5.1	
- Hispanics		1.2	
- Whites		1.3	
Birmingham, UK			
- Whites	1981-83	2.3	Kyle et al
- Asians		1.2	
- Blacks		5.3	
Hamburg, W-Germany	1979-83	2.3	Veelken et al
Southern New Zealand	1979-84	6.3	Nelson et al
Norway	1983-84	2.4	Irgens et al
Sweden	1984-86	0.9	Wennergren et al
Hong Kong	1986-87	0.3	Lee et al
England	1990	1.5	FSID
	1991	1.3	
	1992	0.7	

Listed by year of study.

whites could not be sufficiently explained by socioeconomic factors alone.[16] Kraus et al, however, came to the opposite conclusion: their differences in SIDS rates between American blacks and whites were no longer significant after they controlled their data for potential socioeconomic confounders.[23] Similarly, Mitchell et al, in a nationwide study in New Zealand, found a decrease in odds ratios from 3.8 to 1.4, the latter being no longer significant, when they controlled their results on SIDS rates in Maori versus non-Maori infants for socioeconomic confounders.[24]

Age and Time of Death

One of the most striking epidemiologic features in SIDS is its characteristic age distribution (Fig. 71-2). Occurrence is uncommon in the neonatal period, then a sharp increase in the second month of life, a peak at around 3 to 4 months of age, and a gradual decrease thereafter. Hence, 75% of deaths occur between 2 and 4 months of age, and 95% before 9 months of age.[25] This age distribution is related to gestational, not to postnatal age: in very low birth weight infants (less than 1500 g), the peak incidence occurs about 6 weeks later.[25] Previous beliefs that SIDS is extremely rare in the neonatal period cannot be maintained: approximately 7% of SIDS victims are younger than 1 month of age,[18] and 11% of all neonatal deaths are caused by SIDS.[26]

Throughout the year SIDS occurs primarily in the cold season. In the northern hemisphere, up to 95% of deaths occur between October and April.[27] This seasonal distribution has been related to respiratory tract infections, which show a similar distribution and are often reported to precede death.[28] Infections may also be the explanation for observations of a clustering of deaths, with multiple cases on one day and long "silent" periods on others.[29] This clustering of deaths may coincide with the outbreak of viral or pertussis epidemics in the same region.[30,31] Indirect evidence for the role of respiratory tract infections in SIDS has been given by a report from the National Institute of Health Cooperative Epidemiological Study, which showed that the number of infants immunized against pertussis was significantly smaller in SIDS victims than in a matched control group.[32]

During the week it appears that SIDS tends to occur more commonly on weekends and public holidays.[15,33,34] This has

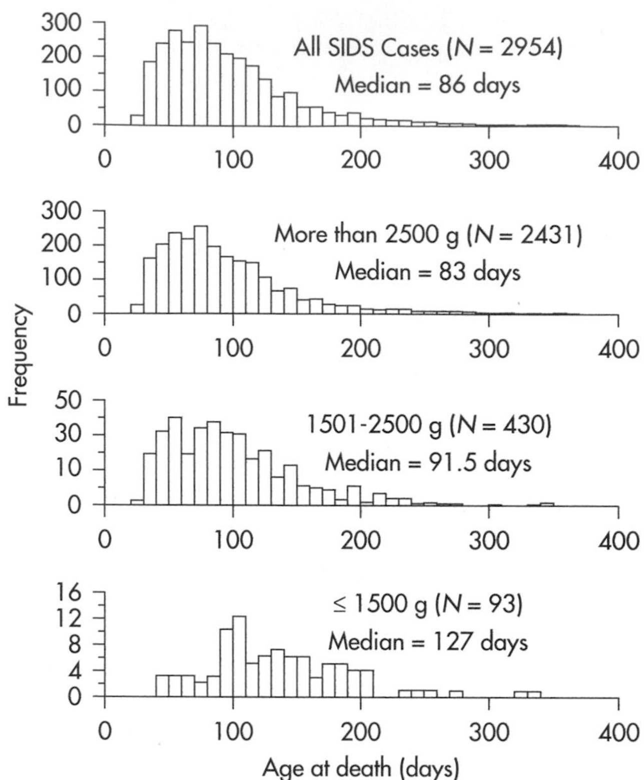

Fig. 71-2. Histograms for age at death for three birth weight groups of SIDS cases in California from 1978-82. (From Grether JK, Schulman J: *J Pediatr* 114:561-567, 1989.)

BOX 7-1
Risk Factors for SIDS

Maternal factors	Infantile factors
young age	male gender
multiparity	low birth weight
smoking during pregnancy	low birth length
maternal drug abuse	premature birth
previous fetal deaths	blood type B
anemia during pregnancy	low Apgar scores
low social class	low hematocrit at 48 hours
low family income	prone sleeping position
short interpregnancy interval	overheating
unmarried mother	not breastfed
late attendance of antenatal clinic	previous cyanotic episode
postnatal depression	previous SIDS in family
attendance to psychiatrist	

Data from Kraus JF, Greenland S, Bulterys M: *Int J Epidemiol* 18:113-120, 1989; Mitchel EA, Taylor BJ, Ford RPK, Stewart AW, Becroft DMO, Thompson JMD, Scragg R, Hassall IB, Barry DMJ, Allen EM, Roberts AP: *J Paediatr Child Health* 28:S3-S8, 1992; Buck GM, Cookfair DL, Michalek AM et al: *Am J Epidemiol* 129:874-884, 1989; Hoffman HJ, Damus K, Hillman L, Krongrad E: *Ann NY Acad Sci* 533:13-20,1988; and Mitchell EA, Thompson JMD, Stewart AW, Webster ML, Taylor BJ, Hassall IB, Ford RPK, Allen EM, Scragg R, Becroft DMO: *J Paediatr Child Health* 28:S13-S16,1992.

been related to the fact that the infants' daily routine and environment are more likely to be disturbed or changed on these days.[33,34] In the recent nationwide study from New Zealand, however, visits to and by friends or relatives, which would certainly disturb the infants' daily routine, appeared to have a protective effect against SIDS.[35] Hence, the mechanisms responsible for the increased occurrence of SIDS on weekends and public holidays remain poorly understood.

SIDS apparently occurs primarily during the night, a time when both parents and infants are most likely to be asleep. For example, in a recent study from Hanover, Germany, 61% of 270 SIDS victims were found in the morning (6 AM to noon).[36] Similarly, in a study that estimated the time of death (not discovery) in 155 SIDS cases, 58% had died between midnight and 8 AM.[37] However, in a recent population based study from Sweden, only 31% of the SIDS victims were found in the morning (6 AM to noon); the peak incidence in that study (33%) was in the afternoon (noon to 6 PM).[20] The reasons for these differences are unclear.

Risk Factors

A large number of factors potentially increasing the risk of SIDS have been identified from epidemiologic studies[23,38-41] (Box 71-1). Many of these risk factors underline the importance of social factors in the pathogenesis of SIDS (although the mechanisms through which these social factors affect the risk of SIDS are poorly understood); others, such as maternal smoking or anemia during pregnancy, suggest that there must already be a disturbance during intrauterine life that puts an infant at risk. In the following, we will concentrate on risk factors that are potentially amenable to modification, namely maternal smoking, not breast feeding, overheating, bed sharing, and the prone sleeping position.

Maternal smoking has long been recognized as a risk factor for SIDS. In a recent study on the influence of maternal smoking on the SIDS incidence in Sweden, a dose-dependent increase in SIDS incidence was observed, which was particularly pronounced in infants who died early (between 7 and 67 days of life).[42] The relative risk for this group was 3.6 if the mothers smoked 10 or more cigarettes per day. It was concluded that smoking is the single most important preventable risk factor for SIDS in countries such as Sweden. Similarly, Mitchell et al found odds ratios of 3.5 for infants whose mothers smoked 1 to 9 cigarettes per day, 3.9 for those who smoked 10 to 19, and 5.9 for those who smoked more than 20 cigarettes per day.[38] Yet another study found adjusted odds ratios of 2.6 for 1 to 10, 2.9 for 11 to 20, and 6.9 for more than 20 cigarettes per day.[43] In addition, there is a further doubling of the risk of SIDS if both parents smoke[44] or if the mother not only smokes but is also anemic.[43,45] Smoking may be related to SIDS via a number of mechanisms, including fetal hypoxia,[43,45] an inhibition of airway growth and development,[46] and an increased susceptibility to respiratory tract infections.[47] Which of these factors is the most relevant with regard to SIDS remains open to debate.

Not breast feeding was only recently confirmed as a risk factor for SIDS in the nationwide study from New Zealand (odds ratio 2.4),[38] and in an analysis of the U.S. Collaborative Perinatal Project (odds ratio 2.0).[23] The beneficial effect of breast feeding may be related to its protective effect on the infants' susceptibility to respiratory tract infections.

Evidence that overheating (arising from overwrapping or high room temperatures) may be a risk factor for SIDS was initially largely circumstantial.[19,48] Recently, two case-control studies found that the level of bedding and clothing was significantly higher among SIDS cases than controls.[49,50] Heavy wrapping may become particularly important if it occurs in combination with other risk factors for SIDS, such as the prone sleeping position[51] or a respiratory tract infection.[52] Thus

Gilbert et al found a relative risk for SIDS of 51.6 for the combined presence of heavy wrapping (more than 10 togs) and a viral infection.[52] In contrast to the data on the prone sleeping position, there is also physiologic evidence that supports the concept that hyperthermia may be a risk factor for SIDS: it has deleterious effects on respiratory control[53,54] and may also impair lung mechanics.[55,56]

Bed-sharing as a risk factor for SIDS was first observed in 1972,[57] but has not received much attention until it was recently confirmed in the study from Mitchell et al,[38] who found that 24% of the SIDS victims, but only 10.5% of the controls, had shared the bed with their parents. These data apparently reconfirm the concept already mentioned in the Bible that accidental suffocation through overlaying may be a mechanism for SIDS, but they can also be interpreted as supporting the hypothesis that hyperthermia, resulting from the infant sleeping close to his parents, may play a role as a trigger for SIDS.

That the prone sleeping position could be a risk factor for SIDS was first reported in 1984,[58] but was not noticed by others until 1989, when a Dutch group, based on results from a retrospective study, started a campaign in their country advising parents to avoid the prone sleeping position.[11] Since then, 17 of 19 retrospective studies investigating the effect of different sleeping positions found that sleeping prone was associated with a significantly increased risk of SIDS.[59] There have, however, been concerns about the retrospective nature of these studies, particularly with regard to recall bias,[60] although the latter was recently shown not to be a major problem in case-control studies of SIDS.[61] The only prospective study published to date, showing an odds ratio of 3.9 for the prone position, is not without problems; it was not population based (sampling a group at high risk because of other epidemiologic factors), and prospective data were only available on 19 of the 29 infants who died.[62]

The issue becomes even more difficult because few physiologic data support the concept that the prone position places an infant at risk.[63,64] In contrast, most physiologic studies suggest that the prone position may even be advantageous in preterm neonates and in infants with respiratory infections, particularly with regard to oxygenation[65-67] and the frequency of apneic pauses.[68,69] The prone position is also an efficient treatment for gastroesophageal reflux,[70] which has repeatedly been accused as a potential trigger for SIDS.[71] Recent data, however, suggest that the prone position can in fact be dangerous to a minority of infants who, for unknown reasons, may be more likely to develop hypercapnia (as a result of rebreathing expired CO_2[63]) or hypoxemia (caused by an unknown mechanism[64]) while sleeping in the prone position.

Most important, however, is the fact that there are now several reports from countries in which public campaigns were launched advising parents to avoid the prone sleep position, which all showed a decrease in SIDS rates by 50% to 70% following these campaigns.[22,72] This decrease was paralleled by a corresponding decrease in overall postneonatal mortality rates and was thus not the result of changes in diagnostic fashions. Although these data still provide no proof for a cause-and-effect relationship between the prone sleeping position and SIDS, they have important practical implications because they demonstrate that public campaigns aimed at avoiding the prone sleeping position can be associated with a major decrease in SIDS rates that occurs without a significant increase in other causes of postneonatal mortality; that is, it does not appear to have any clinically significant side effect. The "back-to-sleep" campaign now finally also launched in the United States[73,74] can thus only be fully endorsed by these authors.

Clinical Risk Groups

In clinical practice, and only partially in accordance with the epidemiologic data just discussed, three major risk groups have been identified. These are (1) infants who have suffered an ALTE, (2) subsequent siblings or surviving twins of SIDS victims, and (3) infants who were born very prematurely (for example, at less than 32 weeks' gestation, or with birth weights less than 1500 g). Particularly the first group is at an extremely high risk of SIDS (up to 13% in one study[75]) but, because the overall incidence of ALTE is comparatively low (about half that of SIDS[20]), this group still contributes to only about 8% to 10% of all SIDS victims.[40]

Infants who have lost a previous sibling from SIDS have a risk about 4 to 6 times that of the total population.[6,77] SIDS siblings also have a higher infant mortality from causes other than SIDS. For example, Guntheroth et al, in a population-based study involving 251,124 live births, found a SIDS rate of 13.0/1000 and an overall infant mortality rate of 20.8/1000 for subsequent siblings (the corresponding rates for the total population of infants were 2.2 and 5.1/1000, respectively).[77] A 2% risk of losing a baby after already suffering the sudden death of another baby is certainly of concern.

The risk of SIDS in preterm infants increases exponentially with decreasing gestational age at birth or birth weight,[16,39] reaching values of up to 24/1000 for those born at less than 32 weeks' gestation.[78] Although it has been questioned whether a sudden unexpected death in an infant with bronchopulmonary dysplasia (BPD) can be classified as SIDS, it is noteworthy that these infants may have a particularly high rate of sudden unexpected deaths (up to 11%).[79] Recently, however, infants with BPD were not found to have an excess risk of SIDS.[80] These conflicting results may be related to a more rigorous use of home oxygen therapy and thus a more effective prevention of unrecognized and untreated hypoxemia in the latter study.[80] In any case, infants who were born prematurely are only a minority (up to 18%) of all SIDS victims.[40] Therefore, because the three clinical risk groups mentioned previously constitute only about 20% of all SIDS victims, any intervention program aiming only at these risk groups is unlikely to achieve a significant reduction of the SIDS incidence in a community.

PATHOLOGY

Intrathoracic Petechial Hemorrhages

As implied by its definition, there is no morphologic finding in SIDS that sufficiently explains the occurrence of death. There are, however, a number of characteristic findings in these infants, some of which are so consistent that they appear to support the concept that SIDS may indeed form a specific disease entity. The most consistent among these findings, first described by Fearn in 1834,[3] are intrathoracic serosal petechiae, which are found on the surfaces of lungs, pericardium, and intrathoracic portion of the thymus. In a recent study involving 1144 sudden unexpected deaths, serosal petechiae were found in 99% of infants who did not have any morphologic finding that could possibly explain death (true SIDS).[81] The distribution of these hemorrhages has led some researchers to suggest that large intrathoracic pressure swings are involved in their production.[82] These large pressure swings may result from breathing efforts against a closed (upper) airway. Thus Krous and Jordan found striking similarities in the distribution of petechiae between SIDS victims and deaths caused by upper airway obstruction,[83] and Campbell and Read observed in rabbits that repeated tracheal occlusion, but not barbiturate-induced apnea, produced pulmonary petechiae.[84] Petechial hemorrhages were also observed by Farber et al[85] and Handforth[86] following repetitive airway obstruction with intermittent recovery in rabbits and rats, respectively. Guntheroth, however, found no petechiae in rats if these were killed by unremitting airway occlusion (total occlusion until death). Only if death was induced by intermittent tracheal occlusions or by the administration of 100% N_2 did petechiae occur.[87] He later reported that lung volume in rats killed by unremitting airway occlusion was 24% smaller than that of rats killed with nitrogen asphyxiation, suggesting that a fully expanded lung might be required to produce petechial hemorrhages.[88]

Riße and Weiler confirmed Guntheroth's findings from animal experiments in observing that infants who had been intentionally suffocated and had thus died very rapidly exhibited much fewer petechiae than those who had died from prolonged asphyxia or SIDS, and concluded from their findings that an episode of prolonged asphyxia is required to produce these bleedings.[89] Marshall[90] and Camps[91] also supported these findings in reporting that abrupt death caused by sudden airway occlusion, unresolving until death, did not produce pulmonary hemorrhages, whereas slower forms of hypoxic death did.

An alternative explanation for the occurrence of petechiae in some but not all cases of death caused by airway obstruction was offered in 1897 by Brouardel, a French pathologist. He occluded the nose and mouth of dogs in whom a window had been placed in the parietal wall of the thorax and saw that petechiae only appeared during the second stage of asphyxia, that is, with the onset of gasping, but not initially, when the animals made vigorous inspiratory efforts against the closed upper airway.[92] These observations were recently confirmed by Winn, who found that when young rats were exposed to an oxygen-free gas they developed petechiae (and frothy pink fluid in their nares) only if there had been gasping, regardless of whether they subsequently recovered or died.[93]

It is thus possible that the petechiae so often observed in SIDS are indicative of a period of prolonged asphyxia (during which gasping occurred) rather than of a specific disease mechanism (such as upper airway obstruction) that has led to death. In this respect it is of interest that Stewart et al observed hemosiderin-containing macrophages in subpleural lung tissues from 13 of 24 consecutive SIDS autopsies, suggesting that these infants had experienced previous asphyxic episodes severe enough to produce petechiae.[94] Finally, it is of considerable concern that parentally induced upper airway obstruction (suffocation) is usually also associated with large gasps before recovery[95] (Fig. 71-3) and may hence produce petechiae very similar to those seen in SIDS.

Blood-Stained Frothy Secretions in the Airway and Lungs

Another characteristic finding in SIDS is the occurrence of froth around the nose and mouth (occasionally blood-stained), which is found in approximately 60% of SIDS victims.[96] This latter phenomenon again may be caused by a combination of pulmonary edema and high transpulmonary pressures (as with vigorous breathing movements) immediately before death.[93,97] Frank nasal or oral bleeding is not a feature of SIDS but is seen in cases of imposed upper airway obstruction.[98]

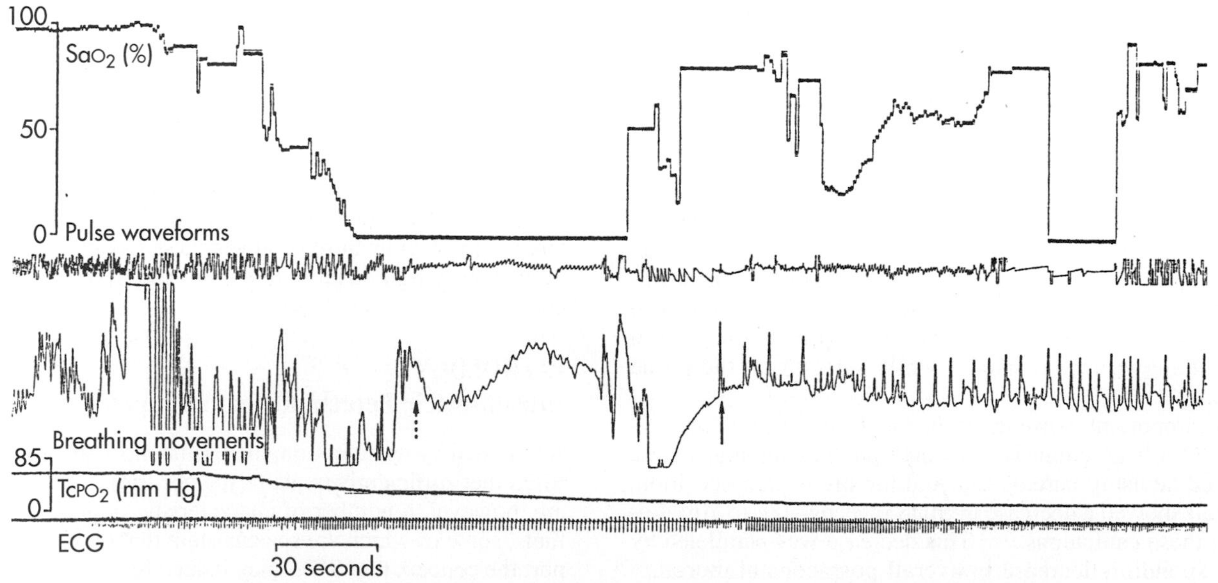

Fig. 71-3. Section from a recording of arterial oxygen saturation (Sa_{O_2}), pulse waveforms, abdominal breathing movements, transcutaneous P_{O_2} (Tc_{PO_2}), and electrocardiogram (ECG) in a 9-month-old infant who was subsequently found to have been repeatedly suffocated by his mother. At the onset of this section there are high-amplitude, irregular breathing movements as the infant struggles vigorously against the imposed upper airway obstruction. This is followed by a fall in Sa_{O_2} and Tc_{PO_2}. Shortly after Sa_{O_2} has reached zero, breathing movements become shallow *(dotted arrow)*. Heart rate subsequently falls to 55 bpm. This episode of apnea/hypopnea is followed by a period of intermittent gasping, beginning some 90 seconds later *(solid arrow)*. Gasping ceases only after blood oxygen levels have returned to normal.

Infection

The majority of SIDS victims (56% to 79%) show histologic evidence of an upper respiratory tract infection,[99,100] and infectious agents, mostly viruses, have been isolated in 40% to 80% of SIDS cases.[30,101] In one study, 55% of SIDS victims, but only 0.8% of controls, had immunoglobulin M antibodies against influenza A.[102] Similarly, grossly increased lung immunoglobulin concentrations have been found in SIDS victims.[103] The histologic changes caused by these agents are apparently not severe enough to explain death as being directly caused by respiratory infection, but the latter may clearly function as a trigger for SIDS. For example, a respiratory tract infection may cause degranulation of eosinophils or proliferation of dendritic cells in the airways, both of which have been found in SIDS,[104,105] resulting in epithelial damage and pulmonary edema and thus a reduced diameter of peripheral airways, which in turn may cause respiratory obstruction and hypoxia.

Hypoxic Tissue Markers

Following the concept that SIDS may be related to the repeated occurrence of apneic pauses, a search for morphologic changes indicative of chronic tissue hypoxia began. As a result, a number of "hypoxic tissue markers" were found. These include the retention of periadrenal brown fat, gliosis of the brainstem, hyperplasia of pulmonary neuroendocrine cells, and an increased wall thickness of both pulmonary arteries and airways.[106-109] Although there has been some debate about the specificity of these hypoxic tissue markers for SIDS,[107] the fact that they are present in SIDS suggests that these deaths may not be a sudden event without antecedent illness. This is also supported by the observation that elevated levels of hypoxanthine are present in the vitreous humor of SIDS victims,[110] indicating that death must have been preceded by an episode of prolonged (4 to 5 hours) tissue hypoxia. In addition, it should be noted that the hypoxic tissue markers found in the lungs of SIDS victims may not only be a result, but also a cause of hypoxia, because they indicate an increased reactivity of the pulmonary airways and vessels in these infants, thereby pointing to a possible pathophysiologic mechanism that might have resulted in or contributed to the development of potentially fatal hypoxia.[97,108]

Intrapulmonary Shunts

Another interesting finding in SIDS, also supporting the concept that prolonged hypoxemia may precede death, is that of intrapulmonary shunts. These were already reported anecdotally some 25 years ago,[111] but have recently been confirmed by Wilkinson and Fagan,[112] who injected microspheres with a known particle size distribution (up to 63 μm) under controlled pressure into the pulmonary arteries of SIDS victims. They found an identical particle size distribution in the liquid flowing out of the pulmonary veins. The authors concluded that large particles must have bypassed the pulmonary capillary bed, a finding best explained by the presence of intrapulmonary arteriovenous shunts.[112] However, because this study was uncontrolled, the implications of their results for the pathophysiology of SIDS remain inconclusive.

Surfactant Abnormalities

In 1982, Morley et al made the chance finding that the surfactant from lungs of SIDS victims contained less phospholipid and dipalmitoylphosphatidylcholine than that from controls.[113] This retrospective observation was subsequently confirmed in four prospective studies.[114-117] However, in a study that investigated the pressure-volume relationships in lungs of SIDS victims and controls, no significant differences were found.[118] Also, postmortem studies have not shown widespread atelectasis in SIDS.[96,119] Nevertheless, surfactant not only prevents the development of atelectasis, but also is crucial for the maintenance of small airway patency and the clearance of lung fluid.[120] The role of surfactant abnormalities in SIDS should therefore be studied in more detail,[121] particularly because the concept that SIDS may be related to a disturbance in surfactant function is supported by physiologic data that suggest that small airway closure or atelectasis may be involved in severe hypoxemic episodes in infants.

Summary of Pathologic Findings in SIDS

The following conclusions can be drawn from the studies summarized in the preceding sections: (1) respiratory tract infections appear to play an important role as a trigger for SIDS; (2) most SIDS victims have suffered tissue hypoxia for some time before death or have an increased reactivity of their pulmonary airways and vessels; (3) the final pathway leading to death apparently involves large intrapulmonary pressure swings, but whether these are caused by upper airway obstruction, lower airway occlusion, or asphyxic gasping is unknown; and (4) recent data on the role of intrapulmonary arteriovenous shunts and surfactant defects are intriguing but deserve further investigation.

PATHOPHYSIOLOGY

Investigations into the pathophysiology of SIDS have been hampered by the fact that the occurrence of death is unpredictable. They have therefore mostly been confined to prospective studies in large numbers of infants, aiming to obtain data in future SIDS victims, and to studies on infants who are known to be at increased risk of SIDS, particularly those who survived a near-death event, that is, an ALTE. Although both approaches have provided invaluable data about the development of respiratory control in infancy, they are unlikely to provide conclusive evidence about the pathogenesis of SIDS. This would only be possible if data were collected during deaths or near-death events. With the introduction of event recorders, which record physiologic signals during alarms on electronic monitors used at home, the potential to collect such data is now available, and preliminary data obtained with these devices suggest that this approach might improve our understanding of the pathophysiology of SIDS itself.

Data Recorded in Future SIDS Victims

The first large population-based study that prospectively collected physiologic data in future SIDS victims was carried out by Southall et al, who performed 24-hour tape recordings of ECG and breathing movements on 9856 infants, 29 of whom subsequently died of SIDS.[122] None of the recordings in the SIDS infants showed a prolonged apneic pause (20 seconds or more), cardiac arrhythmia, preexcitation, or a prolonged QT interval. Compared with surviving matched controls, the SIDS cases did not show significantly increased numbers of short apneic pauses or quantities of periodic breathing.[123] In fact, the SIDS victims who were studied after 1 month of age showed significantly fewer apneic pauses (4 seconds or more) than did the control infants.[124] However, the infants who died exhibited higher mean heart rates[125] and higher levels of sinus tachycardia than the controls.[126]

Since then, this unique data set has been used for more refined analyses by many investigators throughout the world. For example, Waggener et al performed an analysis of the breathing patterns in 10 term future SIDS victims and 10 matched controls.[127] They did not observe abnormal breathing patterns leading to abnormally prolonged, or an abnormally high incidence of, central or obstructive apneas in the SIDS victims and concluded that an instability of the respiratory blood gas feedback control system was not present at the time of the recording in the future SIDS victims. This study, using sophisticated analysis techniques, thus confirmed the previous finding that recordings of breathing movements and ECG cannot serve as predictors for SIDS.[122]

Studies of autonomic cardiovascular control in the SIDS victims produced mixed results. Analysis of overall heart rate variability by power-spectral techniques showed no differences between SIDS cases and controls.[128] More detailed analysis showed, however, that the extent of respiratory sinus arrhythmia was lower in the SIDS victims across all sleep-waking states[129] and that heart rate variability was diminished in the SIDS cases during waking and rapid eye movement (REM) sleep, but not during quiet sleep.[130] More recently, a dynamic analysis of beat-to-beat heart rate variability showed a reduced dispersion of interbeat intervals across all sleep-waking states.[131] These findings indicate a disturbance in autonomic control mechanisms, namely either an increased sympathetic or a reduced vagal tone, or some interaction of the two, in infants who succumb to SIDS. How this disturbance in autonomic control affects the maintenance of vital functions is unknown.

A study on sleep state organization in 22 recordings from 16 term future SIDS victims in the just-mentioned data set and 66 recordings from age-matched controls showed less waking and more sleep during the early morning hours.[132] Interestingly, the future SIDS victims also showed less body movement during REM sleep than did controls. Unfortunately, sleeping position was not recorded in the original study, and it is therefore not clear whether these findings indicate a disturbance in sleep organization or arousal responsiveness, or whether they are related to a higher proportion of future SIDS victims sleeping prone, because the latter position is associated with less motility and longer sleep times.[133,134]

Finally, it should be made clear that the differences identified between SIDS victims and controls were only group differences and could not be used predictively to identify individuals at risk. Some of the studies involved multiple analyses for which statistical corrections were made. Such corrections may have overestimated or underestimated statistical significance.

Another prospective but not population-based study was performed by Kelly et al,[135] who analyzed 12-hour recordings of ECG and impedance pneumography in 17 infants who subsequently died of SIDS, drawn from a group of 11,100 infants referred for nocturnal pneumograms. They found higher mean heart rates, more periodic breathing during quiet time, and more episodes of bradycardia in the SIDS victims. However, the information from this study is limited because some of their infants were siblings of SIDS victims and some had suffered ALTE.

The same critique applies to a large prospective study reported by Kahn et al. They analyzed polygraphic sleep studies in 30 future SIDS victims, taken from a data set of 20,750 infants who had been studied polygraphically in 10 Belgian sleep laboratories between 1977 and 1990.[136] The only two polygraphic differences between the SIDS cases and the controls were an increase in the number of obstructive apneas (defined as a pause in airflow for more than 2 seconds, observed in 23 of 30 future SIDS victims but in only 9 of 60 controls) and, as in the data from Schechtman et al,[132] a decreased number of body movements during sleep (but again, their data were not controlled for sleep position). All other polygraphic parameters (duration of different sleep states, number and duration of apneic pauses, heart and respiratory rates) were not significantly different in the two groups, but significantly more future SIDS victims were reported to have episodes of regurgitation after feeding (9 versus 2) or profuse sweating during sleep (7 versus 0). However, 5 of the 30 future SIDS victims were siblings of SIDS victims and 9 had experienced an ALTE. Therefore, caution must be exercised in extrapolating these data to the pathogenesis of SIDS in infants without such a history.

A number of investigators prospectively recorded ECGs in future SIDS victims to define the incidence of a prolonged QT interval in this group because the latter is associated with an increased susceptibility to potentially fatal ventricular arrhythmias.[137] The results of those studies are controversial. Schwartz[138] found a "markedly prolonged" QT interval in six of nine SIDS victims identified in a population of 8000 infants. In contrast, Southall et al, in the prospective study mentioned previously[122] and in a second prospective study involving standard ECGs on 7254 infants, 15 of whom suffered SIDS, found no abnormal prolongation of the QT interval.[139] Weinstein and Steinschneider[140] were also unable to identify a prolonged QT interval in any of their eight prospectively studied SIDS victims.

An analysis of the relationship between cardiac repolarization and heart rate, as reflected by the relationship between QT and RR interval on the ECG, was also performed by Sadeh et al[141] in recordings from the first 10 infants who died of SIDS in the study from Southall et al[122] and 30 matched controls. They found an inability to shorten the QT interval in response to an increasing heart rate in 5 of the 10 cases and concluded that a prolonged cardiac repolarization may have predisposed these infants to ventricular arrhythmias. The validity of these results, however, was recently questioned in a contemporaneously performed analysis of the same data set by Wynn and Southall, who did not find a difference between recordings from SIDS infants and their surviving controls.[142] Several possible explanations for the differences between their results and those from Sadeh et al were given, including problems with the method used by Sadeh et al for selecting the recording segments from which their RR intervals were analyzed, the use of high-pass filters, and errors in the mathematical treatment of their results.[142]

The results from these prospective studies can be summarized as follows: (1) no marker has yet been identified from physiologic recordings obtained some weeks before death that would identify future SIDS victims with a sensitivity and specificity high enough to justify a specific intervention; (2) short or prolonged cessations of breathing movements, if analyzed some weeks before death, bear no relationship to SIDS; (3) the same applies to cardiac arrhythmias; (4) episodes with an intermittent absence of airflow but continued breathing movements ("obstructive apnea") may be found significantly more often in future SIDS victims than in controls, but this finding awaits confirmation from population-based studies; and (5) indicators suggest a disturbance in autonomic control or sleep state organization in some future victims of SIDS, but the exact mechanism through which these disturbances can lead to sudden death has not yet been determined.

Data Recorded in Infants with a History of ALTE

There is no disease that invariably results in death, and SIDS is no exception to this rule. Hence there have been events during which an infant was about to die, but was found early enough for successful resuscitation. Infants who have suffered such a near-miss death event (ALTE) show striking epidemiologic similarities to those who have died of SIDS.[143] They are therefore widely regarded as a living model for SIDS and have hence been extensively studied. However, there are some problems with this approach. First, as is probably the case with SIDS, a large number of treatable disease entities can cause ALTE. These cannot always be identified from investigations performed after an event has occurred. A proportion of apparently idiopathic ALTE is caused by an identifiable mechanism (such as pneumonia or meningitis) that is temporary and, if identified, can be treated and therefore does not bear any relationship to SIDS itself. Second, it will always be impossible to say whether an infant who was resuscitated by his or her parents would indeed have died without this intervention. Third, certain "abnormalities" identified after ALTE (such as gastroesophageal reflux [GER]) may be coincidental and irrelevant to the ALTE themselves. Therefore, there are some inherent ambiguities in the relationship between SIDS and ALTE, and this must be borne in mind if one draws conclusions from studies performed in infants with ALTE to the pathophysiology of SIDS.

Apnea in Infants with ALTE

Alfred Steinschneider was the first to infer a potential pathomechanism for SIDS from observations made in infants who had experienced an ALTE. He observed prolonged (greater than 15 seconds) cessations in breathing efforts in three infants who had experienced an ALTE and two of their siblings. Two of these five infants (one with ALTE and her brother) subsequently died, and Steinschneider concluded that prolonged apnea is part of the final pathway resulting in SIDS.[144] This paper soon formed the scientific basis for the so-called apnea hypothesis, which was enthusiastically received by the scientific world at its time and resulted in the prescription of thousands of apnea monitors around the world.[145] Recently, however, legal evidence emerged suggesting that the two SIDS infants on whom the apnea hypothesis was primarily based had not died of SIDS but had instead been killed by their mother. This not only highlights the complexity and heterogenicity of the phenomena currently called SIDS and ALTE but also raises doubts about the true relevance of the apnea hypothesis to the pathophysiology of these two phenomena.[146]

Whatever its validity, the apnea hypothesis clearly stimulated many researchers to look for apneas in infants considered to be at risk of SIDS. For example, Kelly et al performed 12-hour home recordings of breathing movements and heart rate in 32 infants with a history of ALTE and found significantly more and longer episodes of periodic apnea in these infants compared with controls.[147] Similarly, Southall et al found larger quantities of periodic breathing and higher numbers of apneic pauses in 77 term infants with ALTE and 157 age-matched controls.[148] In contrast, Oren et al[149] and Guilleminault et al[150] did not find an increased number of apneic pauses or periodic apnea in their 51 and 29 infants, respectively, with ALTE. The latter authors, however, observed an increased number of short (greater than 3 seconds) mixed and obstructive apneas, but this parameter did not help to prospectively identify infants with repeat events.[150] In addition, none of the four investigators found an excessive number of prolonged apneic pauses in their cases.[147-150]

Apneas that were associated with an intermittent closure of the upper airway at the level of the larynx, documented by means of an ultrafine fiberoptic endoscope positioned in the pharynx during spontaneous sleep, were observed by Ruggins and Milner in 3 previously preterm infants with ALTE.[151] These infants were selected from a group of 25 term and preterm infants with a history of ALTE because they had demonstrated some obstructive apneas during an initial routine sleep study. Interestingly, the laryngeal closure occurring in these infants did not appear to happen as a passive collapse of the airway structures, but as a much more abrupt action, suggestive of an active process. The authors speculated that this abrupt closure might have been caused by stimulation of the laryngeal chemoreflex. Although this observation corresponds to prospective data showing an increased number of obstructive apneas in future SIDS victims,[36] it should be noted that this mechanism was only found in 3 of the 25 infants with ALTE enrolled in the study; all 3 had been born at less than 32 weeks' gestation.

Impaired Arousal from Sleep

Based on the hypothesis that SIDS may be related to an impaired arousal responsiveness to hypoxic or hypercapnic stimuli, a number of investigators studied the response to hypoxic or hypercapnic gas mixtures in infants with ALTE. For example, McCulloch et al measured arousal responses in 22 normal and 11 ALTE infants.[152] All infants aroused in response to a stepwise increase in $Fico_2$, but the CO_2 level at which arousal occurred was significantly higher in cases than in controls (a mean of 55.9 versus 48.4 mm Hg). In addition, only one infant with ALTE, but 70% of controls, aroused to hypoxia ($Fio_2 = 0.15$). Van der Hal et al also reported a significantly increased arousal threshold to CO_2 and a failure to arouse to a decrease in Fio_2 in 56 infants with ALTE, who were compared with 9 healthy controls.[153] All control infants, but only 38% of the cases, aroused to hypoxia ($Fio_2 = 0.11$). Interestingly, 42% of those who failed to arouse had subsequent apneas requiring resuscitation, compared with only 5% of those who did not fail to arouse ($p < 0.03$). Subsequent work from the same group, however, demonstrated that a failure to arouse to a hypoxic stimulus is more common in normal infants than previously anticipated, and it was concluded that hypoxic challenge tests do not appear to have any value as a screening tool for SIDS risk.[154]

Nevertheless, the results from these studies are intriguing because they correspond to the observation that future SIDS victims show less motility and fewer arousals during sleep. A reduced number of body movements and brief arousals during sleep have also been observed in infants with ALTE, again suggesting that the arousal response in these infants tends to be blunted.[155] One potential mechanism whereby the arousal response could be blunted is exposure to repeated episodes of hypoxemia,[156] which would be in line with some of the pathologic findings in SIDS victims described previously. These observations point to a potential pathophysiologic mechanism for SIDS, namely an impaired ability of these infants to respond adequately to an intermittent development of hypoxemia and/or hypercapnia during sleep, both of which may therefore progress in some of these infants to become potentially life-threatening.

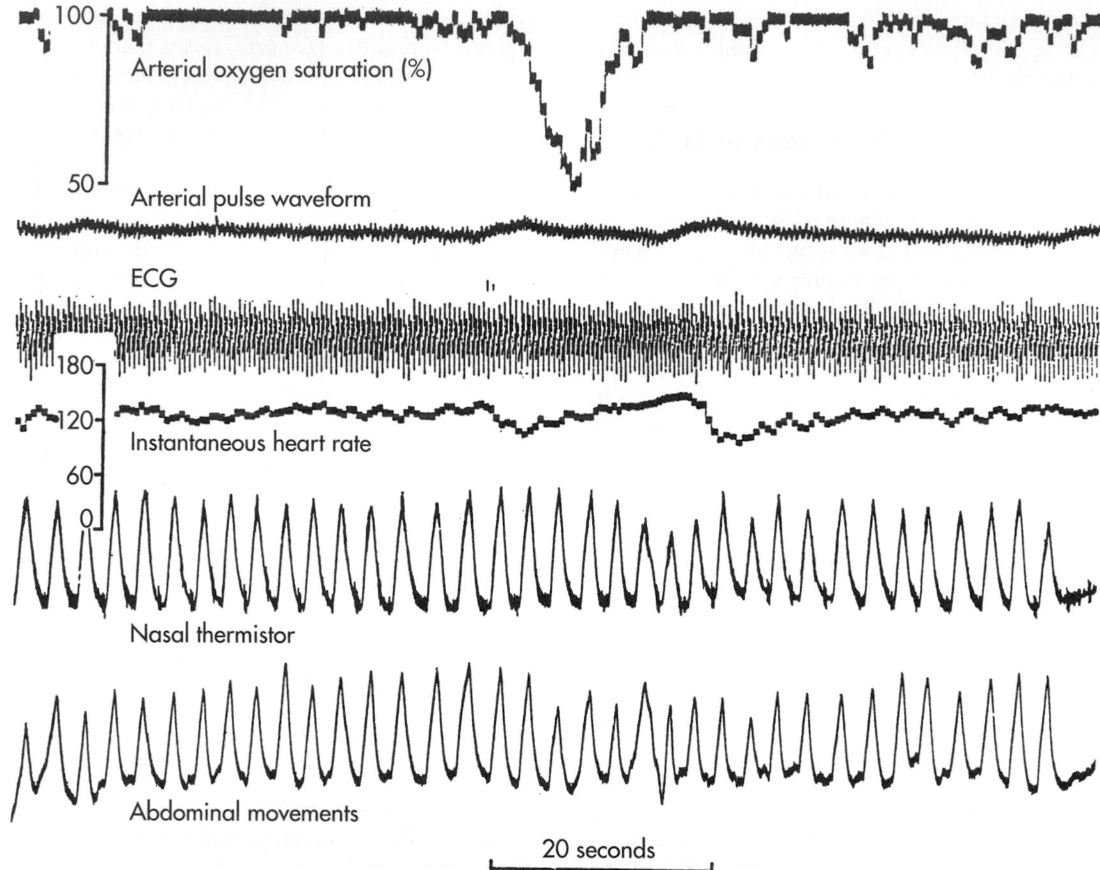

Fig. 71-4. Section from a multichannel recording in a 6-month-old infant who had experienced an apparent life-threatening event. There is a fall in Sao_2 to 50%, lasting 12 seconds, that occurs without any significant change in either breathing movements or nasal airflow and can hence be best explained by a sudden mismatch between ventilation and perfusion in the lung. (From Poets CF, Samuels MP, Southall DP: *Pediatrics* 90:385-392, 1992.)

Ventilation/Perfusion Mismatch and Small Airway Function

Until recently, almost all studies on the pathogenesis of SIDS and ALTE concentrated on the neurologic control of breathing. However, investigations performed during apneic and cyanotic episodes in infants revealed a number of physiologic phenomena that could not be sufficiently explained on the basis of primary disturbances in the central control of the respiratory generators or of upper airway patency. These include (1) the extremely rapid development of hypoxemia during some episodes; (2) the occurrence of sudden hypoxemic episodes despite continuous ventilation (Fig. 71-4); (3) differences in the speed of desaturation between different forms of apneic episodes (Fig. 71-5); (4) the presence of continued breathing efforts and yet absent airflow despite bypass of the upper airway (Fig. 71-6); and (5) evidence that apnea and hypoxemia may begin simultaneously.[157] These observations only become explicable if one assumes that a right-to-left shunt may cause or contribute to hypoxemic episodes in infants and young children. Such a shunt has in fact been demonstrated with continuous intravenous infusions of krypton-81m, an inert gas that normally diffuses completely into the alveoli at first lung passage, in patients with severe cyanotic episodes clinically resembling cyanotic breath-holding spells.[158] At the beginning of a cyanotic episode an increase in background (systemic) activity appeared, suggesting that blood had bypassed gas-exchanging surfaces. Contrast echocardiography, also performed during these cyanotic episodes, showed no right-to-left intracardiac passage of air bubbles. It was thus concluded that a sudden intrapulmonary right-to-left shunt was the explanation for the rapidity with which hypoxemia developed during these episodes.[158]

Intrapulmonary right-to-left shunting may result from the flow of blood through unventilated areas of lung caused by atelectasis or distal airway closure, or from the flow of blood through discrete anatomic pathways that allow direct passage of deoxygenated blood from the pulmonary arteries to the pulmonary veins. The latter possibility has been suggested from postmortem data in SIDS victims,[112] but could not be demonstrated when radioactively labeled microspheres (20 to 50 μm in diameter) were injected during cyanotic breath-holding spells in infants.[159]

Atelectasis and distal airway closure are more likely to occur in infants than in older children. Both can result from a deficient or abnormally functioning surfactant. The latter was recently observed in two children with severe cyanotic episodes, one of whom (a 10-month-old infant) subsequently died suddenly and unexpectedly.[160] These two patients had abnormally low amounts of surfactant, and their surfactant also showed an abnormal surface area to surface tension relationship. The authors speculated that this abnormal function could have affected cardiorespiratory control such that it kept the mechanoreceptors in the distal airways stretched

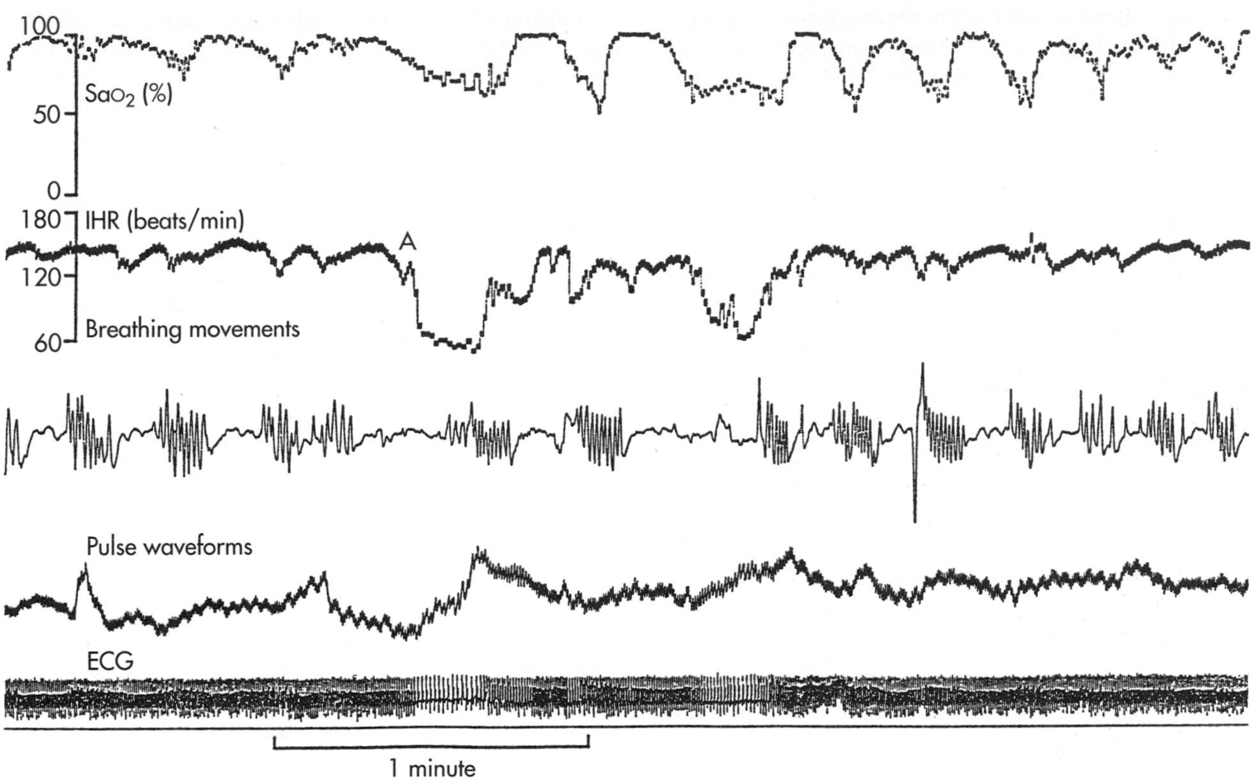

Fig. 71-5. Section from a multichannel recording in a preterm infant, studied at 40 weeks' gestational age and showing periodic apnea. Note the much faster decrease in Sao_2 during the desaturations that follow a severe desaturation that is also associated with a bradycardia (A).

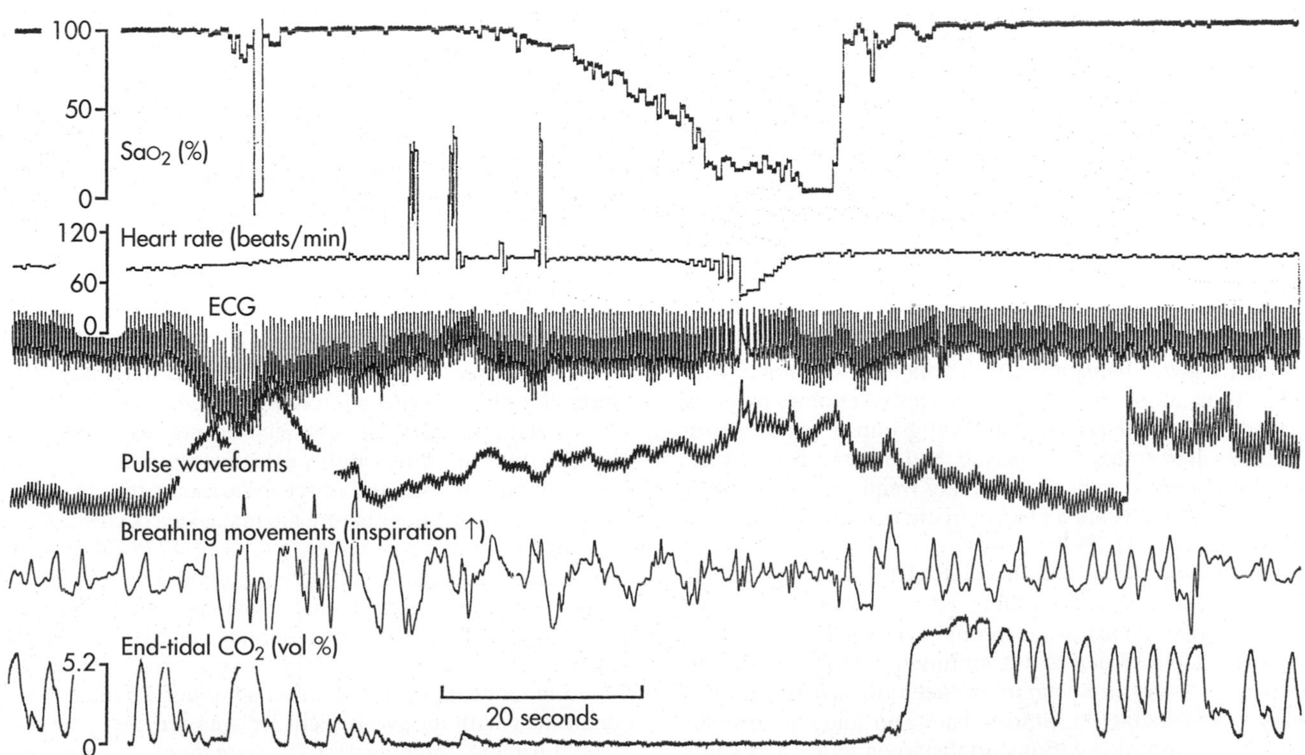

Fig. 71-6. Section from a multichannel physiologic recording in a 2-year-old child with cyanotic breath-holding spells who was breathing through a tracheostomy. There is a hypoxemic episode, lasting 30 seconds, that is associated with continuous breathing movements, but absent airflow, indicating lower airway occlusion (the tracheostomy tube was not blocked). (From Poets CF, Samuels MP, Southall DP: *Pediatrics* 90:385-392, 1992.)

during expiration, thereby signaling to the brainstem that the lung was still fully inflated and inhibiting inspiratory drive at end-expiration[160]; a hypothesis first postulated by Southall and Talbert.[121] The observation that surfactant function may be disturbed in infants with ALTE, and minimal surface tension therefore increased, has since been confirmed in two subsequent studies.[161,162]

Distal airway closure may also occur in infants with normal surfactant because this age group has a tendency to expire to below closing volumes even during tidal breathing.[163] Distal airway closure would be further facilitated if lower lung function is already diminished as a result of, for example, a congenital or acquired reduction in small airway size. The potential role of small airway closure in SIDS was recently summarized in an elegantly written hypothesis paper.[97] This concept is supported by a study from Kao and Keens, who found a lower specific airway conductance in 10 infants with ALTE than in 13 age-matched controls.[164] The methodology used in that study, however, did not indicate whether this reduced conductance was the result of a narrowing of the upper or lower airways. To test the hypothesis that infants with ALTE have a diminished lower airway function, we recently measured V_{max} FRC, a parameter specifically reflecting small airway size, in 22 infants with ALTE and 16 controls of similar age. The cases were carefully selected: all had objective evidence that they had suffered severe prolonged hypoxemia, and all had received cardiopulmonary resuscitation or vigorous stimulation. Median V_{max} FRC in the cases was only about 50% of that in the controls.[165] These data thus confirm the hypothesis that a proportion of infants with ALTE (and possibly also of those who succumb to SIDS) may have an abnormally diminished small airway function and that this may predispose these infants to potentially life-threatening episodes of progressive peripheral bronchial occlusion.[97]

Gastroesophageal Reflux (GER) in Infants with ALTE

In 1978, Herbst et al[166] reported on 14 infants with a history of cyanotic and apneic spells all of whom had severe GER on a barium esophagogram. Five of these infants had a clinically apparent episode of apnea and cyanosis during and immediately following a decrease in esophageal pH. One infant died of SIDS 1 week after the parents had discontinued positional antireflux therapy. Although these data clearly showed that GER may be associated with apneic and cyanotic episodes or even sudden death, it remains questionable how relevant this potential pathomechanism is for the majority of infants with ALTE. For example, in the study by Herbst et al no mention was made about the size of the total group of infants with ALTE seen during the study period, and most of their 14 patients also appeared to have extremely frequent events (up to 10 per day), which is not a characteristic feature in the majority of infants with ALTE.[166]

Nevertheless, the possibility that ALTE or even SIDS is caused by GER remains intriguing, particularly because there are several potential pathways through which GER may cause apnea or cyanosis (such as via stimulation of the laryngeal chemoreflex[167] or via a vagally induced disturbance in pulmonary gas exchange[168]). Unfortunately, no study has investigated the temporal relationship between clinical events (ALTE) and GER, except for the study by Herbst et al.[166] In addition, all but one study investigating the temporal relationship between polygraphically recorded short apnea (not associated with clinical events such as cyanosis) and GER did not demonstrate that such a relationship exists.[169-176] In the one study that did observe such a relationship, all infants had been specifically selected because of a history of apneic spells and frequent regurgitations[176] However, the majority of prolonged apneic spells even in these infants was not associated with regurgitation. Only one study has investigated the temporal relationship between hypoxemia and GER in infants with ALTE.[177] These authors found 60 episodes during which arterial oxygen saturation (Sao_2), measured by pulse oximetry, was less than 90% for more than 3 minutes; 54 of these episodes commenced with a mean latency of 4 minutes after the onset of a drop in esophageal pH to below 4.0. A major problem with this study, however, is that their recordings of Sao_2 were not controlled for movement artifact. Because most episodes of GER occur during wakefulness or active sleep,[171] that is, at times of frequent body movements, it is possible that most of their episodes of apparent hypoxemia were the result of movement artifact, particularly because in our experience true episodes of hypoxemia of the duration described in that study (a mean of 7.3 minutes) are extremely rare, even in symptomatic infants.[178,179]

In summary, apart from some case reports from infants in whom there was direct[166] or indirect[180] evidence that GER may have been involved in the pathogenesis of their ALTE, it remains questionable whether this potential mechanism accounts for a significant proportion of ALTE. This does not imply that GER should not be suspected and possibly treated if there are additional features (such as a history of vomiting immediately before to an ALTE) suggesting GER. Further studies on the temporal relationship between GER and ALTE are urgently required.

Data Recorded During Sudden Deaths or Life-Threatening Events

Two recent studies have analyzed recordings of breathing movements and ECG obtained with event recorders at home during the deaths of three and six infants, respectively.[181,182] All recordings showed a decrease in heart rate preceding any cessation of breathing movements. In the first study, this was interpreted as indicative of a primary cardiac arrhythmia resulting in the death of these infants. However, because there was no information about oxygenation, it was impossible to distinguish between primary bradycardia and one secondary to hypoxemia. Hence the bradycardia may well have been the result of hypoxemia.[183] This was also acknowledged by the authors of the second study, who concluded that additional information about oxygenation would have been essential for the interpretation of the data obtained during these deaths.[182] In one of the recordings during death, reported in the latter study,[182] the infant had bradycardia (heart rate less than 80 bpm) for almost 1 hour before the first apnea occurred (the parents had been desensitized by a total of 1728 false alarms in the 28 days preceding this infant's death and awoke only 2 hours after the first bradycardia alarm). This recording thus confirms data from pathologic studies that SIDS is not always sudden.

Another death of an infant on a cardiorespiratory monitor combined with an event recorder was recently recorded in Grand Rapids, Michigan.[184] The parents of this 3-month-old ex-preterm infant had failed to respond to the monitor alarm. Analysis of the recording showed a gradual decrease in heart rate, probably resulting from hypoxemia, but no initial apnea (Fig. 71-7). Unfortunately, the recording provided no infor-

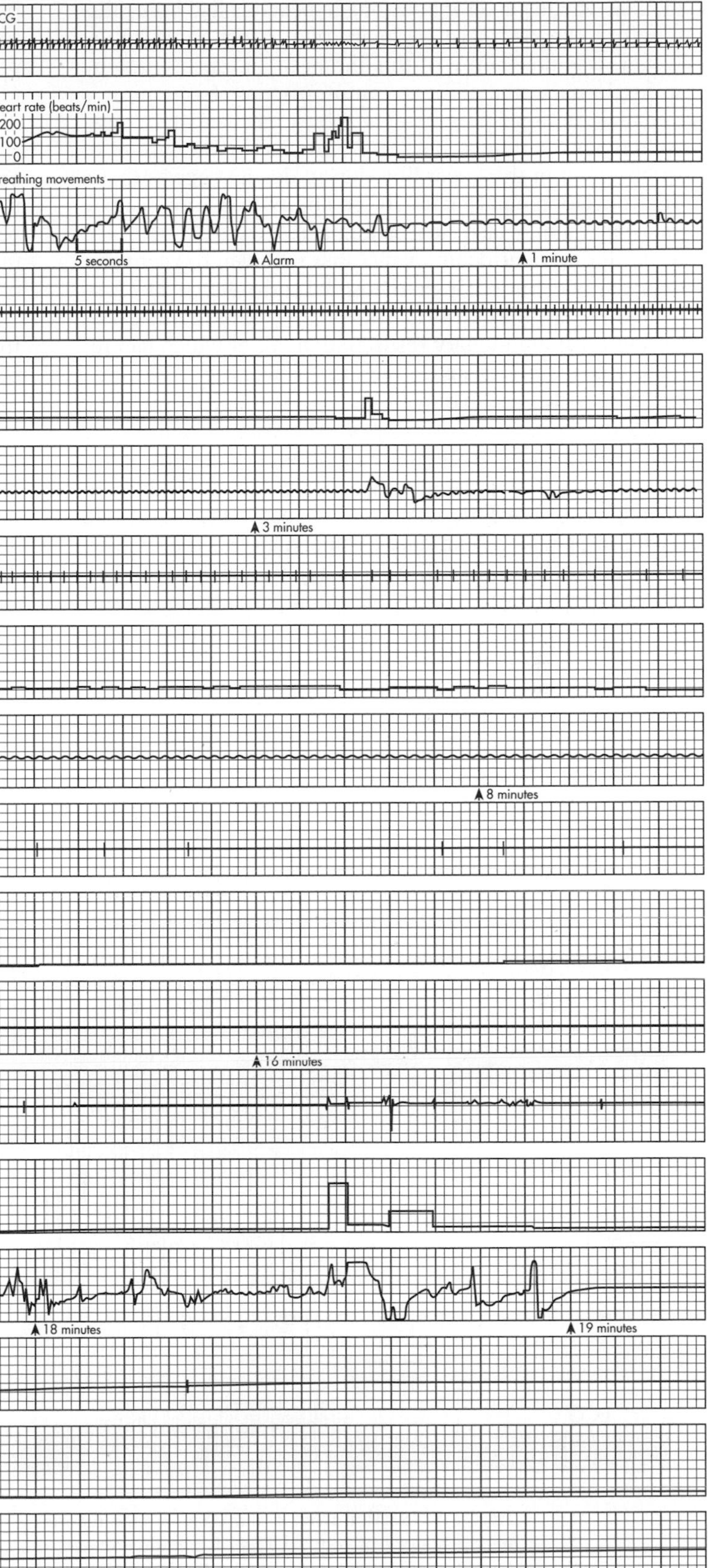

Fig. 71-7. Six 80-second sections from an event recording obtained during the death of a 3-month-old ex-preterm infant whose parents had failed to respond to the monitor alarm. The signals recorded are ECG, heart rate, and breathing movements. There is a gradual decrease in heart rate associated with high-amplitude, irregular breathing movements during the 30 seconds preceding the bradycardia alarm that had triggered the recording. Heart rate then continues to fall to approximately 50 bpm. At this stage breathing movements begin to cease while heart rate remains at 50 bpm. After 148 seconds of apnea two small gasps occur. Following these gasps, apnea again continues, but heart rate only begins to decrease further some 5 minutes into this second apnea, that is, after 8 minutes of recording. Heart rate finally falls to zero following some last respiratory or body movements, which occur 15 minutes after the two gasps, 18 minutes after the onset of recording. (Recording provided by courtesy of RE Bonofiglo, BS, RRT, and E Beaumont, MD).

mation on whether and for how long hypoxemia had been present before the decrease in heart rate. Most remarkable, however, was the failure of this infant to autoresuscitate by gasping. In mice, the ability to autoresuscitate by gasping is age-related, with gasping being a robust mechanism in newborn and adult animals, but not in infants.[185] The failure to gasp observed in this recording during death suggests that a similar developmental hiatus in the ability to autoresuscitate from asphyxia may also exist in humans.

Data during near-death events that included oxygenation were recently recorded, both in hospital and at home, in 77 infants and young children with a history of one or more ALTEs requiring cardiopulmonary resuscitation, all of which had remained unexplained despite a full clinical workup.[186] As mentioned earlier, this group of patients has a particularly high risk of SIDS (up to 13%[75]). A variety of different mechanisms for events were identified from these recordings, including deliberate suffocation by a parent (18 patients, Fig. 71-8), hypoxemia induced by epileptic seizures (10 patients, Fig. 71-9), and fabrication of history and data (Münchhausen syndrome by proxy, 7 patients, Fig. 71-10). Severe hypoxemia of an unidentified mechanism was responsible in 40 patients (truly idiopathic ALTE). In a more detailed analysis of 22 of these unexplained events in 12 patients, there was prolonged severe hypoxemia (a decrease in the transcutaneous pressure of oxygen ($TcPo_2$) to between 4 and 18 mm Hg, and in Sao_2 to 5% to 75%, lasting for 40 to 500 seconds) in all.[187] Only five events (23%), however, involved prolonged apneic pauses (20 seconds or more), and only four (18%) were associated with bradycardia (a decrease in heart rate to less than 60 to 80 beats per minute, depending on age; Figs. 71-11 and 71-12). None of the patients showed a primary cardiac arrhythmia during his or her events.[187]

Clearly, caution must be exercised in drawing conclusions from these mechanisms identified during ALTE to the pathophysiology of SIDS, particularly with regard to the proportions of the different mechanisms identified. It is also important to remember that only a small proportion of SIDS victims (8% to 10%) have previously suffered an ALTE. Nevertheless, the unexpectedly high proportion of infants with parentally induced or fabricated events is extremely worrying, given the epidemiology of SIDS and the close similarities between the risk factors for SIDS and those for child abuse.[188,189] In addition, the mechanisms identified during the

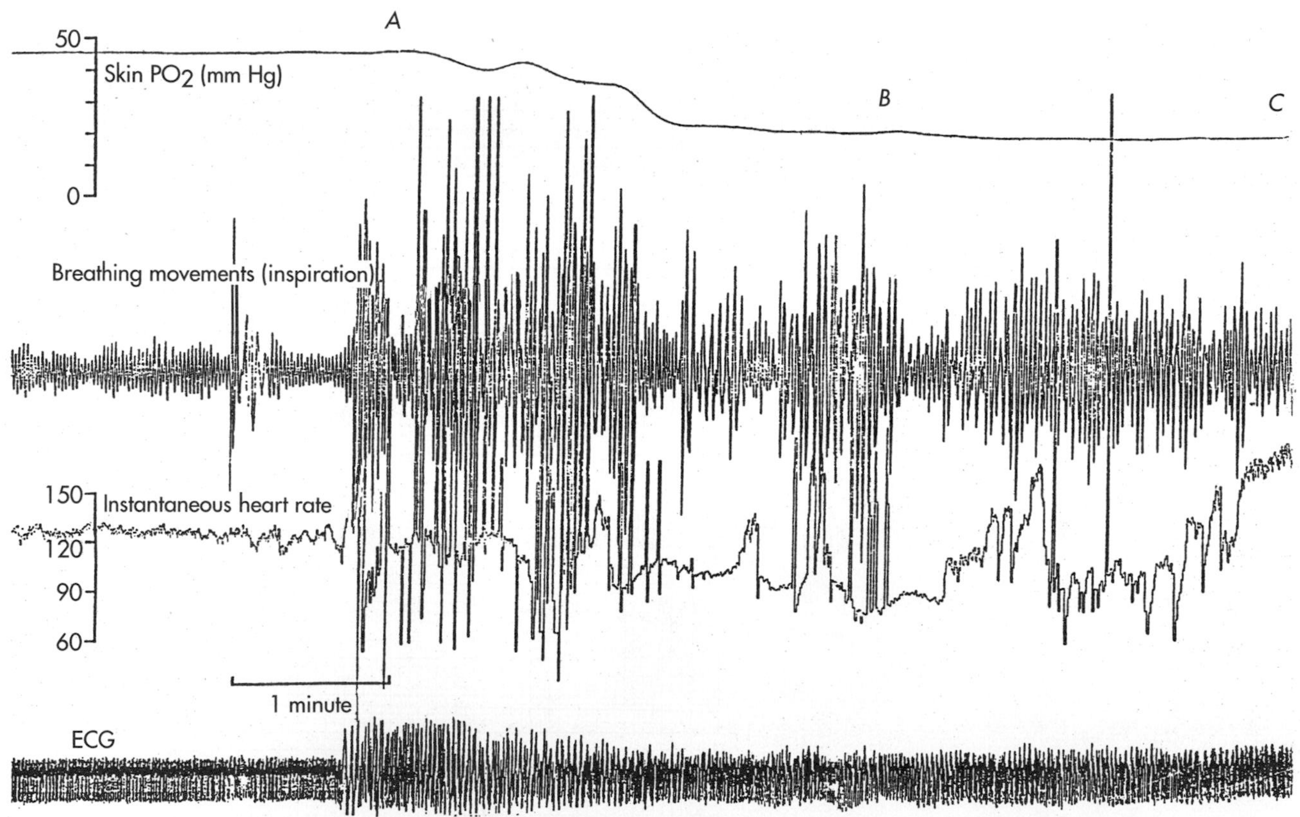

Fig. 71-8. Section from a four channel tape recording performed at home in a 2.5-month-old infant with a history of four ALTEs of unknown cause, showing a severe cyanotic episode necessitating mouth-to-mouth resuscitation by the father, followed by bag and mask ventilation by ambulance personnel. This infant's episodes were subsequently proven by covert video surveillance to be caused by suffocation imposed by the mother. A large-amplitude signal artifact occurs at the onset of the episode *(A),* indicating large body movements while the infant struggles against the sudden airway obstruction. The $TcPo_2$ falls to below 20 mm Hg, coincidental with the heart rate falling to 70 bpm *(B).* Tachycardia occurs at recovery *(C).* (From Samuels MP, et al: *Arch Dis Child* 67:162-170, 1992.)

events that remained unexplained despite being documented on physiologic recordings, particularly the observation that prolonged apnea or bradycardia was only found in about 20% of these idiopathic ALTEs confirms that apnea and bradycardia are not primary mechanisms in their pathogenesis. This observation has major implications for the design of home monitors that aim to identify ALTEs in time for effective resuscitation.

Summary of Physiologic Data in ALTE

Most idiopathic ALTEs appear to be caused by the progressive development of hypoxemia, which may progress until it becomes life-threatening or even fatal because of a failure of these infants to resuscitate themselves by arousal or gasping. This hypoxemia apparently does not, in most instances, result from a primary cessation of respiratory efforts, but is more likely to be caused by some form of upper or lower airway closure (such as obstructive apnea) and may also involve the sudden development of an intrapulmonary right-to-left shunt. The triggers eliciting these airway closures remain unknown.

PREVENTION

Principal Considerations

Because of its unpredictability and relative rarity, strategies aimed at preventing SIDS are bound to be either nonspecific or nonsensitive. Examples for a nonspecific approach are attempts to modify specific child care practices or social behaviors known to be associated with an increased risk of SIDS. Such an attempt is currently being undertaken by the British and the American "back to sleep" campaigns aimed against the prone sleeping position, and by the government of New Zealand in their campaign aimed at encouraging breast feeding and avoiding the prone sleeping position, smoking, and bed sharing. Although the preliminary data from these countries are encouraging, it has not been shown whether the reduction in SIDS rates apparently achieved with these campaigns will persist. This question arises because it is always difficult to infer a cause-and-effect relationship between such campaigns and a reduction in SIDS rates. For example, the campaign by the Department of Health in the UK was partially based on the results from a study from Avon, UK, which claimed a decrease in SIDS rates from

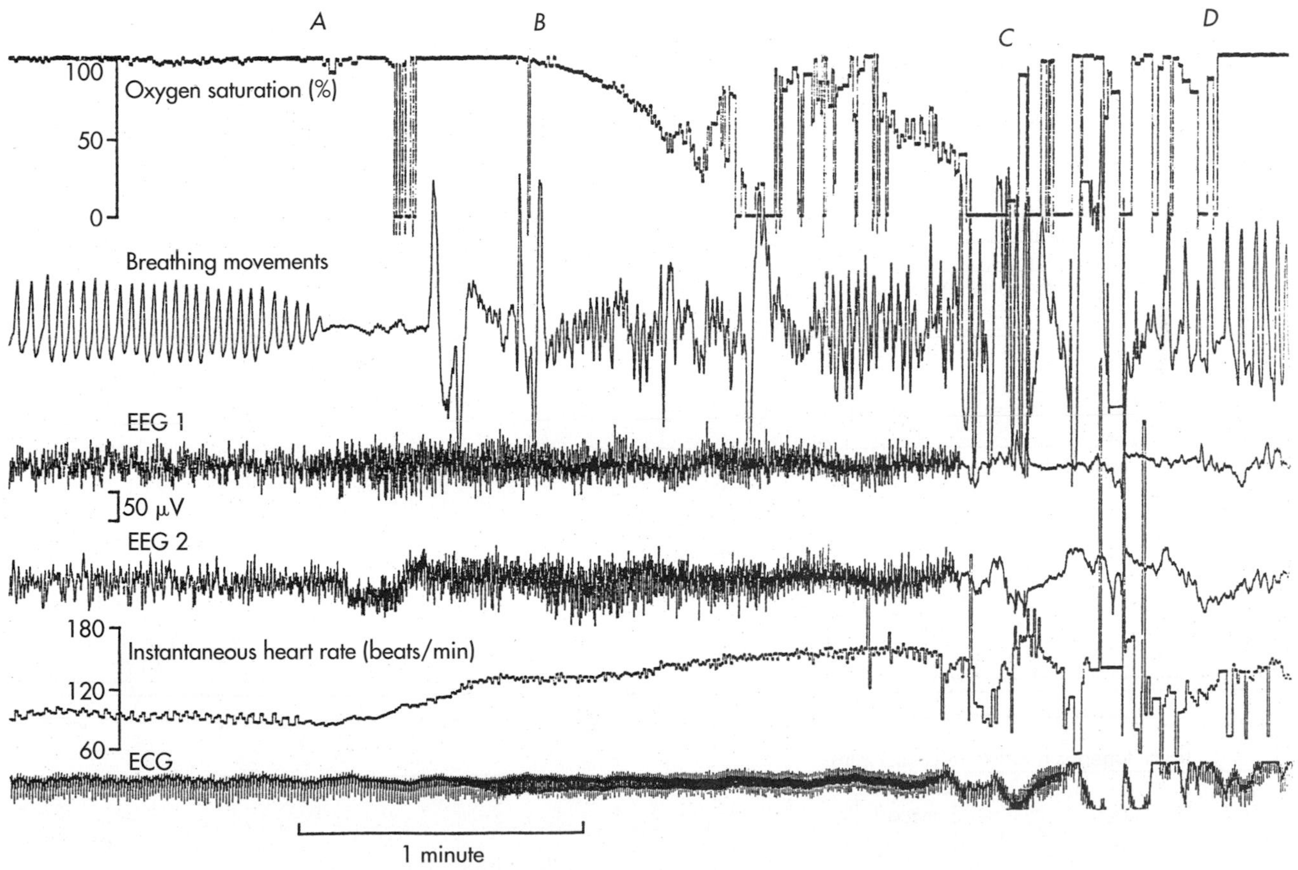

Fig. 71-9. Section from a multichannel recording in an 8-month-old infant with a history of recurrent ALTE of unknown cause. A standard EEG had been normal. Sharp waves appear on the EEG about 10 seconds before the onset of an apneic pause (at *A*). This pause lasts 24 seconds and is not accompanied by a significant fall in Sa_{O_2}. After breathing movements have recommenced (despite continuation of the seizure) hypoxemia develops, lasting 145 seconds (*B* to *D*). Cyanosis occurs and bag-and-mask ventilation is given (*C* to *D*). The instantaneous heart rate signal shows an increase in heart rate commencing with the onset of the apneic pause. Heart rate continues to rise until the end of the seizure (at *C*); it then abruptly falls to below baseline level (80 bpm). The respiratory sinus arrhythmia shown on the instantaneous heart rate signal ceases during the apneic pause, but returns with the reinitiation of breathing movements. EEG 1 = P3-T4, EEG 2 = P4-T3 configuration.

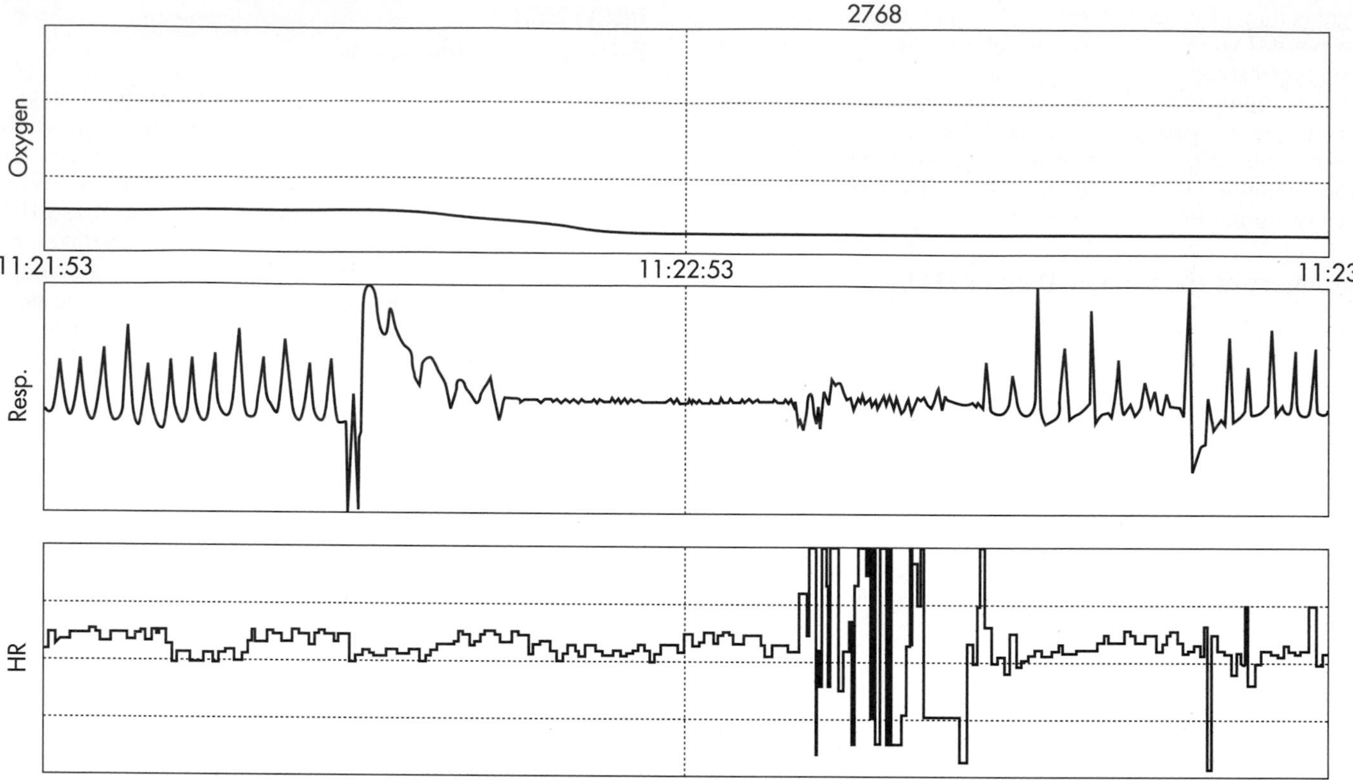

Fig. 71-10. Home event recording of $TcPo_2$, breathing movements, and heart rate in a 7-month-old boy with a history of recurrent ALTE of unknown cause. There is a sharp deflection in the breathing movement signal, which then becomes electronically straight (for 28 seconds) before it abruptly starts to show breathing movements again. During this apparent prolonged apneic pause there continues to be sinus arrhythmia on the instantaneous heart rate signal. The events in this infant were subsequently found to be factitious (Münchhausen syndrome by proxy); the prolonged apneic pause in this recording being caused by the mother temporarily disconnecting the breathing movement sensor.

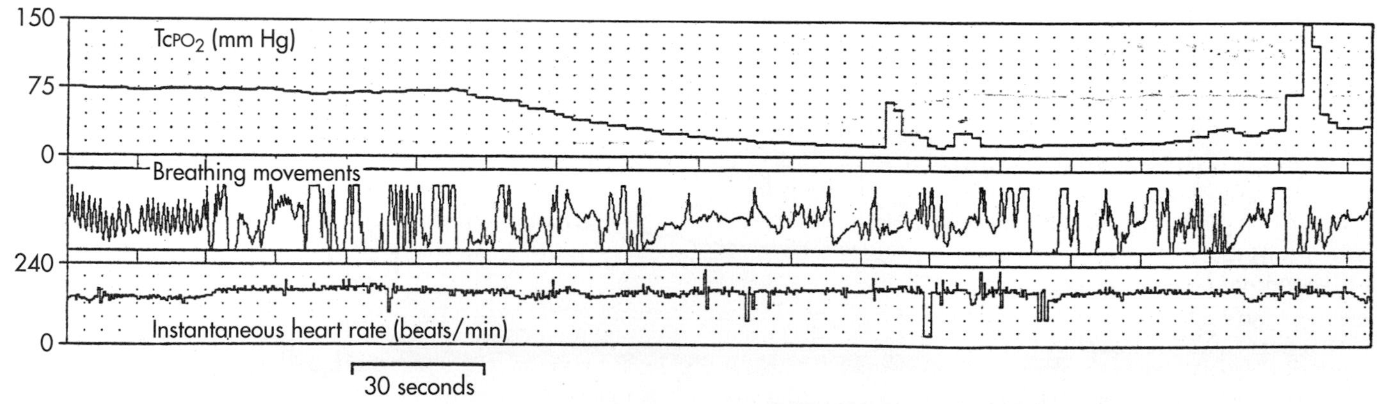

Fig. 71-11. Home event recording in a 6-week-old boy with a history of two ALTEs of unknown cause. There is a fall in $TcPo_2$ from 75 to 12 mm Hg, lasting 3.5 minutes. This is accompanied by irregular breathing movements interrupted by short (4- to 8-second) apneic pauses. Heart rate remains stable throughout the episode. The $TcPo_2$ signal is intermittently disturbed because of poor skin contact during vigorous stimulation by the mother.

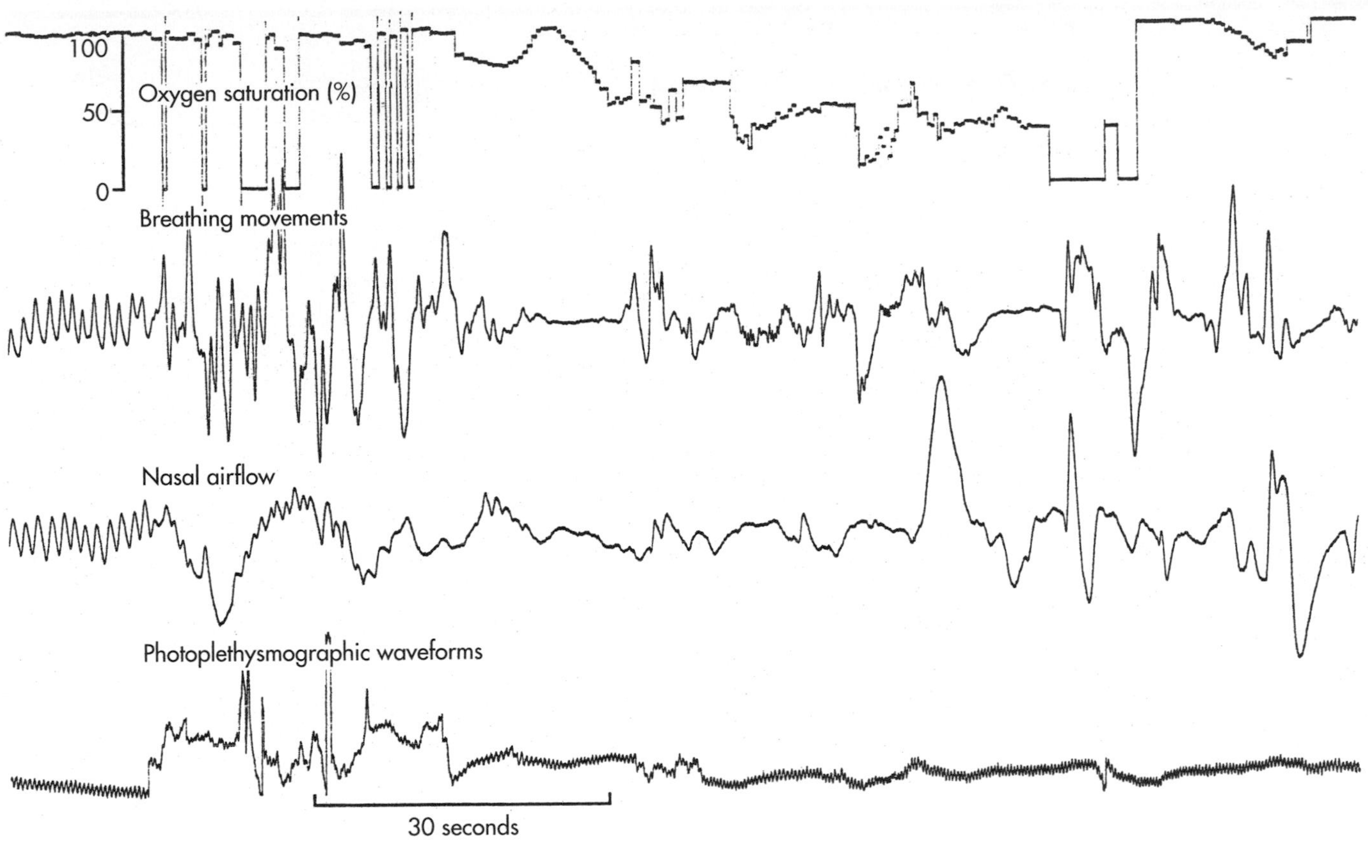

Fig. 71-12. Section from a multichannel recording in the same patient as in Fig. 71-11, recorded after admission to the hospital. There is a decrease in Sa_{O_2}, lasting 70 seconds. This is associated with irregular breathing movements and two short (8 and 7 seconds) apneic pauses. The airflow signal is disturbed, but there is no indication that airflow is absent while breathing movements continue. The infant had a simultaneous EEG recording (not shown in this printout) that was normal. He was later discharged home on additional inspired oxygen; his ALTE never recurred. The cause of his events remains unknown.

3.5/1000 to 1.7/1000 after parents had been instructed to avoid the prone sleeping position.[13] However, data from Scotland, where no such campaigns were launched, also showed a decrease in SIDS rates during the same period (from 2.2/1000 in 1989 to 1.3/1000 in 1991).[190] Similarly, following a recent intervention study in Styria, Austria, a 57% reduction in cot death rates was reported in the study region, but SIDS rates in the surrounding areas also fell by 44% during that period, despite no intervention program being launched in those areas.[191] One explanation for these latter two observations[190,191] could be that information on amenable risk factors had also reached parents in areas where no campaigns had been launched.[192]

An alternative approach to prevent SIDS is to identify individual infants at high risk of SIDS and apply specific preventive measures. Such an approach has been first and most extensively performed in Sheffield, UK, where a predictive risk score for sudden unexpected infant deaths was developed and infants with high scores were regularly seen by a team of health visitors.[193] Although a reduction in overall infant mortality rates was reported, the rate of true SIDS apparently remained unchanged.[194] Moreover, a randomized controlled trial based on this approach was terminated prematurely. A recent meta-analysis of this and other risk scores showed that at least 20% of a population would have to be included to identify 40% to 70% of the SIDS cases in this population.[195] Thus any intervention program that aims to reach at least 50% of all future SIDS victims in a community would have to include very large numbers of infants to even come close to this goal.

Clinical Management of Infants at Risk of SIDS

For the reasons just mentioned, most preventive measures aimed at identifying individual infants at increased risk have been limited to the three clinical risk groups mentioned earlier. In these, the foremost goal is to exclude any treatable disorder potentially resulting in sudden death, particularly in infants with a history of ALTE. The list of diagnoses possibly presenting with an ALTE is long (Box 71-2), and an extensive diagnostic workup is therefore often required in these infants to exclude treatable causes of ALTE. Some suggestions regarding issues that should be covered when obtaining the medical history and organizing the subsequent diagnostic workup in these patients are summarized in Table 71-2.

One of the most difficult issues in the workup of an infant with a history of an ALTE is to determine whether the event described by a parent or caretaker was indeed life-threatening. Recently, concerns have been raised regarding the validity of parental observations of an ALTE. These doubts were based on comparisons between parental observations made in response to monitor alarms and recordings of ECG and breathing movements obtained during these alarms.[196,197] The parental

BOX 71-2
Some Possible Underlying Diagnoses in Patients Presenting with ALTE

Respiratory tract disorders
bronchiolitis
pneumonia
pertussis
tracheoesophageal fistula
aspiration
laryngomalacia; tracheomalacia
Pierre Robin syndrome

Neurologic disorders
meningitis
epileptic seizures
Ondine's curse syndrome (central hypoventilation)
spinal muscular atrophy (Werdnig Hoffmann)
hyperekplexia (startle disease)
Joubert's syndrome
Arnold Chiari malformation
Myopathies

Cardiovascular disorders
long-QT syndrome
cardiac arrhythmias
aortic stenosis
vascular ring

Gastrointestinal disorders
Gastroesophageal reflux
toxic shock syndrome caused by gastroenteritis
Reye's syndrome

Metabolic disorders
medium-chain acyl-CoA deficiency
biotinidase deficiency
ornithine transcarbamylase deficiency
glutaric aciduria type II
systemic carnitine deficiency

Others
cyanotic breath-holding spells
anemia
intentional suffocation (smothering)
Münchhausen syndrome by proxy

observations evaluated in these studies, however, occurred always in response to a monitor alarm, which in itself may cause substantial distress and anxiety. It should therefore not be inferred from these data that parents of infants who are not on a home monitor will also exaggerate the severity of an ALTE, and we would recommend taking parental observations seriously unless objective evidence to the contrary has been obtained during further events.

Because of the importance of obtaining objective data during an ALTE, and because the likelihood of further events is highest during the first 48 hours after the initial event,[75] all infants with a history of an ALTE should be admitted to hospital and immediately connected to a monitor that is combined with an event recorder and can record data on breathing movements, ECG, oxygenation, and preferably also nasal airflow before and after a monitor alarm. If a further event occurs, these recordings may provide important clues to the underlying diagnosis. For example, if an increase in heart rate in association with a severe hypoxemic episode is observed on such an event recording, this may indicate the presence of epileptic seizure–induced hypoxemia as the underlying mechanism. One can then try to confirm this suspected diagnosis by means of long-term EEG recordings, which are otherwise not routinely obtained in infants with ALTE.[198]

If the diagnostic workup summarized in Table 71-2 has failed to identify a treatable cause for the ALTE, a polysomnogram should be performed. This includes a continuous (longer than 6 hours) recording of breathing movements, nasal airflow, ECG, arterial oxygen saturation (and the accompanying light plethysmographic signals), transcutaneous partial pressures of oxygen and carbon dioxide, electrooculogram, and EEG. These recordings occasionally have been valuable in identifying respiratory control disorders such as sleep-related upper airway obstruction or epileptic seizure–induced hypoxemic episodes. However, screening recordings involving only heart rate and breathing movements (so-called pneumograms) have not been shown to have predictive value with regard to SIDS, and it has been recommended that decisions concerning clinical management should not be based on the results of such recordings.[7,199] Screening recordings that include Sao_2, however, may be of value in preterm infants (less than 32 weeks) before discharge from hospital. A considerable proportion of such infants show baseline hypoxemia (Sao_2 less than 95% with Nellcor N200), presumably reflecting subclinical chronic lung disease, which may predispose these infants to ALTE[200] (Figs. 71-13 and 71-14). Treatment with continuous low-dose O_2 (0.2 to 1 L/min) through nasal cannulae appeared, in an uncontrolled study, to reduce the frequency and severity of subsequent ALTE.[201]

In infants in whom a sibling or twin has died of SIDS, clinical investigations apart from a careful medical history and physical examination, an ECG (to exclude long-QT syndrome), and some laboratory tests (such as a full blood count, calcium, glucose, and investigation of the urine for organic acids[202]) should be limited. Because the decision whether these infants should undergo electronic home monitoring cannot be based on the results of a sleep study, the latter should not, in our opinion, be performed on a routine basis in these infants unless they have also been born at less than 32 weeks' gestation, wherein a low baseline Sao_2 may be present.

The next step in the clinical workup of infants at risk of SIDS is the decision as to whether the infant should be started on a home monitor. These devices are the only preventive measure routinely applied to infants at risk of SIDS. However, despite their widespread use (it is estimated that in the United States approximately 45,000 infants are monitored each year[203]), their effectiveness in preventing SIDS has never been proven. The use of these devices should therefore be restricted. According to the guidelines from the National Institutes of Health Consensus Development Conference, monitoring is only medically indicated for infants with a severe ALTE, that is, for those who received vigorous stimulation or resuscitation, symptomatic preterm infants, and siblings of two or more

Table 71-2 Some Suggestions for the Structure of the Medical Interview and the Diagnostic Workup in Patients with ALTE

QUESTION/INVESTIGATION	REASON FOR QUESTION/INVESTIGATION
1. Medical history	
During/after event	
skin color (pale/blue/gray)	estimation of severity of event and necessity for further action
duration of event (seconds/minutes)	
state of consciousness (awake/asleep/unconscious)	
mode of termination (spontaneous/following mild/vigorous stimulation/following CPR)	
time to full recovery (seconds/minutes/hours)	
Immediately before event	
shock, fear, anger	? breath-holding spell
sudden noise followed by startle reaction	? hyperekplexia (startle disease)
coughing, choking, vomiting	? aspiration, TEF ? laryngeal chemoreflex-induced apnea
feeding	? gastroesophageal reflux
turning of eyes, jerky movements, abnormal tongue or mouth movements	? epileptic seizure–induced event
tremor, profuse sweating	? hypoglycemia, hypocalcemia
Hours/days before event	
fever, cold, diarrhea	? infection
abnormal sleepiness or irritability	? meningitis, Reye's syndrome
snoring	? obstructive sleep apnea
stridor	? laryngomalacia or tracheomalacia
wheezing	? bronchiolitis
seizures, turning of eyes, "staring"	? epileptic seizure–induced events
fasting for several hours (± infection)	? medium-chain acyl-CoA deficiency
cyanosis during crying/feeding	? BPD, bronchiolitis, cardiac anomaly
weeks/months before event	
previous events with onset always in presence of the same person	? Münchhausen syndrome by proxy, deliberate suffocation
gradual reduction in spontaneous motor activity	? spinal muscular atrophy, myopathy
profuse sweating	? disorder in autonomic regulation
pertussis or RSV epidemic in the area?	? pertussis, bronchiolitis
prematurity, BPD	? "BPD-spells"
SIDS/ALTE in sibling	inheritable disease (metabolic disorder, long-QT syndrome, startle disease) or parentally induced event more likely
2. Specific features during physical examination	
pallor	? anemia
stridor	? laryngomalacia or tracheomalacia, vascular ring
micrognathia	? Pierre Robin sequence
"TEF-cough"	? tracheoesophageal fistula
wheezing, dyspnea	? bronchiolitis, pneumonia
pronounced second heart tone	? increased PVR, subclinical hypoxemia
heart murmur	? aortic stenosis or other heart defect
muscular hypotonia, no spinal reflexes	? spinal muscular atrophy
chest wall recession	? increased work of breathing (e.g., caused by increased upper airway resistance)
3. Specific laboratory tests	
arterial or capillary blood gas analysis (as soon as possible after event)	estimation of severity of event, ? metabolic disorder, hypoxic/ischemic insult
full blood count including differential	? anemia, infection (e.g., pertussis)
C-reactive protein/ESR	? infection
serum glucose (preferably after fasting period)	? hypoglycemia, metabolic disorder
serum calcium and magnesium	? hypocalcemia, hypomagnesemia
nasal swab, including immunofluorescence	? Pertussis, RSV, adeno virus
organic acids in urine	? medium-chain acyl-CoA deficiency
serum ammonia	? OTCD carrier, glutaric aciduria, carnitine deficiency
4. Further investigations	
electrocardiogram	? long-QT syndrome
chest radiograph	? aspiration, pneumonia, cardiovascular anomaly, BPD
electroencephalogram	? epileptic seizure–induced events
cranial ultrasound/computed tomography	? intracerebral hemorrhage, brainstem abnormalities
sleep study (only if treatable causes of ALTE have been ruled out)	? baseline hypoxemia, hypoventilation, epileptic seizure–induced hypoxemia
home event recording (only if above measures have not helped to identify mechanism)	documentation of further events at home

Note that this list is not complete; in particular, further investigations (e.g., barium swallow, esophageal pH monitoring, echocardiography) may be necessary depending on the results of the initial clinical workup.
BPD, Bronchopulmonary dysplasia; *CPR,* cardiopulmonary resuscitation; *ERS,* erythrocyte sedimentation rate; *OTCD,* ornithine transcarbamylase deficiency; *PVR,* pulmonary vascular resistance; *RSV,* respiratory syncytial virus; *TEF,* tracheo-esophageal fistula.

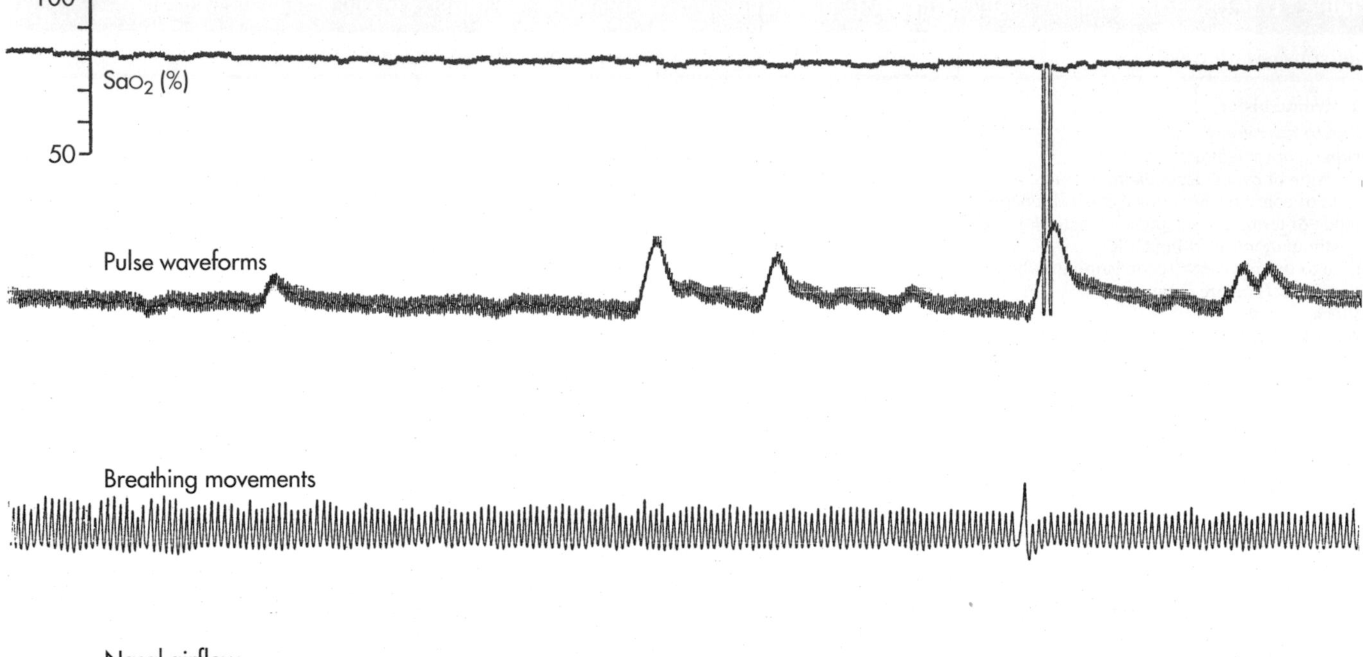

Fig. 71-13. Section from a multichannel recording in a previously preterm infant, born at 31 weeks' gestation and studied at discharge from hospital. There is baseline hypoxemia, with SaO_2 running at 80% to 82% (the 5th centile for baseline SaO_2 in this age group is at 95%). The infant had been ventilated for 3 days after birth, but was considered perfectly well at the time of this recording and this baseline hypoxemia was not suspected clinically.

SIDS victims.[7] For all other infants considered at risk, a decision must be made specific to each infant, and no family should be made to believe that monitoring is necessary. In infants with ALTE, monitoring is recommended until 3 months following the last event or the last true monitor alarm. In SIDS siblings, surviving twins, and premature infants, monitoring should be discontinued at 9 months of corrected age (by this age, 95% of all SIDS deaths have occurred).[25] In preterm infants who are receiving additional inspired oxygen at home and are older than 9 months of age, it is our practice to discontinue monitoring 2 months after they have been weaned off the oxygen. Sometimes, parents find it difficult to stop monitoring their child, particularly if there are repeated alarms of unclear cause. In this situation, the use of documented monitoring (event recording) may be helpful to determine reasons for alarms and to gain a more objective basis for recommendations about discontinuation of monitoring.[204]

Several reports have been made about deaths occurring during monitoring programs, some being attributed to malcompliance[75,205,206] but others occurring despite obviously proper functioning of the monitor.[73,205-208] Deaths caused by electrocution or strangulation have also been reported.[209,210] In a questionnaire study from our institution, which was sent to all members of the British Paediatric Association, 80 deaths were reported in infants on apnea monitors; in 48 of these deaths the infants were reported to have died at home despite the monitor being connected and functioning at the time of death, and 16 additional deaths occurred in infants monitored in hospital (mostly in the low-dependency area of the neonatal unit).[211]

The problems with malcompliance may be explained partially by the fact that home monitors based on impedance cardiorespirography are very prone to false alarms, leading to a severe disturbance of family life.[212] In a recent paper from Weese-Mayer et al, using an event-recording system in combination with a standard cardiorespiratory monitor, 12,980 false alarms were reported during approximately 2100 days of monitoring in 83 infants, giving an average of 6 false alarms per day per infant.[213]

These data clearly suggest that the monitors currently in use on infants at risk of SIDS, which invariably monitor breathing efforts or heart rate, are less than ideally suited for their task. They not only are showing a high rate of false alarms, but are apparently failing to alarm early enough in a proportion of potentially life-threatening events. The latter may be related to the fact that prolonged apneic pauses or bradycardia are not early features of sudden death or near-death events in infants. This was also confirmed in a recent analysis of physiologic data obtained during 69 prolonged

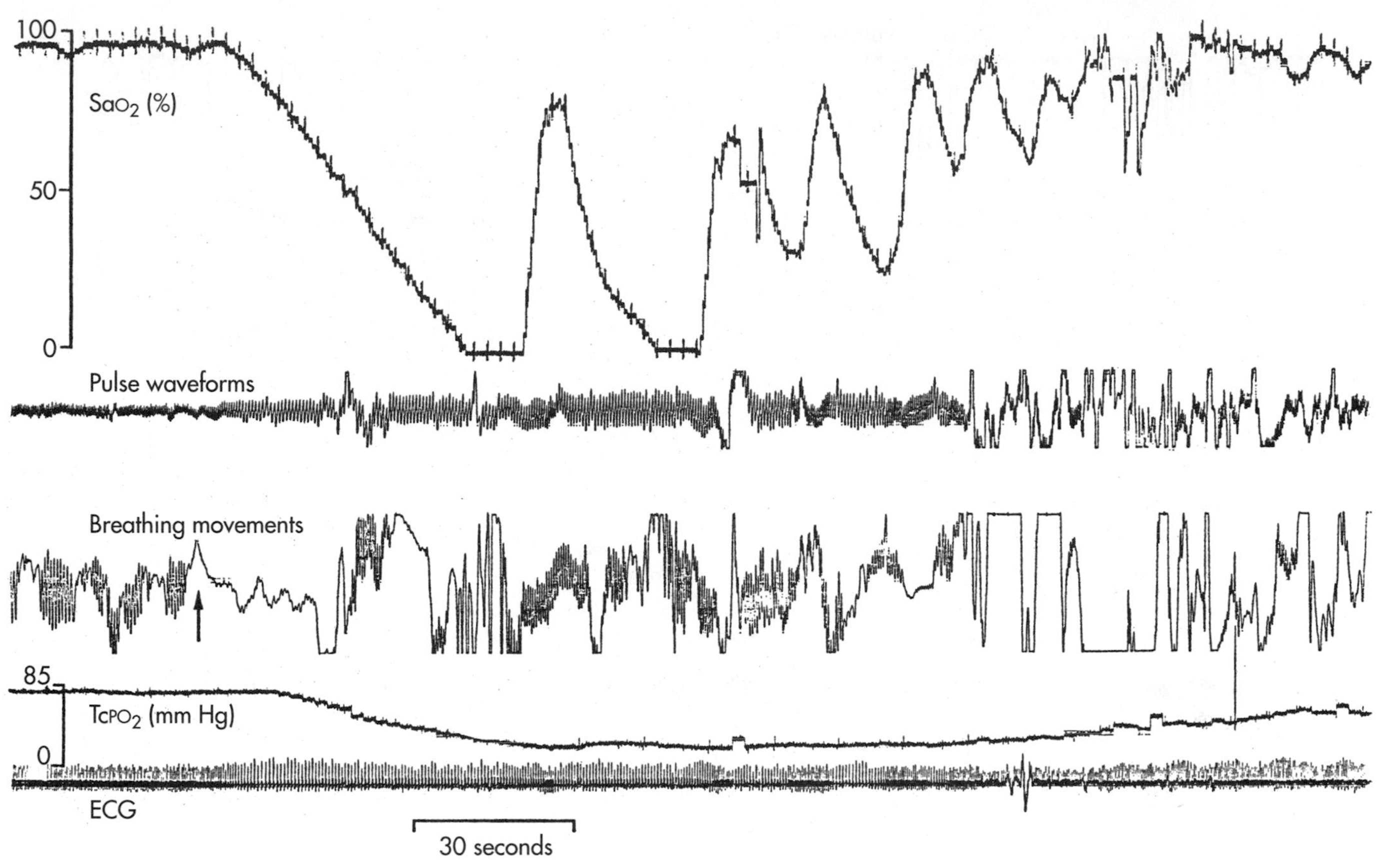

Fig. 71-14. Section from a multichannel recording in a previously preterm infant, born at 28 weeks' gestation and studied at 3 months of age because of a history of frequent cyanotic episodes delaying her discharge from the hospital. The infant had a baseline SaO_2 of only 93%. There is a severe prolonged decrease in SaO_2 and $TcPO_2$, which is accompanied by a 20-second period of apnea/hypopnea (*arrow*) but continues well after breathing movements have resumed. SaO_2 then starts to fluctuate rapidly despite continuous breathing movements. Finally, after 2.3 minutes of hypoxemia, arousal occurs, as indicated by the movement artifacts on the breathing movement, pulse waveform, and ECG signals. Shortly afterward SaO_2 returns to baseline. The ECG shows a decrease in heart rate (from 150 to 105 bpm), but the threshold commonly used for bradycardia (100 bpm) is not reached. Therefore, this episode of prolonged severe hypoxemia would not have been detected by a cardiorespiratory monitor. Note the increase in pulse amplitude during the initial decrease in SaO_2.

hypoxemic episodes, defined as a decrease in SaO_2 to 80% or less for 20 seconds or more or the occurrence of clinically apparent central cyanosis, in 23 infants and young children.[214] Prolonged apneic pauses (20 seconds or more) or bradycardias (heart rate less than or equal to 80 bpm) occurred only during 10% and 28%, respectively, of these episodes. The only recorded signal that would have invariably identified all of these episodes was the transcutaneous PO_2 (the saturation signal from the pulse oximeter was disturbed, because of movement artifact, in 10% of episodes; Fig. 71-15). As a consequence, we began to use a modified transcutaneous PO_2 monitor in infants at risk of hypoxemia or sudden death. Experience with this monitor in over 1100 infants in two centers has shown that it provides reliable and early detection of sudden changes in oxygenation, is safe, and can easily be used by parents at home.[214] However, as with other home monitoring devices, these data are uncontrolled, and there is as yet no proof that home monitoring will reduce the incidence of SIDS.

In infants with recurrent ALTE, it is our practice to routinely combine a $TcPO_2$ monitor with an event recorder that records oxygenation ($TcPO_2$ and SaO_2), ECG, and breathing movements for 20 minutes around a low alarm on the $TcPO_2$ monitor. In the United States, event recorders have chiefly been used to document the frequency and causes of false alarms,[215] investigate the clinical significance of prolonged apneic pauses,[216] or to validate parental perceptions of events.[196,217] We prefer to use these devices as diagnostic tools because a considerable proportion of infants considered to have suffered "idiopathic" ALTE may have a treatable mechanism identified if a further event can be documented by the event recorder. This approach has now also been taken up in the large multicenter Comparative Home Infant Monitoring Evaluation study in the United States, which aims at identifying mechanisms for ALTE and SIDS in infants monitored at home and to compare these findings with polygraphic data obtained prospectively at the time of enrollment of these infants.

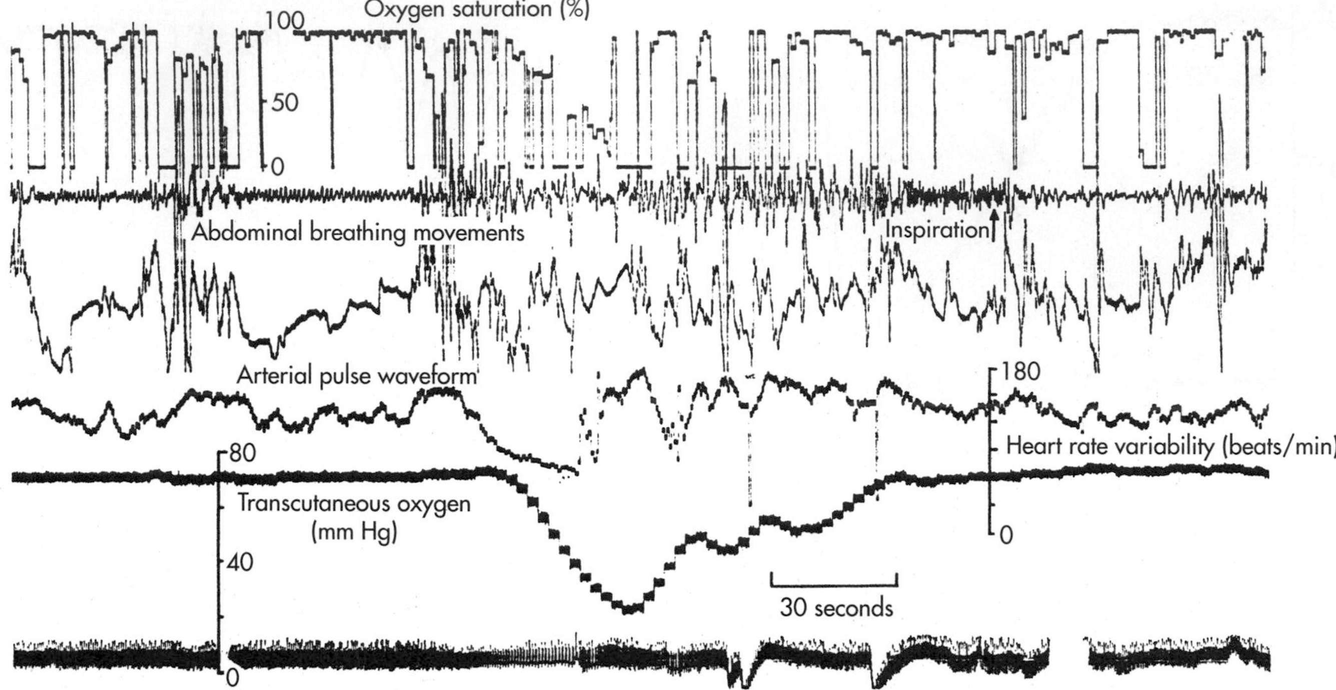

Fig. 71-15. Section from a multichannel recording in a 2-month-old infant during an episode of cyanosis, during which there is a sudden decrease in $TcPo_2$ lasting 90 seconds. This is accompanied by continuous breathing movements, but a decrease in heart rate to 65 bpm. The pulse oximeter signal is lost as a result of movement artifact and would not therefore have identified this event. (From Poets CF, Samuels MP, Noyes JP, Jones KA, Southall DP: *Arch Dis Child* 66:676-682, 1991.)

CONCLUSIONS

The mechanisms responsible for SIDS remain a mystery. However, a growing body of evidence suggests that investigation of its possible pathophysiology should focus on the regulation of the matching between ventilation and perfusion in the lung rather than on the central nervous control mechanisms involved in the regulation of breathing. It is particularly the evidence from physiologic studies (such as lack of primary apnea during deaths and "near-death" events and abnormalities of oxygenation in infants presenting with ALTE) that suggest this. Nevertheless, central nervous mechanisms, such as a reduced arousal responsiveness or a failure of these infants to autoresuscitate via gasping,[218] also appear to be involved in the pathogenesis of SIDS.

It is not yet clear, however, whether an improvement in our understanding of the mechanisms leading to these deaths will enable us to prevent them. In this respect, programs that are based on epidemiologic rather than physiologic data, such as those currently under way in several countries, may be a much more efficient way to reduce the incidence of SIDS in a population, even though the precise roles of the risk factors they are aiming to avoid, such as the prone sleeping position, are poorly understood. Only if the links between the epidemiologic, pathologic, and physiologic characteristics observed in SIDS are elucidated will we fully understand and possibly finally prevent these tragedies.

REFERENCES

1. Sudhoff K: *Internationale Hygiene Ausstellung Dresden,* Dresden Katalog, Item 6375, p 292, 1911.
2. *Allgemeines Gesetzbuch für die preussischen Staaten: Elfter Abschnitt —von den körperlichen Verletzungen,* Berlin, 1791, Königliche Hofbuchdruckerey, p 1282.
3. Fearn SW: Sudden and unexplained death of children, *Lancet* i:246, 1834.
4. Paltauf A: Ueber die Beziehungen der Thymus zum plötzlichen Tod, *Wiener Klin Wochenschr* 2:877-881, 1889; and 3:172-175, 1890.
5. Bergman AB, Beckwith JB, Ray GC, eds: Sudden infant death syndrome: proceedings of the second international conference on causes of sudden death in infants, Seattle, 1970, University of Washington Press, pp 17-18.
6. Huber J: Sudden infant death syndrome: the new clothes of the emperor, *Eur J Pediatr* 152:93-94, 1993.

Terminology

7. National Institutes of Health consensus development conference on infantile apnea and home monitoring, Sept 29-Oct 1, 1986, *Pediatrics* 79:292-299, 1987.

Epidemiology

8. Guyer B, Martin JA, MacDorman MF, Anderson RN, Strobino DM: Annual summary of vital statistics—1996, *Pediatrics* 100:905-921, 1997.
9. Irgens LM, Skjaerven R, Lie RT: Secular trends of sudden infant death syndrome and other causes of post perinatal mortality in Norwegian birth cohorts 1967-1984, *Acta Paediatr Scand* 78:228-232, 1989.
10. Helweg-Larsen K, Knudsen LB, Gregersen M, Simonsen J: Sudden infant death syndrome in Denmark: evaluation of the increasing incidence of registered SIDS in the period 1972 to 1983 and results of a prospective study in 1987 through 1988, *Pediatrics* 89:855-859, 1992.

11. De Jonge GA, Engelberts AC, Koomen-Liefting AJP, Kostense PJ: Cot death and prone sleeping position in the Netherlands, *Br Med J* 298:722, 1989.
12. Engelberts AC, de Jonge GA, Kostense PJ: An analysis of trends in the incidence of sudden infant death in the Netherlands 1969-89, *J Paediatr Child Health* 27:329-333, 1991.
13. Wigfield RE, Fleming PJ, Berry PJ, Rudd PT, Golding J: Can the fall in Avon's sudden infant death rate be explained by changes in the sleeping position? *Br Med J* 304:282-283, 1992.
14. Mitchell EA, Ford RPK, Taylor BJ, Stewart AW, Becroft DMO, Schragg R, Barry DMJ, Allen EM, Roberts AP, Hasall IB: Further evidence supporting a causal relationship between prone sleeping position and SIDS, *J Paediatr Child Health* 28:S9-S12, 1992.
15. Rintahaka PJ, Hirvonen J: The epidemiology of sudden infant death syndrome in Finland in 1969-1980, *Forensic Sci Int* 30:219-233, 1986.
16. Black L, David RJ, Brouillette RT, Hunt CE: Effects of birth weight and ethnicity on incidence of sudden infant death syndrome, *J Pediatr* 108:209-214, 1986.
17. Kyle D, Sunderland R, Stonehouse M, Cummins C, Ross O: Ethnic differences in incidence of sudden infant death syndrome in Birmingham, *Arch Dis Child* 65:830-833, 1990.
18. Veelken N, Ziegelitz J, Knispel JD, Bentele KHP: Sudden infant death syndrome in Hamburg, *Acta Paediatr Scand* 80:86-92, 1991.
19. Nelson EAS, Taylor BJ, Weatherall IL: Sleeping position and infant bedding may predispose to hyperthermia and the sudden infant death syndrome, *Lancet* i:199-201, 1989.
20. Wennergren G, Milerad J, Lagercrantz H, Karlberg P, Svenningsen NW, Sedin G, Andersson D, Grügaard J, Bjure J: The epidemiology of sudden infant death syndrome and attacks of lifelessness in Sweden, *Acta Paediatr Scand* 76:898-906, 1987.
21. Lee NNY, Chan YF, Davies DP, Lau E, Yip DC: Sudden infant death syndrome in Hong Kong: confirmation of low incidence, *Br Med J* 298: 721, 1989.
22. Foundation for the Study of Infant Deaths: *FSID News* no 46, London, 1993.
23. Kraus JF, Greenland S, Bulterys M: Risk factors for sudden infant death syndrome in the U.S.: collaborative perinatal project, *Int J Epidemiol* 18:113-120, 1989.
24. Mitchell EA, Stewart AW, Scragg R, Ford RPK, Taylor BJ, Becroft DMO, Thompson JMD, Hasall IB, Barry DMJ, Allen EM, Roberts AP: Ethnic differences in mortality from sudden infant death syndrome in New Zealand, *Br Med J* 306:13-16, 1993.
25. Grether JK, Schulman J: Sudden infant death syndrome and birth weight, *J Pediatr* 114:561-567, 1989.
26. Polberger S, Svenningsen NW: Early neonatal sudden infant death and near death of fullterm infants in maternity wards, *Acta Paediatr Scand* 74:861-866, 1985.
27. Rajs J, Hammarquist F: Sudden infant death in Stockholm, *Acta Paediatr Scand* 77:812-820, 1988.
28. Guntheroth WG: *Crib death: the sudden infant death syndrome,* New York, 1989, Futura Publishing.
29. Bergmann AB, Ray CG, Pomeroy MA, Wahl PW, Beckwith JB: Studies of the sudden infant death syndrome in King County, Washington. III. Epidemiology, *Pediatrics* 49:860-870, 1972.
30. Uren EC, Williams AL, Jack I, Rees JW: Association of respiratory virus infections with sudden infant death syndrome, *Med J Aust* 1:417-419, 1980.
31. Nicoll A, Gardner A: Whooping cough and unrecognised postperinatal mortality, *Arch Dis Child* 63:41-47, 1988.
32. Hoffman HJ, Hunter JC, Damus K, et al: Diphteria-tetanus-pertussis immunization and sudden infant death: results of the National Institute of Child Health and Human Development cooperative epidemiological study of sudden infant death syndrome risk factors, *Pediatrics* 79:598-611, 1987.
33. Mitchell EA, Stewart AW: Deaths from sudden infant death syndrome on public holidays and weekends, *Aust NZ J Med* 18:861-863, 1988.
34. Kaada B, Sivertsen E: Sudden infant death syndrome during weekends and holidays in Norway in 1967-1985, *Scand J Soc Med* 18:17-23, 1990.
35. Mitchell EA, Nelson KP, Thompson JMD, Stewart AW, Taylor BJ, Ford RPK, Scragg R, Becroft DMO, Allen EA, Hassall IB, Roberts A: Travel and changes in routine do not increase the risk of sudden infant death syndrome, *Acta Paediatr* 83:815-818, 1994.
36. Kleemann WJ, Urban R, Eidam J, Wiechmann B, Tröger HD: Die Auffindesituation beim plötzlichen Kindstod, *Rechtsmedizin* 1:147-151, 1991.
37. Dittmann V, Pribilla O: Zur Epidemiologie des plötzlichen Säuglingstodes im Lübecker Raum, *Z Rechtsmed* 90:277-292, 1983.
38. Mitchell EA, Taylor BJ, Ford RPK, Stewart AW, Becroft DMO, Thompson JMD, Scragg R, Hassall IB, Barry DMJ, Allen EM, Roberts AP: Four modifiable and other major risk factors for cot death: the New Zealand study, *J Paediatr Child Health* 28:S3-S8, 1992.
39. Buck GM, Cookfair DL, Michalek AM, et al: Intrauterine growth retardation and risk of sudden infant death syndrome, *Am J Epidemiol* 129:874-884, 1989.
40. Hoffman HJ, Damus K, Hillman L, Krongrad E: Risk factors for SIDS: results of the National Institute of Child Health and Human Development Cooperative Epidemiological Study, *Ann NY Acad Sci* 533:13-20, 1988.
41. Mitchell EA, Thompson JMD, Stewart AW, Webster ML, Taylor BJ, Hassall IB, Ford RPK, Allen EM, Scragg R, Becroft DMO: Postnatal depression and SIDS: a prospective study, *J Paediatr Child Health* 28:S13-S16, 1992.
42. Haglund B, Cnattingius S: Cigarette smoking as a risk factor for sudden infant death syndrome: a population-based study, *Am J Publ Health* 80: 29-32, 1990.
43. Poets CF, Rudolph A, Schlaud M, Kleemann WJ, Diekmann U, Sens B: Maternal cigarette smoking and sudden infant death Syndrome: results from the lower Saxony perinatal working group, *Eur J Pediatr* 154: 326-329, 1995.
44. Mitchell EA, Ford RPK, Stewart AW, Taylor BJ, Becroft DMO, Thompson JMD, Scragg R, Hassall JB, Barry DMJ, Allen EM, Roberts AP: Smoking and the sudden infant death syndrome, *Pediatrics* 91:893-8906, 1993.
45. Bulterys MG, Greenland S, Kraus JF: Chronic fetal hypoxia and sudden infant death syndrome: interaction between maternal smoking and low hematocrit during pregnancy, *Pediatrics* 86:535-540, 1990.
46. Hanrahan JP, Tager IB, Segal MR, Tosteson TD, Castile RG, van Vunakis H, Weiss ST, Speizer FE: The effect of maternal smoking during pregnancy on early infant lung function, *Am Rev Respir Dis* 145: 1129-1135, 1992.
47. Wright AL, Holberg C, Martinez FD, Taussig LM, Group Health Medical Associates: Relationship of parental smoking to wheezing and nonwheezing lower respiratory tract illnesses in infancy, *J Pediatr* 118:207-214, 1991.
48. Stanton AN: Overheating and cot death, *Lancet* ii:1199-1201, 1984.
49. Fleming PJ, Gilbert R, Azaz Y, Berry PJ, Rudd PT, Stewart A, Hall E: Interaction between bedding and sleeping position in the sudden infant death syndrome: a population based case-control study, *Br Med J* 301:85-89, 1990.
50. Ponsonby AL, Dwyer T, Gibbons L, Cochrane JA, Jones ME, McCall MJ: Thermal environment and sudden infant death syndrome: case-control study, *Br Med J* 304:277-282, 1992.
51. Ponsonby A-L, Dwyer T, Gibbons LE, Cochrane JA, Wang Y-G: Factors potentiating the risk of sudden infant death syndrome associated with the prone position, *N Engl J Med* 329:377-382, 1993.
52. Gilbert R, Rudd P, Berry PJ, Fleming PJ, Hall E, White DG, Oreffo VOC, James P, Evans JA: Combined effect of infection and heavy wrapping on the risk of sudden unexpected infant death, *Arch Dis Child* 67:171-177, 1992.
53. Berterottière D, D'Allest AM, Dehan M, Gaultier C: Effects of increase in body temperature on the breathing pattern in premature infants, *J Dev Physiol* 13:303-308, 1990.
54. Gozal D, Colin A, Daskalovic YI, Jaffe M: Environmental overheating as a cause of transient respiratory chemoreceptor dysfunction in an infant, *Pediatrics* 82:738-740, 1988.
55. Inoue H, Inoue C, Hildebrandt J: Temperature effects on lung mechanics in air- and liquid-filled rabbit lungs, *J Appl Physiol Respir Environ Exercise Physiol* 53:567-575, 1982.
56. Talbert DG: SIDS, surfactant, and temperature (letter), *Lancet* 336:690 1312, 1990.
57. Carpenter RG: Sudden and unexplained deaths in infancy (cot death). In Camps FE, Carpenter RG, eds: *Sudden and unexpected deaths in infancy (cot death),* Bristol, 1972, John Wright pp 7-15.
58. Saternus KS: Plützlicher Kindstod(eine Folge der Bauchlage? In Walther G, Haffner H-T, eds: *Festschrift Horst Leithoff,* Heidelberg, 1985, Kriminalistik Verleg, pp 67-88.

59. Beal SM, Finch CF: An overview of retrospective case-control studies investigating the relationship between prone sleeping position and SIDS, *J Paediatr Child Health* 27:334-339, 1991.
60. Southall D, Stebbens V, Samuels M: Bedding and sleeping position in the sudden infant death syndrome (letter), *Br Med J* 301:492, 1990.
61. Drews CD, Kraus JF, Greenland S: Recall bias in a case-control study of sudden infant death syndrome, *Int J Epidemiol* 19:405-411, 1990.
62. Dwyer T, Ponsonby A-LB, Newman NM, Gibbons LE: Prospective cohort study of prone sleeping position and sudden infant death syndrome, *Lancet* 337:1244-1247, 1991.
63. Kemp JS, Kowalski RM, Burch PM, Graham MA, Thach BT: Unintentional suffocation by rebreathing: a death scene and physiologic investigation of a possible cause of sudden infant death, *J Pediatr* 122:874-880, 1993.
64. Poets CF, Rudolph A, Neuber K, Buch U, von der Hardt H: Arterial oxygen saturation in infants at risk of sudden death: influence of sleep position, *Acta Paediatr* 84:779-782, 1995.
65. Wagaman MJ, Shutack JG, Moomjian AS, Schwartz JG, Shaffer TH, Fox WW: Improved oxygenation and lung compliance with prone positioning of neonates, *J Pediatr* 94: 787-791, 1979.
66. Baird TM, Paton JB, Fisher DE: Improved oxygenation with prone positioning in neonates: stability of increased transcutaneous Po_2, *J Perinatol* 11: 315-318, 1991.
67. Levene S, McKenzie SA: Transcutaneous oxygen saturation in sleeping infants: prone and supine, *Arch Dis Child* 65:524-526, 1990.
68. Heimler R, Langlois J, Hodel DJ, Nelin LD, Sasidharan P: Effect of positioning on the breathing pattern of preterm infants, *Arch Dis Child* 67:312-314, 1992.
69. Kurlak LO, Ruggins NR, Stephenson TJ: Effect of nursing position on incidence, type, and duration of clinically significant apnoea in preterm infants, *Arch Dis Child* 71:F16-F19, 1994.
70. Orenstein SR, Whitington PF: Positioning for prevention of infant gastroesophageal reflux, *J Pediatr* 103:534-537, 1983.
71. Jolley SG, Halpern LM, Tunell WP, Johnson DG, Sterling CE: The risk of sudden infant death from gastroesophageal reflux, *J Pediatr Surg* 26:691-696, 1991.
72. De Jonge GA, Burgmeijer RJF, Engelberts AC, Hoogenboezem J, Kostense PJ, Sprij AJ: Sleeping position for infants and cot death in the Netherlands 1985-1991, *Arch Dis Child* 69:660-663, 1993.
73. Willinger M, Hoffman HJ, Hartford RB: Infant sleep position and risk for sudden infant death syndrome: report of meeting held January 13 and 14, 1994, National Institutes of Health, Bethesda, MD, *Pediatrics* 93:814-819, 1994.
74. Hunt CE: Infant sleep position and sudden infant death syndrome risks: a time for change, *Pediatrics* 94:106, 1994.
75. Oren J, Kelly D, Shannon DC: Identification of a high-risk group for sudden infant death syndrome among infants who were resuscitated for sleep apnea, *Pediatrics* 77:495-499, 1986.
76. Irgens LM, Skjaerven R, Peterson DR: Prospective assessment of recurrence risk in sudden infant death syndrome siblings, *J Pediatr* 104:349-351, 1984.
77. Guntheroth WG, Lohmann R, Spiers PS: Risk of sudden infant death syndrome in subsequent siblings, *J Pediatr* 116:520-524, 1990.
78. Wariyar U, Richmond S, Hey E: Pregnancy outcome at 24-31 weeks' gestation: neonatal survivors, *Arch Dis Child* 64:678-686, 1989.
79. Werthammer J, Brown ER, Neff RK, Taeusch HW: Sudden infant death syndrome in infants with bronchopulnomary dysplasia, *Pediatrics* 69:301-304, 1982.
80. Gray PH, Rogers Y: Are infants with bronchopulmonary dysplasia at risk for sudden infant death syndrome? *Pediatrics* 93:774-777, 1994.

Pathology

81. Haas JE, Taylor JA, Bergman AB, van Belle G, Felgenhauer JL, Siebert JR, Benjamin DR: Relationship between epidemiologic risk factors and clinicopathologic findings in the sudden infant death syndrome, *Pediatrics* 91:106-112, 1993.
82. Beckwith JB: The mechanism of death in sudden infant death syndrome. In Culbertson JL, Krous HF, Bendell RD, eds: *Sudden infant death syndrome. Medical aspects and psychological management,* Baltimore, 1988, The Johns Hopkins University Press, pp 48-61.
83. Krous HF, Jordan J: A comparison of the distribution of petechiae and their significance in sudden infant death syndrome (SIDS), lethal upper airway obstruction and non-SIDS. In Harper RM, Hoffman HJ, eds: *Sudden infant death syndrome. Risk factors and basic mechanisms,* New York, 1988, PMA Publishing, pp 91-100.
84. Campbell CJ, Read DJC: Circulatory and respiratory factors in the experimental production of lung petechiae and their possible significance in the sudden infant death syndrome, *Pathology* 12:181-188, 1980.
85. Farber JP, Catron AC, Krous HF: Pulmonary petechiae: ventilatory-circulatory interactions, *Pediatr Res* 17:230-233, 1983.
86. Handforth CP: Sudden unexpected death in infancy, *Can Med Assoc J* 80:872-873, 1959.
87. Guntheroth WG: The significance of pulmonary petechiae in crib death, *Pediatrics* 52:601-603, 1973.
88. Guntheroth WG: The pathophysiology of petechiae. In Tildon JT, Roeder LM, Steinschneider A, eds: *Sudden infant death syndrome,* New York, 1983, Academic Press, pp 271-278.
89. Riβe M, Weiler G: Vergleichende histologische Untersuchungen zur Genese petechialer Thymusblutungen, *Z Rechtsmed* 102:33-40, 1989.
90. Marshall TK: Significance of petechiae. In Bergmann AB, Beckwith JB, Ray CG, eds: *Sudden infant death syndrome,* Seattle, 1970, University of Washington Press, p 122.
91. Camps FE: Discussion. In Camps FE, Carpenter RG, eds: *Sudden and unexpected deaths in infancy (cot deaths),* Bristol, 1972, Wright & Sons, p 71.
92. Brouardel P: *La Pendaison, la Strongulation, la Suffocation, la Submersion,* Paris, 1897, J-B Bailliere et Fils, p 20.
93. Winn K: Similarities between lethal asphyxia in postneonatal rats and the terminal episode in SIDS, *Pediatr Pathol* 5:325-335, 1986.
94. Stewart S, Fawcett J, Jacobson W: Interstitial haemosiderin in the lungs of SIDS: a histological hallmark of "near-miss" episodes? *J Pathol* 145:53, 1985.
95. Southall DP, Stebbens VA, Rees SV, Lang MH, Warner JO, Shinebourne EA: Apnoeic episodes induced by smothering: two cases identified by covert video surveillance, *Br Med J* 294:1637-1641, 1987.
96. Beckwith JB: The sudden infant death syndrome, *Curr Probl Pediatr* 3:3-35, 1973.
97. Martinez FD: Sudden infant death syndrome and small airway occlusion: facts and a hypothesis, *Pediatrics* 87:190-198, 1991.
98. Berger D: Child abuse simulating "near-miss" sudden infant death syndrome, *J Pediatr* 95:554-556, 1979.
99. Tapp E, Jones DM, Tobin JO'H: Interpretation of respiratory tract histology in cot deaths, *J Clin Pathol* 28:899-904, 1975.
100. Schäfer AT, Lemke R, Althoff H: Airway resistance of the posterior nasal pathways in sudden infant death victims, *Eur J Pediatr* 150:595-598, 1991.
101. Telford DR, Morris JA, Hughes P, Conway AR, Lee S, Barson AJ, Drucker DB: The nasopharyngel bacterial flora in the sudden infant death syndrome, *J Infect* 18:125-130, 1989.
102. Zink P, Drescher J, Verhagen W, et al: Serological evidence of recent influenza virus A (H3N2) infections in forensic cases of the sudden infant death syndrome (SIDS), *Arch Virol* 93:223-232, 1987.
103. Forsyth KD, Weeks SC, Koh L, Skinner J, Bradley J: Lung immunoglobulins in the sudden infant death syndrome, *Br Med J* 298: 23-26, 1989.
104. Howat WJ, Moore IE, Judd M, Roche WR: Pulmonary immunopathology of sudden infant death syndrome, *Lancet* 343:1390-1392, 1994.
105. Haque AK, Mancuso MG: Proliferation of dendritic cells in the bronchioles of sudden infant death syndrome victims, *Modern Pathol* 6:360-370, 1993.
106. Naeye RL: Sudden infant death syndrome, is the confusion ending? *Modern Pathol* 1:169-174, 1988.
107. Valdes-Dapena M: Sudden infant death syndrome: overview of recent research developments from a pediatric pathologist's perspective, *Pediatrician* 15:222-230, 1988.
108. Gillan JE, Curran C, O'Reilly E, Cahalane SF, Unwin AR: Abnormal patterns of pulmonary neuroendocrine cells in victims of sudden infant death syndrome, *Pediatrics* 84:828-834, 1989.
109. Haque AK, Mancuso MG, Hokanson J, Nguyen ND, Nichols MM: Bronchiolar wall changes in sudden infant death syndrome: morphometric study of a new observation, *Pediatr Pathol* 11:551-568, 1991.

110. Rognum TO, Saugstad OD: Hypoxanthine levels in vitreous humor: evidence of hypoxia in most infants who died of sudden infant death syndrome, *Pediatrics* 87:306-310, 1991.
111. Jäykkä S: Precapillary bypass and sudden infant death (letter), *Lancet* ii:1315, 1971.
112. Wilkinson MJ, Fagan DG: Intrapulmonary arteriovenous shunting: a mechanism in sudden unexpected death, *Arch Dis Child* 65:435-437, 1990.
113. Morley CJ, Hill CM, Brown BD, Barson AJ, Davis JA: Surfactant abnormalities in babies dying from the sudden infant death syndrome, *Lancet* i:1320-1322, 1982.
114. Gibson RA, McMurchie EJ: Changes in lung surfactant lipids associated with the sudden infant death syndrome, *Austr Paediatr J* 22 (suppl):77-80, 1986.
115. Hill CM, Brown BD, Morley CJ, Davis JA, Barson AJ: Pulmonary surfactant. II. In sudden infant death syndrome, *Early Hum Dev* 16:153-162, 1988.
116. Gibson RA, McMurchie EJ: Decreased lung surfactant disaturated phosphatidylcholine in sudden infant death syndrome, *Early Hum Dev* 17:145-155, 1988.
117. James D, Berry PJ, Fleming P, Hathaway M: Surfactant abnormality and the sudden infant death syndrome: a primary or secondary phenomenon? *Arch Dis Child* 65:774-778, 1990.
118. Fagan DG, Milner AD: Pressure volume characteristics of the lungs in sudden infant death syndrome, *Arch Dis Child* 60:471-485, 1985.
119. Valdes-Dapena M: The sudden infant death syndrome: pathologic findings, *Clin Perinatol* 19:701-716, 1992.
120. Liu M, Wang L, Li E, Enhorning G: Pulmonary surfactant will secure free airflow through a narrow tube, *J Appl Physiol* 71:742-748, 1991.
121. Southall DP, Talbert DG: Sudden atelectasis apnea braking syndrome. In Hollinger MF, ed: *Current topics in pulmonary pharmacology and toxicology,* New York, 1987, Elsevier, pp 210-289.

Pathophysiology

122. Southall DP, Richards JM, de Swiet M, et al: Identification of infants destined to die unexpectedly during infancy: evaluation of predictive importance of prolonged apnoea and disorders of cardiac rhythm or conduction, *Br Med J* 286:1092-1096, 1983.
123. Southall DP, Richards JM, Stebbens V, Wilson AJ, Taylor V, Alexander JR: Cardiorespiratory function in 16 full-term infants with sudden infant death syndrome, *Pediatrics* 78:787-796, 1986.
124. Schechtman VL, Harper RM, Wilson AJ, Southall DP: Sleep apnea in infants who succumb to the sudden infant death syndrome, *Pediatrics* 87:841-846, 1991.
125. Wilson AJ, Stevens V, Franks CI, Alexander J, Southall DP: Respiratory and heart rate patterns in infants destined to be victims of sudden infant death syndrome: average rates and their variability measured over 24 hours, *Br Med J* 290:497-501, 1985.
126. Southall DP, Stevens V, Franks CI, Newcombe RG, Shinebourne EA, Wilson AJ: Sinus tachycardia in term infants preceding sudden infant death, *Eur J Pediatr* 147:74-78, 1988.
127. Waggener TB, Southall DP, Scott LA: Analysis of breathing patterns in a prospective population of term infants does not predict susceptibility to sudden infant death syndrome, *Pediatr Res* 27:113-117, 1990.
128. Antila KJ, Välimäki IAT, Mäkelä M, Tuominen J, Wilson AJ, Southall DP: Heart rate variability in infants subsequently suffering sudden infant death syndrome (SIDS), *Early Hum Dev* 22:57-72, 1990.
129. Kluge KA, Harper RM, Schechtman VL, Wilson AJ, Hoffman HJ, Southall DP: Spectral analysis assessment of respiratory sinus arrhythmia in normal infants and infants who subsequently died of sudden infant death syndrome, *Pediatr Res* 24:677-682, 1988.
130. Schechtman VL, Harper RM, Kluge KA, Wilson AJ, Hoffman HJ, Southall DP: Heart rate variation in normal infants and victims of the sudden infant death syndrome, *Early Hum Dev* 19:167-181, 1989.
131. Schechtman VL, Raetz SL, Harper RK, Garfinkel A, Wilson AJ, Southall DP, Harper RM: Dynamic analysis of cardiac R-R intervals in normal infants and in infants who subsequently succumbed to the sudden infant death syndrome, *Pediatr Res* 31:606-612, 1992.
132. Schechtman VL, Harper RM, Wilson AJ, Southall DP: Sleep state organization in normal infants and victims of the sudden infant death syndrome, *Pediatrics* 89:865-870, 1992.
133. Hashimoto T, Hiura K, Endo S, Fukuda K, Mori A, Tayama M, Miyao M: Postural effects on behavioral state of newborn infants, *Brain Dev* 5:286-291, 1983.
134. Brackbill Y, Douthitt TC, West H: Psychophysiologic effects in the neonate of prone versus supine placement, *J Pediatr* 82:82-84, 1973.
135. Kelly DH, Golub MD, Carley D, Shannon DC: Pneumograms in infants who subsequently died of sudden infant death syndrome, *J Pediatr* 109:249-254, 1986.
136. Kahn A, Groswasser J, Rebuffat E, et al: Sleep and cardiorespiratory characteristics of infant victims of sudden death: a prospective case-control study, *Sleep* 15:287-292, 1992.
137. Southall DP, Arrowsmith WA, Oakley JR, McEnery G, Anderson RH, Shinebourne EA: Prolonged QT interval and cardiac arrhythmias in two neonates; sudden infant death syndrome in one case, *Arch Dis Child* 54:776-779, 1979.
138. Schwartz PJ: The quest for the mechanisms of the sudden infant death syndrome: doubts and progress, *Circulation* 75:677-683, 1987.
139. Southall DP, Arrowsmith WA, Stebbens V, Alexander JR: QT interval measurements before sudden infant death syndrome, *Arch Dis Child* 61:327-333, 1986.
140. Weinstein SL, Steinschneider A: QTc and R-R intervals in victims of the sudden infant death syndrome, *Am J Dis Child* 139:987-990, 1985.
141. Sadeh D, Shannon DC, Abboud S, Saul JP, Akselrod S, Cohen RJ: Altered cardiac repolarization in some victims of sudden infant death syndrome, *N Engl J Med* 317:1501-1505, 1987.
142. Wynn VT, Southall DP: Normal relation between heart rate and cardiac repolarisation in sudden infant death syndrome, *Br Heart J* 67:84-88, 1992.
143. Kahn A, Blum D, Hennart P, Sellens C, Samson-Dollfus D, Tayot J, Gilly R, Dutruge J, Flores R, Sternberg B: A critical comparison of the history of sudden-death infants and infants hospitalised for near-miss for SIDS, *Eur J Pediatr* 143:103-107, 1984.
144. Steinschneider A: Prolonged apnea and the sudden infant death syndrome: clinical and laboratory observations, *Pediatrics* 50:646-654, 1972.
145. Bergman AB, Beckwith JB, Ray CG: The apnea monitor business, *Pediatrics* 56:1-3, 1975.
146. Little GA, Brooks JG: Accepting the unthinkable, *Pediatrics* 94:748-749, 1994.
147. Kelly DH, Shannon DC: Periodic breathing in infants with near-miss sudden infant death syndrome, *Pediatrics* 63:355-360, 1979.
148. Southall DP, Janczynski RE, Alexander JR, Taylor VG, Stebbens VA: Cardiorespiratory patterns in infants presenting with apparent life-threatening episodes, *Biol Neonate* 57:77-87, 1990.
149. Oren J, Kelly DH, Shannon DC: Pneumogram recordings in infants resuscitated for apnea of infancy, *Pediatrics* 83:364-368, 1989.
150. Guilleminault C, Ariagno R, Korobkin R, et al: Mixed and obstructive sleep apnea and near miss for sudden infant death syndrome: 2. comparison of near miss and normal control infants, *Pediatrics* 64:882-891, 1979.
151. Ruggins NR, Milner AD: Site of upper airway obstruction in infants following an acute life-threatening event, *Pediatrics* 91:595-601, 1993.
152. McCulloch K, Brouillette RT, Guzzetta AJ, Hunt CE: Arousal responses in near-miss sudden infant death syndrome and in normal infants, *J Pediatr* 101:911-917, 1982.
153. van der Hal AL, Rodriguez AM, Sargent CW: Hypoxic and hypercapneic arousal responses and prediction of subsequent apnea in apnea of infancy, *Pediatrics* 75:848-854, 1985.
154. Davidson-Ward SL, Bautista DB, Keens TG: Hypoxic arousal responses in normal infants, *Pediatrics* 89:860-864, 1992.
155. Coons S, Guilleminault C: Motility and arousal in near miss sudden infant death syndrome, *J Pediatr* 107:728-732, 1985.
156. Fewell JE, Konduri GG: Influence of repeated exposure to rapidly developing hypoxaemia on the arousal and cardiopulmonary response to rapidly developing hypoxaemia in lambs, *J Dev Physiol* 11:77-82, 1989.
157. Poets CF, Samuels MP, Southall DP: The potential role of intrapulmonary shunting in the pathogenesis of hypoxemic episodes in infants and young children, *Pediatrics* 90:385-392, 1992.
158. Southall DP, Samuels MP, Talbert DG: Recurrent cyanotic episodes with severe arterial hypoxaemia and intrapulmonary shunting: a mechanism for sudden death, *Arch Dis Child* 65:953-961, 1990.

159. Southall DP, Samuels MP, Poets CF: Prolonged expiratory apnea and intrapulmonary shunting. In Beckerman B, Brouillette B, Hunt CE, eds: *Respiratory control disorders in infants and children,* Baltimore, 1992, Williams & Wilkins, pp 242-251.
160. Hills BA, Masters EB, O'Duffy JF: Abnormalities of surfactant in children with recurrent cyanotic episodes, *Lancet* 339:1323-1324, 1992.
161. Masters IB, Vance J, Hills BA: Surfactant abnormalities in ALTE and SIDS, *Arch Dis Child* 71:501-505, 1994.
162. Poets CF, Martin I, Acevedo C, Neuber K, Rudolph A, von der Hardt H: Abnormally high surface tension of lung surfactant in 2 infants with severe apparent life-threatening events (ALTE), *Pediatr Res* 36:62A, 1994.
163. Macklem PT, Proctor DF, Hogg JC: The stability of peripheral airways, *Respir Physiol* 8:137-150, 1970.
164. Kao LC, Keens TG: Decreased specific airway conductance in infant apnea, *Pediatrics* 76:232-235, 1985.
165. Seidenberg J, Hartmann H, Noyes JP, Poets CF, Samuels MP, Southall DP: Do infants with apparent life-threatening events have decreased airway size? *Eur J Pediatr* 152: 282, 1993.
166. Herbst JJ, Brook LS, Bray PF: Gastroesophageal reflux in the "near miss" sudden infant death syndrome, *J Pediatr* 92:73-75, 1978.
167. Wennergren G, Hertzberg T, Milerad J, Bjure J, Lagercrantz H: Hypoxia reinforces laryngeal reflex bradycardia in infants, *Acta Paediatr Scand* 78:11-17, 1989.
168. Orenstein SR, Orenstein DM: Gastroesophageal reflux and respiratory disease in children, *J Pediatr* 112:847-858, 1988.
169. Walsh JK, Farrell MK, Keenan WJ, Lucas M, Kramer M: Gastroesophageal reflux in infants: relation to apnea, *J Pediatr* 99:197-201, 1981.
170. Newell SJ, Booth IW, Morgan MEI, Durbin GM, McNeish AS: Gastrooesophageal reflux in preterm infants, *Arch Dis Child* 64:780-786, 1989.
171. Kahn A, Rebuffat E, Sottiaux M, Blum D, Yasik EA: Sleep apneas and acid esophageal reflux in control infants and in infants with apparent life-threatening events, *Biol Neonate* 57:144-149, 1990.
172. Paton JY, Nanayakkara CS, Simpson H: Observations on gastrooesophageal reflux, central apnoea and heart rate in infants, *Eur J Pediatr* 149:608-612, 1990.
173. Paton JY, Macfadyen U, Williams A, Simpson H: Gastro-oesophageal reflux and apnoeic pauses during sleep in infancy—no direct relation, *Eur J Pediatr* 149:680-686, 1990.
174. de Ajuriaguerra M, Radvanyi-Bouvet M-F, Huon C, Moriette G: Gastroesophageal reflux and apnea in prematurely born infants during wakefulness and sleep, *Am J Dis Child* 145:1132-1136, 1991.
175. Veereman-Wauters G, Bochner A, van Caillie-Bertrand M: Gastroesophageal reflux in infants with a history of near-miss sudden infant death, *J Pediatr Gastroenterol Nutr* 12:319-323, 1991.
176. Menon AP, Schefft GL, Thach BT: Apnea associated with regurgitation in infants, *J Pediatr* 106:625-629, 1985.
177. See CC, Newman LJ, Berezin S, Glassman MS, Medow MS, Dozor AJ, Schwarz SM: Gastroeosophageal reflux-induced hypoxemia in infants with apparent life-threatening event(s), *Am J Dis Child* 143:951-954, 1989.
178. Stebbens VA, Poets CF, Alexander JA, Arrowsmith WA, Southall DP: Oxygen saturation and breathing patterns in infancy: I. Fullterm infants in the second month of life, *Arch Dis Child* 66:569-573, 1991.
179. Samuels MP, Poets CF, Stebbens VA, Alexander JR, Southall DP: Oxygen saturation and breathing patterns in preterm infants with cyanotic episodes, *Acta Paediatr* 82:875-880, 1992.
180. Leape LL, Holder TM, Franklin JD, Amoury RA, Ashcraft KW: Respiratory arrest in infants secondary to gastroesophageal reflux, *Pediatrics* 60:924-927, 1977.
181. Kelly DH, Pathak A, Meny R: Sudden severe bradycardia in infancy, *Pediatr Pulmonol* 10:199-204, 1991.
182. Meny RG, Carroll JL, Carbone MT, Kelly DH: Cardiorespiratory recordings from infants dying suddenly and unexpectedly at home, *Pediatrics* 93:44-49, 1994.
183. Poets CF, Samuels MP, Southall DP: Sudden severe bradycardia secondary to hypoxemia (letter), *Pediatr Pulmnol* 12:78, 1992.
184. Poets CF, Southall DP: Prone sleep position and SIDS (editorial), *N Engl J Med* 329:425-426, 1993.
185. Jacobi MS, Gershan WM, Thach BT: Mechanism of failure of recovery from hypoxic apnea by gasping in 17- to 23-day-old mice, *J Appl Physiol* 71:1098-1105, 1991.
186. Samuels MP, Poets CF, Noyes JP, Hartmann H, Hewertson J, Southall DP: Diagnosis and management after life threatening events in infants and young children who received cardiopulmonary resuscitation, *Br Med J* 306:489-492, 1993.
187. Poets CF, Samuels MP, Noyes JP, Hewertson J, Hartmann H, Holder A, Southall DP: Home event recordings of oxygenation, breathing movements and electrocardiogram in infants and young children with recurrent apparent life-threatening events, *J Pediatr* 123:693-701, 1993.
188. Oliver JE: Dead children from problem families in NE Wiltshire, *Br Med J* 286:115-117, 1983.
189. Reece RM: Fatal child abuse and sudden infant death syndrome: a critical diagnostic decision, *Pediatrics* 91:423-429, 1993.

Prevention

190. Gibson A, Brooke H, Keeling J: Reduction in sudden infant death syndrome in Scotland (letter), *Lancet* 338:1595, 1991.
191. Einspieler C, Lüscher WN, Kurz R, et al: Der SIDS-Risikofragebogen Graz: II. Prospektive Anwendung bei 6000 Säuglingen, Klin Pädiatr 204:88-91, 1992.
192. Golding J, Fleming P, Parkes S: Cot deaths and sleep position campaigns (letter), *Lancet* 339:748-749, 1992.
193. Carpenter RG, Gardner A, Jepson M, et al: Prevention of unexpected infant death, *Lancet* i:723-727, 1983.
194. Alexander JR, Southall DP: Cot death and the Sheffield score, *Lancet* ii:399, 1986.
195. Peters TJ, Golding J: Prediction of sudden infant death syndrome: an independent evaluation of four scoring methods, *Statistics Med* 5:113-126, 1986.
196. Steinschneider A, Santos V: Parental reports of apnea and bradycardia: temporal characteristics and accuracy, *Pediatrics* 88:1100-1105, 1991.
197. Krongard E: Infants at high risk for sudden infant death syndrome? Have they been identified? —A commentary, *Pediatrics* 88:1274-1278, 1991.
198. Hewertson J, Poets CF, Samuels MP, Boyd SG, Neville BGR, Southall DP: Epileptic seizure-induced hypoxemia in infants with apparent life-threatening events, *Pediatrics* 94:148-156, 1994.
199. Hunt CE, Brouillette RT: Sudden infant death syndrome: 1987 perspective, *J Pediatr* 110:669-678, 1987.
200. Poets CF, Stebbens VA, Alexander JR, Arrowsmith WA, Salfield SAW, Southall DP: Arterial oxygen saturation in preterm infants at discharge from the hospital and six weeks later, *J Pediatr* 120:447-454, 1992.
201. Samuels MP, Poets CF, Southall DP: Abnormal hypoxemia after life-threatening events in infants born before term, *J Pediatr* 125:441-446, 1994.
202. Rinaldo P, O'Shea JJ, Coates PM, Hale DE, Stanley CA, Tanaka K: Medium-chain Acyl-CoA dehydrogenase deficiency. Diagnosis by stable-isotope dilution measurement of urinary n-hexanoylglycine and 3-phenylpropionylglycine, *N Engl J Med* 319:1308-1313, 1988.
203. NIH Consensus Conference on Infantile Apnea and Home Monitoring: U.S. Department of Health and Human Services Publication 87-2905, Bethesda, Md, 1987.
204. Silvestri JM, Weese-Mayer DE, Kenny AS, Hauptman SA: Prolonged cardiorespiratory monitoring of children more than twelve months of age: characterization of events and approach to discontinuation, *J Pediatr* 125:51-56, 1994.
205. Davidson Ward SL, Keens TG, Chan LS, Chipps BE, Carson SH, Deming DD, Krishna V, MacDonald HM, Martin GI, Meredith KS, Merritt TA, Nickerson BG, Stoddard RA, van der Hal AL: Sudden infant death syndrome in infants evaluated by apnea programs in California, *Pediatrics* 77:451-458, 1986.
206. Meny RG, Blackmon L, Fleischmann D, Gutberlet R, Naumburg E: Sudden infant death and home monitors, *Am J Dis Child* 142:1037-1040, 1988.
207. Kelly DH, Shannon DC, O'Connell K: Care of infants with near-miss sudden infant death syndrome, *Pediatrics* 61:511-514, 1978.
208. Rahilly PM: Pneumographic studies: predictors of future apnoeas but not sudden infant death in asymptomatic infants, *Aust Paediatr J* 25:211-214, 1989.
209. Katcher ML, Shapiro MM, Guist C: Severe injury and death associated with home infant cardiorespiratory monitors, *Pediatrics* 78:775-779, 1986.
210. Emery JL, Taylor EM, Carpenter RG, Waite AJ: Apnoea monitors and accidental strangulation (letter), *Br Med J* 304:117, 1992.

211. Samuels MP, Stebbens VA, Poets CF, Southall DP: Deaths on infant 'apnoea' monitors, *J Maternal Child Health* 18:262-266, 1993.
212. Desmarez C, Blum D, Montauk L, Kahn A: Impact of home monitoring for sudden infant death syndrome on family life, *Eur J Pediatr* 146:159-161, 1987.
213. Weese-Mayer DE, Brouillette RT, Morrow AS, Conway LP, Klemka-Walden LM, Hunt CE: Assessing validity of infant monitor alarms with event recording, *J Pediatr* 115:702-708, 1989.
214. Poets CF, Samuels MP, Noyes JP, Jones KA, Southall DP: Home monitoring of transcutaneous oxygen tension in the early detection of hypoxaemia in infants and young children, *Arch Dis Child* 66:676-682, 1991.
215. Nathanson I, O'Donnell J, Commins MF: Cardiorespiratory patterns during alarms in infants using apnea/bradycardia monitors, *Am J Dis Child* 143:476-480, 1989.
216. Weese-Mayer DE, Morrow AS, Conway LP, Brouillette RT, Silvestri JM: Assessing clinical significance of apnea exceeding fifteen seconds with event recording, *J Pediatr* 117:568-574, 1990.
217. Krongrad E, O'Neill L: Near miss sudden infant death syndrome episodes? A clinical and electrocardiographic correlation, *Pediatrics* 77:811-815, 1986.

Conclusions

218. Sanocka UM, Donnelly DF, Haddad GG: Autoresuscitation: a survival mechanism in piglets, *J Appl Physiol* 73:749-753, 1992.

PART THIRTEEN

Structural and Mechanical Abnormalities

CHAPTER 72

Congenital Malformations of the Lungs and Airways

Barry S. Clements

The frequency of congenital lung anomalies is said to range between 7.5%[1] and 18.7%[2] of all congenital malformations, although even the higher figure may be an underestimate because many lesions do not cause symptoms and therefore may remain unrecognized. When they occur, malformations of the respiratory tract are often found in association with other congenital anomalies, particularly those involving the cardiovascular system.

For the purpose of this chapter, it is practical to divide lung malformations into five anatomic subgroups:

1. The lung unit as a whole (unilateral or bilateral),
2. The larynx, trachea, and major bronchi,
3. The small airways and lung parenchyma,
4. The pulmonary vascular and lymphatic systems,
5. The thoracic cage. (In this chapter, only diaphragmatic and thoracic outlet anomalies affecting lung development are discussed. Other thoracic cage anomalies are discussed in Chapter 62.)

CLASSIFICATION

In the past, many classifications of congenital lung malformations have been proposed, although none has gained universal acceptance. These have been based on anatomic localization, histopathologic type, pathogenesis, or extent of lung involvement.[3] In general, lesions involving the lung unit as a whole, or the trachea and the major bronchi, are simply and easily defined, whereas lesions involving the lung parenchyma tend to be more complex, and it is here where consensus on terminology is lacking. In 1966, the American College of Chest Physicians in their catalogue of congenital lung lesions[4] abandoned any attempt at a formal classification and merely produced an inventory of the different malformations. When Landing produced his review on the subject in 1979,[5] he was forced to use the same format. In 1987, an attempt was made to introduce a concept aimed at standardizing the terminology for all lung malformations using a purely descriptive format based on pathogenesis and anatomic content.[6] Although not, strictly speaking, a classification, it enables categorization of all lung lesions depending on their composition and how they are formed. The concept is easily understood if the lung is considered as being composed of a system of tubes or openings, namely, the bronchopulmonary airway (from larynx to alveolus), the arterial supply, the venous drainage, and the lymphatic system. Inosculation is defined as the establishment of communications by means of small openings or anastomoses, especially applied to the establishment of such communications between existing blood vessels or other tubular structures that come into contact. This applies perfectly to the tubular structures composing the lung. Therefore, malinosculation is an abnormal communication of one or more of these tubular components; this forms the basis of all congenital lung malformations. Categorization of these component abnormal communications in a sequential manner thus formulates the malinosculation sequence outlined in the following section.

The Malinosculation Sequence

1. Lesions in which the airway alone is affected—tracheobronchial malinosculation.
2. Lesions in which the airway remains unaffected in the presence of a vascular or lymphatic malformation—pulmonary arterial, pulmonary arteriovenous, or pulmonary lymphatic malinosculation.
3. Lesions in which the airway, together with one or more of the other tubular components of the lung, is affected. These components may include the arterial supply, venous drainage, and the lymphatic channels—bronchovascular or broncholymphatic malinosculation.
4. Lesions in which all components of lung are affected—bronchopulmonary malinosculation.

This categorization is applicable to all *primary* lung anomalies but not necessarily those secondary to thoracic cage malformations. Its major benefit will be seen in categorizing the more complex lesions with more than one abnormal component, when its application becomes particularly important for planning treatment.

ABNORMAL LUNG DEVELOPMENT

The lung is unusual in that its development is incomplete at birth. This has made the study of the pathogenesis of congenital lung malformations both before and after birth difficult compared with malformations elsewhere. There is no doubt that many lung lesions diagnosed in older children and adults bear little resemblance macroscopically or microscopically to the abnormality present at birth (e.g., lesions that have been distorted by chronic air trapping and overdistention, or infection, or both). In the past, numerous theories of abnormal lung development have been suggested and the major ones are considered here.

Vascular Traction

Pryce et al[7] considered the vascular system as playing an important role in pulmonary sequestration. According to his theory, if during lung development a segment of lung retained its systemic vasculature, this aberrant vessel (as it moved caudally with the developing primitive aorta) would apply traction to the lung segment, thus sequestering it from the surrounding lung.

Vascular Theory

This theory stipulated that all abnormal lung development was a result of abnormal vascular development.[8] Although this theory may have some support when applied to conventional bronchovascular malformations (in which the authors claim that the abnormal artery of aortic origin is in reality an aberrant pulmonary artery), it does not explain the pathogenesis of similar pulmonary lesions that have a normal pulmonary artery supply.

Vascular Insufficiency Theory

Abbey-Smith[9] claims that failure of pulmonary vascularization leads to persistence of systemic arterial connections. In addition, the author feels that the systemic pressures found in these aberrant vessels result in the cystic degeneration found in many of the lesions at diagnosis.

Coincidence Theory[10]

The finding of a pulmonary cyst in a 31-mm embryo and a pulmonary segment supplied by a systemic pulmonary artery in another 41-mm embryo led Boyden[10] to suggest that the only way these two lesions could occur simultaneously was by chance.

The Accessory Bud Theory

A supplementary bud arising from the primitive foregut below the normal origin of the lung could constitute a secondary respiratory anlage that may or may not be incorporated within normal lung and may or may not retain a connection with the gut.[11]

None of the just-mentioned theories is really complete and able to explain all lesions. Work by Reid,[12] together with an improved understanding of genetic principles, led Clements[6] to propose a rational sequence of events in lung development that could account for all malformations. This theory takes into consideration all the major principles of normal embryogenesis of the lung that may become disturbed during fetal lung growth:

1. Bronchial branching to terminal bronchiole is complete 16 weeks after conception.[12] An insult affecting lung development in the 8th week of intrauterine life will result in an entirely different lesion to that if the same insult occurred in the 20th week when bronchial branching is complete.
2. Pulmonary vascular development is similar to the pattern of bronchial branching but occurs slightly later.[13]
3. Alveolar development follows formation of the respiratory bronchioles, and later saccules, after the 24th week after conception and continues after birth until 8 to 12 years of age,[12] or possibly later.
4. At any stage during pulmonary development, the rate of growth of individual component tissues, namely the airway, alveoli, arteries, veins, and lymphatics, may not be uniform.[12]
5. In the early stages the tips of the dividing bronchial buds are supplied by a systemic capillary plexus derived from the primitive aorta. This plexus regresses as the lung advances, with the developing pulmonary artery taking over the vascular supply.[9,11]

Bearing these basic principles in mind, a possible explanation for the pathogenesis of most, if not all, congenital lung anomalies has been proposed.[6] This theory discusses the possible pathologic options that would result from an insult to the developing bronchus, emphasizing that it is not necessarily the nature of the insult, but the timing and severity, that is the major determinant of the eventual morphology of the lesion.[12] The insult itself may be undetermined and could take the form of localized trauma, ischemia, infection, adhesions, or any other nonspecific injury. This theory is now discussed and can be followed in Figure 72-1.

1. An insult affecting the development of the bronchus together with its pulmonary artery supply may lead to total arrest of subsequent growth distal to the lesion, resulting in agenesis of that lung, lobe, or segment. The timing determines at which level growth is arrested.
2. If the insult is minor or transient, a localized abnormality followed by normal development of the distal bronchial tree, lung parenchyma, and vasculature may result. This would cause a localized lesion such as bronchial atresia, stenosis, or a bronchogenic cyst.
3. There may be no interference to continued development of the bronchial tree but the pulmonary artery growth may be arrested. Devoid of pulmonary blood supply, continued growth of the developing bronchial branch is supported only by vessels retained from the normally regressing systemic capillary plexus. Growing along with the developing bronchial tree, these systemic vessels become substantial channels, single or multiple, and establish a systemic arterial supply to the area of lung concerned. The sites of origin of these vessels move distally with the caudal shift of the growing primitive aorta from which they arise, resulting in the origin eventually being situated in the lower thoracic or upper abdominal region (Fig. 72-2). Such an anomalous development of an area of "normal" lung with systemic artery supply has been well recognized and also been found in a

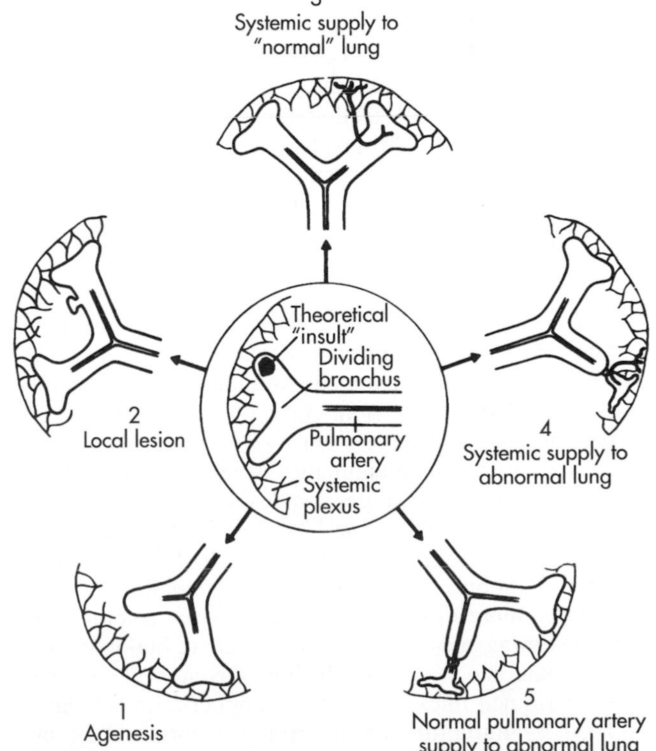

Fig. 72-1. Abnormal lung development. The range of possible outcomes following an insult to the developing lung bud *(center)* are simplistically displayed here as the spokes of a wheel.

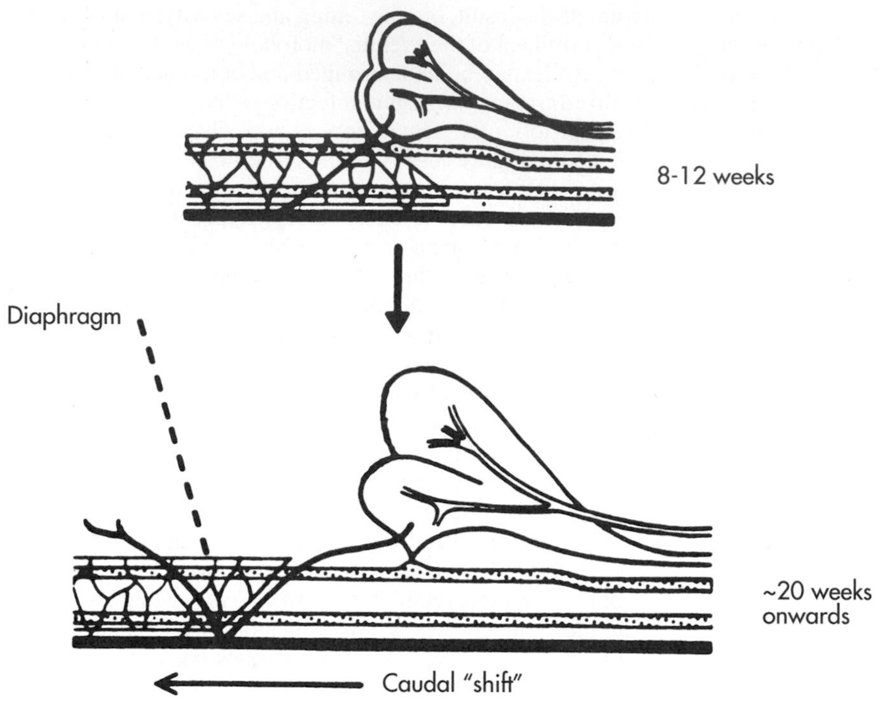

Fig. 72-2. Aberrant systemic arterial development. The origin of an aberrant systemic artery derived from the splanchnic plexus is "dragged" caudally by the rapidly growing primitive aorta and is eventually situated in the lower thorax or upper abdomen.

41-mm embryo.[10] These aberrant arteries are distinct from bronchial arteries, which are found to occur normally in these patients.

4. The insult may be severe enough to disrupt both airway and pulmonary artery development so that a systemic arterial supply is retained to the abnormal area of lung.[14,15] This results in a bronchovascular malinosculation, including such lesions as a classic pulmonary sequestration.
5. Although there may be considerable or complete disruption of the bronchopulmonary connection, the pulmonary artery may continue to develop and supply the abnormal lung segment. This results in such entities as congenital lung cysts and cystic adenomatoid malformations.

Peripheral lesions involving terminal and respiratory bronchioles and alveoli, as in congenital lobar emphysema, suggest a defect occurring late in development. Another important consideration is that lesions normally expected to have only the airway affected (such as those mentioned previously) have been found on a number of occasions to have a systemic arterial blood supply or anomalous venous drainage, supporting the theory that there is an embryologic link between the various forms of malinosculation.[16]

Extrapulmonary lung anomalies develop along a different sequence. In the early stages the developing lung bud with its surrounding mesenchyme lies in close proximity to the primitive foregut from which it is derived.[9,17] Any insult or adhesion in an area where these two developing organs are adjacent is therefore likely to affect both structures, and again the timing and severity of the insult are important to the eventual outcome. Normally the lung develops along genetically determined lines, the dividing epithelial cells being influenced by humoral factors from the surrounding mesenchyme.[18,19] Differentiating lung epithelial cells, drawn by adhesions toward the primitive foregut, may come to lie in mesenchyme, which is not conducive to their normal development. This would result in dysmorphogenesis of the misplaced tissue. Primitive communications between this ectopic tissue and the adjacent organ may develop at any stage.[18,20] Subsequent development of the pleura will sequester this tissue from its parent organ either partially or completely, resulting in extrapulmonary sequestration or ectopic foregut derivatives within the lung. This hypothesis supports the contention that intrapulmonary and extrapulmonary lesions have a similar mode of origin without the need for an accessory lung bud theory.[21-25] It also explains the high incidence of associated foregut anomalies occurring with extrapulmonary lung anomalies.

ABNORMALITIES OF THE LUNG UNIT AS A WHOLE (UNILATERAL AND BILATERAL)

Pulmonary Agenesis and Aplasia

Agenesis and aplasia differ only in the respective absence or presence of a tracheal or bronchial stump. The precise cause (as with all congenital malformations) is unclear[26] but pulmonary agenesis has been observed in monozygotic twins, as well as in rats after the mother has been deprived of vitamin A.[27] Bilateral agenesis is exceedingly rare and may occur in association with anencephaly.[28] Unilateral agenesis, in which there is no formed carina because of absence of a bronchial stump to the missing lung (Fig. 72-3), is almost as rare as lobar agenesis and aplasia, which, when they occur, usually affect the right upper and middle lobes together.[29] Unilateral aplasia (in which a carina and rudimentary bronchial stump are present) is the most common lesion in this group, with over 200 cases described in the literature.[30] Lobar agenesis and aplasia are rarer than complete absence of one lung and, when they occur, usually affect the right upper and middle lobes together.

Embryologically, the tracheobronchial groove appears in the 4th week of fetal life as a median ventral diverticulum of the foregut. The groove deepens to become a tube and an additional longitudinal groove appears in each lateral wall of this

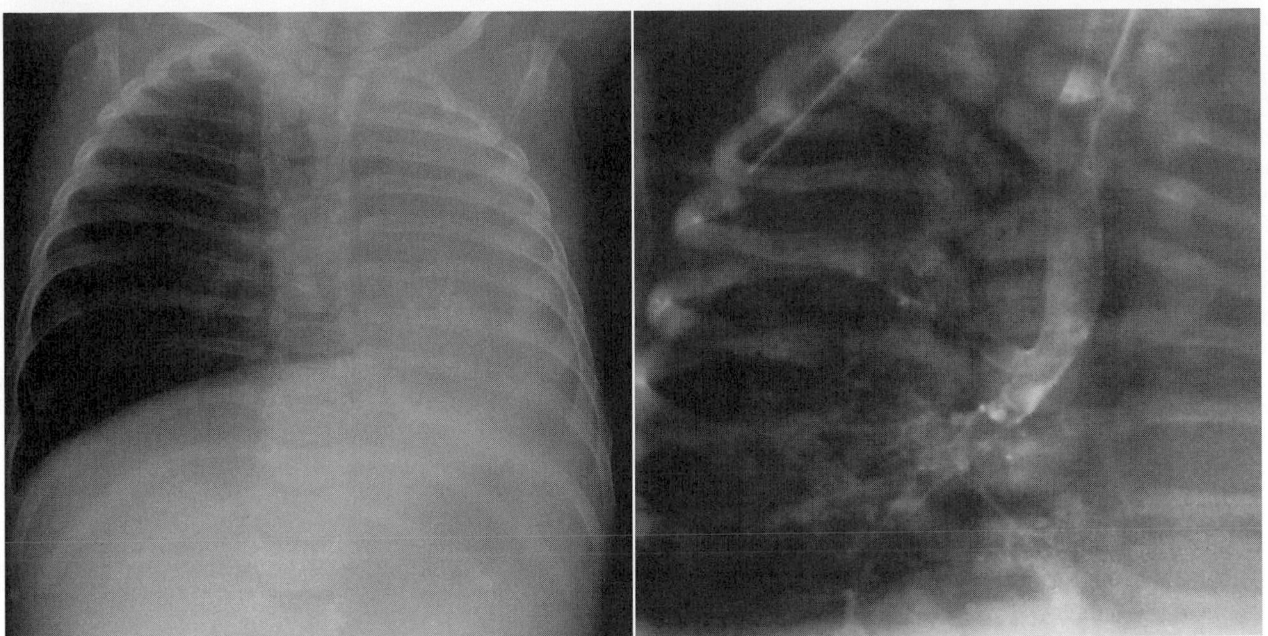

Fig. 72-3. Left lung agenesis. Agenesis of the left lung with absence of the carina and left bronchial stump confirmed on tracheobronchogram. Note the associated vertebral anomaly, a common association with major airway abnormalities.

tube, creating a median ridge that separates the esophagus from the trachea. Before this separation is complete, the lung buds have started developing from the caudal end of what has now become the primitive trachea. The ridges then close to form tubes, with communication retained at the cephalic end, which will become the pharynx.[31] Thus at the 5-mm stage the two main bronchi are formed, complete with vascular supply and lung buds, and it is at this stage that aplasia is likely to occur following major damage to the bud. In total unilateral agenesis or aplasia, the pulmonary artery is always absent and there is agenesis of both sympathetic and parasympathetic plexuses, generally with a lack of parietal pleura.[8] Lesions occur on the left in 70% and equally in male and female patients. About 50% of the patients die in the first year of life. However, there have been several reports of adults dying of other causes who have been found to have absence of a lung, which makes overall incidence estimations impossible.[29] Association with other congenital anomalies, particularly ipsilateral lesions, is common,[29] and in most cases appears to be a major factor determining overall prognosis, particularly anomalies that may compromise the function of the remaining lung, such as cardiovascular anomalies or anomalies within that lung. Associated anomalies include cardiovascular lesions (of which the most common is patent ductus arteriosus[32]),vertebral anomalies (hemivertebra in particular), and rib anomalies.[29] Ipsilateral facial anomalies, including hemiatrophy, abnormal ears, and facial paralysis, and ipsilateral limb anomalies (such as absent radii and rudimentary thumbs) have also been described. Rarer associations include those in the gastrointestinal tract, such as tracheoesophageal fistula, duodenal atresia, anular pancreas, malrotation, and imperforate anus. Defects of the urogenital system include absent ipsilateral kidney, absent ipsilateral ovary, and unicornuate uterus. Cleft lip and palate have also been reported.[29] Combinations of certain of these associated anomalies would classify some patients as having variants of the VATER syndrome.

Clinically, most patients with unilateral pulmonary aplasia or agenesis present in the neonatal period with signs of respiratory distress, which may be compounded by the presence of an associated malformation. Prognosis for survival is considerably different depending on whether the right or left lung is absent. Mortality when the right lung is absent is at least 75%, whereas it is as low as 25% when the left lung is absent.[33] It has been proposed that this is primarily a result of the higher frequency of associated cardiovascular anomalies with right lung absence although it probably also relates simply to the fact that the left lung is the smaller lung, with less effective area for ventilation and perfusion than the right.[34] Patients presenting late usually have readily detectable flattening and reduced movement of the chest wall on the affected side, with reduced air entry on auscultation, although this often sounds surprisingly better than expected. There may be some breathlessness on exertion and the chest wall deformity may be quite pronounced, with an associated secondary scoliosis. The chest radiograph shows the heart, great vessels, and mediastinum drawn over to the side of the abnormality, usually with considerable herniation of the contralateral lung across the mediastinum. The hemithorax is small, with narrowed intercostal spaces. A penetrated film may highlight the absence of carina or a blind-ending main bronchus. Bronchography and bronchoscopy are rarely required to confirm this diagnosis, but may be needed to define additional airway anomalies if they are suspected. Echocardiography and angiography show absence of the pulmonary artery and it is always necessary to exclude other associated cardiovascular lesions. The differential diagnosis includes total atelectasis caused by bronchial obstruction, unilateral emphysema with compression or collapse of the contralateral lung, or severe pulmonary hypoplasia.

Management is limited to supportive treatment (including oxygen if necessary), correcting associated malformations, and the prevention and treatment of respiratory infections. Pulmonary hypertension is a complication that requires particular care and attention. It is more common in these patients simply because a normal blood volume must flow through a reduced pulmonary vascular bed (possibly reduced by as much as 60%). The presence of hypoxia (which is a potent pulmonary vasoconstrictor) or a cardiac left-to-right shunt (which further increases the flow through the already reduced pulmonary vascular bed) will compound this effect and is likely to accelerate the progression of the pulmonary hypertension to irreversible pulmonary vascular disease. These factors should therefore be more aggressively sought and treated in these patients than in patients with a normal-sized pulmonary vascular bed.

Pulmonary Hypoplasia

Pulmonary hypoplasia, unilateral or bilateral, is almost always accompanied by hypoplasia of the corresponding pulmonary vessel. This follows obviously from the second rule of lung embryogenesis, in which the vasculature follows the bronchial development.[13] Hypoplasia as an isolated phenomenon is rare. More commonly, pulmonary hypoplasia is associated with conditions that interfere with lung growth, particularly those that have a restrictive effect, such as maternal oligohydramnios. Other conditions leading to reduction in size of the thoracic cavity in utero with resultant pulmonary hypoplasia include intrathoracic cysts and tumors, cardiomegaly, pleural effusions in anasarca, and thoracic cage anomalies such as the short rib syndromes, which include asphyxiating thoracic dystrophy (Jeune syndrome).[35] Some of the dwarf syndromes may also include small thoracic cages resulting in varying degrees of pulmonary restriction and hypoplasia. In addition, pulmonary hypoplasia is a well-recognized component of Potter syndrome, in which it is found in association with bilateral renal agenesis or dysplasia and a number of dysmorphic features, including hypertelorism, epicanthus, snub-nose, retrognathia, and low positioning of the ears.[36] These patients are stillborn or die soon after birth from respiratory insufficiency. Pulmonary hypoplasia has also been recognized in infants with rhesus disease. Unilateral pulmonary hypoplasia is most commonly found in scoliosis, intrathoracic space-occupying lesions, diaphragmatic hernia (usually left-sided), and Scimitar syndrome (almost universally right-sided). Pathologic examination of a hypoplastic lung shows that both the lung weight and the number of alveoli or terminal air spaces are reduced, usually with a decrease in the number of generations of airways and pulmonary arteries as well.[37]

Clinically, patients with pulmonary hypoplasia may present in early infancy with respiratory distress ranging from mild to severe depending on the degree of hypoplasia. Commonly, particularly in unilateral hypoplasia, it is the associated anomalies that draw attention to the lesion. In severe bilateral hypoplasia the thoracic cage is obviously reduced in size and characteristically bell-shaped, with the base of the chest widening at diaphragmatic level to a normal-sized abdomen. The patient is tachypneic, with restricted chest wall movement, and in respiratory distress. Less severe degrees of hypoplasia—unilateral or bilateral—may present later with persistent tachypnea or disproportionate shortness of breath with exercise. Occasionally, the abnormality is coincidentally noticed on examination or chest radiograph when the patient presents with an intercurrent infection. In unilateral hypoplasia the chest cage appears asymmetric, with diminished air entry and chest expansion on the side of the lesion together with mediastinal shift to that side. The chest radiograph confirms mediastinal deviation and a lung that often appears well aerated despite the reduction in volume. Isotope scanning usually reveals a greater impairment of perfusion than ventilation on the side of the lesion. Bronchoscopy may reveal a smaller airway on one side and bronchography confirms the reduced size of the bronchial branches (often reduced in number as well). Angiography confirms the reduced pulmonary vascular bed. In right-sided hypoplasia, it may be important to establish the pattern of vasculature because of the common association with Scimitar syndrome.[38] In the absence of associated lesions, unilateral pulmonary hypoplasia may be compatible with normal growth, development, and survival. Long-term complications include reduced exercise tolerance, recurrent infections (although not as common as might be expected), and increasing cosmetic chest deformity with scoliosis.

MALFORMATIONS OF THE LARYNX, TRACHEA, AND MAJOR BRONCHI

Abnormalities of the Larynx

Apart from laryngomalacia, which is common and usually benign, the other congenital laryngeal abnormalities discussed in this section, including laryngeal webs, clefts, cysts, and subglottic stenosis, are rare but significant causes of respiratory distress (and possibly life-threatening upper airway obstruction) in the newborn child and infant.

Laryngomalacia

Laryngomalacia is the most common congenital anomaly found in the upper airway. Fortunately, most cases are mild, readily diagnosed clinically, and generally require no more management than parental reassurance. Strictly speaking, it is not a true malformation but represents a delay in the maturation of the supporting structures of the larynx. This causes the larynx to be more collapsible than normal during inspiration, resulting in inspiratory stridor (the most notable symptom associated with this condition), which varies with the inspiratory force at the time. This stridor is usually first noticed in the early neonatal period, with most patients having presented by 6 weeks of age, although some patients appear not to have significant symptoms until up to a few months of age, when the stridor may be made apparent for the first time following an intercurrent upper respiratory tract infection. The stridor is generally more prominent during crying, feeding, and intercurrent respiratory tract infections. A sudden, sharp inspiratory effort often results in a high-pitched loud inspiratory "whoop," which may alarm the parents. Some patients have stridor at rest, and in 10%, a minor expiratory component may occasionally be present as well. Significant airway obstruction in laryngomalacia is rare, although occasionally patients with severe forms may become quite distressed—particularly during intercurrent respiratory tract infections—requiring in-hospital care and, rarely, ventilatory support. The diagnosis in most cases should be based on clinical history and physical examination, with laryngoscopy or bronchoscopy (or possibly upper airway fluoroscopy) reserved for patients with severe or atypical symptoms or those who follow an unusual course. When considering investigating these patients, it should also always be borne in mind that laryngomalacia often coexists with other laryngotracheal malformations, particularly esophageal atresia and tracheoesophageal atresia. Laryngomalacia is generally considered a benign self-limiting condition. Symptoms usually resolve within the first few months and almost always by 2 years of age. However, strong reassurance and ongoing support are often needed to allay parental anxiety. Patients who exhibit significant sleep disturbance, as evidenced on polysomnography, may benefit from administration of positive airway pressure through a closely applied face mask during sleep. However, this form of treatment can be fraught with difficulties and is often not well tolerated, in which case surgical intervention, either epiglottoplasty or tracheostomy, may need to be considered, particularly in cases with severe, potentially life-threatening airway obstruction, or when symptoms are sufficiently severe to interfere with normal growth and development. In the long term, although it is generally accepted that patients who have had laryngomalacia in infancy show no ill effects clinically once their symptoms have subsided, some recent follow-up studies of these patients in late childhood have demonstrated abnormalities of inspiratory flow on pulmonary function testing.[39]

Laryngotracheoesophageal Cleft

A cleft larynx occurs in approximately one in 10,000 to 20,000 live births, comprising less than 1% of all laryngeal anomalies.[40] Male patients are affected more commonly than female patients. Familial occurrences have been reported as well as associations with various syndromes, including G syndrome and Pallister-Hall syndrome. Association with other laryngotracheoesophageal anomalies, particularly esophageal atresia and tracheoesophageal fistula, is high. The most commonly accepted classification divides clefts into four types depending on the length of involvement of the laryngotracheal airway: type 1 extends to the cricoid, type 2 involves the cricoid and may extend to the cervical trachea, type 3 extends to the carina, and type 4 involves one or both main stem bronchi. Embryologically, a laryngeal cleft arises from abnormal separation of the larynx-trachea and the esophagus. At 25 days the laryngotracheal septum develops in the primitive tracheoesophageal groove and begins to fuse in a cephalad direction, thus separating the developing trachea and esophagus. At the same time, cricoid cartilage develops as two lateral centers of chondrification from the sixth branchial arch at the origin of the lung bud from the esophagus. Dorsal fusion of the cricoid plate is complete by day 50 to 54 and laryngeal muscular development ensues. The range of abnormalities seen results from defects in cricoid chondrification or fusion (types 1 and 2) or failure of fusion of the laryngotracheal septum (types 3 and 4). A cleft larynx creates an abnormal communication between the esophagus and the larynx and trachea, thus increasing the likelihood of repeated aspiration of food and saliva into the airway, with resultant symptoms of coughing and choking, respiratory distress, and recurrent pneumonia. Type 1 clefts may be asymptomatic, whereas type 2 clefts can cause problems of varying severity, making diagnosis difficult and often delayed. Increased salivation, stridor, and a low soundless cry are said to be characteristic symptoms that would point to the diagnosis of a cleft, although the triad is rare and more often stridor is absent and the cry is harsh. Therefore, in any neonate or infant who develops respiratory difficulties associated with feeding, the presence of a laryngotracheoesophageal cleft should be considered. The differential diagnosis also includes choanal atresia, esophageal atresia and tracheoesophageal fistula, laryngoesophageal dysmotility syndromes (functional or neurologic), esophageal compression (such as with a vascular ring), and gastroesophageal reflux. Contrast radiography usually demonstrates the abnormal communication, although endoscopy is always necessary to define the extent of the lesion. Endoscopic surgical correction for minor lesions is possible, although many type 1 defects may not require correction, particularly if complicating factors such as gastroesophageal reflux are absent or can be controlled. Timing of surgery for type 2, 3, and 4 lesions depends largely on the overall condition of the child at diagnosis. If the child's respiratory and nutritional status are stable, early repair should be considered. If not, staged repair incorporating tracheostomy initially (with or without gastrostomy and possibly fundoplication), followed by definitive repair when the child is stable, may be best. Overall survival with improved techniques and aggressive treatment is 70%, but is significantly less for patients with extensive type 4 defects and severe associated anomalies. Complications following surgical repair are common and include wound breakdown and tracheoesophageal fistula formation, continuing aspiration and swallowing difficulties, gastroesophageal reflux, tracheobronchomalacia, and chronic respiratory problems.

Laryngeal Atresia and Laryngeal Webs

Laryngeal atresia is a life-threatening malformation requiring immediate diagnosis and treatment. The lesion results from failure of recanalization of the epithelial septum, which forms around 6 weeks gestation, separating the developing esophagus from the tracheal bud, and at 10 weeks is ready to open again into the now-developing primitive laryngeal aditus. Despite the complete lack of communication with the airway, distal lung development and general fetal growth are usually unaffected. These infants present at delivery with evidence of complete airway obstruction—marked chest wall retraction with each attempted breath, no air entry, no cry, and persisting cyanosis. Diagnosis is made on direct laryngoscopy and treatment is immediate perforation of the membrane or emergency tracheotomy. Prognosis is determined largely by the time taken to establish an adequate airway with effective ventilation, although it may also be affected by the presence of associated defects. Subsequent laryngeal function in survivors is usually abnormal, often requiring surgical reconstruction at a later date, particularly to assist with speech. Partial recanalization of the embryologic larynx results in a laryngeal web, of which 75% are glottic with the rest supraglottic or subglottic in location. They are usually situated anteriorly, with a posterior concave glottic opening. Complete webs cause immediate severe respiratory distress soon after delivery, whereas partial webs present with stridor and a hoarse or weak cry and may have varying degrees of respiratory difficulty depending on the degree of obstruction. Diagnosis is made at endoscopy and treatment is excision, although some smaller subglottic webs may respond to dilation.

Laryngeal Cysts

These are usually supraglottic and generally present in the neonatal period (although possibly much later) with hoarse or muffled voice or even aphonia, stridor, and respiratory difficulty. A lateral neck radiograph may show a rounded supraglottic swelling, and at laryngoscopy, a bluish fluid-filled cyst is found, usually in the epiglottic folds. Aspiration relieves symptoms at the time, although resection is necessary to prevent recurrence.

Subglottic Stenosis

The congenital form of subglottic stenosis, similar to laryngeal web and atresia, results from defective recanalization of the larynx, although in subglottic stenosis the defect occurs at the level of, and usually involves, the cricoid cartilage, approximately 2 to 3 mm below the glottis. The most common presenting symptom is stridor, which is worsened by increased respiratory effort and upper respiratory tract infection. In fact, in milder forms the stridor may only be noticed during intercurrent upper respiratory tract infections and be mislabeled as croup. Therefore, recurrent "croup" in infancy should always raise the possibility of a fixed upper airway narrowing such as subglottic stenosis, particularly when the course of the illness and response to treatment are atypical. High-voltage radiographs of the upper airway may help with the diagnosis, and both anteroposterior and lateral views should be requested because the narrowing is often maximal in the anteroposterior direction. Bronchoscopy is the definitive diagnostic tool and is usually necessary to exclude other causes of narrowing in this region, particularly subglottic hemangioma. This lesion may be differentiated clinically from congenital subglottic stenosis in that the history is usually of worsening symptoms with growth of the hemangioma, and on the radiograph the outline of the lesion is generally more ragged. Acquired subglottic stenosis is more common than the congenital form and the diagnosis of the former would be supported by a positive history of laryngeal trauma, the most common of which would be endotracheal intubation, particularly when intubation is prolonged, as in the premature neonate. Treatment is the same for both types. Because subglottic narrowing generally improves with laryngeal growth, a conservative approach using supportive care, particularly during intermittent episodes of "croup," should be the goal in all patients. Surgery should be reserved for patients who fail to cope with this conservative treatment alone, and tracheostomy is the most common first-choice procedure. Most tracheostomized patients can be successfully decannulated within 2 to 3 years, although stridor and varying degrees of breathing difficulties may persist for many years. Dilation techniques and laser resection used in the treatment of subglottic stenosis have had disappointing results and are therefore not generally recommended. In recent years, advances in cricoid reconstruction and cricoid split procedures have allowed these techniques to become more readily available, either as an alternative to tracheostomy or when tracheostomy decanulation has failed. Selection of the appropriate surgical option is determined by the needs of the patient and the level of available expertise.

Abnormalities of the Trachea

Tracheal Agenesis and Aplasia (Atresia)

In tracheal agenesis there is a total absence of the trachea and the main bronchi either communicate directly with each other or arise from the esophagus. In aplasia (or, more correctly, atresia), as a rule the proximal trachea ends in a blind pouch with a distal segment arising from the esophagus before dividing into the two main bronchi. In all types, the lungs are essentially normal, although associated gastrointestinal and genitourinary anomalies are common. Severe respiratory distress occurring immediately after birth is the hallmark of the condition. Correct placement of an endotracheal tube is impossible, although some degree of ventilation may be possible with the tube in the esophagus. When there is no esophageal communication, the lungs are grossly distended with lung fluid.[41] There is no record of survival beyond the first few days of life.

Tracheal Stenosis

Fixed narrowing of the trachea may be intrinsic (congenital or acquired) or result from external compression leading to a fixed constriction. Congenital intrinsic tracheal stenosis has been recognized in a number of forms. Wolman[42] described two types. The first was a short narrowed segment with a trachea of normal caliber above and below; the second involved a tracheal lumen that narrowed progressively as it descended toward the carina in a carrot shape or "rat-tail" trachea. Stenosis is often seen in the segment of trachea distal to the origin of a tracheal bronchus, with the narrowing characteristically extending to the carina, whereas the left and right main bronchi are usually normal in diameter. Various forms of tracheal stenosis have also been associated with other anomalies, including chondrodystrophies such as Ellis van Creveld syndrome, congenital stippled epiphyses, and left pulmonary artery sling syndrome.[43] Other rare causes of short segment stenosis include tracheal webs (found usually just above the carina), tracheal cysts, and sequestered esoph-ageal tissue in the trachea (where the reciprocal may also occur with tracheal remnants sequestered in the esophageal wall leading to esophageal stenosis). Characteristically, patients with tracheal stenosis localized to the extrathoracic portion of the trachea present with stridor, which is usually more prominent during inspiration. Patients with intrathoracic stenosis generally present with wheeze or mixed wheeze and stridor, which is predominantly expiratory. In both instances, when the stenosis is severe and fixed, the added noises may be prominent in both inspiration and expiration. Additional factors, such as associated structural weaknesses in the airway adjacent to the stenosis and the increased pressures this airway is subjected to in the presence of narrowing, also influence the sounds produced during respiration. When narrowing is severe, the breath sounds may be accompanied by significant respiratory distress, whereas in mild cases they may be noticeable only when respiratory load is increased, as with exercise or infection. Penetrated radiographs of the airway may identify a narrowed segment, although usually bronchoscopy is necessary to establish the diagnosis. Respiratory function tests show evidence of fixed obstruction with characteristic flattening of the inspiratory and expiratory portions of the flow-volume loop.

Management is difficult. In some patients the stenosis improves with tracheal growth and conservative symptomatic treatment and support should be the recommended approach when possible. Results of dilation techniques and laser resection of the intraluminal narrowing have been disappointing, with subsequent recurrence of the stenosis the rule. Tracheal surgical techniques, including resection of the narrowed segment, stenting, and tracheal split procedures, remain hazardous, with high morbidity, complication, and mortality rates, and should therefore be reserved for extreme cases and performed only in institutions with available expertise.

The left pulmonary artery sling syndrome is a particularly well-described cause of tracheal stenosis.[44] In this condition, the left pulmonary artery passes initially to the right in front of the carina. It then curls posteriorly over the origin of the right main bronchus before crossing to the left hemithorax between the esophagus and trachea (Figs. 72-4, 72-5). This looping of the aberrant vessel around the carina usually has a strangling effect, resulting in variable degrees of compression and localized narrowing. The compressed area may be malacic or, in

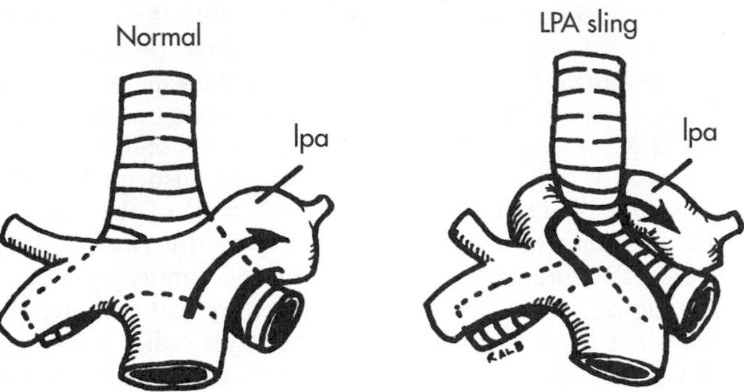

Fig. 72-4. Left pulmonary artery (lpa) sling. Diagram showing the normal and abnormal configuration where the left pulmonary artery curls around the right side of the carina before progressing between the trachea and the esophagus to supply the left lung.

some cases, associated with severe annular constriction of the trachea, which may either be localized to this area or, more commonly, involve the length of the trachea (and possibly major bronchi) in a carrot-shape configuration. When this configuration is present, the tracheal cartilages are characteristically abnormal in that they are increased in number (both in the trachea and major bronchi) and that they take the form of complete annular cartilages—so-called napkin ring cartilages. Although these patients usually present in the first few days of life with severe respiratory distress characterized by inspiratory and expiratory difficulty, some infants surprisingly do not develop significant respiratory difficulties until a few weeks or even several months of age despite an exceedingly narrow trachea. The chest radiograph reveals apparently normal lungs, although the carina and a variable portion of the trachea are not identifiable. Diagnosis can be confirmed at bronchoscopy or with a tracheobronchogram. Long segment tracheal stenosis is usually incompatible with life and not amenable to surgery, whereas a localized constriction may be correctable if the appropriate expertise is available. Decompression of a malacic segment may be achieved by reimplantation of the aberrant left pulmonary artery.

Tracheal Diverticulum

This is an extremely rare anomaly, usually arising from the right posterolateral surface of the trachea, and may give rise to symptoms only late in adult life when it becomes infected. As it is hardly ever found in childhood it has been suggested that it may be an acquired rather than a congenital lesion.

Tracheobronchomegaly (Mounier-Kuhn Syndrome)

This condition is characterized by marked dilation of the trachea and major bronchi, probably as a result of abnormal development of elastic and muscular tissues in the airways.[42,45] Most cases present in adult life but cases have been reported in children as young as 18 months. It is often associated with other congenital defects of the ribs and lung topography.[46] The evidence of an underlying connective tissue abnormality is supported by the finding of this condition coexisting with Ehlers-Danlos syndrome and cutis laxa.[47] Reduced efficiency of airway mucociliary clearance and inefficient cough found in this condition eventually lead to recurrent infection and the development of bronchiectasis, although many of these patients may remain asymptomatic until late adulthood.[48] Marked dilation of the trachea is obvious on the plain radiograph, with the tracheal shadow often being as wide as the vertical bodies. Physiotherapy and aggressive treatment of infection may retard the development of bronchiectasis.

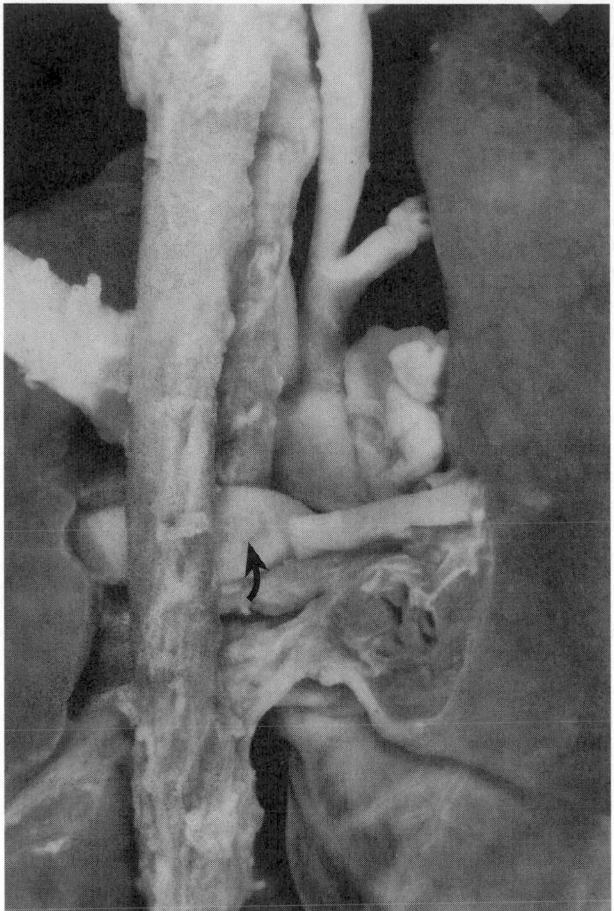

Fig. 72-5. Left pulmonary artery sling. Autopsy photograph showing the posterior view of the left pulmonary artery sling *(curved arrow)* curving over the right main bronchus before passing behind the carina and in front of the esophagus to the left lung. The trachea in this specimen was markedly narrowed, with complete "napkin ring" cartilages, and had the typical "rat-tail" configuration.

Tracheomalacia

The tracheal lumen is maintained by cartilage. Congenital absence, deficiency, or deformation of the cartilage will lead to exaggerated collapse of the airway and symptoms of obstruction. Primary tracheomalacia is rare. When it occurs, it usually takes the form of an abnormal softness of the cartilage, or a shortening of the cartilage rings with a correspondingly large pars membranosa.[49] The Williams-Campbell syndrome is a rare familial severe generalized form of tracheobronchomalacia in which there is marked reduction or absence of cartilage throughout the tracheobronchial airway.[50] Primary tracheomalacia has been found in association with Down syndrome, absence of pectoral muscle, congenital absence of the thumbs, funnel chest, and some congenital heart defects. Most commonly, though, tracheomalacia occurs as a localized abnormality secondary to extrinsic compression such as from a vascular ring[51] or mediastinal cyst. It is also found in virtually all patients with tracheoesophageal fistula, in which the malacic area is not necessarily localized to the site of the fistula but may extend distally to involve the rest of the trachea, bronchi, and peripheral airways. This explains why most of these patients have persisting airway problems postoperatively.[48] Tracheomalacia is usually not associated with laryngomalacia because the larynx does not develop directly from the foregut.

Clinical symptoms usually appear in early infancy and include a harsh loud vibratory cough, rattly chest, dyspnea, wheeze, and possibly stridor. The cough and rattly chest are caused by impaired clearance of normal mucous secretions past the abnormal tracheal segment. Collapse of this malacic segment as a result of increased intrathoracic pressure during expiration causes narrowing of the airway lumen, airway obstruction, and expiratory wheeze. This effect is exaggerated by increased respiratory effort, such as during crying, feeding, or coughing, or during an intercurrent upper or lower respiratory infection, and may lead rapidly to dyspnea and severe respiratory distress.[52] As distress increases, inspiratory difficulty may be noted as well. In its severest form, acute severe obstructive episodes with cyanosis—so-called death attacks—may be seen. These require immediate treatment with oxygen and positive-pressure ventilation, although on occasion this can prove surprisingly difficult to achieve until the abnormal segment is bypassed with an endotracheal tube. Because wheeze is a common symptom in these patients, many are mistakenly treated for asthma for long periods. It is now believed that the incidence of asthma is not higher in patients with tracheomalacia than in the rest of the population, so this diagnosis should always be reconsidered in these patients when they show no convincing response to an adequate trial of appropriate anti-asthma treatment. Other symptoms include a typical barking cough and the "bagpipe sign," a sibilant expiratory note persisting after the end of visible expiration.[53] Marked changes in airway caliber of the malacic segment may be detected on lateral inspiratory and expiratory chest radiographs (Fig. 72-6), although screening is probably more reliable and informative. This is particularly the case in short-segment malacia, in which the difference between the abnormal segment and the remaining normal trachea is readily discernible. When a large segment or the whole of the trachea is involved, it can be difficult to determine whether the degree of airway caliber change is abnormal because the range of "normal" variation, particularly in young infants, is large and may be as high as 50% during conditions of increased respiratory load such as during respiratory infections.[54] Bronchoscopy affords direct visualization of the malacic area and is probably the most commonly used means of confirming the diagnosis. When there is a well-defined localized area of tracheomalacia, an extrinsic lesion compressing the trachea should always be considered, and if at bronchoscopy the abnormal area is seen to pulsate vigorously, a vascular lesion should be suspected. If the pulsation is noted across the anterior wall of the trachea, an aberrant right subclavian artery is the most likely cause. This diagnosis can be confirmed simply by elevating the tip of the bronchoscope, thereby compressing the pulsating mass while palpating the right radial artery for changes in flow and pressure. Pulsations on the posterior tracheal wall usually suggest the presence of a vascular ring. Nonpulsatile lesions compressing the airway include bronchogenic cysts, cystic and solid mediastinal tumors, and enlarged lymph nodes. With all lesions compressing the trachea, computed tomography (CT) is usually necessary to define the anatomy before surgery.

Conservative management is possible in most patients with isolated tracheomalacia. Physiotherapy to improve clearance of trapped secretions, together with antibiotics with intercurrent infections, form the mainstay of treatment. With increasing age, airway function gradually improves as the tracheal diameter increases and the abnormal area stiffens. However, it may be many months or even years before symptoms have cleared.[55] In neonates or young infants with significant ongoing obstructive problems, a period of continuous positive airway pressure can be used to "splint" the airway until airway wall rigidity improves. This positive pressure may be administered through a face mask, nasopharyngeal tube, or endotracheal tube. Patients with severe obstructive problems refractory to conservative measures have a significant morbidity and mortality risk, as high as 80% in some cases,[56] and therefore should be offered surgical treatment. Tracheostomy, with or without continuous positive airway pressure subsequently, is usually the preferred option, although problems may persist when the end of the tracheostomy tube does not extend beyond the malacic segment. Aortopexy and tracheopexy, despite disappointing results in most series, remain surprisingly popular treatment choices.[57] Theoretically, by stitching the anterior wall of the aorta or trachea to the underside of the sternum,

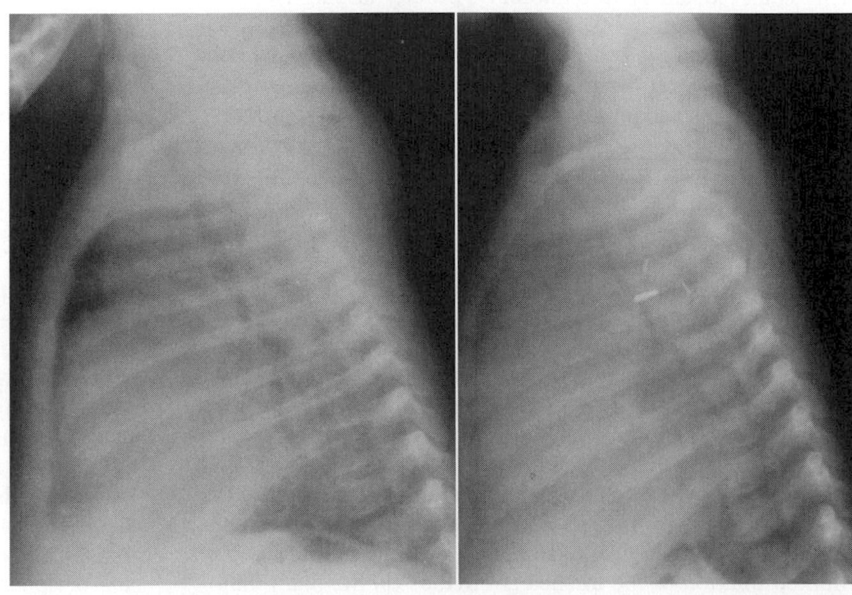

Fig. 72-6. Tracheomalacia. Lateral chest radiographs from a 5-month-old infant with symptoms of persistent expiratory wheeze worsening when distressed, show the abnormally marked collapse of the trachea during expiration *(right)* compared with normal tracheal diameter during inspiration *(left)* which is characteristic of tracheomalacia.

support is provided to the trachea, ideally until spontaneous improvement occurs. Endoscopic placement of expandable stents in the malacic segment[58] has also been tried, although results are very disappointing. The limited initial improvement seen in some of these patients is usually negated by the development of complications caused by the stent, which include erosion and perforation. The more generalized form of the disorder, Williams-Campbell syndrome, is associated with severe obstruction and recurrent infection progressing to bronchiectasis.[50] Other than physiotherapy and antibiotic treatment, no definitive therapy is available for this disorder.

Tracheoesophageal Malformations

Tracheoesophageal fistula and related malformations of the esophagus and trachea occur in approximately 1:3000 live births. The most common types are isolated esophageal atresia and esophageal atresia with tracheoesophageal fistula. Other esophageal malformations, such as esophageal stenosis, duplication, and achalasia, are not directly related to abnormal lung development and are not discussed here.

Esophageal Atresia and Esophageal Atresia with Tracheoesophageal Fistula

The various types of esophageal atresia and tracheoesophageal fistulae form an important group of anomalies causing respiratory distress in the newborn. Esophageal atresia with distal tracheoesophageal fistula is the most common anatomic configuration (85%), with isolated esophageal atresia (5% to 10%), atresia with proximal fistula (less than 5%), and tracheoesophageal fistula without esophageal atresia (H-type fistula, less than 3%) forming most of the rest (Fig. 72-7).

An aberration occurring during early separation of the respiratory-digestive anlage in the fetus forms the basis for these anomalies. Up to 50% of these patients have associated vertebral defects, 25% cardiac defects, and 10% imperforate anus. Many are born prematurely and the incidence is increased in Down syndrome.[30] In esophageal atresia, usually the upper esophageal pouch is of good size, extending approximately one third of the way down the trachea. When the distal esophageal segment is attached to the trachea, it is generally a flimsy structure. Accordingly, ischemia and necrosis of the distal esophagus are constant hazards postoperatively. The distal esophageal attachment is most commonly at the posterior aspect of the tracheal bifurcation. In pure esophageal atresia in which there is no fistulous connection to the trachea or bronchi, the distal esophageal blind end may be a small gastric diverticulum that barely extends above the diaphragm or, more commonly, reach approximately to the proximal end. Classically in esophageal atresia there is a history of maternal polyhydramnios in pregnancy. After birth the baby is unable to swallow its oral secretions, leading to constant drooling of frothy saliva and aspiration, with cough and cyanotic spells, particularly if feeding is attempted before the diagnosis is made. The presence of a distal tracheoesophageal fistula allows passage of refluxed gastric secretions directly into the lung, causing respiratory distress while allowing air to flow easily in the opposite direction into the gastrointestinal tract, leading to gaseous abdominal distention that can further compromise respiration. A gas-filled bowel noted on chest or abdominal radiograph in a baby with respiratory problems and drooling at birth often provide the clue to the presence of a tracheoesophageal fistula with esophageal atresia. The diagnosis is confirmed by failure to pass a nasogastric tube beyond the blind end of the proximal esophageal segment as seen on the chest radiograph (Fig. 72-8). An airless abdomen is presumptive evidence of atresia without a distal fistula. Contrast radiography should be avoided because aspiration is highly likely.

Management is surgical. Preoperatively the upper blind-ending esophageal pouch should be continuously aspirated through an indwelling catheter in order to avoid aspiration. In addition, the baby should be positioned semiupright to minimize gastroesophageal reflux and on his or her side to minimize aspiration. Surgery should be delayed until respiratory complications are controlled because it has been shown that they contribute significantly to postoperative morbidity and mortality. Ligation and division of the tracheoesophageal fistula and end-to-end anastomosis of the two esophageal ends is possible in most patients. When the gap between the two esophageal ends is too large, bougienage may elongate the proximal portion sufficiently to allow end-to-end anastomosis, although overstretching will increase the risk of wound breakdown postoperatively. Therefore, in some patients an interposition graft using either colon or a synthetic material is required.[59]

Postoperative complications are common and troublesome and can be divided into two groups: gastrointestinal and respiratory.[60] Common esophageal complications include wound breakdown with leakage into the mediastinum, anastomotic esophageal strictures requiring intermittent dilations (possibly for many years), swallowing coordination difficulties, and gastroesophageal reflux. Anastomotic strictures occur in one quarter of the patients (usually appearing within 3 months) and are heralded by dysphagia, regurgitation, cough, and recurrent as-

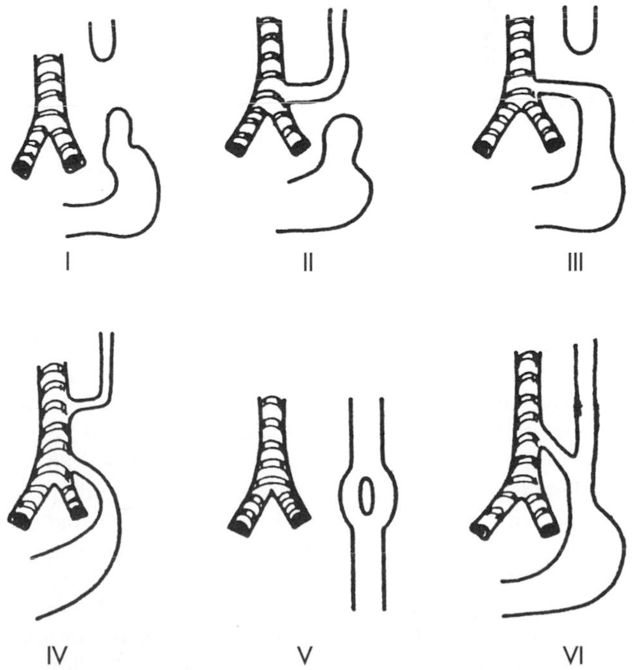

Fig. 72-7. Tracheoesophageal anomalies. Diagrammatic representation of the 6 well-recognized types. Type I (esophageal atresia) and type III (esophageal atresia with distal tracheoesophageal fistula) lesions account for 85% of these anomalies and the others, including type VI (H-type tracheoesophageal fistula), account for virtually all the rest.

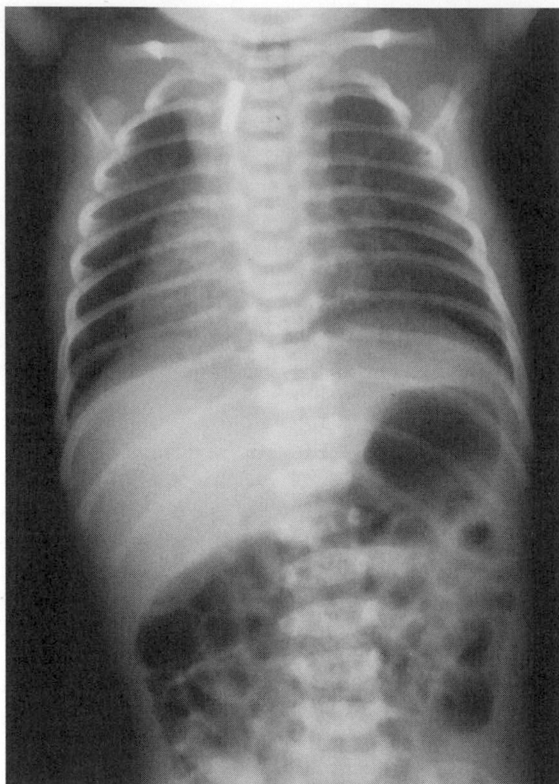

Fig. 72-8. Esophageal atresia with distal tracheoesophageal fistula. Chest radiograph of a newborn boy with choking and respiratory distress following an attempt at his first feeding and inability to pass an orogastric tube shows the tip of the tube ending in the atretic esophageal pouch at the level of the 3rd thoracic vertebra. The gas-filled bowel confirms the presence of a distal tracheoesophageal fistula. The associated dextracardia is a coincidental finding.

piration pneumonia. Respiratory problems include wound breakdown (with recurrence of the fistula occurring in up to 10% of cases), recurrent aspiration, recurrent respiratory infections, a characteristic barking cough, wheeze, dyspnea, and a respiratory rattle. A major contributing factor to these respiratory problems is the tracheomalacia that coexists to a variable degree in virtually all patients with tracheoesophageal fistula. This tracheomalacia may be localized to the site of the fistula or, more commonly, be more widespread. Cough and wheeze are therefore common symptoms in these patients and can be exacerbated at mealtimes, by respiratory infections, or during exercise, and are compounded by increased accumulation of secretions caused by impaired clearance. Severe attacks can lead to acute dyspnea with marked obstruction or even apnea, and in this situation these patients may adopt an attitude of opisthotonos in an effort to support the tracheal wall by putting it on stretch. The wheeze often leads to the misdiagnosis of asthma and because it is now well recognized that the incidence of asthma is not increased in patients with tracheomalacia (whether associated with tracheoesophageal fistula or not), this diagnosis must be reviewed if symptoms fail to show an adequate response to appropriate antiasthma treatment. Consequently, the cornerstones of treatment for postoperative tracheoesophageal fistula patients remain physiotherapy to help clear secretions, antibiotics (either intermittently or prophylactically depending on the frequency of recurrent infections), and treatment of gastroesophageal complications that may be contributing to recurrent respiratory problems. Surgical options are discussed in the section dealing with primary tracheomalacia, and may need to be considered for patients with ongoing severe airway problems. The overall prognosis for survival in children born with the esophageal atresia and tracheoesophageal group of anomalies is approximately 70%, which improves to more than 90% in full-term infants who are otherwise normal.[59]

Tracheoesophageal Fistula without Esophageal Atresia (H-type Fistula)

This particular form of tracheoesophageal fistula is dealt with separately because its clinical features and management differ somewhat from those of the more common types discussed previously. A fistulous connection between an otherwise normal esophagus and trachea occurs in approximately 3% of tracheoesophageal fistulae.[61] Clinically these patients present with a history of recurrent respiratory symptoms (particularly cough and choking with ingested fluids) and recurrent chest infections; gaseous abdominal distention, especially with crying, is another well-recognized feature. The nonspecific nature of the symptoms together with the difficulty in identifying the fistula in many of these patients means that the diagnosis is often delayed and this may result in considerable respiratory morbidity. Plain chest radiographs reveal stigmata of recurrent infection, especially in the right upper and middle lobes, together with gas-filled bowel. Esophagograms in appropriately angled prone positions using fluoroscopy detect most fistulae, although a significant number may be missed; in addition, care must be taken in determining whether the contrast enters the trachea through a fistula or from aspiration. Injection of contrast directly into the esophagus under pressure may occasionally identify a fistula not seen when the contrast is swallowed, although this must be done with care. Esophagoscopy and bronchoscopy are indicated when despite a negative esophagogram, a high index of suspicion of H-type fistula remains clinically. Differential diagnosis includes chronic pulmonary infections, other causes of recurrent aspiration, cystic fibrosis, and vascular rings. Operative ligation and division of the fistulous connection through a transcervical approach is usually sufficient to achieve a satisfactory result. Recurrent fistulae do occur but generally postoperative problems are less severe than with other forms of tracheoesophageal fistula. Morbidity and mortality relate to the degree of preoperative pulmonary disease.

Abnormalities of the Bronchi

Topographic Anomalies

Topographic anomalies of the whole lung such as situs inversus and left mirror image and right mirror image lung (bilateral left or bilateral right lung) have been shown to correlate in almost all instances with topographic anomalies of atrial arrangement (situs inversus, left isomerism, and right isomerism, respectively), and with abdominal aorta and vena caval relationships.[62] Isolated lobar or segmental topographic bronchial anomalies are now often recognized, although most cause no symptoms and are diagnosed coincidentally or at autopsy. Tracheal bronchus, abnormal segmental bronchial branching, supernumerary segmental or lobar bronchi, and bridging bronchi are the most common abnormalities found. Bronchial branching anomalies are also found in the Scimitar syndrome, almost always affecting the right side only.

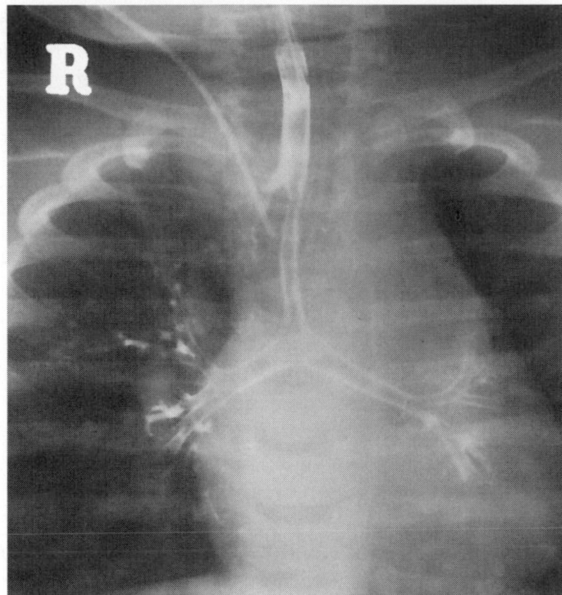

Fig. 72-9. Tracheal bronchus with distal tracheal stenosis. A well-recognized configuration of this anomaly is demonstrated in this bronchogram from a 13-month-old girl with a history of bidirectional wheeze and stridor worsening with infection. It shows the tracheal bronchus (invariably right-sided) arising from the intrathoracic trachea, the subsequent portion trachea stenosed to the carina, normal caliber left and right main bronchi and beyond, and absence of the normal right upper lobe bronchial branch.

Tracheal Bronchus. Tracheal bronchus always occurs on the right, as do 80% of all bronchial topographic anomalies.[63] The abnormal bronchus arises usually from the midintrathoracic region of the trachea and supplies either a segment of the right upper lobe (with the normal right upper lobe branch supplying the rest of the lobe) or the whole right upper lobe (in which case the normal right upper lobe branch is absent; Fig. 72-9). Structural abnormalities such as stenosis and malacia may be found in these bronchi, although the lung segment supplied by this bronchus is usually normal or at least initially so. Poor drainage of this segment often leads to recurrent infection and bronchiectasis in later life and the bronchus itself is more commonly the site of bronchial adenoma, carcinoma, or bronchogenic cysts. The trachea distal to the origin of the tracheal bronchus is often narrowed, usually only to the carina, whereafter the diameter in the left and right main bronchus reverts to normal (Fig. 72-9). Patients usually present with signs and symptoms of persisting right upper lobe infection or tracheal stenosis. The diagnosis is usually made at bronchoscopy or bronchography. Management is directed at improving drainage of the affected segment with physiotherapy and controlling infection with antibiotics. If the segment becomes bronchiectatic and problems persist despite conservative treatment, resection may be necessary. Symptoms caused by any associated tracheal stenosis usually improve with tracheal growth, although if the stenosis is severe, they may prove particularly troublesome and difficult to manage until this occurs.

Bridging Bronchus. A bridging bronchus is an anomalous bronchial branch arising from the left mainstem bronchus and crossing the mediastinum to enter the right lower lobe. In the two cases reported the right lung was bilobed and areas of stenosis in the tracheobronchial tree were present. Both children died of recurrent infection in early infancy.[64,65]

Morphologic Abnormalities

Bronchial Atresia. In bronchial atresia a lobar or segmental bronchus ends blindly, either with an atretic membrane or in a blind pouch, with a short gap to the distal continuation of the airway to that particular lobe or segment. This airway distal to the atresia is always abnormal and the lung parenchyma supplied by it is usually hyperinflated and emphysematous, with reduced alveolar numbers.[66] Ventilation of the segment is thought to occur through the pores of Kohn, which favors inspiration rather than expiration, resulting in gas trapping. It is most commonly found in the left upper lobe,[67] followed by right middle lobe. Characteristically, symptoms are mild or nonexistent and the condition is detected incidentally on chest radiography. The only physical finding may be decreased breath sounds over the affected area. When a major bronchus is atretic and the affected distal lobe is significantly hyperinflated, causing compression of surrounding healthy lung and shift of the mediastinum to the opposite side, symptoms of reduced exercise tolerance and possibly wheeze and shortness of breath may be prominent. The radiographic appearances can be virtually diagnostic, with an ovoid or elongated density extending from the hilar region into an area of hyperlucent lung (Fig. 72-10). The density represents the accumulation of mucus and debris in the distal airway and if extensive, may show branching. CT is commonly used to confirm the diagnosis, whereas bronchography demonstrates the absent or blind-ending bronchus.[68] Surgical excision is indicated only when overdistention of the affected lung segment leads to compromise of surrounding normal lung (as in congenital lobar emphysema) and significant symptoms. Infection in the abnormal segment is not common, and most patients are asymptomatic, requiring no treatment.

Congenital Bronchial Stenosis

Congenital isolated stricture of a bronchus occurs predominantly in mainstem or first-generation bronchi and predisposes to recurrent and chronic infection in the area distal to the narrowing as a result of impaired drainage of secretions.[69] Secondary narrowing is far more common and usually caused by compression by mediastinal cysts, tumors, and vascular anomalies. Apart from infection, these patients may present with recurrent wheeze that does not respond to appropriate antiasthma therapy. The diagnosis is made at bronchoscopy. Surgical resection of the stenosed area usually is precluded by inaccessibility and the small size of the lesion. Chronic infection and bronchiectasis distal to the stenosis usually necessitate resection of the affected lung segment.

Bronchomalacia. Bronchomalacia is most commonly found in association with tracheomalacia and the symptoms, diagnosis, and treatment of these combined lesions are discussed in the section on tracheomalacia. It is defined as abnormal weakness in the airway wall and is found more commonly in premature neonates and patients with Down syndrome, although it may occur in full-term infants. As with tracheomalacia, spontaneous improvement with age is the rule and only patients with significant respiratory problems require treatment in the meantime. Isolated segments of bronchomalacia are rare

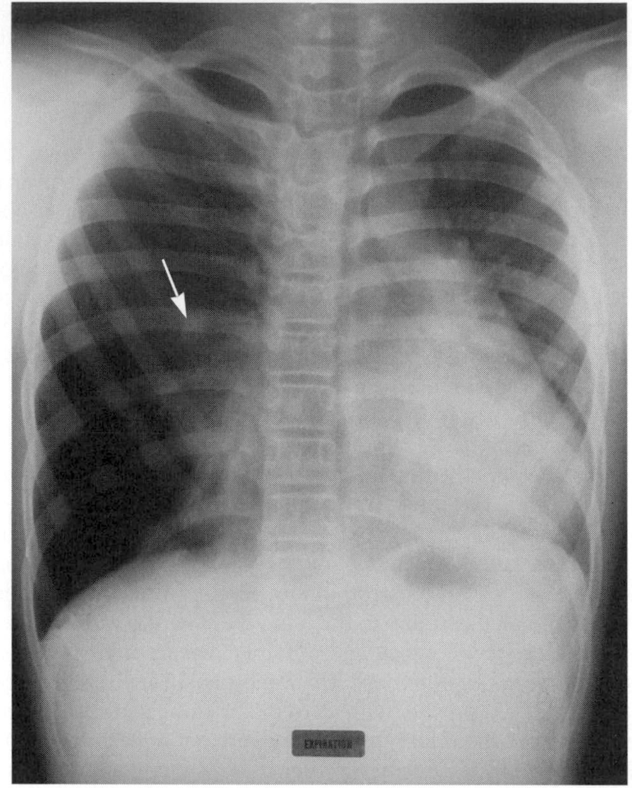

Fig. 72-10. Bronchial atresia. Chest radiograph from a 12-year-old boy with a long history of wheeze and low exercise tolerance compared with his peers, shows hyperinflation of the right middle lobe with compression of the right upper and lower lobes together with mediastinal shift to the left—appearances similar to those seen in congenital lobar emphysema. In this case, the presence of an oval perihilar shadow, called "bullet sign" because of its shape *(arrow)*, suggested the diagnosis of right middle lobe bronchial atresia and this was confirmed on CT and bronchography. The "bullet sign" shadow comprises mucus and debris impacted in the distal atretic bronchial pouch.

and occur most commonly secondary to extrinsic compression. A generalized severe form of bronchomalacia with absence or marked deficiency of airway cartilage, known as Williams Campbell syndrome, is described in the section on tracheomalacia. Bronchomalacia associated with defective cartilage development is also found in affected segments in congenital lobar emphysema.

Bronchogenic Cysts. Bronchogenic cysts account for around 5% of mediastinal masses in infants and children; this percentage is higher in adults. Some are diagnosed incidentally at thoracotomy or at autopsy,[70] which indicates that they may be more common than is normally appreciated. The cyst is usually single and may be very large. In at least 20% of the cases it is totally separated from the bronchopulmonary tree, lying free in the mediastinum or occasionally attached to other structures such as the esophagus, pericardium, or pleura.[12] Bronchogenic cysts have been described in association with other congenital lung anomalies such as sequestration.[71] The cyst is thin-walled, lined with ciliated respiratory epithelium and mucus glands, and surrounded by muscle and fibrous tissue. Very rarely they may have an anomalous arterial supply or venous drainage. Embryologically, the developing bronchus is disrupted at a particular stage and a piece of bronchial tissue separates to form the bronchial cyst. The eventual location and histologic features of the cyst depend primarily on the time of the disruption. A cyst formed during early partition from the foregut is likely to contain some histologic features consistent with its enteric origin.[72]

Bronchogenic cysts are found in five major locations within the thorax:[73]

1. The right paratracheal region (corresponding to the usual site of origin of the tracheal bronchus), 19%;
2. The carinal region (where they are most likely to cause symptoms by airway compression), 51.5%;
3. The hilar region (where the cyst is located on or near a main stem or lobar bronchus and is often latent), 8.6%;
4. Paraesophageal region (usually low near the cardia and may compress the esophagus), 13.8%;
5. Other locations such as pericardial, retrosternal, and paravertebral, 6.9%.

Clinical findings are diverse depending on the location of the cyst. Proximal tracheal compression can cause stridor and respiratory distress. Compression in the carinal area leads to cough, wheeze, atelectasis, overinflation of one or both lungs, or recurrent infections. Compression of a smaller bronchial branch may cause localized signs with recurrent infections and hyperinflation or atelectasis of the distal lung parenchyma. The cyst itself can become infected (usually by contamination through a tracheobronchial communication), leading to acute distention and exacerbation of compression symptoms. Difficulty in swallowing and recurrent vomiting are symptoms of esophageal compression. Many cysts are asymptomatic and may be diagnosed coincidentally on chest radiographs taken for other reasons. They appear as a rounded space-occupying lesion projecting from the mediastinum and often displacing and compressing the lower trachea and bronchus adjacent to the cyst (Fig. 72-11). A barium swallow may demonstrate esophageal compression or a lesion separating the trachea and esophagus. CT is the optimal investigation for identifying, localizing, and defining the cystic mediastinal lesion. Bronchography and bronchoscopy are seldom necessary but may demonstrate compression and displacement of the airway. In symptomatic cases surgical excision is the only treatment.

Other Mediastinal Cysts. Although other mediastinal cystic lesions are not strictly congenital anomalies of the respiratory tract, their close clinical relationship and in some cases similar embryonic origins warrant their inclusion in this chapter. They include enteric duplication cysts, pericardial cysts, benign cystic teratomas, dermoid cysts, thymic cysts, and mediastinal meningoceles.

Cysts of digestive tract origin. Gastroenterogenous cysts (also called enteric duplication cysts) are characterized by their histology, which contains elements of gut tissue including cells from stomach, esophagus, small bowel, pancreas, bile duct, or any combination of these elements.[74,75] Neurenteric cysts are gastroenterogenous cysts that contain neural elements derived through an anterior spinal defect.[76] They arise when abnormal development of the primitive foregut affects closure of the neural canal at the same site, and are found usually in the lower cervical or upper thoracic spine. Cysts of digestive tract origin are rare, forming approximately 1% to 3% of all mediastinal tumors. They are specific in that their wall contains elements of mucosa, muscle, and serous layer, with a mucosal layer histologically similar to a specific segment of the diges-

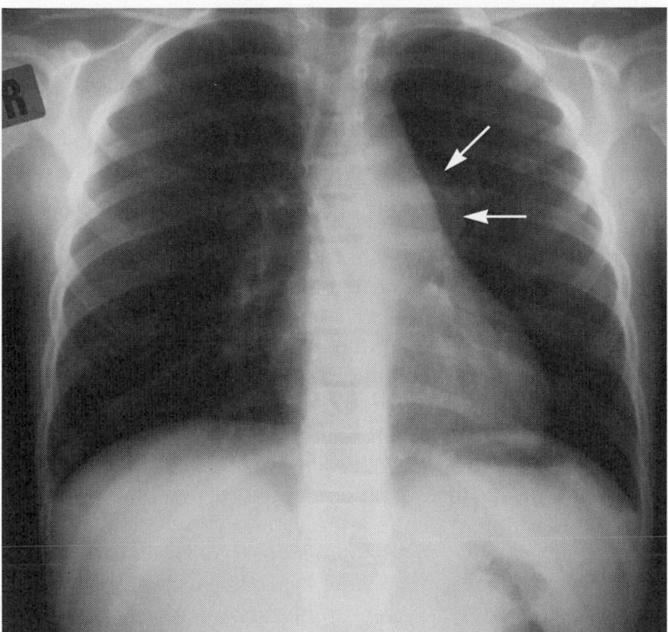

Fig. 72-11. Bronchogenic cyst. The typically rounded hilar mass *(arrow),* seen on this chest radiograph indenting the left main bronchus and lower trachea while deviating the trachea to the right, was confirmed at surgery to be a bronchogenic cyst.

tive tract. Gastric type cysts may secrete hydrochloric acid, pepsin, and renin, whereas others may secrete trypsin and amylase. The location of the cyst does not allow prediction of its mucosal type. Differentiation of a digestive cyst from a bronchogenic cyst is not always possible and some cysts contain both enteric and respiratory elements. Symptoms are related to the site and size of the cyst, the presence of infection, and the contents of the cyst. Gastric cysts present early because of acidic secretions, provoking autodigestion, inflammation, ulceration, or perforation. Other symptoms include hemoptysis, hematemesis, melena, pain, swallowing difficulties, and symptoms of airway compression. Most enteric cysts are found in the lower two thirds of the posterior mediastinum, although they can occur in a variety of other sites, including the rest of the mediastinum, lung parenchyma, and extrathoracic areas.[12] They are often connected to the esophagus or abdominal digestive tracts through the diaphragm by a narrow pedicle or fibrous band. Although the diagnosis may be indicated on the chest radiograph or barium swallow, CT is usually more informative. The associated finding of a vertebral anomaly, such as spina bifida, hemivertebrae, congenital scoliosis, Klippel-Feil syndrome, and particularly vertebral clefts, in a patient with respiratory symptoms, and a mediastinal mass should alert the surgeon to the possibility of a congenital cyst of neurenteric origin (Fig. 72-12). Even in the absence of symptoms, surgical excision should be performed for all of these cysts because of potential risks of hemorrhage, autodigestion, and complications associated with infection.[72]

Pericardial cysts. Pericardial cysts adhere to the parietal pericardium and, although congenital, are almost always diagnosed in adult life. Large cysts may displace the heart or compress lung tissue. They are most commonly situated in the right anterior cardiophrenic angle, where they can be visualized on an oblique chest radiograph. Histologically the cysts are of mesothelial origin. Simple excision, if necessary, is the only therapy.[77]

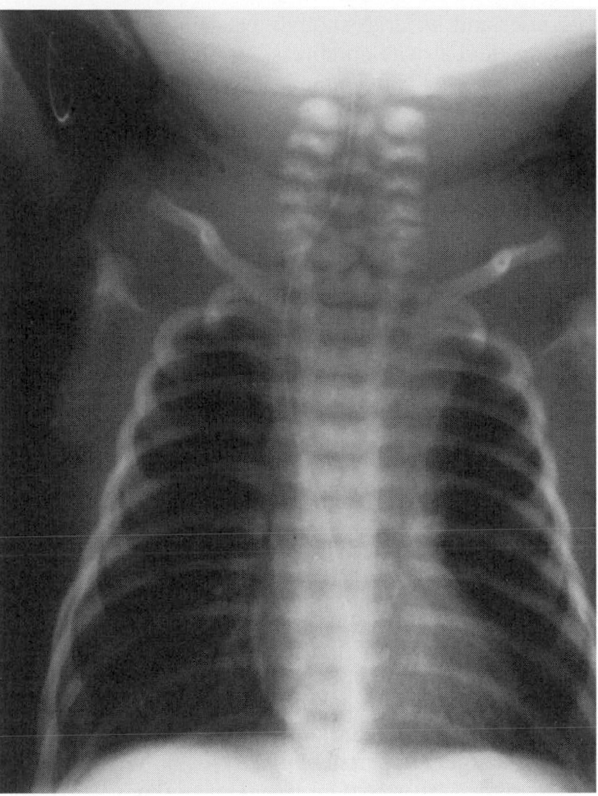

Fig. 72-12. Neurenteric cyst. The presence of a cleft vertebral anomaly underlying a rounded mass indenting the upper trachea and deviating to the right, as seen in this chest radiograph, is characteristic of a neurenteric cyst. The diagnosis was confirmed on histology following surgical resection.

Benign cystic teratoma, dermoid cyst. Teratoma is a tumor of mixed primitive elements containing ectodermal, mesodermal, and endodermal derivatives. It is rarely diagnosed in children. The cystic form is usually benign and lies in the anterior mediastinum as a cystic asymmetric mass, more often on the left than the right. Symptoms are associated mainly with airway and lung compression. A chest radiograph will reveal a well-defined mass and may show diffuse stippled calcification and even teeth. The differential diagnosis includes that of any anterior mediastinal mass including a large thymic cyst, hydatid cyst, or a tumor such as lymphoma. CT scanning is useful to characterize the lesion. Surgical excision is the only treatment. A few teratomas can be malignant. Slightly more than 25% of mediastinal tumors are teratomas.[78]

Thymic cysts and tumors. Thymic cysts are usually small and multiple and rarely cause any symptoms. Occasionally they extend to the thoracic inlet and cause airway compression, making surgical excision necessary.[78] Thymomas, if large enough, may cause symptoms by lung and airway compression. They are usually diagnosed in infancy and surgical removal is curative. Other tumors of thymic origin, such as lymphoma, usually present later in childhood, again with symptoms related to lung and airway compression and a large rounded mass in the anterior upper thorax seen on the chest radiograph. Urgent definitive histologic diagnosis and appropriate treatment are warranted in these cases.

Intrathoracic meningoceles. Diverticulae of spinal meningoceles protruding through neuroforamina adjacent to intercostal nerves may occur. They project into the posterior medial thoracic gutter and, if large enough, cause symptoms related to esophageal and airway compression. They are commonly associated with other spinal abnormalities.[78]

Bronchobiliary Fistula. This is a rare anomaly usually presenting early in infancy because of symptoms produced by the intense inflammatory effect of bile secretions in the bronchial tree. A tract connects the biliary tree to one of the main bronchi, nearly always on the right near the carina.[79] Yellow or green bile-stained sputum associated with cough, atelectasis, and infection forms a distinctive clinical picture in infancy. Early surgery is recommended before extensive autolytic damage occurs.[80] The embryologic origin of the lesion is obscure, although esophageal atresia and tracheoesophageal fistula have been reported in association with the anomaly.[81]

MALFORMATIONS OF THE SMALL AIRWAY AND LUNG PARENCHYMA

Congenital Cystic Lesions of the Small Airway and Lung Parenchyma

Congenital cystic lesions of the lung parenchyma are rare in comparison with acquired cysts, such as those found following infection. Five subgroups are recognized based on current concepts of their embryonic origins.

1. Simple congenital parenchymal cysts, or lung cysts;
2. Parenchymal cysts of digestive tract origin;
3. Congenital cystic bronchiectasis;
4. Cystic adenomatoid malformation, a malformation of the non–cartilage-containing peripheral airway;
5. Cystic lesions within other parenchymal anomalies, such as sequestration.

These distinctions are not always clear and a number of cystic lesions show overlapping features, both within the above subgroups and with other parenchymal lesions. However, until more is known about the pathogenesis of these anomalies, these distinctions remain the most practical.

Simple Congenital Parenchymal Cysts (Lung Cysts)

Most simple parenchymal cysts are thought to represent a localized abnormality or abnormalities of the peripheral bronchioles or terminal bronchopulmonary airway. Cystic dilation may occur locally as a single lesion or involve the lung units distal to the abnormality, resulting in a multicystic lesion. The eventual site of the lesion and its histologic features correlate with the stage in fetal life when the abnormality occurred. Thus simple lung cysts can be divided into bronchogenic, alveolar, and mixed or intermediate types according to their histopathologic features.[82] The cysts may be single (38%) or multiple (62%), but when they are multiple they are usually localized to a segment or lobe, although generalized cystic disease of both lungs occurring as a familial trait has been described.[83] Single cysts are commonly peripheral and most often found in the lower lobe. They may be multilocular, contain fluid, gas, or both, and communicate with the bronchial airway. Aberrant systemic arterial supply and anomalous venous drainage, either singly or together, have been described in simple congenital parenchymal cysts, supporting the concept that these entities may represent variants of a spectrum of bronchopulmonary and bronchovascular anomalies.[84] Histologically, bronchial elements such as cartilage, mucous glands, and smooth muscle can be seen. In general, cysts found more peripherally contain less cartilage and no mucous glands, with bullous alveolar-type cystic lesions forming the most distal end of this spectrum. Infection can distort the lining of the cyst wall, making histologic differentiation from acquired cysts very difficult or impossible.

Clinically, fluid-filled cysts are generally asymptomatic and discovered late, usually by chance. However, air-filled cysts are more likely to present with secondary infections. The infection enters through either rudimentary bronchial communications or the pores of Kohn, and at presentation the patient has systemic signs of sepsis while the chest radiograph reveals a rounded mass lesion, often with an air-fluid level (Fig. 72-13). Enlarging cysts may produce mediastinal shift and

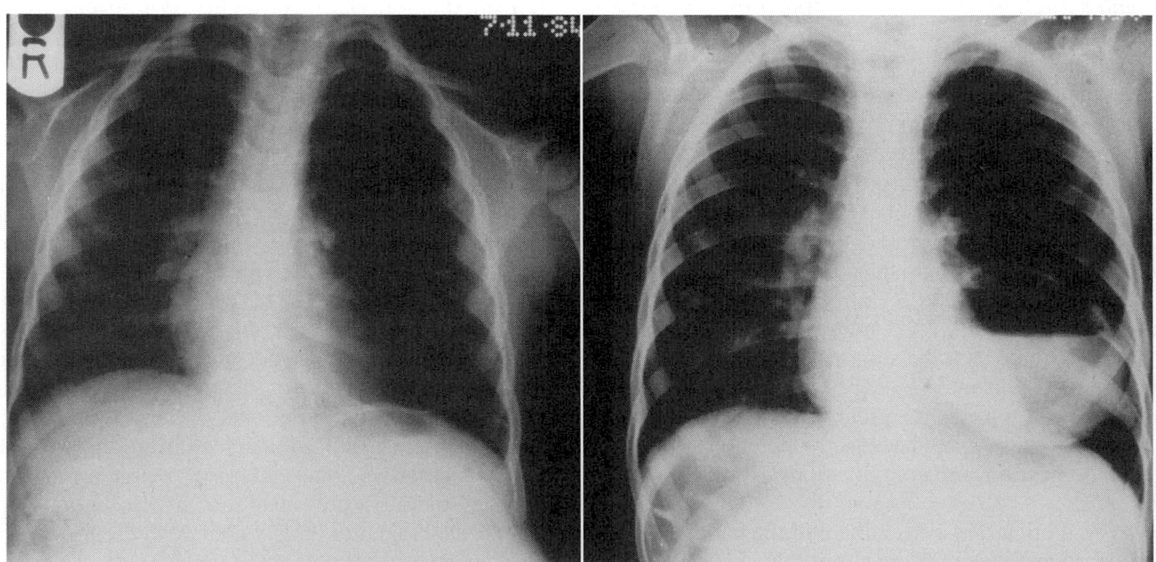

Fig. 72-13. Congenital lung cyst. Chest radiograph showing a large cystic lesion in the left lower lobe *(left)* that became infected forming an abscess with an air-fluid level *(right)*. The infection cleared slowly on prolonged antibiotic therapy, and elective resection of the lesion subsequently confirmed the diagnosis of congenital lung cyst.

symptoms caused by compression of surrounding structures. When quiescent, they are not always readily discernible on the chest radiograph. CT is usually necessary to confirm the diagnosis and define the extent of the lesion. Aortography should be considered, particularly in lower lobe cysts, to rule out the presence of an aberrant arterial supply to the lesion. Sometimes it is difficult to separate larger peripheral cysts, particularly those of the bullous alveolar type, from congenital lobar emphysema on clinical, radiologic, and histologic grounds, although in bullous cystic disease, symptoms of wheeze, evidence of mediastinal shift, and hyperinflation are characteristically less marked. In addition, cyst rupture causing a tension pneumothorax is more common in the bullous alveolar type (Fig. 72-14). Other differential diagnoses include cystic adenomatoid malformation and bronchial atresia; occasionally, gas-filled loops of bowel from a diaphragmatic hernia may simulate the appearance of multiple lung cysts on the chest radiograph and should be suspected if the diaphragmatic silhouette is not visualized. In addition, congenital cysts must be distinguished from those secondary to other diseases because as the management is usually entirely different. Important causes of acquired cysts include infection (particularly the pneumatoceles of staphylococcal pneumonia), Letterer-Siwe disease (eosinophilic granuloma, histiocystosis X), and the abscess cavities of cystic fibrosis. The distinction from pneumatoceles following a staphylococcal pneumonia is critical because these resolve spontaneously once the infection has been treated effectively.[85]

Complications associated with congenital lung cysts are generally serious and include compression of the surrounding lung or an adjacent bronchus, leading to recurrent bronchopneumonia; collapse or hyperinflation of the affected area; rupture leading to pneumothorax and possibly bronchopleural fistula; and infection and abscess formation within the cyst (Fig. 72-13). Thus surgical resection is usually recommended for all congenital parenchymal cysts, even if they are asymptomatic at the time of diagnosis. Surgery is ideally performed electively. If infection is present, adequate treatment should be commenced well before surgery. In addition, consideration should always be given to whether an aberrant arterial supply or venous drainage may be present.

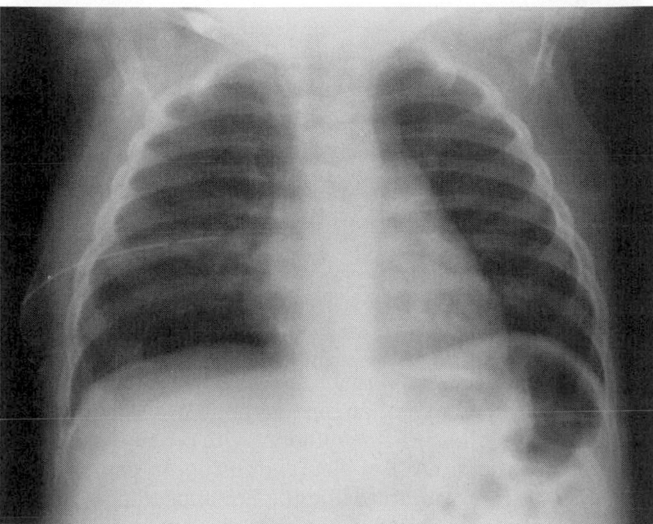

Fig. 72-14. Congenital lung cyst. The intercostal catheter seen on this chest radiograph was inserted to treat a tension pneumothorax caused by rupture of one of the multiple peripheral bullous cysts comprising the multicystic congenital lung cyst in the right lower lobe of this patient. Subsequent recurrent pneumothoraces necessitated surgical removal of the abnormal lobe, which was curative.

Parenchymal Cysts of Digestive Tract Origin

The pulmonary parenchyma is a rare site for cysts of digestive tract origin. More commonly these cysts are located in the mediastinum or form part of a sequestration (intrapulmonary or extrapulmonary). The essential characteristic feature is the presence of cells of enteric origin in the walls of the cysts. It has been suggested that cells arising within abnormally developing bronchi may occasionally retain the ability to develop into any type of epithelium normally derived from the foregut.[86] However, the common finding of a rudimentary connection or fibrous band linking these lesions to the foregut suggests that the more likely explanation for the presence of these foregut cells in the lung is that they are part of ectopic tissue that may have originated as part of an accessory bud of mixed foregut tissue migrating to and being incorporated in error into the normal lung parenchyma and at times retaining some sort of primitive connection to its origins.[17,20] Some researchers argue that the presence of a primitive connection does not necessarily confirm this latter postulate because it has been shown that ectopic or misplaced tissue undergoing dysmorphogenesis can spontaneously form a communication with its parent organ at any stage during development.[18,20] A reciprocal arrangement in which pockets of ciliated respiratory tract epithelium are found in the esophagus is also well recognized.[86] All intrathoracic cysts of digestive origin should be removed surgically before the development of complications.

Congenital Cystic Bronchiectasis

It is debatable whether congenital cystic bronchiectasis should be regarded as a separate entity or as a variant of simple parenchymal cystic disease. It is a localized condition in which multiple small cysts are found in the bronchial wall, distorting the normal bronchial architecture in a particular lung segment. This distortion impairs the normal drainage of secretions, predisposing the abnormal segment to recurrent infection and subsequent bronchiectasis. In the past it has been suggested that infection might be solely responsible for all pathologic changes found in cystic bronchiectasis. However, support for congenital origin of these lesions is gained from the similar distribution of upper and lower lobe cases (in contrast to that of acquired bronchiectasis), the occasional finding of associated vascular or bronchial anomalies, absence of evidence of infection in some cases; and histopathologic features within the cyst wall consistent with its bronchogenic origin.[86] Although infection is the most common presenting feature, many patients simply have a chronic cough or are asymptomatic. The differential diagnosis is that of bronchiectasis caused by other causes and any cystic or solid lesion involving a segment or lobe of the lung, and treatment consists of surgical resection of the affected area in symptomatic cases.

Cystic Adenomatoid Malformation

This is a rare defect of the non–cartilage-containing terminal respiratory structures, probably resulting from an abnormality occurring in the mid to late stages of lung development. One explanation for the pathogenesis of this malformation relates to the postulate of the dual mode of lung development.[86] This states that the endodermal lung bud provides bronchial elements up to and including the terminal bronchioles, whereas the respiratory bronchioles and alveolar elements are of mesodermal origin, deriving from the mesenchyme that surrounds the developing lung bud soon after its appearance. Abnormal terminal bronchiolar development results in failure of these two systems to communicate. Subsequent haphazard proliferation of the terminal bronchiolar elements (interspersed with mesodermal elements) leads to the development of the typical adenomatoid malformation. However, most people now believe that the endodermal lung bud provides all bronchopulmonary elements, including respiratory bronchioles and alveoli, and it may simply be that disruption of humoral factors from the mesenchyme (which also influences connective tissue and capillary plexus development) at a critical stage of terminal airway development results in the abnormal differentiation and proliferation found in these lesions, much like that of a hamartoma.[87] Three types of adenomatoid malformation are recognized based on their morphologic appearances (Fig. 72-15).[88]

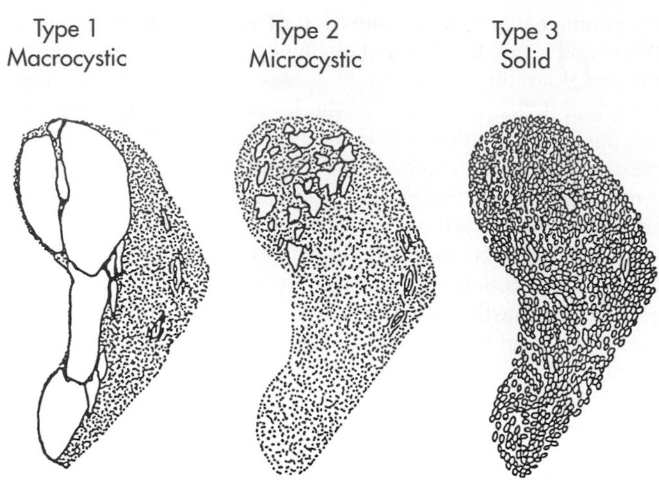

Fig. 72-15. Cystic adenomatoid malformation. Diagrammatic representation of the three pathologic types: macrocystic, microcystic, and solid.

Macrocystic Adenomatoid Malformation. One or more large cysts predominate in this lesion. The cysts are lined with ciliated pseudostratified epithelium, and the walls of the cysts contain smooth muscle and elastic tissue. Bronchiolar and alveolar elements are interspersed among the cysts. This type of adenomatoid malformation has the best prognosis.

Microcystic Adenomatoid Malformation. This lesion has mostly small cysts lined with ciliated cuboidal or columnar epithelium. The intervening solid portions of the lesion are filled with distended respiratory bronchioles and alveolar tissue. Occasionally striated muscle tissue is found outside the cysts.

Solid Adenomatoid Malformation. This lesion consists of a solid airless mass of tissue consisting almost entirely of bronchiolar elements lined by partly ciliated cuboidal epithelium and some alveolar elements. This type of adenomatoid malformation carries the worst prognosis, with many affected infants being stillborn or dying soon after delivery.

Madewell et al[89] found microcystic lesions in 73% of patients, whereas macrocystic and solid lesions accounted for 13% each. The lesions generally affected part or the whole of one lobe, sometimes two lobes, and only rarely the whole lung. Cystic adenomatoid malformation is often associated with other congenital lung lesions but rarely malformations elsewhere in the body, although it has been described in association with renal agenesis.[90] Maternal polyhydramnios is common, and some infants are born hydropic with bilateral pleural effusions and ascites.[90] Cystic adenomatoid lesions sometimes show overlapping features morphologically similar to other congenital lung anomalies such as sequestration and bronchial atresia.[16] Occasionally, there may be an aberrant systemic arterial supply and one extrapulmonary sequestration was found to have histologic features more with cystic adenomatoid malformation supporting the link between cystic adenomatoid malformation and other bronchovascular malinosculations. Clinically, respiratory symptoms appear at birth in 75% of cases and rarely is presentation delayed beyond the neonatal period. Large lesions may cause mediastinal shift, compressing the opposite lung and mediastinal vessels. Rupture of the cyst may produce a pneumothorax. The diagnosis is suggested by the appearance on the chest radiograph of an obvious solid or cystic mass involving part or whole of a hemithorax with possibly mediastinal shift and occasionally a pleural effusion. In patients with the macrocystic form, the radiographic appearances can be strikingly similar to those of simple congenital parenchymal lung cysts (Fig. 72-16), with differentiation possible only on histologic examination. Left-sided lesions with a multiloculated appearance have been mistaken for a diaphragmatic hernia, although in cystic adenomatoid malformation the diaphragm should be readily discernible. Additional differential diagnoses include all other solid or cystic congenital lung le-

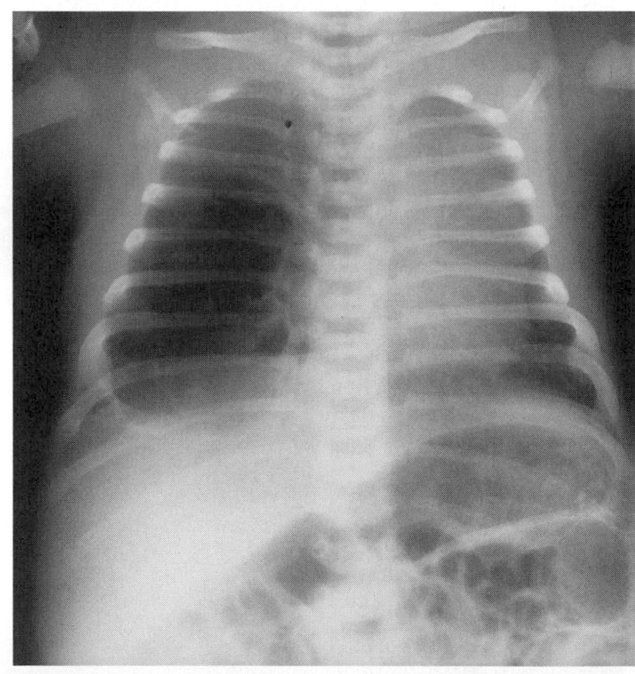

Fig. 72-16. Cystic adenomatoid malformation. The multicystic lesion seen in the right midzone on this chest radiograph of an infant with tachypnea and shortness of breath was shown following surgical resection to be a macrocystic type of cystic adenomatoid malformation involving the right middle lobe.

sions, and possibly infection. The presence of hydrops fetalis in association with solid lung lesions is a poor prognostic sign. Early surgical resection is the treatment of choice in almost all cases.

Cystic Lesions in Other Congenital Parenchymal Anomalies

Cystic areas (either primary or the result of cystic degeneration or infection) are commonly found in a number of other congenital parenchymal lesions (particularly bronchovascular anomalies such as pulmonary sequestration) and in congenital lymphagiectasia.

Congenital Lobar Emphysema

Congenital lobar emphysema is a well-characterized clinical problem in which massive postnatal overinflation of one or more lobes of the lung occurs. The condition is found at birth in 25%, 50% have manifested by 1 month of age, and it is rare for patients to become symptomatic after 6 months of age. It can occur in any lobe but is most common in the left upper lobe, followed by the right upper lobe and right middle lobe. Congenital heart disease is a common accompaniment.[91] The condition is characterized by overdistention and air trapping in the affected lobe, with compression of the remaining lung tissue and displacement of the mediastinum by herniation of the emphysematous lobe across the anterior mediastinum into the opposite chest (Fig. 72-17).[92] These features are uniform at presentation, with the vast majority requiring early surgical intervention because of respiratory embarrassment.[93] Precise understanding of the development of the condition is still lacking. Strictly speaking, the term *emphysema* should be based on morphologic characteristics.[94] A wide range of possible causally associated anomalies have been described in this condition, most of which would not be expected to be associated with true emphysema. The most common associated anomaly, occurring in up to 50% of cases, is a deficiency of bronchial cartilages.[91,95,96] Other abnormalities include extrinsic compression of a bronchus by bronchogenic cyst,[97] bronchial mucosal folds,[98] mucus plugs,[99] polyalveolar lobe,[100] volvulus of a lobe,[101] associated hypoplastic lung,[102] and bronchial atresia or stenosis.[103] Combinations of associated abnormalities have also been described, including abnormal bronchial cartilages and bronchial atresia,[104] and cystic adenomatoid malformation with bronchial atresia.[16] The fact that there is extreme overinflation of the affected segment, producing compression of other intrathoracic structures, suggests that there must be an additional abnormality of alveolar connective tissue in these lesions.[103] True panlobular emphysema has been described in association with this condition[104] and this may account for early presentation with severe respiratory distress. Differential diagnosis can be difficult. Atelectasis with compensatory emphysema may look very similar radiographically. An isotope ventilation scan, using a short–half-life isotope such as krypton-81, should distinguish the two. Normal ventilation occurs in the compensatory emphysema and is absent in congenital lobar emphysema. Occasionally, bronchiolitis, asthma, and foreign body can produce selective overinflation of a lobe. However, this is evident only in expiration. In full inspiration there is no distortion of other intrathoracic structures.

Most infants present in the neonatal period with respiratory distress. Signs include chest asymmetry with hyperinflation and reduced air entry on the affected side, mediastinal shift to the contralateral side, and possibly wheeze. Those presenting later may have varying degrees of respiratory distress and failure to thrive and signs on examination are similar to those of early presenters but less severe. In the past, surgical removal of the affected lobe was the standard recommended treatment, although recent evidence suggests that some of these patients, including some presenting early with severe respiratory distress, may show spontaneous resolution of symptoms, so conservative supportive treatment should be attempted when possible.[105]

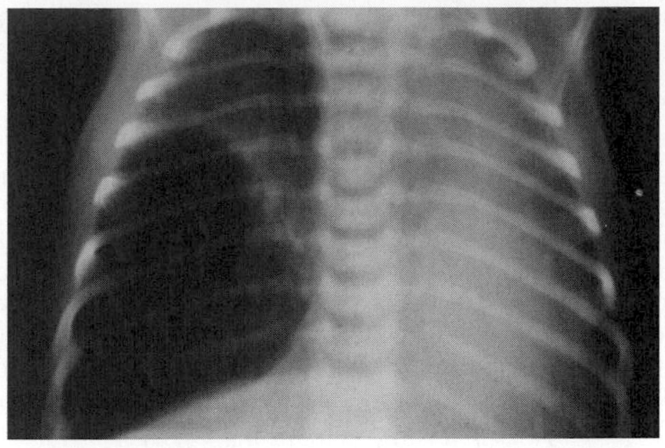

Fig. 72-17. Congenital lobar emphysema. Chest radiograph in an infant with respiratory distress, a hyperexpanded right chest, and reduced air entry in the right lung, showing marked hyperinflation of the right middle lobe, causing compression of the right upper and lower lobes and shift of the mediastinum to the left. The lesion failed to improve with conservative therapy, necessitating surgical resection, which was curative.

Parenchymal Lesions in Which the Airway Is Affected Together with One or More of the Other Tubular Components of Lung, Namely Arterial, Venous, and Lymphatic Channels

Malformations of lung associated with abnormal vasculature (bronchovascular malinosculation) and lymphatic systems (broncholymphatic malinosculation) can all be regarded as variants of a single primary complex of bronchopulmonary malformations (bronchopulmonary malinosculation, when all components are affected). The embryologic support for this concept is discussed earlier in this chapter. *Sequestration spectrum* has been suggested as a collective term for this group of anomalies, although the limits of the spectrum and opinion on which entities should be included have varied.[18,84] In this section, we discuss sequestrations, Scimitar syndrome, and other bronchovascular and broncholymphatic anomalies separately, but with the understanding that differentiation of these lesions is not always clear. Additional confusion may arise when it is realized that vascular anomalies have been described in lung malformations in which normal pulmonary artery supply and venous drainage is generally the rule, as in bronchogenic cysts, congenital parenchymal cysts, cystic adenomatoid malformation, and lobar emphysema. This supports a unifying concept for all lung malformations and emphasizes that the only possible classification that can be applied effectively to these complex lesions is one that incorporates descriptive analysis of component features, as suggested earlier in this chapter.

Pulmonary Sequestration

In 1947, Pryce et al[7] coined the term *sequestration* to describe a disconnected ("dislocated," "ectopic") bronchopulmonary mass or cyst with an anomalous systemic artery supply. It is now well recognized that many of these lesions are not "disconnected," and may have variable communication with the proximal normal tracheobronchial airway. In addition, "sequestered" areas of lung with normal pulmonary artery supply have been described, and both forms may have normal or anomalous venous drainage. Thus a slightly modified version of Pryce's definition would effectively include all sequestration variants, namely "a disconnected or abnormally communicating bronchopulmonary mass or cyst with normal or anomalous arterial supply or venous drainage." The obvious provision that must be made in this definition is that the bronchopulmonary mass does not have features consistent with other specific bronchopulmonary anomalies, such as cystic adenomatoid malformation, lobar emphysema, or simple congenital parenchymal cysts. Since the time of Pryce's definition, sequestrations have been classified as intralobar and extralobar. Again, strictly speaking, these terms are incorrect and should be replaced with *intrapulmonary* (lesions lying within the boundary formed by the pleural layer surrounding the lung) and *extrapulmonary* (ectopic lung tissue lying outside the boundary formed by the pleural layer surrounding the rest of the lung).

Intrapulmonary Sequestration. Intrapulmonary sequestrations form more than 90% of sequestrations, and 60% of these are found in the posterior basal segment of the left lower lobe. The abnormal segment may be accessory when it develops as a supernumerary bronchial anlage with the rest of the lung normal,[75] or it may develop at the expense of one of the bronchial buds in the normal anlage.[7] In almost all instances, the extent of the involvement is segmental or less. Bronchial communication with the normal proximal airway is usually absent or, if present, is abnormal. Alternatively, rudimentary connections may be found linking sequestrations with other bronchi, the surrounding lung parenchyma, or extrapulmonary structures, particularly the esophagus, stomach and small bowel, pancreas, liver, and gallbladder. Communication with surrounding lung is sometimes said to result from rupture of infected tissue or cysts into the neighboring lung substance, although most often the communication is believed to preexist any infection. A well-developed bronchus arising from the esophagus and forming the sole connection to an intrapulmonary sequestration has been described. Similarly, an esophageal bronchus may supply an extrapulmonary sequestration or, very rarely, a normal segment of lung that is disconnected from the normal bronchial airway. A rudimentary connection or fibrous band linking the sequestration to a digestive trace structure may indicate the presence of ectopic foregut tissue within the sequestration. One infant, with ectopic pancreatic tissue sequestered in the right lower lung, had marked distress during feeding, suggesting that the ingestion of milk stimulated secretion of pancreatic enzymes into lung parenchymal tissue causing autodigestion and inflammation.[106]

Intrapulmonary sequestrations may be cystic or noncystic. In lesions with absent bronchial connection, aeration of cystic areas is achieved probably through the pores of Kohn, which are minute accessory airway communications existing probably at alveolar level. Ventilation is extremely inefficient, but the communication is presumably sufficient to provide access for infection—evidence of which is found within almost all sequestrations, usually in the form of bronchiectasis and a scarred, shrunken parenchyma. The aberrant systemic arterial blood supply most commonly arises from the lower thoracic or upper abdominal aorta as a single trunk. Other sites of origin include the subclavian artery, bronchial arteries, intercostal arteries, celiac axis, internal mammary artery, and occasionally the splenic or renal artery. The arteries may be multiple and, rarely, a mixed pulmonary and systemic arterial supply to the abnormal segment may be found.[107,117] Intrapulmonary sequestration with normal pulmonary artery supply has been described.[108] The venous drainage is usually normal to the left atrium, but may be anomalous to the right atrium, vena cava, or azygos systems.[109] The size of the abnormal arteries and veins is sometimes considerable, and with the vascular resistance in these segments sometimes being very low, the blood flow through this anomalous circuit may be high enough to precipitate cardiovascular symptoms or even cardiac failure.[110] Clinically, intrapulmonary sequestrations are generally latent until infection leads to symptoms, usually in mid-childhood but occasionally in late adulthood. Symptoms include fever and cough, and possibly suppuration and hemoptysis. Rarely, lesions with a high blood flow may present with cardiovascular symptoms. Before symptoms occur, the lesion may be discovered coincidentally on chest radiographs taken for another reason. Physical examination reveals signs of consolidation and, possibly, a systolic bruit over the affected area. The chest radiograph may reveal a cystic (Fig. 72-18), reasonably aerated, or solid area of lung parenchyma (Fig. 72-19). When this area fails to clear after a course of appropriate medical therapy, the presence of a malformation such as sequestration should be considered, particularly if the lesion is localized to the posterior basal segment of the left lower lobe, where sequestrations are most commonly found (Figs. 72-18, 72-19). Bronchoscopy usually is not necessary unless an alternative diagnosis such as inhaled foreign body is suspected. Bronchography can be misleading; dye failing to enter a

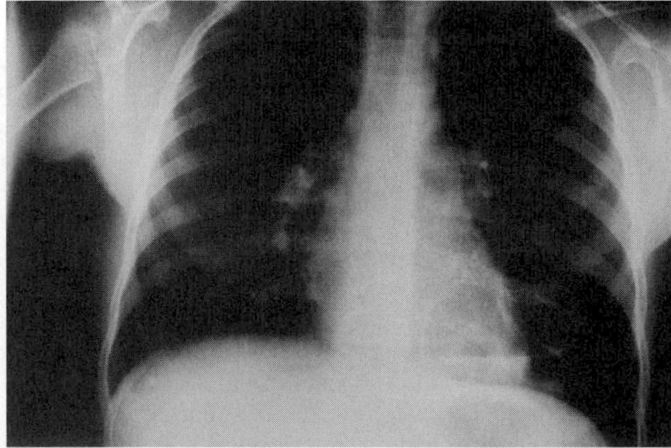

Fig. 72-18. Intrapulmonary sequestration. The multicystic lesion in the left lower lobe seen on the chest radiograph of this patient was causing problems with recurrent infection, leading to fluid-filled cysts with air-fluid levels. At surgical resection, the lesion was found to have a systemic blood supply and histology was compatible with the diagnosis of sequestration.

bronchus is not unique to sequestration and may result from any number of causes, such as a mucus plug, foreign body, bronchial atresia, or simply a technical error. Once the clinical diagnosis is suspected from the history, physical examination, and chest radiograph findings, CT scanning with contrast or angiography is the next investigation of choice. All parenchymal lung lesions should be suspected as having abnormal vasculature, and the unpredictability of the vascular connections necessitates that both the arterial supply and venous drainage be outlined in each case.[107,111,112] Balloon occlusion or embolization of the aberrant systemic arteries at the time of catheterization deserves consideration in all patients with sequestration.[107,111] Some patients may have a considerable shunt through this anomalous circuit,[110,113] to the extent that, once the segment has been removed, the improvement in cardiovascular status may be striking.[112] In addition to the hemodynamic load imposed on the cardiovascular system, some reports have suggested that systemic pressures and flow influence the pathogenesis of these lesions and contribute to the development of cystic degeneration.[9] In support of this, one case report involving an older child describes complete resolution of symptoms, signs, and chest radiograph changes in an abnormal lobe following ligation of the aberrant systemic vascular supply.[114] This lobe had all the features of classical sequestration with apparently no bronchial connection seen on bronchography. On the basis of this and other evidence, it seems reasonable to consider embolization of the systemic arterial supply as the first step in the management of all patients with sequestration because this would allow the option of expectant management for a subsequent reasonable period. An additional benefit would be that if surgical resection later was deemed necessary, the risk of vascular complications at operation, a major source of morbidity and mortality in these patients, would be greatly reduced.[107,111] Infarction of the lung or abnormal segment following occlusion of the aberrant systemic artery supply has been postulated as a potential hazard following aberrant arterial embolization, although it has not been reported.[107,111] This is not entirely surprising because the bronchial circulation to these congenitally abnormal areas is generally found to be normal. Surgical resection of a sequestered segment is not to be taken lightly. Much of the recognized operative morbidity and mortality appears to be caused by unexpected vascular complications encountered during surgery performed without accurate preoperative assessment.[108,115] In the absence of perioperative complications, surgical resection of the abnormal segment is usually curative.

Extrapulmonary Sequestration. The embryogenesis of extrapulmonary sequestration has been discussed earlier. Synonyms for this lesion include accessory lung and Rokitansky lobe. The definition is similar to that of intrapulmonary sequestration except for its location, namely, a bronchopulmonary mass with normal or anomalous arterial supply or venous drainage, situated outside the boundary formed by the pleural layer surrounding the rest of the lung. Extrapulmonary sequestrations occasionally communicate with intrapulmonary structures, or may have a rudimentary connection to a part of the foregut. There is a high association with other congenital anomalies, particularly diaphragmatic hernias, and occasionally intrapulmonary sequestration.[84] Approximately 90% of extrapulmonary sequestrations occur on the left side and a similar percentage have an aberrant systemic arterial supply. The aberrant artery almost always arises within the thorax, most commonly from the thoracic aorta, and is usually small with a low blood flow through the lesion. Venous drainage is characteristically anomalous to the right atrium, vena cava, or azygos systems, but may be normal.[14] Clinical symptoms are usually absent or minor and these lesions are commonly diagnosed coincidentally during investigation of, or surgery for, an associated abnormality. Surgical resection may be necessary in symptomatic cases and is usually not difficult, with a prognosis generally determined by the accompanying anomalies, if present.

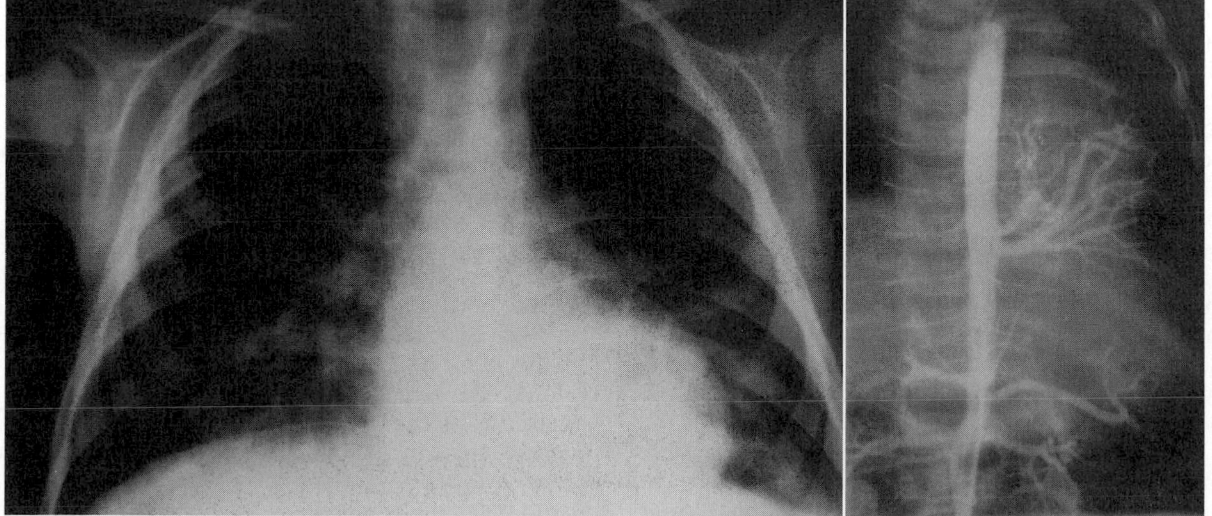

Fig. 72-19. Intrapulmonary sequestration. Chest radiograph showing patchy consolidation in the left lower lobe that failed to clear despite prolonged antibiotic therapy *(left).* The diagnosis of sequestration was suspected and subsequently confirmed when angiography demonstrated the presence of two large aberrant systemic arteries arising from the abdominal aorta and supplying the abnormal segment *(right).* Large arteries such as those seen here should always be considered for embolization before surgery in order to lessen the risk of perioperative hemorrhagic complications.

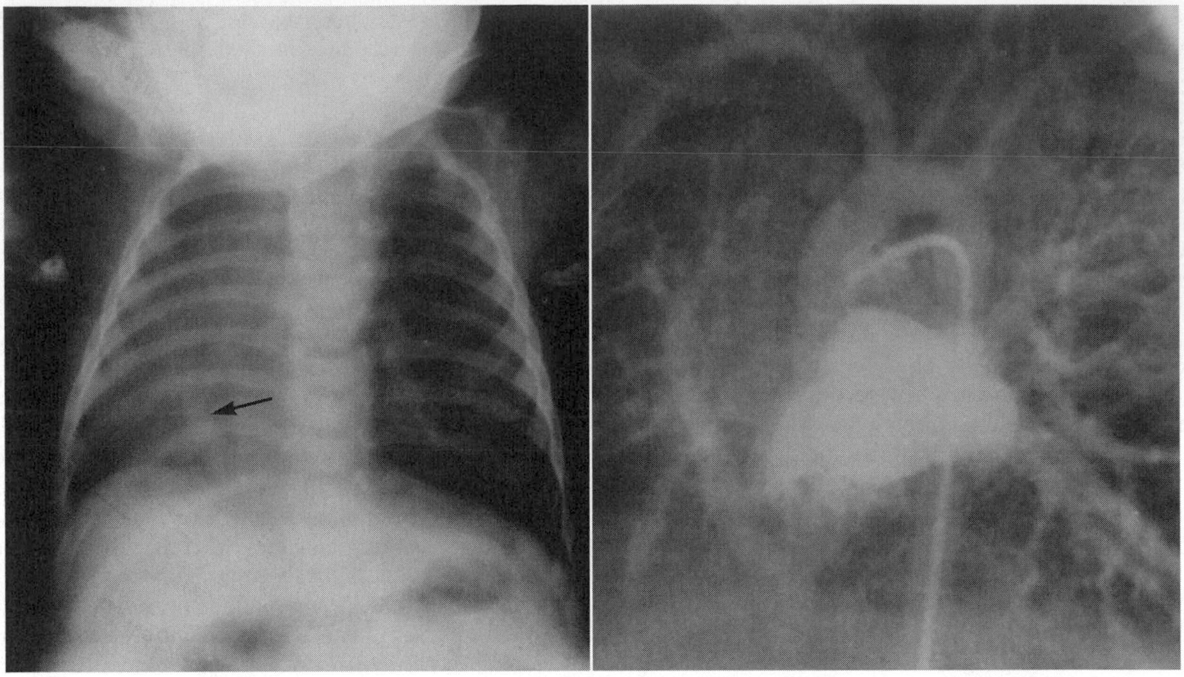

Fig. 72-20. Scimitar syndrome. Chest radiograph *(left)* demonstrating the scimitar-shaped shadow *(arrow)* that represents the anomalous vein and gives the syndrome its name. Angiography *(right)* subsequently confirmed this shadow to be the scimitar vein draining the right lung anomalously to the inferior vena cava.

Scimitar Syndrome. Scimitar syndrome covers a range of anomalies traditionally affecting the right lung, although at least one case has been described on the left. The cardinal feature is partial or hemianomalous venous drainage of the affected lung with one or more associated features, ranging from minor abnormalities of bronchial branching or lobulation to a complex lesion comprising hypoplastic right lung with abnormal lobulation and bronchial branching, dextrocardia, hypoplastic pulmonary arterial supply to the right upper zone, aberrant systemic arterial supply to the right lower zone, and anomalous venous drainage of a major portion or whole of the right lung. The shape of the anomalous vein, which can be visualized on the chest radiograph in at least 40% of cases, is akin to a Turkish scimitar, from which this syndrome derives its name (Fig. 72-20).[116] Because there is a wide range of anatomic variation in Scimitar syndrome, each component feature is discussed separately.

Bronchopulmonary airway. The right lung can be markedly hypoplastic or of normal size. The lung is usually unilobar or bilobar, and if there are three lobes they are abnormally shaped with abnormal bronchial branching patterns. Mediastinal shift is proportional to the degree of right lung hypoplasia. Intrinsic anomalies of the bronchial walls, mainly cartilage and connective tissue, are common but cilial function is normal.

Arterial supply. In over 50% of cases, an aberrant systemic artery is present that usually arises below the diaphragm (most commonly from the celiac axis, abdominal aorta, or hepatic artery) and pierces the diaphragm to supply the right lower zone (Fig. 72-21). Multiple vessels are common, arising sometimes from both the abdominal and thoracic aorta. The aberrant arteries vary in size from minute vessels to substantial channels. Histologically, they are of the elastic pulmonary type and are certainly not bronchial arteries, which have been shown to be normal in these lesions.[10] When the right lower zone has an aberrant systemic supply, the right upper zone is supplied by a hypoplastic right pulmonary artery with abnormal branching patterns, which, together with the left pulmonary artery, may show vascular wall changes consistent with prolonged exposure to pulmonary hypertension, which is commonly found in these patients particularly when pulmonary hypoplasia is marked.[117] In patients with severe right lung hypoplasia an abnormal branch from the right pulmonary artery may be seen traversing the midline into the left hemithorax to supply a crossover segment of right lung or forming part of the isthmus of a horseshoe lung (Fig. 72-22). This phenomenon has been described as a rare variant of Scimitar syndrome[107,111] and is discussed in greater detail later in this chapter. Even in the absence of an aberrant systemic arterial supply, the right pulmonary artery is often abnormal, with minimal to moderate hypoplasia and abnormal branching patterns, although in mild cases this may be difficult to recognize. Very rarely, there is a mixed pulmonary and systemic arterial supply to part or all of the abnormal segment.[107,111]

Venous drainage. One of the most significant features of Scimitar syndrome is that the area drained by the anomalous vein most commonly involves the whole or major portion of the right lung; most interestingly, this area rarely corresponds to that perfused by the aberrant arterial supply (Figs. 72-20, 72-21). The vein usually drains into the inferior vena cava at or below the diaphragm, whereas other sites of anomalous venous entry include directly to right atrium, the superior vena cava, and azygos systems.[118] Occasionally there may be more than one anomalous vein.[107,111,119] A small portion of the right upper lobe may drain normally to the left atrium, and very rarely the whole right lung drains to the left atrium but by an abnormal route. Narrowing at the distal end of the anomalous vein or at its insertion into the vena cava is a rare but important occurrence because it may cause flow obstruction and raised pulmonary venous pressure in the affected lung.

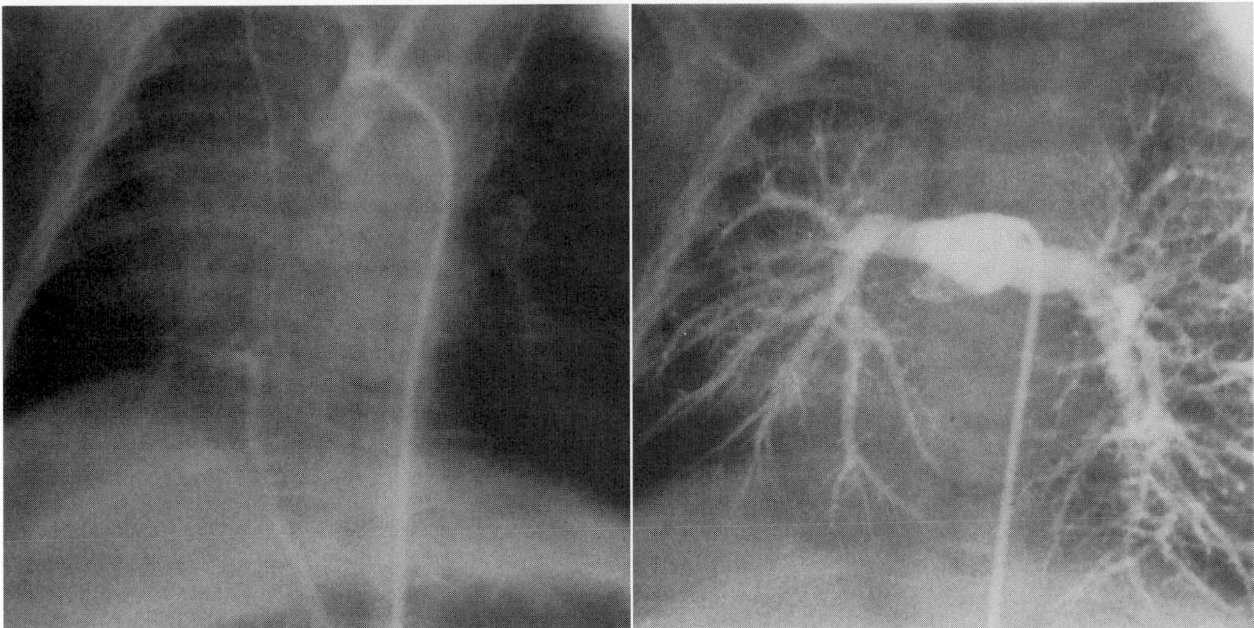

Fig. 72-21. Scimitar syndrome. Arteriography in the patient seen in Fig. 72-20 shows a hyperplastic right pulmonary artery with an abnormal branching pattern *(right)* and an aberrant systemic arterial supply arising from the abdominal artery, piercing the diaphragm, and supplying a segment of the right lower lobe *(left)*. The aberrant artery in this instance is small and not causing any significant hemodynamic disturbance.

Associated congenital lesions. Associated malformations, including diaphragmatic, cardiovascular, gastrointestinal, and other respiratory tract anomalies, are found in over 50% of patients with Scimitar syndrome.[107,111] Cardiac malformations are the most common, with atrial septal defect, patent ductus arteriosus, ventricular septal defect, and tetralogy of Fallot the most commonly recognized.[118] In a number of cases, with the severe form of Scimitar syndrome the right hemidiaphragm is elevated and dome-shaped secondary to marked right lung hypoplasia.[107,111] The diaphragmatic muscle is intrinsically normal, so this is not a true eventration. The dome may contain liver, and on the chest radiograph this gives the appearance of consolidation in the right base. This appearance has been called pseudosequestration.[120] Right-sided diaphragmatic hernia has been described in association with Scimitar syndrome.[119] Bronchogenic cysts and extrapulmonary sequestrations are other respiratory tract anomalies that have been found in association with Scimitar syndrome.[119] Associated gastrointestinal malformations are rare but may include gastric duplication cysts and anal anomalies.

Clinically, patients can be divided into three groups—severe, intermediate, and mild—according to the severity of their presenting symptoms.

Severe form. Patients with the full syndrome usually present in the neonatal period or early infancy with hemodynamic and respiratory problems. On physical examination the child is dyspneic but rarely cyanotic. The right chest may be obviously smaller than the left, in which case air entry and chest wall movement will be noticeably reduced on that side. The apex beat is shifted to the right and a heart murmur may be heard, even in the absence of an associated cardiac defect. Cardiac signs and symptoms may be mild (limited to a tachycardia) or severe, with evidence of pulmonary hypertension or congestive cardiac failure. The ECG is said to be characteristic in some patients, although generally the changes are nonspecific and can be attributed to axis rotation, dextropositioning, and right ventricular overload, in addition to any features of associated cardiac abnormalities. On the chest radiograph, a "white-out" of the right lung, obvious mediastinal shift to the right, narrowing of the right intercostal rib spaces, an elevated right hemidiaphragm, and a hyperinflated left lung all indicate

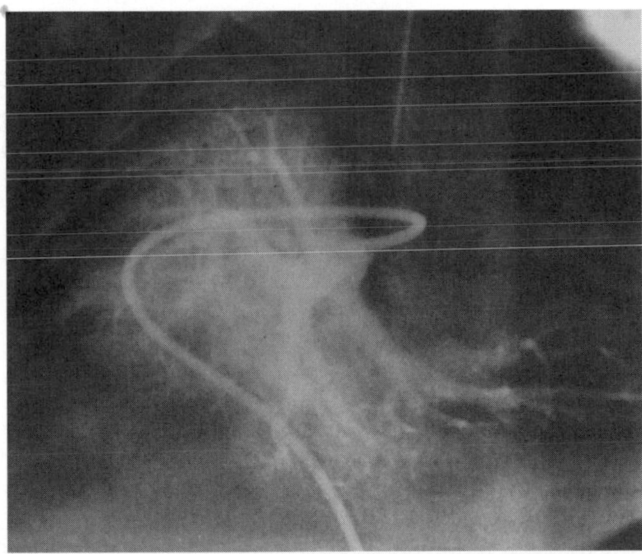

Fig. 72-22. Crossover lung segment. Pulmonary ateriography in this patient with Scimitar syndrome and hyperplastic right lung demonstrates a branch of the right pulmonary artery crossing the midline into the left hemithorax. In some patients this has been shown to supply a segment of lung that represents the isthmus of a horseshoe lung. However, in this patient, who later came to surgery for an associated cardiac anomaly, the segment crossing into the left hemithorax was shown to have no connection with the left lung and therefore represents a crossover lung segment, not the isthmus of a horseshoe lung.

severe right lung hypoplasia. This picture in a neonate is not specific for Scimitar syndrome, but a lucent, small lung with a Scimitar shadow in the right lung would strongly support this clinical diagnosis. Primary right lung aplasia or severe hypoplasia, atelectasis, and infection must be considered in the differential diagnosis. A right-sided eventration or diaphragmatic hernia would tend to shift the mediastinum to the left and therefore should not be confused with this group of lesions. Cardiac catheterization is essential for specific diagnosis and planning of management. Separate pulmonary and aortic contrast injections outline the extent of normal and aberrant arterial supply to the right lung, and on follow-through the anomalous venous drainage is depicted. The hemodynamic mechanisms involved are complicated. The reduction in size of the pulmonary vascular bed leads to increase in the pulmonary vascular resistance. In most patients, the normal pulmonary blood flow is supplemented by an aberrant systemic arterial supply to the right lower zone, hemianomalous venous drainage, and possibly a left-to-right intracardiac shunt. This increased blood flow through the high-resistance pulmonary circuit increases the hemodynamic load on the right ventricle. Blood flow through the anomalous circuit, where the resistance can be very low, can range from trivial to very high, with a pulmonary to systemic shunt ratio of greater than 3:1.[121] It is not surprising therefore that pulmonary artery pressures may range from normal to above systemic.

From the preceding description, it seems that the severity of symptoms and, indeed, the prognosis in this group of patients appears to be related mainly to three factors: the degree of right lung hypoplasia, the flow of blood through the anomalous circuit, and the associated cardiac defects. Most infants presenting in the neonatal period do badly, with a mortality rate of greater than 80%. Ligation of the aberrant systemic arteries is usually the most successful first-stage procedure in infants presenting with hemodynamic problems.[122,123] Balloon occlusion or embolization of the feeding vessels is an attractive alternative to surgical ligation.[107,111,122] Reversal of pulmonary hypertension and cardiac failure with general clinical improvement is now well recognized following this procedure[122-124] and may tide these patients over until they are old enough for definitive repair. The options would then include continued conservative management, correction of anomalous venous return,[38,121] lobectomy, and pneumonectomy. The optimal age for definitive surgery is influenced by the patient's symptoms and the skill and confidence of the surgeon. Reimplantation of the anomalous vein is best deferred until at least 3 years of age and preferably later if symptoms allow. Prognosis for good restoration of function is best when there is a well-developed right lung and right pulmonary artery and the lung has been free from infection. Pneumonectomy under 1 year of age is almost always fatal, and in this age group all efforts should be directed at conservative or staged surgical management. Unfortunately, despite removal of the aberrant systemic supply and correction of any associated cardiac defect that may have been present, many patients who present in infancy continue to do badly. High pulmonary artery pressures may persist, leading to the development of irreversible pulmonary vascular disease. Airway problems predispose to recurrent infections, which may affect both lungs and are usually difficult to treat, often involving resistant organisms such as *Pseudomonas* species. Death may result from cardiac failure or severe pulmonary infection. Encouraging reports, however, indicate that with earlier diagnosis, a better understanding of the hemodynamic and respiratory problems associated with this condition, and improved management techniques, survival will improve.[107,111,122]

Intermediate form. Patients with intermediate forms of Scimitar syndrome typically have a better-developed right lung and right pulmonary artery, with possibly a small associated aberrant systemic arterial supply to the right lower zone. Symptoms are usually those of recurrent infections, which may occasionally result in the development of bronchiectasis. Cardiac symptoms such as dyspnea on effort and signs of right ventricular overload may develop late. The diagnosis is suggested by the history and physical findings and supported by evidence of right lung hypoplasia and the presence of a Scimitar sign on the chest radiograph. A heart murmur may be heard on auscultation. Diagnosis is confirmed with cardiac catheterization. Management options are similar to those of patients in the severe group, with the choice dictated by the severity of the symptoms. Prophylactic occlusion of the systemic arterial supply in patients with no evidence of hemodynamic disturbance also deserves consideration, if only to facilitate subsequent surgery.[107,111]

Mild form. Patients with mild forms of Scimitar syndrome typically have a good-sized right lung with partial or hemianomalous venous drainage and a small or absent aberrant arterial supply. They may be totally asymptomatic or have minor symptoms or recurrent chest infections. Most of these patients are diagnosed in adulthood. Conservative management is usually adequate, although surgical reimplantation of the anomalous vein into the left atrium may be considered in symptomatic patients with a large shunt. Very rarely, a bronchiectatic area requires surgical resection.

Horseshoe Lung and Crossover Lung Segment. Horseshoe lung is an extremely rare malformation in which the left and right lungs are joined by an isthmus across the midline.[5,125] The connection is formed by the pleura and lung connective tissue, with no communication between the left and right bronchopulmonary airway or pulmonary vasculature. Similar anomalies have been described in association with right lung hypoplasia and other features consistent with Scimitar syndrome. In contrast to the typical horseshoe lung, the "isthmus" in these lesions (invariably arising from an abnormal hypoplastic right lung) does not connect to the opposite lung, despite extending well into the left hemithorax. Because no true isthmus is formed, this anomaly cannot be classified as a horseshoe lung, and in one case described, it has been called a crossover lung segment (Fig. 72-22).[107,111] These two conditions, crossover lung segment and horseshoe lung, are obviously closely related, although the distinction is more than academic because it influences surgical management. Both of these anomalies should probably be regarded as variants of Scimitar syndrome.

Other Bronchopulmonary Malformations that May Have Anomalous Vasculature. Bronchopulmonary anomalies that traditionally have a normal pulmonary artery supply and venous drainage are occasionally found to have anomalous vasculature. Examples include bronchogenic cysts, simple parenchymal cysts, cystic adenomatoid malformation, congenital cystic bronchiectasis, and lobar emphysema. These are discussed earlier in this chapter.

PULMONARY VASCULAR OR LYMPHATIC MALFORMATIONS

In this section, isolated malformations of the pulmonary arterial, arteriovenous, venous, and lymphatic systems with no associated abnormality of the bronchopulmonary airway are discussed.

Pulmonary Vascular Anomalies

Abnormalities of the intrapulmonary arteries secondary to congenital heart disease, such as pulmonary artery hypoplasia in tetralogy of Fallot or pulmonary valve atresia, are not considered to be primary abnormalities of lung development and are not discussed here. The pulmonary artery sling syndrome is discussed earlier in the chapter and pulmonary artery hypoplasia, inextricably linked to pulmonary lung hypoplasia, is discussed in the section dealing with abnormalities of the lung unit as a whole. Peripheral pulmonary artery stenoses can occur as isolated phenomena, but are more commonly associated with conditions such as rubella syndrome and Williams syndrome (idiopathic hypercalcemic syndrome of the newborn).

To date, the categorization of primary anomalies of pulmonary venous drainage and their relationship to lung anomalies remains unclear. Embryologically, the pulmonary venous plexus develops from the splanchnic vascular plexus, which lies in the mesenchyme surrounding the developing bronchial tree and foregut. The venous channels formed from this plexus drain into the respective posterior and common cardinal veins, and these in turn communicate freely across the midline with each other and with the vitello-umbilical veins. The connection between the pulmonary venous plexus and the cardinal system of veins is normally lost at an early age when communication is established with the pulmonary veins. The pulmonary veins from each lung grow to fuse with the central stem of the pulmonary vein, which develops from the sinus venosus. The stem of the pulmonary vein later becomes incorporated in the common atrium and, following the development of the interatrial septum, the four pulmonary veins drain into the left atrium.[126] The pulmonary veins normally drain both the pulmonary and bronchial artery systems. When anomalies of pulmonary venous drainage are thought to result from abnormal development of the extrapulmonary parts of the venous system, they are generally regarded as abnormalities of cardiovascular development. When however, the anomalous pulmonary venous drainage is abnormally distributed both in its intrapulmonary and extrapulmonary portion, it could be argued that this anomaly may have originated from a primary maldevelopment of lung mesenchyme. Further confusion arises when anomalies of venous drainage are found in association with malformations of lung parenchyma such as Scimitar syndrome, intrapulmonary and extrapulmonary sequestrations, congenital parenchyma cysts, congenital lymphangiectasia, and, occasionally, cystic adenomatoid malformation, when they are obviously the result of a primary abnormality in lung development and are therefore classified as such. A prime example would be a case of Scimitar syndrome with partial or hemianomalous venous drainage of the right lung, but no detectable associated abnormalities of lung parenchyma. We therefore classify this venous anomaly as a primary maldevelopment of lung. In congenital lymphangiectasia, the commonly associated anomalies of pulmonary venous drainage, interlobular septa, and other connective tissue elements suggests a primary abnormality affecting all or most of the mesenchymal elements during lung development. More information on the embryogenesis of the pulmonary venous drainage in these different circumstances is needed before these anomalies can be categorized properly.

Area of Lung with Systemic Arterial Blood Supply

Isolated aberrant systemic arterial supply to a normal area of lung with no detectable intrinsic abnormality of the bronchopulmonary airway appears to be an extremely rare phenomenon. The embryology is discussed earlier in this chapter. The lesion is said to occur most commonly in the lower lobes, particularly the left lower lobe, and symptoms are mild, with recurrent infections the most common presenting complaint.[127] An aberrant systemic arterial supply to a normally developing segment of lung was described by Boyden[10] in a 41-mm embryo, but postnatally the vascular anomaly almost always coexists with an abnormality of the bronchopulmonary airway or lung parenchyma. This has led to the suggestion that parenchymal abnormalities found in many bronchovascular anomalies are, at least in part, the result of the systemic pressures present in the aberrant artery.[9] Two points refute this postulate: the aberrant systemic artery in intrapulmonary sequestration has been shown to supply a part of the surrounding normal lung with no apparent ill effects[7] and aberrant systemic arteries secondary to congenital heart disease, as in pulmonary atresia, do not cause parenchymal damage, even after many years. Management of patients with systemic arterial supply to an area of normal lung is usually conservative in the absence of complications. Embolization or surgical ligation of the aberrant vessel should be considered if symptoms are present because of a large "shunt" through the anomalous circuit.

Intrapulmonary Arteriovenous Malformations

Pulmonary arteriovenous malformations are fistulous communications between arteries and veins at capillary or arteriolar level resulting from an underlying connective tissue defect in these vessels. These malformations function as a right-to-left shunt delivering unoxygenated blood directly into the systemic circulation. Multiple pulmonary arteriovenous malformations are found in 14% of patients with hereditary telangiectasia,[128,129] an autosomal dominant condition in which telangiectases may occur in any organ in the body. These patients account for approximately half of the cases of pulmonary AV fistula. Primary pulmonary arteriovenous malformations form the majority of the remaining cases, and may be single but are usually multiple. Other forms of fistulous communication in the lung parenchyma occur in hemangiomata (extremely rare) and bronchovascular anomalies such as sequestration and Scimitar syndrome, or secondary to trauma and infection. Symptoms develop in up to 50% of patients with pulmonary arteriovenous malformations but usually only in the second or third decade.[5] They include bleeding with hemoptysis, or cyanosis when a large pulmonary-to-systemic vascular shunt occurs through the malformation. Finger clubbing and polycythemia may be present and a systolic or continuous murmur may be heard over the lesion. Rarely, seeding of emboli from infected lesions can cause cerebral ischemia or abscess formation. Spontaneous rupture of the lesion has been reported.[130]

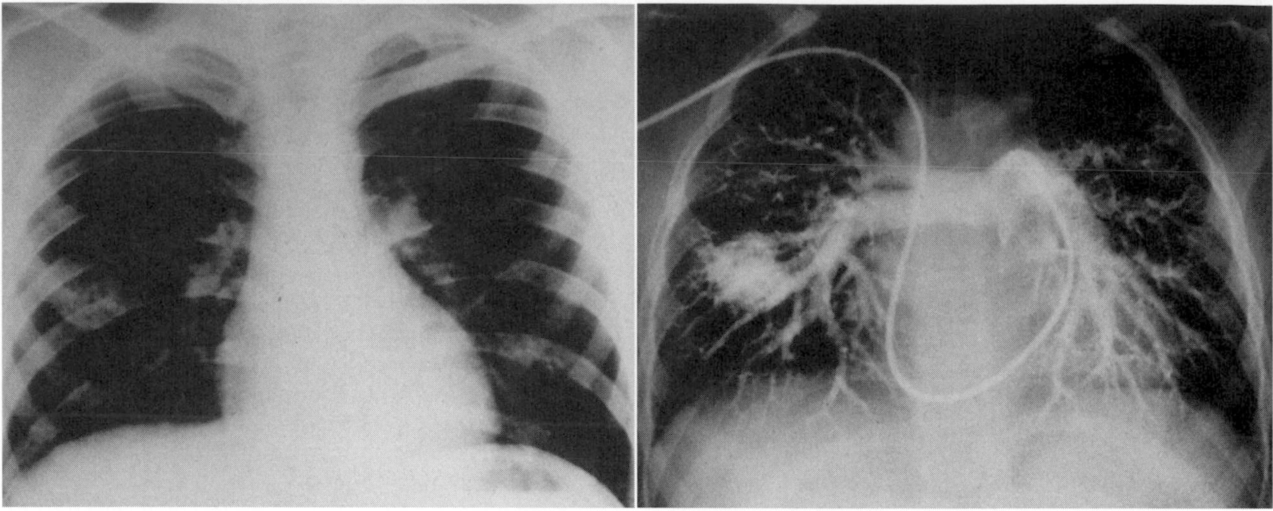

Fig. 72-23. Pulmonary arteriovenous malformation. The chest radiograph *(left)* in a patient with cyanosis, finger clubbing, and a bruit heard in the right chest revealed a rounded parenchymal shadow in the right lung, which was confirmed on pulmonary arteriography *(right)* to represent a large pulmonary arteriovenous malformation.

Evidence of telangiectasis in other organs (such as the skin), epistaxis, or gastrointestinal bleeding suggests the diagnosis of hereditary telangiectasia and relatives should be examined for evidence of telangiectases. Single or multiple nonspecific, poorly defined parenchymal radiodensities may be seen on the chest radiograph, although pulmonary angiography is necessary for definitive diagnosis (Fig. 72-23). In the past, treatment consisted of surgical resection of the arteriovenous malformation or segment of lung involved. Currently, vascular occlusion techniques during cardiac catheterization have proved equally successful and less invasive. Both forms of treatment result in increased blood flow to the remaining lung, and this increase in flow may reveal additional arteriovenous malformations hitherto unnoticed, or impart additional stress on other inherently weak areas, leading to the development of new lesions. In these patients, vascular occlusion of the new lesions can be repeated if clinically indicated. The number of repeats, however, is limited by the accumulative reduction in the size of the pulmonary vascular bed with each attempt. Although the prognosis in patients with multiple pulmonary arteriovenous malformations remains poor, there has been some improvement with the development of these vascular occlusion techniques.

Congenital Lymphangiectasia

Lymphatic development is first seen in the lung from about the 8th week of intrauterine life. By the 14th week, the lymphatic plexuses are well established and from the 20th week, growth of other mesenchymal connective tissue elements predominates, with the pulmonary lymphatics becoming less conspicuous.[131] Congenital lymphangiectasia results from continued proliferation of the lymphatic network beyond the 20th week of intrauterine life. Associated abnormalities such as asplenia, congenital heart disease, and bronchopulmonary and pulmonary vascular anomalies are found in more than half the cases.[132] Usually the lymphangiectatic changes are generalized, with multiple small cysts less than 5 mm in diameter giving a "foam rubber" appearance on cross-section, but noncystic forms are described. Microscopy shows increased numbers of dilated lymphatic channels and often exaggerated lobulation. The absence of muscular hypertrophy in the walls of the dilated lymphatic channels distinguishes primary intrapulmonary lymphangiectasia from dilation secondary to extrapulmonary anomalies of the lymphatic system such as thoracic duct obstruction. Occasionally, large cystic cavities are found, more commonly in the rarer form of lymphangiectasia in which the lesion is limited to a lobe or segment of lung. Generalized lymphangiectasia almost invariably presents soon after birth with tachypnea, intercostal recession, and usually cyanosis. On auscultation, the lungs may sound surprisingly normal. The chest radiograph classically shows a diffuse reticulonodular shadowing throughout the lung fields that fails to clear with time or diuretic treatment. Only symptomatic treatment can be offered to these patients, and more than half die within 24 hours of birth. Some patients may survive to a few weeks of age with severe dyspnea, cyanosis, and recurrent infections.[133] Pulmonary lymphangiectasia is commonly found in association with, or secondary to, obstructed anomalous pulmonary venous return (approximately 30% of cases).[134] The diagnosis becomes manifest when symptoms and chest radiograph changes fail to resolve following surgical correction of the vascular anomaly. The prognosis in this group tends to be slightly better than in the group with isolated generalized pulmonary lymphangiectasia, although it is still very poor. Patients with localized lobar involvement may present later in childhood, usually with infection. These lesions are amenable to surgical resection, although preoperative assessment must include investigations of associated anomalies of pulmonary vasculature.

Pulmonary lymphangiomyomatosis, a condition found only in women after puberty[135] and associated with tuberous sclerosis, is probably not related to congenital lymphangiectasia, although the histologic features may be very similar.

ANOMALIES OF THE THORACIC CAGE

Musculoskeletal abnormalities of the thoracic cage affecting lung development are discussed in Chapter 62. This section deals only with abnormalities of the diaphragm and thoracic outlet that may affect the lung.

Congenital Pneumatocele (Pulmonary Hernia)

Congenital absence of the endothoracic fascia in the cervical thoracic outlet region results in herniation of lung tissue into the neck. This is a rare abnormality presenting in the neonatal period as bilateral supraclavicular masses that increase in size with crying. The infants are usually asymptomatic, although local tenderness and slight dyspnea have been observed. Treatment is usually superfluous. Pulmonary hernias may also be seen in the axilla or in musculoskeletal defects of the thoracic wall, where more commonly they are secondary to trauma.[30]

Diaphragmatic Abnormalities

Diaphragmatic hernias are common congenital lesions representing approximately 8% of major congenital anomalies, whereas other diaphragmatic anomalies such as eventration, duplication, congenital absence, and accessory diaphragm are very rare.[136] The diaphragm is formed by the septum transversum and the dorsal mesentery. The posterolateral zone containing the foramen of Bochdalek is the last to be completed and arrested development in this area could lead to herniation through the widened foramen. Normally the foramen is sealed by pleural and peritoneal membranes around the 6th to 8th week and therefore hernia formation after this stage would be enclosed in a sac. The diaphragmatic muscle is formed by mesoderm developing between the pleuroperitoneal membranes after the 8th week of fetal life. Development of this layer may be insufficient, resulting in an eventration. Diaphragmatic hernias appear at three major sites: foramen of Bochdalek (over 90%), anterior foramen of Morgagni (1% to 5%), and esophageal hiatus (1% to 5%).[137]

Bochdalek Hernia (Posterolateral Hernia)

This is the most common type of congenital hernia, occurring in approximately 4.8 per 10,000 live newborn infants, and represents over 90% of all diaphragmatic lesions. It is found on the left in 80% to 90% of cases, with no hernial sac in 90%, and is twice as common in boys as in girls. It may contain small intestine, colon, stomach, and rarely kidney, liver, and spleen, depending on the affected side. The presence of associated anomalies is high and includes intestinal malrotation,[30] sequestration (often extrapulmonary), and vertebral and cardiovascular anomalies,[119] although the most significant association is pulmonary hypoplasia. During fetal life, invagination of the hernia into the thorax restricts normal lung development by a simple space-occupying effect. A large hernia early in fetal life would lead to severe pulmonary hypoplasia on the affected side and may even restrict growth on the contralateral side.[12] Sudden increase in the size of the hernia late in fetal life would merely compress already well-developed lung, with subsequent good chance of recovery following surgical reduction of the hernia after birth. Therefore, the size of the hernia at diagnosis does not necessarily reflect the extent of intrapartum pulmonary damage, which, as mentioned earlier, is the major determinant of prognosis. This explains why the most reliable prognostic indicator for this condition is the clinical condition of the child at presentation. In general terms, this means that an infant with a diaphragmatic hernia who at 24 hours of age has not required ventilatory assistance has a good prognosis and will almost certainly make a full recovery postoperatively, whereas infants requiring vigorous ventilatory assistance within 24 hours of age and before surgery have severe pulmonary hypoplasia and fare badly.[138]

Clinically, respiratory symptoms usually predominate, with tachypnea, dyspnea, and possibly cyanosis. Increased negative intrathoracic pressure associated with increased inspiratory effort tends to draw more abdominal viscera into the thoracic cavity, aggravating the respiratory difficulties. A scaphoid abdomen may be noted when a significant proportion of the abdominal contents has moved into the thorax. In an infant suspected of having diaphragmatic hernia, early institution of simple emergency measures can considerably improve the baby's condition. Simply positioning the baby upright helps reduce the weight of the abdominal contents compressing the lung, thereby easing respiration. Oxygen should be provided through a face mask or intranasal catheter if the baby is dyspneic or cyanotic. Positive-pressure bagging is contraindicated because this is likely to inflate the stomach, resulting in increased gaseous distention of the abdominal contents within the thorax and further lung compression. Passing a nasogastric tube is imperative, and will help to deflate the abdominal contents in the chest. When there is significant respiratory distress, early tracheal intubation is usually required to provide adequate assisted ventilation. On physical examination of the chest, there may be dullness to percussion on the side of the hernia, with reduced air entry and possibly borborygmi heard on auscultation. The heart and mediastinum are shifted to the opposite side, and the classic triad of dyspnea, cyanosis, and dextrocardia, with or without a scaphoid abdomen, would prompt the diagnosis of congenital diaphragmatic hernia until proven otherwise. Smaller hernias may be asymptomatic early on, presenting later with recurrent pneumonias or intermittent bowel problems such as vomiting and possibly strangulation. Standard chest radiographs should readily provide the diagnosis (Fig. 72-24). Differential diagnosis of clinical and chest radiograph findings includes other causes of cystic or solid space-occupying lesions of the lower, or whole, hemithorax, including cystic adenamatoid malformation, lobar emphysema, multicystic disease of the lung, and digestive tract duplications.

Treatment is always surgical, ideally with the patient stabilized beforehand with adequate ventilatory and cardiovascular support if necessary.[139] Mortality is generally reported to be 30% when surgery is required within the first 24 hours of life, 6% after 24 hours, and 75% in untreated cases.[140] Persistent fetal circulation is a well-recognized complication occurring in patients with diaphragmatic hernia, both preoperatively and postoperatively. Hypoxia, poor peripheral and pulmonary circulation, metabolic disturbances (particularly acidosis), and high pulmonary vascular resistance all contribute to this hazard.[139] Management should be directed at correcting all of these aspects, usually in the order listed, although some of these patients are particularly refractory to treatment. Persisting hypoxia despite nasal or face mask oxygen indicates the need for tracheal intubation and ventilation. Hyperventilation may be necessary, although this should be balanced against the increased risk in these patients of alveolar rupture and air leak, leading to pneumothorax and pneumomediastinum. Circulatory support using appropriate cardiac inotropes may be necessary, followed by pulmonary vasodilators or bicarbonate administration for acid-base correction if clinical improvement has not been achieved.[39] High-frequency ventilation, oscillatory ventilation, and extracorporeal membrane oxygenation are newer techniques used with some success in individual cases refractory to conventional management. Bowel problems postoperatively are usually self-limiting, with normal bowel function and motility restored

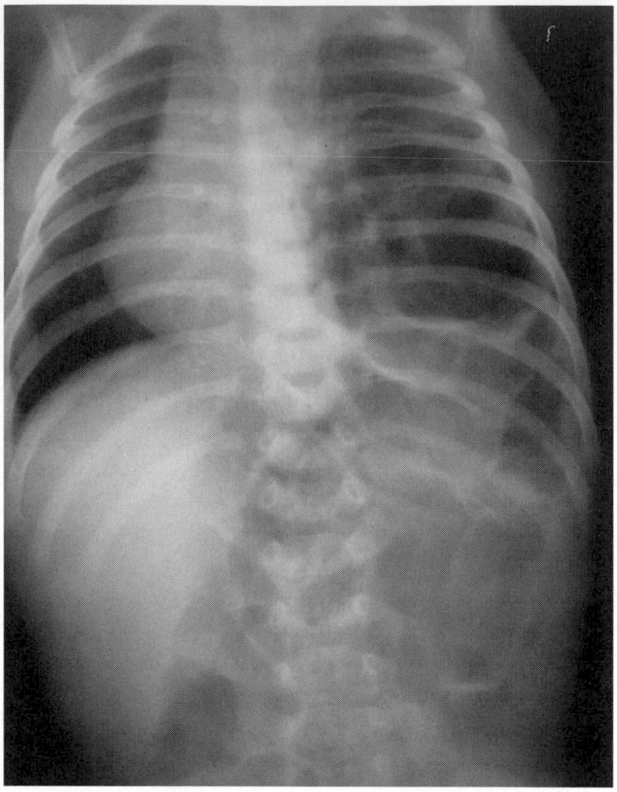

Fig. 72-24. Diaphragmatic hernia. Chest radiograph of a newborn infant showing the characteristic picture seen with a posterolateral diaphragmatic hernia (Bochdalek hernia) with absence of the left diaphragmatic shadow, the left chest filled with gas-filled loops of bowel, and the heart and mediastinum shifted to the right.

within a few days of correction. Occasionally intestinal malrotation is associated with diaphragmatic hernias and can cause persistent obstructive problems. Induction of premature delivery in fetuses diagnosed in utero by ultrasound as having a significant diaphragmatic hernia has been suggested in the past, although there are major doubts as to whether this will improve their prognosis, and it is not recommended. However, techniques for intrauterine fetal surgery are developing rapidly and may be feasible in selected severe cases. Long-term follow-up of survivors of surgery in the neonatal period shows that most of these patients have normal pulmonary function by late childhood apart from a slight reduction in vital capacity (approximately 80% of expected), probably as a result of reduced diaphragmatic efficiency and a mild degree of persisting pulmonary hypoplasia.[141]

Morgagni Hernia (Anterior Diaphragmatic Hernia)

This is the rarest form of diaphragmatic hernia. It projects through a defect found in the anterior portion of the diaphragm around the foramen of Morgagni, which is situated retrosternally. The size of the hernia is restricted because the defect is usually small; it has a sac in 50% of cases and the retrosternal space is bordered laterally by the pleural membranes and above by pericardial adherence to the upper part of the sternum. Occasionally part of the liver, stomach, or transverse colon, or one or two loops of intestine at the most, can be found in the hernia. Cardiorespiratory symptoms are often mild, and the greatest danger is strangulation of the bowel at the narrow hernial orifice. A lateral chest radiograph indicates the diagnosis, which is often difficult to make on anteroposterior films alone (Fig. 72-25). Surgery is indicated even in asymptomatic patients because there is always the risk of small bowel entering the sac and becoming strangulated.[142]

Eventration of the Diaphragm

This results from total or partial absence of muscular development in the septum transversum, resulting in abnormal elevation of one or other hemidiaphragm (more often the left), and as with diaphragmatic hernia, occurs twice as often in boys as in girls. The phrenic nerve may be smaller, but shows no signs of degeneration, which differentiates this lesion from paralysis of the diaphragm secondary to phrenic nerve damage.[143] Clinically, patients with congenital eventration can be divided into three groups according to the severity of their symptoms. The severe form presents in the newborn period, behaving similarly to diaphragmatic hernia, and most of these patients require some form of ventilatory support and possibly surgery if it appears that the child will not cope without artificial ventilation after an unacceptably long period of ventilatory support. A less severely affected group of patients present in infancy with respiratory insufficiency, dysphagia, regurgitation, and failure to thrive. The respiratory problems may be exaggerated in this age group because of increased chest wall compliance, resulting in poor chest cage support. With age, the ribs become more rigid, providing more effective splinting of the chest cage with the help of intercostal and accessory muscles. Once this stage has been reached, these infants may cope sufficiently well with their diaphragmatic weakness to avoid the need for surgery. Consequently, it is worth persevering with conservative treatment for as long as possible in these patients, with particular attention paid to adequate provision of nutrition and calories in order to promote growth. However, some patients may still require surgery before they will begin to thrive normally. Most eventrations are asymptomatic, or, at most, may be associated with a slight increase in respiratory rate and shortness of breath with exercise relative to other children of the same age. Clinical signs can be difficult to elicit but may include reduced air entry and an abnormal percussion note in the area of lung adjacent to the eventration, and ipsilateral paradoxic abdominal muscle wall movement with respiration. A number of eventrations are discovered coincidentally on routine chest radiographs. Others may present with infection in the poorly ventilated area of lung adjacent to the eventration. The infection usually responds well to antibiotics and physiotherapy, although it may recur. On the chest radiograph, the hemidiaphragm is elevated and dome-shaped and fluoroscopy demonstrates minimal displacement, or even paradoxic movement, of the affected side with respiration. Surgical management is not recommended in asymptomatic patients. Surgical treatment following failed conservative management in symptomatic patients (in both the neonatal and infant forms) consists of plication of the diaphragm, which produces a flat rigid membrane and thus eliminates the paradoxic movement of the diaphragm and the space-occupying effect created by the dome. Effectively, this increases the vital capacity, thereby improving ventilatory function. In time, the plicated diaphragm stretches, becoming gradually looser and therefore less efficient. Overall, the effectiveness of the procedure in neonates may only last for a short period (possibly as little as a few weeks in some instances). However, by this time there may be sufficient increase in lung compliance, decrease in

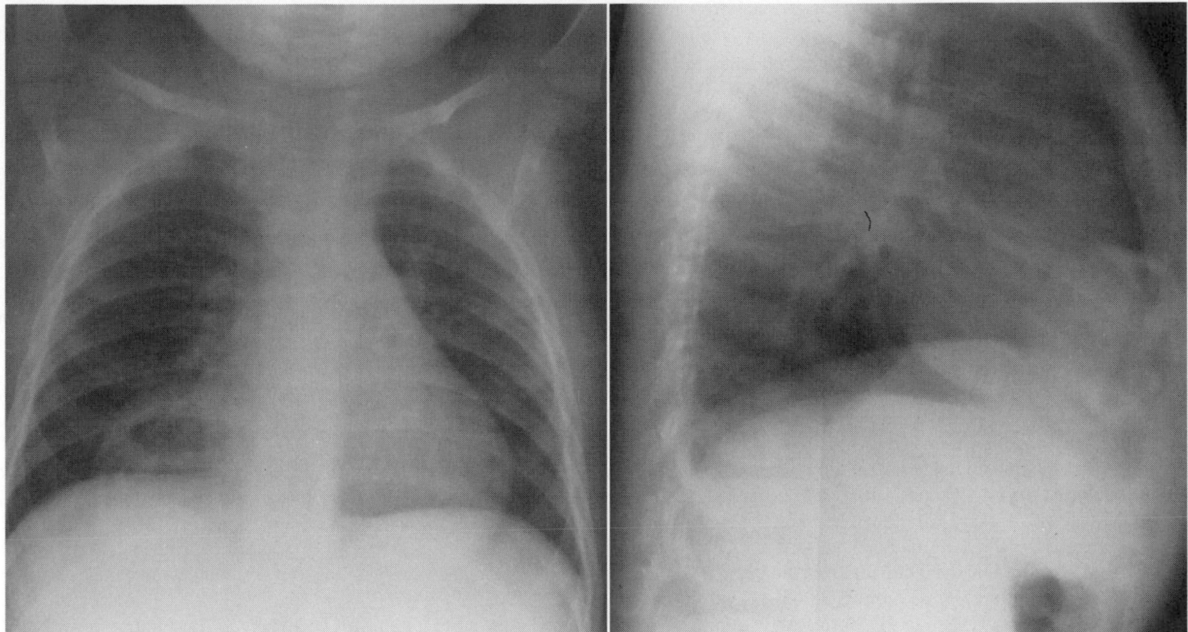

Fig. 72-25. Anterior (Morgagni) diaphragmatic hernia. Anteroposterior chest radiograph showing a rounded shadow at the right heart border *(left),* which on the lateral view showed this shadow to be multiloculated and lying anterior to the heart and immediately behind the sternum. This shadow represents loops of bowel entering the chest through a defect in the anterior foramen of Morgagni, and surgery is recommended in order to avoid the risk of bowel strangulation.

chest wall compliance, and improvement in proficiency of intercostal and accessory muscle function to enable the infant to cope better with the disability. Congenital diaphragmatic eventration is often associated with other malformations of the lung and foregut, including a range of gastrointestinal malformations, pulmonary sequestration, and Scimitar syndrome. In addition, the congenital form must be distinguished from acquired phrenic nerve paralysis as well as from diaphragmatic weakness associated with generalized myopathies or neuropathies, which in neonates can lead to major respiratory difficulties.

Esophageal Hiatus Hernia

Rarely, a defect in the esophageal hiatus is large enough to admit passage of a sac containing stomach high into the thorax. Clinical signs vary from being asymptomatic to including vomiting (92%), recurrent aspiration with repeated respiratory disease (13%), and hematemesis or anemia (25%).[144] Sometimes a rounded radiolucent shadow in the lower mediastinum may be seen on plain anteroposterior chest radiographs to indicate this lesion. Barium swallow confirms the diagnosis and may help in assessing the degree of reflux. pH monitoring and esophagoscopy can be used to assess the extent of secondary esophagitis. Treatment is initially conservative, with posturing, food thickeners, and possibly antacids. When medical treatment fails, surgery is indicated, usually with good results.[145]

Other Diaphragmatic Abnormalities

Congenital absence of the diaphragm is exceptionally rare and generally results in death. Duplication of the diaphragm has been described as a fibromuscular membrane separating one hemithorax into two cavities. It is usually to the right above a hypoplastic middle lobe. Repeated infections are the rule, and the chest radiograph shows a dense band in the right midzone with variable hypoplasia. Associated cardiorespiratory anomalies are common. Persistent symptoms may necessitate surgical resection and lobectomy.

REFERENCES

1. Macintosh R, Merritt KK, Richards MR, Samuels MH, Bellows MT: The incidence of congenital malformation, *Pediatrics* 14:505, 1954.
2. MacGregor AR: The causes of foetal and neonatal death, *Edinburgh Med J* 50:332, 1945.

Classification

3. Dubreuil G, Lacoste A, Raymond R: Les etapes du developpement du poumon humain et de son appareil elastique, *CR Soc Biol* (Paris) 121:244, 1936.
4. Committee on Pulmonary Diseases in Children: American College of Chest Physicians, Congenital pulmonary anomalies and related thoracic conditions, *Dis Chest* 49:441, 1966.
5. Landing BH: Congenital malformations and genetic disorders of the respiratory tract, *Am Rev Respir Dis* 120:150-185, 1979.
6. Clements BS, Warner JO: Pulmonary sequestration and related congenital bronchopulmonary-vascular malformations: nomenclature and classification based on anatomical and embryological considerations, *Thorax* 42:401-408, 1987.

Abnormal Lung Development

7. Pryce DM, Holmes Sellors T, Blair LG: Intralobar sequestration of lung associated with an abnormal pulmonary artery, *Br J Surg* 35:18-29, 1947.
8. de la Rue J, Paillas J, Abelanet R, Chomette G: Les bronchopneumopathies congenitales, *Bronches* 9:114, 1959.
9. Abbey-Smith R: A theory of the origin of intralobar sequestration of lung, *Thorax* 11:10-24, 1956.
10. Boyden EA: Bronchogenic cysts and the theory of intralobar sequestration: new embryologic data, *J Thorac Surg* 35:604-633, 1958.
11. Ellis AG: Congenital absence of a lung, *Am J Med Sci* 154:33, 1917.
12. Reid LM: Lung growth in health and disease, *Br J Dis Chest* 78:113-134, 1984.

13. Stovin PGI: Early lung development, *Thorax* 40:401-404, 1985.
14. Blesovsky A: Pulmonary sequestration, *Thorax* 22:351-357, 1967.
15. Shimuzi K: Pulmonary sequestration with special reference to pathogenesis of polycystic changes, *Trans Soc Pathol Jap* 58:180-186, 1969.
16. Demos NJ, Teresi A: Congenital lung malformations: a unified concept, *J Thorac Cardiovasc Surg* 70:260-264, 1975.
17. Eppinger H, Schavenstein W: Krakbeitene der Lungen, *Ergeb Allg Pathol* 8:267, 1902.
18. Sade RM, Clouse M, Ellis FH: The spectrum of pulmonary sequestration, *Ann Thorac Surg* 18:644-655, 1974.
19. Dameron F: The influence of various mesenchyma on the differentiation of the pulmonary epithelium of the chick embryo in culture in vitro, *J Embryol Exp Morphol* 9:268-274, 1961.
20. Gerle RD, Jaretzki A, Ashley CA, Berne AS: Congenital bronchopulmonary-foregut malformation, *N Engl J Med* 278:1413-1417, 1968.
21. Carter R: Pulmonary sequestration, *Ann Thorac Surg* 7:68-83, 1969.
22. Culiner MM: Intralobar bronchial cystic disease, the "sequestration complex" and cystic bronchiectasis, *Dis Chest* 53:462-469, 1968.
23. Golding MR, Kwon K, Chiu CJ, Nicastri AD: Pulmonary sequestration, *J Thorac Cardiovasc Surg* 54:121-125, 1967.
24. Haller JA, Golladay ES, Pickard LR, Tepas JJ, Shorter NA, Shermeta DW: Surgical management of lung bud anomalies: lobar emphysema, bronchogenic cyst, cystic adenomatoid malformation and intralobar pulmonary sequestration, *Ann Thorac Surg* 28:33-43, 1979.
25. Iwai K, Shindo G, Hajikano H, Tajima H, Morinoto M: Intralobar pulmonary sequestration with special reference to developmental pathology, *Am Rev Respir Dis* 107:911-920, 1973.

Abnormalities of the Lung Unit as a Whole

26. Hislip A, Reid L: Growth and development of the respiratory system—anatomical development. In Davis JA, Dobbing JW, eds: *Scientific foundations of pediatrics,* London, 1974, Heinemann, pp 214-254.
27. Wilson JG, Warkani J: Aortic-arch and cardiac anomalies in the offspring of vitamin A deficient rats, *Am J Anat* 85:113, 1949.
28. Potter EL: Pulmonary pathology of the fetus and the newborn. In *Advances in pediatrics,* vol IV, Chicago, 1952, Year Book Medical Publisher, pp 157-189.
29. Salzberg AM: Congenital malformations of the lower respiratory tract. In Kendig I, Chernick V, eds: *Disorders of the respiratory tract in children,* ed 4, Philadelphia, 1983, WB Saunders, pp 169-213.
30. Booth JB, Berry CL: Unilateral pulmonary agenesis, *Arch Dis Child* 42:361, 1967.
31. Broman I: Zurkenntis der Lungenentwicklun. I Wann und wie entsteht das definitive Lungarenparenchym? *Verh Anat Ges* (Jena) 32:83, 1923.
32. Nicks R: Agenesis of the lung with persistent ductus arteriosus, *Thorax* 12:140, 1957.
33. Shaffer AJ, Rider RV: A note on the prognosis of pulmonary agenesis and hypoplasia according to the side affected, *J Thorac Surg* 33:379, 1957.
34. Lukas DS, Dotter CT, Steinberg I: Agenesis of the lung and patent ductus arteriosus with reversal of flow, *N Engl J Med* 249:107, 1953.
35. Jeune M, Carron R, Beron D, Loaec Y: Polychondrodystrophie avec bloquage thoracique d'evolution fatale, *Pediatrie* 9:390, 1954.
36. Thomas IJ, Smith DW: Oligohydramnios, cause of the non-renal features of Potter's syndrome, including pulmonary hypoplasia, *J Pediatr* 84:811, 1975.
37. Helms P, Stocks J: Lung function in infants with congenital pulmonary hypoplasia, *J Pediatr* 101:918-922, 1982.
38. Yonehiro EG, Hallman GL, Codey DA: Anomalous pulmonary venous return from a hypoplastic right lung to the inferior vena cava (Scimitar syndrome): report of successful correction and review of surgical treatment, *Cardiovasc Res Ctr Bull* 4:106-117, 1966.

Malformations of the Larynx, Trachea, and Major Bronchi

39. Smith GJ, Cooper DM: Laryngomalacia and inspiratory obstruction in later childhood, *Arch Dis Child* 56:345-349, 1981.
40. Dubois JJ, Pokorny WJ, Harberg FJ, Smith RJ: Current management of laryngeal and laryngotracheoesophageal clefts, *J Paediatr Surg* 25:855-860, 1990.
41. Effman EL, Spackman TJ, Berdon WE: Tracheal agenesis, *Am J Roentgenol* 125:767, 1975.
42. Wolman IJ: Congenital stenosis of the trachea, *Am J Dis Child* 61:1263, 1941.
43. Cantrell JR, Gould HG: Congenital stenosis of the trachea, *Am J Surg* 108:297, 1964.
44. Cohen SR, Landing BH: Tracheostenosis and bronchial anomalies associated with pulmonary artery sling, *Ann Otol Rhinol Laryngol* 85:1-9, 1976.
45. Mounier-Kuhn P: Dilation de la trachee constatations radiographiques et bronchoscopiques, *Lyon Med* 150:106, 1932.
46. Fiser F, Tomanek A, Rimanova J, Sedivy RJ: Tracheobronchomegaly, *Scand J Respir Dis* 50:147, 1969.
47. Wanderer AA, Ellis EF, Goltz RW, Cotlon EK: Tracheobronchiomegaly and acquired cutis laxa in a child: physiologic and immunologic studies, *Pediatrics* 44:709, 1969.
48. Van Schoor J, Joos G, Pauwels R: Tracheobronchomegaly—the Mounier-Kuhn syndrome: report of two cases and review of the literature, *Eur Respir J* 4:1303-1306, 1991.
49. Ferguson CF, Neuhauser EB: Congenital absence of lung (agenesis) and other anomalies of the tracheobronchial tree, *Arch Dis Child* 35:182, 1960.
50. Williams H, Campbell P: Generalised bronchiectasis associated with deficiency of cartilage in the bronchial tree, *Arch Dis Child* 35:182, 1960.
51. Lincoln JCR, Deverall PB, Stark J, Aberdeen E, Waterston DJ: Vascular anomalies compressing the oesophagus and trachea, *Thorax* 24:295-306, 1969.
52. Phelan PD, Landau LI, Olinsky A: Respiratory noises. In *Respiratory illness in children,* ed 2, London, 1982, Blackwell Scientific Publications, pp 104-131.
53. Lynch JI: Bronchomalacia in children, *Clin Pediatr* (Phila) 9:279-282, 1970.
54. Wittenborg MH, Gyepes MT, Crocker D: Tracheal dynamics in infants with respiratory distress, stridor and collapsing trachea, *Radiology* 88:653, 1967.
55. Cox WL Jr, Shaw PR: Congenital chondromalacia of the trachea, *J Thorac Cardiovasc Surg* 49:1033, 1965.
56. Cogbill TH, Moore FA, Accurso FJ, Lilly JR: Primary tracheomalacia, *Ann Thorac Surg* 35:538-541, 1983.
57. Blair GK, Cohen R, Filler RM: Treatment of tracheomalacia, eight year's experience, *J Pediatr Surg* 21:781-785, 1986.
58. Mair EA, Parsons DS, Lally KP: Treatment of severe tracheomalacia with expanding endobronchial stents, *Arch Otolaryngol Head Neck Surg* 116:1087-1090, 1990.
59. Waterson DJ, Bonham-Carter RE, Abderdeen E: Congenital tracheo-oesophageal fistula in association with oesophageal atresia, *Lancet* 2:55, 1963.
60. Dudley NE, Phelan PD: Respiratory complications in long-term survivors of oesophageal atresia, *Arch Dis Child* 51:279, 1976.
61. Schneider KM, Becker JM: The "H-Type" tracheo-oesophageal fistula in infants and children, *Surgery* 51:677, 1962.
62. MacCartney FJ, Zuberbuhle JR, Anderson RH: Morphological considerations pertaining to recognition of atrial isomerism, *Br Heart J* 44:657-667, 1980.
63. Atwell SW: Major anomalies of the tracheobronchial tree with a list of the minor anomalies, *Dis Chest* 52:611, 1967.
64. Gonzalez-Crussi F, Padilla L-M, Miller JK, Grosfeld JL: Bridging bronchus, a previously underscribed airway anomaly, *Am J Dis Child* 130(a):1015-1018, 1976.
65. Starshak RJ, Sty JR, Wood G, Kreitzer FV: Bridging bronchus: a rare airway anomaly, *Radiology* 140:95-96, 1981.
66. Simon G, Reid L: Atresia of an apical bronchus of the left upper lobe—report of three cases, *Br J Dis Chest* 57:126, 1963.
67. Meng RL, Jensik RJ, Faber L-P, Matthew GR, Kittle CE: Bronchial atresia, *Ann Thorac Surg* 25:184, 1978.
68. Cohen AM, Solomon EH, Alfidi RJ: Computed tomography in bronchial atresia, *Am J Radiol* 135:1097-1099, 1980.
69. Swenson O: *Paediatric surgery,* ed 2, New York, 1962, Appleton-Century-Crofts.
70. Opsahl T, Berman EJ: Bronchogenic mediastinal cysts in infants. Case report and review of the literature. *Pediatrics* 30:372, 1962.
71. Grewal RG, Yip CK: Intralobar pulmonary sequestration and mediastinal bronchogenic cyst, *Thorax* 49:615-616, 1994.
72. Kirwan WO, Walbaum PR, McCormack RJM: Cystic intrathoracic derivations of the foregut and their complications. *Thorax* 28:424, 1973.
73. Maier HC: Bronchogenic cysts of mediastinum, *Ann Surg* 122:476, 1948.

74. Gross RE: *The surgery of infancy and childhood,* Philadelphia, 1953, WB Saunders.
75. Le Brigand H, Hourtoule R, Merlier M, et al: Sequestration pulmonaire et arteres anomalies. *Poumon* 10:421, 1954.
76. Bremer JL: Dorsal intestinal fistula: accessory neurenteric canal diastematomyelia, *Arch Pathol* 34:132, 1952.
77. Forsec JH, Blake HA: Pericardial celomic cyst, *Surgery* 31:753, 1952.
78. Ellis FH, Dushane JW: Primary mediastinal cysts and neoplasms in infants and children. *Am Rev Tubere Pulm Dis* 74:940, 1956.
79. Sane SM, Sieber WK, Girdany BR: Congenital bronchobiliary fistula, *Surgery* 69:599-608, 1971.
80. Lindahl H, Nyman R: Congenital bronchobiliary fistula successfully treated at the age of three days, *J Pediatr Surg* 21:734, 1986.
81. Kalayoglu M, Olcay I: Congenital bronchobiliary fistula associated with oesophageal atresia and tracheo-oesophageal fistula, *J Pediatr Surg* 11:463, 1976.
82. Cook FN, Blades B: Cystic disease of the lungs, *J Thorac Surg* 23:546, 1952.
83. Lichtenstein H: Congenital multiple cysts of the lung, *Dis Chest* 24: 646, 1953.
84. Thilenius OG, Ruschhaupt DG, Replogle RL, Bharati S, Herman T, Arcilla RA: Spectrum of pulmonary sequestration: association with anomalous pulmonary venous drainage in infants, *Paediatr Cardiol* 4:97-103, 1983.
85. Potts WJ, Riker WL: Differentiation of congenital cysts of lung and those following staphylococcal pneumonia, *Arch Surg* 61:684, 1950.
86. Spencer H: Congenital abnormalities of the lung. In *Pathology of the lung,* ed 4, Oxford 1985, Pergamon Press, pp 79-129.
87. Kwittken J, Reiner L: Congenital cystic adenomatoid malformation of the lung, *Pediatrics* 30:759, 1962.
88. Stocker JT, Madewell JE, Drake RM: Congenital cystic adenomatoid malformation of the lung. Classification and morphologic spectrum, *Hum Pathol* 8:155, 1977.
89. Madewell JE, Stocker JT, Korsower JM: Cystic adenomatoid malformations of the lung: morphologic analysis, *Am J Radiol* 124:436, 1975.
90. Merenstein GB: Congenital cystic adenomatoid malformations of the lung. Report of a case and review of the literature, *Am J Dis Child* 118:772, 1969.
91. Lincoln JCR, Stark J, Subramanian S, Aberdeen E, Bonham-Carter RE: Congenital lobar emphysema, *Ann Surg* 173:55-62, 1971.
92. Nelson RL: Congenital cystic disease of the lung, *J Pediatr* 1:233, 1932.
93. Taber P, Benveniste H, Gans SL: Delayed infantile lobar emphysema, *J Pediatr Surg* 9:245, 1974.
94. Heard BE, Khatchatours V, Otto H, Putov NV, Sobin L: The morphology of emphysema, chronic bronchitis and bronchiectasis: definition, nomenclature and classification, *J Clin Pathol* 32:882, 1979.
95. Binet JP, Nezelof C, Fredet J: Five cases of lobar tension emphysema in infancy: importance of individual malformation and value of postoperative steroid therapy. *Dis Chest* 41:126, 1962.
96. Campbell PE: Congenital labour emphysema: etiological studies, *Aust Paediatr J* 5:226, 1969.
97. Zatzkin HR, Cole PM, Bronsther B: Congenital hypertrophic lobar emphysema, *Surg St Louis* 52:502, 1962.
98. Shafir R, Jaffe R, Kalter Y: Bronchiectasis: a cause of infantile lobar emphysema, *J Pediatr Surg* 11:107, 1976.
99. Murray GF, Talbert JL, Haller JA: Obstructive lobar emphysema of the newborn infant, *J Cardiovasc Surg* 53:886, 1967.
100. Hislop A, Reid L: New pathological findings in emphysema in childhood: 1. Polyalveolar lobe with emphysema, *Thorax* 25:682, 1970.
101. Hislop A, Reid L: New pathological findings in emphysema of childhood: 2. Over-inflation of a normal lobe, *Thorax* 26:190, 1971.
102. Henderson R, Hislop A, Reid L: New pathological findings in emphysema of childhood: 3 unilateral congenital emphysema with hypoplasia and compensatory emphysema of the contralateral lung, *Thorax* 26:195, 1971.
103. Leape LL, Longino LA: Infantile lobar emphysema, *Pediatrics* 34:246-255, 1964.
104. Warner JO, Rubin S, Heard BE: Congenital lobar emphysema: a case with bronchial atresia and abnormal bronchial cartilages *Br J Dis Chest* 76:177, 1982.
105. Eigen H, Lemen RJ, Waring WW: Congenital lobar emphysema: long-term evaluation of surgically and conservatively treated children, *Am Rev Respir Dis* 113:823, 1976.
106. Corrin B, Danel C, Allaway A, Warner JO, Lenney W: Intralobar pulmonary sequestration of ectopic pancreatic tissue with gastropancreatic duplication, *Thorax* 40:630-638, 1985.
107. Clements BS, Warner JO, Shinebourne EA: Congenital bronchopulmonary vascular malformations: clinical application of a simple anatomical approach in 25 cases, *Thorax* 42:409-416, 1987.
108. Telander RL, Lennox C, Sieber W: Sequestrations of the lung in children, *Mayo Clin Proc* 51:578-584, 1976.
109. Flye MW, Conley M, Silver D: Spectrum of pulmonary sequestration, *Ann Thorac Surg* 22:478-482, 1976.
110. Masuda H, Ogata T, Tanaka S, Kikuchi K, Yoshizu H, Takagi K: Blood flow in the abnormal artery of an intralobar sequestration [English abstract], *Nippon Kyobu Geka* 32:2119-2122, 1984.
111. Clements BS, Warner JO: The crossover lung segment: congenital malformation associated with a variant of Scimitar syndrome, *Thorax* 42: 417-419, 1987.
112. Newton Turk L, Lindskog GE: The importance of angiographic diagnosis in intralobar pulmonary sequestration, *J Thorac Cardiovasc Surg* 41:299-304, 1961.
113. Solit RW, Frainow W, Wallace S, Cohn HE: The effect of intralobar pulmonary sequestration on cardiac output, *J Thorac Cardiovasc Surg* 49:844-852, 1965.
114. Makinen EO, Merikanto J, Rikalainen H, Satokari K: Intralobar sequestration occurring without alteration of pulmonary parenchyma, *Paediatr Radio* 10:237-240, 1981.
115. Briccoli A, Mastrorilli M, Spangaro M, et al: La sequestrazione polmonare, *Minerva Chiruge* 37:523-540, 1982.
116. Neill CA, Ferencz C, Sabiston DC, Sheldon H: The familial occurrence of hypoplastic right lung with systemic arterial supply and venous drainage "Scimitar syndrome," *Bull John Hopkins Hosp* 107:1-21, 1960.
117. Haworth SF, Sauer U, Buhlmeyer K: Pulmonary hypertension in Scimitar syndrome in infancy, *Br Heart J* 50:182-189, 1083.
118. Mathey J, Galey JJ, Logeais Y, Santoro E, Vanetti, Maurel A: Anomalous venous return into inferior vena cava and associated broncho-vascular anomalies (the Scimitar syndrome), *Thorax* 23:398-407, 1968.
119. Alivizatos P, Cheatle T, de Leval M, Stark J: Pulmonary sequestration complicated by anomalies of pulmonary venous return, *J Pediatr Surg* 20:76-79, 1985.
120. Macpherson RI, Whytehead L: Pseudosequestration, *J Can Assoc Radiol* 28:17-25, 1977.
121. Honey M: Anomalous pulmonary venous drainage of right lung to inferior vena cava ("Scimitar syndrome"): clinical spectrum in older patients and role of surgery, *Q J Med* 47:463-483, 1977.
122. Dickinson DF, Galloway RW, Massey R, Sankey R, Arnold R: Scimitar syndrome in infancy, *Br Heart J* 47:468-472, 1982.
123. Woody JN, Graham TP, Bradford WD, Sabiston DC, Canent RV: Hypoplastic right lung with systemic blood supply and anomalous pulmonary venous drainage: reversal of pulmonary hypertension with surgical management in infancy, *Am Heart J* 83:82-88, 1972.
124. Litwin SB, Plauth WH, Nadas AS: Anomalous systemic arterial supply to the lung causing pulmonary artery hypertension, *N Engl J Med* 238:1098-1099, 1970.
125. Cipriano P, Swenney LJ, Hutchins GH, Rosenquist GC: Horseshoe lung in an infant with recurrent pulmonary infections, *Am J Dis Child* 118:769-771, 1969.

Pulmonary Vascular or Lympahtic Malformations

126. Anderson RH, Ashley GT: Growth and development of the cardiovascular system: anatomical development. In Davis JA, Dobbing J, eds: *Scientific foundations of pediatrics,* London, 1981, Heinemann Medical.
127. Kirks DR, Otane PE, Free EA, et al: Systemic arterial supply to normal basilar segments of the left lower lobe, *Am J Roentgenol* 126:817-821, 1976.
128. Beresford OD: Hereditary haemorrhagic telangiectasia and pulmonary arteriovenous fistulae, *Br J Dis Chest* 61:219, 1976.
129. Hodgson CH, Burchell HB, Good CA, et al: Hereditary haemorrhagic telangiectasia and pulmonary arteriovenous fistulae: surgery of a large family, *N Engl J Med* 261:625, 1959.
130. Shumacker HB, Waldhausen JA: Pulmonary arteriovenous fistulae in children, *Ann Surg* 158:713, 1963.
131. Maximow AA, Bloom W: *A textbook of histology,* ed 4, Philadelphia, 1942, WB Saunders.

132. France NE, Brown RJK: Congenital lymphangiectases: report of 11 cases with special reference to cardiovascular findings, *Arch Dis Child* 46:528-532, 1971.
133. Felmen AH, Rhatigan, Pierson KK: Pulmonary lymphangiectasia. Observations in 17 patients and proposed classification, *Am J Roentgenol* 116:548, 1972.
134. Laurence KM: Congenital pulmonary cystic lymphangiectasis, *J Pathol Bacteriol* 70:325, 1970.
135. Corrin B, Liebow AA, Friedman PJ: Pulmonary lymphangeomyomatosis: a review, *Am J Pathol* 79:348-382, 1975.

Anomalies of the Thoracic Cage

136. Cantrell JR, Haller JA, Ravitch MM: The syndrome of congenital defects involving the abdominal wall, sternum, diaphragm, pericardium and heart, *Surg Gynecol Obstet* 107:602, 1958.
137. Snyder WH, Greaney EM: Congenital diaphragmatic hernia: 77 consecutive cases, *Surgery* 57:576, 1965.
138. Landau LI, Phelan PD, Gillaim GL, Coombs E, Noblett HR: Respiratory function after repair of congenital diaphragmatic hernia, *Arch Dis Child* 52:282-286, 1977.
139. Nair UR, Entres A, Walker DR: Management of neonatal posterolateral diaphragmatic hernia, *Thorax* 38:254-257, 1983.
140. MacNamara JJ, Eraklis AJ, Gross RE: Congenital postero-lateral diaphragmatic hernia in the newborn, *J Thorac Cardiovasc Surg* 55:55, 1968.
141. Wohl MEB, Griscom NT, Strieder DJ, Schuster SR, Treves S, Zwerding RE: The lung following repair of congenital diaphragmatic hernia, *J Pediatr* 90:405-414, 1977.
142. Barran EM, Houston HE, Lynn HB, O'Connell EJ: Foramen of Morgagni hernias in children, *Surgery* 62:1076, 1967.
143. Thomas VT: Congenital eventration of the diaphragm, *Ann Thorac Surg* 10:180, 1970.
144. Lilly JR, Randolph JG: Hiatal hernia and gastro-oesophageal reflux in infants and children, *J Thorac Cardiovasc Surg* 55:42, 1968.
145. Carre IJ: Management of gastro-oesophageal reflux, *Arch Dis Child* 60:71-75, 1985.

CHAPTER 73

Sleep-Disordered Breathing

Karen A. Waters and Colin E. Sullivan

Obstructive sleep apnea (OSA) is both common and life-threatening[1,2] in children. Remarkably, the level of knowledge about OSA in children has not kept up with the advances of understanding the adult disease counterpart. Extensive research has been conducted with adult OSA and sleep-related hypoventilation,[3] but the majority of research studies and conclusions determined in adult populations have yet to be validated in pediatric groups. Children with severe OSA and sleep-associated hypoventilation may only be brought to medical attention after developing complications of the disease. These complications are largely known through case reports, and include cardiac failure, developmental delay, severe growth failure, respiratory arrest under anesthetic, and daytime respiratory failure.[4,5] Children have been identified as dying suddenly in sleep when affected by this disorder (personal communications), and sudden death is commonly described in congenital anomalies that are now known to be associated with upper airway obstruction, such as Crouzon, Pierre Robin, and Down syndromes, and achondroplasia.[6] Thus it is essential that pediatricians become adept at identifying, assessing, and treating OSA and central hypoventilation in children before these complications occur.

Supported by the National SIDS Foundation of Australia and the National Health and Medical Research Council of Australia.

The authors would like to thank Dr. Margaret-Anne Harris for her critical review of the manuscript and Mr. Simon French and Ms Kellie Tinworth for their assistance with the manuscript preparation.

The dynamics of upper airway respiratory control play an active and fundamental role in protecting normal airway patency. Understanding these mechanisms is crucial to understanding and adequately treating their dysfunction, expressed clinically as OSA. The fact that episodes of airway obstruction are usually confined to sleep is no accident, and normal sleep physiology contributes further to respiratory and upper airway instability, potentiating this dysfunction.

Proper evaluation of sleep-disordered breathing in children requires that it be considered during normal sleep times and within their unique developmental framework.[7] Laboratories that have been established with a specific interest in obtaining detailed all-night sleep studies in infants and children are expanding the understanding of OSA during development.[8] Accurate evaluation of OSA in children, using detailed clinical and investigative procedures, reveals that the expression of OSA in children differs markedly from that of the adult disease.[9,10] The pathophysiology of OSA in children is presumed to be analogous to that of adults, but whereas the underlying mechanisms of OSA in children may be akin to those of adults, the standards set for evaluating severity and likelihood of complications in adult sleep apnea are not discriminatory if used to evaluate children with analogous disorders.[9]

To date, treatment of childhood OSA has essentially consisted of adenoidectomy or tonsillectomy, and this continues to be the appropriate initial treatment. Additional treatment is required in a significant number of children,[11] and nasal mask continuous positive airway pressure (CPAP) has wide application in the pediatric population as a practical and effective means of intervention.

This chapter examines the current knowledge of OSA and sleep-associated hypoventilation in children. First, the pathology and pathophysiology underlying sleep-related upper airway obstruction, as determined in adults and children, are explored. The ways to identify these disorders and their complications, specifically in children, are discussed. The final section explores the treatment modalities available for children and the circumstances in which these treatments should be implemented.

PREVALENCE

OSA can occur in all age groups from infancy to adulthood (Fig. 73-1). The age distribution of children treated for OSA in the David Read Paediatric Sleep Disorders Unit indicates that although the peak age of presentation is 2 to 4 years, the whole spectrum of ages is represented (Fig. 73-1). As an indication of the frequency of OSA in childhood, the David Read Paediatric Sleep Disorders Unit undertook over 700 overnight studies in children less than 16 years of age from a population base of 3.5 million, within 3 years of its establishment. Of these studies, 91% were for the evaluation of sleep-disordered breathing, including 59% for the quantification of OSA and 1.8% to evaluate centralhypoventilation.

Questionnaires have revealed that 12% of children less than 16 years of age snore,[12] and up to 50% of children who habitually snore have OSA.[13] It is also estimated that 15% to 26% of adenotonsillectomies are performed to treat upper airway obstructive symptoms.[14,15] This surgery is performed in 10% to 15% of the population in Western countries.[16] Using these figures, up to 6% of children less than 16 years of age could have OSA, with the rate of adenotonsillectomy for upper airway obstruction in childhood being 1.5% to 3.9% of the population. Specific epidemiologic studies of OSA in childhood place the prevalence at 0.7% to 2.9%.[12,17]

PATHOPHYSIOLOGY

Upper Airway Muscles and Mechanisms of Upper Airway Obstruction

The upper airway extends from the nares to the larynx. From the nasopharynx to the glottis, it is a pliable tube with walls made up of soft tissue supported by muscle.[18] Airway caliber can change with simple events, such as a change in head position.[19] Upper airway reflexes protect airway patency by modulating muscle activity to suit the prevailing respiratory needs. Dysfunction of these oropharyngeal muscles is implicated as the primary defect in adult OSA. The genioglossus and tensor palatini are two muscles that have been extensively studied in this context.[20,21] Activity of these muscles is abnormal in subjects with OSA as compared with controls in basal amplitude and in the timing of phasic (bursts of) muscle activity during the respiratory cycle, even in the awake state.[22,23]

Upper airway patency is maintained by the dynamic interaction of muscle activity and airway size in wakefulness and in sleep,[24] an incessant process that requires responsive muscle function.[25] With sleep onset there is relaxation of all postural muscles, including those of the upper airway. The activity of these muscles, and the reflexes controlling them are reduced dramatically at sleep onset.[22-26]

The mechanism of upper airway obstruction in children has been attributed almost exclusively to structurally small airways.[27-29] This theory has arisen from the many reports of successful reversal of OSA by adenotonsillectomy or tonsillectomy and the strong association of childhood OSA with craniofacial malformations. Population studies are now revealing that, as a group, children with OSA have smaller airway dimensions than children who do not snore.[30] In at least half of the affected children a small upper airway is likely to be the dominant causative factor,[31] but children may have anatomically small airways without any evidence of OSA. For example, acquired bulbar palsy may lead to OSA in previously asymptomatic individuals, and the presence of a hypotonic

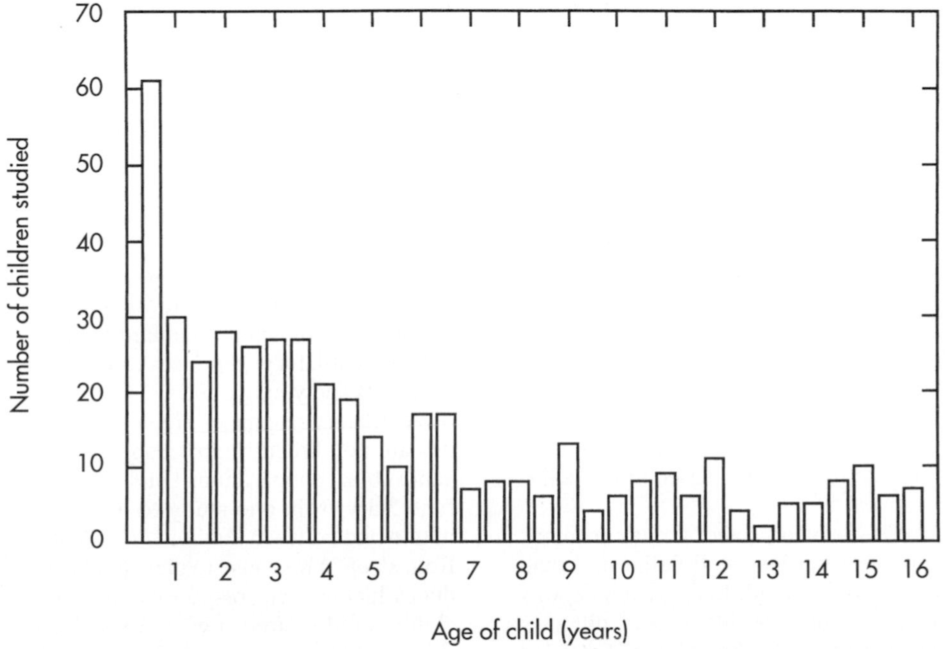

Fig. 73-1. Age distribution of children studied for OSA. Early onset of this disorder in childhood is demonstrated by the fact that 61% of these children were between the ages of 1 and 4 years.

neurologic abnormality can lead to OSA despite normal airway caliber.[32] The dynamic function of the airway should therefore be assumed to play a part in the pathophysiology of all cases of pediatric as well as adult OSA.

Neural Control of the Upper Airway

Respiratory rhythm arises in the brainstem. The cells generating respiratory rhythm have been isolated to the medulla in the region of the pre-bötzinger complex, with close links to the dorsal and ventral respiratory neuron groups.[33] This respiratory network is intimately connected to the neurons that drive the muscles of the respiratory pump (diaphragm and accessory respiratory muscles) and to the upper airway muscles.[34] These respiratory centers are also closely connected to the reticular activating system.[35] The rates of development and myelination are not uniform among these neural centers, and this explains some of the marked changes in respiratory control that take place during development.

The muscles of the upper airway are dynamically controlled throughout the respiratory cycle by connections to and from respiratory neurons. The upper airway muscles show bursts of activity that coincide with normal respiration.[36] Inspiration is associated with activation of upper airway dilator muscles. In lambs, and probably in young infants, there is active breaking at the larynx during expiration.[37,38] Increased respiratory demand results in augmentation of normal respiratory activity, along with the additional recruitment of accessory respiratory muscles, including the sternomastoid and abdominal muscles.[39] Some infants have been shown to lack this response.[40]

Reflexes Protecting the Upper Airway from Upper Airway Obstruction

Intact brainstem reflex pathways are vital for prevention or rapid recovery from sleep-associated airway obstruction. These reflex pathways involve many interconnections between sensory inputs from the oropharynx and chemoreceptors, the respiratory drive, the reticular activating system, and the motor neurons of the upper airway musculature.[41] The afferent supply to the upper airway and larynx is predominantly via the trigeminal, glossopharyngeal, and vagus nerves.

Arousal is an important culmination of upper airway protective mechanisms during sleep,[42] and may occur in response to chemoreceptor, mechanoreceptor, or cutaneous reflexes.[43] In adults, arousal correlates with the degree of increase in respiratory effort regardless of the stimulus,[44,45] and adult patients with OSA have fragmented sleep architecture as a result of the frequent arousals associated with termination of apnea.[3] In children, the actual stimulus to arousal remains unknown, and no correlation has been demonstrated between cortical arousal and increased upper airway muscle tone or apnea. It is possible that arousals in children cannot be seen using traditional investigative procedures[46,47]; certainly, young children often respond to upper airway obstruction with increased motor activity but without cortical arousal.[48]

Local upper airway reflexes also protect airway patency. These responses are important but less well delineated than those acting at spinal or brainstem level. Laryngeal receptors respond directly to increased carbon dioxide (CO_2)[49] and temperature.[50] Rapidly adapting receptors have been identified within the oropharynx, uniquely sensitive to vibration at the frequencies generated by snoring and producing local motor activity.[51] Local receptors in the distribution of the trigeminal nerve respond specifically to respiratory stimuli.[52,53] Reflexes such as the sniff also act locally,[54,55] and may contribute to the occurrence of apnea in infants during upper respiratory tract infections.[56,57]

Presumably, local reflexes are also responsible for triggering increased upper airway muscle activity (measured by electromyography, or EMG) when upper airway obstruction occurs.[58,59] Increased activity occurs in response to upper airway obstruction in adults during both inspiratory and expiratory phases of the respiratory cycle, although the level of response is dependent on sleep/wake state and may be absent in rapid-eye-movement (REM) sleep.[60] This increase in the EMG signals may help to characterize the upper airway obstruction in children.[61] In young infants, genioglossus recruitment with airway occlusion appears to be possible in all sleep states,[40] but the response appears to be less vigorous in infants who have obstructive apnea,[62] and their airway collapses in the presence of a resistive load.[63]

Developmental Aspects of Respiratory and Airway Control: Age-Related Disorders

During infancy, the influences on respiratory control are quite different from those in adults, and inhibitory responses tend to predominate so that upper airway obstruction may produce apnea rather than respiratory stimulation. Laryngeal reflexes can produce life-threatening apnea in young animals, particularly in the presence of infections that damage the upper airway epithelium. Prolonged apnea has been documented in infants in the presence of nasopharyngitis.[56] It is hypothesized that there is associated inflammation or damage to sensory pathways within the epithelium, or damage to the carotid bodies.[57]

One mechanism that may explain these life-threatening apneic responses in otherwise normal infants is a failure to damp the amplitude of an otherwise normal reflex response. Reflexes in the upper airway, along with other spinal motor reflexes, are not under cortical inhibitory control in infancy and upper airway obstruction accompanies central apnea,[64] although increased respiratory effort is generally seen during imposed airway obstruction in term infants.[19,65] Such undamped responses are capable of initiating periodic breathing following a spontaneous apnea or sigh.[66] Whereas the initial apnea is mediated via vagal reflex pathways, for example, following a large breath,[67] other factors contribute to the ongoing respiratory rhythm oscillation.[68]

Brainstem chemoreceptors change with development, and are also affected by environmental factors such as ambient temperature. In adults, standard values are clear and available for the ventilatory responses to hypoxia and hypercapnia.[69,70] In infants and young children, techniques for the measurement of ventilatory responses are not standardized, and adult methods are not directly transferable because they require significant subject cooperation. Thus measurement techniques in infants vary from one study to another, and results may vary within and between studies.[71,72] Infants do consistently arouse from sleep in response to elevated P_{CO_2}, whereas hypoxia produces inconsistent responses and a large number of normal children fail to arouse when exposed to low inspired oxygen (F_{IO_2}).[73] Future studies will be required to provide clearer definitions and reproducibility of the appropriate tests.

RELATIONSHIPS BETWEEN RESPIRATION AND SLEEP

Tone changes associated with sleep are a critical factor in the pathophysiology of OSA. Both tonic activity and reflex responses of upper airway muscles are reduced in sleep, with the most dramatic effects in REM sleep.[74] Sleep onset is associated with reduced upper airway tone (and therefore reduced airway dimensions) and blunted reflex responses to acute events. In this chapter, reflex responses are considered to be at baseline in the awake state, and blunting indicates a reduced response in sleep as compared with the awake state.

Techniques for Evaluating Sleep Breathing

Polysomnography is the name given to a multichannel, physiologic recording performed during sleep. In its complete form, more than 16 variables are measured during the normal period of nighttime sleep. The clear benefit is the amount of information provided. The corollary in pediatrics is the highly demanding process of preparing children with all the attachments necessary for such a recording. Leads must be placed accurately and firmly in order to provide good-quality recordings for an 8- to 10-hour study. The importance of a complete overnight study is that it incorporates all sleep phases, especially the later REM sleep periods, during which OSA is often most severe. The studies may be costly because they are time- and labor-intensive, but this must be balanced against the need for an accurate diagnosis and the fact that inaccurate screening tests probably must be repeated, ultimately increasing the costs involved in obtaining the final diagnosis.

Sleep state is recorded by a combination of electroencephalogram (EEG), eye movements, and muscle (usually genioglossus) tone. The combination of these signals is required to differentiate all sleep states, particularly REM sleep. To record sleep stage, a minimum of one, but usually two to four EEG leads are used. The younger the child, the more channels are likely to be required, and for infants, two EEG leads plus clinical, behavioral observations or video are required. Eye movements and EMG signals are recorded via surface electrodes.

Respiratory recordings include measures of both the effort exerted and the resulting effects. Effort can be recorded using either EMG signals or chest or abdominal displacement. Plethysmography is the most accurate measure of respiration because the signal recorded is proportional to volume and can be calibrated.[75] Impedance recordings, which measure the changes in electrical resistance of the skin between two electrodes during the respiratory cycle, are readily available and commonly used. However, an impedance signal can be misleading with regard to respiratory effort, especially in young infants or in older children with low tidal volumes.

In older children, paradoxic movement of the chest and abdomen reflects tidal volume and can be used as an indicator of the presence or absence of respiratory flow, as well as differentiating central from obstructive apneas. In the very young infant or in older children with neuromuscular disorders, paradoxic movement of the chest and abdomen is so common during normal sleep that airflow and indicators of the blood gases (Po_2 and Pco_2) are an essential component of a sleep study. Airflow may be measured by several methods, including pressure transducer, thermistors, and thermocouples. Oxygenation is usually measured by saturation (Sao_2). Transcutaneous Po_2 may be recorded, but is associated with a slower time-course for change and problems of drift,[76] and is not routinely used for sleep studies. Carbon dioxide levels are most commonly recorded by transcutaneous or end-tidal monitors. More accurate measures require blood gas analysis; these are generally used when noninvasive methods indicate abnormalities.

Specific criteria for scoring respiratory events in adults are not applicable in pediatrics. Adult apneas are scored if they have a duration of 10 seconds or longer. Although this is appropriate in the adult population, it is neither qualitatively nor quantitatively discriminatory in the evaluation of childhood apnea.[9] There are no universal scoring criteria for defining the level of abnormality associated with significant sequelae in childhood. Most laboratories set an arbitrary level of "abnormal" for the apnea indices for clinical purposes, but polysomnography should always be interpreted in the full clinical context of the patient. Apnea definitions that relate to respiratory frequency are the most appropriate across the age ranges in pediatrics. One system in common use is to score respiratory events that disturb two or more consecutive respiratory cycles. The decrease in Sao_2 most commonly used to define a significant event is 3% to 4%, or if the event precipitates an arousal. Fixed flow limitation may not be associated with discrete respiratory events, while still being associated with O_2 desaturation and CO_2 retention because of low respiratory reserve. In these cases, even brief apnea will cause significant desaturation. A rise of 8 mm Hg in CO_2 is generally accepted as the limit of normal for children, as for adults.

Data from polysomnographic studies are recorded with a fixed time base onto polygraphic recording paper or in digital form. Digital storage media are ideal because of the enormous amount of information available in detailed polysomnographic studies. The use of digital systems has greatly enhanced the accessibility of information from the studies and provided more accurate summaries. Commercial packages are now increasingly available with sleep and respiratory analysis capabilities included, but automatic, computerized sleep scoring is not currently suitable for pediatric studies, which always require additional, interactive evaluation of the record.

Characteristics of Normal Sleep

Normal sleep can be divided into five clearly distinguishable sleep states, with predictable sleep state progression during the night. Mature human sleep is divided into stages I to IV and REM sleep.[77] Stages III and IV, also called deep or slow-wave sleep (SWS), are characterized by high-amplitude, low-frequency EEG. REM sleep is characterized by low-amplitude, high-frequency EEG, REMs, and loss of tonic muscle activity seen clearly in the chin (genioglossus) EMG. In older children and in adults sleep is nocturnal, and dominates the early hours of sleep, whereas REM occurs in and SWS dominates the later hours (usually early morning). Stages I and II, also called light sleep, are interspersed throughout the night. In the mature human daytime sleep periods are dominated by light sleep, with little if any REM sleep or SWS occurring at this time.

During infancy, the differentiation of sleep states is less distinct and until the age of approximately 6 months, sleep stages can only be divided into quiet, active, and indeterminate.[78] The distributions of active sleep, which is the equivalent of REM sleep in older individuals, and quiet sleep (equate with SWS in adults) are not dependent on the time after sleep onset. During these first months of life, maturation involves the emergence of the five clear sleep states of adults. Circadian rhythms also mature, and clear distinction between the characteristics of day and night sleep occurs by an average of 3 months of age,[79,80] although sleep may still commence with REM activity. The proportions of the different sleep states change dramatically in the first 6 months of life, and then continue to change over the first years of life; the proportion of SWS increases as the amount of REM sleep declines.[81,82] By early adolescence, children's sleep approximates the adult distribution for stage categories, proportions of the different stages during an overnight sleep period, and nocturnal pattern of progression from an initial predominance of SWS to the later stages of a nocturnal sleep period, when REM sleep emerges and predominates.

Wakefulness is characterized by low-amplitude, high-frequency EEG, the presence of conjugate eye movements, and high muscle tone. Sleep onset is heralded by rolling eye movements, associated with slowing of EEG signal frequency and a decrease in muscle tone. SWS is associated with high-amplitude, low-frequency EEG, absent eye movements, and decreased muscle tone. REM sleep is characterized by low-amplitude, high-frequency EEG, the presence of eye movements, and loss of postural muscle tone. Light sleep stages have the additional characteristics of sleep spindles and K-complexes. These are distinctive EEG patterns seen particularly in stage II sleep. Sleep spindles and K complexes are characteristic of stage II sleep. Sleep spindles are fast (7- to 10-Hz) bursts lasting 3 to 5 seconds and recurring at 30-second intervals. K-complexes are well-delineated negative sharp waves immediately followed by a positive component. The duration of a K complex is no longer than 0.5 seconds. Detailed descriptions of each sleep scoring system are provided in the relevant reference manuals.[77,78]

A diurnal rhythm for sleep-wake states is established by 6 to 12 weeks of age.[82] This is associated with clear differences between daytime and night sleep components. SWS tends to occur early during the night and REM sleep cycles occur with increased frequency in the early morning hours. Light sleep stages are interspersed fairly evenly throughout the night. Significant respiratory disturbances may be isolated to periods of REM sleep.

Sleep-Associated Changes in Cardiorespiratory Patterns

Minute ventilation is under reflex control, even during sleep periods, when it is often lower than in awake states.[83,84] Lung volumes fall to a minimum in REM sleep and ventilatory responses to hypoxia and hypercapnia are at their lowest, so minute ventilation is less for any given CO_2 level,[85] and a rise of 2 to 8 mm Hg of CO_2 is normal. Hypoxic responses are also affected, normal $Sa{O_2}$ variability with sleep is 2% or less, and $P{O_2}$ changes by 2 to 11 mm Hg. Normal children may show central apnea and oxygen desaturation with sleep, but they demonstrate rapid recovery to baseline values.[86,87]

During SWS respiration is almost completely under chemosensory control,[88] and although muscle tone is maintained, arousal responses are lower than in other sleep states. Thus disorders of central respiratory control are most pronounced in SWS. SWS is also characterized by remarkable regularity of cardiorespiratory parameters, with little variability in cardiac or respiratory rate and rhythm and stable tidal volumes. Periodic breathing (recurring cycles of central apnea alternating with normal or increased amplitude breaths) tends to occur in active sleep in infants,[89] although the pattern that generates a very regular, cyclic rhythm is seen most clearly following a sigh in quiet sleep.

During REM sleep the brainstem cardiorespiratory control centers are influenced by input from higher brain structures (basal forebrain or cortex), and this sleep state is characterized by greater tolerance of variability in parameters, including $Sa{O_2}$, $P{CO_2}$, heart rate, and respiratory rate. As a result, minute ventilation may fluctuate, and there is often a relative hyperventilation (fall in $P{CO_2}$). One of the hallmarks of REM sleep is the loss of muscle tone in peripheral muscles, including the accessory respiratory muscles and the muscles of the upper airway; muscle tone is especially low during periods with marked eye movement that are known as phasic REM. Tolerance to the irregularities of cardiorespiratory variables during REM sleep involves less active arousal responses.[44] The hypoxic and hypercapnic ventilatory responses can be difficult to measure, even in adults, but also tend to be lower than in wakefulness. Studies in infants have not consistently found the same decrease in lung volumes as those that occur in adults during REM sleep.[90,91] One remarkable feature of REM sleep in infants and young children is that responsive muscle tone may be maintained.[48] This may be caused by persistence of some immature reflexes or a difference in the nature of REM sleep in the developing brain.

Light sleep (stages I and II) is characterized by a hybrid of these features. The important feature of these sleep states is the relative instability of respiration that can accompany transition between wakefulness and sleep. Perturbation of central control mechanisms, including drive to the upper airway, may be unmasked during this phase. An example of normal, light sleep is shown in Figure 73-2.

Apneic events occur in normal sleep. These are central in type and infrequent, and occur primarily in REM sleep or following sighs in non-REM sleep. Studies in normal children do not reveal obstructive events,[9,92] in contrast to adults, in whom up to five obstructive events per hour is considered normal. When monitoring infants for central apnea, the boundaries of normal are much less clear, but events are abnormal and warrant intervention if they are associated with significant physiologic sequelae, such as marked oxygen desaturation, bradycardia, or disruption of normal sleep architecture. Studies of normal children confirm the presence of occasional prolonged central apneic events, but these are infrequent; in general, if $Sa{O_2}$, $P{CO_2}$, and sleep state are maintained, then the apneic episodes do not warrant intervention.

Sleep-Associated Changes in the Upper Airway

In the upper airway the major change induced by sleep is muscle relaxation resulting in a decrease in airway caliber. Sleep also alters the reflex control of the upper airway, respiratory drive, and sensitivity to a variety of respiratory feedback mechanisms. An airway that maintains adequate functional activity in the awake state can be critically compromised by the fall in muscle tone and less active reflex functions

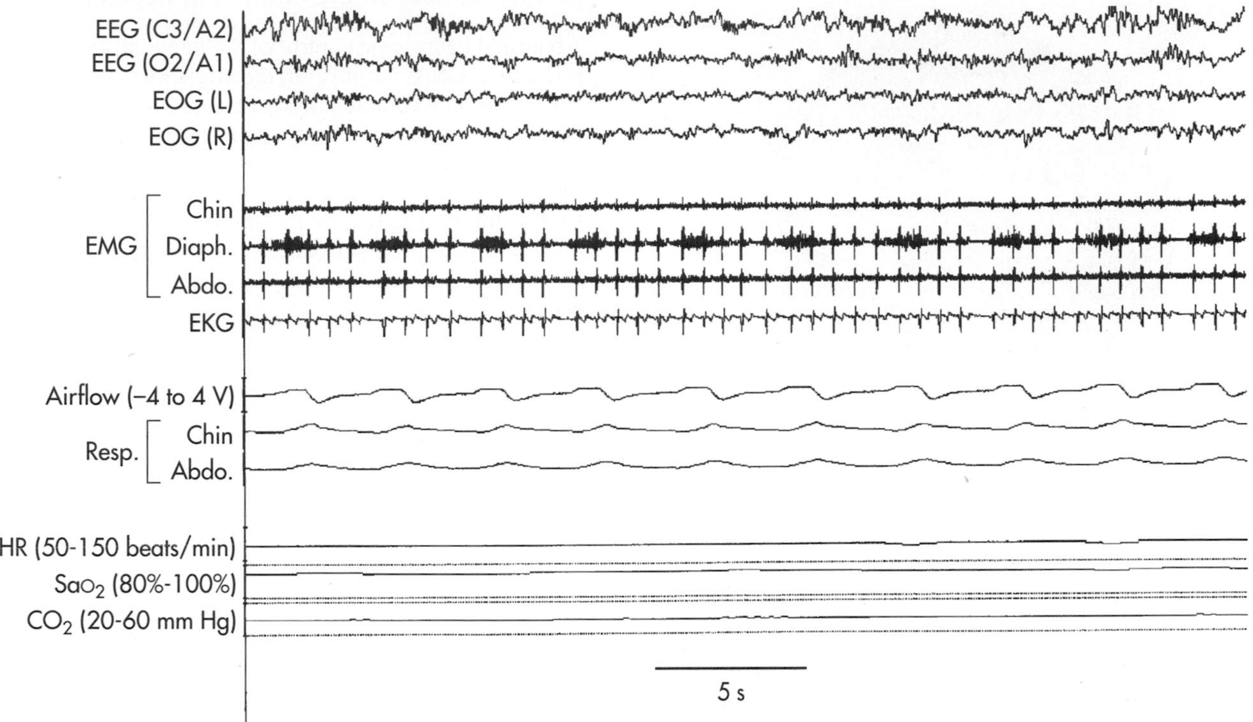

Fig. 73-2. Normal sleep. This study shows normal light sleep (stage II). There is low tonic activity of the chin muscles (genioglossus) and no evidence of active abdominal muscle activity with respiration. In this and subsequent polysomnographic examples, *EOG,* electrooculogram documenting eye movements, *Diaph*, diaphragm; *Abdo*, abdominal; airflow is monitored using a pressure transducer at the nares; *Resp*, respitrace (inductance plethysmography); *bpm*, beats per minute; CO_2 is measured continuously via a transcutaneous electrode.

that coincide with sleep onset. The magnitude of these effects on the upper airway changes with different sleep states. The most pronounced mechanical differences are seen by comparing REM sleep and the awake state.

PATHOLOGY OF OSA

Abnormalities that can underlie sleep-associated respiratory disorders include chronic lung disease, congenital abnormalities that result in facial and upper airway malformations, and congenital or acquired neuromuscular abnormalities. Small facial dimensions or impingement of adenotonsillar tissue into the airway can significantly reduce upper airway dimensions.[93] It has been suggested that a small facial structure or abnormal upper airway is an inherited characteristic in such children,[94] and epidemiologic studies support this.[95] Neuromuscular abnormalities also cause or contribute to OSA, and it is probable that some underlying abnormality in respiratory or upper airway control exists in most cases of sleep-associated obstructive apnea and hypoventilation.

Small Upper Airway

Narrowing of the upper airway can occur at any point from the anterior nares to the larynx. This narrowing may be static or dynamic. Laryngomalacia and large airway stenosis both increase the negative thoracic pressures required to generate inspiratory flow. Lung disease can increase respiratory drive sufficiently to precipitate collapse in an otherwise stable but small airway; the additional work of breathing required to generate adequate gas exchange can create sufficient upper airway loading to precipitate collapse.

Some children clearly have a structurally small upper airway, for example in Down syndrome or craniosynostoses.[96] Not all upper airway obstruction is apparent at birth, and structural abnormalities, even in these congenital syndromes, may be exacerbated with growth. A small airway may be acquired as a result of neuropathically altered growth or chronic nasal obstruction, which has been associated with poor growth of the middle third of the face.[97,98] In other conditions, such as the mucopolysaccharidoses, the airway lumen is crowded by extra soft tissue.[99] A structurally small airway may be further compromised by adenotonsillar hypertrophy. In the presence of reduced airway dimensions, upper airway muscles have been shown to have increased activity in order to maintain a patent airway in the awake state.[20] In this situation, sleep-associated loss of muscle tone may be the critical factor precipitating complete upper airway obstruction.

In the David Read Unit, 49.6% of children assessed for OSA have an underlying syndrome or malformation, or adenotonsillar hypertrophy. The biggest group with a clear structural cause for their upper airway obstruction is the 32% of children studied who had a known congenital syndrome or malformation. Forty percent of children with persisting symptoms after adenotonsillectomy and 70% of the children who required treatment with nasal CPAP therapy are from this group. Thus children with malformations tend to have recalcitrant apnea. An example of the lateral facial profile in such a child is shown in Figure 73-3.

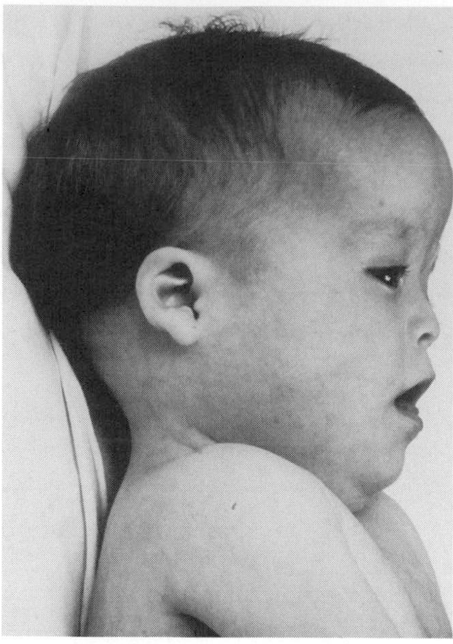

Fig. 73-3. Lateral facial profile of children with obstructive apnea. This child has hypoplasia of the mid third of the face, with extremely small nasal passages, predisposing to the severe upper airway obstruction that was diagnosed on overnight polysomnography and required ongoing treatment with nasal mask CPAP.

Abnormal Neurologic Control of Breathing

Abnormal neurologic control of the upper airway has been implicated in OSA, but it is not clear whether the abnormal control is congenital or acquired secondary to the OSA.[24,100] Abnormalities may occur in the central respiratory drive to the upper airway, or any site along the reflex pathways, the neural input of the upper airway reflexes, the central neural integration of these reflexes, or the motor (output) pathways. The level of blood gas disturbance present before arousal is greatest in adult patients who have abnormal peripheral chemoreceptor activity and low central responses. Maintenance of near normal oxygenation is associated with brisk hypoxic and hypercapnic ventilatory and arousal responses.[101] No studies have confirmed that arousal in response to OSA in children correlates with ventilatory response activity, but in a small group of children with OSA who did not have underlying structural abnormalities, ventilatory responses were normal.[102] Screening studies that measure $Sa{O_2}$ alone may not indicate the level of sleep disturbance present in patients with vigorous arousal in response to upper airway obstruction.

The majority of children with OSA do not appear to arouse in response to either upper airway obstruction or the hypercapnia or hypoxia that result. The pattern of abnormality in these children is preservation of sleep architecture at the expense of oxygenation and CO_2 clearance (Figs. 73-4, 73-5). Children may express the typical "adult" pattern of disease by

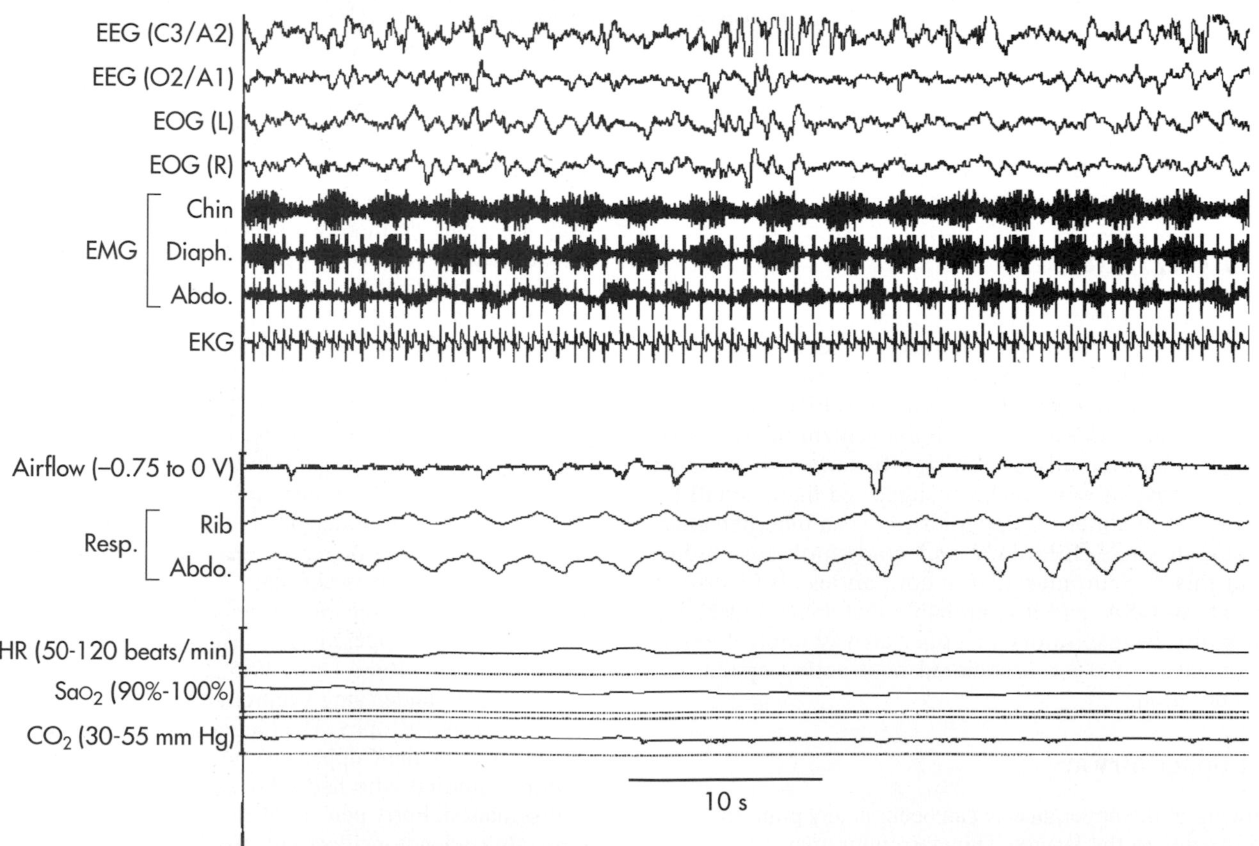

Fig. 73-4. Example of partial upper airway obstruction in SWS. The airflow pattern shows inspiratory flow limitation. There are bursts of activity in the chin (genioglossus) muscles during inspiration and bursts of activity from the abdominal muscles during expiration. There are no discrete respiratory events, reaching criteria for scoring on a polysomnographic report, on this trace.

adolescence. Further studies are needed to determine whether, as hypothesized, the duration of the disease influences its expression and whether onset of OSA during critical periods of development is responsible for secondary changes in respiratory control.

Abnormalities of upper airway reflex pathways may cause OSA, but no published cases demonstrate such an isolated defect. Studies in adults with chronic snoring and OSA suggest that these patients have abnormal reflex control of the airway lumen, although it is not clear whether these abnormalities are the cause or the effect of the disorder.

Central Hypoventilation

Respiratory reflexes can be affected at the level of central brainstem coordination. Alveolar hypoventilation syndromes (known as Ondine's curse) exemplify the most extreme form of abnormal neurologic respiratory control, and result in sleep-associated hypoventilation. In milder cases, including the majority of congenital cases, respiratory control in the awake state approximates normal with normal blood gases. In the most severe cases ventilatory support is required even in the awake state.[103] Two forms of this disorder are recognized: congenital and acquired. These should be considered distinct entities because the majority of congenital cases have no detectable cause. In contrast, when the disorder has commenced in later life, a demonstrable underlying abnormality is more likely and structural lesions in the brainstem, anterior horn cells, or myopathies should be rigorously sought. In the sleep laboratory, acquired central hypoventilation may present with a history of snoring and witnessed apnea indistinguishable from that of OSA. Respiratory infections may precipitate an acute presentation, further imitating the typical history of OSA.[104]

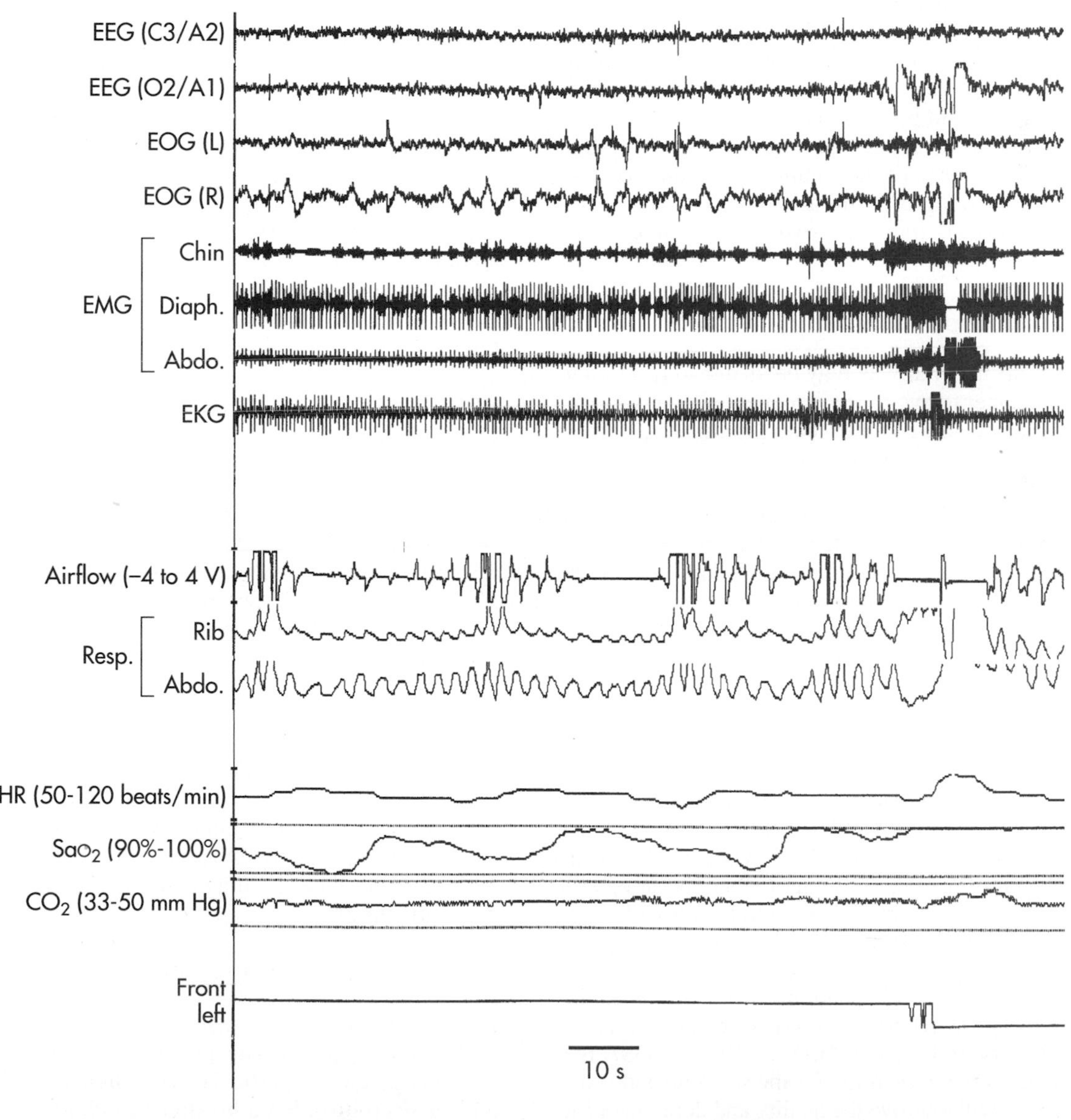

Fig. 73-5. OSA. This example shows intermittent episodes of complete cessation of nasal airflow accompanied by continued and increasing diaphragmatic activity, paradoxic movement of the chest wall and abdomen, and oxygen desaturation. There is no evidence of EEG arousal (burst of alpha activity) until the termination of the third and final event in this example, despite upper airway obstruction and significant oxygen desaturation in the preceding episodes.

In congenital central hypoventilation (Ondine's curse), there is failure of the central coordination of the signals leading to respiratory rate and rhythm generation,[105] despite an anatomically normal airway and brain (including the brainstem). The respiratory defect appears to be isolated in the majority of cases, but may be associated with Hirschsprung disease and nonreactive pupils, suggesting a more generalized serotonergic defect.[106] One distinctive group is patients with acquired central hypoventilation[107] and children with the Arnold-Chiari malformation are a subgroup of these.[108]

Young infants may also have symptoms of noisy breathing and sweating in sleep.[109] Some children who present with apparent life-threatening events (ALTEs) have been demonstrated to have obstructive events on subsequent sleep studies. Children who have subsequently died of the sudden infant death syndrome (SIDS) have had obstructive apneic events demonstrated on sleep studies performed before death,[110] and early epidemiologic studies suggest a positive link between a family history of OSA and SIDS.[111,112] It is widely theorized that the likely underlying cause of SIDS deaths is delayed or abnormal maturation of neural cardiorespiratory control pathways, including the upper airway, creating a risk for death from an insult that would be inconsequential to other infants. Because abnormal neural control may be expressed as OSA, studies may be designed to detect a number of children at risk for SIDS,[113] recognizing that the abnormality may be detectable only during an upper respiratory tract infection or other acute stress.

Muscular Dysfunction

The muscles of the upper airway may be unable to function in a coordinated manner to avoid or overcome upper airway obstruction. This may be the result of local structural malformations, such as congenital clefts that disturb the muscles' insertion or placement, or part of a generalized muscle dysfunction such as the muscular dystrophies. Palatal muscle function is abnormal in association with cleft palate and this remains abnormal after surgery.[114] Structural repair does not restore normal muscle placement or control and may cause a reduction in airway dimensions; postoperatively, these muscles may not be able to prevent upper airway obstruction.[115] Presumably the local sensory perception is also affected, although central respiratory control is not usually affected in isolated clefts.[116]

Most children with abnormal neuromuscular control of the airway have been considered to have normal airway size. Cranial nerve nuclei may be individually affected, and OSA has been seen in association with Moebius syndrome.[117] In the Arnold-Chiari malformation, or syringobulbia, motor control of the cranial nerves is abnormal, but central control of respiration also appears to be affected.[108,118,119] Generalized motor hypotonia contributes to upper airway obstruction in disorders such as Down syndrome.[120,121] The muscular dystrophies, including Duchenne, are generally progressive and ultimately result in respiratory and cardiac failure, of which OSA is a component. Treatment intervention for the sleep-related respiratory dysfunction will improve the quality and duration of life in these patients.[122]

OSA may occur when soft tissue function is abnormal without demonstrable muscle weakness. In Marfan syndrome, in which the only apparent abnormality is poor connective tissue integrity, there is also a high incidence of OSA.[123] It is likely that other syndromes with poor connective tissue integrity, such as Ehler Dhanlos, also have a high incidence of OSA.

The skeletal abnormalities in achondroplasia cause a small foramen magnum. OSA in this group may be a result of compression of the brainstem and upper cervical spinal cord at the level of the foramen magnum.[48,124] However, in achondroplasia it is likely that OSA is caused by mixed pathologies, including a small airway size, and possible connective tissue abnormalities. In achondroplasia, it is therefore important to distinguish the components caused by central control from those attributable to a small or floppy upper airway in order to direct treatment to the predominant abnormality.[125]

Activity of the respiratory accessory muscles is lost during REM sleep in the adult, and functional residual capacity probably falls as a result of the loss of intercostal muscle activity. Any respiratory disorder compensated for by accessory muscle activity in the awake state will show marked decompensation in REM sleep.[126,127]

Complications

The most commonly identified associations with OSA in childhood are failure to thrive (FTT) and pulmonary hypertension. Growth failure may be caused by disturbance of growth hormone secretion or metabolic disturbances.[128,129] Pulmonary hypertension is probably secondary to chronic activation of hypoxic pulmonary vascular responses.[4] Other pathologies that are linked with childhood OSA include obesity, hypersomnolence, and hyperactivity. Much work is still to be done in determining the pathophysiologic consequences of mild to moderate childhood OSA.

PRINCIPLES OF ASSESSMENT

Obstructive apnea appears to be common in children.[12] Clearly, the best way of assessing sleep-related respiratory dysfunction is to study the subject during sleep. The aim of such studies is to find the abnormalities (sleep-associated respiratory dysfunction) and classify them by criteria that are discriminatory between studies and that will also indicate the likelihood of detrimental effects in both the short and long term.

A detailed overnight sleep study provides the most useful diagnostic information. It can be, however, an expensive and time-consuming procedure. Screening procedures are often used to determine which children should undergo sleep studies, and the clinical assessment is the start of this screening process. Until consistent clinical correlates can be found, the sole indicator of risk for OSA is persistent snoring, and the one test that can make the diagnosis with certainty is detailed polysomnography.

CLINICAL CHARACTERISTICS

Public awareness of all aspects of sleep-related upper airway obstruction is limited. This pertains to the disorder in any patient age group, but particularly children. As a result, the history of sleep-disordered breathing in children often must be actively sought. Current experience indicates that even severe sleep-related airway obstruction may be dismissed by parents and doctors, through ignorance about its significance. Standardized questionnaires have been developed to assist in the process of symptom identification and prioritization.[130]

This hidden nature of sleep-associated breathing disorders is partly attributable to the subtlety of associated daytime abnormalities. Normal sleep physiology plays an active role in precipitating the characteristic nocturnal breathing abnormalities, and even severe OSA can be associated with apparently normal daytime function.[7]

The most discriminatory symptoms are breathing difficulty during sleep, witnessed apnea (regardless of reported duration, these are a significant indicator of respiratory abnormalities), persistent snoring, and restless sleep. Disturbed sleep, rhinorrhea, excessive sweating in sleep, and mouth breathing in the awake state are common but not universal features. Upper respiratory tract infections are often reported in children who are shown to have obstructive apnea,[131] but in the clinical setting it can be difficult to distinguish persistent nasal obstruction from recurrent infections on history alone.

Unless there has been a clear precipitating event, the history of sleep-disordered breathing is often intertwined with the developmental history of a child. When syndromes underlie the disorder, the history of sleep-disordered breathing is commonly life-long,[132] and the longer the history, the more likely the parents are to consider the symptoms of OSA a normal characteristic of their child. Symptoms affecting both daytime and nighttime function, including intellectual dysfunction and sleepiness, are often considered part of the inherited syndrome. Such symptoms have, at times, been considered an untreatable and inherently progressive characteristic of the underlying disease itself. There is a great need for education of both lay and medical caretakers of these groups, specifically explaining the symptoms of OSA and its associations.

As children get older their parents are less likely to have witnessed them sleeping on a regular basis, and the sleep history can be difficult to obtain. Other symptoms are seen in association with obstructive apnea, but are not consistently differentiating. These include a history of associated lower respiratory tract disease, enuresis,[133] frequent nausea and vomiting, and behavioral problems. Excessive or daytime sleepiness is unlikely to cause parental concern in prepubertal children, and is variably reported in childhood OSA.[7] Less common presentations, reported anecdotally, include developmental delay, night seizures, costochondritis, cyclic vomiting, hyperactivity or inattentiveness,[12] and morning headaches.[134]

Past history may also give an indication of the severity of upper airway obstruction. There may be a history of anesthetic difficulties.[2] Sedative drugs or muscle relaxants may contribute to upper airway problems.[135] Children with acquired central hypoventilation may have an additional history indicating abnormal ventilatory control, including daytime cyanotic episodes, unusual tolerance of hypoxic environments such as swimming under water, or a neonatal history of cyanotic or severe apneic events.[104] The role of inheritance has not been clarified. Studies do suggest that there is a familial incidence of OSA[95,136] and children with OSA often have one or more parents who are also affected. A genetic link has been proposed,[137] but further studies are needed to confirm the nature of these associations.

Underlying Conditions

Underlying conditions and abnormalities in the current and past history may include atopic disease, especially rhinitis, or nasal abnormalities.[138,139] Any cause of airway narrowing may contribute to the cause of sleep-associated airway obstruction. Causes include choanal stenosis, vocal cord palsy (congenital or acquired), and tracheobronchomalacia. Infants with a history of prematurity have dolicocephaly from positioning that can result in structural facial features predisposing to upper airway obstruction.[140]

Examination

Assessment of the presence and severity of OSA in the awake state is inaccurate in all but the most severely affected adults, and the situation is likely to be the same in children. Careful daytime examination can reveal a wide range of physical features associated with obstructive apnea in children. Increased upper airway (nasal) resistance can result in mouth breathing when awake,[141] and dysphagia may be suggested by a tendency to drool. Such features should raise the suspicion of a small airway, and therefore of the diagnosis of OSA. Ability to breathe through the nose (quietly), and the patency of the nasal airway can be assessed by checking nasal airflow after occluding individual nostrils; definitions of normal nasal patency and size do not exist, but with normal nasal resistance a child should be able to sustain quiet breathing through a single nostril. Careful examination should be made for hypoplasia of the midface or mandible because these are associated with an increased incidence of OSA.[142]

The oropharynx must always be examined for prominent tonsils, the extent of the tonsillar extension behind the tongue, and the presence and quantity of upper airway secretions. Normal tonsils may appear prominent in a small airway.[143] A characteristic "snorer's throat" may be seen in children as well as adults. This includes features of edema and petechiae in the soft tissues of the oropharynx. The palate should specifically be examined for clefts and other clues of submucosal clefts, such as a bifid uvula. The mobility of the palate should be noted, and unusual features such as a long, shawl-like palate or deformity caused by an overlying adenoid mass. The presence of cervical lymphadenopathy supports a diagnosis of recurrent tonsillitis.[144]

Examination of the chest may reveal deformities; Harrison's sulci can be seen with significant upper airway obstruction.[145] Other lower respiratory tract diseases may be associated with respiratory decompensation in sleep, although not necessarily associated with OSA.[122] Intercostal retraction and tracheal tug should be noted, even with quiet respiration. In the presence of other lung disease, and especially if accessory respiratory muscles are being used in wakefulness, the potential exists for the increased respiratory drive to precipitate upper airway obstruction in sleep. Alternatively, the presence of borderline gas exchange when awake can be associated with deterioration in sleep as a result of sleep-associated physiologic changes.[126,127]

Weight abnormalities occur in only a small subgroup of children with OSA. FTT (and a clear growth response following intervention) is variably reported as occurring in 1% to 65% of the children studied for OSA.[146,147] The wide variability in these proportions reflects the differences in definition of FTT that are used, from the requirement of having weight or growth rates less than the 3rd percentile for age to growth across percentiles after treatment. The difficulty is compounded by the short follow-up periods in most studies. Obesity is seen in a much smaller proportion from none at all up to 7%,[11] with around 5% of obese adolescents having OSA.[148]

The most severe complications of OSA in children are pulmonary hypertension and respiratory failure. Any signs that these are present would indicate very severe disease that requires urgent assessment and appropriate medical attention. Clinical features of pulmonary hypertension should be sought, including a loud second heart sound, cardiac murmur of mitral regurgitation, and liver enlargement. These are uncommon, except in the most severe cases.[149] Preexisting cardiac disease with unexplained persistent pulmonary hypertension is another cause of these abnormalities, and OSA should be considered in the differential diagnosis of these cases.

Blood gases should be measured if there is any suspicion of daytime respiratory compromise. In children this test can be difficult and is generally used after indirect assessments have indicated some abnormality. Capillary sampling and transcutaneous monitoring are valuable aids in this assessment.

FURTHER STUDIES

Radiology and Endoscopy

Initial investigations are appropriately directed toward finding the underlying cause or complications of OSA. A lateral airway radiograph is the easiest and most direct means of obtaining valuable information regarding airway caliber, and will show airway-occluding soft tissue (masses). This is a static size of the airway and the relative size of the tonsils and adenoids, so changes with loss of muscle tone in sleep are not assessed. If linked to the respiratory cycle, dynamic differences in airway dimensions can also be determined by radiographs.[150-152]

Nasendoscopy is useful for a dynamic assessment of airway size, and to assess space-occupying lesions,[153] but most children require sedation and the risk of sedation should be weighed against the additional information that will be gained, before undertaking this study. Laryngobronchoesophagoscopy (LBO) will also provide an assessment for underlying causes, and should especially be considered in infants who present at less than 6 months of age. Flexible endoscopy specifically provides a functional assessment of the upper airway and larynx.

More elaborate tests with new technologies are currently expensive, and used predominantly as research tools because they are not validated as a clinical tool for children with OSA. Computed tomography (CT) scan is useful for determining a three-dimensional, static image of airway size. Magnetic resonance imaging (MRI), reconstructed CT images, and acoustic reflection can be used to determine an absolute volume for the airway. If there are concerns about bulbar function or unexplained hypoventilation, MRI is the most useful imaging technique for examining the brainstem, posterior fossa, and upper cervical cord. This is particularly suitable when a diagnosis of Arnold-Chiari malformation or syringomyelia is being considered.

Cardiologic assessment can detect abnormalities sooner than routine clinical examination, so it is appropriate to perform CXR, ECG, and echocardiographic examinations in children with documented OSA and CO_2 retention, or when severe or sustained oxygen desaturation has been documented.

Polysomnography Methods

Overnight sleep studies provide information about respiration during a period of sleep. These studies are usually performed because the history or examination suggest a diagnosis of OSA. Many physiologic studies can be performed during sleep, ranging from dual-channel recording of the output of an oximeter,[154] or studies of movement alone,[155] to comprehensive multichannel physiologic recordings. Overnight oximetry in isolation has poor specificity and sensitivity, so shorter studies or less detailed recordings are unhelpful, and in either case may miss moderate-severity disease.

Studies with increasing levels of sophistication are available, but anything less than full polysomnography cannot diagnose sleep fragmentation, CO_2 retention, and airflow or respiratory efforts. Limited studies provide limited information, but the variables measured may be tailored to specific test outcome requirements. Care must be taken in the design and interpretation of these limited studies if accurate diagnoses are to be expected. Screening studies are most useful if the operator recognizes the limitations of these studies and reserves the option of more detailed studies. Detailed overnight studies are essential to define the exact nature of breathing abnormalities, and should be performed even after a normal screening test if symptoms or signs persist.

Polysomnography Interpretation

The principal aim of an overnight polysomnogram is to evaluate the patterns of respiration in sleep and to quantify the changes in blood gases, levels of arousal, and sleep stage that occur in response to respiratory or other events. Criteria for sleep-stage scoring defined in adults[77] are appropriate in children even though absolute EEG amplitude (in microvolts) tends to be much greater in children. This can limit the capacity of some computer algorithms to score sleep stages accurately in children. Separate, specific criteria have been defined in neonates.

The first stage of interpreting polysomnography is accurate characterization of the sleep-breathing abnormality. Discrete respiratory events are defined as obstructive or central, depending on whether respiratory efforts continue during the apnea. During a central apnea no diaphragmatic movement occurs. An obstructive apnea indicates ongoing respiratory effort without airflow being achieved. During a mixed apnea airflow is absent, with diaphragmatic effort present for only a portion of the event. Respiratory events tend to cluster in REM sleep, and to document the more severe, REM-related events it is essential to monitor the period from midnight to wakefulness.

The immediate significance of an apnea is determined by the physiologic changes it produces. An obstructive event causes reduced or absent airflow despite sustained or increased respiratory efforts, producing hypoxia and increased amplitude of negative intrathoracic pressure swings. Hemodynamic changes include bradycardia or tachycardia and systemic and pulmonary hypertension. Frequent arousals in response to respiratory disturbances are not common in pediatrics, but detailed studies suggest that there is an altered duration and distribution of sleep states in these children as a group.[156] The proportion of the various sleep stages, in particular quiet sleep and REM sleep, should be referred to age-specific tables of normative data to diagnose disturbances of sleep architecture.

The frequency of arousal and the levels of oxygen desaturation seen during the night in children with OSA are higher than in age-matched controls. Children tolerate significant degrees of obstruction if it is stable and partial, and then they do not experience frequent arousals.[157] Understanding the impli-

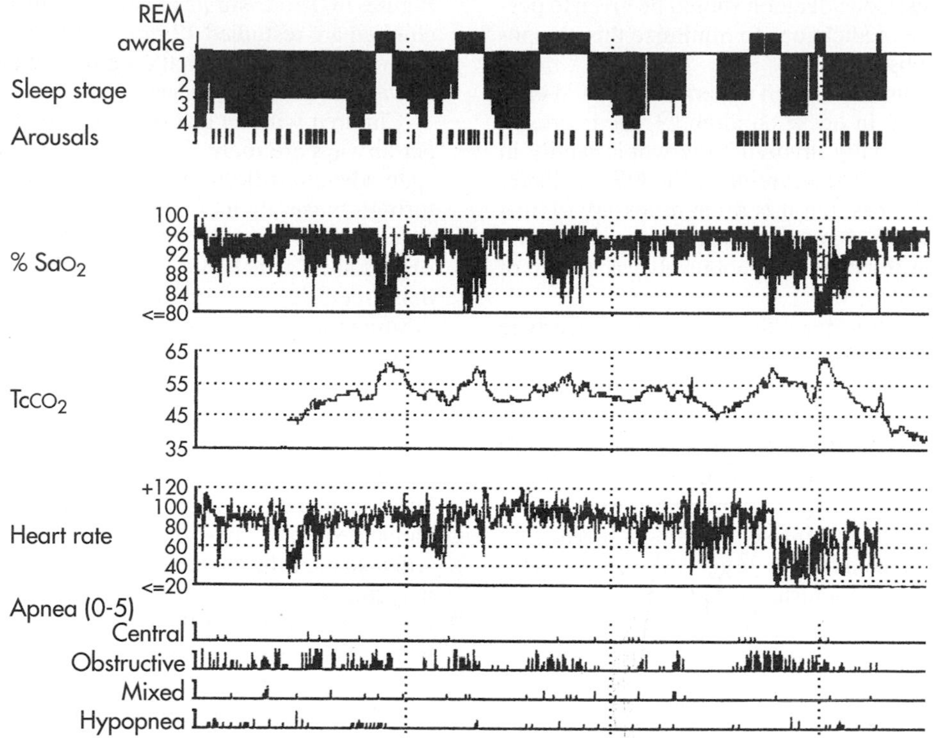

Fig. 73-6. Oxygen saturation and transcutaneous CO_2 recordings in a child with severe, repetitive obstructive apnea. Note that the periods of marked desaturation and CO_2 retention correspond to REM sleep.

cations of partial upper airway obstruction will be one of the keys to understanding the implications of OSA in children.

Young infants do tend to arouse with repetitive apnea[158] and the subsequent sleep disruption can result in significant attenuation of REM sleep. Deprivation of REM sleep during development has been shown to result in permanent behavioral changes, and brain morphologic and biochemical abnormalities in animals.[159] REM sleep deprivation increases neuronal excitability and facilitates seizure activity.[160] It is therefore hypothesized that significant abnormalities are likely to result from REM deprivation in young infants.

Figures 73-5 and 73-6 show recordings of repetitive obstructive apnea on polysomnogram and a summary record of SaO_2 and transcutaneous CO_2, respectively.

MANAGEMENT OPTIONS

It is not yet clear which pathophysiologic components of OSA are operative or dominant in producing the long-term sequelae of OSA in childhood. It is most likely that these severe sequelae are secondary to cumulative effects of severe, repeated hypoxic insults.[161] Sleep deprivation does lead to poor neurologic function and so caution is required before assuming that only the most dramatic sequelae (pulmonary hypertension, FTT, cardiac failure) are present, and only in very severe OSA. Adults, for example, have increased mortality from cardiovascular disease and one of the underlying drives for establishing early detection and treatment of mild to moderate disease in children is the prevention of unknown but equivalent long-term problems. In particular, the risk of neurologic sequelae underpins the desire to treat and thus maximize the neurointellectual outcomes for affected children.

Public Awareness

Public awareness of adult OSA is increasing slowly, despite the availability of effective treatment for the disorder and increasing knowledge of the morbidity and mortality associated with the untreated disease. The disorder in children is less well understood.

Support group networks have been one effective way of disseminating information to the public. A high percentage of children with syndromes and malformations are thought to suffer with OSA and their families often belong to such support associations. Public dissemination of information about the symptoms and signs of the disorder through such networks can help bring affected children to medical attention. Most support groups have newsletters, which are an effective means of distributing such information.

Medical Therapies

Acute deterioration during intercurrent infection is an opportunity to use vasoconstrictive agents in the nose, and oral steroids can acutely reduce lymphadenopathy (including adenotonsillar tissue). Pharmacologic or behavioral management options are limited for the treatment of OSA in children. Special consideration should be give to effective treatment of nasal congestion as part of the overall management of these children. One condition that is particularly amenable to medical treatment is allergic rhinitis, and topical nasal therapy may be effective in a number of these children.

Anticonvulsant therapy, especially the benzodiazepines, may contribute to upper airway discoordination and increase upper airway secretions. Consideration should be given to possible reduction of these medications to minimize this component of upper airway obstruction.

Obesity is not a common problem underlying OSA in children, but OSA can occur in obese children.[162] The treatment of obesity is difficult, usually involving the whole family in long-term intervention.[163] The severity of the OSA is likely to improve after weight loss, but it is often necessary to treat the OSA acutely by other means while commencing such a weight-control program. Obesity does not resolve as a result of effective treatment of OSA.

Chronic and acute respiratory disorders may exacerbate sleep-disordered breathing. Here, the sleep breathing is only one component of a complex problem.[126] Attention should be paid to diagnosing and treating specific conditions (such as frequent coughing), which will cause arousals and disturb sleep,[164] or hypoxia from interstitial lung disease that requires O_2 supplementation during sleep. Maximizing lower respiratory tract function, including aggressive treatment of acute infections, will minimize the additional impact on sleep. Additional treatment, such as nocturnal nasal oxygen, may be necessary during sleep periods.

Surgical Options

The mainstay of surgical treatment for obstructive apnea in children is adenotonsillectomy.[165] Adenotonsillectomy results in significant improvement in 80% of children with obstructive apnea.[11] Both tonsils and adenoids should be removed because adenoidectomy or tonsillectomy alone is commonly followed by failure to improve or subsequent deterioration. Adenotonsillectomy does have associated complications that are more common when it is undertaken to treat OSA,[166,167] such as postoperative apnea, infection, hemorrhage, and risk of sudden death. The size of the tonsils and adenoids clinically does not predict the degree of improvement in upper airway obstruction, even when the glands are not oversized.[143]

Recent studies do not support the initial impression of very high success rates from adenotonsillectomy. As indicated in Figure 73-7, our studies also show that when asymptomatic children are restudied 12 months after their surgery, their respiratory scores reveal that a significant degree of partial upper airway obstruction persists.

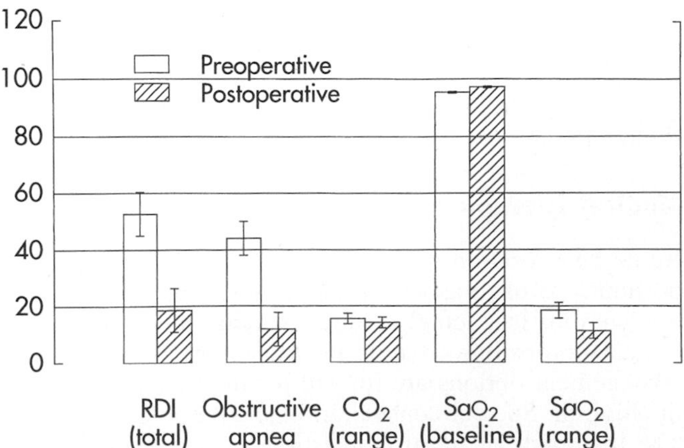

Fig. 73-7. Postoperative evaluation of children following adenotonsillectomy for OSA. The filled bars represent diagnostic polysomnography results for a group of 13 children. The unfilled bars represent the results when these children were recalled for follow-up studies 18 ± 2 months postoperatively. These children were considered well at the time of their studies.

Children with an anatomically small or dysfunctional upper airways are more likely to require ongoing treatment despite adenotonsillectomy[11] and should have follow-up monitoring; these include children with clefts, Pierre-Robin sequence and other craniofacial malformations, or skeletal dysplasias such as achondroplasia.[168] These constituted 70% of those requiring ongoing treatment in the authors' studies, indicating that they are more likely to have severe apnea. Other groups requiring ongoing supervision and intervention are those with diseases that worsen with age, such as mucopolysaccharidoses or muscular dystrophies.

Midface advancement may be used to treat OSA[168] and is being undertaken in skeletal disorders connected with maxillary and mandibular hypoplasia. This surgery is usually implemented on the basis of the cosmetic benefits expected but will also alter the character of the upper airway. Although this may improve the severity of the apnea, in the authors' experience it does not cure the OSA. When this surgery is undertaken, careful perioperative attention should be given to maintaining upper airway patency and normalizing sleep-breathing before and during the operative period.[169,170]

Palatal surgery to correct clefts is known to precipitate OSA, and care of children undergoing this surgery should be cognizant of this. If, after surgery, there is evidence that OSA has become severe, consideration should be given to reopening a previously repaired cleft palate. If pharyngoplasty is combined with cleft repair, then OSA is more likely, possibly as a result of loss of neurologic feedback. As at initial diagnosis, an anatomically good airway size does not preclude OSA.

Uvulopalatopharyngoplasty (UPPP) is mentioned only to caution against its application in children. This surgery is associated with poor long-term response and may have significant complications.[171] Tracheostomy always cures OSA, but because of its own inherent problems, such as loss of speech, and a 5% to 10% mortality rate, it should be considered only after other treatment options have failed.[172]

Diaphragmatic Pacing

This treatment has been available for a little over a decade, and is still developing, so it has potential for future expansion. It is currently used for children who have hypoventilation in the awake state.

Electrical stimulation of the diaphragm, using a small implantable electrode and receiver,[173] can successfully support ventilation in children with inadequate central respiratory drive or high quadriplegia.[174] The signal is transmitted by an antenna placed on the skin, overlying subcutaneously implanted receivers. An electrical impulse is then transmitted to the thoracic phrenic nerve, resulting in diaphragmatic contraction. The stimulus parameters that are most appropriate for children are a low stimulus frequency, short inspiratory time, and moderate respiratory rate.

For diaphragmatic pacing in young children, a tracheostomy is required to prevent pacing-related upper airway obstruction; the larynx does not dilate during inspiration because neurologic feedback is bypassed. Bilateral diaphragmatic pacing is required in children in order to achieve a sufficient level of ventilation. Because of the risk of permanent diaphragmatic and phrenic nerve injury, any additional support (more than 12 to 15 hours per day) requires alternative modes of delivery. The biggest advantage of this mode of treatment is the increased mobility it permits, although backup forms of ventilation should be available at all times. The most significant complications are infection (reported rate 6%), component failure, and mechanical nerve injury. The disadvantages of this mode of ventilation (high cost and the need for a tracheostomy and an external transmitter) mean that for patients who require ventilation only at night, mask ventilation is preferable.[175]

Nasal CPAP and Nasal Mask Ventilation

Nasal mask CPAP has been used for the treatment of adult OSA since 1981,[176] with exponential increase in the number of adult patients using this therapy since that time. The use of CPAP in children is increasing, and although initially hampered by practical difficulties, it is now a useful alternative to tracheostomy[11,177,178] and has potential for much wider use.

Polysomnography is required at the time of commencing CPAP to ensure correction of apnea without causing CO_2 retention. The authors' experience covers use of nasal CPAP in more than 80 children with a success rate of 80%. As seen in Figure 73-8, the age distribution of this group is not confined to the teenage years, confirming that CPAP is a practical treatment alternative for children who do not achieve relief of their upper airway obstruction by adenotonsillectomy. Two important factors in this success have been the development of a widely applicable pediatric nasal mask and head strap (Fig. 73-9), and the use of a behavioral program to introduce the therapy to children. Nasal prongs can be used to deliver the CPAP, as an alternative to the mask, but problems with local pressure effects tend to be greater. Regular reviews with polysomnography are mandatory as the child grows to ensure that treatment is maintained at appropriate therapeutic levels; infants especially require frequent review because of rapid growth and changing airway caliber.

Compliance must be monitored, but successful treatment is usually clear in terms of clinical improvement and is very dependent on family circumstances. Complications may include nasal irritation, with increased nasal discharge or obstruction, and secondary changes in facial growth.

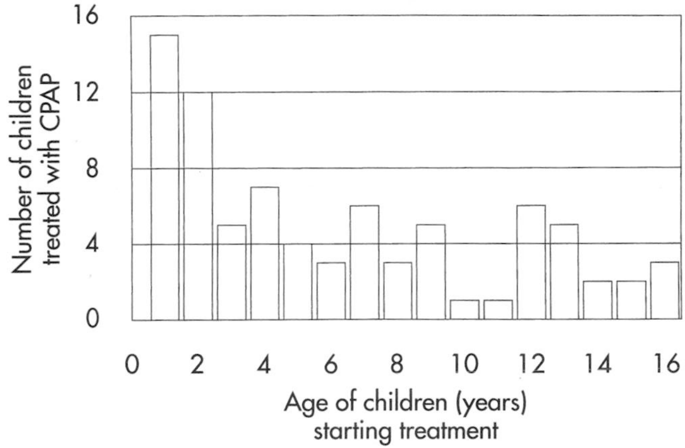

Fig. 73-8. Age distribution of children treated with nasal mask CPAP. There is a high frequency of CPAP correlating with the peak age of presentation of children with sleep-disordered breathing. There are children with sufficient severity of OSA to warrant use of nasal CPAP in all age groups.

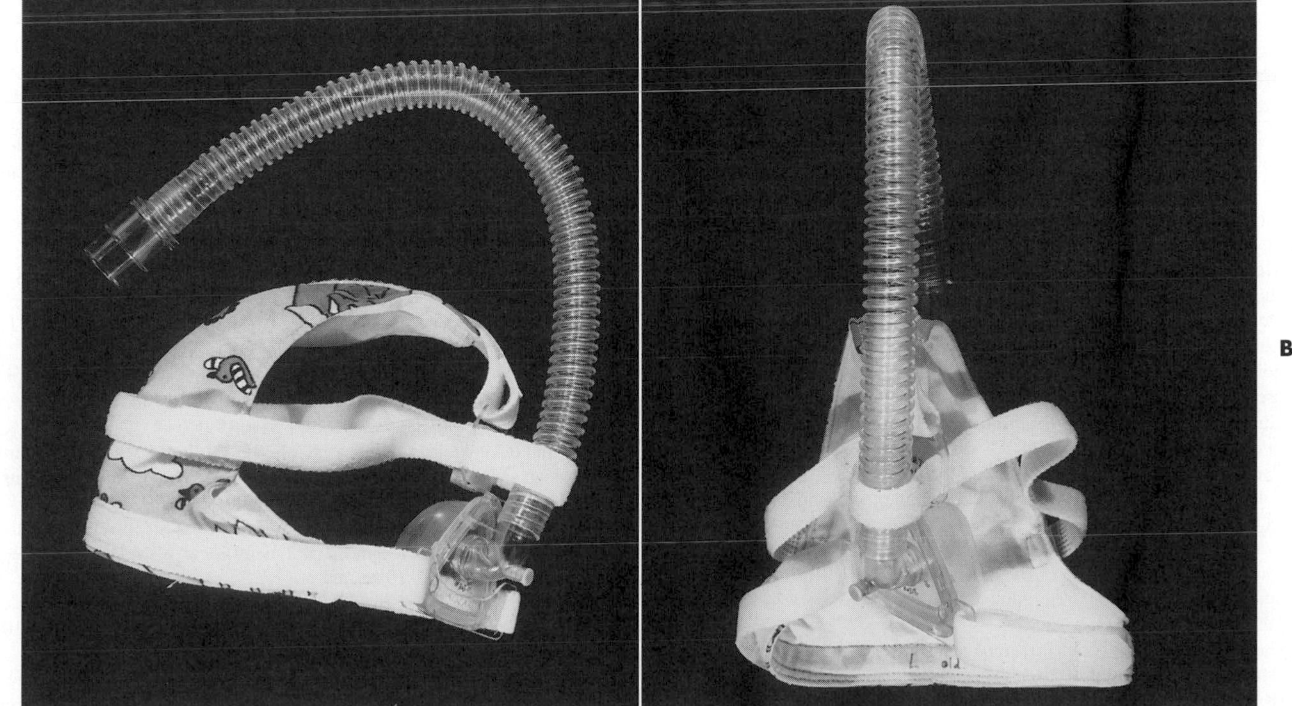

Fig. 73-9. Side (**A**) and front (**B**) view of nose mask and headstrap used in pediatrics. Recent developments in equipment have facilitated the use of nasal masks in young infants and children. Children of all ages may be established on the therapy in the home environment. An important feature is the clear manifold, which allows visualization of the nares.

Bilevel devices effectively provide pressure support ventilation, but they are used in place of CPAP in some clinics to try to improve compliance with therapy, especially in more severe disease. Nasal masks or prongs can also be used for the delivery of nocturnal volume or pressure cycled ventilation, in children who present with acquired central hypoventilation.[179] This mode of treatment delivery circumvents the need for tracheostomy and the authors have successfully used this treatment in the home environment, with children as young as 16 months. Overnight nursing assistance is usually required, as with tracheostomized children ventilated in the home environment,[103] but the need for special daytime care is essentially eliminated. It should be possible to use this technology in even younger infants with congenital central hypoventilation syndrome. Current developments mean that automatically responsive pressure devices will soon be available for all age groups, making both CPAP and nasal mask ventilation more precise and therefore more comfortable to use. The challenge now is to find a more definitive treatment option than CPAP or tracheostomy.

CONCLUSION

We are now able to successfully diagnose and treat OSA or hypoventilation because of advances in the level of knowledge and major technical advances. Children are still seen with very severe disease at the time of presentation. With time, improved knowledge about the consequences of mild to moderate OSA should improve the detection and treatment of the disease. With more refined studies, the precise implications of OSA in children will be elucidated. It is possible that some causative genetic or neurodevelopmental factor will be isolated in the future. Ongoing studies will determine the relationships between SIDS, the childhood syndrome of OSA, and the adult syndrome.

REFERENCES

1. Schechtman FG, Lin PT, Pincus RL: Urgent adenotonsillectomy for upper airway obstruction, *Int J Pediatr Otorhinolaryngol* 24(1):83-89. 1992.
2. Livesey JR, Solomons NB, Gillies EA: Emergency adenotonsillectomy for acute postoperative upper airway obstruction, *Anaesthesia* 46(1): 36-37, 1991.
3. McNamara SG, Cistulli PA, Strohl KP, Sullivan CE: Clinical aspects of sleep apnea. In *Sleep and breathing,* ed 2, New York, 1992, Marcel Dekker, ch 17.
4. Levy AM, Tabakin BS, Hanson JS, Narkewicz RM: Hypertrophied adenoids causing pulmonary hypertension and severe congestive heart failure, *N Engl J Med* 277(10):511, 1967.
5. Guilleminault C, Eldridge FL, Simmons FB, Dement WC: Sleep apnea in eight children, *Pediatrics* 58:23-31, 1976.
6. Pauli RM, Scott CI, Wassman ER, Gilbert EF, Leavitt LA, Ver Hoeve J, Hall JG, Partington MW, Jones KL, Sommer A, Feldman W, Langer LO, Rimoin DL, Hecht JT, Lebovitz R: Apnea and sudden unexpected death in infants with achondroplasia, *J Pediatrics* 104:342-348, 1984.
7. Carroll JL, Loughlin GM: Diagnostic criteria for obstructive sleep apnea syndrome in children [editorial], *Pediatr Pulmonol* 14(2):71-74, 1992.
8. Gaultier C: Obstructive sleep apnea syndrome in infants and children: established facts and unsettled issues, *Thorax* 50:1204-1210, 1995.
9. Rosen CL, D'Andrea L, Haddad GG: Adult criteria for obstructive sleep apnea do not identify children with serious obstruction, *Am Rev Respir Dis* 146(5,1):1231-1234, 1992.
10. Marcus CL, Omlin KJ, Basinki DJ, Bailey SL, Rachal AB, Von Pechmann WS, Keens TG, Ward SL: Normal polysomnographic values for children and adolescents, *Am Rev Respir Dis* 146(5 Pt 1):1235-1239, 1992.
11. Waters KA, Everett FM, Bruderer JW, Sullivan CE: Obstructive sleep apnea: the use of nasal CPAP in 80 children, *Am J Respir Crit Care Med* 152:780-785, 1995.

Prevalence

12. Ali NJ, Pitson DJ, Stradling JR: Snoring, sleep disturbance, and behaviour in 4-5 year olds, *Arch Dis Child* 68(3):360-366, 1993.
13. Zucconi M, Stranbi LF, Pestalozza G, Tessitore E, Smirne S: Habitual snoring and obstructive sleep apnoea syndrome in children: effects of early tonsil surgery, *Int J Pediatr Otorhinolaryngol* 26(3):235-243, 1993.
14. Rosenfeld RM, Green RP: Tonsillectomy and adenoidectomy: changing trends, *Ann Otol Rhinol Laryngol* 99(3 Pt 1):187-191, 1990.
15. Croft CB, Brockbank MJ, Wright A, Swanston AR: Obstructive sleep apnea in children undergoing routine tonsillectomy and adenoidectomy, *Clin Otolaryngol* 15(4):307-314, 1990.
16. Witucki J: Tonsillectomy. Analysis of the data for the 25-year period, *Otolaryngol Polska* 44(4):267-275, 1990.
17. Gislason T, Benediktsdottir B: Snoring, apneic episodes, and nocturnal hypoxemia among children 6 months to 6 years old, *Chest* 107:963-966, 1995.

Pathophysiology

18. Bosma JF: Functional anatomy of the upper airway during development. In Mathew OP, Sant'Ambrogio G, eds: *Respiratory function of the upper airway,* New York, 1988, Marcel Dekker, pp 47-86.
19. Stark AR, Thach BT: Mechanisms of airway obstruction leading to apnea in newborn infants, *J Pediatr* 89(6):982-985, 1976.
20. Mezzanotte WS, Tangel DJ, White DP: Waking genioglossal electromyogram in sleep apnea patients versus normal controls (a neuromuscular compensatory mechanism), *J Clin Invest* 89(5):1571-1579, 1992.
21. Tangel DJ, Mezzanotte WS, White DP: Influence of sleep on tensor palatini EMG and upper airway resistance in normal men, *J Appl Physiol* 70(6):2574-2581, 1991.
22. Hudgel DW, Harasick T: Fluctuation in timing of upper airway and chest wall inspiratory muscle activity in obstructive sleep apnea, *J Appl Physiol* 69(2):443-450, 1990.
23. Wheatley JR, Tangel DJ, Mezzanotte WS, White DP: Influence of sleep on alae nasi EMG and nasal resistance in normal men, *J Appl Physiol* 75(2):626-632, 1993.
24. Cistulli PA, Sullivan CE: Pathophysiology of sleep apnea. In Saunders N, Sullivan CE, eds: *Sleep and breathing,* ed 2, New York, 1992, Marcel Dekker, pp 405-448.
25. Kuna ST, Sant'Ambrogio G: Pathophysiology of upper airway closure during sleep (review), *JAMA* 266:1384-1389, 1991.
26. Ballard RD, Clover CW, White DP: Influence of non-REM sleep on inspiratory muscle activity and lung volume in asthmatic patients, *Am Rev Respir Dis* 147(4):880-886, 1993.
27. Singer LP, Saenger P: Complications of pediatric obstructive sleep apnea, *Otolaryngol Clin North Am* 23(4):665-676, 1990.
28. Guilleminault C, Stoohs R: Chronic snoring and obstructive sleep apnea syndrome in children, *Lung* 168 suppl:912-919, 1990.
29. Editorial: Airway obstruction during sleep in children, *Lancet* 2(8760):1018-1019, 1989.
30. Hultcrantz E, Löfstrand-Tideström B, Ahlquist-Rastad J: The epidemiology of sleep related breathing disorder in children, *Pediatr Otorhinolaryngol* 32(suppl):S63-S66, 1995.
31. Attal P, Lepajolec C, Harboun-Cohen E, Gaultier C, Bobin S: Obstructive sleep apnoea-hypopnoea syndromes in children. Therapeutic results, *Ann Otolaryngol Chir Cervico-Faciale* 107(3):174-179, 1990.
32. Guilleminault C, Stoohs R, Quera-Salva MA: Sleep-related obstructive and nonobstructive apneas and neurologic disorders, *Neurology* 42 (suppl 7,6):53-60, 1992.
33. Duffin J, Ezure K, Lipski J: Breathing rhythm generation: focus on the rostral ventrolateral medulla, *News in Physiological Sciences* 10:133-140, 1995.
34. Otake K, Ezure K, Lipski J, Wong She RB: Projections from the commissural subnucleus of the nucleus of the solitary tract: an anterograde tracing study in the cat, *J Comp Neurol* 324(3):365-378, 1992.
35. Berger AJ, Mitchell RA, Severinghaus JW: Regulation of respiration. The central respiratory controller, *N Engl J Med* 297(3):138-143, 1977.
36. Basner RD, Ringler J, Schwarzstein RM, Weinberger SE, Weiss JW: Phasic electromyographic activity of the genioglossus increases in normals during slow-wave sleep, *Respir Physiol* 83(2):189-200, 1992.

37. Harding R: Function of the larynx in the fetus and newborn, *Annu Rev Physiol* 46:645-59, 1984.
38. Thach BT: Neuromuscular control of the upper airway. In Beckerman RC, Brouillette RT, Hunt CE, eds: *Respiratory control disorders in infants and children,* Baltimore, 1992, Williams and Wilkins, pp 47-60.
39. Mathew OP: Upper airway negative-pressure effects on respiratory activity of upper airway muscles, *J Appl Physiol* 56:500-505, 1984.
40. Cohen G, Henderson-Smart DJ: Upper airway muscle activity during nasal occlusion in newborn babies, *J Appl Physiol* 66:1328-1335, 1989.
41. Mellins RB: Clinical observations of respiratory control. In Haddad GG, Farber JP, eds: *Developmental neurobiology of breathing,* New York, 1991, Marcel Dekker, pp 1-10.
42. Phillipson EA, Sullivan CE: Arousal: the forgotten response to respiratory stimuli, *Am Rev Respir Dis* 118:807-809, 1978.
43. Kimoff RJ, Kozar LF, Yasuma F, Bradley TD, Phillipson EA: Effect of inspiratory muscle unloading on arousal responses to CO_2 and hypoxia in sleeping dogs, *J Appl Physiol* 74(3):1325-1336, 1993.
44. Gugger M, Bogershausen S, Schaffler L: Arousal responses to added inspiratory resistance during REM and non-REM sleep in normal subjects, *Thorax* 48(2):125-129, 1993.
45. Gleeson K, Zwillich CW, White DP: The influence of increasing ventilatory effort on arousal from sleep, *Am Rev Respir Dis* 142(2):295-300, 1990.
46. Mograss MA, Ducharme FM, Brouillette RT: Abstract. Movement/arousals: description, classification and relationship to sleep apnea in children, *Am J Respir Crit Care Med* 150:1690-1696, 1994.
47. McNamara F, Issa FG, Sullivan CE: Arousal pattern following central and obstructive breathing abnormalities in infants and children, *J Appl Physiol* 81(6):2651-2657, 1996.
48. Waters KA, Everett F, Fagan E, Sillence DO, Sullivan CE: Breathing abnormalities in sleep in achondroplasia, *Arch Dis Child* 69:111-117, 1993.
49. Anderson JW, Sant'Ambrogio FB, Orani GP, Sant'Ambrogio G, Mathew OP: Carbon dioxide-responsive laryngeal receptors in dogs, *Respir Physiol* 82(2):217-226, 1990.
50. Sant'Ambrogio G, Mathew OP, Sant'Ambrogio FB: Characteristics of laryngeal cold receptors, *Respir Physiol* 71:287-297, 1988.
51. Henke KG, Sullivan CE: Abstract. Effects of high-frequency oscillating pressures on upper airway muscles in humans, *J Appl Physiol* 75:856-862, 1993.
52. Hwang JC, John WM, Bartlett D Jr: Afferent pathways for hypoglossal and phrenic responses to changes in upper airway pressure, *Respir Physiol* 55:342-354, 1984.
53. Dolfin T, Duffty P, Wilkes D, England S, Bryan H: Effects of a face mask and pneumotachograph on breathing in sleeping infants, *Am Rev Respir Dis* 128:977-979, 1983.
54. Widdicombe J: Nasal and pharyngeal reflexes. Protective and respiratory functions. In Mathew OP, Sant'Ambrogio G, eds: *Respiratory function of the upper airway,* New York, 1988, Marcel Dekker, pp 233-258.
55. Tomori A, Benacka R, Donic V, Tkacova R: Reversal of apnea by aspiration reflex in anaesthetized cats, *Eur Respir J* 4(9):1117-1125, 1991.
56. Steinschneider A: Nasopharyngitis and prolonged sleep apnea, *Pediatrics* 56(6):967-971, 1975.
57. Lindgren C, Grögaard J: Reflex apnea response and inflammatory mediators in infants with respiratory tract infection, *Acta Paediatr* 85:798-803, 1996.
58. Okabe S, Chonan T, Hida W, Satoh M, Kikuchi Y, Takishima T: Role of chemical drive in recruiting upper airway and inspiratory intercostal muscles in patients with obstructive sleep apnea, *Am Rev Respir Dis* 147(1):190-195, 1993.
59. Wilhoit SC, Suratt PM: Effect of nasal obstruction on upper airway muscle activation in normal subjects, *Chest* 92(6):1053-1055, 1987.
60. Henke KG, Dempsey JA, Badr MS, Kowitz JM, Skatrud JB: Effect of sleep-induced increases in upper airway resistance on respiratory muscle activity, *J Appl Physiol* 70(1):158-168, 1991.
61. Jeffries B, Brouillette R, Hunt C: Electromyographic study of some accessory muscles of respiration in children with obstructive sleep apnea, *Am Rev Respir Dis* 129:696-702, 1984.
62. Gauda EB, Miller MJ, Carlo WA, Difiore JM, Johnsen DC, Martin RJ: Genioglossus response to airway occlusion in apneic versus nonapneic infants, *Pediatr Res* 22(6):683-687, 1987.
63. Cohen G, Henderson-Smart DJ: Upper airway stability and apnea during nasal occlusion in newborn infants, *J Appl Physiol* 60(5):1511-1517, 1986.
64. Upton CJ, Milner AD, Stokes GM: Upper airway patency during apnoea of prematurity, *Arch Dis Child* 67(4):419-424, 1992.
65. Milner AD, Saunders RA, Hopkin IE: Apnoea induced by airflow obstruction, *Arch Dis Child* 52:379-382, 1977.
66. Pack AI, Gottschalk A: Mechanisms of ventilatory periodicities, *Ann Biomed Engineering* 21(5):537-544, 1993.
67. Eiselt M, Curzi-Dascalova L, Leffler C, Christova E: Sigh-related heart rate changes during sleep in premature and full-term newborns, *Neuropaediatrics* 23(6):286-291, 1992.
68. Shannon DC, Carley DW, Kelly DH: Periodic breathing: quantitative analysis and clinical description, *Pediatr Pulmonol* 4:98-102, 1988.
69. Read DJC: A clinical method for assessing the ventilatory responses to hypercapnia in normal sleeping humans, *Aust Ann Med* 16:20-32, 1967.
70. Berthon-Jones M, Sullivan CE: Ventilatory and arousal responses to hypoxia in sleeping humans, *Am Rev Respir Dis* 125:623-639, 1982.
71. Cohen G, Henderson-Smart DJ: A modified rebreathing method to study the ventilatory response of the newborn to carbon dioxide, *J Dev Physiol* 14(5):295-301, 1990.
72. Martin RJ, DiFiore JM, Korinke CB, Randal H, Miller MJ, Brooks LJ: Vulnerability of respiratory control in healthy preterm infants placed supine, *J Pediatr* 127(4):609-614, 1995.
73. Ward SL, Bautista DB, Keens TG: Hypoxic arousal responses in normal infants, *Pediatrics* 89(5):860-864, 1992.

Relationships Between Respiration and Sleep

74. Wiegand L, Zwillich CW, Wiegand D, White DP: Changes in upper airway muscle activation and ventilation during phasic REM sleep in normal men, *J Appl Physiol* 71(2):488-497, 1991.
75. Cantineau JP, Escourrou P, Sartene R, Gaultier C, Goldman M: Accuracy of respiratory inductive plethysmography during wakefulness and sleep in patients with obstructive sleep apnea, *Chest* 102(4):145-1151, 1992.
76. Lanigan C, Ponte J, Moxham J: Drift in vivo of transcutaneous dual electrodes, *Adv Exp Med Biol* 220:41-44, 1987.
77. Rechtschaffen A, Kales A, eds: *A manual of standardised terminology: techniques and scoring stages of human subjects.* Los Angeles, 1968, UCLA Brain Information Service/Brain Research Institute.
78. Anders T, Emde R, Parmelee A, eds: *A manual of standardised terminology, techniques, and criteria for scoring of states of sleep and wakefulness in newborn infants.* Los Angeles, 1971, UCLA Brain Information Service, NINDS Neurological Information Network.
79. Hoppenbrouwers T, Jensen D, Hodgman J, Harper R, Sterman M: Respiration during the first six months of life in normal infants. Part II. The emergence of a circadian pattern, *Neuropaediatrie* 10(3):264-280, 1979.
80. Glotzbach SF, Edgar DM, Beoddiker M, Ariagno RL: Biological rhythmicity in normal infants during the first 3 months of life, *Pediatrics* 94(4):482-488, 1994.
81. Coons S: Development of sleep and wakefulness during the first 6 months of life. In Guilleminault C, ed: *Sleep and its disorders in children,* New York, 1987, Raven Press.
82. Hoppenbrouwers T: Sleep in infants. In Guilleminault C, ed: *Sleep and its disorders in children,* New York, 1987, Raven Press.
83. Tepper RS, Skatrud JB, Dempsey JA: Ventilation and oxygenation changes during sleep in cystic fibrosis, *Chest* 84:399-393, 1983.
84. Tabachnik E, Muller NL, Bryan AC, Levison H: Changes in ventilation and chest wall mechanics during sleep in normal adolescents, *J Appl Physiol* 51:557-564, 1981.
85. Ingrassia TS III, Nelson SB, Harris CD, Hubmayr RD: Influence of sleep state on CO_2 responsiveness. A study of the unloaded respiratory pump in humans, *Am Rev Respir Dis* 144(5):1125-1129, 1991.
86. Masters IB, Goes AM, Healy L, O'Neil M, Stephens D, Harris MA: Age-related changes in oxygen saturation over the first year of life: a longitudinal study, *J Paediatr Child Health* 30:423-428, 1994.
87. Hoppenbrouwers T, Hodgman JE, Arakawa K, Durand M, Cabal LA: Transcutaneous oxygen and carbon dioxide during the first half year of life in premature and normal term infants, *Pediatr Res* 31(1):73-79, 1992.
88. Phillipson EA: Control of breathing during sleep, *Am Rev Respir Dis* 118:909-939, 1978.
89. Glotzbach SF, Ariagno RL: Periodic breathing. In Beckerman RC, Brouillette RT, Hunt CE, eds: *Respiratory control disorders in infants and children,* Baltimore, 1992, Williams and Wilkins, pp 142-160.
90. Beardsmore CS, MacGadyen UM, Shakeeb S, Moosavi H, Wimpress SP, Thompson J, Simpson H: Measurement of lung volumes during active and quiet sleep in infants, *Pediatr Pulmonol* 7:71-77, 1989.

91. Henderson-Smart DJ, Read DJC: Reduced lung volume during behavioural active sleep in the newborn, *J Appl Physiol* 46:1081-1085, 1979.
92. Carse EA, Wilkinson AR, Whyte PL, Henderson-Smart DJ, Johnson P: Oxygen and carbon dioxide tensions, breathing and heart rate in normal infants during the first six months of life, *J Dev Physiol* 3:85-100, 1981.

Pathology of OSA

93. Koopmann CF Jr, Moran WB Jr: Surgical management of obstructive sleep apnea. *Otolaryngol Clin North Am* 23(4):787-808, 1990.
94. Guilleminault C, Heldt G, Powell N, Riley R: Small upper airway in near-miss sudden infant death syndrome infants and their families, *Lancet* 2:402-407, 1986.
95. Mathur R, Douglas NJ: Family studies in patients with the sleep apnea-hypopnea syndrome, *Ann Intern Med* 122(3):174-178, 1995.
96. Kakitsuba N, Sadaoka T, Motoyama S, Fujiwara Y, Kanai R, Hayashi I, Takahashi H: Sleep apnea and sleep-related breathing disorders in patients wtih craniofacial synostosis. *Acta Otolarygol* (Stockh) 517(suppl):6-10, 1994.
97. Brodsky L, Adler E, Stanievich JF: Naso- and oropharyngeal dimensions in children with obstructive sleep apnea, *Int J Pediatr Otorhinolaryngol* 17(1):1-11, 1989.
98. Hultcrantz E, Larson M, Hellquist R, Ahlquist-Rastad J, Svanholm H, Jakobsson OP: The influence of tonsillar obstruction and tonsillectomy on facial growth and dental arch morphology, *Int J Pediatr Otorhinolaryngol* 22(2):125-134, 1991.
99. Semenza GL, Pyeritz RE: Respiratory complications of mucopolysaccharide storage disorders, *Medicine* (Baltimore) 67(4):209-219, 1988.
100. Mathew OP: Maintenance of upper airway patency, *J Pediatr* 106:863-869, 1985.
101. Sullivan CE, Grunstein RR, Marrone O, Berthon-Jones M: Sleep apnea—pathophysiology: upper airway and control of breathing. In Guilleminault C, Partinen M, eds: *Obstructive sleep apnea syndrome: clinical research and treatment,* New York, 1990, Raven Press, pp 49-69.
102. Marcus CL, Gozal D, Arens R, Basinski DJ, Omlin KJ, Keens TG, Davidson Ward SL: Ventilatory responses during wakefulness in children with obstructive sleep apnea, *Am J Respir Crit Care Med* 149:715-721, 1994.
103. Weese-Mayer DE, Silvestri JM, Menzies JL, Morrow-Kenny AS, Hunt CE, Hauptman SA: Congenital central hypoventilation syndrome: diagnosis, management, and long-term outcome in thirty-two children, *J Pediatr* 120:381-387, 1992.
104. Del Carmen Sanchez M, Lopez-Herce J, Carrillo A, Moral R, Arias B, Rodriguez A, Sancho L: Late onset central hypoventilation syndrome, *Pediatr Pulmonol* 21:189-191, 1996.
105. Marcus CL, Bautista DB, Amihyia A, Ward SL, Keens TG: Hypercapneic arousal responses in children with congenital central hypoventilation syndrome, *Pediatrics* 88(5):993-998, 1991.
106. Fodstad H, Ljunggren B, Shawis R: Ondine's curse with Hirschsprung's disease, *Br J Neurosurg* 4(2):87-93, 1990.
107. Weese-Mayer DE, Brouillette RT, Naidich TP, McLone DG, Hunt CE: Magnetic resonance imaging and computerized tomography in central hypoventilation, *Am Rev Respir Dis* 137:393-398, 1988.
108. Davidson Ward SL, Jacobs RA, Gates EP, Hart LD, Keens TG: Absent hypoxic and hypercapneic arousal responses in children with myelomeningocele, *J Pediatr* 109:631-634, 1986.
109. Kahn A, Groswasser J, Sottiaux M, Rebuffat E, Sunseri M, Franco P, Dramaix M, Bochner A, Belhadi B, Foperster M: Clinical symptoms associated with brief obstructive sleep apnea in normal infants, *Sleep* 16(5):409-413, 1993.
110. Kahn A, Groswasser J, Rebuffat E, Sottiaux M, Blum D, Foerster M, Franco P, Bochner A, Alexander M, Bachy A, et al: Sleep and cardiorespiratory characteristics of infant victims of sudden death: a prospective case-control study, *Sleep* 15(4):287-292, 1992.
111. Tishler PV, Redline S, Ferrette V, Hans MG, Altose MD: The association of sudden unexpected infant death with obstructive sleep apnea, *Am J Respir Crit Care Med* 153(6):1857-1863, 1996.
112. Mathur R, Douglas NJ: Relation between the sudden infant death syndrome and adult sleep apnoea/hypopnoea syndrome (letter), *Lancet* 344(8925):819-820, 1994.
113. Shechtman VL, Raetz SL, Harper RK, Garfinkel A, Wilson AJ, Southall DP, Harper RM: Dynamic analysis of cardiac R-R intervals in normal infants and in infants who subsequently succumbed to the sudden infant death syndrome, *Pediatr Res* 31(6):606-612, 1992.
114. Marsh JL: Cleft palate and velopharyngeal dysfunction, *Clin Commun Disord* 1(3):29-34, 1991.
115. Ysunza A, Garcia-Velasco M, Garcia-Garcia M, Haro R, Valencia M: Obstructive sleep apnea secondary to surgery for velopharyngeal insufficiency, *Cleft Palate Craniofac J* 30(4):387-390, 1993.
116. Freed G, Pearlman MA, Brown AS, Barot LR: Polysomnographic indications for surgical intervention in Pierre Robin sequence: acute airway management and follow-up studies after repair and take-down of tongue-lip adhesion, *Cleft Palate J* 25(2):151-155, 1988.
117. Gilmore RL, Falace P, Kanga J, Baumann R: Sleep-disordered breathing in Moebius syndrome, *J Child Neurol* 6(1):73-77, 1991.
118. Morley AR: Laryngeal stridor, Arnold-chiari malformation and medullary haemorrhages, *Dev Med Child Neurol* 11:471-474, 1969.
119. Sieben RL, Hamida MB, Shulman K: Multiple cranial nerve deficits associated with the Arnold-Chiari malformation, *Neurology* 21:673-681, 1971.
120. Marcus CL, Keens TG, Bautista DB, von Pechmann WS, Davidson Ward SL: Obstructive sleep apnea in children with Down syndrome, *Pediatrics* 88(1):132-139, 1991.
121. Stebbens VA, Dennis J, Samuels MP, Croft CB, Southall DP: Sleep related upper airway obstruction in a cohort with Down's syndrome, *Arch Dis Child* 66:1333-1338, 1991.
122. Bye PT, Ellis ER, Issa FG, Donnelly PM, Sullivan CE: Respiratory failure and sleep in neuromuscular disease, *Thorax* 45(4):241-247, 1990.
123. Cistulli PA, Sullivan CE: Sleep disorders in Marfan's syndrome, *Lancet* 337:1359-1360, 1991.
124. Pauli RM, Horton VK, Glinski LP, Reiser CA: Prospective assessment of risks for cervicomedullary-junction compression in infants with achondroplasia, *Am J Hum Genet* 56:732-744, 1995.
125. Waters KA, Everett F, Sillence DO, Fagan ER, Sullivan CE: Treatment of obstructive sleep apnea in achondroplasia: evaluation of sleep, breathing, and somatosensory-evoked potentials, *Am J Med Genet* 59:460-466, 1995.
126. Gaultier C: Cardiorespiratory adaptation during sleep in infants and children, *Pediatr Pulmonol* 19:105-117, 1995.
127. Gaultier C: Respiration during sleep in children with chronic obstructive pulmonary disease and asthma. In Guilleminault C, ed: *Sleep and its disorders in children*, New York, 1987, Raven Press, pp 225-229.
128. Waters KA, Kirjavainen T, Jimenez M, Cowell CT, Sillence DO, Sullivan CE: Overnight growth hormone secretion in achondroplasia: deconvolution analysis, correlation with sleep state, and changes after treatment of obstructive sleep apnea, *Pediatr Res* 39(3):547-553, 1996.
129. Marcus CL, Carroll JL, Koerner CB, Hamer A, Lutz J, Loughlin GM: Determinants of growth in children with the obstructive sleep apnea syndrome, *J Pediatr* 125:556-562, 1994.

Clinical Characteristics

130. Brouillette R, Hanson D, David R, Klemka L, Szatkowski A, Fernbach S, Hunt C: A diagnostic approach to suspected obstructive sleep apnea in children, *J Pediatr* 105:10-14, 1984.
131. Frank Y, Kravath RE, Pollak CP, Weitzman ED: Obstructive sleep apnea and its therapy: clinical and polysomnographic manifestations, *Pediatrics* 71(5):737-742, 1983.
132. Mixter RC, David DJ, Perloff WH, Green CG, Pauli RM, Popic PM: Obstructive sleep apnea in Apert's and Pfeiffer's syndromes: more than a craniofacial abnormality, *Plast Reconstr Surg* 86(3):457-463, 1990.
133. Weider DJ, Sateia MJ, West RP: Nocturnal enuresis in children with upper airway obstruction, *Otolaryngol Head Neck Surg* 105(3):427-432, 1991.
134. Guilleminault C: Review. Obstructive sleep apnea syndrome and its treatment in children: areas of agreement and controversy, *Pediatr Pulmonol* 3:429-436, 1987.
135. Biban P, Baraldi E, Pettenazzo A, Fillipone M, Zacchelo F: Adverse effect of chloral hydrate in two young children with obstructive sleep apnea, *Pediatrics* 92(3):461-463, 1993.
136. Redline S, Tishler PV, Tosteson TD, Williamson J, Kump K, Browner I, Ferrette V, Krejci P: The familial aggregation of obstructive sleep apnea, *Am J Respir Crit Care Med* 151(3):382-387, 1995.
137. Yoshizawa T, Akashiba T, Kurashina K, Otsuka K, Horie T: Genetics and obstructive sleep apnea syndrome: a study of human leukocyte antigen (HLA) typing, *Intern Med* 32(2):94-97, 1993.
138. Olsen KD, Kern EB: Nasal influences on snoring and obstructive sleep apnea, *Mayo Clinic Proc* 65(8):1095-1105, 1990.

139. McColley SA, Carroll JL, Curtis S, Loughlin GM, Sampson HA: High prevalence of allergic sensitisation in children with habitual snoring and obstructive sleep apnea, *Chest* 111:170-173, 1997.
140. McGowan FX, Kenna MA, Fleming JA, O'Connor T: Adenotonsillectomy for upper airway obstruction carries increased risk in children with a history of prematurity, *Pediatr Pulmonol* 13(4):222-226, 1992.
141. Leiberman A, Ohki M, Forte V, Fraschetti J, Cole P: Nose/mouth distribution of respiratory airflow in 'mouth breathing' children, *Acta Otolaryngol* 109(5-6):454-460, 1990.
142. Guilleminault C, Stoohs R: Obstructive sleep apnea syndrome in children, *Pediatrician* 17(1):46-51, 1990.
143. Suzuki K, Yamamoto SI, Ito Y, Baba S: Sleep apnea associated with congenital diseases and moderate hypertrophy of tonsils, *Acta Otolaryngol* (Stockh) 523(suppl):225-227, 1996.
144. Contencin P, Nottet JB, Yacoubian K, Soussi T, Nivoche Y, Narcy P: Pharyngolaryngeal fibroscopy under general anesthesia in children. Technique and indications in sleep apnoea and hypopnea, *Ann Otolaryngol Chir Cervicofac* 108(7):373-377, 1991.
145. Castiglione N, Eterno C, Sciuto C, Bottaro G, La Rosa M, Patane R: The diagnostic approach to and clinical study of 23 children with an obstructive sleep apnoea syndrome. *Pediatr Med Chir* 14(5):501-506, 1992.
146. Williams EF III, Woo P, Miller R, Kellman RM: The effects of adenotonsillectomy on growth in young children, *Otolaryngol Head Neck Surg* 104(4):509-516, 1991.
147. Freezer NJ, Bucens IK, Robertson CF: Obstructive sleep apnoea presenting as failure to thrive in infancy, *J Paediatr Child Health* 31:172-175, 1995.
148. Pinhas-Hamiel O, Dolan LM, Daniels SR, Standiford D, Khoury PR, Zeitler P: Increased incidence of non-insulin diabetes mellitus among adolescents, *J Pediatr* 128(5):608-615, 1996.
149. Tal A, Leiberman A, Margulis G, Sofer S: Ventricular dysfunction in children with obstructive sleep apnea: radionuclide assessment, *Pediatr Pulmonol* 4(3):139-143, 1988.

Further Studies

150. Gibson SE, Myer CM, Strife JL, O'Connor DM: Sleep fluoroscopy for localization of upper airway obstruction in children, *Ann Otol Rhinol Laryngol* 105:678-683, 1996.
151. Gunn TR, Tonkin SL: Upper airway measurements during inspiration and expiration in infants, *Pediatrics* 84(1):73-77, 1989.
152. John SD, Swischuk LE: Stridor and upper airway obstruction in infants and children, *Radiographics* 12(4):625-643, 1992.
153. Croft CB, Thomson HG, Samuels MP, Southall DP: Endoscopic evaluation and treatment of sleep-associated upper airway obstruction in infants and young children, *Clin Otolaryngol* 15(3):209-216, 1990.
154. Abdulhamid I, Vauthy PA, Barnett BA, Hufford DR, Reddy RP, Hunt CE: Comparison of 2-channel and 4-channel pneumograms, *Pediatr Pulmonol* 13(2):245-249, 1992.
155. Sadeh A, Lavie P, Scher A, Tirosh E, Epstein R: Actigraphic home-monitoring sleep-disturbed and control infants and young children: a new method for pediatric assessment of sleep-wake patterns, *Pediatrics* 87(4):494-499, 1991.
156. McNamara F, Harris MA, Sullivan CE: Effects of nasal continuous positive airway pressure on apnoea index and sleep in infants, *J Paediatr Child Health* 31(2):88-94, 1995.
157. Guilleminault C, Philip P: Polygraphic investigation of respiration during sleep in infants and children, *J Clin Neurophysiol* 9(1):48-55, 1992.
158. Thoppil CK, Belan MA, Cowen CP, Mathew OP: Behavioural arousal in newborn infants and its association with termination of apnea, *J Appl Physiol* 70(6):2479-2484, 1991.
159. Mirmiran M, Scholtens J, van de Poll NE, Uylings HB, van der Gugten J, Boer GJ: Effects of experimental suppression of active (REM) sleep during early development upon adult brain and behavior in the rat, *Brain Res* 283(2-3):277-286, 1983.
160. Dzoljic MR, Ukponmwan OE, Rupreht J, Haffmans J: Role of the enkephalinergic system in sleep studied by an enkephalinase inhibitor. In Wauquier et al, eds: *Sleep: neurotransmitters and neuromodulators,* New York, 1985, Raven Press.

Management Options

161. Strohl KP, Sullivan CE, Saunders NA: Sleep apnea syndromes. In Saunders NA, Sullivan CE, eds: *Sleep and breathing,* New York, 1984, Marcel Dekker.
162. Silvestri JM, Weese-Mayer DE, Bass MT, Kenny AS, Hauptman SA, Pearsall SM: Polysomnography in obese children with a history of sleep-associated breathing disorders. *Pediatr Pulmonol* 16(2):124-129, 1993.
163. Williams CL, Bollella M, Carter BJ: Treatment of childhood obesity in pediatric practice, *Ann NY Acad Sci* 699:207-219, 1993.
164. Sullivan CE, Kozar LF, Murphy E, Phillipson EA: Arousal, ventilatory and airway responses to bronchopulmonary stimulation in sleeping dogs, *J Appl Physiol* 47:17-25, 1979.
165. Stradling JR, Thomas G, Warley AR, Williams P, Freeland A: Effect of adenotonsillectomy on nocturnal hypoxaemia, sleep disturbance, and symptoms in snoring children, *Lancet* 335(8684):249-253, 1990.
166. Wiatrak BJ, Myer CM III, Andrew TM: Complications of adenotonsillectomy in children under 3 years of age, *Am J Otolaryngol* 12(3):170-172, 1991.
167. Price SD, Hawkins DB, Kahlstrom EJ: Tonsil and adenoid surgery for airway obstruction: perioperative respiratory morbidity, *Ear Nose Throat J* 72(8):526-531, 1993.
168. Edwards TJ, David DJ, Martin J: Aggressive surgical management of sleep apnea syndrome in the syndromal craniosynostoses, *J Craniofac Surg* 3(1):8-10, 1992.
169. Lauritzen C, Lilja J, Jarlstedt J: Airway obstruction and sleep apnea in children with craniofacial anomalies, *Plast Reconstr Surg* 77(1):1-6, 1986.
170. Rosen GM, Muckel RP, Mahowald MW, Goding GS, Ulevig C: Postoperative respiratory compromise in children with obstructive sleep apnea syndrome: can it be anticipated? *Pediatrics* 93(5):784-788, 1994.
171. Carenfelt C, Haraldson PO: Frequency of complications after uvulopalatopharngoplasty (letter), *Lancet* 341(8842):437, 1993.
172. Simma B, Spehler D, Burger R, Uehlinger J, Ghelfi D, Dangel P, Hof E, Fancóni S: Tracheostomy in children, *Eur J Pediatr* 153(4):291-296, 1994.
173. Judson JP, Glenn WL: Radiofrequency electrophrenic respiration. Longterm application to a patient with primary hypoventilation, *JAMA* 203:1033-1037, 1968.
174. Brouillette RT, Marzocchi M: Diaphragm pacing: clinical and experimental results, *Biol Neonat* 65(3-4):265-271, 1994.
175. Moxham J, Shneerson JM: Diaphragmatic pacing, *Am Rev Respir Dis* 148:533-536, 1993.
176. Sullivan CE, Issa FG, Berthon-Jones M, Eves L: Reversal of obstructive sleep apnoea by continuous positive airway pressure applied through the nares, *Lancet* 1:862-865, 1981.
177. Marcus CL, Davidson Ward SL, Mallory GB, Rosen CL, Beckerman RC, Weese-Mayer DE, Brouillette RT, Trang HT, Brooks LJ: Use of nasal continuous positive airway pressure as treatment of childhood obstructive sleep apnea, *J Pediatr* 127:88-94, 1995.
178. Guilleminault C, Pelayo R, Clerk A, Leger D, Bocian RC: Home nasal continuous positive airway pressure in infants with sleep-disordered breathing, *J Pediatr* 127:905-912, 1995.
179. Ellis ER, McCauley VB, Mellis C, Sullivan CE: Treatment of alveolar hypoventilation in a six-year-old girl with intermittent positive pressure ventilation through a nose mask, *Am Rev Respir Dis* 135:188-191, 1987.

Suggested Readings

Beckerman RC, Brouillette RT, Hunt CE, eds: *Respiratory control disorders in infants and children,* Baltimore, 1992,Williams & Wilkins.
Ferber R, Kryger M, eds: *Principles and practice of sleep medicine in the child,* Philadelphia, 1995, WB Saunders.
Saunders N, Sullivan CE, eds: *Sleep and breathing,* New York, 1994, Marcel Dekker.
Thorpy, MJ, ed: *Handbook of sleep disorders,* New York, 1990, Marcel Dekker.

CHAPTER 74

Neuromuscular and Chest-Wall Disorders

Julian Lewis Allen and Mary Ellen B. Wohl

The respiratory system has gas exchange and pump components. Failure of either leads to respiratory failure by different mechanisms (Fig. 74-1).[1] This chapter describes the pump component: normal growth and development of the chest wall, disorders of development of the chest wall, and respiratory muscle weakness.

GROWTH AND DEVELOPMENT OF THE CHEST WALL

Structural Changes with Growth

Major structural changes occur in the chest wall with growth, and these changes have important functional implications for respiratory pump efficiency and function. In infancy, the orientation of the ribs is horizontal; with growth a progressive caudal declination occurs and by the age of 10 years the adult pattern of downward-sloping ribs is achieved[2] (Figs. 74-2, 74-3).

Ossification of the chest wall begins in utero and continues to approximately the 25th year. Vertebral ossification starts by the end of the embryonic period (7th week gestation),[3] and continues to age 25 years. Sternal ossification centers appear by the 5th month of fetal life, although the xiphoid process may not begin ossification until the 3rd year or later (Fig. 74-3*A*); fusion of the individual ossification centers is complete by 25 years (Fig. 74-3*B*). Rib ossification is complete by age 20.[4] Progressive calcification of the costal cartilages can continue into old age (Fig. 74-4).

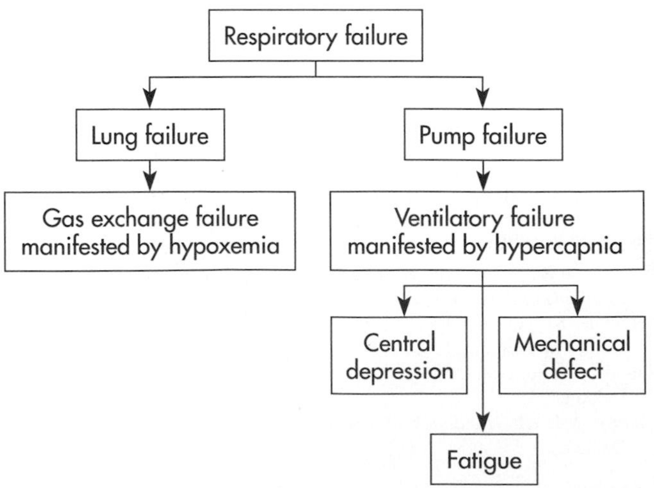

Fig. 74-1. Mechanisms of respiratory failure. (From Roussos C, Macklem PT: *N Engl J Med* 307(13):786-797, 1982.)

Functional Consequences of Developmental Structural Changes of the Chest Wall

Mechanical Properties

Specific chest wall compliance progressively decreases with growth. In the infant, compliance of the chest wall is three to six times that of the lung.[5-8] Chest wall compliance is greater in preterm infants than in full-term infants[8] and decreases further during the first 2 years of life.[9] In school age children, chest wall compliance is approximately twice that of the lung[10]; in the mature adult it is equal to that of the lung and in the elderly it may be half that of the lung[11] (Fig. 74-5).

These changes in chest wall compliance are accounted for by the increasing ossification of the chest wall with age. Increasing muscle mass probably also contributes to this increased stiffening with age.[12-14]

Although it is advantageous to have a highly compliant chest wall during the birthing process, functional disadvantages occur in infancy. The respiratory pump is less efficient in moving tidal volume. The respiratory muscles, by decreasing pleural pressure, expend energy both drawing tidal volume in and distorting the chest wall. This can result in the work performed by the diaphragm exceeding the work performed on the lung up to sevenfold.[15]

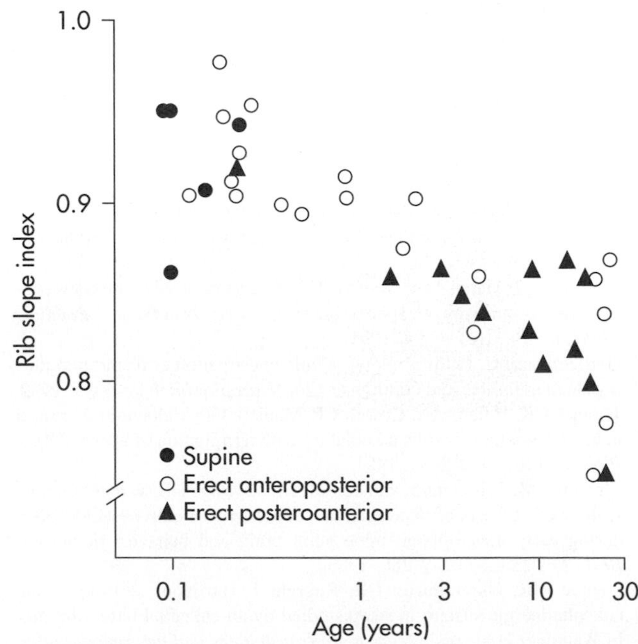

Fig. 74-2. Changes in rib slope index with age. A slope index of 1.0 indicates a horizontal lie of the ribs; lower indices indicate a downward slope. (From Openshaw P, Edwards S, Helms P: *Thorax* 39:624-627, 1984.)

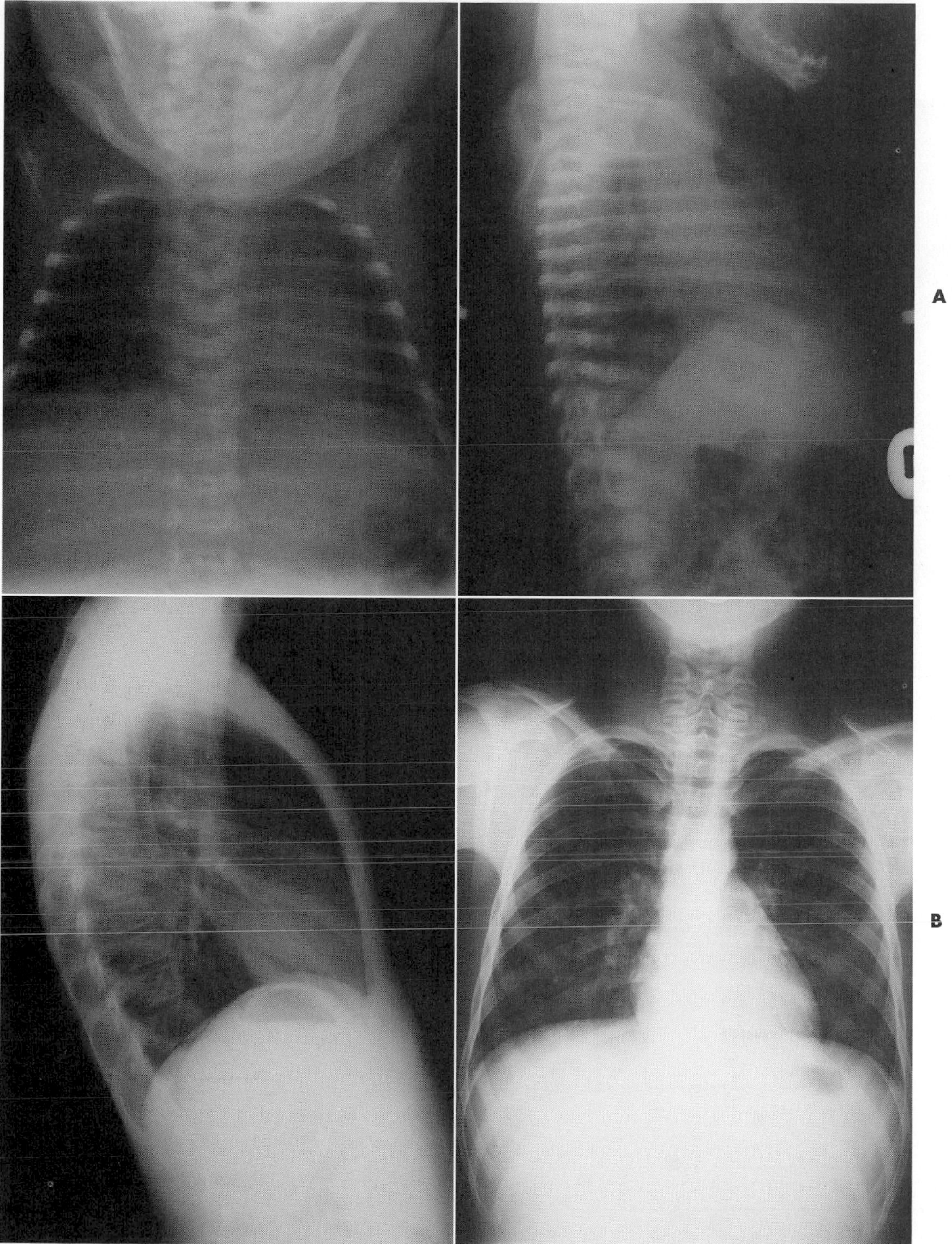

Fig. 74-3. Changes in ribcage morphometry with growth. **A,** Posteroanterior (PA) and lateral chest radiographs of a 4-month-old infant. **B,** PA and lateral chest radiographs of a 14-year-old boy. In the infant the slope of the ribs is nearly horizontal, whereas in the 14-year old there is a downward declination of the ribs. Progressive ossification of the sternal ossification centers can be seen in the lateral

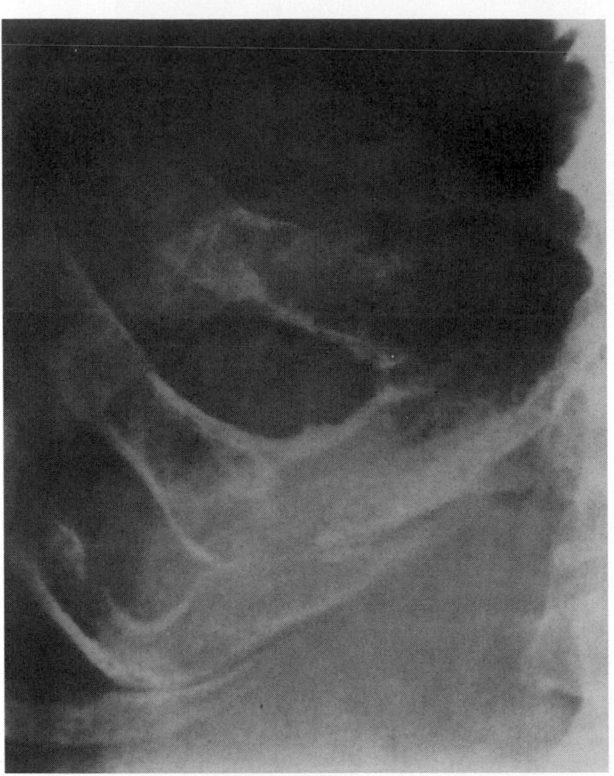

Fig. 74-4. Calcification of the costal cartilages in a 65-year-old man. (From Scott W, Scott P, Treretola S: *Radiology of thoracic skeleton,* Philadelphia, 1991, BC Decker, p 5.)

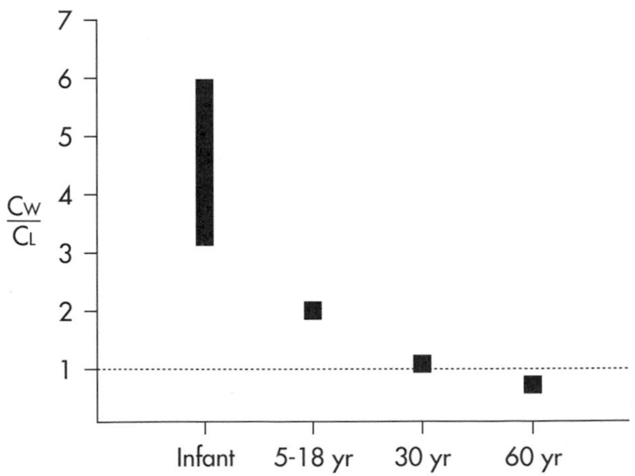

Fig. 74-5. Changes in the ratio of chest wall to lung compliance with aging. Data for infants represent a range from several studies. In infants and children, the chest wall is more compliant than the lungs; in adults the chest wall compliance is close to that of the lungs, and in the elderly it is less than that of the lungs. *Cw,* Wall compliance; *CL,* lung compliance.

Few studies have been done on developmental changes in chest wall resistance. The chest wall accounts for approximately 30% to 35% of total respiratory system resistance in adults.[16] In infants, this figure is 20% to 25%.[9,17]

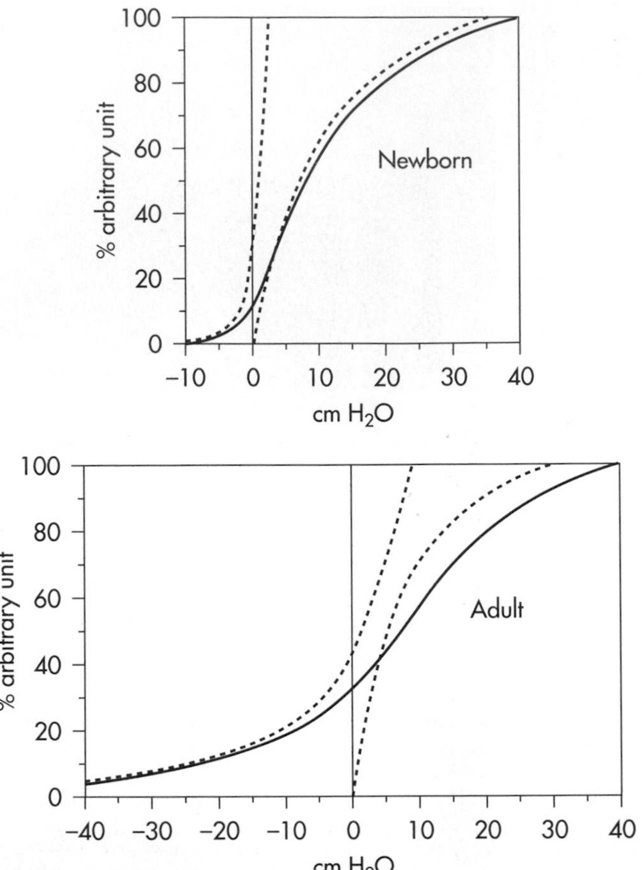

Fig. 74-6. Respiratory system PV curves in the newborn and adult human. The *x*-axis represents pressure and the *y*-axis represents volume. The slope of each curve at a given lung volume represents the compliance at that volume. The solid curve in each diagram is the PV curve of the respiratory system. At a given lung volume, it represents the sum of the pressures resulting from the chest wall PV curve *(left dashed line)* and the lung PV curve *(right dashed line).* Passive end-expiratory lung volume is represented by the point at which the solid curve crosses the volume axis. It is lower in the newborn than in the adult because of the high compliance of the newborn chest wall curve. (From Agostoni E, Mead J: Statics of the respiratory system. In Fenn WO, Rahn H, eds: *Handbook of physiology, respiration,* sect 3, vol 1, Washington, DC, 1964, American Physiological Society, p 401.)

Viscoelastic Properties of the Chest Wall

Respiratory structures are not perfectly elastic. They do not expand and contract along a unique pressure-volume (PV) curve; rather, the elastic recoil pressure of the respiratory system depends not only on volume, but also on volume and time history. Stress relaxation, in which final recoil pressure is slightly less than initial recoil pressure following respiratory system inflation, is one example of this dependence on volume and time history and is a reflection of what are known as respiratory system viscoelastic properties.[18,19] The importance of viscoelastic chest wall properties in human infants and children, and how these properties change with development, are only beginning to be understood.[20]

Maintenance of Functional Residual Capacity

The passive relaxation volume (Vr) is determined by the balance of two opposing forces: the outward recoil of the chest wall and the inward recoil of the lung[21] (Fig. 74-6). The low chest wall re-

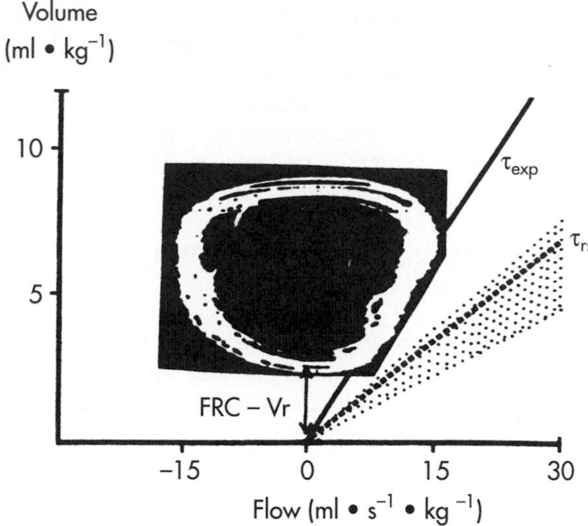

Fig. 74-7. Elevation of EEV by active prolongation of the respiratory system time constant, τ. A tidal flow volume curve is shown on the oscilloscope tracing. The slope of the expiratory limb of this curve ([volume, ml/kg] / [flow, ml/{sec.kg}]) has the units of sec and represents the active expiratory time constant, τ_{exp}. The slope of the dotted line represents the passive time constant of the system (τ_{rs}) following an end-inspiratory occlusion, which activates the Hering-Breuer reflex and therefore relaxes the respiratory muscles. These lines intersect at the passive relaxation volume *(Vr)*. The volume difference between Vr and the active flow volume curve EEV represents difference between functional residual capacity (FRC) and V and reflects active maintenance of FRC. From Mortola JP, Saetta M: *Pediatr Pulmonol* 3:123-130, 1987.

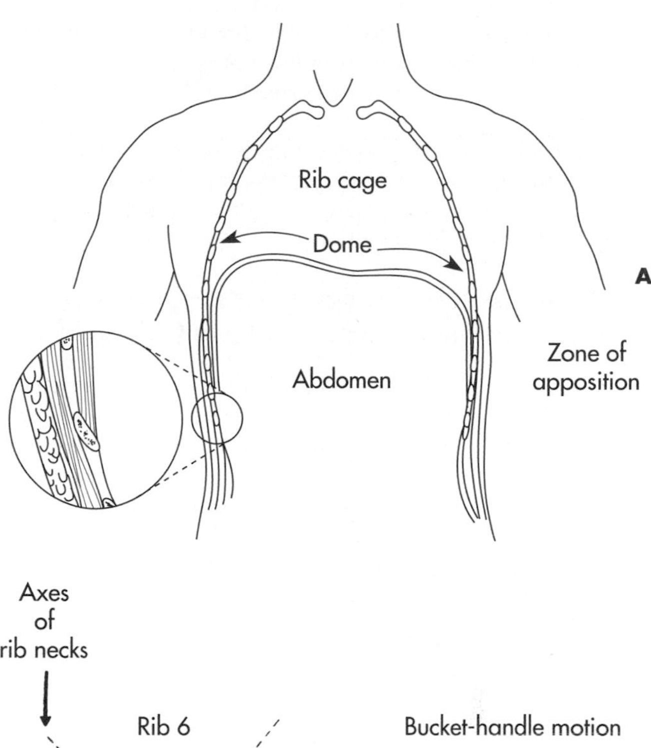

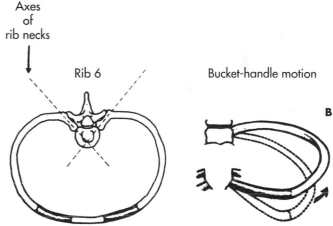

Fig. 74-8. Functional anatomy of the ribcage. **A,** Zone of apposition. (From DeTroyer A, Estenne M: *Clin Chest Med* 9(2):175-193, 1988.) **B,** Bucket handle effect. (From DeTroyer A, Loring SH: Action of the respiratory muscles. In Macklem PT, Mead J, eds: *Handbook of physiology.* The Respiratory System. Mechanics of Breathing, sect 3, Vol III, Part 2, Bethesda, Md, 1986, American Physiological Society, p 453.)

coil of the infant leads to a low Vr, which in turn may predispose the infant to airway closure and atelectasis. Full-term infants therefore adopt a strategy of active maintenance of end-expiratory lung volume (EEV), consisting of an active prolongation of "expiration." This phenomenon can be observed by comparing the active tidal breathing flow volume curve with the passive flow volume curve elicited by relaxing the respiratory muscles with a brief end-inspiratory occlusion, which activates the Hering-Breuer reflex (Fig. 74-7).[22] The active and passive time constants are represented by the slopes of the expiratory limb of these curves. Maintenance of EEV above Vr can be accomplished by increasing the expiratory time constant, τ, of the respiratory system relative to the time actually available for expiration.[23] Expiratory flow is therefore "interrupted" at a lung volume above the relaxed level (Fig. 74-7). Preterm infants also maintain EEV above Vr, but their ability to do so is markedly sleep state–dependent, being less effective in active than in quiet sleep.

The neonate accomplishes active prolongation of expiration by two mechanisms: postinspiratory activity of the inspiratory muscles, such as the diaphragm,[24] and expiratory "braking" by the upper airway muscles.[25-27] Active maintenance of EEV diminishes with age and by the age of 1 to 2 years is no longer present.[28] This may be a result of progressive stiffening of the chest wall, which allows a higher passively determined EEV.[9,29,30]

DEVELOPMENT OF THE RESPIRATORY MUSCLES

Structural and Functional Changes

The diaphragm has three major inspiratory actions.[31,32] First, the diaphragm decreases intrapleural pressure by acting as a piston, thereby causing air to flow in at the mouth and nose. Second, the diaphragm increases intraabdominal pressure. Because a substantial portion of intraabdominal contents actually reside within the ribcage (Fig. 74-8), this increased abdominal pressure causes the lower ribcage to expand. Third, the diaphragm increases lower ribcage dimensions by acting through its area of apposition to the inner ribcage wall to elevate the lower ribs. This elevation of the lower ribs also expands the lower thoracic cross-sectional area by causing the downward-sloping ribs to assume a more horizontal position (bucket handle effect, Fig. 74-8).

The differences between the adult and infant chest wall outlined here would be expected to affect the diaphragm's inspiratory action. Less of the ribcage's contents are intraabdominal and the area of apposition is smaller in the infant than in the older child and adult. Furthermore, diaphragmatic mass is less in the infant.[12] Theoretically, these differences should impair the infant diaphragm's inspiratory action. On the other hand, by the law of LaPlace, the smaller radius of curvature of the infant's diaphragm relative to the adult should improve its pressure generating ability at a given level of tension.

Tidal expiration is primarily driven by the passive elastic recoil of the respiratory system. Neonates, like adults, can recruit abdominal muscles to promote active expiration under conditions of hypercapnia and hypercarbia.[33,34] Such recruitment is highly sleep state–dependent, being much less effective in REM than in NREM sleep.

Developmental Cell Biology of the Respiratory Muscles and Implications for Fatigue Resistance

The mechanical disadvantage imposed by a highly compliant chest wall has been thought to predispose the premature and newborn infant to respiratory muscle fatigue and consequent respiratory pump failure.[35-37] However, the contractile properties and fatigue resistance of respiratory muscles undergo complex changes with development that challenge the notion that the newborn is highly prone to fatigue. Some of these controversial issues have been presented in recent reviews[38,39] and are discussed here.

Developmental Changes in Respiratory Muscle Fiber Type Determined by Histochemistry

Oxidative enzyme and ATPase histochemical staining profiles of muscle unit fibers have been shown to correspond to physiologic classification of motor unit types. Thus fibers classified as type I on the basis of histochemical staining (darkly for oxidative enzymes, lightly for glycolytic enzymes and ATPase after alkaline preincubation) are classified as slow twitch, fatigue resistant. In contrast, type II fibers stain darkly for ATPase and are classified as fast twitch, fatigable. Fatigability as here defined is the ability of individual motor units to maintain force relative to the initial force generated following repetitive activation.[40]

The relative proportion of type I and type II fibers in respiratory muscles changes with development. The percentage compositions of type I fibers in the diaphragm of human premature infants, newborns, and older children (greater than 2 years) are 10%, 25%, and 55%, respectively.[35] A similar developmental pattern was observed in the intercostal muscles.[35] One might infer from this that the premature and newborn infant would be more susceptible to respiratory muscle fatigue than the older child. Indeed, LeSouef et al[36] found that the ability to maintain occlusion pressure during sustained activation of the diaphragm by phrenic nerve stimulation was markedly impaired in newborn compared with older (greater than 30 days) rabbits. They, too, found a paucity of type I fibers in the newborn diaphragm, and concluded that the newborn rabbit diaphragm is highly susceptible to fatigue and that this susceptibility correlated with the fiber type distribution.

Other studies suggest that the picture is not so clear. Maxwell[41] found that the respiratory muscles of premature baboons were highly oxidative and fatigue *resistant.* Factors other than histochemical staining of ATPase and oxidative enzymes may therefore correlate more closely with susceptibility of the respiratory muscles to fatigue. Sieck et al[42] and Watchco et al[43] have demonstrated that although specific force (peak tetanic force output normalized for muscle cross-sectional area) of diaphragmatic fibers increases with postnatal age, fatigue resistance decreases with increasing age. They have further found that fatigue resistance is related not only to oxidative capacity of the muscle (indexed by succinic dehydrogenase [SDH] activity), but also to myosin heavy chain (MHC) phenotype.[44] The neonatal MHC phenotype seems to impart a greater degree of fatigue resistance than do the adult isoforms. Thus fatigue resistance of respiratory muscle during development may relate to a balance between the energetic demands of the muscle contractile proteins (reflected by MHC isoform composition) and its oxidative capacity (reflected by SDH activity).[44]

METHODS FOR ASSESSING CHEST WALL FUNCTION

Chest Wall Motion

The quantitation of chest wall motion yields information about both chest wall function and underlying lung function. The most widely used method to assess chest wall motion is respiratory inductive plethysmography, although strain gauges and magnetometers can be used as well.[45] The magnitude of the ribcage (RC) and abdominal (AB) compartments' contribution to tidal volume can be quantitated, as can timing relationships between the two compartments. Newborn infants breathe predominantly with their abdominal compartments, as opposed to adults, who are primarily ribcage breathers. The ribcage's contribution to tidal breathing during quiet sleep in the newborn is 35% of tidal volume (range 20% to 50%), increasing gradually over the first year to the normal adult value of 65%.[46]

Timing relationships between RC and AB can be conveniently quantitated by plotting RC versus AB motion in a Lissajous, or Konno-Mead figure[47] and calculating the phase angle as an index of thoraco-abdominal asynchrony (TAA) (Fig. 74-9). This phase angle can range from 0° (synchronous RC-AB motion) to 180° (paradoxic RC-AB motion). Normal chest wall motion is synchronous in full-term infants (mean phase angle 8°) (Fig. 74-10) and children (mean phase angle 1.5°) during quiet sleep.[48-50] Chest wall motion becomes more asynchronous as chest wall stiffness decreases and as pleural pressure swings increase. In these circumstances, the chest wall is less able to withstand the decrease in pleural pressure during inspiration, and outward motion of the ribcage can lag behind that of the abdomen or become frankly paradoxic. Thus premature infants normally display asynchronous or paradoxic breathing during quiet sleep (mean phase angle 58°, range 0° to 157°).[51] Infants with bronchopulmonary dysplasia can have markedly asynchronous breathing (Fig. 74-10), the degree of which can be related to the magnitude of abnormality in lung resistance and compliance (Fig. 74-11).[49] Asynchrony improves significantly after bronchodilators in infants with lower airway obstruction[48] and after racemic epinephrine in children with upper airway obstruction.[52] Thus quantitation of asynchrony can be used as a noninvasive indirect index of airway obstruction.

Chest wall motion can also be affected by primary chest wall disease. Patients with neuromuscular disease can display paradoxic breathing. The pattern of RC-AB paradox can give important clues to the underlying disorder. Patients with primary intercostal muscle weakness display inward RC motion during inspiration,[53] whereas patients with primary diaphragmatic paralysis display inward abdominal motion during inspiration.[54,55]

Clinical Assessment of Respiratory Pump Function and Fatigue

Physical Examination of the Chest Wall

Paradoxic motion of the ribcage and abdomen is easy to identify, although lesser degrees of asynchrony may be more difficult to discern. The phase of respiration should be noted in addition to the presence of paradox. Although chest wall paradox

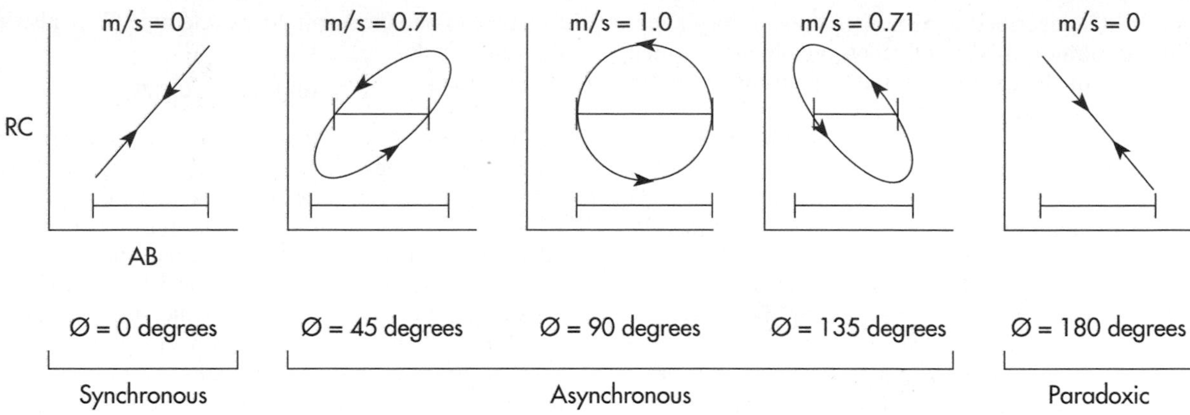

Fig 74-9. Lissajous figures of ribcage (RC) and abdominal wall (AB) motion. Phase angle, Ø, is an index of thoracoabdominal asynchrony. Increasing thoracoabdominal asynchrony is seen as increasing width of the figure up to a phase angle of 90 degrees, and then by a change from a positive to a negative slope between 90 and 180 degrees. For phase angles 0 < Ø < 90 degrees, sin Ø = m/s; for 90 < Ø < 180 degrees, Ø = 180 - μ, where sin μ = m/s (see text). From: Allen JL, Wolfson MR, McDowell K, Shaffer TH: *Am Rev Respir Dis* 141:337-342, 1990.

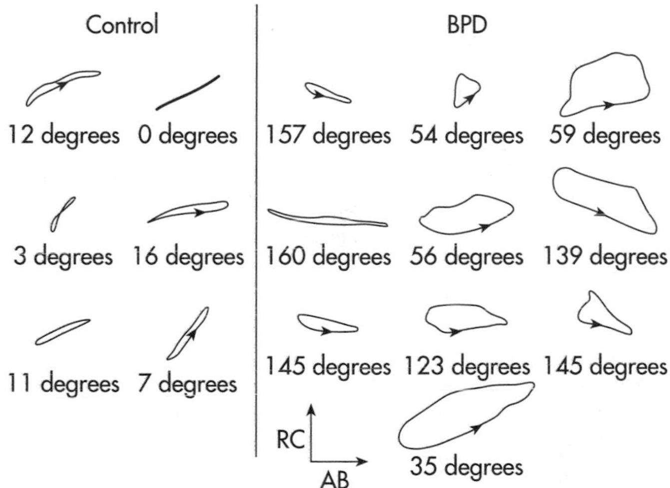

Fig. 74-10. RC-AB Lissajous figures in normal infants *(left)* and infants with BPD, *(right)*. The calculated phase angles are shown. (From Allen JL, Greenspan JS, Deoras KS, Keklikian E, Wolfson MR, Shaffer TH: *Pediatr Pulmonol* 11:37-43, 1991.)

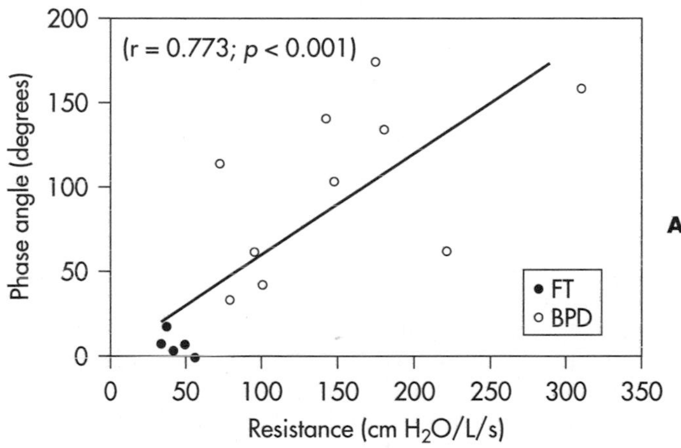

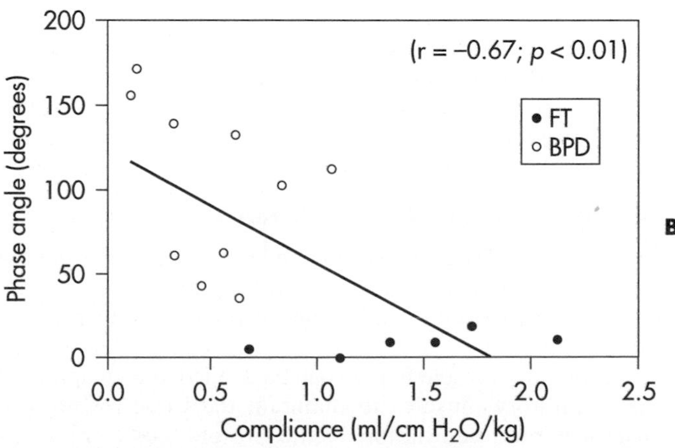

Fig. 74-11. Relationship between thoracoabdominal asynchrony, quantitated by RC-AB phase angle, and lung mechanics. **A,** Phase angle vs. resistance. **B,** Phase angle vs. compliance. *FT,* Full-term control; infants. *BPD,* bronchopulmonary dysplasia. (From Allen JL, Greenspan JS, Deoras KS, Keklikian E, Wolfson MR, Shaffer TH: *Pediatr Pulmonol* 11:37-43, 1991.)

can be observed visually, phase of respiration must often be ascertained by a fingertip held at the mouth or by auscultation. Inward RC motion and outward AB motion during inspiration denotes intercostal muscle or ribcage dysfunction. This pattern is commonly noted in infants with severe airflow obstruction and in some normal premature infants, especially during REM sleep. It is also seen in patients with neuromuscular disease with intercostal muscle weakness but intact diaphragmatic function, such as quadriplegia. Inward AB and outward RC motion during inspiration denotes diaphragmatic dysfunction. It is often noted in adults with severe airflow obstruction and impending diaphragmatic fatigue. It is also seen in patients with phrenic nerve paralysis.

Roussos et al[56] described a pattern of "respiratory alternans" during inspiratory resistive loaded breathing, in which the contributions of the diaphragm and intercostal accessory muscles alternated in time, possibly postponing the onset of fatigue. One would expect this to be reflected in an alternating pattern of RC and AB motion, each compartment's displacement alternating in magnitude. Asynchronous RC/AB motion may also merely reflect the magnitude of the load itself, rather than respiratory muscle fatigue per se.[49,51,57]

Palpation of the abdominal muscles (the rectus abdominis) may reveal active contraction during expiration. This is seen in patients with severe obstructive lung disease, in whom passive recoil of the respiratory system may provide insufficient pressure to overcome expiratory airflow obstruction. It can also be seen in patients with inspiratory muscle weakness who may "actively" expire and "passively" inspire. Active expiration occurs normally during exercise.

Assessment of Respiratory Muscle Strength

Normal adults can develop maximal inspiratory and expiratory pressures against an occluded airway in excess of 100 and 200 cm H_2O, respectively. Maximal inspiratory pressures (Pi_{max}) remain constant throughout development, whereas maximal expiratory pressures (Pe_{max}) increase.[58-61] How much of this increase is related to increasing effort with increasing age versus increasing muscle strength with increasing age is not clear. Occlusion pressures measured during crying in infants and children from the ages of 3 months are nearly constant with age (mean ± SD = 118 ± 21 cm H_2O), and similar to those measured in adults. Pe_{max} increases with increasing age (mean ± SD = 125 ± 35 cm H_2O from 3 months to 3 years[58]; 138 ± 36 cm H_2O from ages 8 to 17 years[61]; nearly 200 cm H_2O in adults). Occlusion pressures are greater in postpubertal boys than girls.[59-61] Because these measurements are sometimes difficult to make, clinicians often accept inspiratory pressures of 80 and expiratory pressures of 100 cm H_2O as evidence of lack of respiratory muscle weakness. Inspiratory respiratory muscle strength and effort can also be inferred by the magnitude of soft tissue recession.

Maximal inspiratory force is sometimes used as an index of ability to wean from mechanical ventilation; such measurements, although reproducible, may not be reliable indicators of true respiratory muscle strength[62] and therefore may not be reliable predictors of successful weaning. Transdiaphragmatic pressure (Pdi) is an index of diaphragmatic strength rather than global respiratory muscle strength. It is more difficult to measure, however, requiring the placement of both gastric and esophageal pressure monitors.

Assessment of Respiratory Muscle Fatigue

Measurement of the tension-time index and frequency pattern assessment of diaphragmatic electromyogram (EMG) activity have been proposed as indicators of impending respiratory muscle failure.

Respiratory muscle fatigue can be defined as an inability of the respiratory muscles to maintain the force required to sustain minute ventilation in the presence of a mechanical load. The development of fatigue is closely linked to the force and duration of muscle contraction. The tension time index (TTI) is a dimensionless product of the ratio of developed transdiaphragmatic pressure (Pdi) to maximal transdiaphragmatic pressure (Pdi_{max}); and the ratio of the inspiratory time (Ti) to the respiratory cycle time (T_{tot}), also known as the "duty cycle."

$$TTI = Pdi/Pdi_{max} \cdot Ti/T_{tot} \tag{1}$$

The TTI has been used in adults to predict the development of fatigue. When the TTI exceeds 0.2, it is highly likely that fatigue will occur. The measurement of the TTI requires the ability to assess Pdi and Pdi_{max}, which can be technically difficult. A few studies have been done in infants and children to determine whether the same values of the TTI are applicable.[63]

Spectral frequency analysis of the surface diaphragmatic EMG during fatiguing loads has been shown to indicate diaphragmatic muscle fatigue in adults.[64] Similarly, in infants diaphragmatic fatigue produces a decrease in the high-frequency power and an increase in the low-frequency power of the EMG.[65] During weaning from mechanical ventilation, the EMG power spectrum remained normal in infants who were able to be weaned successfully, whereas in infants who failed extubation and in whom mechanical ventilation had to be reinstituted, a decrease in the high/low power spectrum ratio occurred before CO_2 retention and clinical deterioration. Because shifts in the diaphragmatic EMG power spectrum may occur in the absence of fatigue,[66] this technique has limited clinical use. Accurate placement of electrodes is critical to adequate recording of power spectra and at present this technique is seldom used for clinical purposes.

TREATMENT OF RESPIRATORY PUMP FATIGUE: GENERAL PRINCIPLES

Respiratory pump fatigue can result from three mechanisms: intrinsic pulmonary disease (such as COPD or interstitial lung disease) that increases the resistive or elastic work of breathing, primary pump pathology (for example, neuromuscular disease) as a result of abnormal respiratory muscle strength, or chest wall deformity (such as kyphoscoliosis) that decreases pump efficiency. All these mechanisms may be thought of in terms of the first half of the TTI, Pdi/P_{max}. Whereas an increased work of breathing increases the quantity (Pdi/P_{max}) by *increasing* Pdi, respiratory muscle weakness and inefficiency increases the quantity (Pdi/P_{max}) by *decreasing* P_{max}. Respiratory pump fatigue has been treated by respiratory muscle rest, respiratory muscle training, and the use of pharmacologic measures.

Respiratory Muscle Rest

Chronic nocturnal ventilation is the most common form of respiratory muscle rest therapy. Although usually used nightly for at least 8 hours, it has also been used three times,[67] and even once[68] per week. The mechanisms by which chronic nocturnal ventilation effects clinical improvement are multifactorial and include respiratory muscle rest[69] and improved inspiratory muscle strength.[70,67] Improvements in arterial blood gases have been demonstrated during assisted ventilation, and after discontinuation of assisted ventilation and throughout the succeeding day.[71,72] This improved gas exchange is a consequence of improved respiratory muscle strength and is likely to also be a consequence of a respiratory control center that has been "reset" by a lower $P{CO_2}$ during the period of assisted ventilation.[73,74] Finally, the increase in tidal volume during nocturnal assisted ventilation may reexpand areas of atelectasis that have developed during nonassisted ventilation, although brief periods of intermittent positive-pressure breathing do not alter lung mechanics.[75] The most common methods of supplying assisted ventilation are negative-pressure ventilation in body ventilators and cuirass, or "raincoat," devices. Recently noninvasive bilevel positive-pressure (BiPAP) ventilators via nasal ventilation have been shown to be a practical means of providing nocturnal ventilatory support in both adults and children.

Respiratory Muscle Training

Training can increase the strength and endurance of skeletal muscle. Strength and endurance training differ (known as "specificity" of training), as do the cellular changes that occur during each type of training. Strength training involves few repetitions of a high-intensity stimulus, and the major cellular response is muscle fiber hypertrophy. Endurance training involves frequent repetitions of a low-intensity stimulus, and the major cellular response is increased oxidative capacity, with increases in oxidative enzymes, number and size of mitochondria, and capillary density.[76]

In normal adults respiratory muscle strength and endurance can be increased by specific training.[77] Respiratory muscle strength training has been most often accomplished with the repetitions of maximal forced respiratory maneuvers or resistive loaded breathing with high inspiratory resistive loads. Endurance training has been accomplished with nonspecific (that is, total body exercise) conditioning and specific conditioning. Specific endurance programs include voluntary isocapneic hyperventilation, resistive loaded breathing, and inspiratory threshold loading.

Respiratory muscle strength training has been shown to increase respiratory muscle strength in patients with COPD,[78] cystic fibrosis,[79] and quadriplegia.[80] Respiratory muscle endurance training has been shown to increase respiratory muscle endurance in patients with COPD,[81] cystic fibrosis,[82,79] and quadriplegia.[80] Inspiratory flow resistive load training has been shown to improve respiratory muscle endurance, but not strength, in premature infants free of lung disease.[83] However, whether this strategy contributes to patient well-being is not known.

A major unresolved question is when respiratory muscles should be exercised and when they should be rested. A general principle is that weak muscles should be exercised and fatigued muscles should be rested.[84,85] It may be difficult, however, to distinguish weakness from fatigue in the clinical setting.

Pharmacotherapy of Respiratory Muscle Fatigue

Theophylline is the most studied pharmacologic agent for respiratory muscle fatigue. In vitro, theophylline produces a dose-dependent increase in peak twitch tension of the diaphragm.[86] In animal models, theophylline increases maximal transdiaphragmatic pressure[87] and improves diaphragmatic force generation after fatigue has developed.[88] In normal humans, theophylline has a potent effect on diaphragmatic contractility[89] and in patients with COPD, theophylline increases diaphragmatic strength and postpones the onset of diaphragmatic fatigue induced by resistive loaded breathing. Results in neo-nates have been conflicting. Mayock et al[90,91] were unable to show an improvement in diaphragmatic contractility or fatigue resistance in the newborn piglet. However, aminophylline increases diaphragmatic excursions in preterm infants,[92] but whether this is a central or peripheral effect is unclear.

STRUCTURAL ABNORMALITIES OF THE CHEST WALL INCLUDING THE DIAPHRAGM

Thoracic Dystrophies

A number of disorders of development of the chest wall exist, many of which are uncommon and result in early death from associated pulmonary hypoplasia or respiratory pump failure.[93] The etiologies of a number of these have recently been elucidated as the genetic control of bone and cartilage growth and development becomes more clearly understood[94] and can replace classifications based on radiographic and morphologic characteristics.[95,96]

Achondroplasia, an autosomal dominant skeletal dysplasia, is one of the most common forms of short-limbed dwarfism. It results from a mutation in the transmembrane domain of fibroblast growth factor receptor 3 (FGFR3).[94] Phenotypically it is associated with developmental abnormalities of the ribs, thorax, long bones, and cranium. The ribs are short and flared and the thorax is shallow. Narrowing of the space between the sternum and vertebral bodies can compress intervening structures such as the trachea.[97] This compression may be related to the posterior ribs bowing around the transverse processes of the spine, thus "pushing" the vertebral bodies anteriorly. The skeletal abnormalities of homozygous offspring are so severe that most die in the first year or two of life.

The respiratory complications of achondroplasia include disordered sleep and obstructive apnea present in about three quarters of subjects.[98] In addition to the obstructive apneas, in part related to the midface hypoplasia, brainstem compression may lead to disorders in the control of breathing.[99,100] In infants and young children, frequent pneumonias, hypoxemia, sudden death, and cor pulmonale occur with some frequency.[101] The small shallow thorax combined with possible pulmonary hypoplasia probably results in breathing at low lung volume, with attendant airway closure, atelectasis, and hypoxemia. Despite the 10% of infants and young children with these complications, most patients with achondroplasia survive into adulthood.

Do patients with achondroplasia have hypoplastic lungs? Two studies in adolescents and adults with achondroplasia addressed the issue of lung size[102,103] and found that lung size is reduced to approximately 70% expected value for height corrected for the abnormal sitting/standing height ratios. When further "corrected" for the size of the cranium, lung volumes are only slightly reduced. Normal tests of airway function and normal residual volume/total lung capacity (RV:TLC) ratios suggest that both lung and thorax are reduced in size, but the mechanics of each are appropriate.[103]

Respiratory muscle weakness secondary to spinal cord compression does occur in older children and adults with achondroplasia and may be associated with pump failure.

Two other mutations in the FGFR3 gene account for the findings in thanatophoric dysplasia, which, like homozygous achondroplasia, is lethal in very early life. These are the most severe mutations of the FGFR3 gene; achondroplasia is less severe and hypochondroplasia (HCH) is the least severe.[104]

Jeune syndrome, or asphyxiating thoracic dystrophy, is a rare autosomal recessive abnormality of endochondral bone formation characterized by a very small, shallow thoracic cage, abnormalities of the pelvis, polydactyly, and abnormal teeth. Severe forms of this disorder are associated with pulmonary hypoplasia and early death.[105] Morphometric measurements on an infant dying at 4 months[106] suggest that the relative stiffness of the chest wall, combined with the mechanical disadvantage of a flat low diaphragm, contributed to pulmonary hypertension and vascular remodeling, the major morphometric finding. A reduction in alveolar number was not observed. In milder cases the thoracic abnormality may be compatible with survival. These patients may go on to develop biliary cirrhosis[107] or diffuse interstitial fibrosis of the kidneys.[108] A variation of this abnormality differing from Jeune syndrome by autosomal dominant inheritance is characterized by laryngeal stenosis, a bell-shaped thoracic configuration, normal stature, absence of polydactyly, and absence of renal disease.[109]

Osteogenesis imperfecta, an inherited disorder of bone formation, usually results from mutations in the genes encoding type I collagen. It is associated with fractures of the bones including the ribs. The common respiratory problems relate to the fractures of the ribs produced by minimal trauma. Tachypnea, related to shallow, rapid respiration because deeper breaths are painful, and increased metabolic rate because of fever related to the inflammatory response to fractures contribute to episodes that clinically are difficult to distinguish from respiratory tract infections. Chest radiographs are often of no help in defining absence or presence of infiltrates because the lung parenchyma is obscured by bone and callus formation.

Lung hypoplasia related to failure of branching of the respiratory tree beyond that usually observed at 10 weeks of gestation has been observed.[110] In view of the multiple genes involved in the mesenchymal interaction with epithelium in the developing airway, there may be some overlap between abnormalities in genetic regulation of cartilage and bone formation and airway branching. This has not been explored.

The mechanical abnormalities of the ribcage, chest, and chest wall in these various thoracic dystrophies have not been studied. One might hypothesize that stiffness of the chest wall in infancy would confer an advantage because there would be less inward displacement of the ribcage with contraction of the diaphragm, particularly during active sleep, but this might be opposed by greater stiffness of ribcage joints increasing chest wall resistance and decreasing compliance. The breathing strategies used, the relative displacements of the abdomen and ribcage, and the relative compliance of the lung and chest wall must be investigated in these disorders before we can understand what respiratory strategies are used by the child or should be provided by caretakers.

Pectus Excavatum

Pectus deformities are among the most common abnormalities of the thorax. Recent data on incidence are not available, but older data give estimates of an incidence of 6 to 8 per 1000 children.[111] The causes of pectus deformities remain obscure, but contributing factors may include upper airway obstruction during chest wall growth, overgrowth of costal cartilage, and underlying mesenchymal abnormalities. The latter is suggested by the association of pectus deformity with other skeletal abnormalities and with mitral valve prolapse.[112]

The nature and extent of physiologic abnormalities associated with pectus deformities is the subject of both controversy and review.[113,114] Recent studies[115,116] support the observations that pectus excavatum produces a mild to moderate restrictive defect manifest by reductions in TLC, vital capacity (VC), and inspiratory capacity (IC). This restrictive defect is loosely associated with radiographic measurements of the magnitude of the pectus. Several studies have shown that although lung volumes increase after surgery done during periods of growth, lung volumes actually decrease when expressed as a percentage of predicted value based on height.[115,117] The relative loss of lung size following surgery appears to be greater in those with only modest reductions in lung volumes preoperatively.[118] The magnitude of restriction that develops with growth following surgery may be substantial.[119]

Most studies report a high incidence of symptoms among patients who seek surgical correction,[115,116] including decreased exercise tolerance and shortness of breath. Efforts to account for these symptoms have focused on cardiac function and respiratory muscle function because the symptoms do not appear to be related to the magnitude of the restrictive defect. The cardiac abnormalities observed before repair include decreased cardiac filling, decreased stroke volume, and impaired left ventricular dynamics.[120,121]

Studies comparing preoperative and postoperative exercise function are difficult to interpret and compare because of limited numbers of subjects, different exercise protocols, different intervals of time after repair, growth, and different parameters evaluated. However, some general conclusions can be drawn. There appears to be limited evidence for increased stroke volume after repair,[121] increased ventricular filling,[122] increased oxygen pulse resulting in a decreased heart rate at the same workload, and increased duration and level of exercise.[116] These changes are modest and have not been observed by all investigators.[123] They are, however, consistent with the relief of ventricular compression following surgery as documented on computed tomography scan by increased space between the sternum and the vertebral column.[124]

Excessive oxygen consumption at high levels of exercise has been observed before[125] and after[123] pectus repair, suggesting the possibility that work of breathing was increased in pectus excavatum at high levels of ventilation. It was hypothesized that this would be related to limited or abnormal ribcage versus abdominal motion. However, in a study of 11 patients with marked pectus excavatum this was not the case.[126]

The surgical techniques used to correct pectus excavatum vary considerably. It is possible that removal of growth centers during surgery may adversely affect chest wall development and may be related to anecdotal reports of restrictive defects in young adults who underwent surgery before growth was complete.[119]

Acquired Thoracic Defects with Respiratory Sequelae

One of the most impressive examples of thoracic deformities occurs in infants with severe rickets. Although now rare, the current warnings about the dangers of sun exposure and emphasis on natural (unsupplemented) foods may lead to a recurrence of this deformity, described in detail in 1921 by Park and Howland.[127] The ribs are soft and compliant and the ends are displaced inward on inspiration leading to symmetric anterior grooves running longitudinally along the chest wall. The chostochondral junctions are swollen and painful, producing the rachitic "rosary" and a fussy, uncomfortable child. The diaphragmatic insertions distort the lower ribs to produce the characteristic Harrison groove. On inspiration, the chest wall is so compliant that inward chest wall displacement rather than lung inflation is thought to have contributed to hypoventilation and ultimate death from respiratory failure in this often fatal disease in the past.

These deformities are now rare but they do occur in infants with severe chronic renal failure, infants with renal tubular disorders including hypophosphatemic familial rickets, and infants treated with some anticonvulsants.

The bony development of the premature infant's chest wall may resemble rickets. Diffuse skeletal abnormalities occur in very-low-birth-weight prematurely born infants at several months of age. Decreased stores of calcium, inadequate supplementation with vitamin D, impaired conversion of vitamin D to its active metabolites secondary to cholestasis, and impaired hepatic function in infants receiving hyperalimentation may all contribute to impairment of bone mineralization, which in turn contributes to the ease of ribcage deformation in prematurely born infants with and without lung disease. Rib fractures may contribute to the development of respiratory failure and impair weaning from ventilatory support.[93]

Although there are a few studies on the effects of therapeutic irradiation delivered in childhood on subsequent development of the lung,[128,129] the effects of therapeutic irradiation on the structure and function of the thorax as a respiratory pump have been essentially unexplored. Radiation in dosages used in therapy can produce abnormalities of developing bone that are related to age and dosage.[130] In young children receiving radiation to the bed of Wilms' tumor, bony changes developed in the vertebrae with lines of growth plate arrest, anterior narrowing and beaking of the vertebral bodies, and impaired vertebral development. In the soft tissues decreased vascularity with muscle and soft tissue fibrosis has been observed. These changes presumably result in the high incidence of spinal deformities reported in the children who received pelvic irradiation.[130]

The studies carried out on young children receiving therapeutic thoracic radiation demonstrate a restrictive defect.[128,129] Although mild scoliosis was observed in some patients, it was not thought to be substantial enough to account for the small lung volumes. The observation that all lung compartments, RV, FRC, and TLC were reduced proportionately argues that the lung and chest wall were both small. Unfortunately, respiratory muscle strength was not investigated in these studies, but our clinical experience has shown that respiratory muscle weakness can be a major contributor to respiratory failure in previously irradiated patients.

Scoliosis

The classic studies of Kafer[131] and Bergofsky[132] detailed the incidence and outcome of severe scoliosis untreated by spinal fusion. In the United States, approximately 1 person in 1000 has a scoliotic curve greater than 35° and 1 out of 10,000 a curve greater than 75°, placing them at risk for respiratory failure. This places about 20,000 patients at risk for respiratory failure caused by scoliosis in the United States.[132] Fortunately, the practice of surveying adolescents for scoliosis and the surgical treatment to prevent further progression of the curve has probably resulted in a decline in scoliosis as a cause of respiratory failure except in children with congenital scoliosis and those whose scoliosis is secondary to neuromuscular disease. However, studies of a cohort of non–surgically treated patients in 1968 followed up 23 years later[133,134] demonstrated increased age-specific mortality in patients with severe scoliosis and those with infantile or juvenile scoliosis. Those with idiopathic scoliosis with onset in adolescence did not appear to be at increased risk of early death.

Scoliosis is associated with a restrictive defect measured as a reduction in TLC or VC.[135] The magnitude of the angle of scoliosis (Cobb Method) is related to the magnitude of restriction but the length of the curve, cephalad location of the curve, and loss of normal thoracic kyphosis together contribute equally to the restriction. Curves greater than 70°, longer than seven vertebra, and located in the upper thorax are likely to be associated with the severest restriction.[136] Congenital scoliosis, defined as spinal deformity with abnormal spinal cord development or congenital rib abnormalities, is associated with further restriction at any given Cobb angle.[137]

Work capacity is modestly reduced in adolescent idiopathic scoliosis.[138] Decreased peripheral musculature manifest by reduced lean body mass and decreased peripheral muscle strength and the restrictive ventilatory defect both contributed to the decrease in work capacity. Whether this decreased work capacity and muscularity is related to an undefined neuromuscular abnormality or to decreased physical activity related to bracing and surgery are not known but physical training does increase work capacity without changing lung function.[139]

Considerable controversy exists over whether Harrington instrumentation improves lung function. A recent metaanalysis of 173 patients indicates an improvement of 2% to 11% of predicted value, which is significant.[140]

Scoliosis in certain circumstances can have profound influence on lung development. Congenital scoliosis, usually associated with neuromuscular weakness, results in a small lung with fewer alveoli. However, these alveoli are of a size appropriate to the child's age.[141] Severe respiratory failure may develop in scoliosis of a milder degree than that usually associated with a restrictive defect in settings of marginal or not easily detectable respiratory muscle weakness, such as myasthenia gravis. Thus it is recommended that maximal inspiratory and expiratory pressures be measured in all patients undergoing pulmonary evaluation related to scoliosis.

Defects in Development of the Chest Wall Muscles

The chest wall considered broadly as the respiratory pump and structures bordering on the lung consists of the thorax, both inspiratory and expiratory musculature, and the abdominal wall. Congenital defects in the structure of the chest wall muscles can affect or be associated with abnormalities in development of the lung and can influence the function of the respiratory pump.

Congenital Diaphragmatic Hernia

Congenital diaphragmatic hernia (CDH) occurs in approximately 1 in 2,000 to 114,000 pregnancies[142,143] and about 40% are associated with severe and often multiple other congenital abnormalities, including neural tube defects, cardiac anomalies, and skeletal, craniofacial, urinary, anterior abdominal wall, and other defects that influence survival.[144,145] Of the 60% without major congenital malformation, the magnitude of the associated pulmonary hypoplasia, in part, determines survival.

CDH, without other major associated developmental abnormalities, results from failure of the pleural peritoneal canal to close during fetal development. Whether the pulmonary hypoplasia, manifest by a decrease in the number of branches of the conducting airways, as well as a decrease in the number of branches of the pulmonary vascular system and a resulting decrease in the number of alveoli and the size of the pulmonary capillary bed is the result of compression of the developing lung by the intestinal tract herniating through the diaphragmatic defect or is the result of a common insult to the developing diaphragm and developing lung is not clear.

A number of investigators[146-153] have studied lung function in school age survivors of CDH. The data are remarkably consistent and demonstrate mild airway obstruction, normal total lung capacity, and some increase in RV:TLC ratios. In studies in which TLC was measured, it was appropriate to the height of the child. However, the major demonstrable residual defect is the decrease in perfusion to the lung on the side of the hernia. This defect probably reflects the developmental truncation of the vascular and airway tree. It is "visible" in the distribution of pulmonary blood flow because distal vessels comprise a substantial resistance on the vascular side and "invisible" in the distribution of ventilation because peripheral airways contribute little to airway resistance and the distribution of ventilation.

The status of the thoracic structures and the thoracic pump has not been extensively investigated. An increased incidence of pectus deformities and scoliosis has been noted[154] and maximal diaphragmatic excursion as estimated from chest radiographs is less on the side of the hernia in older children following repair.[149] Decreased electromyographic signals as recorded by surface electrodes on the hernia side relative to the nonhernia side have also been reported.[150]

Abdominal Wall Defects (Gastroschisis, Omphalocele, Prune Belly Syndrome)

The anterior abdominal wall is part of the respiratory muscle pump, and abdominal wall defects have potential influences on the developing lung. Omphalocoele and gastroschisis occur in approximately 1 in 4000 to 5000 live-born children.[155] Prune belly or Eagle-Barret syndrome is less common. Although this syndrome may be associated with absent or reduced abdominal wall musculature secondary to obstruction of the urinary outflow tract and massive distention of the urinary tract, it may also reflect a mesenchymal defect. These defects allow abdominal contents to extend beyond the usual borders of the anterior abdominal wall.

Limited information on the development of the lung and ribcage is available, but evidence of narrow chest walls, downslanting ribs, and reduced radiographic estimates of lung volume suggests that in some patients pulmonary hypoplasia may contribute to respiratory distress. These observations are supported by the observation that the radial alveolar count, an index of alveolar number, is reduced in children with giant omphaloceles and that lung weight:body weight ratios are reduced in some.[156]

Closure of abdominal wall defects present both respiratory and cardiovascular challenges. Although the size of the entire coeloemic cavity has not been estimated in these conditions, the peritoneal cavity is thought to be small. Thus when the defect is closed abdominal pressure increases. This can be an advantage to the infant in that increased abdominal pressure may elevate and lengthen the diaphragm, thus putting the diaphragm at a more favorable length-tension relationship. However, in the normal infant, contraction of the diaphragm is usually accompanied by modest increases in abdominal pressure and, because the abdominal wall is compliant, displacement of the abdomen outward. Most artificial materials used to close the wall are nondistensible and skin is often under tension. Inspiration in these patients may be associated with large positive swings in intraabdominal pressure, which may prevent venous return to the right side of the heart, compress the inferior vena cava, and impair cardiac output.

Lung function has been measured in some infants before and after surgical closure of abdominal wall defects. Lung volumes as measured by a forced deflation vital capacity maneuver were decreased by about 40% and compliance of the respiratory system was reduced by about 50%, as might be expected.[157]

The major respiratory problems for these children in the postoperative period are related to a small coelomic cavity, a stiff abdominal compartment, positive abdominal pressures, and the absence of functioning anterior abdominal wall expiratory muscles. Although little studied, the anticipated problems include low lung volumes with airway closure, atelectasis, and impaired cough reflex. These patients can be tipped into respiratory failure by any process that contributes to further abdominal filling, such as hepatic enlargement, large formula boluses, and excessive gastrointestinal air or stool.

Prune belly syndrome presents a number of additional respiratory challenges. Some of these patients have generalized muscle weakness related to uremia and to corticosteroids administered following renal transplantation. They have weak or absent abdominal musculature, interfering with cough and forced expiratory maneuvers. A recent study[158] demonstrated very slightly reduced lung volumes, markedly reduced inspiratory and expiratory muscle strength, and impairment in exercise capacity that may be related to the abdominal paradox, which may be related to abnormally large ribcage displacements during exercise. Interpretation of tests of airway obstruction in these patients is difficult because expiratory muscle weakness probably contributes to reduced expiratory flow rates, particularly peak flow.

NEUROMUSCULAR DISEASE

Classification of Neuromuscular Diseases

The respiratory tract is often affected in patients with chronic neuromuscular disease, and respiratory failure is the most common mode of death in these patients. Respiratory tract involvement can be caused by the direct effects of neuromuscular disease on the respiratory muscles, leading to respiratory pump fatigue or diminished cough strength, or a result of the indirect effects of disease on other muscles, such as those of the upper airway (leading to airway obstruction), swallowing mechanism (leading to aspiration of food and saliva), and the gastrointestinal tract (leading to gastroesophageal reflux and aspiration). Scoliosis, a common complication of neuromuscular disease, can further complicate the restrictive lung defect.

Neuromuscular disease can be localized anywhere from the corticospinal tract to the peripheral nervous system and the myoneural junction to the muscle itself (Box 74-1). The ef-

BOX 74-1
Common Neuromuscular Diseases Affecting the Respiratory Tract

Central nervous system

Brain tumors
Head trauma
CNS infections (e.g., meningitis, encephalitis)
CNS hemorrhage of the preterm infant
Degenerative neurologic disorders (e.g., Leigh's encephalopathy, Tay-Sachs, storage diseases)
Cerebral palsy

Spinal cord

Trauma (e.g., cervical cord or high thoracic lesions)
Congenital (e.g., meningomyelocele)

Lower motor neuron

Spinal muscular atrophy

Peripheral nerves and nerve roots

Guillain-Barré

Neuromuscular junction

Botulism (adult and neonatal forms)
Myasthenia gravis (adult and neonatal forms)

Muscle

Muscular dystrophies
Myopathies: congenital, mitochondrial, metabolic, and steroid induced

fects on the respiratory tract depend not only on the nature and location of the abnormality, but also on whether it is acute or chronic. In general, lower motor neuron and more peripheral lesions and acute neurologic illness result in flaccid muscles and poor chest wall stabilization, whereas upper motor neuron lesions and chronic neurologic illness result in tighter muscles and stiffer chest wall ligaments and joints.

Spinal cord trauma is one example of the importance of lesion location. The respiratory effects of low thoracic cord lesions are minimal, although cough and forced expiratory maneuvers that rely on activation of abdominal wall muscles may be impaired. In high thoracic cord and cervical cord lesions, no intercostal muscle activity is apparent and breathing is purely diaphragmatic (abdominal); paradoxic breathing may be evident, with the chest wall caving inward on inspiration. High cervical cord lesions (C3-5) affect the phrenic nerve and therefore the diaphragm; patients with transections of the spinal cord above this level cannot breathe independently.

Respiratory Complications of Neuromuscular Disease

Recurrent Pneumonia

Recurrent pneumonias are a common cause of morbidity in patients with neuromuscular disease. Risk factors include aspiration, poor cough reflex, weak cough because of respiratory and abdominal muscle weakness, and atelectasis caused by low inspiratory capacity. Patients with neuromuscular disease are susceptible to community-acquired organisms but are affected more severely; the choice of antibiotics is similar to that used for patients without neuromuscular disease, but should include antibiotics effective against mouth anaerobic organisms. One exception is patients who are mechanically ventilated or who have respiratory appliances such as tracheostomies, in whom gram-negative organisms are more prevalent. Treatment of underlying conditions with steroids or ACTH may predispose patients to opportunistic infections such as *Pneumocystis carinii.*[159] Treatment should include antibiotics appropriate to the causative organism and supportive care including bronchodilators, chest physiotherapy, and mechanical ventilation when necessary.

Aspiration

Aspiration is the main cause of recurrent pneumonia in patients with neuromuscular disease. The causes of aspiration in these patients are swallowing dysfunction and gastroesophageal reflux. The purpose of a normal swallow is to propel food into the gastrointestinal tract while protecting the respiratory tract. Swallowing is thus a complicated mechanism involving precise timing between various pharyngeal, esophageal, and airway muscles. The presence of a tracheostomy can interfere with normal swallowing function and may therefore be a risk factor for aspiration. Swallowing dysfunction is common in patients with neuromuscular disease, especially in patients with brainstem involvement, central nervous system disease, lower motor neuron disease, disorders of the neuromuscular junction, and primary myopathies. It is less common in patients with thoracic or lower spinal cord trauma and peripheral neuropathies.

Aspiration may also occur during episodes of gastroesophageal (GE) reflux. For reasons incompletely understood, the prevalence of GE reflux is higher in patients with neuromuscular disease than in the general population.

Respiratory Failure

Acute respiratory failure usually occurs in the setting of acute pneumonia.[160] Hypoxic respiratory failure results from severe pneumonia, atelectasis,[161] and resultant ventilation perfusion mismatch. Adult respiratory distress syndrome may occur following massive aspiration. Patients with marginally compensated respiratory muscle strength caused by underlying neuromuscular disease are also more likely to develop respiratory pump failure manifested by worsening hypercarbia. Patients with general muscle weakness caused by myopathies often decompensate during intercurrent systemic illness, such as viral infections. The respiratory muscles are no exception, and even nonpulmonary infections can lead to respiratory failure in this setting.

Chronic respiratory failure complicates end-stage neuromuscular disease. The mechanism of the development of respiratory muscle fatigue in patients with neuromuscular disease can best be understood by consideration of the magnitude of respiratory muscle strength versus the resistive and elastic load. Fatigue occurs in patients with normal respiratory muscle strength when increased elastic or resistive respiratory loads are very great. In patients with neuromuscular disease, modestly increased elastic load resulting from scoliosis and chronic pulmonary fibrosis secondary to aspiration, recurrent pneumonias, and other conditions may produce fatigue. In addition, the decreased chest wall compliance seen in patients with long-standing neuromuscular disease adds to the elastic work of breathing.

Cor Pulmonale

Cor pulmonale is a common end-stage complication of neuromuscular disease, and the genesis is multifactorial. Severe scoliosis can cause restrictive disease severe enough to result in cor pulmonale. Furthermore, patients with neuromuscular disease often develop nighttime hypoxemia. The low FRC that results from stiff chest walls, respiratory muscle weakness, and intrinsic restrictive lung disease is accentuated during REM sleep, when intercostal muscle tone decreases. Prolonged periods of breathing at low FRC can cause airway closure and atelectasis, both of which result in low $\dot{V}/\dot{Q}$ ratios and hypoxemia. Furthermore, the abnormal upper airway muscle control of patients with neuromuscular disease can lead to upper airway obstruction during sleep, hypoxemia, and cor pulmonale.

Nutritional Status

Malnutrition in patients with neuromuscular disease results from underlying chronic illness, swallowing difficulties, and poor appetite, and can accentuate the underlying generalized and respiratory muscle weakness, contributing to respiratory muscle fatigue. Conversely, overnutrition and obesity can place patients at risk for respiratory failure by further reducing lung volume and compliance of the chest wall.

Pathophysiology

Alterations of Lung Function in Neuromuscular Disease

TLC and VC may be normal in mild neuromuscular disease, but are reduced in moderate to severe disease. The reductions in TLC and VC are caused by inspiratory muscle weakness, scoliosis, and chest wall and lung stiffness related to prolonged reduction in tidal volume.[162] RV may be normal or elevated as a result of expiratory muscle weakness. An elevated RV:TLC ratio in patients with neuromuscular disease is therefore not usually a consequence of air trapping. Maximal expiratory flow rates in patients with neuromuscular disease are usually diminished as a consequence of both low lung volumes and decreased expiratory muscle strength. Furthermore, patients with neuromuscular disease often have a characteristic shape of the flow volume curve at low lung volumes, with a precipitous decrease in flows near RV rather than a linear decrease with a decrease in lung volume (Fig.74-12).[163] This phenomenon is a result of the diminished ability of the expiratory muscles to overcome the outward recoil of the chest wall and produce flow limitation at low lung volumes. As is the case in most restrictive lung disease, the FEV_1:VC ratio is normal in patients with neuromuscular disease.

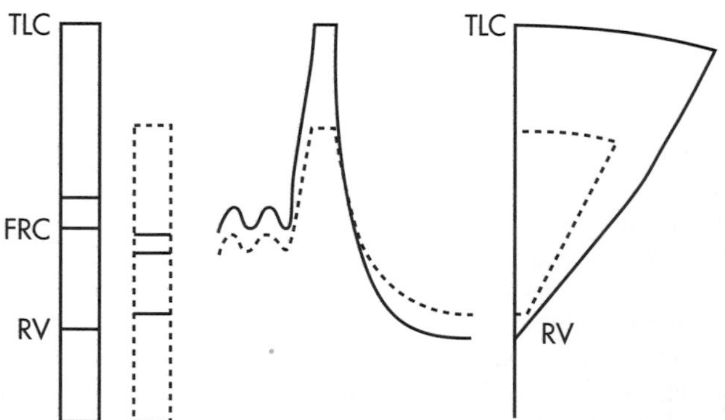

Fig. 74-12. Alterations in lung volumes and flow rates in patients with neuromuscular disease. Lung volumes are represented at left, volume-time spirogram in the center, and flow volume curve at right. In the center figure, time is on the *x* axis and volume is on the *y* axis; in the right figure, flow is on the *x* axis and volume is on the *y* axis. Solid line, normals; dashed line, neuromuscular disease. *TLC,* Total lung capacity; *FRC,* functional residual capacity; *RV,* residual volume.

Lung compliance is reduced in patients with neuromuscular disease.[164] Specific compliance is usually normal, however,[165] suggesting that loss of alveolar number is more important than intrinsic alteration of elastic properties in the genesis of low lung compliance.

Respiratory Muscle Strength

Maximal inspiratory and expiratory pressures are reduced in patients with neuromuscular disease.[58,162,166] The degree of reduction does not seem to correlate with the reduction in general skeletal muscle strength.[167] Respiratory muscle strength is related, however, to the distribution of general muscle weakness, tending to be more severe in patients with proximal muscle weakness and less severe in patients with peripheral muscle weakness.[167] This may be a result of thoracic stabilization by the muscles of the upper limb.

Chest Wall Alterations

Although patients with severe intercostal muscle weakness display patterns of breathing similar to those of preterm infants, suggestive of increased chest wall compliance, passive compliance of the chest wall in adults with neuromuscular disease is usually *reduced.*[168] Preliminary studies in infants with neuromuscular disease, however, demonstrate that the chest wall is more compliant than normal.[169] These studies suggest that intact muscle function is necessary to the development of normal intrinsic chest wall stiffness, but that with time, long-term diminished tidal chest wall excursions lead to chest wall joint contractures, resulting in an abnormally stiff chest wall.

Control of Breathing

Patients with neuromuscular disease may have abnormalities of the respiratory control center as a primary or secondary event. Clearly, brainstem abnormalities can directly affect respiratory control and cause diminished ventilatory responses to hypercarbia and hypoxia, central and obstructive apnea, and excessive periodic breathing. As is the case with chronic lung disease of any sort, long-standing carbon dioxide retention can "reset" the respiratory control center and diminish CO_2 responsiveness. Furthermore, the chronic metabolic alkalosis engendered by long-standing CO_2 retention can blunt respiratory drive in response to increasing CO_2 levels by buffering hydrogen ion and reducing acidosis. Whether patients with neuromuscular disease that is *not* of central origin, such as myopathies, have disordered control of breathing is difficult to ascertain, because most tests of respiratory control depend on intact respiratory system mechanics and muscle strength. For example, assessing the change in minute ventilation during CO_2 rebreathing assumes that such ventilatory changes are not limited by the mechanics of the system, an assumption that is not true in the presence of severe restrictive chest wall disease and muscle weakness. To overcome this limitation, the P_{100} has been suggested as a good index of respiratory drive in patients with lung mechanic abnormalities. By assessing the mouth pressure response to the first 100 ms of an inspiratory occlusion, patients with neuromuscular disease can presumably reach normal values despite respiratory muscle weakness because the normal value of P_{100} (about 2 cm H_2O in adults) is well below the maximal pressures that can be generated by most patients with neuromuscular disease. Although few studies have been reported, it appears the patients with neuromuscular disease have normal P_{100} values, indicating intact respiratory drive.[170,171]

Abnormalities of Cough in Patients with Neuromuscular Disease

A major factor predisposing to recurrent pneumonia in patients with neuromuscular disease is an ineffective cough secondary to weak abdominal and thoracic expiratory muscles. Patients with low thoracic cord lesions and paraplegia can still maintain a fairly effective cough because of intact abdominal muscle strength. Patients with tetraplegia can use the pectoralis major as a muscle of forced expiration and often unconsciously adopt these muscles for coughing.[172]

Approach to the Patient with Neuromuscular Disease

In taking a history from a patient with neuromuscular disease, it is important to ask about recurrent pneumonias, symptoms of gastroesophageal reflux, aspiration of secretions, and symptoms suggesting sleep hypoventilation, obstructive sleep apnea such as daytime hypersomnolence, and snoring. Seizure control should be assessed because uncontrolled seizures may predispose to aspiration pneumonias.

On physical examination, the spine should be carefully assessed for the presence of scoliosis as a possible contributing cause to lung dysfunction. Signs of cor pulmonale should be evaluated and the patient should be examined for clubbing as a possible indication of recurrent suppurative lung infections. Pulmonary function tests including lung volumes should be performed on all patients who can do them. Chest radiographs and assessment of oxygenation and ventilation by either arterial blood gases or pulse oximetry and serum bicarbonate (as an index of the chronic CO_2 retention) should be done. Barium swallow for swallowing function and gastrointestinal anatomy and gastroesophageal reflux studies (scintiscan or pH probe) should be done in patients with histories suggestive of aspiration. Sleeping pulse oximetry or more formal polysomnography should be done in patients with histories suggestive of sleep apnea or in those deemed at risk of sleep hypoventilation by virtue of marginal lung function (VC less than 50%, FEV_1 less than 40% of predicted). Electrocardiography and echocardiography should be done in all patients with baseline or sleeping hypoxemia to evaluate for the presence of cor pulmonale.

Treatment of Pulmonary Complications of Neuromuscular Disease

The treatment of respiratory complications of neuromuscular disease requires an organized approach to their diagnosis and identification. Treatment then follows from the problems that are uncovered by such an approach. Patients with recurrent aspiration pneumonias should have the source of aspiration documented and treated. GE reflux is treated with motility agents such as metoclopramide or cisapride and antacids. If medical management fails, fundoplication may be performed, although the success rate of this procedure in patients with severe neuromuscular disease may be more limited than in the normal population. If aspiration occurs during swallowing, placement of a gastrostomy tube may be indicated to bypass oropharyngeal dysmotility. Before proceeding with this, work with a speech therapist can often identify modes of swallowing that can compensate for the abnormal swallow mechanism and can enable the patient to take at least a part of his or her daily caloric intake by the oral route.

Nocturnal ventilatory support can enhance the quality of life in many patients with nighttime hypoxemia.[173] Supplemental oxygen by nasal cannula may suffice in patients with hypoxemia caused by chronic lung disease. The physiology of chronic respiratory muscle fatigue and its treatment with respiratory muscle rest are discussed earlier in this chapter. The mode of nocturnal ventilatory support chosen depends on the underlying cause of hypoventilation. Central hypoventilation or hypoventilation without an obstructive upper airway component can be treated with negative-pressure ventilation (cuirass or tank respirator) or positive-pressure ventilation by nasal mask (BiPAP). Obstructive apnea can worsen during negative-pressure ventilation, however,[174,175] and should be treated with positive-pressure ventilation only.

General supportive measures should be stressed. Influenza vaccine should be given annually, and patients should receive all routine immunizations, including *Hemophilus influenzae* vaccine, as well as pneumococcal vaccine. For patients with recurrent aspiration, antibiotics to treat common anaerobic mouth organisms (penicillin, clindamycin, amoxicillin-clavulanic acid) should be given either intermittently or prophylactically if aspiration pneumonia is a frequent occurrence. Nutritional supplements are important in maintaining the overall health of the patient and ensuring that malnutrition is not further compromising respiratory muscle function.[175] However, the caloric requirements of patients with neuromuscular disease use a wheelchair may be quite small and obesity is to be avoided. Chest physiotherapy, abdominally assisted coughing, insufflator-exsufflator devices, and inhaled bronchodilators all play important roles in mobilizing lung secretions that accumulate as a consequence of a weak cough mechanism.

In summary, the management of the pulmonary complications of neuromuscular disease depends on defining the cause of these complications (for example, abnormal swallowing with aspiration, gastroesophageal reflux with complications, presence of impaired ventilation, impaired cough, presence of suppurative lung disease, pulmonary hypertension, and cor pulmonale). Careful definition of the extent of impairment then leads to appropriate treatment as the diseases progress.

REFERENCES

1. Roussos C, Macklem PT: The respiratory muscles, *N Engl J Med* 307(13):786-797, 1982 (review).

Growth and Development of the Chest Wall

2. Openshaw P, Edwards S, Helms P: Changes in rib cage geometry during childhood, *Thorax* 39:624-627, 1984.
3. Moore KL: *The developing human. Clinically oriented embryology,* Philadelphia, 1973, WB Saunders, pp 284-287.
4. Warwick R, Williams PL: *Gray's anatomy,* ed 35, Philadelphia, 1973, WB Saunders, p 254.
5. Davis GM, Coates AL, Papageorgiou A, Bureau MA: Direct measurement of static chest wall compliance in animal and human neonates, *J Appl Physiol* 65(3):1093-1098, 1988.
6. Reynolds RN, Etsten BE: Mechanics of respiration in apneic anesthetized infants, *Anesthesiology* 27:13-19, 1966.
7. Richard CC, Bachman L: Lung and chest wall compliance in apneic paralyzed infants, *J Clin Invest* 40:273-278, 1961.
8. Gerhardt T, Bancalari E: Chest wall compliance in full term and premature infants, *Acta Paediatr Scand* 69:359-364, 1980.
9. Papastamelos C, Panitch H, England S, Allen J: Developmental changes in chest wall compliance in early childhood, *J Appl Physiol* 78:179-184, 1995.

10. Sharp JT, Druz WS, Balagot RC, Bandelin VR, Danon J: Total respiratory compliance in infants and children, *J Appl Physiol* 29:775-779, 1970.
11. Mittman C, Edelman NH, Norris AH, Shock NW: Relationship between chest wall and pulmonary compliance and age, *J Appl Physiol* 20(6): 1211-1216, 1965.
12. Leiter JC, Mortola JP, Tenney SM: A comparative analysis of contractile characteristics of the diaphragm and of respiratory system mechanics, *Respir Physiol* 64:267-276, 1980.
13. Davidson MB: The relationship between diaphragm and body weight in the rat, *Growth* 32:221-223, 1968.
14. Kikuchi Y, Stamenovich D, Loring SH: Dynamic behaviour of excised dog rib cage: dependence on muscle, *J Appl Physiol* 70(3):1059-1067, 1991.
15. Heldt GP, McIlroy MB: Distortion of chest wall and work of diaphragm in preterm infants, *J Appl Physiol* 62(1):164-169, 1987.
16. Ferris BG Jr, Mead J, Opie LH: Partitioning of respiratory flow resistance in man, *J Appl Physiol* 19:653-658, 1964.
17. Wohl MEB, Stigol LC, Mead J: Resistance of the total respiratory system in healthy infants and infants with bronchiolitis, *Pediatrics* 43:495-509, 1969.
18. Similowski T, Levy P, Corbeil C, Albala M, Pariente R, Derenne JP, Bates JHT, Jonson B, Milic-Emili J: Viscoelastic behavior of lung and chest wall in dogs determined by flow interruption, *J Appl Physiol* 67(6):2219-2229, 1989.
19. D'Angelo E, Robatto FM, Calderini E, Tavola M, Bono D, Torri G, Milic-Emili J: Pulmonary and chest wall mechanics in anesthetized paralyzed humans, *J Appl Physiol* 70(6):2602-2610, 1991.
20. Freezer NJ, Nicolai T, Sly PD: Effect of volume history in measurements of respiratory mechanics using the interrupter technique, *Pediatr Res* 33:261-266,1993.
21. Agostoni E, Mead J: Statics of the respiratory system. In Fenn WO, Rahn H, eds: *Handbook of physiology: respiration,* sect 3, vol 1, Washington, DC, 1964, American Physiological Society, p 401.
22. Mortola JP, Saetta M: Measurements of respiratory mechanics in the newborn: a simple approach, *Pediatr Pulmonol* 3:123-130, 1987.
23. Vinegar A, Sinnett EE, Leith DE: Dynamic mechanisms determining functional residual capacity in mice, *Mus musculus, J Appl Physiol* 46:867-871, 1979.
24. *J Appl Physiol: Respirat Environ Exercise Physiol* 57(4):1126-1133, 1984.
25. England SJ: Laryngeal function. In Chernick V, Mellins RB, eds: *Basic mechanisms of pediatric respiratory disease: cellular and integrative,* Philadelphia, 1991, BC Decker.
26. Kosch PC, Hutchison AA, Wozniak JA, Carlo WA, Stark AR: Posterior cricoarytenoid and diaphragm activities during tidal breathing in neonates, *J Appl Physiol* 64(5):1968-1978, 1988.
27. Stark AR, Colin BA, Waggener TB, Frantz ID III, Kosch PC: Regulation of end-expiratory lung volume during sleep in premature infants, *J Appl Physiol* 62:1117-1123,1987.
28. Colin AA, Wohl MEB, Mead J, Ratjen FA, Glass G, Stark AR: Transition from dynamically maintained to relaxed end-expiratory volume in human infants, *J Appl Physiol* 67(5):2107-2111, 1989.
29. Devlieger H: *The chest wall in the preterm infant,* Leuven, Belgium, 1987, KU Leuven.
30. Devlieger H, Daniels H, Marchal G, Moerman PH, Casaer P, Eggermont E: The diaphragm of the newborn infant: anatomical and ultrasonographic studies, *J Dev Physiol* 16:321-329, 1991.

Development of the Respiratory Muscles

31. DeTroyer A, Estenne M: Functional anatomy of the respiratory muscles. In Belman MJ, ed: Respiratory muscles: function in health and disease, *Clin Chest Med* 9(2):175-193, 1988 (review).
32. DeTroyer A, Loring SH: Action of the respiratory muscles. In Macklem PT, Mead J, eds: *Handbook of physiology.* The Respiratory System. Mechanics of Breathing, sect 3, vol 3, Part 2, Bethesda, Md, 1986, American Physiological Society, p 453.
33. Watchko JF, Brozanski BS, O'Day TL, Guthrie RD, Sieck GC: Contractile properties of the rat external abdominal oblique and diaphragm muscles during development, *J Appl Physiol* 72(4):1432-1436, 1992.
34. Praud JP, Egreteau L, Benlabed M, Curzi- Dascalova L, Nedelcoux H, Gaultier C: Abdominal muscle activity during CO_2 rebreathing in sleeping neonates, *J Appl Physiol* 70(3):1344-1350, 1991.
35. Keens TG, Bryan AC, Levison H, Ianuzzo CD: Developmental pattern of muscle fiber types in human ventilatory muscles, *J Appl Physiol: Respirat Environ Exercise Physiol* 44(6):909-913, 1978.
36. Le Souef PN, England SJ, Stogryn HAF, Bryan AC: Comparison of diaphragmatic fatigue in newborn and older rabbits, *J Appl Physiol* 65(3): 1040-1044, 1988.
37. Muller N, Volgyesi G, Eng P, Bryan MH, Bryan AC: The consequences of diaphragmatic muscle fatigue in the newborn infant, *J Pediatr* 95(5):793-797, 1979.
38. Watchko JF, Mayock DE, Standaert TA, Woodrum DE: The ventilatory pump: neonatal and developmental issues, *Adv Pediatr* 38:109-134, 1991. (Review)
39. Sieck GC, Fournier M: Developmental aspects of diaphragm muscle cells: structural and functional organization. In Haddad GG, Farber JP, eds: *Developmental neurobiology of breathing,* New York, 1991, Dekker, pp 375-428. (Lung Biology in Health and Disease Series). (Review)
40. Sieck GC: Diaphragm muscle: structural and functional organization. In Belman MJ, ed: Respiratory muscles: function in health and disease. *Clin Chest Med* 9(2):195-210, 1988 (review).
41. Maxwell LC, McCarter RJM, Kuehl TJ, Robotham JL: Development of histochemical and functional properties of baboon respiratory muscles, *J Appl Physiol: Respirat Environ Exercise Physiol* 54(2):551-561, 1983.
42. Sieck GC, Fournier M, Blanco CE: Diaphragm muscle fatigue resistance during postnatal development, *J Appl Physiol* 71:458-464, 1991.
43. Watchko JF, Daood MJ, Vazquez RL, Brozanski BS, LaFramboise WA, Guthrie RD, Sieck GC: Postnatal expression of myosin isoforms in an expiratory muscle-external abdominal oblique, *J Appl Physiol* 73(5):1860-1866, 1992.
44. Watchko JF, Sieck GC: Respiratory muscle fatigue resistance relates to myosin phenotype and SDH activity during development, *J Appl Physiol* 75:1341-1347, 1993.

Methods for Assessing Chest Wall Function

45. American Thoracic Society/European Respiratory Society: Respiratory mechanics in infants: physiologic evaluation in health and disease. A statement of the Committee on Infant Pulmonary Function Testing, *Am Rev Respir Dis* 147:474-496, 1993.
46. Hershenson MB, Colin AA, Wohl MEB, Stark AR: Changes in the contribution of the rib cage to tidal breathing during infancy, *Am Rev Respir Dis* 141:922-925, 1990.
47. Konno K, Mead J: Measurement of the separate volume changes of rib cage and abdomen during breathing, *J Appl Physiol* 22:407-422, 1967.
48. Allen JL, Wolfson MR, McDowell K, Shaffer TH: Thoraco-abdominal asynchrony in infants with airflow obstruction, *Am Rev Respir Dis* 141:337-342, 1990.
49. Allen JL, Greenspan JS, Deoras KS, Keklikian E, Wolfson MR, Shaffer TH: Interaction between chest wall motion and lung mechanics in normal infants and infants with bronchopulmonary dysplasia, *Pediatr Pulmonol* 11:37-43, 1991.
50. Colin AA, Hunter JM, Stark AR, Wohl MEB: Normal infants and children have minimal thoracoabdominal asynchrony assessed by respiratory inductive plethysmography, *Am Rev Respir Dis* 147:A966, 1993. (Abstract)
51. Deoras KS, Greenspan JS, Wolfson MR, Keklikian EN, Shaffer TH, Allen JL: Effects of inspiratory resistive loading on chest wall motion and ventilation: Differences between preterm and full term infants, *Pediatr Res* 32:589-594, 1992.
52. Sivan Y, Deakers TW, Newth CJL: Thoraco-abdominal asynchrony in acute upper airway obstruction in small children, *Am Rev Respir Dis* 142:540-544, 1990.
53. Mortola JP, Sant'Ambrogio G: Motion of the rib cage and the abdomen in tetraplegic patients, *Clin Sci Mol Med* 54:25-32, 1978.
54. DeTroyer A, Kelly S: Chest wall mechanics in dogs with acute diaphragm paralysis, *J Appl Physiol: Respirat Environ Exercise Physiol* 53:373- 379, 1982.
55. Higgenbottam T, Allen D, Loh L, Clark TJH: Abdominal wall movement in normals and patients with hemidiaphragmatic and bilateral diaphragmatic palsy, *Thorax* 32:589-595, 1977.
56. Roussos C, Fixley M, Gross D, Macklem PT: Fatigue of inspiratory muscles and their synergic behaviour, *J Appl Physiol: Respirat Environ Exercise Physiol* 46(5):897-904, 1979.

57. Tobin MJ, Perez W, Guenther SM, Lodato RF, Dantzker DR: Does rib cage abdominal paradox signify respiratory muscle fatigue? *J Appl Physiol* 63(2):851-860, 1987.
58. Shardonofsky FR, Perez-Chada D, Carmuega E, Milic-Emili J: Airway pressures during crying in healthy infants, *Pediatr Pulmonol* 6:14-18, 1989.
59. Cook CD, Mead J, Orzalesi MM: Static volume pressure characteristics of the respiratory system during maximal efforts, *J Appl Physiol* 19:1016-1022, 1964.
60. Gaultier C, Zinman R: Maximal static pressures in healthy children, *Respir Physiol* 51:45-61, 1983.
61. Wagener JS, Hibbert ME, Landau LI: Maximal respiratory pressures in children, *Am Rev Respir Dis* 129:873-875, 1984.
62. Multz AS, Aldrich TK, Prezant DJ, Karpel JP, Hendler JM: Maximal inspiratory pressure is not a reliable test of inspiratory muscle strength in mechanically ventilated patients, *Am Rev Respir Dis* 142:529-532, 1990.
63. Gaultier C: Tension-time index of inspiratory muscles in children, *Pediatr Pulmonol* 23:327-329, 1997.
64. Gross D, Grassino A, Macklem PT: Electromyogram pattern of diaphragm fatigue, *J Appl Physiol* 46:1, 1979.
65. Muller N, Gulston G, Dade C, Whitton J, Froese AB, Bryan MH, Bryan AC: Diaphragmatic muscle fatigue in the newborn, *J Appl Physiol: Respirat Environ Exercise Physiol* 46(4):688-695, 1979.
66. Watchko JF, Standaert TA, Mayock DE,Woodrum DE: Diaphragmatic electromyogram power spectral analysis during ventilatory failure in infants. In Gennser G, Marsal K, Svennigsen N, Lindstrom K, eds: *Fetal and neonatal physiologic measurements. III.* Proceedings of the third international conference on fetal and neonatal physiological measurements, Malmo, Sweden, 1989, Flenhags, Tryckeri, pp 445-449.

Treatment of Respiratory Pump Fatigue: General Principles

67. Cropp A, Dimarco AF: Effects of intermittent negative pressure ventilation on respiratory muscle function in patients with severe chronic obstructive pulmonary disease, *Am Rev Respir Dis* 135:1056-1061, 1987.
68. Gutierrez M, Beroiza T, Contreras G, Diaz O, Cruz E, Moreno R, Lisboa C: Weekly cuirass ventilation improves blood gases and inspiratory muscle strength in patients with chronic airflow limitation and hypercarbia, *Am Rev Respir Dis* 138:617-623, 1988.
69. Rochester DF, Braun NMT, Laine S: Diaphragmatic energy expenditure in chronic respiratory failure: the effect of assisted ventilation with body respirators, *Am J Med* 63:223-232, 1977.
70. Levine S, Henson D, Levy S: Respiratory muscle rest therapy. In Belman MJ, ed: Respiratory muscles in health and disease. *Clin Chest Med* 9(2):297-309, 1988 (review).
71. Carroll N, Branthwaite MA: Control of nocturnal hypoventilation by nasal intermittent positive pressure ventilation, *Thorax* 43:349-353, 1988.
72. Hoeppner VH, Cockroft DW, Dosman JA, Cotton DJ: Nighttime ventilation improves respiratory failure in secondary kyphoscoliosis, *Am Rev Respir Dis* 129:240-243, 1984.
73. Garay SM, Turino GM, Goldring RM: Sustained reversal of chronic hypercapnea in patients with alveolar hypoventilation syndromes. Long-term maintenance with long-term non-invasive mechanical ventilation, *Am J Med* 70:269-274, 1981.
74. Ellis ER, Bye PTP, Bruderer JW, Sullivan CE: Treatment of respiratory failure during sleep in patients with neuromuscular disease. Positive-pressure ventilation through a nose mask, *Am Rev Respir Dis* 135:148-152, 1987.
75. De Troyer A, Deisser P: The effects of intermittent positive pressure breathing on patients with respiratory muscle weakness, *Am Rev Respir Dis* 124:132-137, 1981.
76. Pardy RL, Reid WD, Belman MJ: Respiratory muscle training. In Respiratory muscles: Function in health and disease. *Clin Chest Med* 9(2):287-296, 1988 (review).
77. Leith DE, Bradley M: Ventilatory muscle strength and endurance training, *J Appl Physiol* 41:508-516, 1976.
78. Reid WD, Warren CPW: Ventilatory muscle strength and endurance training in elderly subjects and patients with chronic airflow limitation: a pilot study, *Physiol Can* 36:305-311, 1984.
79. Asher MI, Pardy RL, Coates AL, Thomas E, Macklem PT: The effects of inspiratory muscle training in patients with cystic fibrosis, *Am Rev Respir Dis* 126:855-859, 1982.
80. Gross D, Ladd HW, Riley EJ, Macklem PT, Grassino A: The effect of training on strength and endurance of the diaphragm in quadriplegia, *Am J Med* 68:27-35, 1980.
81. Levine S, Weisser P, Gillen J: Evaluation of a ventilatory muscle endurance training program in the rehabilitation of patients with COPD, *Am Rev Respir Dis* 133:400-406, 1986.
82. Keens TG, Krastins IRB, Wannamaker EM, Levison H, Crozier DN, Bryan AC: Ventilatory muscle endurance training in normal subjects and patients with cystic fibrosis, *Am Rev Respir Dis* 116:853-860, 1977.
83. Tan S, Duara S, Neto GS, Afework M, Gerhardt T, Bancalari E: The effects of respiratory training with inspiratory flow resistive loads in premature infants, *Pediatr Res* 31:613-618, 1992.
84. Aldrich TK: Respiratory muscle fatigue. In Belman MJ, ed: Respiratory muscles: function in health and disease, *Clin Chest Med* 9(2):225-236, 1988. (Review)
85. Braun NMT, Faulkner J, Hughes RL, Roussos C, Sahgal V: When should respiratory muscles be exercised? *Chest* 84:76-84, 1983.
86. Viires N, Aubier M, Murciano D, Marty C, Pariente R: Effects of theophylline on isolated diaphragmatic fibers: a model for pharmacological studies on diaphragmatic contractility, *Am Rev Respir Dis* 133:1060-1064, 1986.
87. Sigrist S, Thomas D, Howell S, Roussos CH: The effect of aminophylline on inspiratory muscle contractility, *Am Rev Respir Dis* 126:46-50, 1982.
88. Howell S, Roussos C: Isoproterenol and aminophylline improve contractility of fatigued canine diaphragm, *Am Rev Respir Dis* 129:118-124, 1984.
89. Aubier M, De Troyer A, Sampson M, Macklem PT, Roussos C: Aminophylline improves diaphragm contractility, *N Engl J Med* 305:249-252, 1981.
90. Mayock DE, Standaert TA, Watchko JF, Woodrum DE: Effect of aminophylline on diaphragmatic contractility in the piglet, *Pediatr Res* 28(3):196-198, 1990.
91. Mayock DE, Standaert TA, Woodrum DE: Effect of methylxanthines on diaphragmatic fatigue in the piglet, *Pediatr Res* 32(5):580-584, 1992.
92. Heyman E, Ohlsson A, Heyman Z, Fong K: The effect of aminophylline on the excursions of the diaphragm in preterm neonates, *Acta Pediatr Scand* 80:308-315, 1991.

Structural Abnormalities of the Chest Wall Including the Diaphragm

93. Wohl MEB, Stark AR, Stokes DC: Thoracic disorders in childhood. In Roussos C, ed: *Lung biology in health and disease: The Thorax. Part C: Disease,* New York, 1995, Marcel Dekker, pp 2035-2070.
94. Francomano C: Clinical implications of basic research: the genetic basis of dwarfism, *N Engl J Med* 332(1):58-59, 1995.
95. International nomenclature of constitutional diseases of bone, *J Pediatr* 98(4):614-616, 1978.
96. Sillence DO, Horton WA, Rimoin DL: Morphologic studies in the skeletal dysplasias, *Am J Pathol* 96:811-870, 1979.
97. Herman TE, Siegel MJ, McAlister WH: Chest wall deformity and respiratory distress in a 17-year-old patient with achondroplasia: CT and MRI evaluation, *Pediatr Radiol* 22:233-234, 1992.
98. Zucconi M, Weber G, Castronovo V, Ferini-Strambi L, Russo F, Chiumello G, Smirne S: Sleep and upper airway obstruction in children with achondroplasia, *J Pediatr* 129(5):743-479, 1996.
99. Mador MJ, Tobin MJ: Apneustic breathing. A characteristic feature of brainstem compression in achondroplasia? *Chest* 97(4):877-883, 1990.
100. Nelson FW, Hecht JT, Horton WA, Butler IJ, Goldie WD, Miner M: Neurological basis of respiratory complications in achondroplasia, *Ann Neurol* 24(1):89-93, 1988.
101. Stokes DC, Phillips JA, Leonardo CO, Dorst JP, Kopits SE, Trojac JE: Respiratory complications of achondroplasia, *J Pediatr* 102:534-541, 1983.
102. Stokes DC, Pyeritz RE, Wise RA, Fairclough D, Murphy EA: Spirometry and chest wall dimensions in achondroplasia, *Chest* 93(2):364-369, 1988.
103. Stokes DC, Wohl MEB, Wise RA, Pyeritz RE, Fairclough DL: The lungs and airways in achondroplasia: do little people have little lungs? *Chest* 98(1):145-152, 1990.
104. Bonaventure J, Rousseau F, Legeai-Mallet L, Le Merrer M, Munnich A, Maroteaux P: Common mutations in the fibroblast growth factor receptor 3 (FGFR 3) gene account for achondroplasia, hypochondroplasia, and thanatophoric dwarfism, *Am J Med Genet* 63(1):148-154, 1996.

105. Finegold MJ, Katzew H, Genieser NB, Becker MH: Lung structure in thoracic dystrophy, *Am J Dis Child* 122:153-159, 1971.
106. Williams AJ, Vawter G, Reid LM: Lung structure in asphyxiating thoracic dystrophy, *Arch Pathol Lab Med* 108:658-661, 1984.
107. Hudgins L, Rosengren S, Treem W, Hyams J: Early cirrhosis in survivors with Jeune thoracic dystrophy, *J Pediatr* 120:754-756, 1992.
108. Donaldson MDC, Warner AA, Trompeter RS, Haycock GB, Chantler C: Familial juvenile nephronophthisis, Jeune's syndrome, and associated disorders, *Arch Dis Child* 60:426-434, 1985.
109. Burn J, Hall C, Marsden D, Matthew DJ: Autosomal dominant thoracolaryngopelvic dysplasia: Barnes syndrome, *J Med Genet* 23:345-349, 1986.
110. Shapiro JR, Burn VE, Chipman SD, Jacobs JB, Schloo B, Reid L, Larsen N, Louis F: Case report: pulmonary hypoplasia and osteogenesis imprefecta type II with defective synthesis of alpha I (1) procollagen, *Bone* 10:165-171, 1989.
111. Clark JB, Grenville-Mathers R: Pectus Excavatum, *Br J Dis Chest* 56:202-205, 1962.
112. Seliem MA, Duffy CE, Gidding SS, Berdusis K, Benson DW Jr: Echocardiographic evaluation of the aortic root and mitral valve in children and adolescents with isolated pectus excavatum: comparison with marfan patients, *Pediatr Cardiol* 13(1):20-23, 1992.
113. Humphreys II GH, Jaretzki III A: Pectus excavatum: late results with and without operation, *J Thorac Cardiovasc Surg* 80(5):686-695, 1980.
114. Shamberger RC, Welch KJ: Cardiopulmonary function in pectus excavatum, *Surg Gynecol Obstet* 166:383-391, 1988.
115. Morshuis W, Folgering H, Barentsz J, van Lier H, Lacquet L: Pulmonary function before surgery for pectus excavatum and at long-term follow-up, *Chest* 105(6):1646-1652, 1994.
116. Quigley PM, Haller Jr JA, Jelus KL, Loughlin GM, Marcus CL: Cardiorespiratory function before and after corrective surgery in pectus excavatum, *J Pediatr* 128(5):638-643, 1996.
117. Derveaux L, Ivanoff I, Rochette F, Demedts M: Mechanism of pulmonary function changes after surgical correction for funnel chest, *Eur Respir J* 1:823-825, 1988.
118. Derveaux L, Clarysse I, Ivanoff I, Demedts M: Preoperative and postoperative abnormalities in chest x-ray indices and in lung function in pectus deformities, *Chest* 95(4):850-856, 1989.
119. Haller JA Jr, Colombani PM, Humphries CT, Azizkhan RG, Loughlin GM: Chest wall constriction after too extensive and too early operations for pectus excavatum, *Ann Thorac Surg* 61:1618-1625, 1996.
120. Bevegard S: Postural circulatory changes during exercise in patients with a funnel chest with special reference to factors affecting stroke volume, *Acta Med Scand* 111:695-713, 1962.
121. Beiser GD, Epstein SE, Stampfer M, Goldstein RE, Noland SP, Levitsky S: Impairment of cardiac function in patients with pectus excavatum, with improvement after operative correction, *N Engl J Med* 287(6):267-272, 1972.
122. Peterson RJ, Young Jr WG, Godwin JD, Sabiston Jr DC, Jones RH: Noninvasive assessment of exercise cardiac function before and after pectus excavatum repair, *J Thorac Cardiovasc Surg* 90(2):251-260, 1985.
123. Morshuis WJ, Folgering HT, Barentsz JO, Cox AL, van Lier HJ, Lacquet LK: Exercise cardiorespiratory function before and one year after operation for pectus excavatum, *J Thorac Cardiovasc Surg* 107(6):1403-1409, 1994.
124. Kaguraoka H, Ohnuki T, Haoka T, Kei J, Yokoyama M, Nitta S: Degree of severity of pectus excavatum and pulmonary function in preoperative and postoperative periods, *J Thorac Cardiovasc Surg* 104(5):1483-1488, 1992.
125. Castile RG, Staats BA, Westbrook PR: Symptomatic pectus deformities of the chest, *Am Rev Respir Dis* 126:564-568, 1982.
126. Mead J, Sly P, Le Souef P, Hibbert M, Phelan P: Rib cage mobility in pectus excavatum, *Am Rev Respir Dis* 13201223-1228, 1985.
127. Park EA, Howland J: The dangers to life of severe involvement of the thorax in rickets, *Bull Johns Hopkins Hosp* 32:101-109, 1921.
128. Wohl MEB, Griscom NT, Traggis DG, Jaffe N: Effects of therapeutic irradiation delivered in early childhood upon subsequent lung function, *Pediatrics* 55(4):507-516, 1975.
129. Littman P, Meadows AT, Polgar G, Burns PF, Rubin E: Pulmonary function in survivors of Wilms tumor, *Cancer* 37:2773-2776, 1976.
130. Riseborough EJ, Grabias SL, Burton RI, Jaffe N: Skeletal alterations following irradiation for Wilm's tumor: with particular reference to scoliosis and kyphosis, *J Bone Joint Surg* 58A(4):526-536, 1976.
131. Kafer ER: Idiopathic scoliosis: gas exchange and the age dependence of arterial blood gases, *J Clinic Invest* 58:825-833, 1976.
132. Bergofsky EH: Respiratory failure in disorders of the thoracic cage, *Am Rev Respir Dis* 119:643-669, 1979.
133. Pehrsson K, Larsson S, Oden A, Nachemson A: Long-term follow-up of patients with untreated scoliosis: a study of mortality, causes of death, and symptoms, *Spine* 17(9):1091-1096, 1992.
134. Pehrsson K, Bake B, Larsson S, Nachemson A: Lung function in adult idiopathic scoliosis: a 20 year follow-up, *Thorax* 46:474-478, 1991.
135. Cooper DM, Rojas JV, Mellins RB, Keim HA, Mansell AL: Respiratory mechanics in adolescents with idiopathic scoliosis, *Am Rev Respir Dis* 130:16-22, 1984.
136. Kearon C, Viviani GR, Killian K: Factors influencing work capacity in adolescent idiopathic thoracic scoliosis, *Am Rev Respir Dis* 148:295-303, 1993.
137. Owange-Iraka JW, Harrison A, Warner JO: Lung function in congenital and idiopathic scoliosis, *Eur J Pediatr* 142:198-200, 1984.
138. Kearon C, Viviani GR, Kirkley A, Killian K: Factors determining pulmonary function in adolescent idiopathic thoracic scoliosis, *Am Rev Respir Dis* 148:288-294, 1993.
139. Bjure J, Grimby G, Nachemson A, Lindh M: The effect of physical training in girls with idiopathic scoliosis, *Acta Orthop Scand* 40:325-333, 1969.
140. Kinnear WJM, Johnston IDA: Does harrington instrumentation improve pulmonary function in adolescents with idiopathic scoliosis?: a meta-analysis, *Spine* 18(11):1556-1559, 1993.
141. Davies G, Reid L: Effect of scoliosis on growth of alveoli and pulmonary arteries and on right ventricle, *Arch Dis Child* 46:623-632, 1971.
142. Philip N, Gambarelli D, Guys JM, Camboulives J, Ayme S: Epidemiological study of congenital diaphragmatic defects with special reference to aetiology, *Eur J Pediatr* 150:726-729, 1991.
143. Wenstrom KD, Weiner CP, Hansom JW: A five-year statewide experience with congenital diaphragmatic hernia, *Am J Obstet Gynecol* 165(4):838-842, 1991.
144. Sweed Y, Puri P: Congenital diaphragmatic hernia: influence of associated malformation on survival, *Arch Dis Child* 69:68-70, 1993.
145. Cunniff C, Jones KL, Jones MC: Patterns of malformation in children with congenital diaphragmatic defects, *J Pediatr* 116(2):258-261, 1990.
146. Chatrath RR, El Shafie M, Jones RS: Fate of hypoplastic lungs after repair of congenital diaphragmatic hernia, *Arch Dis Child* 46:633-635, 1971.
147. Reid IS, Hutcherson RJ: Long-term follow-up of patients with congenital diaphragmatic hernia, *J Pediatr Surg* 11(6):939-942, 1976.
148. Kerr AA: Lung function in children after repair of congenital diaphragmatic hernia, *Arch Dis Child* 52(11):902-903, 1977.
149. Wohl MEB, Griscom NT, Strieder DJ, Schuster SR, Treves S, Zwerdling RG: The lung following repair of congenital diaphragmatic hernia, *J Pediatr* 90(3):405-414, 1977.
150. Khouri-Dagher L, Gaultier C, Gruner M, Boule M, Couvreur J, Grimfeld A, Girard F: Pulmonary function testing in eight children after operation for left congenital diaphragmatic hernia, *Ann Pediatr* 28(6): 385-391, 1981.
151. Freyschuss U, Lannergren K, Frenckner B: Lung function after repair of congenital diaphragmatic hernia, *Acta Pediatr Scand* 73:589-593, 1984.
152. Falconer AR, Brown RA, Helms P, Gordon I, Baron JA: Pulmonary sequelae in survivors of congenital diaphragmatic hernia, *Thorax* 45:126-129, 1990.
153. Delepoulle F, Martinot A, Leclerc F, Riou Y, Remy-Jardin M, Amegassi F, Dubos JP, Lequien P: Long time outcome of congenital diaphragmatic hernia: a study of 17 patients, *Arch F Pediatr* 48:703-707, 1991.
154. Lund DP, Mitchell J, Kharasch V, Quigley S, Keuhn M, Wilson JM: Congenital diaphragmatic hernia: the hidden morbidity, *J Pediatr Surg* 29(2):258-264, 1994.
155. Tan KH, Kilby MD, Whittle MJ, Beattie BR, Booth IW, Botting BJ: Congenital anterior abdominal wall defects in England and Wales 1987-93: retrospective analysis of OPCS data, *Br Med J* 313(7062):903-906, 1996.

156. Argyle JC: Pulmonary hypoplasia in infants with giant abdominal wall defects, *Pediatr Pathol* 9(1):43-55, 1989.
157. Nakayama DK, Mutich R, Motoyama EK: Pulmonary dysfunction after primary closure of an abdominal wall defect and its improvement with bronchodilators, *Pediatr Pulmonol* 12:174-180, 1992.
158. Ewig JM, Griscom NT, Wohl MEB: The effect of the absence of abdominal muscles on pulmonary function and exercise, *Am J Respir Crit Care Med* 153:1314-1321, 1996.

Neuromuscular Disease

159. Quittell LM, Fisher M, Foley CM: Pneumocystis carinii pneumonia in infants given adrenocorticotropic hormone for infantile spasms, *J Pediatr* 110:901-903, 1987.
160. Kelly BJ, Luce JM: The diagnosis and management of neuromuscular diseases causing respiratory failure, *Chest* 99:1485-1494, 1991.
161. Schmidt-Nowara WW, Altman AR: Atelectasis and neuromuscular respiratory failure, *Chest* 85:792-795, 1984.
162. De Troyer A, Borenstein S, Cordier R: Analysis of lung volume restriction in patients with respiratory muscle weakness, *Thorax* 35:603-610, 1980.
163. Vincken WG, Elleker MG, Cosio MG: Flow volume loop changes reflecting respiratory muscle weakness in chronic neuromuscular disorders, *Am J Med* 83:673-680, 1987.
164. Gibson GJ, Pride NB, Newsome Davis J, Loh LC: Pulmonary mechanics in patients with respiratory muscle weakness, *Am Rev Respir Dis* 115:389-395, 1977.
165. De Troyer A, Heilporn A: Respiratory mechanics in quadriplegia: the respiratory function of the intercostal muscles, *Am Rev Respir Dis* 122:591-600, 1980.
166. Black LF, Hyatt RE: Maximal static respiratory pressures in generalized neuromuscular disease, *Am Rev Respir Dis* 103:641-650, 1971.
167. Vincken W, Elleker M, Cosio MG: Determinants of respiratory muscle weakness in stable chronic neuromuscular disorders, *Am J Med* 82:53-58, 1987.
168. Estenne M, Heilport A, Delhez L, Yernault JC, De Troyer A: Chest wall stiffness in patients with chronic respiratory muscle weakness, *Am Rev Respir Dis* 128:1002-1007, 1983.
169. Papastamelos C, Panitch HB, Allen JL: Chest wall compliance in infants and children with neuromuscular disease, *Am J Respir Crit Care Med* 154:1045-1048, 1996.
170. Begin R, Bureau MA, Lupien L, Lemieux B: Control of breathing in Duchenne's muscular dystrophy, *Am J Med* 69:227-234, 1980.
171. Baydur A: Respiratory muscle strength and control of venitlation in patients with neuromuscular disease, *Chest* 99:330-338, 1991.
172. Estenne M, De Troyer A: Cough in tetraplegic subjects: an active process, *Ann Intern Med* 112:22-28, 1990.
173. Garay SM, Turino GM, Goldring RM: Sustained reversal of chronic hypercapnea in patients with alveolar hypoventilation syndrome: long-term maintenance with non-invasive nocturnal mechanical ventilation, *Am J Med* 70:269-274, 1981.
174. Bach JR, Penek J: Obstructive sleep apnea complicating negative pressure ventilatory support in patients with chronic paralytic/restrictive ventilatory dysfunction, *Chest* 99:1386-1393, 1991.
175. Ellis ER, Bye PT, Bruderer JW, Sullivan C: Treatment of respiratory failure during sleep in patients with neuromuscular disease: positive pressure ventilation through a nose mask, *Am Rev Respir Dis* 135:148-152, 1987.
176. Arora NS, Rochester DF: Respiratory muscle strength and maximal voluntary ventilation in undernourished patients, *Am Rev Respir Dis* 126:5-8, 1982.

CHAPTER 75

Ciliary Dysfunction

Jonathan Rutland and Robbert deIongh

A relationship between abnormal ciliary function and respiratory disease was first suggested in the mid-1970s.[1,2] Although an association between bronchiectasis and situs inversus had been noted[3] in 1904, it was not until the 1930s that Kartagener reported a series of patients with sinusitis, situs inversus, and bronchiectasis.[4] In time this became known as Kartagener syndrome. The underlying pathogenesis was not known. In 1975 two groups independently identified sperm immotility and absence of dynein arms in the axonemes of sperm from patients with Kartagener syndrome,[5,6] thus linking male infertility with this syndrome. Subsequent studies of respiratory tract cilia (which have the same axonemal ultrastructure as sperm) revealed defective ciliary motility and deficient dynein arms.[1,2] Initially it was thought that these patients had immotile cilia and the term *immotile-cilia syndrome* was suggested.[7] Subsequent studies demonstrated a wide range of ciliary motility ranging from complete absence to almost normal motility.[8,9] The ciliary motility in these patients was often noted to be uncoordinated or dyskinetic. The term *primary ciliary dyskinesia* (PCD) has gained favor and come into increasing usage in recent years.[10]

A range of ultrastructural abnormalities has been found in patients with PCD. These cause defective ciliary function with resultant impairment of mucociliary clearance. Chronic and recurrent upper and lower respiratory tract disease result.

CILIARY STRUCTURE AND FUNCTION

Cilia are widely distributed throughout the animal kingdom. Throughout the phylogenetic tree there is little variation in the ultrastructural features of cilia. Flagella, including sperm tails, have almost identical internal structure (the axoneme) to that of cilia. When ciliated epithelium is adapted for mucus transport, as in the human respiratory tract, cilia are shorter and more numerous, and beat mainly within a low-viscosity periciliary fluid layer, moving a more viscous overlying mucus layer (Fig. 75-1). The tips of the cilia enter the mucus layer only during the effective stroke and retract beneath the mucus

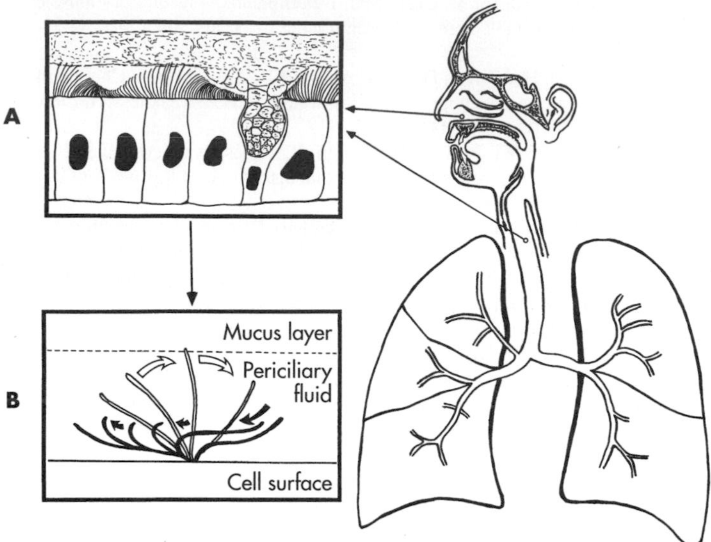

Fig. 75-1. Diagram of the human respiratory tract. Clearance of inhaled particles, secretions, cellular debris, and bacterial products from the upper and lower respiratory tract is carried out by the ciliated epithelium. **A,** A portion of the ciliated epithelium. Cilia on the surface of the epithelial cells beat rhythmically in a wavelike motion that moves the overlying mucus produced by the goblet cells within the epithelium and the subepithelial mucus glands. **B,** The beat cycle of a single cilium. The mucus is moved in the same direction as the effective stroke *(open arrows).* The recovery stroke is shown by the solid arrows.

layer during the recovery stroke so that the mucus is moved in one direction only (Fig. 75-1).

Distribution of Human Cilia

The human tracheobronchial tree is lined by pseudostratified, ciliated epithelium from the larynx down to the level of the terminal bronchiole (Fig. 75-1). The nasal cavity (apart from its most anterior portion) and the paranasal sinuses are also lined by ciliated epithelium, the predominant direction of clearance being toward the oropharynx. Respiratory epithelium undergoes a continual turnover, with cells being replaced approximately once every 4 to 8 weeks. Ciliated cells are present in the middle ear, the eustachian tube, ependyma, and parts of the male (ductuli efferentes) and female (fallopian tubes) genital tracts. Cells with modified cilia are present elsewhere and serve as sensory cells in the olfactory area, the labyrinth, and the retina. Many cell types may carry a single cilium transiently, especially during embryonic life. These may play a role in the orientation of the viscera.[1]

Structure

Human respiratory tract ciliated cells bear 200 to 300 cilia on their surface. Cilia are elongated motile cylindrical projections from the apical cell membrane, approximately 0.25 μm in diameter, which contain microtubules and cytoplasm in continuity with that of the cell. Human tracheal cilia are 5 to 8 μm long, becoming shorter in more distal airways. Ultrastructural examination of a transverse section of a cilium (Fig. 75-2) reveals that the axoneme consists of a characteristic "9+2" structure of nine pairs of microtubules (composed of the proteins, α- and β-tubulin) arranged around two single central microtubules that are surrounded and held together by the central sheath. The peripheral doublets are linked to neighboring doublets by fine filaments (nexin links) composed of a protein called nexin. Radial spokes are thicker filaments that project centrally from the A microtubule and end in a terminal knob, a short distance from the central sheath and central microtubules. Projecting at regular intervals from the A microtubule toward the B microtubule of the adjacent outer doublet are the inner and outer dynein arms, which are curved or hooklike filamentous structures. The dynein arms contain proteins with adenosine triphosphatase (ATPase) activity and, according to the sliding microtubule hypothesis of ciliary bending,[11] attach intermittently to the adjacent B microtubule and change shape, with resultant sliding of doublets in relation to each other. Such a cyclical movement of different microtubule pairs in relation to each other causes ciliary bending, first in one direction and then in the other. The microtubules, radial spokes, and nexin links are considered to form a "skeletal" structure for the cilium. This confers properties of elasticity and rigidity on the cilium and may transfer bending forces through the cilium and help the cilium to resume its initial shape after each beat.

The peripheral doublets extend along the length of the cilium and, at the base, continue into the cell in a modified form, becoming triplets and, in association with several accessory structures, form a basal body. Striated or ciliary rootlets extend from the basal extremity of the basal body into the apical cytoplasm. Together with the basal body they anchor the cilium and maintain the orientation of its direction of beating (Fig. 75-2). Projecting laterally from the basal body in the direction of the active stroke of the cilium is a structure called the basal foot (Fig. 75-2). All basal feet in a cell and in the whole epithelium are normally oriented in approximately the same direction[12] so that the effective strokes of all cilia move in the same direction.

Physiology

Human nasal and tracheal cilia beat at a rate of approximately 10 to 15 Hz (600 to 900 beats/min). Each beat consists of two phases: an effective and a recovery stroke.[11] During the effective stroke, the cilium is extended and moves rapidly around its point of attachment to the cell, extending into and engaging the overlying mucus, thus moving it forward. This is followed by a slower recovery stroke, when the cilium bends on itself and in a different plane to that of the effective stroke, retracting below the mucus layer, within the periciliary fluid, to resume its original position for a short resting phase before the next effective stroke (Fig. 75-1, *B*).

Ciliary beating is coordinated so that each cilium beats slightly later in the beat cycle than the one in front. This results in waves of coordinated beating (metachronal waves), which can be seen over a field of ciliated cells (Fig. 75-1, *A*). Control of the initiation of ciliary beating is thought to be regulated by calcium ion fluxes within the ciliated cell.[13-16] Two other factors that may play a part in ciliary coordination are mechanical stimulation of ciliary activity (as may occur from foreign material) and hydrodynamic forces (which may influence nearby cilia).[11] Electric coupling of the cells via gap junctions may allow transmission of calcium fluxes throughout the epithelium.[13]

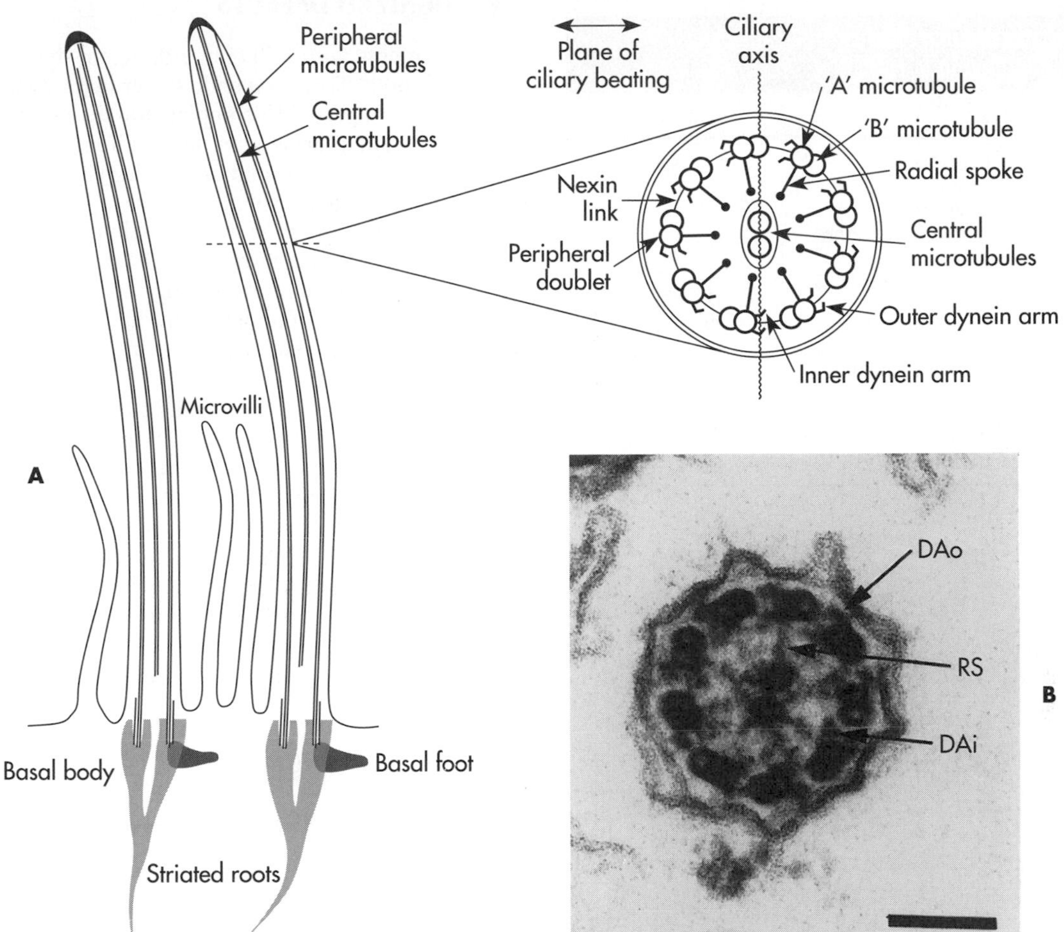

Fig. 75-2. **A,** Diagram of cilia in longitudinal and transverse section showing the organization of the axoneme and the anchoring structures of the cilium: the basal body, the basal foot, and the striated rootlets. **B,** Electronmicrograph of a cilium in transverse section showing normal axonemal structure. Inner *(DAi)* and outer *(DAo)* dynein arms and radial spokes *(RS)* are indicated. Scale bar, 0.1 μm. (**A** Adapted from de Iongh RU, Rutland J: *J Clin Pathol* 42:613-619, 1989; **B** adapted from Rutland J, de Iongh RU: *N Engl J Med* 323:1681-1684, 1990.)

If ciliary beating is impaired or discoordinated, mucus transport is slowed. Effective clearance of mucus requires coordinated ciliary beating, the optimal physicochemical properties of mucus (which is produced by goblet cells and subepithelial glands), and efficient interaction of the cilia with the overlying mucus layer. The direction of ciliary beating must be consistent and the beat patterns must be coordinated and normal. Mucociliary clearance can be measured by the rate of clearance of an inhaled radiolabeled aerosol or, mainly in animal studies, mucus transport rate of a marker can be measured directly.

Analysis of Ciliary Beating and Structure

Human ciliary function, in isolation from the mucous aspects of clearance, may be studied in vitro. Ciliary beating can be recorded and studied in different ways (such as high-speed cinematography or video) but the most commonly used technique in clinical practice is transmitted light microscope photometry.[16] In this technique, light passes through a wet preparation of ciliated epithelium on a slide and the beating cilia interrupt a narrow beam of light. The variations in light intensity caused by the beating cilia across the photometer's field are detected by a photosensitive cell or photometer, transduced into an electric signal, and, after amplification, recorded against time, allowing measurement of ciliary beat frequency. By limiting the area of light entering the photometer it is possible to measure the beat frequency of cilia from an area only a few microns across. In normal ciliated epithelium there is a regular beat pattern, with beat frequency of approximately 10 to 15 Hz.

Internal ciliary structure is studied by electron microscopy. In recent years ciliary ultrastructure has been quantified[17-20] and several distinct types of ciliary ultrastructural defects that lead to respiratory disease have been identified (Table 75-1).[1-7,12,21-30] The orientation of cilia can also be studied and quantified.[12,24,25,31] In various studies, up to 10% of cilia in normal subjects may have ultrastructural defects. These are usually microtubular defects or compound cilia.[17-20]

Quantitative analysis of axonemal ultrastructure is required to identify ultrastructural defects in patients with PCD.[17-20,24,25,31] Confidence in the significance of defects increases when studies can be done on separate occasions or when it is possible to study axonemal structure of cilia from more than one body site or from sperm tails. Because sperma-

Table 75-1 Types of Ciliary Ultrastructural Defects Identified in PCD

	CILIARY DEFECT	REFERENCE
I	Dynein arm defects Inner dynein arms Outer dynein arms Inner and outer dynein arms	1, 2, 5, 6, 7
II	Radial spoke defect	27
III	Microtubule translocation defect	28
IV	Normal ultrastructure but impaired function	29
V	Random ciliary orientation	12, 21, 23
VI	Ciliary aplasia	32, 33
VII	Abnormally long cilia	30
VIII	Abnormally short cilia	31
IX	Abnormal basal bodies	34

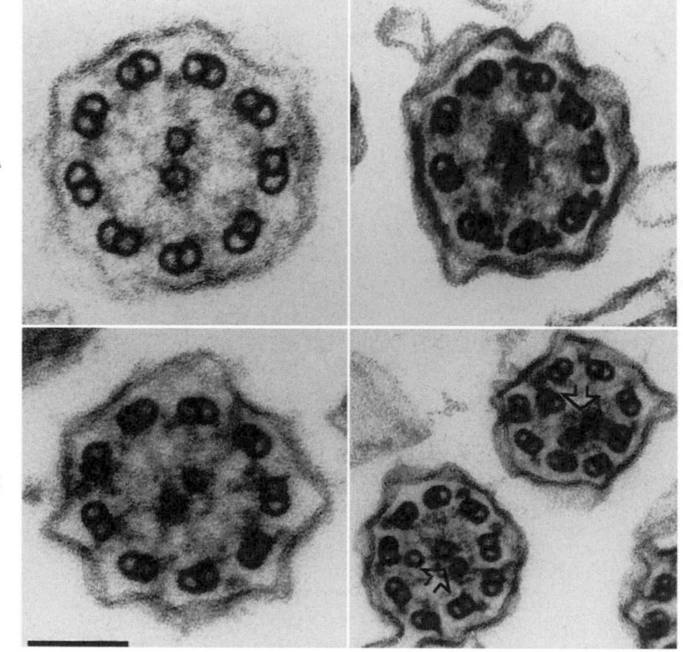

Fig. 75-3. Electronmicrographs of ciliary profiles from four patients with primary ciliary dyskinesia, showing a range of dynein arm defects. **A,** Absence of inner and outer dynein arms; cilia from this patient had no motility. **B,** Absence of inner dynein arms; cilia from this patient had beat frequencies within the normal range. **C,** Absence of outer dynein arms; cilia from this patient had very low motility. **D,** Absence of inner dynein arms and radial spoke defects; cilia from this patient had grossly abnormal beat patterns and reduced beat frequencies. Arrows indicate eccentrically located central tubules, a feature of the radial spoke defect. Scale bar: A-C, 0.10 μm; D, 0.13 μm. (Adapted from de Iongh RU, Rutland J: *Am J Respir Crit Care Med* 151:1559-1567, 1995.)

tozoan and ciliary axonemes may be regulated by different genes,[32] ultrastructural defects in spermatozoa and cilia may not be concordant in some patients. Transitory ciliary defects have been reported in cilia from patients with respiratory tract infection.[33,34] Ideally patients should not be studied at times of acute infection and structural studies should be complemented by measurements of ciliary function.

RECOGNIZED DEFECTS

Most patients with PCD have deficient dynein arms—inner, outer, or both. There is a wide spectrum of dynein arm defects, ranging from partial to complete absence (Fig. 75-3). Defects of outer dynein arms have more effect on motility because there is a positive correlation of ciliary motility with the numbers of outer dynein arm numbers seen by electron microscopy but not with numbers of inner dynein arms.[19] Nevertheless, in patients in whom inner dynein arms are defective, mucociliary clearance is still abnormal, suggesting that although inner dynein arms are sufficient to produce motility in an aqueous in vitro environment, they are ineffective under a mucus load.[19]

A number of other defects have been identified, such as radial spoke defects[21] (Fig. 75-3D) and microtubule translocation defects,[22] in which a peripheral doublet passes to the center of the axoneme to substitute for absent central tubules. Abnormal ciliary orientation has been identified in patients with PCD.[12,19,20,25,31] Patients have been reported in whom axonemal ultrastructure appeared to be normal but ciliary orientation was abnormal[24,25] or ciliary function was abnormal.[23] Abnormally long[28] and short[29] cilia, complete ciliary aplasia,[26,27] and abnormal basal bodies[30] have also been reported (Table 75-1).

CLINICAL FEATURES

Patients with PCD usually present with respiratory tract disease. The clinical features, some of which are shown in Figure 75-4, can range widely in severity and extent. Children appear normal at birth but often present in the neonatal period with respiratory distress or recurrent lower respiratory tract infections. These patients almost always have a chronic cough (often productive) as a result of recurrent and, later, chronic bronchitis. In many this progresses over years to bronchiectasis. The symptoms and clinical findings in these patients are not different from those found in patients with bronchiectasis not caused by defective cilia. However, it should be noted that most patients with bronchitis and most patients with bronchiectasis do not have defective ciliary function or structure.

Upper respiratory tract infections are usual, most patients having chronic sinusitis and recurrent otitis media.[35] Mucopurulent secretions are usually present in the nasal cavity and nasal obstruction, rhinorrhea, postnasal drip, and anosmia are common. Nasal polyps are common.

Males are almost always infertile; spermatozoa are present in normal numbers but have defective motility. Females are usually fertile, despite possible impaired fallopian tube ciliary function.

Malrotation of the internal viscera is common. Patients may have dextrocardia, abdominal situs inversus, or situs inversus totalis. It has been suggested that this may be caused by lack of normal organ rotation thought to be caused by embryonic cilia during closure of the thoracic and abdominal cavities.[1] This results in random rotation of the thoracic and abdominal viscera in patients with PCD.

Radiographs of the paranasal sinuses often reveal mucosal thickening, opacifications, or fluid levels. Chest radiographs may reveal changes consistent with bronchiectasis that can be imaged by thin-section computed tomography (CT) scanning. This is coming into increasing usage in patients who can cooperate. Bronchography can be carried out via fiberop-

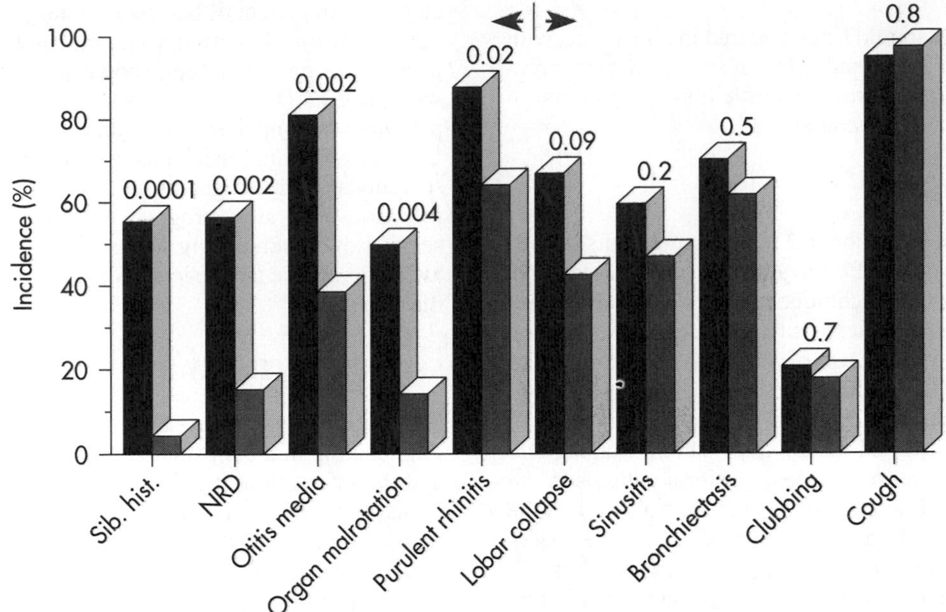

Fig. 75-4. Histogram showing the incidences of clinical features in children with recurrent respiratory tract disease with (n = 39, *solid bars*) or without (n = 28, *hatched bars*) PCD. The p values for each of the comparisons are shown above the bars and the level of significance ($p = 0.05$) is indicated by a vertical line and arrows. Comparisons to the left of the bar were significantly different. *Sib. hist.*, Sibling history; *NRD,* neonatal respiratory distress. (Adapted from Rutland J, Morgan L, Waters KA, van Asperen P, de Iongh RU: *Cilia, mucus and mucociliary interactions,* ch 44; New York, 1998, Marcel Dekker, pp

tic bronchoscopy but is not usually necessary. Both rhinoscopy and bronchoscopy reveal excessive and often purulent secretions.

In most patients the respiratory tract defects progress slowly. Prognosis is good and, for most affected subjects, life expectancy is not impaired.

When measurements of mucociliary clearance are available, this is always reduced. Other investigations of respiratory function reveal abnormalities of variable severity. These may include airway obstruction, gas trapping, and arterial hypoxemia.

Kartagener's original description[4] was of a triad consisting of chronic sinusitis, bronchiectasis, and situs inversus totalis (now commonly interpreted as the presence of any organ malrotation: dextrocardia or situs inversus viscerum). A recent study[36] of the clinical features of patients with recurrent respiratory tract disease caused by PCD compared with patients without PCD showed that although patients who manifested the triad were likely to have PCD (86%), the use of these criteria alone was an insufficient basis for suspecting PCD; of the patients with PCD only 29% presented in this way. A comparison of the clinical features of children (16 years of age or younger) with recurrent respiratory tract infection caused by PCD and not caused by PCD are shown in Figure 75-4. Few of the clinical features were significantly different. These included a sibling history of recurrent respiratory tract infection (but not of any other family history), neonatal respiratory distress (occurring in a term infant without any other apparent cause), otitis media, glue ear, deafness, purulent rhinitis, and organ malrotation (the only component of Kartagener's triad that occurred significantly more often in PCD patients). The incidence of all other clinical features studied, including lobar collapse, sinusitis, bronchiectasis, digital clubbing, and cough, did not differ significantly between the two groups.

GENETICS

PCD is a congenital defect and the structural and functional abnormalities have been shown to be present in cilia from different tissues and also to be similar in affected siblings. Although clinical findings are homogeneous, PCD appears to be caused by a group of heterogeneous genetic disorders, based on the observation of the different ultrastructural defects. Consistent with this, investigation of cilia in other species (sea urchins) has revealed that inner and outer dynein arms have different genetic determinants.[37] In addition, isolation of human axonemal dynein heavy, chain genes indicate that they are located on different chromosomes.[38] Thus it is likely that PCD is caused by specific mutations of several genes resulting in the various structural defects.

The inheritance of PCD is thought to be autosomal recessive (with incomplete penetrance), based on the lack of clinical signs in heterozygous parents, increased incidence of the disease in those of consanguineous parentage, and increased occurrence of the disease in siblings. A study of 38 families with "immotile-cilia" syndrome[39] is consistent with autosomal inheritance.

The incidence of PCD has been estimated to be approximately 1:16,000, based on the assumption that PCD is at least twice as common as Kartagener syndrome.[39] It affects both sexes and has been found in all racial groups. Although the incidence appears to increase with consanguineous parentage, it is not affected by increased parental age. Cytogenetic studies[39] have shown normal karyotypes.

DIAGNOSIS

The presence of PCD should be considered in all patients with recurrent or chronic lower and upper respiratory tract infections when no other cause, such as cystic fibrosis or immunodeficiency, has been demonstrated.

Mucociliary Clearance

Mucociliary clearance is impaired but measurements of pulmonary clearance are not often available in clinical practice. The most commonly used technique involves deposition of inhaled technetium-99 particles (usually as colloid) in central pulmonary airways and the use of a gamma camera to measure the clearance of the radiolabeled particles from the lung. The major disadvantages of this technique are the high cost of the equipment involved and the need for patient training and cooperation to ensure reproducible deposition patterns in the airways. Nasal mucociliary clearance may be gauged with the saccharin technique[40,41] in older children. This involves placement of a small particle of saccharin (approximately 1 mm^3) on the inferior turbinate. The time taken for the particles to be carried posteriorly to the oropharynx, where they stimulate taste receptors, is measured as the nasal clearance time. This is normally less than 30 minutes.[40,41]

Mucociliary clearance is impaired in many respiratory diseases (such as cystic fibrosis, sinusitis, and postviral infections) and a finding of impaired mucociliary clearance alone does not necessarily indicate the presence of a ciliary defect.

Ciliary Function and Ultrastructure

Suitable samples of ciliated epithelium may be obtained by mucosal brushing at bronchoscopy or rhinoscopy.[16] Ciliary beat frequency can be measured in vitro and has been shown to be correlated between the nasal cavity and lower respiratory tract.[42] Similarly, there is concordance between the nasal cavity and lower respiratory tract in ciliary ultrastructure.[43] The use of nasal mucosal brushings avoids the morbidity often associated with the use of nasal biopsy forceps and the requirement for local anesthesia. Ciliary beating may be observed in mucosal brushings suspended in nutrient medium by light microscopy and can be measured by microscope photometry.[16] Ciliary beat pattern and coordination can be observed and filmed but not readily quantified. Mucosal brushings can also be placed into fixative for examination by high-magnification (100,000 to 200,000×) electron microscopy[44] (Figs. 75-2 and 75-3). If possible, abnormalities of structure and function should be studied in more than one body site or on more than one occasion, particularly if the diagnosis is in doubt. In postpubertal male patients, sperm motility and ultrastructure can be determined.

TREATMENT

No specific therapy is available for the management of PCD. For patients who have progressed to bronchiectasis, physical removal of secretions by postural drainage and other forms of physiotherapy is helpful and may limit progression of disease. In acute infective exacerbations, antibiotics and physiotherapy are appropriate. A number of drugs such as β-adrenergic agonists and xanthines have been shown to stimulate ciliary beating in vitro and to increase mucociliary clearance in patients[45] but their efficacy in clinical practice in patients with defective cilia has not been documented. Mucolytics have not been shown to be effective in patients who have PCD. Antitussives are to be avoided because, in patients with impaired mucociliary clearance, cough may be the only remaining mechanism for removing respiratory tract secretions. Early diagnosis and treatment of respiratory tract infections may slow progress to bronchiectasis. Surgical resection of affected lung is rarely necessary and should be avoided because the basic defect is not confined to one part of the lung.

SECONDARY CILIARY DYSFUNCTION

Mucociliary clearance is dependent on adequate numbers of cilia beating in a coordinated pattern, at an appropriate rate, and the interaction of cilia with mucus having optimal rheologic properties. Delayed mucociliary clearance often occurs secondary to respiratory tract diseases, particularly those in which purulent secretions are common, such as bronchiectasis, cystic fibrosis, and sinusitis. During viral and bacterial infections the rheologic properties of mucus may change, becoming less elastic during viral infection[46] or more viscous in bacterial infections.[47] Similarly, viral or bacterial infections may cause changes in the ciliated epithelium, both structural and functional, and thus cause impairment of mucociliary clearance.[48-50] Purulent infection has been shown to cause reduced ciliary beat frequency and abnormal ciliary beat patterns (ciliary dyskinesia).[51] Disruption of ciliary function and structure can also be caused by cell products such as elastases and proteinases liberated by leukocytes in inflammatory lung disease.[52]

Secondary ciliary dyskinesia may result from bacterially produced factors. Organisms that are known to affect ciliary activity or integrity of the ciliated epithelium and thus affect mucociliary clearance include *Pseudomonas aeruginosa, Haemophilus influenzae, Staphylococcus aureus, Mycoplasma pneumoniae, Bordetella pertussis,* and *Streptococcus pneumoniae.*[52]

P. aeruginosa produces a hemolysin and several phenazine derivatives, of which pyocyanin is the most important. It causes slowing of ciliary beating and eventually ciliostasis and epithelial disruption at high concentrations. The hemolysin causes ciliostasis, demembranation of the cilia, cellular disruption and a loss of dynein arms from the axoneme.

Other microorganisms such as *S. aureus* (hemolysin), *B. pertussis* (peptidoglycan), *S. pneumoniae* (pneumolysin), *H. influenzae* (a heat-labile protein and a lipopolysaccharide), and *M. pneumoniae* can produce factors that slow ciliary beating and potentially disrupt the ciliated epithelium.[52-54]

CONCLUSION

Impairment of mucociliary clearance may occur as the result of a congenital defect (PCD) or a secondary ciliary dysfunction. In PCD, impaired mucociliary clearance, affecting particularly the upper and lower respiratory tracts, leads to sinusitis, bronchitis, and bronchiectasis. In such patients a definite diagnosis can be made using studies of ciliary function and structure. No specific effective treatment is available for PCD. Secondary ciliary dysfunction can be caused by a variety of microorganisms.

REFERENCES

1. Afzelius BA: A human syndrome caused by immotile human cilia, *Science* 193:317-319, 1976.
2. Pedersen H, Mygind M: Absence of axonemal arms in nasal mucosa cilia in Kartagener's syndrome, *Nature* 262:494-495, 1976.
3. Siewart AK: Über einem fall von bronchiektasis bei einem patient mit situs inversus viscerum, *Klin Wschr* 41:139-41, 1904.
4. Kartagener M, Horlacher A: Bronchiektasien bei situs viscerum inversus, *Schweiz Med Wschr* 65:782-784, 1935.
5. Afzelius BA, Eliasson R, Johnson ER, Lindholmer C: Lack of dynein arms in immotile human spermatozoa, *J Cell Biol* 66:125-232, 1975.
6. Pedersen H, Rebbe H: Absence of arms in the axoneme of immobile human spermatozoa, *Biol Reprod* 12:541-544, 1975.
7. Eliasson R, Mossberg B, Camner P, Afzelius BA: The immotile-cilia syndrome: a congenital ciliary abnormality as an etiologic factor in chronic airway infections and male sterility, *N Engl J Med* 297:1-6, 1977.
8. Rossman CM, Forrest JB, Lee RMKW, Newhouse MT: The dyskinetic cilia syndrome. Ciliary motility in immotile cilia syndrome, *Chest* 78:580-582, 1980.
9. Pedersen M, Mygind N: Ciliary motility in the "immotile-cilia syndrome". First results of microphot-oscillographic studies, *Br J Dis Chest* 74:239-244, 1980.
10. Sleigh MA: Primary ciliary dyskinesia, *Lancet* 2:476, 1981.

Ciliary Structure and Function

11. Sleigh MA: The nature and action of respiratory tract cilia. In Brain JD, Proctor DF, Reid LM, eds: *Respiratory defence mechanisms. Part I,* New York, 1977, Marcel Dekker, pp 247-288.
12. de Iongh RU, Rutland J: Orientation of respiratory tract cilia in patients with primary ciliary dyskinesia, bronchiectasis, and in normal subjects, *J Clin Pathol* 42:613-619, 1989.
13. Dirksen ER, Sanderson MJ: Regulation of ciliary activity in the mammalian respiratory tract, *Biorheology* 27:533-545, 1990.
14. Sandersen MJ, Dirksen ER: Regulation of ciliary beat frequency in respiratory tract cilia, *Chest* 101 (suppl):69S-71S, 1992.
15. Marano J, Krishnaswamy S, Betrencourt C, Schoevaert D, Provost JM, Volochine B: Control of ciliary beating by calcium: the effects of lindane, a potent insecticide, *Biol Cell* 63:143-150, 1988.
16. Rutland J, Cole PJ: Non-invasive sampling of nasal cilia for the measurement of beat frequency and ultrastructure, *Lancet* 2:564-565, 1980.
17. Fox B, Bull TB, Oliver TN: The distribution and assessment of electron-microscopic abnormalities of human cilia, *Eur J Respir Dis* 64(suppl 127):11-18, 1983.
18. Nielsen MH, Pedersen M, Christensen B, Mygind N: Blind quantitative electron microscopy of cilia from patients with primary ciliary dyskinesis and from normal subjects, *Eur J Respir Dis* 64(suppl 127):19-30, 1983.
19. de Iongh RU, Rutland J: Ciliary defects in healthy subjects, bronchiectasis and primary ciliary dyskinesia, *Am J Respir Crit Care Med* 151:1559-1567, 1995.
20. Rossman CM, Lee RMKW, Forrest JB, Newhouse MT: Nasal ciliary ultrastructure and function in patients with primary ciliary dyskinesia compared with that in normal subjects and in subjects with various respiratory disease, *Am Rev Respir Dis* 129:161-167, 1984.
21. Sturgess JM, Chao J, Wong J, Aspin N, Turner JAP: Cilia with defective radial spokes. A cause of human respiratory disease, *N Engl J Med* 300:53-57, 1980.
22. Sturgess JM, Chao J, Turner JAP: Transposition of ciliary microtubules. Another cause of impaired ciliary motility, *N Engl J Med* 303:318-22, 1980.
23. Greenstone MA, Dewar A, Cole PJ: Ciliary dyskinesia with normal ultrastructure, *Thorax* 38:875-876, 1983.
24. Rutland J, de Iongh RU: Random ciliary orientation. A cause of respiratory tract disease, *N Engl J Med* 323:1681-1684, 1990.
25. Rayner CFJ, Rutman A, Dewar A, Greenstone M, Cole PJ, Wilson R: Ciliary disorientation alone as a cause of primary ciliary dyskinesia syndrome, *Am J Respir Crit Care Med* 153:1123-1129, 1996.
26. De Boeck K, Jorissen M, Wouters K, Van der Scheuren B, Eyssen M, Casteels-Van Daele M, Corbeel L: Aplasia of respiratory tract cilia, *Pediatr Pulmonol* 13:259-265, 1992.
27. Fonzi L, Lungarella G Palatresi R: Lack of kinocilia in the nasal mucosa in the 'immotile-cilia' syndrome, *Eur J Respir Dis* 63:558-563, 1982.
28. Afzelius BA, Gargani G, Romano C: Abnormal length of cilia as a possible cause of defective mucociliary clearance, *Eur J Respir Dis* 66:173-180, 1985.
29. Rautiainen M, Nuutinen J, Collan Y: Short nasal cilia and impaired mucociliary function, *Eur Arch Otorhinolaryngol* 248:271-274, 1991.
30. Lungarella G, De Santi MM, Palatresi R, Tosi P: Ultrastructural observations on basal apparatus of respiratory cilia in immotile cilia syndrome, *Eur J Respir Dis* 66:165-172, 1985.
31. Rayner CF, Rutman A, Dewar A, Cole PJ, Wilson R: Ciliary disorientation in patients with chronic upper respiratory tract inflammation, *Am J Respir Crit Care Med* 151:800-804, 1995.
32. Jonsson MS, McCormick JR, Gillies CG, Gondos B: Kartagener's syndrome with motile spermatozoa, *N Engl J Med* 307:1131-1133, 1982.
33. Carson JL, Collier AM, Hu SCS: Acquired ciliary defects in nasal epithelium of children with acute viral upper respiratory infections, *N Engl J Med* 312:463-468, 1985.
34. Rutland J, Cox T, Dewar A, Cole PJ, Warner JO: Transitory ultrastructural abnormalities of cilia, *Br J Dis Chest* 76:185-188, 1982.

Clinical Features

35. Greenstone M, Cole PJ: Ciliary function in health and disease, *Br J Dis Chest* 79:9-26, 1985. (Review)

Genetics

36. Rutland J, Morgan L, Waters KA, van Asperen P, de Iongh RU: Diagnosis of primary ciliary dyskinesia. In: Baum GL, Priel Z, Liron N, Roth Y, Ostfeld EJ, eds: *Cilia, mucus and mucociliary interactions,* ch 44, New York, 1998, Marcel Dekker, pp 407-428.
37. Gibbons IR: Dynein ATPases, *Cell Motility* 1:87-93, 1982.
38. Chapelin C, Duriez B, Magnino F, Goossens M, Escudier E, Amselem S: Isolation of several human axonemal dynein heavy chain genes: genomic structure of the catalytic site, phylogenetic analysis and chromosomal assignment, *FEBS Lett* 412:325-330, 1997.
39. Sturgess JM, Thompson MW, Czegledy-Nagy E, Turner JAP: Genetic aspects of immotile cilia syndrome, *Am J Med Genet* 25:149-160, 1986.

Diagnosis

40. Rutland J, Cole PJ: Nasal mucociliary clearance and ciliary beat frequency in cystic fibrosis compared with sinusitis and bronchiectasis, *Thorax* 36:654-658, 1981.
41. Canciani M, Barlocco EG, Mastella G, de Santi MM, Gardi C, Lungarella G: The saccharin method for testing mucociliary function in patients suspected of having primary ciliary dyskinesia, *Pediatr Pulmonol* 5:210-214, 1988.
42. Rutland J, Griffin WM, Cole PJ: Human ciliary beat frequency in epithelium from intrathoracic and extrathoracic airways, *Am Rev Respir Dis* 125:100-105, 1982.
43. Verra F, Fleury-Feith J, Boucherat M, Pinchon MC, Bignon J, Escudier E: Do nasal ciliary changes reflect bronchial changes? An ultrastructural study, *Am Rev Respir Dis* 147:908-913, 1993.
44. Rutland J, Dewar A, Cox T, Cole P: Nasal brushing for the study of ciliary ultrastructure, *J Clin Pathol* 35:357-359, 1982.

Treatment

45. Pavia D, Bateman JR, Sheahan NF, Clarke SW: Clearance of lung secretions in patients with chronic bronchitis: effects of terbutaline and ipratropium bromide aerosols, *Eur J Respir Dis* 61:245-253, 1980.

Secondary Ciliary Dysfunction

46. Sakakura Y: Changes of mucociliary function during colds, *Eur J Respir Dis* 64 (suppl 128):348-54, 1983.
47. Wanner A: Clinical aspects of mucociliary transport, *Am Rev Respir Dis* 116:73-125, 1977 (review).
48. Pedersen M, Sakakura Y, Winther B, Brofeldt S, Mygind N: Nasal mucociliary transport, number of ciliated cells and beating pattern in naturally acquired cold, *Eur J Respir Dis* 64(suppl 128):355-65, 1983.
49. Wilson R, Alton E, Rutman A: Upper respiratory tract viral infection and mucociliary clearance, *Eur J Respir Dis* 70:272-9, 1987.

50. Smallman LA, Hill SL, Stockley RA: Reduction of ciliary beat frequency in vitro by sputum from patients with bronchiectasis: a serine proteinase effect, *Thorax* 39:633-667, 1984.
51. Wilson R, Sykes DA, Currie D, Cole PJ: Beat frequency of cilia from sites of purulent infection, *Thorax* 41:453-458, 1986.
52. Wilson R, Cole PJ: The effect of bacterial products on ciliary function, *Am Rev Respir Dis,* 138:S49-S53, 1988 (review).
53. Wilson R, Read R, Thomas M, Rutman A, Harrison K, Lund V, Cookson B, Goldman W, Lambert H, Cole P: Effects of Bordetella pertussis infection on human respiratory epithelium in vivo and in vitro, *Infect Immun* 59:337-345, 1991.
54. Steinfort C, Wilson R, Mitchell T, Feldman C, Rutman A, Todd H, Sykes D, Walker J, Saunders K, Andrew PW, Boulnois GJ, Cole PJ: Effect of Streptococcus penumoniae on human respiratory epithelium in vitro, *Infect Immun* 57:2006-2013, 1989.

SUGGESTED READING

Greenstone M, Cole PJ: Ciliary function in health and disease, *Br J Dis Chest* 79:9-26, 1985 (review).
Rutland J, Morgan L, Waters KA, van Asperen P, de Iongh RU: Diagnosis of primary ciliary dyskinesia. In Baum GL, Priel Z, Liron N, Roth Y, Ostfeld EJ, eds: *Cilia, mucus and mucociliary interactions,* ch 44, New York, 1998, Marcel Dekker, pp 407-428 (review).
Sleigh MA: The nature and action of respiratory tract cilia. In Brain JD, Proctor DF, Reid LM, eds: *Respiratory defence mechanisms,* part I, New York, 1977, Marcel Dekker, pp 247-288.
Sturgess CM, Newhouse MT: Primary ciliary dyskinesia: evaluation and management, *Pediatr Pulmonol* 5:36-50, 1988 (review).
Wilson R: Secondary ciliary dysfunction, *Clin Sci* 75:113-120, 1988 (review).
Wilson R, Cole PJ: The effect of bacterial products on ciliary function, *Am Rev Respir Dis* 138:S49-S53, 1988 (review).

CHAPTER 76

Abnormalities of the Pleural Space

Howard B. Panitch, Caitlin Papastamelos, and Daniel V. Schidlow

The pleural space is bounded by two membranes. The visceral pleura covers the entire surface of the lung and comprises the membrane that separates lobes. The parietal pleura covers the inner surface of the chest wall, the mediastinum, and the diaphragm, and merges with the visceral pleura at the hilar root of the lung. These membranes and the space they define aid in mechanical coupling of the lung and chest wall throughout the respiratory cycle, provide support to lung tissue while allowing the lung to move extensively in relation to the chest wall, and participate in solute and fluid exchange. Pleural membranes form early in gestation. Their role in facilitating organ movement begins prenatally, and pleural lymphatics contribute to the process of fluid reabsorption from airspaces, which occurs after birth.

EMBRYOLOGY AND ANATOMY

The pleural membranes appear early in development, and mesothelial cells can be identified lining the eventual pleural cavity by the 3rd week of gestation.[1,2] The intraembryonic coelom, or primitive body cavity, becomes divided into the pericardial, pleural, and peritoneal cavities during the 2nd month of gestation. All these cavities are lined by visceral and parietal membranes made up of mesothelial cells.[1,2] Lung buds grow into the medial walls of the primitive pleural cavities and become invested by the visceral layer.[1] A similar arrangement occurs with heart, lungs, and intestines, separating them from each other and from the body wall and allowing them to move freely. The formation of a mesothelial cell layer on the surface of motile internal organs and their facing body walls is common to most species of animals.[3]

Pleural membranes are multilayered and vary in thickness among species and regionally within the same animal.[4] There is also regional pleomorphism of mesothelial cells, which range from flat to cuboidal or columnar.[3,5] Mesothelial cells are capable of active transport of small particles (50 nm)[6,7] and of secretion and organization of components of the extracellular matrix, including collagen, elastin, and connective tissue glycoproteins.[8] When stimulated, they are also capable of releasing chemotactic factors for neutrophils.[9] An oligolamellar surface layer with graphite-like lubricant qualities is adsorbed to the mesothelial cell layer.[10]

Microvilli 3 to 6 μm in length appear on the free surfaces of mesothelial cells. They are more slender and less densely packed than microvilli, which have an absorptive function.[11] They are more abundant on the parietal than on the visceral pleura, and caudally compared with cranially on the visceral or the parietal pleura.[3,11] They may be important in entrapping hyaluron-containing glycoprotein—probably excreted by the mesothelial cells—in small compartments created by adjacent microvilli, thereby creating a lubricant layer.[11]

Openings from 2 to 12 μm exist between mesothelial cells on the parietal pleura but not on the visceral pleura.[12] These stomata communicate liquid between the pleural space and underlying lymphatics,[13] and are the route of egress for large particles and blood cells from the pleural space.[12,14] Stomata are most numerous over dilated lymphatic spaces called lacunae that lie just below the mesothelial layer. Respiratory movements help propel fluid and particles from the pleural space into the lacunae, and from there into collecting channels of the lymphatics.[12,14,15] These lymphatics course along the intercostal space, drain into the mediastinum or parasternal or periaortic nodes, into the thoracic duct, and ultimately into the venous circulation. The close apposition of mesothelial and lymphatic cells allows smaller particles (such as ferritin, carbon, protein) and fluid in the pleural space to reach the lacunae directly through intracellular vesicles or intercellular spaces. Thus those particles can be removed more quickly than can cells, which enter the lymphatics only through stomata.[3]

The blood supply of the parietal pleura arises from intercostal arteries, and that of the visceral pleura from the bronchial circulation.[16,17] Although both pleurae are supplied by the systemic circulation, perfusion pressure in the visceral pleura circulation is slightly lower because it drains into the pulmonary veins, which are a low-pressure system.[16] Blood flow to the parietal pleura and its subpleural interstitium is 4 to 5 times higher than flow to the adjacent intercostal muscle, facilitating pleural fluid formation.[18]

Collections of submesothelial macrophages accompanied by a rich vascular network are present in the mediastinal pleura of animals and in the early newborn period in humans.[5,19] These aggregates, called Kampmeier foci, trap bacteria and irritant particles and help protect the mediastinum from infection originating in the pleura.[5]

Under normal conditions, the pleural space contains 0.1 to 0.2 ml/kg of fluid, with a low protein concentration (less than 1.5 g/dl) and approximately 1500 cells/mm^3, with a monocytic predominance.[3,20] No evidence indicates that contact exists between pleural membranes; thus the pleural space can be considered continuous.[21] The fluid within it flows down gravity-dependent gradients.[22] Accordingly, the normal pleural space is approximately 18 μm wide at its least dependent point, and widens to about 20 μm in dependent regions.[21]

PHYSIOLOGY OF THE PLEURAL SPACE

Pressure in the pleural space is subatmospheric. Gases do not accumulate in the pleural space because the *sum* of all partial pressures of gases in venous blood and tissues is lower than atmospheric or alveolar gas. Thus there is a 60-torr pressure gradient that maintains dissolved gases in the venous blood and promotes absorption of gases from the pleural space.

The small amount of fluid contained within the pleural space is the result of a dynamic balance between fluid filtered from subpleural capillaries into the intrapleural space and removal of fluid from the space via lymphatics. Enough fluid must remain in the pleural space to provide lubrication for the lungs to move, but not so much as to uncouple the mechanical forces of the chest wall and the lung.[23]

Controversies exist regarding the direction of pleural fluid flow across the human visceral pleura,[7,20] the permeability of the pleural membranes to fluid,[24,25] and the forces that limit fluid filtration and resorption from the pleural space.[7] Differences in experimental techniques, species differences, and failure to account for the role of spontaneous respiration in resorption of pleural fluid can be cited as the sources of conflicting data.

It has become widely accepted that the visceral pleura in humans derives its blood supply from systemic (bronchial), not pulmonary sources. The Starling forces across both the parietal and the visceral membranes favor filtration of fluid out of the capillaries and into the interstitial spaces.[7] Pleural liquid pressure is lower (more subatmospheric) than interstitial pressure, thus creating a gradient for filtration of fluid into the pleural space.[7,20,23] Furthermore, the pleural membranes present little resistance to transmembrane protein movement.[25] Fluid, cells, and protein are removed from the pleural space by the lymphatics of the parietal pleura via bulk flow rather than by diffusion or ultrafiltration.[7,20] Inspiratory movements probably stretch open the parietal stomata and allow more efficient transfer of fluid, cells, and protein. Thus the rate of pleural fluid or protein uptake into the lymphatics is enhanced by respiratory motion and slowed by general anesthesia or apnea.[7,26]

Both fluid drainage and pulmonary interstitial pressure are determined by the pulmonary lymphatics.[7,27] The lymphatics have a tremendous reserve capability and, in experimental animals, can increase the fluid removal rate to 30 times that of baseline conditions.[13] Pleural drainage rates are higher in newborns than in preterms or adults. In normoxic newborn lambs, pulmonary lymph flow averages 25% more than flow in fetal lambs,[28] probably because the increased interstitial pressure of the liquid-filled fetal lung decreases filtration and because there is a greater surface area for fluid exchange after birth. Similarly, the greater pulmonary lymph flow observed in newborn lambs compared with adult sheep[29] presumably occurs because of higher filtration pressure and larger microvascular surface area for fluid exchange per unit of lung tissue present in the lambs compared with sheep. There is no evidence of developmental changes in microvascular permeability to protein.[29]

Pulmonary lymph flow plays no appreciable role in reducing lung water content before birth, and it is not the major route for removal of lung fluid from potential airspaces. Flow remains constant during labor but it increases transiently in the 2 hours following labor, and accounts for 11% of fluid removal from the lung after birth.[28] Furthermore, increased amounts of fluid were not found in the pleural space in lambs sacrificed during labor or after birth.[28]

In order for abnormal amounts of fluid to collect in the pleural space, the tremendous reserve of the lymphatics must be overcome by increased production of fluid, or removal of fluid must in some way be hampered. Changes in the balance between hydrostatic and oncotic pressures, or in the permeability of the microvascular circulation, as well as obstruction of lymphatic drainage, all can result in an abnormal collection of fluid in the pleural space.

PLEURAL EFFUSION

Clinical Presentation

The severity of the clinical picture is proportional to the size of the effusion. Small effusions are often asymptomatic, whereas large collections can cause respiratory distress, dyspnea, and dry cough. Pain can be localized to the chest or shoulder and worsens with inspiration. Tactile and voice fremitus, as well as breath sounds, are decreased. Dullness to percussion and voice egophony over the area of the effusion can be elicited. Large effusions may cause tachypnea, decreased rib excursion, ipsilateral bulging of the intercostal spaces, and contralateral cardiac and tracheal displacement.[30]

The chest radiograph is the simplest and least expensive method to identify a pleural effusion, but it is not specific. The appearance of pleural effusion depends on the relative position of the patient to the beam.[31] If the patient is supine, small effusions may become undetectable or appear as an "apical cap" of fluid or as diffuse haziness of the hemithorax because of fluid collection behind the lung (Fig. 76-1).[32] Fluid can be visible in the interlobar fissures or appear as a "pleural stripe" of fluid as it displaces the lung away from the chest wall.[33] On radiographs taken in the upright position, blunting of the costophrenic angle occurs. Larger collections create a fluid stripe and shift of the mediastinum to the opposite side. Small

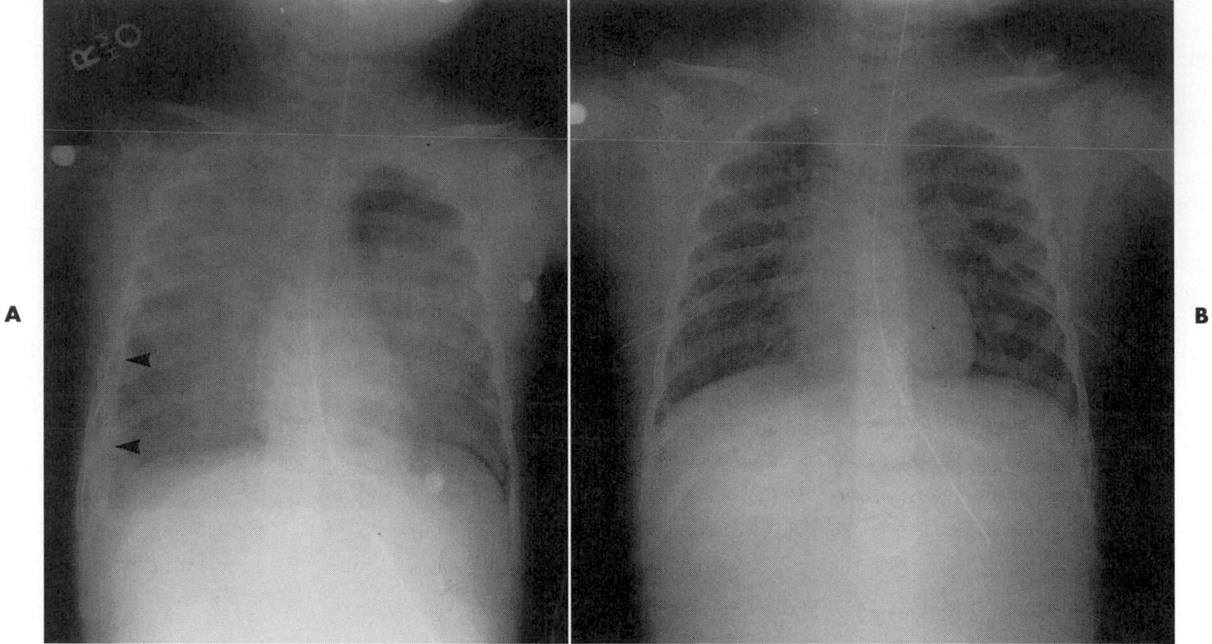

Fig. 76-1. A, Supine chest radiograph of a 7-year-old with group A streptococcal sepsis and adult respiratory distress syndrome. The lungs appear hazy bilaterally. A right-sided effusion is evident because of the blunted costophrenic angle and fluid stripe *(arrows).* Ultrasound examination also demonstrated a small left effusion. **B,** Subsequent radiograph following bilateral placement of chest tubes. The haziness resolved following drainage of a sterile serous exudate.

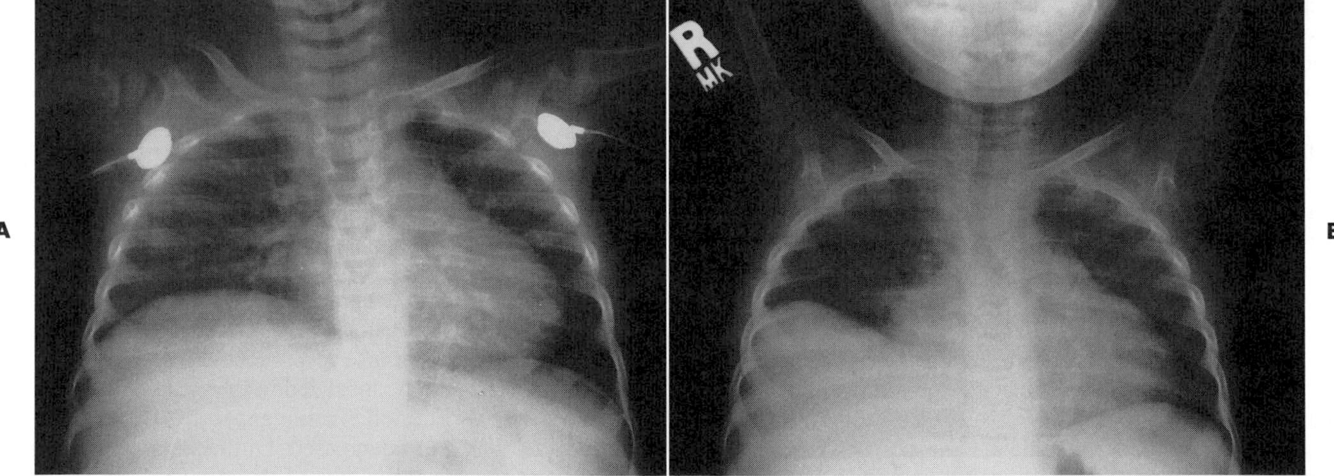

Fig. 76-2. A, Upright radiograph of a 3-year-old following orthotopic liver transplantation. **B,** 1 week later, the patient developed ascites associated with graft rejection. There is a right-sided subpulmonic effusion, with upward and lateral displacement of the hemidiaphragm.

amounts of fluid may appear only as subpulmonic effusions suggested by flattening, lateral displacement and elevation of the apex of the dome of the diaphragm,[34] and concealment of lung vessels below the dome of the diaphragm (Fig. 76-2).[35] An increase in space between the gastric air bubble and the lung also suggests a subpulmonic effusion.[36] Loculated pleural fluid and thickening of the pleural membrane are indistinguishable radiographically, appearing as pleural densities that do not change position on decubitus views.

Occasionally, effusions are not visible on upright radiographs but are visible on decubitus radiographs. Free fluid shifts to the dependent aspect of the hemithorax and layers out as a stripe of fluid (Fig. 76-3). As free fluid shifts position, decubitus views may also expose abnormalities such as mediastinal masses or pulmonary infiltrates covered by pleural fluid on other views. Dependent layering of fluid may not be evident when effusions are so large that they result in opacification of the hemithorax.

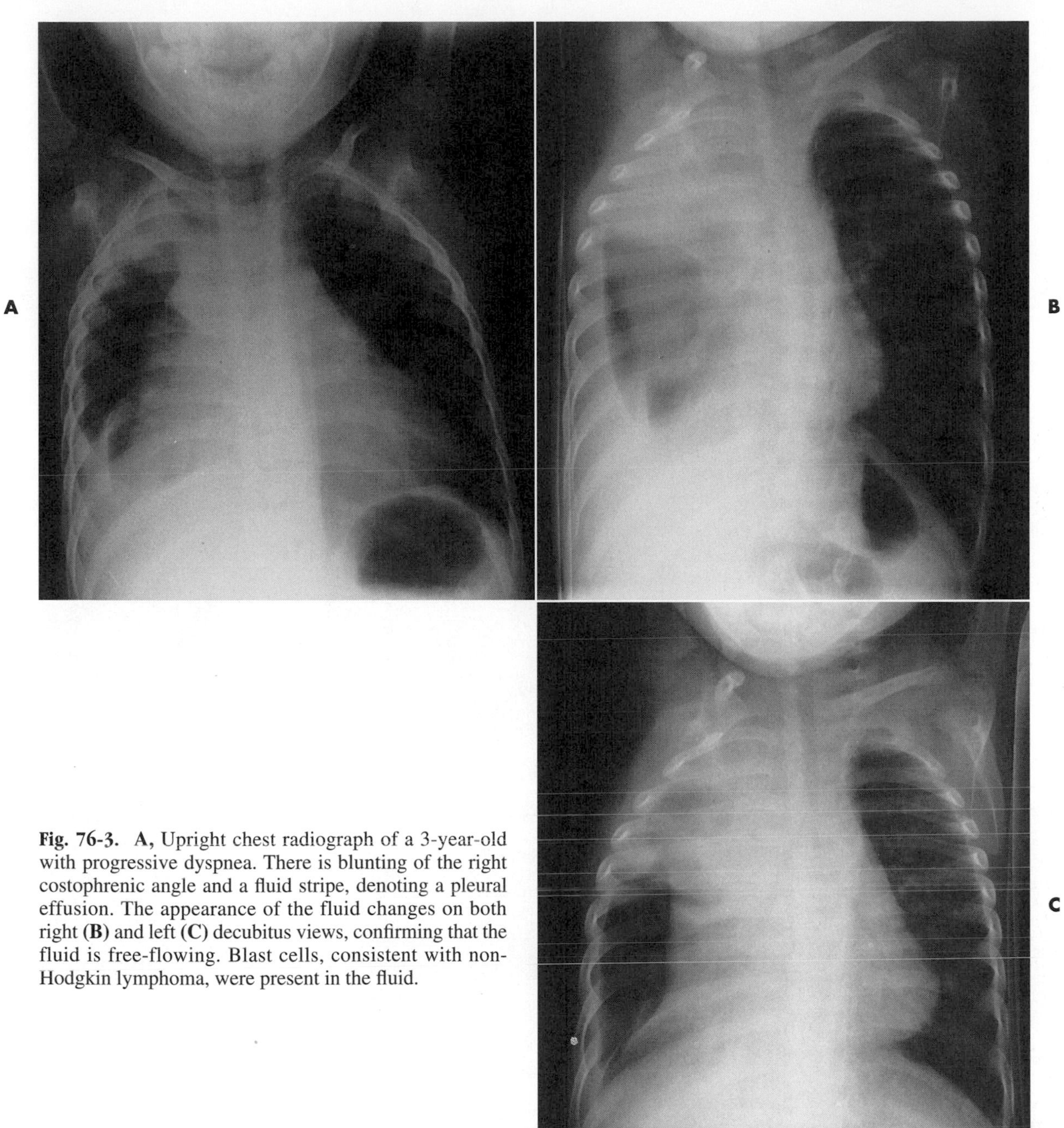

Fig. 76-3. **A,** Upright chest radiograph of a 3-year-old with progressive dyspnea. There is blunting of the right costophrenic angle and a fluid stripe, denoting a pleural effusion. The appearance of the fluid changes on both right **(B)** and left **(C)** decubitus views, confirming that the fluid is free-flowing. Blast cells, consistent with non-Hodgkin lymphoma, were present in the fluid.

Pleural disease can be difficult to distinguish radiographically from parenchymal consolidation, lung abscess, or mediastinal masses. Ultrasound can distinguish pleural effusion from lung abscess[37] or pleural thickening from fluid (Fig. 76-4).[38,39] Computed tomography (CT) is an excellent modality for differentiation of pleural from intraparenchymal processes,[36] but it is more expensive and time-consuming than ultrasound examination.

Diagnosis

The single best method to determine the cause of an effusion is sampling of pleural fluid. Thoracentesis should be performed whenever the cause of the effusion is uncertain. It is unnecessary if the effusion is associated with congestive heart failure, nephrotic syndrome, ascites, or recent initiation of peritoneal dialysis. Small effusions associated with uncomplicated viral or mycoplasmal infection do not require evaluation either. Thoracentesis should be performed in any of these situations, however, if the presentation is atypical, the patient has fever or is in distress, or the effusion persists following treatment.

Thoracentesis may be performed safely when a layer of at least 1 cm of fluid is present dependently on decubitus films, indicating a substantial amount of free fluid.[40] When no fluid shift is present, ultrasound or CT can reveal loculated areas of

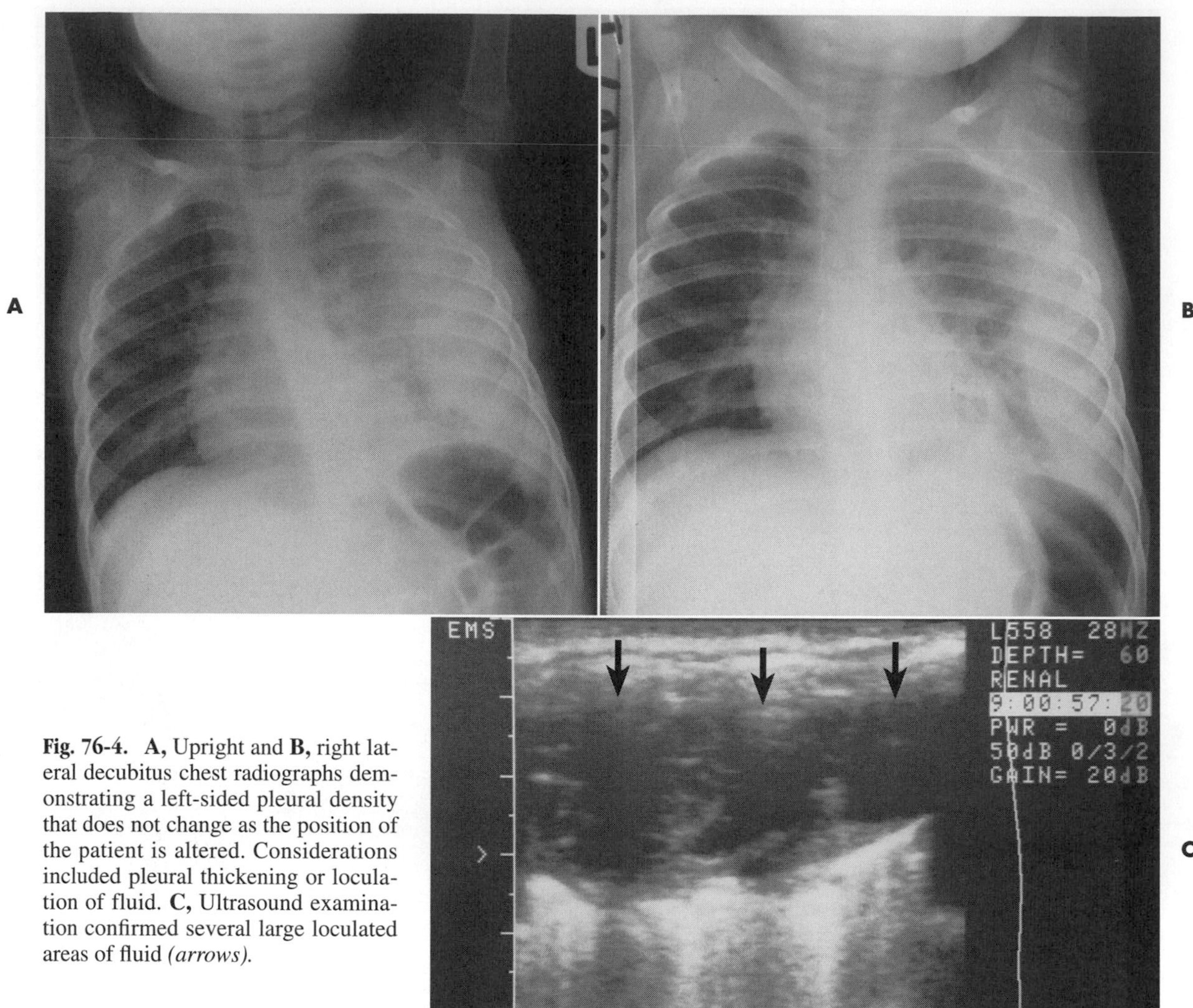

Fig. 76-4. **A,** Upright and **B,** right lateral decubitus chest radiographs demonstrating a left-sided pleural density that does not change as the position of the patient is altered. Considerations included pleural thickening or loculation of fluid. **C,** Ultrasound examination confirmed several large loculated areas of fluid *(arrows).*

fluid amenable to sampling.[38,39,41] Immediate tube thoracotomy is preferred for patients with chest trauma, in whom effusions result from hemothorax or chylothorax and require extended periods of evacuation. Percutaneous pleural biopsy can confirm diagnoses when pleural fluid findings are nonspecific, as in lymphoma, tuberculosis, fungal infection, sarcoid, rheumatoid disease, and echinococcosis.[40,42] Thoracoscopy for guided biopsy of lung and pleura,[43] bronchoscopy, and bronchoalveolar lavage for evaluation of foreign body, tuberculosis, or other pulmonary infections, and open thoracotomy to determine the cause of chylous or lymphocytic effusions, have limited applicability in the evaluation of pleural disease in children.

The most common complications associated with thoracentesis are pneumothorax, pain at the insertion site, and bleeding. Intercostal nerve damage, puncture of the liver or spleen, and secondary empyema occasionally occur.[44-46] Removal of a large amount of pleural fluid, especially in the presence of trapped lung, can cause pulmonary edema.[47] Complication rates have been reported as high as 14% in adults,[44,46] but are markedly reduced in children and adults when the procedure is performed under radiologic guidance,[45,48] even when the patient is being supported by mechanical ventilation.[41,48] Complications of pleural biopsy also include hemothorax, hematoma at the biopsy site, subcutaneous emphysema, air embolism, tumor seeding, and biopsy of extrapleural tissues.[49] Contraindications to performing these procedures are bleeding diathesis, an obliterated pleural space, and anticoagulation therapy.[40]

Pleural Fluid Analysis

The gross appearance of pleural fluid varies with the cause of the effusion. Transudates are serous or straw-colored, whereas chylous effusions are milky. Infecting organisms often yield a characteristic color or odor (Table 76-1). A limited number of laboratory evaluations should be performed on every sample (Table 76-2). Additional studies are often necessary to determine the precise cause of the effusion (Table 76-3). Simple chemical and cellular analysis will determine whether the effusion is transudative or exudative (Table 76-4).[50] Transudates are not associated with inflammation, so their protein and lactose dehydrogenase (LDH) levels are low. In contrast, exudative effusions arise from inflammation of the pleural membranes or lymphat-

Table 76-1 Pleural Fluid Appearance

Grossly purulent fluid	Empyema; rarely pancreatitis, ruptured esophagus
Thick, tan-brown	*S. aureus*
Putrid	Anerobes
Also bloody	Group A *Streptococcus*
Milky fluid	Chylothorax
Bloody fluid	Hemothorax, traumatic thoracentesis, malignancy, tuberculosis, uremia, or empyema due to group A *Streptococcus*
Yellow-green fluid, debris	Rheumatoid arthritis
Black fluid	*Aspergillus nigrans*
"Anchovy" brown fluid	*Entamoeba histolyticum*

Table 76-2 Laboratory Studies to be Obtained in All Cases

Pleural fluid	Protein
	Lactate dehydrogenase (LDH)
	Bacterial culture and Gram stain
	Glucose
	pH
	Differential white blood cell count
	Red blood cell count
	Amylase
Serum	Complete blood cell count with differential
	LDH
	Total protein
	Glucose

From Papastamelos C: Pleural effusions. In Schidlow DV, Smith DS, eds: *A practical guide to pediatric respiratory disorders,* Philadelphia, 1994, Hanley & Belfus, pp 113-126.

Table 76-3 Additional Studies to Be Obtained in Specific Cases

CONDITION	ADDITIONAL STUDIES	COMMENT
Purulent effusion	Blood culture	
	Nasopharyngeal culture	
Lymphocytic effusion	Effusion triglyceride level	Chylothorax contains lymphocyte
	Cytology	
	Pleural fluid culture and stains for acid-fast bacilli and fungi	
	Tuberculin skin test	
	Effusion and serum antinuclear antibody, rheumatoid factor, and complement	
	Fungal titers and skin tests	
Eosinophilic effusion	Fluid bacterial and viral culture	
	Microscopic examination of fluid for ova and scolices	
Bloody effusion	Effusion hematocrit	>50% consistent with hemothorax
	Pleural fluid for hemosiderin-laden macrophages	Absent if blood results from trauma
		Chylothorax can appear bloody
	Effusion triglyceride level	
Effusion with milky appearance	Effusion triglyceride level	

Adapted from Papastamelos C: Pleural effusions, in Schidlow DV, Smith DS, eds: *A practical guide to pediatric respiratory disorders,* Philadelphia, 1994, Hanley & Belfus, pp 113-126.

Table 76-4 Distinguishing Exudates from Transudates

Exudates	Fulfill at least one of the following criteria 1. Pleural fluid/serum LDH >0.6 2. Pleural fluid/serum protein >0.5 3. Pleural fluid LDH >2/3 upper limit of normal serum values 4. Pleural fluid cholesterol >55 mg/dl
Transudates	Fulfill none of these criteria

ics. The associated loss of capillary wall integrity results in elevated cholesterol, protein, and LDH levels.[50,51]

TRANSUDATES

Transudates result from an imbalance of hydrostatic or oncotic pressures. Inflammation is absent, so they contain little protein and few mononuclear cells (less than 500 cells/mm^3).[40] Concentrations of glucose and hydrogen ion resemble those of the serum, and LDH levels are low. The composition of effusions associated with peritoneal dialysis resembles that of the dialysate. Restoration of forces governing pleural fluid homeostasis ultimately resolves transudative effusions; drainage is required only for immediate symptomatic relief. Disorders associated with transudative effusions in children are easily diagnosed, and include atelectasis, left ventricular failure, nephrotic syndrome, free peritoneal fluid, and hypothyroidism.

Alterations in Pleural Pressure

Atelectasis, trapped lung, and upper airway obstruction cause effusions by generating excessive negative pleural pressure.[20] Pleural pressure becomes more negative when lung separates from parietal pleura or when inspiratory effort against an obstruction increases. Atelectasis is the cause of most effusions following upper abdominal surgery.[52]

Left Ventricular Failure

Patients with heart disease develop effusions when left atrial or pulmonary capillary wedge pressure is elevated.[53,54] In contrast, elevation of mean right atrial or pulmonary artery pressure does not cause pleural effusions.[53,54] Effusions are usually bilateral; when they are unilateral they are typically right-sided.[55] Fluid collections that persist for several months can become exudative because of preferential reabsorption of water over protein.[56] Occasionally, repeated thoracentesis or pleurodesis is necessary to control symptomatic effusions resulting from refractory heart failure.[57]

Nephrotic Syndrome

Approximately 20% of patients with nephrotic syndrome develop pleural effusions. A decrease in oncotic pressure from hypoalbuminemia coupled with an increase in hydrostatic pressure from fluid overload favor movement of fluid into the pleural space.[20] Effusions are usually small and bilateral, and resolve following limitation of protein loss and correction of hypervolemia. Thoracentesis is indicated, however, in patients with chest or abdominal pain, fever, pulmonary infiltrates, or unilateral or large effusions. Thoracentesis should be performed if effusions persist despite improvement in renal function, and to rule out infection, thromboembolism, or collagen vascular disease. Therapeutic thoracentesis must be performed with caution because removal of large amounts of pleural fluid can result in hypotension.

Table 76-5 Categories of Effusion

Purulent	>5000 leukocytes/mm³
Lymphocytic	>50% lymphocytes, usually 1000-1500 cells/mm³
Chylothorax	Pleural fluid triglyceride: >110 mg/dl confirms <50 mg/dl excludes 50-110 mg/dl indeterminate
Hemothorax	Pleural fluid hematocrit >50% blood hematocrit
Monocytic	>20% monocytes; usually <5000 cells/mm³ total
Eosinophilic	>10% eosinophils
Elevated amylase	Pleural fluid amylase >serum amylase, or >100 mg/dl

Peritoneal Fluid

Free fluid in the peritoneal cavity can traverse small openings in the diaphragm and enter the pleural space. Urine extravasated into the pleural space (urinothorax) has a pleural fluid/creatinine ratio greater than 1.0[58] and is typically ipsilateral to the obstruction.[20] Effusions caused by ascites occur usually on the right side,[59] whereas effusions secondary to dialysis are usually bilateral and small.[20,60] They occur within the first few days of dialysis, but rarely can occur after several months.[61]

Hypothyroidism

Hypothyroidism has been reported to cause effusions. These are often associated with heart failure, pericardial effusions, or ascites.[62] They respond to thyroid replacement.

EXUDATES

Exudative effusions result from inflammation of the pleura or obstruction of lymphatic flow. Inflammation leads to leakage of fluid and protein from pleural capillaries, and blocks reabsorption of fluid by the lymphatic lacunae of the parietal pleura. Diffuse destruction or obstruction of lymphatic vessels, which occurs in malignancy or granulomatous disease, also can result in pleural fluid accumulation. Inflammatory peritoneal fluid can traverse the diaphragm and enter the pleural space. Pancreatitis and esophageal rupture cause exudates with high amylase levels (over 100 mg/dl).[20,63]

The cause of an exudative effusion often is not evident from the clinical presentation. The diagnosis can be narrowed by the appearance of the fluid and laboratory features, including differential cell count, red blood cell count, and amylase and triglyceride levels. Causes or associated conditions can be categorized by the principal cell type found in the fluid (Table 76-5).

Neutrophilic Predominance (Purulent Effusion)

Purulent effusions contain more than 5000 leukocytes/mm³, although cell lysis occasionally results in lower cell counts.[20] Neutrophils predominate during the acute phase of pleural inflammation, whereas lymphocytes increase in proportion over days to weeks. Bacterial pneumonia is by far the most common cause of purulent effusions in children.[64,65]

Parapneumonic Effusions

Parapneumonic effusions are complications of bacterial pneumonia. They occur most commonly in children under 2 years of age.[66-68] There is often a history of a viral respiratory infection,[67] followed by cough, chest pain, fever, and dyspnea.

Bacterial infection initially causes inflammation of contiguous pleura, with leakage of fluid and protein into the pleural space. This "sympathetic effusion" is sterile,[69] and contains fewer than 10,000 leukocytes/mm³, which are predominantly neutrophils. The LDH is below 1000 IU/L and glucose and pH values are similar to those of serum.[70,71] Eventually, bacteria invade the pleural space, followed by leukocytes. Inflammatory mediators are released and clotting factors and fibroblasts are activated. Characteristics of this pyothorax or empyema include low glucose and pH levels and elevated leukocyte counts and LDH levels.[70,71] The matrix of clotted pleural fluid functions as scaffolding for fibroblasts to form loculations of infected fluid, making antibiotic treatment less effective and drainage difficult.[69-71] As the inflammatory response continues, fibrin and fibroblasts form a dense peel on both pleural surfaces and the remaining pleural fluid becomes a thick, gelatinous mass. The visceral pleural peel contracts, compressing and entrapping the lung. This organizing stage[69] occurs 1 to 3 weeks after the onset of pleural infection.[72] The infection often resolves during this period, but the sequelae of permanent pleural deformity and lung entrapment remain.

The etiologic agent is isolated from pleural fluid or blood in approximately 75% of cases.[68,73-75] Bacteria disappear from the fluid after a few doses of even an oral antibiotic.[73,76] Nasal and pharyngeal cultures can be misleading, because culture of commensal organisms such as pneumococcus, *Staphylococcus aureus,* and Group A *Streptococcus* does not prove causation.

The relative incidence of organisms that cause parapneumonic effusions in the general pediatric population is not known, but it is likely that no one organism accounts for more than 20% of all cases.[77] *S. aureus,* group A streptococcus, and anaerobic bacteria account for only a small number of childhood pneumonias, but they account for a larger proportion of effusions because of their predilection to cause empyema. Conversely, *Streptococcus pneumoniae* accounts for the majority of childhood pneumonias, but seldom causes effusions.[67,77-81] Anaerobes cause effusions in 0.04 to 34% of cases.[65,82,83] This range reflects differences between institutions in the handling of anaerobic culture specimens and inclusion of variable numbers of neurologically impaired children at risk for aspiration in study populations. Organisms typically associated with parapneumonic effusions are listed in Table 76-6.[65,67,68,74,75,77]

Certain bacteria have a predilection to cause pleuropulmonary infection in certain age groups (Table 76-6). Organ-

Table 76-6 Organisms Causing Parapneumonic Effusions in Children

ORGANISM	PEAK AGE	EFFUSION APPEARANCE	ASSOCIATED CONDITIONS	COURSE
S. aureus	<1 year, but prevalent throughout childhood	Thick; tan or brown	Skin infections, postthoracotomy	Loculations, pneumatoceles, bronchopleural fistulae; lung abscess; hydropneumothorax
Pneumococcus	6-12 months, but prevalent throughout childhood			Usually not severe
H. influenzae	6-24 months; rare after 7 years		Meningitis; arthritis; pericarditis	Marked systemic illness but mild pleuropulmonary disease
Group A *Streptococcus*	School age	Serosanguinous or bloody	Pharyngitis; impetigo; following varicella or rubeola infection	Bronchopneumonia; effusions loculate rapidly; prolonged systemic symptoms
Anaerobes	>2 years	Putrid odor	Neurologic impairment, aspiration, foreign body aspiration, dental work, poor dental hygiene	Loculations: bronchopleural fistulae, lung abscess
Gram-negative enterics	Variable		Hospitalized patients; newborns	Underlying diseases and antibiotic resistance result in severe course

Adapted from Papastamelos C: Pleural effusions. In Schidlow DV, Smith DS, eds: *A practical guide to pediatric respiratory disorders,* Philadelphia, 1994, Hanley & Belfus, pp 113-126.

isms causing neonatal empyema include group B *Streptococcus, E. coli,* and *Listeria.*[84] Aerobic multibacterial infection tends to occur in infants under 6 months.[68] Beyond the neonatal period, *S. aureus* is the primary cause of parapneumonic effusions in infants under 1 year of age.[65,67,68,77] Both *Haemophilus influenzae* and pneumococcus are common causes of empyema in infants over 2 months of age, with a peak incidence between 6 and 12 months.[65,68,77] *Pneumococcus* remains a common etiologic agent throughout childhood, whereas empyema related to *H. influenzae* is rare after 7 years of age.[85] Anaerobic infection nearly always occurs after the first year of age,[83,85] when dentition increases the density of anaerobes in the mouth and foreign body aspiration is also more likely. Empyema caused by group A *Streptococcus* occurs most often in school-age children.[77,78]

The clinical picture often indicates the causative organism. A severe course complicated by pneumothorax, pneumatocele, bronchopleural fistula, or lung abscess,[68,81,86] or following thoracotomy or dental abscess, suggests infection caused by *S. aureus.*[80] This organism typically produces severe tissue necrosis and thick pleural fluid. A long period of drainage is necessary to resolve the infection.[68,81,86] Anaerobic bacteria also cause severe necrosis with prolonged fluid production, but distinguishing features include an indolent progression of symptoms over several weeks, fluid with a putrid odor, and association with aspiration, poor dental hygiene, and thoracotomy.[83] Drainage through the chest wall (empyema necessitatis) is characteristic of infection caused by *Actinomyces* sp.[20,80] Prolonged fever, marked systemic illness, bronchopneumonia, and a recent history of impetigo, varicella, measles, or pharyngitis suggest group A streptococcal infection.[78,87,88] Severe systemic illness is also typical of *H. influenza* infection, but pleural and lung involvement is less intense than in infection caused by *Staphylococcus,* group A *Streptococcus,* or anaerobic organisms.[68,77] Comparatively mild systemic and local disease is most likely caused by *Pneumococcus.*

Intravenous antibiotics should be administered in all cases of parapneumonic effusion. They should be continued for at least several days after fever and fluid drainage abate. Orally administered antibiotics should be given for an additional 1 to 2 weeks.

Clinical improvement and defervescence occur within the first few days of treatment in children with sympathetic parapneumonic effusions, whereas those with empyema have a more prolonged recovery. The course is protracted particularly in individuals with empyema caused by *S. aureus,* anaerobic, or group A *Streptococcus* infection, and often requires 3 to 4 weeks of tube drainage and intravenous antibiotic treatment.[65,78,82] Response to therapy is characterized by gradual decrease in blood leukocyte count, respiratory rate, heart rate, quantity of fluid drained, and improvement in air entry and sense of well-being. Radiographic appearance alone is not a good gauge of response because pleural opacification persists for weeks after infection and fluid have cleared.[67,89,90] The presence of loculations or pleural thickening on imaging studies also should not dictate therapy if the patient is clinically improving.

Most parapneumonic effusions resolve with the administration of intravenous antibiotics, and are called uncomplicated, indicating that drainage is not necessary.[70,91-93] Complicated effusions are those that do not resolve with antibiotic treatment alone, but also require drainage for resolution of pleural infection or reexpansion of compressed lung.[70] Effusions that are small and unloculated and have no organisms evident on Gram stain or culture usually resolve without drainage,[70] whereas those that are loculated, large, or grossly purulent, or have bacteria evident on Gram stain are more likely to require drainage.[70,71,92,94,95] Fluid with nearly normal values of LDH, pH, and glucose reflects a mild degree of inflammation and tissue destruction and is more likely to disappear with antibiotic therapy alone.[70] Effusions with abnormal values are more likely to form loculations and pleural peel and to require drainage[95] (Table 76-7). Thoracentesis should be repeated at periodic intervals if intermediate values of glucose and pH are measured; the effusion should be drained if values do not normalize with antibiotic therapy.[96] The presence of chest pain, fever, and leukocytosis does not distinguish complicated from uncomplicated effusions.[70]

Despite these guidelines, the indications for chest tube drainage are controversial because it is not always possible to predict, at the time of presentation, which effusions will require drainage. Furthermore, loculated empyema has been reported in patients with normal initial laboratory values.[71,91,92,95]

Table 76-7 Complicated Versus Uncomplicated Pleural Effusions

	UNCOMPLICATED	COMPLICATED
Size	Small	Large
Gram stain	Bacteria absent	Bacteria present
Fluid appearance	Thin, free flowing	Gross pus, loculated
pH	>7.3	<7.1
Glucose (mg/dl)	>60	<40
Lactose dehydrogenase (IU/L)	<1000	>1000

(From Sahn SA, Light RW: *Chest* 95:945-946, 1989.)

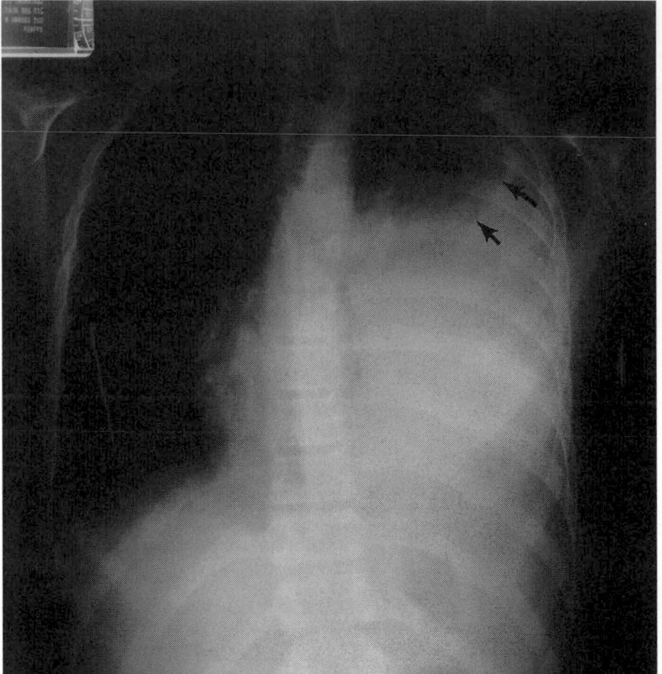

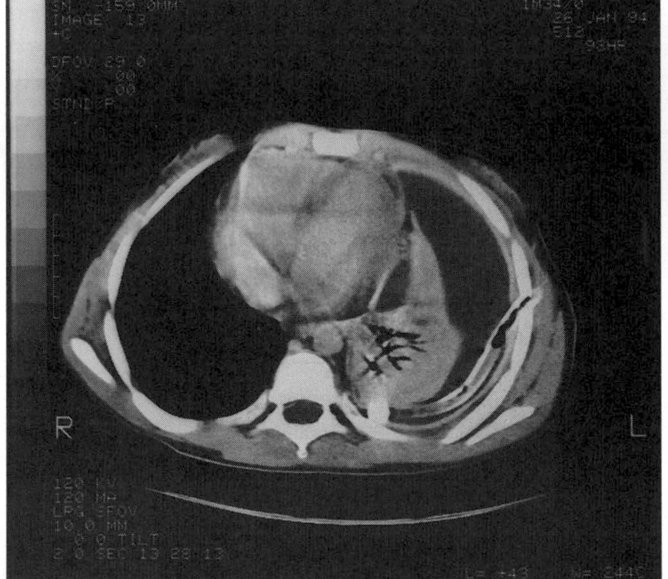

Fig. 76-5. **A,** Upright chest radiograph of a 13-year-old following 10 days of oral antibiotic treatment for low-grade fever and chest pain. There is opacification of most of the left hemithorax and a meniscus *(arrows)* resulting from pleural thickening or collection of fluid. **B,** Following chest tube drainage of 150 ml of serous sterile fluid and intravenous antibiotic therapy, CT of the chest demonstrated persistent compression of the lung by semisolid material. Note the position of the chest tube within the organized effusion. Thoracotomy was performed because of persistent hypoxemia and chest pain. Sterile fibrinopurulent material was removed and the lung reexpanded. The patient was discharged 6 days after undergoing decortication.

Some authors recommend antibiotic therapy alone to treat all effusions, arguing that even grossly purulent and loculated effusions can resolve without drainage.[92,93] If this course of treatment fails, however, drainage can be difficult or impossible because of loculation formation, and open thoracotomy may be required to remove fibrin and pus. We advocate chest tube drainage of all parapneumonic effusions at the time of presentation because the risks of developing complications from undrained empyema fluid are greater than the risks associated with chest tube insertion. With this regimen, fluid is more likely to be drained before loculation formation, thus reducing the need for thoracotomy. Chest tubes are generally well tolerated and can usually be removed in a few days.

Thoracotomy tubes should be removed after little or no fluid drains for a period of 24 hours. The tube itself can act as a stimulus for pleural exudative reaction[67,97] and increases the risk of secondary infection. The location of the tube within the pleural space is usually not a cause of ineffective drainage, as long as the fluid is free flowing. Drainage may cease if suction holes of the tube are outside the pleural space, the tube becomes clogged by pus and debris, or the space becomes loculated.

Loculations are important causes of persistent fever, respiratory distress, and reduced air entry.[70-72,98] After the effusion becomes organized, pleural infection is unlikely to resolve with antibiotics or chest tube placement alone.[72] Open thoracotomy to remove fibrous tissue and infected fluid is curative and results in rapid clinical improvement. Alternative treatment includes the administration of intrapleural urokinase radiologically guided insertion of a new chest tube or pigtail catheter, and thoracoscopic debridement with chest tube placement under direct visualization.[99]

Pleural thickening is a constant feature in cases of empyema, and usually resolves over several months. Rarely, although infection resolves, significant lung compression develops accompanied by persistent fever, hypoxemia, reduced air entry, and respiratory distress (Fig. 76-5). This situation is corrected by removal of the fibrous tissue encasing the lung (decortication).[67,100-103]

Most parapneumonic effusions resolve with no sequelae. Small areas of pleural thickening may persist.[68,80,90,104] Mild restrictive or obstructive abnormalities on lung function tests, up to 7 years after infection, have been reported.[67,89,90,104,105] Most mortality rates range between 6% and 9%.[68] Mortality is highest in young infants and in patients with underlying conditions such as chronic lung disease or malnutrition.

Pancreatitis

Between 3% and 17% of patients with acute or chronic pancreatitis develop effusions.[106] Cough, chest pain, and dyspnea accompany symptoms of acute pancreatitis, whereas patients with chronic pancreatitis often have no abdominal symptoms.[107] Effusions are usually unilateral and left-sided.[106] The pleural fluid is often hemorrhagic,[107,108] and leukocyte counts may reach 50,000/mm^3.[63] Glucose and pH values resemble those of serum. Pleural fluid amylase is elevated, or the pleural fluid:serum ratio is greater than 1.0.[63] Fistulous tracts between pancreatic pseudocysts and the pleural space and mediastinum can occur.[20]

Perforation of the Esophagus

Esophageal perforation following traumatic intubation of the esophagus, endoscopy, esophageal foreign body, or forceful vomiting is also associated with effusions with an elevated amylase level.[109] Patients can present with chest pain, dyspnea, fever, subcutaneous emphysema, and dysphagia.[110] Radiographic signs include mediastinal widening or pneumothorax.[110] The fluid resembles that of a parapneumonic effusion, but with very low pH levels. Secondary anaerobic infection of the pleura is possible.

Pulmonary Infarction

Pulmonary infarction or embolism causes exudates in 80% of instances.[111] Associated conditions include hemoglobinopathies, nephrotic syndrome, and long bone fractures. Patients present with dyspnea and ipsilateral chest pain, and a small ipsilateral effusion that is bloody in two thirds of cases.[111] Leukocyte counts range from a few cells to more than 50,000 leukocytes/mm^3,[111] often with an eosinophilic predominance.[112] Effusions associated with infarction contain the highest number of cells. Hemothoraces require tube drainage. Anticoagulation is not contraindicated.[113]

Pericardial or Myocardial Injury

Pericardial and myocardial lesions can cause effusions and pleuritic chest pain, fever, and dyspnea (Dressler syndrome) within few days to 3 months after the injury.[114] Fluid collections are left-sided or bilateral. Pulmonary infiltration, particularly of the left lower lobe, is common.[114] The fluid is serosanguinous, containing 500-39,000 leukocytes/mm^3. Glucose and pH values resemble those of serum.[114] Treatment includes nonsteroidal antiinflammatory agents or corticosteroids. Chronic pleural thickening rarely develops.[114]

Tuberculosis, connective tissue disease,[115] malignancy, uremia,[116] abdominal abscess,[117] and infections caused by *Actinomyces*[11] or *Nocardia*[119] are usually associated with lymphocytic effusions. On occasion, the fluid may contain a predominance of neutrophils.

Lymphocytic Predominance

Lymphocytic effusions contain fewer than 5000 leukocytes/mm^3, mainly lymphocytes. They should not be confused with chronic purulent effusions in which the cell type changes from neutrophil to lymphocyte, but in which the total cell count is higher. Causes of lymphocytic effusions include malignancy, uremia, connective tissue disease, and mycotic infections. A lymphocyte proportion of over 90% of all cells counted is highly suggestive of tuberculosis[120,121] or lymphoma.

Tuberculosis

Invasion of the pleural space by organisms or bacillus protein follows the rupture of a subpleural focus, direct extension, or hematogenous spread.[20,122] Collections are small and unilateral, and often accompanied by ipsilateral parenchymal disease.[120] Tuberculin antigens activate delayed hypersensitivity, resulting in lymphocyte stimulation, lymphokine release, and activation of macrophages and fibroblasts.

Tuberculous effusions appear serous or serosanguinous. Eosinophils or neutrophils can occasionally predominate.[9,112,120] In about one fifth of cases, pleural glucose decreases as low as 20 to 60 mg/dl; pH can range from 7.0 to 7.3.[20] Tubercle bacilli can be cultured from pleural fluid in 25% to 70% of cases. The organisms are seen on acid-fast smears, however, in fewer than 10% of cases.[120,123,124] Pleural granulomata can be found in biopsy specimens in 55% to 80% of cases.[120,125-127] Combination of these studies is diagnostic in approximately 90% of cases.[20] Other tests that improve the diagnostic yield include ELISA measurements of specific immunoglobulin G to mycobacterial antigen 60 in pleural fluid and serum[128]; determinations of pleural fluid levels of adenosine deaminase (ADA),[129,130] interferon gamma,[130,131] and tuberculosteric acid[132]; and pleural fluid serum lysozyme ratios.[130,133-135] Because of low specificity, these tests are most useful in areas where the prevalence of tuberculosis is high.

Effusions can develop during the first month of antituberculous therapy despite adequate treatment.[136] They usually resolve within 2 months of treatment, and specific therapy is not necessary.[120,137] Corticosteroids are indicated to lessen pleural reaction, but do not reduce the incidence of fibrothorax.[138]

Malignancy

Of all childhood malignancies, lymphoma is the one most commonly associated with pleural effusions.[20] Leukemia, neuroblastoma, chest wall sarcoma (Ewing tumor and rhabdomyosarcoma), Wilms tumor, and hepatoma can occasionally cause effusions. These result from direct invasion of the pleura, diffuse obstruction of lymphatic pathways in the lung, mediastinum, or pleura, or atelectasis or pneumonia resulting from bronchial compression by tumor or adenopathy.

Effusions occur early in the course of non-Hodgkin lymphoma and may be the sole manifestation of the disease.[139,140] Direct pleural invasion is unusual, and mediastinal adenopathy is often absent.[141] In contrast, effusions are a late manifestation of Hodgkin disease,[142] after direct pleural invasion, widespread pulmonary lymphomatous infiltration, and lymphatic obstruction occur.[141] Hilar adenopathy and parenchymal nodules usually are also present.[139,143]

Malignant effusions are usually unilateral. Bloody effusions reflect pleural infiltration, whereas chylous effusions result from lymphatic obstruction.[143,144] Glucose and pH values are normal unless there is diffuse pleural fibrosis or the effusion is long-standing.[145] Pleural fluid cytology is diagnostic in non-Hodgkin lymphoma[140,143,145,146] but immunologic lymphocytic cell marker studies[140] or pleural biopsy are necessary to diagnose effusions from Hodgkin lymphoma.[145,146]

Most effusions resolve following chemotherapy and irradiation. The most common therapy for chronic symptomatic malignant effusions is chemical pleurodesis.[147] When pleurodesis is ineffective, repeated thoracenteses provide only short-term relief; pleuroperitoneal shunts are used to evacuate the pleural space.[148] Chylous effusions respond well to mediastinal radiation and chemotherapy.[143,149] Pleurectomy is effective, but rarely necessary.[147]

Uremia

There is a 20% incidence of unilateral, serosanguinous, predominantly lymphocytic effusions in patients with uremia.[116,150,151] Manifestations include chest pain, fever, cough, and pleural friction rubs. Occasional predominance of neutrophils or eosinophils has been reported.[116,151] Dialysis resolves the effusion; fibrothorax can occur.[116]

Connective Tissue Disease

Rheumatoid arthritis (RA) and systemic lupus erythematosus (SLE) most commonly present with pleural effusions.[115] Immune complex deposition and complement activation, together with inflammatory mediators released by neutrophils and T lymphocytes, damage pleural capillaries and increase capillary permeability.[152,153]

One third of children with RA initially present with asymptomatic pleural effusions along with pericarditis and transient parenchymal infiltrates.[154] Pleuritis can be the sole manifestation of juvenile RA.[155] Approximately 20% of patients under 35 years of age develop pleurisy during the course of their disease.[156] Intermittent chest pain or an acute pneumonia-like syndrome of fever, dyspnea, and chest pain indicates pleural involvement.[157]

The pleural fluid is serous or turbid. Its appearance ranges from yellow-green to milky (from cholesterol) or bloody.[158] Cell counts range from a few hundred to 15,000 cells/mm^3.[159-162] Neutrophils predominate during the acute course and are replaced by lymphocytes with time.[159,162] Glucose measurements less than 50 mg/dl and pH of less than 7.0 are typical.[159] Immunologic findings include rheumatoid factor titers ≥1:320,[163] low complement levels,[160] and higher immune complex levels than in serum.[20] Giant multinucleated or elongated macrophages and a background of granular debris are characteristic.[164]

Effusions resolve spontaneously over several months, occasionally with mild pleural thickening.[156] Severe pleural thickening, however, with constrictive pericarditis and trapped lung can occur.[20]

As many as 60% of children with SLE develop pleural effusions or pleurisy during the course of their disease; the incidence is lower in children receiving corticosteroids.[162,165] Pleuritis with effusion is almost never the initial manifestation of SLE,[166] and lupus pleuritis is usually symptomatic with chest pain, cough, fever, and dyspnea.[161]

The appearance and cell count of lupus effusions are similar to those seen in RA, but glucose and pH values are normal.[161] The fluid contains LE cells,[162] low complement levels,[158] and double-stranded DNA, and the antinuclear antibodies (ANA) titer is greater than 1:160 or higher than serum ANA titers.[161]

Effusions associated with SLE require corticosteroid therapy to resolve.[20] Those caused by drug-induced SLE clear when the offending agent is discontinued.[167]

Fungal Infections

Fungal infections account for less than 1% of all effusions.[168] Because the presentation is nonspecific, however, fungal infection should be considered in every patient with a lymphocytic effusion.

Of the fungi that cause pulmonary disease in humans, the most common to cause effusions are *Coccidioides immitis* and *Candida* sp. Although *Coccidioides* causes disease in normal hosts, *Candida* infects only immunocompromised hosts.[169,170] *Histoplasma capsulatum, Blastomyces dermatitidis, Penicillium marneffei, Paracoccidioides brasiliensis, Cryptococcus neoformans,* and *Aspergillus* all have been reported to cause effusions as well.[169,171]

The course is slow, and most fungal pleuropulmonary infections in normal hosts resolve spontaneously. Diagnostic tests include culture and staining of pleural fluid, skin tests, serology, and assessment of the patient's immune status.[169,172-174] Pleural or lung biopsy may become necessary for a more rapid diagnosis.

Immunocompromised hosts, children with cavitary lesions, or any patient with severe disease should receive antifungal therapy.[169] Therapeutic agents include amphotericin B or ketoconazole, depending on the organism.[169] Chest tube drainage is necessary only when cavitary lung disease and hydropneumothorax exists as a result of coccidiomycosis.[169]

Chylous Effusions

Chylous effusions arise from leakage of chyle from a major lymphatic vessel into the pleural space. The most common cause of chylothorax is injury to the thoracic duct following corrective surgery of vascular malformations,[175] followed by chest or neck trauma, neck hyperextension,[20] or less commonly, coughing, weight-bearing, and vomiting.[40,176,177] Other causes of chylothorax include tumors such as lymphoma, tuberculosis, and sarcoidosis, by obstruction of lymphatic channels or the vena cava.[175]

Chylothorax is the most common cause of pleural effusion in the neonatal period.[30,178] In most cases the cause is unknown and unrelated to birth trauma[178-180]; some cases are associated with thoracic duct atresia or abnormal connections of thoracic lymphatics with the pleural space.[181] Individuals with Down syndrome,[182] Noonan syndrome,[183] extralobar sequestration,[184] and lymphangiomatosis or lymphangiectasia[20,185-189] have a higher incidence of chylothorax.

Clinical presentation includes respiratory distress within the first week of life[30,178,182,190] and exertional dyspnea later in life.[20] Evidence of malignancy or tuberculosis must be sought in children with no history of trauma or chest surgery.

Chyle appears milky because of the presence of chylomicrons, but is serous and straw-colored in neonates and children who are malnourished or have not received enteral feedings.[30,178,191] The glucose and pH levels are comparable to those of serum,[20] and there is a predominance of lymphocytes. Pleural fluid triglyceride levels above 110 mg/dl are diagnostic of chylothorax, whereas levels below 50 mg/dl are highly unlikely to be associated with chylothorax.[191] The diagnosis is confirmed by lipoprotein electrophoresis[192] or by observing a blue discoloration of the effusion 30 to 60 minutes after ingestion of a fat-containing meal dyed with methylene blue.

Treatment consists of tube drainage, measures to control chyle flow, and nutritional support.[176,193-195] Chest tube drainage provides relief of respiratory compromise and quantitation of ongoing chyle leak into the pleural space. Secondary empyema is rare because chyle is bacteriostatic.[196] Enteral feedings with low fat content in the form of medium-chain triglycerides are used to reduce chyle flow because they are absorbed directly from the intestine into the bloodstream and bypass the lymphatics.[197,198] Adequate nutrition must be maintained with either enteral or intravenous alimentation because protein and electrolyte losses can be excessive when large amounts of fluid are drained.[30,186] If chyle leak is not reduced within a few days, oral feedings should be discontinued. Gastric secretions, which stimulate lymph flow, should be reduced by nasogastric tube suctioning. Chylothorax caused by malignancy responds well to mediastinal radiation, and tube drainage is not necessary.[176]

Mortality from chylothorax in the newborn period is high, especially in low-birth-weight infants,[30,180,199,200] and is usually related to associated pulmonary hypoplasia or other congenital malformations.[199] Mortality from chylothorax outside the neonatal period is very low, and is usually a result of underlying congenital heart disease, malignancy, or trauma, rather than the chylothorax itself.[194,201]

Pseudochylothorax, or chyliform effusions, have a milky appearance because of high cholesterol levels (145 to 4500 mg/dl).[202] Pseudochylothorax is most often associated with long-standing effusions (usually more than 5 years) caused by tuberculosis and rheumatoid arthritis.[201] The pathogenesis of elevated cholesterol levels remains unclear, but is not associated with hypercholesterolemia.[201]

Hemothorax

Hemothorax is defined as a collection of fluid with a hematocrit at least 50% that of blood.[40] Most hemothoraces result from trauma, but other causes include erosion of vessels by central venous catheters, pulmonary infarction, malignancy, thrombocytopenia or hemophilia, rupture of a bronchopulmonary sequestration or arteriovenous malformation, or spontaneous rupture of an intrathoracic vessel.[40,203] Hemothorax may become evident radiographically only after several hours following trauma, so radiographs should be repeated periodically after an injury.[204] Concomitant pneumothorax is common.[204]

Management of hemothorax consists of immediate placement of a large-bore thoracotomy tube. Drainage allows the lung to reexpand, to quantify bleeding, and to tamponade surface bleeding by pleural apposition.[205] Suction to the pleural space does not exacerbate bleeding[205] and reduces the incidence of secondary empyema and fibrothorax. Open thoracotomy is indicated if pleural bleeding is copious and persistent after tube placement,[205] or to relieve lung compression by clotted blood.[40] Instillation of streptokinase into the pleural space is an alternative therapy in poor surgical candidates.[206] Small amounts of retained blood may be observed for several months because spontaneous disappearance often occurs.[40] Pleural effusions occasionally occur after removal of chest tubes, and resolve spontaneously without sequelae.[207]

Monocytic Effusions

Viral and *Mycoplasma pneumoniae* infections occasionally result in serous effusions characterized by a predominance of monocytes. Viruses include adenovirus, influenza, herpes, varicella, measles, and cytomegalovirus.[208,209] Small effusions can occasionally occur with viral hepatitis, and may precede the onset of jaundice.[20]

Effusions contain fewer than 5000 cells/mm^3.[208,210,211] Pleural fluid glucose and pH are similar to those of serum. Intranuclear inclusions and multinucleated giant cells in pleural fluid are indicative of infection with the herpes viruses or rubeola.[209]

Viral effusions are usually asymptomatic, are not associated with parenchymal infiltrates, and resolve without therapy.[20,210,211] Effusions caused by *M. pneumoniae* often are associated with an ipsilateral parenchymal infiltrate, and resolve spontaneously. Therapy with erythromycin or doxycycline may hasten resolution.[20]

Eosinophilic Effusions

Pleural fluid eosinophilia (more than 10% eosinophils) results from reactive eosinophilic pleuritis[212] and is most often associated with recent pneumothorax or presence of blood in the pleural space.[40,213] Other causes of eosinophilic effusion include drugs such as dantrolene and nitrofurantoin,[214,215] uremia,[116] fungal and parasitic infections such as histoplasmosis,[216,217] coccidiomycosis,[146] echinococcosis,[218] amebiasis,[146] ascariasis,[146] and paragonamiasis.[219] Some viral infections can cause eosinophilic effusions and may actually be the cause of "idiopathic" eosinophilic effusions.[40,112]

Human Immunodeficiency Virus (HIV) Infection and AIDS

In adults with HIV infection, the most common cause of effusion is aerobic bacterial pneumonia,[220,221] followed by *Pneumocystis carinii* infection in which small lymphocytic exudates and pneumothorax are common.[222,223] Organisms can be detected in the pleural fluid by silver stain.[224,225] Other causes include lymphoma[220,221] and infection with *M. tuberculosis,* atypical mycobacteria,[64] cryptococcus,[226] *Nocardia,* leishmaniasis,[227] or histoplasmosis.[228]

Neonatal Pleural Effusion

Congenital effusions, including chylothorax, occur in approximately 1 in 10,000 to 15,000 births.[180,199] Fetal or congenital hydrothorax has also been reported with Down syndrome,[229] diaphragmatic hernia,[230] congenital heart disease,[231] and hydrops fetalis.[180] Congenital infections can rarely be associated with effusions.[232-234] Polyhydramnios, hydrops fetalis, and pulmonary hypoplasia are commonly associated with congenital effusion.[180,190,199] Mortality is approximately 15% to 36%,[235,236] with a worse prognosis when the effusion is bilateral or present prenatally.[199]

PNEUMOTHORAX

Pneumothorax is defined as the abnormal presence of air in the pleural space outside of the lung. Air enters the pleural space either by disruption of the integrity of the lung parenchyma or the airways with preservation of the continuity of the thoracic wall (closed pneumothorax), or by disruption of the thoracic wall (open pneumothorax). The production of pneumothorax is associated with a variety of causes, which include pulmonary infections,[237-240] chest trauma,[241,242] acute lung injury caused by inhaled physical and chemical agents,[243-247] acute and chronic inflammatory lung diseases,[248-250] neoplastic disease,[239,251-253] and diagnostic and therapeutic procedures[254-259] involving thoracic and high abdominal organs (Table 76-8). Collapse of the lung is also associated with cysts and other malformations of the lung, and with congenital defects of collagen formation such as Marfan syndrome.[260,261] Spontaneous pneumothorax tends to occur more commonly in lanky, asthenic individuals,[262] and more commonly in male than in female patients.

Although the exact mechanism of production of air leaks is poorly understood in many conditions, it is secondary to a defect in the pleural covering, which eventually loses its integrity. Thin subpleural blebs are common in patients with Marfan syndrome and familial spontaneous pneumothorax. In other instances, such blebs develop as a result of destruction of lung parenchyma or by a check valve mechanism secondary to airway obstruction. Blebs are probably quite prevalent among the normal population; it is unclear what triggers the rupture. Sudden changes in atmospheric pressure experi-

Table 76-8 Causes of Pneumothorax

Traumatic	Penetrating or blunt chest trauma
Iatrogenic	Barotrauma (mechanical ventilation)
	Central vein catheterization
	Procedures on the airways (intubation endoscopy-transbronchial biopsy)
	Laparoscopic procedures
	Percutaneous thoracic or abdominal biopsies
Spontaneous	Familial
	Idiopathic
Specific of women	Catamenial (endometriosis)
	Hamman syndrome (during labor and delivery)
Post-infections	Measles
	P. carinii
	Bacterial *(Staphylococcus aureus)*
	Tuberculosis
	Parasitic (ecchinococcal cysts)
After inhalation of toxins	Hydrocarbon inhalation
	Cocaine smoking
	Paraquat toxicity
Congenital malformations	Caustic fumes
	Marfan syndrome
	Congenital lung cysts
	Lymphangiomatosis
Miscellaneous	Foreign body aspiration
	Asthma
	Cystic fibrosis
	Histiocytosis
	Congenital lung malformations (lobar emphysema, etc.)
	Irradiation
	Lymphoma, tumors, and other cancer
	Metastasis

enced during diving or high-altitude flying or sudden changes in intrathoracic pressure such as during coughing spells or asthma attacks are considered predisposing factors in the production of spontaneous pneumothorax. Positive intrapleural pressure associated with labor and delivery (Hamman syndrome) has also been associated with spontaneous pneumothorax in healthy women.[263,264] Many individuals, however, experience such episodes while at rest or during normal activity.

Penetrating injuries to the chest, including diagnostic or therapeutic procedures, disrupt the "vacuum seal" nature of the pleural cavity and allow air to penetrate.[255,257,260] Blunt chest trauma can result in rupture of the esophagus, an airway, or the parenchyma itself, which allows air to escape to the mediastinum and pleural space. Metastatic neoplastic lesions and endometriosis[265] interrupt the integrity of the pleural surface and often that of the underlying lung.[266]

Clinical Manifestations

The cardinal manifestation is sudden chest pain. Tachypnea, dyspnea, tachycardia, and cyanosis are common. The intensity of the symptoms depends on the extent of the collection of air, the patient's threshold of pain, and the degree of respiratory compromise before the occurrence of the problem.

Intense chest pain and difficulty breathing cause anxiety, which worsens the symptoms. The characteristics of the pain are quite variable and may range from localized acute retrosternal pain to an overwhelming pleuritic pain difficult to localize. Ipsilateral shoulder pain is common. Breath sounds, transmission of the voice, and thoracic excursion are decreased. Hyperresonance with percussion becomes evident on the affected side. If the air is under pressure (tension pneumothorax), the mediastinum shifts to the contralateral side, causing displacement of the trachea and the point of maximal cardiac impulse. Because air tries to find a path of least resistance when under tension, air cleaves into the mediastinum and the subcutaneous tissue. Subcutaneous emphysema can be extensive and reach the neck, the abdominal wall, and even the perineum, causing significant deformity of the affected areas. In some cases, pneumothorax appears as an incidental radiographic finding in an asymptomatic patient.

Diagnosis

The most important laboratory examination that confirms the presence of a pneumothorax is the chest radiograph. Frontal and lateral views should be obtained. Expiratory and lateral decubitus views are helpful in detecting small collections of air that are not readily visible in the frontal view. Air rises to the uppermost portion of the thoracic cavity in the affected side, delineating an area of hyperlucency and absent pulmonary markings. Accompanying pneumomediastinum, pneumopericardium, and subcutaneous emphysema can also be present, manifested by collections of air of variable size surrounding the mediastinal structures, heart, and subcutaneous tissue. CT of the chest is a useful technique to detect bullae and blebs in individuals with recurrent pneumothorax, as well as an aid to the detection of air collections when the radiograph is inconclusive.[267,268]

Increased alveolar-arterial oxygen gradient and hemoglobin desaturation can be detected by arterial blood gas measurement and pulse oximetry, respectively. In cases of severe tension pneumothorax with mediastinal and cardiac displacement and rotation, the electrocardiogram may show changes in the amplitude of the QRS complex and the cardiac axis.

In unconscious, heavily sedated or mechanically ventilated patients, sudden decreases in arterial oxygenation, retention of carbon dioxide, and changes in the patterns of ventilation and lung mechanics may be the only manifestations of pneumothorax.

Pneumothorax can be confused with pulmonary cysts such as congenital lobar emphysema, or cystic adenomatoid malformation, and diaphragmatic hernia, particularly in neonates.[269-271] We have witnessed instances in which thoracotomy tubes were inserted into large emphysematous bullae after an erroneous diagnosis. These instances are rare but one should be aware of this possibility. In older children and adolescents, the differential diagnosis includes pleuritis, asthma, and pain of cardiac or psychogenic origin.

Management

The treatment consists of the evacuation of air from the pleural cavity and sealing of the area of leakage. If the collection of air is very small and the patient is minimally symptomatic, one can wait for spontaneous absorption of air. Instances in which the collections of air are larger or the patient is in distress require the insertion of a thoracotomy tube and application of negative pressure by suction (-20 cm H_2O). The lungs should be allowed to reexpand slowly because rapid reexpansion after evacuation of large collections of air can result in pulmonary edema.[272,273] Thus if the pneumothorax is large, it may be best not to apply negative pressure immediately but rather to let air under tension exit slowly and spontaneously over a period of time before the application of suction.[249]

Suction should be maintained until it becomes evident that no air is exiting the thoracic cavity. Suction should then be discontinued and the tube allowed to remain under water seal. If no air leak is evident after 24 hours, the chest tube can be removed. Continuous air leak is a sign of persistent disruption of the pleural surface and lung parenchyma or a bronchopleural fistula requiring surgical correction. The procedure of choice is oversewing or stapling of subpleural blebs and localized pleurodesis. Access to the pleural surface can be achieved by a limited thoracotomy or by thoracoscopy. The latter has emerged as one of the approaches of choice in older children and adults. Thoracoscopy provides a direct access to oversew the blebs and bullae, and induce pleurodesis by physical or chemical means.[274-280] Direct visualization is preferable to blind installation of sclerosing agents via a thoracotomy tube because it allows a better control of the extent of the pleurodesis. Excellent results have been reported, although experience in children is limited. Chemical pleurodesis can be achieved with many agents, including hypertonic glucose solution (30% to 50%), tetracycline,[281] quinacrine,[277] talcum powder,[274,276,278] silver nitrate, fibrin glue,[282,283] autologous blood patches,[284,285] nitrogen mustard, or mechanically by direct abrasion with gauze, scouring pads, or laser-diathermy.

Needle aspiration should be used only when the severity of the patients' symptoms demands immediate action. Heimlich valves allow one-way flow of air out of the lung and are useful as temporizing measures before transport or as a means to control chronic air accumulation. They are used primarily in adults with chronic, intractable pneumothorax and have a limited use in children.

The administration of 100% oxygen as a means of displacing nitrogen and aiding in the reexpansion of the lung is a popular method for the treatment of pneumothorax in the neonatal period. This technique, however, is not as effective in older age groups.

Complications of pneumothorax include bleeding from rupture of bridging blood vessels (hemopneumothorax), infection of the pleural space (rare), and acute cardiovascular collapse. The onset of pneumothorax is associated with a bad prognosis in individuals with chronic lung disease such as cystic fibrosis because it is a manifestation of significant disruption of the lung architecture. The long-term prognosis of spontaneous pneumothorax in individuals who are otherwise healthy is good if the cause is identified and corrected.

REFERENCES

Embryology and Anatomy

1. Moore KL: *The developing human,* ed 2, Philadelphia, 1977, WB Saunders, pp 145-155.
2. Hesseldahl H, Larsen JF: Ultrastructure of human yolk sac: Endoderm, mesenchyme, tubules and mesothelium, *Am J Anat* 126:315-336, 1969.
3. Wang NS: Anatomy and physiology of the pleural space, *Clin Chest Med* 6:3-16, 1985.
4. Suki B, Hantos Z: Viscoelastic properties of the visceral pleura and its contribution to lung impedance, *Respir Physiol* 90:271-287, 1992.
5. Cooray GH: Defensive mechanisms in the mediastinum with special reference to the mechanics of pleural absorption, *J Pathol Bacteriol* 61:551-567, 1949.
6. Fedorko ME, Hirsch JG: Studies on transport of macromolecules and small particles across mesothelial cells of the mouse omentum. I. Morphological aspects, *Exp Cell Res* 69:113-127, 1971.
7. Pistolesi M, Miniati M, Giuntini C: Pleural liquid and solute exchange (state of the art), *Am Rev Respir Dis* 140:825-847, 1989.
8. Rennard SI, Jaurand MC, Bignon J, Kawanami O, Ferrans VJ, Davidson J, Crystal RG: Role of pleural mesothelial cells in the production of the submesothelial connective tissue matrix of lung, *Am Rev Respir Dis* 130:267-274, 1984.
9. Antony VB, Repine JE, Harada RN, Good JT Jr, Sahn SA: Inflammatory responses in experimental tuberculosis pleurisy, *Acta Cytol* 27:355-361, 1983.
10. Hills BA: Graphite-like lubrication of mesothelium by oligolamellar pleural surfactant, *J Appl Physiol* 73:1034-1039, 1992.
11. Andrews PM, Porter KR: The ultrastructural morphology and possible functional significance of mesothelial microvilli, *Anat Rec* 177:409-426, 1973.
12. Wang NS: The preformed stomas connecting the pleural cavity and the lymphatics in the parietal pleura, *Am Rev Respir Dis* 111:12-20, 1975.
13. Broaddus VC, Wiener-Kronish JP, Berthiaume Y, Staub NC: Removal of pleural liquid and protein by lymphatics in awake sheep, *J Appl Physiol* 64:384-390, 1988.
14. Courtice FC, Simmonds WJ: Physiological significance of lymph drainage of the serous cavities and lungs, *Physiol Rev* 34:419-448, 1954.
15. Courtice FC, Simmonds WJ: Absorption of fluids from the pleural cavities of rabbits and cats, *J Physiol* (London) 109:117-130, 1949.
16. Albertine KH, Wiener-Kronish JP, Roos PJ, Staub NC: Structure, blood supply, and lymphatic vessels of the sheep's visceral pleura, *Am J Anat* 165:277-294, 1982.
17. Albertine KH, Wiener-Kronish JP, Staub NC: The structure of the parietal pleura and its relationship to pleural liquid dynamics in sheep, *Anat Rec* 208:401-409, 1984.
18. Townsley MI, Negrini D, Ardell JL: Regional blood flow to canine parietal pleura and internal intercostal muscle, *J Appl Physiol* 70:97-102, 1991.
19. Kampmeier OF: Concerning certain mesothelial thickenings and vascular plexuses of the mediastinal pleura associated with histiocyte and fat cell production, *Anat Rec* 39:201-214, 1928.
20. Sahn SA: State of the art: The pleura, *Am Rev Respir Dis* 138:184-234, 1988 (review).
21. Albertine KH, Wiener KJ, Bastacky J, Staub NC: No evidence for mesothelial cell contact across the costal pleural space of sheep, *J Appl Physiol* 70:123-134, 1991.
22. Miserocchi G, Negrini D, Pistolesi M, Bellina CR, Gilardi MC, Bettinardi V, Rossitto F: Intrapleural liquid flow down a gravity-dependent hydraulic pressure gradient, *J Appl Physiol* 64:577-584, 1988.

Physiology of the Pleural Space

23. Agostoni E, D'Angelo E: Pleural liquid pressure, *J Appl Physiol* 71:393-403, 1991 (review).
24. Negrini D, Reed RK, Miserocchi G: Permeability-surface area product and reflection coefficient of the parietal pleura in dogs, *J Appl Physiol* 71:2543-2547, 1991.
25. Negrini D, Townsley MI, Taylor AE: Hydraulic conductivity of canine parietal pleura in vivo, *J Appl Physiol* 69:438-442, 1990.
26. Miserocchi G, Venturoli D, Negrini D, Gilardi MC, Bellina R: Intrapleural fluid movements described by a porous flow model, *J Appl Physiol* 73:2511-6, 1992.
27. Miserocchi G, Negrini D, Gonano C: Parenchymal stress affects interstitial and pleural pressures in in situ lung, *J Appl Physiol* 71:1967-72, 1991.
28. Bland RD, Hansen TN, Haberkern CM, Bressack MA, Hazinski TA, Raj JU, Goldberg RB: Lung fluid balance in lambs before and after birth, *J Appl Physiol: Respir Environ Exercise Physiol* 53:992-1004, 1982.
29. Bland RD, McMillan DD: Lung fluid dynamics in awake newborn lambs, *J Clin Invest* 60:1107-1115, 1977.
30. Chernick V, Reed MH: Pneumothorax and chylothorax in the neonatal period, *J Pediatr* 76:624-632, 1970.
31. Jay SJ: Diagnostic procedures for pleural disease, *Clin Chest Med* 6:33-48, 1985.
32. Woodring JH: Recognition of pleural effusions on supine radiographs. How much fluid is required? *Am J Roentgenol* 142:59-64, 1984.
33. Rudikoff JC: Early detection of pleural fluid, *Chest* 77:109-111, 1980.
34. Byrk D: Infrapulmonary effusion, *Radiology* 120:33-36, 1976.
35. Schwarz MI, Marmorstein BL: A new radiologic sign of subpulmonic effusion, *Chest* 67:176-178, 1975.
36. Henschke CI, Davis SD, Romano PM, Yankelevitz DF: The pathogenesis, radiologic evaluation, and therapy of pleural effusions, *Radiol Clin North Am* 27:1241-1255, 1989.

37. Doust BD, Baum JK, Maklad NF, Doust VL: Ultrasonic evaluation of pleural opacities, *Radiology* 114:135-140, 1975.
38. Hirsch JH, Rogers JV, Mack LA: Real-time sonography of pleural opacities, *Am J Radiol* 136:297-301, 1981.
39. Lipscomb DJ, Flower CDR, Hadfield JW: Ultrasound of the pleura: an assessment of its clinical value, *Clin Radiol* 32:289-290, 1981.
40. Light RW: *Pleural diseases,* Philadelphia, 1990, Lea & Febiger.
41. Godwin TE, Sahn SA: Thoracentesis: a safe procedure in mechanically ventilated patients, *Ann Intern Med* 113:800-802, 1990.
42. Jacobson ES: A case of secondary echinococcosis diagnosed by cytologic examination of pleural fluid and needle biopsy of pleura, *Acta Cytol* 17:76-79, 1973.
43. Kendall SW, Bryan AJ, Large SR, Wells FC: Pleural effusions: is thorascopy a reliable investigation? A retrospective review, *Respir Med* 86:437-440, 1992.
44. Seneff MG, Corwin RW, Gold LH, Irwin RS: Complications associated with thoracentesis, *Chest* 90:97-100, 1986.
45. Liu P, Daneman A, Stringer DA, Ein SH: Percutaneous aspiration, drainage, and biopsy in children, *J Pediatr Surg* 24:865-866, 1989.
46. Collins TR, Sahn SA: Thoracentesis: clinical value, complications, technical problems, and patient experience, *Chest* 91:817-822, 1987.
47. Ragozzino MW, Greene R: Bilateral reexpansion pulmonary edema following unilateral pleurocentesis, *Chest* 99:506-508, 1991.
48. Grogan DR, Irwin RS, Channick R, Raptopoulos V, Curley FJ, Bartter T, Corwin RW: Complications associated with thoracentesis: a prospective, randomized study comparing 3 different methods, *Arch Intern Med* 150:873-877, 1990.
49. Chretien J, Daniel CJ: Needle pleural biopsy. In Chretien J, Bignon J, Hirsch A, eds: *The pleura in health and disease,* New York, 1985, Marcel Dekker, pp 631-642.
50. Light RW, MacGregor MI, Luchsinger PC, Ball WC: Pleural effusions: the diagnostic separation of transudates and exudates, *Ann Intern Med* 77:507-513, 1972.
51. Valdes L, Pose A, Suarez J, Gonzalez-Jaunatey JR, Sarandeses A, San Jose E, Dobana JMS, Salgueiro M, Suarez JRR: Cholesterol: a useful parameter for distinguishing between pleural exudates and transudates, *Chest* 99:1097-1102, 1991.

Transudates

52. Niehlson PH, Jepsen SB, Olsen AD: Postoperative pleural effusions following upper abdominal surgery, *Chest* 96:1133-1135, 1989.
53. Wiener-Kronish JP, Matthay MA, Callen PW, Filly RA, Gamsu G, Staub NC: Relationship of pleural effusions to pulmonary hemodynamics in patients with congestive heart failure, *Am Rev Respir Dis* 132:1253-1256, 1985.
54. Wiener-Kronish JP, Goldstein R, Matthay RA, Biondi JW, Broaddus VC, Chatterjee K, Matthay MA: Lack of association of pleural effusion with chronic pulmonary arterial and right atrial hypertension, *Chest* 92:967-970, 1987.
55. Race GA, Scheifley CH, Edwards JE: Hydrothorax in congestive heart failure, *Am J Med* 22:83-89, 1957.
56. Pillay VKG: Total protein in serous fluids in cardiac failure, *S Afr Med J* 39:142-143, 1965.
57. Spicer AJ, Fisher JA: Recurring pleural effusion in congestive heart failure treated by pleurodesis, *J Irish Med Assoc* 62:177-178, 1969.
58. Stark DD, Shanes JG, Baron RL, Koch DD: Biochemical features of urinothorax, *Arch Intern Med* 142:1509-1511, 1982.
59. Lieberman FL, Hidemura R, Peters RL, Reynolds TB: Pathogenesis and treatment of hydrothorax complicating cirrhosis with ascites, *Ann Intern Med* 64:341-351, 1966.
60. Chetty KG: Transudative pleural effusions, *Clin Chest Med* 6:49-54, 1985.
61. Milutinovic J, Wuu-Shyang W, Lindholm DD, Lapp NL: Acute massive unilateral hydrothorax: a rare complication of chronic peritoneal dialysis, *South Med J* 73:827-828, 1980.
62. Gottehrer A, Roa J, Stanford GG, Chernow B, Sahn SA: Hypothyroidism and pleural effusions, *Chest* 98:1130-1132, 1990.

Exudates

63. Light RW, Ball WC Jr: Glucose and amylase in pleural effusions, *JAMA* 225:257-259, 1973.
64. Harley RA: Pathology of pleural infections, *Semin Respir Infect* 3:291-297, 1988.
65. Brook I: Microbiology of empyema in children and adolescents, *Pediatrics* 85:722-726, 1990.
66. Santhanakrishnan BR, Thirumoorthy MC, Balagopala RV: Empyema in children: a review of 175 cases, *Indian Pediatr* 9:805-811, 1972.
67. McLaughlin FJ, Goldmann DA, Rosenbaum DM, Harris GBC, Schuster SR, Strieder DJ: Empyema in children: clinical course and long-term follow-up, *Pediatrics* 73:587-593, 1984.
68. Freij B, Kusmiesz H, Nelson JD, McCracken GH: Parapneumonic effusion and empyema in hospitalized children: a retrospective review of 277 cases, *Pediatr Infect Dis J* 3:578-592, 1984.
69. American Thoracic Society: Management of non-tuberculous empyema, *Am Rev Respir Dis* 85:935-936, 1962.
70. Light RW, Girard WM, Jenkinson SG, George RB: Parapneumonic effusions, *Am J Med* 69:507-512, 1980.
71. Potts DE, Taryle DA, Sahn SA: The glucose-pH relationship in parapneumonic effusions, *Arch Intern Med* 138:1378-1380, 1978.
72. Moran JF: Surgical management of pleural space infections, *Semin Respir Infect* 3:383-394, 1988.
73. Munglani R, Kenney IJ: Paediatric parapneumonic effusions: a review of 16 cases, *Respir Med* 85:117-119, 1991.
74. Beg MH, Ahmad SH, Reyazuddin J, Shahab T, Chandra J: Management of empyema thoracis in children: a study of 65 cases, *Ann Trop Paediatr* 7:109-112, 1987.
75. Groff DB, Randolph JG, Blades B: Empyema in children, *JAMA* 195:572-574, 1966.
76. Wasz-hockert O, Takkunen R: Review and follow-up of empyemas in 134 infants and children, *Ann Paediatr* 9:27-41, 1963.
77. Long SS: Pneumonia in older infants, children and adolescents. In Schidlow DV, ed: *A practical guide to pediatric respiratory diseases,* Philadelphia, 1994, Hanley & Belfus, pp 89-98.
78. Molteni RA: Group A beta-hemolytic streptococcal pneumonia, *Am J Dis Child* 131:1366-1371, 1977.
79. Middlekamp JN, Purkerson ML, Burford TH: The changing pattern of empyema thoracis in pediatrics, *J Thorac Cardiovasc Surg* 47:165-173, 1964.
80. Bartlett JG: Bacterial infections of the pleural space, *Semin Respir Infect* 3:308-321, 1988.
81. Chartrand SA, McCracken GH: Staphylococcal pneumonia in infants and children, *Pediatr Infect Dis* 1:19-22, 1982.
82. Brook I, Finegold SM: Bacteriology and therapy of lung abscesses in children, *J Pediatr* 94:10-15, 1979.
83. Fajardo JE, Chang MJ: Pleural empyema in children: a nationwide retrospective study, *South Med J* 80:593-597, 1987.
84. Long SS: Pneumonia in young infants (birth through 3 months). In Schidlow DV, Smith DS, eds: *A practical guide to pediatric respiratory diseases,* Philadelphia, 1994, Hanley & Belfus, pp 83-88.
85. Brook I, Frazier EH: Aerobic and anerobic microbiology of empyema: a retrospective review in two military hospitals, *Chest* 103:1502-1507, 1993.
86. Hochberg L, Kramer B: Acute empyema of the chest in children: a review of 300 cases, *Am J Dis Child* 57:1310-1317, 1939.
87. Kevy SV, Lowe BA: Streptococcal pneumonia and empyema in childhood, *N Engl J Med* 264:738-743, 1961.
88. Basiliere JL, Bistrong HW, Spence WF: Streptococcal pneumonia: Recent outbreaks in military recruit populations, *Am J Med* 44:580-589, 1968.
89. Santosham M, Chipps BE, Strife JL, Moxon ER: Sequelae of *H. influenzae* type b empyema, *J Pediatr* 95:160-161, 1979.
90. Wise MB, Beaudry PH, Bates DV: Long-term follow-up of staphylococcal pneumonia, *Pediatrics* 38:398-401, 1966.
91. Himelman RB, Callen PW: The prognostic value of loculations in parapneumonic pleural effusions, *Chest* 90:852-856, 1986.
92. Poe RH, Marin MG, Israel RH, Kallay MC: Utility of pleural fluid analysis in predicting tube thoracostomy/decortication in parapneumonic effusions, *Chest* 100:963-967, 1991.
93. Berger HA, Morganroth ML: Immediate drainage is not required for all patients with complicated parapneumonic effusions, *Chest* 97:731-735, 1990.
94. Lemmer JH, Botham MJ, Orringer MB: Modern management of adult thoracic empyema, *J Thorac Cardiovasc Surg* 90:849-855, 1985.
95. Sahn SA, Light RW: The sun should never set on a parapneumonic effusion, *Chest* 95:945-946, 1989.
96. Light RW: Management of pleural effusions, *Arch Intern Med* 141: 1339-1341, 1981.

97. Nilsson BS, Broberg S, Larsen F, Diagnosis and treatment of empyema, *Scand J Respir Dis* 102(suppl):202-204, 1978.
98. Orringer MB: Thoracic empyema—back to basics, *Chest* 93:901-902, 1988.
99. Strange C, Sahn SA: The clinicians perspective on parapneumonic effusions and empyema, *Chest* 103:259-261, 1993.
100. Lionakis B, Gray SW, Skandalakis JE, Hoplains WA: Empyema in children: a 25 year study, *J Pediatr* 53:719-725, 1958.
101. Cattaneo SM, Kilman JW: Surgical therapy of empyema in children, *Arch Surg* 106:564-567, 1973.
102. Stiles QR, Lindesmith GG, Tucker BL, Meyer BW, Jones JC: Pleural empyema in children, *Ann Thorac Surg* 10:37-44, 1970.
103. Kosloske AM, Cushing AH, Shuck JM: Early decortication for anaerobic empyema in children, *J Pediatr Surg* 15:422-429, 1980.
104. Hartl H: Pleuropulmonary suppurations, *Prog Pediatr Surg* 10:257-266, 1977.
105. Murphy D, Lockhart CH, Todd JK: Pneumococcal empyema: outcome of medical management, *Am J Dis Child* 134:659-662, 1980.
106. Kaye MD: Pleuropulmonary complications of pancreatitis, *Thorax* 23:297-306, 1968.
107. Cameron JL: Chronic pancreatic ascites and pancreatic pleural effusions, *Gastroenterology* 74:134-140, 1978.
108. Tewari SC, Jayaswal R, Chauhan MS, Kaul SK, Narajanan VA: Bilateral recurrent haemorrhagic pleural effusions in asymptomatic chronic pancreatitis, *Thorax* 44:824-825, 1989.
109. Maultiz RM, Good JT Jr, Kaplan RL, Reller LB, Sahn SA: The pleuropulmonary consequences of esophageal rupture: an experimental model, *Am Rev Respir Dis* 120:363-367, 1979.
110. Bladergroen MR, Lowe JE, Postlethwait RW: Diagnosis and recommended management of esophageal perforation and rupture, *Ann Thorac Surg* 42:235-239, 1986.
111. Bynum LJ, Wilson JE III: Characteristic of pleural effusions associated with pulmonary embolism, *Arch Intern Med* 136:159-162, 1976.
112. Adelman M, Albelda SM, Gottlieb J, Haponik EF: Diagnostic utility of pleural fluid eosinophilia, *Am J Med* 77:915-920, 1984.
113. Simon HB, Daggett WM, DeSanctis RW: Hemothorax as a complication of anticoagulant therapy in the presence of pulmonary infarction, *JAMA* 208:1830-1834, 1969.
114. Stelzner TJ, King TE Jr, Antony VB, Sahn SA: The pleuropulmonary manifestations of the postcardiac injury syndrome, *Chest* 84:383-387, 1983.
115. Sahn SA: Pathogenesis of pleural effusions and pleural lesions. In Cannon GW, Zimmermann GA, eds: *The lung in rheumatic disease,* New York, 1990, Marcel Dekker, pp 27-47.
116. Berger HW, Rammohan G, Neff MS, Buhain WJ: Uremic pleural effusion: a study in 14 patients on chronic dialysis, *Ann Intern Med* 82:362-364, 1975.
117. Carter R, Brewer LA: Subphrenic abscess: a thoracoabdominal clinical complex, *Am J Surg* 108:165-174, 1964.
118. Harrison RN, Thomas DJB: Acute actinomycotic empyema, *Thorax* 34:406-407, 1979.
119. Frazier AR, Rosenow EC III, Roberts GD: Nocardiosis: a review of 25 cases occurring during 24 months, *Mayo Clin Proc* 50:657-663, 1975.
120. Berger HW, Mejia E: Tuberculous pleurisy, *Chest* 63:88-92, 1973.
121. Pettersson T, Riska H: Diagnostic value of total and differential leukocyte counts in pleural effusions, *Acta Med Scand* 210:129-135, 1981.
122. Abrams WB, Small MJ: Current concepts of tuberculous pleurisy with effusion as derived from pleural biopsy studies, *Scand J Respir Dis* 38:60-65, 1960.
123. Sibley JC: A study of 200 cases of tuberculous pleurisy with effusion, *Am Rev Tuberc* 62:314-323, 1950.
124. Falk A: Tuberculous pleurisy with effusion: diagnosis and results of chemotherapy, *Postgrad Med* 38:631-635, 1965.
125. Scerbo J, Keltz H, Stone DJ: A prospective study of closed pleural biopsies, *JAMA* 218:377-380, 1971.
126. Scharer L, McClement JH: Isolation of tubercle bacilli from needle biopsy specimens of parietal pleura, *Am Rev Respir Dis* 97:466-468, 1968.
127. Levine H, Metzger W, Lacera D, Kay L: Diagnosis of tuberculous pleurisy by culture of pleural biopsy specimen, *Arch Intern Med* 126:269-271, 1970.
128. Caminero JA, Rodriguez de Castro F, Carillo T, Diaz F, Rodriguez Bermejo JC, Cabrera P: Diagnosis of pleural tuberculosis by detection of specific IgG anti-antigen 60 in serum and pleural fluid, *Respiration* 60:58-62, 1993.
129. Banales JL, Pineda PR, Fitzgerald JM, Rubio H, Selman M, Salazar-Lezama M: Adenosine deaminase in the diagnosis of tuberculous pleural effusions: a report of 218 patients and review of the literature, *Chest* 99:355-357, 1991.
130. Valdes L, San Jose E, Alvarez D, Sarandeses A, Pose A, Chomon B, Alvarez-Dobano JM, Salguiero M, Rodriguez Suarez JR: Diagnosis of tuberculous pleurisy using the biologic parameters adenosine deaminase, lysozyme, and interferon gamma, *Chest* 103:458-465, 1993.
131. Ribera E, Ocana I, Martinez-Vasquez JM, Rossell M, Espanol T, Ruibal A: High level of interferon gamma in tuberculous pleural effusions, *Chest* 93:308-311, 1988.
132. Yew WW, Chan CY, Kwan SY, Cheun S, French GL: Diagnosis of tuberculous pleural effusions by the determination of tuberculosteric acid in pleural aspirates, *Chest* 100:1261-1263, 1991.
133. Moriwaki Y, Kohjiro N, Itoh M, Nakatsuji Y, Okada M, Ishihara H, Tachibana I, Kokubu T: Discrimination of tuberculous from carcinomatous pleural effusion by biochemical markers: adenosine deaminase, lysozyme, fibronectin, and carcinoembryonic antigen, *Jpn J Med* 28:478-484, 1989.
134. Asseo PP, Tracopoulos GD, Kotsovoulou-Fouskaki V: Lysozyme (muramidase) in pleural effusions and serum, *Am J Clin Pathol* 78:763-767, 1982.
135. Fontan-Bueso J, Verea Hernando H, Perez Garcia Buela J, et al: Dagnostic value of simultaneous determination of pleural adenosine deaminase and pleural lysozyme/serum lysozyme ratio in pleural effusions, *Chest* 93:303-307, 1988.
136. Matthay RA, Neff TA, Iseman MD: Tuberculous pleural effusions developing during chemotherapy for pulmonary tuberculosis, *Am Rev Respir Dis* 109:469-472, 1974.
137. Tani P, Poppius H, Makipaja J: Cortisone therapy for exudative tuberculous pleurisy in the light of the follow-up study, *Acta Tuberc Scand* 44:303-309, 1964.
138. Horne NW: A critical evaluation of corticosteroids in tuberculosis, *Adv Tuberc Res* 15:1-54, 1966.
139. Castellino RA, Bellani FF, Gasparini M, Musumeci R: Radiographic findings in previously untreated children with non-Hodgkin's lymphoma, *Radiology* 117:657-663, 1975.
140. Celikoglu F, Teirstein AS, Krellenstein DJ, Strauchen JA: Pleural effusion in non-Hodgkin's lymphoma, *Chest* 101:1357-1360, 1992.
141. Wong FM, Grace WJ, Rottino A: Pleural effusions, ascites, pericardial effusions and edema in Hodgkin's disease, *Am J Med Sci* 246:678-682, 1963.
142. Fisher AMH, Kendall B, VanLeuven BD: Hodgkin's disease: a radiological survey, *Clin Radiol* 13:115-127, 1962.
143. Xaubet A, Diumenjo MC, Marin A, Montserrat E, Estapa R, Llebaria C, Austi A, Rozman C: Characteristics and prognostic value of pleural effusions in non-Hodgkin's lymphomas, *Eur J Respir Dis* 66:135-140, 1985.
144. Weick JK, Kiely JM, Harrison EG Jr, Carr DT, Scanlon PW: Pleural effusion in lymphoma, *Cancer* 31:848-853, 1973.
145. Jenkins PF, Ward MJ, Davies P, Fletcher J: Non-Hodgkin's lymphoma, chronic lymphatic leukemia and the lung, *Br J Dis Chest* 75:22-30, 1981.
146. Spriggs AI, Van Hegan RI: Cytologic diagnosis of lymphoma of serous effusion, *J Clin Pathol* 34:1311-1325, 1981.
147. Keller SM: Current and future therapy for malignant pleural effusion, *Chest* 103:63S-67S, 1993.
148. Tzeng E, Ferguson MK: Predicting failure following shunting of pleural effusions, *Chest* 98:890-893, 1990.
149. Bruneau R, Rubin P: The management of pleural effusions and chylothorax in lymphoma, *Radiology* 85:1085-1092, 1965.
150. Hopps HC, Wissler RW: Uremic pneumonitis, *Am J Pathol* 31:261-273, 1955.
151. Galen MA, Steinberg SM, Lowrie EG, Lazarus JM, Hampers CL, Merrill FP: Hemorrhagic pleural effusion in patients undergoing chronic hemodialysis, *Ann Intern Med* 82:359-361, 1975.
152. Halla JT, Schrohenloher RE, Volanakis JE: Immune complexes and other laboratory features of pleural effusion, *Ann Intern Med* 92:748-752, 1980.
153. Koster FT, McGregor DD, Mackaness GB: The mediator of cellular immunity: II. Migration of immunologically committed lymphocytes into inflammatory exudates, *J Exp Med* 133:400-409, 1971.
154. Schaler JG, Wedgwood RJ: Juvenile rheumatoid arthritis: a review, *Pediatrics* 50:940-953, 1972.

155. Carr DT, McGuckin WF: Pleural fluid glucose, *Am Rev Respir Dis* 97:302-305, 1968.
156. Walker WC, Wright V: Pulmonary lesions and rheumatoid arthritis, *Medicine* 47:501-519, 1968.
157. Carr DT, Mayne JG: Pleurisy with effusion in rheumatoid arthritis, with reference to the low concentration of glucose in pleural fluid, *Am Rev Respir Dis* 85:345-350, 1962.
158. Joseph J, Sahn SA: Connective tissue diseases and the pleura, *Chest* 104:262-270, 1993.
159. Sahn SA, Kaplan RL, Maulitz RM, Good JT Jr: Rheumatoid pleurisy. Observations on the development of low pleural fluid pH and glucose level, *Arch Intern Med* 140:1237-1238, 1980.
160. Pettersson T, Klockars M, Hellstrom P-E: Chemical and immunological features of pleural effusions: comparison between rheumatoid arthritis and other diseases, *Thorax* 37:354-361, 1982.
161. Good JT Jr., King TE Jr., Antony VB, Sahn SA: Lupus pleuritis: clinical features and pleural fluid characteristics with special reference to pleural fluid antinuclear antibodies, *Chest* 84:714-718, 1983.
162. Orens JB, Martinez FJ, Lynch JP III: Pleuropulmonary manifestations of sytemic lupus erythematosus, *Rheum Dis Clin North Am* 20:159-193, 1994.
163. Levine H, Szanto M, Grieble HG, Bach GL, Anderson TO: Rheumatoid factor in non-rheumatoid pleural effusions, *Ann Intern Med* 69:487-492, 1968.
164. Nosanchuk JS, Naylor B: A unique cytologic picture in pleural fluid from patients with rheumatoid arthritis, *Am J Clin Pathol* 50:330-335, 1968.
165. Jacobs JC: Systemic lupus erythematosus in childhood, *Pediatrics* 32:257-264, 1963.
166. Alarcon-Segovia D, Alarcon DG: Pleuropulmonary manifestations of systemic lupus erythematosus, *Dis Chest* 39:7-17, 1961.
167. Harpey JP: Lupus-like syndromes induced by drugs, *Ann Allergy* 33:256-261, 1974.
168. Storey DD, Dines DE, Coles DT: Pleural effusion. A diagnostic dilemma, *JAMA* 236:2183-2186, 1976.
169. Lambert RS, George RB: Fungal diseases of the pleura: clinical manifestations, diagnosis, and treatment, *Semin Respir Infect* 3:343-351, 1988.
170. Duperval R, Hermans PE, Brewer NS, Roberts GD: Cryptococcus, with emphasis on the significance of isolation of *Cryptococcus neoformans* from the respiratory tract, *Chest* 72:13-19, 1977.
171. Salkin D, Birsner TW, Tarr AD, et al: Roentgen analysis of coccidioidomycosis. In Ajello L, ed: Coccidiomycosis. Tucson, 1967, University of Arizona, pp 63-67.
172. Penn RL, Lambert RS, George RB: Invasive fungal infections: the use of serologic tests in diagnosis and management, *Arch Intern Med* 143:1215-1220, 1983.
173. Kauffman CA, Bergman AG, Severance PJ, McClatchey KD: Detection of cryptococcal antigen, *Am J Clin Pathol* 75:106-109, 1981.
174. Lonky SA, Catanzaro A, Moser KM, Einstein H: Acute coccidioidal pleural effusion, *Am Rev Respir Dis* 114:681-688, 1976.
175. Teba L, Dedhia HV, Bowen R, Alexander JC: Chylothorax review, *Crit Care Med* 13:49-52, 1985.
176. Roy PH, Carr DT, Payne WS: The problem of chylothorax, *Mayo Clin Proc* 42:457-467, 1967.
177. Bower GC: Chylothorax: observations in 20 cases, *Dis Chest* 46:464-468, 1964.
178. Yancy WS, Spock A: Spontaneous neonatal pleural effusion, *J Pediatr Surg* 2:313-319, 1967.
179. Benacerraf BR, Frigoletto FDJ, Wilson M: Successful midtrimester thoracentesis with analysis of the lymphocyte population in the pleural effusion, *Am J Obstet Gynecol* 155:398-399, 1986.
180. John E: Pleural effusion in the newborn, *Med J Aust* 1:102-103, 1974.
181. Van Aerde J, Campbell AN, Smyth JA, Lloyd D, Bryan HM: Spontaneous chylothorax in newborns, *Am J Dis Child* 138:961-964, 1984.
182. Yoss BS, Lipsitz PJ: Chylothorax in two mongoloid infants, *Clin Genet* 12:357-360, 1977.
183. Fisher E, Weiss EB, Michals K, Dubrow IW, Hastrieter AR, Matalon R: Spontaneous chylothorax in Noonan's syndrome, *Eur J Pediatr* 138:282-284, 1982.
184. Dresler S: Massive pleural effusion and hypoplasia of the lung accompanying extralobar pulmonary sequestration, *Hum Pathol* 12:862-864, 1981.
185. Carrington CB, Cugell DW, Gaensler EA, et al: Lymphangioleiomyomatosis. Physiologic-pathologic-radiologic correlations, *Am Rev Respir Dis* 116:977-995, 1977.
186. Berberich FR, Berstein ID, Ochs HD, Schaller RT: Lymphangiomatosis with chylothorax, *J Pediatr* 87:941-943, 1975.
187. Morphis LG, Arcinue EL, Krause JR: Generalized lymphangioma in infancy with chylothorax, *Pediatrics* 46:566-575, 1970.
188. Hunter WS, Becroft DMO: Congenital pulmonary lymphangiectasis associated with pleural effusion, *Arch Dis Child* 59:278-279, 1984.
189. Huber A, Schranz D, Blaha I, Schmitt-Mechelke T, Schumacher R: Congenital pulmonary lymphangiectasia, *Pediatr Pulmonol* 10:310-313, 1991.
190. Doolittle WM, Ohmart D, Egan EA: Congenital bilateral pleural effusions: A cause for respiratory failure in the newborn, *Am J Dis Child* 125:435-437, 1973.
191. Staats BA, Ellefson RD, Bydahn LL, Dines DE, Prakash UBS, Offord K: The lipoprotein profile of chylous and nonchylous pleural effusions, *Mayo Clin Proc* 55:700-704, 1980.
192. Seriff NS, Cohen ML, Samuel P, Schulster PL: Chylothorax: diagnosis by lipoprotein electrophoresis of serum and pleural fluid, *Thorax* 32:98-100, 1977.
193. Strausser JL, Flye MW: Management of non-traumatic chylothorax, *Ann Thorac Surg* 31:520-526, 1981.
194. Milsom JW, Kron IL, Rheuban KS, Rodgers BM: Chylothorax: an assessment of current surgical management, *J Thorac Cardiovasc Surg* 89:221-227, 1985.
195. Rubin JW, Moore HV, Ellison RG: Chylothorax: therapeutic alternatives, *Am Surgeon* 43:292-297, 1977.
196. Lampson RS: Traumatic chylothorax: a review of the literature and report of a case treated by mediastinal ligation of the thoracic duct, *J Thorac Surg* 17:778-791, 1948.
197. Hughes RL, Mintzer RA, Hidvegi DF, Freinkel RK, Cugell DW: The management of chylothorax, *Chest* 76:212-218, 1979.
198. Lichter I, Hill GL, Nye ER: The use of medium-chain triglycerides in the treatment of chylothorax in a child, *Ann Thorac Surg* 4:352-355, 1968.
199. Longaker MT, Laberge JM, Dansereau J, Langer JC, Crombleholme TM, Callen PW, Golbus MS, Harrison MR: Primary fetal hydrothorax: Natural history and management, *J Pediatr Surg* 24:573-576, 1989.
200. Vain NE, Swarner OW, Cha CC: Neonatal chylothorax: a report and discussion of nine consecutive cases, *J Pediatr Surg* 15:261-265, 1980.
201. Sassoon CS, Light RW: Chylothorax and pseudochylothorax, *Clin Chest Med* 6:163-172, 1985.
202. Coe JE, Aikawa JK: Cholesterol pleural effusion, *Arch Intern Med* 108:163-174, 1961.
203. Martinez FJ, Villanueva AG, Pickering R, Becker FS, Smith DR: Spontaneous hemothorax. Report of 6 cases and review of the literature (Review), *Medicine* 71:354-368, 1992.
204. Drumond DS, Craig RH: Traumatic hemothorax: complications and management, *Am Surg* 33:403-408, 1967.
205. Weil PH, Margolis IB: Systematic approach to traumatic hemothorax, *Am J Surg* 142:692-694, 1981.
206. Bergh NP, Ekroth R, Larsson S, Nagy P: Intrapleural streptokinase in the treatment of hemothorax and empyema, *Scand J Thorac Cardiovasc Surg* 11:265-268, 1977.
207. Wilson JM, Boren CH, Peterson SR, Thomas AN: Traumatic hemothorax: is decortication necessary? *J Thorac Cardiovasc Surg* 77:489-495, 1979.
208. Simila S, Ylikorkala O, Wasz-Hockert O: Type 7 adenovirus pneumonia, *J Pediatr* 79:605-611, 1971.
209. Goodman ZD, Gupta PK, Frost JK, Erozan YS: Cytodiagnosis of viral infections in body cavity fluids, *Acta Cytol* 23:204-208, 1979.
210. Fine NL, Smith LR, Sheedy PF: Frequency of pleural effusions in mycoplasma and viral pneumonias, *N Engl J Med* 283:790-793, 1970.
211. Alptekin F: An epidemic of pleurisy with effusion in Bitlis, Turkey. A study of 559 cases, *US Armed Forces Med* J 9:1-11, 1958.
212. Askin FB, McCann BG, Kuhn C: Reactive eosinophilic pleuritis, *Arch Pathol Lab Med* 101:187-191, 1977.
213. Spriggs AI, Boddington MM: *The cytology of effusions,* ed 2, New York, 1968, Grune & Stratton.
214. Petusevsky ML, Faling LJ, Rocklin RE, Snider GL, Merliss AD, Moses JM, Dorman SA: Pleuropericardial reaction to treatment with dantrolene, *JAMA* 242:2772-2774, 1979.

215. Geller M, Flaherty DK, Dickei GA, Reed CE: Lymphopenia in acute nitrofurantoin pleuropulmonary reactions, *J Allergy Clin Immunol* 59:445-448, 1977.
216. Cambell GD, Webb WR: Eosinophilic pleural effusion, *Am Rev Respir Dis* 90:194-201, 1964.
217. Goodwin RA, DesPrez RM: State of the art: Histoplasmosis, *Am Rev Respir Dis* 117:929-956, 1978.
218. Yacoubian HD: Thoracic problems associated with hydatid cyst of the dome of the liver, *Surgery* 79:544-548, 1976.
219. Johnson RJ, Johnson JR: Paragonimiasis in Indochinese refugees: Roentgenographic findings with clinical correlations, *Am Rev Respir Dis* 128:534-538, 1983.
220. Cadranel JL, Chouaid C, Denis M, Lebeau B, Akoun GM, Mayaud CM: Causes of pleural effusion in 75 HIV-infected patients, *Chest* 104:655, 1993.
221. Joseph J, Strange C, Sahn SA: Pleural effusions in hospitalized patients with AIDS, *Ann Intern Med* 118:856-859, 1993.
222. Horowitz ML, Schiff M, Samuels J, Russo R, Shnader J: Pneumocystis carinii pleural effusion. Pathogeneis and pleural fluid analysis, *Am Rev Respir Dis* 148:232-234, 1993.
223. Delorenzo LJ, Huang CT, Maguire GP, Stone DJ: Roentgenographic patterns of Pneumocystis carinii pneumonia in 104 patients with AIDS, *Chest* 91:323-327, 1987.
224. Mariuz P, Raviglione MC, Gould IA, Mullen MP: Pleural Pneumocystis carinii infection, *Chest* 99:774-776, 1991.
225. Jayes RL, Kamerow HN, Hasselquist SM, Delaney MD, Parenti DM: Disseminated pneumocystosis presenting as a pleural effusion, *Chest* 103:306-308, 1993.
226. Grum EE, Schwab R, Margolis ML: Case report: cryptococcal pleural effusion preceeding cryptococcal meningititis in AIDS, *Am J Med Sci* 301:329-330, 1991.
227. Peters BS, Fish D, Golden K, Evans DA, Bryceson ADM, Pinching AJ: Visceral leishmaniasis in HIV infection and AIDS: clinical features and response to therapy, *Q J Med* 77:1101-1111, 1990.
228. Marshal BC, Cox JK, Carroll KC, Morrison RE: Case report: histoplasmosis as a cause of pleural effusion in the acquired immunodeficiency syndrome, *Am J Med Sci* 300:98-101, 1990.
229. Foote KD, Vickers DW: Congenital pleural effusion in Down's syndrome, *Br J Radiol* 59:609-610, 1986.
230. Whittle MJ, Gillmore DH, McNay MB, Turner TL, Raine PA: Diaphragmatic hernia presenting in utero as a unilateral hydrothorax, *Prenat Diagn* 9(2):115-118, 1989.
231. Blott M, Nicolaides KH, Greenough A: Pleuroamniotic shunting for decompression of fetal pleural effusions, *Obstet Gynecol* 71:798-800, 1988.
232. Meyer K, Gergis N, McGravey V: Adenovirus associated with congenital pleural effusion, *J Pediatr* 107:433-435, 1985.
233. Eddleman KA, Levinie AB, Chitkara U, Berkowitz RL: Reliability of pleural fluid lymphocyte counts in the antenatal diagnosis of congenital chylothorax, *Obstet Gynecol* 78:530-532, 1991.
234. Akierman AR, Maycock DE: Group B streptococcal septicemia and delayed onset congenital right-sided diaphragmatic hernia, *Can Med Assoc J* 129:1289-1290, 1983.
235. Hagay Z, Reece EA, Roberts A, Hobbins JC: Isolated fetal pleural effusion: a prenatal management dilemma, *Obstet Gynecol* 81:147-152, 1993.
236. Booth P, Nicolaides KH, Greenough A, Gamsu HR: Pleuroamniotic shunting for fetal chylothorax, *Early Hum Dev* 15:365-367, 1987.

Pneumothorax

237. Beg MH, Reyazuddin, Faridi MM, Ahmad SH, Shahab T: Spontaneous pneumothorax in children—a review of 95 cases, *Ann Trop Paediatr* 8:18-21, 1988.
238. al-Qudah A: Hydatid cyst causing tension pneumothorax in childhood, *Thorac Cardiovasc Surg* 36:287-289, 1988.
239. Chandra KS, Prasad AS, Prasad CE, Murthy KJ, Srinivasulu T: Recurrent pneumothoraces in miliary tuberculosis, *Trop Geogr Med* 40:347-349, 1988.
240. Byrnes TA, Brevig JK, Yeoh CB: Pneumothorax in patients with acquired immunodeficiency syndrome, *J Thorac Cardiovasc Surg* 98: 546-550, 1989.
241. Roux P, Fisher RM: Chest injuries in children: an analysis of 100 cases of blunt chest trauma from motor vehicle accidents, *J Pediatr Surg* 27:551-555, 1992.
242. Unger JM, Schuchmann GG, Grossman JE, Pellett JR: Tears of the trachea and main bronchi caused by blunt trauma: radiologic findings, *Am J Roentgenol* 153:1175-1180, 1989.
243. Daisley H, Barton EN: Spontaneous pneumothorax in acute paraquat toxicity, *West Ind Med J* 39:180-185, 1990.
244. Pezner RD, Horak DA, Sayegh HO, Lipsett JA: Spontaneous pneumothorax in patients irradiated for Hodgkin's disease and other malignant lymphomas, *Int J Radiat Oncol Biol Phys* 18:193-198, 1990.
245. Nash PE, Tachakra SS, Baird H: Pneumothorax following inhalation of caustic soda fumes, *Arch Emerg Med* 5:45-47, 1988.
246. Luque MA 3d., Cavallaro DL, Torres M, Emmanual P, Hillman JV: Pneumomediastinum, pneumothorax, and subcutaneous emphysema after alternate cocaine inhalation and marijuana smoking, *Pediatr Emerg Care* 3:107-109, 1987.
247. Wilkinson KA, Beckett W, Brown TC: Pneumothorax secondary to foreign body inhalation in a 20 month old child, *J Paediatr Child Health* 28:67-68, 1992.
248. Spector ML, Stern RC: Pneumothorax in cystic fibrosis: a 26-year experience, *Ann Thorac Surg* 47:204-207, 1989.
249. Schidlow DV, Taussig LM, Knowles MR: Cystic Fibrosis Foundation consensus conference report on pulmonary complications of cystic fibrosis [Review], *Pediatr Pulmonol* 15:187-198, 1993.
250. Pollack J: Spontaneous bilateral pneumothorax in an infant with bronchiolitis, *Pediatr Emerg Care* 3:33-35, 1987.
251. Bank A, Christensen C: Unusual manifestation of Langerhans' cell histiocytosis, *Acta Med Scand* 223:479-480, 1988.
252. Singla R, Bhagi RP, Singh P, Anand E: Pulmonary metastases from Ewing's sarcoma—presenting as spontaneous pneumothorax in a young child, *Indian J Chest Dis Allied Sci* 30(2):148-53, 1988.
253. Yellin A, Benfield JR: Pneumothorax associated with lymphoma, *Am Rev Respir Dis* 134:590-592, 1986.
254. Casado FJ, Valdivielso SA, Perez JL, Pozo RJ, Monleon LM, Garcia PJ, Ruiz BA, Garcia TM: Subclavian vein catheterization in critically ill children: analysis of 322 cannulations, *Intensive Care Med* 17(6):350-354, 1991.
255. Cohen MB, A-Kader HH, Lambers D, Heubi JE: Complications of percutaneous liver biopsy in children, *Gastroenterology* 102:629-632, 1992.
256. Urschel JD, Parrott JC, Horan TA, Unruh HW: Pneumothorax complicating cardiac surgery, *J Cardiovasc Surg* 33:492-495, 1992.
257. Frazier WD, Pope TL Jr., Findley LJ: Pneumothorax following transbronchial biopsy. Low diagnostic yield with routine chest roentgenograms, *Chest* 97:539-540, 1990.
258. O'Donnell A, Schoenberger C, Weiner J, Tsou E: Pulmonary complications of percutaneous nephrostomy and kidney stone extraction, *South Med J* 81:1002-1005, 1988.
259. Prystowsky JB, Jericho BG, Epstein HM: Spontaneous bilateral pneumothorax—complication of laparoscopic cholecystectomy, *Surgery* 114:988-992, 1993.
260. Bentur L, Canny G, Thorner P, Superina R, Babyn P, Levison H: Spontaneous pneumothorax in cystic adenomatoid malformation. Unusual clinical and histologic features, *Chest* 99:1292-1293, 1991.
261. Warren SE, Lee D, Martin V, Messink W: Pulmonary lymphangiomyomatosis causing bilateral pneumothorax during pregnancy, *Ann Thorac Surg* 55(4):998-1000, 1993.
262. Abolnik IZ, Lossos IS, Gillis D, Breuer R: Primary spontaneous pneumothorax in men, *Am J Med Sci* 305:297-303, 1993.
263. Reeder SR: Subcutaneous emphysema, pneumomediastinum, and pneumothorax in labor and delivery, *Am J Obstet Gynecol* 154:487-489, 1986.
264. Nakamura H, Konishiike J, Sugamura A, Takeno Y: Epidemiology of spontaneous pneumothorax in women, *Chest* 89:378-382, 1986.
265. Dattola RK, Toffle RC, Lewis MJ: Catamenial pneumothorax. A case report, *J Reprod Med* 35:734-736, 1990.
266. Chippindale AJ, Patel B, Eddleston B: Spontaneous pneumothorax with metastatic seminoma, *Br J Radiol* 62:1100-1102, 1989.
267. Mitlehner W, Friedrich M, Dissmann W: Value of computer tomography in the detection of bullae and blebs in patients with primary spontaneous pneumothorax, *Respiration* 59:221-227, 1992.
268. Bridges KG, Welch G, Silver M, Schinco MA, Esposito B: CT detection of occult pneumothorax in multiple trauma patients, *J Emerg Med* 11:179-186, 1993.
269. Fan LL, Strain JD, Foley C, Bailey WC, Stenmark KR, Young LW: Radiologic case of the month. Giant pulmonary cyst simulating pneumothorax, *Am J Dis Child* 142:189-190, 1988.

270. Ekkelkamp S, Vos A: Congenital cystic adenomatoid malformation of the lung: an unusual presentation, *Zeitschr Kinderchirurg* 42:253-254, 1987.
271. Fein JA, Loiselle J, Eberlein S, Wiley JF, Bell LM: Diaphragmatic hernia masquerading as pneumothorax in two toddlers, *Ann Emerg Med* 22:1221-1224, 1993.
272. Mahfood S, Hix WR, Aaron BL, Blaes P, Watson DC: Reexpansion pulmonary edema [Review], *Ann Thorac Surg* 45:340-345, 1988.
273. Matsuura Y, Nomimura T, Murakami H, Matsushima T, Kakehashi M, Kajihara H: Clinical analysis of reexpansion pulmonary edema, *Chest* 100:1562-1566, 1991.
274. Daniel TM, Tribble CG, Rodgers BM: Thoracoscopy and talc poudrage for pneumothoraces and effusions, *Ann Thorac Surg* 50:186-189, 1990.
275. Wakabayashi A: Thoracoscopic ablation of blebs in the treatment of recurrent or persistent spontaneous pneumothorax, *Ann Thorac Surg* 48:651-653, 1989.
276. Tribble CG, Selden RF, Rodgers BM: Talc poudrage in the treatment of spontaneous pneumothoraces in patients with cystic fibrosis, *Ann Surg* 204:677-680, 1986.
277. Rosseel MT: Intrapleural quinacrine instillation for recurrent pneumothorax or persistent air leak, *Ann Thorac Surg* 55:368-371, 1993.
278. Weissberg D, Ben-Zeev I: Talc pleurodesis. Experience with 360 patients, *J Thorac Cardiovasc Surg* 106:689-695, 1993.
279. Inderbitzi R, Furrer M: The surgical treatment of spontaneous pneumothorax by video-thoroscopy, *Thorac Cardiovasc Surg* 40:330-333, 1992.
280. McLaughlin MJ, McLaughlin BH: Thorascopic ablation of blebs using PDS-endoloop in recurrent spontaneous pneumothorax, *Surg Laparasc Endosc* 1:263-264, 1991.
281. Busch E, Barlam BW, Wallace J, Nealon TF: Intrapleural tetracycline for spontaneous pneumothorax in acquired immunodeficiency syndrome, *Chest* 99:1036-1037, 1991.
282. Hansen MK, Kruse-Andersen S, Watt-Boolsen S, Andersen K: Spontaneous pneumothorax and fibrin glue sealant during thoracoscopy, *Eur J Cardio Thorac Surg* 3:512-514, 1989.
283. Berger JT, Gilhooly J: Fibrin glue treatment of persistent pneumothorax in a premature infant, *J Pediatr* 122:958-960, 1993.
284. Dumire R, Crabbe MM, Mappin FG, Fontenelle LJ: Autologous "blood patch" pleurodesis for persistent pulmonary air leak, *Chest* 101:64-66, 1992.
285. Robinson CL: Autologous blood for pleurodesis in recurrent and chronic spontaneous pneumothorax, *Can J Surg* 30:428-429, 1987.

PART FOURTEEN

Miscellaneous Disorders

CHAPTER 77

Atelectasis

Kai-Håkon Carlsen and Bjarne Smevik

Atelectasis was first described by Laennec in 1819[1] from autopsy findings. The term *atelectasis* means imperfect expansion, and comes from Greek: *atelez (ateles)* = imperfect and *ektasiz (ektasis)* = expansion. Atelectasis of the lung (or parts of the lungs) is an incomplete expansion of pulmonary tissue. This may be caused by a congenital defect (congenital or primary atelectasis) or, as in most cases, a collapse of lung tissue (acquired or secondary atelectasis). Atelectasis is defined as "1. incomplete expansion of a lung or portion of a lung, occurring congenitally as a primary or secondary condition, or as an acquired condition. 2. airlessness of a lung that had once been expanded. 3. collapse of a lung."[2]

ETIOLOGY

Atelectasis may be caused by several different conditions, having in common either obstruction of the bronchial lumen, compression of lung tissue, respiratory muscle weakness such as neuromuscular disease affecting the diaphragm and intercostal muscles, or reduction in surface tension of the periciliary fluid lining the respiratory tract. The most important causes of atelectasis are obstructed airways caused by inflammatory processes, as occur in asthma or lower respiratory tract infections, or foreign bodies in the bronchial tree. A short list of the main causes of atelectasis is given in Box 77-1.

DISEASE MECHANISMS

In congenital malformations, parts of the lung tissue may be without communication with the main bronchial tree, precluding the normal aeration of lung tissue at birth. The affected parts of the lung have never been inflated and have not undergone the normal pulmonary adaptation to extrauterine life.[3] Congenital malformations that occlude or indent the bronchial lumen may also lead to secondary atelectasis developing shortly after birth.[4]

Already 100 years ago, Kohn described collateral communicating pores between neighboring alveoli,[5] and also at the preductal level collateral communication between the peripheral bronchioles and adjacent alveoli has been described.[6] These collateral communications help to ensure an even ventilation:perfusion ratio in the lung. At the more proximal bronchial levels no such collateral communications exist, and occlusion of the bronchial lumen therefore leads to trapping of the air in the lung tissue peripheral to the occlusion. By far the most common form of atelectasis is secondary atelectasis, in which normal lung tissue has collapsed as the result of an occluded or compressed bronchial lumen. After occlusion of the bronchial lumen, the trapped air is gradually absorbed into the blood perfusing the occluded lung tissue, with a subsequent collapse of the lung tissue. The rate of absorption into the bloodstream depends on the solubility of the trapped gases. Atmospheric air is absorbed within a few hours, whereas oxygen

BOX 77-1
Causes of Pulmonary Atelectasis

Intraluminal bronchial obstruction
- Foreign body
  - Nuts
  - Plastic objects
  - Misplaced tracheal tube
  - Others
- Bronchial inflammation with mucus plugging
  - Bronchial asthma
  - Infection
    - Bronchiolitis
      - RS virus or other viruses
    - Pneumonia
      - Viral
      - Bacterial
      - Mycoplasma pneumonia
    - Cystic fibrosis
    - Ciliar dyskinesia
    - Immune deficiencies
    - Chronic lung disease of the newborn
    - After repair of esophageal atresia

Bronchial wall involvement
- Airway stenosis after
  - Intubation
  - Aspiration or inhalation injury

Bronchial wall involvement—cont'd
- Tracheobronchial malacia
- Bronchiectasis
- Bronchial tumor
- Other

Compression of bronchi
- Vascular ring
- Lobar emphysema
- Involvement of lymph nodes

Surfactant dysfunction
- Respiratory distress syndrome of the newborn
- Adult respiratory distress syndrome
- Other

Compression of lung tissue
- Pneumothorax
- Cardiac enlargement
- Hemothorax
- Chylothorax
- Lung tumor

Primary atelectasis
- Congenital malformation

is absorbed within minutes.[7] During ventilation with 100% oxygen, atelectasis may therefore develop more rapidly than during normal air breathing. This may partly explain the increased risk of atelectasis during anesthesia.[8] It has been observed that this risk is further increased in the presence of respiratory tract symptoms such as cough.[8]

Hypoxic vasoconstriction of the pulmonary vessels perfusing the affected lung tissue occurs secondary to occlusion of the bronchial lumen.[9] Hypoxic pulmonary vasoconstriction seems to be the major cause of increased vascular resistance in the atelectatic lung tissue, thereby regulating the ventilation:perfusion ratio. Nevertheless, as seen during anesthesia, the magnitude of shunting is related to the atelectatic area.[10] In experimental animal studies, dynamic compliance of atelectatic dog lung lobes increased during inflation with air. This was mainly a result of increased vascular compliance, suggesting that atelectasis results in a stiffer pulmonary capillary bed.[11]

All processes or procedures occluding the bronchial lumen may cause atelectasis. Misplaced tracheal intubation is one example that may cause total collapse of one lung if the distal part of the endotracheal tube is located in a main bronchus (usually the right one). Foreign bodies in the airways may result in complete or partial occlusion of a bronchus. In cases of complete occlusion, atelectasis occurs. However, even when the bronchial lumen initially is only partly occluded, a total occlusion may gradually develop. Some foreign bodies swell when exposed to the humid respiratory mucous membranes, and thereby cause complete obstruction. On the other hand, impaction of a foreign body into the bronchial lumen may initiate inflammatory processes of the respiratory mucous membranes. This inflammation leads to mucosal swelling, which together with increased bronchial secretions and possibly bronchial smooth muscle contraction may cause total obstruction of the bronchial lumen, thereby causing atelectasis.[12]

Among the most common causes of obstruction of the bronchial lumen, leading to atelectasis, are inflammatory processes within the bronchial tree, eosinophilic inflammation caused by asthma,[13,14] infections such as bronchiolitis (caused by respiratory syncytial virus or other viruses),[15] or bacterial pneumonias. In asthma and bronchiolitis the right middle lobe and the lingula segment are the most common localization of atelectasis, so common that this has been given the name middle lobe syndrome.[16] Enlargement of hilar lymph nodes compressing the middle lobe bronchus has been suggested as the probable cause of this preferential localization.[16] The compression enhances the obstruction that is caused by inflammatory mucus, mucosal edema, and bronchial constriction. Positive bacterial culture findings in bronchoalveolar lavage fluid and in sputum from a majority of children with middle lobe atelectasis in asthma[14] or respiratory syncytial virus infections[15] have recently led to a suggested role of bacterial infection in long-standing atelectases of asthma and bronchiolitis.

A number of cytokines and mediators are involved in the airway inflammation in asthma, bronchiolitis, and other respiratory tract illnesses. They have a number of effects on the bronchial mucosa. In addition to increased mucus secretions, edema of the mucous membranes, and bronchial smooth muscle contraction, destruction of bronchial epithelium and cessation of ciliar function with stagnating sticky mucus within the bronchial lumen occur (Fig. 77-1). The airway inflammation leading to destruction of airway epithelium, as in asthma, also affects the periciliary fluid lining the airway epithelium, reducing the effect of surfactant proteins. This further enhances the tendency to bronchial collapse. Illnesses affecting the surfactant function of the airways are known to be complicated by formation of atelectasis. This is the case for respiratory distress syndrome of the newborn, chronic lung disease of the newborn, and the adult respiratory distress syndrome.[17] Aspiration of irritant fluids such as acids and alkali have this effect, as also seen after aspiration of amniotic fluid[18] and meconium aspiration. Bronchoscopy may demonstrate totally obstructed lobar or segment bronchi in atelectasis of lobes or major lung segments. Figure 77-2 shows a totally obstructed left lower lobe bronchus together with the findings in chest radiography and bronchography from an 11-year-old boy with recurrent lower respiratory tract infections resulting from immunoglobulin G subclass deficiency and abnormal cilia structure. Any disease that renders the individual susceptible to respiratory tract infections and to stagnation of mucus increases the risk of atelectasis development. This includes several types of immune deficiencies, congenital or acquired ciliar dysfunction,[19] cystic fibrosis, and others. Furthermore, in the atelectatic lung altered cellular immune function has been described.[20]

Processes affecting the bronchial wall, leading to a narrowing of the bronchial lumen, predispose to atelectasis. This includes airway stenosis complicating long-standing intubation, tracheobronchomalacia, vascular rings, and tumors such as polyps, papillomas, and bronchial carcinoid.[21] Bronchiolitis obliterans gradually causes fibrotic obliteration of bronchi, leading to atelectasis.[22] Bronchiectasis and atelectasis are occasionally present simultaneously, both caused by long-lasting or recurrent airway inflammation. In addition, bronchiectasis may contribute to atelectasis formation by stagnation of bronchial secretions.

Extrapulmonary processes can compress normal lung tissue without affecting the bronchi initially, as is seen in patients with congenital heart defects[23] and cardiomegaly (Fig. 77-3), and sometimes in patients with pneumothorax or hemothorax.

Rounded atelectasis is a special form of atelectasis seen more often in adults than in children. It is thought to be associated with chronic pleural disease, lung fibrosis, or pleural effusions. It consists of infolding of atelectatic lung tissue together with blood vessels, pleura, and bronchi.[24]

Neuromuscular disease of various types commonly causes atelectasis of lung tissue by several mechanisms. Muscular hy-

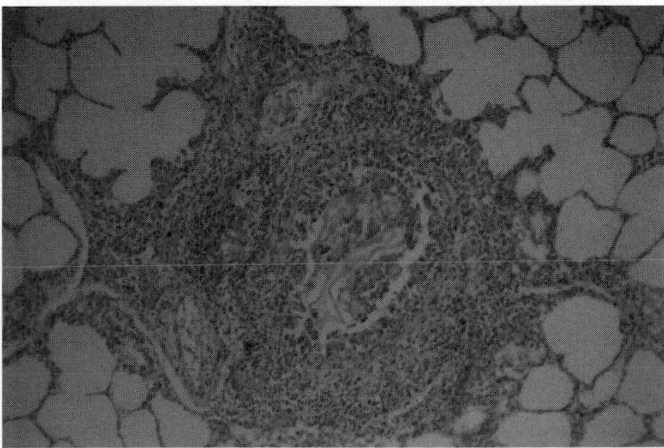

Fig. 77-1. Section of lung tissue from a 20-month-old boy with bronchiolitis. Mucosal and peribronchial inflammation with epithelial destruction and increased intraluminal mucosal secretions and mucus plugging. Hematoxylin-eosin staining. (Courtesy of Aud D. Svindland.)

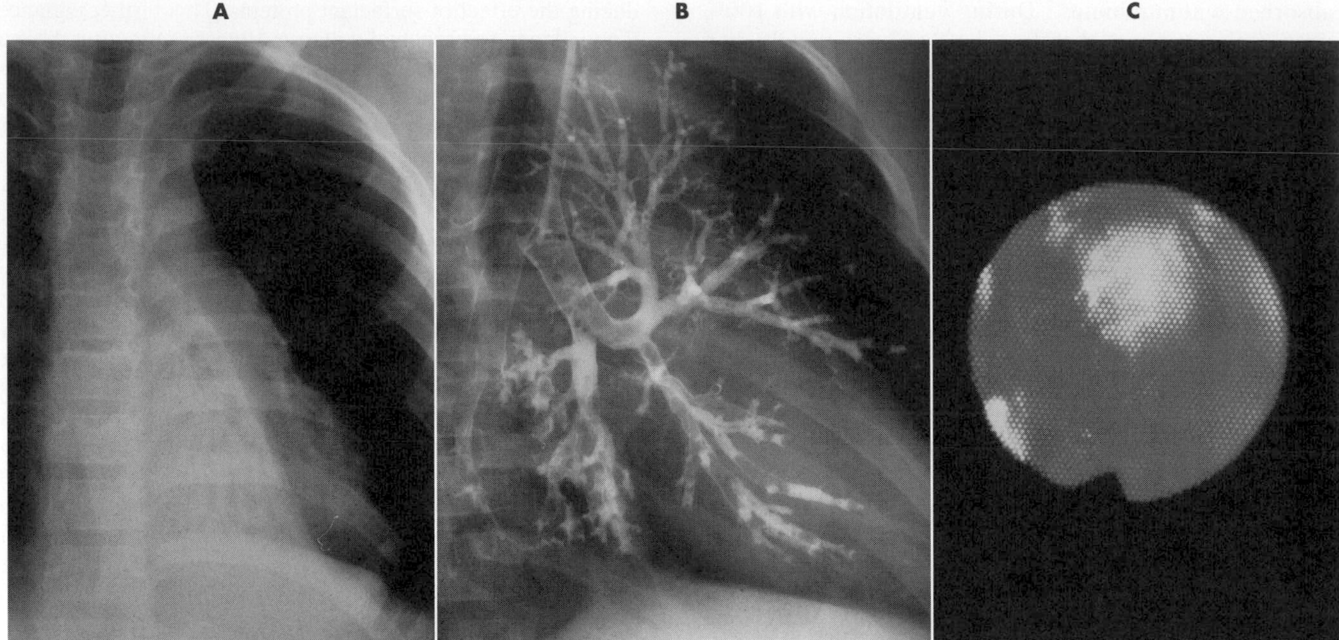

Fig. 77-2. 11-year-old boy with recurrent lower respiratory infections resulting from deficiency of immunoglobulin G_2 and G_4 and abnormal cilial structure. **A,** Radiograph showing atelectasis in left lower lobe. **B,** Bronchography showing pathologic bronchi in left lower lobe with caliber variations and stagnant mucus. **C,** Bronchoscopy showing totally obstructed left lower lobe bronchus. (Courtesy of Nils P. Boye.)

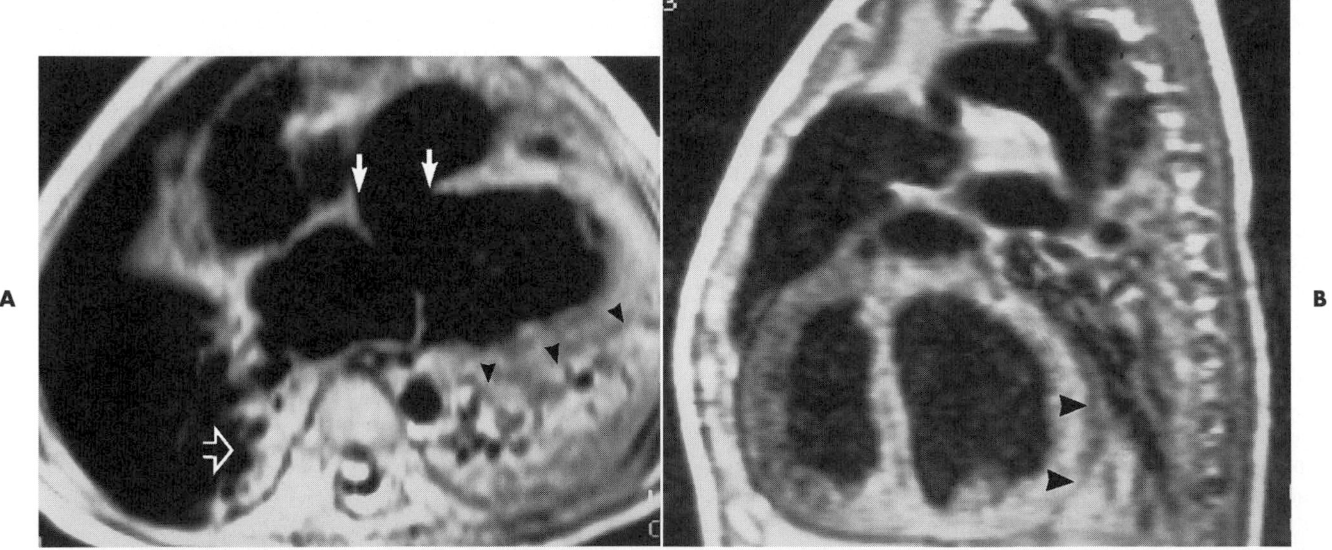

Fig. 77-3. 2-year-old girl with complex congenital heart defect. **A,** Axial T1-weighted magnetic resonance (MR) image showing large ventricular septal defect *(arrows)*. A small atelectasis in the dependent part of the right lung *(open arrow)* was probably induced by general anesthesia. The atelectasis of the left lower lobe *(arrowheads)* was a constant finding in this patient, caused by the enlarged heart. **B,** Parasagittal T1-weighted MR image showing atelectasis of the left lower lobe *(arrowheads)* behind the enlarged heart.

potonia with impaired diaphragmatic movement reduces ventilation and contributes to collapse of lung tissue. Reduced clearing of bronchial secretions and the increased susceptibility to respiratory tract infections further enhance atelectasis formation. Similar mechanisms are seen in acute spinal cord injuries.[25] Hypoventilation may also contribute to the pulmonary collapse, not uncommon during anesthesia in children.[8]

CLINICAL MANIFESTATIONS

The symptoms and signs of atelectasis depend on the extent of atelectasis and the rate of its formation, the age of the patient, and the causative illness. In critically ill infants with respiratory disorders such as respiratory distress syndrome, bronchiolitis, or pneumonia, atelectasis of a lung lobe, occurring suddenly, may cause a severe deterioration. Acute respiratory distress may also occur after aspiration of a foreign body in a previously healthy child. On the other hand, even extensive atelectasis can pass unnoticed clinically. In the case of total obstruction of a bronchus, the hypoxic pulmonary vasoconstriction in the affected lung segment regulates the ventilation:perfusion ratio,[9] thereby minimizing the net result of the atelectasis. However, in the case of atelectasis occurring during anesthesia or in the postoperative period, significant reductions in PaO_2, FEV_1, and FVC have been seen, correlating to size of the atelectatic area.[26]

Symptoms of pulmonary infections may occur because stagnation of secretions predisposes to secondary bacterial infections originating from the atelectatic area.

The clinical signs at examination depend on the size and localization of the atelectatic area. With careful examination an asymmetric expansion of the thorax may be observed with restrained expansion over the atelectatic area. When an entire lung lobe is affected, reduced resonance on percussion and diminished respiratory sounds may be heard at auscultation. In atelectasis of large areas such as an entire lung, displacement of the heart and the mediastinum may take place.

When smaller areas of lung tissue are atelectatic, the clinical signs are scarce and difficult to observe. The diagnosis may depend entirely on chest radiography.

DIAGNOSIS OF ATELECTASIS

The process of diagnosing atelectasis involves first a recognition of the atelectatic tissue and then an attempt at finding the cause of the atelectasis. The diagnosis must be based on an understanding of the etiology, pathophysiology, and anatomy of this phenomenon.

Usually the first imaging modality is chest radiography. Depending on age, clinical condition, and complexity of the process, the study may include frontal, lateral, and oblique views. When lung tissue collapses and atelectasis occurs, the volume of the lung tissue is reduced and the typical changes include elevation of the diaphragm, shift of the mediastinum, and narrowing of the intercostal spaces on the affected side. These signs may be missing when both lungs are affected or when compensatory emphysema develops in parts of the ipsilateral lung. In most cases, biplane chest radiographs give adequate information about the extent of the collapsed lung parenchyma. In the majority of children, repeat chest radiographs suffice to ascertain that the therapy is effective and that the atelectasis has finally cleared. The atelectasis often is seen as an area of increased density. The density may vary with the location and size. An atelectatic lung appears as a radiopaque homogenous hemithorax. A lobar atelectasis is often more dense centrally than in the periphery of the lesion. When volume reduction is pronounced, it often leads to herniation of parts of the contralateral lung across the midline. The lower lobes are most commonly affected by atelectasis.

Different locations and types of atelectasis are associated with certain characteristic radiologic signs:

- Right upper lobe atelectasis in children is often encountered after surgery. The lobe increases somewhat in density and the interlobar fissure may be elevated.
- Left upper lobe atelectasis may produce a density in the upper hilar region on the left side, and the mediastinal structures may be shifted to the left, together with an elevation of the left hemidiaphragm.
- Middle lobe atelectasis is often called right middle lobe syndrome because of its common association with infections or malignancies that cause hilar node enlargement. Middle lobe syndrome is often encountered in children with asthma (Fig. 77-4). The right cardiac contour is indistinct and the atelectasis is usually better recognized on lateral films, where the triangular density points to the hilum with its apex. Compensatory emphysema may produce concave borders.
- Right and left lower lobe atelectases produce a dense triangle medially, with the base at the diaphragm and the apex near the hilum. The heart shadow may obscure this feature unless the radiograph is well exposed. In the lateral projection, the fissure is shifted posteriorly and downward.
- Segmental atelectasis affects parts of a lobe and may be more difficult to delineate. Oblique views are often needed to determine the exact location.
- Focal atelectasis occurs when a subsegmental bronchus is affected, and the density is usually located in the basal lung fields and presents as a thin horizontal or platelike line, often disappearing or "moving" between studies.
- Rounded atelectasis may be confused with a tumor on plain chest films.
- Alveolar atelectasis is commonly encountered in premature babies with the respiratory distress syndrome.

Fluoroscopy may be necessary to determine the exact location of a density and may be helpful in the differential diagnosis. This procedure is also used to localize a suspected foreign body.

Computed tomography (CT) often reveals atelectasis that is not recognized on chest radiographs.[26] The axial projection is preferable when the lesion is located in the periphery of the lungs close to the chest wall, near the heart and great vessels, close to the diaphragm, or in the apical regions. This projection is used in children with malignancies in the search for lung metastases. However, CT of the chest often necessitates general anesthesia in children, and the well-known tendency of general anesthesia to produce dependent atelectasis[27] is of major concern to the pediatric radiologist because lung metastases may be missed (Fig. 77-5). In our experience, general anesthesia produces atelectasis in more than 90% of patients, as opposed to less than 10% when light sedation is used. The CT findings of rounded atelectasis are characteristic: A rounded mass is seen adjacent to a thickened pleural surface in the periphery of the lung, with blurring of the hilar margin caused by the entering vessels and bronchi.[24] CT with a bolus injection of contrast medium may be used to discriminate a tumor from atelectasis.[28] Collapsed lung is appreciably enhanced, whereas tumor enhancement is slow and minimal on rapid sequence CT.[29]

Magnetic resonance (MR) imaging may also clearly depict atelectasis in the axial plane. This modality is superior when the process is located in the apical regions or near the diaphragm because of the ability of MR to produce pictures of equally good quality in any plane. The curved border of the apical and basal portions of the lungs often creates problems with interpretation because of the partial volume effect on CT. However, these problems are not encountered with sagittal and coronal MR views. The MR signal patterns of atelectasis have been described, and obstructive and nonobstructive atelectasis may be differentiated to some extent on the basis of T2

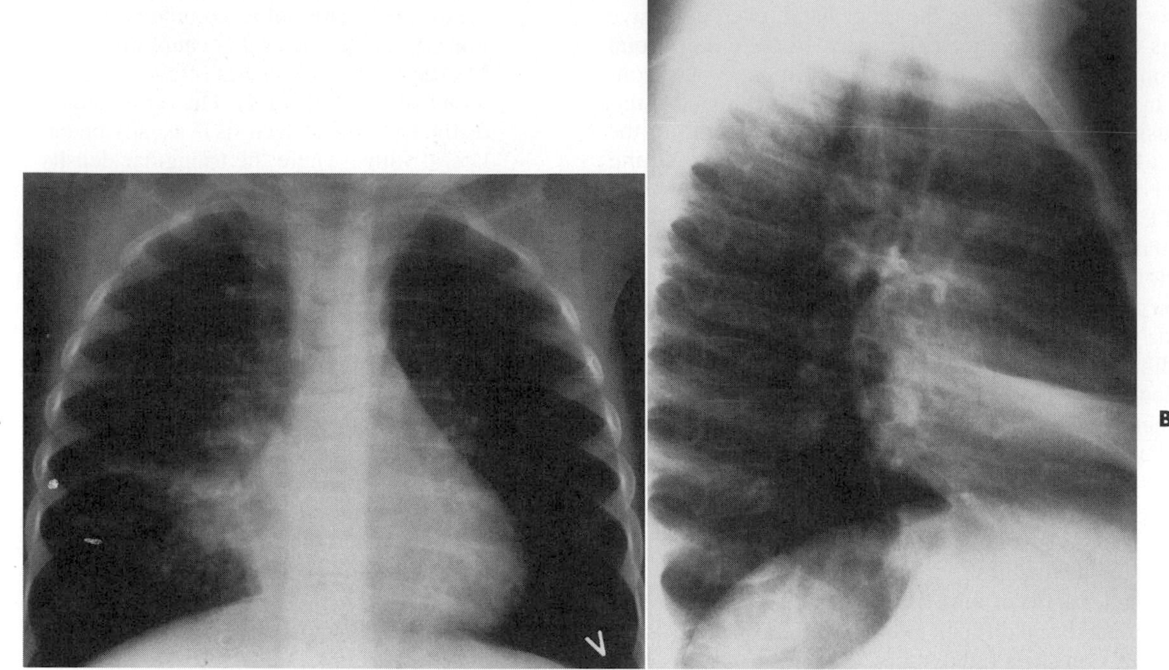

Fig. 77-4. 2-year-old girl with bronchial asthma. **A,** Chest radiography showing atelectasis of the middle lobe. Frontal projection showing blurred right cardiac contour. **B,** Lateral projection showing triangular density pointing its apex toward the hilum.

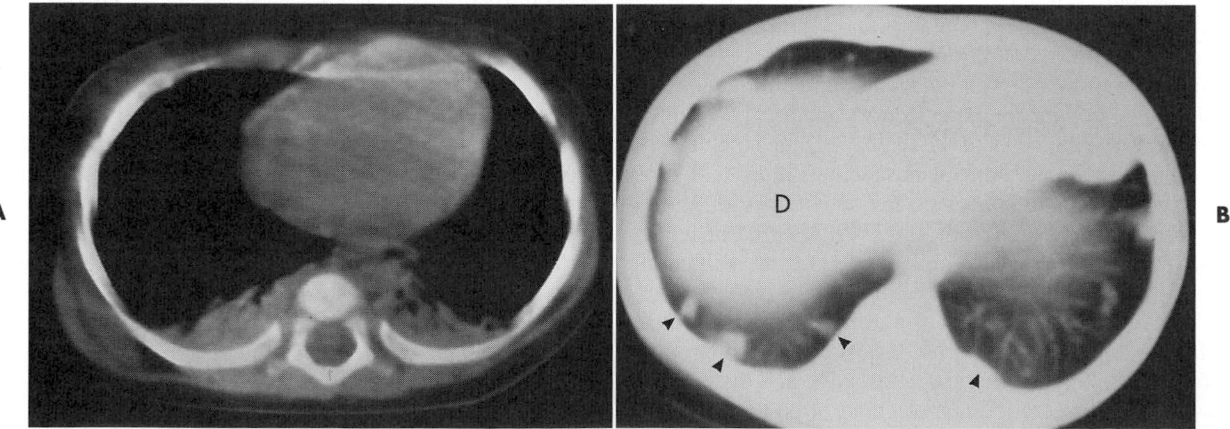

Fig. 77-5. Atelectasis induced by general anesthesia may conceal lung metastases on CT. **A,** 8-month-old boy with typical bilateral atelectases caused by general anesthesia. **B,** 9-month-old girl with peripheral lung metastases *(arrowheads)* from malignant teratoma. *D,* Diaphragm.

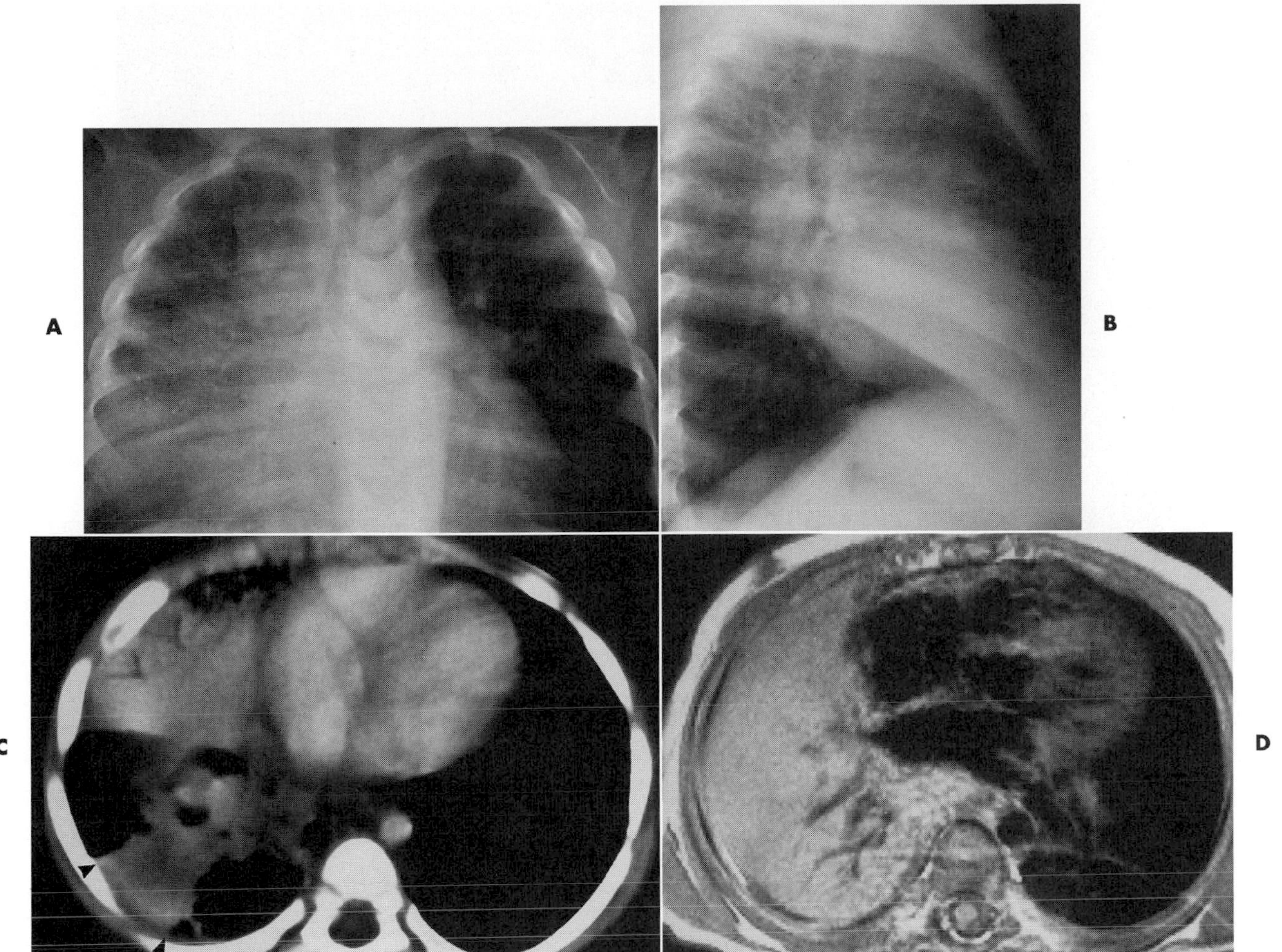

Fig. 77-6. 2-year-old boy with long-standing consolidation of the right middle and lower lobes. **A,** Frontal radiograph showing consolidation mainly of the middle lobe. **B,** Lateral radiograph showing consolidation mainly of the middle lobe. **C,** CT shows additional atelectasis of the right lower lobe *(arrowheads)*. **D,** Axial T1-weighted MR image showing homogenous consolidation anteriorly and atelectasis posteriorly on the right side.

weighted images.[30] Consolidation and atelectasis may produce different patterns on CT and MR (Fig. 77-6).

Ultrasonography of the collapsed lung may be of some benefit when the lesion is combined with pleural effusion or when the density is large enough to provide an acoustic window. An underlying tumor as cause of the atelectasis may then be recognized.[31,32]

Bronchography is useful for the diagnosis of several conditions leading to atelectasis. Bronchomalacia, bronchial stenosis, extrinsic compression, and bronchiectasis may be revealed by this procedure (Fig. 77-7).

Diagnosis of Atelectasis in Neonates

Alveolar atelectasis is an important aspect of the respiratory distress syndrome. Neonates (usually premature infants) with respiratory distress syndrome often need mechanical ventilation, and during intubation the endotracheal tube may inadvertently be situated too low. This may give rise to atelectasis in the contralateral or ipsilateral lung (Fig. 77-8). Other causes of neonatal atelectasis are meconium aspiration and advanced cases of chronic lung disease.[17]

Other Diagnostic Procedures

In order to determine the cause of atelectasis, bronchoscopy by flexible fiberoptic bronchoscopes or rigid bronchoscopes is an important procedure. Foreign bodies in the airways may be diagnosed, localized, and removed via the bronchoscope. Thus bronchoscopy in such cases is the diagnostic and the therapeutic tool of choice.[33] Vascular rings and other narrow areas in the bronchi that predispose to atelectasis may be seen through the bronchoscope. Furthermore, mucus plugs may be visualized and removed by suctioning or by bronchoalveolar lavage followed by suctioning. Biopsies taken through the bronchoscope may occasionally reveal the causal diagnosis of atelectasis, such as ciliar dyskinesia.[19]

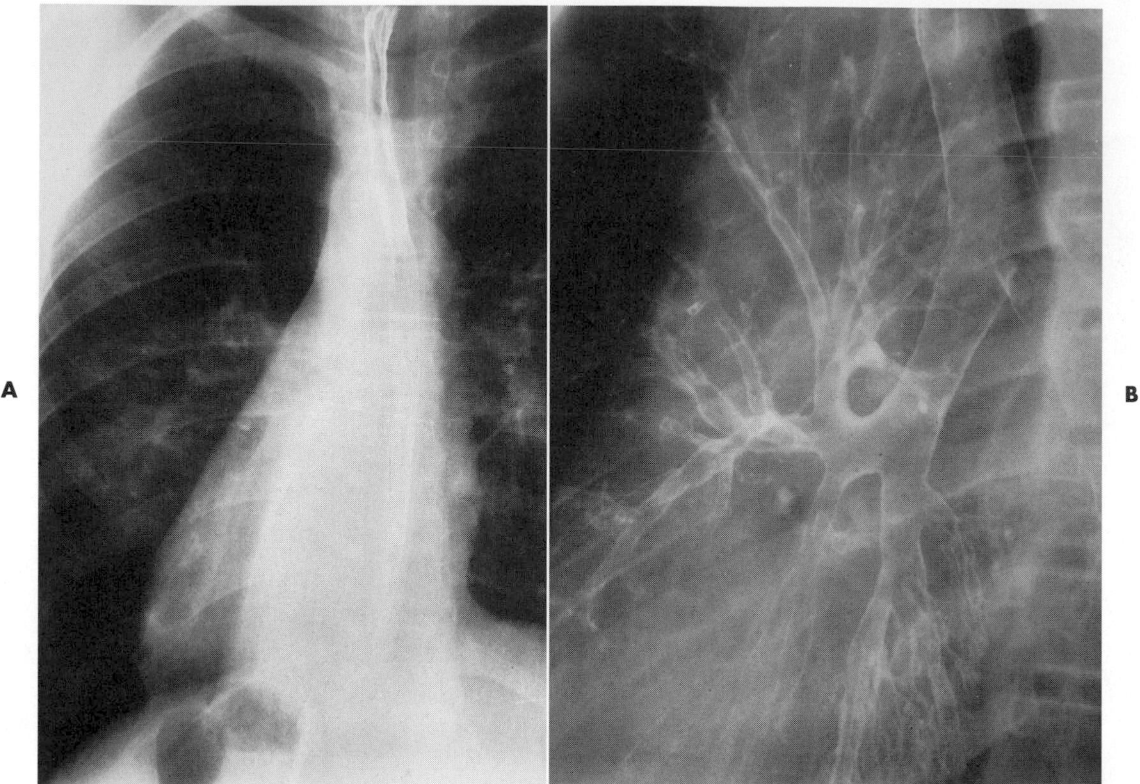

Fig. 77-7. 13-year-old girl with immotile cilia syndrome and situs inversus. **A,** Radiograph showing atelectasis of right lower lobe. **B,** Bronchography showing volume reduction of right lower lobe.

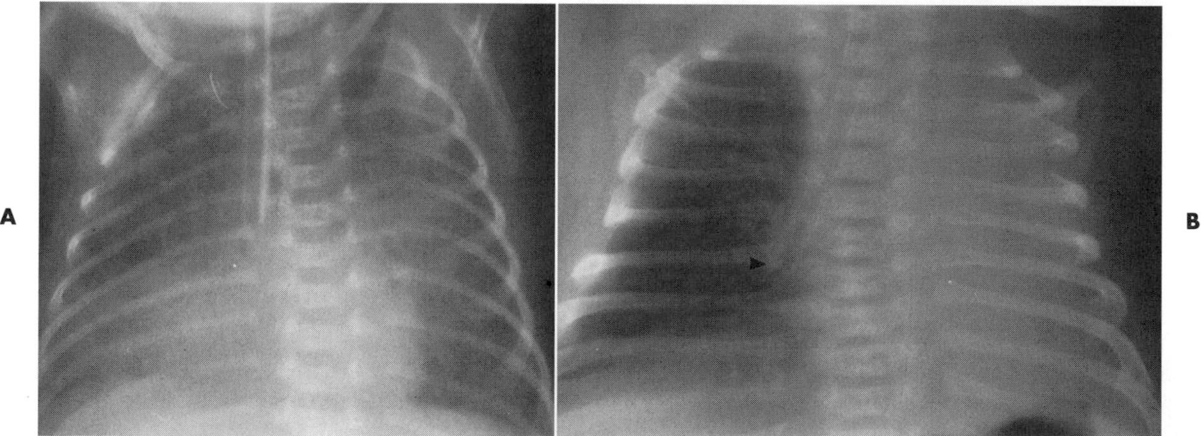

Fig. 77-8. **A,** 9-day-old boy with birth weight 755 g, gestational age 26 weeks. Radiograph showing tracheal tube with tip in right main bronchus and atelectasis of middle lobe. **B,** 8-day-old girl with Kniest syndrome. Tracheal tube with tip into right lower lobe bronchus *(arrowhead)* resulting in atelectasis of left lung.

MANAGEMENT

It is important to remember that atelectasis is not a disease by itself, but a sign of disease. Because many different diseases may lead to atelectasis, the treatment depends on the underlying illness. Primary atelectasis (caused by a congenital malformation) may necessitate surgical intervention according to the primary malformation. Even though atelectasis secondary to malignancies occurs less often in children than in adults, it is important to recognize and treat such an underlying cause.

When atelectasis occurs as a result of airway inflammation such as bronchiolitis, acute attacks of bronchial asthma, or pneumonias, the atelectasis often resolves spontaneously in a few weeks. Inhalation therapy by nebulized bronchodilators such as racemic epinephrine or β_2-agonists and saline may be beneficial in the resolution phase by mobilizing secretions. Such measures are often combined with chest physiotherapy, consisting of positioning, chest vibrations, and suctioning.[34] Measures such as continuous positive airway pressure breathing and positive end expiratory pressure ventilation have also been attempted.[35,36] However, experience shows that physical activity of different kinds may be the most effective physiotherapeutic regimen in mobilizing mucus plugs and resolving atelectasis in children.

Because positive bacterial culture findings from bronchoalveolar lavage or sputum often are present in atelectasis,[14,15] antibiotic treatment may be useful, preferably when bacterial pathogens have been identified.

Although atelectases occurring secondary to pulmonary infections or bronchial asthma usually resolve spontaneously, this is not always the case. Diagnostic or therapeutic procedures such as bronchoscopy may then be needed.

Bronchoscopy is increasingly used in the treatment of atelectasis and is the treatment of choice for removing foreign bodies. Rigid bronchoscopes are usually used.[33] When atelectasis has been present for more than 6 weeks, bronchoscopy is used both for diagnostic and therapeutic measures. In many cases mucus plugs are removed by suctioning and lavage, and the atelectasis resolves.[37] Selective bronchial suctioning in the absence of bronchoscopy has also been used.[38] Attempts at insufflating the atelectatic lung segment have been made using a balloon-tipped catheter introduced through the nostrils, an endotracheal tube,[39] or a fiberoptic bronchoscope.[40] Insufflation has mostly been used in adults. During such procedures it is important to realize that nonatelectatic portions of the lung have higher compliance than the atelectatic portions[11] and that insufflation may result in overexpansion of the normal part of the lung.

In neonates the standard regimen for the removal of atelectases consists of postural drainage with suctioning, and in some cases also selective intubation with suctioning of a major bronchus.[41] Bronchoscopy under direct vision without interrupting the mechanical ventilation has been used with success in 10 cases.[42]

When long-standing atelectasis is a sign of severe lung pathology with formation of bronchiectasis, standard therapeutic measures may be inadequate. Chronic atelectatic portions of the lung are susceptible to recurrent bacterial infections. If there is no other lung disorder, partial lung resection may be useful. This treatment has been used for different causes of atelectasis such as bronchial malformations and stenosis, sequestrations, cysts, lobar emphysema, bronchiectasis, and chronic pneumonia.[43]

Because atelectasis most often is caused by airway inflammation, optimal treatment of the causative disease may be an effective prophylactic measure against atelectasis. This is the case in bronchial asthma with prophylactic antiinflammatory therapy, in immune deficiencies with immunosubstitution, and in cystic fibrosis. In patients with chronic pulmonary symptoms inhalation therapy with nebulized drugs is important in order to facilitate the mobilization of bronchial secretions and to prevent mucus stagnation and plugging.

REFERENCES

1. Laennec RTH: *Diseases of the chest,* ed 4, London, 1819.
2. *Dorland's illustrated medical dictionary,* ed 26, Philadelphia, 1981, WB Saunders.

Disease Mechanisms

3. Sid NS, Shearer LT, Gultekin EK: Retrosternal density: pulmonary underdevelopment or accessory hemidiaphragm, *Pediatr Pulmonol* 11(2):175-180, 1991.
4. Ring-Mrozik E, Hecker WC, Nerlich A, Krandick G: Clinical findings in middle lobe syndrome and other processes of pulmonary shrinkage in children, *Eur J Pediatr Surg.*
5. Kohn HH: Zur Histologie des indurirenden fibrinosen Pneumonie, *Munch Med Wschr* 40:42-45, 1893.
6. Lambert MW: Accessory bronchiolo-alveolar channels, *Anat Rec* 127:472, 1957.
7. Benumof JL: Mechanism of decreased blood flow to atelectatic lung, *J Appl Physiol* 46:1047-1048, 1979.
8. Williams OA, Hills R, Goddard JM: Pulmonary collapse during anesthesia in children with respiratory tract symptoms, *Anesthesia* 47(5):411-413, 1992.
9. Miller FL, Chen L, Malmkvist G, Marshall C, Marshall BE: Mechanical factors do not influence blood flow distribution in atelectasis, *Anesthesiology* 70(3):481-488, 1989.
10. Gunnarsson L, Tokics L, Gustavsson H, Hedenstierna G: Influence of age on atelectasis formation and gas exchange impairment during general anesthesia, *Br J Anesthesia* 66(4):423-432, 1991.
11. Nelin LD, Rickaby DA, Linehan, JH, Dawson CA: Effect of atelectasis and surface tension on pulmonary vascular compliance, *J Appl Physiol* 70(6):2401-2409, 1991.
12. Rothmann BF: Foreign bodies in the larynx and tracheobronchial tree in children. A review of 225 cases, *Ann Otol Rhinol Laryngol* 89:434-436, 1980.
13. Luhr J: Atelectasis in asthma during childhood, *Nord Med* 60:1199, 1958.
14. Springer C, Avital A, Noviski N, Maayan C, Ariel I, Mogle P, Godfrey S: Role of infection in the middle lobe syndrome in asthma, *Arch Dis Child* 67:392-395, 1992.
15. Eriksson J, Nordshus T, Carlsen K-H, Ørstavik I, Westvik J, Eng J: Radiological findings in children with respiratory syncytial virus infection: relationship to clinical and bacteriological findings, *Pediatr Radiol* 16:120-122, 1986.
16. Graham EA, Burford TH, Meyer JH: Middle lobe syndrome, *Postgrad Med* 4:29-34, 1948.
17. McCubbin M, Frey EE, Wagener JDS, Tribbs R, Smith WL: Large airways collapse in bronchopulmonary dysplasia, *J Pediatr* 114:304-307, 1989.
18. Ikeda N, Yamakawa M, Imai Y, Suzuki T: Sudden infant death from atelectasis due to amniotic fluid aspiration, *Am J Forens Med Pathol* 10(4):340-343, 1989.
19. Boutry O, Machillot D, Bellon G, Massonnet B, Dumontel C, Dutailly G, Malou E: Ultrastructure heterogeneity in primary ciliar dyskinesia syndrome, *Ann Pediatr* 37(7):432-436, 1990.
20. Nguyen DM, Mulder DS, Shennib H: Altered cellular immune function in the atelectatic lung, *Ann Thorac Surg* 51(1):76-80, 1991.
21. McDougall JC, Unni K, Gorenstein A, O'Connell EJ: Carcinoid and mucoepidermoid carcinoma of bronchus in children, *Ann Otol Rhinol Laryngol* 89:425-427, 1980.
22. Kargi HA, Kuhn C: Bronchiolitis obliterans. Unilateral fibrous obliteration of the lumen with atelectasis, *Chest* 93(5):11-7-1108, 1988.
23. Stanger P, Lucas RV, Edwards JE: Anatomic factors causing respiratory distress in acyanotic congenital cardiac disease. Special reference to bronchial obstruction, *Pediatrics* 43:760-769, 1969.
24. Carvalho PM, Carr DH: Computed tomography of folded lung, *Clin Radiol* 41:86-91, 1990.
25. Fishburn MJ, Marino RJ, Ditunno JR Jr: Atelectasis and pneumonia in acute spinal cord injury, *Arch Phys Med Rehab* 71(3):197-200, 1990.

Clinical Manifestations

26. Lindberg P, Gunnarson L, Tokics L, Secher E, Lundquist H, Brismar B, Hedenstierna G: Atelectasis and lung function in the postoperative period, *Acta Anesthesiol Scand* 36(6):546-553, 1992.

Diagnosis of Atelectasis

27. Damgaard-Pedersen K, Quist T: Pediatric pulmonary CT-scanning. Anaesthesia-induced changes, *Pediatr Radiol* 9:145-148, 1980.

28. Woodring JH: Determining the cause of pulmonary atelectasis: a comparison of plain radiography and CT, *Am J Roentgenol* 150:757-763, 1988.
29. Onitsuka H, Tsukuda M, Araki A, Murakami J, Torii Y, Masuda K: Differentiation of central lung tumor from postobstructive lobar collapse by rapid sequence computed tomography, *J Thorac Imaging* 6:28-31, 1991.
30. Herold CJ, Kuhlman JR, Zerhouni EA: Pulmonary atelectasis: signal patterns with MR imaging, *Radiology* 178:715-720, 1991.
31. Kelbel von C, Børner N, Schadmand S, Klose KJ, Weilemann LS, Meyer J, Thelen M: Diagnosis of pleural effusions and atelectasis: sonography and radiology compared (German), *Ro Fo* 154:159-163, 1991.
32. Hsu WH, Chianp CD, Hsu JY, Huang WL: Detection of mass lesions in the collapsed lung by ultrasonography, *J Formosan Med Assoc* 91:57-62, 1992.
33. Wood RE, Gauderer MWL: Flexible fiberoptic bronchoscope in the management of tracheobronchial foreign bodies in children: the value of a combined approach with open tube bronchoscopy, *J Pediatr Surg* 19:693-698, 1984.

Management

34. Stiller K, Geake T, Taylor J, Grant R, Hall B: Acute lobar atelectasis. A comparison of two chest physiotherapy regimens, *Chest* 98(6):1336-1340, 1990.
35. Andersen JB, Olesen KP, Eikard B, Jansen E, Quist J: Periodic continuous positive airways pressure, CPAP, by mask in the treatment of atelectasis, *Eur J Respir Dis* 61:20-25, 1980.
36. Fowler AA, Scoggins WG, O'Donohue WJ: Positive end-expiratory pressure in the management of lobar atelectasis, *Chest* 74:497-500, 1978.
37. Wood RE: Clinical application of ultrathin flexible bronchoscopes, *Pediatr Pulmonol* 1:244-248, 1985.
38. Kubota Y, Toyoda Y, Kubota H, Asada A, Sugiyama K: Treatment of atelectasis with a selective bronchial suctioning. Use of a curve-tipped catheter with a guide mark, *Chest* 99(2):510-512, 1991.
39. Susini G, Sisillo E, Bortone F, Salvi L, Moruzzi P: Postoperative atelectasis reexpansion by selective insufflation through a balloon-tipped catheter, *Chest* 102(6):1693-1696, 1992.
40. Tsao TC, Tsai YH, Lan RS, Shieh RS, Shieh WB, Lee CH: Treatment for collapsed lung in critically ill patients. Selective intrabronchial air insufflation using the fiberoptic bronchoscope, *Chest* 97(2):435-438, 1990.
41. Rode H, Millar AJ, Stunden RJ, Cywes S: Selective bronchial intubation for acute post-operative atelectasis in neonates and infants, *Pediatr Radiol* 18(6):494-496, 1988.
42. Shinwell ES: Ultrathin fiberoptic bronchoscopy for airway toilet in neonatal pulmonary atelectasis, *Pediatr Pulmonol* 13(1):48-49, 1992.
43. Hummer HP, Zimmermann T, Vicedom F, Moos P: Surgical indications in persistent atelectasis in early childhood, *Zentralbl Chirurg* 115(24):1533-1542, 1990.

CHAPTER 78

α_1-Antitrypsin Deficiency

Michael Netzel, Kirk Kinberg, George Gwinn, and Robert Townley

HISTORY

Over 35 years ago, the majority of serum trypsin inhibition was localized to the α_1-globulin fraction of plasma.[1] Deficiency of α_1-antitrypsin was first recognized in 1963 when Laurell and Eriksson[2] were routinely surveying and scoring serum protein electrophoresis (SPEP) patterns of hospitalized patients in Sweden. They noted the absence of the α_1-globulin peak in 5 of 1500 patients studied.[2] Subsequent studies of these five patients revealed severe lung disease in three that seemed to be associated with early onset of emphysema.[3] Six years after the initial observation of an association between α_1-antitrypsin deficiency and lung disease in adults, a deficiency of this enzyme inhibitor was noted in some children with familial juvenile cirrhosis and cholestasis.[4] Up to 35% of infants with hepatitis and jaundice may have α_1-antitrypsin deficiency. Since its initial description, a strong association between cigarette smoking and the development of early-onset panacinar emphysema with increased mortality has been observed in α_1-antitrypsin deficiency.[5,6]

PATHOPHYSIOLOGY

α_1-Antitrypsin is a 394-amino-acid glycoprotein with a molecular weight of 52 kilodaltons. It is coded by a single gene on the long arm of chromosome 14. α_1-Antitrypsin is primarily synthesized in and secreted by hepatocytes and makes up approximately 3% of the total mass of serum proteins in a normal adult. Mononuclear phagocytes also produce α_1-antitrypsin to a much smaller extent. On SPEP α_1-antitrypsin accounts for 90% of the area of the α_1-globulin peak (Fig. 78-1). It is a member of the serine proteinase inhibitor (serpin) family and has a broad spectrum of protease inhibitor (PI) activity. α_1-Antitrypsin is responsible for 80% to 90% of serum trypsin inhibitory capacity but is also inhibitory to elastase, collagenase, chymotrypsin, plasmin, thrombin, and other leukocyte and bacterial proteases. In the lung its primary function is to inhibit neutrophil elastase and thereby prevent excessive degradation by proteolysis of the connective tissue elements in the lung architecture. Because of its small molecular size, it diffuses readily into the interstitial fluids from the plasma and in the lung it bathes the alveolar walls after crossing the endothelial-interstitial-epithelial barrier. Its antineutrophil elastase activity protects against the endogenous elastase-like enzymes released by stimulated neutrophils and alveolar macrophages.

α_1-Antitrypsin and Lung Disease

In the normal individual a balance is maintained between proteolytic enzymes and protease inhibitors. Perturbation of this

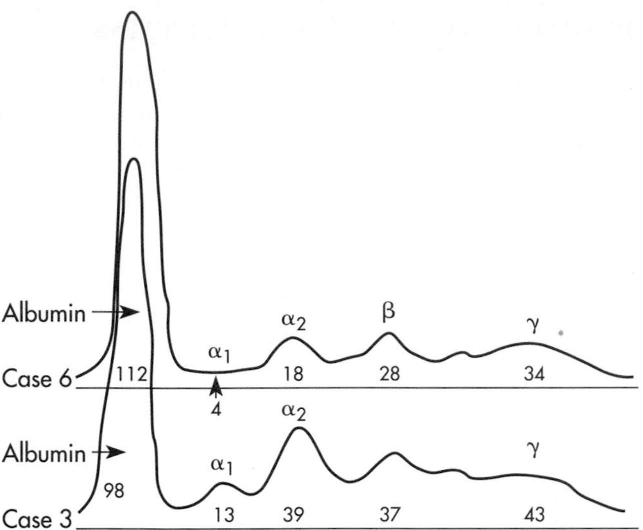

Fig. 78-1. Serum electrophoretic patterns of case 6, proband's sister, and case 3, maternal uncle. Relative amount of protein in peak (numbers) not expressed as percentage. (From Townley RG, Ryning F, Lynch H, Brody AW: *JAMA* 214(2):325-331, 1970.)

balance, either from excessive or unchecked activity of the proteolytic enzymes or from decreased concentration or function of the protease inhibitors, can lead to significant damage of the lung architecture (protease-antiprotease imbalance theory).

Individuals not deficient in α_1-antitrypsin who develop emphysema secondary to cigarette smoke exposure have excessive elastase release by neutrophils. These neutrophils are recruited to the lung because of smoke-induced inflammation and irritation. Cadmium and oxidants in cigarette smoke and oxidative agents released from the inflammatory cells can also inactivate α_1-antitrypsin. The protease-antiprotease imbalance produced is believed to be the cause of the excessive degradation of alveolar walls seen in the common form of emphysema. In α_1-antitrypsin deficiency, which accounts for 1% to 2% of all cases of adult emphysema, even normal levels of neutrophil elastase are unchecked and can lead to destruction of the alveolar walls.

The protease-antiprotease hypothesis is supported by a number of studies. In 1964 Gross et al[7] administered intratracheal papain to rats and produced emphysematous lesions. Others produced similar results using human neutrophil elastase.[8,9] Neutrophil elastase is the major protease in the lower respiratory tract and can degrade elastin, collagen, proteoglycan, and other protein elements of the alveolar walls.[10] Because α_1-antitrypsin is the principal antineutrophil elastase in the lung, it protects the elastin fibers of alveolar septa and bronchiole walls from the neutrophil elastase and other elastase-like enzymes. Deficiency leads to a protease-antiprotease imbalance favoring the destruction of the connective tissue elements in the lung architecture. The principal consequence of the loss of the antiprotease protection in the lower respiratory tract in α_1-antitrypsin–deficient patients is the early onset of panacinar emphysema. In contrast to usual emphysema, the emphysematous changes associated with α_1-antitrypsin deficiency are typically most pronounced in the lower lung zones, presumably because of increased perfusion and therefore concentration of neutrophils.[11] Increased neutrophil elastase activity has been shown in lungs of patients with α_1-antitrypsin deficiency.[12] Factors that can be expected to exaggerate this protease-antiprotease imbalance can accelerate lung destruction in individuals with α_1-antitrypsin deficiency.

Cigarette smoking is the most important risk factor for the development of early-onset emphysema in individuals with α_1-antitrypsin deficiency. Although numerous studies have shown a close correlation between cigarette smoking and emphysema, few researchers have attempted to explain the interaction between cigarette smoke and α_1-antitrypsin–associated lung injury. A series of animal experiments examined the effect of cigarette smoke on α_1-antitrypsin activity.[13] Human neutrophil elastase (HNE) instilled directly into rat tracheas produces emphysema. Carp and Janoff[13] incubated HNE with human α_1-antitrypsin in a test tube. When HNE incubated with α_1-antitrypsin was instilled into rat tracheas, it did not produce emphysema. Interestingly, they found that HNE and α_1-antitrypsin treated with cigarette smoke was again able to cause emphysematous changes. Apparently oxidants in the cigarette smoke inhibit the ability of α_1-antitrypsin to bind with HNE.[13] These experiments underscore how critical it is for children identified as being deficient in α_1-antitrypsin to avoid cigarette smoke to help minimize lung parenchymal damage.

Tobacco smoking can contribute to the protease-antiprotease imbalance in other ways. It increases migration of neutrophils into the airways and increases the number of macrophages and their elastolytic activity.[14] Neutrophils stimulated by smoke can also produce oxidants to inactivate α_1-antitrypsin.

α_1-Antitrypsin and Hepatic Disease

The pathogenic mechanisms of liver disease in α_1-antitrypsin deficiency are unknown. Hepatic damage could result from protease-antiprotease imbalance, although PI null-null individuals with no antiprotease activity do not demonstrate liver disease, or from intracellular accumulation of aggregated protein Z. Accumulation is thought to occur because of a secretory defect resulting from an abnormal primary amino acid structure, incomplete glycosylation, and variant protein folding. The abnormal α_1-antitrypsin molecule accumulates as an insoluble aggregate within the lumen of the hepatic rough endoplasmic reticulum. Diastase-resistant intracytoplasmic globules that are positive on periodic acid–Schiff (PAS) stain are seen in periportal hepatocytes. Immunofluorescence and immunocytochemical studies have shown this material to be antigenically related to α_1-antitrypsin.[3,15]

Other factors may also play a role in the severity of the hepatic disease. α_1-Antitrypsin–deficient hepatic disease is more likely to progress to cirrhosis in male patients or in relatives of other affected individuals. If an α_1-antitrypsin–deficient PI ZZ fetus has a previous sibling with PI ZZ phenotype and no hepatic disease or hepatic disease that resolved, its risk of developing severe hepatic disease is 13%. This risk significantly increases to 40% when a previous sibling with α_1-antitrypsin deficiency had severe hepatic disease.[16] Also, α_1-antitrypsin–deficient infants who were breast fed appeared to have some protection against severe hepatic disease and death in studies by Udall et al,[17,18] possibly because of protease inhibitors in the breast milk binding to intestinal luminal protease enzymes and preventing their crossing to the systemic circulation and thereby contributing to the destruction of the hepatic tissue.

α_1-antitrypsin is an acute-phase reactant, and elevated levels of α_1-antitrypsin are seen in response to infections and inflammatory conditions, suggesting a role in inhibiting proteolytic enzymes released by inflammatory cells. Trauma, hemorrhage, and neoplasms also elevate α_1-antitrypsin levels. Levels are also influenced by estrogens and rise during pregnancy and in women on birth control pills. However, this secretory reserve is not present in individuals with α_1-antitrypsin deficiency. Glucocorticoids can indirectly decrease levels by decreasing inflammation.

α_1-ANTITRYPSIN PROTEASE INHIBITOR PHENOTYPES AND AIRWAY RESPONSIVENESS

Several studies have attempted to correlate various pulmonary pathology with PI phenotypes. Most studies have focused on the generally accepted emphysematous changes associated with α_1-antitrypsin deficient phenotype PI ZZ. However, al-

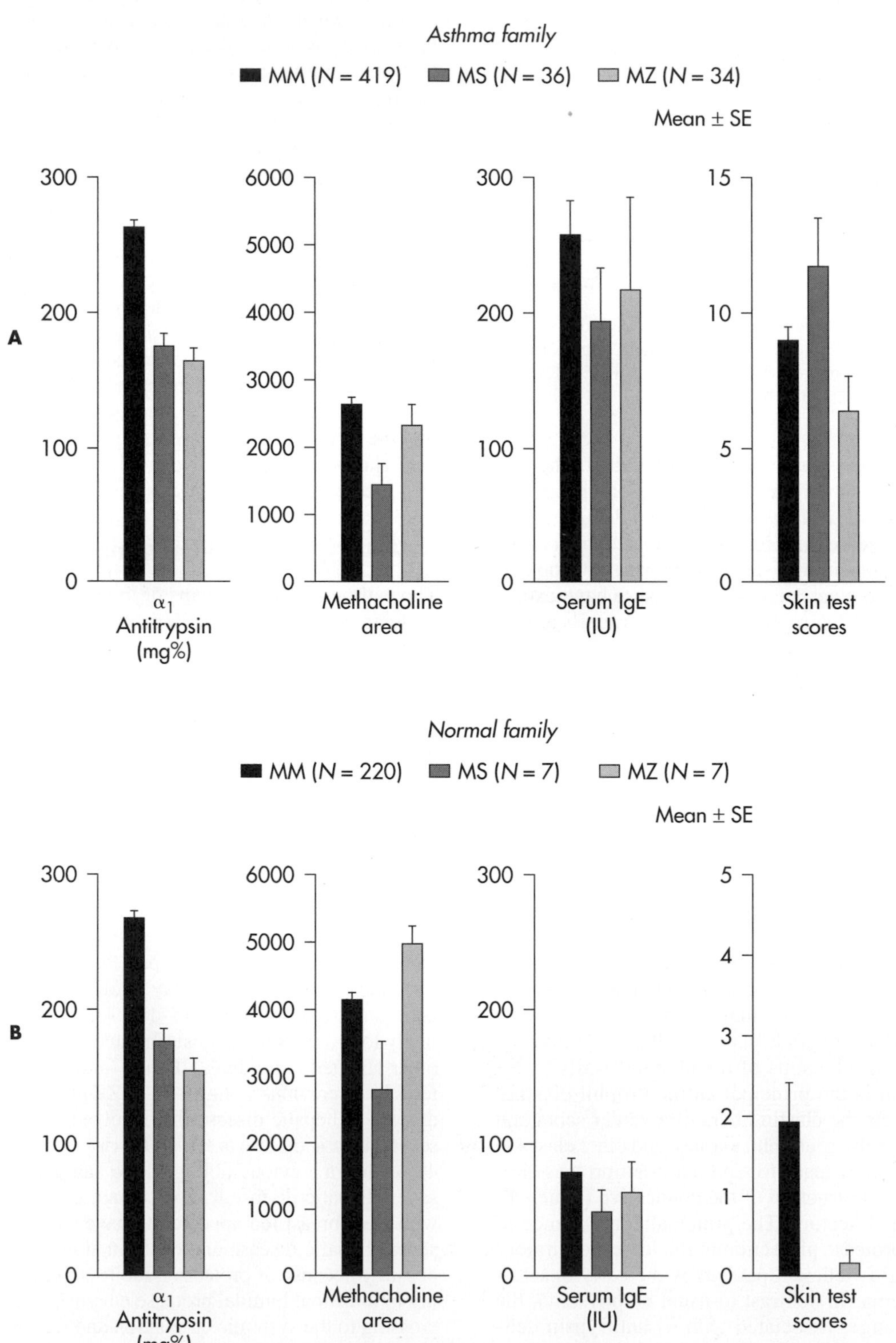

Fig. 78-2. A, Mean values (±SE) in homozygous and heterozygous PI phenotype subjects for α_1-antitrypsin level, methacholine area, serum IgE level, and skin test scores in asthma family members. **B,** Mean values (±SE) in homozygous and heterozygous PI phenotype subjects for α_1-antitrypsin level, methacholine area, serum IgE level, and skin test scores in normal family members. (Data from Townley RG, Southard JG, Radford, P, Hopp RJ, Bewtra AK, Ford L: *Chest* 98:594-599, 1990.)

though still controversial, several disease states also appear to be associated with a variety of the heterozygous states. Townley et al[19] investigated the correlation between PI phenotype (MM, MS, or MZ) in both asthmatic and normal families with respect to variations in methacholine sensitivity. Area under the methacholine dose-response curve was used as a measure of the degree of airway hyperresponsiveness, with lower areas representing higher degrees of hyperresponsiveness. In both asthmatic and normal families the PI MS phenotype was correlated with a significantly greater methacholine-induced bronchial hyperresponsiveness than in PI MM and PI MZ phenotype individuals. This suggests that the PI S allele may be associated with bronchial hyperresponsiveness and asthma[19] (Fig. 78-2). The serum IgE level and total skin test score were not significantly different among the various PI types tested.

Although the PI MM phenotype is associated with normal levels of α_1-antitrypsin, it appears that there may be a functional defect in α_1-antitrypsin in some asthmatic patients. Gaillard et al[20] found that although asthmatic patients had a higher absolute α_1-antitrypsin level, the functional capacity was markedly lower than in normals with the same PI MM phenotype. The study by Gaillard et al[20] suggests that a functional rather than quantitative deficiency of α_1-antitrypsin may play an important role in the inflammatory process characterizing asthma. Interestingly, a high proportion of α_1-antitrypsin–deficient individuals have symptoms suggestive of asthma. Brantley et al[6] in a National Heart, Lung, and Blood Institute (NHLBI) study reported that 20 of 120 (17%) α_1-antitrypsin–deficient individuals had wheezing or a significant response to a bronchodilator. Townley et al[21] noted a similar relationship in their paper in 1970. Although the significance of this is unknown, it does occur more often than expected and is often misdiagnosed as asthma. It also provides an impetus to treat α_1-antitrypsin–deficient patients with maximum bronchodilator therapy.

GENETICS AND EPIDEMIOLOGY

α_1-Antitrypsin gene alleles are inherited in an autosomal codominant fashion, and the α_1-antitrypsin PI phenotype is the result of complete independent expression of the two parental alleles. There are at least 75 known variants, which result from DNA substitutions, deletions, or insertions resulting in single amino acid substitutions or stop codons.[22]

The vast majority are not clinically significant. The PI allele products (normal and deficient) are labeled (A through Z), corresponding to their relative electrophoretic mobility initially in starch or polyacrylamide gels and now on isoelectric focusing (IEF) (Fig. 78-3). Faster-migrating bands are given earlier alphabetic letters and slower bands have later letters. The normal PI M allele is the most common phenotype and has midrange mobility. PI M is found in 90% of individuals of European descent, and α_1-antitrypsin levels are normal. Common α_1-antitrypsin variants include PI S and PI Z. The PI S allelic variant is more common than the PI Z allele and is more prominent in southern Europe, especially Portugal, than elsewhere in Europe and in Puerto Rico. Its allelic frequency is 2% to 4% in white people of northern European descent. The PI Z allele has the slowest electrophoretic mobility. If an allele is not expressed, it is designated null. Genotyping, if necessary, can be accomplished by a variety of techniques, such as the polymerase chain reaction, gradient gel analysis, or allele-specific amplification.

The vast majority of individuals who are severely deficient in α_1-antitrypsin (<15% of normal levels) are homozygous for the allelic variant PI Z and are designated PI ZZ. Most of these PI ZZ individuals are white; the PI Z allele is rarely found in black or Asian populations or Eskimos. The frequency of the PI Z allele in white people of northern European descent is 1% to 2%, in Iranians it is 2.2%, and in New Zealand Maoris it is 8.2%.[23,24] Prevalence of PI ZZ homozygotes has been estimated between 1 in 1670 and 1 in 3500 in populations of European descent. This makes severe hereditary α_1-antitrypsin deficiency only slightly less common than cystic fibrosis and more common than cystinuria and phenylketonuria (Table 78-1). Deficiency of α_1-antitrypsin accounts for 1% to 2% of all cases of emphysema in the United States (approximately 20,000 to 40,000 individuals).[5,24] Not all individuals severely deficient in α_1-antitrypsin with PI ZZ phenotype experience significant clinical sequelae and decreased life spans. The actual percentage is unknown but is thought to be as much as 5%. The

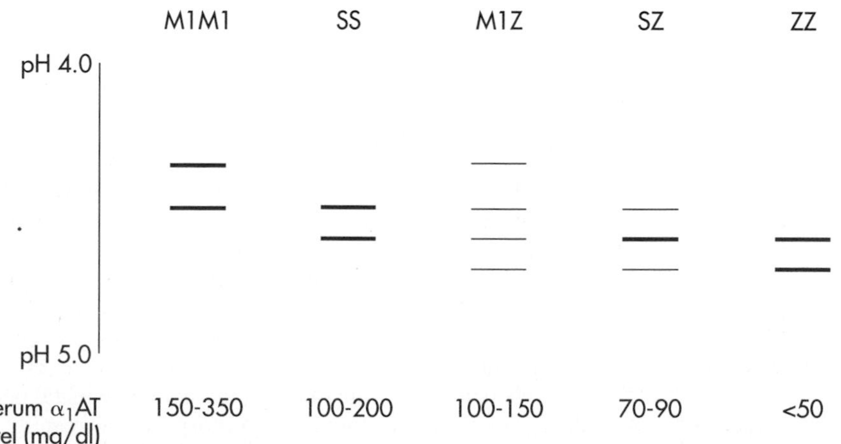

Fig. 78-3. Isoelectric focusing of serum reveals two major α_1-antitrypsin bands between pH 4 and 5; each set is donated by one parent (four bands are present in the MZ PI type). The most common PI type associated with clinically significant α_1-antitrypsin deficiency is ZZ with serum α_1-antitrypsin levels less than 50 mg/dl. (From Gadek JE, Crystal RG. In Stanbury JB, Wyngaarden JB, Fredrickson DS, Goldstein JL, Brown MS, eds: *The metabolic basis of inherited disease,* ed 5, New York, 1983, McGraw-Hill.)

Table 78-1 Prevalence of Inherited Disorders

DISORDER	FREQUENCY
Congenital heart	1/120
Down syndrome	1/700
Cleft lip or palate	1/1000
Cystic fibrosis	1/2000
α_1-Antitrypsin deficiency	1/2500
Phenylketonuria	1/10,000
Cystinuria	1/15,000

Data from Gadek JE, Crystal RG. In Stanbury JB, Wyngaarden JB, Fredrickson DS, Goldstein JL, Brown MS, eds: *The metabolic basis of inherited disease,* ed 5, New York, 1983, McGraw-Hill.

reason for this is unknown but may be related to environmental and other genetic factors, including variations in the expression of the neutrophil elastase gene.

The various α_1-antitrypsin PI types can be categorized into four groups based on enzyme function, IEF pattern, and serum level: normal (normal function and normal levels), deficient (α_1-antitrypsin levels less than normal), null (no detectable α_1-antitrypsin levels), and dysfunctional (normal level but altered function).[25] There is only one known dysfunctional variant (PI Pittsburgh), which forms a molecule homologous to antithrombin III, resulting in death of the patient of hemorrhagic complications. Deficiency alleles are considered clinically significant if they result in α_1-antitrypsin levels less than 35% of normal (80 mg/dl commercial standard or 11 μM true standard). Individuals with α_1-antitrypsin levels below this level are thought to be at higher risk to develop emphysema than the general population. Above this level the lung appears to protect itself adequately. PI ZZ is the most common deficient phenotype of α_1-antitrypsin deficiency with 10% to 20% of normal PI MM levels. Not only is secretion diminished, but the association constant of the PI Z molecule for neutrophil elastase is less than that of the normal PI M molecule, indicating that it is less effective as an elastase inhibitor.[26] Relative deficiency exists in other α_1-antitrypsin PI variants. PI SS homozygotes and PI SZ heterozygotes have α_1-antitrypsin mean levels of 52% and 37% of PI MM serum levels, respectively, and only rarely does the phenotype PI SZ develop early-onset emphysema. PI MS heterozygotes have mean α_1-antitrypsin levels of 80% of normal, whereas PI MZ heterozygotes have intermediate levels between PI ZZ and PI MM of 57%. These phenotypes are not thought to be at increased risk for development of emphysema, although there is some controversy over this issue with respect to PI MZ.[27-30] PI MZ individuals may be at more risk of developing pulmonary disease if they are exposed to various factors over a prolonged period of time that promote inflammation, such as tobacco smoke, infections, pollutants, and other irritants, or if they have other impaired host defenses, such as IgA deficiency.

Rarely observed phenotypes associated with clinically significant deficiency include the nonexpressing homozygous PI null-null, or a heterozygous-deficient allele PI Z-null, and occasional PI SZ heterozygotes with α_1-antitrypsin levels below 11 μM. Deficient null alleles represent fewer than 1% of all α_1-antitrypsin alleles. PI null-null phenotypes have no α_1-antitrypsin to protect their lung connective tissue and are at very high risk of developing emphysema early in life, up to 10 years earlier than individuals with PI ZZ phenotype. Even rarer PI alleles associated with obstructive lung disease and an α_1-antitrypsin deficiency similar to the PI Z allele (<15% of normal serum levels of α_1-antitrypsin) include M_{malton}, M_{duarte}, $M_{heerlen}$, $M_{procida}$, M_{cobalt}, $M_{cagliari}$, and PI P. Other mutations exist and continue to be discovered.

CLINICAL AND NATURAL HISTORY

α_1-Antitrypsin deficiency is mainly a disease of adults. It commonly manifests as dyspnea on exertion associated with early onset of emphysema. However, children can show manifestations of the disease.

α_1-Antitrypsin Pulmonary Disease in Children

In children, chronic progressive respiratory disease associated with α_1-antitrypsin deficiency is rare but may develop. Pulmonary anatomic changes (diffuse airspace and bronchial gland enlargement and slight dilation of small airways) may occur before the development of clinically significant respiratory disease and pathologically significant panacinar emphysema.[31] Infants and children may develop a chronic cough, wheezing, or progressive dyspnea on exertion at any time. If emphysema is complicated by other respiratory diseases and is severe, digital clubbing may occur. Digital clubbing can also occur with familial juvenile cirrhosis, which is another manifestation of α_1-antitrypsin deficiency in children. Significant respiratory disease may be manifested by emphysema alone or emphysema complicated by bronchitis, bronchiectasis, or localized pulmonary cavitation. Liver disease is usually associated with lung disease in children. Children rarely have only respiratory manifestations. α_1-Antitrypsin deficiency in children can be confused with cystic fibrosis, immunodeficiency disorders, and asthma. Physical examination may reveal growth retardation, clubbing, and an increased anteroposterior diameter of the chest in severe cases. Chest roentgenograms may reveal overinflation with depressed diaphragms and hyperlucency of the basilar lung fields.

α_1-Antitrypsin Hepatic Disease in Children

Hepatic disease in children with α_1-antitrypsin deficiency is much more typical than emphysema. Most commonly it manifests as hepatitis with jaundice in the neonate. Although the precise incidence is unknown, it probably occurs in 10% to 20% of children with α_1-antitrypsin deficiency PI ZZ phenotype. The spectrum of liver disease has expanded over the past 25 years to include cases of cryptogenic cirrhosis, chronic active hepatitis, and hepatoma in adults (particularly men), as well as later childhood. However, significant lung and liver disease rarely coexists in adults. Since 1969, when Sharp et al described the association between familial juvenile cirrhosis and α_1-antitrypsin deficiency, 13% to 40 % of children with neonatal cholestatic jaundice have been found to have α_1-antitrypsin deficiency with either PI Z or PI SZ phenotypes.[3,23,32-35] Previously many of these newborns were given a diagnosis of idiopathic neonatal hepatitis with giant cell transformation. A prospective screening study for α_1-antitrypsin deficiency in 200,000 Swedish newborns identified 127 children with the deficiency, 11% of whom had neonatal cholestasis and 6% other signs of liver dysfunction.[36] In the United States, a newborn screening program in Oregon found 21 PI Z homozygous infants out of a total of 107,038 infants screened.

One had neonatal hepatitis and five had hepatomegaly, abnormal liver function tests, or both.[37]

In affected children with PI ZZ, the course of disease can be highly variable. Acholic stools, jaundice, failure to thrive, and hepatomegaly generally appear in the first week to month of life. Often the jaundice disappears by the third or fourth month of life but may persist for up to 8 months. In most children the liver disease disappears; however, in 2% to 3% a more chronic picture may evolve, with the eventual development of familial juvenile cirrhosis and portal hypertension. The course of hepatic disease is variable, although it was initially described as progressive and fatal. Periods of hepatocellular damage alternate with periods of disease inactivity. Prognosis is poorer if the serum glutamic-oxaloacetic transaminase (SGOT) levels remain elevated through the third year of life. The neonatal cirrhosis associated with α_1-antitrypsin deficiency is often fatal,[38] and liver transplantation has been used effectively in treatment.[39] Transplantation changes the patient's PI phenotype to that of the donor. Abnormal liver enzyme levels can also be seen in infants with PI SZ phenotype; however, only 2% of children with the PI SZ phenotype have abnormal liver enzyme levels at age 12.

The low incidence of homozygous PI ZZ phenotype makes long-term follow-up somewhat problematic. Much of what is known about the natural and clinical history of α_1-antitrypsin deficiency comes from epidemiologic studies in Sweden and more recently from the NHLBI reports in the United States. Only two widespread neonatal screenings have been performed, one by Sveger[36] in Sweden and one carried out in the United States.[37] Wall et al[40] studied a cohort of 22 adolescent subjects initially identified in the Oregon neonatal screening program. They found that although some (6 of 21) of the young children with α_1-antitrypsin deficiency had mildly abnormal liver function tests, these tended to resolve by adolescence. No lung damage could be detected by routine pulmonary function testing in the unselected teenagers with α_1-antitrypsin deficiency. However, Wall et al[40] noted that epidemiologic studies routinely show clinically apparent emphysema as early as age 25 but usually between 25 to 40 years of age in α_1-antitrypsin–deficient patients. Something in early adulthood apparently triggers the rapid decline in pulmonary function. Based on epidemiologic evidence Wall et al[40] suggest that cigarette smoking is the major factor responsible for the rapid decline in pulmonary function. Also, because α_1-antitrypsin–deficient nonsmokers develop clinically significant emphysema at a much later age, if at all, than α_1-antitrypsin–deficient individuals who smoke, screening programs to identify individuals with the deficiency and educational intervention to prevent cigarette smoking, decrease exposure to respiratory irritants, and aggressively treat respiratory tract infections would be cost-effective compared with the cost of years of augmentation therapy with human α_1-antitrypsin.

α_1-Antitrypsin Pulmonary Disease in Adults

Adults who develop clinical respiratory manifestations of α_1-antitrypsin deficiency usually do so in the third to fifth decades of life.[5,6,41,42] It usually appears between the ages of 25 and 40 in patients who smoke and between 40 and 50 years in nonsmokers. However, occasionally nonsmokers do well and survive into their seventies and eighties. Other hereditary factors or environmental irritants may play a role.

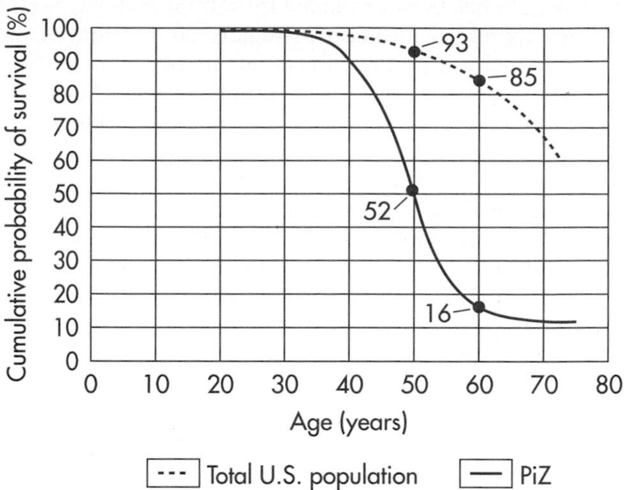

Fig. 78-4. Cumulative probability of survival for 120 adult PI Z homozygotes evaluated at the National Institutes of Health is compared with that of the total U.S. population. All patients in the PI Z group had serum α_1-antitrypsin levels below 80 mg/dl and symptoms of emphysema. The group included men, women, smokers, and nonsmokers. Dots indicate cumulative probability of survival at 50 and 60 years of age for each group. (From Brantley ML, Paul LD, Miller BH, Falk RT, Wu M, Crystal RG: *Am Rev Respir Dis* 138:327-336, 1988.)

In adults the usual presentation is a slowly progressive, severe panacinar emphysema that most often manifests with progressive dyspnea, but other respiratory manifestations may occur. Chronic cough, acute or chronic bronchitis, bronchiectasis, and airway reactivity may add to the clinical picture or be the presenting symptoms. Other factors such as coexisting asthma, lower respiratory tract infections, and other respiratory irritants contribute to the variability of the disease. The onset of dyspnea associated with emphysema and prognosis in nonsmokers with α_1-antitrypsin deficiency is only marginally worse than that of nondeficient individuals who smoke. But significant symptoms and pathology occur 10 to 15 years earlier in α_1-antitrypsin–deficient individuals who smoke. Larsson[5] reported that the average age of onset of symptoms (primarily dyspnea) in nonsmoking individuals with α_1-antitrypsin deficiency was 52, whereas in individuals who smoked it was 40. In his 14-year follow-up of 246 PI ZZ adults in Sweden, 47% of nonsmokers developed emphysema, compared with 85% of smokers with α_1-antitrypsin deficiency. Men and women were equally and similarly affected, unlike persons who are not α_1-antitrypsin deficient. The progression of pulmonary disease in smokers with α_1-antitrypsin deficiency is relentless and often fatal. In 1988 Brantley et al[6] reported information on the clinical course and natural history of individuals with severe α_1-antitrypsin deficiency in the United States (NHLBI). Comparing their population of patients to the total U.S. population, the survival curve shows increased mortality in the α_1-antitrypsin–deficient emphysematous patients, with 52% living to age 50 and only 16% living to age 60 versus 93% and 85%, respectively, of the total population (Fig. 78-4). An important addition is that if the patient smokes, the life expectancy is decreased at least 10 years.

The progressive decline in lung function during aging is accentuated in α_1-antitrypsin deficiency. The destructive lung disease in α_1-antitrypsin deficiency, if untreated by augmentation therapy, is progressive, and the annual rate of decline of lung function has been examined by several authors. Normal nonsmoking adults lose approximately 20 to 30 ml of pulmonary function from their forced expiratory volume (FEV) each year. A smoker who is not α_1-antitrypsin deficient will lose 45 to 90 ml, or 1.5 to 3 times as much (depending on susceptibility) each year.

In contrast, α_1-antitrypsin–deficient patients who do not smoke will lose 80 to 100 ml of lung function from their FEV_1 each year, and those who smoke lose more than 300 ml per year.[43] Buist et al[44] noted that the annual loss in FEV_1 in patients with α_1-antitrypsin deficiency was significantly greater in those who initially had an FEV_1 in the range of 30% to 65% of predicted (111 ml) than in those with an initial FEV_1 less than 30% (45 ml). Similarly, Brantley et al[6] also noted a decrease in the annual rate of decrement in FEV_1 in patients with an initial FEV_1 less than 30% of that predicted. Also, there was a continued increased annual loss of diffusion capacity suggestive of ongoing destruction of the alveolar units even in patients with severe obstructive dysfunction.

On physical examination the anteroposterior diameter may be enlarged (barrel chest). Accessory muscle use and hypertrophy may be evident. There may be decreased breath sound intensity on auscultation. A few expiratory wheezes can occasionally be detected. Percussion of the chest reveals increased tympany and hyperinflation with decreased movement of the diaphragms.

DIAGNOSIS

The diagnosis of α_1-antitrypsin deficiency should be suspected in a number of clinical situations. Because up to 35% of cases of neonatal hepatitis are caused by α_1-antitrypsin deficiency, any infant with liver dysfunction should be evaluated for this deficiency. Correspondingly, older children with hepatic disease or a combination of hepatic and pulmonary disease should also undergo evaluation. Young adults with significant respiratory insufficiency and evidence of obstructive lung disease or individuals between the ages of 30 and 45 with chronic shortness of breath and coughing could have α_1-antitrypsin deficiency. Clinically significant dyspnea associated with abnormal lung function before the age of 45 in individuals who smoke should also prompt evaluation. Dyspnea on exertion is the most common presenting symptom, but acute or chronic bronchitis, increased airway reactivity, mucus hypersecretion, recurrent pneumonias, or pneumothoraces are also associated with α_1-antitrypsin deficiency.[6,45] It may also be manifested by adult liver disease. Emphysema not associated with cigarette smoking or a family history of early-onset emphysema should also prompt an evaluation.

Clinically significant α_1-antitrypsin deficiency should be suspected when the patient has a history suggestive of α_1-antitrypsin deficiency and a flat α_1 region on SPEP. When it is suspected, measurement of serum α_1-antitrypsin levels should be performed, usually by radial immunodiffusion or nephelometry. This test is readily available in most hospital and reference laboratories. When serum levels are less than 35% of normal, more definitive testing should be performed and family studies undertaken to identify others at risk. Accurate prenatal diagnosis can also be accomplished. Phenotyping using IEF patterns will identify the patient's PI type. This test requires skill and experience and is not as widely available locally. Baseline evaluation of patients should also include posteroanterior and left lateral chest roentgenograms; complete pulmonary function tests (PFTs), including spirometry or flow-volume curves before and after a bronchodilator; lung volumes and diffusion capacity; arterial blood gases; and liver function tests (LFTs), including SGOT, serum glutamate pyruvate transaminase (SGPT), total bilirubin, and alkaline phosphatase.

Chest roentgenograms typically show hyperinflation with flattening of the diaphragms and basilar hyperlucency indicative of the panacinar emphysema. The PFTs at time of diagnosis in significantly symptomatic patients usually show moderate to severe obstructive dysfunction, with an FEV_1 less than 30% of that predicted in many. However, with appropriate clinical suspicion at an earlier presentation and an early diagnosis of α_1-antitrypsin deficiency, obstructive dysfunction may be in the mild to moderate range. The diffusion capacity also is reduced commensurate with the amount of lung destruction present. Liver enzymes and bilirubin levels are elevated in 10% to 20% of infants with PI ZZ disease. Measurement of serum α_1-antitrypsin levels should therefore be included in the workup of cholestasis of unknown cause in infants. These LFTs commonly return to normal by the teenage years. In adults, liver enzymes are infrequently elevated (<8%). Liver biopsy in patients with affected livers reveals large intracytoplasmic collections of PAS-positive and diastase-resistant (nonglycogen) protein reactive to anti–α_1-antitrypsin antibody.[3,15] Polycythemia and cor pulmonale are observed in a minority of patients. Ventilation and perfusion scans confirm basilar destructive disease with decreased perfusion and a delay in ventilation washout.

The threshold serum level below which a patient has a higher risk of emphysema than that of the general population is considered to be 80 mg/dl. Below this level the lung is not thought to be adequately protected against protease activity based on the observation that some patients with the PI SZ phenotype have been described with early-onset emphysema. However, many commercial standards overestimate α_1-antitrypsin levels by 35% to 40%, so a true laboratory standard that quantifies the level of α_1-antitrypsin accurately is recommended. To avoid confusion, the true values using pure standards are expressed in micromolar (μM) units. The true standard threshold is therefore 11 μM. Serum levels in patients with α_1-antitrypsin deficiency are usually less than 50 mg/dl (7 μM). The range of α_1-antitrypsin levels for individuals with any combination of normal PI M alleles is 20 to 48 μM (150 to 350 mg/dl), for PI ZZ homozygotes it is 2.5 to 7 μM (20 to 45 mg/dl), and for PI SS homozygotes the range is 13 to 33 μM (100 to 140 mg/dl). Heterozygotes of the phenotype PI SZ have levels ranging from 8 to 19 μM (75 to 120 mg/dl), and with the phenotype PI MZ the range is 12 to 35 μM (90 to 210 mg/dl). Homozygous PI null-null phenotypes have no detectable serum levels (Table 78-2).

TREATMENT

General therapy measures for the pulmonary manifestations of α_1-antitrypsin deficiency are similar to those used in individuals with obstructive lung disease and normal PI phenotypes (Box 78-1). Primary goals are to avoid clinical situations and environmental factors that accelerate lung function loss and to maximize supportive therapy in order to preserve and maximize remaining lung function. Specific therapy involves augmentation of α_1-antitrypsin levels in serum and the lung.

Table 78-2 Threshold Protective Level Concept Based on Epidemiologic Assessment of α_1-Antitrypsin Levels and the Risk for the Development of Emphysema

	SERUM LEVELS		
PHENOTYPE	TRUE LEVELS* (μM)	COMMONLY QUOTED LEVELS† (mg/dl)	EMPHYSEMA RISK COMPARED WITH THAT IN THE GENERAL POPULATION
MM‡	20-48	150-350	No increase
MZ§	12-35	90-210	No increase
SS	15-33	100-140	No increase
SZ	8-19¶	75-120¶	Mildly increased risk
ZZ	2.5-7	20-45	High risk
Null-null‖	0	0	Extremely high risk

Reproduced from the American Thoracic Society: *Am Rev Respir Dis* 140:1494-1497, 1989.
*True levels based on the laboratory standard used by the registry.
†Based on a commonly used commercial standard; these levels are of historic interest only and are 35% to 40% overestimates of the true levels.
‡Includes all combinations of normal M-family alleles, including M1 (Val[213]), M1(Ala[213]), M2, and M3 alleles.
§Includes all combinations of normal M-family alleles with the Z allele.
‖Includes all combinations of null alleles.
¶The threshold protective level of 11 μM (80 mg/dl with a commonly used commercial standard) is based on the knowledge that it is very unusual for SZ heterozygotes to develop emphysema.

BOX 78-1
Therapy for Emphysema Associated with α_1-Antitrypsin Deficiency

General
Smoking cessation
Avoidance of other respiratory irritants
Early antibiotics for infections
Annual influenza vaccinations
One lifetime pneumococcal vaccination
Nutritional support
Physical therapy (pulmonary rehabilitation, breathing techniques)
Bronchodilating medications
Mucolytics, corticosteroids, and home oxygen therapy for selected patients

Specific
α_1-Antitrypsin replacement
Lung transplantation in end-stage disease
Bullectomy in selected patients

Data from Crystal RG: *J Clin Invest* 85: 1343-1352, 1990.

Avoidance of respiratory irritants, in particular cigarette smoking, is of primary importance in reducing the accelerated loss of lung function seen in α_1-antitrypsin deficiency. Smoking cessation should be vigorously pursued, using various techniques as needed, such as pharmacologic withdrawal assistance (nicotine patches or gum, transdermal clonidine), group therapy or counseling, or hypnosis and other behavior modification techniques. Nonsmokers should be strongly encouraged not to start. Patient education regarding the effect of smoking in α_1-antitrypsin deficiency in accelerating the disease course should be emphasized. Although other respiratory irritants that increase the inflammatory cell burden, such as secondhand or sidestream smoke or occupational exposure to dust and gases, have not specifically been shown to play a role in accelerated loss of lung function, it is rational to advise avoidance. Smoking should not be permitted in the households and vehicles of individuals with α_1-antitrypsin deficiency, particularly children with the disease.

Lower respiratory tract infections associated with purulent airway secretions increase the neutrophil burden of the lungs. This exposure may increase the alveolar wall damage in patients with α_1-antitrypsin deficiency. These infections should be treated promptly and aggressively with appropriate antibiotics to reduce the inflammatory cell burden of the lungs. Annual influenza vaccines and one lifetime dose of pneumococcal vaccine (Pneumovax) should be given to all α_1-antitrypsin–deficient individuals with emphysema. Evaluation of immunologic status for deficiency states, and replacement if indicated, may be appropriate in patients with recurrent sinopulmonary infections.

Supportive therapy to maximize remaining lung function is also used in α_1-antitrypsin–deficienct emphysema patients, as in those with obstructive lung disease. Because of the increased work of breathing associated with emphysema, nutritional supplementation can be an important adjunctive treatment to prevent weight loss and cachexia. A pulmonary rehabilitation program to strengthen and improve the endurance of the respiratory muscles, promote increased utilization of available oxygen, and optimize cardiovascular function and conditioning is also important in patients with severe respiratory disease. Breathing techniques (pursed-lip breathing) to attain peak ventilatory potential in severe emphysematous patients may be required. Because airway hyperresponsiveness and some degree of reversibility are often seen in patients with α_1-antitrypsin deficiency, a trial of maximum bronchodilator therapy using β_2-agonists, theophyllines, and anticholinergics is recommended. Additional benefit in selected patients may be derived from mucolytic agents, steroids, or chronic home oxygen therapy (if indicated and the criteria met). Although these general measures provide significant symptomatic relief, unopposed neutrophil elastase activity continues, and the progressive decline in respiratory function is still accelerated compared with normal individuals.

Bullectomy has a very limited role in a highly selected group of α_1-antitrypsin–deficient patients. However, heart-lung transplant (HLT), single-lung transplant (SLT), and double-lung transplant (DLT) have proven successful as techniques have improved and patient selection has expanded, and offer the possibility of resuming an active lifestyle for patients with respiratory failure and an FEV_1 less than 30% of that predicted. All of these procedures—HLT, DLT, and SLT—are

Table 78-3 Effect of Weekly α_1-Antitrypsin Replacement Therapy on Lung and Serum α_1-Antitrypsin Levels and Antineutrophil Elastase Capacity in Patients with PI Type ZZ and Null-Null[a]

	"NORMAL" PIMM	ZZ BEFORE REPLACEMENT	ZZ AFTER REPLACEMENT	NULL-NULL BEFORE REPLACEMENT	NULL-NULL AFTER REPLACEMENT
Serum α_1-antitrypsin level	150-350 mg/dl	<50 mg/dl	163 mg/dl[b]	0	2138 mg/dl[b]
Serum antineutrophil elastase capacity	27 μM	5.4 mM	13 mM[c]	1.2 mM	10.5 mM[d]
ELF α_1-antitrypsin level	3.4 mM	0.46 mM	1.89 mM[e]	0	approx. 1.9 mM[f]
ELF antineutrophil elastase capacity	2.8 mM	0.8 mM	1.65 mM[g]	0.4 mM	approx. 2.2 mM[h]

ELF, (alveolar) epithelial lining fluid.
[a]From Wewers et al[47-49] with weekly α_1-antitrypsin replacement therapy at 60 mg/kg IV.
[b]Average serum α_1-antitrypsin level over 1 month.
[c]Average serum antineutrophil elastate capacity throughout the study.
[d]Trough serum antineutrophil elastase capacity at 7 days after infusion.
[e]Average nadir ELF α_1-antitrypsin levels at day 6 for all patients.
[f]Nadir ELF α_1-antitrypsin at day 6 after infusion.
[g]Average nadir ELF antineutrophil elastase capacity at day 6 for all patients.
[h]Average ELF antineutrophil elastase capacity 6 days after infusion.

comparable and appropriate treatment modalities for patients with end-stage lung disease caused by emphysema. The limiting factor is the supply of donor organs, and for this reason, unless severe cardiac disease is also present, SLT should be the procedure of choice. In one study of 31 lung transplants for emphysema, 13 were for α_1-antitrypsin deficiency.[46] The mean age in the HLT and SLT patients was 46 and 50 years, respectively (range 38 to 60 years). The 2-year survival rate was 79.5% in the HLT and 86.7% in the SLT patients. The major cause of death has been bacterial infection. Infection and rejection remain the two major posttransplant complications. The FEV_1 percentage predicted ranged from 7% to 30% before surgery, and 6 months postoperatively it was 110% for HLT and 52% for SLT.

Because of significant augmentation of C1 esterase (another hepatocyte-produced antiprotease) in hereditary angioedema with danazol, Wewers et al[47] investigated the use of danazol in α_1-antitrypsin–deficient individuals. Danazol, a testosterone derivative without major androgenic properties, has the effect of augmenting α_1-antitrypsin synthesis in some patients, but clinical efficacy is unknown. α_1-Antitrypsin serum levels are increased 50% but are still well below the threshold level of 11 μM (80 mg/dl). Only 60% of men and 25% of women with PI Z α_1-antitrypsin deficiency respond to danazol with increased serum concentrations of α_1-antitrypsin. If intracellular accumulation of aggregated protein Z contributes to the hepatic damage seen in α_1-antitrypsin deficiency liver disease, treatment with danazol to augment hepatic synthesis of α_1-antitrypsin in patients with PI ZZ, PI SZ, and PI MZ could pose an increased risk of hepatic injury. Stanozolol, another testosterone derivative tested, is ineffective in augmenting α_1-antitrypsin production. The use of danazol for augmentation is not justified in α_1-antitrypsin deficiency.

Replacement therapy, although unproven to retard the accelerated decline in respiratory function, offers the potential to limit lung tissue destruction by restoring an adequate protease-antiprotease balance. In 1981 Gadek et al[10] successfully administered a crude preparation of human α_1-protease inhibitor once a week for 4 weeks to five patients with α_1-antitrypsin deficiency. Elevated α_1-antitrypsin levels and neutrophil elastase inhibitory capacity in both serum and bronchoalveolar lavage (BAL) fluid were demonstrated without significant toxity.[10] In 1987 Wewers et al[48] administered a human α_1-protease inhibitor (Cutter Biological) at a dosage of 60 mg/kg weekly for 6 months to 18 PI ZZ α_1-antitrypsin–deficient patients. After replacement, BAL studies demonstrated significantly increased levels of α_1-antitrypsin and functional antineutrophil elastase capacity in the epithelial fluid of the lower respiratory tract compared with levels obtained before replacement[48,49] (Table 78-3). The serum half-life of the administered α_1-protease inhibitor was 4.5 days. More recently, Hubbard et al[50] treated eight PI ZZ and one PI Z-null α_1-antitrypsin–deficient patients with monthly intravenous augmentation therapy of α_1-protease inhibitor (Prolastin, Miles Inc., West Haven, Conn., 80% pure) using a dosage of 250 mg/kg over a period of 12 months. Equivalent augmentation of serum and lung α_1-antitrypsin levels and antineutrophil elastase capacity were obtained, compared with those achieved by Wewers et al[48] with weekly therapy. Nadir lung epithelial lining fluid levels of α_1-antitrypsin remained above a theoretic predicted threshold in this study. The recommended dosage for weekly intravenous replacement therapy with α_1-antitrypsin (Prolastin) is 60 mg/kg. The dosage for monthly administration is 250 mg/kg at a rate of 50 mg/min (concentration of 25 mg/ml). Both weekly and monthly replacement therapy with intravenous infusions of α_1-antitrypsin maintain the serum and epithelial lining fluid levels and the antineutrophil elastase capacity above the threshold required for protection (Fig. 78-5). However, the monthly infusion is more commonly used because it is a more convenient alternative to weekly therapy and it may increase compliance. Serum levels of α_1-antitrypsin using commercial immunologic assays may not reflect the functional capacity, so serum levels should not be used to calculate therapeutic dosage.

Human α_1-antitrypsin (Prolastin) has proven safe and effective in providing increased serum and bronchoalveolar lavage fluid levels and functional antineutrophil elastase capacity. It has been available in the United States since 1988. It is prepared from pooled plasma and is heat treated in solution to 60° C for 10 hours. This process is capable of destroying human immunodeficiency virus (HIV) and hepatitis B viruses, and no instances of viral disease transmission have been documented to date. However, no procedure is considered totally effective in removing viral infectivity; therefore, it is advised to follow the recommendations from the package insert and

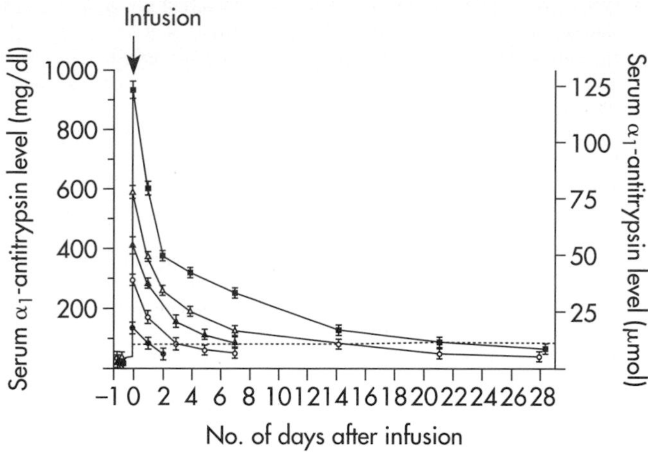

Fig. 78-5. Augmentation of serum α_1-antitrypsin levels. Single infusions of varying amounts of human α_1-antitrypsin were administered to α_1-antitrypsin–deficient individuals on day 0, and serum levels of α_1-antitrypsin were determined at intervals after infusion. Doses of α_1-antitrypsin infused represent amount of active α_1-antitrypsin in preparation. Dashed line indicates threshold level of α_1-antitrypsin based on epidemiologic data; closed circles, 30 mg/kg infusions; open circles, 60 mg/kg infusions; closed triangles, 90 mg/kg infusions; open triangles, 140 mg/kg infusions; and closed squares, 250 mg/kg infusions. (From Hubbard RC, Seller S, Czerski D, Stephens L, Crystal RG: *JAMA* 260:1259-1264, 1988.)

immunize against hepatitis B and screen for HIV before administration of human α_1-antitrypsin as therapy.

Human α_1-antitrypsin replacement therapy is indicated when α_1-antitrypsin levels are below 11 μM or 80 mg/dl in a patient with clinically significant emphysema. There is no upper limit on age or lower limit on lung function; however, it should not be administered while lung function is still in the normal range because a small proportion of patients never develop clinically significant disease within a normal life span. It is not indicated in patients younger than 18 years old except in rare instances when obstructive lung disease is already present. The safety and effectiveness of α_1-antitrypsin replacement therapy in children unfortunately has yet to be established, and it cannot be recommended until further studies are completed. It is also not indicated in patients with liver disease with decreased levels of α_1-antitrypsin and without associated lung disease because the mechanism of liver disease is not amenable to replacement therapy.

Future therapy of α_1-antitrypsin deficiency has many exciting directions of development. The development of synthetic elastase inhibitors for parenteral delivery would obviate obtaining α_1-antitrypsin from pooled serum and reduce the attendant risks. Aerosolized delivery of α_1-antitrypsin (pooled or recombinant), which has shown some promise in animal models, may eliminate the need for parenteral therapy altogether.[51-53] However, the achievement and maintenance of adequate protective interstitial tissue levels using this form of therapy have yet to be accomplished. Gene therapy with the potential to cure the deficiency may eventually be used once safety is ensured and the risks involved minimized.[54-56] Experimental animal studies with adenovirus vectors demonstrate theoretical possibilities of gene therapy in the treatment of α_1-antitrypsin deficiency.[54] An animal model that closely approximates the disease in humans is available (pallid mouse) and may be useful in testing therapeutic interventions and in studying the pathogenesis of α_1-antitrypsin deficiency.[56]

SUMMARY

α_1-Antitrypsin is a protease inhibitor with significant antineutrophil elastase activity and protects the lung architecture from excessive degradation by proteolytic enzymes. It is synthesized primarily in the liver. α_1-Antitrypsin deficiency is mainly a disease of adults, commonly manifesting as dyspnea associated with early-onset emphysema. However, it can manifest in children. It is most commonly associated with hepatic dysfunction in this age group, but respiratory disease does occur. Deficiency can lead to a protease-antiprotease imbalance, which is thought to be responsible for the early-onset panacinar emphysema associated with the disease.

A newsletter, *A_1 News,* is published by the Alpha$_1$ National Association and provides individuals with α_1-antitrypsin deficiency and their families, health care providers, and physicians across the United States, Canada, Mexico, and several other countries information on the diagnosis and treatment of α_1-antitrypsin deficiency, as well as the latest legislative information at both the state and national levels in the United States.

REFERENCES

History

1. Jacobson K: Studies on the trypsin and plasmin inhibitors in human serum, *Scand J Clin Lab Invest* 14(suppl):55-98, 1955.
2. Laurell CB, Eriksson S: The electrophoretic α_1-globulin pattern of serum in α_1-antitrypsin deficiency, *Scand J Clin Lab Invest* 15:312-340, 1963.
3. Eriksson S: Studies in α_1-antitrypsin deficiency, *Acta Med Scand Suppl* 432:1-85, 1965.
4. Sharp HL, Bridges RA, Krivit W, Freier EF: Cirrhosis associated with α_1-antitrypsin deficiency: a previously unrecognized inherited disorder, *J Lab Clin Med* 73:934-939, 1969.
5. Larsson C: Natural history and life expectancy in severe α_1-antitrypsin deficiency, PI Z, *Acta Med Scand* 204:345-351, 1978.
6. Brantly ML, Paul LD, Miller BH, Falk RT, Wu M, Crystal RG: Clinical features and history of the destructive lung disease associated with α_1-antitrypsin deficiency in adults with pulmonary symptoms, *Am Rev Respir Dis* 138:327-336, 1988.

Pathophysiology

7. Gross P, Babyak M, Toker E, Kashak M: Enzymatically produced pulmonary emphysema: a preliminary report, *J Occup Med* 6:481-484, 1964.
8. Janoff A, Sloan B, Weinbaum G, Damiano V, Sandhaus RA, Elias J, Kimbel P: Experimental emphysema induced with purified human neutrophil elastase: tissue localization of the instilled protease, *Am Rev Respir Dis* 115:461-478, 1977.
9. Senior RM, Tegner H, Kuhn C, Ohlsson K, Starcher BC, Peirce JA: The induction of pulmonary emphysema with human leukocyte elastase, *Am Rev Respir Dis* 116:469-475, 1977.
10. Gadek JE, Fells GA, Zimmerman RL, Rennard SI, Crystal RG: Antielastases of the human alveolar structures. Implications for the protease-antiprotease theory of emphysema, *J Clin Invest* 68:889-898, 1981.
11. Tobin MJ, Cook PJ, Hutchinson DC: α_1-antitrypsin deficiency: the clinical and physiological features of pulmonary emphysema in subjects homozygous for PI type Z. A survey of the British Thoracic Association, *Br J Dis Chest* 77(1):14-27, 1983.
12. Weitz JI, Landman SL, Crowley KA, Birken S, Morgan FJ: Development of an assay for in vivo human neutrophil elastase activity. Increased elastase activity in patients with α_1-proteinase inhibitor deficiency, *J Clin Invest* 78:155-162, 1986.
13. Carp H, Janoff A: Possible mechanisms of emphysema in smokers. In vitro suppression of serum elastase-inhibiting capacity by fresh cigarette smoke and its prevention by antioxidants, *Am Rev Respir Dis* 118(3): 617-621, 1978.
14. Carrell RW: Alpha1-antitrypsin: molecular pathology, leukocytes, and tissue damage, *J Clin Invest* 78:1427-1431, 1986.

15. Behrman RE, Vaughan VC, Nelson WE: Alpha1-antitrypsin deficiency. In *Nelson textbook of pediatrics,* ed 13, Philadelphia, 1987, WB Saunders.
16. Langley CE, Berninger RW, Wolfson SL, Talamo RC: An unusual type of α_1-antitrypsin deficiency in a child, *Johns Hopkins Med J* 144:161-165, 1979.
17. Udall JN, Bloch KJ, Walker WA: Transport of proteases across neonatal intestine and development of liver disease in infants with α-l-antitrypsin deficiency, *Lancet* 1:1441-1443, 1982.
18. Udall JN, Dixon M, Newman AP, et al: Liver disease in α-l-antitrypsin deficiency: a retrospective analysis of the influence of early breast- vs. bottle-feeding, *JAMA* 253:2679-2682, 1985.

α_1-Antitrypsin Protease Inhibitor Phenotypes and Airway Responsiveness

19. Townley RG, Southard JG, Radford P, Hopp RJ, Bewtra AK, Ford L: Association of MS PI phenotype with airway hyperresponsiveness, *Chest* 98:594-599, 1990.
20. Gaillard MC, Kilroe-Smith TA, Nogueira C, Dunn D, Jenkins T, Fine B, Kallenbach J: Alpha-l-protease inhibitor in bronchial asthma: phenotypes and biochemical characteristics, *Am Rev Respir Dis* 145:1311-1315, 1992.
21. Townley RG, Ryning F, Lynch H, Brody AW: Obstructive lung disease in hereditary α_1-antitrypsin deficiency, *JAMA* 214(2):325-331, 1970.

Genetics and Epidemiology

22. Guidelines for the approach in the patient with severe hereditary α-l-antitrypsin deficiency, *Am Rev Respir Dis* 140:1494-1497, 1989.
23. Gadek JE, Crystal RG: Alpha$_1$-antitrypsin deficiency. In Stanbury JB, Wyngaarden JB, Fredrickson DS, Goldstein JL, Brown MS, eds: *The metabolic basis of inherited disease,* ed 5, New York, 1983, McGraw-Hill.
24. Dykes DD, Miller SA, Polesky HG: Distribution of α_1-antitrypsin variants, *Adv Hum Genet* 11:1-62, 1981.
25. Crystal RG, Brantly ML, Hubbard RC, Curiel DT, States DI, Holmes MD: The α_1-antitrypsin gene and its mutations. Clinical consequences and strategies for therapy, *Chest* 95:196-208, 1989.
26. Ogushi F, Fells GA, Hubbard RC, Straus SD, Crystal RG: Z-type α_1-antitrypsin is less competent than M_1-type α_1-antitrypsin as an inhibitor of neutrophil elastase, *J Clin Invest* 80:1366-1374, 1987.
27. Mittman C, Lieberman J, Rumsfeld J: Prevalence of abnormal protease inhibitor phenotypes in patients with chronic obstructive lung disease, *Am Rev Respir Dis* 109:295-296, 1974.
28. Horne SL, Tennent RK, Cockcroft DW, et al: Pulmonary function in Pi M and MZ grainworkers, *Chest* 89:795-799, 1986.
29. Cooper DM, Hoeppner V, Cox D, et al: Lung function in α_1-antitrypsin heterozygotes (PI type MZ), *Am Rev Respir Dis* 110:708-715, 1974.
30. Hutchinson DC: The epidemiology of α_1-antitrypsin deficiency, *Lung* 168(suppl):535-542, 1990.

Clinical/Natural History

31. Wagener JS, Sobonya RE, Taussig LM, et al: Unusual abnormalities in adolescent siblings with α-l-antitrypsin deficiency, *Chest* 83:464-468, 1983.
32. Eriksson SG: Liver disease in α_1-antitrypsin deficiency, *Scand J Gastroenterol* 20:907-911, 1985.
33. Cox DW, Smyth S: Risk of liver disease in adults with α_1-antitrypsin deficiency, *Am J Med* 74:221-227, 1983.
34. Cox DW, Mansfield T: Prenatal diagnosis of α_1-antitrypsin deficiency and estimates of fetal risk for disease, *J Med Genet* 24:52-59, 1987.
35. Porter CA, Mowat AP, Cook PI, et al: Alpha$_1$-antitrypsin deficiency and neonatal hepatitis, *Br Med J* 3:435-439, 1972.
36. Sveger T: Liver disease in α_1-antitrypsin deficiency detected by screening of 200,000 infants, *N Engl J Med* 294:1316-1321, 1976.
37. O'Brien MO, Buist NRM, Murphey VVH: Neonatal screening for α_1-antitrypsin deficiency, *J Pediatr* 92(6):1006-1010, 1978.
38. Hussain M, Mieli-Vergani G, Mowat AP: Alpha$_1$-antitrypsin deficiency and liver disease: clinical presentation, diagnosis and treatment, *J Inherit Metab Dis* 14(4):497-511, 1991.
39. van Steenbergen W: Alpha1-antitrypsin deficiency: an overview, *Acta Clin Belg* 48(3):171-189, 1993.
40. Wall M, Moe E, Eisenberg J, Powers M, Buist N, Buist AS: Long term follow up of children with α_1-antitrypsin deficiency, *J Pediatr* 116(2):248-251, 1990.
41. Erikkson S: Alpha-l-antitrypsin deficiency: lessons learned from the bedside to the gene and back again, *Chest* 95:181-189, 1989.
42. Hutchison DCS: Natural history of α-l-protease inhibitor deficiency, *Am J Med* 84(suppl 6A):3-12, 1988.
43. Janus ED, Phillips NT, Carrell RW: Smoking, lung function and α-l-antitrypsin deficiency, *Lancet* 1:152-154, 1985.
44. Buist AS, Burrows B, Eriksson S, Mittman C, Wu M: The natural history of airflow obstruction in PI Z emphysema. Report of an NHLBI workshop, *Am Rev Respir Dis* 127:S43-S45, 1983.

Diagnosis

45. Paul LD: Alpha$_1$-antitrypsin deficiency, *Pulmonary and Critical Care Update* 5(6):1-9, 1989.

Treatment

46. Dennis CM, Briffa NP, Higenbottam TW, et al: Emphysema: heart lung or single lung transplantation? *Eur Respir J* 6:364s, 1993.
47. Wewers MD, Gadek JE, Koegh BA, et al: Evaluation of danazol therapy for patients with PI ZZ α-l-antitrypsin deficiency, *Am Rev Respir Dis* 134:476-480, 1986.
48. Wewers MD, Casolaro MA, Sellers SE, Swayze SC, McPhaul KM, Wittes JT, et al: Replacement therapy for α_1-antitrypsin deficiency associated with emphysema, *N Engl J Med* 316:1055-1062, 1987.
49. Wewers MD, Casolaro MA, Crystal RG: Comparison of α_1-antitrypsin levels and antineutrophil elastase capacity of blood and lung in a patient with the α_1-antitrypsin phenotype null-null before and during α_1-antitrypsin augmentation therapy, *Am Rev Respir Dis* 135:539-543, 1987.
50. Hubbard RC, Seller S, Czerski D, Stephens L, Crystal RG: Biochemical efficacy and safety of monthly augmentation therapy for α_1-antitrypsin deficiency, *JAMA* 260:1259-1264, 1988.
51. Crystal RG: Alpha$_1$-antitrypsin deficiency, emphysema, and liver disease: genetic basis and strategies for therapy, *J Clin Invest* 85:1343-1352, 1990.
52. Hubbard RC, Brantly ML, Sellers SE, Mitchell ME, Crystal RG: Antineutrophil-elastase defenses of the lower respiratory tract in α_1-antitrypsin deficiency directly augmented with an aerosol of α_1-antitrypsin, *Ann Intern Med* 111:206-212, 1989.
53. Hubbard RC, McElvaney NG, Sellers SE, Healy JT, Czerski DB, Crystal RG: Recombinant DNA-produced α_1-antitrypsin administered by aerosol augments lower respiratory tract and neutrophil elastase defenses in individuals with α_1-antitrypsin deficiency, *J Clin Invest* 84:1349-1354, 1989.
54. Rosenfeld MA, Siegfried W, Yoshimura K, et al: Adenovirus-mediated transfer of a recombinant α_1-antitrypsin gene to the lung epithelium in vivo, *Science* 252:431-434, 1991.
55. Crystal RG: Gene therapy strategies for pulmonary disease, *Am J Med* 92(6A):44s-52s, 1992.
56. Martorana PA, Brand T, Gardi C, van Even P, de Santi MM, Calzoni P, Marcolongo P, Lungarella G: The pallid mouse. A model of genetic α_1-antitrypsin deficiency, *Lab Invest* 68(2):233-241, 1993.

CHAPTER 79

Malignant Diseases of the Thoracic Cavity

Edwin C. Douglass

Malignant disease is an uncommon cause of pulmonary pathology in infants and children, but when it does occur, its early recognition is of great importance. The diagnosis of cancer is rare in children younger than 15 years of age. The annual incidence in 1988 was 14.1 per 100,000 children. Survival rates have increased significantly in the last 20 years, from a 5-year survival rate of 55% in 1974 to a projected survival rate in 1994 of 80%. This increase in survival rates is especially true of several tumors involving the chest cavity, such as Hodgkin's and non-Hodgkin's lymphoma, neuroblastoma, and Ewing's sarcoma.[1]

In this chapter, the major manifestations of malignant disease involving the chest cavity will be discussed, first by primary or secondary malignant disease and then by side effects of cancer therapy.

PRIMARY PULMONARY MANIFESTATIONS OF MALIGNANT DISEASE

Cancer of the Lung

Primary cancer of the lung parenchyma and bronchi is extremely rare in childhood. Only about 100 cases have been reported.

Pleuropulmonary Blastoma

This rare pulmonary tumor tends to occur in a subpleural location. It is distinguished by embryonic blastoma and stroma and a propensity for sarcomatous differentiation. Lesions may be intrapulmonary, mediastinal, or pleural.[2] Large lesions (>5 cm) commonly recur or metastasize in spite of pulmonary resection.[3,4] Responses to chemotherapy do occur, but the prognosis is poor.[5] This tumor appears to be associated strongly with a family history of cancer.[6]

Bronchogenic Carcinoma

Most pediatric cases of bronchogenic carcinoma are of the undifferentiated or adenocarcinomatous type, but squamous cell carcinomas have also been reported.[7,8] Long-term survivors of Fanconi's anemia may be particularly prone to develop squamous cell malignancies. Bronchogenic carcinomas may occur in children of any age, but they more typically develop during adolescence.

The management of children with bronchogenic carcinoma should be according to reasonable adult guidelines, with resection of tumors when possible. The prognosis is similarly poor as in adults, but radiation therapy may be of some benefit when the tumor is inoperable.

Bronchial Adenomas

Childhood cases of "bronchial adenomas" have been, in fact, carcinoid tumors or slow-growing malignancies such as mucoepidermoid carcinomas or cylindromas. The treatment of these tumors is surgical resection.[9,10]

Cancer of the Mediastinum

The mediastinum is conventionally divided into anterior, middle, and posterior compartments; however, few tumors are localized to the middle compartment, so tumors will be classified here according to anterior or posterior location (Table 79-1).

Anterior Mediastinum

The most important tumors of the anterior mediastinum occurring in the pediatric age groups are lymphomas and germ cell tumors. Patients with tumor in this location may have symptoms of airway compression such as cough, stridor, or localized wheezing. Very large tumors may cause venous congestion of head, neck, and arms.

Non-Hodgkin's Lymphoma. The mediastinum is the second most common site of non-Hodgkin's lymphoma in childhood. Although large cell lymphomas also occur here, lymphomas in this site are primarily of lymphoblastic histology and T cell origin (Fig. 79-1). Lymphoblastic lymphomas are part of a spectrum of T cell malignancy that ranges from localized lymphoma to lymphoma with bone marrow invasion to T cell acute lymphoblastic leukemia. Pleural effusion is a common finding at diagnosis, and tumor cells may be demonstrated in the pleural fluid.[11] Patients with anterior mediastinal or hilar masses should be evaluated for possible infectious causes, but when these are ruled out, bone marrow aspirate and biopsy should be done before thoracotomy. Lymphoma involves the bone marrow in 15% to 20% of cases, and examination of the marrow may provide diagnostic material without the need for more invasive procedures. The chemotherapy of childhood non-Hodgkin's lymphoma has improved survival dramatically over the last 20 years. More than 70% of children with mediastinal lymphoma will enjoy long-term disease-free survival.[12]

Hodgkin's Disease. Cervical or supraclavicular lymphadenopathy is the usual clinical presentation of Hodgkin's disease, but at least two thirds of patients have mediastinal involvement at diagnosis. One third of patients have systemic symptoms at diagnosis. Staging is based on extent of disease; disease confined above the diaphragm is considered stage II. The majority of cases in childhood are of the nodular sclerosing subtype. Cure rates with combined chemotherapy–radiation therapy are excellent in childhood Hodgkin's disease; even patients with advanced (stage III or IV) disease have a 70% to 90% chance of disease-free survival.[13]

Germ Cell Tumors. This is a collective term for tumors, benign and malignant, that arise from primordial germ cells. A working histopathological classification divides these tumors

Table 79-1 Tumors Originating in the Mediastinum

TYPE	ANTERIOR	POSTERIOR
Malignant (or potentially malignant)	Lymphomas (thymic masses): T cell lymphoma, Hodgkin's disease	Neuroblastoma Neurogenic tumors (nerve sheath tumors, schwannoma)
	Germ cell tumors, teratomas, dermoid	Ewing sarcoma/Peripheral neuroectodermal tumor (PNET)
	Thyroid tumors (rare) Thymomas (rare)	Rhabdomyosarcoma
Benign	Bronchogenic cysts Hygromas Lipomas Lymphangiomas	Bronchogenic cysts Thoracic meningocele

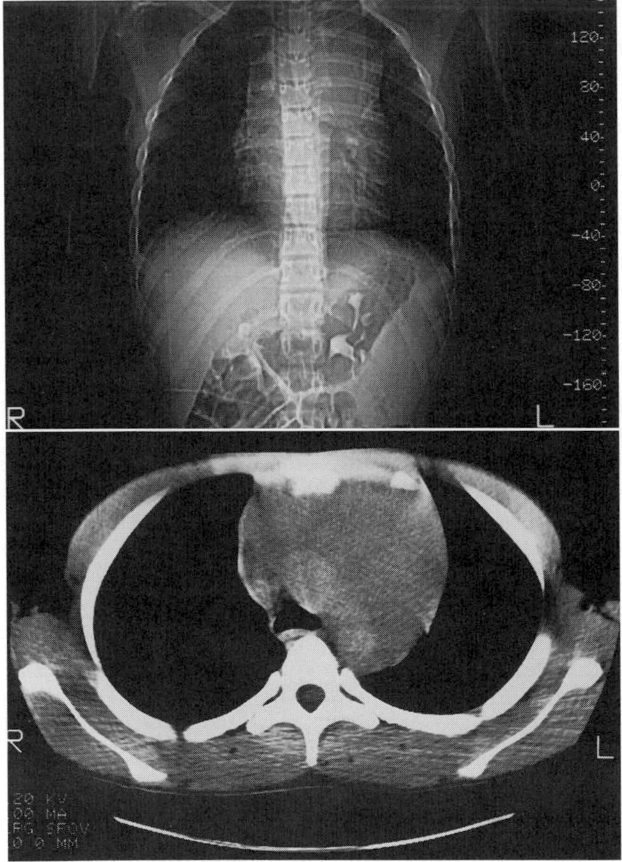

Fig. 79-1. Large anterior mediastinal mass in a 16-year-old adolescent. Bone marrow aspirate revealed 40% lymphoblasts with T cell surface markers.

into the following categories: germinoma, teratoma (mature or immature), embryonal carcinoma, endodermal sinus tumor (yolk sac tumor), choriocarcinoma, gonadoblastoma, and malignant mixed histology. The mediastinum is the third most common site, after sacrococcygeal and gonadal presentations, but only 7% of germ cell tumors occur there. The anterior mediastinum, pericardium, and lung are the main sites of occurrence in the thoracic cavity, and the majority of tumors are mature or immature teratomas. The primary presenting features include dyspnea and chest pain, but as many as 50% of children may be asymptomatic, with the tumor found on a chest radiograph.[14] An interesting syndrome that links the development of hematologic neoplasia (leukemia or malignant histiocytosis) with mediastinal germ cell tumor has been reported.[15] Surgical excision is the primary mode of therapy for benign teratomas. Malignant tumors require chemotherapy. The overall survival rate with modern cisplatin-based chemotherapy regimens for extragonadal germ cell tumors is 40% to 50%.[15]

Thymoma. Any of the previously discussed tumors of the mediastinum can involve the thymus and present a confusing gross and microscopic appearance. A neoplasm of the thymus is not a true thymoma unless it has neoplastic epithelial elements. True thymomas are rare tumors, and only 20% occur in children less than 20 years of age.[17,18] Myasthenia gravis, red cell aplasia, and hypogammaglobulinemia are common clinical findings. Vague symptoms including cough and dysphagia may occur. Surgery is the primary mode of therapy; radiation therapy is added if the tumor is invasive. A subtype of thymic carcinoma that has a histopathologic picture similar to undifferentiated nasopharyngeal carcinoma is associated with Epstein-Barr virus infection. This tumor has a tendency to metastasize but is responsive to chemotherapy.[19]

Posterior Mediastinum

Posterior mediastinal tumors are often asymptomatic but may cause neurologic symptoms. These tumors are commonly dumbbell shaped, with a large intraspinal component in addition to the intrathoracic tumors. Neuroblastoma and Ewing's sarcoma may respond rapidly to cytoreductive chemotherapy and seldom require laminectomy or radiation for relief of early neurologic symptoms.[20] Patients with impending hemiparesis, however, may require surgical intervention to prevent permanent neurologic damage.

Neuroblastoma. Neuroblastomas are derived from cells of the neural crest that form the sympathetic nervous system, including paraspinal ganglia and adrenal medulla (Fig. 79-2). Neuroblastomas may be limited in extent and curable by surgical excision alone, they may undergo spontaneous maturation to benign forms (ganglioneuroma), or they may be very malignant tumors with widespread metastases at diagnosis. Neuroblastomas occur in the thoracic cavity with greater frequency in infants (29%) than in children over 1 year of age (14%).[21] Treatment is based on the age of the child and the stage (extent) of the tumor at diagnosis. Localized tumor completely removed by surgical excision requires no further therapy. Infants with more extensive disease but "good" biologic tumor characteristics (hyperdiploidy, lack of N-*myc* oncogene amplification) have an excellent prognosis with limited chemother-

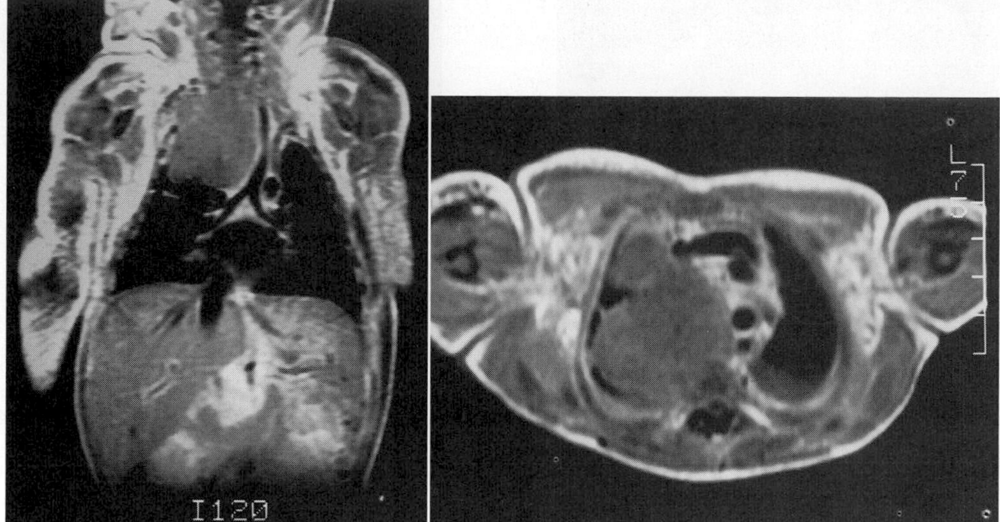

Fig. 79-2. Posterior mediastinal neuroblastoma in a 1-month-old infant. After partial resection the patient achieved a complete response to chemotherapy.

apy and surgery.[22] Older children with widespread disease have a very poor prognosis for long-term disease-free survival.

Ewing's Sarcoma. Ewing's sarcoma is a primitive neoplasm that typically arises in bone; it accounts for about 1% of all childhood cancer. Its peak occurrence is in the second decade of life, without predilection for either sex. The cell of origin remains unknown, although it was originally speculated to originate in endothelial cells. However, most recent evidence points to its origin in a primitive neural cell.[23] Cytogenetic and molecular genetic analyses have demonstrated the close relationship of Ewing's sarcoma to other tumors of presumed neural origin, including extraosseous Ewing's sarcoma, peripheral neuroectodermal tumor (also known as primitive neuroectodermal tumor or peripheral neuroepithelioma), and Askin's tumor[24] (a peripheral neuroectodermal tumor of the chest wall). These tumors may occur in the posterior mediastinal space arising from the vertebral bodies, posterior ribs, or chest wall (Askin's tumor). Approximately 15% of patients have metastatic disease to lung or bone at diagnosis. Multimodal treatment is required with chemotherapy, surgery, and radiation therapy, although radiation therapy and extensive resection may be avoided in resectable rib lesions.[25] With current therapy 60% to 70% of patients with nonmetastatic disease at diagnosis may expect long-term disease-free survival.[26,27] The prognosis is poorer in patients with Ewing's sarcoma that is metastatic at diagnosis, with 30% surviving disease free at 3 years.[28] It is important to distinguish peripheral neuroectoder-mal tumor (Askin's tumor), which carries a worse prognosis than Ewing's sarcoma.[29,30]

Malignant Peripheral Nerve Sheath Tumor (Malignant Schwannoma). These sarcomas, which arise within peripheral nerve or spinal nerve roots, may occur in the posterior mediastinum or the chest wall. Symptoms are those of increasing mass, pain, or nerve deficit. From 20% to 50% of cases occur in children with neurofibromatosis, type I (NF-I, von Recklinghausen's disease), and the incidence in all patients with NF-I may be as high as 5%. These tumors also occur in previously irradiated sites. Complete resection is necessary for cure; chemotherapy and radiation therapy have not been shown to be effective treatment in this tumor. Unfortunately, rates of recurrence, either local or distant, as high as 50% have been found in some series. Age greater than 7 years, large tumor size, and presence of NF-I are adverse prognostic factors.[31,32]

Cancer of the Chest Wall

Both Ewing's sarcoma/PNET and malignant peripheral nerve sheath tumors may involve the chest wall (Fig. 79-3). Other tumors that may originate in the chest wall include rhabdomyosarcoma and mesothelioma.

Rhabdomyosarcoma

Rhabdomyosarcoma is the most common soft tissue sarcoma in childhood and adolescence. The most common sites of occurrence are in the head/neck, pelvis (genitourinary sites), and extremities; however, approximately 10% of cases occur in the trunk, and one half of trunk primaries involve the chest wall.[33] Rhabdomyosarcoma may also involve the posterior mediastinum and thoracolumbar spine. The most important variable in prognosis is the clinical stage at presentation. Tumors that are completely excised by surgery have a much better prognosis than tumors that are unresectable. Radiation therapy plays an important role in the control of local disease, and chemotherapy is necessary to prevent local and metastatic recurrence in all stages of disease. Intrathoracic tumors often grow to a very large size before symptoms such as dyspnea and pain bring patients to medical attention. Although the overall cure rate of rhabdomyosarcoma is approximately 70%, tumors of the chest appear to have a lower survival rate of less than 50%.

Mesothelioma

This tumor of mesothelial surfaces, such as pleura, pericardium, or peritoneum, may be either benign or malignant. Both have been reported in children.[36,37] These tumors are characterized by a pleomorphic histologic appearance and tend to spread over the pleural surface. Surgery is curative in the benign form; malignant mesothelioma, however, carries a poor

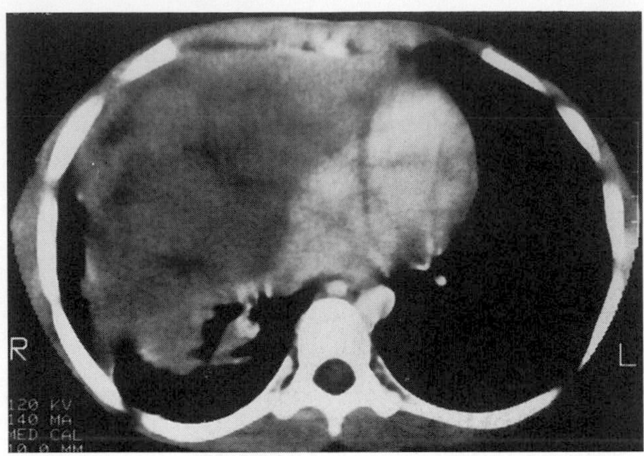

Fig. 79-3. Large PNET (Askin tumor) of the chest wall in an 11-year-old boy. A complete remission was obtained with chemotherapy, radiation therapy, and surgery.

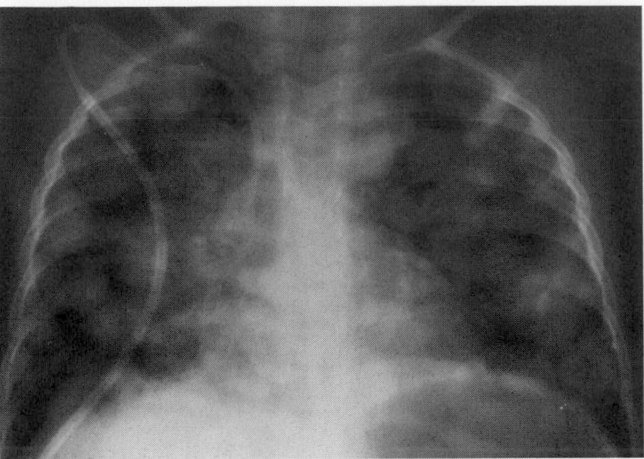

Fig. 79-4. Metastatic Wilms' tumor at diagnosis in a 3-year-old boy.

prognosis, although some responses to chemotherapy have been noted.

PULMONARY MANIFESTATIONS OF METASTATIC DISEASE

Although primary tumors of the lung are rare in the pediatric age group, metastatic disease from other sites is more common. Malignant tumors arising elsewhere in the body may cause pulmonary metastases widespread enough to be symptomatic at diagnosis. The most common childhood tumor to occur in this fashion is Wilms' tumor, in which pulmonary tumors may be numerous enough to give the appearance of pulmonary consolidation (Fig. 79-4). Cure may be possible, however, with radiation therapy and chemotherapy. Adolescents with thyroid carcinoma may develop a miliary picture of pulmonary metastases, which may remain stable for years. In adolescent girls, a picture of multiple pulmonary nodules without an obvious primary may indicate trophoblastic (gestational) choriocarcinoma. Treatment can be complicated by pulmonary hemorrhage. Patients with acute myeloid leukemia or chronic myelocytic leukemia who have white blood cell counts greater than 100,000 are at risk for pulmonary leukostasis. This is a medical emergency that requires early institution of cytoreductive therapy, including chemotherapy and leukapheresis. Other pediatric solid tumors that commonly metastasize to the lung are listed by primary site in Table 79-2. Although 70% of patients with neuroblastoma have stage IV (metastatic) disease to bone and bone marrow, neuroblastoma rarely metastasizes to lung.

Table 79-2 Pediatric Tumors that Metastasize to Lung

PRIMARY SITE	TUMORS
Bone	Osteosarcoma Ewing's sarcoma Chondrosarcoma (rare) Ameloblastoma (very rare)
Musculoskeletal	Rhabdomyosarcoma Soft tissue sarcomas (e.g., synovial sarcoma, malignant fibrous histiocytoma)
Gastrointestinal	Hepatoblastoma/hepatocellular carcinoma Embryonal sarcoma of liver Leiomyosarcoma Adenocarcinoma of colon
Genitourinary	Wilms' tumor Malignant rhabdoid tumor of the kidney Clear cell sarcoma of the kidney Gonadal germ cell tumor Trophoblastic choriocarcinoma

PULMONARY RADIATION FIBROSIS

Radiation injury to the lung occurs in two phases: subacute radiation pneumonitis and late pulmonary fibrosis. The acute phase of radiation pneumonitis can be seen 1 to 4 months after treatment; it typically causes cough, dyspnea, and low-grade fever and is usually self-limited. Damage to type II alveolar cells underlies the pathophysiology of this condition.[38] Late pulmonary toxicity from radiation therapy is caused by the development of interstitial fibrosis with decreased lung compliance.

Whole lung tolerance of radiation therapy is about 18 to 20 Gy, but when chemotherapy (especially actinomycin or bleomycin) is given concurrently, this tolerance is reduced to 15 to 18 Gy. Partial lung volume of irradiation (<30%) can tolerate higher levels of 25 to 30 Gy.[39]

Although children may be exposed to partial lung irradiation during treatment for Ewing's sarcoma/PNET, rhabdomyosarcoma, or Hodgkin's disease, whole lung irradiation is widely used only for the treatment of stage IV (metastatic) Wilms' tumor. Of 153 children who received whole lung irradiation to 12 Gy in the Third National Wilms' Tumor Study, 19 (13%) developed interstitial pneumonitis; however, in four of these cases the cause of the pneumonitis was infectious (varicella, pneumocystis), underscoring the need for a pathologic diagnosis in such cases.[40]

REFERENCES

1. Bleyer WA: What can be learned about childhood cancer from "Cancer Review 1973-1988," *Cancer* 71:3229-3226, 1993.

Primary Pulmonary Manifestations of Malignant Disease

2. Manivel JC, Priest JR, Watterson J, Steiner M, Woods WG, Wick MR, Dehner LP: Pleuropulmonary blastoma. The so-called pulmonary blastoma, *Cancer* 62:1516-1526, 1988.
3. Weinblatt ME, Siegel SE, Isaacs H: Pulmonary blastoma associated with cystic lung disease, *Cancer* 49:669-671, 1982.

4. Fung CH, Lo JW, Yonan TN, Hakimi MM, Chaugus GW: Pulmonary blastoma: an ultrastructural study with a brief review of literature and a discussion of pathogenesis, *Cancer* 39:153-163, 1977.
5. Ozkaynak MF, Ortega JA, Lang W, Gilsanz V, Isaacs H Jr: Role of chemotherapy in pediatric pulmonary blastoma, *Med Pediatr Oncol* 18: 53-56, 1990.
6. Priest J, Watterson J, Dehner L, Friend S, McIntyre L, Strong L, Hausen M, Byrd B, Feussner J, Amylon M: Childhood pleuropulmonary blastoma as a unique marker for familial childhood neoplasms, *Proc Am Soc Clin Oncol* 13:186, 1994 (abstract).
7. Anderson AE, Beuchner HA, Yager I, Ziskind MM: Bronchogenic carcinoma in young men, *Am J Med* 16:404, 1954.
8. La Salle AJ, Andrassy RJ, Stanford W: Bronchogenic squamous cell carcinoma in childhood: a case report, *J Pediatr Surg* 12:519-521, 1977.
9. Verska JJ, Connolly JE: Bronchial adenomas in children, *J Thorac Cardiovasc Surg* 55:411-417, 1968.
10. Leonardi HK, Jung-Legg Y, Legg MA, Neptune WB: Tracheobronchial mucoepidermoid carcinoma: clinicopathological features and results of treatment, *J Thorac Cardiovasc Surg* 76:431-438, 1978.
11. White L, Siegel SE, Quah TC: Non-Hodgkin's lymphomas in children. 1. Patterns of disease and classification, *Crit Rev Oncol Hematol* 13:55-71, 1992.
12. Murphy SB, Fairclough DL, Hutchison RE, Berard CW: Non-Hodgkin's lymphomas of childhood. An analysis of the histology, staging, and response to treatment of 338 cases at a single institution, *J Clin Oncol* 4:186-193, 1989.
13. Leventhal BG, Donaldson SS: Hodgkin's disease. In Pizzo PA, Poplack DG, eds: *Principles and practice of pediatric oncology,* Philadelphia, 1993, JB Lippincott.
14. Dehner LP: Gonadal and extragonadal germ cell neoplasia of childhood, *Hum Pathol* 14:493-511, 1983.
15. Nichols CR, Roth BJ, Heerema N, Griep J, Tricot G: Hematologic neoplasia associated with primary mediastinal germ-cell tumors, *N Engl J Med* 322:1425-1429, 1990.
16. Ablin AR, Krailo MD, Ramsay NKC, Malogolowkin MH, Isaacs H, Ramez RB, Adkins J, Hays DM, Benjamin DR, Grosfeld JL, Leikin SL, Deutsch M, Hammond GD: Results of treatment of malignant germ cell tumors in 93 children: a report from the Childrens Cancer Study Group, *J Clin Oncol* 9:1782-1792, 1991.
17. Dehner LP, Martin SA, Summer HW: Thymus related tumors and tumor-like lesions in childhood with rapid progression and death, *Hum Pathol* 8:53-56, 1977.
18. Furman WL, Buckley PJ, Green AA, Stokes DC, Chieri MD: Thymoma and myasthenia gravis in a 4-year-old child: case report and review of the literature, *Cancer* 56:2703-2706, 1985.
19. Dimery IW, Lee JS, Blick M, Pearson G, Spitzer G, Houg WK: Association of the Epstein-Barr virus with lymphoepithelioma of the thymus, *Cancer* 61:2475-2480, 1988.
20. Hayes FA, Green AA, O'Connor DM: Chemotherapeutic management of epidural neuroblastoma, *Med Pediatr Oncol* 17:6, 1989.
21. Brodeur GM, Castleberry RP: Neuroblastoma. In Pizzo PA, Poplack DG, eds: *Principles and practice of pediatric oncology,* Philadelphia, 1993, JB Lippincott.
22. Look AT, Hayes FA, Shuster JJ, Douglass EC, Castleberry RP, Bowman LC: Clinical relevance of tumor cell ploidy and N-myc gene amplification in childhood study, *J Clin Oncol* 9:581-591, 1991.
23. Lizard-Nacol S, Lizard G, Justrabo E, Ture-Carel C: Immunologic characterization of Ewing's sarcoma using mesenchymal and neural markers, *Am J Pathol* 135:847-855, 1989.
24. Askin FB, Rosai J, Sibley RK, Dehner LP, McAlister WH: Malignant small cell tumor of thoracopulmonary region in childhood: a distinctive clinicopathologic entity of uncertain histogenesis, *Cancer* 43:2438-2461, 1979.
25. Rao BN, Hayes FA, Thompson EL, Kumar APN, Fleming ID, Green AA, Austin BA, Pate SW, Hustin HO: Chest wall resection for Ewing's sarcoma of the rib: an unnecessary procedure, *Ann Thorac Surg* 46:40-44, 1988.
26. Burgert EO Jr, Nesbit ME, Garnsey LA, Gehan EA, Herrman J, Vietti TJ, Caugin A, Tefft M, Evans R, Thomas P, Askin FB, Kissane JM, Pritchard DJ, Neff J, Makley JT, Gilula G: Multimodal therapy for the management of nonpelvic, localized bone: Intergroup Study IESS-II, *J Clin Oncol* 8:1514-1524, 1990.
27. Barbieri E, Emiliani E, Zini G, Maucini A, Toni A, Frezza G, Neri S, Putti C, Babiui L: Combined therapy of localized Ewing's sarcoma of bone: analysis of results in 100 patients, *Int J Radiat Oncology Biol Phys* 19:1165-1170, 1990.
28. Cangir A, Vietti TJ, Gehan EA, Burgert EO Jr, Thomas P, Tefft M, Nesbit ME, Kissane J, Pritchard D: Ewing's sarcoma metastatic at diagnosis: results and comparisons of two intergroup Ewing's sarcoma studies, *Cancer* 66:887-893, 1990.
29. Schmidt D, Herrmann C, Jurgens H, Harris D: Malignant peripheral neuroectodermal tumor and its necessary distinction from Ewing's sarcoma, *Cancer* 63:2251-2259, 1991.
30. Marina N, Etcubanas E, Parham DM, Bowman LC, Green AA: Peripheral primitive neuroectodermal tumor (peripheral neuroepithelioma) in children, *Cancer* 64:1952-1960, 1989.
31. Ducatman RS, Scheithauer BW, Piepgras DG, Reiman HM, Ilstrup DM: Malignant peripheral nerve sheath tumors: a clinicopathologic study of 120 cases, *Cancer* 57:2006-2021, 1986.
32. Meis JM, Enzinger FM, Martz KL, et al: Malignant peripheral nerve sheath tumors (malignant schwannomas) in children, *Am J Surg Pathol* 16:694-707, 1992.
33. Sale PM, Parsons RE, Stevens MM: Diagnosis and behavior of juvenile rhabdomyosarcoma, *Hum Pathol* 14:596-611, 1983.
34. Ortega JA, Wharam M, Gehan EA, Ragab AH, Crist W, Webber B, Wiener ES, Haeberlen V, Maurer HM: Clinical features and results of therapy for children with paraspinal soft tissue sarcoma: a report of the Intergroup Rhabdomyosarcoma Study, *J Clin Oncol* 9:796-801, 1991.
35. Maurer HM, Gehan EA, Beltangady M, Crist W, Dickman PS, Donaldson SS, Fryer C, Hammond D, Hays DM, Herrmann, Heyn R, Jones PM, Lawrence W, Newton W, Ortega J, Ragab AH, Ramez RB, Ruymann FB, Soulef, Tefft M, Webber B, Wiener E, Wharam M, Vietle TJ: The Intergroup Rhabdomyosarcoma Study—II, *Cancer* 71:1904-1922, 1993.
36. Cooper SP, Fraire AE, Buffler PA, Greenberg SD, Langston C: Epidemiologic aspects of childhood mesothelioma, *Pathol Immunopathol Res* 8:276-278, 1989.
37. Brenner J, Sordillo PP, Mogill GB: Malignant mesothelioma in children, *Med Pediatr Oncol* 9:367-373, 1981.

Pulmonary Radiation Fibrosis

38. Rubin P, Shapiro DL, Finkelstein JN, Peuney DP: The early release of surfactant following lung irradiation of alveolar type II cells, *Int J Radiat Oncol Biol Phys* 6:75-77, 1980.
39. Kun LE, Moulder JE: General principles of radiation therapy. In Pizzo PA, Poplack DG, eds: *Principles and practice of pediatric oncology,* Philadelphia, 1993, JB Lippincott.
40. Green DM, Finklestein JZ, Tefft ME, Norkool P: Diffuse interstitial pneumonitis after pulmonary irradiation for metastatic Wilms' tumor, *Cancer* 63:450-453, 1989.

CHAPTER 80

Psychiatric Aspects of Respiratory Symptoms

Marianne Z. Wamboldt and Frederick S. Wamboldt

Soul and body, I suggest, react sympathetically upon each other: a change in the state of the soul produces a change in the shape of the body, and conversely: a change in the shape of the body produces a change in the state of the soul.

Aristotle

This chapter reviews the etiology, pathophysiology, and treatment of three disorders that show prominent concurrence of psychiatric and respiratory symptoms. Before beginning this review it is important to understand current thinking about the interrelationship between psychiatric and respiratory disorders. Just as there are few medical disorders caused by a single gene defect (e.g., Huntington's disease), so too are there few disorders caused by a purely psychologic problem or conflict. Most psychiatric disorders are currently envisioned to have multifactorial etiologies: some amount of genetic contribution, some current imbalance in the biochemical neurotransmitters, some environmental inputs, and some individual cognitive distortions. In examining disorders with intertwined psychiatric and respiratory aspects, one similarly finds etiologic influences across the biopsychosocial continuum. In these cases, the medical problem confronting the pulmonologist usually combines a biogenetic predisposition to certain types of symptoms (e.g., "twitchy airways" or sensitized cough receptors) with environmental inputs, individual beliefs or cognitions, and the response of the medical and family systems to the original symptoms.

Thus it is seldom, if ever, clinically useful to depict a respiratory symptom or symptom complex to a patient or the patient's family as purely emotional or psychiatric. On the contrary, however, once the physiologic component of a symptom is acknowledged, it is often useful to point out that "stress" or other psychologic factors may play a key role in triggering or exacerbating the symptom. As will be seen from the ensuing discussion of the close central nervous system (CNS) connection between centers of respiratory control with affective, anxiety, and cognitive centers, this is especially true for certain common disorders of breathing.

"SOMATIC" ANXIETY DISORDERS: PANIC ATTACKS, PANIC DISORDER, AND HYPERVENTILATION

These common conditions will be discussed together for two reasons. First, there exists great overlap between the phenomenologic and pathophysiologic expression of these conditions, despite the fact that they are not totally overlapping syndromes. Second, principals of effective treatment are more or less the same across these disorders.

In general, all these conditions include some combination of the following clinical paroxysmal signs and symptoms: (1) intense feeling of discomfort or fear; (2) autonomic arousal; (3) vague, diffuse, "atypical" bodily sensations; (4) overbreathing; (5) catastrophic cognitions (e.g., fear of losing control, going crazy, or dying); and (6) avoidance behavior. The onset of these conditions is most common in late adolescence or early adult years, although prepubertal onset has been reported.[1-3] All are prevalent yet underdiagnosed disorders in primary care as well as pulmonology and cardiology specialty clinics. They are major sources of preventable morbidity and mortality in these settings because safe, reliable, and effective treatment strategies exist.

Panic Attacks and Acute Hyperventilation

Panic attacks are an extremely common experience, with one quarter to one third of the U.S. population reporting lifetime occurrence of at least one panic attack.[4,5] The term *panic attack* refers to an acute episode of sudden intense fear or discomfort that rapidly builds in a crescendo fashion over a period of minutes and that is associated with a number of somatic or cognitive symptoms. Accordingly, the diagnostic label *panic attack* is a phenomenologic or descriptive one, implying nothing about etiology or pathophysiology. The specific DSM-IV diagnostic criteria for panic attack are listed in Box 80-1.[6]

Acute hyperventilation, on the other hand, is the physiologic state of overbreathing in which breathing is occurring in excess of metabolic requirements, leading to an acute reduction in $Pa{CO_2}$ and the consistent set of physiologic changes that occur in response to this state. Most typically, acute hyperventilation occurs because of a modest increase in tidal volume (e.g., 750 ml/min) in conjunction with a "normal" respiration rate (e.g., 16 to 17 breaths/min). Hence, clinically significant overbreathing is often not grossly visible.[7]

The multiple physiologic changes that occur during and in immediate response to acute hyperventilation are the proximal cause of many of the somatic and CNS symptoms that occur during a panic attack. The immediate effect of overbreathing is that the $Pa{CO_2}$ drops, blood pH rises, and an acute state of hypocapnic, respiratory alkalosis is induced, typically in 1 minute or less. In response to this state of respiratory alkalosis a variety of secondary physiologic changes occur in a rapid, sequential cascade.[8-11] First, there is a shift in the oxyhemoglobin dissociation curve so that oxygen is bound more tightly (the Bohr effect), resulting in less efficient delivery of oxygen. Second, hypocapnia leads to CNS vasoconstriction. The resulting reduced cerebral flow is assumed to be the cause of a variety of the CNS symptoms observed, such as lightheadedness, dizziness, depersonalization, blurred vision, confusion, and even focal neurologic signs. Third, paresthesias and pain symptoms commonly arise in response to the combination of direct effect of persistent alkalosis on peripheral nerves, mechanical muscle fatigue, and peripheral vasoconstriction and spasm. Fourth, mouth breathing and aerophagia can contribute to the symptoms of dry mouth, abdominal dis-

BOX 80-1
Signs and Symptoms of a Panic Attack

A. A discrete period of intense fear or discomfort,
B. During which four or more of the following symptoms developed abruptly and reached a peak within 10 minutes:
 1. Palpitations, pounding heart, or accelerated heart rate
 2. Sweating
 3. Trembling or shaking
 4. Sensations of shortness of breath or smothering
 5. Feeling of choking
 6. Chest pain or discomfort
 7. Nausea or abdominal distress
 8. Feeling dizzy, unsteady, lighthearted, or faint
 9. Derealization or depersonalization
 10. Fear of losing control or going crazy
 11. Fear of dying
 12. Paresthesia
 13. Chills or hot flashes
C. Other signs/symptoms often associated with panic attacks or hyperventilation:
 1. Electrocardiogram changes (e.g., ST segment depression, T wave inversion)
 2. Musculoskeletal pain, stiffness, "fibrositis"
 3. Weakness, listlessness, exhaustion
 4. Poor concentration, forgetfulness, confusion
 5. Euphoria
 6. Frequent sighing, yawning, thoracic breathing
 7. Dry mouth, aerophagia, flatulence
 8. Blurred vision
 9. Syncope, seizures
 10. Focal neurologic signs and symptoms (often left sided)
 11. Extreme sensitivity to stimulant side effects of medications
 12. Hallucinations (rare)
 13. Tetany (rare)

Criteria A and B are required to make a diagnosis of panic attack using DSM-IV criteria.

tress, and flatulence. Fifth, as the patient attempts to interpret these sensations a variety of catastrophic cognitions can arise, feeding back to lower brain centers and continuing the attack. Finally, this physiologic cascade is mitigated or terminated as renal compensation restores normal arterial pH by increasing bicarbonate excretion and as relative cerebral hypoxia induces vascular dilation restoring CNS blood flow.

Several important long-term effects can occur as a result of the renal compensation of the acute hyperventilation episode that increase the likelihood that a diathesis toward future panic/hyperventilation episodes is maintained. First, although renal compensation restores normal blood pH, both arterial $Paco_2$ and bicarbonate levels remain low. Because the chemoreceptor system's control function for CO_2 is nonlinear (i.e., whereas at $Paco_2$ levels above 35 mm Hg any rise in $Paco_2$ is strongly opposed by the chemoreceptor system promptly increasing ventilation, at $Paco_2$ levels below 35 mm Hg this system provides virtually no change in ventilatory drive), in the "compensated" state, small changes in ventilation can rapidly lower an individual's $Paco_2$ with no opposition from the control system.[8] Furthermore, if episodes of acute hyperventilation continue long enough, continued renal compensation can lead to depletion of the bicarbonate buffer system, thereby amplifying the physiologic effects of low $Paco_2$[11] Hence a vicious cycle can be established in which a few sighs or deep breaths can lead to intensified and continued episodes of acute panic and hyperventilation.[7,8] Indeed, several authors have recently suggested the potential of chronic hyperventilation underlying some states of chronic fatigue and incapacity, such as the "soldier's heart," the "effort syndrome," DaCosta's syndrome, and neurocirculatory asthenia.[11,12]

A key question remains. What is the primary cause of the initial drive toward hyperventilation and the acute episodes? Box 80-2 lists a variety of reported causes. As can be seen from inspection of this list, the site of patient contact, be it in an emergency department, an intensive care unit, or the outpatient office of a pulmonary or psychiatric specialist, is often a major factor in what specific differential diagnoses come to the fore for a specific patient.

Panic Disorder

Panic disorder is diagnosed when there is the presence of recurrent, unexpected panic attacks followed by at least 1 month's duration of persistent concern about having another panic attack, worry about possible implications or consequences of the attacks, or a significant behavioral change as a result of the attacks. Two features of panic disorder should place it near the top of a physician's differential diagnostic list in most patients suffering from recurrent panic attacks or hyperventilation. First, panic disorder is an extremely prevalent condition. Epidemiologic research suggests a lifetime prevalence rate of 2% to 5%.[13,14] Furthermore, panic disorder is estimated as the major clinical problem in 10% to 15% of patients entering primary care as well as pulmonology, cardiology, and gastroenterology subspecialty practices.[15-20] Second, the pathophysiology of panic disorder has become increasingly clear with safe and effective treatments available.[21-24]

The primary lesion in panic disorder appears to be a hyperresponsive brain stem respiratory sensor system.[25] The leading current pathophysiologic model of panic disorder posits that false central "suffocation alarms" arise from the hypersensitive response of ventromedullar chemoreceptors to increasing carbon dioxide lead to prompt activation of the pontine noradrenergic nucleus, the locus ceruleus, thereby increasing minute ventilation twofold to threefold and triggering the physiologic cascade of a panic attack.[21,22,24] In support of this proposition, inhalation of CO_2 or sodium lactate infusion causes increased ventilation, and both challenges are potent and specific panicogens in susceptible individuals. Furthermore, antipanic medication has been shown to be able to block the respiratory stimulatory and panic-inducing effects of these laboratory challenges.[26,27] Interestingly, although acute hyperventilation almost invariably occurs after the triggering of a false suffocation alarm, enforced acute hyperventilation only infrequently (in around 25% of patients with panic disorder) causes a panic attack.[28,29] Furthermore, although approximately 50% of patients with panic disorder have blood gases consistent with chronic, compensated hyperventilation (i.e., low $Paco_2$ and bicarbonate with normal pH), within the false suffocation model of panic disorder such chronic hyperventilation, by resulting in chronically low $Paco_2$, may represent an adaptive response to the central hyperresponsivity to high CO_2.[21] In summary, panic disorder appears best conceptualized as primarily a disorder of brain physiology, not a problem of neurosis, character weakness, or other "deep-seated" psychologic conflict.

Nonetheless, the recurrent panic attacks of panic disorder can be and often are associated with significant psychosocial morbidity. Klein[30] has proposed a temporal and logical sequence for the symptom clusters that are seen in panic disorder. First is the acute panic anxiety elicited during the panic attack. Such anxiety is especially potent given its intense visceral, bodily nature and the sense of inexplicable catastrophe that typically accompanies the episode. Individuals who suffer such an episode usually have no solid, logical explanation of why the event occurred, and therefore with recurrent attacks can feel helpless and confused, and often grasp for answers that will allow them to escape from these attacks.

The second feature, anticipatory anxiety, arises as a response to the intense conditioning stimuli of an acute panic attack. In more common terms, the patient's level of chronic anxiety or "nervousness" rises out of the uncertainty and worry about when the next attack will occur. Three important clinical correlates of this more generalized and chronic anxiety state are that such patients may be more likely (1) to appear to have "excessive stress" or "psychologic overlay" as they enter the health care setting, thereby receiving poorer quality of care[16,23]; (2) to establish a state of chronic hyperventilation, thereby being vulnerable to experience more frequent and intense recurrences[8]; and (3) to have higher cortical learning involved in the pathophysiology of their panic attacks. The relevance of this last point is highlighted by the recent finding from a CO_2 inhalation challenge experiment that panic disorder patients given a false illusion of control during the inhalation protocol were less likely to have a panic attack during the challenge than patients who believed that they had no control over the CO_2 challenge.[31]

Third, up to one third of patients begin to phobically avoid situations that they come to believe trigger acute episodes (e.g., leaving their house, driving their car, or taking baths or showers). Such agoraphobic behavior greatly increases the psychosocial morbidity of panic disorder because of the interpersonal and sociovocational difficulties that arise as the patient's significant others, friends, and employers react to this seemingly "irrational" avoidance behavior.

Finally, significant demoralization or frank depression arises. Indeed, studies suggest that up to three quarters of patients with panic disorder become clinically depressed.[32-34] Suicide rates for patients with panic disorder are among the highest for any psychiatric disorder.[35]

Panic, Hyperventilation, and Asthma

Available information suggests that panic attacks and panic disorder are common comorbid psychiatric disorders in patients with chronic respiratory illness.[36,37] The pulmonologist treating such patients is confronted by the complex intertwining of the "somatic" anxiety disorders and asthma. Hyperventilation (even when isocapnia is maintained) can precipitate bronchial constriction. Indeed, isocapnic hyperventilation has been proposed as a highly specific measure of airway hyperresponsiveness in asthma.[38] Conversely, the $Pa{CO_2}$ increase during an acute asthma attack can trigger a panic attack in patients with panic disorder.[39] Additionally, although the symptoms of air hunger, shortness of breath, chest discomfort, and acute fear are similar across these conditions, the treatments are not. Hence patients with combined panic disorder and asthma may be less adherent with their medication regimen (presumably overusing bronchodilators) and at risk to develop eroded confidence in physicians who prescribe antiasthma medications that do not fully alleviate distress. Additionally, certain asthma treatments, such as beta-agonists, can increase autonomic arousal, thereby precipitating or worsening panic attacks. Accordingly, it is not surprising that a number of clinicians have argued for increased recognition and aggressive treatment of comorbid panic disorder in both pediatric and adult patients with asthma.[39-41]

Principles of Treatment for Panic Attacks, Hyperventilation, and Panic Disorder

Fortunately, acute panic attacks and hyperventilation, as well as more chronic panic disorders, even when complicated by significant agoraphobia, are readily treated. Basic guidelines for treatment follow.

Begin with Education

Panic attacks and episodes of acute hyperventilation are horribly frightening experiences. Patients are generally frightened, confused, and very uncomfortable. They may feel that something is terribly wrong with their bodies. The physician can greatly improve chances of a successful outcome by taking several minutes with the patient to cover the following points, thus providing the patient with a clear, cogent explanation of the panic attack. First, panic attacks are extremely common, even though most people never talk about them. They are not a sign of impending insanity or a flawed character. Second, panic attacks cause a real bodily experience because the brain has given the body a "false alarm," but the body has had no way of knowing that the alarm was not a true one. Third, certain medical problems can cause symptoms similar to those the patient has experienced (see Box 80-2), but these should have been considered, checked, and ruled out by the physician. Fourth, although such attacks may disappear without treatment, safe and effective treatment exists, and it is highly recommended that patients begin these treatments. Such treatment consists of medication and some breathing and behavioral changes, the combination of which will help patients gain control over their attacks over a period of several weeks.

Pharmacological Blockage of Panic

Medication treatment should be instituted to block or blunt the attacks. For the vast majority of patients with panic disorder, the medication of choice is a tricyclic antidepressant (TCA) or selective serotonin reuptake inhibitor (SSRI). Of these, the medications with the most well established record of clinical efficacy are the TCAs (imipramine, desipramine and clomipramine), with a rapidly growing track record for the SSRIs (fluoxetine, sertraline, and paroxetine).[42] A number of other commonly prescribed psychotropic medications, most notably trazadone and buspirone, have little to no antipanic activity. Because a potentially large subset of patients with panic disorder are inordinately sensitive to the stimulatory effects of these antidepressant medications (e.g., agitation, restlessness, insomnia),[42] therapy should begin with low dosages (e.g., fluoxetine 5 to 10 mg every morning or desipramine 10 to 25 mg at bedtime in adults; fluoxetine 5 mg every other day in children). Aggressive use of antidepressant medications is particularly necessary in the case of panic disorder complicated by major depressive disorder because depression appears to significantly diminish the efficacy of the behavioral treatments described in the subsequent two sections.[43,44]

High-potency benzodiazepines (e.g., alprazolam and clonazepam) appear to be equally effective in short-term treatment of panic attacks. Recent reports suggest that these medications can be safe and effective in the context of panic disorder in children with severe asthma.[39] However, given the potential

BOX 80-2
Causes of Hyperventilation

Respiratory Disorders

Asthma
Pneumonia
Pulmonary embolism
Interstitial lung disease
Chronic obstructive lung disease
Respiratory dyskinesia/diaphragmatic flutter
Pulmonary hypertension
Pneumothorax

Central Nervous System and Psychiatric Disorders

Panic disorder (via a hypersensitive medullary "suffocation alarm")
Phobias
Generalized anxiety disorder
Central neurogenic hyperventilation
Hiccup/palatal myoclonus
Central nervous system lesion (especially brain stem; e.g., tumor, post–cerebrovascular accident, meningitis)
Factitious (consciously induced or simulated)

Pharmacologic Agents

Aspirin and other salicylates
Alcohol withdrawal
Neuroleptics (via respiratory dyskinesia)

Other

Chronic, severe pain
Adaptation to higher altitude
Pyrexia/sepsis
Heat exhaustion/heatstroke
Pregnancy/luteal phase of menstrual cycle (via progesterone)
Liver disease/failure

for benzodiazepines to cause tolerance, dependence, and respiratory depression, their use should be limited in individuals with pulmonary illness to patients with very infrequent panic attacks who do not require daily medication, or to the initial weeks of treatment in patients with a more severe disorder while awaiting the response to the antidepressant medication.

Respiratory Control Treatments

Coincident with the start of pharmacologic treatment, patients should be instructed in respiratory control strategies to prevent or limit the hyperventilation that occurs during an attack. Extensive clinical research supports that there are two important aspects to such training.[7,45-51]

First, patients should be informed that once a "false" suffocation alarm occurs, the body's natural response is hyperventilation, and that it is this hyperventilation that causes most of the discomfort experienced during a panic attack/hyperventilation episode. It is to this end that a hyperventilation provocation test (i.e., vigorous, voluntary overbreathing for 1 to 3 minutes to elicit symptoms of hyperventilation and asking the patient to compare these symptoms with those of a panic attack) is most useful. The key is to use the test not so much for diagnosis, but as a step in legitimizing the explanation for symptom production that the patient has been given, thereby fostering a collaborative treatment alliance.

Second, patients benefit from training in slow, regular, diaphragmatic breathing, with specific comments to avoid mouth breathing, thoracic breathing, or excessive sighing or yawning as appropriate. Patients often require practice and the help of a coach (therapist or family member) to remember to commence such breathing during the "heat" of an impending panic attack. Training in more general relaxation techniques is often advocated, although such training is most likely a simple, nonspecific adjuvant therapy.

Finally, effective flooding or desensitization protocols for treatment of panic attacks using CO_2 inhalation or lactate infusions have been described.[51-54] Such repeated provocations of panic attacks probably function similarly to the hyperventilation provocation test in that patients can discover a cause for their distress and thereby gain some sense of control over their panic attacks.

Exposure Therapy of Associated Avoidance Behavior

Given that significant avoidance (agoraphobic) behavior complicates the clinical presentation in up to 30% of patients with panic disorder, in vivo exposure treatment of the avoidance behavior is often required for recovery. Principles of such treatment are well described.[43-45] In essence, exposure treatment involves graduated real-life exposure of the patient to the fear-producing situation until he or she gains tolerance to the discomfort of being in the situation. The patient uses respiratory control techniques to manage the panic experienced during the exposure. Typically, ability for the patient to tolerate the previously dreaded and avoided situation occurs after 2 to 10 repetitions of the exposure.

Additional treatments, such as marital or family therapy, should be considered when appropriate. Treatment ends with a reexplanation of the behavioral "tools," with the explicit prediction that although relapse is possible, any recurrence of symptoms would diminish promptly once the patient reinstitutes the newly learned behavioral control strategies.

VOCAL CORD DYSFUNCTION

Vocal cord dysfunction (VCD) is a recently defined disorder in which the vocal cords paradoxically close on inspiration, producing airflow obstruction at the larynx and causing audible wheeze or stridor. The clinical presentation ranges from mild asthma or croup to total upper airway occlusion. Although usually the arterial blood gases are normal during symptomatic episodes, both hypoxia and hypocapnia have been reported. The acute presentation is often dramatic and misdiagnosed, leading to unnecessary intubation, tracheotomy, or treatment with high doses of corticosteroids.

The clinical syndrome was first documented in 1842 by Dunglison,[55] who described it as an adduction of the laryngeal muscles in hysterical female patients and called it "hysteric croup." The prescribed treatment was "cold water thrown over the face and neck and compound spirit of ammonia held to the nostrils." "Functional upper airways obstruction without organic abnormalities" was described in three patients in 1981,[56] all of whom had acute upper airway obstruction, hypoxia, and tracheotomies. These were the first patients in whom the vocal cord abnormalities were documented by visualization of the adduction of the true and false vocal cords during symptomatic episodes. The term *vocal cord dysfunction* was coined by Christopher et al[57] in 1983, who described five cases of adults in whom paroxysms of wheezing and dyspnea were refractory to standard therapy for asthma. Laryngoscopy confirmed that wheezing was caused by adduction of the true and false vocal cords throughout the respiratory cycle, which was essentially normal when patients were asymptomatic. The patients could not reproduce the vocal cord abnormality voluntarily.

Although the exact prevalence of VCD is unknown, it does not appear to be rare. One reason that it has been thought to be uncommon is that it is often reported under a variety of names, as can be seen in Box 80-3. Additionally, reports have been published in a variety of disparate and nonoverlapping literatures (e.g., anesthesia, otolaryngology, emergency medicine, psychiatry, pulmonology, and pediatrics), thus making it difficult to assimilate a complete clinical picture. Nonetheless, from 1965 through 1995 at least 51 reports of clinical syndromes similar to VCD were published, representing a total of 182 cases.[56-112] Of the reported cases, the majority (83%) have been in female patients. The mean age of the patients is 24 years, with a range of 4 to 74 years of age. One prototypic patient type is described[94] as an overweight woman between the ages of 20 and 40, with a greater than high school education, who works in a medically related field. Another prototypic patient[60] is a child or adolescent with above average IQ and high needs for achievement in academics and sports.

Vocal cord dysfunction can cause stridor, shortness of breath, or wheezing. The syndrome is suspected when the patient does not reveal an organic cause of upper airway obstruction or respond to adequate asthma therapy. The symptoms often start and cease abruptly, and the patient is asymptomatic between attacks. Often patients indicate that they feel throat tightness or that their voice changes during an acute attack. Patients who have "pure" VCD may indicate that bronchodilators do not help their breathing and deny that respiratory symptoms awaken them at night. Although wheezing can sometimes be heard over the larynx, it can be transmitted from the lower airways as well as occur from the larynx; thus the physical examination is unreliable in distinguishing a VCD attack from an asthmatic episode. However, if at the time of acute symptoms the patient is able to hold his or her breath or pant, this is suggestive of VCD because patients suffering an acute asthma attack will be unable to comply. While asymptomatic, patients with pure VCD have normal pulmonary function tests, which may help distinguish them from asthmatics, who often have increased residual volumes, indicating air trapping from small airways closure. During acute symptoms, the patient with VCD may have a truncated inspiratory or expiratory limb of the flow-volume loop, indicating variable obstruction. The ratio of expiratory flow to inspiratory flow at 50% of forced vital capacity is usually greater than 1.5. However, even during an acute VCD attack, the alveolar-arterial oxygen difference is usually normal.

The diagnosis is definitively established by visualization of the vocal cords. Vocal cord dysfunction is characterized by adduction of the anterior two thirds of the vocal cords with a characteristic "posterior chink." Several variations of this classical sign have been defined as well. Of the 182 published cases, 167 documented visualization of the vocal cords. A total of 131 cases (78%) had vocal cord adduction during inspiration only, 19 (11%) during both inspiration and expiration, and 2 (1%) during expiration alone. Another 15 cases (9%) reported normal vocal cord movement. In many of these latter cases, laryngoscopy was performed while the patient was asymptomatic. If the vocal cords are not seen to adduct during an acute attack, the diagnosis of VCD must be seriously questioned. However, in one series approximately half of the unstimulated laryngoscopies done on patients ultimately diagnosed with VCD were normal.[94] Reports of VCD patients have indicated that VCD, like asthma, can be precipitated by stress, exercise, cold air, upper respiratory infections, and inhalation of irritants or methacholine. Many times, the VCD is provoked by bronchial challenges or exercise. One systematic procedure for doing this is suggested in the review by Newman and Dubester.[94] Functional upper airway obstruction has also been described with pharyngeal constriction and abnormal motion of the arytenoid region,[113,114] or "voluntary glottic closure."[66] These patients may or may not also have VCD. Finally, many patients have comorbid asthma and VCD,[60] and one has been reported to have cystic fibrosis and VCD,[106] making the diagnosis very difficult to sort out.

BOX 80-3
Terms Used for Vocal Cord Dysfunction

Adult spasmodic croup[62]
Bilateral abductor vocal cord paresis[111]
Emotional laryngeal wheezing[103]
Episodic laryngeal dyskinesia[102]
Expiratory laryngeal stridor[85]
Factitious asthma[67]
Functional abduction paresis[92]
Functional laryngeal obstruction[99,108]
Functional stridor[82]
Functional upper airway obstruction[56,75,112]
Hysterical croup[55]
Hysterical stridor[111]
Laryngeal spasm[61]
Munchausen's stridor[97,109]
Nonorganic laryngeal obstruction[97]
Nonorganic acute upper airway obstruction[63]
Paradoxic vocal cord adduction[74]
Paradoxic vocal cord motion[87]
Pseudoasthma[66]
Psychogenic stridor[70,83,109]
Psychogenic upper airway obstruction[58]
Psychogenic wheeze[72]

Biogenetic Influences and Vocal Cord Disorder

Patients with VCD closely resemble those with a medical condition described as extrathoracic hyperresponsivity.[115] Extrathoracic airway narrowing was indexed by the maximal mid-inspiratory flow rate (MIF_{50}), and bronchial narrowing assessed by the forced expiratory volume (FEV_1). Bucca et al[115] described a sample of 20 men and 20 women with a 2-month history of episodic dyspnea or cough, but no diagnosis of bronchial asthma. Following a histamine challenge when asymptomatic, all but three of the patients exhibited hyperresponsiveness of the airways: two thirds of these (25 patients) had extrathoracic hyperresponsivity as defined by the provocative concentration of histamine ($PC_{25}MIF_{50}$) being less than 8 mg/ml. The other one third showed lower airway reactivity, as defined by provocative concentration of histamine ($PC_{20}FEV_1$) less than 8 mg/ml. Three patients and 9 controls showed no hyperresponsivity of airways. Results of laryngoscopy revealed that although the glottis was normal at baseline, following histamine challenge there was marked mucosal edema, pharyngoconstriction, and adduction of the vocal cords during inspiration in the extrathoracic hyperresponsivity group, but not in the bronchial hyperreactivity group or controls. Upper airway hyperresponsivity was associated with postnasal drip, dysphonia, and sinusitis, suggesting that it is sustained by chronic inflammatory diseases of the upper respiratory tract. Interestingly, the majority of subjects with upper airway hyperresponsivity were female (77%). The authors note that their group did not appear to have a psychosomatic syndrome, and they had never presented as a medical emergency.

There is some additional suggestion that allergy and inflammation may play a role in extrathoracic airway hyperresponsivity, much as it does in bronchial hyperresponsivity. For example, Zach et al[116] studied 110 children 9 years after each had been hospitalized for recurrent croup. They found a highly significant association between allergy and recurrent croup. Those with recurrent croup also had a family disposition to croup, suggesting some inherited predisposition. Children with recent recurrent croup also showed a plateau deformity of the inspiratory curve following histamine challenge that was significantly greater than that in healthy children and children with asthma.[116] Their flattened flow-volume loops were identical to those of patients with VCD, yet the authors did not mention any increase in psychologic problems among this group. Yet another study documented that chronic postnasal drip in adults is associated with both cough and variable upper airway obstruction, as measured by the FIF_{50}/FEF_{50} ratio and flattened flow-volume loops.[117] In two of these patients, vocal cord edema was noted on laryngoscopy; in the others, the vocal cords were normal. It is possible that these patients have a mild form of upper airway hyperresponsivity, indicating that there is probably a spectrum, with severe VCD at the extreme endpoint.

Psychiatric Disorders and Vocal Cord Disorder

Although previously described as having a purely "psychogenic basis,"[72] the etiologic picture appears to be more complicated as more systematic study of VCD progresses and the reports from differing clinical sites (e.g., primary care versus tertiary care) are collated. The major psychiatric syndromes that have been reported to be associated with VCD are factitious disorder, conversion disorder, and psychologic factors affecting medical condition. These will be discussed in turn.

Factitious Disorder

Factitious disorder, also known as Munchausen's syndrome, is diagnosed when the patient intentionally produces or feigns symptoms in order to assume the sick role. The judgment that a symptom is intentionally produced is made by direct evidence and by excluding other causes of the symptom. The presentation may include fabrication of subjective complaints, self-inflicted conditions, or exaggeration or exacerbation of a preexisting medical condition.[6] The motivation is to assume the sick role. If there is an obvious external incentive (e.g., to be out of jail, economic gain, avoiding legal responsibility), the condition is labeled malingering. In VCD, there is a documented physical abnormality, the paradoxic adduction of the vocal cords. It is doubtful that this can be feigned or purposely induced; for example, in the study by Christopher et al,[57] patients were asked to duplicate their symptoms while the vocal cords were being visualized. The patients were not able to do so. Therefore, in most cases where the vocal cords are seen to have the characteristic posterior chink while the patient is symptomatic, factitious disorder is probably not an accurate diagnosis. Furthermore, factitious disorder is difficult to treat or interrupt, and most patients with the disorder are severely psychologically disturbed. This is not the case in many patients with VCD. However, a patient may feign wheezing or strider at times when the cords are not truly adducted, meeting the criteria of purposeful exaggeration of an existing medical condition. These patients would then be diagnosed as having factitious disorder. It may be possible that in these patients it is actually the pharyngeal muscles that are closing, not the vocal cords per se. Out of the published cases, eight (4%) have been described as factitious disorder. In reviewing the information given in these case reports, it seems that two may be accurately diagnosed, in that evidence is presented that they induced other physical symptoms, lied to health care personnel on several occasions, and left hospitals against medical advice when confronted. However, in the other six cases, the diagnosis is questionable: four were diagnosed without visualization of the vocal cords and before VCD was a well-described syndrome; two others had adduction of vocal cords noted when symptomatic.

Conversion Disorder

Conversion disorder is a diagnosis commonly given to the cases reported as VCD: 25% of the published cases received this diagnosis. The essential feature of conversion disorder is "the presence of symptoms or deficits affecting *voluntary* motor or sensory function that suggest a neurological or other general medical condition. . . . The initiation or exacerbation of the symptom or deficit is preceded by conflicts or other stressors . . . and the symptoms are not intentionally produced or feigned."[6] Most patients with conversion disorders have other symptoms consistent with hysteria. Of note, most patients with VCD did not have the diagnosis of hysterical traits. The diagnosis of conversion disorder should not be given if the symptoms can be fully explained by a neurologic or other general medical condition. Additionally, symptoms of conversion disorders do not generally conform to known anatomic pathways and physiologic mechanisms.[6] These criteria have led some to question whether *conversion disorder* is an accurate description of VCD.[118] The reasoning against conversion disorder is as follows.

First, the diagnosis of VCD is confirmed by evidence of a medical abnormality that conforms to known pathways. The enervation of the musculature involved with upper airway muscles includes cranial nerves 5, 7, 9, and 10 and cervical nerves 1, 2, and 3.[119] Proctor[119] additionally postulates a central nervous system controller of these muscles that can override metabolic demands when necessary for speech, swallowing, cough, and so forth. Given the complexity of timing in the system and the probable enervation from the CNS, it is not surprising that many emotional or cognitive inputs could disrupt the sensitive timing of these muscles. Someone with a basic failure or perversion of the rhythmic neuromuscular activity could have a system that is easily disrupted by emotional inputs. Second, conversion disorders involve symptoms that are under *voluntary* control. In a study of dogs, Aviv et al[120] demonstrated that lung inflation could produce involuntary laryngeal adduction or abduction, depending on the preexisting level of CO_2 and O_2. They studied lightly anesthetized dogs, who were tracheotomized, and administered continuous positive airway pressure (CPAP). They showed that if hyperventilation preceded lung inflation, the vocal cords adducted into laryngospasm. However, if lung inflation was preceded by a 1-minute occlusion of the lower respiratory tract, the vocal cords went into abductor spasm. This study raises the question whether the reflexive adduction of vocal cords may be metabolically determined in part, or, as Proctor suggested, is caused by a misfiring of neurons that control the musculature.

In both instances, however, psychologic factors may contribute to the triggering of the VCD, either through interruption of the timing or through hyperventilation leading to hypocapnia. Thus there is controversy in the literature as to whether VCD should be classified as a conversion disorder. Early reports stating that VCD is a conversion disorder often gave a misdiagnosis.

Psychologic Factors Affecting Medical Condition

Given that strong evidence suggests that vocal cord dysfunction is associated with extrathoracic airway hyperresponsivity and that the previously reported psychiatric diagnoses of conversion disorder and factitious disorder do not accurately describe most cases of VCD, "psychologic factors affecting medical condition" seems to be the most appropriate psychiatric diagnosis for the majority of VCD patients. For reasons given previously, there is likely to be a greater chance that psychologic upset may precipitate or exacerbate this condition more than many other medical conditions. The essential feature of this diagnosis is the presence of specific psychologic or behavioral factors that adversely affect a medical condition.[6] The factors can influence the course of a medical condition (which can be inferred from the close temporal association between the factors and development or exacerbation of a condition), or the factors may precipitate or exacerbate symptoms of a medical condition by eliciting stress-related physiologic responses. In this regard, VCD is similar to asthma. "Psychological factors are known to induce bronchospasm in patients with asthma, yet there is no proof that emotional factors are directly involved in the aetiology of bronchial asthma."[109]

Comorbid Psychiatric Conditions

Is there any evidence that persons suffering from VCD have higher prevalence rates or more severe psychologic problems than the medically ill or non-ill populations? The early, uncontrolled case reports suggested this conclusion. For example, Freedman et al[68] stated, "In our experience, and that of other researchers, VCD appeared as just one symptom of patients suffering from more pervasive psychiatric disturbances." The same group indicated that a high percentage of VCD patients either admitted to or were suspected of having been sexually abused. However, it must be noted that the patients Freedman et al[68] studied were referred to a tertiary center for respiratory illness. Could the conclusion that VCD is associated with severe psychologic problems be an artifact of the sample? In reviewing all of the cases published, many of which were from emergency room or primary care offices, the following psychiatric diagnoses were given (some patients received more than one diagnosis): conversion disorder (19%), "family conflict" (18%), depression (13%), anxiety disorder (13%), factitious disorder (8%), personality disorders (7%), posttraumatic stress disorder (2%), unknown or refused evaluation (9%), no diagnosis (16%). Evidence of prior sexual abuse was not noted in any reports other than Freedman et al[68] (14 of 47 adult patients) and Brugman et al[60] (4 of 37 pediatric patients). Note that not all of the patients were formally evaluated by a psychiatrist and that none were evaluated with a structured psychiatric research interview, the current state of the art. Additionally, these rates are not higher than epidemiologic samples for depression or anxiety disorders. The question of whether conversion disorder and factitious disorder were accurate diagnoses for these patients has already been addressed. The rate for personality disorders, indicating pervasive psychologic problems, is high, but still a minority of the group. In studies in which patients with VCD were compared to patients with moderate to severe asthma, there were no group differences in psychopathology.[57,102] Thus it can be concluded that although the rates of major psychiatric disorders are probably not higher in patients with VCD than patients with other chronic respiratory illnesses, the rates may be higher than in the nonill population. It is likely that emotional factors, such as family conflicts and stress, may precipitate symptoms with this illness more commonly than in other respiratory syndromes. However, it is unlikely that psychologic factors are the sole etiologic factors in this disorder.

Treatment of Vocal Cord Disorder

The importance of making the correct diagnosis is that treatment for VCD differs from those for asthma or organic obstruction of the upper airway. Bronchodilators and antiinflammatory agents are seldom helpful and cause iatrogenic side effects that are problematic. Unless the patient has concomitant asthma, most can be weaned off these medications.

Martin et al[87] emphasize the role of a multidisciplinary team (pulmonologist, otolaryngologist, psychiatrist, and speech therapist) in the evaluation and treatment of adults with these disorders. This is equally important in the pediatric population. The interventions described in the literature for VCD range from simple and quick measures to invasive procedures. The following interventions were tried in the reported cases: explanation and reassurance (27%); behavioral and speech therapy interventions, such as breathing exercises (32%); biofeedback (6%); hypnosis (5%); individual or family psychotherapy (38%); psychotropics, including benzodiazepines and antidepressants (17%); breathing helium-oxygen mixtures (13%); CPAP (one case); botulinum toxin (two cases); bilateral nerve blocks (one case); and posterior fossa cystectomy (one case). Although many patients had been tracheotomized before the diagnosis of VCD was made, five patients still required tracheotomy after the diagnosis was confirmed. A minority of patients (6%) refused any therapy once told they did not have asthma.

In general, the degree of underlying psychopathology and secondary psychologic problems ensuing from having a chronic medical problem predict the ease with which treatments will succeed. Patients who adapt well to being told that their condition is not asthma generally are more willing to pursue appropriate therapy and have a better outcome. Therefore, much care should be taken in explaining the initial diagnosis to the patient. Patients should be told that they do not have asthma, or asthma alone, but another medical condition called vocal cord dysfunction. Viewing the videotape of their own or another patient's vocal cords adducting is often helpful in explaining the medical aspects of this disorder. The shorter the duration from onset of initial symptoms, the more likely it is that a patient will then respond to reassurance and behavioral interventions such as panting or speech therapy. The speech exercises are based on the premise of substituting a voluntary and competing behavior, such as panting or diaphragmatic breathing, whenever the vocal cords adduct. Practiced whenever symptoms are triggered, and coached by supportive persons in the environment, these techniques are very specific and effective. For patients who have many underlying problems, or whose symptom has become incorporated into their self-image and way of dealing with their family conflicts, psychotherapy, in addition to breathing exercises, is often effective in breaking the cycle. The psychotherapy should not be addressed at all underlying problems, but rather focused on the symptom and how to disentangle the VCD from the other issues. Biofeedback, relaxation, and hypnosis can be effective, but they are not as specific and efficient as speech exercises. The more extreme interventions are variably successful. Benzodiazepines, "sedatives," and antidepressants were helpful in some patients for the immediate episode but did not prevent further episodes. Botulinum toxin was used in two cases: one reported good success and the other no help; both were followed for less than 3 months.[69,82]

What is the natural course of VCD? Across all the reported cases, 26 cases reported in the literature gave some indication of follow-up status. The majority of these (73%) reported a good outcome with the use of combinations of education/reassurance, speech or breathing exercises, and psychotherapy. One paper reported a 10-year follow-up on three patients, all of whom were still having recurrent symptoms despite speech therapies and psychotherapies, indicating that some minority of the group may be refractory to treatment.[74]

As opposed to panic disorder and hyperventilation, where solid research exists to guide clinical practice, much more research must be done in VCD. Two areas are particularly important. First, the rates of psychiatric comorbidity must be established, using structured research interviews and appropriate control groups. Second, controlled, prospective outcome studies are needed to establish the efficacy of various multidisciplinary interventions, as well as the subcomponents of these treatments. Given the available information, it appears that patients do better if the condition is diagnosed and explained to them from a collaboration-fostering, biopsychosocial perspective, with multidisciplinary treatment available and offered as clinically appropriate. Left undiagnosed or inappropriately treated, many patients with VCD develop secondary, often iatrogenic problems.

HABIT COUGH

"There are two things not to be hidden: love and a cough."

George Eliot, in *Romola*

Habit cough syndrome, at times also labeled "psychogenic cough,"[121] "the barking cough of puberty,"[122] "honking or psychogenic cough tic,"[123] "operant cough,"[124] or "respiratory tic,"[125] is characterized by a barking or honking cough that is persistent and disruptive to normal activity. By definition, there are no laboratory, radiographic, bronchoscopic, or pulmonary function abnormalities. The patient does not show bronchoconstriction on methacholine challenge test or other provocative tests for asthma. The cough does not respond to usual antitussive therapies, bronchodilators, or antiinflammatory medications. Nonetheless, the cough can become chronic and debilitating, preventing the child from attending school or social activities or impairing the adult's sociovocational functioning. The major morbidity from habit cough is iatrogenic, resulting from misdiagnosis and excessive medical treatment. It is not unusual for children to have been hospitalized for this disorder or to receive extensive evaluations. Two features that distinguish this cough from most of the pulmonary causes of cough is that it usually disappears once the patient is soundly asleep, and it seldom is exacerbated by exertion, as are coughs of most respiratory etiologies.

The prevalence of habit cough seems to be low, but it is not rare. There have been at least 137 cases reported in the pediatric literature[122,123,125-137] and five to seven cases reported for adults.[138,139]

Biogenetic Aspects of Habit Cough

Because the diagnosis of habit cough is essentially a diagnosis of exclusion, care should be taken to exclude all other causes of cough. The differential diagnosis should include cough variant asthma,[140,141] bronchitis, pneumonia, allergic tracheitis, tuberculosis, cystic fibrosis, congenital pulmonary abnormalities, foreign bodies, and other intrinsic and extrinsic pulmonary disorders.[142-145] These pulmonary disorders would usually cause some abnormalities on laboratory, radiographic, or pulmonary function testing. Occasionally, the only abnormality may be noted on bronchoscopic examination, as in localized tracheomalacia.[146]

In understanding the pathophysiology of habit cough, it may be useful to understand its different eponyms because these may reflect different causes, or at least varying degrees of severity. The varying terms that have some differentiating meaning are *habit, tic,* and *psychogenic cough.* Although the initial explanation to the patient and his or her family, as well as the first clinical intervention, in any of these instances may be similar, in general, the major reason to make the distinction between habit, tic, and psychogenic cough is that it is likely that the treatment plan and overall prognosis will differ for each of the different causes.

Habits

Habits are generally semivoluntary activities, often reinforced either because they are self-soothing or because of the response they elicit from people in the environment. Although some habits (e.g., habit cough) disappear during sleep, not all habits do (e.g., bruxism or teeth grinding). In most cases of habit cough, children first develop a cough of infectious etiology, which lingers long after the infection usually should be resolved. Repeated cough continues to irritate the airways and stimulate the cough receptors, lowering the threshold for continued coughing.[142] Another frequently reported source of continued irritation is tobacco smoke exposure. When a simple "suggestive" intervention is given, and patients are shown how to suppress the urge to cough so frequently, the threshold returns to normal and they are "cured."

Tics

Tics are sudden, rapid, recurrent, nonrhythmic, stereotyped motor movements or vocalizations. Like habit cough, tics most often disappear during sleep and are exacerbated by stress, yet are defined as involuntary. Motor tics include coughing, and vocal tics include throat clearing, grunting, barking, and snorting. Occasionally, the first presentation of a tic disorder may be the single motor tic of coughing.[147] Tic disorders involve a spectrum that includes transient tic disorder of childhood on the mild end, chronic motor or vocal tics in the moderate range, and Tourette's syndrome (TS) in the severe range. Transient tic disorder is common, occurring in 5% to 24% of schoolchildren.[148] By definition, tics in this disorder last more than 2 weeks but less than 12 consecutive months. Chronic multiple motor or vocal tics (there may be more than one tic, but all tics are in the same category) appear to represent a mild form of TS because both are transmitted as inherited traits within the same family. The severe end of the spectrum is Tourette's syndrome, in which more than one motor tic and at least one vocal tic occur in the same person, which are not due to the effects of a substance (e.g., stimulants) or a general medical condition (e.g., Huntington's disease or postviral encephalitis).[6] Onset must occur before age 21 (the median age of onset is 7 years), and the tics must be present for at least 1 year. Symptoms that may occur, but do not necessarily occur, include coprolalia, echolalia, and complex motor tics such as touching or picking. Approximately one third of individuals diagnosed with TS have resolution of tics by late adolescence; in another third, the tics diminish markedly; and in the remaining third the tics persist into adulthood.

In a child with habit cough, a tic disorder should be considered once more than one tic is noted, or if there is a family history of tics or other disorders genetically associated with tic disorders. These disorders include obsessive-compulsive disorder, attention deficit/hyperactivity disorder, and learning disorders. The vulnerability to Tourette's disorder is transmitted in an autosomal dominant pattern, with approximately 70% penetrance for female gene carriers and 99% penetrance for male gene carriers. Family members often have transient motor and vocal tics without full-blown Tourette's disorder.[149] Interestingly, in the pediatric reports of habit cough, there is note of some "obsessive-compulsive symptoms" in two of the patients, which is part of the genetic spectrum of tic disorders.[132,133]

The course of the cough symptom over time, comorbid psychiatric conditions, and family history will be most helpful in distinguishing a tic from a habit cough. Of note, antihistamines and sympathomimetic substances have been associated with exacerbation of motor tics in persons with preexisting tic disorders. These widely used agents could potentially bring on a motor tic in a genetically susceptible child and should be discontinued during evaluation of habit cough for that reason.[150]

Psychiatric Aspects of Habit Cough

Psychogenic implies that a symptom is an expression of an underlying, usually unconscious, conflict. Psychoanalysts in the past have postulated that a cough can express this unconscious conflict: "The automatic cough reflex is expropriated by the voluntary muscle system in an effort to protect the ego. Just as weeping serves the dual function of washing irritants out of the eyes and expressing unhappiness, so does the cough share overlapping roles in discharging emotions and clearing the lungs."[139] Early reports on this disorder suggested that the child's cough may be expressing a single, relatively circumscribed conflict (e.g., a way to protest to an overbearing mother).[122] Other reports indicated a more complex motive (e.g., to avoid anxiety-provoking experiences at school).[130] In other cases, the cough was deemed to represent numerous underlying problems and become entrenched as a result of underlying psychopathology.[139] Cohlan and Stone[127] described 33 pediatric patients with habit cough. They noted that 84% had a decreased or absent gag reflex, and 68% lacked a corneal reflex, which they took as evidence of a psychogenic origin, because in certain circles these neurologic signs are viewed as markers of a conversion disorder. Other types of psychologic problems have also been noted in some children with habit cough. In one description of nine cases of psychogenic cough tic, eight of the nine children had school phobia, possibly indicating an anxiety disorder.[130] Several other authors described underlying family conflicts or school phobia and successfully treated the patient with psychotherapy[121,123,135] or antidepressants.[151] These reports indicate that at least some children with habit cough have significant underlying conflicts and need psychotherapeutic help.

On the other hand, the pediatric literature cites numerous examples that in other children, reassurance and simple suggestive therapy are very effective in extinguishing the habit cough, usually within minutes to days and without emergence of other emotional or somatic symptoms.[125,131-133,137] Most of these children are described as being good students, conscientious, and high achievers. These authors use their outcomes to suggest that habit cough is not a sign of underlying psychopathology and could be easily treated with consistent appropriate suggestion therapy.

As with VCD, there is a paucity of objective information with which to judge the actual prevalence of comorbid psychiatric problems in children with habit cough. None of the reports used blinded, objective raters to evaluate the presence of conflicts or psychologic problems. There are no published reports of standardized ratings of emotional or behavioral problems among children with habit cough. None of the studies used control groups to compare rates of conflicts, family problems, or overt psychopathology. Until this is done, it is difficult to say whether habit cough is caused by psychologic problems. It is equally plausible to posit that the cough started for a physiologic reason (e.g., infectious), and continued because of reinforcements from the environment. Like any medical symptom, the cough may be reinforced by environmental reactions, such as being able to stay home from school or receive extra attention from health care personnel, in a manner that serves to maintain the symptom. It is unnecessary to posit that the individual with the cough has any more or less psychopathology than the rest of the population. However, if left untreated, it is possible that the habit cough itself may lead to psychosocial complications that become severe and take on a life of their own (e.g., secondary depression or markedly deficient social skills).[130,138]

Treatment of Habit Cough

What is the natural course of habit cough? In the largest sample of habit cough syndrome reported, Rojas et al[136] followed up 62 patients (34 males and 26 females) an average of 7.9 years after diagnosis. The mean age at diagnosis was 10.5 years, with a range of 4.6 to 15.6 years. Mean duration of cough before diagnosis was 7.6 months, and mean duration until complete resolution was 6.1 months. In their sample, 73% had complete resolution of cough. However, 16 patients were still coughing a mean of 5.9 years after diagnosis. Because none of these patients were given specific treatments for the cough, this may reflect the natural course over time. The authors argue that more direct intervention would most likely shorten the course and limit the morbidity. It is important to clearly inform the patient and family of the diagnosis and intervene in some behavioral way to expedite recovery of these children, so that they do not form secondary problems from an unresolved habit.

Several types of interventions for habit cough and tic cough have been described in the literature. Treatment for simple motor tics is similar to that reported for habit cough. Earlier behavioral techniques tended to be somewhat aversive. For example, there are several reports on the use of electric shock,[126,128] and several more using a "bedsheet" technique.[127,137] In general, although these therapies are effective, they may perhaps be more aversive than is necessary. More recent behavioral therapies have used a combination of education and suggestion, for example, "This cough started with a cold. It has now become a habit in part because each time you cough, it irritates your throat and you are more likely to cough again. We will teach you how to stop doing that." The child is then taught a voluntary behavior that is incompatible with maintenance of the tic cough. Commonly prescribed exercises for tic cough include diaphragmatic breathing, panting, and swallowing.[131,132,152] Finally, the parents are asked to monitor the child's progress (i.e., keep track of how many times an hour the child coughs) and reward the child for decreased coughing. Behavioral therapy is effective for most children with habit cough; overall, habit reversal has been found to reduce tics by 80% to 90%.[153] Pharmacologic interventions are not often used today for transient motor or vocal tics.

Some children and adults have required more intensive psychotherapies, including hypnosis,[129,138,139] and at least one has required antidepressant medication.[151] As in vocal cord dysfunction, the few reported adult cases appeared to have more consistent psychopathology and were more difficult to treat than the pediatric and adolescent cases.[152] Nonetheless, with persistent therapy over 6 to 12 months, the overall morbidity of the disorder was greatly decreased, even if the symptom was not entirely extinguished.[138]

Prognosis and treatment for Tourette's disorder is very different than habit cough or simple transient tic disorder, and the patient suspected of having TS should be referred to a neurologist or psychiatrist. Treatment for TS usually includes psychopharmacologic interventions in addition to psychotherapy focused on behavioral strategies to decrease tics and how to cope with the illness in general. At least 20 agents have been tested for the more severe tics of TS. The most effective are pimozide, haloperidol, and clonidine. These are occasionally used for chronic tics. For example, in one description of nine cases of psychogenic cough tic six of nine children were treated with "tranquilizers" to alleviate symptoms.[130]

Thus habit cough should be in the differential of every cough persisting more than 2 weeks without any laboratory, pulmonary function, or radiographic abnormalities. Children and parents should be informed that the cough does not reflect any dangerous pathology and is indeed a "habit" at this point. Children should then be given a behavioral intervention that teaches them to suppress the cough and that allows a face-saving way out of the now dysfunctional habit/pattern. For most children, this approach is successful. If, however, evidence of more than one tic or strong family history for tic disorder exists, referral to a neurologist or pediatric psychiatrist should be considered. Likewise, if a straightforward behavioral approach is unsuccessful or if comorbid secondary psychiatric problems seem now to contribute to maintenance of the cough, referral to a pediatric psychiatrist or psychologist for further evaluation and treatment would be recommended.

CONCLUSION

This chapter has reviewed three sets of common clinical syndromes that cause interwined respiratory and psychiatric symptoms: panic disorder and hyperventilation, vocal cord dysfunction, and habit cough. In each, a collaborative, potentially multidisciplinary, biopsychosocial orientation toward diagnosis and treatment is indicated because the existing research supports that biogenetic, physiologic, and secondary (and in certain cases underlying) psychiatric factors are associated with the development, course, and outcome of these disorders. As opposed to the notion that these problems are "psychogenic" and "all in the head," this chapter has argued that a clinical approach that acknowledges both the biogenetic and the psychiatric aspects of these problems is more efficacious and conforms more fully to current scientific understanding of these disorders. Given the high prevalence rates, significant degree of preventable morbidity, and availability of effective treatments for these disorders, a clear understanding of the issues related to the disorders discussed in this chapter will foster the clinical success of pulmonologists in what otherwise can be a difficult to treat group of patients.

REFERENCES

"Somatic" Anxiety Disorders: Panic Attacks, Panic Disorder, and Hyperventilation

1. Herman SP, Steckler GB, Lucas AR: Hyperventilation syndrome in children and adolescents: long-term follow-up, *Pediatrics* 67(2):183-187, 1981.
2. Klein DF, Mannuzza S, Chapman T, Fyer AJ: Child panic revisited, *J Am Acad Child Adolesc Psychiatry* 31:112-116, 1992.
3. Black B, Robbins DR: Panic disorder in children and adolescents, *J Am Acad Child Adolesc Psychiatry* 29:36-44, 1990.
4. Salge RA, Beck JG, Logan AC: A community survey of panic, *J Anxiety Disord* 2:157-167, 1988.
5. Von Korff M, Eaton W, Keyl P: The epidemiology of panic attacks and panic disorder: results of three community surveys, *Am J Epidemiol* 122:970-981, 1985.
6. American Psychiatric Association: *Diagnostic and statistical manual of mental disorders,* ed 4, Washington, DC, 1994, American Psychiatric Press.
7. Lum LC: Hyperventilation syndromes in medicine and psychiatry: a review, *J R Soc Med* 80(4):229-231, 1987.
8. Gardner WN, Bass C: Hyperventilation in clinical practice, *Br J Hosp Med* 41(1):73-81, 1989.
9. Gorman JM, Uy J: Respiratory physiology and pathological anxiety, *Gen Hosp Psychiatry* 9(6):410-419, 1987.
10. Missri JC, Alexander S: Hyperventilation syndrome, *JAMA* 240(19):2093-2096, 1978.
11. Nixon PG: The grey area of effort syndrome and hyperventilation: from Thomas Lewis to today, *J R Coll Physicians Lond* 27(4):377-383, 1993.
12. Tavel ME: Hyperventilation syndrome—hiding behind pseudonyms? *Chest* 97(6):1285-1288, 1990.
13. Kessler RC, McGonagle KA, Zhao S, Nelson CB, Hughes M, Eshleman S, Wittchen HU, Kendler KS: Lifetime and 12-month prevalence of DSM-III-R psychiatric disorders in the United States: results from the National Comorbidity Study, *Arch Gen Psychiatry* 51:8-19, 1994.
14. Weissman MM: The epidemiology of panic disorder and agoraphobia. In Hales RE, Francis AJ, eds: *Review of psychiatry,* Washington, DC, 1988, American Psychiatric Press.
15. Katon WJ, Vitaliano PP, Russo J, Jones M, Anderson K: Panic disorder: epidemiology in primary care, *J Fam Pract* 23:233-239, 1986.
16. Katon W: *Panic disorder in the medical setting,* DHHS pub no ADM 89-1629, National Institute of Mental Health, Washington, DC, 1989, US Government Printing Office.
17. Kroenke K: Symptoms in medical patients: an untended field, *Am J Med* 92(suppl 1A):3S-11S, 1992.
18. Kushner MG, Beitman BD: Panic attacks without fear: an overview, *Behav Res Ther* 28(6):469-479, 1990.
19. Sheehan DV: Panic attacks and phobias, *N Engl J Med* 307:156-158, 1982.
20. Goldberg RJ: Clinical presentations of panic: related disorders, *J Anxiety Disord* 2:61-75, 1988.

21. Klein DF: False suffocation alarms, spontaneous panics, and related conditions. An integrative hypothesis, *Arch Gen Psychiatry* 50(4):306-317, 1993.
22. Nutt D, Lawson C: Panic attacks. A neurochemical overview of models and mechanisms, *Br J Psychiatry* 160:165-178, 1992.
23. Pollard CA, Lewis LM: Managing panic attacks in emergency patients, *J Emerg Med* 7(5):547-552, 1989.
24. Papp LA, Klein DF, Gorman JM: Carbon dioxide hypersensitivity, hyperventilation, and panic disorder, *Am J Psychiatry* 150(8):1149-1157, 1993.
25. Gorman JM, Liebowitz MR, Fyer AJ, Stine J: A neuroanatomical hypothesis for panic disorder, *Am J Psychiatry* 146(2):148-161, 1989.
27. Liebowitz MR, Gorman JM, Fyer AJ, Levitt M, Dillon D, Levy G, Appleby IL, Anderson S, Palij M, Davies SO, Klein DF: Lactate provocation of panic attacks. II. Biochemical and physiological findings, *Arch Gen Psychiatry* 42:709-719, 1985.
28. Gorman JM, Papp LA, Coplan JD, Martinez JM, Lennon S, Goetz RR, Ross D, Klein DF: Anxiogenic effects of CO_2 and hyperventilation in patients with panic disorder, *Am J Psychiatry* 151(4):547-553, 1994.
29. Gorman JM, Askanazi J, Liebowitz M, Fyer AJ, Stein J, Kinney JM, Klein DF: Response to hyperventilation in a group of patients with panic disorder, *Am J Psychiatry* 141:857-861, 1984.
30. Klein DF: Anxiety reconceptualized. In Klein DF, Rabkin JG, eds: *Anxiety: new research and changing concepts,* New York, 1981, Raven Press.
31. Sanderson WC, Rapee RM, Barlow DH: The influence of an illusion of control on panic attacks induced via inhalation of 5.5% carbon dioxide–enriched air, *Arch Gen Psychiatry* 46:157-162, 1989.
32. Lesser IM: The relationship between panic disorder and depression, *J Anxiety Disord* 2:3-15, 1988.
33. Barlow DH, Dinardo PA, Vermilyea BB, Blanchard EB: Co-morbidity and depression among the anxiety disorders: issues in diagnosis and treatment, *J Nerv Mental Dis* 174:63-72, 1986.
34. Breier A, Charney DS, Heninger GR: Major depression in patients with agoraphobia and panic disorder, *Arch Gen Psychiatry* 41:1129-1135, 1984.
35. Weissman MM, Klerman GL, Markowitz JS, Ouellette R: Suicidal ideation and suicide attempts in panic disorder and attacks, *N Engl J Med* 321:1209-1214, 1989.
36. Karajgi B, Rifkin A, Doddi S, Killi R: The prevalence of anxiety disorders in patients with chronic obstructive pulmonary disease, *Am J Psychiatry* 147(2):200-201, 1990.
37. Zandbergen J, Bright M, Pols H, Fernandez I, Loof C, Griez EJL: Higher lifetime prevalence of respiratory disease in panic disorders? *Am J Psychiatry* 148(11):1583-1585, 1991.
38. O'Byrne PM, Ramsdale EH, Hargreave FE: Isocapnic hyperventilation for measuring airway hyperresponsiveness in asthma and in chronic obstructive pulmonary disease, *Am Rev Respir Dis* 143(6):1444-1445, 1991.
39. Baron C, Marcotte J: Experience and reason—briefly recorded. Role of panic attacks in the intractability of asthma in children, *Pediatrics* 94(1):108-111, 1994.
40. Wamboldt MZ, Wamboldt FS: Psychosocial aspects of severe asthma. In Szefler SJ,. Leung DYM, eds: *Severe pathogenesis and clinical management,* New York, 1995, Marcel Dekker.
41. Yellowlees PM, Kalucy RS: Psychobiological aspects of asthma and the consequent research implications, *Chest,* 97:628-634, 1990.
42. Coplan JD, Gorman JM, Klein DF: Serotonin related functions in panic-anxiety: A critical overview, *Neuropsychopharmacology* 6(3):189-200, 1992.
43. Marks IM: Cure and care of neurosis, *Psychol Med* 9:629-660, 1979.
44. Marks IM: *Fears, phobias, and rituals: panic, anxiety, and their disorders,* New York, 1987, Oxford University Press.
45. Barlow DH, Cherny JA: *Psychological treatment of panic,* New York, 1988, Guilford Press.
46. Bonn JA, Readhead CPA: Enhanced adaptive behavioural response in agoraphobic patients pretreated with breathing retraining, *Lancet* 2(8404):665-669, 1984.
47. Clark DM, Salkovskis PM, Chalkley AJ: Respiratory control as a treatment for panic attacks, *J Behav Ther Exp Psychiatry* 16(1):23-30, 1985.
48. Grossman P, De Swart JCG, Defares PB: A controlled study of a breathing therapy for treatment of hyperventilation syndrome, *J Psychosom Res* 29(1):49-58, 1985.
49. Hibbert GA, Chan M: Respiratory control: its contribution to the treatment of panic attacks. A controlled study, *Br J Psychiatry* 154:232-236, 1989.
50. Rapee RM: A case of panic disorder treated with breathing retraining, *J Behav Ther Exp Psychiatry* 16(1):63-65, 1985.
51. Wolpe J, Rowan VC: Panic disorder: a product of classical conditioning, *Behav Res Ther* 26(6):441-450, 1988.
52. Van den Hout MA, Van der Molen M, Griez E, Lousberg H, Nansen A: Reduction of CO_2-induced anxiety in patients with panic attacks after repeated CO_2 exposure, *Am J Psychiatry* 144(6):788-791, 1987.
53. Guttmacher LB, Nelles C: In vivo desensitization alternation of lactate-induced panic: a case study, *Behav Res Ther* 15:369-372, 1984.
54. Griez E, Van den Hout MA: CO_2 in the treatment of panic attacks, *Behav Res Ther* 24:145-150,1986.

Vocal Cord Dysfunction

55. Dunglison R: *The practice of medicine,* Philadelphia, 1842, Lea & Blanchard, p 258.
56. Appelblatt NH, Baker SR: Functional upper airway obstruction, a new syndrome, *Arch Otolaryngol* 107:305-306, 1981.
57. Christopher K, Wood RP, Eckert C, Blager F, Raney R, Souhrada J: Vocal-cord dysfunction presenting as asthma, *N Engl J Med* 308(26): 1566-1570, 1983.
58. Barnes S, Grob C, Lachman B: Psychogenic upper airway obstruction presenting as refractory wheezing, *J Pediatr* 80:1067-1070, 1986.
59. Brown TM, Merritt VM, Evans DL: Psychogenic vocal cord dysfunction masquerading as asthma, *J Nerv Ment Dis* 176(5):308-310, 1988.
60. Brugman S, Howell J, Rosenberg D, Blager F, Lack G: The spectrum of pediatric vocal cord dysfunction, *Am Rev Respir Dis* 149(4):A353, 1994.
61. Chawla SS, Upadhyay BK, Macdonnell KF: Laryngeal spasm mimicking bronchial asthma, *Ann Allergy* 53:319-321, 1984.
62. Collett PW, Brancatisano T, Engle LA: Spasmodic croup in the adult, *Am Rev Respir Dis* 127:500-504, 1983.
63. Cormier YF, Camus P, Desmeules MJ: Non-organic acute upper airway obstruction, *Am Rev Respir Dis* 121:147-150, 1980.
64. Corren J, Newman K: Vocal cord dysfunction mimicking bronchial asthma, *Postgrad Med* 92(6):153-156, 1992.
65. Craig T, Sitz K, Squire E, Smith L, Carpenter G: Vocal cord dysfunction during wartime, *Mil Med* 157(11):614-616, 1992.
66. Dailey R: Pseudoasthma: a new clinical entity? *JACEP* 5(3):192-193, 1976.
67. Downing ET, Braman SS, Fox MJ, Corrao WM: Factitious asthma physiological approach to diagnosis, *JAMA* 248(21):2878-2881, 1982.
68. Freedman MR, Rosenberg SJ, Schmaling KB: Childhood sexual abuse in patients with paradoxical vocal cord dysfunction, *J Nerv Ment Dis* 179(5):295-298, 1991.
69. Garibaldi E, La Blance G, Hibbett A, Wall L: Exercise-induced paradoxical vocal cord dysfunction: diagnosis with videostroboscopic endoscopy and treatment with clostridium toxin, *J Allergy Clin Immunol* 91(1):200, 1993.
70. Geist R, Tallet S: Diagnosis and management of psychogenic stridor caused by a conversion disorder, *Pediatrics* 86:315-317, 1990.
71. George MK, O'Connell JE, Batch AJ: Paradoxical vocal cord motion: an unusual cause of stridor, *J Laryngol Otol* 105:312-314, 1991.
72. Goldman: Vocal cord dysfunction and wheezing, *Thorax* 46:401-404, 1991.
73. Hammer G, Schwinn D, Wellman H: Postoperative complications due to paradoxical vocal cord motion, *Anesthesiology* 66(5):686-687, 1987.
74. Hayes JP, Nolan MT, Brennan N, Fitzgerald MX: Three cases of paradoxical vocal cord adduction followed up over a 10-year period, *Chest* 104(3):678-680, 1992.
75. Heiser JM, Kahn ML, Schmidt TA: Functional airway obstruction presenting as strider: a case report and literature review, *J Emerg Med* 8(3):285-289, 1990.
76. Kattan M, Ben-Zvi Z: Stridor caused by vocal cord malfunction associated with emotional factors, *Clin Pediatr* 24:158-160, 1985.
77. Kellman R, Leopold D: Paradoxical vocal cord motion: an important cause of stridor, *Laryngoscope* 92:58-60, 1982.
78. Kemper KJ, Izenberg S, Marvin JA, Heimbach DM: Treatment of postextubation stridor in a pediatric patient with burns: the role of heliox, *J Burn Care Rehabil* 11(4):3379, 1990.
79. Kisoon N, Kronick J, Frewen T: Psychogenic upper airway obstruction, *Pediatrics* 81:714-717, 1988.

80. Kivity S, Bibi H, Schwarz Y, Greif Y, Topilsky M, Tabachnick E: Variable vocal cord dysfunction presenting as wheezing and exercise-induced asthma, *J Asthma* 23(5):241-244, 1986.
81. Kruger M, Acres J, Brownell L: A syndrome of sleep, stridor and panic, *Chest* 80(6):768, 1981.
82. Kuppersmith R, Rosen D, Wiatrak B: Functional stridor in adolescents, *Soc Adoles Med* 14:166-171, 1993.
83. Lacy TJ, McManis SE: Psychogenic stridor, *Gen Hosp Psychiatry* 16(3):213-223, 1994.
84. Liistro G, Stanescu D, Dejonckere P, Rodenstein D, Venter C: Exercise-induced laryngospasm of emotional origin, *Pediatr Pulmonol* 8:58-60, 1990.
85. Logvinoff MM, Lau KY, Weinstein DB, Chandra P: Episodic stridor in a child secondary to vocal cord dysfunction, *Pediatr Pulmonol* 9(1):46-48, 1990.
86. Lund D, Garmel G, Kaplan G, Tom P: Hysterical stridor: a diagnosis of exclusion, *Am J Emerg Med* 11(4):400-402, 1993.
87. Martin R, Blager F, Gay M, Wood R II: Paradoxic vocal cord motion in presumed asthmatics, *Semin Respir Med* 8(4):332-337, 1987.
88. McClean S, Lee J, Sim T, Narajnjo M, Grant J: Intermittent breathlessness, *Ann Allergy* 63:486-488, 1989.
89. McGrath K, Greenberger P, Zeiss C, Patterson R: Factitious allergic disease: multiple factitious illness and familial Munchausen's stridor, *Immunol Allergy Pract* 6(7):263-271, 1984.
90. Michelsen LG, Vanderspek FL: An unexpected functional cause of upper airway obstruction, *Anaesthesia* 43:1028-1030, 1988.
91. Morton N, Barr G: Stridor in an adult. An unusual presentation of functional origin, *Anaesthesia* 44:232-234, 1989.
92. Myears DW, Martin RJ, Eckert RC, Sweeney MK: Functional versus organic vocal cord paralysis: rapid diagnosis and decannulation, *Laryngoscope* 95(10):1235-1237, 1985.
93. Neel E, Posthumus D: Nonorganic upper airway obstruction, *J Adolesc Heath Care* 4(3):178-179, 1983.
94. Newman KB, Dubester SN: Vocal cord dysfunction: masquerader of asthma, *Semin Respir Crit Care Med* 15(2):161-167, 1994.
95. Norman P, Peters S: The problem patient: "asthma" that cleared when patient coughed, *Hosp Pract* 18(11):51-57, 1983.
96. Ophir D, Katz Y, Tavori I, Aladjem M: Functional upper airway obstruction in adolescence, *Arch Otolaryngol* 116:1208-1209, 1990.
97. Patterson R, Schatz M, Horton M: Munchausen's stridor: non-organic laryngeal obstruction, *Clin Allergy* 4:307-310, 1974.
98. Patton H, Dibenedetto R, Downing E, Zeller M, Morgan K: Paradoxic vocal cord syndrome with surgical cure, *South Med J* 80(2):256-258, 1987.
99. Pitchenik AE: Functional laryngeal obstruction relieved by panting, *Chest* 100(5):1465-1467, 1991.
100. Ponder R, Guill M: Severe acute asthma followed by quick reversal, *J Asthma* 30(5):413-415, 1993.
101. Rabin CB: Disturbances of respiration of functional origin, *J Asthma Res* 5(4):295-308, 1968.
102. Ramirez J, Leon I, Rivera LM: Episodic laryngeal dyskinesia—clinical and psychiatric characterization, *Chest* 90(5):716-721, 1986.
103. Rodenstein: Emotional laryngeal wheezing: a new syndrome, *Am Rev Respir Dis* 127:354-358, 1983.
104. Rogers J, Stell P: Paradoxical movement of the vocal cords as a cause of stridor, *J Laryngol Otol* 92:157-158, 1978.
105. Rogers J: Functional inspiratory strider in children, *J Laryngol Otol* 94:669-670, 1980.
106. Rusakow L, Blager F, Barkin R, White C: Acute respiratory distress due to vocal cord dysfunction in cystic fibrosis, *J Asthma* 28(6):443-446, 1991.
107. Selner J, Staudenmayer H, Koepke J, Harvey R, Christopher K: Vocal cord dysfunction: the importance of psychologic factors and provocation challenge testing, *J Allergy Clin Immunol* 79(5):726-733, 1987.
108. Sim TC, McClean SP, Lee JL, Naranjo MS, Grant JA: Functional laryngeal obstruction: a somatization disorder, *Am J Med* 88:293-295, 1990.
109. Skinner DW, Bradley PJ: Psychogenic stridor, *J Laryngol Otol* 103(4): 383-385, 1989.
110. Smith M: Acute psychogenic stridor in an adolescent athlete treated with hypnosis, *Pediatrics* 72:247-248, 1983.
111. Snyder HS, Weiss E: Hysterical strider: a benign cause of upper airway obstruction, *Ann Emerg Med* 18(9):991-994, 1989.
112. Starkman MN, Appelblatt NH: Functional upper airway obstruction: a possible somatization disorder, *Psychosomatics* 25(4):327-333, 1984.
113. Nagai A, Kanemura T, Konno K: Abnormal movement of the arytenoid region as a cause of upper airway obstruction, *Thorax* 47:840-841, 1992.
114. Nagai A, Yamaguchi E, Sakamoto K, Takahashi E: Functional upper airway obstruction, *Chest* 101:1460-1461, 1992.
115. Bucca C, Rolla G, Scappaticci E, Baidi S, Caria E, Oliva A: Histamine hyperresponsiveness of the extrathoracic airway in patients with asthmatic symptoms, *Allergy* 46:147-153, 1991.
116. Zach M, Erben A, Olinsky A: Croup, recurrent croup, allergy, and airways hyper-reactivity, *Arch Dis Child* 56:336-341, 1981.
117. Irwin R, Pratter M, Holland P, Corwin R, Hughes J: Postnasal drip causes cough and is associated with reversible upper airway obstruction, *Chest* 85(3):346-352, 1984.
118. Maricle R: Vocal-cord dysfunction presenting as asthma, *N Engl J Med* 10(19):190-191, 1983.
119. Proctor DF: All that wheezes, *Am Rev Resp Dis* 127:261-262, 1983.
120. Aviv JE, Sanders I, Biller HF: Abductor vocal cord spasm, *Otolaryngol Head Neck Surg* 102(3):233-238, 1990.

Habit Cough

121. Shuper A, Mukamel M, Mimouni M, Lerman M, Varsano I: Psychogenic cough, *Arch Dis Child* 58(9):745-747, 1983.
122. Bernstein L: A respiratory tic: the barking cough of puberty, *Laryngoscope* 78:315-319, 1963.
123. Weinberg E: "Honking": psychogenic cough tic in children, *S Afr Med J* 57(6):198-200, 1980.
124. Munford PR, Liberman RP: Differential attention in the treatment of operant cough, *J Behav Med* 1:289-295, 1978.
125. Berman BA: Habit cough in adolescent children, *Ann Allergy* 24(1):43-46, 1966.
126. Alexander AB, Chai H, Creer TL, Miklich DR, Renne CM, Cardoso RR: The elimination of chronic cough by response suppression shaping, *J Behav Ther Exp Psychiatry* 4:75-80, 1973.
127. Cohlan S, Stone S: The cough and the bedsheet, *Pediatrics* 74(1):11-15, 1984.
128. Creer TL, Chai H, Hoffman A: A single application of an aversive stimulus to eliminate chronic cough, *J Behav Ther Exp Psychiatry* 8:107-109, 1977.
129. Elkins G, Carter B: Hypnotherapy in the treatment of childhood psychogenic coughing: a case report, *Am J Clin Hypn* 29(1):59-63, 1986.
130. Kravitz H, Gomberg R, Burnstine R, Hagler S, Korach A: Psychogenic cough tic in children and adolescents, *Clin Pediatr* 8(10):580-583, 1969.
131. Lavigne J, Davis A, Fauber R: Behavioral management of psychogenic cough: alternative to the "bedsheet" and other aversive techniques, *Pediatrics* 87(4):532-537, 1991.
132. Lokshin B, Lindgren S, Weinberger M, Koviach J: Outcome of habit cough in children treated with a brief session of suggestion therapy, *Ann Allergy* 67:579-582, 1991.
133. Lolin M, Slovis T, Haller J: Fracture of ribs in psychogenic cough, *N Y State J Med* 78(13):2078-2079, 1978.
134. Munford PR, Reardon D, Liberman RP, Allen L: Behavioral treatment of hysterical coughing and mutism: a case study, *J Consult Clin Psychol* 44:1008-1014, 1976.
135. Oberascher G: Psychogene lautausserungen [Psychogenic vocalizations], *Laryngol Rhinol Otol* 65(6):357-358, 1986.
136. Rojas AR, Sachs MI, Yunginger JW, O'Connell EJ: Childhood involuntary cough syndrome: a long term follow-up study, *Ann Allergy* 66:106, 1991.
137. Wolff P: An ingenious way to treat psychogenic cough, *Am J Matern Child Nurs* 13(2):118-120, 1988.
138. Gay M, Blager F, Bartsch K, Emery CF, Rosenstiel-Gross AK, Spears J: Psychogenic habit cough: review and case reports, *J Clin Psychiatry* 48(12):483-486, 1987.
139. Grumet G: Psychogenic coughing: a review and case report, *Compr Psychiatry* 28(1):28-34, 1987.
140. Milgrom H: Cough variant asthma. In Weiss EB, Stein M, eds: *Bronchial asthma: mechanisms and therapeutics,* Boston, 1993, Little, Brown.
141. Gaivez RA: The role of the methacholine challenge in children with chronic cough, *J Allergy Clin Immunol* 79:331-335, 1987.
142. Kamei R: Chronic cough in children, *Pediatr Clin North Am* 38(3):593-605, 1991.

143. Mellis C: Evaluation and treatment of chronic cough in children, *Pediatr Clin North Am* 26(3):553-564, 1979.
144. Morgan WJ, Taussig LM: The child with persistent cough, *Pediatr Rev* 8(8):249-253, 1987.
145. Reisman JJ, Canny GJ, Levison H: The approach to chronic cough in childhood, *Ann Allergy* 61(3):163-171, 1988.
146. Wood RE: Localized tracheomalacia or bronchomalacia in children with intractible cough, *J Pediatr* 116:404-406, 1990.
147. Vogel D: Otolaryngologic presentation of tic-like disorders, *Laryngoscope* 89(9 pt 1):1474-1477, 1979.
148. Singer HS: Tic disorders, *Pediatr Ann* 22(1):22-29, 1993.
149. Hyde TM, Weinberger DR: Tourette's syndrome: model neuropsychiatric disorder, *JAMA* 273:498-501, 1995.
150. Shafii M: The effects of sympathomimetic and antihistaminic agents on chronic motor tics and Tourette's disorder, *N Engl J Med* 315(19):1228-1229, 1986 (letter).
151. Daradkeh T, Sliman N, Aburajab A: Successful management of paroxysms of dry cough by antidepressant chemotherapy and supportive psychotherapy: a case report, *Pharmatherapeutica* 5(4):269-271, 1988.
152. Blager FB, Gay ML, Wood RP: Voice therapy techniques adapted to treatment of habit cough: a pilot study, *J Common Disord* 21(5):393-400, 1988.
153. Peterson AL, Campise RL, Azrin NH: Behavioral and pharmacological treatments for tic and habit disorders: a review, *J Dev Behav Pediatr* 15(6):430-441, 1994.

CHAPTER 81

Pulmonary Manifestations of Systemic Disorders

Laura S. Inselman

Pulmonary physiology and function reflect not only the physiology and function of the lung itself but also that of other tissues and organs of the body. Although the lung's primary roles are the exchange of oxygen and carbon dioxide between the environment and the body and the maintenance of acid-base balance within the body, the lung also has metabolic, endocrinologic, and growth-mediating actions that interact in different ways with other organs. Modifications, dysfunction, and malfunction in other tissues and organs may be reflected in alterations in lung growth, structure, function and physiology. In particular, the lung can be affected by disorders of nutrition; dysfunction of the pancreas, liver, and kidneys; the presence of hemoglobinopathies; and familial dysautonomia.

NUTRITIONAL DISORDERS

Obesity

Obesity, as defined by excessive adipose tissue, may be exogenous (i.e., diet induced) or endogenous (i.e., secondary to an underlying disorder).[1-3] Developmental, biochemical, structural, and functional changes occur in the lung with obesity.[4-16] The lungs of young obese rats fed a high-fat diet are large as measured by the ratio of lung volume to body weight. They have cellular hyperplasia, indicated by elevations in lung deoxyribonucleic acid (DNA) content; enlarged alveoli, measured by alveolar size and alveolar volume; reduced alveolar surface area relative to alveolar volume; and lipid deposits. Alveolar number and septa are normal[4,5] (Table 81-1). Lipid deposits also occur in the diaphragm and intercostal muscles in obese individuals, indicating the direct involvement of these muscles in obesity.[17] Thus obesity affects the lung with biochemical and structural changes, the respiratory muscles with lipid deposits, and the chest wall with the adipose mass.

These effects are observed as alterations in lung function and physiology. The most consistent and characteristic change in lung function is a diminution in the expiratory reserve volume (ERV)[6,7] (Table 81-2). There are also reductions in other lung volumes, maximal voluntary ventilation (MVV), compliance of the lung and chest wall, and flow rates in small airways; elevations in the respiratory rate, minute ventilation $\dot{V}_E$, work of breathing, oxygen consumption ($\dot{V}O_2$), carbon dioxide production ($\dot{V}CO_2$), and the ratio of residual volume (RV) to total lung capacity (TLC) (which reflects the presence of air trapping); and variable diffusing capacity (DLCO) measurements.[6-16] In addition, ventilation-perfusion imbalance and hypoxemia are present.

Obesity itself is associated with eucapnia or hypocapnia.[8] However, severe obesity attenuates the ventilatory response of the brain stem to carbon dioxide and can result in the obesity-hypoventilation syndrome, which is characterized by central sleep apnea, daytime somnolence, hypercapnia, hypoxemia, polycythemia, pulmonary hypertension, and cor pulmonale.[8] In addition, as a result of relaxation of upper airway muscles and soft tissues infiltrated by adipose tissue, obstructive sleep apnea can occur.[8]

Therapy includes dietary, pharmacologic, surgical, and mechanical intervention. Weight loss improves pulmonary function, with restoration of lung volumes toward normal, diminution of ventilation-perfusion imbalance, and reversal of hypercapnia, hypoxemia, and the obesity-hypoventilation syndrome.[8,11,16,18] However, the effect of weight loss on the biochemical and structural changes in the lung in obesity is unknown.

Respiratory stimulants, such as progesterone, theophylline, protriptyline, and buspirone, can improve the central drive to breathe and normalize the arterial carbon dioxide tension in the obesity-hypoventilation syndrome.[8,19-21] Theophylline can also

Table 81-1 Anthropometric, Biochemical, and Structural Alterations in the Lung in Obesity and Malnutrition in the Rat

		MALNUTRITION		
MEASUREMENT	OBESITY	ANTENATAL	BIRTH TO WEANING	POSTWEANING
Body weight	↑	↓	↓	↓
Body length	↑	↓	n/a	↓
Lung weight	↑	↓	↓	↓
Lung volume	↑	↓	↓	↓
Lung weight/body weight	↓	↓	Normal	Normal, ↑
Lung weight/body length	Normal	n/a	n/a	Normal
Lung volume/body weight	↑	n/a	n/a	↑
Lung DNA content	↑	↓	↓	Normal, ↓
Lung protein content	↑	↓	↓	↓
Lung protein/DNA	Normal	Normal	Normal	Normal, ↓
Alveolar number	Normal	↓	↓	Normal, ↓
Alveolar size	↑	n/a	↑	↑
Alveolar volume	↑	n/a	↑	↑
Alveolar surface area	↑	↓	↓	↓
Alveolar surface area/alveolar volume	↓	n/a	↓	↓
Alveolar septa	Intact	Delayed alveolarization	Disruptions	Disruptions

↑, Increased; ↓, decreased; *n/a,* information not available.

Table 81-2 Pulmonary Function Alterations in Obesity and Malnutrition

PULMONARY FUNCTION	OBESITY	MALNUTRITION
Vital capacity	Normal, ↑, ↓	↓
Functional residual capacity	↓	↓
Expiratory reserve volume	↓↓	↓
Residual volume	↑	↑
Total lung capacity	Normal, ↑, ↓	Normal
Residual volume/total lung capacity	↑	↑
Diffusing capacity	Normal, ↑, ↓	n/a
Maximal voluntary ventilation	↓	↓
Airflow rates	↓	Normal
Compliance, lung	↓	↓
Compliance, chest wall	↓	↓
Maximal static inspiratory and expiratory pressures	Normal	↓
Minute ventilation	↑	↓
Work of breathing	↑	↑
Oxygen consumption	↑	↓
Carbon dioxide production	↑	↓
Ventilation-perfusion imbalance	Present	Present

↑, Increased; ↓, decreased; *n/a,* information not available.

increase diaphragmatic contractility and improve pulmonary mechanics and ventilation.[20] However, the side effects and limited efficacy of these medications in these settings curtail their use.[21,22]

If not improved with weight loss, upper airway obstruction in obstructive sleep apnea in obesity may be relieved with surgery, such as a tracheostomy, uvulopalatopharyngoplasty, or dental orthoses.[21,23] In addition, nocturnal distending airway pressure, including continuous positive airway pressure and biphasic positive airway pressure support ventilation, may be used.[21,24] Whereas the continuous mode uses the same pressure throughout the respiratory cycle, the biphasic mode allows variation of the pressure between inhalation and exhalation.

Malnutrition

Malnutrition is characterized by a caloric intake that is inadequate to meet the metabolic requirements of the body.[25] Unlike starvation, which is acute, malnutrition is chronic and can result in either marasmus, which occurs from a deficiency of total calories (including protein), or in kwashiorkor, in which the protein deficit is in excess of the caloric insufficiency.[25] An inadequate quantity of food, an inability to absorb and digest food, or both problems can cause malnutrition.[25]

As with obesity, malnutrition alters lung growth, physiology, structure, and function; the respiratory muscles; and control of breathing.[26-30] In addition, humoral and cellular defense mechanisms of the body and the lung itself and the lung's response to injury and hyperoxia are altered.[31-33] Malnutrition contributes to the pathogenesis of bronchopulmonary dysplasia, cystic fibrosis, and chronic obstructive pulmonary disease[33-35] and the respiratory manifestations of certain neuromuscular diseases such as spinal muscular atrophy, chronic infections, malignancies, and eating disorders, including anorexia nervosa and obesity.[31,36]

Malnutrition causes biochemical and structural modifications in the lung. Although the severity, timing, and duration of the malnutrition determine its effect on lung growth and structure,[37-44] some general principles may be applied. Whether antenatal, early postnatal (i.e., from birth to weaning), or late postnatal (i.e., after weaning), malnutrition in the animal model results in reductions in body weight, lung weight, and lung volume[26,37-42] (see Table 81-1). The ratio of lung weight to body weight is diminished only during antenatal malnutrition, indicating that reduced caloric intake during this period has a greater effect on the lung than on the body.[38] The ratio of lung volume to body weight is increased with late postnatal malnutrition, reflecting the alveolar enlargement and reduction in body weight present at this time.[41]

Normal tissue growth is initially characterized by cell proliferation without cell hypertrophy. This stage is followed by a slowing of cell division while protein accumulates, resulting in new cells that are larger but fewer in number than during the first stage. Finally, cell hypertrophy without cell hyperplasia occurs.[37,38] When compared with controls, animal lungs exposed to antenatal or early postnatal malnutrition have fewer cells as measured by lung DNA content but normal cell size as measured by the ratio of protein to DNA and thus have interference only with cell division.[26,37,38,40] Lungs exposed to postweaning malnutrition may have normal numbers of cells, but these cells may be small, thereby causing alterations during the later stages of tissue growth[38,45] (see Table 81-1). As a result, the lungs in malnutrition are hypoplastic at all stages, whether defined by cell number or cell size.[37,38]

The newborn animal lung exposed to antenatal malnutrition has reduced lecithin and phospholipid content and surfactant activity, increased glycogen content, delayed cellular differentiation and alveolarization, and architectural immaturity.[26-28,42] Although alveolar number is reduced in early postnatal malnutrition[39] and may be decreased or normal in postweaning malnutrition,[42,43] diminished alveolar surface area (both absolute and relative to alveolar volume), enlarged alveoli, disruptions in alveolar septa, loss of elastic recoil, and reduced lung compliance occur during both of these periods and reflect the biochemical abnormalities in these lungs[39-44] (see Tables 81-l and 81-2).

During early and late postnatal malnutrition, pulmonary levels of collagen and elastin as measured by hydroxyproline and desmosine are diminished.[40,43] As a result, lung connective tissue content and structure, which provide the framework for alveolar development and stability, are altered.[39,43]

The respiratory muscles are also affected by malnutrition. Diaphragmatic muscle mass is diminished in malnourished individuals, and diaphragmatic weight, DNA, protein, thickness, and contractile force are reduced in the animal model.[29,45,46] Inspiratory and expiratory respiratory muscles in malnourished patients have decreases in strength and endurance proportional to the loss in body weight and result in part from atrophy of types I and II muscle fibers.[29,47,48] In contrast, acute calorie restriction has little effect on diaphragmatic function and morphology in animals.[48]

Alterations in pulmonary function result from the biochemical and structural changes in the lung and respiratory muscles. Reductions occur in vital capacity (VC), functional residual capacity (FRC), MVV, and forced expiratory volume in 1 second (FEV_1).[29,36] RV and the RV/TLC ratio are elevated, indicating the presence of air trapping and perhaps the alveolar enlargement observed morphologically[29,36,40-41] (see Tables 81-l and 81-2). Maximal respiratory muscle strength measured by inspiratory and expiratory pressures is also reduced.[29] In addition, diminutions in exercise endurance despite normal ventilatory and cardiac responses occur in individuals with anorexia nervosa and likely result from the reduced mass and contractile force of the skeletal and respiratory muscles.[36] The normal hypoxic and to a lesser degree, hypercapnic ventilatory drives controlled by the central nervous system are attenuated with malnutrition and as with respiratory muscle weakness, can cause alterations in ventilation and result in respiratory failure.[30,49]

Pulmonary protective mechanisms, such as the cough reflex, secretory immunoglobulin A (sIgA) levels, pulmonary alveolar macrophage (PAM) number and activity, T cell-mediated immunity, and lung clearance of certain bacteria and viruses, are diminished with malnutrition.[30,32,50,51] Systemic deficiencies in cellular, humoral, neutrophil, complement, and opsonin activity also occur.[30,31,50,52] These changes predispose the lung to acute and chronic infections.

Therapy includes caloric and protein supplementation, which may reverse some alterations. For example, decreases in lung weight and contents of DNA and protein normalize with refeeding after late postnatal malnutrition but persist with refeeding after early postnatal malnutrition, suggesting that the earlier in life the caloric restriction, the more severe and permanent the alterations in the lung despite subsequent refeeding.[38] In addition, adult rats who are refed for 7 to 10 days after a period of caloric restriction have increases toward control values of body and lung weights; lung contents of elastin, hydroxyproline, lecithin, DNA, protein, and, in some studies, the protein/DNA ratio; alveolar surface area but not the ratio of alveolar surface area to alveolar volume; and lung compliance.[38,53-55] Pulmonary elastic recoil pressure remains unchanged, and alveolar enlargement remains although less prominently.[53,54] Thus some biochemical changes reverse, but the morphologic and functional alterations do not, at least in the refed malnourished adult rat.

In malnourished adults with chronic obstructive pulmonary disease, short-term (i.e., 16 to 21 days) and longer-term (i.e., 3 months) caloric supplementation increases $\dot{V}O_2$, $\dot{V}CO_2$, respiratory quotient, and $\dot{V}E$ and improves gas exchange.[30] In addition, respiratory muscle strength, the hypercapnic ventilatory drive, the ability to wean from assisted ventilation, exercise tolerance, lymphocyte number, and delayed cutaneous hypersensitivity responses are augmented.[30,35,56,57] However, improvements do not occur in VC, TLC, FEV_1, MVV, arterial blood gas measurements, humoral immunity, and complement levels.[35,56,57] Similarly, malnourished children with cystic fibrosis have reduced numbers of pulmonary infections and increased MVV and respiratory muscle strength with either short-term (i.e., 1 month) or longer-term (i.e., 6 to 34 months) caloric supplementation.[34,58,59] In addition, lung volumes and airflow rates either improve or decline less rapidly with up to 3 years of nutritional rehabilitation in some of these studies.[58,59]

These observations in both the animal model and the clinical setting are particularly important in intensive care areas, where nutritional needs may be delayed while more acute problems are addressed. Nutritional supplementation in poorly nourished patients can improve lung and respiratory muscle function, ventilation, and local and systemic immunity.

DISORDERS OF THE PANCREAS

Diabetes Mellitus

As a metabolic disorder resulting from dysfunction of the endocrine portion of the pancreas, diabetes mellitus affects many organs in the body with varying degrees of complexity.[60-62] Pulmonary involvement results from abnormalities in collagen, elastin, and the microvasculature in the lung and includes alterations in lung growth, structure, function, and physiology, which are manifested clinically in disease.

The immature diabetic animal has reduced body weight and length compared with controls[63] (Table 81-3). The lungs are small in weight and volume but have high ratios of lung weight to body weight and lung volume to body weight.[63] This reflects a greater effect of diabetes on the body than on the lung and is unrelated to the presence of undernutrition, which often accompanies diabetes in the animal model.[62,63] The lungs are polyalveolar and have an increased number of alveoli, which are small in size, volume, and total surface area, and alveolar septa are intact.[63,64] However, the ratio of alveolar surface area to alveolar volume is elevated and indicates the presence of enhanced alveolar complexity with an increased gas-exchange area, which results from the augmented number of alveoli.[63,64] Despite the increase in alveolar number, the lung content of DNA is reduced, indicating a reduction in cell replication.[63] Thus the diabetic lung is hypoplastic in terms of lung weight, volume, and DNA content but is polyalveolar. These some-

Table 81-3 Alterations in the Lung in Diabetes Mellitus in the Immature Rat

MEASUREMENT	ALTERATION
Body weight	↓
Body length	↓
Lung weight	↓
Lung volume	↓
Lung weight/body weight	↑
Lung volume/body weight	↑
Lung DNA content	↓
Lung protein content	↓
Lung protein/DNA	Normal
Alveolar number	↑
Alveolar size	↓
Alveolar volume	↓
Alveolar surface area	↓
Alveolar surface area/alveolar volume	↑
Alveolar septa	Intact, thickened

↓, Decreased; ↑, increased.

what contradictory observations are explained by the occurrence of alveolar multiplication at the tips, or secondary crests, of newly formed alveoli where DNA and elastin synthesis is high.[63] Thus despite a total decrease in cell multiplication, there appear to be selective areas (i.e., alveolar crests) in the diabetic lung where cell hyperplasia is occurring, resulting in new alveoli.[63] Additional morphologic changes in the lung in both experimental and human diabetes mellitus include thickening of the basal lamina of the alveolar epithelial and capillary basement membrane, collagen and elastin deposits in the interstitium, dilation of the endoplasmic reticulum in alveolar epithelial type II cells, and alterations in secretory granules in Clara cells.[64-68]

Pulmonary levels of collagen and elastin are elevated in immature and adult diabetic rats, reflecting both increased synthesis and diminished degradation of these proteins.[62,63,69] The activity of lysyl oxidase, an enzyme responsible for normal cross-linking of connective tissue proteins, is increased in the lungs of diabetic rats and results in tighter cross-linking of collagen and elastin, rendering them resistant to digestion by proteolytic enzymes and increasing their levels in the lung.[62,65,69] In addition, hyperglycemia-induced nonenzymatic glycosylation of collagen and elastin causes structurally abnormal cross-linking of these proteins.[60,65,66,70] As a result of both the tighter and structurally abnormal cross-linking, alterations occur in the mechanical properties of the lung. For example, stiff lungs in the adult diabetic rat and a reduction in pulmonary elastic recoil in humans with diabetes reflect these biochemical and morphologic changes.[65,66,69]

Although lung growth is somewhat enhanced (at least after birth) in diabetes in terms of alveolar number and relative surface area, antenatal lung growth as observed in the infant of the diabetic mother is delayed. The maternal hyperglycemia associated with diabetes crosses the placenta and stimulates the fetal pancreas to secrete insulin.[71] Pulmonary alterations result from the inhibitory effects of the sustained fetal hyperinsulinemia and are observed biochemically with reduced synthesis, availability, and use of surfactant precursors; morphologically with decreased number of alveolar epithelial type II cells, increased glycogen content in alveolar epithelial type II cells, and reduced air space in relation to the quantity of tissue present; and functionally with diminished lung distensibility.[71] Immaturity of the lung in the infant predisposes to the development of neonatal respiratory distress syndrome (Box 81-1). Both insulin and insulin-like growth factor receptors normally occur in the lung before and after birth, have elevated binding activity in the presence of hyperinsulinemia, and may play a role in the actions of insulin on the lung in the infant of the diabetic mother.[71-73]

BOX 81-1
Respiratory Disorders Associated with Diabetes Mellitus

Neonatal disorder
- Respiratory distress syndrome in infant of diabetic mother

Infectious disorders
- Bacteria: *Staphylococcus aureus, Streptococcus pneumoniae, Escherichia coli, Klebsiella pneumoniae*
- Fungi: zygomycetes (*Mucor, Rhizopus, Absidia* species), *Candida* species, *Aspergillus* species
- Mycobacteria: *Mycobacterium tuberculosis*
- Viruses

Parenchymal disorders
- Adult respiratory distress syndrome
- Pulmonary edema
- Aspiration pneumonia
- Pneumothorax, pneumomediastinum
- Pleural effusion
- Cor pulmonale

Airway disorder
- Autonomic neuropathy: reduced bronchial reactivity, mucus plugging

Chest wall disorder
- Hypokalemic respiratory muscle paralysis

Disorders of control of breathing
- Diminished responses to hypoxia and hypercapnia
- Central hypoventilation
- Central apnea
- Sleep apnea

Disorders of the lung, chest wall, and control of breathing can complicate diabetes mellitus (see Box 81-1). Individuals with diabetes have an increased incidence of severe acute and chronic pulmonary infections. Defective cell-mediated immunity, with quantitative and qualitative dysfunction of lymphocytes and monocytes, and alterations in the activity of polymorphonuclear leukocytes and PAMs in diabetes contribute to the increased frequency and severity of infections.[74,75] Diseases caused by gram-positive bacteria (which grow well in a glucose environment), gram-negative rods, zygomycetes, *Candida* species, and *Mycobacterium tuberculosis* have an increased morbidity and mortality in diabetes.[61]

Mucormycosis (zygomycosis) is an infection caused by the ubiquitous fungi, *Mucor, Rhizopus,* and *Absidia* species, and can result in acute and chronic pulmonary disease in diabetes[61,76] (see Box 81-1). Hyperglycemia and acidemia favor the growth of these fungi by inhibiting the phagocytosis of polymorphonuclear leukocytes and PAMs. Although rhinocerebral mucormycosis occurs more frequently in diabetes, pulmonary involvement has also been observed.[61,76] Inhalation of the spores is the portal of entry to the lung. These fungi invade large airways and blood vessels and cause airway stenosis, thrombosis, ischemic necrosis, and infarction.[61,76] Pulmonary infection occurs as an acute pneumonia; initially the symptoms are fever, dyspnea, and cough, which may be dry or wet sounding, and later they include pleuritic chest pain and hemoptysis, which can be life threatening.[76] Chest radiographs indicate a localized infiltrate or cavity, which then spreads to nearby areas.

The severity of tuberculosis parallels the severity of diabetes.[61] *M. tuberculosis* is more likely to cause cavitary disease, particularly in the lower lobes, in individuals with diabetes than in nondiabetic patients.[61]

The direct effect of acidosis in diabetic ketoacidosis can cause increased pulmonary vascular permeability, pulmonary edema, and adult respiratory distress syndrome (ARDS)[61,65] (see Box 81-1). In addition, the crystalloids and fluids used in the therapy of ketoacidosis can contribute to the development of pulmonary edema and ARDS.[61,77] The gastric stasis and impaired gastric emptying occurring with ketoacidosis can cause gastroparesis, emesis, and aspiration pneumonia.[61] Severe vomiting and deep breathing secondary to acidosis can result in pneumothorax, pneumomediastinum, or both conditions.[61] Diabetic autonomic neuropathy resulting in diminished vagal nerve activity can cause sleep-disordered breathing with diminutions in heart rate and ventilatory responses to hypoxia and possibly hypercapnia and may explain the increased incidence of central hypoventilation and apnea in diabetes.[78,79] Autonomic neuropathy also causes airway abnormalities, including airway hyporeactivity to carbachol and cold air challenge testing and inhaled bronchodilators.[61] Electrolyte imbalance can result in respiratory muscle weakness.[61] The lungs can also be affected in diabetic-related diseases of other organs (i.e., heart failure, pulmonary edema, transudative pleural effusion with cardiac or renal involvement).[61]

Pulmonary function studies in individuals with diabetes have been performed primarily in adults with type I (insulin deficiency, insulin dependency) or type II (end-organ insulin resistance, non-insulin dependency) diabetes mellitus and have produced conflicting results. Investigations have included individuals with a history of cigarette smoking, hyperreactive airway disease, obesity, or all of these and varying degrees of control, duration, and severity of diabetes. Although reductions in VC, forced vital capacity (FVC), TLC, FRC, RV, FEV_1, mean maximum expiratory flow rate, and MVV are inconsistently observed, diminutions in DLCO corrected for alveolar volume (DLCO/VA), alveolar capillary blood volume, and pulmonary elastic recoil pressure have been frequently noted.[64,66,70,79-83]

Reduced pulmonary capillary blood volume, most likely resulting from microangiopathy with thickening of alveolar epithelial and capillary basal lamina, accounts for the diminished DLCO because the membrane component of DLCO is normal.[65,66] Platelet hyperaggregation, which results from reduced synthesis of prostacyclin (an inhibitor of platelet adhesion) and increased synthesis of thromboxane (a stimulant of platelet adhesion), occurs in diabetes and may also contribute to the microangiopathy.[84]

Diminished lung elastic recoil reflects alterations in pulmonary connective tissue.[65,66] Because immobile joints can result from abnormal connective tissue and are associated with the early development of microangiopathy in diabetes, limited joint mobility may be a clinical marker for abnormal lung connective tissue and altered pulmonary function.[61,80,85] Costosternal and costovertebral joint immobility resulting from connective tissue changes may contribute to the reduced lung volumes.[80] In addition, diaphragmatic and inspiratory muscle strength and respiratory muscle endurance are decreased.[81,82]

Pulmonary function changes correlate directly with the duration of diabetes mellitus in some studies.[65,81] In addition, diabetes at its onset may be associated with a faster rate of reduction in lung volumes compared with diabetes of long duration; that is, the rate of change in lung volumes appears greatest early.[70,86] Investigations of control of hyperglycemia in type I diabetes mellitus suggest the presence of normal pulmonary function, including DLCO/VA measurements, with longstanding near-normal serum glucose levels.[60] FVC and FEV_1 are diminished to a lesser extent in type II than in type I diabetes mellitus, suggesting that the milder the disease, the less severe the reductions in lung volumes and that after good biochemical control of diabetes, the rate of decline in lung volumes may decrease.[70,86]

In children who have well-controlled insulin-dependent diabetes and normal lung volumes and airflow rates at rest, exercise testing reveals normal measurements of ventilatory response, anaerobic threshold, and maximal heart rate but reduced work capacity, $\dot{V}O_2$, and oxygen pulse measurements.[87] This suggests the presence of inadequate peripheral oxygen use and subclinical microvascular abnormalities with thickening of the capillary basement membrane in skeletal muscles.[87]

Pulmonary complications in diabetes mellitus are diagnosed by history, physical examination, radiography, and laboratory studies. The presence of ketoacidosis, uncontrolled hyperglycemia, or both conditions in an individual with diabetes and pneumonia should suggest the possibility of a fungal or mycobacterial infection. Pulmonary mucormycosis should be considered in the presence of rhinocerebral disease with a characteristic black eschar.[76] ARDS can develop rapidly in diabetics in the presence of only mild hypoxemia without crackles or radiographic changes initially.[88] Important in the diagnosis of these disorders are stains and cultures of respiratory secretions and blood for bacteria, fungi, mycobacteria, and viruses; immunologic studies for specific viral antigens and antibodies; anteroposterior and lateral chest radiographs; and when indicated, computed tomographic scans.

Therapy includes appropriate antibiotics and antiviral, antifungal, and antimycobacterial agents for the specific etiologic microorganism; thoracentesis for a pleural effusion associated with respiratory distress; supplemental oxygen, assisted ventilation, and vasopressors for ARDS; cardiotonic drugs and diuretics for heart failure and pulmonary edema; correction of electrolyte imbalance; and improved serum glucose control of diabetes. Immunizations with the pneumococcal and influenza vaccines are important in preventing these infections.[61]

Pancreatitis

The more frequent etiologies of pancreatitis in children are listed in Box 81-2.[89-91,91a,91b] Pulmonary disorders associated with acute and chronic pancreatitis are listed in Box 81-3. Although the presence of pleural effusions has been reported in children with pancreatitis, most pleuropulmonary complications of pancreatitis have been described in adults, in whom the majority of cases result from alcoholism, trauma, and cholelithiasis.[89,90,92]

Pleural effusions frequently occur as left sided but may be right sided or bilateral.[93-96] They occur shortly after the onset of acute pancreatitis and are characterized by a serous, serosanguinous, or hemorrhagic exudate with a pH of 7.30 to 7.35, a glucose content similar to that of blood, a predominance of polymorphonuclear leukocytes, and elevations in the pleural/serum ratios of amylase, protein, and lactate dehydrogenase (LDH).[94,95] Fluid resorption correlates with the resolution of acute pancreatitis. However, an effusion persisting more than 14 days usually indicates the presence of chronic pancre-

BOX 81-2
Etiology of Pancreatitis in Children

Cholelithiasis
Congenital anomalies: pancreatic duct, biliary tract
Cystic fibrosis
Diabetes mellitus
Medications: tetracycline, sulfonamides, chlorothiazide, furosemide, corticosteroids, acetaminophen, oral contraceptive agents, immunosuppressive agents
Familial pancreatitis
Hyperparathyroidism
Hypertriglyceridemia
Infections:
- Bacteria: *Mycoplasma pneumoniae*
- Viruses: mumps virus, measles virus, rubella virus, coxsackievirus B, influenza virus type A, hepatitis B virus, Epstein-Barr virus, herpes zoster virus, cytomegalovirus
- Parasites: *Ascaris lumbricoides*
- Fungi: *Aspergillus* species

Malnutrition
Organic acidemias
Polyarteritis nodosa
Porphyria (acute)
Relapsing pancreatitis (acute, chronic)
Toxins: alcohol
Trauma

BOX 81-3
Pulmonary Disorders Associated with Pancreatitis

Acute pancreatitis	Chronic pancreatitis
Pleural effusion	Pancreaticopleural fistula
Empyema	Pancreaticobronchial fistula
Hemidiaphragm elevation	Pancreaticobronchopleural fistula
Atelectasis: left lower lobe	Recurrent pleural effusion
Pneumonia: left lower lobe	Recurrent lobar pneumonia
Pulmonary embolism	Secondary α_1-antitrypsin-deficient emphysema
Pulmonary infarction	
ARDS	
Pulmonary edema	

atic disease, such as a pseudocyst, abscess, or pancreaticopleural fistula, and represents a chronic effusion.[94] When a pancreaticopleural fistula occurs, a sinus tract develops from the apical aspect of the pseudocyst through the diaphragm to the pleural space.[95,96] The resultant pleural effusion may occur after the acute pancreatic symptoms have subsided and characteristically persists despite serial thoracenteses.[95-97] A thickened pleura can develop and encase a chronic effusion but usually resolves within 6 months after the onset of disease.[94]

The etiology and pathogenesis of the fluid have not been defined (Box 81-4). Although transdiaphragmatic channels can exist between the pleural cavity and acutely inflamed pancreas, whose tail normally lies just below the diaphragm, they are only infrequently recognized.[93,94,96] However, the normally occurring diaphragmatic hiatal openings for the esophagus, aorta, and inferior vena cava can allow passage of pancreatic fluid into the mediastinum and pleural space and thereby result in right-sided pleural effusions.[95,96,98] Lymph flow across transdiaphragmatic lymphatic vessels between the pancreas and pleural space may also have a role in the spread of the pancreatic inflammatory exudate.[96,98] In addition, lymphatic drainage

BOX 81-4
Possible Etiologies of Pleural Effusions Associated with Pancreatitis

Passage of inflammatory exudate through the transdiaphragmatic channels between the pancreas and the pleural space
Passage of inflammatory exudate through the esophageal, aortic, and inferior vena caval openings in the diaphragm
Passage of inflammatory exudate in lymph flow through the transdiaphragmatic lymphatic vessels, particularly with impaired diaphragmatic mobility
Passage of inflammatory exudate via retrograde lymph flow into the pleural space, which results from incompetent valves in the lymphatic vessels
Increased pleural vascular permeability resulting from the release of pancreatic chemical mediators

from the pleural space through the collecting lymphatics to the hilar lymph nodes is normally aided by the movement of the diaphragm.[93,94] The pain and inflammation occurring with pancreatitis can impair diaphragmatic mobility, hinder normal lymph flow, and cause pleural fluid to accumulate.[93] In addition, lymphatic valves, which help promote lymph flow in the collecting lymphatic vessels from both the pleural and peritoneal spaces, can become incompetent as a result of inflammatory pancreatic disease.[93] Because lymph flow is bidirectional in these vessels, lymph can then flow back into the pleural space from the peritoneal area.[93,98] Finally, the pancreatic inflammation itself and chemical mediators, such as proteolytic enzymes, prostaglandins, phospholipase A_2, kinins, histamine, and activated complement, which are released by the inflammatory process, can increase the permeability of pleural capillaries, disrupt lymphatic vessels, and promote the formation of pleural fluid.[93,94,99]

Empyema occurs if a bacterial infection results in a pleural effusion (see Box 81-3). *Escherichia coli* and *Staphylococcus aureus* have been isolated in this setting.[96,100] The subdiaphragmatic inflammatory process in the pancreas with its associated pain and limited diaphragmatic mobility can cause elevation of the left hemidiaphragm, lower lobe atelectasis, and pneumonia[94,96,100] (Fig. 81-1). If it is severe, ventilation-perfusion imbalance, intrapulmonary shunting of blood, and hypoxemia can result. Recurrent pneumonia of the left lower lobe suggests the presence of a pancreaticobronchial fistula, and sputum containing amylase associated with an amylase-rich pleural effusion indicates a pancreaticobronchopleural fistula, both of which occur with chronic pancreatitis.[97,101] In addition, pulmonary embolism and infarction result from the release of clotting factors, kinin, and activated complement from the inflamed pancreas.[94,100]

Atelectasis occurs as the inflamed pancreas releases phospholipase A_2, or lecithinase, an enzyme that hydrolyzes dipalmitoyl phosphatidylcholine (lecithin), the main component of the phospholipids in surfactant.[102,103] In addition, pulmonary phospholipid synthesis is reduced.[103] The resultant reduction in surfactant activity increases alveolar surface tension and promotes lung collapse.[102,103]

If the pancreatic inflammatory process is severe, ARDS can occur (see Box 81-3 and Fig. 81-1). The release of multiple chemical mediators, including (in addition to those already mentioned) leukotrienes and pancreatic elastase, increases vascular permeability and promotes the development of

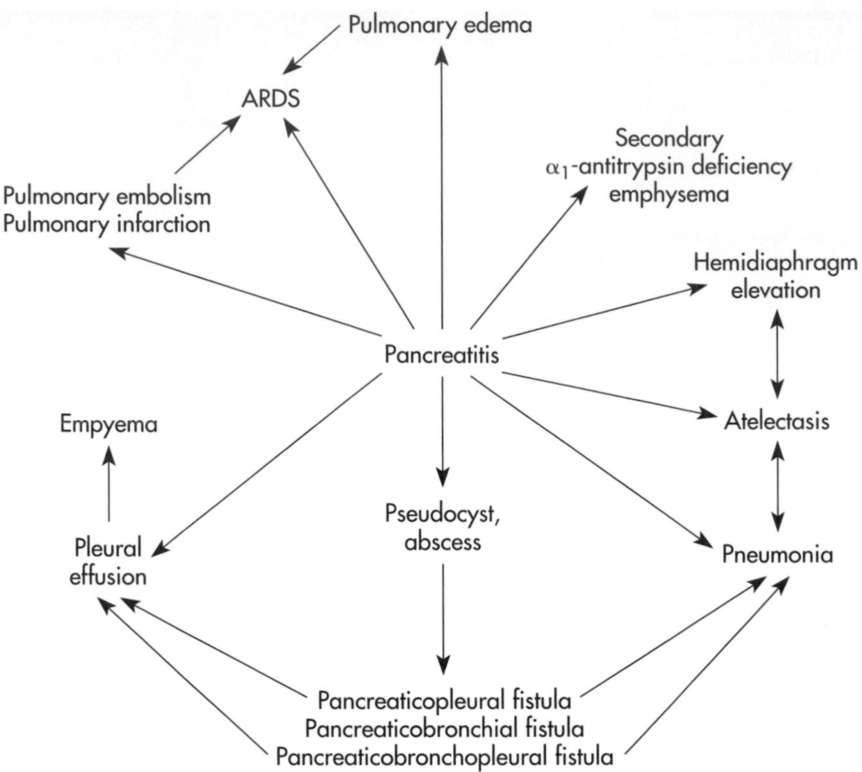

Fig. 81-1. Pancreaticopulmonary disorders.

ARDS.[94,104] High levels of free fatty acids resulting from phospholipid cleavage by phospholipase A_2 and from high serum levels of triglycerides occurring with hypertriglyceridemia by the action of pulmonary lipoprotein lipase also contribute to the lung injury by damaging capillary endothelial cell membranes and thereby increasing vascular permeability.[103,105] In addition, oxygen-free radicals released from activated polymorphonuclear leukocytes play a role.[106,107]

Morphologically, the lung in ARDS secondary to acute pancreatitis has alveolar epithelial type II cell injury with destruction of surfactant-containing lamellar bodies, capillary endothelial cell damage, interstitial and alveolar edema, intravascular and interstitial aggregates of polymorphonuclear leukocytes and platelets, intraalveolar hemorrhage, fibrin deposits, thickening of the alveolar epithelial cell membrane, and distortion of the alveolar architecture.[99,104,107-110] Bronchoalveolar lavage fluid contains increased levels of protein and polymorphonuclear leukocytes, and these lungs weigh more and are stiffer than lungs without ARDS.[99,108]

As a result of trypsin released from the inflamed pancreas, α_1-antitrypsin levels may be decreased and can cause an emphysema-like picture in chronic pancreatitis[111] (see Box 81-3 and Fig. 81-1). Similarly, elastase released from the pancreas also contributes to the development of emphysema.[111]

Hypoxemia without clinical or radiographic manifestations of pulmonary disease can occur during the early stages of acute pancreatitis and may result from intrapulmonary right-to-left shunting of blood.[92,94,111,112] Pulmonary function testing reveals reductions in VC, FEV_1, and TLC in acute pancreatitis, but these measurements are normal in chronic disease.[111,112] However, the DLCO, both absolute and corrected for lung volume, is diminished in acute and chronic pancreatitis.[101,111,112] This may reflect a diminution in the effective gas-exchanging surface, thickening of the alveolar epithelial cell membrane, and reduction in capillary blood volume occurring in the lung even without ARDS as a result of pancreatitis.[111]

The diagnosis of these pancreaticopulmonary disorders is aided by the history, physical examination, and radiographic and laboratory studies. Pancreatitis is associated with sharp, localized midepigastric abdominal pain that is more severe with eating, vomiting, fever, anorexia, abdominal distention and tenderness, lethargy, and malaise.[89-91] The signs and symptoms of pleural effusion, atelectasis, and pneumonia associated with pancreatitis are similar to the signs and symptoms of these conditions without pancreatitis. Pleural effusions are characterized by localized limited chest wall expansion, dullness to percussion, diminished breath sounds, a friction rub, pleuritic pain with splinting, dyspnea, tachypnea, and shallow breathing. Atelectasis is associated with dullness on percussion, localized diminished breath sounds, pectoriloquy, and if large, unilateral tracheal deviation and mediastinal shift. Fever, a wet-sounding cough, crackles, pectoriloquy, and bronchophony indicate the presence of pneumonia.

Anteroposterior and lateral chest radiographs reveal the pleural effusion, which if large, may result in contralateral mediastinal shift. Lateral decubitus films are helpful in evaluating the presence of free-moving pleural fluid. Atelectasis on the chest radiograph may be accompanied by unilateral mediastinal shift. Ultrasonography, computed tomographic scans, and endoscopic retrograde cholangiopancreatographic studies of the pancreas can help in the diagnosis of an abscess, pseudocyst, or fistula.[91,94,97,101]

Measurements of serum phospholipase A_2 concentrations parallel the severity and course of pancreatitis and atelectasis.[113] Pleural fluid amylase levels are elevated in pancreatitis and remain increased after the hyperamylasemia has resolved.[94,98] However, unlike chronic pancreatitis, in which pleural fluid amylase levels are characteristically increased,

Table 81-4 Pulmonary Disorders Associated with Hepatic Disease

HEPATIC DISEASE	PULMONARY DISORDER
Infections	Hilar adenopathy, tracheobronchitis, pneumonia, atelectasis, hyperreactive airway disease, interstitial pneumonitis, interstitial fibrosis, nodules, cysts, pleural effusion, fistulas (hepatopleural, hepatobronchial, biliobronchial)
Primary sclerosing cholangitis	Bronchitis, bronchiectasis
Malignancy	Hilar adenopathy, pneumonitis, nodules, pleural effusion, thromboemboli, lymphangitic carcinomatosis, osteolytic lesions in vertebrae and ribs
α_1-Antitrypsin deficiency	Tracheobronchitis, pneumonia, hyperreactive airway disease, emphysema, pulmonary angiodysplasia
Chronic granulomatous disease of childhood	Hilar adenopathy, pneumonia, atelectasis, pleural effusion, abscess, honeycomb lung, pulmonary hypertension
Cystic fibrosis	Tracheobronchitis, pneumonia, atelectasis, bronchiectasis, hyperreactive airway disease, cysts, bullae, pneumothorax, pulmonary hemorrhage, pulmonary hypertension
Hereditary hemorrhagic telangiectasia (Osler-Weber-Rendu disease)	Pulmonary angiodysplasia
Langerhans' cell histiocytosis	Hilar adenopathy, pneumonitis (lobar, reticulonodular, and interstitial), interstitial fibrosis, pleural effusion, pneumothorax, cysts, bullae, honeycomb lung, pulmonary hypertension
Sarcoidosis	Hilar adenopathy, reticulonodular infiltrates, atelectasis, hyperreactive airway disease, granulomata, bronchial stenosis, interstitial pneumonitis, interstitial fibrosis, pleural effusion, pneumothorax, nodules, cysts, bullae, honeycomb lung, pulmonary hemorrhage, pulmonary hypertension
Chronic active hepatitis	Pneumonia, atelectasis, interstitial pneumonitis, interstitial fibrosis, fibrosing alveolitis, pleural effusion, pulmonary angiodysplasia, pleural vasodilatations, pulmonary hypertension, pulmonary hemorrhage
Cirrhosis (alcoholic, postnecrotic, cryptogenic)	Pneumonia, pleural effusion, pulmonary angiodysplasia, pleural vasodilatations, pulmonary hypertension
Primary biliary cirrhosis	Hyperreactive airway disease, interstitial pneumonitis, interstitial fibrosis, fibrosing alveolitis, granulomata, nodules, pleural effusion, pulmonary angiodysplasia, pulmonary hypertension, rib and vertebral fractures

acute pancreatitis may be initially associated with normal levels of pleural fluid amylase, which rise later as the disease progresses.[95,98] Pleural fluid amylase levels may also be increased in other disorders, including esophageal rupture, pleural fluid metastases, and tuberculosis.[95,98,114] However, in contrast to the pancreatic origin of the amylase in the pleural fluid associated with pancreatitis, the pleural fluid amylase is of salivary origin in these other disorders.[98,114]

Therapy is directed at the specific pulmonary disorder: antibiotics for pneumonia, thoracentesis for an effusion that causes respiratory distress, chest tube drainage and fibrinolytic agents for empyema, chest physical therapy for atelectasis, anticoagulants for pulmonary emboli, and assisted ventilation, supplemental oxygen, and vasopressor agents for ARDS. The pleural effusion usually resorbs as the acute pancreatic inflammation resolves.[95] Repeated therapeutic thoracenteses for a pleural effusion may not be helpful if a fistula is present and allows the effusion to recur. If 2 weeks of medical therapy, including parenteral nutrition; therapeutic pharmacologic suppression of pancreatic secretions using atropine, acetazolamide, cimetidine, or a combination of these drugs; and serial thoracenteses or chest tube drainage, does not resolve the effusion, then surgery to close the fistulous tract is necessary.[92,95,97,98] Pseudocysts are usually removed surgically.[92,94,97]

BOX 81-5
Infections Associated with Hepatopulmonary Disease

Bacteria

Actinomyces israelii
Brucella species
Chlamydia psittacei
Coxiella burnetii
Francisella tularensis
Legionella pneumophila
Leptospira interrogans
Listeria monocytogenes
Mycobacterium tuberculosis, Mycobacterium bovis
Mycoplasma pneumoniae
Rickettsia prowazekii, Rickettsia rickettsii
Treponema pallidum

Viruses

Adenoviruses
Coxsackievirus B
Cytomegalovirus
Hepatitis A, B, and C viruses
Human immunodeficiency virus
Varicella-zoster virus

Parasites

Ascaris lumbricoides
Cryptosporidium species
Echinococcus granulosus
Entamoeba histolytica
Leishmania donovani
Plasmodium species
Schistosoma species
Toxocara canis, Toxocara cati
Toxoplasma gondii

Fungi

Aspergillus species
Blastomyces dermatitidis
Histoplasma capsulatum
Paracoccidioides brasiliensis

DISORDERS OF THE LIVER

Pulmonary disorders can occur with hepatic disease (Table 81-4). Acute hepatic disease associated with lung complications results from infections, medications, and toxins[115,116] (Box 81-5). For example, a pleural effusion can occur with an intrahepatic abscess caused by *Entamoeba histolytica* or a hydatid cyst caused by *Echinococcus granulosus*.[95,98] The pleural effusion associated with *E. histolytica* is composed of blood and liver tissue and has the consistency of chocolate sauce or anchovy paste.[98] The effusion results from direct diaphragmatic irritation by the hepatic lesion, causing increased permeability of diaphragmatic pleural capillaries and transudation of fluid into the pleural space. If the hepatic lesion ruptures through the diaphragm, empyema forms, and the communication may remain patent as a hepatopleural fistula.[95,98] Rupture of the lesion into the airways can result in hepatobronchial and biliobronchial fistulas, with sputum that is dark in color with *E. histolytica* or that has cystlike structures with *E. granulosus*.[95,98] Viral hepatitis also causes an exudative pleural effu-

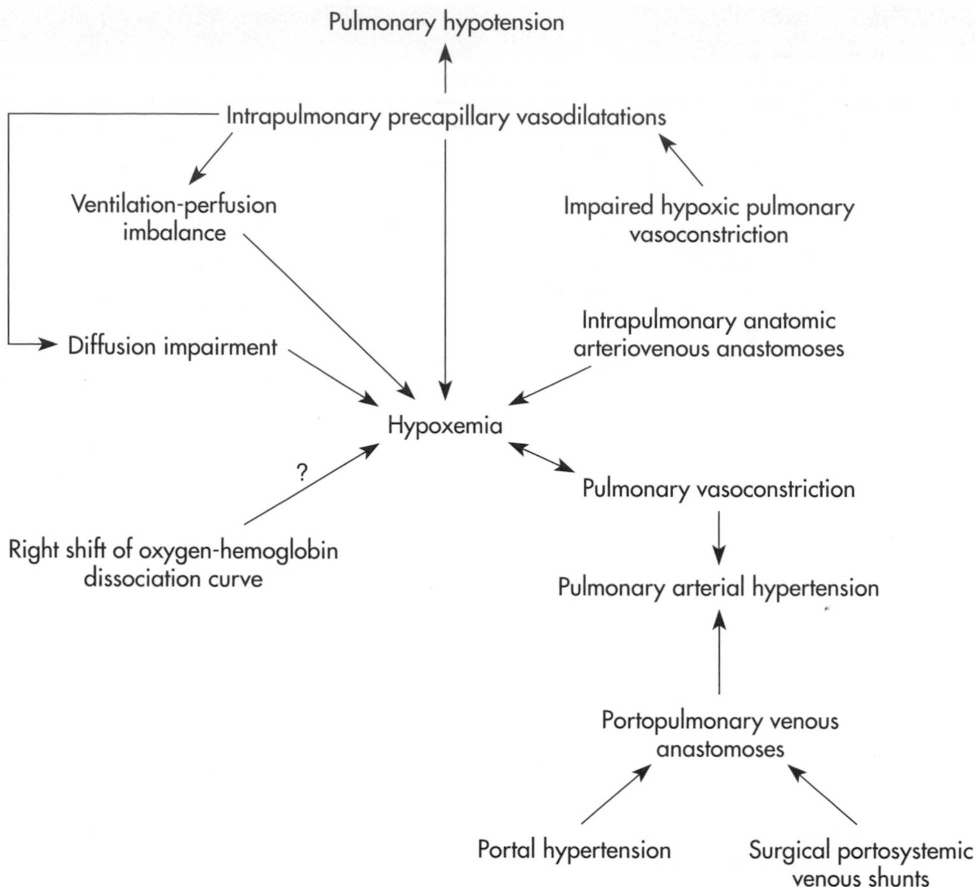

Fig. 81-2. Etiology of hypoxemia in hepatopulmonary disorders.

sion with a predominance of monocytes and without parenchymal disease.[98] If hepatitis B virus is the etiology, the fluid may have the hepatitis B surface and e antigens.[95,98] In addition, hepatitis C virus is associated with interstitial fibrosis.[117] Other infectious agents causing hepatopulmonary disease are listed in Box 81-5, and the pulmonary disorders associated with infections are listed in Table 81-4.

Chronic hepatic disease also causes pulmonary disorders. Primary sclerosing cholangitis results from cholestasis of intrahepatic and extrahepatic bile ducts, causes cirrhosis and liver failure, is frequently seen with inflammatory bowel disease, and is associated with chronic pulmonary infection[115,118] (see Table 81-4). Hepatic malignancies, such as hepatocellular carcinoma, metastasize to the diaphragm and lung either directly or hematogenously from the hepatic vein into the inferior vena cava, right heart, and pulmonary artery and cause parenchymal, pleural, vascular, and lymphatic lesions of the lung and bone disease of the chest wall.[115] Systemic disorders, such as α_1-antitrypsin deficiency, chronic granulomatous disease of childhood, cystic fibrosis, hereditary hemorrhagic telangiectasia, Langerhans' cell histiocytosis, and sarcoidosis, can also result in hepatopulmonary disease. For detailed descriptions of these disorders, the reader is referred to other chapters in this book and literature elsewhere.[115,118,119,119a]

The hepatopulmonary syndrome, which consists of liver disease, pulmonary angiodysplasia, and hypoxemia as defined by a partial pressure of arterial oxygen (PaO_2) of less than 70 mm Hg, is caused by chronic active hepatitis, alcoholic or postnecrotic cirrhosis, and primary biliary cirrhosis[115,120,120a] (see Table 81-4). Portopulmonary anastomoses and pulmonary arterial hypertension may also occur[115,118,120] (Fig. 81-2). Chronic active hepatitis results from viral infections, medication sensitivity or toxicity, or immune dysfunction and is characterized by progressive hepatocytic inflammation and necrosis, cirrhosis, and liver failure.[115,118,121] Hepatic fatty changes, scarring, nodules, and failure occur in postnecrotic cirrhosis.[118] Primary biliary cirrhosis is a chronic granulomatous disorder associated with intrahepatic bile duct inflammation and degeneration, cholestasis, cirrhosis, portal hypertension, hepatic failure, humoral and cellular immunodeficiency, mitochondrial antibodies, keratoconjunctivitis, osteopenia, kyphosis, and rib and vertebral fractures.[115,118,120a,122]

Pulmonary angiodysplasia results from dilation of intrapulmonary precapillary vessels, anatomic pulmonary arteriovenous communications, and an increase in the number of arterioles supplying an alveolus.[115,116,120,123,124] Right-to-left shunting of as much as 70% of the cardiac output occurs.[115,118,125] The precapillary vessels, which are normally 8 to 15 μ in diameter, may dilate to 500 μ in diameter, with subsequent reduction of pulmonary vascular resistance and pulmonary artery pressure and development of pulmonary hypotension.[115,125] The presence of an elevated cardiac output and rapid transit time for blood flow, which results from diminished systemic vascular resistance and increased peripheral blood flow, does not allow adequate oxygenation of venous blood passing through these dilations, and arterial hypoxemia ensues[115,118,126,127] (see Fig. 81-2). With severe liver dysfunction, the hypoxemia may not elicit the normal hypoxic pul-

BOX 81-6
Cardiorespiratory Manifestations of Hepatopulmonary Disorders

Pulmonary manifestations

Adventitious breath sounds
Clubbing
Cough
Cyanosis
Diaphragmatic impairment
Dyspnea
Exercise intolerance
Hemoptysis
Hyperventilation
Hypoxemia
Orthodeoxia
Orthopnea
Paroxysmal nocturnal dyspnea
Platypnea
Precordial chest pain
Respiratory alkalosis
Tachypnea

Cardiac manifestations

Accentuation of pulmonic second sound
Systolic ejection murmur in second or third left intercostal space or over left sternal border

Cardiac manifestations—cont'd

Pulmonary bruit increased by inspiration and Müller's maneuver and decreased by Valsalva maneuver

Electrocardiographic manifestations

Right ventricular hypertrophy
Right axis deviation
Right bundle branch block

Radiographic manifestations

Prominence of main pulmonary arteries
Paucity of peripheral pulmonary vessels
Cardiomegaly

monary vasoconstrictive response, which then augments the pulmonary hypotension and hypoxemia and contributes to ventilation-perfusion imbalance and diffusion impairment.[115,118,128-130] Vasodilations, or spiders, occur not only in the lung parenchyma but also in the pleura and are similar to the cutaneous spiders present in liver disease.[115,116,118,120,123] However, the pleural vasodilations have little blood flow, do not contribute to hypoxemia, and occur in chronic active hepatitis and postnecrotic cirrhosis but not primary biliary cirrhosis.[115,118,123] A circulating nonmetabolized or nondetoxified vasoactive substance or a metabolite whose activity or level is enhanced by the malfunctioning liver may cause these dilations by altering the pulmonary vascular endothelium.[115] Elastase, endotoxin, prostaglandin, substance P, ferritin, thromboxane, and serotonin have been proposed as possible vasoactive substances.[118,125,127,131,132]

The dilated vessels and arteriovenous anastomoses are more numerous at the lung bases than at the apex.[115,118,133] As a result of the effect of gravity on augmenting blood flow through these vessels in the upright position, hypoxemia becomes more pronounced after a change from the supine to standing position.[115,118,133] Orthodeoxia, defined by a decrease in the PaO_2 by more than 10 mm Hg between these two positions, is characteristic and often associated with an increase in dyspnea or platypnea[115,118,133] (Box 81-6).

Paradoxically, pulmonary arterial hypertension can result from portopulmonary venous anastomoses, which develop in the presence of portal hypertension and surgical portosystemic venous shunts (see Fig. 81-2). Instead of blood flowing along its normal pathway from the portal vein to the portal triad, where it combines with oxygenated blood from the hepatic artery, and then flowing through the venous system into the inferior vena cava, it is redirected from the portal vein through the periesophageal, mediastinal, and azygous veins, some of which communicate directly with large extrapulmonary and bronchial veins.[118,134] Although the contribution of these communications to hypoxemia is negligible because of a relatively high oxyhemoglobin saturation of 70% in portal venous blood and only a small amount of blood flow through these anastomoses,[115,118,123,127] pulmonary hypertension does not occur in the absence of portal hypertension and usually develops after portal hypertension is present.[115,131] Pulmonary arterial hypertension results from hypoxemia in the presence of moderately severe liver dysfunction; is associated with intravascular platelet aggregation causing vasoconstriction; has characteristic plexiform lesions consisting of nonfunctional, thin-walled, nonmuscular, saclike dilations of muscular arteries filled with blood, cells, collagen, and elastin; and may be caused by the increased activity of a chemical mediator.[115,129,131,132,134]

Thus pulmonary hypotension, which is associated with precapillary vasodilation and impaired hypoxic pulmonary vasoconstriction, and pulmonary hypertension, which is caused by hypoxemia and portal hypertension, can occur in the hepatopulmonary syndrome[115,135] (see Fig. 81-2). Although the oxygen-hemoglobin dissociation curve is shifted to the right with liver disease because of increased red blood cell (RBC) 2,3-diphosphoglycerate levels, this does not appear to be an important factor in the development of hypoxemia in hepatopulmonary disorders.[118,126,128,130]

The history, physical examination, and laboratory and radiographic studies aid in the diagnosis of these disorders. A family history of early onset lung disease may be present with cystic fibrosis and α_1-antitrypsin deficiency. The presence of the signs and symptoms listed in Box 81-6 should signal a possible hepatopulmonary disorder. The occurrence of orthodeoxia and platypnea should alert the examiner to the presence of pulmonary angiodysplasia.[133]

The underlying hepatic disease is diagnosed with appropriate serologic tests for viral hepatitis, serum liver enzyme levels, and stains, cultures, and histologic studies of liver biopsy material. Abdominal ultrasonography and computed tomographic scans for liver abscesses or cysts; tests for serum α_1-antitrypsin levels and phenotype studies for α_1-antitrypsin deficiency; and cultures of respiratory secretions, a sweat test, and genotype studies for cystic fibrosis are important. Stains and cultures of respiratory secretions, pleural fluid, and blood are necessary to diagnose pulmonary bacterial infections. Langerhans' cell histiocytosis and chronic granulomatous disease are associated with opportunistic infections, including those by *Pneumocystis carinii, S. aureus, Enterobacter* species, *Pseudomonas cepacia,* and *Proteus, Salmonella, Aspergillus, Serratia, Nocardia,* and *Candida* organisms. Samples of bronchoalveolar lavage fluid may be needed for stains and cultures of these organisms.[119] Open lung biopsy aids in the diagnosis of pulmonary angiodysplasia, interstitial lung disease, and pulmonary hypertension.

Anteroposterior and lateral radiographs, ultrasonography, and computed tomographic scans of the chest help in the diagnosis of pneumonia, atelectasis, pleural effusion, abscesses, cysts, bullae, nodules, pulmonary hypertension, interstitial fibrosis, and honeycomb lung. Pulmonary angiodysplasia is diagnosed by pulmonary arteriography, which reveals the dilated precapillaries and the arteriovenous anastomoses at the lung bases in a characteristic spongy pattern that correlates radiographically with the presence of basilar nodular infiltrates.[115,118,120,123] Contrast-enhanced, two-dimensional echocardiography detects the presence of a shunt by scanning the passage of microbubbles in a contrast material. These particles are normally removed in transit through pulmonary capillar-

BOX 81-7
Respiratory Disorders Associated with Renal Failure

Parenchymal disorders

Alveolar hemorrhage
- Goodpasture's syndrome
- Systemic necrotizing vasculitides: Wegener's granulomatosis, Churg-Strauss syndrome, polyarteritis nodosa
- Connective tissue diseases: systemic lupus erythematosus, scleroderma, Behçet's disease
- Henoch-Schönlein purpura
- Medications: penicillamine toxicity

Fibrosing alveolitis
- Renal tubular acidosis

Amyloidosis
- Chronic renal failure, end-stage renal disease

Lymphomatoid granulomatosis
- Chronic renal failure, end-stage renal disease

Metastatic pulmonary calcification
- Renal osteodystrophy, chronic hemodialysis, chronic renal failure, end-stage renal disease

Pulmonary edema ("uremic lung")
- Chronic renal failure, end-stage renal disease

Pneumonia: infectious, uremic pneumonitis
- Acute and chronic renal failure, peritoneal dialysis, end-stage renal disease

Rounded atelectasis
- Chronic renal failure, end-stage renal disease

Airway disorders

Hyperreactive airway disease
- Nephrotic syndrome, peritoneal dialysis, hemodialysis, chronic renal failure, end-stage renal disease

Pleural disorders

Pleural effusion
- Nephrotic syndrome, peritoneal dialysis, chronic renal failure, end-stage renal disease

Chylothorax
- Nephrotic syndrome

Chest wall disorders

Respiratory muscle myopathy ("uremic myopathy")
- Chronic renal failure, peritoneal dialysis, chronic hemodialysis, end-stage renal disease

Fractures: ribs, vertebrae
- Renal osteodystrophy, chronic renal failure, end-stage renal disease

Disorders of control of breathing

Sleep apnea (central, obstructive)
- Chronic renal failure, end-stage renal disease

ies, but in the presence of a right-to-left intrapulmonary shunt, they bypass the capillaries and appear, after several cardiac cycles, in the left side of the heart.[115,118,120,136] Lung perfusion scans using macroaggregated albumin labeled with technetium-99 have particles measuring 20 to 50 μ, which wedge into normal 8- to 15-μ capillaries and do not pass through these vessels. In the presence of arteriovenous fistulas, these particles travel through the fistulas and appear in the systemic circulation of extrapulmonary organs.[115,118,120,137]

Pulmonary function testing reveals reductions in DLCO, variable decreases in lung volumes and airflow rates, increases in $\dot{V}E$, hypoxemia, and hypocapnia.[122,125,135,137,138] Diminutions in the transfer factor cause the diminished DLCO, which occurs as a result of an increase in the pathway for gas diffusion from the alveolus through the vasodilated vessel to the RBC[137,138] and is observed in alveolitis, emphysema, interstitial pneumonitis, and interstitial fibrosis. Ventilation-perfusion imbalance results from pulmonary angiodysplasia, pneumonia, atelectasis, bronchiectasis, and emphysema.

Measurements of lung volumes and compliance may be altered in the presence of ascites complicating liver disease. Peritoneal fluid can raise intraabdominal pressure; elevate and fix the diaphragm; reduce lung volumes, chest wall compliance and MVV; and increase the respiratory rate.[115,118,127,135] In addition, oxyhemoglobin saturation, as measured by pulse oximetry, may be underestimated if the serum total bilirubin level is more than 2.5 mg% because of the interference of bilirubin pigments in the skin with oximetric readings of light transmission.[115,118]

Therapy is directed at the underlying hepatic disorder. However, medications used to treat liver disease can be toxic to the lung. Morrhuate sodium, a sclerosing agent composed of unsaturated fatty acids and cod liver oil, is used in the therapy of esophageal varices associated with portal hypertension and can cause aspiration pneumonia, exudative pleural effusion, bronchospasm, bronchoesophageal fistula, pulmonary hypertension, and ARDS.[95,115,118,127] Penicillamine, a drug used in the treatment of Wilson's disease and primary biliary cirrhosis, can result in bronchospasm, bronchiolitis obliterans, bronchitis, hemorrhagic pleural effusion, interstitial pneumonitis, alveolitis, pulmonary hemorrhage, and a pulmonary-renal syndrome similar to that of Goodpasture's syndrome[118,139] (Box 81-7). Azathioprine, an immunosuppressive agent used after liver transplantation, can cause pulmonary edema and interstitial pneumonitis and fibrosis.[115,118,127] Cyclosporine, another immunosuppressive drug used after liver transplantation, can cause pulmonary edema and ARDS.[115,118,127]

Additional therapy includes the treatment of pulmonary infections with appropriate antimicrobial agents and the relief of dyspnea caused by pleural effusions or ascites with thoracentesis and paracentesis, respectively. Hypoxemia is treated with supplemental oxygen and positioning to reduce the extent of orthodeoxia and platypnea. Percutaneous embolization can be used for the therapy of pulmonary angiodysplasia; hypoxemia improves with this technique.[140] Supplemental oxygen and bronchodilators, which improve airflow and minimize airway resistance and work of breathing, are used in the treatment of pulmonary hypertension. Calcium channel blockers and prostaglandins may also be used.[131] Hypoxemia, clubbing, ventilation-perfusion imbalance, shunts, elevated cardiac output, reduced systemic and pulmonary vascular resistances, abnormal pulmonary function testing, and exercise intolerance may reverse after liver transplantation.[115,126,141]

DISORDERS OF THE KIDNEY

Renal Failure

Acute and chronic renal failure can cause disease involving the lung parenchyma, airways, pleural space, chest wall, and control of breathing centers (see Box 81-7). Pulmonary disease is more likely to be present when the plasma urea concentration is more than 20 mmol/L, or approximately 60 mg%, a level associated with metabolic alterations.[142]

Alveolar hemorrhage occurs in uremia as a result of abnormal coagulation and hypervolemia[143] (see Box 81-7). The coexistence of alveolar hemorrhage and glomerulonephritis produces a spectrum of diseases that affect the pulmonary interstitium and vessels, are frequently identified with immune dysfunction, and compose the pulmonary-renal syndrome[144,145,145a] (Table 81-5). For example, antibasement membrane antibody disease, or Goodpasture's syndrome, is associated with linear deposits of IgG, IgA, IgM, and the third component of complement (C_3) in the basement membranes of renal glomerular capillaries and IgG, IgA, and C_3 in the pulmonary alveolar septa; alveolar hemorrhage, inflammation, and fibrosis; PAMs filled with hemosiderin; focal and diffuse interstitial infiltrates; and acute respiratory failure.[143-145] Pulmonary vasculitis and interstitial necrosis are characteristically absent.[145] The IgG antibodies combine with basement membrane proteins of type IV collagen in renal tubules and glomeruli and in the presence of factors that increase capillary permeability (such as hyperoxia and cigarette smoke), in pulmonary alveoli.[144,145]

Another example is Wegener's granulomatosis, which in addition to glomerulonephritis, is characterized by circulating antineutrophil cytoplasmic IgG antibodies, deposits of IgG and complement in alveolar interstitium and small blood vessels, parenchymal cavitary lesions, localized alveolar hemorrhage, and necrotizing granulomatous vasculitis with infiltration by polymorphonuclear leukocytes, T cells, monocytes, histiocytes, plasma cells, and giant cells[144,145a,146] (see Table 81-5). The pulmonary manifestations of allergic angiitis and granulomatosis, or Churg-Strauss syndrome, include a history of asthma, allergies, or both conditions; vasculitis of the pulmonary arteries, veins, and capillaries of varying sizes; and histologic evidence of asthma, eosinophilic infiltrates, granulomas, and necrotizing vasculitis in the lung.[144,146] Although polyarteritis nodosa is infrequently accompanied by respiratory complications, chronic asthma, alveolar hemorrhage, and necrotizing vasculitis of medium and small pulmonary arteries can occur and probably represent a variant of Churg-Strauss syndrome.[144-146]

Systemic lupus erythematosus is associated with IgG, IgA, IgM, and complement deposition in pulmonary alveolar epithelial and endothelial cells and renal glomerular basement membranes; chronic interstitial pneumonia; hyaline membranes; diffuse alveolar hemorrhage; and pulmonary vasculitis.[143,145,145a,146] Progressive systemic sclerosis, or scleroderma, is characterized by fibrous connective tissue deposition in the lung, which may be inflammatory and immunologic in etiology; pulmonary interstitial fibrosis; and pulmonary hypertension.[146,147] Henoch-Schönlein purpura is associated with alveolar IgA deposition, inflammation, hemorrhage, and widespread pulmonary vasculitis, whereas Behçet's disease is accompanied by deposits of IgG, C_3, and the fourth component of complement (C_4) in pulmonary capillaries and venules; vasculitis of different-sized pulmonary vessels; pulmonary thrombosis and infarction; and pulmonary artery aneurysms invading contiguous airways.[144-146,148,149] In most of these disorders, particularly Goodpasture's syndrome and Wegener's granulomatosis, alveolar hemorrhage occurs early in the course of the glomerulonephritis and may be the presenting manifestation.[145]

Other pulmonary disorders occurring with renal failure include fibrosing alveolitis, which can accompany renal tubular acidosis[150] (see Box 81-7). The combination of these two disorders suggests an underlying systemic disease involving the immune system, particularly because hypergammaglobulinemia and autoantibodies may be present with fibrosing alveolitis.[150] The pulmonary airways, alveolar septa, and blood vessels and kidneys are affected by deposits of amyloid, a glycoprotein, with resultant wheezing, dyspnea, pulmonary hemorrhage, pleural effusion, diffuse reticulonodular infiltrates and nodular lesions on radiographs, and respiratory failure.[144,147] Lymphomatoid granulomatosis, a lymphoproliferative vasculitis of medium and small blood vessels damaged by atypical lymphocytes and plasma cells, causes lung and renal disease, is associated with T cell lymphoma formation with a predominance of CD4+ T cells, and usually occurs in a patient in an already immunocompromised state.[144,146,151] Bilateral pulmonary nodules, particularly at the bases and occasionally with cavitation, are present on chest radiographs, and pulmonary hemorrhage and pneumonia are frequent causes of death.[144,151]

Metastatic pulmonary calcification occurs in chronic renal failure in the presence of hypercalcemia and may result from primary, secondary, or tertiary hyperparathyroidism; hypervitaminosis D; excessive calcium ingestion (milk-alkali syndrome); and other mechanisms of excess calcium that are associated with renal insufficiency, such as bone infections, bone malignancies, and tumors secreting parathyroid-like hormone[152] (see Box 81-7). Calcium deposition in tissues occurs when the calcium-phosphorus product is larger than the solubility constant of calcium-phosphorus in blood[153] (Table 81-6). The lung acts as a reservoir for calcium deposition because of its relatively alkaline environment resulting from the loss of hydrogen ions during ventilation and because of the diminished solubility of calcium salts in areas with a high pH.[153-155] These salts are primarily calcium phosphates, and the occurrence and severity of the calcifications are unrelated to the duration of renal failure or dialysis, degree of parathyroid abnormalities, or extent of elevation of the levels of the calcium-phosphorus product.[155] Metastatic pulmonary calcification appears as diffuse calcium deposits in walls of alveoli, small bronchi, terminal bronchioles, and interstitial blood vessels; may be associated with interstitial thickening, collagen deposition, and fibrosis; can interfere with diffusion across the alveolar-capillary membrane; and can precipitate respiratory failure.[152,155,156] Chronic renal failure is the most frequently occurring entity that causes pulmonary calcification in children.[152]

Pulmonary edema results from fluid retention and hypoproteinemia, which occur as the glomerular filtration rate diminishes, and increased pulmonary capillary permeability[142,157] (see Box 81-7). This contributes to the increased weight of lungs of individuals dying from uremia.[158] The lung fluid is abundant with protein, including fibrin, and, when present radiographically, results in the "uremic lung."[142,158] Uremic pneumonitis can also occur and is associated with lungs that are heavy and indurated and have protein-rich edema fluid, hyaline membranes, alveolar hemorrhage, and fibrin in inflamed pleura.[98,144,159]

Renal failure alters cellular immunity and thus predisposes to pulmonary infection with opportunistic organisms (see Box 81-7). Total lymphopenia, reductions in CD4+ and CD8+ lymphocytes, reversal of the CD4+/CD8+ ratio, diminished

Table 81-5 Pulmonary-Renal Syndrome

SIGNS AND SYMPTOMS			
PULMONARY	**SYSTEMIC**	**LABORATORY FINDINGS**	**CHEST RADIOGRAPHS**
Goodpasture's syndrome			
Hemoptysis, cough, dyspnea, hypoxemia	Glomerulonephritis	Anemia, proteinuria, hematuria, RBC casts, ↑ BUN level, ↑ creatinine level, slightly ↑ ESR, serum antiglomerular basement membrane antibodies, association with HLA-DR2 antigen	Focal or diffuse, bilateral or unilateral interstitial infiltrates; reticulonodular infiltrates; edema; hemorrhage
Wegener's granulomatosis			
Hemoptysis, cough, dyspnea, hypoxemia, pleuritic chest pain, pleural friction rib	Fever, malaise, weight loss, otitis media, hearing loss, uveitis, proptosis, conjunctivitis, arthritis, sinusitis, dermatitis, epistaxis, CNS disease, glomerulonephritis	Anemia, thrombocytosis, ↑ ESR, ↑ creatinine level, ↑ BUN level, RBC casts, hematuria, pyuria, proteinuria, positive RF, circulating immune complexes, ↑ C_3 level, ↑ IgE and IgA levels, chemotaxis and cellular dysfunction, hypergammaglobulinemia, antineutrophil cytoplasmic IgG antibodies, association with HLA-DR2 antigen	Bilateral nodular infiltrates with central cavitation; diffuse alveolar, interstitial, or reticulonodular infiltrates; single nodule; platelike atelectasis; pleural effusion; bronchopleural fistula; hemorrhage
Churg-Strauss syndrome			
Wheezing, hemoptysis, cough, dyspnea, hypoxemia	Allergies, petechiae, purpura, nodular and subcutaneous lesions, seizures, coma, peripheral neuropathy, diarrhea, melena, myocardial and endocardial lesions, glomerulonephritis	Peripheral eosinophilia, slightly ↑ IgE level, ↑ ESR, circulating immune complexes, ↑ BUN level, ↑ creatinine level, hematuria, proteinuria, RBC casts, anemia, ↑ WBC count	Transient diffuse, nodular, or interstitial infiltrates; pleural and pericardial effusions; hemorrhage
Systemic lupus erythematosus			
Hemoptysis, cough, dyspnea, hypoxemia	Fever, malaise, weight loss, CNS disease, alopecia, arthritis, serositis, photosensitivity, nephritis	↓ C_3 level, positive ANA and anti-DNA titers, circulating immune complexes, positive Coombs' test, ↑ ESR, ↑ BUN level, hypergammaglobulinemia, ↑ creatinine level, hematuria, proteinuria, RBC and granular casts, anemia, ↑ or ↓ WBC count	Diffuse unilateral or bilateral infiltrates, interstitial infiltrates, atelectasis, pleural effusion, edema, hemorrhage
Scleroderma			
Hemoptysis, cough, dyspnea, hypoxemia, pleuritic chest pain, pleural friction rub, bibasilar crackles	Sclerosis of skin, telangiectasia, cutaneous calcifications, myositis, arthritis, cor pulmonale, Raynaud's phenomenon, hypertension, esophageal hypomotility, pericardial effusion, renal vascular disease and failure	↑ ESR, ↑ BUN level, ↑ creatinine level, positive RF, positive ANA titer, hypergammaglobulinemia, circulating immune complexes, T cell hyperactivity, proteinuria, hematuria, anemia	Diffuse bilateral interstitial basilar infiltrates, interstitial fibrosis, cystic lesions, honeycomb lung, pleural effusion, calcification, hemorrhage, prominent pulmonary arteries, cardiomegaly
Henoch-Schönlein purpura			
Hemoptysis, cough, dyspnea, hypoxemia	Arthritis, purpura, abdominal pain, melena, glomerulonephritis	↑ ESR, ↑ IgA level , ↑ BUN level, ↑ creatinine level, hematuria, proteinuria, RBC casts, anemia, ↑ WBC count, normal platelet count	Interstitial pneumonitis, hemorrhage, pleural effusion
Behçet's disease			
Hemoptysis, cough, dyspnea, hypoxemia, pleuritic chest pain	Uveitis, ulcers (oral, laryngeal, and genital), fever, subcutaneous nodules, thrombophlebitis, glomerulonephritis	↑ BUN level, ↑ creatinine level, ↑ ESR, hematuria, proteinuria, RBC casts, anemia	Diffuse reticulonodular infiltrates, pleural effusion, infarction, hemorrhage, prominent pulmonary arteries, diffuse bilateral perfusion defects on scan

RBC, Red blood cell; *BUN,* blood urea nitrogen; *ESR,* erythrocyte sedimentation rate; *HLA,* human leukocyte antigen; *CNS,* central nervous system; *RF,* rheumatoid factor; C_3, third component of complement; *WBC,* white blood cell; *ANA,* antinuclear antibodies.

Table 81-6 Serum Calcium and Phosphorus in Untreated Chronic Renal Failure and Hyperparathyroidism

DISORDER	SERUM CALCIUM (mg/dl)	SERUM PHOSPHORUS (mg/dl)	CALCIUM-PHOSPHORUS PRODUCT
Chronic renal failure alone	↓	↑	Normal, ↑, or ↓
Chronic renal failure with secondary hyperparathyroidism	Normal or slightly ↓	↑	Normal, ↑↑, or ↓
Primary hyperparathyroidism alone	↑	↓	Normal, ↑, or ↓
Primary hyperparathyroidism with secondary chronic renal failure*	Normal or ↑	↑	↑↑
Tertiary hyperparathyroidism	↑	↓	↑

↓, Decreased; ↑, increased.
*Individuals with primary hyperparathyroidism and secondary chronic renal failure often have secondary hyperparathyroidism.

Table 81-7 Pleural Effusion Composition in Uremia

TYPE	APPEARANCE	CELLS	GLUCOSE (mg/dl)	PROTEIN (g/dl)	LDH (IU/L)	CREATININE (mg/dl)	COMMENTS
Uremic	Exudate: serous, serosanguinous, hemorrhagic	Lymphocytes	Normal	↑	↑	↑	Unilateral or bilateral
Nephrotic syndrome, congestive heart failure	Transudate: serous	Monocytes, lymphocytes	Normal	↓↓	Normal	None	Bilateral
Chylous	Transudate: white, opalescent	Lymphocytes	Normal	↑	↑	Normal	Cholesterol and triglyceride present, unilateral
Dialysate	Transudate	Monocytes	↑	↓	↓	↓	Unilateral or bilateral

↑, Increased; ↓, decreased.

delayed hypersensitivity reactions, enhanced suppression of T cells by PAMs, and impaired phagocytosis by PAMs secondary to metabolic acidosis occur, but humoral immunity is intact.[160-163] Infections caused by *M. tuberculosis, Legionella pneumophila, S. aureus, Streptococcus pneumoniae, Enterobacter species, Klebsiella* organisms, *Serratia* species, *Mycoplasma pneumoniae,* Epstein-Barr virus, influenza virus type A, echovirus type 9, varicella-zoster virus, herpes simplex virus, cytomegalovirus, human immunodeficiency virus, *P. carinii, Candida* species, *Mucor* species, *Aspergillus* species, *Coccidioides immitis,* and *Histoplasma capsulatum* are present with increased frequency and can affect both the lungs and kidneys.[144,160,161,164]

Transdiaphragmatic movement of ascitic fluid across diaphragmatic openings and pleural capillaries causes a unilateral or bilateral serous, serosanguinous, or hemorrhagic exudative pleural effusion, which has a predominance of lymphocytes, a normal glucose concentration, high protein and creatinine levels, and a ratio of pleural fluid to serum creatinine less than 1.0[95,98,144] (Table 81-7 and Box 81-7). This "uremic" pleural effusion usually occurs with long-standing renal failure (i.e., lasting at least 1 year).[95] It differs from the transudative pleural fluid of nephrotic syndrome and congestive heart failure, which can also occur in uremia; is bilateral and serous; and has predominantly monocytes or lymphocytes with minimal protein and no creatinine.[95,98] Complications of a uremic pleural effusion include a fibrothorax and rounded atelectasis, which occurs when a collapsed lung adjacent to the resolving effusion develops parietal pleural adhesions and tries to expand.[95,98,165] In addition, a chylothorax can occur with the nephrotic syndrome when chylous ascitic fluid passes through diaphragmatic openings or across diaphragmatic lymphatic vessels.[166] This transudative fluid has elevated pleural and ascitic fluid levels of protein, cholesterol, triglyceride, and LDH, most likely resulting from selective absorption of water from the pleural space.[166] Approximately 3% of patients with uremia develop a pleural effusion, although half of these individuals are asymptomatic.[98]

Respiratory muscle weakness occurs in uremia (see Box 81-7), is part of a more generalized myopathy, and is attributed to the presence of large quantities of ascitic fluid, malnutrition, anemia, uremic toxins, elevated parathyroid hormone levels, vitamin D and carnitine deficiencies, aluminum toxicity, and alterations in cellular metabolism affecting protein, fatty acids, and cations.[167,168] Although most studies of respiratory muscle strength in uremia have been performed in individuals receiving dialysis, which contributes to altered muscle function, rats with renal failure as a result of surgical removal of 83% of their kidneys have diaphragmatic dysfunction.[168] In addition, chest wall mechanics are altered by rib and vertebral fractures caused by destructive bone lesions occurring in uremia.

Both central and obstructive sleep apnea can be present in renal failure[21,169] (see Box 81-7). Metabolic acidosis with secondary hyperventilation and hypocapnia, uremic toxins acting on the central nervous system, chemical mediators, diminished airway muscle tone resulting from uremic myopathy, and metabolic cellular alterations may be the etiologies.[21,169]

Dialysis

Complications of peritoneal dialysis include left lower lobe atelectasis and hypoventilation secondary to diaphragmatic immobility and eventration resulting from the large quantities of dialyzing fluid[142] (Box 81-8). A weakened cough with sputum retention can also occur from diaphragmatic immobilization.[142] Other complications include pneumonia and pleural effusion caused by peritonitis and bacteremia; massive hydrothorax resulting from the leakage of dialysate through di-

BOX 81-8
Respiratory Manifestations Associated with Renal Dialysis

Peritoneal dialysis

Atelectasis: left lower lobe
Hypoventilation
Diaphragmatic immobility
Diaphragmatic eventration
Sputum retention
Pneumonia
Pleural effusion
Hydrothorax
Hypoxemia
Ventilation-perfusion imbalance

Hemodialysis

Polymorphonuclear leukocyte sequestration
Complement activation
Anaphylaxis: wheezing
Emboli: air, blood, silicone
Hypoxemia
Ventilation-perfusion imbalance
Hemorrhage: pleural
Pulmonary hypertension
"First-use syndrome"
Abdominal muscle weakness
Metastatic pulmonary calcification

aphragmatic openings, which may occur normally or as defects resulting from the pressure of the repeated instillation of large amounts of fluid into the abdomen; and hypoxemia secondary to ventilation-perfusion imbalance.[142,170,171]

Hemodialysis is associated with intrapulmonary sequestration of polymorphonuclear leukocytes with concomitant peripheral leukopenia; complement activation, particularly of C_3 and the fifth component of complement (C_5); anaphylaxis with wheezing secondary to chemical mediator release; silicone emboli in pulmonary capillaries and PAMs originating from blood pump tubing; hypoxemia resulting from ventilation-perfusion mismatch caused by blood microemboli; air embolism; pleural hemorrhage induced by anticoagulation; pulmonary hypertension secondary to acidosis and chemical mediator release; and metastatic pulmonary calcification[142,144] (see Box 81-8). Hypotension, dyspnea, and chest pain compose the "first-use syndrome" and result from complement activation during an initial hemodialysis with a cuprophane membrane.[142] In addition, abdominal muscle strength, which is important during expiration, can be reduced after hemodialysis because of diminutions in serum levels of potassium and phosphorus.[172]

• • •

As with disorders of other organ systems, the diagnosis of pulmonary diseases associated with renal failure and dialysis is aided by the history, physical examination, and laboratory and radiographic studies. The presence of pulmonary hemorrhage (particularly bilateral alveolar infiltrates) with renal disease, hematuria, RBC casts, an increased serum creatinine level, anemia, hypocomplementemia, elevated antinuclear and anti-DNA antibody titers, arthritis, and purpura should suggest the parenchymal diseases composing the pulmonary-renal syndrome (see Box 81-7 and Table 81-5). Although most of these diseases have been diagnosed in adults, children with some of these disorders have also been identified.[148,149,173,174] Except for Goodpasture's syndrome, the other disorders in this category are accompanied by systemic manifestations.[144,145] The identification of hemosiderin-laden PAMs in bronchoalveolar lavage fluid may aid in the diagnosis of pulmonary hemorrhage, although these cells are also present in other disorders, including congestive heart failure.[145,173] Serial measurements of serum antiglomerular basement membrane antibodies in Goodpasture's syndrome are useful in evaluating the therapeutic response,[144] but the titers do not correlate with the severity or recurrence of pulmonary hemorrhage.[145] In addition, the extent of alveolar hemorrhage does not correlate with the quantity of expectorated blood because alveolar hemorrhage is bleeding within the acinus but can be evaluated by chest radiography, oxyhemoglobin saturation, and hemoglobin levels.[145] If serum antiglomerular basement membrane antibody titers are negative in Goodpasture's syndrome, renal and lung biopsy should be considered to identify IgG antibodies on the basement membranes.[143] In addition, open lung biopsy helps in the diagnosis of these pulmonary diseases.[144,145]

Appropriate stains and cultures of respiratory secretions, pleural fluid, and bronchoalveolar lavage fluid as well as serum titers and rapid antibody and antigen studies for viral infections are important in the diagnosis of the etiology of infectious pneumonias. The uremic pleural effusion is frequently associated with cough, chest pain, dyspnea, fever, and a pleural friction rub.[95,98] Evaluation of a pleural effusion by thoracentesis helps determine whether the fluid is a uremic exudate, chylous, or a transudate. A chylothorax occurring in the nephrotic syndrome suggests a peritoneal etiology of the fluid.[166] An effusion with an elevated glucose level and reduced protein and LDH concentrations reflects the presence of dialysate in the pleural space[170,171] (see Table 81-7). Pleuroperitoneal communications associated with this may be identified by the detection of dialysate stained with methylene blue or by radionuclide scanning of macroaggregated albumin labeled with technetium-99 that passes from the peritoneal to the pleural spaces.[170,171]

Metastatic pulmonary calcification may not be accompanied by symptoms or visualization on anteroposterior and lateral chest radiographs and may require a computed tomographic scan of the chest or open lung biopsy for detection.[155,156] This diagnosis should be considered in an individual with chronic renal failure; persistent pulmonary infiltrates, which may be diffuse, interstitial, fine, or nodular lesions or appear as pneumonia or edema; hypoxemia; and reduced DLCO measurements.[153,154] Fibrosing alveolitis is associated with a reticulonodular pattern on chest radiographs and decreased DLCO measurements and is more definitively diagnosed by open lung biopsy.[150] Alveolar hemorrhage is depicted radiographically as diffuse alveolar and interstitial densities and if chronic, a reticulonodular pattern.[144]

Pulmonary function testing in both acute and chronic uremia reveals reductions in slow vital capacity (SVC), FVC, FEV_1, ERV, TLC, peak expiratory flow rate, DLCO even when corrected for anemia, specific airway conductance, inspiratory and expiratory muscle strength, and PaO_2; elevations in RV; and a normal FRC and FEV_1/FVC ratio.[142,158,167,172] The restrictive ventilatory and gas transfer abnormalities most likely result from interstitial and alveolar edema and fibrin deposits.[175] Metastatic pulmonary calcification causes reductions in VC, DLCO, and PaO_2, which are directly related to the magnitude and extent of the calcium deposits.[156] Wegener's granulomatosis is associated with airflow obstruction and reduced lung volumes and DLCO measurements.[144,146] Decreases in DLCO with normal lung volumes occur in scleroderma and Henoch-Schönlein purpura.[147,148] An elevated DLCO occurs in pulmonary hemorrhage as a result of carbon monoxide binding to the intraalveolar blood, and this finding may help differentiate hemorrhage from pneumonia and pulmonary edema.[144,145] The DLCO may be as high as 30% above base-

Table 81-8 Characteristics of the Sickle Cell Hemoglobulinopathies

DISEASE	HEMOGLOBIN COMPOSITION	GENOTYPE	AMINO ACID CHANGE	HEMOGLOBIN LEVEL (g/dl)	OXYHB CURVE SHIFT
Sickle cell anemia	SS	$\alpha^A\alpha^A\beta^S\beta^S/\alpha^A\alpha^A\beta^S\beta^S$	S: glu → val	6-9 (75%-94% S, 2% A_2, 2%-23% F)	Yes
Sickle cell β-thalassemia	S-thal	$\alpha^A\alpha^A\beta^S\beta^S/\alpha^A\alpha^A\beta^{thal}\beta^{thal}$	S: glu → val	9-11 (75%-90% S, <18% A, 5% A_2, 3%-7% F)	Yes
Sickle cell hemoglobin C disease	SC	$\alpha^A\alpha^A\beta^S\beta^S/\alpha^A\alpha^A\beta^C\beta^C$	S: glu → val C: glu → lys	8-10 (49% S, 49% C, 2% F)	Yes
Sickle cell trait	SA	$\alpha^A\alpha^A\beta^S\beta^S/\alpha^A\alpha^A\beta^A\beta^A$	S: glu → val	14 (36% S, 60% A, 3% A_2, 1% F)	No
Normal	AA	$\alpha^A\alpha^A\beta^A\beta^A/\alpha^A\alpha^A\beta^A\beta^A$	—	>12 (97% A, 2% A_2, 1% F)	No

OxyHb, Oxyhemoglobin; *S,* hemoglobin S; *α,* α chain; *A,* hemoglobin A; *β,* β chain; *glu,* glutamic acid; *val,* valine; *A_2,* hemoglobin A_2; *F,* hemoglobin F; *thal,* thalassemia; *C,* hemoglobin C; *lys,* lysine.

line measurements and return to normal within 48 hours of the acute hemorrhage.[144,145]

Although exercise testing in children with renal failure indicates reductions in work capacity, anerobic threshold, $\dot{V}O_2$, and oxygen pulse, these measurements improve after treatment with recombinant human erythropoietin, suggesting that anemia may contribute to the exercise intolerance.[176] In addition, parathyroidectomy improves inspiratory muscle strength, FVC, and FEV_1, whereas renal transplantation does not reverse diminished DLCO measurements.[142,167]

Peritoneal dialysis results in transient reductions in SVC, FVC, FRC, RV, TLC, and lung compliance, most likely caused by filling the peritoneal cavity with the dialysate and concomitant diaphragmatic elevation.[142,144,175] These measurements return to baseline values with completion of the dialysis. Ventilation and perfusion at the lung bases improve after hemodialysis, but elevations in RV, a diminution in the peak expiratory flow rate, respiratory muscle weakness, and hypoxemia become more pronounced, and ERV, $\dot{V}E$, and the respiratory quotient decrease with this procedure.[142,158,172,177]

Therapy is directed at the underlying renal disease and the associated pulmonary disorders. Corticosteroids, immunosuppressive agents, plasmapheresis to remove antibodies, and renal transplantation are used in the treatment of pulmonary-renal disorders.[143,144,146,147] Supplemental oxygen, assisted ventilation with positive end-expiratory pressure, and corticosteroids are used in the therapy of pulmonary hemorrhage and concomitant hypoxemia, and factors precipitating the hemorrhage (i.e., bleeding disorders, volume overload, bacterial infection) should be diagnosed and treated.[143-146] Metastatic pulmonary calcification can be reduced by dialysis to control serum phosphorus levels, parathyroidectomy to reverse hyperparathyroidism, and renal transplantation.[154] Although central and obstructive sleep apneas are usually addressed with more conventional modalities of therapy,[21] they have resolved in selected individuals who had kidney transplants for treatment of renal failure.[169]

HEMOGLOBINOPATHIES

Sickle Cell Disease

Sickle cell disease comprises three types of anemia—sickle cell anemia (hemoglobin composition, SS), sickle cell β-thalassemia (hemoglobin composition, S-thal), and sickle cell hemoglobin C disease (hemoglobin composition, SC)—that cause varying degrees of pulmonary illness in individuals with these autosomal recessively inherited disorders.[178,178a] Both genes for hemoglobin are altered in these diseases, whereas in sickle cell trait (hemoglobin composition, SA), one gene is abnormal and the other gene has the normal hemoglobin A. Homozygosity for hemoglobin S (SS) causes polymerization and sickling of RBCs at a PaO_2 of 50 mm Hg, whereas heterozygosity (S-thal, SC, SA) causes variable degrees of sickling at lower reductions in PaO_2 levels.[178,179]

Human hemoglobin A is composed of two α chains and two β chains, $\alpha_2\beta_2$ or $\alpha^A\alpha^A\beta^A\beta^A$, each of which has amino acids and a heme group that binds with oxygen[178] (Table 81-8). The α_2 genes are located on chromosome 16, whereas the β_2 genes are on chromosome 11.[178,180] The genetic mutation causing the synthesis of hemoglobin S occurs at the sixth amino acid position in the β chain, where valine is substituted for glutamic acid.[178] Replacement of glutamic acid by lysine at the same position produces hemoglobin C.[178] β-Thalassemia hemoglobin results from decreases (β^+-thalassemia) in or absence (β°-thalassemia) of β chain synthesis caused by impaired messenger ribonucleic acid function or gene transcription or the production of unstable β chains.[178,180] β^+- and β°-thalassemia hemoglobins can combine with hemoglobin S to form S-thal.[178]

RBC sickling, hemolysis, and anemia occur when hemoglobin S is deoxygenated and its molecules are packed closely together.[178] Hemoglobin S has diminished oxygen affinity, and RBCs with hemoglobin S have increased levels of 2,3-diphosphoglycerate.[181-183] As a result, the oxygen-hemoglobin dissociation curve is shifted to the right, causing arterial oxygen desaturation, promoting RBC sickling, and generating the clinical and radiographic manifestations of sickle cell disease[178,182,183] (Boxes 81-9 and 81-10). These occur, in decreasing order of severity, in sickle cell anemia, sickle cell β-thalassemia, sickle cell hemoglobin C disease, and sickle cell trait.[178] Individuals with sickle cell trait do not have alterations in the oxygen-hemoglobin dissociation curve[184] (see Table 81-8).

Hypercoagulability, as evidenced by increased production of thrombin and fibrin and increased activation and use of platelets, also occurs in sickle cell anemia and contributes to the pathophysiology of events that occur during sickling[185] (see Box 81-9). In addition, RBCs with hemoglobin S, as well as with hemoglobin C, are more rigid and less deformable than those with hemoglobin A, even when they have a normal shape and oxygenation.[178] This results in increased viscosity of blood, which contributes to plugging of blood vessels.[178] RBCs

BOX 81-9
Characteristics of Sickle Cell Disease that Predispose to Pulmonary Disorders

- Abnormal hemoglobin levels: right shift of the oxygen-hemoglobin dissociation curve
- Hypoxemia
- Sickling crises: sequestration, vasoocclusive, aplastic, hyperhemolytic
- Hypercoagulability of blood
- Hyperviscosity of blood
- Arteriolar vasculopathy: adherence of RBCs to endothelium, production of vasoactive mediators
- Lung parenchymal injury: synthesis of free oxygen radicals
- Chest wall: small and narrow thorax
- Immune dysfunction: phagocytosis, chemotaxis, opsonin, alternative complement pathway

BOX 81-10
Pulmonary Disorders Occurring in Sickle Cell Anemia

Acute disorders	Chronic disorders
Pneumonia	Chronic lung disease
Pulmonary thromboembolism	Pulmonary arterial hypertension
Pulmonary infarction	Recurrent acute chest syndrome
Bone marrow and fat embolism	Restrictive lung disease
Acute chest syndrome	Cardiac: cardiomegaly, right ventricular strain, cor pulmonale
ARDS	
Pulmonary edema	

Table 81-9 Characteristics of Pneumonia, Pulmonary Vascular Injury, Pulmonary Infarction, Acute Chest Syndrome, and Sickle Cell Chronic Lung Disease (SCLD) in Sickle Cell Disease

PNEUMONIA	PULMONARY VASCULAR INJURY	PULMONARY INFARCTION	ACUTE CHEST SYNDROME	SCLD
Age				
<4 years	All ages	>12 years	All ages	Teenage years, adults
Predisposing factors				
Defective phagocytic, complement, opsonin, polymorphonuclear leukocytic, and chemotactic function; preceding upper respiratory tract infection	Bone marrow necrosis with bone marrow and fat embolism, RBC sickling, increased blood viscosity, hypoxemia, ? pregnancy	Bone marrow necrosis with bone marrow and fat embolism, RBC sickling, pulmonary thrombosis, hypoxemia, pregnancy, preceding upper respiratory tract infection	Presence of hemoglobin S levels >20%,? pulmonary infection with *Chlamydia pneumoniae* and human parvovirus B19, bone marrow necrosis with bone marrow and fat embolism, pulmonary vascular injury, infarction of ribs and sternum	Recurrent episodes of acute chest syndrome
Signs and symptoms				
Fever, chills, cough, malaise, tachypnea, chest wall retractions, flaring of nasal alae, crackles, purulent sputum, pleuritic chest pain, dyspnea	Fever, dyspnea, tachypnea, chest pain, bone pain, fundoscopic changes (including refractile bodies), petechiae, mental depression	Fever, tachypnea, crackles, jaundice, pleuritic chest pain, dyspnea	Fever; cough; tachypnea; dyspnea; rib and sternal tenderness; local soft tissue swelling; pleuritic or chest wall pain; chest wall retractions; flaring of nasal alae; decreased breath sounds; crackles; pain in abdomen, back, and extremities	Progressive dyspnea, exercise intolerance, pleuritic chest pain, hypoxemia, proliferative retinopathy, syncope, fatigue
Laboratory findings				
↑ WBC count, pathogens in cultures of blood and respiratory secretions	Fat globules in sputum, urine, and blood; ↑ fibrin-degradation products	↑ WBC count; fat globules in sputum, urine, and blood; bilirubin level >5 mg/dl; negative cultures; atypical RBCs ("blister" cells) peripherally	↑ WBC count; fat globules in sputum, urine, and blood; positive bone scan; negative cultures; ↑ fibrin-degradation products; thrombocytopenia; serosanguinous pleural fluid	ECG abnormalities
Chest radiographs				
Multilobar, frequently in upper or middle lobes, pleural effusion	Infiltrate, edema, ARDS	May be normal initially, unilateral density, may be wedge-shaped, frequently in lower lobes, pleural effusion, filling defect in lung perfusion scan	May be normal initially, unilateral or multilobar infiltrates, frequently in lower lobes, atelectasis, pleural effusion, edema, ARDS	Diffuse interstitial markings, interstitial edema, prominent pulmonary arteries, filling defects in lung perfusion scan, cardiomegaly
Pulmonary function testing				
↓ lung volumes, hypoxemia	Hypoxemia	↓ lung volumes, hypoxemia	↓ lung volumes, ↓ DLCO, hypoxemia	↓ lung volumes, ↓ DLCO, hypoxemia

↑, Increased; *WBC,* white blood cell; *ECG,* electrocardiogram; *ARDS,* adult respiratory distress syndrome; ↓, decreased; *DLCO,* diffusing capacity.

Table 81-10 Pulmonary Disorders with Hemoglobin S

	S-THAL	SC	SA
Acute disorders			
Acute chest syndrome	X	X	X
ARDS	X	X	X
Bone marrow and fat embolism	—	X	—
Pneumonia	X	X	X
Pulmonary infarction	X	X	X
Chronic disorders			
Chronic lung disease	X	X	—
Pulmonary arterial hypertension	X	X	—
Cardiac: cardiomegaly, right ventricular strain, cor pulmonale	—	X	—

S-thal, Sickle cell β-thalassemia; *SC,* sickle cell hemoglobin C disease; *SA,* sickle cell trait; *ARDS,* adult respiratory distress syndrome.

with hemoglobin S also interact with and adhere to the capillary endothelium, causing the release of vasoactive mediators, which promote the sequence of events leading to vasoocclusive crises.[178,185]

The pulmonary disorders occurring most frequently in sickle cell disease are pneumonia, pulmonary vascular injury, pulmonary infarction, acute chest syndrome, and sickle cell chronic lung disease (SCLD) (Table 81-9 and Box 81-10). Most hospitalizations of individuals with sickle cell anemia result from bacterial pneumonia.[182,186] Functional and anatomic asplenia causes deficient phagocytosis associated with opsonin, polymorphonuclear leukocytes, and PAMs; altered chemotaxis; and an impaired alternative pathway of complement. Because of this, individuals with sickle cell anemia are predisposed to lung infections with encapsulated bacteria *(Haemophilus influenzae, S. pneumoniae), Salmonella typhimurium, S. aureus, Klebsiella* species, *E. coli, Acinetobacter* organisms, *M. pneumoniae,* and *Plasmodium* species.[182,186-191] Pneumonia caused by *L. pneumophila, Cryptococcus neoformans,* and cytomegalovirus has also been identified.[192-194]

Pulmonary vascular injury results from RBC sickling, pulmonary thrombosis, and pulmonary embolism and can cause sudden death if a large vessel is occluded[182] (see Table 81-9). RBC sickling and increased blood viscosity, with subsequent vascular stasis and thrombus formation, predispose to pulmonary thromboembolism and infarction.[182,186,188,195] In addition, during an aplastic crisis, fat from necrotic bone marrow can enter the pulmonary circulation, occlude the pulmonary vasculature, and cause pulmonary infarction.[182,186,188]

The acute chest syndrome causes 25% of deaths in individuals with sickle cell anemia, results from infarction of the ribs and sternum during a vasoocclusive crisis, and may be associated with pulmonary infection with *Chlamydia pneumoniae, M. pneumoniae,* and human parvovirus B19[185,196-199] (see Box 81-10 and Table 81-9). In addition, the acute chest syndrome and ARDS can result from bone marrow and fat embolism to the lungs, which is associated with increased morbidity and mortality in the presence of hypoxemia and intravascular coagulation, both of which readily occur in sickle cell anemia.[179,185,200]

SCLD is accompanied by pulmonary arterial hypertension, cardiomegaly, cor pulmonale, and death[188,201,202] (see Box 81-10 and Table 81-9). Multiple episodes of acute chest syndrome may promote the development of SCLD.[196,202] Hypoxemia in SCLD results from defects in pulmonary perfusion, reductions in diffusion, pulmonary fibrosis, and restrictive lung disease.[185,202] Because the resting PaO_2 and oxyhemoglobin saturation are frequently 70 to 90 mm Hg and 80% to 90%, respectively, ventilation-perfusion imbalance and intrapulmonary shunts may be present.[182,189] Ventilation-perfusion imbalance results from sickling, potentiates hypoxemia, and promotes further sickling.[188] Chronic lung parenchymal injury occurs with the production of free oxygen radicals, and elevated pulmonary vascular resistance results from endothelial hyperplasia of small arterioles caused by sickled RBCs.[202] In addition, the increase in blood flow associated with chronic anemia and myocardial microinfarcts and anoxia occurring with sickling in myocardial blood vessels cause cardiomegaly.[188] Progressive dyspnea, cor pulmonale, and myocardial ischemia ensue.[202]

Sickle cell β-thalassemia, sickle cell hemoglobin C disease, and sickle cell trait are also associated with these pulmonary disorders but to different degrees depending on the amount of hemoglobin S present and the magnitude of increased blood viscosity[195] (Tables 81-8 and 81-10). The likelihood of RBC sickling rises as the level of hemoglobin S increases.[178] The course of the anemia and splenic dysfunction in sickle cell β-thalassemia, sickle cell hemoglobin C disease, and sickle cell trait is milder and has a later onset than in sickle cell anemia, and the risk of pulmonary disorders and their severity are in general less than in sickle cell anemia.[190] Pneumonia occurs in sickle cell β-thalassemia, sickle cell hemoglobin C disease, and sickle cell trait with similar organisms as in sickle cell anemia and may be unusually severe.[190-194,199,203-205] The early onset of splenomegaly in sickle cell hemoglobin C disease appears associated with an increased incidence of infection.[204] Sickle cell hemoglobin C disease is frequently associated with bone marrow and fat embolism, pulmonary vascular injury, pulmonary arterial hypertension, and cor pulmonale, particularly during the third trimester of pregnancy.[182,200,201] This may be a result of a relatively increased hematocrit level in sickle cell hemoglobin C disease compared with sickle cell anemia, with reduced circulatory transit time and elevated blood viscosity.[182] Sickle cell trait has been identified with pulmonary infarction, acute chest syndrome, and ARDS caused by hypoxic-induced sickling.[195,206] Unlike sickle cell β-thalassemia and sickle cell hemoglobin C disease, sickle cell trait is not associated with immune dysfunction.[180,190]

These pulmonary disorders are diagnosed by a history, physical examination, and laboratory and radiographic studies. Pneumonia and pulmonary infarction are often difficult to differentiate, but age, the presence of pathogens in cultures of respiratory secretions and blood, and chest radiographic findings may help[182,186,188] (see Table 81-9). Although a preceding upper respiratory tract infection suggests the occurrence of pneumonia, it can also precipitate sickle cell crisis with a nonpneumonic pulmonary process.[186] Fever and chills suggest pneumonia rather than pulmonary infarction, although children with sickle cell anemia can have high fever and appear quite ill despite lack of objective or laboratory findings of pneumonia.[186] Pneumonia in sickle cell anemia is usually severe, is associated with fever lasting up to 12 days, and tends to resolve slowly despite appropriate antibiotic therapy.[182,186,195]

Pulmonary infarction in sickle cell disease is typically not accompanied by hemoptysis, may have a prolonged course, and is suggested by the presence of acute pulmonary symptoms and an initially normal chest radiograph followed by a radiographic density[182,186,188] (see Table 81-9). The occurrence of extensive jaundice and atypical "blister" RBCs in the peripheral blood also suggests infarction, whereas the white blood cell count is of little diagnostic value because it is elevated in pneumonia and pulmonary infarction and during crises.[182,186] Pneumonia and pulmonary infarction can occur simultaneously because local tissue necrosis secondary to infarction can promote a milieu for bacterial growth.[188] Conversely, hypoxemia resulting from a slow-resolving pneumonia can promote RBC sickling, vascular occlusion, and pulmonary infarction.[195] In addition, pulmonary arterial hypertension may be present if unexplained syncope or dyspnea occurs.[201]

The distinguishing extrapulmonary features of acute chest syndrome include tenderness along the ribs and sternum with localized soft tissue swelling and pain in the abdomen, extremities, and back[196-198] (see Table 81-9). The presence of fat globules in the sputum, urine, and blood during a sickle cell crisis is diagnostic of fat embolism. It occurs in acute chest syndrome, pulmonary vascular injury, and pulmonary infarction, and it is associated with hypoxemia and disseminated intravascular coagulation.[179] Bone marrow infarction can be detected by technetium-99m bone scanning, which initially shows diminished radioactivity in areas of infarction associated with reduced vascularity and later shows increased tracer uptake secondary to augmented bone activity.[179,196,197]

Pulmonary function testing in asymptomatic individuals with sickle cell anemia reveals reductions in SVC, FVC, FEV_1, FRC, ERV, TLC, forced expiratory flow along 25% to 75% of the VC, peak expiratory flow rate, dynamic and specific lung compliance, work capacity, and anerobic threshold; elevations in $\dot{V}E$ and respiratory quotient; and a normal FEV_1/FVC ratio.[182,202,207-211] As SCLD develops, decreases in the FEV_1/FVC ratio also occur.[202] The DLCO is normal before the teenage years and subsequently increases when corrected for anemia and alveolar volume (DLCO/VA), perhaps secondary to an expanded pulmonary capillary blood volume.[202,208,212] However, the DLCO/VA ratio is diminished when compared with control values as a result of a low membrane diffusing capacity.[182,207,208,212]

The reductions in lung volumes, which are unlikely to occur during the first decade of life, reflect the presence of a short and narrow chest wall in relation to standing height and recurrent episodes of pulmonary disease with subsequent pulmonary fibrosis[207,208,213] (see Box 81-9). When these changes occur during the teenage years before the symptoms of SCLD, they can predict later development of SCLD.[202] Sickle cell β-thalassemia and sickle cell hemoglobin C disease are also associated with decreased lung volumes, whereas lung volumes, DLCO, and exercise tolerance in settings of ambient oxygen as low as 18% are normal in sickle cell trait.[208,209,213,214]

Arterial oxygen desaturation during sleep without evidence of central or obstructive apnea can occur in sickle cell anemia and sickle cell trait and may precipitate RBC sickling and crises.[183] In addition, obstructive sleep apnea secondary to enlarged tonsils can contribute to nocturnal arterial oxygen desaturation and complications of these diseases.[215]

Therapy includes appropriate antimicrobial agents for pulmonary infections and should provide coverage for penicillin-resistant *S. pneumoniae, S. aureus,* ampicillin-resistant *H. influenzae, Chlamydia pneumoniae, M. pneumoniae,* and *L. pneumophila.* Antibiotics should be instituted quickly before the clinician knows the specific etiologic diagnosis because infections, particularly pneumococcal pneumonia, can be fulminant and life-threatening in sickle cell anemia.[186,199] Adequate hydration, analgesics, supplemental oxygen administration, correction of acidosis, and folic acid supplementation are important therapeutic adjuncts.[178,186,201] However, supplemental oxygen should be used cautiously because its overuse may reduce erythropoietin synthesis and hemoglobin levels.[178] In addition, vigorous administration of hypotonic saline for hydration, which may alter hydrostatic and oncotic pressures, and narcotics, which may augment vascular permeability, can precipitate pulmonary edema.[189,216] RBC transfusions to maintain a hemoglobin level of 12 g/dl, a hemoglobin A level of at least 30%, a hemoglobin S level of less than 20%, or a combination thereof prevent RBC sickling, improve the oxygen-carrying capacity of hemoglobin, and reduce the incidence of acute chest syndrome, myocardial ischemia, and endothelial hyperplasia leading to SCLD.[185,201,202] In addition, exchange transfusion with hemoglobin A improves the oxygen-carrying capacity of hemoglobin and thus exercise performance.[209]

Additional therapeutic modalities for sickle cell anemia include splenectomy after 2 years of age to prevent sequestration crises; oral penicillin administered prophylactically starting in infancy to reduce the morbidity and mortality of pneumococcal infections; the administration of pneumococcal, influenza, and *H. influenzae* type b vaccines with subsequent boosters of the pneumococcal vaccine to confer immunologic protection against *S. pneumoniae,* influenza virus, and *H. influenzae* type b; and the administration of hepatitis B vaccine because of the necessity for multiple blood transfusions.[178,189,191,217] Pneumococcal infections may occur despite the use of penicillin prophylaxis and pneumococcal vaccine if penicillinase-producing organisms are present or if antibody production is insufficient.[189,191,198,217a] Experimental therapy includes the use of chemotherapeutic agents such as hydroxyurea and 5-azacytidine, which elevate hemoglobin F levels and reduce the incidence and severity of vasoocclusive crises and RBC sickling; bone marrow transplantation; and gene replacement therapy.[178,178a,189,217b] (In early 1998, hydroxyurea became available for routine use in selected individuals with sickle cell disease. It is no longer experimental therapy.)

Thalassemia

The more frequently occurring types of thalassemia are caused by an absence of or reduction in the synthesis of α or β chains.[180] The resultant RBCs have clumps of the unaffected, normally produced chains, which occur in excess, form inclusions, and injure cell membrane integrity.[218] Reduced RBC survival time and intramedullary RBC destruction contribute to the resulting hemolytic anemia, and ineffective erythropoiesis is present.[180,218] Tissue anoxia, increased blood volume, high-output cardiac failure, and infections are characteristic.[180] In addition, excessive iron deposits from chronic hemolysis and repeated blood transfusions cause cardiac and liver failure and pancreatic dysfunction with insulin-dependent diabetes mellitus, which can also contribute to pulmonary disease.[180] The homozygous β-thalassemias (thalassemia major, thalassemia intermedia) are associated with severe microcytic, hypochromic anemia; extramedullary hematopoiesis; hypersplenism; hepatosplenomegaly; lymphadenopathy; growth retardation; bony changes, including frontal and parietal bossing and mandibular and malar prominence; and shortened survival span.[180] The heterozygous β-thalassemias (thalassemia minor, thalassemia minima) produce mild, if any, anemia and clinical manifestations.[180]

Like β-thalassemia, the α-thalassemias are composed of α° (α-thalassemia type 1), in which all four α chains are absent, and α^+ (α-thalassemia type 2), in which at least one α chain is present.[219] Homozygous and heterozygous forms of α-thalassemia occur. The homozygous type has severe anemia and clinical manifestations and a reduced life span, whereas the heterozygous form has milder anemia and clinical features and a normal life span.[219]

Pulmonary disorders occurring in thalassemia are primarily described in β-thalassemia (Box 81-11). Severe pulmonary infections occur in β-thalassemia, particularly because the presence of excess iron impairs cytotoxicity, cellular immunity, and activity of PAMs.[180,220-222] Hemolytic, sequestration, and aplastic crises often secondary to parvovirus B19 infection also occur.[180,223] Recurrent chest pains and pulmonary thromboembolism may be present and appear to be associated with thrombocytosis postsplenectomy.[220] In addition, pulmonary arterial hypertension, cor pulmonale, cardiomyopathy, and dysrhythmias secondary to iron deposits occur and are the usual cause of death.[180,224]

Other pulmonary disorders relate to therapy for β-thalassemia, with serial blood transfusions to maintain a hemoglobin level of at least 10.5 g/dl and use of the iron-chelating agent, deferoxamine.[224-231] Although children with thalassemia intermedia who never receive blood transfusions have elevations in FRC, RV, and the RV/TLC ratio, which indicate the presence of abnormal lung function secondary to the disease,[225] multiple blood transfusions in thalassemia major are associated with restrictive lung disease, small airway obstruction, alterations in DLCO, and hypoxemia. These are observed as reductions in FVC, FEV_1, FRC, ERV, TLC, midmaximal expiratory flow rates, maximal expiratory flow rates at 60% TLC, forced expiratory flow along 25% to 75% of the VC, DLCO corrected for anemia, static and dynamic lung compliance, and PaO_2 and elevations in RV, the RV/TLC ratio, lung elastic recoil pressure, airway resistance, and $\dot{V}E$[224-230] (Table 81-11). These findings are unchanged with diuresis; improve somewhat after splenectomy (i.e., VC and ERV increase and RV decreases); and when measured before and after a blood transfusion, reveal further reductions in FVC and PaO_2 after the transfusion.[229,230] Histologic observations of the lungs in individuals with thalassemia major reveal interstitial fibrosis; subpleural emphysema; vascular congestion and fibrosis; pulmonary angiodysplasia and hemosiderin; iron and lipofuscin deposits in PAMs, epithelial cells, smooth muscle, blood vessels, and interstitial connective tissue; and help explain the restrictive lung disease, reduced DLCO, and hypoxemia.[226,232] In addition, the presence of massive hepatosplenomegaly can impair chest wall mobility and contribute to these reductions in lung volumes.

Exercise testing of individuals with thalassemia major reveals reduced exercise tolerance and hypoventilation, with reductions in anerobic threshold, $\dot{V}E$, $\dot{V}O_2$, oxygen pulse, and ventilatory equivalents for oxygen and carbon dioxide and elevations in end-tidal carbon dioxide, cardiac output, and heart rate.[233,234] Only the anerobic threshold and oxygen pulse increase somewhat after a blood transfusion, most likely resulting from improved arterial oxygenation and enhanced availability of oxygen to exercising muscles.[233,234]

Intravenous infusions of deferoxamine to prevent iron accumulation and hemosiderosis are associated with an acute pulmonary disorder characterized by fever, tachypnea, a dry cough, hypoxemia, bilateral interstitial pneumonitis radiographically and histologic evidence of diffuse alveolar damage, interstitial inflammation and fibrosis, and mast cell proliferation with fixation of IgE antibody observed with immunofluorescence.[231] Pulmonary function testing reveals the presence of restrictive lung disease with reductions in FVC, FEV_1, and TLC as well as air-trapping with elevations in the

BOX 81-11
Pulmonary Disorders Associated with Thalassemia Major

Pneumonia
Chronic pneumonitis
Pulmonary edema
Pulmonary thromboembolism
Pulmonary arterial hypertension
Cardiac: cor pulmonale, right and left ventricular hypertrophy, dysrhythmias, cardiomyopathy

Table 81-11 Correlation of Histologic Features and Functional Abnormalities of the Lung in Thalassemia Major

HISTOLOGIC FEATURES	PULMONARY FUNCTION TESTING
Parenchymal features	
Interstitial fibrosis	↓ lung volumes, ↓ DLCO, ↓ lung compliance, hypoxemia, ↑ $\dot{V}E$
Subpleural emphysema	Air-trapping (↑ RV, ↑ RV/TLC), ↑ elastic recoil, hypoxemia, ventilation-perfusion imbalance
Hemosiderin, iron, and lipofuscin deposits	↓ DLCO, ↓ lung compliance
Ferrugination of interstitial and airway connective tissue	↓ DLCO, ↓ lung compliance, ↓ airflow rates in small airways, ↑ airway resistance
Chronic interstitial pneumonitis	↓ lung volumes, ↓ DLCO, hypoxemia, ventilation-perfusion imbalance
Pulmonary edema	↓ lung volumes, ↓ DLCO, ↓ lung compliance, ↓ airflow rates in small airways, ↑ airway resistance, hypoxemia, ventilation-perfusion imbalance
Vascular features	
Pulmonary angiodysplasia	Hypoxemia, ventilation-perfusion imbalance
Vascular fibrosis	↓ DLCO, hypoxemia, ventilation-perfusion imbalance
Ferrugination of vascular connective tissue	↓ DLCO, ↓ lung compliance
Thromboemboli	Hypoxemia, ventilation-perfusion imbalance
Bone marrow emboli	Hypoxemia, ventilation-perfusion imbalance

↓, Decreased; ↑, increased; *$\dot{V}E$,* minute ventilation; *RV,* residual volume; *TLC,* total lung capacity; *DLCO,* diffusing capacity.

$\dot{V}E$,

RV/TLC ratio.[231] Resolution of these clinical and functional alterations may take as long as 6 months and may be helped with the use of corticosteroids.[231]

In addition to serial blood transfusions and deferoxamine administration, therapy of thalassemia includes splenectomy to relieve symptoms of abdominal pressure resulting from massive splenic enlargement and to control hypersplenism, which is evidenced by an increasing requirement for blood transfusions; the use of oral penicillin prophylaxis in patients who have undergone splenectomy; immunizations with the pneumococcal, *H. influenzae* type b, influenza, and hepatitis B vaccines; daily folic acid supplementation; and bone marrow transplantation, which has been successful in preventing the development of complications of thalassemia major.[180,189,234a] Experimental procedures include gene therapy and the administration of agents such as 5-azacytidine and busulfan, which enhance fetal hemoglobin synthesis, decrease the percentage of abnormal hemoglobin present, and reduce the frequency and severity of the hemolytic anemia.[180,189,219]

FAMILIAL DYSAUTONOMIA

Familial dysautonomia, or Riley-Day syndrome, is an autosomal recessive disorder characterized by abnormalities of the autonomic, sensory, and central nervous systems.[235-237] It is associated with the defective synthesis, transport, and use of nerve growth factor.[235,238] In addition, reduced urinary vanillylmandelic acid levels suggest the presence of a deficient enzyme involved with dopamine catabolism.[236] Histopathologic examination reveals loss of neurons and atrophied nerve fibers in the reticular formation of the pons and medulla; cerebellum; nucleus of the vagus nerve; sympathetic, parasympathetic, and dorsal root ganglia; and along the spinal cord in the spinothalamic tract and posterior columns.[236-238] Characteristic features of familial dysautonomia include a typical facies; dysautonomic crises with episodic vomiting, diaphoresis, hypertension, tachycardia, and skin blotching; recurrent fevers; postural hypotension; swallowing difficulties with excessive salivation and drooling; feeding disturbances; esophageal dysmotility; growth retardation; an absent gag reflex; insensitivity to pain; absence of lacrimation; corneal ulcers; alterations in taste perception, particularly to bitter or sweet substances; nasal speech; ataxia; seizures; and psychomotor retardation.[235-237]

As a result of many of these features, individuals with familial dysautonomia have pulmonary disorders, including recurrent wheezing and pneumonia secondary to the aspiration of secretions from the oropharynx and from gastroesophageal reflux and bronchiectasis caused by repeated pulmonary infections[235,236,239] (Box 81-12). Insensitivity to pain and a poor cough reflex contribute to the inability of the patient to mobilize aspirated material.[235,237] Atelectasis, air-trapping, and pneumothoraces can occur.[235] In addition, kyphoscoliosis contributes to hyperreactive airway disease and alterations in pulmonary function.[235,236,240] Manifestations of respiratory difficulties can also occur in the neonate with familial dysautonomia and include delayed initiation of breathing, difficulty in coordination of sucking with swallowing resulting in aspiration of feedings, and meconium aspiration pneumonitis.[235,241]

Diminished responses to hypoxia and hypercapnia cause abnormalities in control of breathing, including breath-holding with syncope and nonresponsiveness to hypoxia while swimming underwater with subsequent drowning[235,236,240,242] (see Box 81-12). Irregular breathing patterns and apnea can occur during sleep.[235,240]

BOX 81-12
Respiratory Disorders Associated with Familial Dysautonomia

Pulmonary disorders
- Hyperreactive airway disease
- Pneumonia: infectious, aspiration
- Tracheobronchitis
- Bronchiectasis
- Atelectasis
- Pneumothorax

Chest wall disorders
- Kyphosis
- Scoliosis

Disorders of control of breathing
- Delayed initiation of breathing in neonate
- Diminished responses to hypoxia and hypercapnia
- Breath-holding with syncope
- Sleep apnea

Table 81-12 Clinical Tests Used in the Diagnosis of Familial Dysautonomia

	HISTAMINE TEST	METHACHOLINE OR PILOCARPINE TEST	OBSERVATION OF TONGUE
Procedure	Intradermal injection of 1:1000 dilution of histamine phosphate, use 1:10,000 dilution in infant	Instillation of 2.5% methacholine or 0.0625% pilocarpine into conjunctival sac of one eye, comparison of both eyes every 5 minutes for 20 minutes	Examination of tip and sides of tongue for red, vascularized papillae
Normal response	Pain and erythema, development of central wheal with surrounding axon flare of erythema measuring 1-3 cm in radius, wheal and axon flare occur within 10 minutes	No effect	Red, vascularized papillae at tip and sides of tongue
Response in familial dysautonomia	↓↓ pain, absence of axon flare	Meiosis in eye with methacholine or pilocarpine	Absent fungiform papillae with smooth and pale sides and tip of tongue, lack of vascularization
False-negative results	None	None	None
False-positive results	Congenital sensory neuropathy, atopic dermatitis	Disorders with parasympathetic denervation	Present

↓, Decreased.

The history, physical examination, and laboratory and radiographic studies help in the diagnosis of familial dysautonomia. The presence of repeated pneumonias, episodes of cyclic vomiting, temperature instability with recurrent fevers, and mottling of the skin in a child whose family is of Ashkenazi Jewish extraction from eastern Europe suggests the diagnosis.[235,236,241,243] Familial dysautonomia can be diagnosed in the neonate, who is likely to be born full-term in a breech presentation, is small for gestational age, is meconium-stained, is hypotonic, and has respiratory distress, incoordination of suck and swallow, feeding difficulties, lack of weight gain, temperature instability, and mottling of the skin.[235,241,243] Three clinical tests, which can be used as early as 3 days of life, are helpful in confirming the diagnosis[235,236] (Table 81-12). Pulmonary function testing reveals reduced lung volumes, airflow rates, and DLCO measurements and hypoxemia at rest and with exercise, which correlate with the repeated episodes of lung infections.[240] Pneumonia, atelectasis, air-trapping, and pneumothoraces occurring during acute episodes of respiratory distress are observed on chest radiographs. Residual markings from repeated episodes of pneumonia may be present radiographically between these episodes. Fluoroscopic examination of ingested barium may reveal the presence of gastroesophageal reflux and oropharyngeal aspiration of the barium. Salivogram studies with a radioactively labeled contrast material can also help diagnose the presence of aspiration of oropharyngeal secretions.

Therapy includes the use of appropriate antibiotics for lung infections, bronchodilators and antiinflammatory agents for wheezing, chest physical therapy and postural drainage for the mobilization of respiratory secretions, and supplemental oxygen for hypoxemia. Because familial dysautonomia is associated with reduced sympathetic neuronal innervation and augmented sensitivity to sympathomimetic agents,[235,244] β-adrenergic bronchodilators are used with caution. Feeding difficulties are addressed with enteral nutrition, such as a gastrostomy or jejunostomy tube, and if gastroesophageal reflux is present, a fundoplication.[239] Maintenance of a patent airway, often with a tracheostomy and tracheal diversion, is helpful for preventing the aspiration of saliva and for suctioning and clearing secretions. Adequate hydration, appropriate temperature control, and aggressive airway care (including endotracheal intubation, assisted ventilation, antibiotics, and chest physical therapy before, during, and after general anesthesia) help reduce the incidence and severity of postoperative lung infections and atelectasis.[244] An additional preoperative measure includes the use of alternatives to narcotic agents for premedication because of decreased responses to hypoxia and hypercapnia, which may be augmented with narcotics.[244] Gastric decompression and sedation help in the treatment of dysautonomic crises after surgery.[244] With aggressive management, individuals with familial dysautonomia are surviving into adulthood.[235,240,245] However, pulmonary infections, sepsis, cor pulmonale, and respiratory arrest while asleep or precipitated by hypotension remain as frequent causes of death.[235,240,245]

REFERENCES

Nutritional Disorders

1. Hammer LD, Kraemer HC, Wilson DM, Ritter PL, Dornbusch SM: Standardized percentile curves of body-mass index for children and adolescents, *Am J Dis Child* 145:259-263, 1991.
2. Wilber JF: Neuropeptides, appetite regulation, and human obesity, *JAMA* 266:257-259, 1991 (review).
3. Ravussin E, Swinburn BA: Pathophysiology of obesity, *Lancet* 340:404-408, 1992 (review).
4. Inselman LS, Wapnir RA, Spencer H: Obesity-induced hyperplastic lung growth, *Am Rev Respir Dis* 135:613-616, 1987.
5. Inselman LS, Padilla-Burgos LB, Telchberg S, Spencer H: Alveolar enlargement in obesity-induced hyperplastic lung growth, *J Appl Physiol* 65:2291-2296, 1988.
6. Bates DV: *Respiratory function in disease,* ed 3, Philadelphia, 1989, WB Saunders, pp 96, 100-102 (review).
7. Inselman LS, Milanese A, Deurloo A: Effect of obesity on pulmonary function in children, *Pediatr Pulmonol* 16:130-137, 1993.
8. Luce JM: Respiratory complications of obesity, *Chest* 78:626-631, 1980 (review).
9. Bedell GN, Wilson WR, Seebohm PM: Pulmonary function in obese persons, *J Clin Invest* 37:1049-1060, 1958.
10. Douglas FG, Chong PY: Influence of obesity on peripheral airways patency, *J Appl Physiol* 33:559-563, 1972.
11. Emirgil C, Sobol BJ: The effects of weight reduction on pulmonary function and the sensitivity of the respiratory center in obesity, *Am Rev Respir Dis* 108:831-842, 1973.
12. Bosisio E, Sergi M, di Natale B, Chiumello G: Ventilatory volumes, flow rates, transfer factor and its components (membrane component, capillary volume) in obese adults and children, *Respiration* 45:321-326, 1984.
13. Chaussain M, Gamain B, La Torre AM, Vaida P, de Lattre J: Respiratory function at rest in obese children, *Bull Eur Physiopathol Respir* 13:599-609, 1977.
14. Villa MP, Bernardi F, Zappulla F, Testi S, Reggiani L, Tura A, Messina E, Cacciari E: Cardiorespiratory function in obese children, *Minerva Pediatr* 39:95-102, 1987.
15. Mallory GB Jr, Fiser DH, Jackson R: Sleep-associated breathing disorders in morbidly obese children and adolescents, *J Pediatr* 115:892-897, 1989.
16. Thomas PS, Owen ERTC, Hulands G, Milledge JS: Respiratory function in the morbidly obese before and after weight loss, *Thorax* 44:382-386, 1989.
17. Fadell EJ, Richman AD, Ward WW, Hendon JR: Fatty infiltration of respiratory muscles in the Pickwickian syndrome, *N Engl J Med* 266: 861-863, 1962.
18. Browman CP, Sampson MG, Yolles SF, Gujavarty KS, Weiler SJ, Walsleben JA, Hahn PM, Mitler MM: Obstructive sleep apnea and body weight, *Chest* 85:435-436, 1984.
19. Garner SJ, Eldridge FL, Wagner PG, Dowell RT: Buspirone, an anxiolytic drug that stimulates respiration, *Am Rev Respir Dis* 139:946-950, 1989.
20. Aubier M, De Troyer A, Sampson M, Macklem PT, Roussos C: Aminophylline improves diaphragmatic contractility, *N Engl J Med* 305:249-252, 1981.
21. Kimmel PL: Sleep apnea in end-stage renal disease, *Semin Dial* 4:52-58, 1991 (review).
22. Foxworth JW, Reisz GR, Knudson SM, Cuddy PG, Pyszczynski DR, Emory CE: Theophylline and diaphragmatic contractility: investigation of a dose-response relationship, *Am Rev Respir Dis* 138:1532-1534, 1988.
23. Schmidt-Nowara WW, Meade TE, Hays MB: Treatment of snoring and obstructive sleep apnea with a dental orthosis, *Chest* 99:1378-1385, 1991.
24. Sanders MH, Kern N: Obstructive sleep apnea treated by independently adjusted inspiratory and expiratory positive airway pressures via nasal mask: physiologic and clinical implications, *Chest* 98:317-324, 1990.
25. Walker WA, Hendricks KM: *Manual of pediatric nutrition,* Philadelphia, 1985, WB Saunders, p 26.
26. Lechner AJ, Winston DC, Bauman JE: Lung mechanics, cellularity, and surfactant after prenatal starvation in guinea pigs, *J Appl Physiol* 60:1610-1614, 1986.
27. Faridy EE: Effect of maternal malnutrition on surface activity of fetal lungs in rats, *J Appl Physiol* 39:535-540, 1975.
28. Curle DC, Adamson IYR: Retarded development of neonatal rat lung by maternal malnutrition, *J Histochem Cytochem* 26:401-408, 1978.
29. Arora NS, Rochester DF: Respiratory muscle strength and maximal voluntary ventilation in undernourished patients, *Am Rev Respir Dis* 126:5-8, 1982.
30. Rochester DF, Esau SA: Malnutrition and the respiratory system, *Chest* 85:411-415, 1984 (review).

31. Stiehm ER: Humoral immunity in malnutrition, *Fed Proc* 39:3093-3097, 1980 (review).
32. Jakab GJ, Warr GA, Astry CL: Alterations of pulmonary defense mechanisms by protein depletion diet, *Infect Immun* 34:610-622, 1981.
33. Frank L, Sosenko IRS: Undernutrition as a major contributing factor in the pathogenesis of bronchopulmonary dysplasia, *Am Rev Respir Dis* 138:725-729, 1988 (review).
34. Mansell AL, Andersen JC, Muttart CR, Ores CN, Loeff DS, Levy JS, Heird WC: Short-term pulmonary effects of total parenteral nutrition in children with cystic fibrosis, *J Pediatr* 104:700-705, 1984.
35. Whittaker JS, Ryan CF, Buckley PA, Road JD: The effects of refeeding on peripheral and respiratory muscle function in malnourished chronic obstructive pulmonary disease patients, *Am Rev Respir Dis* 142:283-288, 1990.
36. Lands L, Pavilanis A, Charge TD, Coates AL: Cardiopulmonary response to exercise in anorexia nervosa, *Pediatr Pulmonol* 13:101-107, 1992.
37. Brasel JA: Cellular changes in intrauterine malnutrition. In Winick M, ed: *Nutrition and fetal development,* New York, 1974, John Wiley and Sons, pp 13-15 (review).
38. Winick M, Noble A: Cellular response in rats during malnutrition at various ages, *J Nutr* 89:300-306, 1966.
39. Das RM: The effects of intermittent starvation on lung development in suckling rats, *Am J Pathol* 117:326-332, 1984.
40. Kalenga M, Eeckhout Y: Effects of protein deprivation from the neonatal period on lung collagen and elastin in the rat, *Pediatr Res* 26:125-127, 1989.
41. Kerr JS, Riley DJ, Lanza-Jacoby S, Berg RA, Spilker HC, Yu SY, Edelman NH: Nutritional emphysema in the rat: influence of protein depletion and impaired lung growth, *Am Rev Respir Dis* 131:644-650, 1985.
42. Gaultier C: Malnutrition and lung growth, *Pediatr Pulmonol* 10:278-286, 1991 (review).
43. Matsui R, Thurlbeck WM, Fujita Y, Yu SY, Kida K: Connective tissue, mechanical and morphometric changes in the lungs of weanling rats fed a low protein diet, *Pediatr Pulmonol* 7:159-166, 1989.
44. Sahebjami H, Wirman JA: Emphysema-like changes in the lungs of starved rats, *Am Rev Respir Dis* 124:619-624, 1981.
45. Kelsen SG, Ference M, Kapoor S: Effects of prolonged undernutrition on structure and function of the diaphragm, *J Appl Physiol* 58:1354-1359, 1985.
46. Johnson JD, Dunham T: Protein turnover in tissues of the fetal rat after prolonged maternal malnutrition, *Pediatr Res* 23:534-538, 1988.
47. Hards JM, Reid WD, Pardy RL, Pare PD: Respiratory muscle fiber morphometry: correlation with pulmonary function and nutrition, *Chest* 97:1037-1044, 1990.
48. Lewis MI, Steck GC: Effect of acute nutritional deprivation on diaphragm structure and function, *J Appl Physiol* 68:1938-1944, 1990.
49. Doekel RC Jr, Zwillich CW, Scoggin CH, Kryger M, Weil JV: Clinical semi-starvation: depression of hypoxic ventilatory response, *N Engl J Med* 295:358-361, 1976.
50. Martin TR, Altman LC, Alvares OF: The effects of severe protein-calorie malnutrition on antibacterial defense mechanisms in the rat lung, *Am Rev Respir Dis* 128:1013-1019, 1983.
51. Moriguchi S, Sone S, Kishino Y: Changes of alveolar macrophages in protein-deficient rats, *J Nutr* 113:40-46, 1983.
52. Puri S, Chandra RK: Nutritional regulation of host resistance and predictive value of immunologic tests in assessment of outcome, *Pediatr Clin North Am* 32(2):499-516, 1985 (review).
53. Sahebjami H, MacGee J: Changes in connective tissue composition of the lung in starvation and refeeding, *Am Rev Respir Dis* 128:644-647, 1983.
54. Sahebjami H, Vassallo CL: Effects of starvation and refeeding on lung mechanics and morphometry, *Am Rev Respir Dis* 119:443-451, 1979.
55. Sahebjami H, MacGee J: Effects of starvation and refeeding on lung biochemistry in rats, *Am Rev Respir Dis* 126:483-487, 1982.
56. Efthimiou J, Fleming J, Gomes C, Spiro SG: The effect of supplementary oral nutrition in poorly nourished patients with chronic obstructive pulmonary disease, *Am Rev Respir Dis* 137:1075-1082, 1988.
57. Fuenzalida CE, Petty TL, Jones ML, Jarrett S, Harbeck RJ, Terry RW, Hambidge KM: The immune response to short-term nutritional intervention in advanced chronic obstructive pulmonary disease, *Am Rev Respir Dis* 142:49-56, 1990.
58. Levy LD, Durie PR, Pencharz PB, Corey ML: Effects of long-term nutritional rehabilitation on body composition and clinical status in malnourished children and adolescents with cystic fibrosis, *J Pediatr* 107:225-230, 1985.
59. Shepherd R, Cooksley WGE, Cooke WDD: Improved growth and clinical, nutritional, and respiratory changes in response to nutritional therapy in cystic fibrosis, *J Pediatr* 97:351-357, 1980.

Disorders of the Pancreas

60. Ramirez LC, Dal Nogare A, Hsia C, Arauz C, Butt I, Strowig SM, Schnurr-Breen L, Raskin P: Relationship between diabetes control and pulmonary function in insulin-dependent diabetes mellitus, *Am J Med* 91:371-376, 1991.
61. Hansen LA, Prakash UBS, Colby TV: Pulmonary complications in diabetes mellitus, *Mayo Clin Proc* 64:791-799, 1989 (review).
62. Ofulue AF, Thurlbeck WM: Experimental diabetes and the lung. II. *in vivo* connective tissue metabolism, *Am Rev Respir Dis* 138:284-289, 1988.
63. Ofulue AF, Kida K, Thurlbeck WM: Experimental diabetes and the lung. I. Changes in growth, morphometry, and biochemistry, *Am Rev Respir Dis* 137:162-166, 1988.
64. Kida K, Utsuyama M, Takizawa T, Thurlbeck WM: Changes in lung morphologic features and elasticity caused by streptozotocin-induced diabetes mellitus in growing rats, *Am Rev Respir Dis* 128:125-131, 1983.
65. Sandler M: Is the lung a 'target organ' in diabetes mellitus? *Arch Intern Med* 150:1385-1388, 1990 (review).
66. Sandler M, Bunn AE, Stewart RI: Pulmonary function in young insulin-dependent diabetic subjects, *Chest* 90:670-675, 1986.
67. Plopper CG, Morishige WK: Alterations in granular (type II) pneumocyte ultrastructure by streptozotocin-induced diabetes in the rat, *Lab Invest* 38:143-148, 1978.
68. Plopper CG, Morishige WK: Alterations in the ultrastructure of nonciliated bronchiolar epithelial (Clara) cells by streptozotocin-induced diabetes in rats, *Am Rev Respir Dis* 120:1137-1143, 1979.
69. Sahebjami H, Denholm D: Lung mechanics and connective tissue proteins in diabetic Bio-Breeding/Worcester Wistar rats, *J Appl Physiol* 62:1430-1435, 1987.
70. Lange P, Groth S, Mortensen J, Appleyard M, Nyboe J, Schnohr P, Jensen G: Diabetes mellitus and ventilatory capacity: a five year follow-up study, *Eur Respir J* 3:288-292, 1990.
71. Bourbon JR, Farrell PM: Fetal lung development in the diabetic pregnancy, *Pediatr Res* 19:253-267, 1985 (review).
72. Kaplan SA: The insulin receptor, *J Pediatr* 104:327-336, 1984 (review).
73. Stiles AD, D'Ercole AJ: The insulin-like growth factors and the lung, *Am J Respir Cell Molec Biol* 3:93-100, 1990 (review).
74. Mohsenin V, Latifpour J: Respiratory burst in alveolar macrophages of diabetic rats, *J Appl Physiol* 68:2384-2390, 1990.
75. Katz S, Klein B, Elian I, Fishman P, Djaldetti M: Phagocytic activity of monocytes from diabetic patients, *Diabetes Care* 6:479-482, 1983.
76. Sugar AM: Agents of mucormycosis and related species. In Mandell GL, Douglas RG Jr, Bennett JE, eds: *Principles and practice of infectious diseases,* ed 3, New York, 1990, Churchill Livingstone, pp 1962-1969 (review).
77. Oswald GA, Corcoran S, Yudkin JS: Changes in pulmonary venous pressure and albumin concentration during treatment of severe diabetic decompensation, *Diabetes Res* 4:91-94, 1987.
78. Nishimura M, Miyamoto K, Suzuki A, Yamamoto H, Tsuji M, Kishi F, Kawakami Y: Ventilatory and heart rate responses to hypoxia and hypercapnia in patients with diabetes mellitus, *Thorax* 44:251-257, 1989.
79. Williams JG, Morris AI, Hayter RC, Ogilvie CM: Respiratory responses of diabetics to hypoxia, hypercapnia, and exercise, *Thorax* 39:529-534, 1984.
80. Vera M, Suffos R, Carriles M, Güell R, Picasso N, Alvarez MDC: A study of the respiratory function in insulin-dependent diabetic patients with and without limited joint mobility (LJM), *Acta Diabetolog Latin* 27:113-117, 1990.
81. Heimer D, Brami J, Lieberman D, Bark H: Respiratory muscle performance in patients with type 1 diabetes, *Diabetic Med* 7:434-437, 1990.
82. Wanke T, Formanek D, Auinger M, Popp W, Zwick H, Irsigler K: Inspiratory muscle performance and pulmonary function changes in insulin-dependent diabetes mellitus, *Am Rev Respir Dis* 143:97-100, 1991.

83. Bell D, Collier A, Matthews DM, Cooksey EJ, McHardy GJR, Clarke BF: Are reduced lung volumes in IDDM due to defect in connective tissue? *Diabetes* 37:829-831, 1988.
84. Valentovic MA, Lubawy WC: Impact of insulin or tolbutamide treatment on ^{14}C-arachidonic acid conversion to prostacyclin and/or thromboxane in lungs, aortas, and platelets of streptozotocin-induced diabetic rats, *Diabetes* 32:846-851, 1983.
85. Rosenbloom AL, Silverstein JH, Lezotte DC, Richardson K, McCallum M: Limited joint mobility in childhood diabetes mellitus indicates increased risk for microvascular disease, *N Engl J Med* 305:191-194, 1981.
86. Lange P, Groth S, Kastrup J, Mortensen J, Appleyard M, Nyboe J, Jensen G, Schnohr P: Diabetes mellitus, plasma glucose and lung function in a cross-sectional population study, *Eur Respir J* 2:14-19, 1989.
87. Baraldi E, Monciotti C, Filippone M, Santuz P, Magagnin G, Zanconato S, Zacchello F: Gas exchange during exercise in diabetic children, *Pediatr Pulmonol* 13:155-160, 1992.
88. Carroll P, Matz R: Adult respiratory distress syndrome complicating severely uncontrolled diabetes mellitus: report of nine cases and a review of the literature, *Diabetes Care* 5:574-580, 1982 (review).
89. Jordan SC, Ament ME: Pancreatitis in children and adolescents, *J Pediatr* 91:211-216, 1977.
90. Sibert JR: Pancreatitis in children: a study in the North of England, *Arch Dis Child* 50:443-448, 1975.
91. Ghishan FK, Greene HL, Avant G, O'Neill J, Neblett W: Chronic relapsing pancreatitis in childhood, *J Pediatr* 102:514-518, 1983.
91a. Kahler SG, Sherwood WG, Woolf D, Lawless ST, Zaritsky A, Bonham J, Taylor CJ, Clarke JTR, Durie P, Leonard JV: Pancreatitis in patients with organic acidemias, *J Pediatr* 124:239-243, 1994.
91b. Steer ML, Waxman I, Freedman S: Chronic pancreatitis, *N Engl J Med* 332:1482-1490, 1995.
92. Warshaw AL, Richter JM: A practical guide to pancreatitis, *Curr Probl Surg* 21:7-79, 1984 (review).
93. Wilkinson MJ, Robson DK, Basran G: Pleural complications of acute pancreatitis: an autopsy study, *Respir Med* 83:259-260, 1989 (letter).
94. Basran GS, Ramasubramanian R, Verma R: Intrathoracic complications of acute pancreatitis, *Br J Dis Chest* 81:326-331, 1987 (review).
95. Sahn SA: The pleura, *Am Rev Respir Dis* 138:184-234, 1988 (review).
96. Kaye MD: Pleuropulmonary complications of pancreatitis, *Thorax* 23:297-306, 1968 (review).
97. Rotman N, Fagniez P-L: Chronic pancreaticopleural fistulas, *Arch Surg* 119:1204-1206, 1984.
98. Light RW: *Pleural diseases,* Philadelphia, 1983, Lea & Febiger, pp 5-6, 135-137, 142, 151-154, 182, 227 (review).
99. Edelson JD, Vadas P, Villar J, Mullen JBM, Pruzanski W: Acute lung injury induced by phospholipase A_2: structural and functional changes, *Am Rev Respir Dis* 143:1102-1109, 1991.
100. Finley JW: Respiratory complications of acute pancreatitis, *Am Surg* 35:591-598, 1969.
101. Markos J, Tribe AE, McGonigle P: Recurrent lobar infiltrate and chronic pancreatitis, *Med J Aust* 145:94-96, 1986.
102. Idegami K, Mori K, Misumi A, Akagi M: Changes of alveolar stability and phospholipids in pulmonary surfactant in acute pancreatitis, *Jpn J Surg* 13:227-235, 1983.
103. Guice KS, Oldham KT, Wolfe RR, Simon RH: Lung injury in acute pancreatitis: primary inhibition of pulmonary phospholipid synthesis, *Am J Surg* 153:54-61, 1987.
104. Lungarella G, Gardi C, De Santi MM, Luzi P: Pulmonary vascular injury in pancreatitis: evidence for a major role played by pancreatic elastase, *Exp Molec Pathol* 42:44-59, 1985.
105. Kimura T, Toung JK, Margolis S, Bell WR, Cameron JL: Respiratory failure in acute pancreatitis: the role of free fatty acids, *Surgery* 87:509-513, 1980.
106. Chardavoyne R, Asher A, Bank S, Stein TA, Wise L: Role of reactive oxygen metabolites in early cardiopulmonary changes of acute hemorrhagic pancreatitis, *Dig Dis Sci* 34:1581-1584, 1989.
107. Guice KS, Oldham KT, Caty MG, Johnson KJ, Ward PA: Neutrophil-dependent, oxygen-radical mediated lung injury associated with acute pancreatitis, *Ann Surg* 210:740-747, 1989.
108. Berry A, Davies GC, Millar AM, Taylor TV: Changes in the biophysical properties and ultrastructure of lungs, and intrapulmonary fibrin deposition in experimental acute pancreatitis, *Gut* 24:929-934, 1983.
109. Willemer S, Feddersen CO, Karges W, Adler G: Lung injury in acute experimental pancreatitis in rats. I. Morphological studies, *Int J Pancreatol* 8:305-321, 1991.
110. Kerstein MD, Reinitz ER: Influence of hemorrhagic pancreatitis on the lung: an ultrastructural study, *Am Surg* 49:271-274, 1983.
111. Masoero G, Spinaci S, Arossa W, Andriulli A, Gaia E, De Pretis G, Dobrilla G, De La Pierre M: Pulmonary involvement in chronic pancreatitis, *Dig Dis Sci* 29:896-901, 1984.
112. DeTroyer A, Naeije R, Yernault J-C, Englert M: Impairment of pulmonary function in acute pancreatitis, *Chest* 73:360-363, 1978.
113. Schröder T, Lempinen M, Kivilaakso E, Nikki P: Serum phospholipase A_2 and pulmonary changes in acute fulminant pancreatitis, *Resuscitation* 10:79-87, 1982.
114. Otsuki M, Yuu H, Maeda M, Saeki S, Yamasaki T, Baba S: Amylase in the lung, *Cancer* 39:1656-1663, 1977.

Disorders of the Liver

115. Krowka MJ, Cortese DA: Pulmonary aspects of liver disease and liver transplantation, *Clinics Chest Med,* 10:593-616, 1989 (review).
116. Williams A, Trewby P, Williams R, Reid L: Structural alterations to the pulmonary circulation in fulminant hepatic failure, *Thorax* 34:447-453, 1979.
117. Ueda T, Ohta K, Suzuki N, Yamaguchi M, Hirai K, Horiuchi T, Watanabe J, Miyamoto T, Ito K: Idiopathic pulmonary fibrosis and high prevalence of serum antibodies to hepatitis C virus, *Am Rev Respir Dis* 148:266-268, 1992.
118. Krowka MJ, Cortese DA: Pulmonary aspects of chronic liver disease and liver transplantation, *Mayo Clin Proc* 60:407-418, 1985 (review).
119. Ha SY, Helms P, Fletcher M, Broadbent V, Pritchard J: Lung involvement in Langerhans' cell histiocytosis: prevalence, clinical features, and outcome, *Pediatrics* 89:466-469, 1992.
119a. DeRemee RA: Sarcoidosis, *Mayo Clin Proc* 70:177-181, 1995.
120. Krowka MJ, Cortese DA: Hepatopulmonary syndrome, *Chest* 98:1053-1054, 1990 (review).
120a. Neuberger J: Primary biliary cirrhosis, *Lancet* 350:875-879, 1997.
121. Kagalwalla AF, Rahman A, Taleb A, Kagalwalla YA, Ali MM, Yaish H: Pulmonary hemorrhage in association with autoimmune chronic active hepatitis, *Chest* 103:634-636, 1993.
122. Wallaert B, Bonniere P, Prin L, Cortot A, Tonnel AB, Voisin C: Primary biliary cirrhosis: subclinical inflammatory alveolitis in patients with normal chest roentgenograms, *Chest* 90:842-848, 1986.
123. Berthelot P, Walker JG, Sherlock S, Reid L: Arterial changes in the lungs in cirrhosis of the liver-lung spider nevi, *N Engl J Med* 274:291-298, 1966.
124. Oh KS, Bender TM, Bowen A, Ledesma-Medina J: Plain radiographic, nuclear medicine and angiographic observations of hepatogenic pulmonary angiodysplasia, *Pediatr Radiol* 13:111-115, 1983.
125. Andrivet P, Cadranel J, Housset B, Herigault R, Harf A, Adnot S: Mechanisms of impaired arterial oxygenation in patients with liver cirrhosis and severe respiratory insufficiency. Effects of indomethacin, *Chest* 103:500-507, 1993.
126. Eriksson LS, Söderman C, Ericzon B-G, Eleborg L, Wahren J, Hedenstierna G: Normalization of ventilation/perfusion relationships after liver transplantation in patients with decompensated cirrhosis: evidence for a hepatopulmonary syndrome, *Hepatology* 12:1350-1357, 1990.
127. Sherlock S: The liver-lung interface, *Semin Respir Med* 9:247-253, 1988 (review).
128. Daoud FS, Reeves JT, Schaefer JW: Failure of hypoxic pulmonary vasoconstriction in patients with liver cirrhosis, *J Clin Invest* 51:1076-1080, 1972.
129. Schaefer JW, Reeves JT: The lung and the liver, *Chest* 80:526-527, 1981.
130. Rodriguez-Roisin R, Roca J, Agusti AG, Mastai R, Wagner PD, Bosch J: Gas exchange and pulmonary vascular reactivity in patients with liver cirrhosis, *Am Rev Respir Dis* 135:1085-1092, 1987.
131. Silver MM, Bohn D, Shawn DH, Shuckett B, Eich G, Rabinovitch M: Association of pulmonary hypertension with congenital portal hypertension in a child, *J Pediatr* 120:321-329, 1992.
132. Robalino BD, Moodie DS: Association between primary pulmonary hypertension and portal hypertension: analysis of its pathophysiology and clinical, laboratory and hemodynamic manifestations, *J Am Coll Cardiol* 17:492-498, 1991.

133. Robin ED, Laman D, Horn BR, Theodore J: Platypnea related to orthodeoxia caused by true vascular lung shunts, *N Engl J Med* 294:941-943, 1976.
134. Kay JM: Vascular disease. In Thurlbeck WM, Churg AM, eds: *Pathology of the lung,* ed 2, New York, 1995, Thieme, pp 934-955, 974-975 (review).
135. Hourani JM, Bellamy PE, Tashkin DP, Batra P, Simmons MS: Pulmonary dysfunction in advanced liver disease: frequent occurrence of an abnormal diffusing capacity, *Am J Med* 90:693-700, 1991.
136. Hind CRK, Wong CM: Detection of pulmonary arteriovenous fistulae in patient with cirrhosis by contrast 2D echocardiography, *Gut* 22:1042-1044, 1981.
137. Bank ER, Thrall JH, Dantzker DR: Radionuclide demonstration of intrapulmonary shunting in cirrhosis, *Am J Roentgenol* 140:967-969, 1983.
138. Golding PL, Smith M, Williams R: Multisystem involvement in chronic liver disease. Studies on the incidence and pathogenesis, *Am J Med* 55:772-782, 1973.
139. Cooper JAD Jr, White DA, Matthay RA: Drug-induced pulmonary disease. Part 2: Noncytotoxic drugs, *Am Rev Respir Dis* 133:488-505, 1986 (review).
140. Felt RW, Kozak BE, Rosch J, Duell BP, Barker AF: Hepatogenic pulmonary angiodysplasia treated with coil-spring embolization, *Chest* 91:920-922, 1987.
141. Schwarzenberg SJ, Freese DK, Regelmann WE, Gores PF, Boudreau RJ, Payne WD: Resolution of severe intrapulmonary shunting after liver transplantation, *Chest* 103:1271-1273, 1993.

Disorders of the Kidney

142. Bush A, Gabriel R: The lungs in uraemia: a review, *J Royal Soc Med* 78:849-855, 1985 (review).
143. Miller RR: Diffuse pulmonary hemorrhage. In Thurlbeck WM, Churg AM, eds: *Pathology of the lung,* ed 2, New York, 1995, Thieme, pp 365-373 (review).
144. Young KR Jr: Pulmonary-renal syndromes, *Clin Chest Med,* 10:655-675, 1989 (review).
145. Leatherman JW, Davies SF, Hoidal JR: Alveolar hemorrhage syndromes: diffuse microvascular lung hemorrhage in immune and idiopathic disorders, *Medicine* 63:343-361, 1984 (review).
145a. Green RJ, Ruoss ST, Kraft SA, Berry GJ, Raffin TA: Pulmonary capillaritis and alveolar hemorrhage. Update on diagnosis and management, *Chest* 110:1305-1316, 1996.
146. Leavitt RY, Fauci AS: Pulmonary vasculitis, *Am Rev Respir Dis* 134:149-166, 1986 (review).
147. Colby TV, Carrington CB: Interstitial lung disease. In Thurlbeck WM, Churg AM, eds: *Pathology of the lung,* ed 2, New York, 1995, Thieme, pp 632-636, 640, 682-687, 690-693 (review).
148. Chaussain M, de Boissieu D, Kalifa G, Epelbaum S, Niaudet P, Badoual J, Gendrel D: Impairment of lung diffusion capacity in Schönlein-Henoch purpura, *J Pediatr* 121:12-16, 1992.
149. Raz I, Okon E, Chajek-Shaul T: Pulmonary manifestations in Behçet's syndrome, *Chest* 95:585-589, 1989.
150. Mason AMS, McIllmurray MB, Golding PL, Hughes DTD: Fibrosing alveolitis associated with renal tubular acidosis, *Br Med J* 4:596-599, 1970.
151. Rimsza LM, Rimsza ME: Pathological cases of the month. Lymphomatoid granulomatosis, *Am J Dis Child* 147:693-694, 1993.
152. Landing BH: Pulmonary alveolar septal calcinosis, *Pediatr Pathol* 2:363-367, 1984.
153. Smith JC, Stanton LW, Kramer NC, Parrish AE: Nodular pulmonary calcification in renal failure. Report of a case, *Am Rev Respir Dis* 100:723-728, 1969.
154. Mootz JR, Sagel SS, Roberts TH: Roentgenographic manifestations of pulmonary calcifications. A rare cause of respiratory failure in chronic renal disease, *Radiology* 107:55-60, 1973.
155. Wang N-S, Steele AA: Pulmonary calcification. Scanning electron microscopic and x-ray energy-dispersive analysis, *Arch Pathol Lab Med* 103:252-257, 1979.
156. Conger JD, Hammond WS, Alfrey AC, Contiguglia SR, Stanford RE, Huffer WE: Pulmonary calcification in chronic dialysis patients. Clinical and pathologic studies, *Ann Intern Med* 83:330-336, 1975.
157. Rackow EC, Fein IA, Sprung C, Grodman RS: Uremic pulmonary edema, *Am J Med* 64:1084-1088, 1978.
158. Staneseu DC, Veriter C, De Plaen JF, Frans A, Van Ypersele de Strihou C, Brasseur L: Lung function in chronic uraemia before and after removal of excess of fluid by haemodialysis, *Clin Sci Molec Med* 47:143-151, 1974.
159. Hopps HC, Wissler RW: Uremic pneumonitis, *Am J Pathol* 31:261-267, 1955.
160. Benfield M, Michael AF: Immunology of uremia. In Edelmann CM Jr, ed: *Pediatric kidney disease,* ed 2, Boston, 1992, Little, Brown, pp 783-790 (review).
161. Feigin RD, Matson DO: The compromised host. In Feigin RD, Cherry JD, eds: *Textbook of pediatric infectious diseases,* ed 3, Philadelphia, 1992, WB Saunders, pp 960-989 (review).
162. Goldstein E, Green GM, Seamans C: The effect of acidosis on pulmonary bactericidal function, *J Lab Clin Med* 75:912-923, 1970.
163. Alevy YG, Hutcheson P, Mueller KR, Slavin RG: Suppressor alveolar macrophages in experimentally induced uremia, *J Reticuloendothelial Soc* 33:11-20, 1983.
164. Kim Y, Michael AF, Tarshish P: Infection and nephritis. In Edelmann CM Jr, ed: *Pediatric kidney disease,* ed 2, Boston, 1992, Little, Brown, pp 1569-1584 (review).
165. Yao L, Killam DA: Rounded atelectasis associated with end-stage renal disease, *Chest* 96:441-443, 1989.
166. Moss R, Hinds S, Fedullo AJ: Chylothorax: a complication of the nephrotic syndrome, *Am Rev Respir Dis* 140:1436-1437, 1989.
167. Gómez-Fernández P, Agudo LS, Miguel JL, Almaraz M, Dupla MJV: Effect of parathyroidectomy on respiratory muscle strength in uremic myopathy, *Am J Nephrol* 7:466-469, 1987.
168. Tarasuik A, Heimer D, Bark H: Effect of chronic renal failure on skeletal and diaphragmatic muscle contraction, *Am Rev Respir Dis* 146:1383-1388, 1992.
169. Langevin B, Fouque D, Léger P, Robert D: Sleep apnea syndrome and end-stage renal disease. Cure after renal transplantation, *Chest* 103:1330-1335, 1993.
170. Grefberg N, Danielson BG, Benson L, Pitkänen P: Right-sided hydrothorax complicating peritoneal dialysis. Report of 2 cases, *Nephron* 34:130-134, 1983.
171. Chow CC, Sung JY, Cheung CK, Hamilton-Wood C, Lai KN: Massive hydrothorax in continuous ambulatory peritoneal dialysis: diagnosis, management and review of the literature, *NZ Med J* 101:475-477, 1988.
172. Fairshter RD, Vaziri ND, Wilson AF, Fugl-Meyer AR: Respiratory physiology before and after hemodialysis in chronic renal failure patients, *Am J Med Sci* 278:11-18, 1979.
173. Miller RW, Salcedo JR, Fink RJ, Murphy TM, Magilavy DB: Pulmonary hemorrhage in pediatric patients with systemic lupus erythematosus, *J Pediatr* 108:576-579, 1986.
174. Loughlin GM, Taussig LM, Murphy SA, Strunk RC, Kohnen PW: Immune-complex-mediated glomerulonephritis and pulmonary hemorrhage simulating Goodpasture syndrome, *J Pediatr* 93:181-184, 1978.
175. Ahluwalia M, Ishikawa S, Gellman M, Shah T, Sekar T, MacDonnell KF: Pulmonary functions during peritoneal dialysis, *Clin Nephrol* 18:251-256, 1982.
176. Baraldi E, Montini G, Zanconato S, Zacchello G, Zacchello F: Exercise tolerance after anaemia correction with recombinant human erythropoietin in end-stage renal disease, *Pediatr Nephrol* 4:623-626, 1990.
177. Patterson RW, Nissenson AR, Miller J, Smith RT, Narins RG, Sullivan SF: Hypoxemia and pulmonary gas exchange during hemodialysis, *J Appl Physiol* 50:259-264, 1981.

Hemoglobinopathies

178. Ranney HM: The spectrum of sickle cell disease, *Hosp Pract* 27:89-113, 1992 (review).
178a. Bunn HF: Pathogenesis and treatment of sickle cell disease, *N Engl J Med* 337:762-769, 1997.
179. Hutchinson RM, Merrick MV, White JM: Fat embolism in sickle cell disease, *J Clin Pathol* 26:620-622, 1973.
180. Giardina PJ, Hilgartner MW: Update on thalassemia, *Pediatr Rev* 13:55-62, 1992 (review).
181. Charache S, Grisolia S, Fiedler AJ, Hellegers AE: Effect of 2,3-diphosphoglycerate on oxygen affinity of blood in sickle cell anemia, *J Clin Invest* 49:806-812, 1970.
182. Bromberg PA: Pulmonary aspects of sickle cell disease, *Arch Intern Med* 133:652-657, 1974 (review).
183. Scharf MB, Lobel JS, Caldwell E, Cameron BF, Kramer M, De Marchis J, Paine C: Nocturnal oxygen desaturation in patients with sickle cell anemia, *JAMA* 249:1753-1755, 1983.

184. Becklake MR, Griffiths SB, McGregor M, Goldman HI, Schreve JP: Oxygen dissociation curves in sickle cell anemia and in subjects with the sickle cell trait, *J Clin Invest* 34:751-755, 1955.
185. Weil JV, Castro O, Malik AB, Rodgers G, Bonds DR, Jacobs TP: Pathogenesis of lung disease in sickle hemoglobinopathies, *Am Rev Respir Dis* 148:249-256, 1993 (review).
186. Barrett-Connor E: Pneumonia and pulmonary infarction in sickle cell anemia, *JAMA* 224:997-1000, 1973 (review).
187. Powars DR: Natural history of sickle cell disease—the first ten years, *Semin Hematol* 12:267-285, 1975 (review).
188. Smith JA: Cardiopulmonary manifestations of sickle cell disease in childhood, *Semin Roentgenol* 22:160-167, 1987 (review).
189. Vichinsky EP: Comprehensive care in sickle cell disease: its impact on morbidity and mortality, *Semin Hematol* 28:220-226, 1991 (review).
190. Buchanan GR, Smith SJ, Holtkamp CA, Fuseler JP: Bacterial infection and splenic reticuloendothelial function in children with hemoglobin SC disease, *Pediatrics* 72:93-98, 1983.
191. Onwubalili JK: Sickle cell disease and infection, *J Infect* 7:2-20, 1983 (review).
192. Woronow DI, Tenney JH: Legionnaires' disease in a patient with sickle cell anemia, *Md Med J* 30:53-54, 1981.
193. Hardy RE, Cummings C, Thomas F, Harrison D: Cryptococcal pneumonia in a patient with sickle cell disease, *Chest* 89:892-894, 1986.
194. Haddad JD, John JF Jr, Pappas AA: Cytomegalovirus pneumonia in sickle cell disease, *Chest* 86:265-266, 1984.
195. Israel RH, Salipante JS: Pulmonary infarction in sickle cell trait, *Am J Med* 66:867-869, 1979.
196. Rucknagel DL, Kalinyak KA, Gelfand MJ: Rib infarcts and acute chest syndrome in sickle cell diseases, *Lancet* 337:831-833, 1991.
197. Harcke HT, Capitanio MA, Naiman JL: Sternal infarction in sickle-cell anemia: concise communication, *J Nuclear Med* 22:322-324, 1981.
198. Sprinkle RH, Cole T, Smith S, Buchanan GR: Acute chest syndrome in children with sickle cell disease: a retrospective analysis of 100 hospitalized cases, *Am J Pediatr Hematol Oncol* 812:105-110, 1986.
199. Miller ST, Hammerschlag MR, Chirgwin K, Rao SP, Roblin P, Gelling M, Stilerman T, Schachter J, Cassell G: Role of *Chlamydia pneumoniae* in acute chest syndrome of sickle cell disease, *J Pediatr* 118:30-33, 1991.
200. Shelley WM, Curtis EM: Bone marrow and fat embolism in sickle cell anemia and sickle cell-hemoglobin C disease, *Bull Johns Hopkins Hosp* 103:8-25, 1958.
201. Collins FS, Orringer EP: Pulmonary hypertension and cor pulmonale in the sickle hemoglobinopathies, *Am J Med* 73:814-821, 1982.
202. Powars D, Weidman JA, Odom-Maryon T, Niland JC, Johnson C: Sickle cell chronic lung disease: prior morbidity and the risk of pulmonary failure, *Medicine* 67:66-76, 1988.
203. Lobel JS, Sturm R, Carroll WL, Limouze SC: *Mycoplasma* pneumonia in a 15-month-old girl with hemoglobin SC disease, *Am J Pediatr Hematol Oncol* 3:444-446, 1981.
204. Topley JM, Cupidore L, Vaidya S, Hayes RJ, Serjeant GR: Pneumococcal and other infections in children with sickle cell-hemoglobin C (SC) disease, *J Pediatr* 101:176-179, 1982.
205. Pensler MI, Radke JR: ARDS and cerebral infarction complicating *Mycoplasma* pneumonia in sickle cell trait, *Henry Ford Hosp Med J* 28:60-62, 1980.
206. Hasleton PS, Orr K, Webster A, Lawson RAM: Evolution of acute chest syndrome in sickle cell trait: an ultrastructural and light microscopic study, *Thorax* 44:1057-1058, 1989.
207. Miller GJ, Serjeant GR: An assessment of lung volumes and gas transfer in sickle-cell anaemia, *Thorax* 26:309-315, 1971.
208. Pianosi P, D'Souza SJA, Charge TD, Esseltine DE, Coates AL: Pulmonary function abnormalities in childhood sickle cell disease, *J Pediatr* 122:366-371, 1993.
209. Miller DM, Winslow RM, Klein HG, Wilson KC, Brown FL, Statham NJ: Improved exercise performance after exchange transfusion in subjects with sickle cell anemia, *Blood* 56:1127-1131, 1980.
210. Young RC Jr, Rachal RE, Reindorf CA, Armstrong EM, Polk OD Jr, Hackney RL Jr, Scott RB: Lung function in sickle cell hemoglobinopathy patients compared with healthy subjects, *J Natl Med Assoc* 80:509-514, 1988.
211. Bowen EF, Crowston JG, De Ceulaer K, Serjeant GR: Peak expiratory flow rate and the acute chest syndrome in homozygous sickle cell disease, *Arch Dis Child* 65:330-332, 1990.
212. Femi-Pearse D, Gazioglu KM, Yu PN: Pulmonary function studies in sickle cell disease, *J Appl Physiol* 28:574-577, 1970.
213. Stinson JM, McPherson GL: Lung volumes and diffusion capacity in sickle cell trait, *J Natl Med Assoc* 78:505-507, 1986.
214. Weisman IM, Zeballos RJ, Johnson BD: Effect of moderate inspiratory hypoxia on exercise performance in sickle cell trait, *Am J Med* 84:1033-1040, 1988.
215. Robertson PL, Aldrich MS, Hanash SM, Goldstein GW: Stroke associated with obstructive sleep apnea in a child with sickle cell anemia, *Ann Neurol* 23:614-616, 1988.
216. Haynes J Jr, Allison RC: Pulmonary edema. Complication in the management of sickle cell pain crisis, *Am J Med* 80:833-840, 1986.
217. Gaston MH, Verter JI, Woods G, Pegelow C, Kelleher J, Presbury G, Zarkowsky H, Vichinsky E, Iyer R, Lobel JS, Diamond S, Holbrook CT, Gill FM, Ritchey K, Falletta JM: Prophylaxis with oral penicillin in children with sickle cell anemia. A randomized trial, *N Engl J Med* 314:1593-1599, 1986.
217a. Steele RW, Warrier R, Unkel PJ, Foch BJ, Howes RF, Shah S, Williams K, Moore S, Jue SJ: Colonization with antibiotic-resistant *Streptococcus pneumoniae* in children with sickle cell disease, *J Pediatr* 128:531-535, 1996.
217b. Walters MC, Patience M, Leisenring W, Eckman JR, Scott JP, Mentzer WC, Davies SC, Ohene-Frempong K, Bernaudin F, Matthews DC, Storb R, Sullivan KM: Bone marrow transplantation for sickle cell disease, *N Engl J Med* 335:369-376, 1996.
218. Nathan DG, Benz EJ Jr: Pathophysiology of the anaemia in thalassaemia. In *CIBA Foundation Symposium 37 (new series): congenital disorders of erythropoiesis,* New York, 1976, Elsevier, pp 205-220 (review).
219. Gale RP: Prospects for correction of thalassemia by genetic engineering. In Buckner CD, Gale RP, Lucarelli G, eds: *Advances and controversies in thalassemia therapy: bone marrow transplantation and other approaches,* New York, 1989, Alan R Liss, pp 141-159 (review).
220. Edwards JR, Matthay KK: Hematologic disorders affecting the lungs, *Clin Chest Med* 10:723-746, 1989 (review).
221. Caroline L, Kozinn PJ, Feldman F, Stiefel FH: Infection and iron overload in thalassemia, *Ann NY Acad Sci* 165:148-155, 1969.
222. Weinberg ED: Roles of metallic ions in host-parasite interactions, *Bacteriol Rev* 30:136-151, 1966 (review).
223. Serjeant GR, Serjeant BE, Thomas PW, Anderson MJ, Patou G, Pattison JR: Human parvovirus infection in homozygous sickle cell disease, *Lancet* 341:1237-1240, 1993.
224. Grisaru D, Rachmilewitz EA, Mosseri M, Gotsman M, Lafair JS, Okon E, Goldfarb A, Hasin Y: Cardiopulmonary assessment in beta-thalassemia major, *Chest* 98:1138-1142, 1990.
225. Hoyt RW, Scarpa N, Wilmott RW, Cohen A, Schwartz E: Pulmonary function abnormalities in homozygous β-thalassemia, *J Pediatr* 109:452-455, 1986.
226. Cooper DM, Mansell AL, Weiner MA, Berdon WE, Chetty-Baktaviziam A, Reid L, Mellins RB: Low lung capacity and hypoxemia in children with thalassemia major, *Am Rev Respir Dis* 121:639-646, 1980.
227. Fung KP, Chow OKW, So SY, Yuen PMB: Pulmonary function in thalassemia major, *J Pediatr* 111:534-537, 1987.
228. Keens TG, O'Neal MH, Ortega JA, Hyman CB, Platzker ACG: Pulmonary function abnormalities in thalassemia patients on a hypertransfusion program, *Pediatrics* 65:1013-1017, 1980.
229. Lands LC, Woods S, Katsardis C, Desmond K, Coates AL: The effects of diuresis and transfusion on pulmonary function in children with thalassemia major, *Pediatr Pulmonol* 11:340-344, 1991.
230. Bacalo A, Kivity S, Heno N, Greif Z, Greif J, Topilsky M: Blood transfusion and lung function in children with thalassemia major, *Chest* 101:362-365, 1992.
231. Freedman MH, Grisaru D, Olivieri N, MacLusky I, Thorner PS: Pulmonary syndrome in patients with thalassemia major receiving intravenous deferoxamine infusions, *Am J Dis Child* 144:565-569, 1990.
232. Landing BH, Nadorra R, Hyman CB, Ortega JA: Pulmonary lesions of thalassemia major, *Perspect Pediatr Pathol* 11:82-96, 1987.
233. Cooper DM, Hyman CB, Weiler-Ravell D, Noble NA, Agness CL, Wasserman K: Gas exchange during exercise in children with thalassemia major and Diamond-Blackfan anemia, *Pediatr Res* 19:1215-1219, 1985.

234. Grant GP, Graziano JH, Seaman C, Mansell AL: Cardiorespiratory response to exercise in patients with thalassemia major, *Am Rev Respir Dis* 136:92-97, 1987.

234a. Lucarelli G, Galimberti M, Polchi P, Angelucci E, Baronciani D, Giardini C, Andreani M, Agostinelli F, Albertini F, Clift RA: Marrow transplantation in patients with thalassemia responsive to iron chelation therapy, *N Engl J Med* 329:840-844, 1993.

Familial Dysautonomia

235. Axelrod FB, Nachtigal R, Dancis J: Familial dysautonomia: diagnosis, pathogenesis and management, *Adv Pediatr* 21:75-96, 1974 (review).

236. Moses SW, Rotem Y, Jagoda N, Talmor N, Eichhorn F, Levin S: A clinical, genetic and biochemical study of familial dysautonomia in Israel, *Isr J Med Sci* 3:358-371, 1967.

237. Gyepes MT, Linde LM: Familial dysautonomia: the mechanism of aspiration, *Radiology* 91:471-475, 1968.

238. Schwartz JP, Breakefteld XO: Altered nerve growth factor in fibroblasts from patients with familial dysautonomia, *Proc Natl Acad Sci* 77:1154-1158, 1980.

239. Axelrod FB, Schneider KM, Ament ME, Kutin ND, Fonkalsrud EW: Gastroesophageal fundoplication and gastrostomy in familial dysautonomia, *Ann Surg* 195:253-258, 1982.

240. Fishbein D, Grossman RF: Pulmonary manifestations of familial dysautonomia in an adult, *Am J Med* 80:709-713, 1986.

241. Axelrod FB, Porges RF, Sein ME: Neonatal recognition of familial dysautonomia, *J Pediatr* 110:946-948, 1987.

242. Filler J, Smith AA, Stone S, Dancis J: Respiratory control in familial dysautonomia, *J Pediatr* 66:509-516, 1965.

243. Geltzer AI, Gluck L, Talner NS, Polesky HF: Familial dysautonomia: studies in a newborn infant, *N Engl J Med* 271:436-440, 1964.

244. Axelrod FB, Donenfeld RF, Danziger F, Turndorf H: Anesthesia in familial dysautonomia, *Anesthesiology* 68:631-635, 1988.

245. Axelrod FB, Abularrage JJ: Familial dysautonomia: a prospective study of survival, *J Pediatr* 101:234-236, 1982.

Index

C

E

F

M

N

O

Q

R

S

W

X

Y

Z